Equine Neonatal Medicine

Equine Neonatal Medicine

Edited by

David M. Wong
Iowa State University
Ames, Iowa

Pamela A. Wilkins
University of Illinois Urbana–Champaign
Urbana, Illinois

WILEY Blackwell

Published by John Wiley & Sons, Inc., Hoboken, New Jersey.
Published simultaneously in Canada.

Library of Congress Cataloging-in-Publication Data applied for:

Hardback: 9781119617259

Cover Design: Wiley
Cover Image: © Steven Tian

Set in 9.5/12.5pt STIXTwoText by Straive, Pondicherry, India

SKY10065507_012324

Book Dedication

This book is dedicated to my wife, Kristine, and daughters, Olivia, Pip, and Estelle, and their steadfast support of me over the years as an equine veterinarian; to Pam Wilkins, my emergency and critical care mentor and friend; to all my colleagues at the Lloyd Veterinary Medical Center (Iowa State University), Marion duPont Scott Equine Medical Center (Virginia Tech), and New Bolton Center (University of Pennsylvania) – it has been a pleasure to work together through so many foaling seasons with you; and to all the mares and foals that we have had the honor to provide veterinary care to.

David M. Wong

I would like to dedicate this book to those who came before us, the editors of the original Equine Clinical Neonatology book, Anne Koterba, Willa Drummond, and Philip Kosch, and to all our patients and dedicated veterinarians caring for them over the generations since.

Pam A. Wilkins

Contents

List of Contributors

Michelle Abraham, BSc, BVMS, DACVIM
Assistant Professor
University of Pennsylvania
Kennett Square, PA

Emma Adam, BVetMed, PhD, MRCVS, DACVS, DACVIM
Equine Veterinary Research & Outreach
Gluck Equine Research Center
Lexington, KY

Cody Alcott, DVM, DACVIM (LAIM, Neurology)
Owner
Tucson Veterinary Specialists
Tucson, AZ

Monica Aleman, MVZ, PhD, DACVIM (LAIM, Neurology)
Professor
University of California
Davis, CA

Rafael Alzola-Domingo, BVM&S, MSc, Cert AVP, DECVSMR, MRCVS
Equine Surgeon, Veterinary Associate
Troytown Equine Hospital
Kildare, Ireland

Scott Austin, DVM, MS, DACVIM
Clinical Associate Professor
University of Illinois
Urbana, IL

Theresa Beachler, DVM, PhD, DACT
Assistant Professor
Iowa State University
Ames, IA

Daniela Bedenice, Dr. med. vet., DACVIM, DACVECC
Associate Professor
Tufts University
Medford, ME

Darren Berger, DVM, DACVD
Associate Professor
Iowa State University
Ames, IA

Rebecca Bishop, DVM
Equine Surgery Resident
University of Illinois
Urbana, IL

Anthony Blikslager, DVM, PhD, DACVS
Professor
North Carolina State University
Raleigh, NC

Charles Brockus, DVM, PhD, DACVIM, DACVP
Owner
CBCP Consulting
Sparks, NV

Teresa A. Burns, DVM, MS, PhD, DACVIM
Associate Professor
The Ohio State University
Columbus, OH

Christopher Byron, DVM, MS, DACVS
Associate Professor
Virginia Maryland College of Veterinary Medicine
Blacksburg, VA

Undine Christmann, DVM, MPH, PhD, MS, DACVIM
Associate Professor
Lincoln Memorial University
Harrogate, TN

Sarah Colmer, VMD, DACVIM
Neurology Fellow
University of Pennsylvania
Kennett Square, PA

Jennifer Davis, DVM, PhD, DACVIM, DACVCP
Associate Professor
Virginia Maryland College of Veterinary Medicine
Blacksburg, VA

Emma Deane, DVM, DACVECC
Associate Veterinarian
Loomis Basin Equine Medical Center
Penryn, CA

Julie Dechant, DVM, MS, DACVS, DACVECC
Professor
University of California
Davis, CA

Katarzyna A. Dembek, DVM, PhD, DACVIM
Assistant Professor
North Carolina State University
Raleigh, NC

Graeme M. Doodnaught, BSc, BVM&S, DES, MRCVS, DACVAA
Staff Anesthesiologist
Centre Veterinaire Rive-Sud
University of Montreal

Bettina Dunkel, DVM, PhD, DACVIM, DECEIM, DACVECC, MRCVS
Professor
Royal Veterinary College
London, UK

Adam Eatroff, DVM, DACVIM
Associate Veterinarian
ACCESS Specialty Animal Hospitals
Culver City, CA

Kira Epstein, DVM, DACVS, DACVECC
Professor
University of Georgia
Athens, GA

Sara Erwin, DVM
Graduate Student
North Carolina State University
Raleigh, NC

Krista Estell, DVM, DACVIM
Clinical Associate Professor
Marion duPont Scott Equine Medical Center
Virginia Maryland College of Veterinary Medicine
Leesburg, VA

Darien Feary, BVSc, MS, DACVIM, DACVECC
Associate Veterinarian
Randwick Equine Centre
Horsley Park, NSW, Australia

M. Julia B. Felippe, MedVet, MS, PhD, DACVIM
Professor
Cornell University
Ithaca, NY

Gustavo Ferlini Agne, MV, MS, DACVIM
Lecturer
University of Adelaide
Roseworthy, SA

Langdon Fielding, DVM, MBA, DACVECC, DACVSMR
Owner
Loomis Basin Equine Medical Center
Penryn, CA

Constanze Fintl, DVM, EBVS
Associate Professor
Norwegian School of Veterinary Science
Oslo, Norway

Alastair Foote, MA, VetMB, PhD, FRCPath, MRCVS
Clinical Director Rossdales Laboratories
Rossdales Veterinary Surgeons
Newmarket, Suffolk, UK

Ryan Fries, DVM, DACVIM (Cardiology)
Assistant Professor
University of Illinois
Urbana, IL

Paula Galera, DVM, MSc, PhD
Associate Professor
College of Veterinary Medicine
University of Brasilia, Brazil

Brian C. Gilger, DVM, MS, DACVO, DABT
Professor
North Carolina State University
Raleigh, NC

Alexandra Gillen, MA, MS, VetMB, DACVS, DECVS, FHEA, MRCVS
Senior Lecturer
University of Liverpool
Wirral, UK

Elizabeth A. Giuliano, DVM, MS, DACVO
Professor
University of Missouri
Columbia, MO

Jenifer Gold, DVM, DACVIM, DACVECC
Associate Veterinarian
Wisconsin Equine Hospital
Oconomowoc, WI

Ralph Hamor, DVM, MS, DACVO
Clinical Professor
University of Florida
Gainesville, FL

Kelsey A. Hart, DVM, PhD, DACVIM
Associate Professor
University of Georgia
Athens, GA

Bonnie Hay-Kraus, DVM, DACVS, DACVAA
Associate Professor
Iowa State University
Ames, IA

Kate L. Hepworth-Warren, DVM, DACVIM
Assistant Professor
North Carolina State University
Raleigh, NC

Laura D. Hostnik, DVM, MS, DACVIM
Clinical Associate Professor
The Ohio State University
Columbus, OH

Amy L. Johnson, DVM, DACVIM (LAIM, Neurology)
Associate Professor
University of Pennsylvania
Kennett Square, PA

Jamie Kopper, DVM, PhD, DACVIM, DACVECC
Assistant Professor
Iowa State University
Ames, IA

Gabriele Landolt, DVM, MS, PhD, DACVIM
Professor
Colorado State University
Fort Collins, CO

Kara M. Lascola, DVM, MS, DACVIM
Associate Professor
Auburn University
Auburn, AL

Kiho Lee, PhD
Associate Professor
University of Missouri
Columbia, MO

Rudy Madrigal, DVM, DACVIM
Associate Professor
Equine Sports Medicine & Surgery
Weatherford, TX

K. Gary Magdesian, DVM, DACVIM, DACVECC, DACVCP
Professor
University of California
Davis, CA

Dustin Major, DVM, DACVS
Clinical Assistant Professor
Texas A&M University
College Station, TX

Celia Marr, BVMS, MVM, PhD, DEIM, DECEIM, FRCVS
Associate Veterinary Specialist
Rossdales Veterinary Surgeons
Newmarket, Suffolk UK

Bianca Martins, DVM, MS, PhD, DACVO
Associate Professor
University of California
Davis, CA

Annette M. McCoy, DVM, MS, PhD, DACVS
Assistant Professor
University of Illinois
Urbana, IL

Harold McKenzie, DVM, MS, MSc, DACVIM
Professor
Virginia Maryland College of Veterinary Medicine
Blacksburg, VA

Francisco Mendoza, DVM, PhD, MSc, DECIM
Professor
Department of Animal Medicine and Surgery
University of Cordoba
Cordoba, Spain

Bonny Millar, VT, REVN, RVN
Equine Veterinary Nurse
Consultant and VNJ Equine Editor
Gwynedd, UK

James Moore, DVM, PhD, DACVS
Professor
University of Georgia
Athens, GA

Cristobal Navas de Solis, LV, MS, PHD, DACVIM
Assistant Professor
University of Pennsylvania
Kennett Square, PA

Rose Nolen-Walston, DVM, DACVIM
Associate Professor
University of Pennsylvania
Kennett Square, PA

Yvette Nout-Lomas, DVM, MS, PhD, DACVIM, DACVECC
Associate Professor
Colorado State University
Fort Collins, CO

Andrea Oliver, DVM
Resident, Internal Medicine
University of Pennsylvania
Kennett Square, PA

Emil Olsen, DVM, PhD, DACVIM (LAIM, Neurology)
Clinician, Neurology & Equine Internal Medicine
Swedish University of Agricultural Sciences
Uppsala, Sweden

Jon Palmer, DVM, DACVIM
Associate Professor
University of Pennsylvania
Kennett Square, PA

Lindsay M.W. Piel, DVM, PhD
USDA-ARS Veterinary Medical Officer
Washington State University
Pullman, WA

Giorgia Podico, DVM, MSc
Clinical Instructor
University of Illinois
Urbana, IL

Steve Reed, DVM, DACVIM
Shareholder
Rood & Riddle Equine Hospital
Lexington, KY

Heidi Reesink, VMD, PhD, DACVS
Associate Professor
Cornell University
Ithaca, NY

Roxanne M. Rodriguez Galarza, DVM, MS, DACVO
Associate Veterinarian
Animal Eye Care Associates
Cary, North Carolina

Diane Rhodes, DVM, DACVIM
Associate Veterinarian
Loomis Basin Equine Medical Center
Penryn, CA

Eric Rowe, DVM, PhD
Associate Professor
Iowa State University
Ames, IA

Rebecca Ruby, MSc, BVSc, DACVIM, DACVP
Assistant Professor
University of Kentucky
Lexington, KY

Emily Schaefer, VMD, DACVIM
Clinical Assistant Professor
Marion duPont Scott Equine Medical Center
Virginia Maryland College of Veterinary Medicine
Leesburg, VA

Andre Shih, DVM, DACVAA, DACVECC
Associate Veterinarian
Capital Veterinary Specialists
Jacksonville, FL

Nathan M. Slovis, DVM, DACVIM, CHT
Practice Member
Hagyard Equine Medical Institute
Lexington, KY

Sara M. Smith, DVM, MS, DACVO
Veterinary Associate
Eye Specialists for Animals
Denver, Colorado

Brett Sponseller, DVM, PhD, DACVIM
Professor
Iowa State University
Ames, IA

Kim A. Sprayberry, DVM, DACVIM, DACVECC
Professor
Cal Poly University
San Luis Obispo, CA

Danielle Strahl-Heldreth, DVM, MSEd, MSVMS, DACVAA
Clinical Assistant Professor
University of Illinois
Urbana, IL

Ben Sykes, BSc BVMS MSc MBA DipACVIM PhD FHEA
Veterinary Curriculum Development
Southern Cross University
Lismore, NSW, Australia

Ramiro E. Toribio, DVM, MS, PhD, DACVIM
Professor
The Ohio State University
Columbus, OH

Gaby van Galen, DVM, MSc, DES, PhD, DECEIM, DECVECC
Senior Clinician
Goulburn Valley Equine Hospital
Congupna, Victoria, Australia

Ashlee Watts, DVM, PhD, DACVS
Associate Professor
Texas A&M University
College Station, TX

Robin White, DVM, DACVR
Clinical Assistant Professor
Iowa State University
Ames, IA

David Whitley, DVM, MS DACVO
Professor Emeritus
University of Florida
Gainesville, FL

Pamela A. Wilkins, DVM, MS, PhD, DACVIM, DACVECC
Professor
University of Illinois
Urbana, IL

Edwina Wilkes, BVSc, MPHarm, FANZCVS, DVStud
Lecturer in Equine Medicine
Charles Sturt University
New South Wales, Australia

Jarred Williams, DVM, PhD, DACVS, DACVECC
Associate Professor
University of Georgia
Athens, GA

Sharon Witonsky, DVM, PhD, DACVIM
Associate Professor
Virginia Maryland College of Veterinary Medicine
Blacksburg, VA

David Wong, DVM, MS, DACVIM, DACVECC
Professor
Iowa State University
Ames, IA

Kate Wulster Bills, VMD, DACVR
Clinical Assistant Professor
University of Pennsylvania
Kennett Square, PA

Amanda Ziegler, DVM, PhD
Research Assistant Professor
North Carolina State University
Raleigh, NC

Foreword

Anne Koterba, DVM, PhD

It has been quite a few years since Willa Drummond, Philip Kosch, and I published *Equine Clinical Neonatology*—a few decades, in fact! Back then, few hospitals or clinics had space or personnel dedicated to the care of critically ill equine neonates, and there was little advanced training available for clinicians interested in caring for these small patients. But horse owners increasingly demanded improved care and outcomes given economic factors and other considerations, such as the advances already made in human neonatology. When the book was published in 1990, it represented over 10 years of intensive clinical and basic research on the equine neonate. Our "green book" was designed to share what we had learned so that others—including clinicians, students, veterinary nurses, and horse owners—could provide better veterinary care for compromised neonatal foals.

Looking back at that time, I feel our productivity during that decade in terms of advancing the field of equine neonatology was the result of the collaboration of a large team that worked amazingly well together because we were all focused on the goal of improving outcomes for sick foals. These partners included equine organizations that provided important research funding, as well as veterinary clinicians, residents, and basic scientists who worked together in both university and private practice settings to better understand the physiology, pharmacology, and disorders of the equine neonate. A large group of medical specialists, including human neonatologists, respiratory and physical therapists, and nutritionists, volunteered their time and provided important advice and perspectives on accurate identification of disease and treatment of neonates. Veterinary technicians, veterinary students, horse lovers, and community volunteers formed "foal teams" and provided essential around-the-clock intensive nursing care. I still feel very fortunate to have been a part of this innovative collaborative effort.

At the time, our book reflected the state of the art in equine neonatal intensive care. But in the years since, the number of veterinarians, students, and nurses caring for equine neonates has increased greatly. These individuals have expanded our knowledge of the topics we covered in our original book, and this increased understanding of the adaptive physiology from fetus through neonates—along with significant advances in diagnostics, treatments, and nursing care—has greatly improved our neonatal patients' outcomes. Much of this work has contributed to the material covered by this new book.

I want to thank and congratulate David and Pam for taking our concept of the original book and running with it, updating older information and introducing new knowledge. There are now many hospitals and clinicians with space, equipment, and personnel both interested in and capable of delivering high-quality care to equine neonates. This book, like our original, is for the dedicated veterinarians, interested students, and nurses who support them and deliver this care.

Preface

In the year 1990, Drs. Anne Koterba, Willa Drumond, and Philip Kosch edited and published the first and only edition of *Equine Clinical Neonatology*. Many veterinarians refer to this small little green book as *the* reference text for equine neonatal care and without a doubt, over the years, this book has served as an invaluable reference and resource for countless clinicians in their quest to provide veterinary care to neonatal foals. Over the past 30 years, veterinarians and researchers have greatly advanced our understanding of physiology, disease processes, and therapeutic options as it pertains to equine neonatal medicine and critical care. Although many aspects of the foal remain to be studied, the goal of this book is to relay new discoveries and provide clear and comprehensive information on disease processes and their treatment in neonatal foals. This information on equine neonatal care is targeted to veterinary students, practicing veterinarians, and equine veterinary specialists so that we can better serve our patients and their owners.

This textbook is authored by experts in the field of equine perinatology and is organized by body systems; within each system, subtopics such as embryology and anatomy, clinical physiology, diagnostic procedures, congenital disorders, and specific disease processes and treatment are discussed. Furthermore, one section is dedicated to general treatment principles for the equine neonate.

We are incredibly grateful for the expertise and generosity shared by the various contributors to this textbook. Their willingness to spare their time in authoring these chapters and share their individual depth of knowledge and clinical experience form the foundation of knowledge for this textbook and allows us to expand on the information provided by the original neonatal textbook published by Drs. Koterba, Drumond, and Kosch. It is our sincere hope that this text, *Equine Neonatal Medicine*, will prove to be a valuable resource to all those involved in the care of the neonatal foal.

David M. Wong
Pamela A. Wilkins

Part I

The Newborn Foal

Chapter 1 Postpartum Adaptation of the Newborn Foal

Section I Fetal Heart Rate and Fetal ECG

David Wong

Throughout the course of gestation, the maternal and fetal heart rates (FHR) are monitored as a general reflection of health. In the healthy mare, the mean maternal heart rate slowly increases, from 150 days gestation to term [1]. Maternal heart rate in late gestation is relatively constant during the last 15 days of pregnancy with a mean $\pm$ SD heart rate of 53 $\pm$ 1 beats/min prior to parturition. After parturition, heart rate significantly decreases to 42 $\pm$ 1 beats/min (Figure 1.I.1) [2]. The fetal heart is not as easily monitored as the mare but can be measured using fetal electrocardiography (ECG) or ultrasound. Determining the FHR via ECG is a simple parameter used to monitor fetal well-being in the pregnant mare, but this technique has been largely supplanted by determination of FHR through transabdominal ultrasonographic visualization of the fetal heart beat and rate. Acquisition and interpretation of the fetal ECG can be hampered by the larger amplitude of the maternal ECG signal, movement of the mare, small amplitude of the fetal ECG signal, and fetal position. Despite these limitations, most clinicians familiar with fetal ECGs have little difficulty acquiring cardiac activity of the equine fetus [3]. In addition, fetal ECG can be used in a continuous fashion via telemetry, allowing detection of fetal arrhythmias as well as more prolonged monitoring of FHR trends, while the mare is maintained in a quiet stall environment. Fetal ECG can also be used through stage I of labor.

Acquisition of a maternal ECG is initiated first, using a base-apex lead configuration, to differentiate the maternal heart rate and rhythm and confirm the maternal cardiac activity as compared to the fetal cardiac activity obtained via fetal ECG lead placement. A guide to electrode placement for fetal ECG includes the following, keeping in mind that electrode placement may have to be modified based on fetal position: *left arm lead* on the dorsal midline of the mare in the mid-lumbar region; *right arm lead* on the ventral midline 10–15 cm in front of udder; and *neutral lead* anywhere on the trunk of the horse (i.e. left croup) [3]. In late-pregnant mares, the right arm lead may have to be positioned on the right ventral abdomen at a level approximately at the height of the stifle [3]. Electrodes with alligator clips can be used, but electrodes with adhesive pads, reinforced with rapid-drying adhesive glue, can be used for longer or repeated use and is better tolerated by the mare. Conventional and telemetric methods can be used to acquire the ECG tracing. If conventional methods are used, recordings are performed over 10- to 20-minute periods, several times a day. Telemetry allows for continuous monitoring, with paper tracings recorded at approximately 2-hour intervals [4]. Both the maternal and fetal cardiac activity will appear blunted as compared to a maternal base apex lead (Figure 1.I.2) and the tracing can be lost in artifact or background interference. The maximum amplitude of the fetal ECG ranges from 0.05 to 0.1 mV [4].

Volumes of information are available to the obstetrician in regard to monitoring fetal health and viability in human fetuses. In comparison, a trivial amount of published information is available to the equine clinician. However, some of the pertinent information in regard to the fetal response to hypoxia and fetal ECG changes associated with fetal distress and hypoxia in the human fetus can be extrapolated to the equine species, with the disclosed fact that there may be unknown differences between species. Of note, much of the published information in reference to the human fetus's response to hypoxia has been established via experiments performed in fetal sheep.

The clinician should recognize that transient accelerations and decelerations in FHR are present in the healthy fetus. In fact, the presence of intermittent FHR accelerations associated with fetal movement is believed to suggest adequate oxygenation to maintain normal fetal autonomic nervous system function [5]. However, persistent tachycardia or bradycardia can signal fetal distress. One must first recognize that despite the fact that the fetus has twice the

Equine Neonatal Medicine, First Edition. Edited by David M. Wong and Pamela A. Wilkins.

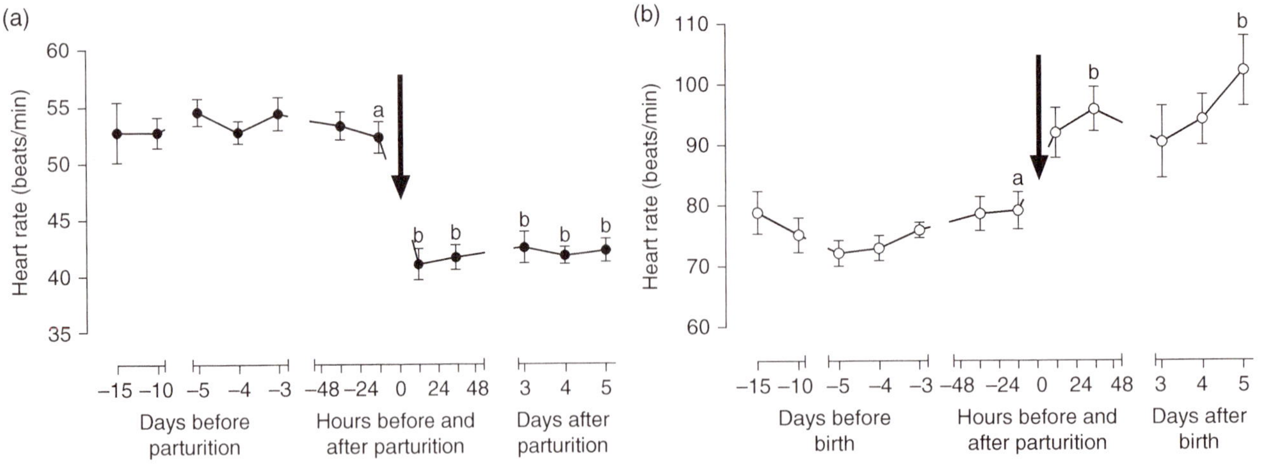

Figure 1.I.1 Maternal (a), fetal and newborn (b) peri-parturient heart rates in the horse. Arrow indicates time of parturition [2].

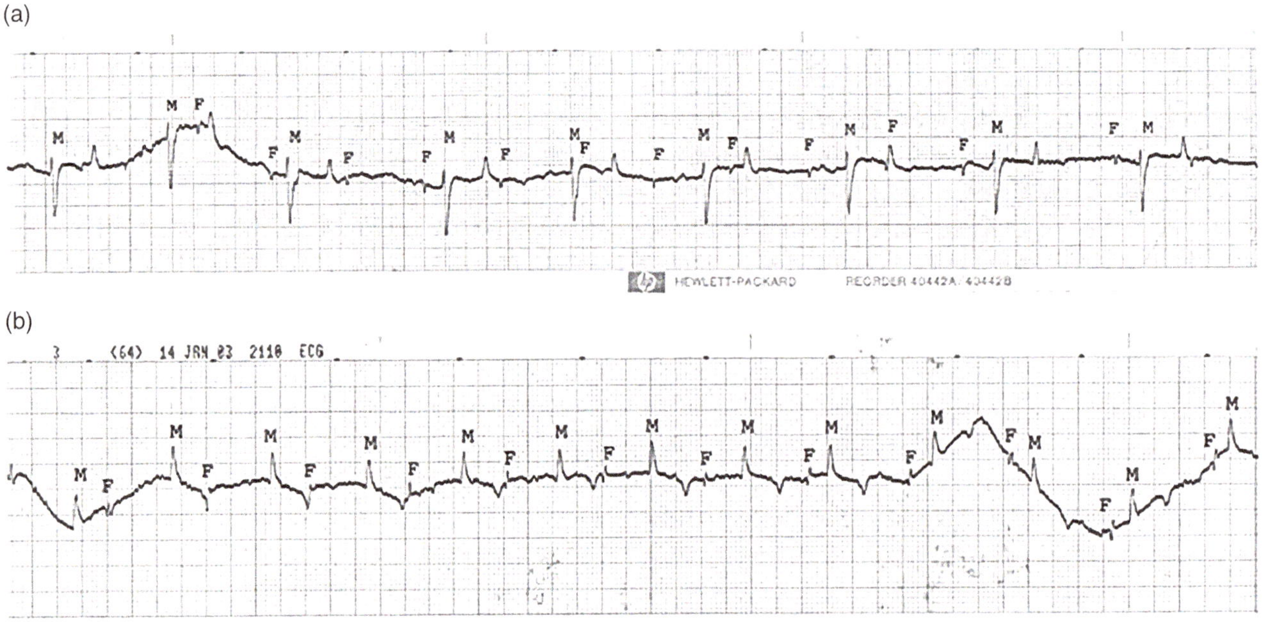

Figure 1.I.2 Fetal and maternal ECG (a). Maternal "M" and fetal "F" signal. Fetal and maternal rates are 48 and 83 beats/min, respectively. In (b), fetal and maternal heart rates are more similar, emphasizing need for careful inspection [4].

oxygen demand as the adult, and yet far lower partial pressures of oxygen and hemoglobin saturations, the fetus has a remarkable ability to compensate for sub-normal provision of oxygen that is necessary to maintain health in the adult [6–8]. In reality, under normal conditions, the fetus has a surplus of oxygen available and is able to survive profound hypoxia for extraordinary periods of time, often without injury [6–8]. This is possible because of the combination of notable fetal anaerobic tolerance and the fetal capacity to establish a coordinated cardiovascular and metabolic defense to hypoxia [8–10]. During episodes of acute hypoxia, peripheral chemoreceptors are stimulated, resulting in a coordinated cardiovascular response designed to sustain perfusion [6–8]. This chemoreflex response balances the severity of the hypoxic insult with the cellular tolerance of the individual [11]. In addition, once initiated, the response is titrated to the hypoxic insult, producing varied responses that are manifested clinically as variable decelerations in FHR [12].

The initial response in the near-term fetus to acute hypoxic challenge is mediated by parasympathetic pathways that result in rapid deceleration in FHR, with the degree of deceleration broadly related to the severity of hypoxia [13–15]. Shallow decelerations in FHR are associated with modest reduction in uteroplacental flow whereas more profound decelerations in FHR suggest near total or total reduction in uteroplacental flow [15, 16]. Fetal bradycardia in response to hypoxic challenge reduces cardiac workload and is likely a defense mechanism present to preserve cardiac glycogen and reduce cardiac stress [17]. Slowing of the FHR may also allow increased exposure of the fetal blood to maternal blood, thus increasing the time for equilibration of dissolved gas from the placenta and improving oxygen content of fetal blood [4, 18, 19]. Regardless of the reduced FHR and concomitant decrease in cardiac output, the fetus maintains blood pressure and normal oxygen delivery to vital organs during moderate hypoxia by peripheral vasoconstriction [6–8, 11, 20]. If mild to moderate hypoxia is sustained, bradycardia is followed by tachycardia, a response that is mediated by increases in circulating catecholamines [21]. Tachycardia allows for ventricular output to contribute to maintaining of blood pressure while allowing peripheral vasoconstriction to abate, consequently permitting more perfusion to peripheral organs to occur [7]. This increase in heart rate does not occur if the hypoxic insult is more severe, in which case bradycardia becomes progressively more profound and is likely related to direct effects of hypoxia on the heart itself [11]. Interestingly, in fetal sheep, age-related differences in the FHR response to hypoxia were observed in that a similar hypoxic challenge that elicited bradycardia followed by tachycardia in near-term fetuses was not observed earlier in gestation; this lack of response might be related to immaturity of neurohormonal regulators and chemoreceptor function [7, 22, 23].

In horses, transcutaneous fetal ECG can be used to evaluate fetal well-being and viability in pregnant mares from approximately 150 days of gestation to parturition. As a general trend, the FHR decreases gradually from 150 days gestation to term (Table 1.I.1). Sporadic episodes of tachycardia are typically observed throughout gestation in the healthy equine fetus and may be associated with fetal movements (Table 1.I.1). Other underlying causes of fetal tachycardia include maternal medications, maternal medical disorders, obstetric bleeding, and fetal tachyarrhythmia [5]. In contrast, fetal bradycardia is not typically observed during normal gestation and, in people, has been associated with maternal hypotension, umbilical cord prolapse, rapid fetal descent, excessive frequent uterine contractions and uterine rupture or fetal congenital heart defects [1, 5]. Thus, substantial and/or prolonged increases or decreases in fetal heart can indicate fetal distress.

The definition of fetal bradycardia and tachycardia remains obscure in the horse with normal FHR ranging from 65 to 115 beats/min in the last months of gestation [4]. During the last weeks of gestation, the baseline FHR ranges from 60 to 75 beats/min with the lower range being 40 to 75 beats/min. In one study, the lowest measured FHR was <70 beats/min in 80% of fetuses evaluated, <60 beats/min in 55%, and <50 beats/min in 14%. In contrast, the highest FHR measured were in the range of 83–250 beats/min, with 86% of fetuses having a FHR >100 beats/min, >120 beats/min in 50% and >200 beats/min in 20% [24]. Thus, if the FHR is <60 or >120 beats/min over a prolonged period of time, repeated evaluation is indicated. One source suggests persistent fetal tachycardia as a heart rate over 200 beats/min at 120–220 days gestation and greater than 110 beats/min from 280 days gestation to parturition; bradycardia is defined as a FHR <60 beats/min at any stage of gestation [25].

Persistent fetal bradycardia usually coincides with late gestation asphyxia, whereas persistent tachycardia may represent early effects of hypoxia, maternal pyrexia, or a prolonged acceleration pattern in a healthy fetus [26]. The fetus is dependent on the placenta for oxygen supply, and a reduction in fetal cardiac activity is the only means to reduce cardiac oxygen consumption. Thus, the primary response to fetal hypoxia is a reduction in heart rate and absence of episodic heart rate increases. Subsequently, persistent tachycardia followed by bradycardia and cardiac

Table 1.I.1 Heart rate, beat-to-beat (RR) interval, and number and duration of accelerations and decelerations in heart rate acquired via equine fetal ECG evaluation at various stages of gestation [3].

Gestational age (days)	170–180	181–220	221–240	280	320	340	1 day prior to parturition
Heart rate (beats/min)	126 ± 2	117 ± 4	101 ± 5	105 ± 4	83 ± 3	79 ± 3	79 ± 1
R-R interval (ms)	481 ± 10	518 ± 15	601 ± 30	578 ± 20	762 ± 41	772 ± 34	764 ± 12
Heart rate accelerations							
Number (number/h)	23 ± 7				22 ± 2		25 ± 3
Duration (heartbeats)	29 ± 11				42 ± 6		35 ± 5
Hear rate decelerations							
Number (number/h)	23 ± 6				27 ± 3		30 ± 3
Duration (heartbeats)	31 ± 12				32 ± 5		23 ± 2

arrest occur as fetal decompensation occurs through the loss of central nervous system control mechanisms [3]. In one report, fetal bradycardia was recorded in an equine fetus 48 hours prior to abortion and reached a nadir of 38 beats/min at 10 minutes prior to abortion [1].

During the last 10–14 days prior to parturition, FHR remains fairly stable, although one report noted increases in FHR 5 days prior to parturition to 5 days after birth [2, 3]. Similar to other studies, the mean ± SD FHR within 24 hours of parturition was 79 ± 3 beats/min and was significantly lower than the heart rate at 48 (96 ± 3 beats/min) and 120 hours of age (102 ± 6 beats/min) in healthy neonatal foals [2]. Unfortunately, FHR and R-R interval do not allow prediction of impending parturition in the horse [3]. In a review of FHR during stage I of labor, a decrease in FHR was observed prior to rupture of the chorioallantois [27]. After rupture of the chorioallantois, 82% (37/45 fetal ECGs) of fetuses demonstrated a gradual decrease or maintenance of the same FHR, whereas 18% had an increase in FHR during stage II [1, 3, 27, 28]. Decelerations in FHR have been associated with brief periods of decreased uteroplacental blood flow during uterine contractions associated with labor in people [5]; however, this has not been directly examined in the horse. Additionally, fetal arrhythmias were detected during stage I of labor in a small number (4/39 fetuses, 10%) of fetal ECGs and included sinus arrhythmia and atrial premature contraction. One fetus with atrial premature contractions was later observed to have atrial fibrillation as a neonatal foal; however, fetal ECG could not be used to predict the presence of neonatal arrhythmias.

Beat-to-beat (R-R interval) variability is another parameter that can be measured when evaluating the fetal ECG. The R-R interval ranges from 0.5 to 4 mm in the equine fetus, with most in the range of 1 mm [4]. The R-R interval variability arises from an intact fetal central nervous system and appropriate functioning of the parasympathetic and sympathetic nervous systems. If there is an absence of variation in R-R interval, loss of the function of the fetal CNS may be present and indicates close observation. Of note, the R-R interval should be measured when the FHR is not accelerating or decelerating and the clinician should be cognizant of the fact that maternal drugs (i.e. sedation) can affect the RR interval [4].

References

1 Colles, C.M. and Parkes, R.D. (1978). Foetal electrocardiography in the mare. *Equine Vet. J.* 10: 32–37.

2 Nagel, C., Erber, R., Bergmaier, C. et al. (2012). Cortisol and progestin release, heart rate and heart rate variability in the pregnant and postpartum mare, fetus and newborn foal. *Theriogenology* 78: 759–767.

3 Nagel, C., Aurich, J., and Aurich, C. (2010). Determination of heart rate and heart rate variability in the equine fetus by fetomaternal electrocardiography. *Theriogenology* 73: 973–983.

4 Wilkins, P.A. (2003). Monitoring the pregnant mare in the ICU. *Clin. Tech. Equine Pract.* 2: 212–219.

5 Walton, J.R. and Peaceman, A.M. (2012). Identification, assessment and management of fetal compromise. *Clin. Perinatol.* 39: 753–768.

6 Martin, C.B. (2008). Normal fetal physiology and behavior, and adaptive responses with hypoxemia. *Semin. Perinatol.* 32: 239–242.

7 Bennet, L. and Gunn, A.J. (2009). The fetal heart rate response to hypoxia: insights from animal models. *Clin. Perinatol.* 36: 655–672.

8 Bennet, L., Westgate, J., Gluckman, P.D. et al. (2003). Fetal responses to asphyxia. In: *Fetal and Neonatal Brain Injury: Mechanisms, Management, and the Risks of Practice*, 2e (ed. D.K. Stevenson and P. Sunshine), 83–110. Cambridge: Cambridge University Press.

9 Gunn, A.J., Quaedackers, J.S., Guan, J. et al. (2001). The premature fetus: not as defenseless as we thought, but still paradoxically vulnerable? *Dev. Neurosci.* 23: 175–189.

10 Gunn, A.J. and Bennet, L. (2008). Timing of injury in the fetus and neonate. *Curr. Opin. Obstet. Gynecol.* 20: 175–181.

11 Bennet, L., Peebles, D.M., Edwards, A.D. et al. (1998). The cerebral hemodynamic response to asphyxia and hypoxia in the near-term fetal sheep as measured by near infrared spectroscopy. *Pediatr. Res.* 44: 951–957.

12 Sameshima, H., Ikenoue, T., Ikeda, T. et al. (2004). Unselected low-risk pregnancies and the effect of continuous intrapartum fetal heart rate monitoring on umbilical blood gases and cerebral palsy. *Am. J. Obstet. Gynecol.* 190: 118–123.

13 Cohn, H.E., Sacks, E.J., Heymann, M.A. et al. (1974). Cardiovascular responses to hypoxemia and academia in fetal lambs. *Am. J. Obstet. Gynecol.* 120: 817–824.

14 Giussani, D.A., Spencer, J.A., Moore, P.J. et al. (1993). Afferent and efferent components of the cardiovascular reflex responses to acute hypoxia in term fetal sheep. *J. Physiol.* 461: 431–449.

15 Itskovitx, J. and Rudolph, A.M. (1982). Denervation of arterial chemoreceptors and baroreceptors in fetal lambs in utero. *Am. J. Phys* 242: H916–H920.

16 Baan, J., Boekkooi, P.F., Teitel, D.F. et al. (1993). Heart rate fall during acute hypoxemia: a measure of chemoreceptor response in fetal sheep. *J. Dev. Physiol.* 19: 105–111.

17 Fletcher, A.J., Gardner, D.S., Edwards, M. et al. (2006). Development of the ovine fetal cardiovascular defense to hypoxemia towards term. *Am. J. Physiol. Heart Circ. Physiol.* 291: H3023–H3034.

18 Cohn, H.E., Piasecki, G.J., and Jackson, B.T. (1980). The effect of fetal heart rate on cardiovascular function during hypoxia. *Am. J. Obstet. Gynecol.* 138: 1190–1199.

19 Jensen, A., Garnier, Y., and Berger, R. (1999). Dynamics of fetal circulatory responses to hypoxia and asphyxia. *Eur. J. Obstet. Gynecol. Reprod. Biol.* 84: 155–172.

20 Richardson, B.S., Carmichael, L., Homan, J. et al. (1993). Cerebral oxidative metabolism in fetal sheep with prolonged and graded hypoxemia. *J. Dev. Physiol.* 19: 77–83.

21 Hanson, M.A. (1997). Do we now understand the control of the fetal circulation? *Eur. J. Obstet. Gynecol. Reprod. Biol.* 75: 55–61.

22 Iwamoto, H.S., Kaufman, T., Keil, L.C. et al. (1989). Responses to acute hypoxemia in fetal sheep at 0.6–0.7 gestation. *Am. J. Phys.* 256 (3 Pt 2): H613–H620.

23 Matsuda, Y., Patrick, J., and Carmichael, L. (1992). Effects of sustained hypoxemia on the sheep fetus at midgestation: endocrine, cardiovascular, and biophysical responses. *Am. J. Obstet. Gynecol.* 167: 531–540.

24 Palmer, J.E. (2000). Fetal monitoring. *Proceedings of the Equine Symposium and Annual Conference*, San Antonio, TX, 39–43. http://nicuvet.com/nicuvet/Equine-Perinatoloy/Reprints/Fetal%20monitoring%20-%20SFT.htm.

25 Knottenbelt, D.C. (2004). Risk category of the foal. In: *Equine Neonatology Medicine and Surgery* (ed. D.C. Knottenbelt, N. Hodstock, and J. Madigan), 29–60. Edinburgh: Sunders.

26 Steer, P.J. (2008). Has electronic fetal heart rate monitoring made a difference? *Semin. Fetal Neonatal Med.* 13: 2–7.

27 Yamamoto, K., Yasuda, J., and Too, K. (1992). Arrhythmias in newborn Thoroughbred foals. *Equine Vet. J.* 24: 169–173.

28 Too, K., Kanagawa, H., and Kawata, K. (1967). Fetal and maternal electrocardiograms during parturition in a mare. *Jpn. J. Vet. Res.* 15: 5–14.

Section II Fetal Circulation and Cardiorespiratory Transition

Cristobal Navas de Solis

Fetal Circulation

Fetal circulation is notably different from what is present in the neonate and adult horse in order to maximize efficiency of blood flow and oxygen delivery during fetal development. Understanding fetal circulation is important to comprehending hemodynamics in utero as well as congenital diseases, but for the clinician, this knowledge is also important in the evaluation of severely ill or premature foals that fail to make the normal transition to extrauterine life. In the fetus, vascular shunts such as the ductus venosus and foramen ovale exists to deliver oxygenated blood from the placenta to the left atrium, while another shunt brings deoxygenated blood to the descending aorta (ductus arteriosus). The critical characteristic of fetal circulation is that gas exchange occurs at the placental interface and not the fetal lungs [1]. Compared to other veterinary species, the difference in partial pressure of oxygen (PO_2) between the uterine vein and umbilical vein is low (0–4 mmHg), resulting in a high umbilical vein oxygen content (48–54 mmHg) [2, 3]. Likewise, the gradients for carbon dioxide (PCO_2) are very low (0–1 mmHg) in the horse, reflecting the greater diffusability of CO_2 compared to O_2 [3]. Umbilical vein oxygenation in the equine fetus is more sensitive to changes in maternal arterial pressure of oxygen (P_aO_2) than in other species. This has been postulated to account for the frequent incidence of perinatal asphyxia in the foal. On the other hand, when maternal P_aO_2 is increased with inhaled oxygen, oxygen concentration in the umbilical vein increases more than in the uterine vein; this characteristic can be used therapeutically in fetal foals with suspected hypoxemia [2].

In other species, a portion of oxygenated blood in the umbilical vein travels to the right atrium through the ductus venosus and caudal vena cava allowing approximately 50% of blood in the umbilical vein to bypass the liver [1]. One theory in regard to the purpose of the ductus venosus is to direct highly oxygenated blood derived from the ductus venosus in such a way that it passes preferentially through the foramen ovale, therefore allowing distribution to the upper body (heart and brain) [4]. A unique feature of the equine fetus is that this species lacks the ductus venosus [3, 5]. The cause for this is uncertain, but one theory put forth is that equine fetal arterial blood has relatively high oxygen tensions and that preferential distribution of umbilical blood contributing to enhanced supply of oxygen to the heart and brain is not necessary [4]. Regardless of the reason, oxygenated blood is preferentially shunted to the left atrium via the valve of the foramen ovale (septum primum). Blood is shunted as higher pressure in the right atrium (due to high volume venous return) keeps the valve over the foramen ovale open, thus allowing blood to flow from right to left atrium [1]. A small amount of blood from the pulmonary veins joins the blood shunted through the foramen ovale; the blood then enters the left ventricle and is ejected and into the aorta to the systemic circulation [6].

Deoxygenated blood that returns to the right atrium from the systemic circulation flows through the tricuspid valve into the right ventricle and is ejected into the pulmonary artery. Due to the high pulmonary vascular resistance of the fetal lungs, most of the right ventricular output is shunted into the descending aorta through the ductus arteriosus. A small part (10–25%) perfuses the lungs to support metabolic needs. The ductus arteriosus connects the pulmonary artery and aorta at the level of the origin of the left subclavian artery and the pulmonary artery bifurcation. For this reason, the brain, heart, and cranial portion of the body receive blood with higher oxygen content during fetal life. For this same reason, selective cyanosis of the caudal extremities is seen in neonates with a patent ductus arteriosus (PDA) and Eisenmenger syndrome. In this situation, the left-to-right shunt causes pulmonary hypertension as blood travels through the ductus arteriosus, eventually reversing the blood flow right-to-left, thereby resulting in

Equine Neonatal Medicine, First Edition. Edited by David M. Wong and Pamela A. Wilkins.

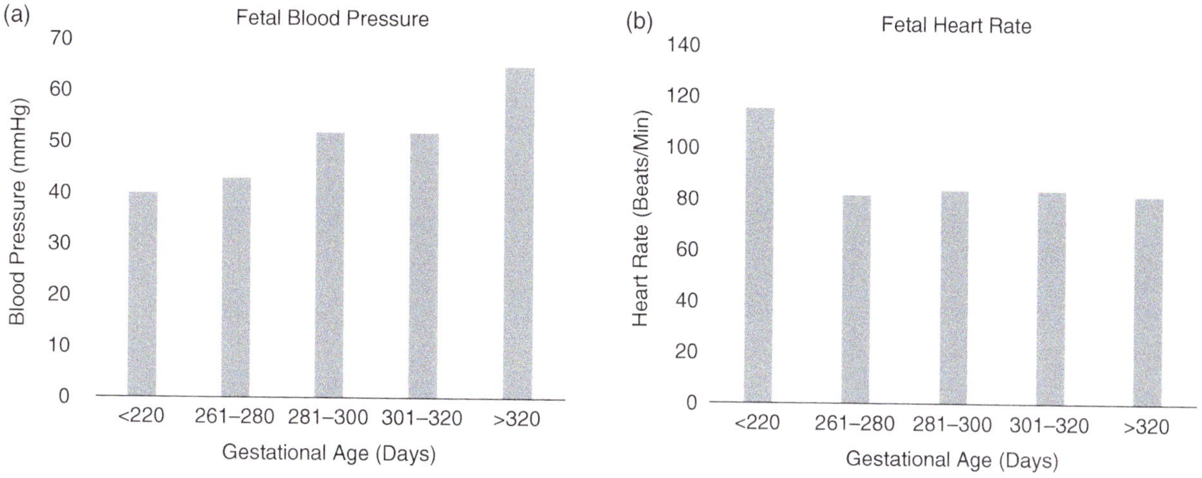

Figure 1.II.1 Mean values of (a) arterial blood pressure and (b) heart rate from fetal ponies at different gestational ages (term ~335 days). $N = 4–9$ individual fetuses at each gestational age. *Source:* Adapted from Fowden et al. [5].

cyanosis. Further details of the physiology and clinical consequences of PDA are explained in Chapter 12. Blood in the descending aorta perfuses the abdominal organs and lower limbs of the fetus, subsequently flowing to the umbilical arteries for gas exchange and transfer of waste products in the placenta [1, 7].

Similar to other species, fetal blood pressure (BP) increases with gestational age in the equine fetus (Figure 1.II.1). The mean BP rises from 30–35 mmHg at 150 days of gestation to 80–90 mmHg at term and is associated with a decline in heart rate from 120 to 80 beats/min [5]. These changes in blood pressure and heart rate occur gradually between 150 and 300 days of gestation and then accelerate as the fetus approaches parturition, with further decreases in heart rate in the last 30 minutes before birth.

Cardiorespiratory Transition

The placenta is a low-resistance vascular bed and the fetal pulmonary circulation is a high-resistance circuit. This is one of the keys to understanding fetal circulation and the changes that occur at birth. It is important to remember, and is intuitive, that different factors can affect gas exchange in the placenta and therefore fetal wellbeing. Maternal diseases such as respiratory disease (resulting in hypoxemia), cardiac diseases (causing low cardiac output and perfusion), nutritional deficiencies, placentitis or placental insufficiency are examples. Congenital diseases, disease in the neonatal period or even cardiovascular dysfunction later in life have been linked to problems in placental circulation [1].

Transition to extrauterine circulation is driven by changes in pulmonary and systemic pressures, oxygenation of pulmonary blood, and prostaglandin metabolism. This transition involves the closure of the aforementioned fetal shunts over the first 1 to 2 weeks of life [6]. At birth the foal is hypoxemic and hypercapnic; this stimulates the first gasping breaths. Compression of the thorax through the birth canal drives fluid out of the airway and the lungs start to inflate [8, 9]. Lung inflation causes a drop in pulmonary resistance, which consequently increases pulmonary blood flow. As pulmonary artery pressure falls below aortic pressure, blood in the pulmonary artery is directed into the lungs rather than the ductus arteriosus, as noted during fetal development. Some blood is shunted from the relatively high aortic pressure into the pulmonary artery, typically lasting 48–72 hours. The shunt created by the ductus arteriosus can often be heard in the neonate as a continuous murmur over the heart base (point of maximal intensity over the pulmonic/aortic valve or somewhat more dorsal under the triceps muscle) but a clinically relevant PDA is rare in the foal [10]. Continuous murmurs should prompt further evaluation in the presence of signs of cardiovascular or respiratory diseases, but benign neglect is acceptable in the first few days of life if the neonatal foal appears clinically healthy. The ductus arteriosus closes progressively under the influence of increased oxygen content in the blood and decreased prostaglandin concentrations. As flow though the ductus arteriosus ceases, a sharp increase in pulmonary circulation increases pulmonary venous return to the left atrium, functionally closing the foramen ovale. Pharmacological closure of selected PDAs, mainly in preterm infants, is often cited in the human literature. Briefly, non-steroidal anti-inflammatory drugs (NSAIDs) or acetaminophen are given to counteract the vascular smooth muscle relaxation induced by PGE_2 on vascular smooth muscle relaxation [11]. Pharmacological therapy has been shown to increase the odds of PDA closure but not change the odds of death, necrotizing enterocolitis, or intraventricular hemorrhage, raising the question of whether this therapy necessarily improves clinical outcomes [12]. The safety, indications, dosages, or efficacy of pharmacological therapy to aid closure of PDAs in neonatal foals has not been explored.

High prostaglandin concentrations, low pulmonary oxygenation, and immaturity of the wall of the ductus arteriosus can predispose to delayed ductal closure in premature neonates. At birth the umbilical cord is severed, which blocks access of peripheral blood to the low-pressure placental bed; thus, systemic vascular resistance rapidly increases. In the majority of neonates, pulmonary vascular resistance drops below systemic vascular resistance within minutes to hours after birth and the arterial ductal shunt becomes left-to-right if the ductus arteriosus remains patent. This means pulmonary hyperperfusion and systemic hypoperfusion, but not cyanosis, are the initial consequences of a PDA [1]. In individuals with severe pulmonary overcirculation, pulmonary vascular remodeling and endothelial damage leads to pulmonary hypertension and shunt reversal (right to left shunt). This is known as Eisenmenger syndrome. Reversed PDA results in poor oxygenation as blood bypasses the lungs and polycythemia develops [13]. Hypoxemia, hypothermia, and acidosis can cause, or contribute to, increased pulmonary pressure and cause reversal to fetal circulation and right-to-left shunting by reopening the foramen ovale and ductus arteriosus. The shunting worsens hypoxemia, which furthers the pulmonary hypertension [14]. Persistent fetal circulation (also called persistent pulmonary hypertension of the newborn) is defined as postnatal persistence of right-to-left ductal or arterial shunting, or both in the presence of elevated right ventricular pressure.

Heart Rate, Rhythm, and Blood Pressure in the Newborn and Neonatal Foal

The heart rate of the healthy equine neonate is approximately 80–100 beats per minute (BPM) [15]. However, heart rate varies considerably in the first hours of life, and different reference intervals can be used for specific time points. The average fetal heart rate decreases progressively during the hour prior to birth from an average of approximately 70 BPM to approximately 60 BPM. Immediately after birth, the average heart rate suddenly increases to approximately 80 BPM, then decreases to approximately 65 BPM after 2 minutes. The heart rate then increases to normal neonatal values of 80–100 BPM over the following 10 minutes [16]. The ranges in heart rate are, however, wide, and ranges of 30–90, 60–200, and 72–133 BPM have been described in the first 1–5 minutes, 6–60 minutes, and 9–43 hours after birth, respectively, in Thoroughbred foals [17]. The difference in rates reported between various studies may be due to breed variation or specific situations of the examination [16–19].

Table 1.II.1 Normal values of heart rate and respiratory rate in equine neonates [20].

Age	Heart rate (/min)	Respiratory rate (/min)	Reference
Birth	70–80	Gasping to 70/min	[10]
1–5 min	30–90		[17]
2–30 min	120–140	50	[10]
6–60 min	60–200		[17]
1–12 h	140–150	40	[10]
12–24 h	110–120	35	[10]
12–24 h	80–120	30–40	[14]
9–43 h	72–133		[17]
24–48 h	90–100	30	[10]
24–48 h	80–100		[14]
48–72 h	60–80	20	[10]
7 d	89–118		[19]
7 d	93–129		[18]
30 d	73–89		[19]
30 d	89–117		[18]
60 d	68–86		[18]
90 d	52–65		[19]
90 d	58–76		[18]
200 d	45–63		[19]
Adult	45–49		[20]

Heart rate is highly dependent on the degree of excitement. It is advisable to obtain the rate when the foal is quiet or sleeping. Reported heart rates for foals in the peripartum period and during the few months of growth are reported in Table 1.II.1. The rhythm is most commonly regular [15] with the exception of the first 15 minutes of life in which there are frequent arrhythmias [21].

Blood pressure (Blood pressure = Cardiac output/Systemic vascular resistance) is often monitored in foals as a surrogate of blood flow. It is important to note that blood pressure does not equate to blood flow or perfusion. Different BP monitors can be used in foals, but oscillometric monitors with the cuff placed over the coccygeal artery are most often used. Positioning the cuff over the metatarsal or median artery can produce analogous measurements, but with some devices this location can produce a less accurate reading [22]. The precision of these devices needs to be assessed in a device-specific manner. Table 1.II.2 provides values in growing ponies using an ultrasonic device [18].

Table 1.II.2 Noninvasive blood pressure values in growing foals.

Age (days)	Systolic (mmHg)	Diastolic (mmHg)	Mean (mmHg)
1	81 ± 10	35 ± 7	50 ± 8
7	104 ± 21	40 ± 14	61 ± 15
14	100 ± 16	41 ± 7	61 ± 6
21	107 ± 28	48 ± 17	68 ± 16
30	114 ± 21	54 ± 13	74 ± 11
60	103 ± 12	53 ± 20	70 ± 6
90	111 ± 15	57 ± 19	75 ± 16

Source: Adapted from Lombard et al. [18].

References

1 Finnemore, A. and Groves, A. (2015). Physiology of the fetal and transitional circulation. *Semin. Fetal Neonatal Med.* 20 (4): 210–216.

2 Palmer, J. (n.d.). *Perinatology*. New Bolton Center, University of Pennsylvania http://nicuvet.com/nicuvet/Learn/Perinatology%20Handout.pdf.

3 Silver, M. (1984). Some aspects of equine placental exchange and foetal physiology. *Equine Vet. J.* 16: 227–233.

4 Barnes, R.J. (1997). Perinatal carbohydrate metabolism and the blood flow of the fetal liver. *Equine Vet. J. Suppl.* 24: 26–31.

5 Fowden, A.L., Giussani, D.A., and Forhead, A.J. (2020). Physiological development of the equine fetus during late gestation. *Equine Vet. J.* 52: 165–173.

6 Sidhu, P.S. and Lui, F. (2020). Embryology, Ductus Venosus. In: *StatPearls*. Treasure Island, FL: StatPearls Publishing https://www.ncbi.nlm.nih.gov/books/NBK547759/https://www.ncbi.nlm.nih.gov/books/NBK547759.

7 Huff, T., Chaudhry, R., and Mahajan, K. (2020). Anatomy, thorax, heart ductus arteriosus. In: *StatPearls*. Treasure Island, FL: StatPearls Publishing https://www.ncbi.nlm.nih.gov/books/NBK470160.

8 Scansen, B.A. (2019). Equine congenital heart disease. *Vet. Clin. North Am. Equine Pract.* 35: 103–117.

9 Saadi, A., Dalir-Naghadeh, B., Hashemi Asl, S.M. et al. (2020). Right to left patent ductus arteriosus, acute bronchointerstitial pneumonia, pulmonary hypertension and cor pulmonale in a foal. *Equine Vet. Educ.* 9: 152–158.

10 Knottenbelt, D.C. et al. (ed.) (2004). Perinatal review. In: *Equine Neonatal Medicine and Surgery E-Book: Medicine and Surgery*, 1–28. Elsevier Health Sciences.

11 Bardanzellu, F., Neroni, P., Dessì, A. et al. (2017). Paracetamol in patent ductus arteriosus treatment: efficacious and safe? *Biomed. Res. Int.* 2017: 1438038.

12 Mitra, S., Florez, I.D., Tamayo, M.E. et al. (2018). Association of Placebo, indomethacin, ibuprofen, and acetaminophen with closure of hemodynamically significant patent ductus arteriosus in preterm infants: a systematic review and meta-analysis. *JAMA* 319: 1221–1238.

13 Navas De Solis, C. and Wesselowski, S. (2020). Equine congenital heart disease and respiratory disease interactions. *Equine Vet. Educ.* 9: 460–464.

14 Paradis, M.R. (ed.) (2006). Cardiac disorders. In: *Equine Neonatal Medicine*, 247–258. W.B. Saunders.

15 Marr, C.M. (2015). The equine neonatal cardiovascular system in health and disease. *Vet. Clin. North Am. Equine Pract.* 31: 545–565.

16 Yamamoto, K., Yasuda, J., and Too, K. (1991). Electrocardiographic findings during parturition and blood gas tensions immediately after birth in thoroughbred foals. *Jpn. J. Vet. Res.* 39: 143–157.

17 Rossdale, P.D. (1993). Clinical view of disturbances in equine foetal maturation. *Equine Vet. J. Suppl.* 14: 3–7.

18 Lombard, C.W., Evans, M., Martin, L. et al. (1984). Blood pressure, electrocardiogram and echocardiogram measurements in the growing pony foal. *Equine Vet. J.* 16: 342–347.

19 Ohmura, H. and Jones, J.H. (2017). Changes in heart rate and heart rate variability as a function of age in Thoroughbred horses. *J. Equine Sci.* 28: 99–103.

20 Wong, D.M. and Wilkins, P.A. (2015). Defining the systemic inflammatory response syndrome in equine neonates. *Vet. Clin. Equine* 31: 463–481.

21 Yamamoto, K., Yasuda, J., and Too, K. (1992). Arrhythmias in newborn thoroughbred foals. *Equine Vet. J.* 24: 169–173.

22 Giguère, S., Knowles, H.A. Jr., Valverde, A. et al. (2005). Accuracy of indirect measurement of blood pressure in neonatal foals. *J. Vet. Intern. Med.* 19: 571–576.

Section III Maturation of the Lung and the Surfactant System

Undine Christmann

A functional lung is characterized by (i) extensive ramification of airways (conducting and respiratory); (ii) large surface area dedicated to gas exchange; (iii) effective vascular and capillary network; and (iv) sophisticated surfactant system that facilitates lung inflation, supports efficient gas exchange, and modulates immune response. The development of these components is tightly regulated during gestation. Maturation of the lung and its surfactant system is essential for the successful transition to extra-uterine life.

Lung Maturation

Pulmonary maturation spans over three different periods: the embryonic period, fetal period, and postnatal period (Table 1.III.1) [1, 2].

Embryonic Period

Lung tissue first becomes visible in the equine embryo between 24 and 49 days of gestation [3, 4]. The development of the lung begins with the formation of a groove (sulcus laryngotrachealis) in the ventral wall of the primitive foregut (Figure 1.III.1a) [1, 2, 5]. This groove deepens and forms the laryngo-tracheal tube, which is lined by endoderm on the inside and mesoderm on the outside. The laryngo-tracheal tube extends caudally and bifurcates into two outpouchings, which represent the origin (primordia) of the lung (Figure 1.III.1b). Airways are subsequently formed by branching morphogenesis. This developmental process generates ramified epithelial trees through repetitive cycles of elongation, growth, and branching into the surrounding mesenchyme. It is tightly coordinated through interactions between epithelial and mesenchymal cells. A principal bronchus develops in the left and right lung primordia and continues to branch out to form secondary (lobar), and tertiary (segmental) bronchi. During this stage, airways are lined by undifferentiated pseudostratified columnar epithelium derived from endoderm. The lamina propria, cartilaginous rings, smooth muscle, blood, and lymphatic vessels originate from the mesoderm. Cartilaginous rings first develop in the central area of the lungs (trachea and principal bronchi) and then continue to form in more distal airways. The pulmonary vasculature also evolves by branching morphogenesis and uses the bronchial tree as a template. The visceral and parietal pleura, derived from mesoderm, enclose the pleural cavity at the end of the embryonic period.

Fetal Period

This period is further subdivided into four stages based on morphological criteria: pseudoglandular, canalicular, saccular, and alveolar stage [1, 2]. These stages overlap as lung maturation starts in the central areas of the lung and continues toward the periphery. Limited studies on pulmonary maturation in the equine fetus preclude detailed information on the duration of overlap between stages [3, 4, 6–8]. The *pseudoglandular stage* ranges from 50 to 190–210 days of gestation in the horse (Table 1.III.1) [5, 6]. During this stage, the structure of the lung mimics an exocrine (tubulo-acinar) gland [1, 2]. An estimated 20 generations of conducting airways form during this stage in the human fetus by branching morphogenesis. The proximal airways are lined by tall columnar epithelial cells while distal airways are covered by cuboidal epithelial cells (Figure 1.III.2a). Cellular differentiation starts in the center of the lung and propagates toward the periphery. Ciliated and goblet cells develop in the airway epithelium. Type 2 epithelial cells, responsible for surfactant production, start to appear during this stage in the equine fetus. Occasional lamellated osmophilic bodies, the precursors of lamellar bodies,

Equine Neonatal Medicine, First Edition. Edited by David M. Wong and Pamela A. Wilkins.

Table 1.III.1 Summary of the major events during lung maturation. Timing in table is referring to days of gestation.

Period	Stage	Timing		Major events
Embryonic	Embryonic	24–50	Branching morphogenesis	Spans from the formation of the laryngotracheal groove to the development of segmental bronchi. Branching morphogenesis Proliferation of epithelial and mesenchymal cells Visceral and parietal pleura form Pulmonary vascular connections are established
Fetal	Pseudoglandular	50–210		The remainder of the conducting airways is formed (bronchi and bronchiole) The lungs resemble a gland lined by cuboidal cells Cellular differentiation starts centrally Ciliated cells, goblet cells, cartilage, smooth muscle, (bronchial glands develop)
	Canalicular	190–300		Canalization of lung parenchyma occurs (respiratory airways and capillaries) Acini contain alveolar ducts and sacculi, the mesenchyma is invaded by capillaries Formation of the future air-blood barrier Cellular differentiation of type 1 and type 2 pneumocytes (appearance of surfactant) Rapid increase in vascular network
	Saccular	300–320		The last generation of airspaces develops as sacculi Sacculi are lined by type 1 and 2 epithelial cells Septa between sacculi contain two networks of capillaries Vascular network expands
Postnatal	Alveolarization (classical)	320+	Alveolarization	Formation of alveoli (approximately 1/3 of alveoli are fully developed at birth in humans) Transition from sacculi to alveoli with secondary septa formation Thinning of alveolo-capillary membrane (capillary endothelium, fused basal lamina, alveolar epithelial cell)
	Alveolarization (continued)	Until adulthood		Septation continues with mature alveolar septa containing a single layer capillary network.
	Microvascular maturation	Until adulthood		Remodeling and maturation of interalveolar septa and capillary bed Thinning of septa from two to one capillary layer Interstitial tissue volume decreases in parallel with alveolarization Maturation of extracellular matrix

become visible around 150 days of gestation in the equine fetus [6]. Cartilage, smooth muscle cells, and bronchial glands start to be established in the bronchial walls.

The *canalicular stage* lasts from 190–210 to 300 days of gestation and is characterized by the development of respiratory airways and formation of the first air-blood barrier [1, 2, 5, 6]. Canaliculi branch out from terminal bronchioles to form acini containing alveolar ducts and sacculi. In parallel, enhanced angiogenesis leads to the creation of a high-density capillary network. The mesenchyme is condensed by growing airways and programmed apoptosis. At the bronchioalveolar duct junction, the epithelium changes from ciliated and club cells to type 1 and 2 epithelial cells. Type 1 epithelial cells are derived from type 2 epithelial progenitor cells and are simple squamous epithelial cells. They spread over the surface of the future gas exchange area in proximity to endothelial cells. Type 2 epithelial cells are cuboidal and initiate surfactant production during this stage in human fetuses. The number of type 2 epithelial cells progressively decreases during this stage as they differentiate into type 1 epithelial cells (Figure 1.III.2b). The number of lamellar bodies found within each remaining type 2 epithelial cell increases.

The *saccular stage* embodies the transition from branching morphogenesis to alveolarization from day 300 to 320 of gestation [5]. During this stage, the future gas exchange area is enlarged through increased numbers of sacculi and condensation of pulmonary mesenchyme [1, 2]. Primary

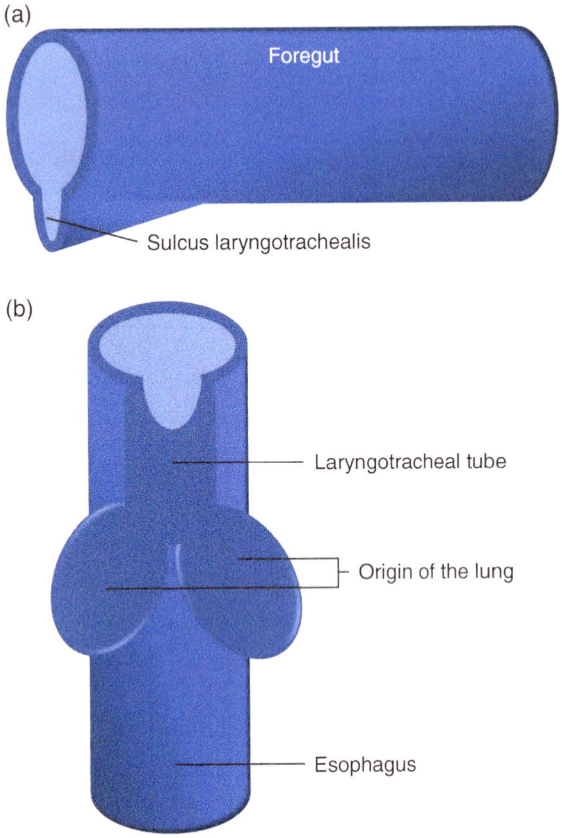

Figure 1.III.1 Lung maturation during the embryonic period. (a) Lung development starts with formation of the laryngotracheal groove in the ventral wall of the primitive foregut. (b) This groove deepens and extends to form the laryngotracheal tube which bifurcates into two outpouchings that become the primordia or origins of the lung.

septa form between airspaces and contain a double-layered capillary bed. Sacculi are lined mostly by type 1 epithelial cells and few type 2 epithelial cells (Figure 1.III.2c). The air–blood barrier consists in type 1 epithelial cells, basement membrane, and endothelial cells. A network of elastic fibers and collagen supports these structures. An incomplete surfactant lining film is present in foals around 300 days of gestation, and this film is sometimes still incomplete at term birth [6].

The process of alveolarization starts during the saccular stage, continues during the last few weeks of the pregnancy, and goes on beyond birth [1, 2, 5]. The *alveolar stage* is marked by formation of sacculi and ultimately alveoli. Initially, primary septa with a double layer of capillaries separate sacculi. These sacculi are subdivided into smaller alveolar units by the growth of secondary septa (Figure 1.III.2d). As the microvasculature matures, the capillary beds become thinner and then fuse into a single layer. In parallel, interstitial tissue volume continues to decrease. In human fetuses, alveolarization and microvascular maturation begin in-utero and continue for several years after birth. The same phenomenon likely occurs in the horse.

Postpartum Period

Alveolarization and microvascular maturation continue through young adulthood in people [1]. The foal is precocial in its development at birth and is born after the process of alveolarization has already started [1, 2]. Similar to what is described in the human medicine, pulmonary maturation in the horse continues after birth. Lung volume and alveolar surface area are known to increase beyond birth in horses [7, 8].

Lung Surfactant Composition

Lung surfactant is produced by type 2 epithelial cells and consists of a complex mixture of phospholipids (80–85%), proteins (5–10%), and other lipids (5–10%) (Figure 1.III.3) [9–11].

Phospholipids

Phospholipids are amphipathic molecules with two different affinities: a polar area attracted to water (hydrophilic) and a nonpolar area that dissolves in lipids or fats (lipophilic) [11, 12]. Phospholipids are composed of a head group (polar) and two tails (nonpolar). The head group determines the phospholipid class. The two fatty acid chains are joined to the headgroup via a glycerol backbone. The variable length and degrees of saturation of fatty acid chains lead to a multitude of different molecular species within each phospholipid class. Phospholipids confer surfactant its surface-active properties as they spread at air–liquid interfaces and form bilayers and numerous other structures. Major phospholipid classes in order of abundancy in lung surfactant include phosphatidylcholine, phosphatidylglycerol, phosphatidylethanolamine, phosphatidy-linositol, and phosphatidylserine [9, 11]. Sphingomyelin, a sphingolipid, is also present in low concentration. There are only a few studies evaluating lung surfactant in the horse so unless specifically indicated, information here refers to people.

Phosphatidylcholine (PC) is zwitterionic and is the major surface-active phospholipid in surfactant (>75% of total phospholipid content) [9, 11]. Diplamitoyl-PC (DPPC) is the predominant molecular species of PC (50%) with two palmitic acid chains (16 carbons in length with no double bonds – 16:0/16:0-PC). Other PC molecular species (25%) in surfactant include 16:0/14:0-PC, 16:0/16:1-PC, 16:0/18:1 PC, and 16:0/18:2-PC. *Phosphatidylglycerol (PG)* is the

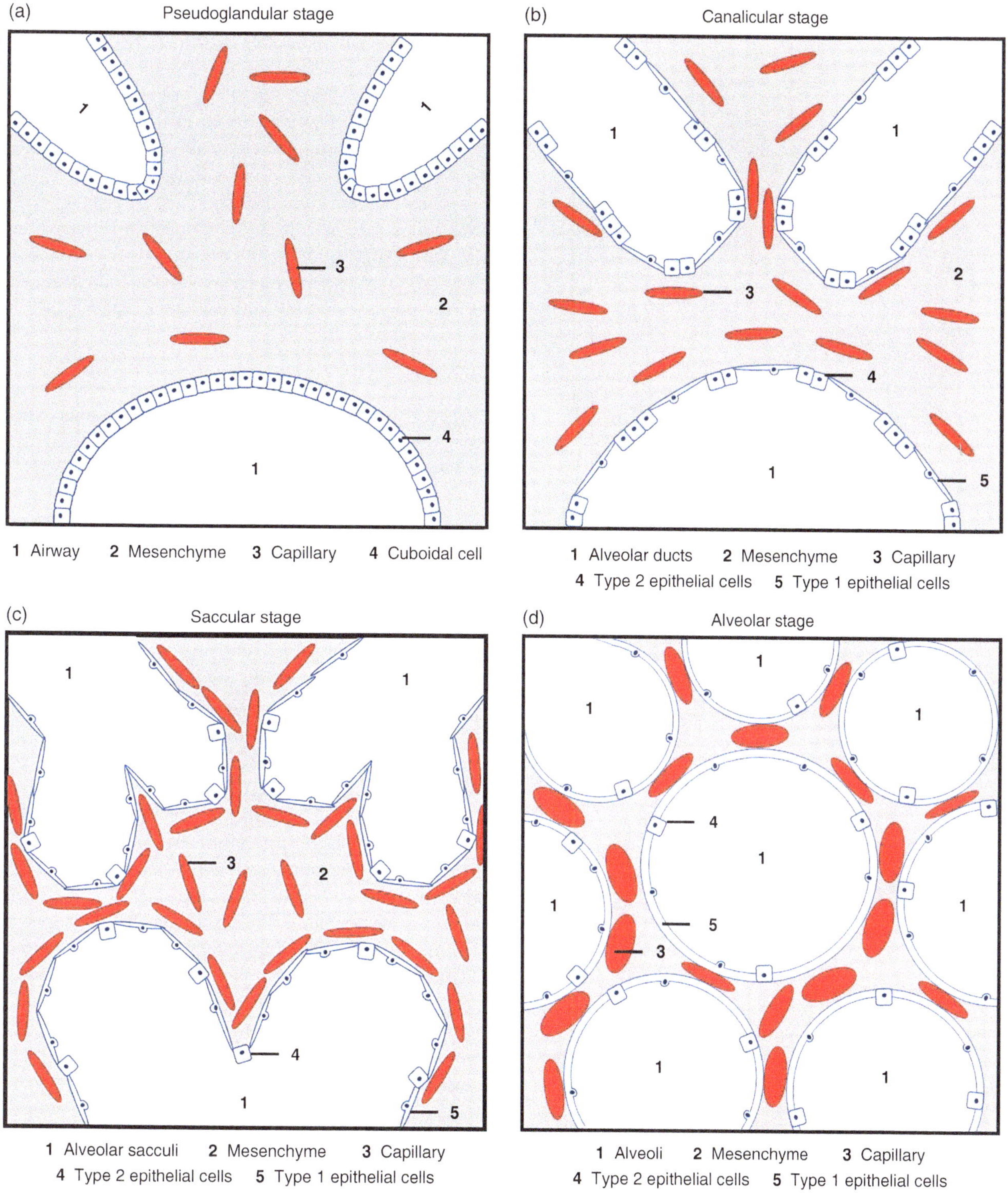

Figure 1.III.2 Lung maturation during the fetal period. Morphological characteristics of the lung during the four different developmental stages are represented. (a) Pseudoglandular stage: airways form by branching morphogenesis, they extend into the mesenchyme containing capillaries, and are lined by cuboidal cells in the distal airways. (b) Canalicular stage: the first air-blood barrier appears as alveolar ducts and sacculi form, mesenchyme is condensed, and a high-density capillary network develops; cellular differentiation from type 2 to type 1 epithelial cells occurs. (c) Saccular stage: transition from branching morphogenesis to alveolarization with an increased number of sacculi, further condensation of the mesenchyme, primary septation with a double-layered capillary bed, and a thin epithelium with mostly type 1 and a few type 2 epithelial cells. (d) Alveolar stage: secondary septa subdivide sacculi into alveoli, interstitial tissue decreases, a single layer capillary bed forms. Microvascular maturation and alveolarization continue in the postnatal period.

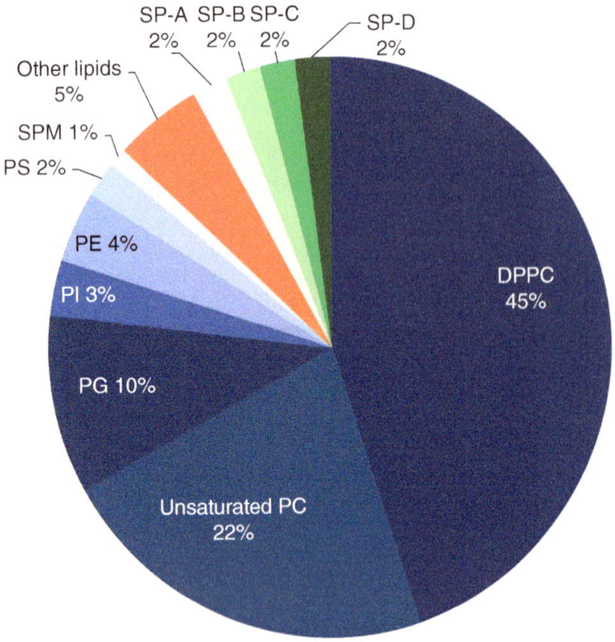

Figure 1.III.3 Lung surfactant composition. Surfactant is a complex mixture of phospholipids (80–85%, represented in different shades of blue), proteins (5–10%, represented in shades of green), and other lipids (5–10%, represented in orange). Phospholipids consist in several major classes (e.g. phosphatidylcholine – PC, phosphatidylglycerol – PG, phosphatidylinositol – PI, phosphatidylethanolamine – PE, phosphatidylserine – PS) that can be further subdivided into multiple subclasses and molecular species based on their fatty acid chain length and degree of saturation (e.g. Dipalmitoyl phosphatidylcholine – DPPC). Surfactant proteins SP-A, SP-B, SP-C, and SP-D are surfactant specific proteins that are either hydrophilic (SP-A and SP-D) or hydrophobic (SP-B and SP-C). The remaining lipids consist in a variety of other lipids.

second most abundant phospholipid class in surfactant but represents a much lower percentage of the total content (10–15%) [9, 11]. Palmitoyl-oleoyl PG or POPG (16:0/18:1-PG) is the dominant molecular species. The concentration of PG is higher in the lung compared to other tissues. PG is an anionic phospholipid and helps in adsorption and spreading of surfactant at the air liquid interface; it is a marker of lung maturity in certain animals including humans. In the neonatal foal, PG accounts for two thirds and PI for one third of anionic phospholipids [13]. In the adult horse, PG is the main anionic phospholipid. *Phosphatidylethanolamine (PE)* is present at a lower percentage than PC and PG (~5%) [9, 11]. PE is zwitterionic phospholipid but molecular species in this phospholipid class are less saturated compared to PC. *Phosphatidylinositol (PI)* is another anionic phospholipid in surfactant and may substitute for PG in some of its functions [9, 11]. In human fetuses, PI peaks around 35 weeks of gestation and then decreases as PG rises. In other species such as pigs and sheep, PI is the major anionic phospholipid in surfactant at birth [12]. In the foal, PI represents one-third of the anionic phospholipids present at birth and decreases significantly in the adult horse [13]. Levels of PI may increase in scenarios where cellular injury or inflammation occurs [9]. *Phosphatidylserine (PS)* and *sphingomyelin (SPM)* are other less-frequent components of lung surfactant [9, 11]. SPM levels remain constant throughout pregnancy and rise with lung injury. Total surface-active phospholipid (lecithin) to sphingomyelin ratio is used as an indicator for of fetal lung maturity (FLM) in human medicine [14].

Proteins

Surfactant contains four surfactant specific proteins: SP-A, SP-B, SP-C, and SP-D. Surfactant proteins are synthesized in the alveoli by type 2 epithelial cells and in the airways by Club cells (formerly known as Clara cells) and submucosal cells (SP-A, SP-B, and SP-D) [9, 11]. *SP-A* and *SP-D* are hydrophilic proteins that are part of the collectin family and participate in the immune defense of the lung [11]. Collectins have common features including an amino-N terminal, a collagen like domain, a neck region, and a carbohydrate recognition domain (Figure 1.III.4a) [12, 15]. SP-A is the most abundant surfactant protein and SP-D is the least lipid bound compared to the other surfactant proteins. *SP-B* and *SP-C* are hydrophobic proteins that are closely associated with surfactant phospholipids [11, 16]. SP-B is essential for survival (SP-B deficiency is lethal) as it plays a crucial role in surfactant metabolism. It consists of a dimer with amphipathic properties that allow interaction with phospholipids (Figure 1.III.4b). SP-C is the smallest and most hydrophobic surfactant protein. It contains a transmembrane helix and two palmitoyl groups that interact with the fatty acid chains in phospholipids (Figure 1.III.4b). It contributes to surfactant stability in close interaction with SP-B and phospholipids.

Surfactant also contains *other lipids* such as cholesterol, cholesterol esters, diglycerides, triglycerides, plasmalogens, and free fatty acids [12]. Their role in surfactant has not been fully characterized. As surfactant goes through a complex cycle of synthesis and recycling, these components are likely byproducts of these processes.

Lung Surfactant Metabolism

Surfactant metabolism includes synthesis, storage, secretion, film adsorption, recycling, clearance, and degradation (Figure 1.III.5) [9, 11, 12]. Surfactant phospholipids are synthesized in the endoplasmic reticulum, mitochondria, and peroxisomes of type 2 epithelial cells. Synthesis

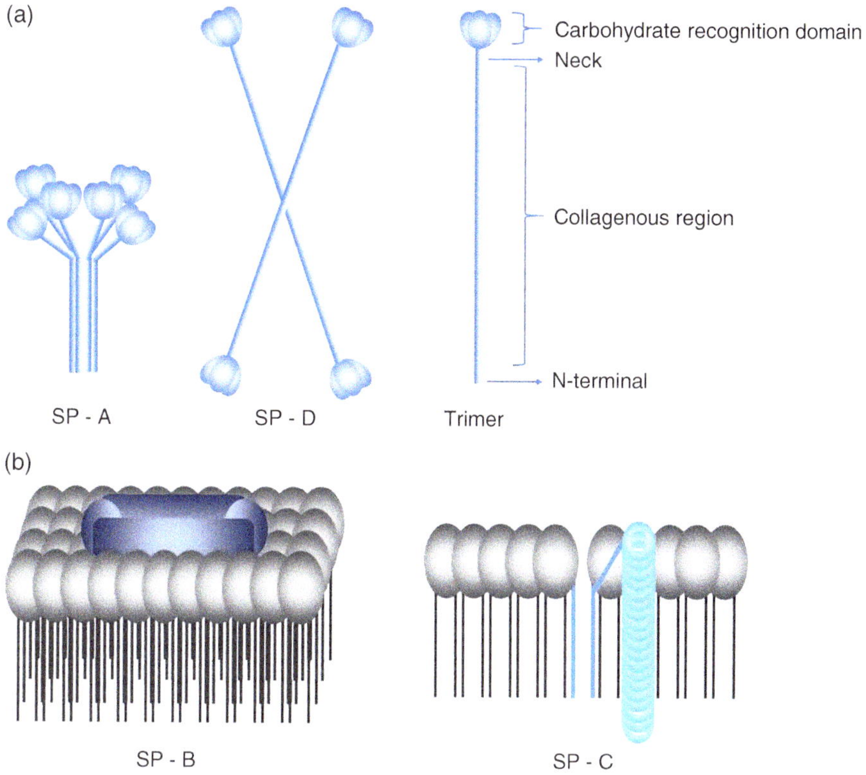

Figure 1.III.4 Surfactant protein structure. (a) Surfactant proteins A (SP-A) and D (SP-D) are hydrophilic and part of the collectin family. They share a common trimer structure with an amino-N terminal, a collagenous domain, a neck region, and a carbohydrate recognition domain. SP-A forms bouquet type structures while SP-D has a cruciform structure. (b) SP-B and SP-C are hydrophobic proteins closely associated with phospholipid structures. SP-B is a dimer that closely interacts with phospholipids. SP-C contains a transmembrane helix with two palmitoyl groups.

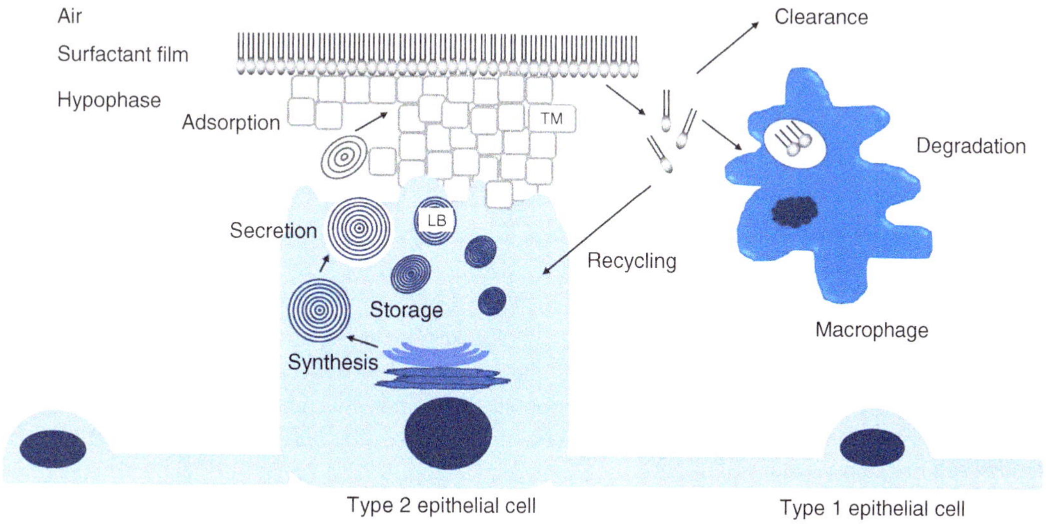

Figure 1.III.5 Surfactant metabolism. Metabolism includes synthesis in type 2 epithelial cells, storage in lamellar bodies (LB), secretion to the alveolar hypophase, where it unravels to form tubular myelin (TM), and adsorption to the air/liquid interface to form a surface tension lowering film. The majority of surfactant undergoes recycling while a smaller portion is cleared toward the small airways or degraded by alveolar macrophages.

is either *de-novo* from various precursors (i.e. free fatty acids) or by molecular remodeling [9]. Proteins are processed in the Golgi apparatus of type 2 epithelial cells. Surfactant is stored in lamellar bodies, which contain tightly packed spirals of phospholipids and associated proteins. Phospholipids and proteins are transported to lamellar bodies directly or via multivesicular bodies. ATP-binding cassette transporters such as ABCA3 are necessary for synthesis and storage of surfactant in type 2 epithelial cells. Surfactant is secreted by exocytosis into the alveolar hypophase (thin fluid layer between the air and epithelial cells). It unravels to form tubular myelin (a cross hatched network of phospholipid bilayers) and other less structured lipoprotein complexes. Surfactant is adsorbed from the alveolar hypophase to the air–liquid interface, where it exerts its function to lower surface tension. The majority of surfactant is recycled to replenish surfactant stores. The remaining fraction is degraded by alveolar macrophages (10–15%) or cleared toward the small airways (2–5%).

Surfactant proteins mediate important steps in this metabolic cycle. SP-A is involved in the conversion of lamellar bodies into tubular myelin and subsequently surface film formation [9]. It mediates surfactant recycling and secretion, and inhibits the activity of secretory phospholipase. SP-B fuses and lyses phospholipid bilayers and is needed for packaging of phospholipids into lamellar bodies, formation of tubular myelin, and creation of the surfactant film at the air-liquid interface. Surfactant at the air–liquid interface is compressed and expanded during the respiratory cycle and its composition is adapted accordingly. Compression (expiration) of the film leads to enrichment in DPPC while less-saturated phospholipids are squeezed out. This allows the generation of extremely low surface tension at the end of expiration. During expansion (inspiration), components are reintegrated into the film to optimize its spreading (Table 1.III.2).

Table 1.III.2 Surfactant components and their function during metabolism.

Surfactant component	Function
DPPC	Achievement of low surface tension
Unsaturated phospholipids	Enhance surfactant spreading
Anionic phospholipids	Surfactant adsorption
Surfactant proteins A, B, and C	Packaging in lamellar bodies, tubular myelin formation, surfactant adsorption

Lung Surfactant Function

Normal Function

Lung surfactant has two main functions: biophysical function to reduce surface tension and modulation of immune function [11, 12].

Biophysical Function

Surface tension is the tension across the surface of a liquid, measured in milliNewton per meter (mN/m) [12, 17]. This tension is created by attractive forces between molecules in the surface layer and the bulk of the liquid and tends to contract the surface area. Surface tension depends on the properties of the liquid, the interface, the temperature and other factors. The surface tension of water is high (70 mN/m), whereas surfactant reaches very low surface tensions (<1 mN/m) at the end of expiration. The amphipathic properties of surfactant allow it to form a layer at the air-liquid interface, to facilitate spreading, and to adapt surface tension throughout the respiratory cycle.

The Law of Laplace states that the transmural pressure (ΔP) to maintain a bubble open is proportional to surface tension (σ) and inversely related to the radius of the bubble, expressed as $\Delta P = 2\sigma/r$ (Figure 1.III.6). A simplified understanding how surface tension acts across an alveolar surface is to apply the Law of Laplace to two theoretical alveoli of different size. If the surface tension in the small alveolus is the same as that in the large alveolus, this leads to the collapse of the small alveolus (atelectasis) and to the expansion of the large alveolus. If the surface tension in the small alveolus is lower than that in the large alveolus, this allows the two alveoli to coexist. Hence, surfactant prevents alveolar collapse, allows for even distribution of ventilation, maintains efficient gas exchange area, improves lung compliance, and reduces work of breathing. Surfactant also balances hydrostatic forces and thereby improves alveolar fluid clearance and counteracts edema formation. It further forms a protective layer over the surface of epithelial cell and facilitates removal of particles and pathogens.

Immune Function

The *host defense function* of surfactant is largely assured by SP-A and SP-D and to a lesser extent by the phospholipid component. SP-A and SP-D opsonize pathogens (i.e. virus, bacteria, fungi) and allergens by binding them via the carbohydrate recognition domain [15]. They also facilitate phagocytosis through opsonization, ligand mediated immune cell activation, and upregulation of cellular receptors involved in microbial recognition. SP-A and SP-D's primary role is to downregulate the immune reaction of the lung and avoid inflammation [18]. However,

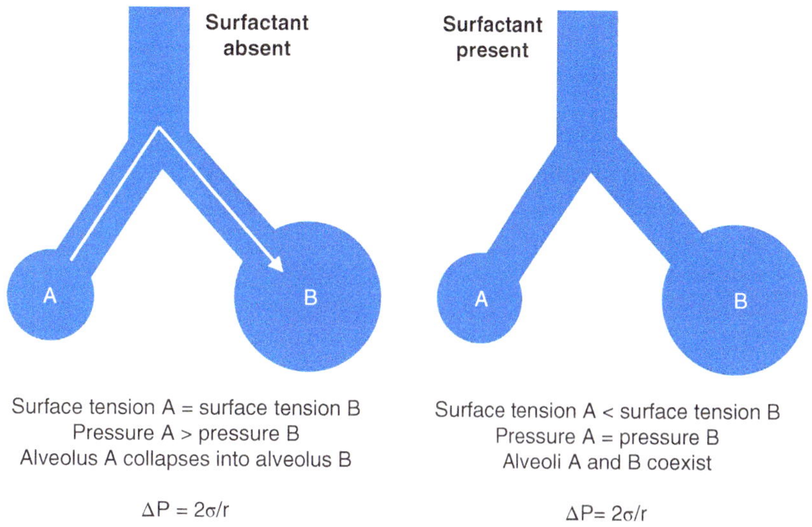

Figure 1.III.6 Biophysical surfactant function. Surfactant lowers the surface tension throughout the respiratory cycle and allows alveoli of different sizes to coexist. This is illustrated by the Law of Laplace $\Delta P = 2\sigma/r$ according to which the transmural pressure (ΔP) to maintain a bubble open is proportional to the surface tension (σ) and inversely related to the radius of the bubble. This simplified representation shows that if σ in alveolus A equals that in alveolus B, then A collapses into B due to the pressure difference between the two. In comparison, if σ is lower in alveolus A versus B, the alveoli coexist.

depending on type and amount of stimulus present, the duration and severity of exposure, and immune cell activation, SP-A and SP-D may upregulate the pulmonary immune defense and promote inflammation.

Abnormal Surfactant Function

Surfactant may not achieve its ability to lower surface tension if lung maturity is insufficient at birth or if type 2 epithelial cells are injured. Surfactant may also be rendered dysfunctional through inactivation, degradation, or injury [10–12].

Surfactant deficiency implies a quantitative and qualitative deficit of surfactant at the air–liquid interface caused by altered surfactant metabolism with impaired synthesis, insufficient pool size, and reduced recycling ability in type 2 epithelial cells [11]. It is due to immaturity of type 2 epithelial cells in premature animals or injury of these cells as a result of inflammation at all ages. Surfactant deficiency and high surface tension play a major role in neonatal respiratory distress syndrome (NRDS) and contribute to the pathophysiology of acute respiratory distress syndrome (ARDS). Low surfactant pool size coupled with altered composition also increases the vulnerability of surfactant to inhibition and degradation, which further exacerbates its inability to lower surface tension.

Surfactant dysfunction or loss of surface activity may be caused by a variety of mechanisms, including inhibition, degradation, and trapping (Table 1.III.3) [11]. Biophysical inhibitors interfere with surfactant film formation and spreading at the air-liquid interface. They are generated through inflammation (i.e. pneumonia, ARDS), aspiration (i.e. meconium, near-drowning), or alveolo-capillary membrane injury. Surfactant degradation occurs via action of enzymes (i.e. proteases, lipases), reactive oxygen species, and other components released in various lung diseases. Other mechanisms leading to surfactant dysfunction include trapping of surfactant through clotting and formation of hyaline membranes.

Table 1.III.3 Mechanisms involved in surfactant deficiency and dysfunction.

Deficiency
Primary or secondary: immaturity/injury of type 2 epithelial cells
– Insufficient pool size
– Slow de-novo synthesis
– Inadequate recycling
– Immature or altered composition
Dysfunction
Surfactant inhibition
– Proteins
○ Edema fluid
○ Plasma proteins (albumin, fibrinogen, hemoglobin)
– Lipids
○ From cell membranes
○ Mediators, byproducts
– Other
○ Meconium
○ Bilirubin
Surfactant degradation
– Proteases
– Phospholipases
– Reactive oxygen species
Surfactant trapping and conversion
– Clots, hyaline membranes
– Increased conversion to inactive forms

Lung Surfactant in the Neonate

Term Neonate

The lung surfactant pool size (lamellar bodies, hypophase, surfactant film) is significantly larger (100 mg/kg) in the term fetus compared to the adult [11, 19]. This allows a smooth transition to breathing air and extra-uterine life and decreases the likelihood of surfactant inactivation and degradation. Neonatal surfactant relative to adult, contains a higher proportion of fluidizing phospholipids (molecular species with shorter or more saturated chain length; 16:0/14:0 PC and 16:0/16:1 PC) to improve surfactant film spreading at the air–liquid interface [20].

Depending on the species, the major anionic phospholipid in surfactant at birth may be PG or PI [12]. In infants, PG is the predominant anionic phospholipid at birth and is used as a marker of lung maturity. In neonatal pigs and sheep, the concentration of PI is higher compared to PG at birth. In term foals, PG corresponds to two-thirds and PI represents one-third of the anionic phospholipids present in surfactant [13]. PG is significantly lower and PI is significantly higher in term foals compared to adult horses. Early studies described maturation of the lung and the surfactant system in the foal [6, 21]. These studies showed that surfactant film may be present at 300 days of gestation but may still be incomplete at birth [6]. Surfactant pool size and detailed surfactant composition have not been evaluated in the equine fetus or postpartum period. Levels of surfactant proteins increase with lung maturation toward the end of gestation [11]. The ability of surfactant to lower surface tension is improved in neonates compared to adults [20]. However, in a study that assessed surfactant isolated from term foals, surface tension was significantly higher in foals compared to adult horses [13]. Mechanisms underlying this difference remain to be determined.

Premature Neonates

Surfactant in the premature lung is immature in several aspects. Pool size is deficient, metabolism is impaired, and composition is altered [11, 19]. The surfactant pool size in the premature lung is significantly lower compared to the term lung (5 mg/kg vs 100 mg/kg) and is rapidly depleted after birth. Recycling mechanisms, normally responsible for regeneration of functional surfactant, are impaired in premature neonates. De novo synthesis is slow and leads to a delay in surfactant release. Surfactant from premature animals contains lower amounts of DPPC, PG, and surfactant proteins SP-A, SP-B, and SP-C compared to term animals. These compositional differences impair the ability to lower surface tension and to deploy enough functional surfactant to the air-liquid interface. Qualitative and quantitative surfactant alterations also make surfactant more vulnerable to inhibition and degradation. Studies that assessed PG levels or lecithin to sphingomyelin ratios in amniotic fluid from premature and term foals did not determine these to be reliable predictors of lung maturity [22–24]. One study described surfactant samples isolated from premature foals ($n = 4$) contained approximately equal percentages of PG and PI after birth indicating immature composition and/or surfactant injury [13]. Further studies are needed to elucidate surfactant maturation in the foal.

Respiratory Distress Syndromes

Neonatal Respiratory Distress Syndrome

Surfactant deficiency plays an important role in the development of NRDS in premature human infants [11, 25]. Surfactant maturation during the last trimester of gestation is crucial for a successful transition to and maintenance of extrauterine life. The likelihood of NRDS decreases with gestational age. Affected infants develop respiratory distress and cyanosis soon after birth and require respiratory support ranging from oxygen supplementation to mechanical ventilation. Surfactant deficiency in premature infants leads to high alveolar surface tension, extensive alveolar collapse, and pulmonary atelectasis. Ventilation perfusion mismatching occurs with hypoxemia, hypercapnia, and respiratory acidosis. Damage to the alveolocapillary membrane induces plasma leakage, fibrin accumulation, and infiltration of inflammatory mediators. These events culminate in the formation of hyaline membranes. Surfactant abnormalities present in preterm infants depend on gestational age (FLM) and degree of secondary dysfunction (Table 1.III.4). In human medicine, prevention against NRDS in high-risk pregnancies consists of treatment with maternal corticosteroids and tocolytics prior to delivery. Tocolytics are used for a short-term delay of delivery and to allow corticosteroids to exert their effect to hasten pulmonary and surfactant maturation. Prophylactic surfactant treatment or early rescue treatment is indicated in premature infants at risk for NRDS (see surfactant treatment).

Acute Respiratory Distress Syndrome

Acute respiratory distress syndrome (ARDS) can occur in patients of all ages [10, 26]. ARDS is the result of either direct injury to the lung or systemic inflammatory response syndrome. ARDS is defined clinically as acute onset of respiratory distress, significant hypoxemia (ratio of arterial oxygenation to inspired oxygen [PaO_2/FiO_2]; with >200

Table 1.III.4 Summary of differences in lung surfactant between premature and term neonates.

Surfactant	Term	Premature
Content		
Pool size	High (100 mg/kg)	Low (5 mg/kg)
Composition		
Saturated/total PC	High	Low
PG	High	Low
PI	Low	Variable
SPM	Unchanged	Unchanged
Surfactant protein	Increases	Low
Function		
Ability to lower surface tension	High	Low
Sensitivity to inactivation	Low	High

but ≤300 mmHg for mild ARDS, >100 but ≤200 mmHg for moderate ARDS, and ≤100 mmHg for severe ARDS), bilateral infiltrates on chest radiographs, and no evidence of left atrial hypertension [26]. Sepsis and multiorgan failure are often associated with ARDS. The pathophysiology of ARDS includes damage to capillary alveolar membrane, influx of protein-rich edema fluid into the alveolus, rise in pulmonary vascular resistance, and severe ventilation/perfusion abnormalities. Surfactant dysfunction in ARDS patients develops through a combination of mechanisms, including surfactant deficiency and dysfunction. The composition of surfactant from ARDS patients is characterized by a decrease in the major surfactant phospholipids PC and PG and an increase of phospholipids released from cellular membranes or infiltrated from plasma such as PI, PE, and SPM [10]. Levels of surfactant proteins decrease in ARDS patients. Treatment of patients with ARDS is complex and includes oxygen administration and ventilatory support, fluid and hemodynamic management, and antimicrobial therapy. Surfactant administration is less efficient in ARDS patients due to ongoing inactivation and degradation.

Respiratory Distress Syndrome in Neonatal Foals

Two distinct syndromes in foals have been described and defined using specific published criteria [27, 28]. *Neonatal equine respiratory distress syndrome (NERDS)* is characterized by surfactant deficiency. A diagnosis of NERDS is based on: (i) persistent hypoxemia and progressive hypercapnia; (ii) presence of known risk factors (gestational length <290 days or <88% of previous pregnancies, induction of parturition, caesarian section); (iii) failure to develop normal immediate postpartum respiratory pattern; (iv) ground glass appearance on lateral radiographs at <24 hours of age; (v) absence of fetal inflammatory response syndrome; and (vi) absence of congenital cardiac abnormalities.

In comparison, *equine neonatal acute respiratory distress syndrome* (EqNARDS) and *equine neonatal acute lung injury* (EqALI; mild ARDS) occurs in foals under <1 week of age and is associated with surfactant dysfunction rather than deficiency [27, 28]. A diagnosis of EqNARDS is based on at least four criteria: (i) acute onset of respiratory distress; (ii) presence of known risk factors (i.e. infection, inflammation, sepsis, aspiration); (iii) absence of cardiogenic pulmonary edema; (iv) evidence of inefficient gas exchange based on age-specific reference values; and (v) presence of diffuse pulmonary inflammation.

Prevention of NERDS and EqNARDS in equine medicine is difficult because of variable gestational lengths in horses, inability to predict lung maturity based on gestational age or FLM testing (see below), limitations in treatment options that hasten pulmonary maturation, and cost of surfactant treatment. The effect of maternal corticosteroids on pulmonary and surfactant maturation in the equine fetus warrants further investigation. Administration of one to three doses of corticosteroids is recommended as an attempt to stimulate fetal lung maturation in the horse. Limited studies suggest that high doses (100 mg) of intramuscular dexamethasone administered to mares around 320 days of gestation reduces gestational length and may stimulate precocious fetal maturation [29, 30]. However, the effect on pulmonary and surfactant maturation remains to be determined. Intramuscular administration of betamethasone and depot corticotropin to the equine fetus using ultrasound guided injection can also be used to prompt pulmonary maturation but may lead to premature delivery [31, 32]. For either option, the risk posed to the mare and fetus must be carefully weighed against the potential benefit.

Fetal Lung Maturity (FLM) Testing

Secretions from the fetal lung are washed into the amniotic fluid throughout pregnancy [14, 33]. The composition of amniotic fluid changes as lung surfactant maturation progresses. Compositional surfactant changes during pregnancy have been well characterized in human medicine (Figure 1.III.7) and were once routinely used to determine FLM in high-risk pregnancies [11]. In recent years, the use of FLM testing has declined and a number of FLM tests are no longer commercially available [14, 33].

This shift occurred because: (i) gestational age is considered a more reliable predictor of readiness for birth and absence of neonatal morbidity; (ii) delaying delivery due to

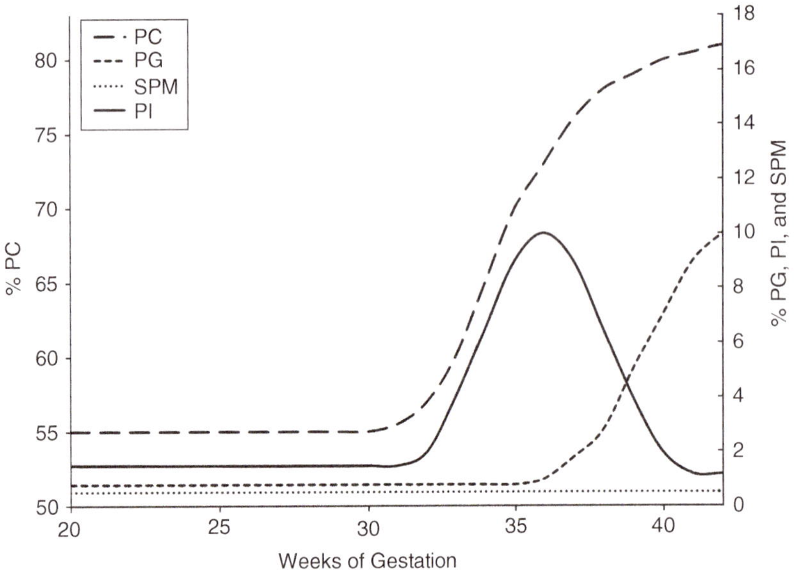

Figure 1.III.7 Fetal lung maturity testing. The composition of amniotic fluid changes as lung surfactant maturation evolves during pregnancy. This graph shows the changes in major phospholipids (PC, PG, PI) and sphingomyelin (SPM) levels in amniotic fluid during human gestation. Amniotic lecithin to sphingomyelin ratio and PG levels were once routinely used in human medicine to predict fetal lung maturity in high-risk pregnancies.

lung immaturity may represent a risk for mother and fetus under certain conditions; (iii) antenatal administration of steroids to hasten pulmonary maturation has become standard in pregnancies where preterm delivery is anticipated or indicated due to medical issues; and (iv) a healthy fetus always benefits from delivery at term if this does not compromise maternal health. There is a strong trend to reduce the number of nonmedically indicated preterm deliveries in human medicine [14, 33].

The lecithin to sphingomyelin (L/S) ratio was one of the first tests used for FLM testing in people [14, 33]. Levels of lecithin (DPPC) in amniotic fluid rise after week 32 of pregnancy whereas levels of sphingomyelin remain unchanged (Figure 1.III.7). L/S is determined by chromatography, which requires technical expertise and time. L/S > 2 is indicative of mature lung surfactant. Results are also influenced by sample contamination with blood or meconium and by sample handling. Phosphatidylglycerol levels in amniotic fluid increase after 35 weeks of pregnancy and can also be used to determine FLM (Figure 1.III.7). PG is measured either by chromatography (levels >2% are indicative of lung maturity) or semiquantitative immunologic slide agglutination. Results are less affected by sample contamination as PG is relatively specific to lung surfactant. Lamellar body (LB) count in amniotic fluid can be performed with standard hematology analyzers using the platelet channel and was used until recently to determine FLM [14, 33]. Counts below 15,000/μl are suggestive of immature lungs, whereas counts >50,000/μl indicate lung maturity. This test is easy to perform, accessible, fast, and inexpensive. Blood contamination can lead to inaccurate counts as the introduction of platelets into a sample leads to false elevation in LB counts. Other tests previously used for determination of FLM include optical density at 650 nm, foam stability index, and surfactant to albumin ratio. FLM prediction has been successfully used in cattle and in sheep [12, 34, 35]. However, in equine medicine, attempts to reliably determine FLM in amniotic fluid using L/S and PG before or at birth have been unsuccessful [22–24]. Lamellar body counts have been performed on amniotic fluid from term foals [36]. Their usefulness in predicting lung maturity remains to be determined.

Treatment

Exogenous surfactant administration was first used for treatment of NRDS in 1980 and has since become part of the standard care for premature infants at risk for NRDS [19, 25, 37]. Exogenous surfactant administration greatly reduced mortality and need for mechanical ventilation in preterm infants. So-called natural and synthetic surfactants are available commercially (Table 1.III.5). Natural surfactants are derived from bovine or porcine lung lavages or minced tissue and contain all surfactant components (phospholipids and proteins). Some preparations have been enhanced in composition and content to decrease administration volume [19]. For example, in poractant alpha (Curosurf), phospholipids are concentrated via chromatography leading to a smaller administration volume compared to other surfactants. Synthetic surfactants consist of select mixtures of components, depending on their generation. The first generation of synthetic surfactants only contained lipids and was not effective in treating NRDS. Components meant to improve adsorption and spreading were added to the second generation of synthetic surfactants (i.e. Exosurf). Third-generation synthetic surfactants have been enhanced with

Table 1.III.5 Commercially available surfactant preparations with their origin, phospholipid and protein content, phospholipid concentration, and suggested dose.

Surfactant	Origin and content	[Phospholipid] (mg/ml)	Suggested dose
Natural			
Beractant (Survanta)	Bovine: minced lung Natural mixture	25 mg/ml	4 ml/kg
Calfactant (Infasurf)	Bovine: calf lung lavage Natural mixture	35 mg/ml	3 ml/kg
Poractant (Curosurf)	Porcine: minced lung Enhanced mixture	80 mg/ml	2.5 ml/kg
Synthetic			
First generation	DPPC	n/a	n/a
Second generation Exosurf (Colfosceril)	DPPC with colfoseril palmitate	13.5 mg/ml	5 ml/kg
Third generation Lucinactant (Surfaxin)	DPPC and POPG with KL4 peptide as SP-B	30 mg/ml	5.8 ml/kg

the addition of SP-B and SP-C analogs (i.e. Lucinactant). While both natural and synthetic surfactant preparations are effective for the treatment of NRDS, natural surfactants have an improved ability to lower surface tension and are more resistant to inactivation and degradation compared to synthetic preparations [19, 25, 37].

Surfactants may be administered prophylactically within 10–30 minutes of delivery to prevent NRDS in infants at high risk. Rescue treatment consists of administration of surfactant <2 hours (early rescue) or between 2 and 12 hours (late rescue) after birth, when certain severity criteria for NRDS are met [25, 37]. Before routine use of continuous positive airway pressure (CPAP), prophylactic surfactant administration was preferred over rescue treatment as it led to improved clinical outcome in preterm infants. However, with routine use of CPAP, this advantage has become less clear. Surfactant treatment (prophylactic or early rescue) should be administered to all infants requiring intubation for stabilization and select rescue treatment given to infants once NRDS meets certain severity criteria. Techniques to administer surfactant include administration through an endotracheal tube (under mechanical ventilation), Intubate Surfactant Extubate (INSURE) (short-term mechanical ventilation), and the Less Invasive Surfactant Administration (LISA) technique (no mechanical ventilation) [19, 25, 37]. During LISA, the infant continues to breathe spontaneously while a small catheter is introduced into the trachea (via laryngoscopic guidance). This treatment is less invasive and corresponds to "supporting transition" to spontaneous breathing in the neonate, which is favored over resuscitation treatment in human medicine [25].

Exogenous surfactant treatment is administered (dose of 100 mg of phospholipid/kg of birth weight) as one or two aliquots [19, 25, 37]. This corresponds to 2.5–5.8 ml/kg depending on the commercial preparation used (Table 1.III.5). In a term neonate, 100 mg/kg is the expected pool size. Exogenously administered surfactant at this dose is integrated into the surfactant metabolism and substitutes for the initial surfactant deficiency. A high initial dose of surfactant is known to reduce the need for repeated administrations [19]. Repeat doses are only recommended in infants that have ongoing signs of NRDS. In infants receiving mechanical ventilation or oxygen supplementation, these settings need to be adjusted following surfactant treatment according to changes in lung compliance and oxygenation status. Level of maturity, severity of NRDS, antenatal steroid administration, timing of surfactant administration, initial dose, and volume of surfactant administered are factors that influence treatment choice and success. Bradycardia, hypotension, endotracheal tube blockage, and oxygen desaturation are the most common side effects of surfactant administration [19, 25, 37].

Surfactant treatment has been reported in foals, but use has been limited by high cost, questionable efficacy, infrequent occurrence of NERDS versus EqNARDS, and presence of surfactant dysfunction rather than deficiency in sick foals [34, 35, 38–40]. Controlled studies evaluating efficacy of exogenous surfactant administration in foals with NERDS do not exist. Surfactant used in equine medicine include (foam-rich) bronchoalveolar lavage fluid (BALF) from a horse donor, organic extracts of surfactant from lung lavages, and on occasion, commercial surfactant preparations. Dose and type of surfactant used were variable, and degree of lung maturity or prematurity were likely different from foal to foal. It is difficult to evaluate the efficacy of surfactant treatment for NERDS under these circumstances.

In the emergent clinical situation, in which a neonatal foal may benefit from exogenous surfactant, collection of surfactant from an adult horse donor may be most expedient. A standard collection procedure has not been established, but surfactant can be collected from an adult horse or immediately after a horse has succumbed from nonpulmonary disease using techniques similar to routine bronchoalveolar lavage (BAL). In this instance, sterile saline (0.5–1 l / live adult horse donor or 3–4 l / deceased horse donor) is administered through a sterile BAL tube or endotracheal tube and diverted into the right and left lung fields to wash the lungs. The fluid is retrieved through the BAL tube. The amount of fluid recovered from a live donor horse will obviously be less than a deceased horse. One report removed the lungs and caudal trachea from a deceased horse to allow for gentle massage and inversion of the lungs to facilitate fluid retrieval [38]. Surfactant can be administered to a foal through a long sterile catheter passed through a nasotracheal tube or a thin catheter introduced into the trachea under endoscopic guidance. The foal is repositioned during administration and positive pressure ventilation applied via mechanical ventilation or with a resuscitation bag prior to and between doses (if surfactant is administered in several doses rather than a single bolus) to distribute surfactant into the distal airways and aid in alveolar recruitment.

The dose of surfactant needed to treat a foal with NERDS is unknown. Following human recommendations of 100 mg/kg, a 45 kg foal would need 4.5 g of surfactant. Even with the most concentrated commercially available surfactant (Poractant or Curosurf), a foal would require 56 ml of Poractant (19–3 ml bottles [80 mg/ml]). In contrast, 300 ml of BALF from a live horse yields approximately 30 mg of phospholipid following concentration via ultracentrifugation at 40 000 × g. Using this approximation, four 300 ml lavages from one live donor would yield 120 mg, and a 5 l whole lung lavage from a deceased horse would yield 500 mg of surfactant. This equates to 35–40 live donor horses or 9–10 deceased horses to produce enough surfactant for a 100 mg/kg dose in a foal. Smaller treatment doses have been described in people but are considered less efficient. The cost associated with commercial surfactant preparations and difficulty with producing enough donor-harvested surfactant may explain the lack of treatment success with exogenous surfactant in foals.

References

1 Schittny, J.C. (2017). Development of the lung. *Cell Tissue Res.* 367: 427–444.
2 Woods, J.C. and Schittny, J.C. (2016). Lung structure at preterm and term birth. In: *Fetal and Neonatal Lung Development* (ed. A.H. Jobe, J.A. Whitsett, and S.H. Abman), 126–137. New York: Cambridge University Press.
3 Rodrigues, R.F., Rodrigues, M.N., Franciolli, A.L. et al. (2014). Embryonic and fetal development of cardiorespiratory apparatus in horses (equus caballus) fom 20 to 115 days of gestation. *J. Cytol. Histol.* 5: 1–10.
4 Franciolli, A.L., Cordeiro, B.M., da Fonseca, E.T. et al. (2011). Characteristics of the equine embryo and fetus from days 15 to 107 of pregnancy. *Theriogenology* 76: 819–832.
5 McGeady, T.A. (2017). Respiratory system. In: *Veterinary Embryology*, 2e (ed. T.A. McGeady, P.J. Quinn, E.S. Fitzpatrick, et al.), 232–239. Wiley Blackwell.
6 Pattle, R.E., Rossdale, P.D., Schock, C. et al. (1975). The development of the lung and its surfactant in the foal and in other species. *J. Reprod. Fertil Suppl.* 23: 651–657.
7 Beech, D.J., Sibbons, P.D., Rossdale, P.D. et al. (2001). Organogenesis of lung and kidney in Thoroughbreds and ponies. *Equine Vet. J.* 33: 438–445.
8 Johnson, L., Montgomery, J.B., Schneider, J.P. et al. (2014). Morphometric examination of the equine adult and foal lung. *Anat. Rec. (Hoboken)* 297: 1950–1962.
9 Agassandian, M. and Mallampalli, R.K. (2013). Surfactant phospholipid metabolism. *Biochim. Biophys. Acta* 1831: 612–625.
10 Griese, M. (1999). Pulmonary surfactant in health and human lung diseases: state of the art. *Eur. Respir. J.* 13: 1455–1476.
11 Weaver, T.E., Nogee, L.M., and Jobe, A.H. (2016). Surfactant during lung development. In: *Fetal and Neonatal Lung Development* (ed. A.H. Jobe, J.A. Whitsett, and S.H. Abman), 141–158. New York: Cambridge University Press.
12 Christmann, U., Buechner-Maxwell, V.A., Witonsky, S.G. et al. (2009). Role of lung surfactant in respiratory disease: current knowledge in large animal medicine. *J. Vet. Intern. Med.* 23: 227–242.
13 Christmann, U., Livesey, L.C., Taintor, J.S. et al. (2006). Lung surfactant function and composition in neonatal foals and adult horses. *J. Vet. Intern. Med.* 20: 1402–1407.
14 Johnson, L.M., Johnson, C., and Karger, A.B. (2019). End of the line for fetal lung maturity testing. *Clin. Biochem.* 71: 74–76.
15 Wright, J.R. (2005). Immunoregulatory functions of surfactant proteins. *Nat. Rev. Immunol.* 5: 58–68.
16 Weaver, T.E. and Conkright, J.J. (2001). Function of surfactant proteins B and C. *Annu. Rev. Physiol.* 63: 555–578.
17 Autilio, C. and Perez-Gil, J. (2019). Understanding the principle biophysics concepts of pulmonary surfactant in health and disease. *Arch. Dis. Child. Fetal Neonatal Ed.* 104: F443–F451.
18 Matalon, S. and Wright, J.R. (2004). Surfactant proteins and inflammation: the yin and the yang. *Am. J. Respir. Cell Mol. Biol.* 31: 585–586.

19 Hentschel, R., Bohlin, K., van Kaam, A. et al. (2020). Surfactant replacement therapy: from biological basis to current clinical practice. *Pediatr. Res.* 88: 176–183.

20 Rau, G.A., Vieten, G., Haitsma, J.J. et al. (2004). Surfactant in newborn compared with adolescent pigs: adaptation to neonatal respiration. *Am. J. Respir. Cell Mol. Biol.* 30: 694–701.

21 Arvidson, G., Astedt, B., Ekelund, L. et al. (1975). Surfactant studies in the fetal and neonatal foal. *J. Reprod. Fertil Suppl.* 23: 663–665.

22 Paradis, M.R. (1987). Lecithin/Sphingomyelin ratios and phosphatidylglycerol in term and premature equine amniotic fluid. *J. Am. Vet. Med. Assoc.* 5: 789–792.

23 Williams, M.A., Goyert, N.A., Goyert, G.L. et al. (1988). Preliminary report of transabdominal amniocentesis for the determination of pulmonary maturity in an equine population. *Equine Vet. J.* 20: 457–458.

24 Williams, M.A., Schmidt, A.R., Carleton, C.L. et al. (1992). Amniotic fluid analysis for ante-partum foetal assessment in the horse. *Equine Vet. J.* 24: 236–238.

25 Sweet, D.G., Carnielli, V., Greisen, G. et al. (2019). European consensus guidelines on the management of respiratory distress syndrome – 2019 update. *Neonatology* 115: 432–450.

26 Force, A.D.T., Ranieri, V.M., Rubenfeld, G.D. et al. (2012). Acute respiratory distress syndrome: the Berlin definition. *JAMA* 307: 2526–2533.

27 Wilkins, P.A., Otten, N.D., and Baumgardner, J.E. (2007). Acute lung injury and acute respiratory distress syndromes in veterinary medicine. Consensus definitions. The Dorothy Havemeyer Working Group on ALI and ARDS in Veterinary Medicine. *J. Vet. Emerg. Crit. Care* 17 (4): 333–339.

28 Dunkel, B. (2020). Acute respiratory distress syndrome and acute lung injury. In: *Large Animal Internal Medicine*, 6e (ed. B.P. Smith, D.C. Van Metre, and N. Pusterla), 564–566. St Louis, MO: Elsevier.

29 Ousey, J.C., Kolling, M., and Allen, W.R. (2006). The effects of meternal dexamethasone treatment on gestational length and foal maturation in Thoroughbred mares. *Anim. Reprod. Sci.* 94: 436–438.

30 Ousey, J.C., Kolling, M., Kindahl, H. et al. (2011). Maternal dexamethasone treatment in late gestation induces precocious fetal maturation and delivery in healthy Thoroughbred mares. *Equine Vet. J.* 43: 424–429.

31 Rossdale, P.D. (1993). Clinical view of disturbances in equine foetal maturation. *Equine Vet. J. Suppl.* 14: 3–7.

32 Rossdale, P.D., McGladdery, A.J., Ousey, J.C. et al. (1992). Increase in plasma progestagen concentrations in the mare after foetal injection with CRH, ACTH or betamethasone in late gestation. *Equine Vet. J.* 24: 347–350.

33 Gillen-Goldstein, J., MacKenzie, A.P., and Funai, E.F. (2019). Assessment of fetal lung maturity. *Up to Date* 1–17.

34 Eigenmann, U.J., Schoon, H.A., Jahn, D. et al. (1984). Neonatal respiratory distress syndrome in the calf. *Vet. Rec.* 114: 141–144.

35 Zaremba, W., Grunert, E., and Aurich, J.E. (1997). Prophylaxis of respiratory distress syndrome in premature calves by administration of dexamethasone or a prostaglandin F2 alpha analogue to their dams before parturition. *Am. J. Vet. Res.* 58: 404–407.

36 Castagnetti, C., Mariella, J., Serrazanetti, G.P. et al. (2007). Evaluation of lung maturity by amniotic fluid analysis in equine neonate. *Theriogenology* 67: 1455–1462.

37 Polin, R.A., Carlo, W.A., and Committee on F, Newborn, American Academy of P (2014). Surfactant replacement therapy for preterm and term neonates with respiratory distress. *Pediatrics* 133: 156–163.

38 Tinkler, S.H., Mathews, L.A., Firshman, A.M. et al. (2015). The use of equine surfactant and positive pressure ventilation to treat a premature alpaca cria with severe hypoventilation and hypercapnia. *Can. Vet. J.* 56: 370–374.

39 Perry, B. (1993). The use of bovine derived surfactant in foals with respiratory distres. In: *11th ACVIM Forum*, 189–192. American College of Veterinary Internal Medicine.

40 Ainsworth, D.M. (2001). Respiratory therapy in foals. In: *19th ACVIM Forum*, 248–249. American College of Veterinary Internal Medicine.

Section IV Onset of Breathing

Kara M. Lascola

The initiation of breathing and establishment of gas exchange are among the first activities of the newborn and are essential for successful adaptation to extrauterine life. In all species, the first spontaneous breath should occur within seconds of birth [1–5] with the establishment of functional residual capacity (FRC) and stabilization of respiratory rate and pattern occurring over the first 30–90 minutes after birth [6–8]. In normal foals, spontaneous breathing is established within 30–60 seconds of birth, with some foals demonstrating attempts to breath as they clear the pelvic canal [9, 10]. Gas exchange and corresponding increases in P_aO_2 and oxygen saturation should stabilize with the first 10 minutes of delivery but in some species, such as foals, this may take several days to reach adult levels (Table 1.IV.1) [1, 11–15].

Preparation for the onset of breathing and the transition from the intrauterine to extrauterine environment relies on a complex series of physiologic changes involving multiple organ systems, of which the most critical include those of the respiratory and cardiovascular systems [1, 2, 16]. In addition to the initiation of breathing, key events that must also occur shortly before and at the time of birth include clearance of fetal lung fluid, secretion of surfactant, establishment of FRC and normal ventilation, and cardiovascular changes to support increased pulmonary blood flow necessary for effective gas exchange [2, 16]. Early recognition of problems and prompt intervention are critical during this transitional period. Thus, understanding what must occur during respiratory transition to the extrauterine environment and familiarity with normal timing of events is essential.

Physiologic Adaptations in the Fetus

Development and maturation of the respiratory system occurs throughout gestation while the fetus is relying entirely on placental support for all gas exchange [1, 2, 16]. Because the fetal lungs do not participate in gas exchange, only a minor portion of fetal cardiac output (approximately 10%) is directed toward the pulmonary circulation [17]. Throughout gestation, the fetal environment remains moderately hypoxic [1, 2, 10, 16]. For example, in the fetal foal, the P_aO_2 of oxygenated placental blood delivered to the fetal foal is 50 mmHg while in the human fetus the P_aO_2 is slightly lower at 30–35 mmHg (saturation 80%) [18, 19]. In response to this relative fetal hypoxia, the pulmonary arteries remain vasoconstricted, resulting in high pulmonary vascular resistance and the shunting of blood flow away from the fetal pulmonary vasculature [1, 16, 20].

During gestation, preparation for the transition to the extrauterine environment involves precise development and maturation of the fetal lung and establishment of the specialized neuronal networks for control of respiration. The development of these neuronal networks within the medullary and pons regions of the brainstem is discussed in section V of this chapter (Control of Breathing). The lungs are one of the last fetal organs to complete maturation, with the majority of the structural development of the airways, alveoli, and parenchyma occurring during the last third of gestation [1, 2]. In some species, including horses, alveolarization continues after birth [21–23]. Fetal lung fluid and surfactant production during gestation also play critical roles in the preparation of the fetal lung for adaptation to breathing at birth [1, 2, 16, 24, 25].

While peri-parturient absorption of fetal lung fluid is critical for normal transition and onset of breathing in the neonate, lung growth, and maturation in the fetus depends on accumulation of fetal lung fluid throughout gestation [24, 25]. Fetal lung fluid, a filtrate of lung interstitial fluid, is high in chloride and low in protein and is secreted via active chloride transport across the airway epithelium of type II alveolar cells [2, 26]. Fluid production begins early in gestation with the rate and volume of secretion increasing until shortly before parturition [2, 25, 27–29]. During very late gestation, it is estimated that the human

Equine Neonatal Medicine, First Edition. Edited by David M. Wong and Pamela A. Wilkins.

Table 1.IV.1 Changes in PaO_2 levels in neonatal foals in lateral recumbency during the first week of life.

Postnatal age	60 min	12 h	24 h	48 h	4 d	7 d
Normal PaO_2 (mmHg)	60.9 ± 2.7	73.5 ± 3.0	67.6 ± 4.4	74.9 ± 3.3	81.2 ± 3.1	90.0 ± 3.1

Source: Adapted from: Wilkins et al. [11].

fetal lung secretes approximately 0.5 l of fluid per day [30] and in fetal sheep, the rate of secretion reaches 4 ml/kg/h [25]. During gestation the accumulation of this fluid within the lung and airways not only increases bronchoalveolar intraluminal pressure and supports the developing airway structures, but also contributes to maintaining increased pulmonary vascular resistance [16, 31]. The production of fetal lung fluid is influenced by hormones (e.g. cortisol), hypoxemia, and fetal breathing movements, also critical for the developing lungs [24].

Surfactant is essential for reducing the work of breathing and for the successful transition to breathing. Surfactant phospholipids and lipophilic proteins (SP-B, SP-C) form a monolayer at the air–liquid interface, lowering alveolar surface tension and allowing for lung inflation at lower pressures [1, 32, 33]. The onset of surfactant production by maturing alveolar type II epithelial cells varies somewhat across species. In humans, production begins at approximately 22 weeks of age [34] while in most foals surfactant production has been detected as early as 100 days of gestation and is thought to be fully developed by 300 days (~88%) of gestation [21, 35–37]. Throughout gestation, surfactant accumulates and is stored in lamellar bodies within type II cells. By the time of parturition, the fetal alveolar surfactant pool may exceed that of an adult by up to 20 times [2, 34]. Secretion of this pool of surfactant coincides with the onset of labor and clearance of fetal lung fluid [38]. Differences in composition of surfactants are described between neonatal foals and adult horses, suggesting incomplete maturation in surfactant at time of birth [39].

Physiologic Transition at Birth

Preparation of the fetus for transition to extrauterine life starts prior to the onset of labor. As previously mentioned, a normal neonatal transition must include clearance of fetal lung fluid, secretion of surfactant, onset of breathing and establishment of normal ventilation, and cardiovascular changes supporting shift from fetal to neonatal circulation. Endocrine adaptations, particularly increases in fetal cortisol, the major regulatory hormone directing final fetal maturation and adaption at birth [2, 40], play a critical role in regulating this transition, as do other chemical and extrauterine stimuli [1, 2, 16]. Prematurity or dysmaturity represents one of the most common reasons why this transition may be impeded, although maternal, fetal, or neonatal infectious or inflammatory conditions and significant in utero hypoxia may also contribute. Depending on the cause, structural or functional immaturity of the respiratory system, surfactant deficiency, delayed clearance of fetal fluid, as well as alterations in adaptations to the endocrine and cardiovascular systems may occur [2, 10, 16, 35].

Complete clearance of fetal lung fluid within a few hours of birth is critical for establishing normal breathing and gas exchange in the neonate. Toward the end of gestation, the production of fluid decreases and the alveolar epithelium adapts to promote fluid absorption before the onset of labor. Fluid absorption dramatically increases during labor leaving a relatively small amount to be cleared postnatally. Complete clearance is typically achieved within a few hours of birth [1]. Cesarean delivery without labor and prematurity both may result in delayed lung fluid clearance and transient tachypnea of the newborn [41, 42]. Fetal endocrine adaptions in late gestation are also critical for initiating clearance of lung fluid [2].

Increased production of fetal cortisol regulates final pulmonary maturation and promotes the transition of the airway epithelium from chloride-mediated secretion to sodium-mediated fluid reabsorption [1, 2, 16, 40]. Cortisol also triggers secretion of thyroid hormones (T3) and increases the expression of pulmonary beta-adrenergic receptors. Together, cortisol, T3, and catecholamines (via beta-receptor stimulation) inactivate chloride-mediated fluid secretion and promote expression and activation of Na^+-K^+ ATPase channels on type II cells within the airway epithelium. Sodium enters the type II cell apical surface, is pumped into the interstitium and then draws water/electrolytes out of alveolar spaces and into the interstitium via passive absorption. The fluid is then cleared from the interstitium via lymphatic or microvascular drainage [2, 29, 43–46]. Increased expression of lung aquaporins (AQP1 & 4) during the periparturient and immediate postpartum period may also play a role in lung fluid clearance [30].

In the immediate postpartum period, additional stimuli contribute to the final clearance of fetal lung fluid. The onset of breathing results in increases in both blood oxygen concentrations and intrapulmonary pressure. Increased PO_2 stimulates further epithelial sodium channel gene expression in the type II cells [45, 46]. The increase in intrapulmonary pressure results in a greater transepithelial pressure gradient, which further drives alveolar fluid absorption [1, 5]. Contrary to earlier theories, thoracic compression associated with passage through the pelvic canal ("thoracic squeeze") most likely plays a very minor role in clearance of fetal lung fluid [47].

At the time of birth and with the onset of breathing, several factors contribute to secretion of the large pool of surfactant stored in the lamellar bodies of the type II alveolar cells. Much of the surfactant is secreted just prior to and at the onset of labor, as clearance of fetal lung fluid is initiated [38]. Specific endocrine triggers include the increased production of fetal cortisol and catecholamine-mediated stimulation of beta 2 adrenergic receptors within the lung [2]. Additionally, after birth the first several deep breaths taken by the newborn result in alveolar stretch and subsequent deformation of the type II cells, which triggers release of surfactant into the alveolar space [2]. Adequate surfactant release during the first respirations allows for uniform expansion of the lung. Without this, both overdistension and atelectasis may develop [2, 48, 49].

Surfactant deficiency is considered a major component of respiratory distress syndrome in preterm infants and also has been reported in premature foals [21, 36, 37]. Depending on the degree of prematurity and other contributing factors, a sufficient pool of surfactant can be achieved within several hours of birth in preterm infants and neonatal lambs in response to endocrine and lung stretch stimuli at the time of delivery [2, 50, 51]. For many premature foals, although surfactant deficiency may contribute, it is probably not the primary cause of respiratory dysfunction, given that surfactant production can be fully developed by 300 days of gestation [35, 36]. Additional factors impede adaptation to breathing and effective gas exchange in premature or dysmature foals (and other newborns). These may include structural and functional immaturity of the respiratory system and in endocrine adaptations as well as incomplete or delayed clearance of fetal lung fluid. Hypoxemia associated with persistent extrapulmonary shunting of blood and poorly reactive pulmonary vasculature, along with increased ventilation perfusion mismatch are other contributors to poor respiratory transition [2, 35, 49].

A successful respiratory transition in the neonate depends on circulatory adaptations that will allow for effective gas exchange in the lung. During gestation, pulmonary vascular resistance is high. Fetal blood flow is shunted away from the pulmonary vasculature through the ductus arteriosus and, as previously mentioned, only a small percentage (10%) of fetal cardiac output is directed toward the lung [1, 16, 17, 20]. In the neonate, the pulmonary vasculature must rapidly transition to accepting almost all cardiac output. Thus, one of the most important adaptations accompanying the onset of breathing in the neonate involves the closure of vascular shunts that directed blood flow away from the pulmonary vasculature during gestation and the subsequent reduction in pulmonary vascular resistance [1, 2, 10, 16].

The increased oxygen tension in the lung and reduction in hypoxia associated with the first respirations are some of the most important triggers for these vascular changes. Oxygen relaxes pulmonary vascular smooth muscle via increased cGMP-dependent protein kinase activity, contributing to the reversal of hypoxia-mediated vasoconstriction [1, 20]. Resolution of hypoxia is also associated with functional closure of the ductus arteriosus and umbilical artery vasoconstriction [1, 20]. As a greater amount of cardiac output is directed toward the lung, the pulmonary vascular resistance further decreases via nitric-oxide–mediated vasodilation [1, 20, 52, 53]. In humans, this transition corresponds to an increase in oxygen saturation from 60% to 90% over the first 10 minutes after birth [54]. Clearance of fetal lung fluid and reductions in airway resistance represent additional physiologic processes that contribute to reducing pulmonary vascular resistance. Increased intravascular fluid volume over the first few hours is attributed to clearance of lung fluid [1, 2] while reduced airway resistance associated with opening of the distal airways in response to breathing provides radial support for the pulmonary vessels [10, 16].

Onset of Breathing

During onset of parturition and immediately afterward, several stimuli are believed to trigger the establishment of the first breaths and adaptation to the extrauterine environment. The important chemical triggers of hypoxemia, hypercapnia, and acidosis are associated with the cessation of placental blood flow and result in stimulation of the respiratory centers in the brainstem. In addition, important extrauterine triggers include thermal (decreased temperature) and tactile stimuli at the time of birth [2–4, 10, 55–57]. Severe in utero hypoxia can impede the transition to spontaneous breathing because of its inhibitory effect on central respiratory control [1].

Newborns inflate their lungs to establish lung aeration at birth by generating large negative pressure breaths. These first breaths should be vigorous and occur within seconds of birth. In newborn rabbits, approximately 50% of lung aeration is achieved in first three breaths [58]. Maintenance of adequate respiratory effort and continued breathing by the neonate is essential to establish FRC and to increase oxygen saturation [2, 46, 59]. During early postnatal breathing, variability in respiratory rate and pattern may be noted and is directed toward the establishment of FRC. Braking maneuvers and expiration against a closed glottis ("grunting") during these initial breathing efforts are not uncommon and can help establish lung expansion and aeration [10, 29, 60]. Deeper breaths with short periods of breath holding are noted and inspiratory volume typically exceeds expiratory volume. Infants that make a normal respiratory transition should establish an appropriate FRC and demonstrate a stable and regular respiratory pattern within the first 90 minutes of birth.

The respiratory transition in foals immediately after birth is similar to other species. Spontaneous breathing in foals should be observed within several seconds of birth [9, 10]. The respiratory rate in the immediate postpartum period is rapid (80 breaths/min), gradually decreasing over first several hours (30–40 breaths/min) with an active component to both the inspiratory and expiratory phases of respiration [9, 10]. Other findings noted on examination may include grunting, expiratory crackles in the dependent lung due to presence of residual fetal fluid, and rarely, slight, rapidly resolving cyanosis [9, 10, 13, 14]. Even with a normal respiratory transition, newborn foals remain relatively hypoxemic with P_aO_2 levels gradually increasing toward those of older foals and adult horses over the first week of life (Table 1.IV.1) [11–15].

References

1 Morton, S. and Brodsky, D. (2016). Featl physiology and the transition to extrauterine life. *Clin. Perinatol.* 43 (3): 395–407.

2 Hillman, N., Kallapur, S.G., and Jobe, A. (2012). Physiology of transition from intrauterine to extrauterine life. *Clin. Perinatol.* 39 (4): 769–783.

3 Ersdal, H.L., Linde, J., Mduma, E. et al. (2014). Neonatal outcome following cord clamping after onset of spontaneous respiration. *Pediatrics* 134: 265–272.

4 Karlberg, P., Cherry, R.B., Escardó, F.E. et al. (1962). Respiratory studies in newborn infants. II: pulmonary ventilation and mechanics of breathing in the first minutes of life, including the onset of respirations. *Acta Pædiatr.* 51: 121–136.

5 Vyas, H., Field, D., Milner, A.D. et al. (1986). Determinants of the first inspiratory volume and functional residual capacity at birth. *Pediatr. Pulmonol.* 2: 189–193.

6 Hooper, S.B., Siew, M.L., Kitchen, M.J. et al. (2013). Establishing functional residual capacity in the non-breathing infant. *Semin. Fetal Neonatal Med.* 18: 336–343.

7 Fisher, J.T., Mortola, J.P., Smith, J.B. et al. (1982). Respiration in newborns: development of the control of breathing. *Am. Rev. Respir. Dis.* 125: 650–657.

8 Michel, A. and Lowe, N.K. (2017). The successful immediate neonatal transition to extrauterine life. *Biol. Res. Nurs.* 19: 287–294.

9 Koterba, A.M. (1990). Physical examination. In: *Equine Clinical Neonatology* (ed. A.M. Koterba, W.H. Drummond, and P.C. Kosch), 71–85. Philadelphia, PA: Lea & Febiger.

10 Wilkins, P.A. (2003). Lower respiratory problems of the neonate. *Vet. Clin. Equine* 19: 19–33.

11 Wilkins, P.A., Otto, C.M., Baumgardner, J.E. et al. (2007). Acute lung injury and acute respiratory distress syndromes in veterinary medicine: consensus definitions: the Dorothy Russell Havemeyer Working Group on ALI and ARDS in veterinary medicine. *J. Vet. Emerg. Crit. Care* 17: 333–339.

12 Hackett, E.S., Traub-Dargatz, J.L., Knowles, J.E. et al. (2010). Arterial blood gas parameters of normal foals born at 1500 metres elevation. *Equine Vet. J.* 42: 59–62.

13 Rossdale, P.D. (1967). Clinical studies on the newborn Thoroughbred foal. I. Perinatal behavior. *Br. Vet. J.* 123: 470.

14 Rossdale, P.D. (1970). The adaptive processes of the newborn foal. *Vet. Rec.* 87: 37–38.

15 Stewart, J.H., Rose, R.J., and Barko, A.M. (1984). Respiratory studies in foals from birth to seven days old. *Equine Vet. J.* 16: 323.

16 Swanson, J.R. and Sinkin, R.A. (2015). Transition from fetus to newborn. *Pediatr. Clin. North Am.* 62: 329–343.

17 Mielke, G. and Benda, N. (2001). Cardiac output and central distribution of blood flow in the human fetus. *Circulation* 103: 1662–1668.

18 Blackburn, S. (2007). *Maternal, Fetal and Neonatal Physiology: A Clinical Perspective*, 3e. St Louis, MO: Elsevier Saunders.

19 Silver, M. and Comline, R.S. (1975). Transfer of gases and metabolites in the equine placenta: a comparison with other species. *J. Reprod. Fertil. Suppl.* 23: 589–594.

20 Gao, Y. and Raj, J.U. (2010). Regulation of the pulmonary circulation in the fetus and newborn. *Physiol. Rev.* 90: 1291–1335.

21 Arvidson, G., Astedt, B., Ekelund, L. et al. (1975). Surfactant studies in the fetal and neonatal foal. *J. Reprod. Fertil. Suppl.* 23: 663–665.

22 Winkler, G.C. and Cheville, N.F. (1985). Morphometry of postnatal development in the porcine lung. *Anat. Rec.* 211: 427–433.

23 Rau, G.A., Vieten, G., Haitsma, J.J. et al. (2004). Surfactant in newborn compared with adolescent pigs: adaptation to neonatal respiration. *Am. J. Respir. Cell Mol. Biol.* 30: 694–701.

24 Hooper, S.B. and Harding, R. (1995). Fetal lung liquid: a major determinant of the growth and functional development of the fetal lung. *Clin. Exp. Pharmacol. Physiol.* 22: 235–241.

25 Harding, R. and Hooper, S.B. (1996). Regulation of lung expansion and lung growth before birth. *J. Appl. Phys.* 81: 209–224.

26 Jain, L. and Eaton, D.C. (2006). Physiology of fetal lung fluid clearance and the effect of labor. *Semin. Perinatol.* 30: 34–43.

27 McCray, P.B. Jr., Bettencourt, J.D., and Bastacky, J. (1992). Developing bronchopulmonary epithelium of the human fetus secretes fluid. *Am. J. Phys* 262: L270–L279.

28 Andersson, S., Pitkanen, O., Janer, C. et al. (2010). Lung fluid during postnatal transition. *Chin. Med. J.* 123: 2919–2923.

29 Jain, L. (1999). Alveolar fluid clearance in developing lungs and its role in neonatal transition. *Clin. Perinatol.* 26: 585–599.

30 Zelenina, M., Zelenin, S., and Aperia, A. (2005). Water channels (aquaporins) and their role for postnatal adaptation. *Pediatr. Res.* 57: 47–53.

31 Lakshminrusimha, S. and Steinhorn, R.H. (1999). Pulmonary vascular biology during neonatal transition. *Clin. Perinatol.* 26: 601–619.

32 Frerking, I., Gunther, A., Seeger, W. et al. (2001). Pulmonary surfactant: functions, abnormalities and therapeutic options. *Intensive Care Med.* 27: 1699–1717.

33 Griese, M. (1999). Pulmonary surfactant in health and human lung diseases: state of the art. *Eur. Respir. J.* 13: 1455–1476.

34 Clements, J.A. (1997). Lung surfactant: a personal perspective. *Annu. Rev. Physiol.* 59: 1–21.

35 Lester, G.D. (2005). Maturity of the neonatal foal. *Vet. Clin. Equine* 21: 333–355.

36 Pattle, R.E., Rossdale, P.D., Schock, C. et al. (1975). The development of the lung and its surfactant in the foal and in other species. *J. Reprod. Fertil. Suppl.* 23: 651–657.

37 Rossdale, P.D., Pattle, R.E., and Mahaffey, L.W. (1967). Respiratory distress in a newborn foal with failure to form lung lining fluid. *Nature* 215: 1498–1499.

38 Faridy, E.E. and Thliveris, J.A. (1987). Rate of secretion of lung surfactant before and after birth. *Respir. Physiol.* 68: 269–277.

39 Christmann, U., Livesey, L.C., Taintor, J.S. et al. (2006). Lung surfactant function and composition in neonatal foals and adult horses. *J. Vet. Intern. Med.* 20: 1402–1407.

40 Liggins, G.C. (1994). The role of cortisol in preparing the fetus for birth. *Reprod. Fertil. Dev.* 6: 141–150.

41 Bland, R.D., Hansen, T.N., Haberkern, C.M. et al. (1982). Lung fluid balance in lambs before and after birth. *J. Appl. Physiol. Respir. Environ. Exerc. Physiol.* 53: 992–1004.

42 Modi, N. (2003). Clinical implications of postnatal alterations in body water distribution. *Semin. Neonatol.* 8: 301–306.

43 Folkesson, H.G., Norlin, A., and Baines, D.L. (1998). Salt and water transport across the alveolar epithelium in the developing lung: correlations between function and recent molecular biology advances. *Int. J. Mol. Med.* 2: 515–531.

44 Tessier, G.J., Lester, G.D., Langham, M.R. et al. (1996). Ion transport properties of fetal sheep alveolar epithelial cells in monolayer culture. *Am. J. Phys* 270 (Part 1): L1008–L1016.

45 Bland, R.D. and Nielson, D.W. (1992). Developmental changes in lung epithelial ion transport and liquid movement. *Annu. Rev. Physiol.* 54: 373–394.

46 O'Brodovich, H.M. (1996). Immature epithelial Na1 channel expression is one of the pathogenetic mechanisms leading to human neonatal respiratory distress syndrome. *Proc. Assoc. Am. Phys.* 108: 345–355.

47 Goldsmith, J.P. (2011). Delivery room resuscitation of the newborn. In: *Neonatal-Perinatal Medicine: Diseases of the Fetus and Infant*, 9e (ed. R.J. Martin, A.A. Fanaroff, and M.C. Walsh), 449–454. St Louis, MO: Elsevier Mosby.

48 Vyas, H., Milner, A.D., and Hopkins, I.E. (1981). Intrathoracic pressure and volume changes during the spontaneous onset of respiration in babies born by cesarean section and by vaginal delivery. *J. Pediatr.* 99: 787–791.

49 Siew, M.L., Te Pas, A.B., Wallace, M.J. et al. (2011). Surfactant increases the uniformity of lung aeration at birth in ventilated preterm rabbits. *Pediatr. Res.* 70: 50–55.

50 Rebello, C.M., Jobe, A.H., Eisele, J.W. et al. (1996). Alveolar and tissue surfactant pool sizes in humans. *Am. J. Respir. Crit. Care Med.* 154: 625–628.

51 Jacobs, H., Jobe, A., Ikegami, M. et al. (1985). Accumulation of alveolar surfactant following delivery and ventilation of premature lambs. *Exp. Lung. Res.* 8: 125–140.

52 Shaul, P.W. (1999). Regulation of vasodilator synthesis during lung development. *Early Hum. Dev.* 54: 271–294.

53 Steinhorn, R.H., Millard, S.L., and Morin, F.C. III (1995). Persistent pulmonary hypertension of the newborn. Role of nitric oxide and endothelin in pathophysiology and treatment. *Clin. Perinatol.* 22: 405–428.

54 Kattwinkel, J., Perlman, J.M., Aziz, K. et al. (2010). Part 15: neonatal resuscitation: 2010 American Heart Association guidelines for cardiopulmonary resuscitation and emergency cardiovascular care. *Circulation* 122: S909–S919.

55 Acworth, N.R.L. (2003). The health neonatal foal: routine examinations and preventative medicine. *Equine Vet. Educ.* 15 (suppl 6): 45–49.

56 Askin, D.F. (2002). Complications in the transition from fetal to neonatal life. *J. Obstet., Gynecol. Neonatal Nurs.* 31: 318–327.

57 Weisbrot, I.M., James, L.S., Prince, C.E. et al. (1958). Acid-base homeostasis of the newborn infant during the first 24 hours of life. *J. Pediatr.* 52: 395–403.

58 Siew, M.L., Wallace, M.J., Kitchen, M.J. et al. (2009). Inspiration regulates the rate and temporal pattern of lung liquid clearance and lung aeration at birth. *J. Appl. Phys.* 106: 1888–1895.

59 Klaus, M., Tooley, W.H., Weaver, K.H. et al. (1962). Lung volume in the newborn infant. *Pediatrics* 30: 111–116.

60 Helve, O., Pitkänen, O., Janèr, C. et al. (2009). Pulmonary fluid balance in the human newborn infant. *Neonatology* 95: 347–352.

Section V Control of Breathing

Kara M. Lascola

In mammalian species, breathing is a rhythmic process whose ultimate purpose represents the uptake of oxygen (O_2) and removal of carbon dioxide (CO_2) from the body [1]. The central control of breathing originates from specialized neuronal networks found within the medullary and pons regions of the brainstem. These networks are established early on in utero and undergo precise development throughout gestation [1–3]. Ultimately, regulation of the pattern, rate, and depth of respiration is involuntary, involving complex interactions between the central respiratory control areas, input from both central and peripheral sites, and output to the muscles of breathing (Figure 1.V.1) [4, 5]. Higher brain centers may provide input in response to changes in temperature or "emotional state," or allow for voluntary control over breathing during activities such as vocalizing, eating, or coughing [5–8]. The reticular activating system also modulates breathing during periods of sleep and arousal [5].

The rate and depth of breathing are tightly regulated to match alveolar ventilation with metabolic rate in order to maintain the partial pressure of CO_2 and O_2 (P_aCO_2, P_aO_2) within a narrow homeostatic range [1, 5, 9, 10]. In response to changing internal and external conditions (e.g. hypercapnia, hypoxemia, bronchoconstriction, postural, or movement changes), sensory afferent signals from central and peripheral chemoreceptors (PCRs) and mechanoreceptors provide input to the respiratory centers within the brainstem, which, in turn, send efferent signals to the muscles of respiration to modify rate and depth of respiration as needed. This adaptability is a critical feature of respiratory control [1, 5].

Respiratory Control Centers in the Brainstem and Generation of Respiratory Rhythm

Synaptic interactions between specific aggregations of neurons located within the medulla and pons are responsible for the central control of respiration (Figure 1.V.1) [5, 6, 8, 10]. Within the medulla, the dorsal respiratory group (DRG; located in the nucleus tractus solitarious) and the ventral respiratory group (VRG; located in the nucleus para-ambiguous, ambiguous, and retroambiguous) comprise the medullary respiratory center [5]. Specific neurons within both the DRG and VRG also comprise the central pattern generator responsible for establishing respiratory rhythmogenesis [5, 11, 12]. Within the pons, the pneumotactic center (PC; rostral pons) and neurons within a poorly defined region in the caudal pons, termed the apneustic center, comprise the pontine respiratory centers [5].

The medullary DRG is composed primarily of inspiratory neurons and controls the basic rhythm of breathing by triggering inspiratory drive [5, 12]. Sensory afferent input from the lungs, airways, PCRs, and proprioceptors is delivered to the DRG by the glossopharyngeal and vagal nerves. In response, the DRG delivers efferent impulses to motor nerves of the diaphragm and external intercostal muscles, resulting in muscle contraction and corresponding changes in tidal volume. At the same time, the inspiratory activity of the DRG stimulates the VRG.

The VRG contains both inspiratory and expiratory neurons as well as the pre-Bötzinger complex, a cluster of

Equine Neonatal Medicine, First Edition. Edited by David M. Wong and Pamela A. Wilkins.

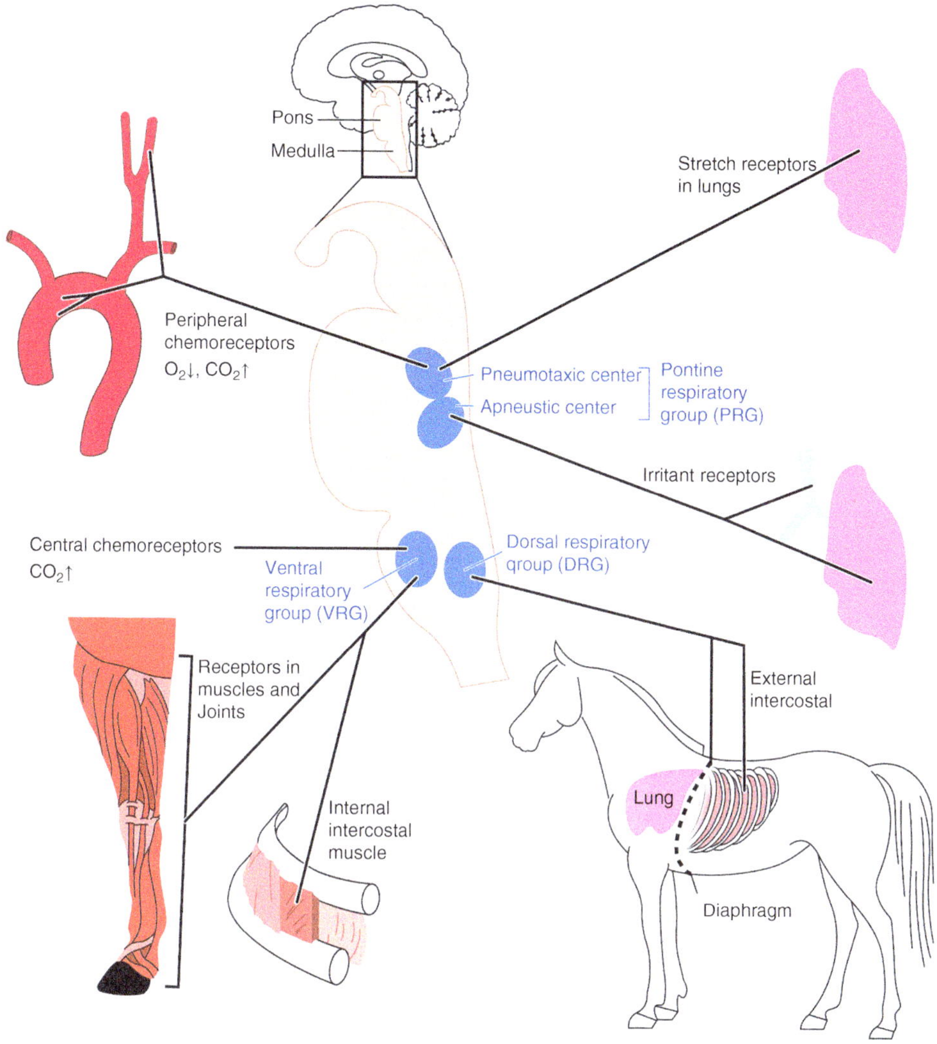

Figure 1.V.1 Overview of control of breathing in the foal. Multiple factors impact respiration, including central respiratory centers (pontine respiratory group, dorsal respiratory group) that interact with central and peripheral receptors that then output to muscles of breathing. See text for further information.

interneurons essential for respiratory rhythmogenesis in mammals [1, 3, 5, 12]. Inspiratory impulses from the VRG travel to laryngeal and pharyngeal muscles (via nucleus ambiguous neurons), as well as to the diaphragm and intercostal muscles (via nucleus retroambiguous neurons). The VRG is important for regulating respiration during exercise and plays a role in initiating expiration [5].

Stimulation from DRG inspiratory activity and input signals from pulmonary stretch receptors leads to activation by the VRG of a separate group of neurons within the medulla, termed the inspiratory cut-off switch [5]. Activation of these neurons initiates expiration by inhibiting inspiratory signaling from the DRG. Input from the pontine PC enhances this activity. Expiratory impulses from the VRG travel from neurons located within the retrotrapezoid nucleus and parafacial respiratory group to the abdominal and external intercostal respiratory muscles [5, 6, 10, 12]. Expiratory activity is modified through input from higher brain centers (cerebrum, thalamus), cranial nerves, and ascending spinal tracts [5].

Respiratory centers in the pons have a modifying effect on medullary respiratory center output but do not play a role in rhythmogenesis [5, 12]. Pneumotaxic center activity influences volume and rate of respiration as well as inspiratory time in response to afferent feedback regarding pulmonary inflation, P_aCO_2, and P_aO_2. Increased pneumotaxic center signaling corresponds to increases in respiratory rate, while decreased signaling results in prolonged inspiratory time and increased tidal volume [5]. The apneustic center stimulates inspiratory neurons within the DRG and VRG to prolong inspiration; its activity is primarily appreciated when damaged [5–7, 12]. Damage to the apneustic center impairs the ability of the medulla to transition from inspiration to expiration and results in apneustic breathing. This abnormal pattern may be observed in foals with neonatal encephalopathy and is characterized by prolonged gasping inspirations and transient expiratory efforts [13].

Defined phases of the respiratory cycle include the inspiratory phase, the post-inspiratory phase (or early expiratory phase), and the expiratory phase [5, 14, 15]. During eupneic breathing, inspiration is primarily active with its length controlled by feedback from pontine PC neurons and pulmonary stretch receptors. In contrast, expiration is primarily passive. Adult horses and dogs represent exceptions in that they have active and passive phases to both inspiration and expiration [16, 17]. In most species, regulation of the duration of expiration during eupneic breathing is the primary determinant of respiratory rate [5]. Research in several species suggests that these phases are controlled through interactions between specific groups of neurons within the medulla. Distinct neuronal firing patterns within each of the respiratory phases by these groups of neurons establishes the eupneic breathing pattern [14]. Influence over neuronal firing via complex feedback mechanisms and neurotransmitter signaling also allows for a large number of potential breathing patterns.

Sensory Afferent Input to the Respiratory Centers

The respiratory centers within the brainstem integrate afferent sensory input from several central and peripheral sites. Most important of these are the chemoreceptors within the brain and arterial vasculature, and the mechanoreceptors, chemoreceptors, and irritant receptors throughout the respiratory tract [1, 9–11]. Peripheral input from other areas may have a variable influence on respiration. Together, this input guides centrally mediated changes in respiratory pattern in response to metabolic changes (pH, P_aCO_2), respiratory disease or pathology, and movement or postural changes.

Central and Peripheral Chemoreceptors

Central chemoreceptors (CRCs) represent a distinct set of neurons within ventral medulla. These receptors act independently from the PCRs. Typically, changes in P_aCO_2 represent the primary stimulus for breathing [1, 5, 10]. While the CRCs do not respond directly to changes in P_aCO_2, they do respond to changes in pH within the cerebrospinal fluid (CSF) and intracerebral interstitial fluid, which correspond closely to changes in P_aCO_2 [5, 10]. The blood-brain barrier (BBB) is highly permeable to CO_2. Hydrolyzation of CO_2 within the CSF and interstitial fluid releases hydrogen ions, thus lowering pH [18]. During respiratory acidosis, CRCs detect this decrease in pH and send signals to the medullary respiratory neurons, resulting in hyperventilation, increased inspiratory, and expiratory muscle activity and corresponding increases in alveolar ventilation. During respiratory acidosis, the response to CO_2 within the brain can be additive as a result of CO_2-mediated cerebral vasodilation and subsequent increased CO_2 delivery [5, 10]. Changes in arterial hydrogen ion and HCO_3 do not have the same effect on the CRCs due to the relative impermeability of the BBB to these acid–base variables.

PCRs include the carotid and aortic bodies located at the bifurcation of the common carotid arteries and the aortic arch, respectively [5, 9]. These chemoreceptors communicate with the medullary respiratory centers via the vagus and glossopharyngeal nerves in response to changes in P_aO_2 and P_aCO_2. Of the two PCRs, the carotid bodies are the more responsive and demonstrate high sensitivity to decreases in P_aO_2 (hypoxemia) [5, 9]. Additionally, although PCRs respond to changes in P_aCO_2, they are less sensitive when compared to central chemoreceptors and contribute approximately 25% of the respiratory response to changes in P_aCO_2 [5]. Metabolic acidosis associated with lactic acid accumulation can also stimulate PCRs leading to a relatively rapid increase in alveolar ventilation.

The PCR-mediated response to decreased P_aO_2 is termed the *hypoxic ventilatory drive* and is associated with increases in minute ventilation through increased respiratory rate and recruitment of inspiratory muscles. This response may not be solely mediated by P_aO_2 – increased sensitivity of these chemoreceptors to hydrogen ions may also contribute [5]. Furthermore, PCRs do not respond to decreases in oxygen content (CaO_2). At relatively normal P_aO_2, oxygen does not play a significant role in respiratory drive and the PCR response increases as P_aO_2 decreases. At P_aO_2 levels <60 mmHg (saturation of hemoglobin [S_aO_2] of 90%), the response increases dramatically but disappears at very low P_aO_2 (<30 mmHg) as respiration becomes suppressed [5, 9, 18]. During severe alkalosis, this response is also diminished.

Together, metabolic acidosis, hypercapnia, and hypoxemia can result in maximal chemoreceptor stimulation, particularly of the PCRs. It is important to consider the response of the chemoreceptors when managing critically ill patients [8], such as septic foals with concurrent pulmonary disease. Signs of respiratory distress in these patients may result from combined acid–base and blood gas abnormalities. Therapeutic strategies directed at correcting one problem (e.g. supplemental oxygen to address hypoxemia) can result in worsening of other problems (e.g. reduced hypoxic ventilatory drive and worsened hypercapnia) [13].

Additional Peripheral Input to Respiratory Centers

Receptors throughout the respiratory tract provide additional sensory input to the respiratory center in response to various mechanical and chemical stimuli. Most of these receptors send information to the medullary respiratory neurons via the vagus nerve [5]. Pulmonary stretch receptors (slow-adapting receptors, SARs) [5, 7, 8, 19] are located within the smooth muscle of the trachea and bronchi. Stimulation of these receptors in response to increased lung volume during inspiration signals the medullary VRG and leads to inhibition of the DRG inspiratory neurons. Along with the pontine PC neurons, this response forms the medullary *inspiratory cutoff switch* [5]. Pulmonary stretch receptors are responsible for the *Hering-Breuer Reflex,* which induces a period of apnea at maximum lung inflation. Hypocapnia enhances pulmonary stretch receptor activity, while hypercapnia diminishes their activity [20]. These receptors may also sense end expiration and thus contribute to onset of inspiratory activity.

Irritant receptors, also referred to as rapidly adapting stretch receptors (RARs) [5, 8, 21], are found in the epithelium throughout the upper and lower respiratory tract. These receptors respond to mechanical stimuli as well as to exogenous (dust, smoke, cold, noxious gas) and endogenous (inflammatory mediators, histamine) irritants, and in the normal resting animal contribute little toward breathing control [5, 13]. In the nasopharynx, stimulation of irritant and chemoreceptors will result in respiratory inhibition, as will stimulation of pressure receptors in pharynx during swallowing. Increased negative pressure detected by laryngeal mechanoreceptors in association with upper airway obstruction will prolong inspiratory time. In response to noxious stimuli or in association with respiratory disease, receptors in the bronchi may directly influence respiratory rate or depth as well as contribute indirectly by causing bronchoconstriction, cough, mucus production, and further release of inflammatory mediators, as is seen in horses with severe asthma [8, 18, 22].

An additional category of receptors, C-fiber receptors, are found within pulmonary tissue often in close association with capillaries. In the past, these receptors were referred to as J (juxtacapillary) receptors [5]. Depending on their location, they may respond to lung hyperinflation, increased pulmonary congestion (edema), as well as a variety of endogenous (e.g. inflammatory mediators) and exogenous chemicals. Stimulation of C-fibers results in a variable outcomes including bronchoconstriction, vasodilation, increased inflammatory cytokine production, vasodilation, and vascular leak [5] and may influence breathing by inducing tachypnea or altering respiratory pattern (e.g. transient apnea followed by rapid shallow breaths).

An additional and relatively minor source of afferent input to the central respiratory system is via mechanoreceptors within respiratory muscles and the thoracic wall, and baroreceptors [5]. Mechanoreceptors within the muscles relay important information regarding the force of muscle contraction and the degree of muscle shortening. For example, input from phrenic nerve activity may provide information regarding inspiratory load. The baroreceptor reflex originates from the carotid sinus and aortic arch and produces hyperventilation in response to hypotension [5].

Efferent Signal from Respiratory Center

Efferent output from the medullary respiratory center is directed toward the muscles of respiration and establishes the rate and depth of respiration during automatic breathing [23]. Contraction and relaxation of these muscles creates pressure gradients allowing for the movement of air into and out of the lungs [18]. Neuronal integration along spinal tracts may modify central neuronal signals through exciting or inhibiting respiratory muscle activity in response to changes in respiratory system compliance or airflow [5]. The major muscle of respiration is the diaphragm [24]. External and internal intercostal muscles and abdominal muscles support and augment diaphragmatic activity. In addition, laryngeal and nasopharyngeal muscles also contribute through control of airflow through the upper respiratory tract. Because these upper respiratory tract muscles are also involved in several nonrespiratory functions, higher brain centers may provide additional input to the respiratory centers in regulating their activity [5].

As mentioned previously, inspiration and expiration in horses are biphasic, with each having an active and passive component [16, 25]. The development of this biphasic respiratory pattern develops over the first year of life in horses and in the neonatal foal, inspiration, and expiration are primarily active and monophasic [25]. In the adult, active inspiration relies on diaphragmatic contraction. Contraction of the external intercostals further drives inspiratory airflow along a negative pressure gradient. During active expiration, contraction of the internal intercostals and abdominal muscles further decreases lung volume beyond what is achieved by the natural recoil of the lung. Damage to these respiratory muscles can significantly affect ventilation resulting in hypoventilation, hypoxemia, and respiratory distress.

References

1 Beyeler, S.A., Hodges, M.R., and Huxtable, A.G. (2020). Impact of inflammation on developing respiratory control networks: rhythm generation, chemoreception and plasticity. *Respir. Physiol. Neurobiol.* 274: 103357.

2 Greer, J.J., Funk, G.D., and Ballanyi, K. (2006). Preparing for the first breath: prenatal maturation of respiratory neural control. *J. Physiol.* 570: 437–444.

3 Del Negro, C.A., Funk, G.D., and Feldman, J.L. (2018). Breathing matters. *Nat. Rev. Neurosci.* 10: 351–356.

4 Cunningham, D.J.C., Robbins, P.A., and Wolf, C.B. Integration of respiratory responses to changes in alveolar partial pressures of CO_2, O_2 and pH. In: *Handbook of Physiology. Section 3, Respiration. Volume II, Control of Breathing* (ed. N.S. Cherniak and J.G. Widdicombe), 475–527. Bethesda, MD: American Physiological Society.

5 Hazari, M.S. and Farraj, A.K. (2015). Comparative control of respiration. In: *Comparative Biology of the Normal Lung* (ed. R.A. Parent), 245–288. Elsevier Inc.

6 Garcia, A.J., Zanella, S., Koch, H. et al. (2011). Chapter 3—Networks within networks: the neuronal control of breathing. *Prog. Brain Res.* 188: 31.

7 Dempsey, J.A. and Smith, C.A. (2014). Pathophysiology of human ventilatory control. *Eur. Respir. J.* 44: 495.

8 Hines, M. (2018). Control of breathing. In: *Equine Internal Medicine*, Clinical Approach to Commonly Encountered Problems, 4e (ed. S.M. Reed, W.M. Bayly, and D.C. Sellon), 232–310. St. Louis, MO: Elsevier.

9 Prabhakar, N.R. and Peng, Y.J. (2017). Oxygen sensing by the carotid body: past and present. In: *Oxygen Transport to Tissue XXXIX*, Advances in Experimental Medicine and Biology, vol. 977 (ed. H. Halpern, J. LaManna, D. Harrison, and B. Epel), 3–8.

10 Guyenet, P.G. and Bayliss, D.A. (2015). Neural control of breathing and CO_2 homeostasis. *Neuron* 87: 946–961.

11 Feldman, J.L., Mitchell, G.S., and Nattie, E.E. (2003). Breathing: rhythmicity, plasticity, chemosensitivity. *Annu. Rev. Neurosci.* 26: 239–266.

12 Feldman, J.L., Del Negro, C.A., and Gray, P.A. (2013). Understanding the rhythm of breathing: so near, yet so far. *Annu. Rev. Physiol.* 75: 423–452.

13 Beech, J. (ed.) (1991). *Equine Respiratory Disorders*. Philadelphia: Lea & Febiger.

14 Lumb, A.B. (2005). *Nunn's Applied Respiratory Physiology*, 6e. Philadelphia, PA: Elsevier.

15 Richter, D.W., Ballanyi, K., and Schwarzacher, S. (1992). Mechanisms of respiratory rhythm generation. *Curr. Opin. Neurobiol.* 2: 788–793.

16 Koterba, A.M., Kosch, P.C., and Beech, J. (1988). The breathing strategy of the adult horse *(Equus caballus)* at rest. *J. Appl. Phys.* 64: 337.

17 Smith, C.A., Ainsworth, D.M., Henderson, K.S. et al. (1989). Differential timing of respiratory muscles in response to chemical stimuli in awake dogs. *J. Appl. Phys.* 66: 392–399.

18 West, J.B. (2012). *Respiratory Physiology: The Essentials*, 9e. Baltimore: Lippincott, Williams & Wilkins.

19 Widdicombe, J. (2006). Reflexes from the lungs and airways: historical perspective. *J. Appl. Phys.* 102: 268.

20 Coleridge, H.M. and Coleridge, J.C.G. (1986). Reflexes evoked from tracheobronchial tree and lungs. In: *Handbook of Physiology. Section 3, Respiration*, Control of Breathing, vol. II (ed. N.S. Chemiack and J.G. Widdicombe), 395–429. Bethesda, MD: American Physiological Society.

21 Widdicombe, J. (2003). Functional morphology and physiology of pulmonary rapidly reacting receptors (RARs). *Anat. Rec. A Discov. Mol. Cell Evol. Biol.* 270: 2.

22 Canning, B.J., Mori, N., and Mazzone, S.B. (2006). Vagal afferent nerves regulating the cough reflex. *Respir. Physiol. Neurobiol.* 152: 223.

23 Smith, L.H. and DeMyer, W.E. (2003). Anatomy of the brainstem. *Semin. Pediatr. Neurol.* 10: 235–240.

24 Lessa, T.B., de Abreu, D.K., Bertasoli, B.M. et al. (2016). Diaphragm: a vital respiratory muscle in mammals. *Ann. Anat.* 205: 122.

25 Koterba, A.M., Wozniak, J.A., and Kosch, P.C. (1995). 1995 Changes in breathing pattern in the normal horse at rest up to age one year. *Equine Vet. J.* 27: 265–274.

Section VI Renal Transition from Fetus to Newborn

Jon Palmer

When trying to understand neonatal organ function, the clinician should always remember that the neonatal period is a time of transition from fetal physiology. Renal function is undergoing rather profound changes as it meets the challenge of supporting independent life. This transition begins several weeks before parturition and is not complete until several weeks after birth. Some aspects of renal transition in the neonatal foal are different from other species, however many aspects are poorly studied in the foal and are assumed to be similar to changes noted in other species. This following section provides a brief summary of the fetal-newborn foal's renal transition.

Renal Perfusion

The fetal kidneys receive approximately 3% of the combined left and right cardiac output due to relatively high vascular resistance resulting in a low glomerular filtration rate (GFR). At the moment of birth there is an immediate increase in renal blood flow to 15% of cardiac output in lambs. Although there is an increase in vascular resistance throughout the body associated with birth, there is actually a relative 86% decrease in renal vascular resistance (as measured in piglets). Simultaneously there is redistribution of renal blood flow from the inner cortex to outer superficial cortex. This is followed, within days to weeks of birth (depending on species), with a further decrease in vascular resistance (both anatomic and vasoactive effect) and rise in systemic blood pressure until blood flow to the kidneys reaches 20% of the cardiac output. This transition is not complete until 3 months in infants [1-3].

The distribution of blood flow to different parts of the kidney also differs between neonates and adults. Renal hemodynamics during the fetal-neonatal transition are controlled by a variety of factors including angiotensin II, the renal sympathetic nervous system (renal sympathetic nerves, intrinsic adrenergic release and circulating adrenergics), prostaglandins (PG), nitric oxide (NO), the Kallikrein-Kinin system, atrial natriuretic factor (ANF), endothelin, and others [4]. Many of these hormones, such as angiotensin II, have additional roles to those generally ascribed to adults. Angiotensin II is an important growth factor required for normal nephrogenesis in addition to its well-established role in tubuloglomerular feedback and autoregulation [5]. Although not studied in animals, in people, angiotensin II concentrations can be decreased with maternal dietary protein restriction during pregnancy leading to decreased neonatal renal mass and development of adult hypertension decades later.

The renal sympathetic nervous system is very important in controlling renal blood flow in the neonate and tends to be more sensitive to the sympathetic nervous system than the adult [6]. Circulating adrenergic hormones play a role, but the dense sympathetic innervation of the kidneys also has an impact on blood flow. The sympathetic control of renal blood flow is part of the baroreceptor reflex that helps the body maintain blood pressure at relatively constant level, but it is important to remember that in the neonate, the baroreceptor is set to maintain a much lower blood pressure threshold which then rises with maturational adaptation [7].

Angiotensin II and adrenergics are the most important renal vasoconstrictors while NO and PGs serve as essential vasodilators [8]. Prostaglandins are very important in normal neonatal renal function [9]. Within the kidney there are cyclooxygenase (COX)-1 receptors in the renal vasculature, glomeruli and collecting ducts whereas the distribution of COX-2 receptors are species dependent. In general, COX-2 receptors increase activity after birth, peaking at 1–2 weeks then decline thereafter and are important in nephrogenesis. During the perinatal period COX-2 inhibitors can cause renal dysgenesis and disruption of nephrogenesis [10]. In general renal PGs result in renal vasodilation

Equine Neonatal Medicine, First Edition. Edited by David M. Wong and Pamela A. Wilkins.

and their renal production increases during the perinatal period. Just as in adults, in pathologic conditions, indigenous PG help protect the kidneys by attenuating renal vasoconstriction such as may be secondary to increased adrenergic tone; however, unlike adults, in neonates normal PG levels are important in maintaining basal renal blood flow as well as in stressed conditions, making non-steroidal anti-inflammatory drugs (NSAIDs) potentially more nephrotoxic. Because intrinsic PG production is important in maintaining normal renal blood flow in neonates the use of NSAIDs in the fetus and neonate, even under nonpathologic conditions, may decrease urine output, cause a significant decrease in blood flow, increase renal vascular resistance and, in the fetus, may result in oligohydramnios [11]. Based on these variables, administration of NSAIDs should be used judiciously in neonates as they may disrupt the important balance of vasodilators and vasoconstrictors, which is important in normal neonatal renal physiology [12].

Development of GFR

The balance between renal vasoconstrictors and vasodilators produces renal vascular resistance and determines GFR. However, in the neonate, as compared to adults, these substances may have different effects, different intrarenal concentrations and even different sites of action. Still, their balance is the major determinate of GFR. Although many factors may be involved, during the renal transitional period the increased renal vascular resistance is mediated by increased activity of angiotensin II and increased sensitivity to catecholamines; counterbalancing these vasoconstrictive substances are critical vasodilators, namely NO and PG. The increase in renal blood flow during the birth transition is primarily mediated by a decrease in vasoconstrictors.

The development of a normal GFR is multifactorial and involves changes in the balance of factors which oppose and promote filtration [13]. There are changes in renal vascular resistance as noted above as well as an increase in nephron mass. In addition, there are modifications of ultrafiltration involving glomerular membrane dynamics, glomerular membrane area and, importantly, the development of concentration gradients in the renal parenchyma.

In lambs there is a dramatic increase in GFR within hours of birth as noted above [14]. This is followed by a much more gradual increase in GFR during the first week. This is caused by functional (rather than morphologic) changes, primarily enhanced glomerular perfusion, but also recruitment of more superficial cortical nephrons. The rate of glomerular filtration depends on starling factors, the rate of flow of plasma into glomerular capillaries, permeability of the capillary wall and total surface area of capillaries. Thus, GFR depends on renal blood flow and glomerular capillary pressure. Transcapillary hydrostatic pressure favors filtration and depends on efferent/afferent capillary resistance.

Tubular Function

Fetal fractional excretion of sodium (Na^+) is 5–15% because of the lack of efficient tubular reabsorption [15]. If this elevated fractional excretion of Na^+ were to continue after birth it would be disastrous to the foal as fresh milk is very deficient of Na^+. In the fetus, more Na^+ absorption occurs in the distal tubules than in the proximal tubules because in the proximal tubules, carrier density is low and even cellular polarization is not fully established. Bulk Na^+ absorption does occur proximally, but due to back leak and inefficient active tubular absorption a higher percent of Na^+ is presented to the distal tubules. At the time of birth in lambs and infants (and perhaps just before birth in the foal) there is an upregulation of Na^+ absorption mechanisms (especially the Na^+/H^+ exchanger) in the distal tubule to capture the Na^+, which has escaped proximal tubular absorption [16]. In lambs there is a dramatic increase in activity of distal tubular absorption mechanisms during the first 24 hours of life [17]. This also appears to occur in foals as reflected by a fractional excretion of Na^+ of 0.31% reported in 3-day-old foals [18]. This upregulation is thought to be a response to the surge in cortisol that occurs in the immediate peripartum period [19, 20]. This results in a rapid decrease in urine Na^+ wasting [21], which is vital for neonates as Na^+ conservation is very important. Fresh milk is very Na^+ poor (mare's milk Na^+ ~ 9-14 mEq/L) [22]. If a foal drinks a generous 20% of its body weight in milk, the foal will receive approximately 1.9 mEq/kg/day of Na^+. The daily Na^+ requirement for growth of a healthy neonate is approximately 1 mEq/kg/day, which indicates that a foal can afford to lose no more than 0.9 mEq/kg/day and still allow normal growth. Almost all the Na^+ loss in the healthy foal is in the urine. The Na^+ conserving mechanisms in the distal tubule and collecting ducts are highly refined, initially always turned on and not responsive to changes in Na^+ intake [23]. This means that unless the foal has a disease that is associated with pathologic Na^+ loss (e.g. Na^+ wasting nephropathy, diarrhea, etc.), it is very easy to Na^+ overload a foal, potentially resulting in edema. Although the author finds it very difficult to restrict Na^+ intake to the expected value of <2.0 mEq/kg/day, the author tries to keep it to no more than 4 mEq/kg/day, which may help prevent the development of edema in most cases. The clinician should be cognizant of the fact that many of the treatments administered to ill neonatal foals contain variable amounts of Na^+. For example, 1 liter of plasma contributes approximately 3 mEq/kg/day of Na^+ (plasma has a variable amount of Na^+ but usually contains 160 to 180 mEq/liter) while the full rate of parenteral nutrition provides approximately 1 mEq/kg/day (contained in the amino acids) [24]. Some drugs are also sodium salts and may be an additional source of Na^+. Of course, if there is pathologic Na^+ loss such as a high renal or GI losses, Na^+ restriction is contraindicated. In addition, some cases may have pathologic retention of water (e.g. neonatal vasogenic nephropathy, syndrome of inappropriate antidiuresis), which can cause a serious hypoosmotic state; in these cases, a choice between the relative dangers of hyposmolarity and Na^+ overload must be weighed [25].

Sodium overloading will result in extracellular volume expansion which will initially result in subclinical edema because of the high compliance of the neonate's interstitium; however, Na^+ overload will eventually result in detectable edema. Once edema is visible, the Na^+ overload is extreme. Hypernatremia will not develop unless there are unusually large insensible losses concurrently [26].

The time frame needed for a neonate to stop indiscriminately conserving Na^+ and begin normal Na^+ regulation in response to intake appears to differ between species. In the face of high Na^+ intakes, based on the author's clinical experience, it appears that neonatal calves begin to respond with renal Na^+ wasting in the first 24 hours of life. Normal foals appear to be slower to begin to respond, and critically ill foals appear to be much slower? often still retaining excess Na^+ inappropriately for 1–2 weeks. These observations are based on the author's clinical observations and therefore require scientific verification.

Beyond Na^+ regulation, other differences in the renal handling of metabolites between neonates and adults exist. For example, the neonate has a higher tubular glucose threshold (depending on species 180–220 mg/dl), thus avoiding glucose spilling as the foal adjusts its insulin responsiveness as glucose control and regulation matures. Phosphate and calcium also have unique fetal and neonatal regulation. They are both transported across the placenta against high concentration gradients to aid in bone calcification. There is a unique Na^+-phosphorus cotransporter in the placenta and neonatal renal tubules which is not modulated by high dietary phosphorus intake; this results in a high rate of renal phosphorus (PO_4) reabsorption in the fetus and neonate. The renal clearance of phosphorus is programmed to be quite low allowing the maintenance of the normal high fetal and neonatal phosphorus levels [27].

Cortisol plays an important role in speeding the maturation of the kidneys and accelerating the renal transition during fetal stress [6]. Rising cortisol levels are associated with an increase in GFR, decrease in PO_4 reabsorption by 50%, and changes in Na^+ reabsorption such as decreasing proximal reabsorption and increasing distal reabsorption resulting in no change to Na^+ fractional excretion. Cortisol also accelerates development of tubular reabsorption capacity of Na^+, potassium, and water as well as distal Na^+ carrier mediated absorption.

Autoregulation is active in the neonate but the range is set to lower perfusion pressure (mean arterial pressure [MAP] 40-60 mmHg). The renal pressure-flow relationship changes with renal maturation. This response is primarily mediated by PG-dependent renin release, causing vasoconstriction at lower levels of perfusion pressure. This is another response that NSAID therapy may disrupt in the neonate [28, 29].

Tubuloglomerular feedback is also present in the fetus and neonate and is controlled by macula densa cells (Figure 1.VI.1). As these cells sense a decrease in sodium chloride delivery to distal tubules, it stimulates a release of angiotensin II from juxtaglomerular cells which in turn constricts efferent arterioles, thereby increasing GFR. This response is mediated by the release of local PGs which also cause vasodilation of the afferent arterioles enhancing the increase in GFR. This response also matures with growth and is maximally sensitive at normal tubular flow ranges. As GFR increases, maximum response and flow range also increase with the relative sensitivity being unaltered during growth.

At birth in the normal foal, calf, kid, and likely other herbivores, the blood creatinine level is high and drops in the first 12–48 hours of life. In the healthy newborn foal, the blood creatinine concentration is usually between 2.0 and 4.0 mg/dL. If the foal has suffered an intrauterine challenge, the blood creatinine at birth can be much higher, often being 8.0–16.0 mg/dL and occasionally reaching 40–60 mg/dL or more. This increase is independent of renal function. If renal function is normal the blood creatinine concentration will drop dramatically after birth reaching < 1.1 mg/dL as quickly as 48–72 hours after birth. Thus, the degree of hypercreatininemia at birth is not a good indication of renal function – rather, the speed at which it returns toward normal serum creatinine concentrations provides much valuable indication of renal function [30].

The fetal fluids appear to be a repository for creatinine. At the time of birth of a healthy foal the creatinine level in amnionic and allantoic fluids ranges from 8 to 12 mg/dL and 120 to 160 mg/dL, respectively. This accumulation of creatinine explains the high birth level in healthy foals, who are working hard to keep their blood creatinine concentrations as low as they do. In the foal suffering intrauterine distress, the extremely high blood creatinine concentrations at birth are likely from the entrainment of creatinine as more fluid is shifted from the fetal fluid reservoir to the fetal interstitium. In addition, stress causing an adrenergic surge may decrease urine production resulting in further retention of creatinine thereby contributing

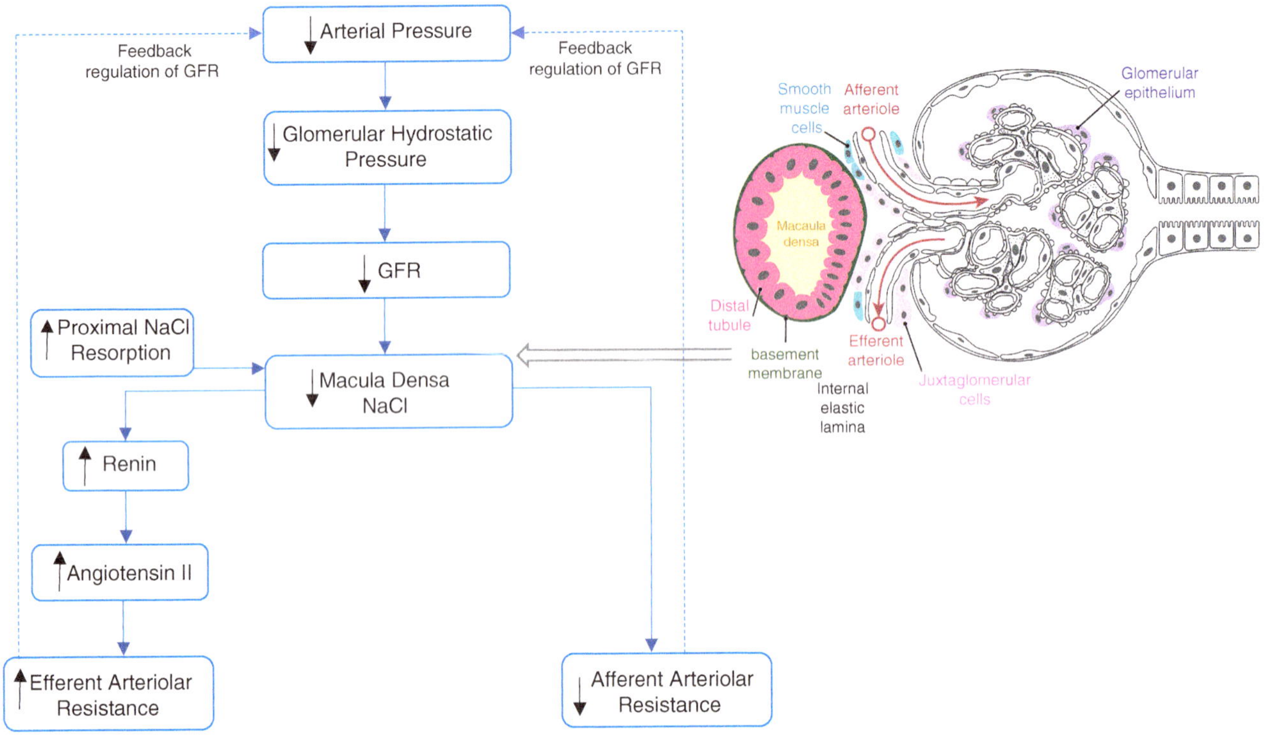

Figure 1.VI.1 Mucula densa cells sense changes in volume delivery to distal tubules; decreased GFR slows flow rate in loop of Henle causing increase resorption of sodium and chloride ions in ascending loop of Henle, thereby decreasing concentration of sodium chloride at macula densa cells. This, in turn, initiates signal from macula densa that cause: (1) increases renin release from juxtaglomerular cells of afferent and efferent arterioles; this, in turn, converts antiogensin I to angiotensin II; angiotensin II constricts efferent arterioles, thereby increases glomerular hydrostatic pressure and returns GFR toward normal; and (2) decreases resistance of afferent arterioles, which raises glomerular hydrostatic pressure and helps return GFR toward normal.

to the often very high birth levels. Therefore, elevated blood creatinine in the newborn foal is typically an indicator of stress induced fetal fluid shifts and not renal compromise. Performing serial measurements of blood creatinine concentrations and observing how rapidly concentrations decrease back to normal neonatal concentrations provides a very powerful, yet simple measure of renal function [30].

The increase in blood creatinine concentrations commonly identified in newborn foals has been called "spurious." [31] This is an unfortunate misnomer as it is not false or fake as *spurious* implies, but rather physiologic when at birth the value is <4.0 mg/dl and pathophysiologic when >4.0 mg/dl. In the healthy foal the blood creatinine concentration decreases rapidly and will often be in what is considered the normal equine range within 12 hours of birth. The blood creatinine concentration usually decreases further reaching the normal neonatal level of 1.1 mg/dl or less (as low as 0.5 mg/dl or less, especially in small or growth restricted foals) by 24 –48 hours. The blood creatinine in healthy foals will remain at this low level until muscle development results in a higher base level, which will differ somewhat with typical muscle mass according to breed.

References

1 Matsell, D.G. and Hiatt, M.J. (2017). Ch 100 Functional development of the kidney in utero. In: *Fetal and Neonatal Physiology*, 5e (ed. R.A. Polin, S.H. Abman, D.H. Rowitch, et al.), 965–976. Elsevier.

2 Solhaug, M.J. and Jose, P.A. (2004). Ch 127 Postnatal maturation of renal blood flow. In: *Fetal and Neonatal Physiology*, 3e (ed. R.A. Polin, W.W. Fox, and S.H. Abman), 1242–1248.

3 Brophy, P.D. and Robillard, J.E. (2004). Ch 126 Functional development of the kidney *in utero*. In: *Fetal and Neonatal Physiology*, 3e (ed. R.A. Polin, W.W. Fox, and S.H. Abman), 1229–1241.

4 Solhaug, M.J., Wallace, M.R., and Granger, J.P. (1990). Role of renal interstitial hydrostatic pressure in the blunted natriuretic response to saline loading in the piglet. *Pediatr. Res.* 28: 460.

5 Almeida, L.F., Tofteng, S.S., Madsen, K. et al. (2020). Role of the renin-angiotensin system in kidney development and programming of adult blood pressure. *Clin. Sci. (Lond.)* 134: 641–656.

6 Robillard, J.E. and Nakamura, K.T. (1988). Hormonal regulation of renal function during development. *Biol. Neonate* 53: 201–211.

7 Johns, E.J. (2005). Angiotensin II in the brain and the autonomic control of the kidney. *Exp. Physiol.* 90: 163–168.

8 Toth-Heyn, P. and Cataldi, L. (2012). Vasoactive compounds in the neonatal period. *Curr. Med. Chem.* 19: 4633–4639.

9 Morris, J.L., Rosen, D.A., and Rosen, K.R. (2003). Nonsteroidal anti-inflammatory agents in neonates. *Paediatr. Drugs* 5: 385–405.

10 Hartleroad, J.Y., Beharry, K.D., Hausman, N. et al. (2005). Effect of maternal administration of selective cyclooxygenase (COX)-2 inhibitors on renal size, growth factors, proteinases, and COX-2 secretion in the fetal rabbit. *Biol. Neonate* 87: 246–253.

11 Drukker, A. (2002). The adverse renal effects of prostaglandin-synthesis inhibition in the fetus and the newborn. *Paediatr. Child Health.* 7: 538–543.

12 Aranda, J.V., Salomone, F., Valencia, G.B. et al. (2017). Non-steroidal anti-inflammatory drugs in newborns and infants. *Pediatr. Clin. North Am.* 64: 1327–1340.

13 Arant, B.S. Jr. (1987). Postnatal development of renal function during the first year of life. *Pediatr. Nephrol.* 1: 308–313.

14 Berry, L.M., Ikegami, M., Woods, E. et al. (1995). Postnatal renal adaptation in preterm and term lambs. *Reprod. Fertil. Dev.* 7: 491–498.

15 Siegel, S.R. and Oh, W. (1976). Renal function as a marker of human fetal maturation. *Acta Paediatr. Scand.* 65: 481–485.

16 Baum, M. (2008). Developmental changes in proximal tubule NaCl transport. *Pediatr. Nephrol.* 23: 185–194.

17 Guillery, E.N., Karniski, L.P., Mathews, M.S. et al. (1994). Maturation of proximal tubule Na^+/H^+ antiporter activity in sheep during transition from fetus to newborn. *Am. J. Physiol.* 267: F537–F545.

18 Brewer, B.D., Clement, S.F., Lotz, W.S. et al. (1991). Renal clearance, urinary excretion of endogenous substances, and urinary diagnostic indices in healthy neonatal foals. *J. Vet. Intern. Med.* 5: 28–33.

19 Guillery, E.N., Karniski, L.P., Mathews, M.S. et al. (1995). Role of glucocorticoids in the maturation of renal cortical Na^+/H^+ exchanger activity during fetal life in sheep. *Am. J. Physiol.* 268: F710–F717.

20 Petershack, J.A., Nagaraja, S.C., and Guillery, E.N. (1999). Role of glucocorticoids in the maturation of renal cortical Na^+-K^+-ATPase during fetal life in sheep. *Am. J. Physiol.* 276: R1825–R1832.

21 Gaucheron, F. (2005). The minerals of milk. *Reprod. Nutr. Dev.* 45: 473–483.

22 Grace, N.D., Pearce, S.G., Firth, E.C. et al. (1999). Concentrations of macro- and micro-elements in the milk of pasture-fed Thoroughbred mares. *Aust. Vet. J.* 77: 177–180.

23 Baum, M. and Quigley, R. (2004). Ontogeny of renal sodium transport. *Semin. Perinatol.* 28: 91–96.

24 Ewalenko, P., Deloof, T., and Peeters, J. (1986). Composition of fresh frozen plasma. *Crit. Care Med.* 14: 145–146.

25 Moritz, M.L. (2019). Syndrome of Inappropriate antidiuresis. *Pediatr. Clin. North Am.* 66: 209–226.

26 Palmer, J.E. (2004). Fluid therapy in the neonate: not your mother's fluid space. *Vet. Clin. North Am. Equine Pract.* 20: 63–75.

27 Jones, D.P. and Chesney, R.W. (1992). Development of tubular function. *Clin. Perinatol.* 19: 33–57.

28 Buckley, N.M. (1986). Maturation of circulatory system in three mammalian models of human development. *Comp. Biochem. Physiol. A Comp. Physiol.* 83: 1–7.

29 Antonucci, R., Zaffanello, M., Puxeddu, E. et al. (2012). Use of non-steroidal anti-inflammatory drugs in pregnancy: impact on the fetus and newborn. *Curr. Drug Metab.* 13: 474–490.

30 Palmer, J.E. (2006). Recognition and resuscitation of the critically ill foal. In: *Equine Neonatal Medicine: A Case-Based Approach* (ed. M.R. Paradis), 135–148. Philadelphia: Elsevier Saunders Inc.

31 Chaney, K.P., Holcombe, S.J., Schott, H.C. II, and Barr, B.S. (2010). Spurious hypercreatininemia: 28 neonatal foals (2000-2008). *J. Vet. Emerg. Crit. Care* 20: 244–249.

Section VII Newborn Physical Examination

Scott Austin

The physical examination is critical to the identification and localization of abnormalities, recognition of complications, and monitoring progression or resolution of disease. Examination should be complete and performed in a systematic manner, regardless of whether it is for a new foal examination or suspected illness. Developing a complete, but concise, method of physical examination ensures that steps are not missed and provides a record that becomes essential when monitoring changes in a foal's condition.

History

The history is important for interpreting examination findings and recognizing potential risk factors for disease. A comprehensive history is imperative, especially if the veterinarian is not familiar with the mare or client. The history includes information about the perinatal period, parturition, and course of events after the foal was born. The mare's reproductive history including number and health of previous foals, length of current and previous pregnancies, vaccination status, travel history, and concurrent medical problems during pregnancy should be collected. It is important to ascertain whether the mare has leaked colostrum prior to delivery or has produced other abnormal foals. It should be determined if parturition was observed and if assistance was needed for delivery, in addition to the time of birth relative to the time of the veterinary examination. Environmental conditions where the foal was born should be determined and caretakers questioned about the foal's behavior since birth and if nursing, urination, and defecation have been observed. Time to standing and first nursing are important to assess the vigor of the foal and document transitional milestones: sternal recumbency by 20 minutes, suckle response by 30 minutes, standing by 60 minutes, and nursing by 2 hours. Larger foals and male foals may take slightly longer to stand and nurse [1, 2].

General Appearance

When examining healthy or non–critically ill foals, the mare and foal should be observed from a distance and nursing behavior, musculoskeletal abnormalities, and resting respiratory rate determined. The mare's attitude toward the foal should be assessed before entering the stall. Some mares will be indifferent, extremely protective, fearful of the foal, or extremely aggressive toward the foal. Maiden mares, older mares, Arabian mares of Egyptian ancestry, and mares that have a history of previously rejecting foals are most likely to reject foals [3]. Normal foals nurse in short bouts (90 seconds) up to 7–10 times per hour. Decrease in nursing or increase in recumbency should prompt a more detailed investigation. Dripping of milk or milk staining on the foal's head indicate inadequate nursing, while foals repetitively udder seeking and butting the mare suggests inadequate milk production. It is important to observe the foal's interactions with its dam and the environment as changes in behavior are an early predictor of sepsis or neurological dysfunction. In health, foals play after eating followed by recumbency and sleep. A decrease in activity or lack of response to external stimuli may be the first signal of illness.

After brief observation of the mare and foal, the foal's vital parameters are collected. Those handling the foal should wear exam gloves to decrease introducing pathogens into the foal's environment. The foal should be examined as to its general appearance and body condition. The normal gait of the neonatal foal, compared to an adult, is characterized by a base-wide stance, mild hypermetria, and a flexed head posture. Poor body condition typified by obvious ribs and bony prominences and a low birthweight may be present with either prematurity or intrauterine growth restriction [4]. In conjunction with gestational length, the physical characteristics of the neonate can determine if the foal is premature, dysmature, or small for

Equine Neonatal Medicine, First Edition. Edited by David M. Wong and Pamela A. Wilkins.

gestational age. Signs of prematurity should be noted and include short, soft hair coat, pliant lips and ears, laxity of the distal limbs, and a domed forehead [4].

Vital Parameters

The order of the examination is not critical if a routine that ensures a complete and comprehensive examination is performed each time. Examination begins with determination of temperature, heart rate, and respiratory rate as these parameters are important determinants in assessment for presence of systemic inflammatory response syndrome (SIRS). The healthy foal's temperature is between 37 and 39 °C (99–102 °F) [2, 4]. Healthy, full-term foals can maintain body temperature at birth but are born with minimal subcutaneous fat and limited energy reserves. Foals that are slow to nurse may become hypothermic secondary to declining activity, low energy reserves, and increased heat loss secondary to a high surface area to body weight ratio. Low body temperature indicates the need for warming and occurs in critical foals with inadequate perfusion, sepsis, or SIRS and in healthy foals when the environmental temperature is low. Elevations in temperature frequently imply infectious disease, but caution should be applied if the temperature is mildly elevated and the foal was recently active such as evading a potential examiner. Altered body temperature is an indication for laboratory assessment of the foal.

At birth, the heart rate is 60–80 beats/min and will increase to 120–150 beats/min during the first 2 hours of life, often associated with the efforts to stand and ambulate. The heart rate should stabilize at 80–100 breaths/min during the first 24 hours of life [4]. Respiratory rate is best determined by observation before entering the stall and should be in the range of 40–60 breaths/min soon after birth and decreases to 12–40 breaths/min within the first 24 hours [4].

Examination of Head

Excessively pliant, floppy ears are consistent with prematurity, and petechiation present inside the pinna is supportive of thrombocytopenia, sepsis, SIRS, or disseminated intravascular coagulation (DIC). Normal mucous membranes should be pink and moist, with a capillary refill time of <2 seconds. Pale mucous membranes are seen with anemia or poor peripheral circulation. The presence of petechia or hyperemia is suggestive of SIRS, and supportive evidence can be garnered by examination of other mucous membranes. Additional signs of decreased perfusion and SIRS include prolonged capillary refill time, cool extremities,

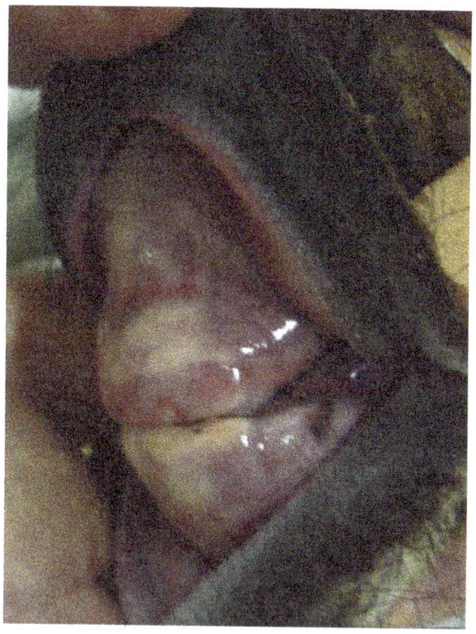

Figure 1.VII.1 Mucous membranes of a neonatal foal demonstrating cyanosis and prolonged capillary refill time. *Source:* Picture courtesy of Dr. Pam Wilkins.

coronary band hyperemia, episcleral injection, and declining activity (Figure 1.VII.1). Icterus is seen with hemolysis, sepsis, neonatal isoerythrolysis, severe liver disease, and infection with equine herpesvirus type-1. Cyanosis is rare and not seen unless P_aO_2 is <40 mmHg and usually associated with severe cardiopulmonary disorders [5].

The incisors characteristically erupt at 6 days, 6 weeks, and 6 months for the central, middle, and corner incisors, respectively. In Miniature Horses and ponies, the middle incisors may not erupt until 4 months, and the corners may not be evident until 12–18 months of age. Dental abnormalities are uncommon except congenital abnormalities such as maxillary prognathism, mandibular prognathism, and wry nose. Mandibular prognathism may be seen in conjunction with congenital goiter. Wry nose may occur as a singular abnormality or in combination with more severe defects such as cleft palate, wry neck, and either mandibular or maxillary prognathism [5]. Severe deviations of the muzzle may interfere with normal nursing and be accompanied by inspiratory noise and breathing problems. The condition should be monitored to assess the development of dental malocclusion. Signs including nasal regurgitation of milk, coughing during nursing, and aspiration pneumonia are seen with cleft palate. The defect may involve both the hard and soft portions of the palate or the soft palate alone (majority). Digital palpation of the hard palate may identify large defects, but endoscopic examination is usually required to confirm defects of the soft palate. Other causes of nasal regurgitation of milk include pharyngeal weakness or incoordination. This condition is usually temporary, and affected foals can be managed by feeding through nasogastric tube until function is present.

The eyes should be examined for corneal ulcers since neonatal foals may not be able to close the eyelids completely, have decreased tear production and corneal sensitivity, and lack a menace response for up to the first 2 weeks of life [6]. The pupillary light response (PLR) is present but slow when the foal is excited or stressed.

During ophthalmic examination, persistent hyaline arteries are visible at the back of the lens, and the optic disc is pale pink or red. Additionally, Y-sutures are present in the lens for a variable period of life and in some instances persist into adulthood. Acquired lesions include subconjunctival and retinal hemorrhages that occur during parturition and typically resolve by 2 weeks of age (Figure 1.VII.2) [7]. The eyes should be examined for cataracts, and the anterior segment should be evaluated for episcleral injection, aqueous flare, hypopyon, and hyphemia, which are often seen in foals with infection (Figure 1.VII.3). Corneal ulcers may be missed during a casual examination since corneal sensitivity is less in the newborn as compared to adults and blepharospasm, tearing, and photophobia are decreased [6]. Additionally, recumbent foals and those with seizures are prone to corneal ulcers and should be stained daily to identify the ulcers and initiate appropriate treatment. Lower lid entropion is often concurrent with dehydration and may contribute to corneal ulcers. Entropion commonly resolves upon correction of dehydration; however, this condition will occasionally require surgical or medical therapy. Entropion can be corrected with several vertical mattress sutures placed in the lower lid or temporary injection of the lower lid with procaine penicillin to roll the lid out. The benefit of penicillin is that it gradually absorbs and may or may not need to be performed again.

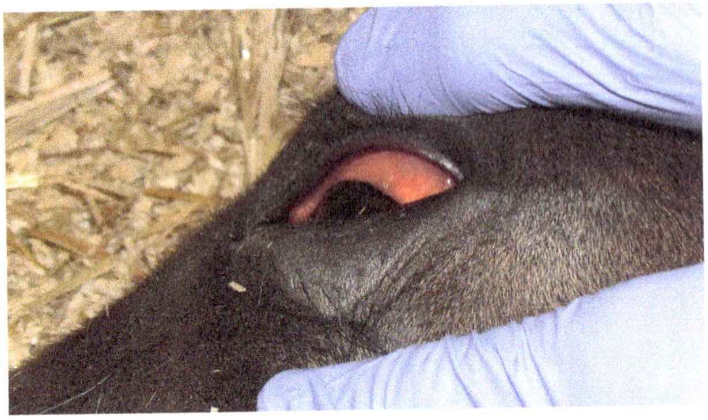

Figure 1.VII.2 Neonatal foal with subconjunctival hemorrhages acquired during parturition. *Source:* Photo courtesy of Dr. David Wong.

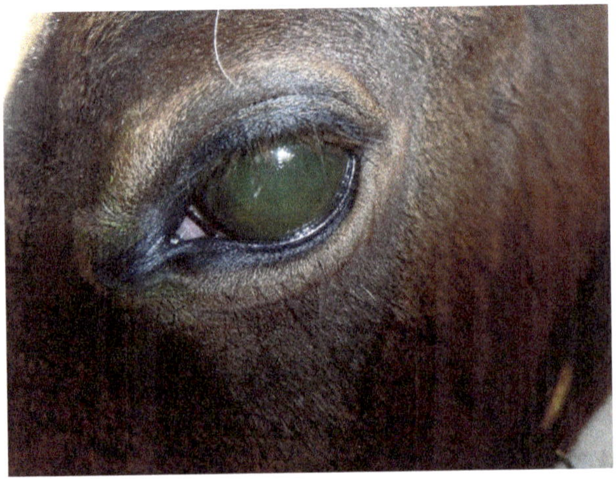

Figure 1.VII.3 Septic foal with aqueous flair. *Source:* Picture courtesy of Dr. Pam Wilkins.

Thyroid enlargement (goiter) may be present at birth and can be secondary to excess or deficient dietary iodine fed during gestation [8–10]. In western Canada and northwest United States, a syndrome of thyroid hyperplasia, mandibular prognathism, and musculoskeletal abnormalities has been recognized; affected foals have hypothyroidism. Risk factors include diets that are high in nitrate or deficient in iodine that affect the developing fetus during pregnancy [11, 12].

Cardiovascular System

Examination of the cardiovascular system includes evaluation of visible mucous membranes, palpation of peripheral pulses, assessment of extremities for warmth, evaluation of limbs for edema, and cardiac auscultation. Dehydration is suspected when mucous membranes are tacky, eyes appear sunken, skin tent is prolonged, and urination is decreased in frequency or amount. Tenting of the skin of the eyelids is a more reliable location to evaluate hydration status than the neck. Poor pulse quality, prolonged capillary refill time (>2 seconds), decreased jugular filling (>2 seconds) and cool ears and distal extremities are signs of decreased peripheral perfusion and warrant further investigation and early intervention. Pale mucous membranes signify anemia or inadequate perfusion, while sepsis is associated with mucous membrane, sclera, ear, and coronary band hyperemia and/or petechiation. Cyanosis should prompt examination of the cardiovascular system and is not typically seen except in congenital cardiac defects with right to left blood flow. In addition to congenital heart defects, cyanosis can be caused by persistent pulmonary hypertension of the newborn (PPHN) and will demonstrate hypoxemia unresponsive to nasal oxygen insufflation.

Peripheral pulses can be felt under the jaw (facial artery), the medial aspect of the elbow (brachial artery), and along the lateral aspect of the metacarpus (greater metatarsal artery). Pulse quality does not always correspond to hypotension, but decreased pulses suggest decreased peripheral perfusion [13]. The limbs and ears should be warm to the touch. If cool, then poor peripheral circulation is a possibility and can be associated with impending shock or other circulatory abnormalities. Blood pressure may be assessed indirectly with an oscillometry or Doppler-based devices placed over the coccygeal artery of the tail or the greater metatarsal artery. With such devices, the mean pressure is 95–101 mmHg during the first 3 days of life [14]. At birth, the heart rate is influenced by vagal tone and varies between 36 and 80 beats/min. Upon standing and over the first 2 hours of life, the heart rate will increase to 120–150 beats/min and will stabilize and remain at 80–100 over the first week of life [15]. Because of the relatively thin body wall, the apex beat and any detected murmurs are louder than in adult horses. Tachycardia increases cardiac output and is expected during periods of exercise or stress. Tachycardia also accompanies sepsis, hypovolemia, anemia, hypoxemia, pain, or primary cardiac disease. Bradycardia can be seen with hypothermia, hypoglycemia, and certain electrolyte abnormalities.

A loud machinery murmur is commonly heard at the left heart base for the first 72 hours of life and is typically associated with a patent ductus arteriosus (PDA) that will close as the transition to normal circulation occurs [15]. Murmurs that are loud (>grade 4/6), pansystolic, bilateral, diastolic, or right-sided are more likely associated with pathological, rather than physiological, causes [16]. In foals that are compromised, the presence of a PDA is more concerning as hypoxemia, septicemia, or endotoxemia, or severe pulmonary disease can trigger reverse flow through the ductus arteriosus. Arrhythmias are frequently heard in newborn foals but resolve spontaneously within the first 15–30 min of life [17]. Arrhythmias are thought to be secondary to high vagal tone and include ventricular premature complexes, ventricular tachycardia, atrial fibrillation, and supraventricular tachycardia. Listening to both sides of the thorax is necessary to detect right-sided murmurs that are more commonly associated with congenital heart defects. If murmurs or arrythmias persist beyond the first week of life, further examination is recommended.

Respiratory System

At birth, the initial respirations are gasping and rapid as the foal attempts to ensure full insufflation of the lungs; the respiratory rate may be as high as 60–80 min. Respirations rapidly decrease to 35–40 breaths/min within the first hour. In ambulatory neonates, examination of the respiratory tract begins from outside of the stall to determine respiratory rate and effort without inducing excitement by catching and restraint. Causes of tachypnea include meconium aspiration, bacterial or viral pneumonia, atelectasis secondary to recumbency, rib fracture, or pleural effusion. Increased respiratory rates can also be observed secondary to nonpulmonary causes such as fever, pain, excitement, exercise, brain disease, respiratory response to metabolic acidosis, and transient idiopathic tachypnea [5].

The nares should be examined for patency and presence of discharge. If respiratory distress or respiratory noise are heard at birth, several uncommon congenital abnormalities should be considered such as stenotic nares, choanal atresia, subepiglottic cyst, or collapsing trachea. Congenital obstruction of nasal passages will result in inspiratory dyspnea, attempts to mouth breath, and flutter of the cheeks during exhalation. Immediate intervention is required to ensure a sufficient airway. Meconium aspiration will result in brown-orange discharge at the nares, and the airways should be suctioned with a soft catheter and dose syringe.

At birth, lung sounds are moist with end-inspiratory crackles. These sounds rapidly resolve as the foal stands. Accurate auscultation can only occur if the foal is standing or at minimum in sternal recumbency for several minutes. Increased harshness with an increase in respiratory rate can be associated with several systemic diseases that do not necessarily affect the lungs, and thoracic auscultation often underestimates possible pathology related to the lungs. Foals with mild to moderate lung disease may simply have decreased sounds or no changes until consolidation becomes severe; however, abnormal lung sounds such as crackles and wheezes are always indicative of pathology. The respiratory pattern and effort are more sensitive indicators than auscultation as to presence of respiratory disease. A gentle in and out motion is characteristic of normal respiration, while exaggerated intercostal movement with synchronous abdominal effort and an expiratory grunt typify dyspnea. Paradoxical movement of the chest and abdomen signify that the foal is approaching respiratory failure [4].

Healthy foals have a regular respiratory pattern while awake but may have an irregular respiratory cycle when sleeping. However, irregular or erratic respiratory patterns in conscious foals or in semi-comatose foals suggest central nervous system disease, metabolic or electrolyte derangements, hypothermia, and disorders in maturation. Irregularities include tachypnea, hypopnea, intermittent apnea, and apneustic breathing. Hypopnea in foals with central nervous system disease can result in severe respiratory acidosis and indicates a need for immediate ventilation or institution of respiratory stimulants such as oral caffeine or doxapram administered as a constant rate infusion [18].

During thoracic auscultation, the chest wall should be examined for possible rib fractures. Clinical signs consistent with rib fractures include localized edema and swelling, palpable crepitus, auscultation of a grinding or click, or subcutaneous emphysema if underlying lung has been punctured. Affected foals may grunt during expiration and avoid lying on the affected side. The most common location is at or just dorsal to the chondrocostal junction over the third to fifth ribs [19]. The location of the fracture increases the likelihood of severe or fatal damage to the underlying heart and lung so affected foals should be handled with care. When fractures are suspected, ultrasound can confirm rib fractures, more readily than radiography, by identification of a "step" in the rib. Additionally, ultrasonography allows evaluation of damage to the underlying lung [19]. Surgery is frequently needed to repair fractures that involve two or more ribs or have visible movement of the chest wall at the site of the fractures.

Gastrointestinal System

The abdomen should be auscultated over all four quadrants (flanks and ventral abdominal wall). Normal borborygmi can be heard every 10–20 seconds, and intestinal sounds are subjectively classified as normal, increased, decreased, or absent. Decreased sounds suggest ileus and can be due to inflammatory, ischemic or obstructive lesions. Increased motility is associate with bowel inflammation or early intestinal obstruction. Splashing sounds are normally heard in the upper right quadrant as fluid enters the cecum, but tympanic sounds or fluid sounds should be considered abnormal. Ballottement and percussion can be used to help identify increased fluid or gas, respectively. Repeated measurement of the abdomen at a marked location can be used to monitor progression of suspected abdominal enlargement.

Internal palpation is limited to digital examination of the rectum. When a foal is suitably relaxed, some abdominal structures can be palpated through the abdominal wall such as meconium impactions, fecaliths, intussusceptions and the urinary bladder or enlargement of the internal umbilical remnants; however, in most foals, ultrasonography is necessary to evaluation internal abdominal structures. Ultrasound can determine motility, intestinal distention, increased thickness of bowel wall, and increase in free fluid within the abdomen. The body wall should be palpated to determine integrity and identify umbilical or inguinal hernias. Inguinal hernias are more common in colts and present as fluctuant swellings that are easily reduced back into the abdomen when the foal is placed in dorsal recumbency. Strangulation of bowel is rare, but damaged bowel can be further investigated using ultrasound to identify a thickened edematous wall.

A nasogastric tube should be passed in foals with signs of abdominal pain or distention of undetermined etiology. When gastric distension is severe, passage of the nasogastric tube through the cardia can be difficult and administration of lidocaine through the tube may facilitate passage into the stomach. Colic signs may resolve or be decreased after removal of accumulated gastric contents. Gastric reflux also may be present in foals not exhibiting colic signs. Causes of gastric distention include gastric outflow obstruction, which may occur secondary to severe gastric/duodenal ulceration, and functional or obstructive lesions of the small intestine. Functional ileus may be seen with a variety of conditions, including sepsis, hypoxic ischemic syndrome, prematurity enteritis, and overfeeding.

Normally, neonates pass dark brown and firm meconium within the first 1–4 hours of life (Figure 1.VII.4). After passage of meconium, feces become yellow and pasty. Some foals exhibit discomfort secondary to retained meconium. While attempting to defecate, affected foals will arch the back, stand with hind legs camped-under, and flag the tail. In contrast, urination is associated with a flat back and the hind legs stretch backward. While straining, the anus will protrude, and a hard pellet of meconium can be felt as it attempts passage through the anus. Digital rectal examination often confirms hard meconium in the rectum. Additional signs include colic and ineffective nursing. As nursing decreases, mares of affected foals will often stream milk. More prolonged obstruction may result in abdominal distention, and continued straining may cause a patent urachus. Affected foals that develop patent urachus should receive antiseptic care of the umbilicus and prophylactic antimicrobials [20].

The passage of feces is infrequent in foals and often not observed, so any observed increase in frequency or softening of feces is suggestive of developing enterocolitis. Signs of colic in a foal include grinding of teeth, rolling, dorsal recumbency, and straining after frequent posturing accompanied by tail flagging. More subtle signs include increased recumbency, with restless repositioning, twisting of head

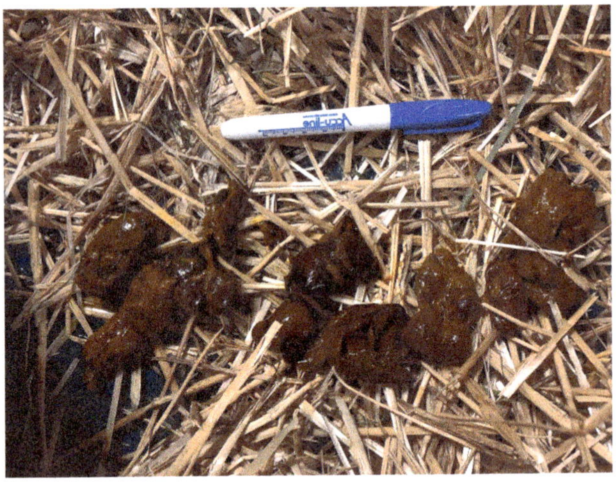

Figure 1.VII.4 Typical appearance of foal meconium. *Source:* Picture courtesy of Dr. Alessandro Migliorisi.

and neck, and frequent stretching. Additionally, increasing abdominal distention may be observed with impending enterocolitis, intestinal obstruction, or urinary bladder rupture. Failure to pass any feces accompanied by clear or white mucous upon digital rectal examination along with colic and progressive abdominal distention increases the suspicion of atresia ani. Similar signs in largely white foals with immediate ancestors exhibiting overo-color pattern is suggestive of lethal white syndrome.

Urogenital System

After birth, the umbilicus breaks at a predetermined location when the mare stands or sufficient traction for other reasons is applied to the cord. The umbilical cord should be allowed to break naturally, but on occasion the placenta may be passed before the cord has broken. Rather than cutting, the umbilical stump should be immobilized close to the body wall, and the cord should be pulled until it breaks at 1–2 cm from the body wall. Sharp transection of the cord does not allow the umbilical vessels to stretch and then retract within the cord and is associated with increased risk of hemorrhage. If hemorrhage occurs, the cord should be ligated or clamped. The umbilicus should be dipped in 0.5% chlorhexidine solution (1 part 2% chlorhexidine solution; 3 parts sterile water) every 8 hours for the first 2–3 days of life. Chlorhexidine has greater residual activity than betadine solution but may cause delay in the drying of the umbilical stump [21, 22].

First urination occurs around 6 hours for colts and 11 hours for fillies with the initial specific gravity around 1.030. Subsequent urinations occur soon after nursing and are much more dilute because of the milk diet. Urine production is 150 ml/kg/d, and the urine specific gravity in hydrated foals should be <1.010 [23]. Red urine is suggestive of passage of blood, hemoglobin, or myoglobin in the urine and should prompt immediate laboratory assessment of the foal to determine the cause. Urinalysis, complete blood count, and serum biochemistry aids in identify possible causes of discolored urine. Urination behavior should be monitored, as rupture of the urinary bladder is not uncommon in foals. Clinical signs include straining, passage of small volumes of urine, progressive enlargement of the abdomen, and progressive inactivity with weakness, which may not be seen until 2–3 days of age. Abdominal ultrasound confirms free fluid within the abdomen, but abdominocentesis and demonstration that the fluid creatinine is double serum creatinine concentrations are necessary to confirm uroabdomen.

The external umbilicus should be examined and inspected for increased moisture, discharge, or enlargement. Sick and recumbent foals frequently develop patency of the urachus, and urine can be seen dribbling from the umbilicus. The patent urachus will normally close after resolution of the inciting cause. The umbilicus should be dipped with 0.5% chlorhexidine solution to decrease bacterial contamination, but insertion of cauterizing agents into the urachus is not recommended. Umbilical hernias are relatively frequent in foals at birth and can be 2–6 cm in length, with most closing by day 4 after birth; however, foals can develop abdominal hernias at 5–8 weeks of age. If the contents are easily reducible, surgery is usually delayed until after weaning. Ultrasonography of the umbilicus is recommended in foals with discharge or enlargement of the external umbilicus, patent urachus, or onset of fever and lethargy. Potential infection of the internal umbilical remnants is suspected when structures are increased in size [24–26]. In normal foals, the umbilical remnants have their largest size at birth and regress linearly over time to 50% of original values by one month. The umbilical remnants continue to regress and are difficult to detect by 5–6 weeks of age [26].

Colts should be examined for the presence of both testicles in the scrotum and if inguinal hernias are present. Most hernias are unilateral, indirect, and easily reducible and rarely result in problems. Patience is recommended as most inguinal hernias will correct spontaneously by 3–4 months of age. If clinical signs of discomfort or the hernia contents appear to be increasing in size, surgical intervention is recommended. For the first month of life, the free portion of the penis is usually fused to the internal lamina of the prepuce, and exteriorization of the penis can be difficult.

Musculoskeletal System

Examination of the musculoskeletal system includes palpation of all joints and growth plates of the limbs. Additionally, the coronary bands should be examined for hyperemia (coronitis) that may be observed in foals with septicemia. Joint distention and periarticular swelling are easiest to detect at the carpi, fetlocks, tarsi, and stifles, but increased fluid in deeper joints such as shoulders, hip, and elbows can be more difficult. Simultaneous palpation of structures on both sides improves the detection of abnormalities. Joint infection should be the primary differential for any distended synovial structure. Aseptic arthrocentesis with a total white cell count of >10,000 cells/μl supports a diagnosis of infection. The tendons are examined for contracture or laxity. Both conditions may negatively affect the foal's ability to nurse and are often associated with failure of passive transfer of antibodies.

Angular limb deformities can be seen in forelimbs, hindlimbs, or both. Most mild-to-moderate deformities spontaneously correct but should be monitored for improvement. Severe flexural deformities or those that are not improving or worsening should be evaluated for surgical intervention (Figure 1.VII.5). Occasionally, luxation of the patella secondary to hypoplasia of the lateral femoral trochlear ridge is identified, and if bilateral, can result in a squatting stance (Figure 1.VII.6).

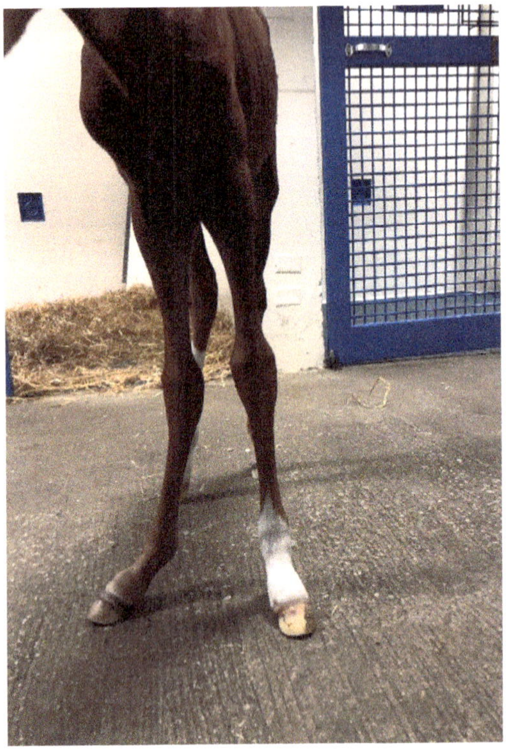

Figure 1.VII.5 Foal with both angular limb deformity and flexor laxity. *Source:* Picture courtesy of Dr. Alessandro Migliorisi.

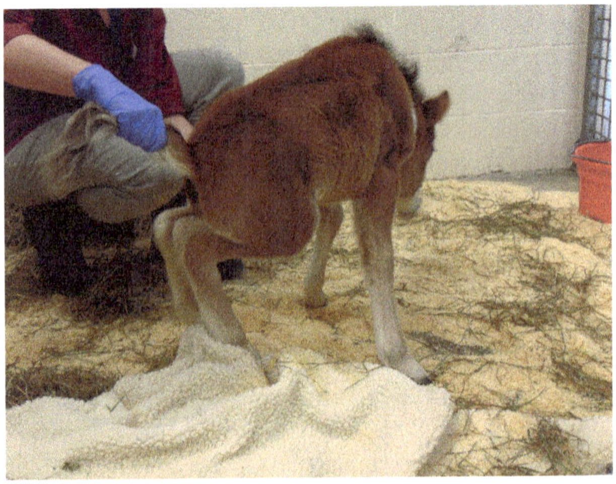

Figure 1.VII.6 Neonatal Miniature Horse foal with bilateral luxating patellas; note the squatting stance as the foal tries to stand. *Source:* Picture courtesy of Dr. David Wong.

Neurological System

Differences in foal behavior, response to restraint, and ambulation must be considered when evaluating the nervous system. Movements are often exaggerated, and foals will often become limp when excessively restrained. During handling, vigorous snapping of the mouth and urination are expressions of submissive behavior. Mouth snapping should not be confused with tooth grinding, teeth clenching, and continuous chewing movements, which are suggestive of pain or seizures. Foals spend a significant portion of time resting, but the foal should be easily aroused, respond to external stimuli, and demonstrate a strong suckle response. Early signs of neurological dysfunction may include loss of suckle, decreasing affinity for the dam, apparent blindness, aimless wandering, intention tremor, seizures, or coma. The head posture of a foal, compared to adults, is more flexed, and movement is jerkier and exaggerated in response to visual, auditory, or tactile stimuli. Cranial nerve evaluation is similar to adults, with a few notable exceptions. The menace response is a learned behavior and is not predictably present until 2 weeks of age. There may be a transition period where foals will demonstrate avoidance by moving their head away from stimulus without blinking. When examining PLR, the pupils should be symmetrical. When excited, foals may have dilated pupils that are poorly responsive to bright light, so caution should be exercised to not overinterpret a lack of PLR in an excited or stressed foal. The pupil of the eye may be oriented ventromedial compared to the palpebral fissure and does not assume the slight dorsomedial angle seen in adult horses until 1 month of age [27]. Cleft palate, weakness, or mild pharyngeal paralysis can result in nasal regurgitation of milk. Careful physical and neurological examination is necessary to determine the cause. Foals with neonatal encephalopathy or severe depression may stand with the tongue hanging out and will be slow to retract the tongue when stimulated.

The foal should be observed for interactions with the dam and environment to evaluate behavior, mental status, and gait. The newborn should be able to right itself into sternal recumbency within minutes of birth. Initial attempts to stand are accompanied by a base wide stance and exaggerated short strides, but the foal rapidly develops a gait typical of adults. A healthy neonate should be aware of people and will return to its dam when approached. When in lateral recumbency, foals demonstrate exaggerated spinal reflexes, and the forelimbs have increased extensor tone. During the first 3 weeks of life, a light pinch of the distal limb will produce an exaggerated flexion response and can be accompanied by a cross extensor response in the opposite limb; this is less obvious in the hind limbs as compared to the forelimbs. Patellar and triceps responses are easily and consistently elicited in foals [27].

Facial grimacing, twitching, chomping, smacking of lips, head and neck rigidity, paddling, abnormal breathing patterns, or repetitive blinking with rapid eye movements are all signs of seizures. The most common cause of neonatal seizures is neonatal encephalopathy, but other causes include congenital malformations, viral and bacterial infections, trauma, metabolic derangements, hepatic encephalopathy, and idiopathic epilepsy. In addition to nervous system causes, hypoglycemia, liver, and electrolyte disorders can also cause seizures. Juvenile seizures may be seen in Arabian foals and congenital narcolepsy has been described in American Miniature Horses, Morgans, Shetlands, and Suffolks. Affected foals exhibit collapse and remain in lateral recumbency for several minutes in a sleep state and then recover without residual signs.

Integument

Close examination of the skin should be made to note abrasions, congenital abnormalities, and discoloration around coronary bands that may suggest septicemia. Recumbent foals need to be examined frequently for pressure necrosis over the bony prominences of the elbows, hocks, stifles, and hips. Additionally, foals with septicemia may have linear dermal necrosis in the crevices of the lateral aspect of the hocks. Hydration can be estimated by evaluation of skin turgor, mucous membrane moisture, corneal moisture, and sunken globes within the orbit. Skin turgor is best assessed by tenting the skin of the upper eyelid since other area in the foal are difficult to interpret.

Viability Assessment and Apgar Score

The above describes physical examination in newborn and neonatal foals, but in 1952, pioneering anesthesiologist Virginia Apgar developed a scoring system to assist doctors and nurses in evaluating cardiopulmonary adaption in infants at 1 and 5 minutes of age. The Apgar score was developed as a convenient method of reporting the status of a newborn immediately after birth and to determine if resuscitation was needed; however, it does not assess the consequence of asphyxia, predict neonatal mortality or neurological outcome, and should not be used for that purpose [28]. The Apgar score has been modified for use in foals with observations also made at 1 and 5 minutes after birth. The 1-minute score is used to recognize intrauterine asphyxia and is used as a semi-quantitative measure of whether resuscitation is necessary (Table 1.VII.1) [29, 30]. A second Apgar score at 5 minutes determines response to therapy and whether more intense interventions are required.

Table 1.VII.1 Modified Apgar score for newborn foals.

Parameter	0 Points	1 Point	2 Points
Muscle tone	Limp extremities	Some flexion of limbs	Sternal
Respiration	Absent	Slow or irregular	≥60 breaths/min, regular
Heart rate	Absent	<60 beats/min	≥60 beats/min
Nasal stimulation	No response	Grimace, slight rejection	Cough or sneeze
Mucous membranes	Cyanotic	Pale pink	Pink

Scores of 0–3 are seen in dead or near dead foals, and cardiopulmonary intervention should be initiated with the realization that if a heartbeat or respirations are not rapidly evident, then attempts at resuscitation should be abandoned. A score of 4–6 indicates severe depression, and stimulation, intubation, and manual ventilation should be undertaken. If heart rate is <60 beats/min, chest compressions are also recommended. A score of 7–8 indicates mild compromise, and foals frequently respond to clearing nostrils and vigorous rubbing. Normal foals will have scores of 9 or 10.

References

1 Rosales, C., Krekeler, N., Tennent-Brown, B. et al. (2017). Periparturient characteristics of mares and their foals on a New Zealand Thoroughbred stud farm. *N. Z. Vet. J.* 65: 24–29.

2 Koterba, A.M. (1990). Physical examination. In: *Equine Clinical Neonatology* (ed. A.M. Koterba, W.H. Drummond, and P.C. Kosch), 71–83. Philadelphia: Lea and Febiger.

3 Vaala, W.E. (2011). Foal rejection. In: *Equine Reproduction*, 2e (ed. A.O. McKinnon, E. Squires, W. Vaala, and D.D. Varner), 117–120. Hoboken: Wiley-Blackwell Publishing.

4 Stoneham, S.J. (2006). Assessing the newborn foal. In: *Equine Neonatal Medicine: A Case-Based Approach*, 1e (ed. M.R. Paradis), 1–13. Philadelphia: Elsevier Saunders.

5 Lester, G.D. and Axon, J.E. (2015). Assessment of the newborn foal. In: *Large Animal Internal Medicine*, 6e (ed. B.P. Smith, D.C. VanMetre, and N. Pusterla), 247–261. St. Louis: Elsevier.

6 Brooks, D.E., Clark, C.K., and Lester, G.D. (2000). Cochet-bonnet aesthesiometer-determined corneal sensitivity in neonatal foals and adult horses. *Vet. Ophthalmol.* 3: 133–137.

7 Barsotti, G., Sgorbini, M., Marmorini, P. et al. (2013). Ocular abnormalities in healthy Standardbred foals. *Vet. Ophthalmol.* 16: 245–250.

8 Osame, S. and Ichijo, S. (1994). Clinicopathological observations on Thoroughbred foals with enlarged thyroid gland. *J. Vet. Med. Sci.* 56: 771–772.

9 Drew, B., Barber, W.P., and Williams, D.G. (1975). The effect of excess dietary iodine on pregnant mares and foals. *Vet. Rec.* 97: 93–95.

10 Miyazawa, K., Motoyoshi, S., and Usui, K. (1978). Nodular goiters of three mares and their foals, induced by feeding excessive amount of seaweed. *Nippon Juigaku Zasshi* 40: 749–753.

11 Allen, A.L., Doige, C.E., Fretz, P.B. et al. (1994). Hyperplasia of the thyroid gland and concurrent musculoskeletal deformities in western Canadian foals: reexamination of a previously described syndrome. *Can. Vet. J.* 35: 31–38.

12 Allen, A.L., Townsend, H.G., Doige, C.E. et al. (1996). A case-control study of the congenital hypothyroidism and dysmaturity syndrome of foals. *Can. Vet. J.* 37: 349–351.

13 Corley, K.T.T. (2002). Monitoring and treating haemodynamic disturbances in critically ill neonatal foals. Part 1: haemodynamic monitoring. *Equine Vet. Educ.* 14: 270–279.

14 Franco, R.M., Ousey, J.C., Cash, R.S.G. et al. (1986). Study of arterial blood pressure in newborn foals using an electronic sphygmomanometer. *Equine Vet. J.* 18: 475–478.

15 Rossdale, P.D. (1967). Clinical studies on the newborn Thoroughbred foal: II heart rate, auscultation and electrocardiogram. *Br. Vet. J.* 123: 521–531.

16 Chope, K. (2006). Cardiac disorders. In: *Equine Neonatal Medicine: A Case-Based Approach*, 1e (ed. M.R. Paradis), 247–258. Philadelphia: Elsevier Saunders.

17 Yamomoto, K., Yasuda, J., and Too, K. (1992). Arrythmias in newborn Thoroughbred foals. *Equine Vet. J.* 23: 169–173.

18 Guigere, S., Sanchez, L.C., Shih, A. et al. (2007). Comparison of the effects of caffeine and doxapram on respiratory and cardiovascular function in foals with induced respiratory acidosis. *Am. J. Vet. Res.* 68: 1407–1416.

19 Wilkins, P.A. and Dolente, B. Body wall tear in late gestational mare and birth resuscitation of a compromised foal. In: *Equine Neonatal Medicine: A Case-Based Approach*, 1e (ed. M.R. Paradis), 22–29. Philadelphia: Elsevier Saunders.

20 Austin, S.M. (2016). Management and treatment of the sick neonate in ambulatory practice. *Equine Vet. J.* 30: 106–112.

21 Madigan, J.E. (1990). Management of the newborn foal. *Proc. Am. Assoc. Equine Pract.* 36: 99–116.

22 Kavan, R.P., Madigan, J.E., and Walker, R. (1994). Effect of disinfectant treatments on bacterial flora of the umbilicus of neonatal foals. *Proc. Am. Assoc. Equine Pract.* 40: 37–38.

23 Brewer, B.D., Clement, S.F., Lotz, W.S. et al. (1991). Renal clearance, urinary excretion of endogenous substances, and urinary diagnostic indices in healthy neonatal foals. *J. Vet. Intern. Med.* 5: 28–33.

24 Reef, V.B. and Collatos, C.A. (1989). Ultrasonography of umbilical structures in clinically normal foals. *Am. J. Vet. Res.* 49: 2143–2146.

25 Franklin, R.P. and Ferrell, E.A. (2002). How to perform umbilical sonograms in the neonate. *Proc. Am. Assoc. Equine Pract.* 48: 261–265.

26 McCoy, A.M., Lopp, C.T., Kooy, S. et al. (2020). Normal regression of the internal umbilical remnant structures in Standardbred foals. *Equine Vet. J.* 52: 876–883.

27 Adams, R. and Mayhew, I.G. (1984). Neurological examination of newborn foals. *Equine Vet. J.* 16: 306–312.

28 Watterberg, K.L., Aucott, S., Benitz, W.E. et al. (2015). American Academy of Pediatrics Committee on Fetus and Newborn and American College of Obstetricians and Gynecologists Committee on Obstetrical Practice. *Pediatrics* 136: 819–822.

29 Knottenbelt, D.C. The foal at delivery. In: *Equine Neonatology* (ed. D.E. Knottenbelt, N. Holstock, and J.E. Madigan), 71. London: Elsevier Ltd.

30 Vaala, W.E. (1994). Peripartum asphyxia. *Vet. Clin. North Am. Equine Pract.* 10: 187–218.

Chapter 2 Principles and Theory of Cardiopulmonary Resuscitation (CPR)

Jon Palmer and David Wong

One of the first modern descriptions of the basic precept of CPR was reported in a 1960 research project involving experimentally induced cardiac arrest in dogs in which chest compressions generated a pulse pressure, recorded by arterial pressure monitoring, thus suggesting cardiac output [1]. Since that time, CPR has greatly advanced and has been repeatedly reevaluated and updated [2, 3]. However, the critical goals during cardiac arrest and CPR have remained the same; those are to improve both cerebral and myocardial blood flow, achieve return of spontaneous circulation (ROSC), and increase survival with an acceptable neurological outcome. When cardiac arrest occurs as a primary event, the average adult person has approximately 2 L of oxygen within the vascular system and in the cells [4]. Estimating the oxygen consumption of the human body to be 250 cm^3/min, the patient at the time of cardiac arrest has approximately 8 minutes worth of oxygen within the body [4]. Unfortunately in pediatric medicine and neonatal foal medicine, respiratory arrest is often primary, leaving less oxygen reserve at the time of cardiac arrest. Thus, the critical need in adult human medicine is to move the oxygen around the body via chest compressions until ROSC is achieved. In pediatric and neonatal foal medicine ventilation is also vital.

Historically, two theories describing the mechanisms by which forward blood flow is achieved during chest compressions have been put forth: the *cardiac pump* and *thoracic pump* theories [5]. The cardiac pump theory suggests that direct compression of the left and right ventricles creates a pressure gradient between the ventricles and the aorta or pulmonary artery, thus causing forward flow of blood. This theory requires that the atrioventricular (AV) valves are closed during cardiac compression. The ventricles then refill during the decompression phase. The thoracic pump theory suggests that the increase in intrathoracic pressure due to chest compressions creates an arteriovenous pressure gradient across the heart, forcing blood to move down the gradient and to flow from the thoracic to systemic circulation. In this theory, the AV valves must be open during cardiac compression with retrograde flow from the right side of the heart to the systemic veins prevented by the venous valves [5].

Although described individually, it is likely that both mechanisms are involved in effective compression-mediated blood flow during CPR. More simplistically, CPR can be divided into two phases, compression and decompression, with each phase providing blood perfusion to specific organ systems. Most of the body's organs are perfused when external chest compressions are provided; these compressions result in forward arterial blood flow from phasic changes in intrathoracic pressure produced by the force generated by the person providing resuscitation [6]. Mechanistically, the increased intrathoracic pressure and reduced thoracic volume created by the chest compressions squeeze the heart and other structures that contain blood within the chest, including the lungs and great vessels. This results in a uniform rise in blood pressure within the intrathoracic vasculature and ejection of blood from the thorax.

In contrast, during the decompression phase of CPR, the chest rebounds to its normal fully expanded position. During this phase, the aortic valve closes under the *vacuum* effect created by the recoiling thoracic cage and maintains an aortic pressure that is higher than the intracardiac pressures that fall quickly behind the closed valve. This intrathoracic negative pressure draws blood from the periphery into the chest, thus filling the heart, lungs, and great vessels in preparation for the next chest compression. Therefore, the better the decompression, the stronger the vacuum is, along with commensurate improved cardiac refilling. This consequently results in more thoracic blood available for subsequent chest compressions.

While the organs of the body are perfused during the compression phase of CPR, it is during the decompression

Equine Neonatal Medicine, First Edition. Edited by David M. Wong and Pamela A. Wilkins.

phase that the heart itself receives blood perfusion. Saving the heart is a critical step in resuscitation. Without it, ROSC cannot occur. The heart is not perfused by blood within the heart chambers, but rather via the coronary arteries. Coronary blood flow is estimated by the coronary perfusion pressure (CPP), which is defined as the difference between the aortic diastolic pressure (DABP; where the coronary arteries originate) and the right atrial diastolic pressure (where the coronary venous blood returns). Right atrial diastolic pressure is estimated via the central venous pressure (CVP) to yield the formula: CPP = DABP − CVP [6, 7]. When the chest is compressed during CPR, the intrathoracic pressure, including the aorta and chambers of the heart, equalize with the compressive force of the hands, thus resulting in no coronary blood flow between the aorta and right atrium. However, during the decompression phase (CPR diastole), the higher aortic pressure above the closed aortic valve compared to the decreasing intrathoracic pressure results in positive CPP. Animal studies have demonstrated excellent correlation between CPP and myocardial blood flow during CPR [8]. It is therefore imperative to allow refilling of the chest and heart to permit adequate myocardial perfusion. Incomplete chest recoil can occur inadvertently from a fatigued resuscitator that unintentionally uses the foal's chest to rest on during the decompression phase of CPR, rather than allowing full chest recoil, and thereby increasing the intrathoracic pressure when it needs to be at its minimum [6].

In adult people with primary cardiac arrest, thoracic compressions are prioritized over ventilation strategies as to focus on continual circulation of blood during the early stages of cardiopulmonary arrest (CPA) [9]. The process of intubation and provision of breaths is associated with a trade-off between cardiac output and delivery of oxygen, but this should be minimized as chest compressions should not be interrupted during the procedure [6]. Hyperventilation also should be avoided as it impairs cardiac output and perfusion because each positive pressure breath increases intrathoracic pressure, compromises chest refilling, and impedes venous return [10]. Hyperventilation has also been associated with higher intrathoracic pressure resulting in increased right atrial diastolic pressure, decreased CPP and lower survival rates [11]. In contrast to adult people, in the majority of foals as in human pediatrics, cardiac arrest is secondary to respiratory arrest [12–14]. Causes of peri-parturient asphyxia in the newborn foal include premature placental separation, early severance or twisting of the umbilical cord, prolonged dystocia, and airway obstruction by fetal membranes [12]. In the neonatal foal, CPA may be associated with sepsis, primary lung disease (hypoxia), hypovolemia, metabolic acidosis, vasovagal reflex, hypoglycemia, and hypothermia [12]. Therefore, unlike adult people, cardiac arrest in foals, as with human pediatrics, is usually secondary to other systemic conditions and not caused by primary cardiac failure, thus explaining the fact that ventricular fibrillation is not as common a presenting arrhythmia in newborn infants (14%) or neonatal foals (20%, see below) [13]. Based on this information, and the ease of intubating the foal's trachea, CPR focusing only on thoracic compressions in not recommended; intubation and ventilation should be attempted as soon as possible, while compressions are being performed [12–14].

Cardiopulmonary Techniques in the Neonatal Foal

The first and most important step in performing CPR is deciding whether resuscitation is appropriate. That is, will it be possible to correct the underlying condition that caused the cardiac arrest? If not and the foal is fated to die again, performing CPR is not a humane treatment. The decision whether resuscitation is futile or may result in long-term survival is best judged by the attending clinician and only if in the clinician's judgment the life may be saved and underlying condition reversed, should the owner be offered the option of CPR as an ancillary treatment. Figures 2.1–2.3 provide quick reference guidelines for CPR.

In general, three possible initiating events can lead to CPA: an asphyxial event, an ischemic event or an arrhythmogenic episode [14]. In neonatal foals, **asphyxial arrest** is most commonly secondary to neonatal encephalopathy leading to respiratory arrest followed by bradycardia and finally cardiac arrest. But there are many other possibilities for the initiating asphyxia, including prolonged Stage II labor, acute, widespread premature placental separation, airway obstruction at birth (e.g. with membranes or meconium), persistent pulmonary hypertension, acute aspiration pneumonia, congenital interstitial pneumonia, acute viral pneumonia, and other conditions. An **ischemic event** is most commonly secondary to septic shock progressing to a nonperfusing bradycardia and finally cardiac arrest. Additional reasons for an ischemic event include critical blood loss, cardiac defects/failure, and acute dehydration, among others. Unlike in adult human medicine, CPA in foals is rarely caused by an intrinsic myocardial event leading to a **nonperfusing arrhythmia**. When this does occur, it is most commonly secondary to a cardiac contusion caused by trauma from a fractured rib.

The primary goal of CPR is the ROSC by returning cardiac perfusion, which will allow the heart to restart. While this primary goal is being achieved, the secondary goal is to preserve the central nervous system (CNS) by maintaining perfusion of the brain. In the vast majority of CPA cases in

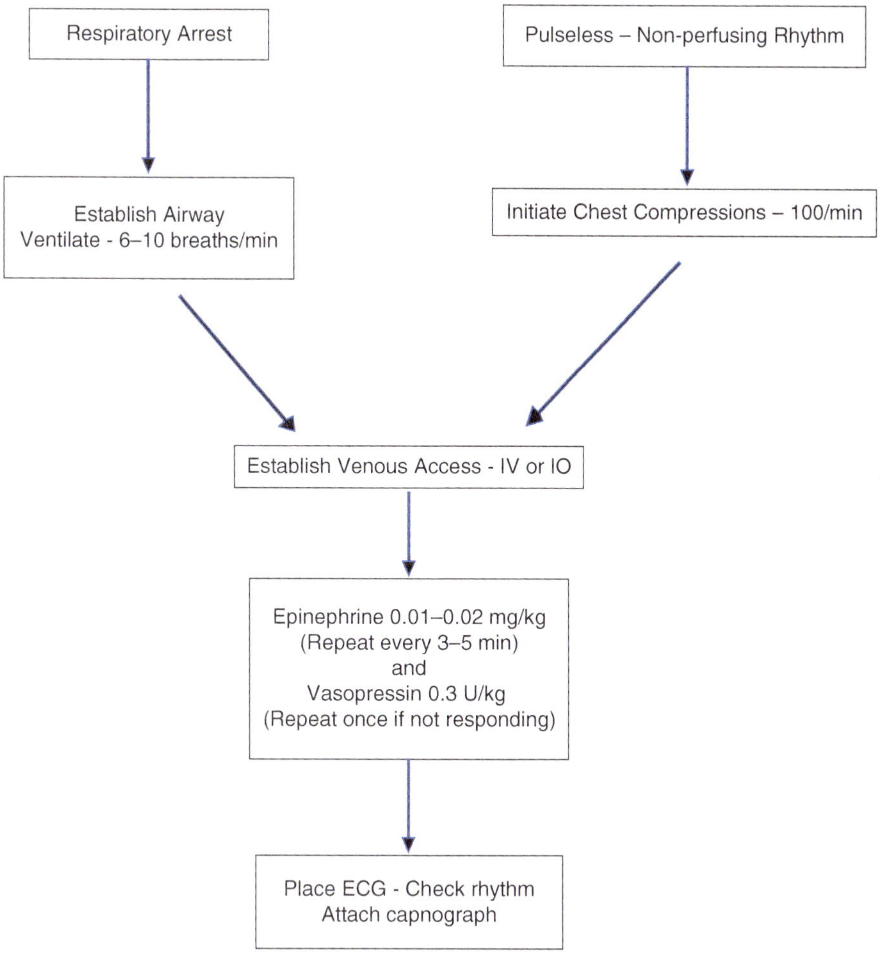

Figure 2.1 CPR suggested scheme.

foals the underlying cause is asphyxial and/or ischemic conditions, which makes establishing ventilation the priority over chest compression (although initiating ventilation and cardiac compressions simultaneously is ideal).

If an endotracheal tube is not readily available, mouth-to-nose ventilation should be initiated. Success depends on minimizing airway resistance by straightening the airway. This can be done with the foal in lateral recumbency by placing one hand on the pole and slightly overextending the head/neck, while placing the other hand on the rostral end of the mandible to fully extend the head and neck. The hand on the mandible can occlude the lower nostril while the resuscitator places their mouth over the upper nostril to give a breath. This positioning allows for an unoccluded path for the forced breath into the lungs. As an alternate method, the resuscitator can enlist the ground's help by rotating the foal's head and neck so that the pole rests on the ground and extend the head as before by placing one hand on the rostral end of the mandible, simultaneously occluding one nostril to allow access to the remaining nostril to give the breath. Now with the freed hand, the resuscitator can place gentle compression on the cricoid cartilage, effectively compressing the esophagus between the cricoid and the spine, and thus preventing any of the delivered breath from traveling down the esophagus. Using either of these techniques, the resuscitator can effectively deliver breaths until the airway can be secured with an endotracheal tube.

Once an endotracheal tube is in place, breaths can be delivered using a self-inflating bag-valve device such as an adult Ambu Bag® or adult Resuscitator Bag (Figure 2.4). The pediatric and infant size self-inflating bags are more appropriate for lambs, kids, and crias. Keep in mind that although ventilation is vital to return of spontaneous circulation, the positive pressure produced in the chest is also detrimental to cardiac return and thus to the cardiac output achievable with chest compressions. If ventilation is improperly administered, it can have a negative effect on outcome as it can result in decreased cardiac return and decreased coronary and cerebral perfusion. The goal is to administer short duration, small volume, infrequent breaths, which will minimally interfere with venous return but at the same time deliver sufficient ventilation for recovery. Since cardiac output achieved in CPR is minimal,

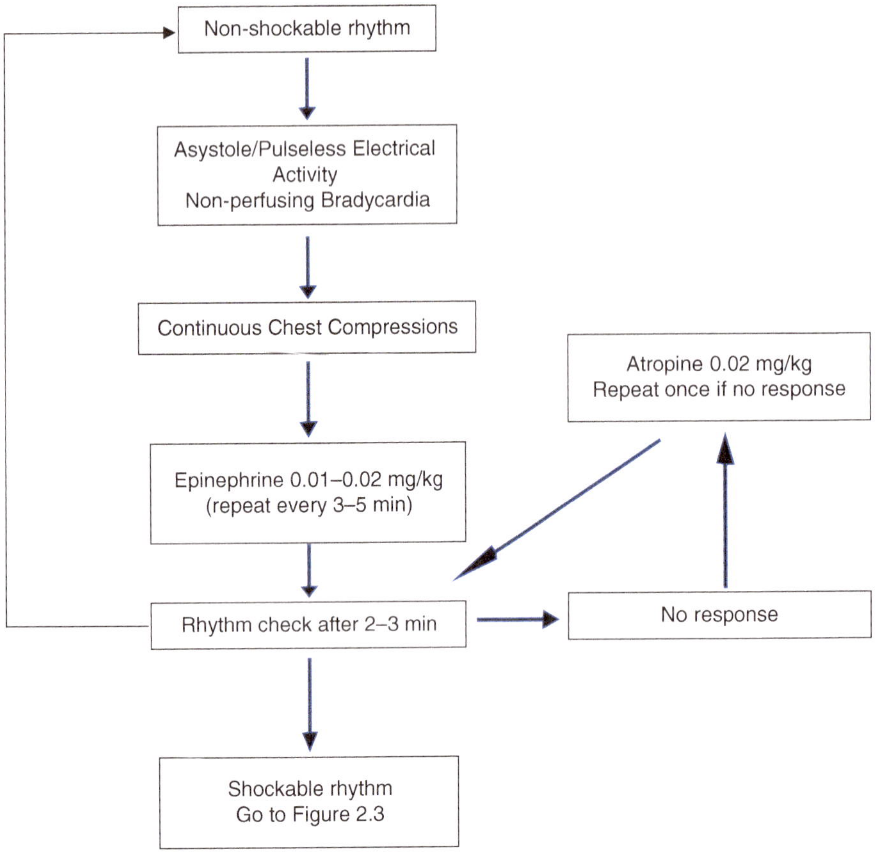

Figure 2.2 CPR suggested scheme for nonshockable rhythm.

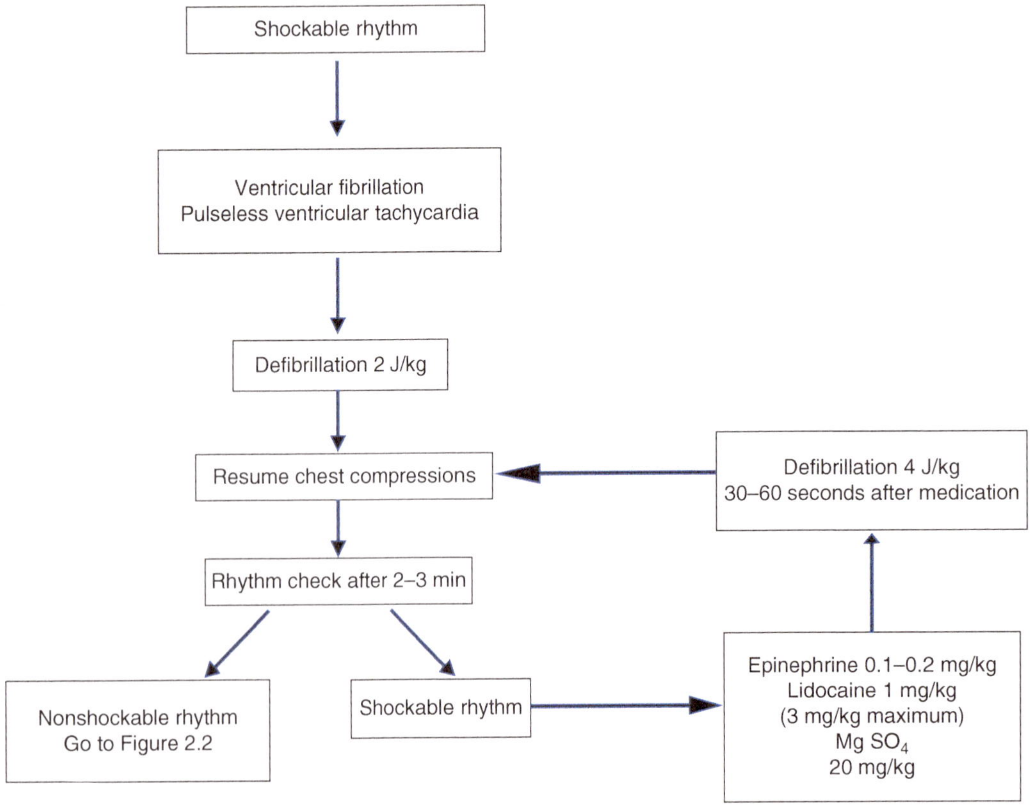

Figure 2.3 CPR suggested scheme for shockable rhythm.

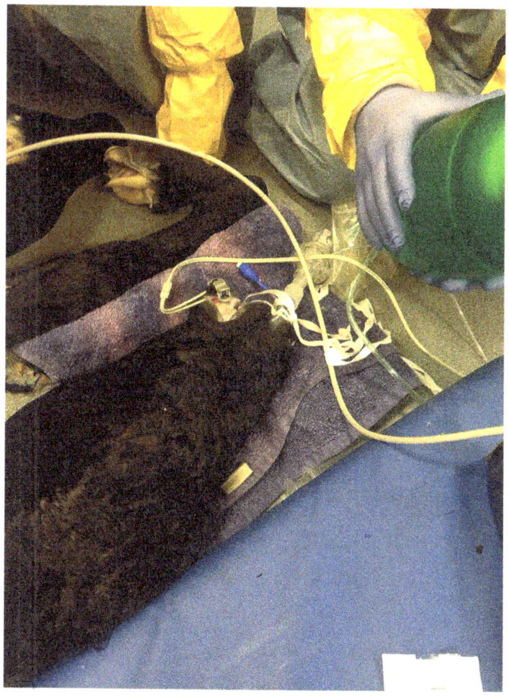

Figure 2.4 Newborn foal receiving cardiopulmonary resuscitation facilitated by an Ambu Bag attached to the foal's endotracheal tube.

deeper, slower breaths will not necessarily increase gas exchange but will decrease cardiac output and thus coronary and cerebral perfusion; however, at the same time some ventilation is vital to allow ROSC.

Ventilation during cardiopulmonary resuscitation should consist of rapid, infrequent breaths with the inspiratory phase <1 second and a rate <8–10 breaths per minute. The individual delivering the breaths can use a watch with a second hand and give a short breath every 10 seconds. This, if followed, would result in 6 breathes per minute, which is an appropriate frequency. Because of the inherent stress of the situation, it is common for resuscitators to provide more frequent breaths. However, if the goal is 1 breath every 10 seconds, then it is unlikely that the rate will be higher than 8–10 per minute, which is the maximum rate that should be allowed. During each delivered breath, close observation of the chest should be made to confirm that the small and short duration breaths are successfully delivered. The controversy about the use of oxygen during CPR remains unresolved so recommendations are difficult to give, but it is clear that lack of availability of oxygen is not a reason to forgo CPR [15].

In almost every case, cardiac arrest in neonatal foals will not be primary but follow respiratory arrest secondary to either asphyxia or ischemia. In these cases, an airway should be established and ventilation initiated as the priority. Chest compression should begin simultaneously or secondarily. When cardiac arrest is primary, cardiac compressions should be initiated immediately, before the airway is secured, but ventilation should be added to the resuscitation efforts as soon as possible. Chest compressions should be started as soon as a nonperfusing rhythm is recognized – do not wait until the heart stops. Once chest compressions are begun, any interruption (e.g. to assess for return of spontaneous cardiac contractions or ECG rhythm, etc.) should be no more than 10 seconds, with at least 2 minutes of continuous chest compressions between interruptions. The mantra of cardiac compression during CPR should be: push hard, push fast, minimize interruptions, and don't overventilate.

Chest Compressions

If the neonate has extreme bradycardia or other nonperfusing cardiac rhythm, cardiac compressions should be initiated. Do not wait until the heartbeat is undetectable. The foal should be placed on a firm surface with its withers against a wall so that it does not move during forceful compressions. Place the palm of the hand with the fist closed over the heart. Place the other hand to reinforce the compressing hand. Compressions should originate from motion of the waist, not the elbows of the attendant (the upper body weight powers compressions resulting in increased endurance). To maximize cardiac output, half of the duty cycle should be compression and half relaxation. This is easiest to achieve with a rapid compression rate of 100–120 per minute. The resuscitator should not be overly ambitious in setting a rate. Too rapid a rate will result in early operator fatigue. If an airway is secured, coordination between ventilation and chest compression is not needed. Cardiac output is enhanced by ventilation superimposed on chest compression, but there is evidence that cardiac perfusion may decrease during the simultaneous ventilation and compression. Cardiac output is heavily dependent on cardiac filling between compressions, which is impeded by positive thoracic pressure such as occurs during positive pressure ventilation. Pausing active chest compressions for more than 3 seconds, as would occur with interposed ventilation with compressions, significantly increases the likelihood of a negative outcome. Routine coordination of chest compression and ventilation can result in increased cerebral pressure, which is contraindicated in cases with hypoxic–ischemic encephalopathy and should be avoided in neonates with possible perinatal hypoxia. There is evidence that rapid respiratory rates during CPR are detrimental, and more effective tissue oxygen delivery will occur at a rate of 1 breath for every 30–60 compressions. Although many of these issues have not been adequately explored in neonatal foals, based on current evidence the authors recommend delivering 100 chest compressions/min with only 4–6 breaths/min without stopping the compressions to deliver positive pressure ventilation. If chest compressions do not increase the heart rate within 30 seconds resulting in a perfusing spontaneous rhythm, administration of medications is indicated.

Vascular Access

Once chest compressions and ventilation are achieved, vascular access should be secured if it is not already available. If vascular access is not already available, because of the lack of vascular fill and movement caused by chest compressions, it can be difficult and time consuming to establish an intravenous catheter. In such cases, intraosseous vascular access is the preferred alternative, if available (Chapter 59 Section VII). When dealing with premature foals with poorly ossified bones or small ruminants, a conventional 16 g or 18 g needle may work to establish intraosseous access. However, when dealing with most newborn foals it is more efficient to use a dedicated interosseous device. These can be hand-driven intraosseous needles, which take some practice placing efficiently, or drill-driven intraosseous needles, which generally can be placed in less than 1 minute. Any drug that can be delivered intravenously can be given through the intraosseous route and will reach the target just as rapidly.

Medications Used in Resuscitation

Epinephrine

During cardiac arrest, vasopressors are used to restore spontaneous circulation by optimizing coronary perfusion while helping to maintain cerebral perfusion. However, these treatments are a double-edged sword as they also cause intense vasoconstriction and increase myocardial oxygen consumption, which could result in more damage. In people, a randomized controlled trial [16] showed epinephrine use was associated with increased ROSC and survival to hospital admission but no improvement in survival to hospital discharge. Although this information may instill confidence in performing CPR in the absence of available epinephrine, it is not strong enough (not to mention species differences) to suggest forgoing epinephrine when it is available.

Despite these downsides, the most valuable pharmacologic aid in resuscitation continues to be epinephrine at a dose of 0.01–0.02 mg/kg, IV (repeat as needed every 3–5 minutes). During chest compression coronary blood flow is restricted to the diastolic period. Diastolic aortic pressure determines coronary perfusion, because during cardiac arrest there is no coronary capillary resistance and central venous pressure is low due to minimal venous return. Epinephrine increases diastolic aortic pressure by simultaneously impeding run off into peripheral tissues (by peripheral arterial constriction) and by increasing aortic tone. The combination of effective chest compression and the action of epinephrine results in a return of coronary perfusion, which is the most important step in resolving cardiac arrest no matter what the cause. Without coronary perfusion, there is no hope of return to a normal cardiac rhythm. Fluid volume loading is contraindicated in neonatal resuscitation unless there is an obvious fluid loss as could occur with significant hemorrhage (umbilical bleeding or bleeding secondary to a fracture).

Stimulation of α-receptors located on vascular smooth muscle causes vasoconstriction which increases aortic diastolic pressure and CPP, which optimizes the chances of achieving ROSC. Potentially harmful effects arise from deleterious changes in cerebral microvascular blood flow leading to worsening of cerebral injury, increased cardiac instability after ROSC and adverse metabolic and immunomodulatory effects [17].

Vasopressin

Vasopressin was explored as an adjunct or alternative to adrenaline in the late 1990s. Early experimental and animal studies suggested that vasopressin was superior to adrenaline, particularly during prolonged resuscitation. However, evaluation in subsequent randomized controlled trials in people produced equivocal results. Vasopressin was recommended in the American Heart Association guidelines from 2000 to 2015, after which its routine use was no longer recommended [18]. The authors have used vasopressin (0.3 U/kg, IV) during CPR in foals with some apparent success (see below) but its true value in resuscitating foals in cardiac arrest is unproven.

Lidocaine

Lidocaine and amiodarone have been used with some success in people with shock-refractory ventricular fibrillation and pulseless ventricular tachycardia [19]. The authors' clinical experience is limited to lidocaine (1.5 mg/kg with a maximum dose of 3 mg/kg), which has been used with some apparent success, but care should be used in dosing to avoid adverse toxic effect.

Atropine

Most foals with extreme bradycardia leading to failure of perfusion have ischemic cardiac disease, which is best treated with cardiac compression and ventilation, not atropine. In these cases, bradycardia can be considered protective until perfusion and ventilation return. Forced tachycardia – as occurs with atropine therapy – will increase oxygen debt without relieving the underlying problem. The possible exception to this is when excess vagal tone has led to a nonperfusing bradycardia, as can occur with extreme GI distension or jugular grove disease.

Defibrillation

Defibrillation is most effective when the electrical impulse travels through the chest from one side to the other. To that end, defibrillation paddles should be placed on opposite sides of the chest, although this is awkward. First, each side of the chest should be clipped and coated with defibrillation gel to allow good and even contact of the paddles with the chest. Trying to defibrillate using the downside of the chest can be very awkward unless a paddle extender or defibrillator pad is used. Care must be taken to ensure that there is no short current through the skin from one paddle to the other or to the ground, which can cause dermal burns and will not allow defibrillation, as the current will not travel through the heart.

When using defibrillation, an initial dose of 2 J/kg is used; if the response is not positive, increase to 4 J/kg. It is important for survival to minimize the time that chest compressions are stopped during each defibrillation episode. Thus, minimize the period of the break from chest contractions to <10 seconds by having the defibrillator charged and ready and the foal ready for defibrillation prior to ceasing chest compressions. This requires having sufficiently trained and experienced staff attending the CPA. Once the shock has been delivered, current resuscitation guidelines direct that chest compressions be promptly resumed for at least 2 minutes before a second equally brief pause is used to check the ECG rhythm. In fact, whenever chest compressions are paused, there should be at least 2 minutes of effective chest compressions before pausing again for any reason.

Monitoring

Capnography is the most useful method of monitoring the effectiveness of CPR. If there is no blood flow through the lungs because of cardiac arrest, then the end-tidal carbon dioxide ($ETCO_2$) will be zero. If chest compressions are effective and blood is propelled through the lungs (and ideally systemically), a measurable $ETCO_2$ will be noted. The $ETCO_2$ value should correlate with the cardiac output produced by the chest compressions. Capnography is a direct measurement of ventilation in the lungs, and it also indirectly measures metabolism and circulation. A decrease in cardiac output will lower the delivery of CO_2 to the lungs and thus cause a decrease in the $ETCO_2$.

The two most useful applications of capnography in CPR are: (i) evaluating the effectiveness of chest compressions, and (ii) identification of ROSC. With effective chest compressions (and when ventilation <10–12 breaths/min) the $ETCO_2$ will be 10–20 mmHg. This is in part due to the very large alveolar dead space ventilation. When ROSC is achieved, the $ETCO_2$ will rise to 30–45 mmHg as more of the ventilated lung is perfused and often much higher as the excessive CO_2 retained during the arrest is excreted. The $ETCO_2$ is a function of cardiac output for any given ventilation. When cardiac output is limited, capnography is a very convenient and readily available noninvasive monitor of pulmonary blood flow. It is also useful in determining the most effective technique of cardiac compression in each individual case. The higher the value, the more effective the cardiac compressions. As the technique required to achieve the best possible cardiac output will vary in each individual foal (depending on chest conformation and duration of the CPA), the use of capnography is useful in adjusting cardiac compression technique to optimize cardiac output. $ETCO_2$ monitoring can also be prognostic. If the $ETCO_2$ is <10 mmHg for >10 minutes, CPR is futile. In these cases, the $ETCO_2$ often drops to 0 during this period.

ECG

An ECG rhythm tracing is vital in directing therapy. As all that is needed is a rhythm tracing, the authors prefer a modified three-lead base-apex with one lead on the withers, one lead on the sternum, and the ground lead either on the withers or sternum. This positioning of the leads results in a relatively flat baseline and large QRS complexes, when present. Although during chest compressions the tracing will only reflect the cardiac compressions, the ECG heart rate will reflect the cardiac compressions, giving the resuscitator valuable feedback. When checking the rhythm, the pause in chest compressions should be no longer than 10 seconds and should be preceded and followed by at least 2 minutes of continuous chest compressions. The short pause for assessment of heart rhythm can be combined with the pause to defibrillate if the resuscitation team is well coordinated.

Blood Gas

Arterial blood gas sampling during CPR is not useful but once a spontaneous rhythm returns, arterial blood gas sampling should be initiated.

Outcome

In people with CPA in which ROSC is subsequently achieved, approximately 25–50% survive to discharge from the hospital. The main causes of hospital deaths are severe brain injury and multi-organ failure [20]. Thus, overall survival rates to hospital discharge are low when considering all patients with CPA, in the range of 0.6–25% [21]. A significant proportion of those who survive to hospital discharge have significant brain damage [17, 22, 23]. Even those with apparently good overall recovery may be left with subtle cognitive impairment [24]. Foals who require CPR at birth have a better chance of survival to hospital discharge than foals requiring CPR later in the neonatal period. In the authors' experience, 54% of foals receiving CPR at birth (6% of high-risk births) will achieve ROSC and 31% will survive; in comparison, 45% of foals receiving CPR outside the immediate peripartum period will achieve ROSC and only 11% will survive to hospital discharge (Tables 2.1–2.6).

In 2013, one of the authors (JP) reported on 20 years of experience with CPR on 83 neonatal foals that received advanced life support between 1993 and 2013 [13]. To be included in the study, foals had to require assisted ventilation and cardiac support (cardiac compressions and/or drugs). Neonates born while their dams were anesthetized or under heavy sedation who required assisted ventilation, but no specific cardiac support, were not included. Approximately half of the cases were resuscitated at birth (2.9% of the 1568 attended births during the time period) and the others ranged from 1 hour to 23 days old (1.4% of 2614 hospitalized critical neonates). The 83 cases had a total of 88 cardiac arrest episodes. CPR resulted in ROSC in approximately half of the episodes (Table 2.1). The rhythm initially identified most often was a nonperfusing bradycardia (heart rate usually estimated at <10/min), half of which were preceded by apnea (Table 2.3). Asystole was the initial nonperfusing rhythm in about 20% of the cases and a nonperfusing ventricular tachycardia or ventricular fibrillation was noted in approximately 10% of foals. During CPR it is common for one arrhythmia to be transformed into another. Almost 70% of cases had a nonperfusing bradycardia at some point during CPR with over half of these associated with initial respiratory failure. ROSC was achieved in over 60% of these cases. A shockable rhythm

Table 2.1 Episodes of cardiac arrest or nonperfusing bradycardia in neonatal foals evaluated over a 20-year period at a tertiary equine hospital [13][a].

RhythmC	Episodes	ROSC[b]	Survival[c]
All episodes	84	41 (49%)	15 (20%)
Cardiac arrest	49 (63%)	17 (35%)	5 (11%)
Nonperfusing bradycardia[d]	29 (37%)	24 (83%)	10 (42%)
Foals requiring CPR at birth[e]	46 (56%)	25 (54%)	12 (31%)
Foals requiring CPR during neonatal period (not in immediate peripartum period)[f]	38 (45%)	17 (45%)	4 (11%)

[a] 84 episodes in neonatal foals of cardiac arrest or non-perfusing bradycardia and outcome after resuscitation #/(%).
[b] ROSC = return of spontaneous circulation.
[c] Survival = survival to hospital discharge (failure to survive because of concurrent problems and not a direct result of cardiac disease except when initial ROSC not achieved); some cases had more than 1 episode.
[d] Nonperfusing Bradycardia (HR usually estimated at <10/min).
[e] Episodes that occurred during birth resuscitation.
[f] Episodes that occurred after birth during the neonatal period.

Table 2.2 Cardiac arrest in the neonatal period (*not associated with birth*) evaluated over a 20-year period at a tertiary equine hospital [13][a].

	Case	ROSC[b]	Survival[c]
All foals requiring CPR during neonatal period (not in immediate peripartum period)[a]	36 (38%)	17 (45%)	3 (9%)
Primary cardiac arrest	15 (42%)	8 (53%)	2 (14%)
Primary respiratory arrest	10 (28%)	5 (50%)	1 (20%)
Primary shock	11 (31%)	4 (36%)	0

[a] 36 episodes at least 1 hour after birth. #/(%).
[b] ROSC = return of spontaneous circulation.
[c] Survival = survival to hospital discharge (failure to survive because of concurrent problems and not a direct result of cardiac disease except when initial ROSC not achieved).

Table 2.3 Initial cardiac rhythm in episodes of cardiac arrest or nonperfusing bradycardia *during birth resuscitation* evaluated over a 20-year period at a tertiary equine hospital [13][a].

Rhythm	Cases	ROSC[b]	Survival[c]
All episodes during birth resuscitation	43	25 (54%)	12 (33%)
Nonperfusing bradycardia	22 (51%)	19 (79%)	10 (59%)
Ventricular fibrillation	3 (7%)	1 (33%)	0
Ventricular tachycardia	3 (7%)	1 (33%)	1 (33%)
Asystole	11 (26%)	1 (9%)	0
Pulseless electrical activity	4 (9%)	2 (50%)	1 (33%)

[a] 43 episodes in neonatal foals of cardiac arrest or nonperfusing bradycardia that occurred during birth (<1 hour old) resuscitation #/(%).
[b] ROSC = return of spontaneous circulation.
[c] Survival = survival to hospital discharge in cases where ROSC was achieved (failure to survive because of concurrent problems and not a direct result of cardiac disease except when initial ROSC not achieved).

Table 2.4 Initial cardiac rhythms occurring during CPR performed *at birth*, evaluated over a 20-year period at a tertiary equine hospital [13][a].

Rhythm	Cases	ROSC[b]	Survival[c]
All cases treated at birth	43	25 (54%)	12 (26%)
Nonperfusing bradycardia[d]	24 (56%)	19 (79%)	10 (53%)
Ventricular fibrillation	9 (21%)	2 (22%)	0
Ventricular tachycardia	7 (16%)	4 (56%)	3 (43%)
Asystole	12 (28%)	1 (8%)	0
Pulseless electrical activity	7 (16%)	2 (29%)	1 (17%)

[a] All rhythms that occurred at any time during 43 episodes of cardiac arrest or nonperfusing bradycardia at birth (<1 hour old) resuscitation of neonatal foals and outcome after resuscitation #/(%).
[b] ROSC = return of spontaneous circulation.
[c] Survival = survival to hospital discharge (failure to survive because of concurrent problems and not a direct result of cardiac disease except when initial ROSC not achieved); some cases had more than 1 episode.
[d] Nonperfusing bradycardia (HR usually estimated at <10/min).

Table 2.5 Initial cardiac rhythm in episodes of cardiac arrest or nonperfusing bradycardia in neonatal foals *not associated with birth*, evaluated over a 20-year period at a tertiary equine hospital [13].

Rhythm	Cases	ROSC[a,b]	Survival[c]
All cases during the neonatal period (excluding birth resuscitation)	35	17 (45%)	3 (8%)
Non-perfusing bradycardia[d]	22 (63%)	11 (50%)	2 (10%)
Ventricular fibrillation	5 (14%)	3 (60%)	0
Ventricular tachycardia	2 (6%)	2 (100%)	0
Asystole	4 (35%)	0	0
Pulseless electrical activity	1 (3%)	1 (100%)	1 (100%)

[a] All rhythms that occurred at any time during 35 episodes of cardiac arrest or nonperfusing bradycardia at least 1 hour after birth in neonatal foals and outcome after resuscitation #/(%).
[b] ROSC = return of spontaneous circulation.
[c] Survival = survival to hospital discharge (failure to survive because of concurrent problems and not a direct result of cardiac disease except when initial ROSC not achieved).
[d] Nonperfusing bradycardia (HR usually estimated at <10/min).

(ventricular tachycardia or ventricular fibrillation) was present at some point in one-third of the cases and ROSC was achieved in 40% of these cases. Asystole was present in approximately 40% of cases, but ROSC was only achieved in 10% of these cases. Pulseless electrical activity (PEA) was detected in approximately 10% of the cases, with ROSC in about 40% of these cases.

When only those cases requiring CPR at birth or within minutes of birth are considered, the most common initial

Table 2.6 Cardiac rhythms occurring during CPR performed in episodes of cardiac arrest or nonperfusing bradycardia in neonatal foals not associated with birth, evaluated over a 20-year period at a tertiary equine hospital [13][a].

Rhythm	Cases	ROSC[b]	Survival[c]
All cases of CPR performed any time during the neonatal period at least 30 min after birth	35 (38)	17 (45%)	3 (8%)
Nonperfusing bradycardia[d]	27 (77%)	14 (52%)	2 (8%)
Ventricular fibrillation	16 (46%)	6 (38%)	0
Ventricular tachycardia	7 (20%)	3 (43%)	0
Asystole	12 (34%)	0	0
Pulseless electrical activity	2 (6%)	2 (100%)	1 (50%)

[a] All rhythms that occurred at any time during 35 episodes of cardiac arrest or nonperfusing bradycardia at least 1 hour after birth in neonatal foals and outcome after resuscitation #/(%).
[b] ROSC = return of spontaneous circulation.
[c] Survival = survival to hospital discharge (failure to survive because of concurrent problems and not a direct result of cardiac disease except when initial ROSC not achieved).
[d] Nonperfusing bradycardia (HR usually estimated at <10/min).

arrhythmia was a nonperfusing bradycardia (about 65% of cases) with half preceded by apnea (Tables 2.3 and 2.4). ROSC was achieved in more than 90% of these cases. Asystole was the initial arrhythmia in about 25% of these cases. ROSC was only achieved in 10% of the cases with asystole. PEA was detected in 10% of the cases with ROSC achieved in half these cases. At some point during the birth resuscitation, approximately 20% of the neonates developed a shockable rhythm. ROSC was achieved in just over half of these cases. ROSC was gained in over 60% of neonates during birth CPR [13].

In cases that arrested 1 or more hours after birth, nonperfusing bradycardia was again the most common rhythm observed in 70% of the cases – occurring at some point during CPR in 80% of the cases (Table 2.5). Approximately half of these cases were preceded by apnea or respiratory failure. ROSC was possible in just under half of these cases. Asystole was the initial arrhythmia in almost a third of the cases and occurred at some point in these cases approximately 45% of the time. ROSC rarely occurred in cases with asystole. Although a shockable rhythm was only present initially in about 20% of cases, it developed sometime during resuscitation efforts in almost half of the cases. ROSC was achieved in about 40% of these cases [13].

When a shockable rhythm was identified (ventricular tachycardia or ventricular fibrillation), conversion was attempted by electrical defibrillation. The details from 37 defibrillation episodes were recorded. A defibrillation episode consisted of one or more shocks interspersed with CPR, which continued until the heart rhythm was converted to a nonshockable rhythm or resuscitation efforts were discontinued. In successful attempts, 1 to 12 shocks were required. In attempts where conversion from fibrillation failed, 3–15 shocks were delivered. The shockable rhythm was converted to a nonshockable rhythm 26 times (70% of the episodes) in 23 of the patients. Of these, ROSC occurred in 27% of the neonates [13].

In cases of CPA occurring in hospitalized neonates after birth, the inciting cause of the arrest appeared to be respiratory failure in approximately 40% of the cases, hypoperfusion from septic shock/cardiogenic shock in approximately 25% of cases, and an apparent primary cardiac event in approximately 25% of cases, with the underlying cause in the remaining 10% of cases being uncertain [13].

Capnography was useful in monitoring effectiveness of cardiac compressions and onset of ROSC but not in predicting futility. Fourteen percent of the cases where ROSC was achieved had an $ETCO_2 \leq 10$ mmHg at one point during CPR and 7% had an $ETCO_2 \leq 5$ mmHg (basically undetectable) at one point during CPR. It is very important to ensure the capnograph is functioning properly if it is being used to decide to discontinue resuscitation efforts as technical problems such as clogged sample lines are common during CPR [13].

In over half the episodes of CPA, resuscitation successfully resulted in ROSC. Of the CPA occurring at birth, ROSC was achieved in 54% of the cases as compared to CPA not occurring at birth, in which ROSC was achieved in 45% of the cases. Of all foals, only 18% were discharged from the hospital. This is not unexpected as CPA primarily occurs in patients with the most severe underlying disease. Of the nonsurvivors, 66% could not be revived during CPR, 21% died or were euthanized because of their underlying disease, 6% were euthanized because of neurologic disease likely as a sequela to the CPA, and 7% were euthanized because of financial considerations [13].

CPR in neonates with CPA can be successful in returning the patient to spontaneous circulation in about half the attempts. Neonates suffering CPA are among the most critical patients, thus survival to hospital discharge is low. However, severe neurologic sequela, a significant morbidity in human medicine, is not common, occurring in only 6% of foals. Revival is most likely in neonates with nonperfusing bradycardia and least likely in neonates with asystole. Many patients have a variety of rhythms during resuscitation. A shockable rhythm may occur in at least a third of the neonates with CPA. These rhythms can be converted with defibrillation in most cases. If defibrillation is not readily available, up to 20% of neonates undergoing birth resuscitation and up to 40% of patients undergoing resuscitation not associated with birth may not be revived [13].

Before CPR is undertaken, the ethics of initiating the treatment needs to be considered. If treatment of the underlying disease processes leading to CPA is futile, then initiating CPR is not humane. In such cases, the decision not to resuscitate the patient if in CPA should be made before the arrest occurs. The authors feel strongly that the clinician, guided by medical knowledge of the severity of the physiologic derangements of the foal, is in a better position than the owner to humanely evaluate the futility of therapy because the owner is emotionally invested.

Post-Resuscitation Care, Complications, and Prognosis

In the authors' experience, outcome of neonatal foals with CPA closely resembles the experience in human neonatology in that CPA frequently occurs only once, with no repeat episodes (96% of our cases only had 1 episode) [25, 26]. Although ROSC may be possible, and if so CPA is unlikely to recur, the underlying disease process(es) that lead to CPA are serious and may not be survivable; thus, the majority of CPA patients do not survive to hospital discharge [26, 27]. Fortunately, unlike adult people, both pediatric patients and foals do not develop post-cardiac arrest syndromes (PCAS) that occur in adult humans. However, it should be emphasized that when CPA occurs in a hospitalized patient, it is a marker of severe illness and because of failure to achieve a normal rhythm, concurrent disease, or owner's election, these patients usually do not survive hospitalization.

With the exception of the case series described above, there have been few reports in neonatal foals with documented postcardiac arrest complications such as acute renal failure and myocardial injury [28, 29]. Azotemia and serum electrolyte derangements were reported in a neonatal foal 24 hours postcardiac arrest with the serum creatinine reaching 10 mg/dl by 72 hours postcardiac arrest [28]. Despite aggressive medical management, the foal was euthanized because of worsening azotemia and oliguria. Microscopic findings noted on postmortem examination were consistent with hypoxic injury and included necrosis and sloughing of the renal tubular epithelial cells, centrilobular necrosis within the liver and neuronal necrosis within the brain [28]. Another case involved a female neonatal foal that was anesthetized for a magnetic resonance imaging of the brain. The foal experienced CPA during the anesthetic recovery period characterized by apnea and ventricular fibrillation.

The foal survived after 48 minutes of aggressive CPR, including external cardiac compressions and cardiac defibrillation. Immediately post-resuscitation, the cardiac troponin I (cTnI) concentration was greatly elevated (29.99 ng/mL, reference range 0.047 ± 0.085 ng/mL); this value decreased to 1.53 ng/mL 5 days later [30]. Interestingly, 16 months later, the filly presented for ventricular tachycardia likely precipitated by a grossly visible area of fibrosis in the left ventricular free wall. Although impossible to prove, the focal myocardial fibrosis may have been caused by myocardial ischemia during CPA and/or myocardial injury sustained during the aggressive and prolonged CPR [29].

Despite the findings of the above two cases, the individuals from our larger group series closely resemble the cases of pediatric CPA reported in people [25]. In human pediatric CPA cases, 82% have been found to have a single cardiac episode rather than repeated episodes closely comparing to our finding of single episodes in 92% of our foals. In the authors' experience, the occurrence of CPA is a marker of severity of illness of the neonatal foal, but not necessarily the cause of mortality except when attempts to return the heart to a normal rhythm fail. The small percentage of foals (<8% in series above) that have recurrent CPA may represent a different population. Unlike adult people where the CPA is usually the primary event, in critical neonatal foals who have CPA secondary to multiorgan dysfunction, it is impossible to determine if comorbidities are exacerbated by, initiated by, or independent of the CPA. This again is similar to human pediatrics [25].

In people, postcardiac arrest monitoring and therapy describe the overarching principles (Table 2.7) of body temperature management, respiratory care, management of appropriate hemodynamics, and treatment of underlying/precipitating systemic disease(s). Targeted temperature management (TTM) via therapeutic hypothermia has been shown to improve neurologic outcome in some prospective trials in people in the early postcardiac arrest period [30]. However, since the vast majority of these patients are responsive and active, the negative effects of anesthesia and required mechanical ventilation to achieve effective TTM are counterproductive and not acceptable. Avoiding hyperthermia, which may be the real danger in these cases, with targeted normothermia being recommended for children postcardiac arrest [33, 34]. Consideration of body temperature with a bias toward hypothermia along with avoidance of hyperthermia is worth consideration in neonatal foals postcardiac arrest.

Careful hemodynamic monitoring is suggested postcardiac arrest, since the cardiovascular system is in a very precarious state and the fact that the brain is very sensitive to additional ischemic episodes. Direct blood pressure monitoring via catheterization of the dorsal metatarsal, facial, radial, or caudal auricular artery (20 gauge, 1.5 in. catheter) is ideal, but may not always be feasible in the neonatal foal. In that instance, indirect blood pressure monitoring via oscillometry can serve to monitor the foal [35]. In one study, oscillometric blood pressure provided an accurate representation of diastolic and mean arterial pressure (MAP) in neonatal foals using an oscillometric bladder around the tail [36]. Optimal blood pressure goals post-arrest in a neonatal foal is dependent on where they are on the transition from low-pressure fetal physiology to pediatric physiology. This transition is not made uniformly in all foals, and there is a population of foals who have low fetal blood pressure for a variable period after birth but maintain good perfusion, resulting in low neonatal blood pressures.

This is a good reminder that blood pressure measurements are an imperfect surrogate of perfusion and should not be confused with the goal. Other indications of perfusion – such as limb warmth, pulse quality, level of arousal, gastrointestinal function, and urine production – should be evaluated when gauging perfusion in the neonatal patient. Once the individual foal's position in the neonatal transition is established, changes in that individual's blood pressure measurements can be helpful in estimating perfusion. Hypotension can be corrected using a balance of volume resuscitation, vasopressors, and inotropes, but great care should be used to prevent volume overload, which can be as damaging as hypoperfusion [31, 32]. Other indicators of blood perfusion, such as blood lactate and central venous oxygen saturation, can also be monitored. There is no evidence to support routine administration of corticosteroids, antiseizure prophylaxis, mannitol, or metabolic protectants after CPA [27]. Additionally, treatment of the primary underlying cause of the CPA should also be addressed.

Table 2.7 Suggested guidelines for neonatal foals in the postcardiac arrest period.

Maintain body temperature within normal range with a bias toward hypothermia.
Maintain normoxemia with P_aO_2 of 70–100 mmHg and/or SpO_2 within 94–97% [31, 32].
Maintain normal pH with the expectation that many critical neonatal foals have a significant metabolic alkalosis, which is balanced by retaining P_aCO_2 resulting in a normal pH (which is the goal).
Maintain organ perfusion with fluid therapy with or without the use of inotropes and vasopressors with great care to avoid fluid overload.
Address original/underlying cause(s) of cardiac arrest.

References

1 Kouwenhoven, W.B., Jude, J.R., and Knickerbocker, G.G. (1960). Closed-chest cardiac massage. *JAMA* 173: 1064–1067.

2 Duff, J.P., Topjian, A., Berg, M.D. et al. (2018). 2018 American Heart Association focused on pediatric advanced life support: an update to the American Heart Association guidelines for cardiopulmonary resuscitation and emergency cardiovascular care. *Circulation* 138: 731–739.

3 Atkins, D.L., de Caen, A.R., Berger, S. et al. (2018). 2017 American Heart Association focused update on pediatric basic life support and cardiopulmonary resuscitation quality: an update to the American Heart Association guidelines for cardiopulmonary resuscitation and emergency cardiovascular care. *Circulation* 137: 1–6.

4 Fowler, R., Chang, M.P., and Idris, A.H. (2017). Evolution and revolution in cardiopulmonary resuscitation. *Curr. Opin. Crit. Care* 23: 183–187.

5 Georgiou, M., Papathanassoglou, E., and Xanthos, T. (2014). Systematic review of the mechanisms driving effective blood flow during adult CPR. *Resuscitation* 85: 1586–1593.

6 Harris, A.W. and Kudenchuk, P.J. (2018). Cardiopulmonary resuscitation: the science behind the hands. *Heart* 104: 1056–1061.

7 Sutton, R.M., Friess, S.H., Maltese, M.R. et al. (2014). Hemodynamic-directed cardiopulmonary resuscitation during in-hospital cardiac arrest. *Resuscitation* 85: 983–986.

8 Halperin, H.R., Tsitlik, J.E., Guerci, A.D. et al. (1986). Determinants of blood flow to vital organs during cardiopulmonary resuscitation in dogs. *Circulation* 73: 539–550.

9 Benner, J.P., Morris, S., and Brady, W.J. (2011). A phased approach to cardiac arrest resuscitation involving ventricular fibrillation and pulseless ventricular tachycardia. *Emerg. Med. Clin. North Am.* 29: 711–719.

10 Fowler, R. and Pepe, P.E. (2002). Prehospital care of the patient with major trauma. *Emerg. Med. Clin. North Am.* 20: 953–974.

11 Aufderheide, T.P., Sigurdsson, G., Pirrallo, R.G. et al. (2004). Hyperventilation-induced hypotension during cardiopulmonary resuscitation. *Circulation* 109: 1960–1965.

12 Jokisalo, J.M. and Corley, K.T.T. (2014). CPR in the neonatal foal. Has RECOVER changed our approach? *Vet. Clin. Equine* 30: 301–316.

13 Palmer, J.E (2013). VET Talks on cutting-edge research in critical care: CPR case series IVECCS. *Proceedings, annual veterinary critical care conference, San Diego, CA.*

14 Palmer, J.E. (2007). Neonatal foal resuscitation. *Vet. Clin. North Am. Equine Pract.* 23: 159–182.

15 Skrifvars, M.B. (2016). Towards interventional trials on the use of oxygen during and after cardiac arrest. *Resuscitation* 101: A3–A4.

16 Jacobs, I.G., Finn, J.C., Jelinek, G.A. et al. (2011). Effect of adrenaline on survival in out-of-hospital cardiac arrest: a randomized doubleblind placebo-controlled trial. *Resuscitation* 82: 1138–1143.

17 Finn, J., Jacobs, I., Williams, T.A. et al. (2019). Adrenaline and vasopressin for cardiac arrest. *Cochrane Database Syst. Rev.* (1): CD003179.

18 Finn, J., Jacobs, I., Williams, T.A. et al. (2020). Adrenaline and vasopressin for cardiac arrest. *Emergencies* 32: 133–134.

19 de Caen, A.R., Berg, M.D., Chameides, L. et al. (2015). Part 12: Pediatric advanced life support: 2015 American Heart Association guidelines update for cardiopulmonary resuscitation and emergency cardiovascular care. *Circulation* 132 (18 Suppl 2): S526–S542.

20 Laver, S., Farrow, C., Turner, D. et al. (2004). Mode of death after admission to an intensive care unit following cardiac arrest. *Intensive Care Med.* 30: 2126–2168.

21 Berdowski, J., Berg, R.A., Tijssen, J.G. et al. (2010). Global incidences of out-of-hospital cardiac arrest and survival rates: systematic review of 67 prospective studies. *Resuscitation* 81: 1479–1487.

22 Corrada, E., Mennuni, M.G., Grieco, N. et al. (2013). Neurological recovery after out-of-hospital cardiac arrest: hospital admission predictors and one-year survival in an urban cardiac network experience. *Minerva Cardioangiol.* 61: 451–460.

23 Kim, Y.J., Ahn, S., Sohn, C.H. et al. (2016). Long-term neurological outcomes in patients after out-of-hospital cardiac arrest. *Resuscitation* 101: 1–5.

24 Nolan, J.P. and Cariou, A. (2015). Post-resuscitation care: ERC–ESICM guidelines 2015. *Intensive Care Med.* 41: 2204–2206.

25 Gupta, P., Pasquali, S.K., Jacobs, J.P. et al. (2016). American Heart Association's get with the guidelines–resuscitation investigators. Outcomes following single and recurrent in-hospital cardiac arrests in children with heart disease: a report from American Heart Association's get with the guidelines registry–resuscitation. *Pediatr. Crit. Care Med.* 17: 531–539.

26 Tress, E.E., Kochanek, P.M., Saladino, R.A. et al. (2010). Cardiac arrest in children. *J. Emerg. Trauma Shock* 3: 267–272.

27 Smarick, S.D., Haskins, S.C., Boller, M. et al. (2012). RECOVER evidence and knowledge gap analysis in veterinary CPR. Part 6: post-cardiac arrest care. *J. Vet. Emerg. Crit. Care* 22: S85–S101.

28 Wong, D.M., Ruby, R.E., Eatroff, A. et al. (2017). Use of renal replacement therapy in a neonatal foal with

post-resuscitation acute renal failure. *J. Vet. Intern. Med.* 31: 593–597.

29 Ruby, R.E., Wong, D.M., Ware, W.A. et al. (2018). Myocardial fibrosis and ventricular tachyarrhythmia in a thoroughbred filly. *J. Equine Vet. Sci.* 70: 107–111.

30 Bernard, S.A., Gray, T.W., Buist, M.D. et al. (2002). Treatment of comatose survivors of out-of-hospital cardiac arrest with induced hypothermia. *N. Engl. J. Med.* 346: 557–563.

31 Walker, A.C. and Johnson, N.J. (2018). Critical care of the post-cardiac arrest patient. *Cardiol. Clin.* 36: 419–428.

32 Randhawa, V.K., Grunau, B.E., Debicki, D.B. et al. (2018). Cardiac intensive care unit management of patients after cardiac arrest: now the real work begins. *Can. J. Cardiol.* 34: 156–167.

33 Moler, F.W., Silverstein, F.S., Holubkov, R. et al. (2015). Therapeutic hypothermia after out-of-hospital cardiac arrest in children. *N. Engl. J. Med.* 372: 1898–1908.

34 Moler, F.W., Silverstein, F.S., Holubkov, R. et al. (2017). Therapeutic hypothermia after in-hospital cardiac arrest in children. *N. Engl. J. Med.* 376: 318–329.

35 Corley, K.T.T. (2002). Monitoring and treating haemodynamic disturbances in critically ill neonatal foals. Part 1: haemodynamic monitoring. *Equine Vet. Educ.* 14: 270–279.

36 Nout, Y.S., Corley, K.T.T., Donaldson, L.L. et al. (2002). Indirect oscillometric and direct blood pressure measurements in anesthetized and conscious neonatal foals. *J. Vet. Emerg. Crit. Care* 12: 75–80.

Chapter 3 The Premature and Dysmature Neonatal Foal

David Wong and Katarzyna A. Dembek

The terms *premature* and *dysmature* are used to describe the immature physical and physiologic characteristics in newborns in relationship to gestational length. The World Health Organization defines a premature infant as a child born alive 21 or more days before the infant's due date (before 37 weeks of pregnancy are completed). In contrast, defining prematurity and dysmaturity in the neonatal foal is more problematic due to the wide variability in gestational length of the equid, which can range from 310 to 388 days [1–4]. The commonly used average gestational length of 340 days in Thoroughbred horses was originally suggested by Rossdale in 1967 [5] and is generally supported by other studies. For example, in a study involving 1,047 births from 652 individual mares of different breeds, the average gestation length was 342.7 days, but the range was quite large, spanning 74 days (range 307–381 days) [6].

Factors that influence gestational length include horse breed (Table 3.1), nutrition, gender of the fetus, and month and season of conception and parturition [4, 6, 9, 23]. Age and parity of the mare along with year of mating can impact gestational length as well [9]. In general, colts have a slightly longer average gestation length of approximately 1.7 to 7 days when compared to fillies and mares that conceive earlier in the breeding season can have a longer pregnancy (up to 10 days longer) as compared to mares bred at the end of the breeding season [3, 9, 14–16]. Of note, pregnancy is typically longer in donkeys, with the mean gestational lengths ranging from 362 to 371 days as compared to horses [18, 19].

Because of the wide variation in the normal gestational length in the mare, defining prematurity and dysmaturity based solely on gestational age could falsely classify a number of appropriately mature foals. Multiparous mares tend to have approximately the same gestational length year-to-year, with some mares consistently delivering healthy newborn foals despite shorter or longer gestational lengths in relation to the standard 340 days gestational length [4]. Therefore, knowledge of gestational length in previously delivered healthy foals may help identify if a foal is premature/dysmature in individual mares. Despite this, a cutoff of 320 days of gestation is a commonly used time point to define premature and dysmature foals and is based on a study that reported significantly lower birth weights and poor outcomes of foals born before this time point [24]. A premature foal is born at 320 gestational days or less and displays physical and physiologic characteristics of immaturity. In contrast, the term *dysmature* in infants has varying definitions and lacks clarity. In particular, confusion among the terms *prolonged pregnancy, post-maturity, intrauterine growth retardation,* and *dysmaturity* occur within the human literature [25–27].

One of the first descriptions of dysmaturity in the United States was published in 1945 in which infants were subdivided into three different stages of severity with placental dysfunction suggested as the underlying etiologic factor [28]. Some physicians refer to dysmaturity in infants as small for gestational age while others refer to dysmaturity as born with absent vernix caseosa (creamy white substance covering the skin of the fetus/infant, unique to humans), dry desquamating skin, and the presence of meconium staining of the amniotic fluid [29]. Still others describe the dysmature infant as having normal body length but reduced weight [27]. The definition of dysmaturity in equine medicine is relatively uniform and is used to define a foal that has had a "normal" gestational length (greater than 320 gestational days), but displays physical and/or physiologic signs of immaturity and is usually undersized [24]. The difference between premature and dysmature foals is tenuous because the physical features of premature and dysmature foals are similar; the distinction between the two is that premature foals are born at 320 gestational days or less. As noted above, because the gestational length of the healthy mare is so variable, the use of a cutoff date of 320 gestational days is quite

Equine Neonatal Medicine, First Edition. Edited by David M. Wong and Pamela A. Wilkins.

Table 3.1 Reported gestational lengths in various horse breeds.

Breed	Mean ± SD gestation (days) (range; if available)	Breed	Mean ± SD gestation (days) (range; if available)
American Saddlebred	340.7 ± 18.5 [7]	Friesian	331.6 [8]
Andalusian	336.8 [9]	Friesian	337.7 ± 9.6 [10]
Arabian	335.5 ± 10.2 [11]	Haflinger	341.3 ± 11.3 [10]
Arabian	340 [9]	Lipizzaner	334 ± 9.8 [12]
Belgian	333.8	Missouri Fox Trotter	342 ± 8.7 [7]
Black Forest Coldblood	344 ± 9.3 [7]	Shetland	337.2 ± 12.4 [10]
Carthusian Spanishbred	338.9 ± 9.6 (319–359) [13]	Standardbred	343.4 [14]
Connemara Pony	345.7 ± 9.8 [7]	Standardbred	349.1 (303–384) [15]
Czech Warmblood	339.2 ± 11.3 (305–392) [16]	Thoroughbred	347 ± 14.4 (306–390) [17]
Donkey (Martina Franca)	371 ± 12 (333–395) [18]	Thoroughbred	344.1 (315–388) [3]
Donkey (Spanish)	362 ± 15 (331–421) [19]	Thoroughbred	350 ± 10 (296–429) [20]
Dutch Freiberger	336.5 (307–361) [21]	Trakehner	336.8 ± 15.6 [22]
Dutch Draught Horse	343.2 ± 10.1 [10]	Welsh Cob	351.3 ± 14.8 [7]
Fjord	342.3 ± 11.4 [10]	Welsh Pony	346.5 ± 12.6 [7]

arbitrary [1]. In fact, a foal born from an individual mare (greater than 320 days gestation) with a naturally longer gestational length may be premature rather than dysmature; thus the terms premature and dysmature are sometimes used interchangeably in equine medicine [1]. A proposed definition of prematurity is a foal that is born prior to the mare's normal gestational length and displays immature physical and physiologic attributes whereas dysmaturity describes a foal that is born at a normal or prolonged gestational length for an individual mare, yet displays physical and physiologic attributes of a premature foal. The terms *fetal growth retardation* or *intrauterine growth retardation* have also been occasionally used in the equine literature and is defined as a condition of pregnancy in which the developing fetus undergoes a pathological process that modifies its growth potential by reducing growth rate [30]. Due to the sparse amount of information available in horses, this term will not be discussed further.

Causes of Prematurity and Dysmaturity

The exact cause(s) of premature and dysmature foals is not known, but placental and/or endocrine insufficiency or dysfunction likely play a role. For instance, when twin foals are born alive, nearly always one or both foals demonstrate clinical signs of prematurity/dysmaturity. Thus, one cause is likely due to a lack of sufficient placental blood flow resulting in insufficient nutrients and substrates necessary for normal fetal growth [31]. Other proposed causes associated with prematurity/dysmaturity include bacterial placentitis, placental edema, premature placental separation, severe prolonged metabolic disturbances (maternal malnutrition), hydrops, fetal infection, congenital abnormalities, and inappropriate induction of labor [32, 33]. Experimental induction of ascending bacterial placentitis resulted in premature parturition in mares, likely due to abnormally regulated cytokine response to infectious stimuli (elevated interleukin [IL]-8, IL-6 in chorioallantois) and progstaglandin (PG) formation (elevated PGE_2 and $PGF_{2}\alpha$ in allantoic fluid) in the mare [34]. Fescue grass infected with the fungal endophyte *Neotyphodium coenophialum* has also been implicated as a cause of dysmaturity in foals [35]. Studies examining the effects of contaminated fescue grass and its impact on neonatal foals have described an increased incidence of weak or stillborn foals [36]. Foals may also appear larger than expected with poor musculature, long fine hair coats, overgrown hooves, and nonerupted or irregular incisor teeth [36, 37]. Of note, consumption of infected fescue grass has also been associated with prolonged gestation, maternal agalactia and a large neonatal skeletal frame. These foals have been referred to as post-term or post-mature foals [35, 36].

Hypothyroidism has also been associated with dysmaturity [29]. Congenital goiter can occur when the mare ingests too much or not enough iodine, or consumes goitrogenic plants, resulting in hypothyroidism in the foal [38–41]. These foals can be weak and have a poor suckle reflex and incomplete ossification of the cuboidal bones [42, 43]. Moreover, a specific syndrome associated with dysmaturity has been reported in Canada, known as thyroid hyperplasia and musculoskeletal deformities (TH-MSD) or congenital hypothyroidism and dysmaturity [42, 44]. The involvement of the thyroid gland in this syndrome implies that thyroid hormone deficiency may be involved in the development of dysmaturity in some foals [45]. Thyroid hormones influence cartilage production and degeneration and promote ossification as well as influence bone development by stimulation of growth hormone [46]. Interestingly, thyroid hormone levels can be either low or normal in foals with TH-MSD when compared with aged matched foals [47]. In some cases, low circulating thyroid hormone results in increased thyroid-stimulating hormone, consequently resulting in hypertrophy and hyperplasia of the thyroid gland and possible development of an enlarged thyroid gland or goiter. In one study, thyroid glands from 25 of 39 affected foals examined histologically were hyperplastic and lacked normal amounts of colloid [42]. Environmental factors associated with hypothyroidism and dysmaturity included the provision of cereal crops (i.e. oats) harvested prior to maturity and lack of mineral supplementation to pregnant mares [48]. Nitrates within the feed were considered a risk factor for the development of dysmaturity syndrome. Abnormalities associated with this syndrome, which is considered present when two or more anomalies are noted, include: mandibular prognathia, inappropriately ossified carpal and tarsal bones, flexural deformities, ruptured common digital extensor tendon(s), incomplete closure of the abdominal wall, and signs of immaturity (despite length of gestation) such as a short silky haircoat, pliable ears, and laxity of tendons and joints. Of interest, in this syndrome, the mean gestational length of affected foals was significantly longer (mean = 358 days; range 330–378 days) when compared to control foals (mean = 339 days; range 322–357 days).

Clinical Signs and Diagnosis of Prematurity/Dysmaturity

Affected neonatal foals display a constellation of clinical signs that can involve one or more body systems. Clinical manifestations of prematurity/dysmaturity include: prominent domed forehead, weak or absent suckle reflex, discolored tongue (red to orange color as opposed to a healthy pink color), short silky hair coat, weak muscle tone and poor muscle development, hypotonia, slow to stand, flexor tendon laxity, increased range of motion of joints (periarticular laxity), incomplete ossification of the cuboidal bones, poor cartilage development of ears/pliant ears, low body temperature, poor thermoregulation, slow respiratory pattern, low lung compliance, gastrointestinal dysfunction, poor or delayed renal function, poor glucose regulation, and small body size/low birth weight (Figure 3.1) [2, 32, 46]. Typically, full-term healthy foals weigh approximately 10% of the dam's body weight; this estimation can be used to help identify low birth weight foals [31].

Diagnosis of prematurity/dysmaturity may be self-evident based on the aforementioned physical characteristics displayed by the newborn foal. Further evidence includes the inability to maintain proper blood pH, low plasma concentrations of cortisol and adrenaline, depressed blood glucose concentrations during the first 2 hours postpartum, and poor response to exogenous ACTH administration (Table 3.2) [1]. In one study, differences in white blood cell counts were noted between term and prematurely induced foals [49]. In term foals, the mean ± SD total white cell, neutrophil count, and lymphocyte count at birth were $8.1 \pm 0.6 \times 10^3/\mu l$, $5.75 \pm 0.30 \times 10^3/\mu l$, and $2.19 \pm 0.34 \times 10^3/\mu l$, respectively, with a neutrophil/lymphocyte (N/L) ratio of >2.5. Comparatively, premature foals (mean gestational length 321 days) counts were $4.9 \pm 0.3 \times 10^3/\mu l$, $1.94 \pm 0.46 \times 10^3/\mu l$, and $2.96 \pm 0.27 \times 10^3/\mu l$, with a N/L count <1.3 [49].

(a) (b) (c)

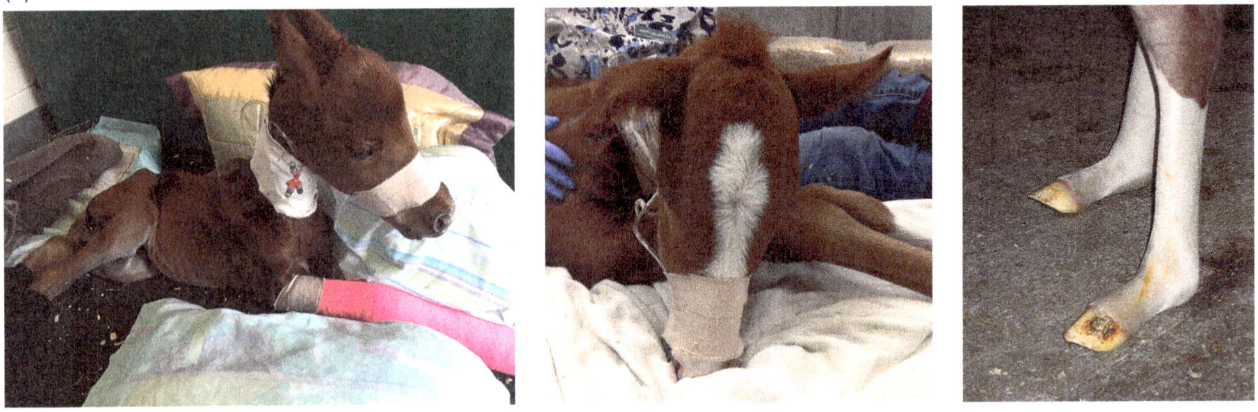

Figure 3.1 Clinical manifestations of prematurity/dysmaturity in neonatal foals including (a) short silky hair coat, small body size and domed forehead, (b) pliant ears, and (c) flexor tendon laxity.

Table 3.2 Suggested criteria used to assess stage of maturity of the newborn foal [1].

	Premature	Full term
Physical		
Gestational age	<320 d	>320 d
Size	Small	Normal or large
Coat	Short and silky	Long
Fetlock	Laxity	Normal extension
Behavior		
1st Stand	>120 min	<120 min
1st Suck	>3 h	<3 h
Suckle reflex	Poor	Strong
Righting reflexes	Poor	Good
Adrenal activity		
Plasma cortisol values first 2 h postpartum	Low concentrations (<30 ng/ml)	Increasing levels (120–140 ng/ml) at 30–60 min post-partum
Plasma ACTH values first 2 h post-partum	Peak values (~650 pg/ml) at 30 min post-partum, declines subsequently	Declining values from peak (300 pg/ml at birth)
Response to synthetic $ACTH_{1-24}$ (dose: 0.125 mg IM)	Poor response shown by a 28% increase in plasma cortisol and no change in neutrophil: lymphocyte ratio	Good response shown by 208% increase in plasma cortisol and widening of N : L ratio
Hematology		
Mean cell volume (fl)	>39	<39
White blood cell count ($\times 10^3/\mu l$)	6.0	8.0
Neutrophil: lymphocyte ratio	<1	>2
Carbohydrate metabolism		
Plasma glucose levels first 2 h postpartum	Low levels at birth (41.4 mg/dl), then declines	Higher levels at birth (73.8 mg/dl) maintained
Plasma insulin levels first 2 h postpartum	Low levels at birth (8.6 µU/ml), declining	Higher levels at birth (16.1 µU/ml), maintained
Acid base status (pH)	<7.25, declining	>7.3, maintaining or rising

Specific Body Systems Affected by Prematurity/Dysmaturity

Endocrine System

Abnormalities in several endocrine systems, such as the hypothalamic–pituitary–adrenal axis (HPAA), thyroid hormones and endocrine pancreas, are associated with premature/dysmature neonatal foals. In the healthy pregnancy, maturation of several organ systems is related to changes in the HPAA that occurs in late gestation. Specifically, fetal cortisol plays a key role in the final development and function of the respiratory, musculoskeletal, neurological, cardiovascular, and immune systems [50]. During the majority of pregnancy, mechanisms are in place to protect the fetus from high concentrations of cortisol with the maturation of the HPAA, and increased cortisol production starting during the last five days of gestation (Figure 3.2). At this point there is an exponential increase in cortisol, particularly in the last 24–36 hours of gestation, that continues into the neonatal period [53]. Cortisol synthesis is regulated by three main enzymes: cholesterol side chain cleavage (P450-scc), 3β-hydroxysteroid dehydrogenase (3β-HSD), and 17α-hydroxylase (P450-17). Cytochrome P450-scc is expressed in the fetal adrenal cortex from as early as 150 days of gestation and 3β-HSD, which synthesizes progesterone from pregnenolone, is present from approximately 280 days of gestation [54–57]. However, P450-17, which is required for cortisol production, is expressed 5 days before birth [54, 57]. This enhanced adrenal activity just prior to birth of the healthy fetus is also reflected postpartum as high plasma cortisol and corticotropin concentrations in healthy-term newborn foals during the first few hours after birth [51]. Premature/dysmature foals have

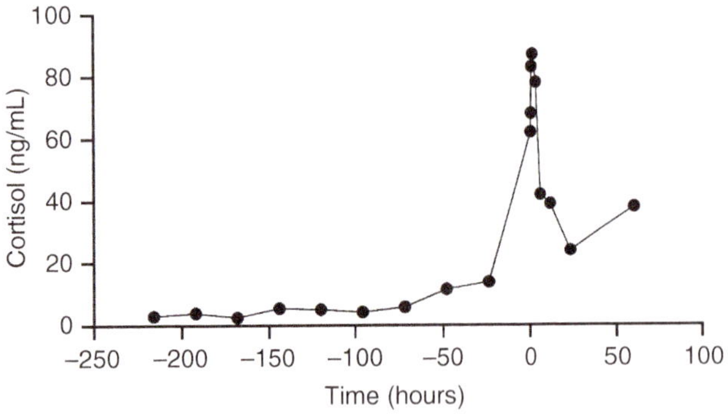

Figure 3.2 Cortisol concentrations in the late-term fetus, at parturition, and in the newborn and neonatal foal. Note the increase in cortisol during the peri-parturient period. *Source:* Adapted from Cudd [51] and Rossdale [52].

lower levels of cortisol and higher endogenous adrenocorticotropic hormone (ACTH) than full-term foals after birth, partially due to the lack of negative feedback [1]. Moreover, these foals show a blunted cortisol response to exogenous ACTH stimulation as compared to healthy foals [58]. Of interest, all three enzymes (P450-scc, 3β-HSD, P450-17) are present at birth and show no change in their expression in the perinatal period in full-term foals. An increased response to exogenous ACTH has been described in late gestation and at birth, with a positive correlation between the cortisol response of the neonatal foal and its gestational age at delivery in healthy foals. This suggests that other factors such as ACTH receptor (MC2R) expression, ACTH metabolism, and adrenal blood flow may be involved in the cortisol response to ACTH in neonatal foals [53, 57]. In other species, fetal maturation is accelerated by administration of glucocorticoids to the dam before birth, and anecdotal reports suggest that dexamethasone administration to pregnant mares at risk of delivering a premature foal may improve fetal outcome [59]. In one study, 100 mg of dexamethasone administered intramuscularly to five pregnant mares at 315, 316, and 317 days of gestation significantly shortened gestational length (322 ± 1.7 days) when compared to the saline control group (335 ± 2.3 days) and likely induced precocious delivery of a viable foal. Thus, late-term mares at risk of delivering a premature foal may benefit from exogenous steroid administration, but further investigation is needed as fetal adrenocortical function is suppressed during maternal dexamethasone treatment, which could, in turn, disrupt the natural HPAA-induced fetal maturation process [59].

The prepartum rise of fetal cortisol also plays an important role in preparing the cardiovascular system for postnatal life. Blood pressure steadily rises during late gestation in fetal sheep, while adrenalectomy of fetal sheep prevents this rise in fetal blood pressure; subsequent infusion of cortisol into the adrenalectomized sheep fetus restores the increase in fetal blood pressure [50]. Therefore, cortisol impacts the fetal and newborn cardiovascular system and may partially explain the hypotension observed in some premature/dysmature foals. In addition, catecholamines have an essential role in the cardiovascular function during the perinatal period in foals. Blood concentrations of adrenaline and noradrenaline gradually increase during late gestation, peak at birth, and return to baseline within 14 days postpartum [60]. In premature foals, noradrenaline levels are higher and adrenaline lower in the first two hours after birth compared to full-term foals. This may be due to lower cortisol concentrations that induce the activity of phenyl-N-methyl-transferase, the enzyme responsible for converting noradrenaline to adrenaline, and an incomplete maturation of the adrenal gland before birth [60]. Catecholamine deficiency may also contribute to neonatal hypotension frequently seen in premature/dysmature and critically ill foals. Therefore, administration of adrenaline or noradrenaline agonists or other vasopressor support may be useful in managing blood pressure and tissue perfusion in equine neonates [54].

Fetal serum thyroid hormone concentrations are low in fetal foals and other species and increase just prior to birth [33, 45]. Additionally, the prepartum rise in plasma cortisol induces de-iodination of T4 to produce the biologically active T3 in fetal sheep [50]. Adequate levels of thyroid hormones are required for a variety of biological functions and likely play a role in the rapid growth and organ development in late gestation and the early postnatal period as well as maintaining neonatal thermogenesis [33, 50]. In healthy-term foals, thyroid hormones such as total T4 and T3 concentrations are as much as 14 times higher than those of healthy adult horses and free T4 and T3 concentrations are five times higher; these concentrations decline over the first few weeks of life (Figure 3.3) [33, 61]. Cortisol and T3 appear to be critical for lung maturation and postpartum reabsorption of lung liquid in the fetal/newborn sheep and might play a similar role in newborn foals [62]. The syndrome of transient hypothyroxinemia of prematurity (THOP) has been described in premature infants and is thought to be caused by an immature hypothalamic–pituitary-thyroid axis [33, 63]. THOP in infants is associated with increased risk of respiratory disease, cerebral white matter damage, and motor and cognitive deficits in infants [33, 63]. Some premature foals have lower concentrations of total T3 and T4 and free T4 shortly after birth compared to healthy and sick neonatal foals and may have thyroid hormone profiles similar to THOP in infants, but further investigation in neonatal foals is necessary [33, 45].

The mechanisms of blood glucose control are not completely developed at birth in neonatal foals. Thus, hypoglycemia is a common finding in both premature/dysmature

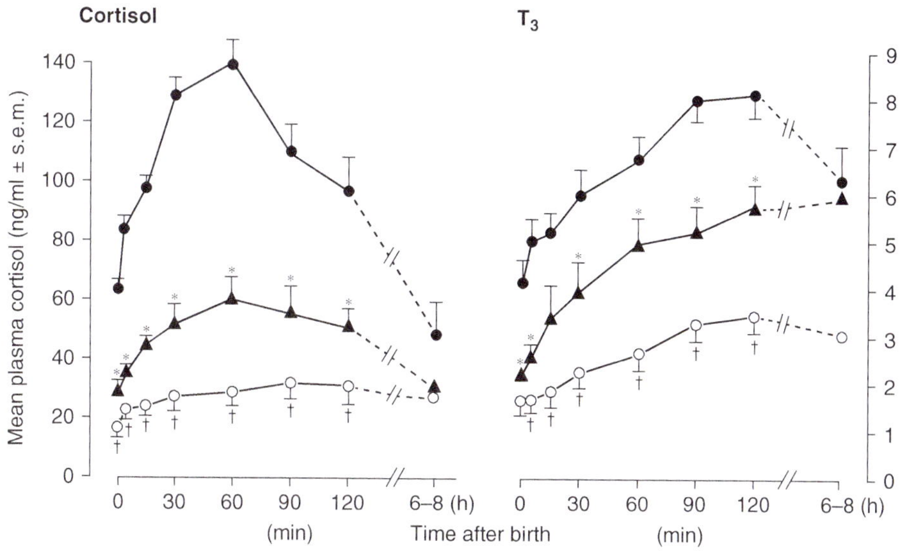

Figure 3.3 Twilight foal is an intermediate state of maturity where multiple last-gestation processes have begun, but complete functional maturity as seen in full-term healthy foals, has not yet been attained [1]. Postpartum changes in plasma cortisol and T_3 in 12 full-term (●), 5 "twilight" (▲) and 6 premature (o) foals. Unpaired *t* tests: premature vs. other three groups. †$P < 0.001$; twilight vs. full-term, *$P < 0.01$.

and full-term foals in the neonatal period. Tissue resistance to insulin also has been described in the first 24 hours after birth in healthy foals [64]. It is possible that the higher concentrations of catecholamines and cortisol may inhibit insulin function and gluconeogenesis in full-term equine neonates. Insulin blood levels are low after birth in premature and critically ill foals [55, 56, 65]. The pancreatic β-cell response to exogenous glucose administration is reduced 2 hours after birth, most likely due to higher-than-normal noradrenaline concentrations in premature foals. Therefore, it is important to closely monitor blood glucose concentrations and maintain euglycemia in premature and dysmature foals.

Musculoskeletal System

Orthopedic consequences of prematurity/dysmaturity, in particular incomplete ossification of the cuboidal bones, is one of the most threatening complications to the long-term wellbeing of premature/dysmature foals because deformation of incompletely ossified cuboidal bones negatively impacts athletic function [66]. Under healthy circumstances, the fetal skeleton begins as a cartilage template, subsequently ossifying as gestation progresses. In the healthy pregnancy, the carpal and tarsal bones are among the last to ossify and are radiographically visible by approximately 300 days of gestation [46, 67, 68]. Ossification of the carpal and tarsal bones begins in the last 2 months of gestation, undergoes a rapid phase in the last 2 weeks of gestation, and continues for approximately 4 weeks after birth [69, 70]. The accessory carpal bone is the first to begin

Table 3.3 Approximate gestational date at which initial appearance of ossification sites of the carpal and tarsal bones are observed [46].

Joint	Structure	Gestational day of first appearance
Carpal bones	Accessory carpal bone	254
	Radial carpal bone	274
	Intermediate carpal bone	264–278
	Ulnar carpal bone	310
	Second, third, fourth carpal bones	280–310
Tarsal bones	Calcaneus	125
	Tuberosity calcaneus	305
	Central, first, second, third, fourth tarsal bones	280–325

ossification in the carpus at approximately 250 gestational days whereas the calcaneus is the first tarsal bone to commence ossification at approximately 125 gestational days (Table 3.3) [46]. Many neonatal foals have a layer of cartilage around the periphery of the cuboidal bones which imparts a rounded radiographic appearance whereas other neonatal foals appear fully ossified at birth; thus there is a considerable degree of variation in the amount of cartilage remaining in the healthy newborn [66, 71].

In contrast to healthy newborn foals, premature/dysmature foals frequently have varying degrees of incomplete ossification of the cuboidal bones of the carpus and tarsus [66, 72]. Because the cuboidal bones are incompletely ossified and malleable, they are susceptible to deformation. As the foal bears weight, loading forces on the incompletely ossified bones causes thinning of the precursor cartilage, which can result in compression, crushing, fragmentation, and ultimately permanent deformation of one or more cuboidal bones that are vital for normal range of joint movement and athletic activities [66, 72]. In the carpus, loading forces are not distributed perpendicularly along the long axis of the forelimb and thus place more bearing forces at certain locations. The lateral aspect of the carpus bears more stress from weight-bearing; therefore, cartilage compression between the ulnar and fourth carpal bones along with the intermediate and third carpal bones can occur, and if severe enough, result in carpal valgus. In contrast, incomplete ossification of the tarsal bones can result in defects in the saggital plane as body weight is transmitted from the long axis of the tibia to the long axis of the third metatarsal bone through the central and third tarsal bones [46, 71]. In some cases, crushing of the central and third tarsal bones can result in collapse of these bones and a characteristic sickle hock appearance (Figure 3.4).

Clinical signs of incomplete ossification may not be immediately apparent, especially if the premature/dysmature foal has other concurrent disease processes such as sepsis or neonatal encephalopathy. Signs of lameness are not frequently noted postpartum, but angular limb deformities such as carpal valgus (knock-kneed) or hyperextension and a broken tarsal axis (sickle-hock) can develop over the first weeks of life if incomplete ossification is unrecognized shortly after birth [72]. Affected foals may display a "bunny-hopping" gait associated with tarsal crushing of the cuboidal bones. Unrecognized cases can predispose the foal to conformational limb deformities, degenerative joint disease, or osteochondrosis dissecans [46, 72]. Diagnosis of incomplete ossification of the cuboidal bones is easily attained by evaluating lateral and anterior–posterior radiographic views of the carpus and tarsus (Figure 3.5). Radiographs should be performed in any neonatal foal that has predisposing factors that would contribute to delivery of a premature or dysmature foal. Adams and Poulus developed a skeletal ossification index to aid in grading the severity of incomplete ossification

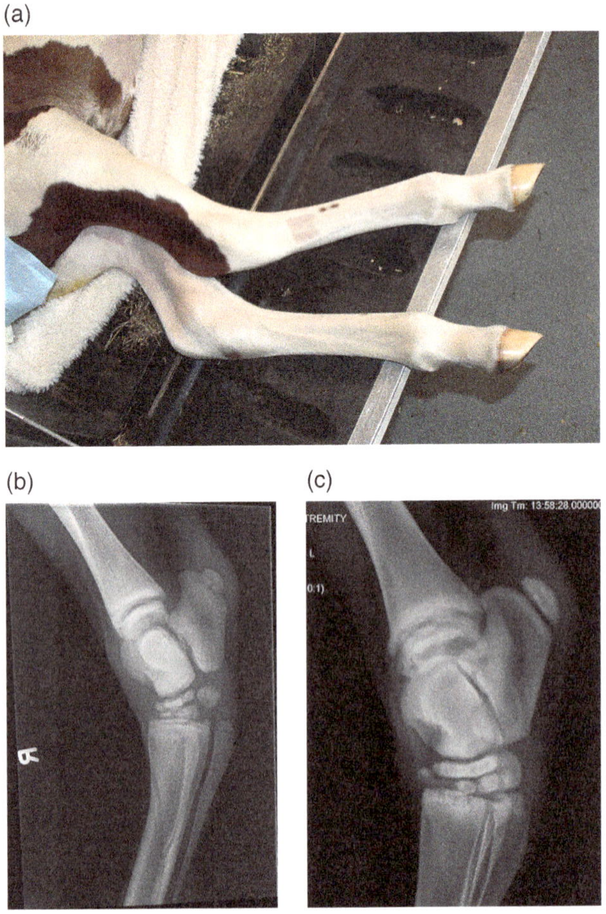

Figure 3.4 A neonatal foal with (a) sickle-hock appearance along with (b and c) corresponding radiographs of the tarsi.

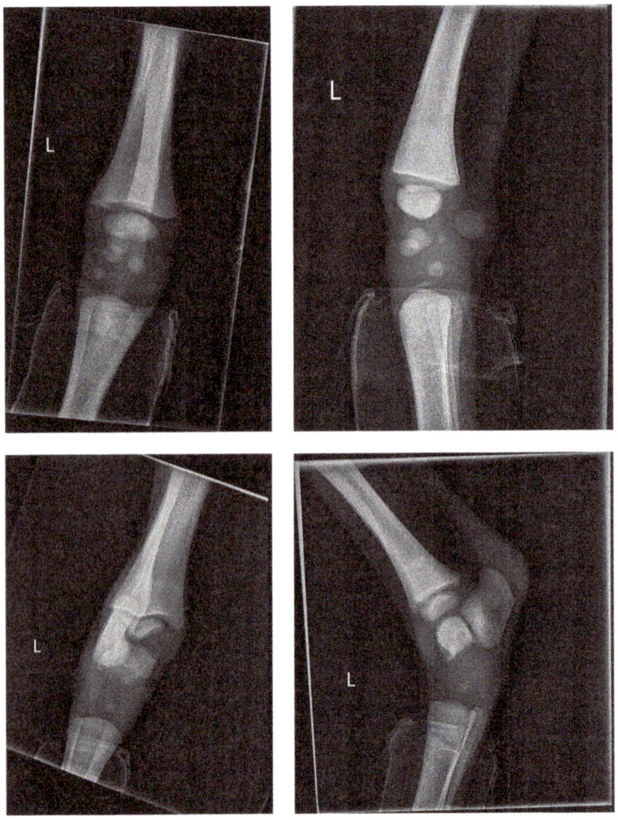

Figure 3.5 Lateral and dorso-palmar/plantar radiographs of a dysmature foal (foal in Figure 3.1a) with severe incomplete ossification of the carpal and tarsal cuboidal bones (grade 1 – skeletal ossification index).

(Table 3.4) and ultrasonographic examination of the tarsus has also been explored but is not widely used [73, 74]. If there is suspicion of hypothyroidism or if the foal has an enlarged thyroid gland, thyroid hormone assays should be evaluated.

Treatment principles of incomplete ossification revolve around maintaining the longitudinal axis of the limb and avoidance of crushing the cuboidal bones until they are sufficiently ossified [75]. Treatment will vary depending on the severity of incomplete ossification as well as other concurrent disease processes. Maintaining extension of the tarsal joint requires substantial muscular effort; as a result of weak muscle tone of the premature/ dysmature foal, compression and crushing of the dorsal portions of the third and central tarsal bones of the tarsus is not uncommon (Figure 3.4) [72]. Conservative therapy of mildly affected foals includes stall confinement, limited weight-bearing, and restriction of activity. Activity can be increased over time as radiographic appearance improves. Splints or tube casts, along with stall confinement and limited activity, can be used in more severe cases to support the limbs in the longitudinal axis while reducing compressive forces associated with weight bearing and ambulation [75]. Wheeled carts with appropriately sized slings can also be used in advanced cases to help reduce the amount of compressive forces on the cuboidal bones while still allowing the foal to suckle from the mare (Figure 3.6). Radiographs should be repeated every 2 weeks until ossification of the cuboidal bones is complete. A positive outcome can be attained in mild-to-moderate cases that are recognized early and treated appropriately; however, a guarded prognosis is warranted for high-performance athletes, especially if there is a large degree of incomplete ossification. Not surprisingly, in a retrospective study involving 22 foals with incomplete ossification of the tarsal bones, an association between severity of radiographic lesions and outcome was documented [72]. Specifically, foals with incomplete ossification and greater than 30% collapse (distance at the point of collapse compared to plantar aspect of

Table 3.4 Skeletal ossification index for neonatal foals [73].

Grade 1	• Some cuboidal bones have no radiographic signs of ossification.
Grade 2	• Some radiographic evidence of ossification is present in all cuboidal bones (excluding the first carpal and first tarsal bones).
	• Proximal epiphysis of either the third metacarpal or metatarsal bones is present, and the physis is radiographically open.
	• Lateral styloid process of the distal radius is absent or barely visible.
	• Malleoli of the tibia absent or barely visible.
Grade 3	• All cuboidal bones are ossified but are small with rounded edges.
	• Joint spaces appear wide.
	• Lateral styloid process and malleoli are distinct.
	• Proximal physis of either the third metacarpal bone or metatarsal bone is radiographically closed.
Grade 4	• All cuboidal bones are shaped like the corresponding bones in the adult.
	• Joint spaces are of expected width.

(a) (b)

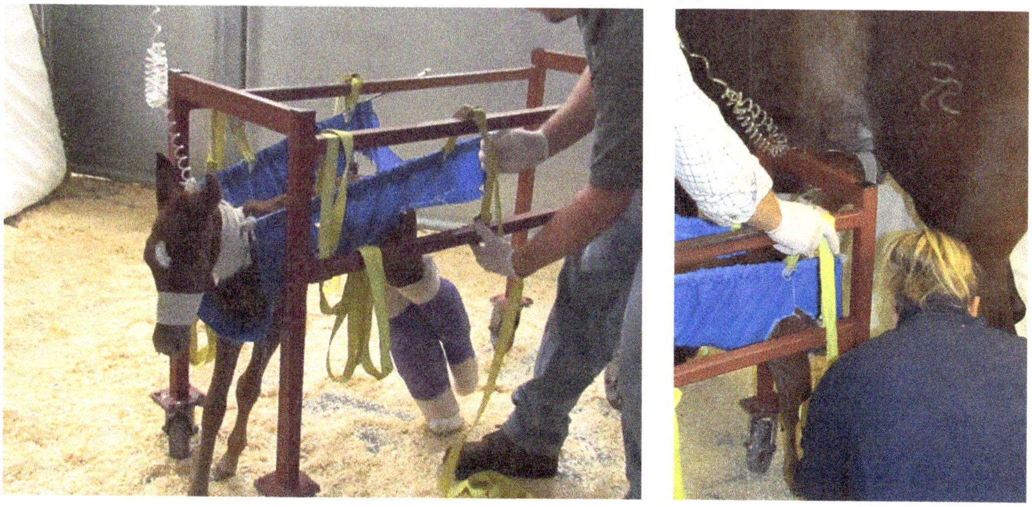

Figure 3.6 (a) Dysmature foal demonstrating small body size and incomplete ossification of the cuboidal bones. The foal only weighed 25 kg (5% of dam's body weight) as compared to the dam's body weight of 475 kg. (b) A wheeled cart and sling were used to help facilitate nursing from the mare.

tarsal bone) of the affected bones had a guarded prognosis for athletic soundness, with only 3/16 (19%) performing as intended. In comparison, 4 of 6 (67%) foals with less than 30% collapse performed as intended [72].

Flexor tendon weakness or laxity is common in healthy neonatal foals and is usually self-correcting. However, a higher association and severity of flexor tendon laxity is present in premature/dysmature neonatal foals [76]. More severe cases can rock back on the hoof wall when standing (Figure 3.1). Despite the severity, many of these cases resolve spontaneously over days to weeks as the musculotendinous structures become stronger. In some instances, placement of heel extensions may help hasten the tendon laxity. When concurrent incomplete ossification of the cuboidal bones is present, a quandary between splinting or casting of the limb to protect the cuboidal bones typically outweighs the fact that the immobilization of the limb will induce further laxity in the flexor tendons.

Respiratory

Premature and dysmature foals can have varying degrees of pulmonary dysfunction or insufficiency and are more susceptible to development of dependent lung atelectasis [32, 77]. These foals tend to have compliant chest walls along with weak respiratory muscles, stiff lungs, altered pulmonary vascular reactivity, a naïve and potentially immature immune system, and a tendency for prolonged or continuous recumbency [32, 77]. These circumstances serve as risk factors for respiratory dysfunction and hypoventilation. In addition, lung stiffness associated with structural immaturity along with high compliance of the immature chest wall results in low end-expiratory lung volume in the newborn foal [78]. If present, surfactant deficiency or dysfunction and high alveolar surface tension can compound lung dysfunction and further decrease end-expiratory lung volume, ultimately contributing to increased work of breathing [78]. Clinically, respiratory dysfunction can manifest as reduced ventilation capacity, tachypnea, hypoxemia, and hypercapnia [32, 77].

Surfactant deficiency is uncommonly recognized disease process in foals but can be associated with premature/dysmature foals [79, 80]. Pulmonary surfactant reduces the alveolar surface tension and allows inflation of the lungs, thereby reducing the work of breathing [81]. In people, *respiratory distress syndrome*, also known as *surfactant dysfunction* or *hyaline membrane disease*, occurs in premature infants and is characterized as a primary surfactant deficiency. Affected infants typically have respiratory distress (tachypnea, nasal flaring, expiratory grunting) at the time of birth that worsens over time along with hypoxemia and apnea. In the equine fetus, evidence of surfactant production was observed at 150 days gestation but maturation of surfactant occurs at or after 300 days of gestation (88% of gestation) and is not always fully developed at full term [82, 83]. Some sources suggest that surfactant maturation is not complete until late gestation, or after birth, based on increased surface tension in newborn foals as compared to adult horses [81, 83]. Surfactant deficiency is not common and does not play a primary role in respiratory dysfunction in most premature/dysmature foals, but the true incidence has not been documented [32, 77, 84]. However, a definition of neonatal equine respiratory distress syndrome (NERDS) has been proposed, with a diagnosis established by meeting a specific set of criteria (Table 3.5) [85].

The incidence of persistent pulmonary hypertension of the newborn (PPHN) in the foal is also unknown, but is presumably low, with only a few reports being documented in the veterinary literature [85–87]. In infants, PPHN affects mainly at-term or post-term newborns, although it can occur in premature infants as well [88]. In brief, PPHN is a syndrome caused by a failure of the circulatory adaptation at birth due to a delay or impairment of the normal decrease in pulmonary vascular resistance that occurs following birth resulting in a state of pulmonary hypertension [88]; the elevated pulmonary vascular resistance causes right-to-left shunt through the ductus arteriosus and/or foramen ovale. Affected individuals consequently have varying degrees of hypoxemic respiratory failure [89]. The limited

Table 3.5 Definition of NERDS: Neonatal Equine Respiratory Distress Syndrome [85].

Etiology: Primary surfactant deficiency due to failure of final fetal pulmonary surfactant maturation. Diagnosis requires meeting all criteria listed below:

1. Persistent hypoxemia, progressive hypercapnia
   a. Hypoxemia defined as $PaO_2 < 60$ mmHg; sample collected with foal in lateral recumbency while breathing room air
2. Appropriate risk factors present: (1 or more of 3)
   a. Very early gestational age: less than 290 d of gestation OR less than 88% of average of dam's previous gestation lengths
   b. Induction of parturition
   c. Caesarian section
3. Failure to develop normal immediate postpartum respiratory patters: development/persistence of paradoxical breathing over first several hours of life, persistent tachypnea
4. At 24 h of age or less "ground glass" appearance of lateral radiograph(s) of lungs taken either standing or in lateral recumbency
5. Absence of evidence of fetal inflammatory response syndrome (FIRS) at birth
   a. Normal white blood cell count, differential and fibrinogen concentration for gestational age
6. Congenital cardiac disease ruled out as cause of hypoxemia

case reports in foals had clinical signs of weakness and inability to suckle along with moderate respiratory distress, tachycardia, tachypnea, nasal flaring, cyanotic membranes, and weakness [85–87]. A loud systolic murmur on the left side of the thorax along with a split-second heart sound coupled with acidemia and hypoxia were also reported in a 10-hour old foal [85–87]. Conditions such as meconium aspiration, sepsis, cesarean delivery, and asphyxia are associated with PPHN, although many cases of PPHN are idiopathic [88]. Treatment includes mechanical ventilation, oxygen supplementation, surfactant replacement therapy, inhaled nitric oxide and/or administration of sildenafil [85–89]. PPHN is further discussed in other sections of the textbook, and a number of reviews are available in infants [86, 88, 89].

Clinical evaluation of the premature or dysmature foal with respiratory dysfunction can reveal increased respiratory rate and effort. Auscultation of the lungs is a worthwhile endeavor, keeping in mind that auscultation is not a sensitive method of evaluating respiratory status in neonatal foals as it is not uncommon for foals with severe pulmonary disease to have normal lung sounds [78]. More objective methods of evaluating respiratory function include collection of an arterial blood sample and measurement of the partial pressure of oxygen (P_aO_2) and carbon dioxide (P_aCO_2) as well as assessment of pH. The P_aO_2 of healthy neonatal foals is lower than that measured in adult horses; thus, age-appropriate reference intervals should be used for comparison (Table 3.6) [90]. Other factors that can contribute to abnormal blood gas parameters in premature/dysmature foals include extrapulmonary shunts, which can account for 30% of cardiac output in comparison to <10% in healthy foals, as well as ventilation-perfusion mismatch, which can occur from dependent atelectasis and poorly reactive pulmonary vasculature [32, 77, 91]. Thoracic radiographs also aid in evaluation of the respiratory system. In foals with surfactant dysfunction or deficiency, radiographs can appear hazy with a ground-glass appearance of the lung field; alternatively, air bronchograms can be present, suggestive of atelectasis and/or hyaline membrane disease [78]. Other radiographic changes associated with hyaline membrane disease include a generalized interstitial density and prominent air bronchograms [78].

Treatment of premature/dysmature foals with respiratory dysfunction includes assessment of systemic oxygenation and, if indicated, administration of unilateral or bilateral humidified intranasal oxygen. Reported fractional inspired oxygen values using unilateral and bilateral nasal canulae have been reported in the healthy neonatal foal to guide therapy (Table 3.7) and oxygen flow rates can be adjusted based on serial arterial blood gas analysis [90]. Recumbent foals should be maintained in sternal recumbency, facilitated with a V-pad or other support to minimize prolonged lateral recumbency and decrease the effects of dependent atelectasis. If the foal is hypercapnic due to hypoventilation secondary to neonatal encephalopathy, a constant rate infusion of doxapram (0.02–0.05 mg/kg/hr) can help increase respiratory rate. Orally administered caffeine (7.5–12 mg/kg loading dose followed by 2.5–10 mg/kg daily dose) can also be used for the same purpose but was less effective than doxapram in one study [86, 92]. If foals continue to have moderate to severe hypoxemia and/or hypercapnia, mechanical ventilator support may be indicated, if available. Mechanical ventilation improves gas exchange by increasing ventilation, improving V/Q matching, decreases intra-pulmonary shunting, and decreases work of breathing [86]. Clinical conditions where mechanical ventilation may be beneficial include PPHN, acute respiratory failure, neonatal encephalopathy-associated central respiratory center failure, weakness associated with prematurity/dysmaturity, central or sepsis-induced hypotension, septic shock, and botulism [86].

Table 3.6 Arterial blood gas values from healthy foals age various ages during the neonatal period [90].

Age (h)	P_aO_2 (mmHg)	S_aO_2 (%)	P_aCO_2 (mmHg)	pH_a
12	64.6 ± 11.6	92.2 ± 4.7	42.4 ± 2.9	7.433 ± 0.015
24	69.9 ± 6.6	94.8 ± 1.7	39.4 ± 2.9	7.445 ± 0.024
36	69.3 ± 12.3	93.4 ± 5.4	41.3 ± 4.0	7.433 ± 0.022
48	72.1 ± 7.7	95.1 ± 1.8	41.0 ± 3.0	7.435 ± 0.017
72	78.8 ± 8.8	96.5 ± 1.3	40.8 ± 2.8	7.441 ± 0.021
96	78.2 ± 7.9	96.3 ± 1.7	38.8 ± 2.9	7.452 ± 0.032
120	78.4 ± 5.9	96.5 ± 1.2	38.5 ± 2.4	7.459 ± 0.020

Other Body Systems

Dysphagia, abnormal thermoregulation, abnormal blood glucose regulation, abnormal gastrointestinal function and congenital cardiac defects may also be observed in premature/dysmature foals. Premature/dysmature foals can have dysphagia associated with pharyngeal dysfunction. In one case series involving 16 neonatal foals with dysphagia, 2 were identified as dysmature and 8/16 (50%) affected foals were premature and/or diagnosed with neonatal encephalopathy [93]. Of these foals, 12/16 (75%) had evidence of aspiration pneumonia. Supportive treatment was provided to include controlled enteral feedings through a feeding tube for several days (median 4 days; range 1–14 days) and antimicrobials. In that report, 15/16 foals were discharged from the hospital and were able to nurse from the mare with no evidence of dysphagia in 14 foals [93].

Table 3.7 Oxygen parameters obtained in healthy foals administered unilateral and bilateral intranasal oxygen at different oxygen flow rates [90].

		Oxygen delivery							
		Unilateral (ml/kg/min)				Bilateral (ml/kg/min)			
Variable	**Baseline**	**50**	**100**	**150**	**200**	**50**	**100**	**150**	**200**
FIO_2 (%)	18.0±0.7	23.0±1.4	30.9±2.1	44.2±5.8	52.6±8.3	30.9±2.6	48.7±6.2	56.4±3.4	74.6±4.2
PaO_2 (mm Hg)	92.5±8.2	135.9±13.2	175.2±14.6	219.6±31.9	269.7±40.8	174.3±26.8	261.2±38.3	307.8±41.0	374.2±58.2
$PaCO_2$ (mm Hg)	47.7±2.8	49.7±2.4	50.5±2.3	50.1±2.8	51.3±3.1	49.8±1.8	51.0±2.2	49.8±2.9	48.6±3.6
SaO_2 (%)	96.7±0.7	98.5±0.3	99.2±0.1	99.4±0.2	99.6±0.1	99.1±0.3	99.6±0.1	99.7±0.1	99.8±0.1

Premature/dysmature foals are also more susceptible to hypothermia, but ambient environmental factors play a role in body temperature [32]. Thermogenic mechanisms are related to circulating T3 concentrations, which is closely related to the maturation of the HPAA; thus normal thyroid hormone concentrations may be absent in premature/dysmature foals, contributing to improper thermoregulation [32, 77]. However, one small study involving three dysmature neonatal foals described the ability of dysmature foals to thermoregulate body temperature and evaluated metabolic rate [94]. In this study, dysmature foals were able to thermoregulate effectively with a mean rectal temperature of 38.2±0.3 °C, similar in magnitude to healthy foals. The reported metabolic rate in the three dysmature foals involved in this study were 114, 174, and 68 W per unit area of body surface (W/m^2) [94]. Body temperature should be carefully monitored in premature/dysmature foals and blankets and warmed IV fluids should be used initially to warm the foal and avoid peripheral vasodilation/cardiovascular compromise that can occur if warming occurs too rapidly. Subsequently heat lamps, forced-air warming devices or warm-water blankets can be utilized to help attain and maintain normothermia.

Affected foals often have difficulty regulating blood glucose and are frequently hypoglycemic because of limited glycogen stores and inadequate gluconeogenic enzyme activity [32, 77]. A constant rate infusion of dextrose solution at 5–8 mg/kg/min may help to maintain adequate blood glucose concentrations [86]; blood glucose concentration should be monitored regularly. In addition, these foals may have incomplete maturation of the gastrointestinal tract, which can manifest as gastric distention, intestinal stasis, gas accumulation, and reduced fecal passage. Small volumes of milk (10–50 ml/hr) should be provided initially to premature/dysmature foals to test the gastrointestinal tract's ability to digest food. Parental nutrition can also be considered if the clinician anticipates a prolonged inability to use the gastrointestinal tract for nutritional management. In addition, failure of passive transfer of immunity should be assessed and treated with a plasma transfusion, if necessary. Little is known about renal function in premature/dysmature foals but the fractional excretion of sodium was higher in newborn premature infants (1–5%) when compared to the term infant (0.3%), suggesting that immature tubular function may be present in some premature infants [95, 96]. One study involving induced-premature foals noted a rapid loss of serum sodium concentrations when administered furosemide, when compared to healthy-term foals [97]. In one report, 6/18 foals with congenital cardiac defects were premature or dysmature; therefore, the heart should be critically evaluated in these foals as well [98].

Prognosis

Limited information is available in regard to the prognosis for survival and athletic potential in premature/dysmature foals but prognosis can be based on a number of factors such as the degree of development of the various organ systems (e.g. respiratory, cuboidal bones), concurrent diseases processes, financial commitment of the owner, and future intended use (performance verse pasture horse). In one study, short-term survival was partially predicted by the total white cell count, neutrophil count, lymphocyte count and N/L ratio. In that study, the N/L ratio of surviving premature foals (12.5±1.7 : 1) was higher than that from healthy-term foals (2.5 : 1) and nonsurviving premature foals (3.2±1.7 : 1) [32, 77]. Outcome was not affected by gestational age, as the gestational length in survivors (born at 311 days) was similar to nonsurvivors (born at 307 days); this suggests that in utero stress or infection may help mature the HPAA and prepare some premature foals for survival after birth [32, 77]. In another study involving induced premature foals, the N/L ratio in surviving foals was initially low (1.1) but increased to 3.16 over the next 18 hours, whereas nonsurviving premature foals remained <1.3 [49]. In regard to future performance, a study evaluated 454 foals and noted that the 44 foals that were premature/dysmature were significantly less likely to race, had fewer starts and wins, and had lower earnings than their maternal siblings [99]. Only 17/34 (50%) of registered foals that were premature/dysmature started a race as compared to 79.5% of their siblings [99]. Incomplete ossification of the cuboidal bones of the carpus and tarsus was a proposed contributing factor to the poor racing performance in the premature/dysmature foals. Most premature/dysmature foals that survive the initial neonatal period will maintain a smaller size as compared to healthy peers for the first year of life, but this size discrepancy can become less apparent as they mature into adults.

References

1 Rossdale, P.D., Ousey, J.C., Silver, M. et al. (1984). Studies on equine prematurity 6: guidelines for assessment of foal maturity. *Equine Vet. J.* 16: 300–302.

2 Rossdale, P.D. (1993). Clinical view of disturbances in equine foetal maturation. *Equine Vet. J. Suppl.* 14: 3–7.

3 Davies Morel, M.C., Newcombe, J.R., and Holland, S.J. (2002). Factors affecting gestation length in the Thoroughbred mare. *Anim. Reprod. Sci.* 74: 175–185.

4 Clothier, J., Hinch, G., Brown, W. et al. (2017). Equine gestational length and location: is there more that the research could be telling us? *Aust. Vet. J.* 95: 454–461.

5 Rossdale, P.D. (1967). Clinical studies on the newborn thoroughbred foal. 1: perinatal behaviour. *Br. Vet. J.* 123: 470–481.

6 McCue, P.M. and Ferris, R.A. (2012). Parturition, dystocia and foal survival: a retrospective study of 1047 births. *Equine Vet. J. Suppl.* 41: 22–25.

7 Heck, L., Clauss, M., and Sanchez-Villagra, M.R. (2017). Gestation length variation in domesticated horses and its relation to breed and body size diversity. *Mammal. Biol.* 84: 44–51.

8 Sevinga, M., Barkema, H.W., Styhn, H. et al. (2004). Retained placenta in Freisian mares: incidence, and potential risk factors with special emphasis on gestational length. *Theriogenology* 61: 851–859.

9 Valera, M., Blesa, F., Dos Santos, R. et al. (2006). Genetic study of gestation length in Andalusian and Arabian mares. *Anim. Reprod. Sci.* 95: 75–96.

10 Bos, H. and Van Dermey, G.J.W. (1980). Length of gestation periods of horses and ponies belonging to different breeds. *Livest. Prod. Sci.* 7: 181–187.

11 Ali, A., Alamaary, M., and Al-Sobayil, F. (2014). Reproductive performance of Arab mares in the Kingdom of Saudi Arabia. *Tierarztl. Prax. Ausg. G Grosstiere Nutztiere* 42: 145–149.

12 Bene, S., Benedek, Z., Nagy, S. et al. (2014). Some effects on gestation length of traditional horse breeds in Hungary. *J. Cent. Eur. Agric.* 15: 1–10.

13 Perez, C.C., Rodriguez, I., Moto, J. et al. (2003). Gestation length in Carthusian Spanishbred mares. *Livest. Prod. Sci.* 82: 181–187.

14 Marteniuk, J.V., Carleton, C.L., Lloyd, J.W. et al. (1998). Association of sex of fetus, sire, month of conception, or year of foaling with duration of gestation in Standardbred mares. *J. Am. Vet. Med. Assoc.* 212: 1743–1745.

15 Dicken, M., Gee, E.K., Rogers, C.W. et al. (2012). Gestation length and occurrence of daytime foaling of Standardbred mares on two stud farms in New Zealand. *N. Z. Vet. J.* 60: 42–46.

16 Rezac, P., Pospisilova, D., Slama, P. et al. (2013). Different effects of month of conception and birth on gestation length in mares. *J. Anim. Vet. Adv.* 12: 731–735.

17 Ewert, M., Luders, I., Borocz, J. et al. (2018). Determinants of gestation length in Thoroughbred mares on German stud farms. *Ann. Reprod. Sci.* 191: 22–33.

18 Carluccio, A., Gloria, A., Veronesi, M.C. et al. (2015). Factors affecting pregnancy length and phases of parturition in Martina Franca jennies. *Theriogenology* 84: 650–655.

19 Galisteo, J. and Perez-Marin, C.C. (2010). Factors affecting gestation length and estrus cycle characteristics in Spanish donkey breeds reared in southern Spain. *Theriogenology* 74: 443–450.

20 Rosales, C., Krekeler, N., Tennent-Brown, B. et al. (2017). Periparturient characteristics of mares and their foals on a New Zealand Thoroughbred stud farm. *N. Z. Vet. J.* 65: 24–29.

21 Giger, R., Meier, H.P., and Kupfer, U. (1997). Length of gestation of Freiberger mares with mule and horse foals. *Schweiz. Arch. Tierheilkd.* 139: 303–307.

22 Flade, J.E. and Frederich, W. (1964). Beitrag zum Problem der Trachtigkeitsdauer und zy ihrer faktoriellen Abhangigkeit beim. *Pferd Arch. Tierz.* 6: 505–520.

23 Howell, C.E. and Rollins, W.C. (1951). Environmental sources of variation in the gestation length of the horse. *J. Anim. Sci.* 10: 789–796.

24 Koterba, A.M. (1993). Definitions of equine perinatal disorders: problems and solutions. *Equine Vet. Educ.* 5: 271–273.

25 Frigoletto, F.D., Tullis, J.L., Reid, D.E. et al. (1971). Hypercoagulability in the dysmature syndrome. *Am. J. Obstet. Gynecol.* 111: 867–873.

26 Szalay, G. (1973). The meaning of dysmature. *Calif. Med.* 118: 41.
27 Sjostedt, S., Engleson, G., and Rooth, G. (1958). Dysmaturity. *Arch. Dis. Child.* 33: 123–130.
28 Clifford, S.H. (1945). Clinical significance of yellow staining of the vernix caseosa, skin, nails and umbilical cord. *Am. J. Dis. Child.* 69: 1945.
29 Ting, R.Y., Wang, M.H., and McNair-Scott, T.F. (1977). The dysmature infant. Associated factors and outcome at 7 years of age. *J. Pediatr.* 90: 943–948.
30 Han, V.K.M. (1993). Pathophysiology, cellular and molecular mechanisms of foetal growth retardation. *Equine Vet. J. Suppl.* 14: 12–16.
31 Platt, H. (1984). Growth of the equine foetus. *Equine Vet. J.* 16: 247–252.
32 Lester, G.D. (2005). Maturity of the neonatal foal. *Vet. Clin. Equine* 21: 333–355.
33 Breuhaus, B.A. (2014). Thyroid function and dysfunction in term and premature equine neonates. *J. Vet. Intern. Med.* 28: 1301–1309.
34 LeBlanc, M.M., Giguere, S., Lester, G.D. et al. (2012). Relationship between infection, inflammation and premature parturition in mares with experimentally induced placentitis. *Equine Vet. J.* 44 (Suppl 41): 8–14.
35 Cross, D.L., Redmond, L.M., and Strickland, J.R. (1995). Equine fescue toxicosis: signs and solutions. *J. Anim. Sci.* 73: 899–908.
36 Monroe, M.S., Cross, D.L., Hudson, L.W. et al. (1988). Effect of selenium and endophyte-contaminated fescue on performance and reproduction in mares. *J. Equine Vet. Sci.* 8: 148–153.
37 Putnam, M.R., Bransby, D.I., Schumacher, J. et al. (1991). Effects of fungal endophyte *Acremonium coenophialum* in fescue on pregnant mares and foal viability. *Am. J. Vet. Res.* 52: 2071–2074.
38 Driscoll, J., Hintz, H.F., and Schryver, H.F. (1978). Goiter in foals caused by excessive iodine. *J. Am. Vet. Med. Assoc.* 173: 858–859.
39 McLaughlin, B.G., Doige, C.E., and McLaughlin, P.S. (1986). Thyroid hormone levels in foals with congenital musculoskeletal lesions. *Can. Vet. J.* 27: 264–267.
40 McLaughlin, B.G. and Doige, C.E. (1981). Congenital musculoskeletal lesions and hyperplastic goitre in foals. *Can. Vet. J.* 22: 130–133.
41 Doige, C.E. and McLaughlin, B.G. (1981). Hyperplastic goiter in newborn foals in Western Canada. *Can. Vet. J.* 22: 42–45.
42 Allen, A.L., Doige, C.E., Fretz, P.B. et al. (1994). Hyperplasia of the thyroid gland and concurrent musculoskeletal deformities in western Canadian foals: reexamination of a previously described syndrome. *Can. Vet. J.* 35: 31–38.
43 Baker, J.R., Wyn-Joines, G., and Eley, J.L. (1983). Case of equine goitre. *Vet. Rec.* 112: 407–408.
44 Gawrylash, S.K. (1004). Thryoid hyperplasia and musculoskeletal deformity in a Standardbred filly in Ontario. *Can. Vet. J.* 45: 424–426.
45 Silver, M., Fowden, A.L., Know, J. et al. (1991). Relationship between circulating tri-iodothyronine and cortisol in the perinatal period in the foal. *J. Reprod. Fertil. Suppl.* 44: 619–626.
46 Coleman, M.C. and Whitfield-Cargile, C. (2017). Orthopedic conditions of the premature and dysmature foal. *Vet. Clin. N. Am. Equine* 33: 289–297.
47 Koikkalainen, K., Knuuttila, A., Karikoski, N. et al. (2014). Congenital hypothyroidism and dysmaturity syndrome in foals: first reported cases in Europe. *Equine Vet. Educ.* 26: 181–189.
48 Allen, A.L., Townsend, H.G., Doige, C.E. et al. (1996). A case-control study of the congenital hypothyroidism and dysmaturity syndrome of foals. *Can. Vet. J.* 37: 349–358.
49 Jeffcott, L.B., Rossdale, P.D., and Leadon, D.P. (1982). Haematological changes in the neonatal period of normal and induced premature foals. *J. Reprod. Fertil. Suppl.* 32: 537–544.
50 Nathanielsz, P.W., Berghorn, K.A., Derks, J.B. et al. (2003). Life before death: effects of cortisol on future cardiovascular and metabolic function. *Acta Paediatr.* 92: 766–772.
51 Cudd, T.A., LeBlanc, M., Silver, M. et al. (1995). Ontogeny and ultradian rhythms of adrenocorticotropin and cortisol in the late-gestation fetal horse. *J. Endocrinol.* 144: 271–283.
52 Rossdale, P., Silver, M., Comeline, R.S. et al. (1973). Plasma cortisol in the foal during the late fetal and early neonatal period. *Res. Vet. Sci.* 15: 395–397.
53 Conley, A.J. (2016). Review of the reproductive endocrinology of the pregnant and parturient mare. *Theriogenology* 86: 355–365.
54 Fowden, A.L., Forhead, A.J., and Ousey, J.C. (2012). Endocrine adaptations in the foal over the perinatal period. *Equine Vet. J. Suppl.* 130–139.
55 Fowden, A.L., Silver, M., Ellis, L. et al. (1984). Studies on equine prematurity 3: insulin secretion in the foal during the perinatal period. *Equine Vet. J.* 16: 286–291.
56 Barsnick, R., Hurcombe, S.D.A., Dembek, K. et al. (2014). Somatotropic axis resistance and ghrelin in critically ill foals. *Equine Vet. J.* 46: 45–49.
57 Fowden, A.L., Forhead, A.J., and Ousey, J.C. (2008). The endocrinology of equine parturition. *Exp. Endocrinol. Diabetes* 116: 393–403.
58 Rossdale, P.D., Silver, M., Ellis, L. et al. (1982). Response of the adrenal cortex to tetracosactrin (ACTH1-24) in the premature and full-term foal. *J. Reprod. Fertil. Suppl.* 32: 545–553.

59 Ousey, J.C., Kolling, M., Kindahl, H. et al. (2011). Maternal dexamethasone treatment in late gestation induces precocious fetal maturation and delivery in healthy Thoroughbred mares. *Equine Vet. J.* 43: 424–429.

60 Silver, M., Ousey, J.C., Dudan, F.E. et al. (1984). Studies on equine prematurity 2: post natal adrenocortical activity in relation to plasma adrenocorticotrophic hormone and catecholamine levels in term and premature foals. *Equine Vet. J.* 16: 278–286.

61 Irvine, C.H. and Evans, M.J. (1975). Postnatal changes in total and free thyroxine and triiodothyronine in foal serum. *J. Reprod. Fertil. Suppl.* 23: 709–715.

62 Wallace, M.J., Hooper, S.B., and Harding, R. (1996). Role of the adrenal glands in the maturation of lung liquid secretory mechanisms in fetal sheep. *Am. J. Physiol.* 270 (1 Pt 2): R33–R40.

63 Van Wassenaer, A.G. and Kok, J.H. (2004). Hypothyroxinaemia and thyroid function after pre-term birth. *Semin. Neonatol.* 9: 3–11.

64 Holdstock, N.B., Allen, V.L., Bloomfield, M.R. et al. (2004). Development of insulin and proinsulin in newborn pony foals. *J. Endocrinol.* 181: 469–476.

65 Barsnick, R.J.I.M., Hurcombe, S.D.A., Smith, P.A. et al. (2011). Insulin, glucagon, and leptin in critically ill foals. *J. Vet. Intern. Med.* 25: 123–131.

66 Haywood, L., Spike-Pierce, D.L., Barr, B. et al. (2018). Gestation length and racing performance in 115 Thoroughbred foals with incomplete tarsal ossification. *Equine Vet. J.* 50: 29–33.

67 Auer, J.A. Angular limb deformities. In: *Equine Surgery* (ed. J.A. Auer), 940–946. Philadelphia: W.B. Saunders Co.

68 Sedrish, S.A. and Moore, R.M. (1997). Diagnosis and management of incomplete ossification of the cuboidal bones in foals. *Equine Pract.* 19: 16–21.

69 Fretz, P.B. (1980). Angular limb deformities in foals. *Vet. Clin. N. Am. Large Anim. Pract.* 2: 125–150.

70 Auer, J.A., Martens, R.J., and Morris, E.L. (1982). Angular limb deformities in foals: I. Congenital factors. *Comp. Contin. Educ. Pract. Vet.* 4: 330–339.

71 McIlwraith, C.W. (1987). Incomplete or defective ossification of carpal or tarsal bones. In: *Adam's Lameness in Horses*, 4e (ed. T.S. Stashak), 419–432. Philadelphia: Lea & Febiger.

72 Dutton, D.M., Watkins, J.P., Walker, M.A. et al. (1998). Incomplete ossification of the tarsal bones in foals: 22 cases (1988–1996). *J. Am. Vet. Med. Assoc.* 213: 1590–1493.

73 Adams, R. and Poulos, P. (1988). A skeletal ossification index for neonatal foals. *Vet. Radiol.* 29: 217–222.

74 Ruohoniemi, M. (1993). Use of ultrasonography to evaluate the degree of ossification of the small tarsal bones in 10 foals. *Equine Vet. J.* 25: 539–543.

75 Leitch, M. (1985). Musculoskeletal disorders in neonatal foals. *Vet. Clin. North Am. Equine Pract.* 1: 189–207.

76 Orsini, J.A. and Kreuder, C. (1994). Musculoskeletal disorders of the neonate. *Vet. Clin. North Am. Equine Pract.* 10: 137–166.

77 Lester, G.D. Outcomes in foals with a gestational age less than 320 days. In: *Proceedings of the Neonatal Septicemia Workshop* (ed. M.R. Paradis), 42–44. Dorothy Russell Havemayer Foundation, Inc.

78 Costa, L.R.R., Eades, S.C., Goad, M.E. et al. (2004). Pulmonary surfactant dysfunction in neonatal foals: pathogenesis and clinical findings. *Comp. Equine* 26: 384–389.

79 Kosch, P.C., Koterbra, A.M., Coons, T.J. et al. (1984). Developments in management of the newborn foal in respiratory distress 1: evaluation. *Equine Vet. J.* 16: 312–318.

80 Vaala, W.E. (1986). Diagnosis and treatment of prematurity and neonatal maladjustment syndrome in newborn foals. *Compend. Contin. Educ. Pract. Vet.* 8: s211–s225.

81 Christmann, U., Livesay, L.C., Taintor, J.S. et al. (2006). Lung surfactant function and composition in neonatal foals and adult horses. *J. Vet. Intern. Med.* 20: 1402–1407.

82 Arvidson, G., Astedt, B., Ekelund, L. et al. (1975). Surfactant studies in the fetal and neonatal foal. *J. Reprod. Fertil.* 23. Suppl: 663–665.

83 Pattle, R.E., Rossdale, P.D., Schock, C. et al. (1975). The development of the lung and its surfactant in the foal and in other species. *J. Reprod. Fertil.* 23 (Suppl): 651–657.

84 Rossdale, P.D., Pattle, R.E., and Mahaffey, L.W. (1967). Respiratory distress in a newborn foal with failure to form lung lining film. *Nature* 215: 1498–1499.

85 Wilkins, P.A. (2003). Lower respiratory problems of the neonate. *Vet. Clin. Equine* 19: 19–33.

86 Palmer, J.E. (2005). Ventilatory support of the critically ill foal. *Vet. Clin. Equine* 21: 457–486.

87 Cottrill, C.M., O'Connor, W.N., Cudd, T. et al. (1987). Persistence of foetal circulatory pathways in a newborn foal. *Equine Vet. J.* 19: 252–255.

88 Cabral, J.E.B. and Belik, J. (2013). Persistent pulmonary hypertension of the newborn: recent advances in pathophysiology and treatment. *J. Pediatr. (Rio J)* 89: 226–242.

89 Matthew, B. and Lakshminrusimha, S. (2017). Persistent pulmonary hypertension in the newborn. *Children (Basel)* 28: 1–14.

90 Wong, D.M., Hepworth-Warren, K.L., Sponseller, B.T. et al. (2017). Measured and calculated variables of global oxygenation in healthy neonatal foals. *Am. J. Vet. Res.* 78: 230–238.

91 Rose, J.R. and Stewart, J. (1983). Basic concepts of respiratory and cardiovascular function and dysfunction in the full term and premature foal. *Proc. Am. Assoc. Equine Pract.* 29: 167–178.

92 Giguere, S., Slade, J.K., and Sanchez, L.C. (2008). Retrospective comparison of caffeine and doxapram for the treatment of hypercapnia in foals with hypoxic-ischemic encephalopathy. *J. Vet. Intern. Med.* 22: 401–405.

93 Holcombe, S.J., Hurcombe, S.D., Barr, B.S. et al. (2012). Dysphagia associated with presumed pharyngeal dysfunction in 16 neonatal foals. *Equine Vet. J.* 44 (Suppl. 41): 105–108.

94 Ousey, J.C., McArthur, A.J., and Rossdale, P.D. (1997). Thermoregulation in sick foals aged less than one week. *Vet. J.* 153: 185–196.

95 Aperia, A., Broberger, O., Herin, P. et al. (1979). Sodium excretion in relation to sodium intake and aldosterone excretion in newborn pre-term and full-term infants. *Acta Paediatr. Scand.* 68: 813–817.

96 Bueva, A. and Guignard, J.P. (1994). Renal function in preterm neonates. *Peadiatr. Res.* 36: 572–577.

97 Pipkin, F.B., Ousey, J.C., Wallace, C.P. et al. (1984). Studies on equine prematurity 4: effect of salt and water loss on the renin-angiotensin-aldosterone system in the newborn foal. *Equine Vet. J.* 16: 292–297.

98 Hall, T.L., Magdesian, K.G., and Kittleson, M.D. (2010). Congenital cardiac defects in neonatal foals: 18 cases (1992–2007). *J. Vet. Intern. Med.* 24 (1): 206–212.

99 Chidlow, H., Giguere, S., and Sanchez, L.C. (2019). Factors associated with long-term athletic outcome in thoroughbred neonates admitted to an intensive care unit. *Equine Vet. J.* 51: 716–719.

Part II

Disorders of the Neonatal Foal

Neonatal Respiratory System

Chapter 4 Embryology and Anatomy of the Respiratory System

David Wong

The main function of the respiratory system is to deliver air/oxygen to red blood cells and remove carbon dioxide from the blood. This is accomplished through a series of conducting airways that connect the atmospheric air with the alveoli, where gas exchange occurs. Included structures in these conducting airways are the nares, nasal cavity, pharynx, larynx, trachea, and bronchioles. Exchange of gas then occurs in the alveoli and alveolar ducts, both of which are lined with extensive pulmonary capillaries that create a massive vascular surface area for oxygen and carbon dioxide diffusion. A detailed review of the embryologic development of the lung is presented in Chapter 1; the section here provides further information about other portions of the respiratory system in the neonatal foal.

The external naris allows a degree of opening and closing of the conducting airways and are supported by the alar cartilages that provide rigidity to the nostril. Muscles attached to the alar cartilages include the *levator nasolabialis*, *dilator naris lateralis*, and *transversus nasi* that allow movement of the external nares. In the equine embryo, the nose, parts of the face rostral to the eyes and dorsal to the mouth are formed by day 20 of gestation, and by day 60 of gestation, the nostrils are formed, including the alar cartilage [1]. Traveling down the conducting airways, the nasal cavity is divided into three passages (dorsal, middle, and ventral meatuses) by the dorsal and ventral turbinates. The ventral meatus has the largest cross-sectional area and provides a direct pathway for airflow between the external nares and the nasopharynx [2]. In the equine fetus, the dorsal and ventral nasal conchae and meatuses are completely formed by 80–100 days gestation [1].

The pharynx (Figure 4.1) delivers air from the caudal portion of the nasal cavity to the larynx and also serves to deliver food and water from the oral cavity to the esophagus. The pharynx does not have rigid support from bone or cartilage and thus remains patent by the actions of muscles associated with the hyoid bone, soft palate, and tongue [3]. Dysfunction of these muscles or related nerves can by associated with pharyngeal collapse. The larynx assists with preventing aspiration of food or water into the lower airways during swallowing and is composed of numerous cartilages, namely the cricoid, thyroid, and arytenoid cartilages. The thyroid and cricoid cartilage are noted by 30 days gestation in the equine embryo and by 45 days of gestation, the larynx and pharynx are formed [1].

Attached to the larynx is the trachea (Figure 4.2), which provides connection between the upper and lower airway. The trachea enters the chest at the thoracic inlet, just above the manubrium of the sternum, and ends at the bronchial bifurcation (carina), which is just dorsal to the left atrium [2]. The trachea is supported by C-shaped cartilages that are connected at the free ends by the trachealis muscle. In the equine embryo, the trachea starts to form from the invagination of the pharyngeal intestine at 21 days of gestation, and by 75 days gestation, the trachea has mucosal epithelium [1].

Beyond the carina (Figure 4.3a) are the openings to the main bronchi, which are distinguished by the presence of cartilage in the walls (typically airways >2 mm). The bronchi are surrounded by lung parenchyma less the first few centimeters. The right main-stem bronchus (Figure 4.3b) forms an almost straight line with the trachea and is one anatomic reason why aspiration pneumonia is more frequently observed in the right lung lobe, while the left bronchus deviates slightly off the trachea (Figure 4.3c) [4]. On both the left and right bronchi, the first bronchus arises from the lateral wall of the main-stem bronchus and is directed toward the cranial portion of the lung. A ventral branch exits the main stem bronchi as well and travels to the corresponding middle lobe. The bronchus to the accessory lobe of the lung originates from the medioventral aspect of the right bronchus. Each main bronchus continues toward the periphery of the lung, with smaller branches forming a series of tributaries throughout the lung.

Equine Neonatal Medicine, First Edition. Edited by David M. Wong and Pamela A. Wilkins.

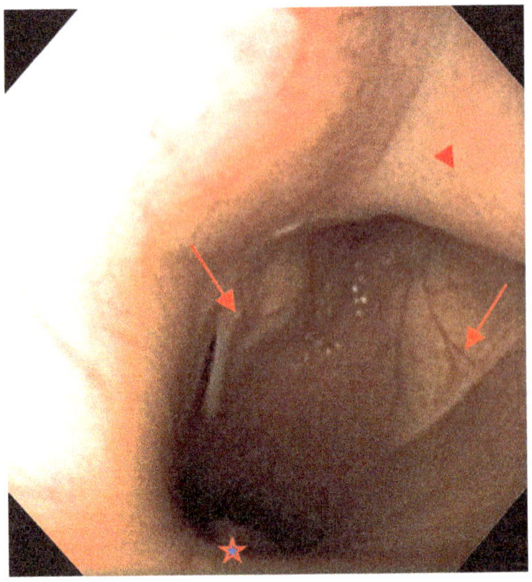

Figure 4.1 Endoscopic view of the pharynx: the caudal portion of the nasal septum can be seen (arrowhead) along with the openings to the guttural pouch (arrows). The tip of the epiglottis can be seen as well (star).

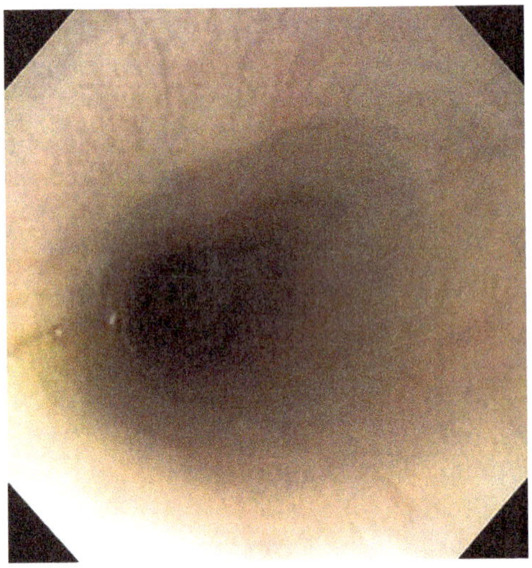

Figure 4.2 Endoscopic view of the trachea in a neonatal foal.

The lungs originate from an invagination of the ventral wall of the primitive intestine in its cranial portion and occur by the fourth week of gestation in the equine embryo [1]. The equine lung is not divided into distinct lobes, with both the left and right lung having similar shape with a ventral notch that accommodates the heart. The right lung lobe is larger than the left due to the accessory lung lobe that fills the area between the heart and diaphragm. Bronchioles, identified by the absence of cartilage in the walls, connect small bronchi to the alveolar ducts and alveoli, where gas exchange occurs. Bronchi and terminal bronchioles are observed by days 50–60 of gestation in the equine fetus. Between days 90 and 105, the primary and secondary bronchi are tubular structures composed of columnar epithelium [1]. Alveolar ducts are extensions of the bronchioles and can form several generations that each have numerous alveoli in their walls [2]. The alveoli are composed of two types of epithelial cells (type I and type II). Bordering alveoli are separated by the alveolar septum, which contains the pulmonary capillaries. Air is separated by the capillary blood by type I epithelial cells, a basement membrane, interstitium, and endothelial cells.

The lung contains two networks of lymphatics: one network surrounds the bronchi, the other is subpleural. These two networks connect to the hilar and mediastinal lymph nodes and drain into the thoracic duct [2]. The entire cardiac output of the right ventricle delivers deoxygenated blood from the right side of the heart through the pulmonary circulation and back to the left atrium. Comparatively, the bronchial circulation, which receives about 2% of the cardiac output, is a branch of the systemic circulation that provides the nutritional blood flow to the walls of the bronchi, large blood vessels, and pleura [5]. The venous drainage from the bronchial circulation returns blood to the azygos vein with a small portion entering the pulmonary veins, adding venous blood to oxygenated blood leaving the pulmonary capillaries [2]. This anatomic configuration

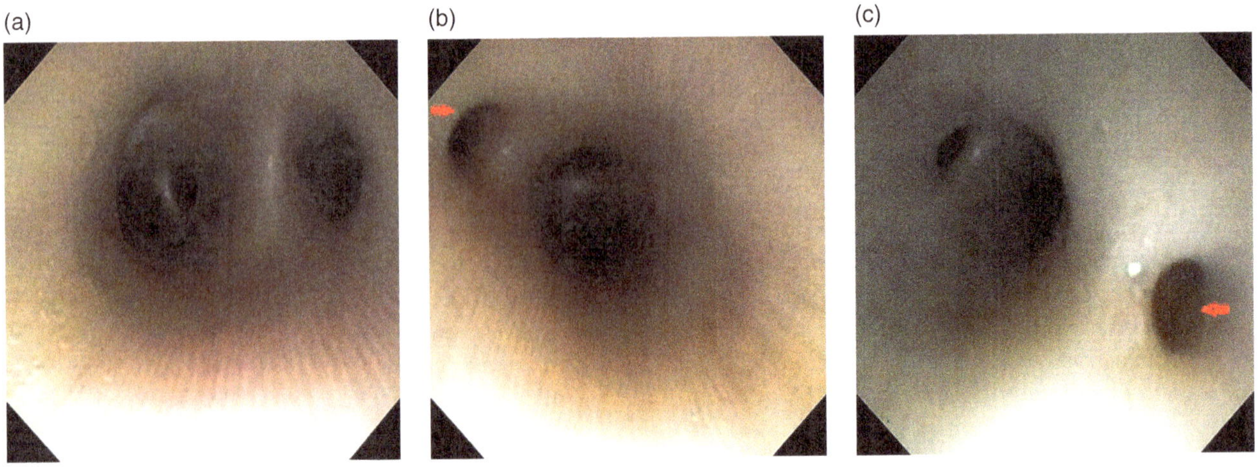

Figure 4.3 (a) Endoscopic image of the carina in a neonatal foal; (b) Right main-stem bronchus; (c) Left main-stem bronchus. Red arrow indicates first bronchus directed toward cranial portion of the lung.

allows blood to be supplied to a region of lung that might have reduced pulmonary circulation, thus allowing blood to enter that region from the bronchial circulation thereby reducing the incidence of ischemia to that particular region of the lung [2].

Surrounding the lungs is the thorax that is composed of 18 ribs that form a relatively rigid cage to protect the intrathoracic organs. Each rib articulates dorsally with the corresponding vertebrae and is extended ventrally by the costal cartilage. The first 8 ribs articulate with the sternum while ribs 9–17 are attached to one another by elastic tissue that forms the costal arch [2]. The 18th rib is a floating rib. The pleurae cover the surface of the thoracic cavity; the visceral pleura covers the lungs and connects with the mediastinal pleura at the hilar region [2]. The parietal pleura – divided into costal, diaphragmatic, and mediastinal sections – covers the ribs, diaphragm, and mediastinal structures, respectively. In some horses, the two pleural compartments communicate through small fenestrations. Moreover, the pleural and peritoneal cavities communicate through diaphragmatic pores and lymphatics [2]. The diaphragm is attached to the thoracic wall along the 8–10 costal cartilages and the costochondral junctions from ribs 10–13 and then to ribs at increasing distances until reaching the last intercostal space.

In the healthy newborn foal, clearance of fetal fluid occurs between 6 and 12 hours of age, based on radiographic evaluation [6, 7]. However, foals may be predisposed to atelectasis because of immaturity of the lung, chest wall compliance, and in some cases surfactant deficiency or function [8, 9].

References

1. Rodrigues, R.F., Rodrigues, M.N., Franciolli, A.L.R. et al. (2014). Embryonic and fetal development of the cardiorespiratory apparatus in horses (Equus Caballus) from 20 to 115 days of gestation. *J. Cytol. Histol.* 5: 1–10.
2. Robinson, N.E. and Furlow, P.W. (2007). Anatomy of the respiratory system. In: *Equine Respiratory Medicine and Surgery* (ed. B.C. McGorum, P.M. Dixon, and J. Schumacher), 3–17. Saunders.
3. Holcombe, S.J., Derksen, F.J., Stick, J.A. et al. (1998). Effect of bilateral blockade of the pharyngeal branch of the vagus nerve on soft palate function in horses. *Am. J. Vet. Res.* 59: 504–508.
4. Carvallo, F.R., Uzal, F.A., Diab, S.S. et al. (2017). Retrospective study of fatal pneumonia in racehorses. *J. Vet. Diagn. Invest.* 29: 450–456.
5. Magno, M. (1990). Comparative anatomy of the tracheobronchial circulation. *Eur. Respir. J.* 12: 557s–562s.
6. Kutasi, O., Horvath, A., Harnos, A. et al. (2009). Radiographic assessment of pulmonary fluid clearance in healthy neonatal foals. *Vet. Radiol. Ultrasound* 50: 584–588.
7. Lamb, C.R., O'Callaghan, W.O., and Paradis, M.R. (1990). Thoracic radiography in the neonatal foal: a preliminary report. *Vet. Radiol. Ultrasound* 31: 11–16.
8. Koterba, A.M., Wozniak, J.A., and Kosch, P.C. (1994). Respiratory mechanics of the horse during the first year of life. *Respir. Physiol.* 95: 21–24.
9. Koterba, A.M., Wozniak, J.A., and Kosch, P.C. (1995). Ventilatory and timing parameters in normal horses at rest up to age one year. *Equine Vet. J.* 27: 257–264.

Chapter 5 Clinical Neonatal Respiratory Physiology

Bettina Dunkel

Gas Exchange in Utero

The equine placenta increases in weight and surface area until term. Fetal villi continue to elongate and branch throughout the second half of gestation, increasing the total exchange area up to fivefold between mid and late gestation [1]. The equine placenta has a unique microcotyledonary circulation with very small intercapillary distances between maternal and fetal vessels (Figure 5.1a) [2]. The distance between the maternal and fetal blood vessels decreases with increasing gestational age to enhance transplacental transfer, particularly oxygen [1]. This is achieved by merging of the fetal vessels' basal lamina with that of the trophoblastic cells and the reduction of maternal epithelium thickness [3]. Together with a high uterine blood flow compared to umbilical blood flow, this results in a minimal PO_2 and PCO_2 gradient across the placenta (Figure 5.1b) [2]. As illustrated in Figure 5.1b, in situations where the mare has a normal PaO_2 concentration (e.g. 90 mmHg, dotted line), the horse has a lower transplacental PO_2 gradient (90 mmHg [maternal] to 50 mmHg [fetal]) when compared to the ewe (90 mmHg [maternal] to 30 mmHg [fetal]); consequently, there is a smaller driving force for the movement of O_2 from dam to fetus in the horse [2]. This smaller difference between maternal and fetal PO_2 suggests an efficient countercurrent blood flow system in the horse. Maternal to fetal O_2 transfer is therefore primarily flow-limited due to the high diffusing capacity of O_2 and the high reaction velocity of the exchange reaction with hemoglobin [4].

In contrast to other species, where fetal hemoglobin has a higher affinity for oxygen, shifting the oxygen dissociation curve to the left, there is no difference between fetal and maternal hemoglobin in horses. Equine fetal red blood cells have lower 2,3-diphosphoglycerate (2,3-DPG) concentrations, which contributes to efficient oxygen unloading to fetal tissues [5]; however, the high uterine flow rate and small diffusion distance are probably most important [2, 6]. The efficient gas transfer across the equine placenta is highlighted by the high umbilical venous PO_2 (50–54 mmHg) compared to other species and a PCO_2 difference across placenta that is close to zero [2]. Fetal arterial PO_2 follows the maternal uterine artery PO_2 in a linear fashion, even when the maternal PaO_2 exceeds 100 mmHg, which is different to other species (Figure 5.1b) [2]. Clinically, this implies that due to the linear relationship, any periods of hypoxia in the mare could predispose the fetus to development of hypoxia. Intranasal oxygen therapy in the mare could help to increase oxygen delivery to the equine fetus, whereas anesthesia of the mare decreases umbilical flow considerably, therefore posing an immediate threat of hypoxemia to the fetus [2]. A similar linear relationship exists between the equine fetal and the mare's plasma glucose concentrations [7], emphasizing that maternal hypoglycemia should be avoided to minimize possible negative side effects on the developing fetus. During short-term maternal fasting, the equine fetus uses proportionately more of their available glucose for oxidative metabolism than other species, suggesting a limited ability to switch to alternative fuels with sudden reduced glucose availability [8].

Pulmonary Development

Detailed information regarding stages of pulmonary development is described in Chapter 1. During lung development, pulmonary epithelial cells actively secrete fluid, which accumulates within the fetal airways. The fluid distension leads to increased intrapulmonary vascular pressure and increased pulmonary vascular resistance [9]. In fetal lambs, the fluid volume filling the lungs is approximately 40–50 ml/kg [10]. The presence of this airway fluid is critical for stimulation of lung growth. In the human

Equine Neonatal Medicine, First Edition. Edited by David M. Wong and Pamela A. Wilkins.

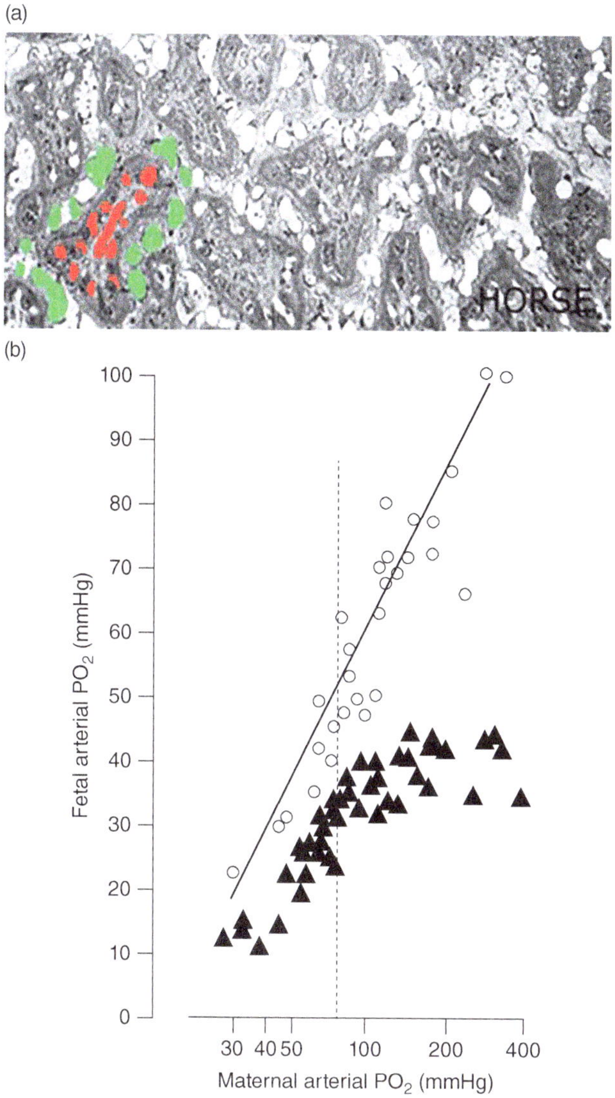

Figure 5.1 (a) Microscopic image from semithin, toluidine blue stained resin section from a late gestation equine placenta with fixative from fetal and maternal sides. Maternal capillaries are highlighted red with their closest fetal capillaries in green. (b) Oxygen gradient across the placentas of the horse (o) and ewe (Δ). PO_2 values are from the fetal umbilical and maternal uterine arteries over a range of experimental conditions. Normal values for maternal arterial blood in ewes and horses lie between 80 and 100 mmHg; mean value (90 mmHg) is indicated by dotted line. The difference in oxygen gradient between the two circulations is always greater in the sheep than in the horse, although the mare can deliver more O_2 at the upper extreme of the maternal range since fetal blood value in the ewe does not increase after the maternal values reach 100 mmHg. *Source:* Images from Wooding and Fowden [2].

fetus, fetal breathing starts at 10 weeks' gestation and is essential for pulmonary development. Hypoxemia in utero inhibits and hyperoxemia stimulates fetal breathing, thereby influencing pulmonary development. In human neonates, clearance of fetal lung fluid begins before birth and is mostly completed by 2 hours of age. Thoracic radiographs in foals suggest complete radiographic clearance of fetal lung fluid within 4 hours after birth [11]. The change from active fluid secretion to fluid absorption by the pulmonary epithelium is initiated before labor under the influence of increased cortisol and thyroid hormone concentrations and continues during and after birth by beta-receptor agonist stimulation and changes in transpulmonary pressure. Clearance of fetal lung fluid decreases pulmonary vascular resistance and increases intravascular fluid volume [9, 12]. However, the liquid initially remains in the surrounding interstitial tissues with a risk of re-entering the alveoli and interfering with gas exchange if efficient breathing and ventilation are not maintained [12].

Cardiorespiratory Transition from Fetus to the Newborn

Umbilical venous blood in the human fetus has an oxygen saturation of 70–80%, which is the highest oxygen saturation in the fetal circulation. In the human fetus, the umbilical vein enters the fetus and splits at the level of the liver with some blood perfusing the hepatic circulation and the remainder entering into the ductus venosus [9]. In contrast to other species, studies in foals indicate that foals do not have a ductus venosus and the entire umbilical venous blood passes through the liver [2, 13]. However, portosystemic shunts have been reported on rare occasion in foals, indicating that some biological variances probably exists [14]. In the human fetus, the oxygenated blood returning to the heart via the inferior/caudal vena cava is preferentially streamed from the right to the left atrium via the foramen ovale to perfuse the coronary and cerebral circulations [15]. The deoxygenated blood returning to the heart via the superior/cranial vena cava is preferentially directed toward the right ventricle and then through the pulmonary artery to the aorta via the ductus arteriosus to the lower part of the body before returning to the low-resistance placenta [9]. The right-to-left shunting of blood across the foramen ovale and ductus arteriosus is enabled by the high pulmonary vascular resistance [15]. Only a small portion of the right ventricular output goes to the lungs via the pulmonary arteries.

In the human fetus, pulmonary blood flow increases during pregnancy and is approximately 21% of the combined ventricular output at 38 weeks [15]. The high pulmonary vascular resistance in the fetus is maintained by the fluid filling the lungs, pulmonary vasoconstriction due to the hypoxemic environment, and presence of vasoactive mediators including thromboxane A2, platelet activating factor, and endothelin 1 [15, 16]. With the first breath, the pulmonary vascular resistance decreases dramatically due to increased oxygen exposure and ventilation. Prostacyclin and nitric oxide (NO) are both potent pulmonary vasodilators mediating pulmonary vasodilation [16]. NO is released from the endothelium when stimulated by increased oxygen tension and sheer stress from increased pulmonary blood flow. Nitric oxide diffuses into the pulmonary arterial smooth muscle cells and stimulates production of the second messenger cyclic guanosine monophosphate (cGMP) from guanosine triphosphate (GTP). Increase in intracellular cGMP initiates a cascade of events that result in NO-mediated relaxation of the pulmonary arterial smooth muscle cells [15]. Cyclic GMP is broken down by phosphodiesterase-5, the predominate phosphodiesterase type present in the lungs. After birth, the pulmonary artery pressure is approximately 40 mmHg with a systemic arterial pressure of approximately 88–100 mmHg. Over the next 2 weeks, the pulmonary artery pressure declines gradually to 20–25 mmHg [16, 17]. The hypertrophied smooth muscle in the fetal pulmonary circulation begins to involute after birth and this is completed at 6–8 weeks.

During the initial postpartum period, neonatal foals remain susceptible to development of pulmonary hypertension during periods of hypoxemia or exposure to other stressors with large inter-individual variations in reactivity of the smooth musculature [18]. Persistent pulmonary hypertension of the neonate (PPHN) has been reported in foals [19] and treatment is extrapolated from babies. Sildenafil, a selective phosphodiesterase 5 inhibitor, is used in PPHN treatment to increase cGMP concentrations in the pulmonary smooth muscle by decreasing its breakdown, thereby promoting smooth muscle relaxation [15]. Other treatments include ventilation with high fractions of inspired oxygen (FiO_2) or inhaled NO to achieve pulmonary vasodilation [20]. However, prior exposure to high FiO_2 can impair the response to inhaled NO, making timing of treatments critical [15].

The occlusion of the umbilical cord results in an increase in systemic vascular resistance. Together with an increasing amount of blood entering the left atrium from the lungs, this leads to an increased pressure within the left atrium [15]. Once the left exceeds the right atrial pressure, the foramen ovale closes [9]. Echocardiographic studies in foals showed no flow across the foramen ovale but continued fluttering of the septum primum into the left atrium was observed until 10 days of age (the end of the study period). Throughout this time, the maximal distance between the septum primum and septum secundum continued to decrease [21]. In human neonates, the flow across the ductus arteriosus reverses to left-to-right flow within 10 minutes after birth, directing blood flow through the pulmonary vasculature. Oxygenation of the ductus arteriosus leads to functional closure, which generally occurs within 72 hours in foals [22, 23]. However, echocardiographic flow through the ductus arteriosus could be visualized in 93% of foals on day 2, 61% on day 5 and 22% on day 10 of life [21].

Pulmonary Function in the Neonate – Gas Exchange

Following birth, the fetal circulation changes to the adult pattern gradually following the pattern described above. This corresponds with a gradual increase in PaO_2 over the first week of life, increasing from approximately 60 mmHg at 1 hour of age to approximately 90 mmHg at 7 days (Chapter 8, Table II.2) [24, 25]. A statistically significant but small decrease in $PaCO_2$ was also observed in neonatal foals during the first days of life [24]. This is likely due to a gradually decreasing intrapulmonary and/or intracardiac right-to-left shunt in the neonate as the change from fetal to adult circulatory pattern is completed [26]. At birth, the process of alveolarization (formation and maturation of distal parts of the lung/alveoli) has already started in foals and, based on stereological techniques, maturation continues after birth with an increase in lung volume until approximately 50 weeks of age and an increase in gas exchange surface area until up to 350 weeks (6.7 years) in Thoroughbreds reported by one study [27–30]. Morphometric measurements suggest that the median alveolar surface area increased with age, from 205, 258, and 630 m^2 in 1-day-old foals, 30-day-old foals, and adults, respectively [30].

Pulmonary Function in Neonate – Mechanics

Research in rabbits shows that during the first breaths, neonates inhale more air than they expire, thereby gradually building a functional residual capacity (FRC) as air replaces the liquid within the lungs [31]. Without any activity of respiratory muscles, the resting or relaxation volume of the respiratory system (V_R; also called elastic equilibrium volume [EEV] or FRC) is determined by the opposing forces of the outward recoil of the chest wall and the inward recoil of the lungs (Figure 5.2). The chest wall recoil is determined by the elastic characteristics of the diaphragm and rib cage, and the inward recoil of the lung is dictated by the viscoelastic properties of the lung. These, in turn, depend on lung tissue properties and the collapsing pressure generated at the alveolar air–liquid interface [10]. In most neonates, the chest wall compliance (change in volume per unit pressure) is higher than the compliance of the lung, favoring a low V_R, which increases the risk of alveolar collapse and makes the infant more vulnerable to development of hypoxia [10, 32]. In most species, neonates therefore use strategies to prevent expiration to V_R by

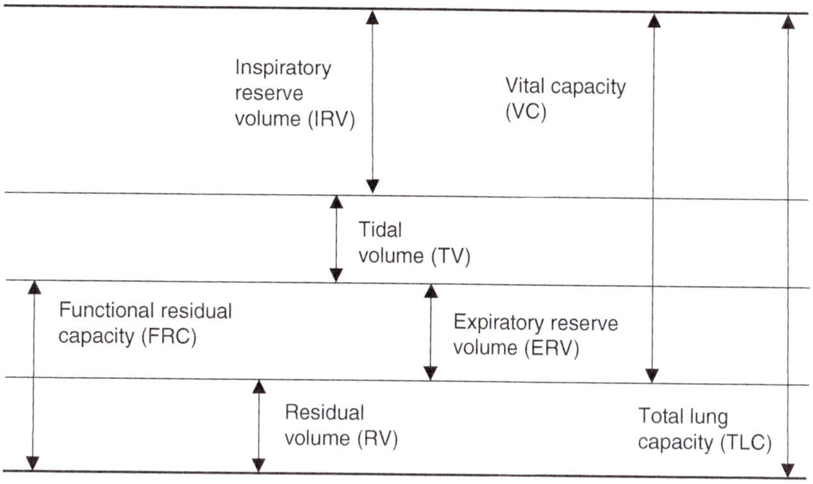

Figure 5.2 Various volumes related to breathing.

increasing the frequency of augmented breaths to improve lung compliance and prolong the expiratory time constant in order to increase the amount of air remaining in the lung at end expiration to help prevent lung collapse [10].

Expiratory braking maneuvers (EBMs) are common in spontaneously breathing neonates of most species and help maintain FRC while the chest wall is still compliant. EBM begin when at least 80% of FRC has accumulated by extending the expiratory flow time and increasing airway pressure during passive expiration [31]. EBMs result from adduction of the glottis or activation of the diaphragm during the middle to late phase of expiratory gas flow to shorten expiration and trapping gas in the lungs [32]. Other respiratory movements that assist in maintaining FRC include grunting and, in babies, crying, in which the infant uses a forced expiratory maneuver against a closed or constricted glottis thereby restricting air loss [31]. An additional mechanism is persistence of inspiratory muscle activity into the expiratory phase, thereby modulating the expiratory flow [32]. This does not seem to be the case in healthy neonatal foals. Due to a stiffer (less compliant) chest wall, the FRC is not as low as in other species and, at least in a standing position, compensatory mechanisms to increase end-expiratory volume are not regularly encountered [33]. This might be different in premature or sick foals with more compliant chest walls where grunting might be used as a method to increase the end-expiratory volume and prevent airway collapse. Surfactant deficiency or dysfunction further compounds this issue by increasing the work of breathing and favoring alveolar collapse [31, 34]. Apneic episodes as they might be observed in sick or premature foals can also contribute to loss of FRC, compound gas exchange, and increase the risk of alveolar collapse and rapid desaturation [32].

Airway tethering, mediated by the elastic components in the alveolar walls surrounding the airways, is an additional crucial mechanism that secures airway patency and maintenance of an adequate FRC [32]. The elastic fibers within the alveolar walls create an extended mesh that exerts a circumferential pull on the intraparenchymal airways transmitting tension from the pleural surface to the individual bronchi. The tension on the system increases during inspiration, resulting in an increasing and decreasing cross sectional area of the airway during inspiration and expiration, respectively, coupling lung volume to airway diameter [32]. In premature neonates, tethering is less effective as alveolarization and the associated parenchymal elastic network are not fully developed yet, leading to decreased airway stability with an increased tendency to closure, increased airway resistance, and a propensity to alveolar collapse in the lung periphery [32]. Limited studies in foals indicate that elastin content of the lungs exponentially increases from 260 days of gestation until birth while collagen showed a linear increase from 100 days up to birth [35]. Ineffective tethering could therefore play a role in premature or dysmature foals.

While neonatal foals have a similar normalized lung volume and compliance compared to neonates of other species, their chest wall compliance is considerably lower. Most neonates – including children, rats, rabbits, cats, dogs, pigs, calves, and goats – have a high chest wall compliance and it has been speculated that the soft and flexible chest wall eases delivery through the birth canal. Mature, healthy foals have a comparatively low chest compliance but it is still significantly greater than in adult horses [33]. Due to their high metabolic rate, neonatal foals have a very high minute ventilation (498–848 ml/min/kg) compared to adult horses (162 ml/min/kg) [33, 34]. In contrast to adult horses, foals show monophasic inspiratory and expiratory pattern with active inspiration and expiration. The active expiration might aid the foal to maintain a high ventilation by promoting fast air movement out of the lungs [33]. Within the first year, the foal makes a transition to the adult biphasic flow pattern using a combination of active and passive inspiration and expiration with most foals showing a biphasic expiration by 3 months [36]. This is associated with a change from breathing from the V_R as a neonate to breathing around V_R as an adult [33, 36]. Chest wall compliance appears to have reached adult levels at 3 months of age and does not appear to be responsible for the changes in breathing pattern. It has been speculated that changes in relative body proportions with an increase in length and depth of the trunk might contribute to the gradual adoption of an adult breathing pattern [36].

In summary, foals undergo a complex in utero development culminating in rapid physiological changes at birth. The flow-dependent glucose and oxygen exchange and linear relationship between maternal and fetal oxygen and glucose make the equine fetus vulnerable to maternal changes in blood flow, PO_2 and glucose concentrations. While in mature foals the well-developed lung and comparatively stiff chest wall rapidly enable an effective gas exchange, this might not be the case in premature and dysmature foals where insufficient or dysfunctional surfactant, a higher chest compliance and insufficient airway tethering can interfere with normal respiratory function.

References

1 Fowden, A.L., Giussani, D.A., and Forhead, A.J. (2020). Physiological development of the equine fetus during late gestation. *Equine Vet. J.* 52: 165–173.

2 Silver, M. and Comline, R.S. (1975). Transfer of gases and metabolites in the equine placenta: a comparison with other species. *J. Reprod. Fertil. Suppl.* 23: 589–594.

3 Robles, M., Loux, S., de Mestre, A.M. et al. (2022). Environmental constraints and pathologies that modulate equine placental genes and development. *Reproduction* 163: R25–R38.

4 Wooding, F.B. and Fowden, A.L. (2006). Nutrient transfer across the equine placenta: correlation of structure and function. *Equine Vet. J.* 38: 175–183.

5 Kitchen, H. and Bunn, H.F. (1975). Ontogeny of equine haemoglobins. *J. Reprod. Fertil. Suppl.* 23: 595–598.

6 Comline, R.S. and Silver, M. (1974). A comparative study of blood gas tensions, oxygen affinity and red cell 2,3 DPG concentrations in foetal and maternal blood in the mare, cow and sow. *J. Physiol.* 242: 805–826.

7 Fowden, A.L. (1997). Comparative aspects of fetal carbohydrate metabolism. *Equine Vet. J. Suppl.* 29: 19–25.

8 Fowden, A.L., Taylor, P.M., White, K.L. et al. (2000). Ontogenic and nutritionally induced changes in fetal metabolism in the horse. *J. Physiol.* 528 (Pt 1): 209–219.

9 Morton, S.U. and Brodsky, D. (2016). Fetal physiology and the transition to extrauterine life. *Clin. Perinatol.* 43: 395–407.

10 Frappell, P.B. and MacFarlane, P.M. (2005). Development of mechanics and pulmonary reflexes. *Respir. Physiol. Neurobiol.* 149: 143–154.

11 Kutasi, O., Horvath, A., Harnos, A. et al. (2009). Radiographic assessment of pulmonary fluid clearance in healthy neonatal foals. *Vet. Radiol. Ultrasound* 50: 584–588.

12 Lista, G., Maturana, A., and Moya, F.R. (2017). Achieving and maintaining lung volume in the preterm infant: from the first breath to the NICU. *Eur. J. Pediatr.* 176: 1287–1293.

13 Silver, M. (1984). Some aspects of equine placental exchange and foetal physiology. *Equine Vet. J.* 16: 227–233.

14 Willems, D.S., Kranenburg, L.C., Ensink, J.M. et al. (2019). Computed tomography angiography of a congenital extrahepatic splenocaval shunt in a foal. *Acta Vet. Scand.* 61: 39.

15 Sankaran, D. and Lakshminrusimha, S. (2022). Pulmonary hypertension in the newborn- etiology and pathogenesis. *Semin. Fetal Neonatal Med.* 27: 101381.

16 Gao, Y. and Raj, J.U. (2010). Regulation of the pulmonary circulation in the fetus and newborn. *Physiol. Rev.* 90: 1291–1335.

17 Thomas, W.P., Madigan, J.E., Backus, K.Q. et al. (1987). Systemic and pulmonary haemodynamics in normal neonatal foals. *J. Reprod. Fertil. Suppl.* 35: 623–628.

18 Drummond, W.H., Sanchez, I.R., Kosch, P.C. et al. (1989). Pulmonary vascular reactivity of the newborn pony foal. *Equine Vet. J.* 21: 181–185.

19 Cottrill, C.M., O'Connor, W.N., Cudd, T. et al. (1987). Persistence of foetal circulatory pathways in a newborn foal. *Equine Vet. J.* 19: 252–255.

20 Lester, G.D., DeMarco, V.G., and Norman, W.M. (1999). Effect of inhaled nitric oxide on experimentally induced pulmonary hypertension in neonatal foals. *Am. J. Vet. Res.* 60: 1207–1212.

21 De Lange, L., Vernemmen, I., van Loon, G. et al. (2022). Echocardiographic features of the ductus arteriosus and the foramen ovale in a hospital-based population of neonatal foals. *Animals (Basel)* 12: 17.

22 Reef, V.B. (1985). Cardiovascular disease in the equine neonate. *Vet. Clin. North Am. Equine Pract.* 1: 117–129.

23 Machida, N., Yasuda, J., Too, K. et al. (1988). A morphological study on the obliteration processes of the ductus arteriosus in the horse. *Equine Vet. J.* 20: 249–254.

24 Wong, D.M., Hepworth-Warren, K.L., Sponseller, B.T. et al. (2017). Measured and calculated variables of global oxygenation in healthy neonatal foals. *Am. J. Vet. Res.* 78: 230–238.

25 Hackett, E.S., Traub-Dargatz, J.L., Knowles, J.E. Jr. et al. (2010). Arterial blood gas parameters of normal foals born at 1500 metres elevation. *Equine Vet. J.* 42: 59–62.

26 Stewart, J.H., Young, I.H., Rose, R.J. et al. (1987). The distribution of ventilation-perfusion ratios in the lungs of newborn foals. *J. Dev. Physiol.* 9: 309–324.

27 Schittny, J.C. (2017). Development of the lung. *Cell Tissue Res.* 367: 427–444.

28 Woods, J.C. and Schittny, J.C. (2016). Lung structure at preterm and term birth. In: *Fetal and Neonatal Lung Development* (ed. A.H. Jobe, J.A. Whitsett, and S.H. Abman), 126–137. New York: Cambridge University Press.

29 Beech, D.J., Sibbons, P.D., Rossdale, P.D. et al. (2001). Organogenesis of lung and kidney in Thoroughbreds and ponies. *Equine Vet. J.* 33: 438–445.

30 Johnson, L., Montgomery, J.B., Schneider, J.P. et al. (2014). Morphometric examination of the equine adult and foal lung. *Anat. Rec. (Hoboken)* 297: 1950–1962.

31 Hooper, S.B., Te Pas, A.B., Lewis, R.A. et al. (2010). Establishing functional residual capacity at birth. *NeoReviews* 11: 1.

32 Colin, A.A., McEvoy, C., and Castile, R.G. (2010). Respiratory morbidity and lung function in preterm infants of 32 to 36 weeks' gestational age. *Pediatrics* 126: 115–128.

33 Koterba, A.M. and Kosch, P.C. (1987). Respiratory mechanics and breathing pattern in the neonatal foal. *J. Reprod. Fertil. Suppl.* 35: 575–585.

34 Gillespie, J.R. (1975). Postnatal lung growth and function in the foal. *J. Reprod. Fertil. Suppl.* 23: 667–671.

35 Barnard, K., Leadon, D.P., and Silver, I.A. (1982). Some aspects of tissue maturation in fetal and perinatal foals. *J. Reprod. Fertil. Suppl.* 32: 589–595.

36 Koterba, A.M., Wozniak, J.A., and Kosch, P.C. (1995). Changes in breathing pattern in the normal horse at rest up to age one year. *Equine Vet. J.* 27: 265–274.

Chapter 6 Examination, Therapeutics, and Monitoring of the Respiratory System

Section I Physical Examination

Pamela A. Wilkins

Obtaining a History

Knowledge of a complete and accurate history, as much as is practical, should be obtained prior to, or during if an emergency, any equine neonate being examined, with particular attention paid to the respiratory tract. Neonatal foals can have widely varied or incomplete histories due to the nature of the breeding business or changes in location associated with the management of pregnant mares and delivery of their foals, making it important to gather as much information as possible. Birth problems such as dystocia or premature placental separation (red bag), postpartum age, and breed, may play a role in the development of respiratory disease and can include problems such as thoracic trauma, neonatal encephalopathy, failure of transfer of passive immunity (FTPI), the presence of congenital defects, inherited problems such as hyperkalemic period paralysis (HYPP), or acquired immunodeficiency syndromes seen in certain breeds, among other conditions.

The local environment may contribute to the development or severity of respiratory disease, with some respiratory diseases associated with a change to a new environment particularly following long-distance transport. It is important to know if certain diseases are either endemic or are an epidemic where the neonate is residing or was transported from; diseases such as influenza, strangles and *Rhodococcus equi* sepsis are frequent infectious pathogens that are possible. If feasible, a thorough vaccination history of the mare should be obtained. Additionally, an accurate history of any administered treatments and the response of the foal to those treatments should be recorded. Dosage of any administered treatment should also be noted as the neonatal foal requires different doses, and in some cases dose frequencies, than older foals or adult horses. Any treatments administered to the dam should also be documented.

Primary Complaints

Thorough examination of the respiratory tract of the neonatal foal should be undertaken in both the "new foal" examination and any examination undertaken due to complaint that the foal is abnormal in any way. Findings or complaints associated with respiratory disease include nasal discharge, not uncommonly milk, present at the nares following nursing, either bilateral or unilateral. Respiratory noise at rest or during exercise may be associated with abnormalities of the upper airway, as can loss of airflow through either nostril or distension of the cheeks during expiration. Other clinical signs that dictate thorough evaluation of the respiratory tract include, but are not limited to, abnormal breathing patterns (tachypnea, hyperpnea, dyspnea, paradoxic breathing), unusual swellings of the face, pharynx or throatlatch regions, any lymphadenopathy, and abnormal or limited movement of the thorax.

Physical Examination

Physical examination begins outside the stall and involves determination of the respiratory rate at rest and evaluation of the general attitude, demeanor, movement, and spontaneous activity of the neonate. The respiratory rate, pattern, and effort are readily determined by observation in the neonate. Entering the stall and restraining the neonatal foal, particularly a healthy foal, commonly results in elevation of the aforementioned parameters due to excitement and effort expended by the foal evading restraint. If possible, take time to assess the foal from outside the stall. Respiratory diseases will not necessarily be obvious at rest, but important clues can be gained from observation prior to attempts at restraint in others.

Equine Neonatal Medicine, First Edition. Edited by David M. Wong and Pamela A. Wilkins.

Table 6.I.1 Respiratory parameters in laterally recumbent newborn and neonatal foals [1].

Value	Birth	15 min	30 min	60 min	4 h	12 h	24 h	48 h	4 d	7 d
Rate (bpm)	71 ± 5.9	58 ± 5.1	53 ± 3.6	40 ± 3.2	57 ± 5.6	32 ± 5.2	42 ± 3.8	44 ± 7.2	46 ± 3.5	42 ± 4.8
PO_2(mmHg)	39.7 ± 2	50.4 ± 3	57.0 ± 2	60.9 ± 3	75.7 ± 5	73.5 ± 3	67.6 ± 4	74.9 ± 3	81.2 ± 3	86.9 ± 2
PCO_2(mmHg)	45.7 ± 1	50.4 ± 2	51.5 ± 2	47.3 ± 2	45.0 ± 2	44.3 ± 1	45.5 ± 2	46.1 ± 1	45.8 ± 1	46.7 ± 1

bpm, breaths per minute; PO_2, partial pressure of PO_2, partial pressure arterial O_2; PCO_2, partial pressure arterial CO_2. Birth blood gas reported from umbilical vein.

The normal resting respiratory rate of a healthy neonatal foal varies widely, depending on time since birth (Table 6.I.1), and can range from up to 70 breaths/min at birth and generally less than 30 breaths/min by 1 month of age [1]. In adult horses at rest there is a small abdominal component during the expiratory phase, which, along with inspiration, is an active process and is considered *eupnea*. Newborn and neonatal foals exhibit greater effort during both inspiration and expiration, in part due to their very compliant chest wall with a relatively less compliant lung, in addition to the challenge of clearing fetal fluids from the lungs in the newborn. Hypoxemia, or low arterial blood partial pressure of oxygen, present at birth gradually resolves as the lung transitions to air breathing and gas exchange (Table 6.I.1).

While the airways of newborn foals are rapidly cleared of liquid to allow the onset of air breathing, initiating a series of physiologic changes enabling the lung to engage in gas exchange, fluid retention within the airways, and gradual opening of airways, creates a veritable cacophony of sounds during auscultation that are in fact expected, normal, and not considered to be of significant concern in the first hours of life in the newborn foal. Radiographically, this airway fluid appears to be cleared from the lungs of healthy foals by 4 hours of age, with the ventral lung clearing first [2]. However, in one study involving CT imaging, investigators identified radiographic patterns and changes in attenuation most consistent with atelectasis that appeared more severe in foals ≤7 days of age than in older neonatal foals [3]. The authors did not suggest that this was due to decreased fetal fluid clearance. Fetal intraluminal fluid is removed by a variety of mechanisms to the interstitial space of the lung, to then be cleared by lymphatics. However, this fluid transiently present in the interstitial space inhibits compliance of the lung, which, when combined with the relatively compliant chest wall, results in the observed increased respiratory effort compared to later in life. While this effort can be considered normal, the uninitiated might consider this to be dyspnea, a breathing pattern that is generally interpreted to reflect difficulty in breathing; the work of breathing is obviously increased, although the rate may be either increased or within normal limits, depending on age. This elevated respiratory rate and effort should resolve with time, and, if it doesn't, must be considered an indication of potential respiratory disease.

Other terms used to describe breathing patterns, include *tachypnea* characterized by rapid rate and shallow depth or low tidal volume; *hyperpnea* with increased frequency and depth of breathing (example would be post-exercise recovery); and *apnea* where there is no discernable breathing. The terms *hypoventilation* and *hyperventilation* require a change in arterial carbon dioxide partial pressure as a component of their definitions and are not appropriate for use describing changes in respiratory rate, effort, or pattern.

Following assessment of the foal at distance, and determination of respiratory rate, effort and pattern, a closer examination is indicated. The clinician should determine that airflow is both present and similar from each nostril. Differences between nostrils can indicate or suggest congenital or acquired abnormalities such as choanal atresia (unilateral of bilateral) or the presence of upper airway masses including pharyngeal cysts. Abnormal respiratory sounds can sometimes be present at rest and may be heard at the nares. The frontal, maxillary, and other sinuses have very low volumes and surface areas in the equine neonate, making percussion irrelevant, although sinuses should certainly be considered if facial deformity is present, particularly over the region of the maxillary sinuses [4]. Observation and palpation of the submandibular area, larynx, pharyngeal, and cervical regions allows for identification of lymph node enlargement, masses, edema, or guttural pouch enlargement, such as seen with empyema or tympany (Figure 6.I.1). Both jugular veins should be examined for patency as obstruction of these vessels may create abnormal upper airway function by interfering with normal recurrent laryngeal nerve or vagosympathetic trunk function. The head and mouth should be examined both visually and by palpation, particularly of the hard palate. While the majority of cleft palate (Figure 6.I.2) cases involve the soft palate and are beyond the point where palpation is practical, oral examination is considered essential [5]. Symmetry of the head is important and wry nose has been known to interfere with breathing and/or create abnormal respiratory noise.

Coughing represents a nonspecific irritation of receptors in the airway is usually a normal protective reflex that allows the foal to clear material from the airway. Cough

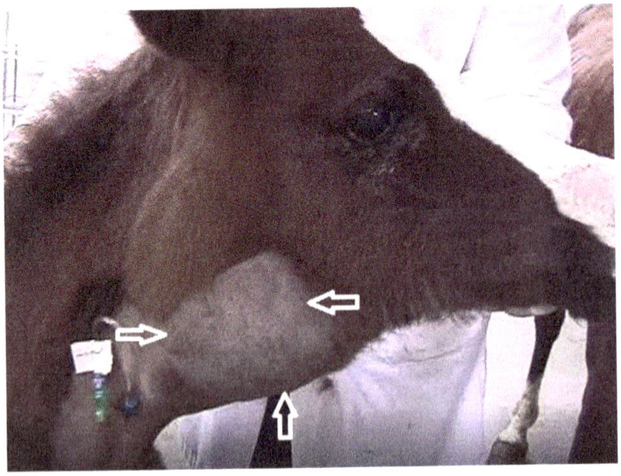

Figure 6.I.1 Guttural pouch tympany in an Arabian foal. Note the severe enlargement of the throatlatch region (arrows). In this case, tympany was associated with dysphagia resulting in a modest accumulation of ingested milk in the guttural pouches. *Source:* Image courtesy of Dr. David Wong, Iowa State University.

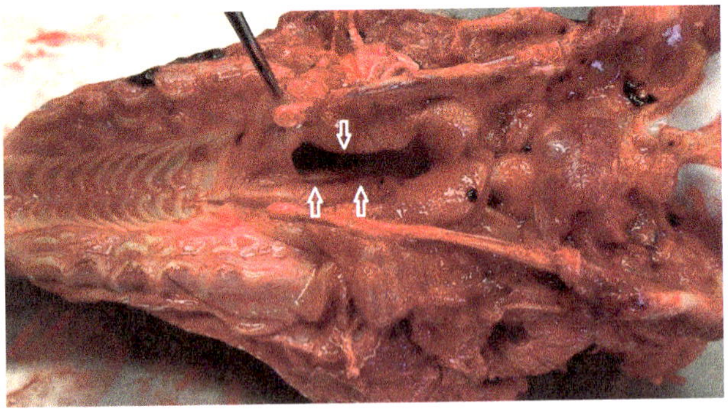

Figure 6.I.2 Postmortem specimen demonstrating a cleft palate (arrows) involving the soft palate. In this image, the mandible has been removed to enhance visualization of the hard and soft palate. *Source:* Image courtesy of Dr. Rebecca Ruby, University of Kentucky.

can be associated with increased mucus production, production of other respiratory secretions, or decreased mucociliary clearance, but is most commonly associated with milk aspiration in newborn and neonatal foals. Coughing and milk appearing at the nostrils of the young foal should prompt further detailed investigation. Auscultation of the trachea while the foal is nursing allows for identification of fluid in the trachea, suggesting milk aspiration that can put the foal at risk of aspiration pneumonia. The dysphagia that results in this finding can be due to abnormal pharyngeal function, pharyngeal laxity, or other upper airway abnormalities, including the dreaded cleft palate [6]. Alternatively, some foals are simply allowing passive regurgitation of milk in the esophagus when dropping their head following nursing. Upper airway endoscopy and thorough examination for pneumonia are indicated in all these cases. While unilateral nasal discharge seems to suggest a source in front of the larynx, bilateral nasal discharge can be of either upper or lower airway origin. While unusual, neonatal foals with severe pneumonia may have nasal discharge, and this should be noted. Hemoptysis and epistaxis are extremely rare in the equine neonate.

Examination of the oral mucous membranes may reveal cyanosis – bluish discoloration of the oral, nasal, or vulvar mucous membranes. Cyanosis does not become apparent until 5 mg/100 ml of deoxygenated hemoglobin, about one-third of the total normal hemoglobin, is present, reflecting a profound decrease in oxygen saturation of hemoglobin and suggestive of severe hypoxemia. Cyanosis also requires that the patient not be anemic, otherwise there is an insufficient quantity of deoxygenated hemoglobin present to give the bluish tint. The clinician is cautioned that all newborns are cyanotic for the first few breaths and only become pink when they have begun the transition to neonatal, as opposed to fetal, cardiorespiratory conditions.

Thoracic palpation and observation for symmetry is the next step of the examination, with the thoracic cage closely evaluated for abnormal swelling or rib profiles, which is suggestive of thoracic trauma and possibly rib fractures. Symmetry is best evaluated by looking at the thorax in its entirety from a "bird's-eye" view, comparing the profile of one side to the other. Following observation, thorough palpation of each rib along its entire length may allow for recognition of partially or fully displaced rib fractures. Although most of these will be found 1–3 cm dorsal to the costochondral junction, and be multiple in number, rib fractures may be located more dorsal and may be present bilaterally [7]. Fractures that are present and not displaced are more difficult to locate and can become displaced later. Areas of trauma may have some swelling present, and pain may be elicited with palpation, but this also may not be immediately present if the trauma was recent. Thoracic ultrasonography, with particular attention paid to the ribs, is considered the diagnostic modality of choice, and is routinely employed as part of the initial examination of foals presenting to some referral hospitals. Further description of rib fractures is discussed in Section III of this chapter.

Auscultation of the thorax, while an important component of the physical examination of the equine neonate, can be variable, sound abnormal when compared to the adult, and yet be normal for a foal. Findings will vary by age of the foal and sounds are much easier to identify due to thin thoracic cage. It is important that auscultation of the thorax take place in as quiet an environment as possible. Additionally, while ideally auscultation of the lung fields should be performed under two breathing conditions: eupnea and hyperpnea, hyperpnea induced by use of a re-breathing bag is not useful in the neonate and, unless quite ill, foals will resist fairly vigorously. It is less stressful to the foal, and more efficient, to move to imaging such as ultrasonography and radiography. Normal breath sounds are produced by turbulence within the tracheobronchial tree and vary considerably depending on location within the lung, breathing pattern, and condition of the animal. Of note, lung sounds do not represent air flow in terminal conducting airways and alveoli and are silent at this location as gas movement here is by diffusion. Bronchial sounds are louder, primarily sounds made in the larger airways, and are best heard over the trachea and base of the lung.

Common abnormalities noted during auscultation include ventral areas of dullness with significant pleural effusion, dorsal areas of dullness or hyperresonance with pneumothorax, and dorsal "harsh" lung sounds. The variation in normal lung sounds is large, and auscultatory findings do not always correlate well with the degree of lung abnormality, particularly in foals. That said, abnormal lung sounds, although they may be transient and not consistently present, are always clinically important. Adventitious lung sounds called crackles are short and discontinuous, while longer continuous sounds are called wheezes. Crackles and wheezes are both commonly identified in the previously "down" lung when foals have recently been recumbent, again due to their very compliant chest wall and probable development of transient atelectasis. Crackles are generated by the sudden pressure equalization when collapsed airway segments open and do not necessarily imply excessive secretions or pulmonary edema. Crackles are commonly end-inspiratory and associated with reinflation of atelectatic lung. Disease processes that generate crackles in neonatal foal, besides resolution of atelectasis, include pneumonia, pulmonary edema, and acute respiratory distress syndrome (ARDS).

Wheezes represent oscillation of airway walls before complete closing (expiratory) or opening (inspiratory). Disappearance of a wheeze after coughing indicates secretory rather than tissue component origin, making wheezes sporadic in nature and of short duration. Disease processes responsible for wheezes include airway stenosis, external airway compression, airway lumen compromise by foreign body, purulent material, cyst or neoplasm, airway wall thickening, and bronchoconstriction. The final type of adventitious sound includes the "rubbing" or "creaking" sounds generated by sliding or stretching of inflamed pleural surfaces, commonly termed *pleural friction rubs*.

Percussion of the thorax is uncommonly performed in neonatal foals but if done is performed by methodically tapping over the intercostal spaces of the thorax using a variety of instruments, including plexors, pleximeters, spoons, fingers, neurologic hammers, and hands. It is an easy way of identifying pleurodynia. While an inexpensive and useful component of physical examination in adult horses, neonatal foals will seldom tolerate the procedure. Thoracic percussion can outline aerated lung immediately beneath the chest wall but will seldom fully delineate the lung field cranially because of the triceps musculature. There is a distinct region of cardiac dullness for all species on the left side. Percussion, if permitted by the foal, will allow delineation of pleural effusion and intrathoracic masses or consolidated lung beneath the pleural surface, but cannot distinguish between them. Ultrasonography has replaced this procedure in neonatal foals, with less stress and better ability to identify disease processes and structures within the thoracic cage.

References

1 Stewart, J.H., Rose, R.J., and Barko, A.M. (1984). Respiratory studies in foals from birth to seven days old. *Equine Vet. J.* 16: 323–328.

2 Kutasi, A., Horvath, A., Harnos, A. et al. (2009). Radiographic assessment of pulmonary fluid clearance in healthy neonatal foals. *Vet. Radiol. Ultrasound* 50: 584–588.

3 Lascola, K.M., O'Brien, R.T., Wilkins, P.A. et al. (2013). Qualitative and quantitative interpretation of computed tomography of the lungs in healthy neonatal foals. *Am. J. Vet. Res.* 74: 1239–1246.

4 Bahar, S., Bolat, D., Dayan, M.O. et al. (2014). Two- and three-dimensional anatomy of paranasal sinuses in Arabian foals. *J. Vet. Med. Sci.* 76: 37–44.

5 Shaw, S.D., Norman, T.E., Arnold, C.E. et al. (2015). Clinical characteristics of horses and foals diagnosed with cleft palate in a referral population: 28 cases (1988–2011). *Can. Vet. J.* 56: 756–760.

6 Holcombe, S.J., Hurcombe, S.D., Barr, B.S. et al. (2012). Dysphagia associated with presumed pharyngeal dysfunction in 16 neonatal foals. *Equine Vet. J. Suppl.* 41: 105–108.

7 Sprayberry, K.A. and Barrett, E.J. (2015). Thoracic trauma in horses. *Vet. Clin. North Am. Equine Pract.* 31: 199–219.

Section II Thoracic Radiography of the Neonatal Foal

Kara M. Lascola

Radiographic imaging remains an important tool for evaluating and diagnosing respiratory disease in neonatal foals. The radiographic appearance of the lungs and other thoracic structures has been previously described in healthy and sick neonatal foals [1–6]. While radiographic patterns observed in foals with pulmonary disease are similar to those described for adult horses and small animal species, there are some unique findings, particularly in the immediate postpartum and neonatal period. As with adult horses, identified patterns include interstitial, alveolar, nodular, and bronchial [1, 4, 6]. While useful for disease characterization and monitoring disease progression, these patterns are not specific to the cause of disease and may also occur in response to nonpathologic changes.

In neonatal foals, radiographic changes have been described for pneumonia (aspiration, viral, bacterial), neonatal equine respiratory distress syndrome (NERDS), and equine neonatal acute respiratory distress syndrome (EqNARDS) [1, 2, 4–7]. Pneumothorax and rib fractures are occasionally identified radiographically, although ultrasound is considered to be superior for detection of fractures [8]. Residual fetal lung fluid in the airways or pulmonary interstitial space and patient related artifacts contribute to the development of the unique nonpathologic changes described in young foals [1–4]. Interpretation of radiographic images in neonatal foals can be complicated because non-pathologic changes or are often difficult to distinguish radiographically from changes associated with pulmonary diseases. Regardless of the underlying cause, interstitial and alveolar radiographic patterns tend to be most commonly identified in young foals [1, 5, 6, 9]. In association with nonpathologic causes, they have been described in healthy foals from 30 minutes to approximately 1 week of age and tend to be most prominent in foals <24 hours of age [1–3].

Radiographic Detection of Fetal Lung Fluid

Production of fetal lung fluid plays a critical role in fetal lung development and maturation. Clearance of this fluid from the airways and interstitium at birth is essential for normal ventilation and gas exchange in the newborn. Fetal lung fluid clearance progresses from the alveolar to interstitial space and is expected to be complete within 2–6 hours after birth [10–13]. Fluid absorption during and immediately after birth is primarily driven by active sodium ion transport across the airway epithelium, followed by passive transport of water and chloride from the airway lumen to the interstitium via paracellular channels [10, 13–15]. Although not completely understood, this immediate shift to fluid absorption is thought to be influenced by a combination of factors, including increases in catecholamines, β-agonists, glucocorticoids, and alveolar PO_2 along with increases in pulmonary blood flow and lymphatic drainage, and, to a varying degree, compression of the chest through the birth canal [13–17]. Preterm and/or cesarean delivery can delay fluid clearance [12, 16–18]. Radiographically, the appearance of fluid varies depending on its location (alveolar or interstitial space) but should gradually resolve over the first several hours after birth.

Radiographic descriptions of presumed clearance of fetal lung fluid are reported for nonsedated foals positioned in lateral recumbency during peak inspiration [1–3]. Radiographically, residual fetal lung fluid appears as a diffuse increase in lung opacity characterized as an interstitial-to-alveolar pattern that often obscures the pulmonary vasculature and soft tissue margins of the lung [1–4]. Radiographic detection of fetal lung fluid in healthy foals has been reported for 4–12 hours after parturition (Figure 6.II.1) [2, 3]. A clearly defined vascular pattern should be

Equine Neonatal Medicine, First Edition. Edited by David M. Wong and Pamela A. Wilkins.

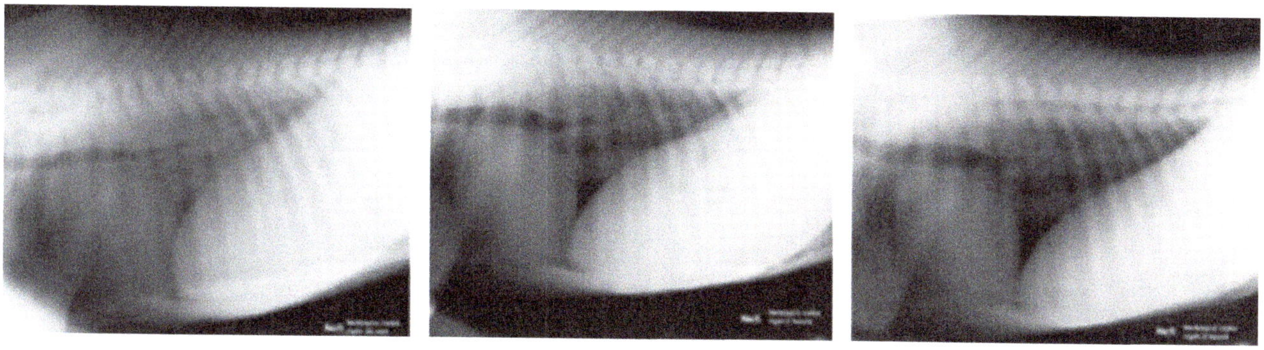

Figure 6.II.1 Series of left-to-right lateral radiographs in a newborn foal performed at 30 minutes (left image), 2 hours (middle image), and 4 hours (right image) of age. Note the fluid absorption pattern and change in radiopacity. The clearing of the ventral quadrants preceded that of the dorsal quadrants [3].

present by 12–24 hours of age [1] and radiographic differentiation of normal versus diseased lung should be possible by 24 hours of age [2]. Resolution of lung opacity progresses gradually from the ventral to the dorsal lung and as residual fluid is cleared from the airways should shift from an alveolar interstitial to primarily an interstitial pattern [2, 3]. This ventral-dorsal pattern of clearance is also reported in calves [19]. To what extent dysmaturity or illness may alter or delay the pattern and timing of clearance of fetal fluid in foals is unknown; however, failure of radiographic changes attributed to fetal lung fluid to resolve within 24 hours of birth should prompt suspicion of concurrent respiratory disease.

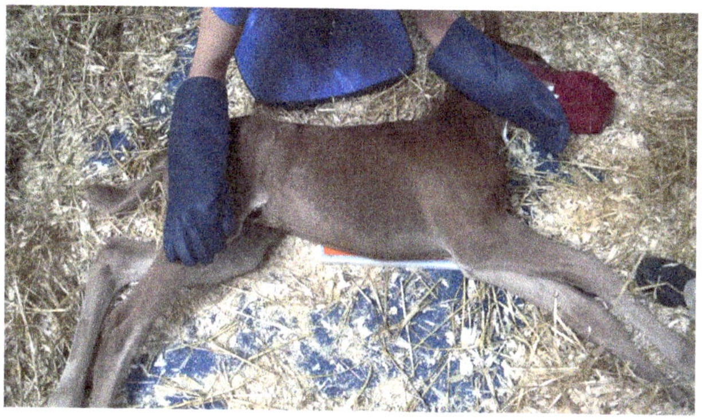

Figure 6.II.2 Nonsedated 14-day-old foal positioned in lateral recumbency for radiographic imaging. Notice the minimal manual restraint and the forelimbs extended cranially to maximize imaging of the cranial lung field. The digital plate is positioned under the foal to capture the cranial lung field.

Patient-Related Artifacts

The most common patient related artifacts observed radiographically in neonatal foals include motion, particularly associated with respiration, and atelectasis. Positioning and the use of sedation influence the development of these artifacts. Lateral views (standing or laterally recumbent) are acquired in the majority of foals. In very young, sick, or debilitated foals, imaging in lateral recumbency is preferred and can be done rapidly with minimal restraint and often no sedation. Lateral views in sternal recumbency and ventro-dorsal views although described, are rarely acquired and may not be tolerated in nonsedated or sick foals [4]. In laterally recumbent foals, acquiring bilateral views at peak inspiration minimizes interference of atelectasis in the dependent lung and optimizes characterization of lung pathology in the nondependent lung field [1, 4]. Evaluation of the craniodorsal lung region is most challenging due to the superimposition of soft tissue structures [1, 4, 6]. Pulling the forelimbs slightly forward improves visualization of the cranial lung field (Figure 6.II.2) [4]. Sedation, in select cases, reduces the chance for movement during image acquisition. In situations where it is necessary, midazolam (0.02–0.1 mg/kg IV or IM) with or without the addition of butorphanol (0.02–0.1 mg/kg IV or IM) can be administered as these drugs are less likely to cause respiratory or cardiovascular side effects in neonatal foals [20]. These medications still have the potential to cause respiratory depression or skeletal muscle relaxation and may contribute to the development of atelectasis [21].

Motion Artifact

Voluntary or involuntary movement of the foal during image acquisition causes motion artifact that can mimic pathologic changes. While these may be more of a problem when using more sensitive imaging modalities, such as computed tomography, they can still impair interpretation on standard radiography. Voluntary movement appears radiographically as blurring or streaking of thoracic structures and can be minimized with proper restraint or sedation. Respiratory motion artifacts appear radiographically as diffuse blurring and are difficult to avoid particularly in neonatal foals with increased respiratory rates. Imaging at peak inspiration minimizes the impact of respiratory motion and has the added benefit of improving contrast

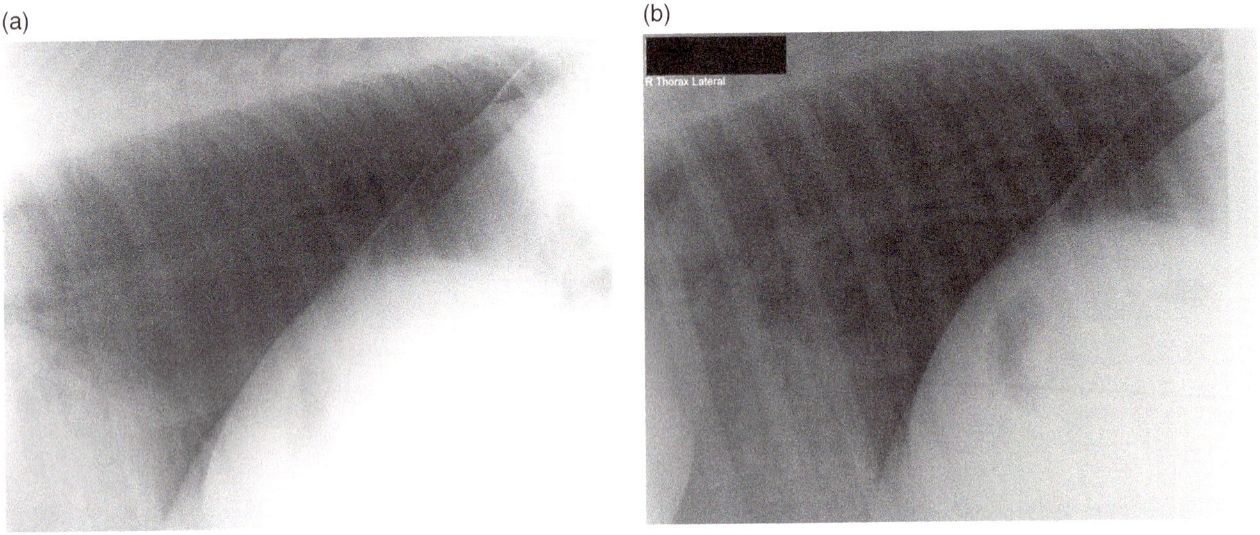

Figure 6.II.3 Standing lateral horizontal beam radiograph of caudodorsal lung taken of a 2-week-old foal during the inspiratory phase of respiration (a) and the expiratory phase of respiration (b). The inspiratory phase is recognized by the flattening of the diaphragm while the expiratory phase is noted by the more domed (curved) appearance of the diaphragm and the appearance of a slight interstitial pattern.

between fully aerated lung and pathological changes (Figure 6.II.3) [4]. In foals imaged during expiration an interstitial lung pattern is observed, which diminishes true contrast between normal aerated lung and pathology [1, 4].

Atelectasis

Atelectasis develops rapidly [22, 23] and is visualized in healthy foals imaged in lateral or sternal recumbency (Figure 6.II.4) [1, 4, 9]. The degree to which atelectasis may progress likely depends on several clinically relevant factors, including duration of recumbency, use of anesthetic or sedative medications, concurrent pulmonary disease, and delivery of supplemental oxygen [4, 22–25]. Age may also play a role among very young foals. Although quantified using CT, sedated foals <7 days of age had more pronounced changes consistent with atelectasis than foals between the ages of 7–14 days of age [24]. Additional factors that may predispose neonatal foals (versus older foals or adults) to the development of

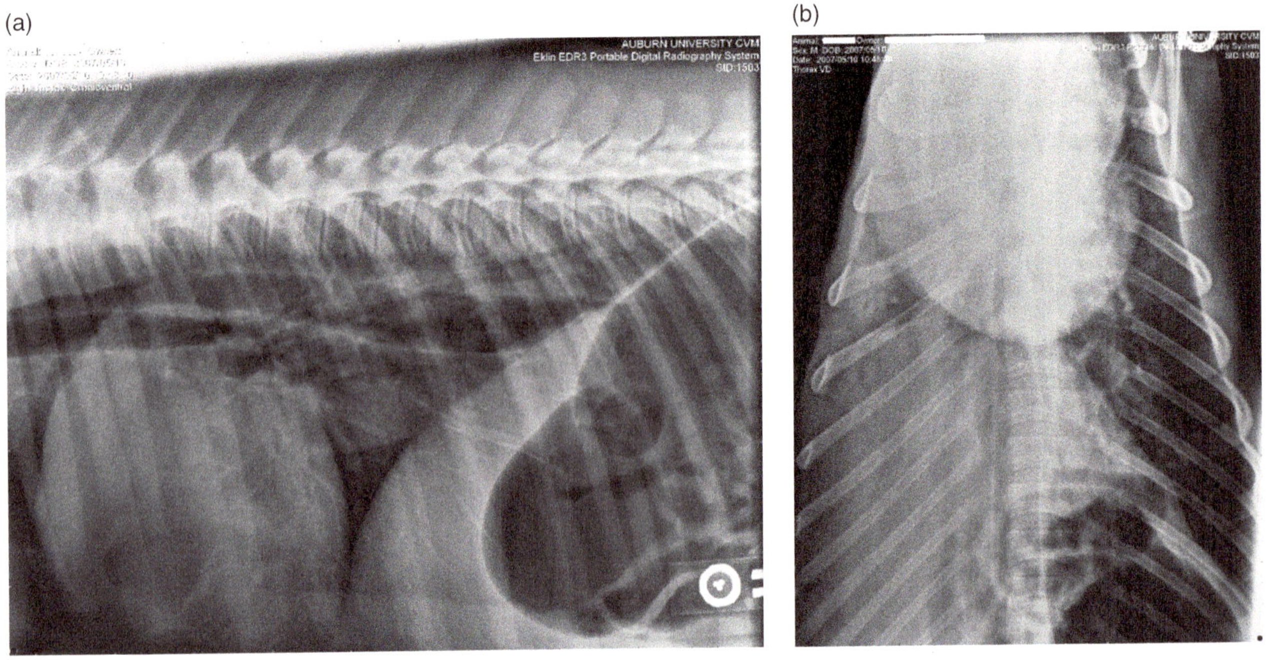

Figure 6.II.4 Three-hour-old QH colt. Radiographs taken on presentation after 1.5-hour transport in right lateral recumbency. Note significant atelectasis of right lung on VD view: (a) lateral view; (b) VD view, no other abnormalities detected.

atelectasis include immaturity in lung and chest wall compliance, and, in sick or sedated foals, increased potential for respiratory muscle fatigue and hypoventilation [4, 25–28].

Interstitial and alveolar radiographic patterns represent regions of atelectatic lung but may also indicate concurrent pulmonary disease. In laterally recumbent foals, dependent atelectasis is most often characterized as a mild-to-moderate interstitial pattern diffusely distributed in the caudodorsal lung [1, 2, 4]. Localized and asymmetric distribution in the perihilar region is also described [1]. In sedated, healthy neonatal foals imaged in sternal recumbency findings are most prominent in the caudoventral lung region where atelectasis is characterized by an alveolar pattern with moderate interstitial changes [9].

In nonsedated recumbent foals imaged while breathing room air, atelectasis is most likely attributed to positional effects [4]. The primary mechanism contributing to development of positional atelectasis is compression of the dependent lung by overlying lung tissue or adjacent thoracic structures and impaired lung expansion [22]. Cranial displacement of the diaphragm and increased pressure from distended abdominal contents may also contribute to positional atelectasis in select cases with concurrent abdominal disease [1]. Positional changes should result in resolution of atelectasis within minutes [1, 22, 25]. Failure to do so may indicate concurrent pulmonary disease.

Absorption atelectasis in response to increases in inspired oxygen (F_iO_2) is well recognized in anesthetized patients [22, 23, 28–30]. Increased F_iO_2 drives oxygen transport across the alveolar membrane resulting in washout of the alveolar nitrogen skeleton, particularly in the presence of low ventilation-perfusion matching, and concurrent hypoventilation [22, 23, 29]. The extent to which supplemental intranasal oxygen contributes to atelectasis formation in recumbent neonatal foals is unknown. Atelectatic changes have been observed in animals with an F_iO_2 as low as 50% and thus may be applicable in sick foals administered intranasal supplemental oxygen at rates ≥150 ml/kg/min prior to and during imaging [4, 30, 31].

Radiographic Changes Associated with Pneumonia and Other Lower Respiratory Tract Diseases

Radiographic patterns may aid in characterization of respiratory disease but can also correlate poorly with clinical severity or lag behind progression or response to treatment [4]. Changes over the course of disease are expected and thus sequential imaging should be performed to best characterize radiographic findings and to monitor disease progression and resolution [4]. Retrospective studies describing radiographic changes in neonatal foals with lower respiratory tract disease identified involvement of the caudodorsal alone or with the caudoventral lung field most frequently, while involvement of the cranioventral lung was identified least frequently [1, 5, 6]. Additionally, increased severity of radiographic changes in the caudodorsal region corresponded to reduced survival of foals [1, 5, 6]. When sequential imaging was available, resolution of radiographic abnormalities most often progressed in a dorsal-to-ventral and caudal-to-cranial direction [5, 6].

In immature foals, NERDS (respiratory distress syndrome or hyaline membrane disease) can present with severe radiographic changes. These foals are presumed to have a primary surfactant deficiency and present at <24 hours of age with clinical signs of severe respiratory distress [32–34]. EqNARDS represents a separate but equally severe clinical syndrome arising secondary to progression of primary pulmonary disease, bacterial sepsis, or perinatal viral disease [7, 33]. Immaturity is not a feature of EqNARDS and foals typically present at >24 hours of age. Both NERDS and EqNARDS carry a poor prognosis and although they represent distinct clinical syndromes, their radiographic characterization is similar [1, 2, 4, 32, 33]. Radiographic changes identified with both syndromes include a diffuse interstitial pattern with an overlying severe, multifocal-to-diffuse coalescing alveolar pattern. Air bronchograms are often noted and the cardiac silhouette and margins of the diaphragm may be obscured, particularly with NERDS. In foals with NERDS radiographic changes are typically distributed throughout all lung fields.

Radiographic changes associated with pneumonia will depend somewhat on the cause of disease. In neonatal foals, aspiration pneumonia most often occurs secondary to aspiration of milk and only rarely to perinatal meconium aspiration (Figure 6.II.5) [32, 33]. Neonatal foals with a poor suckle reflex or dysphagia are at increased risk for aspiration of milk. Radiographically, aspiration pneumonia is characterized by an alveolar pattern primarily in the caudoventral lung with air bronchograms identified in more severe cases [1]. These changes may be localized to the perihilar region with milk aspiration and are generally more severe and more diffusely distributed throughout the lung in foals with meconium aspiration [1, 32]. Radiographic findings associated with pneumonia in neonatal foals secondary to hematogenous spread of bacteria to the lung from sepsis or secondary to viral infection are typically distributed caudodorsally or throughout the entire lung with patterns ranging from interstitial to coalescing alveolar [1, 5–7, 32, 34, 35].

(a) (b)

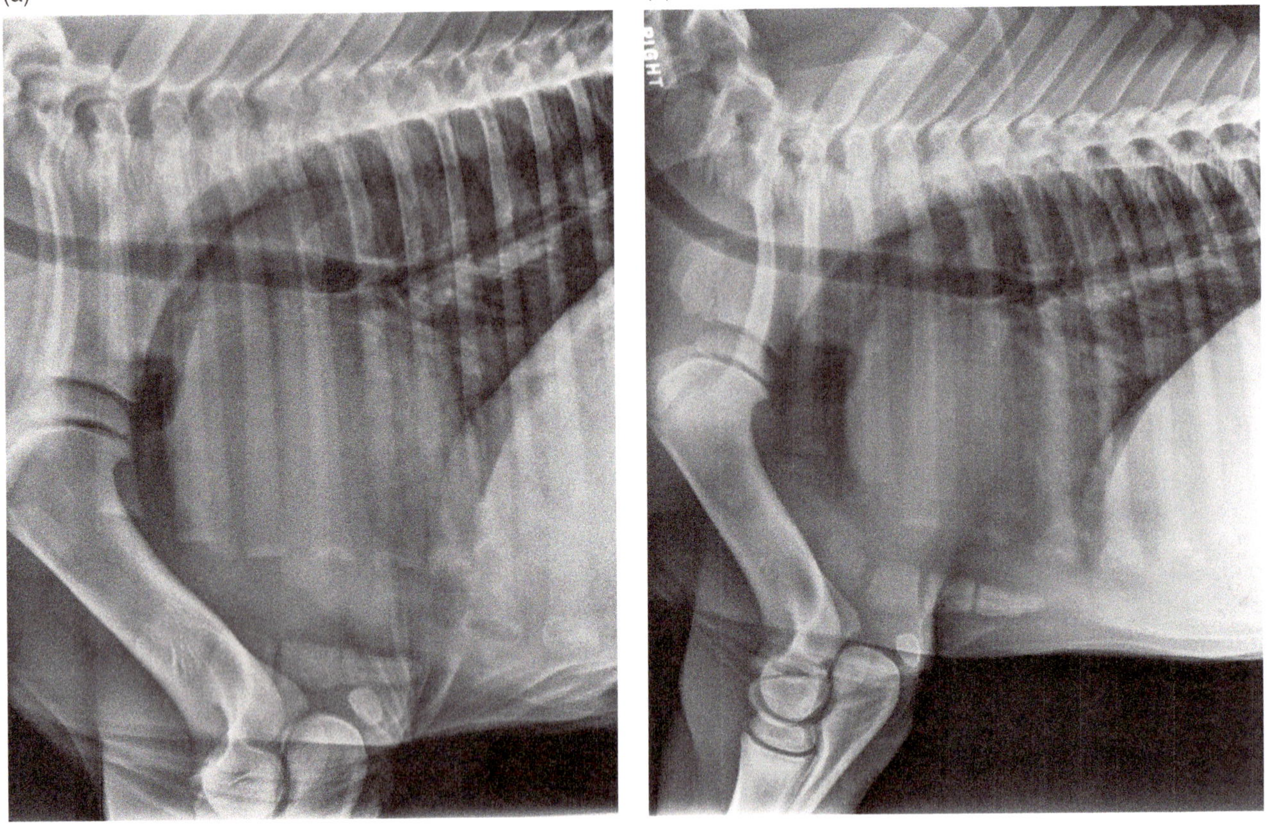

Figure 6.II.5 Standing lateral horizontal beam radiographs of the cranial lung taken in a 10-day-old septic foal with aspiration pneumonia and sepsis. Note alveolar pattern in the caudoventral lung. Additionally, the more caudal forelimb position in image (a) results in superimposition over cranial lung. In image (b) the forelimb is extended forward improving visualization of cranial lung.

Radiographic Identification of Pneumothorax and Rib Fractures

Pneumothorax in neonatal foals develops secondary to thoracic trauma [8] or, in foals with severe pulmonary disease and ruptured pulmonary bullae [4, 36]. Foals present in varying degrees of respiratory distress depending on the severity of air leak and the underlying cause. Radiographic detection is best using horizontal beam radiography with the foal positioned in lateral recumbency [4]. Because of the potential for concurrent parenchymal pathology, rib fractures, or hemothorax, standard lateral views or thoracic ultrasound or CT are recommended. In young foals, the most common cause of rib fracture is trauma associated with parturition. Although fractures can be identified radiographically, detection with thoracic ultrasound or CT is considered superior [4, 8]. In cases where clinical signs of pain or respiratory distress are not present, identification of rib fractures can be an incidental finding. As with pneumothorax, additional imaging is recommended in more severe cases because of the risk for associated damage to other thoracic structures. If surgical correction of complex fractures is necessary, preoperative CT imaging can be useful [37].

References

1 Lester, G.D. and Lester, N.V. (2001). Abdominal and thoracic radiography in the neonate. *Vet. Clin. North Am. Equine Pract.* 17 (1): 19–46.

2 Lamb, C.R., O'Callaghan, M.W., and Paradis, M.R. (1990). Thoracic radiography in the neonatal foal: a preliminary report. *Vet. Radiol.* 31 (1): 11–16.

3 Kutasi, O., Horvath, A., Harnos, A., and Szenci, O. (2009). Radiographic assessment of pulmonary fluid clearance in healthy neonatal foals. *Vet. Radiol. Ultrasound* 50 (6): 584–588.

4 Lascola, K.M. and Joselyn, S. (2015). Diagnostic imaging of the lower respiratory tract in

neonatal foals. *Vet. Clin. North Am. Equine Pract.* 31497–31514.

5 Bedenice, D., Heuwieser, W., Solano, M. et al. (2003). Risk factors and prognostic variables for survival of foals with radiographic evidence of pulmonary disease. *J. Vet. Intern. Med.* 17 (6): 868–875.

6 Bedenice, D., Heuwieser, W., Brawer, R. et al. (2003). Clinical and prognostic significance of radiographic pattern, distribution, and severity of thoracic radiographic changes in neonatal foals. *J. Vet. Intern. Med.* 17 (6): 876–886.

7 Wilkins, P.A. and Lascola, K.M. (2015). Update on interstitial pneumonia. *Vet. Clin. North Am. Equine Pract.* 31 (1): 137–157.

8 Jean, D., Picandet, V., Macieira, S. et al. (2007). Detection of rib trauma in newborn foals in an equine critical care unit: a comparison of ultrasonography, radiography and physical examination. *Equine Vet. J.* 39 (2): 158–163.

9 Schliewert, E.-C., Lascola, K.M., O'Brien, R.T. et al. (2014). Comparison of radiographic and computed tomographic images of the lungs in healthy neonatal foals. *Am. J. Vet. Res.* 76 (1): 42–52.

10 Aherne, W. and Dawkins, M.J.R. (1964). The removal of fluid from the pulmonary airways after birth in the rabbit, and the effect on this of prematurity and pre-natal hypoxia. *Neonatology* 7 (4–5): 214–229.

11 Bland, R.D., Hansen, T.N., Haberkern, C.M. et al. (1982). Lung fluid balance in lambs before and after birth. *J. Appl. Phys.* 53 (4): 992–1004.

12 Silva, L.C.G., Lucio, C.F., Veiga, G.A.L. et al. (2009). Neonatal clinical evaluation, blood gas and radiographic assessment after normal birth, vaginal dystocia or caesarean section in dogs. *Reprod. Domest. Anim.* 44 (Suppl 2): 160–163.

13 Jain, L. and Eaton, D.C. (2006). Physiology of fetal lung fluid clearance. *Semin. Perinatol.* 30: 34–43.

14 Elias, N. and O'Brodovich, H. (2006). Clearance of fluid from airspaces of newborns and infants. *NeoReviews* 7 (2): e88–e94. https://doi.org/10.1542/neo.7-2-e88.

15 Barker, P.M. and Olver, R.E. (2002). Invited review: clearance of lung liquid during the perinatal period. *J. Appl. Phys.* 93 (4): 1542–1548.

16 Katz, C., Bentur, L., and Elias, N. (2011). Clinical implication of lung fluid balance in the perinatal period. *J. Perinatol.* 31 (4): 230–235.

17 Hillman, N., Kallapur, S.G., and Jobe, A. (2012). Physiology of transition from intrauterine to extrauterine life. *Clin. Perinatol.* 39 (4): 769–783.

18 Abdelmegeid, M.K., Kutasi, O., Nassiff, M.N. et al. (2017). Radiographic assessment of pulmonary fluid clearance and lung aeration in newborn calves delivered by elective caesarean section. *Reprod. Domest. Anim.* 52: 939–944.

19 Vannucchi, C.I. and Silva, L.C.G. (2018). Unruh SM, et al calving duration and obstetric assistance influence pulmonary function of Holstein calves during immediate fetal-to-neonatal transition. *PLos One* 13: e0204129.

20 Sinclair, M. (2015). Sedation and anesthetic management of foals. In: *Robinson's Current Therapy in Equine Medicine*, 7e (ed. K.A. Sprayberry and N.E. Robinson), 766–771. Elsevier.

21 Muir, W.W. (2009). Anxiolytics, nonopioid sedative analgesics, and opioid analgesics. In: *Equine Anesthesia: Monitoring and Emergency Therapy*, 2e (ed. W.W. Muir and J.A.E. Hubbell), 185–209. St Louis: Saunders.

22 Magnusson, L. and Spahn, D.R. (2003). New concepts of atelectasis during general anesthesia. *Br. J. Anaesth.* 91: 61–72.

23 Duggan, M. and Kavanagh, B.P. (2005). Pulmonary atelectasis: a pathogenic perioperative entity. *Anesthesiology* 102: 838–854.

24 Lascola, K.M., O'Brien, R.T., Wilkins, P.A. et al. (2013). Qualitative and quantitative interpretation of computed tomography of the lungs in healthy neonatal foals. *Am. J. Vet. Res.* 74 (9): 1239–1246.

25 Lascola, K.M., Clark-Price, S., O'Brien, R.T. et al. (2013). Use of manual alveolar recruitment maneuvers to eliminate atelectasis artifacts identified during thoracic computed tomography of healthy neonatal foals. *Am. J. Vet. Res.* 74 (9): 1239–1246.

26 Koterba, A.M., Wozniak, J.A., and Kosch, P.C. (1994). Respiratory mechanics of the horse during the first year of life. *Respir. Physiol.* 95 (1): 21–41.

27 Koterba, A.M., Wozniak, J.A., and Kosch, P.C. (1995). Ventilatory and timing parameters in normal horses at rest up to age one year. *Equine Vet. J.* 27 (4): 257–264.

28 Serafini, G., Cornara, G., Cavalloro, F. et al. (1999). Pulmonary atelectasis during paediatric anaesthesia: CT scan evaluation and effect of positive end expiratory pressure (PEEP). *Paediatr. Anaesth.* 9: 225–228.

29 Kerr, C.L. and McDonell, W.N. (2009). Oxygen supplementation and ventilatory support. In: *Equine Anesthesia: Monitoring and Emergency Therapy*, 2e (ed. W.W. Muir and J.A.E. Hubbell), 332–352. St Louis: WB Saunders Co.

30 Staffieri, F., De Monte, V., De Marzo, C. et al. (2010). Effects of two fractions of inspired oxygen on lung aeration and gas exchange in cats under inhalant anaesthesia. *Vet. Anaesth. Analg.* 37 (6): 483–490.

31 Wong, D.M., Alcott, C.J., Wang, C. et al. (2010). Physiologic effects of nasopharyngeal administration of supplemental oxygen at various flow rates in healthy neonatal foals. *Am. J. Vet. Res.* 71: 1081–1088.

32 Wilkins, P.A. (2003). Lower respiratory problems of the neonate. *Vet. Clin. North Am. Equine Pract.* 19 (1): 19–33.

33 Wilkins, P.A., Otto, C.M., Baumgardner, J.E. et al. (2007). Acute lung injury and acute respiratory distress syndromes in veterinary medicine: consensus definitions: the Dorothy Russell Havemeyer Working Group on ALI and ARDS in Veterinary Medicine. *J. Vet. Emerg. Crit. Care* 17 (4): 333–339.

34 Vaala, W.E., Hamir, A.N., Dubovi, E.J. et al. (1992). Fatal, congenitally acquired infection with equine arteritis virus in a neonatal thoroughbred. *Equine Vet. J.* 24 (2): 155–158.

35 del Piero, F., Wilkins, P.A., Lopez, J.W. et al. (1997). Equine viral arteritis in newborn foals: clinical, pathological, serological, microbiological and immunohistochemical observations. *Equine Vet. J.* 29 (3): 178–185.

36 Johnson, P.J., LaCarrubba, A.M., Messer, N.T., and DeClue, A.E. (2012). Neonatal respiratory distress and sepsis in the premature foal: challenges with diagnosis and management. *Equine Vet. Educ.* 24 (9): 453–458.

37 Marr, C.M. (2015). The equine neonatal cardiovascular system in health and disease. *Vet. Clin. North Am. Equine Pract.* 31 (3): 545–565.

Section III Thoracic Ultrasonography of the Neonatal Foal

David Wong and Robin White

Thoracic ultrasonography is commonly performed in ill neonatal foals as part of the diagnostic evaluation. The entire thoracic cavity should be examined by using a systematic approach by placing the transducer on both hemithoraces, between each intercostal space (ICS), starting from caudal and moving cranial (or cranial to caudal), working dorsal to ventral. The cranial mediastinum can be visualized cranial to the heart by pulling one of the forelimbs forward and aiming the transducer in as cranial position as possible, angled cranial and toward the opposite shoulder. Rubbing alcohol is needed to generate adequate contact with the skin, but the hair does not necessarily need to be clipped to perform the ultrasound. A 7.5 MHz microconvex or linear transducer generally provides the optimal image quality with a depth setting of 5–10 cm in the neonatal foal. Ideally, the sonogram is performed with the foal standing or in sternal recumbency as excess fluid or intestinal contents within the pleural cavity might lie beneath the air-filled lung and be hidden by the lung field if the foal is in lateral recumbency. Anatomic structures routinely examined via thoracic ultrasonography include the pleural space, lungs, heart, thymus, diaphragm, and ribs.

Thoracic Anatomy

The cranial thorax contains the cranial lung lobes, the caudal portions of the trachea and esophagus, vasculature, fat, and in the neonatal foal, the thymus. The cranial most portion of the thorax lies beneath the triceps and muscles of the lateral thoracic wall. Therefore, ultrasonographic exam through the triceps is necessary to examine the most cranial portions of the lung (Figure 6.III.1a). The heart is covered by the air-filled lung except in the areas of the left and right cardiac notches (ventral at approximately the 3rd to 5th ICS), therefore imaging of the heart should occur in these regions. The cupula of the diaphragm apposes the margin of the caudal heart. Due to gravity, pleural effusion, or consolidated lung, if present, is frequently noted in the area caudal to the cardiac notches and craniolateral to the diaphragm. The liver is the prominent structure ventral to the right caudal lung border while the spleen is the primary organ noted ventral to the diaphragm on the left caudal lung border. The liver can be visualized adjacent to the spleen in the most caudoventral portion of the thorax (Figure 6.III.2). The right accessory lung lobe that surrounds the caudal vena cava is not visualized in the healthy foal nor is the esophagus or trachea.

Ultrasonographic evaluation of the foal's thorax provides information regarding the lungs (e.g. pneumonia, abscess), pleural cavity (e.g. hemothorax, pleural effusion), heart (Chapter 11), diaphragm (e.g. diaphragmatic hernia), thymus, and ribs (e.g. fractures). The ultrasonographic appearance of the lung (pleural) surface in the healthy foal is the same as the adult horse, appearing as a hyperechoic linear (white) echo, with equidistant reverberation artifacts deep to this line (Figure 6.III.1b). The lungs are located between the 3rd to 15th ICS; the cranial lung is observed in the ventral, mid, and dorsal thorax but shifts to the mid and dorsal thorax as the clinician scans caudally toward the abdomen. Air serves as a near-perfect reflector of ultrasound waves because of its low density and slow propagation velocity of sound as compared to soft tissue [1]. Thus, when the sound beam originating from the ultrasound transducer encounters the normal air-filled lung, it subsequently reverberates between the transducer and lung surface. This reverberation artifact creates the characteristic concentric parallel lines ("A" lines) in the image that correspond to multiple reflections of the sound wave between these interfaces.

Equine Neonatal Medicine, First Edition. Edited by David M. Wong and Pamela A. Wilkins.

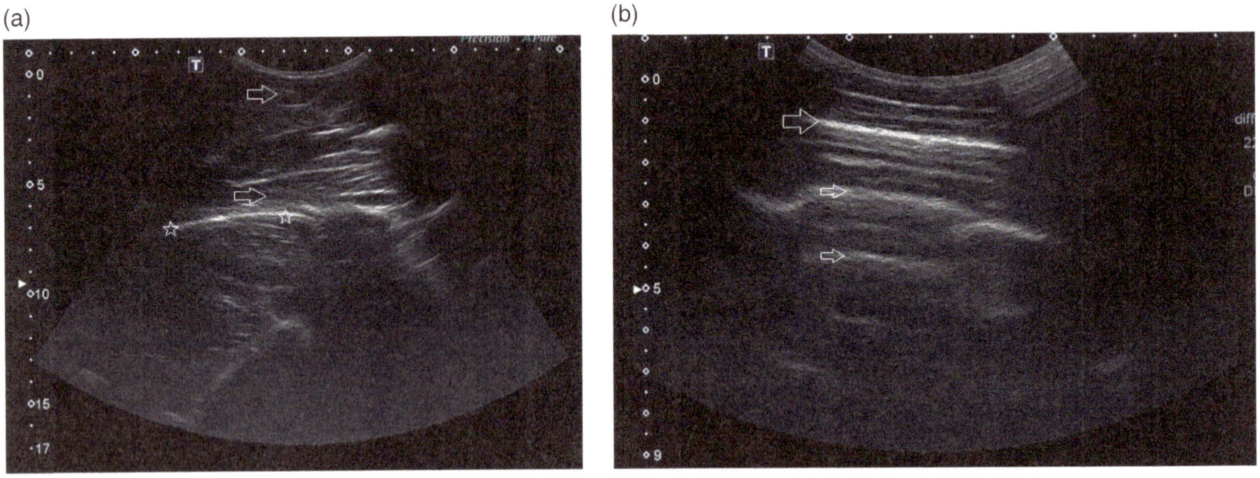

Figure 6.III.1 Thoracic ultrasound in a 3-week-old foal highlighting the lung. (a) Appearance of the pleural surface (stars) of the cranial lung field as imaged through the triceps muscles (arrows). (b) Pleural surface imaged at the 8th ICS (large arrow). Note the normal reverberation artifact caused by the reflective air-filled lung (small arrows).

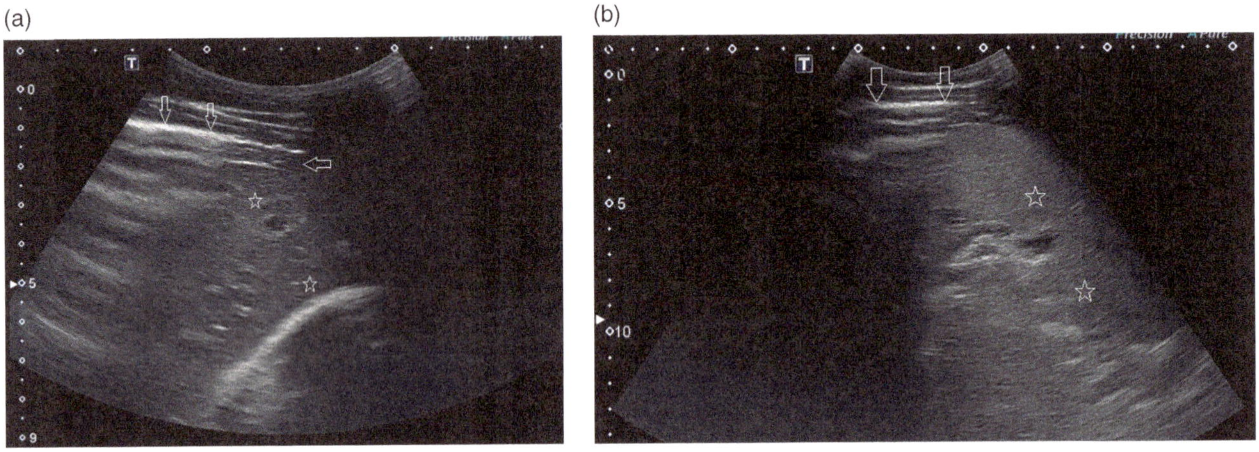

Figure 6.III.2 Thoracic ultrasound in a 3-week-old foal highlighting the interface between the thorax and the abdomen. Cranial is to the left. (a) Appearance of the pleural surface of the caudal lung (vertical arrows), liver (stars), and diaphragm (horizontal arrow) noted on the right side of the foal. (b) Pleural surface of the caudal lung (arrows) and the spleen (stars) noted on the left side of the foal.

Each time the sound reflects back to the ultrasound transducer, another line is recorded deeper in the image because of the time delay [2]. These echoes that form the reverberation lines deep to the pleural surface are artifacts. The "glide sign" or back-and-forth movements of the pleural surface synchronous with respirations should be noted in healthy foals when the transducer is held stationary. In healthy foals there should be no appreciable accumulation of pleural fluid, although a small amount of anechoic fluid may be noted just caudal and ventral to the heart [1].

When the lung surface is irregular due to changes in the peripheral pulmonary parenchyma (i.e. not flat and smooth), small irregularities at the pleural surface result in a reverberation artifact referred to as a "comet tail" ("B" line). Comet tail artifacts are created by the presence of a small area of fluid or cellular infiltrate in the lung periphery [3]. These comet tails appear as a white echogenic streak that originates from the lung surface and traverses deeper into the lung (Figure 6.III.3) and are indicative of variably sized irregularities on the pleural surface [3]. They do not provide information regarding the deeper lung parenchyma and only indicate that the ultrasound has encountered a non-flat subpleural air surface at those sites. The apparently healthy foal may occasionally have a small number of these comet tails, but the clinician should interpret comet tails in light of the number, size, progression, clinical signs, physical examination findings, and potentially other diagnostic tests such as thoracic radiographs.

The thymus can by identified via ultrasound in the foal and appears as a homogenous parenchymatous structure that lies just beneath and medial to the lung in the cranial

(a) (b)

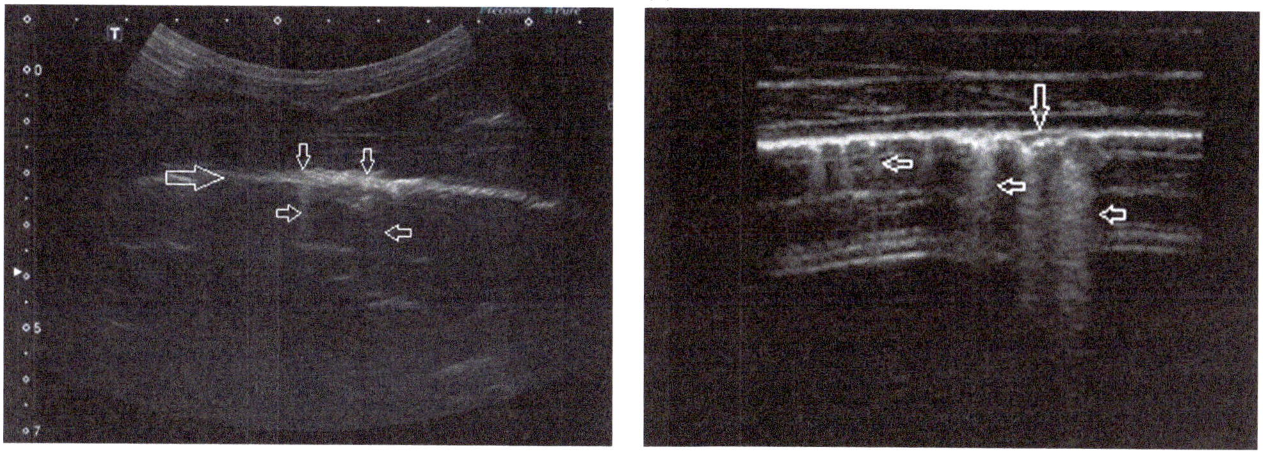

Figure 6.III.3 (a) Pleural surface of a neonatal foal demonstrating the pleural surface (large arrow) along with comet tails (small arrows) created by irregularities on the pleural surface. (b) Neonatal foal with pneumonia demonstrating a series of comet tails (small arrows) and a scant volume of anechoic pleural fluid (large arrow).

mediastinum. Blood vessels may be seen coursing through the thymus (Figure 6.III.4). One study documented normal ultrasonographic features and biometric analysis in 10 healthy foals from birth to 6 months of age [4]. In that study, the thymus was visualized by pulling one of the forelimbs forward and directing the transducer cranial and ventral to the heart in the 2nd to 3rd ICS. The thymus was visible in all age groups, being easier to visualize on the left side, and appeared as a hypoechoic tissue relative to the heart [4]. The diaphragm is also visualized via ultrasonography and appears hypoechoic compared to the pleural surface and is thicker ventrally (Figure 6.III.4). The thickness of the diaphragm, measured at the 12th ICS at the level of the mid-thorax, is noted in Table 6.III.1.

Abnormalities Detected via Thoracic Ultrasound

Pathologic conditions that can be detected via thoracic ultrasonography include pneumonia/pleuropneumonia, pulmonary edema, pulmonary consolidation, superficial pulmonary abscesses, fractured ribs, hemothorax, and pneumothorax. Although the development of pleural fluid is relatively rare in the neonatal foal, when present, fluid is typically located between the thoracic wall and the visceral pleural surface, diaphragm, and/or heart. The fluid can appear anechoic, likely having low cellularity and protein concentration (e.g. transudate), or can have increased echogenicity, which is characteristic highly cellular fluid

(a) (b)

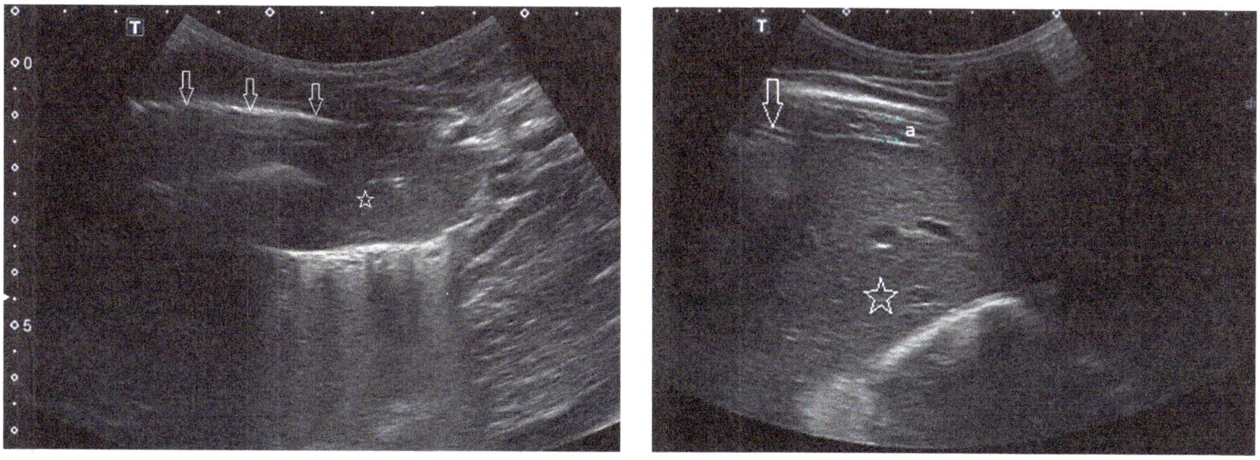

Figure 6.III.4 (a) Sonogram of the thymus (star) in a 4-month-old Standardbred colt imaged in the cranial mediastinum (left 3rd ICS). The overlying pleural lung surface produces an echogenic line at its periphery (arrows). Dorsal is to the right of the image.
(b) Appearance of the diaphragm ("a" marker, 5.3 mm) as imaged from the right side of a healthy foal. Note the pleural surface (arrow) and liver within the image as well (star).

Table 6.III.1 Mean (range) thickness of the diaphragm, measured in centimeters, at various ages in the foal [4].

Age: 1 d	Age: 7 d	Age: 14 d	Age: 21 d	Age: 1 mo	Age: 2 mo
0.5 (0.45–0.55)	0.55 (0.50–0.66)	0.58 (0.50–0.68)	0.59 (0.50–0.68)	0.62 (0.50–0.73)	0.64 (0.60–0.71)
Age: 3 mo	Age: 4 mo	Age: 5 mo	Age: 6 mo		
0.66 (0.59–0.82)	0.73 (0.59–0.84)	0.82 (0.67–0.97)	0.87 (0.73–1.00)		

(e.g. exudate) [5]. Hyperechoic, swirling pleural fluid is characteristic of hemothorax. If there is an accumulation of pleural fluid, the clinician should also determine if there is any cellular debris or fibrin with the latter appearing as linear hyperechoic striations within the fluid. A sample of the fluid can be collected using ultrasound to help guide the sampling from the largest pocket of fluid or area of interest. Differentials for the presence of pleural fluid in the foal include infection of the lung, hemothorax, uroperitoneum resulting in diffusion of peritoneal fluid into the pleural space, penetrating thoracic wound, or a congenital anomaly within the thorax.

Bacterial Pneumonia

Bacterial pneumonia is a common clinical disorder in neonatal foals that develop infection secondary to sepsis or aspiration of foreign material (milk, meconium, other); alternatively, pneumonia can be acquired as a primary condition via inhalation. Ultrasonography is commonly used to identify consolidated lung tissue which refers to a lack of aeration in the pulmonary parenchyma as a result of accumulation of fluid and/or cellular infiltrate [5]. Of note, the appearance of comet tails may precede the ultrasonographic appearance of consolidated lung. Consolidated lung frequently appears as hypoechoic areas of pulmonary parenchyma that retain the lung's normal shape along with a loss of the characteristic bright white line (pleural surface) [3, 5]. Alternatively, the appearance of consolidated lung can range from anechoic to hyperechoic and might highlight lung anatomy that is not normally observed in the healthy foal. For example, pulmonary vessels and air bronchograms may be observed and in more severe cases, the lung can ultrasonographically appear similar to the liver (hepatized lung). Air bronchograms are areas of hypoechoic fluid-filled lung parenchyma with hyperechoic free gas echoes imaged within the bronchial tree (Figure 6.III.5) [3]. Fluid bronchograms may be detected in areas of hepatized lung because there is no air detected within the large or small airways; a fluid bronchogram might appear as a hypoechoic fluid-filled bronchial structure [3]. Pulmonary consolidation occurs when the alveolar tissue is filled with fluid and/or cellular debris, rather than air, and can result from bronchopneumonia, plural pneumonia, pulmonary edema, pulmonary necrosis or neoplasia [1, 3]. Additionally, in foals with pneumonia, thoracic radiography should be performed to provide a global view of the lungs and provide information regarding the deeper parenchyma of the lung that is not accessible via sonography.

Pulmonary Abscesses

Pulmonary abscesses are uncommon in neonatal foals with the exception of infection with *Rhodococcus equi* in older foals (3 weeks to 5 months of age) [6, 7]. *R. equi* causes pyogranulomatous bronchopneumonia and abscessation in foals and is a common cause of morbidity in this age group [8]. Thoracic ultrasonography is frequently used as an early screening tool and to monitor the progression of foals for *R. equi* infection, especially on endemic farms, and has been used to successfully identify clinical and subclinical cases [5–7, 9]. Pulmonary abscesses lack any normal pulmonary architecture and appear as cavitated lesions within the lung parenchyma with an anechoic center and acoustic enhancement of the far wall, indicative of a fluid filled structure (Figure 6.III.6) [1, 3]. Differentiating a pulmonary abscess from an area of lung consolidation can be difficult as both abnormalities can appear as circular hypoechoic areas [3]. Bronchial structures and pulmonary vessels can still be located in foals with severe consolidation whereas these structures are absent in abscesses [3]. In general, pulmonary abscesses in horses are not encapsulated, but foals with *R. equi* are a notable exception [3]. In these foals, a relatively hyperechoic capsule may be noted on ultrasonography surrounding echogenic to anechoic fluid within the pulmonary abscess [3].

Atelectasis

Atelectasis is a common occurrence in ill neonatal foals and can arise from compression of the pulmonary parenchyma during pathologic conditions such as pleural effusion or pneumothorax or from nonpathologic situations

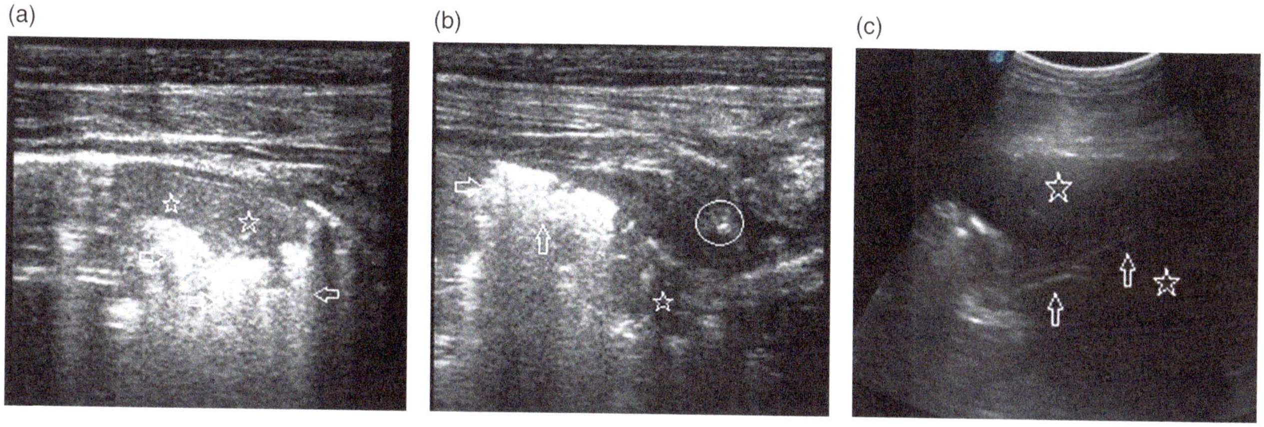

Figure 6.III.5 (a)–(c) Areas of consolidated lung (stars) intermixed with aerated lung (arrows) in a neonatal foal with pneumonia. Note the air bronchogram (circle [b], arrow [c]) characterized by a hyperechoic linear tubular structure surrounded by hypoechoic consolidated lung. *Source:* Figure (c) courtesy of Dr. Kate Hepworth, North Carolina State University.

such as recumbency in the foal. If atelectasis is secondary to pleural effusion, the ventral portion of the lung tip appears as a narrow triangular section of lung in which bronchi and pulmonary vessels are still imaged. As compared to consolidated lung, atelectatic lung appears to float in the pleural fluid (Figure 6.III.7) [5].

Rib Fractures

Rib fractures and costochondral dislocations are common in newborn foals with one report noting that approximately 20% of foals <3 days of age on a large Thoroughbred farm had physical evidence of thoracic trauma [10]. In another study, rib fractures were commonly noted in foals admitted to an equine critical care unit [11]. In this particular study, 29 newborn foals (15 fillies, 14 colts, age range 1–10 days, mean age 2.96 days) were diagnosed with rib fractures during a single foaling season [11]. A comparison was made in establishing a diagnosis of rib fracture(s) between radiography and ultrasonography; thoracic radiographs revealed 10 rib fractures in 5/26 foals (19%) as compared to ultrasonography which located 49 fractures in 19/29 foals (65%) [11]. The authors concluded that ultrasonography is a more accurate than radiography and identifies rib fractures in most patients presented in emergent situations.

Rib fractures are most commonly located close to (e.g. within 3 cm) of the costochondral junction and appear as an interruption (i.e. step defect) in the normally continuous hyperechoic bony surface of the rib, with or without displacement and fragments (Figure 6.III.8) [1]. If the fragment is displaced, the distal portion of the fracture can displace medially or laterally [11, 12]. A hematoma may also be noted surrounding the fracture site. The 2nd through 7th ribs accounted for 69% (34/49) of fractured ribs in one study [11]. This area of the rib cage might be prone to rib fracture(s) because of the inherent shape of the foals chest or from the retention and subsequent focal pressure of a flexed elbow on the thoracic cage during parturition [13]. Other rib abnormalities that might be noted via ultrasonography include abnormal hyperechoic areas on the costochondral junction, medial deformation of the rib near the costochondral junction, abnormal hyperechoic areas involving the ventral part of the rib, irregularity of the rib, and costochondral dislocation [11]. Interestingly, if radiography is used to identify rib fractures, most fractures are identified via a ventro-dorsal radiograph, which allows better evaluation of the rib contours [11].

While many rib fractures may be incidental findings and subclinical, more serious consequences of rib fractures such as pulmonary contusion, hemothorax (Figure 6.III.9), pneumothorax, diaphragmatic hernia, hemopericardium, and death from myocardial laceration have been reported [12]. Another complication of fractured ribs is flail chest; in this situation, several consecutive ribs are fractured, leading to an incompetent segment of thoracic wall. The foal's respiratory efforts are compromised by the failure of the affected rib arcade to lift and participate in the process of inspiration and creating negative pleural pressure [12]. During expiration, the affected rib segment fails to collapse as a unit and impedes the normal development of positive airway pressure. Clinically, flail chest manifests as inward sinking of the affected portion of the chest wall during inspiration.

Pneumothorax

Pneumothorax is rare in the neonatal foal, but can result from penetrating trauma to the thorax (open pneumothorax), from air that originates from the lung parenchyma

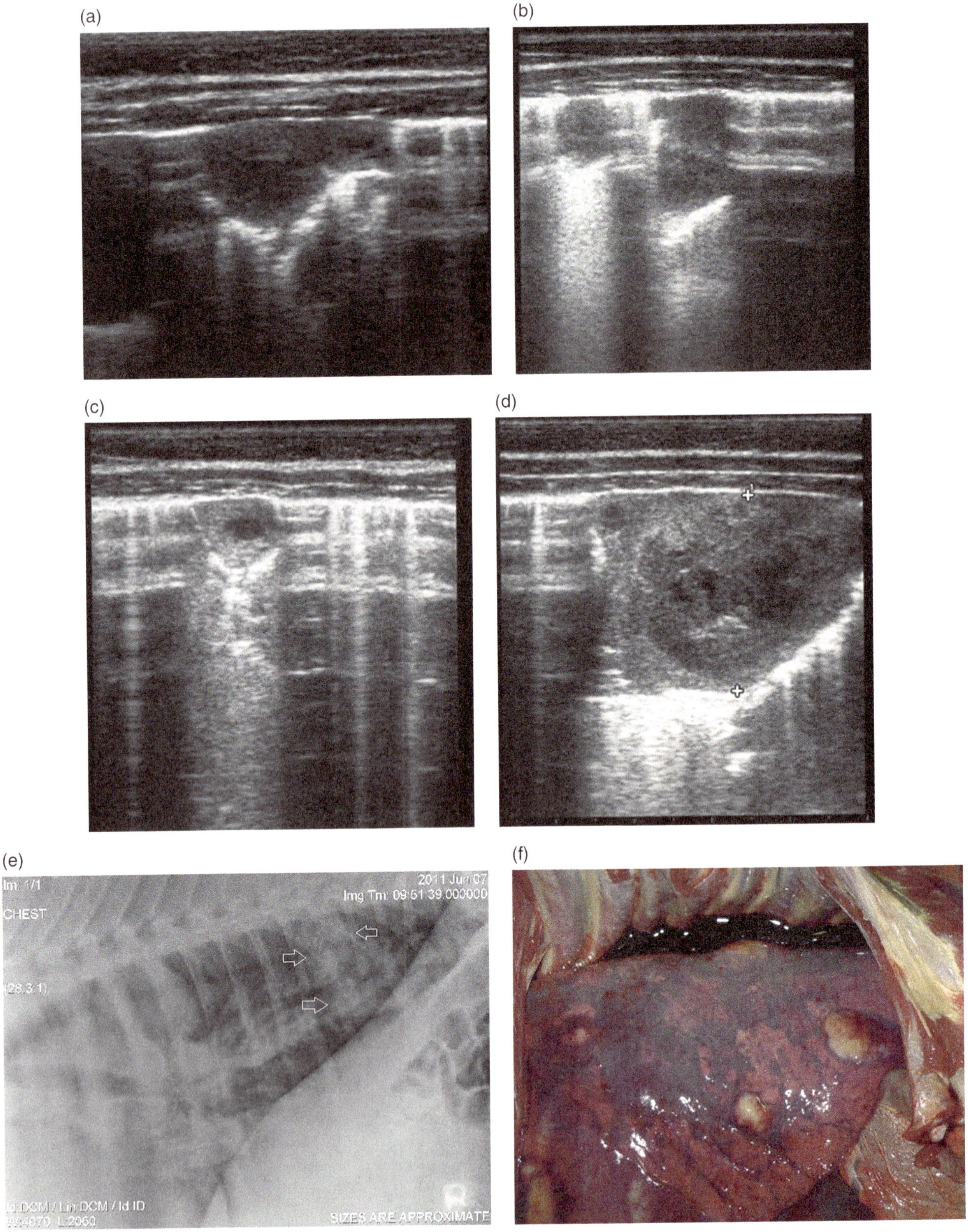

Figure 6.III.6 Various sonographic images of a 6-week-old Thoroughbred foal with signs of respiratory disease that subsequently had growth of *Rhodococcus equi* from a transtracheal wash sample. (a)–(d) Sonogram demonstrating variably sized, well-defined hyperechoic encapsulated nodules with hypoechoic centers. (d) Abscess measuring 2.45 cm. (e) Lateral radiograph of same foal demonstrating diffuse, variably sized abscesses distributed throughout the lung field (arrows). (f) Postmortem image of a different foal that succumbed to *R. equi* pneumonia. Note the appearance of the diffusely distributed pulmonary abscesses in the peripheral portions of the lung.

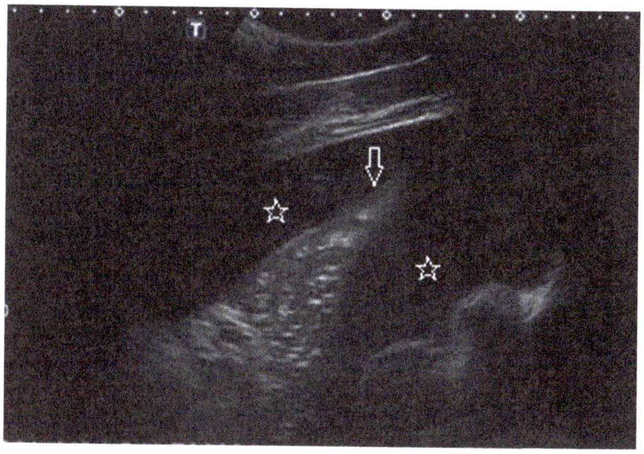

Figure 6.III.7 Atelectasis of the lung tip (arrow) in an adult horse with pleuropneumonia. Note the anechoic fluid surrounding the lung (stars). *Source:* Image courtesy of Dr. Kasia Dembeck, North Carolina State University.

secondary to pneumonia, ruptured bullae, or laceration of the lung from a fractured rib (closed pneumothorax), or secondary to migration of air from a tracheostomy site (air diffuses through facial planes into the thorax) [10, 14]. Pneumothorax is difficult to detect via ultrasonography because the free gas within the pleural space has a similar appearance to the air within the lung (e.g. hyperechoic line with reverberation artifacts) [5]. Careful ultrasonographic examination reveals the absence of the glide sign at the site of the pneumothorax (i.e. dorsal thorax) because the gas in the pleural space prevents the normal gliding of the visceral pleura against the parietal pleura. If available, pneumothorax is easier to detect via a lateral radiograph, but one study demonstrated that ultrasonography is a more sensitive method than radiography in identifying experimentally induced small volume (up to 250 ml) pneumothorax in the adult horse [15].

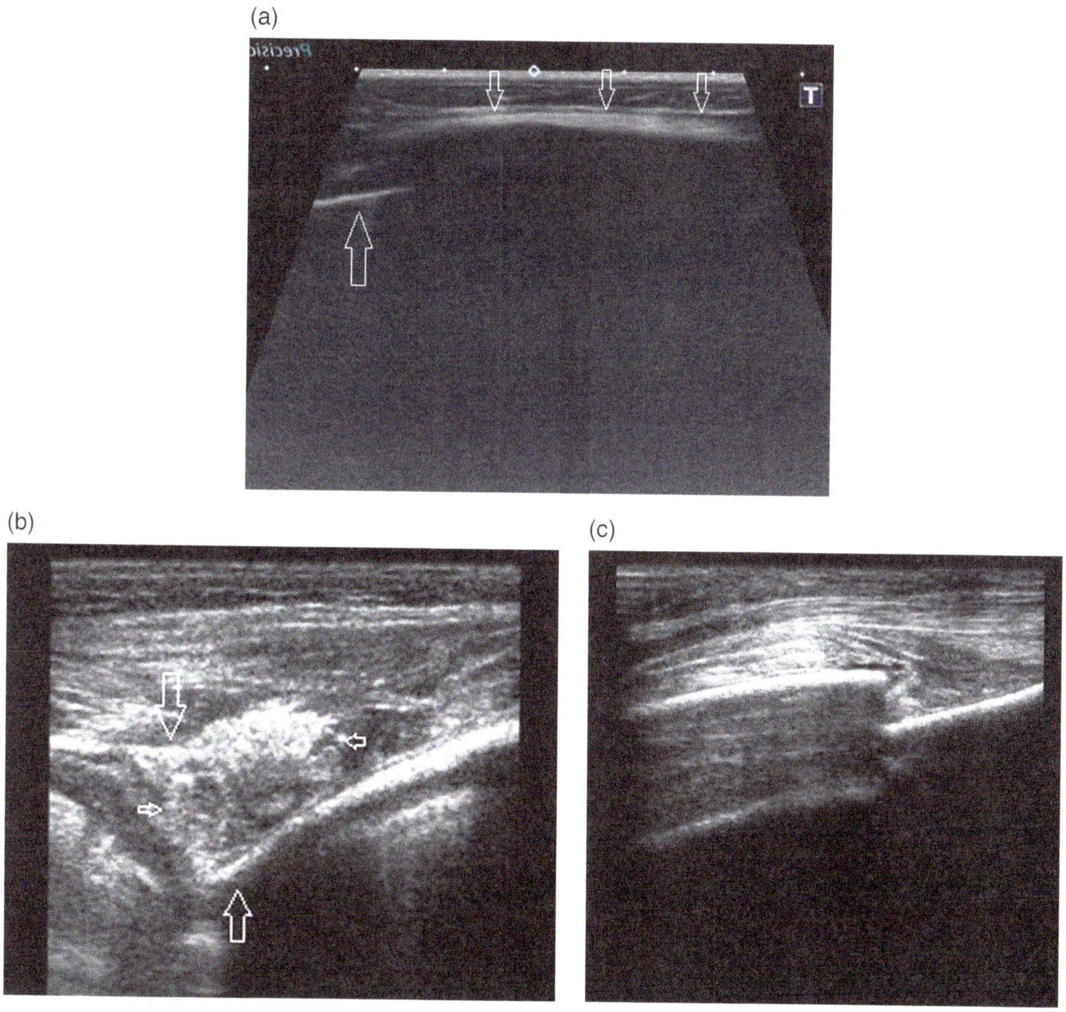

Figure 6.III.8 (a) Sonogram of a normal rib in a 2-day-old neonatal foal. The ultrasound transducer is held parallel to the rib which produces a bright hyperechoic line and casts a shadow deep to the rib (small arrows). A small portion of lung can be seen on the ventral (left) side of the image (large arrow). (b) Image of a neonatal foal with a rib fracture. The ultrasound probe is oriented parallel to the rib and a "step" defect is noted at the fracture site (large arrows). A pocket of heterogeneous fluid with mixed echogenicity, likely a hematoma, is also noted (small arrows). Dorsal is to the right of the image. (c) Rib fracture in a neonatal foal. Note the lateral displacement of the distal portion of the fracture. Dorsal is to the right of the image.

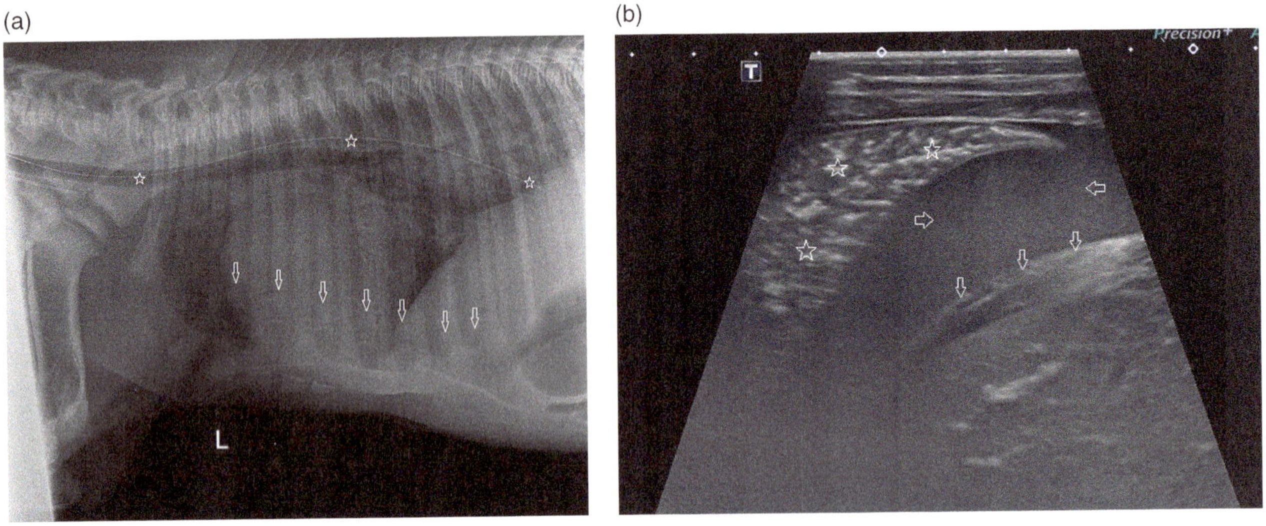

Figure 6.III.9 Four-day-old foal with fractured ribs that occurred secondary to cardiopulmonary resuscitation. (a) Left lateral radiograph noting multiple fractured ribs (arrows) located ventrally, with mild dorsal displacement. A nasoesophageal tube is also observed (stars) along with an alveolar pattern within the caudodorsal lung field. (b) Hemothorax was present (horizontal arrows) in the same foal (ultrasound image acquired day prior to radiographs); note the cellular free fluid within the thorax. The lung (stars) and diaphragm (vertical arrows) are also noted within the image.

References

1 Porter, M.B. and Ramirez, S. (2005). Equine neonatal thoracic and abdominal ultrasonography. *Vet. Clin. Equine* 21: 407–429.

2 Rantanen, N.W. (1998). Thoracic ultrasound. In: *Equine Diagnostic Ultrasonography* (ed. N.W. Rantanen and A.O. McKinnon), 41–46. Baltimore: Williams & Wilkins.

3 Reef, V.B. (2004). Thoracic ultrasonography. *Clin. Tech. Equine Pract.* 3: 284–293.

4 Aleman, M., Gillis, C.L., Nieto, J.E. et al. (2002). Ultrasonographic anatomy and biometric analysis of the thoracic and abdominal organs in healthy foals from birth to age 6 months. *Equine Vet. J.* 34: 649–655.

5 Johns, I. (2020). Use of thoracic ultrasound to investigate respiratory disease. *UK Vet. Equine* 4: 106–111.

6 Huber, L., Gressler, L.T., Sanz, M.G. et al. (2018). Monitoring foals by thoracic ultrasonography, bacterial culture, and PCR: diagnostic of *Rhodococcus equi* subclinical pneumonia in south of Brazil. *J. Equine Vet. Sci.* 60: 104–108.

7 Reuss, S.M. and Cohen, N.D. (2015). Update on bacterial pneumonia in the foal and weanling. *Vet. Clin. Equine* 31: 121–135.

8 Giguere, S. and Prescott, J.F. (1997). Clinical manifestations, diagnosis, treatment, and prevention of *Rhodococcus equi* infections in foals. *Vet. Microbiol.* 56: 313–334.

9 Muscatello, G. (2012). Rhodococcus equi pneumonia in the foal – part 2: diagnostics, treatment and disease management. *Vet. J.* 192: 27–33.

10 Jean, D., Laverty, S., Halley, J. et al. (1999). Thoracic trauma in newborn foals. *Equine Vet. J.* 31: 149–152.

11 Jean, D., Picandet, V., Maciera, G. et al. (2007). Detection of rib trauma in newborn foals in an equine critical care unit: a comparison of ultrasonography, radiography and physical examination. *Equine Vet. J.* 39: 158–163.

12 Sprayberry, K.A., Bain, F.T., Seahorn, T.L. et al. (2001). 56 cases of rib fractures in neonatal foals hospitalized in a referral center intensive care unit from 1997–2001. *AAEP Proc.* 47: 395–399.

13 Reynolds, E.B. (1930). Clinical notes on some conditions met with in the mare following parturition and in the newly-born foals. *Vet. Rec.* 10: 277–281.

14 Boyle, A. (2021). Respiratory distress in the adult and foal. *Vet. Clin. Equine* 37: 311–325.

15 Partlow, J., David, F., Hunt, L.M. et al. (2017). Comparison of thoracic ultrasonography and radiography for the detection of induced small volume pneumothorax in the horse. *Vet. Radiol. Ultrasound* 58: 354–360.

Section IV Advanced Imaging (CT, MRI) of the Neonatal Respiratory System

Kara M. Lascola

Advanced radiographic modalities such as computed tomography (CT) and magnetic resonance imaging (MRI) are increasingly available at academic and select private referral practices and have the potential to improve diagnosis and characterization of respiratory disease in adult horses and foals. When compared to standard radiography or ultrasound, CT and MRI offer the advantage of providing high resolution, three-dimensional (3-D) images with minimal superimposition of overlying structures. Obvious limitations to these modalities include access to equipment, associated costs, standardizations of techniques, and patient size limitations. Size is a particular concern for adult horses or older foals, and to date, use of CT or MRI for the diagnosis of respiratory disease is limited to problems involving the upper airway. When available, the use of CT for diagnosis of sinonasal disorders has become common [1–6] and more recently, the use of MRI for the diagnosis of laryngeal or sinonasal disorders has been described [7–12]. In young foals, imaging of the entire thorax is possible with both CT and MRI [13, 14], and thus, these modalities may offer broader advantages in improving the diagnosis and characterization of pulmonary disease in this age group.

CT Imaging

Although radiography and ultrasonography represent the primary modalities used for diagnosis of respiratory disease in horses, when available, CT provides certain diagnostic advantages, particularly in young foals. Subjective comparison between radiographic and CT images in a small group of foals with pulmonary disease suggested underestimation of the distribution and severity of pathologic changes in the lung on radiographs [13]. CT imaging remains the gold standard in human medicine for diagnosis and characterization of pulmonary disease and has been described for imaging the lungs in healthy foals, and a limited number of neonatal foals with severe pulmonary disease, as well as for a variety of other conditions [13, 15–20].

In the few descriptions of CT images in foals with pulmonary disease, although the type and distribution of patterns described on CT varied from case-to-case, mixed and often, unique patterns were identified in all foals (Figure 6.IV.1) [13]. Similar to what has been described radiographically, imaging changes in surviving foals were subjectively less severe in the caudodorsal lungs [21–23]. Because descriptions of CT images in foals are based on a limited number of cases with severe pulmonary disease, interpretation of CT images from a broader range of cases is needed to provide greater understanding of CT imaging in foals. Appreciation of the potential advantages and limitations of CT imaging in foals is important when considering use of this advanced imaging modality.

Advantages to CT imaging include speed of image acquisition and ability to acquire 3-D images of high detail. With reported scan times for an entire thorax of <1 minute, imaging using short-term sedation is possible [13]. With respect to image quality, CT also provides certain advantages over other available imaging modalities. CT is less impacted by respiratory movement and superimposition of overlying structures, and it is able to better localize disease, characterize lung parenchyma and airways, and differentiate between lung and nonlung thoracic structures [13, 24, 25]. Use of contrast can also improve vascular detail (Figure 6.IV.2). Imaging software allows for 3-D reconstructions of the entire respiratory tract and lung, including vasculature and other thoracic structures [26]. For example, 3-D reconstructions of the rib cage can aid surgical planning for repair of complicated rib fractures [27]. The possibility also exists for quantitative analysis of CT images, which may allow for more objective characterization of identified abnormalities [13, 16–18, 28–34].

Equine Neonatal Medicine, First Edition. Edited by David M. Wong and Pamela A. Wilkins.

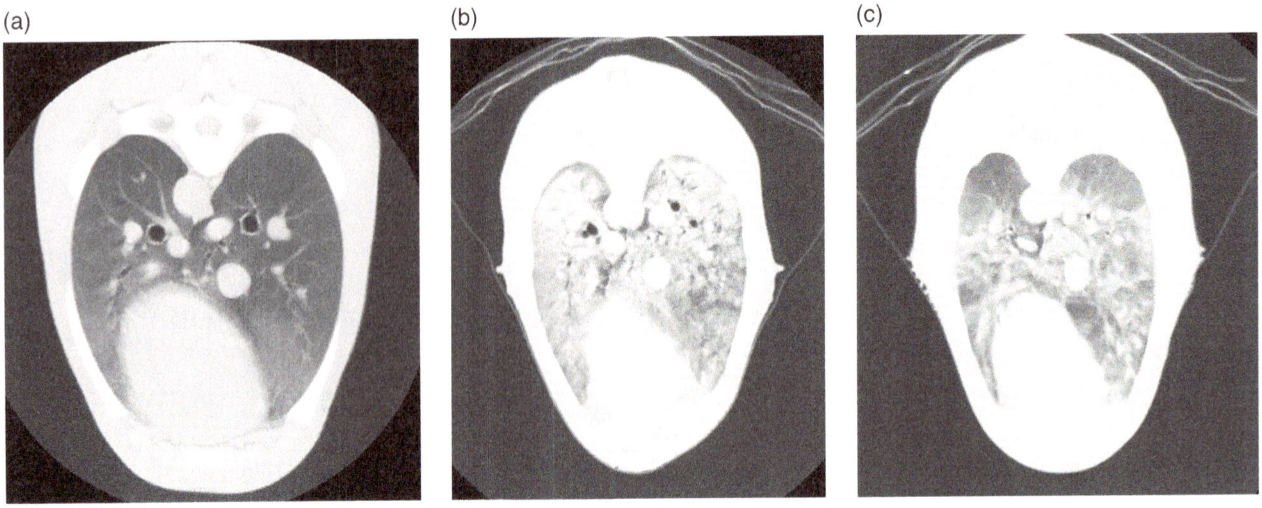

Figure 6.IV.1 Transverse thoracic CT images of (a) a normal 8-day-old foal for comparison; (b) a 4-day-old septic foal with neonatal encephalopathy and suspect meconium aspiration; (c) and a 4-day-old foal with bronchopneumonia and sepsis (*Acinetobacter iwoffi*). In (b), a diffuse hyperattenuating patchy interstitial ground-glass opacity to coalescing alveolar consolidation affects all lung lobes. In (c) there is a "crazy paving" pattern due to interlobular septal thickening surrounding ground glass interstitial pattern and normal lung.

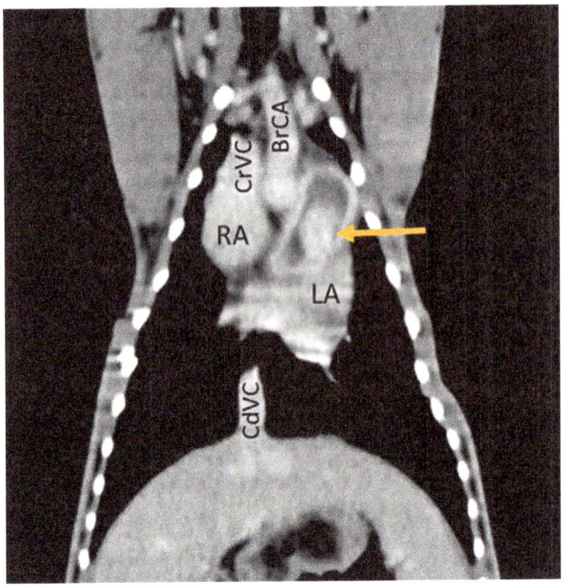

Figure 6.IV.2 Thoracic CT with contrast of a 2-month old miniature foal with a history of fever of unknown origin. A thrombus is identified within the pulmonary artery (arrow). RA = right atrium; LA = left atrium; CrVC = cranial vena cava; BrCA = brachicephalic artery; CdVC = caudal venal cava. *Source:* Image courtesy of Dr. Alisha Gruntman and Dr. Trisha Oura.

In humans, particularly pediatric patients, ionizing radiation exposure remains one of the biggest concerns associated with CT imaging. Depending on the protocol, CT imaging can deliver up to 60 times the radiation dose of a standard chest radiograph [25, 35, 36]. This is less of a concern for veterinary patients given the differences in life span. Instead, cost to owner and availability likely represent the greatest disadvantages associated with CT imaging in veterinary medicine. Although CT units are widely available in veterinary teaching hospitals and some tertiary referral centers, regular access in general practice remains limited for equine patients. Additional considerations for CT imaging are similar to those encountered with standard radiography and include patient positioning and restraint as well as selecting protocols to minimize patient-related artifacts and the need for repetitive scanning.

Ideal positioning for CT is with the foal in sternal recumbency, head toward the gantry, and fore- and hind limbs extended cranially and caudally (Figure 6.IV.3) [13, 17]. The direction toward gantry can be modified if concurrent imaging of limbs is desired. Although imaging in dorsal recumbency has been described in healthy foals [18], it does not provide any clear advantage regarding image quality and is more unsuitable in foals with respiratory compromise. Sedation or general anesthesia is almost always required when imaging foals [13] and may be considered by some to be a potential limitation to CT imaging, particularly in critically ill neonatal foals. The amount and type of sedation required depends on patient age and health status. A single dose of midazolam (0.05–0.1 mg/kg) and butorphanol (0.05 mg/kg) is safe and allows rapid imaging in spontaneously breathing neonatal foals with respiratory disease [13, 16, 17]. Repeat administration of either or both medications, or the addition of propofol (1 mg/kg, IV to effect) may be necessary in healthy or older foals [13, 16, 17]. General anesthesia with or without mechanical ventilation can be used when control of respiration is desired. Supplemental oxygen should be provided as needed but may contribute to the development of atelectasis [13, 18, 28, 37].

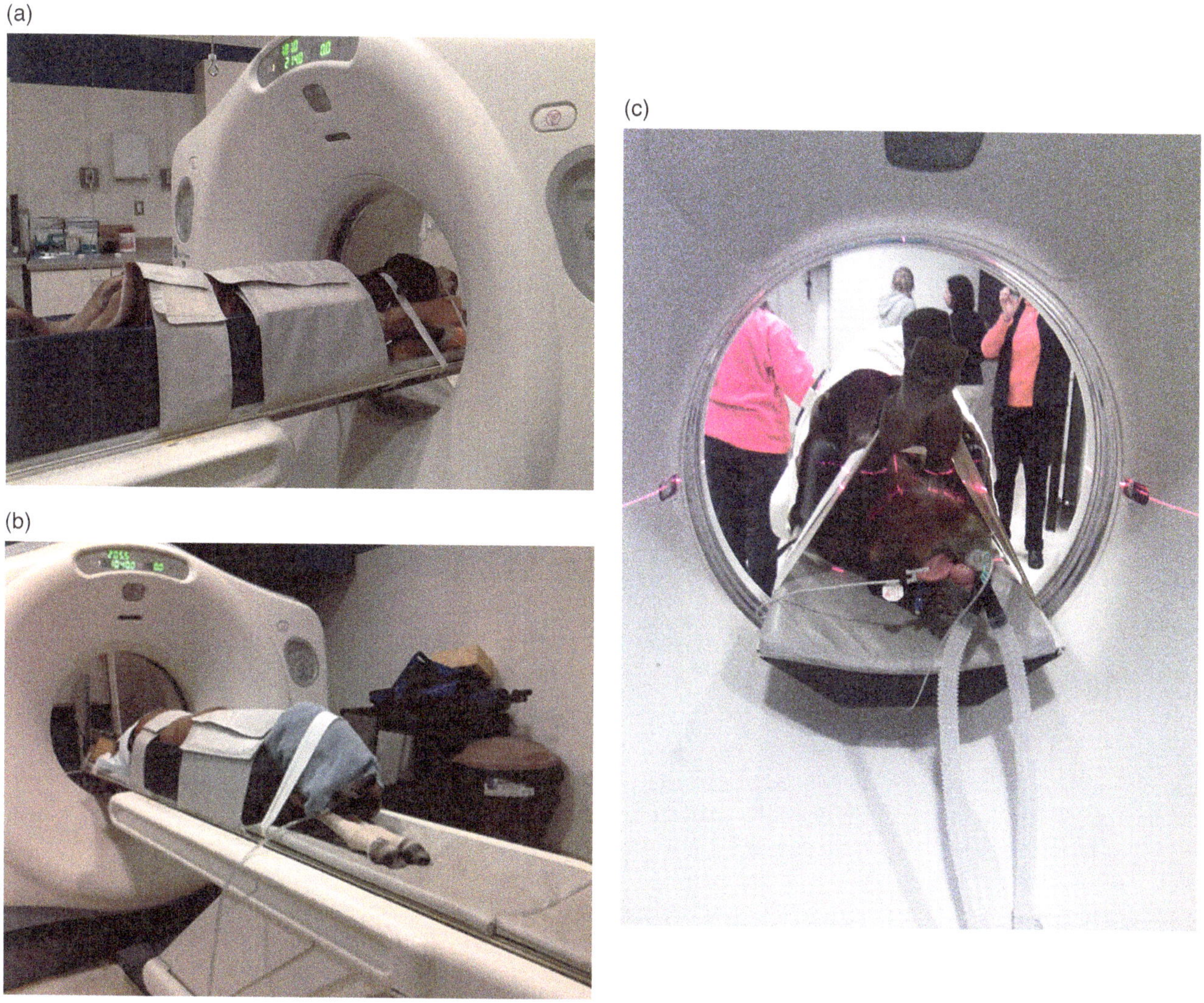

Figure 6.IV.3 Foals positioned for CT imaging (a) sternal recumbency facing gantry; (b) sternal recumbency away from gantry; (c) and dorsal recumbence facing gantry.

Patient-related artifacts encountered with CT imaging include respiratory motion and atelectasis with both having the potential to interfere with image interpretation [34, 38, 39]. In spontaneously breathing healthy foals, motion artifacts were relatively minor on CT [16, 17] but would be expected to be more pronounced in sick foals with tachypnea and other respiratory compromise or abnormalities. Motion artifacts appear as blurring on the axial slice(s) where the motion occurred and tend to be most prominent over the widest part of the thorax [13, 16]. The effect of this blurring on image interpretation can range from mildly obscured margins of thoracic structures to the appearance of a generalized interstitial pattern (Figure 6.IV.4) [13]. Strategies to minimize respiratory motion are limited in spontaneously breathing foals, but motion can be eliminated through the use of controlled apnea in anesthetized and intubated foals [18]. Respiratory gating, primarily described in humans, synchronizes CT slice acquisition to a specific phase of the respiratory cycle and works best in patients with a regular breathing pattern [25]. Other strategies in people, but not suitable for foals, include voluntary breath-hold maneuvers and voluntary spirometry-controlled chest CT [25, 40–43].

Atelectasis is a common finding on CT in neonatal foals [13, 16–18] and also represents a significant concern in sedated pediatric human patients [39, 40]. Reported findings in foals attributable to atelectasis include a gradual and diffuse increase in lung attenuation (opacification) from dorsal to ventral within the lung parenchyma and interstitial and patchy-to-coalescing alveolar patterns with occasional air bronchograms identified ventrally and caudal to the heart in the areas of greatest attenuation [13, 16–18]. Studies in foals and ponies indicate that atelectasis is rapidly detected regardless of whether the animal is under general anesthesia or IV sedation and with or

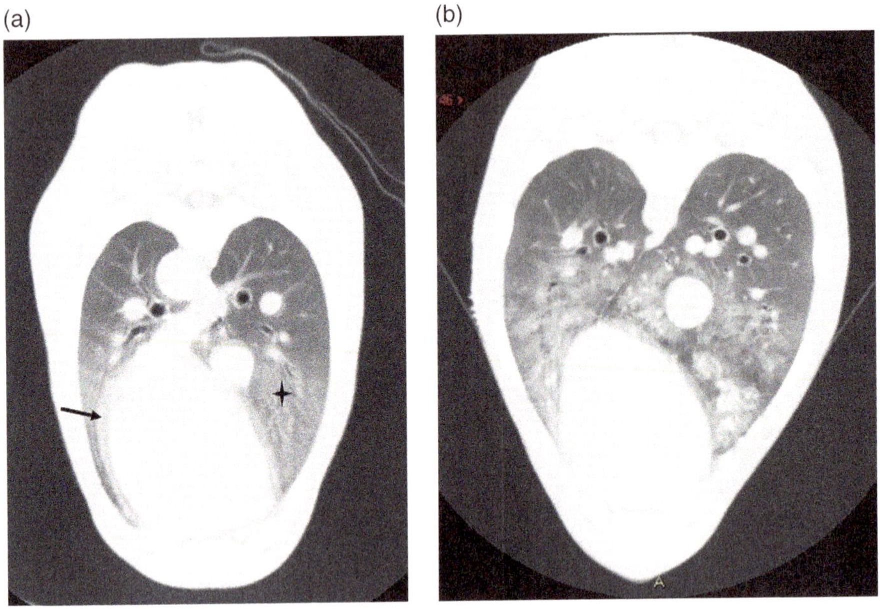

Figure 6.IV.4 Normal transverse CT images of a 10-day-old (a) and 2-day-old (b) foal sedated and positioned in sternal recumbency at the level of the heart. There is slight respiratory motion noted by blurring along the margin of the heart (arrow) and dependent atelectasis noted in the ventral lung fields (star). Note the more pronounced atelectasis in the 2-day-old foal.

without mechanical ventilation [16–18, 44]. Age-related differences for the development of atelectasis have been described in other species [37, 39]. In one study, changes on CT attributed to atelectasis were more pronounced in healthy, sedated foals ≤ 7 days of age when compared to foals > 7 and ≤ 14 days of age (Figure 6.IV.4) [17].

The reasons for which atelectasis develops are similar for both CT and radiographic imaging but may be of greater concern when interpreting CT images [16]. The greater sensitivity of CT imaging in detecting changes associated with atelectasis most likely contributes to this difference. The use of supplemental oxygen (50–100% F_iO_2) may exacerbate the development of atelectasis [18, 28, 37, 39]. Alveolar recruitment maneuvers can be used to reduce or eliminate atelectasis and maximize aeration of normal lung [28, 37, 45–48] and may be voluntary in awake human patients [49]. Manual single breath-hold maneuvers are frequently used in small animal patients [28, 46]. In healthy, anesthetized and spontaneously breathing foals during the first 2 weeks of life, manual single breath hold maneuvers resulted in partial resolution of atelectatic changes identified on CT [18]. The use of recruitment maneuvers during CT imaging has not been described in ill foals.

Subjective interpretation of CT images remains critical in diagnosis and evaluation of ill foals. Quantitative analysis of lung CT images is also possible and can provide benefits in both the clinical and research setting. Quantitative analysis relies on specialized software that objectively measures attenuation values in CT images and categorizes the distribution of those values throughout the lung. Because attenuation is inversely related to aeration and because of the ability to determine the volume of specific regions of attenuation, relative distribution of aeration (hyper-, well-, poorly-, and nonaerated) in a specific lung region or throughout the lung can be determined with the use of sophisticated software. Although best described for use in the research setting [16–18, 28, 44, 50, 51], this type of analysis has been described for clinical use in humans [29–34]. In horses, quantitative analysis has been limited to experimental studies in healthy neonatal foals [16–18] and anesthetized ponies [44] and for retrospective image analysis in a small group of ill foals (Figure 6.IV.5) [13].

MRI

The use of MRI to diagnosis of pulmonary disease in human pediatric patients has increased significantly over the past several years [25, 36, 52–56]. While CT remains the gold standard, there is a greater recognition of the risks associated with ionizing radiation exposure, particularly in pediatric patients, and when repeated imaging is required [35, 36, 52–55]. MRI offers a nonradiation alternative for advanced imaging of the lung, and its use is increasingly described for the diagnosis and characterization of several respiratory conditions in human pediatric patients including congenital malformations, cystic fibrosis, and

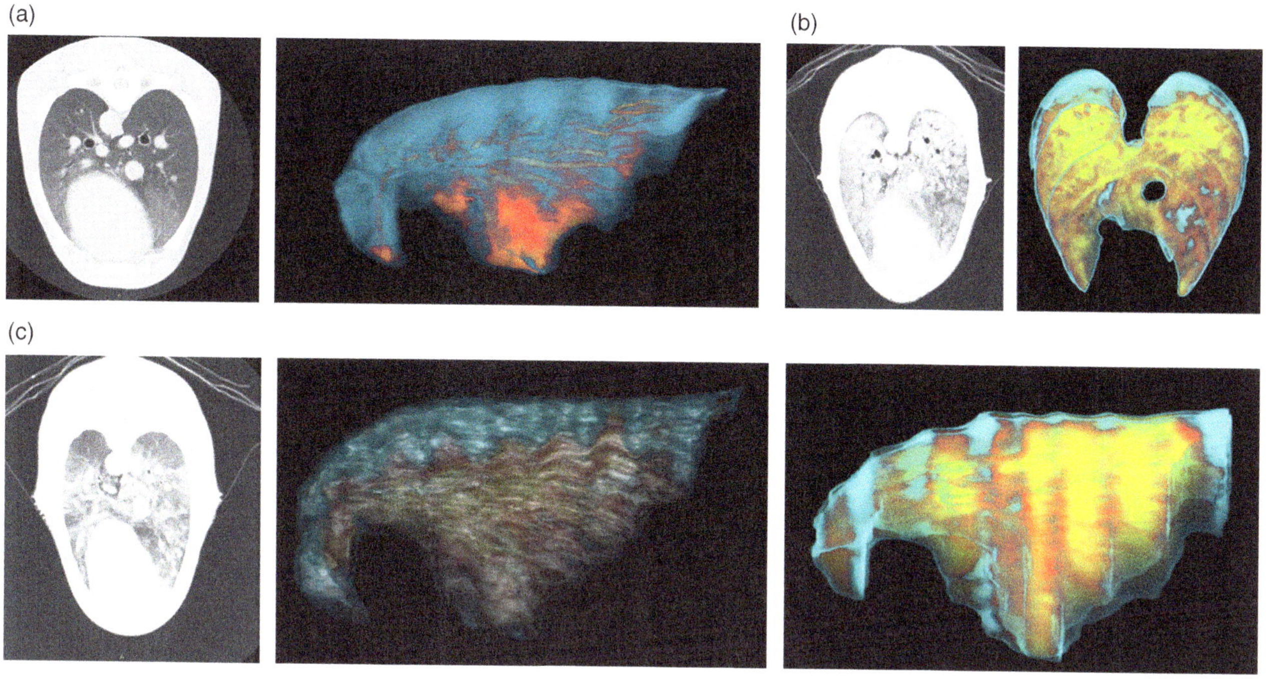

Figure 6.IV.5 Quantitative CT analysis and 3-D attenuation color mapping of foal from image 1 (a = normal; b = suspect meconium aspiration and sepsis; c = bronchopneumonia and sepsis). Areas in blue represent normally aerated lung while areas in orange and red represent poorly and nonaerated lung. In (a), red/orange areas are attributed to positional atelectasis.

inflammatory or infectious diseases such as asthma, chronic bronchitis, pneumonia, and fungal infections [52–62]. Newer MRI systems may provide improved image resolution and soft tissue detail as well as greater flexibility in assessing pulmonary function and structure.

Compared to CT, and to some degree radiography, earlier MRI systems were considered less suitable for lung imaging for reasons related to time required for image acquisition. The low proton density of lung tissue reduces MRI signal intensity, resulting in faster signal decay and an inhomogeneous magnetic environment increases with risk for artifacts [25, 36]. Additionally, high air content and multiple air-tissue interfaces, as well as cardiac and respiratory movement, can all interfere with image acquisition [25, 36, 54]. Recent advances in MRI technology and some specialized protocols have even reduced total scan time to less than 10 minutes [55]. Of greatest significance for the imaging of the lung parenchyma is the introduction of high resolution techniques such as novel ultrashort echo (UTE) and zero echo time (ZTE) sequences [25, 32, 36]. Other advances include respiratory gating capabilities of some systems, superior gradient strength, parallel imaging, volume interpolation, and 3-D reconstruction [25].

Integrating assessment of pulmonary function with morphologic evaluation is useful in characterizing respiratory disease and in monitoring disease progression and response to therapy. Techniques described for assessing pulmonary function during MRI include spirometry and hyperpolarized gas studies [25, 61–64]. Spirometry controlled MRI (as well as CT) is described in awake adult and pediatric human patients and allows for standardization of lung volumes in nonventilated patients during imaging in both the inspiratory and expiratory phases of breathing [63, 65]. Although of limited availability, hyperpolarized gas MRI is described in experimental and clinical studies in humans (adult and pediatric) with asthma, chronic obstructive pulmonary disease (COPD), and cystic fibrosis [57, 61, 63, 65]. Inhaled hyperpolarized gas (129X, 3He) enhances signal intensity and thus special resolution of the lung and airspaces [64, 66]. In addition to enhancing detection and quantification of pathology in the lung, these studies describe functional assessment of lung perfusion, gas exchange, and heterogeneity in ventilation.

Descriptions of the use of MRI for the evaluation of pulmonary disease in foals are lacking. A recent study described the use of gated cardiac MRI in neonatal foals for the assessment of cardiac function [14] and thus the possibility of imaging of the thorax exists (Figure 6.IV.6). Gantry diameter varies among MRI units (60–70 cm) and should be considered when imaging larger foals. Scan time is also expected to be longer compared to CT imaging, and thus general anesthesia would most likely be required. Reports for the use of MRI in foals are primarily limited to single-case reports describing its use in the diagnosis of upper airway and temporohyoid malformation and a few orthopedic or neurologic conditions [67–71].

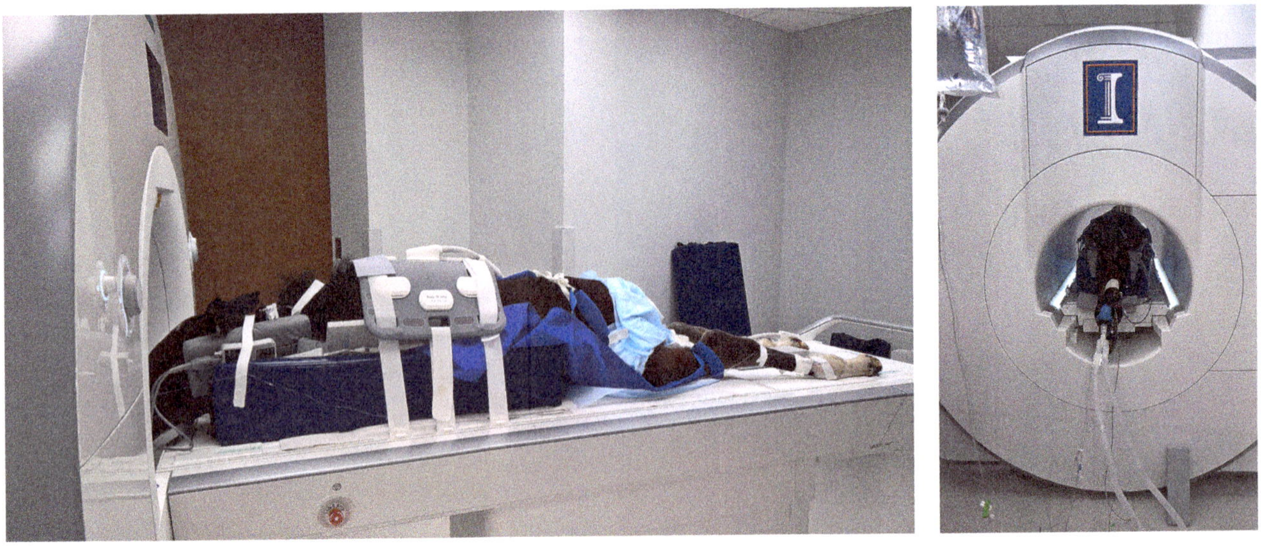

Figure 6.IV.6 Seven-day-old healthy and anesthetized foal positioned in sternal recumbency for cardiac MRI.

References

1 Ostrowska, J., Lindström, L., Tóth, T. et al. (2020). Computed tomography characteristics of equine paranasal sinus cysts. *Equine Vet. J.* 52: 538–546.

2 Dubois, B.B., Dixon, J.J., and Witte, T.H. (2019). Assessment of clinical and computed tomographic findings for association with the outcome of intraoral cheek tooth extraction in horses and ponies. *J. Am. Vet. Med. Assoc.* 255: 1369–1376.

3 Hargreaves, L. and Dixon, J.J. (2018). Computed tomographic description of the highly variable imaging features of equine oromaxillary sinus and oronasal fistulae. *Vet. Radiol. Ultrasound* 59: 571–576.

4 Limone, L.E. and Baratt, R.M. (2018). Dental radiography of the horse. *J. Vet. Dent.* 35: 37–41.

5 Tucker, R., Windley, Z.E., Abernethy, A.D. et al. (2016). Radiographic, computed tomographic and surgical anatomy of the equine sphenopalatine sinus in normal and diseased horses. *Equine Vet. J.* 48: 578–584.

6 Dixon, P.M., Froydenlund, T., Luiti, T. et al. (2015). Empyema of the nasal conchal bulla as a cause of chronic unilateral nasal discharge in the horse: 10 cases (2013–2014). *Equine Vet. J.* 47: 445–449.

7 Tessier, C., Brühschwein, A., Lang, J. et al. (2013). Magnetic resonance imaging features of sinonasal disorders in horses. *Vet. Radiol. Ultrasound* 54: 54–60.

8 Selberg, K. and Easley, J.T. (2013). Advanced imaging in equine dental disease. *Vet. Clin. North Am. Equine Pract.* 29: 397–409.

9 Manso-Díaz, G., Dyson, S.J., Dennis, R. et al. (2015). Magnetic resonance imaging characteristics of equine head disorders: 84 cases (2000–2013). *Vet. Radiol. Ultrasound* 56: 176–187.

10 Careddu, G.M., Evangelisti, M.A., Columbano, N. et al. (2016). Magnetic resonance imaging features of progressive ethmoid hematoma in 2 horses. *Vet. Ital.* 52: 31–35.

11 Kaminsky, J., Bienert-Zeit, A., Hellige, M. et al. (2016). Comparison of image quality and in vivo appearance of the normal equine nasal cavities and paranasal sinuses in computed tomography and high field (3.0 T) magnetic resonance imaging. *BMC Vet. Res.* 19: 12–13.

12 Garrett, K.S., Woodie, J.B., Embertson, R.M. et al. (2009). Diagnosis of laryngeal dysplasia in five horses using magnetic resonance imaging and ultrasonography. *Equine Vet. J.* 41: 766–771.

13 Lascola, K.M. and Joslyn, S. (2015). Diagnostic imaging of the lower respiratory tract in neonatal foals: radiography and CT. *Equine Neonatology* (ed. P.A. Wilkins). *Vet. Clin. N. Am. Eq. Pract.* 31: 497–514.

14 Fries, R., Clark-Price, S.C., Kadotani, S. et al. (2020). Quantitative assessment of left ventricular volume and function by transesophageal echocardiography, ultrasound velocity dilution, magnetic resonance imaging in healthy foals. *Am. J. Vet. Res.* 81: 930–939.

15 Arencibia, A., Corbera, J.C., Ramirez, G. et al. (2020). Anatomical assessment of the thorax in the neonatal foal using computed tomography angiography, sectional anatomy, and gross dissections. *Animals* 10: 1045.

16 Schliewert, E.C., Lascola, K.M., O'Brien, R.T. et al. (2014). Comparison of radiographic and computed tomographic images of the lungs in healthy neonatal foals. *Am. J. Vet. Res.* 76: 42–52.

17 Lascola, K.M., O'Brien, R.T., Wilkins, P.A. et al. (2013). Qualitative and quantitative interpretation of computed

tomography of the lungs in healthy neonatal foals. *Am. J. Vet. Res.* 74: 1239–1246.

18 Lascola, K.M., Clark-Price, S.C., Joslyn, S.K. et al. (2016). The use of manual alveolar recruitment maneuvers to eliminate atelectasis artifacts identified on thoracic computed tomography in healthy neonatal foals. *Am. J. Vet. Res.* 77: 1276–1287.

19 Wion, L., Perkins, G., Ainsworth, D.M. et al. (2001). Use of computerized tomography to diagnose a *Rhodococcus equi* mediastinal abscess causing severe respiratory distress in a foal. *Equine Vet. J.* 33: 523–526.

20 Johnson, P.J., LaCarrubba, A.M., Messer, N.T. et al. (2012). Neonatal respiratory distress and sepsis in the premature foal: challenges with diagnosis and management. *Equine. Vet. Educ.* 24: 453–458.

21 Bedenice, D., Heuwieser, W., Brawer, R. et al. (2003). Clinical and prognostic significance of radiographic pattern, distribution, and severity of thoracic radiographic changes in neonatal foals. *J. Vet. Intern. Med.* 17: 876–886.

22 Bedenice, D., Heuwieser, W., Solano, M. et al. (2003). Risk factors and prognostic variablesfor survival of foals with radiographic evidence of pulmonary disease. *J. Vet. Intern. Med.* 17: 868–875.

23 Lester, G.D. and Lester, N.V. (2001). Abdominal and thoracic radiography in the neonate. *Vet. Clin. North Am. Equine Pract.* 17: 19–46.

24 Alexander, K., Joly, H., Blond, L. et al. (2012). A comparison of computed tomography, computed radiography, and film-screen radiography for the detection of canine pulmonary nodules. *Vet. Radiol. Ultrasound* 53: 258–265.

25 Tiddens, H.A.W.M., Kuo, W., van Straten, M. et al. (2018). Paediatric lung imaging: the times they are a-changin. *Eur. Respir. Rev.* 27: 170097.

26 Kinns, J., Mallinowski, R., McEvoy, F. et al. (2011). Special software applications. In: *Veterinary Computed Tomography*, vol. 1 (ed. T. Schwarz and J. Saunders), 67–74. Chichester: Wiley.

27 Marr, C.M. (2015). The equine neonatal cardiovascular system in health and disease. *Vet. Clin. North Am. Equine Pract.* 31: 545–565.

28 Staffieri, F., De Monte, V., De Marzo, C. et al. (2010). Effects of two fractions of inspired oxygen on lung aeration and gas exchange in cats under inhalant anaesthesia. *Vet. Anaesth. Analg.* 37: 483–490.

29 Gattinoni, L., Caironi, P., Valenza, F. et al. (2006). The role of CT-scan studies for the diagnosis and therapy of acute respiratory distress syndrome. *Clin. Chest Med.* 27: 559–570.

30 Feldhaus, F.W., Theilig, D.C., Hubner, R.H. et al. (2019). Quantitative CT analysis in patients with pulmonary emphysema: is lung function influenced by concomitant unspecific pulmonary fibrosis? *Int. J. Chron. Obstruct. Pulmon. Dis.* 14: 1583–1593.

31 Chiumello, D., Mongodi, S., Algieri, I. et al. (2018). Assessment of lung aeration and recruitment by CT scan and ultrasound in acute respiratory distress syndrome patients. *Crit. Care Med.* 46: 1761–1768.

32 Kim, J., Kim, M.J., Sol, I.S. et al. (2019). Quantitative CT and pulmonary function in children with post-infectious bronchiolitis obliterans. *PLoS One* 14: e0214647. http://dx.doi.org/10.1371/journal.pone.0214647.

33 Stein, J.M., Walkup, L.L., Brody, A.S. et al. (2016). Quantitative CT characterization of pediatric lung development using routine clinical imaging. *Pediatr. Radiol.* 46: 1804–1812.

34 Chen, A., Karwoski, R.A., Gierada, D.S. et al. (2020). Quantitative CT analysis of diffuse lung disease. *Radiographics* 40: 28–43.

35 Migliorettі, D.L., Johnson, E., Williams, A. et al. (2013). The use of computed tomography in pediatrics and the associated radiation exposure and estimated cancer risk. *JAMA Pediatr.* 167: 700–707.

36 Higano, N.S., Hahn, A.D., Tkach, J.A. et al. (2017). Retrospective respiratory self-gating and removal of bulk motion in pulmonary UTE MRI of neonates and adults. *Magn. Reson. Med.* 77: 1284–1295.

37 Magnusson, L. and Spahn, D.R. (2003). New concepts of atelectasis during general anaesthesia. *Br. J. Anaesth.* 91: 61–72.

38 Raju, S., Ghosh, S., and Mehta, A.C. (2017). Chest CT signs in pulmonary disease: a pictorial review. *Chest* 151: 1356–1374.

39 Newman, B., Krane, E.J., Gawande, R. et al. (2014). Chest CT in children: anesthesia and atelectasis. *Pediatr. Radiol.* 44: 164–172.

40 Mansfield, S.A., Dykes, M., Adler, B. et al. (2019). Improving quality of chest computed tomography for evaluation of pediatric malignancies. *Pediatr. Qual. Saf.* 4: e166.

41 Mott, L.S., Graniel, K.G., Park, J. et al. (2013). Assessment of early bronchiectasis in young children with cystic fibrosis is dependent on lung volume. *Chest* 144: 1193–1198.

42 Salamon, E., Lever, S., Kuo, W. et al. (2017). Spirometer guided chest imaging in children: it is worth the effort! *Pediatr. Pulmonol.* 52: 48–56.

43 Otjen, J.P., Swanson, J.O., Oron, A. et al. (2018). Spirometry-assisted high resolution chest computed tomography in children: is it worth the effort? *Curr. Probl. Diagn. Radiol.* 47: 14–18.

44 Reich, H., Moens, Y., Braun, C. et al. (2014). Validation study of an interpolation method for calculating whole lung volumes and masses from reduced numbers of CT-images in ponies. *Vet. J.* 202: 603–607.

45 Gattinoni, L., Caironi, P., Cressoni, M. et al. (2006). Lung recruitment in patients with the acute respiratory distress syndrome. *N. Engl. J. Med.* 354: 1775–1786.
46 Henao-Guerrero, N., Ricco, C., Jones, J.C. et al. (2012). Comparison of four ventilatory protocols for computed tomography of the thorax in healthy cats. *Am. J. Vet. Res.* 73: 646–653.
47 Duff, J.P., Rosychuk, R.J., and Joffe, A.R. (2007). The safety and efficacy of sustained inflations as a lung recruitment maneuver in pediatric intensive care unit patients. *Intensive Care Med.* 33: 1778–1786.
48 Boriosi, J.P., Cohen, R.A., Summers, E. et al. (2012). Lung aeration changes after lung recruitment in children with acute lung injury: a feasibility study. *Pediatr. Pulmonol.* 47: 771–779.
49 Petersen, J., Wille, M.M., Rakêt, L.L. et al. (2014). Effect of inspiration on airway dimensions measured in maximal inspiration CT images of subjects without airflow limitation. *Eur. Radiol.* 24: 2319–2325.
50 Morandi, F., Mattoon, J.S., Lakritz, J. et al. (2004). Correlation of helical and incremental high-resolution thin-section computed tomographic and histomorphometric quantitative evaluation of an acute inflammatory response of lungs in dogs. *Am. J. Vet. Res.* 65: 1114–1123.
51 McEvoy, F.J., Buelund, L., Strathe, A.B. et al. (2009). Quantitative computed tomography evaluation of pulmonary disease. *Vet. Radiol. Ultrasound* 50: 47–51.
52 Singh, R., Garg, M., Sodhi, K.S. et al. (2020). Diagnostic accuracy of magnetic resonance imaging in the evaluation of pulmonary infections in immunocompromised patients. *Pol. J. Radiol.* 85: e53–e61.
53 Kapur, S., Bhalla, A.S., and Jana, M. (2019). Pediatric chest MRI: a review. *Indian J. Pediatr.* 86: 842–853.
54 Sodhi, K.S., Sharma, M., Lee, E.Y. et al. (2018). Diagnostic utility of 3T lung MRI in children with interstitial lung disease: a prospective pilot study. *Acad. Radiol.* 25: 380–386.
55 Sodhi, K.S., Khandelwal, N., Saxena, A.K. et al. (2016). Rapid lung MRI in children with pulmonary infections: time to change our diagnostic algorithms. *J. Magn. Reson. Imaging* 43: 1196–1206.
56 Torres, L., Kammerman, J., Hahn, A.D. et al. (2019). Structure-function imaging of lung disease using ultrashort Echo time MRI. *Acad. Radiol.* 26: 431–441.
57 Tsuchiya, N., Schiebler, M.L., Evans, M.D. et al. (2020). Safety of repeated hyperpolarized helium 3 magnetic resonance imaging in pediatric asthma patients. *Pediatr. Radiol.* 50: 646–655.
58 Gouwens, K.R., Higano, N.S., Marks, K.T. et al. (2020). Magentic resonance imaging evaluation of regional lung Vts in severe neonatal bronchopulmonary dysplasia. *Am. J. Respir. Crit. Care Med.* 202: 1024–1031.
59 Parsons, D. and Donnelley, M. (2020). Will airway gene therapy for cystic fibrosis improve lung function? New imaging technologies can help us find out. *Hum. Gene Ther.* 31: 973–984.
60 Goralski, J.L., Stewart, N.J., and Woods, J.C. (2021). Novel imaging techniques for cystic fibrosis lung disease. *Pediatr. Pulmonol.* 56: S40–S54.
61 Couch, M.J., Thomen, R., Kanhere, N. et al. (2019). A two-center analysis of hyperpolarized ^{129}Xe lung MRI in stable pediatric cystic fibrosis: potential as a biomarker for multi-site trials. *J. Cyst. Fibros.* 18: 728–733.
62 Kaireit, T.F., Sorrentino, S.A., Renne, J. et al. (2017). Functional lung MRI for regional monitoring of patients with cystic fibrosis. *PLoS One* 12: e0187483.
63 Kołodziej, M., de Veer, M.J., Cholewa, M. et al. (2017). Lung function imaging methods in cystic fibrosis pulmonary disease. *Respir. Res.* 18: 96.
64 Flors, L., Mugler, J.P. 3rd, de Lange, E.E. et al. (2016). Hyperpolarized gas magnetic resonance lung imaging in children and Young adults. *J. Thorac. Imaging* 31: 285–295.
65 Young, H.M., Guo, F., Eddy, R.L. et al. (1985). Oscillometry and pulmonary MRI measurements of ventilation heterogeneity in obstructive lung disease: relationship to quality of life and disease control. *J. Appl. Physiol.* 2018 (125): 73–85.
66 Altes, T.A. and Salerno, M. (2004). Hyperpolarized gas MR imaging of the lung. *J. Thorac. Imaging* 19: 250–258.
67 Oey, L., Müller, J.M., von Klopmann, T. et al. (2011). Diagnosis of internal and external hydrocephalus in a warmblood foal using magnetic resonance imaging. *Tierarztl. Prax. Ausg. G Grosstiere Nutztiere* 39: 41–45.
68 Gray, L.C., Magdesian, K.G., Sturges, B.K. et al. (2001). Suspected protozoal myeloencephalitis in a two-month-old colt. *Vet. Rec.* 149: 269–273.
69 Garrett, K.S., Woodie, J.B., Cook, J.L. et al. (2010). Imaging diagnosis--nasal septal and laryngeal cyst-like malformation in a thoroughbred weanling colt diagnosed using ultrasonography and magnetic resonance imaging. *Vet. Radiol. Ultrasound* 51: 504–507.
70 Inui, T., Yamada, K., Itoh, M. et al. (2017). Computed tomography and magnetic resonance imaging findings for the initial stage of equine temporohyoid osteoarthropathy in a thoroughbred foal. *J. Equine. Sci.* 28: 117–121.
71 Martel, G., Forget, C., Gilbert, G. et al. (2017). Validation of the ultrasonographic assessment of the femoral trochlea epiphyseal cartilage in foals at osteochondrosis predilected sites with magnetic resonance imaging and histology. *Equine Vet. J.* 49: 821–828.

Section V Inhalation Therapy

Harold McKenzie

Inhalation Therapy for Neonatal Pneumonia

Pneumonia is a common syndrome in sick neonatal foals, resulting from a variety of insults [1]. Gram-negative bacteria are most commonly involved in neonatal bacterial pneumonia, although Gram-positive and mixed infections occur [2]. Due to the potential for mixed infections, treatment with systemic broad-spectrum antimicrobials is recommended [3]. However, the treatment of bacterial infections of the lower respiratory tract is complicated by the fact that the respiratory epithelium represents a substantial barrier to diffusion of drugs from the systemic circulation into the respiratory compartment [4]. This can result in an impaired response to treatment with systemically administered medications, potentially requiring large dosages be administered to achieve therapeutic levels within the respiratory tract and thus increasing the likelihood of adverse side effects. Aerosol administration can be used to overcome some of these limitations by achieving high drug concentrations within the airway lumen with a rapid onset of action while decreasing the total dose administered and reducing the risk of systemic side effects [5]. These advantages are particularly valuable with drugs such as bronchodilators, where the therapeutic index for systemic administration is narrow, or for drugs with potential systemic toxicity, such as aminoglycosides. Aerosol administration does have limitations, however, including potential difficulties with drug delivery and pulmonary irritation, as well as the expense of the required equipment and time required for administration.

Aerosol Theory

The effect of an aerosolized medication is achieved following deposition of aerosolized particles on the mucosal surface of the respiratory tract. The pattern of deposition of aerosol particles and efficiency of aerosol delivery are influenced by the characteristics of the aerosol itself, including the size distribution of the aerosol particles and aerosol density. These characteristics vary significantly with different delivery systems and drug formulations [6]. The most important characteristic of therapeutic aerosols is the size of individual particles, which dictates the degree to which they will be able to penetrate the respiratory tract. Particles ≥10 μm diameter are deposited within the nasal passages and nasopharynx, while particles <10 μm diameter are deposited within the lower respiratory tract. The optimal particle size range for deep pulmonary deposition is considered to be 1–5 μm [7].

Patient-dependent factors are also important in determining aerosol deposition, including ventilatory parameters and respiratory morphology [7]. The respiratory pattern of the horse is well suited to inhalation therapy because large tidal volumes and high flow rates enhance deep pulmonary deposition of aerosols [8]. Deposition of small particles in the lung periphery may also be enhanced by the relatively low respiratory rate of the resting horse, which increases the residence time of particles within the peripheral airways and may enhance deposition due to sedimentation and diffusion. These advantages may be less prominent in foals due to their higher resting respiratory rates and lower tidal volumes compared to adult horses.

The presence of pulmonary disease is an important consideration in the administration of therapeutic aerosols, because changes in pulmonary function and mechanics associated with pulmonary disease may impair delivery of aerosolized medications to the affected region. Inflammation and airway sensitization are commonly associated with pulmonary disease and can cause bronchoconstriction, mucus hypersecretion, and mucosal edema, resulting in variable degrees of airway obstruction. Airway obstruction increases particle deposition at the site of obstruction but limits delivery of particles beyond the area

Equine Neonatal Medicine, First Edition. Edited by David M. Wong and Pamela A. Wilkins.

of obstruction and diverts airflow to nonobstructed airways, resulting in increased delivery of therapeutic particles to less-affected portions of the lung [7]. The net result is a shift toward more central and decreased peripheral deposition of drug [9]. Administration of an aerosolized bronchodilator to horses with recurrent airway obstruction has been shown to significantly improve pulmonary distribution of a radiolabeled aerosol [10], and in the clinical setting, premedication with albuterol is frequently used prior to nebulization for this reason. Total airway obstruction is generally thought to prevent deposition of aerosol particles in the affected region peripheral to the site of obstruction, and as a result it is believed that no medication will reach a consolidated region of the lung following aerosol administration [11]. Despite this theoretical limitation, experimental models of pneumonia have documented significantly higher concentrations of either amikacin or ceftazidime in consolidated regions of pneumonic lungs following aerosol administration as compared to IV administration, likely due to diffusion of the drugs following deposition in the airway lining fluid [12, 13].

Aerosol Administration

Aerosol delivery of therapeutic substances presents several challenges. The substance to be administered must be available in a formulation that can be delivered to the respiratory tract as an aerosol. The therapeutic agent should be nonirritating, nonallergenic, and lack local toxicity [14]. It must also be capable of exerting its action on the mucosal surface or be absorbed into the respiratory mucosa, but if the therapeutic substance has the potential for systemic toxicity it should be poorly absorbed [14]. The delivery method must be capable of producing particles that are of an appropriate size to deliver the medication to the desired portion of the respiratory tract as well as be able to deliver the total dose in a reasonable period of time with acceptable efficiency. The generation of therapeutic aerosols is accomplished using several different inhalation drug delivery systems. None of these systems, however, is capable of delivering aerosolized medication with very high efficiency, with <10% of the original dose typically being deposited in the lower respiratory tract regardless of delivery system [15].

Devices

Two commonly used aerosol delivery devices in human medicine are metered dose inhalers (MDIs) and dry powder inhalers (DPIs), which generate small volume aerosols of liquids and powders, respectively. These devices have the advantages of being preformulated, prepackaged, and capable of delivering multiple doses, but they require coordination of administration with inhalation. Their prepackaged nature also decreases the risk of introducing microorganisms into the respiratory tract during administration, which is a concern when using nebulizers for aerosol generation. The most commonly used aerosol delivery device for horses is the MDI, and the efficacy of these devices for administration of therapeutic aerosols to horses has been extensively examined [16]. The inability to coordinate activation of these devices with inhalation is addressed in horses and foals by use of closely fitting valved facemasks with an integral spacer[1] or intranasal delivery devices with a spacer[2] (Figure 6.V.1) [17].

MDIs are self-contained devices, consisting of a canister with an integral metering valve. The canister contains the drug and a liquid propellant. The propellant serves as a dispersion medium for the drug, and as an energy source to expel the formulation from the valve as large droplets that

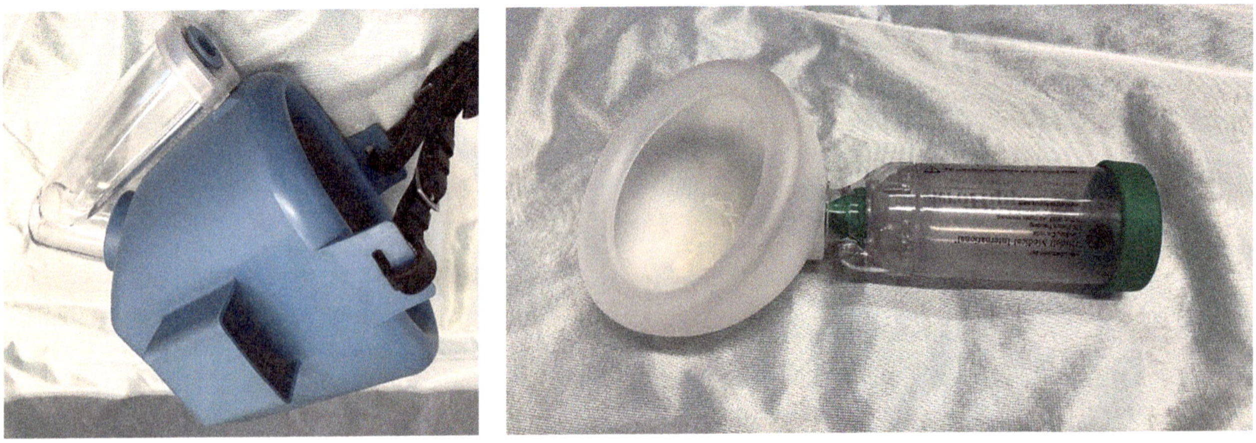

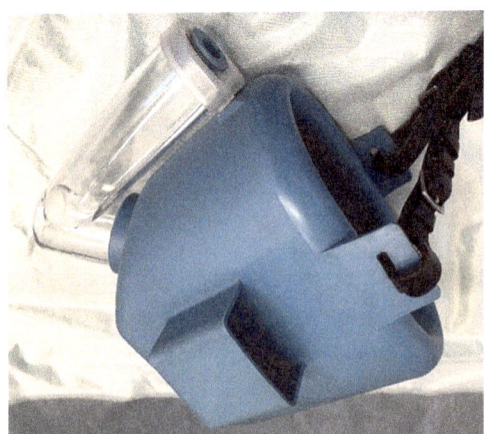

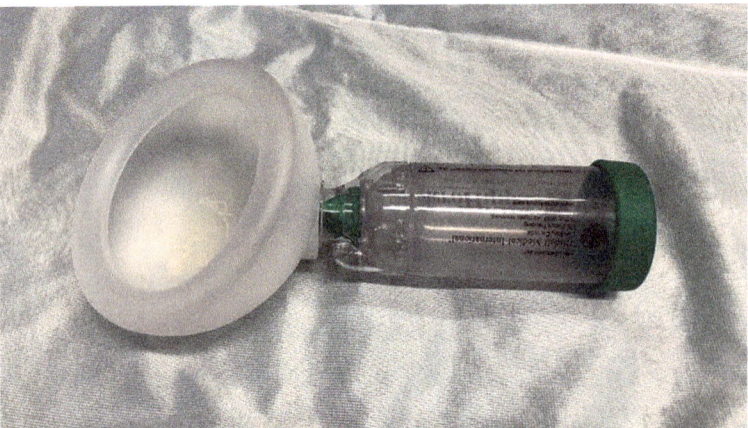

Figure 6.V.1 Equine facemask (Flexineb® facemask, Nortev, Galway, Ireland) configured for use with metered dose inhalers (left). Equine nasal inhalation device (Aerohippus™, Trudell Medical Intl., London, Ont., Canada) with spacer for use with metered dose inhalers (right).

rapidly evaporate following exposure to air, leaving a drug-containing particle of respirable size [18]. Due to the high velocity of the aerosol as it leaves the actuation valve, these devices have been associated with high levels of oral and upper respiratory deposition in human patients [18]. In an effort to avoid this effect, a spacer device is used, with the MDI being actuated into the device, where the particle velocity dissipates, the propellant evaporates further, and the nonrespirable particles impact onto the spacer device, resulting in a decrease in particle size and allowing for increased pulmonary deposition and decreased oropharyngeal deposition (Figures 6.V.1) [18].

The use of MDIs has been extensively investigated in the horse. The pulmonary deposition of radioaerosol generated using a MDI with a spacer and facemask has been evaluated [19] and demonstrated that up to five times more of the dose was deposited in the lung using this device combination than was observed with jet or ultrasonic nebulizers. MDIs are primarily used for administration of β_2 agonist bronchodilators (albuterol/salbutamol, pirbuterol, salmeterol) to horses and have been validated in multiple studies [16, 20]. While administration of anticholinergic bronchodilator ipratropium bromide by DPI has also been validated [21], these devices are not appropriate for use in foals and the MDI formulation is preferred.

Nebulizers

Aerosols are generated from liquids by nebulizers, as compressed-gas driven (jet), ultrasonic, or vibrating mesh in design. Nebulization is considered to be the optimal method of administration when the dose to be delivered exceeds 200 μg [22], and does not require coordination of administration and inhalation, depending only on normal tidal breathing [23]. Nebulizers must be used with a facemask in the conscious foal, with attendant aerosol wastage on the face, facemask, and in the nasal passages and nasopharynx [24]. Jet nebulizers have been widely used in human medicine because they are inexpensive and relatively easy to use. Jet nebulizers are usually limited to reservoir volumes of ≤6 ml, however, and the time required to aerosolize this volume of fluid ranges from 10 to 15 minutes. Jet nebulizers are also relatively inefficient in terms of aerosol delivery, with up to 60% of the dose placed in the device being wasted, and only 15% of the aerosol generated actually being inhaled by the patient [25]. While readily available, jet nebulizers are not preferred for use in foals due to concerns of prolonged administration times and relatively inefficient drug delivery.

Ultrasonic nebulizers generate an aerosol as a result of high frequency vibration of a piezoelectric transducer, and the aerosol produced typically consist of smaller particles more appropriate for inhalation than those produced by jet nebulizers [18]. These devices are also generally capable of producing more aerosol per unit time than jet nebulizers, resulting in shorter treatment times and greater ease of use [26]. These devices cause heating of the aerosol solution during the process of nebulization, which could result in alteration or inactivation of the drug. In addition, ultrasonic nebulizers are expensive and fragile, and are less frequently used clinically at this time. In the US, ultrasonic nebulizers are only available as handheld devices developed for the human market, while an equine specific device that consists of an integral facemask and nebulizer suitable for use in adult horses appears to be available in Europe.[3]

Vibrating mesh nebulizers utilize a rapidly vibrating perforated mesh to generate the aerosol droplets, and these devices have several advantages over jet and ultrasonic nebulizers, including production of an optimal particle size (1–5 μm), more rapid delivery, especially when compared to jet nebulizers, and lower residual volumes, resulting in a greater percentage of the prescribed dose being administered to the patient [27]. These devices are also less likely to alter or degrade medications, as they do not heat or cool the solution being delivered. An equine-specific facemask system with an integral vibrating mesh nebulizer[4] (Figure 6.V.2) is readily available in both foal and adult sizes and is the preferred system for use in foals at this time.

Drug Formulations for Nebulization

The formulation of a therapeutic nebulization solution can have a major impact on the aerosol produced and on the patient response to aerosol administration. The concentration of solute is of major importance, because increased solute concentrations typically result in decreases in aerosol output and

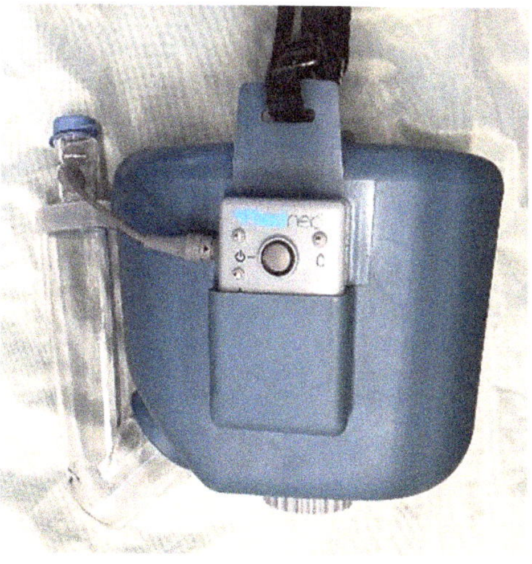

Figure 6.V.2 Equine facemask with integrated vibrating mesh nebulizer (Flexineb® E3, Nortev, Galway, Ireland).

particle size [28]. One study of antimicrobial aerosol generation from medical nebulizers determined that the antimicrobial concentration in a nebulization solution, regardless of the specific antimicrobial, should ideally be 100 mg/ml or less, in a saline solution of 0.23–0.45% concentration, although the choice of diluent may be determined by the drug formulation [28]. Lower antimicrobial concentrations were recommended for ultrasonic nebulizers, with an ideal concentration of approximately 50 mg/ml [28]. The ideal nebulization solution would also be isotonic and have a neutral pH, to minimize the development of coughing and/or bronchoconstriction [28]. A study that characterized the aerosols produced by an ultrasonic nebulizer using antimicrobial solutions appropriate for therapy of equine lower respiratory bacterial infections found that solutions containing 50 mg/ml gentamicin or 25 mg/ml of ceftiofur yielded the optimal combinations of particle size and aerosol density [29]. Vibrating mesh nebulizers are less sensitive to the formulation of the solution, however, and tend to deliver a more dense and uniform aerosol despite differences in drug formulations [27].

Clinical Application: Bronchodilators

Foals with pneumonia may benefit from treatment with aerosolized bronchodilators (Table 6.V.1) because they decrease the work of breathing, improve patient comfort and attitude, and may help prevent reflex bronchoconstriction resulting from aerosol delivery of other medications [30, 31]. β_2 adrenergic agonists (albuterol) are readily used because they are easily administered by the aerosol route. Use of the aerosol route allows for smaller doses, thereby reducing the risk for systemic toxicity. β_2 agonists achieve rapid bronchodilation following aerosol administration and are very effective in relieving bronchospasm or preventing bronchospasm associated with delivery of other aerosolized medications, such as antimicrobials [32]. Additional benefits of β_2 agonists in foals with respiratory disease include enhancement of mucociliary clearance. Two types of β_2 agonists are available, and are characterized by their duration of effect. The most commonly used are short acting β_2 agonists, primarily albuterol (salbutamol), although long-acting compounds such as salmeterol and formoterol are also available. Albuterol is rapidly acting, with onset of clinical effect in as little as 5 minutes, but is typically only active for 1–3 hours [33]. Long-acting compounds have a slower onset of effect, with salmeterol requiring 30–60 minutes to achieve full effect, while clinical efficacy persists for at least 6 hours [34]. While administering these drugs via the aerosol route lessens the likelihood of side effects by decreasing the dosage requirement, the risk is not entirely eliminated. High dosages of these compounds (four to six times the therapeutic dosage) can lead to sweating, trembling, and excitement [35]. Due to the limited duration of activity of albuterol, it can be difficult to maintain effective bronchodilation over time, and its use may be best limited to the treatment of acute bronchoconstriction or intermittent therapy as needed. Long-acting β_2 agonists are less commonly used in foals.

Because the bronchoconstrictive response is autonomically mediated, it is logical to consider the potential application of anticholinergic medications in the control of bronchoconstriction. Ipratropium bromide is a synthetic parasympatholytic bronchodilator that is efficacious in horses suffering from asthma [21], and can be of clinical benefit in foals with severe lower respiratory inflammation. As β_2 agonists and anticholinergics act by different mechanisms, their combined use may result in additive or synergistic effects. This phenomenon has

Table 6.V.1 Potential medications and dosages for aerosol therapy in foals. For MDI drugs, use a spacer device.

Type of medication	Drug	Formulation	Concentration	Dosage	Frequency
Bronchodilator	Albuterol	MDI	90 µg	1–3 µg/kg	q3–8h
		Solution for nebulization	0.083% (2.5 mg/3 ml)	0.025 mg/kg	q6h
	Ipratropium	MDI	17 µg	0.35 µg/kg	q8–12h
		Solution for nebulization	0.02% (0.5 mg/2.5 ml)	2–3 µg/kg	q8–12h
Antimicrobial	Ceftiofur	Injectable	50 mg/ml	2.2 mg/kg	q12–24h
	Gentamicin	Injectable	100 mg/ml	3.3 mg/kg	q24h
	Amikacin	Injectable	250 mg/ml	6–8 mg/kg	q24h
	Cefquinome	Injectable	45 mg/ml	0.4 mg/kg	q12h
	Marbofloxacin	Injectable	100 mg/ml	0.7 mg/kg	q24h
Anti-inflammatory	Fluticasone	MDI	44, 110, 220 µg	2–4 µg/kg	q24h
	Dexamethasone	Injectable	2 or 4 mg/ml	0.01 mg/kg	q24h

For nebulized drugs, dilute to a final volume of 10 ml using an appropriate diluent for the drug (sterile water or saline).

been demonstrated in human patients, where β_2 agonists induce a rapid bronchodilatory response that is subsequently maintained by the anticholinergic compound [36]. There is some suggestion of a synergistic effect in human patients, wherein the combination therapy is more effective in improving pulmonary function both acutely and over time than either compound alone [36]. A combination product containing albuterol sulfate and ipratropium bromide is commercially available as a nebulization solution[5] or MDI,[6] and is clinically effective in equine patients.

Anti-Inflammatory Therapy

The use of aerosolized anti-inflammatory medications is not often indicated in foals with pneumonia, primarily because the drugs available by this route are corticosteroids such as fluticasone or dexamethasone (Table 6.V.1). While there is strong evidence in people and adult horses that inhaled corticosteroids reduce pulmonary inflammation, there are concerns regarding immunosuppressive effects of corticosteroid administration in the face of bacterial infection. Despite this, it is widely accepted that systemic corticosteroids have utility in foals suffering from severe interstitial pneumonia or acute lung injury/acute respiratory distress syndrome [37, 38]. While systemic corticosteroids are likely to be more effective in cases with severe respiratory dysfunction, the use of aerosolized corticosteroids in foals with pneumonia has been described [30, 31].

Aerosolized Antimicrobials

A major limitation of systemic antimicrobial therapy for treatment of lower respiratory infections is the low pulmonary penetration of many antimicrobials. In people, the therapeutic outcome of respiratory infections is more closely associated with airway rather than serum antimicrobial concentrations [39]. Aerosol administration of antimicrobials achieves high antimicrobial concentrations at the respiratory mucosal surface, while minimizing systemic side effects [13]. This mode of antimicrobial delivery also decreases the total dose administered and has a rapid onset of action [40]. This approach does have limitations, however, including potential problems with drug delivery and pulmonary irritation, as well as expense of required equipment and time required for administration [40].

A number of human studies have investigated aerosolized antimicrobial therapy in a variety of types of lower respiratory infections, and in several different clinical settings, including prophylaxis, monotherapy (using only inhaled antimicrobials), adjunct therapy with systemic antimicrobials, and treatment of multidrug resistant pathogens [41]. This treatment modality is effective as an ancillary therapy in preventing the development, or decreasing the severity or duration, of lower respiratory bacterial infections [6]. Moreover, this modality is widely used in human cystic fibrosis patients suffering from chronic *Pseudomonas aeruginosa* infections [6]. The use of inhaled antimicrobials in other conditions, such as ventilator associated pneumonia, is more controversial; currently the primary indication for its use is in patients with multidrug-resistant pathogens or patients not responding to systemic therapy alone [6, 42].

The delivery of gentamicin to the lower respiratory tract of adult horses has been compared following IV and single and repeated aerosol administration (Table 6.V.1) [32, 43]. The gentamicin concentrations in bronchial lavage fluid following aerosol administration were significantly greater than after IV administration for at least 8 hours. Because the maximum bronchial lavage fluid gentamicin concentrations after aerosol administration were approximately 12 times greater than those measured following IV administration, aerosol administration would appear to achieve sufficiently high airway concentrations of gentamicin to be of clinical benefit [43]. This is further supported by one study in which once-daily (6.6 mg/kg) IV gentamicin administration in horses concluded that IV gentamicin administration could not be recommended for treatment of airway infections due to the low concentrations achieved within respiratory secretions [44]. While there are concerns with using IV preparations for aerosol administration, repeated daily aerosol administration of gentamicin to horses for 7 days was not associated with lower respiratory inflammation, drug accumulation, or other adverse effects [32]. A liposomal gentamicin formulation has been studied in foals, using the IV or aerosol route [45]. In that study, liposomal gentamicin achieved higher intracellular concentrations in bronchoalveolar cells than free gentamicin regardless of route of administration, and was well tolerated. Unfortunately, there is not a commercially available liposomal gentamicin formulation at this time. A liposomal amikacin formulation[7] for nebulization is available for human use, but may be cost prohibitive in foals. While no studies have investigated administration of nonliposomal amikacin aerosols (formulated using injectable amikacin) to foals, this therapy is used widely in humans with lower respiratory infections [46, 47] and clinically is well tolerated in foals.

The use of ceftiofur aerosols has been investigated in foals, and this drug may be of greater utility than aminoglycosides in foals with Gram-positive or mixed bacterial pneumonia due to its broad antimicrobial spectrum [48, 49]. Ceftiofur aerosol administration was well tolerated and yielded active drug concentrations in the respiratory tract that were likely to be effective against most strains of *Streptococcus equi zooepidemicus* for up to 24 hours [49]. For organisms with higher MIC values, more frequent administration might be necessary, and this treatment is often utilized clinically at 12-hour treatment intervals for that reason. Other cephalosporins may be administered as aerosols, and ceftazidime is widely used in human medicine for treatment of pneumonia due to multidrug resistant pathogens [50, 51]. A fourth-generation cephalosporin, cefquinome, has been investigated as an aerosolized medication in adult horses [52]. This drug was well tolerated and achieved high local concentrations within the respiratory tract, but the residence time of the drug in the lungs was short, suggesting twice-daily treatment would likely be required [52].

Despite the technical validation of antimicrobial aerosols for delivery to equine patients, there is limited published information on the clinical use of aerosol antimicrobial therapy for treatment of respiratory infections in foals or adult horses. One report (from almost 40 years ago) used aerosolized gentamicin as an adjunct to systemic antimicrobial therapy in a case of bronchopneumonia in a 6-month-old colt [53]. In that report the addition of aerosol antimicrobial therapy was associated with resolution of mucopurulent nasal discharge within 2 days and normalization of respiratory sounds within 7 days of initiation of aerosol therapy. Wilson et al. suggested using aerosolized antimicrobials as an adjunct to systemic antimicrobial therapy for bacterial pneumonia in foals, but no recommendations were made regarding dosage, frequency, or method of administration [54]. More recently, Morresey described the successful use of ceftiofur aerosol therapy as an ancillary treatment in two cases of foal pneumonia, one associated with meconium aspiration and another with milk aspiration [30].

Aerosol administration of antimicrobials has been advocated as an adjunct to parenteral therapy when treating lower respiratory infections in adult horses [55]. This treatment modality was reported in horses with airway infections characterized by the presence of one or more clinical signs of lower respiratory disease, but not exhibiting signs of systemic inflammation or involvement of the pulmonary parenchyma. Aerosol administration of gentamicin (2.2 mg/kg once daily) and/or ceftiofur (2.2 mg/kg twice daily) was effective in reducing the numbers of bacteria present within the airways and resolving the clinical signs of lower respiratory disease in this subset of equine patients. More recently, the use of amikacin by the IV or inhaled route in racehorses with documented lower respiratory tract infections was investigated, and both treatments were equally effective in improving clinical scores and reducing tracheal aspirate neutrophil percentage and bacterial colony forming units [56].

Although controlled studies have not been performed to assess the efficacy of aerosolized antimicrobial therapy in foals, experimental studies in mice, guinea pigs, and piglets have demonstrated the effectiveness of aerosolized antimicrobials, as either the primary or adjunctive therapy in the treatment of bacterial pneumonia [13, 57–61]. The most promising results in large animals come from two studies that used aerosolized ceftiofur as a sole therapy in calves suffering from bacterial pneumonia [62, 63]. Sustronck et al. demonstrated that aerosolized ceftiofur administration in calves with experimental *Pasteurella haemolytica* pneumonia was superior to systemic ceftiofur, with lower mortality rates and more rapid resolution of clinical and hematological parameters in calves treated by the aerosol route [62]. More recently, Joshi et al. compared aerosol and systemic ceftiofur in calves with naturally occurring bovine respiratory disease, and similarly observed that calves treated with aerosolized ceftiofur had lower mortality rates and more rapid clinical and hematological recovery [63].

Limitations

A number of limitations are associated with aerosolized antimicrobials [64]. Most importantly, severe bacterial infections of the respiratory tract often have a systemic component and therefore require systemic antimicrobial therapy. Also, due to concerns regarding the ability of aerosol administration to deliver adequate amounts of medication to poorly ventilated areas of the lung, the administration of antimicrobials by inhalation alone is not appropriate in cases with substantial consolidation or parenchymal involvement. There is an increasing body of evidence, however, that systemic antimicrobial therapy may be effectively augmented by concurrent administration of antimicrobials by the inhaled route.

There are several reports of altered pulmonary mechanics in human patients following aerosol administration of antimicrobials, primarily as the result of bronchoconstriction resulting from irritation induced by the antimicrobial compound, the preservatives or carriers present within the solution, or the tonicity of the solution itself [65]. While repeated administration of gentamicin aerosol to horses was not associated with evidence of bronchoconstriction or a pulmonary inflammatory response, pretreatment with an aerosolized β_2-agonist bronchodilator may attenuate any coughing and bronchoconstriction that may be induced by aerosolized antimicrobials [32].

Treatment Recommendations

Systemic antimicrobial therapy remains the cornerstone of treatment of bacterial pneumonia in foals, but inhalation therapy represents a reasonable ancillary therapy, particularly in more severe cases or those not responding well to standard therapy. Inhaled albuterol can be administered to decrease the severity of bronchoconstriction in foals with pneumonia, decrease work of breathing, and enhance pulmonary penetration of aerosolized medications. Albuterol can be administered using an MDI or a nebulizer. If longer-lasting bronchodilation is desired, ipratropium bromide can be used, either alone or in conjunction with albuterol, and can be delivered by MDI or nebulizer. Aerosolized antimicrobials may shorten the course of the condition. Ceftiofur is a reasonable drug for initial aerosol therapy, unless results of bacterial culture and sensitivity indicate that it is not likely to be efficacious. In cases with substantial Gram-negative involvement, an aminoglycoside, such as gentamicin or amikacin, may be used with ceftiofur. In patients infected with multidrug resistant organisms, the results of bacterial sensitivity testing may indicate other appropriate drug choices for aerosol administration, but care must be taken that any drug used is appropriate for administration by inhalation (Table 6.V.1).

Notes

1 Flexineb® facemask, Nortev, Galway, Ireland.
2 Aerohippus™, Trudell Medical Intl., London, Ont., Canada.
3 SaHoMa®-II inhalation set for horses, Nebutec Intl., Elsenfeld, Germany.
4 Flexineb® E3, Nortev, Galway, Ireland.
5 Combivent® Nebuliser Solution, Boehringer Ingelheim Pharmaceuticals, Inc. Ridgefield, CT USA.
6 Combivent Inhalation Aerosol, Boehringer Ingelheim Pharmaceuticals, Inc. Ridgefield, CT USA.
7 Arikayce®, Insmed, Inc., Bridgewater Township, New Jersey.

References

1 Cohen, N.D. (1994). Causes of and farm management factors associated with disease and death in foals. *J. Am. Vet. Med. Assoc.* 204: 1644–1651.
2 Reuss, S.M. and Cohen, N.D. (2015). Update on bacterial pneumonia in the foal and weanling. *Vet. Clin. North Am. Equine Pract.* 31: 121–135.
3 Magdesian, K.G. (2017). Antimicrobial pharmacology for the neonatal foal. *Vet. Clin. North Am. Equine Pract.* 33: 47–65.
4 Rodvold, K.A., George, J.M., and Yoo, L. (2011). Penetration of anti-infective agents into pulmonary epithelial lining fluid focus on antibacterial agents. *Clin. Pharmacokinet.* 50: 637–664.
5 Duvivier, D.H., Votion, D., Vandenput, S. et al. (1997). Aerosol therapy in the equine species. *Vet. J.* 154: 189–202.
6 Restrepo, M.I., Keyt, H., and Reyes, L.F. (2015). Aerosolized antibiotics. *Respir. Care* 60: 762–761; discussion 771-763.
7 Bennet, W.D. (2019). Particle deposition in the respiratory tract and the effect of respiratory disease. In: *Inhalation Aerosols: Physical and Biological Basis for Therapy* (ed. A. Hickey and H.M. Mansour), 31–40. New York, NY: CRC Press.
8 Rush, B.R. (2003). Aerosolized drug delivery devices. In: *Currenty Therapy in Equine Medicine 5* (ed. N.E. Robinson), 436–440. St Loius: Saunders.
9 Woods, A. and Rahman, K.M. (2018). Antimicrobial molecules in the lung: formulation challenges and future directions for innovation. *Future Med. Chem.* 10: 575–604.
10 Rush, B.R., Hoskinson, J.J., Davis, E.G. et al. (1999). Pulmonary distribution of aerosolized technetium Tc 99m pentetate after administration of a single dose of aerosolized albuterol sulfate in horses with recurrent airway obstruction. *Am. J. Vet. Res.* 60: 764–769.
11 Hiller, F.C. (1992). Therapeutic aerosols: an overview from the clinical perspective. In: *Pharmaceutical Inhalation Aerosol Technology* (ed. A.J. Hickey), 289–306. New York: Marcel Dekker, Inc.
12 Elman, M., Goldstein, I., Marquette, C.H. et al. (2002). Influence of lung aeration on pulmonary concentrations of nebulized and intravenous amikacin in ventilated piglets with severe bronchopneumonia. *Anesthesiology* 97: 199–206.
13 Tonnellier, M., Ferrari, F., Goldstein, I. et al. (2005). Intravenous versus nebulized ceftazidime in ventilated piglets with and without experimental bronchopneumonia: comparative effects of helium and nitrogen. *Anesthesiology* 102: 995–1000.
14 Bassetti, M., Luyt, C.E., Nicolau, D.P. et al. (2016). Characteristics of an ideal nebulized antibiotic for the treatment of pneumonia in the intubated patient. *Ann. Intensive Care* 6: 35.
15 Newman, S.P. (1985). Aerosol deposition considerations in inhalation therapy. *Chest* 88: 152S–160S.
16 Pirie, R.S., McGorum, B.C., Owen, C. et al. (2017). Factors affecting the efficiency of aerosolized salbutamol delivery via a metered dose inhaler and equine spacer device. *J. Vet. Pharmacol. Ther.* 40: 231–238.

17 Cha, M.L. and Costa, L.R. (2017). Inhalation therapy in horses. *Vet. Clin. North Am. Equine Pract.* 33: 29–46.

18 Moraga-Espinoza, D.F., Brunaugh, A.D., Ferrati, S. et al. (2019). Overview of the delivery technologies for inhalation aerosols. In: *Inhalation Aerosols: Physical and Biological Basis for Therapy* (ed. A.J. Hickey and H.M. Mansour), 123–144. New York: CRC Press.

19 Tesarowski, D.B., Viel, L., McDonell, W.N. et al. (1994). The rapid and effective administration of a beta 2-agonist to horses with heaves using a compact inhalation device and metered-dose inhalers. *Can. Vet. J.* 35: 170–173.

20 Bertin, F.R., Ivester, K.M., and Couetil, L.L. (2011). Comparative efficacy of inhaled albuterol between two hand-held delivery devices in horses with recurrent airway obstruction. *Equine Vet. J.* 43: 393–398.

21 Bayly, W.M., Duvivier, D.H., Votion, D. et al. (2002). Effects of inhaled ipratropium bromide on breathing mechanics and gas exchange in exercising horses with chronic obstructive pulmonary disease. *Equine Vet. J.* 34: 36–43.

22 Atkins, P.J., Barker, N.P., and Mathisen, D. (1992). The design and development of inhalation drug delivery systems. In: *Pharmaceutical Inhalation Aerosol Technology* (ed. A.J. Hickey), 155–185. New York: Marcel Dekker, Inc.

23 Hardy, J.G., Newman, S.P., and Knoch, M. (1993). Lung deposition from four nebulizers. *Respir. Med.* 87: 461–465.

24 Votion, D., Ghafir, Y., Munsters, K. et al. (1997). Aerosol deposition in equine lungs following ultrasonic nebulisation versus jet aerosol delivery system. *Equine Vet. J.* 29: 388–393.

25 Rau, J.L., Ari, A., and Restrepo, R.D. (2004). Performance comparison of nebulizer designs: constant-output, breath-enhanced, and dosimetric. *Respir. Care* 49: 174–179.

26 Faurisson, F., Dessanges, J.F., Grimfeld, A. et al. (1995). Nebulizer performance: AFLM study. Association Francaise de Lutte contre la Mucoviscidose. *Respiration* 62 (Suppl 1): 13–18.

27 Ehrmann, S. (2018). Vibrating Mesh Nebulisers – can greater drug delivery to the airways and lungs improve respiratory outcomes? *Eur. Respir. Pulmonary Dis.* 4.

28 Weber, A., Morlin, G., Cohen, M. et al. (1997). Effect of nebulizer type and antibiotic concentration on device performance. *Pediatr. Pulmonol.* 23: 249–260.

29 McKenzie, H.C. (2003). Characterization of antimicrobial aerosols for administration to horses. *Vet. Ther.* 4: 110–119.

30 Morresey, P.R. (2008). How to deliver respiratory treatments to neonates by nebulization. How to deliver respiratory treatments to neonates by nebulization. *AAEP Annual Convention* 54: 520–526 San Diego, CA December 6-10, 2008.

31 Slovis, N.M. Non-*R. equi* pneumonia. *Proceedings of the AAEP Focus Meeting – Focus on the first year of life 2014*, 68–77. American Association of Equine Practitioners: Phoenix, AZ September 11–13, 2014.

32 McKenzie, H.C. 3rd and Murray, M.J. (2004). Concentrations of gentamicin in serum and bronchial lavage fluid after once-daily aerosol administration to horses for seven days. *Am. J. Vet. Res.* 65: 173–178.

33 Derksen, F.J., Olszewski, M.A., Robinson, N.E. et al. (1999). Aerosolized albuterol sulfate used as a bronchodilator in horses with recurrent airway obstruction. *Am. J. Vet. Res.* 60: 689–693.

34 Henrikson, S.L. and Rush, B.R. (2001). Efficacy of salmeterol xinafoate in horses with recurrent airway obstruction. *J. Am. Vet. Med. Assoc.* 218: 1961–1965.

35 Derksen, F.J., Robinson, N.E., and Berney, C.E. (1992). Aerosol pirbuterol: bronchodilator activity and side effects in ponies with recurrent airway obstruction (heaves). *Equine Vet. J.* 24: 107–112.

36 (1997). Routine nebulized ipratropium and albuterol together are better than either alone in COPD. The COMBIVENT inhalation solution study group. *Chest* 112: 1514–1521.

37 Lakritz, J., Wilson, W.D., Berry, C.R. et al. (1993). Bronchointerstitial pneumonia and respiratory distress in young horses: clinical, clinicopathologic, radiographic, and pathologic findings in 23 cases (1984–1989). *JVIM* 7: 277–278.

38 Dunkel, B., Dolente, B., and Boston, R.C. (2005). Acute lung injury/acute respiratory distress syndrome in 15 foals. *Equine Vet. J.* 37: 435–440.

39 Valcke, Y., Pauwels, R., and Van der Straeten, M. (1990). Pharmacokinetics of antibiotics in the lungs. *Eur. Respir. J.* 3: 715–722.

40 Wenzler, E., Fraidenburg, D.R., Scardina, T. et al. (2016). Inhaled antibiotics for Gram-negative respiratory infections. *Clin. Microbiol. Rev.* 29: 581–632.

41 Wong, F.J., Dudney, T., and Dhand, R. (2019). Aerosolized antibiotics for treatment of pneumonia in mechanically ventilated subjects. *Respir. Care* 64: 962–979.

42 Dugernier, J., Reychler, G., Dubus, J.-C. et al. (2017). Aerosolized antibiotics. *Clin. Pulmonary Med.* 24: 183–190.

43 McKenzie, H.C. 3rd and Murray, M.J. (2000). Concentrations of gentamicin in serum and bronchial lavage fluid after intravenous and aerosol administration of gentamicin to horses. *Am. J. Vet. Res.* 61: 1185–1190.

44 Godber, L.M., Walker, R.D., Stein, G.E. et al. (1995). Pharmacokinetics, nephrotoxicosis, and in vitro antibacterial activity associated with single versus multiple (three times) daily gentamicin treatments in horses. *Am. J. Vet. Res.* 56: 613–618.

45 Burton, A.J., Giguere, S., and Arnold, R.D. (2015). Pharmacokinetics, pulmonary disposition and tolerability

of liposomal gentamicin and free gentamicin in foals. *Equine Vet. J.* 47: 467–472.

46 Luyt, C.E., Hekimian, G., Brechot, N. et al. (2018). Aerosol therapy for pneumonia in the intensive care unit. *Clin. Chest Med.* 39: 823–836.

47 Gilbert, D.N. (2019). Nebulized antibiotics for multidrug-resistant ventilator-associated *Pseudomonas aeruginosa* pneumonia. *Crit. Care Med.* 47: 880–881.

48 Meyer, S., Giguere, S., Rodriguez, R. et al. (2009). Pharmacokinetics of intravenous ceftiofur sodium and concentration in body fluids of foals. *J. Vet. Pharmacol. Ther.* 32: 309–316.

49 Fultz, L., Giguere, S., Berghaus, L.J. et al. (2015). Pulmonary pharmacokinetics of desfuroylceftiofur acetamide after nebulisation or intramuscular administration of ceftiofur sodium to weanling foals. *Equine Vet. J.* 47: 473–477.

50 Lu, Q., Yang, J., Liu, Z. et al. (2011). Nebulized ceftazidime and amikacin in ventilator-associated pneumonia caused by *Pseudomonas aeruginosa*. *Am. J. Respir. Crit. Care Med.* 184: 106–115.

51 Quon, B.S., Goss, C.H., and Ramsey, B.W. (2014). Inhaled antibiotics for lower airway infections. *Ann. Am. Thorac. Soc.* 11: 425–434.

52 Winther, L., Baptiste, K.E., and Friis, C. (2011). Antimicrobial disposition in pulmonary epithelial lining fluid of horses, part III. Cefquinome. *J. Vet. Pharmacol. Ther.* 34: 482–486.

53 Rhodes, C.H. and Genetzky, R.M. (1982). Nebulization therapy in the foal. *Iowa State Vet.* 44: 104–108.

54 Wilson, W.D. (1992). Foal pneumonia. In: *Current Therapy in Equine Medicine*, 3e (ed. N. Edward Robinson), 466–473. Philadelphia: WB Saunders.

55 Murray, M.J. (1997). New diagnostic techniques and treatment for lower respiratory disease. *15th Veterinary Medical Forum*, 380–382. 15th ACVIM Forum Lake Buena Vista, FL May 22–25, 1997.

56 Ferrucci, F., Stucchi, L., Salvadori, M. et al. (2013). Effects of inhaled amikacin on racehorses with history of poor performance and comparison with intravenous administration. *Ippologia* 24: 3–9.

57 Makhoul, I.R., Merzbach, D., Lichtig, C. et al. (1993). Antibiotic treatment of experimental *Pseudomonas aeruginosa* pneumonia in Guinea pigs: comparison of aerosol and systemic administration. *J Infect Dis* 168: 1296–1299.

58 Ferrari, F., Lu, Q., Girardi, C. et al. (2009). Nebulized ceftazidime in experimental pneumonia caused by partially resistant *Pseudomonas aeruginosa*. *Intensive Care Med.* 35: 1792–1800.

59 Goldstein, I., Wallet, F., Nicolas-Robin, A. et al. (2002). Lung deposition and efficiency of nebulized amikacin during *Escherichia coli* pneumonia in ventilated piglets. *Am. J. Respir. Crit. Care Med.* 166: 1375–1381.

60 Lin, Y.W., Zhou, Q., Onufrak, N.J. et al. (2017). Aerosolized polymyxin B for treatment of respiratory tract infections: determination of pharmacokinetic-pharmacodynamic indices for aerosolized polymyxin B against *Pseudomonas aeruginosa* in a mouse lung infection model. *Antimicrob. Agents Chemother.* 61.

61 Lin, Y.W., Zhou, Q.T., Cheah, S.E. et al. (2017). Pharmacokinetics/pharmacodynamics of pulmonary delivery of colistin against *Pseudomonas aeruginosa* in a mouse lung infection model. *Antimicrob. Agents Chemother.* 61.

62 Sustronck, B., Deprez, P., Muylle, E. et al. (1995). Evaluation of the nebulisation of sodium ceftiofur in the treatment of experimental *Pasteurella haemolytica* bronchopneumonia in calves. *Res. Vet. Sci.* 59: 267–271.

63 Joshi, V., Gupta, V.K., Dimri, U. et al. (2017). Assessment of nebulisation of sodium ceftiofur in the treatment of calves naturally infected with bovine respiratory disease. *Tropl. Anim. Health Prod.* 49: 497–501.

64 O'Riordan, T. and Faris, M. (1999). Inhaled antimicrobial therapy. *Respir. Care Clin. North Am.* 5: 617–631.

65 Brown, V.A. and Wilkins, P.A. (2006). Advanced techniques in the diagnosis and management of infectious pulmonary diseases in horses. *Vet. Clin. North Am. Equine Pract.* 22: 633–651, xi.

Section VI Ventilator Therapy

Jon Palmer

Abbreviations

CPAP	Continuous positive airway pressure
CSV	Continuous spontaneous ventilation
FRC	Functional residual capacity
PEEP	Positive end expiratory ventilation
PSV	Pressure support ventilation
PC-CMV	Pressure-controlled-continuous mandatory ventilation
PC-IMV	Pressure-controlled-intermittent mandatory ventilation
VC-CMV	Volume-controlled-continuous mandatory ventilation
VC-IMV	Volume-controlled-intermittent mandatory ventilation
VSV	Volume support ventilation
V/Q	Ventilation/Perfusion

Respiratory support, including mechanical ventilation, has been used successfully in neonatal foals for more than 40 years [1, 2]. Using modern mechanical ventilators and principles learned in human medicine, ventilating foals without respiratory failure, such as those suffering from botulism or neonatal encephalopathy–associated central hypercapnia, has become successful, with 80% of such patients surviving to discharge from the hospital and many becoming productive athletes (Figure 6.VI.1) [1–4]. Those with secondary respiratory failure, as with severe sepsis or acute respiratory failure associated with multiorgan dysfunction syndrome remain a major challenge, and successful outcomes are more difficult to achieve.

Mechanical Ventilation

Mechanical positive-pressure ventilation supports and allows manipulation of pulmonary gas exchange; increases lung volume, returning normal functional residual capacity (FRC); decreases work of breathing, allowing ventilatory muscles to rest when fatigued; and decreases oxygen and energy use and perfusion that would be required to support the work of breathing. The main clinical indications for mechanical ventilation in the neonate are persistent pulmonary hypertension, acute respiratory failure, neonatal encephalopathy (associated weakness or central respiratory center failure), weakness associated with prematurity or intrauterine growth restriction (IUGR), fatigue secondary to general weakness or secondary to upper airway obstruction (e.g. pharyngeal collapse, upper airway cysts), central or sepsis-induced hypotension, septic shock, and neuromuscular disorders (i.e. botulism). Acute respiratory failure includes acute respiratory distress syndrome (ARDS), organ dysfunction secondary to sepsis, infectious pneumonia (viral, bacterial, or aspiration pneumonia), noninfectious pneumonia (meconium aspiration, interstitial pneumonia, or aspiration pneumonia), and trauma secondary to fractured ribs. Typically, the goal is to provide respiratory support while therapies for underlying causes of the acute event are initiated [5–7].

The benefits of mechanical ventilation in improving gas exchange by increasing ventilation, improving ventilation/perfusion (V/Q) matching, and decreasing intrapulmonary shunting are well appreciated. Less well appreciated are the benefits of decreasing the work of breathing in cases of

Equine Neonatal Medicine, First Edition. Edited by David M. Wong and Pamela A. Wilkins.

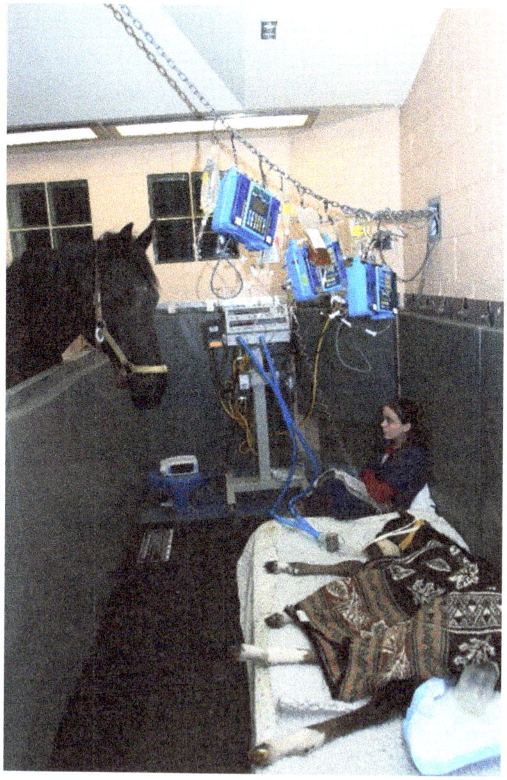

Figure 6.VI.1 Foal receiving positive pressure ventilation with an attendant and mare watching.

pulmonary failure and septic shock. With normal quiet breathing, inhalation is an active process requiring energy, using 3–5% of the oxygen the patient consumes. Exhalation is a passive process that requires no energy. When patients experience respiratory distress, as occurs with primary lung disease or septic shock, oxygen consumption required for the work of breathing increases up to 50% of the available oxygen and diverts perfusion resources as accessory muscles are recruited. Relieving this work of breathing allows redistribution of these oxygen and perfusion resources to support vital organ function. Respiratory support through mechanical ventilation is an important therapeutic modality in treating septic shock (Figure 6.VI.2) [8, 9].

Ventilator Modes

Only select ventilatory modes that form the basis of modern conventional ventilation are discussed here. Many modern conventional ventilators have proprietary modes, often confusing the uninitiated. The best source of information about these special modes is literature from the manufacturer. Most of these proprietary modes remain unproven, being supported only by a physiologic rational or, occasionally, with small and poorly powered studies. A lack of evidence makes it difficult to select one mode over another. The mode used is often selected based on the clinician's experiences as well as the neonate's underlying problem.

Positive-pressure ventilation is classified according to the parameter that is used to terminate inspiration. Common cycling parameters include volume, pressure, flow, and time. With *volume-cycled ventilation*, inspiration is terminated after delivery of a preset tidal volume, irrespective of inspiratory time or the airway pressure during delivery. As the peak pressures in the patient's lungs increase, however, a greater proportion of the preset tidal volume is left behind in the ventilator's circuit. Leaks in the respiratory circuit will result in failure to deliver the set tidal volume. With *pressure-cycled ventilation*, inspiration

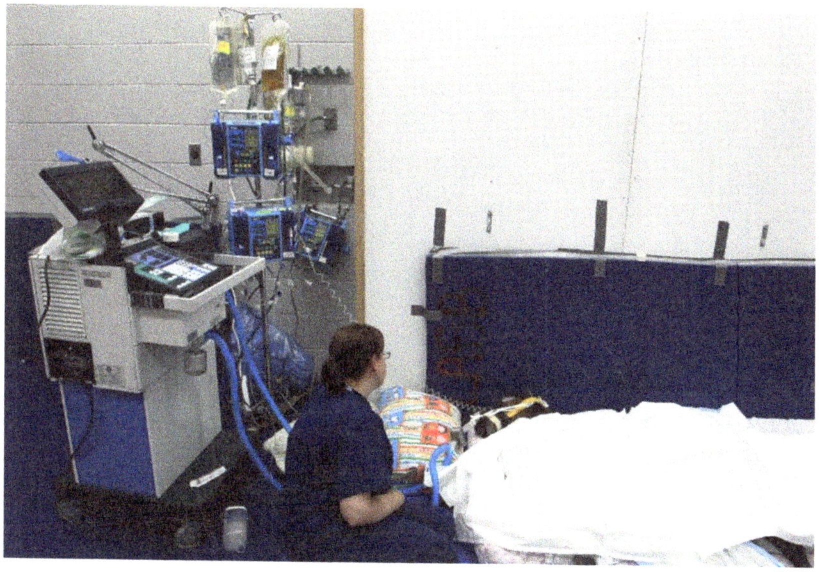

Figure 6.VI.2 Critical foal receiving mechanical ventilation.

ceases when a preset maximum airway pressure is reached, irrespective of the volume delivered, inspiratory time, or inspiratory flow rate. The delivered volume and inspiratory time vary with alterations in lung mechanics; thus, minute ventilation is not assured and may vary with time. With *flow-cycled ventilation*, inspiration is terminated when a particular flow rate is reached. Pressure-support ventilation (PSV) is an example of flow-cycled mechanical ventilation. Here, a preset airway pressure is applied once the machine is triggered and is cycled off after the inspiratory flow decreases to a predetermined percentage of its peak value. Finally, with *time-cycled ventilation*, inspiration is terminated after a preset inspiratory time. The volume of gas delivered, and the resulting airway pressure vary from breath to breath as a function of changes in lung mechanics. Many modern conventional ventilators incorporate variations of all of these ventilator types in one machine as well as several proprietary variations (Table 6.VI.1).

The traditional ventilator modes that can be found on most modern ventilators are volume-controlled or pressure-controlled continuous mandatory ventilation (VC-CMV, PC-CMV), volume-controlled or pressure-controlled intermittent mandatory ventilation (VC-IMV, PC-IMV), and continuous spontaneous ventilation (CSV), all with or without positive end expiratory pressure (PEEP). Subcategories of CSV include PSV and continuous positive airway pressure (CPAP).

With CMV, the ventilator can be set to allow no patient-triggered breaths. In this case, the ventilator delivers breaths at a preset interval, regardless of any ventilatory effort made by the patient. The patient cannot trigger a ventilator breath or take a spontaneous breath through the ventilator circuit. The delivered breath is a result of the preset volume or pressure and is no larger and no smaller. This mode is not appropriate for any conscious foal, because without extremely heavy sedation, the foal fights this mode and there is an absence of synchrony. In general, foals do not require any sedation for successful ventilation as long as they are in synchrony with the ventilatory mode. It is important to avoid sedation with its inherent complications. Sedation is not an acceptable substitute for choosing an appropriate mode and ventilator settings.

Usually with CMV, respiratory efforts by the patient trigger a breath, which will be delivered at the full preset

Table 6.VI.1 Overview of ventilator terms and common ventilator modes.

<u>Positive Pressure Ventilation (PPV) – classified by parameter that terminates inspiration</u>

Volume – inspiration terminated after delivery of preset tidal volume

Pressure – inspiration terminated after delivery of preset maximum airway pressure reached

Flow – inspiration terminated after specific flow rate is reached (pressure support ventilation [PSV] is an example)

Time – inspiration terminated after preset inspiratory time

<u>Common Ventilator Modes (with or without positive end-expiratory pressure [PEEP])</u>

Continuous Mandatory Ventilation (CMV) can be volume controlled or pressure controlled:

Volume controlled continuous mandatory ventilation (VC-CMV)

Pressure controlled continuous mandatory ventilation (PC-CMV)

- Ventilator can be set to allow patient to trigger breaths – ventilator delivers breath at preset volume or pressure. If there is an absence of respiratory effort, ventilator automatically cycles at preset minimum background respiratory rate. Foal receives minimum respiratory rate but can voluntarily breath at higher rate.
- Ventilator can be set to allow no patient triggered breaths – ventilator delivers breaths at preset interval (regardless of ventilatory effort made by patient). Patient cannot trigger breath or take spontaneous breath. Delivered breath given at preset volume or pressure. Mode not appropriate for conscious foal.

Intermittent Mandatory Ventilation (IMV) can be volume or pressure controlled:

Volume-controlled intermittent mandatory ventilation (VC-IMV)

Pressure-controlled intermittent mandatory ventilation (PC-IMV)

- Combination of spontaneous ventilation and CMV. Delivery of mechanical breath is synchronized to support foal's spontaneous breaths at preset rate. If spontaneous breathing occurs at a rate faster than ventilator's set IMV rate, after ventilator delivers preset breath, extra breaths are not supported (but still breath oxygen-rich gas from ventilator circuit). If foal's spontaneous respiratory rate slows or stops, ventilator continues to deliver breaths at IMV rate.

Continuous spontaneous ventilation (CSV)

- Pressure support ventilation (PSV) is an assist flow-cycled mode where breathing is controlled by the foal and peak pressures controlled by the ventilator. PSV supports the foal's spontaneous breaths by helping foal attain a preset peak inspiratory airway pressure each time foal initiates a breath. PSV also decreases work of breathing. Exhalation occurs spontaneously and not augmented by ventilator. Foal has complete control of initiation of breaths, inspiratory time, and tidal volume. IMV and PSV are used together frequently.
- Continuous positive airway pressure (CPAP) refers to maintaining positive airway pressure throughout spontaneous respiration (during exhalation and between breaths).

volume or pressure. In the absence of any respiratory effort, the ventilator automatically cycles at a preset minimum background rate. For example, if the ventilator is set for 12 breaths/minute, the machine delivers a breath every 5 seconds in the absence of spontaneous inspiratory effort. If the patient's inspiratory effort triggers an assisted breath, the ventilator's timer resets for another 5 seconds. The patient is guaranteed to receive a minimum of the set breath rate but can breathe at a higher rate depending on the frequency of effective inspiratory efforts. The initiation of breaths synchronized with spontaneous efforts is welcomed by most foals, but the imposition of a preset breath at a fixed and unforgiving volume or pressure is poorly tolerated.

IMV is a combination of spontaneous ventilation and CMV. The delivery of the mechanical breath is synchronized to support the patient's spontaneous breaths at a preset rate, thus preventing the patient from stacking breaths (a mechanical breath being delivered at the same time as a spontaneous breath). Stacking may result in hyperinflation and volutrauma or barotrauma. If spontaneous breathing occurs at a rate faster than the ventilator's set IMV rate, after the ventilator delivers the preset breaths, extra breaths are not supported. That is, the patient breathes gas from the ventilator circuit without tripping a ventilator breath. These spontaneous extra breaths consist of warmed, humidified, oxygen-enriched gas supplied from the ventilator's circuit but with no preset volume or pressure. If the patient's spontaneous efforts slow or stop, the ventilator continues to deliver breaths by default at the IMV rate. The IMV mode is well tolerated, because breaths above the preset rate are completely controlled by the patient (timing, depth, and duration). The preset breaths are still at a fixed and unforgiving volume or pressure. This mode is often combined with PSV so that the spontaneous breaths have pressure support.

Assisted CSV can be delivered by PSV, which is an assist flow-cycled mode in which breathing is controlled by the foal and peak pressures are controlled by the ventilator. The primary goal of PSV is to support the foal's spontaneous breathing effort while decreasing the work of breathing and providing satisfactory gas exchange. PSV attempts to attain a preset peak inspiratory airway pressure each time the foal initiates inspiratory effort. If the foal's inspiratory effort is strong, the preset airway pressure may never be attained because the inspiratory effort keeps the airway pressure below the pressure goal until the ventilator cycles off. Still, the inspiratory time, inspiratory flow rate, and tidal volume are augmented, whereas the inspiratory work of breathing is reduced. The machine senses the end of inspiration by first measuring the peak inspiratory flow and then waiting until that flow falls to a preset "off-switch" value (typically 25% of the peak flow or some fixed low-inspiratory flow rate). Exhalation is allowed to proceed spontaneously. As a result, a PSV breath is delivered when the ventilator senses a respiratory effort by opening a demand valve at a preset pressure. Gases are forced into the ventilator circuit in an attempt to raise the airway pressure to the preset value, decreasing the work of inspiration. As the foal decides the tidal volume is sufficient, inspiratory flow slows and the demand valve shuts, ending inspiration and allowing expiration. Increasing levels of PSV decrease the work of breathing. Because the foal has complete control of initiation of breaths, inspiratory time, and tidal volume, it readily cooperates with the ventilator; however, because respiratory rate and tidal volume are not controlled, careful monitoring is required. Some new ventilators allow the clinician to set a target tidal volume. These ventilators titrate the delivered airway pressure based on feedback from past tidal volume in a mode often called volume support ventilation (VSV). This allows the ventilator to adjust the pressure delivered on each breath to try to achieve a desired tidal volume. Frequently, IMV and PSV are used together so that spontaneous breaths in IMV are supported, helping to overcome the inherent resistance of the ventilator circuit, and when the predominant mode is PSV, the IMV rate acts as a fail-safe breath rate [10, 11].

There are situations in which PSV can be detrimental. When a foal has severe dyspnea despite ventilation, unless the pressure support is set high, there is an increased risk of alveolar collapse. PSV also may be poorly tolerated in patients that have high airway resistance with long time constants and may not provide sufficient minute ventilation because of the preset high initial flow and terminal inspiratory flow algorithms that are standard on most critical-care ventilators [12]. In patients that have long inspiratory demands, the breath may be terminated too early if the flow rate slows before completion of inspiration. Conversely, the breath may terminate too late in patients that have obstructive airway disease. This can result in a short expiratory time, exacerbating air trapping. New ventilators attempt to solve these problems by using a pressure-targeted time-cycled breath, allowing for control of inspiratory time or control of the pressure slope, with a rapid peak resulting in a higher peak flow, and thus a shorter inspiratory time, and a slow peak initial flow resulting in a longer inspiratory time. A more direct approach used in other ventilators is to allow adjustment of the flow criteria, which causes the inspiratory assist to cycle off [11].

Ventilators often have proprietary modes that combine or modify the traditional modes. One such mode called pressure-regulated volume-control (PRVC) ventilation, which is a mix of volume-control and pressure-control ventilation. This mode is really pressure-controlled breaths with an automatically adjusted pressure-control level. A target tidal volume is set, and the pressure level changes as needed to provide the target volume.

PEEP refers to the maintenance of positive pressure in the airways between ventilator-induced positive-pressure inspiration (during exhalation and between breaths) so that the airway pressure never falls below the set PEEP value. CPAP refers to maintaining positive airway pressure throughout spontaneous respiration (during inspiration and exhalation and between breaths). The terms are usually used synonymously. There is the possibility of subatmospheric pressure during spontaneous inspiration with PEEP depending on the ventilator inspiratory mode. PEEP may be added to any of the ventilation modes discussed previously.

PEEP/CPAP is often effective in treating hypoxemia by decreasing intrapulmonary shunting and V/Q mismatch. Beneficial physiologic affects of PEEP/CPAP are created by an increased transpulmonary pressure, resulting in an increased FRC, stabilization of open alveoli, and improvement in V/Q ratios. PEEP/CPAP affects pulmonary mechanics, cardiovascular stability, and pulmonary vascular resistance. FRC is the volume of gas remaining in the lungs at the end of a normal expiration. At a low FRC (as low volumes in diseased lungs), the compliance is low. At a higher FRC, compliance increases until the alveoli become overdistended, when compliance again decreases. Normal FRC is optimal FRC, which results in optimum compliance and the lowest work of breathing. Lung volume is also related to airway resistance. At low lung volumes airway resistance is high because atelectasis is not resolved, narrowing the airways, and resulting in a high work of breathing. At optimum lung volumes, airway resistance is low as the open alveoli tend to hold open the airways. PEEP/CPAP can improve distribution of ventilation optimizing FRC, and thus increasing lung compliance and decreasing airway resistance. High PEEP/CPAP can have a detrimental effect on the cardiovascular system, compressing right-sided vessels, and decreasing cardiac return, which results in decreased cardiac output. The amount of PEEP/CPAP that is excessive and produces this effect depends on lung compliance. If the lung compliance is low, less intra-airway pressure is transmitted to the plural space and cardiac compromise is less. Hypovolemia exacerbates the negative effect of high PEEP/CPAP. Overdistention of the lung may cause direct pressure on pulmonary arterials and capillaries, increasing pulmonary vascular resistance and pulmonary artery pressure. Low levels of PEEP/CPAP do not resolve atelectasis. Atelectasis results in directing blood away from collapsed alveoli and a regional increase in pulmonary vascular resistance. Optimal PEEP/CPAP optimizes the V/Q ratio. The effects of PEEP/CPAP on cerebral pressure are directly related to the level of positive pressure applied to the airway and the lung compliance affecting blood flow. If the pressure is transmitted to the pleural space and the anterior vena cava, it may result in increased cerebral pressure.

In healthy individuals, the FRC is maintained so that almost all alveoli are open and ventilated. In foals that are weak or fatigued, the FRC can be significantly reduced, resulting in poor ventilatory function. The lung volume begins to decrease to the point at which alveoli collapse during expiration and must be opened on each breath to receive ventilation. Alveoli that repeatedly close in this manner increase the risk of injury from the shear stress and tend to break down surfactant [13, 14]. As the amount of surfactant decreases, it becomes more difficult to open these alveoli on inspiration; eventually, significant atelectasis results in decreasing compliance. This progressive decrease in lung compliance tends to cause collapse of more alveoli. The sum effect of this is progressive atelectasis. Even in those alveoli that are being ventilated, the ventilation is less evenly distributed because alveoli not already open do not open until part way through inspiration. Other alveoli that are already opened accept gas throughout inspiration. This results in maldistribution of ventilation. Also, alveoli that close during expiration only participate in gas exchange during inspiration. Decreased FRC is most effectively treated through initiation of PEEP/CPAP. By increasing the airway pressure during expiration, alveoli tend to stay open, and more alveoli may be recruited on each new inspiration. Full recruitment using PEEP/CPAP requires 15–20 minutes. Optimal PEEP/CPAP can be estimated by producing a PEEP/CPAP grid. By adjusting PEEP/CPAP to 1 cm above and 1 cm below current levels and then allowing maximal recruitment after 10–15 minutes, obtaining a partial pressure of oxygen in arterial blood (P_aO_2) measurement or measuring effective compliance, the optimum PEEP/CPAP can be identified. Because alveolar injury is often quite heterogeneous, PEEP that is appropriate in one region may not be appropriate in another, being suboptimal or excessive. Optimizing PEEP is thus a balance between enrolling the recruitable alveoli in diseased regions without overdistending already recruited alveoli in healthier regions. Another potential detrimental effect of PEEP is that it raises mean and peak airway pressure, potentially contributing to barotrauma or volutrauma [8].

Typical Ventilator Settings

Initial ventilator settings depend on the ventilator make and model, ventilator mode, goal of the intervention, and underlying cause of respiratory failure. The basic parameters to be set in CMV or IMV mode are F_iO_2, tidal volume or peak pressure, breath rate, and a combination of parameters that determine inspiratory characteristics, including inspiratory time/inspiratory flow (set as seconds or % or liters/second; typically begin with 1 second or ⅓ of the respiratory cycle), inspiratory pause (set as % or seconds; also referred to as inspiratory hold), inspiratory rise time (seconds or %; sets the time it takes to reach the preset pressure or flow), depending on the mode. These later parameters in combination with rate determines the inspiratory-expiratory (I/E) ratio. Also, trigger sensitivity (patient effort needed to initiate a breath set as drop of airway pressure or flow rate) and PEEP need to be set. Many ventilator models also allow setting a fail-safe ventilatory rate that is activated if apnea occurs, or a preset minute volume is not achieved. On ventilators offering a PSV mode, the pressure support level can also be set along with other pressure support parameters [5, 8].

Setting the tidal volume is important for successful mechanical ventilation. It is one parameter that has been shown to be important in determining the likelihood of ventilator-induced acute lung injury in human medicine. The National Institutes of Health ARDS Network study in 2000 showed that the use of 6 ml/kg tidal volume resulted in a significantly lower fatality rate than 12 ml/kg [15]. Initially, clinicians were slow to fully embrace the use of these low tidal volumes in ARDS until data became convincing [16–18]. Recently, the use of high tidal volumes in ventilated patients who have no evidence of lung disease at the onset of ventilation has been shown to predispose to ventilatory-associated acute lung injury [19, 20]. Clinicians should be careful not to overinterpret these data when choosing a tidal volume in ventilated foals. It could be dangerous to extrapolate the critical volume based on body weight from one species to another when the ratio of lung volume to body weight differs. High tidal volumes seem to be detrimental because of the resulting volutrauma or barotrauma. This is compounded in situations where damaged lung results in a smaller ventilated lung volume, as in ARDS. The lesson from these clinical studies in people is that the tidal volume should be set as low as practical with the goal of keeping the plateau airway pressure <30 cm H_2O, even at the expense of mild hypercapnia [21]. Thus, tidal volume should be set between 6 and 10 ml/kg as long as the plateau airway pressure <30 cm H_2O when the foal is in synchrony (not fighting the ventilator) [22]. Foals in synchrony with the ventilator and having normal lungs usually will have plateau airway pressure of approximately 20 cm H_2O. Conscious nonsedated foals ventilated using a low tidal volume (e.g. 6 ml/kg) frequently stack breaths so that the effective tidal volume is higher (e.g. 12 ml/kg). The breath stacking can go undetected unless the clinician is quite observant. Sedation, with its associated complications, to achieve a low tidal volume may be more detrimental than a slightly higher tidal volume.

Respiratory rate is often determined by the patient, because most ventilator modes allow the patient to initiate more breaths than the set machine breath rate. The set rate on the machine is in essence a minimum breath rate. For patients that have poor central sensitivity to carbon dioxide (CO_2), the respiratory rate should be set in conjunction with the tidal volume to achieve a desired minute volume adequate to maintain P_aCO_2 in the range that results in an acceptable blood pH. Often, critically ill neonates have an abnormal acid–base balance. Significant metabolic alkalosis is frequently present. The target P_aCO_2 should be the value that returns the pH to a normal value. A P_aCO_2 of 60–65 mmHg may be appropriate if that level is required to buffer a significant metabolic alkalosis, keeping the pH <7.45. This is not permissive hypercapnia with controlled hypoventilation. Permissive hypercapnia is the practice of allowing a P_aCO_2 higher than what is required to correct an acid pH, avoiding the possible lung trauma that could be caused in pursuit of full correction of the pH and allowing more optimal expiratory time. The goal of permissive hypercapnia is to maintain an arterial pH >7.20 but not necessarily >7.35. The practice of permissive hypercapnia is only needed when ventilating foals with significant underlying lung injury. When placing a foal on a ventilator using a mode that requires a set breath rate, an initial rate between 20 and 30 breaths per minute is usually adequate. The rate should be adjusted during the first 30 minutes of ventilation with the aid of capnography, which should be followed up by arterial blood gas (ABG) measurements. In modes where machine-generated breaths are delivered, the parameters that set the inspiratory pattern and time (inspiratory time/peak flow, inspiratory pause/inspiratory hold, inspiratory rise time/slope, etc.) and expiratory parameters setting I : E ratio need to be adjusted. Factors that go into selecting and modifying these settings include pulmonary mechanics, airway resistance, time constants, and airway pressure gradients. There is no clear formula that can be used in setting inspiratory parameters, but it is usually initially set so that the inspiratory time is similar to that of the unventilated patient that has an I/E ratio of approximately 1 : 2; it can then be dynamically adjusted as needed. Improperly set peak flow (speed of inspiration) can be a source of patient-ventilator dyssynchrony when the delivered gas is too rapid or slow for the situation. When airway pressure becomes negative (beyond the trigger point) during inspiration, the patient is demanding gas faster than the ventilator is delivering, which may be because the peak flow is set too low.

The initial F_IO_2 setting is dictated by the preventilation P_aO_2 and the response observed to intranasal oxygen insufflation. If maintaining an acceptable P_aO_2 has not been a problem, beginning with an F_IO_2 of 0.3 should be sufficient. If high intranasal flows have been required to maintain blood oxygen, an F_IO_2 of 0.5 should be initiated. If the foal remains hypoxemic despite high intranasal flows, the initial F_IO_2 should be between 0.8 and 1.0. In all cases, the F_IO_2 should be titrated as directed by arterial blood levels, with the initial measurement within 30 minutes or less of initiating ventilation with the goal of an F_IO_2 <0.5. An initial PEEP of 4–5 cm H_2O is usually adequate if the lungs are normal. Once the foal is stable on the ventilator, the PEEP can be further adjusted by the aid of flow loops or a compliance or P_aO_2 grid can be constructed to ensure that the PEEP is optimal for the patient. In cases with low P_aO_2 values despite high intranasal oxygen flows, a trial with an F_IO_2 of 1.0 can be useful diagnostically in identifying the source of the hypoxemia. If the P_aO_2 is <100 mmHg after 10–15 minutes of ventilation with an F_IO_2 of 1.0, it is likely that the cause of the hypoxemia is a large cardiac shunt rather than an intrapulmonary problem. In most of these cases, the P_aO_2 is often between 20 and 45 mmHg and increases <10 mmHg on an F_IO_2 of 1.0. This clinical rule of thumb has been accurate in this author's experience, predicting the presence of persistent fetal circulation with pulmonary hypertension and a large right-to-left shunt fraction or a significant cardiac malformation resulting in the same. Also, reversion to fetal circulation can easily be detected by this method.

The sensitivity trigger, the patient's inspiratory effort needed to initiate a breath, can be pressure based or flow based. With pressure triggering, the expiratory valve must be closed before the patient generates the preset negative pressure needed to open the flow controller valve. With flow triggering, the inspiratory valve is kept open with a small amount of bias flow and the patient may initiate a breath even if the expiratory valve is still open, allowing for flow-by ventilation. With flow triggering, the patient immediately receives a small amount of flow to satisfy any air hunger, making for a smoother transition to the next breath [8]. Pressure trigger sensitivity is usually set at 2–3 cm H_2O. Care should be taken not to set the trigger value so low that any respiratory movement of the foal or bumping of the respiratory circuit triggers a breath. Increasing the trigger point, and thus making the patient use more effort to trigger a breath, is a common way to judge readiness for weaning and to exercise respiratory muscles in preparation for weaning.

When setting pressure support, the level is dependent on the resistance and compliance of the ventilatory circuit, airway resistance, lung compliance, and inspiratory effort of the patient. In the absence of lung disease, such as in an uncomplicated botulism case, 8–12 cm H_2O is enough to overcome ventilatory circuit resistance and deliver an adequate tidal volume. In cases of low compliance, pressure support as high as 20–25 cm H_2O or higher may be required. Higher pressure support can also be useful in situations in which patient-ventilator dyssynchrony results from a strong patient-derived inspiratory effort that exceeds the rate of gas delivery by the ventilator. Setting the inspiratory time and pressure slope with a rapid peak resulting in a higher peak flow can be helpful in ventilators that allow these adjustments.

All ventilator settings should be adjusted dynamically after initiation of ventilation because success is highly dependent on tailoring the setting to the individual. A combination of simple pulmonary mechanics, end-tidal CO_2 ($ETCO_2$) determination, ventilation pressures, clinical status, and ABG results should form the basis for the adjustments. Having a feel for which combination of ventilatory adjustments improves successful gas exchange and improves ventilatory synchrony while, at the same time, decreasing ventilator-induced lung trauma only comes with experience and forms the basis of the art of successful ventilatory support.

Preconditioning Ventilator Gases

With the upper airway bypassed by tracheal intubation, sufficient heat and moisture must be added to inspired gas mixtures to prevent mucosal injury secondary to drying and cooling. The response of the trachea to such injury is proliferation of goblet cells and production of mucus discharge, which becomes tenacious as it becomes desiccated and can obstruct the airway or endotracheal tube. Active humidifiers use external water sources and electrical power to adjust blended gas mixtures to an intratracheal temperature >35 °C and water content >40 mg/l. When air is fully saturated with water vapor at 37 °C the partial pressure is 47 mmHg which corresponds to a water vapor mass of 44 mg/l. Passive humidifiers use simple heat-moisture exchange (HME) device filters placed on the ventilator side of the endotracheal tube that use heat and moisture trapped from expired gases. HME filters trap heat and moisture from the exhaled air and add both to the next breath as it passes through the filter. These disposable units can usually supply adequate heat and moisture (i.e. warmer than 30–33 °C and higher than 28–32 mg H_2O/l) for most foals receiving mechanical ventilation for only short periods (Figure 6.VI.3). Foals weighing >70 kg or those that have large minute volumes for any reason may need more moisture than can be trapped by large HME filters. In these cases, adding a cold active humidifier to a circuit with an HME filter in place may provide enough moisture to allow effective ventilator gas preconditioning. In this situation, the humidity must be delivered to the HME filter cold so that it passes through the filter to the patient. Once it is warmed by the patient, the moisture is trapped on the patient side of the filter. In addition to the limitation of high minute volume, HME filter use is not effective in hypothermic patients and the presence of airway discharge can obstruct the filter, causing a dangerous situation [3]. An advantage of many HME filters is that they act as an

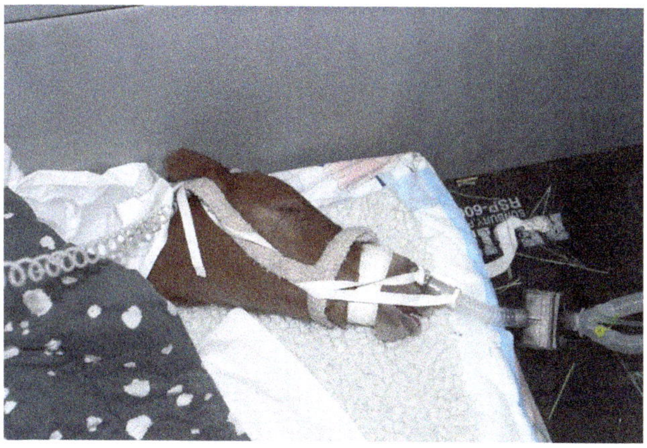

Figure 6.VI.3 Heat moisture exchange (HME) filter is placed between the endotracheal tube and ventilator tubing. The HME filter traps heat and moisture, leaving the foal on expiration and preconditions the gas taken in on the next inhalation.

efficient antimicrobial filter, excluding nosocomial bacteria and viruses from the patient and confining the patient's pathogens to the endotracheal tube and airway. Thus, with this type of HME filter, sterile ventilator circuit tubing is not needed. Without it, the circuit and active humidifier should be sterile and changed at least every 24 hours. The other practical problem with active humidification is the problem of "rainout" in the circuit as the moist warm gas passes through a cool circuit. This requires the addition of water traps in the circuit that require frequent emptying or the addition of heated circuit tubing. The rainout problem is exacerbated by cooler environmental temperatures often found in the equine neonatal intensive care unit (NICU) in the winter.

Preparing to Place a Foal on a Ventilator

The time between the decision to use mechanical ventilation as a therapeutic intervention and initiation of ventilation can be minimized by following a routine for ventilator setup. In clinics in which mechanical ventilation of patients is a rare event, having a ventilator setup checklist, dry runs with the staff practicing setup of the equipment, and sessions covering equipment troubleshooting procedures can minimize confusion and uncertainty during the chaos of implementing therapy in a critically ill foal. Typical equipment needed includes the ventilator, access to oxygen (with minimal interruption of the patient's oxygen insufflation), access to medical-grade compressed air or a compressed-air generator, interface lines, a gas blender (often built into the ventilator), a capnograph with lines and an adaptor, a humidifying device (e.g. HME filter), a ventilator circuit, endotracheal tubes, sterile gloves, sterile lubrication, a means of securing the endotracheal tube, a stethoscope, a self-inflating bag (e.g. Ambubag in case of an emergency), and, most importantly, adequate trained help to restrain the foal, intubate the foal, secure the endotracheal tube, and begin adjusting the ventilator settings as soon as the foal is intubated.

As part of ventilator setup, the circuit and other attachments should be inspected to ensure that everything is in proper working order, and the circuit checked for leaks. This can be done by attaching an artificial lung to the circuit, occluding the exhalation port, and charging the circuit with a manual breath or checking the ventilator's ability to maintain PEEP. It is convenient to select the initial ventilator setting after checking for leaks. It is also important to check the integrity of the endotracheal tube's cuff before intubation. Leaking endotracheal cuffs are a common problem during ventilation. Sterile endotracheal tubes should be used to minimize introduction of nosocomial bacteria during intubation. While checking the cuff, care should be taken to maintain sterility of the tube beyond the cuff inflation port. During setup, a choice about heating and humidifying the delivered gas should be made and implemented.

It is very important that the clinician and patient coordinate their efforts. That is, the ventilator mode and settings are selected in such a way that the foal does not fight ventilation. When the ventilator is set properly, so that the patient comfortably accepts the ventilation, there is no need to sedate the foal. In fact, sedation is contraindicated in ventilating foals and efforts should be made to stand the foal for short periods every two hours when the foal's recumbency is changed (Figure 6.VI.4).

Monitoring During Ventilation

The objective of monitoring during ventilation is to allow dynamic adjustment of mechanical ventilation parameters, to understand and correct underlying pathophysiology, to prevent damage from the act of mechanical ventilation, and to decide if it is time to discontinue mechanical ventilation. Monitoring can take many forms, which vary greatly in sophistication. The following are the most useful monitoring techniques which can be achieved by equipment that should be available in support of mechanical ventilation.

Arterial Blood Gas Measurements

Although noninvasive monitoring, such as pulse oximetry and capnography, can be useful, it is not a substitute for an ABG measurement in a critical neonate. If these noninvasive techniques are being used when an ABG sample is

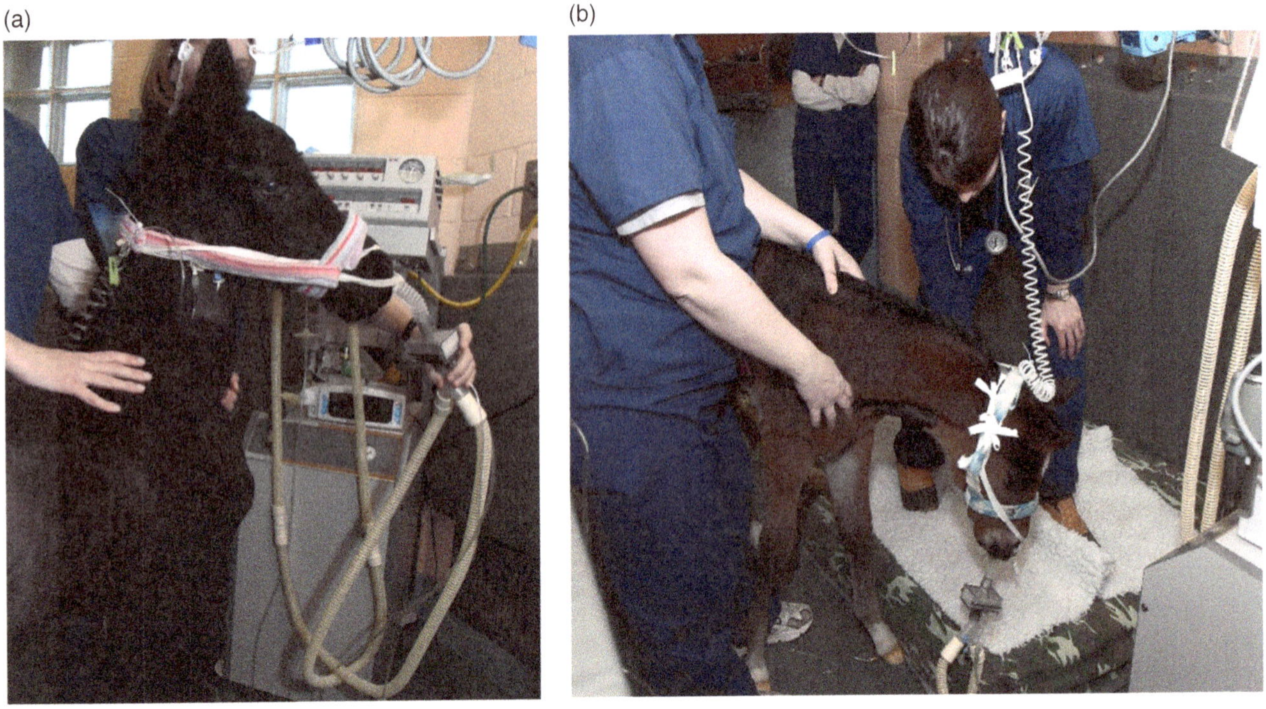

Figure 6.VI.4 When possible, foals should be stood every 2 hours for short periods when changing their recumbency from one side to the other.

drawn, comparison of the results recorded as the syringe is filling and understanding the underlying pathophysiology causing discrepancies between the two monitoring techniques can be useful in understanding the clinical condition of the patient. Whenever an ABG sample is drawn, not only should ventilator settings and other values be recorded to help with dynamic adjustments, but the capnograph reading should also be noted at the same time. An ABG sample should be drawn before initiating ventilation, within 30 minutes or less of beginning of ventilation, and again after 2–3 hours of ventilation. Timing of further ABG samples is dictated by initial results, clinical condition of the patient, and economic considerations. Stable patients without primary pulmonary disease or cardiovascular instability (e.g. botulism cases) may only require one ABG measurement a day. Others may require samples every few hours. The author's goal is to keep the P_aO_2 >60 mmHg and <80–100 mmHg with a S_aO_2 >90% (but <96%) and to keep the pH >7.320 but <7.400.

Capnography

Capnography can be a valuable monitoring technique and should be used continuously during ventilation. It can be useful for simple but vital matters, such as detecting loss of endotracheal cuff integrity, a common problem during ventilation. In this situation, the end-tidal CO_2 ($ETCO_2$) drops to close to 0, as if the foal is apneic, but the cycling of the ventilator suggests that apnea is not the problem. Most of the time, this scenario is caused by a deflated endotracheal cuff with leakage of exhaled gases around the endotracheal tube.

Capnography can also help to diagnose and monitor complex pathophysiologic conditions. In patients that have normal hemodynamics and pulmonary function, the $ETCO_2$ is 2–5 mmHg less than the P_aCO_2, having a strong enough correlation to safely be relied on as a surrogate for P_aCO_2 [23, 24]. In patients that have severe lung disease or hemodynamic instability, the $ETCO_2$ is not a good predictor of P_aCO_2 because the difference between the two measurements varies with changing V/Q relations in the lungs. In these cases, the emphasis should be on more ABG measurements until the V/Q mismatch improves (improved hemodynamics and pulmonary function) and a more consistent relation between $ETCO_2$ and P_aCO_2 is established. Establishment of a consistent relation implies an improvement in the V/Q status of the patient [23–25]. $ETCO_2$ is a function of P_aCO_2, cardiac output, alveolar dead space ventilation (pulmonary perfusion), airway time constants, CO_2 production (metabolic rate), and bicarbonate therapy. Capnography can be used to determine the adequacy of alveolar ventilation, the patency and placement of the endotracheal tube, the relation between alveolar ventilation and pulmonary perfusion, cardiac output, and pulmonary blood flow (especially useful during cardiopulmonary resuscitation), and proper functioning of the ventilator (especially if rebreathing of CO_2 is occurring) [26–30].

The P_aCO_2 is determined by the P_aCO_2 of all perfused alveoli (whether or not they are ventilated), and the $ETCO_2$ represents the PCO_2 of all ventilated alveoli (whether or not they are perfused). As a result, the gradient between P_aCO_2 and $ETCO_2$ reflects alveolar dead space ventilation. Alveolar dead space is the volume of alveoli that are ventilated but not perfused. It represents a failure of pulmonary perfusion and is the other end of the spectrum from shunting or venous admixture in the continuum of V/Q abnormalities. Because the gas leaving alveoli that are ventilated but not perfused does not contain CO_2, it has a diluting effect on the CO_2 leaving other areas of the lung, lowering the $ETCO_2$. The gradient between P_aCO_2 and $ETCO_2$ reflects the percent of alveolar dead space ventilation and can easily be calculated with the following formula: % alveolar dead space = $(P_aCO_2 - ETCO_2/P_aCO_2) \times 100$. The two most common reasons for increased alveolar dead space ventilation are decreased perfusion secondary to decreased cardiac output, and decreased perfusion secondary to increased pulmonary vascular resistance, such as occurs during ventilation with increased alveolar pressure (PEEP level/peak airway pressure/average airway pressure) causing alveolar capillary compression.

Although the P_aCO_2-$ETCO_2$ gradient usually reflects alveolar dead space ventilation, there are also other factors that can affect $ETCO_2$ levels. The $ETCO_2$ is a measure of CO_2 in the last alveoli to empty. If the lungs have uniform conditions throughout most areas, this reflects the average alveoli. However, there are often areas of the lungs with different time constants (reflecting how quickly gas enters and leaves these alveoli). When there are areas of the lungs with long time constants, these alveoli receive less ventilation. The PCO_2 in these alveoli is higher, and gas from these alveoli is the last to leave the lungs and heavily influences the PCO_2 in the end-tidal gas, thus resulting in an $ETCO_2$ that is higher than that of the average alveoli. In fact, in some cases, the $ETCO_2$ may be higher than the P_aCO_2. Thus, the P_aCO_2-$ETCO_2$ gradient underestimates the alveolar dead space ventilation. Inspection of the capnogram readily reveals this situation. This is one of several reasons why, in addition to $ETCO_2$ monitoring, it is important to use capnography, which is the continuous measurement of exhaled CO_2 represented as a graph.

Capnography consists of continuous real-time recording of CO_2 as measured from a sample taken at the ventilator end of the endotracheal tube relative to time or to volume of exhaled gases (Figure 6.VI.5). A volume capnogram is a graph of exhaled CO_2 relative to the volume of gas exhaled. There has been renewed interest in this mode of capnography with the advent of noninvasive cardiac output measurements using CO_2 excretion. Whether or not this technique, which seems to be valuable in patients that have normal physiology, lives up to its promise when applied to critically ill patients remains to be proven. Preliminary animal model data is promising [31]. The clinically more common time capnogram graphs measure exhaled CO_2 relative to time throughout the respiratory cycle. In a time capnogram of a normal individual at the initiation of exhalation the CO_2 is 0 because the first gas to leave the airway exits from anatomic dead space (phase I). As anatomic dead space gas begins to mix with alveolar gas there is a sudden upstroke of the curve (phase II), which is almost at a right angle to the baseline. The upstroke rapidly reaches a plateau (phase III). The end of the plateau marks the end of exhalation, which is the $ETCO_2$. The initial part of inhalation is marked by the downstroke, which rapidly returns to baseline followed by a period with a CO_2 of 0 (phase 0) [32].

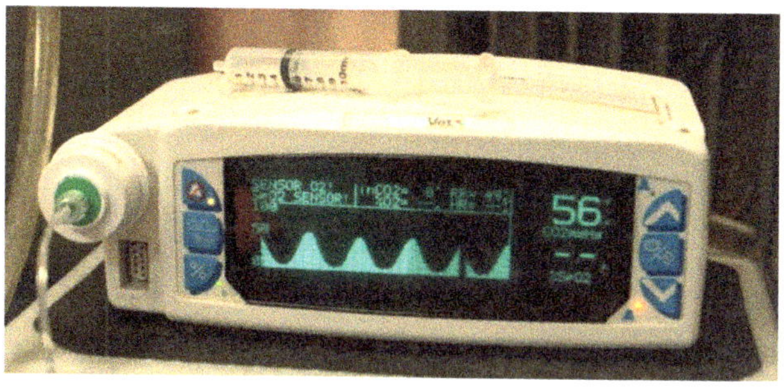

Figure 6.VI.5 Continuous capnography is a valuable ancillary monitoring modality and should be used on all ventilated cases, if possible.

Careful observation of the curve for variations from normal can help characterize abnormalities. An elevated baseline and upstroke (phase II) indicate CO_2 rebreathing if they develop gradually. A sudden increase suggests contamination of the sample cell with water, mucus, or dirt. A prolonged or sloped upstroke that does not meet a clear plateau suggests an obstruction to expiratory gas flow (e.g. bronchospasm, obstructive pulmonary disease, kinked endotracheal tube) or leaks in the breathing circuit [32]. Even in normal patients, the plateau, which is alveolar gas, usually has a slight positive slope, indicating a slight rise in CO_2 during expiration. There are two reasons for this increase. First, because CO_2 is being continuously excreted into alveoli, which are becoming progressively smaller as expiration continues, the last gas emptied from the alveoli has a higher concentration of CO_2. Second, even in normal lungs, there is a wide range of V/Q ratios in different areas of the lungs. Some alveoli have a higher V/Q ratio because they are more readily ventilated (have shorter time constants) and thus have a relatively lower PCO_2. Others have a lower V/Q ratio because of underventilation (longer time constants), resulting in a relatively higher PCO_2. The delayed emptying of these alveoli with a low V/Q (high PCO_2) contributes to the rising slope of the plateau. Factors such as changes in cardiac output, CO_2 production, airway resistance, and FRC may further affect the V/Q status of various areas in the lung, and thus influence the height or slope of the plateau. The presence of a steep slope of this plateau indicates abnormalities in V/Q mismatch of the lung [24]. The V/Q difference can be great enough that the $ETCO_2$ may be higher than the P_aCO_2, which reflects the average perfused alveolar CO_2. When there is a significant slope to the plateau phase, the P_aCO_2-$ETCO_2$ gradient underestimates the amount of alveolar dead space ventilation [33, 34].

Fraction of Inspired Oxygen

It is important to check the accuracy of the F_IO_2 setting on the ventilator periodically by measuring the F_IO_2 at the endotracheal tube. At times, the gas blender of the ventilator may be inaccurate. Most modern ventilators have built-in oxygen sensors and will alarm when there is a discrepancy. Inexpensive handheld oxygen sensors are readily available and convenient for periodic monitoring of the F_IO_2.

Tidal Volume and Minute Volume

It is important to monitor actual tidal volume and minute volume rather than relying on the intended volumes so that leaks or ventilator malfunction will be detected. Also, in ventilator modes like PSV, where the patient sets the tidal volume, which can change at any time, tidal volume monitoring is important. Most modern ventilators have built-in flowmeters, but external flowmeters are available for those that do not. One downfall of common turbine-based flowmeters (where gas moving past the sensor spins a turbine and the volume is measured by counting the revolutions) is that at high respiratory rates, where the expiratory pause is too short to allow the turbine to stop spinning, tidal volume measurements cannot be obtained.

Airway Pressure

Most modern ventilators measure airway pressure, volumes, and flows throughout the respiratory cycle and display both the values and pressure-volume (compliance) loops and flow-volume (resistance) loops. These graphs can be quite useful in adjusting and monitoring ventilator function. If these displays are not available, the most important airway pressures are peak inspiratory pressure (PIP), plateau pressure (PPL), and PEEP or baseline pressure. The PIP is the highest pressure, usually occurring at the end of inspiration, just before the inspiratory pause. The PPL is the pressure after the end of the inspiratory pause when the gases have arrived at equilibrium. If there is no inspiratory pause and if the ventilator does not measure the PPL, the clinician can briefly occlude the expiratory port after full inspiration; the PPL will be the value once the pressure stabilizes. The PEEP or baseline pressure can be measured between respiratory cycles, again, when no air is moving if it is not automatically displayed.

The PIP is the most frequently measured variable of ventilatory function during mechanical ventilation. It depends on lung compliance, airway resistance, and synchrony with the patient. Changes in the magnitude of PIP may reflect any of several potentially detrimental problems related to ventilation. In a practical sense, PIP should be considered an additional vital sign for patients on a ventilator. A sudden decrease in PIP suggests a major leak in the circuit but also can be caused by insufficient gas supply to the ventilator, inadvertent change in settings, unintended extubation, or failure or disconnection of the ventilator. Increases in PIP may indicate endotracheal tube occlusion by secretions or kinking, acute bronchospasm, pneumothorax, lack of patient ventilator synchrony, or conditions causing decreased lung compliance. High PIP may cause barotrauma and acute lung injury. PIP is usually monitored by alarms set at 10 cm H_2O above and below the average PIP of the patient that indicate high values or failure to reach a minimum PIP, both of which require attention. The baseline pressure should be 0 or higher if there is a PEEP, except during patient inspiratory efforts. Failure to maintain PEEP usually suggests a circuit leak.

Compliance and Resistance

With measurement of tidal volume, PIP, PPL, and PEEP, effective compliance and airway resistance can be calculated. Effective compliance is the compliance of the lungs and chest wall combined. Because chest wall compliance rarely changes acutely and effective compliance does not require pleural pressure measurements, effective compliance is a readily attainable and clinically convenient parameter. Static effective compliance can be calculated by dividing the tidal volume by the difference between the PPL and PEEP. It decreases if there is an abnormality of the chest wall (e.g. flail chest) or a decrease in functional alveolar numbers as with pulmonary edema, pneumonia, or atelectasis as well as for other similar reasons. It may also be used to determine the best PEEP and best tidal volume if serial measurements are obtained at trial settings and a response grid is recorded. Dynamic effective compliance can be calculated by dividing the tidal volume by the difference between the PIP and PEEP. Dynamic compliance adds the effects of resistance to static compliance. Dynamic compliance decreases with disorders of the airway, lung parenchyma, and chest wall. Dynamic compliance is less than static compliance when there is increased resistance, such as with secretions in the airways or endotracheal tube, bronchospasm, or endotracheal tube kinking. Changes in airway resistance are most easily detected by monitoring the difference between PIP and PPL. As the difference increases, so does airway resistance. PIP and PPL pressures cannot always be accurately measured with spontaneously initiated breaths, especially in PSV. In the pressure support mode, the airway pressure may be variably decreased by the magnitude of the patient's inspiratory effort. As the patient's effort increases and because the ventilator cycles are based on flow rates and not volume or pressure, the PIP may never reach a value close to that if the patient had the breath delivered by a volume or pressure machine breath. In fact, what is traditionally the measure of PIP (at the end of inspiration) may actually be less than the PPL. Therefore, these measurements should only be made during a ventilator-delivered breath that is not pressure supported.

Endotracheal Tube

Initially, the endotracheal tube should be changed daily or more often in the face of increased airway resistance. Each time the tube is changed, the amount and quality of the discharge in the tube should be monitored. If the discharge is extremely viscous and difficult to clean from the tube, it suggests inadequate preconditioning of ventilator gases (usually too little humidity), which should be corrected. An increased quantity of clear discharge is also an indication of failure of preconditioning of gases. If the discharge becomes dark or sanguineous (in the absence of traumatic intubation), infection should be suspected. In either case, periodic culturing of the lumen of the endotracheal tube when removed is useful. Generally, several species (2–6) of microbes can be recovered, even in the absence of significant disease. These isolates should not be viewed as invaders requiring antimicrobial treatment, but as colonizers that represent the nosocomial population from which the next invader may originate, whether the route is via the respiratory tract, gastrointestinal tract, urinary tract, or IV access. If a secondary infection becomes evident, these culture results give weight to an educated guess of how to modify antimicrobial therapy before definitive culture and sensitivity results are available. Targeting these colonizers with antimicrobials before they invade likely selects for more resistant nosocomial microbes. Recall that cuffed endotracheal tubes provide a degree of protection from aspiration, but this degree of protection is not complete. Studies in human medicine have found gastric contents in the bronchial secretions of approximately 25% of intubated patients [5, 35, 36].

Discontinuing Mechanical Ventilation ("Weaning")

As soon as the foal is started on mechanical ventilation, the clinician should begin to ask if the foal is ready to be weaned. This question should be asked repeatedly until the answer is yes. Because of the threat of secondary nosocomial infections associated with ventilation, it is important to keep the ventilation period as short as possible. Some foals with neonatal encephalopathy can be weaned <24 hours after being placed on a ventilator. Some foals with botulism require 10–14 days of ventilation, and some foals with significant respiratory injury may require a month or more of ventilatory support.

Before attempting to discontinue mechanical ventilation, patients should show cardiovascular and metabolic stability and sepsis, if present, should be controlled. Also, there should be evidence that the original underlying problem which led to the need for mechanical ventilation has resolved or at least improved. No predictor is reliably able to establish when a foal is ready for weaning. Weaning protocols have evolved in human medicine based on clinical evidence [37–39]. There are two methods that the author commonly uses. The preferred method is a spontaneous breathing trial. This involves extubation without further respiratory support except for intranasal oxygen insufflation but with constant observation over a period of 2 hours or more. This trial should not be attempted without extubation, because asking a foal that is just ready to wean to breathe with the extra resistance posed by the endotracheal tube is a formula for weaning failure. As the foal's endotracheal tube is changed daily, there exists the opportunity to assess the foal's readiness to wean during the procedure. This combined with return of general strength and resolution of the reason for mechanical ventilation form the screening procedure for a spontaneous breathing trial. Most foals that have been ventilated <10 days will pass this trial as long as the screening is positive. When the foal fails the spontaneous breathing trial or if the foal has been ventilated for a prolonged period, then a second method used involves having the foal breathe on PSV with a gradual decrease in the level of support, as tolerated. When breathing with minimal to no support, the foal is extubated. As a rule, the author does not sedate ventilated foals, thus avoiding the difficult problem faced by physicians of weaning sedation in conjunction to the ventilator weaning trial. A method previously used in people, but now not recommended based on evidence, is a gradual decrease in the IMV ventilator rate with constant minimal pressure support until the patient is not receiving any mechanical breaths and instead is maintaining minute ventilation requirements spontaneously. The author used this method when first starting ventilation of foals, but also found it anecdotally unsatisfactory. Failure of a weaning trial can be defined by the development of tachypnea, hypoxemia, tachycardia, sustained bradycardia, hypertension, hypotension, or agitation [5].

Summary

Critically ill foals often have respiratory failure and benefit from respiratory support. Some only require intranasal oxygen insufflation, whereas others need full respiratory support with mechanical ventilation. Modern mechanical ventilators developed for human medicine are easily adapted to foals and make mechanical ventilation of foals not only possible but frequently successful. Conventional mechanical ventilation using IMV or PSV (VSV) along with PEEP/CPAP is useful in many foals. Initial ventilator settings are based on the underlying cause of respiratory failure and the usual response of similar cases but must be dynamically adjusted from the outset as dictated by the response of the individual. This dynamic process is aided by constant monitoring of parameters, such as pH, P_aO_2, P_aCO_2, $ETCO_2$, tidal and minute volume, airway pressures, compliance, and resistance. As soon as the foal is started on mechanical ventilation, the clinician should ask if the foal is ready to be weaned. Early weaning is as important as timely initiation of ventilation. Monitoring also aids in deciding when it is appropriate to wean the foal.

References

1 Palmer, J.E. (1994). Ventilatory support of the neonatal foal. *Vet. Clin. North Am. Equine Pract.* 10: 167–185.

2 Palmer, J.E. (2003). Respiratory support of critical equine neonates. In: *American College of Veterinary Internal Medicine Forum Proceedings* (ed. B. Madewell). American College of Veterinary Internal Medicine 2003.

3 Wilkins, P.A. and Palmer, J.E. (2003). Mechanical ventilation in foals with botulism: 9 cases (1989–2002). *J. Vet. Intern. Med.* 17: 708–712.

4 Axon, J.E., Palmer, J.E., and Wilkins, P.A. (1999). Short- and long-term outcome of NICU survivors. *Proc. Am. Assoc. Equine Pract.* 45: 224.

5 Gali, B. and Goyal, D.G. (2003). Positive pressure mechanical ventilation. *Emerg. Med. Clin. North Am.* 21: 453–473.

6 Slutsky, A.S. (1993). Mechanical ventilation. American College of Chest Physicians' Consensus Conference. *Chest* 104: 1833–1859.

7 Esteban, A., Anzueto, A., Frutos, F. et al. (2002). Characteristics and outcomes in adult patients receiving mechanical ventilation: a 28-day international study. *JAMA* 287: 345–355.

8 Fenstermacher, D. and Hong, D. (2004). Mechanical ventilation: what have we learned? *Crit. Care Nurs. Q.* 27: 258–294.

9 Tobin, M.J. (2001). Advances in mechanical ventilation. *N. Engl. J. Med.* 344: 1986–1996.

10 MacIntyre, N.R. (1986). Respiratory function during pressure support ventilation. *Chest* 89: 677–683.

11 MacIntyre, N. (2003). Recent innovations in mechanical ventilatory support. In: *Intensive Care Medicine Annual Update 2003* (ed. J.L. Vincent), 264–271. Springer.

12 Marini, J.J., Crooke, P.S. 3rd, and Truwit, J.D. (1985). Determinants and limits of pressure-preset ventilation: a mathematical model of pressure control. *J. Appl. Phys.* 1989 (67): 1081–1092.

13 Muscedere, J.G., Mullen, J.B., Gan, K. et al. (1994). Tidal ventilation at low airway pressures can augment lung injury. *Am. J. Respir. Crit. Care Med.* 149: 1327–1334.

14 Wyszogrodski, I., Kyei-Aboagye, K., Taeusch, H.W. et al. (1975). Surfactant inactivation by hyperventilation: conservation by end-expiratory pressure. *J. Appl. Phys.* 38: 461–466.

15 The ARDS Network (2000). Ventilation with lower tidal volumes as compared with traditional tidal volumes for acute lung injury and the acute respiratory distress syndrome. *N. Engl. J. Med.* 342: 1301–1308.

16 Ricard, J.D. (2003). Are we really reducing tidal volume–and should we? *Am. J. Respir. Crit. Care Med.* 167: 1297–1298.

17 Weinert, C.R., Gross, C.R., and Marinelli, W.A. (2003). Impact of randomized trial results on acute lung injury ventilator therapy in teaching hospitals. *Am. J. Respir. Crit. Care Med.* 167: 1304–1309.

18 Putensen, C., Theuerkauf, N., Zinserling, J. et al. (2009). Meta-analysis: ventilation strategies and outcomes of the acute respiratory distress syndrome and acute lung injury. *Ann. Intern. Med.* 151: 566–576.

19 Gajic, O., Dara, S.I., Mendez, J.L. et al. (2004). Ventilator-associated lung injury in patients without acute lung injury at the onset of mechanical ventilation. *Crit. Care Med.* 32: 1817–1824.

20 Neto, S., Nagtzaam, L., and Schultz, M. (2014). Ventilation with lower tidal volumes for critically ill patients without

the acute respiratory distress syndrome. *Curr Opin Crit Care* 20: 25–32. http://www.co-criticalcare.com.

21 Kilickaya, O. and Gajic, O. (2013). Initial ventilator settings for critically ill patients. *Crit. Care* 17: 123–126.

22 Bernstein, D.B., Nguyen, B., Allen, G.B. et al. (2013). Elucidating the fuzziness in physician decision making in ARDS. *J. Clin. Monit. Comput.* 27: 357–363.

23 Shankar, K.B., Moseley, H., Kumar, Y. et al. (1986). Arterial to end tidal carbon dioxide tension difference during caesarean section anaesthesia. *Anaesthesia* 41: 698–702.

24 Fletcher, R., Jonson, B., Cumming, G. et al. (1981). The concept of deadspace with special reference to the single breath test for carbon dioxide. *Br. J. Anaesth.* 53: 77–88.

25 Phan, C.Q., Tremper, K.K., Lee, S.E., and Barker, S.J. (1987). Noninvasive monitoring of carbon dioxide: a comparison of the partial pressure of transcutaneous and end-tidal carbon dioxide with the partial pressure of arterial carbon dioxide. *J. Clin. Monit.* 3: 149–154.

26 Maslow, A., Stearns, G., Bert, A. et al. (2001). Monitoring end-tidal carbon dioxide during weaning from cardiopulmonary bypass in patients without significant lung disease. *Anesth. Analg.* 92: 306–313.

27 Weil, M.H., Bisera, J., Trevino, R.P., and Rackow, E.C. (1985). Cardiac output and end-tidal carbon dioxide. *Care Med* 13: 907–909.

28 Ornato, J.P., Garnett, A.R., and Glauser, F.L. (1990). Relationship between cardiac output and the end-tidal carbon dioxide tension. *Ann. Emerg. Med.* 19: 1104–1106.

29 Jin, X., Weil, M.H., Tang, W. et al. (2000). End-tidal carbon dioxide as a noninvasive indicator of cardiac index during circulatory shock. *Crit. Care Med.* 28: 2415–2419.

30 Isserles, S.A. and Breen, P.H. (1991). Can changes in end-tidal PCO_2 measure changes in cardiac output? *Anesth. Analg.* 73: 808–814.

31 Peyton, P.J., Venkatesan, Y., Hood, S.G. et al. (2006). Noninvasive, automated and continuous cardiac output monitoring by pulmonary capnodynamics: breath-by-breath comparison with ultrasonic flow probe. *Anesthesiology* 105: 72–80.

32 Bhavani-Shankar, K., Moseley, H., Kumar, A.Y. et al. (1992). Capnometry and anaesthesia. *Can. J. Anaesth.* 39: 617–632.

33 Nunn, J.F. and Hill, D.W. (1960). Respiratory dead space and arterial to end-tidal carbon dioxide tension difference in anesthetized man. *J. Appl. Phys.* 15: 383–389.

34 Shankar, K.B., Moseley, H., and Kumar, Y. (1991). Negative arterial to end-tidal gradients. *Can. J. Anaesth.* 38: 260–261.

35 Young, P.J., Basson, C., Hamilton, D. et al. (1999). Prevention of tracheal aspiration using the pressure-limited tracheal tube cuff. *Anaesthesia* 54: 559–563.

36 Orozco-Levi, M., Torres, A., Ferrer, M. et al. (1995). Semirecumbent position protects from pulmonary aspiration but not completely from gastroesophageal reflux in mechanically ventilated patients. *Am. J. Respir. Crit. Care Med.* 152 (4 Pt 1): 1387–1390.

37 Bernard, G.R., Artigas, A., Brigham, K.L. et al. (1994). Report of the American-European consensus conference on ARDS: definitions, mechanisms, relevant outcomes and clinical trial coordination. The Consensus Committee. *Intensive Care Med.* 20: 225–232.

38 Girard, T.D. and Ely, E.W. (2008). Protocol-driven ventilator weaning: reviewing the evidence. *Clin. Chest Med.* 29: 241–252.

39 Hooper, M.H. and Girard, T.D. (2009). Sedation and weaning from mechanical ventilation: linking spontaneous awakening trials and spontaneous breathing trials to improve patient outcomes. *Crit. Care Clin.* 25: 515–525.

Chapter 7 Congenital Disorders of the Respiratory System

Andrea Oliver and Rose Nolen-Walston

Introduction

Congenital anomalies of the equine respiratory tract are not common, but the clinician is exposed to these respiratory defects from time to time. The true prevalence of these anomalies is unknown as many of them are not routinely reported. Clinically, congenital defects of the respiratory tract can present with abnormal respiratory noise and difficulty breathing (with some conditions being life-threatening), although other anomalies can be incidental findings. While these respiratory abnormalities are infrequently encountered, awareness of these conditions is important and should be considered when examining neonatal foals.

Condition	Affected breed/ prevalence	Description
Wry nose	Prevalence unknown, but draft breeds and foals of primiparous mares appear to be more commonly affected [1]	Wry nose is a deformity of the incisive, maxillary, nasal, and vomer bones that results in deviation of the nose and upper incisors. Diagnosis is confirmed by physical examination and radiography. Affected foals generally have stridor or stertor due to obstruction of the nasal passages by the deformity. However, most are still able to eat and drink normally [1–3]. Both conservative and surgical treatments have been considered. Deformities <20° can resolve spontaneously; more significant deformities (>20°) require surgical management (Figure 7.1) as described in various case series [1–3].
Nasal atheroma (epidermoid cyst)	Epidermal inclusion cysts are reported to account for 2.5% of referred equine sinonasal disease; however, the true incidence is likely higher due to reduced need to refer these cases [4]. Etiology and heritability are unknown.	Epidermal inclusion cysts, also known as atheroma or atheromata, are soft, fluctuant encapsulated masses that are generally located on the caudal aspect of the false nostril. Most epidermal inclusion cysts are unilateral and 3–5 cm in diameter. Often, they are identified in foals but can also occur in adult horses (Figure 7.2). Rarely, nasal atheromas may partially occlude the airway causing upper respiratory noise. Clinical signs are limited to the presence of a mass on the caudal false nostril. Clinical diagnosis is made based on location and consistency of the mass and can be confirmed by histopathologic evaluation that demonstrates a well differentiated stratified squamous epithelium, thick layer of surface keratin, a variably heavily pigmented basal layer and overlying unremarkable lamina propria. The lumen is filled with keratin flakes and acellular debris. In rare cases, occlusion of the airway may require surgical removal of the mass; however, most masses are moved for cosmesis. The entire cyst lining must be removed to prevent recurrence. A single injection of formalin into the cyst and subsequent removal has been reported [5] which avoids surgical complications related to resection en bloc.

Equine Neonatal Medicine, First Edition. Edited by David M. Wong and Pamela A. Wilkins.

Condition	Affected breed/ prevalence	Description

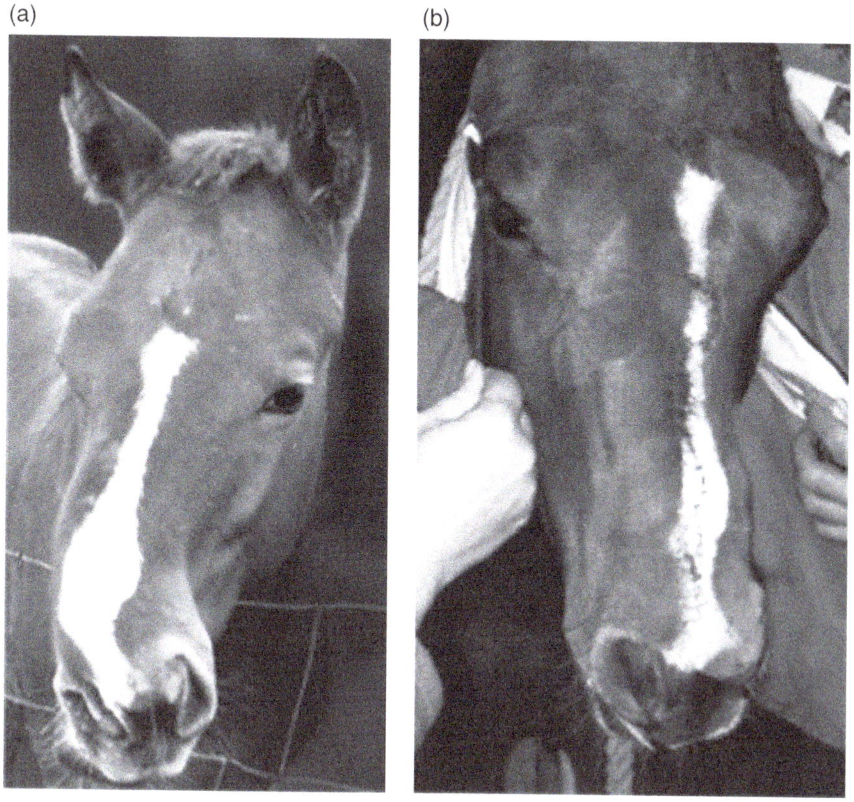

Figure 7.1 A horse with congenital wry nose before (a) and after (b) surgical correction [3].

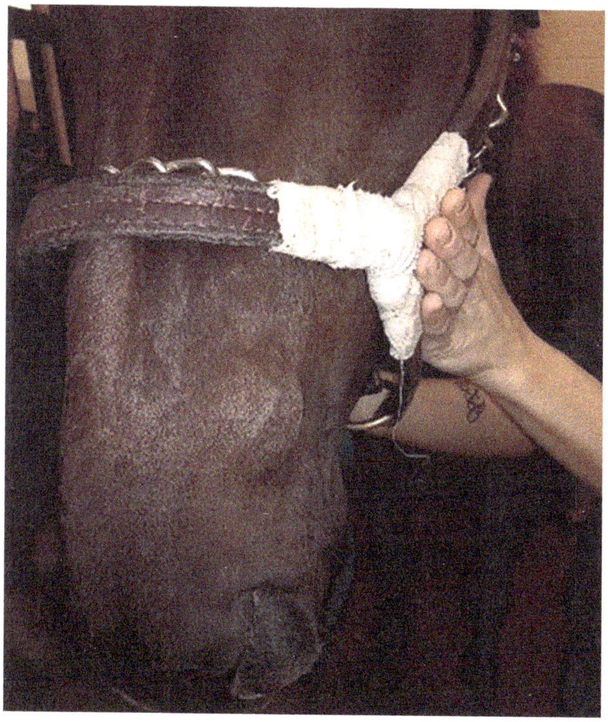

Figure 7.2 Nasal atheroma or epidermal inclusion cyst. *Source:* Image courtesy of Dr. Eric Parente, University of Pennsylvania.

(*Continued*)

Condition	Affected breed/ prevalence	Description
Choanal atresia	Incidence is generally considered to be uncommon in horses; however, may be understated due to the rapidly lethal nature of the disease in cases of bilateral, complete atresia after birth. Heritability in horses is undetermined. In alpacas, candidate genes for inheritance related to suggested human patterns of inheritance have been investigated, though evidence for heritability is incomplete [6]. Breeding of individuals with choanal atresia should be undertaken cautiously.	Choanal atresia develops as the result of an imperforate buccopharyngeal membrane, which causes a partial or complete obstruction of the intersection between the nasal cavity and nasopharynx and can be unilateral or bilateral. Proposed causes include failure of rupture of the buccomucosal membrane, partial or complete persistence of the buccomucosal membrane and/or medial outgrowth of the vertical and horizontal process of the palatine bone. In horses, the obstruction may be osseous, membranous, or osseo-membranous and covered in respiratory epithelium. Ethmoid turbinates are often distorted on the occluded side, and the nasal septum may be deviated toward the occluded side. Foals, particularly with bilateral obstruction, present with respiratory difficulty or distress within hours of birth and reduced airflow is often noted from one or both nostrils. Foals may be cyanotic, depending on the severity of obstruction. Alternatively, unilateral or incomplete obstruction may go unnoticed until adulthood when athletic performance is undertaken, and upper respiratory difficulty or noise is noted. Upper airway endoscopy of the caudal nasal passages may help visualize the obstruction. Contrast radiography can be used to definitively diagnose partial versus complete obstruction of the airway. Partial bilateral obstruction can be difficult to diagnose even with contrast radiography due to the lack of a comparable normal side and paucity of research defining normal choanal measurements. Clinical impression of narrowing in these cases must be compared to normal age matched horses to enable accurate diagnosis. Initial tracheotomy can stabilize foals in respiratory distress while additional diagnostics are undertaken to confirm choanal atresia. Treatment of choanal atresia (both unilateral and bilateral) has been attempted in foals (Figure 7.3), but scar tissue formation has necessitated aggressive and repeated follow-up with additional laser ablation, intranasal laparoscopic resection, and stent placement [7, 8].

(a) (b)

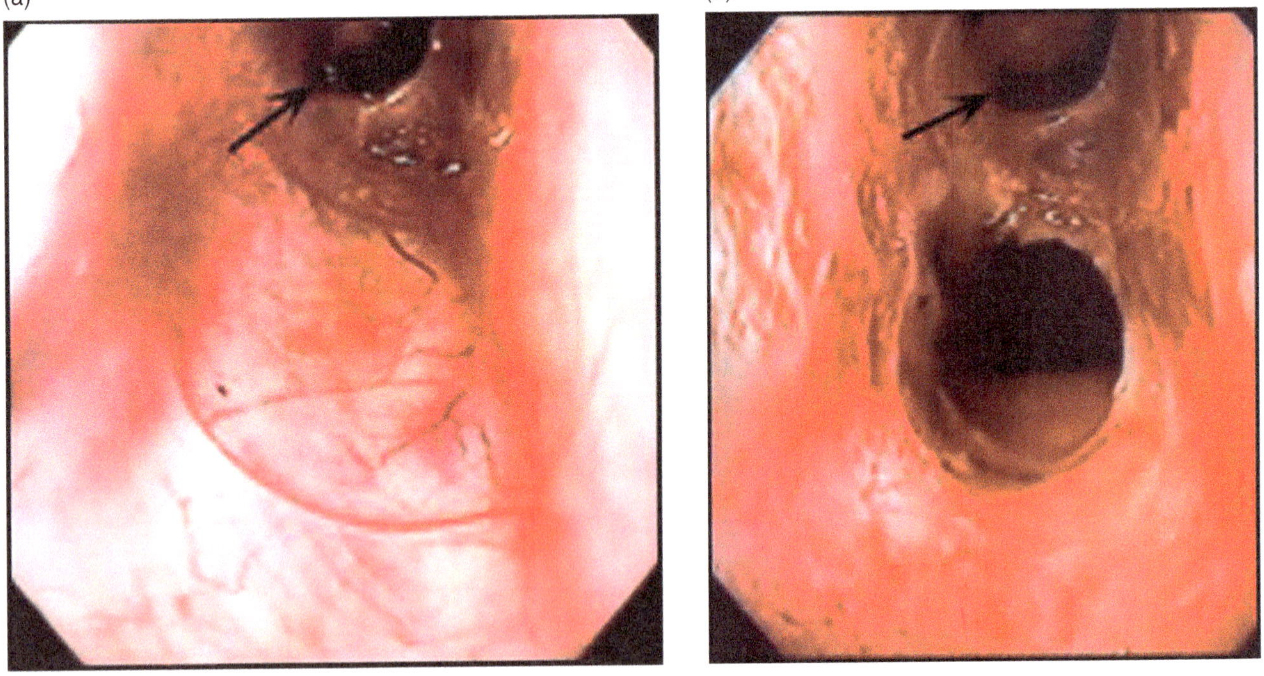

Figure 7.3 Right choana in a foal with bilateral choanal atresia (a) before and (b) after surgery. Arrows indicate the edge of ethmoid recess [7].

Condition	Affected breed/ prevalence	Description
Sinus cyst	In one report of 277 horses, sinus cysts accounted for 13.4% of disease in horses referred for sinonasal disease [4]. Reportedly, it is the third most common equine chronic sinonasal disease. All ages of horses may be affected and there is no breed predilection [9].	Sinus cysts occur in horses at any age, however it is possible that they originate from a congenital error of development and expand as the animal ages. There are several reports of presumed congenital occurrences, one in a 17-day-old foal [10] and one in a 1-year-old Miniature Horse [11]. The true etiology of sinus cysts is undetermined; one proposed theory is that they are linked to the development of progressive ethmoidal hematomas owing to histopathologic similarities and the occasional occurrence of horses affected with both sinus cysts and progressive ethmoidal hematomas. Alternatively, it has been suggested due to common alveolar bone and tooth root involvement that some sinus cysts may have a dental origin. Due to their progressively expansile nature, clinical signs include facial swelling, nasal airway obstruction, abnormal respiratory noise, mucopurulent nasal discharge, epistaxis, ocular discharge and exophthalmos (Figure 7.4). Concomitant local tissue and nerve damage have also led to reports of associated unilateral blindness and headshaking. Paranasal sinus cysts are reported to be the second most common cause of sinusitis in horses. Diagnosis is made via endoscopic visualization of the cyst either in the nasal cavity or caudal to the nasal septum as viewed from the contra-lateral side. A narrowed nasal meatus may be identified. Radiographically, a discrete mass, a diffuse increase in radio-opacity in the sinonasal region, fluid lines, nasal septal deviation, expansion of the ventral conchal sinus and distortion of the dental apices may be identified [12]. More detailed visualization may be possible by way of sinus endoscopy via portals created in the frontomaxillary region of the head. Advanced imaging using CT and MRI provide excellent visualization of cyst capsules [13]. MRI provides the additional benefit of delineation of cystic contents and secondary sinusitis fluid. Fluid obtained from sinus cysts is generally a vivid yellow, translucent, seromucinous substance and is considered pathognomonic for the condition. Surgical removal of the cyst is curative in 80% of cases. Approach is through a standing frontonasal flap, however the cyst may also be drained and removed via sinoscopy portals [11]. In most cases, small portions of the cyst wall adherent to other regional structures are left behind which may account for the reported 19% recurrence rate after removal. In about 50% of cases, cosmetic appearance postoperatively is considered good.

(a) (b)

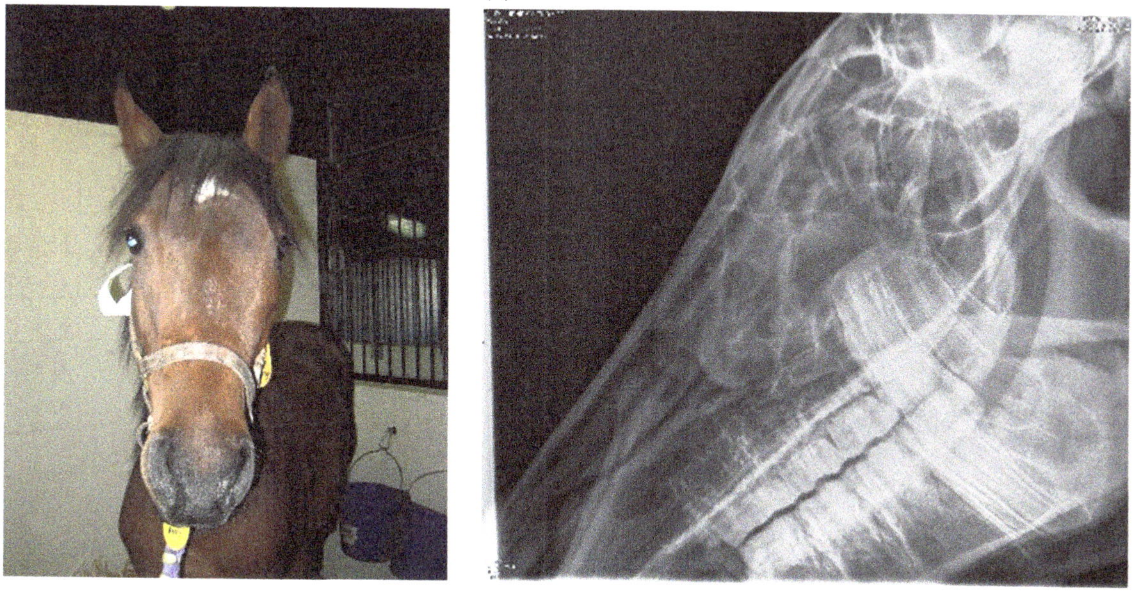

Figure 7.4 (a) Sinus cyst present in the left maxillary sinuses causing outward deviation of the overlying boney structures; (b) Radiographic lateral projection of a sinus cyst located in the maxillary sinuses. *Source:* Images courtesy of Dr. Eric Parente, University of Pennsylvania.

(Continued)

Condition	Affected breed/ prevalence	Description
Guttural pouch tympany	Fillies are two to four times more commonly affected than colts [14, 15]. English Thoroughbreds, Arabian horses, Paint horses, and German Warmbloods (Hanoverians in particular) are overrepresented. For Arabian horses, the incidence has been estimated to be as high as 1 in 555 births [14–17].	This condition is a nonpainful inflation (Figure 7.5) of one or both guttural pouches within the first several weeks of life. Etiology is unknown; however, the disease may arise as a result of either an abnormally large or abnormally functioning mucosal fold that causes development of a one-way valve into the guttural pouch, through which air cannot return into the nasopharynx [18]. Alternatively, paralysis of associated pharyngeal muscles responsible for lifting the mucosal fold and opening the pharyngeal ostium has been suggested. Dyspnea, dysphagia, and respiratory noise may occur as a result of structural displacement caused by the tympanic pouches. One study in German Warmblood foals estimated heritability of guttural pouch tympany at 0.81 ± 0.16 [16, 17]. In Arabian foals, the heritability has been estimated to be 0.49 ± 0.28 [14, 15]. Breed specific quantitative trait loci have been identified in both Arabian and German Warmblood horses [19]. These regions may contain genes that code proteins affecting the development of the mucosal fold at the pharyngeal ostium. In Arabian horses, a polygenic or mixed monogenic-polygenic model has been proposed to be responsible for the trait [15, 16]. Clinical signs of guttural pouch tympany include nonpainful external protrusion of the guttural pouch against the parotid and laryngeal region of the neck, dyspnea, dysphagia, and stridor. Foals may develop aspiration pneumonia secondary to dysphagia [20]. Empyema can occur as a result of mucosal inflammation caused by retained air in the guttural pouches and subsequent swelling. Diagnosis is based upon clinical signs and endoscopic evaluation of the guttural pouches. Treatment is generally undertaken via surgical laser fenestration of the affected guttural pouch into the nasopharynx with or without resection of the mucosal flap [21, 22]. Recurrence after this procedure is approximately 30% [14, 15]. There is one report of development of pharyngeal neuro-muscular dysfunction after this procedure [20]. Success has also been reported in several cases via placement of an indwelling foley catheter through the pharyngeal ostium and into the nasopharynx using endoscopic guidance. The catheter is left in place for 3 weeks. No recurrence of guttural pouch tympany after this procedure was reported [23]. Guttural pouches may have a complete, partial or absent median septum. Attempts should be made to determine this before deciding to treat one or both pouches.

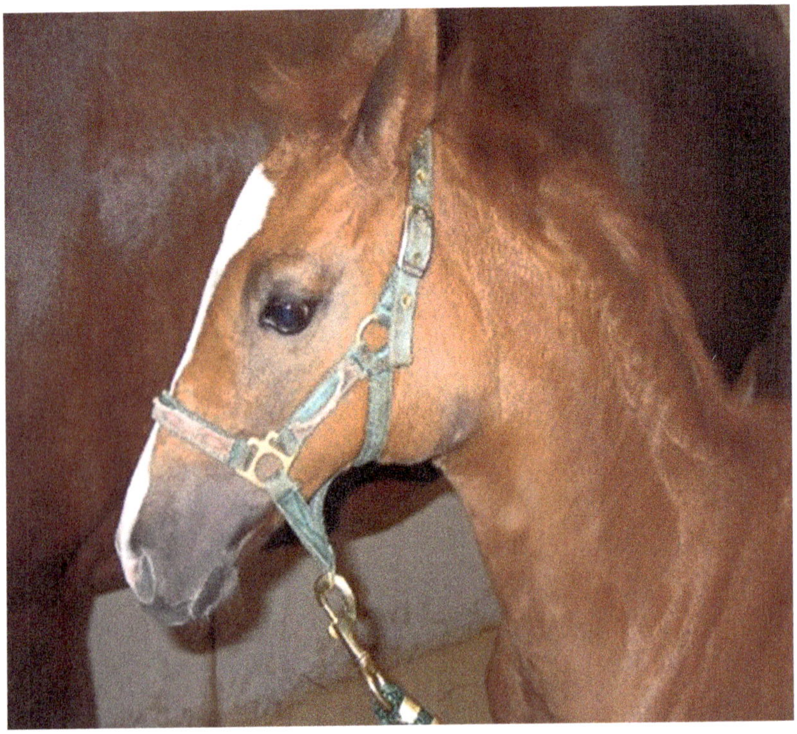

Figure 7.5 Foal with left sided guttural pouch tympany prior to surgical correction. *Source:* Image courtesy of Dr. Eric Parente, University of Pennsylvania.

Condition	Affected breed/ prevalence	Description
Branchial cysts	The branchial arches are embryological structures which derive portions of the head and neck during development. Cysts derived anywhere along these regions are known as branchial arch cysts or cervical lymphoepithelial cysts. Though the true etiology of these cysts is disputed, in general they are presumed to be congenital errors of development during differentiation of the branchial arches. Few case reports seem to indicate that right sided cysts are more common than left and that they are more commonly identified in adults than in neonates or young horses. Heritability has not been established.	Branchial arch cysts generally present as retropharyngeal, non-painful swellings located in the cranial ⅓ of the neck (Figure 7.6). Age at presentation is varied. Though the condition is presumed to be congenital, age distribution at presentation is widely varied [24]. Presenting signs include a visible mass, respiratory stridor, or respiratory distress in foals, whereas in adults, the presenting sign is typically recurrent esophageal obstruction, a visible mass, or respiratory stridor. In all age groups, a firm, nonpainful, spherical mass can generally be palpated in the throat latch. Masses may be slow growing or progress quickly in size over a matter of months. These encapsulated masses may vary in size from 5 to 35 cm in diameter. Advanced imaging may provide high clinical suspicion of branchial arch cysts. They can be identified via ultrasound of the throat latch, radiographs, or magnetic resonance imaging. Video-endoscopy may identify several abnormalities dependent upon the location of the mass. Laryngeal or tracheal displacement, arytenoid displacement, edema, and dysfunction may all be observed. Squamous epithelial cells may be identified after fine needle aspirate of the area, however definitive diagnosis is accomplished via histopathology of the cyst after surgical removal. Treatment is usually performed via surgical resection. Postoperative complications include seroma, transient dysphagia, salivary secretions due to parotid gland trauma, and right sided laryngeal hemiplegia. Laryngeal hemiplegia is a common complication, which may preclude further athletic use and thus, surgical intervention should be approached with caution [25]. Two reports exist of marsupialization and sclerotherapy with a combination of ethanol and iodine with and without the removal of cyst lining, which show mixed success [26, 27].

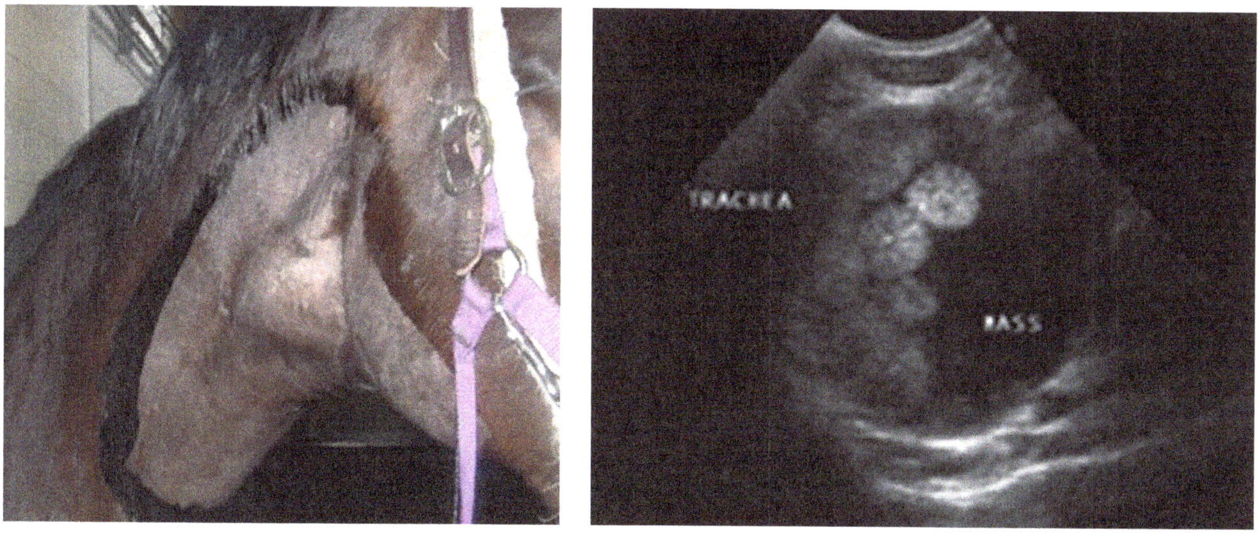

Figure 7.6 Branchial cyst in a mature horse; mass was firm and movable by palpation. The thyroid gland was ventral to the mass. Ultrasound of cyst with hyperechoic structures consistent with blood clots and spherical masses [25].

(Continued)

Condition	Affected breed/ prevalence	Description
Epiglottic, palatal, and pharyngeal cysts	More commonly identified in young horses as they start exercising or during presale resting endoscopy, however they have also been identified in older horses with no prior history of respiratory disease [28–31]. Median age of identification is 4 years old with no particular breed predisposition. Subepiglottic cysts were identified in 0.14% of the Thoroughbred population and accounted for 3% of epiglottic abnormalities in mature non-racehorses [32]. A study of 15 cases revealed that males were twice as likely to be affected as females [33].	Congenital cysts of the upper respiratory tract are most commonly identified in the subepiglottic region or dorsal pharyngeal region. They are usually only identified when young horses start work and develop respiratory noise or exercise intolerance. Occasionally, they are identified incidentally during airway endoscopy. Cysts of the subepiglottic region are thought to be a remnant of the thyroglossal duct which gives rise to the thyroid gland [34]. One case reported a thyroglossal cyst located at the distal end of the thyroglossal duct containing immunohistochemical evidence of thyroglobulin [35]; however, it has also been suggested that they can result from trauma. The less common cysts identified in the dorsal pharyngeal region have been suggested to be an embryologic remnant of Rathke's pouch. Clinical signs include chronic cough, bilateral nasal discharge, dysphagia, abnormal respiratory noise, and secondary aspiration pneumonia, but the majority of subepiglottic cysts carry no apparent clinical signs. When respiratory noise is identified, it is commonly on both inspiration and expiration and tends to be more noticeable while exercising. Diagnosis is made via endoscopy of the upper airway and appear as a soft, mucosa covered, fluctuant mass which diverts and elevates the epiglottis to one side of midline. An epiglottic elevator may be needed to visualize the cyst. Occasionally, intermittent epiglottic entrapment may also be observed (Figure 7.7). Histopathology identifies cyst lining of squamous/cuboidal epithelial cells. Except in the previously described case of a thyroglossal cyst, immunohisto-chemical evidence of thyroid origin is generally absent. Surgical removal, either via a laryngotomy/pharyngotomy approach or transendoscopically, is effective and has a good prognosis for future exercise [32, 34]. In one study, 73% of Thoroughbreds returned to racing after cyst removal. Standing intralesional injection with formalin has also been described as an alternative, cost-effective approach [36].

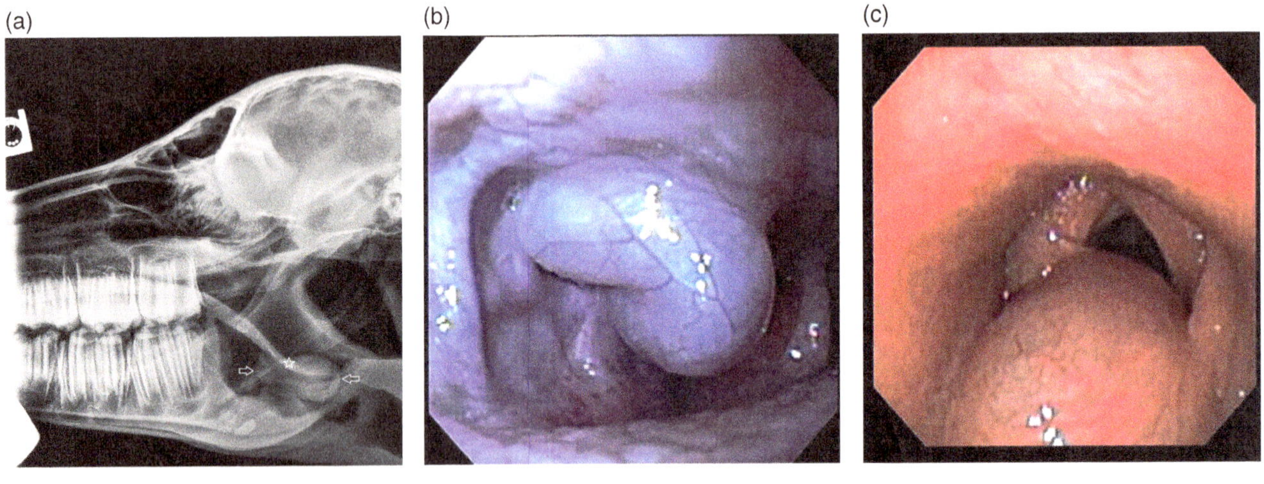

Figure 7.7 Palatal cyst. (a) Lateral radiograph of a palatal cyst (arrows) is it arises from the soft palate (star) causing ventral displacement of the epiglottis. (b) Cyst as visualized endoscopically from the oral cavity. (c) Cyst visualized endoscopically from the nasopharynx. *Source:* Images courtesy of Dr. David Wong, Iowa State University.

Condition	Affected breed/ prevalence	Description
Epiglottic hypoplasia	Incidence of epiglottic hypoplasia is low. In a study of 75 horses with a history of respiratory noise, 2 were reported to have a subjectively hypoplastic epiglottis [37]. Of these horses, one was associated with intermittent dorsal displacement of the soft palate and one was associated with epiglottic flutter. No horses in a study of 23 non-racehorses with epiglottic abnormalities were identified as having epiglottic hypoplasia [32].	Epiglottic hypoplasia is an epiglottis that is either abnormally short or abnormally thin with or without concurrent flaccidity. Etiology is presumed to be the result of a congenital lack of cartilage. Lack of resistance within the epiglottis may predispose the animal to concurrent conditions such as epiglottic entrapment and epiglottic flutter. Epiglottic hypoplasia has also been suggested as a cause for dorsal displacement of the soft palate (DDSP) however, more recent evidence suggests that the condition is likely more complicated and may involve neurologic dysfunction of the pharyngeal branch of the vagus nerve [38–40]. This condition alone generally does not cause clinical signs, however, it may be related to further pharyngeal dysfunction. In this case, clinical signs of epiglottic hypoplasia are the same as those associated with related pharyngeal dysfunction usually identified on work-up for associated respiratory noise or poor performance. Diagnosis is subjectively based on endoscopic observation of a short or flaccid epiglottis (Figure 7.8). Measurements may be taken from a lateral radiograph of the pharyngeal region. In a study of 24 healthy horses, the average thyro-epiglottic distance was 8.76 ± 0.44 cm [41]. Horses with dorsal displacement of the soft palate and epiglottic entrapment were shown to have a significantly shortened thyroepiglottic length [36]. Treatment is only undertaken when concurrent pharyngeal dysfunction is observed. Alterations to the caudal edge of the soft palate are made to prevent entrapment and displacement. Attempts to stiffen or enlarge the epiglottis using polytetrafluoroethylene paste, autografts, allografts, or bovine collagen have been reported with mixed results [42, 43].
Tracheal stenosis, collapse, malformation	Ponies and Miniature Horses appear to be predisposed to tracheal collapse; however, donkeys and mules have also been reported [44]. In one study, 5.6% of Miniature Horses admitted to a referral hospital for respiratory difficulty were diagnosed with tracheal collapse. Radiographic prevalence of subclinical tracheal collapse in healthy Miniature Horses was reported at 14.7% [45]. The average age of affected Miniature Horses was 20 years old, thus, as in dogs, age appears to be a predisposing factor.	Tracheal stenosis/collapse is more often acquired as a result of trauma, airway inflammation, or mass protrusion. Less commonly, congenital anomalies such as chondrodysplasia in younger animals or degenerative chondromalacia is suspected in older animals. Collapse can occur in either the cranial or caudal trachea. Rarely, congenital tracheal obstruction due to tracheal malformation has also been reported. Clinical signs include tachypnea, honking inspiratory noises, increased expiratory effort, and difficulty eating. These signs can be exaggerated by stress, exercise, dusty environments, pregnancy, and eating. Severely affected horses may display respiratory distress, recumbency, collapse, or death. In general signs tend to be progressive. Collapse can occur in the cranial or caudal trachea and may be either dorso-ventral or lateral. Tracheal collapse can be identified by endoscopy, fluoroscopic studies, or radiography. Radiographic reference ranges in Miniature Horses have been established [46]. Endoscopically, the collapsed region can be visualized and in some cases the endoscope may be unable to be passed due to severity. Edema of the pharyngeal region along with prominent arytenoid and epiglottis can often be observed. Occasionally, diagnosis can be made presumptively based on identification of lateral protrusion and flattening of the tracheal rings on palpation. Tracheotomy can be performed for initial stabilization in horses in respiratory distress, however minimal relief is experienced until an endotracheal tube is passed and the airway is opened. Prognosis for recovery without correction is poor. Treatment involves placement of a tracheal stent(s) (Figure 7.9). Post-surgical management of granulation tissue and rostral and caudal collapse is often required long term to maintain patency [47]. In cases where only a short segment of trachea is affected, surgical resection and end to end anastomosis has been attempted with moderate success [48]. Alternatively, conservative management using antitussives and retirement from work can be considered.

(Continued)

Condition	Affected breed/ prevalence	Description

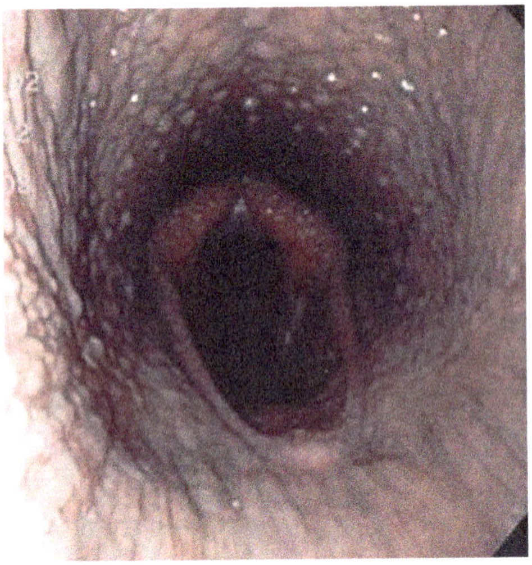

Figure 7.8 Epiglottic hypoplasia and flaccidity visualized endoscopically from the nasopharynx. *Source:* Image courtesy of Dr. Eric Parente, University of Pennsylvania.

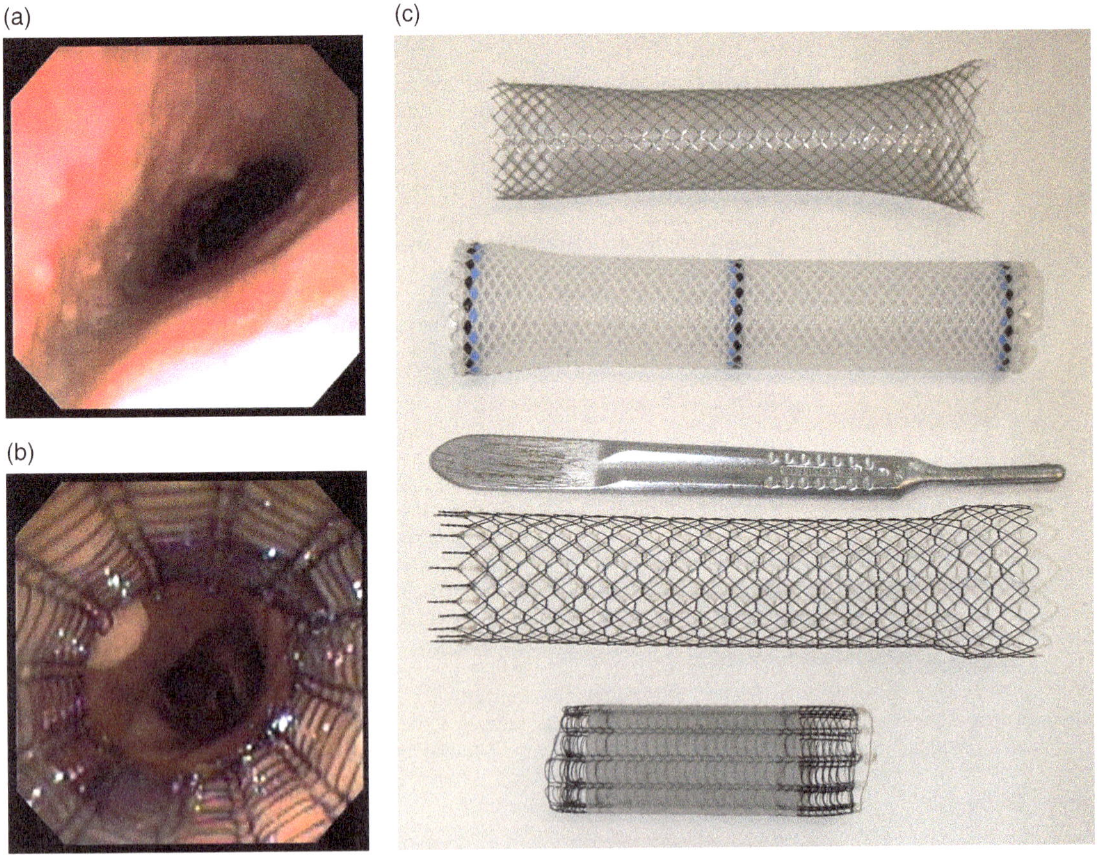

Figure 7.9 Tracheal collapse in a Miniature Horse. (a) An endoscopic view of a collapsing trachea. (b) Placement of an intratracheal stent via endoscopic guidance in the collapsed region. (c) Several tracheal stent options for correction of tracheal collapse. *Source:* Images courtesy of Dr. David Wong.

Condition	Affected breed/ prevalence	Description
Persistent frenulum of the epiglottis	Prevalence is unknown but has been reported in Arabians, Percherons, Shires, Quarter Horses, and Thoroughbreds [49, 50]	Persistent epiglottic frenulum is a restrictive band of tissue that connects the ventral portion of the epiglottis and the base of the tongue. The frenulum leads to dorsal displacement of the soft palate and dysphagia [51]. The cause is presumed to occur because of either: (i) failure of separation of the base of the tongue and epiglottis as they arise from the hypobranchial eminence; (ii) variant of closure of the thyroglossal duct; or (iii) fibrosis of an otherwise normal glossoepiglottic fold and hyoepiglotticus muscle. In a report of four foals, all presented for examination at 1–4 days of age with a history of respiratory distress and milk being seen from the nose or mouth after nursing. Other signs include dysphagia and inflation of the cheeks on expiration and dyspnea. Aspiration pneumonia can also occur, particularly in late diagnosed foals. Diagnosis is via upper airway endoscopy, identifying dorsal displacement of the soft palate followed by oral examination and observation of the persistent frenulum at the base of the epiglottis (Figure 7.10). Successful surgical correction can be performed in by transecting the frenulum under general anesthesia. In the report of four foals, three were reportedly normal 2–4 years after surgery. The fourth died soon after discharge, likely from poor farm management [49, 50].
Laryngeal web	Only one reported case in horses [52]	Laryngeal webs are presumed to arise as the result of morphogenic error of embryonic development in which tissue between the vocal folds fails to atrophy. There is only one report of the condition in horses, however many reports exist in the human literature. This abnormality in a Quarter Horse filly was accompanied by several other congenital laryngeal defects, including laryngeal hypoplasia, epiglottic dysplasia, permanent dorsal displacement of the soft palate and aberrant laryngeal ventricles [51]. Clinical signs include tachypnea and inspiratory/expiratory stertor. Diagnosis is made radiographically or via endoscopic visualization. No reported treatment has been attempted in horses. In humans, endoscopic surgical separation of webs with subsequent keel placement is frequently undertaken.
Paralaryngeal accessory bronchial cyst	Only one reported case in horses [53]	This anomaly has been reported in a 3-year-old Thoroughbred. The cyst was likely of embryonic tracheal origin due to the histopathologic findings of pseudostratified columnar epithelium and underlying epithelium containing few submucosal glands over smooth muscle. Clinical signs included increased inspiratory stridor during exercise. Diagnosis was based on identification of the cyst, along with deformation of the left arytenoid and cricoid cartilages axially during surgical exploration for correction of the laryngeal hemiplegia. Laryngeal radiographs may have identified the structure or potentially careful percutaneous palpation of the region. In humans, bronchogenic cysts are identified radiographically, ultrasonographically, and occasionally via flexible laryngoscope if the cyst is visible from the oral aspect of the laryngeal cartilages. Definitive diagnosis is based on histopathologic evidence of embryonic tracheobronchial involvement. Surgical resection of the cyst wall and contents was curative.

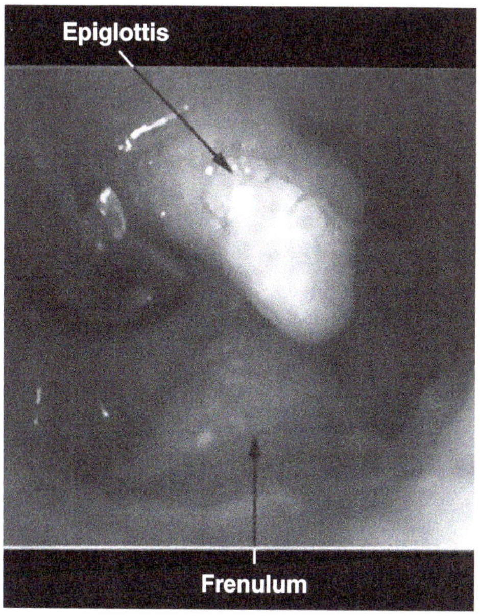

Figure 7.10 Persistent Epiglottic Frenulum [50].

(*Continued*)

Condition	Affected breed/ prevalence	Description
Fourth branchial arch defect (4-BAD)	Thoroughbred racehorses report a 0.5% prevalence of cartilage changes associated with 4-BAD based on palpation of the larynx. Although presumed to be more common in horses, ponies are occasionally reported to be affected [54].	Fourth branchial arch defects are presumed to arise from an error of embryologic development causing abnormalities of the laryngeal cartilages and associated musculature arising from the fourth branchial arch. In humans, the fourth branchial arch forms the thyroid, cricoid, and arytenoid cartilages. The equine larynx is assumed to be analogous. A range of abnormalities may be associated with this condition. Horses may be affected unilaterally or bilaterally; however, right-sided disease appears to be more common, affecting 65% of cases; 25% are reported to be bilaterally affected and the remaining 10% restricted to the left side. Clinical signs are varied, depending on severity and affected structures, but they include upper-respiratory noise, poor performance, exercise intolerance, dyspnea, belching, nasal discharge, coughing, and recurrent colic (presumably as a result of aerophagia). Occasionally, the disease may be identified incidentally on routine presale endoscopy. Horses with 4-BAD may show related endoscopic findings, including rostral displacement of the palatopharyngeal arch, arytenoid collapse, vocal cord collapse, axial deviation of the aryepiglottic fold, and occasionally dorsal displacement of the soft palate. Definitive diagnosis can only be made on necropsy, but a combination of palpation, endoscopy, and radiography can provide enough evidence for diagnosis. On palpation, an unusually large gap between the cricoid and thyroid cartilages is often appreciated. Endoscopically, a combination of rostral displacement of the soft palate and defective arytenoid motility, particularly right sided, should be cause for clinical suspicion. Radiographically, a column of air present in the proximal esophagus, enlargement, and calcification of the arytenoid cartilages and rostrally displaced palatal pillars (dew-drop sign) can be identified. Ultrasonographic evaluation and MRI provide additional visualization of abnormal dorsal extension of the thyroid laminae, absence of the cricoid cartilage articular process and caudal cornu of the thyroid cartilage, and lack of cricothyroid articulation. These findings may help separate 4-BAD from apparent left laryngeal hemiplegia and prevent inappropriate surgical intervention [55]. Horses may also demonstrate concurrent aspiration pneumonia. No treatment exists to restore normal anatomic structure; however, procedures used to restore airway function, such as prosthetic laryngoplasty or noise-eliminating procedures such as ventriculo-chordectomy with laryngeal saccule ablation, can be considered. Abnormal anatomy often complicates prosthetic laryngoplasty and may prevent full abduction of the affected cartilage. Prognosis for athletic function depends on the severity of affliction; however, it is considered to be poor for high-intensity athletic activity.
Accessory lung	Four case reports exist of accessory lung identified in foals	Two of these cases were identified in fetuses on necropsy and two in live foals. Three of the cases were of intrathoracic accessory lung and one was identified in the caudal-cervical region. In one fetal case, the accessory lung was found in conjunction with bronchial hypoplasia and chronic passive congestion of the liver. In the single extrathoracic case, the lesion was found to be associated with an accessory cervical tracheal bronchus and air-filled diverticulum. In this case, successful surgical resection of the diverticulum and closure of the tracheal defect was achieved; however, the foal was euthanized for other unrelated reasons [56]. Accessory lung development is rare in horses and appears to be more common in calves where many more cases are reported. Cause for this condition is undetermined but is suggested to be the be result of embryologic development of an extra lung bud at an abnormal site.
Paratracheal air cyst	There is one existing report of a paratracheal air cyst (PAC) in an American Paint Horse neonate [57].	In humans, congenital PAC is thought to be the result of a malformed supernumerary lung, a high division of the primary lung bud, or a developmental malformation of the membranous posterior portion of the trachea or tracheal rings. Clinical signs include a nonpainful mass and swelling of the cranial ventral neck. Secondary lower respiratory signs, including aspiration pneumonia, were present in this case. This is a commonly reported finding in human cases of PAC. Computed tomography and digital radiography confirmed communication of the cyst with the trachea. On ultrasound, a cyst-like structure was identified, containing air and hyperechogenic material suggestive of purulent debris. Culture of the cystic contents grew *Streptococcus zooepidemicus*. Bronchoscopy in this case was unsuccessful in identifying the origin of this cyst. Tracheal origin of the cyst was confirmed based on histologic identification of squamous epithelium, goblet cells, and occasional ciliated cells. Surgical excision in this case was curative and provided a good cosmetic outcome along with medical treatment for the concurrent lower respiratory disease.

References

1 Vanderplassche, M., Simoens, P., Bouters, R. et al. (1984). Aetiology and pathogenesis of congenital torticollis and head scoliosis in the equine foetus. *Equine Vet. J.* 16: 419–424.

2 DeBowes, R.M. and Gaughan, E.M. (1998). Congenital dental disease of horses. *Vet. Clin. North Am. Equine.* 14: 273–289.

3 Schumacher, J., Brink, P., Easley, J. et al. (2008). Surgical correction of wry nose in four foals. *Vet. Surg.* 37: 142–148.

4 Tremaine, W.H. and Dixon, P.M. (2010). A long-term study of 277 cases of equine sinonasal disease. Part 2: treatments and results of treatments. *Equine Vet. J.* 33: 283–289.

5 Frankeny, R.L. (2003). Intralesional administration of formalin for treatment of epidermal inclusion cysts in five horses. *J. Am. Vet. Med. Assoc.* 223: 221–222.

6 Reed, K.M., Bauer, M.M., Mendoza, K.M. et al. (2010). A candidate gene for choanal atresia in alpaca. *Genome* 53: 224–230.

7 James, F.M., Parente, E.J., and Palmer, J.E. (2006). Management of bilateral choanal atresia in a foal. *J. Am. Vet. Med. Assoc.* 229: 1784–1789.

8 Richardson, J.D., Lane, J.G., and Day, M.J. (1994). Congenital choanal restriction in 3 horses. *Equine Vet. J.* 26: 162–165.

9 Beard, W.L., Robertson, J.T., and Leeth, B. (1990). Bilateral congenital cysts in the frontal sinuses of a horse. *J. Am. Vet. Med. Assoc.* 196: 453–454.

10 Sanders-Shamis, M. and Robertson, J.T. (1987). Congenital sinus cyst in a foal. *J. Am. Vet. Med. Assoc.* 190: 1011–1012.

11 Silva, L.C.L., Zoppa, A.L.V., Fernandes, W.R. et al. (2009). Bilateral sinus cysts in a filly treated by endoscopic sinus surgery. *Can. Vet. J.* 50: 417–420.

12 Gibbs, C. and Lane, J.G. (1987). Radiographic examination of the facial, nasal and paranasal sinus regions of the horse. II. Radiological findings. *Equine Vet. J.* 19: 474–482.

13 Ostrowska, J., Lindström, L., Tóth, T. et al. (2020). Computed tomography characteristics of equine paranasal sinus cysts. *Equine Vet. J.* 52: 538–546.

14 Blazyczek, I., Hamann, H., Ohnesorge, B. et al. (2004). Inheritance of guttural pouch tympany in the Arabian horse. *J. Hered.* 95: 195–199.

15 Blazyczek, I., Hamann, H., Deegen, E. et al. (2004). Retrospective analysis of 50 cases of guttural pouch tympany in foals. *Vet. Rec.* 154: 261–264.

16 Blazyczek, I., Hamann, H., Ohnesorge, B. et al. (2003). Gutteral pouch tympany in German warmblood foals: influence of sex, inbreeding and blood proportions of founding breeds as well as estimation of heritability. *Berliner Und Munchener Tierarztliche Wochenschrift* 116: 346–351.

17 Blazyczek, I., Hamann, H., Ohnesorge, B. et al. (2003). Populations genetische Untersuchung zur Erblichkeit der Luftsacktympanie beim Arabischen Vollblutfohlen [population genetic analysis of the heritability of gutteral pouch tympany in Arabian purebred foals]. *Dtsch. Tierarztl. Wochenschr.* 110: 417–419.

18 Baptiste, K. (1997). Functional anatomy observations of the pharyngeal orifice of the equine guttural pouch (auditory tube diverticulum). *Vet. J.* 153: 311–319.

19 Metzger, J., Ohnesorge, B., and Distl, O. (2012). Genome-wide linkage and association analysis identifies major gene loci for guttural pouch tympany in Arabian and German Warmblood horses. *PLoS One* 7: e41640.

20 McCue, P.M., Freeman, D.E., and Donawick, W.J. (1989). Guttural pouch tympany: 15 cases (1977–1986). *J. Am. Vet. Med. Assoc.* 194: 1761–1763.

21 Bell, C. (2007). Pharyngeal neuromuscular dysfunction associated with bilateral guttural pouch tympany in a foal. *Can. Vet. J.* 48: 192–194.

22 Sparks, H.D., Stick, J.A., Brakenhoff, J.E. et al. (2009). Partial resection of the plica salpingopharyngeus for the treatment of three foals with bilateral tympany of the auditory tube diverticulum (guttural pouch). *J. Am. Vet. Med. Assoc.* 235: 731–733.

23 Caston, S.S., Kersh, K.D., Reinertson, E.L. et al. (2015). Treatment of guttural pouch tympany in foals with transnasal Foley catheter placement. *Equine. Vet. Educ.* 27: 28–30.

24 Glosser, J.W., Pires, C.A.S., and Feibnerg, S.E. (2003). Branchial cleft or cervical lymphoepithelial cysts. *J. Am. Dent. Assoc.* 134: 81–86.

25 Nolen-Walston, R.D., Parente, E.J., Madigan, J.E. et al. (2009). Branchial remnant cysts of mature and juvenile horses. *Equine Vet. J.* 41: 918–923.

26 de Estrada, J. and Schumacher, J. (2013). Treatment of an 18-year-old mare for bilateral, branchial remnant cysts. *Equine. Vet. Educ.* 25: 129–133.

27 Rinnovati, R., Bianchin Butina, B., Bianchi, J. et al. (2018). Marsupialization and sclerotherapy with povidone iodine and ethanol of a branchial remnant cyst in an Arabian filly. *J. Equine. Sci.* 29: 43–46.

28 Haynes, P.F., Beadle, R.E., McClure, J.R. et al. (1990). Soft palate cysts as a cause of pharyngeal dysfunction in two horses. *Equine Vet. J.* 22: 369–371.

29 Koch, D.B. and Tate, L.P. (1978). Pharyngeal cysts in horses. *J. Am. Vet. Med. Assoc.* 173: 860–862.

30 Sinclair, E.A. (2008). Pharyngeal cyst in a 5-year-old Dutch Warmblood. *Can. Vet. J.* 49: 806–808.

31 Stick, J.A. and Boles, C. (1980). Subepiglottic cyst in three foals. *J. Am. Vet. Med. Assoc.* 177: 62–64.

32 Aitken, M. and Parente, E. (2011). Epiglottic abnormalities in mature nonracehorses: 23 cases (1990–2009). *J. Am. Vet. Med. Assoc.* 238: 1634–1638.

33 Salz, R.O., Ahern, B.J., and Lumsden, J.M. (2013). Subepiglottic cysts in 15 horses. *Equine. Vet. Educ.* 25: 403–407.

34 Harvey, C., Raker, C.W., and O'Brien, J.A. (1973). Pharyngeal and laryngeal diseases causing airway obstruction in the dog and horse. *Vet. Surg.* 2: 15–19.

35 Kelmer, G., Kramer, J., Lacarrubba, A.M. et al. (2007). A novel location and en bloc excision of a thyroglossal duct cyst in a filly. *Equine. Vet. Educ.* 19: 131–135.

36 Dougherty, S.S. and Palmer, J.L. (2008). Use of intralesional formalin administration for treatment of a subepiglottic cyst in a horse. *J. Am. Vet. Med. Assoc.* 233: 463–465.

37 Kannegeiter, N. and Dore, M. (1995). Endoscopy of the upper respiratory tract during treadmill exercise: a clinical study of 100 horses. *Aust. Vet. J.* 72: 101–107.

38 Haynes, P.F. (1981). Persistent dorsal displacement of the soft palate associated with epiglottic shortening in two horses. *J. Am. Vet. Med. Assoc.* 179: 677–681.

39 Holcombe, S.J., Derksen, F.J., Stick, J.A. et al. (2010). Pathophysiology of dorsal displacement of the soft palate in horses. *Equine Vet. J.* 31: 45–48.

40 Rehder, R.S., Ducharme, N.G., Hackett, R.P. et al. (1995). Measurement of upper airway pressures in exercising horses with dorsal displacement of the soft palate. *Am. J. Vet. Res.* 56: 269–274.

41 Linford, R.L., O'Brien, T.R., Wheat, J.D. et al. (1983). Radiographic assessment of epiglottic length and pharyngeal and laryngeal diameters in the thoroughbred. *Am. J. Vet. Res.* 44: 1660–1666.

42 Tulleners, E., Stick, J.A., Leitch, M. et al. (1997). Epiglottic augmentation for treatment of dorsal displacement of the soft palate in racehorses: 59 cases (1985–1994). *J. Am. Vet. Med. Assoc.* 211: 1022–1028.

43 Peloso, J.G., Stick, J.A., Nickels, F.A. et al. (1992). Epiglottic augmentation by use of polytetrafluoroethylene to correct dorsal displacement of the soft palate in a Standardbred horse. *J. Am. Vet. Med. Assoc.* 201: 1393–1395.

44 Mair, T.S. and Lane, J.G. (1990). Tracheal obstructions in two horses and a donkey. *Vet. Rec.* 126: 303–304.

45 Aleman, M., Nieto, J.E., Benak, J. et al. (2008). Tracheal collapse in American Miniature Horses: 13 cases (1985–2007). *J. Am. Vet. Med. Assoc.* 233: 1302–1306.

46 Every, L.J., Hostnik, E.T., Hostnik, L.D. et al. (2020). Radiographic tracheal lumen to vertebral ratios in the normal American Miniature Horse. *Equine Vet. J.* 52: 428–434.

47 Wong, D.M., Sponseller, B.A., Riedesel, E.A. et al. (2008). The use of intraluminal stents for tracheal collapse in two horses: case management and long-term treatment. *Equine. Vet. Educ.* 20: 80–90.

48 Tate, L.P., Koch, D.B., Sembrat, R.F. et al. (1981). Tracheal reconstruction by resection and end-to-end anastomosis in the horse. *J. Am. Vet. Med. Assoc.* 178: 253–258.

49 Moorman, V.J., Marshall, J.F., and Jann, H.W. (2007). Persistent dorsal displacement of the soft palate attributable to a frenulum of the epiglottis in a racing Thoroughbred. *J. Am. Vet. Med. Assoc.* 231: 751–754.

50 Yarbrough, T.B., Voss, E., Herrgesell, E.J. et al. (1999). Persistent frenulum of the epiglottis in four foals. *Vet. Surg.* 28: 287–291.

51 Conceição, M.L., Alonso, J.M., Alves, A.L. et al. (2020). Dorsal displacement of the soft palate secondary to persistent frenulum of the epiglottis in neonatal foal. *J. Equine. Vet. Sci.* 87: 102926.

52 Lees, M.J., Schuh, J.C., and Barber, S.M. (1987). A congenital laryngeal web defect in a Quarter Horse filly. *Equine Vet. J.* 19: 561–563.

53 Baxter, G.M., Allen, D., and Farrell, R.L. (1992). Paralaryngeal accessory bronchial cyst as a cause of laryngeal hemiplegia in a horse. *Equine Vet. J.* 24: 67–69.

54 Smith, L.J. and Mair, T.S. (2009). Fourth branchial arch defect in a Welsh section a pony mare. *Equine. Vet. Educ.* 21: 364–366.

55 Garrett, K.S., Woodie, J.B., Embertson, R.M. et al. (2009). Diagnosis of laryngeal dysplasia in five horses using magnetic resonance imaging and ultrasonography. *Equine Vet. J.* 41: 766–771.

56 Davis, D.M., Honnas, C.M., Hedlund, C.S. et al. (1991). Resection of a cervical tracheal bronchus in a foal. *J. Am. Vet. Med. Assoc.* 198: 2097–2099.

57 Zetterstrom, S., Horzmann, K., Yin, J. et al. (2022). Paratracheal air cyst in a foal. *Equine. Vet. Educ.* 34: 187–192.

Chapter 8 Respiratory Disorders

Section I Disorders of Breathing Pattern in the Neonatal Foal

Kara M. Lascola

Precisely timed development of the neuronal, structural, and muscular components of the respiratory system must occur in utero to prepare the newborn foal to take over ventilation and gas exchange in the immediate postpartum period. Neurogenesis within the pontine and medullary respiratory centers (e.g. respiratory center and respiratory pattern generator) is essential for central control of ventilatory drive as is the establishment of sensory and motor neural networks, and development of chemoreceptors, mechanoreceptors, and muscles of respiration [1–3]. Correct development of each of these components and of their appropriate reciprocal interactions is critical. Final maturation of the central respiratory neural networks and chemoreceptors continues after birth. For this reason, neonates, including foals, may be predisposed to developing apneas or other alterations in breathing pattern, particularly in the face of hypoxemia [1, 4]. Furthermore, prematurity, dysmaturity, and hypoxic, inflammatory or other physiologic stressors in the prenatal or perinatal periods can impair or inhibit neural development of respiratory control and potentially the normal transition to extrauterine life [1, 5]. Neonatal apnea, irregularities in respiratory pattern, and transient tachypnea of the newborn (TTN) are thought to arise in response to these stressors in human infants. These conditions are observed in neonatal foals as well, but may differ somewhat in pathophysiology. Recognition of these abnormalities and the possible causes is important in the care of neonatal foals.

Neonatal Apnea

In human infants, neonatal apnea represents a cessation in breathing of ≥20 seconds that may be accompanied by bradycardia and cyanosis [6]. This condition is associated with prematurity but may also develop in association with neonatal encephalopathy (NE) or disorders of various other body systems. The pathophysiologic mechanism associated with neonatal apnea depends somewhat on the underlying cause, but often involves immaturity or impairment in central respiratory control of ventilation. In some premature infants, airflow obstruction secondary to underdevelopment of the upper airway muscles and pharyngeal collapse contributes to these apneic events [6]. Hypercapnia and respiratory acidosis are associated with sustained apneic episodes. Based on experimental studies of NE/hypoxic-ischemic encephalopathy (HIE), cerebral hypoxia and ischemia can damage central and chemoreceptor-mediated recognition of hypercapnia [7, 8]. In severe cases, abnormal cerebral blood flow in response to persistent hypercapnia and acidemia exacerbates cerebral ischemia and can also cause intracranial hemorrhage [9], both of which will worsen damage to the central respiratory center and brain.

In neonatal foals, apnea is recognized as a complication of NE as well as dysmaturity or prematurity [4, 7, 8, 10–12]. The pathophysiologic mechanisms for NE in foals is incompletely defined and most likely multifactorial with wide variability in clinical presentation and disease severity. Mechanisms most likely include neuronal damage (hypoxic, inflammatory), impaired maturation, or imbalance in neurotransmitter or hormonal production in the peri- or prenatal period [10, 11, 13]. The condition of NE is described elsewhere in the textbook. It is assumed that the causes of apnea identified in neonatal foals are similar to those described for HIE in human infants and other species and involve a loss of central regulation of respiration [7, 8, 14, 15].

Neonatal apnea in foals with NE is accompanied by marked reductions in respiratory rate (<4 breaths/minute) as well as hypoxemia, hypercapnia, and respiratory acidosis detected on arterial blood gas analysis [4, 8, 16]. Additional neurologic abnormalities and signs attributed to severe central nervous system (CNS) depression can be noted [7, 14, 15]. Sepsis, hypoglycemia, and hypothermia

Equine Neonatal Medicine, First Edition. Edited by David M. Wong and Pamela A. Wilkins.

can be contributing or independent causes of apnea [1, 17]. Seizure activity and advanced pulmonary disease with respiratory muscle fatigue may also present with altered respiratory rate or pattern [17]. Additional diagnostics should aim to rule out these other conditions.

Medical therapy for apnea is primarily aimed toward improving respiratory drive and normalizing P_aCO_2, but should also address any underlying conditions. Administration of supplemental oxygen improves hypoxemia but will not correct hypercapnia. Pharmacologic treatment with caffeine, a methylxanthine (7.5–12 mg/kg loading dose, then 2.5–5 mg/kg PO daily) or doxapram (0.02–0.05 mg/kg/h IV as continuous rate infusion, CRI) can be attempted [4, 7, 8, 16]. These medications primarily act as central respiratory stimulants but may also improve contractility of the diaphragm (caffeine) or activation of peripheral chemoreceptors (doxapram) [6, 8, 18, 19]. Mechanical ventilation is a more invasive therapeutic intervention reserved for severe cases that do not respond to pharmacologic therapy [15]. The response of foals to caffeine and doxapram is variable [8]. In foals with experimentally induced hypercapnia, doxapram (but not caffeine) improved ventilation [20]. In another study involving foals with a clinical diagnosis of NE, doxapram was also superior to caffeine in correcting hypercapnia but did not correct academia and was not associated with improved survival [8]. Potential side effects associated with these medications include restlessness, excitement, and tachycardia.

Alterations in Respiratory Pattern Associated with Neonatal Encephalopathy (NE)

Alterations in normal respiratory pattern are occasionally identified in foals with NE [7, 14, 15, 17]. These various patterns may reflect damage to the midbrain, pontine, and medullary regions within the brainstem [21, 22]. Although these respiratory abnormalities are not among the most common clinical signs, they do reflect severe disease. In one retrospective study, foals diagnosed with NE that required mechanical ventilation or administration of respiratory stimulants were less likely to survive [23]. In that same study, the majority of nonsurviving foals with histologic evaluation of the brain at necropsy had evidence of neuronal necrosis and degeneration consistent with ischemia. Detailed reports of respiratory abnormalities in foals with NE are limited. Abnormal respiratory patterns may include central hyperventilation, apneustic breathing, cluster breathing, and ataxic breathing, among others (Table 8.I.1). For example, the apneustic center within the pontine region of the brainstem prolongs inspiration via stimulatory input to inspiratory motor neurons elsewhere in the brain stem. When damaged, prolonged inspiratory gasps with only transient expiratory efforts can be observed [12]. Ataxic breathing generally corresponds to complete respiratory failure. Concurrent hypercapnia may or may not be identified with these respiratory pattern abnormalities and can be masked by mechanical ventilation [17]. Treatment includes provision of ventilatory support as needed and addressing underlying causes and other ongoing medical conditions.

Table 8.I.1 Clinical description of various breathing patterns that can be observed in neonates.

Pattern	Description
Central hyperventilation	Prolonged, rapid hyperpnea
Apneustic breathing	Prolonged inspiratory pause without corresponding expiratory pause
Cluster breathing	Episodes of several rapid respirations of varying depth interspersed with pauses of varying length
Ataxic breathing	Irregular inspiratory efforts of varying depth interspersed with periods of apnea

Transient Tachypnea of the Newborn

In neonatal foals, TTN represents an idiopathic syndrome of hyperthermia and tachypnea that is observed most often in Clydesdales, but also reported in Arabian and Thoroughbred breeds [4, 16, 17]. The condition occurs primarily during periods of warm ambient temperatures and humid conditions. There is no reported sex predilection and foals typically have a history of a normal gestation and birth [17]. The exact cause of TTN in foals remains unknown. Immaturity or dysfunction in central or peripheral thermoregulatory mechanisms is considered the most likely cause, but an abnormality with central control of respiratory rate or pattern cannot be ruled out [17].

TTN in foals differs from the condition of the same name observed in newborn infants. In infants, TTN arises secondary to abnormal or delayed clearance of fetal lung fluid [24–27]. Clinical signs appear within a few hours of birth and self-resolve within 24–72 hours with minimal intervention. The most common risk factor is cesarean section, particularly in late preterm infants, however large birth weight, male gender, twin births, and maternal factors may also contribute. The cause of TTN in human infants is primarily attributed to delayed or abnormal Na^+ channel-mediated absorption of fetal lung fluid by Type II pulmonary epithelial cells. Specifically, the Na^+-K^+-ATPase channels may demonstrate diminished activity or immaturity in transport mechanisms.

Clinical signs of TTN in affected foals appear suddenly within a few days of birth and self-resolve within a few days to weeks of onset [4, 15, 16]. Rectal temperatures can reach as high as 108 °F (42.2 °C) and foals can appear to be "panting" with respiratory rates above 80 bpm [17]. Rarely, signs of mild NE can be noted [16]. Diagnosis is presumptive; however, it is important to rule out pathologic causes of fever and tachypnea. Systemic and respiratory system evaluation is recommended and diagnostics may include hematologic evaluation, arterial blood gas analysis, and measurement of markers of inflammation, as well as thoracic radiographs and ultrasound. Treatment is limited to controlling the temperature. Antipyretics are generally not useful; however, body clipping, alcohol baths, and providing a cool environment may help. Foals should be closely monitored for any signs of infection, in which case treatment should be modified accordingly.

References

1 Beyeler, S.A., Hodges, M.R., and Huxtable, A.G. (2020). Impact of inflammation on developing respiratory control networks: rhythm generation, chemoreception and plasticity. *Respir. Physiol. Neurobiol.* 274: 103357.

2 Greer, J.J., Funj, G.D., and Ballanyi. (2006). Preparing for the first breath: prenatal maturation of respiratory neural control. *J. Physiol.* 570: 437–444.

3 Morton, S. and Brodsky, D. (2016). Fetal physiology and the transition to extrauterine life. *Clin. Perinatol.* 43: 395–407.

4 Lester, G.D. (1999). Respiratory disease in the neonatal foal. *Equine Vet. Educ.* 11: 208–217.

5 Dylag, A.M. and Raffay, T.M. (2019). Rodent models of respiratory control and respiratory system development – clinical significance. *Respir. Physiol. Neurobiol.* 268: 103249.

6 Eichenwald, E.C. and AAP Committee on fetus and newborn (2016). Apnea of prematurity. *Pediatrics* 137: e20153757.

7 Vaala, W.E. (1994). Peripartum asphyxia. *Vet. Clin. North Am. Equine Pract.* 10: 187–218.

8 Giguere, S., Slade, J.K., and Sanchez, L.C. (2008). Retrospective comparison of caffeine and doxapram for the treatment of hypercapnia in foals with hypoxic-ischemic encephalopathy. *J. Vet. Intern. Med.* 22: 401–405.

9 Aurora, S. and Snyder, E.Y. (2004). Perinatal asphyxia. In: *Manual of Neonatal Care* (ed. J.P. Cloherty, E.C. Eichenwald, and A.R. Stark), 536–555. Philadelphia, PA: Lippincott, Williams and Wilkins.

10 McKenzie, M.C. (2018). Disorders of foals. In: *Equine Internal Medicine* (ed. S.M. Reed, W.M. Bayly, and D.C. Sellon), 1365–1459. St. Louis, MO: Elsevier.

11 Wong, D., Wilkins, P.A., Bain, F.T. et al. (2011). Neonatal encephalopathy in foals. *Compend. Contin. Educ. Vet.* 33: E5.

12 Beech, J. (ed.) (1991). *Equine Respiratory Disorders*. Philadelphia: Lea & Febiger.

13 Toribio, R.E. (2019). Equine neonatal encephalopathy: facts evidence and opinions. *Vet. Clin. North Am. Equine Pract.* 35: 363–378.

14 Galvin, N. and Collins, D. (2004). Perinatal asphyxia syndrome in the foal: review and a case report. *Ir. Vet. J.* 57: 707–714.

15 MacKay, R.J. (2005). Neurologic disorders of neonatal foals. *Vet. Clin. North Am. Equine Pract.* 21: 387–406.

16 Wilkins, P.A. (2003). Lower respiratory problems of the neonate. *Vet. Clin. North Am. Equine Pract.* 19: 19–33.

17 Koterba, A.M. and Paradis, M.R. (1990). Specific respiratory conditions. In: *Equine Clinical Neonatology* (ed. A.M. Koterba, W.H. Drummond, and P.C. Kosch), 196–197. Philadelphia, PA: Lea & Febiger.

18 Bhatt-Mehta, V. and Schumacher, R.E. (2003). Treatment of apnea of prematurity. *Paediatr. Drugs* 5: 195–210.

19 Stark, A.R. (2004). Apnea. In: *Manual of Neonatal Care* (ed. J.P. Cloherty, E.C. Eichenwald, and A.R. Stark), 388–393. Philadelphia, PA: Lippincott, Williams and Wilkins.

20 Giguère, S., Sanchez, L.C., Shih, A. et al. (2007). Comparison of the effects of caffeine and doxapram on respiratory and cardiovascular function in foals with induced respiratory acidosis. *Am. J. Vet. Res.* 68: 1407–1416.

21 Saito, Y., Hoshimoto, T., Iwata, H. et al. (1999). Apneustic breathing in children with brainstem damage due to hypoxic–ischemic encephalopathy. *Dev. Med. Child Neurol.* 41: 560–567.

22 Friede, R.L. (1990). *Developmental Neuropathology*, 2e, 98–99. Berlin: Springer-Verlag.

23 Lyle-Dugas, J., Giguère, S., Mallicote, M.F. et al. (2017). Factors associated with outcome in 94 hospitalised foals diagnosed with neonatal encephalopathy. *Equine Vet. J.* 49: 207–210.

24 Jain, L. and Eaton, D.C. (2006). Physiology of fetal kung fluid clearance and the effect of labor. *Semin. Perinatol.* 30: 34–43.

25 Bruschettini, M., Moresco, L., Calevo, M.G. et al. (2020). Postnatal corticosteroids for transient tachypnoea of the newborn. *Cochrane Database Syst. Rev.* (3): CD013222. https://doi.org/10.1002/14651858.CD013222.pub2.

26 Hillman, N., Kallapur, S.G., and Jobe, A. (2012). Physiology of transition from intrauterine to extrauterine life. *Clin. Perinatol.* 39: 769–783.

27 Yurdakök, M. (2010). Transient tachypnea of the newborn: what is new? *J. Matern. Fetal Neonatal Med.* 23: 24–26.

Section II Lower Respiratory Tract Disorders

Pamela A. Wilkins, David Wong, Bettina Dunkel, and Brett Sponseller

Lower respiratory tract disorders are common in neonatal foals and can be associated with various routes of disease initiation and numerous etiologies. Pneumonia is a particularly prevalent clinical entity in the neonate and is associated with various potential pathogens. The gold standard for diagnosis of pneumonia is a pathological diagnosis from lung tissue with microscopic evidence of organisms coupled with an inflammatory response [1]. Because it is clinically impractical to obtain lung parenchyma in foals that survive, clinical pneumonia is defined as a lower respiratory tract infection typically associated with fever, respiratory symptoms, and evidence of parenchymal involvement by either physical examination or the presence of infiltrates on thoracic radiography [1–4]. Pneumonia can broadly be classified based on the time and mode of acquisition and includes pneumonia: (i) acquired in utero, (ii) acquired during birth and caused by organisms that colonize the birth canal, or (iii) acquired after birth from environmental pathogens [3, 4]. Bacterial pneumonia is common in foals of all ages, but causative agents can vary with age.

Predisposing factors such as the immature nature of their pulmonary anatomy and physiology and immature host defense mechanisms contribute to the development of lower respiratory diseases in the foal. For example, in one postmortem study, foals did not have evidence of organized lymphoid tissue; additionally, lymphocytes and plasma cells were absent in lung tissue in neonates, suggesting that local humoral immunity within the lower respiratory tract is limited at this age [5]. Other factors such as immaturity of the respiratory ciliary apparatus and modest numbers of pulmonary macrophages might result in decreased bacterial clearance from the respiratory tract [6]. Moreover, immaturity or defects in humoral and cellular function can contribute to inefficient opsonization and phagocytosis of bacteria. Further predisposing factors that might contribute to development of pneumonia include anatomical (e.g. cleft palate) or functional (e.g. dysphagia secondary to hyperkalemic periodic paralysis) defects. Environmental factors and endemic pathogens can also result in increased risk of postnatal respiratory infection.

In the early neonatal period, foals are more likely to have pneumonia as a result of systemic sepsis, but meconium aspiration syndrome (MAS) and in utero infection are also possible in the newborn. Aspiration pneumonia is also relatively common in the neonate while viral, mycotic, or parasitic pathogens are other groups of pathogens that can cause pneumonia at various ages. *Rhodococcus equi* pneumonia, while typically associate with older foals (1–6 months old) is likely introduced into the affected foal's respiratory tract early in the neonatal period [2]. Acute lung injury (ALI), acute respiratory distress syndrome (ARDS), and neonatal equine respiratory distress syndrome (NERDS, also known as hyaline membrane disease) are other processes that impact the foal's lower respiratory tract. Knowledge of these disease processes and causative agents allows specific treatment of foals with lower respiratory tract disorders.

Meconium Aspiration Syndrome (MAS)

Meconium aspiration should be considered in newborn foals and is thought to occur secondary to acute pre- or intrapartum asphyxiation associated with severe fetal distress, subsequent passage of meconium by the fetus, and aspiration of meconium during fetal gasping efforts. Neonates with MAS have marked surfactant dysfunction. Airways and alveoli of affected neonates contain meconium, inflammatory cells, inflammatory mediators, edema fluid, protein, and other debris. MAS can present clinically with different degrees of severity, ranging from a mild form of respiratory

Equine Neonatal Medicine, First Edition. Edited by David M. Wong and Pamela A. Wilkins.

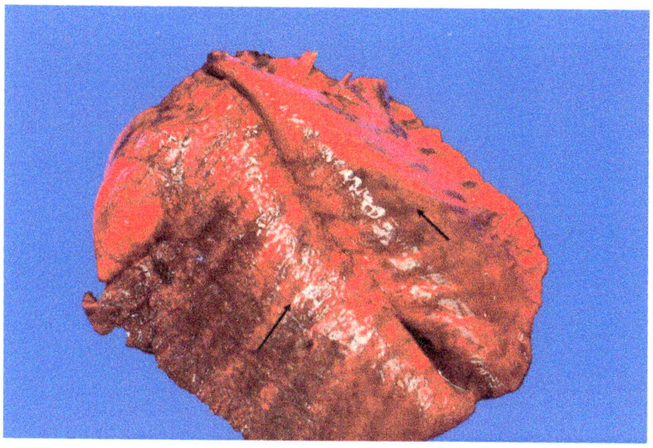

Figure 8.II.1 Lungs from an American Saddlebred fetus, aborted 9 days prior to due date. The lungs are dark red, firm, and fail to collapse with rib impressions present (arrow). Microscopically there was evidence of chronic meconium aspiration resulting in granulomatous pneumonia and mineralization. *Source:* Image Courtesy Dr. Jennifer Janes.

compromise to severe forms resulting in perinatal death (Figure 8.II.1) despite respiratory management up to and including mechanical ventilation and extracorporeal membrane oxygenation (ECMO). However, advances in our knowledge concerning MAS have revealed that many cases of this syndrome in infants may not be causally related to the aspiration of meconium but rather are caused by other pathologic processes occurring in utero, primarily chronic asphyxia and infection. Current treatments being investigated in the management of infants with MAS include surfactant administration, surfactant administration combined with partial liquid ventilation, and surfactant lavage (see Chapter 8, Section III).

Bacterial Pneumonia

As noted, bacterial pneumonia is common in the neonatal foal. One potential route of lower respiratory tract infection is when an organism is acquired in utero. Intrauterine pneumonia, sometimes referred to as early neonatal pneumonia in the human literature, occurs when organisms from an infected mother are transmitted via the transplacental/hematogenous route (rare occurrence) or from fetal aspiration of infected amniotic fluid (more common) [2, 6, 7]. This disease process is frequently associated with chorioamnionitis in pregnant women. Affected infants can present as stillbirth, with low Apgar scores, or with severe respiratory distress at birth. Chorioamnionitis is common in pregnant mares, with bacteria such as *Streptococcus zooepidemicus, Leptospira, Escherichia coli, Pseudomonas*, and *Streptococcus equisimilis* being frequently identified [8]. Anecdotally, it has long been suggested that infectious agents gain access to the fetal foal by infecting the allantoic and amniotic fluids, but less information is available regarding the incidence of fetal infection in mares with chorioamnionitis [8, 9]. In one report involving a single aborted Standardbred fetus (7 months gestation), the fetal lungs had hundreds of small (2–10 mm) irregular foci throughout the lungs in which *R. equi* was subsequently isolated [10]. The authors speculated that the fetus became infected through inhalation or ingestion of amniotic fluid. However, in another study, a group of mares with experimentally induced chorioamnionitis (i.e. *S. zooepidemicus*) had negative bacterial cultures of the fetal fluids despite extensive inflammatory changes and positive bacterial cultures in the fetus and chorioallantois. The investigators suggested that contamination of fetal fluids is not a common primary route of fetal infection. More studies are necessary to better understand the development of fetal infection from mares with chorioamnionitis [8, 9].

In the neonate, bacterial pneumonia is usually secondary to either sepsis or aspiration during sucking whereas older foals can have primary pneumonia. In a study involving 423 bacteremic neonatal foals, 79 foals (19%) were diagnosed with pneumonia while other studies have reported the prevalence of pneumonia in septic foals ranging from 28% to 50% (Figure 8.II.2) [11–14]. In a study involving 38 neonatal foals with confirmed sepsis, 5 foals (13%) presented with respiratory distress and 13 (34%) and 2 (5%) foals had pneumonia or pleuritis, respectively, as a complication of sepsis [13]. In that study, most foals initially had a normal respiratory rate and lung auscultation; as the disease process worsened, respiratory rate and lung sounds became abnormal [13]. Interestingly, 26/29 foals (90%) had respiratory abnormalities noted on necropsy, including pneumonia, pleuritis, atelectasis, emphysema, chronic alveolitis, and meconium aspiration, suggesting that the lower respiratory tract is frequently involved at a clinical or subclinical level in septic foals [13]. The most common bacterial organisms associated with pneumonia in neonates are similar to those that cause sepsis in foals (e.g. *E. coli*, *Klebsiella* spp., *Actinobacillus* spp., *Streptococcus* spp., and *Staphlococcus* spp) [13, 15, 16]. Foals with sepsis can also develop ALI or ARDS as part of the systemic response to sepsis, and this is frequently a contributor to the demise of foals in septic shock (see ARDS/ALI below).

Another frequent cause of bacterial pneumonia in the neonate arises from functional or anatomical disorders of the upper alimentary tract. Aspiration due to poor suck reflex or dysphagia can be associated with neonatal encephalopathy, sepsis, prematurity, hyperkalemic periodic paralysis, or weakness (Figures 8.II.3 and 8.II.4). Aspiration can also be associated with anatomic defects such as cleft palate, subepiglottic cysts, megaesophagus, vascular anomalies resulting in esophageal compression, or other causes of pharyngeal dysfunction. Multiple

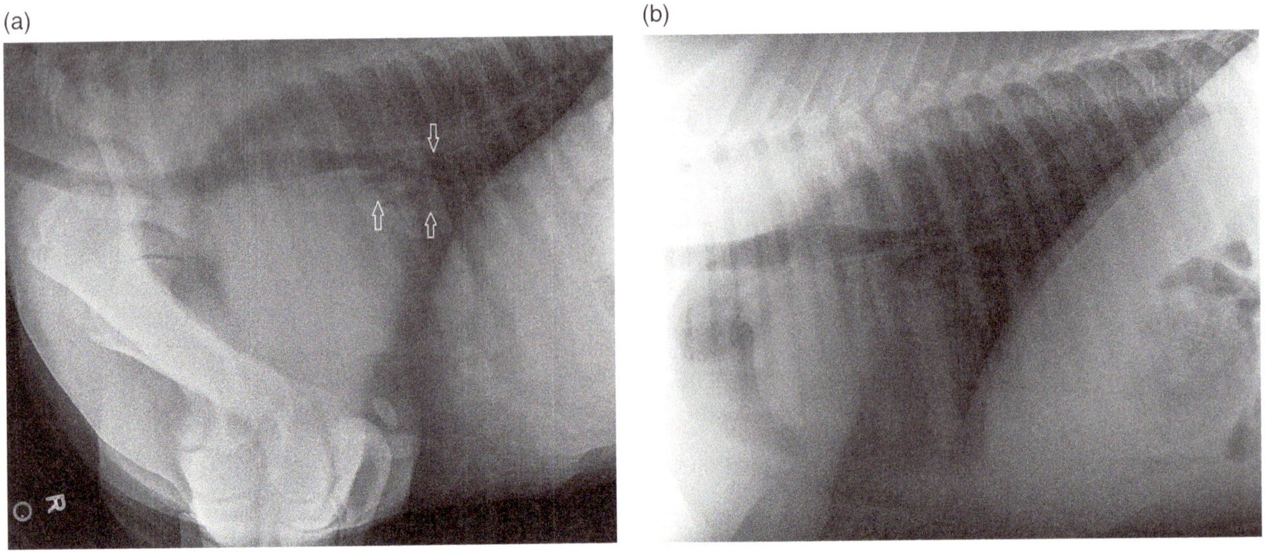

Figure 8.II.2 Lateral radiographs of a 7-day-old Gypsy Vanner colt presented for tachypnea and fever. (a) Within the caudoventral thorax is a patchy region of increase opacity that partially superimposes over the caudal portion of the cardiac silhouette. This consolidated region of pulmonary tissue also contains air bronchograms (arrows). These findings are consistent with bronchopneumonia. (b) Lateral radiograph of the same foal after 10 days of treatment demonstrating radiographic resolution of pneumonia.

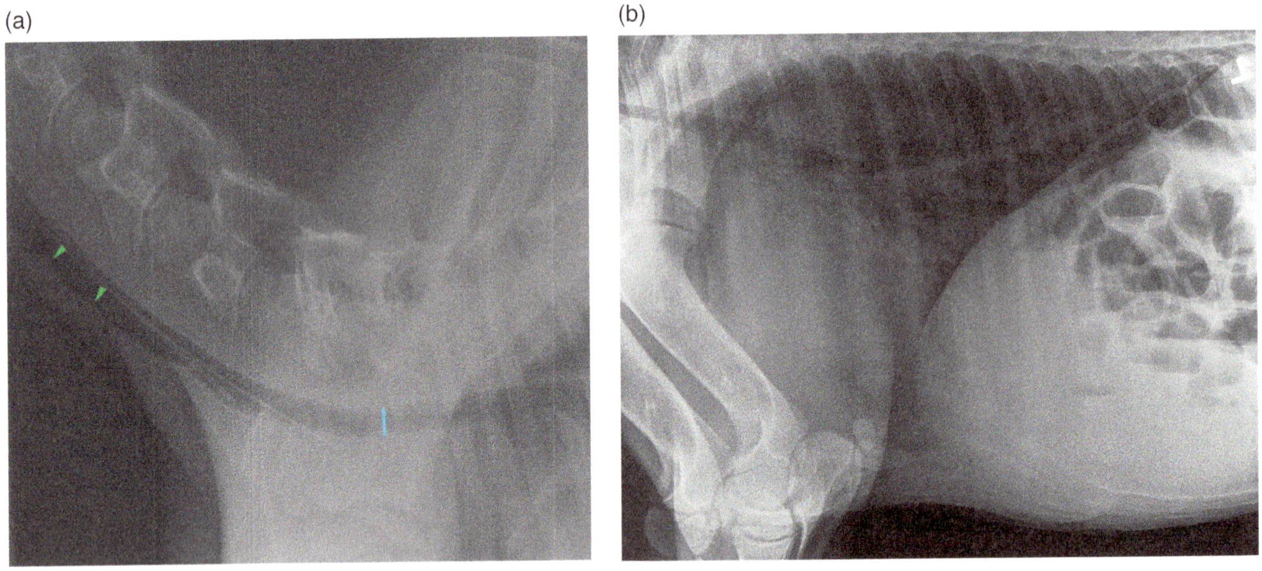

Figure 8.II.3 Lateral radiographs of a 6-day-old Tennessee Walking Horse filly presented with dysphagia and milk dripping from the nares since birth. (a) Tracheal material is observed in the ventral aspect of tracheal lumen (arrowheads). Note an IV catheter is placed in the jugular vein. (b) Moderate heterogenous increased opacity is present in the caudoventral aspect of the lung field partially superimposed with the cardiac silhouette. Ill-defined air-bronchograms are also noted. The alveolar pattern noted in the caudoventral lung is consistent with aspiration pneumonia.

organisms may be isolated from transtracheal aspirates (TTA) with this form of pneumonia. Care must be taken to ensure that aspiration is not iatrogenic in foals being bottle-fed. Foals receiving bottle-feedings should be maintained in sternal recumbency or standing. Additionally, foals with nasoesophogeal tubes in place for feeding should be kept in sternal recumbency or standing for 5 minutes following feeding to prevent passive esophageal regurgitation following changes in position of the head and neck. Some foals with neonatal encephalopathy and poor suck reflexes do not protect their airway well and will aspirate their own saliva, even when not allowed to suck from their dam or a

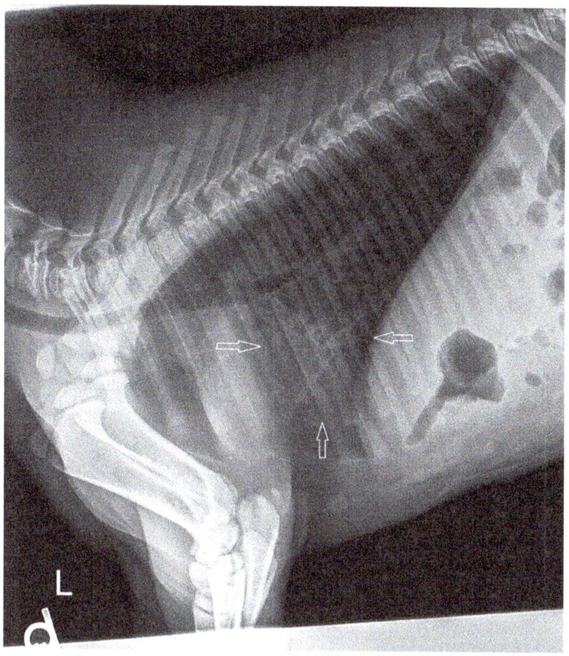

Figure 8.II.4 Lateral radiograph of a 1-day-old Miniature Donkey presented for neonatal encephalopathy. A mild patchy increased opacity in the caudal ventral portion of the lungs (arrows) consistent with pneumonia. The caudal margin of the cardiac silhouette is effaced by increased opacity.

bottle. Auscultation over the trachea while the foal is sucking helps identify occult aspiration in sucking foals. Occult aspiration pneumonia should be suspected in any critically ill neonate that is being bottle-fed, or is sucking on its own, that has unexplained fever, fails to gain weight, or has a persistently increased serum fibrinogen concentration.

Older foals develop bacterial pneumonia via inhalation and frequently secondary to an earlier viral infection. Stressors such as high ambient temperatures, weaning, and transportation serve as risk factors for development of pneumonia in older foals. Auscultation and percussion of the thorax should be performed, but results may not closely correlate with the severity of the disease. The most commonly isolated bacterial organism in this primary pneumonia is *S. zooepidemicus,* which can be isolated alone or as a component of a mixed infection. TTA for culture and cytology is recommended, as mixed Gram-positive and Gram-negative infections are common and antimicrobial susceptibility patterns can be unpredictable. The obtained TTA should be split and submitted for bacterial culture, virus isolation, and cytology. Ascarid larval migration through the lung can mimic bacterial pneumonia. In these cases, the foal might not respond to antimicrobial therapy and should be dewormed with anthelmintics. Deworming of the mare within 1 month of parturition and frequent deworming of the foal will prevent ascarid migration pneumonia in most cases.

R. equi is another common cause of pneumonia in foals between 3 weeks and 6 months of age at endemic farms [15]. Though clinical manifestations of *R. equi* such as pyogranulomatous bronchopneumonia with abscessation are typically not seen until 1–6 months of age (Figure 8.II.5), evidence suggests that foals are susceptible to infection at younger ages and become infected shortly after birth [17]. In an experimental setting, *R. equi* infection was more successful in foals <1 week of age and older foals (3 or 6 weeks old) had significantly lower numbers of bacteria isolated from their lungs when challenged with a specific dose of *R. equi* [17].

The incidence of *R. equi* pneumonia in exposed foals is associated with the infective agent, the foal's environment, and foal-specific factors [15, 18]. Regarding the infective agent, the expression of the virulence-associated plasmid (VapA) by *R. equi* is necessary for the development of pneumonia; additional plasmid-encoded genes might also influence virulence [19, 20]. VapA encodes a temperature-inducible surface-expressed lipoprotein and aids in preventing maturation of the phagasome to the stage of fusion of *R. equi*-containing vacuoles with lysosomes [21]. *R. equi* isolates that do not express VapA do not replicate in macrophages and fail to cause disease in foals. The foal's environment also contributes to the incidence of infection. In one study, the concentration of virulent *R. equi* in air samples over the first 2 weeks of life were higher in stalls or pens of foals that subsequently developed *R. equi* pneumonia versus foals that did not develop pneumonia [22]. In another study, higher airborne concentrations of *R. equi* were observed in stalls as compared to paddocks in horse breeding farms in Kentucky suggesting that foals in this environment are more likely to be exposed to airborne *R. equi* when housed in stalls [23]. Other environmental factors that might contribute to higher exposure *to R. equi* include higher densities of mares and foals [24] and dusty environmental conditions [2]. Finally, an individual foal's immune response and the status of an individual's immune system may contribute to the development of *R. equi* pneumonia [19]. Both the innate and adaptive immune responses are important for controlling *R. equi* infection [19, 21]. For example, total white blood cell (WBC) and neutrophil counts in foals that developed *R. equi* pneumonia were lower (2–4 weeks of age) then age-matched control foals [25], and neutrophil function may be decreased in affected foals, resulting in higher incidence of *R. equi* infection [26].

The incubation period for *R. equi* after experimental infection ranges from approximately 9–28 days and is partially dependent on the challenge dose of bacteria [2]. Once inhaled, *R. equi* is taken up by alveolar macrophages; virulent *R. equi* modifies the phagocytic vacuole that prevents acidification and subsequent fusion with lysosomes [2].

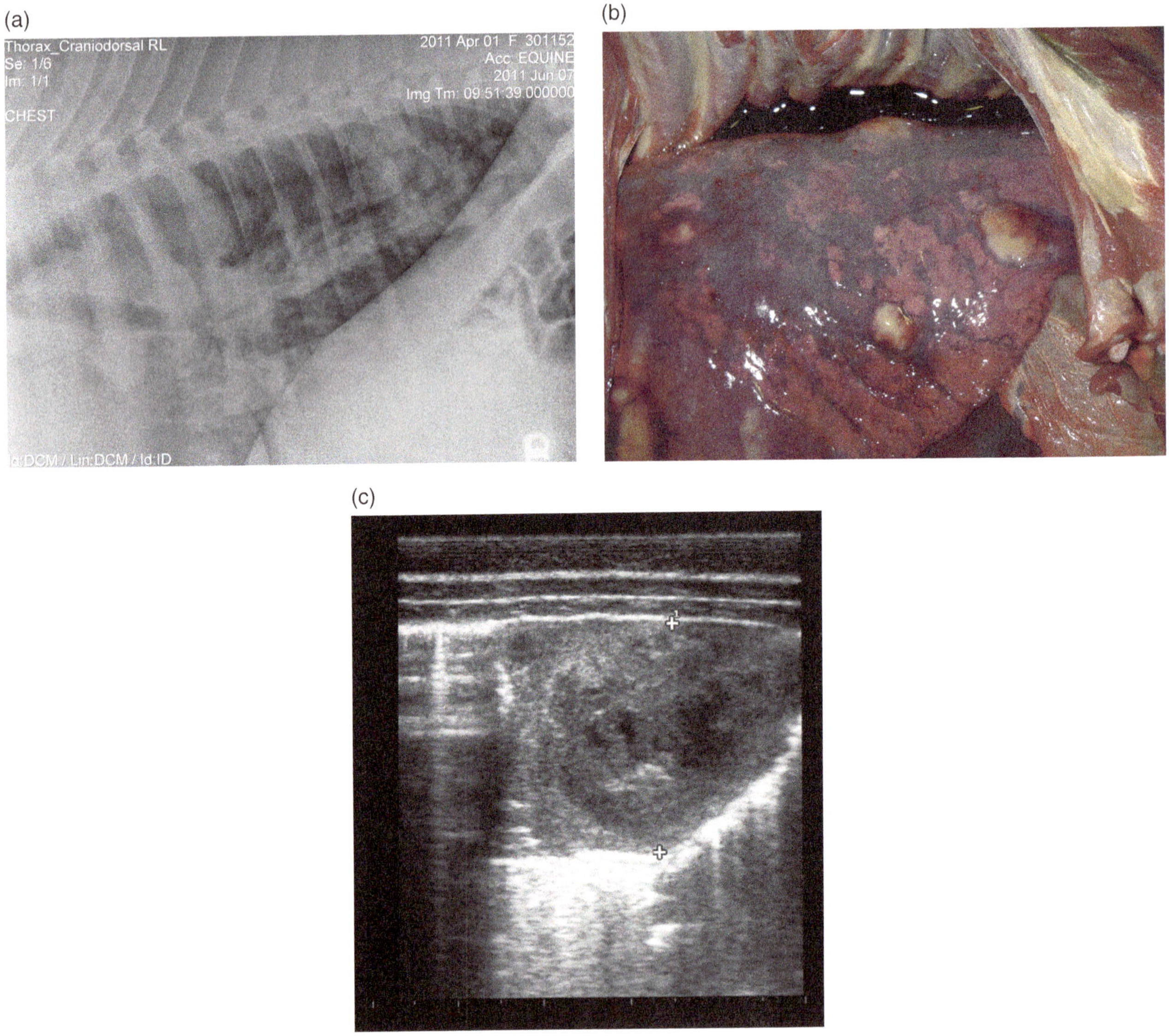

Figure 8.II.5 (a) Lateral radiograph of an 8-week-old foal with *R. equi* pneumonia. Note the areas of increased radiopacity suggestive of abscess formation. (b) Postmortem image of the lung demonstrating multiple *R. equi* abscesses. (c) Ultrasonogram of the thorax (same foal as B) demonstrating appearance of a peripheral lung abscess (24.5mm) caused by R. equi.

The bacteria are able to accommodate survival in the intracellular environment with uncontrolled intracellular replication of *R. equi* leading to necrosis of the macrophage [21]. Foals typically manifest clinical signs of *R. equi* pneumonia between 3 and 24 weeks of age, with most showing signs before 16 weeks of age [21]. The disease course is insidious and progressive with clinical signs variable and dependent on the stage and severity of pulmonary infection. Early clinical signs of infection include fever, lethargy, and cough with more advanced signs consisting of anorexia, tachycardia, tachypnea, nostril flare, and increased respiratory effort [21]. As the disease progresses, weight loss or failure to gain weight and an appearance of ill thrift may become apparent. In one report summarizing 161 cases of *R. equi* pneumonia, the most common clinical signs were cough (71%), fever (68%), lethargy (53%), and increased respiratory effort (43%) [27].

In addition to pneumonia that is associated with *R. equi* infection, a variety of extrapulmonary disorders (EPDs) have been linked to this organism. In one study, 74% of 150 foals with *R. equi* infection also had documented EPD(s) with a median number of 2 EPDs (range 0–9) among all foals [18]. Thus, some foals can have multiple EPDs concurrently; the clinician should also be aware that EPD can occur concurrently with or independent of pneumonia [18]. In fact, an EPDs such as polysynovitis (Figure 8.II.6) might be the first clinical manifestation of *R. equi* infection, prior to any respiratory signs of pneumonia. A list of EPD reported in one study is noted in Table 8.II.1.

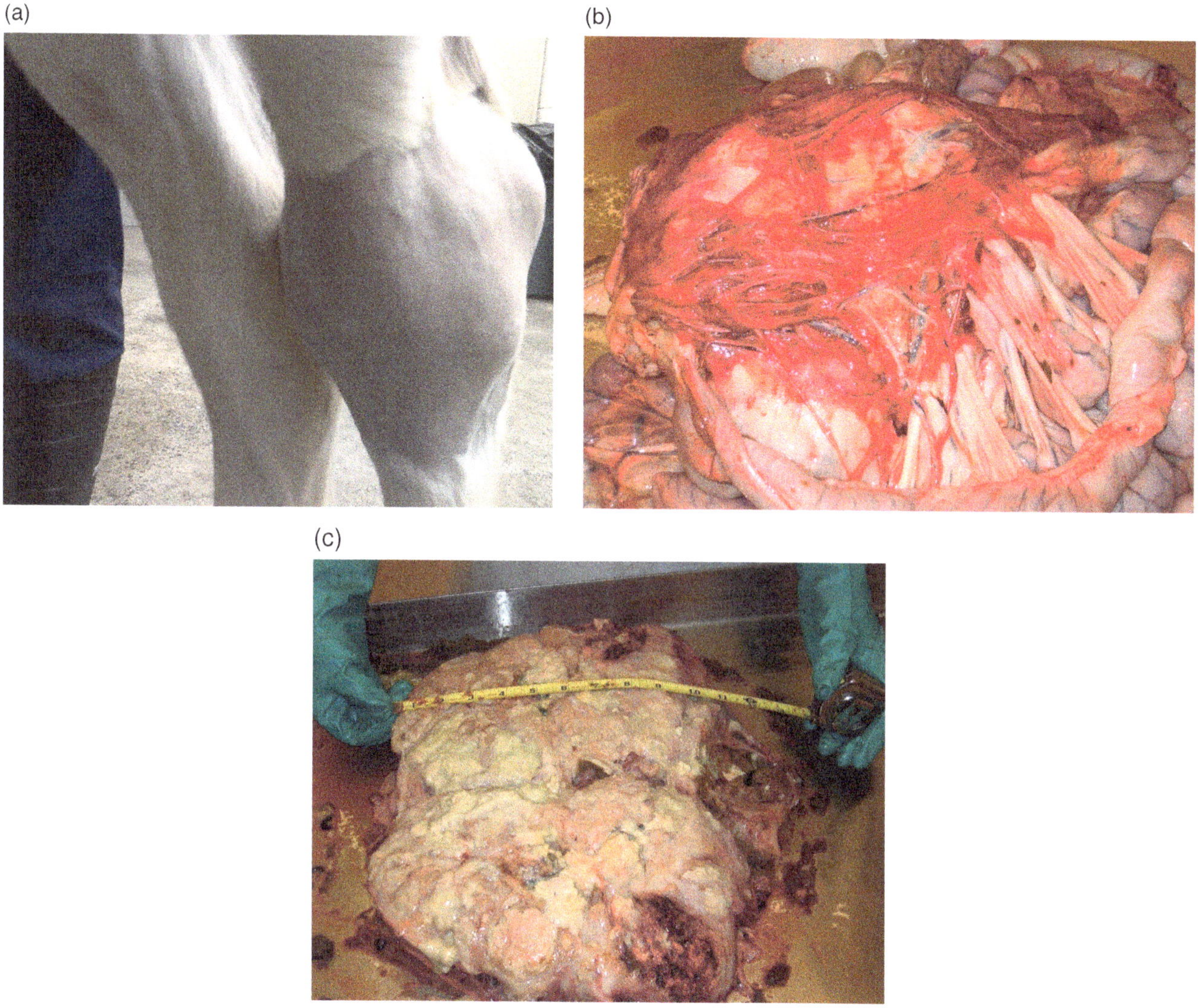

Figure 8.II.6 Extrapulmonary disorders in foals with *R. equi* infection. (a) Belgian foal with immune-mediated polysynovitis. Note the marked distention of the left tarsocrural joint. (b) Large *R. equi* abdominal abscess in a two-month-old foal presented for chronic intermittent colic and weight loss. (c) Same abdominal abscess as in B cut in section measuring approximately 12 in. across.

Table 8.II.1 Frequency of extrapulmonary disorders (EPDs) documented in a population of 150 foals with *R. equi* infection [18].

EPD	No. foals affected (%)	EPD	No. foals affected (%)
Diarrhea	50 (33)	Subcutaneous abscesses	8 (5)
Immune-mediated polysynovitis	37 (25)	Pyogranulomatous nephritis	7 (5)
Ulcerative enterotyphlocolitis	31 (21)	Hyperthermia	6 (4)
Intra-abdominal abscess	25 (17)	Pericarditis	6 (4)
Abdominal lymphadenitis	25 (17)	Osteomyelitis	5 (3)
Uveitis	16 (11)	Pleural effusion	5 (3)
Pyogranulomatous hepatitis	16 (11)	Pleural effusion	5 (3)
Septic synovitis	14 (9)	Granulomatous meningitis	5 (3)
Mediastinal lymphadenitis	12 (8)	Vertebral body osteomyelitis	3 (2)
Peritonitis	11 (7)	Paravertebral abscess	3 (2)
Peripheral lymphadenopathy	11 (7)	Cellulitis/lymphangitis	2 (1)
R. equi bacteremia	11 (7)	Immune-mediated hemolytic anemia	2 (1)

Viral Pneumonia

Viral pneumonia in the neonatal foal raises some distinct features of neonatology that differentiate this period of life from later periods, particularly adulthood, where most of the academic emphasis of host-pathogen interactions occurs. While the neonatal period is primarily viewed as a period of increased susceptibility to pathogens, recognizing and strategically addressing this window of increased susceptibility can yield more successful clinical outcomes regarding foals and general herd health.

Viral infections, such as equine herpesvirus (EHV-1), equine viral arteritis (EVA), and equine infectious anemia virus (EIAV) can be acquired in utero, resulting in severe disease at birth. Depending on risk and the viral pathogen, vaccination of the pregnant mare to favor passive transfer of pathogen-specific colostral antibodies to the neonate can not only aid in mitigating infection of the mare but also yield potential benefit to the fetus and neonate. Several factors can disrupt the desired transfer of maternal antibodies to the neonatal foal, including problems related to the foal (delayed colostral ingestion due to illness of the foal, musculoskeletal problems that interfere with standing to nurse) or maternal problems (premature lactation with colostral loss, decreased quality of colostrum due to age or failure to vaccinate the mare during pregnancy), but even with appropriate levels of protective colostral antibodies transferred from the dam, the foal is still potentially susceptible to many of the same respiratory pathogens that circulate among older horses.

Potential respiratory viruses affecting foals include, but are not limited to, equine adenovirus, EHV (-1, -2, -4, -5), equine rhinitis virus A, equine rhinitis virus B, equine influenza virus (EIV), equine parainfluenza virus, EVA and EIAV. The significance of each virus is context dependent. For example, equine adenovirus is reported sporadically but represents a significant problem in Arabian foals with severe combined immunodeficiency disease [28–30]. However, the most commonly identified causes of viral pneumonia in foals are EHV-1 and -4, EIV, and EVA. EHV-1 is likely the most clinically important in the neonatal period, but outbreaks of EVA in neonates can have equally untoward consequences [31–35].

Viral Entry via the Respiratory Tract

Most equine respiratory viruses enter an epithelial host cell of the respiratory tract and, following replication and budding, infect a neighboring epithelial cell with progeny virions. Host defenses include the mucociliary apparatus that operates by trapping virus particles in a layer of mucus, produced by goblet cells, and propelling the mucus blanket by ciliary action upward to the pharynx. The mucus is either swallowed or coughed out, along with the trapped virus particles. However, some virions may not be trapped in the mucus blanket and gain access to the more distal airways. Virus particles that traffic to the alveoli are often ingested by pulmonary-alveolar macrophages that reside in the alveoli. Nasal and bronchus-associated lymphoid aggregates bolster host defense mechanisms; however, despite these and other host immune defenses of the respiratory system, the respiratory tree represents the most common portal by which viruses gain entry to the host. Viruses have co-evolved with the host and thus it is not surprising that different viral strategies that circumvent host defenses have evolved, including specific attachment of a viral ligand to its cellular receptor, for example, on a respiratory epithelial cell. By binding to the cellular receptor, the virus can attach then potentially gain access to the interior of the epithelial cell and avoid clearance by phagocytes and the mucociliary apparatus, among other mechanisms.

The virus's attachment protein interacts with its corresponding cellular receptor. Receptors tend to be restricted to certain cell types, partially accounting for the tissue and organ tropism observed, and playing a key role in the pathogenesis of the disease caused by the virus. Cell or organ tropism refers to the ability of a virus to selectively infect particular cells, or by extension, organs. Viral attachment to the cellular receptor is a fundamental restriction point for entry and cell infection; other restriction points are also at play.

Respiratory viruses generally have a very short incubation period and can rapidly cause extensive damage to the respiratory epithelium by lateral cell-to-cell spread. Equine influenza (H3N8) is an example of a virus limited to the respiratory epithelium, but can be very virulent, causing significant, acute lung pathology. Once inside the cell, viruses undergo replication and bud; virus particles may either laterally infect a neighboring respiratory epithelial cell or invade other cell types, often gaining access to the blood and lymph systems for dissemination in the body. These two strategies reflect how a particular virus interfaces with the host. For example, if entry and exit of virus promote spread within the same cell type (e.g. respiratory epithelium), as occurs with influenza, then a "quick assault" with no viral persistence is typical. Directional release of virus into the lumen of the respiratory tract facilitates local spread to the surface of neighboring epithelial cells and rapid shedding into the environment. If, however, the virus employs a strategy involving subepithelial spread and buds from the basolateral cell surface, the virus may be disseminated by blood or lymph vessels, seed central organs of replication (e.g. bone marrow, liver spleen or vascular endothelium), and then infect target organs, resulting in a longer infection. Viruses that circulate in blood, and particularly those that circulate free in plasma, encounter vascular endothelial cells and macrophages, cell types that exert especially important roles in determining the subsequent pathogenesis of infection. Subepithelial spread and viremia, either cell free or cell-associated, appear to be important aspects of virus replication that favor fetal infection.

Viral Tropism as a Factor in Placental and Fetal Infection Leading to Perinatal Pneumonia

Viruses that undergo a period of viremia are often phagocytosed and processed for presentation by antigen presenting cells, including monocytes/macrophages or dendritic cells. However, some viruses target macrophages and efficiently replicate in this cell type. From the draining lymph node, viruses may spread to target organs either within a cell or as cell-free virus. The lungs, liver, and spleen are typical target organs infected by viruses egressing from the draining lymph node.

EHV-1, EAV, and EIAV all infect monocytes/macrophages and endothelial cells [32, 36–38]. Carriage of virus inside monocytes/macrophages that emigrate through the walls of small blood vessels, sometimes referred to as the "Trojan horse" mechanism of invasion, is a shared feature of these viruses. In general, cell-associated viruses are more protected from antibodies and other plasma components, including complement, inside a leukocyte where they can reside as "protected passengers." Frequently, cell-associated viruses also gain access to tissues as the leukocytes traffic out of the bloodstream. EHV-1, EAV, and EIAV have the potential to infect fetuses and cause abortion or perinatal pneumonia.

Viruses that gain access to the vasculature may passively exit between or through the endothelium and basement membrane of venules or arterioles, pass through in emigrating leukocytes (Trojan horse mechanism), or directly infect the luminal aspect of endothelial cells with subsequent budding to the basal aspect. EHV-1, EVA, and EIAV can all infect endothelial cells and result in a vasculitis and production of microthrombi at sites of denuded endothelium. Virus-induced endothelial injury leads to coagulation and vascular thrombosis and, if widespread, disseminated intravascular coagulation (DIC). However, it is likely that inflammatory and vasoactive mediators produced by virus-infected macrophages and dendritic cells, including tissue necrosis factor (TNF), also contribute to the pathogenesis of vascular injury. Damaged endothelium is an underlying aspect of abortion in mares infected with EHV-1 and EVA.

Specific Viral Pathogens Associated with Neonatal Pneumonia in the Foal

Equine Herpesvirus-1 (EHV-1)

Monocytes are the main cells that transport EHV-1 during primary infection and serve as the "Trojan horse" since they aid in dissemination of virions to target organs [39]. EHV-1 mediated induction of TNF-α by monocytes increases adhesion of monocytes to endothelial cells via integrins, thereby facilitating infection of target organs, namely the vasculature of the lung, uterus, and endothelium of vessels serving the central nervous system (CNS), especially the sacral segments. Vasculitis and microthrombosis of infected tissues result. Moreover, production of TNF-α by monocytes leads to maturation of monocytes to macrophages with increased production and release of virus [39]. Common clinical signs include mild nasal discharge and fever due to epithelial cell infection and swelling of the submandibular and retropharyngeal lymph nodes [36]. Foals with EHV-1 may be icteric and have petechial hemorrhages, with leukopenia and neutropenia noted on CBC; however, these changes can be encountered in foals with severe sepsis [40]. Once infected leukocytes traffic and adhere to endothelial cells, infection of the uterine microcotyledonary tufts might result in abortion or premature delivery; infection of the fetus may result in fetal death or pneumonia at birth [36]. Transplacental EHV-1 infection in a near-term fetus often results in an infected foal born alive but subsequently succumbing to disease within a few days, regardless of respiratory support and advanced care. EHV-4 causes rhinopneumonitis in young horses but does not appear to be a factor in neonatal pneumonia, perhaps due to lower to absent levels of viremia during infection [41].

Equine Arteritis Virus

EAV replicates in monocytes/macrophages and endothelial cells; viremia is sustained by infection of endothelial cells, monocytes/macrophages and dendritic cells. EAV also replicates in a small subpopulation of $CD3^+$ T cells [42, 43]. CXCL16, an important receptor for EAV, is a type 1 membrane protein expressed on monocytes, macrophages, and endothelial cells [44, 45]. However, evidence indicates that CXCL16 is not the only receptor used. Cell tropism, partially defined by the EAV receptor used, helps to explain the tissues targeted by viral infection, and by extension, the pathology caused by virus replication that leads to a range of disease manifestations. In the case of EAV, the spectrum of disease includes inapparent infection to abortion, fatal hemorrhagic fever, or pneumonia [46]. In neonatal foals, severe interstitial pneumonia has been documented, often with a fatal outcome [47, 48].

Equine Infectious Anemia Virus

EIAV replicates in cells of the monocyte lineage, including macrophages, and endothelial cells [37, 38]. The cellular receptor that mediates EIAV entry into target cells is known as equine lentivirus receptor-1 (ELR1) and is encoded by the TNF receptor superfamily member 14 (*TNFRSF14*) gene, which is expressed on the surface of equine macrophages [49]. Transplacental infection with EIAV is considered exceedingly rare; however, in utero transmission has been documented in an aborted fetus at 8 months gestation [50]. More commonly, foals born to mares infected with EIAV acquire colostral antibodies that result in seropositivity to diagnostic tests, yet these foals may be uninfected [51]. EIAV infection in older horses can cause a bronchointerstitial pneumonia with lymphocytic infiltrates in the alveolar walls, not unlike lentiviral infections in other species [52]. In summary, EIAV infection is a possible, but unlikely, cause of perinatal pneumonia in foals and determination of EIAV infection in neonates should consider acquisition of maternal antibodies to EIAV (p26); demonstration of circulating cell-free virus by RT-PCR would be strong evidence for viral infection of a neonatal foal.

Equine Influenza Virus

EIV is a viral respiratory disease in which replication is limited to the respiratory epithelium. Infection often progresses rapidly and is self-limiting in that it quickly exhausts available epithelial cells to infect. Subepithelial tissues may be found to contain viruses restricted to the respiratory epithelium, pointing out that other restriction points in the virus replication cycle are at play. Virulence and disease severity may vary with upper respiratory tract viral infections, with EIV being notably severe in some instances, leading to ARDS or death, especially in neonates born to unvaccinated, naïve mares [53]. In neonatal foals born to vaccinated mares, EIV tends to be less commonly observed due to acquired passive immunity. In a longitudinal study, serum antibody levels to influenza A waned rapidly within 4 weeks, with 50% of foals being seronegative, demonstrating that passively derived antibodies are short-lived [54]. However, foals consuming colostrum lacking antibodies against EIV are particularly susceptible to infection and severe disease [55]. Collectively, passive immunity appears to be protective throughout the neonatal period, but the duration of protection in foals is brief.

EIV infects and kills ciliated epithelial cells lining the nasopharynx and trachea, producing an upper respiratory disease characterized by a dry, paroxysmal cough, fever, and serous nasal discharge [56]. Shedding of live virus is variable and can persist for 7–10 days. A secondary bacterial pneumonia is frequent due to loss of epithelium and mucociliary clearance mechanisms. Since EIV produces a localized infection, the feto-placental unit is spared, and infection of a neonate would necessarily occur after birth.

Miscellaneous Respiratory Viruses

Less frequently detected viruses in younger horses that have been linked to febrile respiratory disease include EHV-2 and -5, equine adenovirus, equine rhinitis A virus, equine rhinitis B virus, and equine parainfluenza virus [57], all of which do not have commercial vaccines available currently. Nonetheless, circulation of these viruses in the equine population can lead to transfer of protective colostral antibodies to neonates, with waning neutralizing antibody levels by 5–6 months of age. In one longitudinal study, antibodies to equine rhinitis A virus were detected in neonates, waned significantly in weanlings, and were very low or absent in yearlings [58].

Equine Rhinitis A Virus

Equine rhinitis A virus (previously equine rhinovirus 1) – is a picornavirus of the Aphthovirus genus found widely in the equine population. The disease course is characterized by an acute upper respiratory tract infection following a 3- to 8-day incubation period. Clinical signs include nasal discharge and cough with a pharyngitis and lymphadenitis. While clinical signs are limited to the upper respiratory tract, virus may be detected in nasal secretions as well as blood, feces, and urine, consistent with systemic spread. Prolonged shedding is typical and serum antibodies are widely detected in the equine population; however, equine rhinitis A virus is not typically documented as a pathogen in neonates [59].

Equine rhinitis B virus (previously equine rhinovirus 2) – is a picornavirus and the only member of the Erbovirus genus (erbovirus A) with three recognized serotypes. Equine rhinitis B viruses have a worldwide distribution and have been increasingly diagnosed over time in horses of all ages with acute fever and respiratory signs [60]; however, equine rhinitis B virus has not been recognized as a significant pathogen in neonates [59, 61].

Equine adenovirus has been diagnosed as a problem in SCID foals with waning maternal antibodies [28]. Otherwise, it is infrequently detected and has only been reported in immunocompetent horses older than a year of age [57].

Fungal Pneumonia

Although rare, a few case reports have documented various fungal infections, including *Cryptococcus*, *Histoplasma*, *Aspergillus*, and *Coccidioides*, as a cause of pneumonia in the equine fetus or foal [62–65]. In one case, an American Paint horse aborted a 9-month-old fetus and upon necropsy examination, the fetal lungs were firmer than normal along with a large amount of straw-colored fluid within the thorax [62]. Upon culture of the lung sections, *Cryptococcus neoformans* was identified and histologic examination documented moderate, diffuse interstitial pneumonia. Focal hepatic necrosis and suppurative inflammation and necrosis of the spleen was also identified. Although this case resulted in abortion, it is plausible that a newborn foal could be infected with fungi. In another case, *Cryptococcus* was identified in a 1-month-old Arabian foal with severe dyspnea and fever that subsequently died. Histologic examination of the deceased foal revealed severe diffuse interstitial pneumonia with macrophages containing *Cryptococcus* [63]. The following year, the same mare aborted a fetus that had Cryptococcal organisms within the lung; in addition, the fetal membranes contained many of the same organisms [63]. *Histoplasma capsulatum* has also been documented to cause severe granulomatous pneumonia in aborted fetuses or neonatal foals who can display signs of lethargy, weakness, dyspnea, and tachycardia [64]. *Coccidioides immitis* was the cause of severe mycotic pneumonia in a 13-day-old Thoroughbred filly presented for a 7-day history of fever, tachypnea, and leucocytosis [66]. A severe diffuse miliary pattern and pleural irregularities were documented on thoracic radiographs and ultrasound, respectively. The filly was severely hypoxemic (PaO_2 49 mmHg) and was euthanized because of a lack of response to therapy. Upon necropsy, the lungs were diffusely infiltrated with a miliary pattern of multiple, coalescing, firm foci (0.1–0.5 cm in diameter) characterized microscopically by pyogranulomatous inflammation with numerous *C. immitis* observed. The diffuse nature of the foal's lesions was proposed to be due to inhalation from the external environment after birth, aspiration of infected amniotic fluid in utero, or hematogenous spread [66]. In cases of confirmed fungal involvement in the fetus/foal, the mare's reproductive tract should be thoroughly examined as this can serve as a source of infection to the fetus/foal [63, 64, 67]. A few cases of fungal pneumonia from *Candida albicans* and *Pneumocystis carinii* have also been documented in foals with severe systemic disease [68] or immunodeficiency [69, 70]. Antifungals such as voriconazole, amphotericin B, and dapsone have been administered to foals with fungal pneumonia with variable success. The reader is referred to a review of antifungal medications in horses if needed [71].

Parasitic Pneumonia

Clinical pneumonia resulting from parasites is less frequently considered but is a potential cause of respiratory signs in the foal. Parasites such as *Parascaris equorum*, *Dictyocaulus arnfieldi*, *Strongyloides westeri*, and *Strongylus vulgaris* have been implicated as causes of parasitic pneumonia in foals [72–74]. Of these parasites, *P. equorum* is more commonly recognized in the foal as this parasite is typically observed in young horses, particularly weanling age foals. In contrast, *P. equorum* is not commonly observed in healthy adult horses because of their ability to obtain acquired immunity. *P. equorum* has a direct life cycle. The egg is not infective until it contains a larva and embryonation depends on the climate (ideally 25–35 °C, but not above 39 °C) and occurs in 1 week [75]. Interestingly, the larvae can remain viable within soil for up to five years in cool climates [75]. The embryonated eggs are ingested by the foal and the larvae are released from the egg within the small intestine. The larvae then travel through the portal vessels to the liver over the next week and migrate through the liver. This migration results in a fibroblastic reaction that can be seen grossly as white mottling within the liver [76]. The larvae enter the hepatic vein, then travel through the vena cava, heart, and pulmonary artery and capillaries to reach the alveoli. The larvae are present within the bronchi within 16 days of infection and then travel up the trachea via the mucociliary apparatus and are swallowed. The larvae subsequently develop into adults within the small intestine and lay eggs in 7–14 days [73, 75]. *D. arnfieldi* also has a direct life cycle. The infective third-stage larvae are ingested and penetrate the intestinal wall to enter the mesenteric lymphatics. Larvae then migrate to the lungs via the lymphatic system and mature in peripheral bronchi. After approximately 2 months, adults lay eggs in the bronchi; the eggs and larvae ascend by the mucociliary apparatus and are swallowed. The eggs mature to larvae within the host and larvae are then passed in the feces. Once in the environment, maturation to infective larvae occurs within 5–7 days [73]. Larval development is arrested in the horse with patency only occurring in donkeys, mules, and asses. Thus, lungworms should be suspected in horses housed with donkeys or mules.

Although clinical signs of *P. equorum* are more commonly associated with the digestive tract (colic, enteritis, ill-thrift, reduced weight gain), the presence of migrating larvae and adult worms in the lung parenchyma and bronchi can result in an immune-mediated bronchopneumonia. The release of IgE, mast cells, and basophils cause release of histamine and eosinophilic chemotactic factor [75]. Eosinophilic cytoplasmic granules contain major basic protein, peroxidase, and reactive oxygen species that serve to combat the parasite but can also damage the surrounding respiratory cells, thus resulting in an interstitial pneumonia and regions of pulmonary necrosis [75]. The parasites can also directly damage the alveoli and plug bronchioles and small bronchi resulting in adventitial lung sounds. Mucoid to mucopurulent exudate can accumulate as a result of larvae within the lumen [73]. The exudate as well as dead parasites can occlude the small bronchioles and contribute to the development of secondary bacterial infections. Clinical signs of respiratory involvement include coughing, exercise intolerance, and mucopurulent nasal discharge (may occur due to concurrent secondary bacterial infection). Respiratory signs typically develop 11–13 days post-infection and precede intestinal manifestations [76, 77]. Additional nonspecific signs such as anorexia and lethargy have been observed [76]. Other causes of parasitic pneumonia, outside of *P. equorum*, display similar signs such as persistent cough, nasal discharge, lethargy, exercise intolerance, dsypnea, and in some cases fever [75, 78]. Crackles or wheezes might be noted on thoracic auscultation and clinical signs commonly persist despite therapy for nonspecific bacterial respiratory infections [73].

Acute Respiratory Distress Syndrome

ARDS describes severe pulmonary dysfunction and respiratory failure secondary to an exaggerated pulmonary immune response triggered by an intra- or extrapulmonary insult [79]. Injury to the alveolar epithelial–endothelial barrier can occur directly due to pulmonary insults, with primary damage to the lung epithelium, or indirectly due to extrapulmonary insults, with primary damage to the vascular endothelium as a result of systemic inflammation, or, most commonly, both [79]. The definition of ARDS in human medicine has been updated and refined over the years and is currently described as an acute onset of respiratory distress (<1 week after a known insult), combined with the presence of bilateral pulmonary opacities and respiratory failure not fully explained by cardiac failure or fluid overload. Based on the degree of hypoxemia, measured by the ratio of partial arterial oxygen pressure (PaO_2) to the fraction of inspired oxygen (FiO_2), three severities are differentiated in adult human patients: mild (PaO_2/FiO_2 >200 and ≤300 mmHg), moderate (>100 and ≤200 mmHg), and severe ARDS (≤100 mmHg) [80, 81]. The term ALI, initially used to describe a less severe form, is no longer used in people [82] but still used in the definition for veterinary acute lung injury (VetALI) and veterinary acute respiratory distress syndrome (VetARDS) that was published in 2007 [83]. The veterinary definitions were developed during a consensus meeting that predated the more current human (Berlin) definition. Importantly, it included adjustments for physiological differences in arterial oxygenation in foals <1 week of age, which were addressed by different inclusion criteria for this age group [83]. A simplified version of the equine criteria (Tables 8.II.2 and 8.II.3) is based on normal published values [84]. A different disease presentation in neonatal foals with presumed

Table 8.II.2 Normal partial pressures of arterial oxygen (PaO_2) [84, 85] and suggested PaO_2 to fraction of inspired oxygen (FiO_2) ratios for diagnosis of acute respiratory distress syndrome (ARDS) in neonatal foals up to 1 week of age.

Postnatal age	Normal PaO_2 (mmHg) breathing room air	Normal PaO_2/FiO_2 ratio (mmHg)	PaO_2/FiO_2 ratio for ARDS diagnosis (mmHg)
1 h	61 ± 3	>300	<175
12 h	74 ± 3	>350	<200
24 h	68 ± 4	>300	<200
48 h	75 ± 3	>350	<200
4 d	81 ± 3	>400	<250
7 d	90 ± 3	>430	<280

Source: Adapted from Wilkins [83].

Table 8.II.3 Definition of Veterinary Acute Respiratory Distress Syndrome (ARDS) – must meet at least one each of the first four criteria; 5 is a recommended but optional measure.

1) Acute onset (<72 hours) of tachypnea and labored breathing at rest
2) Presence of a known risk factor
   - Inflammation
   - Infection
   - Sepsis
   - Multiple transfusions
   - Smoke inhalation
   - Systemic Inflammatory Response Syndrome (SIRS)
   - Aspiration of stomach contents
   - Severe trauma (long bone fracture, head injury, pulmonary contusion)
3) Evidence of pulmonary capillary leak without increased pulmonary capillary pressure; one or more of the following:
   - Bilateral/diffuse infiltrates on thoracic radiographs
   - Bilateral dependent density gradient on CT
   - Proteinaceous fluid within conducing airways
   - Increased extravascular water
4) Evidence of inefficient gas exchange (any one or more of the following):
   - Hypoxemia without PEEP or CPAP and known FiO_2:
     i) PaO_2/FiO_2 Ratio ≤300 mmHg for ARDS
     ii) Increased alveolar-arterial oxygen gradient
     iii) Venous admixture (noncardiac shunt)
   - Increased "dead-space" ventilation
5) Evidence of diffuse pulmonary inflammation:
   - Transtracheal wash/bronchoalveolar lavage sample neutrophilia
   - Transtracheal wash/bronchoalveolar lavage biomarkers of inflammation
   - Molecular imaging (PET)

Source: Adapted from Wilkins [83].

pulmonary surfactant deficiency (termed neonatal equine respiratory distress syndrome; NERDS) secondary to very early gestational age, induction of parturition, or cesarean section was also included (see below) [83].

ARDS arises as a complication after major infectious or noninfectious bodily injury. The triggering event can be an intrapulmonary (viral or bacterial pneumonia, smoke inhalation, near drowning, food aspiration) or extrapulmonary (trauma, multiple transfusions, systemic inflammatory response, sepsis) insult. During injury or infections, the body mounts a protective response that involves controlled activation of the inflammatory and coagulation system [86, 87]. The pathophysiology of ARDS is centered on dysregulation of this initially protective response. Uncontrolled pulmonary inflammation and coagulation lead to accumulation and activation of leukocytes and platelets in the lungs, altered permeability of the pulmonary endothelial and epithelial barrier, and ultimately accumulation of extravascular protein-rich edema fluid within the alveoli and airways (Figure 8.II.7) [87, 88]. Classically, an initial exudative phase, a fibroproliferative phase, and, if the patient survives, a resolving or fibrotic phase have been described, but these phases are not temporally distinct and largely overlap [89]. The exudative phase is characterized by uncontrolled release of inflammatory mediators and influx of inflammatory cells into the pulmonary tissue. Activated platelets, neutrophils, and alveolar macrophages marginate in the microcirculation and extravasate into the pulmonary tissue where they release inflammatory mediators and agents that amplify inflammation and coagulation [90]. A variety of mediators, pathways, and molecular systems contribute to the breakdown of the alveolar endothelial and epithelial barrier, causing flooding of the alveoli once the edema safety factors are exhausted. The barrier tends to collapse suddenly, resulting in rapid filling of the alveoli with proteinaceous exudate, leukocytes, and red blood cells and destruction of the surfactant layer (Figure 8.II.8) [91]. The rapid onset of pulmonary edema may correspond with the clinically observed acute onset of respiratory distress in some foals. The pro-thrombotic and anti-fibrinolytic environment favors formation of thrombi in the pulmonary microvasculature and deposition of intra-alveolar fibrin-rich hyaline membranes [92]. The fibroproliferative response, which can begin within 24 hours, is characterized by type I pneumocyte necrosis and proliferation of the more resistant type II pneumocytes in an attempt to restore the epithelial surface (Figure 8.II.9) [91, 93]. Fibroblasts invade the pulmonary interstitium and deposit collagen. In people, this can result in fibrosis and permanent impairment of pulmonary mechanics and gas exchange.

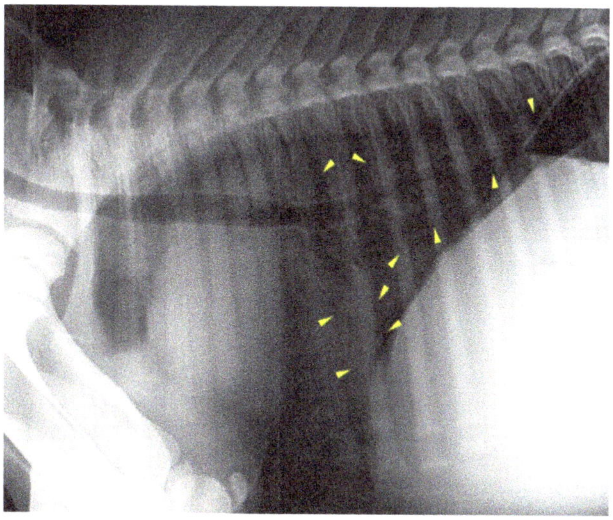

Figure 8.II.7 Right lateral radiograph of a 4-day-old Gypsy Vanner filly. A moderate, diffuse alveolar-interstitial pattern is noted. Air bronchograms are noted diffusely throughout the lung field (arrows). Differential diagnoses included diffuse interstitial pneumonia or pulmonary edema.

Clinically, the extensive pulmonary pathology (Figure 8.II.10) leads to severe hypoxemia with hypo- or hypercapnia caused by ventilation-perfusion (V/Q) mismatch and decreased pulmonary compliance. Alveolar edema creates areas with a low V/Q ratio (adequate perfusion but no ventilation) causing hypoxemia, whereas areas with deceased perfusion generate hypoxemia and eventually hypercapnia by increasing dead space ventilation (high V/Q ratio; adequate ventilation with minimal perfusion) [91]. The coexistence of areas with high and low V/Q ratios adjacent to normal lung tissue makes mechanical ventilation of ARDS patients challenging and predisposes the patient to ventilator-induced lung injury. The resolution of ARDS requires repair of endothelial and epithelial barriers, reabsorption of alveolar edema, and removal of inflammatory exudate and cellular debris [87]. If damage to the pulmonary epithelium is minor, pulmonary edema can be cleared swiftly, pulmonary function improves rapidly, and chances of survival increase. If large areas of alveolar epithelium are destroyed, gradual re-epitheliazation must occur first [87, 94]. Severe damage to the epithelium corresponds with prolonged respiratory failure, slow recovery, and high mortality [95]. Recovering human patients may have complete resolution of pulmonary compromise or may suffer from debilitating residual functional impairment.

In early reports, foals with ARDS were also referred to as acute interstitial or bronchointerstitial pneumonia with the condition described in foals and weanlings up to 7 months of age [53, 96–101]. With increasing understanding of the pathophysiology of ARDS, it is evident that multiple infectious and noninfectious agents are capable of initiating the inflammatory response [96–99]. In foals, the most common risk factor appears to be intrapulmonary

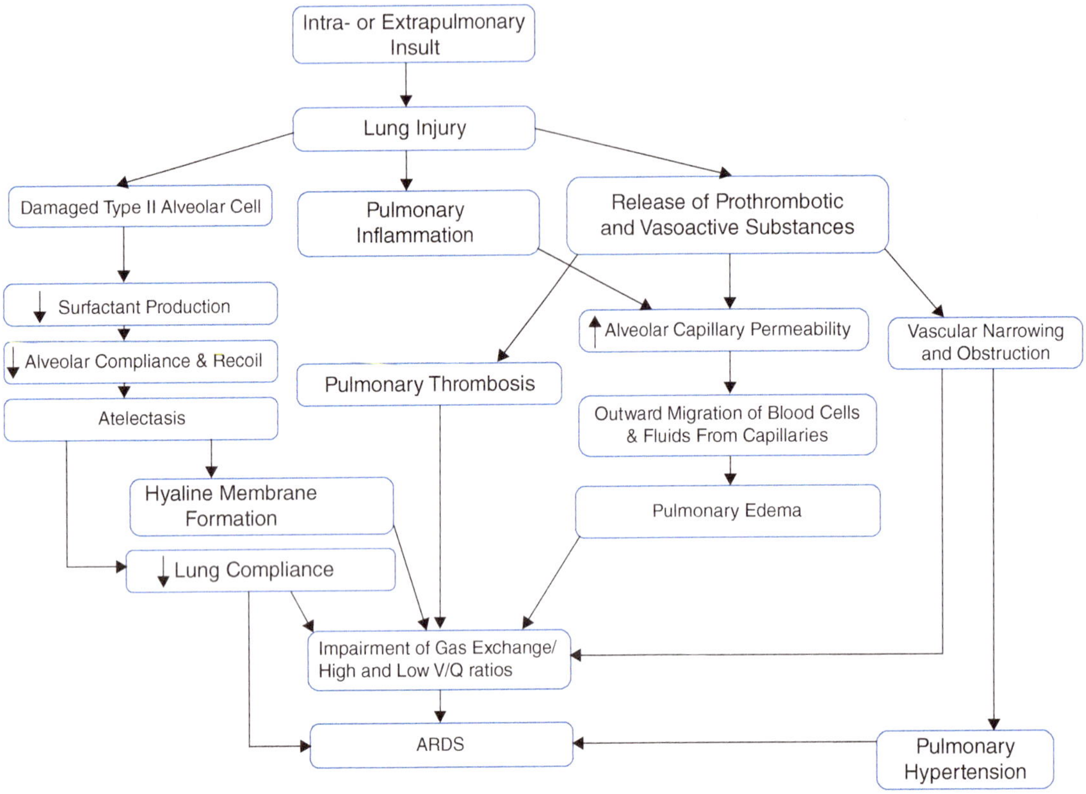

Figure 8.II.8 Schematic representation of some of the mechanisms that contribute to the pathophysiology of ARDS.

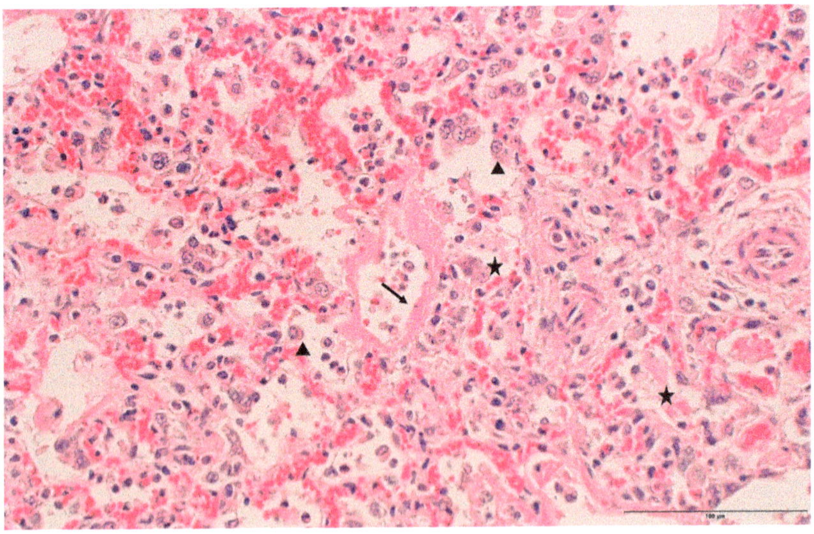

Figure 8.II.9 Microscopic image from a foal with acute respiratory distress syndrome (ARDS). Alveolar walls are frequently lined by amphophilic material referred to as hyaline membranes (arrow) or hypertrophied type II pneumocytes (arrowhead). Alveolar spaces often contain eosinophilic wispy material, macrophages with abundant cytoplasm and scattered neutrophils (star). Source: Image courtesy of Dr. Rebecca Ruby, University of Kentucky.

injury, namely bacterial or, rarely, viral pneumonia [96–102]. It is currently unknown why a small number of foals with bacterial or viral pneumonia develop ARDS while most others with similar primary disease processes do not. In people, environmental and individual risk factors might predispose certain patients to the development of ARDS. Genetic studies have focused on identifying variations in genes linked to the immune response, vascular permeability, fibrosis, inflammation, and immune cell migration that might increase the risk of ARDS [87, 103].

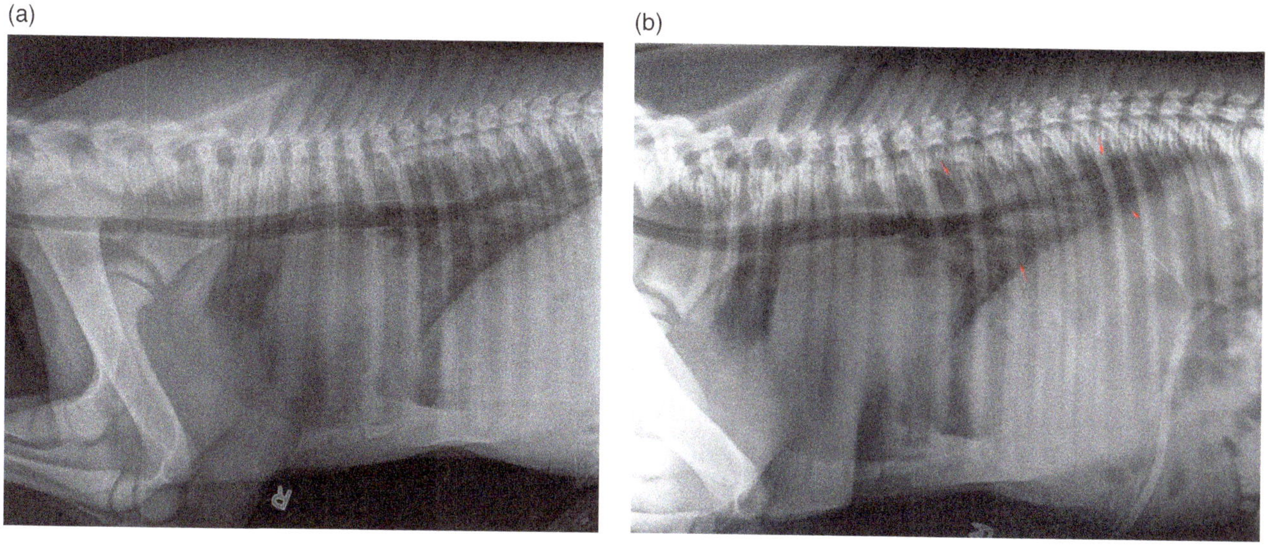

Figure 8.II.10 Four-day-old Paint colt with a history of premature placental separation. (a and b) The foal was recumbent and unable to stand and had increased bronchovesicular lung sounds on auscultation. Respiratory effort increased over the 24 hours prior to acquisition of thoracic radiographs. Increased opacity of the caudal lung field that markedly or completely obscured the pulmonary vessels was noted radiographically with multiple air bronchograms (arrows) noted bilaterally; these findings were consistent with ALI-ARDS and/or immaturity of the lungs.

Neonatal Equine Respiratory Distress Syndrome (NERDS)/Hyaline Membrane Disease

NERDS, previously called hyaline membrane disease, is defined as a distinct disease process from VetALI/VetARDS due to its different pathogenesis [83]. The underlying cause of the progressive respiratory failure is pulmonary immaturity leading to surfactant deficiency and dysfunction. The disease predominately affects foals born or delivered prematurely before surfactant production is fully established [104]. Pulmonary surfactant maturation in foals begins at or after 88% of gestational length (approximately 300 days) but remains incomplete until full term and continues after delivery [105]. Predisposing risk factors include gestational age of 290 days or less or <88% of the dam's average gestation lengths, a history of induced parturition, or cesarean section. Respiratory function can be compromised from birth or might initially appear normal with respiratory difficulties quickly becoming apparent. Over the next 24–48 hours, progressive atelectasis and respiratory failure and fatigue develop [106]. Clinically, persistent tachypnea, nostril flaring, and a paradoxical breathing pattern might be seen. With paradoxical breathing, the chest wall moves inward on inspiration and out on expiration, opposite to the normal movement and can be seen with fatigue of the respiratory muscles or traumatic injury to the chest wall (flail chest). Within 24 hours, a "ground glass" appearance is present on thoracic radiographs, which progresses to a dense interstitial to alveolar pattern with air bronchograms (Figures 8.II.11 and 8.II.12). Arterial blood gas (ABG) analysis identifies persistent hypoxemia (PaO_2

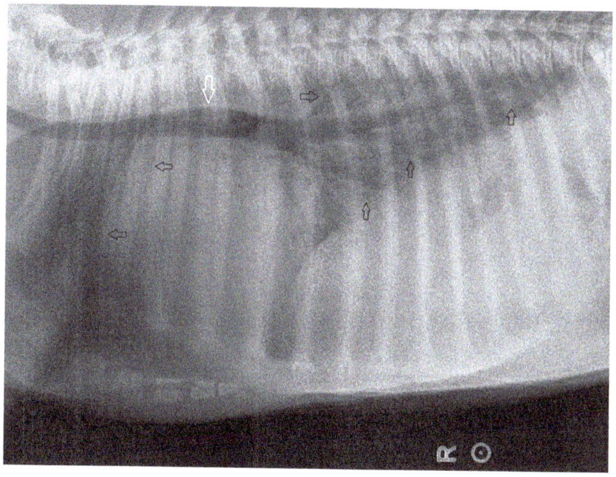

Figure 8.II.11 Newborn Thoroughbred colt with dysmaturity presented for labored breathing and green nasal discharge at birth. A respiratory (PCO_2 132 mmHg) acidemia (pH 6.982) was documented via venous blood gas analysis. A marked diffuse increased opacity in the entire lung field with evidence of air bronchograms throughout (black arrows) was observed via lateral radiograph. The trachea was slightly elevated (white arrow) and the cardiac silhouette appeared enlarged. This diffuse alveolar pattern is consistent with neonatal equine respiratory distress syndrome (NERDS). The foal was euthanized the same day.

<60 mmHg in lateral recumbency on room air) and progressive hypercapnia. This disease can resemble several other respiratory diseases (Table 8.II.4). Based on the 2007 definition [83], the absence of the fetal inflammatory response syndrome at birth and a normal white cell count and fibrinogen concentration for gestational age should be

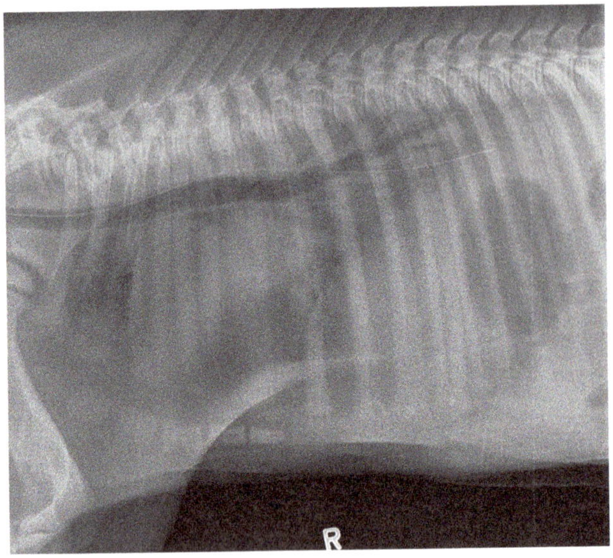

Figure 8.II.12 Four-day-old Thoroughbred filly presented for increased respiratory rate and effort. A diffuse increased opacity of the lung field is present with obscuring of the pulmonary vessels and multiple air bronchograms throughout (diffuse alveolar pattern). The cardiac silhouette is difficult to assess and the terminal trachea and carina appear displaced dorsally. Findings are suggestive of ARDS.

Table 8.II.4 Some causes of respiratory distress in neonatal foals.

Respiratory distress in neonatal foals		
Pulmonary disease	**Upper airway disease**	**Nonrespiratory disease**
Infectious pneumonia (bacterial, viral, fungal, parasitic, aspiration) Acute respiratory distress syndrome Meconium aspiration Pulmonary or pleural hemorrhage Pleural effusion Neonatal equine respiratory distress syndrome (NERDS) Pulmonary hypoplasia	Choanal atresia Stenosis of nares or trachea Epiglottic cyst Guttural pouch tympany/ empyema	Rib fracture Pain or systemic inflammation Anemia (neonatal isoerythrolysis, rib fracture) Congenital or acquired cardiac abnormalities Persistent pulmonary hypertension of the newborn Neurologic disease Acid-base disorders Diaphragmatic hernia Transient tachypnea of the neonate

confirmed and congenital cardiac disease ruled out as a cause of hypoxemia before a diagnosis of NERDS is made.

Evaluation of the Foal with Respiratory Disease

The clinician should be cognizant of the fact that clinical detection of early-stage respiratory disease or mild pneumonia can be difficult as foals are able to compensate for loss of lung function surprisingly well until more advanced disease is present [2, 107]. Thus, clinical signs alone cannot reliably be used to eliminate the suspicion of neonatal pneumonia. Therefore, the foal's respiratory system is best evaluated through a combination of the physical examination, including thorough auscultation of the trachea and lung fields, clinicopathologic data (CBC, serum biochemistry profile, ABG analysis), and diagnostic imaging techniques. Physical examination abnormalities will vary, depending on the severity and cause of respiratory compromise. Prior to restraining the foal, the respiratory rate and effort should be observed. Foals that have respiratory disease might display intermittent cough, a slightly elevated respiratory rate and effort, and intermittent febrile episodes. More advanced cases can display obvious signs of respiratory compromise (tachypnea, dyspnea, increased respiratory effort), nostril flare, poor body condition, and generalized weakness. Caution should be taken in foals with severe respiratory compromise as the stress of handling or performing a procedure (e.g. TTA) can result in deterioration in condition. Auscultation of the trachea might reveal moist sounds suggestive of fluid (milk, mucous, respiratory secretions) within the trachea, and auscultation and percussion of the thorax should be performed, and any noted abnormalities addressed. However, thoracic auscultation can be surprisingly unremarkable in some foals with significant pulmonary disease.

The CBC in foals with pneumonia can reveal leukocytosis and hyperfibrinogenemia, depending on the age of the foal, duration of respiratory disease, and other comorbidities. In one study involving 65 foals with bacterial pneumonia, the mean WBC and neutrophil count was 13,300 (range 5,190–27,890) and 9,000 (753–24,738) cells/μl, respectively; the mean serum fibrinogen concentration was 500 (range 200–900) mg/dl [108]. Interestingly, in that study, foals with *R. equi* pneumonia had significantly higher WBC (21,300, range 6,390–47,700) and neutrophil (17,458, range 2,698–41,976) counts and serum fibrinogen concentrations (700, range 400–1,400) when compared to foals with bacterial pneumonia from pathogens other than *R. equi* [108]. In another study, the diagnostic performance of the WBC count cutoff value of ≥13,000 cells/μl for the detection of early pneumonia was low (sensitivity 42%, specificity

74%) [107] whereas another study noted high diagnostic value of the same cutoff value for the diagnosis of severe (*R. equi*) pneumonia (sensitivity 95%, specificity 61%) [16]. The WBC count can also be used to monitor progression of foals with pneumonia, and serial WBC counts, differentials, and determinations of plasma fibrinogen concentration are useful for monitoring response to therapy with return to normal reference intervals of these parameters suggesting appropriate therapy and clinical improvement.

In foals with parasitic pneumonia, hematology and serum biochemistry results may be normal but leukopenia has been observed in experimental infections (*P. equorum*) and inflammatory alterations such as neutrophilia and hyperfibrinogenemia can be observed if a secondary bacterial component is present [73, 76, 77]. Systemic eosinophilia can be observed in some cases [76, 78]. CBC in foals with ARDS is often representative of the primary disease process, and the WBC can be low or, more commonly, normal or increased [98, 99, 101].

Derangements in the serum biochemistry profile are less predictable, but electrolyte deficiencies and pre-renal azotemia can be detected in some cases and can impact antimicrobial selection. Mild, nonspecific elevations in liver enzyme activity may be evident in foals with parasitic migration through the liver [73, 75]. The ABG evaluation allows the clinician to evaluate the level of alveolar gas exchange and oxygenation and, if present, hypoxemia, and hypercapnia; it also allows the clinician to monitor progression or improvement in gas exchange in foals being treated for respiratory disease. Pulse oximetry is another noninvasive continuous method of monitoring oxygen saturation of blood, but ABG analysis provides a more complete assessment of respiratory function. Moreover, it can be difficult to receive a consistent signal with pulse oximetry, especially in the ambulatory foal.

Diagnostic Imaging

Thoracic radiography and ultrasonography are the main imaging methods used to evaluate the lower respiratory system, although computed tomography has also been used in a limited capacity [109]. A variety of lung patterns have been described in association with various pulmonary disease processes, but a few radiographic findings are unique to the foal. First, healthy newborn foals <24 hours of age can have a diffuse increase in lung opacity characterized by a prominent interstitial-to-alveolar pattern that obscures pulmonary vasculature and soft tissue margins. This radiographic pattern is attributed to a combination of hypoinflation of the lung, residual fetal fluid in the airways, and uptake of fluid from the interstitial space [109]. An additional factor in the neonatal foal is that the thymus fills the mediastinal space cranial to the heart. Also, respiratory motion, particularly those foals with respiratory disease and elevated respiratory rates, causes diffuse blurring of all structures. Finally, atelectasis is readily visualized in neonatal foals imaged in lateral or sternal recumbency [108]. Positional atelectasis can develop over a short period of time (e.g. minutes), especially in the recumbent foal as a result of compression of the dependent lung by overlying lung tissue. Moreover, some foals may be predisposed to atelectasis as a result of immaturity in the lung and chest wall compliance and potential deficiencies in surfactant [108]. Atelectasis in the recumbent foal is characterized by a diffuse, mild to moderate interstitial pattern in the caudoventral lung region of the dependent lung [110]. Therefore, if possible, the foal should be maintained in a standing position for a few minutes prior to acquisition of thoracic radiographs to lessen this effect.

Radiographic lung patterns in neonatal foals are broadly grouped into interstitial, bronchial, alveolar, and nodular and aid in characterizing the respiratory disease (Table 8.II.5) [109, 111]. However, these patterns are not specific to the cause or location of disease histologically and correlate poorly with clinical severity. In general terms, extensive alveolar patterns are suggestive of more severe respiratory disorders (atelectasis, respiratory distress syndrome, pneumonia) whereas interstitial patterns are commonly associated with earlier or milder forms of respiratory disease [112]. General patterns of distribution can also be used to help investigate the type of pulmonary disease. For example, neonatal pneumonia that is secondary to sepsis often results in a diffuse distribution of lung pathology whereas aspiration pneumonia results in a caudoventral distribution [15, 18]. Foals with *R. equi* pneumonia can have a variety of radiographic abnormalities. In one study involving 17 foals with *R. equi* pneumonia, thoracic radiographs were characterized by a structured interstitial pattern with variable-sized nodules or masses consistent with pulmonary abscessation and/or consolidation (Figure 8.II.5) [113]. Pulmonary abscesses were characterized as ill-defined soft tissue nodules, some of which were cavitary. Other radiographic changes included air-bronchograms, increased interstitial infiltrate, hilar lymphadenopathy, and increased soft tissue opacity (mainly cranioventral lung field consistent with consolidative pneumonia) [113]. In comparison, radiographic lung changes associated with parasitic pneumonia may not be discernible but a diffuse increase in bronchointerstitial pattern or evidence of pulmonary abscess formation [73] may be apparent, whereas fungal pneumonia can have a miliary pattern in affected foals [66]. The clinician should also be mindful that radiographic changes lag behind progression or response to treatment.

Interestingly, an older study compared thoracic radiographs of healthy, immature, and septic foals

Table 8.II.5 Summary of radiographic lung patterns possibly observed in neonatal foals with respiratory disease [109, 111].

Interstitial	Characterized by changes in size and shape and increased radiopacity of the interstitium of the lung appearing as a hazy increase in opacity over affected area. An increased lung opacity of irregular linear to lacy appearance, which can appear honeycombed occasionally, can be interspersed within normal lung. Blurring of pulmonary vasculature and airways are more prominent. Can progress to a reticulated pattern or nodule or mass formation with variably defined margins due to infiltrating soft tissue.
Bronchial	Diseases of the bronchi (airways) can result from fluid accumulation or cellular infiltration in the bronchial walls or peribronchial tissue and is commonly seen in conjunction with interstitial disease. Radiographically this results in a thick appearing bronchial wall and a narrower lumen; on cross-section and longitudinal view the thickened bronchus appears as a doughnut or a thick-walled tube, respectively. Isolated bronchial disease can result from acute or chronic bronchitis (e.g. allergic or inflammatory origin) and frequently occurs in conjunction with interstitial lung disease.
Alveolar	Occurs on its own or as a progression of severe interstitial disease. Can be regional or diffuse and appears as a homogenously increased radiopacity of the lungs caused by the replacement of air by fluid in the alveolar spaces. Resultant fluid opacity can be due to cellular infiltration, fluid infiltration (blood, water), lack of air (atelectasis) or a combination of the three. Also characterized by increased soft tissue opacity that causes border effacement with surrounding soft tissue structures and air bronchograms (radiolucent bronchus surrounded by adjacent alveoli that are collapsed or fluid-filled).
Nodular	In neonatal foals, likely represents artifactual concentration of interstitial lung pattern.

(not specifically identified as having bacterial pneumonia) and noted that immature and septic foals had a mild to moderate diffuse increase in bronchial and/or interstitial opacity compared to healthy foals [114]. The interstitial pattern in these foals was described as granular or faintly reticular. In foals with NERDS (hyaline membrane disease), the bronchial structures were obscured by a marked diffuse interstitial or air-space opacity along with widespread air bronchograms (Figure 8.II.11) [114].

Ultrasonography is another imaging modality used to evaluate the lung fields, pleura, and pleural space (Chapter 6) and is most useful for determining abnormalities in the periphery of the lung (e.g. abscess, pulmonary consolidation) or pleural space (effusion). Additionally, ultrasonographic examination of the thorax has been used as a screening tool to identify *R. equi* pneumonia in foals from endemic farms as well as used to monitor response to treatment [115]. In one large study in central Kentucky involving two farms with endemic *R. equi*, foals received an ultrasonographic exam of the thorax every 2 weeks between the ages of 4 and 8 weeks. These screening exams helped identify foals with *R. equi* pneumonia and significantly reduced the incidence of clinical *R. equi* pneumonia and hospitalized cases when compared to years in which screening was not performed, thus suggesting that ultrasonographic screening can facilitate early detection of *R. equi* pneumonia (Figure 8.II.5) [115]. However, when using thoracic ultrasound to screen for *R. equi* pneumonia, clinicians must be selective toward positive cases and which foals receive antimicrobial treatment. For example, in one study where thoracic ultrasonographic screening was performed but where no treatment was instituted in foals based on positive screening test results, the proportion of foals with ultrasonographic evidence of pulmonary lesions was high (80%; 216/270), but only 21% (46/260) of ultrasonographically positive foals required treatment [113].

Diagnosis of bacterial pneumonia is supported by TTA cytology and culture, but blood culture should be obtained in all neonates with systemic signs of sepsis. Results of blood culture aids in early identification of causative organisms involved in pneumonia and allows for rapid institution of directed antimicrobial therapy. The isolated organisms from neonatal foals with sepsis and bacterial pneumonia reflect those commonly isolated in sepsis in newborns: *E. coli*, *Klebsiella* spp., *Actinobacillus equlli*, etc. Bacterial culture also allows for definitive diagnosis and antimicrobial sensitivity testing. Cytology can provide an initial rapid assessment for the presence of intracellular bacteria and if they are Gram-positive or -negative organisms. Cytology might demonstrate abnormally elevated eosinophil counts if parasitic pneumonia is present; the normal eosinophil count as a percentage of total nucleated cells is 0–2%.

If *R. equi* pneumonia is suspected, polymerase chain reaction analysis can be used for detection of VapA. *R. equi* can also be cultured alone or be involved in polymicrobial infections. In one study involving 113 foals with pneumonia, 65% of foals with *R. equi* pneumonia had a mixed bacterial infection [108]. In that study, the authors suggested that WBC counts of >20,000 cell/μl, plasma fibrinogen concentrations >700 mg/dl, cytologic documentation of Gram-positive coccobacilli in TTA samples, and radiological evidence of pulmonary abscessation were highly suggestive of *R. equi* infection. In another study, WBC count cutoffs of 13,000 cells/l and 15,000 cells/l provided sensitivities of 95% and 79%, respectively, and specificities of 61% and 91%, respectively, in the identification of *R. equi*-infected foals housed at farms where the disease was enzootic [16].

Diagnostic tests for suspected cases of viral pneumonia should have blood and tracheal aspirates collected at presentation for virus identification by molecular techniques and isolation; submission of samples for testing for secondary bacterial infections should also be considered. The lungs of foals with EHV-1 or EVA are noncompliant and pulmonary edema is often present. Mechanical ventilation of these cases may prolong life, but death is generally inevitable due to significant lung damage. Foals that are suspected or confirmed as having EHV-1 or EVA should be isolated because they likely are shedding large quantities of virus and pose a threat to other horses, neonates, and pregnant mares. Foals with EVA are generally born to seronegative mares, and treatment with intravenous plasma with a high titer of antibodies against EVA may prove beneficial as passive immunity appears to be protective against this disease in neonates [40].

Fecal parasite examination for parasite eggs or larvae can help identify the presence of the parasite within the host and suggest parasitic pneumonia. Typically, *D. arnfieldi* eggs and larvae usually cannot be recovered from the feces of horses but patent infestations with *P. equorum* may be detected by fecal flotation and examination for eggs. However, the presence of parasites does not indicate a causal relationship to pneumonitis [73]. Of note, donkeys or mules are typically co-housed if horses develop *D. arnfieldi*.

The diagnosis of ARDS is based on the presence of acute (<72 hours) respiratory distress after exposure to a known risk factor with evidence of a pulmonary capillary leak (usually seen as bilateral/diffuse infiltrates on thoracic radiographs; Figures 8.II.13 and 8.II.14), and a PaO_2/FiO_2 ratio <300 mmHg in foals >7 days old. For younger foals, the age specific values detailed in Table 8.II.2 or the 2007 definition should be applied [83]. It is important to note that ARDS is always secondary to another disease process and identifying concurrent bacterial or viral pneumonia is common.

Treatment of Bacterial Pneumonia

Administration of antimicrobials, ideally based on TTA culture and sensitivity results, are the mainstay of treatment for bacterial pneumonia. Initial empiric treatment involves a broad-spectrum bactericidal combination, such as penicillin and amikacin. Antimicrobial therapy can then be altered based on culture and sensitivity patterns of the isolated pathogens. Other supportive therapies include administration of supplemental intranasal oxygen, meeting nutritional requirements, and maintenance of hydration with fluid therapy, if necessary. Intranasal administration of humidified oxygen can be administered via uni- or bilateral nasal cannula(s) at rates ranging from 50 to 200 ml of oxygen/kg/min and targeting a P_aO_2 of 95–100 mmHg or SaO_2 >95%. Anti-inflammatory medications such as flunixin meglumine can be administered to help combat inflammation and fever; alternatively, steroids such as dexamethasone (e.g. 0.03–0.20 mg/kg, q12–24h, IV or PO for 1–9 days) and prednisolone have also been used to quell heightened inflammation within the pulmonary system in severe cases of pneumonia, ALI, ARDS, and interstitial pneumonia [97–99, 116, 117]. Maintaining the foal in a cool and well-ventilated environment is important and some foals also benefit from nebulization with saline, antimicrobials, bronchodilators, and/or steroids (see Chapter 6).

The antiviral drug acyclovir (10–16 mg/kg orally or per rectum 4–5 times per day) has been used in cases of EHV-1 in neonates, with some evidence of efficacy in mildly affected foals or foals affected after birth. Alternatively, the American Association of Equine Practitioners recommends valacyclovir for prophylactic use, dosed at 30 mg/kg q 8 h for 2 days, then 20 mg/kg q 12 h for 1–2 weeks. The higher dose is recommended if the horse remains febrile. Ganciclovir is recommended for horses with clinical disease, dosed at 2.5 mg/kg q 8 h IV for 1 day then 2.5 mg/kg q 12 h IV for 1 week or until resolution of clinical signs. Oseltamivir phosphate (2 mg/kg q 12 h for 5 days) has been found to be effective in horses experimentally inoculated with equine influenza A virus. Treatment reduced the magnitude of virus shedding, reduced fever and mitigated the risk of secondary bacterial pneumonia [118]. Antiviral treatment for influenza infection needs to be used early in infection as the disease is self-limiting; it may be used prophylactically with strong justification.

Plasma products from hyperimmunized horses or colostrum from vaccinated donor mares could be considered for foals from unvaccinated mares or from mares whose vaccination status is unknown. Testing for the risk of neonatal isoerythrolysis is prudent with donor colostrum; commercial plasma producing companies avoid donors with major blood group antigens. Products containing neutralizing antibodies to viral diseases work best as prophylactic aids in disease mitigation.

Parasitic pneumonia is treated with appropriate anthelmentics. *P. equorum* infection can be treated with a variety of anthelmintics such as ivermectin (0.2 mg/kg, PO), moxidectin (0.4 mg/kg, PO [foals>4 months]), fenbendazole (10 mg/kg/d, PO for 5 consecutive days), pyrantel pamoate (6.6 mg/kg, PO), or levamisole (10 mg/kg, PO). Some foals require multiple treatments, and all horses should be dewormed concurrently. In addition, regional and farm resistance to various anthelmintics is a concern [119]. *D. arenfieldi* can be treated with thiabendazole (440 mg/kg/d, PO for 2 days), fenbendazole (15 mg/kg, PO, once), ivermectin (0.2 mg/kg, PO) or moxidectin

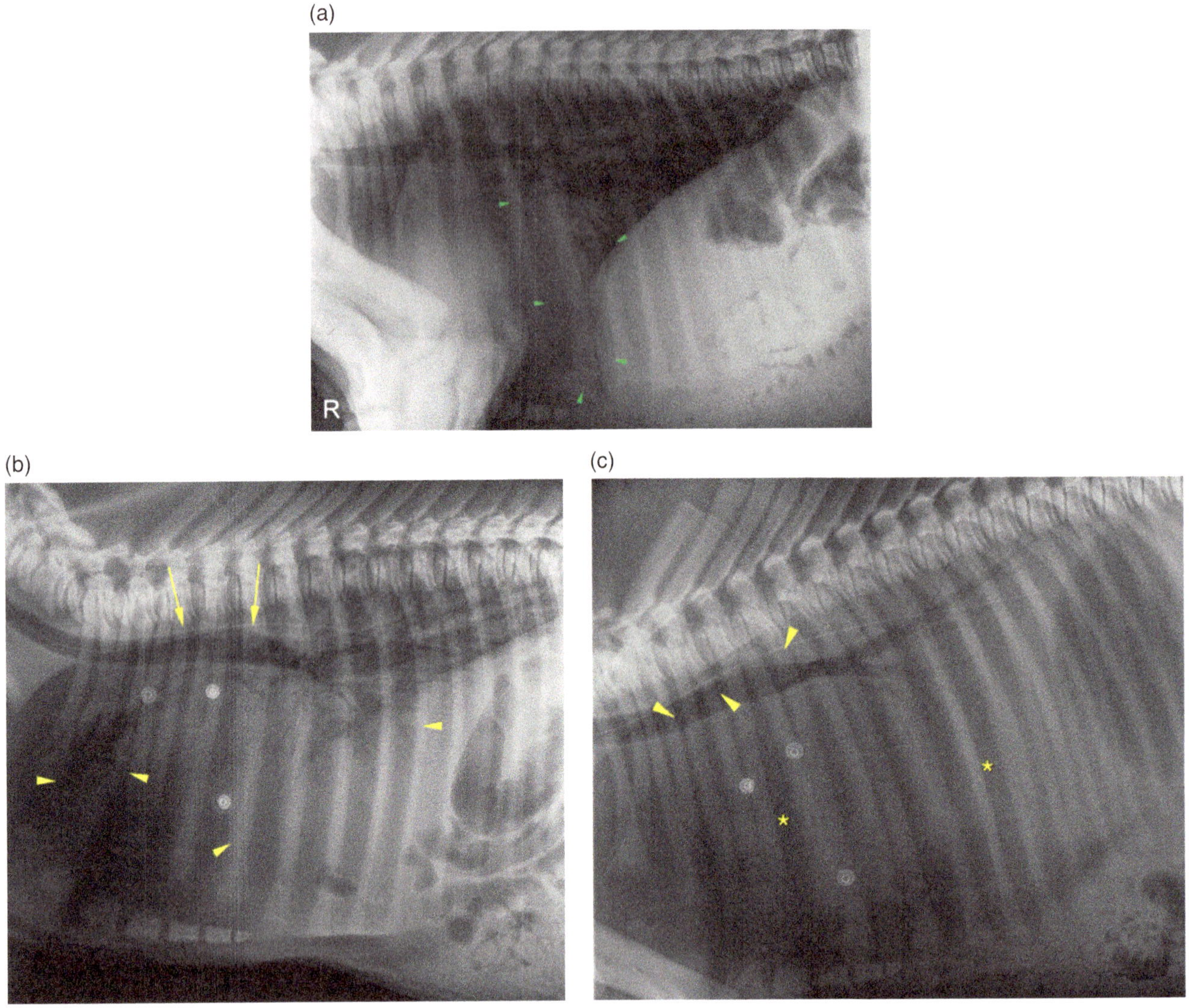

Figure 8.II.13 Serial lateral thoracic radiographs in a foal presented for veterinary care at 7 hours of age for inability to stand and nurse since birth. (a) Image at presentation demonstrating a moderate patchy increased opacity of the caudoventral lung fields (alveolar pattern, green arrows) along with poorly defined air bronchograms. There is partial effacement of the caudal margin of the cardiac silhouette. (b) Image at 24 hours post-admission with a more extensive alveolar pattern (arrowheads) in the caudoventral and caudodorsal lung fields. The trachea is slightly elevated (arrows) along with effacement of the cardiac silhouette. A nasoesophageal tube is also present. (c) Image 48 hours post-admission with marked worsening of the alveolar pattern with complete opacification and consolidation of the entire lung field (asterisk). Air bronchograms are present (consistent with mainstem bronchi) and the trachea, carina, and mainstem bronchi are displaced dorsally. The cranial lung bronchus (arrowheads) is also displaced dorsally and deviated suggestive of cardiac enlargement. These images are consistent with acute respiratory distress syndrome (ARDS). The foal died shortly after the third set of images were acquired. Gross findings on necropsy examination included dark red and firm right and left lung lobes with clear yellow exudate from airways on the cut surface. Microscopically (Figure 8.II.14) the alveolar spaces were filled with neutrophils, sloughed epithelial cells, fibrin, and eosinophilic fluid along with randomly collapsed alveolar spaces (atelectasis).

(0.4 mg/kg, PO) [75]. One way to avoid *D. arnfieldi* in horses is to prevent exposure of foals and their mares to donkey or mules. Removal of manure from pastures decreases parasite burden.

Treatment of ARDS

Treatment of ARDS is directed against the primary disease process and toward providing supportive care – most importantly, oxygen therapy as above. Large-bore tubing systems minimize resistance to airflow, and FiO_2 as high as 75% has been measured at the carina in foals using bilateral flow rates of 10 l/min (20 l/min combined) with bilateral cannulas [120]. Intratracheal oxygen insufflation has been described, achieving results similar to high bilateral intranasal flow rates [121]. Considering the invasive nature of this method and limited benefits, this is rarely indicated. Some foals with ARDS have a large shunt

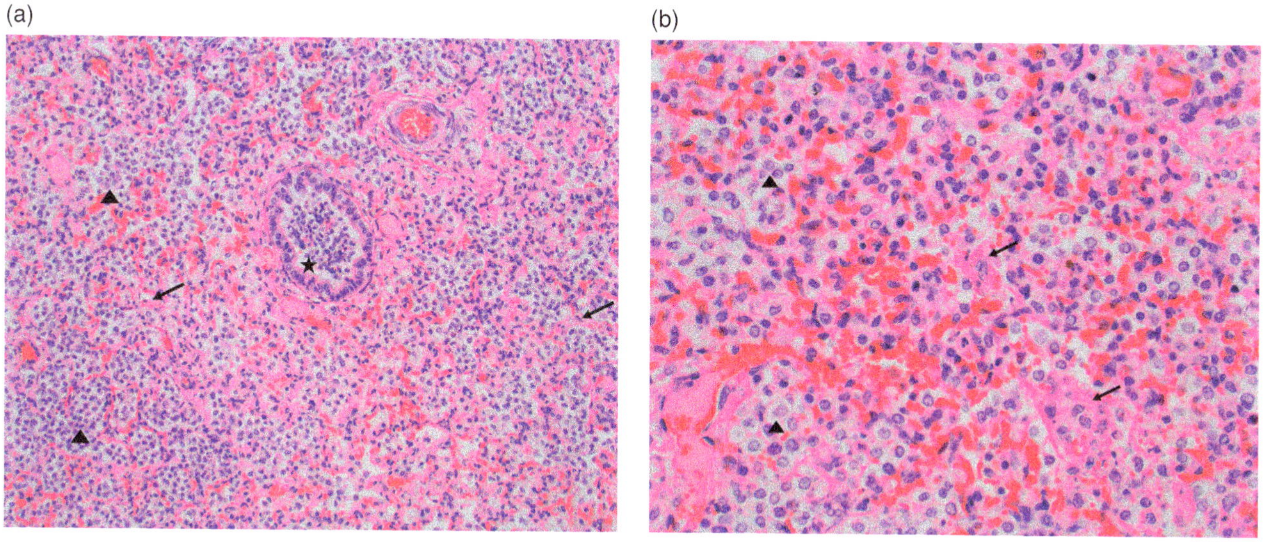

Figure 8.II.14 Same foal is Figure 8.II.13. (a) Lung from a foal with severe bronchopneumonia and ARDS. Bronchioles contain neutrophils, macrophages, and cellular debris (star). Alveolar spaces contain fibrin (arrows) and large numbers of macrophages and neutrophils (arrowheads). (b) Alveolar spaces contain hemorrhage mixed with macrophages and some neutrophils (arrowheads). Throughout the section are aggregates of fibrin (arrows).

fraction and minimal to no response to intranasal oxygen, regardless of flow rate [117]. In these cases choosing the lowest flow rate with the maximal increase in PaO_2 is recommended to minimize chances of oxygen toxicity. Noninvasive ventilation strategies have been investigated including continuous positive airway pressure (CPAP) in foals with pharmacologically induced respiratory depression and nasal high flow oxygen (HFO) therapy in neonatal foals with a variety of diseases requiring respiratory support [122, 123]. Effects on PaO_2 and $PaCO_2$ were comparable to traditional intranasal oxygen therapy and the benefits of these modes of noninvasive ventilation in equine ARDS patients requires further study. Mechanical ventilation of ARDS patients is challenging due to the coexistence of areas with high and low V/Q ratios adjacent to normal and overdistended lung tissue, predisposing the patient to ventilator-induced lung injury. A reduction in mortality in human ARDS has largely been attributed to use of lung-protective ventilation with lower tidal volumes (≤6 ml/kg) [124].

Administration of corticosteroids is still debated in human ARDS patients but the recent meta-analysis found a reduced mortality in adult patients with ARDS with use of methylprednisolone and hydrocortisone but not dexamethasone [125, 126]. Although the same benefits could not be confirmed in children, anecdotal evidence in foals supports the use of corticosteroids. In two reports, all but two foals surviving ARDS received corticosteroids [98, 117]. Use of prednisolone sodium succinate or methylprednisolone at 1–2 mg/kg/d intravenously divided in two to four doses might be indicated. Various other treatments have been trialed in people and largely failed to improve survival [127]. Bronchoconstriction is not a prominent feature of ARDS and bronchodilators are therefore likely of limited use. Judicious intravenous fluid therapy may be necessary in dehydrated patients but overhydration or rapid changes in circulating blood volume should be avoided as capillary hydrostatic pressure is the main determinant of pulmonary edema formation when endothelial and epithelial permeability is increased. Conversely, suboptimal hydration status decreases cardiac output and worsens oxygen delivery to peripheral tissues. Measurement of central venous pressure might aid in determination of the patient's hydration status. If foals are too depressed to nurse or eat, nutritional support is essential as the work of breathing significantly increases energy expenditure.

Treatment of NERDS

Treatment with surfactant and noninvasive or mechanical ventilation is indicated in human neonates with respiratory distress syndrome. Treatments are evolving and currently INtubate-SURfactant-Extubate (INSURE) and Less Invasive Surfactant Administration (LISA) procedures are favored [128]. The INSURE procedure comprises intubation followed by administration of surfactant, early extubation, and CPAP support. With LISA, surfactant is instilled into the trachea via a small-diameter catheter placed orally or nasally into the trachea [128]. Anecdotally, attempts have been to treat foals with NERDS with surfactant with varying results (see Chapter 1). Successful treatment of a premature cria with equine surfactant, obtained by a postmortem lung lavage, and positive pressure ventilation has been reported which would theoretically be feasible in foals [129].

Treatment of *R. equi* Pneumonia

As noted, *R. equi* is a facultative intracellular pathogen that survives and replicates in macrophages. Because of this fact, in vitro antimicrobial activity does not always equate to in vivo efficacy. The combination of a macrolide (erythromycin, azithromycin, or clarithromycin) with rifampin has been a long-standing treatment recommendation for foals with clinical signs of *R. equi* infection. Of these macrolides, erythromycin has been available the longest, but perhaps is the least ideal due to the fact that bioavailability is considerably lower when foals are not fasted (mean $\pm$ SD $26 \pm 15\%$ when fasted, $8 \pm 7\%$ when fed) and the dosing interval is quite frequent (every 6–8 hours) [130]. In comparison, azithromycin and clarithromycin have higher oral bioavailability in the absence of fasting, have prolonged half-lives, and attain much higher concentrations in bronchoalveolar lavage (BAL) cells and pulmonary epithelial lining fluid (PELF) [131–135]. Because of this, azithromycin and clarithromycin are better choices for ease of treatment (less frequent dosing interval, Table 8.II.6) and lower dosages [135, 137]. Some uncertainty arises, however, when considering combination therapy of a macrolide and rifampin as a few studies have documented considerable decreases in plasma, PELF, and BAL cell concentrations of clarithromycin when both medications are administered concurrently [138, 139]; this effect is most likely a result of inhibition of intestinal uptake transporters. Despite the profound decrease in clarithromycin bioavailability associated with concurrent rifampin administration, concentrations of clarithromycin in PELF and BAL cells are well in excess of the MIC against *R. equi* [138, 139]. Based on clinical experience, combination therapy is still regarded as superior to macrolide monotherapy (Table 8.II.6) [135, 137].

Unfortunately, there are no randomized controlled studies comparing treatments in foals with clinical *R. equi* pneumonia. In one retrospective study, the combination of clarithromycin-rifampin was significantly more effective

Table 8.II.6 Recommended dosages for antimicrobial medications used to treat infections caused by *Rhodococcus equi* [136].

Medication	Dose (mg/kg)	Route	Dosing interval
Azithromycin	10	Oral	Every 24 hours for 5 days, then every 48 hours thereafter
Clarithromycin	7.5	Oral	Every 12 hours
Erythromycin	25	Oral	Every 6–8 hours
Gamithromycin	6	Intramuscular	Every 7 days
Rifampin	5	Oral	Every 12 hours

(higher odds of treatment success, fewer febrile days) than erythromycin-rifampin or azithromycin-rifampin, especially in foals with severe radiographic lesions. However, this information must be interpreted with caution as foals were not randomly assigned to treatment groups [137, 140, 141]. There are also occasions in which mixed bacterial infections are isolated from TTA along with *R. equi*, with one study noting that beta-hemolytic *Streptococci* and *E. coli* were the most common bacteria cultured from TTA in foals with *R. equi* [139]. In such cases, the addition of a third antimicrobial may be indicated if there is a Gram-negative pathogen that is resistant to macrolides and rifampin [139]. The duration of antimicrobial therapy is variable and dependent on severity of initial disease, presence or absence of EPDs, and response to therapy. Resolution of clinical signs, normalization of plasma fibrinogen concentration and WBC count, and radiographic or ultrasonographic resolution of lung lesions can be used as guides to direct duration of therapy (generally ranges between 3 and 12 weeks) [136, 140, 141]. Immune-mediated EPDs such as polysynovitis will typically resolve with successful treatment of the accompanying pneumonia but aggressive local therapy (joint lavage, regional limb perfusion) is necessary for foals with *R. equi* septic arthritis or osteomyelitis.

Occasionally, isolates of *R. equi* from foals with clinical disease have resistance to macrolides and rifampin with one study suggesting a 4% resistance rate over a 10-year period [140, 141]. In such cases, the clinician must rely on information from culture and susceptibility testing to identify other potential antimicrobial candidates. In vitro susceptibility to fluoroquinolones, gentamicin, vancomycin, chloramphenicol, tetracycline, and trimethoprim sulfamethoxazole has been documented but some of these medications can have serious side effects (fluoroquinolones-arthropathy) or should be reserved for life-threatening disease (vancomycin) [141]. The clinician should also be cognizant of the fact that many foals have mild subclinical ultrasonographic pulmonary lesions without overt clinical signs of *R. equi* infection and recover without therapy. In fact, studies have documented that administration of antimicrobials to foals with subclinical infection does not hasten resolution as compared to foals that are administered a placebo [141, 142]. Thus, mass antimicrobial treatment of subclinically affected foals is not advised because this can select for antimicrobial resistance over time, which equates to poor antimicrobial stewardship [136].

Intravenous administration of 1–2 l of hyperimmune plasma from horses vaccinated against *R. equi* has been used to reducing the incidence and/or severity of *R. equi* pneumonia in foals on endemic farms in several studies [143–145]. Although the exact mechanism by which hyperimmune plasma incurs protection against *R. equi* infection is not known, provision of anti-*R. equi* antibodies may enhance opsonization and enhance killing of *R. equi* by alveolar macrophages in foals [146, 147]. In a one study, administration of hyperimmunized plasma significantly increased the titers against *R. equi* in foals for over 30 days and appeared to reduce the prevalence of *R. equi* infection as compared to control foals that were not administered hyperimmune plasma [143]. Conversely, no difference in the incidence of *R. equi* pneumonia was observed in clinical trials in which treatment foals received hyperimmunized plasma while untreated foals served as controls [148, 149]. The variable clinical efficacy of *R. equi* hyperimmunized plasma could be due to the method by which plasma donors were immunized, the amount of hyperimmunized plasma administered, timing of administration of hyperimmunized plasma, management conditions, interindividual variability in susceptibility to infection, and/or number of virulent bacteria in the environment [148].

Prognosis

Although the prognosis for survival of neonatal sepsis in foals ranges from 60% to 80%, the prognosis for survival in foals with pneumonia has not specifically been evaluated. In one study that examined thoracic radiographs from neonatal foals, 75 of 128 foals (59%) had radiographic abnormalities within the thorax; of these 75 foals, 49 (65%) were discharged from the hospital [112]. The prognosis of foals with ALI/ARDS is guarded with one case series of 15 foals with ALI/ARDS noting survival in 9 foals, 4 deaths due to respiratory failure, and 2 subject to euthanasia in a moribund state [122]. In foals with lower respiratory disorders, the clinician can attempt to base the prognosis on the degree of involvement of the lung parenchyma, cause, level of veterinary care available, and other comorbidities. In another study, 9 of 23 foals with bronchointerstitial pneumonia/ARDS survived (39%). Ten foals died either at the farm, in transit, or shortly after arriving at the hospital, emphasizing the extremely rapid progression of the disease [98]. Of the foals treated at the hospital, two died and two were euthanized due to the poor prognosis [98].

In comparison, several studies have examined the outcome of foals with *R. equi* infection. With the use of macrolides and rifampin, survival can be as high as 88% in foals with *R. equi* pneumonia [150]. Survival rates at referral hospitals trends lower, ranging from 59% to 72%, as this population of affected foals tend to be more severely affected [136, 151–153]. Isolation of multiple bacteria from TTA along with *R. equi* does not negatively impact prognosis [136]; however, one retrospective study of 150 foals noted that foals with EPD had a significantly lower survival rate (43%) as compared to foals without EPD (82%). The prognosis for foals with large abdominal abscesses is poor but rare cases respond to long-term antimicrobial therapy [21]. Foals with macrolide-resistant *R. equi* infections also have a worse prognosis (sevenfold less than foals infected with susceptible isolates) [136, 140]. The impact of *R. equi* pneumonia on future athletic performance has also been investigated with no significant differences in total earnings, average earning index, and age at first race between horses that had *R. equi* pneumonia as foals and healthy horses [154]. In another student, 54% of foals that survived *R. equi* pneumonia had at least one racing start compared with 65% of their birth cohort suggesting that foals with *R. equi* pneumonia are slightly less likely to race as adults [152, 153]. In that study, those that did race did not have different performance than the rest of the US racing population [152, 153]. Conversely, an Australian study noted that the probability of racing as a 2-year-old was similar between *R. equi*-affected horses and controls but affected horses had less starts and won fewer races than controls [155].

References

1 Walsh, W.F. (1995). Neonatal pneumonia. *Semin. Pediatr. Infect. Dis.* 6: 166–173.

2 Giguere, S. and Prescott, J.F. (1997). Clinical manifestations, diagnosis, treatment, and prevention of *Rhodococcus equi* infections in foals. *Vet. Microbiol.* 56: 313–334.

3 Klein, J.O. and Barnett, E.D. (1998). Neonatal pneumonia. *Semin. Pediatr. Infect. Dis.* 9: 212–216.

4 Gereige, R.S. and Laufer, P.M. (2013). Pneumonia. *Pediatr. Rev.* 34: 438–456.

5 Blunden, A.S. and Gower, S.M. (1999). A histological and immunohistochemical study of the humoral immune system of the lungs in young Thoroughbred horses. *J. Comp. Pathol.* 120: 347–356.

6 Campbell, J.R. (1996). Neonatal pneumonia. *Semin. Respir. Infect.* 11: 155–162.

7 Duke, T. (2005). Neonatal pneumonia in developing countries. *Arch. Dis. Child Neonatal Educ.* 90: F211–F219.

8 Canisso, I., Ball, B.A., Squires, E.L. et al. (2015). Comprehensive review of equine placentitis. *AAEP Proc.* 61: 490–509.

9 Canisso, I.F., Ball, B.A., Scoggin, K.E. et al. (2015). Alpha-fetoprotein is present in the fetal fluids and is increased in plasma of mares with experimentally induced ascending placentitis. *Anim. Reprod. Sci.* 154: 48–55.

10 Fitzgerald, S.D. and Yamini, B. (1995). Rhodococcal abortion and pneumonia in an equine fetus. *J. Vet. Diagn. Investig.* 7: 157–158.

11 Sanchez, L.C., Giguere, S., and Lester, G.D. (2008). Factors associated with survival of neonatal foals with bacteremia and racing performance of surviving Thoroughbreds: 423 cases (1982–2007). *J. Am. Vet. Med. Assoc.* 233: 1446–1452.

12 Stewart, A.J., Hinchcliff, K.W., Saville, W.J. et al. (2002). Actinobacillus sp bacteremia in foals: clinical signs and prognosis. *J. Vet. Intern. Med.* 16: 464–471.

13 Koterba, A.M., Brewer, B.D., and Tarplee, F.A. (1984). Clinical and clinicopathological characteristics of the septicaemic neonatal foal: review of 38 cases. *Equine Vet. J.* 16: 376–383.

14 Freeman, L. and Paradis, M.R. (1992). Evaluating the effectiveness of equine neonatal care. *Vet. Med.* 87: 921–926.

15 Reuss, S.M. and Cohen, N.D. (2015). Update on bacterial pneumonia in the foal and weanling. *Vet. Clin. Equine* 31: 121–135.

16 Giguere, S., Hernandex, J., Gaskin, J. et al. (2003). Evaluation of white blood cell concentration, plasma fibrinogen concentration, and agar gel immunodiffusion test for early identification of foals with *Rhodococcus equi* pneumonia. *J. Am. Vet. Med. Assoc.* 222: 775–781.

17 Sanz, M., Loynachan, A., Sun, L. et al. (2013). The effect of bacterial dose and foal age at challenge on *Rhodococcus equi* infection. *Vet. Microbiol.* 167: 623–631.

18 Reuss, S.M., Chaffin, M.K., and Cohen, N.D. (2009). Extrapulmonary disorders associated with *Rhodococcus equi* infection in foals: 150 cases (1987–2007). *J. Am. Vet. Med. Assoc.* 235: 855–863.

19 Dawson, T.R., Horohov, D.W., Meijer, W.G. et al. (2010). Current understanding of the equine immune response to Rhodococcus equi. An immunological review of *R. equi* pneumonia. *Vet. Immunol. Immunopathol.* 135: 1–11.

20 Wang, X., Coulson, G.B., Miranda-Casoluengo, A.A. et al. (2014). IcgA is a virulence factor of *Rhodococcus equi* that modulates intracellular growth. *Infect. Immun.* 82: 1793–1800.

21 Giguere, S., Cohen, N.D., Chaffin, M.K. et al. (2011). *Rhodococcus equi*: clinical manifestations, virulence, and immunity. *J. Vet. Intern. Med.* 25: 1221–1230.

22 Cohen, N.D., Chaffin, M.K., Kuskie, K.R. et al. (2013). Association of perinatal exposure to airborne *Rhodococcus equi* with risk of pneumonia caused by *R. equi* in foals. *Am. J. Vet. Res.* 74: 102–109.

23 Cohen, N.K., Kuskie, K.R., Smith, J.L. et al. (2012). Association between airborne concentration of virulent *Rhodococcus equi* with location (stall versus paddock) and month (January through June) on 30 horse breeding farms in central Kentucky. *Am. J. Vet. Res.* 73: 1603–1609.

24 Chaffin, M.K., Cohen, N.D., Keith, C.M. et al. (2008). Chemoprophylactic effects of azithromycin against *Rhodococcus equi*-induced pneumonia among foals at equine breeding farms with endemic infections. *J. Am. Vet. Med. Assoc.* 232: 1035–1047.

25 Chaffin, M.K., Cohen, N.D., Martens, R.J. et al. (2004). Hematologic and immunophenotypic factors associated with development of *Rhodococcus equi*. *Vet. Immunol. Immunopathol.* 100: 33–48.

26 McQueen, C.M., Doan, R., Dindot, S.V. et al. (2005). Protective role of neutrophils in mice experimentally infected with *Rhodococcus equi*. *Infect. Immun.* 73: 7040–7042.

27 Chaffin, M.K., Cohen, N.D., Martens, R.J. et al. (2011). Evaluation of the efficacy of gallium maltolate for chemoprophylaxis against pneumonia cause by *Rhodococcus equi* infection in foals. *Am. J. Vet. Res.* 72: 945–957.

28 Ardans, A.A., Pritchett, R.F., and Zee, Y.C. (1973). Isolation and characterization of an equine adenovirus. *Infect. Immun.* 7: 673–677.

29 Moorthy, A.R. and Spradbrow, P.B. (1978). Adenoviral infection of Arab foals with respiratory tract disease. *Zentralbl. Veterinarmed. B* 25 (6): 469–477.

30 Thompson, D.B., Spradborw, P.B., and Studdert, M. (1976). Isolation of an adenovirus from an Arab foal with a combined immunode ficiency disease. *Aust. Vet. J.* 52: 435–437.

31 Del Piero, F., Wilkins, P.A., Lopez, J.W. et al. (1997). Equine viral arteritis in newborn foals: clinical, pathological, serological, microbiological and immunohistochemical observations. *Equine Vet. J.* 29: 178–185.

32 Del Piero, F. (2000). Equine viral arteritis. *Vet. Pathol.* 37: 287–296.

33 Frymus, T., Kita, J., Woyciechowska, S. et al. (1986). Foetal and neonatal foal losses on equine herpesvirus type 1 (EHV-1) infected farms before and after EHV-1 vaccination was introduced. *Pol. Arch. Weter.* 26: 7–14.

34 Gilkerson, J.R., Whalley, J.M., Drummer, H.E. et al. (1999). Epidemiology of EHV-1 and EHV-4 in the mare and foal populations on a Hunter Valley stud farm: are mares the source of EHV-1 for unweaned foals. *Vet. Microbiol.* 68: 27–34.

35 Hartley, W.J. and Dixon, R.J. (1979). An outbreak of foal perinatal mortality due to equid herpesvirus type 1: pathological observations. *Equine Vet. J.* 11: 215–218.

36 Laval, K., Poelaert, K.C.K., Van Cleemput, J.V. et al. (2021). The pathogenesis and immune evasive mechanisms of equine herpesvirus type 1. *Front. Microbiol.* 12: 662686.

37 Maury, W., Oaks, J.L., and Bradley, S. (1998). Equine endothelial cells support productive infection of equine infectious anemia virus. *J. Virol.* 72: 9291–9297.

38 Sponseller, B.A., Sparks, W.O., Wannemuehler, Y. et al. (2007). Immune selection of equine infectious anemia

virus env variants during the long-term inapparent stage of disease. *Virology* 363: 156–165.

39 Laval, K., Favoreel, H.W., Poelaert, K.C.K. et al. (2015). Equine herpesvirus type 1 enhances viral replication in CD172a+ monocytic cells upon adhesion to endothelial cells. *J. Virol.* 89: 10912–10923.

40 Wilkins, P.A. (2003). Lower respiratory problems of the neonate. *Vet. Clin. Equine* 19: 19–33.

41 Crabb, B.S. and Studdert, M.J. (1995). Equine herpesviruses 4 (equine rhinopneumonitis virus) and 1 (equine abortion virus). *Adv. Virus Res.* 45: 153–190.

42 Go, Y.Y., Bailey, E., Cook, D.G. et al. (2011). Genome-wide association study among four horse breeds identifies a common haplotype associated with in vitro CD3+ T cell susceptibility/resistance to equine arteritis virus infection. *J. Virol.* 85: 13174–13184.

43 Balasuriya, U.B., Go, Y.Y., and MacLachlan, N.J. (2013). Equine arteritis virus. *Vet. Microbiol.* 167: 93–122.

44 Sarkar, S., Chelvarajan, L., Go, Y.Y. et al. (2016). Equine arteritis virus uses equine CXCL16 as an entry receptor. *J. Virol.* 90: 3366–3384.

45 Fukumoto, N., Shimaoka, T., Fujumura, H. et al. (2004). Critical roles of CXC chemokine ligand 16/scavenger receptor that binds phosphatidylserine and oxidized lipoprotein in the pathogenesis of both acute and adoptive transfer experimental autoimmune encephalomyelitis. *J. Immunol.* 173: 1620–1627.

46 Plagemann, P.G. and Moennig, V. (1992). Lactate dehydrogenase-elevating virus, equine arteritis virus, and simian hemorrhagic fever virus: a new groupf positive-strand RNA viruses. *Adv. Virus Res.* 41: 99–192.

47 Balasuriya, U.B. (2014). Equine viral arteritis. *Vet. Clin. North Am. Equine Pract.* 30: 543–560.

48 Timoney, P.J., McCollum, W.H., Roberts, A.W. et al. (1986). Demonstration of the carrier state in naturally acquired equine arteritis virus infection in the stallion. *Res. Vet. Sci.* 41: 279–280.

49 Zhang, B., Jin, S., Jin, J. et al. (2005). A tumor necrosis factor receptor family protein serves as a cellular receptor for the macrophage-tropic equine lentivirus. *Proc. Natl. Acad. Sci.* 102: 9918–9923.

50 Kemen, M.J. and Coggins, L. (1972). Equine infectious anemia: transmission from infected mares to foals. *J. Am. Vet. Med. Assoc.* 161: 496–499.

51 McConnico, R.S., Issel, C.J., Cook, S.J. et al. (2000). Predictive methods to define infection with equine infectious anemia virus in foals out of reactor mares. *J. Equine Vet. Sci.* 20: 387–392.

52 Bolfa, P., Nolf, M., Cadore, J.L. et al. (2013). Interstitial lung disease associated with equine infectious anemia virus infection in horses. *Vet. Res.* 44: 113.

53 Patterson-Kane, J.C., Carrick, J.B., Axon, J.E. et al. (2008). The pathology of bronchointerstitial pneumonia in young foals associated with the first outbreak of equine influenza in Australia. *Equine Vet. J.* 40: 199–203.

54 Liu, I.K., Pascoe, D.R., Chang, L.W. et al. (1985). Duration of maternally derived antibodies against equine influenza in newborn foals. *Am. J. Vet. Res.* 46: 2078–2080.

55 Chambers, T.M. (2014). A brief introduction to equine influenza and equine influenza viruses. In: *Animal Influenza Virus* (ed. E. Spackman), 365–370. New York, NY: Springer New York.

56 Tůmová, B. (1980). Equine influenza — a segment in influenza virus ecology. *Comp. Immunol. Microbiol. Infect. Dis.* 3: 45–59.

57 Pusterla, N., Mapes, S., Wademan, C. et al. (2013). Investigation of the role of lesser characterised respiratory viruses associated with upper respiratory tract infections in horses. *Vet. Rec.* 172: 315.

58 Black, W.D., Wilcox, R.S., Stevenson, R.A. et al. (2007). Prevalence of serum neutralising antibody to equine rhinitis A virus (ERAV), equine rhinitis B virus 1 (ERBV1) and ERBV2. *Vet. Microbiol.* 119: 65–71.

59 Back, H., Weld, J., Walsh, C. et al. (2019). Equine rhinitis A virus infection in Thoroughbred racehorses—a putative role in poor performance? *Viruses* 11: 963.

60 Bernardino, P., James, K., Barnum, S. et al. (2021). What have we learned from 7 years of equine rhinitis B virus qPCR testing in nasal secretions from horses with respiratory signs. *Vet. Rec.* 188: 26.

61 Gilkerson, J.R., Bailey, K.E., Diaz-Mendex, A. et al. (2015). Update on viral diseases of the equine respiratory tract. *Vet. Clin. Equine* 31: 91–104.

62 Blanchard, P.C. and Filkins, M. (1992). Cryptococcal pneumonia and abortion in an equine fetus. *J. Am. Vet. Med. Assoc.* 201: 1591–1592.

63 Ryan, M.J. and Wyand, D.S. (1981). Cryptococcus as a cause of neonatal pneumonia and abortion in two horses. *Vet. Pathol.* 18: 270–272.

64 Rezabek, G.B., Donahue, J.M., Giles, R.C. et al. (1993). Histoplasmosis in horses. *J. Comp. Pathol.* 109: 47–55.

65 Hilton, H., Galuppo, L., Puchalski, S.M. et al. (2009). Successful treatment of invasive pulmonary aspergillosis in a neonatal foal. *J. Vet. Intern. Med.* 23: 375–378.

66 Maleski, K., Magdesian, K.G., LaFranco, L. et al. (2002). Pulmonary coccidioimycosis in a neonatal foal. *Vet. Rec.* 151: 505–508.

67 Petrites-Murphy, M.B., Robbins, L.A., Donahue, J.M. et al. (1996). Equine cryptococcal endometritis and placentitis with neonatal cryptococcal pneumonia. *J. Vet. Diagn. Investig.* 8: 383–386.

68 Reilly, L.K. and Palmer, J.E. (1994). Systemic candidiasis in four foals. *J. Am. Vet. Med. Assoc.* 205: 464–466.

69 Perron Lepage, M.F. (1999). A case of interstitial pneumonia associated with *Pneumocystis carinii* in a foal. *Vet. Pathol.* 36: 621–624.

70 Ewing, P.J., Cowell, R.L., Tyler, R.D. et al. (1994). *Pneumocystis carinii* pneumonia in foals. *J. Am. Vet. Med. Assoc.* 204: 929–933.

71 Stewart, A.J. and Cuming, R.S. (2015). Update on fungal respiratory disease in horses. *Vet. Clin. Equine* 31: 43–62.

72 Brown, C.A., MacKay, R.J., Chandra, S. et al. (1997). Overwhelming strongyloidosis in a foal. *J. Am. Vet. Med. Assoc.* 211: 333–334.

73 Burks, B.S. (1998). Parasitic pneumonitis in horses. *Compend. Contin. Educ. Pract. Vet.* 20: 378–383.

74 Turk, M.A. and Klei, T.R. (1984). Effect of ivermectin treatment on eosinophilic pneumonia and other extravascular lesions of late *Strongylus vulgaris* larval migration in foals. *Vet. Pathol.* 21: 87–92.

75 Boyle, A.G. and Houston, R. (2006). Parasitic pneumonitis and treatment in horses. *Clin. Tech. Equine Pract.* 5: 225–232.

76 Srihakim, S. and Swerczek, T.W. (1978). Pathologic changes and pathogenesis of *Parascaris equorum* infection in parasite-free pony foals. *Am. J. Vet. Res.* 39: 1155–1160.

77 Clayton, H.M. (1978). Ascariasis in foals. *Vet. Rec.* 24: 553–556.

78 Henton, J.E. and Geiser, D.R. (1982). Dictyocaulus arenfeldi in foal pneumonia: a case report. *J. Equine Vet. Sci.* 2: 170–171.

79 Gorman, E.A., O'Kane, C.M., and McAuley, D.F. (2022). Acute respiratory distress syndrome in adults: diagnosis, outcomes, long-term sequelae, and management. *Lancet* 400: 1157–1170.

80 Bordes, J., Lacroix, G., Esnault, P. et al. (2014). Comparison of the Berlin definition with the American European consensus definition for acute respiratory distress syndrome in burn patients. *Burns* 40: 562–567.

81 Ranieri, V.M., Rubenfeld, G.D., Thompson, B.T. et al. (2012). Acute respiratory distress syndrome: the Berlin definition. *JAMA* 307: 2526–2533.

82 Bernard, G.R., Artigas, A., Brigham, K.L. et al. (1994). The American-European Consensus Conference on ARDS. Definitions, mechanisms, relevant outcomes, and clinical trial coordination. *Am. J. Respir. Crit. Care Med.* 149: 818–824.

83 Wilkins, P.A., Otto, C.M., Dunkel, B. et al. (2007). Acute lung injury and acute respiratory distress syndromes in veterinary medicine: consensus definitions: the Dorothy Russell Havemeyer Working Group on ALI and ARDS in veterinary medicine. *J. Vet. Emerg. Crit. Care* 17: 333–339.

84 Hackett, E.S., Traub-Dargatz, J.L., Knowles, J.E. et al. (2010). Arterial blood gas parameters of normal foals born at 1500 metres elevation. *Equine Vet. J.* 42: 59–62.

85 Wong, D.M., Hepworth-Warren, K.L., Sponseller, B.T. et al. (2017). Measured and calculated variables of global oxygenation in healthy neonatal foals. *Am. J. Vet. Res.* 78: 230–238.

86 Schultz, M.J., Haitsma, J.J., Zhang, H. et al. (2006). Pulmonary coagulopathy as a new target in therapeutic studies of acute lung injury or pneumonia–a review. *Crit. Care Med.* 34: 871–877.

87 Matthay, M.A., Ware, L.B., and Zimmerman, G.A. (2012). The acute respiratory distress syndrome. *J. Clin. Invest.* 122: 2731–2740.

88 Glas, G.J., van der Sluijs, K.F., Schultz, M.J. et al. (2013). Bronchoalveolar hemostasis in lung injury and acute respiratory distress syndrome. *J. Thromb. Haemost.* 11: 17–25.

89 Butt, Y., Kurdowska, A., and Allen, T.C. (2016). Acute lung injury: a clinical and molecular review. *Arch. Pathol. Lab. Med.* 140: 345–350.

90 Katz, J.N., Kolappa, K.P., and Becker, R.C. (2011). Beyond thrombosis: the versatile platelet in critical illness. *Chest* 139: 658–668.

91 Piantadosi, C.A. and Schwartz, D.A. (2004). The acute respiratory distress syndrome. *Ann. Intern. Med.* 141: 460–470.

92 McVey, M., Tabuchi, A., and Kuebler, W.M. (2012). Microparticles and acute lung injury. *Am. J. Physiol. Lung Cell. Mol. Physiol.* 303: L364–L381.

93 Jain, R. and DalNogare, A. (2006). Pharmacological therapy for acute respiratory distress syndrome. *Mayo Clin. Proc.* 81: 205–212.

94 Mao, M., Xu, X., Zhang, Y. et al. (2013). Endothelial progenitor cells: the promise of cell-based therapies for acute lung injury. *Inflamm. Res.* 62: 3–8.

95 Matthay, M.A., Robriquet, L., and Fang, X. (2005). Alveolar epithelium: role in lung fluid balance and acute lung injury. *Proc. Am. Thorac. Soc.* 2: 206–213.

96 Buergelt, C.D., Hines, S.A., Cantor, G. et al. (1986). A retrospective study of proliferative interstitial lung disease of horses in Florida. *Vet. Pathol.* 23: 750–756.

97 Prescott, J.F., Carman, S., and Hoffman, A.M. (1991). Sporadic, severe bronchointerstitial pneumonia of foals. *Can. Vet. J.* 32: 421–425.

98 Lakritz, J., Wilson, W.D., Berry, C.R. et al. (1993). Bronchointerstitial pneumonia and respiratory distress in young horses: clinical, clinicopathologic, radiographic, and pathological findings in 23 cases (1984–1989). *J. Vet. Intern. Med.* 7: 277–288.

99 Dunkel, B. (2006). Acute lung injury and acute respiratory distress syndrome in foals. *Clin. Tech. Equine Pract.* 5: 127–133.

100 Britton, A.P. and Robinson, J.H. (2002). Isolation of influenza A virus from a 7-day-old foal with bronchointerstitial pneumonia. *Can. Vet. J.* 43: 55–56.

101 Peek, S.F., Landolt, G., Karasin, A.I. et al. (2004). Acute respiratory distress syndrome and fatal interstitial pneumonia associated with equine influenza in a neonatal foal. *J. Vet. Intern. Med.* 18: 132–134.

102 Patterson-Kane, J.C. and Firth, E.C. (2009). The pathobiology of exercise-induced superficial digital flexor tendon injury in Thoroughbred racehorses. *Vet. J.* 181: 79–89.

103 Zheng, F., Pan, Y., Yang, Y. et al. (2022). Novel biomarkers for acute respiratory distress syndrome: genetics, epigenetics and transcriptomics. *Biomark. Med* 16: 217–231.

104 Costa, L.R.R., Eades, S.C., Goad, M.E. et al. (2004). Pulmonary surfactant dysfunction in neonatal foals: pathogenesis and clinical findings. *Compend. Contin. Educ. Vet.* 26: 380–388.

105 Christmann, U., Livesey, L.C., Taintor, J.S. et al. (2006). Lung surfactant function and composition in neonatal foals and adult horses. *J. Vet. Intern. Med.* 20: 1402–1407.

106 Lascola, K.M. and Joslyn, S. (2015). Diagnostic imaging of the lower respiratory tract in neonatal foals. *Vet. Clin. Equine* 31: 497–514.

107 Lester, G.D. and Lester, N.V. (2001). Abdominal and thoracic radiography in the neonate. *Vet. Clin. North Am. Equine Pract.* 17: 19–46.

108 Toal, R.L. and Cudd, T. (1986). Equine neonatal thoracic radiography: a radiographic-pathologic correlation. *Proc. Am. Assoc. Equine Pract.* 32: 117–128.

109 Bedenice, D., Heuwieser, W., Brawer, R. et al. (2003). Clinical and prognostic significance of radiographic pattern, distribution, and severity of thoracic radiographic changes in neonatal foals. *J. Vet. Intern. Med.* 17: 878–886.

110 Ramirez, S., Lester, G.D., and Roberts, G.R. (2004). Diagnostic contribution of thoracic ultrasonography in 17 foals with Rhodococcus equi pneumonia. *Vet. Radiol. Ultrasound* 45: 172–176.

111 Lamb, C.R., O'Callaghan, M.W., and Paradis, M.R. (1990). Thoracic radiography in the neonatal foal: a preliminary report. *Vet. Radiol.* 31: 11–16.

112 McCracken, J.L. and Slovis, N.M. (2009). Use of thoracic ultrasound for the prevention of Rhodococcus equi pneumonia on endemic farms. *AAEP Proc.* 55: 38–44.

113 Cohen, N.D. (2014). *Rhodococcus equi* foal pneumonia. *Vet. Clin. Equine* 30: 609–622.

114 Leclere, M., Magdesian, K.G., Kass, P.H. et al. (2011). Comparison of the clinical, microbiological, radiological and haematological features of foals with pneumonia caused by *Rhodococcus equi* and other bacteria. *Vet. J.* 187: 109–112.

115 Thome, R., Rohn, K., and Venner, M. (2018). Clinical and haematological parameters for the early diagnosis of pneumonia in foals. *Pferdeheikunde* 34: 260–266.

116 Nout, Y.S., Hinchcliff, K.W., Samii, V.F. et al. (2002). Chronic pulmonary disease with radiographic interstitial opacity (interstitial pneumonia) in foals. *Equine Vet. J.* 34: 542–548.

117 Dunkel, B., Dolente, B., and Boston, R.C. (2005). Acute lung injury/acute respiratory distress syndrome in 15 foals. *Equine Vet. J.* 37: 435–440.

118 Yamanaka, T., Tsujimura, K., Kondo, T. et al. (2006). Efficacy of oseltamivir phosphate to horses inoculated with equine influenza A virus. *J. Vet. Med. Sci.* 68: 923–928.

119 Lind, E.O. and Christenson, D. (2009). Anthelmintic efficacy on *Parascaris equorum* in foals on Swedish studs. *Acta Vet. Scand.* 51: 45–48.

120 Wong, D.M., Alcott, C.J., Wang, C. et al. (2010). Physiologic effects of nasopharyngeal administration of supplemental oxygen at various flow rates in healthy neonatal foals. *Am. J. Vet. Res.* 71: 1081–1088.

121 Hoffman, A.M. and Viel, L. (1992). A percutaneous transtracheal catheter system for improved oxygenation in foals with respiratory distress. *Equine Vet. J.* 24: 239–241.

122 Raidal, S.L., McKean, R., Ellul, P.A. et al. (2019). Effects of continuous positive airway pressure on respiratory function in sedated foals. *J. Vet. Emerg. Crit. Care (San Antonio)* 29: 269–278.

123 Floyd, E., Danks, S., Comyn, I. et al. (2022). Nasal high flow oxygen therapy in hospitalised neonatal foals. *Equine Vet. J.* 54: 946–951.

124 Sklar, M.C. and Munshi, L. (2022). Advances in ventilator management for patients with acute respiratory distress syndrome. *Clin. Chest Med.* 43: 499–509.

125 Chang, X., Li, S., Fu, Y. et al. (2022). Safety and efficacy of corticosteroids in ARDS patients: a systematic review and meta-analysis of RCT data. *Respir. Res.* 23: 301.

126 Confalonieri, M., Salton, F., and Fabiano, F. (2017). Acute respiratory distress syndrome. *Eur. Respir. Rev.* 26: 144.

127 Meng, L., Liao, X., Wang, Y. et al. (2022). Pharmacologic therapies of ARDS: from natural herb to nanomedicine. *Front. Pharmacol.* 13: 930593.

128 Chen, I.L. and Chen, H.L. (2022). New developments in neonatal respiratory management. *Pediatr. Neonatol.* 63: 341–347.

129 Tinkler, S.H., Mathews, L.A., Firshman, A.M. et al. (2015). The use of equine surfactant and positive pressure ventilation to treat a premature alpaca cria with severe hypoventilation and hypercapnia. *Can. Vet. J.* 56: 370–374.

130 Lakritz, J., Wilson, W.D., March, A.E. et al. (2000). Effects of prior feeding on pharmacokinetics and estimated bioavailability after oral administration of a single dose of microencapsulated erythromycin base in healthy foals. *Am. J. Vet. Res.* 61: 1011–1015.

131 Davis, J.L., Gardner, S.Y., Jones, S.L. et al. (2002). Pharmacokinetics of azithromycin in foals after IV and oral dose and disposition into phagocytes. *J. Vet. Pharmacol. Ther.* 25: 99–104.

132 Jacks, S., Giguere, S., Gronwall, P.R. et al. (2001). Pharmacokinetics of azithromycin and concentration in body fluids and bronchoalveolar cells in foals. *Am. J. Vet. Res.* 62: 1870–1875.

133 Womble, A., Giguere, S., Murthy, Y.V. et al. (2006). Pulmonary disposition of tilmicosin in foals and in vitro activity against *Rhodococcus equi* and other common equine bacterial pathogens. *J. Vet. Pharmacol.* 29: 561–568.

134 Suarez-Mier, G., Giguere, S., and Lee, E.A. (2007). Pulmonary disposition of erythromycin, azithromycin, and clarithromycin in foals. *J. Vet. Pharmacol. Ther.* 30: 109–115.

135 Giguere, S., Jacks, S., Roberts, G.D. et al. (2004). Retrospective comparison of azithromycin, clarithromycin, and erythromycin for the treatment of foals with *Rhodococcus equi* pneumonia. *J. Vet. Intern. Med.* 18: 568–573.

136 Giguere, S. (2017). Treatment of infections caused by *Rhodococcus equi*. *Vet. Clin. Equine* 33: 67–85.

137 Peters, J., Block, W., Oswald, S. et al. (2011). Oral absorption of clarithromycin is nearly abolished by chronic comedication of rifampicin in foals. *Drug Metab. Dispos.* 39: 1643–1649.

138 Peters, J., Eggers, K., Oswald, S. et al. (2012). Clarithromycin is absorbed by an intestinal uptake mechanism that is sensitive to major inhibition by rifampicin: results of a short-term drug interaction study in foals. *Drug Metab. Dispos.* 40: 522–528.

139 Giguere, S., Jordan, L.M., Glass, K. et al. (2012). Relationship of mixed bacterial infection to prognosis in foals with pneumonia caused by *Rhodococcus equi*. *J. Vet. Intern. Med.* 26: 443–448.

140 Giguere, S., Lee, E., Williams, E. et al. (2010). Determination of the prevalence of antimicrobial resistance to macrolide antimicrobials or rifampin in *Rhodococcus equi* isolates and treatment outcome in foals infected with antimicrobial-resistant isolates of *R. equi*. *J. Am. Vet. Med. Assoc.* 237: 74–81.

141 Venner, M., Rodiger, A., Laemmer, M. et al. (2012). Failure of antimicrobial therapy to accelerate spontaneous healing of subclinical pulmonary abscesses on a farm with endemic infections caused by *Rhodococcus equi*. *Vet. J.* 192: 293–298.

142 Venner, M., Astheimer, K., Lammer, M. et al. (2013). Efficacy of mass antimicrobial treatment of foals with subclinical pulmonmary abscesses associated with *Rhodococcus equi*. *J. Vet. Intern. Med.* 27: 171–176.

143 Higuchi, T., Arakawa, T., Hashikura, S. et al. (1999). Effect of prophylactic administration of hyperimmune plasma to prevent *Rhodococcus equi* infection in foals from endemically affected farms. *Zentralbl. Veterinarmed. B* 46: 641–648.

144 Martens, R.J., Martens, J.G., Fiske, R.A. et al. (1989). *Rhodococcus equi* foal pneumonia: protective effects of immune plasma in experimentally infected foals. *Equine Vet. J.* 21: 249–255.

145 Caston, S.S., McClure, S.R., Martens, R.J. et al. (2006). Effect of hyperimmune plasma on the severity of pneumonia caused by *Rhodococcus equi* in experimentally infected foals. *Vet. Ther.* 7: 361–375.

146 Hietala, S.K. and Ardans, S. (1987). Interaction of *Rhodococcus equi* with phagocytic cells from *R. equi*-exposed and non-exposed foals. *Vet. Microbiol.* 14: 307–320.

147 Hines, S.A., Kanaly, S., Byrne, B.A. et al. (1997). Immunity to *Rhodococcus equi*. *Vet. Mircobiol.* 56: 177–185.

148 Giguere, S., Gaskin, J.M., Miller, C. et al. (2002). Evaluation of a commercially available hyperimmune plasma product for prevention of naturally acquired pneumonia caused by *Rhodococcus equi* in foals. *J. Am. Vet. Med. Assoc.* 220: 59–63.

149 Hurley, J.R. and Begg, A.P. (1995). Failure of hyperimmune plasma to prevent pneumonia caused by *Rhodococcus equi* in foals. *Aust. Vet. J.* 72: 418–420.

150 Hillidge, C.J. (1987). Use of erythromycin-rifampin combination in treatment of *Rhodococcus equi* pneumonia. *Vet. Microbiol.* 14: 337–342.

151 Chaffin, M.K. and Martens, R.J. (1997). Extrapulmonary disorders associated with *Rhodococcus equi* in foals: retrospective study of 61 cases (1988–1996). *Proc. Am. Assoc. Equine Pract.* 43: 79–80.

152 Ainsworth, D.M., Eicker, S.W., Yeager, A.E. et al. (1998). Associations between physical examination, laboratory, and radiographic findings and outcome and subsequent racing performance of foals with *Rhodococcus equi* infection:115 cases (1984–1992). *J. Am. Vet. Med. Assoc.* 213: 510–515.

153 Ainsworth, D.M., Erb, H.N., Eicker, S.W. et al. (2000). Effects of pulmonary abscesses on racing performance of horses treated at referral veterinary medical teaching hospitals: 45 cases (1985–1997). *J. Am. Vet. Med. Assoc.* 216: 1282–1287.

154 Bernard, B., Dugan, J., Pierce, S. et al. (1991). The influence of foal pneumonia on future racing performance. *Proc. Am. Assoc. Equine Pract.* 37: 17–18.

155 Treloar, S.K., Dhand, N.K., and Muscatello, G. (2012). Rhodococcus equi pneumonia and future racing performance of the Thoroughbred. *J. Equine Vet. Sci.* 32: S16–S17.

Section III Meconium Aspiration Syndrome

David Wong and Pamela A. Wilkins

Meconium is composed of substances originating from the fetus and consists of a conglomerate of salivary, gastric, pancreatic and intestinal fluids, mucus, bile, bile acids, triglycerides, cholesterol, free fatty acids, bilirubin, hemoglobin, proteins, cellular debris, fetal wax, blood, and pro-inflammatory cytokines (interleukin [IL]-1β, IL-6, IL-8, tumor necrosis factor [TNF]α) [1, 2]. Meconium-stained amniotic fluid is relatively common in newborn infants and is observed in approximately 10–15% of deliveries; approximately 5% of these infants develop meconium aspiration syndrome (MAS) [3]. Overall, MAS is a well-recognized disease process and accounts for 10% of all causes of respiratory failure in neonatal infants with a mortality of 20% in developing countries [4]. Furthermore, infants with MAS are more likely to develop complications such as sepsis, seizures, and neurologic impairment [5]. MAS in infants is defined by the following criteria: (i) respiratory distress (tachypnea) in a neonate born with meconium-stained amniotic fluid; (ii) need for supplemental oxygen to maintain an oxygen saturation of hemoglobin (SaO_2) ≥92%; (iii) oxygen requirements starting during the first 2 hours of life and lasting at least 12 hours; and (iv) absence of congenital malformations of the airway, lung, or heart [1].

Meconium is released in utero secondary to fetal stress or vagal stimulation due to cord compression, which in turn stimulates peristalsis in the colon and relaxation of the anal sphincter [6]. Some clinicians suggest that chronic in utero insults (e.g. hypoxia, acidosis) may be more important for meconium passage as compared to acute peripartum events [7]. MAS occurs in utero when the fetus aspirates meconium during intrauterine gasping, which is stimulated by fetal hypoxia. MAS can also occur perinatally during the initial breaths immediately after birth of the newborn. In infants, term and post-term fetuses are more likely to pass meconium in response to fetal insults as compared to pre-term infants as it is believed that preterm infants have an immature gastrointestinal system and thus less likely to pass meconium [7]. In addition, primary and secondary causes of meconium stained amniotic fluid have been proposed, with primary meconium defined as meconium occurring at the time of rupture of the fetal membranes; in comparison, secondary meconium staining is described as clear amniotic fluid at the time of fetal membrane rupture that subsequently becomes meconium-stained during partirution [7].

Pathophysiology of Meconium Aspiration Syndrome

The pathophysiology of MAS is complex with the exact mechanisms involved to be further elucidated. However, aspects that contribute to MAS are multifactorial and include mechanical blockage of airways, chemical pneumonitis and direct toxic effects, surfactant dysfunction, persistent pulmonary hypertension of the newborn (PPHN), and activation of the innate immune system and resultant inflammation [1, 7]. With breathing movements, meconium migrates from proximal to distal airways, resulting in partial or complete airway obstruction. Complete airway obstruction results in alveolar atelectasis behind the meconium plug, whereas partial obstruction of the small airways causes a ball valve effect, leading to air trapping, hyperaeration, and air leak into the insersititum [6, 8]. Because of air leak, pneumothorax, pneumomediastinum, or interstitial emphysema can be observed in severe cases. Ventilation/perfusion (V/Q) mismatch also ensues due to meconium particles causing obstruction, atelectasis, and hyperinflation in the small airways [7]. Meconium additionally has direct toxic effects on alveoli and induces a chemical pneumonitis accompanied by alveolar collapse and edema [9].

Equine Neonatal Medicine, First Edition. Edited by David M. Wong and Pamela A. Wilkins.

Further contributing to MAS, meconium changes the viscosity and ultrastructure of surfactant, decreases the levels of surfactant proteins, and accelerates the conversion from large, surface active aggregates into small, less active forms [8]. Type II alveolar cells also produce less surfactant, oxidative stress causes surfactant inactivation, and free fatty acids in meconium displace surfactant [7, 10]. Collectively, these activities result in surfactant dysfunction, increased alveolar surface tension, and decreased lung compliance. The resulting atelectasis causes pulmonary vascular constriction, hypoperfusion, and lung-tissue ischemia [11]. Sloughed respiratory epithelium, protein, edema, and hyaline membrane formation also contribute to respiratory distress [12].

Although meconium is sterile, the fetus/newborn considers meconium to exist “extra-corporally” as its contents are “hidden” in the intestinal tract and normally not recognized by the fetal immune system. This is relevant because of the potential danger that meconium poses to the fetus/newborn lung as meconium contains several signals and ligands that activate the host’s immune system via toll-like receptors and the complement system; consequently, inflammatory cascades are activated and produce cytokines, prostaglandins, and reactive oxygen species (ROS) as well as activate apoptotic pathways [1]. Evidence of the inflammatory response can be noted by the high concentrations of TNF-α, IL-1β, IL-6, and IL-8 that have been measured in meconium-stained amniotic fluid [13].

Meconium itself acts as a potent chemoattractant and induces neutrophil chemotaxis to the lungs within several hours of aspiration [8]. Meconium is also a source of pro-inflammatory mediators such as Il-1, Il-6, and Il-8 and induces inflammation directly and indirectly through stimulation of oxidative burst in neutrophils and alveolar macrophages [8, 14]. These inflammatory mediators cause direct injury to lung parenchyma and vascular endothelium leading to capillary leak of proteinaceous fluid and cells into the alveolar spaces through the alveolocapillary membrane, along with toxic pneumonitis and hemorrhagic pulmonary edema [7]. Cytokines and ROS also injure airway epithelial cells resulting in apoptosis.

Additionally, MAS is often associated with pulmonary vasoconstriction from hypoxia, acidosis, and the vasoconstrictive effects of meconium and other inflammatory substances released during MAS [3, 8]. In fact, postnatal installation of meconium elevated the pulmonary artery pressure and vascular resistance in a concentration-dependent manner in an experimental pig model and was linked with higher concentrations of thromboxane A_2, leukotrienes, prostaglandins, and endothelin-1 [8, 15]. These factors contribute to the development of pulmonary hypertension and PPHN with MAS [3]. In the healthy newborn, pulmonary vascular resistance falls at birth to approximately 10% of fetal values and pulmonary blood flow increases accordingly [16]. Early in the postnatal period, these two changes balance each other out, and the mean pulmonary and systolic pressure remain increased for the first several hours of life [17]. PPHN results when there is a failure of the circulatory pattern to convert to a postnatal circulatory pattern. In this situation, right to left shunting of blood occurs within the lungs and through patent fetal conduits secondary to meconium aspiration (or other factors such as asphyxia or other unknown triggers) [17].

In addition to the above mechanisms involved with MAS, many components of meconium such as bile acids can cause direct injury to umbilical cord vessels and amniotic membranes. This, in turn, causes fetal tissue and organ damage ranging from mild inflammation in the lung, placental membranes, and chorion to severe focal injury of umbilical vessels [18]. Meconium-induced umbilical vessel constriction, vessel necrosis and thrombi production can lead to severe hypoxic–ischemic injury [7].

Clinical Signs and Diagnosis

During parturition, the clinician may note meconium-stained (yellow-brown tinged) fetal membranes providing obvious evidence that MAS may ensue in the newborn foal (Figure 8.III.1a). As a general practice with postpartum mares, clinicians should examine the fetal membranes to identify any areas of potential infection, irregularities, or missing portions of the membranes; meconium staining may be observed at this time as well (Figure 8.III.1b). If the fetal membranes are not available to the clinician, observation of yellow-brown tinged hair coat in the newborn foal may support potential exposure to meconium. Of note, this color observation may not be obvious in bay/brown or dark-colored foals, but the clinician may note meconium staining on their hands as they handle the foal.

Clinical signs of MAS are mainly confined to the respiratory tract and vary in severity, ranging from mild tachypnea to life-threatening respiratory distress (tachypnea, dyspnea, respiratory grunting) and pulmonary hypertension [11]. Additional reported clinical signs in infants with MAS include frothy, yellow-green secretions from the mouth, rapid breathing, intercostal retractions, cyanosis, overinflation of the chest (due to air trapping), rales and rattling in the throat [19]. Other concurrent disease processes such as sepsis or pneumonia may also be present, along with commensurate clinical signs.

Diagnosis of MAS is based on the observation of meconium-stained fetal membranes and/or stained haircoat in the newborn foal along with clinical signs of respiratory disease. Arterial blood gas analysis reveals varying levels of

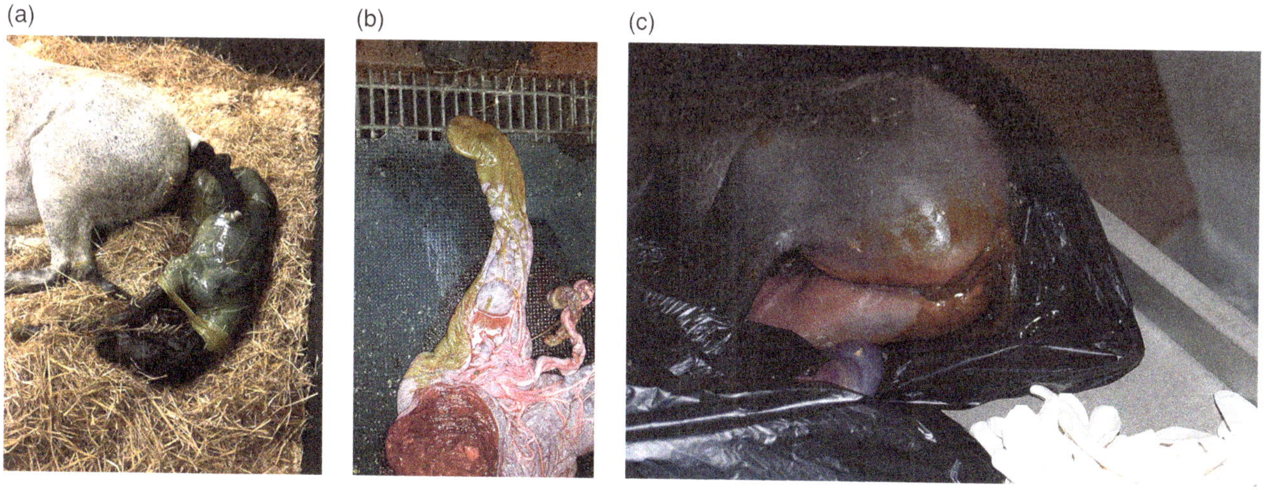

Figure 8.III.1 (a) Newborn Thoroughbred foal with meconium-stained fetal membranes. This foal succumbed to MAS 24 hours after being born. (b) Meconium-stained fetal membranes. *Source:* Images courtesy of Nicki Fewerda, Iowa State University. (c) Mid-gestation aborted fetus, note the meconium staining of the perineum.

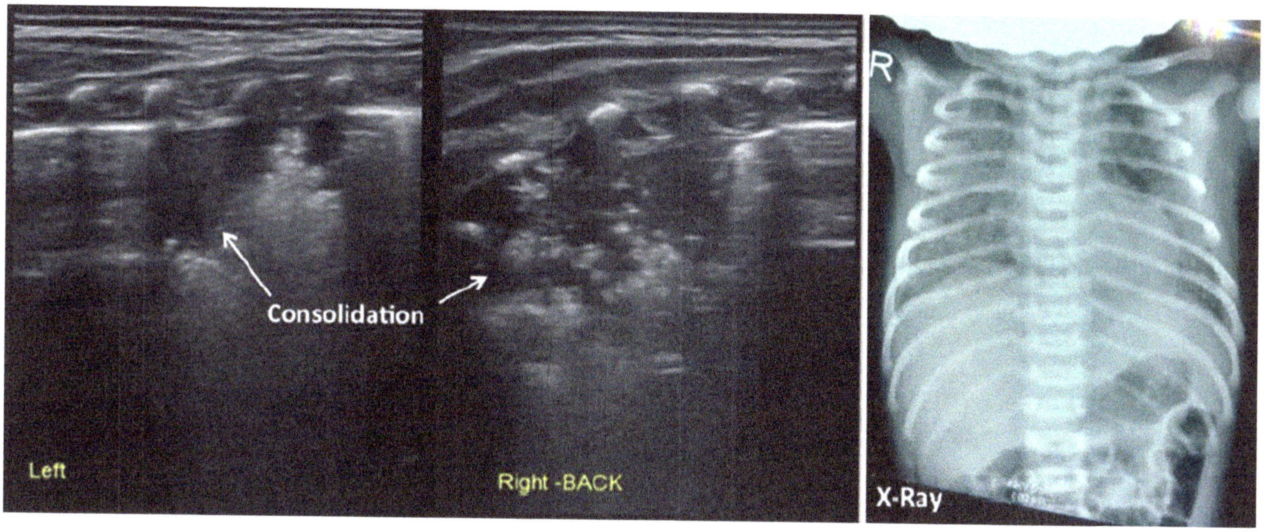

Figure 8.III.2 Ultrasonographic findings in a newborn infant with MAS, born at 39 weeks of gestation. Note the large areas of pulmonary consolidation with air bronchograms and irregular edges in the lungs. The pleural line was abnormal and the A-line disappeared in the consolidated area. Chest radiographs showed patchy and cloudy shadows [20].

hypoxemia, and concurrent diseases may impact other parameters noted on CBC and serum biochemistry profile. Radiography in foals with MAS may note diffuse pulmonary interstitial infiltrates other radiographic descriptions in infants with MAS include patchy and cloudy shadows diffusely within the lungs [11, 20]. Widespread pulmonary pleural irregularities were reported upon ultrasonographic examination of a foal with MAS, while ultrasonographic description of infants with MAS include lung consolidation with air bronchograms, irregular lung edges, pleural line anomalies (disappearance of pleural line, thickened and blurred pleural lines), pleural effusion, and disappearance of A-lines (Figure 8.III.2) [11, 20].

Treatment

Treatment recommendations noted here are primarily based on MAS in infants, as so few cases have been reported in foals. Overall therapeutic themes include pulmonary care (respiratory support, surfactant treatment), attenuation of inflammation (anti-inflammatory medications), prevention of infection (antimicrobials), addressing pulmonary hypertension (vasodilators) if present, and general supportive care (hydration, sedation, and analgesia, if needed) [3].

Oxygen supplementation/respiratory support and IV fluids are cornerstones of treatment of MAS in infants [7].

Monitoring pulse oximetry and/or arterial blood gas analysis with a target S_aO_2 of 90–95% and P_aO_2 of 90 mmHg helps direct the type of respiratory support needed [7]. Respiratory support ranges from the simple provision of intranasal oxygen (8–10 l/min) to mechanical ventilation and/or continuous positive airway pressure. In infants, no other condition poses as much challenge for mechanical ventilation than MAS due to the fact that the lungs of affected infants have areas of atelectasis coexisting with areas of hyperinflation associated with V/Q mismatch and airway compromise [7]. Synchronized intermittent mandatory ventilation or assist/control are preferred mechanical ventilation modes in infants. The goal of mechanical ventilation is to improve oxygenation while simultaneously minimizing barotrauma. Exogenous administration of surfactant is also recommended in infants with MAS requiring $F_iO_2 \geq 50\%$ and can be considered as a therapy in foals (see Chapter 1).

In animal models and newborn infants with MAS, steroids such as hydrocortisone, prednisolone, methylprednisolone, dexamethasone, and budesonide have been administered with the intent of attenuating the inflammatory process that occurs with MAS [8]. Although, systemic steroids may benefit patients with MAS who have lung edema, pulmonary vasoconstriction, and inflammation, various studies have shown no or equivocal improvement in survival; thus, routine steroid therapy for management of MAS is not recommended in infants [8, 21]. Clinicians can also consider the judicious use of nonsteroidal anti-inflammatory medications such as flunixine meglumine in neonatal foals with MAS. The presence of meconium increases the positivity rate of bacterial cultures from amniotic fluid; therefore, most physicians administer prophylactic antimicrobials in MAS in infants and the same may be true for foals with MAS [7].

Antioxidants can be considered in MAS as some of the negative effects are associated with ROS and oxidant injury. N-acetylcysteine has antioxidant, anti-inflammatory and mucolytic effects and has been used as a treatment for MAS in various species, including foals [11]. Administration of N-acetylcysteine can reduce the physical properties and viscosity of meconium via breakage of disulphide bonds between protein molecules [22]. N-acetylcysteine may also inactivate digestive enzymes that exacerbate pulmonary damage after meconium aspiration [11]. In foals with MAS, acetylcysteine (20%) can be administered via nebulizer at a dose of 4–8 mg/kg q 6h [11]. Additionally, N-acetylcysteine can be considered to augment the effects of exogenous surfactant administration as an experimental study using rabbits demonstrated an improved therapeutic effect when both were administered together as compared individually [2].

As noted, MAS can be complicated by pulmonary hypertension and PPHN. The typical approach to treatment of pulmonary hypertension is abolishment of hypoxia and correction of acidosis as both promote vasoconstriction and retention of the fetal circulation pattern; this can be accomplished by maximizing pulmonary exposure to oxygen through ventilation with 100% oxygen, alkalinizing the arterial pH with mild hyperventilation or treatment with bases (increase pH from 7.45 to 7.5), and maintaining systemic blood pressure to counterbalance the increasing pulmonary pressure [3, 17, 23]. Alternatively (or in addition), inhaled nitric oxide (NO) can be used to alleviate hypertension be acting on vascular smooth muscle, causing selective pulmonary vasodilation in ventilated areas of lung, thus decreasing the V/Q mismatch and improving oxygenation in patients [24]. Anecdotal reports have used inhaled NO at concentrations of 5–20 (and up to 40) ppm in ventilatory gas in foals with some purported success [17, 23]. Oral sildenafil (0.5–2.5 mg/kg), a phosphodiesterase-5 inhibitor with some specificity for the pulmonary vasculature, has also been used in foals with some success, but neither of these medications have undergone rigorous pharmacokinetic or pharmacodynamic assessment in the foal [17, 23]. Other vasodilators that have been used in infants with MAS include tolazoline (nonspecific vasodilator); phosphodiesterase inhibitors (hydrolyze cyclic nucleotides and increased intracellular cyclic adenosine monophosphate or cyclic guanosine monophosphate) such as milrinone, dipyridamole, and sildenafil; prostacyclin (pulmonary vasodilator); and magnesium sulfate (smooth muscle relaxant and vasodilator) [3].

Of note, routine intranatal and postnatal endotracheal suctioning of meconium in vigorous infants is no longer recommended. However, prophylactic nasogastric aspiration or suctioning before the newborn nurses has been suggested to reduce the risk of feed intolerance and secondary meconium aspiration in meconium-stained newborn infants, but clear benefit from this practice is lacking [25].

The true incidence of MAS in foals is unknown, but meconium aspiration in newborn foals is not infrequently observed (Figure 8.III.3). Few reports in the equine literature describe treatment and outcome of meconium aspiration, but in one case report, a 1-day-old foal presented soon after birth because of rapid onset of depression and respiratory distress. The respiratory rate at admission was 124 breaths/min with gasping noted, along with a P_aO_2 of 52 mmHg [11]. Parturition was assisted because the mare was diagnosed with placentitis and premature placental separation, and severe meconium staining was noted at birth. Ultrasonographic examination of the lungs noted widespread pulmonary pleural irregularities and thoracic

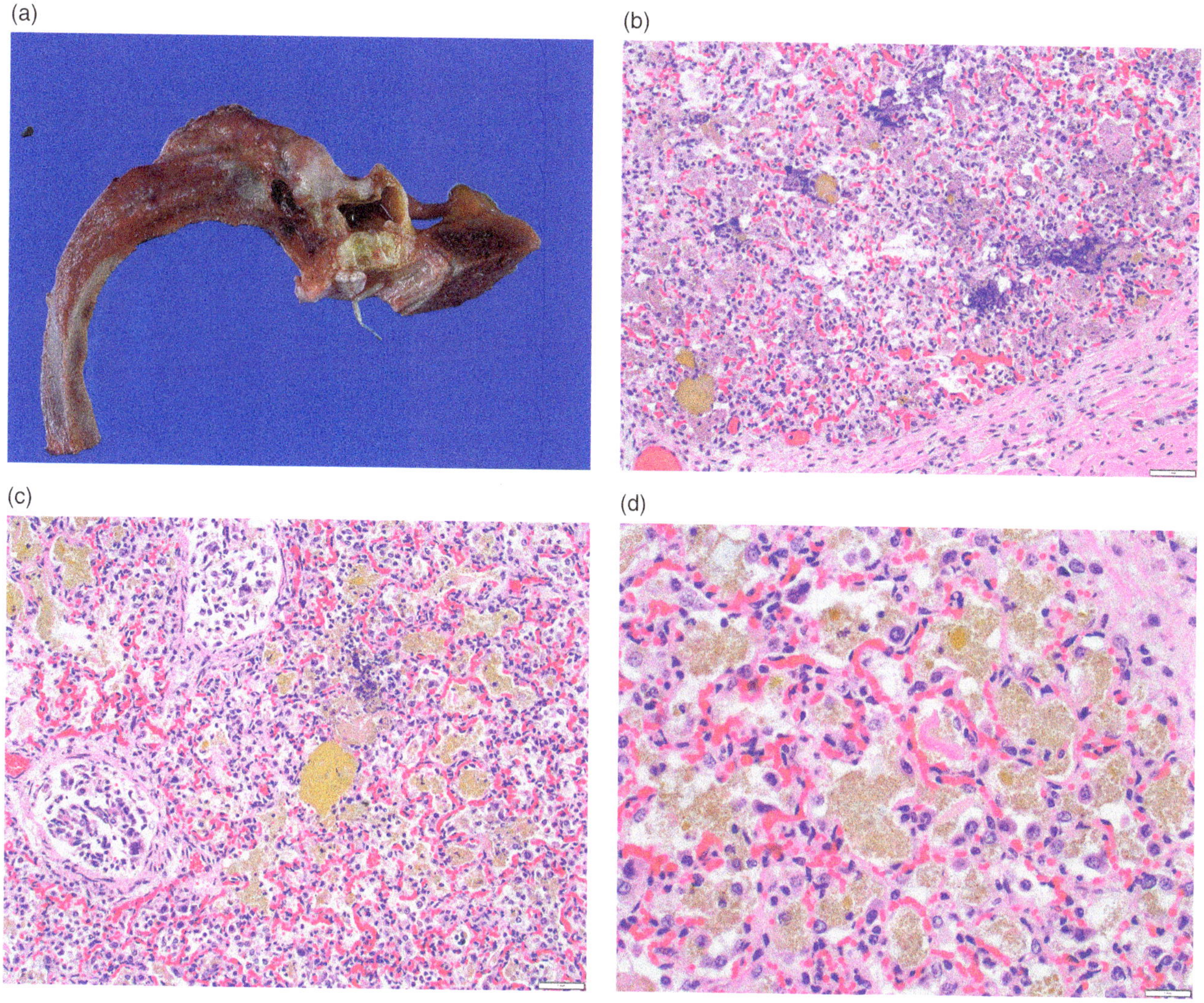

Figure 8.III.3 Images of a 2-day-old Thoroughbred foal with meconium aspiration that presented alert, but with an increased respiratory rate and bronchovesicular sounds. Ultrasonographic examination of the lungs revealed moderate diffuse comet tail lesions bilaterally. The foal's respiratory rate increased significantly over the following 12 hours followed by death. Gross image demonstrating accumulation of meconium and fluid within the tympanic bulla (a). Microscopic examination of the lungs revealed bright yellow concretions (meconium) within the alveolar spaces along with mixed infiltrates of neutrophils, macrophages, fibrin, and sloughed hypereosinophilic cellular debris (b–d). Random alveolar epithelial necrosis and collapsed alveolar spaces were also noted. *Source:* Images courtesy of Dr. Olufemi Fasina, Iowa State University.

radiography displayed a diffuse pulmonary interstitial infiltrate. Treatment included administration of systemic antimicrobials and nebulization therapy using an in-line jet nebulizer and the aerosol administration of ceftiofur (1 mg/kg, q6h), dexamethasone (0.01 mg/kg q12h), N-acetylcsteine (4 mg/kg, q6h), and albuterol sulfate (0.025 mg/kg, q6h); treatments were increased to a total volume of 6 ml using sterile water. Aerosol treatment was continued for 4 days with discontinuation of dexamethasone after 48 hours. The foal's respiratory rate and effort returned to normal (56 breaths/min) and the P_aO_2 improved to 93 mmHg. Thoracic radiographs were repeated on day 5, demonstrating a marked decrease in interstitial infiltrate; the foal was subsequently discharged on systemic antimicrobials.

Prognosis

Unfortunately, there have been no retrospective studies conducted in foals documenting survival rates in neonatal foals with MAS, but prognosis is likely dictated by the amount and severity of MAS. By the time owners seek veterinary intervention of affected foals, many foals are demonstrating significant respiratory compromise and have a guarded prognosis.

References

1 Lindenskov, P.A., Castellheim, A., Saugstad, O.D. et al. (2015). Meconium aspiration syndrome: possible pathophysiological mechanisms and future potential therapies. *Neonatology* 107: 225–230.

2 Kopincova, J., Mokra, D., Mikolka, P. et al. (2014). N-acetylcysteine advancement of surfactant therapy in experimental meconium aspiration syndrome: possible mechanisms. *Physiol. Res.* 63: S629–S642.

3 Asad, A. and Bhat, R. (2008). Pharmacotherapy for meconium aspiration. *J. Perinatol.* 28: S72–S78.

4 Singh, B.S., Clark, R.H., Powers, R.J. et al. (2009). Meconium aspiration syndrome remains a significant problem in the NICU: outcomes and treatment patterns in term neonates admitted for intensive care during a ten-year period. *J. Perinatol.* 29: 497–503.

5 Hutton, E.K. and Thorpe, J. (2014). Consequences of meconium-stained amniotic fluid: what does the evidence tell us? *Early Hum. Dev.* 90: 333–339.

6 Reuter, S., Moser, C., and Baack, M. (2014). Respiratory distress in the newborn. *Pediatr. Rev.* 35: 417–428.

7 Chettri, S., Bhat, B.V., and Adhisivam, B. (2016). Current concepts in the management of meconium aspiration syndrome. *Indian J. Pediatr.* 83: 1125–1130.

8 Mokra, D. and Mokry, J. (2011). Glucosteroids in the treatment of neonatal meconium aspiration syndrome. *Eur. J. Pediatr.* 170: 1495–1505.

9 Tyler, D.C., Murphy, J., and Cheney, F.W. (1978). Mechanical and chemical damage to lung tissue caused by meconium aspiration. *Pediatrics* 62: 454–459.

10 Clark, D.A., Nieman, G.F., Thompson, J.E. et al. (1987). Surfactant displacement by meconium free fatty acids: an alternative explanation for atelectasis in meconium aspiration syndrome. *J. Pediatr.* 110: 765–770.

11 Morresey, P.R. (2008). How to deliver respiratory treatments to neonates by nebulization. *Proceedings from the 2008 AAEP Conference*. 54: 520–526.

12 Srinivasan, H.B. and Vidyasagar, D. (1999). Meconium aspiration syndrome: current concepts and management. *Compr. Ther.* 25: 82–89.

13 Yamada, T., Minakami, H., Matsubara, S. et al. (2000). Meconium-stained amniotic fluid exhibits chemotactic activity for polymorphonuclear leukocytes in vitro. *J. Reprod. Immunol.* 46: 21–30.

14 De Beaufort, A.J., Pelikan, D.M., Elferink, J.G. et al. (1998). Effect of interleukin 8 in meconium on in-vitro neutrophil chemotaxis. *Lancet* 352: 102–105.

15 Holopainen, R., Soukka, H., Halkola, L. et al. (1998). Meconium aspiration induces a concentration-dependent pulmonary hypertensive response in newborn piglets. *Pediatr. Pulmonol.* 25: 107–113.

16 Leffler, C.W., Hessler, J.R., and Green, R.S. (1984). The onset of breathing at birth stimulates pulmonary vascular prostacyclin synthesis. *Pediatr. Res.* 18: 938–942.

17 Wilkins, P.A. (2003). Acute respiratory failure: diagnosis, monitoring techniques, and therapeutics. *Clin. Tech. Equine Pract.* 2: 56–66.

18 Ahanya, S.N., Lakshmanan, J., Morgan, B.L. et al. (2005). Meconium passage in utero: mechanisms, consequences, and management. *Obstet. Gynecol. Surv.* 60: 45–56.

19 Bhatia, B.D., Gupta, V., and Dey, P.K. (1996). Meconium aspiration syndrome: current concepts. *Indian J. Matern. Child Health* 7: 1–7.

20 Liu, J., Cao, H.Y., and Fu, W. (2016). Lung ultrasonography to diagnose meconium aspiration syndrome of the newborn. *J. Int. Med. Res.* 44: 1534–1542.

21 Ward, M. and Sinn, J. (2003). Steroid therapy for meconium aspiration syndrome in newborn infants. *Cochrane Database Syst. Rev.* (4): CD003485. https://doi.org/10.1002/14651858.CD003485.

22 Ivanov, V.A. (2006). Meconium aspiration syndrome treatment – new approaches using old drugs. *Med. Hypotheses* 66: 808–810.

23 Palmer, J.E. (2005). Ventilatory support of the critically ill foal. *Vet. Clin. Equine* 21: 457–486.

24 Walsh, M.C. and Fanaroff, J.M. (2007). Meconium-stained fluid: approach to the mother and the baby. *Clin. Perinatol.* 34: 653–665.

25 Sharma, P., Nangia, S., Tiwari, S. et al. (2014). Gastric lavage for prevention of feeding problems in neonates with meconium-stained amniotic fluid: a randomized controlled trial. *Paediatr. Int. Child Health* 34: 115–119.

Section IV Persistent Pulmonary Hypertension of the Newborn

David Wong and Pamela A. Wilkins

Persistent pulmonary hypertension of the newborn (PPHN), also known as reversion to fetal circulation or persistent fetal circulation, is a well-recognized syndrome in newborn infants and has also been documented, to a much lesser extent, in neonatal foals. In brief, this syndrome is characterized by a structurally normal heart but pulmonary hypoplasia and elevated pulmonary vascular resistance that cases right-to-left shunting through the ductus arteriosus and/or foramen ovale. Ultimately this allows nonoxygenated blood from the pulmonary system to enter the systemic circulation [1, 2]. This section describes the pathophysiology, clinical signs, and potential treatments of PPHN.

Control of Pulmonary Vascular Tone

Control of pulmonary vascular tone and, concomitantly, control of vascular resistance to blood flow, is primarily governed by the arterial musculature. Contraction of the musculature results in reduction of vascular lumen size leading to increased resistance to blood flow; this occurs mainly at the small-caliber arterioles [1]. The clinician must be mindful of the fact that the pulmonary and systemic circulation are two distinct circuits. Moreover, these two circulatory systems may respond differently to different stimuli. For example, hypoxemia causes dilation of the systemic circulation whereas constriction occurs in the pulmonary arteries [1]. The control of vascular muscle is largely determined by factors that are produced by endothelial cells such as nitric oxide (NO), prostacyclin and vascular endothelial growth factor (VEGF), which result in vascular relaxation and thromboxane and prostaglandin $F_2\alpha$ that causes contraction of pulmonary vascular smooth muscle [1]. The composition of the blood, including oxygen and pH, also control pulmonary flow. In the pulmonary system, it is the alveolar oxygen tension rather than an increase in arterial oxygen pressure (P_aO_2) that causes pulmonary vasodilation [1].

The fetal pulmonary circulation is characterized by elevated pulmonary vascular resistance, which is needed to shunt blood right-to-left (i.e. ductus arteriosus, foramen ovale) to the remainder of the fetus. These shunts divert blood from the right atrium to the aorta with only 8–25% of the cardiac output of the right ventricle reaching the lungs [1, 3, 4]. The mechanisms that contribute to the maintenance of this high pulmonary vascular resistance include the presence of fetal lung fluid, low oxygen tension, decreased production of vasodilators (NO, prostacyclin) and increased production of vasoconstrictive molecules (thromboxane, endothelins) [1, 4]. Within minutes of birth, the pulmonary artery pressure rapidly drops to 50% of the systemic pressure and pulmonary blood flow increases approximately 10 times with the onset of respiration in the healthy newborn [1]. The massive decrease in pulmonary vascular resistance after birth is related to expansion of the lungs and alveoli (results in physical expansion of the pulmonary capillary bed), oxygenation of the lungs (stimulates pulmonary arteriolar relaxation), the onset of continuous respiration, and an abrupt increase in pulmonary blood flow [1, 4, 5]. In addition, increased blood flow creates shear stress within the vessel wall; the sheer stress and oxygenation stimulate endothelial nitric oxide synthase (eNOS) to produce NO, consequently relaxing the pulmonary vasculature [4].

PPHN is a syndrome characterized by increased pulmonary vascular resistance and right-to-left shunting of blood through the ductus arteriosus and/or foramen ovale (Figure 8.IV.1) [1]. In contrast to adult people, where primary pulmonary hypertension is defined by a specific pulmonary pressure, PPHN is present (regardless of pulmonary artery pressure) when there is a right-to-left shunt in the absence of a congenital heart abnormality [1]. Although risk factors are not known in mares, maternal conditions

Equine Neonatal Medicine, First Edition. Edited by David M. Wong and Pamela A. Wilkins.

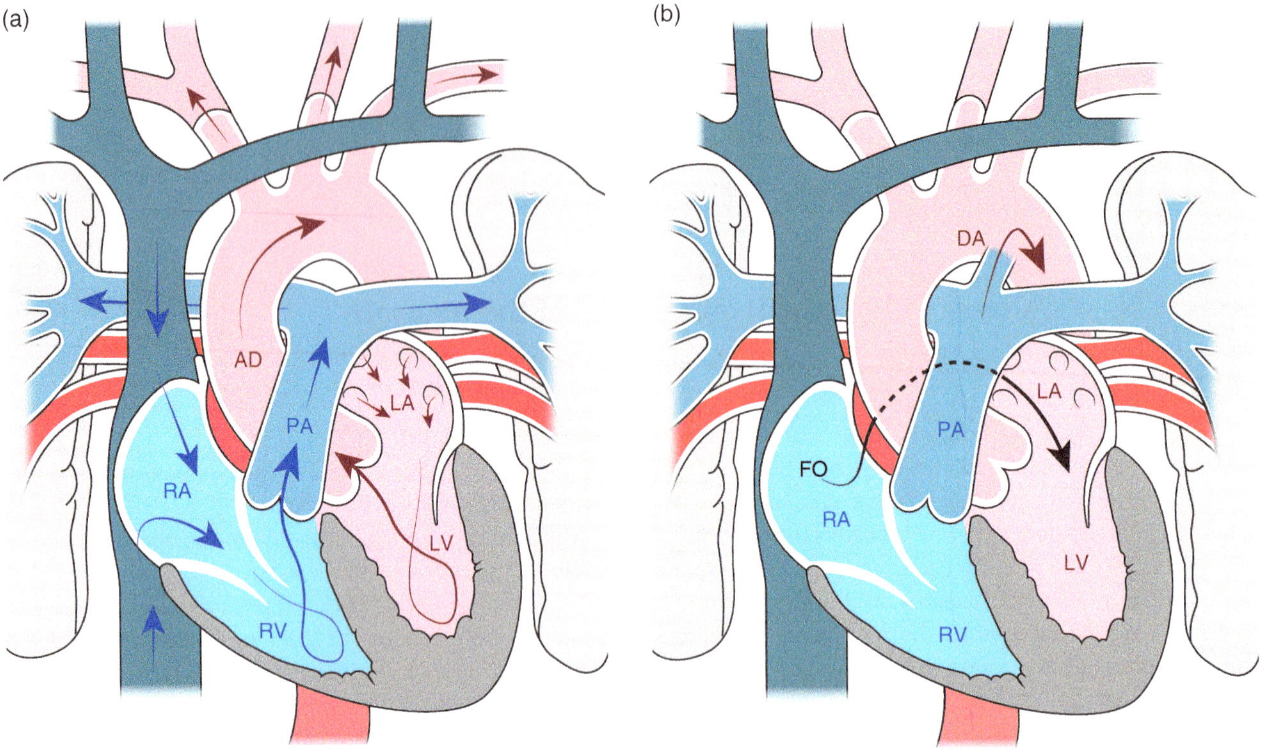

Figure 8.IV.1 Persistent pulmonary hypertension in the newborn (PPHN). (a) Normal circulation in the neonate in which deoxygenated blood enters from the vena cava into the right atrium (RA) passes through the right ventricle (RV) and exits the heart via the pulmonary artery (PA) to the lungs. Blood returns from the lungs via the pulmonary veins into the left atrium (LA) to the left ventricle (LV) and is then pumped to the body via the aorta (AO). (b) With PPHN, the heart is structurally normal but pulmonary hypoplasia and/or elevated pulmonary vascular resistance causes right-to-left shunting of blood through the foramen ovale (FO) and ductus arteriosus (DA), also known as reversion of fetal circulation, ultimately resulting in decreased oxygen delivery to the systemic circulation because of mixing deoxygenated blood with oxygenated blood at the level of the heart. *Source:* Copyright Sara Anais Gonzalez, 2022.

such as obesity, diabetes, asthma, and Black or Asian ethnicity have a higher incidence of PPHN in people [2].

Pathophysiology of PPHN

The pathophysiology of PPHN can be idiopathic or associated with a variety of factors occurring during the perinatal period. Three main types of PPHN described in infants are related to underdevelopment, maldevelopment, or maladaptation of the pulmonary system [4, 6].

Underdevelopment

Some causes associated with *underdevelopment* involve hypoplastic pulmonary vasculature, as seen with congenital diaphragmatic hernia (CDH) and other causes of pulmonary vascular hypoplasia such as oligohydroamnios (secondary to renal disease or chronic leakage of amniotic fluid) or alveolar capillary dysplasia [6, 7]. CDH is an important cause of pulmonary hypoplasia and PPHN in the infant, but infrequently reported in the foal [6, 8, 9]. The molecular and genetic variables resulting in CDH are still unclear, but the lungs of newborn infants with CDH are physically smaller than normal and have a decreased number of airways, decreased number of vascular generations, increased thickness of smooth muscle in the pulmonary arterial walls, reduced number of alveoli, and reduced surfactant production [10, 11]. The affected lung is primarily on the side of the diaphragmatic defect (most often left side) [10]. In conjunction with CDH, the lung development is stalled late in gestation (canalicular or early saccular stage) [10]. Because of the developmental defect in pulmonary vascular growth, there is hypoplasia of the pulmonary vascular bed resulting in increased pulmonary vascular resistance due to an incapacity of the vasculature to accommodate right ventricular cardiac output [1]. Two case reports in foals have described CDH and abnormal lung development; in one case, a full-term Friesian stillborn foal had CDH and the left lung and main bronchus were severely hypoplastic (1/5 the size of the right homolog); the second case was a newborn Quarter Horse filly submitted for necropsy where the left lung had marked volume reduction and CDH, along with several other congenital defects [8, 9, 12].

Maldevelopment

Some causes of PPHN relate to *maldevelopment,* which involves normal lung parenchyma and remodeled pulmonary vasculature. This category includes idiopathic (primary) PPHN in which there is remodeled pulmonary arteries (smooth muscle hyperplasia). Other vascular anomalies that can contribute to PPHN are remodeling of the pulmonary vasculature in which there is histologic characteristics of an increased layer of arterial vascular smooth muscle. This excessive musculature of the vascular wall plays a role in increased pulmonary vascular resistance via decreased vascular lumen size [1]. This vascular remodeling originates from chronic conditions during fetal life, such as placental dysfunction associated with chronic fetal hypoxemia, premature closure of the ductus arteriosus, or fetal exposure to drugs during gestation [1, 4].

Maladaptation

Maladaptation is a category that occurs secondary to parenchymal lung disease, such as meconium aspiration syndrome (MAS), respiratory distress syndrome (RDS), and pneumonia [6, 7]. Diseases such as pneumonia or surfactant deficiency cause decreased alveolar ventilation; this in turn leads to the physiologic response of hypoxic pulmonary vasoconstriction, which attempts to optimize the balance between alveolar ventilation and perfusion by decreasing blood flow to unventilated alveoli. Consequently, there is increased pulmonary vascular resistance. If pulmonary disease involves only a small portion of the lung, pulmonary vascular resistance is not altered; alternatively, if the pulmonary disease is extensive, vascular resistance can increase to a point that induces right-to-left shunt [1].

MAS in the newborn infant is a common cause of the maladaptive form of PPHN in which pulmonary hypertension results as a consequence of airway obstruction, inactivation of surfactant, and chemical pneumonitis from the release of proinflammatory cytokines [13, 14]. The treatment of this category should be aimed at the primary lung condition and not pulmonary vasodilation (i.e. vasoconstriction has protective effect on ventilation/perfusion [V/Q] ratio). Of note, some believe that diseases in this category are incorrectly classified as associated with PPHN because, technically, the primary process is abnormal alveolar ventilation with appropriate vasoconstrictor response of the pulmonary circulation.

Other Conditions

Other conditions associated with PPHN include congenital heart defects (total anomalous pulmonary venous return, left atrial or mitral obstruction, hypoplastic left heart syndrome), polycythemia, hypoglycemia, hypocalcemia, perinatal asphyxia, sepsis, and metabolic acidosis [4]. The underpinning process with perinatal asphyxia, sepsis, or metabolic acidosis is that they cause vasoconstriction. In this instance, the number of vessels, pulmonary structure, and pulmonary vascular branching are normal, but vascular smooth muscle is constricted due to disequilibrium in the balance of vasoactive substances (i.e., vasoconstrictors > vasodilators) caused by an underlying condition (e.g., sepsis) [1]. From a practical standpoint, differentiating the underlying cause of pulmonary vasoconstriction from one another can be clinically difficult.

Infants with PPHN typically present within 12 hours of birth with labile levels of oxygenation that can progress to cyanosis. If pulmonary hypertension is secondary to other conditions, the presentation is complicated by the features of the primary condition [1]. Respiratory distress may be mild unless the pulmonary hypertension is secondary to lung disease such as meconium aspiration. Because of the hypoxemia, infants may be acidemic and hypotensive and remain cyanotic despite administration of high concentrations of oxygen [2]. Auscultation of the heart can reveal increased intensity of the second heart sound (closure of aortic and pulmonary valves) secondary to pulmonary artery hypertension and a systolic murmur of tricuspid regurgitation. PPHN should be considered in neonatal foals in which the level of hypoxemia is disproportionate to the degree of respiratory distress and pulmonary parenchymal findings (i.e. thoracic radiographs, ultrasound) [14]. However, evidence of underlying parenchymal disease (MAS, RDS, pneumonia) may be noted on thoracic radiographs in secondary PPHN [14].

Diagnosis and Treatment

Echocardiography is the standard method of diagnosis of PPHN in infants and is performed to assess for the presence and direction of shunt at the ductus arteriosus and foramen ovale and to evaluate for congenital heart defects. Echocardiography can also be used to estimate right-sided pressures via evaluation of pulmonary artery pressure and right ventricular pressures [1, 4]. Right ventricular function is poor with severe pulmonary hypertension and, in infants, refractory low output from the right and left ventricle is associated with poor outcome [2].

The clinician must recognize that the severity of PPHN can range from mild hypoxemia and minimal respiratory distress to severe hypoxemia and cardiopulmonary instability.

Moreover, treatment recommendations for PPHN in the neonatal foal are extrapolated from recommendations in human neonatology and therefore should be approached with prudence. Treatment consists of addressing the underlying condition (if known) and general measures that allow maintenance of systemic blood pressure, decrease in pulmonary vascular resistance, and ensuring oxygen release to tissues. Supportive care such as correction of electrolyte and metabolic disturbances are also indicated. The heart rate, blood pressure, and oxygen saturation should be monitored frequently, continually if possible, and serial arterial blood gas analysis is necessary in the initial evaluation of the foal as well as response to therapy [2, 14]. Handling of the patient should be kept to a minimum, as slight disturbances could precipitate severe hypoxemia.

Improving Hypoxemia

Efforts should be made to improve oxygenation in patients with PPHN. In foals, intranasal oxygen administration can be used initially (uni- or bilateral nasal canula; 8–12 l/min) with mechanical ventilation used as a potential therapeutic if intranasal oxygen does not improve the delivery of oxygen to tissues. Conservative ventilation strategies with optimal positive end-expiratory pressure (PEEP), relatively low peak inspiratory pressure (PIP) or tidal volume, and permissive hypercapnia are recommended in infants to ensure lung expansion while limiting barotrauma and volutrama [14]. Exogenous surfactant therapy (Chapter 1) may also be beneficial in patients with parenchymal lung disease such as MAS, RDS, pneumonia, or sepsis [14]. In infants, extracorporeal membrane oxygenation (ECMO) is an option for severe cases, but this therapeutic is currently impractical in equine medicine.

Hemodynamic Support

Improvement of systemic blood pressure is one goal of therapy as the size of the right-to-left shunt depends, in part, on systemic blood pressure. However, the most appropriate target blood pressure has not been established in infants. The use of inotropic medications is generally indicated, as myocardial activity is often compromised with PPHN resulting in worsening of the right-to-left shunt at the foramen ovale and decrease in cardiac output from left ventricular impairment [1]. Inotropic and vasopressor agents should be utilized promptly to optimize cardiac function, stabilize systemic blood pressure, and reduce extrapulmonary shunt [1]. These medications have distinct effects, and the preferred choice is controversial. In infants, dopamine is most effective in increasing blood pressure and is most frequently used [1]. However, dopamine can result in pulmonary vasoconstriction at high doses. Other potential inotropic medications to consider are discussed elsewhere in this textbook. Of note, in regard to hemodynamic support, the use of crystalloid and colloid solutions should be used judiciously and only if there is evidence of dehydration, as cases of PPHN already have high right atrial pressure. Excessive fluid administration can cause further increases in right atrial pressure and exacerbate right-to-left shunt.

Pulmonary Vasodilation

The aim of dilating the pulmonary vessels without causing systemic vasodilation and hypotension is a difficult pharmacologic goal (Table 8.IV.1). The standard treatment to induce local (pulmonary) vasodilation in infants with PPHN is inhaled NO [1, 2]. When administered by inhalation, NO reaches the alveoli and diffuses into the vascular smooth muscle of the adjacent pulmonary arteries, consequently resulting in vasodilation by increasing cyclic guanosine monophosphate (cGMP) levels [1]. cGMP activates gated ion channels that inhibit influx of intracellular calcium by opening calcium sensitive potassium channels, resulting in polarization of the membrane and reduced vascular smooth muscle tone [2]. Although inhaled NO continues to disseminate to the pulmonary artery lumen, it is strongly bound to hemoglobin, thereby restricting its effect on the pulmonary circulation without any effect on the systemic circulation; from there it is rapidly converted to methemaglobin. Inhaled NO is preferentially distributed to ventilated portions of the lungs with increased perfusion in those areas. This results in improved V/Q ratios, decreased intra-alveolar shunting, and improved oxygenation [6]. When effective, NO improves oxygenation within a few minutes. The initial inhaled NO concentration recommended in infants with PPHN is 20 ppm as higher concentrations are not more effective and associated with a higher incidence of methemoglobinemia and formation of nitrogen dioxide [1, 16]. Concentrations as low as 5 ppm are effective in some instances, but lower concentrations (2 ppm) are ineffective and reduce the response to subsequent higher doses [17–19]. After initiation of inhaled NO, the dose should be decreased gradually (decrease of 5 ppm/h to 5 ppm) and withdrawn after 1 ppm/4 h; slow weaning of inhaled NO helps prevent rebound vasoconstriction that might occur due to decreased production of endogenous NO. [1] Monitoring of nitrogen dioxide that is generated by the reaction of NO with oxygen is recommended along with daily serum concentrations of methemoglobin (keep <5%).

The use of inhaled NO has been explored in healthy neonatal foals at doses of 20, 40, 80, and 160 ppm [15]. In an experimental setting in neonatal foals, pulmonary hypertension was induced by a drug that mimics thromboxane; inhaled NO at the noted doses attenuated increases in

Table 8.IV.1 Pulmonary vasodilator agents used in infants with PPHN [1, 14].

Drug	Dose	Mechanism of action	Use in PPHN	Use in foals
Nitric oxide	Inhaled 5–20 ppm	Produced in vascular endothelium, causes vasodilation through increase in intracellular cGMP in lung smooth muscle	Selective pulmonary vasodilator; standard treatment	Experimental use at 20, 40, 80, and 160 ppm. Causes dose-dependent vaso-dilation [15]
Prostaglandins	Prostacyclins continuous IV or inhaled Iloprost: inhaled 0.5–2 μg/kg/dose	Produced from arachidonic acid, cause vasodilation by increasing intracellular cAMP in lung smooth muscle	Vasodilation through alternative pathway to NO, may enhance its action; Prostacyclin causes nonspecific pulmonary vasodilation and systemic effects	No information
	Prostaglandin E1 Alprostadil/Prostin continuous nebulization 150–300 ng/kg/min diluted in saline to provide 4 ml/h	Pulmonary vasodilator	Used primarily in adults with pulmonary hypertension	
Sildenafil	IV, PO, or Rectal 0.5–2 mg/kg, q 6h	Inhibits phosphodiesterase 5, responsible for cGMP degradation	May potentiate NO; safe and easy to administer. May worsen oxygenation due to vasodilation of unventilated areas	Anecdotal reports of use in foals; foal-specific dose unknown
Milrinone	IV administration 0.3–0.8 μg/kg/min	Inhibitor of phosphodiesterase 3, responsible for cGMP degradation	May potentiate action of prostaglandins. Improves right cardiac output by reducing afterload.	No information

pulmonary artery pressure in a dose-dependent fashion, with a dose of 160 ppm providing the greatest reduction in pulmonary artery pressure [15]. Of note, NO dilates only preconstricted vessels and does not have an effect on vessels with normal tone; this was documented in healthy foals, as inhaled NO did not impact baseline pressures [15]. In this study, methemoglobin concentrations were always <3% when measured. No negative side effects of inhaled NO were reported, and inhaled NO has been used clinically in foals (4–40 ppm) suspected to have PPHN with some success [20].

Outside of NO, there are no other drugs that restrict vasodilation to the pulmonary circulation, but several do have a predominant effect in PPHN. These include prostaglandins (prostacyclin), sildenafil, and milrinone. Prostacyclin is a potent vasodilator that has been used in adults with pulmonary hypertension, but it frequently causes hypotension as it is not selective for pulmonary vasodilation. However, administered through the inhaled route, it can impart selective pulmonary effects but with a short half-life [1, 21]. Iloprost is a longer-acting prostacyclin analogue with specific effect in pulmonary circulation [22]. Alternatively, sildenafil is a safe, effective, and easily administered vasodilator that acts by inhibiting phosphodiesterase (PDE5) and has been noted to selectively reduce pulmonary vascular resistance with few systemic effects [23]. Sildenafil's vasodilatory effects also extend to poorly ventilated areas of the lungs, which in turn can change the V/Q ratio and increase intrapulmonary shunt, thereby worsening oxygenation [1]. Milrinone causes pulmonary vasodilation by inhibition of PDE3 and also can be effective in reducing pulmonary hypertension in the neonate.

Few cases of PPHN in the foal have been reported [20, 24, 25]. In one case, a 10-hour-old Thoroughbred colt was presented for weakness and inability to suckle. The colt was post-term (gestational length 51 weeks). Clinical examination noted moderate respiratory distress and tachypnea (80 breaths/min; nostril flair), tachycardia (140 beats/min), and cyanotic mucous membranes. The rectal temperature was 101.5 °F (38.6 °C) and the colt was dehydrated, alert, but weak, and could only stand for brief periods before collapsing. Auscultation of the lungs was clear, but a loud, systolic murmur and split-second heart sound was documented. Radiographs of the thorax were normal, as was the white cell count and serum biochemistry. However, the foal had severe hypoxemia with arterial blood gas analysis revealing a pH of 7.26, P_aCO_2 of 27 mmHg, P_aO_2 of 38 mmHg, and hemoglobin saturation of 66%. Intranasal oxygen was administered (12 l/min) with repeat arterial blood gas documenting minimal improvement in oxygenation (pH-7.29; P_aCO_2-24.9 mmHg, P_aO_2-40.6 mmHg, saturation 71%). Despite therapy, the foal's condition deteriorated. Four hours after admission, a contrast bubble cardiac ultrasound examination demonstrated right-to-left shunting at the atrial level; the foal subsequently died shortly thereafter. Postmortem examination noted a patent foramen ovale (12 mm at largest portion), dilated right atrium and ventricle, and a patent ductus arteriosus, findings supportive of PPHN. In summary, foals with clinical findings of respiratory distress, cyanosis, hypoxemia (generally severe with P_aO_2 <50 mmHg), hypercapnia (variable but generally >50 mmHg), and acidemia (while excluding other causes) that persists and worsens despite therapy should be evaluated for PPHN [20, 24].

As reported cases of PPHN are few in equids, recommendations for treatment remain unsubstantiated. Despite this, addressing hypoxemia and acidosis are initial goals as both abnormalities serve to bolster the fetal circulatory pattern [20]. Initial therapy with intranasal oxygen (8–12 l/min) may allow some foals with PPHN to establish neonatal circulatory patterns within a few hours. Failure to improve or worsening of hypoxemic respiratory failure after intranasal oxygen should prompt intubation and mechanical ventilation with 100% oxygen [20]. This will serve both a diagnostic and therapeutic purpose. Ventilation with 100% oxygen may resolve PPHN. If intrapulmonary shunt and altered V/Q relationships are causing the hypoxic respiratory failure, the P_aO_2 should exceed 100 mmHg under these conditions. However, failure to improve P_aO_2 suggests PPHN or a large right-to-left extrapulmonary shunt secondary to congenital cardiac anomaly [20]. Inhaled NO can then be administered at 5–10 ppm in ventilatory gas as a starting dose. Anecdotal experience suggests that foals will require NO treatment for <4–6 hours [20]. Sildenafil is another readily available medication that can be used alone or in conjunction with NO in foals with PPHN.

Too few cases of PPHN in the foal have been reported to provide an accurate prognosis. However, in human infants, the mortality ranges from 4% to 33% and long-term consequences in survivors include neurodevelopmental, cognitive, and hearing abnormalities [14].

References

1 Cabral, J.E.B. and Belik, J. (2013). Persistent pulmonary hypertension of the newborn: recent advances in pathophysiology and treatment. *J. Pediatr.* 89: 226–242.

2 Bendapudi, P., Gangadhara, G., and Greenough, A. (2015). Diagnosis and management of persistent pulmonary hypertension of the newborn. *Paediatr. Respir. Rev.* 16: 157–161.

3 Dakshinamurti, S. (2005). Pathophysiologic mechanisms of persistent pulmonary hypertension of the newborn. *Pediatr. Pulmonol.* 39: 492–503.

4 Puthiyachirakkal, M. and Mhanna, M.J. (2013). Pathophysiology, management, and outcome of persistent pulmonary hypertension of the newborn: a clinical review. *Front. Pediatr.* 1: 1–6.

5 Drummond, W.H., Sanchez, I.R., Kosch, P.C. et al. (1989). Pulmonary vascular reactivity of the newborn pony foal. *Equine Vet. J.* 21: 181–185.

6 Sharma, V., Berkelhamer, S., and Lakshminrushimha, S. (2015). Persistent pulmonary hypertension of the newborn. *Matern. Health Neonatol. Perinatol.* 1: 14. https://doi.org/10.1186/s40748-015-0015-4.

7 Ostrea, E.M., Villanueva, E.T., Natarajan, G. et al. (2006). Persistent pulmonary hypertension of the newborn: pathogenesis, etiology, and management. *Pediatr. Drugs* 8: 179–188.

8 Silva, J.F., Serakides, R., Franca, S.A. et al. (2014). Multiple congenital defects in a newborn foal. *Arq. Bras. Med. Vet. Zootec.* 66: 1671–1675.

9 Tabaran, A.F., Nagy, A.L., Catoi, C. et al. (2015). Congenital diaphragmatic hernia with concurrent aplasia of the pericardium in a foal. *BMC Vet. Res.* 11: 309.

10 Chinoy, M.R. (2002). Pulmonary hypoplasia and congenital diaphragmatic hernia: advances in the pathogenetics and regulation of lung development. *J. Surg. Res.* 106: 209–223.

11 Ameis, D., Khoshgoo, N., and Keijzer, R. (2017). Abnormal lung development in congenital diaphragmatic hernia. *Semin. Pediatr. Surg.* 26: 123–128.

12 Palmer, J.E. (2012). Colic and diaphragmatic hernias in neonatal foals. *Equine Vet. Educ.* 24: 340–342.

13 Konduri, G.G. and Kim, U.O. (2009). Advances in the diagnosis and management of persistent pulmonary hypertension of the newborn. *Pediatr. Clin. North. Am.* 56: 579–600.

14 Swarnam, K., Soraisham, A.S., and Sindhu, S. (2012). Advances in the management of meconium aspiration syndrome. *Int. J. Pediatr.* 2012: 359571.

15 Lester, G.D., DeMarco, V.G., and Norman, W.M. (1999). Effect of inhaled nitric oxide on experimentally induced

pulmonary hypertension in neonatal foals. *Am. J. Vet. Res.* 60: 1207–1212.
16 Committee on Fetus and Newborn (2000). Use of inhaled nitric oxide. *Pediatrics* 106: 344–345.
17 Cornfield, D.N., Maynard, R.C., deRegnier, R.A. et al. (1999). Randomized, controlled trial of low-dose inhaled nitric oxide in the treatment of term and near-term infants with respiratory failure and pulmonary hypertension. *Pediatrics* 104: 1089–1094.
18 Clark, R.H., Kueser, T.J., Walker, M.W. et al. (2000). Low-dose nitric oxide therapy for persistent pulmomary hypertension of the newborn. Clinical Inhaled Nitric Oxide Research Group. *N. Engl. J. Med.* 342: 469–474.
19 Davidson, D., Barefield, E.S., Kattwinkel, J. et al. (1998). Inhaled nitric oxide for the early treatment of persistent pulmonary hypertension of the term newborn: a randomized, double-masked, placebo-controlled, dose response, multicenter study. The I-NO/PPHN Study Group. *Pediatrics* 101: 325–334.
20 Wilkins, P.A. (2003). Acute respiratory failure: diagnosis, monitoring techniques, and therapeutics. *Clin. Tech. Equine Pract.* 2: 55–66.
21 Ewert, R., Schaper, C., Halank, M. et al. (2009). Inhalative iloprost-pharmacology and clinical application. *Expert Opin. Pharmacother.* 10: 2195–2207.
22 Leuchte, H.H. and Behr, J. (2005). Iloprost for idiopathic pulmonary arterial hypertension. *Expert Rev. Cardiovasc. Ther.* 3: 215–223.
23 Vargas-Origel, A., Gomez-Rodriguez, G., Aldana-Valenzuela, C. et al. (2010). The use of sildenafil in persistent pulmonary hypertension of the newborn. *Am. J. Perinatol.* 27: 225–230.
24 Cottrill, C.M., O'Connor, W.N., Cudd, T. et al. (1987). Persistence of foetal circulatory pathways in a newborn foal. *Equine Vet. J.* 19: 252–255.
25 Stoneham, S.J. (1998). Respiratory distress in the neonatal foal. *Equine Vet. Educ.* 10: 242–249.

Section V Pneumothorax and Pneumomediastinum

David Wong

In health, a dynamic relationship exists between the lungs and the thoracic wall. Each lung is covered by a tightly adhered serous membrane known as the visceral pleura. The visceral pleura reflects upon itself at the root of each lung and forms a continuous pleural lining with the mediastinum, diaphragm, and thoracic wall known as the parietal pleura (Figure 8.V.1) [1]. Between the visceral and parietal pleura is a small amount of pleural fluid that facilitates smooth movement of the lung against the thoracic wall and between the lung lobes. The intrapleural pressure is subatmospheric (−5 cm H_2O) at rest and is created by the difference between the elastic recoil forces of the lung and the forces that expand the thorax [1]. Another component of the thoracic cavity is the mediastinum, which is the space between each hemithorax that is enclosed by the mediastinal pleurae. In contrast to the pleural cavities, the mediastinum is not a closed cavity, but rather, is continuous with the fascial planes of the neck cranially and the retroperitoneal space caudally. The thoracic partition of the mediastinum contains the heart, trachea, esophagus, aorta, and thymus. In the horse, the mediastinum is delicate and often fenestrated, allowing communication between each hemithorax as compared to ruminants that have a thick mediastinum that can withstand notable pressure differences between the two pleural cavities [1].

If air enters the pleural space, the intimate interaction between the thoracic wall and lung is lost and the lungs become atelectatic as the thoracic wall expands; this situation impacts both respiratory and cardiovascular function. Pneumothorax develops when atmospheric air or gas enters the pleural space by one of three pathways: pleurocutaneous, pleuropulmonary, or pleuroesophageal [1, 2]. Pleurocutaneous air is typically a result of penetrating trauma to the thoracic wall whereas damage to the trachea, bronchi or lung parenchyma can result in pleuropulmonary air leakage [1]. Pleuroesophageal air leakage is rare and occurs secondary to damage or perforation to the esophagus. There are several methods to classify pneumothorax in people and small animals as it is a well-described disorder in these species. However, it is relatively infrequent in the neonatal foal (Figure 8.V.2) [2, 3]. Broad classifications can be based on pathophysiology (i.e. traumatic, spontaneous, iatrogenic) or physiologic nature (open or closed). Traumatic pneumothorax can be further broken down to open (damage to thoracic wall) or closed (thoracic wall remains intact). Primary spontaneous pneumothorax occurs without the presence of preexisting pulmonary disease with some suggesting that the underlying cause is rupture of a subpleural bleb or bulla (Table 8.V.1) [4]. In comparison, secondary spontaneous pneumothorax occurs with various underlying pulmonary disorders (e.g. pleuropneumonia, bronchopleural fistula) [3, 5]. Tension pneumothorax occurs when there is an ingress of air into the pleural space but no egress (one-way valve effect), resulting in continuous positive intrapleural pressure that can become life-threatening. The accumulation of air exerts mechanical pressure on intrathoracic structures, and the foal loses the ability to compensate through an increase in chest expansion [1]. Once the thorax becomes maximally expanded, the inspiratory muscles cannot perform during the active inspiratory phase resulting in severely compromised respiration that may cease (Table 8.V.1).

In horses and foals, pneumothorax can occur as a result of trauma associated with an open or closed thoracic wound, thoracic surgery, severe pleuropneumonia, rib fractures, thoracocentesis, tracheostomy, severe subcutaneous emphysema, pneumomediastinum, lung biopsy, rupture of alveoli or bronchial structures, or secondary to mechanical ventilation [6–13]. In a retrospective study of 40 cases of pneumothorax in the horse (median age 4.8 years; range 1 day to 20 years), pneumothorax developed secondary to pleuropneumonia (17 horses), open wounds of the thorax (9), close trauma to the thorax (7), surgery on the upper respiratory tract (3), surgery of the

Equine Neonatal Medicine, First Edition. Edited by David M. Wong and Pamela A. Wilkins.

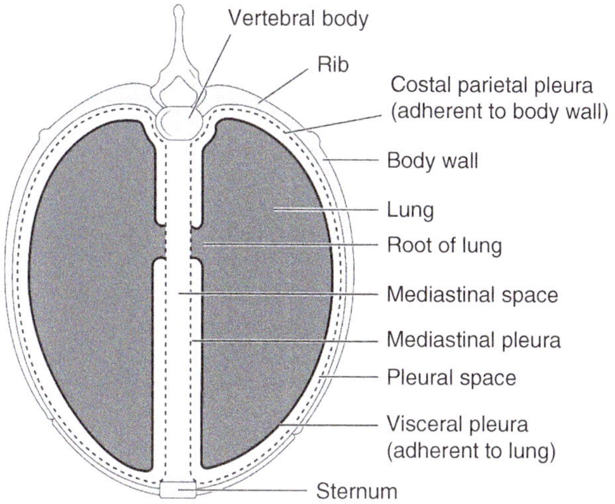

Figure 8.V.1 Cross section of the thoracic cavity detailing the relationship of the visceral and parietal pleura.

thoracic cavity (1), and unknown causes (3) [5]. As just noted, the mediastinum in horses is usually incomplete, with small fenestrations located in the caudal and ventral portions. Because of these fenestrations, pneumothorax can become bilateral, but does not universally occur if the fenestrations become occluded with inflammatory exudate. In the aforementioned retrospective study, pneumothorax was bilateral in 47.5% (19/40) and unilateral in 42.5% (17/40) of horses [5].

Clinical signs and associated degree of respiratory compromise noted with pneumothorax will depend on the amount of collapsed lung and if concurrent pulmonary injury or disease is present. In general, pneumothorax can be tolerated if less than 50% of the lung is collapsed and there is no other underlying injury or pulmonary disease [14]. When small volumes of air are introduced into the pleural cavity, the first response is typically tachypnea, resulting in rapid shallow breaths [1]. If more air enters the pleural cavity, hyperventilation occurs, characterized by an abnormally large amount of air present in the lungs to maintain adequate ventilation. The cardiovascular system is also negatively impacted by pneumothorax because there is a loss of negative intrapleural pressure, resulting in decreased venous return to the heart [1]. Hypoxemia also causes pulmonary vasoconstriction and consequent increased pulmonary vascular resistance, right-sided heart failure and reduced cardiac output [1]. In the retrospective study in 40 horses, clinical signs included tachypnea,

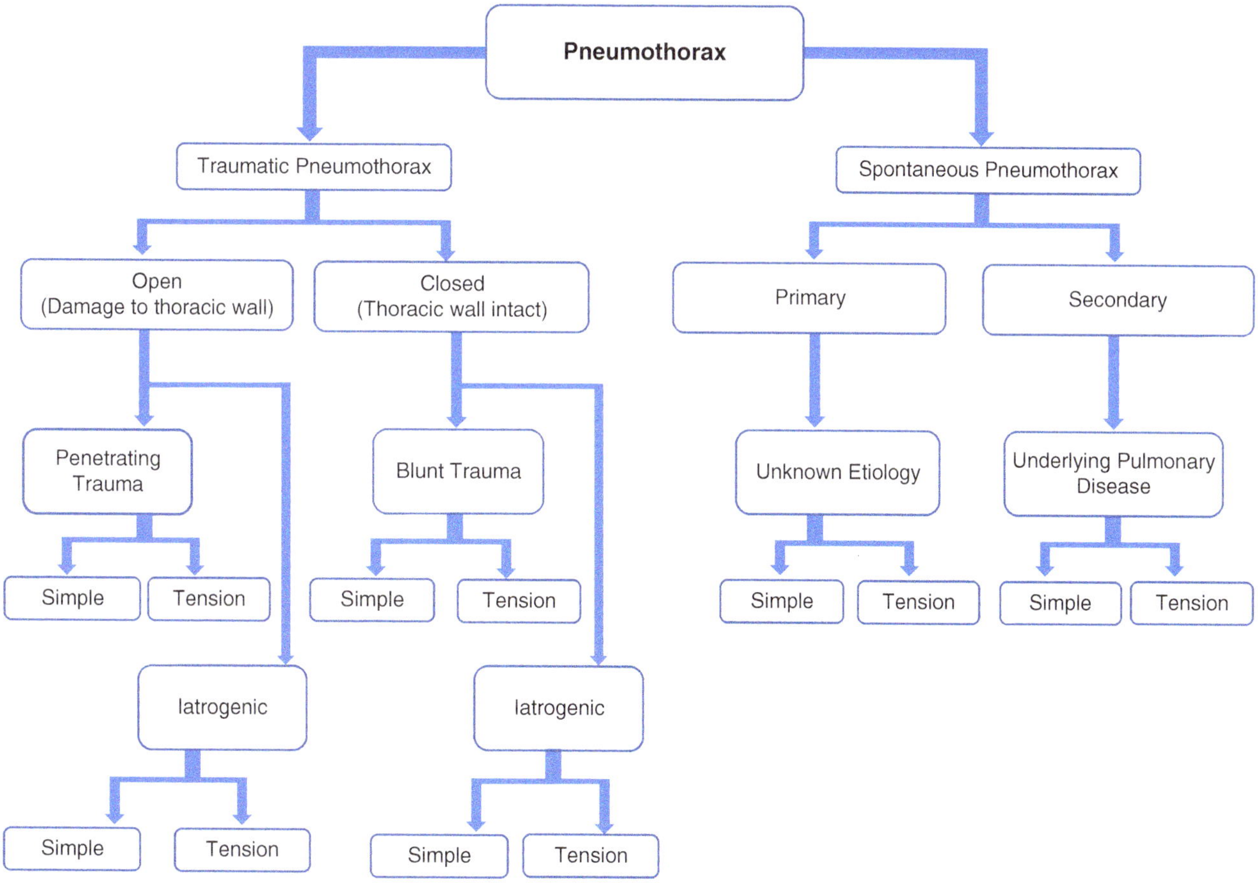

Figure 8.V.2 Classification and causes of pneumothorax.

Table 8.V.1 Description of types of pneumothoraxes.

Traumatic pneumothorax – classified as either open or closed depending on presence or absence of penetrating wound into the thorax.		
Open pneumothorax (rib fractures, bites shearing injuries, lacerations, iatrogenic)	Trauma to thoracic wall causes direct communication between pleural space and external environment.	Air enters pleural space during inspiration and exits during expiration (unless damaged tissue creates a one-way valve and tension pneumothorax).
Closed pneumothorax (blunt trauma, iatrogenic)	Secondary to thoracic damage but intact thoracic wall.	Two theories of how closed pneumothorax occurs: 1) Transmission of energy absorbed by thoracic cage at time of impact to lungs causes rapid compression of air; results in transient increase in airway pressure and shear force damage lung parenchyma and rupture alveoli, thereby resulting in air leakage. 2) Air and body fluids have different densities; tissues in the lung containing air and fluid differ in rate of acceleration and deceleration at time of impact resulting in shear forces that stretch and tear airways, which can result in air leakage.
Spontaneous pneumothorax – air accumulates in pleural space in the absence of trauma or iatrogenic cause.		
Primary spontaneous	Etiology is unknown.	
Secondary spontaneous	Underlying pulmonary disease process is present.	Potential causes: bullous emphysema, pulmonary blebs, pulmonary neoplasia, bacterial or viral pneumonia, migrating foreign body, pulmonary abscess, parasitic granuloma.
Tension pneumothorax – most severe type of pneumothorax that involves progressive accumulation of air in the pleural space resulting in increasing mechanical pressure on intrathoracic structures.		
	Often results from pulmonary damage and continuous leakage of air during inspiration; can result secondary to thoracic wall injury.	Increased intrathoracic pressure results in atelectasis; as the process continues, increased intrapleural pressure exceeds atmospheric pressure resulting in collapse of vascular structures leading to collapse of the vena cava and decreased venous return to heart; if left untreated, death is the final outcome.

dyspnea, cyanosis, absence of lung sounds upon auscultation of the dorsal thorax, fever, tachycardia, lethargy, anxiousness, and cough [5].

Diagnosis

Traumatic pneumothorax is the most common cause of pneumothorax; therefore, suspicion of pneumothorax might start with a history of trauma and abnormalities noted on physical examination [5]. Pneumothorax associated with rib fractures are of particular concern in newborn foals [5, 7, 12]. Determining the cause of spontaneous pneumothorax may be more elusive as the source of air leakage is often not obvious based on history and physical examination. Regardless of if the pneumothorax is traumatic or spontaneous, clinical signs of respiratory compromise should prompt thorough investigation and consideration of pneumothorax. Inconsistent signs of pneumothorax might include absence of bronchovesicular sounds in the dorsal lung field and muted heart sounds on auscultation [14].

Confirmation of pneumothorax can be performed via radiography and ultrasonography in the foal. However, if severe respiratory compromise is present and pneumothorax is highly suspected in the foal, needle thoracocentesis using a three-way stopcock, extension set, and 60 ml syringe should be performed before further diagnostics are performed. Typically, needle thoracocentesis should be performed in the caudal-dorsal lung field while the foal is standing or in sternal recumbency. As the needle is inserted, the syringe is aspirated until free air (if present) is aspirated from the thorax. Alternatively, some clinicians prefer the use of a teat cannula inserted through a small stab incision with a #11 blade [7]. In the absence of obvious traumatic injury to the thorax and once the patient is stable, diagnostic imaging is used to identify evidence of pulmonary disease that could cause pneumothorax. Radiographic imaging of pneumothorax requires differentiation between normal intrapulmonary air and free air in the pleural space. With pneumothorax, the lungs become atelectatic and appear more radiopaque as compared to normal lung. The lungs will appear retracted away from the diaphragm and thoracic vertebrae and free pleural air can be visualized (Figure 8.V.3). Regarding ultrasonography, the acoustic impedance of air is poor, and the normal aerated visceral pleural surface of the lung is characterized by a hyperechoic line that moves during inspiration and expiration when viewed during dynamic ultrasonography (gliding lung sign). Absence of movement of the hyperechoic visceral pleural line

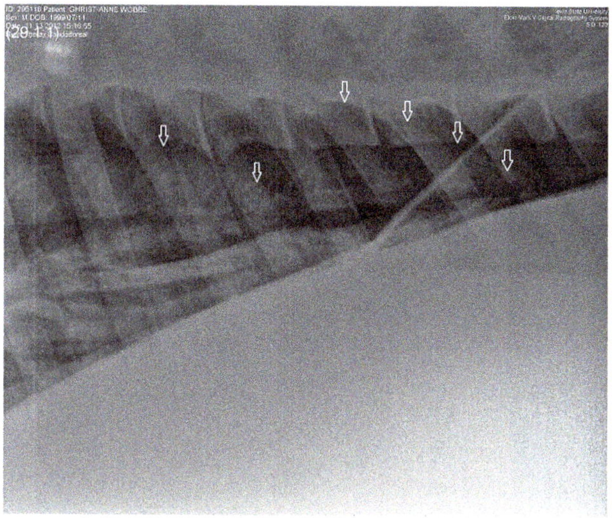

Figure 8.V.3 Lateral radiograph of a horse with pneumothorax. Note the retraction of the normal pulmonary parenchyma, hyperlucency within the caudo-dorsal thorax and visualization of the dorsal caudal borders of both lung lobes (arrows) that are well demarcated by air in the pleural space.

(absence of gliding lung sign) on dynamic ultrasonography is indicative of pneumothorax [15].

Clinicopathologic derangements observed with pneumothorax will depend on the underlying cause and can be within normal reference limits if only associated with acute trauma. Hypercapnia, respiratory acidosis, and hypoxia have been reported in a foal with unilateral pneumothorax secondary to fractured ribs [7].

Treatment of pneumothorax can be conservatively managed if respiratory distress is minimal, and the patient is stable. Intranasal oxygen can be administered as this technique can reduce pneumothorax by up to 80% by forcing nitrogen to diffuse outward [16]. If the pneumothorax is severe and/or respiration is labored, aspiration of air from the pleural space is indicated. This can be accomplished by identifying free air within the caudal dorsal thorax via ultrasonography or radiography, clipping of the hair and sterile preparation of the site. A local anesthetic block is administered and a needle or teat canula (one time use) or appropriately size chest tube (continuous use) is placed to allow suctioning of air using an extension set and 60 ml syringe or a continuous suction unit with water trap. The use of a chest tube is indicated with continued air leak, if underlying pulmonary disease is causing respiratory distress or in patients receiving mechanical ventilation [16]. Medical and, if needed, surgical, treatment of the underlying cause of pneumothorax (if known) is also necessary. Although not reported in foals, in people, some cases of repeated or persistent pneumothorax are treated with pleurodesis and chemical sclerosis. Pleurodesis promotes creation of adhesions between the parietal and visceral pleurae and is performed thoracoscopically or through thoracotomy tubes.

Complications of pneumothorax include recurrence, especially with primary spontaneous pneumothorax. Re-expansion pulmonary edema is also a documented complication in people with chronic atelectasis secondary to pneumothorax that have had pleural air evacuated rapidly [17, 18]. The exact cause of re-expansion pulmonary edema is not known, but increased pulmonary vascular permeability likely plays a factor along with decreased surfactant, hypoxia, and reperfusion injury [17, 18]. Pneumothorax can be a life-threatening process (depending on severity and cause), but if recognized early and treated appropriately, can be treated for a positive outcome.

References

1 Pawloski, D.R. and Broaddus, K.D. (2010). Pneumothorax: a review. *J. Am. Anim. Hosp. Assoc.* 46: 385–397.

2 Kramek, B.A. and Caywood, D.D. (1987). Pnuemothorax. *Vet. Clin. North Am. Small Anim. Pract.* 17: 285–300.

3 Holtsinger, R.H., Beale, B.S., Bellah, J.R. et al. (1993). Spontaneous pneumothorax in the dog. A retrospective analysis of 21 cases. *J. Am. Anim. Hosp. Assoc.* 29: 195–210.

4 Noppen, M. and DeKeukeleire, T. (2008). Pneumothorax. *Respiration* 76: 121–127.

5 Boy, M.G. and Sweeney, C.R. (2000). Pneumothorax in horses: 40 cases (1980–1997). *J. Am. Vet. Med. Assoc.* 216: 1955–1959.

6 Beech, J. (1991). Miscellaneous lung and pleural injuries. In: *Equine Respiratory Disorders* (ed. J. Beach), 220–221. Philadelphia: Lea & Febiger.

7 Borchers, A., van Eps, A., Zedler, S. et al. (2009). Thoracic trauma and post operative lung injury in a neonatal foal. *Equine Vet. Educ.* 21: 186–191.

8 Laverty, S., Lavoie, J.P., Pascoe, J.R. et al. (1996). Penetrating wounds of the thorax in 15 horses. *Equine Vet. J.* 28: 220–224.

9 Burbidge, H.M. (1982). Penetrating thoracic wound in a Hackney horse. *Equine Vet. J.* 14: 94–95.

10 Hance, S.R. and Robertson, J.T. (1992). Subcutaneous emphysema from an axillary wound that resulted in pneumomediastinum and bilateral pneumothorax in a horse. *J. Am. Vet. Med. Assoc.* 200: 1107–1110.

11 Spurlock, S.L., Spurlock, G.H., and Donaldson, L.L. (1988). Consolidating pneumonia and pneumothorax in a horse. *J. Am. Vet. Med. Assoc.* 192: 1081–1082.

12 Jean, D., Laverty, S., Halley, J. et al. (1999). Thoracic trauma in newborn foals. *Equine Vet. J.* 31: 149–152.

13 Marble, S.L., Edens, L.M., Shiroma, J.T. et al. (1996). Subcutaneous emphysema in a neonatal foal. *J. Am. Vet. Med. Assoc.* 208: 97–99.

14 MacPhail, C.M. (2010). Pleural and mediastinal disorders. In: *BSAVA Manual of Canine and Feline Cardiorespiratory Medicine*, vol. 33, 293–100.

15 Partlow, J., David, F., Hung, L.M. et al. (2017). Comparison of thoracic ultrasonography and radiography for the detection of induced small volume pneumothorax in the horse. *Vet. Radiol. Ultrasound* 3: 354–360.

16 Koterba, A.M. and Paradis, M.R. (1990). Specific respiratory conditions. In: *Equine Clinical Neonatology* (ed. A. Koterba, W. Drummond, and P. Kosch), 177–199. Philadelphia: Lea & Fibiger.

17 Soderstrom, M.J., Gilson, S.D., and Gulbas, N. (1995). Fatal reexpansion pulmonary edema in a kitten following surgical correction of pectus excavatum. *J. Am. Anim. Hosp. Assoc.* 31: 133–136.

18 Raptopoulos, D., Papazoglou, L.G., and Patsikas, M.N. (1995). Reexpansion pulmonary edema after pneumothorax in a dog. *Vet. Rec.* 136: 395.

Section VI Diaphragmatic Hernias

David Wong and Pamela A. Wilkins

Diaphragmatic hernias in foals can be a congenital anomaly or arise from a post-trauma diaphragmatic tear. True hernias are characterized by migration of an organ(s) contained within a hernial sac, whereas in the absence of a hernial sac, the term *false hernia* or *rupture* is more accurate [1, 2]. Congenital diaphragmatic hernias (CDH) are musculoskeletal defects defined by the presence of an orifice in the tendinous or muscular part of the diaphragm which subsequently allows migration of abdominal viscera into the thorax [3]. Most CDH (and all acquired diaphragmatic hernias) are false hernias [1, 2]. In foals, CDH occurs infrequently, but when present can be associated with stillbirth, intermittent bowel obstruction, or neonatal colic [4–6]. In several large retrospective studies, CDH was reported as an important congenital malformation leading to abortion and stillbirth in foals [7, 8].

Anatomy of the Diaphragm and Causes of CDH

The diaphragm is composed of two main components, the peripheral muscular portion (pars costalis) and the central tendinous portion [1, 2]. Three foramina perforate the central tendinous portion to allow passage of the caudal vena cava, esophagus, and aorta (Figure 8.VI.1). Embryogenesis of the diaphragm involves four primary embryonal structures, which interact to form the diaphragm [6]. These structures include the septum transversum (forms main primordium of the central tendinous part of the diaphragm), the left and right pleuroperitoneal folds (forms main origin of muscular region), the mesentery of the esophagus (forms crus of diaphragm) and the muscular segment of the latero-dorsal body walls (forms peripheral regions of diaphragm) [6, 9]. The ventral portion of the septum transversum separates the pericardial and peritoneal cavity between the liver and primordial diaphragm [6]. The pleuroperitoneal folds expand and fuse with the septum transversum ventrally and with the caudal mediastinum medially to complete the formation of the diaphragm [6]. The etiology of CDH is uncertain, although theories such as maternal vitamin A deficiency and exposure to pesticides have been proposed [10, 11]. Most cases of CDH are idiopathic, however, the two pleuroperitoneal folds are by far the major contributors to the diaphragm's musculature and their incomplete fusion is likely the main error that produces CDH [12, 13]. Thus, the primary event resulting in CDH is believed to be the destruction of the main mesenchyme primordia from the pleuroperitoneal fold. Incomplete fusion of the pleuroperitoneal fold is based on an embryonal defect of the muscular component of the diaphragm rather than erroneous embryonal migration of myocytes [3].

Although CDH are relatively simple anatomic defects, they can be associated with unilateral lung hypoplasia and malposition of various abdominal viscera into the thoracic cavity [3]. The number of abdominal organs displaced into the thoracic cavity depends on the size of the defect, its location, and the presence of the hernial sac, which prevents visceral displacement [6, 14]. In horses, CDH are typically located in the left dorsal tendinous region of the diaphragm as opposed to retrosternal (Morgagni) [1, 4, 6, 14]; however, CDH can also occur from a failure of fusion of the septum transversum, resulting in a ventrally located hernia [6, 14]. Retrosternal (Morgagni) diaphragmatic hernias are also congenital and have been reported in horses [6]. In people, the foramen of Morgagni is a triangle-shaped space between the muscular portion of the diaphragm that originates from the xiphoid and costal margins and inserts on the central tendinous region of the diaphragm [6]. The space is located ventrally and forms when the septum transversum and pleuroperitoneal folds fail to fuse completely during the development of the diaphragm. This lack of fusion leaves a defect in the diaphragmatic

Equine Neonatal Medicine, First Edition. Edited by David M. Wong and Pamela A. Wilkins.

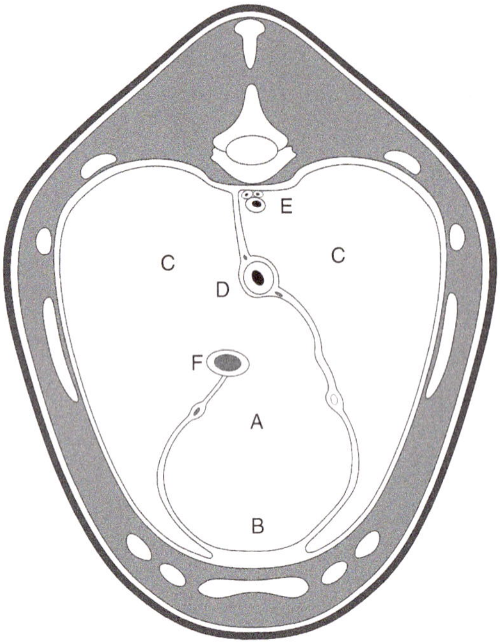

Figure 8.VI.1 Cross-section illustration of the equine diaphragm at the level of the 10th rib. (A) central tendinous portion of diaphragm, (B) pars costalis, (C) bilateral crus muscles, (D) esophagus, (E) aorta; (F) caudal vena cava.

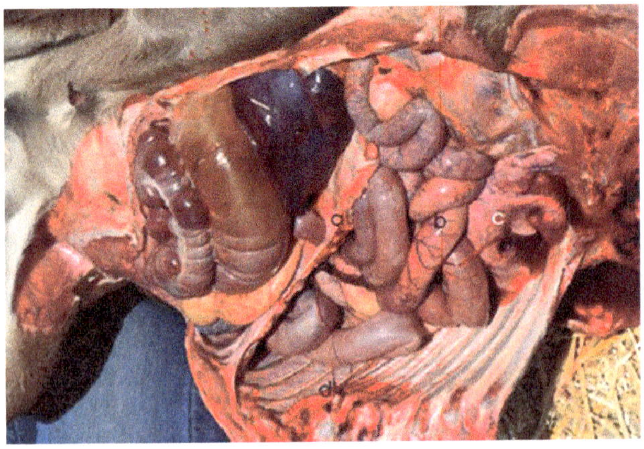

Figure 8.VI.2 Postmortem examination of a neonatal foal in dorsal recumbency demonstrating a traumatic diaphragmatic hernia. Note the small intestine traveling through the diaphragmatic defect (a), distended small intestine in the thoracic cavity (b), compressed lungs (c), and displaced fractured rib, which caused the diaphragmatic defect (d). Cranial is to the right. *Source:* From Palmer [24].

musculature and later develops into the hernial sac; the sac consists of both peritoneum and pleura [6]. CDH can also be associated with more complex congenital malformations involving the cardiovascular, urogenital, nervous, or skeletal systems (Table 8.VI.1) [3, 15–17].

In general, acquired (e.g. post-trauma, strenuous exercise, sudden fall, advanced pregnancy, dystocia) diaphragmatic hernias likely arise when there is a sudden increase in intra-abdominal or intra-thoracic pressure [18–20].

As noted, acquired diaphragmatic hernias do not have a hernial sac and thus the term *diaphragmatic rupture* or *diaphragmatic tear* is more accurate, but due to the prevalence in the literature, *diaphragmatic hernia* is used here [1]. Most acquired hernias are located either at the ventral region of the right or left hemi-diaphragm or in the central portion of the diaphragm, which may be the weakest point at the junction of the muscular and tendinous portions of the diaphragm where there is an interface between two tissues with different mechanical properties [1, 4, 21, 22]. Based on published studies, the left side of the diaphragm is nearly twice as likely to have an acquired lesion as compared to the right [1]. Interestingly, rib fractures may be a source of diaphragmatic laceration and potentially herniation of abdominal viscera in foals [22–24]. In a study of 67 foals with thoracic trauma, 3 foals had diaphragmatic rupture and 2 foals had herniated viscera [23]. In this case series, diaphragmatic rupture occurred as a result of transmural lacerations by fractured ribs in the ventral portion of the diaphragm (Figures 8.VI.1 and 8.VI.2) [23]. Of note, acquired diaphragmatic hernia can occur in the mare secondary to parturition and has been reported in the mare in the immediate (within days) and delayed (4 months) post-parturient period [19, 25].

Table 8.VI.1 Anatomic defects associated with CDH in foals.

Cardiac:	Pericardial aplasia [3]
Respiratory:	Unilateral lung hypoplasia [3, 15]
Musculoskeletal:	Scoliosis, arthrogryposis, hypoplasia of pelvic bones [15, 16]
Urogenital:	Uterus unicornis, unilateral renal agenesis, ureteral agenesis [15, 16]

Clinical Signs

Clinical signs of CDH include acute colic, respiratory distress, exercise intolerance, and lethargy with notable tachycardia and tachypnea on physical examination [4, 13, 21, 22, 26–28]. Decreased respiratory sounds and increased intestinal borborygmi in the affected hemithorax may be observed in some cases [1, 14]. Interestingly, colic has been observed as early as 6 hours after birth in a newborn foal and CDH has also been reported in a newborn foal that was stillborn due to premature placental separation, indicating that herniation can occur prior to birth of the foal [1, 13, 29]. Abdominal pain may result from impaction, incarceration, or strangulation of the intestine in the thorax [1]. Respiratory compromise in foals with diaphragmatic hernias is a result of viscera within the thoracic cavity interfering with normal chest wall and lung expansion, thereby decreasing lung compliance; accompanying alveolar edema and atelectasis causes reduction in total lung capacity and functional residual capacity thus resulting in significant ventilation-perfusion (V/Q) mismatches (hypoxemia, hypercapnia) [29, 30]. Increased intrathoracic pressures and decreased alveolar oxygen tension results in increased pulmonary vascular resistance leading to pulmonary dysfunction and respiratory difficulty or arrest [13]. Potentially, pleural effusion, pneumothorax, loss of diaphragmatic function, and pain during respiration can also contribute to respiratory signs [1]. Severity of clinical signs are reflective of the amount of abdominal viscera that has herniated into the thoracic cavity and whether disturbances in blood flow to the herniated abdominal viscera has been compromised. Some horses with diaphragmatic hernia may exhibit abnormal body postures such as crouching down the hindfeet (dog-sitting) or adopting an exaggeratedly wide forelimb stance [1]. Clinicopathologic changes might include evidence of dehydration (elevated PCV, total protein, lactate), hypoxemia and/or hypercapnia, respiratory acidemia and variable alterations in white cell count [1, 13, 22]. Peritoneal fluid is typically normal, but abnormal results have also been documented [1, 13, 14].

Diagnosis and Treatment

Diagnosis is supported by abdominal and thoracic radiography and/or ultrasonography, which reveals distended loops of amotile small intestine and gas-filled viscera within the thorax (Figure 8.VI.3). Ultrasonography may note gas- and fluid-filled tubular or sacculated structures and excessive pleural fluid in the thorax [1, 13, 19]. Various abdominal organs can be displaced through a diaphragmatic hernia into the thoracic cavity with the small intestine and portions of the large colon being most common; however, the liver lobes, stomach, and spleen have also been reported as herniated organs [4, 13, 22, 31, 32].

On postmortem examination of foals with diaphragmatic hernias, herniated organs can be congested and the caudal lobes of the lung can be atelectatic [13]. Typically, CDH have smooth, rounded edges; show no evidence of scarring or adhesions at the margins of the diaphragmatic defect; and lack hemorrhage, inflammation, or excessive fibrosis (Figure 8.VI.4) [19, 33]. In comparison, acquired diaphragmatic hernias have evidence of trauma or visible laceration of the diaphragm, along with microscopic evidence of inflammation; if the lesion is chronic, the edges of the rent can be fibrotic, thickened, and may be accompanied by visceral adhesions [13, 19].

Surgical intervention is needed to repair diaphragmatic hernias [19]. Surgical access to the diaphragm in the adult horse is difficult, but the smaller size of the foal allows improved accessibility and adequate access to all aspects of the diaphragm [2]. A ventral midline celiotomy is the most common approach, but thoracotomy assisted with thoracoscopy has also been described in a few reports in adult horses [34–36]. In some cases, thoracoscopy has allowed the clinician to identify the location and size of the rent, allowing improved preparation and planning for a ventral midline celiotomy. Repair of the diaphragm should begin in the most inaccessible area (typically most dorsal aspect of lesion) and advance toward the most accessible region using simple continuous or interrupted sutures. Mesh implants have been used in adult horses with large, friable, less accessible diaphragmatic defects [2]. Of note, bilateral pneumothorax can develop intraoperatively as the viscera is returned to the abdominal cavity.

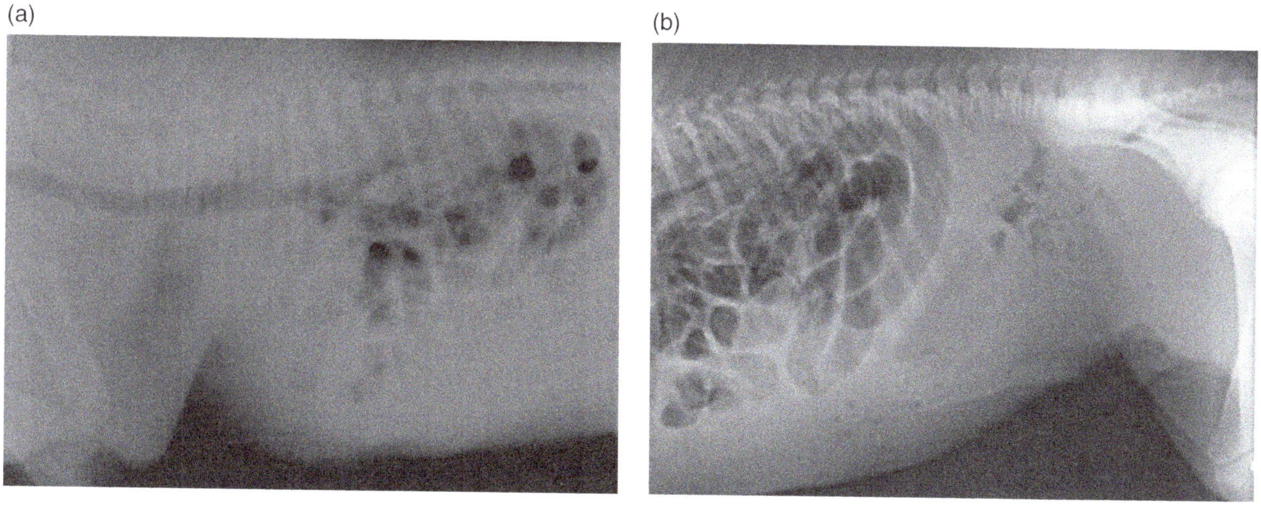

Figure 8.VI.3 (a) Lateral radiographic projection of the thorax demonstrating gas-filled viscera within the thoracic cavity of a 1-day-old Finnhorse colt. (b) Lateral radiographic projection of the abdomen demonstrating cranially displaced gas-filled viscera [13].

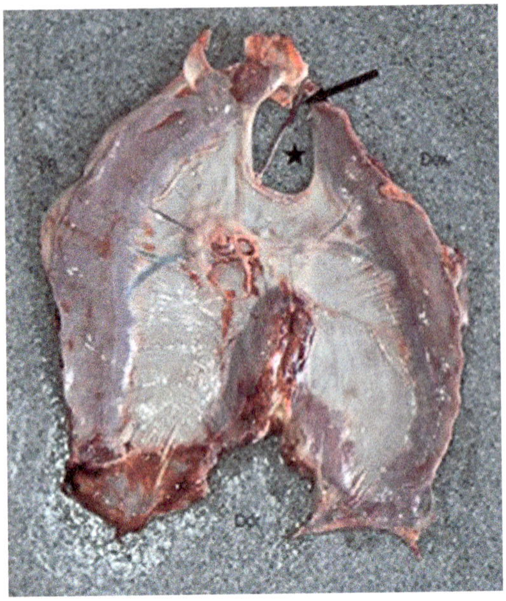

Figure 8.VI.4 Image of a foal's diaphragm (cranial aspect) demonstrating an ovoid hernial opening (7 × 11 cm) located at the sternal part of the diaphragm on the right side (asterisk). The margins of the defect are smooth and round; a round fibrous bundle (5 mm × 15 cm) courses diagonal between the margins of the hernial opening (arrow) [13].

Anesthesia of the foal with a diaphragmatic hernia can be challenging because of hypoventilation and decreased oxygenation [2]. Hypoventilation can result from lung compression by abdominal viscera and the loss of thoracic negative pressure required for lung inflation [2]. Additionally, oxygenation is compromised because of alveolar collapse in the atelectatic lung. Mechanical ventilation using 100% is recommended during repair [2]. After repair of the diaphragm, it may be necessary to evacuate air from the thorax using suction to allow the thoracic cavity to regain normal pressures [22]. Moreover, in some cases in which herniated abdominal viscera has compressed the lungs, it may be difficult to reinflate the lungs after surgical correction with positive pressure ventilation likely needed to facilitate re-inflation [4]. Re-expansion pulmonary edema can result from rapid lung inflation after prolonged collapse in people and small animals, but anecdotal reports suggest that rapid lung inflation does not lead to clinical side effects in horses, regardless of duration of pulmonary collapse [2]. A degree of pneumothorax and pleural effusion is possible after surgery. In surgery of retrosternal hernias in people, removal of the hernial sac is controversial; advocates for removal believe that it is necessary to avoid leaving a loculated space-occupying lesion in the thoracic cavity. In comparison, some surgeons leave the hernial sac in place because it is believed that the sac has no clinical importance and lessens the risk of development of pneumothorax and pneumopericardium and minimizes damage to the lung parenchmyma [6].

Prognosis

Prognosis of diaphragmatic hernia is variable depending on the size and location of the diaphragmatic defect and the presence or absence of devitalized intestine [14]. Historically, the condition carries a guarded to poor prognosis, but survival studies have focused primarily on adult horses [32, 36]. The overall survival rate in one study that evaluated both adult horses (25) and foals (6) was 23% for horses that presented with a diaphragmatic hernia and a surgical success rate of 46% [32]. In another review, the success rate was reported to be 90% (27/30) of horses that recovered from anesthesia [2]. Prognosis may be better in foals than adult horses due to easier access to the diaphragm; in one case series, all foals (3) with diaphragmatic hernias and intestine that required resection and anastomosis recovered from surgery and went on to race [22]. In another study of 6 foals with diaphragmatic hernias, 3 were immediately euthanized on surgical exploration due to the amount of compromised herniated intestine; of the other 3 foals that had surgical correction, 2 died postoperatively and 1 foal survived to discharge and later went on to race [32]. In another retrospective study, young horses (≤2 years old) were more likely to survive than older horses [14].

References

1 Kelmer, G., Kramer, J., and Wilson, D.A. (2008). Diaphragmatic hernia: etiology, clinical presentation, and diagnosis. *Compend. Equine* 3: 28–36.

2 Kelmer, G., Kramer, J., and Wilson, D.A. (2008). Diaphragmatic hernia: treatment, complications and prognosis. *Compend. Equine* 3: 37–46.

3 Tabaran, A.F., Nagy, A.L., Catoi, C. et al. (2015). Congenital diaphragmatic hernia with concurrent aplasia of the pericardium in a foal. *BMC Vet. Res.* 11: 309.

4 Speirs, V.C. and Reynolds, W.T. (1976). Successful repair of a diaphragmatic hernia in a foal. *Equine Vet. J.* 8: 170–172.

5 Cheetham, J. (1998). Congenital diaphragmatic hernia with subsequent incarceration of the left large colon and gastric rupture in a foal. *Equine Vet. Educ.* 10: 239–241.

6 Pauwels, F.F., Hawkins, J.F., MacHarg, M.A. et al. (2007). Congenital retrosternal (Morgagni) diaphragmatic hernias in three horses. *J. Am. Vet. Med. Assoc.* 231: 427–432.

7 Smith, K.C., Blunden, A.S., Whitwell, K.E. et al. (2003). A survey of equine abortion, stillbirth and neonatal death in the UK from 1988 to 1997. *Equine Vet. J.* 35: 496–501.
8 Hong, C.B., Donahue, J.M., Giles, R.C. Jr. et al. (1993). Equine abortion and stillbirth in central Kentucky during 1988 and 1989 foaling seasons. *J. Vet. Diagn. Investig.* 5: 560–566.
9 Sadler, T.W. (2004). Body cavities. In: *Medical Embryology*, 9e (ed. T.W. Salder), 211–222. Philadelphia: Lippincott Williams and Wilkins.
10 Mey, J., Babiuk, R.P., Clugston, R. et al. (2003). Retinal dehydrogenase-2 is inhibited by compounds that induce congenital diaphragmatic hernias in rodents. *Am. J. Pathol.* 162: 673–679.
11 Wilson, J.G., Roth, C.B., and Warkany, J. (1953). An analysis of the syndrome of malformations induced by maternal vitamin A deficiency. Effects of restoration of vitamin A at various times during gestation. *Am. J. Anat.* 92: 189–217.
12 Babiuk, R.P., Zhang, W., Clugston, R. et al. (2003). Embryological origins and development of the rat diaphragm. *J. Comp. Neurol.* 455: 477–487.
13 Tapio, H., Hewestson, M., and Sihvo, H.K. (2012). An unusual cause of colic in a neonatal foal. *Equine Vet. Educ.* 24: 334–339.
14 Hart, S.K. and Brown, J.A. (2009). Diaphragmatic hernia in horses: 44 cases (1986–2006). *J. Vet. Emerg. Crit. Care* 19: 357–362.
15 Silva, J.F., Serakides, R., Franca, S.A. et al. (2014). Multiple congenital defects in a newborn foal. *Arq. Bras. Med. Vet. Zootec.* 66: 1671–1675.
16 Firth, E.C. (1976). Diaphragmatic hernia in horses. *Cornell Vet.* 66: 353–361.
17 Johnson, J.W., Debowes, R.M., Cox, J.H. et al. (1984). Diaphragmatic hernia with a concurrent cardiac defect in an Arabian foal. *J. Equine Vet. Sci.* 4: 225–226.
18 Wimberly, H.C., Andrews, E.J., and Haschek, W.M. (1977). Diaphragmatic hernias in the horse: a review of the literature and an analysis of six additional cases. *J. Am. Vet. Med. Assoc.* 170: 1404–1407.
19 McMaster, M., Spirito, M., and Munsterman, A. (2014). Surgical repair of a diaphragmatic tear in a Thoroughbred broodmare. *J. Equine Vet. Sci.* 34: 1333–1337.
20 Clarke, L.M., Arighi, M., Jamison, J.M. et al. (1987). Clinical diagnosis and surgical repair of a diaphragmatic hernia in a mare. *Can. Vet. J.* 28: 242–244.
21 Edwards, G.B. (1993). Diaphragmatic hernia-a diagnostic and surgical challenge. *Equine Vet. Educ.* 5: 267–269.
22 Santschi, E.M., Juzwiak, J.S., Moll, H.D. et al. (1997). Diaphragmatic hernia repair in three young horses. *Vet. Surg.* 26: 242–245.
23 Schambourg, M.A., Laverty, S., Mullim, S. et al. (2003). Thoracic trauma in foals: postmortem findings. *Equine Vet. J.* 25: 78–81.
24 Palmer, J.E. (2012). Colic and diaphragmatic hernias in neonatal foals. *Equine Vet. Educ.* 24: 340–342.
25 Auer, D.E., Wilson, R.G., Groenendyk, S. et al. (1985). Diaphragmatic rupture in a mare at parturition. *Equine Vet. J.* 17: 331–333.
26 Collobert, C., Gillet, J.P., and Esling, W. (1988). A case of congenital diaphragmatic hernia in a foal. *Vet. Clin. North Am. Equine Pract.* 10: 43–46.
27 Branson, K.R. and Kramer, J. (2000). Anesthesia case of the month. *J. Am. Vet. Med. Assoc.* 216: 1918–1919.
28 Proudman, C.J. and Edwards, G.B. (1992). Diaphragmatic diverticulum (hernia) in a horse. *Equine Vet. J.* 24: 244–246.
29 Jackson, C., Collyer, P.B., and Loynachan, A. (2006). Congenital diaphragmatic eventration in a stillborn foal. *J. Vet. Diagn. Investig.* 18: 412–416.
30 Rush, B.R. Respiratory distress. In: *Equine Internal Medicine*, 2e (ed. R.M. Reed, W.M. Bayly, and D.C. Sellon), 136–142. Philadelphia: Elsevier.
31 Verschooten, F., Oyaert, W., Muylle, E. et al. (1977). Diaphragmatic hernia in the horse: four case reports. *Vet. Radiol.* 18: 45–50.
32 Romero, A.E. and Rodgerson, D.H. (2010). Diaphragmatic herniation in the horse: 31 cases from 2001–2006. *Can. Vet. J.* 51: 1247–1250.
33 Brown, C.C., Baker, D.C., and Barker, I.K. (2007). Alimentary system. In: *Pathology of Domestic Animals*, 5e (ed. K.J.F. Jubb, P.C. Kennedy, and N. Palmer), 1–296. Philadelphia: Elsevier.
34 Vachon, A.M. and Fisher, A.T. (1998). Thoracoscopy in the horse: diagnostic and therapeutic indications in 28 cases. *Equine Vet. J.* 30: 467–475.
35 Malone, E.D., Farnsworth, K., Lennox, T. et al. (2001). Thoracoscopic-assisted diaphragmatic hernia repair using thoracic rib resection. *Vet. Surg.* 30: 175–178.
36 Rocken, M., Mosel, G., Barske, K. et al. (2013). Thoracoscopic diaphragmatic hernia repair in a Warmblood mare. *Vet. Surg.* 42: 591–594.

Section VII Miscellaneous Disorders of the Respiratory System

Constanze Fintl and Pamela A. Wilkins

Pulmonary Hypoplasia

Pulmonary hypoplasia is defined as incomplete development of the lungs, resulting in a reduction in the number or size of the bronchopulmonary segments or pulmonary acini [1]. It is a rare condition in the equine neonate and is usually associated with other defects, principally congenital diaphragmatic hernia (CDH), although pericardial aplasia and pulmonary agenesis have also been reported [2–6]. By comparison, pulmonary hypoplasia is commonly reported in association with CDH in human infants, where the latter condition has a reported incidence of about 1 in 3,000 births [7, 8]. Hypoplastic lung is frequently accompanied by severe pulmonary hypertension and retention of fetal circulatory patterns, having devastating effect on the human neonate with high mortality rates reported despite advanced neonatal intensive care [9].

Congenital diaphragmatic defects are typically reported as either Bochdalek or Morgagni variants, where the former is by far the most common. Bochdalek defects are typically of the left, postero(dorso)lateral diaphragm and are considered most commonly associated with pulmonary hypoplasia and respiratory failure at birth in human neonates [10]. However, there are many variations, and it has been suggested that a more precise classification system would be beneficial in identifying underlying causes [11]. Both Bochdalek and Morgagni defects, as well as other variations, have been reported in the foal [2–6, 12–14].

Because pulmonary hypoplasia and CDH are rare findings in the equine neonate, it is difficult to establish possible underlying causes. In contrast, several different underlying causes of CDH and accompanying pulmonary hypoplasia have been proposed in humans, including genetic, environmental and nutritional factors although not yet fully understood multifactorial conditions are likely [10, 15]. Regardless of the underlying cause of these conditions, it has been proposed that the fetal lung may become hypoplastic as a consequence of herniated abdominal viscera into the thoracic cavity causing physical compression and interference of the developing lung. This includes disruption of fetal breathing movement patterns, which are essential for normal growth and structural maturation of the fetal lungs, as well as the maintenance and circulation of lung fluid [16]. This was experimentally demonstrated in fetal lambs, where conditions similar to the physical compression occurring with CDH were created that reproduced both macroscopic and microscopic findings typically seen with pulmonary hypoplasia [17]. However, subsequent investigations, both teratogenic nitrofen studies in rodents as well as various genetic studies, have instead proposed a so-called "dual-hit" theory where interference with pulmonary development occurs prior to and separate from abnormal diaphragmatic development affecting the ipsilateral lung, even though the underlying primary cause may be the same [18, 19].

Determining factors for survival in human infants with pulmonary hypoplasia and CDH include the presence and degree of pulmonary hypertension. The latter is a result of epithelial dysfunction and subsequent vascular remodeling with a thickening of the pulmonary arterial walls, resulting in a strong contractile response and increased pulmonary vascular resistance [20, 21]. Despite surgical and medical advances, the mortality rates in children remain high and appears to be directly related to the degree of pulmonary hypertension [21, 22].

Newborn foals with pulmonary hypoplasia are likely to present in respiratory distress, similar to human neonates. In the few published reports in equine neonates, the foals were either stillborn or died within 24 hours of birth [3–6]. Respiratory distress and/or apnea were reported to be major presenting or rapidly developing signs with hypercapnia, hypoxemia, and poor response to oxygen supplementation resembling a severe ventilation-perfusion mismatch, shunt, or persistent pulmonary hypertension of

Equine Neonatal Medicine, First Edition. Edited by David M. Wong and Pamela A. Wilkins.

the neonate (PPHN) [3, 5, 6]. In reported cases, immediate resuscitation was necessary but, unfortunately, was unsuccessful in the majority of cases due to the severity of the pulmonary maldevelopment. It seems reasonable to assume that the degree of pulmonary hypoplasia and hypertension may vary, depending on the underlying cause(s) and the degree of lung compression from any herniated abdominal viscera through a diaphragmatic defect as seen in human neonates. The aforementioned causes of severe respiratory signs at or around the time of birth should be fully investigated, with imaging studies becoming requisite.

When presented with a foal with clinical and laboratory findings consistent with unexplained pulmonary hypertension, pulmonary hypoplasia and CDH should be on the list of differential diagnoses, even though it is a rare condition. Ultrasonographic, radiographic, and computed tomographic (CT) imaging of the thoracic and abdominal cavities should demonstrate abnormal lung structure and patterns, loss of usual diaphragmatic anatomy, and/or the presence of herniated abdominal viscera into the thoracic cavity for these diagnoses. Diaphragmatic hernias may of course be traumatic in origin, occurring secondary to lacerations from rib fractures or other forms of trauma surrounding birth [23]. However, thoracic trauma should be evident on clinical examination and ultrasonographic imaging. Successful surgical repair of diaphragmatic defects has been described but is unlikely to solve the problem of lung hypoplasia, although the approach may alleviate some of the respiratory compromise due to limited thoracic space [12, 24, 25].

Unfortunately, foals with pulmonary hypoplasia that survive past parturition have a poor prognosis for survival and typically die soon after presentation. As a genetic component has not been established in the horse, there is no indication that that the problem might recur in subsequent offspring.

Pulmonary Bullae

Pulmonary bullae are rarely reported in the horse and, although well-recognized in other species including in people and dogs, are still considered an uncommon finding [26, 27, 28]. Pulmonary bullae typically form as a consequence of severe alveolar emphysema, which progresses by coalescing with other destroyed alveoli to form a singular or multiple, potentially more severe, emphysematous bullae. Histologically, bullae are characterized by abnormal and permanent enlargement of alveoli resulting from destruction of alveolar septa, and an absence of obvious fibrosis [29]. However, depending on the stage of the disease process, it can be difficult to distinguish alveolar hyperinflation from emphysema. The former is much more common but does not involve the permanent destruction of alveolar walls [29].

With the rarity of occurrence in the horse, it is difficult to firmly establish underlying causes. In humans, lung inflammation from long-term smoking is a common predisposing factor for emphysematous lung injury and subsequent bullae formation, as is alpha-1 antitrypsin deficiency [30, 31]. The latter is inherited in an autosomal codominant manner and results in an imbalance in protease and antiprotease activity, leaving alveolar tissue vulnerable to proteolytic damage by enzymes such as neutrophil elastase [32, 33]. Development of bullae associated with continuous positive airway pressure (CPAP) treatment has also been reported in people, highlighting the possibility of inducing further injury to diseased pulmonary tissue during such treatment [34]. Jakob et al. addressed the challenges of anesthetizing human premature infants, proposing that both CPAP and spontaneous breathing may be sufficient to cause pulmonary emphysema in severely immature lungs, particularly if superimposed on underlying lung disease [35].

Alpha-1 antitrypsin deficiency has not been reported in the horse and clearly other and more relevant underlying causes must be considered in the equine neonate. As pulmonary bullae with confirmed histopathological changes are rarely described in the equine neonate, the search for underlying causes becomes difficult [36]. There are reports of cavitary lesions, evident on thoracic radiographs in both the neonate and adult horse, that have the appearance of pulmonary bullae (Figure 8.VII.1a) [37–42]. Some of these were reported as incidental findings and even spontaneously resolved [39, 42] while in others the observed bullae were considered clinically relevant [36, 38, 40, 41]. The latter foals typically were reported to have concurrent sepsis and respiratory symptoms, where the presence of pulmonary bullae may have been a consequence of the underlying pathophysiological process and/or immaturity of the lungs. Bronchopneumonia resulting in obstruction of the distal airways by inflammatory cells, and increased secretion creating a one-way valve function may be one initiating factor. This could result in air being trapped and subsequent alveolar hyperinflation. If unresolved, destruction of the alveolar walls and emphysema may develop. Given the rarity of bullae and the frequent occurrence of pneumonia in the equine neonate, it seems reasonable to assume that other factors may be involved. Hyperinflation of fragile immature lung tissue may be one such risk factor.

The number and size of the bulla(e) may result in areas of clinically significant compression atelectasis of adjacent lung parenchyma, further adding to the respiratory symptoms. Another possible cause of severe respiratory symptoms is pneumothorax and pneumomediastinum if the bullae or cavitary lesions rupture [15, 38]. In one report, leakage of air

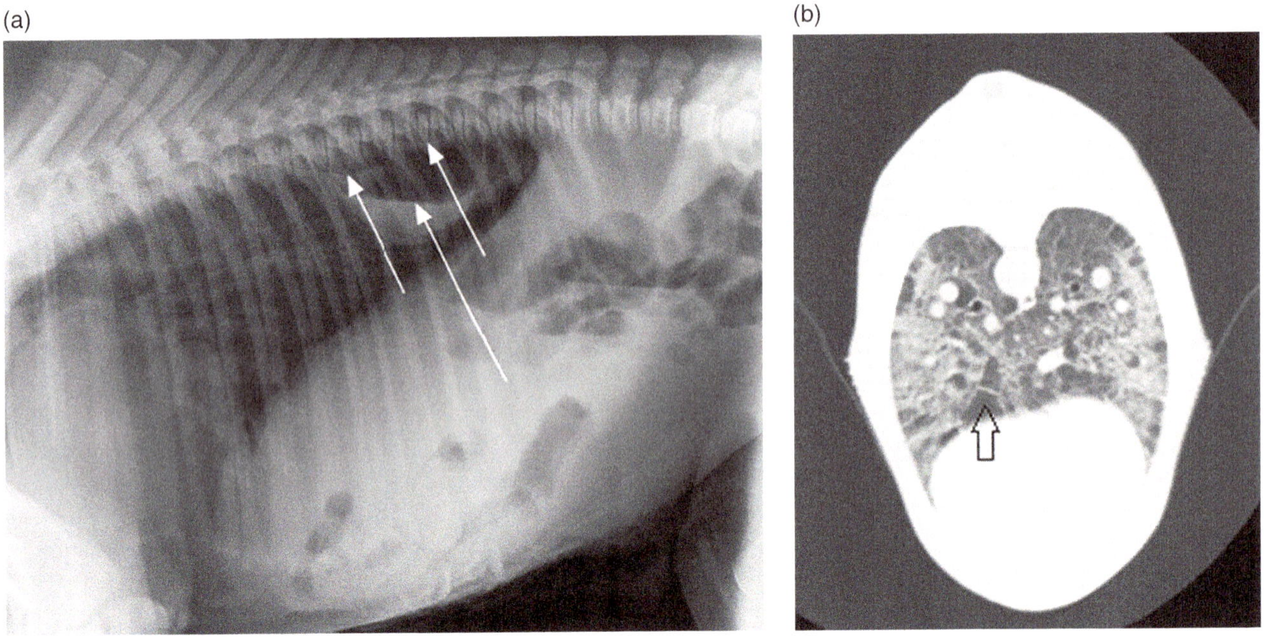

Figure 8.VII.1 (a) Left lateral radiograph of the thorax and abdomen of a standing 12-day-old foal. Note the cavitary lung lesions containing a horizontal fluid line ventrally (arrows) in the caudodorsal lung file. Bullous emphysema with hemorrhage was confirmed on postmortem examination. *Source:* Image from Ackerman et al. [11]. (b) A 6-day-old Quarter Horse colt presented for increased respiratory rate and effort. Computed tomography (CT) imaging documented atypical bullous pneumonia. Patchy heterogenous attenuation is noted within the interstitium along with numerous diffuse, round, well marginated regions of aerated lung noted bilaterally. There is extensive interlobular septal thickening surrounding both a ground glass interstitial pattern and emphysematous lung (arrow). *Source:* Image courtesy of Dr. Kara Lascola, Auburn University.

from ruptured bullae tracked out via the thoracic inlet and emerged subcutaneously resulting in palpable and visible emphysema [38]. There is clearly a need for investigation into these type of pulmonary lesions in order to better understand their origin and pathophysiological development.

Pulmonary bullae are most commonly detected on thoracic radiography as part of the clinical diagnostic investigation, where airway symptoms are present [36, 38–40, 42]. Computed tomography (CT) of the thoracic cavity have also been described providing detailed information on the size and extent of the bullae (Figure 8.VII.1b) [16]. Ultrasonographic evaluation of the thoracic cavity may also reveal bullae or cavitary lesions if they are superficially located, fluid filled, and/or surrounded by atelectatic or consolidated lung tissue [36, 40].

Treatment depends on the degree of respiratory distress caused by the bullae or cavitary lesion and the underlying pulmonary disease process resulting in bullae formation. General intensive supportive treatment and nursing care are required, with more invasive procedures required if pneumothorax develops. It appears prudent to closely monitor foals with respiratory clinical signs closely and provide forms of positive pressure respiratory support with caution. Imaging studies, particularly thoracic radiography and CT, should be repeated if costs are within any financial restriction placed by the owner. It is difficult to provide prognostic information as pulmonary bullae are so rarely reported, although, as described, successful outcomes including spontaneously resolution has been reported.

Rib Fractures

Rib fractures occur commonly in the equine neonate, although treatment opinions may not be clear (conservative or surgical) in some of these cases. Only a limited number of studies exist comparing the outcomes of these two treatment options, as well as reporting on the overall long-term athletic outcome of foals with rib fractures. Rib fractures can potentially cause injury to the underlying structures, including the lung and/or diaphragm resulting in pleural or pulmonary lacerations, pneumothorax, or lung contusions.

Thoracic trauma and rib fractures in foals were described as early as 1930 [43]. Since then, a number of studies have been published reporting on the prevalence and characteristics of these in the equine neonate. Jean and colleagues investigated the incidence of rib fractures on a single large Thoroughbred breeding farm and found that one fifth of neonatal foals had evidence of thoracic trauma, as indicated by thoracic asymmetry and careful physical examination [44]. A subset of these foals had rib fractures confirmed, or strongly suspected, following radiographic evaluation. In spite of the high prevalence, none of the foals suffered clinical complications resulting from thoracic trauma, and with none treated surgically. These findings have been contrasted with an earlier necropsy study, drawing from a large number of breeding farms, documenting that rib fractures were a common cause of death in foals presented for necropsy during their first week of life, accounting for 13% (32 foals) of all life-ending fractures (255 horses) [45]. Similarly, another large retrospective necropsy study found that thoracic trauma lesions were present in 9% of all foals (67/760) examined, with 19/67 (28%) of those foals having the cause of death attributed to rib fractures [46]. Sprayberry et al. found rib fractures to be a common complicating factor in sick newborns presenting for care in a referral setting, directly contributing to the death of the foal in 25% of the cases described [47]. This clearly contrasted the findings of a second report by Jean et al. [48], where rib fractures did not contribute to the death of any foal, including those few foals with clearly displaced rib fractures included in the study. Care must be taken, with the populations under discussion fully considered, prior to drawing any conclusions from comparison of these studies.

While the reported prevalence and potential consequences of rib fractures vary between these different types of studies, there is agreement that the majority of cases are associated with parturition, particularly following difficult and assisted foalings with vaginal delivery in primiparous mares [44, 47]. Malalignment/malpositioning of the foal during parturition in a narrow pelvic canal has been proposed to increase the risk of rib fractures occurring [43, 44].

There does not appear to be a clear sex predilection, or for left- versus right-sided fractures, although bilateral fractures are consistently reported to occur less frequently [44–52]. The majority of fractures are found at approximately 3–4 cm proximal to the costochondral junction, although some may simply be dislocations through the costochondral junction. Typically, the most cranial ribs are affected (except the first rib) with ribs 3–8 reported to be involved in 86% of cases in one study [46]. Although there are reported differences, generally the distal fragment becomes axially displaced predisposing to extensive laceration of thoracic cage contents and potentially resulting in fatal hemorrhage [45–47, 49–52]. In such cases, the pericardial sac or myocardium, major pulmonary vessels, as well the diaphragm, are commonly involved [45–47]. In cases where diaphragmatic lacerations occur, incarceration of herniated intestine in the thoracic cavity may have fatal consequences unless surgically corrected.

Other associated pulmonary lesions such as pleural lacerations, pneumothorax, contusion, and edema may have a more favorable outcome, although they are also a significant cause of morbidity and mortality requiring immediate attention [46, 47, 49–51]. It is well recognized in human medicine that external compressive forces on the rib cage, such as seen with cardiopulmonary resuscitation, can cause mechanical tearing and contusion of lung tissue with, potentially, severe consequence [53]. Focal injury may also affect other parts of the lung through hemorrhage and edema into the distal airways with bronchospasm, increased mucus production, and reduced mucocilliary clearance [54, 55]. Altered surfactant composition has also been detected in injured alveolar tissue [53, 56]. Segmental lung damage can also result in ventilation/perfusion mismatch, intrapulmonary shunts, increases in lung fluid, and loss of lung compliance, all which may be clinically manifested as hypoxemia, hypercapnia, and labored breathing [15, 57]. Depending on the extent and severity of the pulmonary contusion, these pathophysiological processes may deteriorate into further pulmonary dysfunction associated with local and systemic inflammatory responses. Fortunately, they may also resolve within days as seen in both people as well as in experimental animal models [54, 55]. Similar pathophysiological changes were described in a case report by Borcher et al., highlighting the number of possible consequences rib fractures may have on pulmonary function as well as the challenges in separating and identifying the possible causes of the clinicopathological derangement observed [43]. It also highlighted the possible development of acute lung injury and acute respiratory distress syndrome in such cases and the necessity to be able to identity these foals while considering the age-dependent criteria, including PaO_2/FiO_2 ratios [58].

Depending on the extent of the injury, the presenting signs may vary greatly ranging from being very subtle in some foals, to displaying marked respiratory distress and cardiovascular collapse in others. Further indications of pain include a reluctance to move or in a stiff manner and spending more time recumbent than one would expect, often in a sternal position [59]. This quiet behavior may, of course, be indicative of a number of other disease processes commonly encountered in the neonate and, hence, critical clinical evaluation is important. In order to assess the ribs, careful synchronous palpation, ideally in the standing foal, is required. While palpating and comparing the two sides, any signs of asymmetry, crepitus, edema, or discomfort should be identified. The respiratory rate and pattern should also be noted, and particularly signs of paradoxical breathing patterns. This may occur if several sequential ribs are fractured, making the affected area collapse inward during inspiration, being unable to maintain the outward force during the increased intrathoracic negative pressure of the respiratory cycle.

Even with careful and skilled palpation of the ribs, non- or minimally displaced fractures may not be evident and further diagnostic imaging is required. Ultrasonographic examination has proven a much more sensitive imaging modality than radiography for detecting rib fractures, and may also reveal trauma resulting in hemo- and/or pneumothorax with focal atelectasis (Figure 8.VII.2) [44, 47, 48]. In people, computed tomography (CT) was reported to have a higher diagnostic accuracy than radiography in detecting rib fractures in a postmortem study in children, although with a lower specificity resulting in a higher number of false positives [60]. However, imaging modalities including radiography, ultrasonography, and CT may all complement each other while being aware of the strengths and limitations of each one of these.

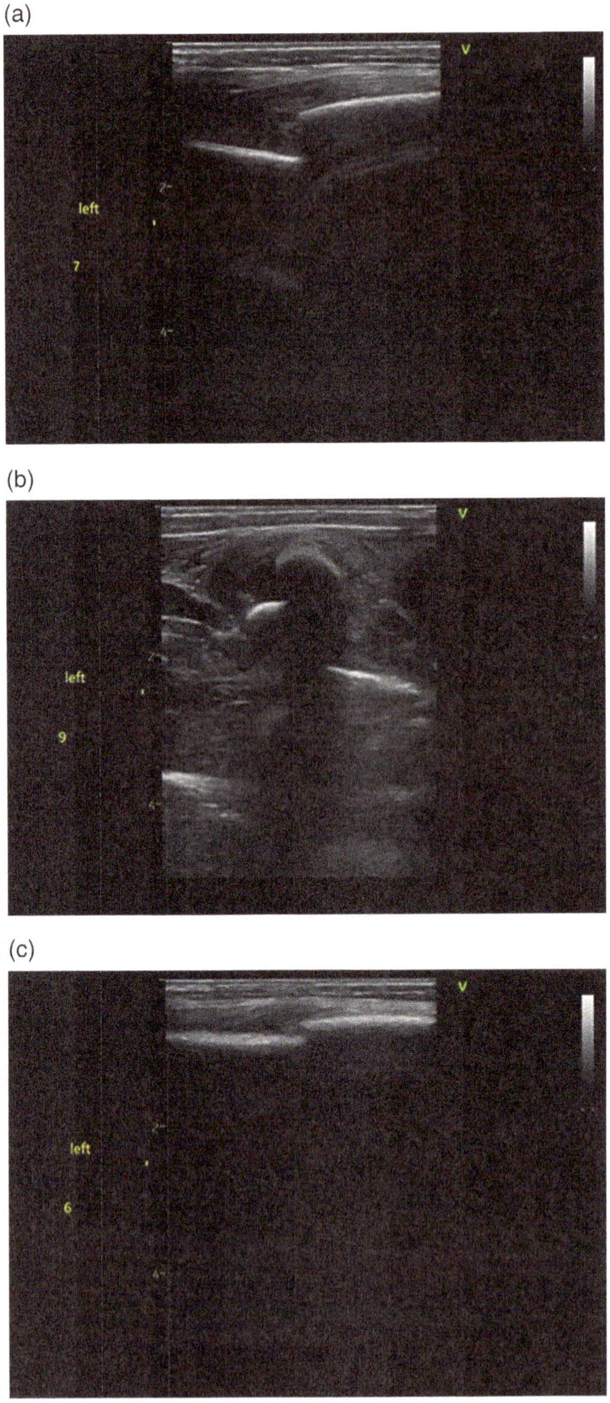

Figure 8.VII.2 (a) Long-axis view of a displaced seventh rib. (b) Short-axis view of a ninth rib revealing a displaced fracture with a surrounding hematoma. (c): A long-axis view of a nondisplaced/minimally displaced fracture of the sixth rib. *Source:* courtesy of Dr. JoAnn Slack.

Rib fractures are frequently managed conservatively. Byars described a conservative treatment protocol that included a 2-week stall rest period during which time analgesic and sedative medication administration was provided as required, making sure that the foal did not become too active risking displacement of the fracture(s) and hence further injury [59]. However, opinions differ as to if and when surgical treatment is indicated. In some cases, the risk of laceration of vital organs from axial displacement of rib fracture edges overlying these, multiple rib fractures interfering with normal breathing patterns, or the identification of already existing intra-thoracic injury, become indications for surgical rib repair and stabilization. The risk of (further) displacement may be of particular concern in equine neonates that are receiving intensive care treatment for other conditions involving frequent handling of the foal, increasing the risk of inadvertent displacement. The value of the foal and expectations of owner and referring veterinarians commonly influence the decision for surgical treatment. The surgical repair and stabilization techniques have evolved, and continue to do so, as have the type of implants utilized. The early percutaneous techniques are now largely replaced by open techniques using reconstruction plates, orthopedic wires, monofilament placement and, most recently, plastic zip-ties [49, 50, 52].

Few studies have evaluated both the short- and long-term outcome of surviving foals with rib fractures, or surviving foals treated conservatively compared to those with surgical repair, with respect to their racing career [25, 61]. These studies demonstrated that both surgical and conservative treatment of neonatal rib fractures had acceptable future racing outcomes in those surviving the initial treatment period. Furthermore, neonates with surgically repaired fractured ribs had a good prognosis for survival with a similar chance of starting a race compared to their maternal siblings [25]. However, in adult people it is well recognized that rib fractures may lead to chronic pain and disability, also reported in horses sustaining injury as adults [62, 63]. Although rib fractures are common in foals and, while life-threatening in some cases, appear uncomplicated in the majority of cases, further follow-up studies of these foals are still required. The high reported prevalence of equine neonatal thoracic trauma also highlights the need for extreme care when handling neonatal foals as nondisplaced fractures may become displaced potentially resulting in severe injury.

Bronchopulmonary Dysplasia

Bronchopulmonary dysplasia (BPD), or chronic lung disease, is one of the most common complications associated with prematurity in human infants. An estimated 48–68% of children born at <28 weeks of gestation are affected [64]. In contrast, only one case report has been described in the premature newborn foal [65]. The term BPD was first used by Northway and colleagues in 1967 to describe a condition in premature infants that developed during or following treatment of acute respiratory distress syndrome. In those babies that did not survive, pulmonary inflammation, bronchial mucosal metaplasia, alveolar emphysema, and fibrosis were typical histopathological findings, depending on the stage of the disease process [66]. Similar findings were also described in the reported foal with varying degrees of inflammation, metaplasia, and regeneration of alveolar and terminal bronchial epithelium as well as segmental fibrinoid degeneration of arteries and arterioles [65].

These early descriptions are no longer considered characteristic of BPD, which might reflect the greater degree of prematurity seen in current cases, and hence earlier stage of lung development, compared to those seen in original studies. Most infants described by Northway et al. [66] were moderate- to late-term premature (32–37 weeks of gestation) while currently, most infants who develop BPD are defined as extremely preterm (<28 weeks of gestation). Current characteristics include impaired pulmonary parenchymal development with deficient alveolarization and dysregulated vascular development leading to increased vascular resistance and pulmonary hypertension [67–69]. Some degree of emphysema and fibrosis can still be evident but with a less heterogeneous distribution than described in the original studies [66, 70–72].

BPD commonly develops when treating acute lung injury in the premature infant; this initiates a cascade of events resulting in an aberrant reparative response and impaired pulmonary development [73]. The initial description by Northway et al. [66] principally attributed BPD development to oxygen toxicity and barotrauma from mechanical ventilation of fragile, premature lungs [66]. Although likely an important contributing factor at that time, as careful oxygen administration and gentler ventilation protocols have been implemented, it is now recognized that BPD is a complex condition that likely has other causes.

Several predisposing factors make the premature infant more susceptible to such aberrant responses to treatment and hence increase the risk of developing BPD. The recognition that (extreme) prematurity is not a normal condition and that complex health problems are likely to accompany these infants has helped broaden the investigation of BPD [73]. Clearly antenatal conditions in human infants differ from those seen in the pregnant mare, although placentitis and placental dysfunction are important and common causes of premature birth in equids [74–76]. There are also differences in the postnatal period between species. Pulmonary inflammation resulting from both pre- and postnatal conditions, including sepsis, remains an important cause of subsequent BPD development in the premature infant [77, 78].

Recently, the influence of intestinal microbiota and the gut-lung axis on the development of BPD has been investigated [78]. One hypothesis is that intestinal dysbiosis disrupts the gut barrier, resulting in metabolic disturbances and local inflammation, which subsequently results in a systemic inflammatory response in which the lungs are also affected [78]. One such possible cause of dysbiosis is antibiotic therapy, routinely used as part of the treatment protocol in both premature foals and infants. Alternatively, the newborn lung is not a sterile environment as previously thought, and the population of bacteria normally present may be disrupted in premature infants paving way for respiratory infections, which accelerate the development of BPD [79]. Indeed, the alveolar epithelial injury described in the one foal reported was later thought to be attributed to a perinatal equine viral arteritis infection [65, 80].

Diagnosis of BPD is challenging due to the lack of well-defined criteria. Prematurity is clearly the single most important factor increasing the risk, although ante-, peri- and postnatal conditions as described are also important to consider.

Historically, the level and duration of oxygen therapy was used as both diagnostic and prognostic criteria [81, 82]. More recently, the mode of respiratory support administered at 36 weeks, regardless of the prior duration or current level of oxygen therapy, appears to better define and predict the outcome of BPD in infants [83]. Clearly, a history of prematurity, and the possible reasons for it, combined with the need for continuing respiratory support are central to the diagnosis and assessment of severity of BPD. Imaging modalities such radiography and computed tomography reflect the histopathological changes in these patients [84, 85].

In infants, the high prevalence of BPD has advanced the development of different treatment strategies, including careful use of oxygen therapy and mechanical ventilation and avoidance of hyperoxia, as well as structural injury from baro-and volutrauma during mechanical ventilation [86, 87]. Hyperoxia may result in acute lung injury, which is characterized by disruption of the alveolar-capillary barrier, influx of inflammatory mediators, vascular leak, and pulmonary edema, ultimately leading to cell death [88, 89]. Premature lungs already predisposed to developing bronchopulmonary dysplasia (BPD), may readily progresses into this condition as a consequence of oxygen toxicity.

Exogenous surfactant therapy is commonly used when treating premature infants. The last trimester (28–40 weeks) is very important for alveolar development and formation as well as maturation of type II pneumocytes enabling surfactant production in people [73, 90]. Alveolar development also occurs late in foals, at around 84% of gestation [91]. However, although type II pneumocytes are differentiated at an early stage, it is not complete until near full term, resulting in smaller amounts and immature composition of surfactant [92, 93]. This makes the premature newborn foal particularly vulnerable to failure of pulmonary function. Bovine surfactant preparation therapy was attempted in the equine case report but had limited success [2]. Corticosteroids, both systemic and inhaled, are also commonly used when treating premature human neonates with BPD [94]. However, there is concern about its use and neurodevelopmental adverse effects, such as cerebral palsy, emphasizing the necessity for its careful use [95, 96].

As mentioned, one of the major problems with BPD is the lack of a recognized working definition. This also makes it challenging to measure outcomes of the different treatment strategies. Clearly there is much to learn about this condition in infants. Although the reporting of BPD in foals is incredibly sparse, this condition might need further attention in premature equine neonates. Certainly, the issues of a careful approach to ventilatory strategies and oxygen therapy as well an awareness of the possible detrimental impact of altered intestinal and pulmonary microflora are important aspects to consider when treating all premature animals. Residual pulmonary damage and possible impact on future athletic use in the horse are also factors to consider. Much more documentation of BPD is required in the neonatal foal.

References

1 Wert, S.E. (2017). Normal and abnormal structural development of the lung. In: *Fetal and Neonatal Physiology*, 5e (ed. R.A. Polin, S.H. Abman, D.H. Rowitch, et al.), 627–641. Elsevier.

2 Palmer, J.E. (2012). Colic and diaphragmatic hernias in neonatal foals. *Equine Vet. Educ.* 24: 340–342.

3 Tapio, H., Hewetson, M., and Sihvo, H.K. (2012). An unusual cause of colic in a neonatal foal. *Equine Vet. Educ.* 24: 334–339.

4 Tăbăran, A.F., Nagy, A.L., Cătoi, C. et al. (2015). Congenital diaphragmatic hernia with concurrent aplasia of the pericardium in a foal. *BMC Vet. Res.* 11: 309.

5 Lanci, A., Ingallinesi, M., Morini, M. et al. (2021). Fetal congenital diaphragmatic hernia and hydramnios in a quarter horse mare. *Vet. Sci.* 8: 201.

6 Loynachan, A.T. (2022). Equine pulmonary agenesis and hypoplasia associated with diaphragmatic herniation. *J. Equine Vet. Sci.* 109: 103855.

7 Langham, M.R., Kays, D.W., Ledbetter, D.J. et al. (1996). Congenital diaphragmatic hernia. Epidemiology and outcome. *Clin. Perinatol.* 23: 671–688.

8 Stege, G., Fenton, A., and Jaffray, B. (2003). Nihilism in the 1990s: the true mortality of congenital diaphragmatic hernia. *Pediatrics* 112: 532–535.

9 Van den Hout, L., Reiss, I., Felix, J.F. et al. (2010). Risk factors for chronic lung disease and mortality in newborns with congenital diaphragmatic hernia. *Neonatology* 98: 370–380.

10 Kardon, G., Ackerman, K.G., McCulley, D.J. et al. (2017). Congenital diaphragmatic hernias: from genes to mechanisms to therapies. *Dis. Model. Mech.* 10: 955–970.

11 Ackerman, K.G., Vargas, S.O., Wilson, J.A. et al. (2012). Congenital diaphragmatic defects: proposal for a new classification based on observations in 234 patients. *Pediatr. Dev. Pathol.* 15: 265–274.

12 Speirs, V.C. and Reynolds, W.T. (1976). Successful repair of a diaphragmatic hernia in a foal. *Equine Vet. J.* 8: 170–172.

13 Cheetham, J. (1998). Congenital diaphragmatic hernia with subsequent incarceration of the left large colon and gastric rupture in a foal. *Equine Vet. Educ.* 10: 239–241.

14 Hart, S.K. and Brown, J.A. (2009). Diaphragmatic hernia in horses: 44 cases (1986–2006). *J. Vet. Emerg. Crit. Care* 19: 357–362.

15 Chandrasekharan, P.K., Rawat, M., Madappa, R. et al. (2017). Congenital diaphragmatic hernia – a review. *Matern. Health Neonatol Perinatol.* 3: 6.

16 Harding, R. (1997). Fetal pulmonary development: the role of respiratory movements. *Equine Vet. J.* 29: 32–39.

17 De Lorimier, A.A. (1967). Hypoplastic lungs in fetal lambs with surgically produced congenital diaphragmatic hernia. *Surgery* 62: 12–17.

18 Keijzer, R., Liu, J., Deimling, J. et al. (1000). Dual hit hypothesis explains pulmonary hypoplasia in the nitrofen model of congenital diaphragmatic hernia. *Am. J. Pathol.* 156: 1299–1306.

19 Ackerman, K.G., Herron, B.J., Vargas, S.O. et al. (2005). Fog2 is required for normal diaphragm and lung development in mice and humans. *PLos Genet.* 1: 58–65.

20 Geggel, R.L., Murphy, J.D., Langleben, D. et al. (1985). Congenital diaphragmatic hernia: arterial structural changes and persistent pulmonary hypertension after surgical repair. *J. Pediatr.* 107: 457–464.

21 Montalva, L., Antounians, L., and Zani, A. (2019). Pulmonary hypertension secondary to congenital

diaphragmatic hernia: factors and pathways involved in pulmonary vascular remodeling. *Pediatr. Res.* 85: 754–768.
22 Wynn, J., Krishnan, U., Aspelund, G. et al. (2013). Outcomes of congenital diaphragmatic hernia in the modern era of management. *J. Pediatr.* 163: 114–119.
23 Schambourgs, M.A., Laverty, S., Mullim, S. et al. (2003). Thoracic trauma in foals: postmortem findings. *Equine Vet. J.* 35: 78–81.
24 Kolus, C.R., MacLeay, J.M., and Hackett, E.S. (2017). Repair of an acquired diaphragmatic hernia with surgical mesh in a foal. *Can. Vet. J.* 58: 145–148.
25 Velloso Álvarez, A., Sandow, C.B., Rodgerson, D.H. et al. (2022). Survival and racing performance after surgical treatment of rib fractures in foals. *Vet. Surg.* 51: 62–67.
26 Silverman, S., Poulos, P.W., and Suter, P.F. (1976). Cavitary pulmonary lesions in animals. *Vet. Radiol.* 17: 134–146.
27 Gattinoni, L., Bombino, M., Pelosi, P. et al. (1994). Lung structure and function in different stages of severe adult respiratory distress syndrome. *JAMA* 271: 1772–1779.
28 Lipscomb, V.J., Hardie, R.J., and Dubielzig, R.R. (2003). Spontaneous pneumothorax caused by pulmonary blebs and bullae in 12 dogs. *J. Am. Anim. Hosp. Assoc.* 39: 435–445.
29 Caswell, J.L. and Williams, K.J. (2016). Respiratory system. In: *Jubb, Kennedy and Palmer's Pathology of Domestic Animals*, 6e, vol. 2 (ed. M. Grant Maxie), 465–591. W.B. Saunders.
30 Fraser, R., Pare, J., Pare, P.D. et al. (1990). *Diagnosis of Diseases of the Chest*, 3e, vol. III, 2107–2112. Philadelphia: WB Saunders.
31 Tuder, R.M., Yoshida, T., Arap, W. et al. (2006). State of the art. Cellular and molecular mechanisms of alveolar destruction in emphysema: an evolutionary perspective. *Proc. Am. Thorac. Soc.* 3: 503–510.
32 Stoller, J.K., Hupertz, V., and Aboussouan, L.S. (2006). Alpha-1 antitrypsin deficiency. In: *Gene Reviews* (ed. M.P. Adam, G.M. Mirzaa, R.A. Pagon, et al.), 1993–2022. Seattle, WA: University of Washington.
33 Gadek, J.E., Fells, G.A., Zimmerman, R.L. et al. (1981). Antielastases of the human alveolar structures. Implications for the protease-antiprotease theory of emphysema. *J. Clin. Invest.* 68: 889–898.
34 Berhane, S., Tabor, A., Sahu, A. et al. (2020). Development of bullous lung disease in a patient with severe COVID-19 pneumonitis. *BMJ Case Rep.* 13: e237455.
35 Jakob, A., Bender, C., Henschen, M. et al. (2013). Selective unilateral lung ventilation in preterm infants with acquired bullous emphysema: a series of nine cases. *Pediatr. Pulmonol.* 48: 14–19.
36 Bezdekova, B., Skoric, M., Pekarkova, M. et al. (2012). Bullous emphysema with haemorrhage in a premature foal. *Equine Vet. Educ.* 24: 447–452.
37 Lavoie, J.P., Fiset, L., and Laverty, S. (1994). Review of 40 cases of lung abscesses in foals and adult horses. *Equine Vet. J.* 26: 348–352.
38 Marble, S.L., Edens, L.M., Shiroma, J.T. et al. (1996). Subcutaneous emphysema in a neonatal foal. *J. Am. Vet. Med. Assoc.* 208: 97–99.
39 Lester, G.D. and Lester, N.V. (2001). Abdominal and thoracic radiography in the neonate. *Vet. Clin. North Am. Equine Pract.* 17: 19–46.
40 Hilton, H., Galuppo, L., Puchalski, S.M. et al. (2009). Successful treatment of invasive pulmonary aspergillosis in a neonatal foal. *J. Vet. Intern. Med.* 23: 375–378.
41 Johnson, P.J., LaCarrubba, A.M., Messer, N.T. et al. (2012). Neonatal respiratory distress and sepsis in the premature foal: challenges with diagnosis and management. *Equine Vet. Educ.* 24: 453–458.
42 Butler, J.A., Colles, C.M., Dyson, S.J. et al. (2017). The thorax. In: *Clinical Radiology of the Horse*, 4e, 639–687. Chichester, West Sussex, UK/Ames, Iowa, USA: Wiley.
43 Reynolds, E.B. (1930). Clinical notes on some conditions met within the mare following parturition and in the newly born foal. *Vet. Rec.* 10: 277.
44 Jean, D., Laverty, S., Halley, J. et al. (1999). Thoracic trauma in newborn foals. *Equine Vet. J.* 31: 149–152.
45 Harrison, L. (1995). Equine fracture cases. *Equine Dis. Quart.* 3: 5.
46 Schambourg, M.A., Laverty, S., Mullim, S. et al. (2003). Thoracic trauma in foals: post mortem findings. *Equine Vet. J.* 35: 78–81.
47 Sprayberry, K.A., Bain, F.T., Seahorn, T.L. et al. (2001). 56 cases of rib fractures in neonatal foals hospitalized in a referral center intensive care unit from 1997–2001. *Proc. Am. Assoc. Equine Pract.* 47: 395–399.
48 Jean, D., Picandet, V., Macieira, S. et al. (2007). Detection of rib trauma in newborn foals in an equine critical care unit: a comparison of ultrasonography, radiography and physical examination. *Equine Vet. J.* 39: 158–163.
49 Bellezzo, F., Hunt, R.J., Provost, R. et al. (2004). Surgical repair of rib fractures in 14 neonatal foals: case selection, surgical technique and results. *Equine Vet. J.* 36: 557–562.
50 Kraus, B.M., Richardson, D.W., Sheridan, G. et al. (2005). Multiple rib fracture in a neonatal foal using a nylon strand suture repair technique. *Vet. Surg.* 34: 399–404.
51 Borchers, A., van Eps, A., Zedler, S. et al. (2009). Thoracic trauma and post operative lung injury in a neonatal foal. *Equine Vet. Educ.* 21: 186–191.
52 Levine, D. (2022). Fractures of the ribs. In: *Fractures in the Horse*, Ie (ed. I. Wright), 739–746. Hoboken, NJ: Wiley.
53 Cohn, S.M. and Dubose, J.J. (2010). Pulmonary contusion: an update on recent advances in clinical management. *World J. Surg.* 34: 1959–1970.

54 Moseley, R.V., Vernick, J.J., and Doty, D.B. (1970). Response to blunt chest injury: a new experimental model. *J. Trauma* 10: 673–683.

55 Demling, R.H. and Pomfret, E.A. (1993). Blunt chest trauma. *New Horiz.* 1: 402–421.

56 Aufmkolk, M., Fischer, R., Voggenreiter, G. et al. (1999). Local effect of lung contusion on lung surfactant composition in multiple trauma patients. *Crit. Care Med.* 27: 1441–1446.

57 Garzon, A.A., Seltzer, B., and Karlson, K.E. (1968). Physiopathology of crushed chest injuries. *Ann. Surg.* 168: 128–136.

58 Wilkins, P.A., Otto, C.M., Baumgardner, J.E. et al. (2007). Acute lung injury and acute respiratory distress syndromes in veterinary medicine: consensus definitions: the Dorothy Russell Havemeyer Working group on ALI and ARDS in veterinary medicine. *J. Vet. Emerg. Crit. Care* 17: 333–339.

59 Byars, T.D. (1997). Fractured ribs in neonatal foals. AAEP report. News and Notes from the AAEP. 13.

60 Shelmerdine, S.C., Langan, D., Hutchinson, J.C. et al. (2018). DRIFT Study Research group. Chest radiographs versus CT for the detection of rib fractures in children (DRIFT): a diagnostic accuracy observational study. *Lancet Child Adolesc. Health* 2: 802–811.

61 Fehin, W.F., Wylie, C.E., Feeney, C. et al. (2017). The future racing performance of neonatal thoroughbreds diagnosed with rib fractures treated both surgically and conservatively. *Equine Vet. J.* 49: 23–23.

62 Witt, C.E. and Bulger, E.M. (2017). Comprehensive approach to the management of the patient with multiple rib fractures: a review and introduction of a bundled rib fracture management protocol. *Trauma Surg. Acute Care Open* 2: e000064.

63 Hall, S., Smith, R., Ramzan, P.H.L. et al. (2023). Rib fractures in adult horses as a cause of poor performance; diagnosis, treatment and outcome in 73 horses. *Equine Vet. J.* 55: 59–65.

64 Stoll, B.J., Hansen, N.I., Bell, E.F. et al. (2010). Eunice Kennedy Shriver National Institute of Child Health and Human Development Neonatal Research Network. Neonatal outcomes of extremely preterm infants from the NICHD Neonatal Research Network. *Pediatrics* 126: 443–456.

65 Freeman, K.P., Cline, J.M., Simmons, R. et al. (1989). Recognition of bronchopulmonary dysplasia in a newborn foal. *Equine Vet. J.* 21: 292–296.

66 Northway, W.H., Rosan, R.C., and Porter, D.Y. (1967). Pulmonary disease following respiratory therapy of hyaline-membrane disease. Bronchopulmonary dysplasia. *N. Engl. J. Med.* 276: 357–368.

67 Armes, J.E., Mifsud, W., and Ashworth, M. (2015). Diffuse lung disease of infancy: a pattern-based, algorithmic approach to histological diagnosis. *J. Clin. Pathol.* 68: 100–110.

68 Higano, N.S., Spielberg, D.R., Fleck, R.J. et al. (2018). Neonatal pulmonary magnetic resonance imaging of bronchopulmonary dysplasia predicts short-term clinical outcomes. *Am. J. Respir. Crit. Care Med.* 198: 1302–1311.

69 Sahni, M. and Bhandari, V. (2020). Recent advances in understanding and management of bronchopulmonary dysplasia. *F1000Res* 9: F1000.

70 Doshi, N., Kanbour, A., Fujikura, T. et al. (1982). Tracheal aspiration cytology in neonates with respiratory distress: histopathologic correlation. *Acta Cytol.* 26: 15–21.

71 Husain, A.N., Siddiqui, N.H., and Stocker, J.T. (1998). Pathology of arrested acinar development in post surfactant bronchopulmonary dysplasia. *Hum. Pathol.* 29: 710–717.

72 Coalson, J.J. (2006). Pathology of bronchopulmonary dysplasia. *Semin. Perinatol.* 30: 179–184.

73 Thébaud, B., Goss, K.N., Laughon, M. et al. (2019). Bronchopulmonary dysplasia. *Nat. Rev. Dis. Primers.* 5: 78.

74 Hartling, L., Liang, Y., and Lacaze-Masmonteil, T. (2012). Chorioamnionitis as a risk factor for bronchopulmonary dysplasia: a systematic review and meta-analysis. *Arch. Dis. Child. Fetal Neonatal Ed.* 97: F8–F17.

75 LeBlanc, M.M., Giguère, S., Lester, G.D. et al. (2012). Relationship between infection, inflammation and premature parturition in mares with experimentally induced placentitis. *Equine Vet. J. Suppl.* 41: 8–14.

76 Kim, C.J., Romero, R., Chaemsaithong, P. et al. (2015). Acute chorioamnionitis and funisitis: definition, pathologic features, and clinical significance. *Am. J. Obstet. Gynecol.* 213: S29–S52.

77 Kim, S.H., Han, Y.S., Chun, J. et al. (2020). Risk factors that affect the degree of bronchopulmonary dysplasia: comparison by severity in the same gestational age. *PLoS One* 15: e0235901.

78 Yang, K., He, S., and Dong, W. (2021). Gut microbiota and bronchopulmonary dysplasia. *Pediatr. Pulmonol.* 56: 2460–2470.

79 Pammi, M., Lal, C.V., Wagner, B.D. et al. (2019). Airway microbiome and development of bronchopulmonary dysplasia in preterm infants: a systematic review. *J. Pediatr.* 204: 126–133.

80 Wilkins, P.A., Del Piero, F., Lopez, J. et al. (1995). Recognition of bronchopulmonary dysplasia in a newborn foal. *Equine Vet. J.* 27: 398.

81 Bancalari, E., Abdenour, G.E., Feller, R. et al. (1979). Bronchopulmonary dysplasia: clinical presentation. *J. Pediatr.* 95: 819–823.

82 Tooley, W.H. (1979). Epidemiology of bronchopulmonary dysplasia. *J. Pediatr.* 95: 851–858.

83 Jensen, E.A., Dysart, K., Gantz, M.G. et al. (2019). The diagnosis of bronchopulmonary dysplasia in very preterm infants. An evidence-based approach. *Am. J. Respir. Crit. Care Med.* 200: 751–759.

84 Oppenheim, C., Mamou-Mani, T., Sayegh, N. et al. (1994). Bronchopulmonary dysplasia: value of CT in identifying pulmonary sequelae. *AJR Am. J. Roentgenol.* 163: 169–172.

85 Mahut, B., De Blic, J., Emond, S. et al. (2007). Chest computed tomography findings in bronchopulmonary dysplasia and correlation with lung function. *Arch. Dis. Child. Fetal Neonatal Ed.* 92: F459–F464.

86 Jobe, A.H. and Bancalari, E. (2001). Bronchopulmonary dysplasia. *Am. J. Respir. Crit. Care Med.* 163: 1723–1729.

87 Isayama, T., Iwami, H., McDonald, S. et al. (2016). Association of noninvasive ventilation strategies with mortality and bronchopulmonary dysplasia among preterm infants: a systematic review and meta-analysis. *JAMA* 316: 611–624.

88 Warner, B.B., Stuart, L.A., Papes, R.A. et al. (1998). Functional and pathological effects of prolonged hyperoxia in neonatal mice. *Am. J. Phys* 275: 110–117.

89 Harijith, A.K. and Bhandari, V. (2016). Hyperoxia in the pathogenesis of bronchopulmonary dysplasia. In: *Bronchopulmonary Dysplasia* (ed. V. Bhandari), 3–26. Philadelphia PA: Humana Press.

90 Schittny, J.C. (2017). Development of the lung. *Cell Tissue Res.* 367: 427–444.

91 Barnard, K., Leadon, D.P., and Silver, I.A. (1982). Some aspects of tissue maturation in fetal and perinatal foals. *J. Reprod. Fertil. Suppl.* 32: 589–595.

92 Arvidson, G., Astedt, B., Ekelund, L. et al. (1975). Surfactant studies in the fetal and neonatal foal. *J. Reprod. Fertil. Suppl.* 23: 663–665.

93 Pattle, R.E., Rossdale, P.D., Schock, C. et al. (1975). The development of the lung and its surfactant in the foal and in other species. *J. Reprod. Fertil. Suppl.* 23: 651–657.

94 Doyle, L.W. (2021). Postnatal corticosteroids to prevent or treat bronchopulmonary dysplasia. *Neonatology* 118: 244–251.

95 Shah, S.S., Ohlsson, A., Halliday, H.L. et al. (2017). Inhaled versus systemic corticosteroids for preventing bronchopulmonary dysplasia in ventilated very low birth weight preterm neonates. *Cochrane Database Syst. Rev.* (10): CD002057. https://doi.org/10.1002/14651858.CD002058.pub3.

96 Shah, S.S., Ohlsson, A., Halliday, H.L. et al. (2017). Inhaled versus systemic corticosteroids for the treatment of bronchopulmonary dysplasia in ventilated very low birth weight preterm infants. *Cochrane Database Syst. Rev.* (10): CD002058. https://doi.org/10.1002/14651858.CD002057.pub4.

Section VIII Nonpulmonary Disease Processes Manifesting as Respiratory Disease

Daniela Bedenice

Respiratory failure can arise from abnormalities in any of the components of the respiratory system, including the airways, alveoli, central nervous system (CNS), peripheral nervous system, respiratory muscles, and chest wall. While primary conditions of the respiratory tract result in clinical and clinicopathologic manifestations of respiratory difficulty, other organ systems outside the respiratory system can manifest as respiratory disease. For example, a variety of metabolic, cardiovascular, and behavioral abnormalities can manifest as respiratory dysfunction. As such, critically ill foals with hypoperfusion secondary to cardiogenic, hypovolemic, or septic shock can present with respiratory distress or failure. This section discusses relevant nonpulmonary causes of respiratory dysfunction in neonatal foals.

Pleural Effusion

Excessive fluid in the thorax causes compressive atelectasis, which can result in respiratory distress. The term *compression atelectasis* refers to incomplete alveolar distension and is used to describe lungs that have collapsed secondary to pneumothorax, space-occupying masses, or excessive fluid in the pleural cavity [1]. The accumulation of pleural fluid has important effects on respiratory system function, by causing a concurrent decrease in lung volume and increase in chest wall volume. Additionally, pleural effusion increases pulmonary resistance and lung stiffness (i.e. elastance), due to alterations in the dynamic properties of the lung. Airway closure may be an important determinant of these alterations. At the same time the elastic recoil and resistance of the chest wall are decreased. These changes result in a restrictive ventilatory effect, chest wall expansion, and reduced efficiency of the inspiratory muscles. However, at least with small to moderate volumes of pleural effusion, the lung may be displaced by the effusion rather than compressed. The magnitude of changes in respiratory system mechanics thus depends on pleural fluid volume and underlying disease of the respiratory system.

The decrease in lung volume is associated with hypoxemia, mainly due to an increase in right-to-left intrapulmonary shunt. Under certain circumstances, large pleural effusions may also impede the filling of the right heart and, by decreasing cardiac output, exaggerate the effects of ventilation/perfusion (V/Q) mismatch and right-to-left shunt. Thoracocentesis may be lifesaving in these cases by increasing cardiac output and oxygenation [2]. However, removal of a relatively large volume of pleural fluid may lead to re-expansion pulmonary edema and, in some cases, to hypovolemia [3]. Re-expansion pulmonary edema after removal of large volumes of pleural effusion is likely caused by the negative pleural pressure and an associated increase in vascular permeability, although an inflammatory process may also be involved [4, 5]. The drainage of pleural fluid results in an increase in lung volume that is considerably less than the amount of aspirated fluid, and hypoxemia may not be readily reversible upon fluid drainage [6].

Pleural effusion is a general term used to describe accumulation of any fluid, transudate or modified transudate, exudate, lymph, blood or chyle, within the thoracic cavity (Figure 8.VIII.1). *Hydrothorax*, or accumulation of serous, clear fluid (transudate), is generally associated with increases in hydrostatic pressure (congestive heart failure [CHF], venous thrombosis, hepatic failure), low colloid oncotic pressure (hypoproteinemia), increased vascular leak (systemic inflammatory response syndrome or sepsis in foals) or less commonly obstruction of lymph drainage [1]. While congenital defects leading to hydrothorax have been described in foals [7], these conditions are considered rare. Both pure transudate (total protein $<2.5\,g/dl$, nucleated cell count $<1.5 \times 10^3\,\mu l$) and modified transudate (total protein $>2.5\,g/dl$) cavitary effusions have been

Equine Neonatal Medicine, First Edition. Edited by David M. Wong and Pamela A. Wilkins.

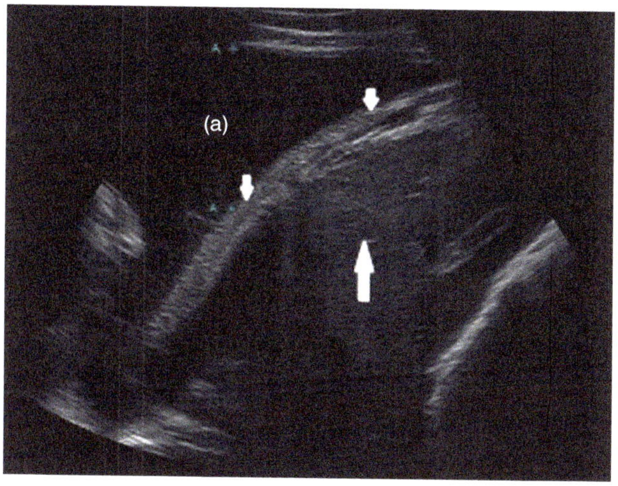

Figure 8.VIII.1 Ultrasonographic exam of a horse with pleural effusion. Note the anechoic fluid (a), diaphragm (arrowheads), and liver (large arrow).

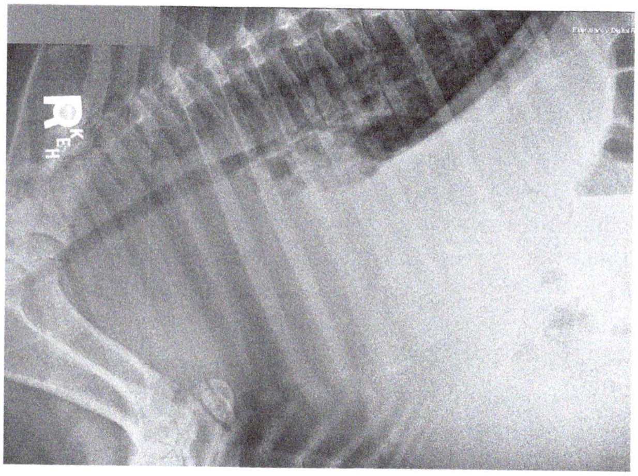

Figure 8.VIII.2 Pleural effusion (hydrothorax) associated with *Anaplasma* infection in a foal.

reported in equids following *Anaplasma* infection [8]. The latter may be considered as an infrequent infectious cause of hydrothorax, even in young foals, as transplacental transmission of *Anaplasma* has been documented in a late gestation mare (Figure 8.VIII.2) [9]. *Chylothorax*, or accumulation of chylous fluid in the mediastinum or pleural cavity, is also an uncommon condition in foals that results from diseases affecting the thoracic or intestinal lymphatic ducts [10]. The rarity of the disease is attributed to the protected location of the thoracic duct and the capacity of lymphatic ducts to heal spontaneously following injury. Chylous fluid (lymph rich in triglycerides) is typically odorless, milky, and opalescent, although microscopic assessment for chylomicrons is recommended to confirm the nature of the fluid [11]. Successful medical management of bilateral chylous effusion has been documented in a neonatal colt with meconium impaction [12].

Hemothorax in neonates can be the result of thoracic trauma (including rib fractures during delivery), vascular erosion, or coagulopathy secondary to systemic conditions such as disseminated intravascular coagulation (DIC), sepsis, neonatal alloimmune thrombocytopenia, and congenital clotting factor deficiencies. Since hemostatic mechanisms of equine neonates are immature at birth, newborn foals may be at particular risk of platelet-associated hemorrhagic disorders during their maturation period [13].

Pleural tissue is readily susceptible to injury through direct implantation of bacteria following penetrating trauma, by hematogenous spread of infection (sepsis), or by direct extension of an adjacent inflammatory process [1]. However, pleural effusion is an uncommon clinical finding in foals with pneumonia. In contrast, pleuropneumonia more frequently develops in foals with severe combined immunodeficiency, where pneumocystis carinii and adenovirus infection are commonly identified respiratory pathogens [14].

Diaphragmatic Hernia

Although rare, diaphragmatic defects have been reported in both foals and adult horses, as a cause of respiratory and gastrointestinal abnormalities (colic) following incarceration of viscera in the thoracic cavity. *Congenital diaphragmatic defects* are thought to result from incomplete fusion of the pleuroperitoneal folds, or from failure of one pleuroperitoneal fold to fuse with the septum transversum. The hernia is usually present in the central tendinous part of the diaphragm associated with the esophageal hiatus [10]. An *acquired defect* may be associated with traumatic rupture of the diaphragm produced by compression of the thorax or abdomen during dystocia, traumatic laceration secondary to displaced rib fractures, or by foreign body penetration. Foals with fractures of the fourth to sixth ribs are most likely to develop serious trauma of the surrounding soft tissues, including diaphragmatic laceration, which can result in life-threatening injury. Repair of diaphragmatic defects using a surgical mesh in neonatal foals has been described [15, 16].

Pulmonary hypoplasia and persistent pulmonary hypertension are major determinants of survival and predictors of long-term morbidity in human infants with *congenital diaphragmatic hernias* [17]. The disturbance of normal pulmonary vascular development is thought to contribute to lung hypoplasia, as angiogenesis is necessary for alveolarization. In affected infants, the lungs ultimately have a reduced surface area for gas exchange due to decreased distal branching and number of alveoli. Additionally, alveolar walls are thicker with structural abnormalities of the pulmonary interstitium [18]. Many affected patients have impaired lung perfusion, which may still be present several years after the surgical repair of *congenital diaphragmatic hernia* in people [19].

Hypoxemia due to abnormal V/Q ratios and increased intrapulmonary shunt also accompanies herniation of alimentary organs into the thorax in patients with *acquired (traumatic) diaphragmatic hernia*. Affected horses often display combined cardiopulmonary and gastrointestinal signs, although work of breathing is sometimes minimized by adopting a rapid shallow breathing pattern. Intrathoracic herniation of the gut generally impairs both ventilation and oxygenation, by reducing both pulmonary compliance (resulting in greater lung stiffness) and functional residual capacity (FRC). If free gas enters the pleural cavity the lung will partially collapse due to pulmonary retractive forces (surface tension and elastic recoil). In acute hypoxemia, maintenance of oxygen transport often depends on compensatory increases in cardiac output resulting in tachycardia [20].

Overall survival rates of conservatively treated horses with diaphragmatic hernia are approximately 11–25%. While surgical correction is reported to increase survival to approximately 46–67% in adult horses [16], only one of six foals undergoing surgery for diaphragmatic hernia survived to hospital discharge in one report (three were euthanized during surgery due to the degree of compromised herniated intestine) [21]. More detailed descriptions of diaphragmatic hernias in the foal are located elsewhere in the textbook.

Congestive Heart Failure (CHF)

CHF usually develops slowly following progressive loss of cardiac pumping efficiency, associated with either volume or pressure overload, or myocardial damage. CHF results in inadequate oxygen delivery by the heart or circulatory system to meet the body's oxygen demands. Left heart failure is generally manifested by pulmonary edema and congestion and is associated with (i) loss of myocardial contractility secondary to myocarditis, myocardial necrosis, or cardiomyopathy; (ii) dysfunction of the mitral and aortic valves; and (iii) several congenital heart diseases. Pulmonary edema hampers gas exchange and (especially in neonates) decreases lung compliance. Right heart failure can result in hepatic congestion and splenomegaly, and generally results in more severe water and sodium retention than left side heart failure. Edema is evident predominantly as ventral subcutaneous edema in horses. Causes of right-sided heart failure include (i) pulmonary hypertension; (ii) cardiomyopathy; and (iii) diseases of the tricuspid and pulmonary valves [1].

Obstructive cardiac lesions in newborns, which may result in CHF include critical or severe aortic, mitral, or pulmonary valve stenosis; hypoplastic left heart syndrome and pathologic elevations in pulmonary or systemic vascular resistance. Certain acquired heart diseases can also produce CHF, including infectious, metabolic, neuromuscular, ischemic, and toxic diseases [22]. CHF in neonates often presents with poor feeding, lethargy, and tachypnea, while cyanosis, dyspnea, hypotonia, and shock are late findings.

Many congenital heart defects and other malformations may ultimately result in CHF. For example, ventricular septal defects (VSD), atrioventricular septal defect (ASD), transposition of the great arteries, or a large patent ductus arteriosus (PDA) are causes of increased pulmonary blood flow, which creates risks for pulmonary hypertension [22]. In children with hemodynamically significant congenital heart defects, a range of pathologic lung function parameters have been identified, resulting in airway obstruction, pulmonary hyperinflation, and decreased lung compliance. The growth of elastic and collagenous tissue may be decreased in affected patients, due to abnormal blood flow during the prenatal and postnatal periods. Significantly impaired lung function is, therefore, caused in part by the pathologic hemodynamics of the lungs and partly by histologic changes in lung tissue [23]. Freezer et al. studied the respiratory mechanics of 15 infants with congenital cardiac anomalies (ASD, VSD, PDA, pulmonary valve stenosis or Tetralogy of Fallot) in the first year of life and noted a significant relationship between pulmonary blood flow and the total respiratory system resistance (Rrs) [24]. This Rrs increased significantly with a rise in mean left atrial pressure, however, dynamic compliance and the sum of airway resistance (Raw) did not. These results suggest that the relationship between Rrs and pulmonary blood flow is due to an increase in the resistive properties of the conducting airways and tissue components.

Central Nervous System (CNS) Lesions

A variety of pharmacologic, structural, and metabolic disorders of the CNS are characterized by depression of the neural drive to breathe, leading to *hypoventilation and hypercapnia*. Examples include neonatal encephalopathy (NE), brain stem disease, overdose of a narcotic or sedative (morphine, barbiturates), septic meningitis, and metabolic disorders such as chronic metabolic alkalosis. Hypoventilation is characterized by hypercapnia and hypoxemia, and can be differentiated from other causes of hypoxemia by the presence of a normal *alveolar-arterial (A-a) PO2 gradient* as expressed in a simplified formula in animals breathing room air: A-a gradient $= 150 - (P_aCO_2/0.8) - P_aO_2$ [25]. The normal

A-a gradient is <15 mmHg in healthy foals breathing room air, and increases with V/Q mismatch, shunt, and severe diffusion impairments [26]. In pure hypercapnic respiratory failure, hypoxemia is easily corrected with oxygen therapy.

Birth Asphyxia (Perinatal Asphyxia Syndrome, Neonatal Encephalopathy)

Birth asphyxia or perinatal asphyxia syndrome (PAS) is a general term used to describe the multi-systemic effects of peripartum blood flow disturbances (perinatal ischemia) or hypoxia, which are associated with cardiopulmonary, endocrine, gastrointestinal, and renal abnormalities, along with neurological and behavioral disturbances in affected foals [27]. Since neurologic abnormalities often predominate, the term NE or neonatal maladjustment syndrome (NMS) is commonly used to describe foals that develop noninfectious neurologic signs in the immediate postpartum period. Controversies about equine NE and NMS relate to the lack of pathophysiologic information. However, pathogenesis can broadly be separated into ischemic/hypoxic (oxygen/energy deprivation, reperfusion, hemorrhage, edema, and inflammation) and nonischemic events (metabolic and endocrine disturbances, neurosteroid imbalances) [28].

Documented respiratory abnormalities in affected foals include irregular respiratory patterns (periodic apnea, abnormally slow respiratory rate), expiratory noises (barkers), and central hypoventilation. Aspiration pneumonia may also develop secondary to dysphagia or lack of normal suckle reflex. Cardiac arrhythmias, edema, poor cardiac output, and systemic hypotension can result from hypoxia of the myocardium. A decrease in pulmonary perfusion may also impair surfactant production, leading to V/Q mismatch and secondary pulmonary atelectasis. However, the most common problem is failure of central respiratory drive associated with variable central depression. Since affected foals do not adequately sense increased P_aCO_2, they do not develop increased respiratory rate or effort. All foals with suspected birth asphyxia should undergo arterial blood gas analysis to monitor for progressive hypercapnia and hypoxemia [29].

Mild cases of periodic apnea can respond adequately to sensory simulation or nasal oxygen insufflation, while more severely affected foal may benefit from short-term mechanical ventilation [29]. The use of xanthine drugs should be considered for their stimulatory effect on respiratory neurons in the brainstem. High blood levels of methylxanthines increase CO_2 responsiveness, but signs of toxicity (tachycardia, diuresis, hyperactivity) may occur [30]. Caffeine, a major metabolite of theophylline, is often used due to its longer half-life and lower toxicity. A loading dose of 10 mg/kg of caffeine followed in 24 hours by 2.5 mg/kg/d with a target blood level of 8–20 μg/kg is recommended in human neonates. In foals, the proposed dose is 10 mg/kg administered orally or per rectum once daily or more frequently based on arterial blood gas results. The full effect of a dose is usually evident within 2 hours [31]. In a retrospective study, nonsurviving hospitalized foals with NE were more likely to receive directed therapy with mechanical ventilation and respiratory stimulants (doxapram and caffeine), likely reflecting the patients' disease severity [32].

Botulism (Neuromuscular Dysfunction)

Disorders of the peripheral nervous system, respiratory muscles, or chest wall (neuromuscular diseases) lead to an inability to maintain minute ventilation appropriate for the rate of CO_2 produced [25]. Concomitant hypoxemia and hypercapnia, therefore, ensues in affected foals. A classic example of a flaccid paralytic syndrome is botulism, caused by *Clostridium botulinum* neurotoxins, which inhibit acetylcholine release at the neuromuscular junction. In horses, botulism is generally associated with Type B toxin, although intoxication with types A and C have also been reported. Ingestion of *C. botulinum* spores that germinate in the intestine and elaborate toxin (toxicoinfectious botulism) is most commonly observed in foals (shaker foal syndrome). Clinical signs include increased episodes and duration of recumbency, muscular trembling, and dysphagia in affected foals. Left untreated, the disease can be rapidly fatal due to respiratory muscle paralysis, usually within 24–72 hours after the onset of clinical signs [33].

A 1991 [34] and 2003 [33] retrospective study of intensively treated foals with botulism reported survival rates of 82% (35/43) and 96.4% (27/28), respectively. The reasons for improved survival in the more recent case series are likely associated with improved intensive care, ventilatory strategies, and early administration of botulinum antitoxin. Neonates have compliant chest walls, and foals with botulism have difficulty maintaining chest volume (impaired ability to hold their lung open with their chest wall) because of loss of intercostal muscle strength. Over time, their lung becomes stiffer secondary to progressive atelectasis, further increasing work of breathing. Nonetheless, foals with botulism and respiratory failure can be successfully mechanically ventilated, with a survival of 87.5% (6/8 foals) following 7.4 ± 1 (range: 1–13) days of mechanical ventilation in one study [35]. Mechanical ventilation of foals with botulism and respiratory failure thus appears to be an effective therapy.

Metabolic Derangements (Acidosis, Hypoglycemia)

Acid-based disturbances can have significant effects on respiratory function, including altered ventilation, perfusion, and oxygen diffusion. For example, ventilatory drive increases in response to acidosis, hypercapnia, and hypoxia, through feedback from arterial chemoreceptors (carotid and aortic bodies) and receptor sites in the medulla oblongata of the brain. As such, neonatal tachypnea may be a symptom (compensatory response) of an underlying metabolic acidosis. Additionally, acidosis may affect pulmonary vascular pressures and perfusion. More specifically, acidosis tends to increase pulmonary vascular resistance and thereby raises pulmonary artery pressure, which can help redistribute blood flow from poorly ventilated regions of lung to better ventilated regions. Acute respiratory acidosis also increases nonelastic resistance in the lungs by a central effect, mediated through the vagus nerve [36]. Acute acidosis increases the rate of oxyhemoglobin dissociation by shifting the oxygen dissociation curve to the right. Therefore, the P_aO_2 required to sustain a given oxygen saturation increases in acute acidosis. This effect may be transient, however, as chronic acidosis reduces the 2,3-diphosphoglycerate (2,3-DPG) concentration in red blood cells after 6–8 hours, thus returning the dissociation curve back toward its normal position [37].

Hypoglycemia is one of the most frequent metabolic abnormalities in the newborn foal and can both be a consequence of or a cause for respiratory dysfunction. For example, the weak, hypoglycemic foal is often unable to generate adequate respiratory muscle activity to maintain tidal volume or functional residual volume [38]. Contrarily, severe respiratory distress from various causes, may also result in hypoglycemia through increased glucose consumption.

Severe Anemia, Hypovolemia

The mechanical properties of the lungs are significantly influenced by changes in pulmonary hemodynamic conditions, including abnormalities in pulmonary blood flow and pressure. Both pulmonary venous congestion and edema usually cause a fall in lung compliance (stiffer lung) and a rise in resistance to air flow, since the pressures of pulmonary blood vessels make an appreciable contribution to lung stiffness and stability of the alveolar architecture [39]. Conversely, hemorrhagic shock and concomitant pulmonary hypovolemia may increase lung compliance and reduce resistance to air flow [40].

Alterations in respiratory mechanical function (i.e. compliance and resistance) related to severe blood loss should be considered in foals with respiratory distress after trauma or during hemorrhage in surgical patients. However, the specific effects of hemorrhagic shock on respiratory system mechanics have been incompletely studied and are controversial. Sprung et al. evaluated the effects of acute hemorrhage on elastic and resistive characteristics of the respiratory system in anesthetized/paralyzed and mechanically ventilated dogs [41]. This protocol was chosen since resistance and compliance of the respiratory system depend on respiratory frequency and tidal volume. The isolated effects of hemorrhage on lung mechanics in spontaneously breathing animals are therefore difficult to interpret because breathing patterns and functional residual capacities vary under these conditions. The authors of the study concluded that the mechanical properties of the respiratory system are only slightly changed during experimentally induced hemorrhagic shock [41]. Initial blood loss did not impact respiratory system compliance and resistance, whereas subsequent shock induced moderate pulmonary mechanical changes. However, it was unlikely that these alterations were large enough to be clinically important during acute hemorrhage in otherwise healthy patients.

Cardiovascular dysfunction and anemia may not only impact the mechanical function of the lung but also alter lung volume and gas exchange. While data in neonatal foals is currently limited, the expected pathophysiological changes associated with volume depletion and expansion are discussed below, based on data in other species.

Cardiovascular Influence on the Resistive Properties of the Lung

Total lung resistance is principally composed of the sum of airway (R_{aw}) and tissue (R_{ti}) resistances, with Raw accounting for 50–90% of total lung resistance at baseline. During bronchoconstriction, however, both airway and tissue resistances increase to varying degrees. More specifically, tissue resistance often increases more than R_{aw} and may be the major determinant of constrictor responses. Baseline R_{aw} is modulated by both the β-adrenergic and nonadrenergic, noncholinergic nervous systems, but tissue resistance and tone are largely independent of nervous system regulation [42]. Martins et al. documented that acute hypovolemia due to hemorrhage resulted in mainly large airway dilation, sparing distal air spaces. The authors suggested that acute bleeding does not increase the mechanical inhomogeneities within the respiratory system, probably due to adrenergic activation [43].

Cardiovascular Effects on Functional Residual Capacity (FRC)

Data from healthy human volunteers has shown a correlation between IV fluid administration and reduction in FRC. For example, a 10% reduction in FRC was documented after administration of a 22 ml/kg IV bolus of saline [44], while a 40 ml/kg bolus of lactated Ringer's solution resulted in a 5–7% decrease in FRC for 8 hours after IV administration [45]. Similarly, a study in neonatal camelids documented that plasma volume expansion (30 ml/kg llama plasma IV) reduced FRC by 11.5% on average [46], which may be attributed to increased pulmonary capillary blood flow, increased interstitial fluid content, and increased lung stiffness. Cardiovascular volume expansion may similarly decrease FRC in neonatal foals.

Cardiovascular Causes of Pulmonary Diffusion Limitations

Diffusion measurements depend on the surface area available for gas exchange, the blood-gas barrier (BGB), and V/Q mismatch. High pulmonary artery pressure is considered a critical factor in the development of BGB failure with subsequent diffusion limitation and impairment of gas exchange. Cardiovascular conditions in foals that may be associated with stress failure of pulmonary capillaries include left ventricular failure, mitral stenosis, some cases of acute respiratory distress syndrome (ARDS), and neurogenic pulmonary edema. Neurogenic pulmonary edema is related to high pulmonary vascular pressures, leading to disruption of both capillary endothelial and alveolar epithelial cells, and high-permeability edema fluid [47].

Pulmonary function is not only impacted by underlying disease, but also by autonomic and cardiovascular effects of common medications. For example, IV sedation with xylazine (α-2 adrenergic agonist) significantly decreased blood pressure (after an initial rise) in healthy neonatal foals [48]. Changes in airflow, upper airway obstruction, and respiratory noise were also noted. Arterial blood gas tensions and pH did not change significantly in healthy foals, although respiratory rate and minute volume decreased, and tidal volume increased after 20 minutes of sedation. Xylazine should thus be avoided in foals with respiratory diseases, including those with upper airway obstructions, and be used with caution in hypovolemic foals, as significant hypotension could ensue [48].

Pain, Excitement, Colic, Fever

Respiratory changes often occur in response to excitement or pain. For example, a breath-hold and expiratory grunt may be observed in response to a sudden onset of acute pain, while hyperventilation may be associated with persistent or uncontrolled pain. These pain-induced increases in minute ventilation result from either deeper breathing or tachypnea, or combination of both [49]. While abdominal pain (colic) can cause primary hyperventilation, notable abdominal distension may result from conditions such as meconium impaction, ileus, intestinal obstruction, gastroenteritis, or uroabdomen, which ultimately impairs ventilation. Significant abdominal distension is a risk factors for the development of abdominal compartment syndrome due to sustained intra-abdominal hypertension. The increase in abdominal pressure not only reduces venous return (decreasing right ventricular preload, stroke volume and cardiac output), but increases V/Q mismatch (impairing oxygenation) and reduces diaphragmatic mobility and ventilatory capacity. An associated rise in airway pressure further contributes to compression of pulmonary capillaries, which in turn increases pulmonary vascular resistance and contributes to pulmonary hypertension [50].

Fever is common in critical illness, since many inflammatory mediators associated with neonatal diseases are pyrogenic. Both fever and hyperthermia may alter pulmonary function through inflammatory pathways or thermoregulatory responses. For example, in animal models of sepsis, fever increases neutrophil-dependent lung injury [51] and augments oxygen toxicity [52]. More specifically, elevated temperatures may worsen lung injury by increasing neutrophil extravasation and vascular leak via effects on the endothelium and increasing epithelial injury [53]. Additionally, leakage of plasma proteins into the alveolar space due to impaired function of the alveolar-capillary barrier may contribute to surfactant alterations [54].

In resting horses, an elevation in core temperature by >1 °C induces hyperventilation [55], accounted for by increases in both tidal volume and frequency of breathing. These thermoregulatory changes in breathing pattern are dependent on hypothalamic integration of peripheral and central sensory information [56] and help regulate body temperature [57].

In summary, a variety of nonpulmonary causes of respiratory abnormalities exist in foals, which can confound the identification of primary lung or airway disease. A strategic patient assessment is necessary to best characterize underlying causes of respiratory dysfunction.

References

1 Lopez, A. (2007). *Syndromes of Cardiac Failure or Decompensation. Pathophysiologic Basis of Veterinary Disease* (ed. M.D. McGavin and J.F. Zachary), 566–568. St. Louis, MO: Mosby Elsevier.

2 Estenne, M., Yernault, J.C., and De Troyer, A. (1983). Mechanism of relief of dyspnea after thoracocentesis in patients with large pleural effusions. *Am. J. Med.* 74: 813–819.

3 Mahfood, S., Hix, W.R., Aaron, B.L. et al. (1988). Reexpansion pulmonary edema. *Ann. Thorac. Surg.* 45: 340–345.

4 Light, R.W., Jenkinson, S.G., Minh, V.D. et al. (1980). Observations on pleural fluid pressures as fluid is withdrawn during thoracentesis. *Am. Rev. Respir. Dis.* 121: 799–804.

5 Suzuki, S., Tanita, T., Koike, K. et al. (1992). Evidence of acute inflammatory response in reexpansion pulmonary edema. *Chest* 101: 275–276.

6 Mitrouska, I., Klimathianaki, M., and Siafakas, N.M. (2004). Effects of pleural effusion on respiratory function. *Can. Respir. J.* 11: 499–503.

7 Bastianello, S.S. and Nesbit, J.W. (1987). The pathology of a case of biliary atresia in a foal. *J. S. Afr. Vet. Assoc.* 58: 89–92.

8 Restifo, M.M., Bedenice, B., Thane, K.E. et al. (2015). Cavitary effusion associated with Anaplasma phagocytophilum infection in 2 equids. *J. Vet. Intern. Med.* 29: 732–735.

9 Dixon, C.E. and Bedenice, D. (2021). Transplacental infection of a foal with *Anaplasma* phagocytophilum. *Equine Vet. Educ.* 33: 62–66.

10 Mair, T.S., Pearson, H., Waterman, A.E. et al. (1988). Chylothorax associated with a congenital diaphragmatic defect in a foal. *Equine Vet. J.* 20: 304–306.

11 Lopez, A. (2007). *Inflammation of the Pleura. Pathophysiologic Basis of Veterinary Disease* (ed. M.D. McGavin and J.F. Zachary), 555–556. St. Louis, MO: Mosby Elsevier.

12 Scarratt, W.K., Wallace, M.A., Pleasant, R.S. et al. (1997). Chylothorax and meconium impaction in a neonatal colt. *Equine Vet. J.* 29: 77–79.

13 Clemmons, R.M., Dorsey-Lee, M.R., Gorman, N.T. et al. (1984). Haemostatic mechanisms of the newborn foal: reduced platelet responsiveness. *Equine Vet. J.* 16: 353–356.

14 Parish, S.M. (2002). *Large Animal Internal Medicine. Immunologic Disorders* (ed. B.P. Smith), 1589–1613. St. Louis: Mosby Co.

15 Speirs, V.C. and Reynolds, W.T. (1976). Successful repair of a diaphragmatic hernia in a foal. *Equine Vet. J.* 8: 170–172.

16 Kolus, C.R., MacLeay, J.M., and Hackett, E.S. (2017). Repair of an acquired diaphragmatic hernia with surgical mesh in a foal. *Can. Vet. J.* 58: 145–148.

17 Guevorkian, D., Mur, S., Cavatorta, E. et al. (2018). Lower distending pressure improves respiratory mechanics in congenital diaphragmatic hernia complicated by persistent pulmonary hypertension. *J. Pediatr.* 200: 38–43.

18 Ameis, D., Khoshgoo, N., and Keijzer, R. (2017). Abnormal lung development in congenital diaphragmatic hernia. *Semin. Pediatr. Surg.* 26: 123–128.

19 Stefanutti, G., Filippone, M., Tommasoni, N. et al. (2004). Cardiopulmonary anatomy and function in long-term survivors of mild to moderate congenital diaphragmatic hernia. *J. Pediatr. Surg.* 39: 526–531.

20 Clutton, R.E., Boyd, C., Richards, D.L. et al. (1992). Anaesthetic problems caused by diaphragmatic hernia in the horse: a review of four cases. *Equine Vet. J. Suppl.* 11: 30–33.

21 Romero, A.E. and Rodgerson, D.H. (2010). Diaphragmatic herniation in the horse: 31 cases from 2001–2006. *Can. Vet. J.* 51: 1247–1250.

22 O'Laughlin, M.P. (1999). Congestive heart failure in children. *Pediatr. Clin. N. Am.* 46: 263–273.

23 Lubica, H. (1996). Pathologic lung function in children and adolescents with congenital heart defects. *Pediatr. Cardiol.* 17: 314–315.

24 Freezer, N.J., Lanteri, C.J., and Sly, P.D. (1985). Effect of pulmonary blood flow on measurements of respiratory mechanics using the interrupter technique. *J. Appl. Phys.* 74: 1083–1088.

25 Harris, D.E. and Massie, M. (2019). Role of alveolar-arterial gradient in partial pressure of oxygen and PaO_2/fraction of inspried oygen ration measurements in assessment of pulmonary dysfunction. *AANA* 87: 214–221.

26 Bedenice, D. (2006). *Neonatal Septic Pneumonia. Equine Neonatal Medicine—A Case-Based Approach* (ed. M. Paradis). Philadelphia, PA: Elsevier.

27 Gold, J.R. (2017). Perinatal asphyxia syndrome. *Equine Vet. Educ.* 29: 158–164.

28 Toribio, R.E. (2019). Equine neonatal encephalopathy: facts, evidence, and opinions. *Vet. Clin. North Am. Equine Pract.* 35: 363–378.

29 Palmer, J.E. (1994). Ventilatory support of the neonatal foal. *Vet. Clin. North Am. Equine Pract.* 10: 167–185.

30 D'Urzo, A.D., Jhirad, R., Jenne, H. et al. (1985). Effect of caffeine on ventilatory responses to hypercapnia, hypoxia, and exercise in humans. *J. Appl. Phys.* 68: 322–328.

31 Palmer, J.E. (2005). Ventilatory support of the critically ill foal. *Vet. Clin. North Am. Equine Pract.* 21: 457–486.

32 Lyle-Dugas, J., Giguere, S., Mallicote, M.F. et al. (2017). Factors associated with outcome in 94 hospitalised foals diagnosed with neonatal encephalopathy. *Equine Vet. J.* 49: 207–210.

33 Wilkins, P.A. and Palmer, J.E. (2003). Botulism in foals less than 6 months of age: 30 cases (1989–2002). *J. Vet. Intern. Med.* 17: 702–707.

34 Vaala, W.E. (1991). Diagnosis and treatment of *Clostridium botulinum* infection in foals: A review of fifty-three cases. *Proc Am. Vet. Intern. Med.* 9: 379–381.

35 Wilkins, P.A. and Palmer, J.E. (2003). Mechanical ventilation in foals with botulism: 9 cases (1989–2002). *J. Vet. Intern. Med.* 17: 708–712.

36 Peters, R.M., Hedgpeth, E.M., and Greenberg, B.G. (1969). The effect of alterations in acid-base balance on pulmonary mechanics. *J. Thorac. Cardiovasc. Surg.* 57 (3): 303–311.

37 Mitchell, J.H., Wildenthal, K., and Johnson, R.L. (1972). The effects of acid-base disturbances on cardiovascular and pulmonary function. *Kidney Int.* 1: 375–389.

38 Carr, E.A. (2007). Respiratory diseases of the foal. In: *Equine Respiratory Medicine and Surgery* (ed. B.C. McGorum), 633–656. Philadelphia, PA: W.B. Saunders Ltd.

39 Cook, C.D., Mead, J., Schreiner, G.L. et al. (1959). Pulmonary mechanics during induced pulmonary edema in anesthetized dogs. *J. Appl. Phys.* 14: 177–186.

40 Cahill, J.M. and Byrne, J.J. (1964). Ventilatory mechanics in hypovolemic shock. *J. Appl. Phys.* 19: 679–682.

41 Sprung, J., Mackenzie, C.F., Green, M.D. et al. (1997). Chest wall and lung mechanics during acute hemorrhage in anesthetized dogs. *J. Cardiothorac. Vasc. Anesth.* 11: 608–612.

42 Ingenito, E.P., Mark, L., Lilly, C. et al. (1995). Autonomic regulation of tissue resistance in the Guinea pig lung. *J. Appl. Phys.* 78: 1382–1387.

43 Martins, M.A., Zin, W.A., Younes, R.N. et al. (1990). Respiratory system mechanics in Guinea pigs after acute hemorrhage: role of adrenergic stimulation. *Crit. Care Med.* 18: 515–519.

44 Hillebrecht, A., Schulz, H., Meyer, M. et al. (1992). Pulmonary responses to lower body negative pressure and fluid loading during head-down tilt bedrest. *Acta Physiol. Scand. Suppl.* 604: 35–42.

45 Holte, K., Jensen, P., and Kehlet, H. (2003). Physiologic effects of intravenous fluid administration in healthy volunteers. *Anesth. Analg.* 96 (5): 1504–1509.

46 Paxson, J., Cunningham, S., Rush, J. et al. (2008). Association of lung function and plasma volume expansion following plasma transfusion in neonatal alpaca crias with failure of passive transfer. *J. Vet. Emerg. Crit. Care* 18: 601–607.

47 West, J.B. (2000). Invited review: pulmonary capillary stress failure. *J. Appl. Phys.* 89: 2483–2489.

48 Carter, S.W., Robertson, S.A., Steel, C.J. et al. (1990). Cardiopulmonary effects of xylazine sedation in the foal. *Equine Vet. J.* 22: 384–388.

49 Jafari, H., Courtois, I., Van den Bergh, O. et al. (2017). Pain and respiration: a systematic review. *Pain* 158: 995–1006.

50 Paal, P., Neurauter, A., Loedl, M. et al. (2009). Effects of stomach inflation on haemodynamic and pulmonary function during cardiopulmonary resuscitation in pigs. *Resuscitation* 80: 365–371.

51 Rice, P., Martin, E., He, J.R. et al. (2005). Febrile-range hyperthermia augments neutrophil accumulation and enhances lung injury in experimental Gram-negative bacterial pneumonia. *J. Immunol.* 174: 3676–3685.

52 Hasday, J.D., Garrison, A., Singh, I.S. et al. (2003). Febrile-range hyperthermia augments pulmonary neutrophil recruitment and amplifies pulmonary oxygen toxicity. *Am. J. Pathol.* 162: 2005–2017.

53 Tulapurkar, M.E., Almutairy, E.A., Shah, N.G. et al. (2012). Febrile-range hyperthermia modifies endothelial and neutrophilic functions to promote extravasation. *Am. J. Respir. Cell Mol. Biol.* 46: 807–814.

54 Krafft, M.P. (2015). Overcoming inactivation of the lung surfactant by serum proteins: a potential role for fluorocarbons? *Soft Matter* 11: 5982–5994.

55 Kaminski, R.P., Forster, H.V., Bisgard, G.E. et al. (1985). Effect of altered ambient temperature on breathing in ponies. *J. Appl. Phys.* 58: 1585–1591.

56 Geor, R.J., McCutcheon, L.J., Ecker, G.L. et al. (1995). Thermal and cardiorespiratory responses of horses to submaximal exercise under hot and humid conditions. *Equine Vet. J. Suppl.* 20: 125–132.

57 White, M.D. (2006). Components and mechanisms of thermal hyperpnea. *J. Appl. Phys.* 101: 655–663.

Neonatal Cardiovascular System

Chapter 9 Embryology and Anatomy of the Heart

David Wong, Kiho Lee, and Celia Marr

The formation of the heart requires multiple critical and time-sensitive steps that must occur in appropriate order to avoid development of congenital heart anomalies. A great deal of complexity surrounds the morphogenesis of the cardiovascular system and has been documented in the human fetus in intricate detail elsewhere [1–3]. An elementary review of the embryonic development of the cardiovascular system will be discussed here as this will aid in the comprehension of many of the congenital heart defects that can occur in the foal. A rudimentary outline of the major events in cardiac development is presented in Table 9.1.

The Cardiovascular System

The cardiovascular system is the first organ system to reach functional maturity, completing structural formation by the 8th week of gestation in the human fetus [3]. Heart development is initiated by the anterior mesoderm and angiogenic cell clusters located in the cardiogenic plate that give rise to the endocardial tubes. The horseshoe-shaped endocardial tubes extend laterally, left, and right. This is followed by the cranial-caudal and lateral folding of the developing embryonic disk, which rotates the position of endocardial tubes and gradually brings the ventral side of the endocardial tubes close to each other, forming a single tube (Table 9.1, Step 1–3). The embryonic heart starts from this single tube within a closed vascular circuit that eventually becomes a four-chambered structure (Figure 9.1). Development of the heart follows the same general pattern in all vertebrates where fusion of the primary heart tube is followed by rightward looping of the newly formed linear tube. The heart is formed by a number of different embryonic cell types, including the cardiac mesoderm (eventually forming the endocardium, myocardium, and Purkinje cells), cardiac neural crest (eventually forming the smooth muscle of the aortic wall), and proepicardial cells (eventually forming the epicardium and coronary arteries) [3]. Subsequently, differentiation of cardiac chambers and valves and development of the conduction system and coronary circulation occurs (Figure 9.2). Internal partitioning of the heart, or cardiac septation, occurs by four concurrent events: atrial septation, formation of endocardial cushions and atrioventricular canal septation, ventricular chamber formation and septation, and truncus septation [1, 6].

Three stages are essential for proper alignment of cardiac structures and normal cardiac septation: looping, convergence, and wedging (Table 9.1, Step 4) [7]. The straight heart tube consists of the truncus arteriosus, bulbus cordis, ventricle, atrium, and sinus venosus, which subsequently turns into specific segments of the heart. Because the size of the primitive heart enlarges faster than its concurrent location within the pericardial cavity, bending of the cardiac tube occurs. The bending of the cardiac tube ventrally and to the right side during cardiac looping is a critical step in the formation of normal cardiac morphology as it brings the future cardiac chambers into relative spatial positions [3]. Cardiac looping positions the junction between the ventricles and the bulbus cordis to point ventrally in the normal heart and is the first sign of the developing left–right asymmetry in vertebrates. Abnormalities in looping result in complex congenital heart malformations such as ventricular inversion [3, 8]. After looping is complete, the embryonic heart is similar in external appearance to the mature organ, but internally remains a single tube. Looping of the cardiac tube establishes two parallel limbs, an inflow and outflow limb, separated by a structure called the inner curvature [9]. During the process of convergence, the two limbs are brought together in a craniocaudal orientation, thus allowing alignment of the outflow tract with the ventricular, atrioventricular (AV), and atrial septa [9]. Proper alignment, or convergence, is necessary for normal septation and valve

Equine Neonatal Medicine, First Edition. Edited by David M. Wong and Pamela A. Wilkins.

Table 9.1 Simplified steps in the fetal development of the heart [2, 4, 5].

1) Formation of the three germ layers	Three germ layers (ectoderm, mesoderm, endoderm) develop via process called gastrulation.
2) Establishment of the first and second heart fields	Progenitor cardiogenic mesodermal cells of primitive streak migrate to form crescent shaped mantle around neural folds, called the first heart field (FHF). The second heart field (SHF) forms from a second progenitor pool of myocardial precursors in the pharyngeal mesoderm (Figure 9.1a).
3) Formation of the heart tube	The heart tube is formed through a complex three-dimensional process, which requires participation from cells derived from all three embryonic germ layers, and eventually settles on the midline as a single endocardial tube (Figure 9.1b).
4) Cardiac looping, convergence, and wedging	Looping results from migration of precursor cells and elongation of the endocardial tube. Convergence describes the movement of the outflow tract and AV canal to a more midline position. Separation of the primitive ventricles and outflow tract into systemic (aorta) and pulmonary trunks are created by wedging, a process in which counterclockwise rotation of the outflow tract occurs along with movement of future aortic valve to a position behind the pulmonary trunk (Figure 9.1c).
5) Formation of the septa (common atrium, AV canal)	The septum primum divides the atrium into right and left sides while the AV canal is partitioned into right and left ventricle by the intraventricular septum via four endocardial cushions (Figures 9.2 and 9.3).
6) Development of the outflow tract	Outflow tract undergoes septation and division by two processes: (i) aorticopulmonary septum partitions the outflow tract giving rise to aorta and pulmonary artery, and (ii) growth and fusion of the proximal outflow tract (endocardial cushions) creates the outlet septum, resulting in separation of left and right ventricular outflow tracts.
7) Formation of cardiac valves	AV valves develop from endocardial cushions (Figure 9.2) while semilunar valves of the aorta and pulmonary artery form during remodeling of the distal outflow tract tissue (truncal endocardial cushions).
8) Formation of vasculature	Vascular system originates from the first heart field where progenitor cells are induced to form cardiac myoblasts that produce paired dorsal aortae. Pharyngeal arches also form, accompanied by aortic arches that connect the aortic sac to bilateral dorsal aortae. There are five paired arches (fifth arch nerve forms) that form vasculature.
9) Formation of the cardiac conduction system (CCS)	Development of CSS occurs simultaneously with cardiac development in the fetus and is comprised of specialized cardiomyocytes directed by gene regulatory networks in a tissue-specific and time-dependent manner to produce nodal and fast conduction phenotypes.

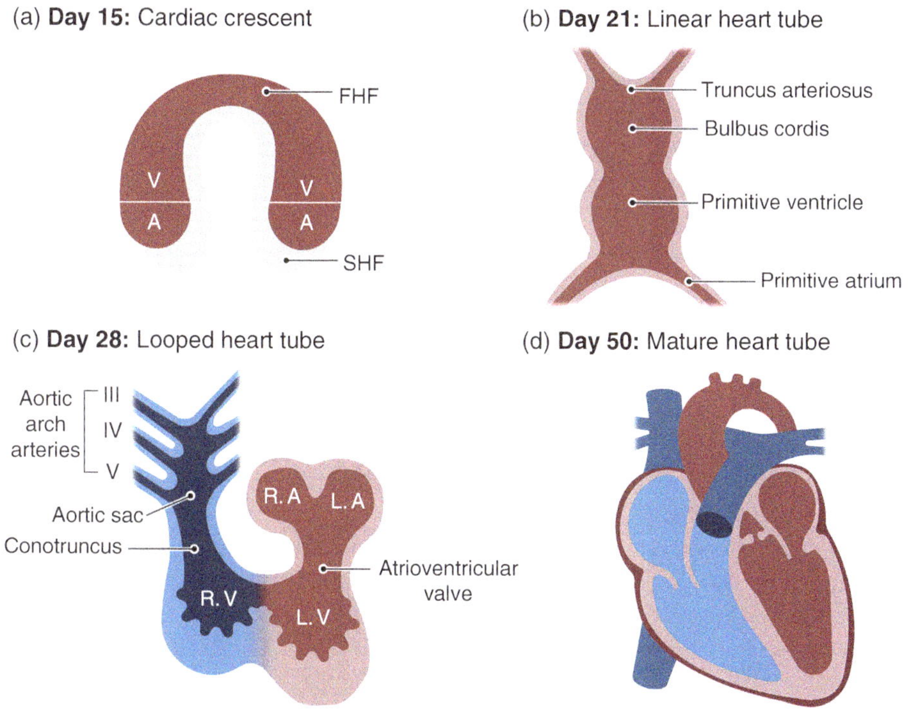

Figure 9.1 Schematic representation of some of the basic events of cardiac embryology in the human fetus. (a) Cardiac crescent at Day 15. First heart field (FHF) is specified to form particular segments of the linear heart tube. The second heart field (SHF) is located medial and caudal to the FHF. (b) Day 21, folding of the embryo establishes a linear heart tube with arterial (truncus arteriosus) and venous (primitive atrium) poles. (c) Day 28, the linear heart tube loops to right to establish the future position of the cardiac regions (atria, ventricles, outflow tract). (d) Day 50, the mature heart has formed. Chambers and outflow tract of heart divided by atrial septum, interventricular septum, two atrioventricular valves and two semilunar valves. *Source:* Adapted from Kloesel [2].

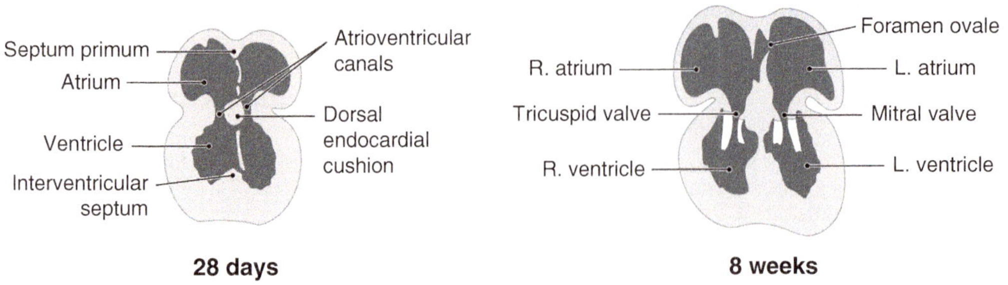

Figure 9.2 Development of the human heart – embryological development of the human heart during the first 8 weeks and the subsequent formation of the four heart chambers.

development [3]. Cardiac malformations resulting from abnormal convergence can result in malalignment between the atrial and ventricular septa, causing congenital defects such as double-inlet ventricle, tricuspid atresia, and ventricular hypoplasia [3]. During the process of wedging, the retraction and rotation of the truncal myocardium results in rotation of the aorta behind, or caudal to, the pulmonary trunk, settling between the two AV valves and establishing mitral-aortic continuity [10]. Concurrently, the conal septum develops via fusion and muscularization of the endocardial cushions of the outflow tract and follows leftward by the rotation of the developing aortic valve, and joins the primitive ventricular septum [3].

Until the process of wedging occurs, the outflow tract remains entirely above the developing right ventricle. In addition, the proliferation of endocardial cushions leads to the formation of the septum intermedium, which divides the AV channel into right and left portions. Malalignment between the outflow tract and ventricles results in failure of fusion of the outlet septum with the primitive ventricular septum creating a ventricular septal defect (VSD). Tetralogy of Fallot is another anomaly that can result from arrest of rotation of the outflow tract at the base of the great arteries [11].

Along with cardiac looping, the primitive atrium is subdivided into right and left chambers by a crescent-shaped fold, called the septum primum (primitive atrial septum), as the structure develops from the dorsal aspect of the common atrium with the free margin extending toward the common AV canal (Table 9.1, Step 5; Figure 9.3) [3]. This occurs early in gestation (22–25 days) in the equine fetus [12]. For a period of time, the atria communicate with one another through a minor opening, termed the ostium primum of Born, which is below the free margin of the septum. This opening is eventually closed by the union of the septum primum with the septum intermedium. By gestational days 30–32 in the equine fetus, the endocardial cushions have fused and form the medial walls of the AV ostia; the ostium primum has closed by this time. The formen ovale (ostium secundum of Born), which persists until birth, reestablishes the communication between the atria through an opening that forms in the upper part of the septum primum and is a pathway for blood to flow from the right atrium to left atrium, largely bypassing the pulmonary circulation because of high pulmonary vascular resistance [3].

The septum secundum grows downward from the upper wall of the atrium and partially fuses with the seputum primum, creating the foramen ovale. After birth, increased oxygen tension from the newborn's extra-uterine breathing allows for increased blood into the lung, thus increasing left atrial pressure and closure of the flap of the foramen ovale (septum primum) against the septum secundum, forming the floor of the fossa ovalis [6]. The foramen ovale can be identified echocardiographically as a mobile septal membrane in newborn foals with failure of complete fusion resulting in a patent foramen ovale.

The aorta and pulmonary artery originate from a single vessel called the conus arteriosus to form the outflow tract (Table 9.1, Step 6). This common trunk, also known as the truncus arteriosus, eventually partitions by migration of the conus arteriosus and development of the conotruncal and spiral septa. Ultimately, these structures twist into appropriate alignment of the great vessels with corresponding ventricular chambers. Failure of these tissues to migrate and/or differentiate appropriately can result in congenital outflow tract defects such as persistent truncus arteriosus (failure of aorta and pulmonary trunk to fully divide), transposition of the great vessels (pulmonary trunk attached to left ventricle, aorta attached to right ventricle), aortic stenosis, and pulmonary stenosis with or without Tetralogy of Fallot.

The endocardial cushions are essential for the formation of the cardiac valves and perform an adhesive role by binding cardiac structures together and acting as scaffolding in which fibroblasts may infiltrate (Table 9.1, Step 7) [13]. Specifically, endocardial cushions close the gap between the atrial and ventricular septa and are important in the septation of the AV canal and AV valves. As the cushions fuse, they divide the AV canal into right and left orifices. The formation of the cardiac valves is intimately related with cardiac septation and development of inflow and

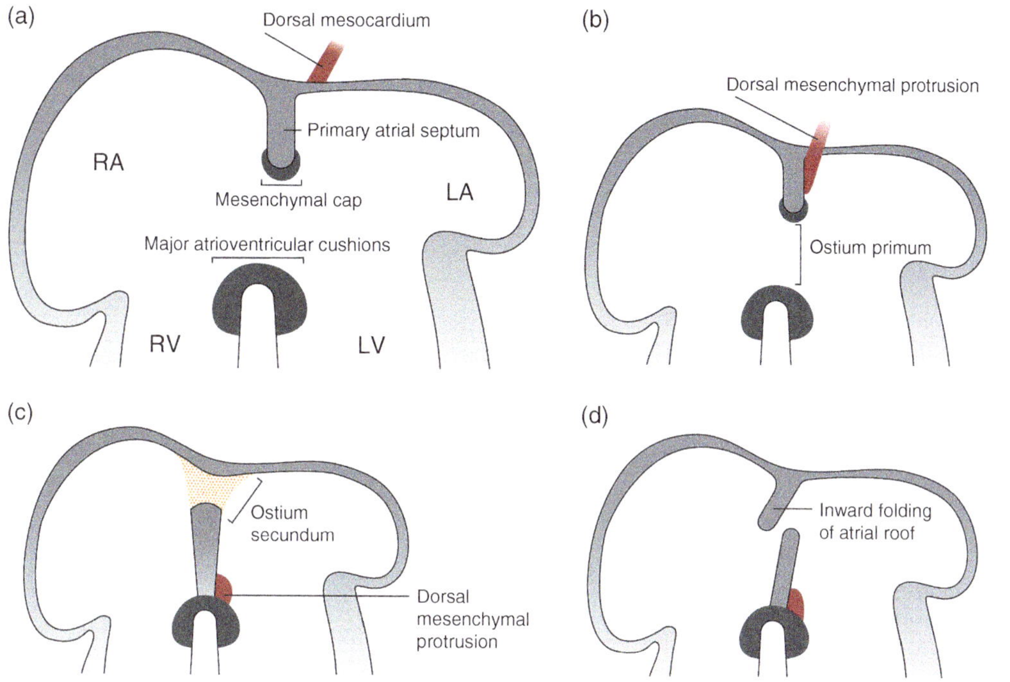

Figure 9.3 Overview of process resulting in atrial septation. (a) Atrial septation begins with formation of the primary atrial septum (septum primum) that extends from the atrial roof downwards toward the major atrioventricular (AV) cushions. The leading edge of the primary atrial septum carries a mesenchymal cap. The venous pole of the heart is attached to the dorsal mesocardium. (b) As the primary atrial septum migrates downward and approaches the major AV cushions, it closes the gap of the ostium primum. Mesenchymal cells from the dorsal mesocardium invade the common atrium and join the downward growing primary atrial septum as the dorsal mesenchymal protrusion. (c) After fusion of the primary atrial septum, the mesenchymal cap, and dorsal mesenchymal protrusion with the major AV cushions, the ostium primum is closed. Simultaneously, part of the cranial septum primum breaks down and forms the ostium secundum. (d) Inward folding of the myocardium from the atrial roof produces the secondary atrial septum (septum secundum), which grows downward to occlude the ostium primum by a flap-valve. *Source:* Adapted from Kloesel [2].

outflow segments [3]. The four cardiac valves share a common origin of the mesenchyme of the endocardial cushions. The tricuspid valve is initially an entirely muscular structure with three walls: a septal wall (made of ventricular septum), inferior wall (made of the inferior wall of developing right ventricle) and the anterior wall (made of a structure called the tricuspid gully) [3]. These three myocardial walls are covered by mesenchymal tissue of the endocardial cushions with the three leaflets of the tricuspid valve forming from delamination (i.e. separation) of these muscular walls. The tendinous cords are formed by fragmentation of the ventricular side of the leaflets and later undergo fibrous transformation whereas the papillary muscles are of myocardial origin [1, 3].

In contrast, the two leaflets of the mitral valve are closely related to the septation process as the aortic valve rotates and positions itself between the developing tricuspid and mitral valve. The aortic valve separates the future anterior leaflet of the mitral valve, which does not have an initial muscular component. This explains why the normal mitral valve does not have a septal attachment and the papillary muscles develop from the free lateral wall of the left ventricle [14]. The mural leaflet delaminates from the inferior wall of the left ventricle similar to the tricuspid valve. The semilunar valves arise from the swelling of subendothelial mesenchymal tissue at the origin of the aortic and pulmonary trunk. The aortic and pulmonary valves develop from mesenchyme of the outflow tract endocardial cushions with fusion of the right and left lateral cushions on midline, forming two symmetrical valve primordia. The two intercalated cushions form the anterior leaflet of the pulmonary valve and the posterior noncoronary leaflet of the aortic valve. The two semilunar valves are therefore morphologically identical but separate structures [15]. Abnormal or excessive fusion of the endocardial cushions can result in the congenital valve defect of the semilunar valves known as bicuspid valves.

The aortic sac, six arterial (aortic) arches, and paired dorsal aortas from the embryonic segments of the branchial arterial system (Table 9.1, Step 8) [1]. As gestation progresses, blood flow gradually shifts caudally in the developing arch system while the first and second arch arteries, which initially carry blood flow from the heart, regress [16]. Remnants of the first pair of arteries form the maxillary artery and external carotid artery. The second arch arteries form the stapedial and hyoid arteries, and the third-arch arteries form the common carotids and proximal portions of the internal carotid arteries [3]. The fourth arterial arches, along with the intersegmental artery, form the distal portion of the right subclavian artery; on the left, the fourth arch forms the definitive left aortic arch. The fifth arterial arch is not a precursor of normal adult structures in the mammals. Finally, the sixth arches form the ductus arteriosus (left arch) and pulmonary artery (right arch) [2, 16, 17]. The post-branchial pulmonary arteries join the arches at the angle between the dorsal and ventral portions; the ventral portions merge and give rise to the main pulmonary artery. The right ventral portion persists as the proximal portion of the right pulmonary artery, whereas the left ventral portion is largely resorbed, contributing only slightly to the left pulmonary artery. The left dorsal portion gives rise to the ductus arteriosus.

The cardiac conduction system (CSS) is an extensive network of specialized electrical tissue that initiates and coordinates the heartbeat. The development of the CSS is composed of highly specialized cardiomyocytes and is governed by gene regulatory networks that are tightly orchestrated in a tissue-specific and time-dependent manner with the structural development of the fetal heart (Table 9.1, Step 9) [4, 18]. Disrupted development of cardiac structures can be accompanied by disturbed formation of the CSS. Thus, some conduction disturbances and cardiac arrhythmias are related to abnormal development of the CSS and originate from anatomical predilection sites. Detailed reviews of the development of the CSS and how disruptions in the development of the CSS in concert with congenital heart anomalies may result in predisposition to cardiac conduction disturbances are available [4, 5].

Table 9.2 Timing of some morphogenetic events in equine cardiogenesis.

Crown-rump length (CRL) in millimeters	Approximate gestational age in days	Morphogenetic events in equine cardiogenesis
5	21	Primitive cardiac loop.
6–8	22–25	Appearance of endocardial cushions in atrioventricular canal, truncus, and conus. Interventricular foramen I. Interatrial septum I and interatrial foramen I and II.
8.5–9.5	26–28	Initial fusion of endocardial cushions in truncus. Presence of aorto-pulmonary septum and primordial of aortic and pulmonary semilunar valves.
11.5–12	30–32	Fusion of atrioventricular endocardial cushions. Closure of interatrial foramen I. Complete separation of aortic and pulmonary trunks. Initial septation of conus.
14–16	33–35	Regression of aortic arches. Completion of conus septum and formation of aortic and pulmonary conuses. Interventricular foramen II.
15–35	36–49	Closure of interventricular foramen II and completion of partitioning of ventricular outflow channel (15–17 mm CRL). Incorporation of pulmonary conus into right ventricle and absorption of aortic conus into left ventricle (15–17 mm CRL). Heart assumes postnatal position (34.5 mm CRL). Definitive arch of aorta (34.5 mm CRL). Interatrial septum II (34.5 mm CRL).

Source: adapted from Vitums [12].

Embryonic Development

The early embryonic development of the equine heart has been examined in some elementary detail (Table 9.2). In one report, 59 equine fetuses were examined at various time points during early gestation, ranging from 21 to 49 days gestation. Results of this study revealed that partitioning of the equine fetal heart begins at a very early stage of cardiogenesis and is completed by approximately 36–38 days gestation. The 28- to 30-day equine embryo has a typical heart shape with partly compartmentalized heart chambers characterized by developing atria and ventricles and a prominent interventricular groove at the apex of the heart. The endocardial cushions and conduction tissue cells can also be identified at this time [19]. Anatomic structures such as easily recognized chambers, cusps of atrioventricular valves, and total separation of the aorta and pulmonary trunk are visible in the 45-day equine fetus.

By around 50–60 days, the major structures of the postnatal heart are formed and, for the remainder of gestation, the fetal circulation includes three shunts. The majority of oxygenated blood entering the fetus via the umbilical vein bypasses the liver via the ductus venosus, which empties into the caudal vena cava, and enters the right atrium (RA). Interestingly, unlike other animals, the equine fetus is devoid of the ductus arteriosus. A proportion enters the left atrium via the foramen ovale. The entrance to this short tunnel is formed by atrial tissue associated with the caudal vena cava

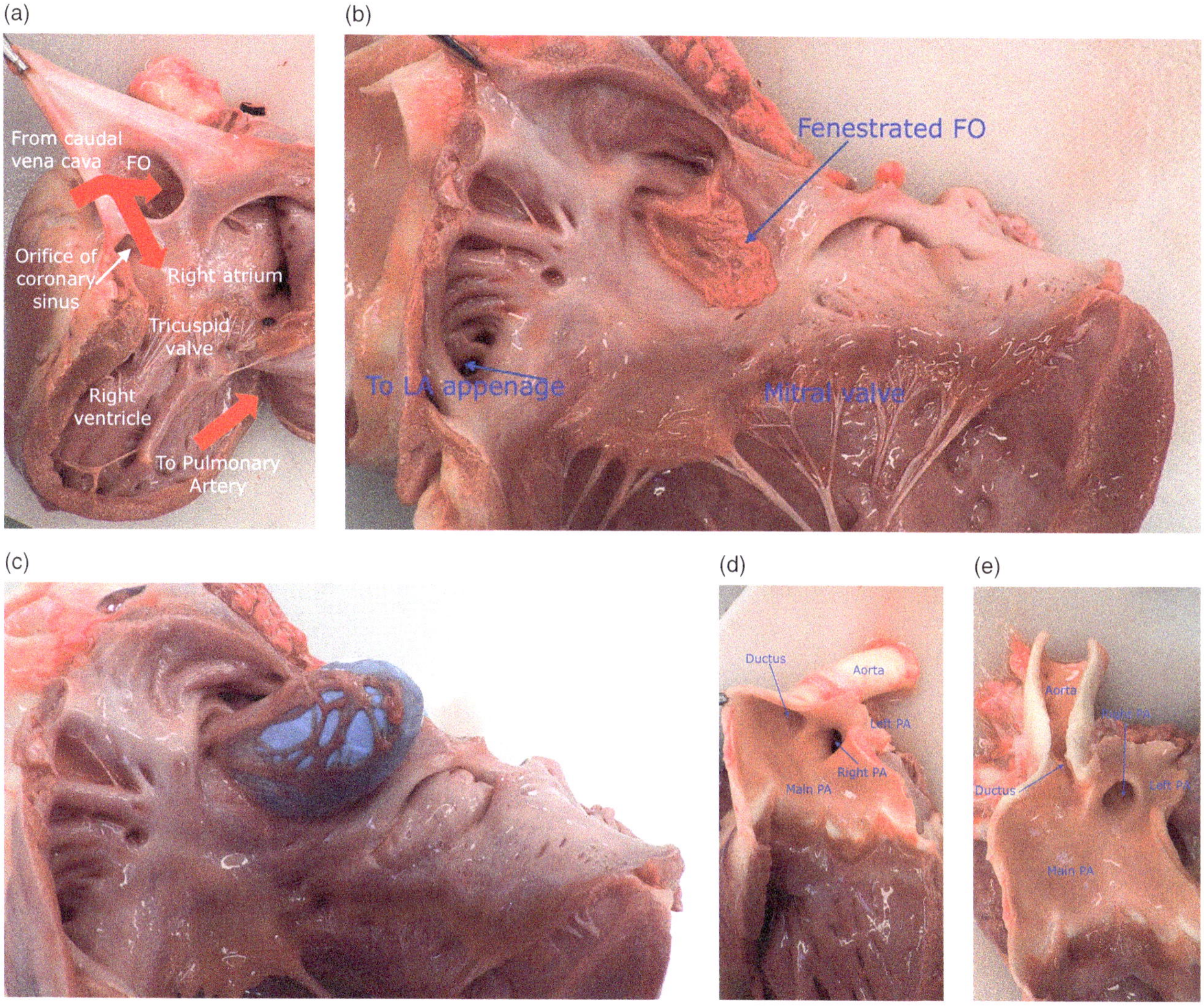

Figure 9.4 In this fresh specimen from a term foal, (a) from the right atrial aspect the foramen ovale (FO) is a large ring-like structure dorsal to the opening of the coronary sinus. The fetal circulation returning from the caudal vena cava and entering each atrium and leaving the right ventricle to the pulmonary artery is indicated (red arrows). (b) When viewed from the left side, the FO consists of a fenestrated sock-like structure, which protrudes into the LA. (c) The pathologist has inserted a finger into the FO to demonstrate its shape. The third shunt, the ductus arteriosus, diverts some of the blood that has entered the pulmonary artery (PA) via the right ventricle into the aorta, thus providing a second route to bypass the fetal lungs. (d) and (e) With the ductus arteriosus and aorta opened, the location of the ductus arteriosus is shown within the main PA connecting to the descending aorta.

and by a ridge of atrial tissue called the *crista dividens*. Blood returning to the heart bifurcates at the crista dividens with some streaming to each atria.

The tube-like FO is covered by a thread-like network of tissue, which is gradually replaced by fenestrations protruding into the left atrium (Figure 9.4) [20]. The third shunt, the ductus arteriosus, diverts some of the blood that has entered the pulmonary artery (PA) via the right ventricle (RV) into the aorta, thus providing a second route to by-pass the fetal lungs (Figure 9.4). Closure of these shunts is the major cardiovascular event as pulmonary circulation is increased, occurring in the first few days of life as the newborn foal adapts for postnatal life.

Development after Birth

After birth, increased oxygen tension from the newborn's extra-uterine breathing allows for increased blood into the lung, thus increasing left atrial pressure and closure of the flap of the foramen ovale (septum primum) against the septum secundum forming the floor of the fossa ovalis [4]. The foramen ovale can be identified echocardiographically as a mobile septal membrane in newborn foals and while fusion is incomplete, the foramen ovale may be patent. This structure gradually recedes and develops into the ovale fossa, a nonpatent ring-like structure within the atrial septum that remains visible into adulthood (Figure 9.5).

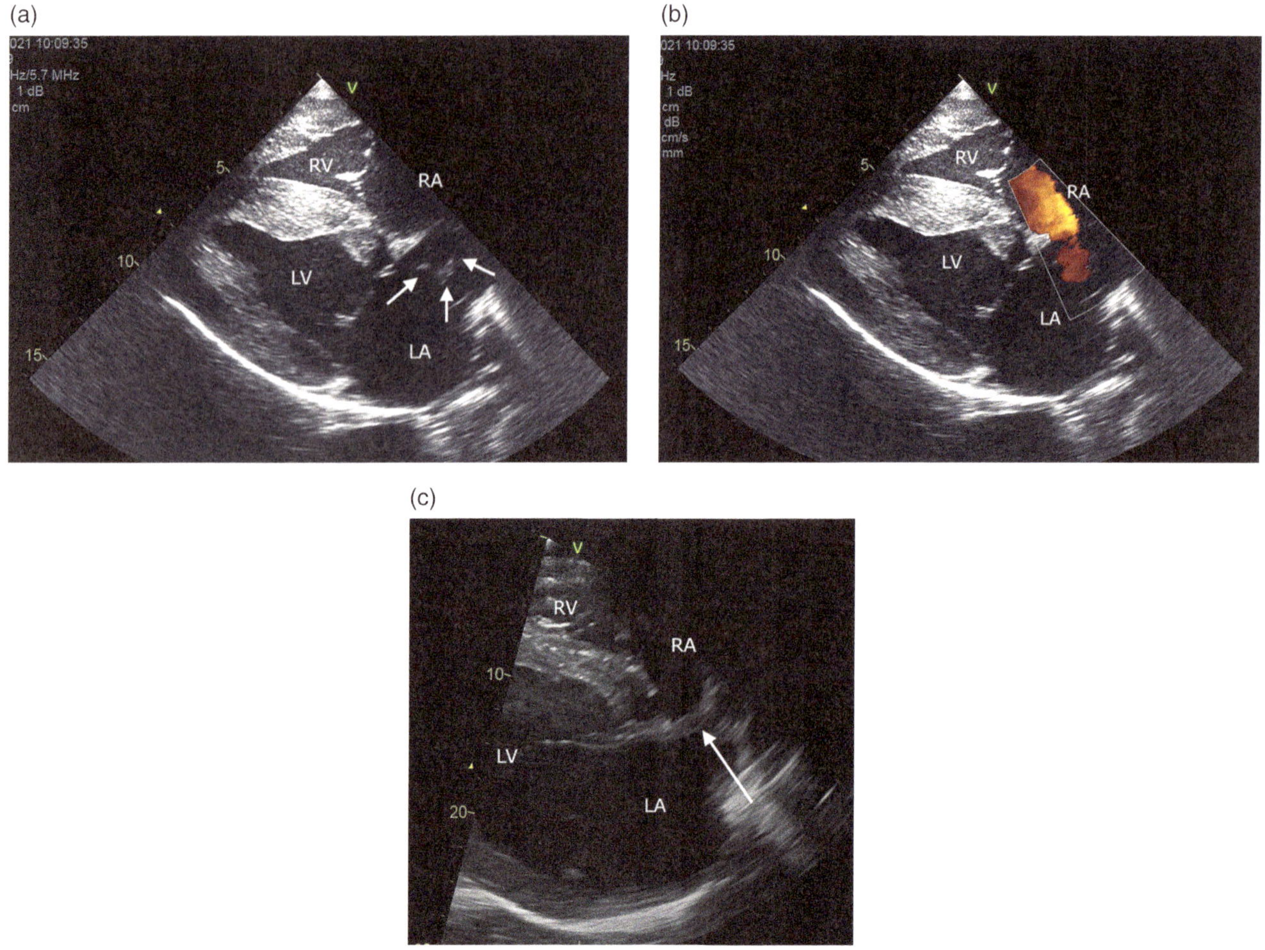

Figure 9.5 Echocardiographic images from newborn and 4-year-old Thoroughbreds. In the newborn, the foramen ovale is a mobile and large flap-like structure (a, arrows) and color-flow Doppler images shows this is patent with flow from left to right indicated by the orange and red signal (b). This tubular structure gradually reduces to form the oval fossa (arrow), a ring-like structure in the inter-atrial septum, which will remain throughout life but is not usually patent (b). RV = right ventricle, RA = right atrium, LV = left ventricle, LA = left atrium.

The ductus arteriosus closes earlier in response to increased arterial oxygen tension. The continuous murmur typically associated with patent ductus arteriosus, over the left heart base is generally no longer audible when foals are around 1 week of age, and in most, this murmur disappears within the first 48 hours of birth.

References

1 Bezold, L.I. Cardiovascular embryology. In: *Oski's Pediatrics: Principles and Practice* (ed. J.A. McMillan, R.D. Feigin, C. DeAngelis, and M.D. Jones). Lipponcott, Williams, and Wilkins.

2 Kloesel, B., DiNardo, J.A., and Body, S.C. (2016). Cardiac embryology and molecular mechanisms of congenital heart disease. *Anesth. Analg.* 123: 551–569.

3 Schleich, J.M., Abdulla, T., Summers, R. et al. (2013). An overview of cardiac morphogenesis. *Arch. Cardiovasc. Dis.* 106: 612–623.

4 Park, D.S. and Fishman, G.I. (2017). Development and function of the cardiac conduction system in health and disease. *J. Cariovasc. Dev. Dis.* 4: 1–16.

5 Jongbloed, M.R.M., Steijn, R.V., Hahurij, N.D. et al. (2012). Normal and abnormal development of the cardiac conduction system; implications for conduction and rhythm disorders in the child and adult. *Differentiation* 84: 1310148.

6 Mathew, P. and Bordoni, B. (2019). *Embryology*. Treasure Island, FL: Heart StatPearls.

7 Kirby, M.L. and Waldo, K.L. (1995). Neural crest and cardiovascular patterning. *Circ. Res.* 77: 211–215.

8 Gitternberger-De Groot, A.C., Bertelings, M.M., Deruiter, M.C. et al. (2005). Basics of cardiac development for the understanding of congenital heart malformations. *Pediatr. Res.* 57: 169–176.

9 Yelbuz, T.M., Wald, K.L., Kumiski, D.H. et al. (2002). Shortened outflow tract leads to altered cardiac looping after neural crest ablation. *Circulation* 106: 504–510.

10 Bajolle, F., Zaffran, S., Kelly, R.G. et al. (2006). Rotation of the myocardial wall of the outflow tract is implicated in the normal positioning of the great arteries. *Circ. Res.* 98: 421–428.

11 Lomonico, M.P., Bostrom, M.P., Moore, G.W. et al. (1988). Arrested rotation of the outflow tract may explain tetralogy of Fallot and transposition of the great arteries. *Pediatr. Pathol.* 8: 267–281.

12 Vitums, A. (1981). The embryonic development of the equine heart. *Zentralbl. Veterinarmed. C* 10: 193–211.

13 Kraus, M.S., Pariaut, R., Alcaraz, A. et al. (2005). Complete atrioventricular canal defect in a foal: clinical and pathological features. *J. Vet. Cardiol.* 7: 59–64.

14 Lamers, W.H., Viragh, S., Wessels, A. et al. (1995). Formation of the tricuspid valve in the human heart. *Circulation* 91: 111–121.

15 Kramer, T.C. (1942). The partitioning of the truncus and conus and the formation of the membranous portion of the interventricular septum in the human heart. *Anat. Rec.* 71: 343–370.

16 Li, S., Wen, H., Liang, M. et al. (2019). Congenital abnormalities of the aortic arch: revisiting the 1964 Stewart classification. *Cardiovasc. Pathol.* 39: 38–50.

17 Noden, D.M. and DeLahunta, A. (1985). *The Embryology of Domestic Animals: Developmental Mechanisms and Malformation*, 212–219. Baltimore: Williams & Wilkins.

18 Moorman, A.F., de Jong, F., Denyn, M.M. et al. (1998). Development of the cardiac conduction system. *Circ. Res.* 82: 620–644.

19 Cottrill, C.M., Sy, H., and O'Connor, W.N. (1997). Embryological development of the equine heart. *Equine Vet. J. Suppl.* 24: 14–18.

20 MacDonald, A.A., Fowde, A.L., Silver, M. et al. (1988). The foramen ovale of the foetal and neonatal foal. *Equine Vet. J.* 20: 255–260.

Chapter 10 Clinical Neonatal Cardiac Physiology

Ryan Fries

Cardiovascular Function in the Equine Perinatal Period

During circulatory development from the embryonic to fetal to neonatal stage, transformation occurs in blood flow, from a single circular system to a double parallel circuit and finally, to a double circulation in series. In the early embryo, all blood enters the heart through a single venous sinus, traverses straight through the heart, and is distributed to the body and placenta by way of the conotruncal bulb and the aortic arches. As partitioning develops, a double circuit is formed with parallel flow and cross-over proximal and distal to the ventricles. Virtually all blood entering the right atrium from the head and forepart of the body is shunted by a muscular fold on the atrial septum, adjacent to the fossa ovalis directly into the right ventricular cavity. This poorly oxygenated blood is pumped by the right ventricle to the pulmonary artery, across the ductus arteriosus, to the descending thoracic aorta en route to the placenta and lower body. The pulmonary vasculature has very high resistance owing to fluid surrounding the vessels and vasoconstriction in response to low blood oxygen content. Only 5–10% of right ventricular and pulmonary artery blood traverses the lungs. Highly oxygenated blood returning from the placenta and umbilical vein enters the right atrium through the postcava. The anatomic relationship of the postcava and the fossa ovalis allows most of this blood to be shunted directly through the fossa ovalis to the left atrium and ventricle. This highly oxygenated blood then enters the root of the aorta where most is distributed to the head and heart. The remainder traverses the aortic isthmus to be mixed with poorly oxygenated blood entering the aorta through the ductus arteriosus. The oxygen-poor blood from the distal postcava is preferentially shunted to the tricuspid valve and enters the right ventricle. Thus, two parallel circuits are present in the fetal period, which deliver highly oxygenated blood to the brain and heart and less oxygenated blood to the placenta.

Abnormalities of cardiac development do not cause functional abnormality in the fetus as long as there is communication between the right and left sides of the circulatory system. However, stenoses and abnormal circulatory patterns may result in reduced flow, causing underdevelopment or hypoplasia of the affected chamber or vessel. Semilunar valve stenoses (e.g. pulmonic stenosis) may cause chamber enlargement proximal to the stenosis due to increased right ventricular workload. Experimentally, left ventricular enlargement may be induced by placing a band on the aortic arch in the fetus; conversely, left ventricular hypoplasia may be caused by inflow obstruction to the left ventricle. Right ventricular enlargement has been produced in fetal lambs by pulmonary artery constriction [1].

At the time of birth and during the early neonatal period, circulatory changes result in the formation of two separate circuits in series. When air is introduced into the lungs, the fluid media surrounding the vasculature is replaced, thus reducing vascular resistance. With exposure to oxygen, the pulmonary vasculature dilates. At the same time, the placental circulation is removed. This increases systemic resistance and prevents right-to-left blood flow through the ductus arteriosus. The musculature of the ductus arteriosus is highly sensitive to oxygen and contracts when exposed to the now increased oxygen content of blood coming from the lungs. In addition, the ductus arteriosus musculature is responsive to prostaglandins that are present at birth, and its closure may be induced by prostaglandin inhibition.

In the fetus, approximately two-thirds of the returning blood enters the right ventricle, causing the right side of the heart to be as large as or larger than the left side. With closure of the ductus arteriosus and reduction in pulmonary resistance, a larger volume of blood now enters the left atrium. This results in increased left atrial pressure and forces the septum primum flap against the septum

Equine Neonatal Medicine, First Edition. Edited by David M. Wong and Pamela A. Wilkins.

secundum. Effective functional closure of the fossa ovalis occurs, completing the formation of two circulatory systems in series.

After septation is complete, the fetus enters a rapid growth phase with a progressive rise in arterial blood pressure. In the sheep, peak systolic pressure at 120–130 days of gestation (of 145 days) is reported to be 45–50 mmHg [2]. In chick embryos, arterial pressure has been reported to be up to 30 mmHg at hatching. In the newborn rat, femoral artery blood pressures using a servonull micro pressure system have been measured; at birth, mean femoral artery pressure was 18 mmHg, increasing to 30 mmHg by 3 days, 50 mmHg by 12 days, and 75 mmHg by 21 days of age [2]. In the newborn, ventricular pressure has been measured by transthoracic puncture of the left and right ventricles with a 21-gauge needle. In newborn puppies, systolic pressure was 35–50 mmHg in the left ventricle and 23–40 mmHg in the right ventricle. Left ventricular pressures rapidly increased to 75--90 mmHg at 3 to 7 days of age, and to 120 mmHg by 3 to 4 weeks of age, while right ventricular pressure remained at 20–30 mmHg [2].

In extra-uterine life, the cardiac cycle is divided into ventricular systole and diastole. Mechanical ventricular systole begins immediately after the QRS complex, with contraction of the ventricular myocardium and closure of the atrioventricular (AV) valves. Pressure within the ventricles rises rapidly, without forward movement of blood (isovolumetric contraction), until the pressures exceed the aorta and pulmonary artery pressures, causing the semilunar valves to open and blood to flow into their respective circulations. Blood flow peaks during the first third of ejection, after which time flow slowly decreases until ejection stops and the semilunar valves abruptly close, marking the end of ventricular systole. Ventricular diastole begins at semilunar valve closure. The ventricular pressures, which have been declining due to relaxation of the myocytes, continues to decline rapidly during early diastole, but ventricular volume remains unchanged because all cardiac valves are closed (isovolumetric relaxation). Once ventricular pressure drops below atrial pressure, the AV valves open and blood passively moves from the atria to ventricles resulting in rapid filling of the ventricles. Temporarily, the atrial and ventricular pressures will equilibrate resulting in minimal or no changes in ventricular pressure or volume (diastasis). Finally, atrial contraction recreates an AV pressure gradient that produces augmented ventricular filling. In the healthy resting horse atrial systole has minimal effects on ventricular filling and cardiac performance. However, the absence of atrial contraction or loss of AV synchrony during exercise can have considerable effects on cardiac performance.

Neonatal Heart Rhythms and Sounds

Heart Sounds

The first step in evaluating heart sounds in the foal involves knowledge of the anatomical position of the heart within the thorax. Positioning of the stethoscope in specific areas on the thorax corresponds to anatomical structures of the heart and great vessels. The pulmonic valve area is located at the left third intercostal space just ventral to the point of the shoulder. Slightly dorsal to this, and located in the left fourth intercostal space, is the aortic valve area. The mitral valve area is the fifth intercostal space just dorsal to a line halfway between the point of the shoulder and the sternum. The tricuspid valve area on the right side is in the ventral third of the thorax in the third to fourth intercostal space [3]. Auscultation of normal heart sounds is best accomplished over the mitral valve area in the neonatal foal. It is normal to hear only the first two heart sounds in the neonate and potentially all four heart sounds in the adult horse.

The first heart sound (S_1) occurs at the onset of ventricular systole and is associated with a palpable apex beat just prior to the rise in arterial pressure; S_1 is louder, longer, and lower pitched than the second heart sound (Figure 10.1). The major audible portion of S_1 is associated with closure of the mitral and tricuspid vales. The sound is not generated by the valve cusps themselves but rather, by the sudden acceleration and deceleration of blood and tensing of the valve cusps, chordae tendinea, and related structures [4]. The first heart sound is loudest in young, thin horses and in those with high sympathetic tone, tachycardia, systemic hypertension, or anemia. S_1 is diminished in obese animals, those with pleural or pericardial effusion, diaphragmatic hernia, shock, myocardial failure, or first-degree AV block. Occasionally, the S_1 is split into two components due to asynchronous closure of the AV valves or accentuation of the later ejection components of S_1. Splitting can occasionally be appreciated at the cardiac apex and mitral valve region. It may be attributed to electrical disturbances (bundle branch block) or to mechanical factors (mitral or tricuspid stenosis) [5, 6]. All these conditions delay either mitral or tricuspid valve closure and produce asynchronous valve closure. It is important to distinguish between a split S_1 and a pre-systolic gallop, ejection sound, and systolic click.

The second heart sound (S_2) is of higher frequency and shorter duration than S_1, and it is heard best at the aortic and pulmonic valve areas [5]. Vibrations contributing to S_2 are produced by early muscular relaxation, blood vibration in the great vessels, and opening of the AV valves; S_2 occurs at the end of ventricular systole, near the end of the T wave on the ECG and corresponds to closure of the semilunar

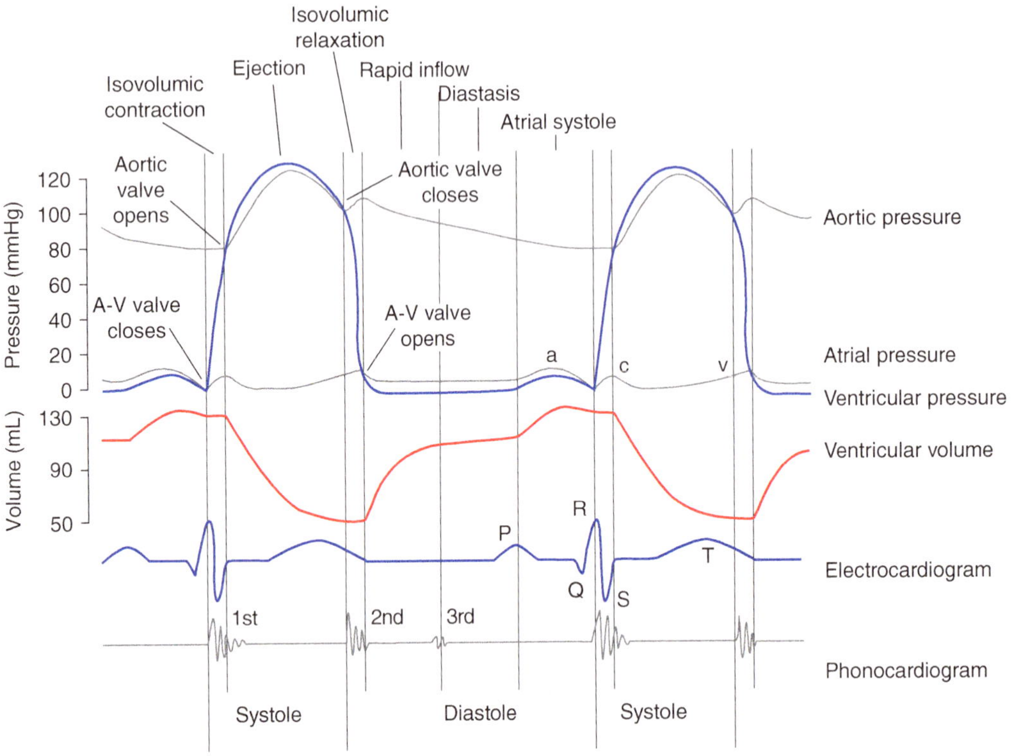

Figure 10.1 Wiggers diagram describing the pressure and volumes changes that occur throughout the cardiac cycle.

(aortic and pulmonic) valves. Aortic valve closure (A_2) precedes pulmonic valve closure (P_2) by a very short interval, which is usually not detectable by ear, causing S_2 to be heard as a single sound. In neonatal foals, the increase in heart rate tends to nullify the increased diastolic filling that occurs during inspiration [7]. Audible splitting during inspiration is occasionally detected in healthy foals. The pulmonic component occurs slightly later in the cardiac cycle than the aortic component. It is best recognized by listening over the pulmonic valve area. Inspiration increases negative intrathoracic pressures, drawing an increased amount of blood into the right ventricle; this requires a longer period for right ventricular ejection, which momentarily delays closure of the pulmonic valve. During expiration, the two components of S_2 approximate each other, and there is no splitting [8]. Pathologic splitting of S_2 is caused by asynchronous closure of the aortic or pulmonic valve, either from hemodynamic abnormalities or electrical disturbances such as bundle branch block, extrasystoles, or ventricular pacing. The most common cause is delayed closure of the pulmonic valve due to pulmonary hypertension. Here, the interval between A_2 and P_2 varies with respiration, as described earlier. In foals with an atrial septal defect, this interval does not vary with respiration, and splitting of S_2 is described as "fixed." Delayed closure of the aortic valve results in "paradoxical splitting" of S_2, which is accentuated during expiration. Aortic stenosis, left bundle branch block, and certain ectopic ventricular beats may delay A_2.

The third heart sound (S_3) is of low frequency and is generated by rapid ventricular filling. It is not heard in most healthy foals, but it is common to auscultate in adult Thoroughbred-type horses [9]. The intensity is determined by the rapidity of early diastolic filling, the pressure in the atrium, and the distensibility of the ventricle during early diastole [10, 11]. The more compliant the ventricle, the less intense the sound. Auscultatable, loud, third heart sounds are abnormal in the neonatal foal and often imply heart failure, especially systolic (myocardial) dysfunction.

The fourth heart sound (S_4) is produced by atrial systole and is inaudible in healthy neonatal foals. Vibrations initiated by forceful ejection of the atrial blood column into an already distended or noncompliant ventricle produce a low-pitched, low-frequency heart sound. When S_4 is audible, the heart sounds may be verbally characterized as *bub-lub-dub;* S_4 is most easily detected using the stethoscope bell positioned near the left cardiac apex.

The normal heart rate of foals immediately after birth is between 30 and 90 beats/minute (bpm) [12]. Over the next few hours, it is common for the heart rate to increase significantly (70–200 bpm), typically corresponding to attempts to rise and ambulate. Gradually the heart rate will decline with age and increased body size until it reaches 25–50 bpm in the mature horse. Identifying normal and abnormal heart sounds can be affected by heart rate.

Types of Murmurs

Foals are often born with low-grade heart murmurs that should disappear within the first 3 days of life [13]. A variety of murmurs may be present after this time frame and could indicate a more severe cardiac condition. The description of heart murmurs requires purposeful auscultation and typically involves six characteristics: 1-grade, 2-timing, 3-point of maximal intensity (PMI), 4-shape, 5-character, 6-duration. The first three characteristics of a murmur are the most clinically relevant:

1) *Grade* indicates the intensity (loudness) of a murmur and whether it can be heard at sights distant to the PMI. Below is an example of murmur grading on a six-point scale:
   - Grade 1/6 – soft, only audible in one anatomical location, may require a quiet environment
   - Grade 2/6 – heard easily when placing stethoscope over PMI
   - Grade 3/6 – loud murmur audible at 1 site distant to the PMI
   - Grade 4/6 – loud murmur audible at ≥2 sites other than the PMI
   - Grade 5/6 – loud with a strong thrill
   - Grade 6/6 – loud with a strong thrill and audible with the stethoscope off chest wall
2) *Timing* of the murmur – systolic, diastolic, or continuous – may require simultaneous auscultation and palpation of an arterial pulse. This can be relatively easily performed in recumbent foals using the median artery near the medial aspect of the elbow.
3) *Location or PMI* is the area where the murmur is loudest but not necessarily to the structure that is affected.
4) *Shape* is the acoustic quality of the murmur, much like an instrument playing a single note. The acoustic quality of the murmur may be described as crescendo (louder at the end), decrescendo (softer at the end), crescendo-decrescendo (loud then soft), or plateau-shaped (equal throughout). This description is particularly important for left-sided systolic murmurs, helping to differentiate mitral regurgitation (often plateau-shaped) from physiologic ejection murmurs (most commonly crescendo-decrescendo).
5) *Character* is the quality of the sound; typically described using familiar terms like blowing, harsh, musical, and honking. These descriptions are rarely diagnostic but can provide addition detail.
6) *Duration* is the length of time the murmur is auscultated. Holo – between the first two heart sound and thus S1–S2 are audible. Pan – extends over S1 and S2 thereby obliterating auscultation of these sounds. If shorter than holo, murmurs can be classified as early, early to mid, mid to late, or late.

Another important key for murmur interpretation is variation in intensity. Neonatal murmurs are often variable, present during excitement or under pharmacologic stressor and absent at a resting/relaxed state. These types of murmurs are referred to as labile. Ejection murmurs are common in neonates and are often labile. Exercise, excitement, pain, sedation with α-2 agonists, or administration of Buscopan® or phenylephrine are common circumstances that would make these murmurs louder. These types of ejection murmurs are typically benign.

Parameters and physiologic considerations that can provide important information regarding cardiac function including cardiac output (CO) and blood pressure. Cardiac output is not routinely measured in clinical equine patients due to expense, practicality, and potential invasiveness, but provides a better measure of hemodynamic status than heart rate, blood pressure, and hematologic values. Various CO measurement techniques have been evaluated in horses and foals. Indicator dilution techniques include transcardiac or transpulmonary thermodilution, lithium dilution, and ultrasound dilution techniques. Dilution techniques require administration of an indicator substance into the venous circulation or the right atrium and subsequent measurement of the indicator substance distal to the heart to determine flow based on versions of the Stewart-Hamilton equation. These methods are intermittent and the most invasive but are considered the most accurate in horses [14, 15]. Both thermodilution and lithium dilution techniques can be used to calibrate pulse waveform analysis methods, which provide a beat-by-beat determination of CO. [15] The indirect Fick principle can also be used to determine CO in foals noninvasively using the partial CO_2 rebreathing method [16]. While this technique is limited to use in foals and very small equine patients, it correlates well with lithium dilution measurements and provides a clinically practical option for CO measurement. Imaging techniques, such as MRI and echocardiography are other possible techniques for evaluating CO in equine patients but require expertise in interpretation [17]. More comprehensive reviews of CO monitoring techniques in equine patients have been published [18–20]. While capnography is not a substitute for CO monitoring, changes in end-tidal CO_2 during stable ventilation may be reflective of changes in pulmonary perfusion and thus CO, and can be helpful to trend during periods of cardiovascular change.

Systemic blood pressure is not a surrogate measure of tissue perfusion; however, hypotension can reflect low perfusion states and is associated with increased risk of myopathy and other potential complications [21, 22]. Blood pressure monitoring is particularly important in foals undergoing inhalational anesthesia, in hemodynamically unstable patients, and in those at risk of cardiovascular complications. By identifying hypotension early, appropriate cardiovascular supportive therapies can be implemented with the goal of minimizing morbidity and mortality. Primary factors determining arterial blood pressure are CO and systemic vascular resistance. Cardiac output is determined by heart rate and stroke volume, while stroke volume is determined by preload, afterload, and contractility. Thus, hypotension may be due to bradycardia, decreased vascular tone, decreased preload, poor contractility, or a combination of these factors. Hypotension is often defined as a mean arterial blood pressure <60 mmHg in dogs [23]. While there is no such consensus reported in equine patients, maintaining a mean arterial blood pressure of ≥70 mmHg reduces the incidence of myopathy in mature halothane-anesthetized horses, with neonatal foals generally tolerating lower blood pressures compared to adult horses [21].

Treatment should be directed at correcting the underlying cause of hypotension. Bradycardia, typically defined as a heart rate <26 bpm in mature horses, is a common finding in horses that are physically fit or following administration of α-2 adrenergic agonists. While anticholinergics effectively elevate heart rate, their administration to hypotensive and bradycardic equine patients should be considered carefully due to resulting reductions in gastrointestinal motility but is often warranted with heart rates <20 beats per minute. The definition of bradycardia in the foal is age dependent (Chapter 1).

Reductions in vascular tone are often associated with systemic inflammatory response syndrome (SIRS), shock, severe sepsis, multiorgan dysfunction syndrome, and endotoxemia. Vasoactive agents, such as phenylephrine, can be administered with the goal of improving vascular tone; however, they should be used judiciously as excessive increases in vascular tone may increase blood pressure at the expense of tissue perfusion [24].

A reduction in preload due to deficits in circulating volume or inadequate venous return is a common source of hypotension in neonatal foals. Correcting volume deficits and ongoing fluid losses should be replaced with a balanced electrolyte solution, with or without the addition of hypertonic saline, synthetic colloids or blood products, depending on the nature and severity of fluid losses, and the presence of other systemic diseases. Myocardial depression and compromised contractility can be caused by several factors. Positive inotropes can effectively improve contractility and elevate blood pressure. Dobutamine is commonly used to increase contractility due to its selectively for β receptors. Other agents with inotropic activity, such as dopamine, norepinephrine, and ephedrine, affect both contractility and vascular tone, and can be used when both are compromised [24].

References

1 Fishman, N.H., Hof, R.F., Rudolph, A.M. et al. (1978). Models of congenital heart disease in fetal lambs. *Circulation* 58: 354–364.

2 Pinson, C.W., Morton, M.J., and Thornburg, K.L. (1991). Mild pressure loading alters right ventricular function in fetal sheep. *Circulation* 68: 947–957.

3 Reef, V.B. (1985). Cardiovascular disease in the equine neonate. *Vet. Clin. North Am.: Equine Pract.* 1: 117–130.

4 Gompf, R.E. (1988). The clinical approach to heart disease: history and physical examination. In: *Canine and Feline Cardiology* (ed. P.R. Fox), 29. New York: Churchill Livingstone.

5 Detweiler, D.K. and Patterson, D.E. (1965). A phonograph record of heart sounds and murmurs of the dog. *Ann. N.Y. Acad. Sci.* 127: 322.

6 Ettinger, S.J. and Suter, P.F. (1970). *Canine Cardiology*, 12. Philadelphia: WB Saunders.

7 Patterson, D.F. and Detweiler, D.K. (1963). The diagnostic significance of splitting of the second heart sound in the dog. *Zentralbl. Veterinarmed.* 10: 121.

8 Perloff, J.K. (1992). Heart sounds and murmurs: physiological mechanisms. In: *Heart Disease: A Text-Book of Cardiovascular Medicine*, 4e (ed. E. Braunwald), 43. Philadelphia: WB Saunders.

9 Blissitt, K. (2010). Auscultation. In: *Cardiology of the Horse* (ed. C.M. Marr and I.M. Bowen), 91–104. Edinburgh: W.B. Saunders.

10 Ravin, A. (1967). *Auscultation of the Heart*, 2e. Chicago: Year Book Medical Publishers.

11 Tilkian, A.G. and Conover, M.B. (1984). *Understanding Heart Sounds and Murmurs*, 2e. Philadelphia: WB Saunders.

12 Rossdale, P.D. (1967). Clinical studies in the newborn thoroughbred foal, heart rate, auscultation and electrocardiogram. *Br. Vet. J.* 123: 521–532.

13 Marr, C.M. (2015). The equine neonatal cardiovascular system in health and disease. *Vet. Clin. North Am. Equine Pract.* 31 (3): 545–565.

14 Linton, R.A., Young, L.E., Marlin, D.J. et al. (2000). Cardiac output measured by lithium dilution, thermodilution, and transesophageal Doppler echocardiography in anesthetized horses. *Am. J. Vet. Res.* 61 (7): 731–737.

15 Shih, A.C., Giguère, S., Sanchez, L.C. et al. (2009). Determination of cardiac output in neonatal foals by ultrasound velocity dilution and its comparison to the lithium dilution method. *J. Vet. Emergency Crit. Care* 19 (5): 438–443.

16 Valverde, A., Giguère, S., Morey, T.E. et al. (2007). Comparison of noninvasive cardiac output measured by use of partial carbon dioxide rebreathing or the lithium dilution method in anesthetized foals. *Am. J. Vet. Res.* 68 (2): 141–147.

17 Young, L.E., Blissitt, K.J., Bartram, D.H. et al. (1996). Measurement of cardiac output by transoesophageal Doppler echocardiography in anaesthetized horses: comparison with thermodilution. *Br. J. Anaesth.* 77 (6): 773–780.

18 Corley, K.T., Donaldson, L.L., Durando, M.M. et al. (2003). Cardiac output technologies with special reference to the horse. *J. Vet. Intern. Med.* 17 (3): 262–272.

19 Shih, A.C., Giguère, S., Sanchez, L.C. et al. (2009). Determination of cardiac output in anesthetized neonatal foals by use of two pulse wave analysis methods. *Am. J. Vet. Res.* 70 (3): 334–339.

20 Shih, A. (2013). Cardiac output monitoring in horses. *Vet. Clin. North Am.: Equine Pract.* 29 (1): 155–167.

21 Grandy, J.L., Steffey, E.P., Hodgson, D.S. et al. (1987). Arterial hypotension and the development of postanesthetic myopathy in halothane-anesthetized horses. *Am. J. Vet. Res.* 48 (2): 192–197.

22 Johnston, G.M., Eastment, J.K., Wood, J.L.N. et al. (2002). The confidential enquiry into perioperative equine fatalities (CEPEF): mortality results of phases 1 and 2. *Vet. Anaesth. Analg.* 29 (4): 159–170.

23 Ruffato, M., Novello, L., and Clark, L. (2015). What is the definition of intraoperative hypotension in dogs? Results from a survey of diplomates of the ACVAA and ECVAA. *Vet. Anaesth. Analg.* 42 (1): 55–64.

24 Dancker, C., Hopster, K., Rohn, K., and Kastner, S.B. (2018). Effects of dobutamine, dopamine, phenylephrine and noradrenaline on systemic haemodynamics and intestinal perfusion in isoflurane anaesthetized horses. *Equine Vet. J.* 50: 104–110.

Chapter 11 Examination, Therapeutics, and Monitoring of the Cardiovascular System

Section I Examination of the Cardiovascular System

Ryan Fries

Physical Examination of the Cardiovascular System

Foals possess a four-chambered heart identical in function and anatomical layout with other mammals [1]. In addition to mechanical pumping, the heart has inherent electrical properties that allow generation and propagation of action potentials through the cells. In the healthy foal, spontaneous depolarization of the sinus node initiates an action potential within the right atrium. Conduction travels throughout both atria and the atrioventricular (AV) node. Subsequently, the action potential enters the specialized conduction tissue, knows as the His Purkinje system. This network is distributed extensively throughout both ventricles and penetrates the entire thickness of the walls. Once excited, there is nearly simultaneous activation of both ventricles resulting in mechanical contraction and pumping of blood [2]. Specific arrhythmias and their consequences related to anesthesia will be discussed later in this chapter.

The cardiac cycle is divided into ventricular systole and diastole. Mechanical ventricular systole begins immediately after the QRS complex, with contraction of the ventricular myocardium and closure of the AV valves. Pressure within the ventricles rises rapidly, without forward movement of blood (isovolumetric contraction), until the pressures exceed the aorta and pulmonary artery pressures, causing the semilunar valves to open and blood to flow into their respective circulations. Blood flow peaks during the first third of ejection, after which time flow slowly decreases until ejection stops and the semilunar valves abruptly close, marking the end of ventricular systole.

Ventricular diastole begins at semilunar valve closure. The ventricular pressures, which have been declining due to relaxation of the myocytes, continues to decline rapidly during early diastole, but ventricular volume remains unchanged because all cardiac valves are closed (isovolumetric relaxation). Once ventricular pressure drops below atrial pressure, the AV valves open and blood passively moves from the atria to ventricles, resulting in rapid filling of the ventricles. Temporarily, the atrial and ventricular pressures equilibrate, resulting in minimal or no changes in ventricular pressure or volume (diastasis). Finally, atrial contraction recreates an AV pressure gradient that produces augmented ventricular filling. In healthy resting foals, atrial systole has minimal effects on ventricular filling and cardiac performance. However, the absence of atrial contraction or loss of AV synchrony on exercising and anesthetized foals can have considerable effects on cardiac performance.

Physical Examination

Auscultation is the principal means to evaluate the equine heart [3]. Auscultation alone can diagnose mitral and tricuspid regurgitation with 53–100% specificity, making auscultation an essential part of evaluation in horses, including neonates [4, 5]. Before a diagnosis of a murmur can be made, it is first necessary to identify normal heart sounds. In all horses, the first two heart sound (S1 and S2) are audible at the level of the apex beat. S1 corresponds to closure of the AV valves at the beginning of systole, while S2 corresponds to closure of the semilunar valves at the end of systole. Diastolic heart sounds are heard in adult Thoroughbred-type horses and less commonly in neonates and smaller horses. There are two diastolic heart sounds, early rapid ventricular filling (S3) and atrial contraction (S4). Murmurs between the first two heart sounds are classified as systolic, while murmurs that occur between S3 and S4 are classified as diastolic. In neonates, congenital

Equine Neonatal Medicine, First Edition. Edited by David M. Wong and Pamela A. Wilkins.

heart defects such as a patent ductus arteriosus have a continuous murmur. Murmurs should be classified based on location (e.g. left apex, left base), intensity (grade 1–6), and timing (systolic, diastolic, or continuous) [6, 7]. In addition to normal heart sounds and murmur detection, auscultation is the primary means of detecting any dysrhythmias. Simply, the neonate's heart rate should be obtained, and the rhythm characterized (regular, regularly irregular, or irregularly irregular). The normal neonate has a sinus heart rate of 70–80 beats/min. Once a dysrhythmia has been detected, further evaluation with an electrocardiogram (ECG) is indicated.

Most neonates with mild to moderate heart disease are subclinical, requiring precise auscultation and palpation to detect heart disease. However, some horses may present with symptoms of heart failure. Clinical signs of heart failure are attributed to a combination of reduced cardiac output (CO) and increased ventricular filling pressures. Depending on the etiology of the cardiac disease, clinical signs may include: tachycardia, weight loss or failure to grow, weakness, exercise intolerance, pale mucous membranes, weak arterial pulses, ataxia, syncope, tachypnea, dyspnea, nasal discharge, coughing, jugular pulsation, distention of peripheral veins, and peripheral edema of the ventrum, distal limbs, or prepuce [8]. Any horse with these clinical signs should be evaluated fully for cardiac disease, including echocardiography, thoracic radiographs, electrocardiography, and if available direct measurement of pulmonary artery and pulmonary capillary wedge pressure.

Electrocardiogram

An ECG is required to definitively diagnosis any dysrhythmia (Figure 11.I.1). In horses, dysrhythmias can be associated with a wide range of cardiac and noncardiac diseases, including valvular disease, congenital defects, pericardial disease, myocarditis, myocardial ischemia, toxicosis, myocardial neoplasia, hypoxia, electrolyte disturbances, autonomic tone, septicemia, endotoxemia, and various drugs [9–15]. An important diagnostic goal in neonates with dysrhythmias is to identity any contributing cardiac or noncardiac disease and the relative risks associated with the arrhythmia.

Due to the extensive Purkinje system throughout the equine myocardium, simultaneous electrical activity within the left and right ventricular myocardium cancels each other out, leaving the electrical activity within the interventricular septum and parts of the left ventricular free wall creating the vectors detectable on a surface ECG. Due to the electrical activity within the equine heart and its orientation within the thorax, cardiac rhythm is often evaluated in lead 1 using a base-apex orientation, as opposed to the frontal plane orientation in humans and small animals. This requires placement of the left forelimb electrode (black) at the level of the apex on the left side of the thorax, with the right forelimb electrode (white) at the top of the right scapular spine, and the left hind limb (red) electrode placed at variable locations distant to the heart. These differences result in equine ECG morphology that has unique characteristics that differ from small animals. Specifically, the P wave may be simple positive, bifid, or biphasic, with a predominantly negative deflection of the QRS complex, and a T wave that is variable in size and orientation (Figure 11.I.1).

Clinicopathologic Parameters to Assess the Heart

A wide range of cardiovascular disorders that result in the impairment of the heart's ability to fill or to pump blood may eventually lead to clinical symptoms. Neonatal foals often present with signs and symptoms that are nonspecific, yielding a wide differential diagnosis, making diagnosis by clinical presentation alone challenging. The evaluation of a patient suspected of having heart disease is traditionally based on clinical assessment with history, physical examination, thoracic radiographs, and echocardiography. However, in isolation, the performance of these diagnostic methods can be limited in accurately diagnosing heart failure. Additionally, these diagnostics may not be indicated for all patients, in particular those in the preclinical stages of disease, when screening is most important. Accordingly, the role of biomarkers to identify the presence of heart disease and heart failure, to risk stratify affected patients, and possibly to serve as a biological tool to guide therapy have been examined.

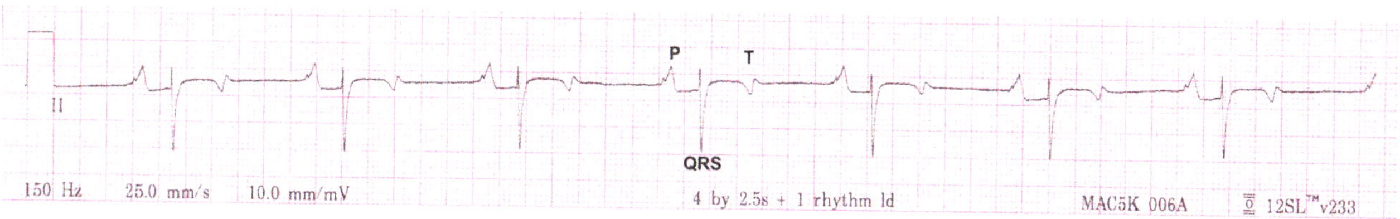

Figure 11.I.1 ECG tracing in a healthy neonatal foal; note the bifid P wave with an estimated heart rate of 45 beats/min.

Cardiac-specific troponins are intracellular proteins that are released into the blood as a consequence of primary or secondary cardiac cell injury or necrosis and have been studied in numerous disease states. Its greatest diagnostic utility is its ability to provide information regarding presence and severity of cardiac injury. Because it is nonspecific marker of cardiac cell injury, it can be increased in a variety of clinical scenarios including myocarditis, severe arrhythmias, or severe systemic diseases. Specific markers of myocardial damage including troponin I (cTnI), troponin T (cTnT), and cardiac isoenzyme of creatine kinase (CKMB) have been well described in neonatal foals. Elevations in these biomarkers indicate myocardial injury and can be associated with wide variety of cardiac and non-cardiac disease. In neonatal foals, these injury markers are elevated during septicemia, indicating myocardial damage; however, it is not associated with decreased survival [16].

B-type natriuretic peptide (BNP) is a hormone that causes renal sodium and water loss, as well as vasodilation. BNP is produced and secreted into the blood by the muscle cells of the heart. Low concentrations of BNP circulate at all times, but the heart increases production and secretion in response to excessive stretching of heart muscle cells. Excessive stretching of heart muscle cells is common in many forms of heart disease and in the setting of heart failure. The secretory granules for BNP have been isolated in the equine atrium, but to date circulating BNP assays have not been validated in the horses [17].

Routine hematology and biochemical analysis in neonatal foals are nonspecific diagnostic tests and rarely provide a diagnosis of heart disease. Rather, these tests are part of a complete evaluation. The heart, as a pump and electrical organ system, is greatly affected by derangements on both hematology and biochemistry. The heart as a pump requires tremendous amounts of oxygen to generate energy in the form of adenosine triphosphate (ATP). In health, the heart's preferred energy producing substrate is fatty acid metabolism. As such, the efficiency of oxidative phosphorylation is greatly affected by oxygen delivery to the heart tissue. In foals, severe anemia can impair oxygen delivery to the heart, reducing the overall energy production, which can lead to decreased myocardial function and even cell death. Foals with impaired myocardial function will have evidence of decreased perfusion secondary to low stroke volume. Compensatory mechanisms are activated to maintain cardiac out, and an increase in heart rate and systemic vascular resistance ensue. If the anemia persists and oxygen delivery is not restored, cellular damage can occur leading to increased circulating cTnI and cTnT. Arrhythmias, in particular ventricular, often manifest when myocardial oxygen delivery is impaired.

The heart possesses the ability to generate spontaneous depolarization and conduct electrical activity through specialized ion channels. By its nature, the heart is electrical and maintains tightly controlled membrane potentials both during rest and excitement of the cell. The resting membrane potential of the heart is primarily determined by control of potassium ions across the cell membrane. Depolarization is achieved through a combination of sodium and calcium ions. Given this tightly controlled balance, small fluctuations in serum ions can have significant impact on membrane excitability and arrhythmogenesis.

Calcium

Hyper- or hypocalcemia predominantly alter the action potential duration. Increased extracellular calcium concentration shortens the ventricular action potential duration by shortening phase 2 of the action potential. In contrast, hypocalcemia prolongs phase 2 of the action potential. These cellular changes correlate with abbreviation and prolongation of the QT interval with hypercalcemia and hypocalcemia, respectively. Severe hypercalcemia can also be associated with decreased T-wave amplitude, sometimes with T-wave notching or inversion.

Potassium

Hyperkalemia is associated with a distinctive sequence of four ECG changes:

1) Widening and lowering of amplitude followed by inversion and eventually disappearance of the P wave;
2) Increase in the amplitude of the T wave;
3) Increase in the QRS interval, with some irregularity in the ventricular rate; and
4) Periods of cardiac arrest that became terminal or followed by ventricular fibrillation [18].

Progressive extracellular hyperkalemia reduces atrial and ventricular resting membrane potentials, thereby inactivating sodium channels, which decreases amplitude and conduction velocity. The QRS begins to widen and P-wave amplitude decreases. Complete loss of P waves may be associated with a junctional escape rhythm (so-called sinoventricular rhythm). In the latter instance, sinus rhythm persists with conduction between the SA and AV nodes and occurs without producing an overt P-wave. Extreme elevations in potassium lead to eventual asystole, sometimes preceded by a slow undulatory "sine-wave" ventricular flutter-like pattern. Electrophysiologic changes associated with hypokalemia, in contrast, include hyperpolarization of myocardial cell membranes and increased action potential duration as result of prolonged repolarization. The major electrocardiographic manifestations are flattened T waves. The prolongation of repolarization with hypokalemia predisposes to torsades de pointes and hypokalemia predisposes to atrial and ventricular tachyarrhythmias.

Magnesium

Specific electrocardiographic effects of mild to moderate isolated abnormalities in magnesium ion concentration are not well characterized. Severe hypermagnesemia can cause atrioventricular and intraventricular conduction disturbances that may culminate in complete heart block and cardiac arrest. Hypomagnesemia is usually associated with hypocalcemia or hypokalemia. Hypomagnesemia can potentiate certain digitalis toxic arrhythmias.

Other Factors

Isolated hypernatremia or hyponatremia does not produce consistent effects on the ECG. Acidemia and alkalemia are often associated with hyperkalemia and hypokalemia, respectively. Systemic hypothermia may be associated with elevation of the ST segment, but this not well described in horses.

Advanced Imaging

Cardiovascular monitoring is important in critically ill neonatal foals for whom hemodynamic derangements are common. These derangements significantly affect tissue perfusion and thus, tissue oxygen delivery [19, 20]. While physical examination and basic hemodynamic monitoring are useful for assessing cardiovascular function, the direct evaluation of cardiac structure and function, including CO, provides the most accurate information and thus can improve patient management [19].

Two-dimensional transthoracic echocardiography (2DE) is well-described in foals and other species and can provide information on both cardiovascular function and morphology. However, accuracy of 2DE is limited by image orientation, geometric assumptions, and boundary tracing errors [21]. Because of this, the estimation of CO demonstrates only a moderate correlation when compared to the diagnostic gold standard [19]. That is, newer, more sensitive, and minimally invasive imaging modalities include 2D-transesophageal echocardiography (TEE) and gated cardiac magnetic resonance imaging (CMR) [22, 23]. TEE has been described in a variety of species, including adult horses, for hemodynamic assessment, cardiac morphology, CO, and volume status and has recently been reported in neonatal foals. TEE has the ability to avoid extra thoracic interference such as ribs, lungs, and hair, but despite these advantages, still suffered from poor reproducibility, was not feasible in all foals, and did not compare favorably with the gold standard. When images of diagnostic quality were successfully acquired, TEE provided superior imaging planes, in particular of the heart base, which in several foals made identifying a patent ductus arteriosus possible that had not been detected by the other modalities or physical examination.

Computed tomography angiography (CTA) allows for minimally invasive assessment of the neonatal thorax. It has been successfully utilized to aid in the diagnosis of thoracic trauma, pulmonary disorders, and congenital heart anomalies [24–27]. To date, CTA has not been used for functional assessment of the heart. Functional CTA requires cardiac gating and sophisticated post-processing equipment that limits widespread usage for functional assessment; nevertheless, this technology provides a robust, repeatable diagnostic modality for the anatomical assessment of the neonatal thorax, including cardiac structures [28]. CMR imaging is considered the gold standard for evaluation of cardiac morphology and measurement of cardiac function and is well-described in humans, dogs, and cats [22, 29–31]. Advantages over echocardiography include cross-sectional images of the heart in any plane avoiding geometric assumptions, improved accuracy, reproducibility, unrestricted field of view, non-ionizing radiation, and the ability to characterized myocardial tissue. It allows cardiologists to view the heart in all planes and can be used to reconstruct a three-dimensional heart. Because of the need for general anesthesia, routine use of CMR is limited, but evaluation of CMR in foals provides valuable information. Recently CMR was described in healthy neonatal foals, and was highly reproduceable, accurate, and easily obtained (Figure 11.I.2) [31]. More importantly, since CMR is not widely available, identifying which modality most accurately agrees with CMR is essential. At this time, 2DE echocardiography obtained from the right parasternal four-chamber view most strongly correlates with CMR for both size and functional assessment of the heart. Despite a strong correlation, dimensions derived from 2DE should not be used interchangeably with CMR and do not replace CMR when accuracy of heart size is paramount.

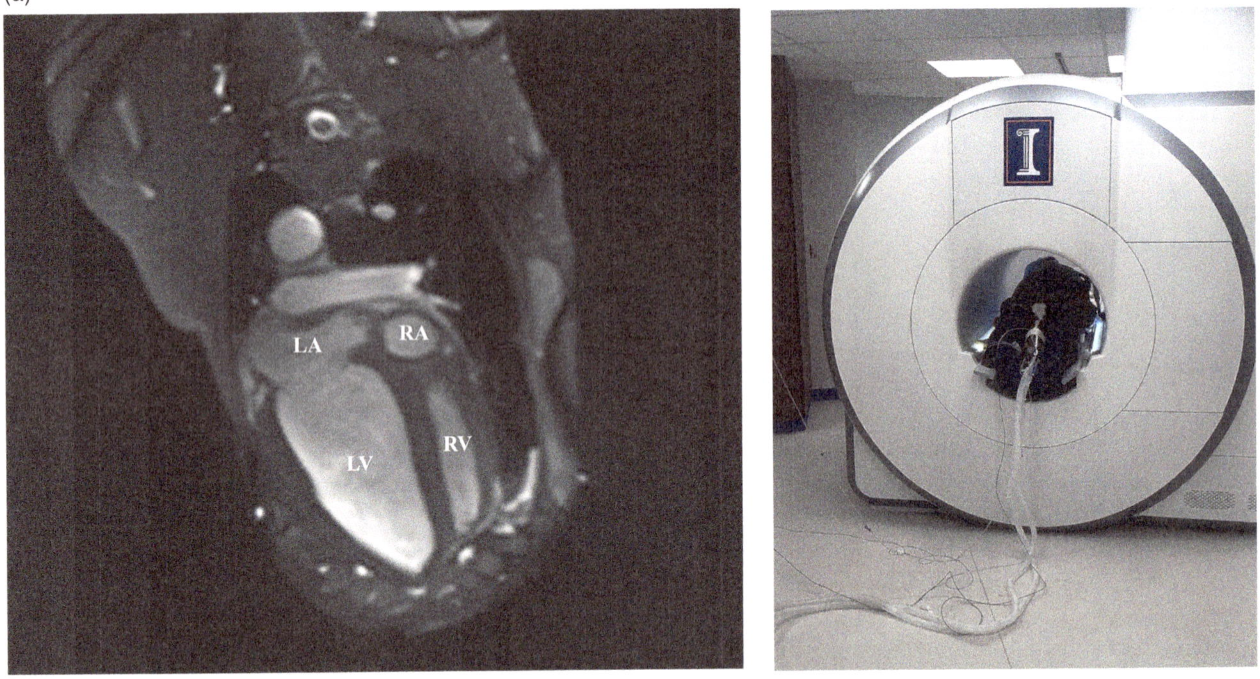

Figure 11.I.2 (a) Four-chamber, long-axis view of the heart acquired using a steady-state free precession sequence in a one-week-old foal (LV, left ventricle; LA, left atrium; RV, right ventricle; RA, right atrium); (b) Cardiac MRI in a one-week-old foal under general anesthesia positioned in sternal recumbency.

References

1 Budras, K.D. (2012). *Anatomy of the Horse*, 6e, 54–57. Schluetersche, Germany: Thieme.
2 Hamlin, R.L. and Smith, C.R. (1965). Categorization of common domestic mammals based upon their ventricular activation process. *Ann. N.Y. Acad. Sci.* 127: 195–203.
3 Bonagura, J.D. (1990). Clinical evaluation and management of heart disease. *Equine Vet. Educ.* 2: 31–37.
4 Naylor, J.M., Yadernuck, L.M., and Oharr, J.W. (2001). An assessment of the ability of diplomates, practitioners, and students to describe and interpret recording of heart murmurs and arrhythmia. *J. Vet. Intern. Med.* 15: 507–515.
5 Young, L.E. and Wood, J.L.N. (2000). The effects of age and training on murmurs and atrioventricular valvular regurgitation in young Thoroughbreds. *Equine Vet. J.* 32: 195–199.
6 Levine, S.A. and Harvey, W.P. (1950). *Clinical Examination of the Heart*, 51. Philadelphia: WB Saunders.
7 Littlewort, M.C.G. (1962). The clinical auscultation of the equine heart. *Vet. Rec.* 74: 1247–1159.
8 Marr, C. (2010). Heart failure, Chapter 19. In: *Cardiology of the Horse*, 2e, 239–252. Edinburgh: WB Saunders.
9 Reef, V.B., Bain, F.T., and Spencer, P.A. (1998). Severe mitral regurgitation in horses: clinical, echocardiographic and pathologic findings. *Equine Vet. J.* 30: 18–27.
10 Reef, V.B. (1993). Pericardial and myocardial disease. In: *The Horse: Diseases and Clinical Management* (ed. C.N. Kobluk, T.R. Ames, and R.J. Geor), 185–197. Edinburgh: Churchill Livingstone.
11 Diana, A., Guglielmini, C., Candini, D. et al. (2007). Cardiac arrhythmias associated with piroplasmosis in the horse: a case report. *Vet. J.* 174: 193–195.
12 Dickinson, C.E., Traub-Dargatz, J.L., Dargatz, D.A. et al. (1996). Rattlesnake venom poisoning in horses: 32 cases (1973–1993). *J. Am. Vet. Med. Assoc.* 208: 1866–1871.
13 Doonan, G., Brown, C.M., Mullaney, T.P. et al. (1989). Monensin poisoning in horses. *Can. Vet. J.* 30: 165–169.
14 Delesalle, C., van Loon, G., Nollet, H. et al. (2002). Tumor-induced ventricular arrhythmia in a horse. *J. Vet. Intern. Med.* 16: 612–617.
15 Reimer, J.M., Reef, V.B., and Sweeney, R.W. (1992). Ventricular arrhythmias in horses: 21 cases (1984–1989). *J. Am. Vet. Med. Assoc.* 201: 1237–1243.

16 Slack, J.A., McGurik, S.M., Erb, H.N. et al. (2005). Biochemical markers of cardiac injury in normal, surviving septic, or nonsurviving septic neonatal foals. *J. Vet. Intern. Med.* 19: 577–580.

17 Mifune, H., Richter, R., and Forssmann, W.G. (1995). Detection of immunoreactive atrial and brain natriuretic peptides in the equine atrium. *Anat. Embryol.* 192: 117–121.

18 Glazier, D.B., Littledike, E.T., and Evans, R.D. (1982). Electrocardiographic changes in induced hyperkalemia in ponies. *Am. J. Vet. Res.* 3: 1934–1937.

19 Shih, A. (2013). Cardiac output monitoring in horses. *Vet. Clin. Equine* 29: 155–167.

20 Mellema, M. (2009). Cardiac output monitoring. In: *Small Animal Critical Care Medicine* (ed. D. Silverstein and K. Hopper), 894–898. Missouri: Saunders Elsevier.

21 Chukwu, E.O., Barasch, E., Mihalatos, D.G. et al. (2008). Relative importance of errors in left ventricular quantitation by two-dimensional echocardiography: insights from three-dimensional echocardiography and cardiac magnetic resonance imaging. *J. Am. Soc. Echocardiogr.* 21: 990–997.

22 Sieslack, A.K., Dziallas, P., Nolte, I. et al. (2013). Comparative assessment of left ventricular function variables determined via cardiac computed tomography and cardiac magnetic resonance imaging in dogs. *Am. J. Vet. Res.* 74: 990–998.

23 Fries, R.C., Gordon, S.G., Saunders, A.B. et al. (2019). Quantitative assessment of two- and three-dimensional transthoracic and two-dimensional transesophageal echocardiography, computed tomography, and magnetic resonance imaging in normal canine hearts. *J. Vet. Cardiol.* 21: 79–92.

24 Barba, M. and Lepage, O.M. (2013). Diagnostic utility of computed tomography imaging in foals: 10 cases (2008–2010). *Equine Vet. Educ.* 25: 29–38.

25 Bauer, S., Livesey, M.A., Bjorling, D.E. et al. (2006). Computed tomography assisted surgical correction of persistent right aortic arch in neonatal foal. *Equine Vet. Educ.* 18: 32–36.

26 Kohnken, R., Schober, K., Godman, J. et al. (2018). Double outlet right ventricle with subpulmonary ventricular septal defect (Taussing-Bing anomaly) and other complex congenital cardiac malformations in an American Quarter Horse foal. *J. Vet. Cardiol.* 20: 64–72.

27 Lascola, K., O'Brien, R.T., Wilkins, P.A. et al. (2013). Qualitative and quantitative interpretation of computed tomography of the lungs in healthy neonatal foals. *Am. J. Vet. Res.* 74: 1239–1246.

28 Arencibia, A., Corbera, J.A., Ramirez, G. et al. (2020). Anatomical assessment of the thorax in neonatal foal using computed tomography angiography, sectional anatomy, and gross dissections. *Animals* 10: 1045.

29 MacDonald, K.A., Kittleson, M.D., Garcia-Nolen, T. et al. (2006). Tissue Doppler imaging and gradient echo cardiac magnetic resonance imaging in normal cats and cats with hypertrophic cardiomyopathy. *J. Vet. Intern. Med.* 20: 627–634.

30 Meyer, J., Wefstaedt, P., Dziallas, P. et al. (2013). Assessment of left ventricular volumes by use of one-, two-, and three-dimensional echocardiography versus magnetic resonance imaging in healthy dogs. *Am. J. Vet. Res.* 74: 1223–1230.

31 Fries, R.C., Clark-Price, S.C., Kadotani, S. et al. (2020). Quantitative assessment of cardiac function and anatomy utilizing transthoracic and transesophageal echocardiography, ultrasound velocity dilution, and gated magnetic resonance imaging in healthy foals. *Am. J. Vet. Res.* 81: 1–10.

Section II Echocardiography

Celia Marr

Echocardiography can provide information on both cardiac structure and function, and is therefore invaluable in assessing foals suspected of having primary cardiac disease, whether congenital or acquired, and in monitoring cardiac function in compromised foals regardless of the underlying disease state and pathogenesis.

Two-dimensional (2DE), M mode and Doppler echocardiography are regarded as the basic modalities that complete a standard echocardiographic examination [1–4], while advanced techniques encompass tissue velocity imaging (TVI), speckle tracking echocardiography (STE) and three-dimensional echocardiography (3DE), the latter being the most relevant technique in equine neonatology because of the additional structural information it provides [5, 6]. Intracardiac echocardiography has been shown to be useful for evaluation of small, doubly committed ventricular septal defects [7] and for evaluation of the foramen ovale [6]. TVI and STE are increasingly used in equine cardiology facilities but foal-specific data are lacking and without these, the clinical application of these advanced echocardiographic tools is currently limited in foals, although doubtless this will change in the future.

Equipment and Techniques

Echocardiographic images are generally most easily obtained using sector or phased array probes, and modern matrix technology has further enhanced the quality of imaging that is readily achievable. Linear or curvilinear formats are not appropriate except where there is no alternative. Due to their smaller size, foals can be imaged using transducers with higher frequencies and lower depth of penetration than adults in which image planes of 30 cm are optimal. The exact depth of imaging used should be modified depending on the size of the foal, but imaging depths of approximately 12–15 cm are a good starting point for 50 kg foals. Frequencies of 6 MHz are usually employed but the echocardiographer should increase the imaging frequency and adjust depth, width, tilt, and focal points for each foal, depending on size, to ensure that the entire heart is visible in one image. Thereafter, as the exam proceeds, reducing the depth and width, adjusting focus, and using tools such as high-resolution zoom can be helpful to optimize imaging of individual structures. An ECG is not essential if the sole purpose of the exam is to assess anatomy, but an integrated ECG system is required to time cardiac events when making measurements and usually is set as a base-apex lead system. In many foals, clipping of the hair coat is necessary. Because most equine clinicians are most familiar with performing echocardiography in the standing adult, it is usually easier to do the same in foals. If this is not possible, positioning in the foal in sternal or near sternal recumbency helps with access to the cardiac window.

Standard Imaging Planes

The standard imaging planes used in foals are identical to those recommended for adults. Beginning the examination, from the right side with a long-axis image of the left and right ventricles and left and right atria, known as the four-chamber view (Figure 11.II.1), provides immediate appraisal information on whether the cardiac anatomy is normal, the heart is the approximate expected size, and there is any pericardial effusion. If the foal has fractured ribs, it is prudent to begin on the nonfractured or least fractured side rather than risk iatrogenic injury

Equine Neonatal Medicine, First Edition. Edited by David M. Wong and Pamela A. Wilkins.

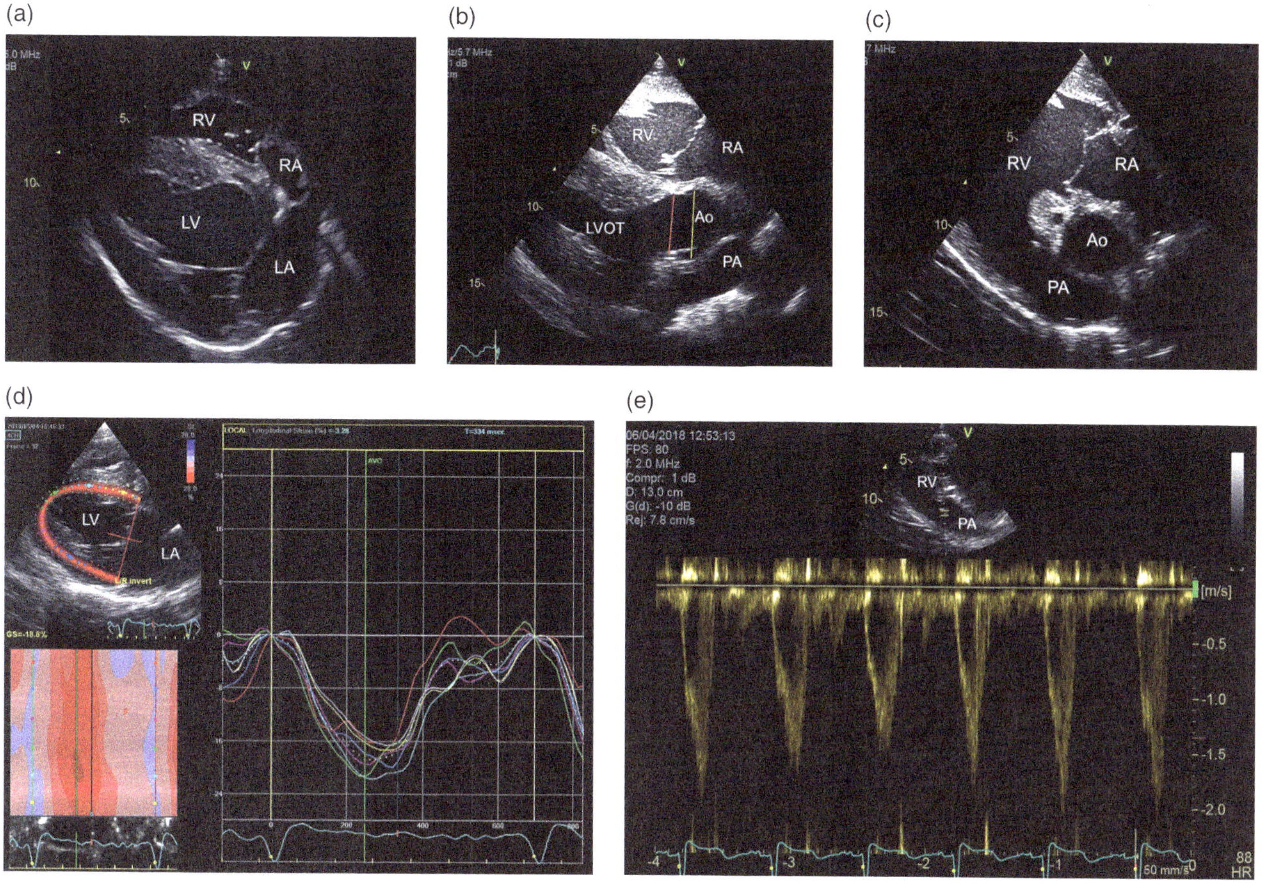

Figure 11.II.1 A series of right parasternal long axis-images from neonatal foals showing (a) Left (LV) and right (RV) ventricles and left (LA) and right (RA) atria. Note that in neonates the RV lumen and wall are relatively large nearing the dimensions of the left. This imaging plane is also known as the four-chambered view. (b) The left ventricular outflow tract (LVOT) and aorta (Ao) with the pulmonary artery (PA) in short-axis to the left of the Ao. The red line indicates the measurement points for the diameter of the aortic root and yellow line the Sinus of Valsalva. For measurement of the sinotubular junction and PA, the imaging plane must be adjusted to achieve better alignment (see Figure 11.II.8). (c) The RA, RV and PA; this image is also known as the right inflow-outflow view. (d) The long-axis image of the LV is used to assess longitudinal strain with speckle tracking echocardiography. The plot on the right displays strain in six segments and on the left lower panel there is an M mode depiction of strain, with locations denoted by the colors shown in the 2D image in the left upper panel. (e) The right inflow-outflow image is useful for orientation and to measure outflow velocities on a spectral trace obtained with pulsed wave Doppler.

as the pressure applied to the thorax during the echocardiographic examination might displace rib fragments (Figure 11.II.2).

Having gained an initial overview from the four chamber view, the 2DE examination is then completed (in an order depending on the clinician's preference) to include: (i) right long-axis images (Figure 11.II.1) of the left ventricular outflow tract to measure the diameters of the aortic root, Sinus of Valsalva and sinotubular junction, and the pulmonary artery; (ii) right long-axis images of right ventricular inflow-outflow tracts to measure the pulmonary artery at the level the valve and sinus; then moving to short-axis by turning the transducer by 90° (Figure 11.II.3); (iii) right short-axis images of the ventricle from apex to base; and (iv) right short-axis images of the heart base showing the aorta, pulmonary artery, atrial septum and tricuspid valve. Right sided images can be supplemented with long and short axis images of the left and right ventricles, the left and right atria, and the aorta (Figure 11.II.4) and pulmonary artery from the left side for more detailed evaluations (Figure 11.II.5). M mode evaluation of the ventricles and aortic valve are useful to derive functional indices that are generated from right short-axis images (Figure 11.II.3). The same basic 2DE images are used to interrogate the valves with color flow Doppler echocardiography (CFD) (Figure 11.II.6) while spectral Doppler images of the aortic and pulmonic outflow tracts can provide additional information on cardiac function (Figure 11.II.1). These basic 2DE imaging planes are also used for interrogation of myocardial velocity and strain with TVI and STE imaging (Figures 11.II.1 and 11.II.3). In foals, unlike adults, it may be possible to obtain near-apical images by placing the ultrasound transducer in a subcostal location (Figure 11.II.4) and due to the more optimal

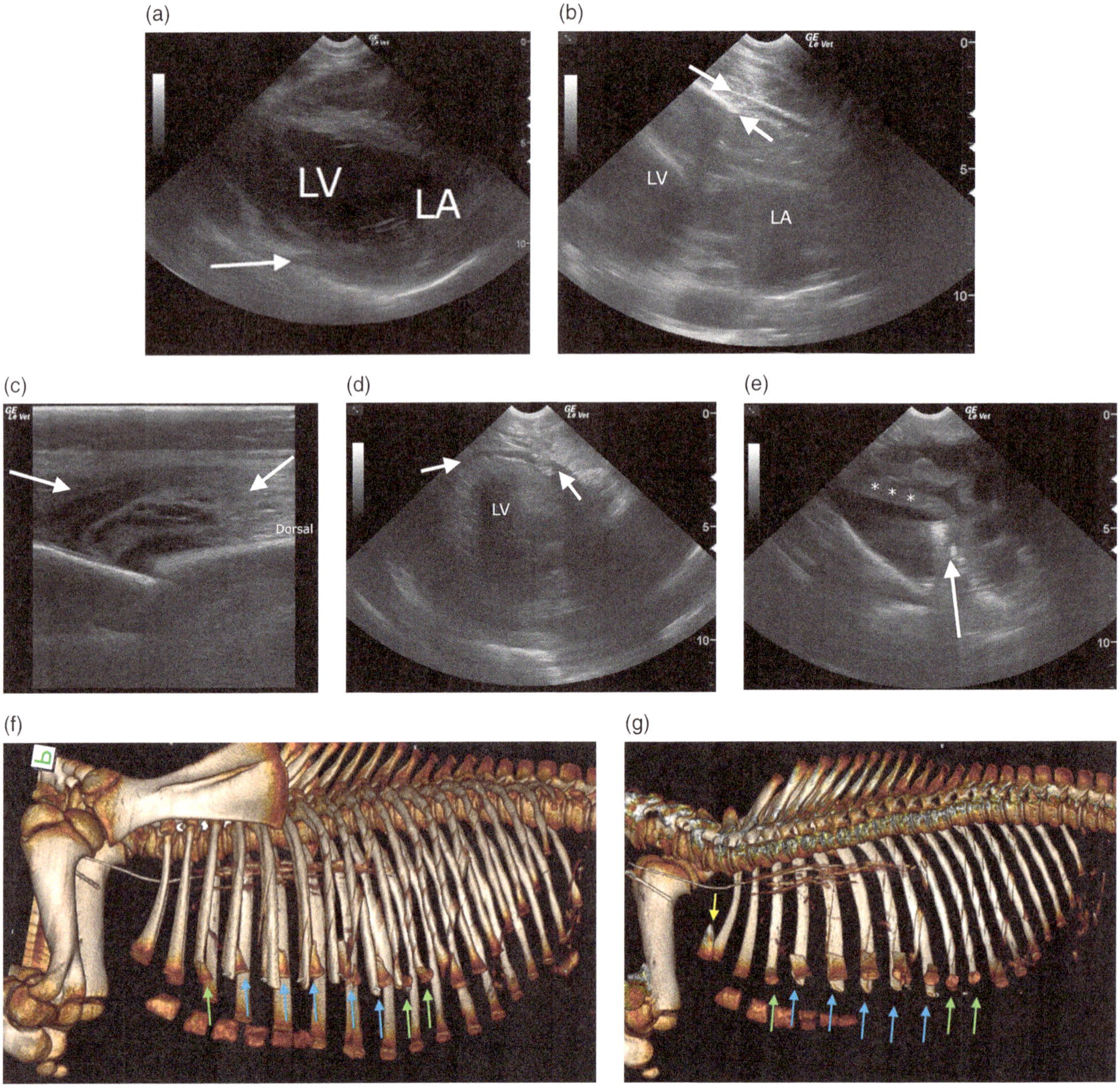

Figure 11.II.2 Ultrasonography is essential for evaluating the consequences of rib fractures. If rib fractures are suspected, it is prudent to begin the echocardiogram on the opposite side of the fracture(s). (a) In this right parasternal long-axis image, a displaced fragment (arrow) can be seen adjacent to the left ventricle (LV). (b) From the left long-axis image of the LV and left atrium (LA), the ventral fragment is displaced medial to the dorsal portion. The arrows indicate how the two fragments overlap. (c) Closeup image of the displaced fragments showing hemorrhage around the fracture site (between arrows). (d) Small amount of fluid within the pericardial sac (arrows) in short-axis image. (e) On both sides of the mediastinum (*) there is free fluid (likely blood) within the pleural cavity that is seen with some irregularity near the ventral aspect of the left lung (arrow). CT images displaying the rib cage for the right lateral aspect (f) and right medial aspect (g) demonstrating multiple rib fractures: there are complete, axial displaced overriding rib fractures (blue arrows) of the right 4th–8th ribs and green stick fractures (green arrows) with distal ends displaced axially of the right 3rd, 9th, and 10th ribs. Note various other lines that are visible across the ribs relate to movement due to respiration, and a portion of the unfractured left first rib (yellow arrow); an intravenous catheter and a nasogastric tube are visible.

alignment this may be useful for spectral Doppler [8], 3DE and TVI; the latter is a Doppler-based technology and is most accurate in determining velocity parallel to the interrogating sound beam. Key features of the echocardiographic examination are summarized in Table 11.II.1.

Echocardiographic Variables

Echocardiographic variables can be loosely classified into those providing information on structure and those that reflect cardiac function. Reference ranges are considered to

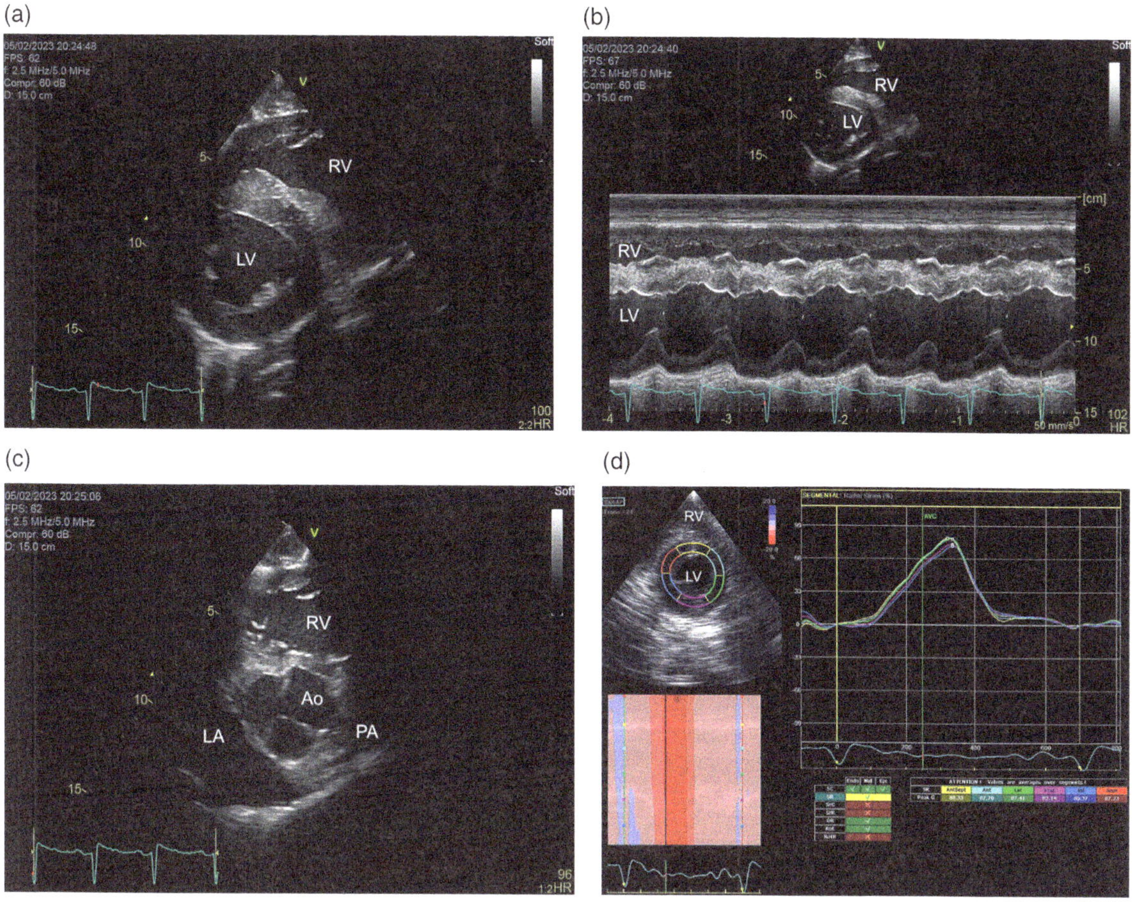

Figure 11.II.3 A series of right parasternal short axis-images from neonatal foals showing (a) left (LV) and right (RV) ventricles at the chordal level. (b) M mode image from the same location, note that the cursor (yellow dotted line) bisects the LV adequately but does not cross the RV at its widest point as a result of the crescent shape of the RV, thus this image is not an accurate means of measuring the RV. (c) The left atrium (LA), aorta (Ao) and pulmonary artery (PA) obtained by moving the imaging plane more dorsally and rotating a few degrees clockwise. (d) Short-axis images of the LV are used to assess radial and circumferential strain with speckle tracking echocardiography. This example shows tracking at the LV apex, the plot on the right displays radial strain in six segments; the left lower panel is an M mode depiction of strain, with locations denoted by the colors shown in the 2D image in the left upper panel. The box lists peak systolic strain measured at the points indicated by the boxes on the plot above.

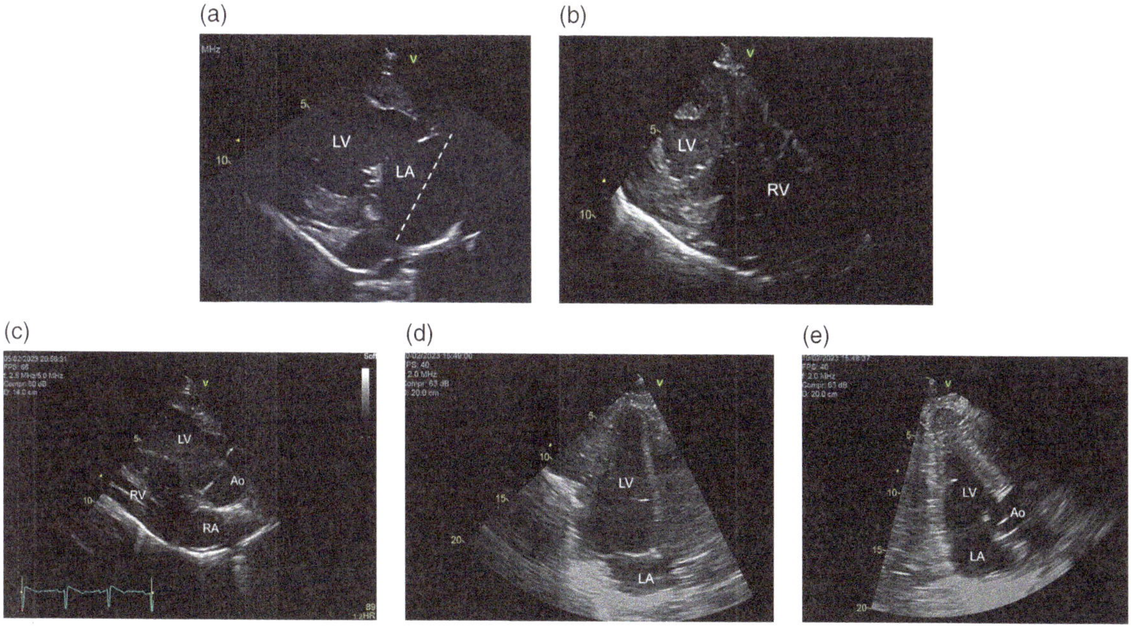

Figure 11.II.4 A series of left parasternal images from neonatal foals. (a) Left ventricle (LV) and left atrium (LA) in long axis. The dotted line indicates measurement of the LA at its maximal diameter. (b) The LV in short axis at the level of the papillary muscles. (c) Image of the aorta (Ao), right ventricle (RV), and right atrium (RA) can be used for spectral Doppler sample volume placement and in adults, this image is used for measurements of the RV and for RV strain, techniques that have yet to be validated in foals. (d) Subcostal image of the LV and LA. (e). Subcostal image of the LV, LA, and Ao.

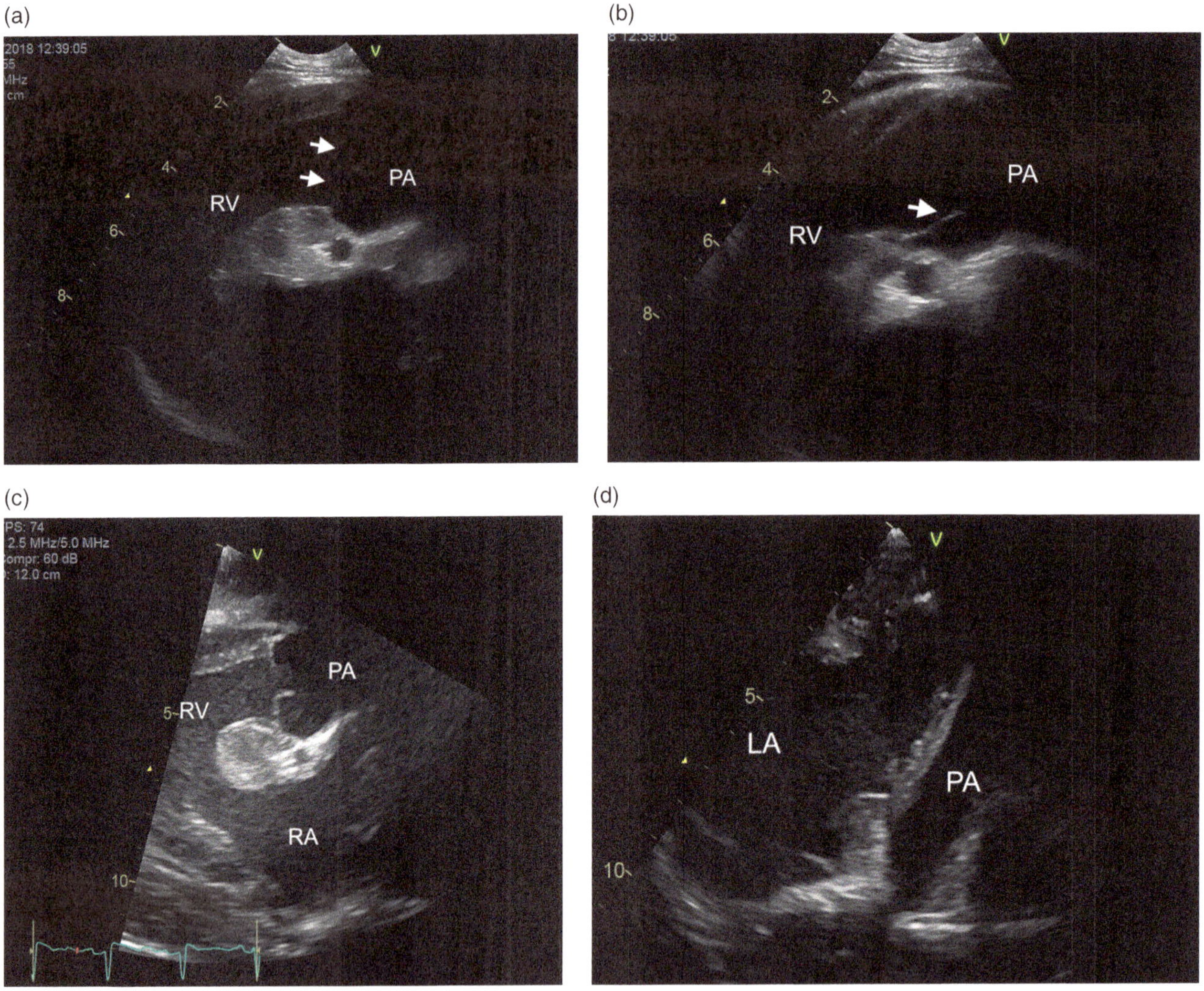

Figure 11.II.5 A series of left parasternal images focusing on the pulmonary artery (PA). (a) From a cranial, long-axis orientation, the pulmonary valve cusps (arrowhead) can be examined. (b) In the same plane, orientating slightly dorsally, more of the PA is visualized. (c) The PA can be examined in a similar plane by placing the transducer on the triceps muscle: this has the advantage of moving the structures of interest out of the near field to optimize focusing and is particularly helpful when only transducers with mid to deep penetration are available. (d) Orientating obliquely and dorsally, the left branch of the PA can be located running dorsally over the left atrium (LA). RV, right ventricle; RA, right atrium.

be breed-specific and data on a wide range of breeds is lacking. Information exists for Thoroughbreds, including a formula developed in foals up to 16 weeks of age to allow for a range of weights [9]. Reference ranges for pony foals are also available [10] but this information is lacking for other breeds. In the absence of breed-specific data, subjective assessment of chamber size is very important; it is useful for the clinician to bear in mind that comparing chambers within an individual can be helpful. For example, the diameter of left atrium, in a left long-axis image plane, should be only slightly larger than the left ventricular internal diameter in a right long-axis four-chambered image plane and, while in the adult the right ventricular internal diameter should be no more than one third of the left ventricle, in the young foal undergoing cardiovascular adaptation the right ventricle is often a little above one third. In the newborn foal, the right ventricular wall is relatively thick compared to adults but neither ventricle should be rounded at the apex. Foals that are hypovolemic may have very empty/small ventricles. In the presence of pericardial effusion, the right and, with increasing severity, the left chambers may be compressed.

Functional indices are used most often to assess individuals that are compromised but have normal cardiac anatomy, and this can be most useful in the presence of hypovolemia and multi-organ failure regardless of the underlying cause.

There are a variety of options available to estimate cardiac output. Doppler estimates are based on measurement of the vessel cross-sectional area (calculated from diameter), the heart rate, and the Doppler spectral

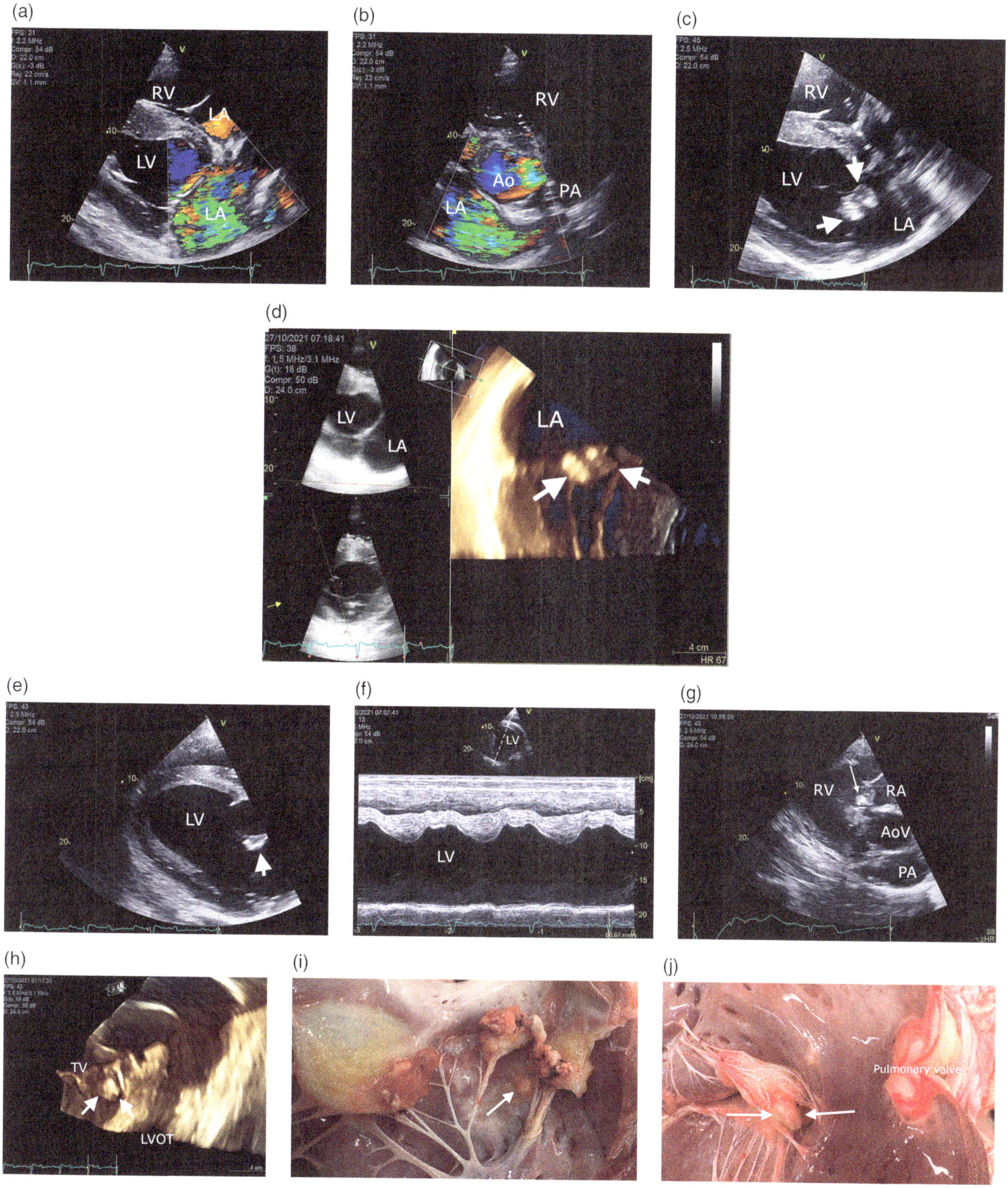

Figure 11.II.6 Long (a) and short (b) axis right parasternal images in which the large area of green signal on color flow Doppler echocardiography, filling the entire left atrium (LA), confirms severe mitral regurgitation in a 5-month-old Thoroughbred presenting with lethargy and fever due to infective endocarditis. (c) Two-dimensional four-chamber and (d) Three-dimensional (3DE) images show large vegetations (white arrows) are present on the mitral valve. In the 3DE image the chorda associated with the right papillary muscle are visible behind the lesions that sit on the lower aspect of both the septal and nonseptal cusps. In the lower left panel, the yellow arrow illustrates the imaging direction and the dotted line, the imaging plane. (e) The apex of the left ventricle (LV) is rounded, and (f) in the M mode image of the LV, the movement of the septum and LV free wall is exaggerated, reflecting volume overload associated with the severe mitral regurgitation. A vegetation (arrow) is visible under the septal cusp of the tricuspid valve in 2DE (g) and 3DE (h) images. Gross postmortem showing (i) vegetations on both main cups of the mitral valve, a mural lesion in the septal wall (arrow) and (j) on the ventricular aspect of the tricuspid valve (arrows), between the septal and angular cusps. LA, left atrium; LV, left ventricle; RA, right atrium; RV, right ventricle; AoV, aortic valve; PA, pulmonary artery.

Table 11.II.1 Commonly used imaging planes for echocardiography in the foal and their key features.

Image plane and imaging mode	Main features in healthy foals	2DE & M mode measurements[a] and techniques	Advanced echocardiography techniques[b]	Specific lesions to rule in or out
Right parasternal long-axis: With transducer positioned in the fourth intercostal space and aligned at approximately 10° from vertical (Figure 11.II.1).				
Four-chamber view, 2DE, 3DE, CFD	Orientating slightly caudally, visualize the right atrium, right ventricle, left atrium and left ventricle. Note the right ventricle can be large relative to the left in healthy foals.	Apply bullet formula for cardiac output.	3DE assessment of valve anatomy and chamber structure and volumetric indices. STE assessment of longitudinal left ventricular strain and displacement, and TVI assessment of left atrial function.	Assess valve anatomy and chamber structure. Expect to see foramen ovale. Check for patency, mitral regurgitation, and pericardial effusion.
Left ventricular outflow view, 2DE, 3DE, CFD	Orientating straight across the chest, visualize the aorta and parts of the left and right ventricle and atria. The right branch of the pulmonary artery lies deep to the aorta. Coronary arteries arise from the aorta.	2DE Aortic diameter diastole = 2.8–3.05 cm	3DE assessment of valve anatomy and chamber structure.	Assess valve and chamber structure and attachments. Look for ventricular septal defects, aortic and tricuspid regurgitation, and pulmonary dilation. Aligning slightly cranially, look for flow from the aorta to the pulmonary artery via the ductus arteriosus.
Right ventricular outflow view, 2DE, CFD, spectral Doppler	Orientating cranially, visualize the right atrium and ventricle and right ventricular outflow tract along with the pulmonary artery branches.	2DE pulmonary artery diameter diastole = 2.83–3.09 cm. Determine pulmonic VTI for cardiac output estimate, right ventricular systolic time intervals and VTI.	TVI assessment of right ventricular function.	Assess valve and chamber structure and attachments. Look for pulmonary regurgitation and pulmonary dilation and use for placement of spectral Doppler cursor/sample volume for pulmonic outflow.
Right parasternal short-axis: With transducer positioned in the fourth intercostal space and aligned at approximately 10° from horizontal (Figure 11.II.3).				
Aortic view, 2DE, M mode, CFD, spectral Doppler	Visualize the aorta, aortic valve cusps, pulmonary artery and its branches. The pulmonary artery branches and coronary arteries arise from the aorta.			Assess valve structure and anatomy of great vessels. Look for doubly committed ventricular septal defect; use to guide M mode cursor placement for aortic M mode and for placement of spectral Doppler cursor/sample volume for pulmonic outflow.

Mitral valve view, 2DE, CFD	Visualize mitral and tricuspid valve cusps.			Assess valve structure, use to assess mitral regurgitation.
Ventricular view, 2DE, M mode, CFD	Visualize left and right ventricles.	Apply bullet formula for cardiac output M mode interventricular. Septal thickness in diastole = 1.47–1.65 cm Left ventricular internal diameter in diastole = 5.09–5.76 cm. Left ventricular free wall thickness in diastole = 1.00–1.19 cm. Interventricular septal thickness in systole = 2.14–2.44 cm. Left ventricular internal diameter in systole = 3.35–3.90 cm. Left ventricular free wall thickness in systole = 1.55–1.84 cm. Fractional shortening percentage = 29.6–36.4. This may be slightly lower in young neonates.	TVI assessment of left ventricular function.	Assess chamber structure and size. Look for pericardial effusion and muscular ventricular septal defects. Use to 2DE image to guide M mode cursor placement for ventricular M mode.
Left parasternal long-axis (Figures 11.II.4 and 11.II.5)				
Left ventricular and atrial view, 2DE, 3DE, CFD, TVI Near-apical and subcostal imaging planes are possible in foals, which may be more appropriate for CFD, 3DE, and TVI than parasternal imaging.	Obtain from fifth intercostal space, orientating roughly vertically. Visualize left atrium and ventricle and caudal vena cava transversely.	2DE Left atrial diameter 5.35–6.02 cm	3DE assessment of valve anatomy and chamber structure, and TVI assessment of left atrial function.	Assess valve structure and chamber size. Use to identify mitral regurgitation.
Aortic view, 2DE, CFD, TVI, spectral Doppler	Obtain from fourth intercostal space, orientating slightly dorsocranially. Visualize aortic outflow, right ventricle and atrium.	Determine aortic VTI for cardiac output estimate	TVI assessment of right ventricular function.	Assess valve structure. Use to identify aortic regurgitation and for placement of spectral Doppler cursor/sample volume for aortic outflow.

(*Continued*)

Table 11.II.1 (Continued)

Image plane and imaging mode	Main features in healthy foals	2DE & M mode measurements[a] and techniques	Advanced echocardiography techniques[b]	Specific lesions to rule in or out
Pulmonic view, 2DE, CFD	Obtain from third intercostal space orientating slightly dorsocranially. Can image through triceps muscle. Visualize pulmonary artery.			Assess valve structure. Use to identify pulmonic regurgitation and subjectively assess pulmonary artery size. Look for retrograde flow in pulmonary artery with patent ductus arteriosus.
Caudal pulmonic view, 2DE (oblique)	Visualize pulmonary artery branches; left courses over left atrial roof.			Assess great vessel anatomy.
Left parasternal short-axis (Figure 11.II.4)				
Left ventricular view, 2DE, 3D, TVI	Obtain from fifth intercostal space, orientating roughly horizontally.		TVI assessment of left ventricular function.	Assess valve structure and chamber anatomy, use to assess mitral regurgitation.

2DE, two-dimensional echocardiography; STE, speckle tracking echocardiography; TVI, tissue velocity imaging; CFD, color flow Doppler echocardiography; VTI, velocity time-integral.
[a] Data represent 95% confidence intervals for healthy Thoroughbred foals aged 1 week and weighing 61.7 ± 6.5 kg (mean + standard deviation) [8].
[b] Foal-specific information is currently lacking.

velocity-time-integral, while there are several options available to estimate volumes from M mode and 2DE measurements of the left ventricle; all make assumptions on ventricular geometry that may lead to errors. Validation studies in healthy anesthetized equine neonates suggest the Bullet method (Figures 11.II.1, 11.II.3, and 11.II.7) is the most appropriate [11]. For this measurement, the left ventricular length is measured, at end systole and diastole, from the four-chambered view (Figure 11.II.1) and the cross-sectional area of the left ventricle is traced, at end systole and diastole, at the chordal level (Figure 11.II.3) [2]. Many ultrasonographic units are equipped to perform this measurement automatically. It is likely that estimates of volumes based on 3DE will be more accurate, but this has yet to be established in foals. It is very important to recognize the limitations of echocardiographic estimates of volume and these measurements are perhaps best used to monitor trends within an individual. The function of the left ventricle can be assessed using fractional shortening, but this commonly used variable is limited insofar that it is a measurement made in one radial plane. STE is easy to perform in adult horses and has shown considerable promise in the identification of myocardial dysfunction in longitudinal, circumferential, and radial planes in adults

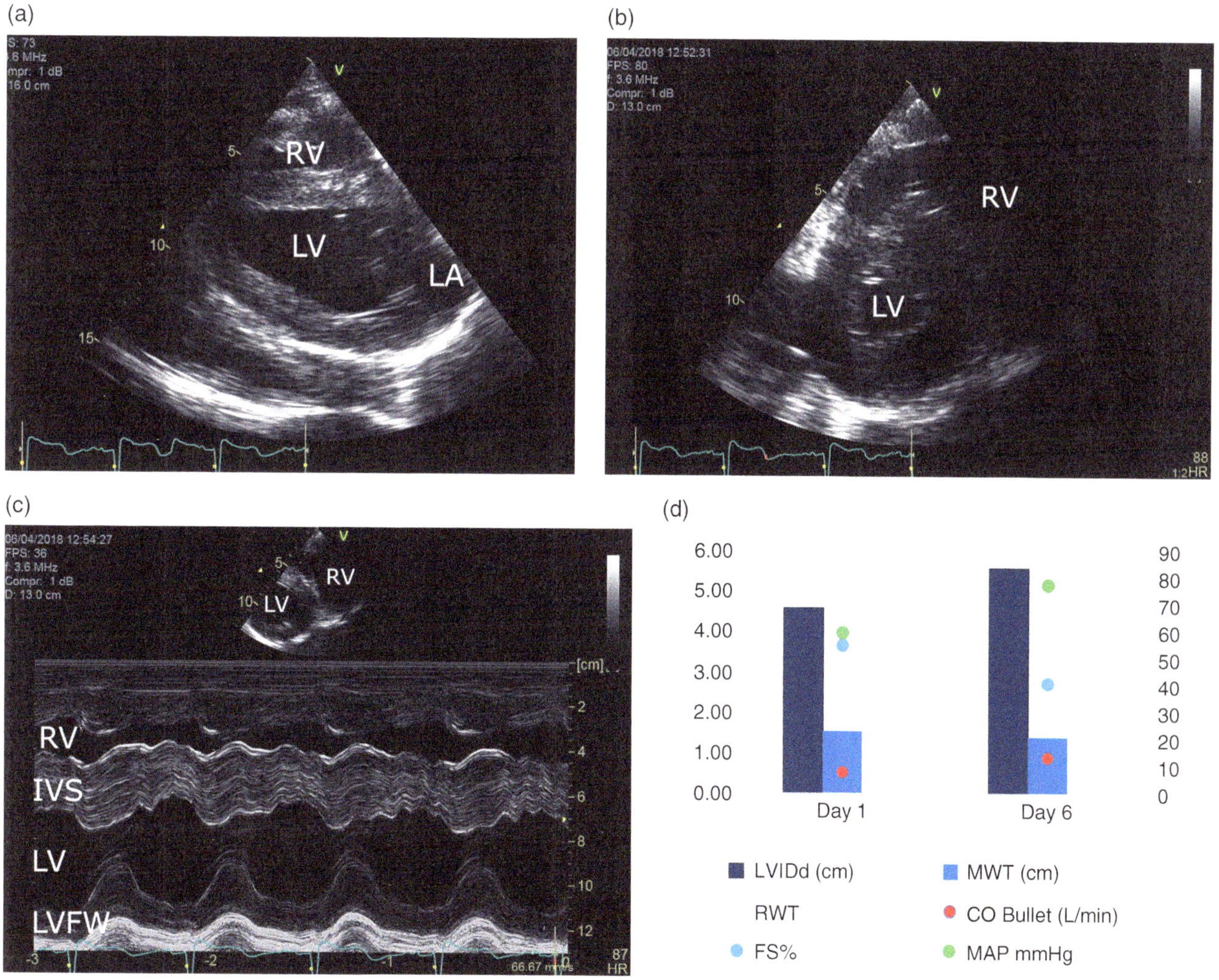

Figure 11.II.7 Echocardiographic images and data from a newborn foal showing signs of neonatal maladjustment and multi-organ failure, including respiratory and gastrointestinal dysfunction. (a) On day 1, four-chamber images of the left (LV) and right (RV) ventricles, and left atrium (LA); subjectively, the left chambers have small diameters. This imaging plane is used to measure the length of the LV to apply the Bullet formula. (b) A short-axis image of the LV and RV show a very small LV diameter. (c) M mode image confirms that the LV free wall (LVFW) and interventricular septum (IVS) are relatively thick. (d) This graph compares data on day 1 and day 6, when the foal's cardiovascular function had stablized. On day 1, cardiac output (CO) and hypovolemia is demonstrated with the high relative (RWT) and mean wall thicknesses (MWT) and low LV internal diameter in diastole (LVIDd). Fractional shortening (FS%) is extremely high, indicating there is little benefit expected if the rate of the dobutamine infusion that the foal is receiving is increased. By day 6, normalization of these variables has occurred. RWT = LVFWd + IVSd/LVIDd; MWT = (LVFWd + IVSd)/2; FS% = (LVIDd − LVIDs)/LVIDd; SV Bullet = (5/6 × LVAd × LVLd) − (5/6 × LVAs × LVLs); CO = SV × HR; SV = stroke volume; LVL = LV length; LVA = LV area.

[12, 13]. Hypohydration results in 'pseudohypertrophy' with decreased left ventricular size and, subjectively the heart appears thickened while relative wall thickness (RWT) is increased (Figure 11.II.7). In adult horses, RWT is a sensitive and specific parameter for identification of hypohydration [14], but this has not been validated in foals. In the hypotensive foal, ventricular assessment can aid in immediate clinical decision-making to gain an understanding on whether ventricular volumes are low and the foal might benefit from changes to the fluid therapy plan; when ventricular movement is very low, this might suggest an inotrope would be helpful or conversely, in the presence of hypotension and exaggerated ventricular movement in a foal already receiving inotropes, seeking to address the problem with pressor agents might be more logical than relying on further increases in inotropic support and volume expansion (Figure 11.II.7).

Pulmonary hypertension leads to dilation of the pulmonary artery, which is most easily recognized by comparing the diameter of the aorta with that of the pulmonary artery seen in the right long-axis left ventricular outflow tract imaging plane (Figure 11.II.8). Pulmonary hypertension can also lead to right ventricular chamber enlargement (Figure 11.II.8), reduced right ventricular systolic function, pericardial effusion [15] and right-to-left shunting of blood across the foramen ovale [6, 16]. Pulmonary

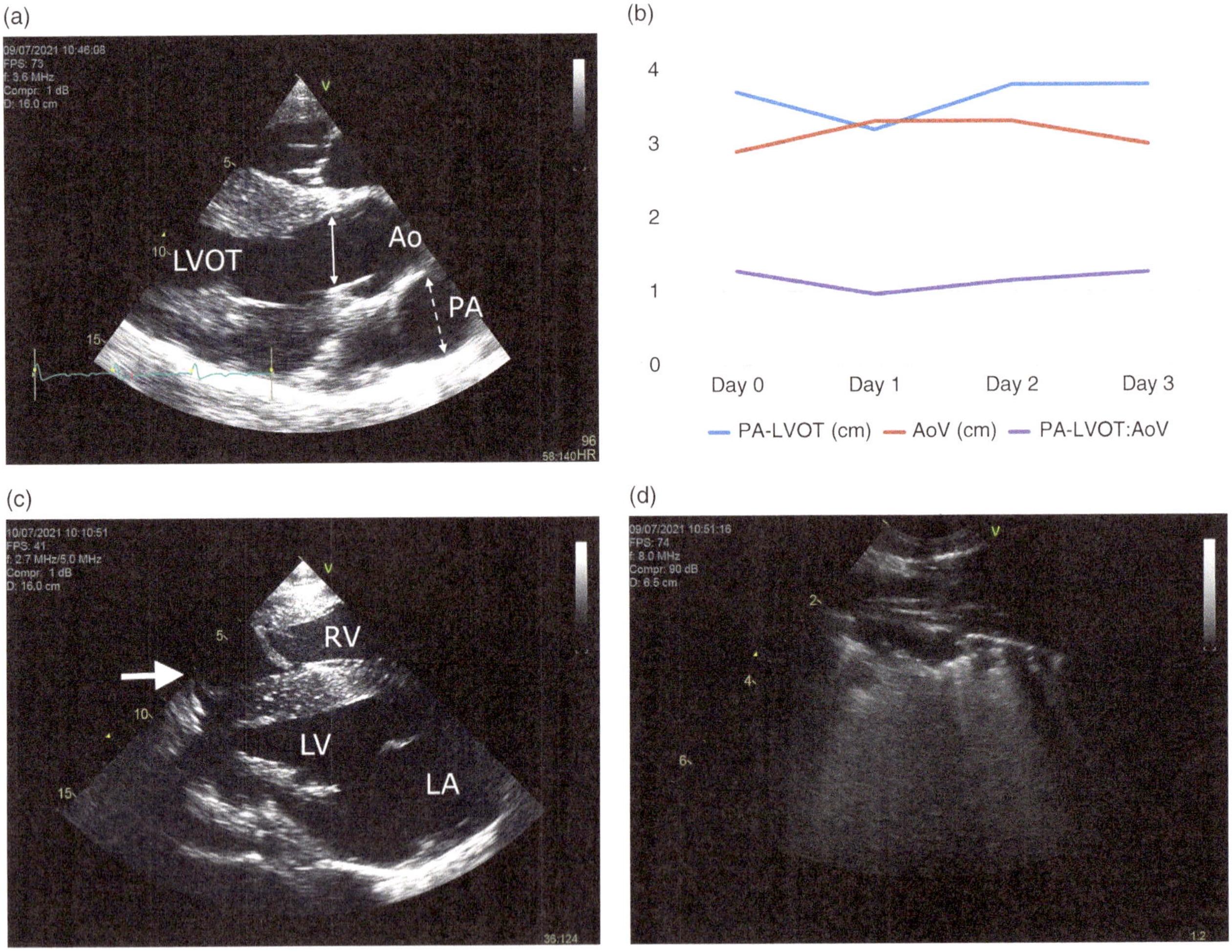

Figure 11.II.8 (a) A long-axis image of the left ventricular outflow tract (LVOT) from a 4-month-old Thoroughbred with severe pneumonia showing how the aortic diameter is measured at the valve level (arrow) and pulmonary artery (PA) diameter is measured in the same image (dashed arrow). (b) From day 0 (admission) to day 1, there was a decrease in PA diameter and the PA-LVOT-Ao ratio in response to therapy with intra-nasal oxygen, furosemide, sildanefil, dexamethasone, rifampin, and clarithromycin; this ratio subsequently increased as a result of pulmonary artery dilation and reduction in the AoV associated with declining cardiac output from day 2 and day 3, reflecting continuing progression of the foal's primary problem. (c) Four-chamber view shows that the apex of the right ventricle (RV) is rounded (arrow) and its wall is hypertrophied with a similar thickness to that of the left ventricle (LV). (d) A representative example of the pulmonary ultrasonographic findings demonstrating multifocal areas of consolidation. PA-LVOT, pulmonary artery diameter from the long-axis image of the LVOT; AoV, aortic diameter at the valve level; PAV RIO, pulmonary artery diameter at the valve level from the right inflow-outflow image; PAS RIO, pulmonary artery diameter at the sinus level from the right inflow-outflow image; PA-LVOT : AoV = ratio of PA & Ao diameters, both measured in the LVOT image.

hypertension is also associated with changes in right ventricular systolic time intervals in human infants and severity and maximal velocities of tricuspid regurgitation [17] can provide similar estimates but have yet to be validated in foals; they are slightly more technically challenging than the simple 2D measures and their repeatability in foal is unknown.

Congenital Cardiac Disease and the Segmental Exam

In assessing the anatomy of the heart when congenital heart disease is suspected, a segmental approach is advocated. Each chamber should be evaluated independently using its inherent echocardiographic characteristics and its connections to other structures confirmed. The specific steps involved in a segmental echocardiographic assessment are summarized in Table 11.II.2.

Acquired Cardiac Disease in Foals

Echocardiography is the primary tool for identification of all forms of structural acquired cardiac disease. Infective endocarditis can affect any valve or involve the chamber walls (mural endocarditis) and multiple sites may be involved (Figure 11.II.6) [57]. Echocardiographically, lesions typically are nodular or vegetative in appearance and the inflammatory process can predispose to additional lesions such as rupture of the chorda tendineae [58]. Vegetations can lead to regurgitation or stenosis, which is best assessed with Doppler echocardiographic techniques (Figure 11.II.6). Based on echocardiography alone, it can be difficult to distinguish dysplasia from chronic endocarditis because both processes can lead to disruption of valvular anatomy. Consideration of accompanying clinical and laboratory findings will often help make this distinction.

Mild pericardial effusion can be the result of sepsis, pulmonary hypertension, or arrhythmia but the main rule

Table 11.II.2 Segmental echocardiographic exam.

Step 1: Atrial morphology and arrangement: The right atrium has a triangular appendage and left atrium is tubular and narrow based. Echocardiographic findings in congenital right atrial diverticulum has been reported [18] and atrial septal defects can occur in isolation [5, 19, 20] or as part of complex conditions [21].

Step 2: Ventricular morphology and arrangement: The right ventricle has coarse apical trabeculations, the leaflet of the atrioventricular valve attaches directly to the septum, moderator band, and septomarginal trabeculations. The left ventricle has fine trabeculations and a smooth upper part of the septum without attachment of the atrioventricular valve. The ventricular morphology can be indeterminate (i.e. a solitary ventricle with no ventricular septum) [22, 23]. Hypoplastic ventricles are complete or incomplete and lack the inlet portion [19, 22, 24, 25].

Step 3: Atrioventricular connections: There are two atria either connected to the appropriate ventricle (concordant) or not (discordant). Biatrial, univentricular connections occur where the atria connect to only one ventricle (double inlet) [22] or one atrium ends blindly in a muscular floor at the atrioventricular junction (artioventricular valve atresia) [26–28]. Usually, the connected ventricle is dominant and the nonconnected ventricle is hypoplastic. Solitary ventricles and uniatrial, biventricular connection can also occur.

Step 4: Atrioventricular valves: Evaluate number of cusps [23, 26, 29, 30], their shape and connections and for regurgitation and stenosis [23, 27, 28, 30–34].

Step 5: Ventriculo-arterial connections: Identify vessels by their specific features: coronary arteries originate from the aorta and the main pulmonary artery branches. If there are two great vessels, these are either connected to the appropriate ventricle (concordant) or not (discordant, i.e. transposition of the great arteries), [34–36] or double outlet [35, 37]. Vessels may be atretic and difficult or impossible to locate [1, 38] or there may be a single vessel (common arterial trunk) [39, 40].

Step 6: Arterial valves: Evaluate number of cusps [1, 41], their shape [42] and connections and examine for regurgitation and stenosis.

Step 7: Associated malformations: Evaluate for the following specific lesions:

- Shunts
  - Atrial, atrioventricular and ventricular septal defects [43, 44]. Both can occur as solitary anomalies but ventricular septal defects are also a common component of complex congenital malformations including Tetralogy of Fallot [45, 46].
  - Patent ductus arteriosus [47]
  - Aorto-pulmonary window [48]
- Outflow tract obstructions [1, 49, 50]
- Coronary abnormalities [51]
- Anomalies of systemic and pulmonary venous connections [52]
- Abnormalities of the aorta [53] and aortic arch [54–56]

outs for pericardial effusion are hemopericardium relating to rib fracture and pericarditis. Rib fractures are extremely common in equine neonates [2, 59]; many will heal with minimal to no clinical consequences provided intrathoracic trauma is minimal. However, when the ribs over the heart are involved, rib fracture can be associated with pericardial contusion and variable degrees of hemopericardium. Foals with hemopericardium can be managed conservatively but consideration should be given to surgical stabilization [60–62], particularly where there are additional risk factors for fatal pericardial hemorrhage such as recumbency and weakness or where echocardiography demonstrates that the pericardial effusion is becoming more severe (Figure 11.II.2). Computed tomography is particularly useful for detailed assessment of the fracture configuration and surgical planning (Figure 11.II.2). Fibrinous pericarditis and cardiac tamponade have been reported occasionally in foals presenting with signs of right heart dysfunction, ventral edema and jugular distension [63, 64].

References

1 Marr, C.M. (2010). Cardiac murmurs: congenital heart disease. In: *Cardiology of the Horse*, 2e (ed. C.M. Marr and I.M. Bowen), 187–200. Edinburgh: Saunders Elsevier.

2 Marr, C.M. (2015). The equine neonatal cardiovascular system in health and disease. *Vet. Clin. North Am. Equine Pract.* 31: 545–565.

3 Reef, V.B. (1985). Cardiovascular disease in the equine neonate. *Vet. Clin. North Am. Equine Pract.* 1: 117–129.

4 Reef, V.B. (1991). Echocardiographic findings in horses with congenital cardiac disease. *Compend. Contin. Educ. Pract. Vet.* 13: 109–117.

5 Redpath, A., Marr, C.M., Bullard, C. et al. (2020). Real-time three-dimensional (3D) echocardiographic characterisation of an atrial septal defect in a horse. *Vet. Med. Sci.* 6: 661–665.

6 Vernemmen, I., Paulussen, E., Dauvillier, J. et al. (2022). Three-dimensional and catheter-based intracardiac echocardiographic characterization of the interatrial septum in 2 horses with suspicion of a patent foramen ovale. *J. Vet. Intern. Med.* 36: 1535–1542.

7 Marr, C.M. and Bain, F.T. (2010). Ventricular Septal Defects. In: *Cardiology of the Horse*, 2e (ed. C.M. Marr and I.M. Bowen), 196. Edinburgh: Saunders Elsevier.

8 Freccero, F., Cordella, A., Dondi, F. et al. (2018). Feasibility of the echocardiographic subcostal view in newborn foals: two-dimensional and Doppler aortic findings. *Equine Vet. J.* 50: 865–869.

9 Collins, N., Palmer, L., and Marr, C.M. (2010). Two-dimensional and M-mode echocardiographic measurements of cardiac dimensions in healthy Thoroughbred foals. *Aust. Vet. J.* 88: 428–433.

10 Lombard, C.W., Evans, M., Martin, L. et al. (1984). Blood pressure, electrocardiogram and echocardiogram measurements in the growing pony foal. *Equine Vet. J.* 16: 342–347.

11 Giguère, S., Bucki, E., and Adin, D. (2005). Cardiac output measurement by partial carbon dioxide rebreathing, 2-dimensional echocardiography, and lithium-dilution method in anesthetized neonatal foals. *J. Vet. Intern. Med.* 19: 737–743.

12 Decloedt, A., Verheyen, T., Sys, S. et al. (2012). Tissue Doppler imaging and 2-dimensional speckle tracking of left ventricular function in horses exposed to lasalocid. *J. Vet. Intern. Med.* 26: 1209–1216.

13 Decloedt, A., Verheyen, T., Sys, S. et al. (2011). Quantification of left ventricular longitudinal strain, strain rate, velocity, and displacement in healthy horses by 2-dimensional speckle tracking. *J. Vet. Intern. Med.* 25: 330–338.

14 Underwood, C., Norton, J.L., Nolen-Walston, R.D. et al. (2011). Echocardiographic changes in heart size in hypohydrated horses. *J. Vet. Intern. Med.* 25: 563–569.

15 El-Kersh, K., Zhao, C., Elliott, G. et al. (2023). Derivation of a risk score (REVEAL-ECHO) based on echocardiographic parameters of patients with pulmonary arterial hypertension. *Chest* (in press).

16 Lakshminrusumha, S. (2012). The pulmonary circulation in neonatal respiratory failure. *Clin. Perinatol.* 39: 655–683.

17 Benatar, A., Clarke, J., and Silverman, M. (1995). Pulmonary hypertension in infants with chronic lung disease: non-invasive evaluation and short term effect of oxygen treatment. *Arch. Dis. Child.* 72: F14–F19.

18 Patterson-Kane, J.C. and Harrison, L.R. (2002). Giant right atrial diverticulum in a foal. *J. Vet. Diagn. Investig.* 14: 335–337.

19 Physick-Sheard, P.W., Maxie, M.G., Palmer, N.C. et al. (1985). Atrial septal defect of the persistent ostium primum type with hypoplastic right ventricle in a Welsh pony foal. *Can. J. Comp. Med.* 49: 429–433.

20 Taylor, F.G., Wotton, P.R., Hillyer, M.H. et al. (1991). Atrial septal defect and atrial fibrillation in a foal. *Vet. Rec.* 128: 80–81.

21 Rahal, C., Collatos, C., and Bildfell, R. (1997). Pentalogy of Fallot, renal infarction and renal abscess in a mare. *J. Equine Vet. Sci.* 17: 604–607.

22 Sedacca, C.D., Bright, J.M., and Boon, J. (2010). Doppler echocardiographic description of double-inlet left ventricle in an Arabian horse. *J. Vet. Cardiol.* 12: 147–153.

23 Kraus, M.S., Pariaut, R., Alcaraz, A. et al. (2005). Complete atrioventricular canal defect in a foal: clinical and pathological features. *J. Vet. Cardiol.* 7: 59–64.

24 Tadmor, A., Fischel, R., and Tov, A.S. (1983). A condition resembling hypoplastic left heart syndrome in a foal. *Equine Vet. J.* 15: 175–177.

25 Musselman, E.E. and LoGuidice, R.J. (1984). Hypoplastic left ventricular syndrome in a foal. *J. Am. Vet. Med. Assoc.* 185: 542–543.

26 Hall, T.L., Magdesian, K.G., and Kittleson, M.D. (2010). Congenital cardiac defects in neonatal foals: 18 cases (1992–2007). *J. Vet. Intern. Med.* 24: 206–212.

27 Bayly, W.M., Reed, S.M., Leathers, C.W. et al. (1982). Multiple congenital heart anomalies in five Arabian foals. *J. Am. Vet. Med. Assoc.* 181: 684–689.

28 Reef, V.B., Mann, P.C., and Orsini, P.G. (1987). Echocardiographic detection of tricuspid atresia in two foals. *J. Am. Vet. Med. Assoc.* 191: 225–228.

29 Duz, M., Philbey, A.W., and Hughes, K.J. (2013). Mitral valve and tricuspid valve dysplasia in a 9-week-old Standardbred colt. *Equine Vet. Educ.* 25: 339–344.

30 Kutasi, O., Voros, K., Biksi, I. et al. (2007). Common atrioventricular canal in a newborn foal-case report and review of the literature. *Acta Vet. Hung.* 55: 51–65.

31 Meurs, K.M., Miller, M.W., Hanson, C. et al. (1997). Tricuspid valve atresia with main pulmonary artery atresia in an Arabian foal. *Equine Vet. J.* 29: 160–162.

32 Honnas, C.M., Puckett, M.J., and Schumacher, J. (1987). Tricuspid atresia in a Quarter horse foal. *Southwestern Vet.* 38: 17–20.

33 McGurrin, M.K., Physick-Sheard, P.W., and Southorn, E. (2003). Parachute left atrioventricular valve causing stenosis and regurgitation in a Thoroughbred foal. *J. Vet. Intern. Med.* 17: 579–582.

34 McClure, J.J., Gaber, C.E., Watters, J.W. et al. (1983). Complete transposition of the great arteries with ventricular septal defect and pulmonary stenosis in a Thoroughbred foal. *Equine Vet. J.* 15: 377–380.

35 Chaffin, M.K., Miller, M.W., and Morris, E.L. (1992). Double outlet right ventricle and other associated congenital cardiac anomalies in an American miniature horse foal. *Equine Vet. J.* 24: 402–406.

36 Sleeper, M.M. and Palmer, J.E. (2005). Echocardiographic diagnosis of transposition of the great arteries in a neonatal foal. *Vet. Radiol. Ultrasound* 46: 259–262.

37 Fennell, L., Church, S., Tyrell, D. et al. (2009). Double-outlet right ventricle in a 10-month-old Friesian filly. *Aust. Vet. J.* 87: 204–209.

38 Young, L.E., Blunden, A.S., Bartram, D.H. et al. (1997). Pulmonary atresia with an intact ventricular septum in a thoroughbred foal. *Equine Vet. Educ.* 9: 123–127.

39 Stephen, J.O., Abbott, J., Middleton, D.M. et al. (2000). Persistent truncus arteriosus in a Bashkir Curly foal. *Equine Vet. Educ.* 12: 251–255.

40 Jesty, S.A., Wilkins, P.A., Palmer, J.E. et al. (2007). Persistent truncus arteriosus in two Standardbred foals. *Equine Vet. Educ.* 19: 307–311.

41 Michlik, K.M., Biazik, A.K., Henklewski, R.Z. et al. (2014). Quadricuspid aortic valve and a ventricular septal defect in a horse. *BMC Vet. Res.* 10: 142.

42 Taylor, S.E., Else, R.W., and Keen, J.A. (2007). Congenital aortic valve dysplasia in a Clydesdale foal. *Equine Vet. Educ.* 19: 4630468.

43 De Lange, L., Vera, L., Decloedt, A. et al. (2021). Prevalence and characteristics of ventricular septal defects in a non-racehorse equine population (2008–2019). *J. Vet. Intern. Med.* 35 (3): 1573–1581.

44 Reef, V.B. (1995). Evaluation of ventricular septal defects in horses using two-dimensional and Doppler echocardiography. *Equine Vet. J.* 27: 86–95.

45 Houe, H., Koch, J., and Bindseil, E. (1996). Tetraology of Fallot in horses. *Dansk Veterinaertidsskrift* 79: 43–45.

46 Cargille, J., Lombard, C., Wilson, J.H. et al. (1991). Tetralogy of Fallot and segmental uterine dysplasia in a three-year-old Morgan filly. *Cornell Vet.* 81: 411–418.

47 Guarda, H.I., Schifferlis, R.C.A., Alvarez, M.L.H. et al. (2005). A patent ductus arteriosus in a foal. *Wien. Tieraztl. Monatsschr.* 92: 233–237.

48 Valdes-Martinez, A., Easdes, S.C., Strickland, K.N. et al. (2006). Echocardiographic evidence of an aortic-pulmonary septal defect in a 4-day-old thoroughbred foal. *Vet. Radiol. Ultrasound* 47: 87–89.

49 Hinchcliff, K.W. and Adams, W.M. (1991). Critical pulmonic stenosis in a newborn foal. *Equine Vet. J.* 23: 318–320.

50 Gehlen, H., Bubeck, K., and Stadler, P. (2001). Valvular pulmonic stenosis with normal aortic root and intact ventricular and atrial septa in an Arabian horse. *Equine Vet. Educ.* 13: 286–288.

51 Karlstam, E., Ho, S.Y., Shokrai, A. et al. (1999). Anomalous aortic origin of the left coronary artery in a horse. *Equine Vet. J.* 31: 350–352.

52 Seco Diaz, O., Desrochers, A., Hoffmann, V. et al. (2005). Total anomalous pulmonary venous connection in a foal. *Vet. Radiol. Ultrasound* 46: 83–85.

53 Reimer, J.M., Marr, C.M., Reef, V.B. et al. (1993). Aortic origin of the right pulmonary artery and patent ductus arteriosus in a pony foal with pulmonary hypertension and right-sided heart failure. *Equine Vet. J.* 25: 466–468.

54 Bauer, S., Livesey, M.A., Bjorling, D.E. et al. (2006). Computed tomography assisted surgical correction of persistent right aortic arch in a neonatal foal. *Equine Vet. Educ.* 18: 32–36.

55 Coleman, M.C., Norman, T.E., and Wall, C.R. (2014). What is your diagnosis? Persistent right aortic arch. *J. Am. Vet. Med. Assoc.* 244: 1253–1255.

56 Viljoen, A., Saulez, M.N., and Steyl, J. (2012). Right subclavian artery anomaly in an adult Friesian horse. *Equine Vet. Educ.* 24: 62–65.

57 Collatos, C., Clark, E.S., Reef, V.B. et al. (1990). Septicemia, atrial fibrillation, cardiomegaly, left atrial mass, and Rhodococcus equi septic osteoarthritis in a foal. *J. Am. Vet. Med. Assoc.* 197 (8): 1039–1042.

58 Reef, V.B. (1987). Mitral valvular insufficiency associated with ruptured chordae tendineae in three foals. *J. Am. Vet. Med. Assoc.* 191: 329–331.

59 Jean, D., Picandet, V., Macieira, S. et al. (2007). Detection of rib trauma in newborn foals in an equine critical care unit: a comparison of ultrasonography, radiography and physical examination. *Equine Vet. J.* 39: 158–163.

60 Bellezzo, F., Hunt, R.J., Provost, R. et al. (2004). Surgical repair of rib fractures in 14 neonatal foals: case selection, surgical technique and results. *Equine Vet. J.* 36: 557–562.

61 Kolus, C.R., MacLeay, J.M., and Hackett, E.S. (2017). Repair of an acquired diaphragmatic hernia with surgical mesh in a foal. *Can. Vet. J.* 58: 145–148.

62 Kraus, B.M., Richardson, D.W., Sheridan, G. et al. (2005). Multiple rib fracture in a neonatal foal using a nylon strand suture repair technique. *Vet. Surg.* 34: 399–404.

63 Alcott, C.J., Howard, J., Wong, D. et al. (2012). Fibrinous pericarditis and cardiac tamponade in a 3-week-old pony foal. *Equine Vet. Educ.* 25: 328–333.

64 Armstrong, S.K., Raidal, S.L., and Hughes, K.J. (2014). Fibrinous pericarditis and pericardial effusion in three neonatal foals. *Aust. Vet. J.* 92: 392–399.

Section III Advanced Cardiac Monitoring in Foals

Andre Shih

The function of the heart is to pump blood through the circulatory system and ensure prompt distribution of oxygen and nutrients to all cells. Simultaneously, circulation of blood facilitates removal of CO_2 and metabolic byproducts from the blood, thereby ensuring cell survival. A thorough physical examination, complemented by basic hemodynamic monitoring (heart rate, pulse quality, mucous membrane color), is sufficient to provide a superficial understanding of perfusion. However, these parameters do not convey the complete clinical picture. Advanced cardiac monitoring techniques attempt to more completely evaluate cardiovascular function through direct and indirect methods and is routinely measured in human medicine during general anesthesia, in critical care units, and during exercise physiology studies. Equine patients have intrinsic characteristics (body size, temperament, unique anatomical features) that make advanced cardiac monitoring challenging such that even for complex anesthetic procedures, some clinicians simply rely on measurements of heart rate and blood pressure (BP).

After heart rate, BP is the most common parameter measured to evaluate cardiac function. BP is the most important determinant of afterload as it influences perfusion pressure and cardiac output (CO) [1]. The clinician must be aware of the fact that although BP is a reliable surrogate of afterload, it does not evaluate cardiac performance. Clinically, monitoring BP helps assess the cardiovascular status of a patient and provides an acceptable assessment of the quality of tissue perfusion at a specific moment. Interestingly, BP in healthy foals varies significantly. In a study in healthy horses, systolic arterial pressure (SAP) ranged between 86–159 mmHg and diastolic arterial pressure (DAP) ranged between 45–97 mmHg. Mean arterial pressure (MAP) is calculated using the formula: $MAP = DAP + \frac{1}{3}(SAP - DAP)$; calculated MAP for previous values yields a MAP between 58 and 117 mmHg [2, 3].

BP is the product of CO and systemic vascular resistance (SVR); the clinician must be cognizant of the fact that BP does not equate to blood perfusion [1, 3]. Ideally BP should be evaluated together with CO or SVR because if BP is used as a sole surrogate for CO, erroneous conclusions can be made. A low CO in a hypotensive patient likely suggests hypovolemia or decreased cardiac function. Patients with low blood pressure may experience high or optimal CO if SVR is low. A high CO in a hypotensive patient suggests decreased vascular tone [4]. Patients with normal to high blood pressure may experience low CO and poor perfusion if SVR is high.

Due to their size and unique anatomical features, equine patients are prone to hypotension, hypoventilation, and tissue ischemia during anesthesia. Hypotension (MAP <70 mmHg) is one of the most common complications in equine anesthesia [5]. Most sedative agents can cause a direct change in SVR. For example, α-2 agonist can cause vasoconstriction and hypertension. Excessive vasoconstriction or vasodilatation makes arterial pressure an unreliable indicator of worsening cardiac performance. Both hypotension and hypertension should be prevented to avoid the negative impact of abnormal tissue perfusion. Due to the size of the adult horse, hypotension can decrease muscle perfusion and put an anesthetized patient at risk of myopathy or neuropathy; these concerns are less relevant in the neonatal foal because of their smaller size and body weight. Severe hypotension can also lead to renal and cerebral ischemia [6]. Conversely, hypertension can lead to retinal damage or intracranial bleeding [7–9]. The clinical significance of hypo- or hypertension depends on the severity and duration of the underlying cause [7–9].

Equine Neonatal Medicine, First Edition. Edited by David M. Wong and Pamela A. Wilkins.

Blood Pressure Measurement Techniques

Invasive Blood Pressure

Invasive blood pressure (IBP) measurement involves canulation of an artery and connecting the catheter to a transducer. IBP allows beat-to-beat real time monitoring, is the gold standard for accuracy, and is routinely performed during equine anesthesia. In foals, the lateral dorsal metatarsal artery can be used during anesthesia while the transverse facial and facial arteries are most used for arterial catheterization in awake animals [10]. Maintaining an arterial catheter for measurement of IBP in healthy foals poses challenges due to the active nature of the foal, however, some critically ill foals are recumbent, nonmobile, and less responsive. Therefore, IBP could be accomplished in critically ill foals, if indicated and desired. Arterial catheterization is correlated with low complication rates (<1%) in human patients; however, when the catheter is removed, pressure should be applied to the catheter insertion site for 2–5 minutes to prevent hematoma formation [11]. Although uncommon, skin infection and complete obstruction of blood flow have been reported [11, 12].

A 20-gauge catheter is used to cannulate the artery in a foal; once catheterization is complete, the catheter is attached to an electronic pressure transducer that displays systolic, diastolic, and MAP (Figure 11.III.1). The intra-arterial catheter should be connected to the BP transducer via a noncompliable fluid filled extension set. The noncompressible fluid column formed by blood and saline creates a hydraulic coupling that places pressure on a diaphragm plate located inside the transducer that is converted into an electrical signal, which is then displayed as BP graphically [13]. The IBP extension set should be visually inspected for air bubbles, kinks, fluid leaks, obstructions, or clots that lead to damping of the system.

Noninvasive BP Techniques

Noninvasive BP techniques (NIBP) are considered adequate for awake and mobile foals in which arterial catheterization is more challenging and is more frequently used to evaluate BP in ill foals. It is also adequate for monitoring the cardiovascular system in stable patients [14]. In general, the techniques available for noninvasive BP monitoring are subdivided into two major methods: ultrasonic Doppler flow (Doppler) and oscillometric.

The ultrasonic Doppler flow detector (Doppler) has been used in veterinary medicine since 1977 for the measurement of BP and is considered inexpensive and easy to use [15, 16]. The Doppler detects blood flow by emitting an ultrasound signal that hits moving red blood cells and receive its echo sound back; it then transduces it into an auditory signal [17]. Doppler BP requires a piezoelectric crystal probe (8.2 MHz) placed over a superficial artery; in neonatal foals the distal limbs can be used while in adult horses the tail is an excellent location (Figure 11.III.2). The cuff is placed on the limb (foal) or near the base of the tail (adult) and the probe placed over the metatarsal or median coccygeal artery, respectively. It is important not to move the probe during cuff inflation. A cuff with a width of 30–40% of the circumference of the limb/tail area is applied

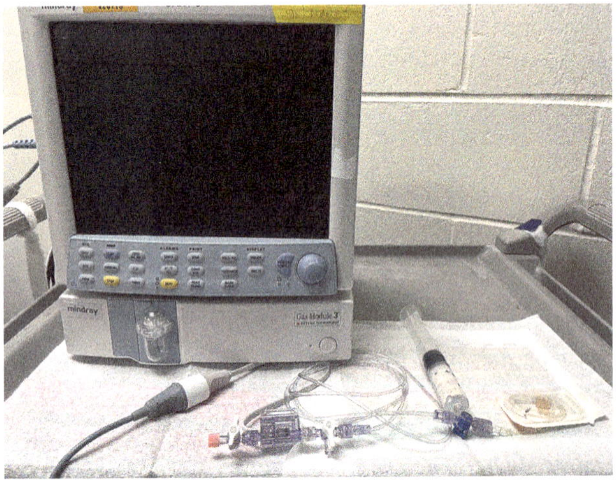

Figure 11.III.1 Equipment needed to measure blood pressure via an arterial catheter (IBP). Once the intra-arterial catheter is placed, it is attached to an electronic pressure transducer that displays the systolic, diastolic, and mean arterial blood pressure. The three-way stopcock is used to flush the catheter with heparinized saline intermittently to prevent clotting of the catheter.

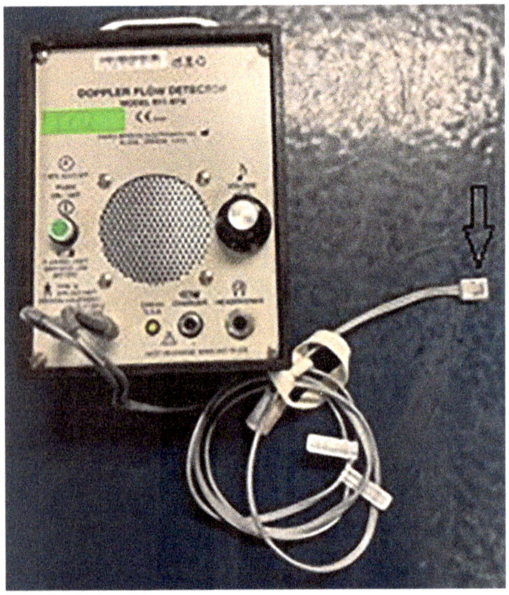

Figure 11.III.2 Doppler flow detector and piezoelectric probe (arrow) used to measure systolic blood pressure from a peripheral artery (e.g. metatarsal artery) in the foal.

proximal to the Doppler probe. The cuff is then inflated with a sphygmomanometer to a pressure high enough to cease the pulsating sounds of the arterial blood flow. The pressure is then slowly released, and the systolic blood pressure (SBP) is identified when the pressure (sound) of arterial pulsation is detected.

The oscillometric method is used in automated NIBP monitors and has been evaluated in foals [18, 19]. This method uses an inflatable cuff or bladder to first obstruct the blood flow from an area over a major peripheral artery. The NIBP device deflates the cuff slowly thus decreasing pressure over the artery. The cuff detects pulsatile amplitude once the pressure is lower than the SAP. The area with higher cuff pressure amplitude is measured as MAP; DAP is calculated through a proprietary algorithm and results are displayed as BP [20, 21]. Peripheral arteries that may be suitable for measuring oscillometric BP in foals include the coccygeal, metatarsal, and median arteries, although the most accurate site can be device dependent [18, 19]. In one study, the investigators concluded that the oscillometric method to determine MAP was best measured with the cuff placed over the coccygeal or dorsal metatarsal artery [18, 19].

Cardiac Output (CO)

In theory, CO is the most important factor to assess cardiovascular function. The reason CO is not routinely measured outside research studies is because it requires specialized equipment and instrumentation that is challenging to accomplish in the clinical setting. CO, defined as the volume of blood pumped out of the heart in the time interval of 1 minute, indicates how well the heart is performing [22]. CO is typically measured in either liters per minute (l/min) or dynes per minute (dm^3/min) [3]. There is significant variation in CO values dependent on patient size and age. CO in healthy neonatal foals is 6.7–7.5 l/min while healthy adult horses the CO is 32–40 l/min [23]. To accommodate for the fact that a bigger animal (e.g. adult horse) has a larger heart chamber, and to make comparisons between variable sized patients, CO is divided by body size and is called the cardiac index (CI). Either the patient's body weight, expressed as $CI_{BW} = CO/BW$ (ml/kg/min), or body surface area (BSA), expressed as $CI_{BSA} = CO/\text{surface area}$ (liters/min/m^2), can be used to express CI [23].

Horses are well-adapted athletic animals, and a knowledge of CO and BP over time is essential for understanding the physiology of exercise and associated BP, heart rate, and cardiac index, which can increase dramatically during exercise. The normal resting CO_{BW} in a healthy adult horse is 72–88 ml/kg/min [24, 25]. During exercise, CO can increase to more than eight times its resting value [24, 25]. Thus, hemodynamic information collected during rest will not predict ramp-up values nor determine exercise performance [24–26].

CO allows for calculation of other cardiovascular parameters for more complete assessment of function. With knowledge of CO and heart rate, one can determine stroke volume (SV). In certain physiological and pathophysiological states, the body's vascular resistance can change. Thus, SVR is calculated from the pressure in the vascular system (difference between MAP and right atrial pressure [RA] divided by CO). Knowledge of SVR allows for safer use of vasopressor and inotrope therapy.

CO, blood hemoglobin concentration, and oxygen saturation of hemoglobin are major factors in determining global tissue oxygen delivery (DO_2) [27]. Shock can be defined as an imbalance between oxygen delivery and oxygen consumption, and many of the supportive care objectives in critical care medicine is to improve DO_2. However, all therapy aimed to increase DO_2 are also associated with some degree of risk. By optimizing DO_2 (using CO monitoring), one can titrate therapy to match the need of the patient, thereby reducing the risk of overzealous treatment [27].

CO Measurement Techniques

Despite significant advantages of CO monitoring, its use is limited in equine medicine due to the invasive nature of many available methods. An excellent review of CO technologies as they pertain to horses is authored by Corley et al. in 2003 [24]; however, newer methods for determination of CO have been established since. When new monitoring techniques are introduced, comparative studies are needed to demonstrate that the measurements are meaningful in different clinical settings and over wide physiological ranges. The choice of the monitoring system depends on the patient (species, size), and the devices and expertise available at a specific hospital. The expertise and familiarity of the operator with the technique represents another critical factor to obtain reliable results with many of the CO monitoring devices available.

There are four basic methods of measuring CO: (i) indicator methods (e.g. pulmonary thermodilution and lithium dilution techniques); (ii) a derivation of Fick's principle; (iii) arterial pulse wave analysis (pulse contour CO); and (iv) imaging diagnostic techniques (e.g. transthoracic echocardiogram, thoracic bio-impedance) [22, 28]. Although there is increasing research into clinically useful methods of monitoring CO in equine patients, limitations remain in the available methods. The methods used to obtain CO are further described below, together with their relevance to equine medicine.

Indicator Methods

Pulmonary Thermodilution

Thermodilution using a pulmonary arterial (PA) catheter (Swan-Ganz technique) remains the accepted clinical gold standard for CO measurement [24]. Thermodilution is one of the few methods capable of determining CO in adult horses and remains a commonly used method for monitoring CO in the research setting involving horses [28, 29]. The Swan-Ganz PA catheter is a double lumen catheter specially designed with a thermistor monitor in the tip. The placement of a pulmonary arterial catheter in a horse is similar to other species. Briefly, the horse is sedated and maintained in a standing position and the area over the distal jugular vein is clipped and aseptically cleaned. An introducer kit (8fr) is placed over the jugular using the Seldinger technique and the Swan-Ganz catheter is fed though the introducer into the distal jugular. The proximal port is connected to a pressure transducer and the pressure waveform, measured in mmHg, is used to monitor the catheter's advancement from the jugular vein (3 mmHg) to right atrium (5/3 mmHg [systolic/diastolic]) followed by the right ventricle (25/5 mmHg) and finally to confirm placement in the proximal PA (25/10 mmHg). Most PA catheters have an inflatable balloon located near the tip of the catheter to facilitate passage from the ventricle to the pulmonary artery. Once properly positioned, the proximal port of the Swan-Ganz PA catheter sits in the right atrium and distal port is located in the PA. Placement of a Swan-Ganz catheter when the animal is in dorsal or lateral position is possible but more challenging. Regular Swan-Ganz catheters designed with dimensions to accommodate an adult person can be used for foals but cannot be used in adult horses. A custom-made Swan-Ganz catheter (>110 cm length) must be specially manufactured to reach and fit the heart of an adult horse. Alternatively, one can use two introducers and two separate catheters with the proximal catheter fed into the right atrium and the distal catheter (e.g. Edward Lifesciences LLC, Irvine, CA) fed into the pulmonary artery.

Once the catheter is properly placed, the thermodilution method involves using thermal energy as an indicator to determine CO. A small bolus of cold, isotonic solution (5% dextrose or 0.9% saline) is injected into the patient's blood proximal to the right ventricle (e.g. right atrium) and the dilution of the indicator (e.g. temperature change) is followed continuously at a point distal to the ventricle (e.g. pulmonary artery). Plotting a graph of the concentration of the indicator against time will produce a concentration-time curve, and the area under the curve (AUC) is calculated. CO is inversely proportional to the AUC and is determined by the Stewart-Hamilton principle (Table 11.III.1).

Table 11.III.1 Common equations associated with cardiovascular monitoring and cardiac output.

Equation	Abbreviated equation
Cardiac output = heart rate (beats/min) × stroke volume (ml)	CO = HR × SV (l/min)
O_2 content = 1.34 × hemoglobin (g/dl) × oxygen saturation (%) + 0.003 × PaO_2 (mmHg)	$CaO_2 = 1.34 \times Hb \times SaO_2 + 0.003 \times PaO_2$ (ml/dl)
O_2 delivery = oxygen content (ml/dl) × cardiac output (l/min)	$DO_2 = CaO_2 \times CO$ (ml/dl/min)
O_2 consumption = O_2 content (arterial) − O_2 content (venous) × cardiac output	$VO_2 = (CaO_2 - CvO_2) \times CO$ (ml/dl/min)
O_2 extraction ratio = O_2 consumption/O_2 delivery	$OER = VO_2/DO_2$
Systemic vascular resistance = (mean art. pressure − cent. venous pressure) × 80/cardiac output	SVR = (MAP − CVP) × 80/CO (dynes/s/cm^{-5})
Pulm. vascular resistance = (pulmonary art. pressure − cent. venous pressure) × 80/cardiac output	PVR = (PAP − CVP) × 80/CO (dynes/s/cm^{-5})
Modified Stewart-Hamilton equation	CO = amount of indicator/ f(concentration indicator × time)

The thermodilution method has several disadvantages, however. The use of a PA catheter carries significant risks, including induction of arrhythmias, damage to the cardiac endothelium, infection, and pulmonary thromboembolism [19–22]. Although rare, the most devastating complication, PA rupture, has a mortality rate of approximately 50%. For these reasons, thermodilution is not routinely used in client-owned foals. Because of these substantial complications, there has been interest in less invasive techniques for CO measurement, such as transpulmonary thermodilution, lithium dilution, and ultrasound velocity dilution techniques. These other indicator methods are, in principle, a modification of thermodilution, and also follow the Stewart-Hamilton principle.

Lithium Dilution (LIDCO)

The LIDCO method has excellent agreement when compared to thermodilution in animal models, is capable of measuring CO in adult horses (including during exercise) and is currently one of the most commonly used methods of determining CO in anesthetized foals [23–25, 30]. The lithium dilution technique (LIDCO, LiDCO ltd. Lake Villa, IL) requires determination of the hemoglobin and serum sodium concentrations. To perform LIDCO, lithium chloride (0.003 mmol/kg) is injected via a central vein, then arterial blood is withdrawn through a lithium sensor placed between the side port of a three-way stopcock and an arterial catheter placed in the metatarsal artery. Blood is collected through a peristaltic pump with a flow rate of 4 ml/min across the sensor. As with the thermodilution method, a graph is plotted of the indicator (in this case, lithium) concentration versus time, and CO is derived from this curve by the Stewart-Hamilton principle [23–25].

For an adult horse, blood removed for one LIDCO determination is minimal (20–40 ml per measurement) and should not be returned to the patient. Drawbacks associated with repeated LIDCO determinations include excessive blood loss and the potential accumulation of the indicator (lithium) in the body, leading to erroneous values and risk of other undesirable effects. Lithium sensors can also react with some drugs used during anesthesia, such as neuro-muscular blocking agents (i.e. Atracurium), resulting in unreliable readings.

Ultrasound Velocity Dilution (UDCO)

UDCO (CO status, Trathaca, NY) is a novel technique for determining CO that resolves some of the disadvantages of previous CO determination methods [31, 32]. UDCO is minimally invasive, does not involve blood loss, and uses a physiologic noncumulative signal (saline solution) [32]. This technique has been used in anesthetized foals and juvenile horses with good success [31]. UDCO also allows the clinician to monitor other preload volumetric variables, such as total end diastolic volume, that can have predictive value for patient fluid responsiveness.

To determine CO using the UDCO technique, an arterio-venous loop is made by attaching tubing between a peripheral (e.g. metatarsal) arterial catheter and a central venous catheter, creating an extracorporeal circuit [31, 32]. Two ultrasound velocity sensors are attached to this circuit; a venous flow sensor is placed upstream from the venous catheter and an arterial flow sensor is placed downstream from the arterial catheter. A small bolus of isotonic saline (0.5–1 ml/kg) is injected into the venous circulation, creating a transient hemodilution, resulting in a change in the velocity of ultrasound in this blood.

CO is calculated as the product of the volume of isotonic saline and the consequent decrease in ultrasound velocity as the saline-diluted blood passes through an ultrasonic sensor. Ultrasound velocity in blood is normally 1560–1590 m/s and is mainly dependent on the levels of red blood cells and protein [32]. Ultrasound velocity in isotonic saline is lower than in blood (1533 m/s). Injection of a saline bolus into the venous system will therefore generate an ultrasound velocity dilution curve due to transient dilution of blood proteins, which results in a decrease in ultrasound velocity in the arterial sample [31–33]. For UDCO to be used in an adult horse, it would require a large amount of fluid (0.5 ml/kg) to be rapidly administered through the small arterio-venous loop. Due to the small diameter/high resistance of the current loop, the UDCO is not currently viable for use in animals >250 kg [31–33].

The Fick Method

This technique is one of the oldest methods of measuring CO. In 1870, Adolph Fick derived this theoretical method, and it was later validated in horses in 1890 [24, 25, 34]. For a substance that is taken up by a tissue (such as oxygen), the Fick principle simply states, "As long as there is no pulmonary and cardiac shunting, the oxygen uptake by the blood (VO_2) is the product of the rate of blood flow through the lungs (CO) and the difference in oxygen content between pulmonary venous and pulmonary arterial blood." In other words, "What went in, minus what came out, must be equal to what was left behind." Pulmonary venous oxygen content is equivalent to systemic oxygen content (CaO_2), while blood collected at the pulmonary artery is known as mixed venous content (CvO_2). Therefore, according to Fick's principle, $VO_2 = CO \times (CaO_2 - CvO_2)$.

The equation can be rearranged as

$$CO = VO_2 / \left(CaO_2 - CvO_2\right)$$

in order to determine CO when the other values are known [25, 34]. Although oxygen content analyzers are available to measure CaO_2, it is more typical for the clinician to measure the partial pressure of oxygen (PO_2), hemoglobin saturation (% Sat), and hemoglobin concentration (Hb) with a gas analyzer and manually calculate systemic oxygen content using the formula:

$$CaO_2 = \left(1.34\,Hb \times Sat\right) + \left(0.003\,PO_2\right)[25].$$

Fick's method has some drawbacks for modern clinical use. Mixed venous blood sampling (to measure CvO_2) requires placement of a pulmonary arterial catheter, which can be associated with complications (noted above), and blood samples from the right atrium and jugular vein are a poor substitute. Furthermore, Fick's method relies on the patient maintaining a stable metabolic state throughout the period of gas collection; the less stable the patient, the less reliable this method becomes [25, 34]. Additionally, oxygen uptake (VO_2) is calculated as $VO_2 = VE\,(FIO_2 - FEO_2)$, where VE = expired minute ventilation volume, FIO_2 = fractional concentration of oxygen in inspired gas, and FEO_2 = fractional concentration of oxygen in expired gas.

Accurate determination of expired minute ventilation volume is difficult in conscious animals and requires a specially designed tight-fitting mask and a cooperative horse. In anesthetized ventilated foals, a commercial spirometer can be used to easily determine expired minute ventilation volume. In adult horses, however, methods for determining expired volume that are sufficiently accurate for the technique to be valid are not readily available [25]. A large animal anesthesia ventilator with a built-in spirometer specifically designed for equine anesthesia (Tafonius Hallowell EMC, Pittsfield, MA) might solve this challenge. To the author's knowledge, validation of Fick's method has not been performed using this machine.

To avoid some of these disadvantages, carbon dioxide (CO_2) production can be used instead of oxygen consumption in a modified Fick's equation. The rate of CO_2 elimination by the lungs (VCO_2) is the product of CO and the difference in CO_2 content between pulmonary venous and pulmonary arterial blood. Mixed blood gas is substituted by having the animal rebreathe exhaled air until the CO_2 tension in the breathing circuit plateaus (NICCO, Respironic Inc./Phillips, Murrysville, PA). This CO_2 tension is theoretically that of mixed venous blood, therefore eliminating the need for a pulmonary arterial catheter. This rebreathing technique has been validated in anesthetized foals and demonstrates good correlation when compared to the LIDCO technique. Unfortunately, the commercially available rebreathing circuits cannot be adapted for adult horses, making it a less than ideal technique for equine medicine.

Pulse Contour Analysis

The concept of deriving CO based on the arterial pressure waveform is not new and is traced back to 1904 [35]. These early attempts, however, had limited success [24, 35]. Calculation of CO based on the contour of the arterial pulse wave, *if accurate,* would offer the advantages of minimally invasive, continuous, beat-to-beat CO. Current arterial wave analysis monitors also display preload volumetric variables, such as stroke volume variation (SVV) and pulse pressure variation (PPV). Both PPV and SSV have predictive value for patient fluid responsiveness [36].

The arterial wave form is a product of the stroke volume force (arterial peak before the dicrotic notch) and the elastic component of the arteries, or Windkessel effect (area after the dicrotic notch) [37]. The stroke volume correlates well with the area of the arterial wave before the dicrotic notch; however, the arterial pressure waveform is dependent on multiple factors, including changes in aortic impedance, SVR, and waveform damping, all of which prevent this from being a straightforward relationship [37].

To adjust for this, most of the available pulse contour CO monitors use a second, more reliable, method to determine true CO, involving a calibration factor. Pulse contour CO monitors that do not have a calibration factor typically use built-in algorithms based on healthy human values, making them less useful in veterinary medicine. Currently, two pulse contour CO monitors have been evaluated in animals: the lithium dilution arterial waveform analysis monitor (PulseCO) and the transpulmonary pulse contour analysis monitor (PiCCO). The PulseCO (LiDCO ltd. Lake Villa, IL) uses the lithium chloride dilution technique for calibration while the PiCCO (Pulsion Medical system, Munich, Germany) uses cold saline transpulmonary thermodilution for calibration (see indicator methods above).

Investigators have compared PulseCO and PiCCO to lithium and thermodilution indicator methods in foals and juvenile horses. In anesthetized neonatal foals, both PiCCO and PulseCO methods were able to monitor CO changes in the same direction (i.e. pulse-wave derived CO increases as CO increases, and vice versa) [25, 31]. However with significant changes in SVR and volume state of the patient, pulse contour technology is less accurate, making the clinical usefulness of both these monitors limited in the presence of severe arrhythmias, severe vasoconstriction, and hemodynamically unstable patients. Furthermore, the manufacturer of the PiCCO device recommends that the arterial catheter be placed in the femoral artery with the catheter tip located in the aorta (central catheterization) to detect central aortic blood pressure. This type of central arterial catheterization is not commonly performed in foals, and the fact that this method requires femoral catheterization makes it clinically impractical in adult horses.

Imaging Techniques

Echocardiogram (Echo)

An advantage of echocardiography over other monitoring techniques is the large amount of hemodynamic information obtained beyond just CO. Cardiac contractility and chamber filling can be rapidly assessed, as well as cardiac valve function and direct visualization of the pericardium [25]. CO can be determined with echocardiography using non-Doppler or Doppler-based methods [24, 25]. Non-Doppler techniques are based on approximate volumetric reconstructions of the left ventricular chamber. The most common method is based on Simpson's rule, wherein the left ventricle is divided into a series of disks stacked from base to apex [38]. Two orthogonal planes are needed to construct the disks, and left ventricular volume is calculated by summing the approximated volumes of the individual disks. Stroke volume is calculated by determining the difference in volume between diastole and systole. The time-consuming nature of the non-Doppler technique can make cardiac output estimation inadequate for rapid assessment in emergent situations. Difficulty with endocardial border definition also can produce largely inaccurate results. For these reasons, non-Doppler techniques are rarely used for clinical purposes.

The real advantage of echocardiography over other CO techniques does not solely rest on the fact that it is a noninvasive technique, but rather, the peculiarity of providing a direct evaluation of cardiac function. The expertise and familiarity of the operator with the technique still represents a critical factor to obtain reliable results with this method, as with other CO monitoring devices available. An example of high operator-dependency is represented by echocardiography compared to other automatic devices that consistently produce results with low inter-operator variability. Lithium dilution, ultrasound velocity dilution, and pulse contour analysis are all less invasive methods than pulmonary thermodilution, but they still require placement of both venous and arterial catheters. In contrast, the echocardiogram is a truly noninvasive techniques available for measurement of CO in both juvenile and adult horses [24, 30].

Measurement of blood velocity (using Doppler ultrasound) and aortic diameter allow estimates of stroke volume and therefore CO. Determining the aortic Doppler velocity can be challenging in adult horses. Another alternative to estimate CO is using the modified Simpson formula. In this method, a two-dimensional view of left ventricle at the widest cross section is acquired, making certain that the endocardial borders are well visualized. Using the geometric assumption that the left ventricular cavity represents a cylinder/cone configuration, the biplane Simpson formula divides the outline of the ventricular chamber into slices. Each slice volume can then be calculated using an algorithm that estimates total ventricular volume (during systole and diastole). In this case, end diastolic volume minus end systolic volume equals stroke volume. CO can then be derived from SV and heart rate. The Simpson method has some built-in error and some variability is expected in results [38]. Although CO by Echo represents significantly less risk to the patient than other methods of CO determination, this method still requires highly trained personnel and expensive equipment. Transthoracic echocardiogram is also more challenging in adult horses once the animal is anesthetized and placed in lateral or dorsal position.

Repeated CO estimation is routinely performed in human anesthesia using transesophageal-echocardiogram (TEE) [24, 30]. This technique is a great option for foals, but currently there is not a commercially available probe that is long enough for TEE in adult horses. A modified echocardiogram probe can be custom made for use in the horse adapted from a 160 cm colonoscope.

Transthoracic Electrical Bioimpedance (TEB)

TEB is a noninvasive method of evaluating changes in the conductivity of the thorax resulting from pulsatile flow of blood within the thoracic cavity [39]. If proven accurate, TEB would be an ideal method for determining CO in horses. TEB can be performed in adult and pediatric horses, and is capable of CO monitoring during anesthesia and during exercise. Determination of CO by this method involves placement of sets of electrodes around the patient's chest. By applying a small, known voltage to the patient and measuring what proportion of the initial voltage reaches distal electrodes, the conductivity (and therefore impedance) of the thorax can be calculated. Changes in thoracic blood volume over time (CO) lead to changes in the bio impedance [39]. In humans, TEB has good correlation and directional tracking, but values were not interchangeable (not complete agreement) with the Fick method. Currently TEB is not widely used, but this method holds promise as a special bio impedance belt is being designed for the equine thorax.

In summary of the methods for determining CO, pulmonary thermodilution, while still the gold standard and commonly used in adult horses in the research setting, is too invasive for routine clinical use. Currently, one of the most commonly used methods in anesthetized foals is lithium dilution. Ultrasound velocity dilution methods and echocardiogram may be valuable options for sick and anesthetized foals but is not widely used or validated currently. The noninvasive method, thoracic bio impedance, is perhaps the most promising for clinical equine use in the future.

Monitoring in Critically Ill Patients

The different types of shock are discussed in other sections of this textbook. However, a brief comment on how monitoring of CO might facilitate categorization of the type of shock as well as treatment and progression of shock states follows. Severe shock and hypovolemic shock represent a major cause of circulatory failure and mortality in foals. *Hyperdynamic shock* is characterized by high HR and high CO, with a massive decrease in SVR leading to evidence of poor microcirculation in tissue beds. A classic example of hyperdynamic shock is the initial stages of septic shock. If not corrected promptly, vasodilation leads to venous blood stasis and a drop in venous return/pre-load which can consequently lead to hypodynamic shock (also called distributive shock). A classic example of distributive shock occurs in the late stages of sepsis where there is a drop in BP, CO, and a decrease in SVR. Alternatively, hypovolemic shock is characterized by a drop in venous return due to loss of intravascular fluid. This can be due to trauma, gastrointestinal disease, or sepsis, among other causes. *Hypovolemic shock* is characterized by a decrease in CO and increase in SVR. Critically ill foals can lose a considerable amount of circulating volume due to third space fluid losses into the gastrointestinal track and from vascular fluid leaking into the interstitium and abdominal cavity due to capillary damage. Knowledge of the type of shock the patient is suffering allows for better treatment methods. Optimizing CO and oxygen delivery and preventing multiple organ ischemic injury decreases morbidity and mortality.

The clinician must also be aware that sole reliance of BP for monitoring of the cardiovascular system in ill foals does not allow for accurate assessment of volume status of the foal [10]. Another difficulty is that not all hypovolemic foals respond to volume loading, and overzealous fluid administration can be extremely harmful to some critically ill foals. Variables traditionally used as indicators of preload to guide fluid resuscitation, such as central venous pressure (CVP), mean arterial blood pressure (MAP), blood lactate concentration, and urine output have been repeatedly shown to be unreliable indicators of fluid status. In comparison, CO monitoring provides global insight as to the adequacy of delivery of blood to the body and can be used to gauge fluid responsiveness and cardiovascular status in ill foals. Thus, evaluation of CO in critically ill foals would help guide therapy, be a better indicator of fluid responsiveness, and theoretically decrease morbidity, but identifying a safe, reliable, accurate, and clinically user-friendly method of determining CO in foals remains elusive.

References

1 Grimm, K.A., Lamont, L.A., Tranquilli, W.J. et al. (ed.) (2015). *Lubb & Jones Veterinary Anesthesia and Analgesia*, 5e. Wiley.

2 Parry, B.W., McCarthy, M.A., and Anderson, G.A. (1984). Survey of resting blood pressure values in clinically normal horses. *Equine Vet. J.* 16: 53–58.

3 Corley, K.T. (2004). Inotropes and vasopressors in adults and foals. *Vet. Clin. Equine Pract.* 20: 77–106.

4 Landry, D.W. and Oliver, J.A. (2001). The pathogenesis of vasodilatory shock. *N. Engl. J. Med.* 345: 588–595.

5 Senior, J.M. (2013). Morbidity, mortality, and risk of general anesthesia in horses. *Vet. Clin. Equine Pract.* 29: 1–18.

6 Venkataraman, R. and Kellum, J.A. (2007). Prevention of acute renal failure. *Chest* 131: 300–308.

7 Brown, S., Atkins, C., Bagley, R. et al. (2007). Guidelines for the identification, evaluation, and management of systemic hypertension in dogs and cats. *J. Vet. Intern. Med.* 21: 542–558.

8 Wityk, R.J. and Caplan, L.R. (1992). Hypertensive intracerebral hemorrhage: epidemiology and clinical pathology. *Neurosurg. Clin. North Am.* 3: 521–532.

9 Bartges, J.W., Willis, A.M., and Polzin, D.J. (1996). Hypertension and renal disease. *Vet. Clin. North Am. Small Anim. Pract.* 26: 1331–1345.

10 Corley, K.T.T. (2002). Monitoring and treating haemodynamic disturbances in critically ill neonatal foals. Part 2: assessment and treatment. *Equine Vet. Educ.* 14: 328–336.

11 Scheer, B.V., Perel, A., and Pfeiffer, U.J. (2002). Clinical review: complications and risk factors of peripheral arterial catheters used for haemodynamic monitoring in anaesthesia and intensive care medicine. *Crit. Care* 6: 1–7.

12 Trim, C.M., Hofmeister, E.H., Quandt, J.E. et al. (2017). A survey of the use of arterial catheters in anesthetized dogs and cats: 267 cases. *J. Vet. Emerg. Crit. Care* 27: 89–95.

13 Ward, M. and Langton, J.A. (2007). Blood pressure measurement. *Contin. Educ. Anesth. Crit. Care Pain* 7: 122–126.

14 Sawyer, D.C., Guikema, A.H., and Siegel, E.M. (2004). Evaluation of a new oscillometric blood pressure monitor in isoflurance-anesthetized dogs. *Vet. Anesth. Analg.* 31: 27–39.

15 McLeish, I. (1977). Doppler ultrasonic arterial pressure measurement in the cat. *Vet. Rec.* 100: 290–291.

16 Gay, C.C., McCarthy, M., Reynolds, W.T. et al. (1977). A method for indirect measurement of arterial blood pressure in the horse. *Aust. Vet. J.* 53: 163–166.

17 Kazamias, T.M., Gander, M.P., Franklin, D.L. et al. (1971). Blood pressure measurement with Doppler ultrasonic flowmeter. *J. Appl. Phys.* 30: 585–588.

18 Giguere, S., Knowles, H.A., Valverde, A. et al. (2005). Accuracy of indirect measurement of blood pressure in neonatal foals. *J. Vet. Intern. Med.* 19: 571–576.

19 Nout, Y.S., Corley, K.T.T., Donaldson, L.L. et al. (2002). Indirect oscillometric and direct blood pressure measurements in anesthetized and conscious neonatal foals. *J. Vet. Emerg. Crit. Care* 12: 75–80.

20 Henneman, E.A. and Henneman, P.L. (1989). Intricacies of blood pressure measurement: reexamining the rituals. *Heart Lung J. Crit. Care* 18: 263–271.

21 Deflandre, C.J.A. and Hellebrekers, L.J. (2008). Clinical evaluation of the Surgivet V60046, a noninvasive blood pressure monitor in anaesthetized dogs. *Vet. Anesth. Analg.* 35: 13–21.

22 Thiele, R.H., Bartels, K., and Gan, T.J. (2015). Cardiac output monitoring: a contemporary assessment and review. *Crit. Care Med.* 43: 177–185.

23 Corley, K.T.T., Donaldson, L.L., and Furr, M.O. (2002). Comparison of lithium dilution and thermodilution cardiac output measurements in anesthetized neonatal foals. *Equine Vet. J.* 34: 598–601.

24 Corley, K.T.T., Donaldson, L.L., Duando, M.M. et al. (2003). Cardiac output technologies with special reference to the horse. *J. Vet. Intern. Med.* 17: 262–272.

25 Shih, A. (2013). Cardiac output monitoring in horses. *Vet. Clin. Equine Pract.* 29: 155–167.

26 Harms, C.A., Wetter, T.J., McClaran, S.R. et al. (1998). Effects of respiratory muscle work on cardiac output and its distribution during maximal exercise. *J. Appl. Phys.* 85: 609–618.

27 Heyland, D.K., Cook, D.J., King, D.B. et al. (1996). Maximizing oxygen delivery in critically ill patients: a methodologic appraisal of the evidence. *Crit. Care Med.* 24: 517–524.

28 Mehta, Y. and Arora, D. (2014). Newer methods of cardiac output monitoring. *World J. Cardiol.* 6: 1022.

29 Muir, W.W., Skarda, R.T., and Milne, D.W. (1976). Estimation of cardiac output in the horse by thermodilution techniques. *Am. J. Vet. Res.* 37: 697–700.

30 Linton, R.A., Young, L.E., Marlin, D.J. et al. (2000). Cardiac output measured by lithium dilution, thermodilution, and transesophageal Doppler echocardiography in anesthetized horses. *Am. J. Vet. Res.* 61: 731–737.

31 Shih, A., Giguere, S., Sanchez, L.C. et al. (2009). Determination of cardiac output in neonatal foals by ultrasound velocity dilution and its comparison to the lithium dilution method. *J. Vet. Emerg. Crit. Care* 19: 438–443.

32 Tsutsui, M., Matsuoka, N., Ikeda, T. et al. (2009). Comparison of a new cardiac output ultrasound dilution method with thermodilution technique in adult patients under general anesthesia. *J. Cardiothorac. Vasc. Anesth.* 23: 835–840.

33 de Broode, W.P. (2020). Advanced hemodynamic monitoring in the neonatal intensive care unit. *Clin. Perinatol.* 47: 423–434.

34 Mathews, L. and Singh, K.R.K. (2008). Cardiac output monitoring. *Ann. Card. Anesth.* 11: 56.

35 Hallowell, G.D. and Corley, K.T.T. (2005). Use of lithium dilution and pulse contour analysis cardiac output determination in anaesthetized horses: a clinical evaluation. *Vet. Anaesth. Analg.* 32: 201–211.

36 Zhang, Z., Lu, B., Sheng, X. et al. (2011). Accuracy of stroke volume variation in predicting fluid responsiveness: a systematic review and meta-analysis. *J. Anesth.* 25: 904–916.

37 Mei, C.C., Zhang, J., and Jing, H.X. (2018). Fluid mechanics of Windkessel effect. *Med. Biol. Eng. Comput.* 56: 1357–1366.

38 Hergan, K., Schuster, A., Fruhwald, J. et al. (2008). Comparison of left and right ventricular volume measurement using the Simpson's mehod and the area length method. *Eur. J. Radiol.* 65: 270–278.

39 Fortin, J., Habenbacher, W., Heller, A. et al. (2006). Non-invasive beat-to-beat cardiac output monitoring by an improved method of transthoracic bioimpedance measurement. *Comput. Biol. Med.* 36: 1185–1203.

Section IV Central Venous Pressure

David Wong

Central venous pressure (CVP) is a reflection of venous blood returning to the heart, venous tone, and cardiac function and is an estimate of preload and right ventricular pressure [1, 2]. By extension, CVP provides information about left ventricular preload based on the assumption that CVP approximates right atrial pressure and thus, right ventricular filling, which ultimately determines left ventricular preload [3]. More simply, CVP serves as an indirect marker of intravascular blood volume. However, CVP is influenced by many factors including compliance of the patient's lungs and intrathoracic pressures [3]. CVP has been used as a tool during fluid resuscitation efforts as well as a guide for assessing fluid therapy in critically ill patients. A few key clinical trials in people have advocated for the use of CVP as a component of early goal-directed therapy, but the usefulness of CVP measurement is not universally accepted nor has the use of CVP and early goal-directed therapy been evaluated in foals [4–9]. Clinical assessment of adequate resuscitation can be difficult in some patients because apparent normalization of some perfusion and physical examination parameters may occur despite continued hypovolemia [3]. For example, in adult horses with experimentally induced blood loss (16 ml/kg) or induced hypohydration, a significant decrease in CVP was measured whereas heart rate and other vital parameters did not change significantly [2, 10]. Therefore, other methods of hemodynamic assessment, such as CVP, may be helpful in some instances. In equine medicine, CVP has been evaluated in several studies, but has not been universally adopted into clinical practice [1, 2, 10–13]. Clinical conditions in which CVP may be useful in foals include hypovolemic or septic shock, heart disease, or renal disease (e.g. anuric or oliguric nephropathy).

The repeatability of CVP measurements in adult horses has been shown to be very good, with consistent head position being an important factor in obtaining reliable readings [14, 15]. To measure CVP in the neonatal foal, a 20- to 30-cm catheter is placed into the jugular vein with the catheter tip passed into the cranial vena cava. The catheter length in neonatal foals can be estimated before insertion of the catheter by measuring the distance from the catheter insertion site to the caudal aspect of the scapula [16]. In one report of 11 neonatal foals with a mean body weight of 52.2 kg, the mean length of the catheter from insertion site to the cranial vena cava was 34.8 cm [16]. Ideally, proper placement is confirmed via thoracic radiography (Figure 11.IV.1) but the identification of oscillations in the CVP measurements that correspond to respiration can also be used to confirm proper location. In adult horses, these oscillations fluctuated by ≤0.5 cmH_2O with respiration, suggesting that the difference in CVP between inspiration and expiration is very slight [14]. Catheters that are placed extra-thoracically will not undergo oscillations in the fluid meniscus with respiration, whereas catheters placed in the right ventricle will demonstrate a higher magnitude of fluctuations and should be retracted into the cranial vena cava [10]. The CVP in healthy neonatal foals ranges from 2.8 to 12 cmH_2O (2.1–8.9 mmHg) with measurements made at end expiration [10, 17, 18]. A factor of 1.36 is used to convert cmH_2O to mmHg. Once the IV catheter is in place, CVP can be measured using a water manometer or an electronic pressure transducer. The specific technique for using a water manometer to measure CVP is discussed in Figure 11.IV.2. Although water manometers are readily available, they tend to overestimate CVP in dogs; thus, some references suggest that electronic pressure transducers are more accurate [3]. Electronic pressure monitors use piezoresistive technology to convert mechanical pressure from the circulation into a measurable electric signal [15]. This method can save time

Equine Neonatal Medicine, First Edition. Edited by David M. Wong and Pamela A. Wilkins.

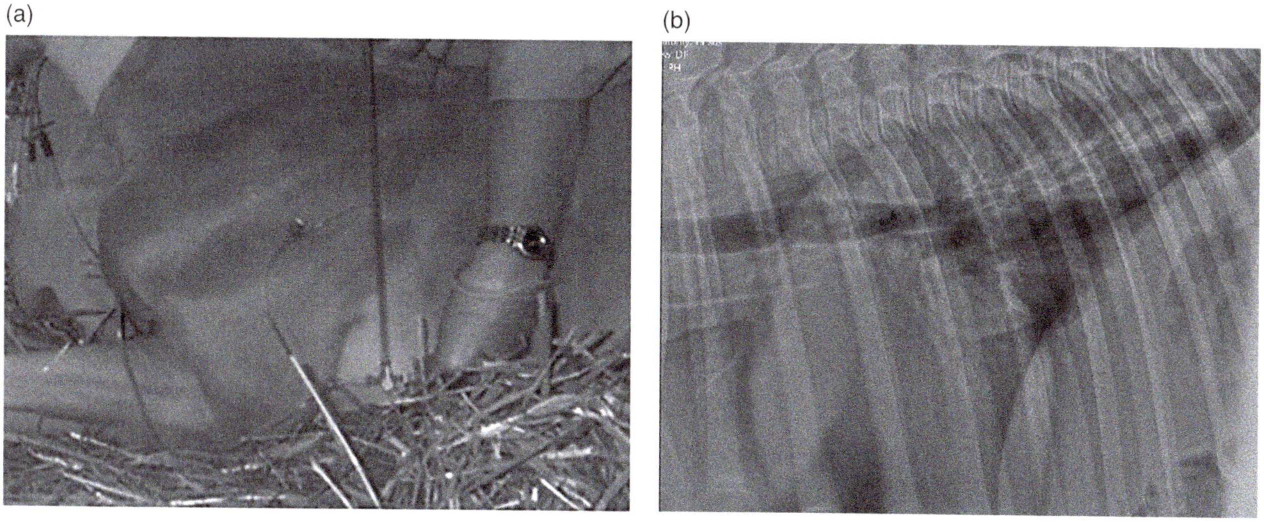

Figure 11.IV.1 (a) Placement of water manometer at level of the heart in a recumbent foal [1]; (b) lateral radiograph demonstrating placement of a central venous catheter in the vena cava of a neonatal foal.

Equipment Required:

- IV catheter (20–30 cm)
- Sterile bag of isotonic fluids (250 ml)
- IV extension set
- Three-way stopcock
- Manometer

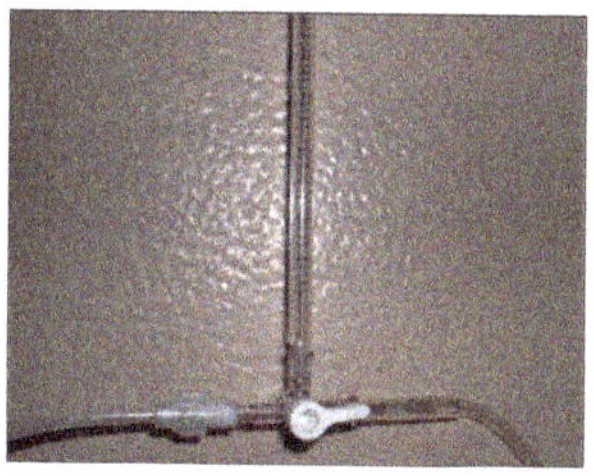

Technique [1]: Estimate the length of the IV catheter to reach the cranial vena cava prior to placement by measuring the distance from the point of IV catheter insertion to the caudal aspect of the foal's scapula [16]. Place the over-the-wire catheter in the jugular vein and verify the position of the catheter within the cranial vena cava via thoracic radiography, if possible. Once appropriate placement is confirmed, suture the catheter to the skin. Attach the fluid administration set to the sterile fluid bag. To measure CVP, attach the end of the administration set (connected to fluid bag) to the lateral port of the stopcock, attach the manometer to the top port of the stopcock and attach an extension set to the other lateral port of the stopcock (Inset Image). Close the stopcock toward the manometer and flush the entire system with sterile fluid; attach the extension set to the foal's IV catheter. Close the stopcock toward the IV catheter and fill the manometer partially with sterile fluid from the fluid bag. Close the stopcock toward the fluid bag and place the bottom of the manometer at the level of the right atrium of the heart (sternal manubrium if lateral; point of the shoulder if sternal). The fluid column within the manometer should oscillate with the respiratory cycle (rise with expiration, drop with inspiration); the fluid column height is equal to the hydrostatic pressure at the end of the catheter and is the CVP, measured in cmH_2O. When taking serial measurements, ensure that the foal is in the same position each time and that the manometer is at the same level; the latter can be facilitated by making a small clipped area on the foal's body to serve as a reference point for serial measurements.

Figure 11.IV.2 Measurement of CVP using a water manometer.

by providing instantaneous readings and can remove inter-reader variation [15]. Interestingly, a study in adult horses noted that CVP was lower, by approximately 2 cmH_2O, when electronic monitors were compared to water manometry. The authors suggested that the difference in readings between devices is clinically minimal [15]. When using a pressure transducer, an extension set is filled with saline and one end of the set is attached to the catheter port, with the other end attached to the pressure transducer (Figure 11.IV.3). The transducer is positioned and zeroed at the level of the sternal manubrium (lateral recumbency) or point of the shoulder (sternal recumbency) [19].

Typically pressure is higher in the smaller veins as compared to the larger veins or right atrium, but a few investigations have examined the use of the jugular venous pressure (JVP) as a surrogate for CVP [19, 20]. One equine study demonstrated that JVP could be used in place of CVP with strong correlation and low bias between the two measurements in laterally recumbent anesthetized adult horses [20]. However, a different study in adult horses noted a statistically greater pressure in the JVP (mean 10.1 cmH_2O [7.4 mmHg]) as compared to right atrial pressure (mean 8.3 cmH_2O [6.1 mmHg]) [19]. The use of JVP in neonatal foals has not been examined, but many

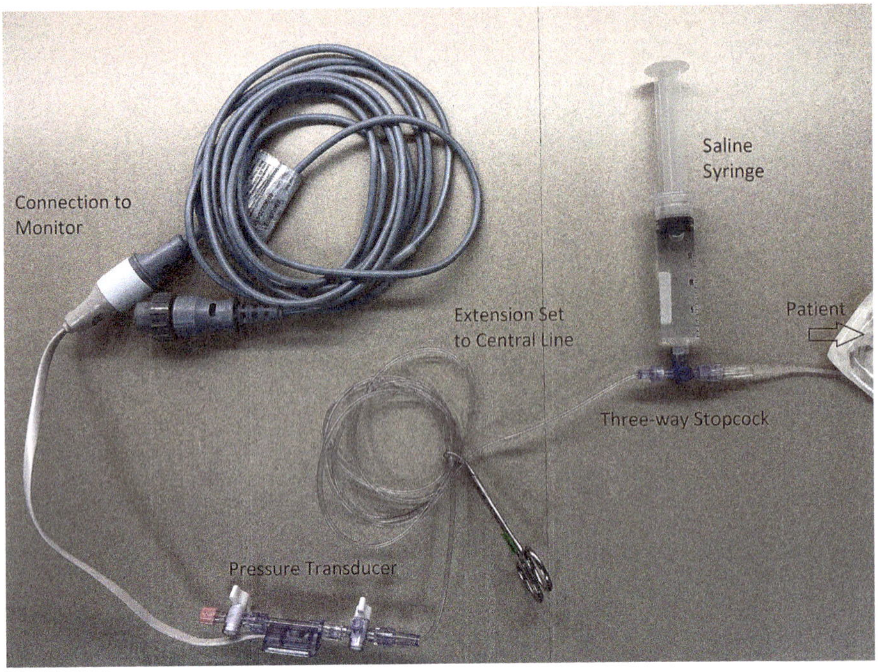

Figure 11.IV.3 Equipment needed for measurement of CVP using an electric transducer. These include pressure transducer with fluid valve, arterial blood pressure tubing or IV fluid extension line, saline syringe, IV fluid line.

IV catheters used in neonatal foals are of sufficient length (20 cm) to reach intra-thoracic placement to the cranial vena cava, thus negating the need to test the JVP [21].

Interpretation of Central Venous Pressure

Interpretation of CVP can be difficult, but it has been used to guide fluid bolus administration during resuscitation as well as help direct fluid therapy in critically ill neonatal foals [10, 11, 21]. The clinician should avoid over-interpreting single CVP measurements as each foal may have a different "normal" value. Rather, one should follow trends and serial changes in CVP measurements and couple those findings with changes in heart rate, pulse quality, extremity temperature, body weight changes and variations in blood parameters, such as blood lactate and packed cell volume, to help guide fluid therapy needs. When clinical examination of the patient's fluid volume status is ambiguous, CVP measurements may help determine if the foal is hypo- or hypervolemic. Subnormal CVP suggests hypovolemia, venodilation, or reduced venous resistance, whereas increased CVP can be caused by hypervolemia (normal cardiac function with excessive fluid administration), cardiac dysfunction (normal blood volume with decreased cardiac function), venoconstriction, increased pleural pressures/pleural effusion, cardiac tamponade, right-sided heart failure, pulmonary hypertension, or increased intra-abdominal pressure [1, 3].

When considering the patient's fluid needs, the clinician must also account for the pressure-volume curve of the ventricles and the fact that it is not linear. The Frank-Starling principle (Figure 11.IV.4a) explains that ventricular stroke volume will increase to a maximum point, but once this point is exceeded, stroke volume remains static (i.e. flat portion of curve) [22]. Patients respond to volume resuscitation on the steep portion of the curve where administration of IV fluids results in an increase in stroke volume. Comparatively, when the ventricles are functioning on the flat portion of the curve, further administration of IV fluids will increase diastolic pressures without increasing stroke volume [3]. Thus, when a high normal CVP is reached in the neonatal foal (10–12 cmH_2O), additional fluid administration should not continue [23]. At this point, the patient's hemodynamic status may be improved by increasing the contractility of the heart or increasing the heart rate. Of note, the correlation between CVP and cardiac stroke volume in critically ill neonatal foals was poor (Figure 11.IV.4b) in one small veterinary report [21].

CVP can also be used in conjunction with a fluid challenge in which 10–15 ml/kg of isotonic crystalloids are administered IV over 5–10 minutes [3, 21]. If the patient has adequate blood volume and normal cardiac function, the CVP should increase by 2–5.4 cmH_2O (1.5–4 mmHg) and then return to baseline over 15 minutes [3]. If the patient is hypovolemic, the CVP should rise transiently (by >2.7 cmH_2O [2.0 mmHg]) or stay static and then rapidly decrease within 5 minutes [3, 12]. In contrast, a large increased in CVP of >5.4 cmH_2O (4 mmHg) with a slow return to baseline over 30 minutes or greater can be seen in hypervolemic animals or in patients with underlying cardiomyopathy [3, 24]. The changes in CVP after a fluid challenge have been described in small animals and people, but in theory should also apply to neonatal foals.

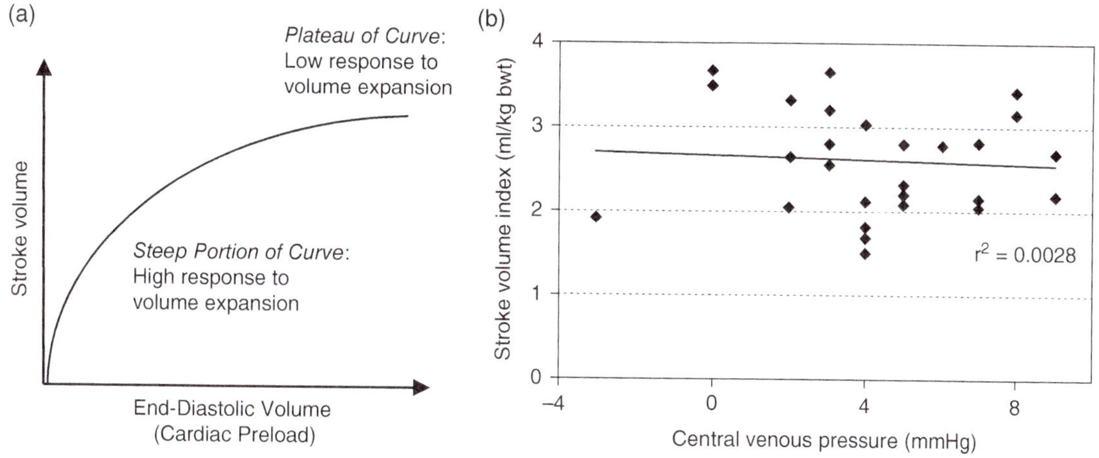

Figure 11.IV.4 Relationship between stroke volume and end-diastolic volume. (a) Demarcated areas show where on the curve there is preload reserve and where on the curve is a low response to volume expansion [3]. (b) Correlation of stroke volume index (stroke volume/body weight) to CVP in critically ill foals [21].

More elaborate CVP waveforms are acquired when using a pressure transducer. These waveforms have primarily been described in people and small animals, although a few reports exist in the neonatal foal [3, 21, 25]. When a pressure transducer is used, it produces a CVP tracing with a number of peaks and troughs, each representing changes in pressure that correlate with the cardiac cycle. The normal CVP tracing has three positive waves, the "a," "c" and "v" waves; and two negative waves, the "x" and "y" waves (Figure 11.IV.5a). The "a" and "c" waves correspond to increases in atrial pressure with the "a" wave corresponding to right atrial contraction and the "c" wave representing closure of the tricuspid valve and protrusion of the valve leaflets into the right atrium during early systole [3]. The "v" wave corresponds to an increase in atrial pressure after tricuspid valve closure (end-diastole). The CVP, measured in mmHg, is the mean of the "a" wave at end expiration, which starts with the PR interval if a concurrent ECG is being used (Figure 11.IV.5b). The "x" descent represents atrial relaxation and filling, which also correlates with tricuspid valve closure and ventricular contraction. The "y" descent is the fall in atrial pressure and ventricular filling after opening of the tricuspid valve.

No specific complications have been documented in foals undergoing CVP measurements, but complications with central lines and CVP measurements in people are relatively infrequent. When they do occur, complications include mechanical (pneumothorax, hemothorax, air embolism), infectious (local or systemic; sepsis, endocarditis, focal abscess), and thrombotic (venous thrombosis, pulmonary embolism) [3, 26]. The use of CVP measurements may be of benefit in guiding fluid therapy in select cases.

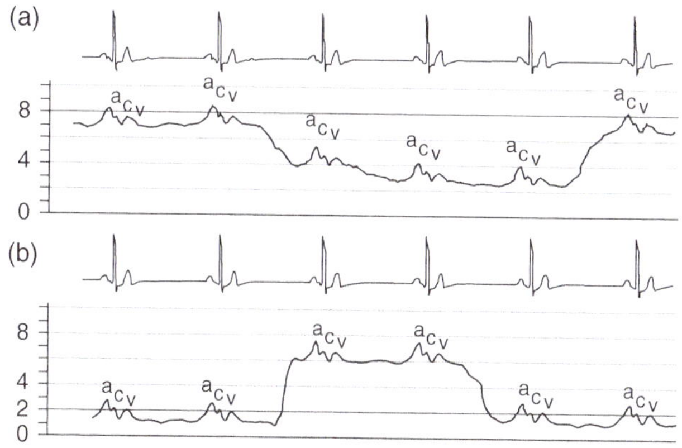

Figure 11.IV.5 (a) Electrocardiogram and CVP recordings from a spontaneously breathing and (b) mechanically ventilated neonatal foal. CVP in the spontaneously breathing foal is measured at end-expiration, just prior to marked decrease in pressure. In this example CVP is 8 mmHg. In contrast, CVP in the mechanically ventilated foal is measured at end-expiration, just prior to the marked increase in pressure. In this example the CVP is 2 mmHg [21].

References

1 Nogradi, N. and Magdesian, K.G. (2018). Measurement of central venous pressure in the neonatal foal. In: *Manual of Clinical Procedures in the Horse* (ed. L.R.R. Costa and M.R. Paradis), 432–435. Hoboken, NJ: Wiley.

2 Nolan-Walston, R.D., Norton, J.L., Navas de Solis, C. et al. (2011). The effects of hypohydration on central venous pressure and splenic volume in adult horses. *J. Vet. Intern. Med.* 25: 570–574.

3 Hutchinson, K.M. and Shaw, S.P. (2016). A review of central venous pressure and its reliability as a hemodynamic monitoring tool in veterinary medicine. *Top. Companion Anim. Med.* 31: 109–121.
4 Rivers, E., Nguyen, B., Havstad, S. et al. (2001). Early goal-directed therapy in the treatment of severe sepsis and septic shock. *N. Engl. J. Med.* 345: 1368–1377.
5 Shoemaker, W.C., Appel, P.L., Kram, H.B. et al. (1988). Prospective trial of supranormal values of survivors as therapeutic goals in high-risk surgical patients. *Chest* 94: 1176–1186.
6 Bishop, M.H., Shoemaker, W.C., Appel, P.L. et al. (1995). Prospective, randomized trail of survivor values of cardiac index, oxygen delivery, and oxygen consumption as resuscitation endpoints in severe trauma. *J. Trauma* 38: 780–787.
7 Jones, A.E., Focht, A., Horton, J.M. et al. (2007). Prospective external validation of the clinical effectiveness of an emergency department-based early goal-directed therapy protocol for severe sepsis and septic shock. *Chest* 132: 415–432.
8 Xu, J.Y., Chen, Q.H., Liu, S.Q. et al. (2016). The effects of early goal-directed therapy on outcome in adult severe sepsis and septic shock patients: a meta-analysis of randomized clinical trials. *Anesth. Analg.* 123: 371.
9 Ren, H.S., Li, M., Zhang, Y.J. et al. (2016). High-volume hemofiltration combine with early goal-directed therapy improves alveolar-arterial oxygen exchange in patients with refractory shock. *Eur. Rev. Med. Pharmacol. Sci.* 20: 355–362.
10 Magdesian, K.G., Fielding, C.L., Rhodes, D.M. et al. (2006). Changes in central venous pressure and blood lactate concentration in response to acute blood loss in horses. *J. Am. Vet. Med. Assoc.* 229: 1458–1462.
11 Corley, K.T., McKenzie, H.C., Amoroso, L.M. et al. (2000). Initial experience with norepinephrine infusion in hypotensive critically ill foals. *J. Vet. Emerg. Crit. Care* 10: 267–276.
12 Corley, K.T.T. (2003). Monitoring and treating the cardiovascular system in neonatal foals. *Clin. Tech. Equine Pract.* 2: 42–55.
13 Hall, L.W. and Nigam, J.M. (1975). Measurement of central venous pressure in horses. *Vet. Rec.* 97: 66–69.
14 Norton, J.L., Nolen-Walston, R.D., Underwood, C. et al. (2011). Repeatability, reproducibility, and effect of head position on central venous pressure measurement in standing adult horses. *J. Vet. Intern. Med.* 25: 575–578.
15 Norton, J.L., Nolen-Walston, R.D., Underwood, C. et al. (2011). Comparison of water manometry to 2 commercial electronic pressure monitors for central venous pressure measurement in horses. *J. Vet. Intern. Med.* 25: 303–306.
16 Wong, D.M., Hepworth-Warren, K.L., Sponseller, B.T. et al. (2017). Measured and calculated variables of global oxygenation in healthy neonatal foals. *Am. J. Vet. Res.* 78: 230–238.
17 Giguere, S., Sanchez, C., Shih, A. et al. (2007). Comparison of the effects of caffeine and doxapram on respiratory and cardiovascular function in foals with induced respiratory acidosis. *Am. J. Vet. Res.* 68: 1407–1416.
18 Thomas, W.P., Madigan, J.E., Backus, K.Q. et al. (1987). Systemic and pulmonary haemodynamics in normal neonatal foals. *J. Reprod. Suppl.* 35: 623–628.
19 Wilstermann, S., Hackett, E.S., Rao, S. et al. (2009). A technique for central venous pressure measurement in normal horses. *J. Vet. Emerg. Crit. Care* 19: 241–246.
20 Tam, K., Rezende, M., and Boscan, P. (2011). Correlation between jugular and central venous pressures in laterally recumbent horses. *Vet. Anesth. Analg.* 38: 580–583.
21 Corley, K.T.T. (2002). Monitoring and treating haemodynamic disturbances in critically ill neonatal foals. Part 1: Haemodynamic monitoring. *Equine Vet. Educ.* 14: 270–279.
22 Marik, P., Monnet, X., and Toboul, J.L. (2001). Hemodynamic parameters to guide fluid therapy. *Ann. Intensive Care* 1: 1–9.
23 Magdesian, K.G. (2015). Fluid therapy for neonatal foals. In: *Equine Fluid Therapy* (ed. L.C. Fielding and K.G. Magdesian), 279–298. Ames, IA: Wiley.
24 Pachtinger, G. (2013). Monitoring of the emergent small animal patient. *Vet. Clin. North Am. Small Anim. Pract.* 43: 705–720.
25 Corley, K.T.T. (2002). Monitoring and treating haemodynamic disturbances in critically ill neonatal foals. Part 2: assessment and treatment. *Equine Vet. Educ.* 14: 328–336.
26 Pittman, J., Sum Ping, J., and Mark, J. (2004). Arterial and central venous pressure monitoring. *Int. Anesthesiol. Clin.* 42: 13–30.

Section V Cardiovascular Medications for the Neonatal Foal

K. Gary Magdesian

Cardiovascular drugs comprise an important component of therapy of the critically ill foal. Several therapeutics are used for hemodynamic support, including inotropes and vasopressors. Though less common in the neonate, occasionally therapeutics are needed as anti-arrhythmic agents or for congestive heart failure (CHF). Finally, anticoagulants are used for their anti-inflammatory and anticoagulant properties during hypercoagulable states such as septic or endotoxic shock.

Inotrope and Vasopressor Therapy

Hemodynamic instability is a common feature of the critically ill foal. Inappropriate vasodilation and reduced cardiac output from compromised myocardial contractility and hypovolemia are common among critical foals. Sepsis and hypoxic-ischemic injury frequently result in hypotension and reduced tissue oxygen delivery, and if prolonged can result in multiple organ dysfunction syndrome (MODS). Fluid therapy is the front-line therapy for treatment of hypovolemia and hypoperfusion. Inotropes and pressors should only begin when adequate fluid replacement has occurred. Fluids expand plasma volume and increase venous return and preload, which result in improved stroke volume and cardiac output. Fluid therapy is discussed in Chapter 62.

After fluid administration, and to avoid fluid overload, the addition of an inotrope is indicated if perfusion remains poor; the goal of inotropes is to maximize myocardial contractility, thereby increasing cardiac output. The final step in the treatment of hypoperfusion, especially when vasodilation and hypotension are present, is the addition of vasopressors to the fluid and inotrope plan. The goal of vasopressor therapy is vasoconstriction to increase peripheral vascular resistance, during states of inappropriate vasodilation such as septic shock. A brief review of adrenergic receptor affinity is below and in Table 11.V.1:

Beta-1 (β_1): Inotropic and chronotropic; e.g. dobutamine
Beta-2 (β_2): Vasodilation and bronchodilation; e.g. albuterol
Alpha-1 (α_1): Vasoconstriction; e.g. phenylephrine
Alpha-2 (α_2): Presynaptic, inhibition of norepinephrine release; transient hypertension followed by hypotension e.g. xylazine

Norepinephrine is nonselective and binds to α_1, α_2, and β_1 receptors, but has greatest affinity for α_1. Epinephrine binds to all four receptors, but is primarily a β_1 agonist at lower doses, such as those used during CPR. Dopamine has dose-dependent effects and can bind to α_1, α_2, β_1, and dopamine receptors. At low doses (2–3 μg/kg/min) it has primary affinity for dopamine receptors, leading to renal, coronary, cerebral, and splanchnic vasodilation. At medium doses (5–10 μg/kg/min) it has β_1 adrenergic affinity and at high doses (>10 μg/kg/min) it has α_1 adrenergic effects. These are generalizations, as there is significant inter-individual variation in dose and receptor affinity type.

Inotropes

Inotropes are indicated for the treatment of cardiogenic shock and heart failure as they improve myocardial contractility. Adrenergic inotropes are primarily β1-agonists. Inotropy and chronotropy are regulated through β1- and β2-adrenergic receptors, respectively. Because heart rate is often already high during sepsis, compounding tachycardia to improve cardiac output is not warranted. Rather, inotropy is the goal of therapy for increasing cardiac output beyond that provided by fluid therapy. A rule of thumb for clinical use, inotropes should not be started until hypovolemia is corrected. Without optimal preload, inotrope therapy could inappropriately increase workload on the myocardium without a concomitant increase in stroke volume. Therefore, fluids should always be administered before and during inotrope therapy.

Equine Neonatal Medicine, First Edition. Edited by David M. Wong and Pamela A. Wilkins.

Table 11.V.1 Inotrope and vasopressor receptor affinities of various drugs for neonatal foals [1].

	Adrenergic				Dopaminergic			
Drug	β_1	β_2	α_1	α_2	1	2	**V1a receptor**	**Starting dosage (titrate carefully to effect)**
Dobutamine	+++	++	+	+	0	0	0	3–5 μg/kg/min (range 2–10 μg/kg/min)
Dopamine	++	+	++	(+)	+++	++	0	5–10 μg/kg/min (affinity varies with dose)
Epinephrine	+++	+++	+++	+++	0	0	0	Mainly for CPR; primarily β_1 at low doses
Norepinephrine	++	0	+++	++	0	0	0	0.05–2.0 μg/kg/min
Phenylephrine	(+)	0	+++	+	0	0	0	
Vasopressin	0	0	0	0	0	0	+++	0.1–0.5 mU/kg/min

strong affinity +++; moderate affinity ++; weak affinity +; possible weak affinity (+); no affinity 0.

Clinical indications for inotropes include low blood pressure and cardiac output in association with clinical signs and laboratory indicators of hypoperfusion. Foals with abnormal perfusion parameters (mentation, pulse quality, extremity temperature, CRT), increased blood lactate concentration, or low indirect blood pressure after adequate fluid replacement may benefit from inotrope therapy, and a trial should be instituted. Another marker for the need for inotropes includes decreased central venous oxygen tension (and increased oxygen extraction ratio [OER]), despite appropriate fluid therapy.

Rule of 6 for calculating how much inopressor should be added to infusion fluids.

6 × body weight (kg) = number of milligrams of drug that is added to 100 ml of infusion fluids.

- Each 1 ml/h infusion the foal will receive 1 μg/kg/min of drug
- Example: Dobutamine dose of 5 μg/kg/min to a 50 kg foal
  - 6 × 50 kg = 300 mg dobutamine added to 100 ml of infusion fluids = concentration of 3 mg/ml (3,000 μg/ml)
  - Dobutamine dose: 5 μg × 50 kg/min = 250 μg/min (for 50 kg foal)
    - Each 1 ml/h infusion results in foal receiving 1 μg/kg/min; if desired dose is 5 μg/kg/min, then the rate would be 5 ml/hour (total dose is 5 ml/hour × 3 mg/ml = 15 mg/hour [15,000 μg/hour] ÷ 60 minutes/hour = 250 μg/minute)

For drugs with infusion rate in the range of 0.1–1 μg/kg/min of drug, 0.6 should replace 6.

- Each 1 ml/h infusion the foal will receive 0.1 μg/kg/min of drug.
- Example: Norepinephrine 0.5 μg/kg/min to 50 kg foal
  - 0.6 × 50 kg = 30 mg norepinephrine added to 100 ml of infusion fluids = concentration of 0.3 mg/ml (300 μg/ml)
  - Norepinephrine dose: 0.5 μg × 50 kg/min = 25 μg/min (for 50 kg foal)
    - Each 1 ml/h infusion results in foal receiving 0.1 μg/kg/min; if desired dose is 0.5 μg/kg/min then the rate would be 5 ml/hour (total dose is 5 ml/hour × 0.3 mg/ml = 1.5 mg/hr [1500 μg/hr] ÷ 60 minutes/hour = 25 μg/minute)

Dobutamine is a β1-receptor adrenergic agonist with less affinity for β2- and α-adrenergic receptors. It is the most common vasoactive catecholamine used in the critically ill foal, indicated when blood pressure and cardiac output remain low after fluid replacement. As pulmonary arterial catheters are not commonly used in sick neonatal foals, cardiac output and systemic vascular resistance (SVR) are often not measured directly. Cardiac output can be estimated noninvasively using echocardiography and the Bullet method (see below).

The dose range utilized for dobutamine is 2–10 μg/kg/min, with the usual starting dose being 3–5 μg/kg/min and then titrated to effect. Dobutamine is fairly safe with the most common side effect being tachycardia. In the event of significant tachycardia or dysrhythmias, the dobutamine dose should be decreased or discontinued. Dobutamine has been shown to increase cardiac index (CI) by 100% and 210% at infusion doses of 4 (low dose) and 8 (high dose) μg/kg/min in hypotensive, anesthetized foals [2]. This improvement was due to both an increase in stroke volume and heart rate. The stroke volume index increased by 64% and 100% and heart rate increased by 17% and 54%, respectively, during the 4 and 8 μg/kg/min infusions [2].

Dobutamine can be diluted in 5% dextrose injection; 5% dextrose and 0.45% sodium chloride injection; 5% dextrose and 0.9% sodium chloride injection; 10% dextrose injection; lactated Ringer's injection; 5% dextrose in lactated Ringer's injection; or 0.9% sodium chloride. Solutions of diluted dobutamine should be used within 24 hours.

Dopamine binds α_1, α_2, β_1 and dopamine-1 receptors depending on administered dose. At low doses it acts on dopamine-1 receptors, causing vasodilation in the renal, splanchnic, cerebral, and coronary beds. Dopamine acts as a β_1 adrenergic agonist through medium doses (5–10 μg/kg/min) and has inotropic effects. Dopamine is less predictable than dobutamine as an inotope, and because of this and concerns over reduced splanchnic circulation at medium-to-higher doses, is not a first-line inotrope. In addition, at β_1 and higher doses, dopamine is more likely to lead to dose-limiting dysrhythmias.

Norepinephrine

While considered primarily a vasopressor through α_1 receptor activity, norepinephrine has some inotropic effect through β_1 adrenergic receptor affinity. In the above study of anesthetized foals, norepinephrine infusion doses of 0.3 and 1.0 µg/kg/min resulted in increases of stroke volume index by 50% and 125%, respectively, which in turn resulted in an increase in CI by approximately the same amount [2].

Other inotropes include isoproterenol and pimobendan. Isoproterenol causes significant tachycardia and decreased arterial pressure in adult horses, thereby making it unacceptable as a means of increasing stroke volume, and should not be used [3]. Pimobendan has been studied in adult horses. It is an inodilator, and IV administration (0.25 mg/kg) resulted in both chronotropic and inotropic effects; intragastric administration did not result in inotropic effects [4]. More data are needed, especially in foals, before it can be recommended for use in this age group.

Vasopressors

Vasopressors are used with the goal of vasoconstriction and improving mean arterial pressure through increases in SVR. They are indicated when fluid replacement and inotrope therapies do not improve perfusion in the form of physical examination findings, plasma lactate concentration, arterial blood pressure, and urine output. Excessive vasoconstriction without optimizing fluid volume and myocardial contractility can actually result in reduced cardiac index through increases in afterload. Use of vasopressors prior to optimizing myocardial contractility and stroke volume can increase afterload to the point of increasing cardiac workload and decreasing cardiac index. Therefore, vasopressors should be used only after inotropes, namely dobutamine, and fluids have been tried and have not successfully improved perfusion. Once vasopressor therapy has been instituted, dobutamine should be continued in order to prevent decreases in cardiac index (CI) secondary to this increased SVR and cardiac work. Vasopressors include norepinephrine, epinephrine (mixed inotrope and pressor effects), phenylephrine, high dose dopamine, and the noncatecholamine vasopressor, arginine vasopressin (AVP). Potential side effects of vasopressor therapy include tachycardia, dysrhythmias, and increased myocardial workload.

Norepinephrine is a first-line pressor used in adult humans with sepsis, and it is preferred over other agents, as noted in the 2021 Surviving Sepsis Campaign Guidelines [5]. In children, either norepinephrine or epinephrine is recommended as a first-line vasopressor, because pressors are not as well studied in that age group [6]. Norepinephrine is one of the best-studied and most commonly used vasopressors in foals as well. While the primary effect of norepinephrine is vasoconstriction due to α_1 adrenergic activity, it also has β_1 affinity, thereby also acting as an inotrope.

Norepinephrine is favored over other pressors in part because splanchnic circulation is better preserved, and it is more potent than dopamine as a vasoconstrictor. In a systematic review and meta-analysis in human patients, norepinephrine resulted in lower mortality and lower risks of arrhythmias compared to dopamine [7]. One retrospective study evaluated norepinephrine infusions in seven foals [8]. The highest dose used in each foal was in the range of 0.1–1.5 µg/kg/min, with a duration of 10.3–84.5 hours [8]. These foals suffered from varying combinations of sepsis, pneumonia, hypoxic-ischemic encephalopathy, and prematurity; all foals had concurrent inotrope infusions in the form of dobutamine or dopamine. Norepinephrine infusions were started in response to decreasing arterial pressures in the presence of continued inotropic support. Norepinephrine administration was associated with an increase in mean arterial pressure in 6/7 foals and all foals experienced an increase in urine output. Three of these foals survived to discharge [8].

Common dosage ranges used for norepinephrine infusions include 0.05–2.0 µg/kg/min, starting with lower infusion rates and titrating to effect. Norepinephrine must be diluted in 5% dextrose in water. It should always be administered along with dobutamine to prevent a reduction in cardiac index from excessive vasoconstriction and afterload.

Vasopressin is used in humans as a vasopressor and has had some use in foals as well. Vasopressin acts as an antidiuretic in the renal tubules through V2 receptors and aids in control of plasma osmolarity and volume as antidiuretic hormone (ADH). It is also a vasoconstrictor through V1a receptors in vascular smooth muscle. It is produced in the hypothalamus but stored and released by the posterior pituitary gland.

During early shock, vasopressin is appropriately increased in human patients, but it rapidly decreases to the normal range within 24–48 hours, even as septic shock persists. This state of normal ADH concentrations during shock has been termed "relative vasopressin deficiency" [5]. Whether relative AVP deficiency also occurs in septic foals remains to be elucidated. A few studies have not suggested a deficiency of AVP in sick foals, but whether there is altered sensitivity to AVP during sepsis remains to be studied [9, 10].

One of the major potential side effects of AVP is a reduction in splanchnic, cardiac, and digital circulation at higher doses in human patients. Vasopressin is therefore generally considered a second-line pressor, when catecholamines fail to improve blood pressure and perfusion. The Surviving Sepsis Guidelines for people states, "For adults with septic shock on norepinephrine with inadequate MAP levels, we suggest adding vasopressin instead of escalating the dose of norepinephrine" [5].

A retrospective study evaluating use of norepinephrine and AVP as pressors in hypotensive critically ill foals found that both increased mean arterial pressures [11]. Both drugs also increased urine output, but only the increase following norepinephrine administration was statistically significantly greater than pre-pressor [11]. AVP resulted in a reduction in heart rate as well, and there were no obvious adverse events noted. Doses used in that study included 0.05–1.75 μg/kg/min for norepinephrine and 0.1–2.5 mU/kg/min for AVP. In adult human patients, a commonly administered dose of AVP is 30 mU/min, which is approximately 0.5 mU/kg/min, because higher doses may have adverse effects on splanchnic circulation [5]. In humans, AVP has been associated with decreased splanchnic or renal perfusion [12, 13]. A study in hypotensive, anesthetized foals also suggested AVP caused a reduction in splanchnic perfusion at doses of 0.3 and 1.0 mU/kg/min as measured by gastric tonometry (CO_2); it did increase MAP through increasing SVR in those foals [2].

In the Surviving Sepsis Campaign guidelines, norepinephrine is strongly recommended as the first-line agent over other pressors [5]. The guidelines also suggest adding vasopressin for adults with septic shock when norepinephrine alone fails to improve mean arterial blood pressure, instead of escalating the dose of norepinephrine (a weak recommendation) [5]. In this regard, AVP has catecholamine-sparing effects, with suggestion of starting vasopressin when norepinephrine dose is in the range of 0.25–0.5 μg/kg/min for at least 4 hours [5]. For children with septic shock, the guidelines suggest either adding vasopressin or further titrating catecholamines when high-dose catecholamines are required. There is no consensus on the optimal threshold for initiation of vasopressin in children [6]. The author suggests doses of vasopressin in foals of 0.1–0.5 mU/kg/min, when perfusion fails to improve with norepinephrine alone. However, in recent times, AVP has been very costly or unavailable.

Phenylephrine primarily has α_1 adrenergic activity, with secondary α_2 and very little to no β_1 activity. The disadvantages as compared to norepinephrine include a longer half-life, making it more difficult to titrate during clinical use [1]. It also causes reflex bradycardia in horses, leading to a decrease in CO. In healthy adult horses, it increased mean arterial pressure through an increase in SVR; however, it decreased CO because of a decrease in heart rate without a concomitant increase in stroke volume [14]. Its use is thus limited in foals, and if used, it should be used concurrent to an inotrope.

Epinephrine is a strong agonist for β_1 and has moderate affinity for α_1 and β_2 adrenergic receptors. At low doses, the β_1 activity predominates and epinephrine acts primarily as an inotrope. It has vasopressor activity as a result of α_1 agonism at higher doses, but its clinical use is markedly limited due to negative effects on splanchnic circulation; splanchnic blood flow is lower with epinephrine as compared to norepinephrine in human patients [1, 15]. Epinephrine may also cause a greater increase in myocardial oxygen consumption than other pressors. For these reasons, epinephrine is not used as a first-line vasopressor in septic human patients, but rather is added only when other pressors fail to improve MAP and perfusion [5]. Other than for CPR, the use of epinephrine in critically ill foals is limited. Dopamine and epinephrine may also be more arrhythmogenic than other vasopressors [5].

Dopamine

As noted above, dopamine has dose-dependent dopamine-1, β_1, and β_2 adrenergic activity, complicating its use. It has vasopressor activity at the higher end of the dose range (10–15 μg/kg/min), through α_1 adrenergic activity. The inter-individual sensitivity to dopamine and varying receptor affinity limits its use, along with reductions in splanchnic circulation. In addition, dopamine has been described as a successful treatment for advanced AV heart block that developed under anesthesia in four foals, which were unresponsive to atropine [16].

In humans with septic shock, norepinephrine is preferred over dopamine [5]. Because of potential negative effects, including reduced splanchnic perfusion at high doses, variable inter-individual receptor affinity giving less predictable effects, and suppression of anterior pituitary hormones in other species (other than cortisol), dopamine is not recommended as a first-line inotrope or pressor for use in foals. In addition, dopamine may depress minute ventilation in some human patients, which would be an undesirable effect in foals where hypoventilation is common [17]. Another disadvantage is that dopamine, like epinephrine, may be more arrhythmogenic than other vasopressors [5].

Fenoldopam is another dopamine-1 receptor agonist. At doses of 0.05 and 0.1 μg/kg/min it significantly increased heart rate, decreased carotid arterial pressure, and increased lateral cecal arterial blood flow in adult horses [18]. In healthy foals, the addition of fenoldopam to norepinephrine did not provide additional benefit to renal function. Norepinephrine alone (0.3 μg/kg/min) or in conjunction with fenoldopam caused an increase in arterial blood pressure, SVR, urine output, and creatinine clearance [19]. The combination also resulted in higher heart rates and lower arterial blood pressure than norepinephrine alone [19]. Fenoldopam requires further study before it can be recommended for use in foals.

Corticosteroids

Hydrocortisone is a glucocorticoid with some mineralocorticoid activity. Physiological doses of corticosteroids may be beneficial for foals with persistent hypotension and hypoperfusion despite inotrope and pressor therapy; this poor response to catecholamines may be associated with adrenal insufficiency or dysfunction. Persistent hypoglycemia may also be present in foals with adrenal dysfunction. High ACTH and low cortisol concentrations are consistent with this syndrome [20]. Healthy foals have cortisol concentrations of 12–14 μg/dl within 2 hours of birth, and that quickly decreases to 2–3.6 μg/dl by 12–24 hours [20]. At 30 minutes postpartum, ACTH concentrations are approximately 300 pg/ml, then approximately 100 pg/ml at 1 hour, and are below 50 pg/ml by 6 hours of age [20, 21]. By a median of 33 hours of age, ACTH concentrations were found to be a median of 4.7 pg/ml with a range of 3.7–8.0 pg/ml in Thoroughbred foals [22]. Cortisol concentrations were 2.1 (1.9–3.1) μg/dl [22]. In the same study, Standardbred foals (median age 30.5 [7.7–58.7] hours) had an ACTH concentration of 8.9 (6.2–12.6) pg/ml and cortisol of 11.5 (7.8–15.7) μg/dl [22].

The 2021 Surviving Sepsis Campaign guidelines recommend, "For adults with septic shock and an ongoing requirement for vasopressor therapy, we suggest using IV corticosteroids." [5] The guidelines state, "The typical corticosteroid used in adults with septic shock is IV hydrocortisone at a dose of 200 mg/d given as 50 mg intravenously every 6 hours or as a continuous infusion. It is suggested that this is commenced at a dose of norepinephrine or epinephrine ≥0.25 μg/kg/min at least 4 hours after initiation" [5]. In the guidelines outlined for children with septic shock, the recommendations for the use of hydrocortisone are vague: "We suggest that either IV hydrocortisone or no hydrocortisone may be used if adequate fluid resuscitation and vasopressor therapy are not able to restore hemodynamic stability (weak recommendation, low quality of evidence)" [6].

There are even fewer data for the use of hydrocortisone in neonatal foals, but hydrocortisone can be attempted in foals with catecholamine-refractory hypotension. For such foals, especially those with persistent hypoglycemia or low plasma cortisol concentrations for age (especially if high ACTH is present), hydrocortisone can be added to the fluid, dobutamine and norepinephrine plan. A dose of 1.3 mg/kg/d of hydrocortisone, divided every 4 hours (i.e. 0.22 mg/kg q 4 h) is approximately twice the daily cortisol production rate of a healthy neonatal foal. A recommended protocol for foals is to administer hydrocortisone at a dose rate of 0.22 mg/kg q 4 h for 2–3 days. This is followed by a decrease in hydrocortisone dose by 50% for 1–2 days, and by 50% again for a total of a 3-day taper [20]. At this dose, the hydrocortisone is generally regarded as immunomodulatory rather than immunosuppressive and can increase the sensitivity of vascular smooth muscle to catecholamines [20].

Practical Use of Inotropes and Vasopressors in Critically Ill Foals

Tissue perfusion is dependent on oxygen delivery and mean arterial blood pressure. Blood pressure can be increased by improvements in either cardiac output or SVR. Treatment strategies should be aimed at increasing cardiac output first, by increasing stroke volume through fluid therapy and increasing cardiac contractility with inotropes. Cardiac output should be maximized before attempting to increase SVR with vasopressors, because excessive vasoconstriction can impede blood flow, even if mean arterial pressure increases. Excessive relative vasoconstriction can increase cardiac workload and resistance to blood flow, thereby decreasing stroke volume and cardiac output. Therefore, the order of cardiovascular support should be fluid administration first, followed with inotropes second, and finally the addition of vasopressors third.

Mean arterial pressure, the most important pressure for organ perfusion, is dependent on cardiac output and SVR. Fluid therapy increases stroke volume through enhancement of preload, whereas inotropes increase stroke volume through enhanced myocardial contractility. Vasopressors increase mean arterial pressure through increases in SVR.

Dobutamine is a safe inotrope with few drawbacks, especially in foals that are volume replete after initial fluid therapy. It is important that blood volume (and preload) be optimized before initiating inotrope (dobutamine) therapy, because inotropic agents increase cardiac work and myocardial oxygen consumption. Inappropriate or unexpected tachycardia in a foal after instituting dobutamine may indicate that the foal is under fluid-resuscitated and would benefit from additional fluids. Mild tachycardia is an expected response. Dobutamine should be started soon after it is determined that fluid therapy alone does not result in adequate perfusion as assessed by clinical

Table 11.V.2 Suggested therapeutic outline for fluid, inotrope, and vasopressor use by the author.

1) Ensure adequate circulating volume with crystalloids. The fluid challenge method of isotonic, balanced electrolyte crystalloid administration is suggested (10–20 ml/kg over 30–60 minutes with reassessment). Begin early antimicrobial administration.
2) If the foal remains in a state of hypoperfusion after adequate fluid replacement based on clinical perfusion parameters, urine output, serial blood lactate concentrations, and arterial blood pressure, begin dobutamine at 2–3 μg/kg/min. Dobutamine dose can be gradually titrated to effect, up to 10 μg/kg/min.
3) If dobutamine fails to improve perfusion, add norepinephrine at 0.05–2.0 μg/kg/min, starting at the lower end of the dosage range and titrating to effect.
4) If norepinephrine fails to successfully improve circulation, add vasopressin at 0.1–0.5 mU/kg/min if available (can titrate up to 2.5 mU/kg/min).
5) Consider physiological doses of hydrocortisone if the above fails to improve blood pressure and perfusion, especially if plasma cortisol concentrations are low and ACTH is high, at 0.22 mg/kg IV every 4 hours for 2–3 days with a 3-day taper period.

perfusion parameters (mentation, mucous membrane color, CRT, extremity temperature, pulse quality), urine output, serial blood lactate concentrations, cardiac index estimation, and serial arterial blood pressure monitoring.

Pressors, starting with norepinephrine, are indicated when perfusion or arterial blood pressure is inadequate despite fluid and dobutamine administration. Finally, hydrocortisone can be tried if norepinephrine does not improve perfusion and the foal is still in shock. An outline of inotrope and vasopressor therapy is noted in Table 11.V.2.

Monitoring Responses to Inotrope and Vasopressor Therapy

The goal of inotrope and vasopressor therapy is to increase oxygen delivery to foals with inadequate perfusion, especially those with septic or endotoxemic shock. Monitoring for responses to inopressor therapy includes a combination of physical examination parameters, urine production, laboratory data, and monitoring tools. Physical examination indicators focus on improvement in perfusion parameters and include mentation, pulse quality, extremity temperature, mucous membrane color, and capillary refill time. Heart rate is another perfusion parameter but is less reliable in neonatal foals.

Urine production is a key component of monitoring the response to vasopressor therapy. An increase in urine production, as evidenced by a measured increase in urine output or indirectly through ultrasonographic evidence of bladder filling, is a positive response to inopressor therapy. It is an important and helpful indicator that organ perfusion, in this case renal, has improved. Any reduction in urine production after pressor therapy has started warrants reassessment of the choice or dose of pressors and fluid volume status.

Laboratory data that are helpful in monitoring for responses to inotrope and vasopressor therapy include serial lactate concentration, OER, and acid base parameters. Plasma lactate concentration may not normalize in foals with sepsis; this occurs because of sepsis itself, which is a form of type B hyperlactatemia. It may not normalize for some time, but the lactate concentration should decrease gradually over the first 24–48 hours of treatment. OER is another tool that can aid in monitoring response to treatment; it reflects the percentage of delivered oxygen that is taken up by the tissues, or in other words, the ratio of oxygen consumption to oxygen delivery. OER is calculated as $SaO_2 - ScvO_2/SaO_2$, where SaO_2 is arterial oxygen saturation and $ScvO_2$ is central venous oxygen saturation. Ideally, the venous saturation would be from a mixed venous sample; however, pulmonary arterial catheters are rarely used. Instead, central venous oxygen can be used, from a central venous catheter placed in neonatal foals. Normal OER is about 18–30%, and values >50% are consistent with shock and inadequate systemic oxygenation in human patients.

More advanced monitoring of inotrope and pressor therapy includes measurement of cardiac index (e.g. through the Bullet method ultrasonographically) and arterial blood pressure measurement (direct or indirect) [23]. The Bullet method of cardiac index (CI) estimation is calculated via the below formula [22]:

Cardiac output (CO) = Stroke volume (SV) × Heart rate (HR)
Cardiac index (CI) = CO/kg bodyweight

SV = (Vd − Vs)
SV = 5/6 (LVAd × LVLd) − 5/6 (LVAs × LVLs)
Vd = left ventricular volume at end diastole
Vs = left ventricular volume at end systole
LVAd = left ventricular area in diastole (short axis)
LVLd = left ventricular length in diastole (long axis)
LVAs = left ventricular area in systole (short axis)
LVLs = left ventricular length in systole (long axis)
Expected CI in neonatal foals = CO/bw (kg) = 150–270 ml/kg/min

Cardiac index, as measured with aortic and pulmonary arterial catheters in foals, increased from 180.5 ± 10.3 to 222.1 ± 21.6 ml/kg/min from day 1 to 14 in healthy, term neonatal foals [24].

To put it simply and in a clinically practical manner, fluid and inotrope therapy should improve stroke volume and cardiac index. Pressor therapy should increase SVR. Because SVR is not measured directly, it can be estimated from the formula MAP = CO × SVR, although MAP and CI are more clinically relevant variables. If MAP and CI are low, treatment should be aimed at fluid volume and inotrope therapy. If MAP and SVR are low, vasopressors should be considered.

Arterial blood pressure is useful as a serial monitoring tool. A single time point is not as clinically useful as are temporal trends. The "normal" arterial pressure for an individual foal may not be known, as this can vary with breed, size of foal, and gestational age. Mean arterial pressure is more important than diastolic or systolic pressure for organ perfusion. While in adult humans a target MAP of 65 mmHg is common, there is no consensus guideline for a specific MAP target for foals. Direct measured MAP in normal foals increased from 84.4 ± 3.7 mmHg at 1 day of age to 101.3 ± 4.4 mmHg at 14 days of age [24]. In sick foals, in general a MAP ≥60–65 mmHg, usually as measured by indirect means, is desired; however, this must be interpreted in light of clinical perfusion parameters, urine output, and serial lactate measurement. Cardiovascular support should not target a specific measured number in foals, but rather an arterial blood pressure that is associated with appropriate urine output, improvements in perfusion parameters, lactate concentration, and cardiac index. For example, 60 mmHg may be an appropriate MAP for perfusion in a given foal, yet represent hypotension for another. It should be kept in mind that the goal of fluid and inopressor therapy is to improve perfusion, not achieve a specific mean arterial pressure number on a monitor per se.

Antiarrhythmics

Pathologic arrhythmias are uncommon in the neonatal foal. Nonetheless, they can develop in foals with underlying heart dysfunction from congenital disorders, those with sepsis or endotoxemia, and those with myocardial disease such as white muscle disease. Transient arrhythmias are common among healthy newborn foals in the early postpartum period. These include atrial premature contractions, wandering pacemaker, sinus arrhythmia, and atrial fibrillation, with ventricular premature contractions and tachycardia being less common. All of these were transient and spontaneously resolved [25, 26]. Another study showed that 64% of healthy newborn foals had sinus arrhythmia, and 60% had APCs. Atrial fibrillation occurred in 30% and VPC in 12%. These arrhythmias spontaneously resolved within 15 minutes of birth [25, 26].

There are no pharmacokinetic or efficacy studies evaluating antiarrhythmic agents in foals. Doses of antiarrhythmics have been extrapolated from adult horses or other species. There are a few individual case reports describing use of antiarrhythmics in foals, primarily for those occurring under general anesthesia. The reader is referred elsewhere for a comprehensive review of the four classes of antiarrhythmic agents based on the Vaughan-Williams classification system [27].

Class I Antiarrhythmic Agents

Class Ia antiarrhythmic agents include quinidine and procainamide. These act as sodium channel blockers in the myocardium, primarily through slowing propagation of action potentials. The class Ia drugs effectively lengthen the refractory period of the cardiac cycle and are indicated for both supraventricular and ventricular arrhythmias. Quinidine is the most commonly used class Ia agent in adult horses, primarily to treat atrial fibrillation. Its use, along with digoxin, has been described in the successful cardioversion of atrial fibrillation in one 3-month-old foal; the atrial fibrillation was secondary to vegetative endocarditis with involvement of the atrial myocardium associated with *Rhodococcus equi* infection [28]. Another case report described unsuccessful cardioversion of atrial fibrillation using quinidine in a 3-month-old foal; the atrial fibrillation was subsequently converted with transcutaneous direct current cardioversion [29].

Class 1b antiarrhythmics include lidocaine and phenytoin. They are effective only against ventricular arrhythmias. They act by shortening the action potential without causing QT prolongation. The class Ib drugs are particularly effective in the presence of damaged myocardial cells, because they bind to refractory sodium channels and prevent re-entry arrhythmias [27].

Lidocaine has not been studied in foals specifically; therefore, its use should be carefully monitored in this age group, because toxic concentrations can be quite variable from horse to horse, and foals may be at increased risk of toxicity due to less-efficient metabolism and increased blood-brain barrier permeability. If used for ventricular tachycardia, a loading dose of serial 0.25 mg/kg boluses can be administered IV, separated by 30–60 seconds, up to a cumulative dose of 1.5–2.0 mg/kg. Following this, the infusion rate is 0.05 mg/kg/min. The foals should be monitored for signs of toxicity, including neurological signs, which can consist of seizures, weakness, muscle fasciculations, excitement, and collapse.

There is one report of cardiovascular collapse in a foal after administration of an unknown amount of lidocaine under anesthesia. The IV line of the pump delivering the lidocaine was accidentally open, allowing delivery of an unknown amount of lidocaine [30]. This was suspected to be a toxic amount, and the foal was successfully treated, including use of a lipid infusion. A second report describes lidocaine use in a foal with an idioventricular rhythm that developed under anesthesia; the rhythm was refractory to lidocaine, but spontaneously converted when the isoflurane was discontinued [31]. The foal appeared to tolerate the lidocaine infusion (loading dose of 2 mg/kg, followed by 0.05 mg/kg/min) [31].

Lidocaine should be used with caution in foals with liver failure, as metabolism will be reduced with prolongation of half-life, increasing the potential for toxicity. In addition, hypokalemia renders lidocaine less effective; therefore, electrolytes should be monitored during therapy.

Phenytoin has a narrow therapeutic index and should be used with caution in foals. The author has used phenytoin in foals that were homozygous for hyperkalemic periodic paralysis and were dysphagic. Therapeutic drug monitoring should ideally be performed for phenytoin because of potential for adverse effects. Effective plasma concentrations of phenytoin range from 5–10 μg/ml, and adverse effects include muscle fasciculations, recumbency, and sedation. Development of these signs warrants dosage reductions.

Class 1c: There are very little data for the use of these drugs in horses in general; these should be avoided in foals, as they can be associated with a narrow safety profile.

Class II antiarrhythmic agents are β-adrenergic antagonists ("β-blockers"), which act through prolongation of phase 4 of the action potential. They reduce sinoatrial pacemaker activity and conduction through the AV nodes, resulting in decreased heart rate. As a virtue of their β-blocking effects, they also have negative inotrope activity. Propranolol is a nonspecific β1- and β2-receptor antagonist, thereby having negative inotropic and chronotropic effects. It is used to treat supraventricular tachycardias (SVT) and ventricular tachycardias (VT) that do not respond to other agents. They can be used for quinidine-induced tachyarrhythmias [27]. Sotalol has both class II and III antiarrhythmic activity and can be used for both SV arrhythmias and VT. It has been studied in adult horses, and can be used orally, however it requires further study before it can be recommended for use in foals. Potential adverse effects of sotalol in horses include sweating and mild colic [32].

Class III antiarrhythmic agents are potassium channel blockers, which suppress the inward potassium current. They prolong phase 3 of the cardiac action potential, as well as the refractory period and are used to treat ventricular arrhythmias. Amiodarone has been used in adult horses for treatment of atrial fibrillation and one report describes treatment of VT in a horse that was refractory to other agents, including lidocaine [33, 34]. Amiodarone can have a variety of adverse effects, including GI, neurological, cardiac, and dermatologic [27]. These drugs have not been studied in foals.

Class IV antiarrhythmic drugs are calcium channel blockers, which act on phase 2 of the cardiac action potential. They are primarily used for SV arrhythmias in other species. Diltiazem has been studied in healthy adult horses and in those with experimental atrial pacing, as a means of controlling ventricular rate during administration of quinidine [35, 36]. There are no data evaluating this class in foals.

Magnesium Sulfate

Intravenous magnesium sulfate is an important antiarrhythmic for ventricular tachycardia, including refractory forms, even when the patient is normomagnesemic. Magnesium is useful for quinidine-induced ventricular arrhythmias, including torsades de pointes. The mechanism of antiarrhythmic action of magnesium is poorly understood but may involve calcium channel-blockage. It is a very safe antiarrhythmic and can potentiate the effects of lidocaine. Along with lidocaine, magnesium represents one of the most clinically useful antiarrhytmics for foals with VT.

Congestive Heart Failure

CHF is uncommon in neonatal foals. Causes include selenium and/or vitamin E deficiency (white muscle disease), congenital cardiac defects, and infectious causes of myocarditis, vegetative endocarditis, and pericarditis. The prognosis is poor when heart failure is clinical, except for cases with potentially reversible causes such as white muscle disease or septic myocarditis and pericarditis. Treatment of CHF in general consists of diuresis, afterload reduction, and possibly inotrope administration.

Treatment of Congestive Heart Failure

Diuretics act as preload reducers. The mechanism of action of loop diuretics includes inhibition of reabsorption of sodium, potassium, and chloride through competitive inhibition of the $Na^+2Cl^-K^+$ cotransporter pump in the thick ascending loop of Henle. These drugs reduce plasma volume and atrial and ventricular pressures, thereby reducing systemic and pulmonary edema.

Furosemide is one of the most important components in the management of clinically apparent CHF. In addition to the noted diuretic actions, it also results in vasodilation, which reduces pulmonary vascular pressures and is another means of improving pulmonary edema. It is highly effective when administered parenterally but has poor oral bioavailability in the adult horse. While the pharmacokinetics of furosemide have not been studied in foals, the author has used 1 mg/kg boluses IV (up to q 8 h), as well as continuous rate infusions (CRI). The CRI administration (0.12 mg/kg/h, after a loading dose of 0.12 mg/kg IV) has resulted in more profound diuresis in adult horses [37]. Longer-term therapy can be accomplished through intramuscular administration (1–2 mg/kg q 6–12 h), but electrolytes should be monitored as hyponatremia, hypochloremia, hypokalemia, hypocalcemia, and hypomagnesemia may develop.

Torsemide, an oral loop diuretic, has been studied in adult horses [38]. A dosing rate of 2 mg/kg orally administered every 12 hours for 6 days resulted in potentially therapeutic concentrations in plasma, and was associated with clinical effects. It caused clinically relevant and rapid diuresis, as well as moderate pre-renal azotemia and electrolyte disturbances including hyponatremia, hypokalemia, and hypochloremia [38]. Mean arterial pressures also decreased from 78 ± 6.1 mmHg to 57.7 ± 8.8 mmHg after the 6 days.

Afterload reduction for horses with CHF can be achieved with the use of angiotensin converting enzyme inhibitors. These act to inhibit the conversion of angiotensin 1 to angiotensin 2, thereby reducing the effects of renin-angiotensin-aldosterone system (RAAS) activation during heart failure. They act to reduce plasma volume and afterload. The ACE inhibitors are commonly used in humans, where they have been shown to reduce the progression of heart failure. Benazapril is currently the most commonly recommended ACE inhibitor for horses, as it has better bioavailability than other ACE inhibitors in adult horses [39]. This class of drugs has not been studied in foals.

Inotropes may be helpful in horses and foals with heart failure, especially if systolic dysfunction is present; the reader is directed to the discussion about dobutamine above, as this would be the most common inotrope used in neonatal foals. Digoxin, an inotrope sometimes used in adult horses, has a narrow therapeutic index and has not been studied in foals. Toxicity can cause lethargy, anorexia, and arrhythmias. Pimobendan, an inodilator discussed next, also has inotrope properties.

Inodilators have both inotropic and afterload reducing effects, through increasing myocardial contractility and peripheral vasodilation, respectively. Phosphodiesterase (PDE) inhibitors such as pimobendan are used to treat canine cardiomyopathies and heart failure, and has improved survival time and delayed clinical signs in animals with subclinical heart failure [40, 41]. There are little data on the use of inodilators in horses, and none in foals to the author's knowledge. A study performed in healthy mature horses showed that IV pimobendan has positive chronotropic and inotropic effects [4].

Anticoagulants During Sepsis

Foals with sepsis commonly experience hypercoagulopathies, with rare risks of thrombosis of major or vital vessels. It also places them at risk for thrombosis of veins that are catheterized. The incidence of coagulopathies in foals with sepsis was reported to be as high as 50% in one study, and they were associated with increased mortality [42]. Widespread fibrin deposition and microthromboses in multiple organs have been found in the capillaries of non-surviving septic foals in another study [43]. Foals with sepsis can develop thromobosis of arteries, including digital vessels, the aorta, and iliac arteries [44, 45]. While aspirin, clopidogrel, unfractioned heparin and low molecular weight heparin (LMWH) have been studied in adult horses, only LMWH has been studied specifically in foals [46]. This is likely the optimal anticoagulant to have been studied in foals, because LMWH has an important place in the treatment of sepsis-associated coagulopathies. In addition to anticoagulant properties, LMWH is anti-inflammatory, including reducing inflammatory cytokine concentrations such as interferon gamma and IL-6 [47].

LMWHs are associated with fewer side effects than unfractioned heparin, including bleeding risk, thrombocytopenia, erythrocyte agglutination, and hematomas at injection sites, including in horses [48]. In the study by Armengou et al., LMWH did not cause thrombocytopenia in healthy or septic foals, and it did not cause prolongation of clotting times even when adequate antifactor-Xa was obtained with 100 IU/kg of dalteparin [46]. A mild decrease in PCV and hemoglobin concentration was observed, but was not clinically significant. None of the 18 healthy or 11 septic foals exhibited any apparent adverse effects of dalteparin in that study, except for one healthy foal, which had a mild jugular hematoma or phlebitis attributed to difficulty in handling the foal and repeated sampling. In that study, plasma antifactor-Xa activity, the laboratory means of monitoring response to LMWH administration, reached prophylactic activity at a dose of 100 IU/kg SC for dalteparin administered daily for three days in foals; the standard adult dose (50 IU/kg daily × 3 days) did not. Of the six septic foals, four achieved antifactor-Xa activity consistent with prophylaxis [46]. Optimal dosing remains to be seen, but 100 IU/kg SC of dalteparin administered daily for 3 days appears to be safe and did not produce bleeding risks, thrombocytopenia, or red blood cell agglutination in foals [46].

References

1 Corley, K.T.T. (2004). Inotropes and vasopressors in adults and foals. *Vet. Clin. North Am. Equine Pract.* 20: 77–106.
2 Valverde, A., Giguere, S., Sanchez, L.C. et al. (2006). Effects of dobutamine, norepinephrine, and vasopressin on cardiovascular function in anesthetized neonatal foals with induced hypotension. *Am. J. Vet. Res.* 67: 1730–1737.
3 Vischer, C.M., Foreman, J.H., Constable, P.D. et al. (1999). Hemodynamic effects of thyroidectomy in sedentary horses. *Am. J. Vet. Res.* 60: 14–21.
4 Afonso, T., Giguere, S., Rapoport, G. et al. (2016). Cardiovascular effects of pimobendan in healthy mature horses. *Equine Vet. J.* 48: 352–356.
5 Evans, L., Rhodes, A., Alhazzani, W. et al. (2021). Surviving sepsis campaign: international guidelines for management of sepsis and septic shock 2021. *Crit. Care Med.* 49: e1063–e1143.
6 Weiss, S.L., Peters, M.J., Alhazzani, W. et al. (2020). Surviving sepsis campaign international guidelines for the management of shock and sepsis-associated organ dysfunction in children. *Pediatr. Crit. Care Med.* 21: e52–e106.
7 Avni, T., Lador, A., Lev, S. et al. (2015). Vasopressors for the treatment of septic shock: systematic review and meta-analysis. *PLoS One* 10: e0129305.
8 Corley, K.T., McKenzie, H.C., Amoroso, L.M. et al. (2000). Initial experience with norepinephrine infusion in hypotensive critically ill foals. *Vet. Emerg. Crit. Care* 10: 267–276.
9 Borchers, A., Magdesian, K.G., Schenck, P.A. et al. (2014). Serial plasma vasopressin concentration in healthy and hospitalised neonatal foals. *Equine Vet. J.* 46: 306–310.
10 Hollis, A.R., Boston, R.C., and Corley, K.T. (2008). Plasma aldosterone, vasopressin and atrial natriuretic peptide in hypovolaemia: a preliminary comparative study of neonatal and mature horses. *Equine Vet. J.* 40: 64–69.
11 Dicky, E.J., McKenzie, H.C., Johnson, A. et al. (2010). Use of pressor therapy in 34 hypotensive critically ill neonatal foals. *Aust. Vet. J.* 88: 472–477.
12 van Haren, F.M.P., Roznedaal, F.W., and van der Hoeven, J.G. (2003). The effect of vasopressin on gastric perfusion in catecholamine-dependent patients in septic shock. *Chest* 124: 2256–2260.
13 Knotzer, H., Pajk, W., Waier, S. et al. (2005). Arginine vasopressin reduces intestinal oxygen supply and mucosal tissue oxygen tension. *Am. J. Physiol. Heart Circ. Physiol.* 289: H168–H173.
14 Hardy, J., Bednarski, R.M., and Biller, D.S. (1994). Effect of phenylephrine on hemodynamics and splenic dimensions in horses. *Am. J. Vet. Res.* 55: 1570–1578.
15 De Backer, D., Creteur, J., Silva, E. et al. (2003). Effects of dopamine, norepinephrine, and epinephrine on the splanchnic circulation in septic shock: which is best? *Crit. Care Med.* 31: 1659–1667.
16 Whitton, D.L. and Trim, C.M. (1985). Use of dopamine hydrochloride during general anesthesia in the treatment of advanced atrioventricular heart block in four foals. *J. Am. Vet. Med. Assoc.* 187: 1357–1361.
17 van de Borne, P., Oren, R., and Somers, V.K. (1998). Dopamine depresses minute ventilation in patients with heart failure. *Circulation* 98: 126–131.
18 Clark, E.S. and Moore, J.N. (1989). Effects of fenoldopam on cecal blood flow and mechanical activity in horses. *Am. J. Vet. Res.* 50: 1926–1930.
19 Hollis, A.R., Ousey, J.C., Palmer, L. et al. (2008). Effects of norepinephrine and combined norepinephrine and fenoldopam infusion on systemic hemodynamics and indices of renal function in normotensive neonatal foals. *J. Vet. Intern. Med.* 22: 1210–1215.
20 Hart, K.A. and Barton, M.H. (2011). Adrenocortical insufficiency in horses and foals. *Vet. Clin. North Am. Equine Pract.* 27: 19–34.
21 Fowden, A.L., Forhead, A.J., and Ousey, J.C. (2012). Endocrine adaptations in the foal over the perinatal period. *Equine Vet. J.* 44 (Suppl 41): 130–139.
22 Lauteri, E., Mariella, J., Beccati, F. et al. (2021). Adrenal gland ultrasonographic measurements and plasma hormone concentrations in clinically healthy newborn Thoroughbred and Standardbred foals. *Animals* 11: 1832–1844.
23 Giguere, S., Bucki, E., Adin, D.B. et al. (2005). Cardiac output measurement by partial carbon dioxide rebreathing, 2-dimensional echocardiography, and lithium-dilution method in anesthetized neonatal foals. *J. Vet. Intern. Med.* 19: 737–743.
24 Thomas, W.P., Madigan, J.E., Backus, K.Q. et al. (1987). Systemic and pulmonary haemodynamics in normal neonatal foals. *J. Reprod. Fertil. Suppl.* 35: 623–628.
25 Yamamoto, K., Yasuda, J., and Too, K. (1991). Electrocardiographic findings during parturition and blood gas tensions immediately after birth in Thoroughbred foals. *J. Vet. Res.* 39: 143–157.
26 Yamamoto, K., Yasuda, J., and Too, K. (1992). Arrhythmias in newborn Thoroughbred foals. *Equine Vet. J.* 23: 169–173.
27 Redpath, A. and Bowen, M. (2019). Cardiac therapeutics in horses. *Vet. Clin. North Am. Equine Pract.* 35: 217–241.
28 Collatos, C., Clark, E.S., Reef, V.B. et al. (1990). Septicemia, atrial fibrillation, cardiomegaly, left atrial mass and Rhodococcus equi septic arthritis in a foal. *J. Am. Vet. Med. Assoc.* 197: 1039–1042.

29 Potter, B.M., Scansen, B.A., Dunbar, L.K. et al. (2017). Transcutaneous direct current cardioversion in a foal with atrial fibrillation. *J. Vet. Cardiol.* 19: 90–105.

30 Vietez, V., Gomez De Seguar, I.A. et al. (2017). Successful use of lipid emulsion to resuscitate a foal after intravenous lidocaine induced cardiovascular collapse. *Equine Vet. J.* 49: 767–769.

31 Pena-Cadahia, C., Manso-Diaz, G., Santiago-Llorentel, I. et al. (2019). Accelerated idioventricular rhythm associated with isoflurane administration in a foal: a case report. *J. Equine Vet. Sci.* 80: 64–68.

32 Broux, B., De Clercq, D., Decloedt, A. et al. (2016). Pharmacokinetics of intravenously and orally administered sotalol hydrochloride in horses and effects on surface electrocardiogram and left ventricular systolic function. *Vet. J.* 208: 60–64.

33 De Clercq, D., van Loon, G., Baert, K. et al. (2007). Effects of an adapted intravenous amiodarone treatment protocol in horses with atrial fibrillation. *Equine Vet. J.* 39: 344–349.

34 De Clercq, D., van Loon, G., Baert, K. et al. (2007). Treatment with amiodarone of refractory ventricular tachycardia in a horse. *J. Vet. Intern. Med.* 21: 878–880.

35 Schwarzwald, C.C., Bonagura, J.D., and Luis-Fuentes, V. (2005). Effects of diltiazem on hemodynamic variables and ventricular function in healthy horses. *J. Vet. Intern. Med.* 19: 703–711.

36 Schwarzwald, C.C., Hamlin, R.L., Bonagura, J.D. et al. (2007). Atrial, SA nodal, and AV nodal electrophysiology in standing horses: normal findings and electrophysiologic effects of quinidine and diltiazem. *J. Vet. Intern. Med.* 21: 166–175.

37 Johansson, A.M., Gardner, S.Y., Levine, J.F. et al. (2003). Furosemide continuous rate infusion in the horse: evaluation of enhanced efficacy and reduced side effects. *J. Vet. Intern. Med.* 17: 887–895.

38 Agne, G.F., Jung, S.W., Wooldridge, A.A. et al. (2018). Pharmacokinetic and pharmacodynamics properties of orally administered torsemide in healthy horses. *J. Vet. Intern. Med.* 32: 1428–1435.

39 Afonso, T., Giguere, S., Rapoport, G. et al. (2013). Pharmacodynamic evaluation of 4 angiotensin-converting enzyme inhibitors in healthy adult horses. *J. Vet. Intern. Med.* 27: 1185–1192.

40 Boswood, A., Haggstrom, J., Gordon, S.G. et al. (2016). Effect of pimobendan in dogs with preclinical myxomatous mitral valve disease and cardiomegaly: the EPIC study – a randomized clinical trial. *J. Vet. Intern. Med.* 30: 1765–1779.

41 Boswood, A., Gordon, S.G., Haggstrom, J. et al. (2018). Longitudinal analysis of quality of life, clinical, radiographic, echocardiographic, and laboratory variables in dogs with preclinical myxomatous mitral valve disease receiving pimobendan or placebo: the EPIC study. *J. Vet. Intern. Med.* 32: 72–85.

42 Bentz, A.I., Palmer, J.E., Dallap, B.L. et al. (2009). Prospective evaluation of coagulation in critically ill neonatal foals. *J. Vet. Intern. Med.* 23: 161–167.

43 Cotovio, M., Monreal, L., Armengou, L. et al. (2008). Fibrin deposits and organ failure in newborn foals with severe septicemia. *J. Vet. Intern. Med.* 22: 1403–1410.

44 Forrest, L.J., Cooley, A.J., and Darien, B.J. (1999). Digital arterial thrombosis in a septicemic foal. *J. Vet. Intern. Med.* 13: 382–385.

45 Moore, L.A., Johnson, P.J., and Bailey, K.L. (1998). Aorto-iliac thrombosis in a foal. *Vet. Rec.* 142: 459–462.

46 Armengou, L., Monreal, L., Delgado, M.A. et al. (2010). Low-molecular-weight heparin dosage in newborn foals. *J. Vet. Intern. Med.* 24: 1190–1195.

47 Litov, L., Petkov, P., Rangelov, M. et al. (2021). Molecular mechanism of the anti-inflammatory action of heparin. *Int. J. Mol. Sci.* 22: 10730.

48 Feige, K., Schwarzwald, C.C., Bombeli, T. et al. (2003). Comparison of unfractioned and low molecular weight heparin for prophylaxis of coagulopathies in 52 horses with colic: a randomized double-blind clinical trial. *Equine Vet. J.* 35: 506–513.

Chapter 12 Congenital Heart Defects

Celia Marr, David Wong, and Alastair Foote

Abbreviations

ACD	atrioventricular canal defect
AOCA	anomalous origin of the coronary artery
AoV	aortic valve
ASD	atrial septal defect
AV	atrioventricular
AVRT	atrioventricular re-entrant tachycardia
CAT	common arterial trunk
CHD	congenital heart defects
DORV	double-outlet right ventricle
IAA	interrupted aortic arch
LA	left atrium
LV	left ventricle
PDA	patent ductus arteriosus
PFO	patent foramen ovale
PMI	point of maximal intensity
PRAA	persistent right aortic arch
RA	right atrium
RV	right ventricle
TOF	tetralogy of Fallot
VSD	ventricular septal defect

The normal cardiac pathway of blood flow (Figure 12.1) is essential to provide the most efficient cardiac output in the neonatal foal. The prevalence of congenital heart defects (CHD) in the foal is unknown, but is considered rare as corroborated by a report in which four CHD were documented in approximately 2,500 fetuses, foals, and adult horses necropsied during a 4-year period [1]. Another report documenting a 3.5% prevalence of CHD in 608 deformed equine fetuses or newborn foals [2] while cardiac involvement was documented in 6 of 38 foals with congenital abnormalities in a survey of 778 fetuses and foals <5 days of age [3]. CHD (all ventricular septal defects, VSD) were diagnosed in 0.3% of horses presented to a University Teaching Hospital [4]. The Arabian, Standardbred, and Welsh Mountain pony may have a higher reported incidence of CDH as compared to other breeds [5–8] and in one European report of VSD prevalence, Warmbloods, and males were overrepresented [9]. However, breed predilections may be driven by factors such as demographics of local horse populations and their access to veterinary services.

Segmental Classification of CHD

Numerous CHD have been described in the equine neonate and include abnormal development of a normal structure (e.g. septal defects, valve atresia), failure of a structure to progress beyond a specific embryonic stage (e.g. common arterial trunk), or modification of the normal blood flow pathway (e.g. coarctation or stenosis). Moreover, many foals with CHD have multiple concurrent congenital cardiac and noncardiac abnormalities [7, 10–12]. Complete reversal of all internal organs, situs inversus, has occasionally been reported in horses; while all organs are found in mirrored locations, the internal morphology of the heart, and other organs, is normal and situs inversus has minimal clinical impact. It is generally detected incidentally when ultrasonography is performed for reasons unrelated to the situs inversus [13–15].

This chapter discusses a variety of CHD documented in the foal but does not cover every individual cardiac anomaly that has been reported as CHD can occur in nearly innumerably different patterns and complexity; this makes categorizing CHD difficult. Historically, reports of equine CHD were invariably single cases and frequently focused on gross anatomical descriptions with minimal clinical information and little attempt to evaluate the pathophysiological mechanisms that anatomical derangements created. However attempts to review the spectrum of CHD seen in horses have been attempted, and in 1964 Rooney and Franks collated and expanded literature on equine

Equine Neonatal Medicine, First Edition. Edited by David M. Wong and Pamela A. Wilkins.

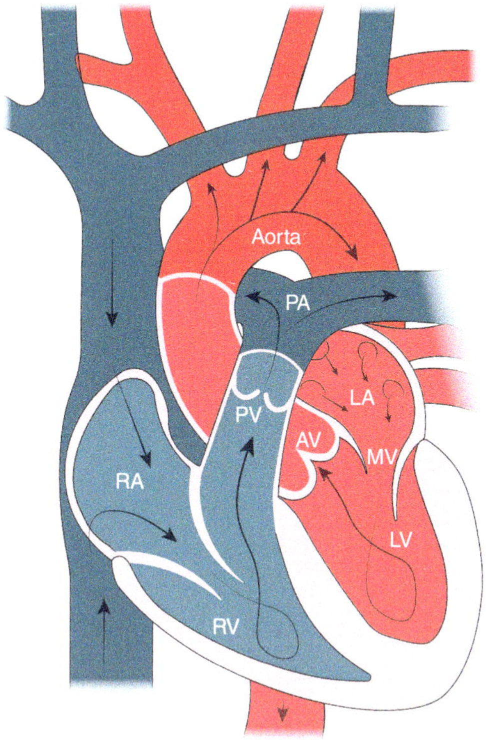

Figure 12.1 Blood flow through the healthy heart; venous blood from the body enters the right atrium (RA), travels through the tricuspid valve into the right ventricle (RV) and is then pumped through the pulmonary valve (PV) and artery (PA) to the lungs where blood is oxygenated. Blood returns to the heart into the left atrium (LA) through the mitral valve (MV) and enters the left ventricle (LV) where it is pushed through the aortic valve (AV) into the aorta and throughout the body. *Source:* Copyright Sara Anais Gonzalez, 2022.

CHD using the terminology of that time [1, 16]. The approach to define CHD in this text is through a sequential segmental approach that analyzes each segment according to blood flow in a sequential fashion (venoatrial connection, atrial morphology, atrioventricular connection, ventricular morphology, ventriculoarterial connection, arterial anomalies, Table 12.1) [27, 125].

Morphological abnormalities can occur in many combinations and in general, while the presence or absence of septal defects together with patency of the ductus arteriosus facilitates shunts, the atrioventricular, and ventriculoarterial connections are key to classifying lesions and determining blood flow patterns where complex disease is present.

Clinical Consequences of CHD

From a clinical perspective, it is helpful to consider a pathophysiological classification based on the consequences of structural defects [125]:

1) Increased pulmonary blood flow (left-to-right shunts without pulmonary obstruction)
2) Decreased pulmonary blood flow (pulmonary obstruction and right-to-left shunt typically resulting in cyanosis)
3) Obstruction to blood progression and no shunts
4) So severe as to be incompatible with postnatal life, likely to show cardiovascular compromise at, or within hours, of birth
5) Minimal clinical impact or silent until adult age
6) Presenting signs related to other body systems

With left-to-right shunting, the clinical impact is largely dependent on the size of the shunt. Small simple shunts (e.g. VSD) [6, 9], patent ductus arteriosus (PDA) [100], and atrial septal defects (ASD) [22] typically lead to mild volume overload of the left chambers, which might be well-tolerated with minimal impact. With larger shunts, left volume overload may be more severe and ultimately pulmonary hypertension and biventricular failure can ensue. Horses are prone to pulmonary artery rupture in the presence of pulmonary hypertension [101] while with marked pulmonary overperfusion, RV failure may be the primary impact [96]. Chronic, high-volume left-to-right shunts can reverse to right-to-left shunting if there is pulmonary vascular remodeling that leads to increased pulmonary vascular resistance sufficient to exceed systemic vascular resistance; this phenomenon is known as Eisenger physiology [27, 126]. Large lesions, such as a large VSD can be associated with bidirectional shunting if pressure between the two ventricles is similar, although usually left-to-right shunting remains dominant.

With right-to-left shunts and decreased pulmonary flow, cyanosis is the hallmark clinical finding and clinical progression is typically driven by the degree of pulmonary obstruction. Obstruction to flow without shunt or stenosis is an unusual isolated lesion in horses and typically stenosis is a component of complex defects; in other species, aortic stenosis is associated with sudden cardiac death [127]. Foals are occasionally born with defects that are incompatible with postnatal life, critical pulmonic stenosis being the best documented [64]. With lesions that remain clinically silent until adulthood the presentation is largely dependent on the level of performance expected of the horse. The clinical impact of CHD is summarized with each specific lesion (Table 12.1).

Venoatrial Connection

Anomalous Pulmonary Venous Return

In people, both total and partial forms of anomalous pulmonary venous return have been reported. To date, only the total form has been reported in horses. In this condition, all pulmonary veins enter the RA (in the partial form,

Table 12.1 Overview of equine congenital heart defects.

Segment and lesion category	Sub-type	Summary	Additional lesions	References	Clinical category
Venoatrial connections					
Anomalous pulmonary venous return		All (total) or some of (partial) pulmonary veins enter right atrium directly or are connected to systemic veins.	Mixed oxygenated and unoxgenated blood enters the left atrium via foramen ovale.	[7, 17, 18]	4
Atrial morphology					
Atrial septal defect (ASD)	Ostium primum ASD	Defect near tricuspid valve.	Usually accompanied by other lesions.	[7, 19–21]	5
	Ostium secundum ASD	Defect near fossa ovale.	Can be reported as isolated lesion.	[22–26]	
	ASD: Sinus venosus	High in the dorsal septum.		[27]	
	Unroofed coronary sinus	At the coronary sinus.		[27]	
Right atrial diverticulum		Large diverticulum communicating with lateral aspect of right atrium.		[28]	3
Atrioventricular (AV) connections					
AV canal defect (ACD, previously common AV canal)	Complete ACD	Interatrial and interventricular shunts with a common AV valve and orifice.		[16, 29–32]	1
	Partial ACD			[19]	1
Tricuspid dysplasia		Malformation of tricuspid valve leads to regurgitation and/or stenosis		[8, 25, 27, 33–35]	3
Mitral dysplasia		Malformation of mitral valve leads to regurgitation and/or stenosis.		[7, 16, 33, 36–38]	3
Tricuspid atresia		Right AV orifice is atretic; systemic venous return enters RA, shunts through a PFO into LA and ventricle. With AV concordance, some flow reaches pulmonary circulation via a VSD.	PFO, VSD hypoplastic right ventricle.	See Table 12.2	2
Double inlet LV		Both atria empty into the LV.	Hypoplastic RV, left-to-right shunt must be present for postnatal life.	[47, 48]	2
Hypoplastic left heart syndrome		Aortic and mitral atresia.	PDA is required for postnatal life.	[23, 49]	4
Ventricular morphology					
Ventricular septal defects (VSD)	Perimembranous VSD	Fibrous continuity between aortic and tricuspid valves.	Perimembranous VSD is frequently associated with aortic valve. Prolapse; all forms can be accompanied by other structural defects and may be required to sustain postnatal life.	[6, 7, 9, 16, 25, 50–53]	1 or 5
	Doubly committed VSD	Fibrous continuity between aortic and pulmonic valves.		[9, 16, 54, 55]	1 or 5
	Muscular VSD	Completely surrounded by muscular tissue.		[7, 9, 16, 50, 56–58]	1 or 5
Ventriculoarterial connections					
Aortic valvular dysplasia		Malformation of aortic valve leads to stenosis and/or regurgitation.		[16, 59–61]	3 or 5
Aortic stenosis		Obstruction below or at the level of the aortic valve.		[7, 16, 62]	3 or 5
Dextroposition of the aorta		Overriding of the aorta; aorta remains to the left of pulmonary artery but sits above both left and right ventricles.	Accompanies VSD and is a component of Tetralogy of Fallot.	[63]	1 or 2

Table 12.1 (Continued)

Pulmonary stenosis	Stenosis is at or below the level of the pulmonary valve.	Reported as isolated lesion; can involve abnormal morphology or number of valve cusps.	[5, 8, 16, 56, 64–66]	2, 3, or 4
Pulmonary atresia	A section of the pulmonary artery is absent.	ASD, PFO, VSD, and/or PDA; right-to-left shunt must be present to sustain postnatal life.	[63, 67–70]	2 or 4
Tetralogy of Fallot (TOF)	Pulmonary stenosis with VSD, overriding aorta, and right ventricular hypertrophy.		[5, 7, 12, 25, 32, 71–80]	2
Pentalogy of Fallot	Tetralogy of Fallot plus PDA or ASD.		[8, 81]	2
Double outlet right ventricle (DORV)	Both pulmonary artery and aorta arise from the right ventricle.	Right-to-left shunt must be present to sustain postnatal life.	[21, 25, 27, 82–85]	2, 4
Great vessel transposition	Aorta originates from RV, pulmonary artery originates from LV ventricle.	Shunts must be present to sustain postnatal life.	[45, 86–88]	2, 4
Common arterial trunk (CAT, previously persistent truncus arteriosus)	Single vessel arises from both ventricles.	Shunts must be present to sustain postnatal life.	[7, 8, 16, 25, 32, 67, 80, 89–94]	2, 4
Aorto-pulmonary septal defect	Communication between aorta and pulmonary artery dorsal to base of heart.		[95]	1
Anomalous origin of pulmonary artery	Systemic pressures in pulmonary circulation leads to pulmonary hypertension.	PDA	[96]	1
Arterial anomalies				
Interruption of the aortic arch (IAA)	Absence of luminal continuity between ascending and descending aorta; found in conjunction with other cardiac defects.		[27, 97, 98]	4
Tubular hypoplasia	Partial IAA		[27]	3
Coarctation of the aorta	The aorta narrows.		[27, 99]	3
Patent ductus arteriosus (PDA)	Ductus arteriosus fails to close.	Often accompanies other morphological abnormalities where PDA can be critical for maintaining postnatal life.	[5, 21, 25, 27, 96, 100–105]	1, 4
PDA with right to left shunt	Ductus arteriosus fails to close.	Right-to-left shunting may be determined by additional morphological abnormalities. Reversal of flow may be due to pulmonary hypertension relating to pulmonary disease or due to other abnormalities such as aortic atresia.	[106]	2
Other congenital conditions affecting the cardiovascular system				
Accessory pathways	Abnormal conducting tissue between atria and ventricles.	Predispose to various forms of supraventricular, junctional, or ventricular tachycardia, including atrial fibrillation.	[107–114]	5
Coronary anomalies	Anomalous origin of coronary vasculature (see individual reports).		[1, 21, 95, 115]	5
Situs inversus	Complete inversion of laterality.		[13–15]	5
Persistent right aortic arch (PRAA)	Vascular ring, formed by right aorta, pulmonary artery, and ligamentum arteriosum, traps esophagus and trachea at base of heart.		[84, 116–121]	6
Other arterial anomalies	See individual reports.		[115, 122, 123]	6
Anomalies of vena cava	See individual reports.		[16, 124]	5

one or two of the pulmonary veins enter the RA and others enter the LA). In people, variations also exist with the pulmonary venous connections returning blood to the RA, vena cava or other systemic veins. The condition may be accompanied by other major cardiac malformations and/or anomalies in other body systems. Given this spectrum of pathology, computed tomographic angiography is recommended for complete evaluation [128, 129].

Anomalous pulmonary venous return entering the RA accompanied by PFO has been reported in one Arabian foal [18] and accompanied by PFO and PDA in one Morgan foal [7]. The condition leads to oxygenated blood returning to the right atrium rather than the left, pressure within the RA rises, and an interatrial connection via a PFO is likely to accompany the anomalous circulation such that there is a mixture of oxygenated and nonoxygenated blood in both atria; the size of the interatrial connection and the degree of pulmonary vascular resistance determines the severity of signs. A small interatrial connection reduces systemic blood flow while increasing pulmonary vascular resistance, which decreases arterial oxygen saturation. In foals, the condition is associated with a presentation early in life with cyanosis and loud bilateral systolic murmurs. Echocardiographically, enlargement of the RA and RV are expected, and the pulmonary veins are absent from their usual location in the LA. Flow mapping techniques, whether Doppler based or using contrast echocardiography, are needed to document the interatrial shunt.

Atrial Morphology

Atrial Septal Defects (ASD) and Patent Foramen Ovale (PFO)

ASDs, in which a true defect of the atrial septum and left-to-right shunting of blood is present, must be differentiated from patent foramen ovale (PFO), which is defined as incomplete anatomical closure of the foramen ovale after birth. Because the foramen ovale is a normal structure, abnormal patency is not regarded as a congenital defect [130]. In the fetus the fossa ovale valve leads to a right-to-left shunt (Figure 12.2) [56, 131]. Some sources view a PFO in foals up to 24–48 hours of age to be a normal finding although the exact age of closure is variable [132–134]. In one report, a foal with a PFO had a normal appearance at birth but was unable to breath and became cyanotic and tachycardic, then subsequently died 2 hours after birth. In this case, necropsy confirmed a large opening in the fenestrae of the fossa ovalis and an opening anterior to the limbus fossa ovalis along the concave lateral margin [135]. However, at this early age, it is possible that the PFO was incidental to the foal's death. PFO can be a component of many complex defects and indeed,

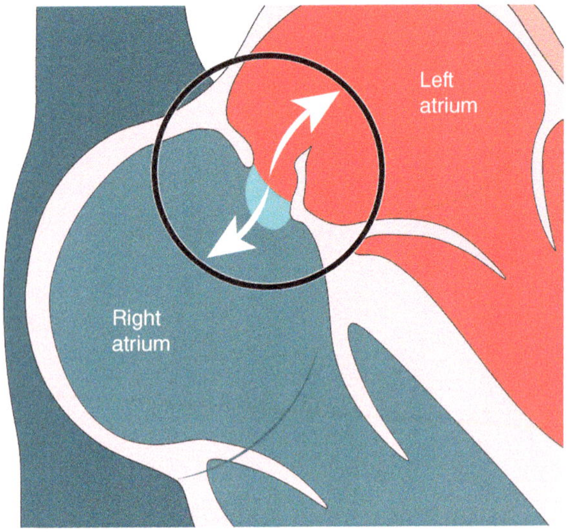

Figure 12.2 Diagram of patent foramen ovale (PFO) in which a small flap-like opening remains between the right and left atrium allowing blood flow to potentially occur between chambers. In the fetus, the direction is right to left, and in postnatal life, the foramen ovale is maintained with pressures in the right exceed the left. *Source:* Copyright Sara Anais Gonzalez, 2022.

the presence of a right-to-left shunt can be essential to survival beyond birth in CHD [7]. PFO is frequently an incidental findings in humans in whom one in four have some degree of anatomical incompetence; under normal physiological conditions, the LA to RA pressure gradient pushes the septum primum against the septum secundum, effectively sealing the PFO such that any shunting is trivial [136]. However, shunting can increase if the interatrial pressure differences are abnormal and it has been suggested that respiratory disease early in life might have resulted in failure of anatomical closure and PFO diagnosed in an adult horse known to have suffered from neonatal dyspnea [130].

ASDs are classified based on their relative location to the interatrial septum and include (Figure 12.3) the tricuspid valve (primum ASD), in the area of the oval fossa (secundum ASD), high in the dorsal atrial septum near either cranial or caudal vena caval inflow (sinus venosus ASD) or near the coronary sinus (coronary sinus ASD) [27]. Overall, ASDs have been infrequently reported in horses, but can represent an isolated defect [22, 25, 27, 137] or, more commonly, be associated with a variety of complex defects. Cases of ASD have been reported in association with VSD [20, 24, 26], tricuspid atresia [1, 8, 39, 40], pulmonic stenosis, pulmonary atresia [67, 69, 70, 89], common atrioventricular canal [16, 29–32], interruption of the aortic arch [97], double outlet RV [21, 82], hypoplastic RV [19], and hypoplastic left heart syndrome [23].

The clinical presentation of ASD depends on its size and presence or absence of concurrent lesions. An isolated ASD may be clinically insignificant, with no obvious murmur [22].

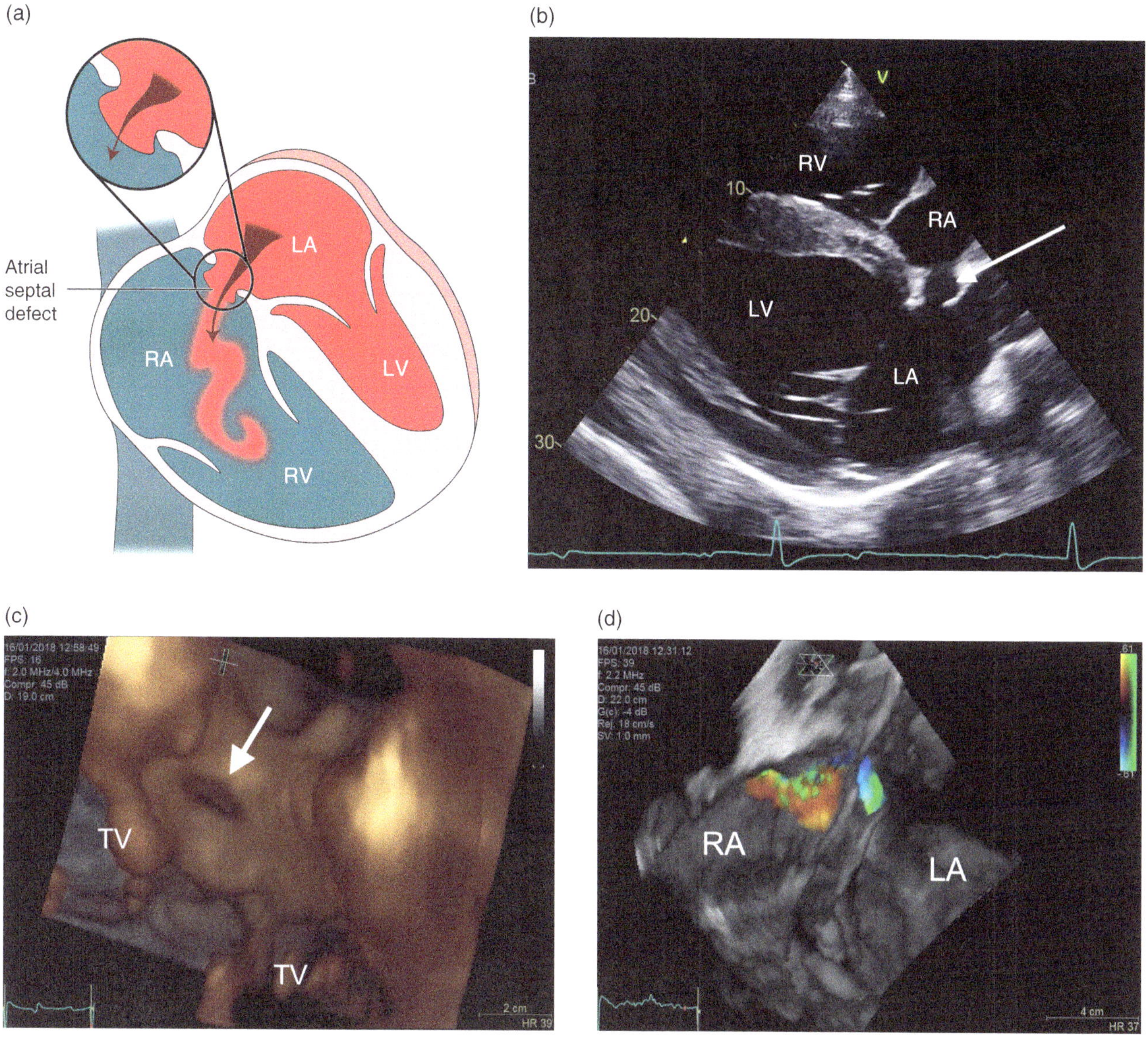

Figure 12.3 (a) Diagram of an atrial septal defect (ASD), which allows left-to-right shunting of blood. *Source:* Copyright Sara Anais Gonzalez, 2022. (b) Long-axis echocardiograph of the right (RV) and left (LV) ventricles and right (RA) and left (LA) atria shows an isolated secundum ASD (arrow) in an adult horse presenting with mild poor performance. (c) 3D echocardiograph, viewing the atrial septum from the right shows the defect (arrow) above a portion of the tricuspid valve (TV). (d) Color-flow Doppler in a 3D image confirms green turbulent flow shunting from LA to RA via the ASD.

Moderate to good exercise capacity may be possible with an ASD as left-to-right shunting of blood decreases as the systemic to pulmonary vascular pressure ratio declines with exercise and, as a result, small ASDs may be underdiagnosed as such cases may not necessarily undergo cardiological investigation in the absence of clear clinical indications. If a large ASD is present, left-to-right shunting may result in right-sided volume overload and pulmonary overcirculation resulting in detection early in life. This situation can generate a murmur at the left heart base and has been termed relative pulmonary stenosis [27]. In addition, atrial fibrillation has also been observed with ASD [20].

Biventricular Atrioventricular Connections

Atrioventricular Canal Defects (ACD)

Atrioventricular canal defects (ACD), sometimes referred to as an AV septal defect, endocardial cushion defect, inter VSD, or common AV valve, is a rare but complex CHD associated with abnormal development of the endocardial cushions, specifically maldevelopment of the atrioventricular septum [16, 29–31]. This malformation involves a low ASD and a high VSD to form a single passageway through which all the cardiac chambers communicate (termed complete ACD). Additionally, because this malformation involves failure of the endocardial cushions to fuse, varying degrees of mitral and tricuspid valve dysplasia may be observed (Figure 12.4). A partial ACD implies that there is only an ASD or only a VSD and that both AV valve annuli are discrete orifices [19, 27]. Further classification of ACD in people is based on the anatomic relationship of the AV leaflets and the ventricular septal crest. Although ACD has been reported in the foal infrequently, it has been suggested that the condition may be more common than generally appreciated since some earlier literature may have misclassified cases [31].

Affected foals can present within the first few weeks of life with tachycardia, tachypnea, and systolic murmurs of moderate to severe intensity (≥ grade 3/6). Echocardiography demonstrates the specific structural changes affecting the interatrial and interventricular portions of the septum and mitral and tricuspid valves. Bidirectional shunts may be present [30–32].

Atrioventricular (AV) Valvular Dysplasia

There is considerable variation in the morphology of the AV valves in healthy horses [138]. The mitral valve consists of two main cusps (septal and nonseptal or parietal) and there can be up to six accessory leaflets with an average of four. The tricuspid valve has three main cusps (septal, parietal, and angular) and up to four accessory cusps with an average of two [138]. Mitral valve dysplasia accounts for 2–8% of CHD in dogs [139, 140] while tricuspid valve dysplasia was reported in 3% [140]. These pathologies are comparatively much less common in horses although their true prevalence is unknown and may be underrepresented in reports based on autopsy surveys. Individual equine case reports of dysplasia of the mitral valve [33, 36, 38, 141] and tricuspid valve [33, 84] have been published. The condition can affect one or both AV valves and dysplasia of the AV valves can also be a component of complex CHD (Figure 12.5) [8, 21, 35]. Mitral and tricuspid valve dysplasia can encompass thickened valve leaflets, abnormally short or long valve leaflets, abnormal chordae tendinae (either too short or too long), and malformed or abnormally located papillary muscles. The cause of AV dysplasia is unknown but likely related to an AV canal defect in the developing heart that results in a failure of proper development of the AV canal [29]. AV valvular dysplasia is generally associated with valvular regurgitation but can lead to stenosis [37].

When severe, AV valve dysplasia can present early in life with one case report described a nine-week-old foal with severe mitral and tricuspid valve dysplasia that presented with lethargy, exercise intolerance, bilateral systolic murmurs, and atrial fibrillation [33]. More often AV valve dysplasia is diagnosed in adulthood particularly when unilateral and/or relating to mild structural changes. Typically, the associated systolic cardiac murmur is loudest over the mitral valve on the left or the tricuspid valve on the right; echocardiographically, it can be difficult to distinguish whether thickening of the valve leaflets is due to dysplasia or inflammation [36]. Other morphological abnormalities such as short chordae tendineae and abnormally located papillary muscles are more definitive indicators that the pathogenesis of valvular regurgitation relates to dysplasia. Echocardiography may also demonstrate enlargement of the RA, RV, LA, and/or LV (depending on which AV valve(s) are affected). Enlargement of all four chambers can be observed if both AV values are affected. The main pulmonary artery and other indications of right-sided overload such as deviation of the intraventricular septum toward the LV were observed in a case of AV valve dysplasia of both AV valves [33]. Color-flow Doppler may reveal a wide jet of turbulent regurgitant blood flow at the AV valve(s). Ultimately, the long-term outcome for cases of AV valve dysplasia depends on the severity of the underlying pathology and resultant regurgitation. In severe cases, the prognosis is poor with postmortem findings in foals including marked dysplasia/hypoplasia of the AV valve(s) and enlargement of the affected chambers of the heart. Evidence of heart failure may be present and includes hydrothorax, ascites, hydropericardium, pulmonary edema, and enlargement of the liver. In mild cases, some level of athletic performance may be achievable. Cases of valvular regurgitation due to dysplasia should be evaluated prognostically based on the criteria that apply to all forms of valvular regurgitation, including assessment of the degree of regurgitation, valvular pathology, chamber enlargement, and presence of concurrent rhythm abnormalities [142].

Univentricular Atrioventricular Connections

The term *univentricular AV connection* is a collective term for hearts in which the atria connect to only one ventricle. This concept groups hearts with double-inlet along with those that have absence of one AV connection and includes tricuspid atresia, double inlet LV, double inlet RV, double inlet indeterminant ventricle, and hypoplastic left heart syndrome [23, 143, 144]. It is rare for there to be a single ventricle; in most of these conditions there is a single receiving ventricle plus a rudimentary second ventricle.

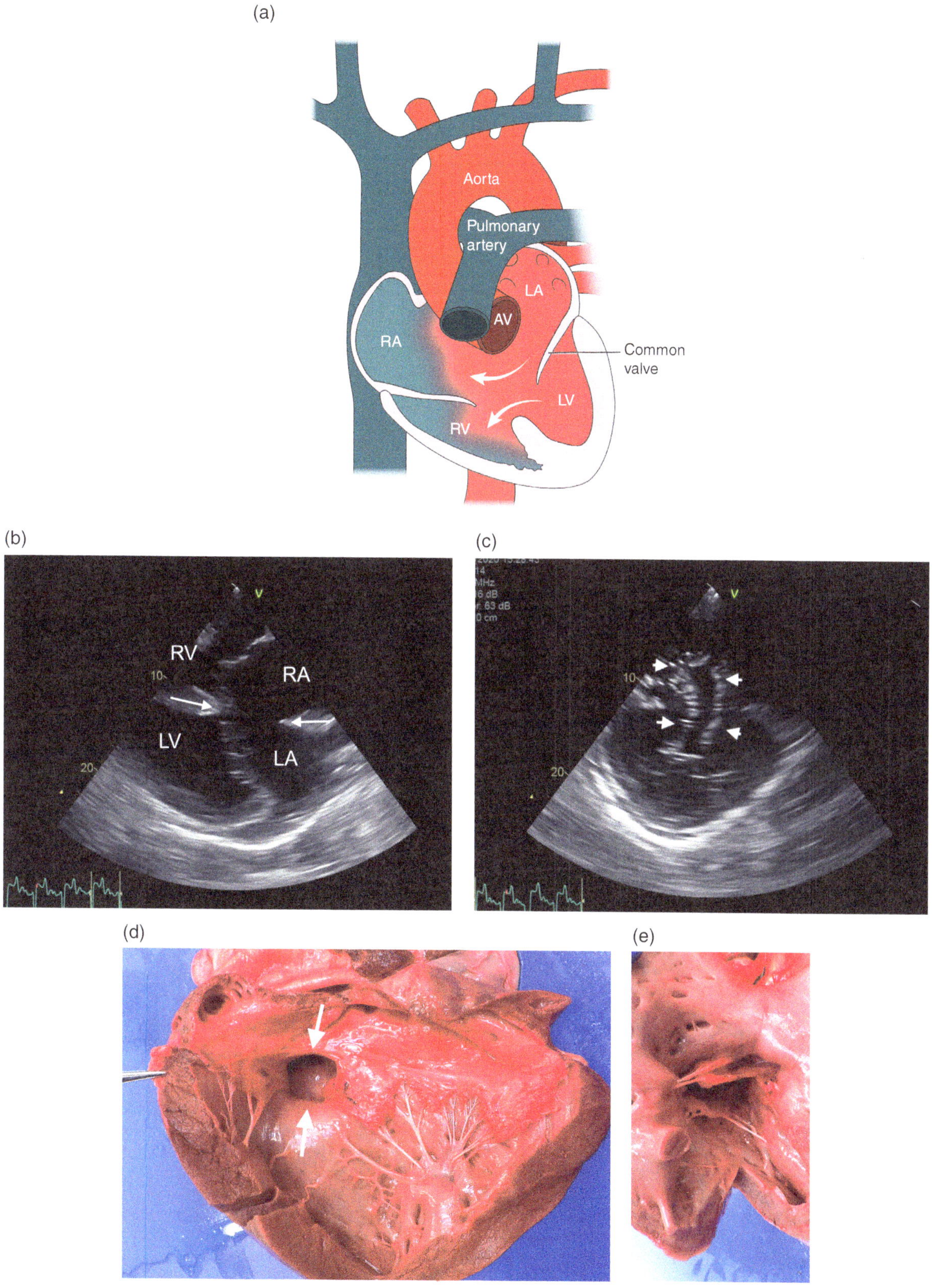

Figure 12.4 (a) Diagram of an atrioventricular canal defect (ACD), which involves a low atrial septal defect and a high ventricular septal defect resulting in a single passageway where all cardiac chambers communicate. *Source:* Copyright Sara Anais Gonzalez, 2022. (b) Long-axis echocardiograph of the right (RV) and left (LV) ventricles and right (RA) and left (LA) atria from a 6-week-old Thoroughbred foal shows the large ventricular and atrial septal defect (between arrows). (c) Short-axis image at the level of the atrioventricular valve shows there are two large cusps of the common valve, traversing the defect (arrowheads). (d) Postmortem specimen from another foal of similar age from the left shows the defect (between arrows) with AV valve cusps traversing it. (e) From the right, the AV valve cusps and their attachments are visible.

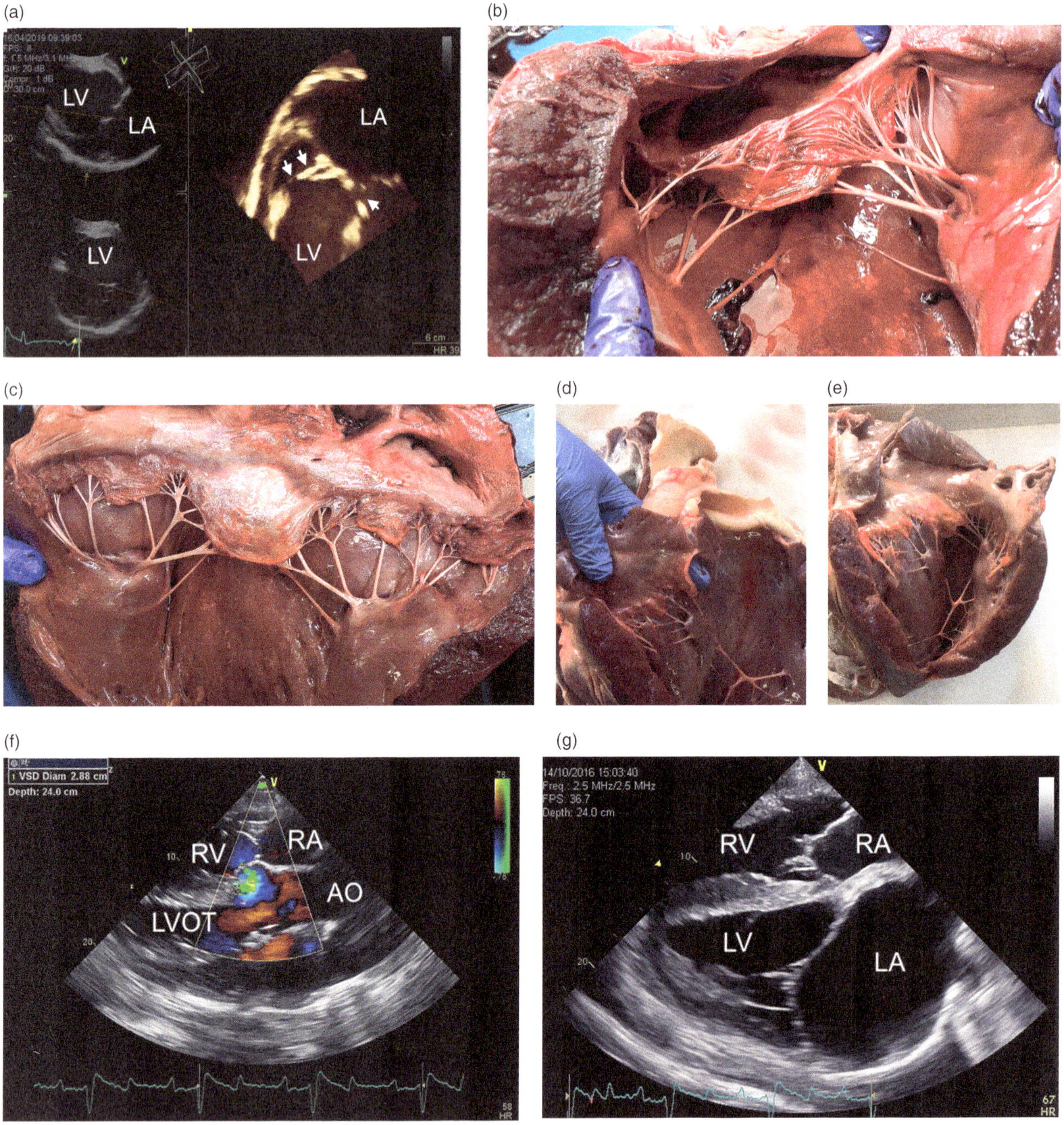

Figure 12.5 Atrioventricular valvular dysplasia. (a) A 3D echocardiograph displaying the left atrium (LA), left ventricle (LV) and mitral valve apparatus in an 18-month-old Thoroughbred with severe mitral regurgitation. The chordae tendinea (arrowheads) are short due to dysplasia. To the left, the 2D images indicate the imaging plane above and below a section at 90° to aid orientation. (b) A similarly aligned postmortem specimen. (c) Examination of the edges of valve cusps show no marked thickening in this case but endocardial jet lesions, confirming regurgitation, are visible across the surface of the septal cusp. (d and e) Postmortem specimens from a 6-month-old Thoroughbred foal confirms the presence of a ventricular septal defect (VSD), into which the pathologist is inserting a finger, and reveals a complex network of false tendons within the left ventricle (also present in the right). The mitral valve is thickened by myxoid stroma likely due to dysplasia; however, it is not certain whether this is a true dysplasia, as this can be seen as secondary remodeling. (f) Long-axis image of the left ventricular outflow tract (LVOT) shows the green shunt through the VSD, which measures 2.88 cm in this plane. (g) Long-axis echocardiograph of the right (RV) and left (LV) ventricles and right (RA) and left (LA) atria shows the LA is markedly enlarged as a result of mitral regurgitation and the mitral valve is thickened. AO, aorta.

Double inlet RV has yet to be reported in horses, while double inlet indeterminant ventricle has not been reported in horses and is extremely rare in people.

Tricuspid Atresia

Tricuspid atresia syndrome is a cyanotic condition typically characterized by a complete lack of communication between the RA and RV (absent tricuspid valve orifice), an enlarged and thickened RA, an interatrial connection (i.e. secundum ASD or PFO), a hypoplastic RV (with or without a VSD), an enlarged mitral valve annulus, and an eccentrically dilated LV (Figure 12.6) [1, 145]. The route of blood flow through the heart involves deoxygenated blood entering the RA, and via a PFO, enters the LA and mixes with oxygenated blood returning from the lungs. This partially oxygenated mixture travels via a left-to-right shunt, either a VSD and/or PDA to the pulmonary trunk. In human infants, tricuspid atresia is classified depending on associated abnormalities. Type 1, the most common form, has normally related great vessels; Type 2 has dextrotransposition of the great arteries; Type 3 refers to any malposition of the great arteries other than dextrotransposition; and Type 4 is accompanied by truncus arteriosus [146, 147]. Tricuspid atresia is sometimes classified as a hypoplastic right heart syndrome because a common feature in all cases is a relative lack of growth of the RV associated with an enlarged LV. However, the severity of right-sided underdevelopment is less apparent in the presence of a VSD. Hypodevelopment of either the pulmonary artery or aorta can also be present, depending on which artery arises from the RV. Importantly, the degree of pulmonary blood flow is critical in determining the degree of cyanosis, and this is determined by the extent of pulmonary obstruction, the presence of a VSD, and the relationship of the great vessels [147, 148].

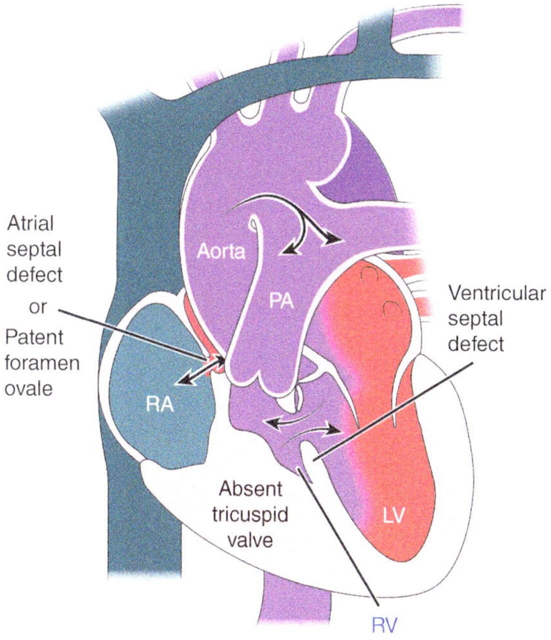

Figure 12.6 Diagram of tricuspid atresia. This defect is characterized by the absence of a tricuspid valve, lack of communication between the RA and RV, an enlarged RA, an interatrial connection (ASD and/or PFO), a hypoplastic right ventricle (RV) with or without a VSD, and enlarged mitral valve annulus and a dilated left ventricle (LV). *Source:* Copyright Sara Anais Gonzalez, 2022.

Fetal hemodynamic adjustments must occur to accommodate structural changes associated with tricuspid atresia, with changes in blood flow depending on the structures involved. In isolated tricuspid atresia with normal great artery position, the entire systemic return of blood can be accommodated through the PFO. Because of the parallel arrangement of the ventricles, shunting of the systemic blood through the foramen ovale is compatible with normal peripheral perfusion throughout gestation. However, in neonatal life, major overload of the LV occurs along with secondary dilation of the aorta due to pulmonary artery hypo-development. The pulmonary circulation is entirely, or in part, provided by retrograde flow through the ductus arteriosus, depending on the presence of a RV, presence and size of the VSD, and/or condition of the pulmonary artery. In cases of tricuspid atresia with transposition of the great arteries, systemic return of blood continues to flow through the PFO as the left side of the heart is overloaded. However, with transposition, the pulmonary artery is dilated while the aorta and aortic arch are relatively hypoplastic (with an increased chance of coarctation of the aorta at birth). In this situation, the aortic arch and its arterial branches going to the head and forelimbs along with the coronary arteries receive blood perfusion by retrograde blood flow from the aortic isthmus and pulmonary artery. In either instance of tricuspid atresia, with or without transposition of the great vessels, the presence of a large VSD will allow passage of blood flow from the left ventricle to the right ventricle, which facilitates some development of the RV. Pulmonary blood flow can be normal or slightly decreased in this situation, depending on the size of VSD.

At birth, arterial oxygen content will primarily depend on the proportion of pulmonary and systemic venous return that enters the LV. In the absence of a VSD, blood flow (and survival) will lie solely on the patency of the ductus arteriosus, which provides the only source of pulmonary flow. In the presence of a VSD, forward pulmonary blood flow can be maintained through the VSD, but development of cardiac failure is possible due to the high cardiac output. If the size of the communication between the RA and LA (i.e. PFO) is relatively small, substantial pooling of blood can occur in the RA with the subsequent development of venous congestion in the neonate. As such, chronic passive congestion of the liver has been reported in foals with tricuspid atresia [7, 44]. If tricuspid atresia is associated with transposition of the great vessels, pulmonary blood flow is normal or increased and the neonate may not have significant cyanosis.

Although tricuspid atresia is considered a rare congenital cardiac abnormality in the foal, several cases have been reported. The Arabian breed is overrepresented, suggesting a potential genetic component [7, 8, 40, 44–46]. The genetic pathways involved in valvulogenesis are complex and not been fully elucidated in people, nor is the dysregulation of genetic control of tricuspid valvulogenesis clearly understood [147]. There are, however, some reports examining familial occurrence [149, 150] and linking specific genetic mutations with tricuspid atresia [151, 152].

Clinical signs and physical examination findings include lethargy, cyanotic mucous membranes, tachycardia, weak peripheral pulses, and tachypnea (Table 12.2) [42]. Consistently reported anatomic features in all foals with tricuspid atresia include the absence of the right atrioventricular (tricuspid) orifice, PFO or ASD, and the presence of a VSD. Other various anomalies associated with tricuspid atresia in foals include enlargement of the RA, small RA, PDA, enlargement of the LV (with LV hypertrophy in some cases), mitral valve annulus dilation, enlargement of the LA, and a small or absent RV. In several reports, a small dimple was observed on the floor of the RA, believed to be a membranous part of the AV septum [44, 46]. Reported vascular anomalies associated with tricuspid atresia in foals include pulmonary artery stenosis, narrowed pulmonary artery, dextroposition of the aorta and pulmonary trunk, anomalous drainage of the vena cava and coronary sinus into the LA, and coarctation (narrowing) of the aorta (Figure 12.7).

Diagnostic procedures utilized in cases of tricuspid atresia in foals include hematology, serum biochemistry analysis, blood gas analysis, radiography, ECG, and echocardiography. Abnormal clinicopathologic findings include polycythemia [40, 44], hypoxemia, and mixed metabolic and respiratory acidemia [7, 8, 40, 44]. Thoracic radiography is often normal with pulmonary edema occasionally reported [40, 45]. Associated ECG abnormalities can include prolongation or enlargement of the P-wave, shortened PR segment, prominent R wave, and ST segment depression [40, 44]. Possible explanations for these ECG changes include RA dilation (shortened PR segment), LV hypertrophy (prominent R-wave) and myocardial ischemia (ST segment depression). Cardiac catheterization may document increased pressures within the RA, and by introducing a catheter to the left side via the interatrial connection increased LA and LV pressures [46].

Echocardiography findings in cases of tricuspid atresia include dilation of the RA, diminutive or absent RV chamber, large LA, large LV, large mitral valve annulus, and thick bands of echoes instead of normal tricuspid valve leaflets [42, 44, 46]. In one report, a single dilated ventricle was identified with significantly reduced systolic function [46]. Additional findings included a thickened and enlarged RA, PFO, and VSD [42, 44, 46]. Contrast echocardiography demonstrated right-to-left shunting of blood at the level of the atria, followed by blood flow into the LV and simultaneous opacification of the RV and aorta [44, 46].

The prognosis for tricuspid atresia is poor, and foals with this anomaly can be found dead or examined within the first few days of life because of severe lethargy and weakness. However, one report describes a foal that was diagnosed with tricuspid atresia that was not euthanized until 7 months of age [44]. Interestingly, in one case, a 1-year-old pony was apparently healthy, but died of peritonitis secondary to rectal rupture [41]. Tricuspid atresia was documented at necropsy, along with a 5 cm PFO and a 2 cm VSD; the pulmonary trunk and aorta were normal, as were the mitral, aortic, and pulmonary valves, suggesting a remote possibility that foals with tricuspid atresia can survive in cases in which there is less complicated anatomic anomalies [41].

Double-Inlet Ventricle

Double-inlet ventricle, a type of univentricular AV connection, is a complex CHD in which both AV valves communicate into a large common or single receiving chamber (Figure 12.8) [47]. The common chamber can be left, right, or mixed ventricular morphology, and the other ventricle, if present, is typically hypoplastic and rudimentary. Few cases have been reported in horses, but in one case, a 4-year-old Arabian gelding was presented for evaluation of both a diastolic and systolic murmur [47]. Echocardiography revealed two distinct AV valves that opened into a large common ventricular chamber, determined to be the morphologic LV. A smaller hypoplastic RV chamber with no AV valve inflow was also reported along with two distinct VSDs. The horse was clinically stable and reportedly the same 1 year after initial exam [47]. Another report described a 2-year-old Thoroughbred filly with a grade V/VI holosystolic murmur best heard over the aortic valve on the left side [48]. The filly had prominent jugular pulses, dark cyanotic mucous membranes, and profound arterial hypoxemia. The filly was euthanized as a 3-year-old, at which time double-inlet ventricle was reported on necropsy [48].

Table 12.2 Case reports of tricuspid atresia in the horse.

References	Breed	Age	Sex	Clinical signs	Murmur
[1]	TB	12 wk	Male	NA	NA
[1]	TB	12 wk	Female	Exercise intolerance from 2 weeks, found dead at 12 weeks	Present, no description provided
[39]	STB	1 d	Male	Found dead approx. 6 hours after birth	NA
[40]	Arabian cross	10 wk	Male	Lethargy, poor body condition, weak	V/V crescendo-decresendo thrill left fourth ICS
[41]	Pony	1 yr	ND	Died from rectal rupture and peritonitis	NA
[42]	Arabian	7 d	Male	Listless since birth, extremely exercise intolerant, cyanosis, esp. with excitement	Present, no description provided
[8]	Arabian	8 d	Male	Weakness, tachycardia, tachypnea, weak peripheral pulses, cyanotic mucous membranes	Pansystolic, left fifth ICS
[43]	Arabian	7 d	ND	Weak, cyanotic mucous membranes	Pansystolic, left heart base with thrill
[44]	Arabian	4 wk	Female	Severe lethargy, small stature, collapse with exertion, weak facial artery pulse, generalized venous distension, cyanotic mucous membranes, tachycardia	IV/V harsh band-shaped pansystolic; left heart base and tricuspid valve area
[44]	ND	10 wk	ND	Severe lethargy, small stature, collapse with exertion, weak facial artery pulse, generalized venous distension, cyanotic mucous membranes, tachycardia	IV/V harsh band-shaped pansystolic; left heart base and tricuspid valve area
[45]	Arabian	6 wk	Female	Poor health since birth, exercise intolerance for 1 month	No description provided
[46]	Arabian	16 d	Female	Lethargy, tachypnea, tachycardia	III/IV continuous, left heart base
[7]	Mini	ND	ND	Tachycardia, cyanotic mucous membranes	≥IV/VI systolic (n = 3) or continuous (n = 1), left heart base
[32]	Mini	2 d	Male	Exercise intolerance, tachycardiac, cyanosis, weak peripheral pulses	VI/VI pansystolic
Summary of current literature	Predisposition in Arabian breed	Usually present in first month	No sex predisposition	Severe cardiovascular compromise with cyanosis	Loud left sided pansystolic murmurs

STB, Standardbred; TB, Thoroughbred; N/A, not applicable; ND, not described.

Ventricular Morphology

Ventricular Septal Defect (VSD)

VSDs are the most commonly observed CHD in horses and have been reported as a single isolated cardiac defect [6] or as part of complex cardiac malformations [7, 9, 21]. The ventricular septum is formed from a number of structures from different cell types. The muscular part of the ventricular septum starts concomitantly with ballooning of the linear heart tube and the development of the bulboventricular groove and continues with proliferation of cells that are localized in the ventricular walls [153]. The membranous part of the ventricular septum is formed by cells of the atrioventricular endocardial cushions. The trabeculae are intraventricular collections of linearly ordered myocytes that fuse with the growing muscular ventricular septum and are derived from myocardial cells of the ventricular walls [153]. As the membranous ventricular septum grows from the atrioventricular endocardial cushion cells it moves toward and fuses with the muscular ventricular septum. Incomplete septation of the ventricles forms a VSD and allows communication of the LV and RV, resulting in mixture of oxygenated and deoxygenated blood and increased blood flow to the lung and LV. This can result in pulmonary edema and dilation and hypertrophy of the LV.

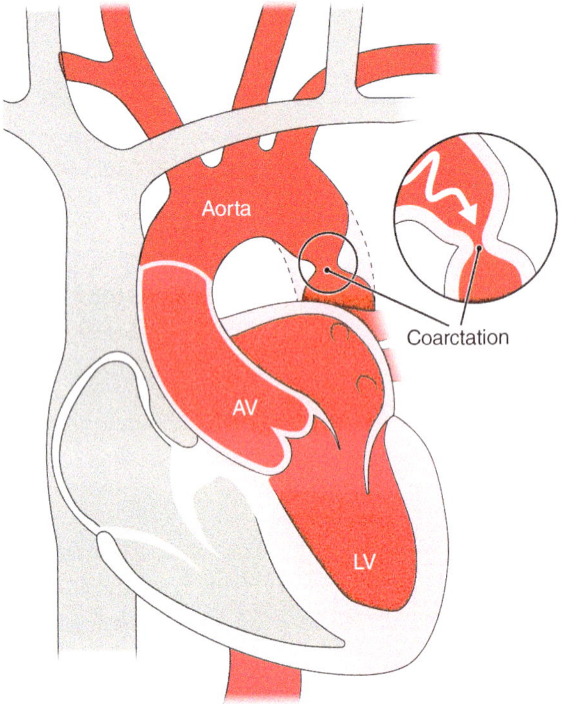

Figure 12.7 Diagram demonstrating coarctation of the aorta, which is characterized by discrete narrowing of the proximal descending aorta resulting in increased afterload. AV, aortic valve; LV, left ventricle. *Source:* Copyright Sara Anais Gonzalez, 2022.

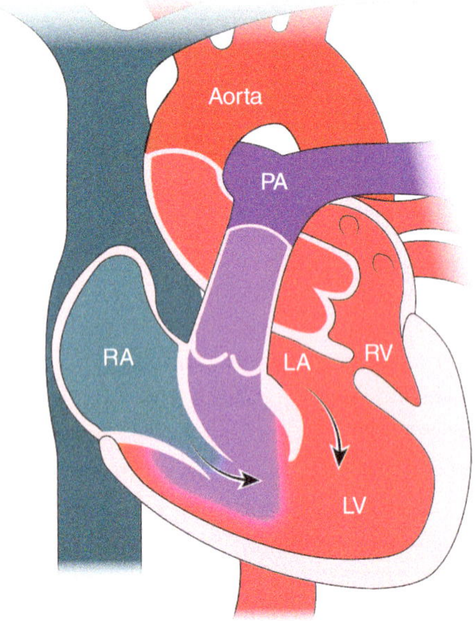

Figure 12.8 Diagram demonstrating double inlet ventricle. In this anomaly, both AV valves communicate into a shared single chamber. In this illustration, the right (RA) and left (LA) atria communicate with the left ventricle (LV) and the right ventricle (RV) is hypoplastic. *Source:* Copyright Sara Anais Gonzalez, 2022.

There are a variety of ways to classify VSDs including by phenotype, geographic location, and degree of septal malalignment [27]. A VSD can be classified as one of the following phenotypes: perimembranous, doubly committed, and muscular (Figure 12.9) [27]. Specifically, perimembranous defects are a fibrous continuity between the aortic and tricuspid valves; doubly committed defects are fibrous continuity between the aortic and pulmonary valves and are also known as subpulmonic, subarterial, supracristal, juxta-arterial, or infundibular defects [9]; and muscular defects, which occur anywhere as long as they are completely surrounded by muscular tissue, can be located within the inlet, trabecular/apical, or outlet septum [27].

To fully describe the VSD, the precise anatomical location that is identifying where in the ventricular septum the VSD is located (as viewed from the RV: centrally, apically, inlet, or outlet), as well as the degree of septal alignment at the borders of the VSD must be defined. The clinical impact of an isolated VSD is dependent on its size. A small VSD, sometimes called restrictive, maintains the normal pressure difference between LV and RV. A moderately sized VSD causes variable degrees of RV hypertension and a large VSD results in equalization of pressures between the LV and RV. The aorta may override a VSD and it is common for the aortic valve to prolapse into the defect with perimembranous lesions (with or without overriding), often leading to aortic regurgitation, which can contribute to LV volume overload (Figure 12.10) [9]. Conversely, some horses with relatively large VSD can appear to benefit from aortic valve prolapse, at least in the short term, if it has the effect of narrowing the shunt size. Eisenmenger syndrome occurs when chronic left to right shunting leads to long-standing pulmonary hypertension, high pulmonary vascular resistance eventually exceeding systemic pressures, and eventually results in reversal of the shunt to right to left and cyanosis. This has been reported rarely in the horse [25]. Interestingly, spontaneous closure of a muscular VSD has been reported in a Quarter Horse Paint colt in which a 1.23×0.95 cm VSD was detected at 2 months of age [57]. Echocardiographic re-evaluation of the colt at 25 months of age revealed that the VSD had closed with a dimple-like irregularity in the myocardium were the VSD was previously located [57].

Clinical signs range from an incidental murmur identified in an otherwise healthy horse to signs of congestive heart failure [6, 9]. The characteristic murmur associated with VSD is a harsh, band-shaped, pansystolic murmur (grade III-VI/VI) with a point of maximal intensity (PMI) over the tricuspid valve area (right cranioventral heart base in the third to fourth intercostal space) [6]. A precordial thrill may be palpated on the right side in association with some murmurs. In addition, a crescendo-decrescendo

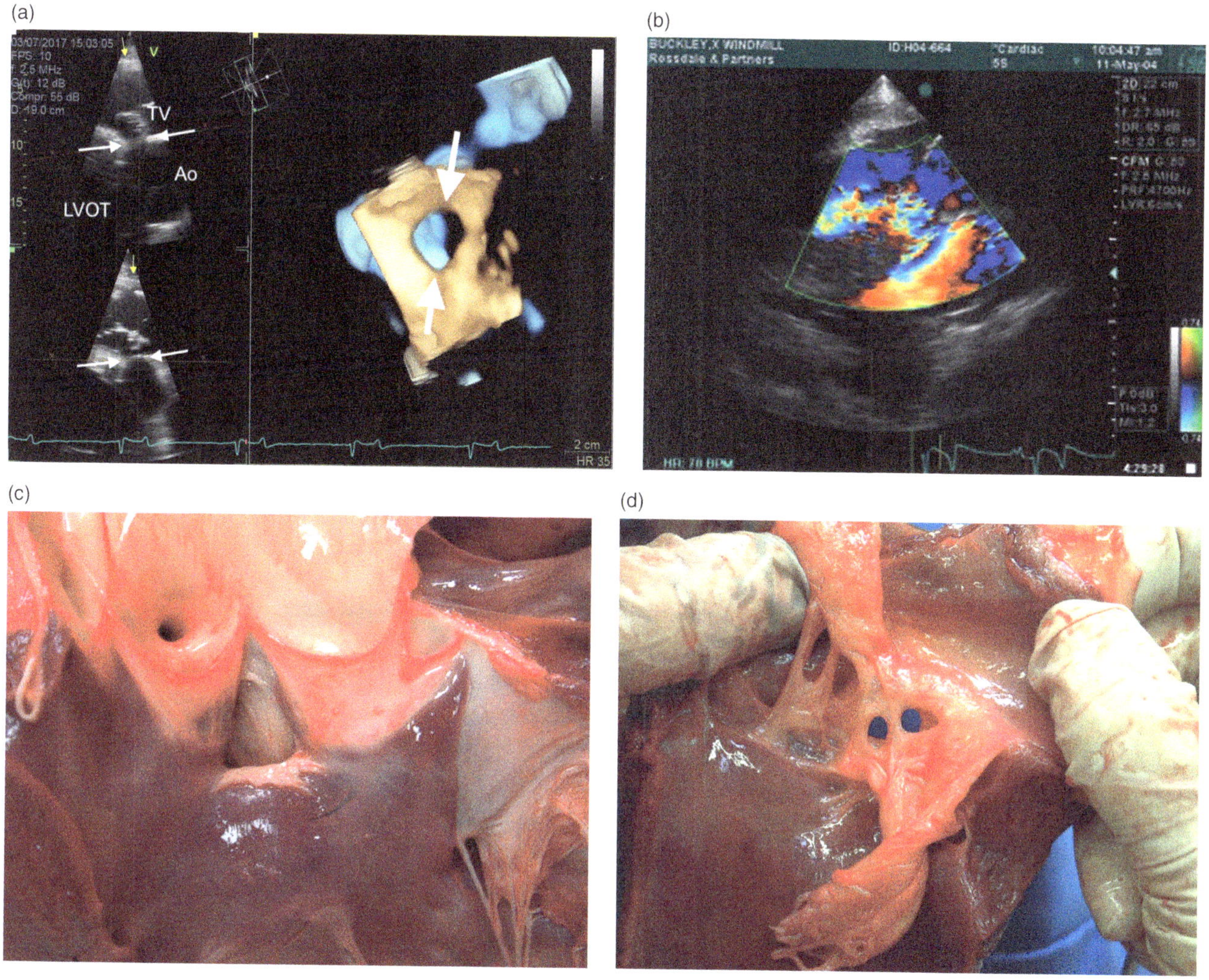

Figure 12.9 (a) The most common form of ventricular septal defect (VSD) is perimembranous: in this 3D echocardiograph, viewing the septum from the right side at the level of the tricuspid valve (TV), the defect is roughly circular (between arrows). To the left, the 2D images indicate the imaging plane above and below a section at 90° to aid orientation. (b) With color-flow Doppler imaging, the shunt speeds up, aliasing through the range of colors from red, yellow, turquoise and blue as it approaches the VSD and then the mosaic pattern within the defect and right ventricle (RV) indicated turbulence. (c) A postmortem specimen showing the perimembranous VSD immediately below the aortic valve. (d) This variation of a perimembranous VSD is comprised of a network of fibrous strands, viewed from under the TV. (e) A short-axis color-flow Doppler echocardiographic image of the heart base showing a shunt, represented by a green, yellow, blue, and red, in a small doubly committed VSD, between the aortic and pulmonic valves (PV). (f) The right heart from a newborn donkey foal, showing severe cardiovascular compromise, in which there is a muscular VSD (between arrows). (g) In this donkey, there was also severe hypoplasia of the aorta with left ventricular outflow obstruction (likely secondary to unequal partitioning of the fetal truncus arteriosus) and left ventricular hypoplasia; the left ventricle is very small in comparison to the right. LVOT, left ventricular outflow tract; RVOT, right ventricular outflow tract.

ejection murmur might be heard over the pulmonary valve on the left (relative pulmonary stenosis murmur), typically softer than the murmur heard in the tricuspid valve area [6].

The majority of VSD in the foal are best imaged ultrasonographically from the right parasternal left ventricular outflow tract view and are usually located in the membranous or perimembranous portions of the septum, while muscular lesions are less commonly observed as isolated lesions. In one retrospective study, 27 horses (age 10 days–18 years) with VSD that were not part of a complex congenital cardiac disorder were evaluated [6]. A VSD was an incidental finding in 14 horses, 10 horses raced or competed successfully, 11 horses had a history of poor performance, 5 horses had stunted growth, and 3 horses presented in congestive heart failure [6]. In this case series, Standardbred and Arabian horses were overrepresented.

Perimembranous VSDs were most commonly detected (85%, Figure 12.9) and were typically observed underneath

(e)

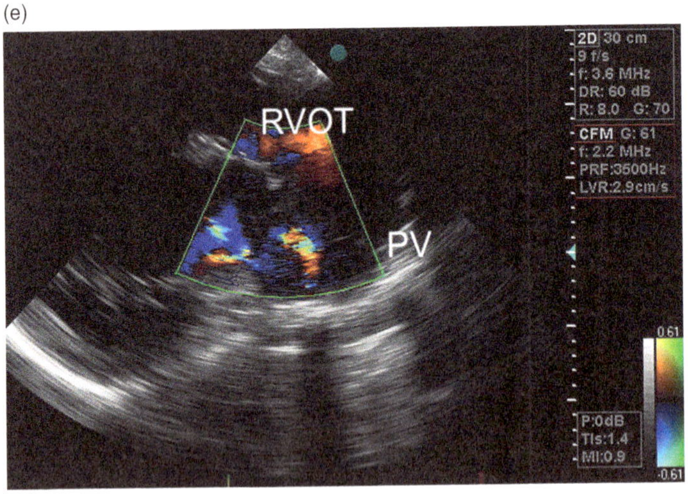

(f)

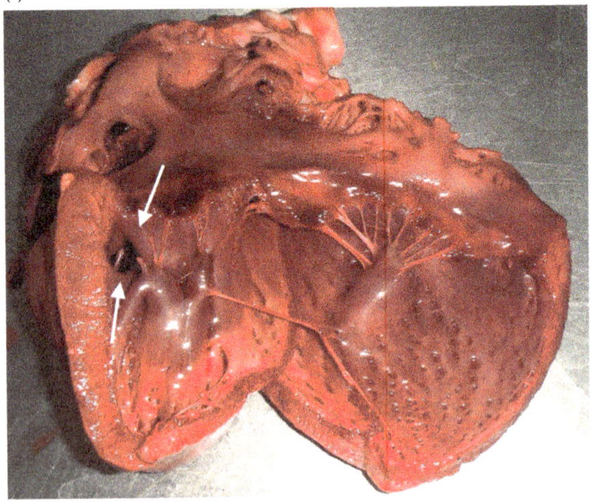

(g)

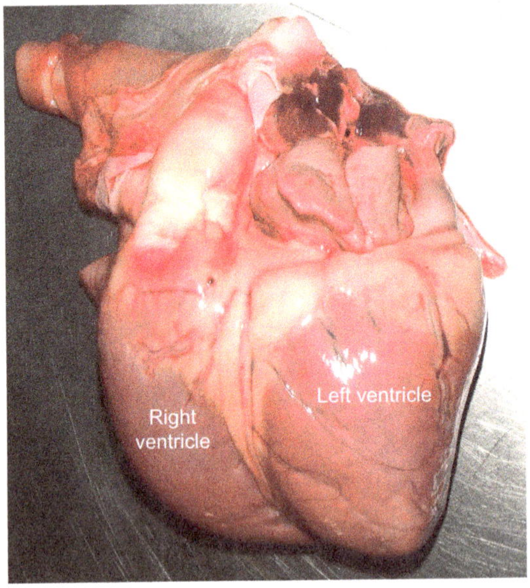

Figure 12.9 (Continued)

the septal leaflet of the tricuspid valve and the right and/or noncoronary leaflet of the aortic valve (Figure 12.10) [6]. VSD size ranged from 1 to 4.6 cm with peak velocity of shunt flow through the VSD ranging from 0 to 5.8 m/s. LV and LA volume overload was frequently detected (85% of horses) while aortic, mitral, tricuspid, or pulmonary valve regurgitation was detected in fewer horses. Horses that were able to compete successfully had a VSD ≤2.5 cm and a peak velocity of shunt flow through the VSD of≥4 m/s [6]. In another study focusing on non-racing breeds, isolated perimembranous VSD accounted for 36 of 42 cases, and 30 of 42 were exercising on a regular basis in lower-level activities. The study confirmed that measuring VSD diameter relative to the diameter of the aortic root (VSD/Ao ratio) is an effective means of evaluating defect size across breeds; in young animals that are not fully grown and have restrictive defects are usually less than approximately one third of the aortic root [5]. A key finding of the pleasure horse VSD study was that it documented that some horses without clinical signs had a higher VSD/Ao ratio and increased left atrial, ventricular, and pulmonary artery size without reported exercise intolerance (if engaged in less physically demanding sports) [9]. A complete echocardiographic assessment of all cardiac structures is critical to determine if the VSD is a component of complex CHD and to identify concurrent valvular pathology and cardiac chamber enlargement in cases with isolated VSD. Due to their lower prevalence, specific guidelines for echocardiographic assessment of doubly committed and muscular VSD are not available.

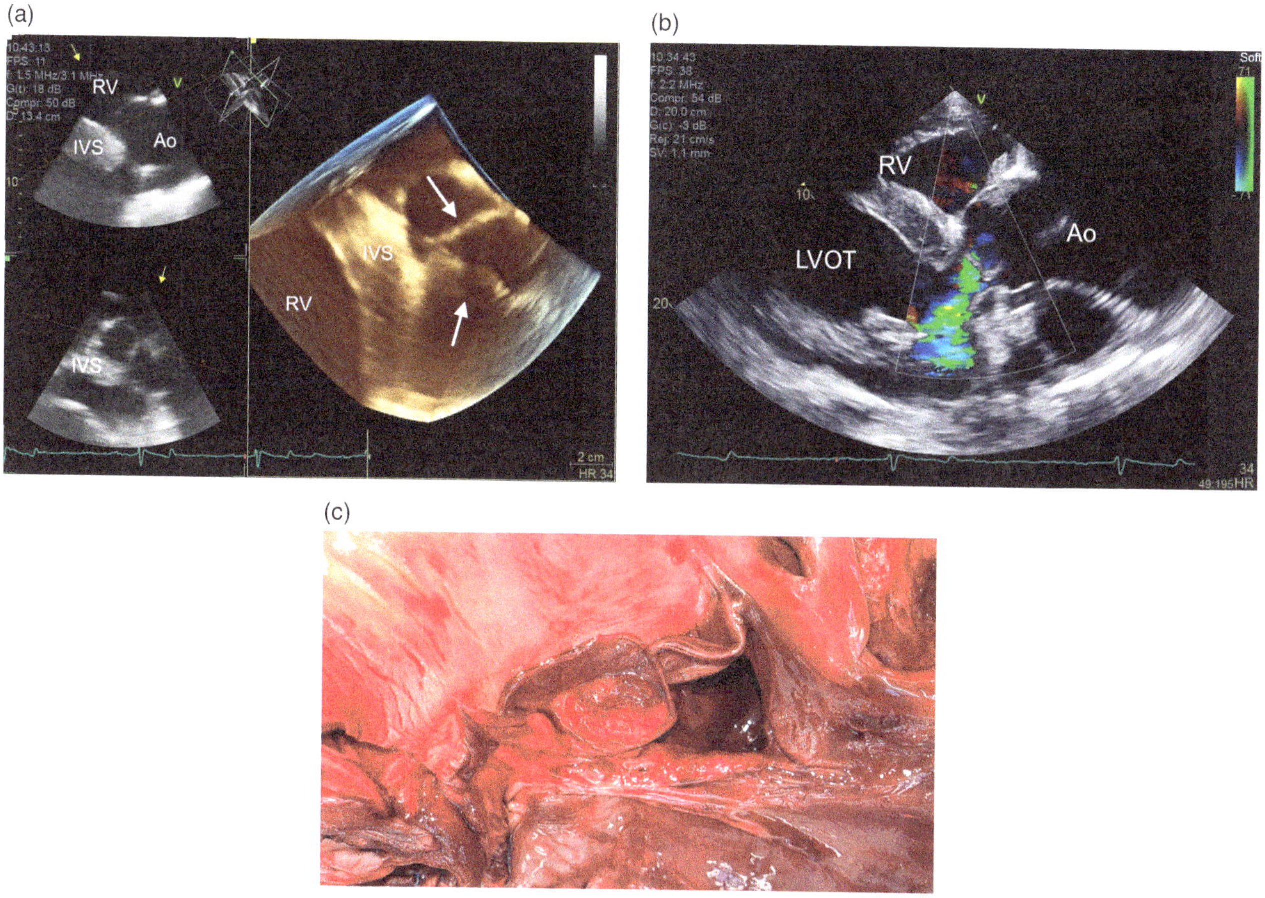

Figure 12.10 (a) 3D echocardiographic image from an adult pony, viewed from the right side looking dorsally toward the defect showing thickened right and noncoronary aortic cusps (arrows) prolapsing into the perimembranous VSD. To the left, the 2D images indicate the imaging plane above and below a section at 90° to aid orientation. (b) Long-axis mid-diastolic image of the left ventricular outflow tract (LVOT) shows the aorta (Ao) is overriding the perimembranous VSD. The large green jet is due to aortic regurgitation. Note there is also a much smaller red and green strand of aortic regurgitation entering the right ventricle (RV) from the overriding Ao. (c) Postmortem specimen from the same pony showing thickening of the aortic valve cusps with the VSD below this. IVS, interventricular septum.

Ventriculoarterial Connections

A sparse number of equine reports have documented anomalies located between the ventricles and their corresponding arteries (ventriculoarterial connections), which can occur as a sole anomaly or, more commonly, in association with complex CHD. These anomalies include pulmonary stenosis, pulmonary atresia, aortic valve dysplasia, and aortic stenosis (Table 12.1).

Pulmonary stenosis has been reported in horses as an isolated lesion [66, 154], but is usually associated with other CHD [7, 40, 64, 65, 70, 86]. Pulmonary stenosis can result from a variety of morphological lesions, including combinations of hypoplasia of the valve, thickening of the valve leaflets, incomplete commissural separation of the leaflets, and asymmetric valve leaflets [66]. In isolated forms of pulmonary stenosis, pure RV pressure overload and RV hypertrophy is present. Obstruction can occur at the pulmonic valve (valvular stenosis) or the distal portion of the RV outflow tract (subvalve or infundibular stenosis). Although infrequently reported, presenting signs in horses include dyspnea, ill thrift, weakness, and a loud heart murmur. In the few reported cases, the murmur was described as a loud systolic crescendo-decrescendo ejection murmur [66] or a holosytolic coarse crescendo murmur; the PMI was at the left heart base (over pulmonic valve) in both instances [66, 154].

Echocardiography may document marked RV concentric hypertrophy and abnormal pulmonary valve leaflets characterized as thin but fused; these leaflets fail to completely open during systole (systolic doming) [154]. The pulmonary valve may be bicuspid [5, 65]. Cardiac catheterization may show a severe marked RV-pulmonary artery pressure gradient along with dilation of the main pulmonary artery. There is one report of successful surgical intervention in pulmonary stenosis in which the foal was treated with balloon valvuloplasty. This procedure widened the opening of the pulmonary valve leaflets and greatly reduced the transvalvular pressures; at 2-year followup, the filly was reported to have normal exercise capacity. Thus, balloon valvuloplasty might serve as a treatment option for isolated pulmonary stenosis [154]. Pulmonary atresia, in combination with other CHD, has been infrequently reported in foals with clinical signs including lethargy, weakness, exercise intolerance, tachycardia, tachypnea, cyanosis, and continuous left-sided murmurs [68, 70].

Aortic valve dysplasia is poorly documented in horses but is characterized by malformed aortic valve cusps that consequently result in valvular incompetence [60, 61] or abnormal numbers of valve cusps [155]. Abnormal aortic valve morphology can also complicate complex CHD [95]. In the few equine cases of aortic valvular dysplasia described as an isolated defect, the valvular insufficiency resulted in increased ventricular filling pressures. Increased pressures on the left side of the heart can cause pulmonary venous congestion and edema (potentially manifesting clinically as tachypnea and lung wheezes), while increased RV and RA pressures cause systemic venous congestion (potentially manifesting as distended jugular veins, ventral edema and enlargement of the liver) [61]. In one report, a 3-month-old Clydesdale filly was presented for lethargy, ill-thrift, and a heart murmur, and upon further examination, clinical signs included cyanotic mucous membranes, weak peripheral pulses, jugular vein distension, tachycardia, and tachypnea [61]. Wheezes were detected on thoracic auscultation and a continuous left-sided systolic (grade III/VI) murmur, and a right-sided holosystolic (grade IV/VI) murmur was detected. Echocardiography demonstrated rounding of the left ventricular apex and enlargement of the LA and LV. The pulmonary artery was larger than the aorta (suggestive of pulmonary hypertension), and the right coronary cusp of the aortic valve appeared abnormal along with a thickened mitral valve. Color-flow Doppler documented moderate to severe regurgitation through the aortic, mitral, and tricuspid valves. Increased liver enzyme activity and an enlarged liver were also observed and attributed to heart failure. The foal was euthanized, with specific postmortem findings including abnormalities of the aortic valve characterized by an asymmetric, partially fibrosed and distorted hypoplastic cranial aortic cusp with no proper commissure adjacent to the right posterior cusp; the latter was mildly thickened [61]. In cases in which aortic regurgitation has been less severe, the prognosis has been slightly more favorable; nevertheless, a poor prognosis is warranted [61, 155]. Aortic stenosis and dextroposition of the aorta have also been rarely reported in the equine literature [7]. Incomplete subaortic stenotic rings are reported as an incidental finding in one pathological description [62]. There are also some older reports in the equine literature suggesting that aortic stenosis was common in horses. However, as a result of knowledge gained from phonocardiographic and echocardiographic studies, this assertion is no longer considered to be relevant and the vast majority of systolic murmurs localized to the aortic valve are now recognized as physiological flow murmurs [156].

Tetralogy of Fallot (TOF)

The four anatomic anomalies associated with tetralogy of Fallot (TOF) are VSD, dextropositioning of the aorta such that it overrides both right and left ventricles, subpulmonary stenosis, and RV hypertrophy (Figure 12.11). Pentalogy of Fallot has also been reported in horses and adds a concurrent PDA [8, 71, 76] or ASD. Development of TOF is believed to occur due to an abnormality in formation of the truncus arteriosus. Because of abnormal growth of the endocardial cushions and underdevelopment of the bulbus cordis, the spiral development of the septum aorticopulmonale and truncobulbare does not take place; this results in overriding of the aortic root, incomplete interventricular septum formation, and stenosis of the pulmonary root [77, 157]. RV hypertrophy is caused by volume and pressure overload related to the aforementioned anatomic defects and is influenced by the degree of RV obstruction (pulmonic stenosis). Hypertrophy can occur in utero in fetal foals with TOF [71, 77].

Horses with TOF can present at variable ages ranging from newborn to several years of age [7, 72, 73]. Clinical signs might include decreased or absent nursing, decreased activity, weakness, exercise intolerance, stunted growth, and possibly syncope [12, 75]. Mucous membrane color can range from pink to cyanotic to purple with tachycardia, tachypnea, and dyspnea also present in some cases [7, 12, 75]. A loud systolic murmur accompanied by a palpable thrill is present in many cases, usually loudest on the left. In one case series, the murmur was described as systolic in four of five foals with TOF and continuous in one of five foals [7]. The PMI was the left heart base and the murmur was graded III-V/VI [7]. Notable hypoxemia (P_aO_2 39–55.8 mmHg) has also been reported in several cases [12, 77]. Echocardiography is the most expedient method to identify TOF ante-mortem although angiography and cardiac catheterization has been used in the past [12, 75, 77]. The prognosis is unfavorable for foals with TOF, although one horse was identified as having TOF at 7 years of age [7, 72].

Double-Outlet Right Ventricle (DORV)

Double-outlet right ventricle (DORV) is characterized by dextropositioning of the aorta (partial transposition) in which both the aorta and the pulmonary artery arise from the RV (Figure 12.12) [21, 25, 83, 84]. This anomaly might

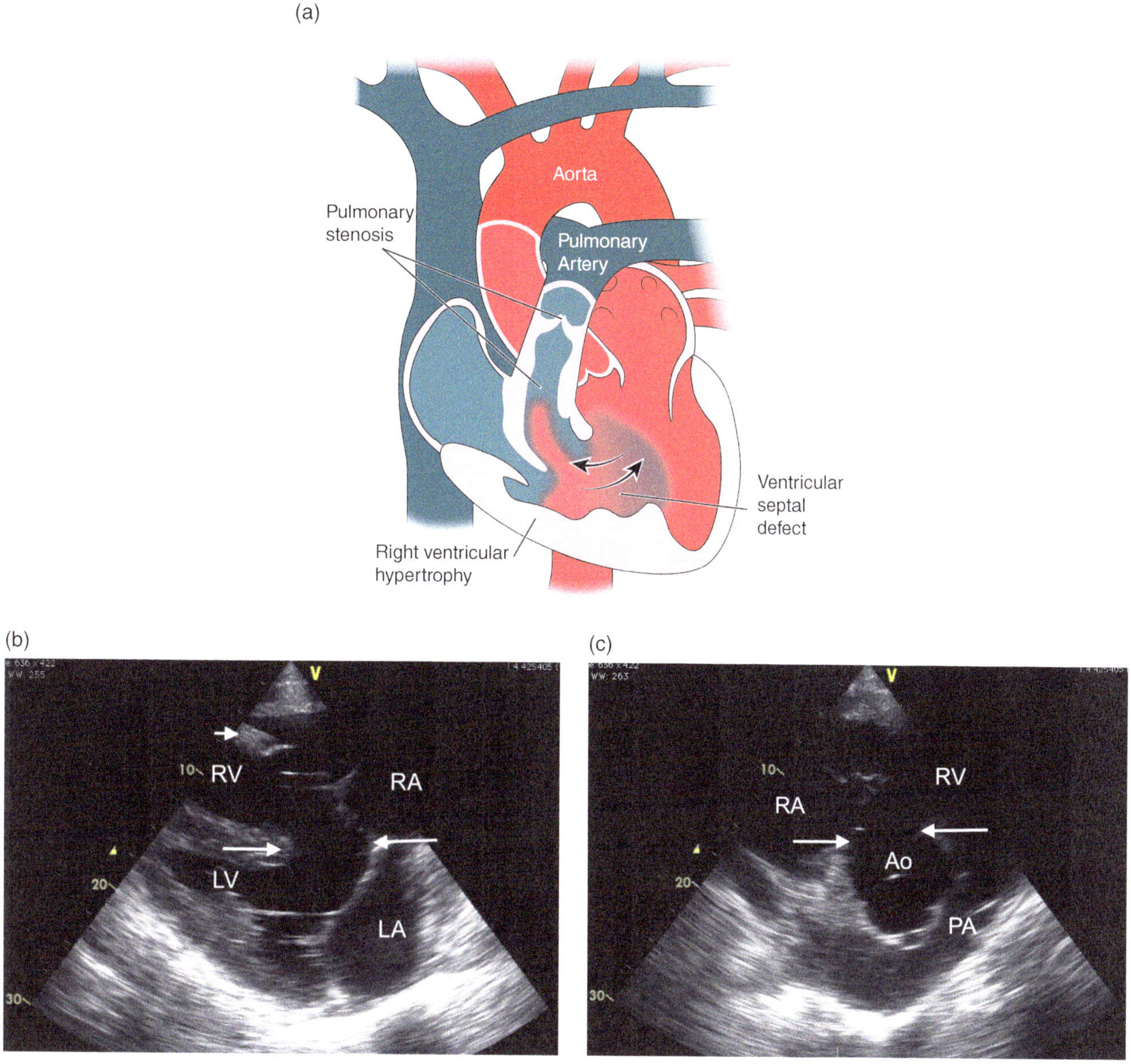

Figure 12.11 (a) Tetralogy of Fallot (TOF), which is characterized by a ventricular septal defect (VSD), dextropositioning (overriding) of the aorta, pulmonary stenosis, and right ventricular (RV) hypertrophy. *Source:* Copyright Sara Anais Gonzalez, 2022. (b) Long-axis echocardiograph of the right (RV) and left (LV) ventricles and right (RA) and left (LA) atria in a 15-month-old Thoroughbred that shows the large VSD (between arrows) and RV hypertrophy: note the RV wall has similar thickness to the LV wall and note the prominent RV papillary muscle (arrowheads). (c) Short-axis image of the heart base shows the VSD (between arrows) and stenotic pulmonary artery (PA): compare its diameter with the adjacent aorta (Ao).

arise from arrest of the normal rotation of the semilunar valve region during embryogenesis [82]. A VSD is typically present in DORV, which provides the LV its only route for transfer of blood from the blind-ended LV to the RV for exit through both great arteries. The VSD can be subaortic, subpulmonary, beneath both great arteries (doubly committed), beneath neither great artery (uncommitted) or absent altogether [82]. More complex CHD have been described with DORV in the horse including ASD, tricuspid valve atresia [21, 82], and PDA [84]. Clinical signs along with physical examination and clinicopathologic findings of DORV in horses include tachycardia, tachypnea, cyanotic mucous membranes, notable systolic murmur (grade V–VI/VI), polycythemia, severe hypoxemia (P_aO_2 24–35 mmHg), hypocapnia (P_aCO_2 36 mmHg) and increased serum cardiac troponin concentrations [82, 83, 85]. Necropsy has demonstrated evidence of congestive heart failure including heart enlargement arising from biventricular dilation and enlargement of the LA along with pulmonary edema, pericardial and pleural effusion, and hepatic congestion [21, 83, 85].

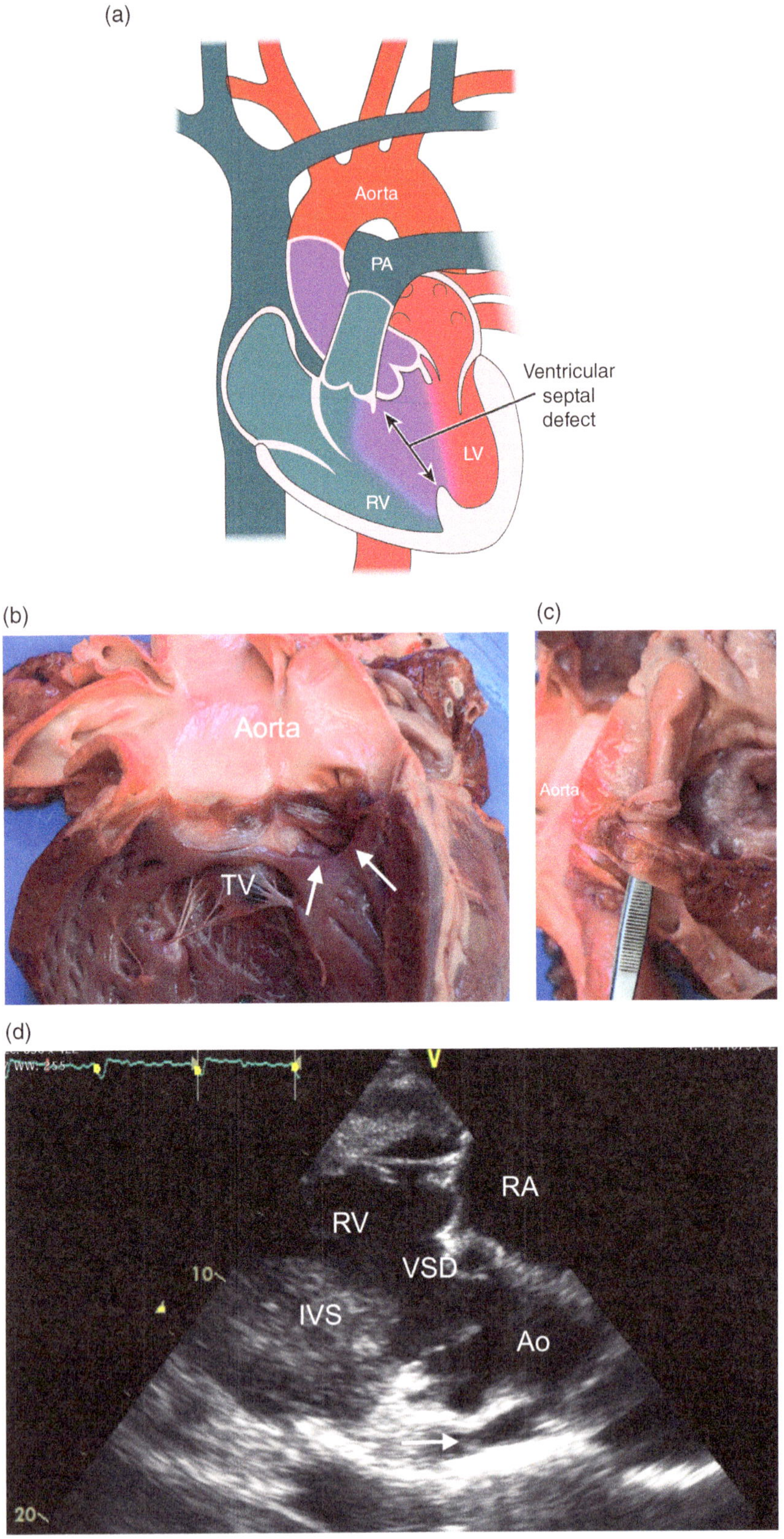

Figure 12.12 (a) Diagram demonstrating double outlet right ventricle characterized by dextropositioning of the aorta (partial transposition) in which both the aorta and the pulmonary artery arise from the right ventricle. *Source:* Copyright Sara Anais Gonzalez, 2022. (b) Four-week-old Suffolk Punch foal, has a large ventricular septal defect (VSD, arrows) and the aorta is exiting the right ventricle. In this pathological specimen, viewed from the right, the pulmonary artery is barely visible (arrowheads). (c) On closer inspection, an extremely stenotic pulmonary artery was identified and is indicated here with the instrument. (d) Similarly, in an oblique long-axis echocardiograph, the aorta (Ao) is overriding a VSD and thus exiting the right ventricle (RV) and a small vessel adjacent to the Ao represents the pulmonary artery (arrow). TV, tricuspid valve; IVS, interventricular septum.

Great Vessel Transposition

Transposition of the great vessels has been infrequently reported in foals, but when present, can arise from abnormal truncus arteriosus partitioning and development [45, 86–88]. Proposed underlying embryonic causes include defective atrioventricular endocardial cushions, incomplete rotation or complete absence of rotation of the truncoconal ridges, or defective primordia of the aortic and pulmonary valves [88]. The primary defect involved with transposition of the great vessels is that the aorta arises from the RV and the pulmonary artery arises from the LV (Figure 12.13) [45]. Complete transposition of the great vessels results in two separate circulations set in parallel (pulmonary and systemic) rather than two circulations set in series [87]. In other words, the right heart and systemic vasculature exist as a separate and parallel circulation to the left heart and pulmonary vasculature [86]. Because of this, intra-cardiac (VSD, PFO) and/or extra-cardiac (PDA, bronchial collateral vessels) shunts must be present to allow for inter-circulatory mixing [87, 88]. Extensive bronchopulmonary anastomotic channels have been reported in a foal with transposition of the great vessels to allow for additional inter-circulatory shunting of blood [86]. The main determinant of systemic arterial O_2 saturation is the degree of blood exchanged between these shunts and the two circulatory patterns, with the larger the shunting, the better the oxygenation [87]. In foals, reported clinical signs and physical examination abnormalities include emaciation, inability to stand, tachycardia (169 beats/min), dyspnea, cough, cyanotic mucous membranes, prolonged capillary refill time, and poor peripheral pulses [87, 88]. Heart murmur(s) are present with a grade V/VI pansystolic band-shaped murmur reported at the tricuspid valve region along with a palpable precordial thrill in a 19-hour-old foal [87]. Severe hypoxemia (P_aO_2 33 mmHg), hypercapnia (P_aCO_2 80.4 mmHg), and respiratory acidosis (pH 7.224) that was minimally responsive to oxygen insufflation were also reported [87]. Echocardiography revealed RV enlargement, a VSD, and bulging of the interatrial septum into the LA (from increased RA pressure) [87]. The aorta and pulmonary artery were similar in size and were arranged in parallel at the heart base, without normal spiraling. The aorta arose from the anatomic RV, whereas the pulmonary artery arose from the anatomic LV. Color-flow Doppler echocardiography demonstrated bi-directional blood flow across a VSD, a PFO with right-to-left atrial flow, and a PDA [87]. Another case described a 2-month-old colt

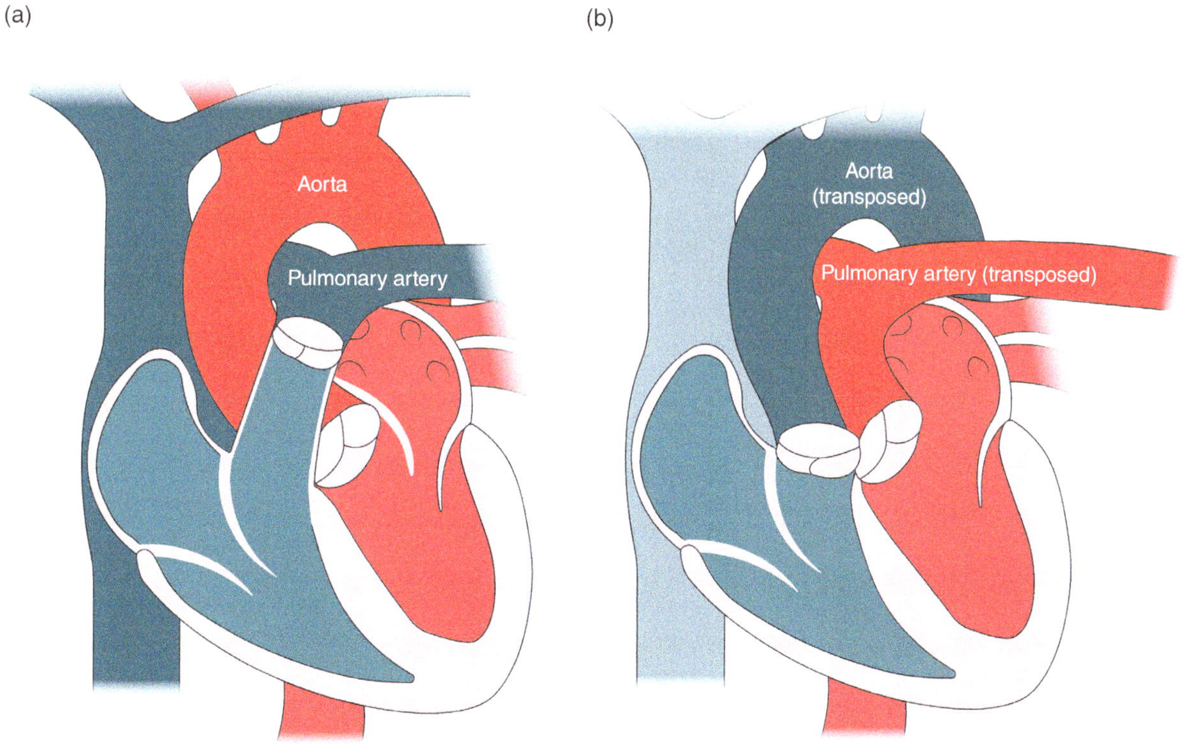

Figure 12.13 (a) Normal orientation of the great vessels and (b) transposition of the great vessels. In this anomaly the aorta arises from the RV and the pulmonary artery from the LV, resulting in two separate circulations in parallel, rather than in series. *Source:* Copyright Sara Anais Gonzalez, 2022.

presented for weakness, cough, cyanotic mucous membranes, and a holostystolic murmur with a PMI over the left fourth and fifth intercostal space. In this case, transposition of the aorta to the RV was present along with a septal defect, RV hypertrophy and an atretic pulmonary trunk [88]; other reports have described transposition of the great arteries with tricuspid atresia [45].

Common Arterial Trunk (CAT)

CAT was previously termed persistent truncus arteriosus [158]. In human cardiology, there are two classification systems. The Collette and Edwards classification system (describes four categories) is based on the branching pattern of the pulmonary arteries and is the system most commonly encountered in veterinary literature. The alternative system is the Van Praagh classification, which considers the presence of absence of a VSD as well as the pulmonary artery morphology. More recently, the *International Pediatric and Congenital Cardiac Code* has sought to clarify the nomenclature and categorized CAT as:

- CAT with aortic dominance and both pulmonary arteries arising from the trunk
- CAT with one branch of the pulmonary artery arising off the common trunk, and one branch of the pulmonary artery isolated
- CAT with pulmonary dominance and aortic arch obstruction

The Collett and Edwards Type IV, where there is pulmonary atresia and the pulmonary arteries arise distally off the aorta (or the lungs are supplied by multiple aortopulmonary collaterals) is now considered a form of TOF [158].

CAT is a rare CHD in the foal where the fetal truncus never partitions, resulting in a single great vessel that serves as the outflow tract for the LV and RV (Figure 12.14). Variations in pulmonary artery origins consistent within the first CAT category include a single hypoplastic main pulmonary artery arising from the truncus then branching [32, 90, 93, 94] and two pulmonary arteries arising separately and directly from the common trunk [90]. It is quite likely that all variations could occur in the horse, but in some case series [7, 8] and earlier pathological reports [16, 25, 67, 89, 91] the specific types of equine CAT described are less clear. In line with classifications now accepted for human cardiology, a case reported in the equine literature as persistent truncus arteriosus type IV (with pulmonary trunk agenesis and pulmonary arteries arising from the descending aorta) should now be classified as TOF [80].

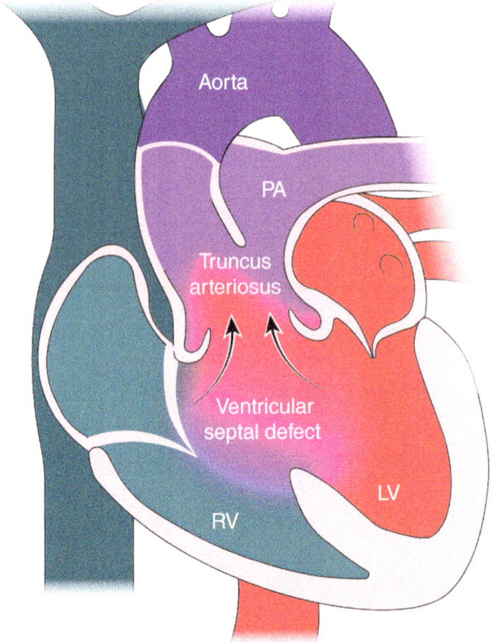

Figure 12.14 Common arterial trunk (also known as persistent truncus arteriosus), which is characterized by a single great vessel (supplies systemic, pulmonic and coronary vessels) that serves as the outflow tract for the left and right ventricles. A VSD allows communication between the left and right ventricle. The lesion is subclassified based on the morphology of the pulmonary supply. In this example, both branches arise from the truncus via a short main artery. *Source:* Copyright Sara Anais Gonzalez, 2022.

With CAT, the LV and RV communicate through a VSD that lies below the single great vessel that supplies the systemic, pulmonic, and coronary vessels [90, 93]. The associated truncal valve may be incompetent or stenotic [126]. There is pulmonary under circulation and right-to-left shunting. Clinical signs and physical examination findings in foals with CAT include tachycardia, tachypnea, exercise intolerance, poor peripheral pulses, cool distal extremities, cyanotic mucous membranes, dyspnea, syncope, and the presence of one or more systolic murmurs (PMI over tricuspid and pulmonic valve area) [92–94]. Severe hypoxemia (P_aO_2 14–31 mmHg) with minimal response to supplemental oxygen therapy may also be documented and may be due to high pulmonary vascular resistance or obstruction to flow at the truncal origin of the pulmonary artery [90, 93, 126]. Echocardiography can typically identify the single great vessel, which can measure 5–6 cm in diameter and overrides the left and right ventricles along with the presence of a VSD. Echocardiographically, it can be difficult to distinguish CTA from TOF with pulmonary atresia [90].

Anomalous Origin of a Pulmonary Artery Branch

There is a single case report of aortic origin of the right pulmonary artery in a 2-month-old pony foal. This CHD arises due to subnormal leftward migration of the right sixth aortic arch to join the left arch. Although the condition leads to left to right shunting, the pulmonary overcirculation and hypertension resulted in right-sided failure in the single equine report. Echocardiographically, care must be taken to differentiate this condition from transposition of the great vessels. With aortic origin of a pulmonary artery branch, the coronary arteries can be expected to arise in the normal location at the base of the aorta and the normal spiral relationship between the aorta and single pulmonary artery connected to the RV is maintained; this is lost with transposition [96]. In humans, anomalous origin of the left pulmonary artery branch is also recognized in association with TOF, but this variation has not been reported in foals.

Arterial Anomalies

Aortic Coarctation, Tubular Hypoplasia, and Interruption of the Aortic Arch (IAA)

Interruption of the aortic arch (IAA) is a rare CHD defined as the absence of luminal continuity between the ascending and descending portions of the aorta. Tubular hypoplasia is a partial form while coarctation consists of a ridge of tissue at the junction of the aortic arch and the descending aorta, at the site of the ductus arteriosus and distal to the brachiocephalic trunk (Figure 12.7) [27]. Coarctation can occur as an isolated lesion [99] but these anomalies commonly occur in conjunction with other cardiac defects such as VSD, PDA, LV outflow track obstruction, bicuspid aortic valve, aberrant right subclavian artery, transposition of the great arteries, single ventricle, and/or truncus arteriosus [21, 27, 45, 98]. The defect in IAA can range from complete interruption of the aortic arch to a cord-like atretic segment present between the ascending and descending aorta [98]. IAA occurs in a preductal (ductus arteriosus) location and, in people, is nearly always associated with a PDA, which supplies blood to the aortic arch distal to the site of interruption. Survival of patients with IAA is dependent on a PDA, as blood flow distal to the site of interruption relies on right-to-left shunting at the ductal level. Constriction or closure of the ductus arteriosus results in systemic hypoperfusion distal to the site of interruption (i.e. abdominal viscera, pelvic limbs). In the presence of an intact atrial and ventricular septum, desaturated blood from the RV will be routed through the PDA and will be distributed to the lower portion of the body resulting in differential cyanosis (pink membranes in the head and face, blue in locations such as the vaginal membranes). However, lesions associated with IAA can modify blood flow such that in the presence of a VSD or ASD, a left-to-right shunt is present, resulting in more saturated blood ejected out the RV and shunted through the PDA to the descending aorta when compared to a patient without intracardiac communication.

While rare in horses [27], one veterinary report described two foals with IAA [97]. Both cases presented in the neonatal period (3 and 9 days old) for clinical signs including cyanosis, weakness, reluctance to suckle, and exercise intolerance. In both cases a grade V/V pansystolic murmur was audible over the left and right thoracic walls along with a palpable thrill, tachycardia, tachypnea, weak pulses, and a prolonged capillary refill time. Hypoxemia (P_aO_2 34.5–43.5 mmHg) and hypercarbia (P_aCO_2 53.5 mmHg) were also measured. Thoracic radiography noted cardiomegaly and a diffuse interstitial pattern of the lung fields with a prominent vascular pattern. In one foal, increased RV pressure (110/10 mmHg) and pulmonary hypertension were present along with increased carotid, aortic, and LV systolic pressures (140 mmHg). In addition, increased LV end-diastolic pressure (50 mmHg) and LA pressure (50/20 mmHg) suggested left-side heart failure. Both foals were euthanized with necropsy examination confirming IAA and pulmonary congestion. One foal had diffuse serosanguineous fluid in the pleural cavity with the descending aorta communicating with the RV via the pulmonary artery and connecting ductus arteriosus. The RV was markedly dilated and a 2 cm VSD and PFO was present. The ascending aorta arose from LV and the ascending and descending aorta were presumptively connected by the left subclavian artery. In the second foal, the descending aorta originated from outflow tract of RV via the ductus arteriosus and pulmonary artery. The RV was hypertrophied and a 2.5 cm VSD was present along with anomalous drainage of cranial vena cava into the LA.

Patent Ductus Arteriosus (PDA)

In the newborn foal, adequate ventilation of the lungs at birth results in a decrease in pulmonary vascular resistance consequently causing the pulmonary arterial pressure to fall below the systemic pressure. Because the ductus arteriosus does not close immediately after birth (Figure 12.15), the blood flow through the ductus arteriosus reverses from the fetal direction (pulmonary trunk to aorta) to the neonatal direction (aorta to pulmonary trunk). This produces a loud continuous murmur best heard on the left side of the thorax between the third and fourth ribs and radiates ventrally [159]. The exact time of closure of the ductus arteriosus is variable in the neonatal foal, but is proposed to close sometime

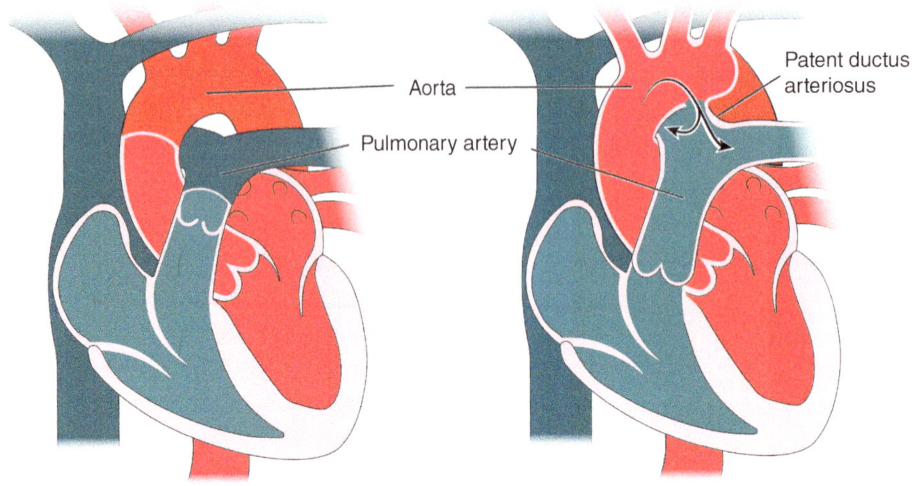

Figure 12.15 Persistent ductus arteriosus (PDA), which connects the main pulmonary artery to the descending aorta. *Source:* Copyright Sara Anais Gonzalez, 2022.

between 2 and 96 hours after birth [160, 161]. In a postmortem study involving aborted equine fetuses and newborn foals, investigators noted that measurements of the ductus arteriosus progressively increased up to 310 days gestation and then decreased in size at 320 and 330 days suggesting that contraction of the ductus arteriosus begins in late gestation [162]. Additionally, in this study, the ductus arteriosus was closed in 3 of 14 foals at one day of age, 2 of 6 at two days of age, and 9 of 9 at three days of age [162]. Another study reported that the ductus arteriosus was physiologically closed in four healthy foals <24 hours old, based on angiography [160]. However, a study in pony foals suggested that although murmurs are confined to the first few days of life, turbulent flow can be detected with Doppler echocardiography in the ductus arteriosus in older foals [163].

PDA has been described in association with a number of different congenital cardiac anomalies [21, 25, 96, 105]. When it occurs as an isolated lesion, its clinical impact is variable, likely depending on the size of the ductus. Some affected individuals will develop heart failure within the first year of life [5, 103, 104] while others may be relatively clinically silent; one aged individual was found dead with PDA, which had not been recognized previously [100]. Although a continuous murmur is classically detected, the murmur can be confined to systole only [5]. With a large PDA, pulmonary overcirculation leads to pulmonary hypertension, which in horses increases the risk of pulmonary artery rupture; one equine case of spontaneous pulmonary artery rupture associated with PDA has been reported [101]. PDA is difficult to identify ultrasonographically due to its location in the descending aorta; however, the diagnosis can be inferred by the identification of retrograde flow entering the pulmonary artery from the aorta [164].

Anomalous Origin of Coronary Arteries (AOCA)

Congenital anomalies of the coronary arteries have been estimated to occur in up to 1% of humans but their true prevalence is unknown as reports have focused on symptomatic patients [165, 166]. Anomalous left coronary artery from the pulmonary artery has a high fatality rate in children but can present with myocardial infarction later in life [167] while AOCA is an important cause of sudden cardiac death in apparently healthy, young human athletes in the United States [168, 169] and as such, perhaps warrants more attention in equine medicine. Nevertheless, equine case reports are sparse. In a single case report of AOCA involving the left coronary artery arising from the right sinus of Valsalva in a yearling that was found collapsed and unable to rise. It was not clear whether the AOCA contributed to this presentation, as clinical details were sparse in this report [115]. In an older report, the origin of left coronary artery was absent and the descending and circumflex branches arose from the right coronary artery in a yearling [1]. Although this coronary artery was considered relevant by the authors, that animal also had valvular lesions, which more likely accounted for its presentation in left-sided failure. Anomalies of coronary and subclavian arteries have also been reported in conjunction with complex CHD [21, 95].

Persistent Right Aortic Arch (PRAA)

PRAA is a CHD in which the right fourth aortic arch forms the aorta rather than the left fourth aortic arch. Because the right fourth aortic arch descends to the right of midline, the left ductus arteriosus (which later becomes the ligamentum arteriosum) forms a vascular ring between the left pulmonary artery and the anomalous right aorta [84, 116, 117, 121]. This consequently results in constriction of the esophagus and trachea within this ring, resulting in variable clinical signs that are dictated by the degree of constriction. Onset of clinical signs varies, ranging from a few days to 14 months of age [116, 117, 119, 121]. Primary clinical signs reported in younger foals include regurgitation of milk through the mouth and nares (particularly when the head is down or the foal is in lateral recumbency), but clinical signs of dysphagia may not occur until the foal begins to ingest more solid food; the later situation may be associated with megaesophagus secondary to the PRAA; several cases have demonstrated an externally dilated and palpable cervical esophagus as well [116, 118, 119]. Other clinical signs include tachycardia, tachypnea, failure to thrive, and aspiration pneumonia [117–119].

Diagnosis of PRAA is supported by compatible clinical signs and endoscopic and radiographic evidence of esophageal dilation in the caudal cervical and cranial thoracic regions [84], along with ventral deviation and narrowing of the intrathoracic trachea. Positive contrast esophagography can reveal contrast medium distending the esophagus to the level of the vascular ring anomaly near the cranial aspect of the heart base along with tapering of the esophageal lumen [84, 117]. It may be difficult or impossible for both the barium and/or the nasoesophageal tube to be passed beyond the constriction. Computed tomography has been used to confirm the presence of PRAA in a neonatal foal and documented a vascular band extending from the pulmonary artery to the cranial aspect of the aorta and the presence of the aortic arch on the right side of the heart as it continued caudally, rather than on the left side [170].

Surgical correction of PRAA has been attempted using a left lateral thoracotomy through the third, fourth, or fifth intercostal space, but many foals died due to complications during surgery or from aspiration pneumonia during the postoperative period [117–119, 121]. If surgical intervention is being considered, the esophagus should be carefully evaluated, as irregularities in the esophagus both cranial (e.g. megaesophagus) and caudal to the PRAA have been demonstrated [116, 118, 119].

Congenital Arrhythmias

Foals frequently have transient arrhythmias at the time of birth, particularly if they are compromised (Figure 12.16). Typically, these arrhythmias are short-lived. Accessory pathways are the result of an additional electrical connection between two parts of the heart, particularly between the atria and ventricles. Three variations exist:

1) The pathway leads to conduction bypassing the AV node, resulting in ventricular pre-excitation or Wolf-Parkinson-White syndrome.
2) The conduction continues normally through the AV node and then spreads via the accessory pathway to re-excite the atria (often associated with re-entrant tachycardia) and is known as ortodromic atrioventricular re-entrant tachycardia (AVRT, Figure 12.16).
3) The less-common form where conduction occurs from the atria, through the accessory pathway to the ventricles, and then backward via the AV node to the atria resulting in antidromic AVRT.

The best-recognized form of congenital arrhythmia in horses is ventricular pre-excitation [107–114]. This is manifested on ECG by a short P-R interval, absence of an isoelectric segment, and possibly a delta wave (Figure 12.16). Pre-excitation may be intermittent and heart-rate dependent; long antegrade effective refractory periods in the pathway will lead to pre-excitation at low heart rates, which is abolished when the heart rate increases and normal antegrade pathways dominate. Ortodromic AVRT is associated with periods of tachycardia and premature P-waves can be identified within the S-T segment (Figure 12.16). Other forms of accessory pathways such as connections within the ventricles, between the AV node and muscle or conducting tissue within the ventricles has been recognized in humans but not yet described in horses.

Accessory pathways between atria and ventricles can increase the risk of supraventricular tachycardia and atrial fibrillation with a rapid ventricular response rate [108]. In one equine case, the presence of pre-excitation was masked, on presentation, by atrial fibrillation and pre-excitation was only diagnosed following transvenous electrocardioversion. However, the authors noted that the presenting heart rate (140 bpm) was atypically high for equine atrial fibrillation, and there was abnormal QRS morphology. A discrete delta wave was not evident, before or after cardioversion, but the authors suggested this might reflect the limitations of surface ECG techniques in horses or arise if the pre-excitation was responsible for only a small portion of total ventricular depolarization [108]. In the absence of major structural defects, the majority of cases of equine atrial fibrillation do not have rapid ventricular response and therefore accessory bypass tracts should be suspected when there are inappropriately fast ventricular rates.

Cells within the accessory pathway are sensitive to autonomic influences and electrolyte imbalance. One equine case appeared to have increased frequency of intermittent pre-excitation related to decreased serum magnesium

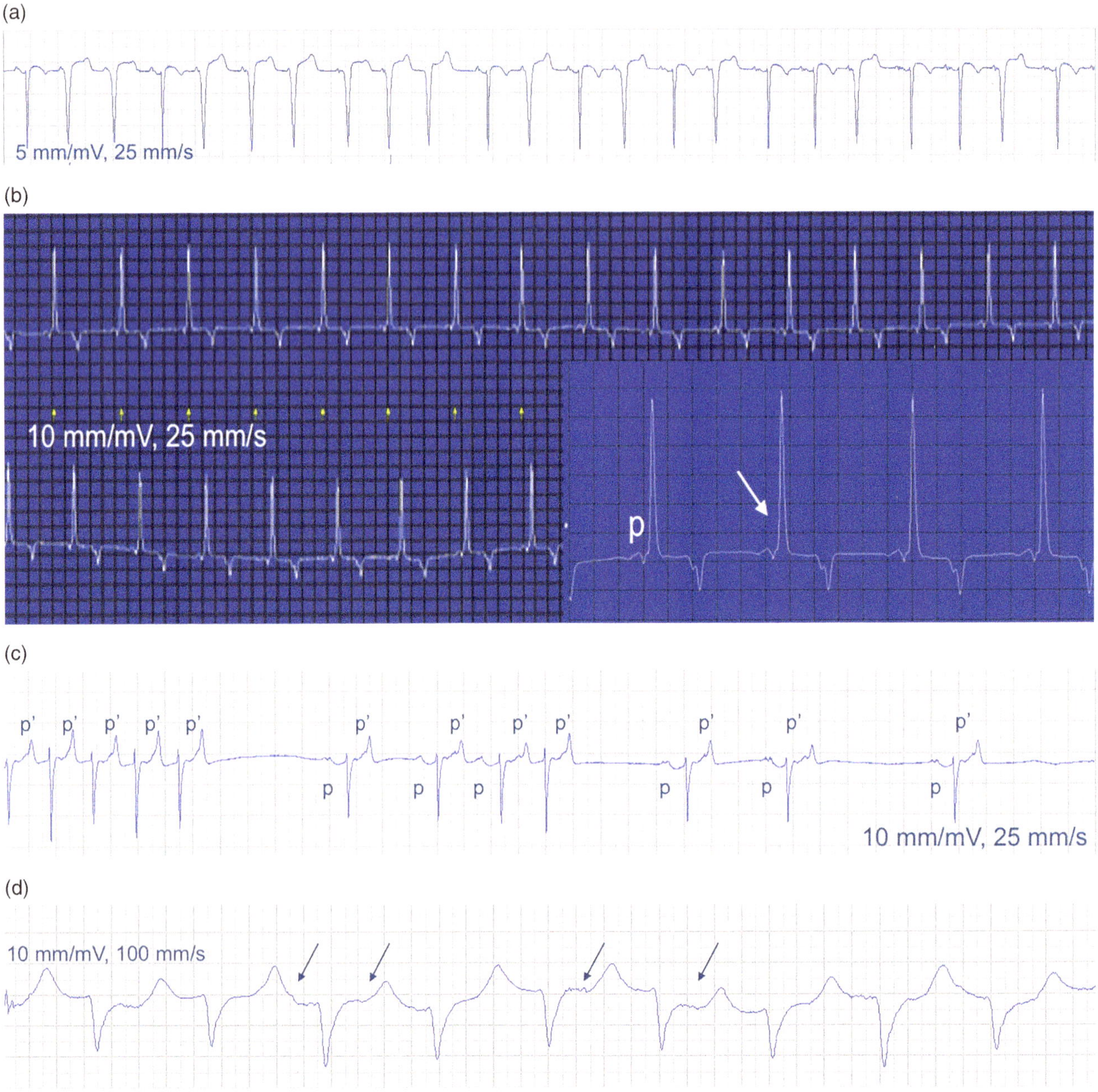

Figure 12.16 (a) Arrhythmias, such as ventricular tachycardia seen here in a hypoxic neonate, are fairly common in the neonatal intensive care unit. In this foal the rhythm resolved as the respiratory dysfunction was addressed. (b) Congenital arrhythmias are much less common and are typically diagnosed in adults. Ventricular pre-excitation (Wolf-Parkinson-White syndrome) occurs when an accessory pathway bypasses the atrioventricular node and is characterized by a short P-R interval and delta wave, a slurring slow rise in the initial portion of the QRS (arrow) in an 8-year-old Warmblood. The ECG inset is magnified to illustrate these features. (c) A run of orthodromic atrioventricular re-entrant tachycardia is seen in this 2-year-old Thoroughbred, and this is followed by two sinus beats, each of which have an additional P′ wave in the S-T segment. On closer inspection, almost every S-T segment contains an additional P wave (P′) due to depolarization traveling back into the atria via an accessory pathway after the ventricles are depolarized via the atrioventricular node. (d) In the same filly, the abnormal P waves in the S-T segment are more difficult to discern during exercise, in this strip, the heart rate is 140 bpm, and arrows indicate deflections in the S-T segment suggesting the accessory pathway is continuing to re-stimulate the atria. All ECGs are recorded on a modified base-apex lead.

concentrations, which resolved with correction of the electrolyte abnormality [113]. Antiarrhythmic drugs in classes Ia (e.g. quinidine, procainamide), Ic (e.g. propafenone, flecanide), and III (e.g. amiodarone, soltalol) are indicated as these prolong refractoriness in the accessory pathway while digoxin and calcium channel blockers are contra-indicated [108].

With 12-lead surface ECG, it may be possible to predict the site of the accessory pathway; however, 3D electrophysiological mapping is required for definitive identification of accessory pathways and, if they can be localized precisely, there is potential to ablate these successfully (G van Loon, personal communication). At this time, there is no available information on breed predisposition or other risk factors for this condition.

Currently, there is insufficient evidence to make firm recommendations regarding the suitability of horses with congenital accessory pathways for use for riding or driving. In humans with accessory pathways, athletic activity is considered a risk factor for life-threatening events and sudden cardiac death [171]. Previous evidence of rapid conduction through an accessory pathway is considered particularly high risk and prompts sports disqualification [172]. Although authors of equine reports express reservation regarding continued use of horses with ventricular pre-excitation for athletic activities, the horses they describe generally were used in sports with no history of poor performance prior to diagnosis [108, 110, 111, 113] and the relationship between accessory pathways and equine sudden cardiac death is currently lacking. Nevertheless, since accessory pathways can lead to rapid, unstable rhythms, current thinking among equine cardiologists is that due to risk of extreme tachycardia, affected horses should not be considered safe to ride or drive [108].

Congenital long Q-T syndromes are reported in humans and relate to alterations in various cardiac ion channels. Action potential duration is altered and ion channel dysfunction increases the risk of early after depolarizations, which, in turn, provide the substrate for unstable ventricular rhythms and Torsade de pointes [173]. At this time, there has been some work exploring the possibility of long Q-T syndromes in Standardbreds [174] and other breeds [175] and some work looking at electrical alterans and relationships between Q-T intervals and heart rate in Thoroughbreds [176], but congenital long Q-T syndromes have not yet been reported in horses.

References

1 Rooney, J.R. and Franks, W.C. (1964). Congenital cardiac anomalies in horses. *Vet. Pathol.* 1: 454–464.

2 Crowe, M.W. and Swerczek, T.W. (1984). Equine congenital defects. *Am. J. Vet. Res.* 46: 353–358.

3 Collobert, C. and Tariel, G. (1993). Congenital abnormalities in foals: results of a seven year postmortem survey. *Pract. Vet. Equine* 25: 105–110.

4 Leroux, A.A., Detilleux, J., Sandersen, C.F. et al. (2013). Prevalence and risk factors for cardiac diseases in a hospital-based population of 3,434 horses (1994–2011). *J. Vet. Intern. Med.* 27: 1563–1570.

5 Marr, C.M. (2010). Cardiac murmurs: congenital heart disease. In: *Cardiology of the Horse*, 2e (ed. C.M. Marr and I.M. Bowen), 187–200. Edinburgh: Saunders Elsevier.

6 Reef, V.B. (1995). Evaluation of ventricular septal defects in horses using two-dimensional and Doppler echocardiography. *Equine Vet. J.* 27: 86–95.

7 Hall, T.L., Magdesian, K.G., and Kittleson, M.D. (2010). Congenital cardiac defects in neonatal foals: 18 cases (1992–2007). *J. Vet. Intern. Med.* 24: 206–212.

8 Bayly, W.M., Reed, S.M., Leathers, C.W. et al. (1982). Multiple congenital heart anomalies in five Arabian foals. *J. Am. Vet. Med. Assoc.* 181: 684–689.

9 De Lange, L., Vera, L., Decloedt, A. et al. (2021). Prevalence and characteristics of ventricular septal defects in a non-racehorse equine population (2008–2019). *J. Vet. Intern. Med.* 35: 1573–1581.

10 Crochik, S.S., Barton, M.H., Eggleston, R.B. et al. (2009). Cervical vertebral anomaly and ventricular septal defect in an Arabian foal. *Equine Vet. Educ.* 21: 207–211.

11 Brommer, H., Ensink, J.M., and Sloet van Oldruitenborgh-Oosterbaan, M.M. (2002). Multiple anomalies in a pony with colic. *Equine Vet. Educ.* 14: 240–242.

12 Cargille, J., Lombard, C., Wilson, J.H. et al. (1991). Tetralogy of Fallot and segmental uterine dysplasia in a three-year-old Morgan filly. *Cornell Vet.* 81: 411–418.

13 Buhl, R., Koch, J., Agerholm, J.S. et al. (2004). Complete situs inversus in a two-year-old standardbred horse. *Vet. Rec.* 154: 600–602.

14 Palmers, K., van Loon, G., Jorissen, M. et al. (2008). Situs inversus totalis and primary ciliary dyskinesia (Kartagener's syndrome) in a horse. *J. Vet. Intern. Med.* 22: 491–494.

15 Turner, S.I. and Jones, R.M. (2004). Complete situs inversus in a horse. *Vet. Rec.* 155: 96.

16 Lilleengen, K. (1934). Hjartmissbildningar hos djuren. *Skand. Vet. Tidsk.* 24: 493–555.

17 Drieux, H., Quinchon, C., and Thiery, G. (1946). Malformation due coeur chez un Poulain. *Rec. Med. Vet.* 122: 491–500.

18 Seco Diaz, O., Desrochers, A., Hoffmann, V. et al. (2005). Total anomalous pulmonary venous connection in a foal. *Vet. Radiol. Ultrasound* 46: 83–85.

19 Physick-Sheard, P.W., Maxie, M.G., Palmer, N.C. et al. (1985). Atrial septal defect of the persistent ostium primum type with hypoplastic right ventricle in a Welsh pony foal. *Can. J. Comp. Med.* 49: 429–433.

20 Taylor, F.G., Wotton, P.R., Hillyer, M.H. et al. (1991). Atrial septal defect and atrial fibrillation in a foal. *Vet. Rec.* 128: 80–81.

21 Kohnken, R., Schober, K., Godman, J. et al. (2018). Double outlet right ventricle with subpulmonary ventricular septal defect (Taussig-Bing anomaly) and other complex congenital cardiac malformations in an American Quarter Horse foal. *J. Vet. Cardiol.* 20: 64–72.

22 Redpath, A., Marr, C.M., Bullard, C. et al. (2020). Real-time three-dimensional (3D) echocardiographic characterisation of an atrial septal defect in a horse. *Vet. Med. Sci.* 6: 661–665.

23 Musselman, E.E. and LoGuidice, R.J. (1984). Hypoplastic left ventricular syndrome in a foal. *J. Am. Vet. Med. Assoc.* 185: 542–543.

24 Spiro, I. (2002). Hematuria and a complex congenital heart defect in a newborn foal. *Can. Vet. J.* 43: 375–377.

25 Buergelt, C.D. (2003). Equine cardiovascular pathology: an overview. *Anim. Health Res. Rev.* 4: 109–129.

26 Reppas, G.P., Canfield, P.J., Hartley, W.J. et al. (1996). Multiple congenital cardiac anomalies and idiopathic thoracic aortitis in a horse. *Vet. Rec.* 138: 14–16.

27 Scansen, B.A. (2019). Equine congenital heart disease. *Vet. Clin. North Am. Equine Pract.* 35: 103–117.

28 Patterson-Kane, J.C. and Harrison, L.R. (2002). Giant right atrial diverticulum in a foal. *J. Vet. Diagn. Investig.* 14: 335–337.

29 Ecke, P., Malik, R., and Kannegieter, N.J. (1991). Common atrioventricular canal in a foal. *N. Z. Vet. J.* 39: 97–98.

30 Kraus, M.S., Pariaut, R., Alcaraz, A. et al. (2005). Complete atrioventricular canal defect in a foal: clinical and pathological features. *J. Vet. Cardiol.* 7: 59–64.

31 Kutasi, O., Voros, K., Biksi, I. et al. (2007). Common atrioventricular canal in a newborn foal-case report and review of the literature. *Acta Vet. Hung.* 55: 51–65.

32 Keen, J.A., Cox, A., Seco Diaz, O. et al. (2010). Complex congenital diseases. In: *Cardiology of the Horse*, 2e (ed. C.M. Marr and I.M. Bowen), 202. Edinburgh: Saunders Elsevier.

33 Duz, M., Philbey, A.W., and Hughes, K.J. (2013). Mitral valve and tricuspid valve dysplasia in a 9-week-old Standardbred colt. *Equine Vet. Educ.* 25: 339–344.

34 Marr, C.M. (2019). Equine acquired Valvular disease. *Vet. Clin. North Am. Equine Pract.* 35: 119–137.

35 van der Luer, R.J. and van der Linde-Sipman, J.S. (1978). A rare congenital cardiac anomaly in a foal. *Vet. Pathol.* 15: 776–778.

36 Young, L.E., Foote, A., Marr, C.M. et al. (2010). Valvular and myocardial diseases. In: *Cardiology of the Horse*, 2e (ed. C.M. Marr and I.M. Bowen), 200. Edinburgh: Saunders Elsevier.

37 McGurrin, M.K., Physick-Sheard, P.W., and Southorn, E. (2003). Parachute left atrioventricular valve causing stenosis and regurgitation in a Thoroughbred foal. *J. Vet. Intern. Med.* 17: 579–582.

38 Schober, K.E., Kaufhold, J., and Kipar, A. (2000). Mitral valve dysplasia in a foal. *Equine Vet. J.* 32: 170–173.

39 Gumbrell, R.C. (1970). Atresia of the tricuspid valve in a foal. *N. Z. Vet. J.* 18: 253–256.

40 Button, C., Gross, D.R., Allert, J.A. et al. (1978). Tricuspid atresia in a foal. *J. Am. Vet. Med. Assoc.* 172: 825–830.

41 van der Linde-Sipman, J.S. and van den Ingh, T.S. (1979). Tricuspid atresia in a foal and a lamb. *Zentralbl. Veterinarmed. A* 26A: 239–242.

42 Hadlow, W.J. and Ward, J.K. (1980). Atresia of the right atrioventricular orifice in an Arabian foal. *Vet. Pathol.* 17: 622–626.

43 Wilson, R.B. and Haffner, J.C. (1987). Right atrioventricular atresia and ventricular septal defect in a foal. *Cornell Vet.* 77: 187–191.

44 Reef, V.B., Mann, P.C., and Orsini, P.G. (1987). Echocardiographic detection of tricuspid atresia in two foals. *J. Am. Vet. Med. Assoc.* 191: 225–228.

45 Zamora, C.S., Vitums, A., Nyrop, K.A. et al. (1989). Atresia of the right atrioventricular orifice with complete transposition of the great arteries in a horse. *Anat. Histol. Embryol.* 18: 177–182.

46 Meurs, K.M., Miller, M.W., Hanson, C. et al. (1997). Tricuspid valve atresia with main pulmonary artery atresia in an Arabian foal. *Equine Vet. J.* 29: 160–162.

47 Sedacca, C.D., Bright, J.M., and Boon, J. (2010). Doppler echocardiographic description of double-inlet left ventricle in an Arabian horse. *J. Vet. Cardiol.* 12: 147–153.

48 Zamora, C.S., Vitums, A., Foreman, J.H. et al. (1985). Common ventricle with separate pulmonary outflow chamber in a horse. *J. Am. Vet. Med. Assoc.* 186: 1210–1213.

49 Tadmor, A., Fischel, R., and Tov, A.S. (1983). A condition resembling hypoplastic left heart syndrome in a foal. *Equine Vet. J.* 15: 175–177.

50 Marr, C.M. and Bain, F.T. (2010). Ventricular septal defects. In: *Cardiology of the Horse*, 2e (ed. C.M. Marr and I.M. Bowen), 196. Edinburgh: Saunders Elsevier.

51 Muylle, E., De Roose, P., Oyaert, W. et al. (1974). An interventricular septal defect and a tricuspid valve insufficiency in a trotter mare. *Equine Vet. J.* 6: 174–176.

52 Pipers, F.S., Reef, V.B., and Wilson, J. (1985). Echocardiographic detection of ventricular septal defects in large animals. *J. Am. Vet. Med. Assoc.* 187: 810–816.

53 Seahorn, T.L.H. (1993). Ventricular septal defect and atrial fibrillation in an adult horse: a case report. *J. Equine Vet. Sci.* 13: 36–38.

54 Lilleegen, K. and Ottoson, P.B. (1935). Ein Fall von Rokitanskyschem Defekt im Sptum aorticum bein Pferd. *Arch. Tierbeilk.* 69: 387–392.

55 McCarthy, K., Ho, S., and Anderson, R. (2000). Ventricular septal defects: morphology of the doubly

committed juxtaarterial and muscular variants. *Images Paediatr. Cardiol.* 2: 5–23.

56 Dufourni, A., Decloedt, A., De Clercq, D. et al. (2018). Reversed patent ductus arteriosus and multiple congenital malformations in an 8-day-old Arabo-Friesian foal. *Equine Vet. Educ.* 30: 315–321.

57 Short, D.M., Seco, O.M., Jesty, S.A. et al. (2010). Spontaneous closure of a ventricular septal defect in a horse. *J. Vet. Intern. Med.* 24: 1515–1518.

58 Ueno, Y., Tomioka, Y., and Kaneko, M. (1992). Muscular ventricular septal defect in a horse. *Bull. Equine Res. Inst.* 29: 15–19.

59 Clark, E.S., Reef, V.B., Sweeny, C.R. et al. (1987). Aortic valvular insufficiency in a one-year-old colt. *J. Am. Vet. Med. Assoc.* 191: 841–844.

60 Gross, D.R., Clark, D.R., McDonald, D.R. et al. (1977). Congestive heart failure associated with congenital aortic valvular insufficiency in a horse. *Southwestern Vet.* 30: 27–34.

61 Taylor, S.E., Else, R.W., and Keen, J.A. (2007). Congenital aortic valve dysplasia in a Clydesdale foal. *Equine Vet. Educ.* 19: 463–468.

62 King, J.M., Flint, T.J., and Anderson, W.I. (1988). Incomplete subaortic stenotic rings in domestic animals: a newly described congenital anomaly. *Cornell Vet.* 78: 262–271.

63 Vitums, A. and Bayly, W.M. (1982). Pulmonary atresia with dextroposition of the aorta and ventricular septal defect in three Arabian foals. *Vet. Pathol.* 19: 160–168.

64 Hinchcliff, K.W. and Adams, W.M. (1991). Critical pulmonic stenosis in a newborn foal. *Equine Vet. J.* 23: 318–320.

65 Critchley, K.L. (1976). An interventricular septal defect, pulmonary stenosis and bicuspid pulmonary valve in a Welsh pony foal. *Equine Vet. J.* 8: 176–178.

66 Gehlen, H., Bubeck, K., and Stadler, P. (2001). Valvular pulmonic stenosis with normal aortic root and intact ventricular and atrial septa in an Arabian horse. *Equine Vet. Educ.* 13: 286–288.

67 Greene, H.J., Wray, D.D., and Greenway, J.A. (1975). Two equine congenital cardiac anomalies. *Irish Vet. J.* 29: 115–117.

68 Krüger, M.U., Wünschmann, A., Ward, C. et al. (2016). Pulmonary atresia with intact ventricular septum and hypoplastic right ventricle in an Arabian foal. *J. Vet. Cardiol.* 18: 284–289.

69 Leinati, L. (1929). Su di un caso raro di malfomazione del cuore in un puledro. *Clin. Vet. (Milano)* 52: 6–10.

70 Young, L.E., Blunden, A.S., Bartram, D.H. et al. (1997). Pulmonary atresia with an intact ventricular septum in a thoroughbred foal. *Equine Vet. Educ.* 9: 123–127.

71 Borst, G.H. (1978). Tetralogy of Fallot in a Belgian foal. *Tijdschr. Diergeneeskd.* 103: 968–970.

72 Gesell, S.B.K. (2006). Tetralogy of Fallot in a 7-year-old gelding. *Pferdeheikunde* 22: 427–430.

73 Houe, H., Koch, J., and Bindseil, E. (1996). Tetraology of Fallot in horses. *Dansk. Veterinaertidsskrift.* 79: 43–45.

74 Keith, J.C. (1981). Tetralogy of Fallot in a Quarter Horse foal. *Vet. Med. Small Anim. Clin.* 76: 889–895.

75 Prickett, M.E., Reeves, J.T., and Zent, W.W. (1973). Tetralogy of Fallot in a thoroughbred foal. *J. Am. Vet. Med. Assoc.* 162: 552–555.

76 Reynolds, D.J. and Nicholl, T.K. (1978). Tetralogy of Fallot and cranial mesenteric arteritis in a foal. *Equine Vet. J.* 10: 185–187.

77 Schmitz, R.R., Klaus, C., and Grabner, A. (2008). Detailed echocardiographic findings in a newborn foal with tetraology of Fallot. *Equine Vet. Educ.* 20: 298–303.

78 Vitale, V., Van Galen, G., Laurberg, M. et al. (2021). Ascending aortic aneurysm associated with tetralogy of Fallot in an adult mare. *Vet. Med. Sci.* 7: 9–15.

79 De Wensvoort, P. (1959). tetalogie van Fallot, met atresia van de arteria pulmonalis bij het hart van eeen Shetland pony. *Tijdschr. Diergeneeskd.* 84: 939.

80 Taulescu, M., Palmieri, C., Leach, J. et al. (2016). Multiple congenital cardiovascular defects including type IV persistent truncus arteriosus in a Shetland pony. *Acta Vet. Hung.* 64: 360–364.

81 Rahal, C., Collatos, C., and Bildfell, R. (1997). Pentalogy of Fallot, renal infacrtion and renal abscess in a mare. *J. Equine Vet. Sci.* 17: 604–607.

82 Chaffin, M.K., Miller, M.W., and Morris, E.L. (1992). Double outlet right ventricle and other associated congenital cardiac anomalies in an American Miniature horse foal. *Equine Vet. J.* 24: 402–406.

83 Fennell, L., Church, S., Tyrell, D. et al. (2009). Double-outlet right ventricle in a 10-month-old Friesian filly. *Aust. Vet. J.* 87: 204–209.

84 Marr, C.M. (2015). The equine neonatal cardiovascular system in health and disease. *Vet. Clin. North Am. Equine Pract.* 31 (3): 545–565.

85 Vitums, A. (1970). Origin of the aorta and pulmonary trunk from the right ventricle in a horse. *Pathol. Vet.* 7: 482–491.

86 McClure, J.J., Gaber, C.E., Watters, J.W. et al. (1983). Complete transposition of the great arteries with ventricular septal defect and pulmonary stenosis in a Thoroughbred foal. *Equine Vet. J.* 15: 377–380.

87 Sleeper, M.M. and Palmer, J.E. (2005). Echocardiographic diagnosis of transposition of the great arteries in a neonatal foal. *Vet. Radiol. Ultrasound* 46: 259–262.

88 Vitums, A., Grant, B.D., Stone, E.C. et al. (1973). Transposition of the aorta and atresia of the pulmonary trunk in a horse. *Cornell Vet.* 63: 41–57.

89 Daniels, vH. (1974). Drei Falle einer Komplexen Herzmissbildung beim Fohlen (Klinische Kurzmitteilung). *Dtsch. Tierarztl. Wochenschr.* 81: 622–623.
90 Jesty, S.A., Wilkins, P.A., Palmer, J.E. et al. (2007). Persistent truncus arteriosus in two Standardbred foals. *Equine Vet. Educ.* 19: 307–311.
91 Rang, H. and Hurtienne, H. (1976). Persistent truncus arteriosus in a 2-year old horse. *Tierarztl. Prax.* 4: 55–58.
92 Sojka, J.E. (1987). Persistent tuncus arteriosus in a foal. *Equine Pract.* 9: 24–26.
93 Stephen, J.O., Abbott, J., Middleton, D.M. et al. (2000). Persistent truncus arteriosus in a Bashkir Curly foal. *Equine Vet. Educ.* 12: 251–255.
94 Steyn, P.F., Holland, P., and Hoffman, J. (1989). The angiographic diagnosis of a persistent truncus arteriosus in a foal. *J. S. Afr. Vet. Assoc.* 60: 106–108.
95 Valdes-Martinez, A., Easdes, S.C., Strickland, K.N. et al. (2006). Echocardiographic evidence of an aortic-pulmonary septal defect in a 4-day-old thoroughbred foal. *Vet. Radiol. Ultrasound* 47: 87–89.
96 Reimer, J.M., Marr, C.M., Reef, V.B. et al. (1993). Aortic origin of the right pulmonary artery and patent ductus arteriosus in a pony foal with pulmonary hypertension and right-sided heart failure. *Equine Vet. J.* 25: 466–468.
97 Scott, E.A., Chaffee, A., Eyster, G.E. et al. (1978). Interruption of the aortic arch in two foals. *J. Am. Vet. Med. Assoc.* 172: 347–350.
98 Sandhu, S.K. and Pettitt, T.W. (2002). Interrupted aortic arch. *Curr. Treat. Options Cardiovasc. Med.* 4: 337–340.
99 Amend, J.F., Ross, J.N., Garner, H.E. et al. (1975). Systolic time intervals in domestic ponies: alterations in a case of coarctation of the aorta. *Can. J. Comp. Med.* 39: 62–66.
100 Carmichael, J.A., Buergelt, C.D., Lord, P.F. et al. (1971). Diagnosis of patent ductus arteriosus in a horse. *J. Am. Vet. Med. Assoc.* 158: 767–775.
101 Buergelt, C.D., Carmichael, J.A., Tashjian, R.J. et al. (1970). Spontaneous rupture of the left pulmonary artery in a horse with patent ductus arteriosus. *J. Am. Vet. Med. Assoc.* 157: 313–320.
102 Hare, T.A. (1931). A patent ductus arteriosus in an aged horse. *J. Pathol. Bacteriol.* 84: 124.
103 Lowe, J.S. (1972). Patent ductus arteriosus in a donkey foal. *N. Z. Vet. J.* 20 (1–2): 15.
104 Glazier, D.B., Farrelly, B.T., and Neylon, J.F. (1974). Patent ductus arteriosus in an eight month old foal. *Irish Vet. J.* 28: 12–13.
105 Reimer, J.M. (1998). Congenital defects and reversions to foetal circulation. In: *Atlas of Equine Ultrasonography* (ed. J.M. Reimer), 138–114. St Louis, MO: Mosby.
106 Saadi, A., Dalir-Naghadeh, B., Hasemi-Asi, S.M. et al. (2020). Right to left patent ductus arteriosus, acute bronchointerstitial pneumonia, pulmonary hypertension and cor pulmonale in a foal. *Equine Vet. Educ.* 32: e153–e158.
107 Delahanty, D.D. and Glazier, D.B. (1959). The Wolff Parkinson White (atrioventricular conduction) syndrome in a horse. *Irish Vet. J.* 13: 205–207.
108 Jesty, S.A., Kraus, M.S., Johnson, A.L. et al. (2011). An accessory bypass tract masked by the presence of atrial fibrillation in a horse. *J. Vet. Cardiol.* 13: 79–83.
109 Muir, W.W. and McGuirk, S.M. (1983). Ventricular preexcitation in two horses. *J. Am. Vet. Med. Assoc.* 183: 573–576.
110 Cooper, S.A. (1962). Ventricular pre-excitation (Wolff-Parkinson-White syndrome) in a horse. *Vet. Rec.* 74: 527–530.
111 Senta, T. and Amada, A. (1967). Wolff-Parkinson-White (ventricular pre-excitation syndrome) in a Thoroughbred. *Japan Racing Association Racehorse Health Research Institute Report* 4: 129–136.
112 Reimer, J.M. (1992). Cardiac arrhythmias. In: *Current Therapy in Equine Medicine*, 3e (ed. N.E. Robinson), 383–392. Philadelphia: W.B. Saunders Co.
113 Viu, J., Armengou, L., Decloedt, A. et al. (2018). Investigation of ventricular pre-excitation electrocardiographic pattern in two horses: clinical presentation and potential causes. *J. Vet. Cardiol.* 20: 213–221.
114 White, N.A. (1977). ECG of the month. *J. Am. Vet. Med. Assoc.* 171: 1236–1238.
115 Karlstam, E., Ho, S.Y., Shokrai, A. et al. (1999). Anomalous aortic origin of the left coronary artery in a horse. *Equine Vet. J.* 31: 350–352.
116 Butt, T.D., MacDonald, D.G., Crawford, W.H. et al. (1998). Persistent right aortic arch in a yearling horse. *Can. Vet. J.* 39: 714–715.
117 Coleman, M.C., Norman, T.E., and Wall, C.R. (2014). What is your diagnosis? Persistent right aortic arch. *J. Am. Vet. Med. Assoc.* 244: 1253–1255.
118 Mackey, V.S., Large, S.M., Breznock, E.M. et al. (1986). Surgical correction of a persistent right aortic arch in a foal. *Vet. Surg.* 15: 325–328.
119 Petrick, S.W., Roos, C.J., and van Niekerk, J. (1978). Persistent right aortic arch in a horse. *J. S. Afr. Vet. Assoc.* 49: 355–358.
120 van der Linde-Sipman, J.S., Goedegebuure, S.A., and Kroneman, J. (1979). Persistent right aortic arch associated with a persistent left ductus arteriosus and an interventricular septal defect in a horse. *Tijdschr. Diergeneeskd.* 104: 189–194.
121 Bartels, J.E. and Vaughan, J.T. (1969). Persistent right aortic arch in the horse. *J. Am. Vet. Med. Assoc.* 154: 406–409.
122 Smith, T.R. (2004). Unusual vascular ring anomaly in a foal. *Can. Vet. J.* 45: 1016–1018.

123 Viljoen, A., Saulez, M.N., and Steyl, J. (2012). Right subclavian artery anomaly in an adult Friesian horse. *Equine Vet. Educ.* 24: 62–65.

124 Cox, V.S., Weber, A.F., and de Lima, A. (1991). Left cranial vena cava in a horse. *Anat. Histol. Embryol.* 20: 37–43.

125 Thiene, G. and Frescura, C. (2010). Anatomical and pathophysiological classification of congenital heart disease. *Cardiovasc. Pathol.* 19: 259–274.

126 Schwarzwald, C.C. (2010). Disorders of the cardiovascular system. In: *Equine Internal Medicine*, 4e (ed. S.M. Reed, W.M. Bayly, and D.C. Sellon), 387–541. St. Louis, MO: Elsevier.

127 O'Grady, M.R., Holmberg, D.L., Miller, C.W. et al. (1989). Canine congenital aortic stenosis: a review of the literature and commentary. *Can. Vet. J.* 30: 811–815.

128 Dyer, K.T., Hlavacek, A.M., Meinel, F.G. et al. (2014). Imaging in congenital pulmonary vein anomalies: the role of computed tomography. *Pediatr. Radiol.* 44: 1158–1168. (quiz 5–7).

129 Files, M.D. and Morray, B. (2017). Total anomalous pulmonary venous connection: preoperative anatomy, physiology, imaging, and interventional management of postoperative pulmonary venous obstruction. *Semin. Cardiothorac. Vasc. Anesth.* 21: 123–131.

130 Vernemmen, I., Paulussen, E., Dauvillier, J. et al. (2022). Three-dimensional and catheter-based intracardiac echocardiographic characterization of the interatrial septum in 2 horses with suspicion of a patent foramen ovale. *J. Vet. Intern. Med.* 36: 1535–1542.

131 Rigatelli, G. (2014). Should we consider patent foramen ovale and secundum atrial septal defect as different steps of a single anatomo-clinical continuum? *J. Geriatr. Cardiol.* 11: 177–179.

132 MacDonald, A.A., Fowden, A.L., Silver, M. et al. (1988). The foramen ovale of the foetal and neonatal foal. *Equine Vet. J.* 20: 255–260.

133 Ottaway, C.W. (1900). The anatomical closure of the foramen ovale in the equine and bovine heart: a comparative study with observations on the foetal and adult states. *Vet. J.* 1944 (100): 111–118.

134 Ottaway, C.W. (1900). The anatomical closure of the foramen ovale in the equine and bovine heart: a comparative study with observations on the foetal and adult states. *Vet. J.* 1944 (100): 130–134.

135 Wilson, A.P. (1943). Persistent foramen ovale in a foal. *Vet. Med. Small Anim. Clin.* 38: 491–492.

136 Kutty, S., Sengupta, P.P., and Khandheria, B.K. (2012). Patent foramen Ovale. The known and the to be known. *J. Am. Coll. Cardiol.* 59: 1665–1671.

137 Spier, S. (1985). Arterial thrombosis as the cause of lameness in a foal. *J. Am. Vet. Med. Assoc.* 187: 164–165.

138 De Silva, M., Tagliavia, C., Galiazzo, G. et al. (2022). Morphological variability of the atrioventricular valve cusps in the equine heart. *Equine Vet. J.* 54: 167–175.

139 Tidholm, A. (1997). Retrospective study of congenital heart defects in 151 dogs. *J. Small Anim. Pract.* 38: 94–98.

140 Oliveira, P., Domenech, O., Silva, J. et al. (2011). Retrospective review of congenital heart disease in 976 dogs. *J. Vet. Intern. Med.* 25: 3.

141 Reimer, J.M. (1998). The heart. In: *Atlas of Equine Ultrasonography* (ed. J.M. Reimer), 379–408. St Louis, MO: Mosby.

142 Reef, V.B., Bonagura, J., Buhl, R. et al. (2014). Recommendations for management of equine athletes with cardiovascular abnormalities. *J. Vet. Intern. Med.* 28: 749–761.

143 Frescura, C. and Thiene, G. (2014). The new concept of univentricular heart. *Front. Pediatr.* 2: 62.

144 Anderson, R.H., Becker, A.E., Tynan, M. et al. (1984). The univentricular atrioventricular connection: getting to the root of a thorny problem. *Am. J. Cardiol.* 54: 822–828.

145 Reef, V.B. (1991). Echocardiographic findings in horses with congenital cardiac disease. *Compend. Contin. Educ. Pract. Vet.* 13: 109–117.

146 Rao, P.S. (2019). Management of congenital heart disease: state of the art-part II-cyanotic heart defects. *Children (Basel)* 6: 4.

147 Sumal, A.S., Kyriacou, H., and Mostafa, A. (2020). Tricuspid atresia: where are we now? *J. Card. Surg.* 35: 1609–1617.

148 Minocha, P.K. and Phoon, C. (2023). *Tricuspid Atresia*. Treasure Island, FL: StatPearls Publishing https://www.ncbi.nlm.nih.gov/books/NBK554495/.

149 Ellesøe, S.G., Workman, C.T., Bouvagnet, P. et al. (2018). Familial co-occurrence of congenital heart defects follows distinct patterns. *Eur. Heart J.* 39: 1015–1022.

150 Kumar, A., Victorica, B.E., Gessner, I.H. et al. (1994). Tricuspid atresia and annular hypoplasia: report of a familial occurrence. *Pediatr. Cardiol.* 15: 201–203.

151 Nozari, A., Aghaei-Moghadam, E., Zeinaloo, A. et al. (2019). A pathogenic homozygous mutation in the Pleckstrin homology domain of RASA1 is responsible for familial tricuspid atresia in an Iranian consanguineous family. *Cell J.* 21: 70–77.

152 Abdul-Sater, Z., Yehya, A., Beresian, J. et al. (2012). Two heterozygous mutations in NFATC1 in a patient with tricuspid atresia. *PLoS One* 7: e49532.

153 Wiegering, A., Rüther, U., and Gerhardt, C. (2017). The role of hedgehog signalling in the formation of the ventricular septum. *J. Dev. Biol.* 5: 4.

154 Junge, H.K., Glaus, T., Matos, J.N. et al. (2021). Balloon valvuloplasty of valvular pulmonary stenosis in a neonatal foal. *J. Vet. Cardiol.* 36: 48–54.

155 Michlik, K.M., Biazik, A.K., Henklewski, R.Z. et al. (2014). Quadricuspid aortic valve and a ventricular septal defect in a horse. *BMC Vet. Res.* 10: 142.

156 Brown, C.M. and Holmes, J.R. (1979). Phonocardiography in the horse: 2. The relationship of the external phonocardiogram to intracardiac pressure and sound. *Equine Vet. J.* 11: 183–186.

157 Rusee, I. and Sinowatz, F. (1991). *Textbook of the Embryology of Domestic Animals*. Berlin, Germany: Verlag Paul Parey.

158 Franklin, R.C.G., Béland, M.J., Colan, S.D. et al. (2017). Nomenclature for congenital and paediatric cardiac disease: the International Paediatric and Congenital Cardiac Code (IPCCC) and the eleventh iteration of the international classification of diseases (ICD-11). *Cardiol. Young* 27: 1872–1938.

159 Amoroso, E.C., Dawes, G.S., and Mott, J.C. (1958). Patency of the ductus arteriosus in the newborn calf and foal. *Br. Heart J.* 20: 92–96.

160 Scott, E.A., Kneller, S.K., and Witherspoon, D.M. (1975). Closure of ductus arteriosus determined by cardiac catheterization and angiography in newborn foals. *Am. J. Vet. Res.* 36: 1021–1023.

161 Rossdale, P.D. (1967). Clinical studies on the newborn thoroughbred foal. II. Heart rate, auscultation and electrocardiogram. *Br. Vet. J.* 123: 521–532.

162 Machida, N., Yasuda, J., Too, K. et al. (1988). A morphological study on the obliteration processes of the ductus arteriosus in the horse. *Equine Vet. J.* 20: 249–254.

163 Livesey, L.C., Marr, C.M., Boswood, A. et al. (1998). Auscultation and two-dimensional, M mode, spectral and colour flow Doppler echocardiographic findings in pony foals from birth to seven weeks of age. *J. Vet. Intern. Med.* 12: 255.

164 Swensson, R.E., Valdes-Cruz, L.M., Sahn, D.J. et al. (1986). Real-time Doppler color flow mapping for detection of patent ductus arteriosus. *J. Am. Coll. Cardiol.* 8: 1105–1112.

165 Angelini, P. and Uribe, C. (2022). Critical update and discussion of the prevalence, nature, mechanisms of action, and treatment options in potentially serious coronary anomalies. *Trends Cardiovasc. Med.* (in press).

166 Molossi, S., Doan, T., and Sachdeva, S. (2023). Anomalous coronary arteries: a state-of-the-art approach. *Cardiol. Clin.* 41: 51–69.

167 Niu, M., Zhang, J., Ge, Y. et al. (2022). Acute myocardial infarction in the elderly with anomalous origin of the left coronary artery from the pulmonary artery (ALCAPA): a case report and literature review. *Medicine (Baltimore)* 101: e32219.

168 D'Ascenzi, F., Valentini, F., Pistoresi, S. et al. (2022). Causes of sudden cardiac death in young athletes and non-athletes: systematic review and meta-analysis: sudden cardiac death in the young. *Trends Cardiovasc. Med.* 32: 299–308.

169 Schiavone, M., Gobbi, C., Gasperetti, A. et al. (2021). Congenital coronary artery anomalies and sudden cardiac death. *Pediatr. Cardiol.* 42: 1676–1687.

170 Bauer, S., Livesey, M.A., Bjorling, D.E. et al. (2006). Computed tomography assisted surgical correction of persistent right aortic arch in a neonatal foal. *Equine Vet. Educ.* 18: 32–36.

171 Książczyk, T.M., Pietrzak, R., and Werner, B. (2020). Management of young athletes with asymptomatic preexcitation – a review of the literature. *Diagnostics (Basel)* 10: 10.

172 Di Mambro, C., Drago, F., Milioni, M. et al. (2016). Sports eligibility after risk assessment and treatment in children with asymptomatic ventricular pre-excitation. *Sports Med.* 46: 1183–1190.

173 El-Sherif, N., Turitto, G., and Boutjdir, M. (2017). Congenital long QT syndrome and torsade de pointes. *Ann. Noninvasive Electrocardiol.* 22: 6.

174 Pedersen, P.J., Kanters, J.K., Buhl, R. et al. (2013). Normal electrocardiographic QT interval in race-fit Standardbred horses at rest and its rate dependence during exercise. *J. Vet. Cardiol.* 15: 23–31.

175 Pedersen, P.J., Karlsson, M., Flethoj, M. et al. (2016). Differences in the electrocardiographic QT interval of various breeds of athletic horses during rest and exercise. *J. Vet. Cardiol.* 18: 255–264.

176 Li, M., Chadda, K.R., Matthews, G.D.K. et al. (2018). Cardiac electrophysiological adaptations in the equine athlete-restitution analysis of electrocardiographic features. *PLoS One* 13 (3): e0194008.

Chapter 13 Cardiovascular Disorders of the Neonatal Foal

Section I Arrhythmias

Cristobal Navas de Solis

Arrhythmias are disorders in the generation or conduction of cardiac electrical impulses. Arrhythmias with increased rates (tachyarrhythmias) can be caused by enhanced automaticity, triggered activity, or reentry mechanisms, whereas arrhythmias with low rates (bradyarrhythmias) are caused by lack of generation or slow or blocked conduction [1]. The pathophysiological and electrophysiological mechanisms responsible for arrhythmias are not commonly elucidated in equine clinical cases, but the potential reasons are the same in the foal and in the adult horse [2]. Certain types of arrhythmias and mechanisms of generation may be more common in the neonate, particularly in the perinatal period [3, 4]. Due to the limited experience with management and scarce literature in equine neonatal arrhythmias, principles of interpretation and therapy for arrhythmias in neonates of other species are often used to manage foals, and these therapies are used in conjunction with clinical experience in adult horses.

Arrhythmias are frequent in the neonatal period in foals and infants. Sinus arrhythmia, single supraventricular premature complexes (SVPCs), single ventricular premature complexes (VPCs), and junctional rhythms are often benign, not having clinical consequences or requiring therapy. However, some arrhythmias may be the consequence of systemic disease, or in particular cases, an early sign of an arrhythmogenic substrate, and should not be disregarded without consideration of the circumstances surrounding the cardiac rhythm. Supraventricular tachycardia (SVT), ventricular tachycardia, and atrioventricular conduction abnormalities are classified as nonbenign arrhythmias [5]. Equine neonatal cardiac and extracardiac diseases that have been associated with arrhythmias include myopathies/cardiomyopathy, sepsis, myocarditis, electrolytes disorders, uroperitoneum, congenital heart disease, severe anemia, respiratory infections, and fractured ribs [6–11].

The basic principles of how to obtain and interpret electrocardiograms (ECG) in foals and adult horses are the same [12]. Age-specific differences in rate, interval durations, and frequency of arrhythmias are summarized in Chapter 1. Electrocardiograms can be obtained with traditional electrocardiography equipment with the same lead positioning used in adult horses [13], digital telemetry, and holter monitors. A base-apex lead is the most common configuration in which the right arm electrode is placed on the right neck in front of the scapula, the left arm electrode is placed caudal to the left elbow over the apex of the heart and the ground electrode is positioned elsewhere, typically over the right jugular groove. With this electrode configuration "Lead I" (right arm to left arm) will display the base-apex ECG trace. Newly developed mobile-health devices have been used in horses [14] and are useful tools for rapid rhythm evaluation. Figure 13.I.1 depicts a foal fitted with a chest band with incorporated electrodes and the ECGs obtained in real time and after processing using electrocardiography software. Mobile-health devices can obtain ECGs of diagnostic quality and make real-time monitoring fast and accessible (Figure 13.I.2). Equipment that allows the use of several leads and continuous monitoring are needed for complex arrhythmias.

Perinatal Period

The first few minutes after birth are a particularly vulnerable period with characteristic physiologic transitions that predispose the foal to arrhythmogenesis; consequently, many perinatal arrhythmias are considered physiologic in the newborn foal and infant [1, 3]. The frequent arrhythmias present during the first minutes of life are most often clinically silent and are only detected in foals monitored closely via ECG or auscultation immediately after birth. In an ECG

Equine Neonatal Medicine, First Edition. Edited by David M. Wong and Pamela A. Wilkins.

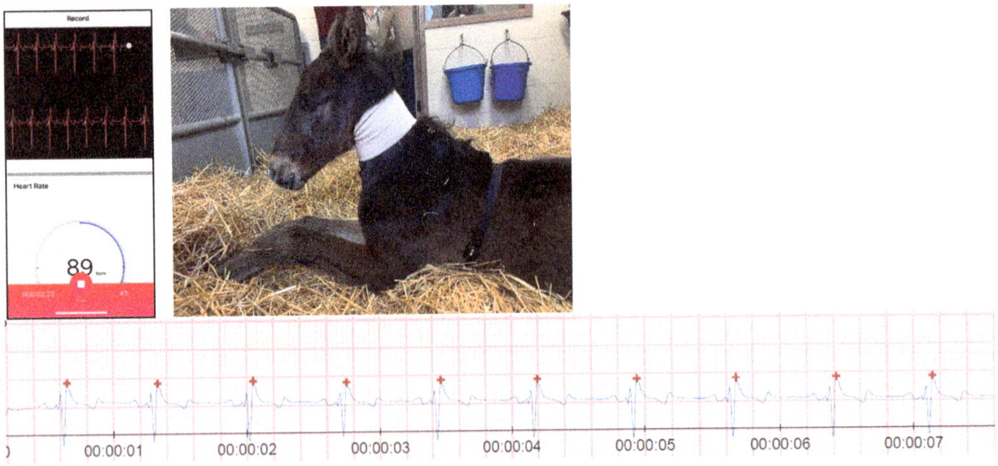

Figure 13.I.1 Normal sinus rhythm in a 2-day-old foal fitted with a wearable ECG designed for human athletes (https://www.w2nd.info). Paper speed is 25 mm/s and gain 10 mm/mV. The top left images shows the real-time display in the mobile phone and the bottom image shows the ECG processed using commercial software [15]. Lead is a modified base-apex lead. "Base" electrode was placed approximately 10 cm lower than the withers in the left side of the horse and apex electrode placed near the sternum.

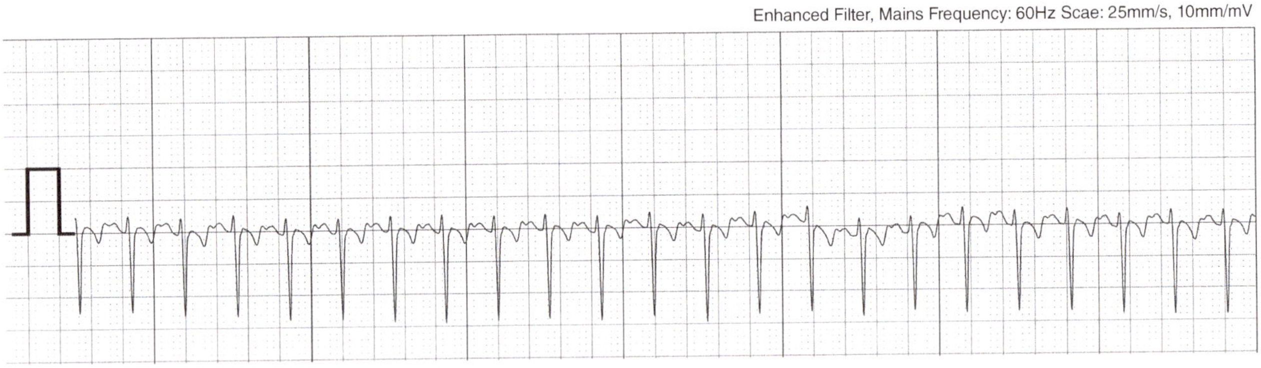

Figure 13.I.2 Sinus tachycardia (heart rate 180/min). Electrocardiogram obtained with a mobile-health device (Alivecor Inc., 444 Castro St #600, Mountain View, CA 94041) in 2-day-old foal presented with myocarditis and necrotizing enterocolitis.

study in foals without known cardiac disease, some type of arrhythmia was found in 96% of foals. Therefore, these arrhythmias were considered part of the adaptive period to the extrauterine environment [3]. Sinus arrhythmia, wandering pacemakers, and SVPC were the most common arrhythmias (Figure 13.I.3). Atrial fibrillation (AF), VPCs, second-degree atrioventricular (AV) block, ventricular tachycardia, and supraventricular- or idioventricular rhythms were less common. Fetal ECGs were not predictive of perinatal arrhythmias and these arrhythmias developed 1–2 minutes before birth coinciding with the compression of the head and umbilical cord in the birth canal that was associated with hypoxemia, hypercapnia, and acidemia [3]. The ST segment was elevated in 90% of foals, further suggesting that myocardial hypoxia could be responsible for a component of the electrocardiographic perinatal changes.

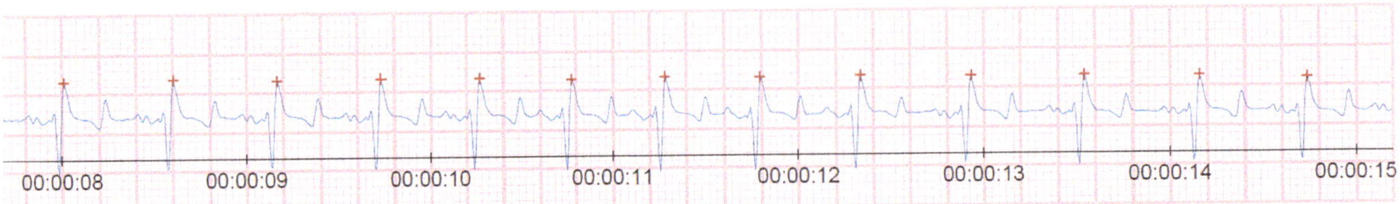

Figure 13.I.3 Electrocardiogram of a 3-day-old foal with sinus arrhythmia and wandering pacemaker. At the time of the electrocardiogram, the foal was clinically normal and with normal clinicopathological findings. Note the variable R-R interval and variable morphology of the P waves. Paper speed is 25 mm/s and gain 10 mm/mV. Lead is a modified base-apex lead. "Base" electrode was placed approximately 10 cm lower than the withers in the left side of the horse and apex electrode placed near the sternum.

All arrhythmias disappeared within 15 minutes of birth, and none of the foals had clinical disorders related to the arrhythmias [4].

Supraventricular Arrythmias

Sinus arrhythmia, wandering pacemaker, junctional rhythms, and some types of atrial ectopy are common in neonates. Up to 25% of healthy children can have these rhythms [1] and these arrhythmias are also common in the foal, although the actual frequency has not been determined beyond the perinatal period. The main predisposing mechanisms to supraventricular arrhythmias (mainly SVPCs and AF) are increased vagal tone, atrial stretch, and myocardial hypoxia. Vagal tone increases immediately after birth, shortening the action potential duration in atrial myocardial cells. Atrial myocardial stretch occurs due to decreased pulmonary vascular resistance causing increased pulmonary flow and increased systemic vascular resistance caused by the stop of placental flow. The myocardial stretch may shorten the refractory period. In addition, transient myocardial hypoxia during adaptation to extrauterine can have an arrhythmogenic effect [16, 17].

Single SVPCs originate from the atria, are often clinically silent, and many times are of uncertain cause. The P wave may be normal or abnormal and the QRS is often normal (Figures 13.I.4 and 13.I.5). However, the amplitude of the QRS and T wave of SVPCs can sometimes change in comparison with sinus beats [18]. SVPCs can be conducted or not conducted to the ventricles, depending on the relationship of the premature complex and the refractory period and most frequently reset the AV node, resulting in a noncompensatory pause. In infants and fetuses, SVPCs resolve in 95% of cases by 1 year of age without development of further signs or arrhythmias [19]. No associations with serious clinical consequences are described in human neonates with SVPCs. Atrioventricular re-entry tachycardia is the most common mechanism of SVT in the newborn. In human fetuses and infants, an immature conduction system causes an increased number of accessory AV pathways making reentrant mechanism the most common cause of SVTs and SVPCs [19]. Central venous catheters are a described cause of SVPCs in the human neonate and clinicians should be cognizant of the fact that 20 cm catheters used frequently in foals can reach the right atrium or even the right ventricle in small foals or in normal sized foals if placed in the lower neck.

AF (Figure 13.I.6) is found rarely in the equine neonate beyond paroxysmal short runs during the first minutes of life [16]. Reports of foals in AF with and without underlying cardiac disease can be found but the incidence seems to be much lower than in the adult horse. Treatment using quinidine and transcutaneous electrical cardioversion has been reported [7, 20, 21].

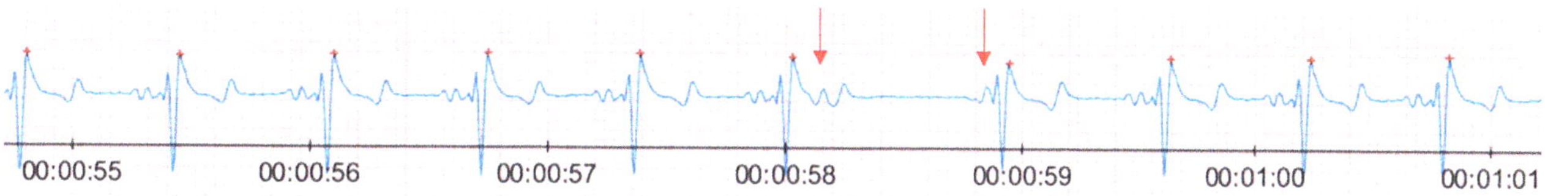

Figure 13.I.4 Nonconducted SVPCs. Electrocardiogram of a 2-day-old foal presented for neonatal isoerythrolysis. There is a premature P wave with different morphology (left red arrow) than the sinus generated complexes and buried in the ST segment (nonconducted SVPC). The following complex also has an abnormal P wave (right red arrow) morphology and short P-R interval. (supraventricular ectopic complex). Paper speed is 25 mm/s and gain 10 mm/mV. Lead is a modified base-apex lead. "Base" electrode was placed approximately 10 cm lower than the withers in the left side of the horse and apex electrode placed near the sternum.

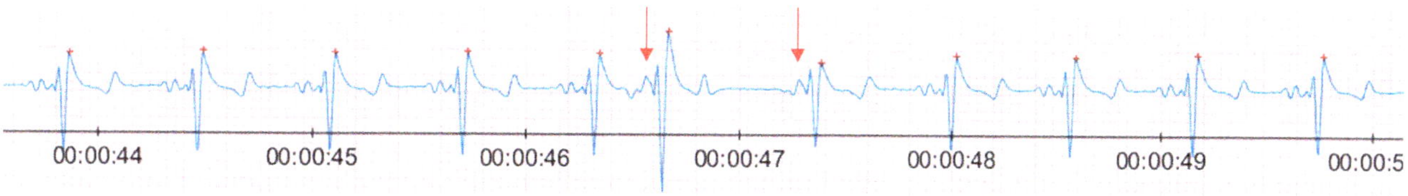

Figure 13.I.5 Supraventricular premature complex. Electrocardiogram of a 2-day-old foal presented for neonatal isoerythrolysis. There is a premature P wave with different morphology (left red arrow) than the sinus generated complexes and buried in the T segment that generates a QRS complex with large amplitude (SVPC). The following complex has also an abnormal P wave morphology (right red arrow) and short P-R interval (supraventricular ectopic complex). Paper speed is 25 mm/s and gain 10 mm/mV. Lead is a modified base-apex lead. "Base" electrode was placed approximately 10 cm lower than the withers in the left side of the horse and apex electrode placed near the sternum.

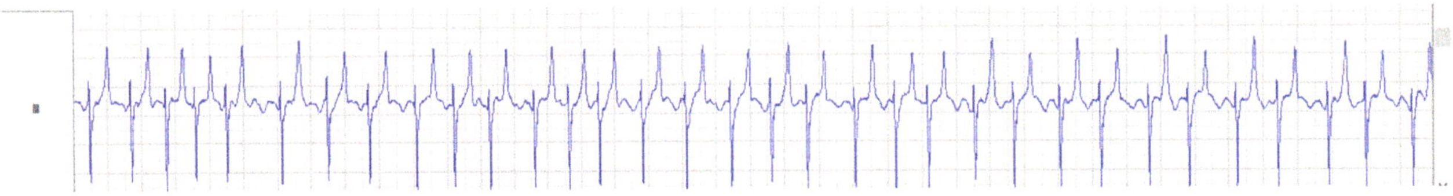

Figure 13.I.6 Atrial fibrillation. Electrocardiogram of a 4-week-old foal. The ECG was obtained with a telemetry unit (Televet Mobile Kit, Engel Engineering Services GmbH, Heusenstamm, Germany). Paper speed is 25 mm/s and gain 10 mm/mV. Lead is a modified base-apex lead. "Base" electrode was placed approximately 10 cm lower than the withers in the right side of the horse and apex electrode placed near the sternum.

Ventricular Arrhythmias

Ventricular arrhythmias originate from the ventricular myocardium. QRS morphology is often aberrant and QRS complexes are wider as conduction is slow via cell-to-cell pathways. In some instances, differentiation from junctional or supraventricular rhythms can be difficult if the impulse is generated near and conducted through the His bundle. When more than one aberrant morphology is found, the rhythm is categorized as multiform, suggesting more widespread myocardial disease and a worse prognosis. Ventricular impulses are not commonly conducted retrograde from the ventricles to the atria and therefore they do not reset the sinoatrial node. For this reason, compensatory pauses are seen in the ECG when single VPCs occur.

VPCs (Figure 13.I.7) are less common in neonates than SVPCs. They can be idiopathic but are more commonly associated with underlying cardiac or noncardiac disease than SVPCs. Approximately 2% of human fetuses and 18% of newborns have VPCs [19]. Continuous ECGs documenting the incidence of asymptomatic VPCs in foals beyond the immediate postnatal period have not been reported. The potential serious consequences of complex ventricular arrhythmias and an undiagnosed arrhythmogenic substrate suggests that the presence of VPCs should not be disregarded [19]. Attention should be directed to identify and monitor cardiac or extracardiac diseases, triggering arrhythmias and to determine if more complex arrhythmias are present [1]. Single, sporadic, monomorphic VPCs can be considered a variation of normal rhythm if investigation for the underlying cause do not reveal cardiac or extra-cardiac abnormalities. Under these circumstances VPCs often disappear spontaneously.

Ventricular tachycardia or idioventricular rhythms (Figures 13.I.8–13.I.10) are uncommon in the neonate, accounting for 5–10% of all tachyarrhythmias in human

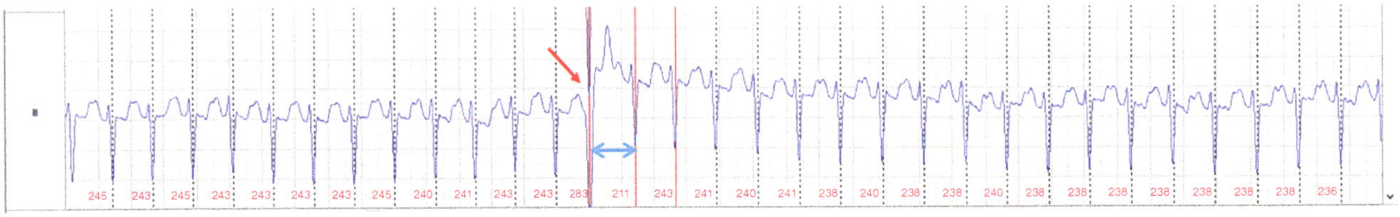

Figure 13.I.7 Sinus tachycardia (heart rate 243/min) and single VPC (red arrow). Electrocardiogram of a 2-day-old foal presented with myocarditis and necrotizing enterocolitis. The red arrow points to a QRS complex that is premature and with aberrant morphology (VPC). The VPC is followed by a compensatory pause (blue arrow). Paper speed is 25 mm/s and gain 10 mm/mV. Lead is a modified base-apex lead. "Base" electrode was placed approximately 10 cm lower than the withers in the left side of the horse and apex electrode placed near the sternum.

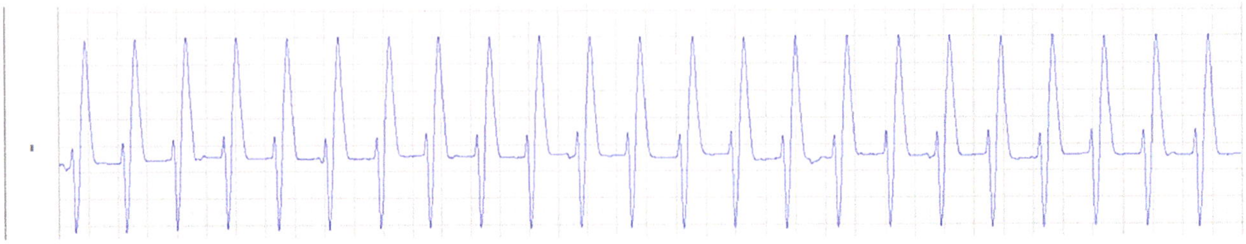

Figure 13.I.8 Idioventricular rhythm. Electrocardiogram of a 2-day old foal presented with myocarditis and necrotizing enterocolitis. Paper speed is 25 mm/s and gain 10 mm/mV. Lead is a modified base-apex lead. "Base" electrode was placed approximately 10 cm lower than the withers in the left side of the horse and apex electrode placed near the sternum.

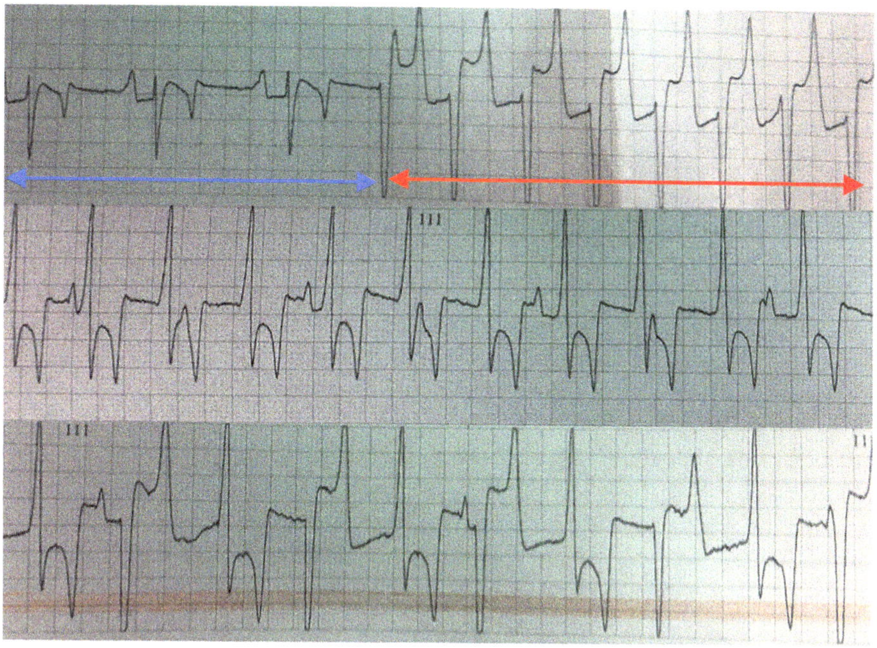

Figure 13.I.9 Multifocal ventricular ectopy in a 2-day-old foal with white muscle disease. The upper strip shows the transition from sinus rhythm (blue arrow) to ventricular tachycardia (red arrow). The middle strip shows a run of ventricular tachycardia with a second morphology, and the third strip shows multifocal ventricular tachycardia. Paper speed is 25 mm/s and gain 10 mm/mV. Lead is a base-apex lead.

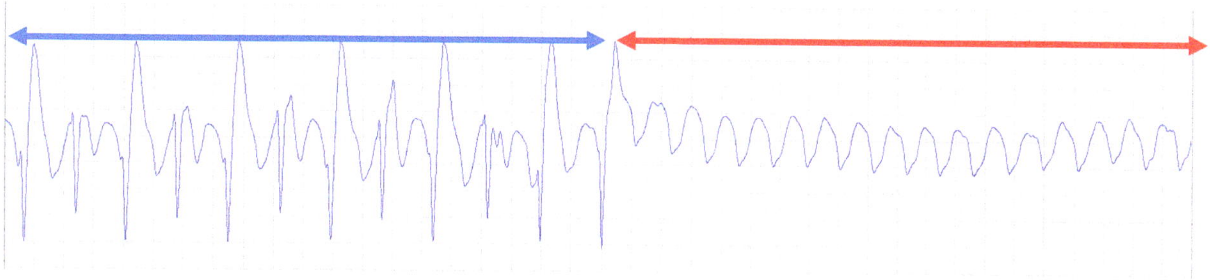

Figure 13.I.10 Idioventricular rhythm (blue arrow) deteriorating into ventricular fibrillation (red arrow). Electrocardiogram of a 2-day-old foal presented with myocarditis and necrotizing enterocolitis. Paper speed is 25 mm/s and gain 10 mm/mV. Lead is a modified base-apex lead. "Base" electrode was placed approximately 10 cm lower than the withers in the left side of the horse and apex electrode placed near the sternum.

neonates [1, 19, 22]. Structural heart disease is found in approximately half of human neonates with ventricular tachycardia and is more frequent than supraventricular arrhythmias or isolated VPCs [19]. Principles for treatment of ventricular arrhythmias in the horse generally apply to the neonate; anti-arrhythmic medications are reviewed in Chapter 11 [23, 24].

Bradyarrhythmias

Bradyarrhythmias include rhythms caused by sinoatrial node dysfunction such as sinus bradycardia or sinus pauses along with second- and third-degree AV block (Figure 13.I.11). Sinus bradycardia is defined as a heartbeat two standard deviations less than the mean and therefore

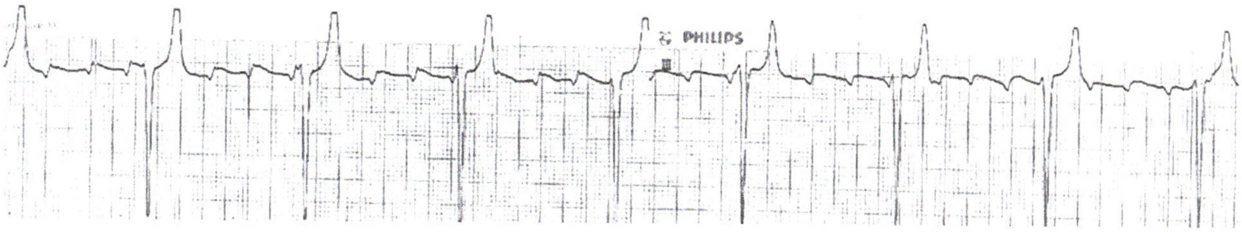

Figure 13.I.11 Thlrd-degree AV block and ventricular escape rhythm in a neonatal foal. Not the dissociated P and QRS complexes Paper speed is 25 mm/s and gain 10 mm/mV. Lead III is displayed.

the rate that defines sinus bradycardia varies with the specific age within the neonatal period [25]. The normal heart rates for the perinatal and neonatal periods are discussed in Chapter 1. Lack of conduction of bigeminal SVPCs is mentioned in people as a cause of bradycardia or pseudo-bradycardia, but this arrhythmia has not been reported in equine neonates. Similar to other rhythms, bradyarrhythmias can be due to cardiac and extracardiac causes and are described in normal neonates in the perinatal period. Sinus bradycardia and sinus pauses can occur in up to 90% of healthy human neonates and are more common in premature and low-weight infants [1]. These arrhythmias were also reported frequently in the immediate postpartum period in foals [4], but their frequency beyond this period is uncertain.

Described secondary causes of bradyarrhythmias include sepsis, central nervous system anomalies, hypothermia, intracranial hypertension, meningitis, hypothyroidism, and electrolyte or metabolic alterations. Intermittent bradycardia associated with apnea and central nervous system immaturity is particularly common in premature neonates [26]. The presence of apnea is recognized in foals associated with neonatal encephalopathy [27, 28] but a syndrome analogous to human bradycardias and sudden infant death syndrome is not commonly reported or recognized. Congenital heart disease is another possible, yet uncommon, cause of bradyarrhythmias [7, 29]. Patients with bradycardias can be asymptomatic or have weakness, syncope, or heart failure. Atropine, isoproterenol, and epinephrine can be useful in the pharmacologic therapy of arrhythmias with consideration for pacemakers in selected cases.

Uroperitoneum

Uroperitoneum deserves specific mention as a cause of arrhythmias in the foal. Atrioventricular conduction disturbances (third-degree and advanced second-degree AV block), VPCs, and ventricular fibrillation are the main arrhythmias of concern with uroperitoneum [30]. Electrolyte abnormalities (hyperkalemia, hyponatremia), acidemia, uremia, along with the effects of inhalant anesthetics and drainage of urine from the abdomen are relevant contributors to arrhythmogenesis. Recent reports have documented a lower incidence of arrhythmias [30, 31] with current management of uroperitoneum; this may be due to more awareness for the need of patient stabilization and use of isofluorane (vs. halothane) as an inhalant anesthetic. Prevention of arrhythmogenic deaths in foals with uroperitoneum may include the control of factors described above, anesthetic protocols to minimize arrythmias, rhythm monitoring and establishing antiarrhythmic drug and resuscitation plans.

Hyperkalemia lowers the resting potential across the cell membrane. Mild hyperkalemia increases tissue excitability, whereas severe hyperkalemia lowers excitability, which may precipitating AV blocks [32]. Despite the classically described role of plasma potassium concentration in arrhythmias [33], arrhythmias in foals with uroperitoneum can occur with normal potassium concentration and the severity of potassium derangements is not always predictive of the rhythm response. Nevertheless, preoperative potassium stabilization is a worthwhile effort. Isotonic saline, glucose infusions to promote insulin production and consequent intracellular uptake of potassium ions, insulin supplementation or sodium bicarbonate administration can be used to control hyperkalemia. Calcium gluconate can also be administered and offers an indirect cardioprotective effect by increasing threshold voltage, restoring the normal resting membrane potential previously increased by hyperkalemia. The use of nebulized β_2-adrenergic agonist has also been used successfully to decrease hyperkalemia [32].

A vagal response is a potential arrhythmogenic mechanism in uroperitoneum and urogenital surgery. Parasympathetic activation and sympathetic inhibition are triggered by pain, reduced venous return to the heart, stimulation of afferent cardiac nerves or noncardiac baroreceptors, and the pull on abdominal organs [30, 34]. An expansion of the abdominal vasculature after abdominal decompression, the use of warm peritoneal lavage solutions, and dorsal recumbency, can also reduce systemic vascular resistance and decrease blood pressure. The decrease in blood pressure causes an increase in heart rate [32, 35] to maintain cardiac output and tissue perfusion. Additionally, the sudden release of the abdominal compartment syndrome has also been suggested to cause a washout of accumulated potassium and waste product from the hypoperfused abdomen, highlighting that arrhythmogenesis during uroperitoneum is a multifactorial process [36].

Therapy

Criteria for pharmacological treatment of arrhythmias in neonates are analogous to the ones used in adults. Monitoring and evaluating for an underlying disease triggering the arrhythmias is the most common approach to arrhythmias in neonates. Specific recommendations for antiarrhythmic drugs are described in Chapter 11. Lidocaine, propranolol, quinidine, magnesium sulfate, amiodarone, propafenone, sotalol, propranolol, metoprolol, and adenosine are drugs commonly mentioned as antiarrhythmic options for foals or human neonates [1, 11]. Extrapolation of drugs and dosages needs to be made with caution as the kinetics, dynamics, interactions, and safety margins of these drugs may be different in horses and humans.

References

1 Drago, F., Battipaglia, I., and Di Mambro, C. (2018). Neonatal and pediatric arrhythmias: clinical and electrocardiographic aspects. *Card Electrophysiol. Clin.* 10: 397–412.

2 van Loon, G. (2019). Cardiac arrhythmias in horses. *Vet. Clin. North Am. Equine Pract.* 35: 85–102.

3 Yamamoto, K., Yasuda, J., and Too, K. (1991). Electrocardiographic findings during parturition and blood gas tensions immediately after birth in Thoroughbred foals. *Jpn. J. Vet. Res.* 39: 143–157.

4 Yamamoto, K., Yasuda, J., and Too, K. (1992). Arrhythmias in newborn Thoroughbred foals. *Equine Vet. J.* 24: 169–173.

5 Ban, J.E. (2017). Neonatal arrhythmias: diagnosis, treatment, and clinical outcome. *Korean J. Pediatr.* 60: 344–352.

6 Reef, V.B. (1985). Cardiovascular disease in the equine neonate. *Vet. Clin. North Am. Equine Pract.* 1: 117–129.

7 Taylor, F.G., Wotton, P.R., Hillyer, M.H. et al. (1991). Atrial septal defect and atrial fibrillation in a foal. *Vet. Rec.* 128: 80–81.

8 Perkins, G., Valberg, S.J., Madigan, J.M. et al. (1998). Electrolyte disturbances in foals with severe rhabdomyolysis. *J. Vet. Intern. Med.* 12: 173–177.

9 Jean, D., Picandet, V., Macieira, S. et al. (2007). Detection of rib trauma in newborn foals in an equine critical care unit: a comparison of ultrasonography, radiography and physical examination. *Equine Vet. J.* 39: 158–163.

10 Katz, L., O'Dwyer, S., and Pollock, P. (2009). Nutritional muscular dystrophy in a four-day-old Connemara foal. *Irish Vet. J.* 62: 119–124.

11 Marr, C.M. (2015). The equine neonatal cardiovascular system in health and disease. *Vet. Clin. North Am. Equine Pract.* 31: 545–565.

12 Mitchell, K.J. (2019). Equine electrocardiography. *Vet. Clin. North Am. Equine Pract.* 35: 65–83.

13 Verheyen, T., Annelies, D., Clercq, D. et al. (2010). Electrocardiography in horses – part 1: how to make a good recording. *Vlaams Diergeneeskundig Tijdschrift* 79: 331–336.

14 Kraus, M.S., Rishniw, M., Divers, T.J. et al. (2019). Utility and accuracy of a smartphone-based electrocardiogram device as compared to a standard base-apex electrocardiogram in the horse. *Res. Vet. Sci.* 125: 141–147.

15 Tarvainen, M.P., Niskanen, J.P., Lipponen, J.A. et al. (2014). HRV – heart rate variability analysis software. *Comput. Methods Programs Biomed.* 113: 210–220.

16 Machida, N., Yasuda, J., and Too, K. (1989). Three cases of paroxysmal atrial fibrillation in the Thoroughbred newborn foal. *Equine Vet. J.* 21: 66–68.

17 Risberg, A.I., Slack, J., Semrad, S.D. et al. (2005). ECG of the month. Sinus rhythm with supraventricular premature complexes. *J. Am. Vet. Med. Assoc.* 226: 527–529.

18 Broux, B., De Clercq, D., Decloedt, A. et al. (2016). Atrial premature depolarization-induced changes in QRS and T wave morphology on resting electrocardiograms in horses. *J. Vet. Intern. Med.* 30: 1253–1259.

19 Sekarski, N., Meijboom, E.J., Di Bernardo, S. et al. (2014). Perinatal arrhythmias. *Eur. J. Pediatr.* 173: 983–996.

20 Potter, B.M., Scansen, B.A., Dunbar, L.K. et al. (2017). Transcutaneous direct current cardioversion in a foal with lone atrial fibrillation. *J. Vet. Cardiol.* 19: 99–105.

21 Collatos, C., Clark, E.S., Reef, V.B. et al. (1990). Septicemia, atrial fibrillation, cardiomegaly, left atrial mass, and *Rhodococcus equi* septic osteoarthritis in a foal. *J. Am. Vet. Med. Assoc.* 197: 1039–1042.

22 Peña-Cadahia, C., Manso-Díaz, G., Santiago-Llorente, I. et al. (2019). Accelerated idioventricular rhythm associated with isoflurane administration in a foal: a case report. *J. Equine Vet. Sci.* 80: 64–68.

23 Redpath, A. and Bowen, M. (2019). Cardiac therapeutics in horses. *Vet. Clin. North Am. Equine Pract.* 35: 217–241.

24 Mitchell, K.J. (2017). Practical considerations for diagnosis and treatment of ventricular tachycardia in horses. *Equine Vet. Educ.* 29: 670–676.

25 McMullen, S.L. (2016). Arrhythmias and cardiac bedside monitoring in the neonatal intensive care unit. *Crit. Care Nurs. Clin. North Am.* 28: 373–386.

26 Wren, C. (2006). Cardiac arrhythmias in the fetus and newborn. *Semin. Fetal Neonatal Med.* 11: 182–190.

27 Lyle-Dugas, J., Giguère, S., Mallicote, M.F. et al. (2017). Factors associated with outcome in 94 hospitalized foals diagnosed with neonatal encephalopathy. *Equine Vet. J.* 49: 207–210.

28 Toribio, R.E. (2019). Equine neonatal encephalopathy: facts, evidence, and opinions. *Vet. Clin. North Am. Equine Pract.* 35: 363–378.

29 Scansen, B.A. (2019). Equine congenital heart disease. *Vet. Clin. North Am. Equine Pract.* 35: 103–117.

30 Richardson, D.W. and Kohn, C.W. (1983). Uroperitoneum in the foal. *J. Am. Vet. Med. Assoc.* 182: 267–271.

31 Dunkel, B., Palmer, J.E., Olson, K.N. et al. (2005). Uroperitoneum in 32 foals: influence of intravenous fluid therapy, infection, and sepsis. *J. Vet. Intern. Med.* 19: 889–893.

32 Marolf, V., Mirra, A., Fouché, N. et al. (2018). Advanced atrio-ventricular blocks in a foal undergoing surgical bladder repair: first step to cardiac arrest? *Front. Vet. Sci.* 5: 96.

33 Fischer, B. and Clark-Price, S. (2015). Anesthesia of the equine neonate in health and disease. *Vet. Clin. North Am. Equine Pract.* 31: 567–585.

34 Nannarone, S., Vuerich, M., Moriconi, F. et al. (2016). Hot peritoneal lavage fluid as a possible cause of vasovagal reflex during two different surgeries for bladder repair in a foal. *J. Equine Vet. Sci.* 36: 5–9.

35 Haga, H.A., Risberg, Å., and Strand, E. (2011). Resuscitation of an anaesthetised foal with uroperitoneum and ventricular asystole. *Equine Vet. Educ.* 23: 502–507.

36 Eddy, V., Nunn, C., and Morris, J.A. (1997). Abdominal compartment syndrome. The Nashville Experience. *Surg. Clin. North Am.* 77: 801–812.

Section II Pathophysiology of Shock Syndromes in the Neonatal Foal

David Wong and Ryan Fries

A primary objective of the cardiovascular system is to ensure delivery of oxygen (DO_2) and other nutrients to the body and facilitate removal of carbon dioxide via the lungs. Through an intricate interplay between neuroendocrine pathways, the cardiovascular system is able to adapt to a number of physiologic demands and disease states to meet the body's oxygen and nutrient demands. Shock is a complex series of pathophysiologic events, resulting from a variety of clinical diseases in the neonatal foal, and represents a final common pathway of circulatory failure in which DO_2 is insufficient to meet the oxygen demand and normal metabolic processes of the body. At the cellular level, inadequate DO_2 results in a shift from aerobic to increased anaerobic metabolism, lactic acidosis, cellular injury/necrosis, and if left untreated, multiorgan failure and death [1]. The underpinning problem of all causes of shock is a decrease in effective blood flow and DO_2 to meet the needs of the tissues.

At a rudimentary level, DO_2 is dependent on cardiac output (CO), which is the product of heart rate (HR) and stroke volume (SV). Stroke volume is impacted by preload, afterload, myocardial contractility, and cardiac rhythm. Equally important to the delivery of oxygen to the tissues is the amount of oxygen contained in the blood. The majority of oxygen in arterial blood is associated with hemoglobin and is therefore dependent on the foal's hemoglobin concentration (Hb; normal value 1-day-old foal 12–16.6 g/dl) and degree of saturation of that hemoglobin with oxygen (SaO_2). Only a small portion of the arterial oxygen content (CaO_2) is comprised of oxygen dissolved in the blood itself ($P_aO_2 \times 0.003$). These variables are expressed as the formula: $DO_2 = CO \times CaO_2$. Other objective measures and approaches that evaluate DO_2 and oxygen consumption in the body are expressed by an assortment of formulas (Table 13.II.1), which provides an overview of the numerous variables that impact DO_2 in states of shock. Although the determination of CO has been explored by several methods in the neonatal foal, routine clinical assessment of CO is not common in the care of critically ill neonatal foals. Of note, assessment of blood pressure (BP) is more readily available in neonatal foals and is commonly monitored during shock states and critical illness [7]. Blood pressure is the lateral force that blood exerts on the blood vessel wall at a specific point within the vascular system and is calculated by the product of CO and systemic vascular resistance (SVR). The clinician must note, however, that blood pressure is not synonymous with blood flow and should not be mistaken for CO. Blood pressure is not a primary determinant of DO_2 but can serve as a sign of poor CO and thus DO_2.

As noted, DO_2 is dependent on blood flow to the tissues and C_aO_2. Blood flow at the tissue level is dependent on several interacting variables. The amount of blood arriving at the arterial side of a tissue is directly dependent on CO, but CO is not divided equally to all tissues. Instead, the amount of blood delivered to a particular tissue bed is regulated by the resistance to flow of that tissue; the resistance is altered by changes in smooth muscle contraction of the arterioles. The resistance at the arterioles also maintains the pressure gradient across the tissue capillary beds. If blood pressure were equal at the arterioles and venules, blood flow would cease [3]. The arteriolar tone thus balances between maintaining a pressure gradient across a tissue bed and not creating excessive resistance to flow. This is expressed via Ohm's law ($Q = P/R$) in which flow (Q) is related to pressure (P) divided by resistance (R); the clinician must be mindful of the fact that low pressure or high resistance will decrease blood flow. In shock states (and other diseases), the resistance over the entire systemic circulation (SVR) can be altered.

With this noted, a reduction in CO is detected by stretch receptors in the aorta and carotid arteries, which then transmit neural signals to the vasomotor center of the medulla oblongata (Figure 13.II.1). Once this signal is

Equine Neonatal Medicine, First Edition. Edited by David M. Wong and Pamela A. Wilkins.

Table 13.II.1 Various formulas and variables related to oxygen delivery in the neonatal foal.

Term	Abbreviation	Formula	Normal value healthy foal
O_2 content arterial blood	C_aO_2	(Hb [g/l] × 1.34 × S_aO_2 [%]) + (P_aO_2 × 0.003)	16.2 ± 0.4 ml O_2/dl (12–120 h old) [2] 15.8 ± 1.3 ml O_2/dl (30-46 h old) [3]
O_2 content central venous blood	$C_{cv}O_2$	(Hb [g/l] × 1.34 × $S_{cv}O_2$ [%]) + ($P_{cv}O_2$ × 0.003)	12.4 ± 0.4 ml O_2/dl [2]
Stroke volume	SV	CO (ml/min)/Heart rate	90.4 ± 5.7 ml (1 d old) [4] 107 ± 6.4 ml (1 d old) [3] 164.2 ± 25.9 ml (14 d old)
Cardiac output	CO	Heart rate × Stroke volume	8.03 ± 0.59 l/min (1 d old) [4] 15.88 ± 1.90 l/min (1 d old) [4]
Cardiac index	CI	CO (ml/min)/BW (kg)	155.3 ± 8.1 ml/kg/min (2 h old) [5] 80.5 ± 10.3 ml/kg/min (24 h old) [4] 222.1 ± 21.6 ml/kg/min (14 d old) [4]
O_2 saturation–arterial	S_aO_2	NA	95.0 ± 1.7% [2]
O_2 saturation–central venous	$S_{cv}O_2$	NA	74.5 ± 1.1% [2]
O_2 delivery	DO_2	CO × C_aO_2	31 ml O_2/kg/min[a]
O_2 consumption	VO_2	(C_aO_2 − C_vO_2) × CO	5.6 ml O_2/kg/min[a]
O_2 extraction	O_2E	C_aO_2 − C_vO_2	3.8 mmHg [2]
O_2 extraction ratio	O_2ER	C_aO_2 − C_vO_2/C_aO_2	21.3 ± 2.0% [2] 18.0 ± 0.02% [3]
Blood pressure	BP	CO × SVR	
Mean arterial pressure	MAP	Systolic BP + 2 × Diastolic BP/3	69–111 mmHg (MAP)
Systemic vascular resistance	SVR	(MAP − CVP) × 80/CO	708 ± 74 dynes/s/cm [6]
Blood flow	Q	Pressure/Resistance (P/R)	
Partial pressure of CO_2–central venous	$P_{cv}CO_2$	NA	44.6 ± 1.1 mmHg [2]
Central venous pressure	CVP	NA	2–9 mmHg [4]

Partial pressure of O_2 or CO_2	Age (h)	P_aO_2 (mmHg)	$P_{cv}O_2$ (mmHg)	P_aCO_2 (mmHg) [2]
	12	64.6 ± 11.6	40.0 ± 5.3	42.4 ± 2.9
	24	69.9 ± 6.6	40.9 ± 4.0	39.4 ± 2.9
	36	69.3 ± 12.3	40.4 ± 3.5	41.3 ± 4.0
	48	72.1 ± 7.7	40.9 ± 3.3	41.0 ± 3.0
	72	78.8 ± 8.8	40.1 ± 3.8	40.8 ± 2.8
	96	78.2 ± 7.9	39.9 ± 6.0	38.8 ± 2.9
	120	78.4 ± 5.9	39.8 ± 3.9	38.5 ± 2.4

[a] Calculated estimated value; intended as a guide only.

received, the sympathetic center is released and the parasympathetic system is suppressed. This, in turn, results in release of epinephrine and norepinephrine from the adrenal medulla, consequently increasing heart rate and contractility along with arterial and venous vasoconstriction. Other physiologic responses to hypotension, aimed at restoring intravascular volume and CO, include release of adrenocorticotropic hormone (ACTH) and vasopressin

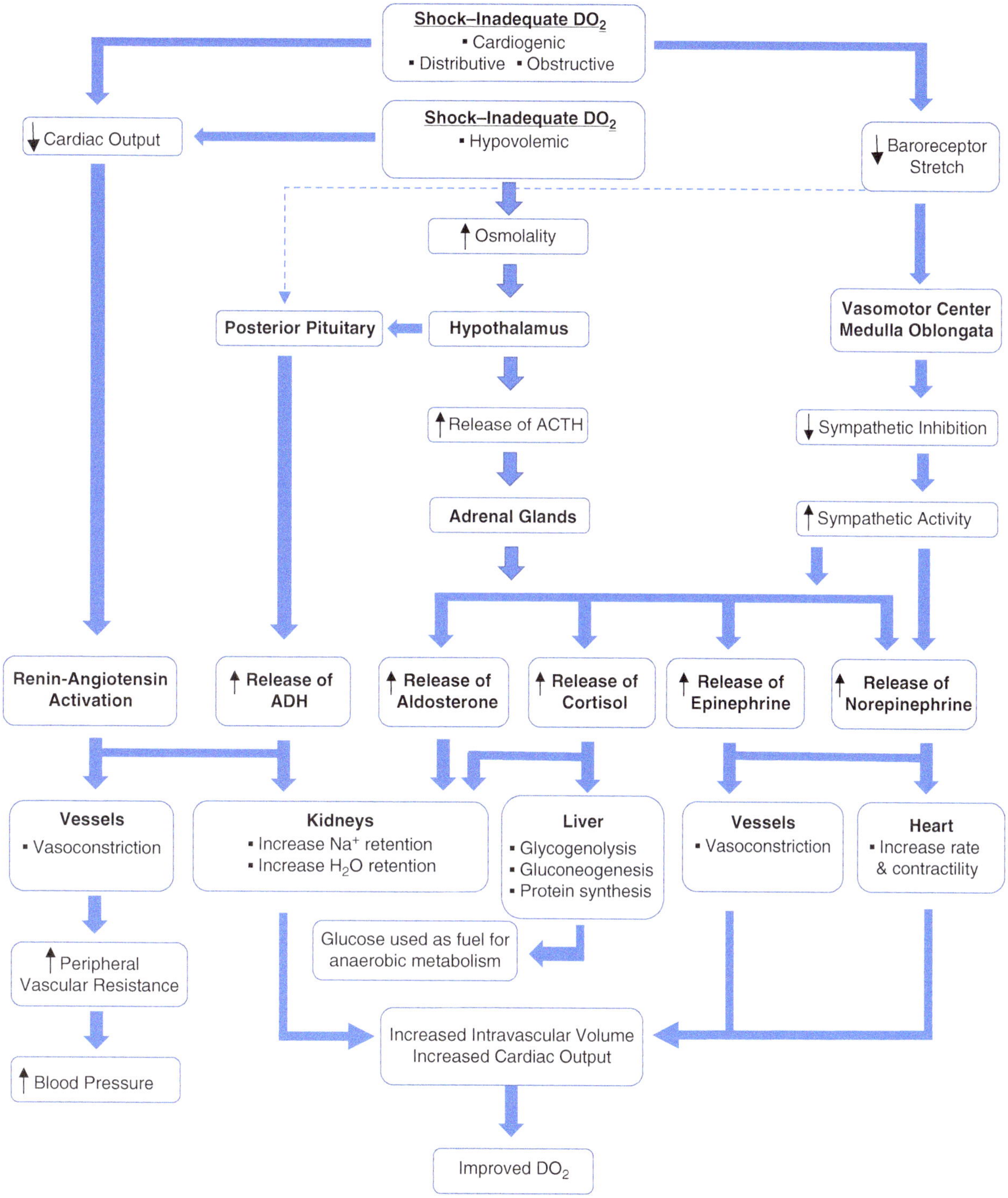

Figure 13.II.1 Overview of neuroendocrine response to shock.

from the anterior and posterior pituitary, respectively. ACTH stimulates release of cortisol from the adrenal gland, which consequently mobilizes substrates for energy production while vasopressin (also called antidiuretic hormone; ADH) promotes retention of water within the collecting ducts of the nephron, thereby contributing to increased intravascular fluid volume. Vasopressin also has potent vasoconstrictive effects to facilitate increased blood pressure [6, 8]. Another neuroendocrine response to decreased CO is the release of aldosterone from the adrenal medulla with the purpose of retaining sodium and water [6]. The goal of these physiologic responses is to reestablish and maintain adequate intravascular volume and blood flow to tissues (e.g. adequate DO_2).

Increases in vasopressin, ACTH, and cortisol have been measured in healthy-term foals in response to experimentally induced hypovolemia, suggesting that these neuroendocrine responses are functional at birth [9]. In addition, some of these hormone profiles have been investigated in foals with sepsis, which ostensibly is the most common cause of shock in the equine neonate. In one study involving 111 neonatal foals, septic foals (51 foals) had significantly higher vasopressin, ACTH, and cortisol concentrations when compared to healthy foals (31), and significantly higher vasopressin and ACTH concentrations when compared to sick, nonseptic foals (29) [10]. In addition, plasma vasopressin and ACTH concentrations were significantly higher in septic foals that died [10]. In another study, septic foals (74 foals) had higher angiotensin-II, aldosterone, cortisol, and ACTH concentrations when compared to healthy foals (34) and higher angiotensin-II and ACTH concentrations when compared to sick, nonseptic foals (59) [11]. Foals were not classified into groups such as severe sepsis or septic shock, but these studies provide evidence that the neuroendocrine response is active, and in many ill foals, hormone concentrations are elevated [6, 10–12].

Types of Shock

A variety of different systems have been used to classify shock, based on differences in pathogenesis and pathophysiology. At a rudimentary level, shock can be viewed via two types: (i) absolute hypovolemic shock in which a lower circulating blood volume is present for a given vascular capacitance (e.g. hemorrhage, diarrhea) or (ii) relative hypovolemic shock where there is expansion of vascular capacitance for a given blood volume (e.g. septic shock) [1]. A more specific system divides shock into four main categories, each of which is primarily related to a specific organ system: hypovolemic, distributive, cardiogenic, and obstructive (Table 13.II.2) [13–15]. Hypovolemic shock is associated with the blood and fluid compartments and is a common cause of shock in foals.

Table 13.II.2 Overview of types of shock [13].

Type of shock	Pathophysiology	General treatment strategy
Hypovolemic	Intravascular volume loss (four subcategories) • **Hemorrhagic shock** – acute hemorrhage without soft tissue injury • **Traumatic hemorrhagic shock** – acute hemorrhage with major soft tissue injury and release of immune system activators • **Hypovolemic shock** – critical reduction in circulating plasma volume without acute hemorrhage • **Traumatic hypovolemic shock** – critical reduction in circulating plasma volume without acute hemorrhage, due to soft tissue injury and release of immune system mediators	Fluid replacement with crystalloids
Distributive	Relative hypovolemia from pathologic redistribution of absolute intravascular volume (three subcategories) • **Septic** – endothelial dysfunction secondary to sepsis results in vasodilation and capillary leak syndrome • **Anaphylactic/anaphylactoid** – histamine mediated vasodilation and maldistribution of fluid from the intravascular to the extravascular space • **Neurogenic** – imbalance of sympathetic and parasympathetic regulation of cardiac action and vascular smooth muscle resulting in vasodilation and hypovolemia	Vasoconstrictors and fluid replacement
Cardiac	Inadequate function of the heart secondary to myocardial dysfunction, mechanical causes, or disorders of heart rhythm	Various, depending on underlying cause (drugs, surgery, interventional)
Obstructive	Elevated resistance caused by obstruction of the great vessels or heart itself	Various, depending on underlying cause

Hypovolemic shock can be further divided into four subcategories: **hemorrhagic**, **traumatic hemorrhagic**, **hypovolemic**, and **traumatic hypovolemic**. Bleeding is the hallmark of hemorrhagic and traumatic hemorrhagic shock with the difference between the two distinguished by the extent of soft tissue damage (e.g. traumatic hemorrhagic shock involves major soft tissue injury). Causes of hemorrhagic and traumatic hemorrhagic shock in neonatal foals are listed in Table 13.II.3, with more common scenarios including rib fractures acquired during parturition that lacerate the lung or heart, bleeding umbilical remnants, and blood loss secondary to cesarean section [16–18]. Shock is triggered by the critical drop in circulating blood volume, coupled with the massive loss of red blood cells, both contributing to tissue hypoxia [13]. Traumatic hemorrhagic shock does not occur commonly in neonatal foals, but might be seen with major soft tissue trauma (e.g. severe kick from adult horse) and results in post-acute inflammation that aggravates the shock state. At the microscopic level, leukocyte-endothelium interactions and disruption of the endothelial membrane-bound proteoglycans and glycosaminoglycans cause microvascular dysfunction (capillary leak syndrome) further contributing to shock [13]. Hypovolemic shock and traumatic hypovolemic shock are characterized by fluid loss without hemorrhage and arise from external or internal fluid losses paired with inadequate fluid intake. Traumatic hypovolemic shock is differentiated by the presence of trauma (e.g. large skin burns or lacerations), and is not a common occurrence in neonatal foals. Conversely, hypovolemic shock arising from diarrhea (primary intestinal infection, secondary to sepsis/endotoxemia), persistent gastrointestinal reflux, or third space sequestration of large quantities of fluid within the abdomen (uroperitoneum, peritonitis) or thorax (pleuropneumonia) can lead to reduction of circulating plasma volume in the foal [15].

Distributive shock (also called vasodilatory shock) is associated with the vascular system and is characterized by a state of relative hypovolemia that results from pathologic redistribution of the absolute intravascular volume [13, 19]. This redistribution arises from loss of regulation of vascular tone with volume being shifted within the vascular system and altered permeability of the vascular system with movement of the intravascular volume into the interstitium. There are three subcategories of distributive shock: septic, anaphylactic/anaphylactoid, and neurogenic [13]. Of these three types, septic (distributive) shock is one of the most common types of shock observed in equine neonates. The term *warm shock* is sometimes used with distributive shock because the vasodilation is coupled with increased CO resulting in the presence of transient blood distributed to the periphery leading to warm extremities [19, 20]. In contrast, cold shock can occur in the later phases of shock and is associated with reduction of myocardial contractility, vasoconstriction, decreased systemic blood flow, prolonged capillary refill time (CRT), increased vascular tone and cold extremities. Interestingly, some studies have documented that neonatal foals that did not have cold extremities on physical examination were more likely to survive when compared to those with cold limbs or ears (odds ratio 12.2) [10, 11]. Other terms describing phases of septic shock such as hyperdynamic and hypodynamic have also been used. These names are based on the hemodynamic pattern of decreased peripheral vascular resistance and increased CO in the hyperdynamic stage followed by loss of plasma volume, increased peripheral vascular resistance, and decreased CO resulting in cold extremities in the hypodynamic stage (e.g. cold shock) [21]. Regardless of nomenclature, septic shock is not only characterized by hypotension due to peripheral vasodilation, but also by a poor response to vasopressor therapy [22]. Sepsis is covered in detail in Chapter 50, with this chapter focusing briefly on the pathogenesis of distributive shock as it relates to sepsis.

The central pathophysiologic tenant of septic (distributive) shock involves endothelial dysfunction leading to dysregulation of vascular tone, reduced peripheral vascular resistance, increased capillary permeability and relative hypovolemia; these variables collectively contribute to reduced pre- and afterload, thus leading to decreased CO. [23] In all forms of distributive shock, plasma catecholamine concentrations are markedly elevated and the renin-angiotensin system is activated [22]. This implies that vasodilation is due to failure of vascular smooth

Table 13.II.3 Causes of Blood Loss in the foal [16].

Hemorrhage	Cesarean section
	Fractured ribs: hemothorax, soft tissue hematoma
	Bleeding from umbilical cord tear or umbilical remnant (external)
	Trauma: ruptured femoral artery, ruptured gastrocnemius tendon, thoracic injury
	Intra-abdominal hemorrhage: ruptured liver or spleen, internal umbilical remnant
	Gastrointestinal tract: bleeding gastric ulcer, hemorrhagic enterocolitis, coagulopathy
	Thrombocytopenia: alloimmune-mediated, immune-mediated, disseminated intravascular coagulopathy

muscle to constrict. Inflammatory mediators (histamine, serotonin, oxygen radicals, lysosomal enzymes) and nitric oxide are modulators of vasodilation and increased capillary permeability and contribute to hypotension and resistance to vasopressor drugs. Inflammatory cytokines such as tumor necrosis factor (TNF)-α, interleukin (IL)-1 and IL-6 increase the expression of the inducible form of nitric oxide synthase (iNOS) [22, 24]. These mediators also cause myocardial depression, further limiting CO and DO_2 [23]. In the initial stages of shock, vasopressin is released and causes vasoconstriction. As shock progresses and worsens, plasma vasopressin concentrations are exhausted. The lack of plasma vasopressin also contributes to vasodilation (Figure 13.II.2). Septic shock is therefore associated with a variety of underlying mechanisms, including endothelial dysfunction, hypovolemia, vasodilation, myocardial dysfunction, mitochondrial dysfunction, and potentially coagulopathies.

The other two causes of distributive shock, anaphylactic/anaphylactoid and neurogenic, occur infrequently in the neonatal foal. In brief, **anaphylactic shock** is associated with widespread histamine-mediated vasodilation, increased capillary permeability, maldistribution of fluid volume, and a shift of fluid from the intravascular to extravascular space. In turn, this results in severe hypotension and cardiovascular collapse [20]. Anaphylaxis is caused by an acute IgE-dependent hypersensitivity reaction regulated by mast cells releasing histamine, proteases, platelet-activating factor, leukotrienes, and other mediators [20]. In comparison, anaphylactoid shock is caused by physical, chemical, or osmotic hypersensitivity reactions that are not IgE-dependent; mediators are released from mast cells and basophilic granulocytes independent of antigen–antibody reaction [15]. Transfusions of blood products (fresh frozen plasma, fresh plasma, whole blood) could potentially result in anaphylactic reactions in neonatal foals, but the incidence is low [25].

Neurogenic shock results from an imbalance between sympathetic and parasympathetic regulation of cardiac function and vascular smooth muscle and is associated with vasodilation with relative hypovolemia (blood volume unchanged). This imbalance produces a lack of vascular tone and can result from three pathophysiologic subsets: (i) direct injury to centers for circulatory regulation as a result of compression (brainstem trauma), ischemia or drugs; (ii) altered afferents to the circulatory center in the medulla oblongata as a response to fear, stress, pain or dysregulated vagal reflexes; or (iii) interruption of descending connections from the bulbar regulatory centers to the spinal cord (trauma to thoracic spine) [13, 20]. A sudden drop in blood pressure and bradycardia (caused by unopposed vagal stimulation in the setting of sympathetic denervation) along with obtunded consciousness can be seen with neurogenic shock [13, 15]. Neurogenic shock is not commonly recognized in the neonatal foal but might be seen with trauma or ischemia to the nervous system.

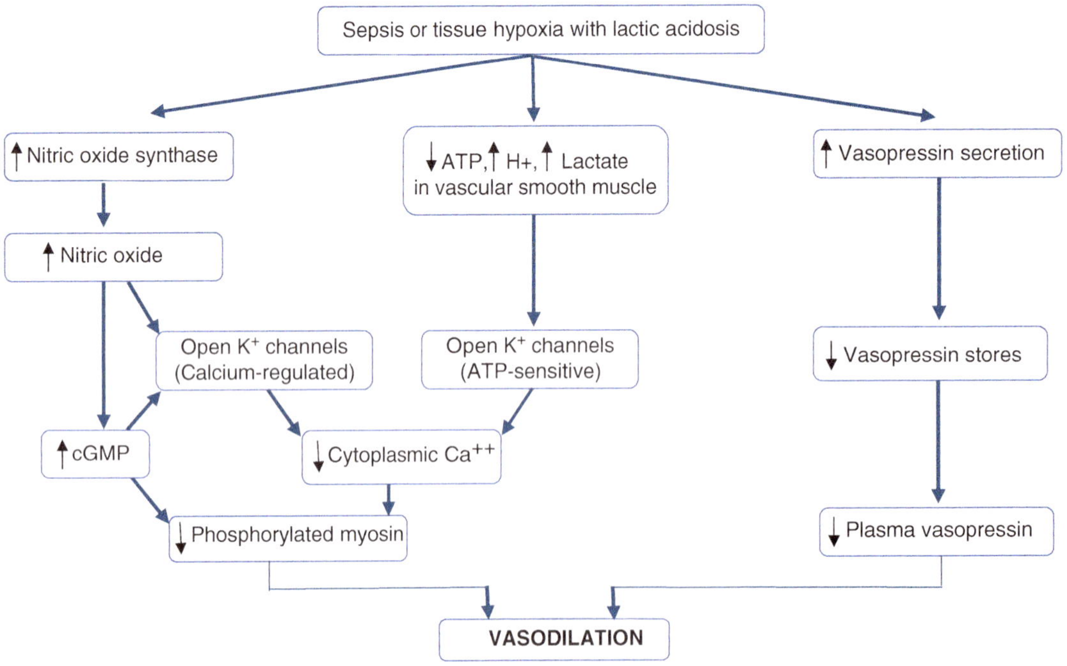

Figure 13.II.2 Mechanisms of vasodilatory shock. Septic shock and states of prolonged shock that result in tissue hypoxia with lactic acidosis increase nitric oxide synthesis, activate ATP-sensitive and calcium-regulated potassium channels in vascular smooth muscle, and lead to depletion of vasopressin. cGMP-cyclic guanosine monophosphate [22].

Cardiogenic shock occurs when cardiac dysfunction results in inadequate CO and insufficient DO_2 to tissues, thereby resulting in inability of the heart to meet resting tissue metabolic demands [26]. Cardiac dysfunction can be due to myocardial, mechanical, or rhythm disorders. Direct myocardial cell injury secondary to peripartum asphyxia or mediators and cytokines released during sepsis are potential causes of cardiac injury in neonatal foals; this situation may or may not result in cardiogenic shock. In one study, septic foals had significantly higher elevations in cardiac troponin (cTnT) and cardiac isoenzyme of creatine kinase (CKMB) compared to healthy foals, but no difference in these cardiac biomarkers was noted between survivors and nonsurvivors in the septic group [27]. Acute fulminant forms of nutritional muscular dystrophy (white muscle disease) are another potential cause of cardiogenic shock in the neonatal foal [28]. Other possible etiologies that could result in cardiogenic shock include primary and secondary cardiomyopathic conditions, pericardial tamponade, myocardial toxins (monensin), and drugs that depress myocardial function (general anesthetics, β-adrenergic blockers) [29]. Congestive heart failure, ischemic injury and necrosis, or metabolic derangement may progress to cardiogenic shock and without therapy; deterioration is inevitable. Clinically, hypotension refractory to volume resuscitation is observed with features of end-organ hypoperfusion requiring pharmacological intervention. Definitions of cardiogenic shock in people include systolic blood pressure <90 mmHg for ≥30 minutes despite adequate volume along with clinical evidence of hypoperfusion (cold extremities, and oliguria) [30–32]. Clinical definitions are less commonly used in equine medicine.

Intravascular volume, which regulates mean circulatory pressures and venous return to the heart is intimately associated with cardiac performance. Decreases in intravascular volume limit venous return to the heart as well as SV and CO. These low-flow states resulting from hypovolemia or cardiac tamponade may have hemodynamic profiles similar to cardiogenic shock with an important exception: the latter has elevated ventricular filling pressures [33]. Therefore, these conditions should not be considered primary cardiogenic shock, but may play a role in the overall assessment of a patient. The heart is the most important component at maintaining CO, determined by heart rate, contractility, and loading conditions.

Abnormalities in rhythm and heart rate may limit CO. Arrythmias such as wandering pacemaker, supraventricular premature complexes, atrial fibrillation, and ventricular premature complexes were not uncommon during the first few hours of the newborn foal but are typically transient and not associated with cardiogenic shock [34]. A low heart rate may limit CO, whereas an increased heart rate can compromise stroke volumes by limiting ventricular filling times. Bradyarrhythmias may indicate structural abnormalities, effects of drugs, hypoxia, or other metabolic stimuli. These types of arrhythmias can represent reflex-mediated responses, as occurs in cases of severe hemorrhagic shock. Tachyarrhythmias may be due to underlying cardiac disease and pharmacologic or environmental stimuli. Alternatively, increases in the heart rate may reflect compensatory responses to maintain CO. Impaired cardiac contractility decreases effective ventricular ejection and compromises SV; abnormalities in valvular function or intracardiac shunts may also limit CO. Finally, the resistance circuit consists of the arteriolar bed, where the major decreases in vascular resistance occur. Arteriolar tone plays an important role in ventricular loading conditions, arterial pressure, and distribution of systemic blood flow. Excessive decreases in arteriolar tone lead to hypotension and limit effective organ perfusion, whereas excessive increases in arteriolar tone impede cardiac ejection by increasing ventricular afterload. Figure 13.II.3 presents potential hemodynamic presentations of cardiogenic shock.

Obstructive shock is not common in neonatal foals, but can arise from blockage of the circulation, including the great vessels or heart itself, resulting in rapid drop in CO and blood pressure [13]. Obstructive shock is characterized by decreased preload and increased afterload and may appear similar to cardiogenic shock but must be distinguished from

		Volume Status	
		Wet	Dry
Peripheral Circulation	Cold	Classic cardiogenic shock (↓CI, ↑SVRI, ↑PCWP)	Euvolemic cardiogenic shock (↓CI, ↑SVRI, ↑PCWP)
	Warm	Vasodilatory cardiogenic shock or mixed shock (↓CI, ↓SVRI, ↑PCWP)	Vasodilatory shock (Not cardiogenic shock) (↑CI, ↓SVRI, ↓PCWP)

CI, cardiac index; PCWP, pulmonary capillary wedge pressure; SVRI, systemic vascular resistance index

Figure 13.II.3 Potential hemodynamic presentations of cardiogenic shock.

each other as the treatments between the two are quite different. Causes of obstructive shock include conditions such as: vena cava compression, tension pneumothorax, pericardial tamponade (impairs diastolic filling and reduced cardiac preload), pulmonary artery embolism, mediastinal mass (increases right-ventricular afterload and reduces left ventricular preload), aortic valve stenosis (increases left ventricular afterload), and thrombosis (atrial or pulmonary) [13]. Although not common, fibrinous pericarditis and pericardial effusion have been reported in neonatal foals and are associated with sepsis and the systemic inflammatory response. In one report, three foals with pericarditis and pericardial effusion had evidence of impairment of cardiac function, as evidenced by tachycardia, tachypnea, and reduced ventricular fractional shortening; two of three foals recovered with pericardiocentesis and medical therapy [35].

In summary, hypovolemic, cardiogenic, and obstructive shock are characterized by low cardiac output and inadequate oxygen transport, whereas in distributive shock, the main deficit lies in the periphery with decreased SVR and altered oxygen extraction. In distributive shock, CO is typically high, but can be low due to associated myocardial depression. Clinically, foals with acute circulatory shock often have a combination of mechanisms contributing to inadequate DO_2 (e.g. foal with distributive shock from sepsis may also have hypovolemia and cardiogenic components from myocardial depression) [36].

Clinical Signs and Stages of Shock

Different schemas have been used to describe phases of shock. A common method of categorizing the progression of shock is compensatory, early decompensatory, and decompensatory (terminal) stages (Tables 13.II.4 and 13.II.5) [20]. The compensatory stage of shock involves baroreceptor mediated release of catecholamines that increase heart rate, SVR, and cardiac contractility to enhance CO [38]. During this stage, activation of the sympathetic nervous system redistributes blood flow to vital organs (brain, heart) and diverts blood away from lower-priority organs (skin, lungs, kidneys, gastrointestinal tract) [38]. In addition, neurohormonal responses (described above) help restore blood volume and pressure (Figure 13.II.1).

With intravascular volume depletion and decreased blood pressure, coupled with decreased renal blood flow, the juxtaglomerular cells in the afferent arteriole in the kidney are stimulated to release renin into the blood. Renin is an enzyme that converts angiotensinogen (produced by liver) to angiotensin I in the plasma [23]. Angiotensin I has mild vasoconstrictive properties; however potent vasoconstrictive properties are associated with angiotensin II, which is converted from angiotensin I in the lungs via angiotensin converting enzyme (ACE). Their vasoconstrictive effects on arterioles increase the peripheral vascular resistance, thereby raising arterial blood pressure. Angiotensin

Table 13.II.4 Clinical stages and associated signs of shock [37].

Clinical stage of shock	Characteristics	Clinical signs
Compensatory	• Increased CO, heart rate and SVR • Neurohormonal response Release of catecholamines, ADH, vasopressin, cortisol • Increased energy demands (hypermetabolic) • Hyperdynamic state	• Normal mentation • Normal blood pressure • Increase in heart and respiratory rate • Hyperemic mucous membranes • CRT <1 s
Early decompensatory	• Redistribution of blood flow to heart and brain • Oxygen consumption dependent on DO_2 • Hyperlactatemia • Varying degrees of tissue hypoxia • Compromise of organ integrity and function Intestine – bacterial translocation Kidney – tubular damage Liver – impaired function	• Depressed mentation • Hypotension • Decreased pulse pressure • Tachycardia • Tachypnea • Pale MM, CRT prolonged • Decreased urine output • Cold extremities
Decompensatory (Terminal)	• Widespread cellular necrosis and multi-organ failure • Sympathetic center lost • Inotropic response lost • Chronotropic response lost	• Obtunded mentation • Bradycardia, despite low CO • Hypotension

CO, cardiac output; SVR, systemic vascular resistance; ADH, antidiuretic hormone; CRT, capillary refill time; MM, mucous membranes; DO_2, oxygen delivery.

Table 13.II.5 Clinical stages of shock [14].

Type of shock	Capillary flow	Cardiac output	Arterial/ arteriolar constriction	Venous/ venular capacity	Ventricular volume	Example
Hypovolemic	↓	↓	↑	↓	↓	Blood or fluid loss
Distributive						
Low resistance	↓	↑	↓	—	↑ —	Early sepsis, spinal shock
High resistance	↓	↓	↑	↑	—	Late sepsis
Cardiogenic	↓	↓	↑	↓↑	↑	
Obstructive	↓	↓	↑	↑—	↓	Pericardial tamponade

also acts directly on the kidneys to cause sodium and water retention. Additionally, angiotensin causes aldosterone to be released from the renal cortex, which subsequently acts on renal tubules to promote further sodium retention and potassium excretion in the urine [23]. With increased sodium, the serum osmolality rises and stimulates osmoreceptors in the hypothalamus; consequently, this signals the posterior pituitary gland to release ADH resulting in renal water retention. In addition to the renin-aldosterone-ADH mechanism, sympathetic activation stimulates catecholamine release from the adrenal medulla and the anterior pituitary gland releases ACTH, which increases production of glucocorticoids such as cortisol; these hormones increase metabolic processes and raise the blood glucose concentration [38]. As blood flow is diverted away from the lungs, pulmonary blood flow is decreased, creating physiologic dead space and ventilation-perfusion mismatch [38]. This may result in hypoxemia and trigger increased rate (clinically represented by tachypnea) and depth of ventilation, resulting in decreased P_aCO_2. The compensatory stage is able to maintain CO in mild to moderate cases of shock for a period of time but requires a hypermetabolic state in which oxygen and energy substrates are consumed at a higher rate. The compensatory phase can be difficult to detect initially as vital parameters can be normal while subtle pathophysiologic disturbances exist [1]. As the early stages of shock progress, nonspecific changes such as tachycardia and tachypnea may be observed in the compensatory phase along with clinicopathologic changes such as hyperglycemia, hypernatremia, hypoxemia, and hypocapnia. A variety of markers have been investigated to aid in detection of the early stages of shock in people, including central venous pressure (CVP), pulmonary capillary wedge pressure (PCWP), base deficit, and lactate and oxygen extraction ratio, but a reliable method remains to be documented [1]. Other blood perfusion parameters targeting nonvital organs (viscera) such as gastric mucosal pH, sublingual capnography, tissue hemoglobin oxygen saturation (S_tO_2) and transcutaneous carbon dioxide and oxygen tensions hold some promise but remain unproven [1]. Contributing to the difficulty in detecting early stages of shock is the variability in an individual patient's compensatory response. When these compensatory mechanisms become exhausted at the cellular level and/or the clinical condition worsens, these responses are unable to restore perfusion and DO_2 and shock progresses.

As CO decreases and autoregulation of blood pressure is lost, a rapid progression from compensatory to decompensatory shock can occur. Left undetected and/or untreated, the intravascular volume remains inadequate, energy stores become depleted, SVR decreases, and cardiac dysfunction occurs, leading into the decompensatory stage. During the early decompensatory stage of shock, redistribution of blood flow is still directed to the brain and heart, but DO_2 and oxygen consumption to other individual tissues is dependent on the amount of blood flow, with anaerobic metabolism, hyperlactatemia, and tissue hypoxia commonly occurring. The metabolic response in nonvital organs to decreased DO_2 varies, depending on the capacity of an organ to autoregulate its blood flow, its basal metabolic demands and ischemic tolerance of its cell populations [39]. The brain and heart have high energy demands and poor ischemic tolerance, but both organs have efficient autoregulatory capacity in low-flow states [39]. In contrast, skeletal muscle is deprived of a considerable amount of blood flow as part of the compensatory response to hypovolemia, but it is resistant to tissue ischemia because of large intracellular glycogen and high energy phosphate stores [39]. Other organs such as the liver, kidneys, and intestines are more severely impacted by shock states due to their low energy reserves and high metabolic needs. Decreased CO and DO_2 to the intestines can result in slowed motility and compromise of the integrity of the intestine resulting in translocation of intraluminal bacteria into the blood stream, while limited perfusion to the kidneys can result in damage to the nephron (tubular necrosis), oliguria, and potentially acute kidney injury. Because the liver is involved in multiple physiologic functions, decreased DO_2 can result in hepatocellular failure and abnormal function impacting metabolism of drugs and hormones, conjugation of bilirubin, filtration of bacteria from the viscera, and metabolism of waste products such as ammonia and lactic acid [38]. Within the lungs, ventilation-perfusion mismatch worsens, alveolar cells become ischemic, surfactant production is reduced (resulting in atelectasis), and pulmonary capillary permeability increases (resulting in pulmonary edema).

If shock progresses without intervention, prolonged tissue hypoxia and vasodilation occurs in all organs, resulting in complete circulatory collapse and multiorgan failure. Widespread cellular necrosis is present, the sympathetic center of the brain is nonfunctional, and there is a loss of chronotropic and inotropic responses. This is the final stage of all types of shock and is referred to as decompensatory (terminal) shock.

The clinician should be cognizant that shock develops over time and that early recognition favors survival. With this in mind, a diagnosis of shock is based on clinical, hemodynamic, and biochemical signs that can be broadly summarized into three components: (i) presence of systemic arterial hypotension (magnitude of hypotension may only be moderate); (ii) presence of clinical signs of tissue hypoperfusion such as cold extremities, decreased urine output, and altered mentation (obtundation, disorientation); and (iii) presence of hyperlactatemia, indicating abnormal cellular metabolism [36].

Treatment and Monitoring of Shock

The treatment of shock can be viewed in four general phases with therapeutic goals and monitoring adapted to each phase and underlying cause(s) [36]. The first (salvage) phase involves rescue therapy to achieve a minimum blood pressure and CO compatible with immediate survival. Interventions such as gaining immediate intravascular access, provision of IV fluids to augment vascular volume, and global assessment of the patient (physical exam, blood lactate, CBC, serum chemistry profile) are initiated; antimicrobial administration for sepsis and/or control of hemorrhage from the umbilicus are examples of actions taken to combat the underlying cause of shock [36]. The goal of the second (optimization) phase is to increase cellular oxygen availability and provide adequate hemodynamic stability; this phase is facilitated by measurements of CO, mixed venous (or central venous) oxygen saturation, and/or serial blood lactate levels as guides. The third (stabilization) phase's objective is to identify and stabilize organ systems involved and to prevent further organ dysfunction. The final (de-escalation) phase encompassing weaning of the foal from therapy (e.g. vasoactive agents, oxygen supplementation) and continued monitoring [36]. More specific therapy and monitoring strategies are described below (Table 13.II.6).

Early and adequate restoration of vascular volume and hemodynamic support in foals with shock is critical to avoid worsening organ dysfunction and failure. A large-bore (14- or 16-gauge) jugular catheter should be placed and fluid resuscitation should commence, even while investigation of the underlying cause is ongoing. Ideally an over-the-wire catheter that is long enough to allow for estimation of CVP in addition to administration of fluid therapy and other medications is placed. Once identified, the cause of shock should be directly addressed (e.g., control of bleeding, administration of antimicrobials and source control for sepsis, slow drainage of uroperitoneum). IV fluid therapy is warranted to improve microvascular blood flow and increase CO. A standard protocol in fluid resuscitation of foals is to administer 20 ml/kg isotonic crystalloid fluid boluses, IV (1 l to 50 kg foal) over 15–20 minutes with subsequent re-evaluation of clinical parameters after each bolus [40]. If after three to four repeated boluses (60–80 ml/kg total) of crystalloids fails to improve hemodynamic status, vasopressors should be considered. Of note, some clinicians challenge the rationale for vasopressor administration based on the fact that β and α-1 adrenergic inotropes increase myocardial and systemic oxygen requirements and possibly increase the severity of ischemic injury in settings of perfusion failure [14]. However, the clinician may not have other therapeutic alternatives. Vasoactive agents are discussed in Chapter 11, but norepinephrine is a first-choice agent in human critical care [36]. Adequate volume resuscitation is the single most important treatment of all types of shock with the exception of cardiogenic shock, in which case fluid therapy should be judiciously employed in light of the underlying cause of cardiogenic shock.

Differences exist between the adult and fetus/neonate in response to isotonic fluid loading. In adults, between 20% and 85% of an isotonic fluid load (dependent partially on state of hypovolemia and dehydration) is retained in the intravascular space 30–60 minutes after infusion [40, 41]. In the fetus, only 6–7% is retained in the vascular space [40]. Poor intravascular retention is due to a high capillary filtration coefficient (allows rapid fluid movement across capillaries) and a large interstitial-to-vascular compliance ratio (allows more extensive fluid movements without resistance) [40]. A neonate is in a transitional phase between fetal and adult fluid dynamics and likely has intravascular fluid retention dynamics between these two extremes. Despite the rapid movement of administered isotonic fluids out of the intravascular space, controversy remains

Table 13.II.6 Overview of treatment and monitoring of shock.

Treatment	
Restoration of intravascular volume/delivery of blood to tissues	
• Volume resuscitation	
• Crystalloids	20 ml/kg, IV boluses over 15–20 minutes; repeat boluses up to a total infusion volume up 60–80 ml/kg
• Colloids	Benefit over crystalloid fluids uncertain; associated with coagulopathies and renal injury in other species
• Plasma	Use if serum IgG <800 mg/dl to support immune system
• Blood	Use if moderate to severe hemorrhage
Support the pump (i.e. heart)	
Vasoactive medications	
• Inopressors	Consider if hemodynamic status does not improve with fluid boluses; First-line choices include:
	Norepinephrine
	Dobutamine
Augmentation of oxygen	
• Mechanical ventilation	Chapter 6
• Oxygen supplementation	Oxygen values in 9 healthy foals using uni- and bi-lateral nasal cannula at various flow rates [2]

		Unilateral nasal canula (ml/kg/min)				Bilateral nasal canula (ml/kg/min)			
Parameter	**Baseline**	**50**	**100**	**150**	**200**	**50**	**100**	**150**	**200**
F_iO_2 (%)	18.0 ± 0.7	23.0 ± 1.4	30.9 ± 2.1	44.2 ± 5.8	52.6 ± 8.3	30.9 ± 2.6	48.7 ± 6.2	56.4 ± 3.4	74.6 ± 4.2
P_aO_2 (mmHg)	92.5 ± 8	135.9 ± 13	175.2 ± 15	219.6 ± 32	269.7 ± 41	174.3 ± 27	261.2 ± 38	307.8 ± 41	374.2 ± 58
P_aCO_2 (mmHg)	47.7 ± 2.8	49.7 ± 2.4	50.5 ± 2.3	50.1 ± 2.8	51.3 ± 3.1	49.8 ± 1.8	51.0 ± 2.2	49.8 ± 2.9	48.6 ± 3.6
S_aO_2 (%)	96.7 ± 0.7	98.5 ± 0.3	99.2 ± 0.1	99.4 ± 0.2	99.6 ± 0.1	99.1 ± 0.3	99.6 ± 0.1	99.7 ± 0.1	99.8 ± 0.1

Address underlying cause of shock	
Antimicrobials	Broad-spectrum antimicrobials in suspected or confirmed sepsis; de-escalate to specific antimicrobials based on blood culture and susceptibility patterns
Antiarrhythmics	Treat according to primary arrythmia
Control hemorrhage	
Adjunctive therapy	
Glucocorticoids	
Analgesics	

Monitoring
General parameters
Vital parameters (heart rate, respiratory rate, rectal temperature)
Serum biochemistry profile (organ function, electrolyte status)
Oxygen delivery and metabolism
Lactate
Pulse oximetry
Central venous oxygen saturation
Arterial blood gas analysis
Assessment of vascular volume
Packed cell volume/total protein
Central venous pressure
Arterial blood pressure
Urine output

regarding the use of crystalloids versus colloids in shock, with no consistent evidence to support one type of fluid over another [14, 15]. As much as 75–80% of infused volume of colloid remains in the vascular space which maintains osmotic pressure (thereby promoting water retention in the vascular space) and increases CO for up to 2 hours but studies in people have not demonstrated a survival benefit between the two types of fluids [15]. Moreover, synthetic colloids have been associated acute kidney injury and coagulopathies [42]. Resuscitation with crystalloids requires more volume as compared to colloids to achieve the same clinical endpoints but are cheaper and more readily available. Thus, crystalloids remain a first-line fluid for initial resuscitation. Blood transfusions should not be used for volume expansion but rather, used if moderate to severe hemorrhage is present as hemoglobin is the main carrier of oxygen, as compared to the amount of oxygen dissolved in blood [15].

Restoration of a mean arterial pressure (MAP) of 65–70 mmHg is an initial goal in people in shock, and can be extrapolated to foals [15, 43]. This target MAP is only a guide and should be evaluated in conjunction with mental status, peripheral perfusion, and urine output in the foal. Tissue hypoperfusion may be present despite normal blood pressure values as blood flow is redirected toward more vital organs. Conversely, hypotension may exist without evidence of organ hypoperfusion. In some vasodilated states, increases in CO maintain vital organ blood flow despite decreased levels of arterial pressure. Pulmonary artery wedge pressure (PAWP) and CVP are indirect measures of ventricular preload but correlate poorly with blood volume, end-diastolic volumes, and fluid responsiveness. CVP is an easier measurement to collect, compared to PAWP, and is an estimate of right atrial pressure and cardiac preload (normal CVP 2–9 mmHg in neonatal foal) and has been used to guide fluid therapy [43]. Normalization of CVP may reflect successful fluid volume resuscitation, whereas elevations in CVP may indicate volume overload. As with measurements of arterial blood pressure, the trend in CVP seen through repeated monitoring is most informative.

Mixed venous oxygen saturation (S_vO_2) can be helpful in assessing the balance between oxygen supply and demand for the entire body but requires placement of a pulmonary artery catheter [36]. In light of this, central venous oxygen saturation ($S_{CV}O_2$), which reflects oxygen saturation from the cranial half of the body, is a more clinically applicable tool to monitor the balance between oxygen delivery and consumption by tissues. In health, $S_{cv}O_2$ is slightly lower than S_vO_2. Decreases in $S_{CV}O_2$ may reflect decreased respiratory function, decreased CO and tissue perfusion, or increased oxygen demand. In goal-directed therapy protocols used in people, normalization of $S_{CV}O_2$ ($S_{cv}O_2 \geq 70\%$) serves as a therapeutic target with one study demonstrating decreased mortality in human patients with septic shock [43]. Values for $S_{CV}O_2$ in healthy foals have been documented (mean $S_{CV}O_2$ 74.5%; Table 13.II.1) but $S_{CV}O_2$ has not been evaluated in critically ill foals, nor has targeted goal-directed therapy using $S_{cv}O_2$.

Evaluation of the foal's blood count, serum IgG concentration and serum biochemistry profile provide information on immune status, electrolyte derangements and organ dysfunction. Assessment of the blood lactate and arterial blood gas analysis provides further information on global oxygen metabolism in the foal. Increased blood lactate levels in low-flow states suggest tissue hypoxia and anaerobic metabolism. With distributive (septic) shock, the pathophysiology of hyperlactatemia is more complex and may involve increased glycolysis, inhibition of pyruvate dehydrogenase along with increased anaerobic metabolism. In all cases, impaired clearance of lactate due to diminished liver function contributes to hyperlactatemia. Blood lactate concentrations in ill neonatal foals has been extensively evaluated. Regardless of final diagnosis, foals with elevated admission blood lactate concentration and/or foals in which lactate does not decrease to within normal reference intervals during the first few days of hospitalization are less likely to survive [44–46]. In a large multi-institutional study of 643 neonatal foals, the mean admission blood lactate was 3.6 mmol/l in foals that survived as compared to 5.5 mmol/l in non-survivors [44, 45]. Only 31% of these foals were categorized as septic, and even fewer were likely in a state of septic shock; however, blood lactate provides the clinician feedback on the global oxygen status of the ill foal.

In the care of people in shock, an arterial catheter is frequently placed to monitor arterial blood pressure and provide an access point for blood sampling. Direct blood pressure trends should be monitored if possible in foals, as opposed to individual readings, combined with other indicators of perfusion to guide therapy. Direct arterial blood pressure measurements are not always feasible in neonatal foals, but if used, the dorsal metatarsal artery is ideal for catheter insertion. Alternatively, indirect measurement of blood pressure (oscillometric) can be used with the realization of the limitations of this technique, such as the fact that vasoconstriction related to compensatory mechanisms that maintain arterial pressure and the use of pharmacologic agents limits the accuracy of noninvasive measurements. Studies in neonatal foals have confirmed that oscillometric measurements of blood pressure provides acceptable MAP measurements when oscillometric cuffs are placed over the coccygeal or dorsal metatarsal arteries [7, 47]. However, blood pressure does not always equate to CO (depends on the cardiovascular status). In one study in neonatal foals, moderate correlation ($r = 0.77$) was noted between MAP and cardiac index in anesthetized foals, but administration of phenylephrine (resulting in vasoconstriction) decreased the correlation substantially [7]. Therefore, the clinician should be aware that arterial pressure can be a poor indicator of blood flow when vascular resistance is altered, such as might occur in states of shock. Urine production should also be monitored, as it is considered a reflection of renal blood flow and hence CO and serves as an indication of adequate organ and tissue perfusion. Urine output in healthy neonatal foals is approximately 6 ml/kg/h (148 ml/kg/d), but this value may be irrelevant in foals receiving IV fluid therapy [3].

Another treatment strategy to bolster DO_2 is administration of humidified oxygen using uni- or bilateral intranasal cannulas. In one study, maximum flow rates of 200 ml/kg/min increased the mean P_aO_2 to 374 mmHg and F_iO_2 to 74.6 in nine healthy neonatal foals [2]. The use of mechanical ventilation is much more commonly utilized in people in shock [36]; mechanical ventilation in foals is more difficult to achieve due to equipment needs, nursing staff, and expertise necessary to effectively implement.

Identifying and treating the underlying etiology of shock is critical in the treatment of shock. The most common causes of shock in foals are hypovolemic and septic shock. Hypovolemic shock in the neonatal foal is commonly associated with severe enterocolitis, which can have multiple causes that result in substantial fluid losses. Diarrhea/enterocolitis can also be associated with progressive weakness and decreased consumption of milk by the foal. Fluid losses and decreased DO_2 can alter electrolyte and acid–base status (increased lactate, metabolic acidemia), resulting in further deterioration of clinical condition. Left untreated, this downward spiral can lead to decompensatory shock. Sepsis is another common cause of shock in the neonatal foal with a complex pathophysiology, ultimately resulting in shock in some cases. Directed therapy of cardiogenic (e.g. pericardiocentesis of cardiac tamponade) or obstructive (e.g. correction of tension pneumothorax) shock, although rare in foals, should occur rapidly, once identified.

In conclusion, shock is a manifestation of inadequate DO_2 to meet tissue demands and has multiple underlying etiologies. It is not an uncommon occurrence in the care of neonatal foals and is most successfully treated with early recognition, aggressive treatment, and careful monitoring.

References

1 Suresh, M.R., Chung, K.K., Schiller, A.M. et al. (2019). Unmasking the hypovolemic shock continuum: the compensatory reserve. *J. Intensive Care Med.* 34: 696–706.

2 Wong, D.M., Hepworth-Warren, K.L., Sponseller, B.T. et al. (2017). Measured and calculated variables of global oxygenation in healthy neonatal foals. *Am. J. Vet. Res.* 78: 230–238.

3 Corley, K.T.T. (2003). Monitoring and treating haemodynamic disturbances in critically ill neonatal foals. Part 1: Haemodynamic monitoring. *Equine Vet. Educ.* 6: 68–77.

4 Thomas, W.P., Madigan, J.E., Backus, K.Q. et al. (1987). Systemic and pulmonary haemodynamics in normal neonatal foals. *J. Reprod. Fertil. Suppl.* 35: 623–628.

5 Shih, A. (2013). Cardiac output monitoring in horses. *Vet. Clin. Equine* 29: 155–167.

6 Hollis, A.R., Boston, R.C., and Corley, K.T.T. (2008). Plasma aldosterone, vasopressin and atrial natriuretic peptide in hypovolaemia: a preliminary comparative study of neonatal and mature horses. *Equine Vet. J.* 40: 64–69.

7 Giguere, S., Knowles, H.A., Valverde, A. et al. (2005). Accuracy of indirect measurement of blood pressure in neonatal foals. *J. Vet. Intern. Med.* 19: 571–576.

8 Demiselle, J., Fage, N., Radermacher, P. et al. (2020). Vasopressin and its analogues in shock states: a review. *Ann. Intensive Care* 10: 9.

9 O'connor, S.J., Gardner, O.J.C. et al. (2005). Development of baroreflex and endocrine responses to hypotensive stress in newborn foals and lambs. *Pflugers Arch.* 450: 298–306.

10 Hucombe, S.D.A., Toribio, R.E., Slovis, N. et al. (2008). Blood arginine vasopressin, adrenocorticotropin hormone, and cortisol concentrations at admission in septic and critically ill foals and their association with survival. *J. Vet. Intern. Med.* 22: 639–647.

11 Dembeck, K.A., Onasch, K., Hurcombe, S.D.A. et al. (2013). Renin-angiotensin-aldosterone system and hypothalamic-pituitary-adrenal axis in hospitalized newborn foals. *J. Vet. Intern. Med.* 27: 331–338.

12 Gold, J., Divers, T., Barton, M.H. et al. ACTH, cortisol and vasopressin levels of septic (survivors and nonsurvivors) in comparison to normal foals. *J. Vet. Intern. Med.* 20: 720.

13 Standl, T., Annecke, T., Cascorbi, I. et al. (2018). The nomenclature, definition and distinction of types of shock. *Dtsch. Arztebl. Int.* 115: 757–768.

14 Weil, M.H. (2004). Personal commentary on the diagnosis and treatment of circulatory shock states. *Curr. Opin. Crit. Care* 10: 246–249.

15 Moranville, M.P., Mieure, K.D., and Santayana, E.M. (2011). Evaluation and management of shock states: hypovolemic, distributive, and cardiogenic shock. *J. Pharm. Pract.* 24: 44–60.

16 Axon, J.E. and Palmer, J.E. (2008). Clinical pathology of the foal. *Vet. Clin. Equine* 24: 357–385.

17 Bellezzo, F., Hunt, R.J., Provost, P. et al. (2004). Surgical repair of rib fractures in 14 neonatal foals: case selection, surgical technique and results. *Equine Vet. J.* 36: 557–562.

18 Schambourg, M.A., Laverty, S., Mullim, S. et al. (2003). Thoracic trauma in foals: post mortem findings. *Equine Vet. J.* 35: 78–81.

19 Kislitsina, O.N., Rich, J.D., Wilcox, J.E. et al. (2019). Shock – classification and pathophysiological principles of therapeutics. *Curr. Cardiol. Rev.* 15: 102–113.

20 Jones, J.G. and Smith, S.L. (2009). Shock in the critically ill neonate. *J. Perinat. Neonatal Nurs.* 23: 346–354.

21 Schumer, W. (1984). Pathophysiology and treatment of septic shock. *Am. J. Emerg. Med.* 2: 74–77.

22 Landry, D.W. and Oliver, J.A. (2001). The pathogenesis of vasodilatory shock. *N. Engl. J. Med.* 348: 588–595.

23 Jadhav, A.P. and Sadaka, F.G. (2019). Angiotensin II in septic shock. *Am. J. Emerg. Med.* 37: 1169–1174.

24 Nguyen, H.B., Rivers, E.P., Abrahamian, F.M. et al. (2006). Severe sepsis and septic shock: a review of the literature and emergency department management guidelines. *Ann. Emerg. Med.* 48: 28–54.

25 Hardefeldt, L.Y., Keuler, N., and Peek, S.F. (2010). Incidence of transfusion reactions to commercial equine plasma. *J. Vet. Emerg. Crit. Care* 20: 421–425.

26 Vahdatpour, C., Collins, D., and Goldberg, S. (2019). Cardiogenic shock. *J. Am. Heart Assoc.* 8: 1–12.

27 Slack, J.A., McGuirk, S.M., Erb, H.N. et al. (2005). Biochemical markers of cardiac injury in normal, surviving, septic, or nonsurviving septic neonatal foals. *J. Vet. Intern. Med.* 19: 577–580.

28 Lofstedt, J. (1997). White muscle disease of foals. *Vet. Clin. N. Am. Equine* 13: 169–185.

29 Gowda, R.M., Fox, J.T., and Khan, I.A. (2008). Cardiogenic shock: basics and clinical considerations. *Int. J. Cardiol.* 123: 221–228.

30 Theile, H., Ohman, E.M., Desch, S. et al. (2015). Management of cardiogenic shock. *Eur. Heart J.* 36: 1223–1230.

31 Carnendran, L., Abboud, R., Sleeper, L.A. et al. (2001). Trends in cardiogenic shock: report from the SHOCK study. *Eur. Heart J.* 22: 472–478.

32 Ponikowski, P. and Jankowska, E.A. (2015). Pathogenesis and clinical presentation of acute heart failure. *Rev. Espan. Cardiol.* 68: 331–337.

33 Haskins, S., Pascoe, P.J., Ilkiw, J.E. et al. (2005). Reference cardiopulmonary values in normal dogs. *Comp. Med.* 2: 156–161.

34 Yamamoto, K., Yasuda, J., and Too, K. (1992). Arrhythmias in newborn thoroughbred foals. *Equine Vet. J.* 24 (3): 169–173.

35 Armstrong, S.K., Raidal, S.L., and Hughes, K.J. (2014). Fibrinous pericarditis and pericardial effusion in three neonatal foals. *Aust. Vet. J.* 92: 392–399.

36 Vincent, J.L. and De Backer, D. (2013). Circulatory shock. *N. Engl. J. Med.* 369: 1726–1734.

37 Toribio, R.E. and Mudge, M.C. (2012). Diseases of the foal. In: *Equine Medicine, Surgery and Reproduction* (ed. T.S. Mair, S. Love, J. Shcumacher, et al.), 423–450. Elsevier.

38 Rice, V. (1991). Shock, a clinical syndrome: an update. Part 2. *Crit. Care Nurs.* 11: 74–85.

39 Haljamae, H. (1993). The pathophysiology of shock. *Acta Anaesthesiol. Scand.* 37: 3–6.

40 Palmer, J.E. (2004). Fluid therapy in the neonate: not your mother's fluid space. *Vet. Clin. Equine* 20: 63–75.

41 Griffel, M.I. and Kaufman, B.S. (1992). Pharmacology of colloids and crystalloids. *Crit. Care Clin.* 8: 235–254.

42 Bayer, O., Reinhart, K., Kohl, M. et al. (2012). Effects of fluid resuscitation with synthetic colloids or crystalloids alone on shock reversal, fluid balance, and patient outcomes in patients with severe sepsis. *Crit. Care Med.* 40: 2543–2551.

43 Rivers, E., Nguyen, B., Havstad, S. et al. (2001). Early goal-directed therapy in the treatment of severe sepsis and septic shock. *N. Engl. J. Med.* 345: 1368–1377.

44 Borchers, A., Wilkins, P.A., March, P.M. et al. (2013). Sequential L-lactate concentration in hospitalized equine neonates: a prospective multicenter study. *Equine Vet. J.* Suppl45: 2–7.

45 Wilkins, P.A., Sheahan, B.J., Vander Werf, K.A. et al. (2015). Preliminary investigation of the area under the L-lactate concentration-time curve (LAC_{area}) in critically ill equine neonates. *J. Vet. Intern. Med.* 29: 659–662.

46 Wotman, K., Wilkins, P.A., Palmer, R.P. et al. (2009). Association of blood lactate concentration and outcome in foals. *J. Vet. Intern. Med.* 23: 598–605.

47 Nout, Y.S., Corely, K.T.T., Donaldson, L.L. et al. (2002). Indirect oscillometric and direct blood pressure measurements in anesthetized and conscious neonatal foals. *J. Vet. Emerg. Crit. Care* 12: 75–80.

Section III Catheter-Associated Thrombophlebitis

Kate L. Hepworth-Warren

Thrombophlebitis is defined as venous thrombosis secondary to inflammation of the vessel wall. Phlebitis can exist alone, whereas thrombophlebitis is inflammation associated with thrombus formation. Thrombophlebitis is a well-known complication of IV catheter placement and is a frequent cause of fevers in hospitalized patients [1–3]. While most of the published data regarding risk factors, potential complications, diagnosis, treatment, and prognosis in cases of thrombophlebitis focus on adult horses or populations of mixed ages, much of the information can likely be extrapolated to foals. In a group of 91 horses diagnosed with jugular thrombophlebitis, 20% were foals presented with neonatal disease, half of which were diagnosed with sepsis [4]. An older study performed bacterial culture on 154 catheters from 99 horses and noted that catheters from foals <4 weeks of age were significantly more likely than adult horses to be contaminated and yield bacterial growth [5]. While sepsis can lead to alterations in coagulation and thus an increased tendency for thrombosis, foals with diseases other than sepsis, including prematurity, diarrhea, pneumonia, and bladder rupture have also developed thrombophlebitis [4].

In one study in people, 48,600 bloodstream infections occurred annually secondary to use of IV catheters [6]. Pathogens implicated most frequently include coagulase-negative *Staphylococci*, *Staphylococcus aureus*, *Enterococcus* species, and *Candida* species [6]. Although large-scale studies have not been performed to identify the frequency of thrombophlebitis and catheter associated infections in horses, in a group of 38 adult horses that underwent colic surgery, the prevalence of thrombophlebitis was 18% with the catheters being in place, for a mean of 3.5 days [7]. In infants, risk-factors for catheter-related bloodstream infections include low birthweight, administration of corticosteroids, administration of antimicrobials, prematurity, type of catheter, insertion site, and presence of disease states that affect the integrity of the skin and gastrointestinal barriers [8]. Some of these factors such as drug administration, prematurity, type, and insertion site of catheter might also serve as risk factors for thrombophlebitis in foals. Given the high prevalence of enteritis and enterocolitis in neonatal foals, it is plausible that altered barrier permeability of the gastrointestinal tract could also play a role in the development of catheter-associated thrombophlebitis in foals.

Pathophysiology/Causes

Thrombosis is incited by a combination of three factors first described by Virchow in 1856 (Virchow's triad). The presence of vessel/endothelial injury, hypercoagulability, and altered (reduced, turbulent, static) venous flow ultimately leads to formation of a thrombus within the affected vessel [1]. Placement of IV catheters can lead to injury of the vessel wall, while an indwelling catheter can irritate the vessel wall or serve as the basis for formation of a fibrin sleeve [9]. In horses, trauma or injury to the vessel appears to be the most important of the three factors [1, 7].

The two locations most likely to be the origin of thrombophlebitis are the insertion site of the IV catheter, and the level of the vein at the tip of the catheter [10]. Septic thrombophlebitis is most likely to originate at the catheter insertion site, whereas nonseptic thrombophlebitis can originate at the insertion site or the tip of the catheter [2]. Data from human medicine indicate that the source of infection typically arises from pathogens on the hands of health care workers and skin of the patients. Microorganisms enter the circulation either intraluminally through injection ports, or extraluminally at the insertion sites [3, 6]. Thrombophlebitis is generally identified within 24–72 hours of catheter placement and is a common cause of fevers in hospitalized patients [3, 9, 10].

Equine Neonatal Medicine, First Edition. Edited by David M. Wong and Pamela A. Wilkins.

Administration of high volumes of fluids and certain drugs can also predispose patients to develop thrombophlebitis. Medications known to be irritating to the vein include glycerol guaiacolate, thiopental, calcium gluconate, phenylbutazone, and oxytetracycline [1]. Thrombophlebitis is also a known complication of administration of parenteral nutrition, owing at least in part, to the hyperosmolar nature of these solutions. In a group of 53 foals that received parenteral nutrition, 15% developed catheter complications that were defined as thrombophlebitis or local sepsis [11]. In infants, the risk of catheter-related infections increases with younger gestational age, longer dwell time of catheter, and administration of blood products and parenteral nutrition [8].

Significant risk factors for thrombophlebitis identified in 50 horses were the presence of endotoxemia (Odds Ratio [OR] 18.48), Salmonellosis (OR 67.52) and treatment with antiulcer medications (ranitidine, bismuth salicylate; OR 31). IV dextrose and age were not significantly associated with development of thrombophlebitis [12]. The presence of fever and/or diarrhea, and administration of "homemade" fluids also increase the risk of thrombophlebitis [7, 13]. Rectal temperature greater than 38.5 °C (101.3 °F) at the time of catheter insertion is associated with a fourfold increase in risk for development of thrombophlebitis in horses [14]. General anesthesia appears to have a protective effect against thrombophlebitis as horses that did not undergo general anesthesia were four times more likely to develop thrombophlebitis than those that were anesthetized [13]. In horses that underwent surgical intervention for colic, increased dwell time of IV catheters was associated with an increased risk of developing thrombophlebitis. Interestingly, in this study, the type of catheter had no significant effect on thrombophlebitis development [7]. Horses with colic that presented with SAA greater than 5 μg/ml were 7.6 times more likely to develop thrombophlebitis [15].

A myriad of pathogens has been cultured from either catheter tips or aspirates from septic thrombophlebitis. In infants, the most commonly isolated microorganisms are coagulase-negative *Staphylococci* [8]. In a group of 99 horses from which 154 catheters were cultured, coagulase-negative *Staphylococcus* species, *Corynebacterium* species, and *Enterobacter* species were the most commonly identified microorganisms [5]. In 46 horses with thrombophlebitis that had a cavitating lesion visible on ultrasound, and subsequent culture of an aspirate, 54.2% of samples yielded aerobic bacterial growth and 8.3% yielded anaerobic bacterial growth. *Pasteurella, Actinobacillus, Klebsiella, and Escherichia coli* were some of the more common Gram-negative organisms identified. Additional isolates included *Klebsiella pneumoniae, Escherichia coli, Enterobacter cloacae, Proteus vulgaris, Enterobacter aerogenes*, and *Pseudomonas putida*. Alpha hemolytic *Streptococcus* species were the most common Gram-positive organisms identified. Others included *S. aureus, Streptococcus intermedius*, and ß-hemolytic *Streptococcus* species. Isolated anaerobes included *Peptostreptococcus magnus, Peptococcus saccharolyticus,* and *Fusobacterium necrophorum* [9].

Diagnosis

Diagnosis of thrombophlebitis is often a clinical diagnosis supported by ultrasonography, laboratory data, and bacterial culture. Clinical signs of thrombophlebitis include fever, firmness of the vein, lack of distention at site of thrombus when the vein is occluded, and a rope or cord-like feel to the vein. Heat and pain may be evident upon palpation and exudate may be visible at the catheter insertion site [3, 4, 9, 16]. The presence of heat, pain, and swelling of the affected vein is significantly associated with a cavitating lesion being visible on ultrasonographic examination [9]. If a catheter is in place when the thrombophlebitis develops, the catheter should be removed carefully and the tip cultured and antimicrobial susceptibility testing performed [1]. Clinicopathologic changes associated with thrombophlebitis include leukocytosis, neutrophilia, and increases in acute phase proteins (serum amyloid A, fibrinogen) [1–3, 17].

In a group of 73 adult horses with thrombophlebitis confirmed via ultrasound, the entire length of the jugular vein was affected in 15 horses (21%), one-third of the vein in 19 horses (26%), and two-thirds of the vein in 7 horses (10%); the extent of the thrombus was not reported in the remaining 32 horses. In the same study, of 57 horse in which the extent of lumen obstruction was recorded, 32 horses (56%) had partial obstruction of the vein and 25 (44%) had complete obstruction of the vein [4]. In more severe cases, congestion of facial veins, facial edema, abscesses, dysphagia, and laryngeal hemiplegia was reported [4, 10]. The inflammation can extend distally from the jugular vein surrounding the catheter to affect the caudal part of the jugular vein or proximally to the external maxillary or linguofacial vein [9].

Ultrasonography can be utilized to confirm the presence of thrombophlebitis, assess blood flow, and monitor progression [1, 9]. Ultrasonographic examination of the affected vein should be performed with the vein occluded distal to the site of concern to allow for visualization of the lumen. A nonseptic thrombus within a vein will appear as relatively uniform echogenic mass inside the lumen (Figure 13.III.1) [3]. In cases of septic thrombophlebitis, the thrombus will appear heterogeneous and hyperechoic areas consistent with gas shadowing, or hypoechoic areas consistent with fluid or necrosis may be present [3, 9]. In some cases, a hyperechoic sleeve of fibrin may be visible

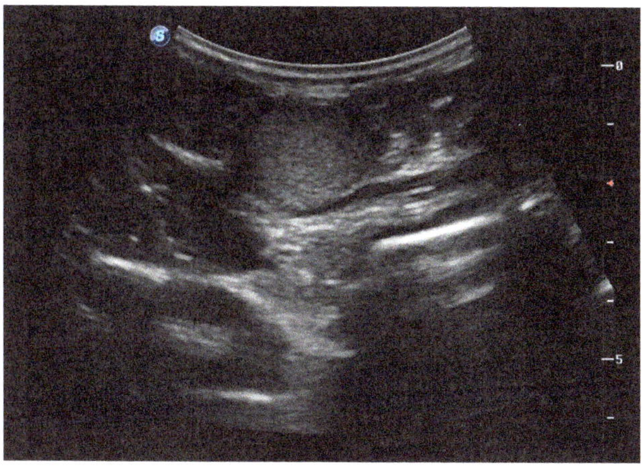

Figure 13.III.1 Uniformly echogenic thrombus within the lumen of the jugular vein.

that formed around the catheter (Figure 13.III.2a–c) [9]. Cavitating lesions may be present, and have a heterogenous appearance with both hypoechoic or anechoic fluid and hyperechoic gas. Generally, the presence of a cavitating lesion is associated with septic thrombophlebitis [9]. When a cavitating lesion is identified, an ultrasound-guided aspirate can be performed to obtain a sample for culture and antimicrobial susceptibility testing [2, 3, 9].

Prevention

While thrombophlebitis can develop in any patient with an indwelling IV catheter, selecting the appropriate catheter and maintaining aseptic technique during placement can decrease the risk. Similarly, monitoring the catheter regularly during hospitalization, keeping the surrounding skin clean and flushing the catheter regularly with heparinized or 0.9% saline can reduce the likelihood of thrombophlebitis and maintain catheter patency [3, 18]. In dogs, no difference was seen in maintaining catheter patency when flushing every 6 hours with 0.9% sodium chloride, or with heparinized saline [19]. Administration of nonsteroidal anti-inflammatory drugs through the catheter has also been associated with a decrease in risk of thrombophlebitis [14]. There can be a delay of 24–48 hours after removal of an IV catheter before clinical evidence of thrombophlebitis is present. Thus, continued monitoring of a vein even after removal of a catheter is critical [10].

Catheter selection is an important component in decreasing the risk of thrombophlebitis. Different materials are inherently more or less thrombogenic. Polyurethane and Teflon™ (polytetrafluorethylene) are most commonly used in equine medicine, although ethylene propylene is sometimes used as well [10]. Generally, catheters made of Teflon™ and ethylene propylene are considered more thrombogenic than catheters made of polyurethane. In a group of 45 horses, the horses in which Teflon™ IV catheters vs polyurethane IV catheters were placed were 2.6 times more likely to develop venous disease [20]. Interestingly, in a group of 38 horses being monitored after colic surgery, there was no statistically significant difference in the incidence of thrombophlebitis between polyurethane and Teflon™ catheters [7]. Another study compared ultrasonographic evidence of thrombophlebitis between horses that had either a polyurethane catheter or a Teflon™ catheter and also found no significant difference between the two materials [21].

Catheters made of Teflon™ are typically placed over-the-needle, and while they are technically simpler to place, they are more rigid and once placed tend to lie adjacent to the vessel wall, making them more irritating and thrombogenic [3, 10, 16]. Polyurethane catheters are more flexible than Teflon™ or ethylene propylene, and thus are either through-the-needle or over-the-wire and placed via the Seldinger technique [3, 18]. Over-the-wire catheters are less

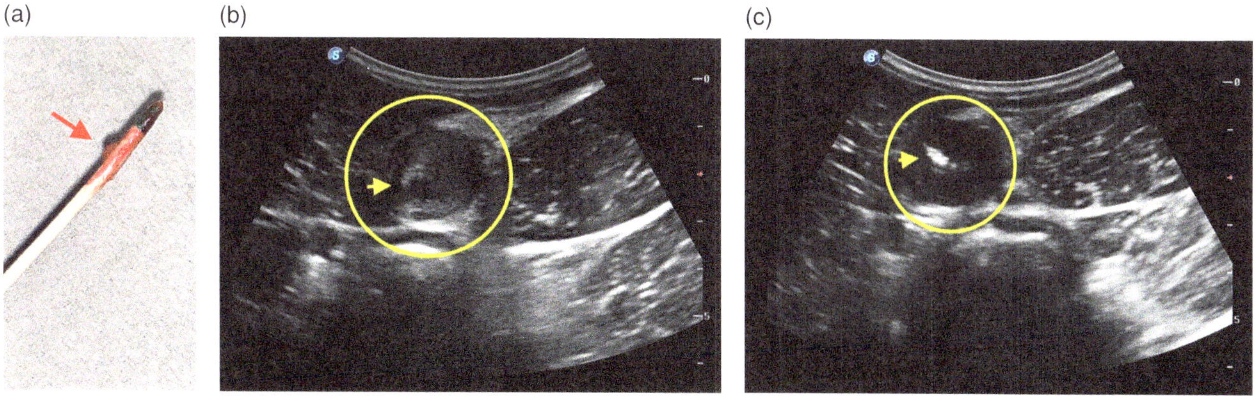

Figure 13.III.2 (a) Fibrin visible at the end of an intravenous catheter after removal from the vein (red arrow). (b) Thrombophlebitis in the jugular vein (yellow circle) with a small hyperechoic region, consistent with a fibrin sleeve, surrounding a hypoechoic region where the catheter was previously in place (yellow arrow). (c) Fibrin (yellow arrow) within the thrombosed jugular vein (yellow circle).

likely to cause endothelial damage during and after placement as they are more flexible than over-the-needle catheters and tend to lie in the lumen as opposed to against the endothelium of the vessel [2, 3, 10, 16, 18]. Additionally, polyurethane catheters are available impregnated with antibiotics, which has been shown to reduce the risk of catheter-related bloodstream infections in human patients [22]. Catheters should be stabilized with either sutures or skin adhesive to minimize movement and secondary irritation to the vein [3, 9]. In addition to selecting the appropriate catheter material, strict adherence to recommendations for length of use should be observed. Short-term catheters, made of ethylene propylene or Teflon™, should be left in place no longer than 24 hours. Medium-term catheters can be left in place for up to 3 days, whereas long-term catheters can be utilized (if managed appropriately) for up to 14 days [18]. Duration of time that catheter is left in place can also impact the risk of thrombophlebitis [2].

Patient restraint to minimize head and neck movement during catheter placement minimizes the chance of contamination and trauma to the vein [18]. In foals, IV catheters are often placed while the foal is in lateral recumbency with a towel or pad placed under the neck to increase access to the jugular vein. Clipping of the hair followed by aseptic preparation of the skin and aseptic placement of the catheter is crucial, especially in critically ill, immunocompromised foals [3, 18, 23]. Clean gloves are recommended for placement of peripheral catheters in human patients, but for central catheters, sterile gloves are recommended for placement [23]. Meticulous management and close monitoring of the catheterized vein is a crucial component in prevention and early identification of thrombophlebitis. Catheters should be flushed every 6 hours with heparinized saline, and the injection port wiped with alcohol and allowed to dry prior to any injection [3, 18]. In order to decrease the risk of needle sticks to health care professionals, needleless connectors have largely replaced injection ports in human medicine and have become increasingly common in veterinary medicine. Subsequently, the use of needleless connectors has been associated with an increased risk of catheter related infections, likely due to inadequate disinfection of the ports prior to injection [24, 25]. A study identified that 50% of needless connectors had bacterial growth from at least 1 of 3 swab samples taken from the connectors in clinical patients [25]. The CDC recommends scrubbing the access ports of needleless connector ports with antiseptic solutions (chlorhexidine, 70% alcohol, povidone iodine, or an iodophor) prior to injection [23]. Evaluation of rates of catheter-related infection in horses and foals associated with needleless injection ports has not been performed, but it is logical that similar issues could arise in foals and thus disinfection of the ports should be performed prior to injection.

In human medicine, dressings placed over the catheter are often utilized to decrease the risk of bacterial colonization, although the efficacy of dressings varies, depending on the type of dressing and the frequency with which it is changed [26]. The Centers for Disease Control (CDC) recommends that catheters in human patients be covered with either sterile gauze or a sterile, translucent semipermeable dressing [23]. No studies directly examining the use of bandages over intravenous catheters in horses have been performed, although given the propensity of critically ill foals to remain recumbent for long periods of time, it is logical that a bandage reduces the risk of contamination [27]. A cyanoacrylate microbial sealant applied to the skin after aseptic preparation and before catheter insertion did not have a significant effect on the likelihood of horses to develop evidence of thrombophlebitis or the likelihood of having a positive bacterial culture from an IV catheter [28]. In human dialysis patients, application of antibiotic ointments at the catheter insertion site was associated with a 75–93% reduction in catheter related bloodstream infections, although only bacitracin/gramicidin/polymyxin B ointment reportedly had this effect [22]. However, the CDC recommends that antibiotic ointments or creams not be utilized in catheters of patients not undergoing dialysis due to the risk of antimicrobial resistance and fungal infections. It is also recommended in human patients that skin surrounding the catheter site be cleansed daily with a 2% chlorhexidine wash [23]. Both the insertion site and the site over the distal tip of the catheter should be palpated multiple times daily for heat, pain, altered firmness, presence of distention when the vein is occluded, and exudate (at insertion site) [3, 10].

Treatment

The goal of therapy for thrombophlebitis is to control pain and inflammation, preserve blood flow through the affected vessel, and treat or prevent infection. Therapeutic options for thrombophlebitis depend on whether infection is present, degree (if any) of blood flow through the affected vessel, and overall health of the patient. Therapies include administration of antimicrobials, aspirin, other non-steroidal anti-inflammatory drugs (systemic and topical), heparin, topical dimethyl sulfoxide (DMSO), application of a poultice, hydrotherapy, and flushing of abscesses [4]. In human medicine, low level laser therapy has been reported to decrease pain and inflammation associated with superficial thrombophlebitis following chemotherapy [29]. Laser therapy has anecdotally been utilized to treat thrombophlebitis in horses, but there is no published information on its efficacy or safety.

In simple cases, where inflammation is localized to the outside of the vein and surrounding tissues, removal of the catheter (ideally with subsequent culture) and topical therapy may suffice. Topical treatment options include application of anti-inflammatories (DMSO, diclofenac), hot compresses to encourage blood flow and drainage, and application of a poultice with drawing agents (e.g. ichthammol) [2, 10]. When septic thrombophlebitis has been identified, broad-spectrum antimicrobial therapy is warranted [10]. As discussed above, infections originating from skin contaminants most commonly involve *Staphylococcus* species [2]. Septic thrombophlebitis originating at the tip of the catheter frequently involves *Actinobacter* [2]. In many foals with indwelling IV catheters, systemic antimicrobial therapy is already being administered; thus, failure to yield bacterial growth from a culture does not rule out the presence of infection [10]. If antimicrobial therapy is not being utilized, then broad-spectrum coverage should be instituted while awaiting culture results.

Antithrombotic agents, including aspirin, heparin, and clopidogrel, have been utilized to prevent additional thrombosis in cases of thrombophlebitis [4, 10, 30]. Aspirin (5 mg/kg, PO, q24h) inhibits platelet cyclooxygenase and has been shown to decrease platelet function in adult horses for up to 24 hours [31, 32]. Clopidogrel (4 mg/kg loading dose PO q24h, followed by 2 mg/kg, PO, q24h) is an antagonist at the platelet P2Y adenosine diphosphate receptor, and decreases platelet aggregation. It is effective at decreasing aggregation of platelets in healthy adult horses; however, the delayed time to onset of effect (3 days) lends to questionable efficacy in preventing additional thrombosis [31]. While both aspirin and clopidogrel have anecdotally been administered to neonatal foals, no studies exist examining their safety, pharmacokinetics, and efficacy in this age group and thus they should be used with caution. Monitoring of coagulation parameters is advised while utilizing these therapies. While the majority of thrombophlebitis cases resolve with medical management, surgical thrombectomy was described in nine horses as a treatment option in horses with septic thrombophlebitis refractory to medical therapy. This procedure was curative in all cases however its application has not been reported in foals [33]. Of note, resolution of thrombophlebitis and re-establishment of blood flow through completely thrombosed veins can require several months of therapy in neonatal foals.

Prognosis and Complications

Thrombophlebitis is often a complication secondary to a primary illness and can lead to potentially fatal complications in the horse including polyarthritis, pneumonia, endocarditis, edema, pulmonary thromboembolism, septicemia, bacteremia, endotoxemia, laryngeal hemiplegia, and airway obstruction secondary to swelling of head and neck [9, 12, 13, 34]. With cephalic vein catheterization, cellulitis, and limb edema can also develop [10].

A review of 91 adult horses that either presented with thrombophlebitis or developed it during hospitalization demonstrated that performance in nonracing animals was not affected by thrombophlebitis. In racing Standardbreds, 84% of horses that had thrombophlebitis returned to racing with no significant differences in their times from those before they developed thrombophlebitis. There was no significant association detected between performance and the presence of unilateral vs bilateral thrombophlebitis, use of antimicrobials, use of aspirin, or the degree of luminal obstruction [4]. In time, thrombosed veins can recanulize and blood flow can return. In other instances, fibrosis and complete occlusion of the vessel occurs, and collateral circulation develops to improve venous drainage to the head [3].

Summary

Thrombophlebitis associated with IV catheters develops frequently in critically ill, hospitalized foals resulting in fevers, swelling, pain, and discharge around the catheter and edema of the head and neck. Changes in the complete blood count and inflammatory proteins can also be observed, as well as more severe complications such as pulmonary embolism. While thrombophlebitis can occur despite every effort to prevent it, utilizing appropriate aseptic technique, catheter selection, and maintenance can decrease the likelihood of its development.

References

1 Dias, D.P.M. and de Lacerdo Neto, J.C. (2013). Jugular thrombophlebitis in horses: a review of fibrinolysis, thrombus formation, and clinical management. *Can. Vet. J.* 54: 65–71.

2 Divers, T.J. (2003). Prevention and treatment of thrombosis, phlebitis, and laminitis in horses with gastrointestinal disease. *Vet. Clin. Equine* 19: 779–790.

3 Tan, R.H.H., Dart, A.J., and Dowling, B.A. (2003). Catheters: a review of the selection, utilization, and complications of catheters for peripheral venous access. *Aust. Vet. J.* 81: 136–139.

4 Moreau, P. and Lavoie, J.P. (2009). Evaluation of athletic performance in horses with jugular vein thrombophlebitis: 91 cases (1988–2005). *J. Am. Vet. Med. Assoc.* 235: 1073–1078.

5 Ettlinger, J.J., Palmer, J.E., and Bencon, C. (1992). Bacteria found on intravenous catheters removed from horses. *Vet. Rec.* 130: 248–249.

6 Wenzel, R.P. and Edmond, M.B. (2006). Team-based prevention of catheter-related infections. *N. Engl. J. Med.* 355: 2781–2783.

7 Lankveld, D.P.K., Ensin, J.M., Van Dijk, P. et al. (2001). Factors influencing the occurrence of thrombophlebitis after post-surgical long-term intravenous catheterization of colic horses: a study of 38 cases. *J. Vet. Med. Assoc.* 48: 545–552.

8 Wu, J. and Mu, D. (2012). Vascular catheter-related complications in newborns. *J. Paediatr. Child Health* 48: E91–E95.

9 Gardner, S.Y., Reef, V.B., and Spencer, P.A. (1991). Ultrasonographic evaluation of horses with thrombophlebitis of the jugular vein: 46 cases (1985–1988). *J. Vet. Med. Assoc.* 199: 370–373.

10 Higgins, J. (2015). Preparation, supplies, and catheterization. In: *Equine Fluid Therapy* (ed. C. Langdon Fielding and K. Gary Magdesian), 129–141. Ames, IA: Wiley Blackwell.

11 Myers, C.J., Magdesian, K.G., Kass, P.H. et al. (2009). Parenteral nutrition in neonatal foals: clinical description, complications and outcomes in 53 foals (1995–2005). *Vet. J.* 181: 137–144.

12 Dolente, B.A., Beech, J., Lindborg, S., and Smith, G. (2005). Evaluation of risk factors for development of catheter-associated jugular thrombophlebitis in horses: 50 cases (1993–1998). *J. Am. Vet. Med. Assoc.* 227: 1134–1141.

13 Traub-Dargatz, J.L. and Dargatz, D.A. (1994). A retrospective study of vein thrombosis in horses treated with intravenous fluids in a veterinary teaching hospital. *J. Vet. Intern. Med.* 8: 264–266.

14 Geraghty, T.E., Love, S., Hughes, K.J. et al. (2009). Assessment if subclinical venous catheter-related diseases in horse and associated risk factors. *Vet. Rec.* 164: 227–231.

15 Westerman, T.L., Foster, C.M., Tornquist, S.J. et al. (2016). Evaluation of serum amyloid A and haptoglobin concentrations as prognostic indicators for horses with colic. *J. Am. Vet. Med. Assoc.* 248: 935–940.

16 Spurlock, S.L., Spurlock, G.H., Parker, G. et al. (1990). Long-term jugular vein catheterization in horses. *J. Am. Vet. Med. Assoc.* 196: 425–430.

17 Aitken, M.R., Stefanovski, D., and Southwood, L.L. (2019). Serum amyloid a concentration in postoperative colic horses and its association with postoperative complications. *Vet. Surg.* 48: 143–151.

18 Chapman, A. (2018). Placement and care of intravenous catheters. In: *Manual of Clinical Procedures in the Horse* (ed. C. LRR and M.R. Paradis), 96–110. Hoboken, NJ: Wiley Blackwell.

19 Ueda, Y., Odunayo, A., and Mann, F.A. (2013). Comparison of heparinized saline and 09% sodium chloride for maintaining peripheral intravenous catheter patency in dogs. *J. Vet. Emerg. Crit. Care* 23: 517–522.

20 Müller, C.D.V.S., Lübke-Becker, A., Doherr, M.G. et al. (2016). Influence of different types of catheters on the development of diseases of the jugular vein in 45 horses. *J. Equine Vet. Sci.* 46: 89–97.

21 Milne, M. and Bradbury, L. (2009). The use of ultrasound to assess the thrombogenic properties of Teflon and polyurethane catheters for short term use in systematically healthy horses. *J. Equine Vet. Sci.* 29: 833–841.

22 Golestaneh, L. and Mokrzycki, M.H. (2018). Prevention of hemodialysis catheter infections: ointments, dressings, locks, and catheter hub devices. *Hemodial. Int.* 22: S75–S82.

23 O'Grady, N.P., Alexander, M., Burns, L.A. (2011). Guidelines for the Prevention of Intravenous Catheter Related Infections. Center for Disease Control. https://www.cdc.gov/infectioncontrol/guidelines/bsi/recommendations.html. (access 2 November 2020).

24 Moureau, N.L. and Flynn, J. (2015). Disinfection of needleless connector hubs: clinical evidence systematic review. *Nurs. Res. Pract.* 2015: 1–20.

25 Slater, K., Cooke, M., Whitby, M. et al. (2017). Microorganisms present on peripheral intravenous needleless connectors in the clinical environment. *Am. J. Infect. Control* 45: 932–934.

26 Ullman, A.J., Cooke, M., and Rickard, C.M. (2015). Examining the role of securement and dressing products to prevent central venous access device failure: a narrative review. *J. Assoc. Vasc. Access* 20: 99–110.

27 Hay, C.W. (1992). Equine intravenous catheterisation. *Equine Vet. Educ.* 4: 319–323.

28 Pasolini, M.P., Passamonti, F., Uccello, V. et al. (2015). Using cyanoacrylate microbial sealant for skin preparation prior to the placement of intravenous catheters in horses. *J. Equine Vet sci* 35: 686–691.

29 Hwang, W.T., Chung, S.H., and Kim, H. (2015). Low-level laser therapy for the treatment of superficial thrombophlebitis after chemotherapy in breast cancer patients: a case study. *J. Phys. Ther. Sci.* 27: 3937–3938.

30 Barr, B. (2018). Pharmacology. In: *Equine Pediatric Medicine*, 2e (ed. W.V. Bernard and B.S. Barr). Boca Raton, FL: Taylor and Francis Group.

31 Brainard, B.M., Epstein, K.L., LoBato, D. et al. (2011). Effects of clopidogrel and aspirin on platelet aggregation, thromboxane production, and serotonin secretion in horses. *J. Vet. Intern. Med.* 25: 116–122.

32 Cambridge, H., Lees, P., Hooke, R.E. et al. (1991). Antithrombotic actions of aspirin in the horse. *Equine Vet. J.* 23: 123–127.

33 Russell, T.M., Kearney, C., and Pollock, P.J. (2010). Surgical treatment of septic jugular thrombophlebitis in nine horses. *Vet. Surg.* 39: 627–630.

34 Lores, M., Cantos, M., De Rijck, M. et al. (2018). Polyarthritis secondary to septic thrombophlebitis in an Arabian mare. *Equine Vet. Educ.* 20: 187–191.

Neonatal Digestive System

Chapter 14 Embryology and Anatomy of the Digestive Tract

David Wong, Rebecca Ruby, and Charles Brockus

An appropriately developed digestive system is vital for the newborn foal's survival as this system allows for the consumption, digestion, and absorption of nutrients. Simultaneously, the digestive tract is an expansive interface between the external environment and host and is under constant exposure to microorganisms and pathogens from the outside world. Thus, a functional system that allows the processing and absorption of nutrients while providing a strong barrier to microorganisms needs to be established at birth, with further maturation as the foal ages.

Embryology of the Digestive System

Embryology of the human digestive tract has been reviewed in detail [1–3], but minimal studies have evaluated this topic in the horse [4, 5]. In the human embryo, there are two major steps in the formation of the gut tube and individual digestive organs and their specialized cell types [6]. During weeks 3–4 of gestation, the embryo folds and the innermost endodermal layer forms the gut tube that communicates ventrally with the yolk sac [3]. The gut tube is divided regionally into the foregut (terminates cranially in the oropharyngeal membrane), midgut, and hindgut (terminates caudally in the cloacal membrane). These membranes eventually rupture and make the gut tube a patent pathway proximally and distally (via the oral cavity and anus, respectively). The endodermal gut tube is surrounded by the lateral plate splanchnic mesoderm that forms the lamina propria, submucosal, and mucosal layers of the gastrointestinal (GI) tract. The midgut elongates and eventually becomes the small intestine, cecum, and ascending and transverse colon. The intestine herniates into the umbilical cord for a portion of gestation and during this process there is rotation around the cranial mesenteric artery, placing the proximal GI tract on the right side and the cecal bud on the left. As the intestines retract back into the abdominal cavity a further 180° of rotation occurs moving the small intestine and cecum to the left and right, respectively. The midgut undergoes rapid elongation in week 5 and forms a hairpin loop around the superior mesenteric artery; the cranial portion of the loop creates the jejunum and parts of the duodenum and ilium while the caudal portion forms the cecum and parts of the colon. A distal portion of the hindgut forms the anorectal canal including the transverse and descending colon. Initially the embryonic gut is supported on a dorsal and ventral mesentery. The ventral mesentery subsequently atrophies, allowing the gut to elongate and partially rotate. The dorsal mesentery contains the mesenchymal layer, which provides the vascular, lymphatic, and neural supply to the intestines. Neural crest cells migrate to the developing gut and form the enteric nervous system and portions of the autonomic (parasympathetic, sympathetic) nervous system that innervate the GI tract. The gut tube is suspended in the peritoneal cavity (intraperitoneal) via the dorsal mesentery and is surrounded by splanchnopleure that forms the visceral peritoneum. Retroperitoneal structures such as the kidneys, adrenal glands, and ureters are not suspended in the abdomen and are "behind" the peritoneal cavity [7].

The stomach forms from a dilation of the foregut. Around week 5 in the human embryo, the stomach wall grows asymmetrically as the dorsal wall grows faster and creates the greater curvature while the ventral wall forms the lesser curvature. During week 7–8, the stomach rotates 90° bringing the greater curvature to the left and lesser curvature to the right, creating a C-shaped loop that also moves the duodenum dorsally.

The pancreas forms as dorsal and ventral pancreatic buds on opposite sides of the foregut. These epithelial buds enlarge and form a treelike ductal system via growth and branching [6]. The left and right lobe of the pancreas arises

Equine Neonatal Medicine, First Edition. Edited by David M. Wong and Pamela A. Wilkins.

from the dorsal and ventral bud, respectively, with the dorsal bud giving rise to the majority of the pancreas. Due to rotation during growth, the developing buds overlap and fuse to result in a single organ with a right and left lobe and body. The minor duodenal papilla is developed from the dorsal lobe and the major duodenal papilla from the ventral lobe. The pancreatic duct from the major duodenal papilla joins with the bile duct to form the common bile duct. In horses both pancreatic ducts persist. By gestational day 50, the pancreatic acini and islets can be identified. The pancreatic endoderm differentiates into cells that perform the duties of the pancreas and include exocrine (function in digestion) and endocrine (produce insulin, glucagon, somatostatin) cells [7]. Individual endocrine cells are identified initially, with islets established later [6].

The embryonic liver develops from an outpouching from the ventral foregut endoderm referred to as the hepatic diverticulum or liver bud [8]. The primitive endodermal cells of this bud (also called hepatoblasts) are bipotential cells with the ability to differentiate into hepatocytes or biliary epithelial cells (cholangiocytes). Kupffer cells, blood vessels, and fibrous tissue are derived from the mesoderm [9]. Early in gestation, hematopoietic stem cells can be found in the liver, marking the shift in hematopoiesis from the yolk sac to the liver. The liver is the main site of hematopoiesis until mid-gestation, after which the bone marrow becomes the primary site of blood cell formation [2]. At birth, the architecture of the liver is well established with portal tracts connected to central veins by plates of hepatocytes [4].

In regard to equine embryogenesis, one study evaluated the digestive tract of 10 embryos and 10 fetuses (Table 14.1) [4]. Between 21 and 25 days gestation, the primitive oral cavity was observed and was composed of disorganized mesenchymal tissue. By Day 25, the tongue was visible and a monogastric stomach was documented. The stomach had distinct and differentiated formation of the epithelium, submucosa, musculature, and serosa by Day 30. The esophagus appeared as a short tube by Day 28 of gestation, and the musculature of the esophagus was noted by Day 38. Intestinal crypts were noted by Day 40 of gestation, and by Day 65, villi of various lengths occurred in the small intestines. By Day 50, the pharynx was noted. With regard to the liver, simple cuboidal capsular epithelium, proliferating endodermal cells, hepatoblasts (later giving rise to hepatocytes), and the formation of a central vein were noted by Day 21 of gestation [4]. At 25 days, the primordial sinusoids and blood cells were differentiated and by Day 30, the liver parenchyma began to organize, and hepatocyte cords began to anastomose. The embryonic hepatocytes developed into long cords into stroma forming plates that were initially three to five cells thick.

Table 14.1 Major embryonic events in the formation of the digestive tract of the equine embryo during the first few weeks of gestation [4].

Age (days)	Crown-rump length (cm)	Weight (grams)	Major events
21	1.6	0.5	Primitive oral cavity, disorganized hepatic parenchyma.
25	1.9	0.8	Disorganized mesenchymal tissue in oral cavity, primordium of stomach. Intestines are small ducts (tubes), pancreatic bud.
28	2.3	1.5	Small tongue, esophagus as short tube.
30	2.5	1.8	Lateral ridges of tongue appear, esophagus has tubular shape, stomach has differentiation of layers, hepatic parenchyma start to organize, pancreas has triangular shape.
35	3.0	2.5	Monogastric stomach but without glands, hepatocytes differentiated.
38	3.3	3.0	Muscular longitudinal fibers in esophagus.
40	3.6	3.5	Connective and muscular tissue in tongue. Intestinal crypts, Kupffer cells in liver. Pancreas is more elongated.
45	4.5	5.5	Final length of esophagus.
50	5.2	8.2	Striated muscle in external muscular layer of esophagus, acini and pancreatic islets.
65	8.4	35.7	Villi various lengths in intestine, mesojejunum, and omentum well differentiated.
75	11.5	116.9	Three sections of pharynx can be distinguished.
105	18.9	391.4	Parietal and visceral peritoneum formed.

Several anomalies in the horse can be linked to embryonic development of the digestive tract. For example, the fetal GI tract rotates around the cranial mesenteric artery in the first stage of gestation. Three types of rotational anomalies have been described: nonrotation, malrotation and reverse rotation [10]. Intestinal nonrotation was reported in a 24-hour male Welsh-Thoroughbred foal. Celiotomy identified abnormal positioning of the intestinal tract, consistent with a 180° rotation (colon remained on left side, small intestine to the right of midline, cecum freely movable with the ileum entering from the right instead of the left). The foal additionally had flexural limb deformities, a body wall hernia and segmentally dilated jejunum. Following surgery, which resected the dilated jejunum and closed the body wall hernia, the foal was reported to be clinically healthy at 15 months of age [11].

Another anomaly known as Meckel's diverticulum has been reported in horses. Embryologically, the connection between the midgut and yolk sac is a narrow vitelline duct that has two associated arteries. This connection becomes Meckel's diverticulum, which is located in the jejunum of adults. Persistence of the vitelline duct forms a fibrous ligament. This band of tissue may persist between the umbilicus and the intestine or be partially formed with attachment to mesentery or intestine without contacting the umbilicus. A persistent vitelline artery is referred to as the mesodiverticular band and will extend from the cranial mesenteric artery to the antimesenteric side of the intestine or Meckel's diverticulum. The band may be observed as an incidental finding or associated with colic due to strangulation or obstruction of entrapped intestine, which may occur with associated volvulus (Figure 14.1) [12]. This can result in colic, peritonitis, or the foal may remain asymptomatic [13].

Mesenteric attachments are critical to maintain arrangement of the intestinal tract. The right dorsal colon has attachments to the body wall, cecum, root of the mesentery, and pancreas, which result in minimal movement of this segment. The right ventral colon attaches to the cecum by the ceco-colic ligament. Mesenteric attachment anomalies include absent, elongated, or shortened segments of tissue that can result in hypermotility of the large intestine leading to displacement and volvulus. An equine case in which there was a lack of retroperitoneal attachment of the cecal base and right dorsal colon was reported to have caused circulation problems in the large colon and cecum resulting in poor growth and colic in a 1.5-year-old Dutch Warmblood. While rare in the literature, two to three cases of mesenteric anomalies are typically identified each year in horses presenting to the University of Kentucky Veterinary Diagnostic Laboratory for necropsy (Dr. Rebecca Ruby, personal observations). Malformations are often identified at the time of colic surgery and, if significant, may be considered incompatible with long-term survival, resulting in euthanasia.

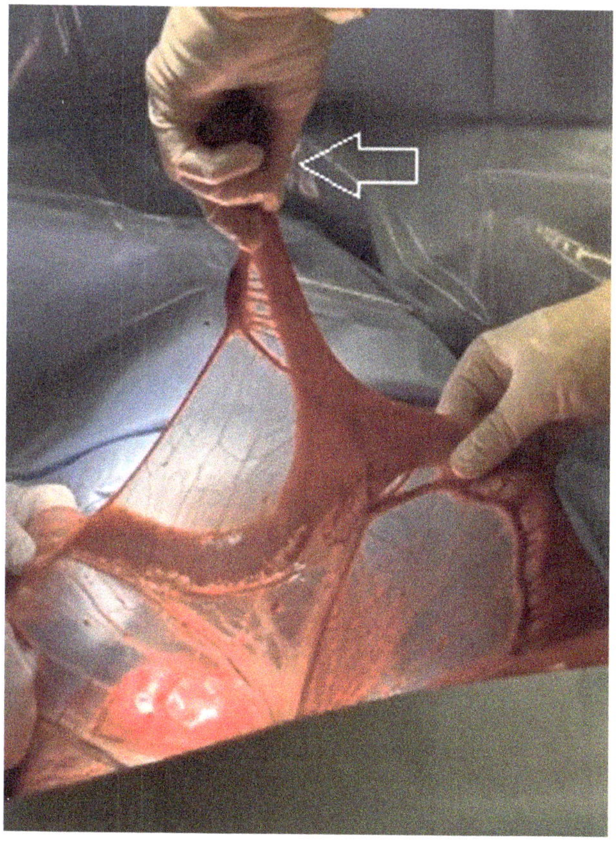

Figure 14.1 Meckel's diverticulum.

Malformations that result in cysts are classified by the structures identified with the cyst's wall (i.e. epithelium, glands, muscular, or cartilage layers). Six types of foregut cysts are recognized based on these features: enteric, enterogastric, esophageal, gastric, bronchogenic, and ciliated foregut. In some cases, cysts will have features of esophageal and bronchogenic development in the cranial and caudal aspects, respectively. This may occur as the trachea arises from the ventral wall of the foregut. The respiratory diverticulum then separates from the foregut, which elongates to form the esophagus. Esophageal cysts have been identified within the duodenum, larynx, and esophagus of horses [14]. Duplication cysts have also been reported in the colon [15].

Anatomy of the Digestive Tract

A basic knowledge of the anatomy of the stomach, intestine, and liver as well as cell types at the microscopic level facilitates understanding of the digestive system in health and disease. The GI tract is composed of the stomach and the small and large intestines. The stomach consists of the upper (squamous) or lower (glandular) regions, with the lower region containing excretory cells including the parietal (oxyntic cells), chief cells, and mucus cells that secrete hydrochloric acid, pepsinogen, and mucus, respectively. Enterocytes line the small intestines, consisting of villi composed primarily of simple columnar epithelial cells with apical microvilli and some goblet cells more abundant in distal regions. In addition, Paneth cells associated with gut immunity and enteroendocrine cells are scattered within the crypts. The large intestines are lined with simple columnar epithelial cells with intestinal crypts and a higher density of goblet cells but lack villi (Figures 14.2–14.4). In the foal, the large intestines are not developed like the

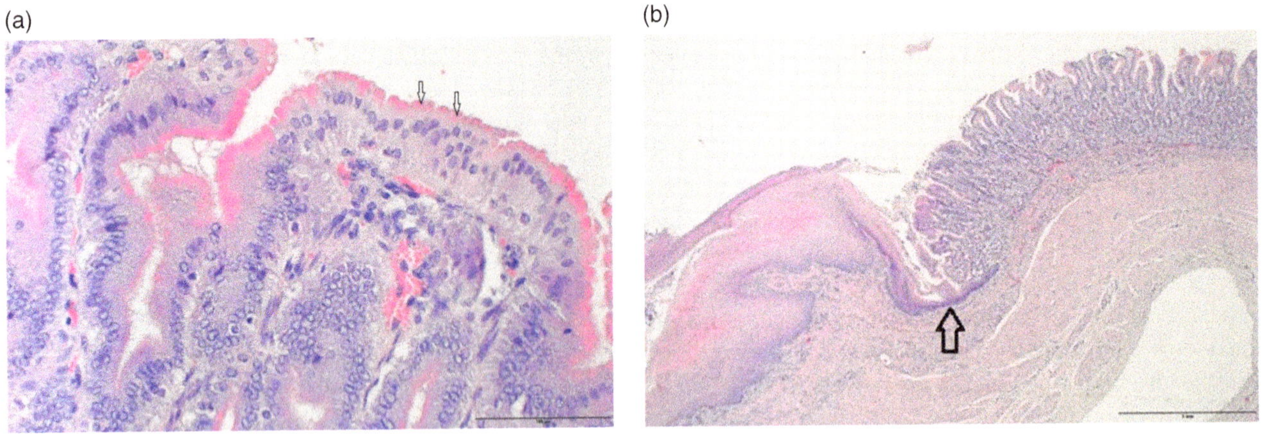

Figure 14.2 (a) Simple columnar epithelium of the stomach (black arrows). (b) Transition from squamous to glandular portion of the stomach (arrow).

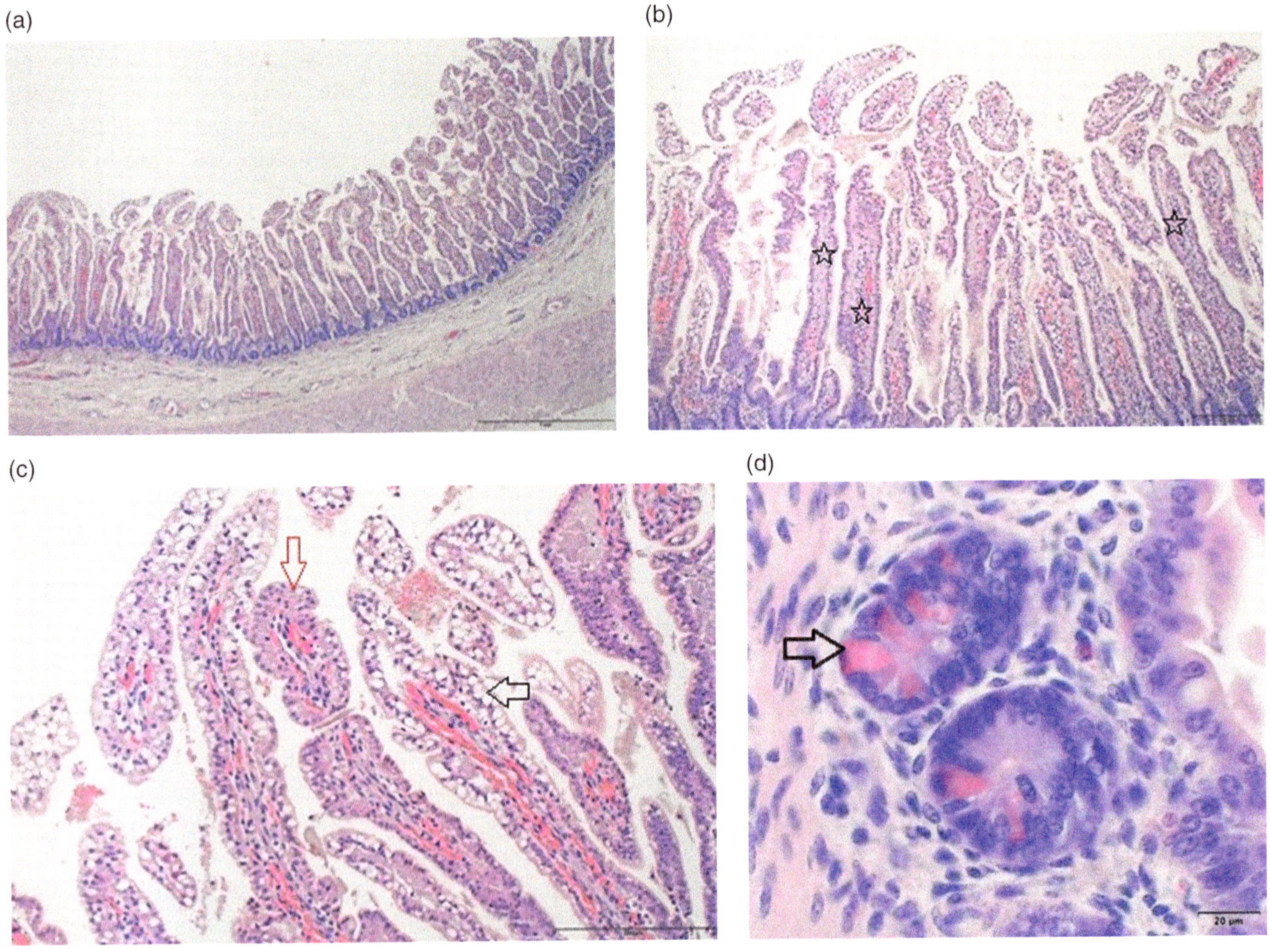

Figure 14.3 (a) Low magnification of jejunum identifying multiple villi; (b) Higher magnification identifying the jejunal villi (stars); (c) High magnification of section of jejunum identifying goblet cells (black arrow) and columnar cells (red arrow); (d) High magnification of Paneth cells of duodenum. Paneth cells are specialized epithelial cells variably present in the small intestine of different species (prominent in the horse) that contain brightly eosinophilic cytoplasmic globules that represent vesicles containing antimicrobial compounds such as defensins.

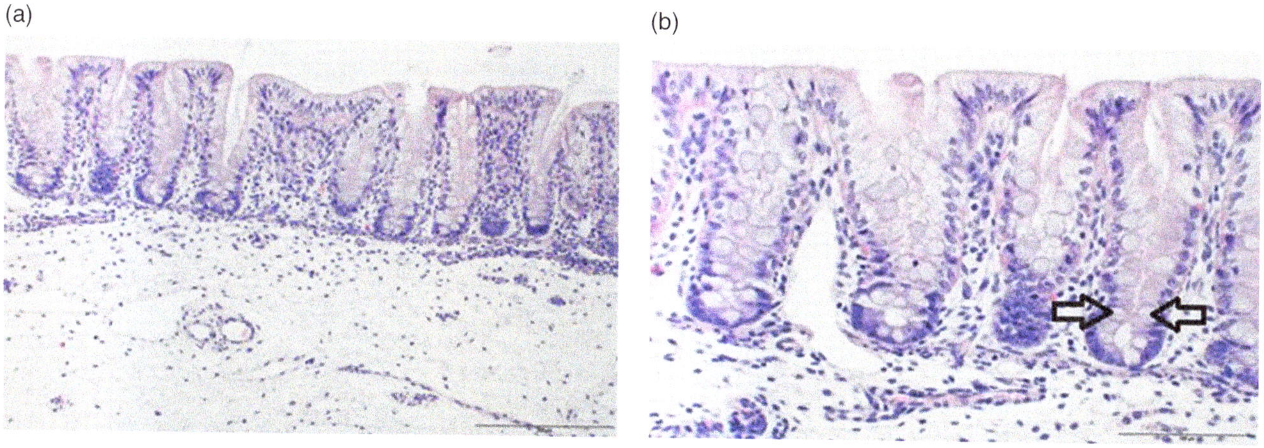

Figure 14.4 (a) Low magnification image of the colonic mucosa. (b) Higher magnification of the mucosa of the large intestine. Note the abundance of lightly stained goblet cells (arrows) within the intestinal crypts.

adult; therefore, they require a lower-fiber diet at young ages (<3 months old).

With regard to the hepatobiliary system, there are four main cell types that comprise the liver: hepatocytes, endothelial cells, Kupffer cells, and stellate cells [16]. The hepatocyte serves as the biosynthetic engine of the liver and has a prominent Golgi system and rough endoplasmic reticulum that allows them to synthesize and secrete proteins. Endothelial cells line the sinusoids and act as a barrier interface between the blood and hepatocytes. Kupffer cells are macrophages within the liver, while stellate cells store fat and vitamin A [16].

The liver can be divided into structural units called hepatic lobules (also called acini), which are polygonal histologic units composed of numerous plates of hepatocytes that radiate toward a central vein (Figure 14.5). At each corner around the perimeter of the hepatic lobule are branches of the hepatic artery, hepatic portal vein, and bile duct (collectively referred to as the hepatic triad), along with lymphatics. Blood from the hepatic arterioles and portal venules mix in the hepatic sinusoids that surround the plates of hepatocytes; this blood bathes the hepatocytes with a mixture of arterial blood along with venous blood that arises primarily from the stomach, intestines, and spleen via the portal system.

In people, approximately 70% of blood flow to the liver is deoxygenated blood from the hepatic portal vein with the remaining 30% being oxygenated blood from the hepatic artery [9]. The sinusoidal blood travels along the plates of hepatocytes toward the central vein, later entering larger hepatic veins that converge near the diaphragm to enter the caudal vena cava. In addition, bile is produced by each hepatocyte which is subsequently secreted into bile canaliculi where are situated between hepatocytes. Bile within each hepatic lobule flows in the opposite direction of blood (i.e. bile moves toward bile duct tributaries at periphery of each lobule). The ducts from each lobe collectively merge to eventually form the left and right hepatic ducts that unite to form the common hepatic ducts leading to the common bile duct. The common bile duct (and pancreatic duct) empties into the proximal duodenum at the major duodenal papilla, which can be noted on endoscopic exam. Opposite the major duodenal papilla lies the minor duodenal papilla that serves as the opening of the accessory pancreatic duct. In summary, hepatocytes can be viewed as having two surfaces: (i) the sinusoidal side that receives and absorbs a mixture of oxygenated blood and nutrients from the portal vein, and (ii) the canalicular side that delivers bile and other products of conjugation and metabolism to the canalicular network that joins the bile ductules [9].

The liver parenchyma can also be divided into three zones based on proximity to the portal triads. Hepatocytes closest to the portal zone (Zone 1; periportal hepatocytes) receive the most oxygen- and nutrient-rich blood and are noted for hepatocyte regeneration, bile duct proliferation, gluconeogenesis, and the presence of a high concentration of enzymes involved in cell respiration [8]. Zone 1 hepatocytes also produce glycogen and other proteins. Zone 3 hepatocytes are closest to the central vein and receive the least oxygen; Zone 3 hepatocytes (perivenular hepatocytes) are involved in detoxification, aerobic metabolism, and glycolysis and contain cytochromes P450. Zone 2 hepatocytes are an intermediate zone.

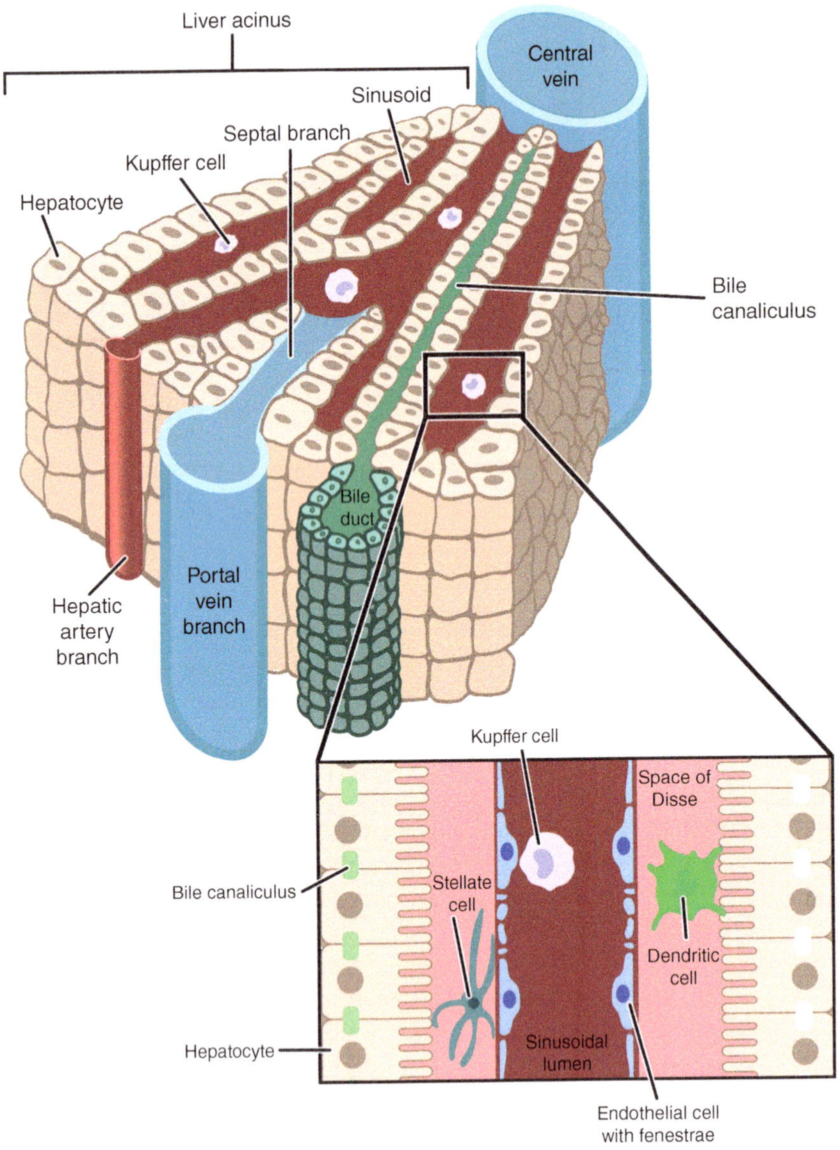

Figure 14.5 Overview of the structural units of the liver. The structural units of the liver are the hepatic lobules that radiate toward a central vein and bile duct (hepatic triad). Blood from the hepatic arterioles and portal venules mix in the hepatic sinusoids that surround the plates of hepatocytes and bathes the hepatocytes with both arterial and venous blood. Bile is produced by hepatocytes and flows in the opposite direction of blood (toward periphery of lobule).

Maturation of the Digestive System

In utero, the fetus must prepare for the transition from a sterile environment and reliance on placental nutrition to the immediate and dramatic functional demands placed on it by a contaminated environment and the pressing need to digest food. Therefore, during fetal development, the GI tract must acquire the capacity to digest food, defend against pathogens, secrete hormones, and detoxify and eliminate toxins produced by metabolism or consumed from the external environment [17]. Some of these functions are also vital prenatally, for example, the ability of the fetus to process large volumes of amniotic fluid swallowed during gestation, which can range from 450 to 750 ml/day in the human fetus [17, 18]. Another essential function at birth is adequate GI motility. The interstitial cells of Cajal (ICC) generate pacemaker activity in the GI tract via generation of slow wave activity. In one equine study, ICC were identified in the fetus at 6 months of gestation and in newborn foals. In this study, a network of ICC was present in the myenteric plexus area of both the small and large intestine at 6 months of gestation; the distribution and density of ICC in the small intestine in the full-term fetus appeared to be similar to the neonatal foal [19]. In contrast, ICC of the distal large intestine continue to colonize the inner aspect of the circular muscle of the intestine after birth [19].

At birth, two physiologic events immediately and dramatically increase blood flow to the GI tract and liver, namely, the blood pressure in the lungs drops dramatically as the newborn's lungs become inflated (blood flow switches from fetal to neonatal circulation pattern) and the newborn's cardiac output, previously traveling to the placenta, is rapidly redistributed to the newborn's vital organs. Thus, within minutes of birth, the venous return from the intestines and liver increases. Upon birth there is also a rapid induction of functions such as transamination, glutamyl transferase, synthesis of coagulation factors, and bile production that occurs [9]. Preterm infants are at heightened risk of hepatic decompensation as their immaturity results in a delay in attaining normal detoxifying and synthetic function. Hypoxia and sepsis are other common causes of liver dysfunction in neonates [9].

As the neonatal foal consumes colostrum and milk, the intestinal tract increases in length and diameter. Differentiation of enterocytes also occurs along with an increase in villus density, height, width, crypt density, and depth [4, 20]. Feeding of the newborn also stimulates the release of gut hormones such as gastrin. In addition to luminal factors that promote postnatal development of the intestines, local and systemic factors promote growth. Outside the basic nutrients in mare's milk, it also contains hormones (steroid hormones, insulin, thyroid hormones), growth factors (epidermal growth factor, insulin-like growth factor), enzymes, and bioactive factors (lactoferrin) that are important for trophic development of the GI tract [21]. The volume, frequency, and type of feeding also influences GI development. For example, newborn animals that are deprived of enteral feed or fed only water have reduced weights and lengths of their GI tract compared to animals that consumed milk. Moreover, the growth and development of the GI tract is less in animals fed milk formula instead of colostrum or milk [21].

One challenge to the GI tract shortly after birth is the fact that it must accept the presence of numerous species of bacteria at high densities. The GI tract's immune system is multifaceted and must be able to differentiate between "good" and "bad" bacteria and contribute to the selection and tolerance of commensal bacteria [17]. Thus, as the GI tract develops, the efficiency of nutritional uptake improves, coinciding with the maturation of microbial colonization and microbial digestion within the intestines [22]. Innate GI defenses include secretion of acid, lysozyme, antimicrobial peptides, and mucus, along with tight junctions that link epithelial cells and provide a physical barrier, activated defense cells (macrophages, neutrophils), and intestinal motility [17]. In comparison, the adaptive immune system of the GI tract relies on organized lymphoid tissue (Peyer's patches, mesenteric lymph nodes), B and T lymphocytes, and antigen presenting cells. A unique feature of the adaptive immune system of the GI tract, as compared to the systemic immune system, is the development of oral tolerance where the GI immune system learns to discriminate between bacteria and antigens that are of low/no risk to those that pose a high risk/virulent.

The liver also plays numerous essential functions in maintaining homeostasis, although the clinician must be cognizant of the fact that the liver is immature at birth. The human neonate has <20% of the hepatocytes that are present in the adult liver, with the liver continuing to grow after birth until it reaches mature size [16]. The percentage of hepatocytes in the neonatal foal, in comparison to the adult horse, is unknown. However, in the newborn foal, the liver is proportionally larger than that of the adult horse, and on fetal ultrasound, the liver is one of the easiest organs to identify. However, the function of the newborn foal's hepatocytes likely still requires maturation for full function.

One of the major functions of the liver is maintenance of blood glucose concentrations. Newborns have labile blood glucose concentrations as they transition from receiving nutrients from the maternal circulation to metabolizing hepatic stores and enteral feedings [8]. The neonatal infant produces glucose at a rate of 4–6 mg/kg/min during the first few days of life; this is accomplished by the liver via glycogenolysis and gluconeogenesis using glycerol, lactate, and volatile fatty acids [8].

The liver is also responsible for bilirubin metabolism. Bilirubin is the byproduct of hemoglobin catabolism from senescent red blood cells. Increased unconjugated bilirubin is common in the first 2 weeks of life in the infant but is typically self-limiting. This hyperbilirubinemia can be caused by increased bilirubin production, deficient conjugation, and/or increased reabsorption of unconjugated bilirubin via the enterohepatic circulation [8].

Production of bile acids also occurs in the liver and is present in the human fetus by 14 weeks of gestation [8]. Although there is increased activity of enzymes involved in bile acid synthesis in late gestation, the capacity to synthesize and excrete bile is immature in the neonatal infant liver, making it susceptible to cholestasis from toxic injury [8, 16]. The liver is also responsible for regulation and production of plasma proteins, acute phase proteins (fibrinogen, amyloid A, hepcidin, albumin), and coagulation factors [16, 23]. Furthermore, the liver must detoxify metabolic byproducts as well as xenobiotics, and it is the primary organ for first-pass metabolism of drugs and excretion of others. Other roles that the liver serves include fatty acid metabolism and store of fat-soluble vitamins (A, D, E, K) and elemental nutrients (iron, copper, selenium, molybdenum).

References

1 Vakili, K. and Pomfret, E.A. (2008). Biliary anatomy and embryology. *Surg. Clin. North Am.* 88: 1159–1174.

2 Diehl-Jones, W. and Fraser, A.D. (2002). The neonatal liver, part 1: embryology, anatomy and physiology. *Neonatal Network* 21: https://doi.org/10.1891/0730-0832.21.2.5.

3 Danowitz, M. and Solounias, N. (2016). Embryology, comparative anatomy, and congenital malformations of the gastrointestinal tract. *Edorium J. Anat. Embryol.* 3: 39–50.

4 Rodrigues, M.N., Carvalho, R.C., Franciolli, A.L. et al. (2014). Prenatal development of the digestive system in the horse. *Anat. Rec.* 297: 1218–1227.

5 Franciolli, A.L.R., Cordeiro, B.M., da Fonseca, E.T. et al. (2011). Characteristics of the equine embryo and fetus from days 15 to 107 of pregnancy. *Theriogenology* 76: 819–832.

6 Montgomery, R.K., Mulberg, A.E., and Grand, J.R. (1999). Development of the human gastrointestinal tract: twenty years of progress. *Gastroenterology* 116: 702–731.

7 Schoenwolf, G.C., Bleyl, S.B., Brauer, P.R. et al. (2009). *Larsen's Human Embryology*, 4e, 1–687. Philadelphia: Churchill Linvingstone.

8 Grijalva, J. and Vakili, K. (2013). Neonatal liver physiology. *Semin. Pediatr. Surg.* 22: 185–189.

9 Beath, S.V. (2003). Hepatic function and physiology in the newborn. *Semin. Neonatol.* 8: 337–346.

10 Wright, J.K., Roesel, J.F., and Lopez, R.R. (1994). Malrotation of the intestine in adulthood. *J. Tenn. Med. Assoc.* 87: 141–145.

11 Dahlberg, J.A., Adam, E.N., Palmer, J.E., and Parente, E.J. (2009). Gastrointestinal nonrotation in a neonatal foal. *Equine Vet. Educ.* 21 (10): 508–512.

12 Freeman, D.E., Koch, D.B., and Boles, C.L. (1979). Mesodiverticular bands as a cause of small intestinal strangulation and volvulus in the horse. *J. Am. Vet. Med. Assoc.* 175: 1089–1094.

13 Abutarbush, S.M., Shoemaker, R.W., and Bailey, J.V. (2003). Strangulation of the small intestines by a mesodiverticular band in 3 adult horses. *Can. Vet. J.* 44 (12): 1005.

14 Loynachan, A.T. (2014). Esophageal cyst in the duodenum of a foal. *J. Vet. Diagn. Invest.* 26 (2): 308–311.

15 Bassage, L.H., Habecker, P.L., Russell, E.A., and Ennulat, D. (2000). Colic in a horse associated with a massive cystic duplication of the ascending colon. *Equine Vet. J.* 32 (6): 565–568.

16 Pineiro-Carrero, V.M. and Pineiro, E.O. (2004). Liver. *Pediatrics* 113: 1097–1106.

17 Buddington, R.K. and Sangild, P.T. (2011). Development of the mammalian gastrointestinal tract, the resident microbiota, and the role of diet in early life. *J. Anim. Sci.* 89: 1506–1519.

18 Neu, J. and Li, N. (2003). The neonatal gastrointestinal tract: developmental anatomy, physiology, and clinical implications. *Neo Rev.* 4: 7–13.

19 Fintl, C., Pearson, G.T., Ricketts, S.W. et al. (2004). The development and distribution of the interstitial cells of Cajal in the intestine of the equine fetus and neonate. *J. Anat.* 205: 35–44.

20 Trahair, J.F. and Sangild, P.T. (1997). Systemic and luminal influences on the perinatal development of the gut. *Equine Vet. J. Suppl.* 29: 40–50.

21 Xu, R.J. (1996). Development of the newborn GI tract and its relation to colostrum intake: a review. *Reprod. Fertil. Dev.* 8: 35–48.

22 Ousey, J.C., Ghatei, M., Rossdale, P.D. et al. (1995). Gut hormone responses to feeding in healthy pony foals aged 0 to 7 days. *Biol. Reprod. Monogr.* 11: 87–96.

23 Divers, T.J. (2015). The equine liver in health and disease. *AAEP Proc.* 61: 66–103.

Chapter 15 Examination of the Digestive Tract

Section I Physical Examination of the Digestive System

David Wong

Diseases involving the digestive system in foals are commonly encountered and include disorders of the oral cavity, esophagus, stomach, small intestine, large intestine, and rectum, as well as other organs that support digestion such as the hepatobiliary system. Initial evaluation of the digestive tract involves a thorough physical examination and is complemented by diagnostic tests and procedures such as assessment of the CBC, serum biochemistry profile, and blood gas analysis. In some instances, diagnostic imaging modalities such as ultrasonography, endoscopy, and advanced imaging (radiography, computed tomography [CT], magnetic resonance imaging [MRI]) of the digestive tract and abdominal cavity can be necessary. Close attention and examination of the cardiovascular system should occur in conjunction with a general physical examination as many foals with digestive diseases (e.g., diarrhea, acute colic) have notable compromise of the cardiovascular system. Vital parameters such as heart rate, rectal temperature and respiratory rate should be collected and compared to age-specific values in healthy foals. Of note, this section discusses general physical examination techniques of the digestive tract whereas the examination and treatment of acute colic is discussed in Chapter 18.

Physical examination of the neonatal foal's digestive system includes an oral examination, abdominal auscultation, transabdominal ballottement, external abdominal palpation, and digital rectal examination. Examination of the oral cavity consists of assessment of the mucous membranes (color, capillary refill time, moistness, perfusion), teeth, tongue, and hard palate, as well as assessment for any congenital defects such as cleft palate (Figure 15.I.1a,b), pronounced disparity in mandibular-maxillary occlusion (brachygnathism, prognathism), or other maxillofacial deformities. Evaluation of the structure and function of the epiglottis and esophagus requires advanced imaging such as endoscopy, radiography (± contrast; Figure 15.I.1c), or fluoroscopy. Passage of a nasogastric tube is indicated in foals with suspected digestive disorders to assess the patency of the esophagus and detect the presence or absence of excessive gastric fluid. Auscultation is a rudimentary and subjective method of assessing motility of the large colon. Decreased or complete absence of intestinal sounds is suggestive of abnormal motility and ileus which can arise from inflammatory, ischemic, or obstructive lesions of the intestinal tract. In comparison, increased frequency and intensity of intestinal borborygmi can suggest enteritis or colitis. Abdominal auscultation in the foal is performed in a similar fashion as that in the adult horse: in the dorsal and ventral right and left flanks. Physical and visual inspection of abdominal contour may identify abdominal distention that might originate from gas or fluid distension of the large (or rarely small) intestine, uroabdomen, abdominal masses/abscess or peritonitis. A very large stomach in the equine neonate may produce a distended appearance of the caudal rib cage when viewed from above. Further, percussion of the abdomen during auscultation can reveal excess gas in the large intestine. Serial measurement of the abdominal circumference, measured at the same location (marked with a small, shaved area of hair) using a flexible tape measure, can provide a more objective and temporal assessment of progressive abdominal distension. Transabdominal ballottement is a technique used to detect masses or an excess volume of peritoneal fluid within the abdominal cavity. In neonatal foals, the abdominal wall is pliable enough to generate a wave with ballottement of the abdomen if a large amount of free fluid or a large mas occupies the abdominal cavity. Furthermore, external abdominal palpation of the neonatal foal's abdomen is possible because of their smaller body size but overall is of limited value; however, palpation may identify masses within the abdomen or disease of the external umbilicus. In addition, the inguinal rings and ventral abdomen also

Equine Neonatal Medicine, First Edition. Edited by David M. Wong and Pamela A. Wilkins.

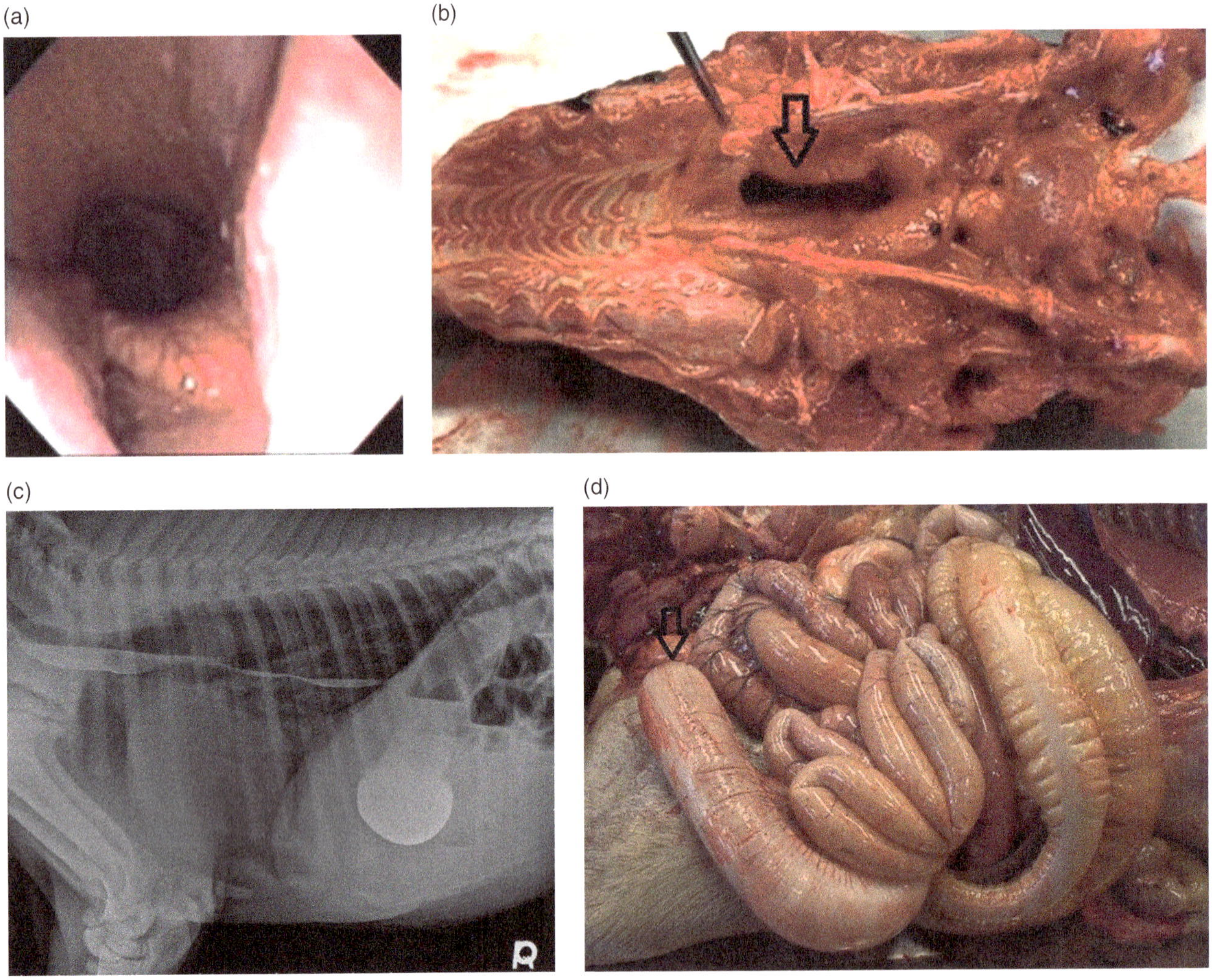

Figure 15.I.1 Various anomalies in the neonatal foal. (a) Endoscopic appearance of a cleft palate in a neonatal foal. (b) Postmortem specimen of a neonatal foal with a cleft palate (black arrow). (c) Lateral thoracic radiograph with contrast administered orally to highlight the esophagus. Note the dilation and contrast within the esophagus at the thoracic inlet. (d) Postmortem specimen of a neonatal foal with atresia ani. Note the blind end of the small colon (black arrow).

should be palpated for hernias. Because of the neonatal foal's size, only digital palpation of the rectum, using a well-lubricated gloved finger, is possible and may help identify abnormalities such as meconium impaction in the rectum. If a digital exam performed in a foal <24 hours of age reveals only mucus and no evidence of meconium, a congenital malformation such as atresia coli and atresia ani (Figure 15.I.1d) should be considered.

Observation of defecation and urination is also an important part of the assessment of the digestive tract. The presence of tenesmus, frequency (or lack) of defecation, and inspection of the feces (taking note of the consistency, smell, and color) are important in the clinical evaluation. Meconium is normally observed around the perineum over the first 24–48 hours. Early in the disease course of enteritis and/or colitis, fecal consistency may be normal, with diarrhea appearing at a later point. Distinguishing tenesmus (dorsoflexed posture, rear limbs under body) from stranguria (ventroflexed posture, limbs stretched out) can be difficult at times but can help rule out involvement of the urinary system. Other diagnostic procedures such as abdominocentesis, radiography, endoscopy, and ultrasonography of the digestive tract are discussed in the following sections.

Clinical Pathology

The hemogram, serum biochemistry profile, and blood gas analysis can provide an overall assessment of the foal's health as well as specifically develop differential diagnoses with regard to digestive system diseases. However, changes in the hemogram in diseases of the digestive tract are frequently nonspecific with alterations associated with sepsis, endotoxemia, and/or the systemic inflammatory response. The WBC and differential count are evaluated to guide the likelihood of a generalized or localized infection. A low-to-normal WBC count characterized by neutropenia, band neutrophils, and toxic changes in the cytoplasm of neutrophils is an indication of bacterial infection, possibly originating from the gastrointestinal tract (enteritis, colitis, intestinal devitalization or perforation, peritonitis) but is also commonly noted with sepsis. Relative polycythemia from hemoconcentration and splenic contraction may also be observed if there are ongoing fluid losses and/or decreased voluntary fluid intake. The serum biochemistry profile can show a variety of derangements, depending on organ system(s) and disease process. With respect to the digestive tract, electrolyte deficiencies such as hyponatremia, hypochloremia, hypokalemia, hypocalcemia, and hypomagnesemia are common, as is prerenal azotemia in neonatal foals with diarrhea. Hypoproteinemia and hypoalbuminemia also might be observed in protein-losing enteropathies, and hypoglobulinemia can be observed from failure of transfer of passive immunity or increased consumption of immunoglobulins due to an infectious disease process. Loss of bicarbonate, sequestration of bicarbonate from pooling of fluid in the intestine, compensatory free water consumption, and electrolyte derangements can result in metabolic acidosis in foals with disorders of the intestinal tract. In addition, hyperlactatemia and hypoglycemia may also be measured and are nonspecific reflections of decreased delivery of oxygen to tissues and decreased caloric consumption/hypermetabolism, respectively.

Section II Abdominocentesis and Cytologic Evaluation of Peritoneal Fluid

David Wong

Abdominocentesis is a common diagnostic procedure performed in foals to help evaluate abdominal disorders such as colic, peritonitis, and uroabdomen. The procedure is performed similar to the adult horse, with some suggesting the use of a teat cannula rather than a single-use hypodermic needle to collect peritoneal fluid in the foal [1]. This suggestion is based on the belief that a teat cannula might decrease the risk of intestinal laceration due to the thin-walled bowel in the foal; however, other studies have used needles (18–20 gauge × 2.5 cm) without complication [1–3]. Abdominocentesis can be performed in the standing foal with the clinician using assistants for proper restraint, however sedatives may be necessary, depending on the temperament and condition of the foal. Alternatively, the procedure can be performed in lateral recumbency and is preferred by some clinicians because of improved restraint.

The abdominocentesis site is preferably selected using ultrasonography to identify pockets of peritoneal fluid, but if ultrasonography is not available, a site just right of midline at the level of the most dependent portion of the abdomen is typically used. The haircoat should be clipped at the abdominocentesis site and disinfected with antiseptic scrub. When using a needle for abdominocentesis, some clinicians prefer to place a small local block of lidocaine (0.5–1 ml) at the insertion site to decrease movement of the foal; a local lidocaine block should always be used when using a teat cannula.

The veterinarian should wear sterile gloves and introduce the needle through the musculature at the selected site, then slowly advance the needle until fluid is obtained [3]. If no fluid is obtained, the clinician can rotate or reposition the needle; attempts to aspirate fluid with a syringe can also be employed. If fluid is still not obtained, an additional needle can be used at a different but local site. If the use of a teat cannula is preferred, a small stab incision using a sterile #15 blade must be made through the musculature at the selected site prior to insertion of the teat cannula. Fluid samples should be collected in EDTA tubes for cytologic analysis and clot tubes if culture is indicated or if biochemical analytes are going to be measured. Of note, it is not uncommon for a small amount of omentum to displace out of the abdomen through the stab incision after the teat cannula is removed; the clinician should sterilely transect any externalized omentum.

Normal reference intervals for peritoneal fluid have been determined in foals at various ages (Table 15.II.1). Peritoneal fluid from healthy foals should be clear, serous, and straw-colored [3]. Many of the parameters evaluated in peritoneal fluid are similar to adult values, with one notable difference being that WBC counts >1,500 cells/μl are considered abnormal in the foal, as compared to >5,000–10,000 cells/μl in adult horses [2, 4]. Cytology of peritoneal fluid is also similar to those of healthy adult horses and should have low cellularity and consist of mononuclear cells with few to no neutrophils or red blood cells.

Peritoneal fluid is frequently normal in foals with enteritis or early stages of mechanical obstruction; the cell count and protein concentration can progressively rise as these conditions progress. Foals with strangulating obstruction of the intestine frequently have elevated peritoneal fluid protein concentrations and nucleated cell counts. Serosanguinous peritoneal fluid suggests devitalized bowel with transudation of leukocytes, erythrocytes, and protein. Elevated nucleated cell counts with degenerate neutrophils and bacteria (Figure 15.II.1) are suggestive of septic peritonitis, which can arise from an abdominal abscess, umbilical remnant infection, or generalized sepsis. Foals with uroperitoneum have large volumes of clear to pale-yellow peritoneal fluid that usually has a relatively low cell count and protein concentration.

Of interest, various coagulation parameters have also been measured in peritoneal fluid as postoperative intra-abdominal adhesion formation is purportedly more

Equine Neonatal Medicine, First Edition. Edited by David M. Wong and Pamela A. Wilkins.

Table 15.II.1 Peritoneal fluid parameters from various aged foals reported as mean ± SD (range) [3, 4].

	32 Foals Mean age 45 days (range 14–75 days)	17 Foals Mean age 68 days (Range 13–134 days)		32 Foals Mean age 45 days (range 14–75 days)
Nucleated cells (/μl)	1418 ± 1077	451 ± 230	Glucose (mg/dl)	136.9 ± 21 (100–178)
Neutrophils (%)	15.3 ± 20.4	43 (2–94)	AST (IU/l)	50 ± 18.9 (28–120)
Lg mononuclear cells (%)	43.8 ± 24.0	54 (5–98)	ALP (IU/l)	43.6 ± 22 (13–82)
Sm mononuclear cells (%)	22.3 ± 24.5		LDH (IU/l)	46.5 ± 22 (23–108)
Eosinophils (%)	0	4 (one foal)	Creatinine (mg/dl)	1.39 ± 0.22 (0.91–1.87)
Total protein (gm/dl)	1.8 ± 0.7	1.2 ± 0.3	Sodium (mEq/l)	133.6 ± 2.18 (128–137)
Red blood cells (/μl)	12 070 ± 15 219		Chloride (mEq/l)	98.7 ± 4.16 (92–106)
			Potassium (mEq/l)	4.2 ± 0.36 (3.6–4.9)
			Fibrinogen (mg/dl)	<200

Note: ALP – alkaline phosphatase; AST – aspartate aminotransferase; LDH – lactate dehydrogenase.

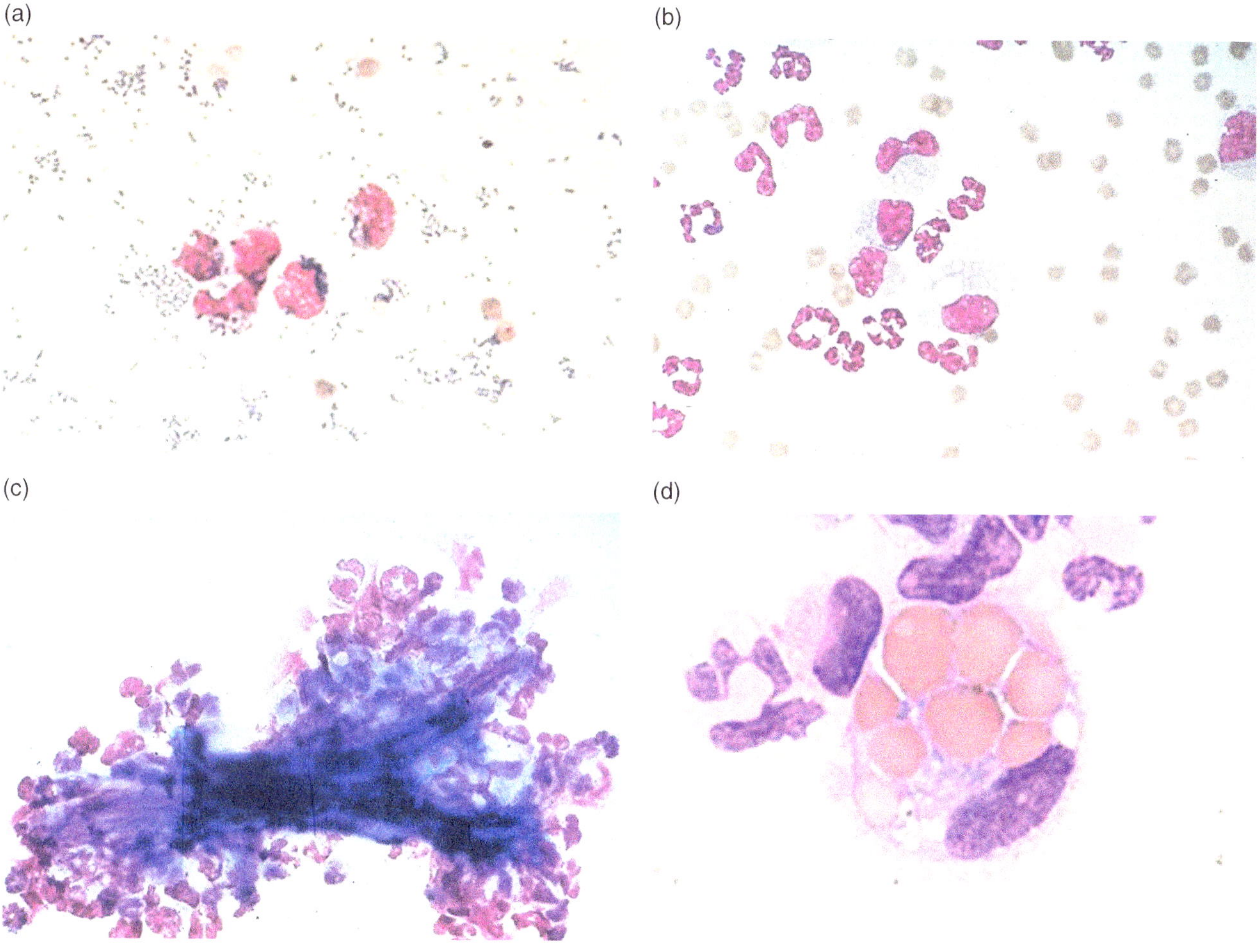

Figure 15.II.1 Various abdominal fluid samples from horses. (a) Sample contains numerous degenerate neutrophils and numerous bacteria associated with septic purulent inflammation. (b) Inflammatory abdominal fluid sample indicated by numerous nondegenerate neutrophils along with fewer macrophages. (c) Sample demonstrates numerous degenerate neutrophils surrounding a plant particle, suggestive of gastrointestinal compromise. (d) Macrophage phagocytosing mature erythrocytes, consistent with a hemorrhagic abdominal effusion.

Table 15.II.2 Median (interquartile range) values of antiplasmin activity, D-dimer concentration, fibrinogen concentration, and plasminogen activity in the abdominal fluid of horses with (n = 16 foals, 19 adults) and without (25 foals, 20 adults) colic [5].

Variable	Antiplasmin (% of control)	D-dimer (ng/ml)	Fibrinogen (mg/dl)	Plasminogen (% of control)
Foals without colic	14 (5.5–22.5)	677 (192–1796)	11 (5–24)	20 (16–32)
Foals with colic	41 (23–67)	3179 (935–3664)	48 (12–85)	46 (24–64)
Adults without colic	20 (15–26)	339 (64–694)	12 (5–22)	22 (14–40)
Adults with colic	42 (25–52)	2727 (2016–3627)	45 (16–59)	37 (22–45)

common in foals that require surgical abdominal exploration for acute abdominal pain compared to adult horses. In one study, coagulation factors were compared between adult horses and foals with the intent of identifying hemostatic imbalances that suggested differences in peritoneal environment that would promote higher frequency of intra-abdominal adhesion formation in foals compared to adults [5]. In this study, no differences in antiplasmin, D-dimer, fibrinogen, and plasminogen were measured (Table 15.II.2) between healthy foals and adult horses and foals and adult horses that required exploratory celiotomy for colic [5].

Complications of abdominocentesis are very low but include enterocentesis and perforation or laceration of the gastrointestinal tract or spleen. Peritonitis and abdominal well cellulitis can rarely occur after enterocentesis [6]. As noted, if a teat cannula is used, omentum can prolapse through the abdominocentesis site [2].

References

1 Tulleners, E.P. (1983). Complications of abdominocentesis in the horse. *J. Am. Vet. Med. Assoc.* 182: 232–2341.

2 Bartmann, C.P., Freeman, D.E., Glitz, F. et al. (2002). Diagnosis and surgical management of colic in the foal: literature review and a retrospective study. *Clin. Tech. Equine* 1 (3): 125–142.

3 Behrens, E., Parraga, M.E., Nassiff, A. et al. (1990). Reference values of peritoneal fluid from healthy foals. *Equine Vet. Sci.* 10: 348–352.

4 Grindem, C.B., Fairley, N.M., Uhlinger, C.A. et al. (1990). Peritoneal fluid values from healthy foals. *Equine Vet. J.* 22: 359–361.

5 Watts, A.E., Fubini, S.L., Todhunter, R.J. et al. (2011). Comparison of plasma and peritoneal indices of fibrinolysis between foals and adult horses with and without colic. *Am. J. Vet. Res.* 72: 1535–1540.

6 Siex, M.T. and Wilson, J.H. (1992). Morbidity associated with abdominocentesis – a prospective study. *Equine Vet. J. Suppl.* 13: 23–25.

Section III Ultrasonographic Examination of the Neonatal Foal Abdomen

Kim A. Sprayberry and David Wong

Comprehensive evaluation of the neonatal foal with signs of abdominal disease incorporates physical examination, imaging, and clinicopathologic assessment. Used in combination with radiography or as a stand-alone imaging modality, ultrasound evaluation of the abdominal cavity can be a high-yield diagnostic test. Because the newborn foal is not a hindgut fermenter, the gastrointestinal (GI) segments can usually be imaged effectively because of fewer gas interfaces to reflect the acoustic beam before it can enter a soft-tissue organ. Sonographic imaging is not affected by intracavitary fluid effusions and reveals abnormalities of both soft tissue and bony origin. This makes many abdominal conditions in foals amenable to sonographic investigation, including colic, hemorrhage, and urinary tract disorders.

Preparing for the Ultrasound Examination

The acoustic beam emitted from the ultrasound transducer is halted by air trapped in the hair coat; therefore, the area to be scanned should be either clipped or wetted with warmed rubbing alcohol. Alcohol displaces the air between and beneath hairs and creates an interface for transfer of the acoustic beam into the body in the presence of hair. If the hair is clipped, ultrasound coupling gel is applied to the skin. Clipping the haircoat is generally recommended and facilitates higher image resolution, but the author prefers not to clip hair for examining foals, especially in cold climates. Application of water to the hair will not yield the same result and is not helpful for ultrasound imaging. Rubbing alcohol should be warmed by preplacing one to two plastic bottles in a bucket of hot water (not in a microwave oven) for a few minutes before applying to the foal's skin. The alcohol is applied in a unidirectional fashion (in direction of hair growth); rubbing against the nap introduces air and defeats the purpose of applying the alcohol.

Clipping of the hair is recommended for ultrasound of superficial structures such as the umbilicus, as the higher-frequency transducers used to image these structures perform best in the absence of hair. After the ultrasound examination, the foal should be toweled dry as clipping and applying alcohol greatly increases evaporative heat transfer and even healthy foals may struggle with thermodynamic homeostasis.

A high-frequency transducer such as a 4–9 MHz microconvex array is recommended when evaluating finer abdominal structures, such as the small intestinal wall or umbilical structures; however, any size probe, including a macroconvex probes, will yield valuable information. To evaluate the abdomen thoroughly and expediently, a systematic approach from caudal to cranial and ventral to dorsal is used. Many neonatal abdominal ultrasounds are performed in clinically ill patients; as such, lateral recumbency is easily attained.

Sonographic Survey of the Abdomen

Beginning in the cranial-most aspect of the abdomen, at intercostal (ICS) space 7 on the left side, the first structure to be encountered, lying in contact with the diaphragm, is the liver. Just caudal (ICS 6–12 depending on the volume of gastric contents) lies a curvilinear arc that represents the greater curvature of the stomach (Figure 15.III.1). The liquid contents of the neonatal stomach enable viewing of the luminal contents. By about 7 days of age [1], gas echoes fill the stomach, limiting evaluation to the mural structures. Immediately caudal to and in contact with the stomach lies the cranial pole of the spleen, which has a solid, stromal architecture and soft-tissue echogenicity. The spleen should be more echogenic than the liver; the difference is easily appreciated where the caudal edge of the left liver lobe lies in contact with the stomach and cranial pole of the

Equine Neonatal Medicine, First Edition. Edited by David M. Wong and Pamela A. Wilkins.

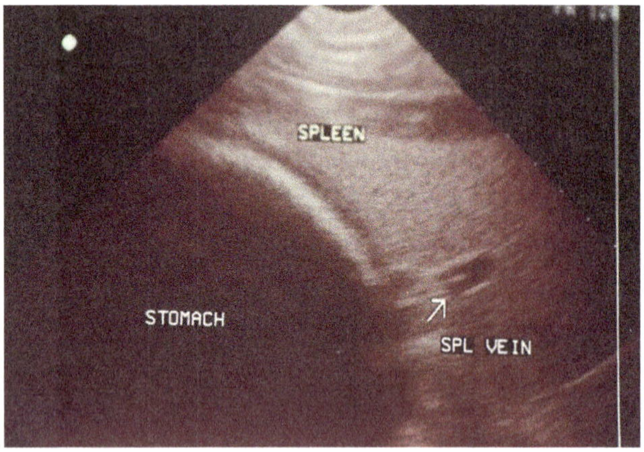

Figure 15.III.1 Sonogram of structures in the left cranial region of the abdomen in a healthy foal. Notice the proximity between the stomach and spleen, and the tight radius of curvature of the stomach.

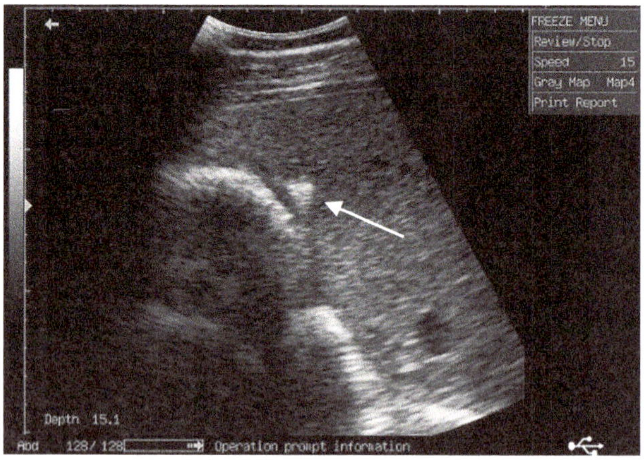

Figure 15.III.2 Sonogram from the cranial region of the right side of the abdomen in a healthy foal. The duodenum (white arrow) is in a contractile state, lying between the white curvilinear arcs of the right dorsal colon and the more echogenic liver. Close inspection of the duodenum reveals the hypoechoic outer wall segments and the hyperechoic mucosa, bunched up by contractile motility.

spleen, in ICS 8–10 on the left side. The spleen can be viewed from ICS 7 back to the paralumbar fossa area, depending on the state of splenic contraction or engorgement at the time of examination. The left kidney is a hypoechoic structure lying axial to the spleen from ICS 15 to the caudal border of the paralumbar fossa and can be recognized by the typical oblong shape and the corticomedullary anatomic pattern with the echogenic cortex, hypoechoic medulla, and hyperechoic renal pelvis. In the groin area ventral to the paralumbar fossa and in the area caudal to the fossa, segments of jejunum can often be seen. Large colon segments occupy most of the ventral abdomen in all quadrants and, unlike in older foals and adult horses, will be filled with fluid rather than with a sonoreflective gas layer. The urinary bladder is viewed in the caudoventral aspect of the abdomen.

On the right side of the body, again proceeding cranial-to-caudal, the first structure seen on the abdominal side of the diaphragm, in ICS 7–14, is the liver. The liver lies in the cranioventral and middle regions of the abdomen in these rib spaces and is also seen in the dorsal abdomen at its caudal-most extent in ICS 14. Bile ducts and hepatic blood vessels can be seen in the liver parenchyma, and the sharpness of the lobe edges and echogenicity of the parenchyma can be appreciated. Caudal and ventral to the liver in ICS 7–12, the examiner will see a long white curvilinear echo corresponding with the right dorsal colon. Beginning about ICS 10, the duodenum can be viewed in transverse section lying dorsal to the surface of the right dorsal colon and the ventral and caudal margin of the liver (Figure 15.III.2). To appreciate the structure, it may be necessary to keep the transducer still and observe for the relaxation-contraction cycle of the duodenum, as duodenal motility is typically intermittent. The duodenum can be seen as far caudally as the cranial margin of the paralumbar fossa, lying ventral to the right kidney and dorsal to the base of the cecum. Moving the transducer ventrally from the right kidney, the examiner can view portions of the cecal body and ventral large colon segments.

While surveying visceral structures, several primary aspects of anatomy and function should be noted: the mural width of the small and large intestine walls; the appearance of the walls, whatever the thickness (is there a hypoechoic band, indicating edema, within the wall layers, is there hyperechoic mucosa); degree of distention and motility of various segments; the nature of the luminal contents; and the contractility patterns, in any discrete segment and in the context of overall intestinal motility. Particularly with gastrointestinal disorders, which can be fulminant and rapidly changing, serial imaging of an ill foal whose condition is labile can be helpful. The sonographic observations should also be interpreted in light of ongoing changes in physical status, clinicopathology test values, and response to treatment. Response to initial treatment can itself be an important diagnostic factor, because surgical and medical lesions of the GI tract can manifest very similarly in foals.

Diseases of the Abdomen

Gastrointestinal (GI) Tract Disease

The major morbid conditions affecting the GI tract of compromised newborn foals – prematurity, asphyxia-related injury, and septicemia – can all induce injury and dysfunction, including diarrhea, in the GI tract [2, 3]. All can lead to motility impairment and functional failure of the blood-mucosal barrier; these two problems are responsible for many of the clinical signs and abnormalities affecting the compromised neonate. The GI tract constitutes a significant potential portal of entry for microbes and a vulnerable target for bacteremic showering by pathogens that entered the body by another route [3].

Gastroduodenal Ileus

The most common indicator of GI tract injury from sepsis or hypoxic-ischemic insult in a foal is motility failure. Gastroduodenal ileus results in a distended, hypomotile stomach and duodenum filled with milk or residual fluid that is not proceeding in the aboral direction (Figures 15.III.3 and 15.III.4). When the stomach is seen distended and atonic on the left side of the abdomen, the duodenum will usually be found in a similar state on the right side. Normal small intestinal mural thickness in foals is ≤3 mm [1, 4, 5]. As mentioned, the qualitative appearance of the viscus wall should be noted, even if the mural width is normal. Scanning a bowel segment with a higher-frequency probe is needed to distinguish the layers of the bowel wall; if available, this should be performed to confirm the following normal echo patterns [4, 6]:

> hyperechoic mucosal surface → hypoechoic mucosa → hyperechoic submucosa → hypoechoic muscularis propria → hyperechoic serosa

Appearance of hypoechoic edema in the bowel wall even before there is thickening of the overall dimensions may be seen with strangulating lesions, for instance, and the appearance of hyperechoic gas echoes within the wall

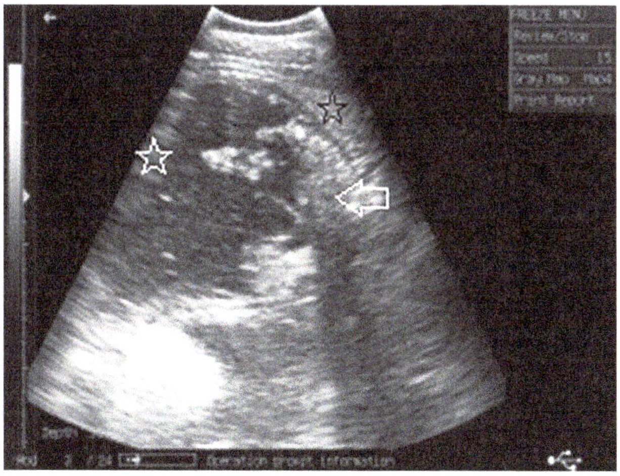

Figure 15.III.3 Stomach of a healthy foal that has suckled recently. Clotting of milk can be seen lying along the greater curvature (arrow). Notice the slice of reverberation artifact generated by aerated lung to the left side of the image (white star), and the stomach's immediate proximity to the spleen (black star).

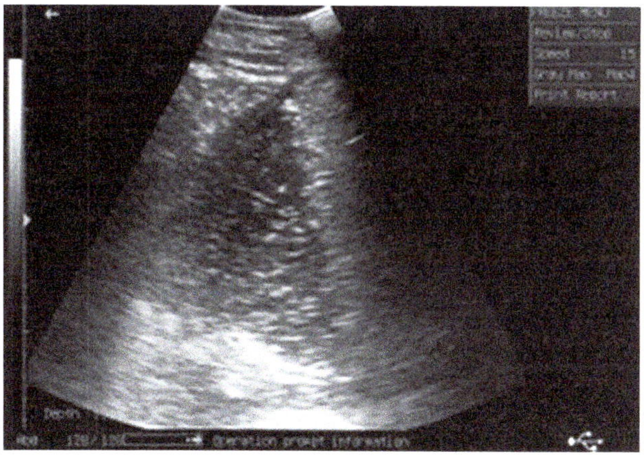

Figure 15.III.4 gastric distension from delayed gastric emptying in a neonatal foal with enteritis and ileus. This stomach is filled with gassy liquid chyme from the foal's last milk meal. Notice the linear interface between the echogenic material (right) and gassy material (hypoechoic area with white gas echoes on the left); such an interface suggests delayed emptying and settling of contents into their respective phases.

layers is diagnostic for pneumatosis intestinalis and necrotizing enterocolitis [7].

Detection of distension and delayed emptying of the stomach and duodenum facilitates treatment decisions:

1) *Distension and atony necessitate placement of an indwelling feeding tube to facilitate decompression.* This may be necessary every few hours. Enteral feeding should be withheld or restricted until contractility is restored.
2) *Persistent gastric engorgement and absence of propulsive contractions in a neonate prompt longer-term care decisions.* This could be referral to a hospital or discussing with the owner the logistics of home care for the foal. Foals that cannot tolerate enteral feeding need partial or total parenteral nutrition, prokinetic agents, and gastroprotectants in addition to antimicrobials and intravenous fluids. Incorporating imaging into morning and evening physical examinations can help determine the return of contractility and when to begin introducing enteral feeding.

Gastritis and ulcer formation in neonatal foals is a multifactorial and complex clinical entity (Chapter 17), but visceral hypoperfusion secondary to sepsis-associated hypotension or from failure to maintain euhydration likely constitute risk factors for gastritis that are unrelated to luminal acidity alone, as ulcers can develop and progress to the point of gastric perforation even while foals are receiving gastroprotectants and anti-ulcer drugs. Reflux of duodenal fluids into the stomach may also injure the mucosa by contact with bile acids and pancreatic secretions. Ulcer formation proceeding to gastric perforation can be clinically silent, especially in recumbent, obtunded

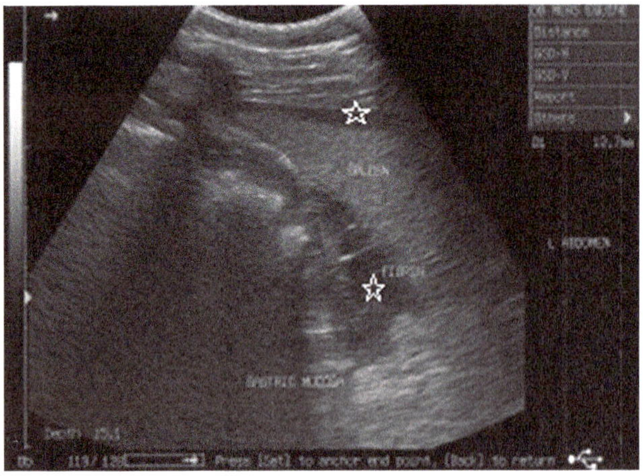

Figure 15.III.5 Sonogram of the left cranial region of the abdomen of a foal with severe sepsis and the complication of deep gastric ulceration. A local accumulation of free peritoneal fluid can be seen between the spleen and body wall and between the stomach and spleen (white stars), and adhesion formation is underway as denoted by the fibrin strands extending between the stomach and spleen. On necropsy the gastric wall section depicted here, in the region of the ulcers, was inflamed across its width and exudative on the serosal surface, although it was not yet anatomically ruptured.

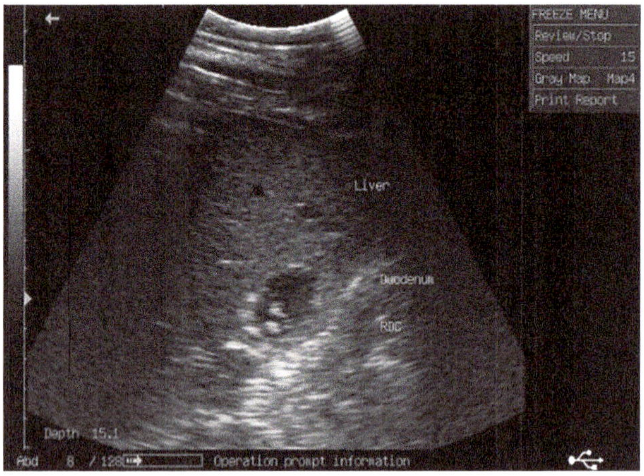

Figure 15.III.6 Duodenitis and ileus as a feature of severe enteritis in a foal with *Clostridium perfringens* type A. This sonogram is from the right side in mid-abdomen. Notice the thickened duodenal wall and gassy luminal contents. Although this duodenum is open and appears patent, ileus creates pseudo-obstruction, and delayed gastric emptying, and reflux can be anticipated. In real time, sonography would indicate little to no effective peristaltic contractions in the duodenum at this site.

foals. Gastric endoscopy is necessary for diagnosis of gastric ulcers, but sonographic imaging of the area in the left cranial abdomen where the liver, stomach, and spleen lie in contact can reveal gastric wall edema and serositis as local effects of severe ulcerative gastritis and incipient perforation (Figure 15.III.5).

Enteritis and Enterocolitis

Bacterial and viral pathogens can cause enteritis or enterocolitis in foals beginning on the first day of life. The sonographic hallmark of enteritis of any etiology is the combination of distension, hypomotility (although hypermotility may be seen in the prodromal stages), intestinal walls of normal or thickened width, and hypoechoic to echogenic gassy luminal contents (Figure 15.III.6). The luminal surface can be hyperechoic due to small gas bubbles trapped between the villous tips. When hyperechoic shadows extend into this typically hypoechoic submucosal layer, necrotizing enteritis or enterocolitis should be considered. This extension of gas bubbles into the submucosa is termed *pneumatosis intestinalis* (Figure 15.III.7) and can progress to extensive intestinal damage that may result in viscus rupture. In a retrospective study of 89 foals with GI disease, *pneumatosis intestinalis* was negatively associated with outcome and was the only ultrasonographic sign with prognostic value [7]. Radiographically, this lesion appears as a radiolucent region within the wall of the small and/or large intestines. With severe enteritis, transudative to exudative fluid may also accumulate in the peritoneal fluid,

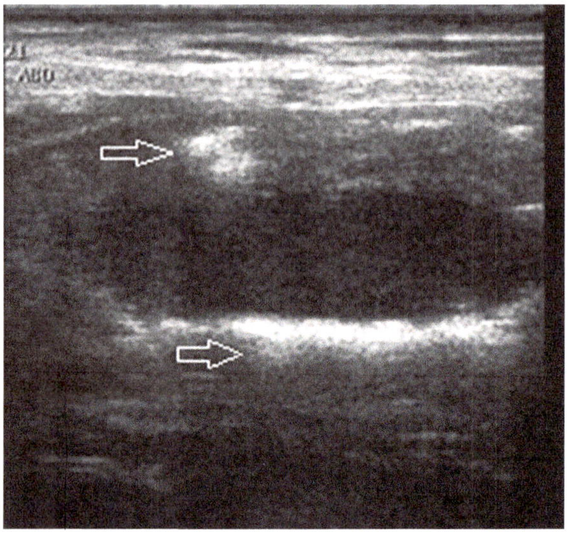

Figure 15.III.7 Ultrasonographic image of intramural hyperechoic gas echoes (arrows) within the small intestine of a foal. *Source:* Image courtesy of Dr. Cristobal Navas de Solis, University of Pennsylvania.

setting the foal up for fibrous adhesions in the weeks to months following resolution of the enteritis. Distended small intestinal segments are easy to find and are the dominant feature in the affected foal's abdomen (Figure 15.III.8). Enteritis and enterocolitis in newborn foals are severe systemic diseases, often attended by dehydration, pain, and marked acid-base and metabolic alterations. Common

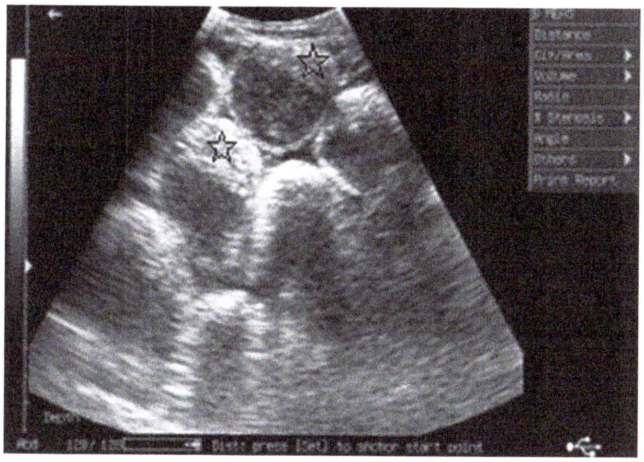

Figure 15.III.8 Sonogram from a neonatal foal with ileus secondary to rotaviral enteritis. Notice the nesting of jejunal segments, the distension, and the ventral settling of luminal contents (stars) seen with motility failure (ventral is upward in this image). This image was obtained in the left caudal region of the abdomen.

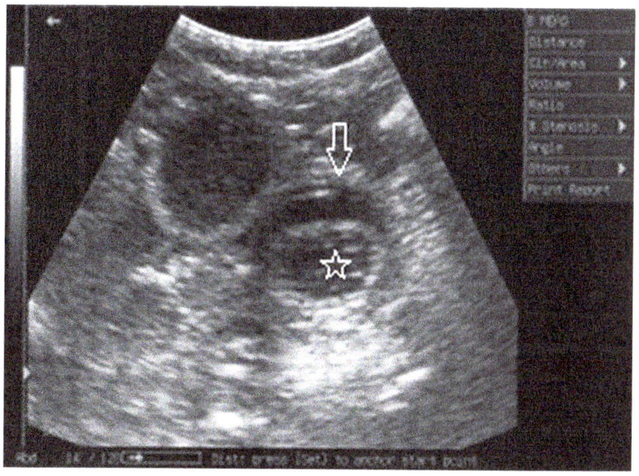

Figure 15.III.9 Sonogram of jejunojejunal intussusception in a week-old foal with enteritis. The fluid-filled intussusceptum segment (star) can be seen surrounded by the intussuscipiens segment (arrow).

causes in neonatal foals include bacterial infection (*Clostridium perfringens* type A or C, *Clostridium difficile*, *Enterococcus durans*, and *Salmonella* spp) and viral infection (rotavirus, coronavirus). Less common pathogens reported in diarrheic foals include *Aeromonas hydrophila*, *Bacteroides fragilis*, *Cryptosporidium parvum*, and adenovirus [3]. Features of mucosal barrier compromise may be noted along with fever, but fever in neonatal foals is not a reliable clinical finding and its absence should not be relied on to rule out illness.

Strangulation

The sonographic appearance of strangulated small intestine is similar to that of enteritis/enterocolitis [8], but venous congestion in the strangulated bowel wall leads to progressive increase in mural width and engorgement of mesenteric vasculature over time. Some causes of intestinal strangulation in neonatal foals include volvulus; incarceration through a mesenteric rent or congenital anomaly such as Meckel's diverticulum; herniation through the inguinal ring; or a rupture in the diaphragm. Because the initial appearance of strangulated small intestine may resemble that of enteritis, a global assessment of the foal is necessary to determining whether the foal requires surgical intervention. Analysis of peritoneal fluid, clinicopathologic results, physical status, and response to analgesics help make this determination.

Intussusception

Intestinal intussusception can occur in neonatal foals but is more common in foals several months of age and older. Development of intussusception arises from differences in motility between neighboring segments of bowel, and may be associated with enteritis, administration of the prokinetic neostigmine, and parasitism. Intussuscepted intestine has an easily recognizable sonographic appearance formed from the concentric layering of one bowel segment (intussusceptum) inside an outer segment (intussuscipiens; Figure 15.III.9) [9, 10]. Types of intussusceptions include jejunojejunal, ileal-ileal, ileocecal, cecocolic, or cecocecal [10]. Clinical signs and severity of colic depend on length of involved bowel segment and whether the mesenteric blood vessels attached to the intussusceptum are obstructed. Diagnosis of an intussusception typically warrants surgical correction, and in older foals and horses, this is likely true. However, a report [6] detailing the existence of intussusceptions as an incidental finding in healthy, asymptomatic Standardbred foals suggests that in neonates, surgery is not always needed. The findings in that study corroborate observations by the author, who has observed one or more jejunojejunal intussusceptions arising in hospitalized foals and resolving spontaneously (unpublished data).

Most causes of colic in neonatal foals are associated with medical problems of the GI tract. In a recent retrospective study [8] of colic in 137 neonatal foals (<30 days of age; median age, 2 days) at a referral hospital, 89% of foals had conditions that were managed medically. In that population of 137 foals, enterocolitis, meconium-related colic, and transient colic of undetermined cause, but managed medically, were the most common diagnoses. In the 11% of foals that underwent surgery for colic, small intestine strangulating obstruction was the most frequent diagnosis, with volvulus, intussusception, and mesenteric rent comprising most of these cases.

Meconium Impaction (Retention)

Meconium is a sterile concretion of intestinal cells and secretions that accumulates in the intestine during gestation and becomes sufficiently tenacious or inspissated in some newborn foals that it becomes impacted in the large intestine or rectum resulting in obstruction. Ultrasound is sensitive at detecting the impacted colon segment and the length or extent of the retained luminal material (Figure 15.III.10). Meconium is usually detected in the caudal part of the abdomen. In a retrospective study [8], ultrasound was helpful in distinguishing large from small intestinal disease, and, within a given portion of the intestine, the nature of the disease. Distended, hypodynamic small intestine was seen more frequently with strangulating lesions, enterocolitis, and necrotizing enterocolitis than with meconium-associated colic. In the large intestine, fluid distension was seen more frequently with enterocolitis and necrotizing enterocolitis than with meconium retention. Thickening of the bowel wall was also sensitively detected: Mural thickening in the small intestine was seen with strangulating obstructions, enterocolitis, and necrotizing enterolitis, but not with meconium-associated, transient medical colic, or other forms of colic. Thickening of the large intestine wall was seen only in foals with necrotizing enterocolitis. The fact that mural thickening was seen with strangulating small bowel lesions and with inflammatory bowel lesions underscores how sonography can be useful at detecting the site of abnormality but must be supported with physical exam and clinicopathologic data when establishing a diagnosis. For example, in the scenario of colic in the neonatal foal with thickened small intestine walls, fever, leukopenia, abnormal serum electrolyte values, and fluid accumulating in both the small and large intestine point toward enterocolitis. Severity of pain and response to pain controlling medications is also clinically useful. In the aforementioned study [8], neonates with a strangulating small intestine lesion (usually volvulus) were significantly more likely to have severe and continuous pain than foals with medical colic; fewer foals with strangulating lesions responded to analgesics compared to foals with medical colic.

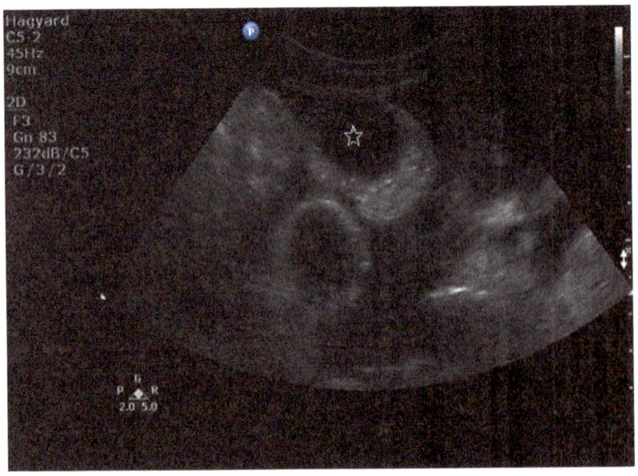

Figure 15.III.10 Sonogram from the caudal region of the abdomen in a 1-day-old foal with failure to pass meconium. Despite its solid physical consistency, meconium images as hypoechoic to anechoic material. In this view, the small colon is seen in transverse section and the round, dark, anechoechoic areas (star) are meconium balls.

A protocol of focused abdominal scanning for use in emergent cases has been reported [11]. The technique, deemed fast localized abdominal sonography in horses, has been used to good effect in human [12] and small animal [13] medicine. Abdominal imaging is limited to assessing visceral structures and free peritoneal fluid volume at seven locations, which were determined from earlier reports of sites that were fruitful for scanning in horses with colic. In this 2011 report of horses with colic [11], use of the focused technique could be quickly learned, and enabled quick evaluation (mean exam time, 10.7 minutes) with acceptable sensitivity, specificity, and predictive values in horses whose clinical condition made performing a complete abdominal survey impossible. Foals' small size usually means that a full survey of the abdomen can be undertaken relatively quickly but use of the focused protocol may be helpful.

Urinary Tract Abnormalities

Umbilical Remnant Anatomy

Overlap exists among clinical signs of GI and urinary tract disease, as colic and diarrhea can be seen in diseases of both systems. Ultrasound can help discern possible sources of disease. The umbilical cord should rupture approximately 1–2 in. from the abdominal wall [14], at which time the vascular structures inside the cord contract and occlude further blood flow. Inside the umbilical cord are four structures that can be assessed sonographically: two umbilical arteries, one umbilical vein, and the urachus, all bundled into a single cord by an outer adventitial covering.

The maximum normal cord length in Thoroughbreds is <84 cm (range, 36–83 cm; mean, 55 cm), with up to four twists along its length [15]. Cord length is relevant because an abnormally long cord can become excessively torsed or wrapped around the fetus' trunk or limbs in utero, strangulating or impinging the structures within it. Upstream dilatation and pressure in the urachus and bladder created by cord impingement can predispose to higher-than-normal intravesicular volume, and bladder rupture, during parturition. A short umbilical cord increases the degree of traction placed on the placenta during parturition and can cause premature placental separation and foal death if a human attendant is not present. Short cord length can also place tension on the foal's urachus during passage through the birth canal, increasing the risk for tearing and urine leakage postpartum. Cord length can be subjectively appreciated during sonographic monitoring of the pregnant mare.

In the fetal vasculature, the umbilical arteries arise as branches of the pudendal arteries, which are themselves branches of the internal iliac arteries. From their origins on the pudendal arteries in the dorsocaudal aspect of the abdomen, the umbilical arteries flow cranially and ventrally toward the bladder, where each travel on its respective side along the lateral aspect of the bladder. From its entry site at the umbilical stalk, the umbilical vein courses cranially along abdominal midline until entering the liver. In the weeks following birth, the umbilical vein atrophies and becomes the cordlike round ligament of the liver, running through the fatty connective tissue of the falciform ligament. The umbilical arteries also undergo involution to become the round ligaments of the bladder. The urachus is not a walled tubular structure but is the potential space running along the umbilical blood vessels and bound by the adventitial layer. In the fetus, the urachus conducts urine from the fetal bladder to the allantoic cavity. At birth, it should involute and close and urine should be voided through the urethra.

Because the bladder lies close to the ventral abdominal wall in neonates, the umbilical arteries are still amenable to ultrasonography. High-resolution images are needed for determining the dimensions of small structures such as arteries and vein, and this is one study for which the author routinely clips the hair around the base of the umbilicus, between the base and the groin, and between the base and the liver. Foals can be scanned standing, in lateral recumbency, or in a semidorsal recumbent position. Transducer frequencies of 6–10 MHz yield useful images for evaluation of the umbilical remnants.

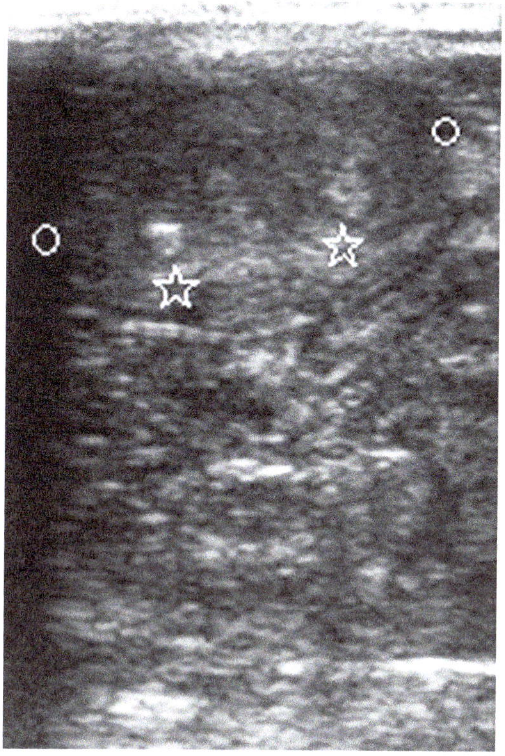

Figure 15.III.11 Sonogram of the internal umbilical remnants obtained at the posterior aspect of the base of the umbilicus in a healthy 24-hour-old foal. The two umbilical artery remnants (stars) are seen in transverse section. The tissue space lying between the two arteries is the remnant of the urachus, which conducted urine from the fetal bladder through the umbilical cord into the allantoic space during gestation. The length of the overall structure at this location (white dots indicate measuring points) should be ≤2.5 cm.

Omphalophlebitis

The umbilical arteries and vein should be imaged along their full length. The transducer is placed on the cranial aspect of the umbilical stalk and the umbilical vein is observed in the transverse plane and longitudinal plane running from the umbilical base cranially toward the liver. It should be <1 cm in diameter throughout its length, with some narrowing about halfway between the base and the point where the vein merges into the liver [5, 16]. The umbilical arteries are observed by placing the probe caudal to the umbilical base. At this juncture, the arteries and urachus are seen together in an oblong grouping, and the long axis diameter should be <2.5 cm (Figure 15.III.11). Moving the probe caudally along midline, the urachus will disappear and the arteries will diverge laterally along the bladder wall. When imaged separately, each umbilical artery remnant in transverse section should be <1 cm. It is easier to discern the arteries when the bladder contains urine. Of the umbilical structures, the urachus is the most commonly infected [17]. Infection appears as soft-tissue or echogenic material in the urachal lumen or in the tissue space around the arteries and/or urachus. Umbilical infections are first noticed by thickening, edema, or exudate at the umbilical stalk (Figure 15.III.12). Infection can cause the urachus to become patent again and drip urine. Infection that tracks internally from the base can cause cellulitis of the subcutaneous tissues and peritonitis. Internal structures can be infected even if the external portion of the stalk appears normal. Development of a urachal diverticulum (Figure 15.III.13) is also possible, although uncommon. Umbilical vein infections can track cranially and enter the liver; this condition typically manifests in foals several weeks to months old, manifesting as an unthrifty foal (Figure 15.III.14).

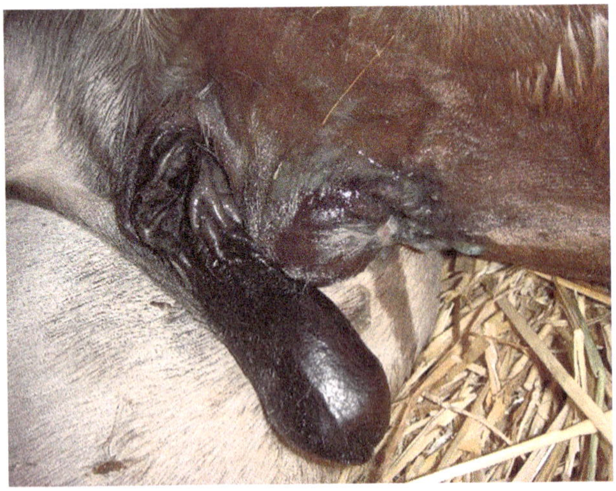

Figure 15.III.12 Umbilical area in a 2-week-old colt with omphalitis. Notice the edema surrounding and involving the umbilical base, and the moisture from draining exudate.

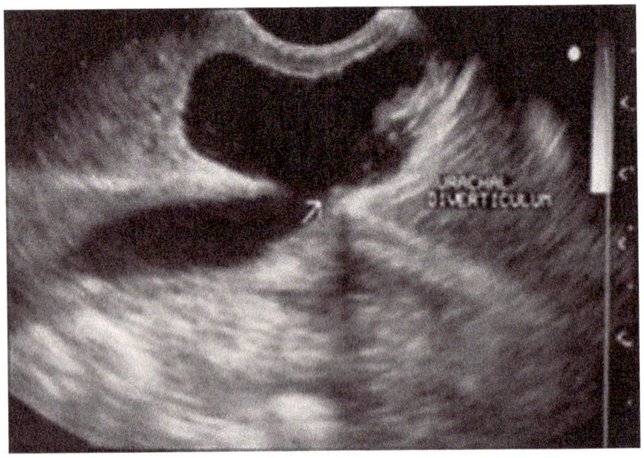

Figure 15.III.13 Sonogram of a urachal diverticulum in a newborn foal. Notice the anechoic urine at the ventral abdomen (top of the image), which communicates with the apex of the bladder (arrow). *Source:* Image courtesy of Dr. Fairfield Bain.

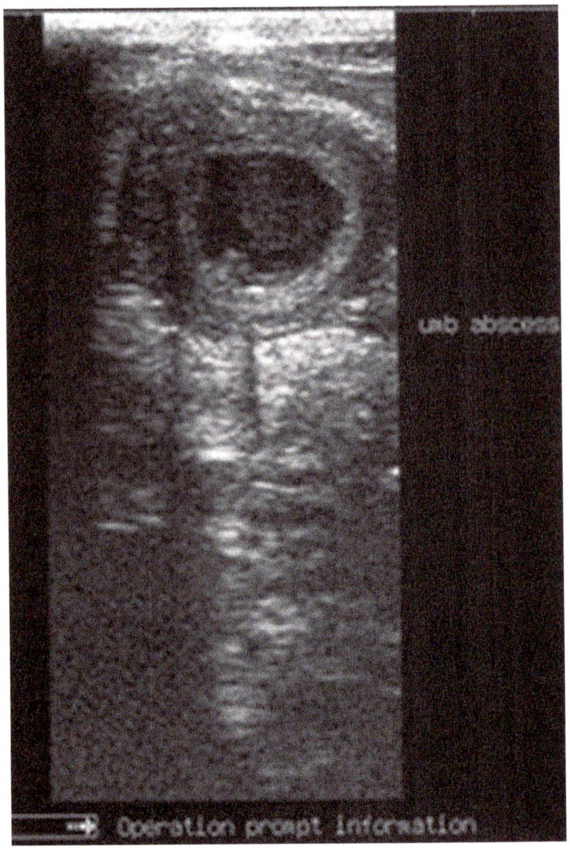

Figure 15.III.14 Sonogram of the umbilical vein in a 4-week-old foal that had omphalophlebitis as a neonate. Treatment had led to apparent resolution of infection at the externally visible umbilical stalk, but ultrasound revealed persistence of infection in this internal part of the vascular remnant. Exudative fluid is seen as the hypoechoic fluid in the lumen of the vascular structure, and the thickened walls of the structure are easily appreciated. This image was acquired on ventral midline 6 cm cranial to the umbilical base.

Uroperitoneum

Leaking of urine into the peritoneal cavity may result from rupture of the bladder, urachus, ureters, or urethra, but bladder and urachal rupture are most common. Underlying conditions associated with uroperitoneum include parturition-associated trauma, congenital anomalies, postpartum traumatic injury, strenuous exercise, focal necrosis of the bladder wall, and urachal infection [18, 19]. Uroperitoneum develops as the foal begins forming urine with abdominal distension and attendant clinical signs becoming noticeable 1–3 days of age with urachal or bladder rupture, and 5–10 days of age with ureteral rupture. Foals with uroperitoneum have some combination of colic, tenesmus, tachycardia, injected or congested mucous membrane appearance, dehydration, diarrhea, failure to nurse, lethargy, abdominal distension, frequent urinary posturing, and stranguria. As abdominal fluid volume increases, foals adopt rapid, shallow breathing as tidal volumes become smaller from impaired diaphragmatic contraction [20]. These signs have overlap with those of birth asphyxia and sepsis. Foals with bladder rupture usually continue to pass some urine through the urethra as well as through the bladder rent into the abdomen, and owners may report that the foal has, in fact, been urinating.

The hallmark sonographic appearance of uroperitoneum is voluminous anechoic to hypoechoic fluid in which viscera and mesentery are floating (Figure 15.III.15). Some foals with uroperitoneum also develop pleural effusion [21]. If uroperitoneum is chronic or associated with rupture of an infected or necrotic urachus, the peritoneal fluid will be more cellular in appearance from an influx of leukocytes. Identifying the rupture site in the bladder

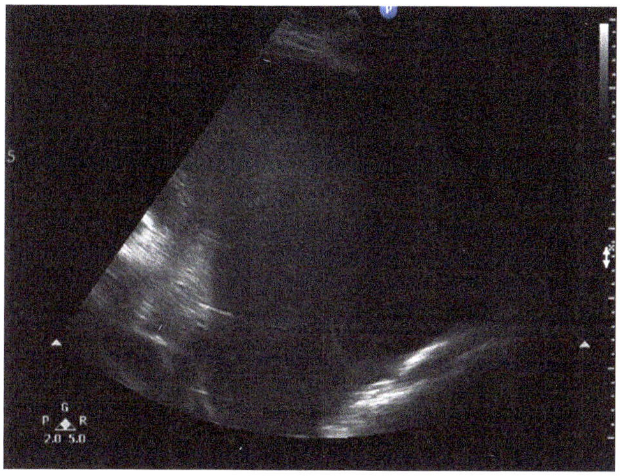

Figure 15.III.15 Sonogram of the abdomen of a 2-day-old foal with ruptured bladder and uroabdomen. Image was obtained with a microconvex transducer imaging at 4–6 MHz, placed midabdomen. Top of the image is the ventral surface of the abdomen. Hypoechoic fluid is seen filling the entire abdomen, with a few visceral margins seen floating dorsally (bottom of image).

wall is not always possible but can be appreciated in a partially filled bladder. Hyponatremia, hypochloremia, hyperkalemia, azotemia, and metabolic acidosis may be reported, and confirmation of uroperitoneum is obtained by comparing creatinine concentration in abdominal fluid with serum creatinine (uroperitoneum abdominal fluid creatinine ≥2 times serum creatinine concentration).

Imaging of the foal with uroperitoneum should go beyond detection of the abdominal fluid, to identify the site of urinary tract rupture. Bladder rupture and urachal rupture or leaking can usually be seen with ultrasound; ureteral rupture is considered after bladder and urachal rupture are ruled out, and contrast radiography, with or without surgical exploration, is usually needed to confirm ureteral injury. Because accumulation of urine in the abdomen with ureteral rent is slow and a week or longer may pass before the foal is examined, the blood changes are more longstanding and can be more severe. Rupture of the urethra near its origin at the bladder trigone is an uncommon cause of uroabdomen. Urethral rent in the more distal, intrapelvic segments will cause azotemia but the leaked urine dissects into the retroperitoneal tissue planes and causes edema in the prepuce and inguinal area, rather than uroabdomen. Urethral rents are diagnosed with contrast radiography or urethral endoscopy.

The traditionally reported [22] gender predilection toward males was not noted in two more recent retrospective studies on uroperitoneum [23, 24]. Moreover, the clinical presentation and serum biochemical abnormalities classically associated with uroperitoneum may be different in hospitalized foals that are receiving intravenous fluids, in which uroperitoneum arises as one of multiple systemic abnormalities rather than foals referred with uroperitoneum as the primary problem [23]. In hospitalized foals, clinical signs can be masked by a neurologically depressed state, and administration of intravenous fluids prevents or blunts the hyponatremia, hypochloremia, and hyperkalemia typically associated with uroperitoneum [22, 25]. Administration of fluids does not impact the development of high serum creatinine concentration or the usefulness of determining the peritoneal fluid: serum creatinine ratio (ratio ≥2). Use of ultrasound can facilitate early diagnosis and intervention before biochemical changes can fully develop. In a 2005 retrospective study [24], the rent in the bladder wall was ventrally located about as frequently as it was dorsal.

Sepsis and focal infections, in the urogenital tract [26] and elsewhere in the body, are risk factors for uroperitoneum, irrespective of whether a foal is hospitalized [23, 24]. In these foals, rupture of the bladder or urachal remnant is related to infection or necrosis rather than to traumatic rupture during parturition. It is not uncommon to detect uroperitoneum in a septic or bed-ridden foal one or more days into hospitalization when it was not present at admission. It is advisable to place and properly maintain an indwelling urinary catheter in nonambulatory foals to prevent urine stasis and pressure in the bladder; broad-spectrum antimicrobials are also important. Daily to twice daily sonographic imaging of the abdomen enables detection of even a modest volume of free peritoneal fluid, days before abdominal distension, colic, or other clinical signs become evident. The bladder is the most common site of rupture followed by the urachus. Practical guides on scanning of the bladder and umbilical remnants are available [27].

The term *navel ill* has traditionally been used to describe septic polyarthritis thought to result from pathogens gaining entrance to the body through the umbilicus. Although the umbilicus can serve as an access point for pathogens, it is now recognized that the GI tract and other portals are often the chief entry point, and the umbilical structures can become infected by bacteremia along with other tissues. The most common reported bacterial isolates from omphalitis or omphalophlebitis specimens are *Escherichia coli* and *Streptococcus zooepidemicus* [17, 28, 29]. Infection with *C. perfringens*, either from direct invasion from the environment or bacterial translocation from the intestinal tract, can also occur [28]. A 2007 report [30] revealed *Clostridium sordelli* as a cause of fulminant omphalitis, peritonitis, and death in eight foals.

Bladder rupture is surgically managed by primary closure of the rent. Aftercare includes placement of an indwelling urinary catheter for 2–3 days following surgery, to prevent bladder distension and challenging of the suture line in the immediate postoperative period. Even so, dehiscence and re-rupture a few days to first week following surgery is an occasional complication and can be managed by a second surgical repair or by replacing an indwelling urinary catheter and allowing the suture line to heal by second intention. In situations in which surgical repair is not possible, bladder wall rents can electively be managed conservatively, with an indwelling catheter, antimicrobials, and serial monitoring of serum biochemistry and ultrasonography. This regimen has yielded favorable results [31] and is most likely to be successful when the rent is not large and involves the more dorsal aspects of the bladder. Nonsurgical management of bladder rupture in four adult horses was recently reported [32].

Other Bladder Disorders

Ultrasonography can distinguish between other problems affecting the lower urinary tract resulting in clinical signs that overlap with those of uroperitoneum. Hematoma formation within the bladder, ascribed to tearing of the intraabdominal portion of the umbilicus, has been reported and is not an uncommon finding (Figure 15.III.16) [33]. In some instances, the resulting thrombus can be large and obstruct urine flow leading to stranguria in the foal. Megavesica is another cause of abdominal enlargement and stranguria, but not uroperitoneum, although it is speculated that some cases of bladder rupture occur secondary to undetected megavesica [34, 35]. Foals with this syndrome of bladder atony and enlargement have been reported, but the cause is not understood. Urine dribbles from the urethra, either passively or during straining, and ultrasound reveal a grossly dilated but intact bladder distended with urine.

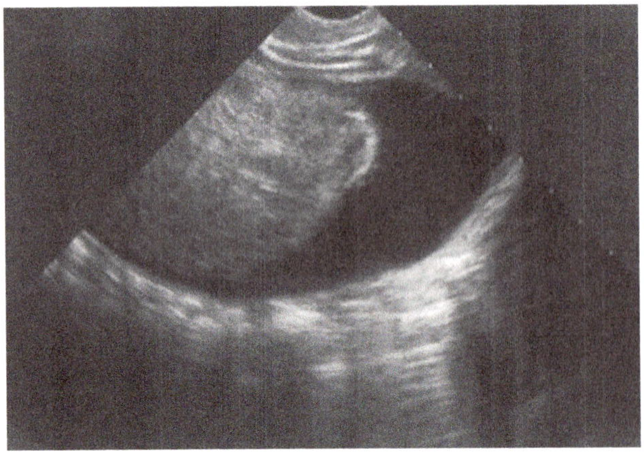

Figure 15.III.16 Ultrasonogram of the bladder of a Thoroughbred colt with pigmenturia and stranguria. Note the homogenous echogenic mass in the ventral bladder, presumably a cystic hematoma [33].

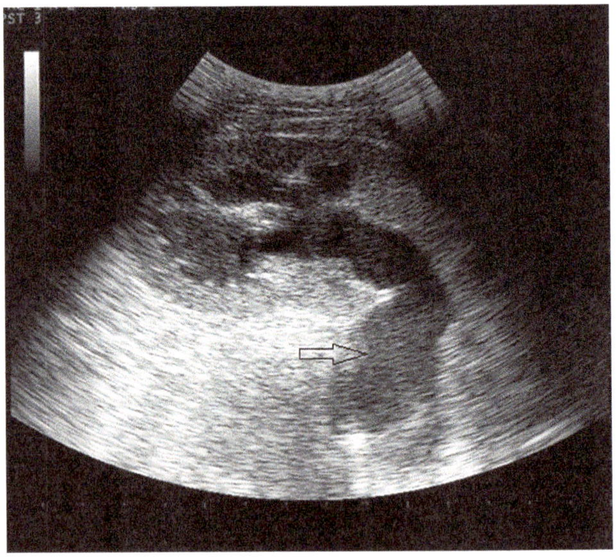

Figure 15.III.17 Sonogram of congenital hydroureter in a neonatal foal. Notice the distended ureter exiting the kidney (black arrow). *Source:* Image courtesy of Dr. Fairfield Bain.

Renal Disease

The kidneys are easily imaged in foals. Renal dysfunction is not unusual in foals and can be associated with shock, hypoperfusion, septic injury, and toxicosis from administration of nephrotoxic medications. Congenital renal conditions are uncommon in foals, but polycystic kidney disease, renal agenesis, hydroureter (Figure 15.III.17), and renal/glomerular hypoplasia [36] are occasionally reported. A recent case report [34] detailed a diffuse, bilateral alteration of renal parenchyma in a 9-day-old Thoroughbred foal that was histologically characterized as diffuse cystic renal dysplasia. Kidneys can have an unremarkable sonographic appearance while being in functional failure; clinicopathologic testing should be done as the primary means of determining renal function.

Summary

Sonographic imaging of the abdomen brings a visual component to the clinical assessment of the compromised neonatal foal and can be invaluable for confirming or ruling out many of the differential diagnoses that could be causing the observed clinical or clinicopathologic alterations. The quality of care and speed with which it can be initiated can be significantly augmented with this safe, fast, noninvasive, and highly informative imaging modality.

References

1 Aleman, M., Gillis, C.L., Nieto, J.E. et al. (2002). Ultrasonographic anatomy and biometric analysis of the thoracic and abdominal organs in healthy foals from birth to age 6 months. *Equine Vet. J.* 34: 649–655.

2 Magdesian, K.G. (2005). Neonatal foal diarrhea. *Vet. Clin. North Am. Equine Pract.* 21: 295–312.

3 Hollis, A.R., Wilkins, P.A., Palmer, J.E. et al. (2008). Bacteremia in equine neonatal diarrhea: a retrospective study (1990–2007). *J. Vet. Intern. Med.* 22: 1203–1209.

4 Reef, V.B. (1998). Pediatric abdominal ultrasonography. In: *Equine Diagnostic Ultrasound* (ed. B.V. Reef), 364–403. Philadelphia: WB Saunders.

5 Abraham, M., Reef, V.B., Sweeney, R.W. et al. (2014). Gastrointestinal ultrasonography of normal Standardbred neonates and frequency of asymptomatic intussusceptions. *J. Vet. Intern. Med.* 28: 1580–1586.

6 Porter, M. and Ramirez, P. (2005). Equine neonatal thoracic and abdominal ultrasonography. *Vet. Clin. North Am. Equine Pract.* 21: 407–429.

7 de Solis, N.C., Palmer, J.E., Boston, R.C. et al. (2012). The importance of ultrasonographic pneumatosis intestinalis in equine neonatal gastrointestinal disease. *Equine Vet. J.* 44 (Suppl): 64–68.

8 MacKinnon, M.C., Southwood, L.L., Burke, M.J. et al. (2013). Colic in equine neonates: 137 cases (2000–2010). *J. Am. Vet. Med. Assoc.* 243: 1586–1590.

9 Bernard, W.V., Reef, V.B., Reimer, J.M. et al. (1989). Ultrasonographic diagnosis of small-intestinal intussusception in three foals. *J. Am. Vet. Med. Assoc.* 194: 395–397.

10 McGladdery, A.J. (1996). Ultrasonographic diagnosis of intussusception in foals and yearlings. *Proc. Am. Assoc. Equine Pract.* 40: 239–240.

11 Busoni, V., De Busscher, V., Lopez, D. et al. (2011). Evaluation of a protocol for fast localized abdominal sonography of horses (FLASH) admitted for colic. *Vet. J.* 188: 77–82.

12 Soundappan, S.V.S., Holland, A.J.A., Cass, D.T. et al. (2005). Diagnostic accuracy of surgeon-performed focused abdominal sonography (FAST) in blunt paediatric trauma. *Injury – Int. J. Care Injured* 36: 970–975.

13 Boysen, S.P., Rozanski, E.A., Tidwell, A.S. et al. (2004). Evaluation of a focused assessment with sonography for trauma protocol to detect free abdominal fluid in dogs involved in motor vehicle accidents. *J. Am. Vet. Med. Assoc.* 225: 1198–1204.

14 Morresey, P.R. (2014). Umbilical problems. *Proc. Am. Assoc. Equine Pract.* 60: 18–21.

15 Whitwell, K.E. (1975). Morphology and pathology of the equine umbilical cord. *J. Reprod. Fertil. Suppl.* 23: 599–603.

16 Reef, V.B. and Collatos, C. (1988). Ultrasonography of umbilical structures in clinically normal foals. *Am. J. Vet. Res.* 49: 2143–2146.

17 Reef, V.B., Collatos, C., Spencer, P.A. et al. (1989). Clinical, ultrasonographic, and surgical findings in foals with umbilical remnant infections. *J. Am. Vet. Med. Assoc.* 195: 69–72.

18 Hackett, R.P. (1984). Rupture of the urinary bladder in neonatal foals. *Compend. Contin. Educ. Pract. Vet.* 6: S488–S492.

19 Robertson, J.T. and Embertson, R.M. (1988). Surgical management of congenital and perinatal abnormalities of the urogenital tract. *Vet. Clin. North Am. Equine Pract.* 4: 359–379.

20 Wilkins, P.A. (2004). Respiratory distress in foals with uroperitoneum: possible mechanisms. *Equine Vet. Educ.* 16: 293–295.

21 Wong, D.M., Leger, L.C., Scarratt, W.K. et al. (2004). Uroperitoneum and pleural effusion in an American paint filly. *Equine Vet. Educ.* 16: 290–293.

22 Richardson, D.W. and Kohn, C.W. (1983). Uroperitoneum in the foal. *J. Am. Vet. Med. Assoc.* 182: 267–271.

23 Kablack, K.A., Embertson, R.M., Bernard, W.V. et al. (2000). Uroperitoneum in the hospitalised equine neonate: retrospective study of 31 cases, 1988–1997. *Equine Vet. J.* 32: 505–508.

24 Dunkel, B., Palmer, J.E., Olson, K.N. et al. (2005). Uroperitoneum in 32 foals: influence of intravenous fluid therapy, infection, and sepsis. *J. Vet. Intern. Med.* 19: 889–893.

25 Behr, M.J., Hackett, R.P., Bentinck-Smith, J. et al. (1981). Metabolic abnormalities associated with rupture of the urinary bladder in neonatal foals. *J. Am. Vet. Med. Assoc.* 178: 263–266.

26 Lores, M., Lofstedt, J., Martinson, S. et al. (2011). Septic peritonitis and uroperitoneum secondary to subclinical omphalitis and concurrent necrotizing cystitis in a colt. *Can. Vet. J.* 52: 888–892.

27 Franklin, R.P. and Ferrell, E.A. (2002). How to perform umbilical sonograms in the neonate. *Proc. Am. Assoc. Equine Pract.* 48: 261–265.

28 Hyman, S.S., Wilkins, P.A., Palmer, J.E. et al. (2002). *Clostridium perfringens* urachitis and uroperitoneum in 2 neonatal foals. *J. Vet. Intern. Med.* 16: 489–493.

29 Adams, S.B. and Fessler, J.F. (1987). Umbilical cord remnant infections in foals: 16 cases (1975–1985). *J. Am. Vet. Med. Assoc.* 190: 316–318.

30 Ortega, J., Daft, B., Assis, R.A. et al. (2007). Infection of the intestinal umbilical remnant in foals by *Clostridium sordelli*. *Vet. Pathol.* 44: 269–275.

31 Lavoie, J.P. and Harnagel, S.H. (1998). Nonsurgical management of ruptured urinary bladder in a critically ill foal. *J. Am. Vet. Med. Assoc.* 192: 1577–1580.

32 Peitzmeier, M.D., McNally, T.P., Slone, D.E. et al. (2016). Conservative management of cystorrhexis in four adult horses. *Equine Vet. Educ.* 28: 631–635.

33 Arnold, C.E., Chaffin, K.M., and Rush, B.R. (2005). Hematuria associated with cystic hematomas in three neonatal foals. *J. Am. Vet. Med. Assoc.* 227: 778–780.

34 Rijkenhuizen, A. (2012). Megavesica and bladder rupture in foals. *Equine Vet. Educ.* 24: 404–407.

35 Toth, T., Liman, J., Larsdotter, S. et al. (2012). Megavesica in a neonatal foal. *Equine Vet. Educ.* 24: 396–403.

36 Brown, C.M., Parks, A.H., Mullaney, T.P. et al. (1988). Bilateral renal dysplasia and hypoplasia in a foal with an imperforate anus. *Vet. Rec.* 122: 91–92.

Section IV Endoscopy of the Digestive Tract

David Wong and Emily Schaefer

In the neonatal foal, portions of the digestive tract can be visualized via endoscopy, including the pharynx, esophagus, stomach, duodenum, and rectum/small colon. These structures are typically accessible in the neonatal foal (e.g. ~50 kg) using a 1 m endoscope with a diameter of 9 mm or less; however, smaller patients such as miniature donkeys or American Miniature Horse foals may require a smaller-diameter pediatric endoscope or ureteroscope while draft breed foals may require an endoscope that is 1.5–2 m in length. Physical restraint might be sufficient and is recommended for evaluation of the upper airway and pharyngeal region, but sedation might be necessary.

Palate and Pharynx

Endoscopy of the pharynx is readily accomplished in the neonatal foal with passage of the endoscope through the nasal passage via the ventral meatus. As the endoscope is advanced, it will enter the pharynx, providing visualization of the soft palate, openings to the guttural pouches, dorsal pharyngeal recess (Figure 15.IV.1a), and larynx (Figure 15.IV.1b). A cleft palate defect that involves the hard palate can be easily recognized via visual and digital examination of the oral cavity (Figure 15.IV.1c), but endoscopy is needed to visualize a cleft palate involving the soft palate (Figure 15.IV.1d). The entire oropharynx should be inspected via endoscopy when evaluating the upper portion of the digestive tract. Anatomic defects of this portion of the digestive tract might result in dysphagia with evidence of milk in the oropharynx suggestive of this. Disorders that can be observed in the oropharynx include cleft palate involving the soft palate (Figure 15.IV.1d), palatal cyst (Figure 15.IV.1e,f), and subepiglottic cysts. If a functional disorder in deglutition is suspected, examining the pharynx immediately after the foal has nursed may provide some clues as to the origin of dysphagia.

Esophagus

Esophagoscopy is easily accomplished in the foal as the clinician passes the endoscope toward the stomach. The esophageal opening lies dorsal to the arytenoid cartilages and is entered by placing gentle pressure as the endoscope is positioned slightly lateral to the dorsal aspect of the corniculate process of the arytenoid cartilage. The entire length of the esophagus is examined using intermittent air insufflation to expand the lumen (Figure 15.IV.2a,b). Some clinicians prefer to examine the stomach first, and then examine the esophagus as the endoscope is retracted toward the pharynx while simultaneously insufflating the esophagus with air.

The esophagus is a continuation of the laryngopharynx and is composed of four tissue layers:

1) *Tunica adventitia*. The outer fibrous sheath that loosely attaches the esophagus to surrounding structures thus allowing freedom of movement and expansion during swallowing.
2) *Tunica muscularis*. The muscular layer arranged in two layers of fibers that are oriented spirally and consist of striated muscle in the proximal two-thirds of the esophagus and transitions to smooth muscle in the distal one-third.
3) *The submucosa*. This is the next layer, followed by the mucosal layer.
4) *Mucosa*. The mucosal layer (tunica mucosa) lines the esophageal lumen. The mucosa should lie in longitudinal folds when not dilated with air and appear smooth and glistening with a pale pink to whitish-gray color when the esophagus is dilated with air.

Proximally, the cervical esophagus resides along the median plane and at approximately the fourth cervical vertebra, the esophagus typically deviates laterally to lie on the left lateral aspect of the neck coursing in close proximity to the trachea.

Equine Neonatal Medicine, First Edition. Edited by David M. Wong and Pamela A. Wilkins.

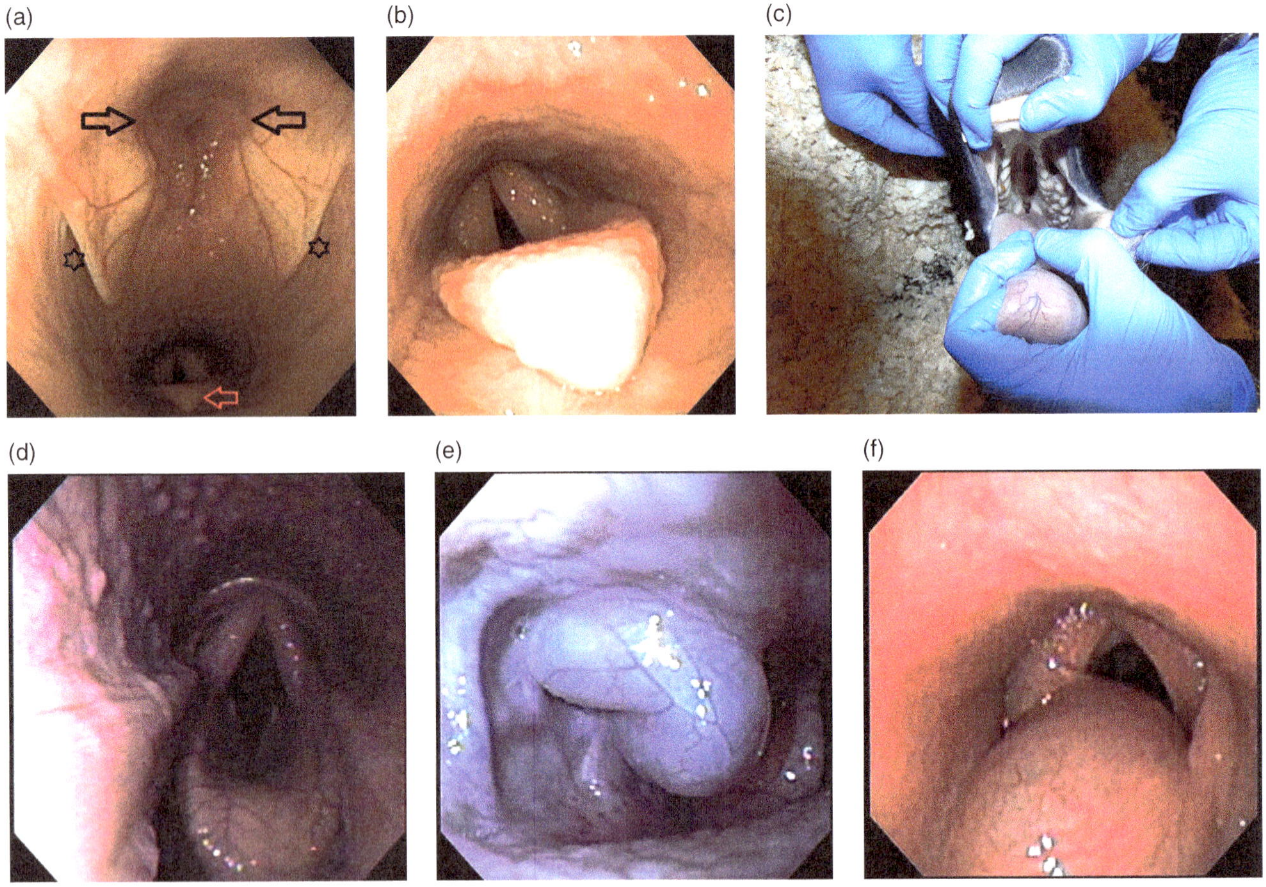

Figure 15.IV.1 (a) Endoscopic view of the pharynx demonstrating the openings to the guttural pouches (stars), dorsal pharyngeal recess (black arrows), larynx, and epiglottis (red arrow). (b) Closer image of the epiglottis and larynx. (c) Oral view of a neonatal foal with a cleft palate involving the hard palate; (d) Endoscopic view of a cleft palate involving the soft palate, just rostral to the larynx; (e) Endoscopic view of a palatal cyst noted from the perspective of the oral cavity and (f) pharynx.

The endoscopist may note frequent peristaltic waves over time. As the esophagus enters the thoracic inlet, the thoracic portion of the esophagus deviates back to the median plane, dorsal to the trachea. The abdominal portion of the esophagus is short and terminates at the lower esophageal sphincter and enters the stomach. Disorders of the esophagus in neonatal foals are rare but include esophageal strictures (Figure 15.IV.2c–e), megaesophagus, esophageal ectasia, esophageal erosions and ulcers, and foreign bodies, all of which might be observed via endoscopy.

Stomach and Duodenum

Gastric ulceration is frequently encountered in foals. Affected foals with may have poor appetite, intermittent colic, and diarrhea; alternatively, no overt clinical signs may be observed [1, 2]. Gastric ulceration is reviewed in Chapter 17, with this section focusing on how to perform the gastroscopy procedure.

In preparation for gastroscopy, suckling foals should not be allowed to nurse for at least 3 hours prior to the procedure; older foals that are consuming solid feed may need to be fasted 8–10 hours prior to gastroscopy to ensure that the stomach is relatively empty. The clinician can judge whether sedation is necessary, but it is often not required, especially in ill foals. The endoscope is passed in standard fashion through the ventral meatus and into the esophagus as described above. Upon reaching the stomach, air is insufflated through the endoscope to allow visualization of the nonglandular and glandular portions of the gastric surface. Remaining gastric contents should be rinsed from the walls of the stomach to allow for complete inspection. When first entering the stomach, the greater curvature of the stomach will be seen (Figure 15.IV.3a,b). As the endoscope is advanced, it will typically follow the contour of the greater curvature, at which point the lesser curvature

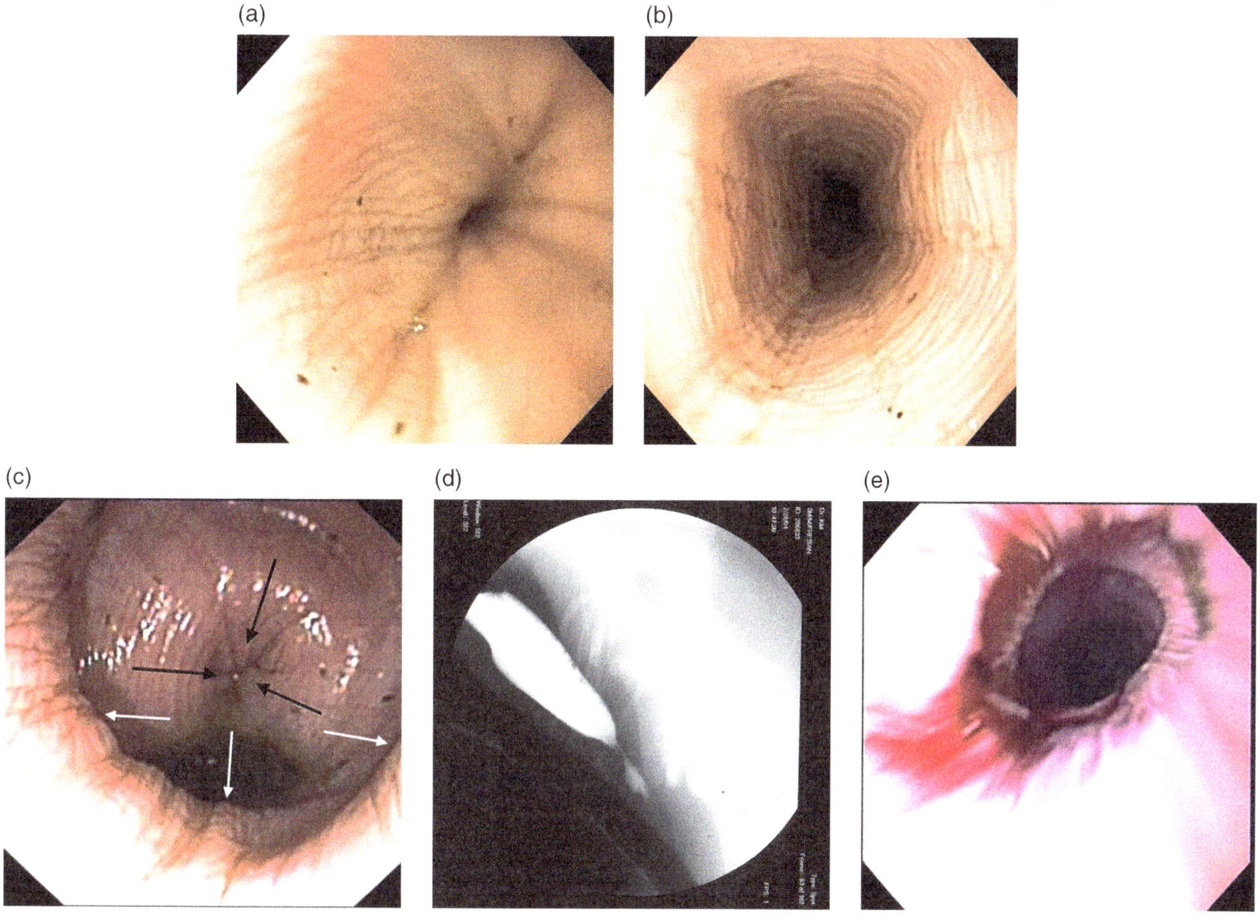

Figure 15.IV.2 Endoscopic view of the esophagus (a) before and (b) after dilation with air. (c) Esophageal stricture, note the area of stricture (black arrows) and dilated esophagus (white arrows) proximal to the stricture. (d) Same foal as in (c), Fluoroscopic image of contrast material in the dilated esophagus, rostral to the esophageal stricture. (e) Image of stricture after esophageal bouginage. Note the hemorrhage secondary to the bouginage procedure.

(Figure 15.IV.3c) and cardia of the stomach will be observed. Continued advancement of the endoscope will allow visualization of the pylorus (Figure 15.IV.3d,e). Once the pylorus is identified, the endoscopist will note a central "black hole" to which the tip of the endoscope is passed through (pyloric orifice). Once the scope is inside the duodenal ampulla, progression of the endoscope should be very slow and is enhanced by the peristaltic movement of the gastrointestinal tract. In some adult horses, passage of the endoscope into the duodenum (Figure 15.IV.3f) can be difficult and this difficulty is further increased because of the small size of the foal. When the endoscopic exam is complete, the endoscopist should evacuate the insufflated air within the stomach through the biopsy channel of the endoscope using a portable suction unit or 60 ml syringe.

As the endoscopist visualizes the stomach, the squamous mucosa of the nonglandular portion of the foal's stomach is relatively thin and should appear somewhat pale and pink to white. The margo plicatus provides a landmark between the junction of the squamous and glandular gastric mucosa. The glandular mucosa will appear darker pink to red and should be smooth. Within the stomach, milk may appear as strands of curdled milk or a conglomeration of curdled milk and gastric fluids giving a more yellow appearance. If the endoscopist is able to reach the small intestine, the duodenal mucosa should have a uniform red-brown to pink color and have a velvet-like appearance (Figure 15.IV.3f); the major duodenal papilla is the common outlet of the hepatic and pancreatic ducts and may be visualized at the end of the duodenal ampulla; the accessory pancreatic duct lies further aboral and on the opposite side of the major duodenal papilla.

Direct imaging of the stomach may reveal significant pathology that requires intervention and allows the clinician to evaluate severity of gastric ulcerative disease (Figures 15.IV.3g–i).

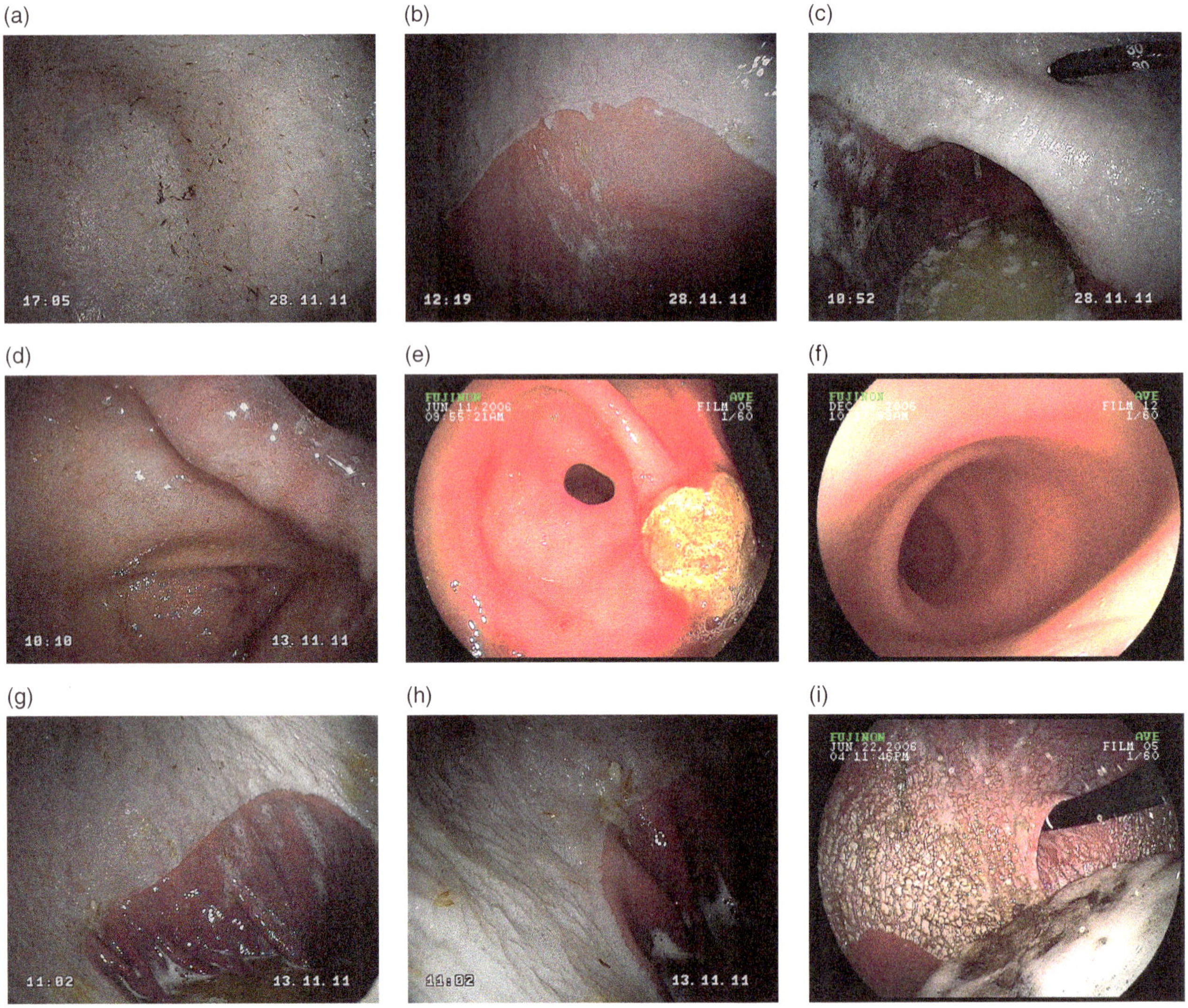

Figure 15.IV.3 Endoscopic view of the stomach of a healthy neonatal foal; (a) entering the stomach, (b) greater curvature and margo plicatus, and (c) lesser curvature looking toward pylorus. Endoscopic image the pylorus with the orifice (d) closed and (e) open. (f) Endoscopic image of the duodenum in a healthy neonatal foal. (g–i) Varying severities of gastric ulcers in neonatal foals. *Source:* Images courtesy of Dr. Mike Hewston (a–d, g, h), Royal Veterinary College and Dr. Chris Sanchez (e, f, i), University of Florida.

There have been multiple studies evaluating prevalence of ulcerative disease in healthy and ill foals [1–3]. By combining the results of these studies, we learn that healthy foals <1 month old may experience subclinical squamous ulceration and up to 8% glandular mucosal ulceration. By contrast, foals with systemic disease may experience glandular ulceration up to 40% of the time, and those with gastrointestinal (GI) diseases are significantly more likely to experience glandular ulceration [4]. Additionally, gastroscopy may reveal incidental gastric ulcers and, because many foals with glandular ulceration have additional GI lesions, the diagnostic expedition should not stop with ulcer diagnosis [5]. The true prevalence of duodenal ulcers is unknown but has been reported in neonatal foals.

Colon

Colonoscopy is infrequently performed in the foal but has aided in the diagnosis of atresia coli and colonic hamartomas in several case reports involving neonatal foals [6–8]. Colonoscopy might also be of benefit if the clinician suspects an obstruction or stricture of the distal portion of the colon. A 1 m endoscope will be sufficient to visualize the mucosa of the rectum and small colon, which should appear pink and glistening. N-butylscopolammonium bromide (0.3 mg/kg, IV) imparts anticholinergic effects by competitively inhibiting muscarinic receptors and has been used to facilitate smooth muscle relaxation and examination of the small colon in foals with atresia coli [6].

References

1 Murray, M.J., Murray, C.M., Sweeney, H.J. et al. (1990). Prevalence of gastric lesions in foals without signs of gastric disease: an endoscopic survey. *Equine Vet. J.* 22 (1): 6–8.

2 Murray, M.J., Grodinsky, C., Cowles, R.R. et al. (1990). The progression of gastric lesions in young Thoroughbred foals: an endoscopic study. *J. Am. Vet. Med. Assoc.* 196: 1623–1627.

3 Furr, M.O., Murray, M.J., and Ferguson, D.C. (1992). The effects of stress on gastric ulceration, T3, T4, reverse T3 and Cortisol in neonatal foals. *Equine Vet. J.* 24 (1): 37–40.

4 Elfenbein, J.R. and Sanchez, L.C. (2012). Prevalence of gastric and duodenal ulceration in 691 nonsurviving foals (1995–2006). *Equine Vet. J.* 44 (s41): 76–79.

5 Wilkins, P.A. (2004). Disorders of foals. *Equine Intern. Med.* 1381–1440.

6 Hunter, B. and Belgrave, R.L. (2010). Atresia coli in a foal: diagnosis made with colonoscopy aided by N-butylscopolammonium bromide. *Equine Vet. Educ.* 22: 429–422.

7 Mejia, S., Hurcombe, S.D.A., Rodgerson, D.H. et al. (2021). Retrograde intussusception of the descending colon secondary to multiple colonic hamartomas in a neonatal foal. *Equine Vet. Educ.* 33: e12–e16.

8 Nappert, G., Laverty, S., Drolet, R. et al. (1992). Atresia coli in 7 foals (1964–1990). *Equine Vet. J. Suppl.* 13: 57–60.

Section V Radiography of the Alimentary Tract

Sarah Colmer, Kate Wulster Bills, and David Wong

Diseases of the alimentary tract are relatively common in the foal, with dysphagia, esophageal disorders, abdominal pain (colic), abdominal distension, and enterocolitis being some of the primary clinical complaints encountered. Abdominal radiography can aid in the diagnosis of these clinical concerns and can also help facilitate investigations in foals with clinical signs of stranguria or tenesmus. Although ultrasonography is the primary method for evaluation of the gastrointestinal (GI) tract, radiography can be used alone or in conjunction with other modalities, such as ultrasonography and endoscopy, to evaluate the upper alimentary tract and augment the evaluation of the GI tract and abdomen in ill foals with alimentary disorders. Radiography can be especially useful in foals considering the diminutive size of the foal's abdomen, compared to the adult horse, which lends itself to improved radiographic imaging of the GI tract in an efficient and economical capacity. Radiographs can provide information regarding deglutition, esophageal disease, abdominal organ position, degree of gastric or intestinal distension, potential site of GI obstruction, and the nature of obstructive material. Serial radiography can also document the progression or resolution of various causes of acute abdominal pain. Additionally, contrast studies of the alimentary and urinary tracts can provide valuable information regarding luminal size and transit time.

Technique

Adequate radiographs can be obtained in foals up to 500 pounds (230 kg) if proper radiographic equipment is available. This includes a grid and adequate mAs (5–28) and kVp (75–95). A 14-in. × 17-in. detector is usually large enough to accommodate the abdomen of most neonatal foals. Radiographic exposure factors to acquire abdominal radiographs from a typical neonatal Thoroughbred foal is 85 kVP and 20 mAs, using a 10 : 1 focused grid and focal distance of 40 in. with the beam centered on the last rib [1, 2]. High-quality images can be obtained with a portable generator with the following technique; 75 kVp, 2 mAs or 80 kVp, 4 mAs with a 6 : 1 grid (Figure 15.V.1). These settings serve as guidelines as the technique may need to be modified based on the size of the foal and equipment used. Radiographs of the alimentary tract can be performed with the foal standing or in lateral recumbency and is dependent on the patient's condition, the area of interest, compliance of the patient, and radiographic images required. A foal also may be required to stand to facilitate contrast studies of the esophagus or upper GI tract. The preferred position to acquire abdominal radiographs is standing as to allow evaluation for fluid lines within the GI tract; however, some ill foals or those that demonstrate more severe clinical signs of colic or pain may be unable to remain standing during radiographic acquisition. Obtaining images in various positions (e.g., left/right standing, left/right recumbency, ventrodorsal) can aid in the diagnosis, but acquisition in such positions may not always be feasible. Unlike adult horses, ventrodorsal radiographs are possible in the neonatal foal but can be difficult to acquire due to patient cooperation and may also pose negative consequence to the cardiopulmonary system [2]; therefore, this positioning should only be performed in the context of the individual foal. Ventrodorsal radiographs may be most useful if attempting to image the pylorus, sigmoid loop, descending segments of the duodenum, cecal base, and aspects of the colon [2].

Normal Radiographic Anatomy

In the healthy foal, a small amount of gas is expected in the stomach, small intestine, and small colon; less frequently, gas can be observed in the cecum and rectum. Small

Equine Neonatal Medicine, First Edition. Edited by David M. Wong and Pamela A. Wilkins.

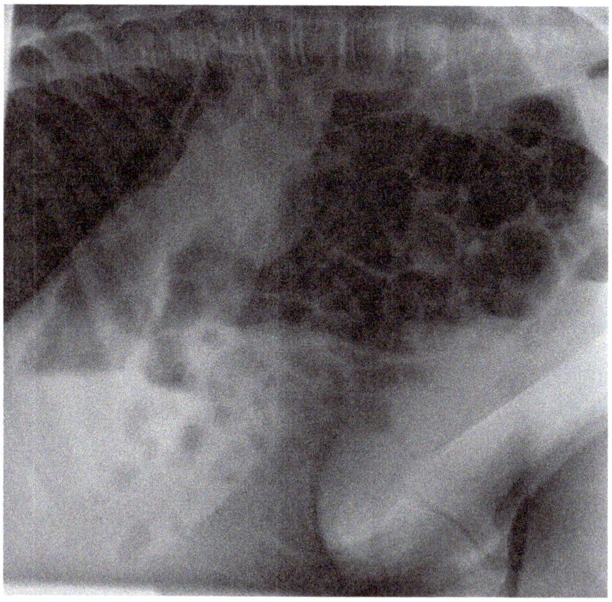

Figure 15.V.1 Lateral radiograph of a normal 7-day-old, 54 kg foal taken with a portable generator with the following technique: 80 kVp, 4.2 mAs and 6 : 1 grid.

intestinal loops are difficult to individually identify radiographically in the healthy foal but occupy the majority of the abdomen [1]. More specifically, in the healthy foal, standing lateral radiographs of the abdomen are characterized by: (i) a gas cap over fluid and ingesta within the stomach, (ii) small collections of gas in the small intestine in the cranial and mid-central abdomen, (iii) gas caps over fluid and ingesta in the cecum and large colon within the caudodorsal abdomen, (iv) small amounts of gas in the small colon, and (v) inconsistent gas in the rectum within the pelvis (Figure 15.V.2) [1]. The stomach can typically be seen in the cranial abdomen with the pylorus on the right side. The small intestine can often be identified throughout the abdomen with thin and smooth walls devoid of sacculation [2]. The length of the first lumbar vertebra (L1) can be used to determine pathologic distension of the small intestine in that the diameter of the small intestine should be less than the length of L1 [1]. The cecum is located in the right caudal abdomen and can be identified in light of its prominent haustra [2]. The colon is located in the ventral abdomen and is also identifiable by accompanying haustra. The small colon can be seen in the left caudal abdomen. A general lack of peritoneal fat results in decreased serosal detail and therefore, decreased contrast of intrabdominal organs compared to adult equids [2]. As described later, contrast (e.g. barium) studies can be helpful in identifying various aspects of the alimentary and urinary tracts. Radiography of the GI tract should be complemented with abdominal ultrasonography, keeping in mind that gas distention of the intestines can preclude complete ultrasonographic examination of abdominal organs.

Dysphagia

Radiography can be used to evaluate some scenarios of dysphagia in the foal. Although congenital abnormalities of the larynx and epiglottis are rare in horses, epiglottic hypoplasia and restrictive membranous frenulums have been reported, yielding dorsal displacement of the soft palate and subsequent oronasal reflux after nursing [3]. Endoscopy and radiographic methods have been implemented, where radiographs can be utilized to determine thyroepiglottic length [4].

Esophageal Radiology

Esophageal radiographs can be used from a diagnostic and therapeutic standpoint. One use of radiography of the proximal alimentary tract is to confirm placement of a feeding tube in the esophagus as opposed to the trachea. Endoscopy of the pharynx can also be used for this purpose. This can be particularly useful if the foal has been sedated, which can negatively impact swallowing and thus make passage of the feeding tube more difficult. Some hospitals use palpation alone to presume proper placement; however, others require imaging confirmation of proper placement of a feeding tube in neonatal foals prior to use of the tube (e.g., enteral milk feedings). A lateral radiograph of the upper alimentary tract is a rapid method to accomplish this goal with the clinician confirming the tube's location (Figure 15.V.3). If there is a question of proper placement of the feeding tube because of superimposition with the caudal cervical or cranial thoracic trachea, inclusion of the pharynx within the radiographic image can help mitigate this concern.

Diagnostically, esophageal conditions in newborn foals are uncommon; however, radiographs (and in some cases, contrast studies) can be used to investigate some congenital disorders. Esophageal stenosis [5] has been identified in foals, which can be caused by a vascular ring anomaly secondary to a persisting right aortic arch, among other vascular aberrations [6]. Stenosis secondary to acquired esophageal obstruction ("choke," as it is known colloquially) tends to occur rarely, given the liquid diet of newborn foals as opposed to their adult counterparts, though it can occur. Esophageal ectasia (dilation) has also been diagnosed in newborn foals as a congenital consequence, though in some cases it can be associated with decreased ganglionic cells in the myenteric plexus of the proximal esophagus [7, 8]. If recent and repeated placement of a feeding tube has been performed, some foals may exhibit transient esophageal dilation [2]. Gastric outflow obstruction may result in reflux and thus the appearance of esophageal dilation with a combination of fluid and gas on radiographs of the esophagus. Duplication of the cervical

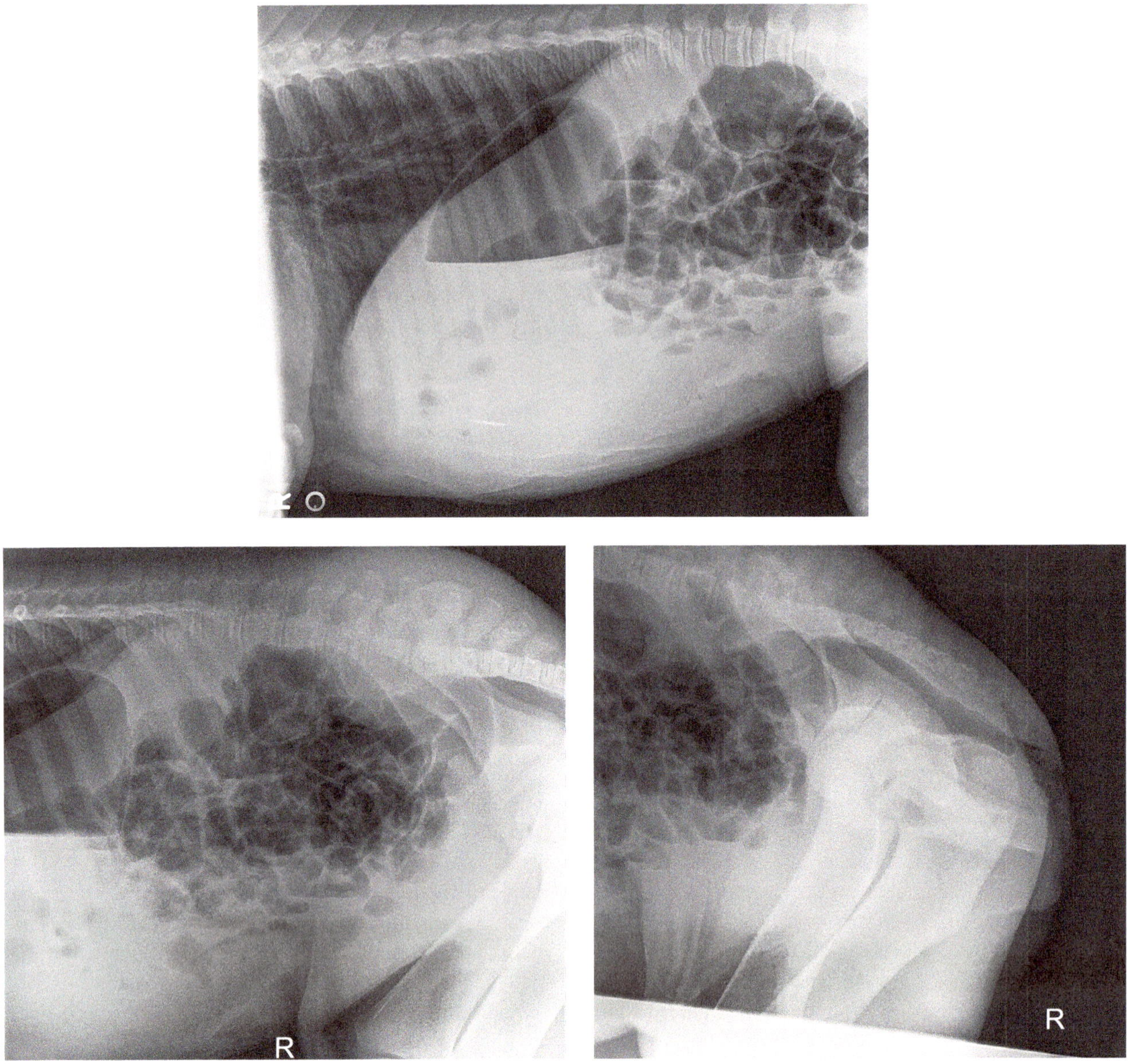

Figure 15.V.2 Lateral radiographs of a healthy 1-day-old neonatal foal. A gas cap is observed over fluid within the stomach, areas of small intestine contain gas, and some gas within the rectum is noted; no abnormalities were identified in this radiographic series.

portion of the esophagus has been identified in one Quarter Horse filly [9], identified as a fluid- and gas-filled mass via radiography and ultrasonography.

Radiographs can be used to help identify functional or anatomic abnormalities of the pharynx (e.g. dysphagia) or esophagus (e.g. stricture, dilation) and are best performed by feeding barium mixed with food or administering barium suspension via feeding tube into the proximal portion of the cervical esophagus (Figure 15.V.4). Radiographs should be performed immediately after ingestion or esophageal administration of contrast media. Esophageal strictures or dilations are typically easily observed with contrast media highlighting the affected region, whereas identifying the cause of dysphagia may be more elusive.

Radiography of the Stomach

A variety of radiographic findings within the abdomen combined with details surrounding the clinical picture can help the clinician develop a list of differential diagnoses. Abdominal radiographs that display a large, distended, gas- and fluid-filled stomach without intestinal distension aborally can be due to gastric ulcer disease, gastric outflow obstruction (e.g., pyloric stenosis secondary to ulceration or proximal small intestinal obstruction), or gastric atony [1, 10]. Ulcers at the gastroduodenal junction are a relatively common cause of delayed gastric emptying in foals [11]. Endoscopy is used to confirm a diagnosis of gastric ulceration, however barium-contrast radiography can

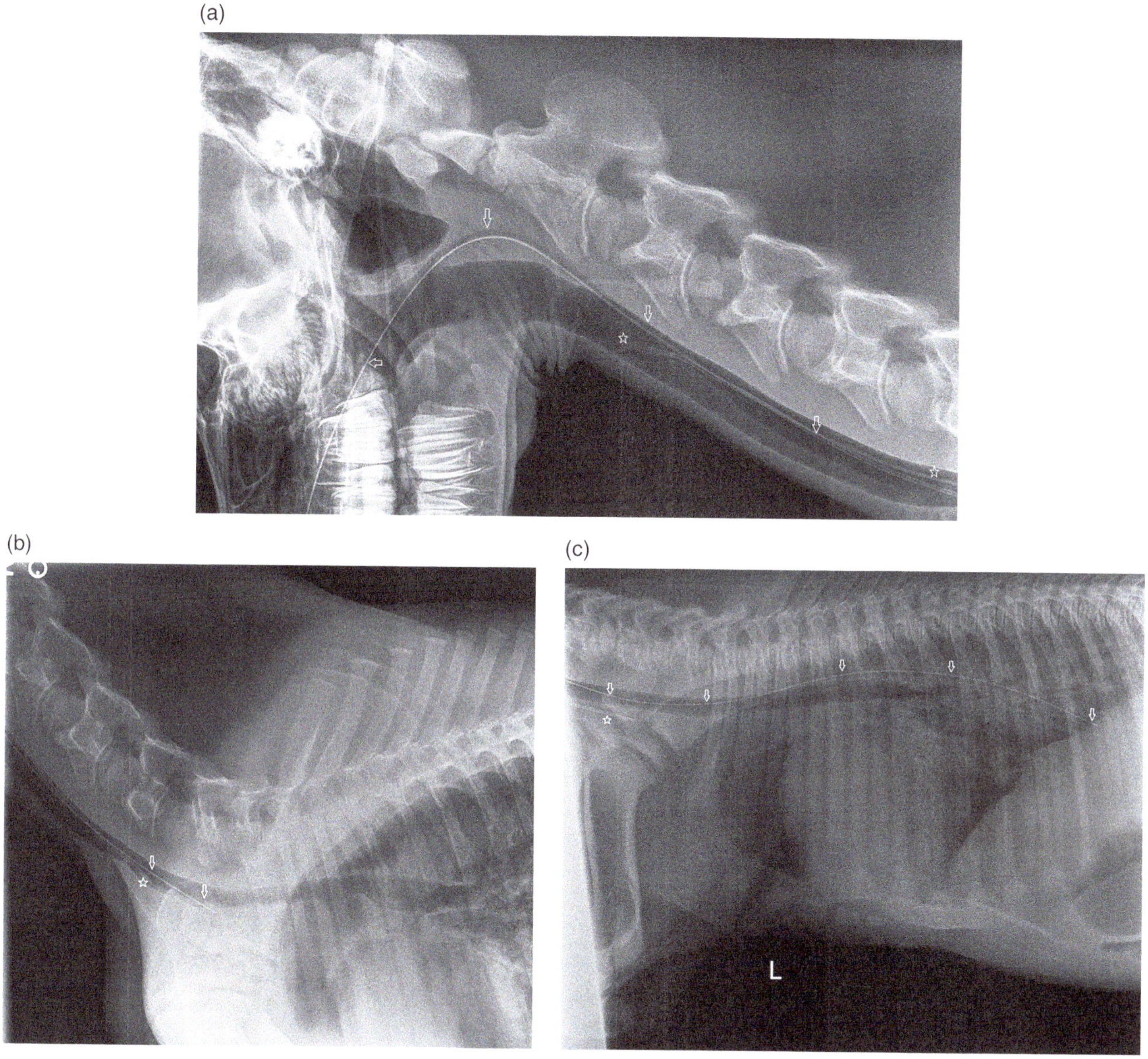

Figure 15.V.3 Lateral radiographs demonstrating placement of a feeding tube (arrows) in the (a) upper esophagus, (b) thoracic inlet, and (c) distal esophagus in a neonatal foal. An IV jugular catheter (star) can also be noted in these images.

be used to confirm delayed gastric emptying (see below for *general considerations for contrast studies* and Figure 15.V.5). The normal gastric emptying time ranges between 30 and 120 minutes though emptying often occurs immediately after administration of barium in normal foals.

Small and Large Intestinal Distension

In general, gas distension of the small intestine in foals is a nonspecific finding and can be observed in a variety of disorders such as enteritis, peritonitis, or intestinal obstruction and is characterized radiographically by intraluminal gas-fluid interfaces [10]. Radiography can be useful in cases of foals with colic and intestinal distension, however the clinical decision regarding whether a lesion can be managed medically or requires surgical intervention relies most strongly on history, accompanying signs, clinicopathologic findings, and degree of pain and response to attempts to control it.

Small intestinal obstruction may appear radiographically as multiple uneven, intraluminal gas-fluid interfaces and/or large, distended, inverted U-shaped loops of small intestine with hairpin turns, often with multiple-level fluid lines (Figures 15.V.6 and 15.V.7) [10, 12]. As mentioned, the normal small intestinal diameter should be less than the length of the first lumbar (L1) vertebra [13]. Radiographically, ileus may appear as diffuse, mild, small

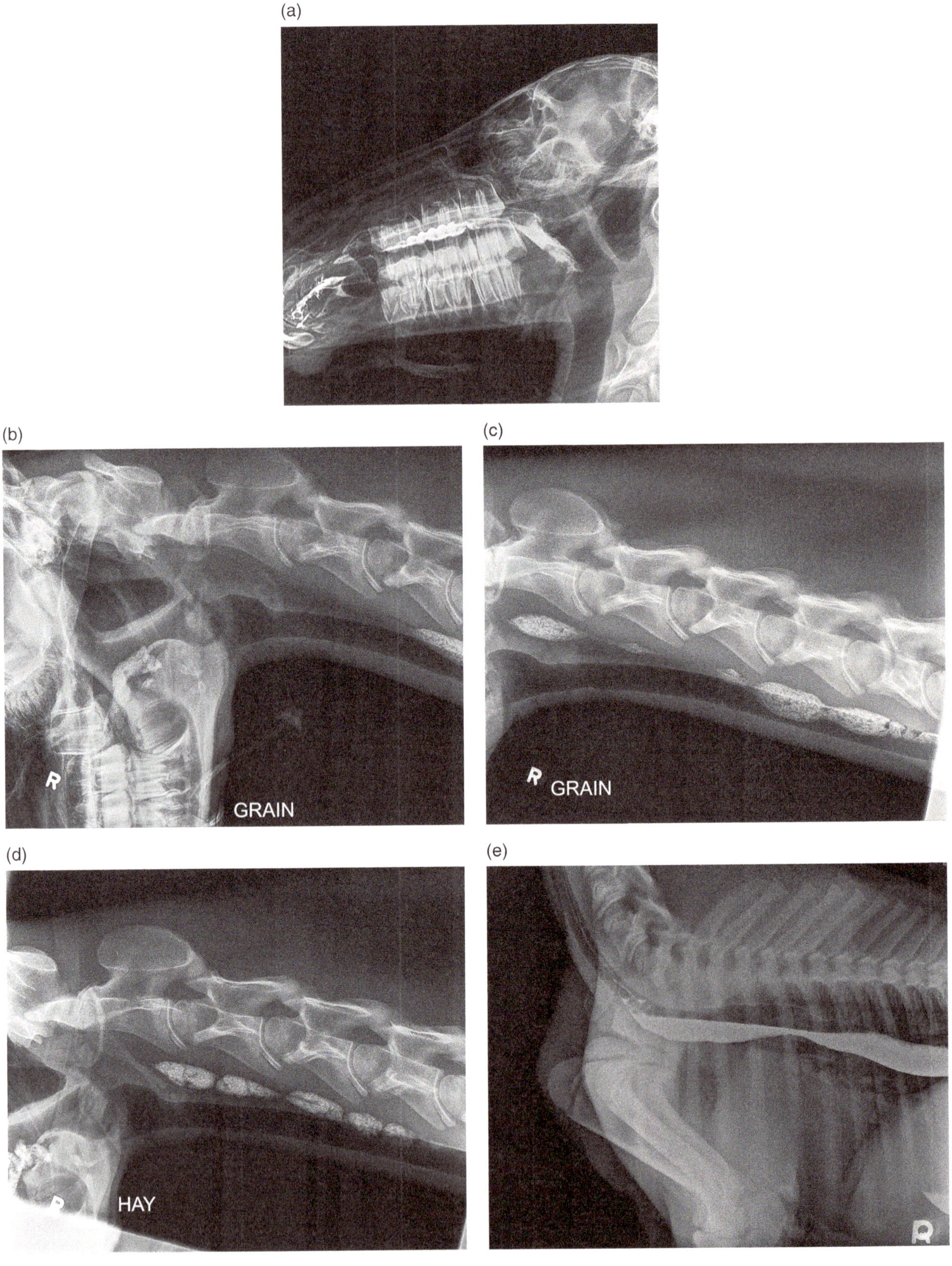

Figure 15.V.4 (a–d) Various contrast media studies of the oropharynx and esophagus in a 1-month-old Saddlebred foal with dysphagia noted since birth. (a) Lateral radiograph of the mouth during voluntary ingestion of contrast media. (b) Lateral radiograph of the oropharynx, epiglottis, and proximal esophagus immediately after feeding grain mixed with contrast media. (c) Same as (b) at the level of the mid-cervical esophagus. (d) Lateral radiograph of same foal fed hay mixed with contrast media. (e) Lateral radiograph of a 5-day-old Thoroughbred foal presented for milk regurgitation from the nares. Note the accumulation of contrast media in the thoracic esophagus, characteristic of esophgaeal dysmotility.

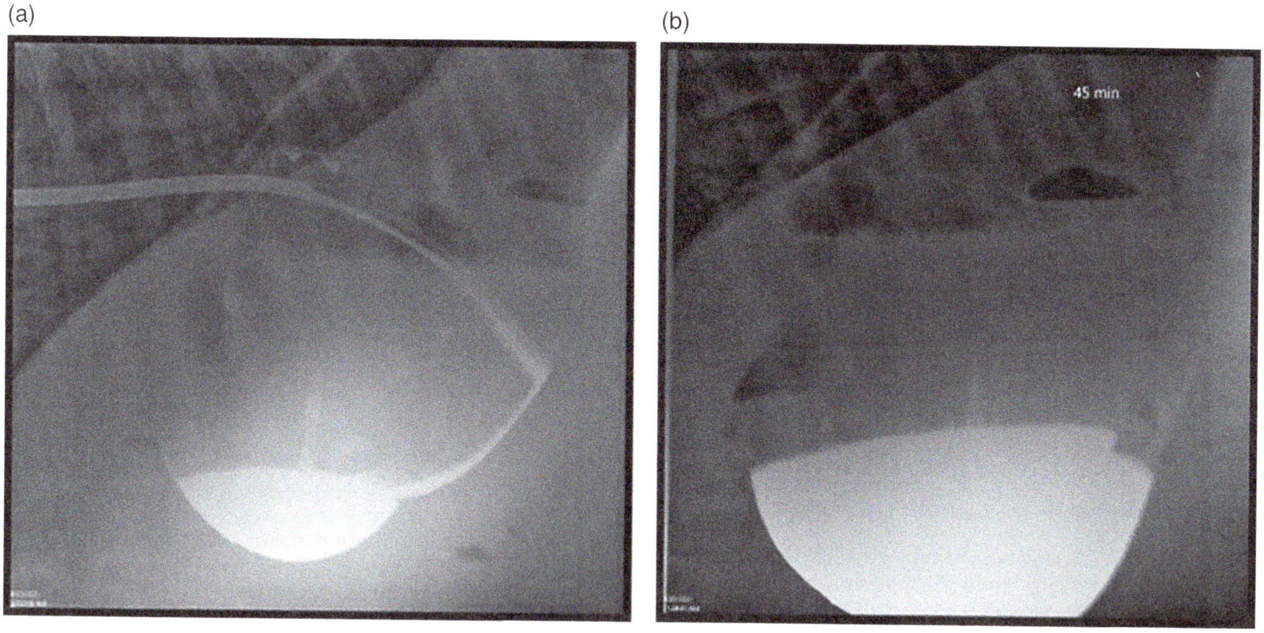

Figure 15.V.5 Lateral radiographs of a 2-month-old Percheron foal presenting for intermittent fever, colic, and hyporexia following administration of 750 ml barium via nasogastric tube at (a) time zero (b) and 45 minutes. The stomach is markedly distended with gas and dependent fluid prior to contrast administration with a small contribution of the initial barium administration. Note the absence of contrast in the small intestines at 45 minutes, indicative of delayed gastric emptying.

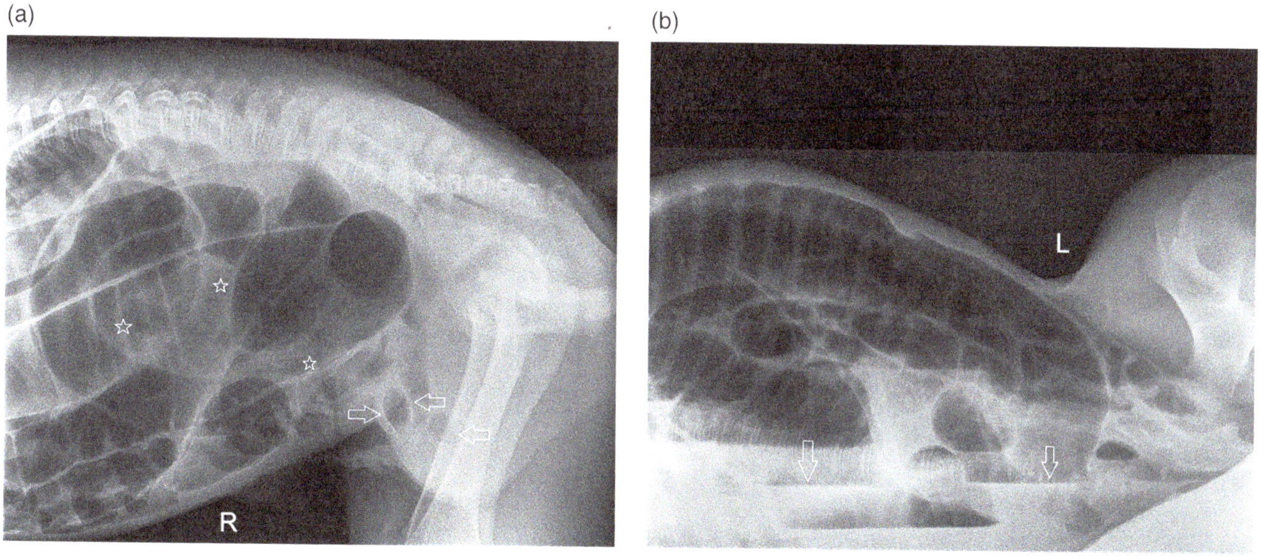

Figure 15.V.6 A 36-hour-old Dutch Harness Horse presented for signs of colic. (a) Severe gas dilation of the large and small intestine occupies the majority of the abdomen. The diameter of multiple small intestinal loops is much greater than the length of the L1 vertebra. Fecal material (presumed meconium) is noted in the large colon (stars) and a few gas-filled loops of small intestine are noted in the inguinal/scrotal region (arrows). (b) Ventrodorsal radiograph of the same foal. Note the gas disention within the small intestine and colon and multiple fluid-gas interfaces (arrows).

intestinal distension involving the entire intestinal length. Ileus has a variety of causes and is common in ill foals secondary to sepsis and asphyxia among other conditions.

If large bowel obstruction is present, the large intestine is distended, and the colon may appear displaced within the abdomen (Figures 15.V.6 and 15.V.8). Gas distension of the large bowel is typically more pronounced in foals with large intestinal obstruction as compared to foals with enteritis [10]. Large colon distension can be observed in foals with ileus, meconium impactions, large colon displacements, and atresia coli/ani. Colonic torsion can be identified as a nonhaustrated viscus in contact with the ventral abdominal wall [14]. More commonly than torsions or rotations are infectious and inflammatory

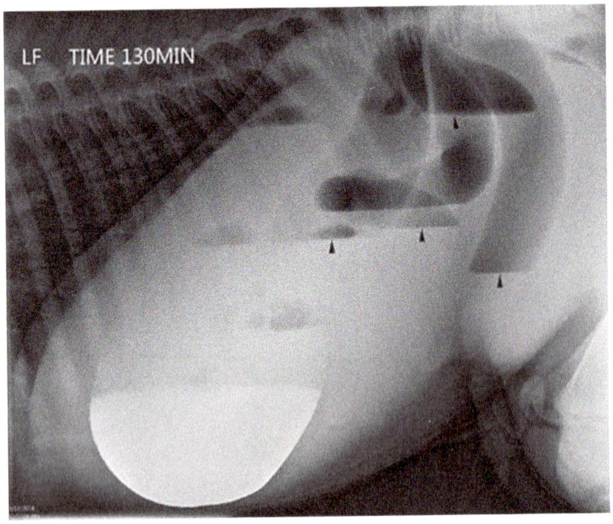

Figure 15.V.7 An 11-day-old Thoroughbred filly presented for signs of colic. Images acquired 130 minutes following barium administration via nasogastric tube. Lack of aboral movement of contrast from the stomach into the small intestines. Moderate to marked small intestinal distension with multiple-level fluid lines (black arrows).

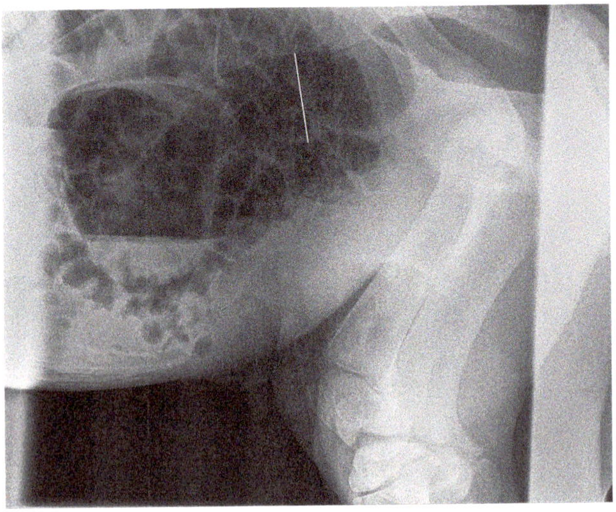

Figure 15.V.8 Lateral image of the caudal abdomen of a 1-day-old Morgan filly with transient signs of colic illustrating gas distended colon (bar) along with gas within the rectum. A fluid line is noted in a structure in the cranial abdomen (possibly the diaphragmatic flexure of the colon). In this image, a conclusive cause of distension is not identified with the clinical signs of colic resolving with medical therapy.

conditions of the large bowel in foals. Variations of distension with gas and fluid are seen in these radiographically.

Meconium impactions are a common cause of colic in newborn foals and can be secondary to anatomy (narrow pelvic canal), congenital abnormalities (atresia), or dehydration, among other causes. Meconium is considered "retained" when it has not been passed within 12 hours of birth. Impaction generally occurs in the small colon and/or rectum where it can be digitally palpated. However, when the transverse colon or right dorsal colon are affected, lateral radiographs may reveal granular, spherical masses within the intestine [15]. Ultrasonography can be more useful for identification of meconium and should be used prior to radiography (Figure 15.V.9).

When no meconium staining is observed in a foal exhibiting colic signs, atresia ani, recti, or coli should be

(a) (b)

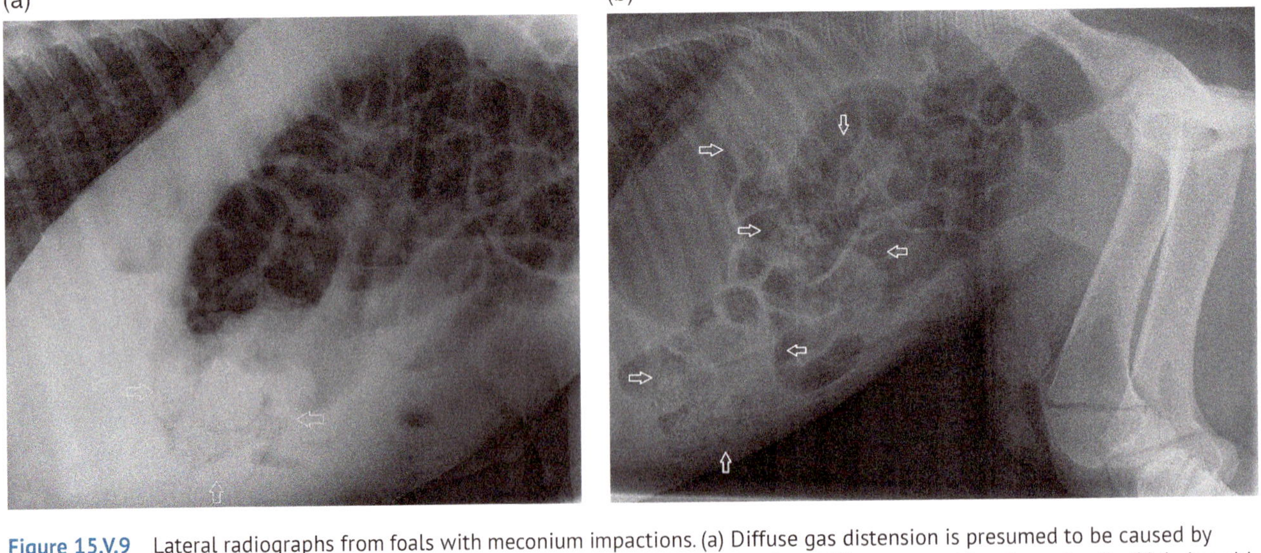

Figure 15.V.9 Lateral radiographs from foals with meconium impactions. (a) Diffuse gas distension is presumed to be caused by meconium material in the cranio-ventral abdomen (arrow) in a 2-day-old Standardbred filly presented for signs of colic. (b) 1-day-old Hackney colt presented for mild signs of colic. Lateral radiograph of abdomen indicates a region of mixed soft tissue and gas material consistent with fecal material (meconium) within the mid-abdomen (arrows) along with moderate gas distention of portions of the small intestine, stomach, large colon, and rectum.

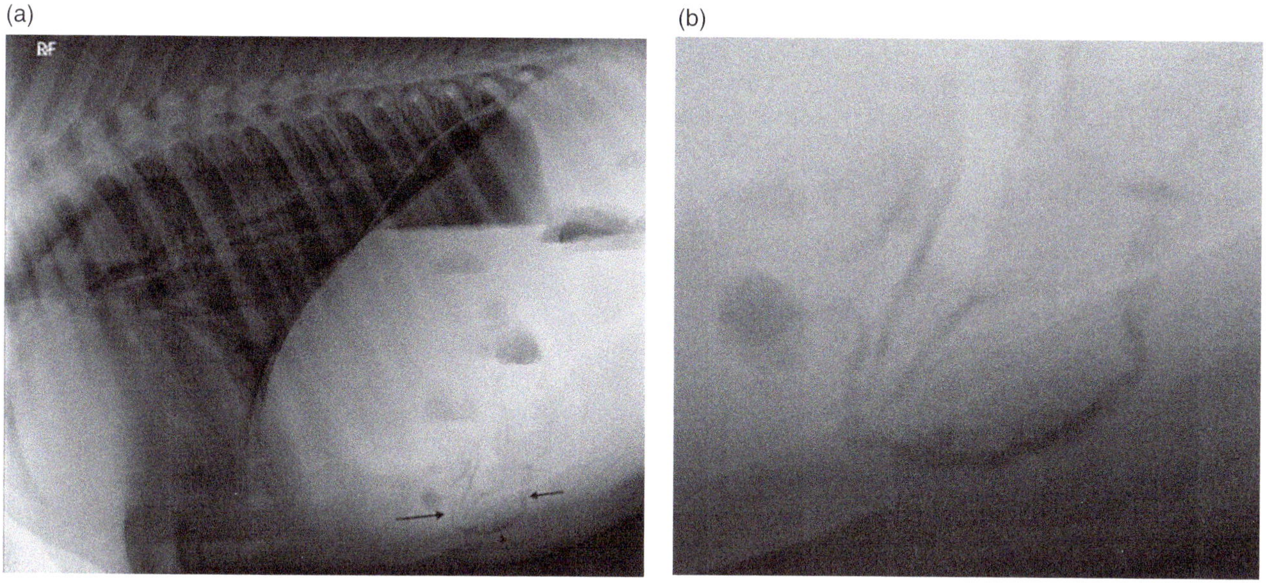

Figure 15.V.10 Lateral radiographs of an 11-day-old Thoroughbred filly presented for signs of colic. (a) Note the irregular gas accumulation within a small intestinal segment within the cranial abdomen on survey radiographs (arrows); (b) a magnified image of same area. The stomach is mildly distended with fluid and gas.

considered. Atresia ani and atresia recti can be diagnosed with relative ease (i.e., digital palpation); however, atresia coli involving a blind-ended terminus of the colon may be amenable to radiographic identification [16]. Radiographs with contrast can be implemented using a barium enema to identify a truncated colon in some cases, but in others the barium may fail to reach the terminus and render the study nondiagnostic [16].

Free peritoneal fluid and ingesta or sand can be noted on abdominal radiography as a consequence of a compromised mucosal barrier secondary to many aforementioned conditions. Pneumoperitoneum, which can occur with bowel rupture (e.g., gastric or colonic perforation) or previous abdominocentesis or abdominal surgery, appears radiographically as a gas cap in the dorsal aspect of the abdominal cavity in the standing foal [1]. In these cases, small volumes of gas tend to accumulate adjacent to the dorsal margin of the diaphragm. Increased conspicuity of serosal surfaces of the intestine may be present in a foal with pneumoperitoneum [13].

Diarrhea

Abdominal radiography can be used to investigate select causes of diarrhea. One example is examination for foreign material within the GI tract such as sand, gravel, or foreign bodies (e.g., wire) that might cause diarrhea in the foal. Small intestinal distension can be seen with *Clostridia* and *Salmonella* associated diarrhea in the foal, although large intestinal distension is more likely in these cases [2]. Necrotizing enterocolitis can also occur commonly in foals that are premature or experienced some period of hypoxia [2]. These cases may radiographically present with gas, fluid, or a combination of these findings within the intestinal wall. Pneumatosis intestinalis or emphysematous enteritis is also a possible finding, which is defined as the trapping and production of gas within the bowel wall and may appear as gas opacities (localized, fragmented, linear, or diffuse lucent regions) in foals with necrotizing enterocolitis (Figure 15.V.10) [2]. Pneumatosis intestinalis can be better imaged ultrasonographically than radiographically in some cases [10, 12]. This finding can be observed in a variety of clinical settings, including intestinal volvulus and other sources of GI ischemia in addition to enterocolitis.

General Considerations for Radiographic Contrast Studies of the Neonatal Gastrointestinal Tract

Contrast radiography (e.g., barium) administered orally or via feeding tube can be used to evaluate foals with dysphagia, or suspected disorders of the esophagus, gastric emptying, intestinal motility, or intestinal obstruction. Alternatively, retrograde contrast enemas can be administered to assess the rectum, small colon, and portions of the large colon in the neonatal foal. In these procedures, a survey radiograph of the abdomen is performed of the area of interest to confirm that the proper radiographic technique is utilized. Sedation should be avoided, if possible, as to not interfere with motility of the alimentary tract. One may need to increase exposure factors by 10% to compensate for the radiodense contrast media [12].

When performing a contrast study of the GI tract, the neonatal foal is ideally fasted for 4 hours (12 hours in older foals on solid feed) and any excess gas or fluid is removed from the stomach via placement of a nasogastric tube [2]. Barium (5–10 ml/kg) is subsequently administered via a feeding tube and a series of standing lateral radiographs are acquired immediately after barium administration and at approximately 5, 15, 30, 60, and 90 minutes with additional radiographs collected at later times if necessary (e.g., every 2 hours until contrast media has reached the small colon) (Figure 15.V.11) [2]. In a healthy foal, the stomach's width is typically half the vertical length of the stomach and the stomach is usually empty within 2 hours of administration [17]. Contrast media is observed entering the duodenum almost immediately post-contrast administration, and contrast media should clear the small intestine within 3 hours of administration [2, 10, 13, 17]. The cecum is usually visible within 1–2 hours after barium administration and a gas cap is typically observed in the cecal base, large sacculations (haustra) can be identified, and the base of the cecum is located in the right caudal abdomen and the apex near the xiphoid [2, 10, 13, 17]. Transit of contrast material through the large colon is rapid with contrast media noted within the transverse colon by 3 hours post-administration; complete elimination of barium should be noted by 36 hours in neonatal foals [2, 13]. A diagnosis of delayed gastric emptying is supported if minimal to no contrast media aboral to the stomach or duodenum is observed 30–90 minutes after contrast administration (Figures 15.V.5, 15.V.7, 15.V.11, and 15.V.12). Alternatively, extra-luminal filling defects of the proximal duodenum are suggestive of duodenal stricture [10]. Failure of the contrast media to pass through a segment of the intestine is suggestive of obstruction at that location [13]. Of note, a contrast study should not be performed in the presence of severe small intestinal distension.

If large intestinal distension is observed on noncontrast radiographs, retrograde contrast radiography can be attempted to potentially identify the site of obstruction [13]. Examples of intestinal disorders that can be identified with retrograde contrast enemas include obstruction of the rectum, small colon (e.g. meconium impaction) or transverse colon, and right displacement of the colon [13]. During this imaging procedure, foals might require sedation to limit movement and control visceral pain caused by the primary disease process. A soapy-water enema is used to evacuate any feces from the rectum, and a lubricated Foley catheter (30 French with balloon) is passed approximately 2–3 in. into the rectum and the balloon is inflated [18]. Barium sulfate suspension (approximately 200–500 ml 30% wt/vol) is infused via gravity flow while a radiograph is acquired immediately after instillation of the barium [2, 12]. If more than several hundred milliliters of contrast media flows easily into the small colon of the neonatal foal, the small colon is likely not obstructed [13]. Volumes of contrast media up to 20 ml/kg of body weight, administered via gravity flow per rectum, have been suggested to evaluate the large colon [2].

In the healthy foal, retrograde barium enemas can be followed cranially where the barium reaches the transverse colon in the mid-abdomen; contrast media then enters the right dorsal colon, where dilation is observed [13]. Contrast media subsequently continues cranially in the right dorsal colon until it reaches the left dorsal colon, where contrast media then traces caudally. The contrast media can then outline the pelvic flexure and then course cranially via the left ventral colon [13]. Ventrodorsal radiographs might facilitate contrast studies and outline similar structures as noted via lateral radiographs. In foals with atresia coli, the contrast media will be observed to stop abruptly at the affected site (Figure 15.V.13). If atresia coli is located proximal to the transverse colon, more contrast media might have to be administered to identify the affected region [13]. Meconium obstructions can be highlighted during contrast studies, as the meconium is silhouetted by the media. Barium enemas have proven to be a reliable test for the diagnosis of obstruction of the large, transverse, or small colon [19] but the clinician should remain mindful that rupture of the intestinal tract is a rare, but potential, fatal complication of this procedure.

Although gastroscopy has largely supplanted this method, double-contrast studies have also been described to evaluate the gastric wall and detect gastric ulceration in older foals [20]. In this technique, the foal is fasted and sedated, and barium (2.2 ml/kg) is administered into the stomach via feeding tube; the stomach is then distended with air. A right lateral standing radiograph with the beam centered at the 12th rib is acquired with right and left lateral recumbent and ventrodorsal projections serving as optional views. In the healthy standing foal, the gastric wall appears thin, and the barium uniformly coats the gastric mucosa, which appears smooth.

Diaphragmatic Hernia

Although diaphragmatic herniation in the foal is uncommon [21], it has been reported in congenital [22] and traumatic contexts [23]. As opposed to the etiology in adult counterparts, neonatal diaphragmatic hernias caused by trauma are more often associated with lacerations secondary to fractured rubs rather than blunt trauma. Neonatal diaphragmatic hernia has presented with dyspnea and exercise intolerance in one foal under the age of 12 weeks [24]; however, other reports tend to present most

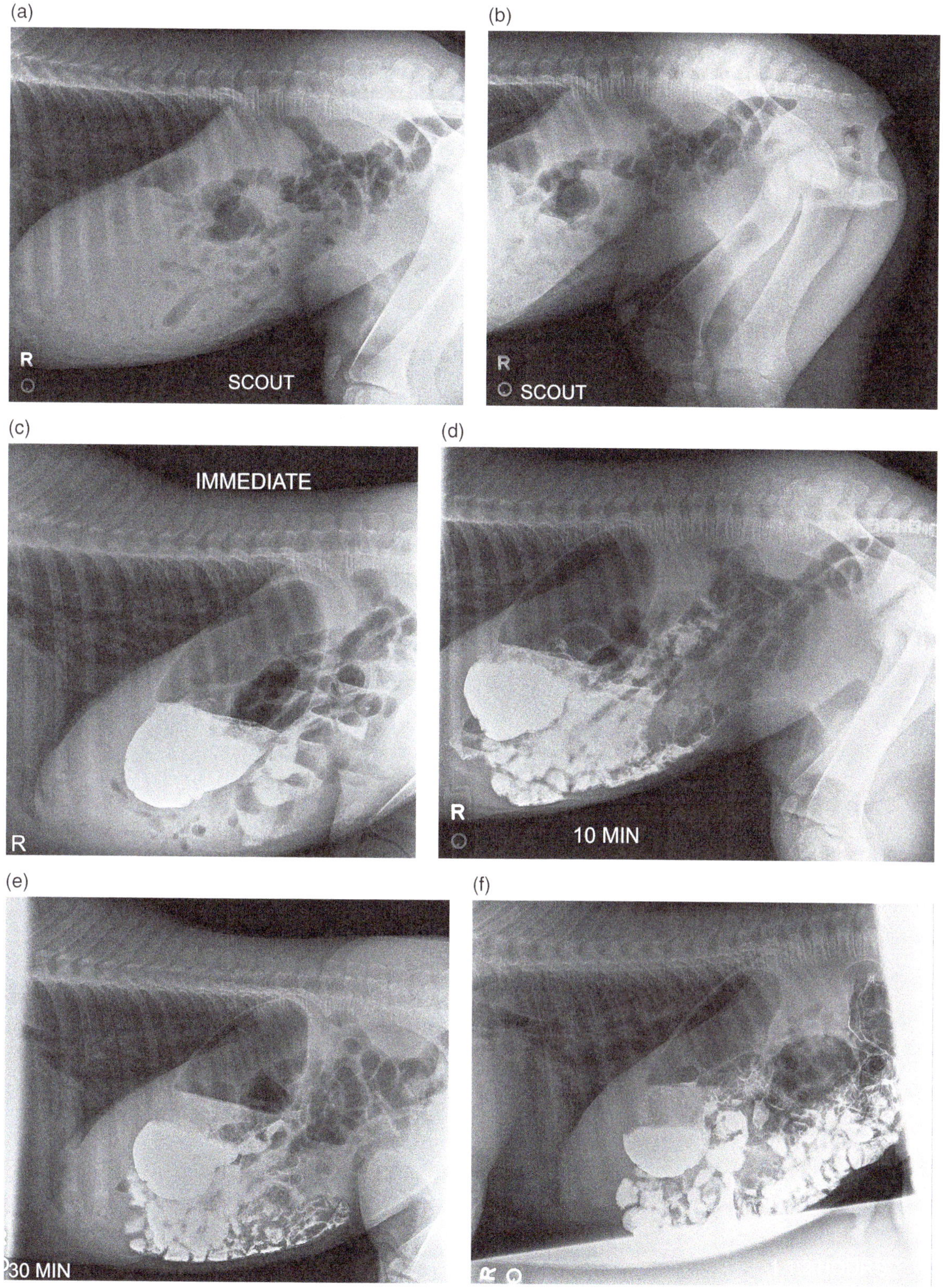

Figure 15.V.11 Seven-day-old Arabian colt presented for a 5-day history of mild colic. A contrast study was performed to determine if there was delayed gastric emptying. (a and b) Survey radiographs noting gas within the stomach, small intestine, and large colon prior to contrast media administration. (c) Following contrast media administration, approximately one-third of the lumen of the stomach is filled with media along with immediate presence of contrast media within the adjacent small intestinal loops. A gas cap is present in the dorsal portion of the stomach. (d) At 10 minutes, there is a moderate amount of contrast media in the small intestine with numerous overlying loops of partially filled small intestine. There is a slightly irregular contour of the ventral curve of the stomach noted. (e and f) At 30 minutes and 1.5 hours, there is contrast media filling the majority of the small intestine. (g and h) At 2.5 hours, there is contrast media within the lumen of the large colon. A moderate amount of contrast media remains within the ventral portion of the stomach. There is also semi-formed ingesta in the rectum. The normal gastric emptying time ranges between 30 and 120 minutes.

(g) (h)

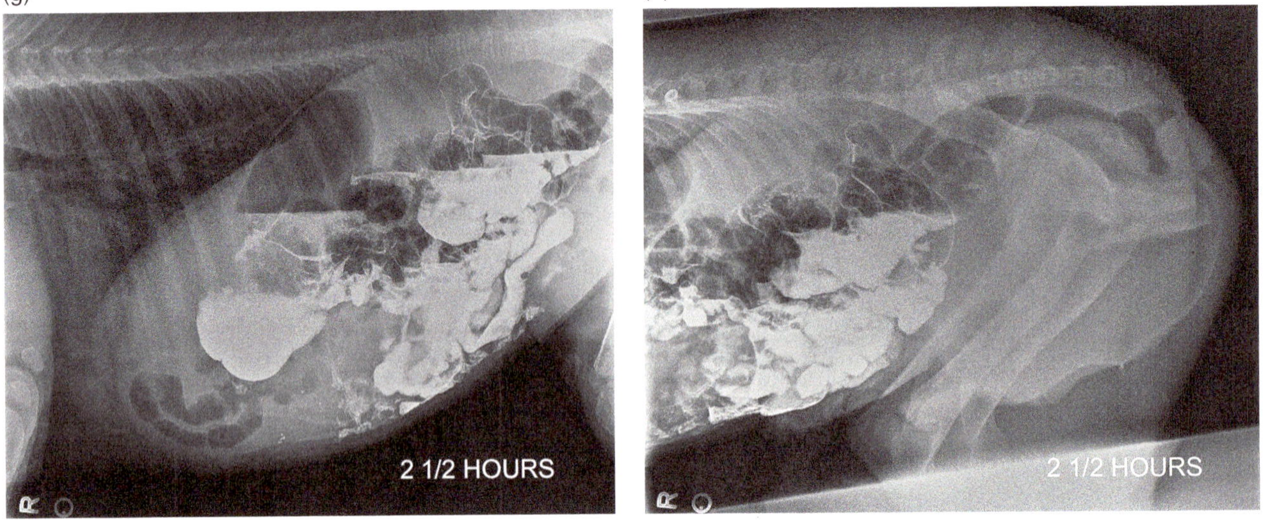

Figure 15.V.11 (Continued)

(a) (b)

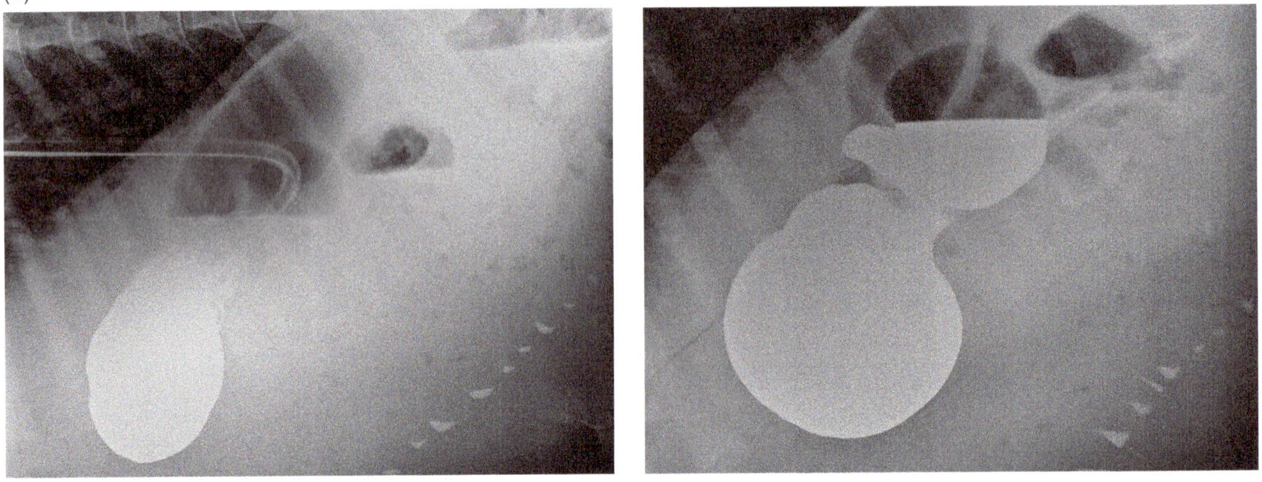

Figure 15.V.12 Lateral radiographs of a 4-month-old Thoroughbred colt presented for chronic colic in which a contrast study of the GI tract was performed evaluate gastric emptying. (a) Contrast media is administered via NG tube into the stomach, Time 0. (b) 70 minutes after administration, contrast media is still noted in the stomach without passing into the duodenum. Ultrasound confirmed severe duodenal thickening and ulceration, consistent with duodenal stricture and secondary outflow obstruction.

(a) (b)

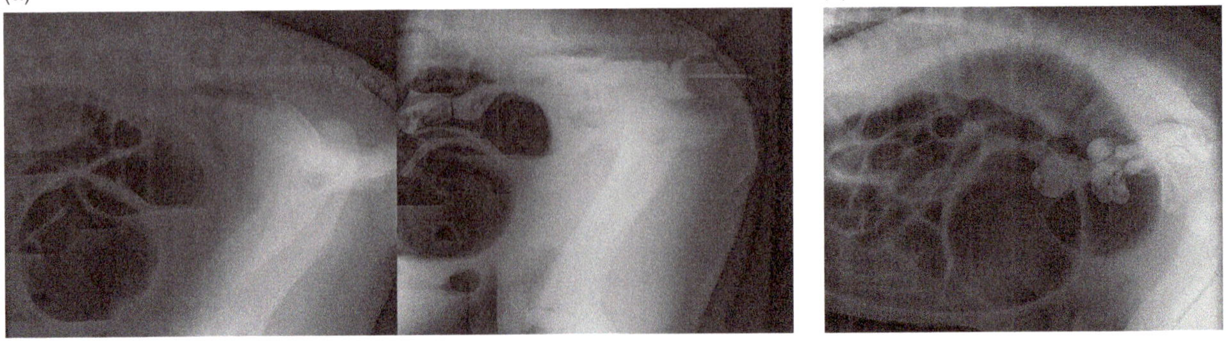

Figure 15.V.13 Survey and contrast radiographs of a 2-day-old Thoroughbred filly with atresia coli. (a) Note the marked small intestinal and large colonic gas distension on survey images. (b) Using a Foley catheter, barium was administered into the rectum. Barium occupies the aborad aspect of the small colon before abrupt cessation is noted with smooth oral tapering.

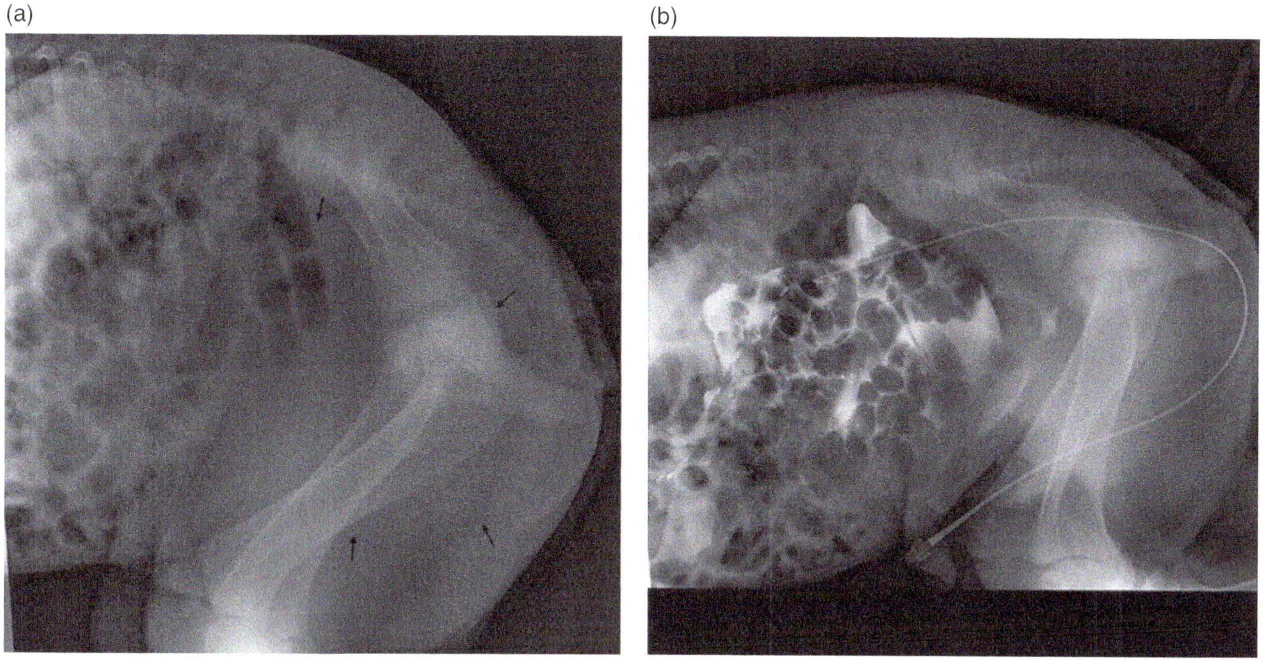

Figure 15.V.14 Three-day-old Irish Sport horse colt presented for stranguria. (a) Image demonstrating gas within the lumen of a retrograde urinary catheter (arrows). (b) Image following administration of nonionic iodinated contrast medium with distribution into the peritoneal cavity due to urinary bladder rupture.

commonly with signs of colic. A lateral radiograph taken in lateral recumbency revealed multiple gas-filled loops of small intestine within the thoracic cavity, and absence of the cardiac silhouette was observed. Ultrasonography can also be used in conjunction with radiographs and may be a more sensitive imaging modality. The most common radiographic sign of diaphragmatic hernia is pleural effusion, although it is not a finding specific to herniation.

Inguinal Hernia

Inguinal hernias can often be incidental and without clinical consequence, but occasionally incarcerated bowel can be present. If an inguinal hernia is not reducible or if there is evidence of strangulation, surgical correction is recommended [25]. Ultrasonography is recommended; however, lateral radiographs of the inguinal region may be helpful in identifying incarcerated bowel or mesentery (Figure 15.V.4).

Urinary Tract

Contrast cystography can be used to detect bladder or urachal rupture. Although plain radiographs are not of particular use when evaluating the urinary tract in horses, contrast studies can harbor utility, particularly cystography. Urine leakage can occur by way of the bladder, ureters, or urachus [25]. Historically, pollakiuria is often but not always described. Abdominal distension may be present in these cases. Ultrasonography is often a useful diagnostic in investigating bladder rupture and urachal leakage in foals. It has largely supplanted the need for contrast radiography, but the latter has been used successfully. Castagnetti et al. described retrograde positive-contrast cystography using 50 ml of diluted contrast media through a urinary catheter and performed a lateral abdominal radiograph revealing contrast media within the peritoneum and outside of the bladder (Figure 15.V.14) [26].

References

1 Fischer, A.T., Kerr, L.Y., and O'Brien, T.R. (1987). Radiographic diagnosis of gastrointestinal disorders in the foal. *Vet. Radiol. Ultrasound* 28: 42–48.

2 Lester, G.D. and Lester, N.V. (2001). Abdominal and thoracic radiography in the neonate. *Vet. Clin. North Am. Equine Pract.* 17: 19–46.

3 Yarbrough, T.B., Voss, E.D., Herrgesell, E.J. et al. (1999). Persistent frenulum in the epiglottis in four foals. *Vet. Surg.* 28: 287–291.
4 Tulleners, E.P. (1991). Correlation of performance with endoscopic and radiographic assessment of epiglottic hypoplasia in racehorses with epiglottic entrapment corrected by use of contact neodymium:yttrium aluminum garnet laser. *J. Am. Vet. Med. Assoc.* 198: 621–626.
5 Clabough, D.L., Roberts, M.C., and Robertson, I. (1991). Probable congenital esophageal stenosis in a thoroughbred foal. *J. Am. Vet. Med. Assoc.* 199: 483–435.
6 Smith, T.R. (2004). Unusual vascular ring anomaly in a foal. *Can. Vet. J.* 45: 1016–1018.
7 Barber, S.M., McLaughlin, B.G., and Fretz, P.B. (1983). Esophageal ectasia in a quarterhorse colt. *Can. Vet. J.* 24: 46–49.
8 Rohrback, B.W. and Rooney, J.R. (1980). Congenital esophageal ectasia in a Thoroughbred foal. *J. Am. Vet. Med. Assoc.* 177: 65–67.
9 Gaughan, E.M., Gift, L.J., and Frank, R.K. (1992). Tubular duplication of the cervical portion of the esophagus in a foal. *J. Am. Vet. Med. Assoc.* 201: 748–750.
10 Chaffin, M.K. and Cohen, N.D. (1999). Diagnostic assessment of foals with colic. *Proc. Annu. Conv. Am. Assoc. Equine Pract.* 45: 235–242.
11 Bezdekova, B., Wohlsein, P., and Venner, M. (2020). Chronic severe pyloric lesions in horses: 47 cases. *Equine Vet. J.* 52: 200–204.
12 Furr, M. (2017). Imaging of the foal with colic and abdominal distension. In: *The Equine Acute Abdomen*, 3e (ed. A. Blikslager, N. White, J. Moore, and T. Mair), 418–421. Hoboken, NJ: Wiley.
13 Fischer, A.T. (1997). Advances in diagnostic techniques for horses with colic. *Vet. Clin. North Am. Equine Pract.* 13: 203–219.
14 Cudd, T.A., Toal, R.L., and Embertson, R.M. (1987). The use of clinical findings, abdominocentesis, and abdominal radiographs to assess surgical versus non-surgical abdominal disease in the foal. In: *Proc. 33rd Annual Convention of the American Association of Equine Practice*, 41–53.
15 Burbidge, C. (2012). Meconium impaction in the equine neonate. *Vet. Nurs. J.* 27: 194–197.
16 Young, R.L., Linford, R.L., and Olander, H.J. (1992). Atresia coli in the foal: a review of six cases. *Equine Vet. J.* 24: 60–62.
17 Campbell, M.L., Ackerman, N., and Peyton, L.C. (1984). Radiographic gastrointestinal anatomy of the foal. *Vet. Radiol.* 25: 194–204.
18 Cudd, T.A. (1990). Gastrointestinal system dysfunction. In: *Equine Clinical Neonatology* (ed. A.M. Koterba, W.H. Drummond, and P.C. Kosch), 367–442. Phildelphia: Lea & Febiger.
19 Fischer, A.T. and Yarbrough, T.Y. (1995). Retrograde contrast radiography of the distal portions of the intestinal tract in foals. *J. Am. Vet. Med. Assoc.* 207: 734–737.
20 Traub, J.L., Gallina, A.M., Grant, B.D. et al. (1983). Phenylbutazone toxicosis in the foal. *Am. J. Vet. Res.* 44: 1410–1418.
21 Blood, D.C. and Henderson, J.A. (1974). *Veterinary Medicine*, 4e, 175 and 98. London: Bailliere and Tindall.
22 Tăbăran, A.F., Nagy, A., Cătoi, C. et al. (2015). Congenital diaphragmatic hernia with concurrent aplasia of the pericardium in a foal. *BMC Vet. Res.* 11: 309.
23 Palmer, J.E. (2012). Colic and diaphragmatic hernias in neonatal foals. *Equine Vet. Educ.* 24: 340–342.
24 Speirs, V.C. and Reynolds, W.T. (1976). Successful repair of a diaphragmatic hernia in a foal. *Equine Vet. J.* 8: 170–172.
25 Richardson, D.W. (1985). Urogenital problems in the neonatal foal. *Vet. Clin. North Am. Equine Pract.* 1: 179–188.
26 Castagnetti, C., Mariella, J., Pirrone, A. et al. (2010). Urethral and bladder rupture in a neonatal colt with uroperitoneum. *Equine Vet. Educ.* 22: 132–138.

Section VI Oral Lactose Tolerance Test and Oral Glucose Absorption Test

David Wong

Although clinically infrequently implemented, the oral lactose tolerance test (OLTT) has been described in foals to determine if a foal has lactose maldigestion. Lactase is a disaccharidase produced by small intestinal mucosal cells and hydrolyzes the primary milk carbohydrate lactose to monosaccharides glucose and galactose [1]. This hydrolytic process is needed for milk digestion in the foal. Lactase is present in the small intestine of the fetal foal from the third month of gestation, peaking at birth, and then waning around 4–6 months of age and is usually insignificant by the time of weaning; horses over 3 years of age are unable to hydrolyze lactose [2, 3]. Maldigestion and diarrhea can occur secondary to milk intolerance in the foal due to lactase deficiency. Lactase deficiency in foals can be primary or more commonly secondary to enteric disease, such as *Clostridium difficile* or rotaviral infection [4–6]. Diagnosis of lactose intolerance is frequently based on clinical suspicion, but the OLTT can be used to confirm the diagnosis.

The OLTT is an indirect assay that evaluates changes in blood glucose concentration after lactose is administered orally. After a 4-hour fast, the OLTT is performed by administered 1 g/kg of lactose monohydrate in a 20% water solution via nasogastric tube. Blood is collected before dosing (time 0) and at 30, 60, 90, 120, 180 minutes after dosing to measure glucose concentrations. In one study, mean plasma glucose concentrations in foals increased from 99.7 mg/dl at time 0 to 176.8 by 90 minutes post-lactose administration [1]. The study documented that the mean plasma glucose concentration in all foals (6–92 days of age) should increase by at least 35 mg/dl (mean increase ± 2 SD) within 90 minutes [1]. More specifically, in six neonatal foals (mean age 7 days), there was a 57.6 mg/dl increase of plasma glucose after lactose administration.

The oral glucose absorption test (OGAT) is another diagnostic test used to evaluate small intestinal absorption of glucose, hepatic glucose update, and endocrine function of the pancreas in horses. In healthy horses, the plasma glucose concentration doubles (peak), compared with baseline concentration, by 120 minutes (Phase I) after administration of 1 g/kg body weight of dextrose (20% solution) administered via a nasogastric tube; subsequently the plasma glucose should return to baseline concentrations after 4–6 hours (Phase II) [5, 7–9]. A decreased or flattened plasma glucose concentration curve suggests reduced intestinal absorption and implies considerable morphologic or functional alterations of the small intestine [5, 9, 10]. Total small intestinal malabsorption is defined as a failure of plasma glucose concentration to increase by >15% above baseline concentrations 120 minutes after oral glucose administration; in comparison, partial malabsorption is defined as glucose concentrations that are >15% but <85% of the baseline glucose concentration at 180 minutes [9]. The OGAT is impacted by the rate of gastric emptying, mucosal cell transport function, intestinal transit time, dietary history, patient age, length of fast before testing and degree of excitement, pain or stress experienced by the foal [9–11]. The OGAT has been used to serially monitor small intestinal function of foals with *Lawsonia intracellularis* infection, but could also be used to evaluate small intestinal dysfunction or serially monitor other diseases that impact small intestinal function [12].

Equine Neonatal Medicine, First Edition. Edited by David M. Wong and Pamela A. Wilkins.

References

1 Martens, R.J., Malone, P.S., and Brust, D.M. (1985). Oral lactose tolerance test in foals: techniques and normal values. *Am. J. Vet. Res.* 46: 2163–2165.

2 Roberts, M.C., Hill, F.W.G., and Kidder, D.E. (1974). The development and distribution of small intestinal disaccharidases in the horse. *Res. Vet. Sci.* 17: 42–48.

3 Roberts, M.C. (1975). The development and distribution of mucosal enzymes in the small intestine of the fetus and young foal. *J. Reprod. Fertil. Suppl.* 23: 717–723.

4 Weese, J.S., Parsons, D.A., and Staempfli, H.R. (1999). Association of *Clostridium difficile* with enterocolitis and lactose intolerance in a foal. *J. Am. Vet. Med. Assoc.* 214: 229–232.

5 Sweeney, R.W. (1987). Laboratory evaluation of malassimilation in horses. *Vet. Clin. N. Am. Equine Pract.* 3: 507–514.

6 Roberts, V.L.H., Knottenbelt, D.C., Williams, A. et al. (2008). Suspected primary lactose intolerance in neonatal foals. *Equine Vet. Educ.* 20: 249–251.

7 Firshman, A.M. and Valberg, S.J. (2007). Factors affecting clinical assessment of insulin sensitivity in horses. *Equine Vet. J.* 39: 567–575.

8 Roberts, M.C. and Hill, F.W. (1973). The oral glucose tolerance test in the horse. *Equine Vet. J.* 5: 171–173.

9 Mair, T.S., Hillyer, M.H., Taylor, F.G. et al. (1991). Small intestinal malabsorption in the horse: an assessment of the specificity of the oral glucose tolerance test. *Equine Vet. J.* 23: 344–346.

10 Roberts, M. (1985). Malabsorption syndromes in the horse. *Compend. Contin. Educ. Pract. Vet.* 7: S637–S646.

11 Kempter, D.L., Perkins, G.A., Schumacher, J. et al. (2000). Equine lympho-plasmacytic enterocolitis: a retrospective study of 14 cases. *Equine Vet. J.* 32 (Suppl): 108–112.

12 Wong, D.M., Alcott, C.J., Sponseller, B.A. et al. (2009). Impaired intestinal absorption of glucose in 4 foals with *Lawsonia intracellularis* infection. *J. Vet. Intern. Med.* 23: 940–944.

Section VII Liver Biopsy

David Wong

Liver biopsy is an infrequent diagnostic test needed in the neonatal foal, but has been used to help characterize neonatal hepatic tumors [1]; investigate portosystemic shunts [2],toxic hepatopathies [3], and elevated liver enzyme activity [4]; identify infectious organisms (e.g. *Clostridium piliforme*, Equine Herpesvirus-1, bacterial cholangiohepatitis) [5, 6]; and collect liver samples in the research setting [7, 8].

A few methods have been described to perform liver biopsy in the foal, but ultrasound guided biopsy collection is the safest and most reliable. Foals should be sedated adequately to prevent sudden movements that are common in the awake foal [8, 9]; other clinicians choose to collect biopsy samples under general anesthesia [7, 10].

In one research project in which liver biopsies were collected, foals were sedated with xylazine and butorphanol and anesthetized with ketamine. Foals were then placed in left lateral recumbency and the appropriate biopsy site was selected from the right flank using transabdominal ultrasound guidance. Similar to biopsy techniques in the adult horse, the skin over the biopsy site is clipped and aseptically prepared and typically a 14-gauge Tru-cut or spring activated biopsy instrument is used [7, 10]. Other techniques have included laparoscopic-guided biopsy collection using a 14-gauge Tru-cut biopsy needle under general anesthesia [7]. Biopsy samples should be submitted for histopathologic and/or microbiological culture. Minimal side effects of liver biopsy have been reported.

Complications associated with liver biopsy in the horse appear to be relatively rare with hemorrhage being the most common complication [11]. In one study involving 66 horses between 1 and 30 years of age, the most common complications were subclinical bleeding (three horses) and a diaphragmatic hematoma (one horse). Interestingly, at least one coagulation profile abnormality was detected in 58% of the 43 horses with histopathologically confirmed liver disease suggesting that abnormalities in coagulation are common in the horse but are not correlated with complications (i.e. hemorrhage) in adult horses; a similar study investigating complications of liver biopsies is not available in foals, but clinicians should consider evaluating coagulation profiles in foals prior to biopsy [11].

References

1 Hepworth-Warren, K.L., Wong, D.M., Galow, N.L. et al. (2014). Metastatic tumor in pregnancy: placental germ cell tumor with metastasis to the foal. *J. Equine Vet. Sci.* 34: 1134–1139.

2 Buonanno, A.M., Carlson, G.P., and Kantrowitz, B. (1998). Clinical and diagnostic features of portosystemic shunt in a foal. *J. Am. Vet. Med. Assoc.* 192: 387–389.

3 Acland, H.M., Mann, P.C., Robertson, J.L. et al. (1984). Toxic hepatopathy in neonatal foals. *Vet. Pathol.* 21: 3–9.

4 Haggett, E.F., Magdesian, K.G. et al. (2011). Clinical implications of high liver enzyme activity in hospitalized neonatal foals. *J. Am. Vet. Med. Assoc.* 239: 661–667.

5 Borchers, A., Magdesian, K.G., Halland, S. et al. (2006). Successful treatment and polymerase chain reaction (PCR) confirmation of Tyzzer's disease in a foal and clinical and pathologic characteristics of 6 additional foals (1986–2005). *J. Vet. Intern. Med.* 20: 1212–1218.

6 Hess-Dudan, F. (1994). Four possible causes of hepatic failure and/or icterus in the newborn foal. *Equine Vet. Educ.* 6: 310–315.

7 Pearce, S.G., Firth, E.C., Grace, N.D. et al. (1997). Liver biopsy techniques for adult horses and neonatal foals to assess copper status. *Aust. Vet. J.* 75: 194–198.

Equine Neonatal Medicine, First Edition. Edited by David M. Wong and Pamela A. Wilkins.

8 Gee, E.K., Grace, N.D., Firth, E.C. et al. (2000). Changes in liver copper concentration of Thoroughbred foals from birth to 160 days of age and the effect of prenatal copper supplementation of their dams. *Aust. Vet. J.* 78: 347–353.

9 Setlakwe, E.L., Sweeney, R., Engiles, J.B. et al. (2014). Identification of Bartonelle henselae in the liver of a Thoroughbred foal with severe suppurative cholangiohepatitis. *J. Vet. Intern. Med.* 28: 1341–1345.

10 Elfenbein, J.R., Giguere, S., Meyer, S.K. et al. (2010). The effects of deferoxamine mesylate on iron elimination after blood transfusion in neonatal foals. *J. Vet. Intern. Med.* 24: 1475–1482.

11 Johns, I.C. and Sweeney, R.W. (2008). Coagulation abnormalities and complications after percutaneous liver biopsy in horses. *J. Vet. Intern. Med.* 22: 185–189.

Section VIII Diagnostic Tests and Fecal Analysis in the Neonatal Foal with Diarrhea

Emily Schaefer

The wide variety of gastrointestinal (GI) diseases that affect foals warrants individualized treatment plans in addition to nonspecific supportive care, and therefore attaining a diagnosis is a critical precursor to therapy. This section reviews the diagnostic steps available for evaluating feces in the diarrheic foal. Following diagnostics, a specific as well as generalized approach to the treatment of inflammatory GI diseases is warranted.

Fecal Molecular Testing

Molecular testing for infectious pathogens, including genetic and antigenic materials, has greatly improved the diagnostic ability over the last several decades. Polymerase chain reaction (PCR) and enzyme-linked immunosorbent assays (ELISA) are the predominant molecular testing types in veterinary medicine and are used to diagnose numerous infectious etiologic agents associated with diarrhea in the foal. As such, this section is disease-based to provide an orderly summation of the available information. The molecular testing modalities in equine neonatal diarrhea are summarized in Table 15.VIII.1.

Types of Infectious Diseases

Rotavirus

For years, electron microscopy (EM) of ultracentrifugated fecal material was the gold standard of identification. However, EM has low sensitivity with a threshold of detection of 10^7 viral particles/mL of feces and requires specialized equipment and trained personnel [2]. Immunofluorescence of tissue samples only detect virus within epithelial cells for the short time they are present on the villous surface, or 4–6 hours after the onset of diarrhea, thereby reducing its utility. Enzyme-linked immunosorbent assay (ELISA) based on the VP6 protein, a highly conserved protein of the intermediate capsid and most abundant rotaviral particle, is available for fecal testing. Though this stall side test can provide rapid results, some variations exist between human and equine VP6 proteins, reducing the accuracy of some commercially available ELISA rotavirus kits [3].

PCR testing is the most sensitive and specific test and comes in several forms. A one-step multiplex reverse transcriptase quantitative polymerase chain reaction (rt-qPCR) demonstrates 100% sensitivity and 99.2% specificity for the G14 VP7 protein, which is found in the outer capsid of equine rotavirus (Group A) [2, 4, 5]. In the same study, the PCR based on the NSP3 protein had excellent diagnostic accuracy for equine rotavirus (100% sensitivity and specificity), and the G3 protein (which is present in vaccine strains but not in wild type infections) PCR had a 92.7% sensitivity and 100% specificity. These findings suggest that detection of equine rotavirus antigen via NSP3 positive results with a negative G3 or G14 type should be considered a positive diagnostic test but should be followed up with Sanger sequencing for epidemiological and vaccine response surveillance. Additionally, an insulated isothermal RT-PCR is available as a "stall side" test with a portable PCR reader that shows 91.7% agreement with a commercial reverse transcriptase RT-PCR [6].

Pregnant mares mount serologic responses to both G3 and G14 strains of rotavirus when vaccinated, but serum was not collected from the foals in this study [7]. Another study demonstrated that vaccination of the dam resulted in protective titer levels to G3 rotavirus strains in the foal, but not to G14 strains, which may explain the recent rise in rotavirus infections in Kentucky [4, 8–10]. Serology may be of little diagnostic utility due to the relatively ubiquitous nature of rotavirus and vaccination on many breeding farms.

Equine Neonatal Medicine, First Edition. Edited by David M. Wong and Pamela A. Wilkins.

Table 15.VIII.1 Testing methodologies for infectious disease pathogens in equine neonatal diarrhea.

Etiologic Agent	Age Range	Clinical Signs	Test
Salmonella	Any	Endotoxemia, colic, hemorrhagic diarrhea	24 h selenite enrichment fecal culture, blood culture, PCR
C. difficile	Any	Diarrhea, colic, fever	PCR, toxin ELISA
C. perfringens	2 h–2 wk	Colic, fever, hemorrhagic diarrhea with foul odor	PCR, β toxin ELISA, netF toxin PCR
Rotavirus	3–60 d	Yellow diarrhea, fever	Fecal ELISA, PCR
Coronavirus	2 d–2 wk	Soft manure to diarrhea, fever	PCR, postmortem intestinal immuno-histochemistry, convalescent titers
Rhodococcus equi	3 wk–6 mo	Diarrhea, poor growth	VapA fecal PCR
Equine Adenovirus 2	2 wk–9 mo	Diarrhea, may have respiratory and other mucosal epithelium affected	Inclusion bodies on electron microscopy
Cryptosporidium parvum	2–21 d	Chronic, intermittent, self-limiting diarrhea	Acid-fast stained fecal smear
Strongyloides westeri	7–14 d, patent infections up to 6 mo	Acute-chronic diarrhea, hypoalbuminemia	Fecal flotation >2000 embryonated eggs per gram [1]
Others	Any	Diarrhea	By exclusion and fecal culture, ideally
E. coli, Bacteroides, Aerococcus, Aeromonas, Enterococcus			Koch's postulates would be satisfied for definitive diagnosis

Clostridium perfringens Type A and C

Due to the ubiquitous nature of *Clostridium perfringens*, positive culture of fecal material alone is not diagnostic. In the foal, the most common pathogenic strains are types A and C, both of which carry the *cpa* gene for the alpha toxin, but only type C carries the *cpb* gene for the beta toxin. Documentation of the elucidated toxin or associated gene is required to attribute clinical signs to GI inhabitation. This is most often done by toxin ELISA for alpha and beta toxins. Alpha toxin alone is considered to be nonpathogenic. While unusually high concentrations of alpha toxin can be hemolytic, resulting in intravascular hemolysis and icterus, the occasional pathogenicity of type A strains has thus far not had a definitive etiology. However, type A strains may contain a newly discovered pore-forming toxin (PFT) called netF that has been associated with signs of necrotizing enterocolitis in foals [11, 12]. A PCR primer has been developed, showing that netF is contained on a conjugative plasmid with netE, along with a second conjugative plasmid that contains genes *cpe* and *cpb2*, and a third conjugative plasmid that contains the genetic code for a bacteriocin, which is suspected to enhance intestinal colonization [13]. In a study by Gohari et al., *C. perfringens* type A isolated from dogs with necrotizing hemorrhagic gastroenteritis and foals with necrotizing enteritis was cytotoxic to experimental equine ovarian cells, whereas strains positive for *cpa*, *cpb*, *cpb2*, and/or *cpe* did not show cytotoxicity. In an elegant investigative process, researchers were able to show that retention of the netF gene with concurrent mutation of other suspected toxin genes netE and netG did not reduce cytotoxicity of the strain. When a mutant strain including netF complementation (i.e. the netF gene was returned to the strain) was evaluated, cytotoxicity to equine ovarian cells returned. In addition, investigators noted that with trans-conjugation with the netE/netF plasmid without the cpe plasmid, cytoxicity was also returned. Finally, a netF plasmid, with no other toxin genes, was electrophorated into a nonpathogenic strain of *C. perfringens,* which then became cytotoxic to the equine ovarian cells. These studies demonstrated that netF alone was responsible for cytotoxicity, not netE, netG, or cpe [14]. However, though clear netF-induced cytotoxicity to equine ovarian cells was demonstrated, Koch's postulates were not fulfilled for necrotizing enteritis of neonatal foals, and therefore netF could not be included in the expanded toxinotyping scheme proposed by Rood et al. (Table 15.VIII.2) [15]. At this time, the nomenclature will continue as netF+ type A *C. perfringens* until such time that Koch's postulates are fulfilled and a new toxinotype is designated. For diagnostic purposes, necrotizing enterocolitis in neonatal foals is most likely to be either beta toxin-containing type C, or netF+ type A *C. perfringens* (Table 15.VIII.1). In Ontario, Canada, netF+ strains of type A were not found in 135 fecal samples from 88 foals aged <1 week

Table 15.VIII.2 Toxin-based typing scheme for classification of *Clostridium perfringens* strains.

Toxinotype	a	ß	e	i	CPE	NetB
A	+	–	–	–	–	–
B	+	+	+	–	–	–
C	+	+	–	–	±	–
D	+	–	+	–	±	–
E	+	–	–	+	±	–
F	+	–	–	–	+	–
G	+	–	–	–	–	+

CPE, *Clostridium perfringens* enterotoxin.
Source: Adapted from Rood et al. [15].

to 4 months that had positive fecal cultures for *cpa+ C. perfringens*, suggesting that this pathogenic strain is not ubiquitous in healthy foals [16]. Thorough diagnostics, including toxin ELISA and a panel for other infectious causes of diarrhea should be performed.

Clostridium difficile Toxins A or B

Typical findings of necrotizing enteritis, such as mesocolonic edema, fluid GI contents, and diarrhea, are suggestive but not definitively diagnostic. Considering that some healthy foals carry *Clostridium difficile* and shed it in their feces, bacterial presence alone may be misleading when attempting to diagnosis GI disease in the neonate. Microbial identification can be performed by fecal culture or ELISA for microbial antigen, which has improved sensitivity compared to the fecal culture. Once *C. difficile* has been identified, the production of toxins must be confirmed. Antigen ELISA (TechLab, Blacksburg, VA) is diagnostic for both toxins, though has a lower sensitivity in foal fecal samples as compared to human samples [17–19]; PCR is available for detection of tcdA and tcdB genes, which has a 91.6% sensitivity, and is the preferred screening test [20, 21]. If the PCR is positive, then the bacterial strain is capable of elucidating toxin, but does not confirm clinical disease due to elucidated toxin. If the presence of elucidated toxins is confirmed via ELISA, then the diarrhea can be attributed to *C. difficile* enteritis.

Rhodococcus

As the second-most common extrapulmonary disorder of *Rhodococcus* infection [22], diarrhea results from ulcerative enterotyphlocolitis associated with lymphatic spread of bacterial infection that begins in the Peyer's patches of the small intestine, namely the ileum [22–24]. Clinical signs can include diarrhea, weight loss, and rarely, colic [25]. Antemortem diagnosis of *Rhodococcus equi*-associated enterocolitis is difficult because bacterial identification in feces is not definitive [26]. As is true for Rhodococcal pneumonia diagnosis, identification of the virulence-associated protein A (vapA) via polymerase chain reaction is a necessary but not always sufficient component of diagnosis.

Salmonella

Fecal culture is inherently difficult to perform, given the bacterial load of normal manure. Therefore, culture should be performed on selective media with a specific target in mind. In other words, fecal culture can be performed on specific media (e.g., brilliant green agar) to enhance the chances of identifying *Salmonella* or *Clostridial* species. Though PCR can quickly and easily give a positive diagnosis for presence of bacteria, culture more specifically identifies serotypes when attempting to identify outbreaks or nosocomial infections. Culture also provides antimicrobial sensitivity, which can be used to justify antimicrobial use, as well as recognize similar antibiograms between positive patients, which may be suggestive for infectivity between patients. For example, oral vancomycin has been used in critically ill horses with colitis caused by metronidazole-resistant *C. difficile* infections.

Equine Coronavirus

Viral isolation is rarely used in clinical practice due to the need for specialized equipment and trained personnel. However, it remains the gold standard for identification of enteric viral infections, such as equine coronavirus, rotavirus, and adenovirus. Today, RT-PCR is predominantly used for equine coronavirus and has superseded viral isolation in all but academic pursuits [27–30].

Cryptosporidium parvum

Though not a common cause of disease in equine neonates, *Cryptosporidium parvum* should remain a differential in diarrheic foals <1 month of age. Acid-fast stain is taken up by oocytes in feces and produces a characteristically bright red stain that is easily appreciated on fecal smear.

Parasite Testing

Helminth infestation as cause of diarrheic disease is rarely reported in foals. Previous reports have described severe disease as a result of patent infestation with small intestinal mucosal edema resulting in hypoalbuminemia, diarrhea, and lethargy with subjectively high burdens of *Strongyloides westeri* and embryonated eggs noted on postmortem examination [31]. In the United Kingdom, a significant association with disease was found in foals with greater than 2000 eggs/g of feces [32]. The primary route of infection for foals is nursing, as the parasite is excreted from the mammary gland with lactation. Therefore, appropriate anthelminthic administration to the mare with ivermectin immediately postpartum greatly reduces exposure to nursing foals [33–35]. The eggs seen on fecal flotation are typically ovoid, thin-shelled, and larvated, which is in contrast to the expected morula within the *Strongylus* spp. eggs (Figure 15.VIII.1).

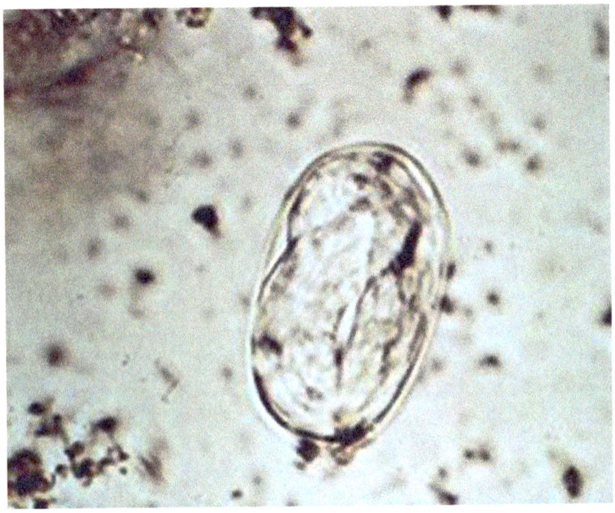

Figure 15.VIII.1 Typical ovoid, thin-shelled and embryonated egg of *Strongyloides westeri*.

Fecal Occult Blood

Immunochemical fecal blood testing is used to aid colorectal cancer diagnosis in humans, in conjunction with colonoscopy [36–38]. The available equine fecal occult blood test (Succeed)® can be used to detect albumin or hemoglobin in feces. In an abattoir study, the test's accuracy of diagnosing gastric and colonic ulcers was 62% and 64%, respectively, with an unacceptably low (83%) confidence level [39]. The test's specificity was reportedly 100%, though notably 97% of horses were diagnosed with gastric, colonic, or both types of ulceration at necropsy, and the sensitivity was only 64%. In light of these findings, many clinicians have not adopted this diagnostic test in suspected cases GI ulceration. Previously, an NSAID toxicity study demonstrated extremely poor sensitivity of fecal occult blood in detecting GI disease in horses [40]. However, when accompanied by ancillary diagnostics, some clinicians may use a positive test to aid diagnosis of GI neoplasia in the horse [41]. To the author's knowledge, there have been no studies evaluating the utility of occult blood testing in the feces of equine neonates. However, frank blood in the feces of a foal should increase index of suspicion for necrotizing enterocolitis or clostridial GI infection [42, 43].

References

1 Fielding, C.L. (2015). Diarrhea in foals. In: *Robinson's Current Therapy in Equine Medicine*, 7e (ed. K. Sprayberry and N.E. Robinson), 722–725. St. Louis, MO: Elsevier.

2 Bailey, K.E., Gilkerson, J.R., and Browning, G.F. (2013). Equine rotaviruses—current understanding and continuing challenges. *Vet. Microbiol.* 167: 135–144.

3 Mino, S., Kern, A., Barrandeguy, M. et al. (2015). Comparison of two commercial kits and an in-house ELISA for the detection of equine rotavirus in foal feces. *J. Virol. Methods* 222: 1–10.

4 Carossino, M., Barrandeguy, M.E., Li, Y. et al. (2018). Detection, molecular characterization and phylogenetic analysis of G3P[12] and G14P[12] equine rotavirus strains co-circulating in central Kentucky. *Virus Res.* 255: 39–54.

5 Carossino, M., Barrandeguy, M.E., Erol, E. et al. (2019). Development and evaluation of a one-step multiplex real-time TaqMan® RT-qPCR assay for the detection and genotyping of equine G3 and G14 rotaviruses in fecal samples. *Virol. J.* 16: 49.

6 Soltan, M.A., Tsai, Y.-L., Lee, P.-Y.A. et al. (2016). Comparison of electron microscopy, ELISA, real time RT-PCR and insulated isothermal RT-PCR for the detection of Rotavirus group A (RVA) in feces of different animal species. *J. Virol. Methods* 235: 99–104.

7 Nemoto, M., Tsunemitsu, H., Murase, H. et al. (2012). Antibody response in vaccinated pregnant mares to recent G3BP[12] and G14P[12] equine rotaviruses. *Acta Vet. Scand.* 54: 63.

8 Barrandeguy, M., Parreño, V., Lagos Mármol, M. et al. (1998). Prevention of rotavirus diarrhoea in foals by parenteral vaccination of the mares: field trial. *Dev. Biol. Stand.* 92: 253–257.

9 Powell, D.G., Dwyer, R.M., Traub-Dargatz, J.L. et al. (1997). Field study of the safety, immunogenicity, and efficacy of an inactivated equine rotavirus vaccine. *J. Am. Vet. Med. Assoc.* 211: 193–198.

10 Slovis, N.M., Elam, J., Estrada, M. et al. (2014). Infectious agents associated with diarrhoea in neonatal foals in central Kentucky: a comprehensive molecular study: infectious agents associated with foal diarrhoea in central Kentucky. *Equine Vet. J.* 46: 311–316.

11 Gohari, I.M., Parreira, V.R., Timoney, J.F. et al. (2016). NetF-positive *Clostridium perfringens* in

neonatal foal necrotizing enteritis in Kentucky. *Vet. Rec.* 178: 216.

12 Gohari, I.M., Unterer, S., Whitehead, A.E. et al. (2020). NetF-producing *Clostridium perfringens* and its associated diseases in dogs and foals. *J. Vet. Diagn. Investig.* 32: 230–238.

13 Gohari, I.M., Kropinski, A.M., Weese, S.J. et al. (2016). Plasmid characterization and chromosome analysis of two netF+ *Clostridium perfringens* isolates associated with foal and canine necrotizing enteritis. *PLoS One* 11: e0148344.

14 Gohari, I.M., Parreira, V.R., Nowell, V.J. et al. (2015). A novel pore-forming toxin in type A *Clostridium perfringens* is associated with both fatal canine hemorrhagic gastroenteritis and fatal foal necrotizing enterocolitis. *PLoS One* 10: e0122684.

15 Rood, J.I., Adams, V., Lacey, J. et al. (2018). Expansion of the *Clostridium perfringens* toxin-based typing scheme. *Anaerobe* 53: 5–10.

16 Finley, A., Gohari, I.M., Parreira, V.R. et al. (2016). Prevalence of netF-positive *Clostridium perfringens* in foals in southwestern Ontario. *Can. J. Vet. Res.* 80: 242–244.

17 Magdesian, K.G., Hirsh, D.C., Jang, S.S. et al. (2002). Characterization of *Clostridium difficile* isolates from foals with diarrhea: 28 cases (1993–1997). *J. Am. Vet. Med. Assoc.* 220: 67–73.

18 Arroyo, L.G., Staempfli, H., and Weese, J.S. (2007). Molecular analysis of *Clostridium difficile* isolates recovered from horses with diarrhea. *Vet. Microbiol.* 120: 179–183.

19 Uzal, F.A., Diab, S.S., Blanchard, P. et al. (2012). *Clostridium perfringens* type C and *Clostridium difficile* co-infection in foals. *Vet. Microbiol.* 156: 395–402.

20 Keessen, E.C., Hopman, N.E.M., van Leengoed, L.A.M.G. et al. (2011). Evaluation of four different diagnostic tests to detect *Clostridium difficile* in piglets. *J. Clin. Microbiol.* 49: 1816–1821.

21 Kuhl, S.J., Tang, Y.J., Navarro, L. et al. (1993). Diagnosis and monitoring of *Clostridium difficile* infections with the polymerase chain reaction. *Clin. Infect. Dis.* 16 (Suppl 4): S234–S238.

22 Reuss, S.M., Chaffin, M.K., and Cohen, N.D. (2009). Extrapulmonary disorders associated with *Rhodococcus equi* infection in foals: 150 cases (1987–2007). *J. Am. Vet. Med. Assoc.* 235: 855–863.

23 Prescott, J.F. (1991). *Rhodococcus equi*: an animal and human pathogen. *Clin. Microbiol. Rev.* 4: 15.

24 Yager, J.A. (1987). The pathogenesis of *Rhodococcus equi* pneumonia in foals. *Vet. Microbiol.* 14: 225–232.

25 Giguère, S., Cohen, N.D., Chaffin, K.M. et al. (2011). *Rhodococcus equi*: clinical manifestations, virulence, and immunity. *J. Vet. Intern. Med.* 25: 1221–1230.

26 Giguère, S., Cohen, N.D., Chaffin, K.M. et al. (2011). Diagnosis, treatment, control, and prevention of infections caused by *Rhodococcus equi* in foals. *J. Vet. Intern. Med.* 25: 1209–1220.

27 Mattei, D.N., Kopper, J.J., and Sanz, M.G. (2020). Equine coronavirus-associated colitis in horses: a retrospective study. *J. Equine Vet. Sci.* 87: 102906.

28 Nemoto, M., Oue, Y., Murakami, S. et al. (2015). Complete genome analysis of equine coronavirus isolated in Japan. *Arch. Virol* 160: 2903–2906.

29 Pusterla, N., Vin, R., Leutenegger, C.M. et al. (2018). Enteric coronavirus infection in adult horses. *Vet. J.* 231: 13–18.

30 Berryhill, E.H., Magdesian, K.G., Aleman, M. et al. (2019). Clinical presentation, diagnostic findings, and outcome of adult horses with equine coronavirus infection at a veterinary teaching hospital: 33 cases (2012–2018). *Vet. J.* 248: 95–100.

31 Lucena, R.B., Fighera, R.A., and Barros, C.S.L. (2012). Mortalidade em potros associada ao parasitismo por *Strongyloides westeri*. *Pesqui. Vet. Bras.* 32: 401–404.

32 Netherwood, T., Wood, J.L.N., Townsend, H.G.G. et al. (1996). Foal diarrhoea between 1991 and 1994 in the United Kingdom associated with *Clostridium perfringens*, rotavirus, *Strongyloides westeri* and *Cryptosporidium* spp. *Epidemiol. Infect.* 117: 375–383.

33 Mallicote, M., House, A.M., and Sanchez, L.C. (2012). A review of foal diarrhoea from birth to weaning. *Equine Vet. Educ.* 24: 206–214.

34 Magdesian, K.G. (2005). Neonatal foal diarrhea. *Vet. Clin. North Am. Equine Pract.* 21: 295–312.

35 Oliver-Espinosa, O. (2018). Foal diarrhea. *Vet. Clin. North Am. Equine Pract.* 34: 55–68.

36 Sokoro, A., Shafer, L.A., Darr, M. et al. (2020). Utility of fecal immunochemical test vs guaiac fecal occult blood test for assessment of gastrointestinal bleed in hospitalized patients. *Clin. Chim. Acta* 500: 202–207.

37 Yuan, S.Y., Wu, W., Fu, J. et al. (2019). Quantitative immunochemical fecal occult blood test for neoplasia in colon cancer screening. *J. Dig. Dis.* 20: 78–82.

38 Kościelniak-Merak, B., Radosavljević, B., Zając, A. et al. (2018). Faecal occult blood point-of-care tests. *J. Gastrointest. Cancer* 49: 402–405.

39 Pellegrini, F.L. (2005). Results of a large-scale necroscopic study of equine colonic ulcers. *J. Equine Vet. Sci.* 25: 113–117.

40 MacAllister, C.G., Morgan, S.J., Borne, A.T. et al. (1993). Comparison of adverse effects of phenylbutazone, flunixin meglumine, and ketoprofen in horses. *J. Am. Vet. Med. Assoc.* 202: 71–77.

41 Knottenbelt, D. and Leverhulme, P. (2014). Gastrointestinal neoplasia. In: *XX Sive International Congress*, 152–160. Milano: Italian Association of Equine Veterinarians.

42 Palmer, J.E. (1985). Gastrointestinal diseases of foals. *Vet. Clin. North Am. Equine Pract.* 1: 151–168.

43 Wilkins, P.A. (2004). Disorders of foals. In: *Equine Internal Medicine*, 2e (ed. S. Reed, W. Bayly, and D. Sellon), 1381–1440. St. Louis MO: Saunders.

Section IX Nutritional Support

Bettina Dunkel

Providing adequate nutrition is an essential part of supportive care for the compromised neonate. Review of feeding of the neonatal foal is presented in Chapter 58; this chapter focuses on nutritional support in foals with disorders of the alimentary tract. Ideally, the foal is allowed to nurse from the dam free choice to meet nutritional needs. Unfortunately, foals with disorders of the alimentary tract are frequently unable to nurse and/or cannot tolerate any or insufficient amounts of enteral nutrition. A nutritional plan is thus an essential part of treatment, whether this includes enteral or parenteral nutrition (PN), or a combination thereof, and how many calories should be provided, in what form and what monitoring is necessary.

Energy Requirements

Assuming milk intake of 20–30% of the foal's body weight and a caloric content of 500–600 kcal/l of mare's milk, a healthy, active, growing foal consumes approximately 100–180 kcal/kg/d. This intake supports an average weight gain of 1.0–1.3 kg/d for a 50 kg foal [1–3]. Critically ill patients are frequently recumbent and, if hospitalized, kept in a thermoneutral environment, which decreases the caloric needs significantly. The actual resting energy requirements or expenditure (REE) in critically ill patients are best determined by indirect calorimetry as disease can result in hyper- or hypometabolic stages. In addition, large inter- and intra-individual differences exist, making use of static formulas prone to error [4]. The caloric requirements of critically ill equine neonates have been determined [2]. Using open-circuit calorimetry, REE was reduced by approximately one-third in premature foals and foals suffering from neonatal encephalopathy (mean of 40.8 kcal/kg/d) compared with healthy age-matched controls (mean of 75 kcal/kg/d) [2]. A second study, in which ill and healthy foals were sedated with diazepam to perform indirect calorimetry using a metabolic cart, REE ranged from 40–50 kcal/kg/d [5]. Only slight differences between ill, recovering, and healthy foals were noted, but large inter-individual variances existed [5]. The most recent study measured REE in unsedated critically ill and healthy foals but, particularly in healthy foals, measurements were obtained after nursing to ensure patient compliance (Jose-Cunilleras, personal communication). In critically ill foals, REE was 50 kcal/kg/d on admission and increased in surviving foals to 68 kcal/kg/d, which was similar to the values measured in healthy control foals (65 kcal/kg/d) [6]. In people, REE increases by 10–27% in the immediate postprandial period, depending on the size and composition of the meal [7, 8]. In the aforementioned study, it could not be established whether the increase in REE in recovering foals was associated with increased enteral intake prior to measurements or a true effect of recovery. Provision of 40–50 kcal/kg/d is therefore an appropriate target rate for ill equine neonates.

Enteral Nutrition

Enteral nutrition is the most physiologic and preferable route of providing nutrition, has a low cost, and is easy to administer. In critically ill people, additional presumed benefits include improved intestinal health and integrity, reduced incidence of sepsis and possibly infections, shorter length of hospital stay, and decreased mortality [9]. However, foals with a compromised alimentary tract may preclude this route of nutrition, at least in the initial stages of treatment. If a foal is ambulatory and has a strong suckle reflex, it can be allowed to nurse from the mare. However, dysphagia from presumed pharyngeal weakness or dysfunction is not uncommon in compromised foals and predisposes to the development of aspiration pneumonia [10]. Foals should therefore be observed carefully while nursing,

Equine Neonatal Medicine, First Edition. Edited by David M. Wong and Pamela A. Wilkins.

with some clinicians auscultating the trachea while the foal is drinking to detect gurgling sounds suggestive of milk aspiration. Coughing is not always observed in neonates of many species despite aspiration of milk. If milk is exiting the nostrils, pharyngeal dysfunction should be suspected and endoscopy performed to identify if the nasopharynx is anatomically normal or if there are signs of pharyngeal weakness, flaccidity, collapse, inflammation, persistent dorsal displacement of the soft palate, or arytenoid paralysis (See "Dysphagia," Chapter 17) [10]. Cleft palate should also be ruled out, although this is less common compared to pharyngeal dysfunction [11]. Foals should not be allowed to nurse until pharyngeal function is normal. Time to resolution varied from 1–14 day (median 4 days) in one study, but rarely, dysfunction might persist [10].

If a sufficient suckle reflex is not present or the foal is unable to stand, enteral nutrition is best provided via an indwelling feeding tube. Due to the substantial risk of aspiration, recumbent neonates might benefit from feedings via an indwelling feeding tube, even if a suckle reflex is present, until they have gained sufficient strength to stand and nurse from the mare. A soft, small diameter feeding tube allows the foal to suck with the tube in place and can be used to supplement the foal enterally if an adequate intake is not yet achieved by nursing alone. Mare's milk is the best source of nutrition if available. If the mare is not producing enough milk, or there is inadequate nursing care to collect milk from the mare every 2–3 hours, mare's milk replacer or goat's milk can be used instead, but indigestion (e.g., bloating, reflux, diarrhea) may occur [12]. Some clinicians believe that colostrum, if available, is better tolerated than mare's milk and is the most suitable source of nutrition for the first enteral feedings of a foal recovering from severe illness.

Few compromised equine neonates tolerate sufficient quantities of enteral nutrition to meet daily caloric requirements; thus, some degree of parenteral support might be necessary to avoid malnutrition. Ill neonatal foals with gastrointestinal (GI) disorders often have significant fluid deficits and are frequently hyporexic. Moreover, ill neonatal foals with enteritis, colitis, hypoxic-ischemic injury to the GI tract and ileus pose additional challenges when considering enteral nutrition. The provision of enteral nutrition to foals with some GI disorders can exacerbate the disease process and the clinician must carefully deliberate if feeding milk via tube feeding will cause further complications such as nasogastric reflux, abdominal distension, worsening diarrhea, and colic. Colic signs can be subtle, particularly if the foal is weak or mentally obtunded, and sometimes only become apparent when restlessness, stretching, and shifting into a more dorsal position is observed. In cases of ileus, characterized by persistent gastric reflux and/or amotile intestines (via ultrasound), enteral nutrition should be avoided and these foals should receive PN until the GI tract demonstrates more normal motility.

Foals with enteritis/colitis can be allowed to suckle from the mare, but often, weak to no effort to voluntarily consume milk is noted. The clinical decision to institute enteral or parenteral nutrition thus remains. A reality of neonatal care is that the amount of financial investment of the foal's owner may not allow PN, outside perhaps the use of intravenous dextrose infusions; in these cases, enteral feedings may be the only option. If any doubt exists whether enteral nutrition will be tolerated in a foal with GI disease, trial feeding of very small (2–3% body weight/day) amounts of milk and careful observation of the foal's comfort after feedings provides an indication of whether larger volumes of milk are likely to be tolerated. Ideally, this should be accompanied by some form of parenteral support until sufficient caloric intake via the enteral route is guaranteed to prevent a negative energy balance and catabolism.

The best time to introduce enteral nutrition, the amount that should be fed, and how quickly the amount can be increased are subject to intense debates in both human and equine critical care. Currently, there are no evidence-based guidelines in people, and certainly none in foals, with most choices being opinion-driven. Maintaining a flexible approach and selecting an enteral or parenteral route (or combination of both) according to the clinical situation, hemodynamic status, GI function, disease processes, and financial resources available is the best option until firm evidence is available.

One of the most feared complications associated with enteral nutrition is necrotizing enterocolitis (NEC), particularly in preterm human neonates. NEC has been reported in foals but remains poorly characterized compared to the disease in human neonates. An association with prematurity, blood in the feces, gastric reflux, and abdominal distension was described in one study but predisposing factors remain ill-defined, and it is unknown whether enteral feeding plays any part in the pathogenesis of NEC in foals [13].

In general, the initial volume of milk to feed the foal depends on the degree of compromise and disease process present. In less severe cases, feedings of 5–10% of the foal's body weight/d with relatively quick increases in volume within 2–3 days to the full feeding volume (25% of body weight/day) administered every 1–4 hours may be achievable. In preterm human infants, enteral feeding has, in the past, often been delayed or kept to a minimum (trophic feeding; 1–20 ml/kg/d) to decrease the risk of NEC [14]. Later studies and meta-analyses seem to favor early enteral nutrition with more rapid advancements in volume in stable preterm neonates without increasing the risk of NEC, but controversy still continues [14]. A cautious and conservative approach, beginning with small volumes of enteral feedings, is therefore prudent in premature and compromised foals. Currently, there is no evidence in human neonates to support continuous over bolus feeding, and most clinicians find bolus administration more convenient. Any foal not receiving 40–50 kcal/kg/d via enteral feeding should be supplemented with at least intravenous glucose or, ideally, PN.

Milk intolerance may occur secondary to lactose intolerance after enteric infections that diminish the brush border enzymes, such as rotavirus or Clostridia [15, 16]. Of note, primary lactose intolerance has been suspected in two foals [17]. Lactose intolerance should be considered if milk and milk substitutes are persistently tolerated poorly, despite otherwise improving general health. Oral lactase therapy, as drops or tablets, with doses being extrapolated from recommendations for children appears to help in these cases [17, 18]. Daily weighing of the foal is an essential part of monitoring the success of the nutritional treatment plan and consistent daily weight gain should be observed [1–3].

Parenteral Nutrition

Parenteral nutritional (PN) is often needed in ill neonatal foals, including foals with GI disorders, as they commonly do not consume enough milk voluntarily and tube feedings of milk may overwhelm the diseased intestinal tract. PN can be provided in the form of a glucose infusion, glucose-amino acid solutions, or a glucose-amino acid-lipid combination. The glucose oxidation rate in human pediatric patients ranges from 4–8 mg/kg/min, and similar rates are recommended for equine neonates [19–21]. Glucose can be provided as 5%, 10%, or 50% dextrose solution via an infusion pump, usually in addition to maintenance fluids. Dextrose concentrations of up to 25% have been administered to adult equine patients via the jugular vein without complications [22], but lower concentrations are advisable to avoid unnecessary irritation of the veins. Using the approach outlined above, dextrose alone can provide 20–40 kcal/kg/d (1 g glucose = 3.4 kcal). However, the low caloric density and high osmolarity of the solution make it difficult to provide sufficient energy via dextrose alone for prolonged periods of time. PN should be considered in neonatal foals if full enteral nutrition is not anticipated within 48–72 hours. Principles of PN are described in Chapter 58 [1, 23–25], but in brief, glucose and lipids in varying ratios (40–70% of energy requirements met by glucose and 30–60% by lipids) are used to provide the caloric requirements of the patient, while amino acids are supplied to facilitate protein synthesis and minimize endogenous protein catabolism [21, 26]. This approach is well tolerated in most equine patients [21, 22, 26]. Lipids are provided in emulsions most commonly consisting of long-chain fatty acids made from soybeans. The emulsions are iso-osmolar, decreasing the hyperosmolarity of the parenteral solution and making it less irritating to peripheral veins. A 10% lipid emulsion contains 0.9–1.1 kcal/ml, whereas a 20% solution provides 1.8–2 kcal/ml. Additionally, the use of lipids in parenteral formulas can potentially reduce the occurrence of hyperglycemia and hypercapnia. While healthy nursing foals consume approximately 5–6 g/kg/d of protein, amino acids at a rate of 2–3 g/kg/d are often used in parenteral formulations for compromised equine neonates [21, 27]. A parenteral solution providing 10 g/kg/g glucose, 2 g/kg/d amino acids, and 1 g/kg/d lipids can be formulated by mixing 1000 ml of 50% dextrose in water with 1000 ml of 10% amino acid solution and 500 ml of 10% lipid emulsion under sterile conditions in a flow hood (Table 15.IX.1). The final infusion rate for a 50 kg foal is 104 ml/h and provides 53 kcal/kg/d. Potassium chloride and multivitamins can be added to the solution as needed. The starting infusion rate is usually 25–50% of the target rate, which is then gradually increased over 24–48 hours to the full rate [28]. Blood glucose concentrations should be monitored every 4–6 hours initially. This can be reduced to twice daily monitoring when the patient's blood glucose concentration remains stable. Once the condition of the patient improves and enteral nutrition meets at least 50% of the REE, parenteral nutrition is gradually decreased and discontinued over 24–48 hours, depending on the enteral intake at the time.

The most common complication encountered in foals receiving PN is hyperglycemia. One study reported blood glucose concentrations >180 mg/dl (10 mmol/l) in 62% of foals receiving PN [28]. Other complications included phlebitis in 6% and hyperlipidemia (plasma triglyceride concentrations >55 mg/dl; 0.6 mmol/l) in 11% of foals [28]. More recent publications suggest that glucose and triglyceride concentrations vary significantly in healthy nursing foals [29, 30]. Triglyceride concentrations of up to, and occasionally exceeding, 200 mg/dl (2.25 mmol/l) were

Table 15.IX.1 Example of how to calculate total parenteral nutrition for a 50-kg foal using a 50% dextrose solution, 10% amino acid solution and 10% lipid solution in a 3-l mixing bag.

Dextrose: 10 g/kg/d × 50 kg = 500 g dextrose; 500 g = 1000 ml of 50% dextrose (50% dextrose = 500 mg/ml)
Amino acids: 2 g/kg/d × 50 kg = 100 g = 1000 ml of 10% amino acid solution (10% amino acid solution = 100 mg/ml)
Lipids: 1 g/kg/d × 50 kg = 50 g = 500 ml of 10% lipid solution (10% lipid solution = 100 mg/ml)
Total volume: 2500 ml/d with a final target rate of 104 ml/h provides 53 kcal/kg/d

documented in healthy foals [29, 31]; thus, the percentage of true hyperlipidemia as a complication of PN might be lower. Hyperglycemia has been associated with a worse prognosis in critically ill people, foals, and adult horses [32–34]. While tight glucose control 80–110 mg/dl (4.4–6.1 mmol/l) using intensive insulin therapy has been advocated in human critical care for some time [35, 36], benefits of this treatment strategy for critically ill people are still debated [32]. In light of the fact that almost all studies identified an increased risk of hypoglycemia with intense insulin therapy, most current suggestions favor a more lenient approach [37, 38]. Serial measurements of glucose concentrations in healthy foals after birth, 24–48 hours old, and 10–12 days old showed wide hourly variations [30]. Concentrations remained largely >90 mg/dl (5 mmol/l) and increased up to 241 mg/dl (13.4 mmol/l) in individual foals [30] highlighting the fact that marked fluctuations in glucose concentrations are normal in healthy nursing foals. In contrast, hypoglycemia (<90 mg/dl; 5 mmol/l) was not observed in nursing foals >24–48 hours old with the lowest measured blood glucose concentration being 52 mg/dl (2.9 mmol/l) in foals <24 hours old [30]. Moreover, hypoglycemia did not occur in healthy 4-day-old foals (glucose concentrations remained >79 mg/dl; 4.4 mmol/l) [39] in which feed was withheld for 24 hours, suggesting that hypoglycemia (glucose concentrations <50 mg/dl; 2.8 mmol/l) should be interpreted as a sign of disease, particularly sepsis and systemic inflammation [34].

It is also worth noting that in critically ill people and adult horses with GI disease, blood glucose, and lactate concentrations are significantly correlated as lactate can be converted into glucose in the Cori cycle and vice versa [40]. The same could be true for foals [41–43], highlighting the importance of considering both parameters together.

From a practical point, tight glucose control is associated with a significant increase in workload for nursing staff and successful tight glucose control without exposing the patient to substantial risks of iatrogenic hypoglycemia is difficult in most equine intensive care units. Benign neglect could therefore be reasonable unless hyperglycemia is severe or osmotic diuresis occurs. Glucosuria is easily identified by use of urinary dipsticks and signifies the need for intervention to avoid dehydration. Continuous rate infusion of regular insulin is indicated in these cases. Because reduction of the glucose or parenteral nutrition infusion rate is counterproductive as the energy requirements of the foals will not be met, decreasing the amount of glucose and increasing the amount of lipids and/or amino acids in the PN could be considered to decrease the glucose load. Recommended insulin infusion rates range from 0.001–0.2 IU/kg/h, beginning at a low rate followed by titration to effect under frequent monitoring of blood glucose concentration [1, 20, 28]. In people, insulin is classified as a high-alert medication and is frequently associated with preventable patient harm from hypoglycaemia. Insulin administration should therefore be carried out by experienced personnel and the patient must be carefully supervised. Easily accessible instructions for emergency administration of IV glucose in case of a hypoglycemic crisis is useful.

Immunonutrition, defined as provision of specific nutrients that have the potential to modulate the activity of the immune system, is a much debated topic in adult and pediatric human critical care [44]. The term has also become associated with attempts to improve the clinical course of critically illness via exogenous supply of nutrients through parenteral or enteral routes [45]. Due to the lack of proven benefits, use of immunonutrition is currently not recommended in critically ill children [4] and the same is true for foals until more information is available. Further information on feeding of the neonatal foal via enteral and parenteral routes is located in Chapter 58.

References

1 Paradis, M. (2003). Nutritional support: enteral and parenteral. *Clin. Tech. Equine Prac.* 2: 87–95.

2 Ousey, J., Holdstock, P., and Rossdale, P. (1996). How much energy do sick neonatal foals require compared to healthy foals? *Pferdeheilkunde* 12: 231–237.

3 Ousey, J.C., Prandi, S., Zimmer, J. et al. (1997). Effects of various feeding regimens on the energy balance of equine neonates. *Am. J. Vet. Res.* 58: 1243–1251.

4 Mehta, N.M., Skillman, H.E., Irving, S.Y. et al. (2017). Guidelines for the provision and assessment of nutrition support therapy in the pediatric critically ill patient: Society of Critical Care Medicine and American Society for Parenteral and Enteral Nutrition. *JPEN J. Parenter. Enteral Nutr.* 41: 706–742.

5 Paradis, M. (2001). Nutrition and indirect calorimetry in neonatal foals. *Proceedings of the 19th American College of Veterinary Internal Medicine Forum*, Lakewood CO, 245–247.

6 Jose-Cunilleras, E., Viu, J., Corradini, I. et al. (2012). Energy expenditure of critically ill neonatal foals. *Equine Vet. J. Suppl.* 44: 48–51.

7 de Graaf, M., van Lieshout, M., van den Berg, P.T.M. et al. (2018). Indirect calorimetry: challenging the 5 hours fasting requirement. *Clin. Nutr.* 37: S223.

8 Raben, A., Agerholm-Larsen, L., Flint, A. et al. (2003). Meals with similar energy densities but rich in protein, fat, carbohydrate, or alcohol have different effects on energy expenditure and substrate metabolism but not on appetite and energy intake. *Am. J. Clin. Nutr.* 77: 91–100.
9 Gostynska, A., Stawny, M., Dettlaff, K. et al. (2019). Clinical nutrition of critically ill patients in the context of the latest ESPEN guidelines. *Medicina (Kaunas)* 55: 770–785.
10 Holcombe, S.J., Hurcombe, S.D., Barr, B.S. et al. (2012). Dysphagia associated with presumed pharyngeal dysfunction in 16 neonatal foals. *Equine Vet. J. Suppl.* 44: 105–108.
11 Shaw, S.D., Norman, T.E., Arnold, C.E. et al. (2015). Clinical characteristics of horses and foals diagnosed with cleft palate in a referral population: 28 cases (1988–2011). *Can. Vet. J.* 56: 756–760.
12 Paradis, M.R. (2012). Feeding the orphan foal. *AAEP Proc.* 58: 402–406.
13 de Solis, C.N., Palmer, J.E., Boston, R.C. et al. (2012). The importance of ultrasonographic pneumatosis intestinalis in equine neonatal gastrointestinal disease. *Equine Vet. J. Suppl.* 44: 64–68.
14 Kwok, T.C., Dorling, J., and Gale, C. (2019). Early enteral feeding in preterm infants. *Semin. Perinatol.* 43: 151159.
15 Weese, J.S., Parsons, D.A., and Staempfli, H.R. (1999). Association of Clostridium difficile with enterocolitis and lactose intolerance in a foal. *J. Am. Vet. Med. Assoc.* 214: 229–232, 205.
16 Sweeney, R.W. (1987). Laboratory evaluation of malassimilation in horses. *Vet. Clin. North Am. Equine Pract.* 3: 507–514.
17 Roberts, V.L.C., Knottenbelt, D.C., Williams, A. et al. (2008). Suspected primary lactose intolerance in neonatal foals. *Equine Vet. Educ.* 20: 249–251.
18 Sloet van Oldruitenborgh-Oosterbaan, M.M. (2008). Lactose intolerance in foals. *Equine Vet. Educ.* 20: 252–255.
19 Palmer, J.E. (2004). Fluid therapy in the neonate: not your mother's fluid space. *Vet. Clin. North Am. Equine Pract.* 20: 63–75.
20 Wilkins, P.A. (2004). *Disorders of Foals*, 2e. St. Louis, Missouri: Saunders.
21 Spurlock, S.L. and Ward, M.V. (1991). Parenteral nutrition in equine patients: principles and theory. *Compend. Contin. Educ. Pract. Vet.* 13: 461–468.
22 Spurlock, S.L. (1990). Providing parenteral nutritional support for equine patients. *Vet. Med.* 85: 883–890.
23 Dunkel, B.M. and Wilkins, P.A. (2004). Nutrition and the critically ill horse. *Vet. Clin. North Am. Equine Pract.* 20: 107–126.
24 Buechner-Maxwell, V.A. (2005). Nutritional support for neonatal foals. *Vet. Clin. North Am. Equine Pract.* 21: 487–510, viii.
25 Koterba, A.M. and Drummond, W.H. (1985). Nutritional support of the foal during intensive care. *Vet. Clin. North Am. Equine Pract.* 1: 35–40.
26 Lopes, M.A. and White, N.A. 2nd (2002). Parenteral nutrition for horses with gastrointestinal disease: a retrospective study of 79 cases. *Equine Vet. J.* 34: 250–257.
27 Hansen, T.O. (1990). *Nutritional Support: Parenteral Feeding*. Philadelphia: Lea & Febiger.
28 Krause, J.B. and McKenzie, H.C. 3rd. (2007). Parenteral nutrition in foals: a retrospective study of 45 cases (2000–2004). *Equine Vet. J.* 39: 74–78.
29 Berryhill, E.H., Magdesian, K.G., Kass, P.H. et al. (2017). Triglyceride concentrations in neonatal foals: serial measurement and effects of age and illness. *Vet. J.* 227: 23–29.
30 Berryhill, E.H., Magdesian, K.G., Tadros, E.M. et al. (2019). Effects of age on serum glucose and insulin concentrations and glucose/insulin ratios in neonatal foals and their dams during the first 2 weeks postpartum. *Vet. J.* 246: 1–6.
31 Duncan, N.B., Johnson, P.J., Crosby, M.J. et al. (2020). Serum chemistry and hematology changes in neonatal stock-type foals during the first 72 hours of life. *J. Equine Vet. Sci.* 84: 102855.
32 Gunst, J., De Bruyn, A., and Van den Berghe, G. (2019). Glucose control in the ICU. *Curr. Opin. Anaesthesiol.* 32: 156–162.
33 Hollis, A.R., Boston, R.C., and Corley, K.T. (2007). Blood glucose in horses with acute abdominal disease. *J. Vet. Intern. Med.* 21: 1099–1103.
34 Hollis, A.R., Furr, M.O., Magdesian, K.G. et al. (2008). Blood glucose concentrations in critically ill neonatal foals. *J. Vet. Intern. Med.* 22: 1223–1227.
35 van den Berghe, G., Wouters, P., Weekers, F. et al. (2001). Intensive insulin therapy in the critically ill patients. *N. Engl. J. Med.* 345: 1359–1367.
36 Verbruggen, S.C., Joosten, K.F., Castillo, L. et al. (2007). Insulin therapy in the pediatric intensive care unit. *Clin. Nutr.* 26: 677–690.
37 Zhao, Y., Wu, Y., and Xiang, B. (2018). Tight glycemic control in critically ill pediatric patients: a meta-analysis and systematic review of randomized controlled trials. *Pediatr. Res.* 84: 22–27.
38 Bhatia, A. and Salas, A.A. (2018). Does tight glycaemic control with insulin therapy in the early neonatal period improve long-term outcomes? *Acta Paediatr.* 107: 2032–2033.
39 Buchanan, B.R., Sommardahl, C.S., Rohrbach, B.W. et al. (2005). Effect of a 24-hour infusion of an isotonic electrolyte replacement fluid on the renal clearance of electrolytes in healthy neonatal foals. *J. Am. Vet. Med. Assoc.* 227: 1123–1129.

40 Rubin, R.P. (2021). Carl and Gerty Cori: a collaboration that changed the face of biochemistry. *J. Med. Biogr.* 29: 143–148.

41 van Beest, P.A. and Spronk, P.E. (2014). Lactate and glucose in critically ill patients: what goes around, comes around. *Crit. Care Med.* 42: 1545–1546.

42 Kaukonen, K.M., Bailey, M., Egi, M. et al. (2014). Stress hyperlactatemia modifies the relationship between stress hyperglycemia and outcome: a retrospective observational study. *Crit. Care Med.* 42: 1379–1385.

43 Dunkel, B., Mason, C.J., and Chang, Y.M. (2019). Retrospective evaluation of the association between admission blood glucose and l-lactate concentrations in ponies and horses with gastrointestinal disease (2008–2016): 545 cases. *J. Vet. Emerg. Crit. Care* 29: 418–423.

44 Walsh, V. and McGuire, W. (2019). Immunonutrition for preterm infants. *Neonatology* 115: 398–405.

45 Calder, P.C. (2003). Immunonutrition. *BMJ* 327: 117–118.

Section X Prokinetic Therapy in Foals

Anthony Blikslager, Sara Erwin, and Amanda Ziegler

Foals are susceptible to many of the intestinal obstructive disorders noted in adult horses, such as impactions and strangulating obstructions, which are associated with alterations in intestinal motility. However, intestinal motility has not been studied in great detail in the foal, limiting our knowledge of the usage of prokinetic drugs largely to extrapolation from the adult horse (Table 15.X.1). Nonetheless, there are some important distinctions between the intestinal enteric nervous system of the neonatal and adult horse, which may affect efficacy of prokinetic medications.

Enteric Nervous System

Normal intestinal physiology, including gut motility, is modulated intrinsically and extrinsically by an extensive enteric nervous system [7]. The intrinsic enteric nervous system is composed of neurons and glia arranged into two major plexuses, the myenteric and submucosal plexus, as well as an abundance of neuronal and glial elements throughout the lamina propria [8]. The enteric nervous system arises in early development from the embryonic vagal and sacral neural crest, and migrates rostro-caudally [9]. Following completion of linear migration throughout the length of the gastrointestinal (GI) tract, neural crest cells migrate inward radially, forming the two concentric myenteric and submucosal plexuses [9]. Although enteric innervation is established during embryonic development, neural plasticity persists into the postnatal period and is thought to be influenced by colonization of the gut by bacteria after birth as well as alterations in populations of microbiota as the diet changes [10]. Studies testing this hypothesis have shown that germ-free mice have a reduced number of enteric neurons and associated deficits in gut-motility when compared to normally colonized mice [11]. Similarly, studies assessing foal fecal microbial populations from birth to weaning show changes in microbiome as the diet changes from liquid to solid [10]. Foals also exhibit maternal coprophagy as a normal behavior from 5 days to 19 weeks-of-age, with the highest incidence during the first 2 months. This behavior is thought to be stimulated by the presence of deoxycholic acid in the mare's feces that the foal may be deficient in, and is required for gut immunocompetence and myelination of the nervous system. Coprophagy may also further colonize the gut with normal bacterial flora [12]. Although not technically "prokinetic," it is conceivable that alteration of foals' diets, possibly including pre- and probiotics, may result in earlier maturation of the enteric nervous system, and a more robust motility response following intestinal obstruction.

Within the enteric nervous system, there are up to 10 times as many glial cells as neuronal cells, but this highly complex and extensive network of glia is restricted to just the outer plexuses at the time of birth [13]. These glial cells are then driven to migrate luminally into all the layers of the gut wall establishing a complete network during early postnatal development. This is thought to occur in response to microbial colonization at birth, which is in turn thought to be driven by intestinal content [14]. The precise signaling mechanisms inducing glial cell migration into the lamina propria remain to be fully elucidated, and the relative role of this developing network of enteric glial cells in intestinal motility and disease in foals remains largely undefined and is the subject of ongoing study.

Diseases Where Prokinetic Therapy May Be Indicated

Adynamic Ileus

In foals, adynamic ileus, referring to functional obstruction of the intestinal tract, has been noted as the primary cause of colic in 9 of 20 (45%) foals taken to surgery for persistent

Equine Neonatal Medicine, First Edition. Edited by David M. Wong and Pamela A. Wilkins.

Table 15.X.1 Medications that might serve as prokinetics in neonatal foals. The clinician should use these medications with caution as minimal research has been performed to thoroughly investigate their use in foals. Many of these doses were extracted from information available from adult horses or case reports.

Drug	Indication for use	Mechanism of action	Dose
Lidocaine	Ileus, POI	Exact mechanism unknown	• 1.3 mg/kg, IV, followed by 0.05 mg/kg/min, IV [1, 2]
Bethanechol	Promote gastric emptying (gastro-duodenal ulcers/stricture, gastric outflow obstruction, gastro-esophageal reflux), POI	Parasympathomimetic	• 0.025 mg/kg, SC once, then 0.35 mg/kg PO, q 8 h [2, 3] • 0.22–0.45 mg/kg, PO, q 6–8 h [4] • 0.02 mg/kg, SC, q 6 h [5]
Metoclopramide	Promote gastric and/or small intestinal motility, POI	5-HT_4 agonist; 5-HT_3 Antagonist, dopaminergic (D2) antagonist	• 0.1 mg/kg, IV, q 6 h in 1 l saline over 1 h [3] • 0.02–0.04 mg/kg/h, IV, CRI [4] • 0.6 mg/kg, PO, q 4–6 h [4] • 0.25 mg/kg, PO, q 8 h [5] • 0.10–0.20 mg/kg, SC, q 6 h [5]
Cisapride	Promote gastric and/or small Intestinal motility, POI	5-HT_4 agonist, 5-HT_3 antagonist	• 0.1 mg/kg, IM [6]
Erythromycin	Promote gastric or small intestinal motility, POI	Motilin receptor agonist	• 0.5–2 mg/kg, IV, q 6 h in 1 l saline over 45 min [3]
Neostigmine	Enhance cecal and colonic motility Relieve abdominal tympany	Cholinesterase inhibitor	• 0.005–0.01 mg/kg, SC [4] • 1 mg/50 kg foal SC, q 1–8 h; IV if severe distension [5]

POI, Postoperative ileus; HT, Hydroxytryptamine.

colic [15] and in a more recent study in 1 of 67 foals taken to surgery [16]. Functional obstruction of the small intestine as the primary source of colic in neonatal surgical patients, in the absence of other nonobstructive conditions like enteritis, is a diagnosis of exclusion (i.e., no other apparent cause of colic with the presence of distended small intestine noted pre- or postoperatively). Prokinetic therapy is indicated for treatment of adynamic ileus in adult equine patients, but very little data exists to either support or refute use of prokinetic medications in foals. Most reports simply indicate usage of supportive therapy, such as IV fluids. According to recent surveys, lidocaine is the most commonly used prokinetic in adult horses [17, 18], but its use in foals has been limited to a perceived benefit in terms of analgesia [1].

Gastroduodenal Ulceration

Neonates with gastroduodenal ulcers, particularly when accompanied by some level of duodenal stricture, may benefit from prokinetic therapy to enhance gastric emptying. One prokinetic medication that has been advocated for this purpose is bethanechol at a dosage of 0.025 mg/kg, SC, once, followed by 0.35 mg/kg, PO, q8h. Bethanechol is a synthetic parasympathomimetic that acts on M2 and M3 muscarinic receptors, and has the advantage of not being broken down by acetylcholinesterase. Bethanechol has been studied in equine tissues in vitro and has been shown to trigger dose-dependent increase in spontaneous contractility of equine adult duodenum, jejunum, cecum, and large colon [2, 3].

Gastric Outflow Obstruction

Although this syndrome is typically noted in older suckling foals, neonates may also suffer from gastric outflow obstruction. The pathogenesis is thought to be related to gastroduodenal ulceration, and subsequent obstruction at the level of the pylorus. Treatment is typically surgical bypass. One problem that has been identified as significantly affecting the prognosis is postoperative ileus, presumably partially related to the nonanatomical configuration of the surgical bypass, but also to intra-abdominal inflammation [19]. Although the use and results of prokinetic therapy is limited in foals with gastric outflow obstruction [1, 19, 20], one report noted that 2 of 40 foals were administered metoclopramide at a dose of 0.1 mg/kg, IV, q6h [19]. Metoclopramide is a 5-HT_4 agonist, a 5-HT_3 antagonist, and a D_2 dopaminergic antagonist that has a dosage in adult horses of 0.04 mg/kg/h, IV, CRI [6]. A study of foal tissues revealed that 5-HT-positive cells were located in the stomach and pylorus of foals, suggesting an active role of 5-HT and its receptors in the proximal GI tract, and therefore the likelihood of activity of metoclopramide in foals [21].

Additionally, 5-HT_4 receptors have been identified in the duodenum of foals. The usage of metoclopramide in adult horses has been limited because of extrapyramidal side effects [6], and monitoring for these clinical signs has also been suggested for foals [4]. Cisapride also has activity at 5-HT receptors, and antagonizes 5-HT_3 receptors, and is a putative 5-HT_4 agonist. However, its use in normal pony foals at a dosage of 0.1 mg/kg IM had no effect on the rate of gastric emptying of a liquid meal [22]. Additionally, cisapride is no longer commercially available due to cardiac side effects in human patients, but has been compounded by some pharmacies. There is also the possibility that bethanechol, as mentioned previously for gastroduodenal ulceration, may serve as viable prokinetic for postoperative neonatal patients following pyloric bypass surgery.

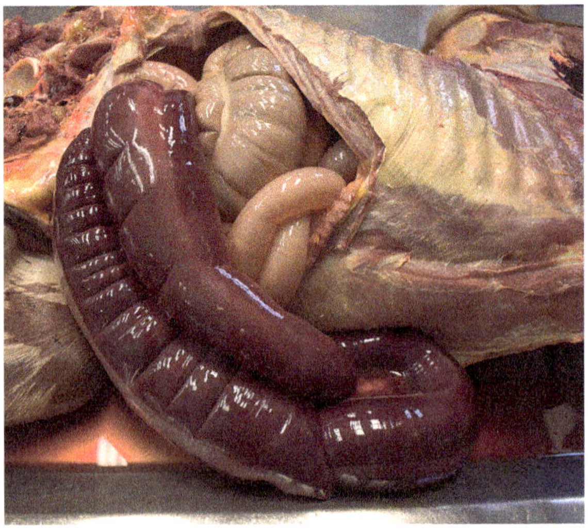

Figure 15.X.1 Postmortem appearance of a large colon volvulus in a 2-day-old foal. Note the devitalized area of colon.

Ileocolonic Aganglionosis (Lethal White Foal Syndrome)

This disease is characterized by a lack of ganglia in the ileum and large intestine because of a failure of migration of neural cell progenitors from the neural crest into the distal intestinal tract. Therefore, treatment of this disease with prokinetic drugs is futile without the neural receptors that initiate or modify intestinal motility. For example, one study found that the 5-HT_4 receptor, which is triggered by 5-HT_4 agonists such as cisapride, is absent in the foal colon with enteric aganglionosis [23]. Additionally, another study found that extrinsic neural innervation in foals with ileocolonic aganglionosis was reduced [24], further reducing viable targets for pharmacological therapy such as neostigmine.

Meconium Impaction

The most common cause of intestinal obstruction in foals is meconium impaction. This form of obstruction is usually managed medically, although refractory cases may require surgery to resolve the obstructing mass of meconium [25]. Medical management includes the use of enemas, which can include dilute soap solutions, dilute mineral oil, acetylcysteine, or formulated sodium phosphate enemas [26]. While the use of prokinetic drugs has not been specifically advocated for the use of enemas, in human pediatric patients, use of saline as an enema has been shown to stimulate motility [27].

Strangulating Obstruction

Causes of strangulating obstruction in the foal include small and large intestinal volvulus and other rare causes of strangulation such as entrapment by an ovarian ligament or a mesodiverticular band. Small intestinal volvulus is the most common reported cause of surgical colic in foals [16, 28], although large intestinal volvulus (Figure 15.X.1) was more common if the foal population was restricted to neonates [15]. The prevalence of postoperative ileus following small intestinal strangulating obstruction in adult horses is approximately 10–20% in studies since the 1990s [29–33], but this has not been determined for neonatal foals. Current treatments for postoperative ileus in adults are centered on anti-inflammatory therapy with both nonsteroidal anti-inflammatory drugs, primarily flunixin meglumine (0.25 mg/kg, IV, q8h–1.1 mg/kg, IV, q12h), and lidocaine (1.3 mg/kg slow IV bolus, followed by 0.05 mg/kg/min by controlled rate infusion). An alternative anti-inflammatory that has been evaluated in adult horses for prevention of postoperative ileus is dexamethasone (0.1 mg/kg, IV during surgery) [34]. Although dexamethasone reduced the incidence of postoperative ileus, findings were deemed inconclusive without a randomized clinical trial. Lidocaine was originally believed to serve as a prokinetic by reducing inhibitory sympathetic neural input, but is currently thought to relate to a reduction in inflammation [35, 36]. However, the mechanisms by which lidocaine exerts any "prokinetic" action are unclear, and the efficacy of lidocaine in horses with postoperative ileus has been questioned using a rigorous multivariable approach assessing two cohorts of a total of 318 horses [37].

Another interesting finding related to the use of flunixin meglumine and lidocaine in horses with experimental strangulating obstruction is that flunixin paradoxically causes an increase in intestinal permeability to lipopolysaccharide, likely related to its inhibitory action on mucosal epithelial repair, which increases rather than reduces inflammation [38, 39]. Neonatologists are aware of the potential adverse effects of NSAIDs on intestinal mucosal barrier function, and studies showing flunixin-induced delayed mucosal repair in adults suggest cautious and judicious use of flunixin meglumine in foals. In experimental adult studies, concurrent administration of lidocaine ameliorated the negative effects of flunixin on intestinal permeability, thereby reducing inflammation [40]. Neonatal foals can develop strangulating obstruction, and it is likely that some of the factors thought to play a role in postoperative ileus in horses play a role in ileus in foals, particularly inflammation associated with ischemia/reperfusion injury and surgical manipulation [41]. Whether lidocaine reduces inflammation in foals with ileus, and/or serves as a prokinetic is not currently known. However, there is some limited evidence that lidocaine provides consistent analgesia in foals suffering from colic [1].

References

1 Furr, M.O. (2017). Medical management of colic in the foal. In: *The Equine Acute Abdomen*, 3e (ed. A.T. Blikslager, N.A. White, J.N. Moore, and T.S. Mair), 422–425. Hoboken, NJ: Wiley.

2 Marti, M., Mevissen, M., Althaus, H. et al. (2005). In vitro effects of bethanechol on equine gastrointestinal contractility and functional characterization of involved muscarinic receptor subtypes. *J. Vet. Pharmacol. Ther.* 28: 565–574.

3 Barr, B.S. (2006). Duodenal stricture in a foal. *Vet. Clin. North Am. Equine.* 22: 37–42.

4 Magdesian, K.G. (2015). Foals are not just mini horses. In: *Equine Pharmacology* (ed. C.B.B. Cole and L. Maxwell), 99–117. Ames, Iowa: Wiley Blackwell.

5 Slovis, N.M. (2003). Gastrointestinal failure. *Clin. Tech. Equine Pract.* 2: 79–86.

6 Wong, D.M., Davis, J.L., and White, N.A. (2011). Motility of the equine gastrointestinal tract: physiology and pharmacotherapy. *Equine Vet. Educ.* 23: 88–100.

7 Uesaka, T., Young, H.M., Pachnis, V. et al. (2016). Development of the intrinsic and extrinsic innervation of the gut. *Dev. Biol.* 417: 158–167.

8 De Giorgio, R., Giancola, F., Boschetti, E. et al. (2012). Enteric glia and neuroprotection: basic and clinical aspects. *Am. J. Gastrointest Liver Physiol.* 303: G887–G893.

9 Lake, J.I. and Heuckeroth, R.O. (2013). Enteric nervous system development: migration, differentiation, and disease. *Am. J. Gastrointest Liver Physiol.* 305: G1–G24.

10 De La Torre, U., Henderson, J.D., Furtado, K.L. et al. (2019). Utilizing the fecal microbiota to understand foal gut transitions from birth to weaning. *PLoS One* 14: e0216211.

11 Obata, Y. and Pachnis, V. (2016). The effect of microbiota and the immune system on the development and organization of the enteric nervous system. *Gastroenterology* 151: 836–844.

12 Crowell-Davis, S.L. and Houpt, K.A. (1985). Coprophagy by foals: effect of age and possible functions. *Equine Vet. J.* 17: 17–19.

13 Vales, S., Touvron, M., and Van Landeghem, L. (2018). Enteric glia: diversity or plasticity? *Brain Res.* 1693 (Pt B): 140–145.

14 Kabouridis, P.S. and Pachnis, V. (2015). Emerging roles of gut microbiota and the immune system in the development of the enteric nervous system. *J. Clin. Invest.* 125: 956–964.

15 Adams, R., Koterba, A.M., Brown, M.P. et al. (1988). Exploratory celiotomy for gastrointestinal disease in neonatal foals: a review of 20 cases. *Equine Vet. J.* 20: 9–12.

16 Vatistas, N.J., Snyder, J.R., Wilson, W.D. et al. (1996). Surgical treatment for colic in the foal (67 cases): 1980–1992. *Equine Vet. J.* 28: 139–145.

17 Lefebvre, D., Hudson, N.P., Elce, Y.A. et al. (2015). Clinical features and management of equine postoperative ileus (POI): survey of diplomates of the American Colleges of Veterinary Internal Medicine (ACVIM), Veterinary Surgeons (ACVS) and Veterinary Emergency and Critical Care (ACVECC). *Equine Vet. J.* 48: 714–719.

18 Van Hoogmoed, L.M., Nieto, J.E., Snyder, J.R. et al. (2004). Survey of prokinetic use in horses with gastrointestinal injury. *Vet. Surg.* 33: 279–285.

19 Zedler, S.T., Embertson, R.M., Bernard, W.V. et al. (2009). Surgical treatment of gastric outflow obstruction in 40 foals. *Vet. Surg.* 38: 623–630.

20 Bryant, J.E. and Gaughan, E.M. (2005). Abdominal surgery in neonatal foals. *Vet. Clin. North Am. Equine* 21: 511–535.

21 Fink, C., Tatar, M., Failing, K. et al. (2006). Serotonin-containing cells in the gastrointestinal tract of newborn foals and adult horses. *Anat. Histol. Embryol.* 35: 23–27.

22 Baker, S.J. and Gerring, E.L. (1994). Gastric emptying of four liquid meals in pony foals. *Res. Vet. Sci.* 56: 164–169.

23 Giancola, F., Rambaldi, A.M., Bianco, F. et al. (2017). Localization of the 5-hydroxytryptamine 4 receptor in equine enteric neurons and extrinsic sensory fibers. *Neurogastroenterol. Motil.* 29 (7).

24 Giancola, F., Gentilini, F., Romagnoli, N. et al. (2016). Extrinsic innervation of ileum and pelvic flexure of foals with ileocolonic aganglionosis. *Cell Tissue Res.* 366: 13–22.

25 Hughes, F.E., Moll, H.D., and Slone, D.E. (1996). Outcome of surgical correction of meconium impactions in 8 foals. *J. Equine Vet. Sci.* 16: 172–175.

26 McCue, P.M. (2006). Meconium impaction in newborn foals. *J. Equine Vet. Sci.* 26: 152–155.
27 Gomez, R., Mousa, H., Liem, O. et al. (2010). How do antegrade enemas work? Colonic motility in response to administration of normal saline solution into the proximal colon. *J. Pediatr. Gastroenterol. Nutr.* 51: 741–746.
28 Stephen, J.O., Corley, K.T., Johnston, J.K. et al. (2004). Small intestinal volvulus in 115 horses: 1988–2000. *Vet. Surg.* 33: 333–339.
29 Holcombe, S.J., Rodriguez, K.M., Haupt, J.L. et al. (2009). Prevalence of and risk factors for postoperative ileus after small intestinal surgery in two hundred and thirty-three horses. *Vet. Surg.* 38: 368–372.
30 Cohen, N.D., Lester, G.D., Sanchez, L.C. et al. (2004). Evaluation of risk factors associated with development of postoperative ileus in horses. *J. Am. Vet. Med. Assoc.* 225: 1070–1078.
31 Roussel, A.J., Cohen, N.D., Hooper, R.N. et al. (2001). Risk factors associated with development of postoperative ileus in horses. *J. Am. Vet. Med. Assoc.* 219: 72–78.
32 Blikslager, A.T., Bowman, K.F., Levine, J.F. et al. (1994). Evaluation of factors associated with postoperative ileus in horses: 31 cases (1990–1992). *J. Am. Vet. Med. Assoc.* 205: 1748–1752.
33 Freeman, D.E., Hammock, P., Baker, G.J. et al. (2000). Short- and long-term survival and prevalence of postoperative ileus after small intestinal surgery in the horse. *Equine Vet. J. Suppl.* 32: 42–51.
34 McGovern, S.E., Allen, S.E., and Bladon, B.M. (2017). Evaluation of dexamethasone to prevent postoperative ileus in 66 horses with and without resection. *Equine Vet. Educ.* 29: 12.
35 Cook, V.L. and Blikslager, A.T. (2008). Use of systemically administered lidocaine in horses with gastrointestinal tract disease. *J. Am. Vet. Med. Assoc.* 232: 1144–1148.
36 Cook, V.L., Jones Shults, J., McDowell, M.R. et al. (2009). Anti-inflammatory effects of intravenously administered lidocaine hydrochloride on ischemia-injured jejunum in horses. *Am. J. Vet. Res.* 70: 1259–1268.
37 Salem, S.E., Proudman, C.J., and Archer, D.C. (2016). Has intravenous lidocaine improved the outcome in horses following surgical management of small intestinal lesions in a UK hospital population? *BMC Vet. Res.* 12: 157.
38 Cook, V.L., Meyer, C.T., Campbell, N.B. et al. (2009). Effect of firocoxib or flunixin meglumine on recovery of ischemic-injured equine jejunum. *Am. J. Vet. Res.* 70: 992–1000.
39 Tomlinson, J.E., Wilder, B.O., Young, K.M. et al. (2004). Effects of flunixin meglumine or etodolac treatment on mucosal recovery of equine jejunum after ischemia. *Am. J. Vet. Res.* 65: 761–769.
40 Cook, V.L., Jones Shults, J., McDowell, M. et al. (2008). Attenuation of ischaemic injury in the equine jejunum by administration of systemic lidocaine. *Equine Vet. J.* 40: 353–357.
41 Little, D., Tomlinson, J.E., and Blikslager, A.T. (2005). Post operative neutrophilic inflammation in equine small intestine after manipulation and ischaemia. *Equine Vet. J.* 37: 329–335.

Section XI Endotoxemia in the Neonatal Foal

David Wong and James Moore

Endotoxemia is a well-described pathophysiologic process impacting adult horses and foals. Although the term *endotoxemia* strictly refers to the presence of endotoxin in the blood, it frequently is used to describe the clinical syndrome observed in response to activation of the animal's inflammatory and immune systems. Complete descriptions of the molecular pathways and mediators associated with endotoxemia are available elsewhere [1–3], with an abbreviated review of the pathophysiological processes in foals presented here, along with potential therapies.

Role of Endotoxin

Endotoxin is the lipopolysaccharide (LPS) component of the outer cell envelope of Gram-negative bacteria and is comprised of three portions: an outer polysaccharide (O-antigenic) region, a unique core region, and an inner hydrophobic fatty acid-rich region, called lipid A. The latter component is highly conserved among Gram-negative bacteria. The majority of deleterious effects associated with endotoxin arise from the lipid A moiety [2]. Endotoxin is liberated from the outer membrane of Gram-negative bacteria as a result of rapid proliferation or lysis of microorganisms, with the source of bacteria being endogenous (e.g., leakage from intestinal tract) or exogenous (e.g., sepsis) [2]. When endotoxin gains access to the circulation, it is recognized by the innate immune system and can either interact with circulating proteins and blood cells or be removed by macrophages in the liver, spleen, and pulmonary vasculature [1, 3]. In the circulatory system, endotoxin binds to LPS-binding protein (LBP), which facilitates endotoxin's interaction with monocytes and macrophages within the peripheral blood. LBP is synthesized by the liver and in health is present in trace amounts. During the acute phase response to inflammatory stimuli, such as sepsis, circulating concentrations of LBP can increase as much as 100-fold [4].

LBP functions to shuttle LPS to the host's inflammatory cells, where it transfers LPS to the cell surface receptor cluster of differentiation antigen 14 (CD14), a pattern-recognition receptor primarily located on mononuclear phagocytes. LBP can also interact with soluble forms of CD14 that are released from the surface of mononuclear phagocytes. In doing so, cells lacking CD14, such as endothelial and epithelial cells, can initiate and participate in the inflammatory response [5]. Although CD14 is a cell surface receptor attached to the exterior of the cell, it lacks a transmembrane component. Therefore, toll-like receptors (TLR), in collaboration with myeloid differentiation factor 2 (MD2) transmits the extracellular signal into a cytoplasmic signal. Specifically, TLR-4 is responsible for communicating the presence of LPS from CD14 to the interior of the cell. Once the signal is transmitted into the cell, mobilization of a variety of intracellular pathways such as nuclear factor K (NF-KB) and mitogen-activated protein kinase initiate DNA transcription, consequently resulting in the generation of a multitude of pro-inflammatory substances [1].

The macrophage is the major effector cell in the innate immune system and plays a vital role in the pathophysiology of endotoxemia in foals. The majority of clinical and clinicopathologic changes associated with endotoxemia arise from the plethora of pro-inflammatory mediators produced and their subsequent binding to specific receptors on target cells, resulting in the activation of specific genes [1]. These genes encode for proteins (adhesion molecules, proteases, acute phase proteins), enzymes (cyclooxygenase, nitric oxide synthase), and cytokines. Notable mediators associated with endotoxemia include interleukin-1 (IL-1), IL-6, and tumor-necrosis factor-α (TNF-α), amongst many others. These three cytokines are pyrogens

Equine Neonatal Medicine, First Edition. Edited by David M. Wong and Pamela A. Wilkins.

and have the capacity to stimulate the liver to produce acute phase proteins [1]. The acute phase response elicits a local response (e.g., local inflammation) and systemic reaction (e.g., fever, leukocytosis, cytokine production, complement) with the ultimate goal of facilitating removal of the pathogen from the body. Acute phase proteins include molecules such as serum amyloid A (SAA), fibrinogen, C-reactive protein, haptoglobin, and ceruloplasmin, among others.

Endotoxin in the Equine Neonate

Endotoxemia has been widely discussed in equine medicine due to its common involvement with disorders such as strangulating intestinal lesions, pleuropneumonia, peritonitis, enterocolitis, and retained fetal membranes in adult horses. In the neonatal foal, endotoxemia is most commonly associated with sepsis, although it also may be involved in septic peritonitis, colitis, and pneumonia [6]. In one study, very low concentrations of LPS were detected in plasma from healthy neonatal foals ($n = 7$; 1–6 days of age), with a median concentration of 2.61 endotoxin units (EU)/ml (range 1.61–3.50) [7]. In comparison, the median plasma LPS concentration in six foals with Gram-negative sepsis was 78.06 EU/ml (range 0.76–2696) and 2.73 EU/ml (range 0.59–4.04) in eight potentially septic foals with negative blood cultures or Gram-positive isolates [7]. In a different study, endotoxin was detected in 50% of foals (15/30 septic foals) with a mean value of 243 ± 640 pg endotoxin/ml [8].

Acute-phase response proteins have been detected in septic neonatal foals, but they have not been able to consistently predict sepsis [9–11]. For example, circulating concentrations of SAA, which induces cytokine production and serves as a chemotactic for neutrophils, are frequently increased in foals with endotoxemia and sepsis [12]. In an induced model of bacterial placentitis, septic newborn foals had higher SAA concentrations compared to control and ill foals, and these values increased over the first 48 hours of life in septic foals. At birth, concentrations of SAA in septic foals ($n = 9$) were mildly elevated 0.5 mg/l (range 0–589) and increased to 66 mg/l (range 3.6–631) and 330 mg/l (range 20–963) at 24 and 48 hours of age, respectively [9]. In another study, the median SAA concentration in healthy 2-day-old foals was 4.9 mg/l as compared to 280 mg/l in septic foals [10]. Plasma concentrations of fibrinogen also increase, but do so at a slower rate, starting at 2 days after stimulation and peaking at 6 days [10]. Fibrinogen may be elevated in newborn foals with in utero infection, with one study demonstrating a fibrinogen concentration of 640 ± 320 mg/dl (range 300–1100 mg/dl; normal 200 ± 70) in eight foals <12 hours of age born from mares with chorioamnionitis. In contrast, no differences were detected in fibrinogen concentrations between septic and healthy foals born to mares with experimentally induced placentitis [9, 13]. In a different study, septic neonatal foals had a significantly increased fibrinogen concentrations when compared to age-matched healthy foals [8].

C-reactive protein is a downstream mediator of the acute phase response and plays an active role in the inflammatory process by binding to microorganisms and triggering the classical complement pathway [14]. In one study, no statistical difference in C-reactive protein concentrations was identified between healthy (15 mg/ml, range 0–336), sick, nonseptic (6 mg/ml, range 0–260), and septic foals (39 mg/ml, range 0–240) [11]. Haptoglobin, a protein produced by the liver that inhibits iron uptake by microbes by binding hemoglobin, is increased in septic infants. However, haptoglobin concentrations were lower in septic foals (1190 mg/ml, range 238–3200) when compared to critically ill (1619 mg/ml, range 392–3200) and healthy foals (1627 mg/ml, range 601–3224) [11].

Clinical Signs of Endotoxemia

LPS has been infused IV to healthy neonatal foals at varying doses to document the responses associated with experimentally induced endotoxemia (Figure 15.XI.1) [15–19]. Signs associated with LPS infusion are listed in Table 15.XI.1.

A topic that has received relatively little attention in equine medicine, but relevant to this textbook, is the impact of endotoxemia on the fetus and the fetal inflammatory response syndrome (FIRS). The fetal immune system has limited functional capacity due to gestational immaturity as well as the need for stimulation for it to develop; thus, the fetal immune response relies largely on innate immunity, as adaptive immune cells are not mature [20]. However, it is not uncommon for a fetus to be exposed to chorioamnionitis and develop a systemic inflammatory response known as FIRS [21]. FIRS occurs when the fetus comes in direct contact with infected amniotic and/or inflammatory cell transfer from uteroplacental circulation [21]. If the inflammatory response becomes systemic in the fetus, plasma IL-6 concentrations increase and neutrophils and macrophages become activated [20]. Clinically, FIRS is defined in people by fetal plasma IL-6 concentration > 11 pg/ml while subclinical cases are characterized by microscopic evidence of funisitis and vasculitis.

Although intrauterine infection is the leading cause of preterm birth in women, the presence of bacteria in the amniotic fluid does not always result in preterm delivery or induce chorioamnionitis [22]. Infectious challenges to the fetus occur in the pregnant mare, most notably with placentitis, and can result in abortion or delivery of a premature, ill, or healthy foal [9]. If born premature, the foal may have

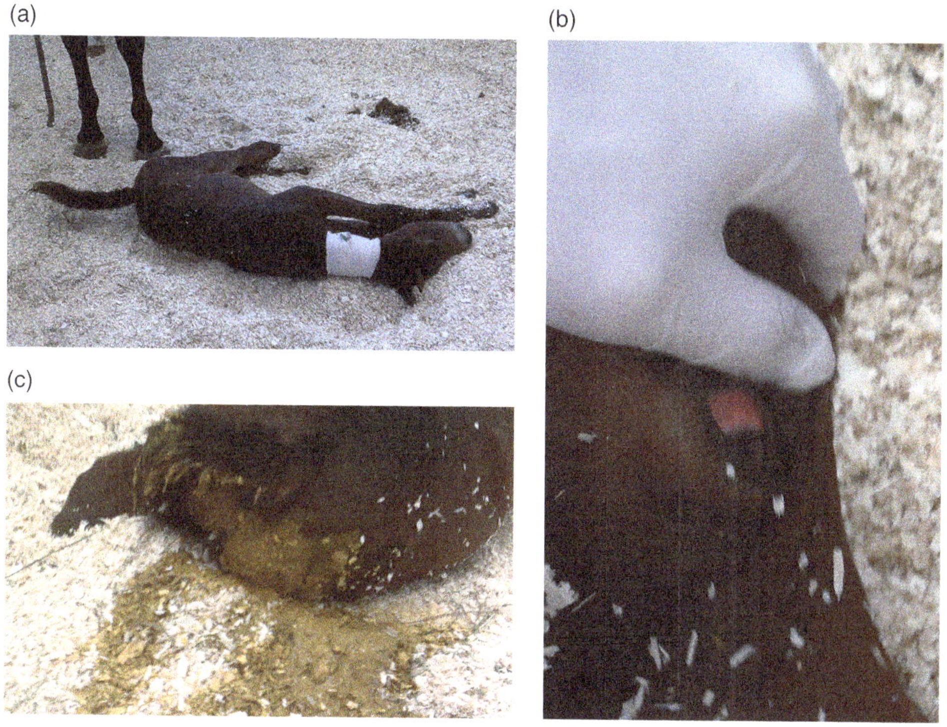

Figure 15.XI.1 Neonatal foal demonstrating clinical signs of colic (a), hyperemic scleral vessels (b) and diarrhea (c) noted within 1 hour of IV administration of LPS (0.5 μg/kg).

Table 15.XI.1 Clinical signs and hemodynamic changes associated with infusion of LPS to neonatal foals.

System	Signs and Hemodynamic Changes
General	Fever, frequent urination, recumbency
Digestive	Abdominal pain, diarrhea
Neurologic	Marked lethargy (low head carriage, lack of awareness of environment, loss of suck reflex)
Cardiovascular	Congestion of mucous membranes, injection of scleral vasculature. Tachycardia can be observed but heart rate can be unchanged or decreased. Increases in pulmonary artery pressure, pulmonary wedge pressure, right atrial pressure, aortic pressure, systemic vascular resistance, and pulmonary vascular resistance may occur, as well as hyperlactatemia (6–8 mmol/l). Effects of LPS on the cardiovascular system are dose dependent.
Respiratory	Variable changes in respiratory rate, both increased and decreased rates have been reported post-LPS infusion along with decreased P_aO_2.
Hematological	Biphasic change in white blood cell count characterized by initial leucopenia (primarily neutropenia) for first 6–8 hours after LPS infusion, followed by neutrophilic leukocytosis 12–48 hours after LPS infusion. Mild to marked decrease in lymphocyte count noted during infusion along with increased PCV (33 ± 3% at baseline to 36–38% over a 12-hour period after LPS infusion).
Coagulation	Increase in PT and APTT and decreased platelet count
Biochemical	Decreased blood glucose with varying degrees of hypoglycemia (35–50 mg/ml post-LPS infusion).

Note: PCV = packed cell volume; APTT = activated partial thromboplastin time; PT = prothrombin time

precocious development or be physiologically and anatomically immature. Bacteria that invade the fetal membranes release LPS and/or exotoxins, resulting in activation of the innate immune system. This results in the production of inflammatory mediators including cytokines, chemokines, prostaglandins, and metalloproteases that cause uterine contraction, biochemical and structural changes of the cervix and weakening of the fetal membranes [20]. In health, prostaglandins produced in the amnion are inactivated by prostaglandin dehydrogenase, thereby preventing uterine contractions. Infection of the chorion inhibits prostaglandin dehydrogenase activity resulting in higher prostaglandin concentrations, which consequently stimulate premature uterine contractions [23]. Additionally, metalloproteases causes cervical ripening and degradation of the chorioamniotic membrane, causing it to rupture [21]. In pregnant women, FIRS leads to increased production of fetal and placental corticotrophin releasing hormone (CRH), which in turn increases cortisol production and stimulates placental prostaglandin synthesis and myometrial contractility [24, 25]. FIRS has not been extensively examined in equine medicine, but information from other species indicates that intrauterine inflammation may have beneficial or detrimental effects on multiple organ systems. It is possible that equine fetuses exposed to LPS and inflammation in utero might have altered development of their organs, resulting in positive or negative outcomes, but further research is needed.

Lungs

Preterm infants exposed to chorioamnionitis have advanced lung function for their gestational age and reduced incidence of respiratory distress syndrome (RDS) [26, 27]. Experimentally induced intrauterine inflammation via intra-amniotic LPS injection in sheep results in increased pulmonary surfactant and improved lung function and may explain the decreased incidence of RDS in infants [27, 28]. This precocious development may result from direct action of proinflammatory mediators on the lung, rather than secretion of corticosteroids via the hypothalamic-pituitary-adrenal (HPA) axis [23]. Conversely, detrimental effects of LPS-induced chorioamnionitis include anatomical changes of the lung characteristic of bronchopulmonary dysplasia [29].

Central Nervous System

Intrauterine inflammation has been linked to perinatal brain injuries, such as cerebral palsy, periventricular leukomalacia, and intraventricular hemorrhage [21, 30, 31]. FIRS may play a part in the development of some cases of neonatal encephalopathy in foals, but direct evidence of this is not available [32]. Possible mechanisms of fetal inflammatory cytokine-induced brain injury include: (i) direct effect on cerebral vasculature causing hypoperfusion and ischemia, (ii) activation of the coagulation cascade and capillary thrombosis with necrosis of white matter, (iii) activation of microglia causing toxic effects on oligodendrocytes and myelin, (iv) increased permeability of the blood-brain-barrier allowing passage of microbial products and cytokines into cerebral tissues, (v) increased production of nitric oxide synthase, cyclooxygenase and free radicals, and/or (vi) direct cytotoxic effects [21, 30–32].

Intestines

Intrauterine inflammation may negatively impact the intestines as reflected by the fact that chorioamnionitis and prenatal inflammation are risk factors for necrotizing enterocolitis in infants [33]. Injection of LPS to pregnant mice results in significantly increased incidence of this condition in neonatal mice and is dependent on endogenous production of TNF-α. Decreased intestinal microvascular density, endothelial cell proliferation, and decreased expression of vascular endothelial growth factor (VEGF) and VEGF receptor 2 were noted in neonatal mice suggesting that inflammation impairs development of intestinal microvasculature, thereby predisposing to necrotizing enterocolitis [33].

Heart

Exposure of the fetus to inflammation in utero impairs cardiac function (increased left ventricular dilation) and development of the myocardium. As evidence of this, human neonates with FIRS have reduced mean and diastolic blood pressures [21].

Retina

An association between chorioamnionitis, FIRS, and retinopathy of prematurity exists in infants. The exact mechanism is unknown, but a direct sensitizing of the developing retina to oxygen-induced changes in VEGF availability and subsequent vascular development or systemic hypotension resulting in retinal hypoperfusion or ischemia has been suggested as potential causative factors [21, 34]. Direct exposure of the developing retina to circulating products of infection and inflammation and/or oxidative damage may also participate in the pathogenesis of retinopathy of prematurity [34].

Treatment of Endotoxemia

An expansive array of treatments has been examined to counteract the negative impact of LPS on the host. Overarching strategies target: (i) elimination of the source of LPS; (ii) blocking interactions of LPS with the host immune system; and (iii) counteracting the inflammatory cascade induced by LPS. Foundational therapies in foals such as IV fluid therapy and antimicrobials have remained consistent over time. Nonsteroidal anti-inflammatory drugs (NSAID) are nearly always administered to adult horses with endotoxemia, but their use in neonatal foals with endotoxemia is controversial due to increased risk of adverse effects [35]. Therapies that may provide some benefit are discussed below, but efficacy of many therapies in uncertain (Table 15.XI.2).

Fluid Therapy

Varying severities of hypovolemia and decreased oxygen delivery to tissues occur with endotoxemia due to the

Table 15.XI.2 Potential therapies for endotoxemia in the foal.

Fluid therapy	20 ml/kg boluses	Clinical and objective re-assessment required after each bolus; maximum dose 80 ml/kg [37].
Antimicrobials	Numerous	Awareness of potential worsening of clinical signs due to bacteriolysis and release of LPS.
Flunixin meglumine	0.25 mg/kg, q 8–12 h	Correct blood volume deficits prior to administration, if possible, to decrease incidence of nephrotoxicity [35]
Hyperimmunized plasma	1–3 l (50 kg foal)	No conclusive data to support its use [19, 60].
Polymyxin B	6000 IU/kg, IV q 8–12 h	Clinical studies needed to determine if polymyxin B improves survival in septic foals; potential for renal or neurologic toxicity, but neither reported in foals [16, 63].
Pentoxifylline	7.5–10 mg/kg, PO q 12 h; 7.5 mg/kg bolus injection, then 3 mg/kg/h for 3 h, IV	Inhibits TNF-α production in equine blood and cultured equine macrophages [65, 68, 70, 71]. Stimulates production of anti-inflammatory cytokine IL-10, suppresses neutrophil activation, inhibits NF-KB in other species [88]. No studies conducted in neonatal foals.
Lidocaine	1.3 mg/kg bolus, followed CRI of 0.05 mg/kg/min, IV	Evaluated as a therapy for experimental endotoxemia in adult horses; further studies needed in neonatal foals [72].
DMSO	0.02–1 g/kg diluted to ≤10% solution, IV q 12–24 h	Efficacy in treatment of endotoxemia unknown; may reduce adhesion formation in foals with small intestinal ischemia [75].
Corticosteroids	Hydrocortisone 1.3 mg/kg/d, IV total dose divided into q4h treatments	Low-dose hydrocortisone decreased LPS-induced inflammation without impacting neutrophil function in an ex vivo model in neonatal foals and might improve clinical condition (e.g., hypotension not responsive to fluid and vasopressors) in foals with critical illness related corticosteroid insufficiency (CIRCI) [79].
Ketamine	Step-wise infusion rate of 4.8, 3.6, 3.0, and 2.4 mg/kg/h, IV in 10-minute intervals, followed by CRI of 1.5 mg/kg/h	No positive impact on clinical, hematological or inflammatory mediators in experimentally induced endotoxemia in adult horses [85].

profound impact that LPS has on the cardiovascular system, coupled with the underlying disease and lack of normal fluid/milk intake in ill neonatal foals (see also Chapter 62, "Fluid Therapy"). Endotoxemia can also cause alterations in vascular and intestinal permeability that can result in protein loss [36]. Therefore, restoration and maintenance of circulatory volume and optimizing global oxygen delivery is a fundamental treatment goal. This is accomplished by IV administration of isotonic polyionic electrolyte solutions. One to four individual fluid boluses of 20 ml/kg, administered over 10–20 minutes per bolus, can be used in hypovolemic foals, followed by reevaluation of subjective clinical (mentation, pulse quality, extremity temperature) and objectively measured (blood L-lactate, blood pressure, heart rate, urine output, PCV) parameters at regular intervals to determine further fluid needs [37]. Reevaluating these parameters after each 20 ml/kg bolus allows the clinician to limit the amount of IV fluids given to restore appropriate fluid volume without causing fluid overload. Natural or synthetic colloids can be used in foals with low colloid oncotic pressure.

Antimicrobials

Antimicrobials have been a cornerstone of treatment of endotoxemia related to sepsis in the neonatal foal, as clearance of invading microbes is essential for recovery. Discussions regarding sepsis and antimicrobial selection are found in Chapters 50 and 61, respectively. Pertinent to this chapter, LPS is released during rapid bacteriolysis, and enters the circulation resulting in endotoxemia. Combination therapy of different classes of antimicrobials are frequently used to provide broad-spectrum coverage with antimicrobial de-escalation employed if blood culture and susceptibility results are available. Administration of antimicrobials can result in Gram-negative bacteriolysis, consequently resulting in increased LPS in the blood and exacerbation of the inflammatory response [38]. In vitro studies have demonstrated increased release of LPS when Gram-negative bacteria are exposed to different antimicrobials, with some clinical studies in people demonstrating a survival benefit when a combination of an aminoglycoside and β-lactam is administered [39]. Additionally, lower antibiotic-induced release of LPS has been demostrated in vitro when an aminoglycoside was administered along with cefuroxime, with a beneficial effect possibly related to decreased LPS release and reduced inflammatory response [40, 41]. The results of other studies have not been conclusive. In a porcine model of sepsis, *Escherichia coli* was infused to 36 anesthetized pigs that received cefuroxime, a combination of cefuroxime and tobramycin, or saline; no differences were noted in plasma LPS concentrations in vivo, but antimicrobial-treated pigs had higher IL-6 concentrations, leukocyte activation, and decreased pulmonary compliance compared to controls [38].

Few studies of this concept have been performed in foals, but one in vitro foal model investigated which antimicrobial(s) would minimize LPS release using *E. coli* isolates: (i) amikacin alone, (ii) amikacin and ampicillin, or (iii) ampicillin, (iv) imipenem, or (v) ceftiofur alone. In that study, amikacin alone or combined with ampicillin resulted in significantly less LPS activity compared to monotherapy with ampicillin, imipenem, or ceftiofur [6]. The β-lactam antimicrobials generated 2–25 times more LPS activity than amikacin, with ceftiofur inducing the greatest release of LPS (Figures 15.XI.2 and 15.XI.3) [6]. This result

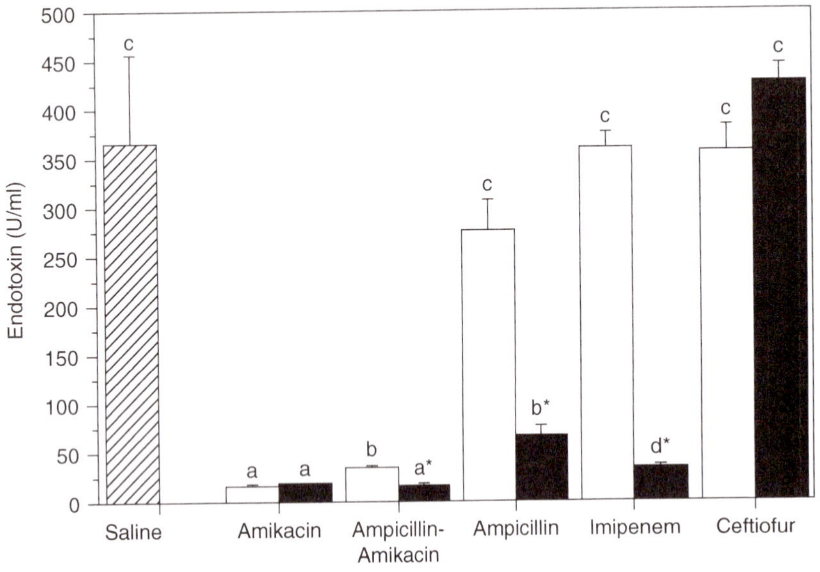

Figure 15.XI.2 Mean ± SE endotoxin activity of mononuclear cells isolated from six healthy foals that were incubated for 6 hours with *E. coli* isolate and each antimicrobial at 2× MIC (white bars), 20× MIC (black bars) or saline (gray bar). (a–d) Values with different letters differ significantly within that concentration ($P<0.05$) [6].

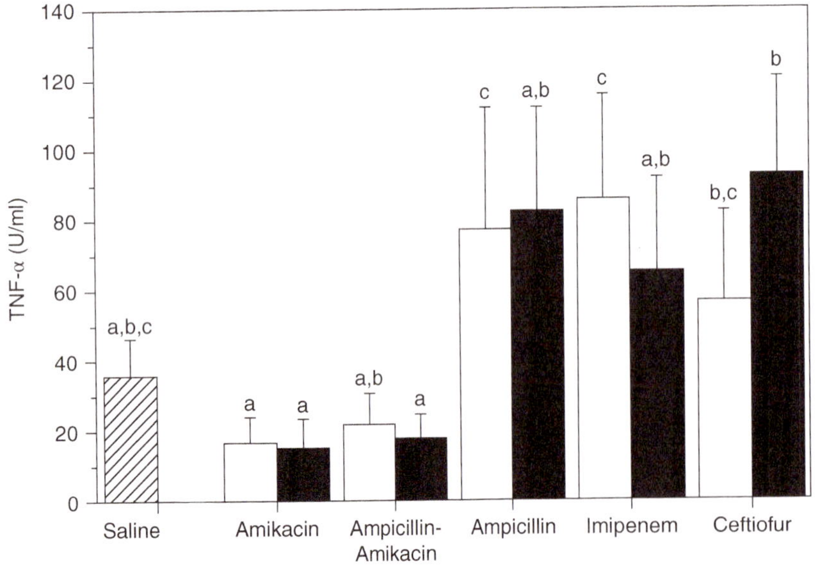

Figure 15.XI.3 Mean ± SE TNF-α activity released from mononuclear cells isolated from six healthy foals that were incubated for 6 hours with *E. coli* isolate and each antimicrobial at 2× MIC (white bars), 20× MIC (black bars) or saline (gray bar). [a–c]Values with different letters differ significantly within that concentration ($P<0.05$) [6].

was attributed to the fact that antimicrobials active against the cell wall of Gram-negative bacteria promote release of LPS during bacterial killing, as compared to antimicrobials having other mechanisms of action. The investigators concluded that the amount of LPS released and subsequent TNF-α activity was dependent on the mechanisms of action of the antimicrobial used [6]. Another small study examined the same concept in an in vivo model involving ill foals [42]. Neonatal foals ($n = 14$) that received a β-lactam alone (ceftiofur), had a significant increase in LPS concentration (0.16 ± 0.23 EU/ml) 12 hours after antimicrobial administration when compared to admission values (0.07 ± 0.1 EU/ml), whereas foals that received a combination of a β-lactam and aminoglycoside did not have an increase in serum LPS concentration. Differences in clinical signs and clinicopathologic parameters were not evaluated over time [42]. Other studies suggest that LPS release after aminoglycoside administration is minimal and that aminoglycosides are capable of neutralizing LPS activity, similar to polymyxin B; thus, aminoglycosides should be considered in appropriate cases of equine neonatal sepsis [6, 43–45]. It is not known if differing levels of LPS release after administration of specific antimicrobials impacts clinical outcome. Although specific antimicrobials, including β-lactams, are frequently required to facilitate clearance of bacterial pathogens, clinicians should be aware that antimicrobial therapy might result in initial worsening of clinical condition, clinicopathologic parameters, and hemodynamic variables as a result of bacteriolysis and liberation of LPS in some septic foals [6, 42].

Nonsteroidal Anti-inflammatory Drugs (NSAIDs)

As briefly noted, one component of the LPS-initiated inflammatory cascade is increased cyclooxygenase (COX) activity. Cyclooxygenase occurs in two isoforms (COX-1 and COX-2) that participate in conversion of arachidonic acid into prostaglandins, thromboxane, prostacyclin, and other compounds [46]. Many clinical signs associated with endotoxemia are mediated, in part, by products of COX. Therefore, blocking the production of these mediators via administration of NSAIDs (which inhibit COX activity) provides anti-inflammatory, antipyretic, and antithrombotic effects, which may ameliorate some negative effects of endotoxemia in the neonatal foal. However, NSAIDs are associated with the development of gastrointestinal ulcers and renal injury, particularly in the neonatal foal. These negative side effects can be exacerbated by hemodynamic derangements and multiple organ dysfunction that are commonly present in critically ill neonatal foals. Thus, these variables, coupled with the fact that many vital functions of cardiorespiratory transition from fetal to neonatal life are prostaglandin dependent, results in sparing clinical use of NSAIDs, especially in the foals <5–7 days of age [47].

If NSAIDs are used, the dosing regimen in neonatal foals is different than adults due to the foal's higher volume of distribution (e.g., greater total body water and extracellular fluid compartment) and altered kinetics (e.g., longer drug clearance, longer half-life) [48–50]. Flunixin meglumine has longer drug disposition and lower clearance in 1-day-old foals compared to older (10–11- and 27–28-day-old) foals and adult horses [48, 51, 52]. Phenylbutazone and ketoprofen are infrequently used in critically ill neonatal foals, but the few studies available for this age group suggest a larger volume of distribution, longer serum half-life and lower total clearance of the drug compared to adult horses [49, 50, 53]. The selective COX-2 inhibitors, meloxicam and firocoxib, may provide anti-inflammatory and analgesic effects with fewer complications. Drug clearance of meloxicam is more rapid in neonatal foals compared to adult horses. In one study, administration of meloxicam at 0.6 mg/kg every 12 hours for 3 weeks was well tolerated in neonatal foals and a dose of 1.8 mg/kg every 12 hours for 7 days did not result in side effects [54]. Oral administration of firocoxib to neonatal foals at the adult therapeutic dose of 0.1 mg/kg every 24 hours for 9 days was cleared faster and had a shorter half-life compared to adults. In addition, bioavailability of firocoxib was lower in foals compared to adults, thereby necessitating more frequent or higher dosages [55]. Ibuprofen has been studied in 5- to 10-week-old foals at 10 and 25 mg/kg, administered orally every 8 hours for 6 days, and was reported to be safe in this age group (see Chapter 63 NSAIDs) [56].

Hyperimmune Plasma

Hyperimmune plasma has been used in horses and foals to provide anti-lipid A antibodies to patients with presumed endotoxemia, with the intent of binding LPS and preventing its downstream interaction with host cells. Administration of hyperimmune plasma decreased mortality in horses with endotoxic shock and reduced TNF-α activity, but few studies involving foals are available [57–59]. In a study of 40 foals with presumed or suspected sepsis, 22 foals received hyperimmune plasma and 18 foals received regular plasma. No difference in survival rate was reported between groups, but the study did not examine trends in vital parameters, inflammatory mediators or clinicopathologic parameters that may have identified more specific differences between groups, rather than survival alone [60]. In another study involving 3- to 5-month-old foals ($n = 6$), Salmonella antiserum was associated with higher respiratory rates and plasma concentrations of IL-6 and TNF-α activity compared to controls, but the number of foals in this study was very small [19].

In human neonates, Intravenous Immunoglobulin (IVIG) has been examined as a treatment for sepsis and a method of reducing the impact of LPS on the patient. Polyclonal immunoglobulin is composed of pooled serum containing different immunoglobulins, primarily IgG and IgM, but not necessarily directed at specific antigen sites [61, 62]. This treatment has direct antibacterial effects through pathogen recognition and increased clearance. It also has anti-inflammatory properties through its ability to scavenge bacterial toxins and pro-inflammatory cytokines, immune cell depletion, blockade of activating receptors and modulating Fc receptors [62]. Large studies and reviews in human neonatal sepsis suggest that IV administration of immunoglobulin did not decrease mortality [61]. Currently, there are too few studies available to make specific recommendations about the efficacy of this approach in neonatal foals.

Polymyxin B

Polymyxin B is a bactericidal antimicrobial at high doses that binds the lipid A component of LPS at lower doses. In one study, 14 neonatal foals were administered 6000 U/kg of polymyxin or an equal volume of saline IV, immediately after LPS administration. The treatment group had significantly lower blood lactate, TNF-α, and thromboxane B_2 concentrations and higher blood glucose concentrations and attitude scores when compared to the control group at various times during the study [16]. Although polymyxin B can cause nephrotoxic and neurotoxic effects, no evidence of these side effects was detected. In another study involving 3- to 5-month-old foals administered 6000 U/kg of polymyxin B, IV prior to LPS injection resulted in significantly lower plasma TNF-α and IL-6 activity as well as lower rectal temperature and respiratory rates in foals when compared to control foals [19]. Studies investigating the ability of polymyxin B to attenuate endotoxemia in adult horses have revealed similar overall positive results [63, 64]. There is a need to determine if polymyxin B improves clinical course of disease or survival in horses and foals. Interestingly, polymyxin B has been used to neutralize LPS in septic human patients, but polymyxin B is highly toxic to people [62]. To circumvent toxicity, physicians have used extracorporeal circuits (continuous renal replacement therapy units) in which the dialysis filter contains fibers coated with polymyxin B to avoid the drug from entering the patient's bloodstream.

Pentoxifylline

Methyl xanthine derivatives, such as pentoxifylline, suppress inflammatory cytokine production by macrophages via phosphodiesterase inhibition and resultant elevation of intracellular cyclic adenosine monophosphate (cAMP) [65]. Pentoxifylline has been suggested as a potential anti-inflammatory in foals to treat neonatal encephalopathy, severe acute pancreatitis, and sepsis, but the efficacy is unknown in foals [32, 66–68]. Pentoxifylline, used as an adjunct to antimicrobials in septic neonatal infants, decreased all-cause mortality in a systematic review [69]. In an in vitro model in adult horses, pentoxifylline significantly inhibited production of TNF-α and IL-6 activity in blood exposed to LPS, in a dose-dependent fashion [70]. However, a follow-up in vivo study demonstrated only limited benefit (lower respiratory rate and temperature) in adult horses administered pentoxifylline after LPS injection as compared to saline control [71]. Pentoxifylline is rapidly eliminated after IV administration, necessitating constant rate infusions in horses [65]. In adult horses, oral absorption of the drug is rapid, but similar studies examining either oral absorption of pentoxifylline or its effectiveness in foals administered LPS has yet to be performed [65].

Lidocaine

Lidocaine has been administered to adult horses for its purported pro-kinetic, analgesic, and anti-inflammatory effects and has been examined as a medication to ameliorate experimentally induced endotoxemia [72, 73]. In one small study, LPS was administered intraperitoneally and either lidocaine (bolus 1.3 mg/kg, followed by continuous rate infusion of 0.05 mg/kg/min), or an equal volume of saline was administered after LPS injection. In that study, lidocaine-treated horses had significantly better clinical scores and lower serum and peritoneal fluid TNF-α activity when compared to controls [72]. Further studies, including the use of lidocaine in neonatal foals, are needed to evaluate its effectiveness as a treatment for endotoxemia in adult horses and foals.

Dimethyl Sulfoxide (DMSO)

Historically, DMSO has had ubiquitous use in equine practice based on its oxygen-free radical scavenging and anti-inflammatory properties [74]. Foals with neonatal encephalopathy and disease processes associated with endotoxemia (e.g., neonatal sepsis, strangulating intestinal lesions) have been treated with DMSO [32, 75]. The rationale for DMSO use is to combat the cellular damage that occurs when reactive oxygen species are released during endotoxemia [17]. Moreover, DMSO reduces platelet aggregation, which may combat hypercoagulability, microthrombi formation, and ischemia at the microvascular level commonly associated with endotoxemia [17]. While reduced fever was noted in one study in which DMSO was administered to LPS-challenged horses, there were minimal effects on clinical signs induced by LPS administration [74]. Because its effectiveness is questionable, the use of DMSO has declined in equine neonatal medicine in recent years [76, 77].

Corticosteroids

Low doses of corticosteroids provided beneficial effects in experimental endotoxemia in horses and foals but their use is controversial in neonatal endotoxemia and sepsis [78, 79]. Corticosteroids provide anti-inflammatory effects through inhibition of NF-Kβ, reducing neutrophil activation, and downregulating production and release of pro-inflammatory cytokines [62, 77]. Exogenously administered corticosteroids might provide additional benefit in some neonatal foals with endotoxemia and sepsis that have dysfunction of their HPA axis, characterized by inadequate cortisol response to illness. This syndrome has been called critical illness–related corticosteroid insufficiency (CIRCI) [79–83]. Hypotensive septic foals that are unresponsive to administration of fluid therapy and vasopressors may have CIRCI and might benefit from corticosteroid administration, which provides favorable vascular and hemodynamic effects. A short tapering dose of hydrocortisone at 1.3 mg/kg/d, divided every 4 hours, IV, has been suggested for treatment of CIRCI in foals [81]. This dose significantly reduced LPS-induced expression of TNF-α, IL-6, IL-8, and IL-1β while not impacting neutrophil phagocytosis or reactive oxygen species production in an ex vivo foal model [81]. It should be noted that the global initiative on sepsis (Surviving Sepsis Campaign) suggests that IV administration of hydrocortisone should not be used to treat children with septic shock if fluid resuscitation and vasopressor therapy are able to restore hemodynamic stability. However, this was a weak recommendation with low quality of evidence [84]. Corticosteroids can impart positive physiologic effects (e.g. help increase blood pressure) in critically ill neonatal foals, but should be used judiciously and with caution.

Ketamine

The dissociative anesthetic agent ketamine also has immunomodulating and anti-inflammatory effects that have been demonstrated in experimental endotoxemia in rats and in vitro studies using equine macrophages [85–87]. Ketamine down-regulates NF-kB signaling and decreases inflammatory cytokine production [85]. In one study of experimentally induced endotoxemia in adult horses, ketamine failed to attenuate the clinical, hematological, or inflammatory mediator (TNF-α, thromboxane B_2) production associated with LPS, when compared to saline-treated horses [85]. Studies in neonatal foals investigating ketamine's impact on endotoxemia have not been conducted.

Mares with Placentitis

Treatment of mares with placentitis is clearly indicated to improve the health of the fetus/newborn foal. In one study of experimentally induced placentitis (*S. zooepidemicus*) in pregnant mares (295–303 days gestation), 33% of foals born to mares that were treated with antibiotics, NSAIDs, progesterone, or estrodial were septic as compared to 100% of foals born septic in which the mare received no treatment [9].

Therapies to treat endotoxemia are constantly evolving. Below are brief discussions of other therapies that have been investigated in horses but have yet to be applied clinically.

Phospholipid Emulsion (PLE)

Lipoproteins produced by the body are composed of apolipoproteins, cholesterol, triglycerides, and phospholipids [88]. Lipoproteins bind and neutralize LPS, thereby lessening the negative effects of LPS on the host (e.g. attenuates fever, tachycardia, leukopenia) [88]. Because of these positive attributes, protein-free phospholipid-rich emulsions were developed to reduce the impact of LPS. In experimentally induced endotoxemia in adult horses, infusion of a phospholipid-rich emulsion significantly lowered rectal temperature, heart rate, and serum TNF-α concentrations and increased total leukocyte counts in treated horses, as compared to controls [88]. However, mild to moderate hemolysis was observed in horses treated with the emulsion within 1–2 hours of initiation of its administration. In a similar study, a lower dose of the emulsion was administered over a shorter period of time to determine whether the effects of LPS administration would still be attenuated while preventing hemolysis [89]. This follow-up study demonstrated that many of the adverse effects of LPS were prevented or ameliorated, but mild-to-moderate hemolysis was still observed in 3/6 horses [89]. The reason for the increased fragility of erythrocytes after administration of the emulsion is unknown.

Lipid A Analogue E5564

Synthetic analogues of the lipid A region, such as E5564 (based on the lipid A structure of *Rhodobacter sphaeroides*) serve as synthetic TLR-4 antagonists and prevent in vitro and in vivo induction of cellular mediators and improve survival in LPS-challenged mice [90]. In an in vitro study, E5564 was evaluated in an LPS model using adult horse blood and monocytes. This treatment resulted in a dose-dependent inhibition of TNF-α production and procoagulant activity was documented [91]. No further equine studies are available.

Anti-Cytokine Therapy

Few studies have evaluated the possibility of attenuating the inflammatory response by administration of antibodies directed against inflammatory cytokines such as TNF-α in horses. One study administered murine and rabbit TNF-α antibodies after LPS administration to adult horses and noted that TNF-α activity was decreased in vitro, but no beneficial effects were noted in horses in vivo [92]. In another study, administration of monoclonal antibody against TNF-α reduced plasma TNF-α activity and significantly improved clinical scoring, heart rate, PCV and plasma total protein, when compared to control horses [93]. This therapy has not been examined in neonatal foals.

Mesenchymal Stem Cells

Mesenchymal stem cells have the ability to proliferate and differentiate when inserted into injured tissue and initiate tissue repair. In addition, these cells exhibit immunomodulatory and immunosuppressive effects that may aid in the treatment of endotoxemia and sepsis [62, 94]. Mesenchymal stem cells also inhibit proliferation of T and B cells, differentiation of monocytes to immature dendritic cells and prevent production of TNF-α by dendritic cells. Furthermore, these cells inhibit proliferation of resting NK cells and thereby reduce cytokine release [95]. Studies using animal models have noted that administration of these cells decreases pro-inflammatory cytokines when compared to controls and improve survival rate [96, 97]. The use of mesenchymal stem cells in endotoxemic neonatal foal remains to be explored to address key questions such as dose, route, optimum timing of administration and their efficacy.

Other Compounds That May Attenuate the Effects of LPS

Several other drugs have been examined to reduce the detrimental impact of LPS in horses. Ethyl pyruvate is a stable derivative of pyruvate that has anti-inflammatory properties. Specifically, it inhibits NF-KB and the production of reactive oxygen species [77, 98]. An in vitro model of endotoxemia in horses, IV administration of ethyl pyruvate significantly decreased pain scores, TNF-α and IL-6 expression as compared to control horses. Other drugs that have been examined to combat endotoxemia include rolipram, azithromycin and metformin. Rolipram is a phosphodiesterase inhibitor and may reduce cytokine production; azithromycin is a macrolide antimicrobial that inhibits NF-KB; and metformin is a biguanide used in the treatment of metabolic syndrome but also has anti-inflammatory effects through inhibition of high-mobility group box-1 [99]. In an in vitro model, these drugs produced a concentration-dependent inhibition of TNF-α production from equine leukocytes and rolipram and azithromycin showed a concentration-dependent inhibition of IL-1β [99, 100]. Tyloxapol is a liquid polyether alcohol used as a surfactant to liquify and remove mucus from bronchopulmonary secretions. It also blocks lipolytic activity of plasma and breakdown of triglyceride-rich lipoproteins and has been used as a detergent to treat endotoxemia in horses [100]. Pretreatment of adult horses with IV tyloxapol prevented fever and leucopenia in an LPS-model in horses. Further in vivo studies of these medications are needed in horses and foals.

References

1 Werners, A.H., Bull, S., and Fink-Gremmels, J. (2005). Endotoxaemia: a review with implications for the horse. *Equine Vet. J.* 37: 371–383.

2 Moore, J.N. and Morris, D.D. (1992). Endotoxemia and septicemia in horses: experimental and clinical correlates. *J. Am. Vet. Med. Assoc.* 200: 1903–1914.

3 Moore, J.N. (2001). A perspective on endotoxemia. *AAEP Proc.* 47: 61–74.

4 Tobias, P.S. and Ulevitch, R.J. (1993). Lipopolysaccharide binding protein and CD14 in LPS dependent macrophage activation. *Immunobiology* 187: 227–232.

5 Fujihara, M., Muroi, M., Tanamoto, K. et al. (2003). Molecular mechansims of macrophage activation and deactivation by lipopolysaccharide: roles of the receptor complex. *Pharmacol. Ther.* 100: 171–194.

6 Bentley, A.P., Barton, M.H., Lee, M.D. et al. (2002). Antimicrobial-induced endotoxin and cytokine activity in an in vitro model of septicemia in foals. *Am. J. Vet. Res.* 63: 660–668.

7 Breuhaus, B.A. and DeGraves, F.J. (1993). Plasma endotoxin concentrations in clinically normal and potentially septic equine neonates. *J. Vet. Intern. Med.* 7: 296–302.

8 Barton, M.H., Morris, D.D., Norton, N. et al. (1988). Hemostatic and fibrinolytic indices in neonatal foals with presumed septicemia. *J. Vet. Intern. Med.* 12: 26–35.

9 Borba, L.A., Nogueira, C.E.W., Bruhn, F.R.P. et al. (2020). Peripheral blood markers of sepsis in foals born from mares with experimentally ascending placentitis. *Vet. Rec.* 187: 29–37.

10 Stoneham, S.J., Palmer, L., Cash, R. et al. (2001). Measurement of serum amyloid A in the neonatal foal using a latex agglutination immunoturbidimeteric assay: determination of the normal range, variation with age and response to disease. *Equine Vet. J.* 33: 599–603.

11 Zabrecky, K.A., Slovis, N.M., Constable, P.D. et al. (2015). Plasma C-reactive protein and haptoglobin concentrations in critically ill neonatal foals. *J. Vet. Intern. Med.* 29: 673–677.

12 Eklund, K.K., Niemi, K., and Kovanen, P.T. (2012). Immune functions of serum amyloid A. *Crit. Rev. Immunol.* 32: 335–348.

13 Koterba, A.M., Brewer, B.D., and Tarplee, F.A. (1984). Clinical and clinicopathological characteristics of the septicaemic neonatal foal: review of 38 cases. *Equine Vet. J.* 16: 376–383.

14 Sproston, N.R. and Ashworth, J.J. (2018). Role of C-reactive protein at sites of inflammation and infection. *Front. Immunol.* 9: 754.

15 Lavoie, J.P., Madigan, J.E., Cullor, J.S. et al. (1990). Haemodynamic, pathological, haematological and behavioural changes during endotoxin infusion in equine neonates. *Equine Vet. J.* 22: 23–29.

16 Wong, D.M., Sponseller, B.A., Alcott, C.J. et al. (2013). Effects of intravenous administration of polymyxin B in neonatal foals with experimental endotoxemia. *J. Am. Vet. Med. Assoc.* 243: 874–881.

17 Sykes, B.W. and Furr, M.O. (2005). Equine endotoxaemia – a state-of-the-are review of therapy. *Aust. Vet. J.* 83: 45–50.

18 Allen, G.K., Green, E.M., Robinson, J.A. et al. (1993). Serum tumor necrosis factor alpha concentrations and clinical abnormalities in colostrum-fed and colostrum-deprived neonatal foals given endotoxin. *Am. J. Vet. Res.* 54: 1404–1410.

19 Durando, M.M., MacKay, R.J., Linda, S. et al. (1994). Effects of polymyxin B and Salmonella typhimurium antiserum on horses given endotoxin intravenously. *Am. J. Vet. Res.* 55: 921–927.

20 Helmo, F.R., Alves, E.A.R., Moreira, R.A. et al. (2018). Intrauterine infection, immune system and premature birth. *J. Matern. Fetal Neonatal Med.* 31: 1227–1233.

21 Galinsky, R., Polglase, G.R., Hooper, S.B. et al. (2013). The consequences of chorioamnionitis: preterm birth and effects on development. *J. Pregnancy* 2013: 412831.

22 Van Well, G.T.J., Daalderop, L.A., Wolfs, T. et al. (2017). Human perinatal immunity in physiological conditions and during infection. *Mol. Cell Pediatr.* 4: 4.

23 Westover, A.J. and Moss, T.J.M. (2012). Effects of intrauterine infection or inflammation on fetal lung development. *Clin. Exp. Pharmacol. Physiol.* 39: 824–830.

24 Goldenberg, R.L., Haugh, J.C., and Andrews, W.W. (2000). Intrauterine infection and preterm delivery. *N. Engl. J. Med.* 342: 1500–1507.

25 Yoon, B.H., Romero, R., Jun, J.K. et al. (1998). An increase in fetal plasma cortisol but not dehydroepiandresterone sulfate is followed by the onset of preterm labor in patients with preterm premature rupture of the membranes. *Am. J. Obstet. Gynecol.* 179: 1107–1114.

26 Thomas, W. and Speer, C.P. (2011). Chorioamnionitis: important risk factor or innocent bystander for neonatal outcome? *Neonatology* 99: 177–187.

27 Moss, T.J.M., Nitsos, I., Ikegami, M. et al. (2005). Experimental intrauterine ureaplasma infection in sheep. *Am. J. Obstet. Gynecol.* 192: 1179–1186.

28 Sloboda, D.M., Challis, J.R.G., Moss, T.J.M. et al. (2005). Synthetic glucocorticoids. Antenatal administration and long-term implications. *Curr. Pharm. Des.* 11: 1459–1472.

29 Goldenberg, R.L., Andrews, W.W., Soepfert, A.R. et al. (2008). The Alabama preterm birth study umbilical cord blood ureaplasma urealyticum and Mycoplasma hominis cultures in preterm newborn infants. *Am. J. Obstet. Gynecol.* 198: e1–e5.

30 Khwaha, O. and Volpe, J.J. (2008). Pathogenesis of cerebral white matter injury of prematurity. *Arch. Dis. Fetal Neonatal Educ.* 93: F153–F161.

31 Leviton, A., Paneth, N., Reuss, M.L. et al. (1999). Maternal infection, fetal inflammatory response, and brain damage in very low birth weight infants. *Pediatr. Res.* 46: 566–575.

32 Wong, D.M., Wilkins, P.A., Bain, F.T. et al. (2011). Neonatal encephalopathy in foals. *Compend. Contin. Educ. Vet.* 33: E1–E10.

33 Yan, X., Managlia, E., Tan, X.D. et al. (2019). Prenatal inflammation impairs intestinal microvascular development through a TNF-dependent mechanism and predisposes newborn mice to necrotizing enterocolitis. *Am. J. Physiol. Gastrointest. Liver Physiol.* 317: G57–G66.

34 Lee, J. and Dammann, O. (2012). Perinatal infection, inflammation, and retinopathy or prematurity. *Semin. Fetal Neonatal Med.* 17: 26–29.

35 Castagnetti, C. and Mariella, J. (2015). Anti-inflammatory drugs in equine neonatal medicine. Part I: nonsteroidal anti-inflammatory drugs. *J. Equine Vet. Sci.* 35: 475–480.

36 Goligorsky, M.S. and Sun, D. (2020). Glycocalyx in endotoxemia and sepsis. *Am. J. Pathol.* 190: 791–798.

37 Palmer, J.E. (2004). Fluid therapy in the neonate: not your mother's fluid space. *Vet. Clin. Equine* 20: 63–75.

38 Skorup, P., Maudsdotter, L., Tano, E. et al. (2018). Dynamics of endotoxin, inflammatory variables, and organ dysfunction after treatment with antibiotics in an *Escherichia coli* porcine intensive sepsis model. *Crit. Care Med.* 46: e634–e641.

39 Kumar, A., Safdar, N., Kethireddy, S. et al. (2010). A survival benefit of combination antibiotic therapy for serious infectious associated with sepsis and septic shock is contingent only on the risk of death: a meta-analytic/meta-regression study. *Crit. Care Med.* 38: 1651–1664.

40 Sjolin, J., Goscinski, G., Lundholm, M. et al. (2000). Endotoxin release from *Escherichia coli* after exposure to

tobramycin: dose-dependency and reduction of cefuroxime-induced endotoxin release. *Clin. Microbiol. Infect.* 6: 74–81.

41 Goscinski, G., Lundholm, M., Odenholt, I. et al. (2003). Variation in the propensity to release endotoxin after cefuroxime exposure in different Gram-negative bacteria: uniform and dose-dependent reduction by the addition of tobramycin. *Scand. J. Infect. Dis.* 35: 40–46.

42 Atherton, R.P. and Furr, M. (2006). Endotoxin release after antimicrobial treatment in sick foals is mediated by antimicrobial class. *J. Equine Vet. Sci.* 26: 356–363.

43 Artenstein, A.W. and Cross, A.S. (1989). Inhibition of endotoxin reactivity by aminoglycosides. *J. Antimicrob. Chemother.* 24: 826–828.

44 Prins, J.M., Kuijper, E.J., Mevissen, M.L. et al. (1995). Release of tumor necrosis factor alpha and interleukin 6 during antibiotic killing of *Escherichia coli* in whole blood: influence of antibiotic class, antibiotic concentration, and presence of septic serum. *Infect. Immun.* 63: 2236–2242.

45 Kusser, W.C. and Ishiguro, E.E. (1989). Effects of aminoglycosides and spectinomycin on the synthesis and release of lipopolysaccharide by *Escherichia coli*. *J. Antimicrob. Chemother.* 24: 826–828.

46 Hanna, V.S. and Hafez, E.A.A. (2018). Synopsis of arachidonic acid metabolism: a review. *J. Adv. Res.* 11: 23–32.

47 Heymann, M.A. (1999). Control of the pulmonary circulation in the fetus and during the transitional period to air breathing. *Eur. J. Obstet. Gynecol.* 84: 127–132.

48 Semrad, S.D., Sams, R.A., and Ashcraft, S.M. (1993). Pharmacokinetics of and serum thromboxane suppression by flunixin meglumine in healthy foals during the first month of life. *Am. J. Vet. Res.* 54: 2083–2087.

49 Wilcke, J.R., Crisman, M.V., Sams, R.A. et al. (1993). Pharmacokinetics of phenylbutazone in neonatal foals. *Am. J. Vet. Res.* 54: 2064–2067.

50 Wilke, J.R., Crisman, M.V., Scarratt, W.K. et al. (1998). Pharmacokinetics of ketoprofen in healthy foals less than twenty-four hours old. *Am. J. Vet. Res.* 59: 290–292.

51 Crisman, M.V., Wilcke, J.R., and Sams, R.A. (1996). Pharmacokinetics of flunixin meglumine in healthy foals less than twenty-four hours old. *Am. J. Vet. Res.* 57: 1759–1761.

52 Carrick, J.B., Papich, M.G., Middleton, D.M. et al. (1989). Clinical and pathological effects of flunixin meglumine administration to neonatal foals. *Can. J. Vet. Res.* 53: 195–201.

53 Crisman, M.V., Wilcke, J.R., Sams, R.A. et al. (1991). Concentrations of phenylbutazone and oxyphenbutazone in post-parturient mares and their neonatal foals. *J. Vet. Pharmacol. Ther.* 13: 330–334.

54 Raidal, S.L., Edwards, S., Pippia, J. et al. (2013). Pharmacokinetics and safety of oral administration of meloxicam to foals. *J. Vet. Intern. Med.* 27: 300–307.

55 Kvaternick, V., Pollmeier, M., Fischer, J. et al. (2007). Pharmacokinetics and metabolism of orally administered firocoxib, a novel second generation coxib, in horses. *J. Vet. Pharmacol. Ther.* 30: 208–217.

56 Breuhaus, B.A., DeGraves, F.J., Honore, E.K. et al. (1999). Pharmacokinetics of ibuprofen after intravenous and oral administration and assessment of safety of administration in healthy foals. *Am. J. Vet. Res.* 60: 1066–1073.

57 Spier, S.J., Lavoie, J.P., Cullor, J.S. et al. (1989). Protection against clinical endotoxemia in horses by using plasma containing antibody to an Rc mutant *E. coli* (J5). *Circ. Shock.* 28: 235–248.

58 Forbes, G., Church, S., Savage, C.J. et al. (2012). Effects of hyperimmune equine plasma on clinical and cellular responses in a low-dose endotoxaemia model in horses. *Res. Vet. Sci.* 92: 40–44.

59 Gaffin, S.L. and Wells, M.T. (1987). A morphological study of the action of equine anti-lipopolysaccharide plasma on Gram-negative bacteria. *J. Med. Mircobiol.* 24: 165–168.

60 Morris, D.D. and Whitlock, R.H. (1987). Therapy of suspected septicemia in neonatal foals using plasma containing antibodies to core lipopolysaccharide (LPS). *J. Vet. Intern. Med.* 1: 175–182.

61 Alejandria, M.M., Lansand, M.A., Dans, L.F. et al. (2013). Intravenous immunoglobulin for treating sepsis, severe sepsis and septic shock. *Cochrane Database Syst. Rev.* (16): CD001090. https://doi.org/10.1002/14651858.CD001090.pub2.

62 Heming, N., Lamothe, L., Ambrosi, Z. et al. (2016). Emerging drugs for the treatment of sepsis. *Expert Opin. Emerging Drugs* 21: 27–37.

63 Morresey, P.R. and Mackay, R.J. (2006). Endotoxin-neutralizing activity of polymyxin B in the blood after IV administration in horses. *Am. J. Vet. Res.* 67: 642–647.

64 Parviainen, A., Barton, M.H., and Norton, N.N. (2001). Evaluation of polymyxin B in an ex vivo model of endotoxemia. *Am. J. Vet. Res.* 62: 72–76.

65 Liska, D.A., Akucewich, L.H., Marsella, R. et al. (2006). Pharmacokinetics of pentoxifylline and its 5-hydroxyhexyhl metabolite after oral and intravenous administration of pentoxifylline to healthy adult horses. *Am. J. Vet. Res.* 67: 1621–1627.

66 Ollivett, T.L., Divers, T.J., Cushing, T. et al. (2012). Acute pancreatitis in two five-day-old Appaloosa foals. *Equine Vet. J.* 44 (Suppl 41): 96–99.

67 Sanchez, L.C. (2005). Equine neonatal sepsis. *Vet. Clin. Equine* 21: 273–293.

68 Magdesian, K.G. (2015). Foals are not just mini horses. In: *Equine Pharmacology* (ed. C. Cole, B. Bentz, and L. Maxwell), 99–117. Wiley Blackwell.

69 Pammi, M. and Haque, K.N. (2015). Pentoxifylline for treatment of sepsis and necrotizing enterocolitis in neonates. *Cocrhane Database Syst. Rev.* (3): CD004205. https://doi.org/10.1002/14651858.CD004205.pub3.

70 Barton, M.H. and Moore, J.N. (1994). Pentoxifylline inhibits mediator synthesis in an equine in vitro whole blood model of endotoxemia. *Circ. Shock.* 44: 216–220.

71 Barton, M.H., Moore, J.N., and Norton, N. (1997). Effects of pentoxifylline infusion on response of horses to in vivo challenge exposure with endotoxin. *Am. J. Vet. Res.* 58: 1300–1307.

72 Peiro, J.R., Barnabe, P.A., Daioli, F.A. et al. (2010). Effects of lidocaine infusion during experimental endotoxemia in horses. *J. Vet. Intern. Med.* 24: 940–948.

73 Malone, E., Ensink, J., Turner, T. et al. (2006). Intravenous continuous infusion of lidocaine for treatment of equine ileus. *Vet. Surg.* 35: 60–66.

74 Kelmer, G., Doherty, T.J., Elliot, S. et al. (2008). Evaluation of dimethyl sulphoxide effects on initial response to endotoxin in the horse. *Equine Vet. J.* 40: 358–363.

75 Sullins, K.E., White, N.A., Lundin, C.S. et al. (2004). Prevention of ischaemia-induced small intestinal adhesions in foals. *Equine Vet. J.* 36: 370–375.

76 Schleining, J.A. and Reinertson, E.L. (2007). Evidence for dimethyl sulphoxide (DMSO) use in horses. Part 2: DMSO as a parenteral anti-inflammatory agent and as a pharmacological carrier. *Equine Vet. Educ.* 19: 598–599.

77 Frauenfelder, H.C., Fessler, J.F., Moore, A.B. et al. (1982). Effects of dexamethasone on endotoxin shock in the anesthetized pony: hematologic, blood gas and coagulation changes. *Am. J. Vet. Res.* 43: 405–411.

78 Hart, K.A. and Barton, M.H. (2011). Adrenocortical insufficiency in horses and foals. *Vet. Clin. North Am. Equine Pract.* 27: 19–34.

79 Gold, J.R., Divers, T.J., Barton, M.H. et al. (2007). Plasma adrenocorticotropin, cortisol, and adrenocorticotropin/cortisol ratios in septic and normal-term foals. *J. Vet. Intern. Med.* 21: 791–796.

80 Couetil, L. and Hoffman, A. (1998). Adrenal insufficiency in a neonatal foal. *J. Am. Vet. Med. Assoc.* 212: 1594–1596.

81 Hart, K.A., Barton, M.H., Vandenplas, M.L. et al. (2011). Effects of low-dose hydrocortisone therapy on immune function in neonatal horses. *Pediatr. Res.* 70: 72–77.

82 Wong, D.M., Vo, D.T., Alcott, C.J. et al. (2009). Baseline plasma cortisol and ACTH concentrations and response to low-dose ACTH stimulation testing in ill foals. *J. Am. Vet. Med. Assoc.* 234: 126–132.

83 Weiss, S.L., Alhazzani, W., Flori, H.R. et al. (2020). Surviving sepsis campaign international guidelines for the management of septic shock and sepsis-associated organ dysfunction in children. *Crit. Care Med.* 21: e52–e106.

84 Coimbra, R., Melbostad, H., Loomis, W. et al. (2005). Phosphodiesterase inhibition decreases nuclear factor-kappa B activation and shifts the cytokine response toward anti-inflammatory activity in acute endotoxemia. *J. Trauma* 59: 575–582.

85 Alcott, C.J., Sponseller, B.A., Wong, D.M. et al. (2011). Clinical and immunomodulating effects of ketamine in horses with experimental endotoxemia. *J. Vet. Intern. Med.* 25: 934–943.

86 Tanighuchi, T., Takemoto, Y., Kanakura, H. et al. (2003). The dose-related effects of ketamine on mortality and cytokine responses to endotoxin-induced shock in rats. *Anesth. Analg.* 97: 1769–1772.

87 Lankveld, D.P.K., Bull, S., Van Dijk, P. et al. (2005). Ketamine inhibits LPS-induced tumor necrosis factor-alpha and interleukin-6 in an equine macrophage cell line. *Vet. Res.* 36: 257–262.

88 Winchell, W.W., Hardy, J., Levine, D.M. et al. (2002). Effect of administration of a phospholipid emulsion on the initial response of horses administered endotoxin. *Am. J. Vet. Res.* 63: 1370–1378.

89 Moore, J.N., Norton, N., Barton, M.H. et al. (2007). Rapid infusion of a phospholipid emulsion attenuates the effects of endotoxaemia in horses. *Equine Vet. J.* 39: 243–248.

90 Rossignol, D.P. and Lynn, M. (2002). Antagonism of in vivo and ex vivo response to endotoxin by E5564, a synthetic lipid A analogue. *J. Endotoxin Res.* 8: 483–488.

91 Figueiredo, M.D., Moore, J.N., Vandenplas, M.L. et al. (2008). Effects of the second-generation synthetic lipid A analogue E5564 on responses to endotoxin in equine whole blood and monocytes. *Am. J. Vet. Res.* 69: 796–803.

92 Barton, M.H., Bruce, E.H., Moore, J.N. et al. (1998). Effect of tumor necrosis factor antibody given to horses during early experimentally induced endotoxemia. *Am. J. Vet. Res.* 59: 792–797.

93 Cargile, J.L., MacKay, R.J., Dankert, J.R. et al. (1995). Effect of treatment with a monoclonal antibody against equine tumor necrosis factor (TNF) on clinical, hematologic, and circulating TNF responses of miniature horses given endotoxin. *Am. J. Vet. Res.* 56: 1451–1459.

94 MacDonald, E.S. and Barrett, J.G. (2020). The potential of mesenchymal stem cells to treat systemic inflammation in horses. *Front. Vet. Sci.* 6: 507.

95 Peroni, J.F. and Borjesson, D.L. (2011). Anti-inflammatory and immunomodulatory activities of stem cells. *Vet. Clin. North Am. Equine Pract.* 27: 351–362.

96 Mei, S.H., Haitsma, J.J., Dos Santos, C.C. et al. (2010). Mesenchymal stem cells reduce inflammation while enhancing bacterial clearance and improving survival in sepsis. *Am. J. Respir. Crit. Care Med.* 182: 1047–1057.
97 Gonzalez-Rey, E., Anderson, P., Gonzalez, M.A. et al. (2009). Human adult stem cells derived from adipose tissue protect against experimental colitis and sepsis. *Gut* 58: 929–939.
98 Jacobs, C.C., Holcombe, S.J., Cook, V.L. et al. (2013). Ethyl pyruvate diminishes the inflammatory response to lipopolysaccharide infusion in horses. *Equine Vet. J.* 45: 333–339.
99 Bauquier, J.R., Tudor, E., and Bailey, S.R. (2014). Anti-inflammatory effects of four potential anti-endotoxaemic drugs assessed in vitro using equine whole blood assays. *J. Vet. Pharmacol. Ther.* 38: 290–296.
100 Longworth, K.E., Smith, B.L., Staub, N.C. et al. (1996). Use of a detergent to prevent initial responses to endotoxin in horses. *Am. J. Vet. Res.* 57: 1063–1066.

Chapter 16 Congenital Disorders of the Equine Gastrointestinal Tract

Kate L. Hepworth-Warren

Introduction

Congenital anomalies of the equine gastrointestinal (GI) tract are very rare clinical findings. Of the reported congenital abnormalities that involve the oral pharynx, GI tract, or hepatobiliary systems, umbilical hernias have been reported the most frequently and are the second most common congenital defect in foals overall [1]. The prevalence of many of the other anomalies described in this chapter is unknown, as many have only been documented via sporadic case reports. Many of the defects affecting the GI tract can lead to abdominal pain, but others have been identified either on postmortem examination or during exploratory celiotomy as incidental findings. Certain conditions are seen with much higher frequency in certain breeds, such as esophageal ectasia/megaesophagus in Friesians and overo lethal white foal syndrome (ileocolonic aganglionosis) in Paint Horses [2, 3]. Other conditions have been reported only once or twice and the true prevalence is unknown. While many of these abnormalities are infrequently encountered, they should be considered when examining neonatal foals, especially foals that exhibit signs of colic. The table below reviews some of the congenital gastrointestinal conditions in foals and affected breeds.

Condition	Affected breed/ prevalence	Description
Oral/dental conditions		
Cleft palate	Cleft palate is the most common craniofacial defect in horses. It was identified in 4% of a group of 608 congenitally deformed foals, and other studies have identified similar prevalence – ranging from 1% to 4% [2, 4]. In one study, Quarter Horses were the most represented breed, but the proportion of horses with cleft palates was not significantly different than the proportion of this breed admitted to the hospital [4].	Cleft palate (Figure 16.1) results from a failure of the palate to fuse around day 47 of gestation. Most cleft palates occur in the caudal half or two-thirds of the soft palate. Causes are ill defined, but could be genetic or environmental factors, maternal drug administration, vitamin and mineral deficiencies, and toxic plants. Clinical signs are usually associated with dysphagia. Coughing is observed and milk is present at the nares shortly after nursing. Foals often develop secondary aspiration pneumonia. Definitive diagnosis requires endoscopic examination of the pharynx as many defects are located too far caudally to be reached by digital palpation. Surgical repair is difficult, but has been performed successfully in smaller defects (typically those that involve ≤20% of the soft palate) [2, 4, 5].

(*Continued*)

Equine Neonatal Medicine, First Edition. Edited by David M. Wong and Pamela A. Wilkins.

Condition	Affected breed/ prevalence	Description
Cleft palate continued...		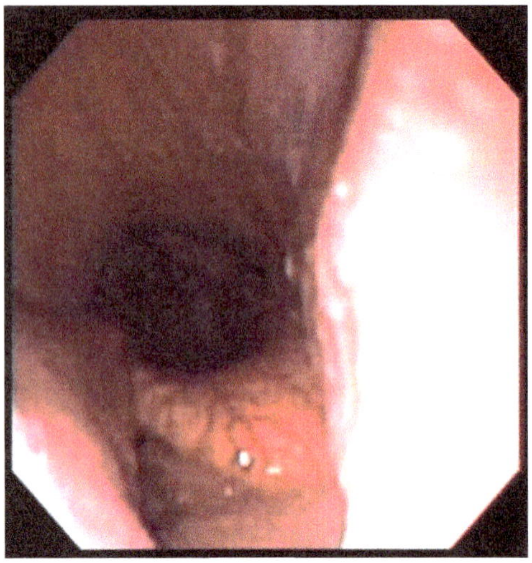 **Figure 16.1** Congenital cleft palate in a newborn foal.
Bifid tongue with mandibular cleft	This defect is very rare in nonequid species and has only been reported in 3 mule foals and a donkey foal, never in horses [6].	Bifid tongue also known as glossoschisis, cleft or snake tongue, is an abnormality that leads to a longitudinal fissure at the tip of the tongue extending caudally (Figure 16.2). It develops when the growth of the lateral lingual structures that serve to cover the tuberculum impar is interrupted [8]. Clinical signs include difficult or complete inability to suckle. Bifid tongue was present in one mule foal in conjunction with a mandibular cleft, where the two sides of the mandible failed to fuse. In two other mule foals, a mandibular cleft alone was identified. Surgical correction was attempted in two of the three cases to repair the mandibular cleft and was successful up to 15 d post-surgery in one foal when it was lost to follow-up. The other foal died on the fifth day after surgery and the third did not receive treatment [6–8]. 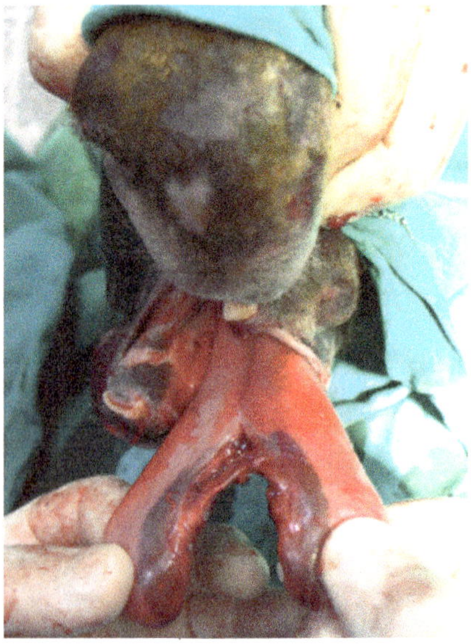 **Figure 16.2** Preoperative frontal view of the glossoshisis. Aksoy et al. [7].

Condition	Affected breed/ prevalence	Description
Cheiloschisis (hare lip)	There are few reports in horses without associated palatal abnormalities, but it has been documented in one donkey foal and two horse foals [9].	Cause of the lesion is unknown. It is visible on physical examination and can be associated with other congenital deformities such as cleft palates, thus endoscopy is generally warranted (Figure 16.3). Another foal was reported at 2d of age, and surgical correction was performed. The foal did well immediately postoperatively but was found dead 15d later [7, 9]. 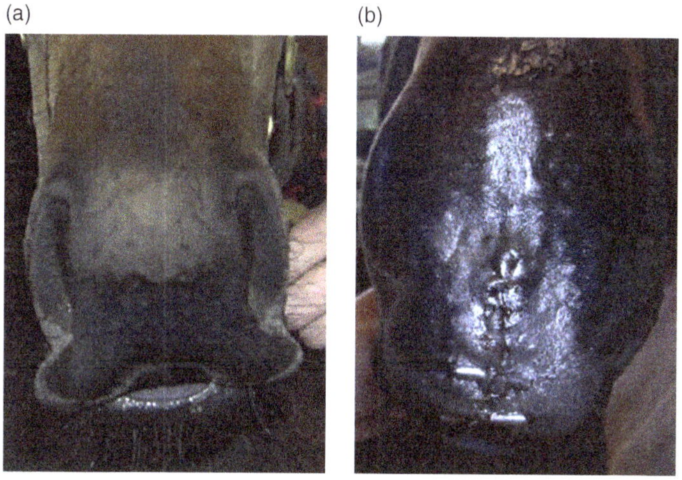 **Figure 16.3** Cheiloschisis in a horse before (a) and after (b) surgical correction. Watkins et al. [9].
Persistent lingual frenulum	Unknown	Persistent lingual frenula often present with other craniofacial deformities. The primary clinical sign is difficulty suckling [7]. Surgical correction is a relatively straightforward procedure.
Congenital Glossocheilognath-ochisis	There is one report in the literature a 2-day-old mixed-breed filly [7].	Congenital glossocheilognathoschisis (Figure 16.4) is a congenital midline cleft of the lower lip, mandible, and tongue combined with bilateral persistent frenula lingua. In the one reported case, physical examination and radiographs confirmed the diagnosis. Surgical correction was performed and foal did well immediately postoperatively, but died 14d later [7]. 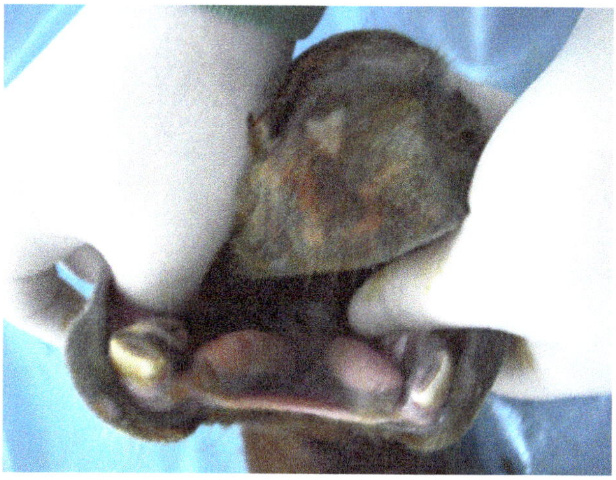 **Figure 16.4** Glossocheilognathoschisis in a 2-day-old colt. Aksoy et al. [7].

(Continued)

Condition	Affected breed/ prevalence	Description
Brachygnathia (parrot mouth)	The exact prevalence is unknown, although it is considered to be a rare anomaly. Anecdotally, it may be more common in Quarter Horses [10].	Brachygnathia (Figure 16.5) is an abnormal shortness of the jaw, wherein the mandible appears shorter than the maxilla – thus creating an "undershot" jaw with no occlusal contact between the upper and lower incisors [10]. Generally considered a congenital condition but can also be acquired while a foal is growing. Diagnosis is via physical examination and radiographs. Surgical treatment to correct the defect has been performed [10]. 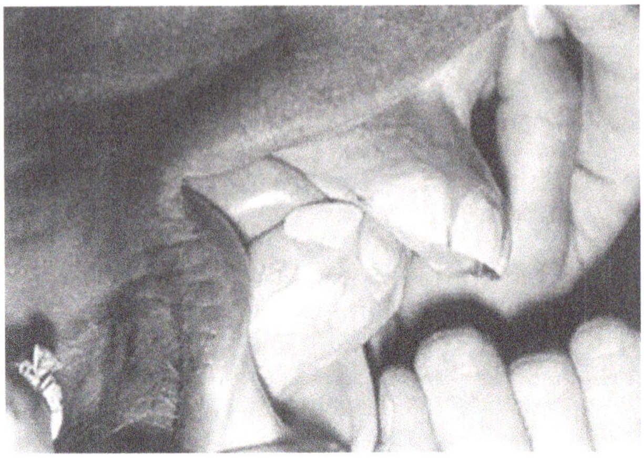 **Figure 16.5** Brachygnathia in a horse. Debowes [10].
Odontoma	Unknown	Odontomas are congenital dental tumors. They are classified by the presence of epithelial or mesenchymal cells and the degree of differentiation. Complex odontomas have been reported in young horses and contain the components of a tooth, but in a disorganized structure. Lesions usually present as firm nonpainful swellings and diagnosis is confirmed by radiographs. Treatment involves surgical removal of mass [10, 11].
Prognathia (sow mouth)	Prognathia is rare, but is most commonly in Miniature Horses and ponies. The exact prevalence unknown [10].	Prognathia is also called sow mouth or monkey mouth, where the mandible appears longer than the maxilla. Surgical correction can be performed by application of a mandibular tension band. The condition can be hereditary, so affected animals should not be used for breeding [10].
Persistent frenulum of the epiglottis	The prevalence is unknown. Persistent epiglottic frenula have been reported in 2 Arabians, 1 Percheron, and 1 Shire [12].	A persistent epiglottic frenulum (Figure 16.6) is a restrictive band of tissue connecting the ventral portion of the epiglottis and the base of the tongue. The frenulum leads to dorsal displacement of the soft palate and dysphagia. In a report of four foals, all presented for examination at 1–4 d of age with a history of respiratory stress and milk being seen either coming from the nose or mouth after nursing. Diagnosis can be confirmed via upper airway endoscopy. Successful surgical correction was performed in all four foals, three of which were reportedly normal 2–4 yr after surgery. The fourth died soon after discharge, likely as a consequence of poor husbandry on the farm [12].

Condition	Affected breed/ prevalence	Description
Persistent frenulum of the epiglottis continued...		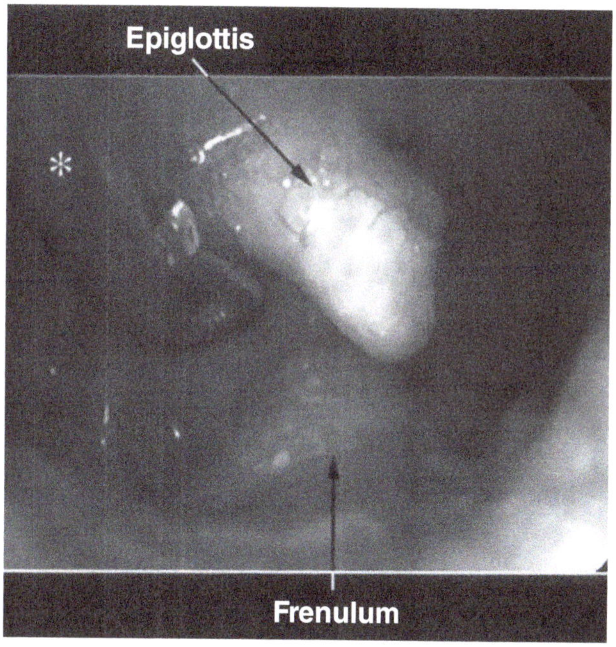 Figure 16.6 Oral endoscopic view of a foal with persistent frenulum. The epiglottis is being elevated with a blunt probe (asterisk). Yarbough et al. [12].
Esophagus		
Esophageal ectasia/ Megaesophagus	Friesians are thought to be predisposed to megaesophagus, although exact prevalence is unknown. The condition has also been reported in Arabians, Akhal Tekes, Thoroughbreds, Appaloosas, Warmbloods, and Quarter Horses [2, 13–17].	Ectasia is the dilation or expansion of a hollow tube, and is a synonym for megaesophagus [2, 13]. Congenital megaesophagus has been described in association with persistent right aortic arch, esophageal stricture, and aganglionosis [2, 13, 18]. Clinical signs are similar to those seen with cleft palate, where milk is visible at the nares after nursing. However, it was suggested in one report that there may be a delay in the accumulation of milk at the nares and it may occur as a result of low head positioning in ectasia as compared to a cleft palate. Foals may also have secondary aspiration pneumonia. Diagnosis is via physical examination, esophagoscopy, and contrast radiography. The cause is unknown, but in one report it appeared to resolve spontaneously with age [14, 16, 17].
Esophageal cyst/ duplication cyst/ intramural inclusion cyst	Unknown	Esophageal cysts are a type of congenital foregut malformation that results from a defect in the budding or division of the primitive foregut. They typically occur in close association with the respiratory or gastrointestinal tract, but can also be found in the mediastinum, retroperitoneum, or inside other organs [19]. They are defined as esophageal by the components of the cyst wall- namely the lining epithelium, the glands and muscular layer [19–23].

(Continued)

Condition	Affected breed/ prevalence	Description
Esophageal stricture, stenosis (secondary to persistent right aortic arch), diverticula	Unknown. Stricture has been reported in Thoroughbreds, Appaloosas, Haflingers, and ponies [13, 15, 24, 25].	Esophageal strictures and stenosis can occur as a primary defect, or secondary to vascular ring abnormalities that entrap the esophagus. The most commonly reported vascular abnormality associated with esophageal stricture/stenosis is a persistent right aortic arch (Figure 16.7). Clinical signs are noted shortly after birth and involve milk coming from the nose and mouth after nursing. Esophageal stricture has also been reported in concert with megaesophagus cranial to the stricture. Diagnosis of a congenital defect is usually made when signs are noted shortly after birth, although acquired strictures/stenosis cannot be ruled out. Diagnosis is made via esophagoscopy and contrast radiography. Surgical correction, either by removal of vascular abnormalities or balloon dilation of a primary esophageal stricture, have been performed successful [15, 24–29].

(a) (b)

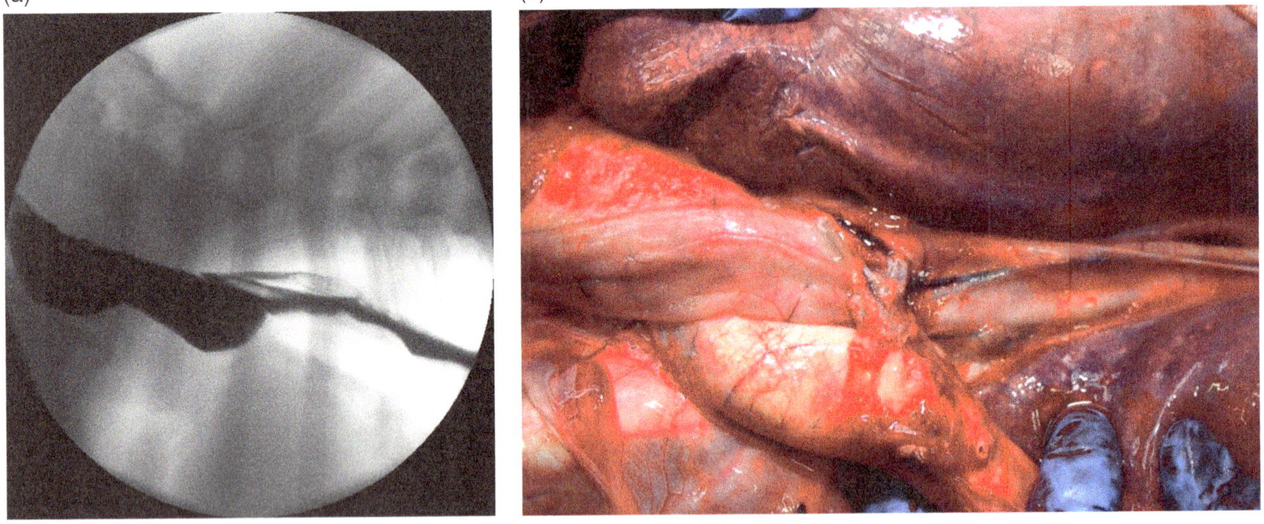

Figure 16.7 Fluoroscopic image depicting pooling of contrast material within the esophagus (a) secondary to a persistent right aortic arch (b) in a neonatal foal. *Source:* Images courtesy of Dr. Edwina Wilkes, Charles Sturt University.

Hernias: diaphragmatic, umbilical, or inguinal	Umbilical hernias are the second most common congenital defect in horses. They are more common in females [1]. Inguinal and scrotal hernias are reported more frequently in Standardbreds and Tennessee Walking Horses, whereas umbilical hernias are more common in Quarter Horses and Thoroughbreds [1].	Umbilical, inguinal, scrotal, and diaphragmatic hernias have been described as congenital defects in foals [1, 30–33]. Congenital diaphragmatic hernias occur due to failure of fusion of the diaphragm during development, from intrauterine rupture, or rupture during parturition. Rib fractures are commonly associated with diaphragmatic hernias that occur during parturition. The left dorsal tendinous region of the diaphragm is the most commonly affected in congenital hernias, although Morgagni hernias, which affect the right retrosternal portion of the diaphragm, have also been reported in horses [30–33]. This opening then allows for abdominal organs to move into the thoracic cavity. In three horses with Morgagni hernias, the large colon became incarcerated in the hernia. Foals with diaphragmatic hernias typically present with acute colic and evidence of respiratory distress. Diagnosis can be difficult but is achieved with ultrasound and radiography. Surgical correction for the more common type of diaphragmatic hernias has been attempted, but outcome is poor. Two of the three horses with Morgagni hernias had successful surgical hernia repairs and the third was managed with conservative management [33].

Condition	Affected breed/ prevalence	Description
Hernias: diaphragmatic, umbilical, or inguinal continued...		Inguinal and scrotal hernias are often visible shortly after birth and present as a fluctuant swelling. They are generally reducible when the foal is moved into dorsal recumbency, but intestine can be incarcerated and repair of the hernia should be performed. A variety of techniques for surgical correction have been described. Umbilical hernias are relatively common, and smaller lesions can resolve spontaneously. Intestine can become strangulated in the lesion, and should be suspected in patients presenting with colic that also have a nonreducible umbilical hernia that may be warm, painful, firm, or swollen [1]. Diagnosis is by manual palpation and ultrasound of the hernia sac. Prognosis following surgical reduction is good [1].
Gastrointestinal nonrotation	There is only one reported case in the literature involving a Welsh-Thoroughbred foal [34].	Gastrointestinal nonrotation occurs during the first stage of gestation, where the intestine only rotates 180° instead of 270°. This results in a "left-sided colon" as the colon stays on the left side of the abdomen and the small intestine is on the right side after development is finished. The only reported case was a 24-hr-old foal that was presented for evaluation and repair of a body wall hernia that had acute colic. The abnormality in the GI tract was identified during emergency exploratory celiotomy. In addition to the malpositioning of the GI tract, there was a large segment of diluted jejunum that was resected during surgery. The foal refluxed for 5 d postoperatively, but was reportedly doing well at 15 mo of age [34].
Stomach		
Gastric hypoplasia	This has been reported in one Thoroughbred filly [35].	A severely hypoplastic stomach was identified at necropsy in a Thoroughbred filly. The filly presented at 2 d of age for weakness and dehydration. It improved with intravenous fluids, but milk was noted streaming from its mouth when it suckled. Nasogastric intubation was difficult and the tube could not be passed to a normal extent. The foal failed to improve and was euthanized. At necropsy, the stomach measured 95 mm long and 55 mm wide [35].
Pyloric stenosis	Congenital pyloric stenosis has been reported in Thoroughbreds, and an Italian Saddle Horse [36, 37].	While acquired pyloric stenosis has been reported in foals secondary to gastric ulceration and gastritis, congenital stenosis is rarely reported [36]. In the first report, a Thoroughbred filly was presented for evaluation of colic at 2 mo age. Signs had first developed at 6 wk of age, when the filly began eating solid feed. Exploratory celiotomy identified pyloric stenosis with a nearly empty intestinal tract. Pyloroplasty was performed and the filly was reportedly doing well 6 mo after surgery. While not utilized in this report, the use of abdominal radiography and endoscopy were discussed. Another group has utilized computed tomography to diagnose pyloric stenosis in two foals [36, 37].
Small intestine		
Meckel diverticulum	A postmortem study of 15,000 horses identified Meckel's diverticulum in five horses; the population was mostly Thoroughbreds, so prevalence may be different in other breeds. The anomaly has been reported in Quarter Horses, Standardbreds, Tennessee Walking Horses, pit ponies, Highland ponies, and Icelandic ponies [34, 38, 39].	Meckel's diverticulum is an embryological remnant of the omphalomesenteric duct that forms near the distal portion of the jejunum or proximal jejunum. The diverticulum is a blind extension of the affected portion of small intestine that may also have a fibrous attachment to the umbilicus (vitello-umbilical band) [32, 40]. The presence of the diverticulum can lead to signs of colic, and the diverticulum is typically found either during exploratory laparotomy or postmortem examination [32, 34, 38]. The presence of the diverticulum can lead to strangulation of small intestine when there is also a mesodiverticular band or vitelloumbilical band present, although strangulation has been reported in their absence in two horses [39].

(*Continued*)

Condition	Affected breed/ prevalence	Description
Intestinal polyp	Congenital intestinal polyps have only been reported in a Trakehner foal and a Thoroughbred foal, with the latter being identified in the small colon [41, 42].	Polyps have been identified in both the small and large intestine in foals and have been associated with signs of colic (Figure 16.8). In one case, intestinal polyps were identified on postmortem examination in the jejunum of a foal that also developed a secondary intussusception. Euthanasia was elected due to the severity of colic signs and client's declination of surgery [41]. In another foal, a polyp obstructing the small colon, with secondary rupture of the small colon was identified during exploratory celiotomy. That foal was euthanized intra-operatively [42]. Intestinal polyps have been reported in older horses that led to weight loss and recurrent colic, but it is unclear if they were congenital [43, 44]. 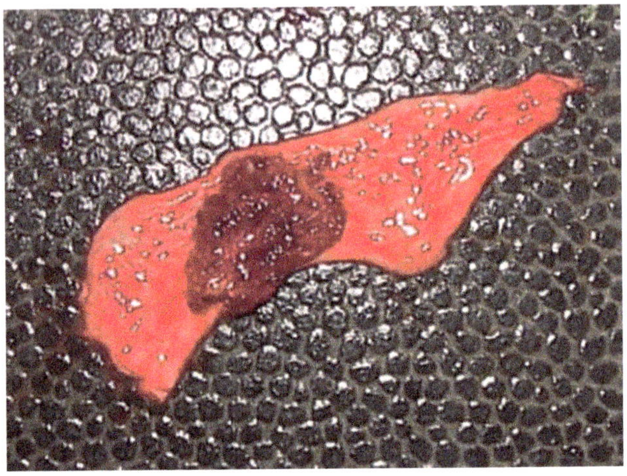 **Figure 16.8** Hyperplastic poly from a 3-day-old Trakehner-cross foal. A dark red pedunculated filamentous mass (5 × 15 × 5 mm) was identified on the mucosa at the leading edge of the intussusceptum. Gold et al. [41].
Mesenteric attachment defects	True prevalence is unknown as some lesions may not cause clinical signs, and thus go unidentified. Any breed can be affected; some in which defects have been reported include Friesians, Quarter Horses, Warmbloods, and Arabians [45–49].	Mesenteric attachment defects are among the most common congenital abnormalities of the equine gastrointestinal tract (Figure 16.9). Of these, mesodiverticular bands are the most common and are typically identified either during exploratory celiotomy or necropsy following an episode of colic [49]. Occasionally, they are identified as incidental findings [49]. Mesodiverticular bands are remnants of the vitelline duct that can cause obstruction or strangulation of small intestine through a tear in the band, or a small intestinal volvulus at the site of the band [47, 49]. Mesenteric attachment abnormalities often lead to signs of colic, but signs may not always present at a young age [49–51]. While abnormalities are more commonly identified in foals, they have also been diagnosed in older animals with history ranging from chronic recurrent colic with unthriftiness, to no previous episode of abdominal pain [32, 45–50]. Other mesenteric attachment abnormalities have sporadically been reported that have been associated with both the small intestine and large colon [32]. Reported abnormalities include an absent retroperitoneal attachment to the cecum and large colon, a mesenteric band attached to the ileocecal fold, and abnormal length of the ceco-colic ligament, ileocecal, ascending mesocolon, and the attachment of the right dorsal colon to the cecum [46–48].

Condition	Affected breed/ prevalence	Description
Mesenteric attachment defects continued...		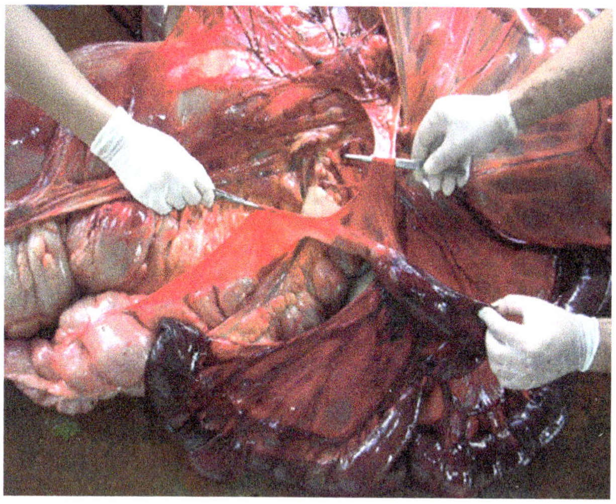 **Figure 16.9** Postmortem appearance pf an anomalous band (right forceps) attached to the root of the mesentery and to the ileocecal fold (left forceps). A space between the band and the underlying mesentery is identified (right forceps). Dearo et al. [47].
Colon		
Atresia coli	Rare anomaly of the intestinal tract. Records of 7565 foals identified only 41 cases of atresia coli in one review [52]. Older literature may have higher numbers as cases of colonic aganglionosis were historically categorized as atresia coli [52]. Atresia coli does not appear to have a sex or breed predilection [52].	Intestinal atresia is exceedingly rare, but when it occurs is most commonly identified in the colon [52, 53]. Atretic lesions of the intestine are classified as either Type 1 (membrane atresia, where a diaphragm or membrane separates the bowel lumen), Type 2 (cord atresia, where there is a thin cord of connective tissue between two segments of bowel with or without mesentery), Type 3a (blind end atresia, where there is complete separation of the two segments of bowel with no mesenteric attachment), Type 3b (similar to Type 3a, but intestinal segment distal to defect is coiled), and Type 4 (multiple types of atresia) [52, 54, 55]. Neonatal foals with atresia coli present within the first few days of life with signs of acute colic. Initially, many are presumed to have meconium impactions, but the absence of fecal staining results in additional investigation. Many foals with atresia coli have a normal anal opening, although digital palpation identifies an empty rectum [52]. Diagnostics should include abdominal radiographs, including the use of contrast, proctoscopy, abdominal ultrasound, and peritoneal fluid analysis [52, 54]. Lesions can be identified definitively during exploratory surgery or on postmortem examination, and concurrent congenital anomalies of other structures are sometimes present [32]. Successful surgical repair has been reported, but failure of the anastomosis is common [56, 57]. Prognosis is generally poor [52, 54].
Ileocolonic aganglionosis/overo lethal white foal syndrome (OLWS)	OLWS affects primarily American Paint Horses and Quarter Horses, but it has rarely been reported in Thoroughbreds. There is >94% incidence of OLWS heterozygotes in the frame overall, highly white calico overo, and frame blend overo color patterns. Many non-white animals are also heterozygotes [3, 58].	Ileocolonic aganglionosis, or overo lethal white foal syndrome (OLWS) is genetic disease that occurs due to a mutation the endothelin B receptor gene. It is analogous to Hirchsprung disease in humans. It is an autosomal recessive trait that leads to foals that are either all white or nearly all white in color (Figure 16.10) and have complete absence of myenteric and submucosal ganglia starting in the distal small intestine and going to the large colon [3, 59]. Affected foals generally show signs of colic (rolling, progressive abdominal distention, absent fecal output) within 12–24h of birth and die shortly thereafter due to an inability to move ingesta through the gastrointestinal tract [3, 59, 60]. Diagnosis is often clinical in the case of a white foal that fails to pass meconium, although additional diagnostics including abdominal radiographs, ultrasound, and contrast studies can be useful adjuncts. Genetic testing via hair samples is the only way to identify carriers [59–62]. There is no treatment available and prognosis is poor [3].

(*Continued*)

Condition	Affected breed/ prevalence	Description
Ileocolonic aganglionosis/overo lethal white foal syndrome (OLWS) continued...		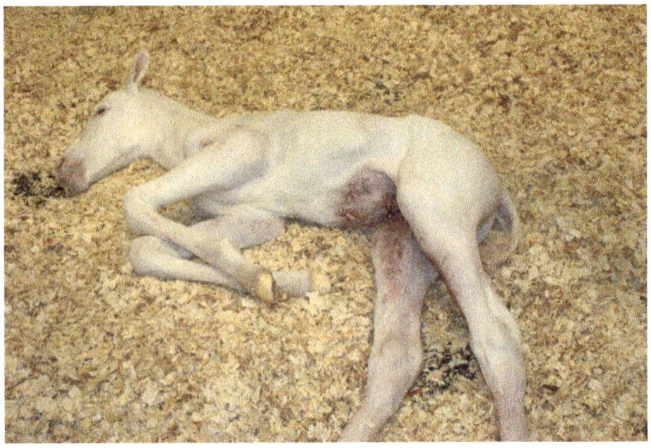 **Figure 16.10** Ileocolonic aganglionosis in a foal that demonstrated signs of colic within 24 hours of birth.
Anomalies of the ascending colon	Prevalence is unknown as there are only sporadic reports [62, 63].	In the one report, a 4-mo-old Standardbred colt was presented for evaluation of colic. Due to unrelenting pain, exploratory laparotomy was performed where the colon was noted to be abnormal. The ventral colon was present, but the pelvic flexure and dorsal colon were absent. The colt recovered uneventfully from anesthesia, and despite poor weight gain and repeated episodes of mild colic, remained otherwise healthy, and was in training 18 mo after surgery [63]. Congenital hypoplasia of the dorsal colon, that resulted in an extra flexure was reported in a Quarter Horse filly that ultimately had exploratory surgery at 17 mo of age following a history of chronic colic that began at 6 mo of age. Additional reported anomalies in the ascending colon include stellate shape, T-shaped, and an extra loop [62]. Diagnosis is typically via exploratory surgery or postmortem examination [62, 63].
Duplication cyst of the ascending colon	There is only one report in the literature, in a 27-yr-old Thoroughbred mare [64].	There has been a report of a duplication cyst within the ascending colon of an adult horse. The horse presented at 27 yr of age with signs of acute colic. The cyst was identified during exploratory celiotomy and originated from the right ventral colon, measuring 30 × 50 × 80 cm. The mass was resected and the mare recovered uneventfully and was doing well 2.5 yr after surgery. Of note is the advanced age of this horse at the time of diagnosis, and the absent history of previous episodes of colic [64].
Rectum/anus		
Atresia ani/rectal atresia	The prevalence is unknown, but both atresia recti and atresia ani are very rare anomalies. In two studies of surgical findings from 20 and 119 foals undergoing exploratory celiotomy, atresia ani was identified in 1 foal in each study [42, 65]. No specific breed predilection has been described, but donkeys as well as horses have been reported [55, 66].	Atresia ani (Figure 16.11) and recti are defects that occur due to failure of normal embryological development that leads to a lack of normal portions of the anus and rectum. Atresia ani can occur simultaneously with congenital defects of the urinary tract (i.e. hypospadias) [27, 67]. Anal atresia has a similar classification system to that for intestinal atresia described above. Type 1 is described as congenital anal stenosis. Type 2 is an imperforate anus alone. Type 3 is an imperforate anus in combination with cranial termination of the rectum as a blind pouch. Type 4 is discontinuity of the proximal rectum with normal anal and terminal rectal development [67]. Diagnosis of atresia ani is more straightforward than atresia coli and can be confirmed via digital rectal examination. Prognosis after surgical correction is good, although the anal sphincter may not have normal function [32].

Condition	Affected breed/ prevalence	Description
Atresia ani/rectal atresia continued...		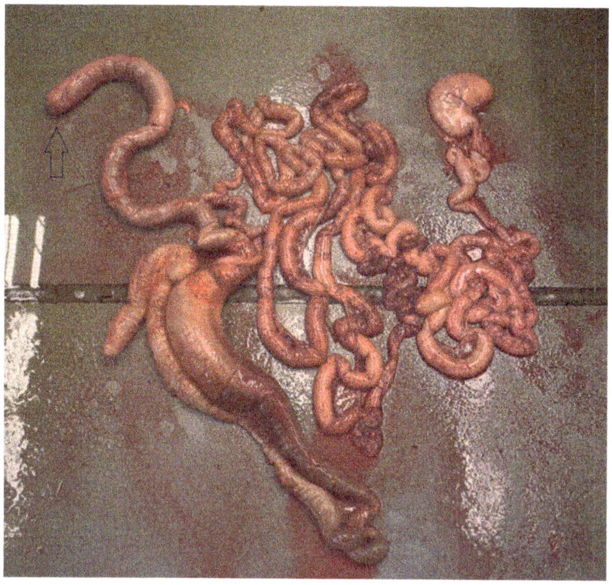 **Figure 16.11** Postmortem specimen of the gastrointestinal foal with atresia ani. Note the blind end (arrow) at the end of the intestinal tract. *Source:* Image courtesy of Dr. Rebecca Ruby, University of Kentucky.
Rectal/colonic hamartomas	Hamartomas of the rectum and colon have been reported in two Thoroughbred and one Paint foal [68–70].	Hamartomas are non-neoplastic nodules of mature cells that are frequently present at birth and grow until the host stops growing. Two cases of rectal hamartomas and one case of colonic hamartomas have been reported in foals [68–70]. Interestingly, of the three cases, the colonic hamartoma and one of the rectal hamartomas were associated with the development of secondary intussusception [68, 70]. Two of the three foals described were <24 hr of age when signs were first noted, and the third was 3 wk of age. Presenting complaints included hematochezia, tenesmus, rectal prolapse with a visible mass, and acute colic. Diagnosis was via histopathology from masses removed via either proctoscopy, exploratory laparotomy, or in one case from tissue that was sloughed naturally. Surgical resection of the mass was performed in all three cases, but only the foal that did not have a secondary intussusception survived long term [68–70].
Congenital lacteal obstruction	Congenital lacteal obstruction has been described in draft breeds, particularly Shires, but the true prevalence is unknown [27].	The lacteal system in the small intestinal mesentery is obstructed and becomes enlarged and then overflows into the peritoneal cavity after a milk meal. Affected animals may display mild signs of colic, inappetence, and abdominal distention. It is diagnosed via ultrasound and subsequent abdominocentesis where a milky white to pinkish peritoneal fluid is identified. If <25% of the jejunum is affected, it can be resected and animals can have a normal life expectancy [27].
Colt foal narrow pelvis syndrome	This defect can affect any breed, but has been reported more in Thoroughbred colts. Prevalence is unknown [27].	Colt foal narrow pelvis syndrome describes a congenital anomaly wherein foals are born with an exceptionally narrow pelvis that leads them to be more prone to developing meconium impactions. Digital rectal examination will confirm presence of meconium within the rectum, but the finger may not even pass into the rectum. A radiographic study of the pelvis using barium as contrast will confirm the narrow pelvis. Foals should be treated as a standard meconium impaction, and care should be taken not to force entry into the rectum and to ensure the meconium is liquefied to allow passage [27].

(*Continued*)

Condition	Affected breed/ prevalence	Description
Hepatobiliary		
Biliary atresia	There is only one reported case in a Guelder foal [71].	In the reported case, the foal was normal for the first 24 hr after birth. At 2 d of age, the foal had not passed normal meconium, but pale gray feces were noted. Mild signs of colic developed and a meconium impaction was diagnosed. Feces remained gray and claylike in character, and chemical analysis was performed, which identified complete absence of bile components. Serial serum biochemistry profiles documented increased activity of ALP, LDH, SDH, GGT and increased unconjugated bilirubin. The foal died at 6 d of age and postmortem examination identified both intra- and extrahepatic biliary atresia. The cause is unknown [71].
Portosystemic vascular anomalies/ shunt	Portosystemic shunts are rare anomalies in foals, the prevalence of which is unknown [72].	Portosystemic shunts (PSS) are vascular anomalies that redirect blood from the portal circulation away from the liver and back into systemic circulation. These shunts can either be congenital or acquired, and can be either intrahepatic or extrahepatic. Foals with congenital PSS begin to show signs between 2 and 6 mo of age, which may include poor growth and nonspecific neurologic signs attributable to hepatic encephalopathy (blindness, ataxia, depression) [72]. Diagnosis of PSS is supported by hyperammonemia and increased serum bile acids and has been confirmed with a multitude of advanced imaging techniques, including computed tomography angiography, mesenteric vein portography, splenic portography, transcolonic sodium pertechnetate Tc99m scintigraphy, ultrasonography, and "bubble grams" [72–74]. Surgical correction has been reported for both intra- and extrahepatic PSS in foals by either surgical ligation, transvenous coil embolization, or cellophane banding of the shunt [72].
Hyperammonemia of Morgan Horses	Congenital hyperammonemia has been reported in two related Morgan foals [75].	Congenital hyperammonemia was reported in two Morgan weanlings who shared the same sire and the dams were sisters. In both foals, clinical signs developed within a few weeks of weaning and included abnormal behavior, unthriftiness, and poor growth. The first foal was hospitalized three times over 2 mo and had marked hyperammonemia (>200 μg/ml; reference 13–108 μg/ml) each time, despite being treated with lactulose and being maintained on a low protein diet. Neurologic signs consistent with hepatic encephalopathy were noted, and the filly was ultimately euthanized. The second filly presented with profound depression, circling, and aimless walking. Marked hyperammonemia (321 μg/ml) and moderate hyperbilirubinemia were identified. Treatment was declined and the filly was euthanized. Necropsy identified nonspecific hepatic changes. In the first filly, acute changes in the liver were consistent with a toxic or infectious insult but did not correlate with the chronic history of clinical abnormalities. In the second filly, severe hepatic lipidosis and plasmacytic/lymphocytic hepatitis was identified. Because necropsy was unable to explain the severe hyperammonemia seen in either case, serum form both fillies and urine from the first were submitted for amino acid profiles that identified significantly increased glutamate and ornithine and lower arginine concentrations when compared to healthy foals. Urine from the first filly was suspected to have a peak in homocitrulline. The condition identified in these two foals was considered to likely be an inherited condition similar to hyperornithinemia-hyperammonemia-homocitrullinuria syndrome in humans that is likely caused by defective mitochondrial transporter protein that leads to interrupted synthesis of urea. In humans, clinical signs become evident shortly after weaning from breast milk and patients have histories of intermittent hyperammonemia in association with high-protein diets [75].
Congenital hyperbilirubinemia	The majority of cases of congenital hyperbilirubinemia have been in Thoroughbreds, but the prevalence is unknown [76].	Persistent hyperbilirubinemia has been identified in otherwise healthy horses that is considered to be due to a congenital deficiency in bilirubin uridine diphosphate-glucuronyl transferase activity that limits conjugation of bilirubin within the liver. Affected animals have total bilirubin values between 9 and 16 mg/dl, most of which is unconjugated. Affected animals have normal hepatic enzyme activity, normal appetite, and normal serum bile acids and were healthy with extended follow-up [76].

References

1 Bartmann, C.P., Freeman, D.E., and Glitz, G. (2002). Diagnosis and surgical management of colic in the foal: literature review and a retrospective study. *Clin. Tech. Equine Pract.* 1: 125–142.
2 Crowe, M.W. and Swerczek, T.W. (1985). Equine congenital defects. *Am. J. Vet. Res.* 46: 353–358.
3 Finno, C.J., Spier, S.J., and Valberg, S.J. (2009). Equine diseases caused by known genetic mutations. *Vet. J.* 179: 336–347.
4 Shaw, S.D., Norman, T.E., Arnold, C.E. et al. (2015). Clinical characteristics of horses and foals diagnosed with cleft palate in a referral population: 28 cases (1988–2011). *Can. Vet. J.* 56: 756–760.
5 Kirkham, L. and Vasey, J.R. (2002). Surgical cleft soft palate repair in a foal. *Aust. Vet. J.* 80: 143–146.
6 Rifai, S., Bouyad, H., Kay, G. et al. (2006). Bifid tongue and mandibular cleft in three mule foals. *Vet. Rec.* 158: 97–98.
7 Aksoy, O., Kilic, E., Kacar, C. et al. (2007). Congenital Glossocheilognathoschisis and persistent frenula linguae in a foal: a case report. *J. Equine Vet. Sci.* 27: 277–280.
8 Surej, K.L., Kurien, N.M., and Sivan, M.P. (2010). Isolated congenital bifid tongue. *Natl. J. Maxillofac. Surg.* 1: 187–189.
9 Watkins, A., Abuja, G., Javsicas, L. et al. (2017). Cheiloschisis: surgical repair of cleft lip in a Thoroughbred foal. *J. Equine Vet. Sci.* 58: 20–23.
10 DeBowes, R.M. and Gaughan, E.M. (1998). Congenital dental disease of horses. *Vet. Clin. Equine* 14: 273–289.
11 Griffin, C. (2013). The gold standard of dental care: the juvenile horse. *Vet. Clin. Equine* 29: 487–504.
12 Yarbrough, T.B., Voss, E., Herrgesell, E.J. et al. (1999). Persistent frenulum of the epiglottis in four foals. *Vet. Surg.* 28: 287–291.
13 Bezdekova, B., Skoric, M., and Pekarkova, M. (2015). Congenital triple oesophageal strictures in a neonatal colt. *Equine Vet. Educ.* 27: 227–229.
14 Wong, D.M., Ruby, R.E., Van Eerde, E. et al. (2020). Oesophageal ectasia as a cause of dysphagia and regurgitation in a neonatal foal. *Equine Vet. Educ.* 32: 45–49.
15 Butt, T.D., MacDonald, D.G., and Crawford, W.H. (1998). Persistent right aortic arch in a yearling horse. *Can. Vet. J.* 39: 714–715.
16 Rohrbach, B.W. and Rooney, J.R. (1980). Congenital esophageal ectasia in a Thoroughbred foal. *J. Am. Vet. Med. Assoc.* 177: 65–67.
17 Barber, S.M., McLaughlin, B.G., and Fretz, P.B. (1983). Esophageal ectasia in a Quarter Horse. *Can. Vet. J.* 24: 46–49.
18 Bezdekova, B. (2012). Esophageal disorders in horses – a review of literature. *Pferdeheilkunde* 28: 187–192.
19 Loynachan, A.T. (2014). Esophageal cyst in the duodenum of a foal. *J. Vet. Diagn. Invest.* 26: 308–311.
20 Matsuda, K., Qiu, Y., Furuse, T. et al. Bronchogenic and esophageal cyst with laryngeal malformations in a Thoroughbred foal. *Vet. Pathol.* 47: 351–353.
21 Orsini, J.A., Sepesy, L., Donawick, W.J. et al. (1988). Esophageal duplication cyst as a cause of choke in the horse. *J. Am. Vet. Med. Assoc.* 193: 474–476.
22 Scott, E.A.A., Snoy, P., Prasse, K.W. et al. (1993). Intramural esophageal inclusion cysts in three horses. *Vet. Surg.* 22: 135–139.
23 Peek, S.F., de Lahunta, A., and Hackett, R.P. (1995). Combined oesophageal and tracheal duplication cyst in an Arabian filly. *Equine Vet. J.* 27: 475–478.
24 Tillotson, K., Traub-Dargartz, J.L., and Twedt, D. (2003). Balloon dilation of an oesphageal stricture in a one-month-old Appaloosa colt. *Equine Vet. Educ.* 15: 67–71.
25 Stewart, K.A. and Reinertson, E.L. (1983). Congenital esophageal stricture in a pony foal. *Mod. Vet. Pract.* 64: 753–754.
26 Clabough, D.L., Roberts, M.C., and Robertson, I. (1991). Probable congenital oesophageal stenosis in a Thoroughbred foal. *J. Am. Vet. Med. Assoc.* 199: 483–485.
27 Knottenbelt, D.C., Holdstock, N., and Madigan, J.E. (2004). *Equine Neonatology Medicine and Surgery*. Philadelphia PA: Saunders.
28 Mackey, V.S., Large, S.M., Breznock, E.M. et al. (1986). Surgical correction of a persistent right aortic arch in a foal. *Vet. Surg.* 15: 325–328.
29 Ryan, C.A. and Sanchez, C. (2005). Nondiarrheal disorders of the gastrointestinal tract in neonatal foals. *Vet. Clin. Equine* 21: 313–332.
30 Rubio-Martínez, L.M. (2015). Diaphragmatic hernias in horses. *Equine Vet. Educ.* 27: 396–397.
31 Tabaran, F., Nagy, A.L., Catoi, C. et al. (2015). Congenital diaphragmatic hernia with concurrent aplasia of the pericardium in a foal. *BMC Vet. Res.* 11: 309–316.
32 Epstein, K.L. (2014). Congenital causes of gastrointestinal disease. *Equine Vet. Educ.* 26: 345–346.
33 Pauwels, F.F., Hawkins, J.F., MacHarg, M.A. et al. (2007). Congenital retrosternal (Morgagni) diaphragmatic hernias in three horses. *J. Am. Vet. Med. Assoc.* 231: 427–432.
34 Dahlberg, J.A., Adam, E.N., Palmer, J.E. et al. (2009). Gastrointestinal nonrotation in a neonatal foal. *Equine Vet. Educ.* 21: 508–512.
35 Pearson, A.B. and Murfitt, C.G. (1988). Hypoplasia of the stomach in a Thoroughbred foal. *N. Zeal. Vet. J.* 36: 158.

36 Barth, A.D., Barber, S.M., and McKenzie, N.T. (1980). Pyloric stenosis in a foal. *Can. Vet. J.* 21: 234–236.

37 Rabbogliatti, V., Di Giancamillo, M., De Zani, D. et al. (2018). Helical Hydyo-Computed Tomography in the diagnosis of pyloric stenosis in two foals. *Proceeding of Veterinary and Animal Science Days 2018*, Milan, Italy (6–8 June).

38 Sprinkle, F.P., Swercek, T.W., and Crowe, M.W. (1984). Meckel's diverticulum in the horse. *J. Equine Vet. Sci.* 4: 175–176.

39 Barakzai, S.Z., Swain, J.M., and Else, R.W. (2003). Two cases of small intestinal strangulation involving Meckel's diverticulae. *Equine Vet. Educ.* 15: 291–294.

40 Verwilghen, D., van Galen, G., Busoni, V. et al. (2010). Meckel's diverticulum as a cause of colic: 2 cases with different morphological features. *Netherlands J. Vet. Sci.* 135: 452–455.

41 Gold, J.R., Belgrave, R.L., and Haldorson, G.J. (2006). Congenital intestinal polyp associated with intussusception in a 3-day-old foal. *Equine Vet. Educ.* 18: 116–119.

42 Adams, R., Koterba, A.M., and Brown, M.P. (1988). Exploratory celiotomy for gastrointestinal disease in neonatal foals: a review of 20 cases. *Equine Vet. J.* 20: 9–12.

43 Patterson-Kane, J.C., Sanchez, L.C., Mackay, R.J. et al. (2000). Small intestinal adenomatous polyposis resulting on protein-losing enteropathy in a horse. *Vet. Pathol.* 37: 82–85.

44 Younkin, J.T., Kim, I.J., Lutter, J.D. et al. (2020). Small intestinal adenomatous polyps resulting in chronic obstruction in a 3-year-old Quarter Horse gelding. *Equine Vet. Educ.* 32: 18–21.

45 Robert, M.P., Benamou-Smith, A.E., Cadore, J.L. et al. (2008). Recurrent colics in a 9-year-old Arabian stallion due to several congenital anomalies. *Equine Vet. Educ.* 20: 567–571.

46 Bosch, G. and Van der Velden, M.A. (2004). Impaired growth and colic caused by congenital defects in the mesenteric attachments of caecum and colon in a yearling. *Equine Vet. Educ.* 16: 116–120.

47 Dearo, A.C.O., de Moraes, M.G., Araújo, J.C.O. et al. (2014). Strangulatiom of the small intestine by an anomalous congenital band in a yearling. *Equine Vet. Educ.* 26: 640–644.

48 Knowles, E.J. and Mair, T.S. (2009). Colonic volvulus with defects of the mesenteric attachments in a yearling Friesian colt. *Equine Vet. Educ.* 21: 396–400.

49 Edwards, G.B. (2004). Congenital abnormalities of the equine gastrointestinal tract. *Equine Vet. Educ.* 6: 119.

50 Abutarbush, S.M., Shoemaker, R.W., and Bailey, J.V. (2003). Strangulation of the small intestines by a mesodiverticular band in 3 adult horses. *Can. Vet. J.* 33: 1005–1006.

51 Wefel, S., Mendez-Angulo, J.L., and Ernst, N.S. (2011). Small intestinal strangulation caused by a mesodiverticular band and diverticulum on the mesenteric border of the small intestine in a horse. *Can. Vet. J.* 52: 884–887.

52 Nappert, G., Laverty, S., Drolet, R. et al. (1992). Atresia coli in 7 foals (1964–1990). *Equine Vet. J. Suppl.* 13: 57–60.

53 van der Gaag, I. and Tibboel, D. (1980). Intestinal atresia and stenosis in animals: a report of 34 cases. *Vet. Pathol.* 17: 565–574.

54 Young, R.L., Linford, R.L., and Olander, H.J. (1992). Atresia coli in the foal: a review of six cases. *Equine Vet. J.* 24: 60–62.

55 Teixeira, L.G., Spasiani, J.P., Meirelles, A.E.W.B. et al. (2010). Rectal atresia in a newborn donkey. *Equine Vet. Educ.* 22: 434–437.

56 Schneider, J.E., Leipold, H.W., White, S.L. et al. (1981). Repair of congenital atresia of the colon in a foal. *Equine Vet. Sci.* 1: 121–126.

57 Prange, T. (2013). Small colon obstructions in foals. *Equine Vet. Educ.* 25: 293–296.

58 Santschi, E.M., Purdy, A.K., Valberg, S.J. et al. (1998). Endothelin receptor B polymorphism associated with lethal white foal syndrome in horses. *Mamm. Genome* 9: 306–309.

59 Hultgren, B.D. (1982). Ileocolonic aganglionosis in white progeny of overo spotted horses. *J. Am. Vet. Med. Assoc.* 180: 289–292.

60 Vonderfecht, S.L., Trommershausen Bowling, A. et al. (1983). Congenital intestinal aganglionosis in white foals. *Vet. Pathol.* 20: 65–70.

61 Santschi, E.M., Vrotsos, P.D., Purdy, A.M. et al. (2001). Incidence of the endothelin receptor B mutation that causes lethal white foal syndrome in white-patterned horses. *Am. J. Vet. Res.* 62: 97–103.

62 Robinson, K.A., Manning, S.T., Barber, S.M. et al. (2017). Congenital hypoplasia of the dorsal colon in a Quarter Horse filly with chronic, intermittent colic. *Equine Vet. Educ.* 29: 270–273.

63 Koenig, J.B., Rodriguez, A., Colquhoun, K. et al. (2007). Congenital colonic malformation ("short colon") in a 4-month-old Standardbred foal. *Can. Vet. J.* 48: 420–423.

64 Bassage, L.H., Habecker, P.L., and Russell, E.A. (2000). Colic in a horse associated with a massive cystic duplication cyst of the ascending colon. *Equine Vet. J.* 32: 565–568.

65 Cable, C.S., Fubine, S.L., Erb, H.N. et al. (1997). Abdominal surgery in foals: a review of 119 cases (1977–1994). *Equine Vet. J.* 29: 257–261.

66 Nelson, B.B., Ferris, R.A., McCue, P.M. et al. (2015). Surgical management of atresia ani and perineal hypospadias in a miniature donkey foal. *Equine Vet. Educ.* 27: 525–529.

67 Toth, F. and Schumacher, J. (2015). An overview of anal atresia and hypospadias in equids. *Equine Vet. Educ.* 27: 530–532.
68 Dunkel, B., Shokek, A.B., and Wilkins, P.A. (2004). Congenital cystic polypoid rectal hamartoma in a newborn foal. *Vet. Pathol.* 41: 700–702.
69 Salazar, T., Caldwell, F., Joiner, K. et al. (2011). Laparoscopic assisted surgical removal of a congenital rectal hamartoma in a foal. *Equine Vet. Educ.* 23: 55–61.
70 Mejia, S., Hurcombe, S.D.A., Rodgerson, D.H. et al. (2021). Retrograde intussusception of the descending colon secondary to multiple colonic hamartomas in a neonatal foal. *Equine Vet. Educ.* 33: 12–16.
71 van Der Luer, R.J.T. and Kroneman, J. (1982). Biliary atresia in a foal. *Equine Vet. J.* 14: 91–93.
72 Gold, J.R. (2017). Portosystemic shunts: a diagnostic challenge. *Equine Vet. Educ.* 29: 249–251.
73 Hug, S.A., Guerrero, T.G., Makara, M. et al. (2012). Diagnosis and surgical cellophane banding of an intrahepatic congenital portosystemic shunt in a foal. *J. Vet. Intern. Med.* 26: 171–177.
74 Woodford, N.S., Hotson Moore, A., Renfrew, H. et al. (2017). Surgical management of an extrahepatic portosystemic shunt in a foal: a multidisciplinary problem. *Equine Vet. Educ.* 29: 243–248.
75 McConnico, R.S., Duckett, W.M., and Wood, P.A. (1997). Persistent hyperammonemia in two related Morgan weanlings. *J. Vet. Intern. Med.* 11: 264–266.
76 Divers, T.J. (2015). The equine liver in health and disease. In: *AAEP Annual Convention*, 66–103. Las Vegas, NV: Am Assoc Equine Pract.

Chapter 17 Gastrointestinal Disorders

Section I Causes of Dysphagia in the Neonatal Foal

David Wong

The swallowing function develops during fetal life as the primitive esophagus delivers swallowed amniotic fluid to the stomach via a primary peristaltic reflex. This reflex is generated by coordination with the pharyngeal phase of swallowing and relaxation of the esophageal sphincters [1]. Neonatal suckling and swallowing is not fully developed until after birth and is characterized by an oral, pharyngeal, and esophageal phase that involves more than 30 nerves and muscles in the infant [2]. The oropharynx has one of the most abundant and diverse sensory inputs of the entire body with cranial nerves V, VII, IX, X, and XII providing the majority of afferent input to the brainstem swallowing center (rostral nucleus tractus solitarius) from the oropharynx [2]. The ability to suckle and swallow is associated with coordinated events, including closure of the glottis, relaxation of the cricopharyngeus muscle that allows opening of the cranial esophageal sphincter, and reflex inhibition of breathing [3, 4].

The oral phase of swallowing involves mixing of the food bolus with salivary enzymes, lingual-palatal coordination, and protection of the airway via the epiglottis, whereas the pharyngeal phase involves propulsion of the bolus and airway protection. This is followed by the esophageal phase that moves the food bolus to the stomach via peristalsis [1]. Besides pure transit of food boluses to the stomach, the esophagus also has an important supportive function in protecting the airway. The esophagus and airways share similar innervation via the vagus nerve with communication between afferent and efferent neuronal pathways that modulate sensory-motor function and facilitate safe swallowing and simultaneous airway protection [5]. The vagal neural pathways involved in swallowing and airway protection are directly and indirectly influenced by neurosensory and neuromotor pathways within the supranuclear regulatory centers, basal ganglia, cerebrum, and cerebellum [1]. These pathways can be impacted by perinatal events such as prematurity, inflammatory conditions, or coexisting medical conditions (Figure 17.I.1) that can contribute to dysphagia.

Clinical Signs

Dysphagia, or difficulty swallowing, is defined as any defect in the ingestion or transport of endogenous secretions, food, or water from the oral cavity to the distal esophagus and can arise from abnormalities in the oral, pharyngeal, or esophageal phase of swallowing [6]. Dysphagia can present with slightly different clinical signs, depending on its origin [7]. Dysphagia that occurs during the oral phase can be associated with congenital anomalies, absent oral reflexes, weak and/or uncoordinated suckle, immature biting and/or chewing, poor bolus propulsion, and/or poor bolus containment. Dysphagia associated with the pharyngeal phase can be associated with a delayed or absent swallow reflex along with suckle, swallow, and breathing incoordination resulting in food boluses that infiltrate the larynx resulting in aspiration and choking, thereby causing feed material to appear in the nares and/or lower airway [4, 7]. Nasal regurgitation of feed is particularly prevalent in dysphagic equids due to the position for the soft palate relative to the larynx and the minimal and dynamic nature of the hypopharynx [4].

As breathing and swallowing share a common space in the pharynx, problems in either of these processes, or lack of synchronization between processes, can affect the ability to protect the airway [7]. In adults, coughing occurs as a result of chemical or mechanical stimulation of the laryngeal and tracheal mucosa, which thereby initiates the laryngeal reflexes via afferent branches of the superior laryngeal nerve [4]. In neonates in other species, stimulation of these chemoreflexes causes swallowing, apnea, and glottis closure, but cough is uncommon and may not develop for weeks to months [4, 8]. The age at which foals develop a cough reflex is unknown, but the absent or limited nature of the cough reflex in neonatal

Equine Neonatal Medicine, First Edition. Edited by David M. Wong and Pamela A. Wilkins.

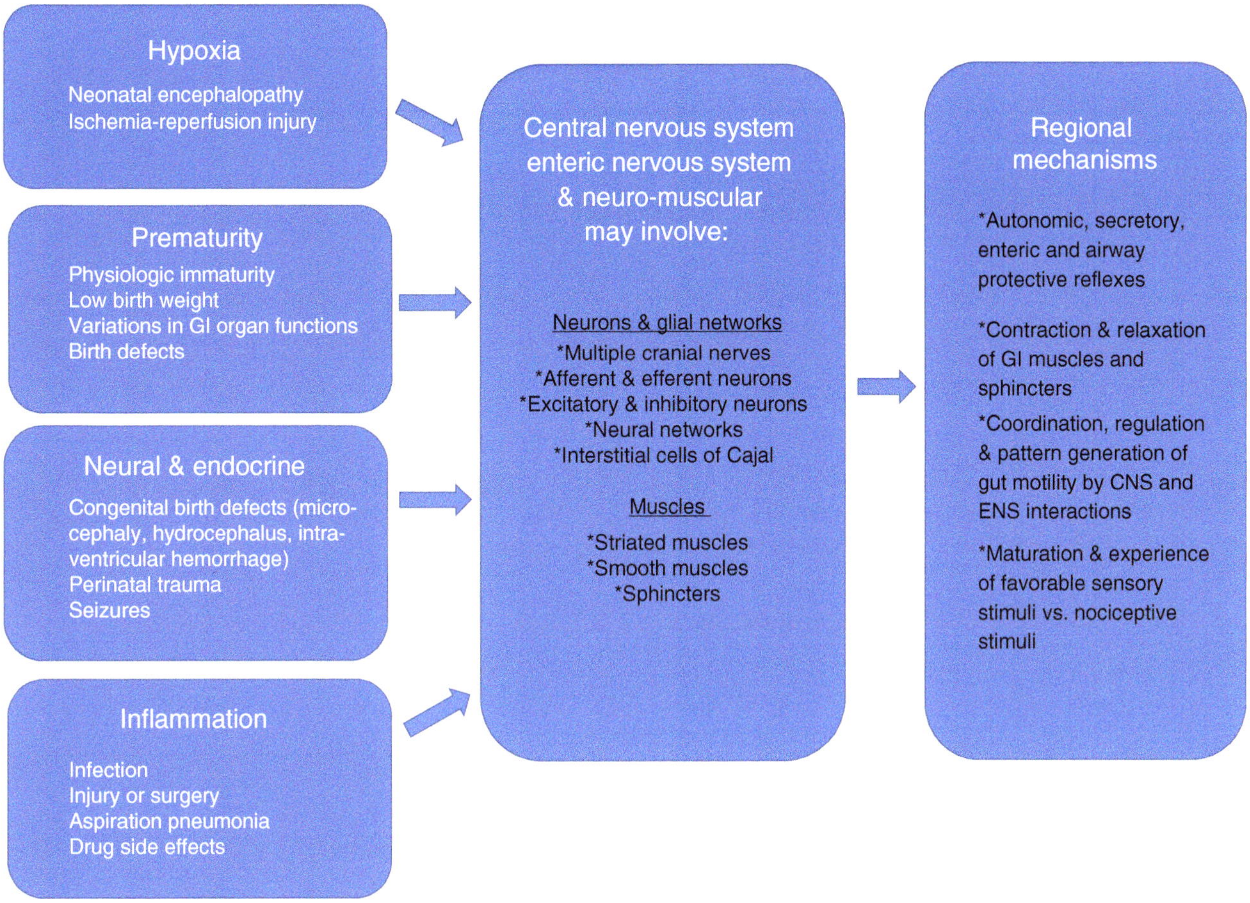

Figure 17.I.1 Contributory factors and potential central and regional mechanisms associated with neonatal dysphagia [1] CNS, central nervous system; ENS, enteric nervous system.

foals places dysphagic foals at high risk for aspiration pneumonia. Because aspiration events are commonly silent, the clinician should not rely on the presence of cough as evidence alone of aspiration of feed in dysphagic foals [7]. However, aspiration of milk is supported by a tracheal gurgle or rattle upon auscultation of the trachea while the foal suckles [4, 9].

Dysphagia in the foal is not uncommon and can result from a variety of causes (Table 17.I.1). Clinical signs of dysphagia can include the presence of milk from one or both nostrils, coughing during or immediately after ingestion of milk, dribbling, or drooling milk from the mouth and the presence of a tracheal gurgle or rattle due to aspiration of milk into the trachea [16]. In addition to these signs, foals with dysphagia associated with esophageal disease may have milk regurgitation when the head is lowered or while recumbent [30]. Evidence of aspiration pneumonia such as tachypnea, tachycardia, fever, respiratory distress, and/or cough may be observed, and other clinical signs related to the primary disease process (e.g. sepsis, nutritional myodegeneration, etc.) may be present. Older foals with dysphagia might also have a failure to thrive due to decreased availability of nutrients coupled with potential aspiration pneumonia.

Although dysphagia in neonatal foals is not unusual in clinical practice, the veterinary literature citing such cases is limited to individual case reports or small case series. A number of these reports describe congenital disorders in which diagnosis was not difficult. However, one relatively larger case series described pharyngeal dysfunction as a cause of dysphagia in 16 neonatal foals [4]. Pharyngeal dysfunction can cause dysphagia as a result of pharyngeal weakness, incoordination, or a combination of motor and sensory under development (central or peripheral in origin) with risk factors in human neonates including prematurity, low birth weight, and periparturient hypoxic episodes [1, 6]. In the report in 16 neonatal foals, the mean age at presentation to the hospital was 2.9 days (range 0.5–12 days) [4]. In this cohort of foals, 2 were dysmature, 1 was premature, and 6 had evidence of neonatal encephalopathy. Failure of transfer passive immunity was noted in 5/12 (42%) and aspiration pneumonia was noted in 12/16 (75%) of foals. Sepsis was not detected in 9 foals in which blood culture was submitted. Endoscopy of the nasopharynx was normal in 4 foals, but characterized as weak, flaccid, collapsed,

Table 17.I.1 Disorders associated with dysphagia in the foal.

Category	Specific diseases
Anatomic/congenital disease	Cleft Palate [10, 11]
	Subepiglottic, pharyngeal, or soft palate cyst [12–14]
	Persistent frenulum of the epiglottis [15]
	Choanal atresia [16]
	Persistent right aortic arch [17]
	Guttural pouch tympany [18, 19]
	Megaesophagus [20]
	Esophageal stricture [21]
	Microcephaly[a] [7]
	Hydrocephalus[a] [7]
Generalized weakness	Prematurity [7]
	Sepsis (causing central stupor, weakness, and/or pain)
	Hypoglycemia
	Electrolyte abnormalities
	Respiratory disease
	Infectious disease (e.g. in utero EHV infection)
	Any disease that depresses general mentation
Primary muscle disease	Nutritional myodegneration (white muscle disease) [22, 23]
	Hyperkalemic periodic paralysis [24]
Central neurologic disease	Neonatal encephalopathy (hypoxic–ischemic encephalopathy) [4]
	Cerebrovascular accident /Vascular hamartoma [25]
	Head trauma [26]
	Seizures
Peripheral neurologic disease	Botulism [27]
	Guttural pouch mycosis [28]
Trauma/injury	Tracheal intubation
	Tongue infection, laceration
	Fractured or luxated jaw
	Pharyngeal/laryngeal trauma
	Esophageal trauma
Miscellaneous causes	Dorsal displacement of the soft palate [29]
	Pharyngeal dysfunction [4]
	Esophageal ectasia [30]

[a] Congenital disease associated with dysphagia in human infants that might cause dysphagia in foals.

and/or inflamed in 12 foals. Dorsal displacement of the soft palate was persistent in 2 foals and frequent in another foal, whereas 2 other foals had complete left-sided arytenoid paralysis and 2 foals had slow or sluggish movement of the arytenoid cartilages. Milk was noted in the guttural pouch (1 foal) and trachea (5 foals), and evidence of aspiration pneumonia was noted on radiographic (7/8 foals) or ultrasonographic (12/16 foals) examination of the thorax.

Diagnosis

The diagnostic evaluation of the dysphagic foal should start with a complete physical examination with particular attention directed at detection of macroscopic congenital anomalies or trauma/injury within the oral and nasal cavities. A CBC may reflect evidence of aspiration pneumonia (neutrophila or neutropenia, hyperfibrinogenemia), may be altered from sepsis, or may be within reference

(a) (b)

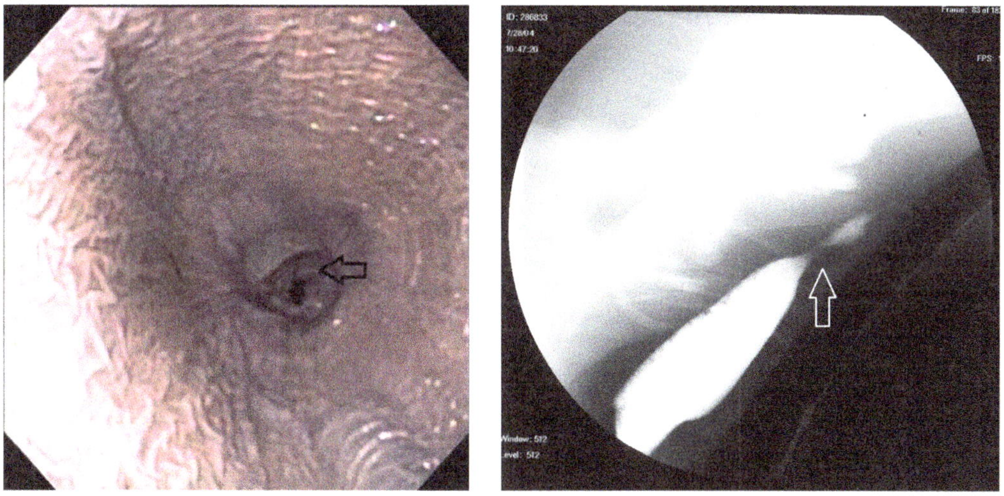

Figure 17.I.2 Neonatal foal presented for dysphagia. Endoscopy (a) and fluoroscopy (b) identified an esophageal stricture (arrows) as the cause of dysphagia.

(a) (b)

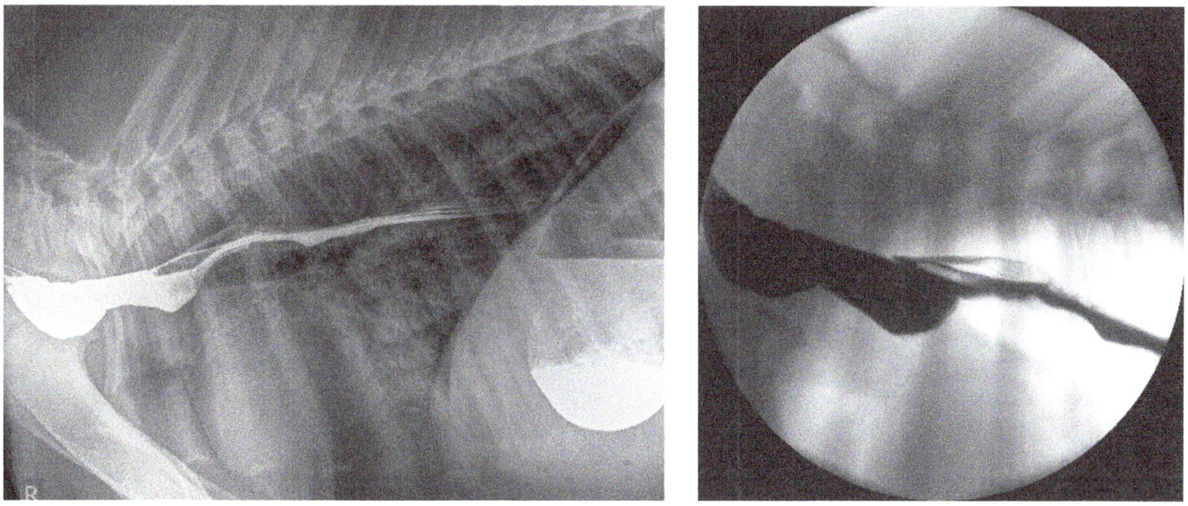

Figure 17.I.3 Neonatal foal presented for dysphagia after nursing. Contrast study of the esophagus identified pooling of contrast material and dilation of the esophagus in the cranial thorax via (a) radiography and (b) fluoroscopy. A diagnosis of persistent right aortic arch was established on postmortem examination. *Source:* Images courtesy of Dr. Edwina Wilkes, Charles Sturt University.

intervals depending on the age and condition of the foal. Serum biochemistry profile can highlight metabolic or electrolyte aberrations or other underlying primary diseases or comorbidities. Endoscopy and/or radiography of the nasopharynx, guttural pouches, oral cavity, trachea, and esophagus should be performed (Figure 17.I.2) to detect anatomic anomalies or trauma associated with dysphagia. Contrast studies may be necessary in some instances to determine the flow of ingested feed (Figure 17.I.3). Thoracic imaging should be performed to assess for the presence of aspiration pneumonia. In more elusive cases, advanced imaging such as magnetic resonance imaging (MRI) or computed tomography (CT) may be necessary to evaluate for head trauma, cerebrovascular accidents, and persistent right aortic arch.

Treatment

Treatment of dysphagia depends on the underlying cause. Medical management of foals with megaesophagus, esophageal stricture, esophageal ectasia, botulism, neonatal encephalopathy, and guttural pouch mycosis have been described whereas surgical correction of cleft palate, subepiglottic/pharyngeal cysts, persistent frenulum of the epiglottis, choanal atresia, persistent right aortic arch, guttural pouch tympany, and dorsal displacement of the soft palate have been documented with variable success. Time and supportive care are needed for foals with pharyngeal dysfunction and in cases of idiopathic dysphagia. In the case series described above, supportive treatment included controlled enteral feeding through a nasogastric tube in 11/16 foals (69%) or muzzling of the foal with intermittent periods in which the foal was allowed to suckle from the mare for 12–48 hours (5/16 foals). In that case series, foals receiving enteral nutrition via nasogastric tube were transitioned to suckling from the mare within 5.5 ± 4.6 days (median 4 days, range 1–14 days) with minimal to no evidence of dysphagia or aspiration [4]. One foal showed no improvement, remained dysphagic after 7 days of controlled feeding, and was euthanized. The 5 foals that did not receive controlled feedings suckled successfully after 2 days (range 0–5 days).

Supportive care includes broad spectrum antimicrobials and nonsteroidal anti-inflammatory drugs. Physical therapy may hasten recovery of pharyngeal dysphagia by strengthening the pharyngeal muscles [4]. This can be accomplished by milking the mare's udder (empty the udder) and subsequently allowing the foal to suckle for short periods of time with the intent of strengthening the pharyngeal muscles and improving coordination. A high survival RATE was noted in the aforementioned case series with the majority of foals (15/16; 94%) being discharged from the hospital, nursing from the mare with no (14/16) or mild (1/16) evidence of dysphagia 7 ± 6 days (range 0–22 days) after admission. Long-term follow-up revealed that 13/15 foals were alive, with one foal euthanized 3 weeks after hospital discharge from severe aspiration pneumonia. No evidence of lower airway disease or dysphagic was reported in 12/13 foals. Of note, anecdotal observations by the author indicate that dysphagia can take a longer time to resolve (>1–2 weeks), with some foals improving once they are transitioned to forage.

References

1 Jadcherla, S. (2016). Dysphagia in the high-risk infant: potential factors and mechanisms. *Am. J. Clin. Nutr.* 103 (Suppl): 622S–628S.

2 Raol, N., Schrepfer, T., and Hartnick, C. (2018). Aspiration and dysphagia in the neonatal patient. *Clin. Perinatol.* 45: 645–660.

3 Derkay, C.S. and Schechter, G.L. (1998). Anatomy and physiology of pediatric swallowing disorders. *Otolaryngol. Clin. North Am.* 31: 397–404.

4 Holcombe, S.J., Hurcombe, S.D., Barr, B.S. et al. (2012). Dysphagia associated with presumed pharyngeal dysfunction in 16 neonatal foals. *Equine Vet. J.* 44Suppl 41: 105–108.

5 Goyal, R.K., Padmanabhan, R., and Sang, Q. (2001). Neural circuits in swallowing and abdominal vagal afferent-mediated lower esophageal sphincter relaxation. *Am. J. Med.* 111 (Suppl 8A): 95S–105S.

6 Grobyoski, J.D. (1965). The swallowing mechanism of the neonate. *Pediatrics* 35: 445–452.

7 Dodrill, P. and Gosa, M.M. (2015). Pediatric dysphagia: physiology, assessment, and management. *Ann. Nutr. Metab.* 66 (suppl 5): 24–31.

8 Thatch, B.T. (2007). Maturation of cough and other reflexes that protect the fetal and neonatal airway. *Pulm. Pharmacol. Ther.* 20: 365–370.

9 Yarbrough, T.B., Voss, E., Herrgesell, E.J. et al. (1999). Persistent frenulum of the epiglottis in four foals. *Vet. Surg.* 28: 287–291.

10 Kirkham, L. and Vasey, J.R. (2002). Surgical cleft soft palate repair in a foal. *Aust. Vet. J.* 80: 143–146.

11 Shaw, S.D., Normal, T.E., Arnold, C.E. et al. (2015). Clinical characteristics of horses and foals diagnosed with cleft palate in a referral population: 28 cases (1988–2011). *Can. Vet. J.* 56: 756–760.

12 Stick, J.A. and Boles, C. (1980). Subepiglottic cyst in three foals. *J. Am. Vet. Med. Assoc.* 177: 62–64.

13 Sullivan, E.K. and Parente, E.J. (2003). Disorders of the pharynx. *Vet. Clin. Equine* 19: 159–167.

14 Haynes, P., Beadle, R., McClure, J. et al. (1990). Soft palate cysts as a cause of pharyngeal dysfunction in two horses. *Equine Vet. J.* 22: 369–371.

15 Yarbrough, T.B., Voss, E.D., Herrgesell, E.J. et al. (1999). Persistent frenulum of the epiglottis in four fouls. *Vet. Surg.* 28: 287–291.

16 Buechner-Maxwell, V. (2012). Practical approach to nutritional support of the dysphagic foal. *Proceedings 58th Annual AAEP Convention* 8: 412–424.

17 Coleman, M.C., Norman, T.E., and Wall, C.R. (2014). What is your diagnosis? Persistent right aortic arch. *J. Am. Vet. Med. Assoc.* 244: 1253–1255.

18 Bell, C. (2007). Pharyngeal neuromuscular dysfunction associated with bilateral guttural pouch tympany in a foal. *Can. Vet. J.* 48: 192–194.

19 Sparks, H.D., Stick, J.A., Brakehoff, J.E. et al. (2009). Partial resction of the plica salpingopharyngeus for the treatment of three foals with bilateral tympany of the auditory tube diverticulum (guttural pouch). *J. Am. Vet. Med. Assoc.* 235: 731–733.

20 Broekman, L.E.M. and Kuiper, D. (2002). Megaesophagus in the horse. A short review of the literature and 18 own cases. *Vet. Q.* 24: 199–202.

21 Knottenbelt, D.C., Harrison, L.J., and Peacock, P.J. (1992). Conservative treatment of oesophageal stricture in five foals. *Vet. Rec.* 131: 27–30.

22 Dill, S.G. and Rebhun, W.G. (1985). White muscle disease in foals. *Compend. Contin. Educ. Pract. Vet.* 7: 627.

23 Lofstedt, J. (1997). White muscle disease of foals. *Vet. Clin. North Am. Equine* 13: 169–185.

24 Traub-Dargatz, J.L., Ingram, J.T., Stashak, T.S. et al. (1992). Respiratory stridor associated with polymyopathy suspected to be hyperkalemic periodic paralysis in four Quarterhorse foals. *J. Am. Vet. Med. Assoc.* 201: 85–89.

25 Borel, N., Grest, P., Junge, H. et al. (2014). Vascular hamartoma in the central nervous system of a foal. *J. Vet. Diagn. Invest.* 26: 805–809.

26 Feary, D.J., Magdesian, K.G., Aleman, M.A. et al. (2007). Traumatic brain injury in horses: 34 cases (1994–2004). *J. Am. Vet. Med. Assoc.* 231: 259–266.

27 Wilkins, P.A. and Palmer, J.E. (2003). Botulism in foals less than 6 months of age: 30 cases (1989–2002). *J. Vet. Intern. Med.* 17: 702–707.

28 Chidlow, H.B. and Slovis, N.M. (2017). Guttural pouch mycosis in two foals. *Equine Vet. Educ.* 29: 213–218.

29 Shappell, K.K., Caron, J.P., Stick, J.A. et al. (1989). Staphylectomy for treatment of dorsal displacement of the soft palate in two foals. *J. Am. Vet. Med. Assoc.* 195: 1395–1398.

30 Wong, D.M., Ruby, R.E., Van Eerde, E. et al. (2020). Oesophageal ectasia as a cause of dysphagia and milk regurgitation in a neonatal foal. *Equine Vet. Educ.* 32: 45–49.

Section II Gastroduodenal Ulcer Syndrome and Ileus in the Foal

Ben Sykes

Diagnostics – Endoscopy

Endoscopy is a valuable diagnostic aid for the investigation of upper gastrointestinal (GI) tract disease in the neonatal foal. In the neonate, gastroscopy is uncommon, and the focus is primarily on examination of the pharynx and esophagus, whereas gastroscopy is more commonly performed in older foals. This reflects the relative importance of esophageal and gastric diseases in the neonate and older foal populations, respectively. In addition, endoscopy is also a useful adjunct for confirming correct placement of indwelling nasogastric tubes.

Equipment Required

No special endoscopy equipment is required, but videoendoscopic equipment is preferred as it allows for the procedure to be completed as quickly as possible. A standard 9 mm outer diameter endoscope is suitable for most foals, although a smaller diameter pediatric endoscope may be required for pony or Miniature Horse foals. An insertion length of 1 m is suitable for examination of the pharynx and esophagus of the neonatal foal while a longer 2 m insertion length is required for gastroscopy. Further information on endoscopy of the esophagus and upper GI tract can be found in Chapter 15.

Special Considerations

In general, endoscopy of the foal is well tolerated. However, foals with respiratory compromise may experience additional difficulties with respiratory function during the procedure. To partially accommodate for this, the provision of oxygen supplementation via the biopsy channel can be used when performing endoscopy of the upper respiratory tract of foals with respiratory compromise. If performing gastroscopy, the period of starvation required is dependent on the age and diet of the foal. In neonates the period of starvation is minimal (<1–2 hours) as their milk-based diet is rapidly cleared from the stomach. Older foals consuming roughage-based diets require longer durations of fasting, typically 12 hours; however, foals of this age (>14 days) have significantly greater energy reserves and tolerate starvation well.

Diseases of the Esophagus

A wide range of congenital esophageal diseases have been described in the neonatal foal including stenosis or stricture [1, 2], ectasia [3–5], esophageal cysts [6], and vascular ring anomalies such as fourth brachial arch defects [7, 8]. As such, although pharyngeal weakness is a more common presentation [9], structural diseases should be considered in all neonatal foals with unexplained dysphagia or nasal reflux of milk. Congenital conditions become less commonly recognized and acquired conditions such as esophageal laceration [10], stricture [11–13] or ulceration [14, 15] become more common as foals age.

Acquired esophageal disease is most attributed to trauma, typically ingested foreign bodies, but esophageal ulceration may occur secondary to delayed gastric emptying (Figure 17.II.1). As such gastroscopy is required in unexplained cases of esophageal ulceration to rule out causative gastric disease. Esophageal ulceration attributed to Equine Herpes Virus-2 has also been reported [14].

Treatment of esophageal disease is dependent on the inciting cause and specific disease process. Supportive care with esophageal rest utilizing feeding via an indwelling nasogastric tube is beneficial in the acute stages while the return of small, frequent meal feeding within 24–48 hours may be advantageous to debride ulcerative lesions and reduce the risk of stricture formation. The use of mucosal

Equine Neonatal Medicine, First Edition. Edited by David M. Wong and Pamela A. Wilkins.

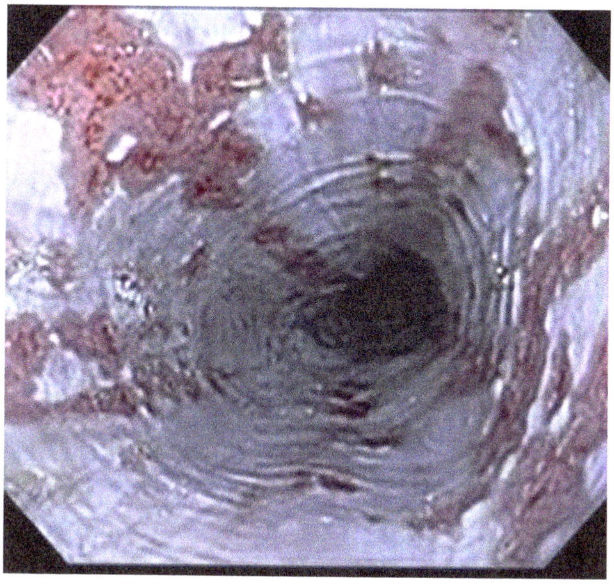

Figure 17.II.1 Esophageal ulcers secondary to gastric reflux in a neonatal foal. *Source:* Photo courtesy of D. Wong, Iowa State University.

barrier protectants such as sucralfate is logical (10–20 mg/kg PO q6–8h). Both surgical [13] and nonsurgical [11, 12] management of esophageal stricture has been reported.

Diseases of the Stomach

Equine Gastric Ulcer Syndrome

Equine Gastric Ulcer Syndrome (EGUS) is a well-recognized condition in the foal. The prevalence of disease varies substantially between age groups, as does the lesion type observed. Although rare, congenital EGUS affecting the squamous mucosa has been reported in the foal [16]. Early studies reported the prevalence of EGUS in healthy foals of approximately 50% [17, 18], while more recent studies [19, 20] reported lower prevalences possibly reflecting improved management practices over ensuing decades. During the first month of life the prevalence of EGUS is approximately 15% in both healthy and hospitalized foals [19, 20]. Between 1 and 3 months of age the prevalence in both healthy and hospitalized foals increases to approximately 32% [19, 20]. Within these age groups there is no difference between healthy foals [19] and those presented for postmortem [20], and squamous lesions dominate, making up the majority of observed lesions. Beyond 3 months of age the prevalence of EGUS decreases in healthy foals to <15% [19] but remains high at approximately 33% in sick foals until 6 months of age before decreasing to <15% [20]. Importantly, although squamous lesions remain more prevalent in foals ≥4 months of age, a greater proportion of glandular and duodenal lesions are observed as foals age [19, 20].

The pathophysiology of EGUS in the foal is poorly studied but is assumed to be similar to adult horses. Equine squamous gastric disease (ESGD) primarily results from acid injury to the squamous mucosa which has inherently poor defense mechanisms [21]. The mean baseline intra-gastric pH of healthy foals of 2.9–4.2 [22] is higher than the pH of <2 typically recorded in the ventral stomach of adult horses [23–26]. This is likely attributable to the frequent nursing behavior of foals with both milk and saliva acting as buffers against gastric acid. Accordingly, systemically healthy foals that have restricted nursing behavior may have higher intra-gastric acid load and, as such, are predisposed to ESGD. Further, neonatal foals do not have the stratification of pH that is present in the adult horse stomach, where the pH is <2 ventrally and increases to approximately 7 at the level of the cardia [23–27]. As such, increased intra-gastric acid loads are likely to result in increased ulcerogenic potential in this population. In contrast, critically ill neonates (≤4 days of age) often have altered gastric acid production, such that they often have pH neutral or alkaline intra-gastric conditions [28].

The pathophysiology of equine glandular gastric disease (EGGD) is poorly understood but is believed to result from a breakdown of normal defense mechanisms [21]. The histopathology of EGGD in foals is poorly described, but in adults, true ulcerative lesions are rare, with lesions more accurately classified as erosive gastritis rather than true ulcerative lesions [21]. Importantly, this classification separates erosive glandular gastritis, the dominant presentation of EGGD in foals, from perforating ulceration or gastroduodenal ulcer disease (GDUD), which present as specific diseases (discussed below).

When considering treatment or prophylaxis of EGUS, it is important to distinguish between the two. Where a clear and clinically significant lesion is identified, treatment is warranted. In contrast, where no distinct lesion is present or clinical significance is questionable, a risk–benefit analysis should be performed on each individual case. This is particularly important for prophylaxis where the benefits are often unclear along with growing concerns over the potential for adverse side effects as discussed below. The effects of age and differentiation between ESGD and EGGD lesions also have important implications for assessing the value of prophylaxis and the means of therapeutic intervention in specific populations.

Routine prophylaxis of EGUS in healthy foals is not justified. In sick foals <30 days of age, prophylaxis has no demonstratable effect on EGUS prevalence [29], and, combined with the low prevalence of disease at this age, the benefit of prophylaxis in this population is questionable

Table 17.II.1 Relative benefit of EGUS prophylaxis in sick foals of different ages with or without gastrointestinal disease.

Disease state	<1 mo of age	1–3 mo of age	≥4 mo of age
Gastrointestinal disease	Low	Medium	High
Non-gastrointestinal disease	Low	Low	Medium

(Table 17.II.1). At 1–3 months of age, EGUS prevalence increases, and it is likely that the pathophysiology of disease more closely represents that of adults than the neonatal population. As such, the relative benefit of prophylaxis increases in this age group. This is particularly true in foals with a primary diagnosis of GI disease, which are reported to have increased EGUS risk [20]. In populations where glandular disease, in particular GDUD, is more prevalent (specifically foals ≥2–4 months of age) the benefits of routine prophylaxis in sick foals increase further. Moreover, as sick foals ≥4 months of age are more likely to have EGUS than healthy counterparts [19, 20], it appears that disease related factors may contribute to increased prevalence, further justifying the use of prophylaxis in this population. Both selective and nonselective nonsteroidal anti-inflammatory drugs (NSAIDs) have been demonstrated to induce ESGD and EGGD lesions at commonly used therapeutic doses in adult horses [30], and it is logical that a similar effect occurs in foals. This has led to a recommendation to provide prophylaxis in foals receiving NSAIDs, although this is not without risk (discussed below).

Conversely, the risk of prophylaxis for EGUS in foals has been questioned, with increasing concerns raised over the safety of omeprazole in this population. Similar to studies in people, a multicenter equine study demonstrated increased risk of nonspecific diarrhea, but not infectious diarrhea, in neonatal foals receiving anti-ulcer medication, especially acid-suppressive therapy, when compared with those that did not [31]. In the same study, an increased risk of nonspecific diarrhea was also observed with sucralfate administration [31], suggesting that its use is not without risk contrary to a common perception otherwise. Importantly, this study focused on foals ≤14 days of age and an increased risk of diarrhea associated with EGUS prophylaxis has not been demonstrated in older foals. Given the significant differences in intestinal microflora of foals as they age, with their microflora resembling that of adults by 60-days of age [32], the author does not believe that extrapolation of the risk of prophylaxis from the neonatal population to foals ≥1 month of age is appropriate. As such, the author's threshold for therapeutic intervention is lower in foals ≥1 month of age than neonates.

More recently concerns have been raised over the use of omeprazole and the potential for increased fractures in performance horses [33]. While initial research focused on administration during the horse's performance career, a study in people demonstrated a prolonged increased risk of fracture in children treated with proton pump inhibitors (PPIs), such as omeprazole, at <1 year of age [34]. Importantly, an increased fracture risk was observed following treatment with either PPIs or H_2-receptor antagonist drugs, such as ranitidine, with as little as <30 days of treatment, and the increased fracture risk persisted for the entirety of the study's 13-year follow-up period [34]. Similar findings have also been reported in young adult people (aged 18–29 years old) receiving PPIs [35]. Although not demonstrated in an equine population to date, the study raises concerns for the injudicious use of acid suppressive drugs in the foal population, the majority of whom are expected to compete as athletes.

Administration of omeprazole is commonly recommended to prevent against NSAID-induced gastric disease. However, while a study in adult horses demonstrated that concurrent omeprazole therapy was effective in ameliorating the development of EGGD in horses receiving phenylbutazone over a 14-day period, a higher rate of intestinal complications (i.e. impaction, diarrhea, colic, ulcerative, and necrotizing enterocolitis) was observed in the omeprazole/phenylbutazone group, with 75% (6/8) of horses affected compared to the phenylbutazone group with 25% (2/8) of horses affected with complications [36]. This study provides further evidence to refute the common notion that omeprazole administration is risk free and reinforces the need for administration to be considered on a risk–benefit basis rather than blanket recommendations.

Lastly, a further risk to consider relates to the association of acid suppressive medications (H_2-receptor antagonists, PPIs) with systemic infection. Gastric acidity is a primitive innate defense mechanism of the body that decreases the density of orally ingested microorganisms that travel from the stomach into the intestines [37]. In the normal gastric acidity of pH <4, most microorganisms do not survive [38]. In people, increasing the stomach pH decreases the gastric acid barrier and increases the number of microorganisms that survive in the stomach and intestinal tract, thus potentially increasing the risk of systemic infection and necrotizing enterocolitis [37, 39]. In one study, infants fed acidified milk formula or maternal breast milk had lower intragastric pH and significantly lower gastric bacterial colonization [40]. Acid-suppressive agents may also directly inhibit leukocyte activity and blunt the immune response to infection [38, 41]. In one study, administration of H_2-receptor blockers or PPIs was significantly associated with the occurrence of late-onset sepsis in preterm infants [37]. Other studies have demonstrated that the use of H_2-receptor antagonists or PPIs is a risk factor for Gram-negative septicemia [42, 43]. Studies examining the association between acid suppressive medications and infection have not been performed in foals, but the findings from human medicine provide further evidence for the potential of side effects to occur.

Considering the above, the author does not advocate for routine EGUS prophylaxis in sick foals. In foals ≥1 month of age, a risk–benefit assessment is made on an individual case basis, with the default recommendation of avoiding EGUS prophylaxis. The exceptions being foals ≥1 month of age with other GI disease [20] and any sick foal ≥4 months of age [19, 20] where the risk of EGUS, and in particular glandular disease, increases and as such the relative value of prophylaxis increases. The routine administration of acid suppressive medications to prevent NSAID-induced gastric disease is not recommended. Where concerns persist regarding the potential for NSAID-induced gastric disease, the author's preference is to use sucralfate for this specific purpose [44].

In contrast to the conservative approach to prophylaxis outlined above, it is important to emphasize that treatment of clinical EGUS remains an important aspect of case management where clinical signs of EGUS are present, or the clinical index of suspicion is high. In such cases, the risk–benefit equation clearly shifts, especially in foals ≥1 month of age toward demonstratable benefit of treatment over the theoretical risks of either GI, systemic or orthopedic disease.

Clinical signs of EGUS in foals are often vague and vary widely between age groups. Anecdotally, restlessness, bruxism, inappetence, intermittent low-grade colic, and laying in dorsal recumbency have been associated with EGUS in neonates while overt colic, inappetence and diarrhea are more common in older foals. Definitive diagnosis requires gastroscopy but given the relatively high prevalence of EGUS in clinically healthy foals, especially those ≥1 month of age, a response to appropriate treatment remains important for assigning clinical significance and discounting other differentials with nonspecific clinical signs. The author's preference is to treat based on clinical suspicion and to reserve gastroscopy for refractory cases or those where obtaining a definitive diagnosis is critical for case management.

The principles of treatment in foals with EGUS are the same as adults [21, 45]. Acid suppression remains a cornerstone of treatment especially in foals ≤3 months of age where squamous lesions predominate [19, 20]. Recent studies in adult horses have supported the use of monotherapy with 100% ESGD [26, 46] and 75% EGGD [26] healing with 2–4 weeks of potent acid suppressive therapy alone. Accordingly, the focus of management of EGUS in foals should primarily be on ensuring adequate acid suppression is achieved.

Omeprazole remains the most widely used acid suppressive drug because of its ability to rapidly induce long lasting (>22 hours) acid suppression in foals [22, 47] making once daily use at a dose of 2–4 mg/kg feasible and appealing from a case management perspective. In contrast to adults, neonatal foals consume a milk based diet, thus no adjustment to diet to accommodate feed-induced decreases in bioavailability is required [28]. However in older foals consuming roughage based diets, drug administration should occur after a brief overnight fast and 30–60 minutes prior to feeding *as per* current recommendations for adult horses [48]. Omeprazole is an acid-labile drug and where increased dwell time in the stomach is suspected, such as in pyloric outflow obstruction or where esophageal ulceration suggests delayed gastric outflow, systemic (IV or IM) administration of either omeprazole or esomeprazole at 0.5 mg/kg, or pantoprazole at 1.5 mg/kg [49], once daily is preferred [50–52]. Alternatively, ranitidine, a H_2-receptor antagonist, can be used at 5 mg/kg orally q 8 hours [53] where PPIs are unavailable or unsuitable. However, unlike omeprazole in which efficacy in sick and healthy foals is similar, it has been documented that, when compared with healthy foals, sick neonatal foals respond less effectively to ranitidine [28], decreasing its utility in this population.

Sucralfate is a popular adjunctive treatment to omeprazole, and it is appealing due to its perceived favorable safety profile compared with acid suppressive drugs. The use of sucralfate has not been associated with subsequent increased fracture risk in people but, similar to acid suppressive drugs, it is associated with increased risk of noninfectious diarrhea in foals [31]. Further, it is important to recognize that its clinical efficacy is poorly documented in foals. In one study, sucralfate had some protective effects on high-dose phenylbutazone induced disease [44], while in another it had no demonstrable benefits on naturally occurring EGUS in weanling foals [54]. Accordingly, as discussed above, the author's preference is to treat with acid suppressive drugs, primarily omeprazole, and to use sucralfate as an adjunctive treatment where glandular disease is suspected, in populations where EGGD is more prevalent (i.e. foals ≥4 months of age with GI disease), or in cases where NSAID toxicity is suspected. Sucralfate can also be used in cases in which the response to acid suppression has been suboptimal, as it can offer additional relief of clinical signs in the early stages of treatment, and in foals with concurrent hindgut disease, such as diarrhea, where it may also be beneficial.

The response to treatment is generally good with an excellent long-term prognosis. Gastric perforation and exsanguination [55] are rare complications. The pathophysiology of such lesions likely differs from typical EGUS lesions described above, and more likely represent infarctive or malperfusion related disease rather than acid injury [29]. Further supporting this hypothesis is that anecdotally such severe manifestations of EGUS appear to becoming less common as the overall level of supportive, and in particular hemodynamic, care has dramatically improved over time.

Gastroduodenal Ulcer Disease and Pyloric Stenosis

GDUD is a distinct disease entity affecting foals, typically between 2–4 months of age [56], although it has been reported as a congenital defect in foals [57] and an acquired disease in foals as young as 4–5 days of age [56, 58]. Although the exact cause of GDUD is unknown, inflammation, scarring, and granulation tissue associated with ulceration can cause mechanical and functional obstruction of the bowel [56]. Affected foals demonstrate poor growth for their age with a pot-bellied appearance, and typically present with bruxism, ptyalism, and teeth grinding or with overt colic with spontaneous reflux of gastric contents [59]. Diagnosis is most commonly confirmed by gastroscopy, although examination of the duodenum may not be possible in foals with extensive pyloric stricture. Extensive ESGD and esophageal ulceration is a common finding in foals with GDUD, and its presence supports a concurrent diagnosis of delayed gastric emptying alongside the primary diagnosis. Transcutaneous abdominal ultrasonography is a useful adjunctive diagnostic to document the extent of the disease and identify any concurrent pathology. In selected cases, contrast radiography with liquid barium may add additional diagnostic information (i.e. delayed gastric emptying). If contrast radiography is performed, the stomach is decompressed via nasogastric tube and barium (10 ml/kg) is administered with the foal standing and ideally unsedated. Lateral radiographs are then performed at approximately 5, 15, 30, 60, and 90 minutes after administration. Gastric outflow obstruction is present if minimal or no contrast material is observed aboral to the stomach or duodenum after 30–90 minutes [56].

Early surgical intervention is warranted, as the risk of developing secondary complications, such as aspiration pneumonia, is high. Surgical intervention involves bypass of the affected region with the specific technique chosen dictated by the lesion type and surgeon preference [58, 60]. Surgeons are referred to specific equine surgical textbooks and retrospective studies [56, 58, 60] for intricate details of surgical interventions but some reported surgical techniques for the treatment of gastric outflow obstruction include gastroduodenostomy, gastrojejunostomy with or without jejunojejunostomy, duodenojejunostomy, and pyloroplasty [56]. In brief, gastroduodenostomy is suggested when pyloric obstruction and/or obstruction of the proximal 1–2 cm of duodenum is noted, provided the duodenum distal to the obstruction can be aligned with the stomach without excessive tension. Gastrojejunostomy is suggested when obstruction is at the level of the duodenum and when additional involvement is suspected in cases of pyloric obstruction.

Surgical intervention was previously considered to be hazardous with a poor prognosis, with older reports noting higher mortality rates associated with postoperative complications such as full thickness ulceration and peritonitis, cholangiohepatitis, aspiration pneumonia, stricture of stapled anastomoses, and small intestinal volvulus around the anastomosis site, resulting in high early postoperative mortality [59, 60]. More recently short-, and long-term (≥2 years) survival rates have been more favorable at 97.5% and 69%, respectively [56], further supporting early surgical intervention where possible. Case selection is important with foals with isolated pyloric stenosis having a significantly higher survival rate than those with duodenal involvement [58, 60]. A summary of 40 foals that underwent surgical correction of gastric outflow obstruction is noted in Table 17.II.2.

Where medical therapy is attempted, systemic (IV or IM) therapy with omeprazole [50, 51], esomeprazole [52], or pantaprazole [49] is preferred as the increased dwell time associated with delayed gastric emptying leads to degradation of acid-labile oral PPIs that markedly reduces their efficacy. The use of sucralfate is logical as per the treatment of EGUS (described above), and it may be particularly important in duodenal ulceration where the impact of acid suppressive medication is likely to be minimal. Dietary intervention is also an important element of medical management and affected foals should be restricted to milk only diets wherever possible until documented improvement in gastric emptying is evident.

Motility Disorders and Ileus in the Neonatal Foal

Nonobstructive ileus is a common disorder of neonatal foals, especially those that are recumbent with multiple comorbidities. In human medicine, GI motility disorders are associated with increased duration of ICU stay and mortality [61], and anecdotally a similar effect is seen in equine neonatology.

Obstructive and postoperative ileus are covered elsewhere, but they are relatively uncommon in the neonatal foal. In contrast, nonobstructive, or functional, ileus is common. In human intensive care units the incidence of nonobstructive ileus is as high as 80% [62], and the author's clinical impression is that a high percentage of recumbent foals are affected to varying degrees. Consequences of

Table 17.II.2 Summary of 40 foals that underwent surgical correction of gastric outflow obstruction [56].

Signalment:
- Foals included in study: 40 foals (age range 5–180 d; mean ± SD – 82 ± 37 d)

Historical abnormalities:

• Diarrhea (12/40; 30%)	• Colic (3/40; 7.5%)	• Chronic gastric ulceration (2/40; 5%)
• Pneumonia (1/40; 2.5%)	• Small intestinal volvulus (1/40; 2.5%)	

Physical examination abnormalities:

• Bruxism (38/40; 95%)	• Ptyalism (31/40; 77.5%)	• Fever (>101.5°F; 18/40; 45%)
• Abnormal lung sounds (9/40; 22.5%)	• Diarrhea (9/40; 22.5%)	• Tachycardia (9/40; 22.5%)
• Abdominal distention (4/40; 10%)	• Nasogastric reflux (30/40; 75%; volume 1–10 l)	

Diagnostic imaging:
- Ultrasound examination (17 foals): 12/17 (71%) gastric distension, 5/17 (29%) duodenal abnormalities
- Endoscopic examination (23 foals): 20/23 (87%) linear erosions of esophagus, 17/23 (74%) gastric ulcers
- Barium study (38 foals): 31/38 (82%) no barium aboral to stomach within 90 min of administration

Surgical findings:

• Pyloric abnormalities 8/40 (20%)	• Duodenal lesions 22/40 (55%)	• Pyloric & duodenal lesions 10/40 (25%)

Specific duodenal abnormalities causing obstruction of pylorus (32/40; 80%):

• Mural thickening (14/40; 35%)	• Fibrosis (18/40; 45%)	• Serosal discoloration (4/40; 10%)
• Proximal distension (8/40; 20%)	• Distension of common bile duct (11/40; 28%)	

Postoperative treatment:

• Enteral nutrition withheld 1–10 d (mean 2.3 d)	• Antimicrobial medications 2–10 d (mean 8 d)
• Anti-ulcer medications 7–60 d (mean 25 d)	• Heparin (30 foals) 1–6 d (mean 3 d)
• Flunixin meglumine (23 foals) 1–7 d (mean 3.8 d)	

Non-surgical complications:

• Ileus (10/40; 25%)	• Diarrhea (10/40; 25%)	• Pneumonia (9/40; 23%)
• Incisional infection (6/40; 15%)	• Peritonitis (3/40; 7.5%)	• Thrombophlebitis (2/40; 5%)
• Persistent azotemia (1/40; 2.5%)		

Outcome:
- Short-term survival: discharged from hospital 39/40 (97.5%); deceased foal had suppurative pancreatitis
- Long-term survival (>2 yr): available for 36 foals – 25/36 (69%)
- Competed as racehorse 19/40 (48% of all foals); 19/25 (76% of foals that survived long-term)

nonobstructive ileus include abdominal distention, colic, and intolerance of enteral feeding resulting in failure to meet nutritional needs or a requirement for parental nutrition. In people, ileus is also associated with an increased risk of aspiration pneumonia.

The pathogenesis of nonobstructive ileus is complex and incompletely understood. Activation of inhibitory sympathetic inputs and release of inflammatory mediators, both systemically and locally, have deleterious impacts on GI motility [61, 63]. A range of risk factors have been described in human medicine with hypoperfusion of the GI tract, potentially further exacerbated by the use of vasopressors [61], a central factor of particular relevance to the critically ill foal. Excessive IV fluid therapy, which may cause intestinal wall edema and electrolyte abnormalities (particularly potassium and magnesium) are other key factors in human medicine [61, 62] and are relevant to equine neonatology. Opioid administration is an additional risk factor identified in human medicine [64] that warrants consideration in the neonatal foal.

In addition to nonobstructive ileus, other factors associated with decreased GI motility may have an impact on outcome in the critical care setting. The lower esophageal sphincter, together with the diaphragmatic crura, provides an important defense mechanism that prevents regurgitation of gastric contents into the oropharynx under normal physiological conditions [61]. In people, lower esophageal sphincter pressure and esophageal peristalsis are decreased in critical illness, leading to increased "silent" regurgitation events that may be further exacerbated by the presence of esophageal feeding tubes [61]. Collectively, these factors are present in critically ill foals, and it is logical to presume that these processes may result in increased risk of secondary aspiration pneumonia in this population. It has previously been believed that the use of acid suppressive drugs, such as PPIs, increase the risk of aspiration pneumonia due to alterations in intra-gastric defense mechanisms. However, a recent meta-analysis in human critical care found no association between PPI use and increased risk of aspiration pneumonia [65], making this factor less of a concern.

Management of nonobstructive ileus focuses on high-quality supportive care. The judicious use of fluid therapy, close monitoring of electrolytes (particularly potassium and magnesium) with supplementation when indicated, and overall effective hemodynamic support with sparing use of vasopressors are central to management. Specific pharmaceutical intervention is unlikely to be effective, and despite years of intensive research, there is no consensus in human medicine for the management of nonobstructive ileus beyond a focus on high-quality supportive care [63]. Opioids should be avoided in affected, or at-risk, patients. Instead, where additional analgesia is required, the use of lidocaine (1.3 mg/kg IV bolus over 15 minutes, followed by 50 μg/kg/min [3.0 mg/kg/h]) may serve as an alternative. Despite lidocaine achieving lower concentrations in foals than adult horses [66] the author's clinical impression is that it remains a valuable and well-tolerated approach to analgesia.

Given the high incidence of nonobstructive ileus in recumbent patients and the challenges faced when dealing with enterally intolerant patients, it is tempting to completely avoid enteral feeding in critically ill recumbent foals. However, blanket avoidance of enteral feeding is deleterious as early enteral nutrition is well recognized in human medicine as a critically important strategy to maintain GI motility and perfusion, and mucosal barrier defenses [61, 62]. Considering this, a case-by-case risk assessment should be performed with a preference toward enteral feeding whenever possible, even if only in limited quantities.

In practice, assessment of the foal's overall status should lend particular attention to the cardiovascular status and GI tract (borborygmi, abdominal distension, colic). In questionable cases abdominal ultrasound is a useful adjunct for assessing intestinal distension and motility. Enteral nutrition should not be used in foals with evidence of abdominal bloating, active colic, immotile distended intestine on ultrasound, or those with uncontrolled hypotension.

Barring those exceptions, enteral nutrition is attempted via an indwelling nasogastric tube starting at 5% bwt/d given as q1–2h feedings (approximately 100 ml/h in 50 kg foal). If well tolerated, and the foal is otherwise stable, then feeding is increased to 10% body weight/d after 6–8 hours with subsequent increases dictated by clinical needs and tolerance of enteral feeding. If the increase is not tolerated, or if concerns persist regarding motility at the rate of 10% body weight/d, then the original rate of 5% per day is maintained if tolerated, and the foal's nutritional and volume needs supplemented parentally (Chapter 15). Appropriate positioning, in sternal recumbency with an elevated head, and gentle handling that avoids increasing intra-abdominal pressure are expected to reduce the risk of secondary aspiration pneumonia.

References

1 Clabough, D.L., Roberts, M.C., and Robertson, I. (1991). Probable congenital esophageal stenosis in a Thoroughbred foal. *J. Am. Vet. Med. Assoc.* 199: 483–485.

2 Berlin, D., Shaabon, K., and Peery, D. (2015). Congenital oesophageal stricture in an Arabian filly treated by balloon dilation. *Equine Vet. Educ.* 27: 230–236.

3 Rohrbach, B.W. and Rooney, J.R. (1980). Congenital esophageal ectasia in a Thoroughbred foal. *J. Vet. Med. Assoc.* 177: 65–67.

4 Wong, D.M., Ruby, R.E., Van Eerde, E. et al. (2020). Oesophageal ectasia as a cause of dysphagia and milk regurgitation in a neonatal foal. *Equine Vet. Educ.* 32: O45–O49.

5 Barber, S.M., McLaughlin, B.G., and Fretz, P.B. (1983). Esophageal ectasia in a Quarterhorse colt. *Can. Vet. J.* 24: 46–49.

6 Matsuda, K., Qui, Y., Furuse, T. et al. (2010). Bronchogenic and esophageal cyst with laryngeal malformations in a Thoroughbred foal. *Vet. Pathol.* 47: 351–353.

7 Smith, T.R. (2004). Unusual vascular ring anomaly in a foal. *Can. Vet. J.* 45: 1016–1018.

8 Mackey, V.S., Large, S.M., Breznock, E.M. et al. (1986). Surgical correction of a persistent right aortic arch in a foal. *Vet. Surg.* 15: 325–328.

9 Holcombe, S.J., Hurcombe, S.D., Barr, B.S. et al. (2012). Dysphagia associated with presumed pharyngeal dysfunction in 16 neonatal foals. *Equine Vet. J.* 44: 105–108.

10 Abutarbush, S.M. (2011). Esophageal laceration and obstruction caused by a foreign body in 2 young foals. *Can. Vet. J.* 52: 764–767.

11 Nijdam, P., Elmas, C., and Fugazzola, M.C. (2017). Treatment of an esophageal stricture in a 1-month-old Miniature Shetland colt. Case reports. *Vet. Med.* 2–5.

12 Mira Hernández, J., Posada Arias, S., Castillo Franz, C.A. et al. (2016). Dilation of a proximal esophageal stricture by endoscopically and radiologically guided balloon in a Falabella foal. *Rev. Med. Vet. (Bogota)* 31: 85–95.

13 Gideon, L. (1984). Esophageal anastomosis in two foals. *J. Am. Vet. Med. Assoc.* 184: 1146–1148.

14 Vengust, M., Baird, J.D., van Dreumel, T. et al. (2008). Equid herpesvirus 2-associated oral and esophageal ulceration in a foal. *J. Vet. Diagn. Investig.* 20: 811–815.

15 Gross, T.L. and Mayhew, I.G. (1983). Gastroesophageal ulceration and candidiasis in foals. *J. Am. Vet. Med. Assoc.* 182: 1370–1373.

16 Lewis, S. (2003). Gastric ulceration in an equine neonate. *Can. Vet. J.* 44: 420–421.

17 Murray, M.J., Grodinsky, C., Coweles, R.R. et al. (1990). Endoscopic evaluation of changes in gastric lesions of Thoroughbred foals. *J. Am. Vet. Med. Assoc.* 196: 1623–1627.

18 Murray, M.J., Murray, C.M., Sweeney, H.J. et al. (1990). Prevalence of gastric lesions in foals without signs of gastric disease: an endoscopic survey. *Equine Vet. J.* 22: 6–8.

19 Okai, K., Taharaguchi, S., Orita, Y. et al. (2015). Comparative endoscopic evaluation of normal and ulcerated gastric mucosae in thoroughbred foals. *J. Vet. Med. Sci.* 77: 449–453.

20 Elfenbein, J.R. and Sanchez, L.C. (2012). Prevalence of gastric and duodenal ulceration in 691 nonsurviving foals (1995–2006). *Equine Vet. J.* 44: 76–79.

21 Sykes, B.W.W., Hewetson, M., Hepburn, R.J.J. et al. (2015). European College of Equine Internal Medicine Consensus Statement-Equine Gastric Ulcer Syndrome in adult horses. *J. Vet. Int. Med.* 29: 1288–1299.

22 Sanchez, L.C., Murray, M.J., and Merrit, A.M. (2004). Effect of omeprazole paste on intragastric pH in clinically normal neonatal foals. *Am. J. Vet. Res.* 65: 1039–1041.

23 Merritt, A.M., Sanchez, L.C., Burrow, J.A. et al. (2010). Effect of GastroGard and three compounded oral omeprazole preparations on 24 h intragastric pH in gastrically cannulated mature horses. *Equine Vet. J.* 35: 691–695.

24 Sykes, B.W., Underwood, C., and Mills, P.C. (2017). The effects of dose and diet on the pharmacodynamics of esomeprazole in the horse. *Equine Vet. J.* 49: 637–642.

25 Sykes, B.W., Underwood, C., Greer, R. et al. (2017). The effects of dose and diet on the pharmacodynamics of omeprazole in the horse. *Equine Vet. J.* 49: 525–531.

26 Sykes, B.W., Kathawala, K., Song, Y. et al. (2017). Preliminary investigations into a novel, long-acting, injectable, intramuscular formulation of omeprazole in the horse. *Equine Vet. J.* 49: 795–801.

27 Husted, L., Sanchez, L.C., Baptiste, K.E. et al. (2009). Effect of a feed/fast protocol on pH in the proximal equine stomach. *Equine Vet. J.* 41: 658–662.

28 Sanchez, L.C., Lester, G.D., and Merritt, A.M. (2001). Intragastric pH in critically ill neonatal foals and the effect of ranitidine. *J. Am. Vet. Med. Assoc.* 218: 907–911.

29 Barr, B.S., Wilkins, P.A., Del Piero, F. et al. (2000). Is prophylaxis for gastric uclers necassary in critically ill equine neonates? A retrospective study of necropsy cases 1989–1999. *J. Vet. Int. Med.* 14: 328.

30 Richardson, L.M., Whitfield-Cargile, C.M., Cohen, N.D. et al. (2018). Effect of selective versus nonselective cyclooxygenase inhibitors on gastric ulceration scores and intestinal inflammation in horses. *Vet. Surg.* 47: 784–791.

31 Furr, M., Cohen, N.D., Axon, J.E. et al. (2012). Treatment with histamine-type 2 receptor antagonists and omeprazole increase the risk of diarrhoea in neonatal foals treated in intensive care units. *Equine Vet. J.* 44: 80–86.

32 Costa, M.C., Stämpfli, H.R., Allen-Vercoe, E. et al. (2016). Development of the faecal microbiota in foals. *Equine Vet. J.* 48: 681–688.

33 Pagan, J.D., Petroski-Rose, L., Mann, A. et al. (2020). Omeprazole reduces calcium digestibility in Thoroughbred horses. *J. Equine Vet. Sci.* 86: 1–5.

34 Malchodi, L., Wagner, K., Susi, A. et al. (2019). Early acid suppression therapy exposure and fracture in young children. *Pediatrics* 144: 1–9.

35 Freedberg, D.E., Haynes, K., Denburg, M.R. et al. (2015). Use of proton pump inhibitors is associated with fractures in young adults: a population-based study. *Osteoporos. Int.* 26: 2501–2507.

36 Ricord, M., Andrews, F.M., Yniguez, F.J.M. et al. (2021). Impact of concurrent treatment with omeprazole on phenylbutazone-induced equine gastric ulcer syndrome (EGUS). *Equine Vet. J.* 53: 256–363.

37 Manzoni, P., Sanchez, R., Meyer, M. et al. (2018). Exposure to gastric acid inhibitors increases the risk of infection in preterm very low birth weight infants but concomitant administration of lactoferrin counteracts this effect. *J. Pediatr.* 193: 62–67.

38 Chung, E.Y. and Yardley, J. (2013). Are there risks associated with empiric acid suppression treatment of

infants and children suspected of having gastroesophageal reflux disease? *Hosp. Pediatr.* 3: 16–23.

39 Costarino, A.T., Dai, D., Feng, R. et al. (2015). Gastric acid suppressant prophylaxis in pediatric intensive care: current practice as reflected in a large administrative database. *Pediatr. Crit. Care Med.* 16: 605–612.

40 Carrion, V. and Egan, E.A. (1990). Prevention of neonatal necrotizing enterocolitis. *J. Pediatr. Gastroenterol. Nutr.* 11: 317–323.

41 Zedtwitz-Liebenstein, K., Wenisch, K., Patruta, S. et al. (2002). Omeprazole treatment diminishes intra- and extracellular neutrophil reactive oxygen production and bactericidal activity. *Crit. Care Med.* 30: 1118–1122.

42 Graham, P.L., Begg, M.D., Larson, E. et al. (2006). Risk factors for late onset gram-negative sepsis in low birth weight infants hospitalized in the neonatal intensive care unit. *Pediatr. Infect. Dis. J.* 25: 113–117.

43 Vincent, J.L., Bihari, D.J., Suter, P.M. et al. (1995). The prevalence of nosocomial infection in intensive care units in Europe: results of the European prevalence of infection in intensive care (EPIC) study. *J. Am. Med. Assoc.* 274: 639–644.

44 Geor, R.J., Petrie, L., Papich, M.G. et al. (1989). The protective effects of sucralfate and ranitidine in foals experimentally intoxicated with phenylbutazone. *Can. J. Vet. Res.* 53: 231–238.

45 Rendle, D. (2018). Recommendations for the management of equine glandular gastric disease. *UK-Vet. Equine.* 2: 2–11.

46 Gough, S., Hallowell, G., and Rendle, D. (2020). A study investigating the treatment of equine squamous gastric disease with long-acting injectable or oral omeprazole. *Vet. Med. Sci.* 6: 235–241.

47 Javsicas, L.H. and Sanchez, L.C. (2008). The effect of omeprazole paste on intragastric pH in clinically ill neonatal foals. *Equine Vet. J.* 40: 41–44.

48 Sykes, B.W. (2019). Courses for horses: rethinking the use of proton pump inhibitors in the treatment of equine gastric ulcer syndrome. *Equine Vet. Educ.* 31: 441–446.

49 Ryan, C.A., Sanchez, L.C., Giguere, S. et al. (2010). Pharmacokinetics and pharmacodynamics of pantoprazole in clinically normal neonatal foals. *Equine Vet. J.* 37: 336–341.

50 Jenkins, C.C., Frazier, D.L., Blackford, J.T. et al. (2010). Pharmacokinetics and antisecretory effects of intravenous omeprazole in horses. *Equine Vet. J.* 24: 84–88.

51 Haven, M.L., Dave, K., Burrow, J.A. et al. (1999). Comparison of the antisecretory effects of omeprazole when administered intravenously, as acid-stable granules and as an oral paste in horses. *Equine Vet. J. Suppl.* 31: 54–58.

52 Videla, R., Sommardahl, C.S., Elliott, S.B. et al. (2011). Effects of intravenously administered esomeprazole sodium on gastric juice pH in adult female horses. *J. Vet. Intern. Med.* 25: 558–562.

53 Holland, P.S., Brumbaugh, G.W., Ruoff, W.W. et al. (1997). Plasma pharmacokinetics of ranitidine HCl in foals. *J. Vet. Pharmacol. Ther.* 20: 447–452.

54 Borne, A.T. and MacAllister, C.G. (1993). Effect of sucralfate on healing of subclinical gastric ulcers in foals. *J. Am. Vet. Med. Assoc.* 202: 1465–1468.

55 Traub-Dagartz, J., Bayly, W., Riggs, M. et al. (1985). Exsanguination due to gastric ulceration in a foal. *J. Am. Vet. Med. Assoc.* 186: 280–281.

56 Zedler, S.T., Embertson, R.M., Bernard, W.V. et al. (2009). Surgical treatment of gastric outflow obstruction in 40 foals. *Vet. Surg.* 38: 623–630.

57 Kol, A., Steinman, A., Levi, O. et al. (2005). Congenital pyloric stenosis in a foal. *Isr. J. Vet. Med.* 60: 59–62.

58 Orsini, J.A. and Donawick, W.J. (1986). Surgical treatment of gastroduodenal obstructions in foals. *Vet. Surg.* 15: 205–213.

59 Venner, M. (2004). Pyloric stenosis: a rare disease with a typical anamnesis. *Equine Vet. Educ.* 16: 176–177.

60 Campbell-Thompson, M.L., Brown, M.P., Slone, D.E. et al. (1986). Gastroenterostomy for treatment of gastroduodenal ulcer disease in 14 foals. *J. Am. Vet. Med. Assoc.* 188: 840–844.

61 Aderinto-Adike, A.O. and Quigley, E.M.M. (2014). Gastrointestinal motility problems in critical care: a clinical perspective. *J. Diagn. Dis.* 15: 335–344.

62 Caddell, K.A., Martindale, R., McClave, S.A. et al. (2011). Can the intestinal dysmotility of critical illness be differentiated from postoperative ileus? *Curr. Gastroenterol. Rep.* 13: 358–367.

63 Bauer, A.J., Schwarz, N.T., Moore, B.A. et al. (2002). Ileus in critical illness: mechanisms and management. *Curr. Opin. Crit. Care* 8: 152–157.

64 Nguyen, T., Frenette, A.J., Johanson, C. et al. (2013). Impaired gastrointestinal transit and its associated morbidity in the intensive care unit. *J. Crit. Care* 28: 537.

65 Alshamsi, F., Belley-Cote, E., Cook, D. et al. (2016). Efficacy and safety of proton pump inhibitors for stress ulcer prophylaxis in critically ill patients: a systematic review and meta-analysis of randomized trials. *Crit. Care* 20.

66 Ohmes, C. (2014). *The Disposition of Lidocaine During a 6-Hour Intravenous Infusion to Young Foals*. Kansas State University.

Section III Enteritis, Colitis, and Diarrhea

Nathan M. Slovis

Gastrointestinal (GI) failure is associated with a variety of disorders in foals and can manifest as diarrhea, ileus, abdominal pain, obstipation, and weight loss. Clinical syndromes associated with GI failure include enteritis, colitis, meconium impactions, and necrotizing enterocolitis (NEC). Numerous noninfectious and infectious agents are responsible for enteritis and colitis in the neonatal foal. Formulating a diagnostic plan is important when trying to determine if an infectious agent is responsible for the GI disorder. Common infectious causes of enteritis in neonates include rotavirus, coronavirus, *Salmonella, Clostridium perfringens A* and *C*, *Clostridium difficile,* and *Enterococcus durans/hirae*. This chapter reviews common causes, pathogenesis, clinical manifestations, diagnosis, and treatment for noninfectious and infectious equine neonatal diarrhea.

Formulating a Diagnostic Plan

The goal of the diagnostic plan for detecting pathogenic organisms is threefold:

1) Determine if the pathogenic organism can be detected (Qualitative testing).
2) If the pathogenic organism can be detected, how much is present (Quantification).
3) If the pathogenic organism can be detected, identify the (bacterial) organism and its antibiogram.

Diagnostic methods for pathogen detection in foals with diarrhea include microscopy, bacterial culture, immunological (ELISA – enzyme linked imunnosorbent assay), and molecular methods (PCR – polymerase chain reaction). The effectiveness of a proper diagnostic plan depends on appropriate sample collection. Clinicians must be cognizant of safety precautions when collecting fecal samples; all sample collections should be obtained while wearing gloves and placed in a leak-proof container to prevent environmental contamination during transport. Samples should be at least 1 g (size of an adult's thumb nail) or four fecal swabs with adequate manure staining of the swabs. Most pathogens resulting in foal diarrhea can cause a wide spectrum of overlapping clinical syndromes that make it difficult to decide which organism(s) to test for. PCR is a molecular technique that amplifies a DNA fragment via enzymatic replication and has advantages over conventional laboratory diagnostic techniques because results are quick, accurate, affordable, and have high sensitivity and specificity. Multiplex PCR is available and offers testing for a variety of enteric pathogens using one fecal sample. This is preferred over single pathogen testing, as a study has documented that the rate of coinfections in cases of diarrhea in foals is not uncommon [1]. If there are multiple cases of diarrhea on a farm, pooling of fecal samples from several foals, and performance of multiplex PCR on the combined sample is more cost-effective. If a pathogen from a pooled fecal sample is detected, it can be assumed that the pathogen is the causative agent. The author routinely performs pooled fecal testing for enteric pathogens and acknowledges that pooling fecal samples for equine enteric pathogens has been validated only for *Salmonella enterica* and not the other pathogens [2].

Noninfectious Diarrhea

Foal Heat Diarrhea

Foal heat diarrhea is experienced by up to 80% of healthy foals at 1–2 weeks of age [3]. Mares experience their first post-foaling estrus known as "foal heat" during a similar time, thus forming an assumed association between the two [4]. Most foals remain bright and alert, maintain normal hematology and laboratory results, and continue to

Equine Neonatal Medicine, First Edition. Edited by David M. Wong and Pamela A. Wilkins.

nurse while experiencing foal heat diarrhea [5]. Orphaned foals and foals kept on milk replacer experience a similar episode of diarrhea as foals kept on the mare, thereby ruling out the mare or her milk as a cause [6]. Although the origin is still uncertain, one theory for foal heat diarrhea is the development of GI flora associated with the ingestion of other feeds and the natural tendency of coprophagy [3, 6]. Other possible causes have been studied and ruled out. For example, one study observed the GI and endocrine function of 11 foals, 10 of which experienced foal heat diarrhea. There was no relationship found between diarrhea and any of the following theories: IgG concentrations in foal plasma, viral, parasitic, or bacterial pathogens, lactose digestion, or intestinal gas production [7]. In Ocala, Florida, fecal composition of 10 foals was evaluated during foal heat and fecal osmolality and volatile fatty acid concentrations were observed to drop abruptly at the onset of diarrhea while electrolyte concentrations were noted to increase simultaneously, suggesting that foal heat diarrhea may be caused by small intestinal hypersecretion [7]. Another study investigated the presence of yeast as a cause, which was also ruled out. Cultured yeasts have been associated with contamination from the environment in which the foals were living rather than being the cause of diarrhea [3].

Foal heat diarrhea rarely requires treatment and foals naturally recover on their own. In severe cases, IV fluids may be needed to replace fluid losses. A study performed in Poland across four stud farms noted that bentonite clay in the form of paste given to foals for 3 consecutive days, starting on the first day of diarrhea, significantly reduced the duration and severity of foal heat diarrhea. Bentonite clay has absorptive properties that reduces fecal fluid level, and in this study, suggested that foal heat diarrhea can be caused by disturbances in the intestinal osmotic balance [8].

Nutritional

Nutrition plays a large role in fecal composition. Diarrhea of nutritional etiology is more often seen in foals receiving milk replacer, especially when the replacer is prepared incorrectly using a concentration higher or lower than manufacture's recommendations [5]. Foals fed milk replacer tend to have looser feces compared to consumption of mare's or goat's milk. The author adds goat milk to milk replacer (ratio of 1 : 10) to help reduce diarrhea. In addition, mares that are high milk producers may cause their foal to be overfed. This can result in a large amount of undigested lactose reaching the large intestine where fermentation leads to osmotic diarrhea [6]. Primary lactose intolerance is a rare cause of diarrhea, but if present milk intake for these foals should be restricted [5]. Foals with lactose intolerance usually continue to have diarrhea until weaned from the mare. These foals continue to gain bodyweight, but fecal consistency is not normal until they are removed from the mare (Table 17.III.1). Supplementation with lactase enzyme (6000 Food Chemical Codex [FCC] units/50-kg foal, PO, q3–8h) is indicated in foals with suspected lactase deficiency (Figure 17.III.1). Lactose intolerance can be confirmed with a lactose tolerance test (Chapter 15), but this test is usually unnecessary as supplementation is inexpensive and practical [5, 9].

Table 17.III.1 Causes of lactose intolerance.

- Lactose malabsorption:
  - Physiological problem that arises from the consumption of too much lactose and the capacity for lactase to hydrolyze it (to glucose and galactose).
    Example: overfeeding or incorrectly prepared milk replacer.
- Secondary lactase deficiency (Figure 17.III.1)
  - A lactase deficiency that results to injury of the brush border (location of lactase enzyme).
    Example: during enterocolitis.
- Primary Lactase deficiency
  - Low or completely absent lactase concentrations

Sand Accumulation/Pica

Through natural coprophagy, some foals ingest large amounts of sand or dirt, whose abrasive characteristics are irritating to the GI mucosa [6]. The continuous intake of sand (and dirt) with feed without its equivalent excretion in stool may result in accumulation in the digestive tract and can result in digestive disorders. Sand colic is the most common symptom of sand intake, as the accumulating sand can cause mechanical irritation of the GI mucosa, decrease peristalsis, and narrow the intestinal lumen. Colic is the most common clinical sign of sand intake; however, foals can present with diarrhea, with or without colic [6, 10]. Sand ingestion can affect foals as young as 1 week of age, but is more common in older foals and adult horses [11]. Sand accumulation predominantly affects horses in geographical areas with sandy (light) soils and little rain and almost exclusively affects foals/horses that spend most of their time on poor condition pastures in dry areas or in paddocks and stalls with dirt floors. Hay collected from fields with numerous molehills may also contain excessive amounts of sand and may be associated with this pathology [10]. Diagnosis is easily made with gentle manual (digital) palpation of the rectum and evaluation of the feces. Abdominal radiography is definitive for radiodense material such as sand. Recently, serial monitoring of the evacuation of sand through ultrasonography has been described [12]. In the authors' opinion, the sedimentation test using a rectal glove is the quickest and easiest diagnostic method and due to its simplicity, can be carried out in the field. However, the amount of sand excreted in the

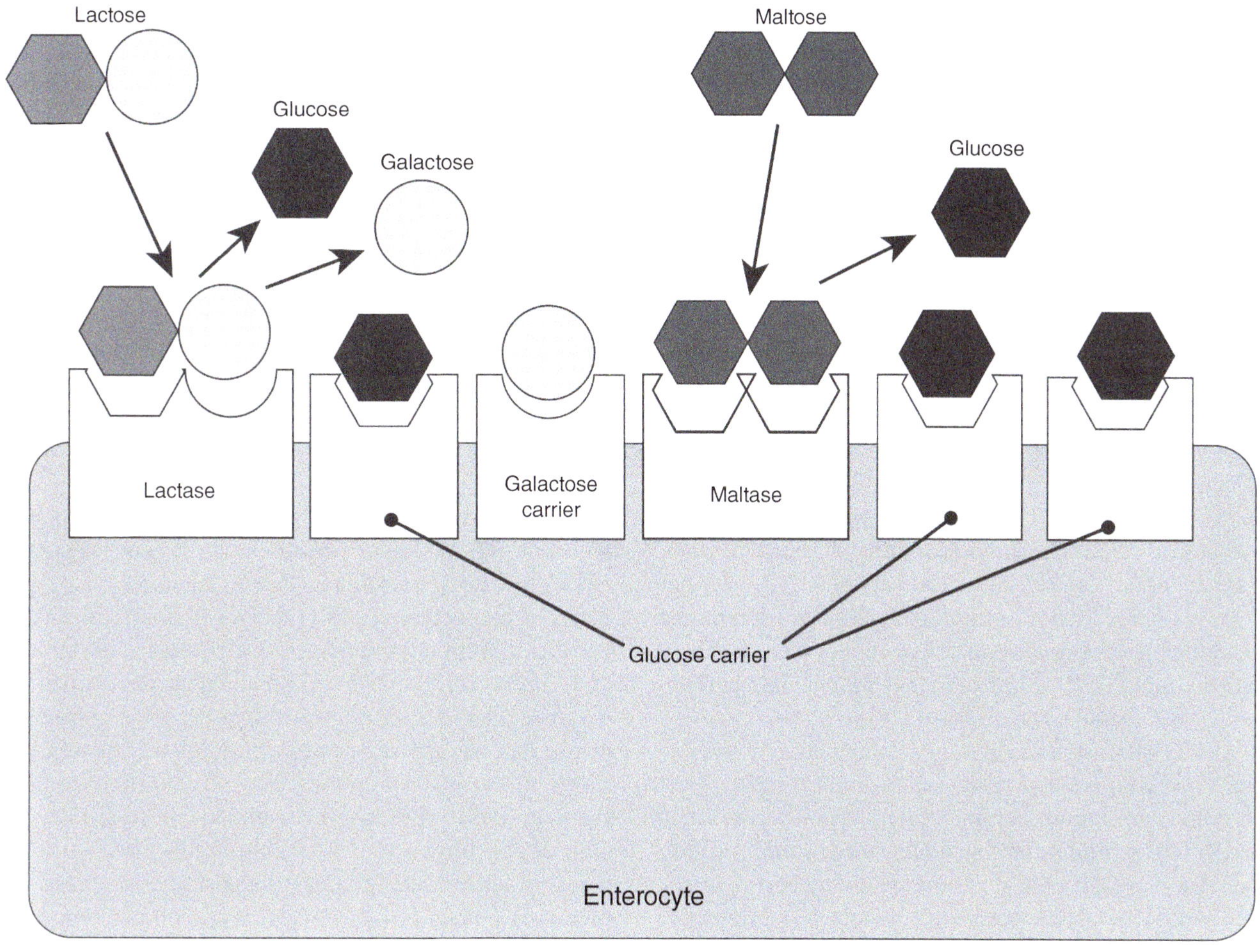

Figure 17.III.1 Schematic of brush border on the enterocyte and the digestive enzymes lactase and maltase.

stool is not an accurate indicator of the amount of sand accumulated in the GI tract [10]. Abdominal ultrasonography was the most reliable and practical diagnostic tool used in this study, hence, both diagnostics should be used concurrently to improve accuracy [12].

Treatment of foals with sand accumulation includes supportive care consisting of enteral laxatives, including mineral oil and, when severe, IV fluid therapy with appropriate analgesics may be necessary. The author has also used psyllium hydrophilic mucilloid in eliminating sand impactions.

Necrotizing Enterocolitis and Pneumatosis Intestinalis

Perinatal asphyxia syndrome (PAS) can cause equine neonatal encephalopathy, resulting in neurological deficits ranging from hypotonia to grand mal seizures. Foals affected with PAS can also experience GI disturbances ranging from mild ileus, delayed gastric emptying, gastroduodenal reflux, and intolerance to enteral feeding to colic, abdominal distension, severe bloody diarrhea, and NEC (Figure 17.III.2). In one foal study, the presence of

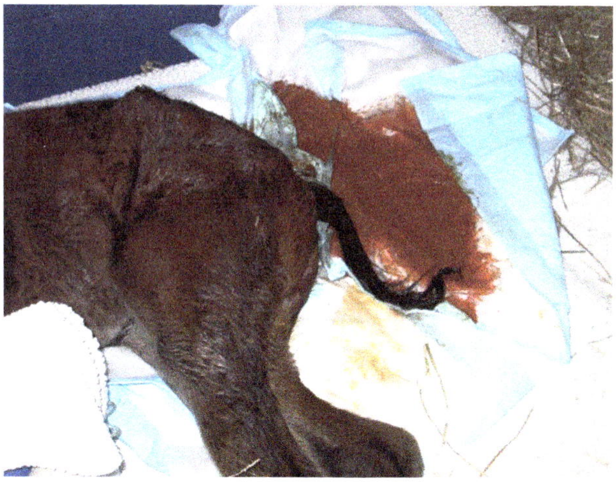

Figure 17.III.2 Neonatal foal with severe bloody diarrhea possibly associated with necrotizing enterocolitis (NEC).

necrotizing GI disease was significantly associated with prematurity, blood in the feces, gastric reflux, and abdominal distension [13]. It has been postulated that when the preterm infant is stressed by periods of hypoxia or hypotension, blood flow is redistributed via input from the adrenergic system away from the splanchnic bed. During reperfusion, oxygen-free radicals are generated and cause tissue damage that is typically seen with reperfusion injury. If the hypoxic event is severe enough, NEC can occur, resulting in bloody diarrhea, pneumatosis intestinalis (PI), ascites, and/or intestinal perforation.

The complete pathogenesis of NEC in infants in unclear, and although a similar syndrome has been noted in foals, even less is known in regard to NEC in equids [13, 14]. In infants, NEC is associated with necrotic injury to the mucosal and submucosal layers of the GI tract, GI inflammation, and bacterial invasion of the bowel wall [5, 13]; any region of the GI tract (stomach to rectum) can be affected by NEC, but the distal small intestine and proximal colon are more commonly involved [5]. In infants, symptoms of NEC include abdominal distension, ileus, hematochezia, emesis, and signs of sepsis [5]. NEC has been rarely reported in foals, but clinical signs of reported cases included ileus, gastric reflux, intolerance of enteral feeding, and PI radiographically [14]. In two foals, perforation of the ventral colon occurred [14].

NEC is believed to result from a combination of interactions revolving around the developmental immaturity of the neonate, GI mucosal injury, enteral feeding, and bacterial invasion. Most infants with NEC are preterm, suggesting that the lack of GI maturation is important in the development of NEC. Premature infants may experience decreased GI perfusion due to vasoconstriction, hypotension, and thrombosis [5]. In one case report of NEC in two foals, one foal was preterm and the other was full term but likely exposed to hypoxia during a prolonged delivery [14]. Mucosal injury from hypoxic–ischemic injury, free radical damage, impaired circulation dynamics to the GI tract, or combination thereof, is the second factor in the development of NEC. The initial ischemia-induced mucosal injury in the immature infant is believed to predispose infants to bacterial invasion of the bowel wall; in turn, milk serves as a substrate for bacterial proliferation and infection. Abnormal intestinal gas originating from bacterial proliferation can result in the development of subsequent PI. Based on limited information, foals with NEC should not be fed enteral feedings but rather partial or total parenteral nutrition (PPN/TPN) to meet nutritional needs. Antimicrobials targeting anerobic overgrowth along with broad-spectrum antimicrobials to attenuate sepsis should be administered [5, 14].

PI, the presence of intramural gas, is not a diagnosis or clinical disease, but rather a physical or radiographic finding that is highly indicative of an underlying pathological process [13]. One retrospective study of PI in foals described the ultrasonographic appearance of PI as hyperechoic echoes casting a dirty shadow within the bowel wall consistent with intramural gas (Figure 17.III.3a). Ileus and abnormal peritoneal fluid defined on ultrasound as diffuse hypomotility and distension of the GI viscera (Figure 17.III.3b) and hypoechoic to echoic peritoneal fluid or increased amount of peritoneal fluid (Figure 17.III.3c), respectively, was noted in some cases of PI [13]. In that report, PI was most frequently imaged as scattered hyperechoic foci within the intestinal wall, but large clusters of hyperechoic foci within the bowel wall was also imaged in some foals. Intramural gas was imaged in the small intestine in 58% (11/19) of foals, the large intestine in 32% (6/19), and in both the small and large intestine in 10.5% (2/19) [13].

The pathogenesis of PI is a multifaceted phenomenon with several possible mechanisms by which gas forms within the wall of the GI tract and include intraluminal GI gas and bacterial production of gas [15]. Two mechanisms enable bacteria to form intramural gas: direct invasion of the wall by bacteria and alteration of intraluminal gas content by bacteria. Direct gas diffusion and direct invasion of bacteria across mucosa can occur with injury to the mucosa. As stated earlier, PI is a multifaceted phenomenon because there are many disorders that can alter mucosal integrity without the formation of PI. PI can be diagnostic for NEC when other clinical findings support the diagnosis of NEC [16]. A diagnosis of PAS ileus is presumptive when the patient has a history of peripartum asphyxia (placentitis, premature placental separation, dystocia, cesarean section, umbilical cord problem), negative fecal diagnostics for infectious diseases, and distended small intestine with decreased motility noted on ultrasonography (Figure 17.III.3b). Treatment for NEC and PI includes "resting" the intestinal tract and utilization of PPN or TPN. Treating the underlying disease with antimicrobials is also warranted.

Infectious Diarrhea

Rotavirus

Foals are most susceptible to viral diarrhea during the neonatal, perinatal, and suckling periods by virtue of being immunological naïve [17]. *Rotavirus* is a genus within the family Reoviridae. By electron microscopy, rotavirus is approximately 70–80 nm in size and has the appearance of a wheel (*rota*, derived from the Latin word for "wheel") with short spokes radiating from a wide central hub (Figure 17.III.4).

Rotaviruses are double stranded, ribonucleic acid (RNA), nonenveloped viruses subdivided into several groups (A

(a)

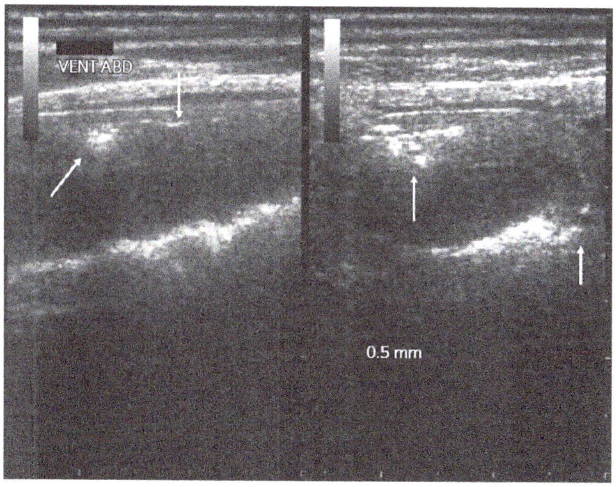

(b)

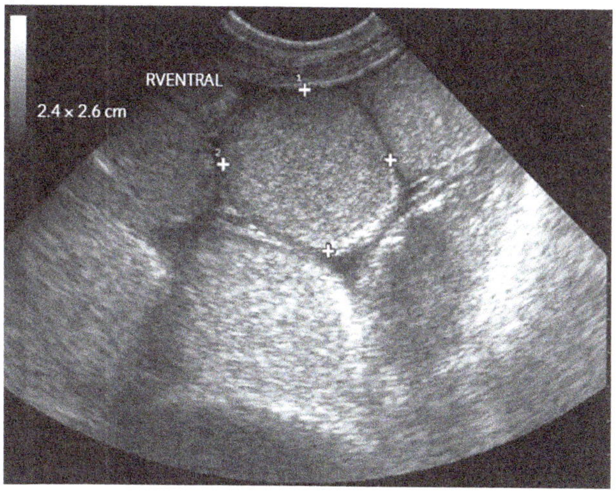

(c)

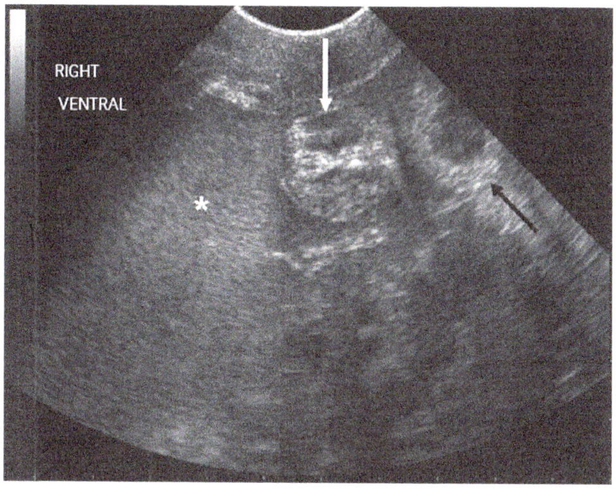

Figure 17.III.3 (a) Sonogram of ventral abdomen from foal with enterocolitis. Note hyperechoic intramural gas echoes (arrows) with a loop of thickened small intestine (5 mm). The gas echoes are imaged in mutually perpendicular longitudinal (left) and transverse (right) panes. (b) Sonogram of abdomen obtained from a foal with enterocolitis. Note the distended loops of small intestine consistent with ileus. (c) Sonogram of ventral abdomen of foal with enterocolitis. Note the increased amount of echoic peritoneal fluid (asterisk) surrounding loops of ileum (white arrow) and jejunum (black arrow). *Source:* From Navas de Solis 2012 [13].

through G) based on differences in the group-specific inner capsid protein, VP6. Three rotavirus groups (A, B, and C) cause disease in people compared to only two groups that affects horses (Group B) [19]. Equine rotavirus can be further subdivided using neutralizing antibodies to the VP4 and VP7 outer capsid proteins into P (Proteinase sensitive, VP4 positive) and G (Glycoprotein, VP-7 positive) serotypes [20]. Five P serotypes (P1, P6, P7, P12, and P18) and eight G serotypes (G1, G3, G5, G8, G10, G13, G14, and G16) have been identified in horses [20].

In 2017, Dr. Udeni Balasuriya processed 108 diarrhea samples from foals <6 months of age from 38 farms in central Kentucky. Of these diarrheal samples, 23/108 (21%) were positive for equine rotavirus type A [21]. Further assessment detected that 17/23 (74%) were the G14 strain, 6/23 (26%) were the G3 strain, and one foal was coinfected with both. Previous studies conducted in Kentucky noted that 100% of equine rotavirus type A were the G3 strain. This is particularly disturbing because various genetic and antigenic variants of G3 and G14 are circulating in the horse population in central Kentucky, and they significantly differ from the vaccine strain currently used in the field.

Starting in February 2021, there has been an increase in frequency of diarrhea in neonatal (24–72 hour old) foals in central Kentucky whose dams had been immunized with a commercial inactivated equine rotavirus group A (ERVA) vaccine. Diagnostic investigation of fecal samples collected from seven foals with severe watery to hemorrhagic diarrhea did not detect evidence of diarrhea-associated pathogens including ERVA. Based on Illumina-based metagenomic sequencing, a novel equine rotavirus group B (ERVB) was identified in fecal specimens from affected foals in the absence of any other known enteric pathogens [22]. The

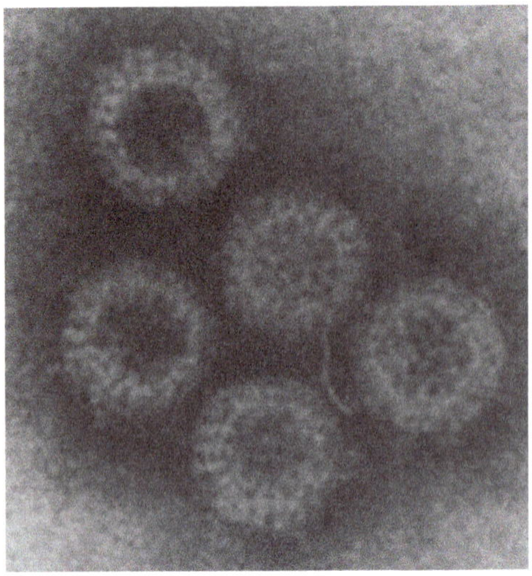

Figure 17.III.4 Rotavirus particles as seen by negatively stained electron microscopy. *Source:* From Rodger et al. [18].

complete protein-coding sequence of the ERVB was determined; interestingly, the sequence of all 11 segments had >96% protein sequence identity with group B rotaviruses previously identified in calves and goats. Furthermore, phylogenetic analysis demonstrated clustering of the ERVB with group B rotaviruses of ruminant origin, particularly with caprine and bovine strains from the United States. Subsequent analysis of 33 foal diarrheic samples by RT-qPCR identified 23 rotavirus B-positive cases (69.69%). These observations suggest that the ERVB originated from ruminants. It is in circulation in horses in the United States and has been associated with outbreaks of neonatal foal diarrhea during the 2021 and 2022 foaling season in Kentucky. Farms that were experiencing increased cases in 2021 were not affected as severely as the naïve farms. Studies are currently ongoing by Dr. Emma Adam (Maxwell H. Gluck Equine Research Center, University of Kentucky) to determine if the mares are a source of infection for the foals and if older foals can be affected with this virus. Farms that have been affected have reported that foaling outside and limiting human handling for the first 5 days of life has significantly reduced morbidity. Emergence of the ruminant-like group B rotavirus in foals warrants further investigation due to the significant impact of the disease in neonatal foals and its economic impact on the equine industry.

Clinical Signs

Clinical signs of disease, including diarrhea, lethargy, anorexia, and abdominal tympani, have been reported in foals <6 months old and most often foals <3 months old [23]. A 3-year study of horse farms in central Kentucky during the 1980s noted that rotavirus was the most common cause of diarrhea in foals [22]. Rotavirus is species specific with an incubation period of 1–2 days. In healthy animals, the brush border epithelium of the small intestine synthesizes disaccharides to monosaccharides (glucose and galactose), which are absorbed in the gut. With rotaviral infection, the virus invades the intestinal epithelium on the sides and tips of the villi of the small intestine. Enterocyte destruction of the brush border villi results in decreased lactase formation, consequently resulting in undigested lactose. This sugar remains in the lumen of the gut, osmotically attracting more fluid. This effect is compounded as bacteria in the large intestine ferment lactose into acetate, propionate, and butyrate, which increase osmolality of the colonic contents [9]. Of note, intestinal crypt cells are not affected and continue to replicate, eventually replacing the tip cells destroyed by the virus, resulting in self-limiting disease. Foals infected with rotavirus may shed the virus for up to 10 days while some horses may shed the virus for up to 8 months; the virus can persist in the environment for up to 9 months [24, 25]. As the virus is highly contagious, rotavirus infections can occur as outbreaks on farms with transmission occurring directly (foal-to-foal contact) or indirectly (personnel or fomites).

Diagnosis

Diagnosis requires detection of the virus in feces via electron microscopy, enzyme-linked immunoassay (ELISA), PCR, and/or latex agglutination virogen rotatest.[1] In a study by the author, human specific rotavirus antigen detection (Rotatest) was compared with an equine specific real-time PCR (IDEXX Equine Diarrhea Panel RealPCR™) and demonstrated the inadequacy of using some human diagnostic tests in veterinary medicine (false negatives). Analysis of 35 samples with the human specific rotavirus immunoassay resulted in no positive results. Within that same group of samples, 13 were positive when real-time PCR was used. Real-time PCR was confirmed by resequencing VP4 and VP7 genes with outside primers. Sequences showed 98% identities to equine rotavirus isolates deposited in GenBank. These results suggest that the immunoassay with human specificity may not detect some equine isolates.

Treatment

Treatment is generally empirical and symptomatic, including precautionary antibiotics and anti-ulcer medications (sucralfate 1 g per 50 kg PO q6h and/or omeprazole 1–4 mg/kg PO q24h). Lactase[2] (6000 FCC lactase U/50 kg PO q3–8h for 10–14 days) has been used to improve digestion of milk lactose. Antidiarrheal medications such as 1.75% bismuth subsalicylate (0.5–1 ml/kg PO q6–24 h in 50 kg foal) might help reduce intestinal inflammation and provide secondary toxin adsorption and resorption when combined with activated charcoal (1 g/kg q24h). Neostigmine (1 mg SQ q1–8h, or IV if severe tympany) is often used to help relieve

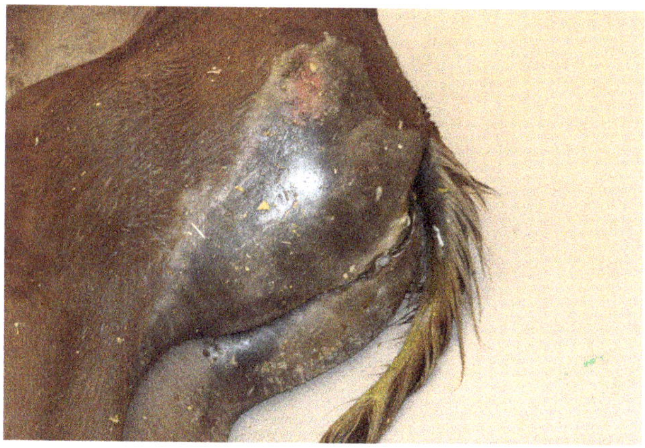

Figure 17.III.5 Foal with severe diarrhea resulting in scalding and alopecia of the perineal region.

GI tympany. Intravenous fluid therapy is necessary to correct hydration and electrolyte imbalances, if noted. A novel adjunctive treatment used for viral causes of diarrhea is administration of oral Bentonite clay [26].[3] Supportive care and hygiene are necessary for foals with diarrhea to avoid pressure ulcers, perineal scalding (Figure 17.III.5), and secondary infections. Stalls should have deep bedding and be kept as clean as possible. Baby oil, baby power, zinc oxide ointment, or diaper rash ointments can be applied to the help prevent perineal dermatitis. Rotaviral diarrhea has a low mortality and high morbidity in foal populations.

Prevention of Rotavirus Disease

Prevention of disease includes proper hygiene and use of phenol disinfectants or peroxygens, as bleach in ineffective at killing rotavirus. A commercial modified live vaccine[4] is available for use in mares prior to foaling (administered at 8, 9, and 10 months of gestation) to help accentuate colostral antibodies [23]. One vaccine study compared 100 foals from vaccinated mares to 65 foals from unvaccinated mares; in this study, 30% of foals from vaccinated mares developed diarrhea as compared to 80% of foals from unvaccinated mares [27]. Of note, foals from vaccinated mares can still become infected with rotavirus although clinical signs may be attenuated. This was demonstrated in the aforementioned study in which duration of diarrhea was shorter in foals from vaccinated mares (1.8 days verses 7.3 days). Another important variable in that study was there was 80% shedding from diarrheic foals from unvaccinated mares as compared to 0% shedding in foals from vaccinated mares [27]. A different field study noted that the rotavirus vaccine was safe and immunogenic when administered to mares at 8, 9, and 10 months of gestation. Furthermore, a lower incidence of rotaviral diarrhea in foals born to vaccinated mares as compared to unvaccinated mares, but this difference was not statistically significant [23].

Coronavirus

Equine coronavirus (ECoV) was isolated and characterized in 2000 but described as an infectious agent in ill foals in 1976 [28–30]. Several studies and case reports have identified coronaviruses in foals with enteric disease, but the pathogenicity and its etiologic role in enteric disease have not been examined. A recent prevalence study in central Kentucky by the author clearly shows that healthy foals without signs of GI disease are equally infected with equine coronavirus as ill foals. This finding suggests low pathogenicity of ECoV in foals. However, when analyzed as a coinfecting agent, EcoV was significantly associated with diseased animals. Specifically, all EcoV infections in the GI disease group were associated with coinfections (15/15), while foals in the healthy group were mostly mono-infected (8/10) [1]. This supports the theory that certain viruses act primarily as immunosuppressing agents, allowing opportunistic infections to take place [31]. Opportunistic infections can be of different origin, including bacterial or protozoal, as shown in this study. Coinfection data in piglets indicate that coronavirus and bacterial coinfections have a significant effect on the magnitude of the inflammatory immune response and the amount of tissue damage compared to animals infected with a single pahogen [32]. Furthermore, in young turkeys, coronavirus and enteropathogenic *Escherichia coli* (EPEC) were shown to synergistically interact and cause severe growth depression and high mortality when compared to mono-infected turkeys [33]. In this study, turkeys infected first with coronavirus and then with EPEC developed numerically greater mortality, significantly lower survival probability, and increased frequency of attaching and effacing lesions than that observed in turkeys inoculated with EPEC prior to turkey coronavirus or simultaneously inoculated with these agents. These observations not only suggest a role for coronavirus in foals but they also suggest diagnostic value of detecting ECoV in apparently healthy foals to assess their susceptibility for potentially detrimental coinfections. In coronavirus-infected healthy foals, the focus could be directed toward epidemiological aspects to reduce the likelihood of coinfections. Additional studies are needed to determine ECoV virulence factors and the relative importance as a coinfecting agent to contribute to GI disease in foals.

Diagnosis

Diagnosis of ECoV is based on PCR, virus isolation or electron microscopy.

Treatment

Refer to rotavirus infection. An ultra-purified Bentonite clay is available for use in horses that has the same composition as a product being investigated for human rotavirus or coronavirus [29].[3]

Clostridium difficile

C. difficile is the agent that causes antibiotic-associated pseudomembranous colitis in people. It has also been identified as a significant nosocomial pathogen for equids as well as human patients. First described in 1935 by Hall and O'Toole, this Gram-positive anaerobic bacillus was named "the difficult clostridium" because it resisted early attempts at isolation and grew very slow [34]. The organisms were found in stool specimens from healthy human neonates (up to 50%), which led to its classification as a commensal and was subsequently ignored as a potential pathogen. In the 1960s and 1970s antibiotic-associated pseudomembranous colitis became a major clinical problem, which was attributed to mucosal ischemia or viral infection. In 1977, Larson et al. reported that stool specimens from affected patients contained a toxin that produced cytopathic changes in tissue culture cells [35]. *C. difficile* was identified as the source of the cytotoxin. It is now clear that *C. difficile* is responsible for virtually all cases of human pseudomembranous colitis and 20% of the cases of antibiotic induced colitis.

Pathogenesis of antibiotic-associated diarrhea/colitis begins with disruption of colonization resistance (disruption of the normal colonic flora) of *C. difficile*. Colonization occurs by the oral-fecal route. *C. difficile* forms heat-resistant spores that can persist in the environment for years. These spores survive the acid environment of the stomach and convert to vegetative forms in the colon. Environmental contamination by *C. difficile* is particularly common in human hospitals with isolation rates of 11.7–29% [36]. Health care personal may carry bacteria on their hands, under rings, or on stethoscopes, but fecal carriage by staff is rare. High rates of infection can be isolated from stalls (hospital rooms), scales, thermometers, and surgical preparation rooms [36]. *C. difficile* has also been implicated in an outbreak of colitis among horses at veterinary teaching hospitals [36, 37].

When established in the colon, pathogenic strains of *C. difficile* produce toxins that cause diarrhea and colitis. Strains that do not produce toxins are not pathogenic. Two large exotoxins, toxin A (enterotoxin) and toxin B (cytotoxin), are produced by *C. difficile* (Table 17.III.2). Toxins A and B act synergistically and cause fluid secretion, mucosal damage, and intestinal inflammation. Toxin A is also a chemoattractant for human neutrophils *in vitro* [42]. A third toxin, an actin-specific adenosine diphosphate (ADP)-ribosyltransferase (binary toxin), has been identified in certain strains of *C. difficile* isolated from human patients. The role and pathogenesis of binary toxin is unclear, but it may act synergistically with toxins A and B [38, 39]. The toxic effects appear to follow binding of toxins to membrane receptors. After binding to its intestinal receptor, toxin A enters the cell and alters the actin cytoskeleton, leading to cell rounding. Toxin B causes identical rounding.

In human medicine *C. difficile* is generally acquired in the hospital setting. Neonatal colonization is common but almost invariably asymptomatic despite stool cytotoxin levels being similar to those in adults with severe colitis. Over 50% of healthy human infants have transient colonies of toxicogenic *C. difficile*. Baverud et al. demonstrated that neither *C. difficile* nor cytotoxin B was found in the fecal flora of 56 healthy foals ranging in age from 14 days to 4 months (foals were not receiving antibiotics) [43]. Similarly, a small percentage of foals are reported to be asymptomatic carriers, with rates ranging from 0–3%. Reported rates of asymptomatic carriers in adult horses are similar to people (<1–15% of healthy adults) and range from 0% to 4% [9, 39]. This organism, therefore, is most likely a minor and uncommon component of the usual GI tract flora. Diarrhea and fatal hemorrhagic NEC have been reported to occur in neonatal foals infected with toxigenic strains of *C. difficile*, and the organism can be considered a primary pathogen in foals, not requiring prior antimicrobial use for development of disease [39].

Clinical Signs

Clinical signs of *C. difficile* in foals range from low-grade diarrhea to severe watery to hemorrhagic diarrhea to fulminate colitis with ileus. Foals with severe colitis can become anorexic and dehydrated. In addition to diarrhea, foals become tachypneic, which may be secondary to discomfort associated with enteritis, pyrexia, metabolic acidosis, or anxiety of hospitalization. Hypoproteinemia is also a feature of *C. difficile* secondary to the effects of toxins A and B leading to extravasation of plasma proteins. Metabolic acidosis is also consistent with Clostridial enterocolitis and hypovolemia or intestinal loss of bicarbonate. Hyponatremia may also be attributed to GI losses as well as excess free water associated with water consumption by foals.

Diagnosis

Diagnosis of *C. difficile* infection requires demonstration of *C. difficile* toxins in the stool. Fecal PCR that incorporates primers for genes of toxins A and B can also be utilized. The cytotoxin assay that uses tissue cell culture is the gold standard for diagnosis and most sensitive test (sensitivity 94–100%, specificity 90%), detecting as little as 10 pg of toxin B. This test is not commonly used because it is time consuming and costly. Alternatively, two enzyme immunoassays are available to detect toxin: (i) toxin A/toxin B (*C. difficile* TOX A/B test, Techlab®, Blacksburg VA, USA) and (ii) antigen of *C. difficile* and toxin A (TRIAGE® Micro; BIOSITE, San Diego CA 1-888-BIOSITE). These tests have good sensitivity (69–87%) and specificity (99–100%).

Table 17.III.2 Toxins associated with *Clostridium difficile* and *Clostridium perfringens*.

Clostridium difficile [38, 39]

Toxins	Characteristics of toxin
▪ Toxin A (enterotoxin)	▪ Fluid secretion, mucosal damage and increase permeability, intestinal inflammation, chemoattractant for neutrophils
▪ Toxin B (cytotoxin)	▪ Fluid secretion, mucosal damage and increase permeability, intestinal inflammation
▪ Binary toxin (ADP-ribosyltransferase)	▪ Role unclear; acts synergistically with Toxins A and B

Diagnosis	Tests available
▪ Identify *C. difficile* toxins in stool	▪ Cytotoxin assay ▪ PCR with primers for toxin A and B genes ▪ Toxin A/Toxin B (*C. difficile* TOX A/B test, Techlab®, Blacksburg VA) ▪ Antigen of *C. difficile* and toxin A (TRIAGE Micro; BIOSITE, San Diego, CA)

Clostridium perfringens [40]

Typed as A, B, C, D, E, F, and G strains, based on production of one or more exotoxins

Typing of isolates performed using PCR analysis for toxin gene sequences after isolates are cultured.

Toxins	Characteristics of toxin
▪ α	▪ Main virulence factor of gas gangrene in primarily people
▪ β	▪ Responsible for necrotizing enteritis and enterotoxemia in neonates
▪ ε	▪ Main toxin involved in enterotoxemia of sheep and goats
▪ ï	▪ Causes enteritis in rabbits
▪ Enterotoxin (CPE)	▪ Responsible for human food-poisoning
▪ Necrotic B-like (NetF)	▪ Causes necrotic enteritis

- Types A and C are most commonly associated with diarrhea in foals <10 d of age
  - Type A produces α toxin, variably produces enterotoxin
  - Type C produces α and β toxins, variably produces enterotoxin
- Type C causes severe hemorrhagic diarrhea, with higher mortality than Type A [41].

Diagnosis	Test available
▪ Identification of toxins AND isolation of Organism from intestinal contents/feces	▪ PCR that identifies toxins ▪ *C. perfringens* enterotoxin ELISA (Techlab, Blacksburg VA)

Diagnostic testing laboratories

- UC Davis PCR Laboratory offers Foal Diarrhea Panel on feces or rectal swab and includes: *C. difficile* toxins A and B, equine coronavirus, *Lawsonia intracellularis*, *Salmonella* spp., Cryptosporidium spp., equine rotavirus, *Rhodococcus equi*, *C. perfringens* (antigen and toxins α, β, β-2, NetF, CPE)
- Antech offers Acute Diarrhea Panel on feces and includes: Fecal culture, *C. perfringens* enterotoxin, *C. difficile* toxins A and B

C. difficile TOX A/B test (Techlab) has been validated for use in feces of horses [44]. PCR that incorporates primers to detect the genes for toxin A and B can be used for diagnosis.

The author has evaluated fecal samples that were *C. difficile* ELISA antigen positive and toxin negative and compared these results to bacterial culture. *C. difficile* was isolated from 54% of the antigen positive, toxin negative samples. All recovered isolates from the antigen positive and toxin negative samples were toxigenic, possessing genes encoding toxins A and B. Of those, 32% also possessed genes encoding binary toxin, all of which were classified as ribotype 078; ribotype 012 ($n = 6$, 27%), ribotype 020 ($n = 2$, 9.1%), ribotypes 056, 508, 689, AI-37, AI-82/1 ($n = 1$ each) and two ribotypes not present in the accessible databases were also found. In that study, the 54% toxigenic (confirmed with PCR of the culture) recovery rate of *C. difficile* from antigen positive, toxin negative samples were similar to the 63% rate from a recent study in people [44]; thus these results represent a diagnostic challenge. Over-diagnosis can lead to failure to investigate the true cause or unnecessary treatment, while underdiagnosis results in missed treatment and infection control intervention. These results indicate that the presence of toxigenic *C. difficile* was not uncommon in samples, suggesting the results were due to lower sensitivity of the toxin

ELISA compared to the antigen ELISA or lack of production of toxins in the gut. Differentiating these two is difficult. While the clinical relevance of antigen positive, toxin negative results require further study, foals in this study all had enteritis consistent with *C. difficile* infection and few foals had other potential causes of disease identified. As a disease that is potentially treatable and a pathogen that requires infection control, the presence of toxigenic *C. difficile* in a foal with signs consistent with *C. difficile* infection likely warrants treatment and use of appropriate infection control measures. Therefore, in the presence of clinical signs consistent with *C. difficile* infection in foals, it is prudent to consider an antigen positive, toxin negative result to be supportive of *C. difficile* infection [45].

Treatment

Therapy is aimed at eradicating *C. difficile* from the intestinal tract, with oral metronidazole being the drug of choice. Foals <6 months of age are dosed at 10–15 mg/kg PO q8–12h [46]. The response rate for *C. difficile* in people administered metronidazole is 98%. Patients who cannot tolerate oral medication because of ileus may receive the same dose per rectum or IV at 10 mg/kg q6–8h. Excretion of the drug into bile and exudation from the inflamed colon results in bactericidal levels in the feces [42]. Metronidazole resistant strains of *C. difficile* have been isolated in which case vancomycin has been used; there are even reports of metronidazole inducing colitis. Treatment should be continued for 5 days past resolution of diarrhea. A substantial number of human patients (10–20%) will have a relapse of *C. difficile* diarrhea. Various approaches have been suggested for the management of relapses, including a slow tapering dose of metronidazole, bacteriotherapy with the use of nasogastric fecal transfaunation or fecal enemas, oral administration of nontoxigenic *C. difficile* and treatment with the yeast *Saccharomyces boulardii,* which may compete with *C. difficile* toxin A for binding sites on the intestinal epithelium [47]. *S. boulardii* anecdotally is administered to foals at dose of 5 billion colony-forming units PO, q12h. An adjunctive treatment plan used for both viral and bacterial causes of diarrhea is Bentonite clay. Bentonite is effective because it bonds to a variety of toxins and prevents the absorption of toxins by coating the intestinal wall [48]. Additionally, hyperimmunized *C. difficle Toxin A and B* plasma is available[5] but the efficacy of this treatment in resolving diarrhea/toxic insult is currently anecdotal [41].

Clostridium perfringens

C. perfringens is a relatively ubiquitous bacterium associated with enteric diseases in a number of diverse species [40]. It is widespread in the soil and found in the alimentary tract of nearly all warm-blooded species. *C. perfringens* is a frequent postmortem invader in tissues of the alimentary tract of bloating cadavers. Therefore, caution must be exercised when drawing conclusions based on the presence of organisms in the tissues of deceased animals. Types of *C. perfringens* are differentiated (major types: A, B, C, D, E, F, and G) based on production of four major toxins; alpha, beta, epsilon, and iota (Table 17.III.2). In addition, isolates may have the gene known as *C. perfringens* enterotoxin (CPE) and necrotic B-like (NetF) toxin [49]. It is produced by sporulating bacteria in an alkaline environment and is released upon lysis. This toxin is resistant to proteolytic enzymes and binds and inserts on the brush border membrane, causing pore formation in cells leading ultimately to cell lysis. Enterotoxin can be produced by all types of *C. perfringens*, but is most commonly associated with type A. Many factors are involved in the production of enterotoxin by *C. perfringens*. In one study the prevalence of CPE in feces of adult horses with diarrhea was 16% and detected in only 10% of the horses with colic, regardless of whether they had diarrhea [50]. Studies investigating CPE in feces of adult horses and foals with diarrhea have produced variable results. CPE has been detected in feces of 7–33% of adult horses with diarrhea and 28% of the foals with diarrhea [40, 50, 51]. Furthermore, out of 843 *C. perfringens* type A isolates from dogs, people, and horses that were genotyped, only 62 (7.3%) contained the CPE gene [51].

Other toxins have been associated with an unassigned type of *C. perfringens* that produces α-toxin and a β2-toxin and was isolated from piglets with necrotic enterocolitis and horses with enterocolitis [52]. Since the α-toxin, which is produced by all types of *C. perfringens* including non-pathogenic type A strains, is not considered a primary cause of digestive lesions, it was suggested that the β2-toxin, which is present in this new type of *C. perfringens*, is responsible for the lesions. In one study, β2-toxin was found in 52% of the horses with typical and atypical typhlocolitis; to a lesser extent, they were also isolated from horses with other intestinal disorders, representing 37% of isolates [52]. β2-toxinigenic *C. perfringens* has not been found in healthy horses or horses hospitalized for reasons other than intestinal disease [52]. Recently, a novel spore-forming toxin, NetF, has been strongly associated with necrotizing enteritis in foals [53].

Pathogenesis of *C. perfringens* arises from production of one or more of the four major exotoxins or enterotoxin. The factors that cause disease are not clear but are believed to be related to alterations of the normal intestinal flora that allows overgrowth of *Clostridia*. Proposed causes include diet changes, antibiotic therapy, stress, or concurrent infection. In adult ponies, enterocolitis has been produced when antibiotics (clindamycin or lincomycin) were administered orally with a fecal cocktail containing *Clostridium* [54]. However, fecal cocktail alone did not cause disease.

Other host factors that may play a role in the development are age, immunity, and presence or absence of intestinal receptors for *C. perfringens* toxins. β-toxin producing types of *C. perfringens* (Type C) appear to cause enterocolitis in neonatal animals only. The digestive enzyme trypsin is produced by older animals and can inactivate the toxin.

Neonatal animals have less developed digestive enzyme production, thus may be more susceptible to disease caused by this toxin [54]. Most affected foals in one study had serum IgG concentrations of >800 mg/dl, indicating adequate passive transfer; this finding supports the theory that trypsin inhibitors in the dam's colostrum, which protects immunoglobulins from GI breakdown, may potentially allow the β-toxin of *C. perfringens* type C to persist in foals with adequate passive transfer and allows type C bacteria to overgrow.

Clinical Signs and Diagnosis

Clinical disease occurs in foals <5 days of age with a history of obtundation, colic and/or diarrhea for less than 24 hours (Figure 17.III.6). Foals usually present dehydrated with severe colitis; some may develop ileus with evidence of colonic distention. Definitive diagnosis of equine clostridial enterocolitis requires both identification of toxins *and* isolation of the organism from intestinal contents. Isolation of the organism without analysis for toxins is inappropriate because of the possibility of isolating non-enterotoxigenic *C. perfringens* type A, which can be isolated from normal horse manure. In a study of fecal shedding of *C. perfringens* in 128 broodmares and foals, *C. perfringens* was isolated from 90% of healthy 3-day-old foals; 85% were identified as type A and 12% of samples had type A with the β2-toxin gene isolated [55]. *C. perfringens* in which the enterotoxin gene was identified occurred

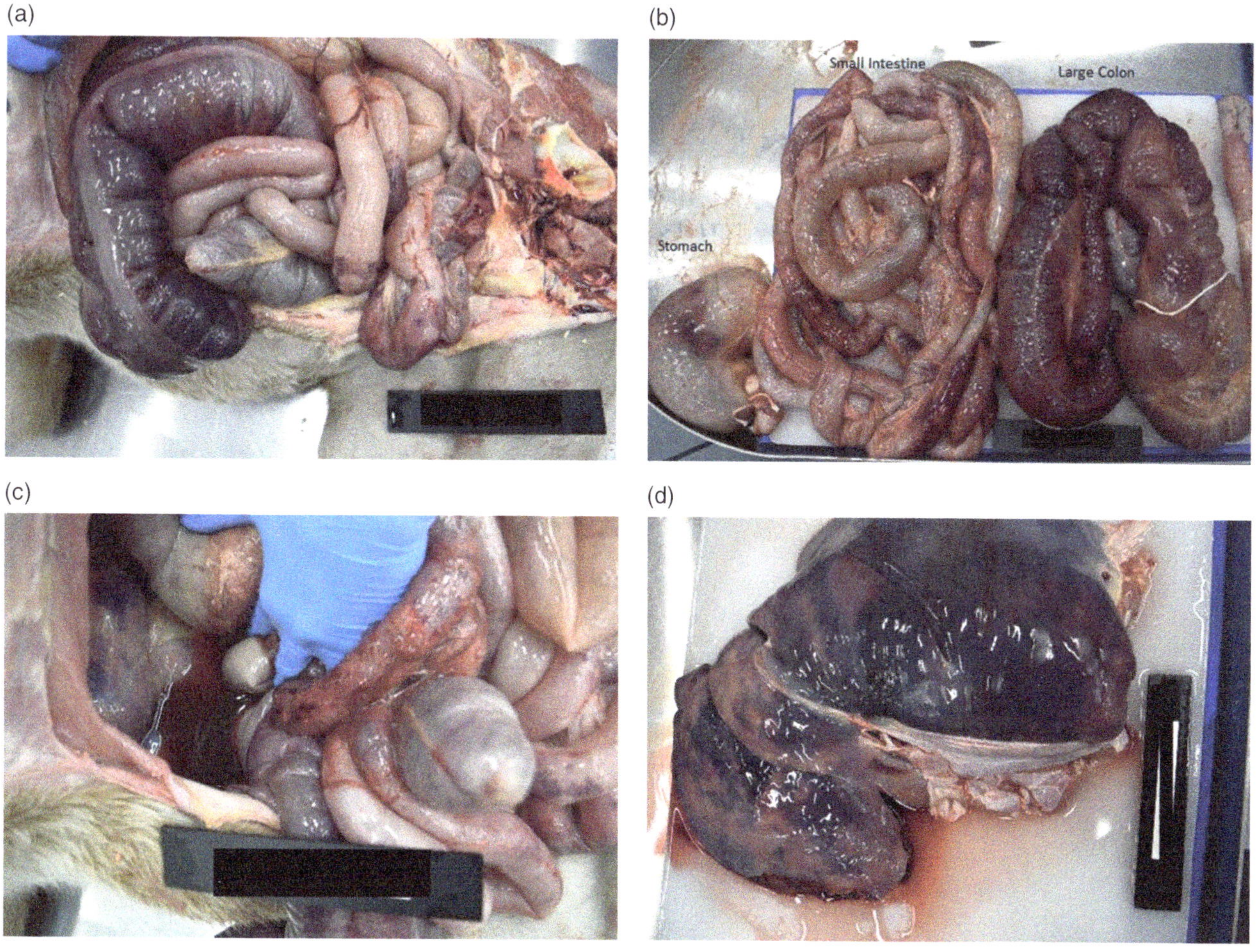

Figure 17.III.6 Postmortem images from a 3-day-old Warmblood foal with acute (<18 hour) onset of hemorrhagic diarrhea that was subsequently diagnosed with *Clostridium perfringens* enterocolitis. (a and b) The small intestine, especially distal jejunum and ileum, along with the large colon was markedly hemorrhagic and edematous and had diffuse patchy petechiation and ecchymoses; the lumen also contained hemorrhagic fluid. (c) The abdominal cavity contained 2 l of sanguineous fluid. (d) The liver was swollen and mottled on the capsular surface and extended into the parenchyma. *Source:* Images courtesy of David Wong, Iowa State University.

in 2.1% of samples whereas *C. perfringens* type C was identified in <1% of samples [55].

A presumptive diagnosis can be supported (until culture and toxin analysis) by demonstration of abundant Gram-positive bacteria in a fecal smear. However, this is an insensitive test as *C. perfringens* can be isolated from 59% of samples in which no Gram-positive rods are seen [55]. The diagnosis is supported by culture of fecal Clostridia and further verifying the isolates as *C. perfringens* by PCR that incorporates primers for classification of *C. perfringens* types A, B, C, D, and E, as well as genes for β2-toxin, NetF and enterotoxin (CPE). PCR can also be performed on fecal swabs or feces to detect toxigenic *C. perfringens,* and toxin detection kits are commercially available for identification of *C. perfringens* enterotoxin (*C. perfringens* enterotoxin test, ELISA, Techlab, Blacksburg, VA USA).

Treatment

Treatment of *C. perfringens* infection is a medical emergency. Even with high levels of intensive care, many foals can succumb to infection with *C. perfringens* type C. Additionally, human neonates with Clostridiosis are at higher risk for developing peritonitis. When there is a large volume of peritoneal exudate, the prognosis is grave and euthanasia is recommended. If attempted, aggressive treatment is aimed at controlling abdominal pain, septic shock, Clostridial infection and toxin production, along with maintenance of nutrition. Oral metronidazole at a dose of 10–15 mg/kg q6–8h (dose depends on severity) for foals and 15 mg/kg q6–8h for adult horses is indicated. If ileus is present and the foal is intolerant to oral feeding, IV metronidazole is recommended (10 mg/kg IV q6h). Ileus with marked colonic distention (if present), can be treated with neostigmine (1 mg SQ q 1–8 h, or IV if severe tympany) to help relieve GI tympany (2 mg for foals >250 pounds, subcutaneously). Subjectively, foals administered hyperimmunized plasma appear to have more rapid resolution of diarrhea compared to foals not treated with hyperimmunized plasma. Bentonite clay can also be used to adsorb α, β, and β-2 exotoxins without interfering with absorption equine colostral antibodies [56].

Numerous prophylactic measures can be instituted on farms with a history of *C. perfringens*-associated enterocolitis. Optimal hygiene efforts to ensure cleanliness of the foaling stall and mare (clean udder before and after birth, clean perineal and hind limb region) at parturition should be undertaken to decrease the degree of exposure of the foal to pathogens in the feces [41]. Some farms have halted outbreaks of foal diarrhea by foaling mares out in pasture. Specific preventative methods addressing *C. perfringens* include immunizing mares with a toxoid vaccine (aluminum hydroxide adsorbed culture supernatant plus recombinant β2-toxoid). Hagyard Equine Medical Institute has developed (2007) a vaccine against *C. perfringens* Type A that carries genes for α, β-2, NetF and CPE. Other oral enteric protectants include oral and/or IV administration of *C. perfringens* hyperimmunized plasma,[6] as noted. Specific immune treatments for *C. perfringens* types C and D provide some protection against α-toxin but generally provides inadequate protection against *C. perfringens* type A organisms.

Salmonella

Salmonella are Gram-negative, facultative, anaerobic bacteria, which usually access the intestinal tract via fecal-oral route. *Salmonella* commonly infects foals between 12 hours and 4 months of age with young foals being more susceptible because of a less sophisticated or less well-established GI microflora. The most common source of exposure and infection in the foal is another horse. Often the mare herself in an asymptomatic carrier. In fact, mares have been shown to shed *Salmonella* at or shortly after parturition despite having as many as 19 negative cultures before foaling [57]. Observation of parturition reveals that all mares defecate during stage 2 labor and that contamination of fetal membranes and the perineum/udder of the mare is possible if *Salmonella* is in the feces. During udder seeking foals will have extensive contact with the perineum and therefore may be at risk of *Salmonella* ingestion.

Once *Salmonella* has overcome host defense mechanisms (gastric acidity, intestinal flora, peristalsis, intestinal mucus, lactoferrin) the bacteria migrate through enterocytes and access the lamina propria where they stimulate an inflammatory response. Both phagocytized and free *Salmonella* organisms travel via the lymphatics to regional lymph nodes where they persist in stimulating an inflammatory response. *Salmonella* can also reach the circulation from efferent lymphatics. The neonatal foal's predisposition toward bacteremia and septicemia may be partially related to factors such as delayed gut closure at birth, immature cellular immune response, and decreased complement activity. *Salmonella* enterotoxins, cytotoxins and generalized inflammation within the bowel induce secretions of fluid from the intestinal epithelium.

Clinical Signs and Diagnosis

Clinical signs of *Salmonellosis* are variable, ranging from mild enteritis to severe illness, voluminous diarrhea, and septic shock. Diagnosis of *Salmonella* is demonstrated by positive fecal or blood cultures. Some foals present with fever of unknown origin with no signs of diarrhea and subsequently have positive blood and fecal cultures for *Salmonella*. Intermittent shedding of *Salmonella* is common and therefore a minimum of three to five consecutive fecal cultures taken 24 hours apart is recommended. Identification of *Salmonella* in fecal samples via PCR is also readily available.

Treatment

Treatment principles are nonspecific and aimed at maintaining hydration and electrolyte balance. Antibiotic therapy, although believed to not alter clinical course of diarrhea or shedding of organisms, should be initiated in attempts to prevent bacteremia. Polymyxin B (6 000 IU/kg IV q8h) diluted in 1 l of fluids, flunixin meglumine (0.25 mg/kg IV q8h), and pentoxifylline (7.5 mg/kg PO q12h) can reduce the effects of endotoxemia. Bismuth subsalicylate (1–3 ml/kg PO q4–8h) is also commonly used as a gastroprotectant and for its anti-endotoxic and anti-prostaglandin properties. J-5 hyperimmunized plasma may also be administered to aid in decreasing systemic endotoxemia. In addition, administration of high volumes of equine plasma (1–4 l in 50 kg foal) may be necessary to increase the serum albumin/protein concentrations in extremely hypoproteinemic foals (serum albumin <1–1.2 g/dl). Plasma administration will not only help reduce external edema but likely decreases intestinal edema that occurs secondary to hypoalbuminemia. Foals with *Salmonellosis* (or other forms of severe diarrhea/colitis) can have a decreased or absent appetite, thus parenteral nutrition is indicated in some cases. As the neonatal foal does not have an abundance of endogenous energy reserves, parenteral nutrition may be needed to provide maintenance calories. Foals will also catabolize endogenous proteins to provide an energy source, further contributing to hypoproteinemia, if supplemental nutrition is not provided to these debilitated foals.

Prevention of *Salmonella*

Prevention of *Salmonella* consists of proper hygiene. Prior to the foal nursing, the udder and perineal regions of the mare should be thoroughly washed with dilute chlorohexidine or ivory soap and water. During a *Salmonella* outbreak, foals should be administered 6–8 oz. of colostrum prior to contact with the mare. An experimental inactivated bacterin (*Salmonella typhimurium* and *Newport*) vaccine has been developed by Hagyard Equine Medical Institute and Dr. John Timoney at the Gluck Research Center (Lexington, KY) and has been used on endemic farms since 2007.

Enterococcus durans/hirae (Group D Streptococcus)

E. durans is a Gram-positive coccus in the alimentary tract and has been implicated as a cause of enteritis in foals, piglets, calves, and puppies. The author has documented *E. durans* as a cause of diarrhea in five of seven foals that developed diarrhea during the first 10 days of life [58].

In a study in Australia, *E. durans,* isolated from a foal that had severe diarrhea, was experimentally infected in seven foals via nasogastric intubation. All seven foals developed profuse watery diarrhea within 24 hours of inoculation with varying degrees of depression, anorexia, abdominal tenderness, and dehydration [59]. The pathogenesis of diarrhea and enteric disease remains unknown. Diarrhea induced by *E. durans* is not associated with enterotoxin production or substantial mucosal injury. However, decreased activity of brush border digestive enzymes such as lactase and alkaline phosphatase suggest that there is a direct mechanical interference with digestion and absorption at the brush border [59]. Recent molecular assessment by the author of the *E. durans,* isolated from sick foals in central Kentucky revealed that bacterium may actually be *E. hirae*.

Treatment of *E. durans* diarrhea has not been adequately investigated, but in the author's experience, β-lactam antimicrobials such as ampicillin or penicillin appear to help decrease the duration of diarrhea. The ideal treatment is to improve husbandry on the farm.

Protozoa

Cryptosporidium parvum is a protozoal pathogen with *significant* zoonotic potential. Diarrhea can result when oocytes (infective when shed) are ingested. *C. parvum* typically occurs in immunocompromised (often hospitalized) foals but has been reported in an immunocompetent adult [60, 61]. The infection is often noted in Arabian foals with combined immunodeficiency or foals that have secondary immunosuppression associated with chronic, catabolic disease. There have been rare outbreaks of diarrhea in equine neonates that were immunocompetent. The author has documented *C. parvum* in both healthy foals as well as foals with diarrhea in central Kentucky. The majority of cases involving *C. parvum* were coinfections, thus questioning the clinical significance of *Cryptosporidium* in the feces of ill foals [1].

Diagnosis is based on detection of oocysts in fecal samples. Kinyoun acid-fast stain, immunoflourescence, flow cytometry and fecal PCR are useful. *Eimeria* and *Giardia* spp. may be noted in fecal samples, but the pathogenicity of these organisms in the neonate has not been conclusively documented.

Treatment of *C. parvum* is largely supportive, but specific drug therapy with the oral aminoglycoside paromomycin (100 mg/kg PO q24h for 5 days) or nitazoxanide (2 g PO q12h for 3 days) can be used. Efficacy and safety have not been established in foals but nitazoxanide was effective in calves [62].

Strongyloides westerii

One of the most common parasites of foals is *Strongyloides westerii*; however, it likely rarely causes diarrhea based on the fact that foals passing high egg counts can be asymptomatic [5]. One study noted that this parasite may be suspected as a cause of diarrhea when >2000 eggs/g of feces were detected [63]. The source of infection in most foals is mare's milk. The period of heaviest shedding in milk occurs 2–3 weeks after parturition. Prevention of *S. westerii* includes targeted deworming of the mare with ivermectin 2–3 days post foaling.

Lawsonia intracellularis

Lawsonia intracellularis is not associated with diarrhea in neonatal foals, but rather, causes proliferative enteropathy in weanling age foals [64]. *L. intraceullaris* is an obligate intracellular Gram-negative bacterium that will not be discussed at length here, but the clinician should suspect infection in 4–9-month-old foals presented with nonspecific signs including lethargy, pyrexia, anorexia, weight loss, and colic, along with signs of hypoalbuminemia such as peripheral/ventral edema, poor body condition, and diarrhea. Ultrasonography of the intestines may demonstrate notable thickening of the intestinal wall (>3 mm) supporting the diagnosis, which can be confirmed using fecal PCR or serologic assays [64]. Treatment of proliferative enteropathy includes supportive care (IV fluids, colloids, plasma transfusions, parenteral nutrition) and antimicrobial therapy such as the macrolides (azithromycin 10 mg/kg, PO, q24h; or clarithromycin 7.5 mg/kg, PO, q12h), IV tetracycline (oxytetracycline 6.6 mg/kg, IV, q12h × 5 days then oral antimicrobial), oral tetracycline (doxycycline 10 mg/kg, PO, q 12h for 14 days or longer; or minocycline 4 mg/kg, PO, q12h for 14 days or longer), or chloramphenicol (44–55 mg/kg, PO, q6–8h × 14 days or longer) [64].

Infectious Control Measures for Neonates with Diarrhea

Isolation from the Remainder of the Population

Foals that have clinically recovered from an episode of diarrhea or that continue to pass soft feces may potentially shed infectious organisms in their feces and therefore should be isolated from healthy animals. This isolation period is most easily managed in a stall for most farm situations. In general, a minimum period of 30 days isolation is recommended for foals diagnosed with *Salmonella* and a period of 14 days after normalization of feces in foals infected with *rotavirus* and *Clostridium*. Those diagnosed with *Salmonella* should be recultured prior to returning to the healthy population. Additionally, the recovering foal should not be placed in stressful situations or activities (long-distance transportation, elective veterinary procedures) as this may induce the recurrence of diarrhea or the shedding of infectious organisms.

Handling the Affected Individual

As noted, infectious organisms may be present in the feces of clinically recovered foals, and thus these foals should be handled with care to avoid spreading or carrying infected feces from the isolation area to the remainder of the farm population. Farm personnel should wear gloves, boots, and protective gowns when handling the affected foal to avoid cross-contamination. Protective articles of clothing may then be removed and either discarded or saved stall-side for use when re-entering the stall. Additional actions include footbaths and hand washing (soap and water or hand disinfectants), but these control measures are effective only if consistently and stringently used. Farm personnel should remember that infectious organisms are not visible and may be in feces that have contacted the horse's tail and then spread to other parts of the body or stall walls, feed containers, water buckets (e.g. a water hose submerged in a contaminated water bucket can conceivably carry infectious organisms to other water buckets) and grooming tools. Farm personnel should be informed that many of the infectious diseases that cause diarrhea in foals may cause illness in humans.

Manure Disposal

Foals that have clinically recovered from an episode of diarrhea or that continue to pass soft feces have the potential to shed infectious organisms in their feces; therefore, feces and contaminated bedding material should not be spread on pastures where other horses or farm animals (dogs, cats, cattle) may come in contact and potentially consume the material. Ideally, feces and contaminated bedding should be discarded at a landfill. Composting may be effective in killing infectious organisms if the compost material reaches adequate temperatures and if the material remains unused for several months.

Cleaning and Disinfection

Stall cleaning must begin with complete removal of all bedding and fecal material. In some cases, it may be necessary to scrape the fecal material from the floor or walls. Pressure washing may aerosolize organisms, facilitating spread to other stalls or rafters above the contaminated stall; therefore, this type of equipment should not be used for cleaning when infectious organisms are likely. After thoroughly removing all fecal material, the walls and floor (if solid) should be scrubbed with detergent (i.e. Tide) and water, and then rinsed. After thorough cleaning, the walls and floor should be sprayed with a suitable disinfectant for the suspected agent.

A number of disinfectants can be considered. Phenolic compounds such as Wex-Cide, Biophene, Tek-Trol, or 1-Stroke will kill bacteria (e.g. *Salmonella*) and viruses (e.g. rotavirus) and this class of disinfectants is effective in the presence of organic material such as mucus, blood, and manure; however, these compounds are corrosive. Chlorine-containing compounds are corrosive and will cause discoloration. Additionally, these agents are inactivated by organic material; therefore, thorough cleaning must take place before these agents can be used. These agents are ineffective against rotavirus. Iodophors are corrosive and inactivated by organic material. They should not be mixed with chlorine-containing compounds for disinfection. Quaternary ammonium compounds (e.g. Roccal-D, Virkon-S, Madisan 75) are noncorrosive. They are not as effective against enterobacteriaceae and can be incompatible with many soaps and detergents and are inactivated by organic material. Peroxygens (Rescue and Virkon) will kill bacteria and viruses and are considered to be effective in the presence of organic material.

Return to the Farm Population

The time required for a foal to return to the healthy farm population without being a source of infection or contamination to the environment varies, depending on the infectious agent. Foals infected with *Salmonella* may shed the bacteria for unknown periods of time. The best (and most widely accepted) method for determining how long a *Salmonella*-infected foal will shed and how long the foal should be isolated is to submit feces for microbiologic culture. Approximately 60% of recovered horses from Salmonellosis have negative fecal cultures by 30 days after recovery, and approximately 90% are negative by 60 days (Dr. Brandy Burgess personal communication of preliminary data). Because it is impossible to predict the degree to which an infected horse sheds *Salmonella*, the infected horse should be isolated from other horses for a minimum of 30 days. After this period, the author uses a series of three fecal cultures. These fecal samples may be submitted once daily or once weekly. Regardless of the technique, negative results on three consecutive cultures should be obtained prior to reintroducing this horse into the herd. It is generally accepted that horses infected with rotavirus may shed the virus for a period of 14 days after normalization of feces. A similar isolation period is recommended for horses infected with *Clostridium and Enterococcus* spp.

Treatments

Antimicrobials

Broad-spectrum antimicrobial usage is recommended in sick neonatal foals with diarrhea, due to the increased risk of bacterial translocation across damaged or denuded epithelium. In one study, 50% of foals presenting to a referral hospital with diarrhea were bacteremic; 57% and 43% of foals had Gram-negative and Gram-positive bacteria isolated, respectively [65]. The author utilizes an antimicrobial program that has broad-spectrum activity against both Gram-negative and Gram-positive bacteria. An example used in a foal with diarrhea and normal renal parameters includes ampicillin (20–25 mg/kg IV q6–8h) or potassium penicillin (20,000 IU IV q 6h) and amikacin (25 mg/kg IV q24–30h) or gentamicin (12 mg/kg IV q36h; foals ≤2 weeks of age). A third-generation cephalosporin such as ceftiofur (5–10 mg/kg IV q 12h) or ceftazidime (20–50 mg/kg IV q6–8h) should be used if the foal has evidence of renal injury (e.g. azotemia).

Hemodynamic Control

The goal of fluid therapy in foals of all ages is to expand vascular volume to restore and maintain cardiovascular function, thereby improving organ perfusion and blood pressure while correcting dehydration and disturbances of acid–base balance, osmolality, and electrolytes. The initial formulation of a fluid plan should be based on clinical examination of the foal (Table 17.III.3) and laboratory parameters. The author assesses water deficit to calculate the quantity of fluids needed to correct the deficit:

$$\text{Water deficit (l)} = \text{Percentage dehydration} \times \text{Body weight (kg)}$$

Thus, a 10% dehydrated foal weighing 50 kg has a fluid deficit of 5 l. Foals that present without significant acid–base or electrolyte abnormalities and mild to moderate dehydration (5–10%) typically receive an initial 1 l of crystalloid fluid, such as lactated ringers or Normosol, over 1 hour followed by reevaluation. The initial fluid replacement will commonly improve attitude and

Table 17.III.3 Estimation of degree of dehydration in neonatal foals.

Dehydration (%)	Skin tent (s)	Mucous membrane moisture	CRT (s)	PCV (%)	TP (g/l)
5	2–3	Moist	1–2	32–40	65–70
10	3–5	Sticky	2–4	36–48	70–75
15	>5	Dry	>4	>48	>75

appetence. A foal that may not have been nursing on presentation may commence milk consumption, leading to correction of some of the fluid deficit. Rarely do foals require all the deficit be replaced via IV fluids. In fact, doing so may lead to overhydration, which, in compromised foals, could result in generalized edema.

Fluid therapy is discussed in Chapter 62. In brief, IV fluids are commonly required for successful supportive care of the diarrheic neonate. A 50 kg foals with diarrhea can safely be given 4–6 l of isotonic crystalloids per day. The goal of fluid therapy is to administer crystalloid fluids to replace free water loss and control electrolyte and acid/base imbalances. For example, in hypersecretory diarrhea in which bicarbonate is lost, isotonic bicarbonate (150 ml 8.4% sodium bicarbonate in 850 ml sterile water) may need to be supplemented in the fluid plan by replacing half of the deficit over 6 hours and the remaining half of the bicarbonate deficit over the following 12–24 hours. Colloid therapy (hyperimmune plasma) can be considered to increase oncotic pressure, provide immunotherapy in the form of immunoglobulins, and replace clotting factors lost to consumption or small protein loss in the GI tract. If septic shock is diagnosed, pressor agents (dobutamine, norepinephrine) are necessary to increase perfusion to vital organs.

Nutrition

Damaged epithelial cells are less effective at absorbing nutrients and the increased metabolic burden of pinocytosis can have negative effects on the health of these cells, resulting in exacerbated osmotic diarrhea and colic signs. At the initial signs of diarrhea accompanied by abdominal discomfort or distension, GI rest (30 seconds nursing q2h) or complete cessation of milk intake for 6–24 hours, may be warranted. Intravenous fluid and carbohydrate administration is warranted in these foals.

Parenteral nutrition is a temporary option for foals that are hospitalized with a GI ailment or intolerance to enteral nutrition. TPN usually contains varying amounts of carbohydrates, lipids, proteins (essential and nonessential amino acids) and electrolytes [66]. Though beneficial, it is not a long-term solution, and frequent increments of minimal enteral nutrition for these foals should still be implemented if possible. This will provide local nutrition to enterocytes and is important in preserving normal GI physiology [5, 66].

Identifying the cause of a foal's diarrhea is important; a foal with diarrhea but no additional abnormalities of the GI tract can often be allowed to continue normal food/milk consumption, but foals whose diarrhea is a result of ileus, sepsis, or colic will benefit from restriction of enteral nutrition [66]. Adding parenteral nutrition is dependent on age and length of time the foal will be restricted from enteral nutrition [66].

Gastroprotectants

Gastric ulcer prophylaxis is used variably in cases of enterocolitis. Omeprazole (1 mg/kg PO q24h), ranitidine (1.5 mg/kg IV q8h), pantoprazole (1.5 mg/kg IV q24h), or sulcralfate (10–20 mg/kg PO q6–8h) may be used for prevention of ulcers in foals. However, the benefit of prophylaxis is unproven and the incidence of gastric ulceration in neonates at one hospital appeared unrelated to administration of ulcer prophylaxis. There is additional concern that human ICU patients treated with ulcer prophylaxis may be more likely to develop respiratory or GI infections [67, 68]. The net benefit of antacid medication in neonatal foals remains elusive. An association between rotaviral infection and a syndrome of severe gastroduodenal ulceration resulting in stricture formation or duodenal perforation has been suggested, but studies have not been performed in foals to test this hypothesis. However, empirical treatment with low doses of gastroprotectants after recovery from rotaviral diarrhea might be warranted.

Sucralfate is a topical gastroprotectant that provides benefit in numerous ways. This aluminum hydroxide and sucrose derivative provides an adherent topical barrier to prevent acid contact, act as a local prostaglandin E_2 analog, thereby increasing blood flow and mucus production and encourages epithelialization by binding fibroblast growth factor [69]. Other oral drugs should not be administered within two hours of sucralfate administration to reduce the decreased absorption caused by binding with other medications. The author tends to not use gastric ulcer prophylaxis, but rather starts treatment if the foal has clinical signs of decreased nursing behavior, bruxism, or low-grade colic. If prophylactic treatment is warranted, the author utilizes sulcralfate.

Anti-diarrheals

A mainstay of diarrheal treatment includes adsorbents and clay-like substances intended to absorb excess water and potential toxins before they are absorbed by the gut (Table 17.III.4). They include di-tri-octahedral smectite, bismuth subsalicylate, kaolin/pectin, and sometimes charcoal in the older foal. Bismuth subsalicylate coats the GI epithelium and may provide local anti-inflammatory effects when metabolized to salicylate. In an *in vitro* model, bismuth subsalicylate inhibited bacterial growth of *C. difficile* and *E. coli* and prevented invasion of enterocytes by the GI virus, norovirus, and promoted prostaglandin E_2 release [70–72]. It is important to note that bismuth subsalicylate will produce dark feces that may be mistaken for hematochezia.

Lactase

Due to the destructive effects of many infectious agents, especially rotavirus, on the brush border of the

Table 17.III.4 Common anti-diarrheal treatments used in foals.

Anti-diarrheal	Dose	Mechanism	Comment
Di-tri-octahedral smectite	30g in a thin paste PO q 6–12h	Binds intraluminal Clostridal toxins, absorbs water	Reduce dose as diarrhea subsides to prevent intraluminal obstruction
	3.2g of ultra-purified Bentonite PO q6–12h[a]		
Bismuth subsalicylate	0.5–1.0ml/kg PO q6–12h	Cyclooxygenase inhibitor	May produce dark feces

[a] Relieve™, Resolvet, Lexington KY 40361.

epithelium, it is important to supplement the disaccharidase lactase. This provides a means for the foal to utilize the primary carbohydrate source, lactose. Lactaid can be administered orally at a dose of 3000–9000 FCC units PO or dissolved in milk if bucket fed, every 6 hours to as frequently as 3000 FCC units every 2 hours in severe cases or those foals transitioned to milk replacer. Exogenous supplementation of lactase provides the small bowel with the capacity to digest the disaccharide and subsequently absorb it. Tablets can be purchased at drug stores and administered at a rate of 1–2 tablets per 50kg foal (60–120FCC units lactase/kg bodyweight) as frequently as necessary. For most foals, one tablet (3000 FCC units) every 4–6 hours is sufficient.

Probiotics

A wide range of commercial probiotic products is available and includes *Lactobacillus plantarum* and *Bifidobacterium animalis*. These two bacterial species have promising *in vitro* effects of inhibiting growth of both *C. difficile* and *C. perfringens* at pHs as low as 4.0 and in the presence of up to 0.3% bile [43]. However *in vivo* studies have demonstrated mixed results, ranging from increased weight gain and decreased incidence of diarrhea, to no effect on incidence or duration of diarrhea in foals or fecal shedding of *C. difficile* and *C. perfringens* during 3 weeks of administration, to a potential exacerbated effect of probiotics on the severity of diarrhea, requiring veterinary intervention [73, 74]. The author currently uses fecal transfaunations in foals that have severe dysbiosis.

Conclusions

Equine practitioners have always considered the availability of a correct etiologic diagnosis, particularly in contagious infections, to make early decisions on patient care and management, to address appropriate treatment, and to allow timely notification and discussion of management improvements regarding prevention of disease spread a priority. Over the past years, both the understanding and characterization of existing and new equine infectious agents as well as the development of rapid, comprehensive, and affordable molecular diagnostic tools has experienced rapid development. Recent advances in diagnostic technology have allowed for the development of various Equine Point of Care Diagnostics (EPOCD). EPOCD provide results in <1hour, and in some instances, <1minute. Advantages of EPOCD include rapid implementation of treatment and reduced guesswork of the cause of diarrhea. This in turn allows optimal care with the goal of better clinical outcomes. Several PCR point-of-care systems have recently entered the veterinary market. Companies such as Fluxergy LLC (Irvine California USA), Horiba's POCKIT Central PCR System (Japan) and Credo Biomedical's QubeMDx (Singapore) offer a variety of Veterinary PCR assays. Credo's QubeMDx PCR does not offer any equine testing currently but does offer canine and feline infectious disease testing. Fluxergy is unique in that they have been concentrating on primarily equine PCR POC technology. These advances will not only help practitioners make an accurate diagnosis but will be utilized to discover new pathogens affecting the foal's alimentary tract.

Notes

1 Rotazyme, Abbott Laboratories, North Chicago, IL 60064; Wampole Laboratories, Cranberry, NJ 08512.
2 LACTAID®, McNeil Consumer Healthcare, Fort Washington, PA 19034 USA.
3 Relieve™, Resolvet, Lexington, KY 40361.
4 Equine Rotavirus Vaccine, Zoetis Parsippany, NJ 07054.
5 Lake Immunogenics Clostridium difficle Toxin a and B Antibody Select HI Plasma, Ontario, NY 14519 USA.
6 Lake Immunogenics *Clostridium perfringens* Type A, C & D Antibody Select HI Plasma, Ontario, NY 14519 USA.

References

1 Slovis, N.M., Elam, J., Estrada, M. et al. (2014). Infectious agents associated with diarrhea in foals in central Kentucky. *Equine Vet. J.* 46: 311–316.
2 Pusterla, N., Byrne, B.A., Maples, S. et al. (2014). Investigation of the use of pooled faecal and environmental samples following an enrichment step for the detection of *Salmonella enterica* by real-time PCR. *Vet. Rec.* 174: 252.
3 Sgorbini, M., Nardoni, S., Mancianti, F. et al. (2008). Foal-heat diarrhea is not caused by the presence of yeasts in gastrointestinal tract of foals. *J. Equine Vet. Sci.* 28: 145–148.
4 Gianini, M., Sutter, O., Burger, D. et al. (2000). Gastrointestinal and endocrine function during "foal heat diarrhoea" in healthy foals. *J. Reprod. Fertil. Suppl.* 56: 717–724.
5 Magdesian, K.G. (2005). Neonatal foal diarrhea. *Vet. Clin. North Am. Equine Pract.* 21: 295–312.
6 Mallicote, M., House, A.M., and Sanchez, L.C. (2012). A review of foal diarrhoea from birth to weaning. *Equine Vet. Educ.* 24: 206–214.
7 Masri, M.D., Merritt, A.M., Gronwall, R. et al. (1986). Faecal composition in foal heat diarrhoea. *Equine Vet. J.* 18: 301–306.
8 Pieszka, M., Luszczyński, J., Hedrzak, M. et al. (2016). The efficacy of kaolin clay in reducing the duration and severity of 'heat' diarrhea in foals. *Turk. J. Vet. Anim. Sci.* 40: 323–328.
9 Weese, J.S., Parsons, D.A., and Staempfli, H.R. (1999). Association of *Clostridium difficile* with enterocolitis and lactose intolerance in a foal. *J. Am. Vet. Med. Assoc.* 214: 229–232.
10 Siwińska, N., Luczka, A., Zak, A. et al. (2019). Assessment of sand accumulation in the gastrointestinal tract and its excretion with stool in silesian foals. *Pol. J. Vet.* 22: 337–343.
11 McAuliffe, S.B. (2004). Abdominal ultrasonography of the foal. *Clin. Tech. Equine Pract.* 3: 308–316.
12 Korolainen, R. and Ruohoniemi, M. (2002). Reliability of ultrasonography compared to radiography in revealing intestinal sand accumulations in horses. *Equine Vet. J.* 34: 499–504.
13 Navas de Solis, C., Palmer, J.E., Boston, R.C. et al. (2012). The importance of ultrasonographic pneumatosis intestinalis in equine neonatal gastrointestinal disease. *Equine Vet. J.* 44: 64–68.
14 Cudd, T. and Pauly, T.H. (1987). Necrotizing enterocolitis in two equine neonates. *Compend. Contin. Educ. Pract. Vet.* 9: 88–96.
15 St. Peter, S.D. (2003). The spectrum of pneumatosis intestinalis. *Arch. Surg.* 138: 68.
16 MacKinnon, M.C., Southwood, L.L., Burke, M.J. et al. (2013). Colic in equine neonates: 137 cases (2000–2010). *J. Am. Vet. Med. Assoc.* 243: 1586–1595.
17 Byars, T.D. (2002). Diarrhea in foals. In: *Manual of Equine Gastroenterology* (ed. T. Mair, T. Divers, and N. Duscharme), 493–495. Philadelphia: WB Saunders CO.
18 Rodger, S.M., Holmes, L.H., and Studdert, M.J. (1980). Characteristics of the genomes of equine rotaviruses. *Vet. Microbiol.* 5: 243–248.
19 Estes, M. and Cohen, J. (1989). Rotavirus gene structure and function. *Microbiol. Rev.* 53: 410–449.
20 Wilson, W.D., East, N., Rowe, J.D. et al. (2009). Use of biologics in the prevention of infectious diseases. In: *Large Animal Internal Medicine* (ed. B.P. Smith), 1586. St. Louis: Mosby.
21 Balasuriya, U. (2020). Baton Rouge, LA. Personal communication.
22 Uprety, T., Sreenivasan, C.C., Hause, B.M. et al. (2021). Identification of a ruminant origin group B rotavirus associated with diarrhea outbreaks in foals. *Viruses* 13: 1330.
23 Powell, D.G., Dwyer, R.M., Traub-Dargatz, J.L. et al. (1997). Field study of the safety, immunogenicity, and efficacy of an inactivated equine rotavirus vaccine. *J. Am. Vet. Med. Assoc.* 211: 193–198.
24 Conner, M.E. (1983). Detection of rotavirus in horses with and without diarrhea with electron microscopy and rotazyme test. *Cornell Vet.* 73: 280–287.
25 Conner, M.E. and Darlington, R.W. (1980). Rotavirus infection in foals. *Am. J. Vet. Res.* 41: 1699–1703.
26 Darlington, J.W. (2006). Modified nano-bentonite anti-viral activity against the herpes simplex virus type 1, rhinovirus type 37, and rotavirus. *19th International Conference of Antiviral Research*. San Juan, Puerto Rico, May 7–11, 2006.
27 Barrandguy, M., Parreno, V., Lagos Marmol, M. et al. (1998). Prevention of rotavirus diarrhea in foals by parenteral vaccination of the mares: field trial. *Dev. Biol. Stand.* 92: 253–257.
28 Guy, J.S., Breslin, J.J., Breuhaus, B. et al. (2000). Characterization of a coronavirus isolated from a diarrheic foal. *J. Clin. Microbiol.* 38: 4523–4526.
29 Bass, E.P. and Sharpee, R.L. (1975). Coronavirus and gastroenteritis in foals. *Lancet* 25: 822.
30 Zhang, J., Guy, J.S., Snijder, E.J. et al. (2007). Genomic characterization of equine coronavirus. *Virology* 369: 92–104.
31 D'Armino Monforte, A., Cozzi-Lepri, A., and Castagna, A. (2009). Risk of developing specific AIDS-defining illnesses in patients coinfected with HIV and hepatitis C virus with or without liver cirrhosis. *Clin. Infect. Dis.* 15: 612–622.

32 Brockmeier, S.L., Loving, C.L., Nicholson, T.L. et al. (2008). Coinfection of pigs with porcine respiratory coronavirus and Bordetella bronchiseptica. *Vet. Microbiol.* 128: 36–47.

33 Pakpinyo, S., Ley, D.H., Barnes, H.J. et al. (2003). Enhancement of enteropathogenic *Escherichia coli* pathogenicity in young turkeys by concurrent turkey coronavirus infection. *Avian Dis.* 47: 396–405.

34 Hall, I.C. and O'Toole, E. (1935). Intestinal flora in new-born infants with a description of a new pathogenic anaerobe, Bacillus difficilis. *Am. J. Dis. Child.* 49: 390–402.

35 Larson, H.E., Price, A.B., Honour, P. et al. (1978). *Clostridium difficile* and the aetiology of pseudomembranous colitis. *Lancet* 311: 1063–1066.

36 Weese, J.S., Staempfli, H.R., and Prescott, J.F. (2000). Isolation of environmental *Clostridium difficile* from a veterinary teaching hospital. *J. Vet. Diagn. Invest.* 12: 449–452.

37 Madewell, B.R., Tang, Y.J., Jang, S. et al. (1995). Apparent outbreaks of *Clostridium difficile*-associated diarrhea in horses in a veterinary medical teaching hospital. *J. Vet. Diagn. Invest.* 7: 343–346.

38 Magdesian, G., Hirsh, D., Jang, S. et al. (1997). *Clostridium difficile* and horses: a review. *Rev. Med. Microbiol.* 8: S46–S48.

39 Magdesian, G., Hirsh, D., Jang, S. et al. (2002). Characterization of *Clostridium difficile* isolates from foals with diarrhea: 28 cases (1993–1997). *J. Am. Vet. Med. Assoc.* 220: 67–73.

40 Weese, J.S., Staempfli, H.R., and Prescott, J.F. (2001). A prospective study of the roles of *Clostridium difficile* and enterotoxigenic *Clostridium perfringens* in equine diarrhoea. *Equine Vet. J.* 33: 403–409.

41 East, L.M., Dargatz, D.A., Traub-Dargatz, J.L. et al. (2000). Foaling-management practices associated with the occurrence of enterocolitis attributed to *Clostridium perfringens* infection in the equine neonate. *Preventive Vet. Med.* 46: 61–74.

42 Kelly, C.P., Pothoulakis, C., and LaMont, J.T. (1994). Clostridium difficile colitis. *N. Engl. J. Med.* 330: 257–262.

43 Baverud, V., Franklin, A., Gunnarsson, A. et al. (1998). *Clostridium difficile* associated with acute colitis in mares when their foals are treated with erythromycin and rifampicin for Rhodococcus equi pneumonia. *Equine Vet. J.* 30: 482–488.

44 Medina-Torres, C.E., Weese, J.S., and Staempfli, H.R. (2010). Validation of a commercial enzyme immunoassay for detection of clostridium difficle toxins in feces of horses with acute diarrhea. *J. Vet. Intern. Med.* 24: 628–632.

45 Slovis, N., Justin, E., and Weese, N. (2019). Evaluation of *Clostridium difficile* antigen positive toxin ELISA negative results in foals. *J. Vet. Intern. Med.* 33: 2358.

46 Swain, E. (2014). Pharmacokinetics of Metronidazole in Foals. *Proc Annu Conv Am Assoc Equine Pract.* 318.

47 Desrochers, A.M., Dolente, B.A., Roy, M.F. et al. (2005). Efficacy of *Saccharomyces boulardii* for treatment of horses with acute enterocolitis. *J. Am. Vet. Med. Assoc.* 227: 954–959.

48 Weese, J.S. and Cote, N.M. (2003). Evaluation of in vitro properties of di-tri-octahedral smectite on clostridial toxins and growth. *Equine Vet. J.* 35: 638–641.

49 Navarro, M., McClane, B.A., and Uzal, F.A. (2018). Mechanisms of action and cell death associated with *Clostridium perfringens* toxins. *Toxins* 10: 212.

50 Donaldson, M.T. and Palmer, J.E. (1999). Prevalence of *Clostridium perfringens* enterotoxin and *Clostridium difficile* toxin A in feces of horses with diarrhea and colic. *J. Am. Vet. Med. Assoc.* 215: 358–361.

51 Bueschel, D., Walker, R., Woods, L. et al. (1998). Enterotoxigenic *Clostridium perfringens* type A necrotic enteritis in a foal. *J. Am. Vet. Med. Assoc.* 213: 1305–1307.

52 Herholz, C., Miserez, R., Nicolet, J. et al. (1999). Prevalence of beta2-toxigenic *Clostridium perfringens* in horses with intestinal disorders. *J. Clin. Microbiol.* 37: 358–361.

53 Mehdizadeh, G., Parreira, V.R., Timoney, J.F. et al. (2016). NetF-positive *Clostridium perfringens* in foal with necrotizing enteritis in Kentucky. *Vet. Rec.* 178: 216.

54 Traub-Dargatz, J.L. and Jones, R.L. (1993). Clostridia-associated enterocolitis in adult horses and foals. *Vet. Clin. North Am. Equine Pract.* 9: 411–421.

55 Tillotson, K., Traub-Dargatz, J.L., Dickinson, C.E. et al. (2002). Population-based study of fecal shedding of *Clostridium perfringens* in broodmares and foals. *J. Am. Vet. Med. Assoc.* 220: 342–348.

56 Lawler, J.B., Hassel, D.M., Magnuson, R.J. et al. (2008). Adsorptive effects of di-tri-octahedral smectite on *Clostridium perfringens* alpha, beta, and beta-2 exotoxins and equine colostral antibodies. *Am. J. Vet. Res.* 69: 233–239.

57 Madigan, J.E., Walker, R.L., Hird, D.W. et al. (1990). Equine neonatal salmonellosis: Clinical observations and control measures. *Proc. Annu. Conv. Am. Assoc. Equine Pract.* 1: 371–375.

58 Williams, N.J., Slovis, N.M., Browne, N.S., Troedsson, M.H.T., Giguère, S., Hernandez, J.A. et al. (2022). Enterococcus durans infection and diarrhea in Thoroughbred foals. *J. Vet. Intern. Med.* 36(6): 2224–2229. doi:10.1111/jvim.16568.

59 Tzipori, S. and Hayes, J. (1984). *Streptococcus durans*: an unexpected enteropathogen of foals. *J. Infect. Dis.* 150: 589–593.

60 Perrucci, S., Buggiani, C., Sgorbini, M. et al. (2011). *Cryptosporidium parvum* infection in a mare and her foal with foal heat diarrhoea. *Vet. Parasitol.* 182: 333–336.

61 Synder, S.P. and England, J.J. (1978). Cryptosporidiosis in immunodeficient Arabian foals. *Vet. Pathol.* 15: 12–17.

62 Schnyder, M., Kohler, L., Hemphill, A. et al. (2009). Prophylactic and therapeutic efficacy of nitazoxanide against *Cryptosporidium parvum* in experimentally challenged calves. *Vet. Parasitol.* 160: 149–154.

63 Netherwood, T., Wood, J.L.N., Townsend, H.G.G. et al. (1996). Foal diarrhoea between 1991 and 1994 in the United Kingdom associated with *Clostridium perfringens*, rotavirus, Strongyloides westeri, and Cryptosporidium sp. *Epidemiol. Infect.* 117: 375–383.

64 Page, A.E., Slovis, N.M., and Horohov, D.W. (2014). *Lawsonia intracellularis* and equine proliferative enteropathy. *Vet. Clin. Equine* 30: 641–658.

65 Hollis, A.R., Wilkins, P.A., Palmer, J.E. et al. (2008). Bacteremia in equine neonatal diarrhea: a retrospective study (1990–2007). *J. Vet. Intern. Med.* 22: 1203–1209.

66 Barr, B. (2016). Nutritional management of the foal with diarrhoea. *Equine Vet. Educ.* 30: 100–105.

67 Kappstein, I., Schulgen, G., Friedrich, T. et al. (1991). Incidence of pneumonia in mechanically ventilated patients treated with sucralfate or cimetidine as prophylaxis for stress bleeding: bacterial colonization of the stomach. *Am. J. Med.* 91: S125–S131.

68 Dinsmore, J.E., Jackson, R.J., and Smith, S.D. (1997). The protective role of gastric acidity in neonatal bacterial translocation. *J. Pediatr. Surg.* 32: 1014–1016.

69 Masuelli, L., Giovanni, T., Turriziani, M. et al. (2010). Topical use of sucralfate in epithelial wound healing: clinical evidence and molecular mechanisms of action. *Recent Pat Inflamm Allergy Drug Discov* 4: 25–36.

70 Pitz, A.M., Park, G.W., Lee, D. et al. (2015). Antimicrobial activity of bismuth subsalicylate on *Clostridium difficile*, *Escherichia coli* O157: H7, norovirus, and other common enteric pathogens. *Gut Microbes* 6: 93–100.

71 Keogan, D.M. and Griffith, D.M. (2014). Current and potential applications of bismuth-based drugs. *Molecules* 19: 15258–15297.

72 Mahony, D.E., Lim-Morrison, S., Bryden, L. et al. (1999). Antimicrobial activities of synthetic bismuth compounds against *Clostridium difficile*. *Antimicrob. Agents Chemother.* 43: 582–588.

73 Schoster, A., Staempfli, H.R., Abrahams, M. et al. (2015). Effect of a probiotic on prevention of diarrhea and *Clostridium difficile* and *Clostridium perfringens* shedding in foals. *J. Vet. Intern. Med.* 29: 925–931.

74 Weese, J.S. and Rousseau, J. (2005). Evaluation of Lactobacillus pentosus WE7 for prevention of diarrhea in neonatal foals. *J. Am. Vet. Med. Assoc.* 226: 2031–2034.

Section IV Peritonitis

David Wong and Charles Brockus

Anatomy of the Peritoneum

The peritoneum is a thin serous semipermeable membrane derived from the mesoderm lining the body cavity of the primitive embryo; full reviews of peritoneal embryogenesis are available elsewhere [1–3]. The peritoneum has varying definitions, with one indicating that the peritoneum is composed of a mesothelial cell layer, basal lamina, and submesothelial stroma (Figure 17.IV.1) [4]. In contrast, a more simplistic definition includes a single layer of mesothelial cells, with the basal lamina and submesotheial stroma not incorporated into the structure [4]. Two layers of peritoneum line the abdomen, the parietal layer (lining the abdominal wall) and the visceral layer (lining the abdominal viscera). The narrow space between these two layers is the peritoneal cavity [5]. The peritoneum is essential for maintaining intra-abdominal homeostasis and serves as an extensive serous membrane that lines the abdominal cavity, a portion of the pelvic inlet and almost all the abdominal viscera with the exception of a small portion of the liver that is attached directly to the diaphragm (area nuda hepatis) [4]. Of note, the peritoneum covers the intestines and contributes to the mesentery, which consists of connective tissue, adipocytes, intestinal vasculature, lymphatics, and two layers of mesenteric peritoneum [4]. Blood supply to the parietal peritoneum arises from arteries of the abdominal wall and parietal pelvic arteries, whereas blood supply to the visceral peritoneum originates from mesenteric, coeliac, and visceral pelvic arteries [4]. Venous blood is drained via the portal vein (visceral peritoneum) and inferior vena cava (parietal peritoneum). The subserous surface of the peritoneum is attached to the body wall, and viscera and the omenta divide the peritoneal cavity into two regions: one created by the greater omentum and another by the lesser omentum. The two regions communicate via the epiploic foramen. In the colt, the peritoneum is a closed sac as compared to the filly, in which two small abdominal orifices allow the fallopian tubes to communicate with the uterus. These small orifices allow communication, indirectly, to the external environment.

Peritoneal fluid is an ultrafiltrate of plasma and contains water, electrolytes, solutes, proteins, and cells [1]. It is primarily produced by the peritoneal capillaries and is renewed every 1–2 hours [6]. The peritoneum and its associated fluid facilitates frictionless movement between abdominal organs; serves as a physiological barrier; permits exchange of nutrients; allows selective fluid and cell transport; participates in immune induction, modulation and inhibition; removes pathogens; and partakes in reparative events [2, 5]. In health, peritoneal fluid has low volume, cellularity, and total protein concentration with its composition being dictated by: (i) capillary hydrostatic pressure, (ii) plasma oncotic pressure, (iii) conditions impacting vascular permeability and lymphatic flow, and (iv) any pathophysiologic process impacting the mesothelial surfaces [7].

Peristaltic movements of the intestines along with movement of the diaphragm and abdominal body wall disseminate peritoneal fluid throughout the abdominal cavity. In general, gravity directs peritoneal fluid ventrally and the negative intra-abdominal pressure generated by the diaphragm during inspiration directs peritoneal fluid cranially. Peritoneal fluid is drained from the mesothelial lining of the peritoneal cavity through lymphatic channels between mesothelial cells, or stomata, into the celiac, superior mesenteric, and periportal lymph nodes. The lymphatic fluid is then transported to the thoracic duct by efferent visceral lymphatics and back into the intravascular space. The muscular portion of the diaphragm also has a high concentration of lymphatic stomata and facilitates peritoneal drainage to the mediastinal lymph nodes [3, 4, 8, 9]. Rapid removal of intra-abdominal microbes occurs

Equine Neonatal Medicine, First Edition. Edited by David M. Wong and Pamela A. Wilkins.

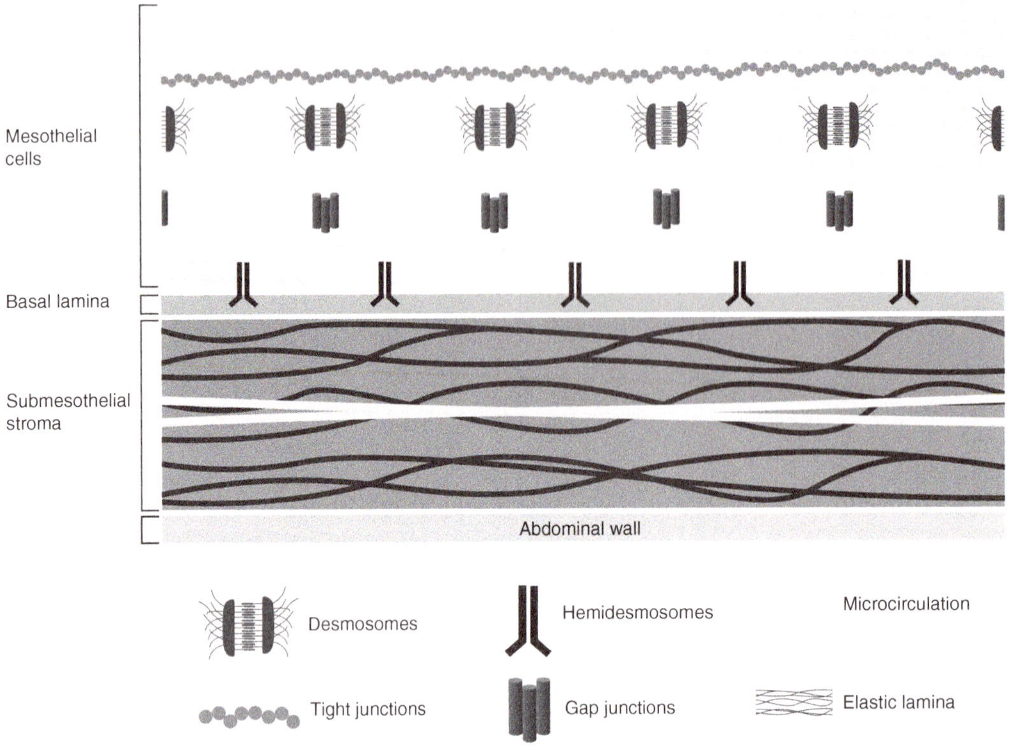

Figure 17.IV.1 Schematic representation of the peritoneum. The mesothelial layer it the innermost layer of the peritoneum and is in contact with the abdominal cavity. The basal lamina is less than 100 nm thick but supports the mesothelial cells via an extracellular matrix, composed primarily of collagen type IV and laminin; the collagen fiber network serves as a skeleton for the basal lamina, whereas laminin provides binding sites for adhesion of mesothelial cells via hemi-desmosomes. The submesothelial stroma supports both the mesothelial cell layer and basal lamina and is composed of collagen type I fibers, laminin, fibronectin, proteoglycans, glucosaminoglycans, fibroblasts, adipocytes, blood and lymph vessels, along with nerves [4].

through these lymphatics and plays a central role in the pathophysiology of abdominal infections, as uncontained contamination can result in bacteremia and sepsis [3].

Interestingly, the relatively porous nature of the diaphragm may be one explanation of the clinical finding of secondary pleural effusion in foals with primary effusive diseases of the abdominal cavity, as reported in foals with uroabdomen [10–13]. Additionally, the greater omentum has specific areas, called milky-spots, that are specialized areas of tissue with abundant populations of leukocytes. These milky-spots have lymphoid-associated properties and are essential in T-cell responses [2]. Together, lymphatic stomata and milky-spots serve to clean the abdominal cavity during an inflammatory process. The stomata serve as a physical protective mechanism via drainage of bacteria and inflammatory residues, and milky-spots regulate the inflammatory response and eliminate the inflammatory agent [2].

Under healthy conditions, monocytes and macrophages are the primary cell within the peritoneal fluid, but mesothelial cells have the ability to initiate immune responses as well as control the balance between coagulation and fibrinolysis within the peritoneal cavity [5]. With peritoneal injury (e.g. bacterial infection, surgical injury), damage-associated molecular patterns (DAMPs) and pathogen-associated molecular patterns (PAMPs) are released by dying cells and invading microorganisms, respectively, resulting in recruitment, proliferation, and activation of cells that contribute to tissue repair [5]. Mesothelial cells play a vital role in cell-signaling pathways and are an important source of pro-inflammatory mediators which subsequently recruit phagocytes and neutrophils into the peritoneal cavity. Neutrophils arrive within 2–4 hours and remain the prominent cell type within the peritoneum for 48–72 hours [3]. Bacterial destruction by the host's immune system releases lipopolysaccharide (LPS) which further stimulates the pro-inflammatory response [3]. Similar to the concept of sepsis and the systemic inflammatory response syndrome (SIRS), some consider peritonitis as both and infectious and inflammatory process in which, despite clearance of the inciting cause within the peritoneum via medical and/or surgical therapy, the overall morbidity and mortality of the disease process might be related to the continued systemic inflammation and organ injury [3]. In addition, peritoneal injury activates the coagulation cascade with the final outcome being the production of fibrin that is deposited on the injured peritoneal surface. While fibrin deposition is part of the normal process of containing the area of damage/infection and tissue repair, fibrinolysis is also necessary for adequate peritoneal healing. This balance between fibrin deposition and fibrinolysis are crucial for peritoneal healing [4]. Fibrinolysis is governed by the conversion of plasminogen to plasmin, as the latter enzyme is needed to degrade fibrin. Mesothelial cells produce enzymes that promote (tissue-plasminogen activator [tPA], urokinase plasminogen activator [uPA]) and inhibit (plasminogen-activator inhibitor [PAI]) the conversion of plasminogen to plasmin [14]. When fibrin is not degraded completely and inflammation continues, such as the case when the initial triggering factor persists, fibrin forms a scaffold for fibroblasts and capillary ingrowth, thus allowing peritoneal adhesion formation.

Accumulation of peritoneal fluid (ascites) develops when pathologic disturbances in peritoneal fluid equilibrium are present. Excess accumulation of peritoneal fluid can be categorized as a transudate (total protein [TP] < 2.5 g/dl; total nucleated cell count [TNCC] < 1500 cells/μl), modified transudate (TP 2.5–5 g/dl; TNCC 1000–7000 cells/μl) or exudate (TP > 3.5 g/dl; TNCC > 7000 cells/μl). The type of peritoneal fluid that develops is dictated by the underlying pathophysiologic process. For example, hepatic disease resulting in increased portal pressure can result in higher peritoneal capillary pressures, thus causing formation of a relatively low protein transudate. In comparison, peritonitis results in increased permeability of the capillary endothelium in the submesothelial layer of the peritoneum resulting in an exudate, as albumin leaks out of capillaries and inflammatory cells infiltrate into the area [15]. Regardless of the cause, increased intra-abdominal fluid in cases of moderate to severe ascites can decrease the absorptive capacity of the peritoneal surface and lymphatic system [16].

Types of Peritonitis

Peritonitis is a specific cause of peritoneal injury and is defined as inflammation of the peritoneum resulting in exudation of fibrin, serum, inflammatory cells, and pus. It can be classified as acute or chronic, localized or diffuse, septic or aseptic, and primary or secondary [17]. **Primary peritonitis** is a spontaneous pathologic event that results from bacterial translocation, hematogenous spread, or iatrogenic contamination of the abdomen in the absence of a macroscopic defect in the gastrointestinal (GI) tract [3]. In contrast, **secondary peritonitis** occurs as a result of direct contamination of the peritoneum by spillage from the urogenital or GI tracts or associated solid organs [3]. A third category, **tertiary peritonitis**, is described in people and refers to secondary peritonitis that persists or recurs for more than 48 hours after an attempt at surgical source control [3]. With peritonitis, the initial insult (e.g. bacterial contamination) results in release of inflammatory mediators such as histamine and serotonin from peritoneal macrophages and mast cells, which subsequently causes increased vascular permeability and transudation of proteins and fluid into the peritoneal cavity [17]. Macrophages also release chemotactic factors that promote neutrophil migration and adhesion, along with other mediators such as platelet-aggregating factor, tumor necrosis factor-α (TNFα), interleukin-1 (IL-1), IL-6, IL-8, monocyte chemoattractant protein 1, and prostaglandins and leukotrienes, all contributing to a sustained inflammatory response within the peritoneum [17, 18]. As neutrophils migrate into the peritoneal cavity, lysosomal degranulation and degradative enzymes are released as these neutrophils die. These events damage mesothelial cells, resulting in depleted fibrinolysis; thus, fibrin is produced to seal off bacterial contamination and heal defects within the peritoneal cavity [17]. Ideally, the foal's inflammatory and immune response successfully clears the cause of the peritonitis resulting in resolution of inflammation, restoration of the mesothelium, and subsequent fibrinolysis. However, if inflammation persists, abdominal adhesions and abscesses can occur. Causes of peritonitis in the foal are noted in Table 17.IV.1.

Table 17.IV.1 Causes of peritonitis in the foal.

Localized infection that invades abdominal cavity
Umbilical remnant infection, uroperitoneum [19–28]
Enterocolitis (*Salmonella*, *Clostridium*) [29, 30]
Intestinal ischemia
Disseminated infections
Neonatal sepsis [22, 28, 31–33]
Rhodococcus equi (typically older foals, 1–4 mo of age) [34, 35]
Gastrointestinal perforation or secondary to abdominal surgery
Perforated gastric ulcer [36, 37]
Duodenitis [38, 39]
Duodenal ulceration or stricture [39, 40]
Surgery procedures for acute colic or urogenital disorders [41–45]
Chemical insults (bile, urine, pancreatic enzymes)
Acute pancreatitis [46, 47]
Chyloperitoneum [48, 49]

Clinical Signs of Peritonitis

Clinical signs of peritonitis are variable, with some signs reflecting the innervation of the peritoneum, which has two distinct patterns to the parietal and visceral peritoneum. The parietal peritoneum is innervated by the phrenic, thoraco-abdominal, subcostal, lumbosacral, and obturator nerves and is sensitive to pressure, temperature, and laceration [3, 4]. These stretch, temperature, and pain receptors are very sensitive and have a relatively low threshold, with people describing the discomfort associated with parietal peritonitis as sharp, constant, well-localized pain [4, 50]. In contrast, innervation of the visceral peritoneum occurs through the splanchnic and vagus nerves and the celiac and mesenteric plexus and are sensitive only to chemical irritation and stretch/distention and insensitive to pain [3]. An ill-defined and paroxysmal colic pain is described in people with visceral peritonitis [50]. Veterinarians cannot determine the specific type of pain or discomfort a foal might experience with peritonitis, but the description in people provides awareness to the types of discomfort that may occur. General clinical signs and physical examination findings of peritonitis in the foal include lethargy, colic, tachycardia, tachypnea, fever, and diarrhea [51–53]. More specific clinical signs can be associated with explicit types of peritonitis as described below.

Localized infections can occasionally invade the abdominal cavity and are typically extensions from umbilical remnant or GI infections. Tearing of the umbilical cord at birth opens up a potential path for infection until complete atrophy and loss of the external remnant occurs, particularly if there is poor hygiene of the navel and/or the foal's environment [19]. The infection can remain localized to the umbilical structures, but peritonitis can develop if localized infection and necrosis extends beyond the confines of these structures [54]. Review of diseases of the umbilical remnants is found in Chapter 27. However, signs of septic peritonitis associated with omphalophblebitis include lethargy, decreased nursing, stranguria, fever, and possibly abdominal distension and respiratory compromise if uroabdomen is also present. Acute death, without prodromal signs, was reported in foals with *Clostridium sordellii* omphalitis and peritonitis [19]. Severe enterocolitis can also result in peritonitis in some cases. In one case series, 8/27 (30%) neonatal foals with Clostridial diarrhea had evidence of peritonitis on necropsy examination [29]. Fibrinonecrotic and necrohemorrhagic enterocolitis was commonly identified in foals with severe disease along with microscopic changes such as denuded, ulcerated, and necrotic villi and mucosa of the small intestine. These pathologic findings can result in bacterial translocation and development of peritonitis [29, 30]. Diarrhea was observed in these cases. Disseminated infections such as occurs with neonatal sepsis can result in peritonitis, although generalized clinical signs associated with sepsis, such as lethargy, inappetence, dehydration, diarrhea, and shock may predominate [31].

Perforation of the GI tract (perforated gastric or duodenal ulcer, intestinal perforation, secondary to abdominal surgery) results in gross contamination of the abdominal cavity. Gastric ulcers may be subclinical, but foals with clinical ulcers can have variable clinical signs such as diarrhea, poor appetite, poor growth, rough hair coat, potbellied appearance, bruxism, dorsal recumbency, excessive salivation, decreased suckling, and colic [55]. Foals with gastric perforation (or any other type of intestinal perforation) may not show any prodromal signs, but once perforation occurs, profound depression, tachycardia, abdominal distention, colic, shock and death ensue (Figure 17.IV.2) [55]. In a case series of 8 foals with perforated gastric ulcers, the mean age at presentation was 48 days (range 19–90 days) with consistent clinical signs including fever, diarrhea, dyspnea, and diarrhea [36]. Upon necropsy examination, gastric perforation was noted in two areas: the margo plicatus (5/8 foals) and at the pyloric region (3/8 foals) [36].

Chemical insults, such as occurs with severe acute pancreatitis, is rarely described in neonatal foals but this condition can be suspected in foals with acute neurological signs (seizures), hypovolemic shock, and abdominal crisis associated with a chylous-hemorrhagic peritonitis, diarrhea and lipemic serum [46, 47]. Hypertriglyceridemia (53.4 mmol/l, rr 0.15–0.86 mmol/l) and increased serum amylase (34–155 u/l, rr < 4 u/l) and lipase activity (326–449 u/l rr, <39 u/l) were reported in foals with acute pancreatitis [46, 47]. Peritoneal effusion was noted, and abdominal fluid analysis revealed orange, turbid fluid with normal to slightly elevated TNCC ($2.3 \times 10^3/\mu l$, $rr < 1.5 \times 10^3/\mu l$), increased total protein (4.2–5.6 g/dl), and elevated abdominal fluid amylase (79–729 u/l, rr < 14 u/l) and lipase activity (1300–1746 u/l, rr 36 u/l) [46, 47]. All reported cases of foals with acute pancreatitis did not survive. Chyloperitoneum is also uncommonly reported in equine neonates, but can result in chemical peritonitis as chyle is irritating to the abdomen and contains elevated levels of fibrinogen that favors peritoneal adhesion formation [48, 49]. Underlying causes of chyloperitoneum (chyloabdomen) include congenital defects of the lymphatic system, intestinal lymphangiectasia, trauma, abnormal permeability, obstruction or hypoplasia of the mesenteric lymphatic vessels, malignancy, inflammatory lesions, abdominal surgery, or idiopathic [48, 49, 56–58]. Intestinal lymphangectasia as a cause of chyloperitoneum has been reported in neonatal foals and is suspected to occur when pressure in the mesenteric and/or intestinal lymph vessels increase (Figure 17.IV.3) [48, 49, 56]. If the lacteals in the intestinal villi rupture, lymph (including chylomicrons, lymphocytes, and proteins) leaks into the intestinal lumen, whereas rupture of the mesenteric lymphatics or cisterna chyli results in escape of chlye into the abdominal cavity [48, 49]. Foals with intestinal lymphangectasia present with signs of colic and may be tachycardic. Lymphopenia and hypoalbuminemia may be noted

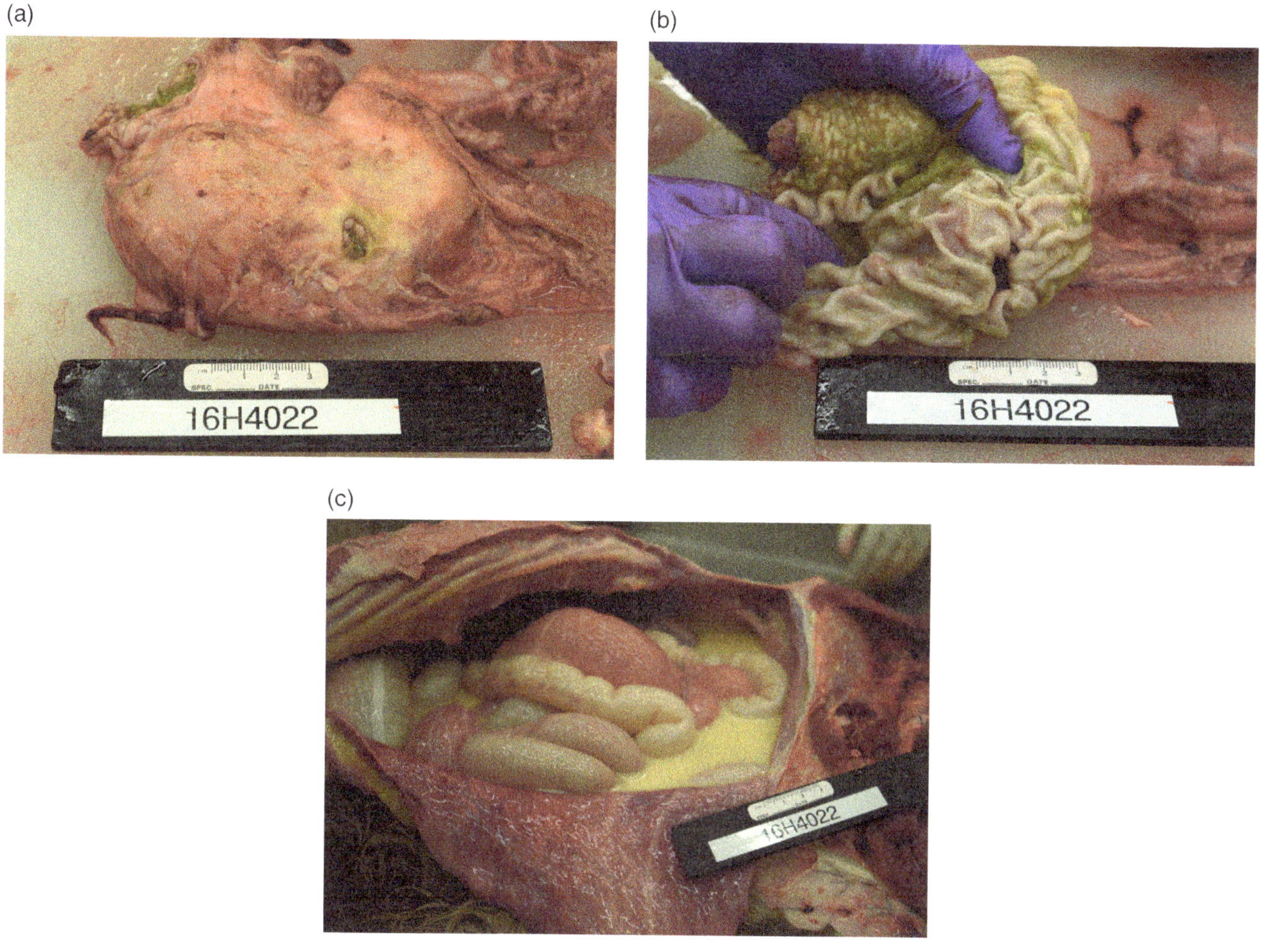

Figure 17.IV.2 Gastric perforation in a neonatal foal. (a) Serosal and (b) mucosal images of gastric perforation. (c) Resultant peritonitis and excess peritoneal fluid and milk within the abdominal cavity. Ruler = 3 cm.

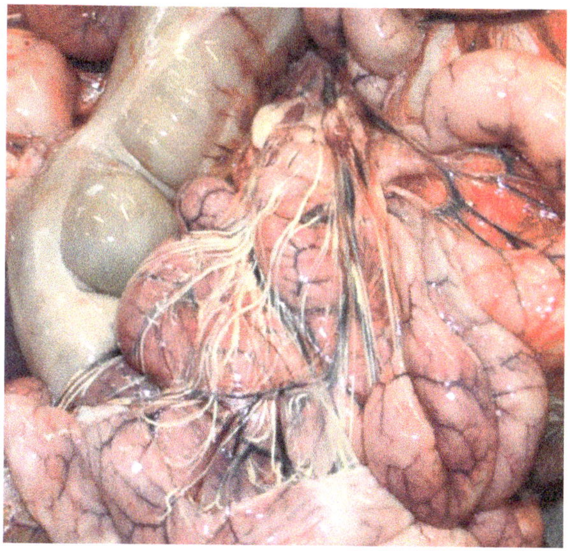

Figure 17.IV.3 Postmortem image of a neonatal foal with dilated lacteals observed in the abdomen as an incidental finding. The foal was euthanized for a congenital heart anomaly. *Source:* Image courtesy of Dr. Edwina Wilkes, Charles Sturt University.

due to enteric protein loss [58]. Abdominal ultrasound notes excess free fluid within the abdomen with abdominocentesis yielding odorless, white to yellow opaque fluid [48]. The color of the abdominal fluid does not clear with centrifugation as compared to markedly purulent exudates that separate the white cells from the remainder of the abdominal fluid [49, 58]. Elevated TNCC (range: 8.0 to 23.2×10^3 cells/μl), total protein (4.9 g/dl) and triglyceride concentrations (range: 397–1496 mg/dl; rr < 110 mg/dl) were measured in the peritoneal fluid of affected foals [48, 49, 57]. Given time, lymphatic vessels mature and medical management with broad-spectrum antimicrobials, anti-inflammatories and supportive care resulted in positive outcomes in foals [48]. Reduction of fat intake, provision of a medium-chain triglyceride-based diets, and drainage of chylous fluid is suggested in people [48, 59]. Medium-chain triglycerides are recommended as they are absorbed directly into the portal venous circulation thereby avoiding lacteal overload. Fortuitously, foals do not require a change in diet as mare's milk contains large amounts of medium-chain fatty acids [60]. However, exploratory celiotomy and surgical

Table 17.IV.2 Peritoneal fluid values from 17 healthy foals (age range 13–134 days) [62].

Mean age	WBC ($\times 10^3/\mu l$)	Neutrophils ($\times 10^3/\mu l$)	Mononuclear cells ($\times 10^3/\mu l$)	RBC ($\times 10^3/\mu l$)	Protein (gm/dl)	Specific gravity	BUN (mg/dl)
68 days	0.451 ± 0.322	0.230 ± 0.318	0.211 ± 9.152	4.3 ± 5.3	1.2 ± 3	1.013 ± 0.0015	5.48 ± 1.56

Table 17.IV.3 Peritoneal fluid values from 32 healthy Thoroughbred foals (age range 14–75 days) [63].

Mean age	WBC ($\times 10^3/\mu l$)	Neutrophils (%)	Large mononuclear cells (%)	Small mononuclear cells (%)	RBC count ($\times 10^3/\mu l$)	Protein (mg/dl)
45 days	1.418 ± 1.077	15.3 ± 20.4	43.8 ± 24.8	22.3 ± 24.5	12.070 ± 15.219	1.8 ± 0.7

correction of a physical lesion associated with damage to the lymphatics may be necessary in some foals to resect affected segments of intestine [49, 56].

Diagnosis

Diagnosis of peritonitis in the neonatal foal is based on elevated abdominal fluid TNCC and total protein concentration (Table 17.IV.4). A site to the right of midline along the ventral abdomen, approximately 5–8 cm caudal to the xiphoid, is a good starting point for abdominocentesis, but ultrasonographic examination of the abdomen is suggested to determine volume, character, and location of free fluid. Peritoneal fluid can be collected from the ventral abdomen in the foal in either a standing or laterally recumbent position using an 18-gauge, 1-in. needle or teat cannula, after sterile preparation of the skin at the centesis site. Of note, because the use of a teat cannula requires a small skin incision with a scalpel, it is not uncommon for a small amount of omentum to exit the abdomen through the incision after the procedure is complete [61]. Thus, the use of an 18-gauge needle may lend to fewer complications.

Peritoneal fluid parameters from healthy foals have been reported in two studies with notable similarities and differences compared to adult horses. The abdominal fluid in both adult horses and foals is pale yellow to yellow in color, is clear to slightly turbid, and has a total protein concentration <2.0 g/dl [17, 62–64]. However, the TNCC in peritoneal fluid from healthy foals (Tables 17.IV.2, 17.IV.3, and 17.IV.4) is lower than that of adult horses ($5.0–10.0 \times 10^3/\mu l$). Therefore, in foals, TNCC $> 1.5 \times 10^3$ to $3.0 \times 10^3/\mu l$ should be considered elevated [62, 63]. Cytologic examination of abdominal fluid from foals with peritonitis reveals suppurative inflammation with a predominance of degenerate neutrophils and the possibility of intra- or extra-cellular bacteria. Gram staining can be performed in attempts to identify bacteria, but only 27–32.5% of samples submitted were Gram-stain positive in adult horses with peritonitis [50, 51, 65]. As well, samples should be submitted for bacterial culture, but expect moderate sensitivity, with positive growth noted in 8.5–41% of samples in adult horses with peritonitis [50–52, 65]. In one study, samples submitted in blood culture bottles had a higher return of bacterial growth (54%) as compared to sterile plastic tubes (21%) in adult horses with peritonitis, suggesting that blood culture medium might lend to improved sensitivity [52, 66]. Another variable to consider is that recent abdominal surgery will alter peritoneal fluid analysis, including marked increases in TNCC and protein concentration even after simple abdominal procedures in adult horses [67, 68].

Other diagnostics that support a diagnosis of peritonitis include alterations in the complete blood count (CBC),

Table 17.IV.4 Peritoneal fluid values from 32 healthy Thoroughbred foals (age range 14–75 days) [63].

Parameter	Mean ± SD (range)	Parameter	Mean±SD (range)	Parameter	Mean ± SD (range)
Glucose (mg/dL)	136.9±21 (100–178)	ALP (IU/l)	43.6 ±15.15 (13–82)	Creatinine (mg/dl)	1.39 ±0.22 (0.91–1.87)
Chloride (mEq/l)	98.7±4.16 (92–106)	AST (IU/l)	50±18.9 (28–120)	LDH (IU/l)	46.5±22 (23–108)
Sodium (mEq/l)	133.6±2.18 (128–137)	Potassium (mEq/l)	4.2±0.36 (3.6–4.9)		

ALP, alkaline phosphatse; AST, aspartate aminotransferase, LDH, lactate dehydrogenase.

including leukocytosis or leukopenia and hyperfibrinogenemia, elevated concentrations in serum amyloid A (SAA) and changes in serum biochemistry profile such as azotemia, metabolic acidosis and electrolyte imbalances. Elevation in peritoneal fluid L-lactate can also be observed with peritonitis [52].

Treatment

Determining the underlying cause of peritonitis is the first step in formulating a treatment plan, as therapy will vary depending on the cause (Figure 17.IV.4). General treatment principles include restoration of fluid, protein and electrolyte balances, antimicrobial therapy, anti-inflammatory and

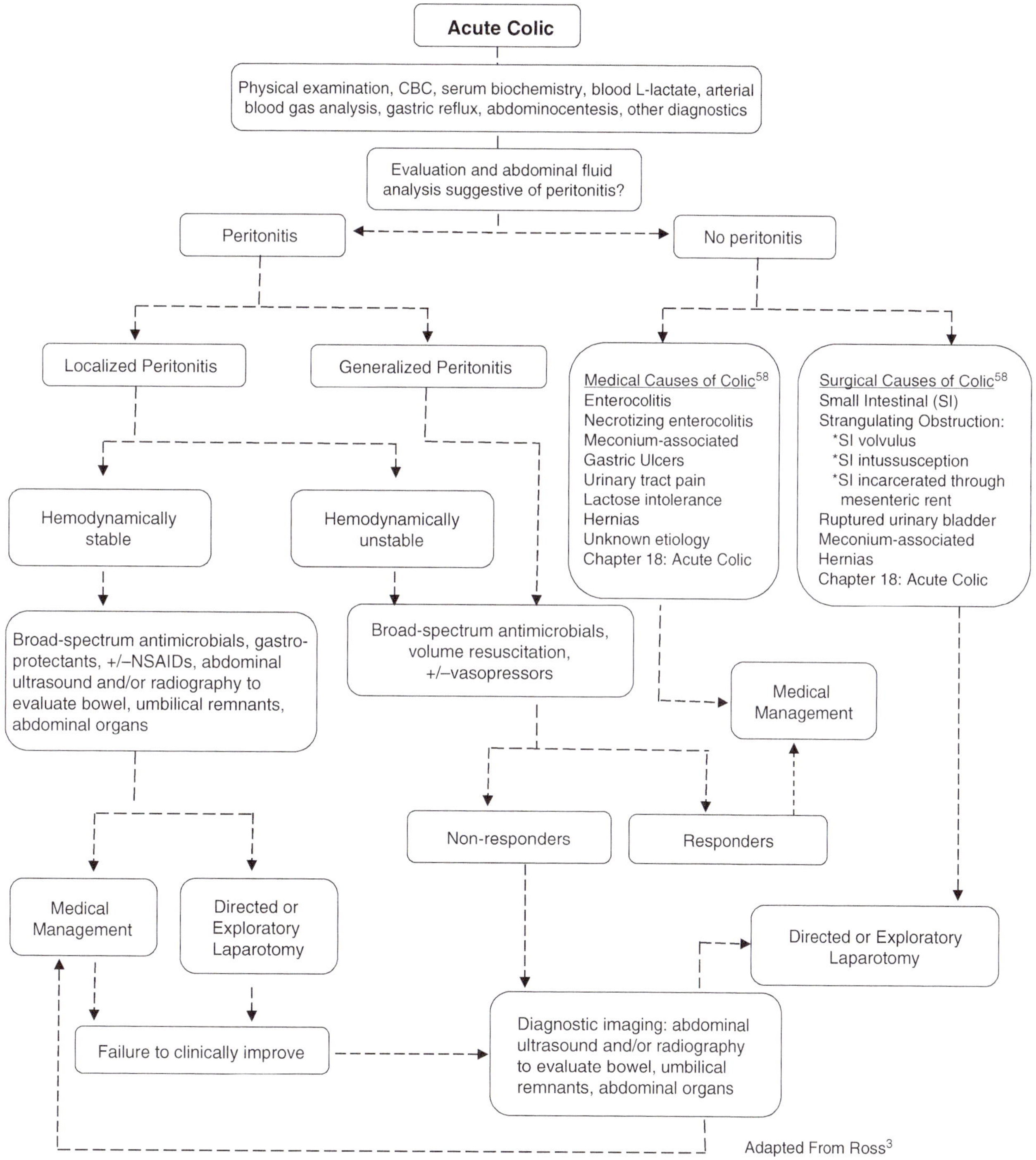

Figure 17.IV.4 Diagnostic and therapeutic outline for a foal with acute colic. *Source:* Adapted from Ross et al. [3].

anti-endotoxic therapy, removal of bacteria, prevention of adhesions, and supportive care [17, 51, 53, 65].

Hypovolemia may be present due to fluid shifts into the peritoneal cavity and inadequate milk intake that commonly occurs in ill neonatal foals. Thus, volume resuscitation and restoration of adequate blood pressure is an initial therapeutic goal. Fluid resuscitation includes bolus IV administration of 20 ml/kg of isotonic fluids over 10–15 minutes [69]. Blood pressure and other indications of perfusion (pulse quality, extremity temperature, urine production, improved mental status) should be reevaluated after each bolus. If these parameters remain inadequate, repeated 20 ml/kg boluses can be administered up to a total volume of 60–80 ml/kg. If perfusion parameters are still not improved, inopressor therapy, such as dopamine, dobutamine, vasopressin, or norepinephrine should be initiated (Chapter 11) [69]. If hypoproteinemia is present, administration of natural (plasma) or synthetic (hydroxyethyl starch solutions) colloids should be considered. Additionally, peritonitis is often associated with deficiencies in calcium, sodium, potassium, and chloride [20, 29]. Therefore, oral and/or IV supplementation and periodic re-assessment of these electrolytes is necessary. It is important to consider adequate volume resuscitation in neonatal foals prior to drainage of fluid from the abdomen, as severe accumulation of abdominal fluid can result in increased intra-abdominal pressure (a function of internal organ mass, abdominal fluid volume and wall compliance), abdominal hypertension, and possibly abdominal compartment syndrome, all of which can exacerbate existing hypovolemic shock [70]. Maintenance IV fluids should be instituted once volume is restored.

Administration of broad-spectrum antimicrobials is indicated in neonatal foals with peritonitis and can be based on bacterial culture and antibiotic sensitivity results of the peritoneal fluid, umbilical remnants, or blood samples. If these samples are negative, or if empirical antimicrobial selection is the only option, combinations of beta-lactams (ceftiofur, ampicillin, potassium penicillin) and aminoglycosides (amikacin, gentamicin) are viable broad-spectrum options [17]. De-escalation of antimicrobials should be instituted if bacterial antimicrobial sensitivity testing is available. Parenterally administered antimicrobials should be instituted for 7–10 days followed by oral antibiotics for another 7–14 days, or longer if indicated.

Judicious use of nonsteroidal anti-inflammatory drugs (NSAIDs) and/or analgesics may be needed to combat endotoxemia and pain. Flunixin meglumine (0.25–1.1 mg/kg, IV or PO every 12 hours) has been a mainstay of anti-inflammatory treatment in equids, however the predilection for gastric ulcers with the use of NSAIDs must be considered in the neonatal foal; if used, a lower dose (0.25–0.5 mg/kg) administered 2–3 times/day is suggested along with administration of gastroprotectants [37, 71]. The use of opioids such as butorphanol, can be used as an analgesic in foals (0.05–0.1 mg/kg, IV or IM, as needed) [72, 73]. Other medications to combat endotoxemia include hyperimmune plasma (20 ml/kg, IV), pentoxyifylline (8–10 mg/kg, PO every 12 hours), and polymyxin B (6,000 units/kg diluted in 20 ml of 0.9% NaCl, slow IV, every 8–12 hours), although these treatments have not been universally accepted as treatments for endotoxemia in foals [46, 74–76].

Nutritional support is an important consideration in ill neonatal foals with oral or parenteral options available. If the foal voluntarily suckles an appropriate amount and frequency, no nutritional supplementation may be necessary. However, if the foal has decreased or absent suckling behavior (e.g. low daily body weight gain), the clinician must decide if nasogastric tube feedings of mare's milk (or artificial milk) or parenteral nutrition is indicated. The clinician must determine if the foal can tolerate PO nutritional support, as certain circumstances such as severe enterocolitis or compromised GI tract may be contra-indications for PO nutrition. Alternatively, calories can be provided via IV dextrose solution using 4–8 mg/kg/min of dextrose as a guide [69]. If voluntary caloric intake is anticipated to remain low for more than 24 hours, partial parenteral nutrition should be formulated and administered (Chapter 58).

Determining the need for surgical management can be ambiguous (primary peritonitis from sepsis) or obvious (secondary peritonitis from extension of an umbilical remnant infection). Physical examination parameters and results of diagnostic tests should be considered collectively to decide if surgery is indicated. Severity of pain, degree of abdominal distension, and/or confirmed sources of infection may favor a surgical approach [61]. If surgery is indicated, the goals in cases of secondary peritonitis have remained relatively unchanged over time and include: (i) eliminate septic focus, (ii) remove necrotic tissue, and (iii) drain purulent material [3]. Measures should be taken to prevent abdominal adhesions and include therapies such as NSAIDs, dimethyl sulfoxide (DMSO), broad-spectrum antimicrobials, systemic heparin, intra-abdominal (intra-operative) carboxymethylcelluose, and omentectomy. Minimal prospective studies have investigated these therapies individually or in combination, but a full review of colic in the foal and prevention of adhesions is found in Chapter 18 [61, 77–79].

Peritoneal drainage and lavage are frequently used in adult horses with peritonitis and may be indicated in some neonatal foals with peritonitis. Management of a peritoneal lavage system can be more difficult in the foal because of the frequency in which foals lay down and rise, leading to potential dislodgement and/or contamination of the lavage system. Peritoneal drainage and lavage can be used in cases of peritonitis that do not require surgery (e.g. septic peritonitis), or alternatively, a lavage system can be placed at the time of exploratory surgery to allow for lavage postoperatively. Abdominal drainage and lavage removes excess fluid, bacteria, bacterial products, fibrin, blood, and other foreign materials from the abdominal cavity and may decrease the incidence of intra-abdominal adhesions [17]. Lavage catheters are typically placed in the ventral abdomen using ultrasound guidance to identify a fluid pocket and reduce the risk of bowel perforation. Once the area is identified, the skin is clipped and aseptically prepared, and lidocaine is used to desensitize the skin, subcutaneous tissue, and underlying muscle. A scalpel blade is used to incise the skin and underling tissue, but ideally should not penetrate into the abdominal cavity. A thoracic drain/catheter is typically placed through the incision and into the abdominal cavity, then secured in place using purse-string and finger-trap suture patterns. A closed system, using a sterile collection bag, should be utilized to allow for continued drainage while inhibiting the risk of retrograde travel of fluid or contaminants. Alternatively, a one-way Heimlich valve can be used. The catheter should be secured and covered with a sterile bandage. Sterile, warmed, balanced electrolyte solution (Lactate Ringer's solution, 0.9% saline) can be used as the lavage fluid using a volume of 500–1000 ml in a 50 kg foal. This fluid is retained in the abdomen for 15–25 minutes, then recovered.

The volume of the effluent should be measured in efforts to gauge the amount of fluids administered and removed from the patient. This process can be performed 1–4 times/day and continued for 3–5 days or until peritoneal fluid becomes clear. Of note, peritoneal catheters frequently become clogged with omentum, thus reducing the effectiveness of peritoneal drainage and lavage.

Summary

The incidence of peritonitis in the neonatal foal is relatively low, with one large retrospective study in 137 neonates documenting septic peritonitis in 1.5% (2 foals) of neonates presented for colic; 1 foal had a perforated gastric ulcer and the other a ruptured urachus [79]. Large retrospective studies establishing the prognosis of neonatal foals with peritonitis have not been performed, but prognosis will ultimately vary with underlying cause. Foals with gross contamination of the abdominal cavity from a ruptured GI structure have a grave prognosis [21, 37, 38]. Moreover, foals with severe acute pancreatitis, albeit rare, also have a poor prognosis [46, 47]. Conversely, foals with septic peritonitis from generalized sepsis or from an umbilical remnant or urinary structure typically have fair-to-good prognosis.

References

1 Blackburn, S.C. and Stanton, M.P. (2014). Anatomy and physiology of the peritoneum. *Semin. Pediatr. Surg.* 23: 326–330.
2 Isaza-Restrepo, A., Martin-Saavedra, J.S., Velez-Leal, J.L. et al. (2018). The peritoneum: beyond the tissue – a review. *Front. Physiol.* 9: 738.
3 Ross, J.T., Matthay, M.A., and Harris, H.W. (2018). Secondary peritonitis: principles of diagnosis and intervention. *BMJ* 361: k1407.
4 Kastelein, A.W., Vos, L.M.C., de Jong, K.H. et al. (2019). Embryology, anatomy, physiology and pathophysiology of the peritoneum and the peritoneal vasculature. *Semin. Cell Dev. Biol.* 92: 27–36.
5 Capobianco, A., Cottone, L., Monno, A. et al. (2017). The peritoneum: healing, immunity, and diseases. *J. Pathol.* 243: 137–147.
6 Krediet, R.T., Lindholm, B., and Rippe, B. (2000). Pathophysiology of peritoneal membrane failure. *Perit. Dial. Int.* 20 (Suppl. 4): S22–S42.
7 DeHeer, H.L., Parry, B.W., and Grndem, C.B. Peritoneal fluid. In: *Diagnostic Cytology and Hematology of the Horse*, 2e (ed. R.L. Cowell and R.D. Tyler), 127–162. Mosby.
8 Maddaus, M.A., Ahrenholz, D., and Simmons, R.L. (1988). The biology of peritonitis and implications for treatment. *Surg. Clin. North Am.* 68: 431–443.
9 Peroni, J.F. (2017). Diagnosis and treatment of peritonitis and hemoperitoneum. In: *The Equine Acute Abdomen* (ed. A.T. Blikslager, N.A. White, J.N. Moore, and T.S. Mair), 361–375. Wiley Blackwell.
10 Wong, D.M., Leger, L.C., Scarratt, W.K. et al. (2004). Uroperitoneum and pleural effusion in an American Paint filly. *Equine Vet. Educ.* 16: 290–293.
11 Behr, M.J., Hackett, R.P., Bentinck-Smith, J. et al. (1981). Metabolic abnormalities associated with rupture of the urinary bladder in neonatal foals. *J. Am. Vet. Med. Assoc.* 178: 263–266.
12 Hackett, R.P. (1984). Rupture of the urinary bladder in neonatal foals. *Compend. Contin. Educ. Pract. Vet.* 6: S488–S494.
13 Richardson, D.W. and Kohn, C.W. (1983). Uroperitoneum in the foal. *J. Am. Vet. Med. Assoc.* 182: 267–270.
14 Sikkink, C.J., Reijnen, M.M., Falk, P. et al. (2005). Influences of monocyte-like cells on the fibrinolytic activity of peritoneal mesothelial cells and the effect of

sodium hyaluronate. *Fertil. Steril.* 82 (Suppl. 2): 1072–1077.

15 Sangisetty, S.L. and Miner, T.J. (2012). Malignant ascites: a review of prognostic factors, pathophysiology and therapeutic measures. *World J. Gastrointest. Surg.* 4: 87–95.

16 Moore, C.M. and Van Thiel, D.H. (2013). Cirrhotic ascites review: pathophysiology, diagnosis and management. *World J. Hepatol.* 5: 251–263.

17 Davis, J.L. (2003). Treatment of peritonitis. *Vet. Clin. Equine* 19: 765–778.

18 Riese, J., Schoolmann, S., Denzel, C. et al. (2002). Effect of abdominal infections on peritoneal and systemic production of interleukin 6 and monocyte chemoattractant protein-1. *Shock* 17: 361–364.

19 Ortega, J., Daft, B., Assis, R.A. et al. (2007). Infection of internal umbilical remnant in foals by *Clostridium sordellii*. *Vet. Pathol.* 44: 269–275.

20 Dunkel, B., Palmer, J.E., Olson, K.N. et al. (2005). Uroperitoneum in 32 foals: influence of intravenous fluid therapy, infection and sepsis. *J. Vet. Intern. Med.* 19: 889–893.

21 Adams, R., Koterba, A.M., Cudd, T.C. et al. (1988). Exploratory celiotomy for suspected urinary tract disruption in neonatal foals: a review of 18 cases. *Equine Vet. J.* 20: 13–17.

22 Platt, H. (1973). Septicaemia in the foal. A review of 61 cases. *Br. Vet. J.* 129: 221–229.

23 Adams, S.B. and Fessler, J.F. (1987). Umbilical cord remnant infections in foals: 16 cases (1975–1985). *J. Am. Vet. Med. Assoc.* 190: 316–318.

24 Bain, A.M. (1963). Common bacterial infections of fetuses and foals and association of infection with the dam. *Aust. Vet. J.* 39: 413–416.

25 Hymann, S.S., Wilkins, P.A., Palmer, J.E. et al. (2002). Clostridium perfringens urachitis and uroperitoneum in 2 neonatal foals. *J. Vet. Intern. Med.* 16: 489–493.

26 Swerczek, T.W. (1980). Toxicoinfectious botulism in foals and adult horses. *J. Am. Vet. Med. Assoc.* 176: 217–220.

27 Lores, M., Lofstedt, J., Martinson, S. et al. (2011). Septic peritonitis and uroperitoneum secondary to subclinical omphalitis and concurrent necrotizing cystitis in a colt. *Can. Vet. J.* 52: 888–892.

28 Hoffman, A.M., Staempfli, H.R., and Willan, A. (1992). Prognostic variables for survival of neonatal foals under intensive care. *J. Vet. Intern. Med.* 6: 89–95.

29 East, L.M., Savage, S.J., Traub-Dargatz, J.L. et al. (1998). Enterocolitis associated with Clostridium perfringens infection in neonatal foals: 54 cases (1988–1997). *J. Am. Vet. Med. Assoc.* 212: 1751–1756.

30 Edwards, P.R. (1934). Salmonella aertrycke in colitis of foals. *J. Infect. Dis.* 54: 85–90.

31 Koterba, A.M., Brewer, B.D., and Tarplee, F.A. (1984). Clinical and clinicopathological characteristics of the septicaemic neonatal foal: review of 38 cases. *Equine Vet. J.* 16: 376–383.

32 Monterio, F., Wong, D.M., Scarratt, W.K. et al. (2006). Listeria monocytogenes septicaemia in 2 neonatal foals. *Equine Vet. Educ.* 18: 27–31.

33 Cotovio, M., Monreal, L., Armengou, L. et al. (2008). Fibrin deposits and organ failure in newborn foals with severe septicemia. *J. Vet. Intern. Med.* 22: 1403–1410.

34 Zink, M.C., Yager, J.A., and Smart, N.L. (1986). *Corynebacterium equi* infections in horses, 1958–1984: a review of 131 cases. *Can. Vet. J.* 27: 213–217.

35 Giguere, S. and Prescott, J.F. (1997). Clinical manifestations, diagnosis, treatment and prevention of *Rhodococcus equi* infections in foals. *Vet. Mircobiol.* 56: 313–334.

36 Rooney, J.R. (1964). Gastric ulceration in foals. *Pathol. Vet.* 1: 497–503.

37 Becht, J.L. and Byars, T.D. (1986). Gastroduodenal ulceration in foals. *Equine Vet. J.* 18: 307–312.

38 Acland, H.M., Gunson, D.E., and Gillette, D.M. (1983). Ulcerative duodenitis in foals. *Vet. Pathol.* 20: 653–661.

39 Orsini, J.A. and Donawick, W.J. (1986). Surgical treatment of gastroduodenal obstructions in foals. *Vet. Surg.* 15: 205–213.

40 Zedler, S.T., Embertson, R.M., Bernard, W.V. et al. (2009). Surgical treatment of gastric outflow obstruction in 40 foals. *Vet. Surg.* 38: 623–630.

41 Vatistas, N.J., Snyder, J.R., Wilson, W.D. et al. (1996). Surgical treatment for colic in the foal (67 cases): 1980–1992. *Equine Vet. J.* 28: 139–145.

42 Modransky, P.D., Wagner, P.C., Robinette, J.D. et al. (1983). Surgical correction of bilateral ectopic ureters in two foals. *Vet. Surg.* 12: 141–147.

43 Coleman, M.C., Slovis, N.M., and Hung, R.J. (2009). Long-term prognosis of gastrojejunostomy in foals with gastric outflow obstruction: 16 cases (2001–2006). *Equine Vet. J.* 41: 653–657.

44 Cable, C.K., Fubini, S.L., Erb, H.N. et al. (1997). Abdominal surgery in foals: a review of 119 cases (1977–1994). *Equine Vet. J.* 29: 257–261.

45 Adams, R., Koterba, A.M., Brown, M.P. et al. (1988). Exploratory celiotomy for gastrointestinal disease in neonatal foals: a review of 20 cases. *Equine Vet. J.* 20: 9–12.

46 Ollivett, T.L., Divers, T.J., Cushing, T. et al. (2012). Acute pancreatitis in two five-day-old Appaloosa foals. *Equine Vet. J.* 44 (Suppl. 41): 96–99.

47 Taintor, J., Sartin, E.A., Waldridge, B.M. et al. (2006). Acute pancreatitis in a 3-day old foal. *J. Vet. Intern. Med.* 20: 210–212.

48 Cesar, F.B., Johnson, C.R., and Pantaleon, L.G. (2010). Suspected idiopathic intestinal lymphangiectasia in two foals with chylous peritoneal effusion. *Equine Vet. Educ.* 22: 172–178.
49 May, K.A. and Good, M.J. (2007). Congenital lymphangiectasia and chyloperitoneum in the foal. *Equine Vet. Educ.* 19: 16–18.
50 Mair, T.S., Hillyer, M.H., and Taylor, F.G.R. (1990). Peritonitis in adult horses: a review of 21 cases. *Vet. Rec.* 126: 567–570.
51 Dyson, S. (1983). Review of 30 cases of peritonitis in the horse. *Equine Vet. J.* 15: 25–30.
52 Odelros, E., Kendall, A., Hedberg-Alm, Y. et al. (2019). Idiopathic peritonitis in horses: a retrospective study of 130 cases in Sweden (2002–2017). *Acta Vet. Scand.* 61: 18.
53 Henderson, I.S.F., Mair, T.S., Keen, J.A. et al. (2008). Study of the short- and long-term outcomes of 65 horses with peritonitis. *Vet. Rec.* 163: 293–297.
54 Elce, Y.A. (2006). Infections of the equine abdomen and pelvis: perirectal abscesses, umbilical infections, and peritonitis. *Vet. Clin. Equine* 22: 419–436.
55 Andrews, F.M. and Nadeau, J.A. (1999). Clinical syndromes of gastric ulceration in foals and mature horses. *Equine Vet. J.* 31 (Suppl. 29): 30–33.
56 Campbell-Beggs, C.L., Johnson, P.J., Wilson, D.A. et al. (1995). Chyloabdomen in a neonatal foal. *Vet. Rec.* 137: 96–98.
57 Hanselaer, J.R. (1983). Chyloabdomen and ultrasonographic detection of an intra-abdominal abscess in a foal. *J. Am. Vet. Med. Assoc.* 183: 1465–1467.
58 Morresey, P.R. (2010). Intestinal lymphangiectasia and chyloperitoneum. *Equine Vet. Educ.* 22: 179–181.
59 Campisi, C., Bellini, C., Eretta, C. et al. (2006). Diagnosis and management of primary chylous ascites. *J. Vasc. Surg.* 43: 1244–1248.
60 Breckenridge, W.C. and Kuksus, A. (1967). Molecular weight distributions of milk fat triglycerides from seven species. *J. Lipid Res.* 8: 473–478.
61 Bryant, J.E. and Gaughan, E.M. (2005). Abdominal surgery in neonatal foals. *Vet. Clin. Equine* 21: 511–535.
62 Grindem, C.B., Fairley, N.M., Uhlinger, C.A. et al. (1990). Peritoneal fluid values from healthy foals. *Equine Vet. J.* 22: 359–361.
63 Behrens, E., Parraga, M.E., Nassiff, A. et al. (1990). Reference values of peritoneal fluid from healthy foals. *Equine Vet. Sci.* 10: 3348–3352.
64 Bach, L.G. and Ricketts, S.W. (1974). Paracentesis as an aid to the diagnosis of abdominal disease in the horse. *Equine Vet. J.* 6: 116–122.
65 Hawkins, J.F., Bowman, K.F., Roberts, M.C. et al. (1993). Peritonitis in horses: 67 cases (1985–1990). *J. Am. Vet. Med. Assoc.* 203: 284–288.
66 Lye, W.C., Wong, P.L., Leong, S.O. et al. (1994). Isolation of organisms in CAPD peritonitis: a comparison of two techniques. *Adv. Perit. Dial.* 10: 166–168.
67 Hanson, R.R., Nixon, A.J., Gronwall, R. et al. (1992). Evaluation of peritoneal fluid following intestinal resection and anastomosis in horses. *Am. J. Vet. Res.* 53: 216–221.
68 Santschi, E.M., Grindem, C.B., Tate, L.P. et al. (1988). Peritoneal fluid analysis in ponies after abdominal surgery. *Vet. Surg.* 17: 6–9.
69 Palmer, J.E. (2004). Fluid therapy in the neonate: not your mother's fluid space. *Vet. Clin. Equine* 20: 63–75.
70 Brosnahan, M.M., Holbrook, T.C., Gilliam, L.L. et al. (2009). Intra-abdominal hypertension in two adult horses. *J. Vet. Emerg. Crit. Care* 19: 174–180.
71 Wichtel, M.E., Buys, E., DeLuca, J. et al. (1999). Pharmacologic considerations in the treatment of neonatal septicemia and its complications. *Vet. Clin. North Am. Equine* 15: 725–746.
72 Arguedas, M.G., Hines, M.T., Papich, M.G. et al. (2008). Pharmacokinetics of butorphanol and evaluation of physiologic and behavioral effects after intravenous and intramuscular administration to neonatal foals. *J. Vet. Intern. Med.* 22: 1417–1426.
73 McGowan, K.T., Elfenbein, J.R., Robertson, S.A. et al. (2013). Effect of butorphanol on thermal nociceptive threshold in healthy pony foals. *Equine Vet. J.* 45: 503–506.
74 Wong, D.M., Wilkins, P.A., Bain, F.T. et al. (2011). Neonatal encephalopathy in foals. *Compend. Contin. Educ. Vet.* E1–E10.
75 Wong, D.M., Sponseller, B.A., Alcott, C.J. et al. (2013). Effects of intravenous polymyxin B in neonatal foals with experimental endotoxemia. *J. Am. Vet. Med. Assoc.* 243: 874–881.
76 Baskett, A., Barton, M.H., Norton, N. et al. (1997). Effect of pentoxifylline, flunixin meglumine, and their combination on a model of endotoxemia in horses. *Am. J. Vet. Res.* 58: 1291–1299.
77 Sullins, K.E., White, N.A., Lundin, C.E. et al. (2004). Prevention of ischaemia-induced small intestinal adhesions in foals. *Equine Vet. J.* 36: 370–375.
78 Mueller, P.O., Hunt, R.J., Allen, D. et al. (1995). Intraperitoneal use of sodium carboxymethylcellulose in horses undergoing exploratory celiotomy. *Vet. Surg.* 24: 112–117.
79 MacKinnon, M.C., Southwood, L.L., Burke, M.J. et al. (2013). Colic in equine neonates: 137 cases (2000–2010). *J. Am. Vet. Med. Assoc.* 243: 1586–1595.

Section V Meconium Impaction

David Wong

Meconium consists of sterile mucilaginous material in the intestine of the late-term fetus and is composed of a mixture of cellular debris, intestinal gland secretions, bile, and ingested amniotic fluid [1, 2]. Meconium is firm and pasty with a dark greenish brown or black color and is typically evacuated in the newborn foal within 3 hours of birth. The average time to initial passage of meconium in 22 healthy foals was 53 ± 35 minutes and is considered retained if the foal makes frequent attempts but fails to produce meconium by 12–36 hours of age [2, 3]. Meconium impaction is one of the most common causes of colic in the newborn foal, reportedly involving 1.5% of all newborn foals, and may require varying levels of veterinary intervention [4]. In a large retrospective study of 137 neonatal foals presenting to a referral hospital for signs of colic, the three most common causes were enterocolitis (27%), meconium-associated (20%), and transient medical colic (19%) [5]. The underlying cause of meconium impaction in the foal is unknown, but the intrinsic consistency of the material and narrow pelvic inlet may contribute to the condition. Meconium plug syndrome has been described in newborn infants as a benign cause of bowel obstruction without a specific underlying etiology; however, some reports link meconium plug to Hirschsprung's disease, maternal hypermagnesemia (used as a tocolytic), or cystic fibrosis [6]. No such links to meconium impaction in foals and an underlying disease process have been established.

The majority of impactions are located in the small colon near the pelvic inlet (low impaction) but also can be situated in the right dorsal or transverse colon (high impaction) [2, 3, 7]. Male foals may have a higher incidence than fillies, possibly due to the colts smaller pelvic inlet where the ischiatic arch is approximately two-thirds the diameter of the female and the pubis is convex as compared to concave in the female [3, 8]. In one study, colts were affected twice as often as fillies and in another study, six of eight foals requiring abdominal surgery to alleviate meconium impaction were colts [1, 2]. Other potential contributing factors predisposing to meconium impaction include maternal malnutrition, delayed consumption of colostrum (which serves as a laxative and stimulates the gastrocolic reflex), dehydration, intestinal disease, or hypomotility of the colon [4]. Medical disorders that compromise the foal – such as septicemia, prematurity, neonatal encephalopathy, and dystocia – might result in secondary ileus that can likewise delay the evacuation of meconium.

Clinical Signs

Clinical signs of meconium impaction are variable with early signs (6–24 hours old) manifesting as reduced frequency of sucking and increased recumbency [2]. Other signs such as restlessness, tail swishing, and/or elevation, frequent posturing to defecate, and tenesmus may also develop. Mild to severe signs of colic may be present along with abdominal distention as the condition persists and progresses. Some clinicians differentiate meconium-associated colic into one of two clinical situations: meconium impaction and meconium retention [5].

Other clinical signs associated with meconium impaction also include persistent signs of colic, decreased to absent fecal production, and identification of meconium via digital rectal examination, abdominal palpation, or ultrasonographic examination [5]. In contrast to meconium impaction, meconium retention occurs when meconium is not passed and retained within the large intestine for up to 2 weeks of age, and on rare occasions for 4 weeks or more (J. Palmer, personal communication). Meconium retention can result from excessive meconium formation in utero, impaired intestinal motility associated with intrauterine distress (asphyxia, hypoxic-ischemic insult, placenitis), sepsis, prematurity, or secondary to prolonged recumbency, dehydration or

Equine Neonatal Medicine, First Edition. Edited by David M. Wong and Pamela A. Wilkins.

Table 17.V.1 Clinical findings and treatment results of 44 foals with meconium impaction [1].

Clinical signs	Number of foals (%)	Treatment	Number of foals (%)
Disinterest in suckling	44 (100)	Acetylcysteine enema	41 (93.2)
Straining to defecate	44 (100)	Administration of 1 enema	24 (58.5)
Absence of milk feces	43 (97.7)	Administration of 2 enemas	12 (29.3)
Digital palpation of meconium	40 (90.9)	Administration of 3 enemas	5 (12.2)
Colic	39 (88.6)		
Abdominal distention	27 (61.4)	Impaction resolved ≤6 hours	24 (58.5)
Tachypnea (RR > 40 breaths/min)	27 (61.4)	Impaction resolved 7–12 hours	8 (19.5)
Restlessness	22 (50)	Impaction resolved 13–24 hours	7 (17.1)
Tachycardia (HR > 120 beats/min)	12 (27.3)	Impaction resolved >24 hours	2 (4.9)
Abdominal palpation of meconium	12 (27.3)		
Ruptured urinary bladder	3 (6.8)	IV fluids	32 (72.7)
Decreased borborygmi	1 (2.3)	Analgesics	25 (56.8)
Rectal temperature > 101.8 °F	1 (2.3)	Phosphate or soapy water enema	8 (18.2)
Bladder atony	1 (2.3)	Surgery	3 (6.8)

changes in motility from administered drugs. Foals with meconium retention are typically unaware of its presence but may have episodic signs of colic [5]. These differentiating terms are not universally used, with the majority of clinicians referring to the clinical disorder associated with persistent signs of colic as meconium impaction. Table 17.V.1 summarizes clinical signs of meconium impaction in 44 foals referred to a tertiary veterinary hospital for treatment.

Diagnosis

Diagnosis of meconium impaction is based on signalment, clinical signs, and the presence of firm stool upon digital palpation of the rectum. However, meconium can be retained more proximal than digital palpation allows, thus the absence of a palpable firm fecal mass does not rule out impaction. Rectal temperature is typically normal unless other disease processes such as sepsis are present, but tachycardia and tachypnea can be noted. Occasionally, the foal may develop a patent urachus due to excessive tenesmus. Results of a CBC and biochemistry profile are normal unless other underlying or concurrent disease processes are present. Gas distention of the large colon or cecum can manifest as abdominal distention with an audible "ping" potentially heard on auscultation and percussion in more severe cases. Deep abdominal palpation can be performed when the foal is sleeping or sedated in the area dorsal to the bladder, which may reveal a firm distinct mass of meconium. Ultrasonography and radiography can be used to

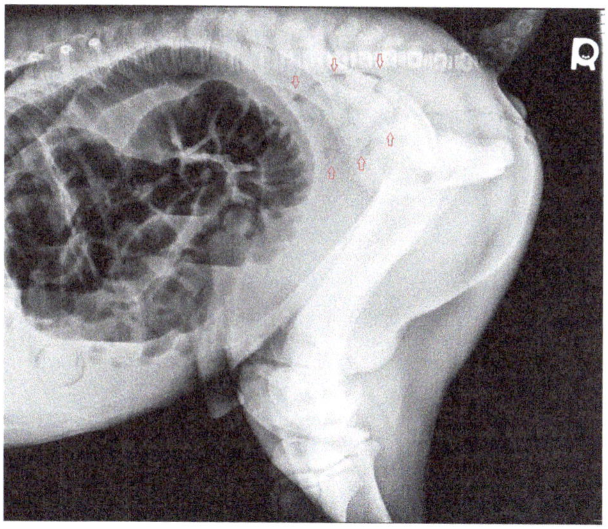

Figure 17.V.1 Lateral radiograph of a 12-hour-old foal presenting for abdominal distension and colic. Note the generalized gas distension of the intestines and meconium within the pelvic inlet (arrows).

further evaluate foals with clinical signs of colic, including those with meconium impaction. Other diseases that can result in similar clinical signs as meconium impaction include atresia coli, ruptured urinary bladder, congenital aganglionosis, enterocolitis, colon torsion, and small intestinal volvulus.

Severe generalized gas distention of the large colon can be documented on lateral radiography of the abdomen (Figure 17.V.1). Meconium appears as granular contents in the ascending or descending colon. Contrast studies using barium enemas, administered via a Foley catheter placed in the rectum, may facilitate identification of meconium obstruction. In particular, one study in neonatal foals described the technique of retrograde contrast radiography in which a Foley catheter is inserted into the rectum, the Foley's bulb is inflated, and up to 20 ml/kg of 30% wt/vol barium sulfate suspension is administered via gravity flow (flow stopped when suspension begins to travel around the Foley balloon or the foal struggles) [9]. This technique outlines the transverse colon and, depending on the amount administered, other portions of the large colon can be evaluated, including meconium impaction (Figure 17.V.2) and atresia coli [9].

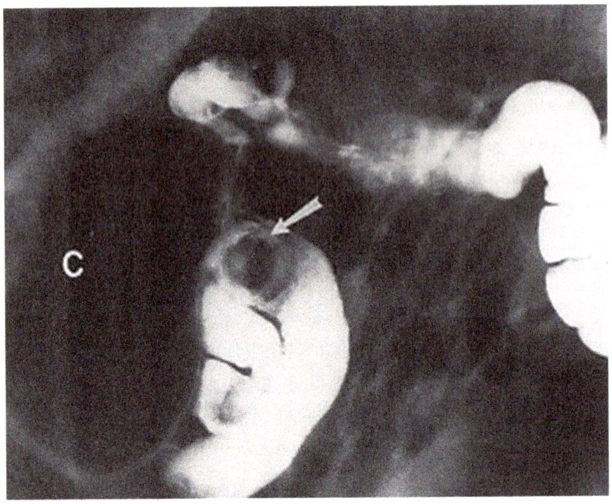

Figure 17.V.2 Lateral radiograph of a 1-day-old fold. Retrograde contrast agent stops at the proximal aspect of the small colon. Meconium (arrow) is silhouetted by contrast agent along with gas distension within the large colon (C) oral to the obstruction. *Source:* Image from Fisher [9].

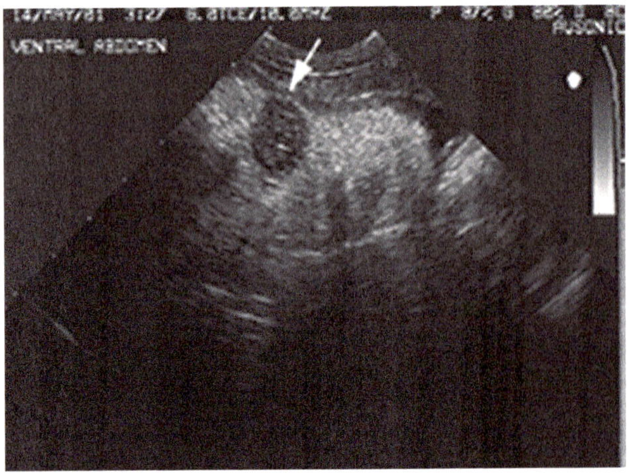

Figure 17.V.3 Abdominal ultrasound of a foal with meconium retention in the large intestine. Note the hypoechoic appearance of the meconium (arrow) surrounded by echoic milky ingesta in the large colon. *Source:* Image from McAuliffe [10].

Upon ultrasound of the abdomen, meconium appears as an intraluminal mass with hyperechoic, hypoechoic, or mixed echogenicity (Figure 17.V.3) along with fluid or gas present proximal to the obstruction [10, 11]. Meconium in the small colon may appear as a row of fecal balls surrounded by the intestine in the caudal abdomen whereas meconium in the large colon may appear more amorphous.

Treatment

Most foals with meconium impaction are treated with medical management, which includes administration of analgesics such as flunixin meglumine (0.25–0.5 mg/kg, IV, q 12 hours), diazepam (0.05–0.2 mg/kg, IV as needed), and/or butorphanol (0.01–0.04 mg/kg, IV as needed), IV fluids to establish normal hydration and soften the feces, oral laxatives such as mineral oil (60–120 ml via feeding tube) if the foal is older than 24 hours of age, and enemas.

Two main types of enemas are routinely used to facilitate passage of meconium in the neonatal foal. Commercially available phosphate enemas (Fleet enema; 4.5 oz) are effective but should not be administered more than twice in a 24-hour period to avoid hyperphosphatemia [2]. Alternatively, or in addition, warm soapy water enemas can be used. In this instance 500 ml of warm water is combined with ½ teaspoon of mild liquid dish soap and 250–500 ml is administered per rectum using a Foley catheter or similar and gravity flow. Caution should be exercised as repeated enemas of any type can be irritating to the rectal mucosa. Irritation in itself results in active colonic secretion that might help loosen the impaction, but too much irritation can increase the likelihood of traumatic perforation or serve as a portal for bacterial translocation and sepsis.

If meconium impaction persists, refractory cases can be administered acetylcysteine retention enemas. Of note, in one study involving 42 neonatal foals with colic, 42 foals received a warm soapy water enema and an acetylcysteine retention enema was only needed subsequent to a soapy water enema in 7 (17%) of foals, but not all 42 foals had meconium impaction [5]. Acetylcysteine does not dissolve the meconium but cleaves disulfide bonds in the mucoprotein molecules of meconium, thereby decreasing the overall tenacity and making the outer surface of the meconium slippery [2]. The acetylcysteine enema is also hypertonic (4%) and draws fluid into the bowel, which may soften the meconium and help detach it from the bowel wall [1]. Commercially available acetylcysteine enemas are available (EZ-pass; Animal Reproduction Systems, Chino CA), but can also be produced stall-side by adding 20 g of sodium bicarbonate (baking soda) and 8 g of acetylcysteine to 200 ml of water. This produces a 4% acetylcysteine solution at a pH of 7.6; increasing the pH of the solution increases the inherent mucolytic activity. Alternatively, acetylcysteine is available as a 20% solution, and 40 ml of this solution can be mixed with 160 ml of water and 20 g of sodium bicarbonate [1]. Because acetylcysteine requires several minutes of contact time with the meconium, sedation of the foal and elevation of the hindquarters is recommended to keep the foal in lateral recumbency. A Foley catheter with a large bulb is then inserted 3–5 cm into the rectum and the bulb is slowly inflated with 20–30 ml of water to occlude the rectum. Subsequently, 100–200 ml of the 4% acetylcysteine is administered by gravity flow and retained in the rectum by clamping the Foley catheter with hemostats for 20–45 minutes. The Foley catheter's balloon is deflated and the catheter is removed. The foal can then resume normal activity. In a retrospective study of 44 foals referred to an equine hospital for meconium impaction, affected foals were between 10 and 96 hours of age at presentation (mean ± SD: 29.6 ± 17.5 hours), with 3 foals older than 48 hours (50, 72, and 96 hours of age) [1]. In this study, an average of 1.5 acetylcysteine enemas were used and resolved the impaction in all foals without complications, even after administration of three enemas in five foals. Resolution occurred within 24 hours in 95% of foals treated (Table 17.V.1). Acetylcysteine retention enemas may not be as effective with high meconium impactions due to the more proximal location and inability for the enema to fully reach these locations [3]. Interestingly, administration of acetylcysteine via nasogastric tube has been reported to decrease stool viscosity within 6 hours in infants and might serve as a possible treatment for high impactions, but this route of administration has not been investigated in foals [12].

The prognosis of meconium impaction is very good with medical therapy resolving the majority of cases. The use of warm soapy water enemas and acetylcysteine retention enemas has largely supplanted the need for surgery [1, 5]. However surgical correction has been pursued when there is a lack of response to medical therapy coupled with progressively worsening clinical signs of abdominal distension and continuous abdominal pain [3, 13]. In one study involving 27 foals with meconium impaction, 24 (89%) were treated successfully with medical management and 3 (11%) required surgical intervention, wherein another study involving 20 neonatal foals requiring exploratory celiotomy for colic, only 1 foal was diagnosed with meconium impaction [5, 13]. In another study, 8 of 53 neonatal foals subject to exploratory celiotomy for colic had meconium impaction [14]. In a study specifically evaluating meconium impactions in 24 foals, 8 required surgical correction [3]. A ventral midline celiotomy was performed in all 8 foals, and in 6 foals manual massage of the impaction along with simultaneous administration of an enema resolved the impaction. An enterotomy at the pelvic flexure was necessary in the 2 other foals. The location of the impaction was at the pelvic inlet in 5 foals, and 1 at each of the following locations: transverse colon, dorsal colon, and proximal descending colon [3]. All foals recovered from surgery and were discharged, with follow-up available in 7 foals; 4 of 7 foals were used for their intended purpose of racing while 2 foals were euthanized due to recurrent severe colic caused by serosal adhesions. One foal was euthanized due to unrelated orthopedic disease [3]. In another study in which surgical correction of meconium impaction was needed, 3/3 foals were discharged from the hospital [5]. This information thus emphasizes that surgical correction can result in a successful outcome but should be pursued as a last resort because secondary intestinal adhesion formation is a complication of exploratory celiotomy in the foal. Another variable to consider is that a number of the aforementioned retrospective studies examining surgical options for meconium impaction were performed prior to wide use of acetylcysteine retention enemas, which has likely decreased the need for surgical intervention.

References

1 Pusterla, N., Magdesian, K.G., Maleski, K. et al. (2004). Retrospective evaluation of the use of acetylcysteine enemas in the treatment of meconium retention in foals: 44 cases (1987–2002). *Equine Vet. Educ.* 16: 133–136.

2 McCue, P. (2006). Meconium impaction in foals. *J. Equine Vet. Sci.* 26: 152–155.

3 Hughes, F.E., Moll, D.H., and Slone, D.E. (1996). Outcome of surgical correction of meconium impactions in 8 foals. *J. Equine Vet. Sci.* 16: 172–175.

4 Semard, S.D. and Shaftoe, S. (1992). Gastrointestinal diseases of the neonatal foal. In: *Current Therapy in Equine Medicine*, 3e (ed. L. Mills), 446–447. Philadelphia: W.B. Saunders Co.

5 MacKinnon, M.C., Southwood, L.L., Burke, M.J. et al. (2013). Colic in equine neonates: 137 cases (2000–2010). *J. Am. Vet. Med. Assoc.* 243: 1586–1595.

6 Cuenca, A.G., Ali, A.S., Kays, D.W. et al. (2012). "Pulling the plug" – management of meconium plug syndrome in neonates. *J. Surg. Res.* 175: e43–e46.

7 Burbidge, C. (2012). Meconium impaction in the equine neonate. *Vet. Nurs. J.* 27: 184–197.

8 Martens, R.J. (1982). Pediatrics. In: *Equine Medicine and Surgery*, 3e (ed. R.L. Mannsmann and E.S. McAllister), 333–334. Santa Barbra: American Veterinary Publications.

9 Fischer, A.T. and Yarbrough, T.Y. (1995). Retrograde contrast radiography of the distal portions of the intestinal tract in foals. *J. Am. Vet. Med. Assoc.* 207: 734–737.

10 McAuliffe, S.B. (2004). Abdominal ultrasonography of the foal. *Clin. Tech. Equine Pract.* 3: 208–316.

11 Orsini, J.A. (1997). Abdominal surgery in foals. *Vet. Clin. North Am. Equine* 13: 393–413.

12 Paradiso, V.F., Briganti, V., Oriolo, L. et al. (2011). Meconium obstruction in absence of cystic fibrosis in low birth weight infants: an emerging challenge from increasing survival. *Ital. J. Pediatr.* 37: 55.

13 Cudd, T.C. and Baker, W.A. (1988). Exploratory celiotomy for gastrointestinal disease in neonatal foals: a review of 20 cases. *Equine Vet. J.* 20: 9–12.

14 Cable, C.S., Fubini, S.L., Erb, H.H.N. et al. (1997). Abdominal surgery in foals: a review of 119 cases (1997–1994). *Equine Vet. J.* 29: 257–261.

Section VI Hernias

Annette M. McCoy

A hernia is most simply defined as protrusion of an organ through the wall of a body cavity that would normally contain it. In neonatal foals, abdominal hernias are commonly encountered at the umbilicus and in the inguinal region, termed umbilical and inguinal hernias, respectively. In cases in which abdominal viscera are found within the scrotum rather than being retained in the inguinal region, the abnormality may be termed a scrotal hernia. Each of these hernia types may be congenital or acquired within the first few weeks of life. In one study of 19 foals diagnosed with a palpable umbilical defect at birth, only one had a persistent hernia past five days of age (a true "congenital" hernia), while 12 foals developed umbilical hernias at 5–8 weeks of age [1].

In a "true" hernia, the defect through which the viscera exit the abdomen is called the hernial ring, and the hernia contents lie within the hernial sac, which is lined by peritoneum. A hernia may be termed "ruptured" or "false" if the orifice through which the organ protrudes is not natural, such as a rent in the body wall or vaginal tunic. In this situation, there is no peritoneal lining. In many cases, the contents of abdominal hernias in young foals are easily replaced within the abdomen by manual manipulation (so-called reducible hernia). The contents of a hernia are considered incarcerated when they cannot be easily replaced within the abdomen. Incarcerated viscera may or may not become strangulated. If only the antimesenteric surface of an intestinal segment is incarcerated, the hernia is called a parietal or Richter hernia. These are relatively rare, but isolated cases have been reported [2].

Congenital hernias, both umbilical and inguinal, are suspected to have a hereditary component, although to date there is no conclusive evidence substantiating this assumption. One retrospective study of 168 foals treated at a single hospital found that Thoroughbreds were at higher risk for umbilical hernias than Standardbreds [3]. In the same study, females were twice as likely as males to be affected with an umbilical hernia [3]. However, a smaller prospective study of nonhospitalized Dutch Warmblood foals did not show a significant sex difference [1]. Interestingly, in the cohort of Dutch Warmblood foals, there were clear sire predilections for the development of umbilical hernias [1]. Inguinal (and scrotal) hernias are, not surprisingly, overwhelmingly reported in males [4–7], although there is a case report of a congenital inguinal hernia in a Thoroughbred filly [8]. One report demonstrated a high rate of inguinal hernias (4.6%) at the time of castration in a large population of draft horses, and speculated that genetic predisposition could contribute to this [9]. The following information describes common hernias in foals.

Umbilical Hernia

In early embryonic development, the abdominal contents are located extra-abdominally within the coelomic cavity. As gestation progresses, the intestines retract back into the abdominal cavity and the peritoneal ring narrows and then seals. If the body wall overlying the closed peritoneal ring does not close, this allows viscera to protrude into a hernial sac [1]. Suggested predisposing factors for umbilical hernias that develop after the first few days of life include weakening of the linea alba at the umbilical scar and increased intra-abdominal pressure [1]. The condition is considered common, with a prevalence of 0.5–2% of foals in most reports [3, 10–12]. However, this is likely an underestimation, since it is based on hospitalized populations. A single report in a nonhospitalized population of normal

Equine Neonatal Medicine, First Edition. Edited by David M. Wong and Pamela A. Wilkins.

foals reported a prevalence of 29.5% [1]. Diagnosis is made by observation of a swelling at the umbilicus and palpation of viscera within the hernial sac (Figure 17.VI.1). Ultrasound may be useful to confirm the diagnosis and evaluate the health of related umbilical structures. Foals with strangulated hernia contents typically present with signs of colic [12, 13]. Formation of an enterocutaneous fistula secondary to an incarcerated umbilical or Richter's hernia has been infrequently reported [13–16].

Small congenital umbilical defects often resolve within a few days without treatment [1]. Hernias <2–3 cm in diameter may resolve spontaneously or with daily digital reduction within the first few months of life. Nonsurgical treatment options for nonincarcerated umbilical hernias include placement of an Elastrator ring or hernia clamp [10, 12, 17]. Complications reportedly associated with these procedures include accidental incarceration of bowel and premature dislodging of the device [10, 17]. A belly bandage is not recommended due to the tendency to slip out of position [12]. Herniorrhaphy is recommended if the hernia is large, nonreducible, or fails to resolve spontaneously by 6–12 months of age. Open herniorrhaphy allows examination of viscera, which is particularly important when the hernia contents have been incarcerated, to determine if resection and anastomosis is required. Mesh repair of large defects has been reported [10, 18]. Herniorrhaphy typically results in a good outcome, with only minor complications reported [10]. More serious complications have been associated with incarcerated and strangulating hernias although overall outcome is still good for these cases [10, 16].

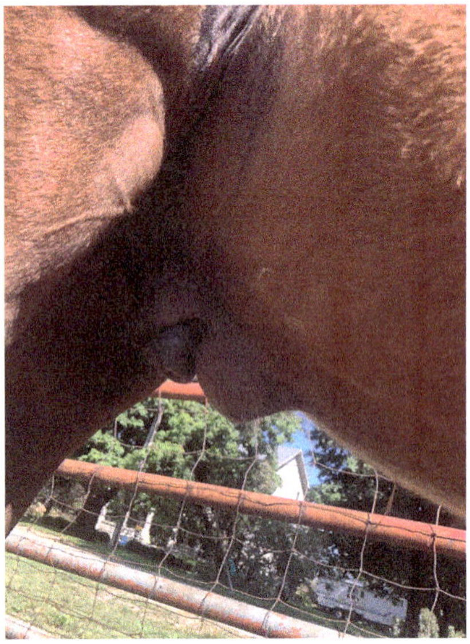

Figure 17.VI.1 Typical appearance of a reducible umbilical hernia in a young colt.

Inguinal (Scrotal) Hernia

Herniated viscera travels through the vaginal ring into the vaginal process, which is continuous with the peritoneum, before traversing the inguinal canal, through the deep and superficial inguinal rings. Herniated bowel may stay within the vaginal process (parietal tunic), or it may exit into the subcutaneous space through a rent in the vaginal process, in which case it is referred to as a ruptured inguinal hernia (Figure 17.VI.2). If the rent occurs in the peritoneum such that the bowel traverses the inguinal canal external to the vaginal process, the condition is referred to as an inguinal rupture. Diagnosis is made by observation of a swelling in one or both inguinal regions and palpation of viscera within the swelling. Ultrasound may be useful to confirm the diagnosis. Foals with a ruptured inguinal hernia/inguinal rupture often present with signs of depression and/or colic even if the hernia contents are not strangulated [4]. Small hernias may be unrecognized and present a risk for evisceration at the time of routine castration [9].

Small reducible hernias generally resolve without intervention within the first 6 months of life. Daily manual reduction of the hernia may help to resolve the condition more quickly and promotes early recognition of any changes in the condition [19]. For larger hernias, a truss may be necessary to maintain hernia reduction. This is constructed of gauze rolls aligned over the superficial inguinal ring, held in place by elastic tape placed in a figure-8 pattern around the pelvis [19, 20]. The truss should be reset every 5–7 days and resolution should be

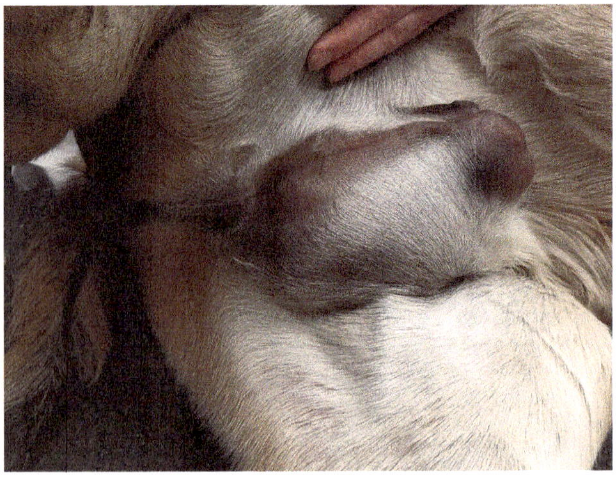

Figure 17.VI.2 Left-sided ruptured inguinal hernia in a 1-day-old Thoroughbred colt. The colt presented for signs of mild colic and the hernia was nonreducible.

expected in 10–14 days if this conservative approach is going to be successful [20]. In cases where the hernia does not spontaneously resolve as expected, enlarges, or is nonreducible, herniorrhaphy is recommended. Unilateral castration and surgical closure of the inguinal ring is typically performed after the viscera is returned to the abdomen [20], although a testicle-sparing laparoscopic technique has been reported [21]. A number of different surgical approaches for inguinal hernias have been reported, including an open inguinal approach (Figure 17.VI.3), with or without the addition of a ventral midline incision, and laparoscopy [4, 20]. Laparoscopic closure of the internal inguinal and vaginal rings in foals has been achieved using intracorporeal suturing [6] and staples [5]. Mesh closure via an open approach has also been reported for a very large inguinal hernia [8]. Reported complications are generally mild and include swelling and seroma or abscess formation at the surgery site [4, 6]. However, severe complications or death may occur if damaged bowel is not recognized as compromised at the time of the initial surgery [4]. Additional information regarding inguinal hernias is in Chapter 18.

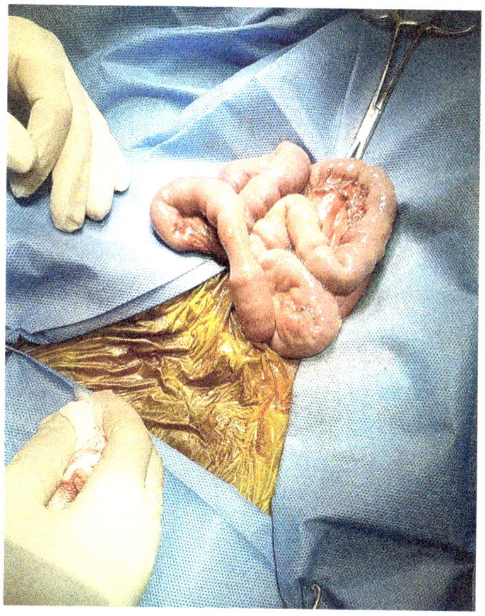

Figure 17.VI.3 Intra-operative image of the foal in 17.IV.2. A skin incision has been made in the left inguinal region revealing several loops of jejunum in the subcutaneous space. All intestine was viable and replaced into the abdomen via the rent in the vaginal process.

References

1 Enzerink, E., van Weeren, P.R., and van der Velden, M.A. (2000). Closure of the abdominal wall at the umbilicus and the development of umbilical hernias in a group of foals from birth to 11 months of age. *Vet. Rec.* 147: 37–39.

2 Avison, A. (2019). Richter's hernia in a 3-month-old colt – a rare event. *Can. Vet. J.* 60: 651–653.

3 Freeman, D.E. and Spencer, P.A. (1991). Evaluation of age, breed, and gender as risk factors for umbilical hernia in horses of a hospital population. *Am. J. Vet. Res.* 52: 637–639.

4 van der Velden, M.A. (1988). Ruptured inguinal hernia in new-born colt foals: a review of 14 cases. *Equine Vet. J.* 20: 178–181.

5 Klohnen, A. and Wilson, D.G. (1996). Laparoscopic repair of scrotal hernia in two foals. *Vet. Surg.* 25: 414–416.

6 Caron, J.P. and Brakenhoff, J. (2008). Intracorporeal suture closure of the internal inguinal and vaginal rings in foals and horses. *Vet. Surg.* 37: 126–131.

7 Spurlock, G.H. and Robertson, J.T. (1988). Congenital inguinal hernias associated with a rent in the common vaginal tunic in five foals. *J. Am. Vet. Med. Assoc.* 193: 1087–1088.

8 Moorman, V.J. and Jann, H.W. (2009). Polypropylene mesh repair of a unilateral, congenital hernia in the inguinal region in a Thoroughbred filly. *Can. Vet. J.* 50: 613–616.

9 Shoemaker, R., Bailey, J., Janzen, E. et al. (2004). Routine castration in 568 draught colts: incidence of evisceration and omental herniation. *Equine Vet. J.* 36: 336–340.

10 Riley, C.B., Cruz, A.M., Bailey, J.V. et al. (1996). Comparison of herniorrhaphy versus clamping of umbilical hernias in horses: a retrospective study of 93 cases (1982–1994). *Can. Vet. J.* 37: 295–298.

11 Fretz, P.B., Hamilton, G.F., Barber, S.M. et al. (1983). Management of umbilical hernias in cattle and horses. *J. Am. Vet. Med. Assoc.* 183: 550–552.

12 Orsini, J.A. (1997). Management of umbilical hernias in the horse: treatment options and potential complications. *Equine Vet. Educ.* 9: 7–10.

13 Markel, M.D., Pascoe, J.R., and Sams, A.E. (1987). Strangulated umbilical hernias in horses: 13 cases (1974–1985). *J. Am. Vet. Med. Assoc.* 190: 692–694.

14 Rijkenhuizen, A., van der Velden, M.A., and Back, W. (1997). Incarcerated umbilical hernia with enterocutaneous fistulae in two foals. *Equine Vet. Educ.* 9: 3–6.

15 Sommerfeld, T.C., Röcken, M., Al Nem, M., and Geburek, F. (2020). Surgical management of an enterocutaneous umbilical fistula caused by an incarcerated Richter's hernia in a one-year-old Quarter Horse filly. *Equine Vet. Educ.* 32: 68–72.

16 Freeman, D.E., Orsini, J.A., Harrison, I.W. et al. (1988). Complications of umbilical hernias in horses: 13 cases (1972–1986). *J. Am. Vet. Med. Assoc.* 192: 804–807.
17 Greenwood, R.E.S. and Dugdale, D.J. (1993). Treatment of umbilical hernias in foals with Elastrator rings. *Equine Vet. Educ.* 5: 113–115.
18 Kawcak, C.E. and Stashak, T.S. (1995). Predisposing factors, diagnosis, and management of large abdominal wall defects in horses and cattle. *J. Am. Vet. Med. Assoc.* 206: 607–611.
19 Toth, F. and Schumacher, J. (2019). Abdominal hernias. In: *Equine Surgery*, 5e (ed. J.A.S. Auer, J.A. Stick, J.M. Kummerle, and T. Prange), 645–659. St. Louis, MO: Elsevier, Inc.
20 Richardson, D.W. (1985). Urogenital problems in the neonatal foal. *Vet. Clin. North Am. Equine Pract.* 1: 179–188.
21 Marien, T., van Hoeck, F., Adriaenssen, A., and Segers, L. (2000). Laparoscopic testis-sparing herniorrhaphy: a new approach for congenital inguinal hernia repair in the foal. *Equine Vet. Educ.* 13: 32–35.

Section VII Intestinal Hyperammonemia

Bettina Dunkel

Ammonium (NH_4^+) is produced in all tissues of the body during the metabolism of amino acids and various compounds that contain nitrogen. It is also produced in the intestinal tract by urease-producing bacteria by converting urea to NH_4^+. Because increased blood concentrations of NH_4^+ are toxic to the central nervous system, NH_4^+ is removed from the body by conversion to urea in the liver. Hyperammonemia (HA) develops when the liver's urea cycle cannot convert NH_4^+ into nontoxic urea effectively. This occurs when the NH_4^+ load is excessive due to increased production, increased absorption from the intestinal tract, when portal blood flow from the intestines is compromised or bypasses the liver, or when urea cycle functions are impaired [1]. By far, the most common cause of HA in horses is decreased clearance secondary to severe hepatic disease with subsequent development of hepatic encephalopathy. More recently, a syndrome of increased blood NH_4^+ concentrations in the absence of hepatic disease has been described. Increased blood NH_4^+ concentrations are thought to originate from the intestinal tract; therefore the syndrome is referred to as intestinal HA.

Intestinal HA is presumed to be caused by either overgrowth of urease-producing bacteria in the large or small intestine or increased absorption of NH_4^+ from the intestinal tract because of altered permeability of the intestinal barrier. In the intestine, NH_4^+ can be produced by breakdown of urea, luminal amino acids, or proteins by urease-producing bacteria. This occurs mainly in the large intestine, but cases of HA in horses with predominately small intestinal disease have also been observed [2]. Urease-producing bacteria include many enterobacteriaceae, in particular *Proteus mirabilis*, *Pseudomonas* spp., *Klebsiella* spp., *Staphylococcus* spp., *Corynebacterium* spp., *Ureaplasma ureolyticum*, and *Proteus penneri*. Apart from two horses with intestinal HA from which *Clostridium sordelli* was isolated from the feces of one horse and *Clostridium perfringens* from the feces of the other, no other potential pathogens have been identified in horses with intestinal HA [3, 4].

Typically, individual horses are affected, but small outbreaks involving multiple animals have been suspected [2, 5]. The syndrome has been reported in a variety of horse and pony breeds across all age groups but predominately in adult horses [3]. In foals, HA has been associated with portosystemic shunts, suspected enzymatic defects in Morgan foals, and thrombosis of the portal vein [6–10]. Intestinal HA in foals has been described in a case series that included 10 foals and weanlings ranging from a few hours to 9 months of age [2].

Hyperammonemia is defined as increased blood NH_4^+ concentration of >60 µmol/l, but reference values for foals are lacking [2, 3, 11, 12]. Neonatal foals have been suggested to have low NH_4^+ production in the colon compared to mature horses due to the presumed lower number of bacteria in the neonatal intestine [11, 13]. However, human neonates have slightly higher NH_4^+ concentrations on the first day of life with <100 µmol/l being considered normal [14]. Studies have identified a rich and diverse intestinal bacterial population in newborn foals highlighting the need for determination of normal NH_4^+ values in foals of different ages [15]. Of the 10 foals included in the case series, ages were 3 days, 3 weeks, 1 month ($n = 2$), 4 months, and 9 months ($n = 2$) old with an average age of 3 months [2]. Three neonatal foals <24 hours were also included but the presentation was slightly different (see below).

Clinical Signs

The case history of foals with intestinal HA is often nonspecific but gastrointestinal disease, depression, and fever are frequently noted and no common predisposing factors have been identified. Most foals have or develop diarrhea with or without colic but intestinal stasis could also play a

Equine Neonatal Medicine, First Edition. Edited by David M. Wong and Pamela A. Wilkins.

role as three neonates presented with signs of meconium impaction and a 3-month-old foal presented with a history of constipation [2]. Intestinal HA has also been observed in a 2-month-old colt following resection of 3 m of small intestine (Dunkel, unreported data). Clinical signs and laboratory values are similar to changes observed in mature horses and largely indicative of intestinal disease with moderate to severe cardiovascular compromise. Common findings included depression, weakness, abdominal pain, diarrhea, fever, tachycardia, and evidence of hypovolemia and systemic inflammation. Neurologic signs might be present during the initial evaluation, develop during the course of disease, or be the only clinical signs at presentation. Ataxia, central blindness, aimless wandering, head pressing, and seizures are most commonly observed in foals (Dunkel, unreported data). Laboratory findings include hemoconcentration, azotemia, metabolic acidosis with increased blood lactate concentrations, hyper- or hypoglycemia, and electrolyte abnormalities. Ammonium concentrations reported in foals with intestinal HA ranged from 70 to 483 μmol/l with a mean concentration of 213 μmol/l. The three neonatal foals mentioned above were 3–12 hours old and showed mild to moderate neurological signs (seizures) and concurrent colic, attributed to meconium impactions. Those foals had comparatively low blood NH_4^+ concentrations of 67–116 μmol/l with neurological signs resolving following resolution of the meconium impaction and all survived to discharge.

Diagnosis of intestinal HA is based on increased blood NH_4^+ concentration in the absence of significant hepatic disease and other causes of HA. The concentration of blood NH_4^+ necessary to cause neurologic signs has not been determined, but is probably also influenced by concurrent disease processes, electrolyte abnormalities, and potential release of other neurotoxic mediators. Ammonium can be measured stall-side with a handheld device that uses individual reagent strips (PocketChem™ BA; Arkray USA, Inc. Edina, MN 55439). The analyser is designed for human whole blood but does not perform well with whole equine blood. However, a centrifuged equine heparin or EDTA plasma sample can produce acceptable correlation with a reference laboratory machine, provided a stall side centrifuge is available. If whole-blood ammonium concentrations are required, the concentration can be calculated from the plasma concentration using the following formula: Plasma ammonia concentration × Hct (% e.g. 0.33) = blood ammonia concentration (Leguillette R., unpublished data). The limited range of 8–285 μmol/l might also be a limitation in cases of severe HA. If stall-side analysis is not possible, blood NH_4^+ concentrations can be determined in EDTA- or heparin-anticoagulated blood. Plasma should be immediately separated and stored at 4 °C (39.2 °F) on ice for analysis within an hour. The latter situation is ideal, but analysis after storage for up to 6 hours may also yield acceptably accurate results. If samples cannot be processed within this time, separated plasma should be frozen (−20 °C) for analysis, optimally within 48 hours. However, analysis after freezing at −20 °C for up to 7 days can also be useful, with only minimal, clinically insignificant, increases in NH_4^+ occurring from storage. Increased NH_4^+ concentrations can also be detected in cerebrospinal fluid and aqueous humor if blood samples cannot be obtained *ante mortem* or have been handled suboptimally. The NH_4^+ concentration in human cerebrospinal fluid remains stable for up to 48 hours if stored at 4 °C (39.2 °F). *Postmortem* examination might reveal no or very few gross and histopathological lesions in any organ system, as was the case in the foal that presented for constipation. Alternatively, severe gastrointestinal pathology such as ulcerative or necrotizing enterocolitis may be noted. A clinical diagnosis of intestinal HA can be supported by *postmortem* histopathological changes such as astrocyte swelling in the acute form of HA or Alzheimer type II astrocytosis with more chronic HA. These microscopic changes were noted in foals with intestinal HA. Three foals in the case series of 10 foals had evidence of bacteremia with bacteria being isolated from multiple organs *postmortem*.

Other differential diagnoses for foals with HA include congenital or acquired portosystemic shunts, inherited disorders in Morgan foals similar to hyperornithinemia, hyperammonemia, and homocitrullinuria in people, portal vein obstruction by a thrombus or tumor, urea toxicity, and black locust (*Robinia pseudoacacia*) toxicity [9, 16, 17]. In people, intestinal bleeding (which could be regarded as a form of intestinal HA), infection with urease-producing bacteria at other body sites, renal failure, malnutrition, total parenteral nutrition, and cardiac arrest are known causes of HA [18]. It is worthwhile to note that blood NH_4^+ concentrations can also be significantly increased following exercise (up to 150 μmol/l) and after generalized seizure activity (mean concentration 76 μmol/l but up to 500 μmol/l reported in people) [19].

Treatment

In people, treatment of HA aims to reduce the generation and uptake of NH_4^+, improve endogenous detoxification systems, or both. Nonabsorbable disaccharides, antimicrobials, and probiotics are used in attempts to decrease bacterial production and absorption of NH_4^+ in the intestine, but their efficacy is disputed [20]. In adult horses, use of neomycin (10–100 mg/kg, PO, q6h) and lactulose (0.3 ml/kg, PO, q6-12h) has been advocated, but their beneficial effects are equally questionable. Oral neomycin has the potential to cause diarrhea in horses, and probiotics in foals have repeatedly been associated with the development of diarrhea [21–23]. Lactulose is metabolized by colonic bacteria to organic acids, which decrease the large intestinal pH. The lower pH favors conversion of ammonia (NH_3) to NH_4^+ thereby trapping the molecule in the intestinal lumen and preventing absorption [24]. Although administration of lactulose significantly reduced plasma NH_4^+ in healthy horses, the mean numeric decrease was small (3.0 μmol/l). Moreover, fecal pH had a tendency to increase, rather than decrease, and one in seven horses developed laminitis [24]. Intravenous infusion of hypertonic saline (2–4 ml/kg) as a bolus to decrease intracranial pressure has anecdotally resulted in rapid improvement in some cases with intestinal HA but should be used with care in foals. In people, other avenues are being explored that support endogenous NH_4^+-detoxifying metabolic pathways, notably glutamine synthesis and the urea cycle. The deamidation of glutamine to glutamate by the enzyme phosphate-activated glutaminase in intestinal enterocytes contributes to intestinal ammoniagenesis, producing one mole of NH_3 per mole of glutamine. Metformin has been suggested for its inhibitory effects on enterocyte glutaminase to decrease intestinal NH_3 production [20]. Glutaminase activity in the equine small intestine has been described; this could be a therapeutic option in horses if metformin is proven to be effective in inhibiting the equine enzyme [25]. Control of neurologic signs and prevention of self-trauma may require repeated sedation, given either as boluses or continuous intravenous infusion. Administration of activated charcoal, mineral oil, or other agents aimed at decreasing intestinal absorption of potential toxins might be useful if ingestion of toxic substances is suspected.

Prognosis

The prognosis for foals with intestinal HA depends largely on the underlying cause and ability to control neurologic signs and prevent self-trauma. Survival in the case series involving 10 foals was 50% (three died, two were euthanized). Excluding the three neonates with meconium impaction, survival was 29% [2]. In most horses, demise or recovery occurred within 24–72 hours, but cases of intestinal HA persisting for longer than 10 days have also been observed with a positive outcome (Dunkel, unpublished data). Even horses with severe neurologic abnormalities may recover if the neurologic symptoms can be controlled and structural gastrointestinal lesions are absent or mild. Recovery is usually complete, and no long-term complications or recurrence have been reported.

References

1 Walker, V. (2012). Severe hyperammonaemia in adults not explained by liver disease. *Ann. Clin. Biochem.* 49: 214–228.

2 Dunkel, B., Chaney, K.P., Dallap-Schaer, B.L. et al. (2011). Putative intestinal hyperammonaemia in horses: 36 cases. *Equine Vet. J.* 43: 133–140.

3 Desrochers, A.M., Dallap, B.L., and Wilkins, P.A. (2003). *Clostridium sordelli* infection as a suspected cause of transient hyperammonemia in an adult horse. *J. Vet. Intern. Med.* 17: 238–241.

4 Stickle, J.E., McKnight, C.A., Williams, K.J. et al. (2006). Diarrhea and hyperammonemia in a horse with progressive neurologic signs. *Vet. Clin. Pathol.* 35: 250–253.

5 Fielding, C.L., Higgins, J.K., Higgins, J.C. et al. (2015). Disease associated with equine coronavirus infection and high case fatality rate. *J. Vet. Intern. Med.* 29: 307–310.

6 Ness, S.L., Kennedy, L.A., and Slovis, N.M. (2013). Hyperammonemic encephalopathy associated with portal vein thrombosis in a Thoroughbred foal. *J. Vet. Intern. Med.* 27: 382–386.

7 Buonanno, A.M., Carlson, G.P., and Kantrowitz, B. (1988). Clinical and diagnostic features of portosystemic shunt in a foal. *J. Am. Vet. Med. Assoc.* 192: 387–389.

8 Fortier, L.A., Fubini, S.L., Flanders, J.A. et al. (1996). The diagnosis and surgical correction of congenital portosystemic vascular anomalies in two calves and two foals. *Vet. Surg.* 25: 154–160.

9 McCornico, R.S., Duckett, W.M., and Wood, P.A. (1997). Persistent hyperammonemia in two related Morgan weanlings. *J. Vet. Intern. Med.* 11: 264–266.

10 Willems, D.S., Kranenburg, L.C., Ensink, J.M. et al. (2019). Computed tomography angiography of a congenital extrahepatic splenocaval shunt in a foal. *Acta Vet. Scand.* 61: 39.

11 Axon, J.E. and Palmer, J.E. (2008). Clinical pathology of the foal. *Vet. Clin. North Am. Equine Pract.* 24: 357–385, vii.

12 Sharkey, L.C., DeWitt, S., and Stockman, C. (2006). Neurologic signs and hyperammonemia in a horse with colic. *Vet. Clin. Pathol.* 35: 254–258.

13 Southwood, L.L. (2013). Normal ranges for hematology and plasma chemistry and conversion table for units. In: *Practical Guide to Equine Colic*, 1e (ed. L.L. Southwood), 339–342. Wiley.

14 Colombo, J.P., Peheim, E., Kretschmer, R. et al. (1984). Plasma ammonia concentrations in newborns and children. *Clin. Chim. Acta* 138: 283–291.

15 Costa, M.C., Stampfli, H.R., Allen-Vercoe, E. et al. (2016). Development of the faecal microbiota in foals. *Equine Vet. J.* 48: 681–688.

16 Vanschandevijl, K., van Loon, G., Lefere, L. et al. (2010). Black locust (*Robinia pseudoacacia*) intoxication as a suspected cause of transient hyperammonaemia and enteral encephalopathy in a pony. *Equine Vet. Educ.* 22: 336–339.

17 Patton, K.M., Peek, S.F., and Valentine, B.A. (2006). Gastric adenocarcinoma in a horse with portal vein metastasis and thrombosis: a novel cause of hepatic encephalopathy. *Vet. Pathol.* 43: 565–569.

18 Sakusic, A., Sabov, M., McCambridge, A.J. et al. (2018). features of adult hyperammonemia not due to liver failure in the ICU. *Crit. Care Med.* 46: e897–e903.

19 Nakamura, K., Yamane, K., Shinohara, K. et al. (2013). Hyperammonemia in idiopathic epileptic seizure. *Am. J. Emerg. Med.* 31: 1486–1489.

20 Matoori, S. and Leroux, J.C. (2015). Recent advances in the treatment of hyperammonemia. *Adv. Drug Delivery Rev.* 90: 55–68.

21 Strobel, C., Gunther, E., Romanowski, K. et al. (2018). Effects of oral supplementation of probiotic strains of Lactobacillus rhamnosus and Enterococcus faecium on diarrhoea events of foals in their first weeks of life. *J. Anim. Physiol. Anim. Nutr. (Berl.)* 102: 1357–1365.

22 Schoster, A., Staempfli, H.R., Abrahams, M. et al. (2015). Effect of a probiotic on prevention of diarrhea and Clostridium difficile and *Clostridium perfringens* shedding in foals. *J. Vet. Intern. Med.* 29: 925–931.

23 Weese, J.S. and Rousseau, J. (2005). Evaluation of Lactobacillus pentosus WE7 for prevention of diarrhea in neonatal foals. *J. Am. Vet. Med. Assoc.* 226: 2031–2034.

24 Scarratt, W.K. and Warnick, L.D. (1998). Effects of oral administration of lactulose in healthy horses. *J. Equine Vet. Sci.* 18: 405–408.

25 Duckworth, D.H., Madison, J.B., Calderwood-Mays, M. et al. (1992). Arteriovenous differences for glutamine in the equine gastrointestinal tract. *Am. J. Vet. Res.* 53: 1864–1867.

Chapter 18 The Acute Abdomen in the Neonatal Foal

Alexandra Gillen

Introduction

Colic in the neonate has numerous etiologies, both congenital and acquired. A complicating factor in the diagnosis and treatment of foals with signs of colic is that many exhibit concurrent disease; thus, evaluation of all body systems is important. Most cases of neonatal colic require medical rather than surgical intervention but differentiating between medical and surgical causes is challenging due to overlap in clinical signs and the possibility of surgical lesions developing during medical management [1]. Additionally, neonatal diseases often progress rapidly, therefore accurate assessment and timely intervention are crucial.

Evaluation of the Neonate with Colic

History

The medical history is useful in assessing the foal and in some cases suggesting potential diagnoses. The age of the foal should be accurately determined as the precise age can suggest specific causes of colic. Observation of clinical signs (e.g. nursing frequency, ease of defecation, presence of urination) is also beneficial. As with all neonates, information relating to overall health, including whether parturition progressed normally, serum IgG concentration, and if other medical concerns have been detected should be obtained. Interestingly, in one study, 64% of neonates evaluated for colic had a concurrent systemic disease [1].

Physical Examination

Initially, examine the foal from a distance to observe behavior and degree of discomfort (Figure 18.1). Foals with colic frequently exhibit signs such as repeated positioning in lateral or dorsal recumbency. The mucous membrane color, capillary refill time, temperature, heart rate, respiration rate, and gastrointestinal (GI) borborgymi should be assessed. The thorax should be auscultated, joints and ribs palpated, eyes and umbilicus examined, and abdomen assessed for presence of hernias. The degree of abdominal distention should be evaluated and monitored for progression [2]. The value of external abdominal palpation is variable; however, it can be useful in neonatal foals [2]. A digital rectal examination allows assessment for the presence, consistency, and color of feces (i.e., meconium or genuine feces), and the presence of mucus. Some foals may require sedation for examination.

Passage of a Nasogastric Tube

Although a foal's stomach can be visualized ultrasonographically, passage of a nasogastric tube is recommended. A volume of reflux >250 ml should be interpreted with concern; however, common sense is required in interpretation of smaller volumes of reflux in smaller foals [3]. Passage of an endoscope into the stomach may be needed to overcome difficulties of passing a nasogastric tube where the stomach is particularly distended [3].

Clinicopathologic Data

The following laboratory analysis is recommended to gain a comprehensive picture of the foal's condition but can be adjusted based on clinician preference and presenting clinical signs: point-of-care blood L-lactate and glucose, CBC, serum biochemistry profile, serum IgG, arterial or venous blood gas analysis (dependent on ventilation/oxygenation status), and blood culture. Although MacKinnon et al. noted minimal association between the need for surgical intervention and presenting signs or ultrasonographic findings, foals requiring surgery had a lower plasma

Equine Neonatal Medicine, First Edition. Edited by David M. Wong and Pamela A. Wilkins.

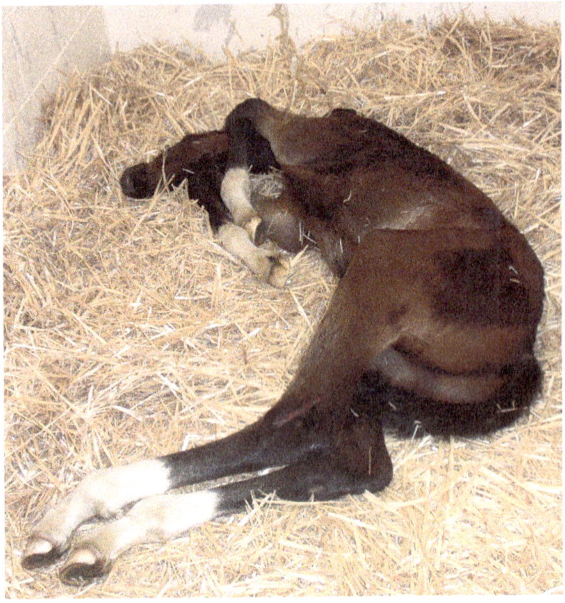

Figure 18.1 Foals frequently exhibit marked colic signs, including rolling from lateral to dorsal recumbency. *Source:* Image courtesy of Scone Equine Hospital.

chloride concentration (92.8 ± 7.0 mmol/l) compared to medically managed foals (96.2 ± 6.1 mmol/l) [1].

Abdominocentesis

The procedure for performing abdominocentesis is in Chapter 15; indications include if peritonitis, uroabdomen, or compromised intestine is suspected, or in cases of colic where a diagnosis is lacking. In brief, ultrasonography performed prior to abdominocentesis helps identify free abdominal fluid and decreases the risk of enterocentesis [4]. The author prefers to perform abdominocentesis in lateral recumbency in neonates, and standing in older foals, however, the procedure can be performed in either orientation. Regardless of technique, it is imperative for the foal to be adequately restrained. Although use of a teat cannula can result in omental herniation, it is preferred in neonates as it reduces the risk of enterocentesis. If a hypodermic needle is used, an 18- to 20-gauge 1-in. needle is appropriate [2]. The location to perform abdominocentesis is the same as for an adult (slightly right of midline, most dependent point of abdominal wall), however, this can be adjusted depending on ultrasonographic findings (Table 18.1). If enterocentesis occurs, broad-spectrum antimicrobials along with metronidazole should be administered [3].

Ultrasonography (See Chapter 15)

Abdominal ultrasonography is completed using a 5 or 7.5 MHz linear, curved linear (convex) or sector probe. A depth of 5–10 cm is required, depending on the size of the foal [3]. The author prefers not to clip the hair of foals, particularly in more urgent situations; application of 70% isopropyl alcohol to the skin is sufficient to allow quality ultrasonographic images to be obtained [5]. The foal can be examined standing or in lateral recumbency, however, unless the degree of discomfort or malaise dictates otherwise, the examination is easier in the standing foal [5]. In most neonates, the clinician can observe the structures noted in Table 18.2 [2–10].

Table 18.1 Common fluid parameters used to assess neonatal foals with colic.

- The following abdominocentesis parameters should be obtained (values in healthy foals):
  - Total protein (<2.5 g/dl)
  - White blood cell count (<1.5 × 10^3 cells/μl)
  - Lactate (<2 mmol/l; may be slightly higher in foals less than 12 hours of age)
  - Other parameters that can be assessed:
    - Creatinine (see *Uroperitoneum*)
    - Cytology – performed in cases of suspected gastrointestinal rupture (see *Equine Gastric Ulceration Syndrome*) or where a diagnosis has not been reached.
    - Red blood cells (*hemoabdomen*)

Radiography

Abdominal radiography is an ancillary test used to aid in the diagnosis of some foals with colic (Table 18.3). Ideally a lateral radiograph is obtained in the standing position; however, radiographs obtained in lateral recumbency can be diagnostic [3].

Following initial plain radiography, serial and/or contrast radiographs can be obtained; however, contrast studies are contraindicated in the presence of marked small intestinal distention. When performing a contrast study, the technique should be increased by 10% [3, 10]. If a lesion is suspected in the upper GI tract (e.g. duodenal stricture or delayed gastric emptying), the following method can be used for further evaluation:

- Fast foal for 2 hours
- Administer 5 ml/kg of 10% barium sulfate suspension via nasogastric tube [3]
- Serial radiographs are obtained at 5, 15, and 30 minutes, and then at 2-hour intervals until contrast medium has reached the small colon [3]. Alternatively, perform radiography at 30-minute intervals until contrast medium reaches the small colon [10].

In normal foals, the contrast should begin to enter the duodenum within 15–30 minutes and the stomach should be empty within 2 hours and should not become dilated [5, 10]. The small intestine should be empty of contrast

Table 18.2 Abdominal structures typically visible via ultrasonography in the neonatal foal [2–10].

Structure	Location	Observation/interpretation
Stomach	• Approximately 10th intercostal space, halfway up the lateral body wall	• Observed as a curvilinear echo • May see gas or fluid if abnormal
Duodenum	• Right 15th intercostal space, caudomedial margin of liver	• Ensure full contraction is observed
Small intestine	• Ventral abdomen and inguinal regions	• Can be visualized in healthy foals • Normally flaccid with good motility and minimal intramural content • Wall thickness <3 mm, except ileum (4–5 mm) • Wall thickness may not appreciably change with enteritis but usually increases in strangulating lesions • If distension (>3 cm diameter) and lack of motility observed, consider strangulation • Intussusception will appear as concentric rings (Figure 18.7)
Large and small colon	• Ventral and lower left side of abdomen	• Gaseous ingesta is normal • Meconium appears hypoechoic • Fluid may indicate colitis • Wall thickness should be <3 mm • Intussusception will appear as concentric rings
Peritoneum	• Cranioventral abdomen; if effusion marked can see fluid in all ventral locations	• Uroperitoneum usually anechoic fluid • Anechoic or echogenic fluid with/without gas can be consistent with GI rupture (see EGUS) • Fibrinous reaction may be observed with peritonitis
Diaphragm	• Cranial abdomen	• Evaluate for suspected ruptured diaphragm

Table 18.3 Abdominal structures typically visible via radiography in the neonatal foal [3, 5, 9, 10].

Stomach	• Situated in cranial abdomen • Appears comparatively larger in neonates (compared to older foals) due to small cecum and colon • Usually gas or fluid filled
Small Intestine	• Distended small intestine is abnormal and an obstructive lesion should be suspected
Large Intestine	• Small gas caps are considered normal • Marked gaseous distention is suggestive of an obstruction
Diaphragm	• Evaluate thorax for evidence of abdominal contents in the thoracic cavity

after 3 hours and contrast should be visible in the cecum and large colon approximately 2 hours following contrast administration [2, 3, 10].

Retrograde contrast studies can be used to evaluate the caudal part of the GI tract (e.g. atresia coli, colon obstruction), but administration should be stopped if discomfort or backflow is observed. If tapering of the contrast in the small colon is observed, an insufficient amount of contrast may have been infused to reach the transverse colon [2]. To perform a retrograde contrast study, a barium sulfate suspension (180 ml) is administered as an enema under gravity via a foley catheter [3]. In the author's experience, the foley balloon typically does not need to be inflated, however, others prefer to follow this protocol [10]. Radiography is then performed with the foal standing, immediately after instillation of the barium suspension. In some cases of atresia coli, a ventrodorsal view may be beneficial.

Diagnostic Endoscopy (See Chapter 15)

A lubricated 1-m endoscope (10 mm diameter) is used with sedation often required. Once the stomach is reached, mild distention with air allows better visualization; however, air should be removed following examination. If milk is not withheld, visualization of parts of the stomach may be impaired, but the stomach should be empty if milk is withheld for 2 hours [2, 3]. The endoscope can be advanced into the duodenum for evaluation of ulceration, erosions, or stricture. The endoscope should be removed slowly to allow thorough evaluation of the esophagus.

Advanced Imaging

Computed tomographic (CT) evaluation of neonates with colic is rarely necessary and reserved for cases of continued colic where a diagnosis has not been established. There are some reports of challenging diagnoses being made with CT, such as an intra-abdominal abscess [11]. The majority of neonates can undergo CT evaluation in sternal recumbency with sedation alone, but general anesthesia may be required [12].

Exploratory Celiotomy

Although general anesthesia and abdominal surgery in a neonate should not be undertaken lightly, delaying surgical intervention can result in increased risk of devitalized bowel developing. In the event of persistent colic signs and a lack of diagnosis, exploratory celiotomy may be necessary to ascertain and resolve the source of colic. However, surgery is necessary in the minority of cases of foals presenting for colic as exemplified by one study that reported that 89% of neonates admitted to a referral hospital were managed medically [1].

Conditions Causing Abdominal Discomfort in the Neonate

There are numerous causes of the acute abdomen in the neonate (Table 18.4), many of which are similar to causes of colic in adults. However, there are several conditions which are specific to the neonate.

Conditions of the Stomach Causing Colic

Equine Gastric Ulceration Syndrome (Chapter 17)

Gastric ulceration in the foal is common with an estimated prevalence of 25–50% [13]. Clinical signs included colic, unthrifty appearance, increased recumbency, bruxism, and ptyalism [14, 15]. Foals typically show more severe disease compared to adult horses, with more pronounced endoscopic findings, increased involvement of the duodenum (Figure 18.2), increased risk of stricture, and increased risk of GI perforation [15]. One method of grouping gastric ulceration in foals is into four clinical syndromes: [16] subclinical, clinical, perforating, and gastric outflow obstruction (secondary to pyloric stricture). Murray, provides a different but more detailed list of syndromes (Table 18.5) [15].

Table 18.4 Potential causes of colic in the foal categorized by anatomical location.

Region of GI tract	Condition	Age of foal (neonate or older)
Stomach	Equine gastric ulcer syndrome	Any age but neonates very susceptible
	Gastric outflow obstruction	Usually older
	Gastric rupture	Any age but neonates very susceptible
	Gastric endoparasitism	Usually older
	Gastric abscessation	Any age
Small Intestine	Small intestinal volvulus	Any age
	Scrotal/ruptured inguinal hernia	Neonates but can be older
	Inguinal hernia	Usually older but neonates may require surgical intervention
	Diaphragmatic hernia	Any age
	Umbilical hernia	Usually older but neonates may require surgical intervention
	Meckel's diverticulum	Any age
	Mesodiverticular band	Any age
	Mesenteric defects	Any age
	Intussusception (jejunojejunal, jejunoileal and ileocaecal)	Any age
	Chyloperitoneum	Neonates
	Small intestinal impaction (e.g. Ascarids)	Usually older
	Lactose intolerance	Any age
	Enteritis	Any age
	Necrotizing enteritis	Any age
	Abscess	Usually older
Cecum	Jejunocecal intussusception	Usually older
	Cecocolic intussusception	Usually older
	Atresia cecum	Neonates
Large and small colons	Meconium retention	Neonates
	Atresia coli	Neonates
	Ileocolonic aganglionosis	Neonates
	Large colon displacement/torsion	Any age
	Small colon fecalith/impaction	Usually older
	Diarrhea	Any age

Table 18.4 (Continued)

Region of GI tract	Condition	Age of foal (neonate or older)
Rectum and anus	Atresia recti/ani	Neonates
	Rectal prolapse	Any age but usually younger
Other causes	Peritonitis	Any age
	Uroperitoneum	Neonates but can occur in older foals
	Ovarian torsion	Neonates
	Hemoperitoneum	Any age
	Ovarian stalk obstruction of the intestine	Neonates
	Ruptured spleen	Any age
	Fractured ribs	Neonates but can occur in older foals
	Bile duct obstruction	
	Liver abscessation	
	Acute hepatic necrosis	
	Ovarian artery rupture	Neonate
	Ascites	
	Blunt abdominal trauma	Any age

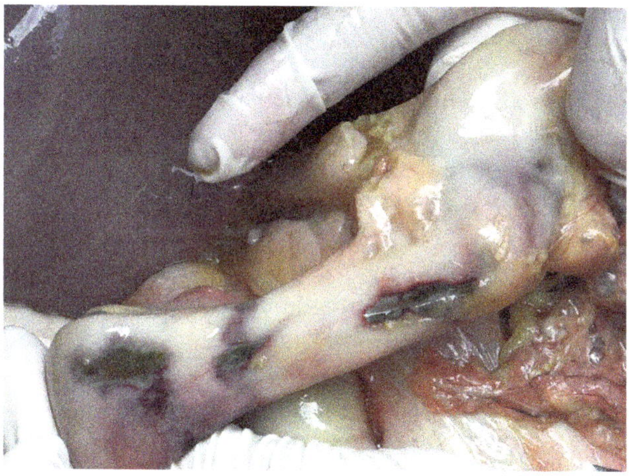

Figure 18.2 Intraoperative image of neonatal foal with duodenal ulcerations. *Source:* Image courtesy of Scone Equine Hospital.

Gastroscopy may be necessary in some hospitalized foals but should be performed as a matter of urgency in foals where a diagnosis of colic has not been made or when equine gastric ulcers syndrome (EGUS) is suspected [16]. The presence of comorbidities is common and a thorough

Table 18.5 Clinical syndromes associated with gastric ulceration in the neonatal foal as described by Murray [15].

Syndrome	Characteristics
Mild gastric erosions	• Frequently no clinical signs • Often heal spontaneously but progression possible
Stress-induced gastric lesions	• Consider in any foal that has another medical condition which may result in discomfort, reduced nursing or a change in management
Sudden onset, severe gastric ulcers	• Mostly observed in gastric antrum and pylorus • Less commonly observed in squamous mucosa
Duodenal ulceration and duodenitis	• Ulceration can result in stricture of the pylorus and duodenum
Gastric outflow obstruction	• Sequelae include colic, further ulceration, and potential for esophageal ulceration and megaesophagus
Gastric or duodenal perforation with peritonitis	• Minimal clinical signs may be apparent prior to perforation; perforations may sometimes be sealed by omentum; however, if this occurs, the prognosis is frequently hopeless
Pyloric ulceration	• Can lead to stricture and delayed gastric emptying
Duodenal ulceration	• Can lead to stricture and delayed gastric emptying
Gastro-esophageal reflux	• Can results in esophageal ulceration
Pyloric duodenal stricture	• Can result in delayed gastric emptying

evaluation of the patient is necessary. Ultrasonographic evaluation and contrast radiography can be beneficial in evaluating gastric and duodenal motility. Although blood sucrose can aid in the diagnosis of EGUS in weanling foals, this test has not been validated in neonates [17] and is unlikely to replace gastroscopy.

A variety of treatment options have been used for gastric ulceration (Chapter 17). In brief, medications such as omeprazole, ranitidine, and cimetidine, as well as mucosal protectants, such as sucralfate are commonly used. The clinician should be aware that, in certain cases, prophylactic treatment of hospitalized neonates can be associated with an increased incidence of diarrhea [18].

Severe cases of gastric ulceration can result in GI perforation (Figure 18.3). By the time ultrasonographic changes (increased peritoneal fluid, ± fibrinous reaction) are observed, the prognosis is hopeless; for the welfare of the foal, a rapid diagnosis must be made. Ultrasonography can

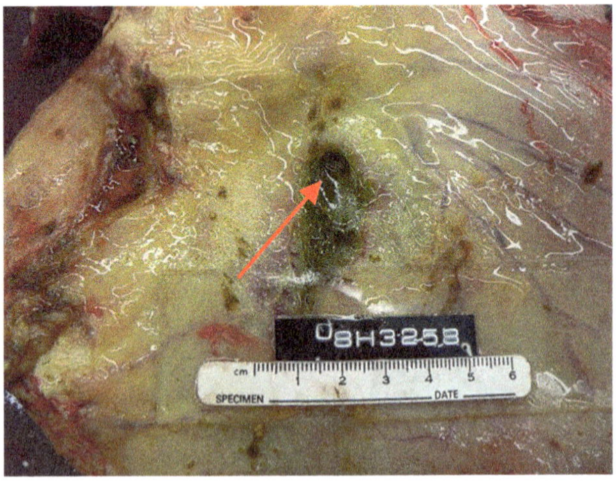

Figure 18.3 Gastric perforation (arrow), noted from the serosal side, during postmortem examination. *Source:* Image courtesy of David Wong, Iowa State University.

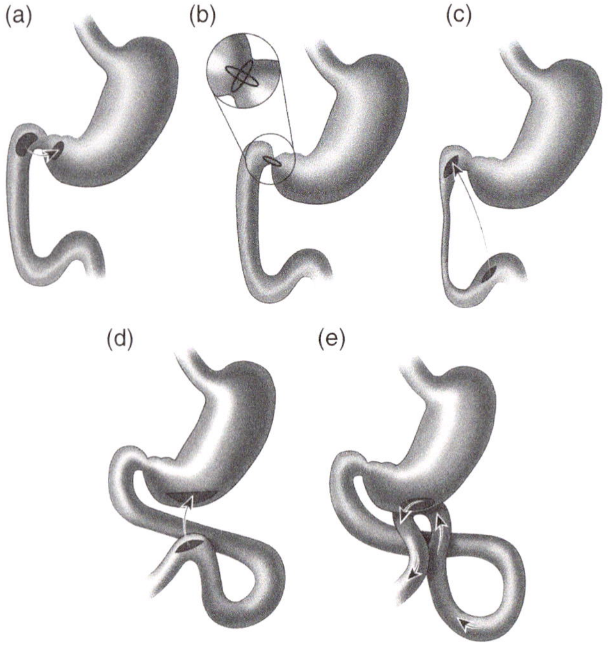

Figure 18.4 (a) Gastroduodenostomy to bypass a pyloric or proximal duodenal stricture. (b) Heineke-Mikulicz pyloroplasty involves a full-thickness, 4-cm long, longitudinal incision over the pyloric stenosis and closed transversely to expand the pylorus. (c) Duodeno-jejunostomy to bypass a duodenal stricture. (d) Gastrojejunostomy to bypass a duodenal stricture. (e) Gastrojejunostomy and jejunojejunostomy, the latter to allow contents of the duodenum and proximal jejunum to drain back into the jejunum [23].

be more reliable than evaluation of abdominal fluid as the fluid sample may reveal an inflammatory reaction secondary to gastric or duodenal perforation, but a relatively normal white blood cell count can be obtained in some cases [3, 15]. Moreover, cytology may be required to make a definitive diagnosis. Alternatively, if a rupture is suspected, exploratory celiotomy can confirm the diagnosis and is the preferred course of action if insufficient information is available to support euthanasia.

Gastric outflow obstruction typically occurs in foals 2–6 months of age and is usually a result of gastric ulceration, however, cases involving a cyst in a 21-day-old foal, a primary melanoma in a 2-month-old foal, and muscular hypertrophy can demonstrate similar clinical signs [19–22]. The foals with masses were euthanized whereas the foal with muscular hypertrophy was managed surgically. Cases of gastric outflow obstruction present in a similar manner to foals with gastric ulceration and are diagnosed via endoscopy or contrast radiography. Medical therapy includes decompression of the stomach, antiulcer medications, broad-spectrum antimicrobials, prokinetics and intravenous fluids [19]. If clinical improvement is not observed within 2–3 days, or if severe colic signs persist, surgical intervention should be performed to bypass the pylorus (Figure 18.4) [24–26]. Surgical options include the modified Heineke-Mikulicz technique, gastroduodenostomy (with or without a partial gastrectomy), gastrojejunostomy (with or without a jejunojejunostomy) and duodenojejunostomy (with or without a jejunojejunostomy). A jejunojejunostomy is recommended to reduce the likelihood of retrograde flow of ingesta from the jejunum into the stomach [29]. The specific procedure depends on the location of the obstruction and is described in brief in Table 18.6 [24]. A modified Heineke-Mikulicz technique at the pylorus to relieve pyloric stenosis in a 2-month-old filly has been described [22, 27]. This was followed by incising the hepatoduodenal ligament to mobilize the duodenum. A similar procedure was described in three foals, two of which went on to race; the remaining foal was euthanized due to a small intestinal volvulus and adhesions [28].

Gastrojejunostomy is indicated if the pyloric obstruction involves more than the first 1–2 cm of the duodenum (Figure 18.5) [24]. This procedure is performed by taking a segment of jejunum, approximately 20 cm aboral to the duodenocolic ligament, for the anastomosis. The jejunum is then aligned along the avascular portion of the stomach by situating the oral portion to the left, and the aboral portion to the right, creating a left-to-right anastomosis [24, 30]. The procedure for the anastomosis itself is similar to the gastroduodenostomy, with the exception of creating a 7–8 cm stoma (Table 18.6) [19, 24].

Aftercare following a gastrojejunostomy, or variation of this procedure, is extensive and includes non-steroidal anti-inflammatory drugs (NSAIDs), broad spectrum antimicrobials, antiulcer therapy, IV fluids, nutritional support, and intermittent gastric decompression. Contrast radiography

Table 18.6 Gastroduodenostomy procedure. As described by Khatibzadeh and Brown [24].

- A cranial ventral midline celiotomy is performed. This can be extended to a J-shape if required.
- The abdomen is packed off and stay sutures are placed in the stomach.
- The duodenal anastomosis site is located oral to the common duodenal papilla and entrance of the common bile duct.
  - Use 2-0 absorbable suture material on a taper needle in a Lembert pattern to position the duodenum on the stomach by suturing the seromuscular portion of the duodenum to the seromuscular portion of the stomach.
  - A 3 cm full thickness incision is made in the stomach and duodenum and the far cut edges of the stomach and duodenum are sutured together in a simple continuous pattern; the same suture pattern is performed on the near cut edges.
  - A continuous Lembert pattern is used to suture the seromuscular portion of the duodenum to the seromuscular portion of the stomach.
  - A three-layer technique (seromuscular, muscular, and mucosal layers), or creation of a gastrojejunostomy stoma using a gastrointestinal anastomosis (GIA) stapling device, is also possible; however, due to the increased time needed to suture three layers, and the difficulty of maneuvering stapling devices in the limited space of the foal's abdomen, the majority of clinicians prefer the two-layer method [19].
- The packing is removed and the abdomen lavaged

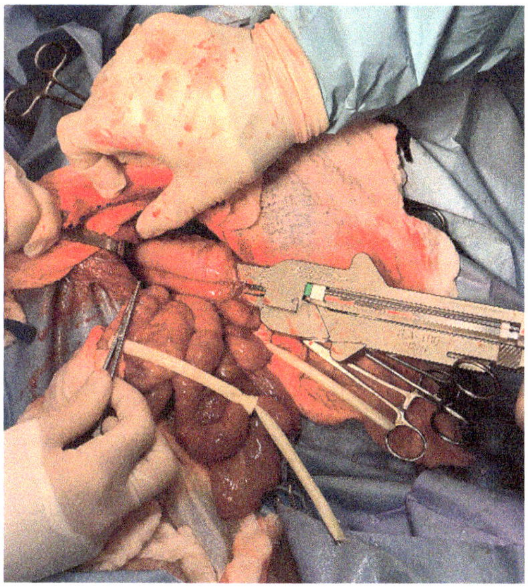

Figure 18.5 Gastrojejunostomy in a foal using a stapling device to create an anastomosis between the stomach and jejunum; note the positioning of the jejunum to maintain a left-to-right flow of ingesta. *Source:* Cole Sandow, Hagyards Equine Medicine Institute, Lexington, KY.

should be performed 24 hours postoperatively to evaluate the bypass [31]. Up to 1 week may be necessary for gastric emptying to occur consistently and intensive support should be provided during this period before the foal is allowed to nurse [32]. The owner should be advised that the foal will require long-term antiulcer medication and the procedure carries a fair to guarded prognosis. One report noted that 46% of patients survived to discharge [29] while another reported 69% of patients alive 2 years following surgery [30]. Common complications include surgical site infection, sepsis, ileus, anastomotic leakage, and anastomotic stricture [32].

Gastric Endoparasitism

Gastric endoparasitism is uncommon in neonates but infection with *Gasterophilus* species can be considered [15]. Parasites can be detected via endoscopy and treatment with ivermectin is effective [15]. Although rare, gastric rupture has been reported [15].

Gastric Abscessation

Gastric abscessation is uncommon, but can occur with ulceration, *Rhodococcus equi* infection, bacteremia, foreign body, or septic peritonitis [15]. Together with colic, foals may exhibit fever, neutrophilia, hyperfibrinogenemia, and anemia [15]. Although a partial gastrectomy has been described, the prognosis is poor [29].

Conditions of the Small Intestine Causing Colic

Small intestinal lesions can be divided into congenital and acquired lesions (Table 18.7). In general, small intestinal obstruction is a common indication for exploratory celiotomy in foals with colic [33]. Many of these lesions are strangulating lesions with Cable et al. reporting 44% of foals that required surgery had a small intestinal strangulating

Table 18.7 Congenital and acquired lesions of the small intestine associated with colic in the neonatal foal.

Congenital	Acquired
• Vitelline anomalies Meckel's diverticulum Mesodiverticular band	• Volvulus • Small intestinal impaction • Ascarids
• Mesenteric defects	• Intussusception
• Chyloabdomen	• Enteritis
• Scrotal (ruptured inguinal) hernia	• Necrotizing enterocolitis
• Inguinal hernia	• Lactose intolerance
• Diaphragmatic hernia (traumatic or congenital)	• Abscess

obstruction [2]; MacKinnon et al. reported slightly higher numbers, with 11 out of 19 (58%) surgical cases having small intestinal strangulating obstruction [1]. Foals with small intestinal strangulating obstructions present with overt colic signs, distended loops of small intestine on ultrasonographic evaluation, and abnormal peritoneal fluid obtained on abdominocentesis. Unfortunately, enteritis and enterocolits can present with similar clinical findings, however, the peritoneal fluid typically remains normal [1]. Of note, in the early stages of small intestinal strangulating obstruction, foals may not exhibit changes in peritoneal fluid. In one study, 55% of neonates with small intestinal strangulating lesions exhibited severe pain whereas only 3% of those with enterocolitis exhibited the same level of discomfort [1]. In the same study, 55% of neonates with small intestinal strangulating lesions exhibited continuous pain but only 5% of foals demonstrated continuous pain with enterocolitis; however, 18% of neonates with necrotizing enterocolitis demonstrated either severe or continuous pain.

Vitelline Anomalies

Meckel's diverticulum is a blind extension, or fibrous band, at the antimesenteric surface of the distal jejunum or ileum [34–36]. Although more commonly documented in older foals (2–7 months), Meckel's diverticulum can cause colic in the neonates [37, 38]. Signs of colic arise from either impaction of the diverticulum or strangulation of the small intestine around Meckel's diverticulum [27]. Presenting signs and clinical examination findings are consistent with a small intestinal obstruction prompting surgical intervention. Treatment requires resection and anastomosis of the small intestine [38].

A mesodiverticular band is located in the distal jejunum and extends from one side of the mesentery to the antimesenteric surface of the small intestine, to form a variably sized pocket [27]. Mesodiverticular bands are often incidental findings, but can be a source of colic later in life, thus the merits of removal should be considered [27, 39]. A mesodiverticular band can cause colic due to shortening of the mesentery, which consequently results in focal narrowing of the lumen [27]. Alternatively, colic can arise from a mesenteric rent forming within the mesenteric fold resulting in small intestinal strangulation and volvulus.

Presenting signs and clinical examination findings are consistent with small intestinal obstruction, and sometimes strangulation, prompting exploratory celiotomy. Any strangulated small intestine should be resected and the mesodiverticular band removed. In some cases, the band creating a pocket in which intestine can become entrapped can simply be transected, provided that blood supply to the small intestine is not disrupted [27, 40]; however, this method of correction is not appropriate in all cases. In the author's opinion a resection an anastomosis should be performed when: a concurrent mesenteric rent is present, where a transection of the band alone would result in disruption of small intestinal blood supply, or where shortened mesentery is present and transection of the band alone would not provide resolution.

Mesenteric Rents

Mesenteric rents may be congenital or acquired and can lead to incarceration of small intestine. Foals have clinical findings consistent with small intestinal obstruction or strangulation. Surgical intervention is required with the incarcerated segment resected if necessary. Mesenteric defects should be repaired via ventral midline celiotomy to reduce the likelihood of further colic episodes [27]. In order to reduce the risk of mesenteric tearing, the author uses 4-0 USP (1.5 M) monofilament suture in a combination of simple continuous and simple interrupted sutures to close mesenteric defects in the neonate.

Chyloperitoneum

Chyloperitoneum is uncommon, but when it occurs, foals appear normal for the first 12–36 hours of life [41]. Once signs of abdominal distention start, foals often remain in lateral recumbency. Ultrasonography demonstrates a large quantity of fluid in the peritoneal space; depending on the location of the lesion, the duodenum may be distended. Abdominocentesis yields white fluid with a marked hypertriglyceridemia (4.9–16.9 mmol/l [434–1495 mg/dl]) [42, 43]. The abdominal fluid cell count is frequently within normal reference intervals; however, total protein concentrations cannot be accurately evaluated [41]. Other abnormalities are associated with dehydration from reduced nursing. Most cases of chyloperitoneum are managed surgically [44], however, successful outcomes have been reported in a few cases provided medical therapy with antimicrobials, analgesics, and IV fluids [42, 43]. With laparotomy, the abdomen contains white opaque fluid, variable lengths of discolored duodenum and jejunum, and white and distended mesenteric lymphatics of affected segments of intestine. Resection of the affected intestine, either via end-to-end jejunojejunal anastomosis, or a gastrojejunostomy (depending on location of pathology), can result in a successful outcome [42].

Volvulus

Volvulus is reported as the most common cause of surgical colic in foals and occurs in horses of any age; foals are most commonly affected at <3–4 months of age [1, 45–47]. Foals with small intestinal volvulus are typically (but not always) afebrile which aids the clinician in distinguishing volvulus from enteritis [41, 47]. In one study, only 2/9 (22%) patients with small intestinal strangulating lesions had a positive response to analgesia, whereas all patients with enterocolitis had improvement in clinical signs following administration of analgesia [1]. Although patients with small intestinal strangulating lesions typically have abdominal distention, the same is true of patients with meconium-associated colic and necrotizing colitis. Abdominal distention due to small intestinal strangulating lesions can lead to secondary dyspnea [41]. In addition, patients with small intestinal strangulating obstruction or necrotizing enteritis were more likely to exhibit abnormal mucous membrane color compared to other types of colic. In one study, 90% of neonates with strangulating obstruction of the small intestine exhibited distended small intestine on ultrasonography compared to 67% of patients with enterocolitis and 65% of patients with necrotizing enteritis [1]. The majority of enteritis cases demonstrated fluid-filled intestine, which was not present in foals with strangulating obstructions. In contrast to adults, small intestinal thickness does not reliably distinguish between patients with strangulating obstruction and enterocolitis or necrotizing colitis [1, 3].

The fact that volvulus can occur secondary to enteritis is well-documented and emphasizes the need for vigilant monitoring of foals with enteritis, or other abdominal inflammatory conditions; surgical intervention should be considered in cases where a strangulating lesion cannot be ruled out [48]. Prompt surgical intervention, prior to alterations in abdominal fluid, may reduce the need for resection and anastomosis. Small intestinal volvulus must be managed surgically via correction of the volvulus and resection of the affected segment if necessary. Prognosis for recovery is fair to good with one report noting 8/9 foals recovering from surgery and surviving to discharge [1]. The remaining foal had a large quantity of nonviable intestine and was euthanized while under anesthesia. None of these cases had volvulus nodosus, which is a more severe and difficult to resolve form of volvulus, typically occurring in foals 2–7 months of age [27].

Small Intestinal Impaction

Parascaris equorum most commonly causes small intestinal obstruction however, infestation has also been associated with intussusception, abscessation, and rupture of the small intestine [27]. Affected foals often appear in poor condition, suggesting heavy parasite burden. Although impaction can occur at any time, it is most associated with anthelmintic treatment, and hence frequently occurs at approximately 5 months of age [49, 50]. However, younger foals (2–4 months old) are more susceptible to small intestinal rupture [41, 51].

Foals with acute colic due to ascarids exhibit moderate to severe colic signs with abdominal distention observed secondary to small intestinal distention. Ultrasonographic evaluation reveals distended loops of small intestine, and, in some cases the presence of ascarids (Figure 18.6a and b) [52]. Ascarids may also be observed in the feces as well as gastric reflux, obtained via nasogastric tube; if either of these occurrences are observed, ascarid impaction should be suspected. In addition, following rupture, ascarids may be observed in the peritoneal cavity [52]. Other indications of intestinal rupture include large quantities of abdominal fluid on ultrasonographic evaluation and cardiovascular compromise.

Resolution of ascarid impactions typically requires surgical intervention [27]. Impactions are usually located in the ileum but numerous sites can be affected and multiple enterotomies may be required [41]. Initially attempts to massage the impaction into the cecum should be pursued, however, the ileocecal valve can make this difficult in large impactions [27]. Once the impaction has been massaged into the cecum, the cecum can be evacuated via a typhlotomy [27, 49, 53]. A distal jejunal enterotomy, and in some cases multiple enterotomies, are required in severe cases [54]. Enterotomies are performed on the antimesenteric border of the intestine following draping of the abdominal incision; closure of enterotomy is accomplished using 3–0 or 2–0 (2 or 3 M) poliglecaprone on a taper needle in a double layer Cushing pattern, taking care not to cause narrowing of the intestinal lumen. A distal jejunal enterotomy is appropriate for resolution of ileal impactions as this enables the clinician to maintain the enterotomy site further away from the surgical site to maintain sterility. In the majority of cases, a resection is not required, however, if devitalized intestine is present, resection and anastomosis should be performed [46]. Ascarids can be present in the stomach, therefore anthelmintic treatment is required postoperatively [3, 53].

The prognosis for foals requiring surgery is considered guarded with reported postoperative mortality rates as high as 92% [27, 45, 46, 49], but these reports included patients with bowel rupture present at the time of surgery. More recent studies suggest lower mortality rates of 20–21% [27, 50, 55]. Even with improved survival rates, undetected ascarid-induced damage in the intestinal wall, particularly in the part of the ileum that cannot be visualized, failure to remove all worms at surgery, and risk of adhesions are contributing factors to postoperative morbidity and mortality [27, 50, 53]. Prevention of ascarid impaction is possible with a deworming program starting in foals at 4–6 weeks of age [27, 56]. Highly parasitized foals should be treated with a slow acting drug such as a benzimidazole [45].

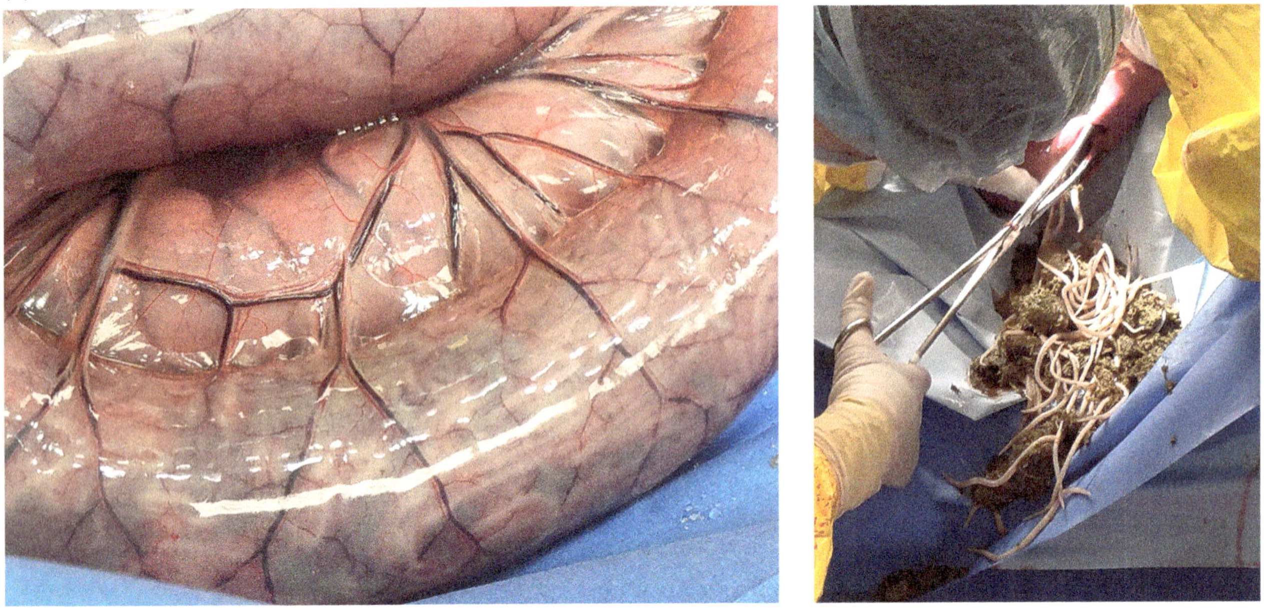

Figure 18.6 (a) Impaction of the jejunum with ascarids. Note the ability to visualize the ascarids through the wall of the small intestinal lumen. (b) Ascarids being evacuated via a jejunal enterotomy. *Source:* Images courtesy of Dr. David Wong, Iowa State University.

Intussusception

Intussusceptions most commonly occur at 3–12 months of age and can occur in neonates at a variety of locations in the small intestine including jejunojejunal, ileoileal, jejunoileal, and ilelocecal [1, 27, 46]. Foal intestine are particularly prone to intussusception and even when normal intestinal motility is observed during surgery, short segments of small intestine frequently intussuscept and resolve spontaneously; this is considered normal in foals [27]. Such occurrences can also be observed ultrasonographically; therefore, the ultrasound probe should be held over a specific loop of intestine for several seconds if an intussusception is suspected [57].

Clinical signs are variable with degree of discomfort and quantity of distended small intestine present depending on the length and location of the intussusception, as well as the chronicity of the lesion [41, 58]. Abdominal fluid analysis in this situation may be normal, but alterations in white blood cell count, total protein and lactate also can be observed [59]. A pathognomonic ultrasonographic finding of an intussusception is the appearance of concentric rings with a bull's-eye appearance when the intussusception is viewed in cross-section (Figure 18.7) [27, 60]. If this is observed, surgical intervention may be required [27].

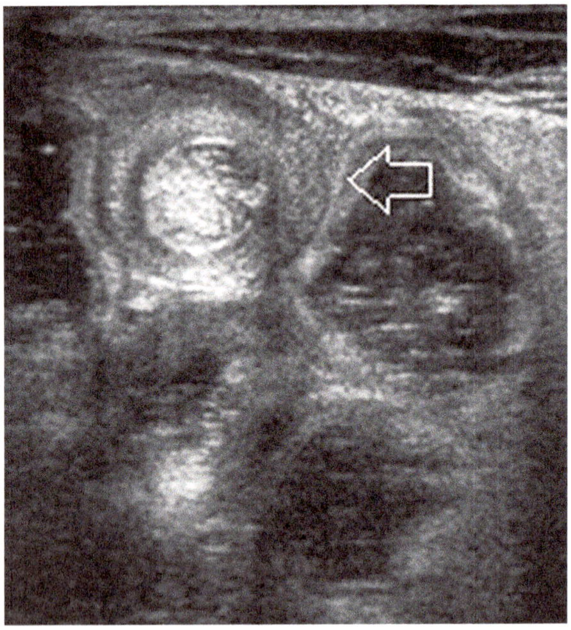

Figure 18.7 Bull's-eye appearance noted on abdominal ultrasound of jejunojejunal intussusception (arrow). *Source:* Image courtesy of Jessica Partlow, Scone Equine Hospital.

Once the lesion is located via surgical intervention, reduction is achieved by massaging the distal part of the intussuscipiens and placing gentle traction on the intussusceptum [27]. In cases of long or chronic intussusceptions, other techniques can be utilized. With jejunojejunal intussusception (Figures 18.7 and 18.8) the entire intussusception can be removed via resection [58]; jejunocecostomy can be performed following resection if

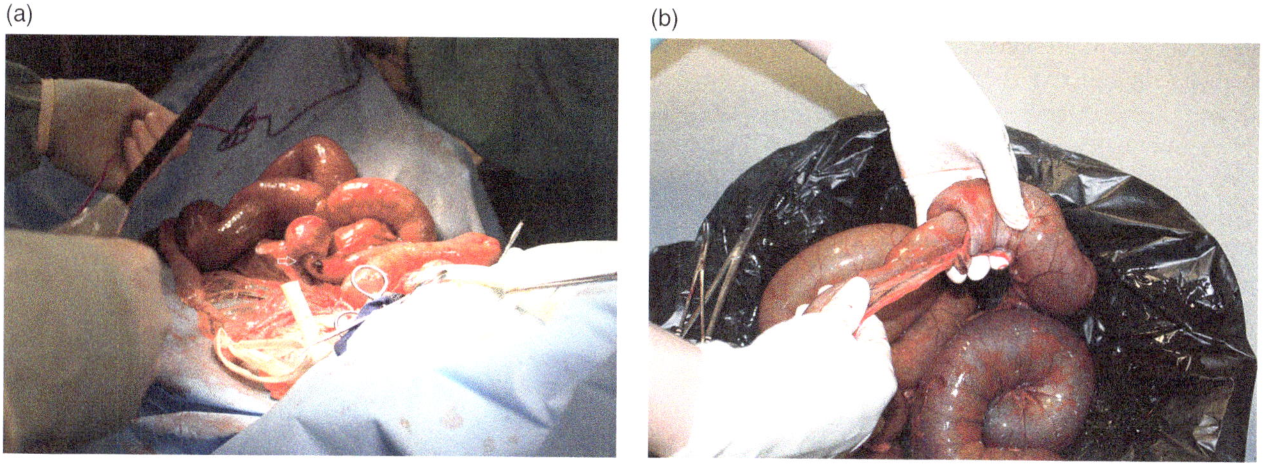

Figure 18.8 Jejunojejunal intussusception (a) (arrow) intraoperatively and (b) after surgical resection. *Source:* Image courtesy of David Wong, Iowa State University.

the mesentery is too short. Cases of ileoileal or ileocaecal intussusception can be treated with a myotomy and the intussusceptum removed via a typhlotomy [27, 61, 62]. More specifically, as described by Freeman [27], the jejunum proximal to the intussusception is transected using a gastrointestinal anastomosis (GIA) that is performed as close to the ileocecal junction as possible [63, 64]. A 10 cm incision is made in the cecum to allow the intussusception to be exteriorized and the outer part of the intussusception is incised to expose the inner loop of ileum. Subsequently, the inner loop is pulled through the incision in the outer layer until the transected end of the jejunum is situated distal to the site where the planned transection is to be performed. A thoracoabdominal (TA-90) stapler is then applied across the inverted ileum within the cecum and the intussusception is removed. The typhlotomy incision is closed in a double layer Cushing pattern using 2-0 to 3-0 USP (2 or 3 M) poliglecaprone on a taper needle. A jejunocecostomy or an ileocecal bypass can be performed to restore intestinal continuity [27]. Foals with cecocecal intussusception may require a partial cecal resection, which has been documented in foals (6–7 months of age) [58].

The prognosis for recovery from an intussusception postoperatively is typically favorable but is lower in cases where reduction is particularly difficult [27, 59]. *Anaplocephala perfoliata* and *Eimeria Leukarti* have been implicated in the pathogenesis of intussusceptions, therefore affected foals should be treated with pyrantel pamoate and praziquantel [65]. In addition, anthelmintic treatment should be considered in foals sharing the same pasture providing they are at least 4 weeks of age [56]. As an aside, a retrograde intussusception of the small colon has been diagnosed secondary to a hamartoma in a neonatal foal, but the foal was euthanized due to a poor prognosis [66].

Enteritis and Necrotizing Enterocolitis

Enteritis and enterocolitis (Chapter 18) are common in the neonatal foal and are typically treated medically. Of note, small intestinal volvulus can occur following enteritis [48]. Enterocolitis was the most common reason for admission of neonates with colic, with enterocolits and necrotizing entrocolitis being diagnosed in 27 and 16% of foals, respectively [1]. Foals with enterocolitis and necrotizing colitis presented at a median age of 2.5 and 2 days, respectively [1]. Necrotizing enterocolitis (Figure 18.9) has similar clinical signs as enterocolitis but carries a worse prognosis due to gas forming bacteria colonizing the bowel wall, resulting in gas accumulation within the intestinal wall [3].

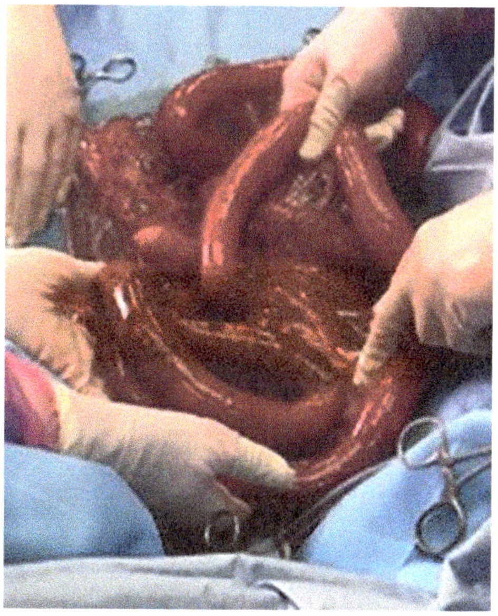

Figure 18.9 Necrotizing enterocolitis noted in a neonatal foal at the time of surgery. *Source:* Image courtesy of Cajsa Isgren, Leahurst Equine Hospital.

Differentiating between enterocolitis and small intestinal strangulating lesions is challenging. Variables such as degree of pain (e.g. 3% of enterocolitis cases and 18% of necrotizing enterocolitis cases had marked colic signs compared to 55% with small intestinal strangulating obstructions), duration of pain/discomfort (enterocolitis cases were less likely to exhibit continuous discomfort compared to intestinal strangulating obstructions), and response to analgesia (enterocolitis cases were responsive to analgesia whereas foals with small intestinal strangulating obstruction were non-responsive) can be used to help in differentiation [1]. The majority (82–97%) of cases of enterocolitis and necrotizing enterocolitis are managed with medical therapy [1]. However, difficulty ruling out small intestinal strangulating obstructions are well documented and is a common reason for surgical intervention [1, 24]. The prognosis for necrotizing enteritis is guarded to poor [24, 41, 45].

Abscess

Colic due to abscessation of the umbilical remnants usually occurs in foals <6 weeks of age whereas mesenteric abscessation occurs between 2 and 6 months of age [41]. Although both *Streptococcus spp.* and *Rhodococcus equi* are frequently implicated, many foals do not exhibit signs of pulmonary infection (Figure 18.10) [24]. Other than mild colic signs, clinical findings may include weight loss, pyrexia, and hyperfibrinogenemia [41]. Abscessation can be diagnosed ultrasonographically, particularly large abscesses situated ventrally, or via CT [11, 45]. Gastric abscessation resulting in filling defects can also be observed using contrast radiography in some cases [3].

Surgical treatment involves bypass, resection, or marsupialization, which is only possible in some cases [24]. Abscessation of the umbilical stump can be resolved with surgical intervention in most cases. Treatment also includes antimicrobials (broad-spectrum or based on culture and sensitivity results). Placement of an abdominal drain and peritoneal lavage can also be performed. Medical treatment with rifampin and azithromycin or clarithromycin along with gallium maltolate can be successful in selected cases of abscessation due to *Rhocodoccus equi* infection [67].

Surgical Techniques

Intestinal resection and anastomosis (IRA) is performed in a similar manner in foals and adults but the friable nature of the mesentery and increased risk of adhesions in foals warrants extra care when handling the intestine [24]. The author recommends a monofilament suture of 3-0 or 4-0 USP (1.5–2 M) to be used in a combination of simple interrupted and simple continuous patterns to close any mesenteric defects. Copious quantities of sterile saline, and in some cases carboxymethycellulose can be used to aid in manipulation of the intestine. The procedure to perform a handsewn end-to-end jejunojejunostomy is noted in Table 18.8 [27].

Prognosis for Small Intestinal Lesions

In one study, neonates with small intestinal strangulating obstruction and necrotizing enterocolitis were less likely to survive to discharge (36%) than foals with meconium-associated colic (100%), enterocolitis (86%), or medical causes (85%) of colic [1]. Another study reported a higher

(a) (b)

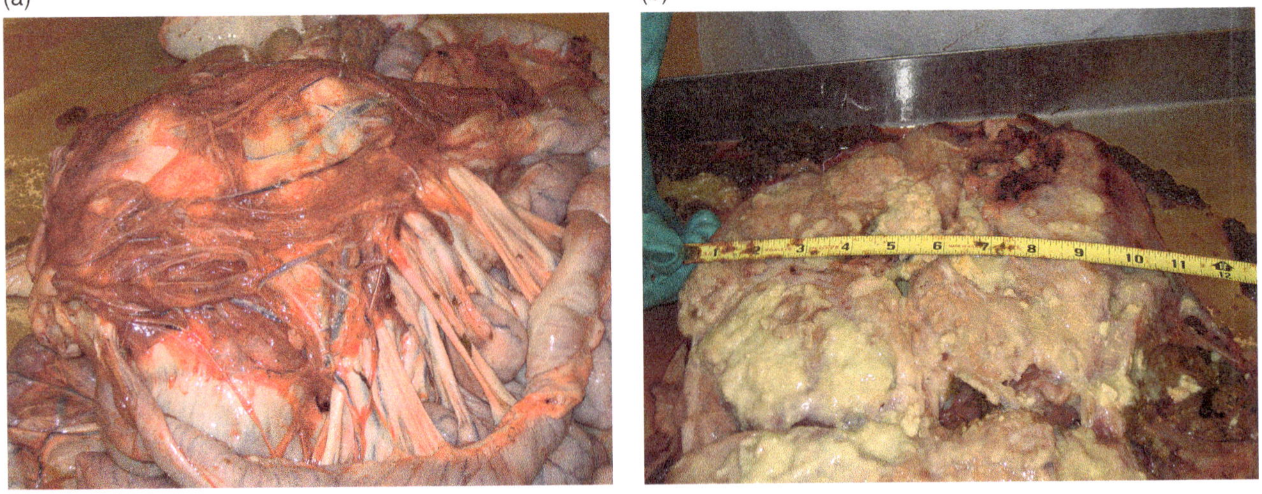

Figure 18.10 Large *Rhodococcus equi* abdominal abscess noted in a foal presented for weight loss and chronic colic. (a) Abscess with mesentery adhered to mass; (b) abscess cut in half and measuring approximately 12 in. long. *Source:* Images courtesy of David Wong, Iowa State University.

Table 18.8 Procedure for end-to-end jejunojejunostomy as described by Freeman [27].

- Following resolution of lesion and decompression of the small intestine, the bowel is arranged in its correct orientation.

The author prefers to decompress the small intestine into the cecum and perform a typhlotomy if necessary; however, other techniques, such as decompression via small intestinal enterotomy or via the cut end of a small intestinal segment following ligation and transection of the mesentery are alternative options [27].

- The region of resection is identified; remove the strangulated bowel and at least 1 vascular arcade of healthy bowel either side of the strangulated bowel.
- The mesenteric vessels are ligated:
  - 3-0 USP (2 M) poliglecaprone or other absorbable suture is used to double ligate the first nonstrangulated mesenteric vessel oral to the strangulated bowel, level with proposed line of mesenteric resection. Repeat procedure for each mesenteric vessel to be ligated. A hemostat is applied to the mesenteric vessel 2 cm distal to the ligature. A Ligasure Vessel Sealing instrument is not recommended in neonates due to a perceived risk of adhesion formation; however, literature proving this theory is lacking. The distal ligature at the first ligated mesenteric vessel is not cut; the short end of the ligature is left longer than normal (5 cm) and is secured with a hemostat. The long end is used to gather the trimmed edge of the mesentery [27].
  - The mesenteric vessel is transected distal to the distal ligature using Metzenbaum scissors and the trimmed mesenteric edge is gathered.
  - Where possible, the line of mesenteric resection should remain at a constant distance from the bowel, aiming for the bifurcation of the major mesenteric arteries to reduce the likelihood of mesenteric shortening.
  - Once the mesentery is gathered and the bowel is decompressed, the two ends of the suture used to gather the mesentery are tied together. Gathering the mesentery prior to intestinal resection largely prevents bowel rotation when the two transected ends are sutured together [68].
  - A large arcuate artery, no more than 4 cm from its origin from the major mesenteric vessel, is left to supply the anastomosed ends. The chosen arcuate artery is ligated marginally beyond the proposed intestinal transection site.
  - The mesentery is transected parallel, but at least 5 cm distant from the major mesenteric vessel that will supply each end of the anastomosis. Leaving adequate mesentery is essential to ensure the mesenteric defect can be closed at the end of the anastomosis.
  - A penrose drain is tied 20–30 cm proximal and, in some cases, 20–30 cm distal to the proposed intestinal transection sites to reduce ingesta at the anastomosis site. The healthy intestine and penrose drains can be returned to the abdomen while the anastomosis is performed.
  - Several methods of transecting the intestine to remove nonviable bowel exist. The author places doyen clamps no more than 60° from the mesenteric attachment. A No. 10 scalpel blade is used to cut oral to the proximal clamp and aboral to the distal clamp, so the tissue held within the clamp is removed together with the resected bowel. Some surgeons prefer not to use clamps while others choose to transect the bowel with Metzenbaum scissors [27].
  - Stay sutures (3-0 USP/2 M poliglecaprone or polydioxanone) incorporating the seromuscular layer of the small intestine are placed in a Lembert pattern to appose the mesenteric and anti-mesenteric edges of the transected intestine. The mesenteric segment should be apposed first.
  - There are several methods available for performing the anastomosis, including single-layer and two-layer continuous patterns; the author recommends placing sutures in an interrupted modified Lembert pattern, approximately 5 mm apart [27]. If a continuous suture is preferred, this must be interrupted at the mesenteric and antimesenteric surfaces to prevent a purse-string effect.
  - Lavage the bowel with sterile saline.
  - The remaining mesenteric defect is closed using 3-0 or 4-0 USP (1.5–2 M) in a combination of simple interrupted and simple continuous sutures to reduce the likelihood of mesenteric tearing.

two-year survival rate (69%) in foals that had non-strangulating small intestinal lesions, compared to strangulating lesions (19%) [46]. Thus, small intestinal strangulating lesions have a lower likelihood of survival compared to other types of colic, with the exception of necrotizing enterocolitis and certain congenital conditions such as atresia coli. Although reduced survival rates are reported in foals with small intestinal strangulating lesions, in one report, all foals with small intestinal strangulating obstruction that recovered from surgery survived to discharge, with 1 foal euthanized under general anesthesia [1]. Another factor to consider is the implications of performing a resection and anastomosis, and particularly a more involved procedure such as jejunocecostomy, in a foal and the high incidence of adhesion formation. Although not a strangulating obstruction, ascarid impactions may have a lower short-term survival (8–80%) due to the possibility of bowel rupture, peritonitis, adhesion formation, and a failure to remove all worms at surgery [2, 3, 24, 46, 50].

Cecum

Disorders of the cecum leading to acute colic in the neonate are rare but include cecocolic and cecocecal intussusception, cecal atresia, cecal impaction, and cecal perforation/rupture.

Cecocolic and Cecocecal Intussusception

The etiology of intussusceptions of the cecum and colon are identical to small intestinal intussusceptions, however a case of cecocolic intussusception has been associated with *Eimeria leukarti* [69]. Cecocecal and cecocolic intussusceptions can have acute, subacute, and chronic forms [70]. Diagnosis of cecal intussusceptions is similar to that of the small intestine. Specific abnormalities may not be observed on examination, particularly in more chronic cases. Moreover, the clinician should not rely on abdominocentesis alterations as the peritoneal fluid may be normal [70, 71]. However, identification of a bull's eye lesion ultrasonographically is pathognomonic and should prompt surgical intervention [72].

Treatment of cecal intussusceptions follow similar principles of those involving the small intestine with manual reduction successful in approximately 30% of cases involving the cecum [72]. Following reduction, a partial typhlectomy may be required if there is vascular compromise. A partial typhlectomy can be performed using the following steps: [70] isolate the cecum from the abdomen and drape off the incision; double ligate the lateral and medial cecal vessels using 0 USP (3.5 M) polyglactin 910; apply a Doyen intestinal clamp proximal to the intended incision site; sharpy transect the cecum proximal to the compromised wall (distal to the Doyen clamp); close in a double layer inverting pattern (first layer may be full thickness, second layer should be partial thickness and inverting) using 2-0/0USP (3/3.5 M) absorbable suture.

If manual reduction is not possible, a typhlotomy (cecocecal intussusception) or a right ventral colotomy (cecocolic intussusception) can be performed to aid in reduction [70]. If reduction is still not possible, the surgeon should resect as much of the cecum as possible; this can be followed by a complete cecal bypass [70] but reports in neonates are lacking. Postoperatively, administration of IV fluids and NSAIDs along with broad spectrum antimicrobials for at least 1 week is important due to the presence of compromised intestine and the risk of contamination [70]. Foals that remain comfortable can nurse 24 hours postoperatively; IV nutrition should be considered until this time.

Cecal Impaction and Cecal Rupture

Cecal impaction can occur in horses of all ages [73]. Foals with cecal impaction may only exhibit mild colic signs and diagnosis is rarely obtained preoperatively. This highlights the importance of considering surgical intervention in cases of persistent colic where a diagnosis has not been reached. Cecal impaction can be resolved by via typhlotomy or cecal bypass procedure (Table 18.9) [70].

In one study, 7 foals (age range 1–6 months) with cecal perforation or rupture were all suspected of having a cecal impaction preceding rupture [75]. In addition, 6/7 foals had undergone general anesthesia, (5 for orthopedic disease) [75]. In another report, cecal rupture in a foal occurred 7 days after an orthopedic surgery [73]. Rupture has also been documented following general anesthesia and endoscopy in a foal [76]. Thus, cecal impaction should be considered if a foal has been anesthetized and is exhibiting signs of abdominal discomfort.

Table 18.9 Typhlotomy and cecal bypass procedure as described by Sherlock [70].

- Typhlotomy
  - The cecum is exteriorized and manipulated to the right side of the incision (procedure can also be performed with the cecum situated to the left side of the incision).
  - Drape off abdomen and place stay suture at the distal end of the typhlotomy site to enable control of the site and reduce contamination.
  - A 5 cm incision is made between the lateral and ventral bands of the cecum.
  - A stomach tube and pump are used to gently aid in evacuation of the impaction. Alternatively, a 60 ml syringe can fit onto the end of a foal stomach tube to gently administer water into the cecum via the typhlotomy.
  - The typhlotomy site is closed in a double layer inverting pattern (e.g. Cushing pattern) using 2-0 USP (3 M) poliglecaprone or other absorbable suture.
- Cecal bypass is recommended in cases of type II (cecal motility disorder resulting in fluid accumulation) cecal impaction in adult horses [74]. It is suspected that, given the frequency of cecal rupture in foals, this procedure may be a viable option if a type II cecal impaction is encountered during surgery. However, documented cases in neonates are lacking.

Because more foals present with cecal rupture (suspected or confirmed to be secondary to cecal impaction) compared to cecal impaction, it can be assumed that initial clinical signs are mild. Unfortunately, the inability to perform a transrectal examination in foals greatly hinders obtaining a diagnosis resulting in delayed surgical intervention and cecal rupture. This also suggests that cecal impactions in foals, particularly when they occur following orthopedic surgery, typically require surgical rather medical intervention.

Clinical signs of cecal rupture are variable. Some foals exhibit colic signs prior to systemic signs of endotoxic shock [70]. Diagnosis is based on clinical signs, ultrasonography (increased abdominal fluid, marked fibrinous reaction over time) and abdominal fluid derangements. As with gastric rupture secondary to ulceration, white blood cell and total protein levels may remain within reference limits in early stages, but gradually increase [70]. Cytological evaluation can aid in detection. A definitive diagnosis is made via exploratory laparotomy or postmortem examination. The sparse number of published cases of cecal impaction in foals makes evaluation of prognosis difficult. However, the literature suggests that early surgical intervention is preferable. Should cecal rupture occur, the prognosis is hopeless [72, 75].

Diseases of the Large and Small Colon

The majority of conditions affecting the neonatal small colon involve an obstruction and include meconium retention, atresia coli and ileocolic aganglionosis.

Meconium Retention

A full discussion of meconium retention is in Chapter 17 but is briefly discussed here. Meconium impaction is a common causes of colic in the neonate, occurring in 27 of 75 cases of neonatal colic in one report [1]. Meconium has a dark brown color and sticky consistency and is usually passed within the first 24 hours of birth. Passage of a lighter yellow-brown material indicates that complete passage of the meconium has occurred [77]. Differential diagnoses for meconium impaction include ruptured bladder, rectal irritation, congenital atresia and ileocolonic aganglionosis.

Meconium retention is more common in colts. Clinical signs include repetitive posturing to defecate and tail flagging, without production of feces. This can progress to straining to defecate, abdominal distention and colic. Digital palpation may reveal the presence of meconium in the rectum. In addition, many foals pass some meconium if an enema is administered, aiding diagnosis. If no meconium is produced, congenital atresia should be considered. Impaction is suspected based on the age (<24–48 hours of age) and clinical signs, with confirmation achieved via ultrasonography and plain and contrast radiography. Most cases are managed medically, but surgery may infrequently be necessary [1]. Treatment includes analgesics, aiding passage of meconium via enemas, and correction of dehydration if necessary.

Warm water/soap enema(s) or a commercial phosphate (e.g. Fleet) enema can be used but the neonatal rectum is very delicate and can tear if excessive volume or force is used during administration. General guidelines include volumes of 250–350 ml of a warm water and soap enema via gravity flow using a soft flexible Foley catheter; this procedure can be repeated in 1–2 hours if meconium is not passed. Phosphate enemas (100 ml) should only be repeated a maximum of twice in 24 hours, however, smaller doses of phosphate enema can be given more frequently (i.e. a total of two commercial enemas over a period of 24 hours). If meconium is not passed following two to three separate enemas, an acetylcysteine retention enema can be performed.

In cases where overt colic signs are continuous and abdominal distention is increasing, surgical intervention should be considered [32, 77]. During exploratory celiotomy, the region of the impaction is manually massaged, sometimes with the aid of fluid being injected proximal to the impaction in the small colon and rectum; the large colon can sometimes also be involved [31]. In rare cases, an enterotomy is required on the antimesenteric taenia of the small colon to enable evacuation of the meconium. To perform this procedure, exteriorize the small colon while the location for enterotomy is moved away from the incision and draped off; place stay sutures at either end of the proposed incision site on the antimesenteric band. This aids control of the small colon and reduces contamination. A No.10 scalpel blade is used to make a 5 cm incision and fluid is gently introduced via the enterotomy taking care to avoid contamination of the abdominal incision; the enterotomy is closed using 3-0 USP (2 M) polyglicaprone on a taper needle in two layers using a Cushing pattern. It is essential that over-inversion does not occur; as a guide, the author recommends attempting to keep both layers of the Cushing closure on the antimesenteric tenial band to prevent excessive inversion. Impactions in the large colon may require a pelvic flexure enterotomy to introduce fluid and evacuate the impaction. In rare cases, when the intestine is compromised, a resection may be required [32].

The prognosis for foals that require surgical intervention to treat meconium impaction is good, providing surgical intervention is not delayed; the prognosis for survival is decreased if intestinal resection is needed [1]. In a one report, all cases (3) requiring surgical intervention survived to discharge [1] whereas in another report, 88% of cases treated surgically survived to discharge [2].

Atresia Coli

Intestinal atresia has a reported incidence of 0.44% [78]. Atresia coli is diagnosed within the first few days of life and can occur in both sexes [79]. A lack of blood supply to a particular segment of the large colon or cecum during development leads to a failure of development of that part of the GI tract [32]. There are three types of atresia: [32]

- Type 1 – Membrane atresia: a membranous tissue separating two adjacent segments of normal bowel
- Type 2 – Cord atresia: an atretic segment consisting of a fibrous band
- Type 3 – Blind end atresia: a missing segment between two blind ending segments of bowel (Figure 18.11)

Clinical signs of atresia coli or atresia cecum include progressive abdominal distention and colic. In addition, regardless of enema administration, there is no evidence of fecal staining or meconium production [80]; this lack of fecal staining can assist with differentiating between meconium impaction and atresia coli. Proctoscopy can also be utilized in the diagnosis of atresia coli but this is rarely required [79]. Radiography can reveal the absence of a complete colon with a gas distended stump. A barium enema may also result in the appearance of a blind ending stump [78, 80–82]. Caution should be used in over-interpretation of a barium enema as a tapering of the contrast column suggests insufficient contrast administration, rather than atresia coli [3].

Although surgical interventions are the only treatment option, the anomaly has a poor prognosis as the proximal

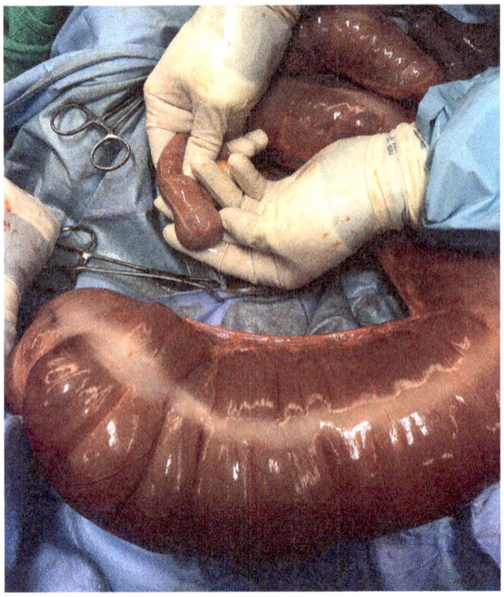

Figure 18.11 Blind end atresia coli. Note the distention oral to the blind end. *Source:* Image courtesy of Cole Sandow, Hagyard Equine Medical Institute, Lexington KY.

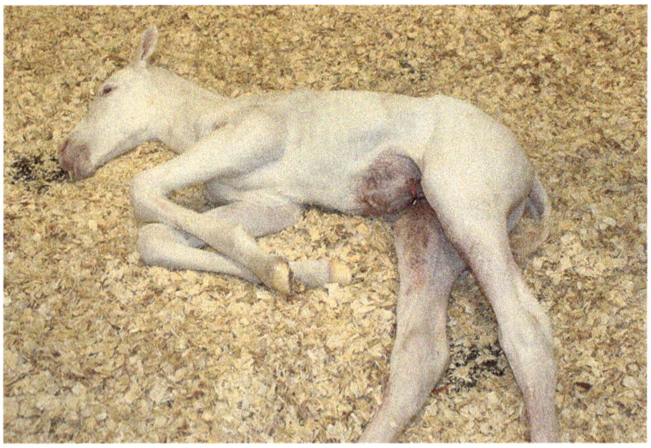

Figure 18.12 Neonatal foal with ileocolonic aganglionosis demonstrating signs of colic at 12 hours of age. *Source:* Image courtesy of David Wong, Iowa State University.

and distal segments of bowel are often insufficiently formed to create an adequate anastomosis, resulting in failure of the anastomosis site [46, 80, 81]. However, successful reports have been published [82]. Postoperative feeding should begin slowly as initiation of motility in the distended oral segment may be delayed [77].

Nappert et al. (1992) and Young et al. (1992) report surgical correction in 3 and 2 foals, respectively, all of which were eventually euthanized due to ileus, adhesions, and peritonitis [78, 80]. Successful surgical correction of a type 2 atresia was performed via a stapled side-to-side anastomosis, with the foal considered normal 22 months postoperatively [82]. Although a permanent colostomy is another possible treatment option, it is unlikely to be successful [79]. When considering surgical treatment, the clinician should consider the likelihood of concurrent congenital abnormalities as one report noted that 50% of the foals evaluated had congenital abnormalities including cardiac and brain defects [80].

Ileocolonic Aganglionosis

Approximately 25% of foals, of both sexes, born from an overo-overo breeding will exhibit the recessive genetic condition known as overo lethal white syndrome (Figure 18.12) [3]. The condition is most common in American Paint horses but has been reported in other breeds [79]. Postmortem histopathology reveals a lack of myenteric ganglia in the ileum, cecum, and colon of affected foals [32, 79]. Similar to atresia coli, affected foals present at 24–48 hours of age with progressive abdominal distention and colic [32]. Although there is no proper fecal production, administration of an enema may result in some fecal staining; this may assist in differentiation of the condition from atresia coli, in which no fecal production occurs [79]. In such cases, it is common to make a diagnosis based on clinical signs and breeding history, and the fact that the foal has no skin pigmentation [32]. Although theoretical solutions exist, the lack of neurons in the myenteric plexus results in the strong recommendation of euthanasia once a presumptive diagnosis is made [79]. Allele-specific testing is available and heterozygotes should not be bred.

Other Congenital Abnormalities of the Large Colon

In addition to atresia coli, duplications and malformations of the colon can also occur; there are at least three recorded types of colonic duplications including simple cysts, diverticula, and tubular colonic duplications [83]. Although these conditions are congenital, affected horses can present at any age [84]. T-shaped and short colon malformations of the large colon have been described in 24-month old foals. The lesions were managed with and without resection respectively [85, 86]. Another case reported a congenital mesocolon defect resulting in small intestinal herniation; this was resolved by suturing the defect closed. Congenital malformations should be considered in foals with unexplained colic [87].

Large Colon Displacement/Torsion

Large colon displacements are uncommon in neonates, however, 4 cases of large colon displacement in 3 foals (age range 3–10 weeks) have been reported [88]. In all cases, the displacements were corrected via a ventral midline celiotomy, without the need for a pelvic flexure enterotomy. All foals survived to discharge, although one foal required a repeat laparotomy for recurrence of the condition; in this latter foal, a third episode occurred at 18 months of age, at which point the horse was euthanized. The other foals developed normally.

Large colon volvulus in neonatal foals is uncommon with 5 foals reported in a case series of 67 foals [46]. Another report noted 4 cases of 360° large colon volvulus out of 119 foals [2] whereas a 720° large colon volvulus was noted in a 1-day-old foal that was euthanized during surgery as a partial large colon resection was declined by the owner [89]. Overall, the majority of foals treated for large colon volvulus were euthanized [2, 46, 89–91] but 2 foals have been documented as surviving to discharge [46, 90].

Small Colon Fecaliths and Impaction with Feed Material

Impactions of the small colon can occur in foals as young as 7 days old and are most frequently documented in American Miniature Horses and pony foals [92–94]. Similar to other large intestinal obstructions, straining to defecate and reduced or no fecal output are initially observed leading to abdominal distention and colic. Due to the firm nature of these impactions, medical intervention is less likely to be effective [46, 92, 95]. Impactions of the small colon can be resolved surgically by any of the following methods:

- Gentle administration of a warm-water enema while the impaction is manually broken down via transluminal massage
- Removal of fecalith via a small colon enterotomy (as described with meconium impactions)
- If a fecalith is present in a section of the small colon that cannot be exteriorized, the obstruction should be retropulsed into the large colon and removed via a large colon enterotomy

Foals typically recover well following surgical intervention for small colon impaction with one reported citing a 78% survival to discharge [46].

Rectum and Anus

Atresia Ani/Recti

Foals with atresia ani and atresia recti present in the first few days of life in a similar manner as foals with atresia coli: abdominal discomfort, absent fecal passage, and gas distention of the large colon [31]. Alternatively, a lack of an anus may be noted soon after birth and prompts veterinary attention. Abdominal radiography can reveal gas distention of the large colon and retrograde administration of contrast documents a blind ending small colon in atresia recti. In atresia ani, skin will be present where the anus should be, but in some cases, the location of the anus can be determined due to a change in the contour of the skin or a thinning of the skin over the anus (Figure 18.13). The severity of atresia ani can vary with some foals missing several inches of anus. The amount missing directly affects prognosis [3]. As with atresia coli, concurrent congenital abnormalities are not uncommon [3, 32, 96].

Surgery is needed in a timely manner as delayed surgical intervention results in increasing large colon distention. In foals with an intact anal ring and a lack of skin perforation, surgical correction can be performed under general anesthesia in sternal recumbency. A 2×1 cm elliptical incision, with the long axis oriented vertically is made through the persistent anal membrane. A change in contour of the skin can direct the clinician to the correct location in some cases. The terminal rectum is retracted caudally and opened, prior to suturing to the skin. To ensure correct orientation is maintained, four simple interrupted sutures at 12, 3, 6, and 9 o'clock are placed, prior to placing the remaining interrupted sutures [79]. Urethral or vaginal fistulae with the rectum can often be present; these should be corrected with a 2-layer inverting closure (Figure 18.13). In more advanced cases, surgical correction is more complex and rarely successful [3, 32]. Furthermore, there is no guarantee of normal anal function.

Rectal Prolapse

Rectal prolapse is typically not a cause of acute colic in the foal, however, conditions such as enteritis can occasionally result in rectal prolapse due to repeated straining (Figure 18.14) [97].

Hernias

Abdominal hernias do not always result in colic; however, any foal that has both a hernia and signs of colic should be investigated promptly due to the potential presence of strangulated intestine. The types of congenital hernias in foals include umbilical, inguinal, and scrotal (further information in Chapter 17).

Umbilical Hernias

Congenital umbilical hernias develop during gestation, are slightly more common in fillies than colts, and have a higher incidence in Thoroughbreds and Quarter Horses (Figure 18.15) [98–100]. An umbilical hernia is diagnosed via external palpation and should be reducible. If the hernia cannot be reduced, intestinal strangulation or presence of

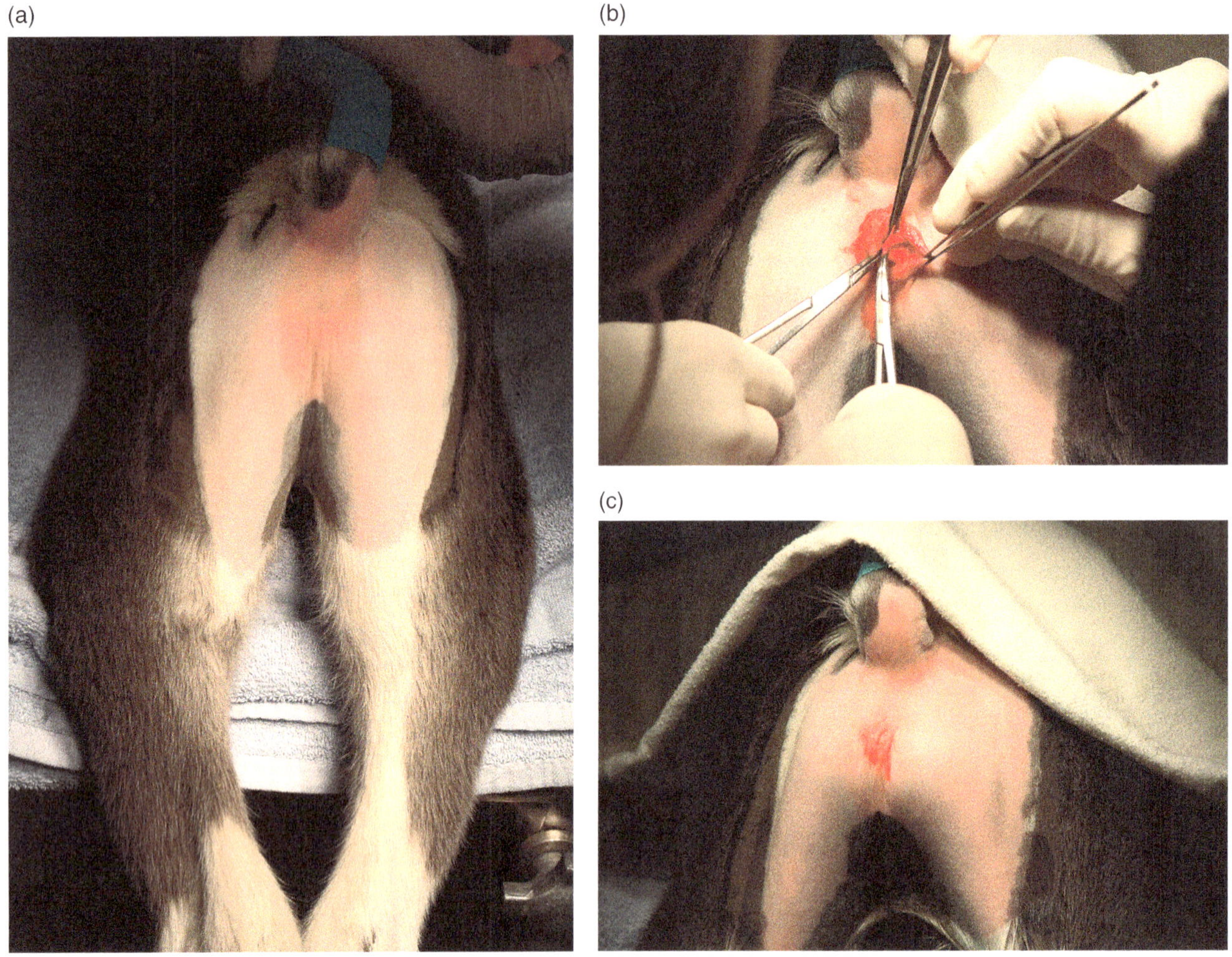

Figure 18.13 (a) Atresia ani in a newborn foal. (b) Surgical repair of atresia ani. (c) Postoperative appearance of atresia ani. *Source:* Images courtesy of Dr. Stephanie Caston Iowa State University.

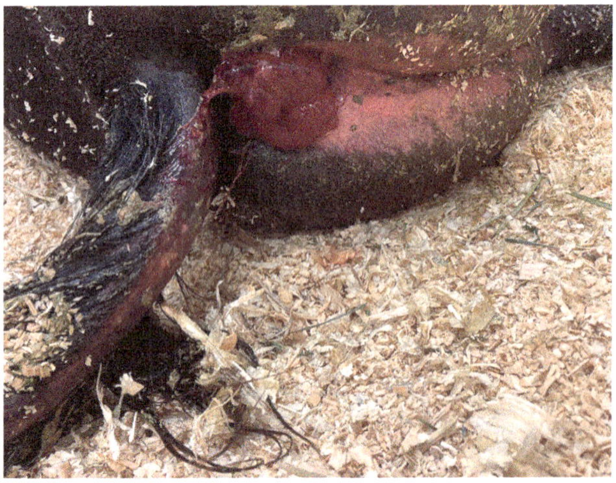

Figure 18.14 Neonatal foal with colitis secondary to Salmonellosis; rectal prolapse occurred after several days of profuse watery diarrhea and repeated tenesmus. *Source:* Image courtesy of David Wong, Iowa State University.

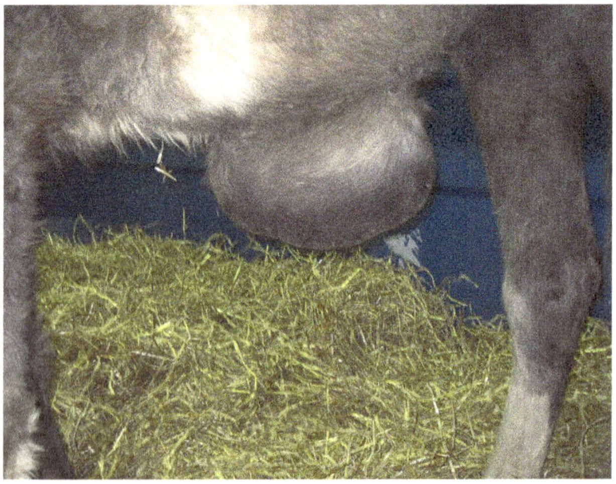

Figure 18.15 A large umbilical hernia in a foal. *Source:* Image courtesy of Scone Equine Hospital.

abscessation should be considered. Ultrasonography is used to identify intestine or omentum within the hernia sac, and aids in detection of abnormalities of the umbilical remnants. With nonreducible hernias, peritoneal fluid may be obtained via needle centesis of the hernia providing fluid can be obtained without affecting the viscera. Although peritoneal fluid may exhibit abnormalities, in early stages of disease abdominal fluid can be normal. Differential diagnosis includes abscessation of the umbilical remnants [100]. Incarcerated umbilical hernias can also result in enterocutaneous fistulae, which are managed surgically [101].

Umbilical hernias ≤3 cm in diameter often resolve spontaneously over 6–12 months; however, the caregiver must reduce the hernia several times per day [100]. If an umbilical hernia becomes nonreducible, strangulation of the intestine should be suspected, and immediate surgical intervention should be performed if ultrasonographic evaluation supports diagnosis of intestinal strangulation. Immediate surgical management is recommended in any nonreducible hernia. Hernias >3 cm diameter, or those that do not resolve by 12 months of age should also be managed surgically on an elective basis [100].

Herniorrhaphy can be performed in an open or closed fashion, however, if incarceration of the bowel is suspected, an open approach is necessary. The author prefers an open approach in all hernia repairs to reduce the likelihood of bowel perforation or performing an inadvertent intestinal pexy but opening the peritoneal cavity can increase the likelihood of adhesion formation. Correction of an umbilical hernia is described in Table 18.10 [100].

Postoperative management incudes stall rest for 4 weeks followed by small paddock turnout. An abdominal bandage can be placed and changed every 2–4 days for 2 weeks postoperatively, or longer if incisional complications occur and depending on the health of the incision. It is important to ensure the bandage is not placed too tightly due to the compliance of a foal's chest.

Table 18.10 Surgical correction of an umbilical hernia as described by Toth and Schumacher [100]. Please see Table 18.12 for management of umbilical remnants.

- A fusiform incision is made around the umbilicus and redundant skin excised.
- Dissection, if performed, is done using Metzenbaum scissors until the hernia ring can be visualized. This will increase the safety of the procedure when entering the abdomen.
- The hernia sac is entered and contents inspected. If the abdomen cannot be entered safely (common when intestine is incarcerated) a small incision can be made cranial to the hernia on ventral midline.
- The hernia is reduced and intestine inspected. If a resection is required, this is performed as described previously.
- The hernia is closed using 1–2 USP (3.5–5 M) polyglactin 910 in an appositional pattern. The author uses a taper needle unless the hernia ring is particularly well developed and prefers a simple continuous pattern; other choices such as an inverted cruciate pattern are also valid options.
- The skin and subcutaneous tissues are closed routinely.

Inguinal and Scrotal Hernias

In most inguinal hernias, the intestine remains within the vaginal tunic (indirect hernia). A scrotal hernia, or ruptured inguinal hernia, occurs when the parietal tunic is ruptured and the intestine (typically small intestine) is present in the subcutaneous tissues (Figure 18.16). Clinical appearance and ultrasonography can be used to determine whether any small intestine is present within the parietal tunic or subcutaneous tissues. A scrotal or ruptured inguinal hernia frequently becomes rapidly larger over the first 12 hours of life if left untreated.

Inguinal hernias are more common in Standardbreds, draft breeds, and Tennessee Walking Horses, which have larger inguinal rings [102]. An indirect inguinal hernia in which the parietal tunic is intact is rarely a source of colic unless either rupture of the parietal tunic or incarceration of the intestine occurs. Small congenital indirect hernias can be managed in a similar way as small umbilical hernias, that is manual reduction several times per day. Alternatively, a well-padded truss can be constructed in a figure-of-eight fashion around and between the hind limbs, but this requires close monitoring and is not always well-tolerated by foals (Figure 18.17) [3].

Scrotal or ruptured indirect inguinal hernias are most common in Standardbreds and Tennessee Walking Horses and usually present within the first 12 hours of life with an inguinal hernia that is increasing in size. Such foals often exhibit mild abdominal discomfort [102]. On presentation, the hernia can have an irregular contour due to the presence of intestine in the subcutaneous space; this can help with differentiation with an indirect hernia with small intestinal strangulation. Ultrasonography confirms rupture of the parietal tunic and the presence of intestine in the subcutaneous tissues [32]. Immediate surgical intervention should be performed as described, but in larger ruptured indirect hernias, the large quantity of small intestine in the subcutaneous tissues can make hernia reduction difficult without a small ventral midline incision. These cases have a good prognosis and foals can be managed routinely postoperatively.

In larger hernias, particularly those in which the hernia contents appear to be dissecting down the inner thigh, surgical repair is necessary (Figure 18.18). Strangulation of intestine in an inguinal hernia is uncommon in a neonate, but should the hernia be nonreducible or overt colic signs

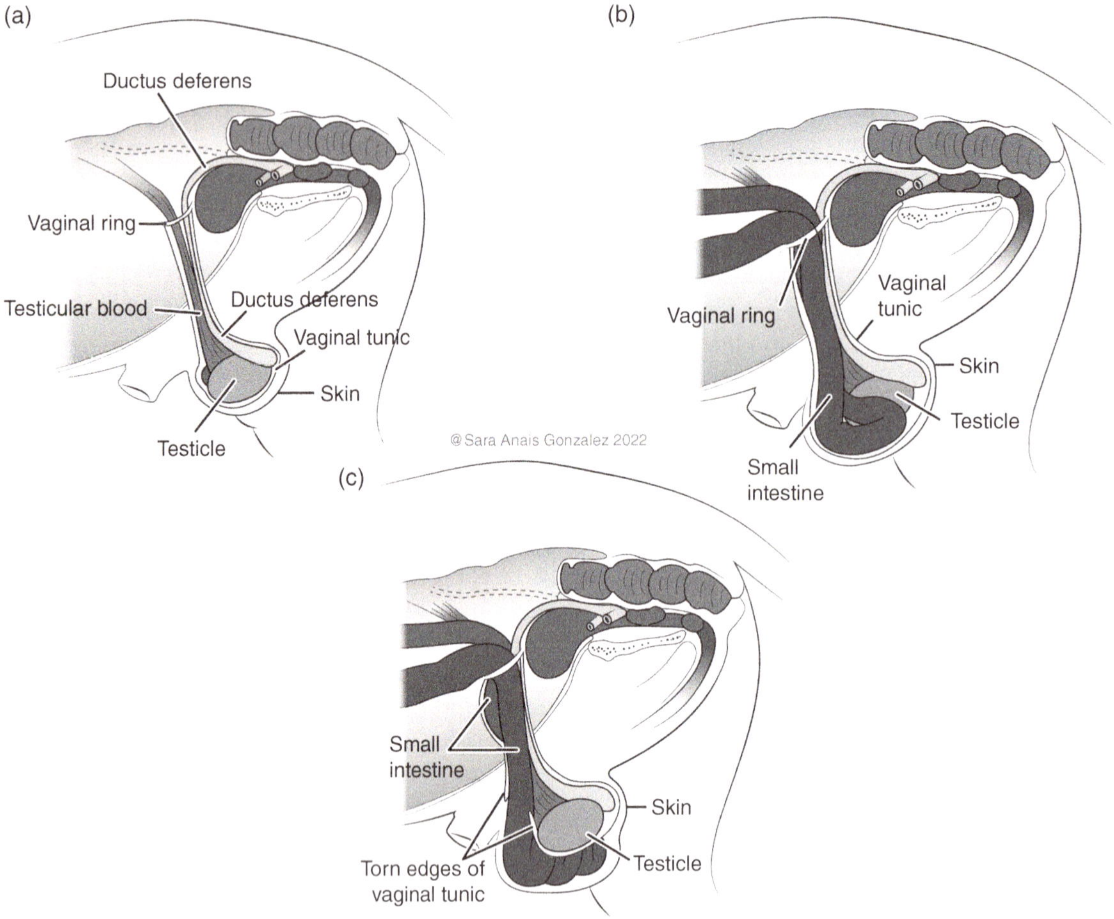

Figure 18.16 (a) Normal inguinal structures. (b) Indirect inguinal hernia. (c) Direct inguinal hernia. The difference between direct and indirect hernias is that the tunic has ruptured in direct hernias, thus allowing bowl to escape into the subcutaneous position [23].

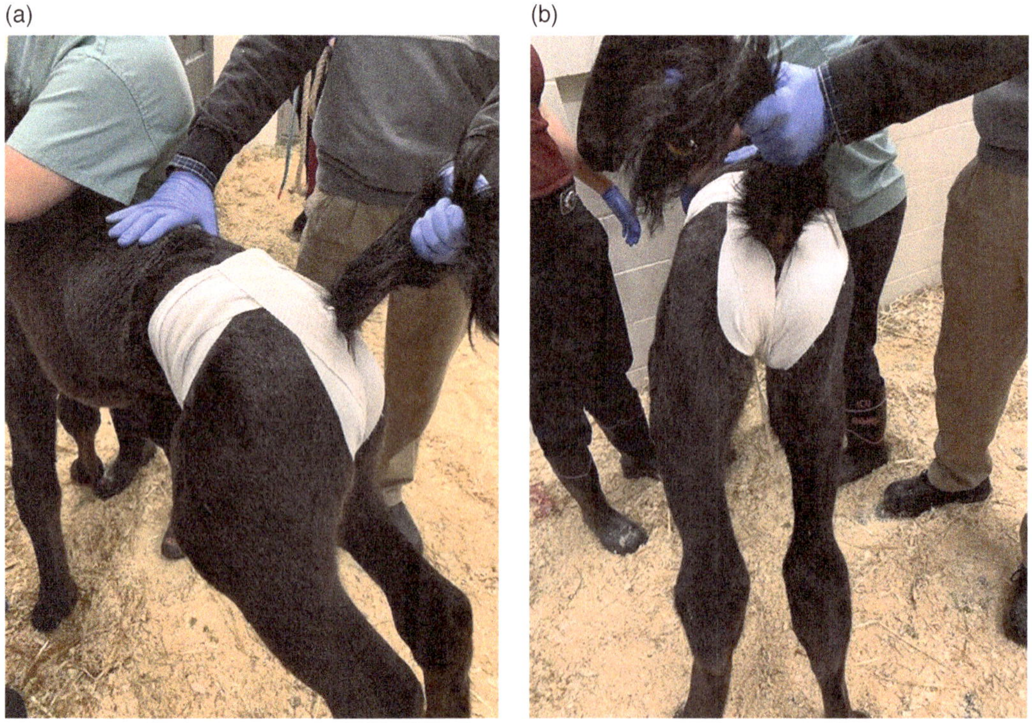

Figure 18.17 A 7-day-old Percheron colt with a figure-of-eight truss and between the hind limbs. *Source:* Images courtesy of David Wong, Iowa State University.

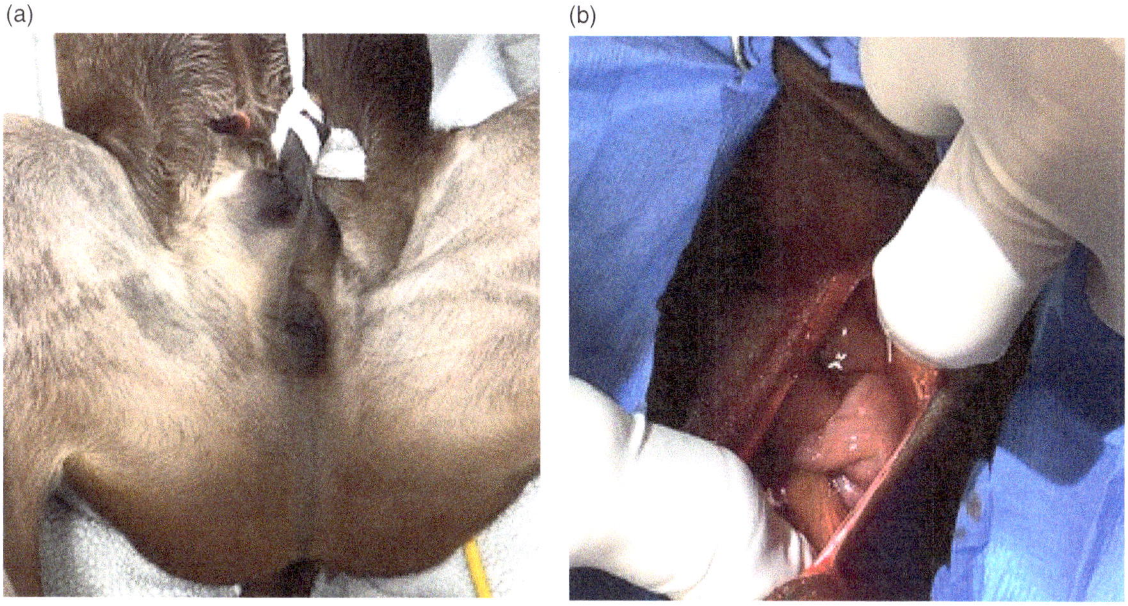

Figure 18.18 (a) Preoperative image of a ruptured inguinal hernia. (b) Intra-operative image of a ruptured inguinal hernia. Note presence of small intestine in the subcutaneous space. *Source:* Images courtesy of Cole Sandow, Hagyard Equine Medical Institute.

are observed, an exploratory celiotomy should be performed. Recall that the inguinal rings in young foals are friable and re-herniation can occur. Inguinal herniation in neonates can be surgically managed (Table 18.11).

Postoperatively, foals can nurse provided that strangulated intestine was not present. Foals should be maintained on stall rest for 2–4 weeks. Foals with incarcerated small intestine should be managed as discussed in the section on small intestinal postoperative management.

Diaphragmatic Hernias

Congenital diaphragmatic hernias are usually located in the left dorsal tendinous portion of the diaphragm (Figure 18.19) [103]. Although congenital hernias are present from birth, clinical signs may occur at any age from 6-hours of age to adult [104, 105]. Acquired diaphragmatic hernias are frequently a result of trauma and should be considered in foals with rib fractures [31, 100]. Retrosternal, or Morgagni hernias, are a form of congenital hernia that results from a failure of fusion of the septum transversum and pleuroperitoneal folds [100].

Foals with diaphragmatic hernias can present with abdominal pain, respiratory distress, or a combination of both. Respiratory distress can be marked, and emergency provision of intranasal oxygen and rapid surgical intervention may be required. Visualization of abdominal contents within the thoracic cavity via ultrasonography in a foal is usually sufficient to make a diagnosis of a diaphragmatic herniation; however, radiography can provide a more concrete diagnosis [3, 100].

Table 18.11 Surgical correction of an inguinal hernia.

- In dorsal recumbency, an attempt is made to reduce the hernia.
- A No. 10 scalpel blade is used to incise the skin close to the inguinal ring, taking care to protect the herniated small intestine. Metzenbaum scissors and finger dissection are then used to gain access to the inguinal ring and the small intestine can be returned to the abdomen.
- In cases of small intestinal strangulation, or particularly large ruptured inguinal (scrotal) hernia, a small ventral midline incision is made to assist with returning the small intestine to the abdomen.
- Inguinal ring closure is performed as follows:
  - Although castration makes the surgical procedure less technically challenging, the testicles can be maintained if the foal is intended for breeding.
  - The external inguinal ring is closed using 0 to 1 USP (3.5–4 metric) polyglactin 910 in a simple continuous, interrupted inverted cruciate, or mayo mattress suture pattern. The author chooses to form a loop in the standing end of the suture and tying a knot to hold the loop in place. This negates having to tie a knot to start the closure of the inguinal ring, where there is often tension on the tissues. The suture size can vary depending on the size of the foal and the thickness of the external inguinal ring. A taper needle can be used to close the inguinal rings to reduce the likelihood of tearing of the tissues when the needle is placed.
  - Be mindful of the proximity of the caudal superficial epigastric vessels.
  - The subcutaneous tissue and skin are closed in a routine fashion.

Treatment necessitates a ventral midline incision, beginning just caudal to the xiphoid and extending caudally. The author has found a J-shaped incision beneficial for dorsally located defects, however, a Finochetto rib

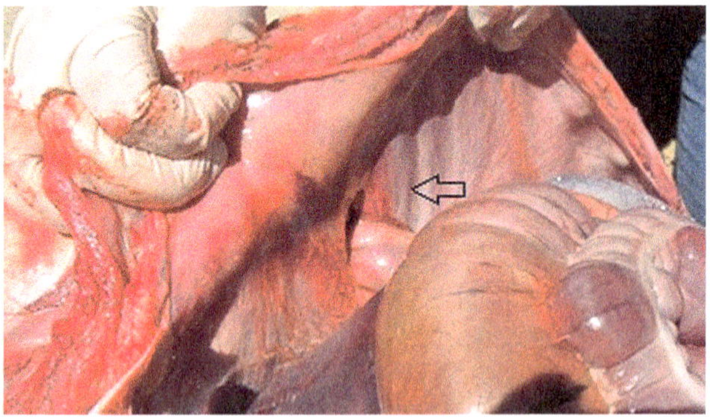

Figure 18.19 Postmortem image of a diaphragmatic hernia with small intestinal entrapment (arrow). *Source:* Image courtesy of Scone Equine Hospital.

retractor can also aid in visualization of the defect [100]. The majority of defects in neonates can be closed by direct suturing, using either a continuous or interrupted appositional pattern. A modified Roeder knot can be used to close dorsally located defects; alternatively, the forwarder knot is another logical choice [106]. Large defects can be closed by suturing a mesh to the edges of the defect and negative thoracic pressure must be re-established at the end of the procedure [9].

Complications associated with general anesthesia in adults with diaphragmatic hernias are well documented and the anesthetist should be mindful of similar complications in foals [107]. Factors other than anesthetic complications contributing to a negative prognosis include involvement of >50% of the small intestine, a larger size hernia, and a dorsal location of the hernia [100, 108]. However, diaphragmatic hernias in horses <2 years of age have an improved prognosis compared to adults [108].

Peritonitis

Peritonitis in foals can be caused by localized infection invading the abdominal cavity, disseminated infections, chemical insults, or GI perforation. Localized infection invading the abdominal cavity, due to uroperitoneum or ischemic intestine, and GI perforation, are discussed in this chapter. Further discussion of peritonitis is provided in Chapter 17.

Uroperitoneum

Uroperitoneum can be associated with signs of colic (Chapter 27). Of note, megavesica is an uncommon condition in neonatal foals with an uncertain pathogenesis. In people, the most common cause (in male fetuses) is bladder outflow obstruction due to a posterior urethral valve; one report in foals suggests that megavesica was related to an abnormal umbilical remnant. Potential abnormalities include a fibrous ligament being present instead of a normal urachus and umbilical torsion [109, 110]. Foals present with bladder and abdominal distention, with or without a ruptured bladder [111, 112]. Megavesica, even without bladder rupture, requires surgical intervention. Adams et al. reported management of a case of megavesica by resecting half of the excessively distended bladder with the foal surviving to discharge [111]. Toth et al. describe a similar successful case with follow-up to 15 months following resection of 50% of the cranial portion of the bladder [110]. Another report advises thorough evaluation for other abnormalities, due to experience of a foal with megavesica and a developmental defect in the distal small colon [113]. An additional differential diagnosis is temporary bladder distention that can occur in foals with perinatal asphyxia syndrome [111, 114, 115]. The condition can be managed with a temporary indwelling catheter.

Ovarian Torsion

Ovarian torsion should be considered in neonatal fillies exhibiting marked abdominal discomfort, without evidence of pain attributed to the GI tract. Although rare, one report describes an infarction of the left ovary, secondary to a 720° torsion of the mesovarium in a 1-week-old filly [116]. Following ligation of the ovarian pedicle and removal of the ovary, the filly recovered successfully. The filly was examined 2 years postoperatively and was noted to be clinically normal. A similar report describes a successful case in a 7-day-old filly, with the torsion being assumed to be secondary to an ovarian hematoma [117].

Hemoperitoneum

Rupture of a granulosa theca cell tumor in a neonate has been reported to cause hemoperitoneum. The foal presented with abdominal distention, colic, and anemia with an enlarged left ovary was found during exploratory laparotomy [118].

Ovarian Stalk Obstruction of the Intestine

Although rare, a case of ovarian strangulation as a cause of small colon obstruction has been reported in a 7-day-old Arabian filly [119]. The foal had not defecated for 6 days; therefore, radiography was utilized to estimate the location of the obstruction. The ovarian strangulation was resolved during exploratory laparotomy and the foal was reportedly healthy 6 months postoperatively.

Ruptured Spleen

A ruptured spleen should be considered in cases of hemoabdomen in a neonate. One report describes a 45-day-old foal that presented with abdominal discomfort and hemoabdomen [120]. As exploratory celiotomy revealed a large tear in the visceral surface of the spleen, splenectomy was performed without rib resection. The only complication observed was a lateral body wall hernia, which was repaired with a polypropylene mesh 10 weeks postoperatively.

Fractured Ribs

Clinical signs in cases of fractured ribs will typically lead to evidence of respiratory difficulty or an abnormal breathing movement. This condition can, however, result in signs of abdominal discomfort (Chapter 37).

Bile Duct Obstruction

Duodenal ulceration can lead to strictures at the site of the biliary openings. Affected foals typically have a history of malaise and present with signs of delayed gastric outflow [25]. Depending on the location of the stricture, medical treatment may be effective and includes intravenous omeprazole, ranitidine/cimetidine, sucralfate, misoprostol and bethanechol (0.025 mg/kg subcutaneously q4hrs) [3]. Patients refractory to medical therapy or those with chronic conditions, may require surgical intervention where a bypass procedure is performed.

Other Conditions

Other causes of colic in neonatal foals include liver abscessation (Chapter 19), which often requires marsupialization of the vein (see below), acute hepatic necrosis, ovarian artery rupture, ascites, and blunt abdominal trauma. Such conditions should be considered when clinical findings support these differentials.

Surgical Approach and Closure of the Abdomen

The abdomen of a foal is entered in a similar manner as adults, however, depending on the location of the lesion, or the need to resect umbilical remnants, some differences exist. The umbilicus should be oversewn or covered securely prior to skin preparation. If the surgeon wishes to avoid the umbilical remnants, an incision can be made more cranially. The skin is incised along the ventral midline using a No. 10 scalpel blade and the subcutaneous tissues are gently incised until the linea alba is visualized or palpated. A new No. 10 scalpel blade is used at the caudal aspect of the incision in a subtle back and forth motion on the linea alba until the linea alba is penetrated sufficiently to insert a finger into the abdomen. The finger is then used to separate the linea alba from any other tissues in the abdomen, including the umbilical vein. Using Russian forceps or the handle of Adson-Brown forceps (or similar), the linea alba is raised and the blade used to incise a short distance along the linea alba. A finger is inserted into the abdomen and the remaining linea alba is separated from the deeper tissues. The process of incising the linea alba with a scalpel blade, while using the handle of the thumb forceps to protect the viscera, is repeated until the linea alba has been opened along the length of the incision.

Alternatively, if the umbilical remnants are to be resected, the surgical site is prepared and draped, and a small elliptical skin incision is made around the umbilicus. Metzenbaum scissors and blunt dissection are used until the body wall surrounding the umbilicus is visualized. The author chooses to enter the abdomen just lateral to the umbilical sac. Once the abdomen has been entered, Metzenbaum scissors are used to excise the umbilical sac, taking care to isolate and double ligate the umbilical vein using 2-0 USP (3 M) absorbable suture material. The incision in the skin and linea alba can be extended craniad, taking care to avoid the remnants of the umbilical vein (the remainder of the umbilical remnant removal process is described below). If the cardiovascular status of the foal allows, the author removes the umbilicus during abdominal surgery.

The abdomen is closed in three layers. The linea alba is apposed using 1 USP (3.5 M) polyglactin 910 in a simple continuous suture pattern. A slightly larger size (2 USP [5 M]) may be required in larger foals. Other absorbable suture materials are considered appropriate. Some surgeons choose to place sutures in an interrupted inverted cruciate pattern. The subcutaneous tissues are apposed using 2-0 USP (2 M) absorbable suture material on a taper needle in a simple continuous pattern and the skin is apposed with 2-0 USP (2 M) poliglecaprone on a reverse cutting needle, taking care not to interfere with the linea alba sutures. A simple continuous, ford-interlocking suture pattern, or modified subcuticular pattern can be chosen, however, the author places a continuous horizontal mattress pattern in the skin, with the intention of not removing the sutures unless incisional complications occur.

The author performs an umbilical resection (Table 18.12) in neonatal foals undergoing exploratory celiotomy, providing the foal is stable and the additional surgical time to

Table 18.12 Surgical procedure for umbilical remnant resection.

- In dorsal recumbency, the umbilicus is oversewn/securely covered and clamped prior to skin preparation.
- Once the surgical site is prepared and draped, a small elliptical skin incision is made around the umbilicus.
- Metzenbaum scissors and blunt dissection are used until the body wall surrounding the umbilicus is visualized.
- The author enters the abdomen just lateral to the umbilical sac; however, a cranial approach, avoiding the umbilical vein can also be used. Once the abdomen has been safely entered, Metzenbaum scissors are used to excise the umbilical sac, taking care to isolate and double ligate the umbilical vein using 2-0 USP (3 M) absorbable multifilament suture material. The author uses polyglactin 910. The vein should be ligated proximal to any diseased portion. This may require extension of the ventral midline incision. Marsupialization of the vein may be required.
- The umbilical arteries are dissected free from the lateral ligaments of the bladder if this enables more accurate ligation. It is essential to preserve the lateral branches of the internal pudendal arteries supplying the bladder [112].
- The umbilical arteries are double ligated using 2-0 USP (3 M) absorbable multifilament suture material. Larger suture material may be needed where arterial abnormalities exist. The author uses polyglactin 910. The arteries should be ligated proximal to any diseased tissue. If the arteries are normal, they can be ligated at the level of the apex of the bladder. The most proximal arterial ligations can be used as stay sutures to maintain position of the bladder. Alternatively, stay sutures can be placed in the bladder itself.
- While maintaining the position of the stay sutures, the urachus is transected with Metzenbaum scissors.
- The site of urachal transection is closed with a double layer Cushing pattern using 2-0USP (3 M) absorbable suture material; the author uses poliglecaprone.
- The abdominal incision is closed routinely.
- The affected umbilical segments can be submitted for bacterial culture and antimicrobial susceptibility.

If the umbilical vein infection extends to the liver, resulting in an inability to ligate and remove the vein proximal to any diseased areas, the umbilical vein stump should be marsupialized.

- While the linea alba/umbilical incision is still open, a stab incision is made using a new No. 10 scalpel blade approximately 5 cm to the right of the linea alba. The stab incision should be made either at level of the cranial aspect of the incision or further cranial to allow as much of the affected vein as possible to be removed.
- The umbilical vein is freed from its attachments to the abdominal wall to allow it to be maneuvered.
- A large clamp is inserted through the stab incision and placed on the transected end of the umbilical vein to prevent abdominal contamination. The clamp and vein are withdrawn through the stab incision.
- Alternatively, the umbilical vein can be marsupialized at the cranial edge of the ventral midline incision.
- The umbilical vein is sutured to the skin in a simple interrupted pattern using an absorbable suture material. The author uses polyglactin 910 to avoid suture material cutting through the vein wall, however, multifilament suture material is not ideal for placement in the skin.
- The umbilical vein should protrude from the skin for 2–3 cm.
- The stoma will gradually heal by second intention. The site will typically heal after 14 days when the sutures can be removed. At 60 days, the body contour typically returns to normal, with no need to close the marsupialization site.

perform a cystoplasty is not detrimental. This allows any concurrent disease, such as patent urachus and/or umbilical remnant infection, to be treated at the same time as exploratory laparotomy. The prognosis for umbilical resections is good when infections are localized. Hepatic involvement or concurrent sepsis worsens the prognosis [24].

Postoperative Care

Incisional Care

A stent bandage can be sutured over the incision during the recovery period; alternatively, gauze swabs can be placed over the incision followed by an adhesive drape. Either option can be difficult to remove in more exuberant foals. An abdominal bandage can be placed but are prone to slippage and are frequently soiled from urine in colts [24]. It is essential to ensure abdominal bandages are not placed too tightly due to a risk of reducing thoracic expansion during respiration.

Abdominal Drain

In some circumstances, such as peritonitis or an abdominal abscess, an abdominal drain facilitates treatment; however, if the abdomen is thoroughly lavaged, this is rarely necessary [24]. Drains can be placed as follows:

- Prior to closing the linea alba, a stab incision is made at least 5 cm, but ideally further (depending on the size of the foal) from the linea alba. The stab incision should be located cranially, at the most dependent part of the abdomen when the foal is standing. If a drain is being placed for an abscess, the location of the abscess may dictate drain placement. The stab incision is placed through the skin and abdominal musculature. Some clinicians choose to offset the skin and muscle incisions

- A 20-26Fr chest drain is placed through the stab incision, with a hand inserted via the ventral midline incision to protect the viscera [24]. The trocar is removed when the drain enters the abdomen; the drain is positioned cranially in the abdomen. The author performs an omentectomy and places the end of the drain cranial to the liver to reduce the chances of the drain becoming blocked.
- 1USP (3.5 M) polypropylene or other nonabsorbable monofilament suture material is used to perform a purse-string suture in the skin around the drain, followed by a finger-trap suture to secure the drain.
- A Heimlich valve, or condom with an incision at the end is placed over the drain. The drain should be clamped closed during anesthetic recovery to prevent the recovery floor from becoming slippery due to the presence of peritoneal fluid.

Medications

Postoperatively, most foals receive broad-spectrum antimicrobials, NSAIDs, IV fluids, anti-ulcer medications, analgesics, and nutritional support. General guidelines are as follows, but may differ based on clinician preference [24]:

- Flunixin meglumine (0.25–1 mg/kg) IV BID for 3–5 days, possibly longer, depending on condition treated.
- Potassium penicillin G (22 000 IU/kg) IV QID for 3–5 days or longer, depending on the condition treated.
  - If IV penicillin is not available, ceftiofur (5–10 mg/kg) IV/IM BID is a viable alternative.
  - Amikacin is a possible alternative if available.
- Gentamicin sulfate (11–15 mg/kg if <2 weeks of age; 6.6 mg/kg if >2 weeks of age) IV SID for 3–5 days or longer, depending on the condition treated. Amikacin can be used instead of gentamicin.
- Isotonic polyionic IV fluids to correct dehydration:
  - Electrolyte abnormalities should be corrected.
  - Dextrose solution can be added as needed, especially if the foal has undergone gastric or small intestine surgery and nursing is temporarily withheld.
- Anti-ulcer medications, such as omeprazole (2–4 mg/kg PO q24h) and sucralfate (1–2 g per 50 kg foal BID-TID) should be considered during hospitalization or for longer periods in certain conditions [24].
- An IV lidocaine infusion (1.3 mg/kg over 15 minutes, followed by 0.05 mg/kg/min) can be considered in foals with small intestinal lesions, or foals that are anticipated to be uncomfortable postoperatively.
- IV nutrition is required in foals treated for conditions such as gastric outflow obstruction, where nursing is not permitted postoperatively (Chapter 58).

Feeding

As a general guide, foals with small intestinal or gastric lesions should only be allowed restricted nursing postoperatively. This may require separating the foal from the mare in the stall or placing a muzzle on the foal. The mare's udder can become sore if foals repeatedly try to nurse while wearing a muzzle. Nursing can be gradually increased when ultrasonographic examinations show improved small intestinal motility. Patients following a gastric bypass procedure require radiographic evaluation prior to a return to nursing. Foals with large intestine or other sources of abdominal discomfort are typically allowed to nurse immediately postoperatively with the majority of foals keen to nurse soon after surgery.

Stabling

Mares and foals should be confined to stall rest for up to 4 weeks postoperatively, depending on the length of the incision, number of surgical sites, presence of hernias preoperatively, and healing of the body wall. Hand walking should be performed 3–4 times daily during this time, providing the foal is not overexuberant. Foals are confined to small paddock rest with the mare for another 4–8 weeks after the period of stall rest. Normal turnout in a large paddock and with other horses should not occur until at least 2–3 months postoperatively, and the surgical sites should be considered healed with no evidence of discharge or herniation prior to turnout.

Long-Term Prognosis Following Surgical Intervention

For foals undergoing exploratory laparotomy, the likelihood of future athletic performance should be considered. In a report on exploratory laparotomy in Thoroughbred foals, 75% of foals that survived to discharge went on to race [121]. If more than 1 colic surgery is necessary, the prognosis for racing is reduced to 25%, however, all foals were considered in this calculation [121]. Moreover, 78% of horses with nonstrangulating lesions went on to race, whereas only 14% of those with strangulating lesions began a racing career [121]. Interestingly, once a racing career had commenced, there was no difference in racing career length or earnings between those that had undergone exploratory laparotomy as a foal and control subjects.

Adhesions

Adhesion formation following exploratory laparotomy is common in all equids (Figure 18.20), but neonates <30 days old are particularly prone to forming

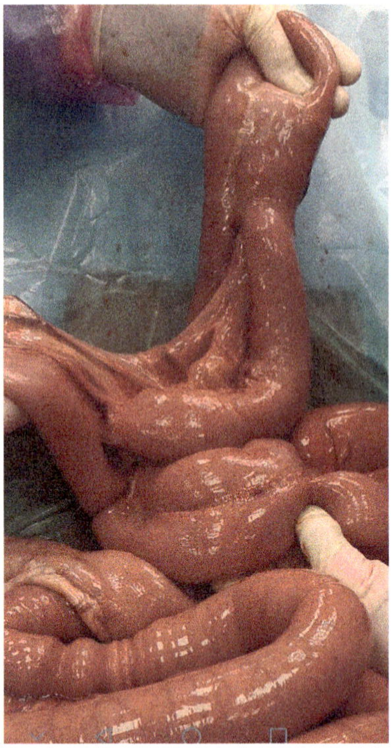

Figure 18.20 Multiple adhesions of the small intestine of a foal.

adhesions [122, 123]. In one study, 33% of foals that were evaluated postoperatively developed adhesions [2]. In this case series, only 48% of foals showed clinical signs associated with adhesions, the remainder were considered subclinical.

Much research effort has been placed on methods to minimize the likelihood of development of intra-abdominal adhesions in foals.

These techniques include:

- Prompt intervention in any case of suspected intestinal strangulation
- Strict adherence to Halsted's principles and ensuring copious lavage of the bowel [27, 31]
- Performing an omentectomy
- Intraperitoneal carboxymethylcellulose has shown promise in adults [124] and foals [1].

When adhesions are encountered intra-operatively, the prognosis is poor, with survival rates ranging from 0 to 20% [23, 121, 122]. Adhesions can be gently separated with those detected early being easier to separate; however, the author's opinion is that they are no less likely to reoccur than adhesions that are more established. Some clinicians advocate complete resection of the affected segment of bowel to ensure complete removal of the adhesions. Unfortunately, although breakdown of adhesions and supportive therapy postoperatively can be attempted, the owners should be advised of a poor to guarded prognosis if repeat celiotomy is required due to the presence of adhesions. Despite this, occasional successful cases with survival to discharge and commencement of race training have been documented [121].

References

1 MacKinnon, M.C., Southwood, L.L., Burke, M.J. et al. (2013). Colic in equine neonates: 137 cases (2000–2010). *J. Am. Vet. Med. Assoc.* 253: 1586–1595.

2 Cable, C.S. (2002). Clinical evaluation of the foal. In: *Manual of Equine Gastroenterology* (ed. T. Mair, T. Divers, and N. Ducharme), 449–462. London: Saunders, Elsevier.

3 Furr, M. (2017). Diagnosis of colic in the foal. In: *The Equine Acute Abdomen*, 3e (ed. A.T. Blikslager, N.A. White II, J.N. Moore, and T.S. Mair). New Jersey, USA: Wiley.

4 Tulleners, E.P. (1983). Complications of abdominocentesis in the horse. *J. Vet. Med. Assoc.* 182: 232–234.

5 Neal, H.N. (2003). Foal colic: practical imaging of the abdomen. *Equine Vet. Educ.* 15: 263–270.

6 Porter, M.B. and Ramierez, S. (2005). Equine neonatal thoracic and abdominal ultrasonography. *Vet. Clin. Equine* 21: 407–429.

7 Reef, V.B. (1998). *Equine Diagnostic Ultrasound*. Philadelphia: Saunders.

8 Reimer, J.M. and Bernard, W.V. (1998). *Abdominal Sonography of the Foal*. Baltmore, MD: Williams & Wilkins.

9 Romero, A.E. and Rodgerson, D.H. (2010). Diaphragatic herniation in the horse: 31 cases (2001–2006). *Can. Vet. J.* 51: 1247–1250.

10 Campbell, M.L., Ackerman, N., and Peyton, L.C. (1984). Radiographic gastrointestinal anatomy of the foal. *Vet. Radiol. Ultrasound* 25: 194–204.

11 Barba, M. and Lepage, O.M. (2013). Diagnostic utility of computed tomography imaging in foals: 10 cases (2008–2010). *Equine Vet. Educ.* 25: 29–38.

12 Lascola, K.M., O'Brien, R.T., Wilking, P.A. et al. (2013). Qualitative and quantitative interpretation of computed tomography of the lungs in healthy neonatal foals. *Am. J. Vet. Res.* 74: 1239–1246.

13 Wilson, J.H. (1986). Gastric and duodenal ulcers in foals: a retrospective study. In: *Proceedings of the Second Equine Colic Rsearch Symposium*, 126–129. Athens, GA: Center for Continuing Education.

14 Murray, M.J., Murry, C.M., Sweeney, H.J. et al. (1990). Prevalence of gastric lesions in foals without signs of gastric disease: an endoscopic survey. *Equine Vet. J.* 22: 6–8.

15 Murray, M.J. (2002). Stomach diseases of the foal. In: *Manual of Equine Gastroenterology* (ed. T. Mair, T. Divers, and N. Ducharme), 449–462. London: Saunders, Elsevier.

16 Camacho-Luna, P., Buchanan, B., and Andrews, F.M. (2018). Advances in diagnostics and treatment in horses and foals with gastric and duodenal ulcers. *Vet. Clin. North Am. Equine Pract.* 34: 97–111.

17 Hewetson, M., Venner, M., Volquardsen, J. et al. (2018). Diagnostic accuracy of blood sucrose as a screen test for equine gastric ulcers syndrome (EGUS) in weanling foals. *Acta Vet. Scand.* 60: https://doi.org/10.1186/s13028-018-0377-5.

18 Furr, M., Cohen, N.D., Axon, J.E. et al. (2012). Treatment with histamine-type 2 receptor antagonists and omeprazole increase the risk of diarrhea in neonatal foals treated in intensive care units. *Equine Vet. J. Suppl.* 41: 80–86.

19 Blikslager, A.T. and Wilson, D.A. (2018). Stomach and duodenum. In: *Equine Surgery*, 5e (ed. J.A. Auer, J.A. Stick, J. Kummerle, and T. Prange). Missouri: Elsevier.

20 Loynacham, A.T. (2014). Esophageal cyst in the duodenum of a foal. *J. Vet. Diagn. Invest.* 26: 308–311.

21 Caston, S.S. and Fales-Williams, J.A. (2013). Primary malignant melanoma in the esophagus of a foal. *Equine Vet. Educ.* 22: 387–390.

22 Barth, A.D., Barber, S.M., and McKenzie, N.T. (1980). Pyloric stenosis in a foal. *Can. Vet. J.* 21: 234–246.

23 Mueller, E. (2004). Advances in prevention and treatment of intra-abdominal adhesions in horses. *Clin. Tech. Equine Pract.* 1: 163–173.

24 Khatibzadeh, S.M. and Brown, J.A. (2017). Surgical management of colic in the foal. In: *The Equine Acute Abdomen*, 3e (ed. A.T. Blikslager, N.A. White, J.N. Moore, and T.S. Mari). New Jersey, USA: Wiley.

25 Sprayberry, K.A. (2003). Gastric outflow obstruction in young horses. In: *Current Therapy in Equine Medicine*, 5e (ed. N.E. Robinson), 101–103. Philadelphia: Saunders.

26 Aronoff, N., Keegan, J.G., Johnson, P.J. et al. (1997). Management of pyloric obstruction in a foal. *J. Am. Vet. Med. Assoc.* 210: 902–905.

27 Freeman, D. (2018). Small intestine. In: *Equine Surgery*, 5e (ed. J.A. Auer, J.A. Stick, J. Kummerle, and T. Prange). Missouri: Elsevier.

28 Kent, A.V., Slone, D.E., Clark, K.E. et al. (2020). Heineke-Mikulicz pyloroplasty for the treatment of pyloric stenosis secondary to gastroduodenal ulceration. *Equine Vet. Educ.* 32: 540–544.

29 Orsini, J.A. and Donawick, W.J. (1986). Surgical treatment of gastroduodenal obstructions in foals. *Vet. Surg.* 15: 205–231.

30 Zedler, S.T., Embertson, R.M., Bernard, W.V. et al. (2009). Surgical treatment of gastric outflow obstruction in 40 foals. *Vet. Surg.* 38: 623–630.

31 Bryant, J. and Gaughan, E. (2005). Abdominal surgery in neonatal foals. *Vet. Clin. North Am. Equine Pract.* 21: 511–535.

32 Furr, M. (2017). Specific diseases of the foal. In: *The Equine Acute Abdomen*, 3e (ed. A.T. Blikslager, N.A. White, J.N. Moor, and T.S. Mair). Hoboken, NJ: Wiley.

33 Bartmann, C.P., Glitz, F., von Oppen, T. et al. (2001). Diagnosis and surgical management of colic in the foal. *Pferdejeilkunde* 17: 676–680.

34 Sprinkle, T.P., Swerczel, T.W., and Crowe, M.W. (1984). Meckel's diverticulum in the horse. *J. Equine Vet. Sci.* 4: 175–176.

35 Hooper, R.N. (1989). Small intestinal strangulation caused by Meckel's diverticulum in a horse. *J. Am. Vet. Med. Assoc.* 194: 943–944.

36 Freeman, D.E., Koch, D.B., and Boles, C.L. (1979). Mesodiverticular bands as a cause of small intestinal strangulation and volvulus in the horse. *J. Am. Vet. Med. Assoc.* 175: 1089–1094.

37 Verwildgen, D.R., van Galen, G., Busoni, V. et al. (2010). Meckel's diverticulum as a cause of colic: 2 foals with different morphological features. *Tildschrift voor diergeneeskunde* 135: 452–455.

38 Barakzai, S.Z., Swain, J.M., Else, R.W. et al. (2003). Two cases of small intestinal strangulation involving Mechel's diverticula. *Equine Vet. Educ.* 15: 291–294.

39 Edwards, G.B. (2004). Congenital abnormalities of the equine gastrointestinal tract. *Equine Vet. Educ.* 16: 119.

40 Abutarbush, S.M., Shoemaker, R.W., and Bailey, J.V. (2003). Strangulation of the small intestines by a mesodiverticular band in 3 adult horses. *Can. Vet. J.* 44: 1005–1006.

41 Orsini, J.A. (2002). Small intestinal diseases associated with colic in the foal. In: *Manual of Equine Gastroenterology* (ed. T. Mair, T. Divers, and N. Ducharme), 449–462. London: Saunders, Elsevier.

42 Edwards, G.B., Scholes, S.R., Edwards, S.E.R. et al. (1994). Colic in four neonatal foals associated with chyloperitoneum and congenital segmental lymphatic aplasia. *Proceedings of the fifth equine colic research symposium*, Athens, GA, 35 September 6–28th, 1994. Athens, Georgia USA.

43 Cesar, F.B., Johnson, C.R., and Pantaleon, L.G. (2010). Suspected idiopathic intestinal lymphangiectasia in two foals with chylous peritoneal effusion. *Equine Vet. Educ.* 22: 172–178.

44 May, K.A. and Good, M.J. (2007). Congenital lymphangiectasia and chyloabdomen in a foal. *Equine Vet. Educ.* 19: 16–18.
45 Orsini, J.A. (1997). Abdominal surgery in foals. *Vet. Clin. N. Am. Equine Pract.* 13: 393–413.
46 Vatistas, N.J., Snyder, J.R., Wilson, W.D. et al. (1996). Surgical treatment for colic in the foal (67 cases): 1980–1992. *Equine Vet. J.* 28: 139–145.
47 Stephen, J.O., Corley, K.T.T., Johnson, J.K. et al. (2004). Small intestinal volvulus in 115 horses: 1988–2000. *Vet. Surg.* 33: 333–339.
48 Southwood, L.L. (2009). Colic surgery in the equine neonate: not your typical cause of colic and are we doing better with treatment? *Equine Vet. Educ.* 20: 513–515.
49 Southwood, L.L., Ragle, C.A., and Snyder, J.R. (1996). Surgical treatment of ascarid impactions in horses and foals. *Proc. Am. Assoc. Equine Pract.* 42: 258–261.
50 Tatz, A.J., Segev, G., and Steinmen, A. (2012). Surgical treatment for acute small intestinal obstruction caused by Parascaris Equorum infection in 15 horses (2002–2011). *Equine Vet. J. Suppl.* 43: 111–144.
51 Arroyo, L.G., Quesada, R.J., and Medina-Torres, C.E. (2011). What is your diagnosis? *J. Am. Vet. Med. Assoc.* 239: 435–436.
52 Nielsen, M.K. and Donoghue, E.M. (2016). An ultrasonographic scoring method for transabdominal monitoring of ascarid burdens in foals. *Equine Vet. J.* 48: 380–386.
53 Southwood, L.L., Baxter, G.M., and Bennet, D.G. (1998). Ascarid impaction in young horses. *Compend. Contin. Educ. Pract. Vet.* 20: 100–106.
54 Davis, H.A. and Munsterman, A. (2012). Ileal impaction and jejunal enterotomy in a 4-month-old Arabian filly. *Can. Vet. J.* 53 (1): 71–74.
55 Cribb, N.C., Cote, N.M., and Boure, L.P. (2006). Acute small intestinal obstruction associated with Parascaris equorum infection in young horses: 25 cases (1985–2004). *N. Z. Vet. J.* 54: 338–343.
56 Blikslager, A.T. (2019). Colic prevention to avoid colic surgery: a surgeon's perspective. *J. Equine Vet. Sci.* 76: 1–5.
57 Abraham, M., Reef, V.B., and Sweeney, R.W. (2014). Gastrointestinal ultrasonography of normal Standardbred neonates and frequency of asymptomatic intussusceptions. *J. Vet. Intern. Med.* 28: 1580–1586.
58 Edwards, G.B. (1986). Surgical management of intussusception in the horse. *Equine Vet. J.* 18: 313–321.
59 Ford, T.S., Freeman, D.E., and Ross, M.W. (1990). Ileocecal intussusception in horses: 26 cases (1981–1988). *J. Am. Vet. Med. Assoc.* 196: 121–126.
60 Bernard, W.V., Reef, V.B., and Reimer, J.M. (1989). Ultrasonographic diagnosis of small-intestinal intussusception in three foals. *J. Am. Vet. Med. Assoc.* 194: 385–397.
61 Greet, T.R.C. (1992). Ileal intussusception in 16 young thoroughbreds. *Equine Vet. J.* 24: 81–83.
62 Homey, E.D. and Funk, K.A. (1971). Ileal myotomy in the horse. *Mod. Vet. Pract.* 52: 49–50.
63 Beard, W. (1998). Nonreducible intussusception. In: *Current Techniques in Equine Surgery and Lameness 2nd* (ed. N.A. While and J.N. Moore), 280–282. Philadelphia: Saunders.
64 Beard, W., Bryne, B.A., and Henninger, R.W. (1992). Ileocecal intussusception corrected by resection within the cecum in two horses. *J. Am. Vet. Med. Assoc.* 200: 1978–1980.
65 Proudman, C.J. (2003). Intestinal tapeworm infestation. In: *Current Therapy in Equine Medicine*, 5e (ed. N.E. Robinson), 158–160. Philadelphia: Saunders.
66 Mejia, S., Hurcombe, S., Rodgerson, D. et al. (2019). Retrograde intussusception of the descending colon secondary to multiple colonic hamartomas in a neonatal foal. *Equine Vet. Educ.* 33: e12–e16.
67 Shaw, S., Arroyo, L., zur Linden, A. et al. (2020). Medical management of a large intra-abdominal mass caused by *Rhodococcus equi* in a foal. *Equine Vet. Educ.* 33: 477–481.
68 Freeman, D.E. (1997). Surgery of the small intestine. *Vet. Clin. North Am. Equine Pract.* 13: 261–301.
69 White, M.R., Crowell, W.A., and Guy, B.L. (1988). Cecocolic intussusception in a foal with Eimeria leukarti infection. *Equine Pract.* 10: 15–18.
70 Sherlock, C. (2018). Caecum. In: *Equine Surgery*, 5e (ed. J.A. Auer, J.A. Stick, J. Kummerle, and T. Prange). Missouri: Elsevier.
71 Boussauw, B.H., Domingo, R., Wilderjans, H. et al. (2001). Treatment of irreducible cecocolic intussusception in horses by jejuno(ileo)colostomy. *Vet. Rec.* 149: 16–18.
72 Martin, B.B., Freeman, D.E., Ross, M.W. et al. (1999). Cecocolic and cecocecal intussusception in horses: 30 cass (1976–1996). *J. Am. Vet. Med. Assoc.* 214: 80–84.
73 Plummer, A.E., Rakestraw, P.C., Hardy, J. et al. (2007). Outcome of medical and surgical treatment of cecal impaction in horses: 114 cases (1994–2004). *J. Am. Vet. Med. Assoc.* 231: 1378–1385.
74 Aitken, M.R., Southwood, L.L., Ross, B.W. et al. (2015). Outcome of surgical and medical management of cecal impaction in 150 horses (1991–2011). *Vet. Surg.* 44: 540–546.
75 Tabar, J.J. and Cruz, A.T. (2009). Cecal rupture in foals – 7 cases (1996–2006). *Can. Vet. J.* 50: 65–70.
76 Edwards, J.F. and Ruoff, W.W. (1991). Idiopathic cecal rupture in foals after anesthesia for gastric endoscopy. *J. Am. Vet. Med. Assoc.* 198: 1421–1422.
77 Bernard, W.V. (2002). Large and small colon diseases associated with colic in the foal. In: *Manual of Equine Gastroenterology* (ed. T. Mair, T. Divers, and N. Ducharme). London: Saunders, Elsevier.

78 Nappert, G., Laverty, S., Drolet, R. et al. (1992). Atresia coli in 7 foals (1964–1990). *Equine Vet. J. Suppl.* 13: 57–60.

79 Santschi, E.M. (2004). Rectum and anus. In: *Manual of Equine Gastroenterology* (ed. T. Mair, T. Divers, and N. Ducharme), 491–492. Edinburgh: Saunders.

80 Young, R.L., Lindford, R.L., and Olander, H.J. (1992). Atresia-coli in the foal: a review of 6 cases. *Equine Vet. J.* 24: 60–62.

81 Cho, D. (1986). Blind-end atresia colic in two foals. *Cornell Vet.* 76: 11–15.

82 Skov Hansen, S., Mattei, C., Treffenbery, H. et al. (2020). Successful outcome after surgical correction of large colon atresia in a colt foal. *Equine Vet. Educ.* 33: 433–437.

83 McPherson, A.G., Trapnell, J.E., and Arith, G.R. (1969). Duplication of the colon. *Br. J. Surg.* 56: 138–142.

84 Southwood, L.L. (2018). Large colon. In: *Equine Surgery*, 5e (ed. J.A. Auer, J.A. Stick, J. Kummerle, and T. Prange), 591–621.

85 Trope, G.D. and Steel, C.M. (2010). T-shaped malformation of the ventral colon in a Thoroughbred filly with colic. *Aust. Vet. J.* 88: 322–325.

86 Koenig, J.B., Rodriguez, A., Colquhoun, J.K. et al. (2007). Congenital colon malformation ("short colon") in a 4-month-old Standardbred foal. *Can. Vet. J.* 48: 420–422.

87 Steenhaut, M., van Huffel, X., and Gasthuys, F. (1991). Agenesis of the mesocolon causing colic in a foal. *Vet. Rec.* 129: 54–55.

88 Hennessy, S.E. and Fraser, B.S.L. (2012). Right dorsal displacement of the large colon as a cause of surgical colic in three foals in New Zealand. *N. Z. Vet. J.* https://doi.org/10.1080/00480169.2012.694406.

89 Du Preez, S., Trope, G.D., Owens, C. et al. (2018). Volvulus of the large colon in a neonatal foal. *Equine Vet. Educ.* 30: 306–311.

90 Adams, R., Koterba, A.M., Brown, M.P. et al. (1988). Exploratory celiotomy for gastrointestinal disease in neonatal foals: a review of 20 cases. *Equine Vet. J.* 20: 9–12.

91 Lillich, J.D., Goggin, J.M., Valentino, L.W. et al. (2000). Volvulus of the large colon in a foal. *Equine Vet. Educ.* 12: 18–19.

92 McClure, J.T., Kobulk, C., Volter, K. et al. (1992). Fecalith impaction in four Miniature foals. *J. Am. Vet. Med. Assoc.* 200: 205–207.

93 Haupt, J.L., McAndrews, A.G., Chaney, K.P. et al. (2008). Surgical treatment of colic in the Miniature Horse: a retrospective study of 57 cases (1993–2006). *Equine Vet. J.* 40: 364–367.

94 Dart, A.J., Snyder, J.R., Pascoe, J.R. et al. (1992). Abnormal conditions of the equine descending (small) colon: 102 cases (1979–1989). *J. Am. Vet. Med. Assoc.* 200: 971–978.

95 Prange, T. (2013). Small colon obstructions in foals. *Equine Vet. Educ.* 25: 293–296.

96 Baker, G., Hyppa, T., and Wilson, D.A. (1987). Covered anus with anobulbar fistula in an Arabian foal. *Vet. Surg.* 16: 82.

97 Manuka, A., Virami, N., Kurrupusamy, S. et al. (2011). Rectal prolapse and enteritis in a foal. *Online J. Vet. Res.* 15: 462–467.

98 Enzerink, E., van Weeren, P.R., and van der Velden, M.A. (2000). Closure of the abdominal wall at the umbilicus and the development of umbilical hernias in a group of foals from birth to 11 months of age. *Vet. Rec.* 147: 37–39.

99 Freeman, D.E. and Spencer, P.A. (1991). Evaluation of age, breed and gender as risk factors for umbilical hernia in horses of a hospital population. *Am. J. Vet. Res.* 52: 637–639.

100 Toth, F. and Schumacher, J. (2018). Abdominal hernias. In: *Equine Surgery* (ed. J.A. Auer, J.A. Stick, J. Kummerle, and T. Prange), 645–659. Missouri: Elsevier.

101 Rijkenhuizen, A., Van der Velden, M., and Back, W. (1997). Incarcerated umbilical hernia and enterocutaneous fistulae in two foals. *Equine Vet. Educ.* 9: 3–6.

102 Blikslager, A.T. (2010). Ischemic disorders of the intestinal tract. In: *Equine Internal Medicine*, 3e (ed. S.M. Reed, W.M. Bayly, and D.C. Sellon), 876–882. St Louis: Saunders, Elsevier.

103 Rubio-Martinez, L.M. (2015). Diaphragmatic hernias in horses. *Equine Vet. Educ.* 27: 396–397.

104 Tapio, H., Hewetson, M., and Sihvo, H.K. (2012). An unusual cause of colic in a neonatal foal. *Equine Vet. Educ.* 24: 334–339.

105 Palmer, J.E. (2012). Colic and diaphragmatic hernias in neonatal foals. *Equine Vet. Educ.* 27: 340–342.

106 Rocken, M., Mosel, G., and Barske, K. (2013). Thoracoscopic diaphragmatic hernia repair in a warmblood mare. *Vet. Surg.* 42: 591–594.

107 Clutton, R.E., Boyd, C., and Richards, D.L. (1992). Anesthetic problems caused by diaphragmatic hernia in the horse: a review of four cases. *Equine Vet. J. Suppl.* 11: 30–33.

108 Hart, S.K. and Brown, J.A. (2009). Diaphragmatic hernia in horses: 44 cases (1986–2006). *J. Vet. Emerg. Crit. Care* 19: 357–362.

109 Dubs, B. (1976). Megavisica due ot the absence of an urachus in a newborn foal. *Schweiz Arch. Teirheilkd* 18: 393–395.

110 Toth, T., Liman, J., Larsdotter, S. et al. (2012). Megavesica in a neonatal foal. *Equine Vet. Educ.* 24: 396–403.

111 Adams, R., Koterba, A.M., Cudd, T.A. et al. (1988). Exploratory celiotomy for suspected urinary tract disruption in neonatal foals: a review of 18 cases. *Equine Vet. J.* 20: 13–17.

112 Rossdale, P.D. and Greet, T.R.C. (1989). Megavesica in a newborn foal. *Int. Soc. Vet. Perinatol. Newsl.* 2: 10.

113 Schott, H.C. and Woodie, J.B. (2018). Bladder. In: *Equine Surgery*, 5e (ed. J.A. Auer, J.A. Stick, J. Kummerle, and T. Prange), 1129–1145.

114 Kablack, K.A., Embertson, R.M., and Bernard, W. (2000). Uroperitoneum in the hospitalized equine neonate: retrospective study of 31 cases (1988–1977). *Equine Vet. J.* 32: 505–508.

115 Dunkel, B., Palmer, J.E., Olson, K.N. et al. (2005). Uroperitoneum in 32 foals: influence of intravenous fluid therapy, infection and sepsis. *J. Vet. Intern. Med.* 19: 889–893.

116 Valk, N., Dawis, E.W., and Blackford, J.T. (1998). Ovarian torsion as a cause of colic in a neonatal foal. *J. Am. Vet. Med. Assoc.* 213: 1454–1456.

117 Bartmann, C.P., Glitz, F., Lorber, K. et al. (2000). Colic associated with ovarian torsion in a neonatal foal. *Tierarztl. Prax.* 28: 57–59.

118 Green, S.L., Sprecht, T.E., and Dowling, S.C. (1988). Hemoperitoneum caused by rupture of a juvenile granulosa cell tumor in an equine neonate. *J. Am. Vet. Med. Assoc.* 193: 1417–1419.

119 Evard, J.H., Fischer, A.T., and Greenwood, L.D. (1988). Ovarian strangulation as a cause of small colon obstruction in a foal. *Equine Vet. J.* 20: 217–218.

120 Garcia-Seeber, F., McAuliffe, S.B., McGovern, F. et al. (2008). Splenic rupture and splenectomy in a foal. *Equine Vet. Educ.* 20: 367–370.

121 Santschi, E.M. (2000). Colic surgery in 206 juvenile thoroughbreds: survival and racing results. *Equine Vet. J. Suppl.* 32: 32–36.

122 Watts, A. (2001). Comparisons of plasma and peritoneal indices of fibrinolysis between foals and adult horses with or without colic. *J. Am. Vet. Med. Assoc.* 72: 1535–1540.

123 Baxter, G., Broome, T., and Moore, J. (1989). Abdominal adhesions after small intestinal surgery in the horse. *Vet. Surg.* 18: 409–414.

124 Munsterman, A., Kottwitz, J., and Hanson, R. (2016). Meta-analysis of the effects of adhesion barriers on adhesion formation in the horse. *Vet. Surg.* 45: 587–595.

Chapter 19 Hepatobiliary Diseases

Krista Estell

Liver disease in foals may be due to a primary hepatic insult or occur secondary to other disease processes. Clinical signs of liver disease may be subtle initially, and difficult to differentiate from other comorbidities such as sepsis or neonatal encephalopathy. A serum biochemical analysis that includes analytes that evaluate the liver should be performed for neonates presenting with critical illness, particularly those that have icterus or fail to respond to initial medical therapy. Age-specific reference intervals should be used for foals when interpreting the serum biochemistry profile as healthy neonatal foals have higher concentrations of ϒ-glutamyltransferase (GGT), bile acids, bilirubin, and triglycerides compared to adult horses (Table 19.1). Normal reference intervals for ammonia have not been established in neonatal foals, but previous reports suggest a range between 7 and 63 μmol/l [3–7].

Congenital Liver Anomalies

Congenital liver anomalies occur infrequently in foals as compared to other domestic species [8]. Clinical signs of congenital hepatic disease in foals include icterus, failure to thrive, lethargy, encephalopathy, and yellow or pale-colored feces. Clinicopathologic derangements are specific to the type of hepatic disease present, and in some instances, liver enzyme activity may be normal or only slightly elevated. Severe liver disease should be suspected if liver function tests are abnormal, or if hyperammonemic encephalopathy is present. Hyperammonemia and elevated bile acids are fairly specific indicators of hepatic dysfunction, and if present warrant further investigation. Documented congenital liver anomalies in foals include portosystemic shunt (PSS), biliary atresia, congenital hepatic fibrosis (CHF), and hepatic tumors.

Portosystemic Shunt

PSS, an anomalous communication between the portal venous circulation and systemic circulation that bypasses the liver, has been reported in the equine literature in various case reports (Table 19.2). The majority of PSS documented in foals are extrahepatic, though an intrahepatic shunt has also been reported (Figure 19.1) [3, 10]. The higher incidence of extrahepatic PSS in the equid may relate to the fact that most intrahepatic PSS stem from defective closure of the embryonic ductus venosus (which the equine fetus does not have) as compared to extrahepatic PSS, which connect the splanchnic vascular system with the vena cava or azygous vein [11–13]. Other intrahepatic PSS communications occur between the portal vein and hepatic vein or caudal vena cava [6]. Extrahepatic shunts are an abnormal functional vascular communication between the embryonic vitelline veins (which form the entire extrahepatic portal system) and the cardinal venous system (which contributes to all nonportal abdominal veins) [11]. This results in a shunting vessel between the portal vein or its contributors (e.g. left gastric, splenic, mesenteric, or gastroduodenal vein) and the caudal vena cava or azygous vein.

In health, the abdominal organs are connected to the splanchnic vascular bed (gastrointestinal tract, pancreas, spleen) and supply efflux blood to the portal vein. The portal vein then delivers blood that contains nutrients, toxins, and bacteria absorbed from the intestine to the liver. In horses with PSS, blood bypasses the liver and normal hepatic function and toxins and metabolites such as ammonia, aromatic amino acids, absorbed bacteria, and endotoxins distribute to the systemic circulation [11]. This anomalous circulation results in abnormal clinical features in foals, including small or unthrifty stature, lethargy, variable signs

Equine Neonatal Medicine, First Edition. Edited by David M. Wong and Pamela A. Wilkins.

Table 19.1 Foal and adult serum enzyme activity and organic molecule concentrations associated with the liver [1, 2].

Age	ALP	GGT	SDH	AST	ALT	Total bilirubin	Conj. bilirubin	Unconj. bilirubin	Cholesterol	Triglyceride	Bile acids
<12 h	152–2835	13–39	0.2–4.8	97–315	0–47	0.9–2.8	0.3–0.6	0.8–2.5	111–432	24–88	21.7–81.7
Days											
1	861–2671	18–43	0.6–4.6	146–340	0–49	1.3–4.5	0.3–0.7	1.0–3.8	110–562	30–193	26.0–74.3[a]
3	283–1462	9–40	0.6–3.7	80–580	0–52	0.5–3.9	0.2–0.8	0.2–3.3	142–350	63–342	
5	156–1294	8–89	0.8–5.3	–	–	1.2–3.6	0.1–0.7	0.8–2.8	127–361	52–340	
7	137–1169	14–164	0.8–5.2	237–620	4–50	0.8–3.0	0.3–0.7	0.5–2.3	139–445	30–239	16.7–29.4
14	182–859	16–169	0.6–4.3	240–540	1–9	0.7–2.2	0.3–0.6	0.5–1.6	164–287	39–200	11.3–30.6
21	146–752	16–132	1.0–8.4	226–540	0–45	0.5–1.6	0.2–0.5	0.2–1.1	74–276	34–124	7.2–18.4
28	210–866	17–99	1.2–5.9	252–440	5–47	0.5–1.7	0.1–0.6	0.4–1.2	83–233	45–155	9.0–17.1
Months											
2	201–741	8–38	1.1–4.6	282–484	7–57	0.5–2.0	0.2–0.5	0.3–1.5	98–242	10–148	
3	206–458	0–27	1.1–3.9	282–480	8–65	0.4–2.0	0.1–0.7	0.4–1.4	110–226	28–151	
4	124–222	0–27	1.5–4.4	280–520	8–65	0.3–1.0	0.1–0.6	0.2–0.4	91–207	14–148	
5	105–239	0–30	1.3–4.8	225–420	0–65	0.3–1.8	0.1–0.7	0.1–1.1	51–137	14–57	
6	155–226	0–26	0.3–3.3	300–620	7–20	0.3–1.3	0.1–0.7	0.1–0.6	83–173	35–76	
9	158–232	0–26	0.3–3.3	246–728	4–27	0.3–1.1	0.1–0.7	0.2–0.6	11–187	38–86	
12	–	–	–	283–720	5–20	0.4–1.4	0.1–1.0	0.2–0.6	–	–	
Adult	64–214	5–28	0.5–3.0	149–267	4–10	0.5–1.8	0.2–0.7	0.3–1.0	58–109	6–44	4–11.5
Units	IU/l	IU/l	IU/l	IU/l	IU/l	mg/dl	mg/dl	mg/dl	mg/dl	mg/dl	μmol/l

ALP-Alkaline phosphatase; GGT-Gamma-glutamyl transferase; SDH-Sorbitol dehydrogenase; AST-Aspartate transaminase; ALT-Alaine transaminase; Conj-Conjugated; Uncong-Unconjugated.
[a] 2-day-old foal.

Table 19.2 Reported cases of portosystemic shunts in foals.

Signalment	Clinical signs	Laboratory values	Imaging findings	Treatment and outcome
5-wk-old Belgian colt [4]	Episodic disorientation, recumbency, thrashing, nonresponsive to auditory stimuli, apparently blind, throws head and lunge violently	• Blood ammonia 380 µmol/L (control 40) • Total bile acids 86 µmol/L(< 20) • Total bilirubin 12.0 mg/dL (0.3-3.5) • GGT 21 U/L (10–59) • BUN 42 mg/dL (10–27) • Hypoglycemia 20 md/d	• US: large vessel appeared to communicate with caudal vena cava • Pos. Contrast portography: intrahepatic portocaval shunt outlined by contrast agent flowing from portal vein to caudal vena cava without parenchymal perfusion	• Surgery: shunt ligated with suture • Shunt ligation loosened within 16 d; religation unsuccessful; foal euthanized
8-wk-old Dutch Warmblood colt [7]	Episodic apathy and ataxia, gnashing, circling, apparently blind, depression, hypermetria alternated with dysmetria of all four limbs, bilateral horizontal nystagmus, ptosis, variable menace reflex	• Blood ammonia 117 µmol/L (11–55) • Total bile acids 53 µmol/L (1–8.6) • Unconjugated bilirubin 168 mol/L (<35)	• CT angiography: abnormal vessel identified looping from portal vein to caudal vena cava. Abnormal vessel looped to left and caudally, entering left side of caudal vena cava, cranial to left renal vein. Length of shunt approx. 5 cm.	• Surgery: shunt ligation planned, but surgical complication resulted in euthanasia
6-mo-old Quarter Horse filly [5]	Severe depression, ataxia, blindness, small stature, circling, head tilt, facial nerve paresis	• Increased GGT • Total bilirubin 2.8 mg/dL • Blood ammonia 176 µg/dL (<108) • Bile acids 51.7 µmol/L	• Nuclear hepatic scintigraphy: decreased portal circulation - Intra-operative mesenteric portography: extrahepatic shunt, multiple vascular communications between cranial mesenteric and portal veins to azygous vein	• Foal euthanized
5-mo-old Belgian filly [4]	Small for breed and age, clumsiness, acutely blind, head pressing, circling, staggering, dragging of feet, small for age	• Blood ammonia 179 µmol/L (control 21 µmol/L) • Total bile acids 83 µmol/L (< 20) • Total bilirubin 1.7 mg/dL (0.3–3.5) • GGT 29 U/L (1059) • BUN 11 mg/dL (1027)	• Pos. Contrast Portography: large portocaval shunt delineated by contrast agent. No filling of portal veins within the liver was observed	• Surgery: shunt ligated with suture • Clinical improvement. • Persistent increased blood ammonia (100 µmol/L), bile acids (24 µmol/L). Foal remained healthy, no recurrence of signs for2 yr after ligation

(Continued)

Table 19.2 (Continued)

Signalment	Clinical signs	Laboratory values	Imaging findings	Treatment and outcome
9-wk-old Arab mix filly [6]	Intermittent episodes circling, incoordination, absence of menace reflex, apparent blindness, inability to nurse, lethargy, unresponsive, ptyalism, bruxism noted soon after birth. Further signs were apathy, circling, ataxia, hypermetric gait (forelimbs), high head carriage	• Blood ammonia 208 μmol/L (<50) • Total bilirubin 4.8mg/dL (0.52.3) • Lactate 3.7 mmol/L (<2)	• CT angiography: abnormal vessel originated from intrahepatic portion of portal vein, entering most ventral aspect of caudal vena cava, just caudal to diaphragm • Echocardiography with transsplenic injection of agitated saline: immediate contrast in right atrium and ventricle -Intra-operative ultrasound: see Figure 19.2	• Surgery: shunt ligated with cellophane • Clinical improvement within 22 d; • 6 wks after surgery: • Blood ammonia mildly increased (54 μmol/l), bile acid normal (5 μmol/l) • Foal bright alert at 7 months postsurgery
5-wk-old Miniature Horse filly [3]	Hypersalivation, trismus, poor appetite, hyper-aesthesia, aimless wandering, blindness. Developed generalized pruritis, head-pressing, marked ataxia, hind-limb stiffness, hypermetria, disorientation, difficulties locating dam, no menace reflex, absent pupillary light reflexes	• Blood ammonia 92 μmol/L (7.6–63.2) • Total bile acid 54.6 μmol/L (<15)	• Ultrasound: liver reduced in size, hepatic portal vein and caudal vena cava identified. Abnormal vessel arising from prehepatic portal vein, looped dorsally and caudally to merge with caudal vena cava near right renal vein. • Intra-operative mesenteric portovenogram: single extrahepatic PSS identified curving dorsally into caudal vena cava. Cranial to origin of shunt, portal vein markedly reduced diameter	• Surgery: shunt ligated with suture. • Clinical improvement with foal growing to normal size
11-mo-old Thoroughbred gelding [9]	Poor weight gain, lethargy, decreased appetite, aimless walking, mentation was unresponsive to violent and aggressive	• Blood ammonia 2.6 μg/mL (0.12–0.57 μg/mL) • Total bilirubin 2.1μg/dL (1.4 μg/dL)	• None performed	• Euthanasia, arteriovenous anomaly and thrombosis of portal vein • Shunting may have been from thrombosis rather than congenital PSS

Normal ranges for analytes reported in parenthesis.

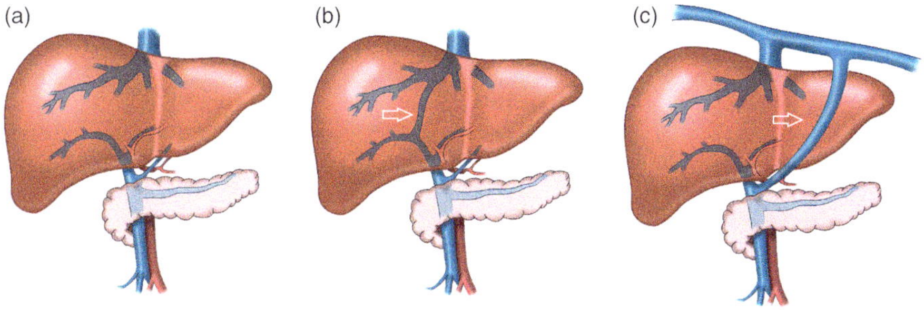

Figure 19.1 Overview of the anatomy of a normal liver (a) and of livers with intrahepatic (b) or extrahepatic (c) portosystemic shunts (PSS). (a) No connection of blood vessels in the liver is present, resulting in blood flow through the hepatic sinusoids; (b) In an intrahepatic PSS, blood bypasses the liver sinusoids and is therefore not subject to hepatic metabolism. The intrahepatic shunt represents an abnormal connection of the portal vein with the systemic circulation within the liver. (c) In an extrahepatic PSS, the aberrant connection is located outside the liver.

of encephalopathy (blindness, wandering, head-pressing, cranial nerve abnormalities), and ataxia. Though the PSS is present at birth, signs may not become apparent until weeks to months of age, after transition to forage and grain, which are higher in protein than milk. Neonatal foals also have a relatively low amount of ammonia produced by the colon, as compared to older foals; this fact may also help explain the absence of clinical signs until the foal is older (6–12 weeks of age) [2, 14].

Diagnosis of PSS is made using a combination of hematology, serum biochemical data, and advanced diagnostic imaging. Foals with PSS are hyperammonemic, with values up to four times greater than age-matched controls (Figure 19.2) [4]. Serum bile acids are elevated, though liver enzyme activity may be within normal reference intervals or only mildly increased [3, 5]. Foals may also have microcytic, normochromic red cells, and may be anemic [4]. Some cases have an elevated total white blood cell count and inflammatory leukogram [3, 4]. Because liver mass and function are supported primarily by hepatic perfusion, decreased portal perfusion of the liver can result in a microhepatica, which has been noted on ultrasound in foals with PSS. Microscopic examination of the liver includes hepatocyte atrophy and arteriolar proliferation in the area of the portal triad, consistent with PSS findings in other species [5]. The anomalous shunt may be visualized ultrasonographically (Table 19.1) arising from the prehepatic portal vein, bypassing the liver, and joining with the caudal vena cava [3, 4]. Advanced diagnostic imaging such as nuclear hepatic scintigraphy, computed tomography angiography (Figures 19.3 and 19.4), transrectal portoscintigraphy, and intra-operative mesenteric portography (via catheterization and contrast injection of a jejunal vein and fluoroscopy) have been used to identify PSS in foals [3–7, 14].

Treatment of PSS in foals begins with medical management of hepatic encephalopathy with lactulose, nutritional support, and treatment of any comorbidities. The benzodiazepine antagonist sarmazenil may be useful in managing

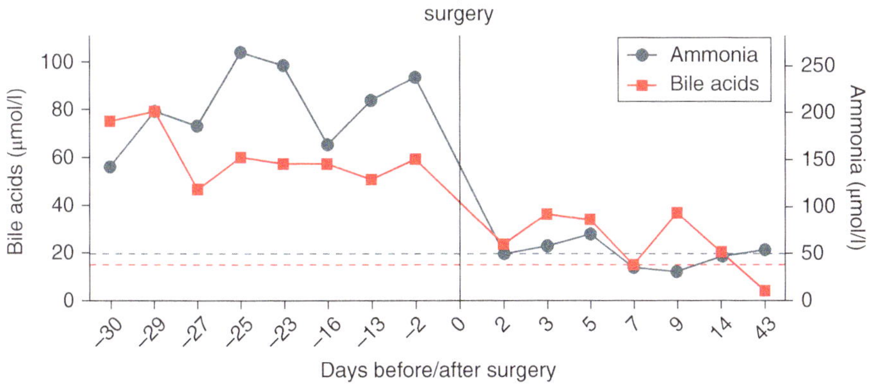

Figure 19.2 Trend of bile acid and ammonia concentrations in a 9-week-old Arabian filly before and after surgery to correct a PSS. The filly presented with a history of intermittent episodes of circling around the mare, incoordination, absence of menace reflex, apparent blindness, inability to nurse, lethargy, unresponsiveness, ptyalism, and bruxism starting soon after birth. The upper limits of the reference interval for bile acids and ammonia concentrations are indicated by horizontal dotted lines [6].

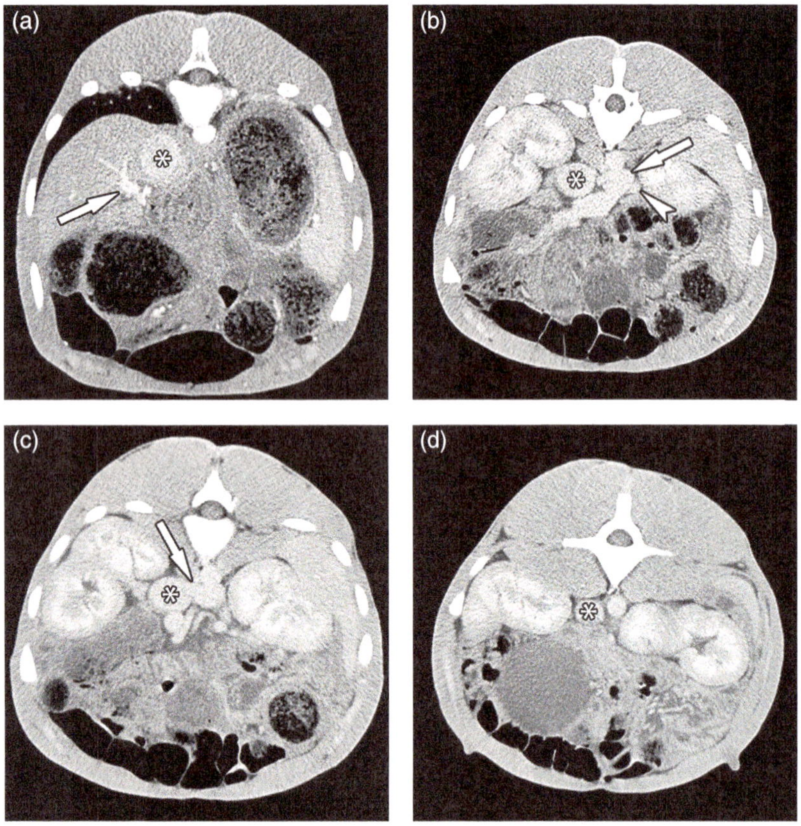

Figure 19.3 CT images of a congenital extrahepatic portosystemic shunt in a 2-month-old Dutch Warmblood colt presented for episodic neurologic signs. Letters (a, b, c, d) denote right side of patient; a to d is cranial to caudal. (a) Cranial to shunt, remaining portal vein (arrow) enters liver and the caudal vena cava (asterisk) appears normal size, shape, and position. (b) A broad and short abnormal vessel arises from the combined caudal and cranial mesenteric veins (arrow) at the level of the junction of the splenic vein (arrowhead) and mesenteric veins. (c) Shunt (arrow) merges with caudal vena cava (asterisk) on left side. (d) Caudal to the shunt, the caudal vena cava is visible (asterisk) [7].

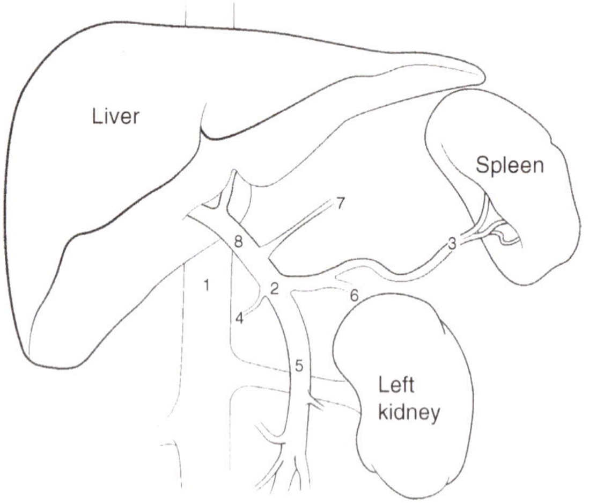

Figure 19.4 Anatomic illustration of the extrahepatic portocaval shunt. At the level of the junction of the splenic and portal vein, a shunting vessel loops to the left and caudally before merging with the caudal vena cava, just cranial to the left renal vein: (1) caudal vena cava; (2) portal vein; (3) splenic vein; (4) caudal mesenteric veins; (5) cranial mesenteric veins; (6) splenocaval shunt; (7) gastroduodenal vein; (8) remaining portal branch to liver [7].

seizures induced by hyperammonemia [6]. After patient stabilization, careful surgical planning to ligate the PSS is explored. Different surgical approaches have been described in the literature including shunt ligation and coil embolization [3, 4, 7, 15]. A single case report describes surgical cellophane banding for the correction of an intrahepatic PSS In an Arabian foal [6].

Portal Vein Thrombosis and Acquired Portosystemic Shunt

A single case report describes a thrombosed portal vein resulting in the development of a PSS in conjunction with *Rhodococcus equi* lymphadenitis [16]. The foal was initially presented at four days of age with diarrhea, which responded to standard medical management. The foal presented again at 73 days of age with clinical signs of encephalopathy. Clinicopathologic abnormalities were consistent with PSS with the addition of severe thrombocytosis and hyperfibrinogenemia. The foal was euthanized due to persistent encephalopathy. At postmortem exam, a large thrombus that completely occluded the portal vein was identified. Portal vein occlusion resulted in the development of collateral circulation that bypassed the liver with subsequent hyperammonemic encephalopathy.

Congenital Biliary Atresia

Another rare condition reported in foals, biliary atresia involves absence of the biliary tract or biliary lumen in all or part of the biliary tree [17, 18]. In one reported involving a Guelder foal, clinical signs included colic in the neonatal period along with depression, weakness, dull haircoat, and failure to gain weight noted by 4 weeks of age. The feces was clay-like and appeared gray in color (acholic feces), which is associated with the absence of bile secretion into the small intestine (e.g. bile needed to emulsify dietary fat before it can be absorbed). Elevations in bilirubin, alkaline phosphatase, sorbitol dehydrogenase, and GGT suggested liver disease. Unfortunately, the foal died after a needle biopsy of the liver was attempted. Necropsy documented emaciation, marked icterus throughout the body, dilated abdominal vasculature, and an enlarged, pale, and very firm liver. In addition, the entrance to the bile duct and the main bile duct to the liver and the duodenum were absent. Microscopic exam noted increased amounts of connective tissue, proliferation of bile ductules and small islands of hepatic cells distributed throughout the parenchyma of the liver.

Congenital Hepatic Fibrosis

Congenital hepatic fibrosis (CHF) is a developmental disorder that has been described in Spanish Purebred, Swiss Franches-Montagnes, and Swiss Freiberger horses [19–21]. This disorder occurs when there is defective remodeling of the embryological ductal plate, abnormal branching of the intrahepatic portal veins, and progressive hepatic fibrosis [22]. Clinical signs of CHF in foals include small stature, colic, icterus, encephalopathy, lethargy, and abdominal distention with yellow, oily feces. Interestingly, microscopic findings of Alzheimer type 2 cells along with gliosis and spongiosis of the thalamus and white mater of the cerebral cortex are findings compatible with hepatic encephalopathy and have been reported in affected Swiss Freiberger foals with CHF (Figures 19.5–19.7) [21].

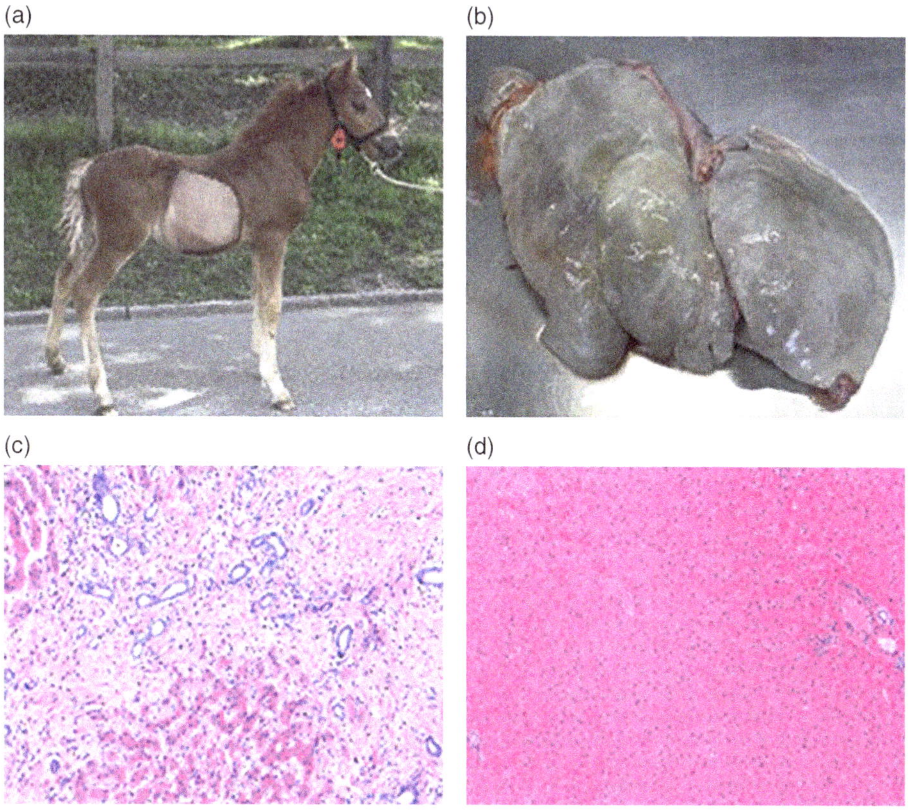

Figure 19.5 Congenital liver fibrosis in Franches-Montagnes horses. (a) Two-month-old affected foal that was small for its age and displayed a potbelly. (b) Enlarged and gray-colored liver of affected foal with macroscopically visible cysts. (c) Histologic image of liver with marked proto-portal bridging fibrosis and abundant dilated bile ductules surrounded by inflammatory cells within fibrotic tissue (H&E, 400×). (d) Histologic image of liver demonstrating small bile ducts in portal areas and absence of fibrosis (H&E 400×) [11].

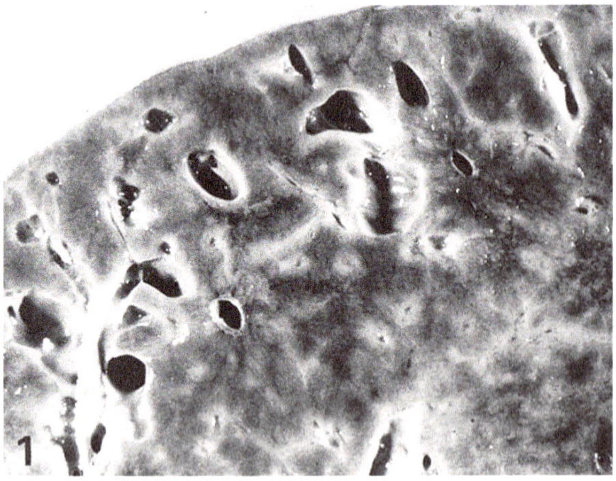

Figure 19.6 (Left). Liver of a Swiss Freiberger foal with congenital hepatic fibrosis. The cut surface displays a prominent reticular pattern and multiple macroscopically visible, irregular cysts [21].

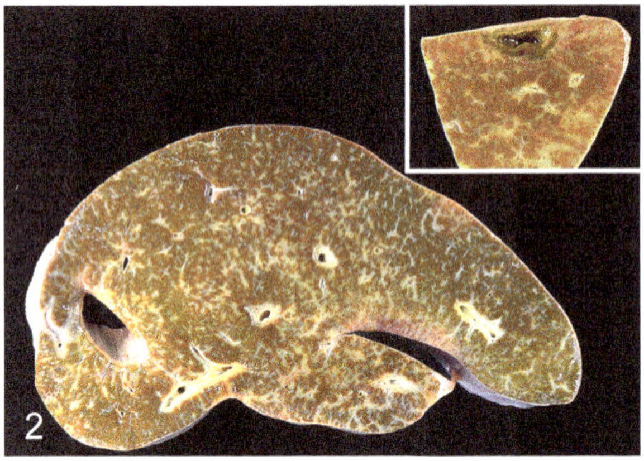

Figure 19.7 Congenital hepatic fibrosis in a foal. Liver exhibits prominent reticular pattern with greenish-yellow discoloration within the parenchyma separated by bridging fibrotic bands. Inset: 2 cm diameter subcapsular cyst [20].

Abdominal ultrasound reveals hepatomegaly, heterogenous hyperechogenicity, and potentially multiple cystic lesions within the hepatic parenchyma. Clinicopathologic abnormalities are typical for severe liver disease, though bile acid concentration and neutrophil count are reported to be exceptionally high in cases of CHF [19].

Congenital Hepatic Tumors

Neoplastic disease of the equine fetus and neonate is uncommon. Liver-specific tumors such as hepatoblastomas, which are malignant hepatic neoplasms, have been reported at necropsy of fetuses and euthanized neonatal foals [23, 24]. Hepatoblastomas may be large and may metastasize to the brain and other tissues [9, 15]. Histopathologically, they are epithelial/mesenchymal in nature, may be necrotic, and encapsulated. In one report, a 10-month-old Thoroughbred foal presented for anorexia and alternating constipation and diarrhea; on physical examination, tachycardia, dyspnea, venous congestion, and fever was recorded. Notable clinicopathologic derangements included elevations in RBCs (17.7×10^3/ml; rr, 6.5–13×10^3/ml), PCV (60.8%), serum creatinine and total bilirubin concentrations. The foal ultimately died as a result of the hepatoblastoma (Figure 19.8) [25]. Other hepatic neoplasms to consider in the foal include hepatocellular carcinoma, mixed hamartoma, and mesenchymal hamartoma [26].

Another unusual clinical scenario in which the liver can be impacted by neoplasia is disseminated forms of cancer, with some potentially arising from metastasis of placental neoplasia to the fetus/foal [27–34]. If the placenta develops neoplasia, it is possible that some neoplastic cells can reach the fetal circulation, with the fetal liver being the first organ to receive these cells via the umbilical vein. Further dissemination of neoplastic cells beyond the liver

(a)

(b)

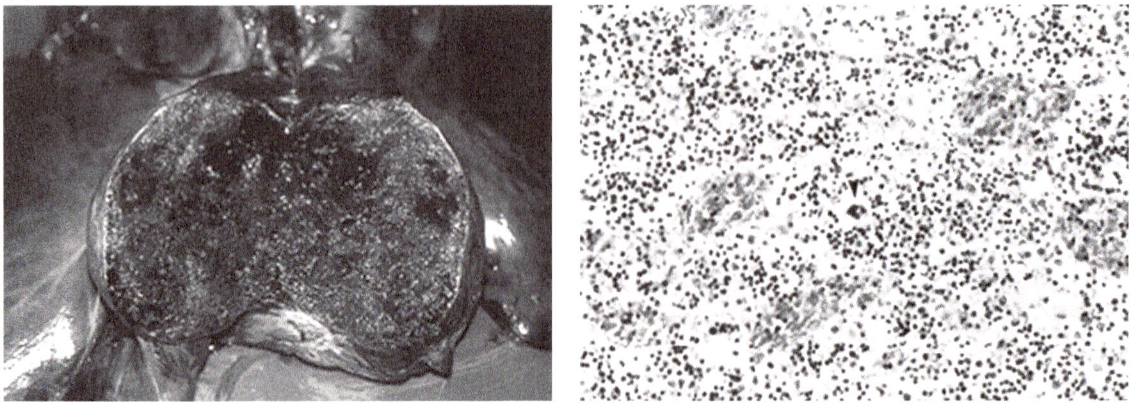

Figure 19.8 (a) Sectioned foal's liver displaying a well-demarcated neoplastic mass (hepatoblastoma) in the quadrate lobe. Variegated hemorrhagic and necrotic areas are evident on the cut surface. (b) Microscopic evaluation of hepatoblastoma revealing large areas of extramedullary hemopoiesis comprising red blood cells, erythroblastic cells, and myeloblastic cells. A megakaryocyte is present (arrowhead). H&E × 200 [25].

is possible and has been observed in other fetal or neonatal neoplasms that have metastasized to brain, bone, lung, and skin [30, 31, 34]. In one report, a 52-day-old Quarter Horse filly presented with a history of urine dribbling, intermittent fever, decreased nursing, hind-limb weakness, prolonged recumbency and difficulty rising [32]. Elevations in liver enzyme activity (AST 985 IU/L, rr 282–484 IU/L; GGT 95 IU/L, rr 8–38 IU/L) and bilirubin (58.14 μmol/L, rr 8.55–34.2 μmol/L) prompted further evaluation of the liver. Diagnostic imaging of the liver, including ultrasonography and computed tomography, revealed heterogenous masses of varying size diffusely distributed throughout the liver parenchyma (Figure 19.9). The filly was euthanized with the masses subsequently identified as mixed germ cell tumors. Interestingly, the same type of tumor was identified in the placenta of the foal (previously evaluated microscopically shortly after birth). The ataxia noted in the foal was caused by a fracture of the sacral vertebral body, which was also infiltrated with neoplastic cells of the same type. A similar type of report involving placental metastasis has been reported in a 10-week-old Arabian foal that presented for acute colic, abdominal distension,

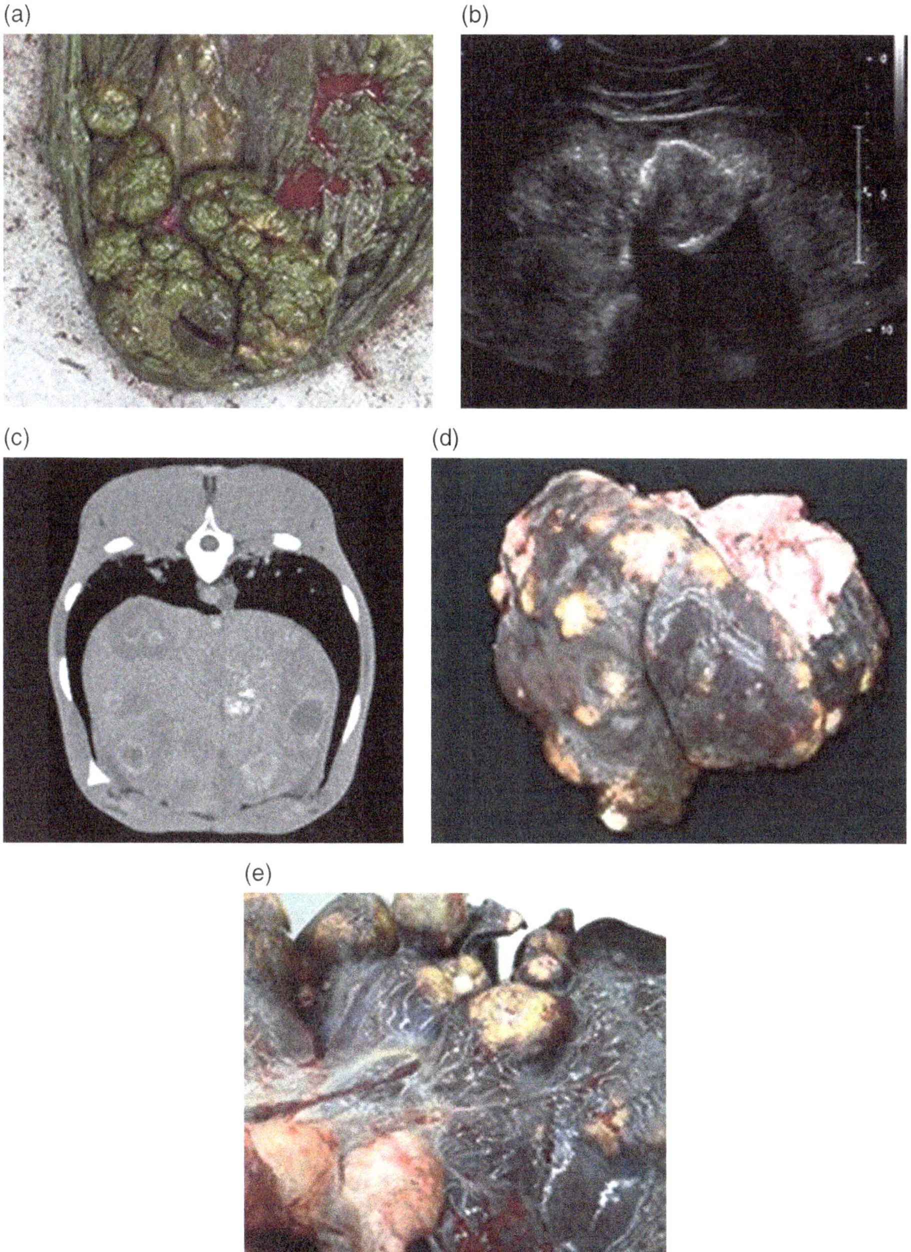

Figure 19.9 (a) Placenta from a mare demonstrating multiple masses determined to be a mixed germ cell tumor. (b) Ultrasonographic image of a liver mass from a 52-day-old foal in which placental masses were noted post-parturition. (c) Computed tomographic image of multiple liver masses. (d) and (e) Gross appearance of the liver of the foal with multiple masses distributed throughout parenchyma. Masses determined to be mixed germ cell tumors, similar to placental masses [32].

tachycardia, and dehydration [29, 33]. Ultimately, teratocarcinoma was identified throughout the liver, omentum, spleen, and sublumbar lymph nodes of the foal. Although rare, if abnormal masses are identified in the fetal membranes of a post-parturient mare, repeated evaluation for metastasis to the foal may be warranted.

Congenital Errors of Metabolism

Glycogen Branching Enzyme Deficiency

Glycogen branching enzyme deficiency (GBED) is an invariably fatal autosomal recessive disease reported in Quarter Horses and Paint Horses. In affected horses, a mutation in glycogen branching enzyme 1 (GBE1) results in an inability of the foal to store glycogen and efficiently mobilize adequate amounts of glucose to provide energy for normal activity. Abnormal glycogen accumulates in the skeletal and myocardial muscle, and to a lesser extent in the liver, with the amount of abnormal glycogen inclusions increasing with age of the foal [35, 36].

Neonates typically present within the first week of life with clinical signs of weakness, lethargy, and flexural deformities, though GBED has also been associated with late-term abortion and premature parturition. With supportive care and nutritional management, foals have been reported to survive for several weeks before experiencing sudden death, often during exercise [35]. Clinicopathologic abnormalities include leukopenia, intermittent severe hypoglycemia, and elevations in creatine kinase, aspartate aminotransferase (AST), and GGT. A diagnosis of GBED can be made by histopathologic analysis of skeletal or cardiac muscle and liver, which shows basophilic inclusions within myocytes and hepatocytes after standard H&E staining. Periodic acid Schiff's staining reveals abnormal accumulation of glycogen within these tissues (Figure 19.10).

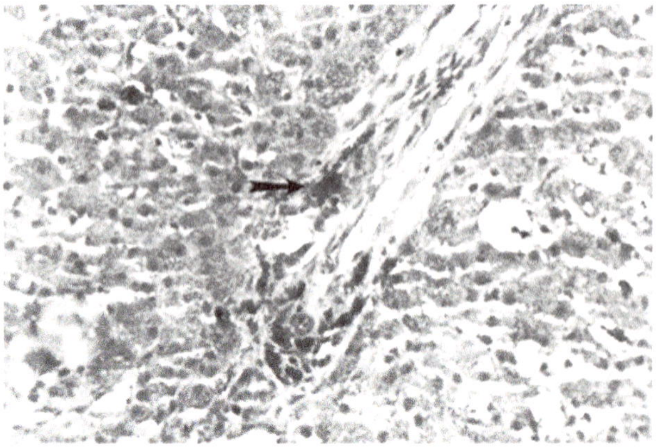

Figure 19.10 Periodic acid Schiff's (PAS) stain of the liver from a foal with GBED. Note accumulation of PAS-positive material (arrow) in connective tissue elements near portal triad (860×) [35].

Genetic testing for a nonsense mutation at codon 34 in exon 1 of the *GBE1* gene can identify affected foals in the antemortem period and can also identify heterozygote carrier horses [37]. The American Quarter Horse Association has made efforts to eliminate GBED and other heritable diseases by requiring genetic screening of breeding stock prior to registration. Prior to genetic screening, the *GBE1* allele was present in the Quarter Horse breed at a frequency of 8.3% and in Paint Horses at 7.1% [38].

Lipid Storage Myopathy/Congenital Multiple Acyl-CoA Dehydrogenase Deficiency

A congenital lipid myopathy similar to acquired multiple acyl-CoA dehydrogenase deficiency (MADD) has been described in a neonatal Paint filly [39]. In infants, MADD is most often caused by a deficiency of one of the two electron transfer flavoproteins that transfer electrons from acyl-CoA dehydrogenases to the respiratory chain; these deficiencies are usually caused by inherited genetic mutations [39]. The filly displayed clinical signs similar to GBED, including lethargy, obtundation, and generalized weakness along with clinicopathologic derangements such as mildly increased liver and muscle enzyme activity and persistent hypoglycemia despite nutritional supplementation. To help determine if a myopathy was present, muscle biopsy of the semimembranosus was performed, which subsequently indicated a lipid storage myopathy based on numerous large densely packed lipid droplets in oil red O stains of frozen sections. The filly was subsequently euthanized.

Hyperammonemia in Morgan Foals

A seemingly rare inherited mitochondrial condition has been reported to affect Morgan foals. It is hypothesized that these foals have a defective mitochondrial transporter protein, resulting in an impaired urea cycle and the accumulation of ammonia and the amino acid ornithine [40]. Affected foals typically present soon after weaning (typically at least 3 months of age before signs are observed) with variable signs of ill-thrift and encephalopathy as a result of hyperammonemia. In addition to elevated ammonia, foals have increased bile acids, SDH, AST, and bilirubin with low blood urea nitrogen. The liver is generally unremarkable ultrasonographically and histopathologically. A serum amino acid profile will show elevation in ornithine and glutamine as a result of the error in metabolism.

Bacterial Hepatitis

Hepatic disease may result as a complication of sepsis due to direct bacterial infection of the liver during periods of bacteremia, or secondary to septic shock and multiple organ dysfunction syndrome [41]. Bacterial sepsis is common in neonatal foals with microorganisms such as *Escherichia coli, Actinobacillus* spp. and *Streptococcus* spp. being frequently isolated from blood [42]. *Actinobacillus equuli* has been cultured from liver specimens collected at necropsy in foals but other specific bacteria, not commonly associated with neonatal sepsis such as *Listeria monocytogenes, Leptosira interrogans*, and *Bartonella henselae,* have also been reported to cause hepatitis [43–47]. People with sepsis can have varied clinical patterns of liver dysfunction associated with infection. One such pattern is sepsis-induced hypoxic hepatitis (also known as hypoxic liver injury), which is triggered by inadequate oxygen supply, reduced blood flow due to decreased arterial and/or increased venous pressures and/or lack of oxygen carriers [48, 49]. Microthrombi can also impair perfusion of the liver. This underlying injurious mechanism is characterized by increased serum AST and alanine aminotransferase (ALT) activities [48, 49]. Another pattern of liver dysfunction is sepsis-induced cholestasis (also known as sclerosing cholangitis or ischemic-like cholangiopathy) and results from either impaired bile formation at the hepatocellular level or from defective bile flow at the level of small or large bile ducts. Sclerosing cholangitis is characterized by inflammation, fibrosis, and destruction of bile ducts resulting from inflammation-mediated impairment of hepatocellular transport systems and disruption of tight junctions [48]. A third pattern of liver dysfunction associated with sepsis is secondary sclerosing cholangitis characterized by inflammation, fibrosis, and destruction of bile ducts and is triggered by ischemia of biliary cells. Biliary epithelial cells are exceptionally susceptible to hypoxia, which initiates apoptosis and necrosis. Severe systemic hypotension and the systemic inflammatory response syndrome are risk factors for secondary sclerosing cholangitis. A hallmark characteristic of secondary sclerosing cholangitis is early formation of biliary casts that fill the intrahepatic ductal system [48].

Although these specific types of liver dysfunction have not been specifically examined in the septic neonatal foal, evidence of liver injury during sepsis in foals is supported by a large retrospective study in foals that examined 147 neonatal foals with high serum GGT and/or SDH activity and compared them to hospitalized control foals without elevations in liver enzyme activity [47]. In this study, foals with elevated liver enzyme activity were significantly more likely to have sepsis and were also significantly more likely to die or be euthanized (odds ratio 2.22) compared to control foals [47]. More specifically, of the 410 neonatal foals evaluated over the study period, 147 (36%) had high liver enzyme activity; in this cohort, septic foals were significantly more likely (66/130 [51%]) than nonseptic foals (70/255 [27%]) to have increased liver enzyme activity. Further evidence of hepatic injury secondary to sepsis is revealed by the fact that hepatic sinusoids from septic foals have fibrin deposits, attributed to disseminated intravascular coagulation secondary to sepsis [50].

Bacterial cholangitis or cholangiohepatitis may also occur due to primary gastrointestinal disease, including gastrointestinal enteritis, meconium impaction, strangulating or obstructive intestinal lesions, ileus, and severe gastroduodenal ulceration [51]. Inflammation or injury of the small intestine may cause outflow obstruction of the major duodenal papilla and cholestasis, or in cases of small intestinal obstruction, reflux of the duodenal contents into the common bile duct [50].

Clinical signs of bacterial hepatitis may be difficult to differentiate from those signs associated with neonatal sepsis. Persistent or exceptional elevation in liver enzyme activity and bilirubin and bile acid concentrations after initiation of antimicrobial therapy and improvement in hemodynamic status should trigger the possibility of hepatitis as a differential. Ultrasonographic evaluation of the liver should be performed as changes in the echogenicity of the parenchyma reflect hepatitis. The liver should be fully evaluated in all cases of omphalophlebitis to identify liver abscesses, which may occur in the absence of significant elevation in liver enzymes (Figure 19.11).

Treatment of bacterial hepatitis includes broad-spectrum intravenous antimicrobial therapy and nutritional support. The combination of ampicillin and amikacin is likely the most effective for neonatal sepsis, though anaerobic coverage in the form of metronidazole should be considered if clostridial enteritis is suspected [42].

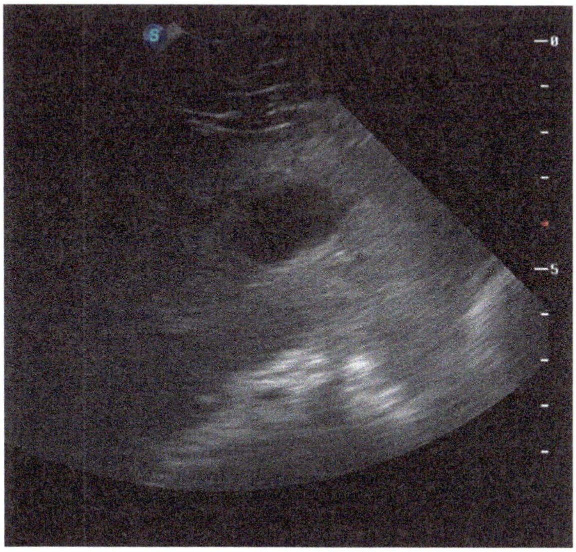

Figure 19.11 Ultrasound examination of the liver of a foal with a hepatic abscess.

Tyzzer's Disease

Tyzzer's disease is an infectious enterohepatic syndrome caused by the bacteria *Clostridium piliforme*, a Gram-negative, spore-forming anaerobe. The suspected route of infection in foals is ingestion of *C. piliforme* spores shed by carrier horses or other affected foals. The exact pathogenesis of Tyzzer's disease is unknown, but infection with the intracellular bacteria causes a severe hepatitis with widespread hepatocyte necrosis, liver dysfunction, and overwhelming sepsis. Risk factors for infection include age and resident status of the mare, with foals born to young mares or mares new to the property at higher risk. Additional risk factors include feeding of high-protein diets and birth in late spring [52].

Tyzzer's disease may affect a single foal or occur as an outbreak and should be considered in cases of peracute death in neonates. Clinical signs include lethargy, temperature dysregulation, colic, diarrhea, and signs of encephalopathy. Classic clinicopathologic derangements include severe hypoglycemia, increased hepatic enzyme activity and markers of hepatic function, leukopenia, and metabolic acidosis [52, 53]. The disease is generally rapidly progressive and nearly always fatal. Chances of survival may improve if intensive treatment with antimicrobials, intravenous fluids, parenteral nutrition, and anti-inflammatories is initiated early [53]. Antimicrobial treatment in surviving foals has included parenteral ampicillin or potassium penicillin in conjunction with an aminoglycoside followed by enteral trimethoprim sulfamethoxazole.

Liver tissue is necessary for definitive diagnosis of Tyzzer's disease. For a rapid, specific diagnosis, *C. piliforme* DNA can be detected using PCR of liver tissue [53]. Histopathologic evidence of filamentous bacteria within hepatocytes, coagulation necrosis of hepatic tissue, and degenerate hepatocytes surrounded by inflammatory cells is consistent with Tyzzer's disease [52]. Silver-type stains may be necessary for detection of *C. piliforme*. Grossly, the liver appears large with multifocal areas of discoloration. Bacterial culture of the liver samples may yield no growth despite evidence of overwhelming infection [53].

Viral Hepatitis

Equine Herpesvirus-1

Equine herpes virus 1 (EHV-1) is endemic in horse populations and may cause late-gestation abortion and neonatal disease. Foals are infected in-utero from repeated cell-associated viremia in the dam; thus, clinical signs are observed immediately after birth [51]. Clinical signs of congenital EHV-1 infection in foals that are born alive frequently involve the liver as part of a severe multiorgan infection. Liver enzyme activity can be elevated and the foal may be icteric along with severe neutropenia [14]. In one retrospective study involving 14 foals with EHV-1 infection, liver enzyme activity was not increased despite profound hepatic necrosis [54]. Interstitial pneumonia is another component of EVH-1 infection in foals, thus respiratory signs may be apparent (Figure 19.12). Treatment with the antiviral medications valacyclovir or acyclovir may be considered in addition to standard treatment for neonatal sepsis in cases where EHV-1 is suspected. Prognosis is poor in neonatal foals born with EHV-1 infection (14/14 foals with EHV-1 infection died in aforementioned study), although foals with milder infections may survive [51]. Areas of necrosis and evidence of viral inclusion bodies are often seen within the liver on necropsy examination [54–56].

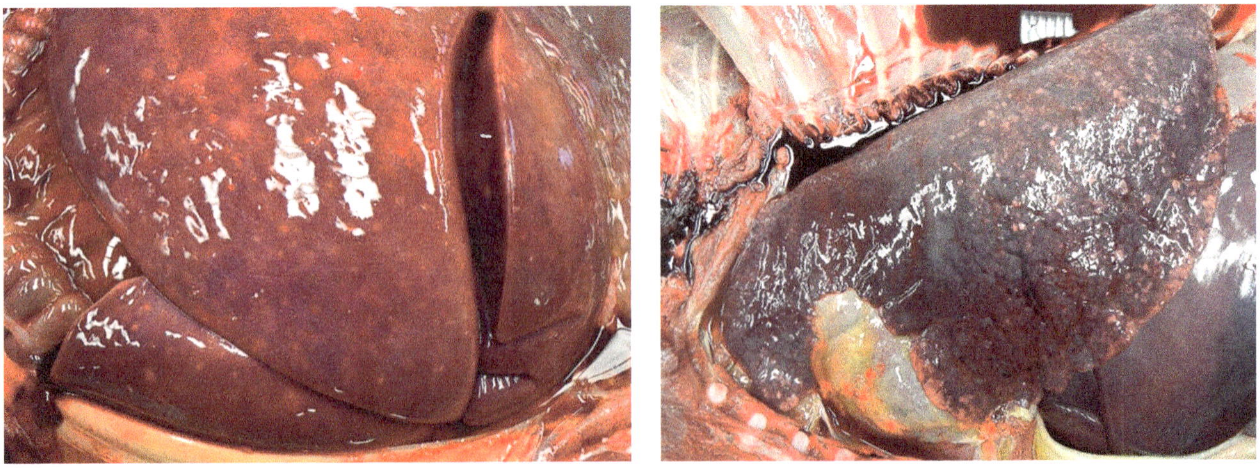

Figure 19.12 Gross appearance of the liver and lung of a neonatal foal with EHV-1 demonstrating multifocal areas of necrosis (small yellow/tan foci) throughout the parenchyma of both organs. *Source:* Photo courtesy of Dr. Rebecca Ruby, MSc, BVSc, DACVP, DACVIM.

Equine Hepacivirus and Equine Parvovirus

Recent clinical studies have identified viral causes of hepatitis in adult horses. Specifically, equine parvovirus has been shown to cause subclinical hepatitis and is suspected to be the causative agent of Theiler's disease, also known as serum sickness. Equine hepacivirus (nonprimate hepacivirus) has recently been shown to cause mild or subclinical hepatitis, not associated with the administration of equine biologic agents [57]. Though there are no reports thus far of equine hepacivirus or parvovirus hepatitis in neonates, vertical transmission of the viruses is suspected. Equine hepacivirus has been identified in aborted fetal tissues and chorioallantois using PCR, though vertical transmission could not be documented for equine parvovirus-hepatitis [58, 59].

Toxic Hepatitis

Neonatal Isoerythrolysis

Neonatal isoerythrolysis (NI) occurs when maternal antibodies absorbed from colostrum bind to foal red blood cells resulting in their destruction. One of the hallmark signs of NI is icteric mucous membranes (Figure 19.13). Hepatic failure in foals with NI has been observed sporadically in foals [14]. The cause of hepatic failure is unknown, but could be related to severe hypoxia, iron overload, immune reactions resulting from blood transfusion(s) and/or bile stasis caused by the inability to secret increased amounts of conjugated bilirubin. Neonatal foals are particularly susceptible to iron overload from multiple transfusions because they have lower concentrations of iron-binding proteins when compared to adult horses [14]. Conjugated bilirubin can approach 50% of the total bilirubin, suggestive of bile stasis. Most foals recover from hepatic damage after several weeks [14]. The central nervous system can also be rarely affected in cases of NI. Because hyperbilirubinemia can be severe in some cases of NI (>27 mg/dl) due to hemolysis and decreased uptake as a result of hypoxic liver damage, the unconjugated bilirubin pigment can be deposited in the basal nuclei of the brain causing the syndrome kernicterus and the development of obtundation and seizures (Chapter 35).

A serum biochemical analysis that includes evaluation of liver enzyme activity should be performed in foals presenting with NI to identify foals that have liver damage in addition to hyperbilirubinemia secondary to hemolysis. While most cases of NI can be treated with conservative management and isotonic fluid therapy, foals with severe NI and hypoxia may require one or more blood transfusions. A retrospective study noted that foals that received blood transfusions of 4 L or more were more likely to develop liver failure and hypothesized that these foals were suffering from hepatic iron overload and subsequent toxicity [60]. Treatment with deferoxamine (1 g SC q12h), a drug that increases renal iron excretion, may help prevent iron toxicity in foals that require multiple blood transfusions [61]. Plasma exchange has been used as a treatment for hyperbilirubinemia in foals with NI at risk of developing kernicterus and could also likely help cases at risk of iron toxicity [62, 63].

(a) (b) (c)

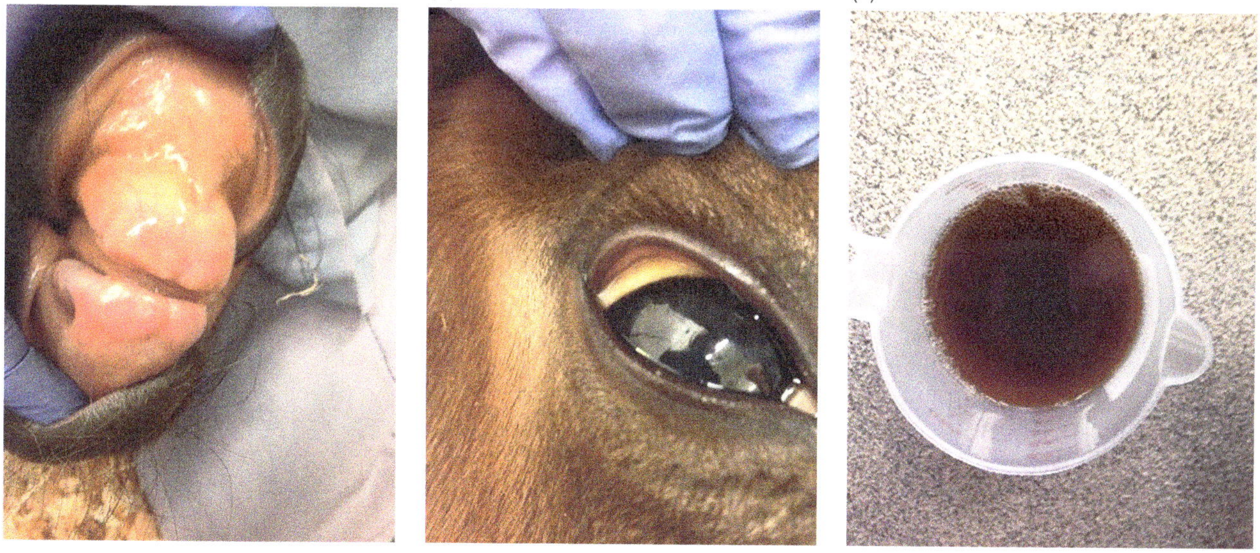

Figure 19.13 Foal with neonatal isoerythrolysis (NI) demonstrating icterus of the (a) mucous membranes and (b) sclera, along with (c) hemoglobinuria.

Iron Toxicity

Enteral supplementation of iron (ferrous fumarate) has been reported to cause severe and fatal hepatitis in neonates two to five days after administration. Iron is concentrated within mitochondria of hepatocytes where it disrupts oxidative phosphorylation, forms free radicals, and eventually causes cellular death. Clinical signs of iron toxicity are consistent with liver failure and included icterus, ataxia, head-pressing, and encephalopathy [64–66]. Histopathology of the liver demonstrates massive or periportal hepatocellular necrosis with lobular collapse, cholestasis, and moderate to severe bile ductule proliferation [66]. Iron is particularly well-absorbed in the first 12–24 hours of life, and all iron-containing products should be avoided during this time period. The clinician should be very cautious in the use of oral administration of any medication to foals less than 24 hours of age because of the potential for increased bioavailability and possible hepatotoxicity [14, 51, 64].

Drug-Induced Liver Injury

Several commonly used drugs including phenobarbital, histamine blockers, rifampin, metronidazole, macrolides, and sulfa antimicrobials have the potential to cause drug-induced liver injury (DILI). There are multiple different mechanisms of DILI documented in human medicine, including cytochrome p450 function alterations, mitochondrial transport inhibition, bile acid transporter inhibition, direct DNA damage, immune-allergenic responses, or a combination of these mechanisms [67–70]. One particular drug combination, doxycycline and rifampin, has rarely been associated with liver damage and possible hemolysis in foals [71]. Liver values should be monitored, particularly with long-term use of these drugs, and elevations in liver enzymes should prompt drug discontinuation.

Miscellaneous Causes of Liver Disease

Infrequently, obstructive and/or ascending cholangitis or cholangiohepatitis can occur secondary to ileus, enteritis, or healing duodenal ulcers in foals [14, 51]. If scarring occurs at the opening of the bile ducts, a hepaticojejunostomy can be attempted, but prognosis is guarded. If the obstruction is distal to the opening of the bile ducts, duodenojejunostomy can be curative. Orally administered barium can be seen ascending the biliary ducts in these cases [14].

Umbilical vein infections (omphalophlebitis) that extend to the liver are uncommon but can occur [14]. These foals may be febrile, tachycardic, lethargic, and have evidence of infection in other body systems (e.g. septic arthritis). Transabdominal ultrasound can reliably identify the enlarged umbilical vein. Omphalophlebitis causing liver abscesses requires long-term medical management with antimicrobials but surgical intervention should be strongly considered to remove the umbilicus. If the infection extends into the liver, the vein should be either marsupialized to the ventral body wall or the remnant portion in the liver cauterized and left open to drain (Figure 19.14) [14]. Prognosis is typically good.

Peripartum asphyxia can result in hypoxic–ischemic injury, commonly involving the central nervous system (neonatal encephalopathy), kidneys, and/or gastrointestinal tract. Less commonly, hepatopathies can occur from peripartum hypoxic–ischemic episodes. Affected foals exhibit icterus from biliary stasis and hepatic dysfunction and increased liver enzyme activity may be noted [51].

Another cause of hepatic injury in foals is parasitic migration (e.g. *Parascaris equorum, Strongylus* species) through the liver [72–74]. Larvae can be first observed microscopically in the liver by 24-hours post-infection [72, 74]. Clinical signs of parasitic migration are often non-specific with one study noting coughing, anorexia, rough haircoat, and weight loss seven days after foals were experimentally infected with *P. equorum* eggs [72]. Mild anemia, eosinophila, and leukopenia may be noted on CBC and postmortem examination findings with parasitic migration can include hemorrhage, edema, and white or yellow necrotic foci in the lungs, liver, and bronchial and hepatic lymph nodes. Migration of parasites through the liver typically does not cause overt liver disease in foals, with

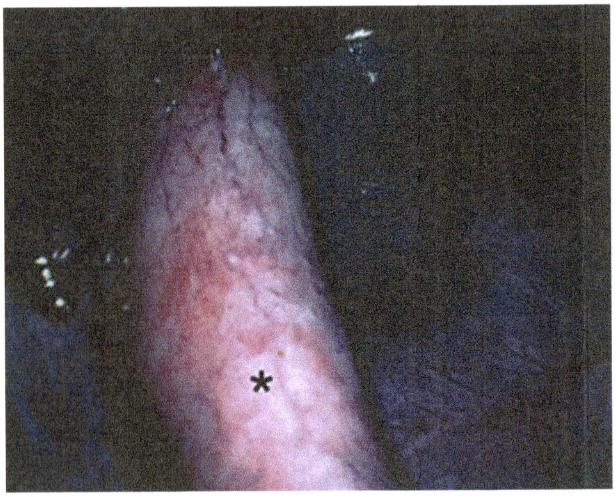

Figure 19.14 Foal with an infected and enlarged umbilical vein (*), extending into the liver. The umbilical vein was removed laparoscopically and the remaining portion of the vein entering the liver was marsupialized to an opening in the body wall. *Source:* [14].

clinical signs attributed to damage of other organ systems such as the intestines.

Potential Drugs Used with Liver Disease

Little information is available regarding drugs that facilitate recovery of liver injury in the horse or foal. However, anecdotal reports have suggested the use of certain medications that might aid in treatment of liver disease in the equid. Ursodeoxycholic acid (ursodiol) is a hydrophilic bile acid that is normally present in human bile at low (~3% of total bile acids) concentrations [75]. It is specifically used to encourage dissolution of cholesterol-rich stones and treat cholangitis and cholestasis in people as well as act as an anti-inflammatory and choleretic agent that increases bile production [75]. The mechanisms of action by which ursodiol is beneficial in liver disease may be related to three major mechanisms:

1) Protection of cholangiocytes against cytotoxicity of hydrophobic bile acids
2) Stimulation of hepatobiliary secretion, and
3) Protection of hepatocytes against bile acid-induced apoptosis [75]

One or all of these mechanisms may be of importance in individual cholestatic disorders and different stages of cholestatic liver disease. A common disturbance in all forms of cholestasis is impairment of bile formation, which subsequently results in retention of bile acids and other toxic biliary constituents in the liver; this leads to hepatocyte injury and further impairment of bile formation and hepatocellular apoptosis. Ursodiol stimulates biliary secretion of bile acids and other organic anions and prevents cholestasis induced by bile acids [75]. Thus, ursodiol (15 mg/kg, PO, q12h) might help protect the liver as well as promote production of bile. It has been used in cholangiohepatitis in adult horses with no obvious signs of toxicity [76]. Of note, administration of ursodiol may increase serum bile acid concentrations [73].

S-adenosylmethionine (SAMe) is an endogenous molecule produced primarily by the liver as a byproduct of methionine metabolism and plays a critical role in the transsulfuration process in the generation of glutathione [77]. Glutathione is an antioxidant and free radical scavenger and may serve as a physiologic defense mechanism against oxidative stress in hepatocytes [77]. SAMe is administered to patients as a nutritional supplement with purported beneficial effects include anti-inflammatory and antioxidant effects as well as playing a role in cellular replication and protein synthesis. SAMe has been administered to dogs and cats (20 mg/kg/d PO) as an adjunct treatment of necroinflammatory, metabolic and cholestatic hepatopathies [77]. Bioavailability or efficacy is unknown in the foal.

Milk thistle extract has been used by people as a home remedy for liver disease. Milk thistle extract contains 60–70% silymarin, which is composed of a mixture of flavonolignans such as silibinin (major active component), isosilibinin, silidianin, and silichristin [78]. Milk thistle extract is believed to exert antioxidant, anti-inflammatory, and antifibrotic effects [77, 79]. Overall, the oral bioavailability across species is low, and this holds true for horses as well. In one study, doses of 6.5, 13, and 26 mg/kg silibinin were administered to adult horses over seven consecutive days for each dose; bioavailability in horses was 0.6–2.9% and silibinin did not accumulate when given at these doses over the seven days at each dose [80]. No toxicity was observed in horses. The efficacy of milk thistle is unknown in horses.

Other medications that might be beneficial in liver disease include dimethyl sulfoxide (DMSO), pentoxifylline, and vitamin E. Use of DMSO has been reported in people with brown pigment stones as it is a direct solubilizer of calcium bilirubinate; DMSO has been recommended as an adjunctive therapy in some cases of equine cholangiohepatitis and cholelithiasis [76, 81]. Pentoxifylline (8.5 mg/kg, PO, q 12h) has also been used in horses with liver disease for its anti-inflammatory and antifibrotic effects. Vitamin E (α-tocopherol) is an antioxidant commonly used in horses and foals as it is a lipid-soluble component of cell membranes. Vitamin E inhibits lipid peroxidation and modulates intracellular signaling pathways that rely on reactive oxygen intermediates. It may be of some benefit in foals (5–10 IU/kg, PO, q24h) with liver disease [76].

References

1 Bauer, J.E. (1990). Normal blood chemistry. In: *Equine Clincial Neonatology* (ed. A.M. Koterba, W.H. Drummond, and P.C. Kosch), 602–614. Philadelphia: Lea & Fibiger.

2 Barton, M.H. and LeRoy, B.E. (2007). Serum bile acid concentrations in healthy and clinically ill neonatal foals. *J. Vet. Intern. Med.* 21: 508–513.

3 Woodford, N.S., Hotson Moore, A., Renfrew, H. et al. (2017). Surgical management of an extrahepatic portosystemic shunt in a foal: a multidisciplinary problem. *Equine Vet. Educ.* 29: 243–248.

4 Fortier, L.A., Fubini, S.L., Flanders, J.A. et al. (1996). The diagnosis and surgical correction of congenital

portosystemic vascular anomalies in two calves and two foals. *Vet. Surg.* 25: 154–160.
5 Buonanno, A.M., Carlson, G.P., and Kantrowitz, B. (1988). Clinical and diagnostic features of portosystemic shunt in a foal. *J. Am. Vet. Med. Assoc.* 192: 387–389.
6 Hug, S.A., Guerrero, T.G., Makara, M. et al. (2012). Diagnosis and surgical cellophane banding of an intrahepatic congenital portosystemic shunt in a foal. *J. Vet. Intern. Med.* 26: 171–177.
7 Willems, D.S., Kranenburg, L.C., Ensink, J.M. et al. (2019). Computed tomography angiography of a congenital extrahepatic splenocaval shunt in a foal. *Acta Vet. Scand.* 61: 39.
8 Martin, R.A. (1993). Congenital portosystemic shunts in the dog and cat. *Vet. Clin. N. Am. Small* 23: 609–623.
9 Beech, J., Dubielzig, R., and Bester, R. (1977). Portal vein anomaly and hepatic encephalopathy in a horse. *J. Am. Vet. Med. Assoc.* 170: 164–166.
10 Hillyer, M.H., Holt, P.E., Barr, F.J. et al. (1993). Clinical signs and radiographic diagnosis of a portosystemic shunt in a foal. *Vet. Rec.* 132: 457–460.
11 Van Steenbeek, F.G., van den Bossche, L., Leegwater, P.A.J. et al. (2012). Inherited liver shunts in dogs elucidate pathways regulating embryonic development and clinical disorders of the portal vein. *Mamm. Genome* 23: 76–84.
12 Silver, M. (1984). Some aspects of equine placental exchange and foetal physiology. *Equine Vet. J.* 16: 227–233.
13 Fowden, A.L., Giussani, D.A., and Forhead, A.J. (2020). Physiological development of the equine fetus during late gestation. *Equine Vet. J.* 52: 165–173.
14 Divers, T.J. and Perkins, G. (2003). Urinary and hepatic disorders in neonatal foals. *Clin. Technol. Equine Pract.* 2: 67–78.
15 Martens, A., Nollet, H., Saunders, J.H. et al. (2009). Successful minimal invasive coil embolisation of a portosystemic shunt in a foal. In: *Proceedings of the ECVS 18th Annual Scientific Meeting*, 176–179. Nantes, France: American College of Veterinary Surgeons.
16 Ness, S.L., Kennedy, L.A., and Slovis, N.M. (2013). Hyperammonemic encephalopathy associated with portal vein thrombosis in a thoroughbred foal. *J. Vet. Intern. Med.* 27: 382–386.
17 Van Der Luer, R.J.T. and Kroneman, J. (1982). Biliary atresia in a foal. *Equine Vet. J.* 14: 91–93.
18 Bastianello, S.S. and Nesbit, J.W. (1986). The pathology of a case of biliary atresia in a foal. *J. S. Afr. Vet. Assoc.* 57: 117–120.
19 Drogemuller, M., Jagannathan, V., Welle, M.M. et al. (2014). Congenital hepatic fibrosis in the Franches-Montagnes horse is associated with the polycystic kidney and hepatic disease 1 (PKHD1) gene. *PLoS One* 9: e110125.
20 Molin, J., Asin, J., Vitoria, A. et al. (2018). Congenital hepatic fibrosis in a purebred Spanish horse foal: pathology and genetic studies on PKHD1 gene mutations. *Vet. Pathol.* 55: 457–461.
21 Haechler, S., Van den Ingh, T.S., Rogivue, C. et al. (2000). Congenital hepatic fibrosis and cystic bile duct formation in Swiss Freiberger horses. *Vet. Pathol.* 37: 669–671.
22 Gunay-Aygun, M., Gahl, W.A., and Heller, T. (2014). *Congenital Hepatic Fibrosis Overview*. U.S. National Library of Medicine.
23 de Vries, C., Vanhaesebrouck, E., Govaere, M. et al. (2013). Congenital ascites due to hepatoblastoma with extensive peritoneal implantation metastases in a premature equine fetus. *J. Comp. Pathol.* 148: 214–219.
24 Loynachan, A.T., Bolin, D.C., Hong, C.B. et al. (2007). Three equine cases of mixed hepatoblastoma with teratoid features. *Vet. Pathol.* 44: 211–214.
25 Cantile, C., Arispici, M., Abramo, F. et al. (2001). Hepatoblastoma in a foal. *Equine Vet. J.* 33: 214–216.
26 Beeler-Marfisi, J., Arroyo, L., Caswell, J.L. et al. (2010). Equine primary liver tumors: a case series and review of the literature. *J. Vet. Diagn. Invest.* 22: 174–183.
27 Durham, A.C., Pillitteri, C.A., San Myint, M. et al. (2012). Two hundred three cases of equine lymphoma classified according to the World Health Organization (WHO) classification criteria. *Vet. Pathol.* 59: 86–93.
28 Haley, P.J. and Spraker, T. (1983). Lymphosarcoma in an aborted equine fetus. *Vet. Pathol.* 20: 647–649.
29 Bockenstedt, M., Fales-Williams, A., and Haynes, J. (2015). Equine placental mixed germ cell tumor with metastasis to the foal. *Vet. Pathol.* 52: 360–363.
30 Wilsher, S. and Allen, W.R. (2012). Factors influencing placental development and function in the mare. *Equine Vet. J.* 44 (Suppl 41): 113–119.
31 Lennox, T.J., Wilson, J.H., Hayden, D.W. et al. (2000). Hepatoblastoma with erythrocytosis in a young female horse. *J. Am. Vet. Med. Assoc.* 216: 718–721.
32 Hepworth-Warren, K.L., Wong, D.M., Galow, N.L. et al. (2014). Metastatic tumor in pregnancy: placental germ cell tumor with metastasis to the foal. *J. Equine Vet. Sci.* 34: 1134–1139.
33 Allison, N., Moeller, R.B., and Duncan, R. (2004). Placental teratocarcinoma in a mare with possible metastasis to the foal. *J. Vet. Diagn. Invest.* 16: 160–163.
34 Loynachan, A.T., Bolin, D.C., Hong, C.B. et al. (2010). Drs Loynachan et al Respond. *Vet. Pathol.* 47: 1005–1006.
35 Valberg, S.J., Ward, T.L., Rush, B. et al. (2001). Glycogen branching enzyme deficiency in Quarter Horse foals. *J. Vet. Intern. Med.* 15: 572–580.
36 Sponseller, B.T., Valberg, S.J., Ward, T.L. et al. (2003). Muscular weakness and recumbency in a Quarter Horse colt due to glycogen branching enzyme deficiency. *Equine Vet. Educ.* 15: 182–188.
37 Ward, T.L., Valberg, S.J., Adelson, D.L. et al. (2004). Glycogen branching enzyme (GBE1) mutation causing

equine glycogen storage disease IV. *Mamm. Genome* 15: 570–577.

38 Wagner, M.L., Valberg, S.J., Ames, E.G. et al. (2006). Allele frequency and likely impact of the glycogen branching enzyme deficiency gene in Quarter Horse and Paint Horse populations. *J. Vet. Intern. Med.* 20: 1207–1211.

39 Pinn, T.L., Divers, T.J., Southard, T. et al. (2017). Persistent hypoglycemia associated with lipid storage myopathy in a paint foal. *J. Vet. Intern. Med.* 32: 1442–1446.

40 McConnico, R.S., Duckett, W.M., and Wood, P.A. (1997). Persistent hyperammonemia in two related Morgan weanlings. *J. Vet. Intern. Med.* 11: 264–266.

41 Cotovio, M., Monreal, L., Armengou, L. et al. (2008). Fibrin deposits and organ failure in newborn foals with severe septicemia. *J. Vet. Intern. Med.* 22: 1403–1410.

42 Theelen, M.J.P., Wilson, W.D., Edman, J.E. et al. (2014). Temporal trends in prevalence of bacteria isolated from foals with sepsis: 1979–2010. *Equine Vet. J.* 46: 169–173.

43 Le'on, A., Pronost, S.P., Tapprest, J. et al. (2006). Identification of pathogenic Leptospira strains in tissues of a premature foal by use of polymerase chain reaction analysis. *J. Vet. Diagn. Invest.* 18: 218–221.

44 Pirs, T., Zdovc, I., Gombac, M. et al. (2005). Listeria monocytogenes septicemia in a foal. *Slovak. Vet. Res.* 42: 49–53.

45 Setlakwe, E.L., Sweeney, R., Engiles, J.B. et al. (2014). Identification of *Bartonella henselae* in the liver of a thoroughbred foal with severe suppurative cholangiohepatitis. *J. Vet. Intern. Med.* 28: 1341–1345.

46 Warner, S.L., Boggs, J., Lee, J.K. et al. (2012). Clinical, pathological, and genetic characterization of listeria monocytogenes causing sepsis and necrotizing typhlocolitis and hepatitis in a foal. *J. Vet. Diagn. Invest.* 24: 581–586.

47 Haggatt, E.F., Magdesian, K.G., and Kass, P.H. (2011). Clinical implications of high liver enzyme activities in hospitalized neonatal foals. *J. Am. Vet. Med. Assoc.* 239: 661–667.

48 Strnad, P., Tacke, F., Koch, A. et al. (2017). Liver-guardian, modifier and target of sepsis. *Nat. Rev. Gastroenterol. Hepatol.* 14: 55–66.

49 Caraballo, C. and Jaimes, F. (2019). Organ dysfunction in sepsis: an ominous trajectory from infection to death. *Yale J. Biol. Med.* 92: 629–640.

50 Buote, M. (2003). Cholangiohepatitis and pancreatitis secondary to severe gastroduodenal ulceration in a foal. *Can. Vet. J.* 44: 746–748.

51 Magdesian, K.G. (2006). Liver failure in the foal. In: *Equine neonatal medicine: a case-based approach* (ed. M.R. Paradis), 221–229. Philadelphia: Elsevier Saunders.

52 Swerczeck, T.W. (2013). Tyzzer's disease in foals: retrospective studies from 1969 to 2010. *Can. Vet. J.* 54: 876–880.

53 Borchers, A., Magdesian, K.G., Halland, S. et al. (2006). Successful treatment and polymerase chain reaction (PCR) confirmation of Tyzzer's disease in a foal and clinical and pathologic characteristics of 6 additional foals (1986–2005). *J. Vet. Intern. Med.* 20: 1212–1218.

54 Perkins, G., Ainsworth, D.M., Erb, H.N. et al. (1999). Clinical, haematological and biochemical findings in foals with neonatal equine herpesvirus-1 infection compared with septic and premature foals. *Equine Vet. J.* 31: 422–426.

55 Marenzoni, M.L., Bietta, A., Lepri, E. et al. (2013). Role of equine herpesviruses as co-infecting agents in cases of abortion, placental disease and neonatal foal mortality. *Vet. Res. Commun.* 37: 311–317.

56 Murray, M.J., del Piero, F., Jeffrey, S.C. et al. (1998). Neonatal equine herpesvirus type 1 infection of a thoroughbred breeding farm. *J. Vet. Intern. Med.* 12: 36–41.

57 Tomlinson, J.E., Van de Walle, G.R., and Divers, T.J. (2019). What do we know about hepatitis viruses in horses? *Vet. Clin. N. Am. Equine* 35: 351–362.

58 Pronost, S., Fortier, C., Marcillaud-Pitel et al. (2019). Further evidence for in utero transmission of equine hepacivirus to foals. *Viruses* 11: 10.3390/v11121124.

59 Tomlinson, J.E., Jager, M., Struzynab, A. et al. (2020). Tropism, pathology, and transmission of equine parvovirus-hepatitis. *Emerg. Microbes Infect.* 9: 651–663.

60 Polkes, A.C., Giguere, S., Lester, G.D. et al. (2008). Factors associated with outcome in foals with neonatal isoerythrolysis (72 cases, 1988–2003). *J. Vet. Intern. Med.* 22: 1216–1222.

61 Elfenbein, J.R., Giguere, S., Meyer, S.K. et al. (2010). The effects of deferoxamine mesylate on iron elimination after blood transusion in neonatal foals. *J. Vet. Intern. Med.* 24: 1475–1482.

62 Broux, B., Lefere, L., Deprez, P. et al. (2015). Plasma exchange as a treatment for hyperbilirubinemai in 2 foals with neonatal isoerythrolysis. *J. Vet. Intern. Med.* 29: 736–738.

63 Carlsson, M., Cortes, D., Jepsen, S. et al. (2009). Severe iron intoxication treated with exchange transfusion. *BMJ Case Reports* 2009: https://doi.org/10.1136/bcr.01.2009.1445.

64 Divers, T.J., Warner, A., Vaala, W.E. et al. (1983). Toxic hepatic failure in newborn foals. *J. Am. Med. Assoc.* 183: 1407–1413.

65 Mullaney, T.P. and Brown, C.M. (1988). Iron toxicity in neonatal foals. *Equine Vet. J.* 20: 119–124.

66 Acland, H.M., Mann, P.C., Divers, T.J. et al. (1984). Toxic hepatopathy in neonatal foals. *Vet. Pathol.* 21: 3–9.

67 National Library of Medicine (2012). *LiverTox: Clinical and Research Information on Drug-Induced Liver Injury.* Bethesda, MD: National Institute of Diabetes and

Digestive and Kidney Diseases https://www.ncbi.nlm.nih.gov/books/NBK547852.

68 Kancherla, D., Gajendran, M., Vallabhaneni, P. et al. (2013). Metronidazole induced liver injury: a rare immune mediated drug reaction. *Case Rep. Gastrointest. Med.* 2013: 568193.

69 Kim, J.H., Shik Nam, W., Joo Kim, S. et al. (2017). Mechanism investigation of rifampicin-induced liver injury using comparative toxicoproteomics in mice. *Int. J. Mol. Sci.* 18: 1417.

70 Woodhead, J.L., Yang, K., Oldach, D. et al. (2019). Analyzing the mechanisms behind macrolide antibiotic-induced liver injury using quantitative systems toxicology modeling. *Pharm. Res.* 36: 48.

71 Venner, M., Astheimer, K., Lammer, M. et al. (2013). Efficacy of mass antimicrobial treatment of foals with subclinical pulmonary abscesses associated with *Rhodococcus equi*. *J. Vet. Intern. Med.* 27: 171–176.

72 Srihakim, S. and Swerczek, T.W. (1978). Pathologic changes and pathogenesis of *Parascaris equorum* infection in parasite-free pony foals. *Am. J. Vet. Res.* 39: 1155–1160.

73 Brown, P.J. and Clayton, H.M. (1979). Hepatic pathology of experimental *Parascaris equorum* infection in worm-free foals. *J. Comp. Pathol.* 89: 115–123.

74 McCraw, B.M. and Slocombe, J.O.D. (1974). Early development of and pathology associated with *Strongylus edentatus*. *Contin. J. Compend. Med.* 28: 124–138.

75 Paumgartner, G. and Beuers, U. (2002). Ursodeoxycholic acid in cholestatic liver disease: mechanisms of action and therapeutic use revisited. *Hepatology* 36: 525–531.

76 Divers, T.J. (2015). The equine liver in health and disease. *AAEP Proc.* 61: 66–103.

77 Vandeweerd, J.M., Cambier, C., and Gustin, P. (2013). Nutraceuticals for canine liver disease: assessing the evidence. *Vet. Clin. Small Anim.* 43: 1171–1179.

78 Flatland, B. (2003). Botanicals, vitamins, and minerals and the liver: therapeutic applications and potential toxicities. *Compend. Contin. Educ.* 25: 514–524.

79 Twedt, D.C. (2001). A review of traditional and not so traditional therapies for liver disease. In: *Proceedings, 19th Annual American College of Veterinary Internal Medicine Forum*, 610–612. Denver, CO: ACVIM.

80 Hackett, E.S., Mama, K.R., Twedt, D.C. et al. (2013). Pharmacokinetics and safety of silibinin in horses. *Am. J. Vet. Res.* 74: 1327–1332.

81 Igimi, H., Asakawa, S., Tamura, R. et al. (1994). DMSO preparation as a direct solubilizer of calcium bilirubinate stones. *Hepatogastroenterology* 41: 65–69.

Neonatal Endocrine System

Chapter 20 Endocrine Physiology in the Neonatal Foal

Ramiro E. Toribio, Katarzyna A. Dembek, Laura D. Hostnik, and Teresa A. Burns

The ontogeny of multiple organs and body systems in the equine embryo and fetus requires coordinated endocrine differentiation and maturation to modulate development. Additionally, in health, several homeostatic systems are functional and work in synchrony during the transition from intra- to extrauterine life and in response to physiological needs, stressors and illnesses to maintain the foal viable during this critical period. The endocrinology of the equine pregnancy differs from other species. Endocrine maturation in the equine fetus occurs at different stages, with most taking place a few days before parturition and continuing after birth. In addition, gestational length in the mare is variable and early foaling or induction can result in a premature, dysmature, maladapted, or septic foal. Delayed differentiation or abnormal endocrine response to postpartum challenges can lead to organ dysfunction, especially systems that rely on hormones secreted in late pregnancy for proper differentiation. For example, cortisol promotes skeletal, cardiovascular, respiratory, thyroid gland, adrenomedullary and pancreatic development; thyroid hormones are essential for neurologic, skeletal, respiratory, adrenal, and pancreatic function; and catecholamines influence the function of the adrenal gland cortex. Inappropriate hormone secretion during development (e.g. prematurity, maladaptation) or in response to diseases (e.g. sepsis) can be devastating to newborn foals. Therefore, an overview of general aspects of endocrinology as well as foal-specific information enhances our understanding of equine neonatal physiology, facilitates our ability to interpret clinical and laboratory findings, and influences therapies and prognosis. A summary of abbreviations used in this section is below:

Abbreviations

$1,25(OH)_2D_3$	1,25-Dihydroxyvitamin D_3
$25(OH)D_3$	25-Hydroxyvitamin D_3
3β-HSD	3β-Hydroxysteroid dehydrogenase
ACE	Angiotensin-converting enzyme
ACTH	Adrenocorticotropic hormone
ADH	Anti-diuretic hormone
ADM	Adrenomedullin
AMPA	α-Amino-3-hydroxy-5-methyl-4-isoxazolepropionic acid
ANF	Atrial natriuretic factor
ANG-II	Angiotensin II
ANP	Atrial natriuretic peptide
AVP	Arginine vasopressin
BDNF	Brain-derived neurotropic factor
BNP	Brain natriuretic peptide
Ca	Calcium
Ca^{2+}	Ionized or active calcium
CBG	Corticosteroid-binding globulin
Cl^-	Chloride
CNS	Central nervous system
CRH	Corticotropin-releasing hormone
CT	Calcitonin
DHEA	Dehydroepiandrosterone
DHEAS	DHEA sulfate
DIT	Diiodotyrosine
DOC	Deoxycorticosterone
EGF	Epidermal growth factor
EIA	Enteroinsular axis
ET-1	Endothelin-1
FFA	Free fatty acid

Equine Neonatal Medicine, First Edition. Edited by David M. Wong and Pamela A. Wilkins.

FGF-23	Fibroblast growth factor-23
fT_3	Free T_3
fT_4	Free T_4
GABA	Gamma-aminobutyric acid
$GABA_AR$	GABA type A receptor
GH	Growth hormone
GHIH	Growth hormone inhibiting hormone
GHRH	Growth hormone releasing hormone
GIP	Glucose-dependent insulinotropic polypeptide
GLP-1	Glucagon-like peptide-1
GLP-2	Glucagon-like peptide-2
HPAA	Hypothalamic–pituitary–adrenal axis
HPTA	Hypothalamic–pituitary-thyroid axis
IGF-1	Insulin-like growth factor-1
K^+	Potassium
LPS	Lipopolysaccharide
MC2R	Melanocortin type 2 receptor
Mg	Magnesium
Mg^{2+}	Ionized or active magnesium
MIT	Monoiodotyrosine
mPRs	Membrane progesterone receptors
Na^+	Sodium
NCX	Na^+/Ca^{2+} exchanger
NE	Neonatal encephalopathy
NEFA	Non-esterified fatty acids
NIS	Sodium Iodide symporter
NMDA	N-Methyl-D-aspartate
NMDAR	NMDA receptor
NO	Nitric oxide
NTIS	Nonthyroidal illness syndrome
PMCA	Plasma membrane Ca2+ ATPase
PO_4	Phosphorus or phosphate
POMC	Proopiomelanocortin
PP	Pancreatic polypeptide
PTH	Parathyroid hormone
PTHrP	Parathyroid hormone-related protein
PVN	Paraventricular nucleus
RAAS	Renin-angiotensin-aldosterone system
rT_3	Reverse T_3
T_3	Triiodothyronine
T_4	Thyroxine
TBPA	Thyroid-binding prealbumin
TCa	Total calcium
TH	Thyroid hormone
THDOC	Tetrahydrodeoxy-corticosterone
TMg	Total magnesium
TRH	Thyrotropin-releasing hormone
TSH	Thyroid stimulating hormone
tT_3	Total T_3
tT_4	Total T_4

Section I The Hypothalamic-Pituitary-Adrenal Axis and Steroid Hormones

Ramiro E. Toribio, Katarzyna A. Dembek, Laura D. Hostnik, and Teresa A. Burns

The Hypothalamic-Pituitary-Adrenal Axis (HPAA)

The hypothalamic-pituitary-adrenal axis (HPAA) is a complex regulatory system that modulates numerous functions (metabolism, pain, hunger, thirst, blood pressure, electrolyte balance, autonomic activity, immunity, sexual behavior, fetal maturation), as well as the stress response to assure organ function and survival. The HPAA consists of the hypothalamus, which secretes corticotrophin-releasing hormone (CRH) and arginine vasopressin (AVP) that stimulate the pituitary gland to release adrenocorticotropic hormone (ACTH), which stimulates the adrenal cortex to secrete glucocorticoids (cortisol), mineralocorticoids (aldosterone), sex steroids (androgens and progestogens), and steroid precursors [1–4]. The HPAA plays a central role in the transition from intra- to extrauterine life in equine neonates [5] and is activated during perinatal illnesses; HPAA dysfunction has been documented in critically ill and premature foals [3, 6–9].

Corticotropin-Releasing Hormone and Arginine Vasopressin

Under stress or physiological needs, the hypothalamus secretes CRH and AVP. CRH (41 amino acids) is synthesized by parvocellular neurons in the paraventricular nucleus (PVN) of the hypothalamus and released in the portal system of the median eminence to bind CRH receptors (CRH-1) on pituitary corticotropes to elicit synthesis and secretion of ACTH and other proopiomelanocortin (POMC)-derived peptides. In other species, the placenta is also a source of CRH that is released into fetal circulation, perhaps to directly promote cortisol synthesis [10]. CRH stimulates the adrenal cortex and enhances the adrenocortical response to ACTH to increase the synthesis of dehydroepiandrosterone (DHEA) and cortisol [10]. Whether a similar process occurs in the equine fetus is unknown. However, both CRH and ACTH injections to equine fetuses increased progestagen concentrations in the mare [11]. Factors that modulate CRH secretion include brain-derived neurotropic factor (BDNF), cytokines, lipopolysaccharides (LPS), glucocorticoids, neurosteroids, nitric oxide (NO), glutamate (via N-methyl-D-aspartate [NMDA] receptors), gamma-aminobutyric acid (GABA; through GABA receptors), angiotensin II, endocannabinoids, opioids and other factors. CRH plays a permissive role in HPAA regulation during chronic stress, while AVP is a dynamic modulator of ACTH release in response to CRH [1, 12].

Arginine Vasopressin

Arginine vasopressin (nine amino acids) is synthesized by magnocellular and parvocellular neurons (vasopressinergic) located in the PVN and supraoptic nucleus. Magnocellular neurons project to the neurohypophysis where AVP (and oxytocin) is stored to be released in response to hypotension, hyperosmolality, and angiotensin-II. These are the pressor and blood volume-regulatory functions of AVP. A subset of neurons (mainly parvocellular) release AVP in the portal system of the median eminence to bind V3 receptors on pituitary corticotropes to stimulate ACTH secretion [2, 13–15]. These are the HPAA-modulatory functions of AVP. Factors that promote AVP secretion include hypovolemia, hyperosmolality, angiotensin-II, BDNF, neurosteroids, pain, stress, and inflammation (cytokines, LPS, NO) [13, 14]. AVP from the neurohypophysis mediates vasoconstriction via V1 receptors on vascular smooth muscle and aquaporin-facilitated

Equine Neonatal Medicine, First Edition. Edited by David M. Wong and Pamela A. Wilkins.

water reabsorption in the renal collecting tubules via V2 receptors to maintain blood pressure, blood volume, and osmolality. In the equine fetus, plasma AVP concentrations increase with gestational age and are correlated with cortisol concentrations [16]. Plasma AVP concentrations do not change with age in healthy foals [17]. Plasma AVP and CRH concentrations increase in sick foals during critical illness and hypotension [6, 18–20].

Adrenocorticotropic Hormone

Adrenocorticotropic hormone (39 amino acids) is the main pituitary stress hormone derived from post-translational processing of POMC. The primary action of ACTH is to maintain adrenocortical size, structure, and function, therefore, HPAA activity. Through the melanocortin type 2 receptor (MC2R), ACTH stimulates steroidogenesis, increasing the synthesis and secretion of cortisol and, to a lesser extent, other adrenocortical steroids [9]. Cytokines, LPS, thyrotropin-releasing hormone (TRH), glucocorticoids, endocannabinoids, hypoglycemia, and NO also influence ACTH secretion. In the equine fetus, changes in ACTH secretion and glucocorticoid response increase over time [5, 21]. Plasma ACTH concentrations are high in critically ill foals [3, 6–9].

Cortisol

Cortisol is synthesized in response to ACTH stimulation. It binds to glucocorticoid receptors present in most cells and has a multitude of functions including immune modulation, neuromodulation, energy homeostasis, maintenance of vascular tone and blood pressure, tissue differentiation, behavior, and mediates the systemic stress response. Cortisol also increases gluconeogenesis, glycemia and lipolysis, and inhibits insulin-mediated glucose uptake and lipogenesis [2, 14]. By promoting fat and amino acid mobilization, cortisol makes these substrates available to meet energy demands in response to stress or physiological needs. Endogenous glucocorticoids have anti-inflammatory and immunosuppressive effects, which are central to their immune-modulatory effects [2, 14]. Cortisol has direct and indirect negative feedback effects on the hypothalamus and pituitary gland by decreasing the secretion of CRH, ACTH, and AVP. In regard to equine fetal development, cortisol concentrations increase at the end of gestation, which is essential for organ maturation and differentiation that are crucial in the transition to extrauterine life [2, 5, 13, 22]. This is evident for the musculoskeletal, gastrointestinal, respiratory, and endocrine systems [5, 23–27]. Most critically ill foals have elevations in cortisol concentrations [3, 6–9].

Sex Steroids

Sex steroids, including progestogens, androgens, and estrogens, are classified by their main roles in reproductive function. Estradiol (estrogen) and progesterone (progestogen) are the major hormones produced by the ovary and testosterone (androgen) by the testis. In variable degrees and depending on the species, progestogens, androgens, and estrogens are also produced by the fetal adrenal glands, fetal gonads, and the fetoplacental unit. The equine fetal adrenal gland and gonads release large amounts of progestogens and androgens into circulation that are processed by the fetomaternal unit into metabolites (progestogens, androgens, estrogens) that are subsequently transferred to fetal and maternal circulation to exert specific functions. The role of sex steroids in the pathogenesis of perinatal disorders is poorly understood, however, high progesterone, androgen, and estrogen concentrations have been measured in premature, maladjusted, and septic foals [3, 9, 28–35]. Androgen precursors have been proposed as markers of adrenal insufficiency in foals [3, 9, 30, 35].

In people and animals, CRH, ACTH and cortisol are secreted in a circadian fashion, mediated by inputs from the pineal gland and suprachiasmatic nucleus of the hypothalamus. The highest hormone concentrations are measured in the morning and lowest in the evening [1, 36]. Of interest, a circadian rhythm for cortisol secretion was observed in horses, but not neonatal foals (<5 days old) [37, 38]. The mean 24-hour cortisol concentration was lower in foals; however, daily endogenous cortisol production was higher in foals than horses, suggesting increased cortisol clearance in foals [37]. ACTH is released in irregular (time and amplitude) peaks that occur about 10 times per hour in the horse [1, 12].

The HPAA, Steroids, and Equine Fetal Maturation

In foals, the adrenal glands lie retroperitoneally on the medial cranial pole of each kidney. Fetal adrenal weight increases at the end of gestation from 60 mg/kg of body weight at 300 days gestation to 100 mg/kg at term [5, 39]. The adrenal glands develop from two separate embryological tissues: the medulla is derived from neural crest cells in proximity to the dorsal aorta, while the cortex develops from intermediate mesoderm (urogenital ridge) [40]. The adrenal cortex consists of three zones: the outermost *zona glomerulosa* secretes mineralocorticoids (aldosterone) in response to angiotensin II, hyperkalemia, and changes in extracellular fluid osmolality (sodium [Na^+], chloride [Cl^-]); the *zona fasciculata* secretes glucocorticoids (cortisol) in response to ACTH stimulation; and the *zona reticularis* produces sex steroids [2, 38, 41]. These steroids are synthesized from cholesterol. Functions of the adrenal cortex include maintenance of fluid and electrolyte balance, immune modulation, energy metabolism, and tissue differentiation. Removal or destruction of the adrenal glands leads to death unless exogenous steroids are administered [1, 41].

The main circulating adrenocortical steroids include cortisol, aldosterone, DHEA, pregnenolone, progesterone, and 17α-hydroxyprogesterone. Other steroids can be measured during pregnancy in maternal and fetal circulation. Some of these steroids are neuroactive or can be used as precursors in other organs (placenta, brain). *Cortisol* (glucocorticoid) has a multitude of functions related to immunity, energy regulation, vascular tone, blood pressure, and tissue differentiation. *Aldosterone* (mineralocorticoid) is central to blood pressure regulation through renal Na^+ and Cl^- reabsorption and potassium [K^+] excretion. *Progestogens* (aka progestagens) serve as steroid precursors but also have other functions, including regulation of neuronal and glial activity and immune modulation. *Androgens* have masculinizing affects, are anabolic, have neuroactive properties, and serve as precursors to other steroids, including estrogens. DHEA can modify the stress response and immune function by antagonizing the effect of glucocorticoids [42]. *Estrogens* are not a major product of the adrenal gland, but can be measured during pregnancy in the dam and fetus. In the brain, pregnenolone, progesterone, and DHEA can be converted into neuroactive steroids (e.g., allopregnanolone, tetrahydrodeoxycorticosterone [THDOC]) [3, 29]. Elevated concentrations of neurosteroids may contribute to the pathogenesis of neonatal encephalopathy (NE) in foals [3, 30, 35, 43].

In foals, maturation of the HPAA occurs late in gestation and continues in the first week of life [3, 5, 21, 38, 40, 41, 44–47]. Before day 300 of gestation, ACTH has minimal effect on adrenocortical steroidogenesis [5, 21, 44]. Thereafter, there is a slow increase in cortisol concentrations, but ACTH mainly stimulates progestogen synthesis [5]. Approximately 5 days before foaling, cortisol concentrations start increasing in parallel with increases in ACTH concentrations [5, 44], reaching maximum values 30–60 minutes after birth to subsequently decrease to baseline by 24 hours of age [5, 44, 47]. Foals are also born with high concentrations of deoxycorticosterone, a precursor of aldosterone, that also has mineralocorticoid activity [30]. Immediately after birth, cortisol response to ACTH is highest and returns to baseline after 3–5 days of age [5]. Of interest, the cortisol response to the stress of hypoglycemia in 12-hour-old foals is minimal, noticeable by 3 days of age, and highest at 1 week of age [5]. This is probably related to increasing capacity of the pituitary gland to secrete ACTH days after birth [48]. These postnatal dynamic changes in cortisol response to stress further indicate that the HPAA continues to adapt and mature after birth in the foal. This is also relevant to energy homeostasis. A complication of timing of birth and maturity is evident in term versus premature foals, where cortisol concentrations are several fold higher in term compared to premature foals at birth and over time [5, 26, 27, 47]. This likely impairs function of many body systems (e.g., energy regulation, tissue perfusion) with negative implications to survival.

In equids, the fetal peripartum ACTH and cortisol peaks occur immediately after birth while in other species this occurs before birth [5, 21, 27]. In the last week of gestation there is a major fetal adrenocortical enzymatic shift leading to a cortisol rise together with a reduction in progestogen concentrations [5, 44, 49–53]. These endocrine changes are also noted in the pregnant mare, where progestogens increase in the last 2 weeks of pregnancy reflecting endocrine activity of the uteroplacental unit [5, 44, 49–55]. In maternal circulation, progestogens peak 2–4 days before foaling then rapidly drop while cortisol peaks just before foaling [54, 55]. These progestogens consist of pregnenolone, progesterone, 5α-dihydroprogesterone, allopregnanolone, 20α-dihydroprogesterone, and 3β, 20α-dihydroprogesterone [55]. From birth until 3 months of age, there are minimal changes in cortisol concentrations, but ACTH concentrations increase during this time [48]. Therefore, it is important to use age-specific reference intervals when assessing HPAA function in neonatal foals (Tables 20.I.1 and 20.I.2) [2].

Chronological variations in adrenocortical steroid synthesis and secretion result from sequential changes in steroidogenic enzyme expression [5, 63]. In the equine fetal adrenal cortex, from day 150 until birth there is an incremental expression of enzymes involved in the conversion of cholesterol to pregnenolone (cholesterol side-chain cleavage enzyme; P450scc), pregnenolone to progesterone (3β-Hydroxysteroid dehydrogenase; 3β-HSD), and downstream synthesis of glucocorticoids, androgens, and estrogens (cytochrome P450 17A1; CYP17A1) [63, 64]. The equine fetal adrenal gland produces corticosterone and deoxycorticosterone in early to mid-gestation and cortisol synthesis later on, indicating the presence of 3β-HSD, but minimal activity of terminal enzymes for glucocorticoid synthesis (e.g., CYP17A1) [64]. Expression is negligible before day 280 but high after day 310 [63]. This expression parallels increased activity of enzymes involved in catecholamine synthesis in the adrenal medulla [63].

The adrenal gland represents two endocrine organs with different embryological origins (neural crest – medulla; coelomic epithelium/mesoderm – cortex) and functions that are highly interactive. Adrenocortical and chromaffin cells have a close relationship during development and after birth. Cortisol influences the differentiation of

Table 20.I.1 Blood concentrations of total cortisol, free cortisol, CBG, ACTH, AVP and CRH in healthy foals (mean ± SD)

Age	<4h	4–12h	12–24h	36–48h	48–96h	5–7 days	14 days
Total cortisol	10.2 ± 2.3 μg/dl [56] 32 ± 9.6 ng/ml [48]	2.7 ± 1.3 μg/dl [7]	3.6 ± 1.6 μg/dl [7] 27.2 ± 7.8 ng/ml [48] 52.7 ± 27.3 nmol/l [57] 2.76 (0.8–28.4) [3][a] 52 (10–1100) nmol/L [6] 4.05 ± 3.02 μg/dl [8] 8.6 (2.6–14.5) ng/ml [58] [b]	2.6 ± 1 μg/dl [7] 29.8 ± 6 ng/ml [48]	2.5 ± 0.6 μg/dl [59] 28.5 ± 7 ng/ml [48]	2 ± 0.8 μg/dl [7] 26.5 ± 3.9 ng/ml [48]	24.9± 6.2 ng/ml [48]
Free cortisol	6.0 ± 1.8 μg/dl [60]		1.9 ±1.5 μg/dl [60]	1.1 ± 0.5 μg/dl [60]		0.6 ± 0.3 μg/dl [60]	
CBG	45.9 ± 2.2 nM [45]						
ACTH	285.5 ± 284.8 pg/ml [56] 16 ± 7.1 pg/ml [48]	28.8 ± 20.9 pg/ml [7]	19.6 ± 5.3 pg/ml [56] 23.7 ± 5.7 pg/ml [48] 24.4 (10–279) pg/ml [3][a] 16.6 ± 6.3 pg/ml [57] 5.2 (3–140) pmol/L [6] 44.16 ± 42.75 pg/ml [8] 18.2 (15.3–31.1) pg/ml [58][b]	32.7 ± 26.4 pg/ml [56] 34.7 ± 7.2 pg/ml [48]	37.9 ± 13.5 pg/ml [48]	33.8 ± 23.1 pg/ml [56] 36.4 ± 7.8 pg/ml [48]	26.8 ± 5.3 pg/ml [48]
AVP	4.8 ± 1.7 pg/ml [17]		4.6 (2.2–60) pmol/L [6] [a] 10.2 (2.15–35.7) pg/ml [61][c] 1.66 (0.38–52.85) pmol/l [18][a] 2.9 (0–79.0) pmol/l [19][a]	0 (0–5.7) pmol/L [19][a]	5.5 ± 2.9 pg/ml [17] 0 (0–3.6) pmol/l [19] [a]	6.2 ± 2.6 pg/ml [17]	6.2 ± 2.7 pg/ml [17]
CRH			12.09 ± 5.8 pg/ml [62]				

CBG = corticosteroid-binding globulin; ACTH = adrenocorticotropic hormone; AVP = arginine vasopressin; CRH = corticotropin-releasing hormone.
[a] Median and range
[b] Median and interquartiles
[c] Median and 25–75th percentile

Table 20.I.2 Published studies on ACTH stimulation tests in healthy neonatal foals

Author	Age	N	ACTH dose	Delta cortisol 30 min (μg/dl)	Delta cortisol 60 min (μg/dl)
Hart et al [59]	3–4 days	10	10 μg	2.4 ± 1	
	3–4 days	10	100 μg	5.0 ± 2.2	
	3–4 days	6	250 μg	5.6 ± 2.1	
Hart et al [56]	Birth	11	10 μg	3.6 ± 2.0	
	12–24 h	10	10 μg	5.5 ± 2.1	
	36–48 h	10	10 μg	3.5 ± 1.7	
	5–7 days	11	10 μg	1.3 ± 0.6	
	Birth	11	100 μg	6.4 ± 4.1	
	12–24 h	10	100 μg	9.4 ± 3.5	
	36–48 h	10	100 μg	6.8 ± 3.4	
	5–7 days	11	100 μg	3.5 ± 1.3	
Wong et al [48]	Birth	13	0.1 μg/kg	8.36 ± 1.42	5.8 ± 1.11
	3 days	13	0.1 μg/kg	3.68 ± 0.64	2.29 ± 0.4
	5 days	13	0.1 μg/kg	3.49 ± 0.66	2.41 ± 0.33
	7 days	13	0.1 μg/kg	3.42 ± 0.51	2.27 ± 0.48
	14 days	13	0.1 μg/kg	3.37 ± 0.66	2.24 ± 0.46
	21 days	13	0.1 μg/kg	3.53 ± 0.45	2.38 ± 0.39
Dembek et al [9]	< 48 h	13	10 μg	125 (1.3 to 316) [a]	

[a] Median and range (percent change from baseline cortisol 30 after ACTH stimulation)

chromaffin cells in the medulla and enzymes involved in catecholamine synthesis such as phenylethanolamine N-methyltransferase that are cortisol-dependent in the horse [16, 63]. At least in other species, the presence of chromaffin cells facilitates the effect of ACTH and CRH on cortisol production as part of the intra-adrenal CRH-ACTH system [10, 65]. As noted, catecholamine secretion at the end of gestation in the equine fetus parallels cortisol concentrations [5, 16, 40, 66–68]. These coordinated changes in enzymatic expression and interactions among endocrine systems are essential in preparing the fetus for birth and explain many abnormalities observed in premature or dysmature foals.

In most species, 80–90% of circulating cortisol is bound to corticosteroid-binding globulin (CBG), which functions as a reservoir and protects against excessive amounts of free cortisol. Unbound or free steroids are biologically active, and important to be in equilibrium with protein-bound fractions. In the equine fetus, as ACTH and cortisol increase, CBG concentrations decrease to its lowest value at birth, with a large fraction of free plasma cortisol (30–60%) [37, 38]. This amplifies exposure of fetal tissues to higher concentrations of bioactive cortisol [38, 40]. At birth, plasma CBG concentrations are lower in foals compared to other species [45]. However, after birth CBG concentrations increase in foals while in other species, they decrease [37, 38, 40]. It is possible that plasma cortisol binding capacity in foals may be supplemented by unidentified proteins [45].

During development, progestogens, directly or as precursors, play major roles in organ differentiation. They are processed by uteroplacental tissues into other progestogens, androgens, estrogens, and neuroactive steroids that are transferred to both fetal and maternal circulation [5, 28, 31, 49–51]. As gestation advances, progestogens in the fetal adrenal cortex serve as glucocorticoid precursors. In addition to the adrenal gland, the fetal gonads are a source of steroid precursors [5, 69–72]. The function of many of these steroids remain unknown.

Temporal changes in adrenocortical cortisol response to exogenous ACTH have been documented in newborn foals using low and high ACTH doses [2, 48, 56]. Foals born prematurely often have poor cortisol response to exogenous ACTH and may have high ACTH concentrations that could be explained by reduced adrenocortical sensitivity to ACTH and decreased inhibitory effects of glucocorticoids over the hypothalamus and pituitary gland [5, 26, 27, 41, 44, 73]. The importance of glucocorticoids at the end of gestation is evident in foals from mares treated with dexamethasone that are born earlier and are small but often viable [74].

These foals usually have normal cortisol concentrations, indicating that their hypothalamus and pituitary gland may be refractory to glucocorticoids at the end of pregnancy, similar to premature foals. After birth, these foals may have reduced adrenocortical response to ACTH that could indicate adrenal insufficiency [74]. This provides insight into the importance of coordinated HPAA function, fetal maturity, and delivery. The reduced inhibitory effect of glucocorticoids over the HPAA during development was demonstrated in a study where mares had similar progestagen increases in response to betamethasone, ACTH, and CRH injections to their fetuses indicating that maternal increases in progestogens before foaling are the result of fetal adrenocortical activity [11]. It also suggests that fetal glucocorticoids influence progestagen synthesis in the fetus and fetoplacental unit. The fetal gonads contribute to circulating steroids in the fetus and mare, but their function seems to be more important earlier in gestation.

Foals are born with high concentrations of cortisol, pregnenolone, progesterone, 17α-hydroxyprogesterone, deoxycorticosterone, DHEA, DHEAS, testosterone, androstenedione, 5α-dihydrotestosterone, 17β-estradiol, and estrone sulfate, which decline rapidly by 1–5 days of age [3, 9, 20, 29–35]. In one study in healthy newborn foals, progesterone and pregnenolone dropped by 24 hours compared to DHEA, DHEAS, and deoxycorticosterone that decreased to low values by 72–96 hours [30]. In another study focused on androgens, DHEAS, androstenedione, testosterone, and 5α-dihydrotestosterone decreased by 72 hours [35]. Of interest, progesterone, androgens, and estrogens remained elevated in proportion to severity of illness [3, 29, 32–35], suggesting increased adrenocortical production or reduced steroid clearance [34, 35]. Allopregnanolone concentrations at birth are low and change minimally in healthy foals after birth, however, increase in sick foals and those with NE [20]. In contrast, progestogens, androgens, and estrogens remain elevated in sick foals, and their concentrations as well as time to decrease have been associated with disease severity and mortality [3, 9, 20, 29–35].

Equine Pregnancy and Relevance to the Foal

The endocrinology of equine pregnancy has unique features compared to other species [53, 69]. In the pregnant mare, progesterone and 17α-hydroxyprogesterone concentrations increase and remain elevated until week 25 of gestation, when they decrease to negligible values [69, 71]. Thereafter, other progestogens (pregnenolone, 5α-dihydroprogesterone, 20α-dihydroprogesterone, 3β,20α-dihydroprogesterone, allopregnanolone) rise steadily, reflecting adrenocortical function, fetal gonad size, and placental enzymatic activity. Pregnenolone, progesterone, 5α-dihydroprogesterone, and allopregnanolone are the highest progestogens (progestagens; pregnanes) in equine fetal circulation, while 5α-dihydroprogesterone, 20α-dihydroprogesterone, 3β,20α-dihydroprogesterone, and allopregnanolone are the main hormones in maternal circulation, consistent with increased placental 5α-reductase activity [50, 53, 69–71, 75].

Throughout gestation, equine fetal gonads are the major source of pregnenolone, while fetal adrenal glands are the chief contributors to progesterone in fetal circulation [70]. In addition to progestogens, fetal gonads also produce androgens, in particular DHEA that is converted to other androgens (e.g. testosterone) and estrogens by the fetoplacental unit [50, 53, 69–71]. This has implications to equine fetal biology, as it places the gonads as a major contributor to progestogens, androgens, and other steroids to the fetus and mare. The role of these gonadal steroids on the HPAA and fetal development remains unclear. It is well documented that ACTH stimulates adrenocortical steroidogenesis in the equine fetus, neonate, and horse [2, 9, 56, 59, 76], but at least in other species, ACTH also stimulates the fetal gonads [77]. Considering that the gonads and adrenal cortex share their embryological origin and express similar enzymatic machinery, one can speculate that the gonads of the equine fetus may be part of the system that regulates development and programming, in particular in mid-gestation.

As noted, 5–7 days before foaling, there is an adrenocortical enzymatic shift from progestogen to glucocorticoid synthesis, reflected as a drop in progestogens with a parallel increase in fetal ACTH and cortisol concentrations indicating maturation of the HPAA [5]. This is a highly coordinated process, and interference with fetoplacental or adrenocortical function could keep progestogens elevated after birth with implications for fetal to neonatal transition and adaptation to extrauterine life [28, 78]. In support of this concept as it relates to placental disease, blockade of 5α-reductase activity in late-pregnant mares increases progesterone concentrations [53, 79]. As discussed next, increased progestogen concentrations could potentially alter neurological function in the neonate.

Neurosteroids and Neuroactive Steroids

Extensive evidence from other species indicate that progestogens, androgens, and estrogens with neuroactive properties contribute to fetal neuronal plasticity and high concentrations of progestogens in the central nervous system (CNS) are protective and induce a sleep-like state [28, 80–83]. A similar process likely occurs in the equine fetus since progestogen concentrations are high in fetal and maternal circulations at the end of pregnancy, drop rapidly after birth [49, 50, 54, 55, 69, 72], and allopregnanolone has sedative properties in foals [43]. There is valid speculation that steroid imbalances are involved in the pathogenesis of equine NE [3, 28, 29, 35, 43].

Neurosteroids promote neurogenesis, neuronal plasticity, and programming, enhance axon, and dendrite growth, organize neuronal circuits, influence glial cell development and function, facilitate energy conservation, and are neuroprotective. They modulate the HPAA and stress response through CRH and AVP synthesis, protect against glucocorticoid excess that could lead to neurological disorders, and mitigate cerebral hypoxic, ischemic, and traumatic injury [81–85]. Neurosteroids and neuroactive steroids include steroids synthesized from cholesterol in the nervous system and steroid metabolites from peripheral tissues (adrenal gland, gonads, placenta) [3, 81, 83, 85–88]. Neurons and glial cells can synthesize de novo neurosteroids from cholesterol and circulating steroids can readily cross the blood brain barrier to be metabolized in the CNS into neuroactive steroids [28, 80, 81]. The effects of neurosteroids are not mediated by classical intracellular steroid receptor interactions that modulate gene transcription because they are minimally active at cytosolic and nuclear receptors [89]. Rather, their activity is through cell membrane receptors and ion channels [89], which explains their rapid effects when given exogenously (Figure 20.I.1).

Progestogens and neuroactive steroids are positive allosteric modulators of GABA type A ($GABA_A$) receptors and to a lesser extent, the N-Methyl-D-aspartate (NMDA), α-amino-3-hydroxy-5-methyl-4-isoxazolepropionic acid (AMPA), kainate, glycine, serotonin, and sigma 1 (σ1) receptors [87–91]. In the CNS, there are also membrane progesterone receptors (mPRs) [92, 93]. Activation of $GABA_A$ receptors results in Cl^- entry and cell membrane hyperpolarization, reducing neuronal excitability [87, 76–78]. A number of sedatives, anticonvulsants, anxiolytics,

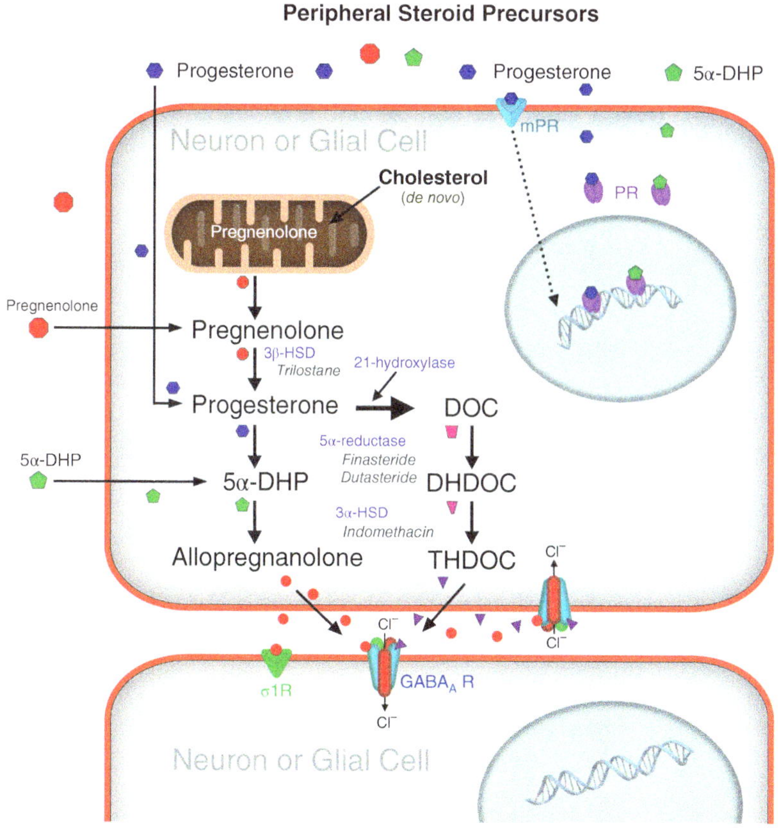

Figure 20.I.1 Synthesis of neurosteroids in the central nervous system. Neurons and glial cells (astrocytes in particular) have the enzymatic machinery for de novo synthesis of neuroactive steroids from cholesterol. These cells can also uptake progestogens and androgens (not shown) from peripheral circulation to convert them into steroid metabolites that affect neuronal function. Neuroactive steroids bind cell membrane ($GABA_AR$, mPR) and intracellular (PR) receptors. Progestogens act through traditional nuclear receptors but their neuroactive properties are mainly through cell membrane receptors ($GABA_AR$, mPR, σ1R). Drugs such as trilostane, finasteride, and indomethacin can inhibit steroidogenic enzymes and have been proposed to treat foal disorders such as NMS. 3α-HSD = 3α-hydroxysteroid dehydrogenase; 3β-HSD = 3β-hydroxysteroid dehydrogenase; 5α-DHP = 5α-dihydroprogesterone; DHDOC = dehydrodeoxycorticosterone; DOC = deoxycorticosterone; THDOC = allotetrahydrodeoxycorticosterone; $GABA_AR$ = γ-aminobutyric acid (GABA) type A receptor; mPR = membrane progesterone receptor; NMS = neonatal maladjustment syndrome; PR = progesterone receptor; σ1R = sigma-1 receptor. *Source:* Image courtesy of Dr. R. E. Toribio, College of Veterinary Medicine, The Ohio State University.

and anesthetics (benzodiazepines, barbiturates, propofol, etomidate, ethanol) work through $GABA_A$ receptors. Allopregnanolone, progesterone, 5α-dihydroprogesterone, pregnanolone, deoxycorticosterone (DOC), and THDOC are potent agonists of $GABA_A$ receptors [91, 94]. Of these, allopregnanolone is considered the main agonist. While emphasis has been placed on the neuroactive properties of progestogens, certain androgens and estrogens also modulate neuronal and glial function and can be considered neurosteroids [95].

Dehydroepiandrosterone is an androgen precursor that can be modified by nervous tissue to more active compounds. Androstanediol is a good illustration of an androgen that potentiates function of $GABA_A$ receptors [83]. Simple steroid modifications can completely change steroid actions. For example, pregnenolone and DHEA have minimal activity over $GABA_A$ receptors; however, their sulfate esters (pregnenolone sulfate; DHEA sulfate) are negative allosteric modulators of $GABA_A$ and glycine, but positive modulators of NMDA receptors [90, 91]. These sulfated steroids are found in high concentrations in equine fetal and neonatal circulation. Through these receptors, neurosteroids exert multiple actions, including neuronal plasticity, glial cell function, energy conservation, neuroprotection, and HPAA modulation [81–85]. Allopregnanolone is a potent neurosteroid that increases during pregnancy and in the fetal brain of multiple species to promote neural development, protect neurons against injury, and induce a sleep-like state while neurons and glial cells differentiate [85]. As noted, it is possible that similar events occur in the equine fetus considering the following:

- Allopregnanolone concentrations are very high in term-pregnant mares and their fetuses [49, 50, 55, 69].
- Major changes in fetal progestogen and glucocorticoid concentrations take place in the last week of pregnancy [5, 50].
- Endogenous pregnanes have sedative effects in foals [43].
- Progestogens may keep late-term fetuses in an unconscious state and facilitate their arousal after birth [96].
- A new generation of anesthetic drugs are based on pregnane precursors [97].

Increased concentrations of pregnenolone, progesterone, 17α-hydroxyprogesterone, allopregnanolone, androstenedione, DHEA sulfate, testosterone, dihydrotestosterone, 17β-estradiol, and estrone sulfate have been measured in critically ill, premature, and NE foals [3, 28–35, 78]. It is reasonable to assume that abnormally high steroids from fetal adrenal glands, gonads, placenta, and perhaps the CNS – as well as steroid imbalances in the CNS – contribute to abnormalities observed in sick newborn foals [28, 78]. It remains to be determined if they promote disease progression or are protective. In other words, they could be proxies for underlying pathophysiological processes.

As mentioned, neurons and glial cells have the enzymatic machinery for neurosteroid synthesis and processing. Of particular interest is 5α-reductase, which is required for conversion of progesterone to 5α-dihydroprogesterone and allopregnanolone, and testosterone to 5α-dihydrotestosterone. This enzyme is inhibited by dutasteride and finasteride, drugs used in men to treat benign prostatic hyperplasia, prostate cancer, and pattern baldness. They have been used anecdotally in foals with NE to reduce neurosteroid synthesis with inconclusive results [78]. One must be cautious with this approach as some of these steroids may be protecting brain cells, and altering their balance could be detrimental.

References

1 Hurcombe, S.D. (2011). Hypothalamic-pituitary gland axis function and dysfunction in horses. *Vet. Clin. North Am. Equine Pract.* 27: 1–17.

2 Hart, K.A. and Barton, M.H. (2011). Adrenocortical insufficiency in horses and foals. *Vet. Clin. North Am. Equine Pract.* 27: 19–34.

3 Dembek, K.A., Timko, K.J., Johnson, L.M. et al. (2017). Steroids, steroid precursors, and neuroactive steroids in critically ill equine neonates. *Vet. J.* 225: 42–49.

4 Annane, D., Pastores, S.M., Arlt, W. et al. (2017). Critical illness-related corticosteroid insufficiency (CIRCI): a narrative review from a Multispecialty Task Force of the Society of Critical Care Medicine (SCCM) and the European Society of Intensive Care Medicine (ESICM). *Intensive Care Med.* 43: 1781–1792.

5 Fowden, A.L., Forhead, A.J., and Ousey, J.C. (2012). Endocrine adaptations in the foal over the perinatal period. *Equine Vet. J. Suppl.* 44: 130–139.

6 Hurcombe, S.D., Toribio, R.E., Slovis, N. et al. (2008). Blood arginine vasopressin, adrenocorticotropin hormone, and cortisol concentrations at admission in septic and critically ill foals and their association with survival. *J. Vet. Intern. Med.* 22: 639–647.

7 Hart, K.A., Slovis, N.M., and Barton, M.H. (2009). Hypothalamic-pituitary-adrenal axis dysfunction in hospitalized neonatal foals. *J. Vet. Intern. Med.* 23: 901–912.

8 Gold, J.R., Divers, T.J., Barton, M.H. et al. (2007). Plasma adrenocorticotropin, cortisol, and adrenocorticotropin/cortisol ratios in septic and normal-term foals. *J. Vet. Intern. Med.* 21: 791–796.

9 Dembek, K.A., Johnson, L.M., Timko, K.J. et al. (2019). Multiple adrenocortical steroid response to administration of exogenous adrenocorticotropic hormone to hospitalized foals. *J. Vet. Intern. Med.* 33: 1766–1774.

10 Xing, Y., Lerario, A.M., Rainey, W., and Hammer, G.D. (2015). Development of adrenal cortex zonation. *Endocrinol. Metab. Clin. North Am.* 44: 243–274.

11 Rossdale, P.D., McGladdery, A.J., Ousey, J.C. et al. (1992). Increase in plasma progestagen concentrations in the mare after foetal injection with CRH, ACTH or betamethasone in late gestation. *Equine Vet. J.* 24: 347–350.

12 Alexander, S.L., Irvine, C.H., and Donald, R.A. (1996). Dynamics of the regulation of the hypothalamo-pituitary-adrenal (HPA) axis determined using a nonsurgical method for collecting pituitary venous blood from horses. *Front. Neuroendocrinol.* 17: 1–50.

13 Badiu, C. (2019). Williams textbook of endocrinology. *Acta Endocrinol. (Buchar)* 15: 416–416.

14 Barrett, K.E., Barman, S.M., Boitano, S. et al. (2016). *Ganong's review of medical physiology*. New York: New York: McGraw Hill Education.

15 Goncharova, N.D. (2013). Stress responsiveness of the hypothalamic-pituitary-adrenal axis: age-related features of the vasopressinergic regulation. *Front. Endocrinol. (Lausanne)* 4: 26.

16 Giussani, D.A., Forhead, A.J., and Fowden, A.L. (2005). Development of cardiovascular function in the horse fetus. *J. Physiol.* 565: 1019–1030.

17 Wong, D.M., Vo, D.T., Alcott, C.J. et al. (2008). Plasma vasopressin concentrations in healthy foals from birth to 3 months of age. *J. Vet. Intern. Med.* 22: 1259–1261.

18 Dembek, K.A., Hurcombe, S.D., Stewart, A.J. et al. (2016). Association of aldosterone and arginine vasopressin concentrations and clinical markers of hypoperfusion in neonatal foals. *Equine Vet. J.* 48: 176–181.

19 Borchers, A., Magdesian, K.G., Schenck, P.A. et al. (2014). Serial plasma vasopressin concentration in healthy and hospitalised neonatal foals. *Equine Vet. J.* 46: 306–310.

20 Dembek, K.A. (2016). Hypothalamic-pituitary-adrenal axis dysfunction in critically ill foals. PhD thesis. The Ohio State University, Columbus, Ohio.

21 Rossdale, P.D., Ousey, J.C., and Chavatte, P. (1997). Readiness for birth: an endocrinological duet between fetal foal and mare. *Equine Vet. J. Suppl.* 29: 96–99.

22 Fowden, A.L., Giussani, D.A., and Forhead, A.J. (2020). Physiological development of the equine fetus during late gestation. *Equine Vet. J.* 52: 165–173.

23 Fowden, A.L., Silver, M., Ellis, L. et al. (1984). Studies on equine prematurity 3: Insulin secretion in the foal during the perinatal period. *Equine Vet. J.* 16: 286–291.

24 Rossdale, P.D. (1993). Clinical view of disturbances in equine foetal maturation. *Equine Vet. J. Suppl.* 25: 3–7.

25 Rossdale, P.D., Ousey, J.C., Silver, M., and Fowden, A. (1984). Studies on equine prematurity 6: Guidelines for assessment of foal maturity. *Equine Vet. J.* 16: 300–302.

26 Silver, M., Fowden, A.L., Knox, J. et al. (1991). Relationship between circulating tri-iodothyronine and cortisol in the perinatal period in the foal. *J. Reprod. Fertil. Suppl.* 44: 619–626.

27 Silver, M., Ousey, J.C., Dudan, F.E. et al. (1984). Studies on equine prematurity 2: Post natal adrenocortical activity in relation to plasma adrenocorticotrophic hormone and catecholamine levels in term and premature foals. *Equine Vet. J.* 16: 278–286.

28 Toribio, R.E. (2019). Equine Neonatal Encephalopathy: Facts, Evidence, and Opinions. *Vet. Clin. North Am. Equine Pract.* 35: 363–378.

29 Aleman, M., Pickles, K.J., Conley, A.J. et al. (2013). Abnormal plasma neuroactive progestagen derivatives in ill, neonatal foals presented to the neonatal intensive care unit. *Equine Vet. J.* 45: 661–665.

30 Aleman, M., McCue, P.M., Chigerwe, M. et al. (2019). Plasma concentrations of steroid precursors, steroids, neuroactive steroids, and neurosteroids in healthy neonatal foals from birth to 7 days of age. *J. Vet. Intern. Med.* 33: 2286–2293.

31 Houghton, E., Holtan, D., Grainger, L. et al. (1991). Plasma progestagen concentrations in the normal and dysmature newborn foal. *J. Reprod. Fertil. Suppl.* 44: 609–617.

32 Rossdale, P.D., Ousey, J.C., McGladdery, A.J. et al. (1995). A retrospective study of increased plasma progestagen concentrations in compromised neonatal foals. *Reprod. Fertil. Dev.* 7: 567–575.

33 Muller, V., Curcio, B.R., Toribio, R.E. et al. (2019). Cortisol, progesterone, 17alphaOHprogesterone, and pregnenolone in foals born from mare's hormone-treated for experimentally induced ascending placentitis. *Theriogenology* 123: 139–144.

34 Swink, J.M. (2020). Sex steroids and the effect of in-utero altrenogest exposure in neonatal foals. Master's thesis. College of Veterinary Medicine, The Ohio State University, Columbus, Ohio.

35 Swink, J.M., Rings, L.M., Snyder, H.A. et al. (2021). Dynamics of androgens in healthy and hospitalized newborn foals. *J. Vet. Intern. Med.* 35: 538–549.

36 Spencer, R.L. and Deak, T. (2017). A users guide to HPA axis research. *Physiol. Behav.* 178: 43–65.

37 Hart, K.A., Dirikolu, L., Ferguson, D.C. et al. (2012). Daily endogenous cortisol production and hydrocortisone pharmacokinetics in adult horses and neonatal foals. *Am. J. Vet. Res.* 73: 68–75.

38 Cudd, T.A., LeBlanc, M., Silver, M. et al. (1995). Ontogeny and ultradian rhythms of adrenocorticotropin and cortisol in the late-gestation fetal horse. *J. Endocrinol.* 144: 271–283.

39 Ousey, J.C. (2004). Peripartal endocrinology in the mare and foetus. *Reprod. Domest. Anim.* 39: 222–231.

40 Fowden, A.L. and Silver, M. (1995). Comparative Development of the Pituitary-Adrenal axis in the Fetal Foal and Lamb. *Reprod. Domest. Anim.* 30: 170–177.

41 Silver, M. and Fowden, A.L. (1995). Sympathoadrenal and other endocrine and metabolic responses to hypoglycaemia in the fetal foal during late gestation. *Exp. Physiol.* 80: 651–662.

42 Beishuizen, A. and Thijs, L.G. (2003). Endotoxin and the hypothalamo-pituitary-adrenal (HPA) axis. *J. Endotoxin Res.* 9: 3–24.

43 Madigan, J.E., Haggettt, E.F., Pickles, K.J. et al. (2012). Allopregnanolone infusion induced neurobehavioural alterations in a neonatal foal: is this a clue to the pathogenesis of neonatal maladjustment syndrome? *Equine Vet. J. Suppl.* 109–112.

44 Silver, M. and Fowden, A.L. (1994). Prepartum adrenocortical maturation in the fetal foal: responses to ACTH. *J. Endocrinol.* 142: 417–425.

45 Irvine, C.H. and Alexander, S.L. (1987). Measurement of free cortisol and the capacity and association constant of cortisol-binding proteins in plasma of foals and adult horses. *J. Reprod. Fertil. Suppl.* 35: 19–24.

46 LeBlanc, M. (1996). Equine perinatology: What we know and what we need to know. *Anim. Reprod. Sci.* 42: 189.

47 Nathanielsz, P.W., Rossdale, P.D., Silver, M. et al. (1975). Studies on fetal, neonatal and maternal cortisol metabolism in the mare. *J. Reprod. Fertil. Suppl.* 23: 625–630.

48 Wong, D.M., Vo, D.T., Alcott, C.J. et al. (2009). Adrenocorticotropic hormone stimulation tests in healthy foals from birth to 12 weeks of age. *Can. J. Vet. Res.* 73: 65–72.

49 Holtan, D.W., Houghton, E., Silver, M. et al. (1991). Plasma progestagens in the mare, fetus and newborn foal. *J. Reprod. Fertil. Suppl.* 44: 517–528.

50 Ousey, J.C., Forhead, A.J., Rossdale, P.D. et al. (2003). Ontogeny of uteroplacental progestagen production in pregnant mares during the second half of gestation. *Biol. Reprod.* 69: 540–548.

51 Ousey, J.C., Fowden, A.L., Rossdale, P.D. et al. (2001). Plasma progestagens as markers of feto-placental health. *Pferdeheilkunde* 17: 574–578.

52 Ousey, J.C., Rossdale, P.D., Fowden, A.L. et al. (2004). Effects of manipulating intrauterine growth on post natal adrenocortical development and other parameters of maturity in neonatal foals. *Equine Vet. J.* 36: 616–621.

53 Fowden, A.L., Forhead, A.J., and Ousey, J.C. (2008). The Endocrinology of equine parturition. *Exp. Clin. Endocrinol. Diabetes* 116: 393–403.

54 Nagel, C., Erber, R., Bergmaier, C. et al. (2012). Cortisol and progestin release, heart rate and heart rate variability in the pregnant and postpartum mare, fetus and newborn foal. *Theriogenology* 78: 759–767.

55 Legacki, E.L., Corbin, C.J., Ball, B.A. et al. (2016). Progestin withdrawal at parturition in the mare. *Reproduction* 152: 323–331.

56 Hart, K.A., Heusner, G.L., Norton, N.A. et al. (2009). Hypothalamic-pituitary-adrenal axis assessment in healthy term neonatal foals utilizing a paired low dose/high dose ACTH stimulation test. *J. Vet. Intern. Med.* 23: 344–351.

57 Stewart, A.J., Wright, J.C., Behrend, E.N. et al. (2013). Validation of a low-dose adrenocorticotropic hormone stimulation test in healthy neonatal foals. *J. Am. Vet. Med. Assoc.* 243: 399–405.

58 Armengou, L., Jose-Cunilleras, E., Rios, J. et al. (2013). Metabolic and endocrine profiles in sick neonatal foals are related to survival. *J. Vet. Intern. Med.* 27: 567–575.

59 Hart, K.A., Ferguson, D.C., Heusner, G.L. et al. (2007). Synthetic adrenocorticotropic hormone stimulation tests in healthy neonatal foals. *J. Vet. Intern. Med.* 21: 314–321.

60 Hart, K.A., Barton, M.H., Ferguson, D.C. et al. (2011). Serum free cortisol fraction in healthy and septic neonatal foals. *J. Vet. Intern. Med.* 25: 345–355.

61 Hollis, A.R., Boston, R.C., and Corley, K.T. (2008). Plasma aldosterone, vasopressin and atrial natriuretic peptide in hypovolaemia: a preliminary comparative study of neonatal and mature horses. *Equine Vet. J.* 40: 64–69.

62 Dembek, K. (2017). Corticotropin releasing hormone in foals with adrenal insufficiency. *J. Vet. Intern. Med.* 31: 1340.

63 Han, X., Fowden, A.L., Silver, M. et al. (1995). Immunohistochemical localisation of steroidogenic enzymes and phenylethanolamine-N-methyl-transferase (PNMT) in the adrenal gland of the fetal and newborn foal. *Equine Vet. J.* 27: 140–146.

64 Chavatte, P., Rossdale, P.D., and Tait, A.D. (1995). Corticosteroid Synthesis by the Equine Fetal Adrenal. *Biol. Reprod.* 52: 13–20.

65 Silverman, M.N., Pearce, B.D., Biron, C.A. et al. (2005). Immune modulation of the hypothalamic-pituitary-adrenal (HPA) axis during viral infection. *Viral Immunol.* 18: 41–78.

66 Forhead, A.J., Broughton Pipkin, F., and Fowden, A.L. (2000). Effect of cortisol on blood pressure and the renin-angiotensin system in fetal sheep during late gestation. *J. Physiol.* 526 (Pt 1): 167–176.

67 Forhead, A.J., Broughton Pipkin, F., Taylor, P.M. et al. (2000). Developmental changes in blood pressure and the renin-angiotensin system in pony fetuses during the second half of gestation. *J. Reprod. Fertil. Suppl.* 56: 693–703.

68 Giussani, D.A., Forhead, A.J., Gardner, D.S. et al. (2003). Postnatal cardiovascular function after manipulation of fetal growth by embryo transfer in the horse. *J. Physiol.* 547: 67–76.

69 Conley, A.J. (2016). Review of the reproductive endocrinology of the pregnant and parturient mare. *Theriogenology* 86: 355–365.

70 Legacki, E.L., Ball, B.A., Corbin, C.J. et al. (2017). Equine fetal adrenal, gonadal and placental steroidogenesis. *Reproduction* 154: 445–454.

71 Legacki, E.L., Scholtz, E.L., Ball, B.A. et al. (2016). The dynamic steroid landscape of equine pregnancy mapped by mass spectrometry. *Reproduction* 151: 421–430.

72 Hamon, M., Clarke, S.W., Houghton, E. et al. (1991). Production of 5 alpha-dihydroprogesterone during late pregnancy in the mare. *J. Reprod. Fertil. Suppl.* 44: 529–535.

73 Rossdale, P.D., Silver, M., Ellis, L. et al. (1982). Response of the adrenal cortex to tetracosactrin (ACTH1-24) in the premature and full-term foal. *J. Reprod. Fertil. Suppl.* 32: 545–553.

74 Ousey, J.C., Kolling, M., Kindahl, H. et al. (2011). Maternal dexamethasone treatment in late gestation induces precocious fetal maturation and delivery in healthy Thoroughbred mares. *Equine Vet. J.* 43: 424–429.

75 Scholtz, E.L., Krishnan, S., Ball, B.A. et al. (2014). Pregnancy without progesterone in horses defines a second endogenous biopotent progesterone receptor agonist, 5alpha-dihydroprogesterone. *Proc. Natl. Acad. Sci. U. S. A.* 111: 3365–3370.

76 Ousey, J.C., Rossdale, P.D., Dudan, F.E. et al. (1998). The effects of intrafetal ACTH administration on the outcome of pregnancy in the mare. *Reprod. Fertil. Dev.* 10: 359–367.

77 O'Shaughnessy, P.J., Fleming, L.M., Jackson, G. et al. (2003). Adrenocorticotropic hormone directly stimulates testosterone production by the fetal and neonatal mouse testis. *Endocrinology* 144: 3279–3284.

78 Toribio, R.E. and Madigan, J.E. (2019). Equine neonatal maladjustment syndrome/neonatal encephalopathy: Evidence for the etiology and treatment. ACVIM Forum, Phoenix, AZ.

79 Wynn, M.A.A., Ball, B.A., Legacki, E. et al. (2018). Inhibition of 5alpha-reductase alters pregnane metabolism in the late pregnant mare. *Reproduction* 155: 251–258.

80 Belelli, D. and Lambert, J.J. (2005). Neurosteroids: endogenous regulators of the GABA(A) receptor. *Nat. Rev. Neurosci.* 6: 565–575.

81 Brunton, P.J. (2015). Programming the brain and behaviour by early-life stress: a focus on neuroactive steroids. *J. Neuroendocrinol.* 27: 468–480.

82 Brunton, P.J., Russell, J.A., and Hirst, J.J. (2014). Allopregnanolone in the brain: protecting pregnancy and birth outcomes. *Prog. Neurobiol.* 113: 106–136.

83 Reddy, D.S. and Estes, W.A. (2016). Clinical Potential of neurosteroids for CNS Disorders. *Trends Pharmacol. Sci.* 37: 543–561.

84 Kawarai, Y., Tanaka, H., Kobayashi, T. et al. (2018). Progesterone as a Postnatal Prophylactic Agent for Encephalopathy Caused by Prenatal Hypoxic Ischemic Insult. *Endocrinology* 159: 2264–2274.

85 Hirst, J.J., Kelleher, M.A., Walker, D.W. et al. (2014). Neuroactive steroids in pregnancy: key regulatory and protective roles in the foetal brain. *J. Steroid Biochem. Mol. Biol.* 139: 144–153.

86 Melcangi, R.C., Giatti, S., Pesaresi, M. et al. (2011). Role of neuroactive steroids in the peripheral nervous system. *Front. Endocrinol. (Lausanne)* 2: 104.

87 Tuem, K.B. and Atey, T.M. (2017). Neuroactive Steroids: Receptor Interactions and Responses. *Front. Neurol.* 8: 442.

88 Longone, P., di Michele, F., D'Agati, E. et al. (2011). Neurosteroids as neuromodulators in the treatment of anxiety disorders. *Front. Endocrinol. (Lausanne)* 2: 55.

89 Reddy, D.S. (2010). Neurosteroids: endogenous role in the human brain and therapeutic potentials. *Prog. Brain Res.* 186: 113–137.

90 Laube, B., Maksay, G., Schemm, R., and Betz, H. (2002). Modulation of glycine receptor function: a novel approach for therapeutic intervention at inhibitory synapses? *Trends Pharmacol. Sci.* 23: 519–527.

91 Wang, M. (2011). Neurosteroids and GABA-A Receptor Function. *Front. Endocrinol. (Lausanne)* 2: 44.

92 Thomas, P. and Pang, Y. (2012). Membrane progesterone receptors: evidence for neuroprotective, neurosteroid signaling and neuroendocrine functions in neuronal cells. *Neuroendocrinology* 96: 162–171.

93 Dressing, G.E., Goldberg, J.E., Charles, N.J. et al. (2011). Membrane progesterone receptor expression in mammalian tissues: a review of regulation and physiological implications. *Steroids* 76: 11–17.

94 Olsen, R.W. (2018). GABAA receptor: Positive and negative allosteric modulators. *Neuropharmacology* 136: 10–22.

95 Mouton, J.C. and Duckworth, R.A. (2021). Maternally derived hormones, neurosteroids and the development of behaviour. *Proc. Biol. Sci.* 288: 20202467.

96 Diesch, T.J. and Mellor, D.J. (2013). Birth transitions: pathophysiology, the onset of consciousness and possible implications for neonatal maladjustment syndrome in the foal. *Equine Vet. J.* 45: 656–660.

97 Goodwin, W.A., Keates, H.L., Pasloske, K. et al. (2011). The pharmacokinetics and pharmacodynamics of the injectable anaesthetic alfaxalone in the horse. *Vet. Anaesth. Analg.* 38: 431–438.

Section II Energy and Growth Hormones

Ramiro E. Toribio, Katarzyna A. Dembek, Laura D. Hostnik, and Teresa A. Burns

Energy Hormones

The energy regulatory systems are complex and comprise multiple axes (pancreatic, enteroinsular, somatotropic, bone-pancreas, orexigenic, hypothalamic–pituitary–adrenal, thyroid). Several organs and cells with endocrine functions are involved in energy homeostasis, including the pancreas (α and β-cells), fat (adipocytes), hypothalamus (multiple nuclei), pituitary gland (pars distalis), adrenal gland (cortex, medulla), stomach (glandular cells), intestine (K and L cells), thyroid gland (follicular cells), liver (hepatocytes), and bone (osteoblasts). Disorders of energy regulation are common in critically ill and dysmature foals. Despite the frequency and clinical relevance of energy dysregulation in hospitalized foals, few studies have evaluated hormones involved with energy metabolism in sick newborn foals [1–5].

The equine fetus is highly dependent on maternal transfer of glucose [6], with major increases in glucose utilization from mid-gestation to 300 days, matching umbilical glucose uptake, but not total energy demands [6, 7]. Per body weight, glucose utilization decreases steadily after day 180 of pregnancy, in part due to maximal placental transfer capacity [6]. It is feasible that the reduced rate of glucose transfer to the equine fetus at the end of gestation, together with restricted uterine space and endocrine changes around this period, contribute to the duration of pregnancy [6, 8].

An infrequently discussed energy source for the equine fetus is L-lactate, with significant increases occurring in late pregnancy [6, 7]. As glucose transfer reaches its limit, L-lactate from placental origin fills part of this energy gap. Glucose and free fatty acid (FFA) concentrations are lower, while L-lactate concentrations are higher in fetuses compared to their dams in most mammalian species, including the horse [6, 9]. Foals are born with high L-lactate and nonesterified fatty acids (NEFA) but low glucose concentrations [6, 10–16]. Fructose concentrations are high in the equine fetus, but its source and metabolic fate are uncertain [17]. The equine placenta is lipid permeable, in particular to FFAs [18], but also synthesizes lipids from glucose in late gestation to be used by the fetus [7, 19–21].

Fructose, lipids, and amino acids may be valuable sources of energy for the fetus; however, based on oxygen utilization and nutritional studies, it appears that after glucose, lipids may be the next most important fuel for the equine fetus in late pregnancy [6, 7, 19, 21, 22].

Based on urea production by equine fetuses, amino acid oxidation could account for up to 15% of oxygen consumption, which may be more important when mares are in a negative balance [6]. This energy dynamic is relevant during the transition to extrauterine life. Equine fetuses in late gestation have low capacity to produce glucose, and glycogenic capacity is limited due to low hepatic and renal glycogenic enzyme activity [23]; therefore, foals are often born hypoglycemic, with minimal energy reserves (low glycogen and adipose tissue) and limited time to adapt [6, 9, 11, 15, 23, 24]. Hepatic and renal glucose 6-phosphatase activity as well as hepatic and skeletal glycogen content increase rapidly after birth, with foals having values similar to horses within 24 hours [23]. This is likely driven by increases in cortisol, thyroid hormones, catecholamines and glucagon concentrations around the same time [19, 25].

Maintaining normoglycemia immediately after birth can be challenging; thus, rapid caloric intake and utilization in are essential for survival. This requires functional endocrine systems that rapidly regulate energy homeostasis. In addition, the gastrointestinal tract must be functional to handle the rapid load of nutrients from colostrum and milk. The foal must become efficient at converting lactose into galactose and glucose, translocate glucose into cells to become a rapid source of energy, use it efficiently, store it,

Equine Neonatal Medicine, First Edition. Edited by David M. Wong and Pamela A. Wilkins.

and reduce energy waste. There are many aspects of energy homeostasis in the equine neonate that remain unclear, in particular processes involved in gluconeogenesis, glycogenolysis, glycogenesis, and lipolysis. Fatty acids and amino acids in colostrum and milk may be important fuels and could have regulatory functions in the transition to extrauterine life. This is noted when contrasting equine colostrum and milk composition [26, 27]. In addition, mare's colostrum contains cytokines and growth factors that play important biological functions, including gastrointestinal development, immunity, and endocrine modulation.

The Endocrine Pancreas

The islet of Langerhans is the functional unit of the endocrine pancreas. Five cell types are present in the islets (α, β, δ, ε, and γ cells) and secrete glucagon (α-cells), insulin, amylin, and C-peptide (β-cells), and somatostatin (δ-cells); ε-cells produce ghrelin, and γ (PP)-cells release pancreatic polypeptide (PP). Insulin and glucagon are the primary pancreatic hormones.

Insulin is the main hormone-controlling energy metabolism and storage. Its actions involve three major substrates (carbohydrates, proteins, and fats) and three major tissues (liver, skeletal muscle, and adipose tissue). Insulin secretion is stimulated by hyperglycemia, certain amino acids, cortisol, growth hormone (GH), and cholinergic stimulation, while it is suppressed by hypoglycemia, somatostatin, ghrelin, and adrenergic agonists. In the liver, insulin decreases glycogenolysis, gluconeogenesis, and ketogenesis, but promotes glycogenesis, glycolysis, and fatty acid synthesis. In adipose tissue, insulin decreases lipolysis and stimulates fatty acid uptake, synthesis, and esterification. In skeletal muscle, insulin increases glucose and amino acid uptake, protein synthesis, and glycogen synthesis, but decreases proteolysis and amino acid output. Glucagon has opposing actions to insulin on energy metabolism with its main targets being the liver and adipose tissue. Its main function is to increase glucose concentrations during hypoglycemia by promoting glycogenolysis and gluconeogenesis. In adipose tissue, it enhances lipolysis. Glucagon secretion is stimulated by hypoglycemia, catecholamines, acetylcholine, cholecystokinin, and glucose-dependent insulinotropic polypeptide (GIP). Glucagon synthesis is suppressed by insulin, somatostatin, and hyperglycemia. The significance of insulin is evident being the only hormone that prevents against hyperglycemia, while glucagon, epinephrine, and cortisol avert hypoglycemia. There is evidence that neurogenic factors modulate both α and β-cell function.

The equine fetal pancreas develops early, with a pancreatic bud being evident by day 25, that acquires a triangular shape by day 30 and becomes elongated by day 40 of gestation [28]. Pancreatic acini and islets are observed in equine fetuses around day 50 [28]. By days 270–300 of gestation equine fetuses secrete insulin in response to glucose stimulation and the hypoglycemic actions of insulin are evident by 2 weeks before birth [29–32]. Equine fetuses also secrete insulin in response to amino acids, arginine in particular [32]. The rise in fetal plasma cortisol concentrations affect the insulin response to glucose, but it does not influence the response to arginine [32], indicating that different insulin-stimulating pathways are functional in equine fetal β cells at the end of pregnancy. Equine fetuses with higher cortisol concentrations have a faster and greater β-cell insulin response [32]. The effect of arginine on insulin concentrations continues after birth [33], suggesting that amino acids in milk play a role in energy homeostasis and metabolism.

A poorly understood variable about foals is how the method of delivery (spontaneous vs. induced vs. dystocia) influences the endocrine pancreas in the immediate postpartum period. For example, one study found that foals born to oxytocin-induced mares had two to threefold greater insulin response to exogenous glucose and arginine compared to spontaneously delivered foals [33]. Differences in pancreatic endocrine response were associated with higher cortisol concentrations in induced foals, suggesting HPAA activation from fetal stress or mechanisms to rapidly adapt to extrauterine life [33]. This also indicates that the method of delivery may compromise glucoregulatory mechanisms and adaptation to nutrition in the immediate postpartum period, with potential negative consequences after birth [33]. This topic deserves investigation as it is assumed that the response to nutrition is similar between foals, regardless of method of delivery or adverse perinatal events.

Because insulin is a central energy regulatory hormone, it is essential for foals to use glucose and other substrates immediately after birth as sources of energy for a multitude of metabolic processes. Insulin also has functions beyond energy homeostasis. Foals are born with a functional pancreas that rapidly secretes insulin in response to nursing as well as enteral and parenteral carbohydrates and amino acids [32, 34–37]. In the newborn foal, in addition to promoting glucose disposal and lipogenesis, insulin-induced hypoglycemia activates the adrenal medulla, adrenal cortex, and adenohypophysis to release cortisol, catecholamines, and GH, and increases FFA and lactate concentrations [31], perhaps to enhance availability of other sources of energy.

Basal insulin concentrations change minimally in the equine fetus at the end of gestation [19], but the β-cell response to exogenous glucose increases from 270 days of gestation to term [34, 36]. In one study, resting insulin concentrations were similar between pre-suckle (before colostrum), 1–2 and 10- to 12-day-old healthy foals [24]. Insulin concentrations before birth, at birth, and 1 week after birth were lower in foals compared to their dams [24, 36]. Duration and frequency of nursing were negatively associated with insulin concentrations in these foals [24].

One proposal is that foals are born in an insulin resistant state due to peripartum increases in cortisol concentrations [31, 35, 38]; however, this effect may be short lasting based on recent work from our lab, demonstrating that low doses of insulin (0.02 IU/kg, IV) have hypoglycemic effects in 1- to 3-day-old foals [39]. Insulin caused hypoglycemia in 2- to 4-day-old foal born to mares that experienced illness during pregnancy [40], although in this study a higher insulin dose (0.05 IU/kg, IV) was used. Taking into consideration time from birth, a study noted minimal insulin response to hyperglycemia in 2-hour-old foals [15], suggesting that perhaps other endocrine factors that peak around this time, such as cortisol and epinephrine, interfere with insulin secretion [29, 41]. This is in contrast to a study that documented poor hypoglycemic effect of exogenous insulin in newborn foals, even at high doses [31]. These findings indicate evolutionary adaptations geared at preserving energy and shifting glucose intracellularly as soon as it enters circulation, likely to be used in various metabolic activities, including locomotion and thermogenesis.

The intrauterine environment and caloric intake by the dam might influence insulin secretion in the foal [15, 35, 40, 42]. No difference in insulin sensitivity was noted between foals born to mares fed high- or low-starch diets, however, over time foals from high-starch diet dams had reduced insulin sensitivity [42]. Nutrient restriction in mid-pregnancy from illness enhanced insulin sensitivity in foals born to mares in moderate compared to high body condition [40]. Another study in newborn foals found no difference in insulin secretion between control and overfed mares, however, foals from overfed mares had increased islet number and size [15]. Foals overgrown in utero had higher basal insulin concentrations and greater β-cell response to glucose [35]. This suggests that nutritional programing of fetal β cells is influenced by the nutrition plane of the mare, maternal diseases and intrauterine growth rate.

The functionality of the HPAA is important in the maturation of the equine endocrine pancreas and thyroid gland. Equine fetuses in a low cortisol environment have poor insulin response to hyperglycemia compared to those with normal or high cortisol levels [32]. Of interest, this cortisol effect was not evident to arginine challenge, hinting that cortisol is more important for β-cell maturation and carbohydrate sensing, which would enable β cells to regulate glycemia in the immediate postnatal period [32].

Immunoreactive glucagon is present in the equine fetus after day 260 of pregnancy, increases steadily after 320 days, reaching peak concentrations at birth [19, 43]. Hypo- or hyperglycemia do not influence fetal plasma glucagon concentrations in the equine fetus [43]. Equine fetal α cells respond rapidly to IV arginine infusion, but the response is not affected by glucose concentrations [43]. The mechanisms involved in glucagon release in the equine fetus in response to hypoglycemia do not appear to develop until birth [43]. This difference between α and β-cell response to glucose implies that in preparation for extrauterine life, a functional β-cell is necessary for rapid glucose disposal. One can speculate that gluconeogenic mechanisms may not be as mature and a glucagon response to amino acids may be important to promote gluconeogenesis immediately after birth considering the minimal hepatic energy reserves in newborn foals [23]. It is also possible that catecholamines contribute to glucagon secretion near term in anticipation for postpartum hypoglycemia as both epinephrine and norepinephrine peak around the same time [19].

A study in newborn healthy foals showed minimal changes in glucagon concentrations in response to fasting for 180 minutes while insulin concentrations decreased steadily until foals were allowed to nurse [44]. In response to nursing, glucagon concentrations doubled within 30 minutes, which was surprising finding. In the same foals, insulin concentrations increased to threefold prenursing values [44]. The fact that both α and β cells had a rapid response to nursing indicates that there are regulatory mechanisms in the equine neonatal endocrine pancreas that remain to be elucidated – in particular when these hormones are considered counterregulatory. It is possible that milk carbohydrates, together with incretins, promoted insulin release while milk amino acids or fatty acids triggered glucagon secretion. In addition, the rise in glucagon could enhance β-cell insulin secretion. Another factor is GIP, an intestinal peptide high in concentrations in newborn foals that stimulates glucagon secretion [4]. This information identifies knowledge gaps in equine pancreatic biology. For example, in most species α_2-adrenoreceptor activation inhibits insulin secretion and both α_2- and β-adrenoreceptors promote glucagon release. In horses, α_2-adrenergic stimulation also inhibits insulin secretion, however, a study showed that α_2-adrenergic stimulation also suppresses glucagon secretion, which was unexpected [45]. The point is that, similar to the parallel insulin and glucagon response to nursing in newborn foals [44], insulin and glucagon followed a comparable secretory pattern from α_2-adrenergic stimulation in horses.

Hypoglycemia from insulin administration activates the sympathoadrenal system in the equine fetus at the end of gestation, which is characterized by an increase in plasma noradrenaline but not adrenaline [30]. This effect is independent of HPAA activation [30], and perhaps involves the adrenal medulla [31]. One can speculate that this is a stress response to hypoglycemia and a compensatory mechanism to promote glycogenolysis and gluconeogenesis, indicating that at this stage of development, this regulatory system is functional. Of interest, immediately after birth, the catecholamine response to hypoglycemia is poor, but after day 7, epinephrine increases but the norepinephrine response is poor [30, 31]. This highlights differing responses of the adrenergic system to hypoglycemia (epinephrine increase) compared to hypotension (norepinephrine increase) [29–31, 46]. It also appears that the adrenocortical response to hypoglycemia is low at birth but increases over time [31]. Again, catecholamines promote gluconeogenesis, glycogenolysis, and lipolysis, contributing to energy homeostasis in the equine neonate.

In the neonatal foal, hypoglycemia is more frequent than hyperglycemia, and both are linked to mortality [2, 47]. Septic foals often have low insulin [1, 2], but increased glucagon, triglyceride, and NEFA concentrations [1, 2], which likely reflects metabolic balance and energy needs. Glucagon increases blood glucose concentrations by promoting gluconeogenesis and glycogenolysis, which in sick foals could be an appropriate response. Low insulin concentrations in septic foals are likely a response to hypoglycemia; however, in foals with hyperglycemia, low insulin values should be considered inadequate. These foals are unable to regulate glycemia and may require insulin therapy. This is also an indication of disease severity that often results in death.

The enteroinsular axis (EIA) comprises intestinal factors that stimulate the endocrine pancreas to secrete insulin and include GIP (K cells), glucagon-like peptide-1 (GLP-1; L cells) and glucagon-like peptide-2 (GLP-2; L cells). These factors are known as incretins and represent the basis for new generation drugs used to treated diabetes. GLP-1 and GIP have synergistic actions over β cells enhancing insulin secretion; however, GLP-1 inhibits while GIP stimulates glucagon release [48]. GLP-2 has more enterotrophic actions, appears to be more relevant in regulating nutrient absorption, maintaining mucosal morphology, and energy balance [49]. At least in humans, the EIA is more important than glucose in promoting insulin secretion [50].

Newborn foals have a functional EIA and its response to nutrients differs from horses [4, 51], likely due to diet and influenced by endocrine changes that occur in the peripartum period [4]. In one study, enteral glucose (1000 mg/kg) and lactose (1000 mg/kg) administration promoted a weak insulin release, with minimal effect on GLP-1 and GIP secretion [4]. In the same study, IV glucose had no effect on incretin secretion. Of interest, nursing was a strong stimulator of the EIA, with a rapid increase in GLP-1, GIP, insulin, and glucagon concentrations [4, 44]. This indicates that in addition to carbohydrates, other factors in milk (e.g. amino acids, fatty acids) mediate communication between the intestine and the endocrine pancreas. This information could have clinical relevance in future strategies to manage critically ill or orphan foals in that without proper enteroinsular activation, foals could develop hyperglycemia, in part due to a poor insulin response. This could be a potential explanation for the low insulin concentrations measured in septic foals [2], and may contribute to hyperglycemia or poor glucose control.

Information on the EIA in sick foals is minimal. A study showed that septic foals have high GLP-1 and GLP-2, but low insulin concentrations, despite normo- to hyperglycemia [52], indicating a disconnect between the intestine (incretins) and insulin secretion (β cells), which could promote glucose intolerance in critically ill foals (e.g. hyperglycemia in premature or septic foals). Of interest, plasma GIP concentrations in septic foals were lower compared to healthy foals and followed a pattern to insulin [52]. Based on low GIP, together with increased GLP-1 and GLP-2 concentrations, it was proposed that different mechanisms could contribute to reduced insulin secretion in critically ill foals [52].

Growth Hormone, IGF-1, Ghrelin, Leptin, and Adiponectin

The somatotropic axis (hypothalamic–pituitary-somatotropic axis) consists of GH from the pituitary gland and insulin-like growth factor-1 (IGF-1; somatomedin-1), mainly from the liver. Growth hormone-releasing hormone (GHRH) and growth hormone-inhibiting hormone (GHIH; somatostatin) from the hypothalamus, and ghrelin from the stomach and brain, are important regulators of GH secretion. In addition to growth, this system is relevant to energy homeostasis, in particular during food deprivation, where it makes different substrates available to be used as fuels. Hypoglycemia is a potent stimulus for GH release.

Many of the peripheral actions of GH are mediated by IGF-1; therefore, an increase in GH is followed by elevations in IGF-1 levels. IGF-1 also suppresses GH secretion. GH also counteracts the effects of insulin on glucose and lipid metabolism during fasting or negative energy balance states [53–55]. In the liver, GH stimulates glucose production via gluconeogenesis and glycogenolysis. In adipose tissue, GH has lipolytic actions that are direct and indirect through its anti-insulin properties, resulting in FFA release. Together, these actions support growth and metabolic needs. Growth hormone has anti-insulin properties, while IGF-1 has insulin-like actions [55–58]. Of interest, GH shares anabolic properties with insulin, which are likely mediated by IGF-1. Growth hormone increases insulin concentrations by interfering with its peripheral actions, by promoting hyperglycemia, and by directly stimulating its synthesis and secretion [59]. After birth, blood concentrations of GH and IGF-1 increase over time in healthy foals [16, 60]. In one study, donkey foals had higher IGF-1 concentrations after birth than horse foals [61]. Ghrelin is mainly produced by gastric glandular cells in response to anorexia to promote hunger, is a potent GH secretagogue, but also inhibits insulin secretion [62]. Small amounts are also produced in the small intestine, pancreas, and brain.

Disturbances of the somatotropic axis have been documented in critically ill foals [3]. A study found increased GH, but reduced IGF-1 concentrations in septic foals, suggesting impaired somatotropic axis signaling [3]. This phenomenon, termed *somatotropic axis resistance* [3], may be equivalent to insulin resistance in horses; its clinical implications are unclear, but likely relevant to energy homeostasis. This is supported by the fact that some foals with high GH concentrations also have increased ghrelin concentrations, indicating that the pituitary component of the axis remains functional during critical illness. Therefore, current information points to impaired GH signaling at the hepatocyte level. This is likely a consequence of systemic inflammation or endotoxemia, which are frequent in septic foals. These findings are in contrast to premature foals, in which IGF-1 concentrations were high [63]. It is plausible that increased GH concentrations, through its insulin-blocking actions, interferes with glucose uptake and promotes glycogenolysis, gluconeogenesis, and lipolysis in critically ill foals. This could explain some metabolic abnormalities in hospitalized foals – in particular, increased NEFA and triglyceride concentrations [1, 2].

Leptin is an adipocyte-derived hormone (adipokine) considered to be the main regulator of satiety (anorexigenic factor; high leptin suppresses hunger) and its blood concentrations correlate with total body fat in horses and other species [64, 65]. Leptin increases insulin sensitivity and insulin hepatic extraction, decreases insulin secretion (adipoinsular axis), and glucose concentrations [66, 67]. As part of this regulatory system, insulin stimulates leptin secretion by adipocytes. Thus, a key function of the adipoinsular axis is to inhibit insulin secretion to reduce adipogenesis. In newborn foals, leptin concentrations rise after birth to decline a few days later [68].

No differences in blood leptin concentrations were identified between healthy and sick foals [2]. However, leptin concentrations were lower in septic foals that died [2]. The role of leptin in disorders of newborn foals remains unclear, but likely important considering its actions on various aspects of energy homeostasis. In other species, insulin increases leptin secretion, suggesting that low leptin in critically ill foals could be, in part, reflecting low insulin concentrations [2].

Adiponectin is another adipocyte-derived peptide hormone (adipokine) that is negatively correlated with body fat mass in horses and other species and known to increase insulin sensitivity [65, 69]. Adiponectin promotes the cell membrane translocation of GLUT4, increases insulin sensitivity, glycolysis, and fatty acid oxidation [69].

In neonatal foals, blood adiponectin concentrations were not different between healthy, sick nonseptic and septic foals [70]. Therefore, its role in the pathogenesis of energy dysregulation and systemic inflammation in neonates is unclear.

References

1 Armengou, L., Jose-Cunilleras, E., Rios, J. et al. (2013). Metabolic and endocrine profiles in sick neonatal foals are related to survival. *J. Vet. Intern. Med.* 27: 567–575.

2 Barsnick, R.J., Hurcombe, S.D., Smith, P.A. et al. (2011). Insulin, glucagon, and leptin in critically ill foals. *J. Vet. Intern. Med.* 25: 123–131.

3 Barsnick, R.J., Hurcombe, S.D., Dembek, K. et al. (2014). Somatotropic axis resistance and ghrelin in critically ill foals. *Equine Vet. J.* 46: 45–49.

4 Rings, L.M., Swink, J.M., Dunbar, L.K. et al. (2019). Enteroinsular axis response to carbohydrates and fasting in healthy newborn foals. *J. Vet. Intern. Med.* 33: 2752–2764.

5 Himler, M., Hurcombe, S.D., Griffin, A. et al. (2012). Presumptive nonthyroidal illness syndrome in critically ill foals. *Equine Vet. J. Suppl.* 44 (Suppl. 41): 43–47.

6 Fowden, A.L., Taylor, P.M., White, K.L. et al. (2000). Ontogenic and nutritionally induced changes in fetal metabolism in the horse. *J. Physiol.* 528 (Pt 1): 209–219.

7 Vaughan, O.R. and Fowden, A.L. (2016). Placental metabolism: substrate requirements and the response to stress. *Reprod. Domest. Anim.* 51 (Suppl. 2): 25–35.

8 Fowden, A.L., Ralph, M.M., and Silver, M. (1994). Nutritional regulation of uteroplacental prostaglandin production and metabolism in pregnant ewes and mares during late gestation. *Exp. Clin. Endocrinol.* 102: 212–221.

9 Girard, J., Pintado, E., and Ferre, P. (1979). Fuel metabolism in the mammalian fetus. *Ann. Biol. Anim. Biochem. Biophys.* 19: 181–197.

10 Fowden, A.L., Forhead, A.J., White, K.L. et al. (2000). Equine uteroplacental metabolism at mid- and late gestation. *Exp. Physiol.* 85: 539–545.

11 Aoki, T. and Ishii, M. (2012). Hematological and biochemical profiles in peripartum mares and neonatal foals (heavy draft horse). *J. Equine Vet. Sci.* 32: 170–176.

12 Pirrone, A., Mariella, J., Gentilini, F. et al. (2012). Amniotic fluid and blood lactate concentrations in mares

and foals in the early postpartum period. *Theriogenology* 78: 1182–1189.

13 Cruz, R.K.S., Alfonso, A., Souza, F.F. et al. (2017). Evaluation of neonatal vitality and blood glucose, lactate and cortisol concentrations in foals of the Paint Horse breed. *Pesqui. Vet. Bras.* 37: 891–896.

14 Linhares Boakari, Y., Alonso, M.A., Vallone Riccio, A. et al. (2021). Evaluation of blood glucose and lactate concentrations in mule and equine foals. *J. Equine Vet. Sci.* 101: 103369.

15 Bradbery, A.N., Coverdale, J.A., Hartz, C.J. et al. (2021). Effect of maternal overnutrition on predisposition to insulin resistance in the foal: maternal parameters and foal pancreas histoarchitecture. *Anim. Reprod. Sci.* 227: 106720.

16 Panzani, S., Comin, A., Galeati, G. et al. (2012). How type of parturition and health status influence hormonal and metabolic profiles in newborn foals. *Theriogenology* 77: 1167–1177.

17 Silver, M. (1984). Some aspects of equine placental exchange and foetal physiology. *Equine Vet. J.* 16: 227–233.

18 Stephenson, T., Stammers, J., and Hull, D. (1993). Placental transfer of free fatty acids: importance of fetal albumin concentration and acid-base status. *Biol. Neonate* 63: 273–280.

19 Fowden, A.L., Giussani, D.A., and Forhead, A.J. (2020). Physiological development of the equine fetus during late gestation. *Equine Vet. J.* 52: 165–173.

20 Stammers, J.P., Silver, M., and Fowden, A.L. (1988). Effects of nutrition on uterine and umbilical venous plasma lipids in chronically catheterised mares in late gestation. *Equine Vet. J. Suppl.* 20: 37–40.

21 Stammers, J.P., Hull, D., Silver, M. et al. (1994). Release of lipid from the equine placenta during in vitro incubation. *Placenta* 15: 857–872.

22 Stammers, J.P., Hull, D., Silver, M. et al. (1995). Fetal and maternal plasma lipids in chronically catheterized mares in late gestation: effects of different nutritional states. *Reprod. Fertil. Dev.* 7: 1275–1284.

23 Fowden, A.L., Mundy, L., Ousey, J.C. et al. (1991). Tissue glycogen and glucose 6-phosphatase levels in fetal and newborn foals. *J. Reprod. Fertil. Suppl.* 44: 537–542.

24 Berryhill, E.H., Magdesian, K.G., Tadros, E.M. et al. (2019). Effects of age on serum glucose and insulin concentrations and glucose/insulin ratios in neonatal foals and their dams during the first 2 weeks postpartum. *Vet. J.* 246: 1–6.

25 Silver, M., Fowden, A.L., Knox, J. et al. (1991). Relationship between circulating tri-iodothyronine and cortisol in the perinatal period in the foal. *J. Reprod. Fertil. Suppl.* 44: 619–626.

26 Buechner-Maxwell, V.A. (2005). Nutritional support for neonatal foals. *Vet. Clin. North Am. Equine Pract.* 21: 487–510.

27 Barreto, I., Urbano, S.A., Oliveira, C.A.A. et al. (2020). Chemical composition and lipid profile of mare colostrum and milk of the quarter horse breed. *PLoS One* 15: e0238921.

28 Rodrigues, M.N., Carvalho, R.C., Franciolli, A.L. et al. (2014). Prenatal development of the digestive system in the horse. *Anat. Rec. (Hoboken)* 297: 1218–1227.

29 Fowden, A.L., Forhead, A.J., and Ousey, J.C. (2012). Endocrine adaptations in the foal over the perinatal period. *Equine Vet. J. Suppl.* 44: 130–139.

30 Silver, M. and Fowden, A.L. (1995). Sympathoadrenal and other endocrine and metabolic responses to hypoglycaemia in the fetal foal during late gestation. *Exp. Physiol.* 80: 651–662.

31 Silver, M., Fowden, A.L., Knox, J. et al. (1987). Sympathoadrenal and other responses to hypoglycaemia in the young foal. *J. Reprod. Fertil. Suppl.* 35: 607–614.

32 Fowden, A.L., Gardner, D.S., Ousey, J.C. et al. (2005). Maturation of pancreatic {beta}-cell function in the fetal horse during late gestation. *J. Endocrinol.* 186: 467–473.

33 Holdstock, N.B., Allen, V.L., and Fowden, A.L. (2012). Pancreatic endocrine function in newborn pony foals after induced or spontaneous delivery at term. *Equine Vet. J. Suppl.* 44: 30–37.

34 Fowden, A.L., Silver, M., Ellis, L. et al. (1984). Studies on equine prematurity 3: insulin secretion in the foal during the perinatal period. *Equine Vet. J.* 16: 286–291.

35 Forhead, A.J., Ousey, J.C., Allen, W.R. et al. (2004). Postnatal insulin secretion and sensitivity after manipulation of fetal growth by embryo transfer in the horse. *J. Endocrinol.* 181: 459–467.

36 Fowden, A.L., Barnes, R.J., Comline, R.S. et al. (1980). Pancreatic beta-cell function in the fetal foal and mare. *J. Endocrinol.* 87: 293–301.

37 Fowden, A.L., Ellis, L., and Rossdale, P.D. (1982). Pancreatic beta cell function in the neonatal foal. *J. Reprod. Fertil. Suppl.* 32: 529–535.

38 Holdstock, N.B., Allen, V.L., Bloomfield, M.R. et al. (2004). Development of insulin and proinsulin secretion in newborn pony foals. *J. Endocrinol.* 181: 469–476.

39 Kinsella, H.M., Hostnik, L.D., Snyder, H.A. et al. (2022). Comparison of insulin sensitivity between healthy neonatal foals and horses using minimal model analysis. *PLoS One* 17: e0262584.

40 Ousey, J.C., Fowden, A.L., Wilsher, S. et al. (2008). The effects of maternal health and body condition on the endocrine responses of neonatal foals. *Equine Vet. J.* 40: 673–679.

41 Melchert, M., Aurich, C., Aurich, J. et al. (2019). Controlled delay of the expulsive phase of foaling affects sympathoadrenal activity and acid base balance of foals in the immediate postnatal phase. *Theriogenology* 139: 8–15.

42 George, L.A., Staniar, W.B., Treiber, K.H. et al. (2009). Insulin sensitivity and glucose dynamics during pre-weaning foal development and in response to maternal diet composition. *Domest. Anim. Endocrinol.* 37: 23–29.

43 Fowden, A.L., Forhead, A.J., Bloomfield, M. et al. (1999). Pancreatic alpha cell function in the fetal foal during late gestation. *Exp. Physiol.* 84: 697–705.

44 Kinsella, H.M., Hostnik, L.D., Rings, L.M. et al. (2021). Glucagon, insulin, adrenocorticotropic hormone, and cortisol in response to carbohydrates and fasting in healthy neonatal foals. *J. Vet. Intern. Med.* 35: 550–559.

45 Box, J.R., Karikoski, N.P., Tanskanen, H.E. et al. (2021). The effects of an alpha-2-adrenoceptor agonist, antagonist, and their combination on the blood insulin, glucose, and glucagon concentrations in insulin sensitive and dysregulated horses. *Vet. J.* 269: 105610.

46 O'Connor, S.J., Gardner, D.S., Ousey, J.C. et al. (2005). Development of baroreflex and endocrine responses to hypotensive stress in newborn foals and lambs. *Pflugers Arch.* 450: 298–306.

47 Hollis, A.R., Furr, M.O., Magdesian, K.G. et al. (2008). Blood glucose concentrations in critically ill neonatal foals. *J. Vet. Intern. Med.* 22: 1223–1227.

48 Seino, Y., Fukushima, M., and Yabe, D. (2010). GIP and GLP-1, the two incretin hormones: similarities and differences. *J. Diabetes Investig.* 1: 8–23.

49 Amato, A., Baldassano, S., and Mule, F. (2016). GLP2: an underestimated signal for improving glycaemic control and insulin sensitivity. *J. Endocrinol.* 229: R57–R66.

50 Holst, J.J. (2019). The incretin system in healthy humans: the role of GIP and GLP-1. *Metabolism* 96: 46–55.

51 de Laat, M.A., McGree, J.M., and Sillence, M.N. (2016). Equine hyperinsulinemia: investigation of the enteroinsular axis during insulin dysregulation. *Am. J. Physiol. Endocrinol. Metab.* 310: E61–E72.

52 Rings, L.M., Kamr, A.M., Kinsella, H.M. et al. (2022). The enteroinsular axis during hospitalization in newborn foals. *Domest. Anim. Endocrinol.* 78: 106686.

53 Houssay, B.A. (1936). Carbohydrate metabolism. *N. Engl. J. Med.* 214: 971–986.

54 Moller, N. and Jorgensen, J.O. (2009). Effects of growth hormone on glucose, lipid, and protein metabolism in human subjects. *Endocr. Rev.* 30: 152–177.

55 Jorgensen, J.O., Krag, M., Jessen, N. et al. (2004). Growth hormone and glucose homeostasis. *Horm. Res.* 62 (Suppl 3): 51–55.

56 Yuen, K.C. and Dunger, D.B. (2007). Therapeutic aspects of growth hormone and insulin-like growth factor-I treatment on visceral fat and insulin sensitivity in adults. *Diabetes Obesity Metab.* 9: 11–22.

57 Moller, N., Jorgensen, J.O., Abildgard, N. et al. (1991). Effects of growth hormone on glucose metabolism. *Horm. Res.* 36 (Suppl 1): 32–35.

58 Kim, S.H. and Park, M.J. (2017). Effects of growth hormone on glucose metabolism and insulin resistance in human. *Ann. Pediatr. Endocrinol. Metab.* 22: 145–152.

59 Vijayakumar, A., Yakar, S., and Leroith, D. (2011). The intricate role of growth hormone in metabolism. *Front. Endocrinol. (Lausanne)* 2: 32. https://doi.org/10.3389/fendo.2011.00032.

60 Stewart, F., Goode, J.A., and Allen, W.R. (1993). Growth hormone secretion in the horse: unusual pattern at birth and pulsatile secretion through to maturity. *J. Endocrinol.* 138: 81–89.

61 Panzani, S., Carluccio, A., Faustini, M. et al. (2017). Comparative study on Insulin-Like Growth Factor I (IGF-I) plasma concentrations in newborn horse foals, donkey foals and calves. *Open Access Text* 1: 1–6.

62 Poher, A.L., Tschop, M.H., and Muller, T.D. (2018). Ghrelin regulation of glucose metabolism. *Peptides* 100: 236–242.

63 Panzani, S., Castagnetti, C., Prandi, A. et al. (2013). Insulin-like growth factor I: could it be a marker of prematurity in the foal? *Theriogenology* 79: 495–501.

64 Buff, P.R., Dodds, A.C., Morrison, C.D. et al. (2002). Leptin in horses: tissue localization and relationship between peripheral concentrations of leptin and body condition. *J. Anim. Sci.* 80: 2942–2948.

65 Kearns, C.F., McKeever, K.H., Roegner, V. et al. (2006). Adiponectin and leptin are related to fat mass in horses. *Vet. J.* 172: 460–465.

66 Amitani, M., Asakawa, A., Amitani, H. et al. (2013). The role of leptin in the control of insulin-glucose axis. *Front. Neurosci.* 7: 51.

67 Paz-Filho, G., Mastronardi, C., Wong, M.L. et al. (2012). Leptin therapy, insulin sensitivity, and glucose homeostasis. *Indian J. Endocrinol. Metab.* 16: S549–S555.

68 Berg, E.L., McNamara, D.L., and Keisler, D.H. (2007). Endocrine profiles of periparturient mares and their foals. *J. Anim. Sci.* 85: 1660–1668.

69 Barsnick, R.J. and Toribio, R.E. (2011). Endocrinology of the equine neonate energy metabolism in health and critical illness. *Vet. Clin. North Am. Equine Pract.* 27: 49–58.

70 Barsnick, R.J., Hurcombe, S.D., Saville, W.J. et al. (2009). Endocrine energy response in septic foals: insulin, leptin and adiponectin. ACVIM Forum.

Section III Thyroid Hormones

Ramiro E. Toribio, Katarzyna A. Dembek, Laura D. Hostnik, and Teresa A. Burns

Thyroid hormones (THs) – specifically thyroxine (T_4) and triiodothyronine (T_3) – are pleiotropic factors that regulate essential processes including growth, tissue differentiation, thermogenesis, body weight, energy metabolism, as well as function of multiple endocrine systems. An understanding of TH biology is important in the diagnosis, treatment, and prognosis of thyroidal and nonthyroidal disorders in the foal.

Thyroid Hormone Physiology

The thyroid gland has two embryological origins: the endoderm of the primitive larynx that gives origin to the follicular cells that secrete THs and the ultimobranchial body of the fourth pharyngeal pouch that contains neuroendocrine cells (from the neural crest) that give rise to the C-cells (parafollicular cells) that secrete calcitonin, which participates in calcium homeostasis.

THs promote cell growth, differentiation, thermogenesis, and energy metabolism [1]. Receptors for THs are present in almost every cell in the body and stimulate oxidative phosphorylation, oxygen consumption, carbohydrate, protein, and lipid metabolism, carbohydrate absorption, lipolysis, insulin and catecholamine sensitivity, and many other functions. In other words, TH increase the basal metabolic rate, with high TH concentrations promoting a hypermetabolic state due to increased energy expenditure; the opposite occurs with low TH concentrations. THs also contribute to differentiation of other endocrine systems (e.g. adrenal gland, pancreas). Therefore, they are crucial for fetal and neonatal development and survival [2]. In the adult, THs are not essential but important for organ function [3].

Secretion of THs is controlled by the hypothalamic–pituitary-thyroid axis (HPTA). The hypothalamus secretes thyrotropin-releasing hormone (TRH) that stimulates the pituitary pars distalis to release thyroid-stimulating hormone (TSH), which in turn promotes synthesis and secretion of THs by follicular cells of the thyroid gland. Subsequently, THs suppress TRH and TSH secretion (negative feedback). TRH is also a releasing factor for prolactin and ACTH [4–8]. Circulating THs include total T_4 (tT_4), free T_4 (fT_4), total T_3 (tT_3), free T_3 (fT_3), and reverse T_3 (rT_3). Of these, free T_3 is the active hormone. Synthesis and release of THs are mainly controlled by TSH and iodine availability. The regulation of TSH is linked to concentrations of free (unbound) THs (fT_4 and fT_3) [2, 9]. The actions of THs are genomic and nongenomic. In the genomic actions, T_3 binds cytoplasmic receptors (TRα and TRβ) creating a TH/receptor complex that translocates to the nucleus to function as a transcription factor to increase or decrease gene expression. For nongenomic actions, T_3 and T_4 bind cell membrane receptors (e.g. $\alpha v\beta 3$ integrin) that trigger a signal transduction cascade that modulates gene transcription [10].

A major function of thyroid gland follicular cells is to actively trap iodine against a concentration gradient (30–40 fold) [2, 9]. Iodine is absorbed in its soluble form (iodide; I^-) via the intestinal mucosa, moist body surfaces, and broken skin [2]. Subsequently, iodide is transported and concentrated into the thyroid gland by a Na^+/I^- symporter (NIS) that is coupled to a Na^+ gradient generated by Na^+/K^+-ATPase to promote I^- accumulation [11, 12]. Pendrin mediates the transport of I^- across the thyrocyte to the cell-to-colloid interface [12]. Once in the follicular lumen, trapped I^- is oxidized to iodine by thyroperoxidase to be incorporated into tyrosine residues of thyroglobulin forming inactive precursors (monoiodotyrosine [MIT]; diiodotyrosine [DIT]). These precursors are coupled to form T_4 and T_3. Thyroglobulin is a large glycoprotein containing MIT, DIT, T_3, and T_4 that is stored in the follicular colloid [13]. Upon demand, colloid is endocytosed by follicular cells and proteases cleave T_3 and T_4 from thyroglobulin and transferred to systemic circulation [2, 9]. Most TH

Equine Neonatal Medicine, First Edition. Edited by David M. Wong and Pamela A. Wilkins.

released into circulation is T_4 and its concentration in equine blood is 20 times higher than T_3 [14].

Conversion of T_4 (prohormone) to T_3 (active hormone) occurs through removal of an iodine from the outer ring. All circulating T_4 derives from the thyroid gland while only 10–20% of T_3 is directly secreted by the thyroid gland [1]. Enzymes responsible for the production of T_3 and rT_3 are also responsible for their inactivation. Three deiodinases (selenoproteins) are responsible for conversion of T_4 to T_3 [15]. Type I deiodinase is found in peripheral tissues (liver, kidney) and responsible for most of the conversion of T_4 to T_3 (T_3 neogenesis) and to rT_3. In the fetus, T_3 neogenesis is minimal due to low type I deiodinase activity, which during development predominantly converts T_4 to rT_3. Near birth, there is an enzymatic switch due to increasing cortisol concentrations resulting in high T_3 concentrations in newborn foals [16–21]. Type II deiodinase is found in the thyroid gland, adipose tissue, central nervous system, reproductive tract, and pituitary gland [22, 23]. Type III deiodinase is present in the placenta and developing fetal brain; its key function is to regulate T_3 availability during development by inactivating T_4 and T_3. It also prevents excessive access of maternal THs to the fetus. The generation of inactive rT_3 by type I and III deiodinases is essential in TH homeostasis. TH metabolites are processed through conjugation, enter the enterohepatic circulation, and most are excreted in urine. Most iodine is recycled to the thyroid gland. The equine mammary gland concentrates iodine at higher concentrations than plasma, making colostrum and milk major sources of iodine in the early neonatal period. [24] Iodine concentrations are higher in colostrum than milk [24]. Serum iodine concentrations in foals at birth are much higher than their mares, decrease over time, and correlate with tT_4 concentrations [24].

Secretion of THs is influenced by age, physiological status, hormones, iodine availability, season, caloric intake, exogenous compounds, and diseases [1]. Foals are born with very high TH concentrations that are 10–20 times higher compared to horses and their dams but decrease rapidly in the 2 weeks after birth to reach adult values by 30–180 days of age [20–23, 25, 26]. Plasma TH concentrations in newborn foals increase for 120 minutes after birth and follow a pattern similar to cortisol concentrations [23]. TH concentrations are higher in young donkeys compared to older ones [27]. The maturation of the equine thyroid gland endocrine system depends on a functional HPAA [23]. ACTH promotes equine fetal TH secretion, likely through adrenocortical production of glucocorticoids, as there is a positive correlation between fetal cortisol and TH concentrations in late pregnancy and immediately after birth [23].

Reduced or excessive iodine availability, excess of compounds that interfere with NIS activity (e.g. perchlorate, thiocyanate, nitrate) or inhibit iodide oxidation and coupling (e.g. thiouracil, thiopental, methimazole), as well as consumption of plants that contain goitrogenic substances (e.g. *Brassica* family) can result in TH deficiency [1, 2]. In general this is not a serious concern for pregnant mares but could be for the developing fetus. Several drugs used in equine practice (e.g. dexamethasone, phenylbutazone) reduce TH concentrations in horses [28, 29], but effects on TH concentrations in foals remains to be elucidated.

In blood, THs circulate bound to plasma proteins. Thyroxine-binding globulin (TBG) is the major protein (70% of T_4 and T_3 are bound to TBG), transthyretin (thyroid-binding prealbumin; TBPA), and albumin. In horses, percent circulating T_4 bound to TBG, TBPA, and albumin were 61%, 22%, and 17%, respectively [30]. T_3 is bound to TBG and albumin but not TBPA. Binding of THs to proteins is reversible, and these proteins act as TH reservoirs. Changes in protein concentrations may change TH concentrations. Only free, unbound THs cross cell membranes to exert biologic actions [1]. T_3 is much more potent than T_4 and it has a shorter half-life, which is important for proper homeostatic control. The half-life of T_4 in horses is approximately 50 hours [31].

Due to their type of placentation in people a large proportion of fetal THs come from placental transfer [22, 23, 32], thus, maternal THs are central to fetal development at the end of gestation. This does not occur in horses with their epitheliochorial placentation, which depend on transplacental transfer of iodine for de novo fetal synthesis of T_4 and T_3 [22]. In the horse, impaired fetal TH synthesis can delay tissue differentiation that, if severe or prolonged, leads to congenital hypothyroidism [1, 22, 33]. In the developing fetus, T_4 and T_3 concentrations are low, while concentrations of inactive rT_3 are high, reflecting maturation of the HPTA and coordination with the deiodinase system [23, 32]. While the physiological significance of low T_3 concentrations throughout gestation is unknown, it might be an ontogenic adaption to avoid excessive thermogenesis, preserve energy and facilitate the anabolic state of the growing fetus [32]. The rapid rise in THs at the end of gestation and immediately postpartum support the importance of coordination between different endocrine systems to accelerate adaptation to the harsh conditions from the new environment.

Considering their pleiotropic functions, low TH concentrations in the developing fetus and newborn foal can have negative consequences [33–37]. A number of studies have documented congenital abnormalities in foals due to TH deficiency [33–37]. This is evident in foals with congenital hypothyroidism, which have musculoskeletal anomalies (tendon rupture, bone dysgenesis, angular/flexural deformities), prognathism, respiratory failure, inappropriate nervous tissue development, and other abnormalities.

Studies have shown that premature, septic, and maladjusted foals often have low TH concentrations linked to disease severity and mortality [23, 26, 38–40]. This condition, known as *euthyroid sick syndrome* or *nonthyroidal illness syndrome* (NTIS), refers to low TH concentrations in sick patients. It is important to note that low TH concentrations in a sick foal or horse (NTIS) is not equivalent to hypothyroidism, and its implications remain unclear.

References

1 Toribio, R.E. (2018). Thyroid gland. In: *Equine Internal Medicine*, 4e (ed. S.M. Reed, W.M. Bayly, and D.C. Sellon), 1058–1069. St. Louis, Missouri: Elsevier.
2 Kaneko, J.J. (1989). Thyroid function. In: *Biochemistry of Domestic Animals*, 4e (ed. J.J. Kaneko), 630. San Diego: Academic Press.
3 Breuhaus, B.A. (2011). Disorders of the equine thyroid gland. *Vet. Clin. North Am. Equine Pract.* 27: 115–128.
4 Beech, J., Boston, R., Lindborg, S. et al. (2007). Adrenocorticotropin concentration following administration of thyrotropin-releasing hormone in healthy horses and those with pituitary pars intermedia dysfunction and pituitary gland hyperplasia. *J. Am. Vet. Med. Assoc.* 231: 417–426.
5 Gentry, L.R., Thompson, D.L., and Stelzer, A.M. (2002). Responses of seasonally anovulatory mares to daily administration of thyrotropin-releasing hormone and (or) gonadotropin-releasing hormone analog. *J. Anim. Sci.* 80: 208–213.
6 Pruett, H.E., Thompson, D.L., Cartmill, J.A. et al. (2003). Thyrotropin releasing hormone interactions with growth hormone secretion in horses. *J. Anim. Sci.* 81: 2343–2351.
7 Thompson, D.L. Jr., Godke, R.A., and Nett, T.M. (1983). Effects of melatonin and thyrotropin releasing hormone on mares during the nonbreeding season. *J. Anim. Sci.* 56: 668–677.
8 Thompson, D.L. and Nett, T.M. (1984). Thyroid stimulating hormone and prolactin secretion after thyrotropin releasing hormone administration to mares – dose-response during anestrus in winter and during estrus in summer. *Domest. Anim. Endocrinol.* 1: 263–268.
9 Ingbar, S.H. (1985). The thyroid gland. In: *Williams' Textbook of Endocrinology*, 7e (ed. J.D. Wilson and D.W. Foster), 682. Philadelphia: W.B. Saunders.
10 Hammes, S.R. and Davis, P.J. (2015). Overlapping nongenomic and genomic actions of thyroid hormone and steroids. *Best Pract. Res. Clin. Endocrinol. Metab.* 29: 581–593.
11 Dai, G., Levy, O., and Carrasco, N. (1996). Cloning and characterization of the thyroid iodide transporter. *Nature* 379: 458–460.
12 Fong, P. (2011). Thyroid iodide efflux: a team effort? *J. Physiol.* 589: 5929–5939.
13 Yen, P.M. (2001). Physiological and molecular basis of thyroid hormone action. *Physiol. Rev.* 81: 1097–1142.
14 Abraham, G., Allersmeier, M., Schusser, G.F. et al. (2011). Serum thyroid hormone, insulin, glucose, triglycerides and protein concentrations in normal horses: association with topical dexamethasone usage. *Vet. J.* 188: 307–312.
15 Bates, J.M., Spate, V.L., Morris, J.S. et al. (2000). Effects of selenium deficiency on tissue selenium content, deiodinase activity, and thyroid hormone economy in the rat during development. *Endocrinology* 141: 2490–2500.
16 Chen, C.L. and Li, W.I. (1986). Effect of thyrotropin releasing hormone (TRH) on serum levels of thyroid hormones in thoroughbred mares. *J. Equine Sci.* 6: 58.
17 Chen, C.L., McNulty, M.E., and McNulty, B.A. (1984). Serum levels of thyroxine and triiodothyronine in mature horses following oral administration of synthetic thyroxine (Synthroid®). *J. Equine Vet. Sci.* 4: 5.
18 Irvine, C.H. (1967). Thyroxine secretion rate in the horse in various physiological states. *J. Endocrinol.* 39: 313–320.
19 Irvine, C.H. (1984). Hypothyroidism in the foal. *Equine Vet. J.* 16: 302–306.
20 Irvine, C.H. and Evans, M.J. (1975). Postnatal changes in total and free thyroxine and triiodothyronine in foal serum. *J. Reprod. Fertil. Suppl.* 709–715.
21 Malinowski, K., Christensen, R.A., Hafs, H.D. et al. (1996). Age and breed differences in thyroid hormones, insulin-like growth factor (IGF)-I and IGF binding proteins in female horses. *J. Anim. Sci.* 74: 1936–1942.
22 Forhead, A.J. and Fowden, A.L. (2014). Thyroid hormones in fetal growth and prepartum maturation. *J. Endocrinol.* 221: R87–R103.
23 Silver, M., Fowden, A.L., Knox, J. et al. (1991). Relationship between circulating tri-iodothyronine and cortisol in the perinatal period in the foal. *J. Reprod. Fertil. Suppl.* 44: 619–626.
24 Lopez-Rodriguez, M.F., Cymbaluk, N.F., Epp, T. et al. (2020). A field study of serum, colostrum, milk iodine, and thyroid hormone concentrations in postpartum draft mares and foals. *J. Equine Vet. Sci.* 90: 103018.
25 Panzani, S., Comin, A., Galeati, G. et al. (2012). How type of parturition and health status influence hormonal and metabolic profiles in newborn foals. *Theriogenology* 77: 1167–1177.

26 Muller, V., Toribio, R.E., Dembek, K. et al. (2020). Serum cortisol and thyroid hormone concentrations and survival in foals born from mares with experimentally induced ascending placentitis. *J. Vet. Intern. Med.* 34: 1332–1338.
27 Mendoza, F.J., Perez-Ecija, R.A., Toribio, R.E. et al. (2013). Thyroid hormone concentrations differ between donkeys and horses. *Equine Vet. J.* 45: 214–218.
28 Messer, N.T., Ganjam, V.K., Nachreiner, R.F. et al. (1995). Effect of dexamethasone administration on serum thyroid hormone concentrations in clinically normal horses. *J. Am. Vet. Med. Assoc.* 206: 63–66.
29 Ramirez, S., Wolfsheimer, K.J., Moore, R.M. et al. (1997). Duration of effects of phenylbutazone on serum total thyroxine and free thyroxine concentrations in horses. *J. Vet. Intern. Med.* 11: 371–374.
30 Larsson, M., Pettersson, T., and Carlstrom, A. (1985). Thyroid hormone binding in serum of 15 vertebrate species: isolation of thyroxine-binding globulin and prealbumin analogs. *Gen. Comp. Endocrinol.* 58: 360–375.
31 Katovich, M., Evans, J.W., and Sanchez, O. (1974). Effects of season, pregnancy and lactation on thyroxine turnover in the mare. *J. Anim. Sci.* 38: 811–818.
32 Chung, H.R. (2014). Adrenal and thyroid function in the fetus and preterm infant. *Korean J. Pediatr.* 57: 425–433.
33 Allen, A.L., Townsend, H.G., Doige, C.E. et al. (1996). A case-control study of the congenital hypothyroidism and dysmaturity syndrome of foals. *Can. Vet. J.* 37: 349–351.
34 Doige, C.E. and McLaughlin, B.G. (1981). Hyperplastic goitre in newborn foals in Western Canada. *Can. Vet. J.* 22: 42–45.
35 Irvine, C.H. and Evans, M.J. (1977). Hypothyroidism in foals. *N. Z. Vet. J.* 25: 354.
36 Koikkalainen, K., Knuuttila, A., Karikoski, N. et al. (2014). Congenital hypothyroidism and dysmaturity syndrome in foals: first reported cases in Europe. *Equine Vet. Educ.* 26: 181–189.
37 Allen, A.L., Fretz, P.B., Card, C.E. et al. (1998). The effects of partial thyroidectomy on the development of the equine fetus. *Equine Vet. J.* 30: 53–59.
38 Himler, M., Hurcombe, S.D., Griffin, A. et al. (2012). Presumptive nonthyroidal illness syndrome in critically ill foals. *Equine Vet. J. Suppl.* 44 (Suppl. 41): 43–47.
39 Breuhaus, B.A. (2014). Thyroid function and dysfunction in term and premature equine neonates. *J. Vet. Intern. Med.* 28: 1301–1309.
40 Pirrone, A., Panzani, S., Govoni, N. et al. (2013). Thyroid hormone concentrations in foals affected by perinatal asphyxia syndrome. *Theriogenology* 80: 624–629.

Section IV Hormones Involved in Blood Pressure and Blood Volume Regulation

Ramiro E. Toribio, Katarzyna A. Dembek, Laura D. Hostnik, and Teresa A. Burns

Blood Pressure (Vasopressor)

In the transition from intra- to extrauterine life, the foal must have functional homeostatic systems that maintain tissue perfusion to ensure survival. A negative fluid balance (dehydration), insufficient secretion of factors to restore blood volume (volume expansion), poor vascular response to vasoconstrictors (refractory vessels; vasoplegia), vasopressor imbalances (insufficient vasoconstrictor or excessive vasodilator secretion), and reduced cardiac output can have devastating consequences.

Foals have a high extracellular fluid water content and a diet rich in water but poor in Na^+. Foals ingest up to 25% of their body weight in milk, requiring rapid water absorption and elimination, but also efficient Na^+ retention. A reduction in fluid consumption or excessive elimination rapidly leads to dehydration and hypoperfusion, which are linked to foal mortality [1–4]. Dehydration, hypotension, hypoperfusion, and disorders of water and Na^+ balance are common in critically ill foals [1–4]. The response to volume depletion and hypotension is complex and involves hormones from the hypothalamus, pituitary gland (adeno- and neurohypophysis), adrenal gland (cortex and medulla), kidneys, liver, heart, and endothelium.

The mechanisms that control cardiovascular differentiation and ontogenic increase in arterial blood pressure in the equine fetus mature closer to birth compared to other species, in part due to steady activation of the HPAA [5–7]. Elevations in plasma cortisol concentrations have been associated with vasopressors and arterial blood pressure in near-term fetuses in a number of species [5–10]. There is strong correlation between norepinephrine and arginine vasopressin (AVP) with cortisol concentrations and blood pressure in equine fetuses [6]. This increase in plasma cortisol concentrations indicates that cardiovascular maturation is a glucocorticoid-dependent process [5–10]. The rate of fetal growth outside the normal trajectory could influence cardiovascular function and blood pressure in the equine neonate and may be more evident in premature and sick foals [10]. The vascular response to pressors such as phenylephrine, angiotensin II (ANG-II), and AVP increases with gestational age, suggesting developmental expression of their receptors are behind many of these dynamic changes [11].

Adrenergic System

The adrenal medulla is functionally part of the sympathetic nervous system and consists of chromaffin cells (pheochromocytes) that are modified post-ganglionic neurons controlled by pre-ganglionic fibers [12, 13]. These cells secrete catecholamines (epinephrine, norepinephrine, dopamine) and other peptides (enkephalin, neuropeptide Y, substance P) in response to autonomic stimulation from the splanchnic nerve and circulating factors (e.g. glucose, cytokines). They are considered stress hormones central to the "fight or flight" response of the sympathetic nervous system during stressful conditions. Catecholamines exert diverse physiological actions by binding to alpha (α1, α2), beta (β1–β3) adrenergic and dopaminergic (D1–D5) receptors, with a plasma half-life of approximately 1–2 minutes [14].

Catecholamines cause vasoconstriction, enhance cardiac and skeletal muscle contractility, increase heart rate, respiratory rate and blood pressure, relax smooth muscle in the gastrointestinal, urinary, and respiratory tracts, induce mydriasis, enhance aerobic glycolysis and oxygen consumption, increase blood glucose by promoting glycogenolysis, gluconeogenesis, and glucagon release, but inhibit insulin secretion, induce lipolysis, enhance thermogenesis, and attenuate the release of mediators from mast cells and

Equine Neonatal Medicine, First Edition. Edited by David M. Wong and Pamela A. Wilkins.

basophils during type I hypersensitivity reactions. The differential actions between epinephrine and norepinephrine are dictated by receptor affinity and distribution. In the neonate, catecholamines regulate blood pressure, improve cardiac function, stimulate pulmonary surfactant release and absorption of pulmonary fluids, and increase energy metabolism [2, 15]. Norepinephrine promotes vasoconstriction in most organs; however, epinephrine dilates the blood vessels in skeletal muscle and the liver and causes bronchodilation [12, 13, 16].

Similar to the HPAA, maturation of equine cardiovascular function occurs in late pregnancy and continues in the early postnatal period [3, 17, 18]. The equine fetal adrenal gland doubles in weight in the last month of gestation, from 60 mg/kg of fetal weight at day 300 to 100 mg/kg at term [8]. This increase is mainly due to growth of the adrenal cortex, in particular the zona fasciculata, which is responsible for cortisol secretion [8]. This maturation process likely influences differentiation of chromaffin cells, in particular the expression of cortisol-dependent enzymes involved in catecholamine synthesis [19]. In other species, the presence of chromaffin cells facilitates the effect of ACTH and corticotropin-releasing hormone (CRH) on cortisol production as part of the intra-adrenal CRH-ACTH system [20, 21]. These are examples where two endocrine systems within a gland show dependency, which could be relevant to conditions such as prematurity and sepsis. In other words, timely HPAA maturation influences the synthesis and secretion of vasopressors and the response of blood vessels to vasoactive compounds. Clinically, this is evident in premature foals that are often hypotensive and may have signs of tissue hypoperfusion [2, 3, 11].

At the end of gestation, the equine fetus has an increase in arterial blood pressure and blood flow with a decrease in vascular resistance and heart rate that are associated with elevations in plasma epinephrine, norepinephrine, AVP, and cortisol concentrations [6]. A reduction in oxygen delivery to uteroplacental tissues, combined with elevations in AVP and norepinephrine concentrations and the increased expression of their receptors, contribute to the rise in arterial blood pressure in the near term fetus [6, 11]. A functional HPAA at the end of gestation facilitates maturation of the sympathoadrenal system in the equine neonate [6].

In the equine fetus, epinephrine and norepinephrine increase steadily until term [6]. After birth, the adrenergic response to the stress of hypotension is stronger for norepinephrine compared to epinephrine and remains unchanged for at least 2 weeks after birth [11]. In regard to cardiovascular function, norepinephrine is the dominant catecholamine in newborn foals and might be a better vasopressor candidate in critically ill hypotensive foals [11, 15]. This is supported by studies showing that the equine fetal adrenal medulla secretes both epinephrine and norepinephrine in response to hypoxia, but norepinephrine is the predominant catecholamine released; this persists after birth [22]. Epinephrine, but not norepinephrine, increases within 30 minutes of normal foaling, suggesting that epinephrine may be more important for adaptive events immediately after birth [15], perhaps to enhance pulmonary ventilation, protect against hypoxia, and promote energy availability. The equine fetal adrenal medulla has higher norepinephrine content than epinephrine that can be rapidly released from hypoxia [22], and may explain differences observed after birth [11]. In addition, cardiovascular sympathetic sensitivity increases after birth in foals, which contributes to their rapid response to hypotension [11], a serious complication to illness in foal [1–4]. Healthy foals in the first week of life have a rapid sympathetic and adrenocortical response to the stress of being separated from their mares, with increases in epinephrine, norepinephrine, and cortisol concentrations [23].

Information on catecholamine concentrations in premature or septic foals is lacking; however, norepinephrine is a frequently used vasopressor in critically ill hypotensive foals, many of which respond appropriately with increases in mean arterial pressure [24, 25].

Arginine vasopressin (AVP; anti-diuretic hormone [ADH]; 9 amino acids) is a neuropeptide hormone synthesized by magnocellular and parvocellular neurons in the paraventricular and supraoptic nuclei of the hypothalamus. Magnocellular AVP neurons mainly project to the posterior pituitary gland, while parvocellular neurons project to the median eminence [26]. In the neurohypophysis, AVP is stored and released in response to hypotension and increased plasma osmolality. AVP is a potent vasoconstrictor, and a major function is to maintain blood pressure via vasoconstriction and renal water retention. AVP interacts with V1 receptors in vascular smooth muscle causing vasoconstriction, V2 receptors in the renal collecting ducts to promote water reabsorption via aquaporin channels, and V3 receptors in the pituitary gland to increase synthesis and secretion of ACTH (corticotropin) [12].

AVP is one of the main hormones regulating extracellular fluid tonicity and functions to correct hypotension (blood pressure balance) and hyperosmolality (Na^+ balance); it also mediates ACTH secretion from the pituitary gland in response to stress (AVP released in the median eminence) in the horse [27, 28]. In other words, AVP potentiates the stimulatory effects of CRH on ACTH secretion and may provide a mechanism to escape glucocorticoid inhibition on the HPAA [28]. AVP enhances vascular response to catecholamines, especially in acute shock to maintain organ perfusion.

In the equine fetus, plasma AVP concentrations increase with gestational age and are correlated with cortisol concentrations [6]. Similarly, the pressor response to exogenous AVP is higher near term [11]. Newborn foals have a rapid endogenous AVP response to the stress of hypotension [11]. No age-related changes in plasma AVP concentrations were detected in healthy foals from birth to 3 months of age [29]. These findings indicate that the vasopressinergic system in foals is mature at birth. In the clinical setting, this information justifies the use of AVP and its analogs as alternative vasopressors in hypotensive foals nonresponsive to catecholamines. The use of glucocorticoids in these animals should be considered. Plasma AVP concentrations increase in critically ill and hypotensive foals [1, 2, 30]. In addition, AVP concentrations have been associated with activation of the HPAA [1, 2]. This supports the physiological role of AVP in maintaining tissue perfusion and modulating the stress response. Plasma AVP concentrations can decrease with severe septic or hypovolemic shock, suggesting hormonal depletion. Exogenous AVP and synthetic analogues are used to provide hemodynamic support to people with catecholamine-refractory hypotension, and occasionally are also used in hypotensive septic foals [12, 24].

The Renin-Angiotensin-Aldosterone System's (RAAS) main function is to maintain blood volume and tissue perfusion by increasing intravascular fluid volume, systemic vascular resistance, arterial blood pressure and cardiac output [3, 31]. Hypotension and hyponatremia are strong stimulators of the RAAS [16]. Renin is a proteolytic enzyme released by the kidneys in response to sympathetic activation (β1-adrenoceptors), renal artery hypotension (sensed by juxtaglomerular apparatus via prostaglandins), and reduced Na^+, Cl^-, and K^+ in the renal distal tubules [16, 32]. An increase of these electrolytes in the distal tubules promotes local adenosine release, causing vasoconstriction of the afferent arteriole to decrease renin secretion. Renin cleaves angiotensinogen to angiotensin I, which is converted in the lungs by angiotensin-converting enzyme (ACE) into angiotensin II (ANG-II; 8 amino acids), a potent vasoconstrictor that also induces aldosterone and AVP secretion, renal Na^+ reabsorption, thirst, and facilitates catecholamine release [33]. Aldosterone is secreted by the zona glomerulosa of the adrenal gland cortex in response to hyperkalemia, ANG-II and ACTH [16, 32]. Aldosterone increases renal Na^+ reabsorption and K^+ elimination, thus, increasing water retention, blood pressure and tissue perfusion. It binds to mineralocorticoid receptors to stimulate expression of genes involved in renal Na^+, K^+, and water transport, including Na^+ and K^+ channels, Na^+/K^+-ATPase, and aquaporins [16, 32]. Reclamation of Na^+ and water by aldosterone and efferent arteriolar vasoconstriction by ANG-II aim at improving blood volume and perfusion to vital organs and offset hypotension from septic, hypovolemic and neurogenic shock [3, 16, 32]. AVP is usually released simultaneously with aldosterone to complementary expand the intravascular compartment and blood pressure.

Plasma ACE and angiotensinogen concentrations increase toward term in the equine fetus and are associated with gestational age, blood pressure, and plasma cortisol concentrations [7]. Plasma ANG-II and renin concentrations were correlated in equine fetuses, but were not associated with gestational age [7]. However, exogenous ANG-II increased heart rate and blood pressure in a dose-dependent manner that was associated with gestational age and cortisol concentrations in equine fetuses [11]. The increase in pulmonary ACE activity in term fetuses may be induced by the prepartum surge in cortisol [34]. This suggests that premature delivery disrupts pulmonary ACE activity that potentially alters their response to hypovolemia and hypotension [34]. At birth, newborn foals have a functional RAAS that is responsive to changes in blood volume, Na^+, K^+, and hypotension, characterized by increases in ACE activity, renin substrate (angiotensinogen), ANG-II, and aldosterone concentrations [7, 34–36]. The RAAS is more responsive to hypovolemia/hyponatremia in newborn foals than horses [31]. Low concentrations of renin, ANG-II, and aldosterone have been measured in critically ill foals [3]. ANG-II analogs are used as a new non-catecholamine pressor option for people with vasodilatory shock [37]. As previously mentioned, exogenous ANG-II increases blood pressure in the equine fetus [11], but analogs have not been evaluated in sick foals.

Natriuretic Peptides

Atrial natriuretic peptide (ANP; 28 amino acids) or atrial natriuretic factor (ANF) is secreted by the cardiac atria in response to atrial wall stretching from hypertension, increased intravascular volume, corticosteroids, alpha-adrenergic agonists, and hypoxia [38, 39]. It is a potent natriuretic, diuretic, and hypotensive factor and an endogenous antagonist of the RAAS [38, 39]. It reduces intravascular volume and extracellular fluid by decreasing renal reabsorption of Na^+ (natriuresis) and water (diuresis). Its natriuretic and diuretic actions result from increased glomerular filtration rate and reduced renal Na^+ reabsorption [31, 39]. Brain natriuretic peptide (BNP; 32 amino acids) is secreted by cardiac ventricular muscle cells with actions similar to ANP using the same receptors but is less effective than ANP. Because BNP has a longer half-life than ANP, N-terminal pro-brain natriuretic peptide (NT-proBNP) is used clinically and in research settings to assess heart function. The role of natriuretic peptides in equine disorders is unclear. One study found no differences in ANP concentrations in hospitalized foals before and after fluid resuscitation, but concentrations were different in horses [31]. BNP concentrations were not different in horses with various cardiac pathologies [40], but information in healthy or sick foals is lacking.

Endothelin-1 (ET-1; 21 amino acids) is a potent vasoconstrictor peptide that plays a major role in regulation of vascular tone [41]. It is produced by endothelial cells in response to hypoxia, epinephrine, ANG-II, AVP, cytokines, and endotoxemia [41]. Its secretion is reduced by nitric oxide (NO), prostacyclin, and ANP. Endothelin-1 acts through four receptors (ET_A, ET_{B1}, ET_{B2}, ET_C) [41] and counters vasodilators such as NO. While increased ET-1 concentrations are important to maintain tissue perfusion in certain pathological conditions, it can also interfere with proper blood flow and tissue oxygenation, in part by reducing NO synthesis. In healthy foals, big ET-1 (ET-1 precursor) concentrations increase immediately after birth, stay elevated for the first 3 days to gradually decrease, and remain constant after day 4 [42]. Increases in big ET-1 concentrations were documented in sick foals [42]. Other endothelin isoforms (ET-2, ET-3) are found in circulation and are vasoconstrictors, but ET-1 is considered the main form; information is not available in equids. Of relevance to neurological, gastrointestinal, and skin physiology, the ET_B receptor is important for neural crest cell migration, and mutations cause lethal white syndrome [43].

Adrenomedullin (ADM; 52 amino acids) is a potent vasodilator expressed by numerous tissues and participates in blood pressure regulation [44]. Its vasodilatory effects are mediated in part through NO release. ADM is also important to endothelial barrier development and stability [45]. ADM increases in response to various chronic conditions as well as endotoxemia and septic shock [45]. Experimental treatment with ADM has shown benefits in hypertension, heart failure, septic shock, endotoxemia, ischemia/reperfusion injury, and endothelial integrity [44, 46]. It may reduce systemic inflammation and could be protective against endotoxin-induced organ damage [46]. Plasma ADM concentrations were higher in critically ill compared to healthy foals, but were not associated with disease severity or mortality [47].

References

1 Hurcombe, S.D., Toribio, R.E., Slovis, N. et al. (2008). Blood arginine vasopressin, adrenocorticotropin hormone, and cortisol concentrations at admission in septic and critically ill foals and their association with survival. *J. Vet. Intern. Med.* 22: 639–647.

2 Dembek, K.A., Hurcombe, S.D., Stewart, A.J. et al. (2016). Association of aldosterone and arginine vasopressin concentrations and clinical markers of hypoperfusion in neonatal foals. *Equine Vet. J.* 48: 176–181.

3 Dembek, K.A., Onasch, K., Hurcombe, S.D. et al. (2013). Renin-angiotensin-aldosterone system and hypothalamic-pituitary-adrenal axis in hospitalized newborn foals. *J. Vet. Intern. Med.* 27: 331–338.

4 Dembek, K.A., Hurcombe, S.D., Frazer, M.L. et al. (2014). Development of a likelihood of survival scoring system for hospitalized equine neonates using generalized boosted regression modeling. *PLoS One* 9: e109212.

5 Fowden, A.L., Forhead, A.J., and Ousey, J.C. (2012). Endocrine adaptations in the foal over the perinatal period. *Equine Vet. J. Suppl.* 44: 130–139.

6 Giussani, D.A., Forhead, A.J., and Fowden, A.L. (2005). Development of cardiovascular function in the horse fetus. *J. Physiol.* 565: 1019–1030.

7 Forhead, A.J., Broughton Pipkin, F., Taylor, P.M. et al. (2000). Developmental changes in blood pressure and the renin-angiotensin system in pony fetuses during the second half of gestation. *J. Reprod. Fertil. Suppl.* 56: 693–703.

8 Fowden, A.L. and Silver, M. (1995). Comparative development of the pituitary-adrenal axis in the fetal foal and lamb. *Reprod. Domest. Anim.* 30: 170–177.

9 Forhead, A.J., Broughton Pipkin, F., and Fowden, A.L. (2000). Effect of cortisol on blood pressure and the renin-angiotensin system in fetal sheep during late gestation. *J. Physiol.* 526 (Pt 1): 167–176.

10 Giussani, D.A., Forhead, A.J., Gardner, D.S. et al. (2003). Postnatal cardiovascular function after manipulation of fetal growth by embryo transfer in the horse. *J. Physiol.* 547: 67–76.

11 O'Connor, S.J., Gardner, D.S., Ousey, J.C. et al. (2005). Development of baroreflex and endocrine responses to hypotensive stress in newborn foals and lambs. *Pflugers Arch.* 450: 298–306.

12 Hurcombe, S.D. (2011). Hypothalamic-pituitary gland axis function and dysfunction in horses. *Vet. Clin. North Am. Equine Pract.* 27: 1–17.

13 Ehrhart-Bornstein, M. and Bornstein, S.R. (2008). Cross-talk between adrenal medulla and adrenal cortex in stress. *Ann. N.Y. Acad. Sci.* 1148: 112–117.

14 Cohen, G., Holland, B., Sha, J. et al. (1959). Plasma concentrations of epinephrine and norepinephrine during intravenous infusions in man. *J. Clin. Invest.* 38: 1935–1941.

15 Melchert, M., Aurich, C., Aurich, J. et al. (2019). Controlled delay of the expulsive phase of foaling affects

sympathoadrenal activity and acid base balance of foals in the immediate postnatal phase. *Theriogenology* 139: 8–15.

16 Barrett, K.E., Barman, S.M., Boitano, S. et al. (2016). *Ganong's Review of Medical Physiology*. New York: McGraw Hill Education.

17 Ousey, J.C. (2004). Peripartal endocrinology in the mare and foetus. *Reprod. Domest. Anim.* 39: 222–231.

18 Forhead, A.J., Ousey, J.C., Allen, W.R. et al. (2004). Postnatal insulin secretion and sensitivity after manipulation of fetal growth by embryo transfer in the horse. *J. Endocrinol.* 181: 459–467.

19 Han, X., Fowden, A.L., Silver, M. et al. (1995). Immunohistochemical localisation of steroidogenic enzymes and phenylethanolamine-N-methyl-transferase (PNMT) in the adrenal gland of the fetal and newborn foal. *Equine Vet. J.* 27: 140–146.

20 Xing, Y., Lerario, A.M., Rainey, W., and Hammer, G.D. (2015). Development of adrenal cortex zonation. *Endocrinol. Metab. Clin. North Am.* 44: 243–274.

21 Silverman, M.N., Pearce, B.D., Biron, C.A. et al. (2005). Immune modulation of the hypothalamic-pituitary-adrenal (HPA) axis during viral infection. *Viral Immunol.* 18: 41–78.

22 Comline, R.S. and Silver, M. (1971). Catecholamine secretion by the adrenal medulla of the foetal and new-born foal. *J. Physiol.* 216: 659–682.

23 Niezgoda, J. and Tischner, M. (1995). Intensity of stress reactions during short-term isolation of mothers from foals. *Biol. Reprod.* 52: 107–111.

24 Dickey, E.J., McKenzie, H., Johnson, A. et al. (2010). Use of pressor therapy in 34 hypotensive critically ill neonatal foals. *Aust. Vet. J.* 88: 472–477.

25 Corley, K.T. (2002). Monitoring and treating haemodynamic disturbances in critically ill neonatal foals. Part 2: assessment and treatment. *Equine Vet. Educ.* 14: 328–334.

26 Aguilera, G., Subburaju, S., Young, S. et al. (2008). The parvocellular vasopressinergic system and responsiveness of the hypothalamic pituitary adrenal axis during chronic stress. *Prog. Brain Res.* 170: 29–39.

27 Livesey, J.H., Donald, R.A., Irvine, C.H. et al. (1988). The effects of cortisol, vasopressin (AVP), and corticotropin-releasing factor administration on pulsatile adrenocorticotropin, alpha-melanocyte-stimulating hormone, and AVP secretion in the pituitary venous effluent of the horse. *Endocrinology* 123: 713–720.

28 Antoni, F.A. (2019). Magnocellular vasopressin and the mechanism of "Glucocorticoid Escape". *Front. Endocrinol. (Lausanne)* 10: 422.

29 Wong, D.M., Vo, D.T., Alcott, C.J. et al. (2008). Plasma vasopressin concentrations in healthy foals from birth to 3 months of age. *J. Vet. Intern. Med.* 22: 1259–1261.

30 Borchers, A., Magdesian, K.G., Schenck, P.A. et al. (2014). Serial plasma vasopressin concentration in healthy and hospitalised neonatal foals. *Equine Vet. J.* 46: 306–310.

31 Hollis, A.R., Boston, R.C., and Corley, K.T. (2008). Plasma aldosterone, vasopressin and atrial natriuretic peptide in hypovolaemia: a preliminary comparative study of neonatal and mature horses. *Equine Vet. J.* 40: 64–69.

32 Badiu, C. (2019). Williams textbook of endocrinology. *Acta Endocrinol. (Buchar)* 15: 416–416.

33 Harrison-Bernard, L.M. (2009). The renal renin-angiotensin system. *Adv. Physiol. Educ.* 33: 270–274.

34 O'Connor, S.J., Fowden, A.L., Holdstock, N. et al. (2002). Developmental changes in pulmonary and renal angiotensin-converting enzyme concentration in fetal and neonatal horses. *Reprod. Fertil. Dev.* 14: 413–417.

35 Broughton Pipkin, F., Ousey, J.C., Wallace, C.P. et al. (1984). Studies on equine prematurity 4: effect of salt and water loss on the renin-angiotensin-aldosterone system in the newborn foal. *Equine Vet. J.* 16: 292–297.

36 Broughton Pipkin, F., Rossdale, P.D., and Frauenfelder, H. (1982). Changes in the renin-angiotensin system of the mare and foal at parturition. *J. Reprod. Fertil. Suppl.* 32: 555–561.

37 Bussard, R.L. and Busse, L.W. (2018). Angiotensin II: a new therapeutic option for vasodilatory shock. *Ther. Clin. Risk Manage.* 14: 1287–1298.

38 Potter, L.R., Yoder, A.R., Flora, D.R. et al. (2009). Natriuretic peptides: their structures, receptors, physiologic functions and therapeutic applications. *Handb. Exp. Pharmacol.* 191: 341–366.

39 McGrath, M.F., de Bold, M.L., and de Bold, A.J. (2005). The endocrine function of the heart. *Trends Endocrinol. Metab.* 16: 469–477.

40 van Maanen, J.M., van Dijk, A., Mulder, K. et al. (1994). Consumption of drinking water with high nitrate levels causes hypertrophy of the thyroid. *Toxicol. Lett.* 72: 365–374.

41 Kowalczyk, A., Kleniewska, P., Kolodziejczyk, M. et al. (2015). The role of endothelin-1 and endothelin receptor antagonists in inflammatory response and sepsis. *Arch. Immunol. Ther. Exp. (Warsz)* 63: 41–52.

42 Giordano, A., Castagnetti, C., Panzani, S. et al. (2015). Endothelin 1 in healthy foals and in foals affected by neonatal diseases. *Theriogenology* 84: 667–673.

43 Santschi, E.M., Purdy, A.K., Valberg, S.J. et al. (1998). Endothelin receptor B polymorphism associated with lethal white foal syndrome in horses. *Mamm. Genome* 9: 306–309.

44 Beltowski, J. and Jamroz, A. (2004). Adrenomedullin – what do we know 10 years since its discovery? *Pol. J. Pharmacol.* 56: 5–27.

45 Geven, C., Kox, M., and Pickkers, P. (2018). Adrenomedullin and adrenomedullin-targeted therapy as treatment strategies relevant for sepsis. *Front. Immunol.* 9: 292.

46 Saito, R., Shimosawa, T., Ogihara, T. et al. (2012). Function of adrenomedullin in inflammatory response of liver against LPS-induced endotoxemia. *APMIS* 120: 706–711.

47 Toth, B., Slovis, N.M., Constable, P.D., and Taylor, S.D. (2014). Plasma adrenomedullin concentrations in critically ill neonatal foals. *J. Vet. Intern. Med.* 28: 1294–1300. https://doi.org/10.1111/jvim.12358.

Section V Hormones Involved in Calcium, Phosphorus, and Magnesium Regulation

Ramiro E. Toribio, Katarzyna A. Dembek, Laura D. Hostnik, and Teresa A. Burns

Calcium, Phosphorus, and Magnesium

Calcium (Ca), phosphorus (phosphate; PO_4), and magnesium (Mg) are essential minerals with structural and nonstructural functions. Their demands are higher for growing foals. Therefore, precise endocrine homeostatic systems to regulate their extracellular concentrations are vital [1, 2] and include parathyroid hormone (PTH), calcitonin (CT), vitamin D, fibroblast growth factor-23 (FGF-23), and parathyroid hormone-related protein (PTHrP). Other hormones such as insulin, catecholamines, and arginine vasopressin (AVP) can influence PO_4 and Mg concentrations but are not considered central to their regulation.

PTH increases renal reabsorption of Ca and Mg, enhances renal excretion of PO_4, stimulates renal 1α-hydroxylase activity and vitamin D activation, and promotes bone resorption. CT decreases plasma Ca and PO_4 concentrations, increases urinary Ca and PO_4 excretion, and inhibits osteoclastic bone resorption. It is protective against hypercalcemia and excessive bone resorption. Hypocalcemia stimulates and hypercalcemia suppresses PTH synthesis and secretion, while the opposite occurs with CT release [1]. PTHrP has multiple functions and works through the PTH receptor; its role in Ca metabolism is important in the developing fetus as well as making Ca available during lactation. Vitamin D, through its active metabolite, $1,25(OH)_2D_3$ (calcitriol), increases intestinal absorption and renal reabsorption of Ca and PO_4, promotes bone remodeling, stimulates FGF-23 secretion, suppresses PTH synthesis and secretion, has immune regulatory actions, modulates cell proliferation and differentiation, and has antibacterial properties. FGF-23 is involved in Ca, PO_4, and vitamin D regulation and considered the main PO_4-regulating hormone. It suppresses 1α-hydroxylase activity and $1,25(OH)_2D_3$ synthesis and prevents PO_4 reabsorption, resulting in phosphaturia, and also inhibits PTH secretion [1].

Hypocalcemia, hypomagnesemia, and hyperphosphatemia are frequent disorders in critically ill foals [3–5]. Abnormally high PTH, high FGF-23, and low vitamin D concentrations have been associated with disease severity and mortality in critically ill newborn foals [3–5]. No differences in CT and PTHrP concentrations between healthy and sick foals have been documented [3–5].

Calcium

Calcium has structural (mechanical) and nonstructural (ionic) functions, and its extra- and intracellular concentrations are influenced by physiological and pathological conditions. Calcium is essential for a multitude of physiological processes, including muscle contraction, neuromuscular excitability, blood coagulation, enzyme activation, hormone secretion, cell division, and cell membrane stability. It is also involved in processes leading to cell injury and cell death (necrosis, apoptosis). Due to its importance in intra- and extracellular processes, maintenance of steady Ca concentrations is essential.

Calcium represents approximately 1.5% of body weight, with most (99%) located in the skeleton (hydroxyapatite), 1% in the intracellular compartment, and 0.1% in the extracellular fluid (Figure 20.V.1). This distribution is influenced by age, physiological status, and physical activity, but information in foals is lacking. Total calcium (TCa) in circulation is bound to proteins (albumin), in a free/ionized or active form (Ca^{2+}), and chelated to anions (lactate, phosphate, bicarbonate, sulfate, citrate). Calcium requirements are higher in growing equids [1]. Intestinal absorption and reabsorption of Ca are higher in neonates compared to adult animals to match increased bone apposition rate during growth, especially in the early neonatal period [1, 10, 11].

Equine Neonatal Medicine, First Edition. Edited by David M. Wong and Pamela A. Wilkins.

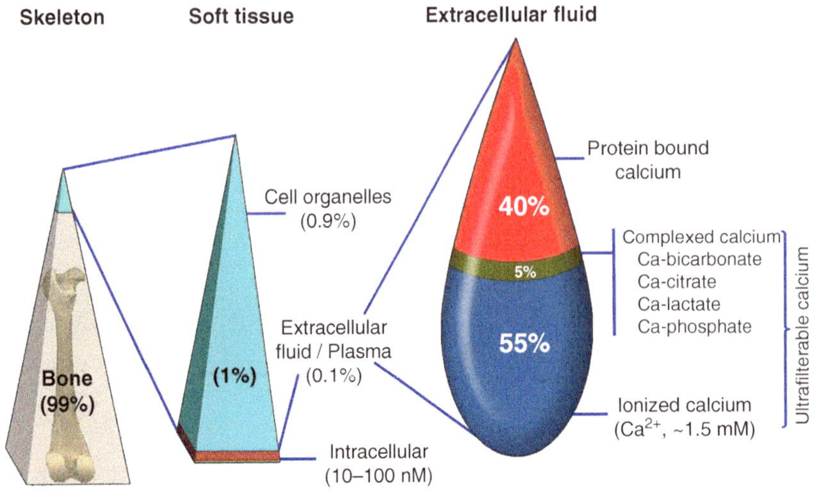

Figure 20.V.1 Calcium distribution in the body and extracellular compartment. The skeleton contains approximately 99% of the total body calcium (Ca) with the remaining 1% present in the cell membrane, organelles, and the extracellular fluid. In blood, Ca exists bound to proteins, as a free or ionized form (Ca^{2+}) and complexed to anions. In horses, Ca^{2+} represents ~55% of the total blood Ca concentration. Foals have slightly lower blood Ca concentrations than horses but total Ca to Ca^{2+} proportions are similar to horses [6–9]. *Source:* Image courtesy of Dr. R. E. Toribio, College of Veterinary Medicine, The Ohio State University.

Calcium concentrations in body fluids are reported in mg/dl or mmol/l. The atomic weight of Ca is 40 and its valence is 2+; therefore, 1 mEq of Ca is equal to 20 mg (0.5 mmol) of Ca. Conversion factors are: mmol/l = mg/dl × 0.25; mg/dl = mmol/l × 4. Dietary Ca is reported as %, g/kg, or parts per million (ppm; mg/kg).

Extracellular Ca concentrations are regulated by PTH, CT, and 1,25-dihydroxyvitamin D_3 ($1,25(OH)_2D_3$; calcitriol). Low extracellular Ca^{2+} stimulates PTH secretion, which promotes renal reabsorption of Ca^{2+}, synthesis of $1,25(OH)_2D_3$, as well as bone resorption. Hypercalcemia promotes CT release, which increases renal excretion of Ca^{2+} and inhibits osteoclast activity to reduce bone resorption. Calcitriol inhibits parathyroid cell function and PTH secretion but increases intestinal absorption and renal reabsorption of calcium.

Blood concentrations of TCa and Ca^{2+} are lower in foals (TCa = 10–13 mg/dl; Ca^{2+} = 4.1–7 mg/dl) than adult horses (TCa = 11–13.2 mg/dl; Ca^{2+} = 5.8–7 mg/dl) [3, 5–7]; thus, it is important to use age-specific reference ranges. Foals with hypoproteinemia can have low TCa concentrations, but do not have signs of hypocalcemia because Ca^{2+} concentrations are normal [1, 12]. Hypocalcemia is frequent in critically ill equine patients (foals and horses) [4, 7, 13]. Hypercalcemia is less frequent but occasionally occurs in sick foals [1].

Phosphorus

Similar to Ca, phosphorus has structural (mechanical) and nonstructural (ionic) functions, and its concentrations in the extra- and intracellular compartments are influenced by physiological and pathological conditions. Phosphorus is essential for energy homeostasis, intermediary metabolism of carbohydrates, fats, and proteins, oxidative phosphorylation, enzyme activity, electrolyte transport, oxygen transport, cell membrane stability, neuromuscular excitability, muscle contraction, nucleic acid metabolism, gene transcription, and cell proliferation [1].

Phosphorus (phosphate) represents ~1% of the body weight, with most (85%) located in bone matrix (hydroxyapatite), 15% in blood and soft tissues, and <0.1% in extracellular fluid. In blood, phosphate exists in organic (70%) and inorganic (30%) forms [1] (Figure 20.V.2). Organic phosphate is bound to lipids, proteins, and blood cells, but only inorganic phosphate (PO_4) is measured. Blood PO_4 concentrations are higher in foals compared to horses (30–40% higher). Foals also have a higher % of phosphorus in the extracellular compartment, which is estimated at 0.2% (Toribio, personal communication). This indicates that foals have a higher inorganic to organic fraction (~40%) of phosphorus in circulation. This is driven by growth, increased bone apposition rate, energy storage and use, phosphorylation processes (signaling), and bound to organic compounds (proteins, nucleic acids, lipids) that require PO_4.

The atomic weight of phosphorus is 31; for unit conversion, 1 mmol/l = 3.1 mg/dl (1 mmol = 31 mg); mg/dl × 0.32 = mmol/l (1 mg/dl = 0.32 mmol/l; 1 mg = 0.032 mmol); 1 mmol/l = 1.8 mEq/l. Dietary phosphorus is reported as %, g/kg, or parts per million (ppm; mg/kg).

Extracellular PO_4 concentrations are regulated by PTH, $1,25(OH)_2D_3$, FGF-23, insulin, growth hormone, and

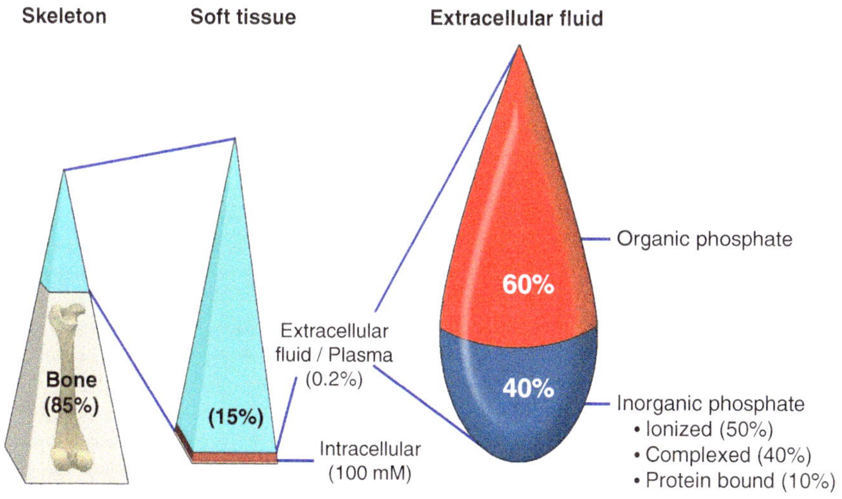

Figure 20.V.2 Phosphorus distribution in the body and extracellular compartment. The skeleton contains approximately 85% of the total body phosphorus with the remaining 15% present in soft tissues and the extracellular fluid. In blood, phosphorus exists in organic (70%) and inorganic (30%) forms. Inorganic phosphorus (phosphate; PO_4) is present in an ionized form, bound to proteins, and complexed to cations such as Ca^{2+} and Mg^{2+}. In foals, a higher % of phosphorus is in the extracellular compartment. *Source:* Image courtesy of Dr. R. E. Toribio, College of Veterinary Medicine, The Ohio State University.

insulin-like growth factor-1 (IGF-1) [1, 14, 15]. Hyperphosphatemia stimulates PTH and FGF-23 secretion and inhibits $1{,}25(OH)_2D_3$ synthesis [1]. Both PTH and FGF-23 promote renal PO_4 excretion, while $1{,}25(OH)_2D_3$ stimulates intestinal absorption and renal reabsorption of PO_4. Growth hormone and IGF-1 increase PO_4 concentrations in growing animals [14, 15]. Due to increased intestinal absorption and growth, blood concentrations of PO_4 are higher in foals (4.4–8.4 mg/dl; 1.4–2.7 mmol/l) than horses (2–5.6 mg/dl; 0.65–1.8 mmol/l) [3–5, 7, 16]. High PO_4 concentrations in foals parallel increased alkaline phosphatase activity, which reflects enhanced intestinal absorption, osteoblast activity and bone apposition rate [1, 17]. Phosphorus requirements are higher in growing equids [1] and intestinal absorption and renal reabsorption are more efficient in young animals [11, 18].

Information on the prevalence of disorders of phosphorus in sick foals is minimal; however, depending on the condition and metabolic status, they develop hypophosphatemia and hyperphosphatemia. Hyperphosphatemia is more frequent in critically ill foals, associated with disease severity and acid–base status [4], while hypophosphatemia occurs in foals with hyperglycemia, hyperlipemia, parenteral nutrition, from insulin administration, and less commonly in septic foals. Hypophosphatemia is often associated with hypomagnesemia and hypokalemia.

Magnesium

Magnesium (Mg) functions are mainly regulatory and concentrations in the extra- and intracellular compartments are influenced by physiological and pathological conditions. Mg participates in a multitude of physiological processes, including enzymatic activation, energy generation and use, oxidative phosphorylation, intermediary metabolism of carbohydrates, fats, and proteins, nucleic acid metabolism, ion transport, cell membrane stability, neuromuscular excitability, muscle contraction, cell proliferation, immune cell function, and Ca homeostasis. Over 600 enzymatic reactions require Mg [19].

Extracellular Mg concentrations are not under tight hormonal homeostatic control as occurs with Ca, and plasma Mg concentrations depend on intestinal absorption, renal excretion, and bone exchange. However, various hormonal and nonhormonal factors influence extracellular Mg concentrations. For example, PTH, AVP, glucagon, β-adrenergic agonists, and epidermal growth factor (EGF) increase renal Mg^{2+} reabsorption, while hypercalcemia decreases renal Mg^{2+} reabsorption [20]. [2, 21] Insulin promotes Mg^{2+} shift to the intracellular compartment [22].

The body contains 0.05% Mg by weight, of which 60% is in the skeleton, 38% in soft tissues, and 1–2% in the extracellular fluid [2]. Total magnesium (TMg) in the extracellular compartment exists bound to proteins (albumin), free/ionized/active (Mg^{2+}), and chelated to anions [2] (Figure 20.V.3). It is unclear if there are differences in body Mg content between foals and horses, but extracellular concentrations are comparable. Daily Mg requirements are higher in foals compared to horses [2]. Intestinal absorption and renal reabsorption of Mg are higher in young animals [23]. Feeding Mg-deficient diets to foals and young horses results in low serum Mg concentrations and total body Mg depletion [24, 25] along with soft tissue mineralization [25].

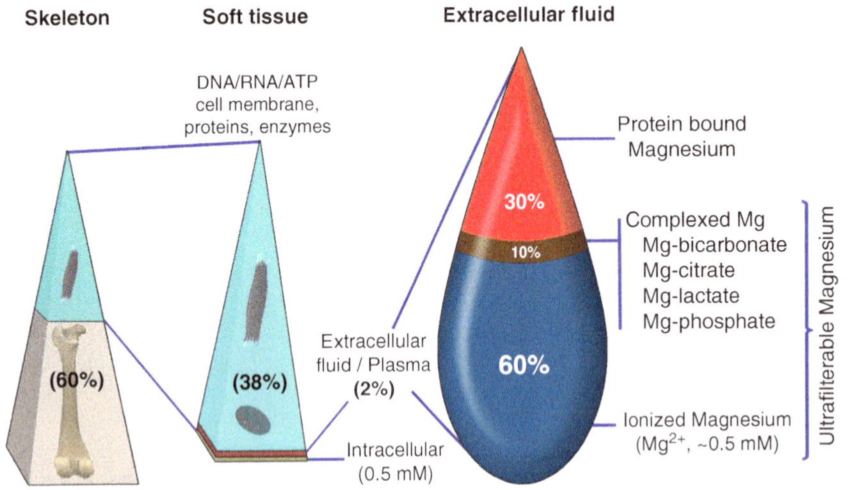

Figure 20.V.3 Magnesium distribution in the body and extracellular compartment. Around 60% of the total body Mg is in the skeleton, 38% in soft tissue, and 2% in the extracellular fluid. In horses, 60% of Mg exists as a free or ionized form (Mg^{2+}), 30% is bound to proteins, and 10% is complexed to anions [6, 7, 9, 21]. *Source:* Image courtesy of Dr. R. E. Toribio, College of Veterinary Medicine, The Ohio State University.

Mg concentrations are higher in the intracellular compartment, where it binds to negatively charged molecules (ATP, GTP, DNA, RNA), enzymes, and other proteins. Any ATP-dependent reaction also requires Mg^{2+} because inside the cell ATP is complexed with Mg^{2+} (ATP·Mg^{2+} complex) [19, 26, 27]. Mg^{2+} is necessary for the activity of the Na^+/K^+-ATPase, Mg^{2+}-ATPase, H^+/K^+-ATPase pump (proton pump), plasma membrane Ca^{2+} ATPase (PMCA), Na^+/Ca^{2+} exchanger (NCX), N-methyl-D-aspartate (NMDA) receptor (NMDAR), Ca^{2+} channels, and other proteins involved in neuronal and glial function. The neuroprotective actions of Mg^{2+} are in part due to its ability to compete with Ca^{2+} and Na^+ at proteins that increase intracellular Ca^{2+} concentrations (e.g. NCX, NMDAR, Ca^{2+} channels, Na^+ channels). At high concentrations, Mg^{2+} also blocks Na^+ channels, which affects the function of excitable tissues. Mg^{2+} may protect brain cells against free radical injury, neurotoxicity, and inflammation [28]. Its ability to interfere with cell membrane proteins and nerve conduction is one explanation for its neuromodulatory and putative analgesic actions.

Magnesium concentrations in body fluids are reported in mg/dl, mEq/l, or mmol/l. The atomic weight of Mg is 24.3 and its valence is 2+, therefore, 1 mEq of Mg is equal to 12.15 mg (0.5 mmol) of Mg. Conversion factors are: mmol/l = mg/dl × 0.41; mg/dl = mmol/l × 2.43; mg/dl = mEq/l × 1.21; mmol/l = mEq/l × 0.5. Dietary Mg is reported as %, g/kg, or parts per million (ppm; mg/kg).

Blood concentrations of TMg and Mg^{2+} are similar between foals (TMg = 0.54–1.1 mmol/l; Mg^{2+} = 0.46–0.8 mmol/l) and horses (TMg = 0.53–1.2 mmol/l; Mg^{2+} = 0.46–0.8 mmol/l) [2, 3, 6, 7, 29]. Hypomagnesemia is frequent in septic foals, but rarely diagnosed because values are not included in most chemistry profiles [2, 3]. Measurement of TMg and Mg^{2+} concentrations is increasing in equine practice, which aids in the implementation of Mg-replacement therapies in ill foals. Similar to hypophosphatemia, hypomagnesemia is a common finding in foals receiving enteral or parenteral energy supplementation as these ions are highly interactive, in particular in processes involving transmembrane ion transport and energy expenditure [2]. Measurement of plasma Mg^{2+} concentration is better to assess the functional Mg status in the extracellular compartment [2]. Intracellular Mg concentration provides a better assessment of the total body Mg content, although this is only done for research purposes [2].

Calcium- and Phosphorus-Regulating Hormones

Parathyroid Hormone

As previously mentioned, PTH, CT, $1,25(OH)_2D_3$ are the main calcium-regulating hormones. PTH (84 amino acids) is produced by chief cells of the parathyroid glands, which derive from the endoderm of the third and fourth pharyngeal pouches. Horses have four parathyroid glands with variable locations [30]. The cranial parathyroid glands are usually located dorsolaterally to the cranial pole of the thyroid gland and along the thyroid artery but can be around or within the thyroid gland. The caudal parathyroid glands are located near the bicarotid trunk, cranial to the thymus, or within the thymus in young horses. The parathyroid glands consist of chief cells, oxyphil cells, and clear cells, representing different stages of the same parenchymal cells. The chief cells are the most active [1].

The actions of PTH on renal tubular cells and osteoblasts are mediated by the PTH1 receptor [1]. In the kidneys, PTH enhances Ca and Mg reabsorption (distal nephron; paracellular transport), inhibits Na/PO_4 cotransporters to reduce PO_4 reabsorption (proximal tubules), and increases 1α-hydroxylase activity (tubular cells) to increase $1,25(OH)_2D_3$ synthesis [1, 12]. In bone, PTH promotes osteoclast-mediated bone resorption (via osteoblasts) and stimulates secretion of FGF-23 by osteocytes [31]. Serum PTH concentrations are similar between healthy newborn foals and horses [3–5, 32, 33]. Both low and high PTH concentrations have been measured in critically ill foals, with high PTH concentrations associated with mortality [4, 5]. A number of foals with high PTH do not have hypocalcemia, suggesting that other mechanisms, including hyperphosphatemia and systemic inflammation, may be at play [4].

Calcitonin

Calcitonin (32 amino acids) is synthesized by parafollicular cells (C-cells) of the thyroid gland [34]. The thyroid gland has two embryological origins: the endoderm of the primitive larynx gives origin to follicular cells that secrete thyroid hormones and the ultimobranchial body of the fourth pharyngeal pouch that contains neuroendocrine cells (from the neural crest) that give rise to C-cells that secrete calcitonin [1]. Secretion of CT is controlled by several factors, with Ca^{2+} and gastrin playing main roles [1, 12, 35]. High Ca and gastrin concentrations stimulate CT secretion while the opposite occurs with low concentrations [1, 35]. CT decreases plasma Ca and PO_4 concentrations by suppressing osteoclastic bone resorption and increasing urinary excretion of Ca and PO_4 [1]. The role of CT in equine neonates is unclear, but likely has unique regulatory aspects considering their diet is rich in Ca [1, 3]. A major function of CT is to prevent excessive maternal bone loss during lactation [36]. Basically, CT inhibits bone resorption in an equilibrium with PTHrP produced by the mammary gland that functions as PTH to increase Ca release from bone to be transferred to milk. Postprandial increases in CT are mediated by gastrin as a preemptive mechanism to avoid hypercalcemia after a meal. Equine C cells are highly responsive to hypercalcemia [35]. From limited studies, CT concentrations are lower in healthy foals compared to horses [3, 35], and might facilitate bone apposition.

Vitamin D

Vitamin D is a pleiotropic factor with classical and nonclassical functions. The actions of vitamin D are mediated by the vitamin D receptor found in organs involved in Ca and PO_4 regulation (*classical;* intestine, bone, kidney, parathyroid gland), but also other locations (*nonclassical;* skin, pancreas, immune system, reproductive organs) [1, 37]. Vitamin D increases intestinal absorption and renal reabsorption of Ca and PO_4 by promoting their transcellular transport [37]. In bone, $1,25(OH)_2D_3$ promotes bone remodeling; both bone formation and resorption are vitamin D-dependent processes [1]. Vitamin D stimulates FGF-23 secretion by osteocytes and suppresses PTH synthesis and secretion as part of its regulatory system [1, 31]. Nonclassical functions of vitamin D include immune regulation, modulation of cell proliferation and differentiation, and antibacterial properties [37]. Active vitamin D is synthesized in a multistep process.

In horses, vitamin D derives from dietary sources (vitamin D_2 or ergocalciferol from fungi and plants) and from cutaneous activation of 7-dehydrocholesterol into cholecalciferol (vitamin D_3). From the skin, vitamin D_3 is transported to the liver to be hydroxylated by 25-hydroxylase to 25-hydroxyvitamin D_3 [$25(OH)D_3$]. From the liver, $25(OH)D_3$ is transported to the kidney to be converted by 1α-hydroxylase to the active metabolite of vitamin D, 1,25-dihydroxyvitamin D_3 [$1,25(OH)_2D_3$; calcitriol]. Vitamin D_2 (ergocalciferol) is a major source of vitamin D for horses [1, 38]; however, its relevance in foals, based on their diet, remains unclear. Except for cutaneous activation, other steps for vitamin D_2 are similar to vitamin D_3. Blood concentrations of $1,25(OH)2D_3$ are regulated by PTH, Ca^{2+}, PO_4, 1,25(OH)2D, and FGF-23. Low PO_4 and PTH increase whereas high Ca^{2+}, PO_4, $1,25(OH)_2D$, and FGF-23 concentrations suppress renal 1α-hydroxylase activity and $1,25(OH)_2D_3$ synthesis. PTH and FGF-23 (FGF-23/klotho axis) are the main regulators of vitamin D synthesis [39, 40]. Vitamin D concentrations are lower in healthy foals compared to horses [16]. Low concentrations of vitamin D metabolites are associated with disease severity and mortality in critically ill newborn foals [4, 5].

FGF-23

FGF-23 is a recently discovered factor produced by osteocytes in response to PTH, PO_4, and $1,25(OH)_2D_3$ [31]. FGF-23 plays central functions in Ca, PO_4, and vitamin D regulation. In fact, FGF-23 is considered the main PO_4^- regulating hormone (phosphatonin) [31]. In renal tubular cells, FGF-23 binds to its receptor and klotho to suppress 1α-hydroxylase activity and $1,25(OH)_2D_3$ synthesis [31, 39, 40]. FGF-23 inhibits Na/PO_4 cotransporters reducing PO_4 reabsorption [31, 39, 40]. These combined actions result in phosphaturia. In addition, under physiological conditions FGF-23 inhibits PTH secretion [41]. Abnormalities in FGF-23 and klotho have been associated with disease severity, hypovitaminosis D, and PO_4 disturbances in sick foals [4].

Parathyroid Hormone-Related Protein

Parathyroid Hormone-Related Protein (PTHrP) has a multitude of functions during fetal development and adult life. Its actions are paracrine, autocrine, intracrine, and endocrine. It is mainly a paracrine factor, but in the developing fetus also has endocrine actions [42–44]. PTHrP is central to fetal Ca homeostasis, functioning as PTH and promoting transplacental Ca transport. PTHrP binds the PTH1 receptor [43, 44], which explains its pathological PTH-like endocrine effects [1, 12]. PTHrP is required for mammary gland development and lactation [42, 43]. High PTHrP concentrations are found in milk of lactating mares [45]. Its functions in milk are unclear, but it enhances Ca transport into milk and perhaps promotes intestinal Ca absorption in the newborn [1]. During lactation PTHrP released into maternal circulation promotes osteoclastic activity to meet Ca demands for milk production [42]. PTHrP concentrations in healthy foals are low to undetectable and no different to horses [3]. High-serum PTHrP concentrations are considered pathologic in horses and in general associated with malignancies (HHM; humoral hypercalcemia of malignancy). Serum PTHrP concentrations were not different between healthy and sick foals [3].

As mentioned above, endocrine control of Mg is not as precise as for Ca^{2+} and PO_4, but its extracellular concentrations can be influenced by various hormones, including PTH, vitamin D, insulin, AVP, aldosterone, glucagon, β-adrenergic agonists, and EGF [2, 46]. These hormones mainly increase renal Mg reabsorption, but some (insulin, β-adrenergic agonists) also promote its shift to the intracellular compartment [46].

References

1 Toribio, R.E. (2018). Disorders of calcium and phosphorus. In: *Equine Internal Medicine*, 4e (ed. S.M. Reed, W.M. Bayly, and D.C. Sellon), 1029–1052. St. Louis, Missouri: Elsevier.

2 Toribio, R.E. (2018). Magnesium and disease. In: *Equine Internal Medicine*, 4e (ed. S.M. Reed, W.M. Bayly, and D.C. Sellon), 1052–1058. St. Louis, Missouri: Elsevier.

3 Hurcombe, S.D., Toribio, R.E., Slovis, N.M. et al. (2009). Calcium regulating hormones and serum calcium and magnesium concentrations in septic and critically ill foals and their association with survival. *J. Vet. Intern. Med.* 23: 335–343.

4 Kamr, A.M., Dembek, K.A., Hildreth, B.E. et al. (2018). The FGF-23/klotho axis and its relationship with phosphorus, calcium, vitamin D, PTH, aldosterone, severity of disease, and outcome in hospitalised foals. *Equine Vet. J.* 50: 739–746.

5 Kamr, A.M., Dembek, K.A., Reed, S.M. et al. (2015). Vitamin D metabolites and their association with calcium, phosphorus, and PTH concentrations, severity of illness, and mortality in hospitalized equine neonates. *PLoS One* 10: e0127684.

6 Berlin, D. and Aroch, I. (2009). Concentrations of ionized and total magnesium and calcium in healthy horses: effects of age, pregnancy, lactation, pH and sample type. *Vet. J.* 181: 305–311.

7 Toribio, R.E., Kohn, C.W., Chew, D.J. et al. (2001). Comparison of serum parathyroid hormone and ionized calcium and magnesium concentrations and fractional urinary clearance of calcium and phosphorus in healthy horses and horses with enterocolitis. *Am. J. Vet. Res.* 62: 938–947.

8 Kohn, C.W. and Brooks, C.L. (1990). Failure of pH to predict ionized calcium percentage in healthy horses. *Am. J. Vet. Res.* 51: 1206–1210.

9 Lopez, I., Estepa, J.C., Mendoza, F.J. et al. (2006). Fractionation of calcium and magnesium in equine serum. *Am. J. Vet. Res.* 67: 463–466.

10 Beggs, M.R. and Alexander, R.T. (2017). Intestinal absorption and renal reabsorption of calcium throughout postnatal development. *Exp. Biol. Med. (Maywood)* 242: 840–849.

11 Wilkens, M.R. and Muscher-Banse, A.S. (2020). Review: regulation of gastrointestinal and renal transport of calcium and phosphorus in ruminants. *Animal* 14: s29–s43.

12 Toribio, R.E. (2011). Disorders of calcium and phosphate metabolism in horses. *Vet. Clinic. North Am. Equine Pract.* 27: 129–147.

13 Hurcombe, S.D., Toribio, R.E., Slovis, N. et al. (2008). Blood arginine vasopressin, adrenocorticotropin hormone, and cortisol concentrations at admission in septic and critically ill foals and their association with survival. *J. Vet. Intern. Med.* 22: 639–647.

14 Caverzasio, J. and Bonjour, J.P. (1992). IGF-1 and phosphate homeostasis during growth. *Nephrologie* 13: 109–113.

15 Haramati, A., Mulroney, S.E., and Lumpkin, M.D. (1990). Regulation of renal phosphate reabsorption during development: implications from a new model of growth hormone deficiency. *Pediatr. Nephrol.* 4: 387–391.

16 Pozza, M.E., Kaewsakhorn, T., Trinarong, C. et al. (2014). Serum vitamin D, calcium, and phosphorus concentrations in ponies, horses and foals from the United States and Thailand. *Vet. J.* 199: 451–456.

17 Kamr, A.M., Dembek, K.A., Gilsenan, W. et al. (2020). C-terminal telopeptide of type I collagen, osteocalcin, alkaline phosphatase, and parathyroid hormone in healthy and hospitalized foals. *Domest. Anim. Endocrinol.* 72: 106470.

18 Vorland, C.J., Lachcik, P.J., Aromeh, L.O. et al. (2018). Effect of dietary phosphorus intake and age on intestinal phosphorus absorption efficiency and phosphorus balance in male rats. *PLoS One* 13: e0207601.

19 de Baaij, J.H., Hoenderop, J.G., and Bindels, R.J. (2015). Magnesium in man: implications for health and disease. *Physiol. Rev.* 95: 1–46.

20 Long-Jun, D., Bapty, B., Ritchie, G., and Quake, G.A. (1998). Glucagon and arginine vasopressin stimulate Mg2+ uptake in mouse distal convoluted tubule cells. *Am. J. Physiol. Cell Physiol.* 274 (2): F328–F335, https://journals.physiology.org/doi/full/10.1152/ajprenal.1998.274.2.F328.

21 Toribio, R.E., Kohn, C.W., Rourke, K.M. et al. (2007). Effects of hypercalcemia on serum concentrations of magnesium, potassium, and phosphate and urinary excretion of electrolytes in horses. *Am. J. Vet. Res.* 68: 543–554.

22 Paolisso, G. and Barbagallo, M. (1997). Hypertension, diabetes mellitus, and insulin resistance: the role of intracellular magnesium. *Am. J. Hypertens.* 10: 346–355.

23 Barbagallo, M., Veronese, N., and Dominguez, L.J. (2021). Magnesium in aging, health and diseases. *Nutrients* 13: 463. https://doi.org/10.3390/nu13020463.

24 Stewart, A.J., Hardy, J., Kohn, C.W. et al. (2004). Validation of diagnostic tests for determination of magnesium status in horses with reduced magnesium intake. *Am. J. Vet. Res.* 65: 422–430.

25 Harrington, D.D. (1975). Influence of magnesium deficiency on horse foal tissue concentration of Mg, calcium and phosphorus. *Br. J. Nutr.* 34: 45–57.

26 Jahnen-Dechent, W. and Ketteler, M. (2012). Magnesium basics. *Clin. Kidney J.* 5: i3–i14.

27 Wolf, F.I., Torsello, A., Fasanella, S. et al. (2003). Cell physiology of magnesium. *Mol. Aspects Med.* 24: 11–26.

28 Weglicki, W.B. (2012). Hypomagnesemia and inflammation: clinical and basic aspects. *Annu. Rev. Nutr.* 32: 55–71.

29 Mariella, J., Isani, G., Andreani, G. et al. (2016). Total plasma magnesium in healthy and critically ill foals. *Theriogenology* 85: 180–185.

30 Krook, L. and Lowe, J.E. (1964). Nutritional secondary hyperparathyroidism in the horse. *Pathol. Vet.* 65: 26–56.

31 Lanske, B. and Razzaque, M.S. (2014). Molecular interactions of FGF23 and PTH in phosphate regulation. *Kidney Int.* 86: 1072–1074.

32 Toribio, R.E., Kohn, C.W., Hardy, J. et al. (2005). Alterations in serum PTH and electrolyte concentrations and urinary excretion of electrolytes in horses with induced endotoxemia. *J. Vet. Intern. Med.* 19: 223–231.

33 Toribio, R.E., Kohn, C.W., Sams, R.A. et al. (2003). Hysteresis and calcium set-point for the calcium parathyroid hormone relationship in healthy horses. *Gen. Comp. Endocrinol.* 130: 279–288.

34 Toribio, R.E., Kohn, C.W., Leone, G.W. et al. (2003). Molecular cloning and expression of equine calcitonin, calcitonin gene-related peptide-I, and calcitonin gene-related peptide-II. *Mol. Cell. Endocrinol.* 199: 119–128.

35 Rourke, K.M., Kohn, C.W., Levine, A.L. et al. (2009). Rapid calcitonin response to experimental hypercalcemia in healthy horses. *Domest. Anim. Endocrinol.* 36: 197–201.

36 Woodrow, J.P., Sharpe, C.J., Fudge, N.J. et al. (2006). Calcitonin plays a critical role in regulating skeletal mineral metabolism during lactation. *Endocrinology* 147: 4010–4021.

37 Dusso, A.S., Brown, A.J., and Slatopolsky, E. (2005). Vitamin D. *Am. J. Physiol. Renal. Physiol.* 289: F8–F28.

38 Azarpeykan, S., Dittmer, K.E., Gee, E.K. et al. (2016). Influence of blanketing and season on vitamin D and parathyroid hormone, calcium, phosphorus, and magnesium concentrations in horses in New Zealand. *Domest. Anim. Endocrinol.* 56: 75–84.

39 Martin, A., David, V., and Quarles, L.D. (2012). Regulation and function of the FGF23/klotho endocrine pathways. *Physiol. Rev.* 92: 131–155.

40 Kuro-o, M. (2010). Overview of the FGF23-Klotho axis. *Pediatr. Nephrol.* 25: 583–590. https://doi.org/10.1007/s00467-009-1260-4.

41 Silver, J., Rodriguez, M., and Slatopolsky, E. (2012). FGF23 and PTH–double agents at the heart of CKD. *Nephrol. Dial. Transplant.* 27: 1715–1720.

42 Wysolmerski, J.J. (2012). Parathyroid hormone-related protein: an update. *J. Clin. Endocrinol. Metab.* 97: 2947–2956.

43 Wysolmerski, J.J. and Stewart, A.F. (1998). The physiology of parathyroid hormone-related protein: an emerging role as a developmental factor. *Annu. Rev. Physiol.* 60: 431–460.

44 Martin, T.J., Sims, N.A., and Seeman, E. (2021). Physiological and pharmacological roles of PTH and PTHrP in bone using their shared receptor, PTH1R. *Endocr. Rev.* 42: 383–406.

45 Care, A.D., Abbas, S.K., Ousey, J. et al. (1997). The relationship between the concentration of ionised calcium and parathyroid hormone-related protein (PTHrP[1-34]) in the milk of mares. *Equine Vet. J.* 29: 186–189.

46 Dai, L.J., Ritchie, G., Kerstan, D. et al. (2001). Magnesium transport in the renal distal convoluted tubule. *Physiol. Rev.* 81: 51–84.

Chapter 21 Endocrine Disorders in Foals

Katarzyna A. Dembek, Laura D. Hostnik, Teresa A. Burns, and Ramiro E. Toribio

Sepsis, neonatal encephalopathy, and dysmaturity are common disorders in newborn foals, with sepsis being the main cause of death. While the focus tends to be on clinical findings, laboratory abnormalities, and causative pathogens, the underlying processes for many of these disturbances are endocrine in nature. Cortisol and thyroid hormones are central to development and differentiation and therefore maturity at birth. Cortisol is essential for skeletal, cardiovascular, pulmonary, thyroid gland, and pancreatic development and function, and in the stress response. Equally important, thyroid hormones are crucial in tissue differentiation, metabolism, and thermogenesis. Thus, inappropriately low cortisol and thyroid hormone concentrations at critical stages of development can hamper the function of multiple body systems resulting in energy dysregulation, cardiovascular and respiratory dysfunction, tissue hypoperfusion, electrolyte disturbances, musculoskeletal abnormalities, a poor stress response, a pro-inflammatory state, and many other disorders. Endocrine energy dysregulation is frequent and linked to disease severity in critically ill foals. In addition, disturbances in the somatotropic axis occur in critically ill foals, but consequences remain unclear. Morover or a synonym, steroids with neuroactive properties may influence disease progression, and calcium, phosphorus, and magnesium dyshomeostasis is often overlooked in foals. Understanding how endocrine dysregulation contributes abnormalities observed in hospitalized foals could enhance diagnostic, therapeutic, and prognostic abilities.

Abbreviations

ACE	Angiotensin-converting enzyme
ACTH	Adrenocorticotropic hormone
ADH	Anti-diuretic hormone
ADM	Adrenomedullin
AI	Adrenal insufficiency
AMPA	α-amino-3-hydroxy-5-methyl-4-isoxazole propionic acid
ANF	Atrial natriuretic factor
ANG-II	Angiotensin II
ANP	Atrial natriuretic peptide
AVP	Arginine vasopressin
BDNF	Brain-derived neurotropic factor
BNP	Brain natriuretic peptide
Ca	Calcium
Ca^{2+}	Ionized or active calcium
CBG	Corticosteroid-binding globulin
CHDS	Congenital hypothyroidism and dysmaturity syndrome
CIRCI	Critical illness-related corticosteroid insufficiency
Cl^-	Chloride
CRH	Corticotropin-releasing hormone
CRI	Continuous rate infusion
CT	Calcitonin
DHEA	Dehydroepiandrosterone
DHEAS	DHEA sulfate
DIT	Diiodotyrosine
DOC	Deoxycorticosterone
EGF	Epidermal growth factor
EIA	Enteroinsular axis
ET-1	Endothelin-1
FFA	Free fatty acid
FGF-23	Fibroblast growth factor-23
fT_3	Free T_3
fT_4	Free T_4
GABA	Gamma-aminobutyric acid
$GABA_AR$	GABA type A receptor
GH	Growth hormone
GHIH	Growth hormone inhibiting hormone
GHRH	Growth hormone releasing hormone
GIP	Glucose-dependent insulinotropic polypeptide

Equine Neonatal Medicine, First Edition. Edited by David M. Wong and Pamela A. Wilkins.

GLP-1	Glucagon-like peptide-1
GLP-2	Glucagon-like peptide-2
GLUT4	glucose transporter type 4
HPAA	Hypothalamic-pituitary-adrenal axis
HPTA	Hypothalamic-pituitary-thyroid axis
IGF-1	Insulin-like growth factor-1
K^+	Potassium
LPS	Lipopolysaccharide
MC2R	Melanocortin type 2 receptor
Mg	Magnesium
Mg^{2+}	Ionized or active magnesium
$MgSO_4$	Magnesium sulfate
MIT	Monoiodotyrosine
mPRs	Membrane progesterone receptors
Na^+	Sodium
NCX	Na^+/Ca^{2+} exchanger
NE	Neonatal encephalopathy
NEFA	Non-esterified fatty acids
NIS	Sodium iodide symporter
NMDA	N-methyl-D-aspartate
NMDAR	NMDA receptor
NMS	Neonatal maladjustment syndrome
NO	Nitric oxide
NTIS	Non-thyroidal illness syndrome
PCT	Procalcitonin
PMCA	Plasma membrane Ca^{2+} ATPase
POMC	Proopiomelanocortin
PO_4	Phosphorus/phosphate
PP	Pancreatic polypeptide
PTH	Parathyroid hormone
PTHrP	Parathyroid hormone-related protein
PVN	Paraventricular nucleus
QUICKI	quantitative insulin-sensitivity check index
RAI	Relative adrenal insufficiency
SIADH	Syndrome of inappropriate antidiuretic hormone
SIRS	Systemic inflammatory response syndrome
TBPA	Thyroid-binding prealbumin
TCa	Total calcium
TH	Thyroid hormone
THDOC	Tetrahydrodeoxy-corticosterone
TMg	Total magnesium
TRH	Thyrotropin-releasing hormone
TSH	Thyroid stimulating hormone
T_3	Triiodothyronine
T_4	Thyroxine
tT_3	Total T_3
tT_4	Total T_4
RAAS	Renin-angiotensin-aldosterone system
rT3	Reverse T3
$1,25(OH)_2D_3$	1,25-dihydroxyvitamin D_3
$25(OH)D_3$	25-hydroxyvitamin D_3
3β-HSD	3β-Hydroxysteroid dehydrogenase

Section I Disorders of the Hypothalamic Pituitary Adrenal Axis and Neurosteroids

Katarzyna A. Dembek, Laura D. Hostnik, Teresa A. Burns, and Ramiro E. Toribio

Disorders of the Hypothalamic Pituitary Adrenal Axis (HPAA)

The HPAA is a complex neuroendocrine system that modulates multiple physiological functions (metabolism, pain, hunger, thirst, blood pressure, autonomic activity, immunity, tissue differentiation) as well as the stress response. The HPAA maintains homeostasis under physiological and pathological conditions [1, 2] and consists of the hypothalamus, which secretes corticotropin-releasing hormone (CRH) and arginine vasopressin (AVP); the pituitary gland, that in response to CRH and AVP releases adrenocorticotropin hormone (ACTH); and the adrenal gland cortex, that upon ACTH stimulation, secretes glucocorticoids (cortisol), mineralocorticoids (aldosterone), sex steroids, and steroid precursors (pregnenolone, dehydroepiandrosterone) [1, 2]. Cortisol acts on intracellular glucocorticoid receptors to modulate multiple functions (metabolic, immune, neuromodulatory, behavioral). Cortisol has direct and indirect negative feedback effects on the hypothalamus and pituitary gland by decreasing the synthesis and secretion of CRH, AVP, and ACTH. The role of CRH on the HPAA is mainly permissive during chronic stress, while at least in horses, AVP is a dynamic modulator of ACTH release [3, 4]. The pituitary gland and adrenal cortex in healthy foals are responsive to exogenous AVP and CRH with rapid increases in ACTH and cortisol concentrations [5, 6].

Relative Adrenal Insufficiency (RAI)/ Critical Illness-Related Corticosteroid Insufficiency (CIRCI)

Dysfunction of the HPAA results in adrenal insufficiency, which can have devastating consequences. Depending on which level of the HPAA is affected, adrenal insufficiency is classified as primary, secondary, or tertiary. In *primary* adrenal insufficiency the failure is in the adrenal gland cortex, *secondary* occurs at the level of the pituitary gland, and *tertiary* insufficiency refers to failure of the hypothalamus to secrete CRH and AVP. In most critically ill patients the adrenal continues to respond to ACTH (response can be inappropriate), thus the term relative adrenal insufficiency (RAI) or critical illness-related corticosteroid insufficiency (CIRCI) is preferred [7, 8]. RAI and CIRCI are defined as inappropriate cellular corticosteroid activity for the severity of illness and is characterized by insufficient glucocorticoid production or their actions. In addition to HPAA dysfunction, it also encompasses tissue resistance to glucocorticoids (decreased activity) or increased conversion of cortisol to cortisone (increased inactivation) [9–12]. CIRCI is a common complication of sepsis, septic shock, severe pneumonia, acute respiratory distress, trauma, postoperative surgery, and other critical illnesses in people and neonatal foals [8, 9, 11, 13–15]. Conditions leading to RAI occur at any level of the HPAA, but steroid deficiency ultimately leads to systemic abnormalities from this condition. Reduced glucocorticoid actions exacerbate the pro-inflammatory state due to reduced anti-inflammatory and immunomodulatory effects. Some animals have aldosterone deficiency, which contributes to other disturbances, mainly related to perfusion from volume depletion. RAI has been documented in foals and horses but the pathogenesis in non-critically ill horses (chronic adrenal insufficiency) is different than RAI of acute illness [10, 12, 16].

Types and Definitions of Adrenal Insufficiency (AI)

A variety of terms describe adrenal disorders, as noted below:

- Irreversible adrenal insufficiency, hypoadrenalism, or hypoadrenocorticism (Addison's disease) results from

Equine Neonatal Medicine, First Edition. Edited by David M. Wong and Pamela A. Wilkins.

failure of the adrenal gland cortex to produce steroid hormones (mineralocorticoids and glucocorticoids) [1].

- RAI is a transient form of adrenal insufficiency that occurs in critically ill patients. In RAI, the adrenal cortex still responds to ACTH, glucocorticoid secretion is reduced, and there is inadequate cellular cortisol activity for the severity of the patient's illness from insufficient glucocorticoid receptor-mediated downregulation of pro-inflammatory transcription factors [8, 13, 17]. Mineralocorticoid concentrations can also be low [18].
- CIRCI is a term proposed instead of RAI because it considers clinical findings, an exaggerated pro-inflammatory response from cortisol deficiency, and tissue refractoriness to corticosteroids [9].
- ACTH to cortisol dissociation or ACTH/cortisol imbalance (ACI) has been proposed in critically ill patients instead of CIRCI because it does not suggest adrenocortical insufficiency [7, 13, 19]. It also has been proposed that hypercortisolemia from reduced cortisol biodegradation may lead to ACTH suppression in the absence of adrenocortical dysfunction [19].
- Iatrogenic adrenal insufficiency is the most common type of adrenal insufficiency in adult horses and is caused by chronic administration of exogenous steroids (glucocorticoids, anabolic steroids) resulting in HPAA suppression [20, 21].
- Adrenal insufficiency can also be classified based on the level of the HPAA that is affected [1]:
  - ✓ *Primary AI:* damage or dysfunction of the adrenal gland cortex.
  - ✓ *Secondary AI:* impaired ACTH secretion by the pituitary gland (pars distalis).
  - ✓ *Tertiary AI:* reduced CRH and/or AVP secretion from the hypothalamus into the median eminence.

In neonatal foals, the most recognized form of adrenal insufficiency is RAI or CIRCI [10, 13]. Studies note that adrenocortical dysfunction is common in ill foals and linked to disease severity and mortality [8, 13–15, 22]. In one study, 40% of septic foals had HPAA dysfunction [8] and in another study, high ACTH/cortisol ratio, consistent with RAI, was common in nonsurviving septic foals [14]. High AVP/ACTH and ACTH/cortisol ratios in ill foals also support HPAA dysfunction at the pituitary and adrenal levels [14, 15]. AVP is a major secretagogue for ACTH in the horse, and a high AVP/ACTH ratio suggests decreased ACTH response to AVP stimulation (pituitary insufficiency) [3, 15]. Similarly, high ACTH/cortisol and ACTH/aldosterone ratios indicate reduced adrenocortical response to ACTH in critically ill foals [8, 14, 18].

Both low and high cortisol concentrations have been associated with nonsurvival in septic foals [8, 14, 18]. Low cortisol concentrations in premature foals do not appear to be due to ACTH deficiency, as ACTH concentrations are often elevated in these foals, suggesting that primary AI occurs in premature foals [23]. This might impact other endocrine systems (thyroid gland, endocrine pancreas) as well as cardiovascular function that rely on appropriate glucocorticoid concentrations at the end of pregnancy for proper differentiation and function. Another study demonstrated that exogenous AVP and CRH stimulate ACTH and cortisol secretion in healthy foals and these methods might be useful to help determine the pathogenesis of RAI in sick foals [5, 6].

In addition to cortisol, other adrenal steroids and steroid precursors have been studied in foals [7, 13, 24, 25]. In one study, critically ill foals with high progesterone concentrations at admission were more likely to die [7]. In that study, dehydroepiandrosterone (DHEA) sulfate (DHEAS) was a good indicator of AI in hospitalized foals [7]. The response of multiple adrenal steroids (cortisol, aldosterone, progesterone, 17α-hydroxyprogesterone, DHEAS, pregnenolone) to administration of 10 μg of ACTH was investigated in healthy and hospitalized foals. Interestingly, the 17α-hydroxyprogesterone response to ACTH stimulation was a good predictor of disease severity and mortality in hospitalized foals [13]. An explanation for the altered adrenal steroid and steroid precursor response to ACTH stimulation in nonsurvivors is unclear. A shift in adrenal steroidogenesis secondary to inflammatory factors has been proposed in ex vivo models. However, studies measuring multiple adrenal steroids as well as pro and anti-inflammatory cytokines are limited in ill foals [7, 13]. Possible shifts in the adrenocortical enzymatic machinery may reduce glucocorticoid synthesis with accumulation of precursors such as progesterone and 17α-hydroxyprogesterone [13].

Pathophysiology

The pathogenesis of RAI/CIRCI in horses and other species is unclear, but likely multifactorial – including decreased production of CRH, AVP, ACTH, and cortisol, along with interactions between the HPAA with other organs and body systems [7, 9–11, 16]. The equine adrenal gland is highly vascular; during critical illness, it is highly susceptible to hypoperfusion, hemorrhages, and necrosis, and has been observed in septic nonsurviving foals (Figure 21.I.1) [8, 18]. Depending on severity, this could affect all adrenocortical layers, altering multiple steroids and their local and systemic balance. Prolonged hypotension and hypoperfusion from sepsis and septic shock may lead to irreversible adrenocortical damage in critically ill foals, similar to Waterhouse-Friderichsen syndrome in people [9–11]. Multiple mechanisms can directly or indirectly cause adrenocortical dysfunction, including: (i) inappropriately low CRH, AVP, and ACTH release; (ii) adrenocortical resistance to ACTH; (iii) impaired adrenocortical steroidogenesis; (iv) tissue

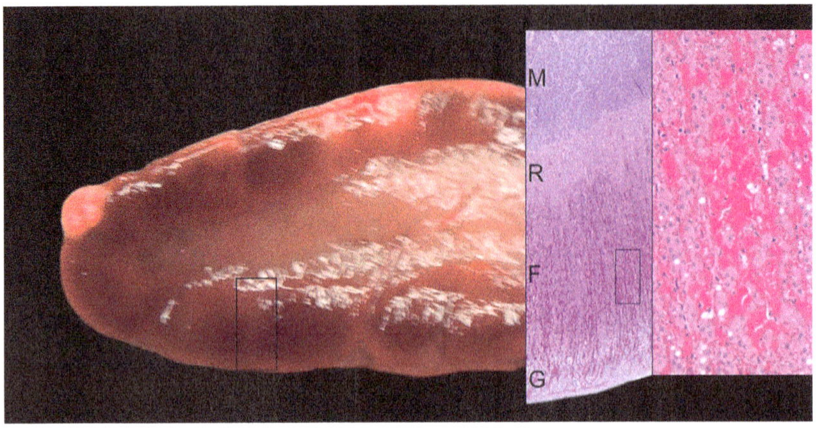

Figure 21.I.1 Adrenal gland from a septic foal with relative adrenal insufficiency. Gross cross section showing adrenocortical congestion and hemorrhage affecting all cortical layers. Histologically, there is hemorrhage, thrombosis, and adrenocortical necrosis (M, medulla; R, zona reticularis; F, zona fasciculata; G, zona glomerulosa). Despite disease severity this foal had relatively low serum cortisol and aldosterone concentrations, with high plasma ACTH concentrations consistent with primary adrenal insufficiency. *Source:* Image courtesy of Dr. R. E. Toribio, College of Veterinary Medicine, The Ohio State University.

resistance to cortisol and aldosterone; (v) increased or reduced cortisol metabolism; and (vi) decreased concentrations of bioactive ACTH [9, 10, 13, 15, 26, 27]. Reduced cortisol metabolism has been documented in critically ill people, resulting in high cortisol concentrations that suppress ACTH secretion, and thus, its trophic actions on the adrenal cortex [19]. This is a different phenomenon that could alter HPAA function.

The exaggerated proinflammatory response that occurs in foals with systemic inflammatory response syndrome (SIRS) and sepsis can be, in part, attributed to adrenocortical failure and suppression of the HPAA [8, 13]. However, experimental and clinical data suggest that tissue resistance to glucocorticoids may contribute to HPAA dysregulation [9, 11, 28]. One study found that nonsurviving horses with SIRS had lower glucocorticoid binding affinity compared to survivors, suggesting that in addition to HPAA dysfunction, impaired glucocorticoid receptor activity contributes to their proinflammatory state [28]. A decrease in cortisol breakdown rather than an increase in cortisol production has been suggested as a major contributor to hypercortisolemia in critically ill human patients [19]. These patients also had lower ACTH concentrations that, according to the authors, were a consequence of cortisol-mediated suppression of ACTH synthesis and secretion [19, 26]. Therefore, ACTH to cortisol dissociation or imbalance (ACI) has been used to describe this phenomenon. Cortisol, as most steroids, circulates in free and protein-bound fractions that are affected by health and disease. Free cortisol is the active form, and high free cortisol concentrations in equine fetal circulation in late pregnancy is important for its fetal pleiotropic actions. Foals are born with a high percentage of free cortisol (58% of total) compared to horses (5–7% of total) [29]. However, in response to disease and low proteins, disruption of this balance could be detrimental. Critically ill foals have low free and total cortisol responses to cosyntropin stimulation (RAI) [29].

Prolonged ACTH suppression can have adverse effects on the integrity of the HPAA that ultimately results in adrenal insufficiency. These observations are in contrast to critically ill newborn foals with RAI that often have increased ACTH and low cortisol concentrations with increased ACTH/cortisol ratios [8, 13–15]. However, information on adrenocortical steroid metabolism in neonatal foals is limited.

Clinical and Laboratory Findings

Clinical signs of RAI are related to (or masked by) the primary illness and include neutropenia, fever, hypotension, hypovolemia, and tissue hypoperfusion. Laboratory abnormalities include hypoglycemia, electrolytes abnormalities (e.g. hyponatremia, hyperkalemia), and an exacerbated SIRS [9–11]. The functions of other body systems also is likely altered due to steroid imbalances. An equine neonatal SIRS criteria has been proposed to assist with clinical classification [30].

Diagnosis

The diagnosis of RAI in critically ill foals is challenging because many signs and laboratory findings are nonspecific. However, persistent hypoglycemia, hyponatremia, hemodynamic instability, and hypotension refractory to fluid and vasopressor therapy should raise suspicion of RAI [8, 10]. Diagnosis is confirmed using the cosyntropin (synthetic $ACTH_{1-24}$) stimulation test, which is practical if cortisol concentrations can be measured on-site. The test is performed by administering a low (10 µg) or high (100 µg) dose of cosyntropin [13, 22, 29, 31, 32]. After baseline sample collection, cosyntropin (10 or 100 µg) is administered IV, and additional samples collected at 30, 60, and 90 minutes but two sample collections (0, 30 minutes) can be diagnostic [13]. In foals with a functional adrenal cortex, cortisol concentrations are expected to double by 30 minutes [13]. It is important to use response reference values based on ACTH dose [13, 22, 29, 31, 33]. Further diagnostic details are noted as follows.

Neurosteroids and Neuroactive Steroids

Extensive evidence suggests that a number of progestogens, androgens, and estrogens have neuroactive properties [34]. Neurons and glial cells synthesize de novo neurosteroids from cholesterol and circulating steroids that can cross the blood brain barrier to be metabolized in the central nervous system (CNS) into neuroactive steroids [35–37]. Neurosteroids and neuroactive steroids promote neurogenesis, neuronal plasticity, and programming; enhance axon and dendrite growth; organize neuronal circuits; influence glial cell development and function; facilitate energy conservation; and are neuroprotective [35, 38]. They modulate the HPAA and stress response through CRH and AVP synthesis, protect against glucocorticoid excess that could lead to neurological disorders, and mitigate cerebral hypoxic, ischemic, and traumatic injury [35, 38–41].

Neurosteroid imbalances have been associated with psychiatric, behavioral, cognitive, and sleep disorders in people [40]. High concentrations of progestogens in the CNS are protective and can induce a sleep-like state [35–37, 40, 41]. A similar process might occur in the equine fetus since progestogen concentrations are high in fetal and maternal circulations at the end of pregnancy, drop rapidly after birth [42–47], and allopregnanolone has sedative properties in foals [48]. Steroid imbalances may be involved in the pathogenesis of equine neonatal encephalopathy (NE) [7, 25, 37, 48, 49].

Neuroactive steroids are positive allosteric modulators of the gamma-aminobutyric acid type A ($GABA_A$) receptor ($GABA_AR$) and, to a lesser extent, the N-Methyl-D-aspartate (NMDA), α-amino-3-hydroxy-5-methyl-4-isoxazolepropionic acid (AMPA), kainate, glycine, serotonin, and sigma 1 (σ1) receptors [34, 50–53]. In the CNS, there are also membrane progesterone receptors (mPRs) [54, 55]. Allopregnanolone, progesterone, 5α-dihydroprogesterone, pregnanolone, deoxycorticosterone (DOC), and tetrahydrodeoxycorticosterone (THDOC) are potent agonists of $GABA_AR$ [53, 56]. Of these, allopregnanolone is the main neurosteroid. A number of androgens and estrogens modulate neuronal and glial function [57]. Some estrogens have anti-oxidant properties and are neuroprotective. Of interest, many estrogens are in high concentration in equine fetal and maternal circulation [58].

Dehydroepiandrosterone (DHEA) is an androgen precursor that can be modified in the CNS to compounds that potentiate or suppress $GABA_AR$ activity [40, 52, 53]. Minor modifications to steroids can shift their actions. For example, pregnenolone and DHEA have minimal activity over $GABA_AR$, but their sulfate esters are positive modulators of NMDA receptors (NMDAR) [52, 53]. These sulfated steroids are found in high concentrations in equine fetal and neonatal circulation [7, 13, 24]. Allopregnanolone concentrations are high in pregnant mares and their fetuses [42, 44, 45, 47], perhaps to modulate the HPAA and to keep the fetus in a sleep-like state until birth [59].

Increased concentrations of pregnenolone, progesterone, 17α-hydroxyprogesterone, allopregnanolone, androstenedione, DHEAS, testosterone, dihydrotestosterone, 17β-estradiol, and estrone sulfate have been measured in critically ill, premature, and NE foals [7, 8, 13, 24, 25, 37, 49, 60–65]. Abnormally high steroids in circulation and steroid imbalances in the CNS could contribute to disorders of ill newborn foals [37, 63]. However, it is uncertain whether they promote disease progression or are protective. These steroids could be proxies for underlying pathological processes and severity of illness, and their concentrations could have prognostic value [7, 13, 24, 25, 49]. The fact that progestogens activate $GABA_AR$ and their concentrations are high in critically ill foals might explain the lethargy and behavioral changes observed in sick newborn foals [7, 25, 64].

Neuroactive Steroids and Foal Disorders

In addition to cortisol, foals are born with high progestogen, androgen, and estrogen concentrations that decrease rapidly in the first 1–4 days of age, depending on the steroid [24, 49, 61, 62, 66]. As noted, HPAA activation in foals is associated with increased cortisol, and to lesser extent, aldosterone concentrations [18, 67]. Studies have shown that ill foals have imbalances of other steroids [7, 13, 24, 49, 60, 61, 67, 68]. Progestogen, androgen, and estrogen concentrations were increased in critically ill foals, and persistent elevations were associated with disease severity and mortality [7, 13, 24, 49, 60–62, 67]. The mechanisms behind this steroid increase remain elusive, but they might relate to asynchrony between parturition and the fetal physiological drop at birth, intrauterine disease, disease severity, and reduced clearance.

A number of mechanisms have been proposed in the pathogenesis of NE; however, mechanistic information is lacking [37]. Increased concentrations of steroids with neuroactive properties have been documented in hospitalized foals, including those with sepsis and NE [7, 13, 24, 25, 49, 61, 62, 67]. Progestogen metabolites such as allopregnanolone and THDOC have been proposed to be central to the pathogenesis of NE, in particular in foals with a normal delivery that develop signs of NE hours to days later [7, 25, 37, 62]. In these foals, it is possible that despite being mature, the physiological decrease in progestogens just before birth is delayed, remaining elevated, thus inducing a sedated state [7, 25, 37, 62]. One can speculate that part of the behavior of ill foals is explained by steroid imbalances. In fact, allopregnanolone has sedative properties in foals [48] and new anesthetics (e.g. alfaxolone) are based on progestogen precursors [37]. Conversion of progesterone to 5α-dihydroprogesterone and allopregnanolone is mediated by 5α-reductase, which is inhibited by dutasteride and finasteride. Anecdotal reports have used these drugs to treat foals with NE with inconclusive results. Caution must be used with this approach because increases in some of these steroids might be a protective mechanism [63].

References

1 Newell-Price, J.D.C. and Auchus, R.J. (2020). The adrenal cortex. In: *Williams Textbook of Endocrinology*, 14e (ed. S. Melmed, R.J. Auchus, A.B. Goldfine, et al.), 480–541. Philadelphia: Elsevier.

2 Barrett, K.E., Barman, S.M., Boitano, S. et al. (2016). *Ganong's Review of Medical Physiology*. New York: McGraw Hill Education.

3 Alexander, S.L., Irvine, C.H., and Donald, R.A. (1996). Dynamics of the regulation of the hypothalamo-pituitary-adrenal (HPA) axis determined using a nonsurgical method for collecting pituitary venous blood from horses. *Front. Neuroendocrinol.* 17: 1–50.

4 Keenan, D.M., Alexander, S., Irvine, C. et al. (2009). Quantifying nonlinear interactions within the hypothalamo-pituitary-adrenal axis in the conscious horse. *Endocrinology* 150: 1941–1951.

5 Elder, E.M., Wong, D.M., Johnson, K. et al. (2022). Assessment of the hypothalamic-pituitary-adrenocortical axis function utilitizing a vasopressin stimulation test in healthy foals. *Proceedings of the 2022 ACVIM Forum*. Austin, TX: American College of Veterinary Internal Medicine.

6 Johnson, K., Peterson, J., Kopper, J. et al. (2023). The hypothalamic-pituitary-adrenal axis response to ovine corticotropin-releasing-hormone stimulation tests in healthy and hospitalized foals. *J. Vet. Intern. Med.* 37: 292–301.

7 Dembek, K.A., Timko, K.J., Johnson, L.M. et al. (2017). Steroids, steroid precursors, and neuroactive steroids in critically ill equine neonates. *Vet. J.* 225: 42–49.

8 Hart, K.A., Slovis, N.M., and Barton, M.H. (2009). Hypothalamic-pituitary-adrenal axis dysfunction in hospitalized neonatal foals. *J. Vet. Intern. Med.* 23: 901–912.

9 Annane, D., Pastores, S.M., Arlt, W. et al. (2017). Critical illness-related corticosteroid insufficiency (CIRCI): a narrative review from a Multispecialty Task Force of the Society of Critical Care Medicine (SCCM) and the European Society of Intensive Care Medicine (ESICM). *Intensive Care Med.* 43: 1781–1792.

10 Hart, K.A. and Barton, M.H. (2011). Adrenocortical insufficiency in horses and foals. *Vet. Clin. North Am. Equine Pract.* 27: 19–34.

11 Marik, P.E. (2009). Critical illness-related corticosteroid insufficiency. *Chest* 135: 181–193.

12 Levy-Shraga, Y. and Pinhas-Hamiel, O. (2013). Critical illness-related corticosteroid insufficiency in children. *Horm. Res. Paediatr.* 80: 309–317.

13 Dembek, K.A., Johnson, L.M., Timko, K.J. et al. (2019). Multiple adrenocortical steroid response to administration of exogenous adrenocorticotropic hormone to hospitalized foals. *J. Vet. Intern. Med.* 33: 1766–1774.

14 Gold, J.R., Divers, T.J., Barton, M.H. et al. (2007). Plasma adrenocorticotropin, cortisol, and adrenocorticotropin/cortisol ratios in septic and normal-term foals. *J. Vet. Intern. Med.* 21: 791–796.

15 Hurcombe, S.D., Toribio, R.E., Slovis, N. et al. (2008). Blood arginine vasopressin, adrenocorticotropin hormone, and cortisol concentrations at admission in septic and critically ill foals and their association with survival. *J. Vet. Intern. Med.* 22: 639–647.

16 Hurcombe, S.D. (2011). Hypothalamic-pituitary gland axis function and dysfunction in horses. *Vet. Clin. North Am. Equine Pract.* 27: 1–17.

17 Annane, D., Pastores, S.M., Rochwerg, B. et al. (2017). Guidelines for the diagnosis and management of critical illness-related corticosteroid insufficiency (CIRCI) in critically ill patients (part I): Society of Critical Care Medicine (SCCM) and European Society of Intensive Care Medicine (ESICM) 2017. *Intensive Care Med.* 43: 1751–1763.

18 Dembek, K.A., Onasch, K., Hurcombe, S.D.A. et al. (2013). Renin-angiotensin-aldosterone system and

hypothalamic-pituitary-adrenal axis in hospitalized newborn foals. *J. Vet. Intern. Med.* 27: 331–338.

19 Boonen, E., Vervenne, H., Meersseman, P. et al. (2013). Reduced cortisol metabolism during critical illness. *N. Engl. J. Med.* 368: 1477–1488.

20 MacHarg, M.A., Bottoms, G.D., Carter, G.K. et al. (1985). Effects of multiple intramuscular injections and doses of dexamethasone on plasma cortisol concentrations and adrenal responses to ACTH in horses. *Am. J. Vet. Res.* 46: 2285–2287.

21 Dowling, P.M., Williams, M.A., and Clark, T.P. (1993). Adrenal insufficiency associated with long-term anabolic steroid administration in a horse. *J. Am. Vet. Med. Assoc.* 203: 1166–1169.

22 Wong, D.M., Vo, D.T., Alcott, C.J. et al. (2009). Baseline plasma cortisol and ACTH concentrations and response to low-dose ACTH stimulation testing in ill foals. *J. Am. Vet. Med. Assoc.* 234: 126–132.

23 Silver, M., Ousey, J.C., Dudan, F.E. et al. (1984). Studies on equine prematurity 2: post natal adrenocortical activity in relation to plasma adrenocorticotrophic hormone and catecholamine levels in term and premature foals. *Equine Vet. J.* 16: 278–286.

24 Aleman, M., McCue, P.M., Chigerwe, M. et al. (2019). Plasma concentrations of steroid precursors, steroids, neuroactive steroids, and neurosteroids in healthy neonatal foals from birth to 7 days of age. *J. Vet. Intern. Med.* 33: 2286–2293.

25 Aleman, M., Pickles, K.J., Conley, A.J. et al. (2013). Abnormal plasma neuroactive progestagen derivatives in ill, neonatal foals presented to the neonatal intensive care unit. *Equine Vet. J.* 45: 661–665.

26 Boonen, E. and Van den Berghe, G. (2016). MECHANISMS IN ENDOCRINOLOGY: new concepts to further unravel adrenal insufficiency during critical illness. *Eur. J. Endocrinol.* 175: R1–R9.

27 Jellyman, J.K., Valenzuela, O.A., Allen, V.L. et al. (2015). Neonatal glucocorticoid overexposure programs pituitary-adrenal function in ponies. *Domest. Anim. Endocrinol.* 50: 45–49.

28 Hoffman, C.J., McKenzie, H.C. 3rd, Furr, M.O. et al. (2015). Glucocorticoid receptor density and binding affinity in healthy horses and horses with systemic inflammatory response syndrome. *J. Vet. Intern. Med.* 29: 626–635.

29 Hart, K.A., Barton, M.H., Ferguson, D.C. et al. (2011). Serum free cortisol fraction in healthy and septic neonatal foals. *J. Vet. Intern. Med.* 25: 345–355.

30 Wong, D.M., Ruby, R.E., Dembek, K.A. et al. (2018). Evaluation of updated sepsis scoring systems and systemic inflammatory response syndrome criteria and their association with sepsis in equine neonates. *J. Vet. Intern. Med.* 32: 1185–1193.

31 Hart, K.A., Heusner, G.L., Norton, N.A. et al. (2009). Hypothalamic-pituitary-adrenal axis assessment in healthy term neonatal foals utilizing a paired low dose/high dose ACTH stimulation test. *J. Vet. Intern. Med.* 23: 344–351.

32 Wong, D.M., Vo, D.T., Alcott, C.J. et al. (2009). Adrenocorticotropic hormone stimulation tests in healthy foals from birth to 12 weeks of age. *Can. J. Vet. Res.* 73: 65–72.

33 Hart, K.A., Ferguson, D.C., Heusner, G.L. et al. (2007). Synthetic adrenocorticotropic hormone stimulation tests in healthy neonatal foals. *J. Vet. Intern. Med.* 21: 314–321.

34 Reddy, D.S. (2010). Neurosteroids: endogenous role in the human brain and therapeutic potentials. *Prog. Brain Res.* 186: 113–137.

35 Brunton, P.J. (2015). Programming the brain and behaviour by early-life stress: a focus on neuroactive steroids. *J. Neuroendocrinol.* 27: 468–480.

36 Belelli, D. and Lambert, J.J. (2005). Neurosteroids: endogenous regulators of the GABA(A) receptor. *Nat. Rev. Neurosci.* 6: 565–575.

37 Toribio, R.E. (2019). Equine neonatal encephalopathy: facts, evidence, and opinions. *Vet. Clin. North Am. Equine Pract.* 35: 363–378.

38 Hirst, J.J., Kelleher, M.A., Walker, D.W. et al. (2014). Neuroactive steroids in pregnancy: key regulatory and protective roles in the foetal brain. *J. Steroid Biochem. Mol. Biol.* 139: 144–153.

39 Kawarai, Y., Tanaka, H., Kobayashi, T. et al. (2018). Progesterone as a postnatal prophylactic agent for encephalopathy caused by prenatal hypoxic ischemic insult. *Endocrinology* 159: 2264–2274.

40 Reddy, D.S. and Estes, W.A. (2016). Clinical potential of neurosteroids for CNS disorders. *Trends Pharmacol. Sci.* 37: 543–561.

41 Brunton, P.J., Russell, J.A., and Hirst, J.J. (2014). Allopregnanolone in the brain: protecting pregnancy and birth outcomes. *Prog. Neurobiol.* 113: 106–136.

42 Conley, A.J. (2016). Review of the reproductive endocrinology of the pregnant and parturient mare. *Theriogenology* 86: 355–365.

43 Hamon, M., Clarke, S.W., Houghton, E. et al. (1991). Production of 5 alpha-dihydroprogesterone during late pregnancy in the mare. *J. Reprod. Fertil. Suppl.* 44: 529–535.

44 Holtan, D.W., Houghton, E., Silver, M. et al. (1991). Plasma progestagens in the mare, fetus and newborn foal. *J. Reprod. Fertil. Suppl.* 44: 517–528.

45 Legacki, E.L., Corbin, C.J., Ball, B.A. et al. (2016). Progestin withdrawal at parturition in the mare. *Reproduction* 152: 323–331.

46 Nagel, C., Erber, R., Bergmaier, C. et al. (2012). Cortisol and progestin release, heart rate and heart rate variability

in the pregnant and postpartum mare, fetus and newborn foal. *Theriogenology* 78: 759–767.

47 Ousey, J.C., Forhead, A.J., Rossdale, P.D. et al. (2003). Ontogeny of uteroplacental progestagen production in pregnant mares during the second half of gestation. *Biol. Reprod.* 69: 540–548.

48 Madigan, J.E., Haggettt, E.F., Pickles, K.J. et al. (2012). Allopregnanolone infusion induced neurobehavioural alterations in a neonatal foal: is this a clue to the pathogenesis of neonatal maladjustment syndrome? *Equine Vet. J. Suppl.* 344: 109–112.

49 Swink, J.M., Rings, L.M., Snyder, H.A. et al. (2021). Dynamics of androgens in healthy and hospitalized newborn foals. *J. Vet. Intern. Med.* 35: 538–549.

50 Longone, P., di Michele, F., D'Agati, E. et al. (2011). Neurosteroids as neuromodulators in the treatment of anxiety disorders. *Front. Endocrinol. (Lausanne)* 2: 55.

51 Tuem, K.B. and Atey, T.M. (2017). Neuroactive steroids: receptor interactions and responses. *Front. Neurol.* 8: 442.

52 Laube, B., Maksay, G., Schemm, R., and Betz, H. (2002). Modulation of glycine receptor function: a novel approach for therapeutic intervention at inhibitory synapses? *Trends Pharmacol. Sci.* 23: 519–527.

53 Wang, M. (2011). Neurosteroids and GABA-A receptor function. *Front. Endocrinol. (Lausanne)* 2: 44.

54 Thomas, P. and Pang, Y. (2012). Membrane progesterone receptors: evidence for neuroprotective, neurosteroid signaling and neuroendocrine functions in neuronal cells. *Neuroendocrinology* 96: 162–171.

55 Dressing, G.E., Goldberg, J.E., Charles, N.J. et al. (2011). Membrane progesterone receptor expression in mammalian tissues: a review of regulation and physiological implications. *Steroids* 76: 11–17.

56 Olsen, R.W. (2018). GABAA receptor: positive and negative allosteric modulators. *Neuropharmacology* 136: 10–22.

57 Mouton, J.C. and Duckworth, R.A. (2021). Maternally derived hormones, neurosteroids and the development of behaviour. *Proc. Biol. Sci.* 288: 20202467.

58 Conley, A.J. and Ball, B.A. (2019). Steroids in the establishment and maintenance of pregnancy and at parturition in the mare. *Reproduction* 158: R197–R208.

59 Diesch, T.J. and Mellor, D.J. (2013). Birth transitions: pathophysiology, the onset of consciousness and possible implications for neonatal maladjustment syndrome in the foal. *Equine Vet. J.* 45: 656–660.

60 Houghton, E., Holtan, D., Grainger, L. et al. (1991). Plasma progestagen concentrations in the normal and dysmature newborn foal. *J. Reprod. Fertil. Suppl.* 44: 609–617.

61 Muller, V., Curcio, B.R., Toribio, R.E. et al. (2019). Cortisol, progesterone, 17alphaOHprogesterone, and pregnenolone in foals born from mare's hormone-treated for experimentally induced ascending placentitis. *Theriogenology* 123: 139–144.

62 Swink, J.M.(2020). Sex steroids and the effect of in-utero altrenogest exposure in neonatal foals. Masters thesis. College of Veterinary Medicine, The Ohio State University.

63 Toribio, R.E. and Madigan, J.E. (2019). Equine neonatal maladjustment syndrome/neonatal encephalopathy: Evidence for the etiology and treatment. *Proceedings of the 2019 ACVIM Forum*. Phoenix, AZ: American College of Veterinary Internal Medicine

64 Rossdale, P.D., Ousey, J.C., McGladdery, A.J. et al. (1995). A retrospective study of increased plasma progestagen concentrations in compromised neonatal foals. *Reprod. Fertil. Dev.* 7: 567–575.

65 Toribio, R.E. (2011). Endocrine dysregulation in critically ill foals and horses. *Vet. Clin. North Am. Equine Pract.* 27: 35–47.

66 Muller, V., Toribio, R.E., Dembek, K. et al. (2020). Serum cortisol and thyroid hormone concentrations and survival in foals born from mares with experimentally induced ascending placentitis. *J. Vet. Intern. Med.* 34: 1332–1338.

67 Dembek, K.A., Hurcombe, S.D., Stewart, A.J. et al. (2016). Association of aldosterone and arginine vasopressin concentrations and clinical markers of hypoperfusion in neonatal foals. *Equine Vet. J.* 48: 176–181.

68 Hollis, A.R., Boston, R.C., and Corley, K.T. (2008). Plasma aldosterone, vasopressin and atrial natriuretic peptide in hypovolaemia: a preliminary comparative study of neonatal and mature horses. *Equine Vet. J.* 40: 64–69.

Section II Disorders of Energy and Growth Hormones

Katarzyna A. Dembek, Laura D. Hostnik, Teresa A. Burns, and Ramiro E. Toribio

Energy Metabolism

Different organs and systems with endocrine function are involved in energy homeostasis, including the pancreas (islet of Langerhans), gastrointestinal (GI) tract, hypothalamus, pituitary gland, thyroid gland, liver, and adipose tissue. Despite the importance of energy availability in the survival of the newborn foal, information regarding endocrine dynamics in response to illness for these systems is scarce. Glucose, lactate, and free fatty acids (FFAs; non-esterified fatty acids [NEFAs]) are major sources of energy for cellular metabolism in utero and after birth. Newborn foals have limited energy reserves and low blood glucose concentrations, thus voluntary nursing or caloric supplementation is needed within a few hours of birth to survive [1]. Thereafter, resting blood glucose concentrations are higher in neonatal foals compared to horses, with wide variations due to intermittent nursing [2–4]. This is relevant when defining normoglycemia and hyperglycemia. For example, a few minutes after nursing, a newborn foal's blood glucose concentration can be 220–250 mg/dl. Enteral dextrose and lactose administration also increase glucose concentrations, but the increase is more robust with nursing [2, 3]. Fasting of healthy foals for up to 4 hours results in minimal decrease in glucose concentrations, seldom causing hypoglycemia [2, 3]. This indicates that hypoglycemic ill foals have severe energy depletion and homeostatic systems are not coping with demands.

Endocrine Pancreas

The main pancreatic hormones include insulin (beta cells), glucagon (alpha cells) and somatostatin (delta cells). *Insulin* regulates energy conservation and the main stimuli for secretion includes glucose, amino acids, and intestinal hormones (incretins). Fatty acids potentiate insulin secretion while hypoglycemia, catecholamines, and somatostatin suppress insulin secretion. Under physiological conditions, insulin promotes glucose and fatty acid transport into cells, increases glycolysis and glycogenesis, and inhibits lipolysis, glycogenolysis, gluconeogenesis, and glucagon secretion. Insulin also stimulates leptin secretion by adipocyte tissue, likely to modulate hunger. In turn, leptin inhibits insulin secretion (adipoinsular axis). Thus, fluctuations in insulin concentrations are essential to balance energy storage and disposal. Insulin concentrations in healthy foals are similar to horses [3–7] and is effective at lowering blood glucose concentrations in healthy foals [5, 8, 9].

Hyperglycemia, amino acids, lactose, and milk stimulate insulin secretion in healthy foals [3, 6–12]. Incretins include glucagon-like peptide 1 (GLP-1), GLP-2, and gastric inhibitory peptide (GIP), of which GLP-1 and GIP are the main insulin secretagogues. This dynamic system is known as the *enteroinsular axis* (EIA; incretins and insulin) and is functional in newborn foals [2]. There is evidence that the EIA is more important to stimulate insulin secretion than enteral nutrients, including glucose [13].

Glucagon prevents tissue glycopenia by making energy substrates available during negative energy balances or increased energy needs by promoting glycogenolysis, gluconeogenesis, and lipolysis, and by inhibiting glycolysis and fatty acid synthesis. Glucagon secretion is stimulated by hypoglycemia, fasting, exercise, protein-rich meals, catecholamines, and sympathetic islet innervation. In contrast to insulin, high-glucose concentrations inhibit glucagon secretion. In the immediate postpartum period, milk ingestion promotes both insulin and glucagon secretion in foals. The reasons for this phenomenon are unclear but could be a transient adaptation to extrauterine life to make energy readily available to assure survival while at the same time conserving energy for other needs [3].

Equine Neonatal Medicine, First Edition. Edited by David M. Wong and Pamela A. Wilkins.

Somatostatin inhibits synthesis and secretion of both insulin and glucagon, which is part of an autoregulatory paracrine mechanism to control secretion of these hormones. Glucose as well as local factors promote somatostatin release. Other somatostatin functions beyond the pancreas include suppression of growth hormone (GH), prolactin, and thyroid-stimulating hormone (TSH) secretion, inhibition of pancreatic exocrine secretion, and delaying gastric emptying. Vagal stimulation inhibits somatostatin secretion. Somatostatin circulates in very low concentrations (paracrine factor). Foals are born with low somatostatin concentrations that increase thereafter, likely in response to energy intake and growth [14]. Information in sick foals is lacking.

FFAs are released from adipose tissue in response to negative energy balance or stressful conditions that activate lipolytic pathways. A small fraction of FFAs come from intestinal absorption and various tissues. They are produced through breakdown of triacylglycerols mediated by lipases, yielding glycerol and FFAs. The liver is a major site of FFAs metabolism to be oxidized, stored, or released as other type of substrates. FFAs circulate in low concentrations in healthy foals [15, 16].

Triglycerides are mainly produced in the liver through re-esterification of glycerol and FFAs. They are released into circulation at a steady rate as very low-density lipoproteins (VLDLs), but concentrations can increase from energy demands, stress, or reduced removal of VLDLs. Serum triglyceride concentrations vary widely in healthy foals and are within adult reference ranges at birth, increase by 1–2 days of age, and remain higher than horses for up to 6 weeks of age [5, 15–18]. Healthy foals can have serum triglyceride values of 100–200 mg/dl in the first week of life, although most have concentrations <50 mg/dl [17, 18]. Foals from some breeds (e.g. Andalusian, Paso Fino, draft breeds, ponies, donkeys) have higher resting triglyceride concentrations immediately after birth (R. Toribio, personal communication).

Disorders of the Endocrine Pancreas

Understanding endocrine pancreatic biology is valuable as energy disorders, including hypoglycemia and hypertriglyceridemia are common in ill foals. This information could influence treatments. Hypoglycemia in sick newborn foals can reflect anorexia, limited energy storage, access to nursing, bacteremia, organ dysfunction, and endocrine dysregulation. Illnesses alter the synthesis and secretion of pancreatic hormones in newborn foals [5] but pancreatic hormones are rarely measured. Measurement of blood glucose concentrations is a method to monitor energy balance in sick foals. Septic and premature foals often have low glucose and insulin concentrations compared to healthy foals [5, 6, 8, 15], which is contrary to what occurs in adult horses and calves [19, 20]. Moreover, premature foals have lower plasma glucose and insulin concentrations compared to full-term foals [8], potentially as a consequence of immature beta cells that depend on cortisol in late pregnancy to achieve full differentiation [10]. Both low and high glucose and insulin concentrations have been associated with foal mortality [2–5, 21]. Low insulin concentration is considered an appropriate response to hypoglycemia, but also a mechanism to indirectly promote release of energy substrates into circulation through glycogenolysis, gluconeogenesis, lipolysis, and glucagon secretion [2]. High insulin concentration in septic nonsurviving foals is likely similar to what occurs in horses with endotoxemia-induced hyperinsulinemia [20]. Thus, assessing insulin concentrations in hospitalized foals may have prognostic value [5]. Lipolysis and increased glucagon concentrations have been documented in septic foals [5, 15].

Most critically ill foals are insulin sensitive because insulin administration decreases their glucose concentrations, and the majority have a high quantitative insulin-sensitivity check index (QUICKI), a proxy measurement of insulin sensitivity [5]. However, depending on disease severity, they have varying degrees of insulin sensitivity, which in part is dictated by high cortisol concentrations in septic foals, which promotes insulin resistance [22, 23]. Septic foals that develop hyperglycemia often have high insulin secretion, suggesting that most have a functional endocrine pancreas, although some may have insulin resistance – in particular, those with severe sepsis [5]. Foals that are unresponsive to exogenous insulin administration have a poor prognosis for survival. Serum glucagon concentrations were higher in septic (~tenfold) and sick-nonseptic (~twofold) compared to healthy foals and linked to disease severity [5], which is an appropriate response to energy restriction and stress. Hyperglucagonemia activates processes leading to glucose, fatty acid, and triglyceride release, which have been documented in hospitalized foals [5, 15, 17].

Lipid derangements occur in critically ill foals and foals with acute pancreatitis [5, 17, 24, 25]. Serum triglyceride and FFA concentrations were high in septic and nonsurviving foals and negatively associated with glucose concentrations [5, 15, 17]. Serum triglyceride concentrations were positively correlated with glucagon concentrations [5]. This parallel increase likely reflects disease severity, stress, and low insulin, combined with hyperglucagonemia to promote energy delivery. Unfortunately, for many foals this response is not enough to prevent death. To further promote energy availability, these foals also have HPAA activation, characterized by increased ACTH and cortisol concentrations [15, 22, 23]. Glucagon acts in synergy with cortisol and epinephrine to promote hepatic glucose output. Septic and nonsurviving hospitalized foals have higher serum triglyceride concentrations compared to healthy foals [5, 15, 17]. Hypertriglyceridemia is also a complication of parenteral nutrition and is associated with foal mortality [26].

The Enteroinsular Axis

Healthy newborn foals have a functional EIA comprised of GLP-1, GLP-2, and GIP, of which GLP-1 and GIP are the main insulin secretagogues [2]. Milk and nursing in healthy foals elicit a rapid release of GLP-1, GIP, and insulin [2]. EIA imbalances occur in ill foals and is linked to disease severity and outcome [6]. In one study, hospitalized and septic foals had higher plasma GLP-1 and GLP-2, but lower GIP concentrations than healthy and sick nonseptic foals [6]. Over time, plasma GLP-1 and GLP-2 remained elevated longer in hospitalized and septic compared to healthy foals [6]. This study noted that septic and nonsurviving foals had lower insulin concentrations and hospitalized foals with low insulin and high plasma GLP-1 and GLP-2 concentrations were more likely to die [6]. Low plasma GIP together with increased GLP-1 and GLP-2 concentrations suggests that different mechanisms contribute to reduced insulin secretion in critically ill foals, including impaired intestinal production (GIP, proximal intestine) and pancreatic endocrine resistance to incretins (GLP-1, GLP-2; distal intestine). These imbalances likely contribute to energy dysregulation in sick foals [6].

Leptin and Adiponectin

Leptin and adiponectin are adipocyte-derived hormones (adipokines) released in response to different stimuli and have unique functions that affect multiple body systems. Information on these hormones in foals is minimal. *Leptin* regulates satiety and suppresses hunger (anorexigenic factor), increases insulin sensitivity and insulin hepatic extraction and decreases insulin secretion (adipoinsular axis) and glucose concentrations [27, 28]. As part of this regulatory system, insulin stimulates leptin secretion by adipocytes. A function of the adipoinsular axis is to inhibit insulin secretion to reduce adipogenesis. Blood leptin concentrations correlate with total body fat and body condition score in horses [29, 30] but are not associated with fat depth and body condition score in foals; this may be an adaptive mechanism to promote feed intake for rapid growth [31]. In newborn foals, leptin concentrations rise after birth and decline a few days later [31]. Postpartum hyperlipidemia and hyperleptinemia in mares did not affect lipid status and plasma leptin concentrations in their foals [16]. However, increased leptin concentrations in pregnant mares was associated with decreased foal birthweight [32]. In other studies, blood leptin concentrations were not different between healthy and sick foals [5], but leptin concentrations were lower in nonsurviving septic foals [5]. Insulin increases leptin secretion, suggesting that low leptin in critically ill foals could be in part reflecting low insulin concentrations [5], perhaps to indirectly stimulate hunger (low leptin results in hunger). In addition to promoting energy intake, another function could be to protect against systemic inflammation [33]. The fact that low leptin concentration was associated with nonsurvival in sick foals aligns with studies in other species where leptin administration is protective against sepsis and endotoxemia [33]. *Adiponectin* promotes cell membrane translocation of GLUT4, increases insulin sensitivity, glycolysis, and fatty acid oxidation, and is negatively correlated with body fat mass in horses [30, 34]. Serum adiponectin concentrations were not different between healthy, sick nonseptic and septic foals; thus, its role in energy dysregulation and systemic inflammation in sick foals remains unclear [35].

Somatotropic Axis

The somatotropic axis includes GH from the pituitary gland and insulin-like growth factor-1 (IGF-1), primarily from the liver. Growth hormone-releasing hormone (GHRH) and growth hormone-inhibiting hormone (GHIH; somatostatin) from the hypothalamus regulates GH secretion. In addition, ghrelin from the stomach and brain and hypoglycemia are potent stimulators of GH release. In addition to growth, this system is essential to energy homeostasis, especially during food deprivation – which, in conjunction with other regulatory systems, makes different substrates available to be used as fuels.

Most peripheral actions of GH are mediated by IGF-1. An increase in GH results in elevations in IGF-1 concentrations; IGF-1 suppresses GH secretion (negative feedback). GH counteracts the effects of insulin on glucose and lipid metabolism [36–38]. GH increases insulin concentrations by interfering with its actions, by promoting hyperglycemia, and by stimulating its synthesis and secretion [39]. In the liver, GH stimulates gluconeogenesis and glycogenolysis to increase glucose output. In adipose tissue, directly and indirectly through its anti-insulin properties, GH promotes lipolysis and fatty acid release. Ghrelin is produced by gastric glandular cells in response to gastric emptiness and energy restriction, promotes hunger (orexigenic factor) and GH release, and inhibits insulin secretion [40]. Small amounts are also produced in the small intestine, pancreas, and brain. Ghrelin has anti-inflammatory properties; higher concentrations may improve survival [24].

Disturbances of the somatotropic axis occur in critically ill foals [24]. Increased GH but reduced IGF-1 concentrations were measured in septic foals, suggesting impaired somatotropic axis signaling [24]. This phenomenon (termed *somatotropic axis resistance*) was characterized by a high GH : IGF-1 ratio [24], but clinical implications are unclear. Blood ghrelin concentrations increase in foals in response to illness [24], consistent with a response to energy deprivation, perhaps to directly promote hunger and indirectly make glucose available through GH secretion [24]. In addition, this could be a protective mechanism against systemic illness.

The fact that most sick foals with high GH concentrations also have increased ghrelin concentrations indicates that the pituitary component of this axis is functional during critical illness. This also suggests that impaired GH signaling at the hepatocyte level is central to the pathogenesis of somatotropic axis resistance, likely from systemic inflammation or endotoxemia, which are frequent in septic foals. This is in contrast to premature foals, where IGF-1 concentrations were high [41]. It is possible that increased GH concentrations, through its insulin-blocking actions, interferes with glucose uptake and promotes glycogenolysis, gluconeogenesis, and lipolysis in critically ill foals. This could also explain some metabolic abnormalities such as increased FFA and triglyceride concentrations in hospitalized foals [5, 15, 17].

Diagnosis

The diagnosis of underlying causes of energy derangements in ill foals is often undetermined. Often, it is secondary to disease severity, anorexia, or lack of access to nursing. In premature foals, delayed intestinal and endocrine pancreas differentiation are central to energy disorders.

References

1 Fowden, A.L., Mundy, L., Ousey, J.C. et al. (1991). Tissue glycogen and glucose 6-phosphatase levels in fetal and newborn foals. *J. Reprod. Fertil. Suppl.* 44: 537–542.

2 Rings, L.M., Swink, J.M., Dunbar, L.K. et al. (2019). Enteroinsular axis response to carbohydrates and fasting in healthy newborn foals. *J. Vet. Intern. Med.* 33: 2752–2764.

3 Kinsella, H.M., Hostnik, L.D., Rings, L.M. et al. (2021). Glucagon, insulin, adrenocorticotropic hormone, and cortisol in response to carbohydrates and fasting in healthy neonatal foals. *J. Vet. Intern. Med.* 35: 550–559.

4 Berryhill, E.H., Magdesian, K.G., Tadros, E.M. et al. (2019). Effects of age on serum glucose and insulin concentrations and glucose/insulin ratios in neonatal foals and their dams during the first 2 weeks postpartum. *Vet. J.* 246: 1–6.

5 Barsnick, R.J., Hurcombe, S.D., Smith, P.A. et al. (2011). Insulin, glucagon, and leptin in critically ill foals. *J. Vet. Intern. Med.* 25: 123–131.

6 Rings, L.M., Kamr, A.M., Kinsella, H.M. et al. (2022). The enteroinsular axis during hospitalization in newborn foals. *Domest. Anim. Endocrinol.* 78: 106686.

7 Smyth, G.B., Young, D.W., and Duran, S.H. (1993). Maturation of insulin and glucose responses to normal feeding in foals. *Aust. Vet. J.* 70: 129–132.

8 Fowden, A.L., Silver, M., Ellis, L. et al. (1984). Studies on equine prematurity 3: insulin secretion in the foal during the perinatal period. *Equine Vet. J.* 16: 286–291.

9 Kinsella, H.M., Hostnik, L.D., Snyder, H.A. et al. (2022). Comparison of insulin sensitivity between healthy neonatal foals and horses using minimal model analysis. *PLoS One* 17: e0262584.

10 Fowden, A.L., Gardner, D.S., Ousey, J.C. et al. (2005). Maturation of pancreatic {beta}-cell function in the fetal horse during late gestation. *J. Endocrinol.* 186: 467–473.

11 Holdstock, N.B., Allen, V.L., Bloomfield, M.R. et al. (2004). Development of insulin and proinsulin secretion in newborn pony foals. *J. Endocrinol.* 181: 469–476.

12 Holdstock, N.B., Allen, V.L., and Fowden, A.L. (2012). Pancreatic endocrine function in newborn pony foals after induced or spontaneous delivery at term. *Equine Vet. J. Suppl.* 30–37.

13 Holst, J.J. (2019). The incretin system in healthy humans: the role of GIP and GLP-1. *Metabolism* 96: 46–55.

14 Murray, M.J. and Luba, N.K. (1993). Plasma gastrin and somatostatin, and serum thyroxine (T4), triiodothyronine (T3), reverse triiodothyronine (rT3) and cortisol concentrations in foals from birth to 28 days of age. *Equine Vet. J.* 25: 237–239.

15 Armengou, L., Jose-Cunilleras, E., Rios, J. et al. (2013). Metabolic and endocrine profiles in sick neonatal foals are related to survival. *J. Vet. Intern. Med.* 27: 567–575.

16 Kedzierski, W., Kusy, R., and Kowalik, S. (2011). Plasma leptin level in hyperlipidemic mares and their newborn foals. *Reprod. Domest. Anim.* 46: 275–280.

17 Berryhill, E.H., Magdesian, K.G., Kass, P.H. et al. (2017). Triglyceride concentrations in neonatal foals: serial measurement and effects of age and illness. *Vet. J.* 227: 23–29.

18 Barton, M.H. and LeRoy, B.E. (2007). Serum bile acids concentrations in healthy and clinically ill neonatal foals. *J. Vet. Intern. Med.* 21: 508–513.

19 Kenison, D.C., Elsasser, T.H., and Fayer, R. (1991). Tumor necrosis factor as a potential mediator of acute metabolic and hormonal responses to endotoxemia in calves. *Am. J. Vet. Res.* 52: 1320–1326.

20 Toribio, R.E., Kohn, C.W., Hardy, J. et al. (2005). Alterations in serum PTH and electrolyte concentrations and urinary excretion of electrolytes in horses with induced endotoxemia. *J. Vet. Intern. Med.* 19: 223–231.

21 Rings, L.M., Swink, J., Dembek, K. et al. (2019). Enteroinsular axis response of healthy and hospitalized equine neonates. *ACVIM Forum* E36: 2435.

22 Dembek, K.A., Timko, K.J., Johnson, L.M. et al. (2017). Steroids, steroid precursors, and neuroactive steroids in critically ill equine neonates. *Vet. J.* 225: 42–49.

23 Dembek, K.A., Onasch, K., Hurcombe, S.D. et al. (2013). Renin-angiotensin-aldosterone system and hypothalamic-pituitary-adrenal axis in hospitalized newborn foals. *J. Vet. Intern. Med.* 27: 331–338.

24 Barsnick, R.J., Hurcombe, S.D., Dembek, K. et al. (2014). Somatotropic axis resistance and ghrelin in critically ill foals. *Equine Vet. J.* 46: 45–49.

25 Ollivett, T.L., Divers, T.J., Cushing, T. et al. (2012). Acute pancreatitis in two five-day-old Appaloosa foals. *Equine Vet. J. Suppl.* 96–99.

26 Myers, C.J., Magdesian, K.G., Kass, P.H. et al. (2009). Parenteral nutrition in neonatal foals: clinical description, complications and outcome in 53 foals (1995–2005). *Vet. J.* 181: 137–144.

27 Amitani, M., Asakawa, A., Amitani, H. et al. (2013). The role of leptin in the control of insulin-glucose axis. *Front. Neurosci.* 7: 51.

28 Paz-Filho, G., Mastronardi, C., Wong, M.L. et al. (2012). Leptin therapy, insulin sensitivity, and glucose homeostasis. *Indian J. Endocrinol. Metab.* 16: S549–S555.

29 Buff, P.R., Dodds, A.C., Morrison, C.D. et al. (2002). Leptin in horses: tissue localization and relationship between peripheral concentrations of leptin and body condition. *J. Anim. Sci.* 80: 2942–2948.

30 Kearns, C.F., McKeever, K.H., Roegner, V. et al. (2006). Adiponectin and leptin are related to fat mass in horses. *Vet. J.* 172: 460–465.

31 Berg, E.L., McNamara, D.L., and Keisler, D.H. (2007). Endocrine profiles of periparturient mares and their foals. *J. Anim. Sci.* 85: 1660–1668.

32 Smith, S., Marr, C.M., Dunnett, C. et al. (2017). The effect of mare obesity and endocrine function on foal birthweight in Thoroughbreds. *Equine Vet. J.* 49: 461–466.

33 Vallejos, A., Olivares, P., Varela, D. et al. (2018). Preventive leptin administration protects against sepsis through improving hypotension, tachycardia, oxidative stress burst, multiple organ dysfunction, and increasing survival. *Front. Physiol.* 9: 1800.

34 Barsnick, R.J. and Toribio, R.E. (2011). Endocrinology of the equine neonate energy metabolism in health and critical illness. *Vet. Clin. North Am. Equine Pract.* 27: 49–58.

35 Barsnick, R.J., Hurcombe, S.D., Saville, W.J. et al. (2009). Endocrine energy response in septic foals: Insulin, leptin and adiponectin. *Proceedings of the 2009 ACVIM Forum*. Montreal, Canada: American College of Veterinary Internal Medicine.

36 Houssay, B.A. (1936). Carbohydrate metabolism. *N. Engl. J. Med.* 214: 971–986.

37 Moller, N. and Jorgensen, J.O. (2009). Effects of growth hormone on glucose, lipid, and protein metabolism in human subjects. *Endocr. Rev.* 30: 152–177.

38 Jorgensen, J.O., Krag, M., Jessen, N. et al. (2004). Growth hormone and glucose homeostasis. *Horm. Res.* 62 (Suppl 3): 51–55.

39 Vijayakumar, A., Yakar, S., and Leroith, D. (2011). The intricate role of growth hormone in metabolism. *Front. Endocrinol. (Lausanne)* 2: 32.

40 Poher, A.L., Tschop, M.H., and Muller, T.D. (2018). Ghrelin regulation of glucose metabolism. *Peptides* 100: 236–242.

41 Panzani, S., Castagnetti, C., Prandi, A. et al. (2013). Insulin-like growth factor I: could it be a marker of prematurity in the foal? *Theriogenology* 79: 495–501.

Section III Disorders of Thyroid Hormones

Katarzyna A. Dembek, Laura D. Hostnik, Teresa A. Burns, and Ramiro E. Toribio

Introduction

Thyroid hormones (THs) – including thyroxine (T_4) and triiodothyronine (T_3) – modulate cell growth, differentiation, thermogenesis, and energy metabolism. THs also facilitate differentiation of other endocrine systems (adrenal gland, pancreas) and are essential for fetal development and survival. The secretion of THs is controlled by the hypothalamic–pituitary-thyroid axis (HPTA) [1]. The hypothalamus secretes thyrotropin-releasing hormone (TRH) that stimulates the pituitary pars distalis to release thyroid-stimulating hormone (TSH), which in turn promotes synthesis and secretion of THs (total T_4 [tT_4], free T_4 [fT_4], total T_3 [tT_3], free T_3 [fT_3], reverse T_3 [rT_3]) by follicular cells of the thyroid gland. Of these, free T_3 is the active hormone. TH concentrations are influenced by age, physiological status, season, caloric intake, exogenous compounds, iodine deficiency or excess, and diseases. TH and iodine concentrations are several-fold higher in newborn foals compared to horses [2, 3]. Due to their multitude of functions, TH deficiency in the developing fetus and newborn can be detrimental. Similarly, the interactions between THs and glucocorticoids during development seem to be important in foals. Appropriate cortisol concentrations at the end of gestation influence TH concentrations and maturity in the developing fetus and newborn foal [4].

Hypothyroidism is the clinical manifestation of TH deficiency that in foals often occurs at critical stages of development. Hypothyroidism results from diseases that affect thyroid gland function, exogenous compounds that interfere with TH synthesis, and less frequently by disorders of the hypothalamus or pituitary gland. In foals, it is mainly the consequence of reduced TH synthesis and secretion. This condition is sporadic, rarely affecting multiple foals in a farm, and usually linked to nutrition. An exception is congenital hypothyroidism and dysmaturity syndrome (CHDS) in which multiple foals can be affected. Whether sporadic or congenital hypothyroidism, most foals do not recover because crucial stages of developmental are passed. Tests to evaluate thyroid gland function may be within normal limits, making confirmation of TH deficiency challenging [5]. Thus, diagnosis of hypothyroidism is based on clinical assessment and epidemiology – in particular, farms with a history of having dysmature foals or diagnosed with hypothyroidism.

Causes

Many causes of hypothyroidism in foals are nutritional. Hypothyroidism and goiter in foals have been associated with iodine deficiency and ingestion of excessive amounts of iodine (i.e., particular kelp-supplemented rations), compounds that interfere with iodine uptake by the thyroid gland (e.g. perchlorate, thiocyanate, nitrate) or compounds that inhibit iodide oxidation and coupling (e.g. thiouracil, methimazole); consumption of goitrogenic plants (e.g. *Brassica* family) that result in TH deficiency are also potential causes of hypothyroidism [1, 6–10]. Mares may or may not be affected [10]. Feeding 40 mg or more of iodine daily can produce this syndrome [11]. Sodium and potassium iodide used to treat fungal and bacterial infections, granulomatous conditions, hyperthyroidism, and as expectorants, have potential to cause congenital hypothyroidism in foals. Prolonged use in adult horses may cause iodism or hyperthyroidism. Several drugs used in equine practice (e.g. dexamethasone, phenylbutazone) reduce TH concentrations in horses [12, 13], but effects on TH concentrations in the developing fetus or newborn foal is unknown. Although information is lacking, at theory,

Equine Neonatal Medicine, First Edition. Edited by David M. Wong and Pamela A. Wilkins.

selenium deficiency can reduce TH concentrations because deiodinases are selenium-dependent proteins.

Clinical Signs

Most foals are affected at birth with clinical signs related to interference with essential functions of THs in tissue maturation and differentiation during pre- and postnatal development. Signs include prematurity, inability to stand, long curly haircoat, weakness, lethargy, weak suckle reflex, respiratory insufficiency and distress, incoordination, cold intolerance, hypothermia, physeal dysgenesis, incomplete ossification, hypoplastic carpal and tarsal bones, collapse of cuboidal bones, rupture of extensor tendons, forelimb contracture, prognathism, delayed incisor eruption, growth retardation, feeding intolerance, energy dysregulation, hypoperfusion, and death [5, 7–11, 14–23]. Functions of other endocrine systems (e.g. HPAA, endocrine pancreas) may be affected. Some foals may have thyroid gland enlargement (goiter), but this is an inconsistent finding. Many of these signs are present in premature or critically ill foals, making diagnosis of hypothyroidism challenging. To add complexity, sick foals often have low TH concentrations due to disease, which is not equivalent to hypothyroidism.

Diagnosis

Thyroid hormone deficiency may occur at different stages of development, and thyroid function may return to normal after the insult. Thus, a foal with clinical evidence of hypothyroidism could have normal TH concentrations. The lack of TH negative feedback to pituitary thyrotropes results in excessive TSH secretion, leading to thyroid follicular cell hyperplasia, and in fetuses or foals with prolonged TH deficit, goiter may be observed. Foals with clinical evidence of hypothyroidism, with or without an enlarged thyroid gland are suspects. Thyroid gland enlargement does not imply hypo- or hyperthyroidism.

Clinical presentation, age, and concurrent diseases are considerations when interpretating TH concentrations. Resting TH concentrations in newborn foals are 10- to 20-fold higher than horses and decrease rapidly in the first 2 weeks of life (Table 21.III.1) [2, 3, 15]; thus, age-specific ranges should be used. Measuring TH from age-matched healthy foals, horses, or their dams in parallel may be helpful. Low TH concentrations have been measured in premature, septic, and maladjusted foals [24–28]; however, this does not indicate hypothyroidism, but a systemic response to disease. Thus, relying on resting TH concentrations in the diagnosis of hypothyroidism can be challenging and misleading [25, 27]. Serum rT_3 concentrations in premature and septic foals may be lower, similar, or higher than in term foals [26, 27, 29]. Unfortunately, rT_3 concentrations are not routinely measured.

Treatment

Treatment of hypothyroidism is palliative; the benefits of TH supplementation have not been evaluated in foals. Several analogs to T_3 and T_4 are available. It is also important to consider the TH status of the mare as well as other animals at the farm, including pregnant mares. See below for further treatment information.

Congenital Hypothyroidism and Dysmaturity Syndrome in Foals (CHDS)

CHDS is a form of hypothyroidism characterized by thyroid gland hyperplasia, congenital musculoskeletal deformities, organ dysfunction, and high mortality rates. Multiple foals can be affected from a farm or region, with the condition initially recognized in western Canada and the northwestern United States [14, 17, 23, 30–34]. Other cases have been reported in other parts of Canada, the United States [35–37], Finland [38], and Chile (anecdotal reports) [34]. In the cases described in Canada, up to 100% of newborn foals were affected [33], with no sex or breed predilection [31].

The etiology remains unknown. Foals with CHDS had a history of prolonged gestation and mares grazed irrigated

Table 21.III.1 Total and free T4 and T3 in foals and adult horses housed in a temperate environment (mean ± SD) [15].

Age	n	Total T4 (nM)	Free T4 (pM)	n	Total T3 (nM)	Free T3 (pM)
Adult	31	22 ± 5	35 ± 9	59	1.20 ± 0.18	10.4 ± 1.1
Foal (cord)	8	557 ± 108	195 ± 76	5	8.13 ± 2.1	21.8 ± 7.5
Foal (4–6 days)	6	143 ± 66	76 ± 29	6	14.44 ± 6.8	41.6 ± 19.2

pastures, were fed greenfeed, and did not leave their home farm [33]. Nitrates were proposed as a cause because they can cross the placenta, impair thyroid gland function, and were found in high concentrations in these areas [39]. Nitrate and nitrite levels can be high in greenfeed, and plants such as alfalfa, ryegrass, timothy, wheat, oats, rye, and barley can accumulate high quantities of nitrates. These plants are also low in iodine content. Nitrate levels can be high in irrigated areas from use of fertilizers, feedlots, and dairy farms [33]. TH concentrations in foals with CHDS are low or within the normal range, and their response to TSH stimulation is poor [18]. Adrenocortical function is normal in affected foals [40], supporting the importance of THs in musculoskeletal differentiation.

The clinical presentation of CHDS varies from weak but mature foals to clinical signs primarily revolving around dysmaturity (weakness, floppy ears, short silky hair coat, tendon laxity, pulmonary insufficiency, hydrocephalus, and defects in abdominal wall) [33]. Musculoskeletal abnormalities include angular and flexural limb deformities, rupture of digital extensor tendons, delayed ossification of the cuboidal bones, osteochondrosis, and prognathism [31–34]. Foals can be born apparently healthy, but develop skeletal lesions days to weeks later [22]. Goiter is unusual; however, there is thyroid gland hyperplasia [32]. The prognosis for CHDS is poor, and most foals die or are euthanized within days [34, 38]. Foals that survive can develop other abnormalities – in particular orthopedic disorders. There are no specific treatments for CHDS except for medical support. Control should be oriented at identifying and controlling environmental and management risk factors.

Nonthyroidal Illness Syndrome (Euthyroid Syndrome)

Diseases, systemic inflammation, starvation, and stressful conditions suppress the HPTA, lowering THs. This phenomenon is known as *euthyroid sick syndrome* or *nonthyroidal illness syndrome (NTIS)* [41]. Low TH concentrations under these conditions does not imply hypothyroidism. In people, NTIS is associated with disease severity and mortality [41–45] and has been documented in a number of species [46, 47]. NTIS is common in sick foals as low concentrations of tT_3, fT_3, tT_4, and fT_4 have been measured in premature, septic, and maladjusted foals [24–28]. Sick foals born to mares with experimentally induced placentitis had lower TH concentrations than healthy foals [24] and serum concentrations of tT_3, fT_3, fT_4, and TSH were lower in hospitalized and premature foals that died compared to survivors [24, 25, 27]. TH and TSH concentrations were negatively correlated, but rT_3 positive correlated with the sepsis score [25, 27]. Serum rT_3 concentrations in premature and septic foals may be lower, similar, or higher than in term foals, but more often are lower [26, 27, 29].

Multiple mechanisms are involved in the pathogenesis of NTIS. Reduced activity of the hypothalamic and pituitary component of the HPTA are involved [41, 44], as administration of TRH to human patients with NTIS increases TSH, T_4, and T_3 release [48]. The involvement of the pituitary gland is evident because these patients often have normal TSH despite low TH concentrations [44]. There is also evidence of suppressed TRH secretion [49] as well as reduced generation of T_3, increased formation of rT_3, down-regulation of deiodinases, and reduced function of TH transporters and receptors [42–44]. Cytokines, glucocorticoids, and leptin are candidates in the pathogenesis of NTIS. IL1-β, IL-6, and TNF-α suppress TRH, TSH, T_4 and T_3 synthesis and secretion, and increase rT_3 concentrations. These cytokines are commonly increased in critically ill foals. A reduction in leptin concentrations is also important in the pathogenesis of NTIS. This may also be the case in sick foals, since low leptin concentrations have been measured in septic nonsurviving foals [50]. Evidence that patients with NTIS are hypothyroid at the cellular level is mixed [41]. In other words, low TH concentrations do not equate to hypothyroidism. There is controversy on the impact of NTIS in critically ill human patients due to its association with disease severity [41–45], but there is more consensus that NTIS from feed restriction could be beneficial and adaptive to reduce energy expenditure and catabolism [45].

The value of TH replacement therapy has not been evaluated in hospitalized foals but should be considered in foals with evidence of dysmaturity and severe sepsis. This issue remains contentious in human medicine where some believe that replacement therapy may be harmful because exogenous TH may inhibit the HPTA, leading to additional complications. Conversely, others advocate for replacement therapy [42]. Part of the argument comes from leukocyte function that relies on intracellular availability of THs, which is regulated by deiodinases [44]. NTIS decreases deiodinase activity in neutrophils and macrophages, reducing T_3 generation and bacterial killing capacity [44]. In addition to T_3 and T_4 supplementation, other therapies including TRH infusion to stimulate the pituitary gland have been proposed [44, 45].

Hyperthyroidism

Hyperthyroidism (thyrotoxicosis) has not been documented in newborn foals, although exposure to iodine-containing compounds could result in hyperthyroidism. The risk appears higher for hypothyroidism in foals born to mares with prolonged iodine exposure.

References

1 Toribio, R.E. (2018). Thyroid gland. In: *Equine Internal Medicine*, 4e (ed. S.M. Reed, W.M. Bayly, and D.C. Sellon), 1058–1069. St. Louis, Missouri: Elsevier.

2 Panzani, S., Comin, A., Galeati, G. et al. (2012). How type of parturition and health status influence hormonal and metabolic profiles in newborn foals. *Theriogenology* 77: 1167–1177.

3 Lopez-Rodriguez, M.F., Cymbaluk, N.F., Epp, T. et al. (2020). A field study of serum, colostrum, milk iodine, and thyroid hormone concentrations in postpartum draft mares and foals. *J. Equine Vet. Sci.* 90: 103018.

4 Silver, M., Fowden, A.L., Knox, J. et al. (1991). Relationship between circulating tri-iodothyronine and cortisol in the perinatal period in the foal. *J. Reprod. Fertil. Suppl.* 44: 619–626.

5 Irvine, C.H. (1984). Hypothyroidism in the foal. *Equine Vet. J.* 16: 302–306.

6 Kaneko, J.J. (1989). Thyroid function. In: *Biochemistry of Domestic Animals*, 4e (ed. J.J. Kaneko), 630. San Diego: Academic Press.

7 Conway, D.A. and Cosgrove, J.S. (1980). Equine goiter. *Irish Vet. J.* 34: 29–31.

8 Drew, B., Barber, W.P., and Williams, D.G. (1975). The effect of excess dietary iodine on pregnant mares and foals. *Vet. Rec.* 97: 93–95.

9 Driscoll, J., Hintz, H.F., and Schryver, H.F. (1978). Goiter in foals caused by excessive iodine. *J. Am. Vet. Med. Assoc.* 173: 858–859.

10 Eroksuz, H., Eroksuz, Y., Ozer, H. et al. (2004). Equine goiter associated with excess dietary iodine. *Vet. Hum. Toxicol.* 46: 147–149.

11 Baker, J.R., Wyn-Jones, G., and Eley, J.L. (1983). Case of equine goitre. *Vet. Rec.* 112: 407–408.

12 Messer, N.T., Ganjam, V.K., Nachreiner, R.F. et al. (1995). Effect of dexamethasone administration on serum thyroid hormone concentrations in clinically normal horses. *J. Am. Vet. Med. Assoc.* 206: 63–66.

13 Ramirez, S., Wolfsheimer, K.J., Moore, R.M. et al. (1997). Duration of effects of phenylbutazone on serum total thyroxine and free thyroxine concentrations in horses. *J. Vet. Intern. Med.* 11: 371–374.

14 Doige, C.E. and McLaughlin, B.G. (1981). Hyperplastic goitre in newborn foals in Western Canada. *Can. Vet. J.* 22: 42–45.

15 Irvine, C.H. and Evans, M.J. (1975). Postnatal changes in total and free thyroxine and triiodothyronine in foal serum. *J. Reprod. Fertil. Suppl.* 709–715.

16 Irvine, C.H. and Evans, M.J. (1977). Hypothyroidism in foals. *N. Z. Vet. J.* 25: 354.

17 McLaughlin, B.G., Doige, C.E., Fretz, P.B. et al. (1981). Carpal bone lesions associated with angular limb deformities in foals. *J. Am. Vet. Med. Assoc.* 178: 224–230.

18 McLaughlin, B.G., Doige, C.E., and McLaughlin, P.S. (1986). Thyroid-hormone levels in foals with congenital musculoskeletal lesions. *Can. Vet. J.* 27: 264–267.

19 Shaver, J.R., Fretz, P.B., and Doige, C.E. (1979). Skeletal manifestations of suspected hypothyroidism in two foals. *J. Equine Med. Surg.* 3: 269.

20 Vivrette, S.L., Reimers, T.J., and Krook, L. (1984). Skeletal disease in a hypothyroid foal. *Cornell Vet.* 74: 373–386.

21 Murray, M.J. (1990). Hypothyroidism and respiratory insufficiency in a neonatal foal. *J. Am. Vet. Med. Assoc.* 197: 1635–1638.

22 McLaughlin, B.G. and Doige, C.E. (1982). A study of ossification of carpal and tarsal bones in normal and hypothyroid foals. *Can. Vet. J.* 23: 164–168.

23 McLaughlin, B.G. and Doige, C.E. (1981). Congenital musculosketal lesions and hyperplastic goitre in foals. *Can. Vet. J.* 22: 130–133.

24 Muller, V., Toribio, R.E., Dembek, K. et al. (2020). Serum cortisol and thyroid hormone concentrations and survival in foals born from mares with experimentally induced ascending placentitis. *J. Vet. Intern. Med.* 34: 1332–1338.

25 Breuhaus, B.A. (2014). Thyroid function and dysfunction in term and premature equine neonates. *J. Vet. Intern. Med.* 28: 1301–1309.

26 Dudan, F.E., Ferguson, D.C., and Little, T.V. (1987). Circulating serum thyroxine (T4), triiodothyronine (T3) and reverse T3 (rT3) in neonatal term and preterm foals. *5th Annual Verinary Medical Forum*. San Diego, CA.

27 Himler, M., Hurcombe, S.D., Griffin, A. et al. (2012). Presumptive nonthyroidal illness syndrome in critically ill foals. *Equine Vet. J. Suppl.* 44 (Suppl 41): 43–47.

28 Pirrone, A., Panzani, S., Govoni, N. et al. (2013). Thyroid hormone concentrations in foals affected by perinatal asphyxia syndrome. *Theriogenology* 80: 624–629.

29 Breuhaus, B.A. and LaFevers, D.H. (2005). Thyroid function in normal, sick and premature foals. *Proceedings of the 23rd ACVIM Forum*. Baltimore, MD: American College of Veterinary Internal Medicine

30 McCall, C.A., Potter, G.D., Kreider, J.L. et al. (1987). Physiological-responses in foals weaned by abrupt or gradual methods. *J. Equine Vet. Sci.* 7: 368–374.

31 Allen, A.L., Doige, C.E., Fretz, P.B. et al. (1994). Hyperplasia of the thyroid gland and concurrent musculoskeletal deformities in western Canadian foals: reexamination of a previously described syndrome. *Can. Vet. J.* 35: 31–38.

32 Allen, A.L. (1995). Hyperplasia of the thyroid gland and musculoskeletal deformities in two equine abortuses. *Can. Vet. J.* 36: 234–236.

33 Allen, A.L., Townsend, H.G., Doige, C.E. et al. (1996). A case-control study of the congenital hypothyroidism and dysmaturity syndrome of foals. *Can. Vet. J.* 37: 349–351.
34 Allen, A.L. (2014). Congenital hypothyroidism in horses: looking back and looking ahead. *Equine Vet. Educ.* 26: 190–193.
35 Borchers, A., Magdesian, K.G., Schenck, P.A. et al. (2014). Serial plasma vasopressin concentration in healthy and hospitalised neonatal foals. *Equine Vet. J.* 46: 306–310.
36 Schott, H.C., Bayly, W.M., Reed, S.M. et al. (1993). Nephrogenic diabetes insipidus in sibling colts. *J. Vet. Intern. Med.* 7: 68–72.
37 Ousey, J.C. (2004). Peripartal endocrinology in the mare and foetus. *Reprod. Domest. Anim.* 39: 222–231.
38 Koikkalainen, K., Knuuttila, A., Karikoski, N. et al. (2014). Congenital hypothyroidism and dysmaturity syndrome in foals: first reported cases in Europe. *Equine Vet. Educ.* 26: 181–189.
39 van Maanen, J.M., van Dijk, A., Mulder, K. et al. (1994). Consumption of drinking water with high nitrate levels causes hypertrophy of the thyroid. *Toxicol. Lett.* 72: 365–374.
40 Card, C.E. and Manning, S.T. (2000). Response of newborn foals with thyroid musculoskeletal disease to adrenocorticotrophic hormone (ACTH). *J. Reprod. Fertil. Suppl.* 709–715.
41 De Groot, L.J. (1999). Dangerous dogmas in medicine: the nonthyroidal illness syndrome. *J. Clin. Endocrinol. Metab.* 84: 151–164.
42 De Groot, L.J. (2006). Non-thyroidal illness syndrome is a manifestation of hypothalamic-pituitary dysfunction, and in view of current evidence, should be treated with appropriate replacement therapies. *Crit. Care Clin.* 22: 57–86, vi.
43 DeGroot, L.J. (2003). 'Non-thyroidal illness syndrome' is functional central hypothyroidism, and if severe, hormone replacement is appropriate in light of present knowledge. *J. Endocrinol Invest.* 26: 1163–1170.
44 Fliers, E. and Boelen, A. (2021). An update on non-thyroidal illness syndrome. *J. Endocrinol. Investig.* 44: 1597–1607.
45 Van den Berghe, G. (2014). Non-thyroidal illness in the ICU: a syndrome with different faces. *Thyroid* 24: 1456–1465.
46 Peterson, M.E., Davignon, D.L., Shaw, N. et al. (2020). Serum thyroxine and thyrotropin concentrations decrease with severity of nonthyroidal illness in cats and predict 30-day survival outcome. *J. Vet. Intern. Med.* 34: 2276–2286.
47 Nishii, N., Okada, R., Matsuba, M. et al. (2019). Risk factors for low plasma thyroxine and high plasma thyroid-stimulating hormone concentrations in dogs with non-thyroidal diseases. *J. Vet. Med. Sci.* 81: 1097–1103.
48 Van den, B.G., de Zegher, F., Baxter, R.C. et al. (1998). Neuroendocrinology of prolonged critical illness: effects of exogenous thyrotropin-releasing hormone and its combination with growth hormone secretagogues. *J. Clin. Endocrinol. Metab.* 83: 309–319.
49 Fliers, E., Guldenaar, S.E., Wiersinga, W.M. et al. (1997). Decreased hypothalamic thyrotropin-releasing hormone gene expression in patients with nonthyroidal illness. *J. Clin. Endocrinol. Metab.* 82: 4032–4036.
50 Barsnick, R.J., Hurcombe, S.D., Smith, P.A. et al. (2011). Insulin, glucagon, and leptin in critically ill foals. *J. Vet. Intern. Med.* 25: 123–131.

Section IV Disorders of Hormones Involved in Blood Pressure and Volume Regulation

Katarzyna A. Dembek, Laura D. Hostnik, Teresa A. Burns, and Ramiro E. Toribio

Disorders of the Renin-Angiotensin-Aldosterone System (RAAS)

The main function of the RAAS is maintenance of tissue perfusion via increasing blood pressure and intravascular fluid volume [1, 2]. A decrease in sodium (Na^+) and chloride (Cl^-) concentrations consistent with hypovolemia and reduced glomerular filtration is sensed in the distal tubules by the macula densa of the juxtaglomerular apparatus, resulting in local prostaglandin and nitric oxide (NO) release that causes vasodilation of the afferent arterioles, which thereby increases glomerular filtration and promotes renin release [3, 4]. The juxtaglomerular apparatus also detects drops in blood pressure through stretch-sensitive baroreceptors to release renin. Renin is a proteolytic enzyme that cleaves hepatic angiotensinogen to angiotensin I (ANG-I), which is primarily converted in the lungs by angiotensin-converting enzymes (ACE) into ANG-II. ANG-II is a potent vasoconstrictor that also causes aldosterone secretion from the adrenal gland cortex, arginine vasopressin (AVP) from the posterior pituitary gland, and triggers thirst. Aldosterone secretion is also activated by hyperkalemia and ACTH [3, 4]. The actions of ANG-II are mainly mediated by the ANG-II type 1 receptor in the blood vessels, heart, kidney, adrenal cortex, lung, hypothalamus, neurohypophysis, basal ganglia, and brainstem. Aldosterone is the main adrenocortical mineralocorticoid that increases renal reabsorption of Na^+ and water and eliminates potassium (K^+). In the distal nephron, aldosterone binds to mineralocorticoid receptors to stimulate the expression of genes involved in Na^+, K^+, and water transport, including Na^+ and K^+ channels, Na^+/K^+-ATPase, and aquaporins [3, 4]. Reabsorption of Na^+ (and water) by aldosterone, as well as efferent arteriolar vasoconstriction by ANG-II, help maintain volume and perfusion to organs and offset hypotension associated with septic, hypovolemic and neurogenic shock [1, 3, 4].

Newborn foals have a functional RAAS that is more responsive to hypovolemia/hyponatremia than adult horses [1, 2]. Of interest, aldosterone concentrations were higher in neonatal foals compared to adults during hypovolemia and after fluid resuscitation. This difference may reflect relative insensitivity of the distal tubules to aldosterone in the perinatal period or an evolutionary adaptation of the foal that develops in a low Na^+ environment and ingests a low Na^+ diet [2, 5]. Therefore, it must be very efficient at retaining Na^+, which likely is mediated by aldosterone. Septic foals have a substantial aldosterone and ANG-II response to sepsis, inflammation, endotoxemia, and hypoperfusion [1, 6, 7]. Critically ill foals with low aldosterone concentrations were more likely survive in one study [1]. Inappropriately low cortisol and aldosterone concentrations characterized by high ACTH/cortisol and ACTH/aldosterone ratios were documented in septic foals, suggesting relative adrenal insufficiency (RAI) is not restricted to the zona fasciculata, but also affects the zona glomerulosa and zona reticularis. Currently, there are no recommendations for aldosterone replacement therapy in critically ill foals [1]. Because foals with RAI often have inappropriately low cortisol and aldosterone secretion, hydrocortisone is the glucocorticoid of choice for replacement therapy because it also has mineralocorticoid properties. Fludrocortisone is a synthetic mineralocorticoid used in other species with Addison's disease, but there is no information on its use in sick foals. Isoflupredone is another glucocorticoid with mineralocorticoid activity used in veterinary medicine. In support of its aldosterone-like effect, prolonged use of isoflupredone can cause hypokalemia in cattle and horses.

Disorders of Vasopressin

AVP is a neural hormone synthesized in the hypothalamus and transported down axons to the posterior pituitary lobe (neurohypophysis) to be stored and subsequently released

Equine Neonatal Medicine, First Edition. Edited by David M. Wong and Pamela A. Wilkins.

in response to hypovolemia or hyperosmolality [4]. There are three types of AVP receptors: V1, V2, and V3. The vasoconstrictor effects of AVP are mediated by V1 receptors in blood vessels. V2 receptors mediate anti-diuretic effects by promoting translocation of aquaporins (water channels) from cytoplasmic endosomes to the luminal cell membrane of the principal cells in the collecting ducts. V3 receptors mediate ACTH secretion in the anterior pituitary. There is evidence that AVP is the main ACTH-releasing hormone in adult horses, late-term fetuses, and foals [8–11]. Normal values for AVP concentrations have been published for healthy foals <3 months old with minimal changes over time [7, 12].

Plasma AVP concentrations increased and were associated with hypoperfusion and nonsurvival in critically ill foals [1, 2, 6, 7, 13]. Common causes for hypervasopressinemia in sepsis include decreased blood pressure and blood volume, increased blood osmolality, ANG-II, stress and HPAA activation, as well as proinflammatory cytokines and endotoxin. An interaction of both osmotic-related and non-osmotic–related mechanisms are likely involved in enhanced AVP release in critically ill foals [1, 6]. One study showed no change in AVP response after fluid resuscitation in hypovolemic foals, suggesting a depletion of vasopressin stores or physiological differences in neonatal foals compared to adult horses. These differences may impact treatment of hypovolemia in critically ill foals and require further investigations [2]. AVP and analogs are used to treat hypotension in critically ill foals (Chapter 11).

In one study, a higher AVP/ACTH ratio was found in septic compared to sick nonseptic and healthy foals [6]. This suggested pituitary dysfunction (pars distalis); however, to confirm this hypothesis, CRH and AVP stimulation might be a better test to assess pituitary corticotrope function and HPAA integrity in critically ill foals. The CRH and AVP stimulation tests were evaluated in healthy and hospitalized neonatal foals [8, 14] with administration of CRH (1 μg/kg, IV) eliciting rapid ACTH and cortisol responses in foals [14]. AVP (2.5–7.5 IU/foal, IV) resulted in a strong ACTH and cortisol response that was even higher than the CRH stimulation test [8, 14]. This information suggests that AVP and CRH stimulation tests may be valuable to assess HPAA function in hospitalized foals.

AVP Deficiency and Syndrome of Inappropriate Antidiuretic Hormone Secretion (SIADH)

Diabetes insipidus (DI) is a rare equine condition resulting from inadequate AVP secretion (central or neurogenic DI) or inadequate renal response to AVP (nephrogenic DI). Psychogenic DI (psychogenic polydipsia) is a common cause of polyuria and polydipsia in horses with the occasional foal also developing this condition. Clinical findings in affected horses include polyuria without renal dysfunction, hyposthenuria, and increase serum osmolality [15, 16]. DI is poorly documented in newborn foals. The fact that foals ingest large amounts of liquid makes the diagnosis of DI challenging. However, it is not unusual for sick foals to develop hypernatremia, which could be an ontogenic adaptation to retain Na^+ to maintain blood volume, in part mediated by high aldosterone concentrations [1], but in some instances could be related to insufficient AVP secretion (neurogenic DI) or renal refractoriness to AVP (nephrogenic DI). Nephrogenic DI was documented in two sibling colts with a history of polyuria and polydipsia since birth [17].

SIADH is caused by excessive AVP secretion. In people, this syndrome results from brain injury, cerebral inflammation, or drugs (e.g. antidepressants, thiazides, citalopram, carbamazepine, clofibrate, morphine). High levels of AVP results in excessive water retention leading to serum hypoosmolality, hyponatremia, and urine hyperosmolality [3]. Horses and foals with brain pathologies may develop signs and laboratory abnormalities consistent with SIADH, but AVP concentrations are not routinely measured, limiting clinical recognition and diagnosis. In addition, as part of the stress response in ill foals, plasma AVP concentrations are often elevated [1, 6]. There are anecdotal reports of horses with no history of systemic illness that develop laboratory abnormalities suggestive of SIADH (D. Gomez, personal communication).

Other Pressor Systems

Adrenergic System

The adrenal medulla is part of the sympathetic nervous system consisting of chromaffin cells (pheochromocytes) that secrete catecholamines (epinephrine, norepinephrine, dopamine) in response to autonomic stimulation and circulating factors (e.g. glucose, cytokines). These are stress hormones central to the "fight or flight" response. Catecholamines are also produced in other tissues (e.g. central nervous system, enteric nervous system) and cause vasoconstriction, enhance cardiac and skeletal muscle contractility, increase heart and respiratory rates, increase blood pressure, relax smooth muscle in the GI, urinary, and respiratory tracts, enhance aerobic glycolysis and oxygen consumption, increase blood glucose, inhibit insulin secretion, induce lipolysis, enhance thermogenesis, and attenuate type I hypersensitivity reactions. The maturation of the equine adrenergic system occurs in late pregnancy and continues in the early postnatal period [1, 18, 19]. The HPAA influences the synthesis and secretion of catecholamines and vascular response to vasoactive factors. This is evident in premature foals that are often hypotensive and may have signs of tissue hypoperfusion [1, 7, 20].

Cardiovascular sympathetic sensitivity increases after birth in foals, which is essential to face challenges such as volume depletion and hypotension that are frequent during critical illness [1, 6, 7]. Information on catecholamine concentrations in hospitalized foals is lacking. Systemic inflammation in foals with severe disease cause adrenocortical hemorrhage and necrosis; however, it is unclear to what extent damage to the adrenal medulla impairs catecholamine production, therefore, blood pressure and other functions. Hypotension and hypoperfusion are frequent in ill foals and often require treatment with catecholamine analogs. The importance of the adrenergic system is evident in foals that are refractory to catecholamine therapy (e.g. norepinephrine), consistent with receptor downregulation [21, 22]. Glucocorticoid therapy may improve pressor response in many of these foals.

Natriuretic Peptides

Atrial (ANP) and brain natriuretic peptide (BNP) are secreted by the cardiac atria and ventricle, respectively, in response to wall stretching, increased intravascular volume, corticosteroids, hypoxia, and alpha-adrenergic agonists [23, 24]. They are part of the cardiovascular homeostatic system and have natriuretic, diuretic, and hypotensive properties. One study found no differences in ANP concentrations in hospitalized foals before or after fluid resuscitation, but concentrations were different in horses [2]. Plasma ANP concentrations were higher in septic compared to healthy newborn foals (R. Toribio, personal communication). BNP concentrations were not different in horses with various cardiac pathologies [25], but information in healthy or sick foals is lacking.

Endothelins

Endothelin-1 (ET-1) is a potent vasoconstrictor peptide important in regulating vascular tone [26] and is produced by endothelial cells in response to hypoxia, epinephrine, ANG-II, AVP, cytokines, and endotoxemia [26]. Secretion is reduced by NO, prostacyclin, and ANP. Increased in big ET-1 concentrations were found in sick foals [27].

Adrenomedullin

Adrenomedullin (ADM) is a strong vasodilator expressed by a multitude of tissues [28]. ADM increases in response to endotoxemia and septic shock [29]. Plasma ADM concentrations were higher in critically ill foals, but were not associated with disease severity or mortality [30].

References

1 Dembek, K.A., Onasch, K., Hurcombe, S.D.A. et al. (2013). Renin-angiotensin-aldosterone system and hypothalamic-pituitary-adrenal axis in hospitalized newborn foals. *J. Vet. Intern. Med.* 27: 331–338.

2 Hollis, A.R., Boston, R.C., and Corley, K.T. (2008). Plasma aldosterone, vasopressin and atrial natriuretic peptide in hypovolaemia: a preliminary comparative study of neonatal and mature horses. *Equine Vet. J.* 40: 64–69.

3 Newell-Price, J.D.C. and Auchus, R.J. (2020). The adrenal cortex. In: *Williams Textbook of Endocrinology*, 14e (ed. S. Melmed, R.J. Auchus, A.B. Goldfine, et al.), 480–541. Philadelphia: Elsevier.

4 Barrett, K.E., Barman, S.M., Boitano, S. et al. (2016). *Ganong's Review of Medical Physiology*. New York: McGraw Hill Education.

5 Hart, K.A. and Barton, M.H. (2011). Adrenocortical insufficiency in horses and foals. *Vet. Clin. North Am. Equine Pract.* 27: 19–34.

6 Hurcombe, S.D., Toribio, R.E., Slovis, N. et al. (2008). Blood arginine vasopressin, adrenocorticotropin hormone, and cortisol concentrations at admission in septic and critically ill foals and their association with survival. *J. Vet. Intern. Med.* 22: 639–647.

7 Dembek, K.A., Hurcombe, S.D., Stewart, A.J. et al. (2016). Association of aldosterone and arginine vasopressin concentrations and clinical markers of hypoperfusion in neonatal foals. *Equine Vet. J.* 48: 176–181.

8 Elder, E.M., Wong, D.M., Johnson, K., et al. (2022). Assessment of the hypothalamic-pituitary-adrenocortical axis function utilitizing a vasopressin stimulation test in healthy foals. *Proceedings of the 2022 ACVIM Forum*. Austin, TX: American College of Veterinary Internal Medicine.

9 Evans, M.J., Marshall, A.G., Kitson, N.E. et al. (1993). Factors affecting ACTH release from perifused equine anterior pituitary cells. *J. Endocrinol.* 137: 391–401.

10 Fowden, A.L., Forhead, A.J., and Ousey, J.C. (2012). Endocrine adaptations in the foal over the perinatal period. *Equine Vet. J.* 44: 130–139.

11 Giussani, D.A., Forhead, A.J., and Fowden, A.L. (2005). Development of cardiovascular function in the horse fetus. *J. Physiol.* 565: 1019–1030.

12 Wong, D.M., Vo, D.T., Alcott, C.J. et al. (2008). Plasma vasopressin concentrations in healthy foals from birth to 3 months of age. *J. Vet. Intern. Med.* 22: 1259–1261.

13 Borchers, A., Magdesian, K.G., Schenck, P.A. et al. (2014). Serial plasma vasopressin concentration in healthy and hospitalised neonatal foals. *Equine Vet. J.* 46: 306–310.

14 Johnson, K., Kopper, J., Hsu, W. et al. (2021). Cortisol and adrenocorticotropin (ACTH) response to corticotropin-releasing-hormone (CRH) stimulation tests in healthy and hospitalized foals. *Proceddings of the 2021 ACVIM Forum*. Virtual conference: American College of Veterinary Internal Medicine.

15 Hurcombe, S.D. (2011). Hypothalamic-pituitary gland axis function and dysfunction in horses. *Vet. Clin. North Am. Equine Pract.* 27: 1–17.

16 Schott, H.C. (2011). Water homeostasis and diabetes insipidus in horses. *Vet. Clin. North Am. Equine Pract.* 27: 175–195.

17 Schott, H.C., Bayly, W.M., Reed, S.M. et al. (1993). Nephrogenic diabetes insipidus in sibling colts. *J. Vet. Intern. Med.* 7: 68–72.

18 Ousey, J.C. (2004). Peripartal endocrinology in the mare and foetus. *Reprod. Domest. Anim.* 39: 222–231.

19 Forhead, A.J., Ousey, J.C., Allen, W.R. et al. (2004). Postnatal insulin secretion and sensitivity after manipulation of fetal growth by embryo transfer in the horse. *J. Endocrinol.* 181: 459–467.

20 O'Connor, S.J., Gardner, D.S., Ousey, J.C. et al. (2005). Development of baroreflex and endocrine responses to hypotensive stress in newborn foals and lambs. *Pflugers Arch.* 450: 298–306.

21 Dickey, E.J., McKenzie, H., Johnson, A. et al. (2010). Use of pressor therapy in 34 hypotensive critically ill neonatal foals. *Aust. Vet. J.* 88: 472–477.

22 Corley, K.T. (2002). Monitoring and treating haemodynamic disturbances in critically ill neonatal foals. Part 2: assessment and treatment. *Equine Vet. Educ.* 14: 328–334.

23 Potter, L.R., Yoder, A.R., Flora, D.R. et al. (2009). Natriuretic peptides: their structures, receptors, physiologic functions and therapeutic applications. *Handb. Exp. Pharmacol.* 341–366.

24 McGrath, M.F., de Bold, M.L., and de Bold, A.J. (2005). The endocrine function of the heart. *Trends Endocrinol. Metab.* 16: 469–477.

25 van Maanen, J.M., van Dijk, A., Mulder, K. et al. (1994). Consumption of drinking water with high nitrate levels causes hypertrophy of the thyroid. *Toxicol. Lett.* 72: 365–374.

26 Kowalczyk, A., Kleniewska, P., Kolodziejczyk, M. et al. (2015). The role of endothelin-1 and endothelin receptor antagonists in inflammatory response and sepsis. *Arch. Immunol. Ther. Exp.* 63: 41–52.

27 Giordano, A., Castagnetti, C., Panzani, S. et al. (2015). Endothelin 1 in healthy foals and in foals affected by neonatal diseases. *Theriogenology* 84: 667–673.

28 Beltowski, J. and Jamroz, A. (2004). Adrenomedullin–what do we know 10 years since its discovery? *Pol. J. Pharmacol.* 56: 5–27.

29 Geven, C., Kox, M., and Pickkers, P. (2018). Adrenomedullin and adrenomedullin-targeted therapy as treatment strategies relevant for sepsis. *Front. Immunol.* 9: 292.

30 Toth, B., Slovis, N.M., Constable, P.D. et al. (2014). Plasma adrenomedullin concentrations in critically ill neonatal foals. *J. Vet. Intern. Med.* 28: 1294–1300.

Section V Disorders of Calcium, Phosphorus, and Magnesium Homeostasis

Katarzyna A. Dembek, Laura D. Hostnik, Teresa A. Burns, and Ramiro E. Toribio

Disorders of Calcium, Phosphorus, and Magnesium Homeostasis

Calcium

Calcium (Ca) has structural (mechanical) and nonstructural (ionic) functions, and its extra- and intracellular concentrations are influenced by physiological and pathological conditions. Calcium is essential for numerous physiological processes including muscle contraction, neuromuscular excitability, blood coagulation, enzyme activation, hormone secretion, cell division, and cell membrane stability. In excitable tissue, including muscle fibers, neurons, and conduction systems, Ca modulates the action potential, blocks sodium entry, and is required for muscle contractility. Maintaining extracellular Ca concentrations within a narrow limit is essential for cell function. Calcium nutritional needs are higher in foals than horses [1].

Total calcium (TCa) in blood exists bound to proteins (albumin), in a free/ionized or active form (Ca^{2+}), and chelated to anions (lactate, phosphate, bicarbonate, sulfate, citrate). Extracellular Ca concentrations are regulated by parathyroid hormone (PTH), calcitonin (CT), and 1,25-dihydroxyvitamin D_3 (1,25$(OH)_2D_3$; calcitriol). Low Ca^{2+} stimulates PTH secretion, which promotes renal reabsorption of Ca^{2+}, synthesis of 1,25$(OH)_2D_3$, as well as bone resorption. Calcitriol inhibits parathyroid cell function and PTH secretion. Blood concentrations of TCa and Ca^{2+} are lower in foals than horses [2–5]. TCa is reported in most biochemistry profiles, but Ca^{2+} is less frequently measured. Acidosis reduces Ca binding to albumin thus increasing Ca^{2+} concentrations [6]. Foals with hypoproteinemia can have low TCa concentrations (pseudohypocalcemia), but Ca^{2+} concentrations can be normal [6, 7]. Conversion factors for Ca are: mmol/l = mg/dl × 0.25; mg/dl = mmol/l × 4.

Phosphorus

Similar to Ca, phosphorus has structural (mechanical) and nonstructural (ionic) functions. Phosphorus is essential for energy homeostasis, intermediary metabolism of carbohydrates, fats, and proteins, oxidative phosphorylation, enzyme activity, electrolyte transport, oxygen transport, cell membrane stability, neuromuscular excitability, muscle contraction, nucleic acid metabolism, gene transcription, and cell proliferation. Additionally, phosphorus is important to the movement of magnesium (Mg) and K^+ across the cell membrane. In other words, phosphorus, Mg, and K^+ are highly interactive ions. Phosphorus concentrations are higher in foals than horses [3–5, 8] and phosphorus nutritional needs are also higher in foals [1]. In blood, phosphorus exists in organic (70%) and inorganic (30%) forms [6]. Most phosphorus in the extracellular fluid is inorganic (PO_4; phosphate), which is the form measured by chemistry analyzers [6, 9, 10]. Conversion factors for PO_4 are: 1 mmol/l = 3.1 mg/dl; mg/dl × 0.32 = mmol/l; 1 mmol/l = 1.8 mEq/l.

Magnesium

Magnesium functions are mainly regulatory and concentrations in the extra- and intracellular compartments are influenced by physiological and pathological conditions. It has antioxidative properties. Mg participates in the following [11–13]:A

- Enzymatic activation, and energy generation and use
- Oxidative phosphorylation
- Intermediary metabolism of carbohydrates, fats, proteins, and nucleic acid
- Ion transport
- Cell membrane stability, cell proliferation, and immune cell function

Equine Neonatal Medicine, First Edition. Edited by David M. Wong and Pamela A. Wilkins.

- Neuromuscular excitability and muscle contraction
- Calcium homeostasis

Magnesium is required for the activity of the Na^+/K^+-ATPase, Na^+/Ca^{2+} exchanger (NCX), N-methyl-D-aspartate (NMDA) receptor (NMDAR), Ca^{2+} channels, and other proteins involved in neuronal and glial function. Mg has neuroprotective actions because it competes with Ca^{2+} and Na^+ at proteins that increase intracellular Ca^{2+} concentrations. This is the rationale for administering magnesium salts (e.g. $MgSO_4$) to foals with neonatal encephalopathy and brain trauma. Mg also contributes to the structural functions of Ca and PO_4; it facilitates mineral deposition and stabilizes hydroxyapatite and bone structure. Mg also reduces inflammation, leukocyte activation, free radical injury, and neurotoxicity [12, 13]. Hypomagnesemia and body Mg depletion can interfere with Ca homeostasis, energy regulation, cardiovascular function, and neuromuscular activity [7, 14]. In contrast to Ca, extracellular Mg is not under tight hormonal control and its concentrations depend on intestinal absorption, renal excretion, and bone exchange [14–16].

Like TCa, extracellular total magnesium (TMg) is bound to proteins (albumin), free/ionized/active (Mg^{2+}), and chelated to anions [14]. Mg concentration is higher in the intracellular compartment, where it binds to negatively charged molecules. Any reaction that requires energy also requires Mg^{2+} because inside the cell ATP is complexed with Mg^{2+} ($ATP{\cdot}Mg^{2+}$) [11, 17, 18]. Blood concentrations of TMg and Mg^{2+} are similar between foals and horses [2, 3, 5, 14, 19]. Plasma Mg^{2+} concentration provides a better assessment of the functional Mg status in the extracellular compartment. Intracellular Mg concentration is better to estimate the total body Mg content. Conversion factors for Mg are: mmol/l = mg/dl × 0.41; mg/dl = mmol/l × 2.43; mg/dl = mEq/l × 1.21; mmol/l = mEq/l × 0.5.

Calcium and Phosphorus-Regulating Hormones

Parathyroid Hormone (PTH)

PTH is released in response to hypocalcemia or hyperphosphatemia and targets renal tubules and osteoblasts. In the kidneys, PTH enhances Ca and Mg reabsorption, inhibits PO_4 reabsorption, and increases 1α-hydroxylase activity to promote $1{,}25(OH)_2D$ synthesis [6, 7]. In bone, PTH increases osteoclast-mediated bone resorption (via osteoblasts) and stimulates secretion of FGF-23 by osteocytes [20]. Serum PTH concentrations are similar between healthy newborn foals and horses [3, 4, 8, 21, 22]. Both low and high PTH concentrations have been measured in ill foals with high PTH concentrations associated with mortality [4, 8]. Increase in PTH concentrations is an expected response to hypocalcemia and hyperphosphatemia, which occurs in critically ill foals [3, 4, 8]. In addition, hypovitaminosis D, which is a frequent finding in sick foals, further enhances PTH secretion because physiologically, vitamin D inhibits parathyroid chief cell function and PTH synthesis. In normocalcemic foals with high PTH, in addition to hyperphosphatemia, hypovitaminosis D and systemic inflammation may be involved [8]. This is relevant in critically ill foals where high PTH concentrations have been associated with disease severity and mortality. *Equine familial isolated hypoparathyroidism* was the first identified equine mutation that interferes with parathyroid gland development and PTH synthesis; this condition has a grave prognosis but to date, has only been diagnosed in Thoroughbred foals [23].

Calcitonin (CT)

CT is synthesized by parafollicular cells (C-cells) of the thyroid gland [24]. High Ca and gastrin concentrations stimulate CT secretion while the opposite occurs with low concentrations [6, 25]. CT decreases plasma Ca and PO_4 concentrations by suppressing osteoclastic bone resorption and increasing urinary excretion of Ca and PO_4 [6]. High CT concentrations were proposed as a potential cause of hypocalcemia in foals, but this is unlikely because serum CT concentrations were lower in sick compared to healthy foals [3], which is the expected response from low Ca concentrations. Procalcitonin (PCT) is a product of the calcitonin gene (unrelated to Ca homeostasis) that under normal conditions is in very low blood concentrations but rapidly released in response to systemic inflammation by leukocytes, hepatocytes, and other cells [24]. The function of PCT is to modulate inflammation and is used in as a marker of disease severity in human medicine [26]. Plasma PCT concentrations were higher in septic compared to healthy foals and associated with disease severity [27].

Vitamin D

In horses, vitamin D is derived from plants (vitamin D_2; ergocalciferol) and cutaneous activation of 7-dehydrocholesterol into cholecalciferol (vitamin D_3) [6]. In the liver, vitamin D_3 is hydroxylated to 25-hydroxyvitamin D_3 [$25(OH)D_3$], which is transported to the kidney to be converted by 1α-hydroxylase to $1{,}25(OH)_2D_3$ (calcitriol), the active metabolite of vitamin D_3. Vitamin D_2 is a major source of vitamin D for horses [6, 28] and follows similar hepatic and renal processing steps as vitamin D_3 [6]. Blood concentrations of 1,25(OH)2D (both D_2 and D_3 metabolites) are regulated by PTH, Ca^{2+}, PO_4, 1,25(OH)2D, and FGF-23. Vitamin D promotes intestinal absorption and renal reabsorption of Ca and PO_4, modulates bone remodeling, and suppresses PTH synthesis. It also has nonclassical functions, including immune regulation, antimicrobial and anti-inflammatory properties, promotes epithelial and endothelial integrity, and facilitates energy metabolism. Vitamin D concentrations are lower in healthy foals compared to horses [4, 29].

Hypovitaminosis D is rarely diagnosed because vitamin D metabolites are not routinely measured in the clinical setting. Hypovitaminosis D is highly prevalent in critically ill foals and associated with mortality [4, 8]. In one study, 63% of hospitalized foals had low $25(OH)D_3$ concentrations [4]. Explanations for low vitamin D concentrations in sick foals include decreased milk intake, protein loss, reduced vitamin D binding proteins, hepatic injury, renal dysfunction, PTH resistance, increased activity of the FGF-23/klotho axis (see below), and excessive vitamin D inactivation [6, 8]. PTH resistance is a compelling explanation considering that despite having high PTH concentrations many sick foals have low $1,25(OH)_2D$ concentrations and hyperphosphatemia [3, 4, 8]. Dysregulation of the FGF-23/klotho axis also seems a likely contributor to hypovitaminosis D in sick foals [8]. Septic foals have high concentrations of FGF-23, which is a potent inhibitor of 1α-hydroxylase and vitamin D activation [8]. Information of inactivation of vitamin D metabolites in most domestic animals is lacking.

Due to its multiple actions, vitamin D deficiency can contribute to hypocalcemia, bone abnormalities, disruption of epithelial and endothelial integrity, increased risk of bacterial infections from reduced antibacterial peptides, impaired immune response, energy dysregulation, and a pro-inflammatory state. The potential value of vitamin D replacement therapy in hospitalized foals should be considered as there have been many clinical trials evaluating the benefits of vitamin D therapy in hospitalized adults and children, some with positive results [30–36].

Calcium Disorders

Disorders of calcium homeostasis include hypo- and hypercalcemia, of which hypocalcemia is more frequent in foals whereas hypercalcemia is generally associated with a worse prognosis.

Hypocalcemia

Hypocalcemia is frequent in ill equine patients [5, 8, 37] affecting up to 50% of foals with sepsis [8]. Mechanisms that contribute to hypocalcemia during systemic inflammation include calciuresis, intracellular Ca accumulation, impaired Ca mobilization, Ca chelation (e.g. hyperphosphatemia), parathyroid gland dysfunction, reduced tissue response to PTH, hypovitaminosis D, and Mg depletion [6]. In addition to critical illness, newborn foals may present with signs of hypocalcemia from a condition known as idiopathic hypocalcemia [23]. Renal loss of Ca seems unlikely based on studies in horses with enterocolitis and endotoxemia, which have low urinary fractional excretion of Ca [5, 21]. PTH concentrations in critically ill foals are variable with most foals with hypocalcemia having an appropriate PTH response [3, 4, 8]. However, some hypocalcemic foals have low to normal PTH concentrations (inappropriate PTH secretion), hyperphosphatemia and hypomagnesemia, suggesting a form of secondary hypoparathyroidism [3, 4, 8]. There are also normocalcemic foals with exaggerated PTH secretion, which could reflect a response to systemic inflammation, hyperphosphatemia, or low vitamin D [4, 8]. Hypovitaminosis D is highly prevalent in critically ill foals [4]. Based on the prevalence of hyperphosphatemia in critically ill foals, it is possible that many develop PO_4-induced hypocalcemia (chelation).

Clinical Signs

Signs of hypocalcemia include hyperexcitability, seizures, convulsions, tremors, fasciculations, stiff gait, tetany, dysrhythmias, synchronous diaphragmatic flutter, ileus, and recumbency. These signs can be exacerbated with hypomagnesemia.

Equine familial isolated hypoparathyroidism (idiopathic hypocalcemia) is a condition in foals born hypocalcemic or develop hypocalcemia in the immediate postpartum period, are refractory to medical treatment, can be hypomagnesemic, and inevitably die [6, 23]. A non-sense mutation of the *RAPGEF5* gene was identified in Thoroughbred foals with refractory hypocalcemia [23]. This mutation appears to interfere with parathyroid gland development and affected foals have persistent hypocalcemia, hypomagnesemia, hyperphosphatemia, and low to inappropriately normal PTH concentrations. In other words, this is a form of primary hypoparathyroidism. Clinical signs include hyperexcitability, seizures, tremors, stiff gait, tetanic contractions, synchronous diaphragmatic flutter, and recumbency [23]. Genetic testing is available at the UC Davis Veterinary Genetic Laboratory.

Hypercalcemia

Approximately 20% of hospitalized foals have hypercalcemia [8]. Idiopathic hypercalcemia has been reported in a subset of sick foals [6]. Some affected foals have a history of placental disease, dystocia, or perinatal asphyxia but the cause of this condition is unknown. Proposed mechanisms in sick foals include increased PTH and PTHrP, reduced CT concentrations, and hypervitaminosis D [6] – in particular in foals with normal renal function. In foals with low or normal PTH concentrations, high PTHrP levels is a possibility [3], considering its importance in the developing fetus and transplacental Ca transport. Hurcombe et al. did not find differences in PTHrP concentrations between healthy and hospitalized foals [3]. Decreased CT concentrations were documented in sick foals, but many of these foals had hypocalcemia [3]. High vitamin D concentrations as a cause of hypercalcemia in sick foals is unlikely since approximately 5% of hospitalized foals have vitamin D concentrations above normal [4]. Increased PTH concentrations in response to hyperphosphatemia or systemic inflammation can contribute to hypercalcemia, although most foals with these abnormalities are hypocalcemic [3, 4, 8]. Prolonged hypercalcemia can lead to hypomagnesemia due to increased renal excretion of Mg [16].

Diagnosis

Most foals with low tCa and Ca^{2+} concentrations do not show overt signs of hypocalcemia; however, signs can be evident with severe hypocalcemia. Low Mg concentrations can exacerbate signs of hypocalcemia, so measurement of Mg concentrations in hypocalcemic foals is recommended. Ideally, Mg^{2+} concentrations should be measured, but TMg also provides valuable information. Foals can remain hypocalcemic if the underlying disease process persists, but they usually respond to medical treatment. See below for additional diagnostic information.

Phosphorus Disorders

Disorders of phosphorus are poorly documented in sick foals but hypo- and hyperphosphatemia can occur depending on the condition and metabolic status [3, 4, 8]. The definition of these abnormalities is based on healthy foal reference values [6]. Studies in critically ill foals note that hyperphosphatemia is more frequent than hypophosphatemia [4, 8].

Hypophosphatemia

Hypophosphatemia develops from reduced intestinal absorption of PO_4, increased urinary excretion of PO_4, and shift of PO_4 to the intracellular compartment (redistribution). The opposite occurs with hyperphosphatemia. Hypophosphatemia occurs in foals with hyperglycemia, hyperlipemia, in those receiving enteral and parenteral nutrition or insulin administration, and less commonly, from sepsis. In foals receiving enteral or parenteral nutrition, increased intracellular demands for carbohydrate phosphorylation and ion shifts, in part driven by increased insulin concentrations, reduces extracellular PO_4 concentrations. This phenomenon is similar to refeeding syndrome. Increased PTH concentrations can also be a potential cause of hypophosphatemia by promoting PO_4 renal excretion; however, this would be unusual because PO_4 concentrations in most of these foals are normal or elevated [4, 8], suggesting they have PTH resistance. Hypophosphatemia may develop from respiratory or metabolic alkalosis, although this situation occurs infrequently in foals. Alkalosis stimulates glycolysis due to increased phosphofructokinase activity, glucose phosphorylation, and intracellular PO_4 demands. Parenteral nutrition, hyperglycemia, and insulin administration can also lead to hypomagnesemia and hypokalemia by shifting these ions to the intracellular compartment. In addition, hypophosphatemia could contribute to hypomagnesemia and hypokalemia due to their transcellular interdependency. In foals under nutritional management, it is important to assess PO_4, Mg, and K^+ concentrations. FGF-23 and PTH are phosphaturic hormones that reduce renal reabsorption of PO_4, and may contribute to the development of hypophosphatemia since both hormones are often increased in critically ill foals [3, 4, 8, 38]. Hypovitaminosis D, which is highly prevalent in hospitalized foals and linked to mortality [4, 8], is an unlikely cause of hypophosphatemia because most sick foals with low vitamin D concentrations are hyperphosphatemic [4, 8].

Hyperphosphatemia

Hyperphosphatemia is common in hospitalized foals but mechanisms for development are unclear. Potential causes include metabolic acidosis (e.g. lactic acidosis) that shifts PO_4 to the extracellular compartment, cell lysis, hypoinsulinemia – which shift PO_4 to the extracellular compartment – as well as acute renal injury and renal refractoriness to PTH and FGF-23 that impair renal PO_4 excretion. Cell lysis can occur in foals with severe sepsis, hypoperfusion, or hemolysis. Phosphate containing enemas can also cause hyperphosphatemia in foals, although infrequent. Hypervitaminosis D is an unlikely cause of hyperphosphatemia because most critically ill foals have low concentrations of vitamin D metabolites [4, 8].

Clinical Signs

Signs of hypophosphatemia in foals are not specific and are difficult to determine in recumbent or weak animals. Signs relate to PO_4 regulatory functions on ion transport, cell membrane stability, and energy metabolism [7]. They include muscle weakness, fasciculations, tremors, neuromuscular excitability, dysrhythmias, and ileus, as well as cell membrane fragility and lysis from impaired glucose use, reduced ATP synthesis, and altered cell membrane action potential [6, 39, 40]. Hypophosphatemia may impair leukocyte function and predispose to infections [40]. Signs of hyperphosphatemia are mainly linked to hypocalcemia due to Ca chelation and include hyperexcitability, tetany, muscle fasciculations, ileus, and dysrhythmias. In addition to PO_4, it is important to measure Mg and K^+ concentrations as these ions are highly interactive.

Diagnosis

The diagnosis of hypo- and hyperphosphatemia is based on foal-specific reference values since clinical signs are vague. Blood concentrations of PO_4 are higher in foals (4.4–8.4 mg/dl; 1.4–2.7 mmol/l) than horses (2–5.6 mg/dl; 0.65–1.8 mmol/l) [3–5, 8, 29]. High PO_4 concentrations in foals parallel increased alkaline phosphatase activity [6, 38]. Hypophosphatemia is often missed because PO_4 values could be in the normal range of horses. In addition to PO_4, it is important to assess Mg and K^+ concentrations because these ions are highly interactive. Laboratory abnormalities (e.g. hypomagnesemia) should also be considered as well as concurrent treatments, especially those related to energy supplementation. Hyperphosphatemia can be overlooked under the premise that PO_4 concentrations are higher in foals. In foals with hyperphosphatemia, it is important to assess the acid-base status (acidosis), Ca concentrations, and other electrolytes. Sepsis-mediated hypoparathyroidism could contribute to hyperphosphatemia.

Treatment

Most phosphorus disorders are addressed by treating the underlying condition. Parenteral supplementation with PO_4 salts is indicated in foals with severe hypophosphatemia, ideally via phosphate salts administered as a CRI (see below) [39]. Potassium or sodium phosphate are available, but if unavailable, enemas that contain monobasic and dibasic sodium phosphate can be given via nasogastric intubation or rectally. Treatment of hyperphosphatemia is not specific and includes addressing the underlying process, correcting acid-base status, and Ca supplementation.

Magnesium Disorders

Magnesium disorders in foals include hypo- and hypermagnesemia. Hypomagnesemia is frequent in hospitalized foals [3, 14], but often missed because TMg and Mg^{2+} values are not included in most biochemistry profiles [3, 14].

Hypomagnesemia

Causes of hypomagnesemia include sepsis, GI disease, acute renal injury, tissue sequestration, shift to the intracellular compartment, and endocrine abnormalities [14]. Hypomagnesemia could be a consequence of other abnormalities such as hypophosphatemia, hypercalcemia, hyperglycemia, hyperinsulinemia, hypervasopressinemia, intestinal disease, renal injury, and prolonged fluid therapy [6, 14, 16, 41]. Alkalosis also can decrease Mg^{2+} concentrations [14]. Mg modulates inflammation, leukocyte activation, and protects against free radical injury and neurotoxicity [12, 13]. Mg deficiency is permissive to increases in intracellular Ca^{2+} concentrations, which primes cells to a pro-inflammatory response, releasing IL-1β, IL-6, TNF-α, and acute phase proteins as well as excessive free radical production and oxidative injury that results in systemic inflammation [12, 13, 42, 43]. In addition, intracellular Ca^{2+} activates proteases and cytotoxic cascades that may lead to apoptosis or necrosis [6]. Mg is neuroprotective by blocking Ca^{2+} entry through the NMDAR, thus depressing excitotoxicity. Information on the role of Mg in equine inflammatory conditions is scarce [5, 44–46].

Hypomagnesemia could contribute to the pro-inflammatory state observed in critically ill foals considering that cytokines are often increased in equine patients with evidence of systemic inflammation and endotoxemia [5, 21, 47, 48]. Hypomagnesemia and total body Mg depletion could interfere with Ca homeostasis, energy regulation, cardiovascular function, and neuromuscular activity [7, 14]. This deserves study, as some abnormalities in sick foals could be exacerbated by low Mg concentrations.

The potential cause-effect relationships between hypomagnesemia with electrolyte and endocrine abnormalities in foals remain to be elucidated. Hypomagnesemia is often associated with hypokalemia and hypophosphatemia, especially in foals receiving enteral or parenteral nutrition. Any reaction that requires energy, meaning PO_4, also requires Mg^{2+}. Hyperinsulinemia shifts Mg^{2+} to the intracellular compartment, but also increases the activity of the Na^+/K^+-ATPase, which requires PO_4 and Mg^{2+} to move K^+ intracellularly. In addition, it is well documented that Ca regulation depends on Mg for PTH secretion and receptor activation. Total body Mg depletion can result in a form of hypoparathyroidism that does not improve until Mg status is corrected [14]. Therefore, Mg concentrations should be measured in sick foals as it may influence therapy and outcome [14].

Clinical Signs

Signs of hypomagnesemia and Mg depletion include muscle weakness, tremors, seizures, spasticity, cardiac dysrhythmias, synchronous diaphragmatic flutter, and ileus. Hypokalemia, hypocalcemia, and hypophosphatemia can also be present, with some signs occurring as a combination of these electrolyte abnormalities. On electrocardiography, the P-R interval could be prolonged, with a wide QRS complex and tall T waves. Tetany has been reported in horses and ponies [49, 50], and in foals fed Mg-deficient diets [44]. Affected foals exhibited hyperexcitability, muscular tremors, ataxia, profuse sweating, hyperpnea, collapse, and convulsions [44]. On necropsy, these foals had severe mineralization of the aorta and pulmonary artery [44, 45].

Hypermagnesemia

Hypermagnesemia is rare in foals and might occur from cell lysis (e.g. rhabdomyolysis, hemolysis), but is often iatrogenic. High Mg concentrations may be seen in horses with chronic renal failure, which is unlikely in newborn foals. Clinical signs of hypermagnesemia are not specific and, at least in horses, may reduce neuromuscular activity, have calming effects, reduce physical activity, and decrease blood pressure through its Ca^{2+} and Na^{+} channel and receptor-blocking properties [51–53].

Diagnosis

The diagnosis of hypo- and hypermagnesemia is based on blood TMg and Mg^{2+} concentrations. Hypomagnesemia is frequent in septic foals, but often missed because Mg is not included in all chemistry profiles [3, 14]. Due to the implications of hypomagnesemia, measurement of Mg concentrations is recommended in hospitalized foals – in particular, those with hypocalcemia, receiving enteral or parenteral nutrition, with hypophosphatemia and hypokalemia, or having signs of neuromuscular excitability. Hypermagnesemia is seldom diagnosed in foals.

Treatment

Intravenous (IV) administration of $MgSO_4$ is indicated in foals with hypomagnesemia, hypocalcemia, extended fasting, prolonged fluid therapy, and electrolyte abnormalities associated with enteral or parenteral nutrition and hyperglycemia (hypokalemia, hypophosphatemia, hypomagnesemia). Administration is also considered in foals with neurological disorders (NE, seizures, cerebral and spinal trauma) [14, 54]. Evidence that Mg therapy is beneficial for acute neurological disorders in foals is lacking; however, physiological and pathophysiological information from other species justify its use.

References

1 (U.S.) NRC, Horses CoNRo (2007). *Nutrient Requirements of Horses*, 6th revised ed. Washington, D.C: National Academies Press.
2 Berlin, D. and Aroch, I. (2009). Concentrations of ionized and total magnesium and calcium in healthy horses: effects of age, pregnancy, lactation, pH and sample type. *Vet. J.* 181: 305–311.
3 Hurcombe, S.D., Toribio, R.E., Slovis, N.M. et al. (2009). Calcium regulating hormones and serum calcium and magnesium concentrations in septic and critically ill foals and their association with survival. *J. Vet. Intern. Med.* 23: 335–343.
4 Kamr, A.M., Dembek, K.A., Reed, S.M. et al. (2015). Vitamin D metabolites and their association with calcium, phosphorus, and PTH concentrations, severity of illness, and mortality in hospitalized equine neonates. *PLoS One* 10: e0127684.
5 Toribio, R.E., Kohn, C.W., Chew, D.J. et al. (2001). Comparison of serum parathyroid hormone and ionized calcium and magnesium concentrations and fractional urinary clearance of calcium and phosphorus in healthy horses and horses with enterocolitis. *Am. J. Vet. Res.* 62: 938–947.
6 Toribio, R.E. (2018). Disorders of calcium and phosphorus. In: *Equine Internal Medicine*, 4e (ed. S.M. Reed, W.M. Bayly, and D.C. Sellon), 1029–1052. St. Louis, Missouri: Elsevier.
7 Toribio, R.E. (2011). Disorders of calcium and phosphate metabolism in horses. *Vet. Clin. North Am. Equine Pract.* 27: 129–147.
8 Kamr, A.M., Dembek, K.A., Hildreth, B.E. et al. (2018). The FGF-23/klotho axis and its relationship with phosphorus, calcium, vitamin D, PTH, aldosterone, severity of disease, and outcome in hospitalised foals. *Equine Vet. J.* 50: 739–746.
9 Caverzasio, J. and Bonjour, J.P. (1992). IGF-1 and phosphate homeostasis during growth. *Nephrologie* 13: 109–113.
10 Haramati, A., Mulroney, S.E., and Lumpkin, M.D. (1990). Regulation of renal phosphate reabsorption during development: implications from a new model of growth hormone deficiency. *Pediatr. Nephrol.* 4: 387–391.
11 de Baaij, J.H., Hoenderop, J.G., and Bindels, R.J. (2015). Magnesium in man: implications for health and disease. *Physiol. Rev.* 95: 1–46.
12 Weglicki, W.B., Phillips, T.M., Freedman, A.M. et al. (1992). Magnesium-deficiency elevates circulating levels of inflammatory cytokines and endothelin. *Mol. Cell. Biochem.* 110: 169–173.
13 Kramer, J.H., Misik, V., and Weglicki, W.B. (1994). Magnesium-deficiency potentiates free radical production associated with postischemic injury to rat hearts: vitamin E affords protection. *Free Radic. Biol. Med.* 16: 713–723.

14 Toribio, R.E. (2018). Magnesium and disease. In: *Equine Internal Medicine*, 4e (ed. S.M. Reed, W.M. Bayly, and D.C. Sellon), 1052–1058. St. Louis, Missouri: Elsevier.
15 Paolisso, G. and Barbagallo, M. (1997). Hypertension, diabetes mellitus, and insulin resistance: the role of intracellular magnesium. *Am. J. Hypertens.* 10: 346–355.
16 Toribio, R.E., Kohn, C.W., Rourke, K.M. et al. (2007). Effects of hypercalcemia on serum concentrations of magnesium, potassium, and phosphate and urinary excretion of electrolytes in horses. *Am. J. Vet. Res.* 68: 543–554.
17 Jahnen-Dechent, W. and Ketteler, M. (2012). Magnesium basics. *Clin. Kidney J.* 5: i3–i14.
18 Wolf, F.I., Torsello, A., Fasanella, S. et al. (2003). Cell physiology of magnesium. *Mol. Asp. Med.* 24: 11–26.
19 Mariella, J., Isani, G., Andreani, G. et al. (2016). Total plasma magnesium in healthy and critically ill foals. *Theriogenology* 85: 180–185.
20 Lanske, B. and Razzaque, M.S. (2014). Molecular interactions of FGF23 and PTH in phosphate regulation. *Kidney Int.* 86: 1072–1074.
21 Toribio, R.E., Kohn, C.W., Hardy, J. et al. (2005). Alterations in serum PTH and electrolyte concentrations and urinary excretion of electrolytes in horses with induced endotoxemia. *J. Vet. Intern. Med.* 19: 223–231.
22 Toribio, R.E., Kohn, C.W., Sams, R.A. et al. (2003). Hysteresis and calcium set-point for the calcium parathyroid hormone relationship in healthy horses. *Gen. Comp. Endocrinol.* 130: 279–288.
23 Rivas, V.N., Magdesian, K.G., Fagan, S. et al. (2020). A nonsense variant in Rap Guanine Nucleotide Exchange Factor 5 (RAPGEF5) is associated with equine familial isolated hypoparathyroidism in Thoroughbred foals. *PLos Genet.* 16: e1009028.
24 Toribio, R.E., Kohn, C.W., Leone, G.W. et al. (2003). Molecular cloning and expression of equine calcitonin, calcitonin gene-related peptide-I, and calcitonin gene-related peptide-II. *Mol. Cell. Endocrinol.* 199: 119–128.
25 Rourke, K.M., Kohn, C.W., Levine, A.L. et al. (2009). Rapid calcitonin response to experimental hypercalcemia in healthy horses. *Domest. Anim. Endocrinol.* 36: 197–201.
26 Assicot, M., Gendrel, D., Carsin, H. et al. (1993). High serum procalcitonin concentrations in patients with sepsis and infection. *Lancet* 341: 515–518.
27 Bonelli, F., Meucci, V., Divers, T. et al. (2015). Evaluation of plasma procalcitonin concentrations in healthy foals and foals affected by septic systemic inflammatory response syndrome. *J. Equine Vet. Sci.* 35: 645–649.
28 Azarpeykan, S., Dittmer, K.E., Gee, E.K. et al. (2016). Influence of blanketing and season on vitamin D and parathyroid hormone, calcium, phosphorus, and magnesium concentrations in horses in New Zealand. *Domest. Anim. Endocrinol.* 56: 75–84.
29 Pozza, M.E., Kaewsakhorn, T., Trinarong, C. et al. (2014). Serum vitamin D, calcium, and phosphorus concentrations in ponies, horses and foals from the United States and Thailand. *Vet. J.* 199: 451–456.
30 Amrein, K., Schnedl, C., Holl, A. et al. (2014). Effect of high-dose vitamin D3 on hospital length of stay in critically ill patients with vitamin D deficiency: the VITdAL-ICU randomized clinical trial. *JAMA* 312: 1520–1530.
31 McNally, D., Amrein, K., O'Hearn, K. et al. (2017). Study protocol for a phase II dose evaluation randomized controlled trial of cholecalciferol in critically ill children with vitamin D deficiency (VITdAL-PICU study). *Pilot Feasibility Stud.* 3: 70.
32 Martin, A., David, V., and Quarles, L.D. (2012). Regulation and function of the FGF23/klotho endocrine pathways. *Physiol. Rev.* 92: 131–155.
33 Kuro-o, M. (2010). Overview of the FGF23-Klotho axis. *Pediatr. Nephrol.* 25: 583–590.
34 Wysolmerski, J.J. (2012). Parathyroid hormone-related protein: an update. *J. Clin. Endocrinol. Metab.* 97: 2947–2956.
35 Wysolmerski, J.J. and Stewart, A.F. (1998). The physiology of parathyroid hormone-related protein: an emerging role as a developmental factor. *Annu. Rev. Physiol.* 60: 431–460.
36 Martin, T.J., Sims, N.A., and Seeman, E. (2021). Physiological and pharmacological roles of PTH and PTHrP in bone using their shared receptor, PTH1R. *Endocr. Rev.* https://doi.org/10.1210/endrev/bnab005.
37 Hurcombe, S.D., Toribio, R.E., Slovis, N. et al. (2008). Blood arginine vasopressin, adrenocorticotropin hormone, and cortisol concentrations at admission in septic and critically ill foals and their association with survival. *J. Vet. Intern. Med.* 22: 639–647.
38 Kamr, A.M., Dembek, K.A., Gilsenan, W. et al. (2020). C-terminal telopeptide of type I collagen, osteocalcin, alkaline phosphatase, and parathyroid hormone in healthy and hospitalized foals. *Domest. Anim. Endocrinol.* 72: 106470.
39 DiBartola, S.P. and Willard, M.D. (2005). Disorders of phosphorus: hypophosphatemia and hyperphosphatemia. In: *Fluid, Electrolyte and Acid-Base Disorders in Small Animal Practice*, 3e, 195–209. Philadelphia, PA: Elsevier Saunders.
40 Amanzadeh, J. and Reilly, R.F. Jr. (2006). Hypophosphatemia: an evidence-based approach to its clinical consequences and management. *Nat. Clin. Pract. Nephrol.* 2: 136–148.
41 Dai, L.J., Ritchie, G., Kerstan, D. et al. (2001). Magnesium transport in the renal distal convoluted tubule. *Physiol. Rev.* 81: 51–84.

42 Nielsen, F.H. (2018). Magnesium deficiency and increased inflammation: current perspectives. *J. Inflamm. Res.* 11: 25–34.

43 Weglicki, W.B. (2012). Hypomagnesemia and inflammation: clinical and basic aspects. *Annu. Rev. Nutr.* 32: 55–71.

44 Harrington, D.D. (1974). Pathological features of magnesium deficiency in young horses fed purified rations. *Am. J. Vet. Res.* 35: 503–513.

45 Harrington, D.D. (1975). Influence of magnesium deficiency on horse foal tissue concentration of Mg, calcium and phosphorus. *Br. J. Nutr.* 34: 45–57.

46 Stewart, A.J., Hardy, J., Kohn, C.W. et al. (2004). Validation of diagnostic tests for determination of magnesium status in horses with reduced magnesium intake. *Am. J. Vet. Res.* 65: 422–430.

47 Bueno, A.C., Seahorn, T.L., Cornick-Seahorn, J. et al. (1999). Plasma and urine nitric oxide concentrations in horses given below a low dose of endotoxin. *Am. J. Vet. Res.* 60: 969–976.

48 Seethanathan, P., Bottoms, G.D., and Schafer, K. (1990). Characterization of release of tumor necrosis factor, interleukin-1, and superoxide anion from equine white blood cells in response to endotoxin. *Am. J. Vet. Res.* 51: 1221–1225.

49 Meyer, H. and Ahlswede, L. (1977). Magnesium metabolism in the horse. *Zentralbl. Veterinarmed. A* 24: 128–139.

50 Green, H.H., Allcroft, W.M., and Montgomerie, R.F. (1935). Hypomagnesemia in equine transit tetany. *J. Comp. Pathol. Ther.* 48: 74–79.

51 Schumacher, S.A., Toribio, R.E., Lakritz, J. et al. (2019). Radio-telemetric assessment of cardiac variables and locomotion with experimentally induced hypermagnesemia in horses using chronically implanted catheters. *Front Vet. Sci.* 6: 414.

52 Schumacher, S.A., Toribio, R.E., Scansen, B. et al. (2020). Pharmacokinetics of magnesium and its effects on clinical variables following experimentally induced hypermagnesemia. *J. Vet. Pharmacol. Ther.* 43: 577–590.

53 Houston, M. (2011). The role of magnesium in hypertension and cardiovascular disease. *J. Clin. Hypertens. (Greenwich)* 13: 843–847.

54 Toribio, R.E. (2019). Equine neonatal encephalopathy: facts, evidence, and opinions. *Vet. Clin. North Am. Equine Pract.* 35: 363–378.

Section VI Diagnosis and Treatment of Endocrine Disorders

Laura D. Hostnik, Teresa A. Burns, Katarzyna A. Dembek, and Ramiro E. Toribio

Endocrine disorders in the perinatal period can compromise the survival of the equine neonate. Clinical and laboratory findings can be suggestive of endocrine dysregulation that can be associated with disease severity and outcome. The diagnosis and treatment of certain endocrinopathies can be difficult due to lack of validated endocrine tests, turnaround time, result interpretation, implementation of therapies aligned with results, and clinical findings, and cost. Certain disorders can be suspected based on historical information and clinical findings (e.g. multiple foals with evidence of dysmaturity). Others can be readily assessed via serum biochemistry profile (e.g. hypocalcemia, hypoglycemia) and treated promptly, although information regarding underlying cause may not be available. In other instances, there is evidence of an endocrinopathy associated with critical illness (e.g. hypoglycemia, refractory hyperglycemia, hyponatremia), and treatment is empirical. The diagnosis and treatment of disorders of endocrine systems that require dynamic testing for confirmation (e.g. adrenal gland, thyroid gland) can be challenging, but accomplished. Certain endocrine systems are central to fetal development and the neonatal transition; information on foals is scarce, and many parameters cannot be easily assessed in practice, although imbalances in these endocrine axes may explain abnormalities observed. Although briefly discussed above, the goal of this section is to provide a more detailed overview of the diagnosis and treatment of equine neonatal endocrinopathies.

Diagnosis and Treatment of Hypothalamic-Pituitary-Adrenal Axis Disorders

Diagnosis of RAI/CIRCI

The clinical relevance of RAI or CIRCI as well as the criteria to diagnose CIRCI are controversial issues in human and veterinary medicine due to conflicting data from clinical studies [1–3]. Methods to diagnose RAI/CIRCI include baseline serum cortisol concentrations, cortisol-to-ACTH ratios, cortisol response to stimulation with synthetic ACTH (cosyntropin), CRH and AVP, insulin-induced hypoglycemia, and the metyrapone test [3–5]. Baseline cortisol concentrations, the cosyntropin test, and ACTH/cortisol ratio have been studied in healthy and septic foals [1, 2, 6–10]. Baseline cortisol concentrations provide a rapid method to assess adrenocortical function in neonatal foals. Cortisol concentrations change over time in healthy neonatal foals; therefore, age-related variations need to be considered when assessing HPAA function [9, 11]. Hart et al. reported basal cortisol concentrations in healthy foals at birth, 24 hours, 48 hours, and 5–7 days old [9, 11]. Interpretation of a single random cortisol concentration can be difficult because multiple factors (e.g., feeding, drugs, disease severity, environmental conditions) can influence cortisol concentrations in healthy animals and people. Therefore, measurement of cortisol and other steroid concentrations in conjunction with ACTH provides a better assessment of HPAA integrity. Evaluation of other adrenocortical steroids that are not controlled by a precise HPAA feedback mechanism may give a better evaluation of adrenocortical secretory capacity during critical illness [2, 12, 13].

One study in hospitalized foals showed an association of low dehydroepiandrosterone sulfate (DHEAS) concentration with RAI and suggested that DHEAS could be a good indicator of adrenal dysfunction in equine perinatal disorders [12]. High ACTH/cortisol and ACTH/aldosterone ratios in critically ill foals may suggest CIRCI; however, specific cut-off values are not well defined because of the wide ranges of these ratios [1, 6–8]. In addition, high ACTH/progesterone and ACTH/DHEAS ratios were associated with nonsurvival and disease severity in hospitalized foals, supporting the clinical value of assessing adrenal dysfunction or CIRCI [12].

Equine Neonatal Medicine, First Edition. Edited by David M. Wong and Pamela A. Wilkins.

Diagnosis of CIRCI in critically ill people and foals is improved by utilizing dynamic tests such as the ACTH stimulation test. In general, ACTH doses used to assess adrenocortical function in foals are divided into high 100 μg (1–2 μg/kg or higher) and low 10 μg (0.01–0.2 μg/kg) dose protocols [1, 2, 8, 14]. After blood collection for baseline cortisol concentrations, ACTH is administered IV or IM, and additional blood samples are collected 30 and 90 minutes post-stimulation [1, 2, 8, 14]. High-dose ACTH produces maximal cortisol release; therefore, it is considered supraphysiologic and may be less sensitive in the diagnosis of CIRCI. On note, the high-dose ACTH stimulation test (250 μg/kg) remains the most commonly used diagnostic test for RAI in critically ill people but the sensitivity is low [3, 15]. Delta cortisol (difference in cortisol concentration between 30 minute and baseline sample) is highly variable in healthy and critically ill foals, and diagnostic cutoff points have not been established; however, an increase from baseline cortisol concentrations less than one- to twofold at 30 minutes after low-dose ACTH stimulation and less than three- to fourfold 90–120 minutes after high-dose ACTH stimulation may be indicative of CIRCI in foals (Table 21.VI.1) [1, 2, 8, 9, 14]. A combined low- and high-dose ACTH stimulation test seems to provide a better assessment of HPAA function but is not practical for clinical use [9].

Of note, disease severity affects free and total cortisol concentrations as well as cosyntropin-stimulated total and free cortisol concentrations in critically ill foals [17]. Interestingly, basal and cosyntropin-stimulated free cortisol concentrations were no better than total cortisol concentrations at predicting disease severity and mortality [17]. This suggests that basal or cosyntropin-stimulated free cortisol offers no advantage compared to basal or cosyntropin-stimulated total cortisol to diagnose RAI. The AVP and CRH stimulation tests will likely help in the diagnosis of RAI in sick foals [18, 19].

The response of multiple adrenocortical steroids and steroid precursors to the ACTH stimulation test has been described in critically ill foals [2]. Impaired response of 17α-OH-progesterone and cortisol to 10 μg of ACTH was associated with non-survival. The authors proposed that the 17α-OH-progesterone response to ACTH might have prognostic value for disease severity and death in equine perinatal diseases [2]. Insulin-induced hypoglycemia, the metyrapone (11β-hydroxylase inhibitor) test, and CRH and AVP stimulation tests assess integrity of the entire HPAA. There are no data on ACTH and cortisol responses to metyrapone administration in healthy or sick foals. Therefore, this test is not recommended for the diagnosis of CIRCI in equine neonates [4, 5]. The CRH and AVP stimulation tests have also been evaluated in healthy and hospitalized neonatal foals [18, 19]. Administration of ovine CRH (1 μg/kg, IV) elicited rapid ACTH and cortisol responses in healthy foals [19]. AVP (2.5–7.5 IU/foal, IV) resulted in a strong ACTH and cortisol response that was higher than the CRH stimulation test [18, 19]. These results support the value of the AVP and CRH stimulation tests for assessment of HPAA function in foals. Cortisol and ACTH cut-off values for this test remain to be determined.

In conclusion, baseline cortisol concentration can be used as the primary method for assessment of adrenocortical function in sick foals. If cortisol concentrations are <13.5 μg/dl at birth, <6.7 μg/dl at 12–24 hours, <4.4 μg/dl at 36–48 hours, and < 2.7 μg/dl 5–7 days of age, CIRCI can be suspected [11]. In patients with borderline cortisol concentrations, performing an ACTH stimulation test may be reasonable [1, 4]

Treatment of RAI

Therapy of RAI is centered at addressing the primary problem(s), but steroid replacement therapy should be considered (Figure 21.VI.1). Hydrocortisone (commercial cortisol) is preferred because it is short acting, endogenously produced, and has been evaluated in foals [20]. Dexamethasone is the next choice and is readily available. A low-dose course of hydrocortisone (<400 mg/d for >3 days at full dose IV) is recommended in people with vasopressor-unresponsive septic shock [15, 21, 22]. Bolus administration of hydrocortisone has been associated with hyperglycemia and hypernatremia in ICU patients; therefore, CRI rather than bolus injection is preferred [3, 15]. Boonen et al. suggested treatment of critically ill human patients for adrenal failure if they have unexplained vasoplegia, overwhelming inflammation, or coma for more than 6 days with basal plasma cortisol of <6 μg/dl and an incremental cortisol response to an ACTH stimulation test (250 μg) of <6 μg/dl [23, 24]. Similar criteria have not been developed for critically ill foals. Recommendations for hydrocortisone use in septic foals are based on daily endogenous production in healthy foals [11]. There is no ideal diagnostic test for CIRCI in foals, therefore, a short course of tapering replacement therapy with hydrocortisone (1–3 mg/kg/d, IV, divided every 4 hours) is recommended in foals with signs of CIRCI, such as vasopressor-unresponsive hypotension, hypoglycemia, or persistent SIRS [11]. Combined therapy with hydrocortisone, thiamine, and ascorbic acid seems beneficial in critically ill people [25]. Hypovitaminosis C is common in hospitalized foals [26], and supplementation with ascorbic acid, thiamine, and hydrocortisone warrants further investigation in this population.

Table 21.VI.1 ACTH stimulation test results in healthy and hospitalized neonatal foals (cortisol, μg/dl unless indicated otherwise).[a,b]

Author	Age	N	ACTH dose	Delta cortisol 30 min	Delta cortisol 60 min
ACTH stimulation test in hospitalized foals					
Wong et al. [8]	<24 h	6	0.1 μg/kg	43.5 ± 31.3[a]	28.7 ± 28.5
	1–56 d	18	0.1 μg/kg	17.4 ± 24.8[a]	0.6 ± 21.5
Hart et al. [1]	<7 d	58	10 μg	4.5 ± 5	—
	<7 d	58	100 μg	7.6 ± 7.8	—
Dembek et al. [2]	<48 h	11	10 μg	24 (−88 to 345.8)[b]	—
Hart et al. [1]	<4 h	9	10 μg	1.5 ± 3.5	—
	4–30 h	18	10 μg	6.7 ± 5.5	—
	30 h–3 d	27	10 μg	4.6 ± 5.0	—
	3–7 d	4	10 μg	5.3 ± 6.9	—
	<4 h	9	100 μg	4.6 ± 6.6	—
	4–30 h	18	100 μg	13 ± 10.3	—
	30 h–3 d	27	100 μg	7.3 ± 5.1	—
	3–7 d	4	100 μg	2.1 ± 6.2	—
ACTH stimulation test in healthy foals					
Hart et al. [16]	3–4 d	10	10 μg	2.4 ± 1	—
	3–4 d	10	100 μg	5.0 ± 2.2	—
	3–4 d	6	250 μg	5.6 ± 2.1	—
Hart et al. [9]	Birth	11	10 μg	3.6 ± 2.0	—
	12–24 h	10	10 μg	5.5 ± 2.1	—
	36–48 h	10	10 μg	3.5 ± 1.7	—
	5–7 d	11	10 μg	1.3 ± 0.6	—
	Birth	11	100 μg	6.4 ± 4.1	—
	12–24 h	10	100 μg	9.4 ± 3.5	—
	36–48 h	10	100 μg	6.8 ± 3.4	—
	5–7 d	11	100 μg	3.5 ± 1.3	—
Wong et al. [10]	Birth	13	0.1 μg/kg	83.6 ± 14.2[a]	58.0 ± 11.1[a]
	3 d	13	0.1 μg/kg	36.8 ± 6.4[a]	22.9 ± 4.0[a]
	5 d	13	0.1 μg/kg	34.9 ± 6.6[a]	24.1 ± 3.3[a]
	7 d	13	0.1 μg/kg	34.2 ± 5.2[a]	22.7 ± 4.8[a]
	14 d	13	0.1 μg/kg	33.7 ± 6.6[a]	22.4 ± 4.6[a]
	21 d	13	0.1 μg/kg	35.3 ± 4.5[a]	23.8 ± 3.9[a]
Dembek et al. [2]	<48 h	13	10 μg	125 (1.3–316)[b]	—

[a] ng/ml.
[b] Median and range (percent change from baseline cortisol 30 minutes after ACTH stimulation).

Diagnosis and Treatment of Energy Regulation Disorders

Endocrine Pancreas

Pancreatic endocrine dysfunction is common in ill foals [27] but evaluation of the pancreas is rarely performed. This may have clinical relevance for the diagnosis and treatment of hospitalized foals. Septic foals often have lower glucose and insulin concentrations compared to healthy foals, and high insulin concentrations have been linked to mortality [27]. The quantitative insulin-sensitivity check index (QUICKI) was higher in sick foals (both septic and sick nonseptic) compared to healthy foals (suggesting insulin sensitivity) and low insulin concentrations in these foals could be an evolutionary adaptation to reduced

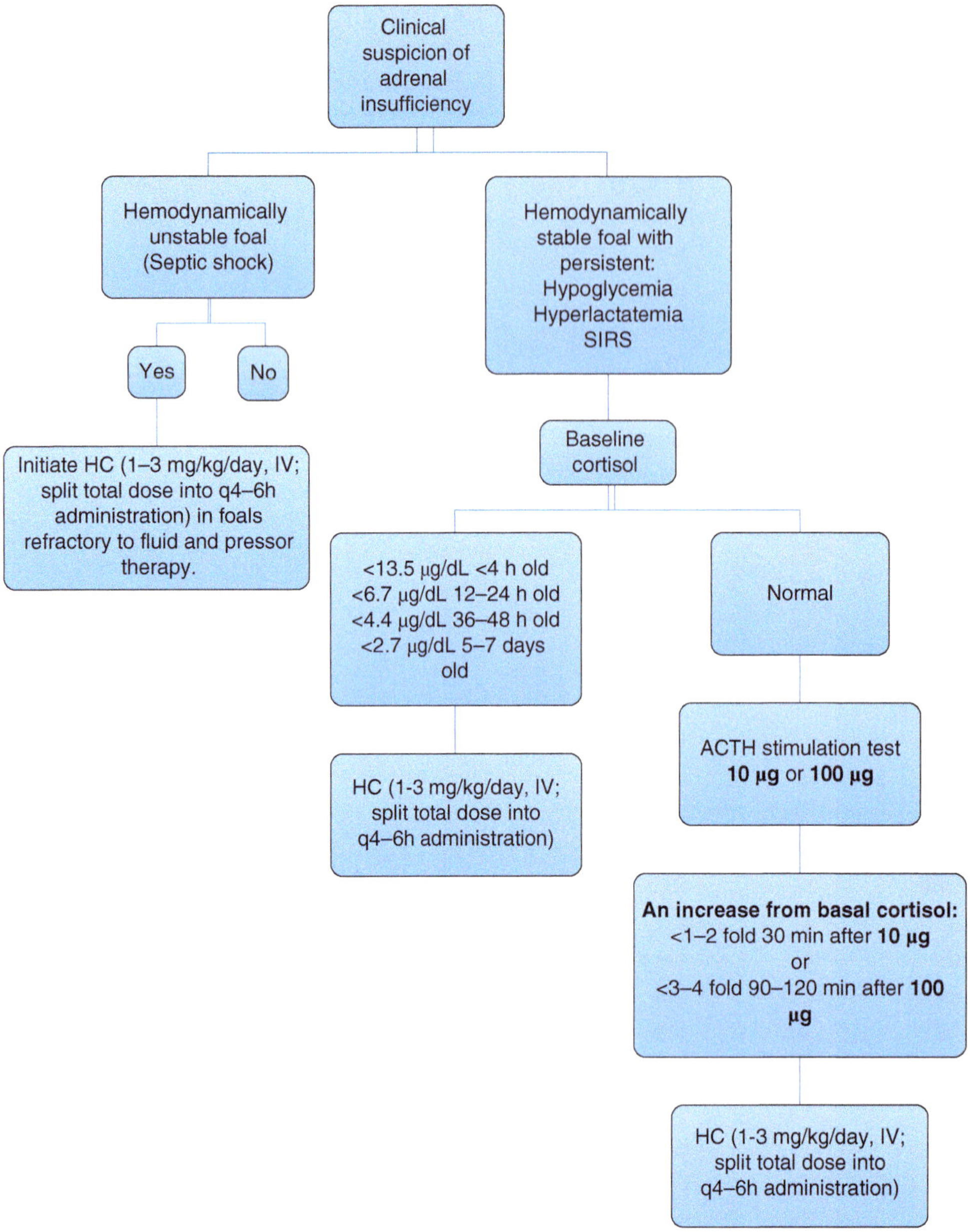

Figure 21.VI.1 Algorithm for the management of the foal with suspected adrenal insufficiency (HC = hydrocortisone).

energy intake and systemic inflammation. Glucagon concentrations were also higher in septic foals [27]. Healthy foals have a responsive enteroinsular axis (EIA) in the immediate postnatal period [28], and incretin dysregulation likely occurs in critically ill neonatal foals [29].

Pancreatic β Cell

Glucose

Measuring basal insulin and glucose concentrations is a nonivasive method to evaluate insulin and glucose dynamics in sick and healthy neonatal foals [27, 28, 30, 31]. Blood glucose concentrations in neonatal foals are consistently higher than adult values after suckling [28, 30, 31], although wide hourly variations occur, likely due to intermittent nursing. Defining hyperglycemia is relative because glucose concentrations of 200–250 mg/dl are normal in healthy newborn foals after nursing [28, 32]. Blood glucose concentrations increase in response to suckling, enteral and parenteral dextrose administration, and enteral lactose administration [28] but the most robust increase occurs in response to direct nursing from the mare. With up to 4 hours of fasting, blood glucose concentrations decrease marginally over time, and healthy foals did not become hypoglycemic [28].

Insulin

Insulin lowers blood glucose concentrations in healthy foals in the immediate postpartum period, and insulin concentrations are often low in septic and premature foals [27, 33]. It is speculated that sick foals exhibit an adaptive response to hypoglycemia and likely systemic inflammation by reducing insulin secretion rather than developing cytokine or stress-induced insulin resistance. Higher insulin concentration in septic foals on admission was associated with mortality, indicating that nonsurviving hospitalized foals exhibit insulin dysregulation [27]. According to studies, insulin concentrations in healthy foals are within normal adult reference ranges (<20 μIU/ml; Table 21.VI.2) [27, 28, 30, 31, 34], although foal values were lower in mares up to 12 days postpartum [35]. Premature foals have lower plasma glucose and insulin concentrations than term foals [33] but no difference in glucose and insulin concentrations was shown between younger and older foals within the first 10–12 days of age [31, 36]. However, one study found lower insulin concentrations in foals 1 day, 1 week, and 1 month of age compared to foals of 3 months of age [34]. These differences in insulin concentrations between foals and adult horses suggest that changes in pancreatic β-cell function occur over time.

Proxy Measurements of Insulin Sensitivity and Secretion

There are few studies on proxy measurements of insulin sensitivity in foals. One study investigated the glucose-to-insulin ratio (G/I) in foals at 1–2 days and 10–12 days of age and also compared these ratios to postpartum mares [31]. The G/I was significantly higher in foals compared to mares in both age groups. Insulin concentrations trended higher in 10–12-day old foals (although not significantly), and the G/I was significantly higher in younger foals. This suggests that there are small, if any, changes in insulin sensitivity within the first 10 days of life [31]. Another study comparing proxy measurements between healthy foals 24–72 hours of age and adult horses revealed that proxies for insulin sensitivity (QUICKI), the homeostatic model assessment of insulin resistance (HOMA-IR), and the reciprocal square root of insulin (RISQI) were not different between foals and horses. However, the modified insulin-to-glucose ratio (MIRG) was significantly lower in foals compared to horses [32]. This study confirmed findings from previous studies that G/I was significantly higher in foals compared to adults [32].

Table 21.VI.2 Normal insulin and glucose concentrations in neonatal foals (median and range).

References	Age	Glucose (mg/dl)	Insulin (μIU/ml)
Barsnick et al. [27]	18–24 h	148 (110–182)	4.9 (3.2–13)
Rings et al. [28]	≤4 d	140 (123–160)	10.7 (6–16.7)
Berryhill et al. [31]	Post-suckle	114 (67–242)	11.43 (5.85–25.09)
Berryhill et al. [31]	1–2 d	169 (121–227)	8.50 (4.32–18.4)
Berryhill et al. [31]	10–12 d	167 (133–202)	12.26 (6.55–30.24)
Kinsella et al. [30]	24–60 h	166 (160–184)	8.3 (5.2–11.7)

Dynamic Insulin Sensitivity Testing

Dynamic tests evaluating insulin sensitivity are documented in the equine fetus and neonate [26, 32, 33, 36, 37]. As noted, the equine fetus exhibits an insulin response to IV glucose in late gestation. The magnitude of the insulin response is higher in fetuses with higher cortisol concentrations [38]. Term neonates exhibit similar incremental increases in insulin in response to exogenous glucose infusion, while premature neonates show a smaller and delayed insulin response to glucose [33]. Glucose concentrations peaked at the end of a 5-minute glucose infusion in both induced and spontaneously born neonatal pony foals. Glucose concentrations decreased to baseline or below baseline values by 30 minutes in 5- and 9-day-old foals but remain elevated at 60 minutes in 1-day-old foals. Insulin concentrations peaked 5–15 minutes after glucose administration in all foals and fell to baseline or below by 60 minutes, except on the first day of life [37]. This dynamic testing indicates differences in insulin sensitivity in newborn (first day of life) compared to days 5 and 9. The prolonged duration of the insulin and glucose curves (larger area under the curve [AUC] values) suggests decreased insulin sensitivity in the first day of life. This might be due to hypercortisolemia in the immediate perinatal period, inducing insulin resistance and promoting β-cell proliferation [37]. These results contradict studies assessing baseline insulin, glucose, and proxy measurements of insulin sensitivity, which suggest that neonatal foals are insulin sensitive. However, in humans and adult horses, dynamic testing methods, including the frequently sampled IV glucose tolerance test (FSIGTT), are more sensitive than baseline measurements for detecting insulin resistance [39, 40]. The insulin-modified FSIGTT was performed in healthy Standardbred foals 24–72 hours of age and revealed significantly higher insulin sensitivity values compared to adults; this suggests that neonates are actually quite insulin sensitive, even in the early neonatal period [32]. Glucose effectiveness and the acute insulin response to glucose were not significantly different from adult values [32]. This may indicate reduced insulin clearance is responsible for increased glucose and insulin AUC values, but more studies are needed.

Pancreatic α Cell

Glucagon concentrations have been evaluated in neonatal foals at baseline and in response to dynamic tests, including IV arginine and dextrose, enteral carbohydrates (dextrose and lactose), and mare's milk [28, 30, 37]. Glucagon concentrations increase in late gestation, peak at birth, then decrease progressively [41]. Glucagon concentrations are higher in septic and sick nonseptic foals compared to healthy foals [27]. The α cells are responsive to arginine infusion from late gestation into the newborn period [37, 42]. However, α cells are less responsive to changes in glucose concentrations in the fetal foal [42]. No changes in glucagon concentrations were observed when foals were fasted for 4 hours. In these foals, glucose concentrations decreased over time, but foals remained euglycemic [30], suggesting that the change in glycemia was not significant enough over a 4-hour fast to promote glucagon secretion. A significant decrease in glucagon concentration was observed in foals administered enteral lactose, but not after enteral or IV dextrose administration. Surprisingly, once allowed to nurse ad libitum, glucagon concentrations increased three- to fourfold within 30 minutes, along with profound increases in glucose and insulin concentrations [30].

Enteroinsular Axis (EIA, Incretin Hormones)

The EIA comprises intestinal factors that stimulate insulin secretion, including glucose-dependent insulinotropic polypeptide (GIP) and glucagon-like peptide-1 (GLP-1). Healthy foals (<4 days of age) have a functional EIA characterized by a rapid secretion of GIP and GLP-1 in response to ingestion of mare's milk [28]. However, GIP concentrations decreased when foals were muzzled and administered enteral lactose and dextrose. GLP-1 concentrations decreased in response to enteral lactose and dextrose, except for when foals were administered 1000 mg/kg oral dextrose; under these conditions, a significant increase in GLP-1 was observed [28]. Despite the minimal incretin response to enteral lactose and dextrose, a robust response was observed once foals were allowed to nurse, demonstrating a functional EIA that may be responsive to other substrates in mares' milk (e.g. galactose, lipids, or amino acids), or the increase may be related to a more prolonged fast (four hours) prior to ad libitum nursing (compared to a 1-hour fast prior to administration of enteral dextrose and lactose). The act of suckling also may produce neuroendocrine responses that enhance release of GI hormones in foals, as occurs in infants [43]. The increase in GLP-1 and GIP in response to nursing was greater than that of adult horses, which may indicate that foals have a greater incretin secretory capacity compared to adults [28]. Human neonates have higher resting GLP-1 concentrations than adults, which might play a role in maturation of the enteroendocrine system and pancreatic β cells [44, 45].

Leptin, Adiponectin, Ghrelin, Triglycerides, and the Somatotropic Axis

Evaluation of hormones involved in energy metabolism (including leptin, adiponectin, and ghrelin) has been reported in horses but little is known about their roles in neonatal foals in health and disease. Studies have compared leptin, adiponectin, and ghrelin in healthy, sick nonseptic, and septic equine neonates and suggests their involvement in diseases of foals (at least as biomarkers of severity of disease, but also potentially as therapeutic targets). As noted, septic foals have lower concentrations of insulin and glucose and higher concentrations of glucagon upon admission compared to healthy foals [27]; however, higher insulin and lower leptin concentrations were associated with mortality. Leptin concentrations are not correlated to increases in fat depth and body condition score in foals as reported in horses, which might be an adaptive mechanism to promote feed intake for rapid growth [46]. Although leptin concentrations are high in mare's colostrum, levels drop within hours and do not appear to be correlated with foals' serum leptin concentrations [46]. In one study, postparturient hyperleptinemia and hyperlipidemia in mares did not affect lipid and leptin concentrations in foals [47]. Adiponectin is negatively correlated with body condition in horses and other species. Blood adiponectin concentrations were not different between sick and healthy foals in one study [48], but adiponectin's role in energy dysregulation in foals remains unclear.

Growth hormone (GH) and insulin-like growth factor-1 (IGF-1) concentrations increase in foals over time [49, 50]. Evidence of somatotropic axis (ghrelin, growth hormone, and IGF-1) resistance characterized by high GH and low IGF-1 concentrations (high GH/IGF-1 ratio) was shown in ill foals and associated with hypoglycemia, hypertriglyceridemia, and mortality in foals with severe disease [51]. Serum ghrelin concentrations were high in septic compared to healthy and sick nonseptic foals indicating an appropriate ghrelin response to negative energy balance from anorexia, causing hypoglycemia and hypertriglyceridemia [51]. In other species, higher ghrelin concentrations may improve survival, possibly due to its anti-inflammatory properties [51] but this has not been observed in sick foals.

Lipid derangements (hypertriglyceridemia, hyperlipemia) occur in critically ill foals and foals with acute pancreatitis [27, 51–53]. Serum triglyceride concentrations can be measured with concentrations varying widely in healthy foals and are influenced by breed [54]. Serum triglycerides are within adult reference ranges at birth, increase by 1–2 days of age, and remain higher than horse reference ranges up to 6 weeks of age [52, 55]. Healthy foals can have serum triglyceride values as high as 100–200 mg/dl (1.13–2.26 mmol/l) in the first week of life [52, 55]. Hospitalized septic foals have higher serum triglyceride concentrations compared to healthy foals [51], and in one study, nonsurviving foals had higher triglycerides than surviving foals [52]. Hypertriglyceridemia can be a complication of parenteral nutrition (PN) in neonatal foals; its cause is not clearly understood, and elevated triglyceride concentrations have been associated with nonsurvival [56].

Treatment of Energy Disorders

Depending on the condition involved, different feeding strategies can be used for managing sick foals. The type of disease, metabolic parameters (glycemia, triglycerides), acid-base and electrolyte status, maturity, GI function, type of feeding (enteral, parenteral), tolerance to enteral feeding, type of diet (mare's milk, replacer), feeding approach (nursing, tube feeding, or pan), and cost are considerations when creating a nutritional plan (Chapter 58). Blood glucose monitoring (every 4–8 hours) in foals is important, particularly those with sepsis, as low glucose and insulin concentrations are common [48]. Enteral nutrition using mare's milk or commercial mare's milk replacer should be implemented in foals with a functional GI tract that are unable to suckle.

In ill foals, feeding begins at 5–10% of body weight/day (split into 12–24 feedings, every 1–2 hours). The amount is increased based on the foal's illness, response to treatment, estimated energy requirements, and tolerance to enteral feeding. Resting energy requirements (RER) for healthy foals are 150–165 kcal/kg/d of digestible energy from milk for rapid growth for the first 10–11 days of life [57]; however, RER for ill foals is lower at approximately 50 kcal/kg/d (10% body weight in mare's milk/day) [58]. Thus, goals for enteral nutrition in sick neonates should be adjusted based on clinical condition and estimated energy expenditure. For foals with severe illness, hypoglycemia, or intolerance to enteral nutrition, PN should be employed to initially provide 25–30% RER, increasing to 50% RER prior to transitioning to enteral feeding. This is accomplished with IV dextrose administration or total or partial PN solutions. Initial dextrose support is administered at a rate of 4–8 mg/kg/min, starting at the lower rate and increasing gradually or quickly based on blood glucose monitoring and energy requirements.

The addition of amino acids to PN (Chapter 58) is beneficial (1 g of protein = 4 kcal of energy) and recommended to provide 4–6 g of protein per 100 kcal of energy [59]. Commercial solutions contain 2.75–8% of amino acids combined with 5–20% dextrose. Energy density can be increased by adding lipids (1 g of lipids = 9 kcal) but lipids increase cost, destabilize some solutions, and are contraindicated with hypertriglyceridemia or hepatic dysfunction [59]. Monitoring blood glucose, electrolyte, and triglyceride concentrations during PN administration is important, as exogenous dextrose can lead to hyperglycemia and electrolyte shifts that could result in hypokalemia, hypomagnesemia, and hypophosphatemia. Hyperglycemia is controlled with concurrent administration of regular insulin (IV or IM; 0.1 IU/kg or preferably as a CRI 0.1–1 IU/kg/h). Monitoring of blood glucose concentrations is necessary when administering insulin as hypoglycemia is common; the insulin dose is titrated to effect, and infusion of dextrose-containing fluids concurrently is recommended for foals receiving insulin as a CRI [32]. Little is known regarding incretins in hospitalized foals, although some sick foals have a dysregulated EIA that could interfere with insulin secretion [29]. Therapeutics, including incretin analogues or dipeptidyl peptidase-4 inhibitors increase insulin concentrations in people with type 2 diabetes mellitus and may have applications in foals with pancreatic endocrine dysregulation and hyperglycemia. A GLP-1 analogue was safe and effective in reducing postprandial insulin in a group of horses, likely by increasing insulin sensitivity but these medications have not been fully evaluated in horses and foals [60].

The mainstay of therapy for foals with hyperlipemia is administration of enteral and/or PN. For severe hyperlipemia, the addition of PN is critical. Complications of PN include hyperglycemia, thrombophlebitis, and hyperlipemia [56]; therefore, total PN in the face of severe hyperlipemia is controversial, and the use of partial PN without lipids is preferred. The risk of insulin-induced laminitis is much lower in neonates than horses. Administration of regular insulin as intermittent bolus doses (IV or IM; 0.1 IU/kg) or a CRI (0.1–1 IU/kg/h) is appropriate for the management of hyperlipemia, hyperglycemia, or refractory hyperkalemia. Some authors recommend a starting CRI for regular insulin of 0.0025 to 0.01 IU/kg/h with steady increases every 2 to 4 h to 0.2 I U/kg/h, even higher rates until normoglycemia is restored [121]. Hypertriglyceridemia associated with milk feeding should not be mistaken for hyperlipemia, where the timing of blood sample collection in relation to nursing should be taken into account during evaluation of the serum triglyceride concentrations (triglycerides concentrations can vary hourly by over 100 mg/dl in nursing foals) [52]; ideally, serum triglycerides concentrations are monitored regularly during treatment, and regular biochemical evaluation is indicated, as lipid infiltration may interfere with organ function (liver and kidney, in particular).

Diagnosis of Thyroid Hormone Disorders

TH includes triiodothyronine (T_3), thyroxine (T_4), and reverse T_3 (rT_3). Both T_4 and T_3 are found in circulation bound to plasma proteins (albumin, thyroxine-binding globulin, transthyretin) and unbound or free. Therefore, THs include total T_4 (tT_4), free T_4 (fT_4), total T_3 (tT_3), and free T_3 (fT_3). The free hormone is the active fraction and better reflects thyroid gland function. Most TH secreted by the thyroid gland is T_4, which is converted in peripheral tissues into T_3 by deiodinases. Free T_3 is much more potent than fT_4. Both, total (tT_4, tT_3) and free (fT_4, fT_3) TH concentrations should be measured in suspect cases, noting the foal's age; ideally, an age-matched sample from a healthy foal from the same farm or area is submitted concurrently, although this may not always be possible. Disorders of the thyroid gland in the equine neonate include nonthyroidal illness syndrome (NTIS; "euthyroid sick syndrome"), congenital goiter, and congenital hypothyroidism and dysmaturity syndrome (CHDS).

Identification of foals requiring evaluation of HPTA function can be difficult, and priority given to those displaying clinical signs consistent with thyroid dysfunction. Given the variable presentation and severity of these disorders in foals, they are often underdiagnosed. Other conditions should be ruled out before performing functional tests (TSH and TRH-stimulation tests) to confirm the diagnosis of hypothyroidism. TH deficiency may occur at different stages of development, and thyroid function may return to normal after the insult. Therefore, a foal with clinical evidence of hypothyroidism could have normal TH concentrations. Clinical abnormalities such as prematurity or dysmaturity, inability to stand, long/curly haircoat, weakness, lethargy, weak suckle reflex, respiratory insufficiency/distress, cardiovascular insufficiency, incoordination, cold intolerance, hypothermia, physeal dysgenesis, incomplete ossification, collapse of cuboidal bones, rupture of extensor tendons, angular and flexural deformities, prognathism, delayed incisor eruption, growth retardation, energy dysregulation, and goiter are suggestive of hypothyroidism. Most foals are clinically affected at birth, although signs may go unnoticed early on in some foals.

The lack of TH negative feedback to pituitary thyrotropes results in excessive TSH secretion, leading to thyroid follicular cell hyperplasia, and in fetuses or foals with prolonged TH deficit, thyroid gland enlargement (goiter). The presence of goiter does not necessarily indicate hypothyroidism, and foals without goiter can also have hypothyroidism. Foals with clinical evidence of hypothyroidism, with or without enlarged thyroid glands, are suspects. Some foals with goiter survive, suggesting that their TH deficiency was transient. The nutritional program should be examined; feed and pasture analysis are recommended. Both iodine deficiency and excess can lead to signs of hypothyroidism. Foals born to mares ingesting excessive amounts of iodine often have goiter [61]. Other conditions should be ruled out (e.g., branchial cysts) before performing functional tests (TSH or TRH-stimulation tests) to confirm the diagnosis of hypothyroidism.

Iodine concentrations in healthy newborn foals are much higher than those of adult horses [62]. Foals with selenium or vitamin E deficiency can display signs that resemble hypothyroidism [63]. In theory, selenium deficiency can contribute to hypothyroidism because deiodinase enzymes are selenium-dependent proteins [64]. Therefore, assessment of iodine and selenium status of mares and foals, as well as feedstuffs, may be warranted. This is even more important in farms or areas where multiple foals are born prematurely or with signs of hypothyroidism. An example is western Canada and northwestern United States, where congenital hypothyroidism can be endemic on some farms. Nitrates have been proposed as a potential cause because they can cross the placenta, interfere with thyroid gland iodide uptake, and are found in high concentrations in these areas [65]. Other compounds that interfere with iodine transport can alter thyroid gland function.

The clinical presentation and foal's age should be considered when interpreting TH concentrations. TH concentrations in the equine fetus are low until late gestation, increasing significantly around parturition (TH approximately 10 times adult horse concentrations) [66]. This perinatal increase in HPTA activity supports the importance of THs in normal fetal-to-neonatal transition, particularly with respect to respiratory, cardiovascular, and endocrine functions. Adult horse reference values should not be used as resting TH concentrations in newborn foals are higher and decrease rapidly in the first 2 weeks of age reaching adult values around 1 month of age (Table 21.VI.3) [49, 62, 72]. Providing reference values for foals is challenging due to the rapid drop in TH concentrations [49]. Most times, single measurements are not diagnostic, and use of dynamic tests to assess HPTA function is indicated (Box 21.VI.1). Studies demonstrate that premature, septic, and maladjusted foals often have low TH concentrations that are linked to disease severity and mortality (known as euthyroid sick syndrome or NTIS) [66–68].

Congenital Hypothyroidism and Dysmaturity Syndrome (CHDS)

Diagnosis of CHDS is based on clinical signs including prematurity/dysmaturity, inability to stand, long and curly haircoat, lethargy, weak suckle reflex, myxedema,

Table 21.VI.3 Reference ranges for hypothalamic-pituitary-thyroid axis factors in neonatal and adult equids.

Age	tT_4	fT_4	tT_3	fT_3	TSH	References
1 d	260.5 nmol/l (191–318)	97.5 pmol/l (49–144)	8.2 nmol/l (6–11.8)	10 pmol/l (5.6–24.2)	0.24 ng/ml (0.1–0.68)	[66]
1–2 d	712 nmol/l (295–1012)	50.2 pmol/l (27–70)	7.9 nmol/l (3.2–9.5)	21.2 pmol/l (6.9–34.3)		[67]
4 d	231.7 ± 61.8 nmol/l	1.2 ± 0.4 ng/dl	7.8 ± 4.2 nmol/l	3.4 ± 1.1 pg/ml		[68]
28 d	30.6 ± 17.4 nmol/l		3.1 ± 0.4 nmol/l			
Birth	394.8 ± 140.8 nmol/l		9.6 ± 4.8 nmol/l			[49, 68]
1 d	249.5 ± 82.7 nmol/l		11 ± 2.8 nmol/l			
3 d	178.9 ± 74 nmol/l		9 ± 3.5 nmol/l			
7 d	100.7 ± 79.7 nmol/l		7 ± 2.4 nmol/l			
14 d	29.6 ± 0.6 nmol/l		2.4 ± 0.1 nmol/l			
1 d	207 μg/dl		6.7 ng/ml			[69]
1 mo	26 μg/dl		1.6 ng/ml			
6 mo	35 μg/dl		0.9 ng/ml			
Adult horses	12.9 ± 5.6 nmol/l	12.2 ± 3.5 pmol/l	0.99 ± 0.51 nmol/l	2.07 ± 1.14 pmol/l	0.40 ± 0.29 ng/ml	[70]
Adult donkeys	3.53 ± 0.25 μg/dl	0.44 ± 0.02 ng/dl	67.1 ± 2.9 ng/dl	1.81 ± 0.1 pg/ml		[71]

respiratory distress, cardiovascular insufficiency, incoordination, cold intolerance, physeal dysgenesis, incomplete ossification and collapse of cuboidal bones, contracture and rupture of tendons, angular and flexural deformities, prognathism, delayed incisor eruption, energy dysregulation, goiter, and death [72, 75–89]. Having multiple foals in a farm or area indicates that management and environmental factors are likely involved. Necropsy may demonstrate incomplete tissue differentiation, including pulmonary atelectasis, incomplete ossification of cuboidal bones, prognathism, tendon abnormalities, and thyroid gland enlargement. On histology, there could be thyroid follicular hyperplasia with small amounts of colloid, adenohypophysis hyperplasia, pulmonary atelectasis, collapsed alveoli, immature pneumocytes that fail to produce surfactant, and delayed bone matrix deposition [90, 91]. Other tissues could have evidence of delayed development or secondary lesions.

Box 21.VI.1 Dynamic Tests for HPTA Function in Equine Neonates

TRH Stimulation Test Protocol [73]

- Measure baseline serum tT_4, fT_4, tT_3, and fT_3 concentrations, administer 0.5 mg TRH IV
- Measure concentrations at two- and four-hours post-administration
- *Interpretation*: serum tT_3 and fT_3 concentrations should increase by 40–60% two hours post-administration, and tT_4 and fT_4 should increase by 7–30% four hours post-administration

TSH Stimulation Test Protocol [74]

- Measure serum [tT_3] at baseline, administer 5 IU TSH IV
- Measure serum [tT_3] at one- and three-hours post-administration
- *Interpretation*: [tT_3] should increase by at least 50% over baseline by three hours in normal foals

Testing of Thyroid Gland Function

The simplest method to assess thyroid function is measurement of resting TH concentrations (total and free). This approach is useful but often difficult to interpret. To provide a comprehensive assessment of HPTA function, in addition to baseline TH concentrations, dynamic tests are indicated (Box 21.VI.1). For the TRH-stimulation test, 0.5 mg of TRH is administered IV with TH measured at baseline, and 2, and 4 hours later [66]. In foals with normal thyroid function, T_3 and T_4 increase two- to threefold over baseline values. The TSH-stimulation test is not performed in clinical practice due to reagent availability and cost. Similar to resting TH measurements, it is recommended to perform this test in parallel with an age-matched healthy foal, considering the rapid changes in TH concentrations that occur after birth [49].

There are no commercially available tests to measure equine TSH concentrations. Serum fT_3 and fT_4 concentrations are better reflections of thyroid gland activity. TH concentrations are measured in foals via immunoassays

(ELISAs, radioimmunoassays, immunochemiluminescence) and equilibrium dialysis [66, 67, 92] with equilibrium dialysis considered the best method to measure fT_4 and fT_3 concentrations. Since these methods can yield variable results for the same sample, using a single certified laboratory or method for serial or comparative testing is important for accurate interpretation [93]. Serum is the preferred sample to measure TH concentrations, although plasma may be appropriate for some assays. Hemolyzed or lipemic samples, as well as those from patients that have received TH therapy, should be avoided for diagnostic purposes.

Clinical signs of HPTA dysfunction can be present in the face of normal TH concentrations because TH deficiency may have occurred previously during critical periods of fetal development. In foals with low TH concentrations or clinical abnormalities consistent with TH deficit, sequential monitoring of TH values and other abnormalities (e.g. serial radiography for ossification of the cuboidal bones) is recommended. Hypothyroidism in foals carries a poor prognosis, even after TH replacement therapy. Dynamic tests for HPTA evaluation in foals have been described, including TSH and TRH stimulation tests (Box 21.VI.1) [66].

Various drugs and systemic illnesses affect the results and interpretation of thyroid function testing in horses. While similar influences are assumed to occur in foals, they have not been evaluated in neonates. For example, glucocorticoids suppress HPTA function in horses at the thyroid, pituitary, and hypothalamic levels, but in foals, these drugs may actually enhance the conversion of T_4 to T_3 in the peripartum period as part of the processes of maturation and readiness for birth [93]. Noting medications that the foal has historically or currently received is recommended during evaluation of test results.

NTIS is a centrally mediated decrease in TH concentrations [67, 94]. Criteria for diagnosis in neonatal foals include low serum T_3 concentrations, accompanied by low, normal, or elevated serum T_4 concentrations [93] and preserved response to TRH stimulation regarding release of TSH, T_4, and T_3 (Box 21.VI.1). NTIS has been documented in foals and characterized by low serum fT_3, fT_4, and TSH concentrations. The sepsis score in foals was inversely correlated to TH and TSH concentrations, and rT_3 concentrations positively correlated to the sepsis score [66, 67]. Non-surviving sick foals had lower TH concentrations compared to survivors [67]. Premature and sick neonatal foals have lower TH concentrations than healthy neonates, but the response to dynamic testing differs; premature foals had low T_4 concentrations and a blunted response to TRH stimulation when compared to normal and non-premature sick foals [66]. Diurnal variability in TH concentrations has been reported in other species, but this does not occur in neonatal foals [95].

Environmental conditions can influence equine neonatal thyroid function. Foals born to mares grazing *Neotyphodium coenophialum*-infested fescue pasture had lower serum T_3 concentrations than control foals born to mares unexposed to endophyte-infested pasture (serum T_4 and rT_3 concentrations were not different between these foal populations) [96]. Foals with neonatal maladjustment syndrome had lower TH concentrations at birth than healthy foals; however, this had no apparent prognostic value [68]. Foals born via spontaneous delivery had higher T_3 and T_4 concentrations in the first week of life than foals born to pharmacologically induced mares, suggesting that conditions surrounding parturition can influence TH concentrations. This may warrant generation of TH reference ranges for induced foals or foals of dystocia [49]. The iodine content of mares' colostrum and milk correlate with neonatal tT_4, tT_3, and serum iodine concentrations [62], and TSH concentration in mare's milk is highest on the day of birth with a nadir at Day 61 [46]. Donkey and mule foals may display differences in TH concentrations when compared to horse and pony foals; thus, they should be evaluated against species-specific reference ranges [71, 97]. Collectively, these studies emphasize the importance of considering environmental and contextual factors when evaluating a clinical patient suspected of a disorder of the HPTA.

Treatment of TH Disorders

Treatment of hypothyroidism is palliative, and the benefits of TH supplementation have not been prospectively evaluated in sick foals. Studies on therapeutic protocols for foals with hypothyroidism are lacking. Candidates for supplementation with analogs to T_4 (levothyroxine) and T_3 (liothyronine) include foals with clinical manifestations of congenital hypothyroidism supported by dynamic testing. Advantages of commercial T_3 (liothyronine sodium) over T_4 (levothyroxine sodium) is that the conversion of T_4 to T_3 is not required, and faster effects are anticipated. Oral levothyroxine at 20–50 µg/kg/d and liothyronine at 1 µg/kg/d have been proposed for foals with hypothyroidism [61]. One author suggested T_4 orally at $10 \times 0.22 \times$ body weight (kg) $\times 0.08 \times$ plasma [T_4] (µg/l) or 2.5 mg/d for a 1- to 3-day-old 50 kg foal [75, 98]. This dose is based on the physiological T_4 secretion rate [75, 98]. Because the conversion of T_4 to T_3 can be slow, an initial treatment of T_3 at one third the T_4 dose, preferably parenterally, is recommended [75]. Another protocol is $0.176 \times$ body weight (kg) $\times$ desired T_4 concentration in µg/l/d [61]. Measurement of TH concentrations is recommended to ensure that they are returning to age-specific ranges. More important is that foals show clinical improvement. Administration of selenium should be considered in affected and suspect foals.

It is also important to measure TH concentrations in pregnant mares at the farm. Nutritional evaluation of broodmare diets, particularly iodine content and supplementation (such as kelp-based products), should be performed if hypothyroidism is confirmed in a foal born on the property. If there is iodine deficiency at the farm level, animals should receive iodine at 0.007–0.008 mg/kg of body weight or 0.35 mg/kg of dry matter per day, and 0.4 mg/kg of dry matter for late pregnant mares [99]. Nitrate content of the diet and water should be evaluated, as well as access to goitrogenic plants (such as kale, soybeans, cabbage, rape, turnips, etc.). Replacement therapy for foals with NTIS, similar to people, remains controversial and information is scarce [66, 84].

Diagnosis and Treatment of Blood Pressure Disorders

Diagnosis and Treatment of Renin-Angiotensin-Aldosterone System (RAAS) Disorders

This section does not provide therapy specific to hypotension as consequences of critical illness (Chapter 11) but is limited to approaches to diagnose endocrine disorders affecting blood pressure and perfusion. The RAAS helps maintain tissue perfusion by increasing blood pressure and intravascular fluid volume. Although healthy newborn foals have a functional RAAS, some critically ill foals with evidence of hypotension have inappropriately low aldosterone concentrations (high ACTH/aldosterone ratio), suggesting mineralocorticoid insufficiency in critically ill foals [7, 100, 101]. Most of these foals also had reduced cortisol concentrations, indicating that RAI affects different layers of the adrenal cortex and, therefore, different homeostatic systems. Clinically, this can be suspected in foals that fail to regulate electrolyte concentrations, often developing hyponatremia and hyperkalemia associated with hypotension or hypoperfusion. These foals often have RAI that may contribute to hypoglycemia and a pro-inflammatory state. Unlike cortisol, measurement of aldosterone concentrations is not readily available. Some foals with hypoperfusion have inappropriately low angiotensin-II (ANG-II) concentrations [7] that, in addition to impairing vasoconstriction, reduces aldosterone and AVP secretion. ANG-II is a strong stimulator of aldosterone synthesis and secretion.

Because foals with RAI may also have inappropriately low aldosterone secretion, administration of hydrocortisone is recommended because it has glucocorticoid and mineralocorticoid properties. Fludrocortisone is a synthetic steroid with mineralocorticoid activity that is commonly used to treat adrenal insufficiency in people. A combination of hydrocortisone and fludrocortisone therapy resulted in lower mortality in people with septic shock [102]. Isoflupredone is a glucocorticoid with aldosterone-like effects that can cause hypokalemia after prolonged use and can be considered in foals suspected of having low aldosterone concentrations. Currently, there are no established recommendations for aldosterone replacement therapy in critically ill foals [7]. Most critically ill foals have increased AVP concentrations, which is an appropriate response to hypoperfusion [7, 100, 103–105]. However, some have low AVP concentrations that contribute to disease severity and poor outcome. AVP and analogs are used to treat hypotension in critically ill foals.

Information on other vasoregulatory factors in critically ill foals is scarce and far from having diagnostic value, although disorders can be suspected. For example, adrenomedullin is a potent vasodilator and its concentrations were higher in critically ill foals, although not associated with disease severity or mortality [106]. Big endothelin-1 concentrations were higher in sick foals [107]. Association between natriuretic peptides and disease severity in hospitalized foals remains to be determined.

Disorders of Calcium, Phosphorus, and Magnesium

Calcium (Ca), phosphorus (PO_4), and magnesium (Mg) are highly interactive mineral ions that participate in numerous cellular functions. Due to their chemical configurations, they have structural and ionic properties and are highly interactive. Demands for these ions are higher in the neonate and decrease over time. Precise endocrine homeostatic systems are necessary to regulate their extracellular concentrations [108, 109]. Disorders of Ca, Mg, and PO_4 have received less attention in foals than in horses but hypocalcemia, hypomagnesemia, and hyperphosphatemia are frequent in critically ill foals [110–112].

Diagnosis of Calcium Disorders

The diagnosis of hypocalcemia is based on measurement of tCa and Ca^{2+} concentrations. Blood concentrations of tCa and Ca^{2+} are lower in healthy foals (tCa = 10–13 mg/dl; Ca^{2+} = 4.1–7 mg/dl) compared to horses (tCa = 11–13.2 mg/dl; Ca^{2+} = 5.8–7 mg/dl) [108, 110, 111, 113, 114], emphasizing use of foal-specific reference values. Most chemistry analyzers measure tCa and phosphorus. Heparinized blood collected under anaerobic conditions is preferred to measure Ca^{2+} and Mg^{2+} concentrations, although some analyzers also use serum. Sequential measurements are important to assess disease progression and response to treatment.

Measurement of PTH concentrations can be considered in foals with refractory hypocalcemia as they can have primary or secondary hypoparathyroidism. Secondary hypoparathyroidism is more common from systemic inflammation or hypomagnesemia. Most foals with hypocalcemia have an appropriate PTH response [110–112] but some have low to normal PTH concentrations (inappropriate PTH secretion), hyperphosphatemia, and hypomagnesemia, supporting secondary hypoparathyroidism [110–112]. These foals have hyperphosphatemia, with values above normal for a foal [112]. Thoroughbred foals unresponsive to treatment could have equine familial isolated hypocalcemia (genetic testing sent to UC Davis Veterinary Genetic Laboratory) [114]. Although the condition has been diagnosed in Thoroughbred foals, it can potentially be present in other founding breeds.

Hypovitaminosis D, which is prevalent in critically ill foals, can contribute to the pathogenesis of hypocalcemia [111]. Measurement of vitamin D, CT, and FGF-23 concentrations is not readily available. Few conditions justify measurement of PTHrP in foals; its pathological actions (endocrine) have been limited to horses (humoral hypercalcemia of malignancy). One consideration could be persistent hypercalcemia, especially if there is hypophosphatemia.

Treatment of Calcium Disorders

Replacement therapy via parenteral calcium supplementation should be considered in foals with mild hypocalcemia but implemented when severe hypocalcemia is present. A standard treatment protocol is to add 10–20 ml of 23% calcium gluconate per liter of parenteral fluids (~50–100 mg/kg) and administer as boluses or preferably as a CRI [108]. Depending on severity, some foals require higher doses or more rapid administration (e.g., 5–10 ml of 23% calcium gluconate over 5–10 min). Calcium chloride is another option, but it can cause irritation if inadvertently administered within the subcutaneous tissue. Oral administration of calcium salts (e.g., calcium carbonate) is rarely done in newborn foals due to disease severity, requiring faster availability of calcium. Measurement of Ca^{2+} and Mg^{2+} concentrations is recommended to optimize dosing. In foals that are refractory to calcium replacement therapy and have persistent clinical signs, IV administration of magnesium sulfate ($MgSO_4$) should be considered (dosing protocols below) as Mg depletion impairs calcium homeostasis. Long-term management of older foals with refractory hypocalcemia may require oral administration of Ca salts (e.g., calcium carbonate) and Mg salts (e.g., Mg oxide, citrate). Different forms of chelated Ca and Mg are available for people. Given that vitamin D metabolite concentrations are often low in septic foals [112], work is ongoing to evaluate the appropriateness of this therapy in critically ill foals. In foals with refractory hypocalcemia and questionable parathyroid gland function, treatment with calcitriol should be considered. This could potentially be beneficial to enhance immunity but should be a short-term therapy, as calcitriol inhibits parathyroid gland function.

Hypercalcemia is rare in newborn foals, and treatment should be oriented at promoting calciuresis (e.g., furosemide) and identifying the underlying cause. Most of these foals have a poor prognosis.

Diagnosis of Phosphorus Disorders

The diagnosis of hypophosphatemia in foals relies on idnitifcation on blood biochemistry. In addition to PO_4 measurement, it is important to assess Mg and K^+ concentrations as these ions are highly interactive. The diagnosis of hypo- and hyperphosphatemia is based on foal-specific reference values. Blood concentrations of PO_4 are higher in foals (4.4–8.4 mg/dl; 1.4–2.7 mmol/l) than horses (2–5.6 mg/dl; 0.65–1.8 mmol/l) [110–113, 115]. High PO_4 concentrations in foals parallel increased alkaline phosphatase activity [108, 116]. Conversion factors for PO_4 are: 1 mmol/l = 3.1 mg/dl; mg/dl × 0.32 = mmol/l; 1 mmol/l = 1.8 mEq/l.

In foals, hypophosphatemia is defined as serum PO_4 concentrations <4 mg/dl (1.3 mmol/l) and severe hypophosphatemia <3 mg/dl (1 mmol/l). Hypophosphatemia is often missed when PO_4 values are in the normal range for horses. Consideration of the clinical presentation, other laboratory abnormalities as well as previous treatments are important. Enteral and parenteral nutrition can be associated with hypophosphatemia due to increased intracellular PO_4 demands for glucose phosphorylation. In foals with hypomagnesemia or hypokalemia, evaluating PO_4 concentrations is highly recommended. Increased insulin concentrations in response to carbohydrates may contribute to these abnormalities by promoting their shift to the intracellular compartment.

Treatment of Phosphorus Disorders

Most phosphorus disorders are addressed by treating the underlying condition. Parenteral supplementation with PO_4 salts is indicated in foals with severe hypophosphatemia. There are different phosphate formulations available (Tables 21.VI.4 and 21.VI.5). The IV route is preferred to treat hypophosphatemia in critically ill foals. Potassium phosphate is the salt of choice if hypokalemia is present but sodium phosphate is a good alternative (Table 21.VI.5). When these solutions are not available, enemas containing monobasic and dibasic sodium phosphate can be given via nasogastric intubation (Table 21.VI.5). While they can be administered rectally, this route should be avoided for this purpose unless enteral or parenteral options are not feasible.

Table 21.VI.4 Products used for parenteral supplementation of phosphate in people and animals.

Product	Composition/ml	Phosphorus/ml	Potassium/ml	Sodium/ml	Presentation	Company
Potassium phosphate[a]	236 mg of K_2HPO_4 224 mg of KH_2PO_4	3 mmol or 93 mg	4.4 mmol or 170 mg	0	5, 15, 50 ml	American Reagents, Inc. Fresenius Kabi USA
Sodium phosphate[a]	142 mg of Na_2HPO_4 276 mg of NaH_2PO_4	3 mmol or 93 mg	0	4 mmol or 92 mg	5, 15, 50 ml	American Reagents, Inc. Fresenius Kabi USA Hospira, Inc
Phosphaid[b,c]	200 mg of NaH_2PO_2	2 mmol or 60 mg	0	46 mg	100 ml	Vedco, Inc
Phos-Aid[b,c]	200 mg of NaH_2PO_2	2 mmol or 60 mg	0	46 mg	100 ml	Neogen, Inc.
Phos P 200[b,c]	200 mg of NaH_2PO_2	2 mmol or 60 mg	0	46 mg	100 ml	Phoenix, Inc.
CMPK[b,d]	5 mg of NaH_2PO_2 16 mg of KCl	1.5 mg	0.4 mmol or 16 mg	0.16 mmol or 3.7 mg	500 ml	Vedco, Inc.

K_2HPO_4 = dibasic potassium phosphate/KH_2PO_4 = monobasic potassium phosphate.
Na_2HPO_4 = dibasic potassium phosphate/NaH_2PO_4 = monobasic potassium phosphate.
[a] For human use.
[b] Approved for cattle. Contains phosphinic acid (hypophosphorous acid [H_3PO_2]; sodium hypophosphite [NaH_2PO_2]).
[c] Recommended dose for cattle is 1 ml/25–50 kg (50–100 lb) of body weight.
[d] Formulated to treat hypocalcemia, hypomagnesemia, and hypophosphatemia in cattle. Suggested dose for adult cattle is 500 ml/360–450 kg (800–1000 lb) of body weight IV. Contains calcium, magnesium, phosphate, and potassium salts. Other formulations containing phosphorus include Norcalciphos (Zoetis, Inc) and Cal-Phos (Vedco, Inc).

Table 21.VI.5 Products used for enteral supplementation of phosphate in people and small animals.[a,b]

Product	Phosphorus/ml	Potassium/ml	Sodium/ml	Presentation	Company
Neutra-Phos	250 mg (8.1 mmol)	278 mg (7.1 mmol)	164 mg (7.1 mmol)	Per tablet or 75 ml solution	Baker Norton
Neutra-Phos-K	250 mg (8.1 mmol)	566 mg (14.2 mmol)	0	Per tablet or 75 ml solution	Baker Norton
K-Phos-Neutral	250 mg (8.1 mmol)	45 mg (1.1 mmol)	298 mg (13 mmol)	Per tablet	Beach
Fleet Phospho-soda	129 mg (4.15 mmol)	0	110 mg (4.8 mmol)	Per 45 ml oral solution	Fleet
Fleet Enema[c,d]	43 mg (1.38 mmol)	0	37 mg (1.6 mmol)	Per 118 ml	Fleet
Fleet Enema Extra[c,d]	25 mg (0.8 mmol)	0	23 mg (1 mmol)	Per 197 ml	Fleet
Fleet Pedia-Lax[e]	43 mg (1.38 mmol)	0	37 mg (1.6 mmol)	Per 59 ml	Fleet

[a] Other formulations are available in the market.
[b] Sodium and potassium phosphate salts (chemical grade) can be used via nasogastric intubation in horses.
[c] Phosphate enemas contain monobasic (19 g) and dibasic (7 g) sodium phosphate in 118 ml or monobasic (19 g) and dibasic (7 g) sodium phosphate in 197 ml solution.
[d] Phosphate enemas are often used intravenously in ruminants to treat hypophosphatemia. There are anecdotal reports of their used in horses.
[e] Pediatric enemas contain monobasic (9.5 g) and dibasic (3.5 g) sodium phosphate in 59 ml.

There are anecdotal reports of their use IV with no apparent complications (R.E. Toribio, personal communication), but this route should be used as a last resort. Phosphate content in enemas varies (Table 21.VI.5). Chemical grade sodium or potassium phosphate via nasogastric intubation is another option to consider (R.E. Toribio, personal communication). It is advisable to administer phosphate salts as a CRI. In small animals, rates of 0.01–0.06 mmol/kg/h are considered safe [117]. In people, rates of 0.08–0.16 mmol/kg/h are recommended, but rates up to 0.6 mmol/kg/h are indicated for severe hypophosphatemia (PO_4 < 1 mg/dl; <0.32 mmol/l). The dose required to restore normophosphatemia is often twice the deficit because these animals have total body PO_4 depletion and PO_4 will rapidly shift to the intracellular compartment, in particular when receiving energy supplementation [108]. In foals receiving IV Ca or Mg, a different line should be used for PO_4 supplementation to avoid precipitation.

Diagnosis of Magnesium Disorders

The diagnosis of hypo- and hypermagnesemia is based on blood tMg and Mg^{2+} concentrations. Hypomagnesemia is frequent in septic foals but often missed because Mg is not included in most chemistry profiles [109, 110]. The analytical principles to measure blood Ca concentrations also apply to Mg. Blood concentrations of tMg and Mg^{2+} are similar between foals (tMg = 0.54–1.1 mmol/l; Mg^{2+} = 0.46–0.8 mmol/l) and horses (tMg = 0.53–1.2 mmol/l; Mg^{2+} = 0.46–0.8 mmol/l) [109, 110, 113, 118, 119]. Hypoalbuminemia can result in pseudohypomagnesemia and acidosis reduces Mg binding to albumin increasing Mg^{2+} concentrations [109]. To measure Mg^{2+} concentrations, blood is collected in heparinized syringes or tubes under anaerobic conditions (do not use EDTA tubes). Some analyzers can measure Mg^{2+} in serum. Ideally measure both Ca^{2+} and Mg^{2+} simultaneously. Similar to hypophosphatemia, hypomagnesemia is common in foals receiving enteral or parenteral energy supplementation because these ions are highly interactive, in particular in processes involving transmembrane ion transport as well as energy storage and expenditure [109]. Conversion factors for Mg are: mmol/l = mg/dl × 0.41; mg/dl = mmol/l × 2.43; mg/dl = mEq/l × 1.21; mmol/l = mEq/l × 0.5.

Treatment of Magnesium Disorders

IV administration of $MgSO_4$ is indicated in foals with hypomagnesemia, refractory hypocalcemia, extended fasting, prolonged fluid therapy, and electrolyte abnormalities associated with enteral or parenteral nutrition and hyperglycemia (hypokalemia, hypophosphatemia, hypomagnesemia). $MgSO_4$ is also used to treat brain trauma and neonatal encephalopathy [109, 120]. A CRI of $MgSO_4$ (40–60 mg/kg/IV, loading dose over 5–10 min; 50–150 mg/kg/d/IV, CRI) is a good starting point for supplementation of Mg in sick foals [109, 120]. One practical approach is to add 2 g of $MgSO_4$ per liter of isotonic solution and administer intermittently (250–1000 ml IV, every 4-6 hours). If $MgSO_4$ is not available, $MgCl_2$ can be used, but the dose must be reduced by half because these salts are not equivalent and Mg content in $MgCl_2$ is higher. Per molecular weight, $MgSO_4$ has 9.7% of Mg (100 mg provides 9.7 mg of elemental Mg), while $MgCl_2$ has 25.5% of Mg (100 mg provides 25.5 mg of elemental Mg) [109]. Sequential measurement of Ca and Mg concentrations is recommended to adjust dosing.

Enteral administration of Mg salts in newborn foals is risky due to GI and systemic complications (e.g. diarrhea, hypermagnesemia, sedation). It is hard to justify enteral Mg administration in newborn foals, even in those with meconium impaction, but enteral administration can be used with caution in older foals with intestinal impactions (R.E. Toribio, personal communication). It is unknown how fast and how much Mg equine neonates can absorb. However, older foals with refractory hypocalcemia can be supplemented with oral Mg salts (e.g. sulfate, oxide, citrate). Hypermagnesemia is rare in sick foals and most often associated with cell lysis or iatrogenic administration of Mg salts. Treatment should be aimed at promoting diuresis and identifying the underlying cause.

References

1 Hart, K.A., Slovis, N.M., and Barton, M.H. (2009). Hypothalamic-pituitary-adrenal axis dysfunction in hospitalized neonatal foals. *J. Vet. Intern. Med.* 23: 901–912.

2 Dembek, K.A., Johnson, L.M., Timko, K.J. et al. (2019). Multiple adrenocortical steroid response to administration of exogenous adrenocorticotropic hormone to hospitalized foals. *J. Vet. Intern. Med.* 33: 1766–1774.

3 Annane, D., Pastores, S.M., Rochwerg, B. et al. (2017). Guidelines for the diagnosis and management of critical illness-related corticosteroid insufficiency (CIRCI) in critically ill patients (part I): Society of Critical Care Medicine (SCCM) and European Society of Intensive Care Medicine (ESICM) 2017. *Intensive Care Med.* 43: 1751–1763.

4 Hart, K.A. and Barton, M.H. (2011). Adrenocortical insufficiency in horses and foals. *Vet. Clin. North Am. Equine Pract.* 27: 19–34.

5 Hurcombe, S.D. (2011). Hypothalamic-pituitary gland axis function and dysfunction in horses. *Vet. Clin. North Am. Equine Pract.* 27: 1–17.

6 Gold, J.R., Divers, T.J., Barton, M.H. et al. (2007). Plasma adrenocorticotropin, cortisol, and adrenocorticotropin/cortisol ratios in septic and normal-term foals. *J. Vet. Intern. Med.* 21: 791–796.

7 Dembek, K.A., Onasch, K., Hurcombe, S.D.A. et al. (2013). Renin-angiotensin-aldosterone system and hypothalamic-pituitary-adrenal axis in hospitalized newborn foals. *J. Vet. Intern. Med.* 27: 331–338.

8 Wong, D.M., Vo, D.T., Alcott, C.J. et al. (2009). Baseline plasma cortisol and ACTH concentrations and response to low-dose ACTH stimulation testing in ill foals. *J. Am. Vet. Med. Assoc.* 234: 126–132.

9 Hart, K.A., Heusner, G.L., Norton, N.A. et al. (2009). Hypothalamic-pituitary-adrenal axis assessment in healthy term neonatal foals utilizing a paired low

dose/high dose ACTH stimulation test. *J. Vet. Intern. Med.* 23: 344–351.

10 Wong, D.M., Vo, D.T., Alcott, C.J. et al. (2009). Adrenocorticotropic hormone stimulation tests in healthy foals from birth to 12 weeks of age. *Can. J. Vet. Res.* 73: 65–72.

11 Hart, K.A., Dirikolu, L., Ferguson, D.C. et al. (2012). Daily endogenous cortisol production and hydrocortisone pharmacokinetics in adult horses and neonatal foals. *Am. J. Vet. Res.* 73: 68–75.

12 Dembek, K.A., Timko, K.J., Johnson, L.M. et al. (2017). Steroids, steroid precursors, and neuroactive steroids in critically ill equine neonates. *Vet. J.* 225: 42–49.

13 Aleman, M., McCue, P.M., Chigerwe, M. et al. (2019). Plasma concentrations of steroid precursors, steroids, neuroactive steroids, and neurosteroids in healthy neonatal foals from birth to 7 days of age. *J. Vet. Intern. Med.* 33: 2286–2293.

14 Stewart, A.J., Wright, J.C., Behrend, E.N. et al. (2013). Validation of a low-dose adrenocorticotropic hormone stimulation test in healthy neonatal foals. *J. Am. Vet. Med. Assoc.* 243: 399–405.

15 Annane, D., Pastores, S.M., Arlt, W. et al. (2017). Critical illness-related corticosteroid insufficiency (CIRCI): a narrative review from a Multispecialty Task Force of the Society of Critical Care Medicine (SCCM) and the European Society of Intensive Care Medicine (ESICM). *Intensive Care Med.* 43: 1781–1792.

16 Hart, K.A., Ferguson, D.C., Heusner, G.L. et al. (2007). Synthetic adrenocorticotropic hormone stimulation tests in healthy neonatal foals. *J. Vet. Intern. Med.* 21: 314–321.

17 Hart, K.A., Barton, M.H., Ferguson, D.C. et al. (2011). Serum free cortisol fraction in healthy and septic neonatal foals. *J. Vet. Intern. Med.* 25: 345–355.

18 Elder, E.M., Wong, D.M., Johnson, K., et al. (2022). Assessment of the hypothalamic-pituitary-adrenocortical axis function utilizing a vasopressin stimulation test in healthy foals. *ACVIM Forum*. Austin, Texas.

19 Johnson, K., Peterson, J., Kopper J., et al. (2023). The hypothalamic-pituitary-adrenal axis response to ovine corticotropin-releasing-hormone stimulation tests in healthy and hospitalized foals. *J. Vet. Intern. Med.* 37: 292–301.

20 Hart, K.A., Barton, M.H., Vandenplas, M.L. et al. (2011). Effects of low-dose hydrocortisone therapy on immune function in neonatal horses. *Pediatr. Res.* 70: 72–77.

21 MacHarg, M.A., Bottoms, G.D., Carter, G.K. et al. (1985). Effects of multiple intramuscular injections and doses of dexamethasone on plasma cortisol concentrations and adrenal responses to ACTH in horses. *Am. J. Vet. Res.* 46: 2285–2287.

22 Beltowski, J. and Jamroz, A. (2004). Adrenomedullin–what do we know 10 years since its discovery? *Pol. J. Pharmacol.* 56: 5–27.

23 Boonen, E., Vervenne, H., Meersseman, P. et al. (2013). Reduced cortisol metabolism during critical illness. *N. Engl. J. Med.* 368: 1477–1488.

24 Boonen, E. and Van den Berghe, G. (2016). MECHANISMS IN ENDOCRINOLOGY: new concepts to further unravel adrenal insufficiency during critical illness. *Eur. J. Endocrinol.* 175: R1–R9.

25 Wong, D.M., Young, L., and Dembek, K.A. (2021). Blood thiamine (vitamin B(1)), ascorbic acid (vitamin C), and cortisol concentrations in healthy and ill neonatal foals. *J. Vet. Intern. Med.* 35: 1988–1994.

26 Bradbery, A.N., Coverdale, J.A., Hartz, C.J. et al. (2021). Effect of maternal overnutrition on predisposition to insulin resistance in the foal: maternal parameters and foal pancreas histoarchitecture. *Anim. Reprod. Sci.* 227: 106720.

27 Barsnick, R.J., Hurcombe, S.D., Smith, P.A. et al. (2011). Insulin, glucagon, and leptin in critically ill foals. *J. Vet. Intern. Med.* 25: 123–131.

28 Rings, L.M., Swink, J.M., Dunbar, L.K. et al. (2019). Enteroinsular axis response to carbohydrates and fasting in healthy newborn foals. *J. Vet. Intern. Med.* 33: 2752–2764.

29 Rings, L.M., Kamr, A.M., Kinsella, H.M. et al. (2022). The enteroinsular axis during hospitalization in newborn foals. *Domest. Anim. Endocrinol.* 78: 106686.

30 Kinsella, H.M., Hostnik, L.D., Rings, L.M. et al. (2021). Glucagon, insulin, adrenocorticotropic hormone, and cortisol in response to carbohydrates and fasting in healthy neonatal foals. *J. Vet. Intern. Med.* 35: 550–559.

31 Berryhill, E.H., Magdesian, K.G., Tadros, E.M. et al. (2019). Effects of age on serum glucose and insulin concentrations and glucose/insulin ratios in neonatal foals and their dams during the first 2 weeks postpartum. *Vet. J.* 246: 1–6.

32 Kinsella, H.M., Hostnik, L.D., Snyder, H.A. et al. (2022). Comparison of insulin sensitivity between healthy neonatal foals and horses using minimal model analysis. *PLoS One* 17: e0262584.

33 Fowden, A.L., Silver, M., Ellis, L. et al. (1984). Studies on equine prematurity 3: insulin secretion in the foal during the perinatal period. *Equine Vet. J.* 16: 286–291.

34 Smyth, G.B., Young, D.W., and Duran, S.H. (1993). Maturation of insulin and glucose responses to normal feeding in foals. *Aust. Vet. J.* 70: 129–132.

35 Hoffman, C.J., McKenzie, H.C. 3rd, Furr, M.O. et al. (2015). Glucocorticoid receptor density and binding affinity in healthy horses and horses with systemic inflammatory response syndrome. *J. Vet. Intern. Med.* 29: 626–635.

36 Holdstock, N.B., Allen, V.L., Bloomfield, M.R. et al. (2004). Development of insulin and proinsulin secretion in newborn pony foals. *J. Endocrinol.* 181: 469–476.

37 Holdstock, N.B., Allen, V.L., and Fowden, A.L. (2012). Pancreatic endocrine function in newborn pony foals after induced or spontaneous delivery at term. *Equine Vet. J. Suppl.* 30–37.

38 Fowden, A.L., Gardner, D.S., Ousey, J.C. et al. (2005). Maturation of pancreatic {beta}-cell function in the fetal horse during late gestation. *J. Endocrinol.* 186: 467–473.

39 Dunbar, L.K., Mielnicki, K.A., Dembek, K.A. et al. (2016). Evaluation of four diagnostic tests for insulin dysregulation in adult light-breed horses. *J. Vet. Intern. Med.* 30: 885–891.

40 Muniyappa, R., Lee, S., Chen, H. et al. (2008). Current approaches for assessing insulin sensitivity and resistance in vivo: advantages, limitations, and appropriate usage. *Am. J. Physiol. Endocrinol. Metab.* 294: E15–E26.

41 Fowden, A.L., Forhead, A.J., and Ousey, J.C. (2012). Endocrine adaptations in the foal over the perinatal period. *Equine Vet. J.* 44: 130–139.

42 Fowden, A.L., Forhead, A.J., Bloomfield, M. et al. (1999). Pancreatic alpha cell function in the fetal foal during late gestation. *Exp. Physiol.* 84: 697–705.

43 Uvnas-Moberg, K., Widstrom, A.M., Marchini, G. et al. (1987). Release of GI hormones in mother and infant by sensory stimulation. *Acta Paediatr. Scand.* 76: 851–860.

44 Padidela, R., Patterson, M., Sharief, N. et al. (2009). Elevated basal and post-feed glucagon-like peptide 1 (GLP-1) concentrations in the neonatal period. *Eur. J. Endocrinol.* 160: 53–58.

45 Diaz, M., Garcia-Beltran, C., Lopez-Bermejo, A. et al. (2018). GLP-1 and IGF-I levels are elevated in late infancy in low birth weight infants, independently of GLP-1 receptor polymorphisms and neonatal nutrition. *Int. J. Obes.* 42: 915–918.

46 Berg, E.L., McNamara, D.L., and Keisler, D.H. (2007). Endocrine profiles of periparturient mares and their foals. *J. Anim. Sci.* 85: 1660–1668.

47 Kedzierski, W., Kusy, R., and Kowalik, S. (2011). Plasma leptin level in hyperlipidemic mares and their newborn foals. *Reprod. Domest. Anim.* 46: 275–280.

48 Barsnick, R.J., Hurcombe, S.D., Saville, W.J. et al. (2009). Endocrine Energy Response in septic Foals: Insulin, Leptin and Adiponectin. *ACVIM Forum.*

49 Panzani, S., Comin, A., Galeati, G. et al. (2012). How type of parturition and health status influence hormonal and metabolic profiles in newborn foals. *Theriogenology* 77: 1167–1177.

50 Stewart, F., Goode, J.A., and Allen, W.R. (1993). Growth hormone secretion in the horse: unusual pattern at birth and pulsatile secretion through to maturity. *J. Endocrinol.* 138: 81–89.

51 Barsnick, R.J., Hurcombe, S.D., Dembek, K. et al. (2014). Somatotropic axis resistance and ghrelin in critically ill foals. *Equine Vet. J.* 46: 45–49.

52 Berryhill, E.H., Magdesian, K.G., Kass, P.H. et al. (2017). Triglyceride concentrations in neonatal foals: serial measurement and effects of age and illness. *Vet. J.* 227: 23–29.

53 Ollivett, T.L., Divers, T.J., Cushing, T. et al. (2012). Acute pancreatitis in two five-day-old Appaloosa foals. *Equine Vet. J. Suppl.* 44: 96–99.

54 Pongratz, M.C., Junge, H.K., Riond, B. et al. (2016). Validation of the Accutrend Plus point-of-care triglyceride analyzer in horses, ponies, and donkeys. *J. Vet. Emerg. Crit. Care (San Antonio)* 26: 682–690.

55 Barton, M.H. and LeRoy, B.E. (2007). Serum bile acids concentrations in healthy and clinically ill neonatal foals. *J. Vet. Intern. Med.* 21: 508–513.

56 Myers, C.J., Magdesian, K.G., Kass, P.H. et al. (2009). Parenteral nutrition in neonatal foals: clinical description, complications and outcome in 53 foals (1995–2005). *Vet. J.* 181: 137–144.

57 Oftedal, O.T., Hintz, H.F., and Schryver, H.F. (1983). Lactation in the horse: milk composition and intake by foals. *J. Nutr.* 113: 2096–2106.

58 Jose-Cunilleras, E., Viu, J., Corradini, I. et al. (2012). Energy expenditure of critically ill neonatal foals. *Equine Vet. J. Suppl.* 44: 48–51.

59 Buechner-Maxwell, V.A. (2005). Nutritional support for neonatal foals. *Vet. Clin. North Am. Equine Pract.* 21: 487–510. viii.

60 Stefanovski, D., Robinson, M.A., and Van Eps, A. (2022). Effect of a GLP-1 mimetic on the insulin response to oral sugar testing in horses. *BMC Vet. Res.* 18: 294.

61 Breuhaus, B.A. (2011). Disorders of the equine thyroid gland. *Vet. Clin. North Am. Equine Pract.* 27: 115–128.

62 Lopez-Rodriguez, M.F., Cymbaluk, N.F., Epp, T. et al. (2020). A field study of serum, colostrum, milk iodine, and thyroid hormone concentrations in postpartum draft mares and foals. *J. Equine Vet. Sci.* 90: 103018.

63 Muirhead, T.L., Wichtel, J.J., Stryhn, H. et al. (2010). The selenium and vitamin E status of horses in Prince Edward Island. *Can. Vet. J.* 51: 979–985.

64 Bates, J.M., Spate, V.L., Morris, J.S. et al. (2000). Effects of selenium deficiency on tissue selenium content, deiodinase activity, and thyroid hormone economy in the rat during development. *Endocrinology* 141: 2490–2500.

65 van Maanen, J.M., van Dijk, A., Mulder, K. et al. (1994). Consumption of drinking water with high nitrate levels causes hypertrophy of the thyroid. *Toxicol. Lett.* 72: 365–374.

66 Breuhaus, B.A. (2014). Thyroid function and dysfunction in term and premature equine neonates. *J. Vet. Intern. Med.* 28: 1301–1309.

67 Himler, M., Hurcombe, S.D., Griffin, A. et al. (2012). Presumptive nonthyroidal illness syndrome in critically ill foals. *Equine Vet. J. Suppl.* 44 (Suppl 41): 43–47.

68 Pirrone, A., Panzani, S., Govoni, N. et al. (2013). Thyroid hormone concentrations in foals affected by perinatal asphyxia syndrome. *Theriogenology* 80: 624–629.

69 Malinowski, K., Christensen, R.A., Hafs, H.D. et al. (1996). Age and breed differences in thyroid hormones, insulin-like growth factor (IGF)-I and IGF binding proteins in female horses. *J. Anim. Sci.* 74: 1936–1942.

70 Breuhaus, B.A. (2002). Thyroid-stimulating hormone in adult euthyroid and hypothyroid horses. *J. Vet. Intern. Med.* 16: 109–115.

71 Mendoza, F.J., Perez-Ecija, R.A., Toribio, R.E. et al. (2013). Thyroid hormone concentrations differ between donkeys and horses. *Equine Vet. J.* 45: 214–218.

72 Irvine, C.H. and Evans, M.J. (1975). Postnatal changes in total and free thyroxine and triiodothyronine in foal serum. *J. Reprod. Fertil. Suppl.* 23: 709–715.

73 Newell-Price, J.D.C. and Auchus, R.J. (2020). The adrenal cortex. In: *Williams Textbook of Endocrinology*, 14e (ed. S. Melmed, R.J. Auchus, A.B. Goldfine, et al.), 480–541. Philadelphia: Elsevier.

74 Barrett KE, Barman SM, Boitano S, Brooks HL, Weitz M, Kearns BP, Ganong WF, McGraw-Hill E. Ganong's Review of Medical Physiology. New York: McGraw Hill Education, 2016.

75 Irvine, C.H. (1984). Hypothyroidism in the foal. *Equine Vet. J.* 16: 302–306.

76 Conway, D.A. and Cosgrove, J.S. (1980). Equine goiter. *Irish Vet. J.* 34: 29–31.

77 Drew, B., Barber, W.P., and Williams, D.G. (1975). The effect of excess dietary iodine on pregnant mares and foals. *Vet. Rec.* 97: 93–95.

78 Driscoll, J., Hintz, H.F., and Schryver, H.F. (1978). Goiter in foals caused by excessive iodine. *J. Am. Vet. Med. Assoc.* 173: 858–859.

79 Eroksuz, H., Eroksuz, Y., Ozer, H. et al. (2004). Equine goiter associated with excess dietary iodine. *Vet. Hum. Toxicol.* 46: 147–149.

80 Baker, J.R., Wyn-Jones, G., and Eley, J.L. (1983). Case of equine goitre. *Vet. Rec.* 112: 407–408.

81 Doige, C.E. and McLaughlin, B.G. (1981). Hyperplastic goitre in newborn foals in Western Canada. *Can. Vet. J.* 22: 42–45.

82 Irvine, C.H. and Evans, M.J. (1977). Hypothyroidism in foals. *N. Z. Vet. J.* 25: 354.

83 McLaughlin, B.G., Doige, C.E., Fretz, P.B. et al. (1981). Carpal bone lesions associated with angular limb deformities in foals. *J. Am. Vet. Med. Assoc.* 178: 224–230.

84 McLaughlin, B.G., Doige, C.E., and McLaughlin, P.S. (1986). Thyroid-hormone levels in foals with congenital musculoskeletal lesions. *Can. Vet. J.* 27: 264–267.

85 Shaver, J.R., Fretz, P.B., and Doige, C.E. (1979). Skeletal manifestations of suspected hypothyroidism in two foals. *J. Equine Med. Surg.* 3: 269.

86 Vivrette, S.L., Reimers, T.J., and Krook, L. (1984). Skeletal disease in a hypothyroid foal. *Cornell Vet.* 74: 373–386.

87 Murray, M.J. (1990). Hypothyroidism and respiratory insufficiency in a neonatal foal. *J. Am. Vet. Med. Assoc.* 197: 1635–1638.

88 McLaughlin, B.G. and Doige, C.E. (1982). A study of ossification of carpal and tarsal bones in normal and hypothyroid foals. *Can. Vet. J.* 23: 164–168.

89 McLaughlin, B.G. and Doige, C.E. (1981). Congenital musculoskeletal lesions and hyperplastic goitre in foals. *Can. Vet. J.* 22: 130–133.

90 Allen, A.L. (2014). Congenital hypothyroidism in horses: looking back and looking ahead. *Equine Vet. Educ.* 26: 190–193.

91 Koikkalainen, K., Knuuttila, A., Karikoski, N. et al. (2014). Congenital hypothyroidism and dysmaturity syndrome in foals: first reported cases in Europe. *Equine Vet. Educ.* 26: 181–189.

92 Muller, V., Toribio, R.E., Dembek, K. et al. (2020). Serum cortisol and thyroid hormone concentrations and survival in foals born from mares with experimentally induced ascending placentitis. *J. Vet. Intern. Med.* 34: 1332–1338.

93 Toribio, R.E. (2018). Thyroid gland. In: *Equine Internal Medicine*, 4e (ed. S.M. Reed, W.M. Bayly, and D.C. Sellon), 1058–1069. St. Louis, Missouri: Elsevier.

94 Hilderbran, A.C., Breuhaus, B.A., and Refsal, K.R. (2014). Nonthyroidal illness syndrome in adult horses. *J. Vet. Intern. Med.* 28: 609–617.

95 Komosa, M., Flisinska-Bojanowska, A., and Gill, J. (1990). Development of diurnal rhythm in some metabolic parameters in foals. *Comp. Biochem. Physiol. A Comp. Physiol.* 95: 549–552.

96 Boosinger, T.R., Brendemuehl, J.P., Bransby, D.L. et al. (1995). Prolonged gestation, decreased triiodothyronine concentration, and thyroid gland histomorphologic features in newborn foals of mares grazing Acremonion coenophialum-infected fescue. *Am. J. Vet. Res.* 56: 66–69.

97 Mendoza, F.J., Toribio, R.E., and Perez-Ecija, A. (2019). Metabolic and endocrine disorders in donkeys. *Vet. Clin. North Am. Equine Pract.* 35: 399–417.

98 Breuhaus, B.A. (2020). Thyroid gland: congenital hypothyroidism in foals. In: *Large Animal Internal Medicine*, 6e (ed. B.P.V.M. Smith, D.C. Van Metre, and N. Pusterla), 1368. Elsevier.

99 (U.S.) NRC, Horses CoNRo (2007). *Nutrient Requirements of Horses*, 6e. Washington, D.C: National Academies Press.

100 Hollis, A.R., Boston, R.C., and Corley, K.T. (2008). Plasma aldosterone, vasopressin and atrial natriuretic peptide in hypovolaemia: a preliminary comparative

study of neonatal and mature horses. *Equine Vet. J.* 40: 64–69.

101 Dembek, K.A., Onasch, K., Hurcombe, S.D. et al. (2013). Association of hyperlactatemia with aldosterone and arginine vasopressin concentrations and clinical indicators of hypoperfusion in hospitalized foals. *J. Vet. Intern. Med.* 27: 655–656.

102 Annane, D., Renault, A., Brun-Buisson, C. et al. (2018). Hydrocortisone plus fludrocortisone for adults with septic shock. *N. Engl. J. Med.* 378: 809–818.

103 Hurcombe, S.D., Toribio, R.E., Slovis, N. et al. (2008). Blood arginine vasopressin, adrenocorticotropin hormone, and cortisol concentrations at admission in septic and critically ill foals and their association with survival. *J. Vet. Intern. Med.* 22: 639–647.

104 Dembek, K.A., Hurcombe, S.D., Stewart, A.J. et al. (2016). Association of aldosterone and arginine vasopressin concentrations and clinical markers of hypoperfusion in neonatal foals. *Equine Vet. J.* 48: 176–181.

105 Borchers, A., Magdesian, K.G., Schenck, P.A. et al. (2014). Serial plasma vasopressin concentration in healthy and hospitalised neonatal foals. *Equine Vet. J.* 46: 306–310.

106 Toth, B., Slovis, N.M., Constable, P.D. et al. (2014). Plasma adrenomedullin concentrations in critically ill neonatal foals. *J. Vet. Intern. Med.* 28: 1294–1300.

107 Giordano, A., Castagnetti, C., Panzani, S. et al. (2015). Endothelin 1 in healthy foals and in foals affected by neonatal diseases. *Theriogenology* 84: 667–673.

108 Toribio, R.E. (2018). Disorders of calcium and phosphorus. In: *Equine Internal Medicine*, 4e (ed. S.M. Reed, W.M. Bayly, and D.C. Sellon), 1029–1052. St. Louis, Missouri: Elsevier.

109 Toribio, R.E. (2018). Magnesium and disease. In: *Equine Internal Medicine*, 4e (ed. S.M. Reed, W.M. Bayly, and D.C. Sellon), 1052–1058. St. Louis, Missouri: Elsevier.

110 Hurcombe, S.D., Toribio, R.E., Slovis, N.M. et al. (2009). Calcium regulating hormones and serum calcium and magnesium concentrations in septic and critically ill foals and their association with survival. *J. Vet. Intern. Med.* 23: 335–343.

111 Kamr, A.M., Dembek, K.A., Reed, S.M. et al. (2015). Vitamin D metabolites and their association with calcium, phosphorus, and PTH concentrations, severity of illness, and mortality in hospitalized equine neonates. *PLoS One* 10: e0127684.

112 Kamr, A.M., Dembek, K.A., Hildreth, B.E. et al. (2018). The FGF-23/klotho axis and its relationship with phosphorus, calcium, vitamin D, PTH, aldosterone, severity of disease, and outcome in hospitalised foals. *Equine Vet. J.* 50: 739–746.

113 Toribio, R.E., Kohn, C.W., Chew, D.J. et al. (2001). Comparison of serum parathyroid hormone and ionized calcium and magnesium concentrations and fractional urinary clearance of calcium and phosphorus in healthy horses and horses with enterocolitis. *Am. J. Vet. Res.* 62: 938–947.

114 Rivas, V.N., Magdesian, K.G., Fagan, S. et al. (2020). A nonsense variant in Rap Guanine Nucleotide Exchange Factor 5 (RAPGEF5) is associated with equine familial isolated hypoparathyroidism in Thoroughbred foals. *PLos Genet.* 16: e1009028.

115 Pozza, M.E., Kaewsakhorn, T., Trinarong, C. et al. (2014). Serum vitamin D, calcium, and phosphorus concentrations in ponies, horses and foals from the United States and Thailand. *Vet. J.* 199: 451–456.

116 Kamr, A.M., Dembek, K.A., Gilsenan, W. et al. (2020). C-terminal telopeptide of type I collagen, osteocalcin, alkaline phosphatase, and parathyroid hormone in healthy and hospitalized foals. *Domest. Anim. Endocrinol.* 72: 106470.

117 DiBartola, S.P. and Willard, M.D. (2005). Disorders of phosphorus: hypophosphatemia and hyperphosphatemia. In: *Fluid, Electrolyte and Acid-Base Disorders in Small Animal Practice*, 3e (ed. S. DiBartola), 195–209. Philadelphia, PA: Elsevier Saunders.

118 Berlin, D. and Aroch, I. (2009). Concentrations of ionized and total magnesium and calcium in healthy horses: effects of age, pregnancy, lactation, pH and sample type. *Vet. J.* 181: 305–311.

119 Mariella, J., Isani, G., Andreani, G. et al. (2016). Total plasma magnesium in healthy and critically ill foals. *Theriogenology* 85: 180–185.

120 Toribio, R.E. (2019). Equine neonatal encephalopathy: facts, evidence, and opinions. *Vet. Clin. North Am. Equine Pract.* 35: 363–378.

121 Kinsella, H.M. Hostnik, L.D., and Toribio, R.E. (2022). Energy endocrine physiology, pathophysiology, and nutrition of the foal. *J. Am. Vet. Med. Assoc.* 260(S3): S83–S93.

Neonatal Urinary System

Chapter 22 Embryology and Anatomy of the Urogenital System

David Wong, Eric Rowe, and Rebecca Ruby

Embryology of the Urogenital System

Minimal information is available regarding the development of the equine fetal kidney and urinary system; thus, much of the knowledge concerning embryology of the kidney and other components of the urinary system in the equine fetus is garnered from other species. In overview, the development of the urogenital system starts from the nephrogenic cord that divides into nephrotomes. This subsequently gives rise to pronephric and then mesonephric (transitory) kidneys. The metanephric kidneys then appear as permanent organs from the metanephrogenic mass (mesenchymal component) that contributes to nephron formation and the ureteric bud (epithelial component) that produces the collecting ducts, calices, renal pelvis, and ureter [1]. A more detailed yet general description of this process follows. The reader is directed to more comprehensive descriptions of the embryogenesis of the urogenital system if further information is desired [1, 2].

The urinary system originates from the dorsal body wall of the developing embryo as a longitudinal elevation of intermediate mesoderm referred to as the urogenital ridge. This ridge flanks the aorta on both sides and gives rise to the urinary (nephrogenic ridge or cord) and gonadal (gential ridge) systems (Figure 22.1). The intermediate mesoderm initially divides into a metameric set of cell masses called nephrotomes in the cervical and thoracolumbar regions [1]. Early in gestation, the primitive kidneys (pronephroi, pleural of pronephros) are noted as elevations along the cervical region of the developing embryo [2]. These structures are transitory and nonfunctional, composed of epithelial buds that extend ventromedially and pronephric ducts that extend caudally. As gestation progresses, the rudimentary pronephroi degenerate while the pronephric ducts persist and become incorporated into the second set of kidneys, mesonephros, and become the mesonephric (Wolffian) duct (Figure 22.2) [2]. These mesonephroi are functional until the permanent kidneys develop. Mesonephric tubules begin to emerge on either side of the vertebral column along the length of the mesonephric ducts [2]. The cranial tubules regress while the remaining caudal tubules form cup-like pouches that extend medially toward loops of capillaries that originate from the aorta. Collectively, these structures eventually form the renal corpuscle that consist of the cup-like glomerular capsule and capillary plexus.

Further through gestation, the metanephroi (definitive kidneys) begin to develop from the metanephric diverticulum (ureteric bud) and the metanephrogenic mass (Figures 22.2 and 22.4). The metanephric diverticulum begins as an outgrowth from the caudal part of the mesonephric duct near the cloaca. As the metanephric divertculum becomes larger, they invade the metanephrogenic mass. Penetration of the metanephric mesenchyme results in repetitive branching of the metanephric diverticulum, which eventually forms the renal collecting ducts, calyces, renal pelvis, and ureter (Figure 22.3). The distal portion of the diverticulum induces the metanephric mesenchyme to condense, thereby forming the metanephric vesicles [2]. These vesicles subsequently develop into a series of metanephric tubules, which develop into the nephron (glomerulus, proximal and distal convoluted tubules, and the nephron loop [descending and ascending loops]). The metanephroi begin to function as the distal convoluted tubule adjoins the collecting tubule. During this time in gestation, the number of glomeruli continue to increase, forming approximately 10 million nephrons in each kidney in the newborn foal [3]. In most species, nephrogenesis stops by or shortly after birth, with further nephron maturation occurring postnatally.

The fetal kidneys then begin to ascend from the pelvic region up alongside both sides of the aorta, where they reach their final destination along the dorsal abdominal wall in the lumbar region. As the kidneys move toward

Equine Neonatal Medicine, First Edition. Edited by David M. Wong and Pamela A. Wilkins.

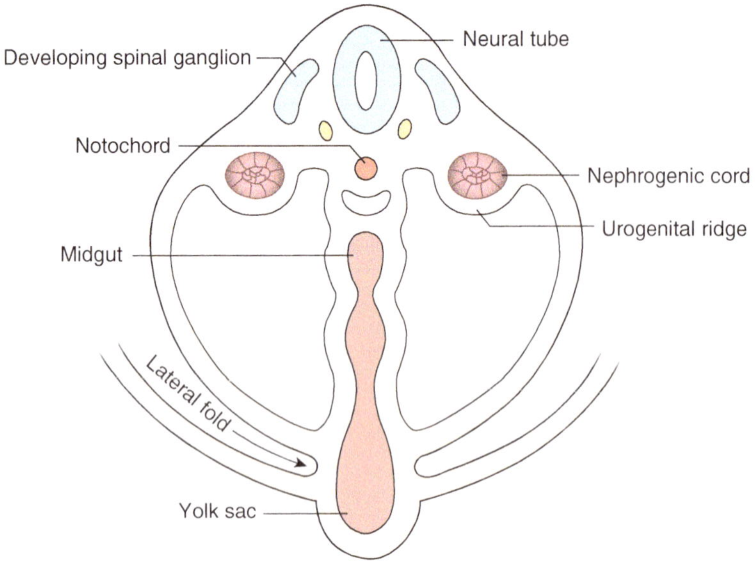

Figure 22.1 Transverse section demonstrating development of the urogenital ridge from the intermediate mesoderm.

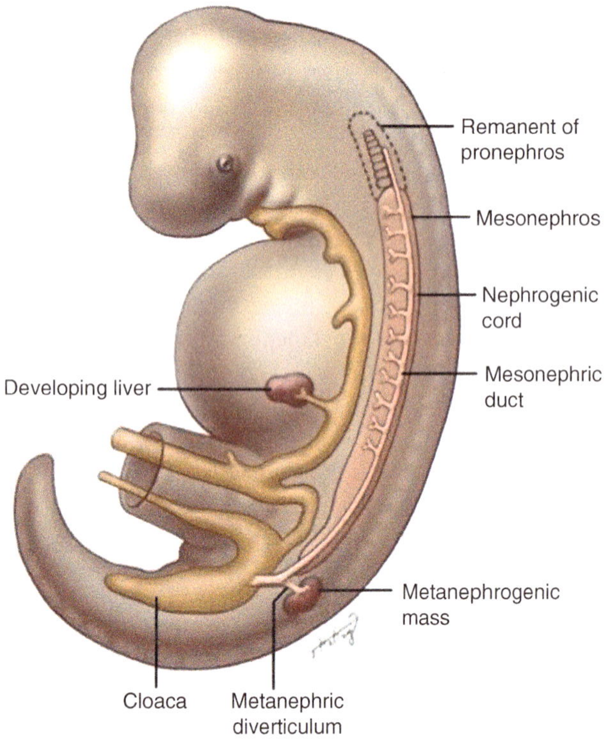

Figure 22.2 Drawing of the development of the nephric system. Lateral drawing of an embryo showing the different stages of kidney development.

their permanent location, the original blood supply (common iliac arteries) disappears and is replaced by the primary arterial supply originating from the abdominal aorta (e.g. renal artery). However, accessory renal arteries arising from the caudal mesenteric, testicular, ovarian, or deep circumflex iliac artery may remain [4].

The urinary bladder is formed as a dilated proximal portion of the allantois and is separated from the hindgut by a craniocaudal growth of the urorectal septum (Figure 22.4) [5, 6]. This septum divides the rectum from the urogenital sinus; the latter structure eventually develops into part of the urinary bladder and all of the urethra. Prior to this separation, the shared space for the developing hindgut and urogenital sinus is the cloaca. In early development, the cloaca is closed by the cloacal membrane, necessitating an alternate route for urine elimination because both the mesonephric and metanephric kidneys are producing urine. This is where the urachus (the intraembryonic part of the allantoic stalk) and allantoic stalk provide the route of urine elimination. After separation of the cloaca by the urorectal septum, the cloacal membrane persists for a time as the urogenital and anal membranes until they both eventually breakdown. After that time, urine can exit through the urogenital sinus.

In the process of development, the metanephric diverticulum (future ureter) does not directly enter the future site of the urinary bladder; instead, it is connected by the mesonephric duct (Figure 22.4) [5]. The metanephric diverticulum is incorporated into the urogenital sinus by growth and expansion of the sinus. Both the mesonephric duct and metanephric diverticulum are now directly opening into the site of the future caudal bladder and cranial urethra, respectively. Differential growth in the dorsal wall of the urogenital sinus will bring the metanephric diverticulum (ureter) into the bladder and move the mesonephric duct (ductus deferens of the male) into the urethra. Failure of this process to occur can result in an ectopic ureter.

The fate of the mesonephric tubules and mesonephric ducts varies based on the sex of the fetus. In both sexes,

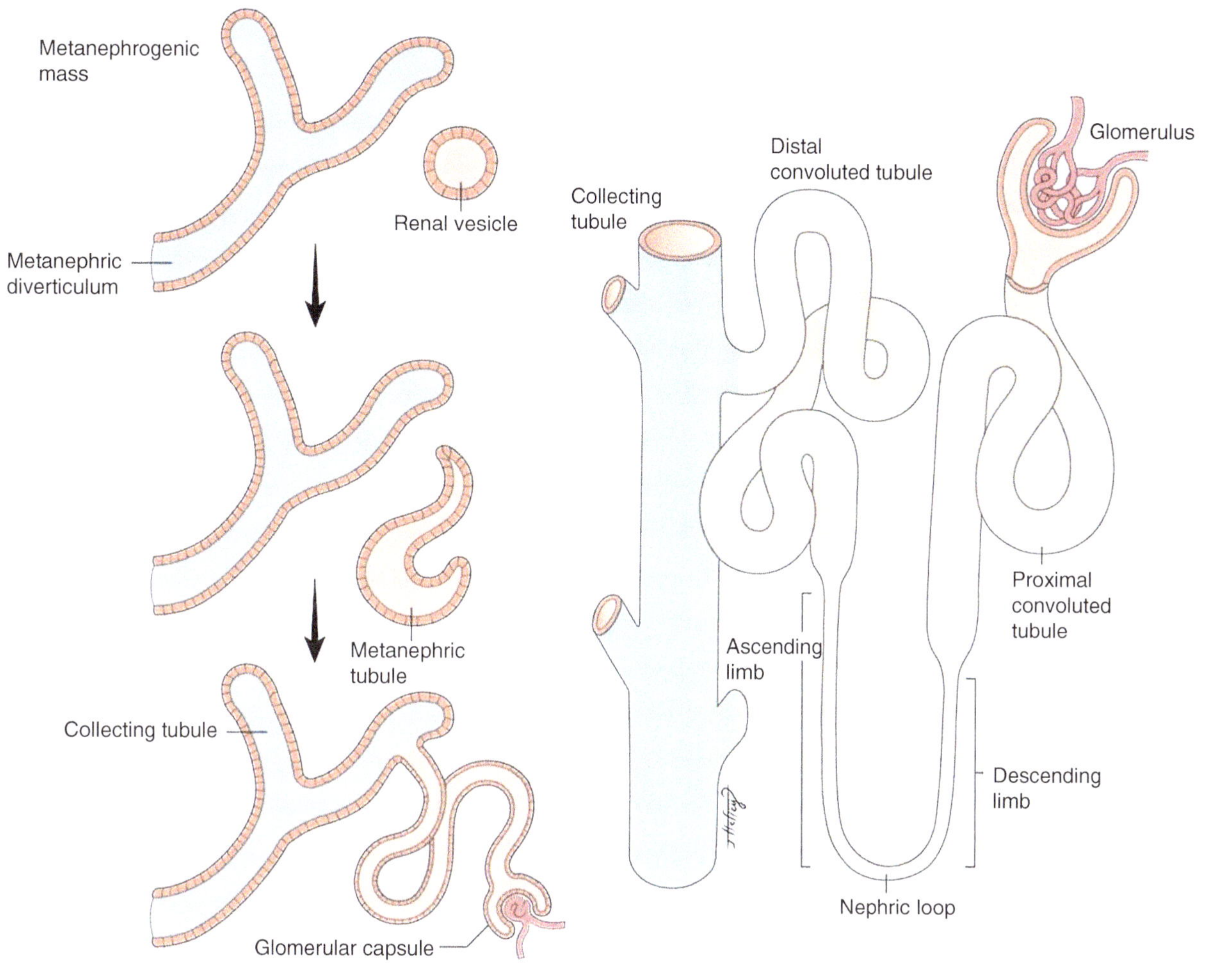

Figure 22.3 Metanephros development from the metanephric diverticulum and metanephrogenic mass with the final adult nephron shown on the right. The collecting duct is derived from the diverticulum, while the remainder of the nephron from the mass. *Source:* Adapted from Noden and De Lahunta.

paired paramesonephric ducts (Mullerian ducts) arise and parallel the mesonephric ducts. In the male fetus, sexual differentiation of the gonads and resultant production of anti-Mullerian hormone and androgenic hormones results in regression of the paramesonephric ducts [4]. The duct system of the male reproductive tract is appropriated from the mesonephros and mesonephric (Wolffian) ducts. In addition, androgenic steroids stimulate these structures to develop into the ductus deferens, epididymis, and seminiferous tubules. In comparison, in the female fetus, the paired paramesonephric ducts fuse distally to form the vagina and uterine body while proximally they remain separate to become the uterine horns and oviducts [4].

As noted, minimal information is available regarding the development of the urinary system in the fetal foal. Histologically, equine nephrons are similar to other mammals, but the diameter and epithelial height of the tubule and collecting ducts are comparatively larger [4]. In one study involving 16 equine fetuses and 20 foals, the volume of the kidney was documented to increase both pre- and postnatally until 50–90 weeks of postnatal life [3]. Nephrogenesis, in terms of glomerular number, increased prenatally and appeared to be complete by 30–40 weeks of gestation in pony fetuses [3]. In Thoroughbred fetuses, the glomerular number continued to increase up to birth [3]. This study estimated that the equine kidney has approximately 10 million glomeruli/kidney (20 million total in both kidneys) [3]. Another small study involving Thoroughbred foals with intrauterine growth retardation (IUGR) noted microanatomical deficits such as deficiency in glomerular volume in the kidneys of affected foals [7]. Only six foals with IUGR were evaluated, but it is possible that there is altered or deficient organogenesis in foals with IUGR that might explain some of the physiological incompetence noted in affected foals [7]. A different study documented the glucogenic capacity of the fetal kidney (and

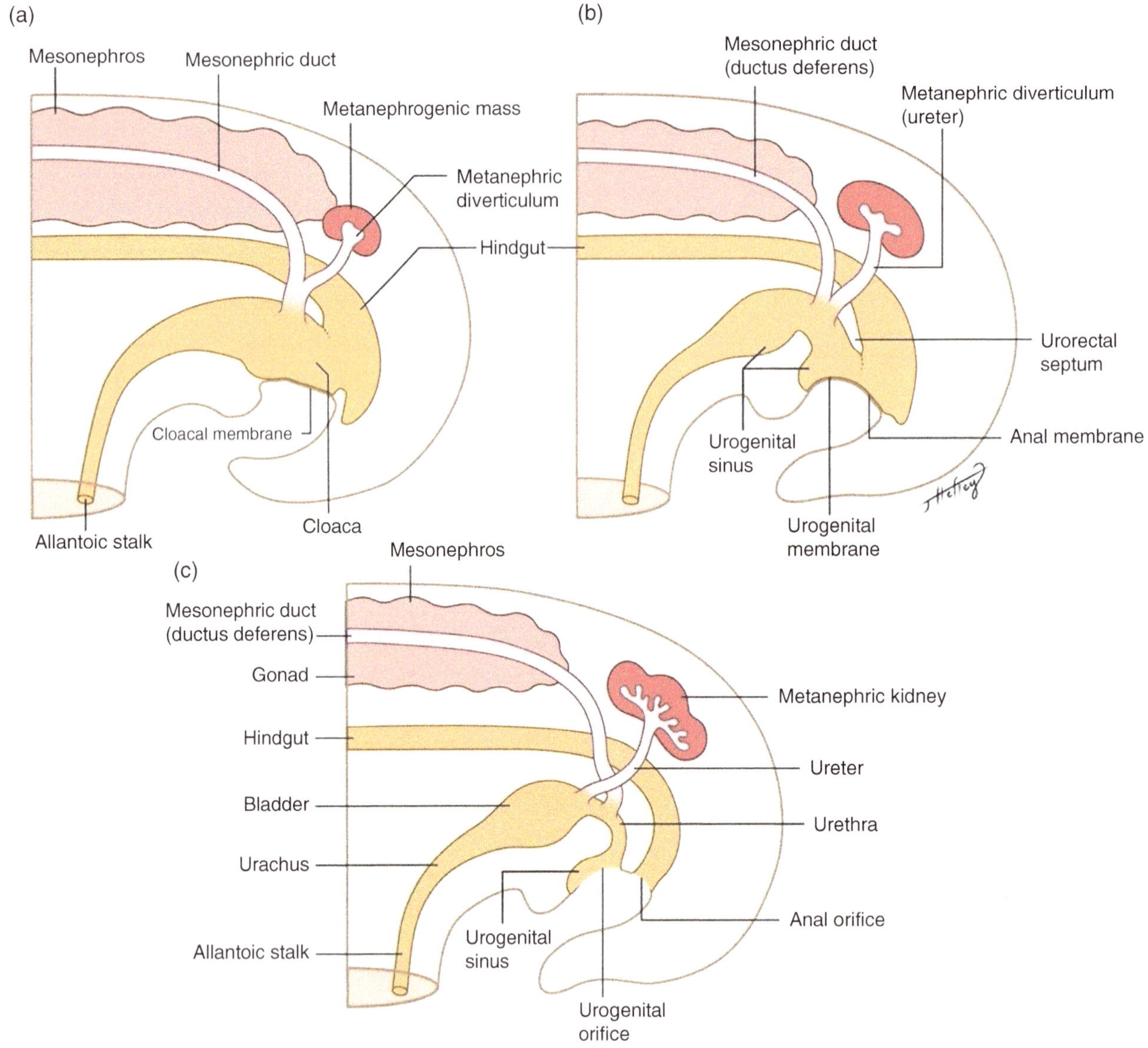

Figure 22.4 Illustrations demonstrating the separation of the urogenital sinus and rectum, incorporation of the ureter into the bladder, and transposition of the ureter and ductus deferens. (a), (b), and (c) occur at different time points in development, with (a) being earlier and (c) later. *Source:* Adapted from Noden and De Lahunta.

liver) and measured activity of glucose-6-phosphate, fructose diphosphatase, phosphoenolpyruvate carboxykinase, aspartate transferase, and alanine transferase from the fetal kidney and liver as early as 100 days gestation in equine fetuses [8].

Anatomy of the Kidney

The newborn foal's kidneys (Figure 22.5) are located retroperitoneally along the dorsal abdominal wall and weigh approximately 175 g in the average newborn foal, as compared to 500–600 g in the adult horse [4, 9, 10]. The foal's kidney can exhibit some internal lobations, but these lobations are not present in the adult horse kidney [11]. In the horse, the right kidney is further cranial than the left kidney and is horseshoe-shaped; the right kidney is located just below the dorsal extent of the last two to three ribs and the first lumbar transverse process and embedded within the liver. Much of the right kidney's ventral surface is attached to the base of the cecum in the horse with the pancreas noted medially and the caudal pole contacting the descending duodenum [12]. The left kidney is more elongated than the right and is located further caudal than the right kidney and can be palpated rectally in adult horses. The kidneys' blood vessels, nerves, lymphatics, and renal pelvis are located on the medial aspect of each kidney and enter and exit at an indentation called the hilus. Retroperitoneal connective tissue is formed around the

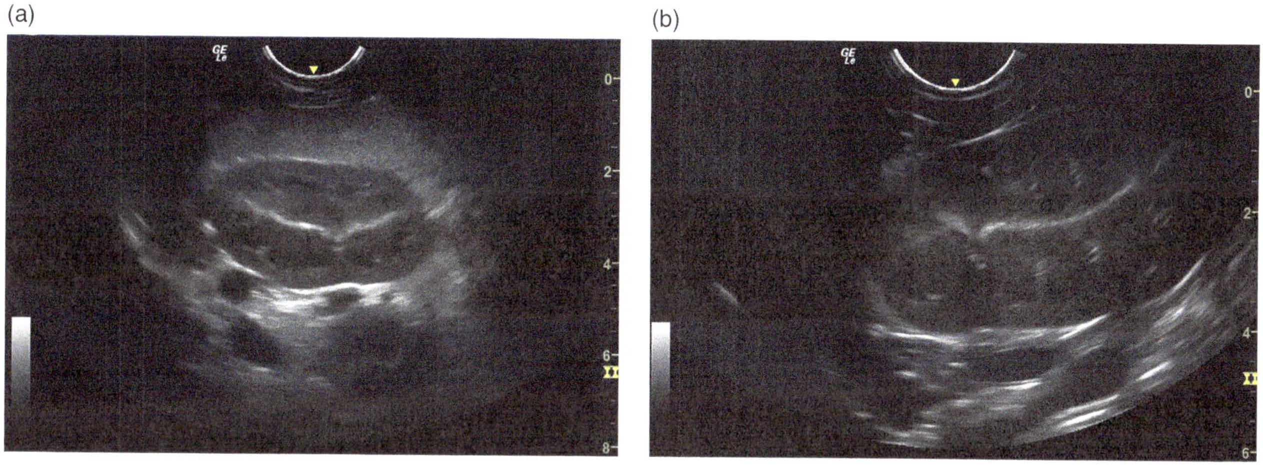

Figure 22.5 Ultrasonographic images of the left (a) and right (b) kidneys in a neonatal foal. Note the spleen between the body wall and kidney when imaging the left kidney.

kidneys and forms layers of fascia and adipose tissue. The renal capsule is a smooth fibrous layer that encapsulates the kidney and is in immediate contact and tightly fitted to the underlying kidney parenchyma. Around the renal capsule is perirenal fat. As noted, the arterial blood supply to the kidneys originates from the abdominal aorta via the renal arteries. As the renal arteries course toward the kidneys, these vessels give off various nonrenal branches that perfuse the renal capsule and ureters. The renal veins arise from a number of small branches exiting the renal hilum that eventually converge on the caudal vena cava [2]. The lymphatic drainage from the kidneys and ureters consolidate into the lumbar lymph nodes.

The equine kidneys receive approximately 22% of the cardiac output of which 90% is directed toward the cortex and the remaining 10% toward the medulla [11]. Because of this high blood flow, the kidneys appear brownish red due to the extensive blood volume that passes through the network of vessels. In cross-section of the kidney, two obvious sections are visible: the inner medulla (approximately 45% of the area of the kidney) and the outer cortex that is slightly wider (slightly >50%) in the horse (Figure 22.6) [4].

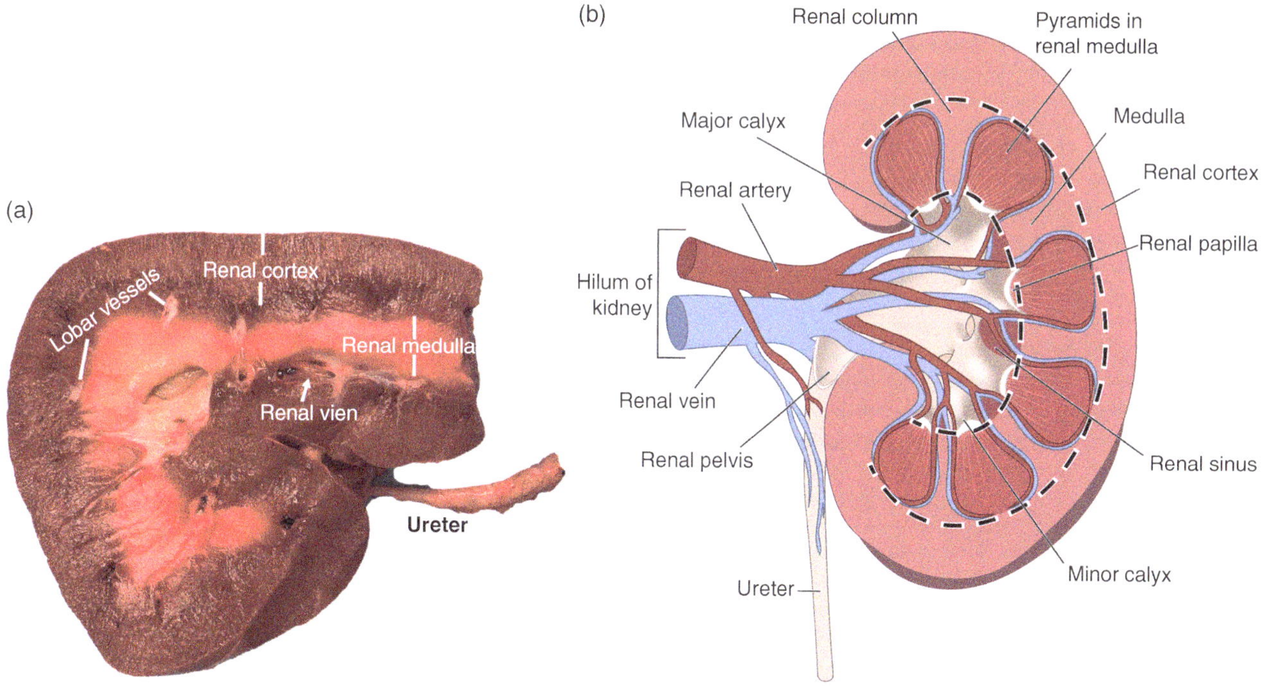

Figure 22.6 Postmortem (a) and schematic (b) images of the kidney from a horse noting some of the gross anatomical details of the kidney.

In one study, the proportional volumes of the renal structural subcomponents, namely the cortex, medulla, and renal pelvis, were determined as 54.0, 44.1, and 1.9, and 57.1, 41.4, and 1.5 in the right and left adult kidneys, respectively [9]. The cortex contains the initial portion of the nephron called renal corpuscles along with various segments of the tubule system (convoluted and straight tubules, collecting tubules, collecting ducts). The medulla is composed of primarily tubules and ducts that are surrounded by interstitium and drain urine toward the renal pelvis. In horses, the corticomedullary junction is less obvious than other species but is a deep red color, in contrast to the paler medulla and red-brown cortex (Figure 22.6). Cortical nephrons are located more superficially in the cortex and have short tubular loops that make a shallow dive into the medulla. In comparison, juxtamedullary nephrons are located deep in the cortex (near the corticomedullary junction) and their tubules extend deep into the medulla. In people, the cortical nephrons comprise approximately 75% of the nephrons and have a primary role in filtration of plasma whereas the juxtaglomerular nephrons are important for concentrating or diluting urine. The medulla contains structures similar to the cortex but are referred to as part of the medulla. Within the medulla are straight tubules and collecting ducts that are accompanied by a capillary network oriented in parallel to the tubules and ducts called the vasa recta. The equine kidney consist of 40–60 pyramids, which are subdivisions of the renal parenchyma (cone-shaped arrangement of renal tubules in the medulla), and are arranged in four parallel rows [4]. At the tip of each pyramid is the papilla that projects into the renal pelvis and consists of large collecting ducts (ducts of Bellini) [10]. The corticomedullary junction undulates along renal pyramids and renal columns.

The structural and functional unit of the kidney is the nephron, which is responsible for producing urine and is composed of a renal corpuscle and renal tubule. The renal corpuscle is composed of the glomerulus within Bowman's capsule and has a vascular pole that includes an afferent and efferent arteriole and a urinary pole in which the proximal tubule arises (Figure 22.7). The glomerulus is composed of capillary endothelial cells, visceral epithelial cells, mesangial cells, intercellular matrix, and a basement membrane [10]. The glomerular capillary endothelial cells have fenestrae (pores) while the visceral epithelial cells contain podocytes (foot-like processes) that extend to the basement membrane. The spaces between the podocytes are filtration slits where final plasma filtration occurs [10]. These components (endothelial cells, podocytes, slit pores) are covered with negative charges that serve to repel the passage of large negatively charged molecules such as proteins. Mesangial cells serve to provide structural support to the glomerulus but are not part of the filtration barrier. The proximal tubule consists of cuboidal cells with striated cytoplasm on the basal side and a brush border on the luminal side. The proximal tubule straightens out and continues as the loop of Henle (intermediate tubule), distal tubule, connecting tubule, and collecting ducts (cortical, outer medullary, and inner medullary collecting ducts). More specifically, the proximal convoluted tubule has a tortuous course through the renal cortex and then enters the medulla as the thick descending limb of the loop of Henle. The tubule continues as the thin descending limb, makes a hairpin turn, and traverse back toward the cortex as the thin ascending limb. As it enters the cortex, it transitions to the thick ascending limb of the loop of Henle and subsequently contacts the vascular pole of its renal corpuscle. Here the epithelial cells of the tubule near the afferent arteriole of the glomerulus are modified to form the macula densa. Continuing, the tubule forms the distal convoluted tubule, then the connecting tubule, which then empties into the collecting duct (Figure 22.3). The collecting ducts form minor calyces that are then followed by major calyces; the major calyces join the renal pelvis, which eventually flows into the ureter.

At the junction of the thick ascending loop of Henle and the distal convoluted tubule is the juxtaglomerular apparatus, which consists of a vascular component (afferent and efferent arterioles, extraglomerular mesangium) and the macula densa (Figure 22.7) [13]. Tubuloglomerular feedback is a mechanism by which the kidney regulates blood flow and glomerular filtration rate (GFR) to nephrons and ultimately influences extracellular fluid and sodium balance. In short, the composition of the tubular fluid at the juxtaglomerular apparatus are sensed by the macula densa; because fluid composition in the distal tubule is a function of GFR, an increase in sodium, potassium, and chloride indicates elevated GFR. When this is sensed by the mucula densa, it increases extracellular adenosine concentrations thereby causing vasoconstriction of the afferent arteriole and decreases renin release, thereby decreasing GFR [10]. Conversely, decreased concentrations of sodium and chloride in the distal tubule results in increased interstitial prostaglandins which increases renin release, ultimately resulting in increased aldosterone and vasopressin concentrations that facilitate renal sodium and water resorption [10].

As noted, urine produced in the kidney flows into the dilated proximal portion of the ureter called the renal pelvis. In the horse, two tubular terminal recesses enter the relatively small renal pelvis [12]. Urine departs the renal pelvis via the proximal ureter, and in the horse, these structures (renal pelvis, ureter) are lined with mucous glands and goblet cells that secret a thick viscous mucus; this mucus is commonly observed in the urine of healthy horses. Urine travels down the ureters with the distal

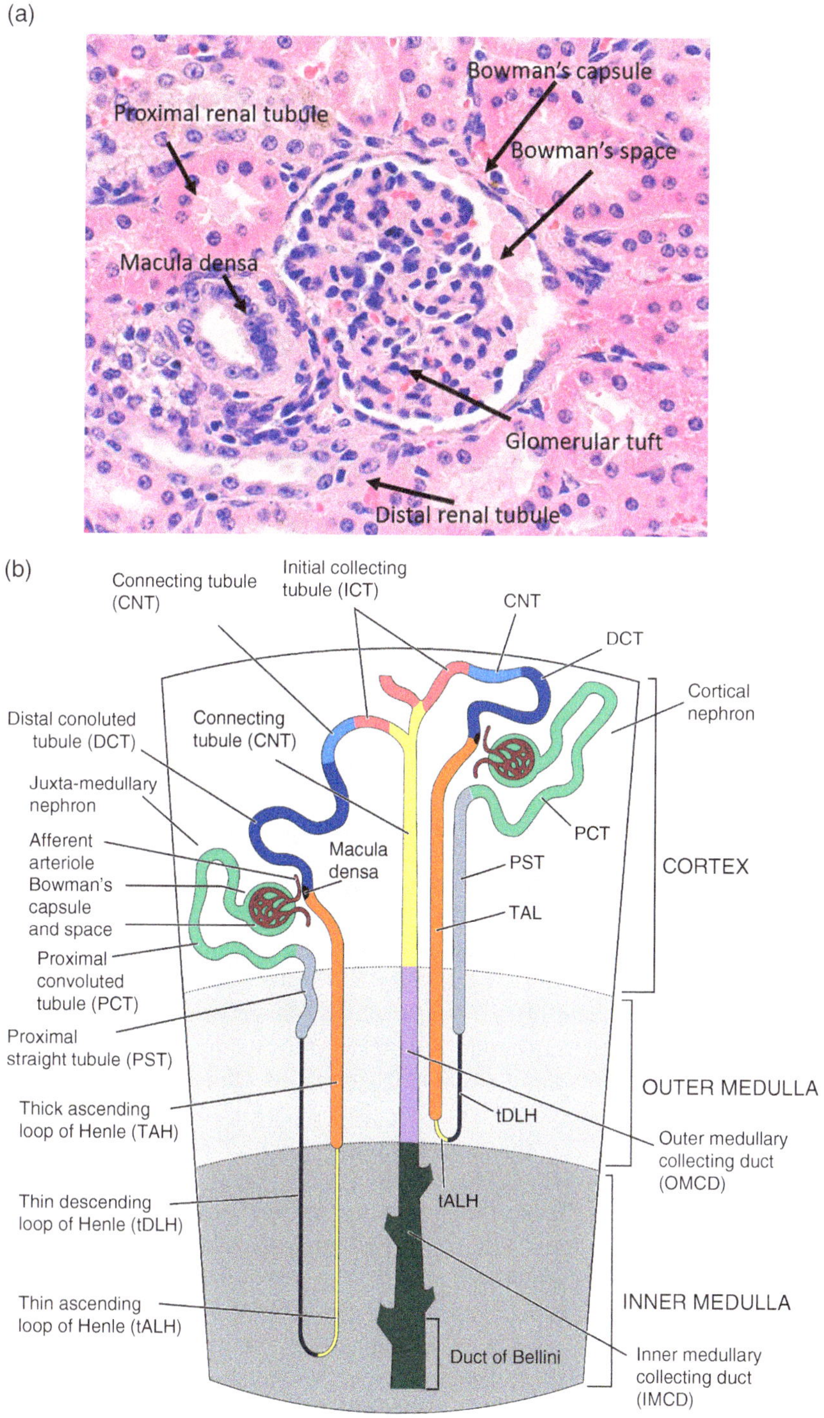

Figure 22.7 Microscopic (a) and schematic (b) anatomy of the kidney nephron demonstrating the glomerulus and various components of the tubule system in the neonatal foal.

portion of the ureter coursing within the bladder wall [4]. This anatomic arrangement helps create a one-way valve to prevent vesicoureteral reflux when the bladder becomes distended. The bladder consists of the cranial blind end (apex), the body of the bladder, and the neck (caudal end leading to the urethra). The bladder is located on the pelvic floor and in the foal, is attached to the ventral abdominal wall via the urachus and the remnants of the paired umbilical arteries, giving the bladder an elongated form [10]. In utero, the urachus is a tubular connection between the primitive bladder and the allantoic sac. As the foal ages, these structures become the median ligament (urachus) and lateral and round ligaments (umbilical arteries) of the bladder.

Blood enters the hilus of the kidney via the renal artery and undergoes a series of divisions to supply the glomeruli. The renal artery divides into the interlobar arteries that enter the parenchyma between adjacent lobes and radiate toward the cortex. At the corticomedullary junction, each interlobar artery gives rise to the arcuate arteries, which run between the cortex and medulla [12]. Arcuate arteries give rise to interlobular arteries that enter the cortex and traverse toward the renal capsule [12]. The afferent arterioles that supply blood to individual glomeruli arise from branches of the cortical interlobular arteries [11]. Blood enters and exits the glomeruli via the afferent and efferent arteriole, respectively; both afferent and efferent arterioles play a critical role in maintaining glomerular perfusion pressure and GFR. Of note, efferent arterioles from juxtamedullary nephrons descend into the medulla via the vasa recta, which are unique bundles of vessels that form a second capillary network around the tubules (peritubular capillaries) [10, 11]. The vasa recta comprise part of the countercurrent mechanism that is vital for water reabsorption, solute exchange, and maintenance of a hyperosmotic medullary interstitium. Blood then leaves the kidney via the renal vein at the hilus of each kidney. The kidney therefore has two capillary networks, glomerular and peritubular, that are arranged in series: the high hydrostatic pressure of the glomerular capillaries promotes fluid filtration as compared to the low hydrostatic pressure of the peritubular capillaries that allows fluid and electrolyte reabsorption [10].

The kidneys receive neural input from the sympathetic nervous system that originates from the thoracolumbar spinal cord via the aorticorenal and celiacomesenteric ganglia [10]. These nerve fibers form the renal plexus along the renal arteries [2]. The autonomic innervation to the kidney controls blood flow (regulates vascular resistance), controls tubular cell function, activates the juxtaglomerular cells (renin secretion), and sets the sensitivity of the tubuloglomerular feedback [10]. Renal blood flow is complex and dependent on cardiac output and regulation via a number of extrinsic and intrinsic factors (Table 22.1). Extrinsic factors include the sympathetic nerves, typically via circulating catecholamines; when sympathetic nerve fibers are stimulated (e.g., excitement, shock), vasoconstriction occurs, and thus renal blood flow and GFR decrease. Other circulating hormones that can cause vasoconstriction of the renal vasculature include angiotensin II, vasopressin, and endothelin I [11]. In comparison to these extrinsic factors, intrinsic factors include autoregulation via the afferent and efferent arterioles that control blood flow by myogenic responses and tubuloglomerular feedback [11]. There appears to be minimal parasympathetic innervation to the kidney.

Table 22.1 Vasoactive factors that impact renal blood flow and glomerular filtration rate [10].

Vasodilators	Vasoconstrictors
Acetylcholine	Epinephrine
Dopamine	Norepinephrine
Prostaglandin E2, I2	Vasopressin
Natriuretic peptides	Angiotensin II
Nitric oxide	Endothelin I
Bradykinin	Thromboxane

Autonomic innervation of the ureters, bladder, and urethra is also important to facilitate ureteral peristalsis and micturition. The ureteral smooth muscle receives sympathetic (celiac ganglion), and parasympathetic (pelvic nerve) innervation and the horse has both α_1- and β_2-adrenoreceptors that cause contraction and relaxation, respectively when stimulated by norepinephrine. The urinary bladder is innervated by the hypogastric nerve (sympathetic nerve supply) with preganglionic fibers arising from lumbar spinal segments L1–L4 to synapse in the caudal mesenteric ganglion [10]. Postganglionic fibers supply the bladder (β_2-adrenergic receptors) and proximal urethra (mainly α_1-, some α_2-adrenergic receptors). In horses, β_2-adrenergic receptors are noted throughout the bladder and induce detrusor muscle relaxation, which allows bladder filling; α_1-adrenoreceptors (to a lesser extent α_2-adrenoreceptors) are noted throughout the internal urethral sphincter and induce contraction and continence. The sacral segments of the spinal cord provide the parasympathetic innervation to the urinary bladder via the pelvic nerve. Striated muscle of the external urethral sphincter and trigone is innervated by a branch of the pudendal nerve that originates from sacral cord segments S1–S2 and is critical in the tonic voluntary control of continence.

References

1 Zweyer, M. (2014). Embryology of the kidney. In: *Radiological Imaging of the Kidney*, 2e (ed. E. Quaia), 3–16. New York: Springer.

2 McBride, J.M. (2015). Embryology, anatomy, and histology of the kidney. In: *The Kidney* (ed. D. Hansel, C. Kane, G. Pancer, and S. Chang), 1–18. New York: Springer.

3 Beech, D.J., Sibbons, P.D., Rossdale, P.D. et al. (2001). Organogenesis of lung and kidney in thoroughbreds and ponies. *Equine Vet. J.* 33: 438–445.

4 Schott, H.C., Waldridge, B., and Bayly, W.M. (2018). Disorders of the urinary system. In: *Equine Internal Medicine*, 4e (ed. S.M. Reed, W.M. Bayly, and D.C. Sellon), 888–990. St. Louis, MO: Elsevier.

5 Noden, D. and De Lahunta, A. (1985). *The Embryology of Domestic Animals* (ed. D.M. Noden and A. De Lahunta). Baltimore: Williams and Wilkins.

6 McGeady, T. (2006). Urinary system. In: *Veterinary Embryology* (ed. T. McGeady, P. Quinn, E. FitzPatrick, and M. Ryan), 240–205. Blackwell Publishing.

7 Holdstock, N.B., Rossdale, P.D., Beech, D.J. et al. (2001). Miroanatomical development of the equine kidney and defects associated with intra-uterine growth retardation. *Pferdeheilkunde* 17: 659–661.

8 Fowden, A.L., Mijovic, J., Ousey, J.C. et al. (1992). The development of gluconeogenic enzymes in the liver and kidney of fetal and newborn foals. *J. Dev. Physiol.* 18: 147–142.

9 Bolat, D., Bahar, S., Tipirdamaz, S. et al. (2013). Comparison of the morphometric features of the left and right horse kidneys: a stereological approach. *Anat. Histol. Emrbyrol.* 42: 448–452.

10 Toribio, R.E. (2007). Essentials of equine renal and urinary tract physiology. *Vet. Clin. Equine* 23: 533–561.

11 Divers, T.J. (2022). Relevant equine renal anatomy, physiology, and mechanisms of acute kidney injury: a review. *Vet. Clin. Equine* 38: 1–12.

12 Nickel, R., Schummer, A., Seiferle, E., and Sack, W.O. Urogenital system. In: *The Viscera of the Domestic Mammals*, 2e (ed. A. Schummer, R. Nickel, and W.O. Sack), 282–304. Berlin: Verlag Paul Parey.

13 Barajas, L. (1079). Anatomy of the juxtaglomerular apparatus. *Am. J. Phys* 237: 333–343.

Chapter 23 Clinical Neonatal Renal Physiology

Jon Palmer

When trying to understand neonatal organ function, the clinician should always remember that the neonatal period is a time of transition from fetal physiology. Renal function is undergoing rather profound changes as it meets the challenge of supporting independent life. This transition begins several weeks prior to parturition and is not complete until several weeks after birth. Some aspects of this transition in the neonatal foal are different from other species. However, many aspects are poorly studied in the foal and are assumed to be similar to the changes noted in other species. It is well to remember that although the fetal kidneys are functional, the true workhorse balancing fluids and electrolytes, excreting waste, and preforming excretory and nutritional balancing in the fetus is the fetal-maternal placenta. Otherwise apparently healthy full-term equine fetuses can be born without detectable renal tissue (personal observation), suggesting that all vital functions of the fetal kidney can be performed by other tissues (such as the placenta) until birth. This is indeed amazing, considering the variety of functions that the neonatal kidney must assume at birth (e.g. glomerular filtration; salt and water reabsorption; acid–base homeostasis; regulation of blood pressure; tubular secretion; endocrine functions including vitamin D, calcium, and phosphate metabolism; erythropoiesis; immune regulation; and circulating drug and toxin metabolism) [1]. Despite the fact that normal renal function is not vital to fetal survival, the development of normal kidney function originates in utero as soon as nephrogenesis begins and continues into the neonatal period; it is evident that fetal kidney function affects normal fetal development in some aspects and is linked to the normal development of other fetal organ systems such as the lung and genitourinary systems.

Fetal renal function is not sufficient to balance all the metabolic requirements of the growing fetus, nor does it need to be, given the interposition of the placenta and maternal-fetal membranes. Nevertheless, the contribution of fetal kidneys to fluid and electrolyte homeostasis gradually increases as gestation progresses, so that the kidneys are prepared to replace the placenta at the time of birth. Alteration of normal kidney development and therefore normal kidney structure and function by factors such as placental insufficiency, protein restriction, or in utero exposure to toxins (e.g. inhibitors of prostaglandin synthesis, corticosteroids, or inhibitors of the renin-angiotensin-aldosterone axis) affects not only fetal development but also postnatal kidney function. Abnormal fetal kidney development and fetal kidney function therefore may result in postnatal physiologic consequences. This chapter provides a brief summary of the foal's renal physiology with reference to fetal development.

Renal Perfusion

The intrarenal distribution of blood flow changes during gestation as a result of a centrifugal pattern of new glomerular development. The hemodynamic evolution of the fetal kidney is characterized by a shift from a low-flow, high-resistance organ, with most of the blood supply to the inner cortex, to a high-flow, low-resistance organ, with most of the blood flow supplying the outer cortex [2].

The fetal kidneys receive approximately 3% of the combined left and right cardiac output due to higher relative vascular resistance resulting in a low glomerular filtration rate (GFR). At birth there is an immediate increase in renal blood flow to 15% of cardiac output in lambs. Although there is an increase in vascular resistance throughout the body associated with birth, there is less of an increase in the renal vasculature resulting in an 86% relative decrease renal vascular resistance (as measured in piglets). Simultaneously, there is a redistribution of blood flow from

Equine Neonatal Medicine, First Edition. Edited by David M. Wong and Pamela A. Wilkins.

the inner cortex to outer superficial cortex. This is followed within days to weeks of birth (depending on species) with a further decrease in vascular resistance (both anatomic and vasoactive effect) and rise in systemic blood pressure until the blood flow to the kidneys reaches 20% of the cardiac output. This transition is not complete until 3 months in infants but is likely to occur primarily within days of birth in foals [3, 4].

The distribution of blood flow to different parts of the kidney differs between neonates and adults. Renal hemodynamics during the fetal–neonatal transition are controlled by a variety of factors including angiotensin II, the renal sympathetic nervous system (renal sympathetic nerves, intrinsic adrenergic release, and circulating adrenergics), prostaglandins (PG), nitric oxide (NO), the Kallikrein-Kinin system, atrial natriuretic factor (ANF), endothelin, and others. Many of these hormones, such as angiotensin II, have roles in addition to those generally thought about in adults. Angiotensin II is an important growth factor required for normal nephrogenesis in addition to its well-established role in tubuloglomerular feedback and autoregulation. Although not studied in animals, in people, levels can be decreased with maternal dietary protein restriction during pregnancy leading to decreased neonatal renal mass and development of adult hypertension decades later [1].

The renin-angiotensin system (RAS) plays a major role in controlling systemic blood pressure in the fetus by maintaining systemic and renal vascular resistance. The RAS directly regulates GFR in the fetal kidney by control of vascular tone. The expression of renin, angiotensin-converting enzyme (ACE), and angiotensin II are upregulated in the fetal kidney, more so than in the postnatal and mature adult kidney. Also, angiotensinogen and ACE expression and activity increase more during late gestation. Angiotensin II preferentially increases efferent arteriolar tone, resulting in an increase in glomerular capillary hydrostatic pressure and an increase in single nephron GFR (SNGFR). The effects of angiotensin II on the renal vasculature are mediated through the type 1 angiotensin (AT1) receptor, which itself is upregulated in the renal vasculature during fetal kidney maturation [5–8].

The renal sympathetic nervous system is very important in controlling renal blood flow in the neonate, as renal blood flow tends to be more sensitive to the sympathetic nervous system in foals as compared to the adult. Circulating adrenergics play a role, but so does the dense sympathetic innervation of the kidneys. The high renal vascular resistance seen in the fetus is due to a combination of increased sympathetic nervous system activity, increased α1 receptor activity, and increased secreted catecholamines. This preferentially increases the afferent arteriolar tone of the fetal glomerulus, with a consequent decrease in glomerular capillary hydraulic pressure and a decrease in SNGFR. The sympathetic control of renal blood flow is part of the baroreceptor reflex, but it is well to remember that in the neonate the baroreceptor is set at a much lower blood pressure threshold that rises with maturational adaptation. Circulating catecholamine levels fall immediately after birth, with a corresponding increase in GFR. The effects of the sympathetic nervous system on the renal vasculature and therefore on fetal GFR appear to be mediated in part through the stimulation of renin release. In lambs with renal denervation, there is an associated decrease in circulating plasma renin activity associated with the stress of birth [9–11].

Endothelin is another vasoconstrictor that is upregulated in the fetal kidney. Endothelin production is stimulated by angiotensin II, bradykinin, epinephrine, and shear stress. Its sources are thought to include the vascular endothelium, the glomerulus, and distal tubular epithelial cells. Both endothelin and its receptor (ETR) are increased during fetal life but decrease early in the neonate's life [12].

Angiotensin II and adrenergics are the most important renal vasoconstrictors, while NO and PG serve as the most important vasodilators. Prostaglandins are very important in normal neonatal renal function both in their role as renal vasoregulators and in determining normal kidney development. There are cyclooxygenase (COX)-1 receptors in the renal vasculature, glomeruli, and collecting ducts. The distribution of COX-2 receptors are species dependent. In general COX-2 receptors increase activity after birth, peaking at 1–2 weeks, then decline and are important in nephrogenesis. During the perinatal period COX-2 inhibitors can cause renal dysgenesis and disruption of nephrogenesis. In general, renal PGs result in renal vasodilation and their renal production increases during the perinatal period. Just as in adults, in pathologic conditions indigenous PG help protect the kidneys by attenuating renal vasoconstriction such as may be secondary to increased adrenergic tone; unlike adults, in neonates, normal PG levels are important in maintaining basal renal blood flow as well as in stressed conditions, making nonsteroidal anti-inflammatory drugs (NSAIDs) potentially more toxic. Intrinsic PG production is important in maintaining normal renal blood flow in neonates. The use of NSAIDs in the fetus and neonate even under nonpathologic conditions may decrease urine output, cause a significant decrease blood flow, increase renal vascular resistance, and in the fetus may result in oligohydramnios. The use of NSAIDs in neonates may disrupt the important balance of vasodilators and vasoconstrictors, which is important in normal neonatal renal physiology. Clinical observation shows that when PG inhibitors, such as flunixin, are given to a neonatal foal, urine production may decrease dramatically and inappropriately for approximately 18 hours. During this period, any urine produced will have a very high specific gravity. This effect appears more marked and reliably present in critically ill foals, perhaps because of increased sympathetic tone, and usually disappears within 48 hours of birth. A similar effect has been observed in preterm infants, but in infants it also may result in long-term renal injury. Although the author has not noted this in foals, the possibility of long-term injury is a good reason to avoid NSAIDs during at least the first 48 hours of a foal's life [13, 14].

Development of GFR

The balance of renal vasoconstrictors and vasodilators produces renal vascular resistance and determines GFR. In the neonate, as compared to adults, these substances may have different effects, have different intrarenal levels, and even different sites of action. Still, their balance is the major determinate of GFR. Although many factors may be involved, during the transition the increased renal vascular resistance is mediated by increased activity of angiotensin II and increased sensitivity to catecholamines. Counterbalancing this effect is mediated by the critical vasodilators, namely, NO and PG. The increase in renal blood flow during the birth transition is primarily mediated by a decrease in vasoconstrictors.

The development of a normal GFR is multifactorial and involves changes in the balance of factors that oppose or promote filtration. There are changes in renal vascular resistance as noted, along with an increase in nephron mass. There is also a modification of ultrafiltration involving glomerular membrane dynamics and glomerular membrane area as well as the important development of concentration gradients in the renal parenchyma [15].

In lambs there is a dramatic increase in GFR within hours of birth. This is followed by a much more gradual increase in GFR during the first week. This is caused by functional changes (not morphological changes) – primarily enhanced glomerular perfusion but also recruitment of more superficial cortical nephrons. The rate of glomerular filtration depends on Starling factors, the rate of flow of plasma into glomerular capillaries, the permeability of the capillary wall, and total surface area of capillaries. Thus, GFR depends on renal blood flow and glomerular capillary pressure. Transcapillary hydrostatic pressure favors filtration and depends on efferent/afferent capillary resistance [15, 16].

Tubular Function

Fetal fractional excretion of sodium (Na^+) is 5–15% because of the lack of efficient tubular reabsorption [15, 17]. If this were to continue after birth, it would be disastrous, as mare's milk has very low Na^+ concentration. In the fetus, more Na^+ absorption occurs in the distal tubules than in the proximal tubules. In the proximal tubules, carrier density is low, and even cellular polarization is not fully established [18]. Bulk Na^+ absorption does occur proximally [19]. At the time of birth in lambs and infants (perhaps just before birth in the foal), there is an upregulation of Na^+ absorption mechanisms (especially the sodium/hydrogen exchanger) in the distal tubule [20]. In lambs there is dramatically increased activity during the first 24 hours of life. This upregulation is thought to be a response to the peripartum cortisol surge. This results in a rapid decrease in urine Na^+ wasting, which is vital for neonates as Na^+ conservation is very important. As noted, fresh milk is very Na^+ poor (mare's milk Na^+ 9–14 mEq/l); if a foal drinks a generous 20% of body weight in milk, the foal receives approximately 1.9 mEq/kg/d of Na^+. Sodium growth requirement for a normal neonate is about 1 mEq/kg/d, which means a foal can afford to lose no more than 0.9 mEq/kg/d and still allow normal growth. Almost all the normal Na^+ loss is in the urine. The Na^+ conserving mechanisms in the distal tubule/collecting ducts are highly refined, initially always turned on and not responsive to changes in Na^+ intake. This means that unless the foal has a pathologic Na^+ loss (e.g. Na^+ wasting nephropathy, diarrhea, etc.) it is very easy to Na^+ overload a foal, resulting in edema. Although the author finds it very difficult to restrict Na^+ intake to the expected <2.0 mEq/kg/d, attempts to keep it to no more than 4 mEq/kg/d should be made and might help avoid edema in most cases. One liter of plasma contributes about 3 mEq/kg/d (frozen plasma produced by plasmapheresis has a variable amount of Na^+ but usually 160–180 mEq/l) and full rate of parenteral nutrition contains about 1 mEq/kg/d of Na^+ (in the amino acids). Some drugs are also Na^+ salts and may be an additional source. Of course, if there is a pathologic Na^+ loss such as a high renal or intestinal loss, Na^+ restriction would be contraindicated. In addition, some cases may have pathologic retention of water (e.g. neonatal vasogenic nephropathy, syndrome of inappropriate antidiuresis), which can cause a serious hypoosmotic state where a choice between the relative dangers of hypoosmolality and Na^+ overload must be weighed.

Sodium overloading will result in extracellular volume expansion, which will initially be subclinical because of the high compliance of the neonate's interstitium but will eventually result in detectable edema. Once edema is visible, the Na^+ overload is extreme. Hypernatremia will not develop unless there are unusually large insensible losses concurrently.

The time frame needed for a neonate to stop indiscriminately conserving Na^+ and begin normal Na^+ regulation in response to intake differs between species. In the face of high Na^+ intakes, based on the author's clinical experience, it appears that neonatal calves begin to respond with renal Na^+ wasting in the first 24 hours of life. Normal foals appear to be slower to begin to respond and critically ill foals appear to be much slower, often still retaining excess Na^+ inappropriately for 1–2 weeks. These observations are based on the author's casual clinical observations and may therefore not be accurate.

Beyond Na^+ regulation, there are other differences between neonates and adults in the renal handling of metabolites. Glucose has a higher tubular maximum (depending on species 180–220 mg/dl), avoiding glucose spilling as the neonate adjusts its insulin responsiveness and learning glucose control [21, 22]. Phosphate and calcium also have unique neonatal and fetal regulation. They are both transported across the placenta against high-concentration gradients to aid in bone calcification [23]. There is a unique Na^+-phosphorus cotransporter in the placenta and neonatal renal tubules that is not modulated by high dietary phosphorus intake and results in a high rate of renal phosphorus reabsorption in the fetus and neonate. The renal clearance of phosphorus is programed to be quite low allowing the maintenance of the normally high fetal and neonatal phosphorus levels [24].

Cortisol plays an important role in speeding the maturation of the kidneys, accelerating the renal transition during fetal stress. Rising cortisol levels are associated with an increase in GFR, decrease in phosphorus reabsorption by 50%, and changes in Na^+ reabsorption, decreasing proximal reabsorption and increasing distal reabsorption, resulting in no change to Na^+ fractional excretion. Cortisol also accelerates development of tubular reabsorption capacity of Na^+, potassium (K^+), H_2O, as well as a distal Na^+ carrier-mediated absorption [25].

Autoregulation of blood pressure is active in the neonate, but the range is set to lower perfusion pressure (mean arterial pressure [MAP] 40–60 mmHg). The renal pressure-flow relationship changes with renal maturation. This response is primarily mediated by PG-dependent renin release causing vasoconstriction at lower levels of perfusion pressure. This is another response that NSAID therapy may disrupt in the neonate.

Tubuloglomerular feedback is also present in the fetus and neonate and is controlled by macula densa cells (Figure 23.1) [26]. As those cells sense a decrease in NaCl delivery to distal tubules, it stimulates release of angiotensin II form juxtaglomerular cells, which in turn constricts efferent arterioles increasing GFR. This response is mediated by the release of local PGs, which also causes vasodilation of the afferent arterioles enhancing the increase in GFR. This response also matures with growth. It is maximally sensitive at normal tubular flow ranges. As GFR increases, maximum response and flow range also increases, with the relative sensitivity being unaltered during growth.

At birth in the normal foal, calf, kid, and likely other herbivores, the blood creatinine level is high and drops in the first 24–48 hours of life [27]. At birth in the healthy foal, the creatinine is usually between 2.0 and 4.0 mg/dl. If the foal has suffered an intrauterine challenge the birth creatinine can be much higher, often being 8.0–16.0 mg/dl and occasionally being 40 mg/dl or more. This increase is independent of renal function. If renal function is normal, the level

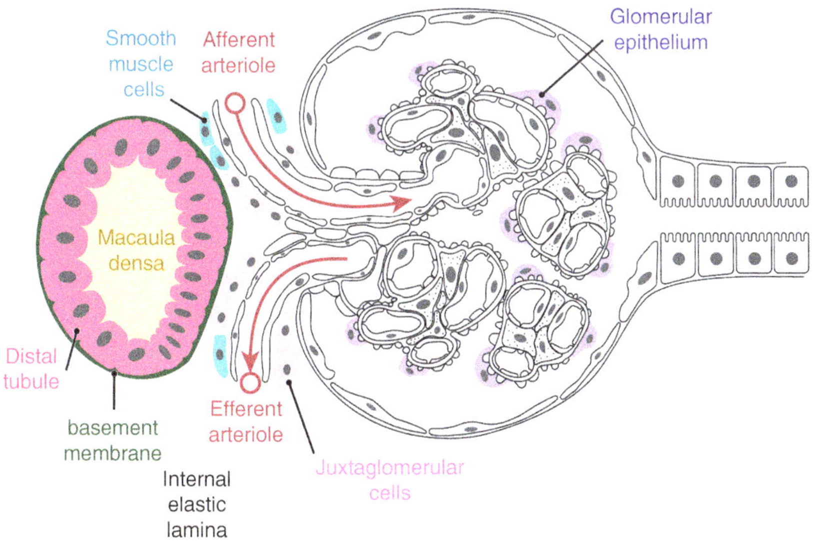

Figure 23.1 Structures of the juxtaglomerular apparatus, demonstrating its possible feedback role in the control of nephron function.

will drop dramatically after birth reaching <1.1 mg/dl as quickly as 48–72 hours. Thus, the degree of elevation in serum creatinine concentration at birth is not a good indication of renal function, but how rapidly it decreases is.

The fetal fluids appear to be a repository for creatinine. At the time of birth of a healthy foal the creatinine level in amnionic fluid ranges from 8 to 12 mg/dl and the creatinine level in allantoic fluid ranges from 120 to 160 mg/dl. This accumulation of creatinine explains the high birth level in normal foals, who are working hard to keep their blood levels as low as they do. In the foal suffering intrauterine distress, the extremely high levels are likely from the entrainment of creatinine as more fluid is shifted from the fetal fluid reservoir to the fetal interstitium. Thus, elevated creatinine is an indicator of stress-induced fetal fluid shifts and not renal compromise. Measurement of serial blood creatinine levels and watching how rapidly it drops to normal neonatal levels provides a very powerful, yet simple measure of renal function.

Neonatal Vasomotor Nephropathy (NVN)

Neonatal vasomotor nephropathy (NVN) is a fairly common and important but seldom described renal disease of equine neonates [28, 29]. In order to achieve normal GFR there is a careful balance of renal afferent and efferent arteriolar tone. Although many mediators may be involved in this balance, the major contributors are the vasoconstrictors such as angiotensin II and adrenergics (circulating epinephrine or norepinephrine, local renal derived adrenergics, or renal sympathetic tone) and vasodilators such as PG and NO. NVN describes the disease caused by an imbalance of these vasoconstrictors and vasodilators. The author notes this problem occurring most often secondary to a failure of the renal birth transition, but it can also occur in the face of hypovolemia/hypoperfusion, stress, hypertension, autonomic dysfunction, pressor therapy, and NSAID therapy. Clinical signs include sudden onset of oliguria, where urine that is passed has a very-high-specific gravity, and the foal's creatinine either slows its decrease from birth levels or in rare cases will increase mildly. In foals, the fractional excretion of Na^+ is usually very low unless tubular damage accompanies vasogenic nephropathy. In other species the fractional excretion of Na^+ may be high in some individuals. The problem resulting in NVN is thought to be caused by the inappropriate vasoconstriction of afferent arterioles or inappropriate vasodilation of efferent arterioles or a combination of both. Generally, the decrease in blood supply to tubular cells is not enough to cause damage, as reflected by the production of concentrated urine. When the abnormal blood flow pattern is reversed, normal renal function returns.

Healthy foals have a somewhat different urine production pattern in the perinatal period compared with other species. In most species, neonates produce dilute urine shortly after birth. In infants, about half the babies born are reported to pass urine before they leave the delivery room. But normal foals generally do not pass urine in the first 12 hours of life despite their fluid intake; additionally, the first urine produced has a specific gravity on the high end of the scale. Once they begin to urinate, they usually pass more urine regularly and, with each subsequent urination, their urine specific gravity drops until within a few hours it is usually <1.002. With NVN the neonate may not urinate until 48 or even 72 hours after birth. If urine is produced it will be very concentrated (often higher than a refractometer will report specific gravity). This inappropriate antidiuresis results in fluid overload.

Therapy of NVN consists of several, what may seem contradictory, trials. If there is any indication that hypovolemia is resulting in an appropriate antidiuresis then a volume trial may be in order. If there is not an immediate response to the volume trial, then it should be discontinued as it will lead to more fluid overload. Likewise, if there are any clinical signs of hypoperfusion then an inotrope/pressor trial might be in order, but if this is the wrong approach it will only exacerbate the problem. Usually, it is quite evident from the physical exam that these are not part of the problem. If the problem is primarily afferent vasoconstriction, then a furosemide trial might be in order, not for its tubular effect, but rather, it will induce renal PG production. If furosemide works in reversing the vasogenic disorder, then one or two doses (0.5–1 mg/kg) will result in a sustained diuresis, which will continue without additional doses. However, if only the traditional tubular effect of furosemide is noted, the diuresis will only last 4–6 hr and then the concentrated urine will return. If repeat doses of furosemide are used, the adverse effects of significant electrolyte imbalances (Na^+, K^+, Cl^-, Ca^{++}) and their accompanying adverse effects might occur [30, 31].

If one or two doses of furosemide does not resolve the NVN then the author prefers fluid restriction and time as long as perfusion is adequate. As the author's maintenance fluid rate is based on guesses of normal urine output and insensible losses, which the author believes each account for about half the needs, the author begins the foal who is not making urine on a half-maintenance rate until they make urine, or if there is evidence of fluid overloaded, consider starting with quarter-fluid rate until the overload lessens. Once they return to normal urine output and isosthenuric urine, the author returns them to normal maintenance fluid rate. Throughout this period, the foal's weight should be monitored closely. In general, there is no parenchymal damage or functional impairment noticed once NVN resolves and the fluid overload is corrected.

References

1 Matsell, D.G. and Hiatt, M.J. (2017). Functional development of the kidney in utero. In: *Fetal and Neonatal Physiology*, 5e (ed. R. Polin, S. Abman, D. Rowitch, and W. Benitz), 965–976. Elsevier, Inc.

2 Satlin, L.M.W.C. and Schwartz, G.J. (2003). Development of function in the metanephric kidney. In: *The Kidney: From Normal Development to Congenital Disease* (ed. P.D. Vize, A.S. Woolf, and J.B.L. Bard), 267–325. London: Academic Press.

3 Gruskin, A.B., Edelmann, C.M., and Yuan, S. (1970). Maturational changes in renal blood flow in piglets. *Pediatr. Res.* 4: 7–13.

4 Aperia, A., Broberger, O., Herin, P. et al. (1977). Renal hemodynamics in the perinatal period. A study in lambs. *Acta Physiol. Scand.* 99: 261–269.

5 Wolf, G. (2002). Angiotensin II and tubular development. *Nephrol. Dial. Transplant.* 17: 48–51.

6 Robillard, J.E., Weismann, D.N., Gomez, R.A. et al. (1983). Renal and adrenal responses to converting-enzyme inhibition in fetal and newborn life. *Am J Physiol* 244: R249–R256.

7 Tufro-McReddie, A., Harrison, J.K., Everett, A.D. et al. (1993). Ontogeny of type 1 angiotensin II receptor gene expression in the rat. *J. Clin. Invest.* 91: 530–537.

8 Kakuchi, J., Ichiki, T., Kiyama, S. et al. (1995). Developmental expression of renal angiotensin II receptor genes in the mouse. *Kidney Int.* 47: 140–147.

9 DiBona, G.F. and Kopp, U.C. (1997). Neural control of renal function. *Physiol. Rev.* 77: 75–197.

10 Pupilli, C., Gomez, R.A., Tuttle, J.B. et al. (1991). Spatial association of renin-containing cells and nerve fibers in developing rat kidney. *Pediatr. Nephrol.* 5: 690–695.

11 Smith, F.G., Smith, B.A., Guillery, E.N. et al. (1991). Role of renal sympathetic nerves in lambs during the transition from fetal to newborn life. *J. Clin. Invest.* 88: 1988–1994.

12 Abadie, L., Blazy, I., Roubert, P. et al. (1996). Decrease in endothelin-1 renal receptors during the 1st month of life in the rat. *Pediatr. Nephrol.* 10: 185–189.

13 Guignard, J. and Gouyon, J.B. (2012). *Glomerular Filtration in Neonates. Polin R Nephrology and Fluid/Electrolyte Physiology: Neonatology Questions and Controversies*, 117–135. Philadelphia: Elsevier.

14 Akima, S., Kent, A., Reynolds, G.J. et al. (2004). Indomethacin and renal impairment in neonates. *Pediatr. Nephrol.* 19: 490–493.

15 Seikaly, M.G. and Arant, B.S. (1992). Development of renal hemodynamics: glomerular filtration and renal blood flow. *Clin. Perinatol.* 19: 1–13.

16 Hill, K.J. and Lumbers, E.R. (1988). Renal function in adult and fetal sheep. *J. Dev. Physiol.* 10: 149–159.

17 Schmidt, U. and Horster, M. (1977). Na-K-activated ATPase: activity maturation in rabbit nephron segments dissected in vitro. *Am. J. Physiol.* 233: F55–F60.

18 Baum, M. and Quigley, R. (2004). Ontogeny of renal sodium transport. *Semin. Perinatol.* 28: 91–96.

19 Quigley, R. and Baum, M. (2002). Developmental changes in rabbit proximal straight tubule paracellular permeability. *Am. J. Physiol. Renal Physiol.* 283: F525–F531.

20 Beck, J.C., Lipkowitz, M.S., and Abramson, R.G. (1991). Ontogeny of Na/H antiporter activity in rabbit renal brush border membrane vesicles. *J. Clin. Invest.* 87: 2067–2076.

21 Falcão, M.C., Leone, C.R., and Ramos, J.L. (1999). Is glycosuria a reliable indicator of adequacy of glucose infusion rate in preterm infants? *Sao Paulo Med. J.* 117: 19–24.

22 Jagła, M., Szymońska, I., Starzec, K. et al. (2018). Preterm glycosuria – new data from a continuous glucose monitoring system. *Neonatology* 114: 87–92.

23 Karlén, J., Aperia, A., and Zetterström, R. (1985). Renal excretion of calcium and phosphate in preterm and term infants. *J. Pediatr.* 106: 814–819.

24 Senterre, J. and Salle, B. (1988). Renal aspects of calcium and phosphorus metabolism in preterm infants. *Biol. Neonate* 53: 220–229.

25 Robillard, J.E. and Nakamura, K.T. (1988). Hormonal regulation of renal function during development. *Biol. Neonate* 53: 201–211.

26 Turner, A.J., Brown, R.D., Boyce, A. et al. (2015). Fetal tubuloglomerular feedback in an ovine model of mild maternal renal disease. *Physiol. Rep.* 3: e12448.

27 Palmer, J.E. (2006). Chapter 7: Recognition and resuscitation of the critically ill foal. In: *Equine Neonatal Medicine, A Case-Based Approach* (ed. M.R. Paradis), 121–134. Philadelphia: Elsevier Saunders.

28 Gouyon, J.B. and Guignard, J.P. (1989). Insuffisance rénale vasomotrice du nouveau-né. Physiopathologie et traitement [Vasomotor kidney failure in the newborn infant. Physiopathology and treatment]. *Arch. Fr. Pediatr.* 46: 137–141.

29 Tóth-Heyn, P., Drukker, A., and Guignard, J.P. (2000). The stressed neonatal kidney: from pathophysiology to clinical management of neonatal vasomotor nephropathy. *Pediatr. Nephrol.* 14: 227–239.

30 Cattarelli, D., Spandrio, M., Gasparoni, A. et al. (2006). A randomised, double blind, placebo controlled trial of the effect of theophylline in prevention of vasomotor nephropathy in very preterm neonates with respiratory distress syndrome. *Arch. Dis. Child. Fetal Neonatal Ed.* 91: F80–F84.

31 Dubourg, L., Drukker, A., and Guignard, J.P. (2000). Failure of the loop diuretic torasemide to improve renal function of hypoxemic vasomotor nephropathy in the newborn rabbit. *Pediatr. Res.* 47: 504–508.

Chapter 24 Examination, Therapeutics, and Monitoring of the Urinary System

Section I Examination of the Urinary System

Emma Deane and Langdon Fielding

Clinical signs of dysfunction of the urogenital tract in foals typically present within the first few days to weeks of life. Commonly encountered urogenital abnormalities include ruptured bladder, patent urachus, omphalophlebitis, and congenital malformations. Evaluation of the urogenital system begins with a careful physical examination along with diagnostic tests including hematology, serum biochemistry analysis, urinalysis, and enzymuria. If indicated, diagnostic imaging such as ultrasound, endoscopy, and radiography are used to evaluate for specific conditions. Some foals will require urinary catheterization and monitoring of urine output with a closed urinary system. This chapter reviews common diagnostics and therapeutics used to evaluate the urogenital system in foals.

Physical Examination of the Urogenital System

Early detection of urogenital dysfunction in foals can be difficult. As with any disorder, a complete physical examination is indicated with special attention directed to mentation, behavior, assessment of the external umbilical structures, and perfusion parameters. Foals with azotemia or oliguria may present with altered mentation, including obtundation and decreased reactivity to stimuli. Reduced nursing frequency may also be observed, and foals may have dried milk accumulated on the muzzle or forehead. The dam may exhibit engorged mammary glands or spontaneous mammary excretion of milk indicative of decreased consumption by the foal.

Urogenital dysfunction commonly results in varying degrees of stranguria which manifests as dorsoventral flexion of the spine and increased frequency and decreased volume of urination. Owners often confuse straining to urinate with straining to defecate, which presents as dorsal extension of the spine (rounding of the back). External abdominal palpation also should be included as part of the examination. Abdominal distension, pain on abdominal palpation, and increased abdominal fluid may be present in foals with urogenital dysfunction. In cases of uroabdomen, a fluid wave might be palpable with ballottement of the abdomen, but failure to palpate a fluid wave does not eliminate ascites or uroabdomen. The external umbilicus should be examined for surrounding soft tissue swelling, enlargement, patent urachus, purulent discharge, and hernias. Any abnormalities with the external umbilicus warrant ultrasonographic evaluation of the external and internal umbilical structures. Umbilical hernias are commonly detected during a neonatal exam and are generally 1–2 cm in size. Palpation of a hernia ring within the body wall of a foal should be considered a normal variant. In one report, approximately half of the foals examined had a palpable umbilical ring at birth [1]. The hernia ring typically resolves within 1 month of age and should not be classified as a true hernia until then.

Parameters that identify perfusion, dehydration, and fluid overload should be closely monitored. Signs of poor perfusion include poor jugular fill and pulse quality, increased heart rate, pale mucous membranes, cold extremities, prolonged capillary refill time, decreased mentation, and decreased urination. Foals with urogential disease, particularly those involving the kidney, may be at risk of fluid overload, which can manifest as subcutaneous edema involving the triceps, axilla, ventral abdomen, submandibular space, and distal limbs. Fluid can also accumulate in the lungs or body cavities.

Urine production is one of the best indicators of urogenital health and function in foals. Due to the high milk diet, foals produce 5–10 times the amount of urine compared to their adult counterparts on a per kilogram body weight basis.

A healthy foal produces approximately 148 ml/kg/d of urine [2]. A foal's first urination occurs between 8 and 12 hours after birth with colts urinating earlier than fillies [3]. The urination is often concentrated with a

Equine Neonatal Medicine, First Edition. Edited by David M. Wong and Pamela A. Wilkins.

specific gravity >1.030 soon after birth, and rapidly decreases over the next several hours to days [2, 4]. The rate at which urine specific gravity decreases varies greatly per individual due to environmental and maternal factors as well as milk consumption.

Foals typically have hyposthenuric urine because of their milk diet with normal urine specific gravity in 4-day-old foals ranging between 1.001 and 1.010 [2]. The healthy equine neonate will also have marked but transient proteinuria during the first 48 hours after birth. Urinary pH in foals is more acidic than adult horses (mean pH of <7), and epithelial cells and calcium oxalate crystals are also more prevalent [4]. Comorbidities in neonates are common; therefore, if a urogenital problem is suspected, the foal should be examined for signs of sepsis, neonatal encephalopathy, and other common neonatal disorders.

Hematology/Biochemistry Analysis

Alterations in hematology and serum biochemical parameters encountered with urogenital tract disease depend on the segment of urogenital tract affected and type of pathology. Common hematological abnormalities include leukocytosis and hyperfibrinogenemia, which are suggestive of an inflammatory or infectious disease process [5]. Anemia may be associated with chronic renal disease due to decreased erythropoietin production by the interstitial fibroblasts in the kidneys. Progressive anemia has been associated with polycystic kidney disease and failure in a 9-day-old foal [6]. Commonly used markers of renal function include serum creatinine and blood urea nitrogen (BUN), which are measured to assess glomerular filtration rate (GFR). Azotemia may not occur until approximately 70–75% of the nephrons become nonfunctional; therefore, they are not ideal indicators of early changes in GFR [4]. Foals <24 hours old without renal disease may have elevated serum creatinine concentrations as a result of placentitis or placental insufficiency [7, 8]; if renal function is normal, the elevated creatinine will normalize by 3–5 days of age [4]. BUN values on day 1 and 2 of life reflect maternal BUN levels and are not indicative of neonatal renal function [9, 10].

Similar to adult horses, renal disease in neonates can be classified as prerenal, renal, or postrenal. However, this classification scheme fails to address the fact that prerenal and postrenal causes of azotemia often lead to direct renal damage. Prerenal azotemia is a result of decreased renal perfusion, which occurs with dehydration and hypotension. Renal azotemia can result from sepsis, other inflammatory conditions, tubular damage, ischemia, and toxicities (e.g. nonsteroidal anti-inflammatory drugs, aminoglycosides, tetracyclines, hemoglobin from neonatal isoerythrolysis). Postrenal causes of renal disease or azotemia include urachal tearing, urinary obstruction, ruptured bladder, and urachal rents.

Electrolyte derangements are frequently encountered in foals with urogenital disease. In the case of acute kidney injury and uroperitoneum, common electrolyte abnormalities include hyponatremia, hypochloremia, hyperkalemia, and metabolic acidosis. This may vary, however, in foals receiving IV fluid therapy, making electrolyte abnormalities more subtle [11].

Symmetric dimethylarginine (SDMA) is a relatively new biomarker for detection of acute kidney injury in horses, although it is commonly used in people and small animals as a marker of acute renal disease [12]. SDMA is a methylated form of arginine and is a byproduct of catabolism; it is found throughout the body in all nucleated cells [12]. Approximately 90% of SDMA is excreted through the kidneys [13] and is less affected by extrarenal factors (sex, age, body weight) compared to creatinine [14]. Healthy foals have higher mean serum SDMA concentrations compared to healthy adults, and the values decrease with age in foals (Table 24.I.1) [14]. Foals with renal dysfunction have higher SDMA concentrations than foals with presumed "spurious" hypercreatinemia and sick hospitalized foals had higher SDMA concentrations than healthy foals at comparable time points [15].

Table 24.I.1 Median concentrations of symmetric dimethylarginine (SDMA) and serum creatinine (sCr) from healthy foals and their mares at various ages [15].

	Foal			Mare		
Time point	N	SMDA (μg/dl) (range)	sCr (mg/dl) (range)	N	SDMA (μg/dl) (range)	sCr (mg/dl) (range)
Birth	112	70 (7–100)	1.8 (1–7.9)	79	10 (3–20)	1.0 (0.6–2.2)
1–4 d	87	49 (5–100)	1.1 (0.6–3.3)	61	9 (2–20)	0.8 (0.6–1.4)
5–10 d	80	26 (5–37)	0.9 (0.1–1.5)	61	8 (3–17)	0.8 (0.6–1.6)
20+ d	78	18 (6–27)	1.0 (0.6–2.0)	54	7 (1–15)	0.8 (0.6–1.1)

Urinalysis

A urinalysis should be performed if urinary tract disease is suspected in the foal. However, given that most foals presenting to intensive care units have conditions that may affect the renal system, a urinalysis is considered part of the standard database for sick neonates. Care should be taken with interpretation of a single time point and serial assessments may be more helpful due to the wide variation between foals in the first 4 days of life [2, 4]. Normal values have been reported in foals after this time period (Table 24.I.2) [2, 4].

As with adults, a positive blood result on urine dipstick in neonatal foals can indicate the presence of red blood cells, hemoglobin, or myoglobin. Hemoglobinuria can occur with intravascular hemolysis and may be present in foals with neonatal isoerythrolysis. Hematuria may be present in the first urination or subsequent urinations due to trauma from parturition or be associated with urinary catheterization. Myoglobinuria is less common but seen in cases of severe white muscle disease or other causes of rhabdomyolysis.

Assessing Renal Function

Measurement of serum creatinine and BUN are used to assess renal function; however, as noted, azotemia may not develop until 75% of the nephrons are no longer functioning. Therefore, these markers are poor indicators of early renal dysfunction. Plasma disappearance curves and clearance studies used to assess the GFR are more sensitive detectors of smaller declines in renal function. Plasma disappearance curves of inulin is considered the gold standard to assess renal function or GFR. Clearance studies of creatinine, inulin and radionucleotides to measure GFR have been well described but are infrequently used in the clinical setting [16].

The urinary clearance of several substances can be directly compared to urinary clearance or excretion of creatinine. A substance that is poorly filtered (larger molecule) or is reabsorbed (e.g. sodium, chloride) will have lower clearance values than creatinine. A substance that is eliminated by glomerular filtration and tubular secretion (e.g. potassium) will have higher clearance value compared to serum creatinine. Comparing clearance of a substance to creatinine eliminates the need for timed urine collection because urine flow is no longer necessary in the calculation. This calculation is best performed on matched serum and urine samples, but creatinine and blood electrolytes are relatively stable.

Fractional excretion measurements may be performed to assess renal tubular function. In infants, fractional excretion of sodium is used in premature newborns to assess renal function [17]. Increased fractional excretion of sodium suggests subclinical or early tubular disease. Fractional excretion values for sodium, potassium, chloride, calcium, and phosphorus have been reported in foals at 4 days of age (Table 24.I.3) [2].

Table 24.I.2 Urine specific gravity and osmolality in healthy foals from birth to 4 days of age; Mean ± SD (range) [4].

Parameter	0–6 h	12 h	24 h	48 h	4 d
Urine specific	1.025 ± 0.008	1.026 ± 0.018	1.007 ± 0.010	1.004 ± 0.003	1.004 ± 0.005
Gravity	(1.008–1.035)	(1.003–1.041)	(1.001–1.031)	(1.001–1.012)	(1.001–1.016)
Urinary osmolality	527 ± 173	544 ± 285	161 ± 238	143 ± 98	138 ± 131
(mOsm/kg)	131–658	81–781	48–750	51–314	58–432
	7 d	**14 d**	**28 d**	**42 d**	**56 d**
Urine specific	1.006 ± 0.005	1.007 ± 0.005	1.007 ± 0.006	1.004 ± 0.003	1.010 ± 0.013
Gravity	(1.002–1.015)	(1.002–1.014)	(1.000–1.016)	(1.001–1.012)	(1.001–1.038)
Urinary osmolality	173 ± 145	165 ± 100	194 ± 154	126 ± 78	250 ± 253
(mOsm/kg)	55–416	71–365	42–441	43–279	44–740

Table 24.I.3 Fractional excretion measurements in 96-hour-old foals [2].

Sodium	Potassium	Chloride	Phosphorous	Calcium
0.31 ± 0.18%	13.26 ± 4.49%	0.42 ± 0.32%	3.11 ± 3.81%	2.85 ± 3.26%

Enzymuria

Enzymuria, the measurement of urinary enzyme activity, has been studied as an early indicator of renal disease [18]. It is not commonly used in equine practice due to its lack of specificity; however, it may have application when used as serial measurements for detection of early renal tubular disease. Importantly, enzymuria is best used in acute renal damage as adult horses with chronic renal disease can have decreased or normal enzyme activity [5].

Renal tubules have high metabolic activity and excrete a wide range of substances. Excretion is facilitated by enzymes located in lysosomes on the brush border of the tubular epithelial cells [5]. Increased activity of the lysosomal and brush border enzymes can be induced by inflammation and damage to the tubular epithelial cells. Enzymuria may be an early indicator of tubular damage and may precede the onset of azotemia. This may be particularly helpful with ischemia, as the tubular epithelial cells are particularly sensitive to ischemic insult [19].

Enzymes that might be elevated in urine secondary to tubular damage include N-acetyl-beta-D-glucosaminidase (NAG), gamma-glutamyl transferase (GGT), alkaline phosphatase (ALP), lactate dehydrogenase (LDH), and kallikrein. Values for these enzymes in the urine have been established in healthy adult horses [19]. Of these enzymes, GGT is the most clinically measured enzyme and, along with NAG and ALP, is associated with proximal tubule injury. The values are typically reported as a ratio (GGT : Creatinine), to correct for dilutional effects. Urine GGT activity has a high sensitivity for the detection of subclinical renal tubular damage but is not a good predictor for the development of acute renal failure. LDH is associated with distal tubule injury [20]. The urinary activity of both GGT and ALP has been studied in healthy foals [4]. Both enzymes increase significantly during the first 48 hours of life, with considerable variation among foals. The activity of these enzymes then decreases over the next 7 weeks [4]. In healthy foals <14 days of age, the urinary GGT : creatinine ratio is 12.5–46.15 [4]. Elevations of urine GGT : creatinine ratio above 25 are suggestive of proximal tubular injury, however the test lacks specificity. Elevations of urinary GGT : creatinine ratio are expected in foals that are receiving systemic aminoglycoside therapy. This increase, however, does not correlate with the severity of renal injury [21].

Abdominocentesis

Abdominocentesis is a reliable test for uroperitoneum, which is supported by a peritoneal-to-serum creatinine ratio of >2 : 1 [22]. Common causes or urinary tract rupture in foals includes parturition, rupture secondary to omphalophlebitis, and neurogenic dysfunction. Primary rupture of the bladder or urachus is the most common with ureteral rupture being uncommon. Bladder rupture during parturition is reported to be more common in colts than fillies. It is hypothesized that the anatomy of the male urethra (longer and narrow) results in increased urethral resistance during parturition when intra-abdominal pressure is increased. This results in increased resistance to bladder emptying for colts compared to fillies and may predispose them to bladder or urachal rupture. This has recently been disputed based on small case numbers in early reports resulting in a gender bias [11].

The diagnostic criteria for uroperitoneum include increased free abdominal fluid in combination with a peritoneal to peripheral creatine ratio >2 : 1. There have also been reports of uroperitoneum diagnosed based on the identification of calcium carbonate crystals in the peritoneal fluid [23]. Peritoneal fluid should be collected for cytological evaluation and bacterial culture as uroperitoneum may be associated with sepsis.

Diagnostic Imaging

Endoscopy/Cystoscopy

A pediatric endoscope or bronchoscope is typically required (diameter: 5.0 mm; working length: 84 cm) for endoscopic evaluation of the urethra and bladder in foals. Endoscopy can be used for visualization of bladder rents [24]. In foals, the dorsal bladder wall is a more common site of bladder rupture; however, ventral bladder wall tears have been described [25].

Umbilical Ultrasound

Ultrasound of the umbilicus can be performed with a microconvex or linear transducer with foals scanned standing or in lateral recumbency. Imaging frequencies ranging from 6 to 10 MHz are recommended [26]. To improve the image, the hair should be clipped along the ventral abdomen in a strip from the xyphoid to the umbilical stump and from the umbilical stump to the sheath or udder. There are eight views that are recommended for an umbilical ultrasound exam: three of the umbilical vein, one of the umbilical stump, and four of the urachus and umbilical arteries (Table 24.I.4) [27]. The umbilical vein is visualized along its length on ventral midline from the umbilicus, running cranially to the liver. The diameter should be <1 cm and the vein may narrow as it progresses toward the liver. Three cross sectional measurements should be taken. The first measurement approximately 1 cm cranial to the umbilical stump, then halfway between the liver and umbilicus, and the third measurement where the vein curves to enter the

Table 24.I.4 Average umbilical measurements for foals (age range 6 hours to 4 weeks) [27].

Structure	Measurement
Umbilical vein	
Cranial to umbilical stalk	0.61 ± 0.20 cm
Midway between umbilicus and liver	0.52 ± 0.19 cm
At the liver	0.6 ± 0.19 cm
External umbilical stump	1.5 cm
Internal umbilical stump (urachus and umbilical arteries to apex of the bladder)	1.75 ± 0.37 cm
Umbilical arteries	0.85 ± 0.21 cm

liver. A cross sectional view of the external umbilical stump should be assessed at the level of the body wall. At 24 hours of age, the average diameter of the umbilical stump is 15 mm; by day 7, it decreases to 12.5 mm [27]. The urachus and umbilical arteries are scanned from the umbilical stalk to the apex of the urinary bladder and along either side of the bladder [27]. The urachus is the most central structure of the umbilical stump adjacent to the body wall and tracks caudally to the apex of the bladder. The umbilical arteries run caudally from the umbilicus and terminate along the caudodorsal aspect of the bladder, becoming the broad ligaments of the bladder. At the base of the body wall, the umbilical arteries and urachus are adjacent to each other. Once the umbilical arteries diverge and track laterally along the bladder, the average size is <1 cm in diameter. Mild asymmetry between the umbilical arteries may be normal, but significant divergence warrants monitoring or further investigation. There is a significant reduction in vessel diameter within the first 7 days of life and enlargement of these structures necessitates additional scrutiny if correlated with clinical signs or laboratory findings. Further information regarding umbilical remnant ultrasound is discussed in Chapter 27.

Kidney and Bladder Ultrasound

Transabdominal assessment of the right and left kidneys and bladder are performed with a microconvex or curvolinear abdominal probe. Visualization of the ureters is difficult transabdominally unless there is severe distension and renal pelvis dilation [28]. The right kidney is curvilinear or heart shaped and is best visualized during inspiration as the cranial pole of the kidney is obscured by the caudal lung lobe. The left kidney is bean-shaped and consistently seen with the probe placed in the paralumbar fossa or 17th intercostal space in a laterally recumbent foal. The right kidney can be seen in the 15th and 16th intercostal space (Table 24.I.5). The renal cortex, medulla, renal pelvis, renal artery and vein, and arcuate vessels are identifiable structures in both the left and the right kidneys.

Table 24.I.5 Ultrasonographic measurements of the equine neonatal kidney [28].

Anatomical location and view		Mean ± SD
Right kidney	Width	9.57 ± 0.54 cm
	Length – dorsal	8.35 ± 0.64 cm
	Length – sagittal	8.72 ± 0.93 cm
Left kidney	Width	7.67 ± 0.61 cm
	Length – dorsal	9.90 ± 0.66 cm
	Length – sagittal	9.40 cm (n = 1)

Radiography

Abdominal radiographs in foals can be performed standing or in lateral recumbency; however, renal radiography is not commonly performed due to lack of imaging detail. Due to the lack of retroperitoneal and intrabdominal fat and the variable ingesta volume, radiographic visualization of the kidneys can be limited. The kidneys are seen as overlapping soft tissue opacities adjacent to the caudal thoracic and proximal lumbar vertebrae. Gas accumulation in the stomach or adjacent bowel enhances visualization by providing contrast, but radiographs provide limited information other than size, shape, position, and opacity [29].

Excretory Urography or Intravenous Pyelography

Excretory urography (EU) or intravenous pyelography (IVP) is a type of contrast study used to assess the entire urinary tract. In human and small animal medicine, EU/IVP is less utilized with the advent of imaging modalities such as ultrasound, computed tomography (CT), or magnetic resonance imaging (MRI). It remains, however, an excellent diagnostic tool for assessment of the entire urinary track, specifically the renal pelvis and ureters. In human medicine, the majority of EU/IVP is performed to assess hematuria and for pre- and post-treatment imaging of nephrolotihiasis [30].

A nonorganic iodide is given IV as a bolus and is excreted by the kidneys. This results in radiographic opacification of the renal and urinary structures at different time points. Sequential radiographs are taken to evaluate the parenchyma of the kidneys, renal pelvis, ureters, and urinary bladder. In small animal practice, ultrasound has largely replaced EU/IVP for assessing the urinary track, but it can be vital in the assessment of vascular, renal, or ureteral ruptures along with the diagnosis of ectopic ureters [31–34]. CT-EU has replaced traditional radiographic EU in small animal practice due to its ease of use and improved spatial and temporal detail, as there is no superimposition.

Contrast Radiography

Retrograde urethrogaphy is used to evaluate the urethra and bladder using a positive contrast medium. This is most applicable in foals for assessment of urethral and/or bladder rupture as extravasation or intrabdominal accumulation of the contrast medium will be seen. It can also be used to assess strictures, urethral trauma, urethral obstruction, and urethral calculi.

Scintigraphy

Additional renal imaging modalities have been performed in adult horses, including renal scintigraphy, although the author found no reports of renal scintigraphy in foals [29].

Advanced Imaging

CT and MRI are useful to confirm abnormalities detected via ultrasound, detect complex malformations, evaluate the collecting system, or for vascular abnormalities. These imaging modalities can be important for early detection of conditions such as renal calculi, infection, and malignancies [35]. MRI of the foal's urinary tract can be used to further assess the renal parenchyma. In humans, renal MRI is used to assess renal volume and is more accurate than three-dimensional ultrasound renal volume measurements. Renal volume has been shown to be positively correlated with renal function in human neonates [36]. MRI has also been used to assess nephron function in acute kidney injury (AKI).

Urinary Bladder Catheterization, Closed System Urine Collection

Urinary Bladder Catheterization

Urinary catheterization is commonly performed in recumbent, critically ill foals and foals with anuria or oliguria to monitor urine output and the response to fluid therapy (Table 24.I.6). Additional conditions that may warrant catheterization include patent urachus, an atonic bladder associated with neonatal encephalopathy or any condition that results in prolonged recumbency in the neonatal foal (e.g. sepsis).

Urinary catheter placement in colts is similar to adult horses. The penis is exteriorized from the sheath and the glans penis and urethral opening cleaned with soap or chlorhexidine solution. Care should be taken when exteriorizing the penis as colts can have a persistent frenulum that can make exteriorization challenging. If a persistent frenulum is present, it can be carefully broken down. Once clean, the catheter is lubricated with a sterile, water-soluble lubricant and is inserted into the urethra (Figure 24.I.1). If the catheter has a guide wire, it should be removed from the catheter prior to placement, lubricated, and replaced. This will ease removal and prevent bunching or kinking of the urinary catheter once placed. Once the urinary catheter is in place, a syringe is attached to the catheter and light suction applied to confirm placement as evidenced by collection of urine. This sterile urine sample can be submitted for bacterial culture if indicated.

The urinary catheter is then secured in place. Foley urinary catheters should have the Foley balloon inflated with sterile saline. If a urinary catheter without a Foley balloon is used, the catheter can be sutured to the glans penis with a purse-string suture pattern followed by a Chinese finger-trap pattern. Alternatively, the catheter can be secured to the glans penis using stay sutures secured to white tape placed over the catheter in a butterfly pattern. This may reduce the risk of bladder rupture during spontaneous urination around the catheter and can reduce trauma to the glans penis. Infusion of a local anesthetic such as lidocaine into the glans penis can improve patient comfort during the procedure. A Foley catheter is recommended as the balloon inflation is sufficient to keep the catheter in place and reduces trauma to the glans penis. This technique can be used in ambulatory foals. Depending on the behavior of the foal, sedation may be required for urinary catheter placement.

Table 24.I.6 Recommended urinary catheter size [37].

	Diameter	Length
Colt	5–8 Fr Foley	54 cm
Filly	8–12 Fr Foley	33 cm

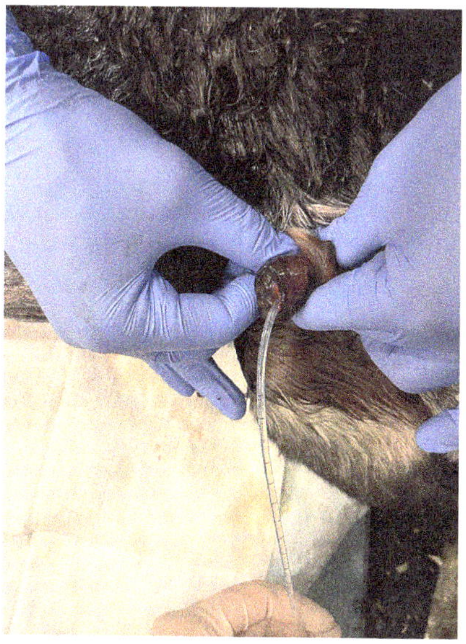

Figure 24.I.1 Placement of a urinary catheter in a colt.
Source: Image courtesy of David Wong, Iowa State University.

Urinary catheterization of the filly is more challenging because the clinician cannot visualize the urethral opening, thus the catheter is placed blindly. The perineum and vulva are cleaned in the same way as the colt. For placement, one hand is responsible for the catheter and the other hand has a finger inserted on the vestibular floor. The catheter is advanced on the ventral floor of the vestibule and should enter the urethra and pass into the bladder. Once the urinary catheter is in place, a syringe is attached to the catheter and suction applied to confirm placement. A sterile laryngoscope with a light source can be used to visualize the urethral orifice, if needed. The catheter is secured by inflating the Foley catheter or suturing the catheter to the vulvar lips. A non-Foley catheter can be secured in a similar fashion to the colts with a purse string and Chinese finger-trap combination. Alternatively, white tape can be made into a butterfly pattern and securing to the body wall with two simple interrupted sutures.

The urinary catheter should be connected to a device to prevent air aspiration. For ambulatory foals, a one-way valve (Heimlich valve) or a small slit in the fingertip of a sterile glove can be used and secured to the end of the catheter with tape. The latter must be changed every 24 hours and monitored closely. If the slit is too large, the one-way valve action will fail, thereby increasing the risk of air aspiration. For down foals, a urinary collection bag can be secured to the abdomen or the hind limb. If the foal is inactive, the collection bag can simply be placed on the floor of the stall next to the foal bed.

Catheter Care

Complications of urinary catheterization include urinary tract infection, cystitis, occlusion with debris (mucous, sedimentation, crystallization), incorrect placement, balloon failure, air embolism, and swelling or cellulitis of the external urethra and genitalia. Foals with an indwelling urinary catheter are typically treated with broad-spectrum antimicrobials, with preference to those that concentrate in the urine (e.g. sulfamethoxazole, beta-lactams). Catheters should be removed as soon as possible to reduce the risk of complications. For foals with a history of difficulty voiding urine, it is advisable to temporarily obstruct the catheter to assess the foal's ability to urinate prior to its removal.

Closed System Urinary Collection

A closed system for urine collection is indicated in recumbent foals (Figure 24.I.2), cases in which fluid balance and monitoring is required, and cases of oliguria or anuria. The system allows the clinician to quantify urine production.

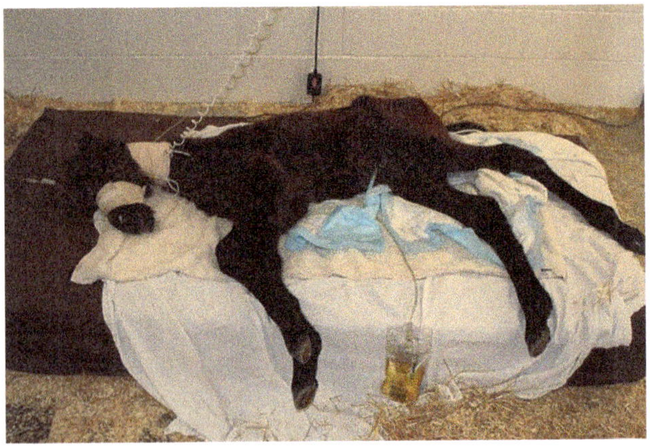

Figure 24.I.2 Ill neonatal foal with closed urinary collection system. *Source:* Image courtesy of David Wong, Iowa State University.

For down foals, a urinary collection bag can be secured to the abdomen or hind limb. All ends should be cleaned once daily with dilute chlorhexidine and the urine collection bag should be emptied regularly or when full and the volume of urine recorded [37].

Therapeutics

Increasing Urine Production

Fluid therapy for polyuric renal disease should be titrated to supply maintenance fluids as well as account for increased fluid losses. Fluid therapy for oliguric or anuric renal failure should be titrated carefully. It is important to be judicious with fluid administration while avoiding dehydration, especially if the foal is receiving furosemide or dopamine. Fluids are indicated to correct dehydration and hypovolemia and to induce diuresis. Placement of a urinary catheter and urinary collection system is helpful for fluid monitoring [20]. Serial body weight measurements should be performed every 12–24 hours to monitor for large fluctuations in weight gain, which suggests fluid overloading.

There are several pharmacological interventions available for patients in anuric or oliguria renal failure that aid in increasing urine production. Commonly used medications include diuretics, dopaminergics, and positive ionotropes. Furosemide, a loop diuretic, is the most common drug used in anuric or oliguric patients to increase urine production. Furosemide acts on the thick ascending loop of Henle where it inhibits the $Na^+/K^+/2Cl^-$ co-transporter resulting in natriuresis and diuresis. Furosemide also decreases renal metabolic demands and is generally well tolerated [20]. Furosemide is administered as a single bolus at a dose of 0.5–1.0 mg/kg IV q8–12 h to 1–2 mg/kg every

30–120 minutes over 6 hours [38, 39]. Alternatively, furosemide can also be administered as a constant rate infusion (CRI) using a loading dose of 0.12 mg/kg IV, followed by CRI of 0.12 mg/kg/h (dosing based on adult horses). [40] Electrolyte monitoring is important with furosemide administration, as it can cause hypokalemia and metabolic acidosis as a sequel to its natriuretic effects. Hypovolemia and hypotension should be corrected in the foal with adequate fluid administration prior to diuretic therapy to avoid profound dehydration. The use of furosemide in humans with acute renal failure has not been shown to reduce mortality [41].

Osmotic diuretics such as mannitol are considered if improvement is not made with furosemide. Mannitol is a potent osmotic diuretic but should be avoided in anuric renal failure. Other potential benefits of mannitol include increased renal blood flow by inducing synthesis of PGE_2 and increasing release of atrial natriuretic peptide [42, 43]. Mannitol may be effective in treating renal tubular obstruction and swelling of tubular cells. A dose of 0.25–1.0 g/kg IV as a 20% solution over 20 minutes has been used in foals [8].

Dopamine is administered as a CRI to increase urine production. The effects of dopamine are dose-dependent. At low doses (<2 μg/kg/min), dopamine stimulates dopaminergic receptors and results in increased urine production via natriuresis [44]. Low to moderate doses (2–10 μg/kg/min) of dopamine stimulate β-adrenergic receptors to improve cardiac function, whereas high doses (>10 μg/kg/min) stimulate α-adrenergic receptors resulting in vasoconstriction [45–47]. High doses should be avoided due to the risk of decreased renal blood flow and decreased GFR. In human medicine the use of dopamine is controversial in cases of renal failure [48]. Dobutamine should be considered as a positive inotrope if cardiac dysfunction or hypotension are contributors to decreased renal blood flow. In horses, doses of 2.5 and 5 μg/kg/min showed improved cardiac output with some dysrhythmias detected at the higher dose [49]. Reported doses for dobutamine range from 3 to 5 μg/kg/min [5, 50].

Antimicrobials

The most common microorganisms associated with omphalitis and omphalophlebitis are Gram-negative enteric and nonenteric bacteria, *Streptococcus,* and occasionally anaerobes [51–53]. For renal or urinary tract infections, broad-spectrum antimicrobials are recommended, preferably those that are excreted in the urine. These include beta-lactams or trimethoprim sulfas combined with amikacin for adequate Gram-negative coverage. The use of aminoglycosides depends on the presence of normal renal function. The most common antimicrobial for anaerobic infection is metronidazole.

Pain Management

NSAID therapy should be used judiciously in foals, even those with adequate renal function. Phenazopyridine can be administered (4 mg/kg PO, q 8–12 hours) for urinary tract pain. This medication anesthetizes the urinary tract epithelium and provides significant urinary tract pain relief. Phenazopyridine loses efficacy within 72 hours but can be used for acute urinary tract pain. Other medications to consider include butorphanol and a CRI of lidocaine.

Further information regarding medications used for treatment of the urinary system are noted in the next section.

References

1 Enzerink, E., van Weeren, P.R., and van der Velden, M.A. (2000). Closure of the abdominal wall at the umbilicus and the development of umbilical hernias in a group of foals from birth to 11 months of age. *Vet. Rec.* 147: 37–39.

2 Brewer, B.D., Clement, S.F., Lotz, W.S. et al. (1991). Renal clearance, urinary excretion of endogenous substances, and urinary diagnostic indices in healthy neonatal foals. *J. Vet. Intern. Med.* 5: 28–33.

3 Knottenbelt, D.C. (2004). Perinatal review. In: *Equine Neonatology Medicine and Surgery* (ed. N. Knottenbelt, N.B. Holdstock, and J.E. Madigan), 1–27. London: WB Saunders.

4 Edwards, D., Brownlow, M., and Hutchins, D. (1990). Indices of renal function: values in eight normal foals from birth to 56 days. *Aust. Vet. J.* 67: 251–254.

5 Walridge, B. (2018). Disorders of the urinary system. In: *Equine Internal Medicine* (ed. S.M. Reed, W.M. Bayly, and D.C. Sellon), 1140–1247. St. Louis, MO: Elsevier.

6 Medina-Torres, C.E., Hewson, J., Stämpfli, S. et al. (2014). Bilateral diffuse cystic renal dysplasia in a 9-day-old Thoroughbred filly. *Can. Vet. J.* 55: 141–146.

7 Morresey, P.R. (2005). Prenatal and perinatal indicators of neonatal viability. *Clin. Tech. Equine Pract.* 4: 238–249.

8 Vaala, W.E. (1999). Peripartum asphyxia syndrome in foals. *Proc. Am. Assoc. Equine Pract.* 45: 247–253.

9 Schmitz, D.G., Joyce, J.R., and Reagor, J.C. (1982). Serum biochemical values in Quarter Horse foals in the first 6 months of life. *Equine Pract.* 4: 24–30.

10 Rumbaugh, G.E. and Adamson, P.J.W. (1983). Automated serum chemical analysis in the foal. *J. Am. Vet. Med. Assoc.* 183: 769–772.

11 Kablack, K.A., Embertson, R.M., Bernard, W.V. et al. (2000). Uroperitoneum in the hospitalised equine neonate: retrospective study of 31 cases, 1988–1997. *Equine Vet. J.* 32: 505–508.
12 Paltrinieri, S., Giraldi, M., Prolo, A. et al. (2018). Serum symmetric dimethylarginine and creatinine in Birman cats compared with cats of other breeds. *J. Feline Med. Surg.* 20: 905–912.
13 Nijveldt, R.J., Teerlink, T., Van Guldener, D. et al. (2003). Handling of asymmetrical dimethylarginine and symmetrical dimethylarginine by the rat kidney under basal conditions and during endotoxemia. *Nephrol. Dialysis Transplant.* 18: 2542–2550.
14 Siwinska, N., Zak, A., Slowikowska, M. et al. (2020). Serum symmetric dimethylarginine concentration in healthy horses and horses with acute kidney injury. *BMC Vet. Res.* 16: 396.
15 Bozorgmanesh, R., Magdesian, G., Offer, K. et al. (2019). Equine neonatal symmetric dimethylarginine in sick neonates with hypercreatininemia. *J. Vet. Emerg. Crit. Care.* 29: S30.
16 Brewer, B.D., Clement, S.F., Lotz, W.S. et al. (1990). A comparison of inulin, para-aminohippuric acid, and endogenous creatinine clearances as measures of renal function in neonatal foals. *J. Vet. Intern. Med.* 4: 301–305.
17 Escobedo-Chávez, E., Carvallo-Herrada, R., Thompson-Chagoyan, O. et al. (1990). Kidney function in the newborn infant of 32 to 36 weeks gestation: the usefulness of the excreted sodium fraction. *Bol. Med. Hosp. Infant Mex.* 47: 756–759.
18 Westhuyzen, J., Endre, Z.H., Reece, G. et al. (2003). Measurement of tubular enzymuria facilitates early detection of acute renal impairment in the intensive care unit. *Nephrol. Dialysis Transplant.* 18: 543–551.
19 Breshears, M.A. and Confer, A.W. (2017). The urinary system. In: *Pathologic Basis of Veterninary Disease* (ed. M.D. McFavin and J.F. Zachary), 617–681.e1. St. Louis, MO: Mosby:https://doi.org/10.1016/B978-0-323-35775-3.00011-4.
20 McKenzie, H.C. III (2018). Disorders of foals. In: *Equine Internal Medicine* (ed. S.M. Reed, W.M. Bayly, and D.C. Sellon), 1365–1459. St. Louis, MO: Elsevier.
21 McKenzie, H.C. and Furr, M.O. (2003). Aminoglycoside antibiotics in neonatal foals. *Compend. Contin. Educ. Vet.* 25: 457–469.
22 Aumann, M., Worth, L.T., and Drobatz, K.J. (1998). Uroperitoneum in cats: 26 cases (1986–1995). *J. Am. Anim. Hosp. Assoc.* 34: 315–324.
23 Morley, P. and Desnoyers, M. (1992). Diagnosis of ruptured urinary bladder in a foal by the identification of calcium carbonate crystals in the peritoneal fluid. *J. Am. Vet. Med. Assoc.* 200: 1515–1517.
24 Stephen, J., Harty, M., Hollis, A. et al. (2009). A non-invasive technique for standing surgical repair of urinary bladder rupture in a post-partum mare: a case report. *Ir. Vet. J.* 62: 734–736.
25 Behr, M.J., Hackett, R.P., Bentinck-Smith, J. et al. (1981). Metabolic abnormalities associated with rupture of the urinary bladder in neonatal foals. *J. Am. Vet. Med. Assoc.* 178: 263–266.
26 Sprayberry, K.A. (2015). Ultrasonographic examination of the equine neonate, thorax and abdomen. *Vet. Clin. North Am. Equine Pract.* 31: 515–543.
27 Reef, V.B. and Collatos, C. (1988). Ultrasonography of umbilical structures in clinically normal foals. *Am. J. Vet. Res.* 49 (12): 2143–2146.
28 Hoffmann, K.L., Wood, A.K.W., and Mccarthy, P.H. (2010). Ultrasonography of the equine neonatal kidney. *Equine Vet. J.* 32 (2): 109–113.
29 Matthews, H.K. and Toal, R.L. (1996). A review of equine renal imaging techniques. *Vet. Radiol. Ultrasound* 37: 163–173.
30 Heuter, K.J. (2005). Excretory urography. *Clin. Tech. Small Anim. Pract.* 20: 39–45.
31 Rademacher, N. (2019). Diagnostic imaging of the urinary tract. *Vet. Clin. North Am. Small Anim. Pract.* 49: 261–286.
32 Beccati, F., Cercone, M., Angeli, G. et al. (2015). Imaging diagnosis - use of multiphase computed tomographic urography in the diagnosis of ureteral tear in a 6-day-old foal. *Vet. Radiol. Ultrasound.* 57: E10–E15.
33 Coleman, M.C., Chaffin, M.K., Arnold, C.E. et al. (2011). The use of computed tomography in the diagnosis of an ectopic ureter in a Quarter Horse filly. *Equine Vet. Educ.* 23: 597–602.
34 Blikslager, A.T., Green, E.M., MacFadden, K.E. et al. (1992). Excretory urography and ultrasonography in the diagnosis of bilateral ectopic ureters in a foal. *Vet. Radiol. Ultrasound* 33: 41–47.
35 Ramanathan, S., Kumar, D., Khanna, M. et al. (2016). Multi-modality imaging review of congenital abnormalities of kidney and upper urinary tract. *World J. Radiol.* 8: 132–141.
36 Kim, H.C., Yang, D.M., Jin, W., and Lee, S.H. (2010). Relation between total renal volume and renal function: usefulness of 3D sonographic measurements with a matrix array transducer. *Am. J. Roentgenol.* 194: W186–W192.
37 Nogradi, N. and Magdesian, K. (2017). Urinary catheter placement in the neonatal foal. In: *Manual of Clinical Procedures in the Horse* (ed. L.R.R. Costa and M.R. Paradis), 452–456. Hoboken, NJ: Wiley Blackwell.
38 Wong, D., Wilkins, P.A., Bain, F.T. et al. (2011). Neonatal encephalopathy in foals. *Compend. Contin. Educ. Vet.* 33: E5.

39 Divers, T. and Perkins, G. (2003). Urinary and hepatic disorders in neonatal foals. *Clin. Tech. Equine Pract.* 2: 67–78.

40 Johansson, A.M., Gardner, S.Y., Levine, J.F. et al. (2003). Furosemide continuous rate infusion in the horse: evaluation of enhanced efficacy and reduced side effects. *J. Vet. Intern. Med.* 17: 887–889.

41 Shilliday, I.R., Quinn, K.J., and Allison, M.E. (1997). Loop diuretics in the management of acute renal failure: a prospective, double-blind, placebo-controlled, randomized study. *Nephrol. Dialysis Transplant.* 12: 2592–2596.

42 Yu, C.C., Chen, S.M., and Young, T.K. (1993). The effect of mannitol on antidiuretic and natriuretic actions of ADH in rats. *Chin. J. Phys.* 36: 181–186.

43 Johnston, P.A., Bernard, D.B., Perrin, N.S. et al. (1981). Prostaglandins mediate the vasodilatory effect of mannitol in the hypoperfused rat kidney. *J. Clin. Invest.* 68: 127–133.

44 Armando, I., Villar, V.A., and Jose, P.A. (2011). Dopamine and renal function and blood pressure regulation. *Compr. Physiol.* 1: 1075–1117.

45 Dancker, C., Hopster, K., Rohn, K. et al. (2018). Effects of dobutamine, dopamine, phenylephrine and noradrenaline on systemic haemodynamics and intestinal perfusion in isoflurane anaesthetized horses. *Equine Vet. J.* 50: 104–110.

46 Goldberg, L.I. (1985). Dopamine: receptors and clinical applications. *Clin. Physiol. Biochem.* 3: 120–126.

47 De Backer, D., Biston, P., Devriendt, J. et al. (2010). Comparison of dopamine and norepinephrine in the treatment of shock. *N. Engl. J. Med.* 362: 779–789.

48 Lauschke, A., Teichgräber, U.K., Frei, U. et al. (2006). Low-dose dopamine worsens renal prefusion in patients with AKI. *Kidney Int.* 69: 1669–1674.

49 Trim, C.M., Moore, J.N., and White, N.A. (1985). Cardiopulmonary effects of dopamine hydrochloride in anaesthetised horses. *Equine Vet. J.* 17: 41–44.

50 Hollis, A.R., Ousey, J.C., Palmer, L. et al. (2006). Effects of norepinephrine and a combined norepinephrine and dobutamine infusion on systemic hemodynamics and indices of renal function in normotensive neonatal thoroughbred foals. *J. Vet. Intern. Med.* 20: 1437–1442.

51 Russell, C.M., Axon, J.E., Blishen, A. et al. (2008). Blood culture isolates and antimicrobial sensitivities from 427 critically ill neonatal foals. *Aust. Vet. J.* 86: 266–271.

52 Marsh, P.S. and Palmer, J.E. (2001). Bacterial isolates from blood and their susceptibility patterns in critically ill foals: 543 cases (1991–1998). *J. Am. Vet. Med. Assoc.* 218: 1608–1610.

53 Wilson, W.D. and Madigan, J.E. (1989). Comparison of bacteriologic culture of blood and necropsy specimens for determining the cause of foal septicemia: 47 cases (1978–1987). *J. Am. Vet. Med. Assoc.* 195: 1759–1763.

Section II Medications Acting on the Urinary System

David Wong and Jennifer Davis

Safe and effective drug administration to neonatal foals is based on the combined knowledge of the developing physiological characteristics of the foal receiving the medication and the pharmacokinetics (PK) and pharmacodynamics (PD) of individual drugs. As one can imagine, there is a variety of physiologic changes that occur within the first week, first month, and first year of life of the growing foal. In regard to the neonatal period, there are notable changes in organ function, body composition, cellular function, and metabolic activity that can impact drug metabolism [1]. Because of the rapidly changing physiology, there can be a large degree of PK and PD variability between foals early in life.

Medications specifically targeting the urinary tract are seldom needed in the care of critically ill neonatal foals. However, perhaps the most frequent disease process encountered in ill foals is acute kidney injury (AKI) that occurs secondary to hypoxia–ischemia or as a consequence of sepsis. Compromised renal function can be documented clinically by measuring increased serum creatinine concentrations or decreased urine production. The best method to support renal function is prevention (e.g. maintenance of adequate fluid volume, avoidance of hypotension) or immediate treatment of hypovolemia and hypotension, but this is not always possible.

When faced with a foal with AKI, carefully titrated fluid therapy is indicated; if the foal remains oliguric or anuric, administration of medications that may promote renal perfusion is warranted. However, the clinician should note that neither diuretics such as furosemide nor other pharmacologic agents (dopamine, fenoldopam, mannitol) that aim to improve renal perfusion have been shown to improve outcome in human studies of renal failure [2, 3]. Other medications used to treat the urinary system include antimicrobials to treat urinary tract infections, medications used to stimulate detrusor function, and dyes that aid in identifying physical defects within the urinary tract.

Dopamine

Dopamine is an endogenous catecholamine (immediate metabolic precursor of norepinephrine and epinephrine) that has widespread effects on neural (neurotransmitter) and non-neural (endocrine or paracrine agent) tissues. Dopamine occurs as a natural neurotransmitter in the brain, but other receptors are located peripherally; these receptors are subtyped into D_1 and D_2 (central nervous system) and DA_1 and DA_2 (peripheral) receptors, respectively [4]. DA_1 receptors are most abundantly located in the adrenal cortex and in renal, splanchnic, coronary, and cerebral vascular beds. When receptors are stimulated by dopamine, smooth muscle relaxation occurs, and it is by this mechanism that renal arteriolar vasodilation and increased renal blood blow occurs. DA_1 receptors are also present in the brush-border and basolateral membranes of the proximal tubules and, when stimulated, induce changes in tubular ion fluxes and increase renin release [4]. DA_2 receptors are located in the carotid body, gastrointestinal tract, and anterior pituitary gland and are found presynaptically on adrenergic nerve terminals and in sympathetic ganglia; activation results in inhibition of norepinephrine release [5–7].

Exogenous dopamine exerts complex effects via dose-dependent stimulation of dopaminergic and α- and β-adrenergic receptors. Low doses of dopamine (0.5–2 μg/kg/min) stimulate receptors of the cardiovascular system, kidneys, and adrenergic nerve endings. At intermediate doses (2–6 μg/kg/min), the effects of cardiac β_1- and β_2-adrenergic receptor stimulation are also present. Intermediate doses can also augment renal perfusion by increasing cardiac output via stimulation of cardiac β_1 receptors [7]. At higher doses (6–10 μg/kg/min), activation of the cardiovascular and α_1- and α_2-adrenergic receptors are apparent [4]. For the purposes of this chapter, the effects of lower doses (1–5 μg/kg/min) will be emphasized as they stimulate

Equine Neonatal Medicine, First Edition. Edited by David M. Wong and Pamela A. Wilkins.

peripheral DA_1 and DA_2 receptors resulting in increased renal, mesenteric, and coronary blood flow [8]. For many years, low doses of dopamine were administered to patients with decreased renal perfusion (e.g. AKI/failure), as stimulation of renal vascular receptors was believed to increase renal blood flow by approximately 20–40% [4]. However, the use and efficacy of dopamine has been increasingly challenged and is no longer recommended for renal protection in people [9, 10].

Despite this, equine clinicians have used low-dose dopamine to try to promote renal perfusion when rehydration alone is unsuccessful. In healthy horses administered a low dose of dopamine, renal blood flow, and urine volume increased [11]. Specifically, at dopamine doses of 2.5 and 5.0 μg/kg/min, renal blood flow significantly increased during administration, whereas urine volume significantly increased when 5.0 μg/kg/min of dopamine was administered. Arterial blood pressure and heart rate were not impacted by dopamine administration, but transient arrythmias were noted in healthy horses [11]. The use of dopamine has been reported in a variety of adult horses and foals with AKI, but the true benefit (if any) is unknown [12–15]. If used, dopamine should be diluted in isotonic saline, 5% dextrose, or lactated Ringer's solution. Avoid mixing with solutions containing bicarbonate or other alkaline solutions. The dose should be carefully titrated from a starting point of 1–3 μg/kg/min in foals.

Fenoldopam Mesylate

Fenoldopam mesylate is a selective DA_1 receptor agonist used to treat hypertension in people. At low-dose rates of 0.03–0.05 μg/kg/min, fenoldopam increases renal blood flow and urine output, although renal responses vary between species. In a small study in healthy 3- to 5-day-old foals, the systemic and renal effects were evaluated in response to a low (0.04 μg/kg/min) and high (0.4 μg/kg/min) dose of fenoldopam [16]. In that study, low-dose fenoldopam did not significantly affect hemodynamic variables but the high dose produced a significant decrease in mean (MAP), systolic (SAP), and diastolic arterial pressure (DAP) and a moderate increase in heart rate. With regard to renal function, administration of low-dose fenoldopam significantly increased urine output (153 ± 110 ml) and tended to increase creatinine clearance (5930 ± 2470 ml/min) when compared to saline control (53 ± 47 ml; 3270 ± 2290 ml/min, respectively) [16]. Based on this study, low-dose fenoldopam has the potential clinical application for prophylaxis or treatment of AKI in neonatal foal.

In people, perioperative treatment with fenoldopam was associated with a significant reduction in AKI after major surgery but did not change hospital mortality [17]. In comparison, in a study in critically ill dogs and cats, fenoldopam administration did not have significant impact between treated and control groups with regard to survival, length of hospital stay, adverse effects, or changes in creatinine, blood urea nitrogen or sodium concentrations [18]. Fenoldopam can be considered in foals with AKI, but further study in foals is necessary to determine if it could help prevent or treat AKI in foals.

Furosemide

Furosemide is a short-acting loop diuretic with the primary site of action at the thick ascending limb of the loop of Henle. Furosemide is highly protein bound (98%) and thus only a small amount of the drug is filtered through the glomerulus; therefore, delivery of the majority of drug to the tubules is by tubular secretion [19]. Consequently, the pharmacological effect of furosemide is not realized until it reaches the proximal tubule by tubular secretion through the vasa recta [20]. Because of this fact, decreased renal blood flow and/or compromised proximal tubular epithelial cell function that can be associated with AKI might limit furosemide entry into the nephron. Furthermore, tubular obstruction by cellular debris, pigments, or crystals can inhibit tubular flow and the amount of furosemide that is able to reach the thick ascending limb of the loop of Henle. Once the drug reaches the lumen of the tubules, it reversibly binds to the $Na^+/K^+/2Cl^-$ cotransport mechanism of the thick ascending loop of Henle and inhibits active reabsorption of these ions [20]. Furosemide also reduces reabsorption of sodium and chloride in the proximal and distal tubules (uncertain mechanism) [20]. An additional benefit of furosemide in regard to AKI is its ability to increase renal blood flow, likely from prostaglandin-mediated vasodilation [19]; increased prostaglandin production probably occurs through stimulation of the renin-angiotensin pathway [20]. This particular property forms part of the rationale for the use of furosemide to treat AKI after hypoxia, hypovolemia, hypotension, and resulting vasomotor nephropathy [20].

In human neonates there is remarkable interindividual variability in the kinetic parameters of furosemide. For example, the half-life ($t_{1/2}$) is 6–20-fold longer, clearance is 1.2–14-fold smaller, and volume of distribution (V_d) is 1.3–6 fold larger than adults [19]. These differences have not been directly compared between neonatal foals and adult horses, but some likely exist. The traditional IV bolus dose of furosemide is 1 mg/kg every 12 hours, but this dose may not be sufficient in sick infants.

In addition to the aforementioned barriers that furosemide must overcome to be effective, in neonates with AKI, retained organic acids can compete with furosemide for

Table 24.II.1 Diuretics classified according to mechanism of action.

Class	Drug	Mechanism of action	Comments
Osmotic diuretics	Mannitol	Increase extracellular fluid, renal blood flow Freely filtered, not reabsorbed Increase water diuresis Increase natriuresis	Avoid in anuric renal failure, cerebral hemorrhage May crystallize at cool temperatures
Carbonic anhydrase inhibitors	Acetazolamide	Inhibit proximal tubular H+ secretion Increase HCO_3 excretion Increase water and sodium excretion	Mild diuretic effects Use is typically reserved for foals with hyperkalemic periodic paralysis
Loop diuretics	Furosemide Bumetanide	Inhibit NaCl active reabsorption Increased natriuresis	Very potent, high-ceiling diuretic
Thiazides	Hydrochlorothiazide Chlorothiazide	Inhibit NaCl active reabsorption Increase water excretion	Avoid in patients with hypercalcemia and azotemia
K^+-sparing diuretics	Spironolactone	Inhibit sodium reabsorption in cortical collecting duct	Avoid in patients with hyperkalemia

proximal tubular secretion resulting in only 10–20% of the drug being secreted into the tubular lumen [21]. Thus, larger doses (2–5 mg/kg, IV) have been suggested in AKI in people, adult horses, and foals (e.g. 1–2 mg/kg, repeated every 30–120 minutes for up to 6 hours or until urine production is increased) before it can be concluded that the treatment is ineffective [7, 8, 22]. Dosing of furosemide either as intermittent IV boluses or continuous rate infusions (CRIs) has also been compared in infants [19]. Most studies noted no significant difference in urinary output between the two methods of administration over a 24-hour period. However, some investigators felt that CRI of furosemide was superior to intermittent administration because it offered a more constant urinary flow and more controlled diuresis following cardiac surgery [19]. In other reports, use of CRI of furosemide was not suggested in cases of AKI unless there was good urine output after the initial bolus dose of furosemide [20]. CRI of furosemide (loading dose 0.12 mg/kg, CRI 0.12 mg/kg/h) has been compared to intermittent bolus dosing (1 mg/kg, IV, q8h) in healthy adult horses with somewhat similar results as those noted in human studies [23]. Overall urine volume in horses was not significantly greater in the CRI group, but the CRI group produced a more uniform urine flow, had decreased fluctuations in plasma volume, and induced higher urine volume production during the first 8 hours of the infusion when compared to intermittent bolus dosing [23]. Whether a CRI of furosemide improves outcome in foals with AKI is unknown, but the use of furosemide, either solely or in addition to dopamine, remains an option to enhance urine production in oliguric/anuric AKI. Of note, if using a CRI, infusion sets should be protected from light to prevent photochemical degradation of the furosemide during infusion [23].

Furosemide has a wide margin of safety and negative effects were not observed in healthy horses given doses of up to 16 mg/kg, IV [7]. However, the clinician should be aware of the fact that furosemide produces a rapid decrease in plasma and blood volumes and concomitant increase in total protein concentration. Other side effects of furosemide administration include hyponatremia, hypokalemia, and hypochloremic alkalosis; hypercalciuria and development of renal calculi can occur with long-term furosemide therapy. In people, furosemide is potentially ototoxic, especially in patients receiving other ototoxic drugs such as aminoglycosides, but this has not been demonstrated in foals. Furosemide administration has been associated with increased incidence of patent ductus arteriosus which may be secondary to furosemide's ability to stimulate renal synthesis of prostaglandin E2 [19]. Other diuretics that could be potentially utilized in foals are noted in Table 24.II.1 keeping in mind that diuretics must be coupled with judicious fluid therapy and careful monitoring of electrolyte and acid–base parameters.

Adenosine Antagonists

Theophylline and its related salt aminophylline are methylxanthines that also act as adenosine antagonists and have been used to prevent or treat AKI by inhibiting renal vasoconstriction [24]. Adenosine is a tissue hormone involved in metabolic control of organ function and local matching of blood flow with energy consumption (i.e. adenosine concentrations increase with negative energy balance) [25]. In the kidney, the metabolic burden and demand for energy largely falls on the renal cortex, which expends energy to perform tubular electrolyte transport [25]. During periods of negative energy balance, or in cases of hypoxia, the kidney increases adenosine to lower glomerular filtration rate (GFR), through afferent arteriolar vasoconstriction [26].

Adenosine is also a mediator of tubuloglomerular feedback [27]. In this mechanism, the macula densa senses tubular NaCl load in the thick ascending limb and induces a change in afferent arterial tone. In other words, with increasing solute load in the renal tubule, energy depletion is accompanied by release of adenosine. Subsequently, adenosine stimulates preglomerular vasoconstriction, resulting in a reduction in solute flow (via decreased GFR) and maintaining energy balance [27].

Low doses of nonspecific adenosine antagonists such as theophylline or aminophylline inhibit vasoconstriction produced by adenosine, whereas higher doses block type IV phosphodiesterase thereby lowering the breakdown of cyclic adenosine monophosphate (cAMP), which promotes renal vasodilation and renal perfusion [5, 27, 28]. In one systemic review, a single dose of prophylactic theophylline administered to term neonates with severe birth asphyxia decreased the incidence of AKI by 60% compared to placebo and decreased serum creatine levels from days 2–5; no significant difference in mortality was noted between groups [5]. Conversely, another systemic review of aminophylline administered in children with AKI did not document significant differences in incidence of AKI, serum creatine clearance rate, urine output, and all-cause mortality [27]. Although not widely investigated in foals with AKI, an aminophylline dose of 5 μg/kg as a slow infusion over 12 hours has provided anecdotal clinical success in foals with AKI [8]. PK/PD studies involving theophylline/aminophylline have been sporadically examined in adult horses for treatment of equine asthma, but not for the purpose of preventing or treating AKI [8, 29, 30]. In six healthy adult horses, IV aminophylline administered at a dose of 9.94 mg/kg (as theophylline) resulted in theophylline plasma concentrations of 11.51 ± 1.5 μg/ml [29]. Theophylline has wide variation in metabolism and a narrow therapeutic window. Typically, theophylline/aminophylline therapy is short term (1–2 days) and thus toxicity at this dosage is not common; however, if the drug is continued for a more prolonged period, serum theophylline concentrations should be measured and maintained at <15 μg/ml to avoid toxicity [5, 8]. Toxicity in horses typically involves central nervous system (CNS) excitement.

Interestingly, caffeine is also an adenosine receptor antagonist that has been evaluated for its renoprotective effects in preterm infants; in some studies AKI was less frequent when caffeine was administered within the first postnatal week [24, 31, 32]. To the authors' knowledge, caffeine has not been examined in foals for the purpose of prevention or treatment of AKI.

Mannitol

Along with furosemide and dopamine, mannitol (0.25–1 g/kg as a 20% solution administered over 15–20 minutes, IV) has been suggested as a treatment for oliguric AKI that is refractory to volume replacement therapy with the goal of increasing renal perfusion and urine production. Mannitol is a six-carbon, linear, simple sugar that is only mildly metabolized by the body and excreted primarily by the kidneys when administered IV. Mannitol administration increases plasma osmolality thereby causing a shift of fluid into the intravascular space and increasing the circulating volume, renal blood flow, and GFR. Additionally, because mannitol does not undergo renal tubular reabsorption, it increases intratubular osmotic pressure and enhances free water excretion. Mannitol also scavenges oxygen radicals. In addition to potentially augmenting diuresis in AKI, mannitol has been used to treat increased intracranial pressure as well as reduce intraocular pressure in people. However, mannitol can cause significant osmotic injury to the tubules resulting in acute tubular necrosis and/or oxidative stress resulting in damage to the renal tubular epithelial cells, thereby decreasing its use in clinical practice [33]. Moreover, retrospective studies have not demonstrated renal protective characteristics in a variety of major surgeries [34].

Mannitol has been used in foals with AKI in attempts to enhance urine production in cases of AKI, but the risks of administration with AKI are not inconsequential and should be carefully considered prior to administration. With regards to administration, crystals may form in mannitol solutions especially if the solution is chilled. These crystals can be dissolved by warming the bottle in hot water at 80 °C and shaking periodically. When infusing 25% mannitol concentrations, administration should include a filter.

Antimicrobials

Primary urinary tract infections are relatively uncommon in neonatal foals, but ascending infections via the urachus are frequently encountered in ill neonates [35–37]. In one study involving 52 foals that had cultures performed on umbilical remnants, 58 Gram-positive isolates were cultured as compared to 53 Gram-negative isolates [37]. In that study, *Streptococcus* (23 isolates), *Enterococcus* (15), and *Staphylococcus* (11) species were the most common Gram-positive organisms while *Escherichia coli* (12), *Vibrio* (12), and *Klebsiella* (6) species were the most common Gram-negative organisms [36]. *E. coli* and beta-hemolytic *Streptococci* were the most common isolates in 33 foals in another study of foals with umbilical remnant infections [35]. In light of this information, use of broad-spectrum antimicrobial combinations in foals with umbilical infections, similar to those used in sepsis (Chapter 50) in foals, is recommended unless culture and sensitivity results allow more targeted antimicrobial therapy. Common therapies include combinations of beta-lactams and aminoglycosides, assuming normal renal function. In foals that are otherwise healthy but develop umbilical abscessation, broad-spectrum oral antimicrobial therapy with a drug that accumulates and has high activity in abscesses, such as chloramphenicol, may be successful.

Miscellaneous Medications

Phenazopyridine

Phenazopyridine is an over-the-counter azo dye that is commonly used to provide urinary tract analgesia in people and horses with urinary tract pain [38–41]. It is not recommended in small animals due to potential adverse effects. Phenazopyridine is primarily excreted in the urine where it exerts a topical analgesic effect on the urinary mucosa. The exact mechanism of action is unknown, and the pharmacokinetic properties, efficacy, and safety have not been examined in horses. However in people, it is rapidly excreted by the kidneys, with as much as 65% of the dose being excreted unchanged within the urine [42]. Phenazopyridine has been used in horses and foals to help alleviate urinary tract pain for conditions such as urolithiasis, sabulous, hemorrhagic or ulcerative cystitis, and post-operative bladder repair (e.g. ruptured urinary bladder) [40, 41, 43, 44]. One report in horses used a dose of 4 mg/kg, by mouth, every 6–8 hours for up to 72 hours; the authors of that report did not note any adverse effects as described in people or small animals, but caution should still be maintained when using in horses with concurrent renal injury/disease [40]. Of note, administration of phenazopyridine causes the urine to appear orange-red tinged soon after administration.

Potential side effects and complications of phenazopyridine administration in people include yellow skin discoloration, hemolytic anemia, methemoglobinemia, hepatitis, nausea, vomiting, and diarrhea [45]. A rare but significant adverse effect of phenazopyridine is acute renal failure and acute interstitial nephritis, especially in patients with preexisting renal disease [45]. Postulated mechanisms of nephrotoxicity with administration include direct toxic effects on renal tubules (from triaminopyridine, a metabolite of phenazopyridine), secondary to hemolytic anemia, or secondary to methemoglobinemia [45]. Methemoglobinemia has been reported as a side effect in cats and dogs, and hepatotoxicity, rhabdomyolysis and keratoconjunctivitis sicca in dogs [38, 39]. No adverse effects have been reported regarding the use of phenazopyridine in foals, but clinicians should remain cognizant of the potential complications noted in people and avoid its use in foals with underlying renal disease.

Bethanechol

Bethanechol is used in people with reduced strength or duration of detrusor contraction consequently resulting in failure to completely empty the urinary bladder [46]. The M3 muscarinic receptor is responsible for contraction of the bladder muscle and is necessary for voiding urine. With normal bladder function, the receptor is activated by the neurotransmitter acetylcholine released by parasympathetic nerves. Bethanechol is a parasympathomimetic drug that acts directly on the muscarinic receptor and stimulates stronger contraction of the urinary bladder smooth muscle and increases intravesicular pressure [7, 46]. Bethanechol also increases ureteral peristalsis and relaxes the bladder neck and external uretheral sphincter [7]. Bethanechol has no effect when the bladder is completely atonic or areflexic, however, if the detrusor muscle is capable of generating weak contractions, the drug may be of benefit [7]. Bethanechol is also used as a prokinetic drug as it stimulates gastrointestinal smooth muscle.

The PK of bethanechol in horses is not known, but it has been used in adult horses to ostensibly facilitate bladder emptying in horses with sabulous cystitis [47, 48, 49]. Although not commonly needed in neonatal foals, bethanechol has been used to treat bladder atony after ruptured bladder repair [49]. In one particular case, a 3-day-old foal had classic signs of uroperitoneum and underwent routine surgical repair of a bladder tear. Postoperatively, the foal did not pass urine despite having a large fluid-filled bladder. A urinary catheter was placed to facilitate passage of urine, but each time the urinary catheter was removed, voluntary urine voiding was absent, and the bladder became distended. In this case, 0.4 mg/kg of bethanechol was administered by mouth twice daily, which apparently facilitated voluntary urination. The foal was kept on a 10-day tapering course of bethanechol, which purportedly facilitated bladder emptying; the foal had no further complications [49]. The exact cause of the bladder atony was not known, but proposed causes included bladder trauma, generalized peritonitis, and/or celiotomy [49].

Methylene Blue

Methylene blue has been used as a sterile solution to help identify anatomic defects in the urinary tract, rather than for medicinal purposes, in some neonatal foals. For example, sterile methylene blue helped identify a ureteral defect in a 6-day-old Oldenberg colt that had a 5 mm ureteral tear [50]. Methylene blue was also used to evaluate the security of the defect after it was surgically repaired by injecting the dye into the ureter [50]. Transabdominal ultrasonography and abdominal fluid creatinine concentrations are used in the majority of cases to identify other anatomic defects. However, when those tests are unavailable, methylene blue (10 ml) can be injected through a sterile catheter inserted into the bladder. If a defect is present, dye should be detected in the peritoneal fluid within 15 minutes [51, 52].

Prazosin

Prazosin is a sympatholytic drug that blocks the alpha-1 adrenergic receptors of the trigone and urethral smooth muscle (urethral sphincter), resulting in low urinary outflow tract opening pressure. During the urine storage phase of micturition, stimulation of alpha-1 receptors in the neck of the bladder and proximal urethra narrows the bladder outlet, thus maintaining continence [53]. Voluntary urination occurs with simultaneous contraction of the detrusor muscle and relaxation of the urethral sphincter. Prazosin has been used in people and small animals with urinary retention originating from a variety of causes, including increased sympathetic activity secondary to any surgical procedure [53]. Prazosin has also been used to treat inappropriate contraction of the bladder neck or muscular urethra during the voiding phase of micturition resulting in obstruction of normal urine flow (functional outlet obstruction), in cases of detrusor-sphincter dyssynergia that can be secondary to spinal trauma or disc disease (upper motor neuron bladder), or cases of increased urethral tone in dogs and cats with postobstructive voiding dysfunction [53, 54]. The proposed benefit of prazosin in these clinical situations of urinary retention is that it facilitates relaxation of urethral smooth muscle, allowing the voiding phase of micturition to proceed [55].

Prazosin has been used anecdotally in foals with detrusor-sphincter dyssynergia or in rare cases where foals do not urinate after surgical repair of a ruptured bladder. Pharmacokinetic and pharmacodynamic information is not available in foals/horses but in dogs, an oral dose of 0.1 mg/kg (range 0.1–1.2 mg/kg) daily in divided doses every 8 hours has been used [55, 56]. Prazosin has been administered at a dose of 0.025 mg/kg, IV to adult horses as a potential therapy for laminitis, but minimal effects were noted in laminar microcirculatory blood flow [57, 58]. The clinician should be aware of the dearth of knowledge regarding prazosin in foals as well as potential side effects including hypotension and sedation. Vascular smooth muscle is rich in alpha-1 receptors and hypotension is a potential side effect of prazosin administration due to alpha-1 blockade [53]. Sedation and reduction in blood pressure was documented in an experimental study in dogs administered prazosin, but the level of hypotension was not clinically detectable [53].

Phenoxybenzamine and Diazepam

Phenoxybenzamine is a nonselective, noncompetitive alpha-adrenergic antagonist that has been historically used in companion animals to improve urine voiding. Alternatively, diazepam has been used to promote urine voiding in people and dogs [56]. Diazepam is a centrally acting skeletal muscle relaxant that decreases the tone within the external urethral sphincter through potentiation of the inhibitory amino acid gamma-aminobutyric acid [56]. These medications have not been evaluated for the purpose of facilitating micturition in the neonatal foal but may be potential therapeutic options.

References

1 Allegaert, K., van de Velde, M., and van den Anker, J. (2014). Neonatal clinical pharmacology. *Paediatr. Anaesthesia* 24: 1–14.

2 Guignard, J.P. and Lacobelli, S. (2021). Use of diuretics in the neonatal period. *Peidatr. Nephrol.* 36: 2687–2695.

3 De Vriese, A.S. and Bourgeois, M. (2003). Pharmacologic treatment of acute renal failure in sepsis. *Curr. Opin. Crit. Care* 9: 474–480.

4 Seri, I. (1995). Cardiovascular, renal, and endocrine actions of dopamine in neonates and children. *J. Pediatr.* 126: 333–344.

5 Bhatt, G.C., Gogoia, P., Bitzan, M. et al. (2019). Theophylline and aminophylline for prevention of acute kidney injury in neonates and children: a systemic review. *Arch. Dis. Child* 104: 670–679.

6 Cheung, P.Y. and Barrington, K.J. (1996). Renal dopamine receptors: mechanisms of action and developmental aspects. *Cardiovasc. Rev.* 31: 2–6.

7 Schott, H.C. Drugs acting on the urinary system. In: *Equine Clinical Pharmacology* (ed. J.J. Bertone and L.J.K. Horspool), 155–175. Edinburgh: Saunders.

8 Divers, T.J. and Perkins, G. (2003). Urinary and hepatic disorders in neonatal foals. *Clin. Tech. Equine Pract.* 2: 67–78.

9 Bellomo, R., Wan, L., and May, C. (2008). Vasoactive drugs and acute kidney injury. *Crit. Care Med.* 36: 179–186.

10 Dellinger, R.P., Levy, M.M., Carlet, J.M. et al. (2008). Surviving Sepsis Campaign: International guidelines for management of severe sepsis and septic shock: 2008. *Crit. Care Med.* 36: 296–327.

11 Trim, C.M., Moore, J.N., and Clark, E.S. (1989). Renal effects of dopamine infusion in conscious horses. *Equine Vet. J.* 21: 124–128.

12 Divers, T.J., Whitlock, R.H., Byars, T.D. et al. (1987). Acute renal failure in six horses resulting from haemodynamic causes. *Equine Vet. J.* 19: 178–184.

13 Matsuda, H., Matsuda, K., Muko, R. et al. (2021). Short-term infusion of ultralow-dose dopamine in an adult horse with acute kidney injury: a case report. *Vet. Anim. Sci.* 12: 1000176.

14 Goer, R.J. (2007). Acute renal failure in horses. *Vet. Clin. North Am. Equine Pract.* 23: 577–591.

15 Vivrette, S., Cowgill, L.D., Pascoe, J. et al. (1993). Hemodialysis for treatment of oxytetracycline-induced acute renal failure in a neonatal foal. *J. Am. Vet. Med. Assoc.* 203: 105–107.

16 Hollis, A.R., Ousey, J.C., Palmer, L. et al. (2006). Effects of fenoldopam mesylate on systemic hemodynamics and indices or renal function in normotensive neonatal foals. *J. Vet. Intern. Med.* 20: 595–600.

17 Gillies, M.A., Kakar, V., Parker, R.J. et al. (2015). Fenoldopam to prevent acute kidney injury after major surgery-a systemic review and meta-analysis. *Crit. Care.* 19: 449.

18 Nielsen, L.K., Bracker, K., and Price, L.L. (2015). Administration of fenoldopam in critically ill small animal patients with acute kidney injury: 28 dogs and 34 cats (2008–2012). *J. Vet. Emerg. Crit. Care* 25: 396–404.

19 Pacifici, G.M. (2013). Clinical pharmacology of furosemide in neonates: a review. *Pharmeaceuticals* 6: 1094–1129.

20 Moghal, N.E. and Shenoy, M. (2008). Furosemide and acute kidney injury in neonates. *Arch. Dis. Child Fetal Neonatal Ed.* 93: F313–F316.

21 Brater, D.C. (1992). *Diuretic Pharmacokinetics and Pharmacodynamics* (ed. C.J. van Boxtel, N.H.G. Holoford, and M. Danhof), 253–275. Amsterdam: Elsevier.

22 Prandota, J. (1991). High doses of furosemide in children with acute renal failure. A preliminary retrospective study. *Int. Urol. Nephrol.* 23: 383–392.

23 Johansson, A.M., Gardner, S.Y., Levine, J.F. et al. (2003). Furosemide continuous rate infusion in the horse: evaluation of enhanced efficacy and reduced side effects. *J. Vet. Intern. Med.* 17: 887–895.

24 Starr, M.C., Charlton, R.J., Guillet, R. et al. (2021). Advances in neonatal acute kidney injury. *Pediatrics* 148: 1–14.

25 Vallon, V. and Osswald, H. (2009). Adenosine receptors and the kidney. *Handb. Exp. Pharmacol.* 193: 443–470.

26 Bhatt-Mehta, V. and Nahata, M.C. (1989). Dopamine and dobutamine in pediatric therapy. *Pharmacotherapy* 9: 303–314.

27 Alsaadoun, S., Rustom, F., Hassan, H.A. et al. (2020). Aminophylline for improve acute kidney injury in pediatric patients: a systemic review and meta-analysis. *Int. J. Health Sci.* 14: 44–51.

28 Thomas, N.J. and Carcillo, J.A. (2003). Theophylline for acute renal vasoconstriction associated with tacrolimus: a new indication for an old therapeutic agent? *Pediatr. Crit. Care Med.* 4: 392–393.

29 Goetz, T.E., Munsiff, I.J., and McKiernan, B.C. (1989). Phamracokinetic disposition of an immdieate-release aminophylline and a sustained-release theophylline formulation in the horse. *J. Vet. Pharmacol. Therap.* 12: 369–377.

30 Kowalzcyk, D.F., Beech, J., and Littlejohn, D. (1984). Pharmacokinetic disposition of theophylline in horses after intravenous administration. *Am. J. Vet. Res.* 45: 2272–2275.

31 Carmody, J.B., Harer, M.W., Denotti, A.R. et al. (2016). Caffeine exposure and risk of acute kidney injury in a retrospective cohort of very low birth weight neonates. *J. Pediatr.* 172: 63–68.

32 Sivasaranappa, S.B. and Anjum, A.C.A. (2020). A clinical study of acute kidney injury and caffeine citrate in preterm neonates. *Indian J. Child Health* 7: 230–233.

33 Shi, J., Quan, J., Li, H. et al. (2018). Renal tubular epithelial cells injury induced by mannitol and its potential mechanism. *Renal Fail.* 40: 85–91.

34 Waskowski, J., Pfortmueller, C.A., Erdoes, G. et al. (2019). Mannitol for prevention of peri-operative acute kidney injury. A systemic review. *Eur. J. Vasc. Endovasc. Surg.* 58: 130–140.

35 Reef, V.B., Collatos, C., Spenser, P.A. et al. (1989). Clinical, ultrasonographic, and surgical findings in foals with umbilical remnant infections. *J. Am. Vet. Med. Assoc.* 195: 69–72.

36 Oreff, G.L., Tatz, A.J., Dahan, R. et al. (2017). Surgical management and long-term outcome of umbilical infection in 65 foals (2010-2015). *Vet. Surg.* 46: 962–970.

37 Codina, L.R., Were, S.R., and Brown, J.A. (2019). Short-term outcome and risk factors for post-operative complications following umbilical resection in 82 foals (2004–2016). *Equine Vet. J.* 3: 323–328.

38 Slatter, D.H. (1973). Keratoconjunctivitis sicca in the dog produced by phenazopyridine hydrochloride. *J. Small Anim. Pract.* 14: 749–771.

39 Harvey, J.W. and Kornick, H.P. (1976). Phenazopyridine toxicosis in the cat. *J. Am. Vet. Med. Assoc.* 169: 327–331.

40 Abuja, G.A., Garcia-Lopez, J.M., Doran, R. et al. (2010). Pararectal cystotomy for urolith removal in nine horses. *Vet. Surg.* 39: 654–659.

41 Judy, C. and Galuppo, L. (2002). Endoscopic assisted disruption of urinary calculi using a holmium YAG laser in standing horses. *Vet. Surg.* 31: 245–250.
42 Zelenitsky, S.A. and Zhannel, G.G. (1996). Phenzopyridine in urinary tract infections. *Ann. Pharmacother.* 30: 866–868.
43 Smith, F.L., Madigan, K.G., Michel, A.O. et al. (2018). Equine idiopathic hemorrhagic cystitis: clinical features and comparison with bladder neoplasia. *J. Vet. Intern. Med.* 32: 1202–1209.
44 Aleman, M., Neito, J.E., and Higgins, J.K. (2011). Ulcerative cystitis associated with phenylbutazone administration in two horses. *J. Am. Vet. Med. Assoc.* 239: 499–503.
45 Singh, M., Shailesh, F., Tiwari, U. et al. (2014). Phenazopyridine associated acute interstitial nephritis and review of literature. *Renal Fail.* 36: 804–807.
46 Moro, C., Phelps, C., Vineesha, V. et al. (2022). The effectiveness of parasympathomimetics for treating underactive bladder: a systemic review and meta-analysis. *Neurourol. Urodynamics* 41: 127–139.
47 Rendle, D.I., Durham, A.E., Lloyd, D. et al. (2008). Long-term management of sabulous cystitis in five horses. *Vet. Rec.* 162: 783–787.
48 Zakia, L.S., Gomez, D.E., Kenney, D.G. et al. (2021). Sabulous cystitis in the horse: 13 cases (2013–2020). *Can. Vet. J.* 62: 743–750.
49 Booth, T.M., Howes, D.A., and Edwards, G.B. (2000). Bethanechol-responsive bladder atony in a colt foal after cystorrhaphy for cystorrhexis. *Vet. Rec.* 147: 306–308.
50 Morisset, S., Hawkins, J.F., Frank, N. et al. (2002). Surgical management of a ureteral defect with ureterorrhaphy and of ureteritis with ureteroneocystostomy in a foal. *J. Am. Vet. Med. Assoc.* 220: 354–358.
51 Hawkins, J.F. (2010). Evaluation and treatment of the foal with uroperitoneum. *Equine Vet. Educ.* 22: 139.
52 Adams, R., Koterba, A.M., Cudd, T.C. et al. (1988). Exploratory celiotomy for suspected urinary tract disruption in neonatal foals: a review of 18 cases. *Equine Vet. J.* 20: 13–17.
53 Fischer, J.R., Lane, I.F., and Cribb, A.E. (2003). Urethral pressure profile and hemodynamic effects of phenoxybenzamine and prazosin in non-sedated male beagle dogs. *Can. J. Vet. Res.* 67: 30–38.
54 Gonullu, N.N., Dulger, M., Utkan, N.Z. et al. (1999). Prevention of postherniorrhaphy urinary retention with prazosin. *Am. Surg.* 65: 55–58.
55 Diaz Espineira, M.M., Wiehoff, F.W., and Nickel, R.F. (1998). Idiopathic detrusor-urethral dyssnergia in dogs: a retrospective analysis of 22 cases. *J. Small Anim. Pract.* 39: 264–270.
56 Barnes, K.H., Aulakh, K.S., and Liu, C. (2019). Retrospective evaluation of prazosin and diazepam after thoracolumbar hemilaminectomy in dogs. *Vet. J.* 253: 105377.
57 Galey, F.D., Twardock, A.R., Goetz, T.E. et al. (1990). Gama scintigraphic analysis of the distribution of perfusion of blood in the equine foot during black walnut (Juglans nigra) – induced laminitis. *Am. J. Vet. Res.* 51: 688–695.
58 Adair, H.S., Schmidhammer, J.L., Goble, D.O. et al. (1997). Effects of acepromazine maleate, isoxsurpine hydrochloride and prazosin hydrochloride on laminar microcirculatory blood flow in healthy horses. *J. Equine Vet. Sci.* 17: 599–603.

Section III Renal Replacement Therapies

David Wong and Adam Eatroff

Renal replacement therapy (RRT) includes extracorporeal modalities such as *intermittent hemodialysis (IHD)* and *continuous renal replacement therapy (CRRT)* and intracorporeal methods such as peritoneal dialysis (PD) [1]. The general goals of RRT are to: (i) eliminate solutes and fluid retained during renal injury until the kidney regains partial or complete function and/or (ii) remove toxins (e.g. medications, myoglobin) from the body.

The main indication for RRT in people is treatment of acute kidney injury (AKI) and chronic kidney disease but RRT has also been used to treat electrolyte or acid–base abnormalities, toxicities, and fluid overload [1]. If the main goal of RRT is toxin removal, the toxin ideally should be of low molecular weight (<1500 Daltons), have a small volume of distribution and have minimal protein binding, provided that conventional IHD is being used [2].

While RRT is a mainstay of treatment in people and to a lesser extent small companion animals, RRTs are infrequently utilized in the equine neonate. This is due, in part, to the lack of availability of specialized equipment and trained clinicians and staff. However, with advancement of equine critical care and growth of more advanced equine hospitals, RRT may become more widely available and used. Alternatively, PD does not require any specialized equipment and serves as a viable and available option in foals. Clinical scenarios in which RRT might be used in the neonatal foal include treatment of AKI secondary to sepsis or cardiopulmonary resuscitation and toxicities. This chapter provides a brief overview of RRT and reviews its limited use in equids. More complete reviews of equipment, techniques, and prescriptions for RRT are available elsewhere.

IHD and CRRT extract and circulate the patient's blood through an extracorporeal circuit with the intent of removing unwanted solutes and/or water (e.g. volume overload secondary to AKI) using the principles of diffusion, convection, and adsorption. The magnitude of solute transfer is associated with the force(s) imposed across a semi-permeable membrane, the physical and chemical characteristics of the solute(s) and the structural properties of the semi-permeable membrane [2].

Diffusion of solutes (primary mechanism used in intermittent dialysis) occurs by thermal motion of molecules in the blood and dialysate causing a random encounter with the membrane and transfer through porous channels [2]. These random events are proportional to the concentration gradient and thermodynamic potential of the solute on each side of the membrane with net solute transfer directed from a solution of higher concentration to the solution of lower concentration or thermodynamic potential [1]. Diffusion may add or remove solute to the patient's blood, depending on the relative concentrations in dialysate and plasma. The molecular weight of each solute is a major factor that dictates the diffusive potential of each solute. Small solutes (e.g. urea, 60 Daltons) diffuse faster than larger solutes (e.g. creatinine, 113 Daltons) and generally decrease faster within the plasma of patients undergoing dialysis. The permeability of the membrane and surface area available for diffusion also govern rate of diffusion [3].

Convective transport of solutes (primary mechanism used in hemofiltration) is another means of removing solutes and water and is achieved through a pressure gradient in the process of ultrafiltration, rather than relying on a concentration gradient that governs diffusion. Ultrafiltration drives water through the membrane via a hydrostatic pressure gradient, and diffusible solutes, dissolved in the water, are carried through the membrane by solvent drag [1]. Factors such as transmembrane hydrostatic pressure gradient, hydraulic permeability, surface area, and sieving coefficient of the membrane determine the rate of ultrafiltration and solute transfer [2]. Convection has a greater ability for fluid removal and transfer of middle and large molecular weight solutes that have limited diffusibility.

Equine Neonatal Medicine, First Edition. Edited by David M. Wong and Pamela A. Wilkins.

The third mechanism of removing solutes from blood is *adsorption* in which solutes attach to a material surface. Adsorption occurs in IHD and CRRT but is most efficient in the process of hemoperfusion, where blood is exposed directly to an adsorbent that selectively or nonselectively binds solutes or toxins [2].

Extracorporeal modalities (IHD, CRRT) require vascular access, typically provided by an IV dual-lumen dialysis catheter and administration of an anticoagulant to limit clotting of blood in the extracorporeal circuit. **IHD** is primarily a diffusive process that is instituted for 3–6 hours per session, or longer depending on the body weight of the foal, and repeated at variable schedules contingent on patient needs and clinical condition. An advantage of IHD is its overall efficiency, permitting near normalization of blood composition and volume in a single treatment. However, IHD results in large swings in solute concentration and fluid volume during and between treatments that may not be tolerated well in hemodynamically unstable patients. Another disadvantage of IHD is the requirement of purified water treatment equipment to generate ultrapure dialysate solution on-site.

CRRT utilizes one or more modalities (diffusion, convection, adsorption), depending on treatment prescribed, to provide a slow and continuous rate of solute and water removal over a more prolonged period of time (18–24 hrs/day). Critically ill patients that are intolerant to large changes in solutes or hemodynamics benefit from the slower process of CRRT. The basic modalities of CRRT (Figure 24.III.1) include slow continuous ultrafiltration (SCUF – primarily used to remove excess fluid volume), continuous venovenous hemofiltration (CVVH – primarily used to remove toxins), continuous venovenous hemodialysis (CVVHD – akin to hemodialysis using diffusion as the main mechanism of solute removal) and continuous venovenous hemodiafiltration (CVVHDF – a combination of convective and diffusive therapies). Advantages of CRRT include slower changes in solute concentrations, more stable blood pressure, and the fact that the dialysate and replacement fluids are commercially produced and stored in sterile bags, thereby negating the need for dedicated water purification equipment.

Renal Replacement Therapy for AKI

A few cases have implemented RRT for the treatment of AKI in neonatal foals [4, 5]. In one case, a 4-day-old foal with oxytetracycline-induced AKI received IHD treatments over 4 days after failing to respond to medical treatment with IV fluids, furosemide and dopamine [4]. Vascular access was established, and the foal was anesthetized on three separate occasions. The extracorporeal blood flow rate was maintained between 214 and 330 ml/min and the dialysate flow rate at 500 ml/min. Initial creatinine and blood urea nitrogen (BUN) concentrations were 7.8 and 117 mg/dl, respectively, and decreased to 6.2 and 69 mg/dl and further decreased to 3.7 and 19 mg/dl, respectively, after 11 days of hospitalization. Ultrafiltration of excess plasma water also effectively corrected peripheral and pulmonary edema, along with electrolyte imbalances; the foal was reportedly healthy at 2 years of age [4]. Another case used CRRT in a 3-day-old Thoroughbred filly that presented as a newborn foal in cardiopulmonary arrest (Figure 24.III.2) [5]. Cardiopulmonary cerebral resuscitation was administered to the foal, which revived the patient. However, AKI, characterized by azotemia (creatinine 10 mg/dl; BUN 63 mg/dl), fluid retention (weight gain of 9.1 kg over 48 hours), and oliguria, developed. A 6-hour CRRT session was delivered utilizing an extracorporeal blood flow rate between 50 and 280 ml/min, dialysate rate of 62 ml/kg/h, replacement fluid rate of 62 ml/kg/h and a fluid removal rate from the patient of 300–600 ml/h [5]. Ultimately the foal did not recover from the AKI but the CRRT session decreased the creatinine and BUN to 6.7 and 42 mg/dl, respectively, and removed 1700 ml of fluid from the patient, corresponding to 1.1 kg loss in body weight, after the 6-hour session [5].

Peritoneal Dialysis

PD is a more available, affordable, and perhaps more feasible modality that can be used to remove unwanted solutes and water from patients. In contrast to IHD and CRRT, solutes and water are removed from the patient by instilling a dialysate into the abdominal cavity via a PD catheter. Plasma solute concentrations, including uremic toxins, equilibrate with those of the dialysate across the peritoneum and are subsequently drained from the abdomen, carrying along with it solute. Net movement of plasma water, typically into the dialysate, also occurs depending on the osmotic gradient between the plasma and dialysate. This process is repeated several times a day to meet clinical needs. Hyperosmotic solutions are also infused into the peritoneum, which draws excess water from the circulation into the peritoneal cavity; the ultrafiltrate is then drained. With PD, movement of solutes and fluid between the blood and peritoneal cavity occurs across the blood capillary wall, though the interstitium and across the highly permeable mesothelium [6]. The capillary endothelium is the primary barrier to trans-peritoneal solute and water movement and determines the amount of solute transported to the interstitium and peritoneal cavity [3, 6]. The processes of diffusion, convection, and ultrafiltration take part in transporting fluids and solutes across the peritoneal membrane and can

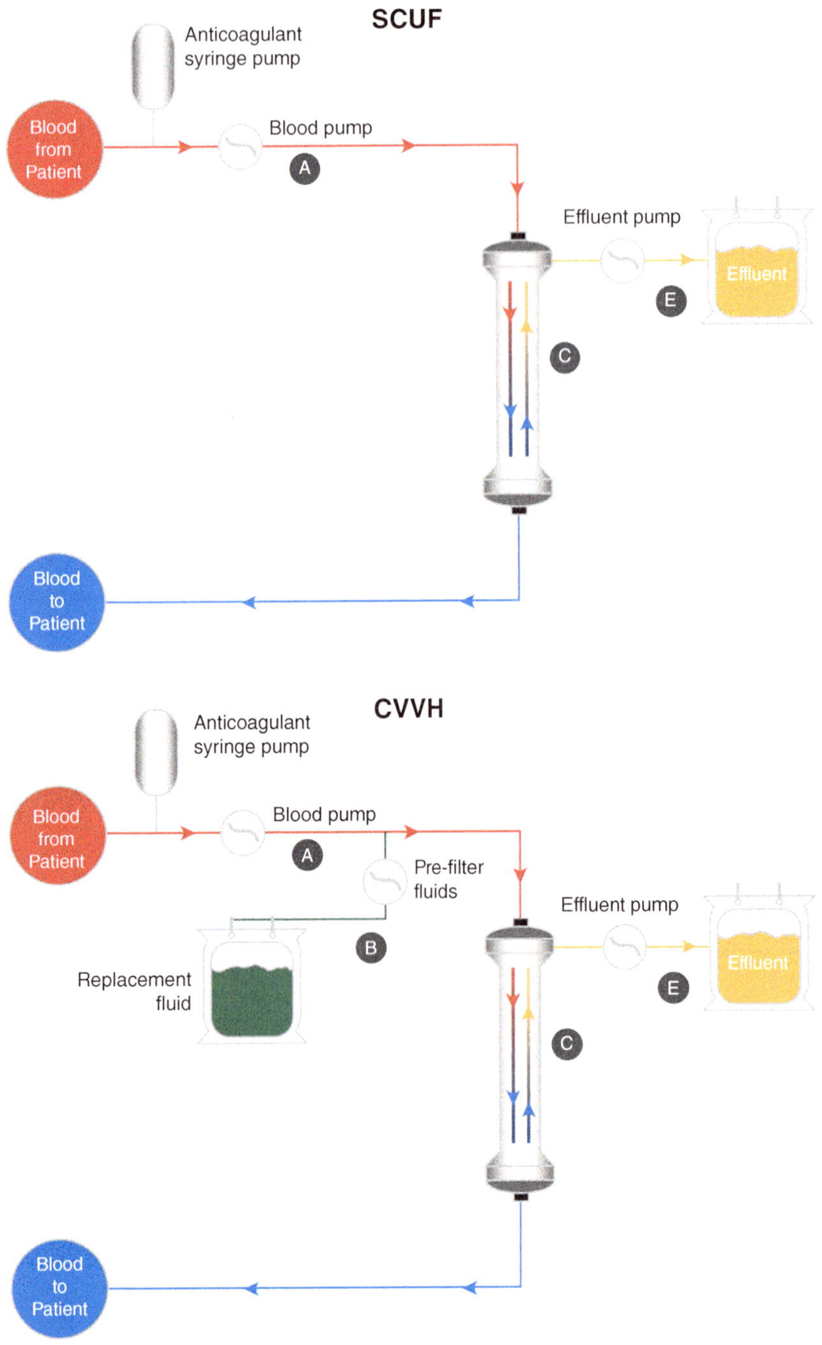

Figure 24.III.1 Continuous renal replacement modalities. Slow continuous ultrafiltration (SCUF) is purely a convective modality where the blood enters the dialyzer, is divided into thousands of straw-like semipermeable membranes, and is exposed to positive transmembrane pressure that forces ultrafiltrate out, which is then discarded as effluent. Hemoconcentrated blood is returned to the patient. SCUF is used to remove excess fluid, for example a patient with nondiuretic responsive congestive heart failure. Continuous venovenous hemofiltration (CVVH) is similar to SCUF, but sterile replacement fluids are added back into the circuit to supplant the ultrafiltrate removed. With continuous venovenous hemodialysis (CVVHD), blood enters the dialyzer and straw-like semipermeable membranes, which are bathed in dialysate that flows countercurrent to blood flow. Toxins that are in high concentration in the blood (e.g. creatinine) diffuse across the membrane and enter the dialysate, whereas substances high in concentration in the dialysate (e.g. sodium) diffuse into the blood. The dialysate is then discarded in the effluent. Continuous venovenous hemodiafiltration (CVVHDF) combines the diffusive properties of hemodialysis and the convective properties of ultrafiltration by bathing the blood entering the straw-like membranes in dialysate while also exposing the blood to positive transmembrane pressure. Diffusion removes smaller uremic toxins and electrolytes while ultrafiltration facilitates removal of larger molecules and fluid.

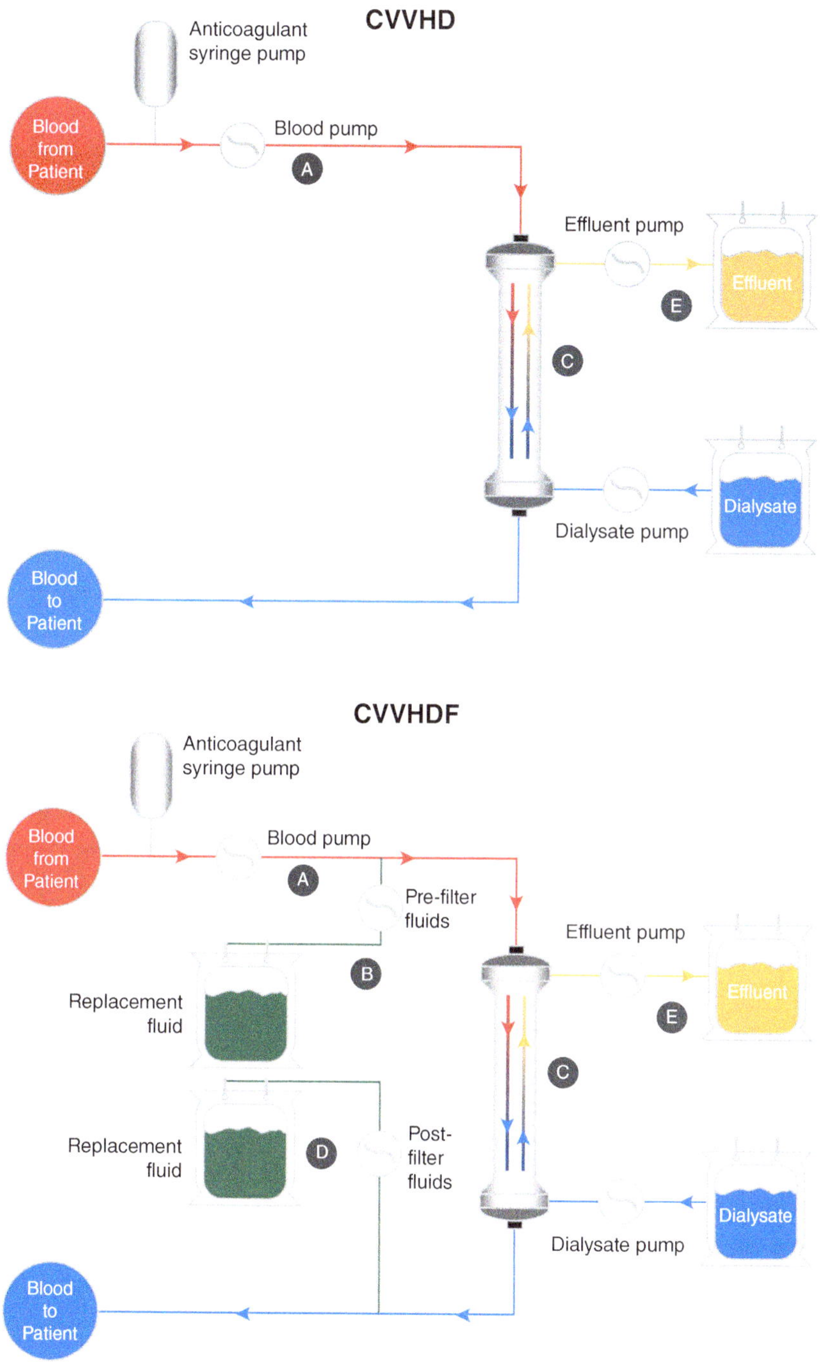

Figure 24.III.1 (Continued)

be viewed by the three pore model. In this model, the major trans-capillary exchange route for water and small solutes is through small pores, 40–55 Å in diameter, formed by clefts between endothelial cells [3, 6]. These small pores represent more than 90% of the pore surface area and restrict the movement of protein but allows passage of low molecular weight substances such as urea, creatinine, and glucose [3]. Ultra-small pores (4–6 Å in diameter) are aquaporin I channels that account for approximately 50% of ultrafiltration and are located within peritoneal capillary and mesothelial cells; they function to transport only water [3]. Large pores (100–300 Å in diameter) are few in number (0.01% of total pore population) and correspond to inter-endothelial clefts and allow passage of macromolecules such as albumin [3, 6].

Only one case of PD has been reported in a neonatal foal, but further cases have been described in older horses [7–9]. A 6-day-old Paint colt was presented for uroabdomen

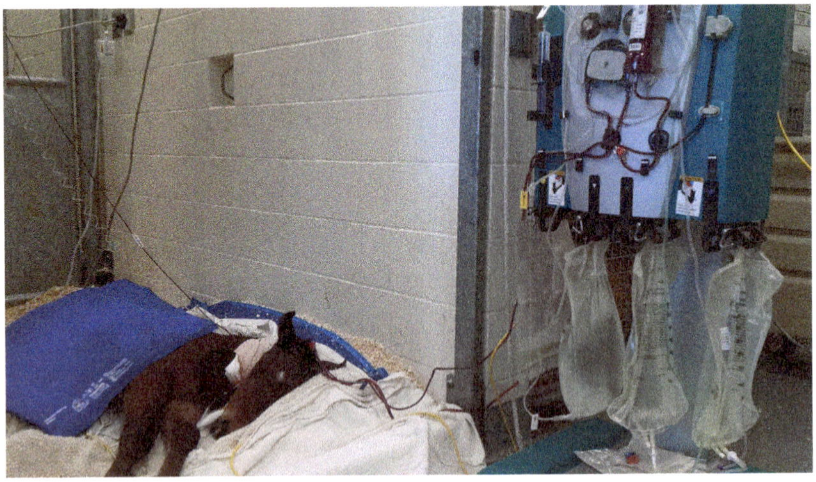

Figure 24.III.2 Neonatal foal with acute kidney injury receiving continuous renal replacement therapy.

and was initially profoundly depressed with marked hyponatremia (104 mEq/l), hypochloremia (73 mEq/l) and hyperkalemia (7.6 mEq/l). Prior to surgery, an 11 French PD catheter was placed in the ventral abdomen, the peritoneal fluid was allowed to drain, and 2 l of hypertonic dialysate was infused and allowed to dwell for 1 hour. Subsequently, the abdomen was allowed to drain for 2–3 hours. Dialysate was infused and removed a total of 9 times over 36 hours using a total of 18 l of dialysate; at this point, the electrolyte abnormalities were corrected and the foal underwent surgical correction of the ruptured bladder [9]. Successful implementation of intermittent PD as an adjunctive therapy for AKI in a yearling Thoroughbred and a 6-month-old Thoroughbred has also been reported using similar techniques [8]. Continuous-flow PD also has been documented in a 15-year-old Paso Fino with AKI refractory to standard medical therapy. Once daily intermittent PD was used initially, but because of a lack of response, continuous-flow PD was initiated. A spiral fenestrated catheter was placed in the left flank via peritoneoscopy for inflow of dialysate and a 28-french thoracic tube was placed in the ventral abdomen for outflow [7]. Approximately 3 l/h of dialysate was administered for 72 hours with the effluent collected via a closed collection system. The azotemia slowly resolved and the horse was discharged after 23 days of hospitalization [7]. The effectiveness and practical implementation of continuous-flow PD in the neonatal foal is unknown and its success is likely dependent on the foal's temperament along with the clinician and staff's ability to provide constant care.

As PD is more readily available than extracorporeal methods, a more detailed description of the methods of implementing PD follows. The clinician should realize, however, that there is no standard protocol established in neonatal foals and much of the information presented here is extrapolated from small animal and human patients. Thus, close observation of clinical cases and modifications of protocols are warranted. For administration of PD, a purpose-specific dialysis catheter (e.g. straight, pigtail-curled, swan-neck, fluted-T) is aseptically placed percutaneously into the abdomen, under sedation or IV anesthesia, through the ventral abdominal musculature to the right of midline [10]. Ultrasound guidance can be used to select the insertion site and avoid damage to abdominal organs. A thoracic drain can be used if a dialysis catheter is not available [8]. Prior to placement, the clinician can consider cutting additional fenestrations into the thoracic drain using a sterile blade to provide additional drainage ports as it is not uncommon for the omentum to obstruct outflow. Laproscopic or open surgical placement techniques of dialysis catheters have been described in people, with the latter allowing for omentectomy that may help prevent omental entrapment of the catheter [10]. However, these techniques may not be as feasible in the neonatal foal. The catheter is then sutured in place using a purse-string suture pattern followed by a Chinese fingertrap suture pattern. A sterile closed exchange system utilizing a Y-type system (e.g. T-U-R Y-set, ICU Medical, Lake Forest, IL) can be used to administer and remove the dialysate. The catheter and insertion site can be protected by using sterile gauze and held in place with elastic tape. Broad-spectrum antibiotics should be considered because of the increased risk of developing peritonitis. Commercially available dialysate or sterile polyionic fluids should be warmed in an incubator to 38 °C and used as dialysate; commercially available Lactated Ringer's solution and Normosol-R have been used in equine cases [7, 8]. If part of the goal is to remove fluid overload in the patient, dextrose can be added to the dialysate to create a 1.5% dextrose solution, which will increase ultrafiltration [8]. The addition of heparin (500 U/l of dialysate) may help minimize formation of fibrin clots within the abdomen and dialysis catheter [11]. The appropriate amount of dialysate to administer to a neonatal foal is unknown, but a dose of 30–40 ml/kg is suggested in small animals and corresponds to volumes used in reported equine cases [8, 11]. Aseptic technique for administration of dialysate is essential to minimize risk of peritonitis and the drain first-infuse later method has been suggested in people and small animals. Specifically, a small amount of fresh dialysate is flushed into the drainage bag and then the peritoneal cavity is drained so that any contaminants introduced during the connection procedure are flushed into the drainage bag [3]. After drainage, fresh dialysate is administered into the peritoneal cavity via gravity flow over 10–15 minutes and left in (dwell time) for 30–40 minutes or longer. In small animals, this process is continually repeated every 1–2 hours for the first 12–24 hours according to patient needs and response, but this treatment intensity may not be practical in neonatal foals. Approximately 90–100% of the dialysate is ideally recovered, but a one-way (Heimlich) valve can be attached to the catheter if small volumes are returned [8]. Care should be taken to record both the infusion volume, as well as the drainage volume, to ensure that fluid is not accumulating in the peritoneal space, which may result in intra-abdominal hypertension or fluid overload.

Intermittent PD was successfully implemented in two horses using a dialysis frequency of twice daily for 4–6 days, but higher frequencies may be needed, depending on severity of AKI and patient response [8]. In people, PD is typically needed for a minimum of 48–72 hours if not longer to treat refractory AKI and should be continued until kidney function and urine output is adequate to maintain the patient without dialysis.

The efficacy of treatment can be monitored by evaluating the BUN and serum creatinine concentrations and calculating hourly urea reduction rate (URR). The URR (typically expressed in terms of percentage) represents the percentage decrease of urea over a designated period of therapy using the formula: $URR = preBUN - postBUN/preBUN \times 100$.

A theoretical concern for too rapid a reduction in BUN concentrations exists, which has prompted (in small animal hemodialysis) general guidelines of maximum hourly URR of 5–10% of the initial urea concentration. However, the likelihood of greater hourly reductions is low, given the relative inefficiency of solute removal in PD, compared to IHD. While creatinine clearance is generally better utilized to determine native kidney function, the clearance of creatinine in PD is less predictable, thus resulting in less utility for assessing solute clearance. This is due to less uniform transport of creatinine across the peritoneal membrane in individuals.

Complications with PD are common but manageable. Catheter flow problems, catheter site leaks, hypoalbuminemia, peritonitis, pleural effusion, dyspnea (from increased abdominal pressure), and changes in hydration status and electrolyte abnormalities have been reported in small animals. Similar complications, such as peritonitis, catheter failure, and development of subcutaneous edema, have been reported after catheter removal in horses [8, 9]. Tables 24.III.1 and 24.III.2, adopted from small animal PD [11], can be used as a guide to implement and adjust PD in the neonatal foal. Although RRT is infrequently used in the neonatal foal, the clinician should consider these treatment options in severely affected foals where medical therapy of AKI has proven ineffective.

Table 24.III.1 Provision and adjustment of dialysate prescription for treatment of AKI [11].

1) Provide warm (38 °C) dialysate at 30–40 ml/kg; decrease volume to 15–20 ml/kg if dialysate leaks around catheter site or if colic or increased respiratory effort is noted.
2) If evidence of overhydration is noted (inappropriate increase in body weight, recovery of less than 90% infused volume, elevated central venous pressure):
   a) Evaluate for catheter obstruction by omentum of fibrin.
   b) Consider dialysate with higher dextrose concentration to facilitate ultrafiltration.
3) If evidence of dehydration (poor skin turgor, decreased body weight):
   a) Discontinue hyperosmotic dialysate.
   b) Supplement patient with IV fluids.
4) If hypokalemia is present, add KCl to dialysate at a level equal to desired serum potassium (e.g. 3–4 mEq/l) and/or consider IV KCl supplementation diluted in IV fluids.
5) If hyperglycemia is present:
   a) Discontinue hyperosmotic dextrose solutions if ultrafiltration is not required.
   b) Begin insulin therapy; insulin can be added to dialysate. People on 1.5% dextrose dialysate receive 0.175 U regular insulin/kg of body weight for short dwell times (<4 hours). Monitor blood glucose carefully.
6) If there is hypoalbuminemia that is suspected to be related to PD and not concurrent disease:
   a) Evaluate for peritonitis.
   b) Evaluate caloric intake and nutritional support to patient.
7) If there is evidence of peritonitis (cloudy effluent, fever, colic, diarrhea, hypoalbuminemia):
   a) Gram stain and culture effluent.
   b) Ensure appropriate systemic antimicrobials are administered.
8) If unexplained respiratory distress is noted, evaluate for pleural effusion.

Table 24.III.2 Suggested guidelines for management of peritoneal dialysis in a foal.

Date	Time	Exchange number	Dialysate composition or type	Volume dialysate infused (ml)	Dwell time (min)	Volume dialysate drained (ml)	Fluids administered (ml, enteral, parenteral)	Urine volume (ml)[a]	Net volume per hour	Patient BUN	Patient body weight	Comments

[a] Estimated or measured urine volume.

References

1 Fleming, G.M. (2011). Renal replacement therapy review: past, present and future. *Ogranogenesis* 7: 2–12.
2 Cowgill, L.D. and Guillaumin, J. (2013). Extracorporeal renal replacement therapy and blood purification in critical care. *J. Vet. Emerg. Crit. Care* 23: 194–204.
3 Ross, L.A. and Labato, M.A. (2013). Current techniques in peritoneal dialysis. *J. Vet. Emerg. Crit. Care* 23: 230–240.
4 Vivrette, S., Cowgill, L.D., Pascoe, J. et al. (1993). Hemodialysis for treatment of oxytetracyline-induced acute renal failure in a neonatal foal. *J. Am. Vet. Med. Assoc.* 203: 105–107.
5 Wong, D.M., Witty, D., Alcott, C.J. et al. (2013). Renal replacement therapy in healthy adult horses. *J. Vet. Intern. Med.* 27: 308–316.
6 Rippe, B. (1993). A three-pore model of peritoneal transport. *Perit. Dial. Int.* 13 (Suppl. 2): S35–S38.
7 Gallatin, L.L., Couetil, L.L., and Ash, S.R. (2005). Use of continuous-flow peritoneal dialysis for the treatment of acute renal failure in an adult horse. *J. Am. Vet. Med. Assoc.* 226: 756–759.
8 Han, J.H. and McKenzie, H.C. (2008). Intermittent peritoneal dialysis for the treatment of acute renal failure in two horses. *Equine Vet. Educ.* 20: 256–264.
9 Kritchevsky, J.E., Stevens, D.L., Christopher, J. et al. (1984). Peritoneal dialysis for presurgical management of ruptured bladder in a foal. *J. Am. Vet. Med. Assoc.* 185: 81–82.
10 Peppelenbosch, A., van Kuijk, W.H.M., Bouvy, N.D. et al. (2008). Peritoneal dialysis catheter placement technique and complications. *NDT Plus* 1 (Suppl. 4): iv23–iv28.
11 Dzyban, L.A., Labato, M.A., Ross, L.A. et al. (2000). Peritoneal dialysis: a tool in veterinary critical care. *J. Vet. Emerg. Crit. Care* 10: 91–102.

Chapter 25 Congenital Urogenital Disorders

Jamie Kopper and David Wong

Evaluation of the equine neonatal urinary system for congenital disorders should include a careful physical examination, serum biochemistry evaluation, and urinalysis. Additional diagnostics, depending on initial findings, include transcutaneous ultrasonographic (i.e. kidneys, bladder, and associated umbilical structures) and/or endoscopic evaluation of the urinary tract. This chapter describes some of the more commonly documented congenital urinary disorders in the horse.

Renal Agenesis

Renal agenesis is a congenital defect that refers to the complete absence of one or both kidneys. Foals with unilateral renal agenesis may not present with any abnormalities on physical examination or serum biochemical evaluation, as approximately 50% loss of renal tubular function must be present before urine concentrating abilities are lost, and loss of approximately 65–75% of tubular function must be present before azotemia is detected. Thus, with one normal functioning kidney, a foal may be able to concentrate/dilute urine or could have isosthenuric urine but should not be azotemic. Renal agenesis is most commonly identified on transcutaneous abdominal ultrasonographic evaluation or, later in life, due to the development of azotemia when the remaining kidney suffers acute injury or chronic disease leading to further evaluation (Figure 25.1). Short-term, unilateral renal agenesis may have little clinical consequence to the foal, assuming that the other kidney is functioning appropriately. However, in the absence of one kidney the clinician and owners should take particular care to avoid nephrotoxic medications to preserve the function of the remaining kidney for as long as possible. Initial identification of renal agenesis often occurs secondary to diagnostic investigations due to other abnormalities in adult horses – for example a 4-year-old Quarter Horse with contralateral ureterolith [1]. Unilateral renal agenesis may occur as a sole abnormality, or in combination with additional congenital abnormalities [1]. Thus, once a congenital abnormality has been identified, the foal should be carefully examined for additional renal and nonrenal abnormalities.

Renal Dysplasia and Hypoplasia

Renal dysplasia is a congenital condition reported in a variety of breeds [2–11] and is characterized by relative immaturity of the renal tissues at birth, indicating failure of appropriate maturation from fetal to functional neonatal renal tissue (Figure 25.2). Histologic findings indicative of renal dysplasia include the persistence of structures that are inappropriate for the foal's stage of development. These microscopic findings include undifferentiated or primitive mesenchyme, persistence of immature glomeruli, blind-ended collecting tubules, atypical tubular epithelium, and primitive metanephric ducts [12]. In other species, the development of renal dysplasia has been associated with familial predispositions, fetal infection, teratogenesis, in utero urinary tract obstructions, and administration of medications such as aminoglycosides, corticosteroids, and angiotensin converting enzyme inhibitors to the mother during gestation [12–14]. To the authors' knowledge, similar predispositions have not been identified in the horse.

In horses, renal dysplasia appears to affect a variety of breeds, both sexes, and can affect either one or both kidneys [11]. Furthermore, the disease can be diffuse or segmental, leading to varying degrees of renal dysfunction [11]. With severe diffuse renal dysplasia, affected foals might be identified at a young age due to severe azotemia and associated clinical signs; however, many are not recognized until they are older foals or adults. Clinicopathologic findings vary but generally include some degree of azotemia (mild to severe),

Equine Neonatal Medicine, First Edition. Edited by David M. Wong and Pamela A. Wilkins.

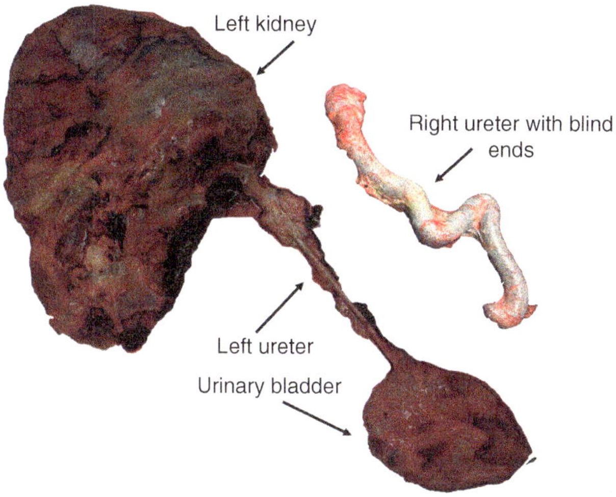

Figure 25.1 Yearling Thoroughbred colt initially presented for leukocytosis and azotemia. Upon ultrasonographic examination, right-sided renal agenesis was identified. Necropsy demonstrated an enlarged and atypical left kidney with areas of fibrosis and a nephrolith. The right kidney was absent and the right ureter markedly enlarged with two blind endings. *Source:* Image courtesy of Dr. Jennifer Janes, University of Kentucky.

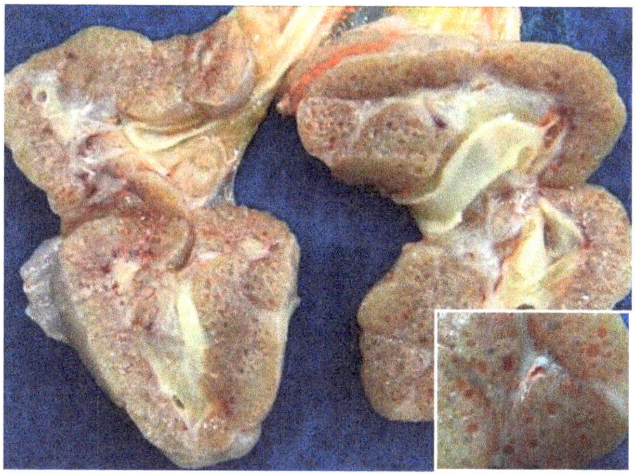

Figure 25.2 Postmortem image of the kidneys of a 9-day-old Thoroughbred filly with diarrhea, lethargy, and renal dysfunction. Diffuse cystic lesions of both kidneys were identified on ultrasonographic examination with postmortem evaluation identifying congenital nephropathy compatible with bilateral diffuse cystic renal dysplasia. Note the bilateral pyelic ectasia, ureteral dilation, lack of corticomedullary differentiation, and sponge-like appearance of the renal parenchyma. Inset: close-up view showing multiple cysts [2].

hyponatremia, hypochloremia, and hyperkalemia. The majority of cases have ultrasonographic abnormalities such as small kidneys, an indistinct corticomedullary junction, and increased echogenicity [11] but in general these findings are nonspecific. Ultimately, a diagnosis is made via microscopic examination of a renal biopsy sample or histopathology obtained at necropsy. However, depending on whether the dysplastic tissue is affecting both kidneys and the diffuseness of the dysplastic tissue, biopsies may not accurately reflect the abnormalities. Thus, a normal biopsy does not positively rule out this disease.

There is no specific treatment for renal dysplasia other than supportive care (i.e. fluid therapy, electrolyte correction, etc.). Prognosis is ultimately dependent on the percentage of affected nephrons and additional renal insults (i.e. acute on chronic conditions), but in general, the prognosis is poor.

Renal hypoplasia is similar to renal dysplasia in that it is the result of a reduction of metanephrogenic tissue or incomplete transformation of nephron formation by the metanephric duct [15]. However, unlike renal dysplasia, renal hypoplasia is characterized by actual loss of renal mass, which has been defined as a 50% decrease in one kidney versus the other, or an overall decrease in renal mass by 30%. Foals with unilateral hypoplasia (and without concurrent renal diseases) may not show clinical signs of disease early in life and have been reported to have hypertrophy of the other kidney to compensate [12, 16].

Renal Cysts

Renal cysts can be congenital or acquired secondary to obstructive disorders, drug therapy, and/or chemical insult [12, 16]. Congenital cysts can be differentiated from acquired cysts based on the lack of associated scarring. Congenital cysts can vary in size (microscopic to macroscopic) and contain clear fluid. Renal cysts can arise from any part of the nephron and are usually incidental findings on postmortem examinations.

Polycystic Kidney Disease

Unlike renal cysts, where the animal has one or a few renal cysts that appear to be without clinical consequence, polycystic kidney disease (PKD) is characterized by numerous variably sized cysts throughout the cortex and medulla leading to obliteration of the normal renal parenchyma and ultimately the development of chronic kidney disease (Figure 25.3) [15]. In addition to the presence of renal cysts, affected foals may also have similar cysts within the bile ducts and pancreas [12, 18]. In people and cats, there are autosomal recessive and dominant variants of PKD, with the infantile congenital form being rare in people. The majority of reports of horses with PKD are middle-aged horses that were evaluated due to clinical signs associated with progressive chronic kidney disease [17–21]. However, PKD has been rarely reported as a cause of neonatal death [12]. In middle-aged horses with PKD, it is sometimes unclear whether this started as a congenital abnormality that progressed to

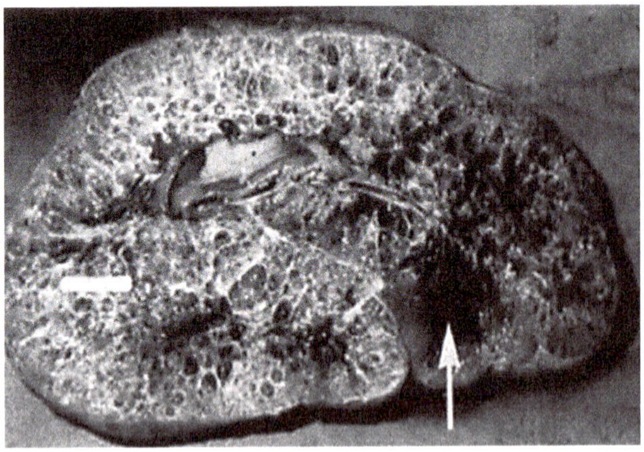

Figure 25.3 Cut surface of polycystic left kidney (scale 3 cm) from a 9-year-old mare. Arrow indicates grossly normal renal parenchyma [17].

chronic renal failure, thereby resulting in clinical signs that prompt veterinary evaluation, or was an acquired form that emerged later in life. Characteristic ultrasonographic findings in foals (and adult horses) include numerous variably sized round hypoechoic areas scattered throughout the renal parenchyma.

Vascular Anomalies

Vascular anomalies associated with the equine urinary tract are rare; however, when reported [22, 23] they are often associated with clinical signs and findings including (intermittent) hematuria or hemoglobinuria, abdominal pain, hydronephrosis, or partial ureteral obstruction [22, 23]. Intermittent hematuria and hemoglobinuria are thought to occur when the vascular anomaly lies close to the urine collecting system [24, 25]. Diagnosis of vascular anomalies associated with the urinary tract relies on a combination of diagnostic tests, including ultrasonographic evaluation, contrast imaging such as computed tomography or a nephrogram, and cystoscopy (which may identify unilateral pigmenturia coming from the ureter or the affected side). Depending on the degree of blood loss associated with hematuria, treatment options include continued monitoring or, if significant blood loss is a concern, unilateral nephrectomy or renal embolization [15, 22].

Nephrogenic Diabetes Insipidus

Nephrogenic diabetes insipidus results from a lack of sensitivity of the cortical and medullary collecting duct epithelial cells to vasopressin. Consequently, the kidney is unable to concentrate urine, resulting in the production of large volumes of hyposthenuric urine (≤1.003) leading to profound polyuria and polydipsia. This condition is rare in horses but has been reported in two young Thoroughbred siblings [26] in which two colts were presented for a history of polyuria and polydipsia. A diagnosis of nephrogenic diabetes insipidus was established through a combination of diagnostic tests, including confirmation of polyuria and polydipsia through monitoring water intake and urine output, ruling out other causes of hyposthenuria, polyuria, and polydipsia by confirming normal serum biochemistry results, calculating normal urine fractional electrolyte excretions, and obtaining normal resting serum cortisol and thyroxine levels. Subsequently, the ability of the cortical and medullary collecting ducts to concentrate urine was evaluated by a water deprivation test, which did not result in concentration of urine despite achieving notable dehydration and subsequent failure to increase urine osmolality by administration of intravenous hypertonic saline. Finally, a diagnosis of nephrogenic diabetes insipidus was confirmed by administration of exogenous vasopressin (0.30 U/kg), which only resulted in a slight decrease in hyposthenuria (1.003–1.008). In these cases, both colts were euthanized. Interestingly, the affected colts were two full siblings, and a third half-sibling (filly) was suspected to also have nephrogenic diabetes insipidus based on owner reported polyuria and polydipsia. This evidence would support an x-linked inherited disorder, which is also reported in people.

Hydroureter and Hydronephrosis

Hydroureter (dilation of one or both ureters) and hydronephrosis (dilation of the renal pelvis) are infrequent findings in neonatal foals and may occur in conjunction with additional congenital abnormalities [10, 27]. Hydroureter and hydronephrosis can both be identified via transcutaneous abdominal ultrasound (Figure 25.4). Hydroureter is frequently coupled with severe hyponatremia that is often associated with neurologic sequela (i.e. obtunded mentation, head pressing, seizures). In foals with hydroureter, a fluid-filled (hypoechoic) ureter is easily identified exiting the associated kidney and can frequently be followed to its entrance into the bladder. Likewise, foals with hydronephrosis will have a large, dilated fluid-filled (hypoechoic) renal pelvis. While hydroureter in the adult horse is frequently associated with an acquired physical obstruction of the ureter (i.e. ureterolith), this is rarely the case in foals where it appears to be due to a neurogenic and/or developmental defect.

The foal's mentation will likely improve in response to careful sodium correction (0.5–1 mEq/l/h and by no more than 12 mEq/l/d) and temporary bladder and/or ureteral catheterization. Administration of low-dose alpha-agonists can be attempted to promote ureteral motility. However, long-term success is not usually favorable unless a physical obstruction affecting urine flow is identified and can be corrected.

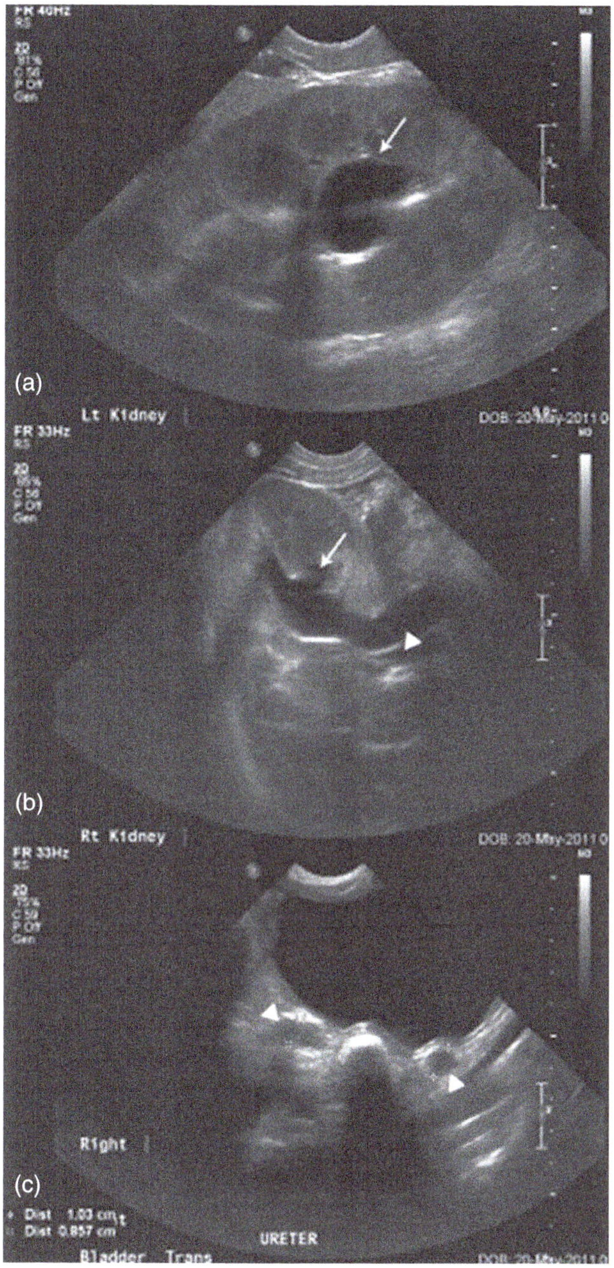

Figure 25.4 Transcutaneous ultrasonograms of a neonatal Warmblood colt with hydronephrosis and hydroureter. (a) Left kidney with dilated renal pelvis (arrow). (b) Right kidney with dilated renal pelvis (arrow) and ureter (arrowhead). (c) Horizontal transverse cross-section of the ureters and bladder showing ureteral dilation proximal to entry into bladder. Ureters marked with arrowheads [28].

Ureteral Ectopia

Ectopic ureters are rare, but most frequently identified in fillies, and can be unilateral or bilateral. This congenital abnormality occurs due to abnormal embryologic development of the metanephric bud [28]. Depending on the location of the ureteral openings, affected foals usually have some degree of urinary incontinence, which may be recognized by the owners due to urine scalding of the skin. If only one ureter is affected, or the ureters are located caudally within the bladder but still within the urethral sphincter, the foal may still be able to urinate normally despite having evidence of urinary incontinence. If this is the only congenital abnormality related to the urinary tract system, affected foals should not be azotemic or show other evidence of urinary tract dysfunction.

A diagnosis of ectopic ureters is made via endoscopic evaluation of the vagina and bladder to identify the location of the ureteral openings. Agents that discolor the urine, such as azosulfamide or sodium fluorescein, can assist in identifying aberrant ureteral openings [29, 30]. Additional diagnostic modalities such as ultrasonography, excretory pyelography, and nuclear scintigraphy have also been reported to aide in the diagnosis of ectopic ureters. Surgical correction via ureterocystostomy has been reported and can be attempted to relocate the affected ureter(s) to a more correct position within the dorsal bladder wall [30, 31].

Ureteral Tears

Ureteral defects, or tears, can be an unusual but reported congenital source of uroperitoneum or retroperitoneal accumulation of urine in the foal [32–37]. Suspicion of a ureteral defect(s) is based on the presence of uroperitoneum, as described elsewhere in this text. However, upon further evaluation of the source of uroperitoneum, the foal will have an intact bladder and urachus. Unfortunately, identifying ureteral tears on surgical exploration of the abdomen can be challenging [35]. Additional diagnostics include excretory urogram by the use of 60% diatrizoate meglumine at a dose of 182 mg/kg IV [37]. Of note, urograms may be more challenging with a higher risk for nondiagnostic findings in foals that are nursing adequately or on intravenous fluid therapy due to hyposthenuria [37]. Alternatively, nephropyelocentesis and antegrade urography can also be considered [37]. Briefly, nephropyelocentesis and antegrade urography has been described [37] by placing a 22-gauge 3.5 in. spinal needle into the desired renal pelvis under ultrasound guidance, and confirming placement by acquisition of urine and injection of contrast medium. Fluoroscopy and sequential radiographs can be used to evaluate the location and trajectory of the ureters and path of urine flow. Surgical correction involving ureterorrhaphy has been described [37]; at long-term follow-up (2 years), the horse was reported to be healthy. Alternatively, if the defect is unilateral and a repair is unable to be performed, unilateral nephrectomy can also be considered [38].

Rectourethral and Rectovaginal Fistulae

Rectourethral and rectovaginal fistulas result from failure of the urorectal fold to fully separate the fetal primitive distal colon from the urogenital sinus [15]. Affected foals are most commonly presented for evaluation of concurrent atresia ani with clinical signs including colic and straining to defecate. The diagnosis in fillies is easier to confirm by observing passage of feces through the vagina and digital palpation of a fistula in the dorsal vaginal vault. In colts, fecal material may be observed from the urethral opening, but this occurs less commonly due to the comparatively long and narrow urethra. Thus, a diagnosis is often made via positive contrast urethrogram and observing contrast material in both the urethra and rectum. Surgical correction of the fistula and associated congenital abnormalities (i.e. atresia ani) can be pursued [39, 40]. However, given the evidence that these defects are hereditary in humans, owners should be counseled against using affected animals for breeding.

Megavesica

Megavesica is a rarely reported congenital fetal syndrome caused by morphological or functional obstruction of the urethra or urachus, leading to urine retention and secondary developmental abnormalities, including distention of the upper and lower urinary tract. In horses, feti continue to drain urine through the urachus until the time of parturition, whereas in humans the urachus regresses mid- to late gestation, resulting in urine drainage through the urethra [41–43]. Thus, in horses, obstruction or malformation of the urethra can lead to fetal urine retention in utero. Of the few equine descriptions of megavesica in the literature, appropriate voiding of a thin-walled urinary bladder has been impeded by a fibrous ligament in place of the urachus [44], incomplete development of the bladder wall and urachus [45], and urinary bladder diverticulum [46]. In all cases, restoration of the foal's ability to void urine was achieved by transection of the fibrous ligament [44], repair of the defect [46], or resection of the abnormally.

References

1 Johnson, B.D., Lingborg, D.J., Heitman, J.M. et al. (1976). A horse with one kidney, partially obstructed ureter, and contralateral urogenital anomalies. *J. Am. Vet. Med. Assoc.* 169: 217.

2 Medina-Torres, C.E., Hewson, J., Stampfli, S. et al. (2014). Bilateral diffuse cystic renal dysplasia in a 9-day-old Thoroughbred filly. *Can. Vet. J.* 55: 141–146.

3 Plummer, P.J. (2006). Congenital renal dysplasia in a 7-month-old quarter horse colt. *Vet. Clin. North Am. Equine Pract.* 22: e63–e69.

4 Wooldridge, A.A., Seahorn, T.L., Williams, J. et al. (1999). Chronic renal failure associated with nephrolithiasis, ureterolithiasis, and renal dysplasia in a 2-year-old quarter horse gelding. *Vet. Radiol. Ultrasound* 40: 361–364.

5 Anderson, W.I., Picut, C.A., King, J.M. et al. (1988). Renal dysplasia in a standardbred colt. *Vet. Pathol.* 25: 179–180.

6 Ronen, N., van Amstel, S.R., Nesbit, J.W. et al. (1993). Renal dysplasia in two adult horses: clinical and pathological aspects. *Vet. Rec.* 132: 269–270.

7 Gull, T., Schmitz, D.G., Bahr, A. et al. (2001). Renal hypoplasia and dysplasia in an American miniature foal. *Vet. Rec.* 149: 199–203.

8 Brown, C.M., Parks, A.H., Mullaney, T.P. et al. (1988). Bilateral renal dysplasia and hypoplasia in a foal with an imperforate anus. *Vet. Rec.* 122: 91–92.

9 Zicker, S.C., Marty, G.D., Carlson, G.P. et al. (1990). Bilateral renal dysplasia with nephron hypoplasia in a foal. *J. Am. Vet. Med. Assoc.* 196: 2001–2005.

10 Jones, S.L., Langer, D.L., Sterner-Kock, A. et al. (1994). Renal dysplasia and benign uteropelvic polyps associated with hydronephrosis in a foal. *J. Am. Vet. Med. Assoc.* 204: 1230–1234.

11 Jaramillo-Morales, C. and Magdesian, K.G. (2022). Renal dysplasia in horses: 25 cases (1991–2021). ACVIM Forum Abstract 2022.

12 Maxie, M.G. and Newman, S.J. (2007). Urinary system. In: *Jubb, Kennedy and Palmer's Pathology of Domestic Animals*, 5e (ed. M.G. Maxie), 438–444. San Diego, CA: Elsevier.

13 Barr, M. (1994). Teratogen update: angiotensin-converting enzyme inhibitors. *Teratology* 50: 399–409.

14 Hulton, S.A. and Kaplan, B.S. (1995). Renal dysplasia associated with in utero exposure to gentamicin and corticosteroids. *Am. J. Med. Genet.* 58: 91–93.

15 Schott, H.C., Waldridge, B., and Warwick, B.M. (2018). Disorders of the urinary system. In: *Equine Internal Medicine*, 4e (ed. S.M. Reed, W.M. Bayly, and D.C. Sellon), 888–990. San Diego, CA: Elsevier.

16 Jones, T.C. and Hunt, R.D. (1983). The urinary system. In: *Veterinary Pathology* (ed. T.C. Jones, R.D. Hung, and V.W. King), 1111–1148. Philadelphia: Lea & Febiger.

17 Bertone, J.J., Traub-Dargats, J.L., Fettman, M.J. et al. (1987). Monitoring the progression of renal failure in a horse with polycystic kidney disease: use of reciprocal of serum creatinine concentration and sodium sulfanilate clearance half-time. *J. Am. Vet. Med. Assoc.* 191: 565.

18 Chandler, K.J., Johnston, H.M., and Murphy, D.M. (2003). Polycystic kidney disease in an aged pony. *Vet. Rec.* 153: 754–756.

19 Ramsay, G., Rothwell, T.L., Gibson, K.T. et al. (1987). Polycystic kidneys in an adult horse. *Equine Vet. J.* 19: 243–244.

20 Scott, P.C. and Vasey, J. (1986). Progressive polycystic renal disease in an aged horse. *Aust. Vet. J.* 63: 92.

21 Aguilera-Tejero, E., Estepa, J.C., Lopez, I. et al. (2000). Polycystic kidneys as a cause of chronic renal failure and secondary hypoparathyroidism in a horse. *Equine Vet. J.* 32: 167.

22 Latimer, F.G., Magnus, R., and Duncan, R.B. Jr. (1991). Arterioureteral fistula in a colt. *Equine Vet. J.* 23: 483–484.

23 Schott, H.C., Barbee, D.D., Hines, M.T. et al. (1996). Clinical vignette. Renal arteriovenous malformation in a quarter horse foal. *J. Vet. Intern. Med.* 10: 204–206.

24 Crotty, K.L., Orihuela, E., and Warren, M.M. (1993). Recent advances in the diagnosis and treatment of renal arteriovenous malformations and fistulas. *J. Urol.* 150: 1355.

25 Takaha, M., Matsumoto, A., Ochi, K. et al. (1980). Intrarenal arteriovenous malformation. *J. Urol.* 124: 315.

26 Schott, H.C., Bayly, W.M., Reed, S.M. et al. (1993). Nephrogenic diabetes insipidus in sibling colts. *J. Vet. Intern. Med.* 7: 68–72.

27 Gilday, R.A., Wojnarowicz, C., Tryon, K.A. et al. (2015). Bilateral renal dysplasia, hydronephrosis and hydroureter in a septic neonatal foal. *Can. Vet. J.* 56: 257–260.

28 Chaney, K.P. (2007). Congenital anomalies of the equine urinary tract. *Vet. Clin. North Am. Equine Pract.* 23: 691–696.

29 MacAllister, C.G. and Perdue, B.D. (1990). Endoscopic diagnosis of unilateral ectopic ureter in a yearling filly. *J. Am. Vet. Med. Assoc.* 197: 617–618.

30 Gettman, L.M., Ross, M.W., and Elce, Y.A. (2005). Bilateral ureterocystostomy to correct left ureteral atresia and right ureteral ectopia in an 8-month-old Standardbred filly. *Vet. Surg.* 34: 657–661.

31 Modransky, P.D., Wagner, P.C., Robinette, J.D. et al. (1983). Surgical correction of bilateral ectopic ureters in two foals. *Vet. Surg.* 12: 141–147.

32 Stickle, R.L., Wilcock, B.P., and Husemann, J.L. (1975). Multiple ureteral defects in a Belgian foal. *Vet. Med. Small Anim. Clin.* 70: 819.

33 Robertson, J.T., Spurlock, G.H., Bramlage, L.R. et al. (1983). Repair of ureteral defect in a foal. *J. Am. Vet. Med. Assoc.* 183: 799.

34 Divers, T.J., Byers, T.D., and Spirito, M. (1988). Correction of bilateral ureteral tears in a foal. *J. Am. Vet. Assoc.* 183: 799.

35 Cutler, T.J., MacKay, R.J., Johnson, C.M. et al. (1997). Bilateral ureteral tears in a foal. *Aust. Vet. J.* 75: 413.

36 Jean, D., Marcoux, M., and Louf, C.F. (1998). Congenital bilateral distal defect of the ureters in a foal. *Equine Vet. Educ.* 10: 17.

37 Morisset, S., Hawkins, J.F., Frank, N. et al. (2002). Surgical management of a ureteral defect with ureterorrhaphy and of ureteritis with ureteroneocystostomy in a foal. *J. Am. Vet. Med. Assoc.* 220: 354.

38 Bryant, J.E. and Gaughan, E.M. (2005). Abdominal surgery in neonatal foals. *Vet. Clin. Equine* 21: 511–535.

39 Gideon, L. (1977). Anal agenesis with rectourethral fistula in a colt: a case report. *Vet. Med.* 72: 238–240.

40 Kingston, R.S. and Park, R.D. (1982). Atresia ani with an associated urogenital tract anomaly in foals. *Equine Pract.* 4: 32–34.

41 Bourdelat, D., Husson, S., Soisic, F. et al. (1998). Embryological study of the mechanism of antenatal lower urinary tract obstruction. *Ann. Urol.* 32: 253–268.

42 Lye, S.J., Freitag, C.L., and Challis, J.R. (1988). Ovine fetal urachus – physiological and hormonal control of its contractile activity. *Am. J. Phys* 254: F25–F31.

43 Koterba, A.M. (1990). Physical examination. In: *Equine Clinical Neonatology* (ed. A.M. Koterba), 77. Philadelphia: Lea & Febinger.

44 Dubs, B. (1976). Megavesica due to the absence of an urachus in a newborn foal. *Schweiz. Arch. Tierheilkd.* 118: 393–395.

45 Rossdale, P.D. and Greet, T.C. (1989). Mega vesica in a newborn foal. *ISVP News* 2: 10–13.

46 Tóth, T., Liman, J., Larsdotter, S. et al. (2012). Megavesica in a neonatal foal. *Equine Vet. Educ.* 24: 396–403.

Chapter 26 Renal Disorders in Neonatal Foals

Langdon Fielding

A variety of renal disorders have been described in neonatal foals (Table 26.1) and are discussed in this chapter. In a simple classification, renal disorders can be categorized as acute kidney injury (AKI), and infectious, congenital, and traumatic causes. Of primary importance, AKI is most common in foals and is a focus for equine neonatologists. Typical causes of AKI in human patients such as sepsis, ischemia, and toxicity occur alone or in combination in many of the sick foals presenting to equine neonatal ICUs. It is no surprise that the clinical decisions and monitoring in equine neonatal ICUs revolve around renal function. The first part of this chapter focuses on the causes of and risk factors for AKI in equine neonates, while the remainder discusses other less common renal disorders.

Types of Acute Kidney Injury

AKI can be defined as a sudden or abrupt decrease in renal function that often has multifactorial causes, including sepsis, ischemia, and toxicity [1]. The term *acute kidney injury* has largely replaced the term *acute renal failure (ARF)* as there is increased recognition that ARF represents a later stage of kidney injury, and the entire spectrum of disease is more completely described by AKI. There are numerous potential criteria for AKI in humans, but a straightforward checklist was established in 2013 by the *Kidney Disease: Improving Global Outcomes* (KDIGO) foundation [2]. In general, most definitions focus on a combination of an increase in creatinine and decrease in urine production. More recently, the definition was modified with specific criteria that were used as part of the *Assessment of Worldwide Acute Kidney Injury Epidemiology in Neonates* (AWAKEN) study, which characterized AKI in a large number of human neonates (Table 26.2) [3]. By far, the most important finding from the AWAKEN trial and similar research projects was to confirm that neonatal AKI often goes unrecognized, particularly in the early stages. In general, clinicians do not understand the early signs and risk factors for AKI and do not modify treatments until renal injury is more advanced.

Some risk factors associated with neonatal AKI in people include placental insufficiency (prenatal), exposure to nephrotoxic drugs and/or delivery complications resulting in hypoxia/asphyxia (perinatal), and sepsis, nephrotoxin exposure, and prematurity (postnatal) [4]. Additional criteria or definitions of AKI have also been proposed based on refinements from continued research [5]. These refinements recognize that cutoffs for AKI may need to be gestational age-specific and may use either an absolute change in creatinine or a percentage change as the criteria.

A complete review of renal physiology is beyond the scope of this chapter, however changes in renal blood flow impact glomerular filtration and oxygen delivery to the filtering units of the kidney. Renal blood flow is modulated by the afferent and efferent arterioles, which can be affected by numerous factors that are altered during AKI and depend on the inciting cause. In morphologic studies, the proximal tubule is often the most affected segment in AKI [6]. Sepsis, ischemia, and toxicities can independently or in conjunction lead to direct damage to the nephron as well as changes in renal blood flow and filtration. As this injury progresses, the patient advances through the stages of AKI starting with primarily reversible disease and ending with complete kidney failure and chronic kidney disease.

Following birth, human neonates have an increase in renal blood flow, filtration, and tubular function. In horses, there is some evidence that there may be less difference between neonates and adults than the discrepancies observed between human neonates and adults [7–10]. Regardless of the underlying physiology, equine neonates appear to be at high risk for AKI, and three factors (sepsis, ischemia, and toxicities) are likely to be associated with

Equine Neonatal Medicine, First Edition. Edited by David M. Wong and Pamela A. Wilkins.

Table 26.1 Renal disorders reported in neonatal foals.

Acute kidney injury (AKI)	Other renal disorders
Sepsis-associated AKI (S-AKI)	Infectious causes (*Actinobacillus equuli*, Leptospirosis, etc.)
Toxin-associated AKI (ToxAKI)	Congenital abnormalities
Ischemic AKI (I-AKI)	Trauma

Table 26.2 Neonatal Kidney Disease: Improving Global Outcomes (KDIGO) criteria for diagnosing acute kidney injury.

Stage	Serum creatinine	Urine output
0	No change or increase <0.3 g/dl	≥0.5 ml/kg/h
1	Increase in serum creatinine level of ≥0.3 mg/dl within 48 h or rise in serum creatinine level ≥ 1.5–1.9 times the reference serum creatinine level within 7 d	<0.5 ml/kg/h for 6–12 h
2	Rise in serum creatinine level ≥ 2–2.9 times the reference serum creatinine level within 7 d	<0.5 ml/kg/h for >12 h
3	Serum creatinine level ≥ 3 times the reference serum creatinine level or serum creatinine level > 2.5 mg/dl or receipt of renal replacement therapy	<0.3 ml/kg per hour for >24 h or anuria for >12 h

this increased risk. For these three inciting causes, the paths to disease and the sections of the nephron affected can be quite different.

Of additional interest, the crosstalk that potentially occurs between the kidney with AKI and other organs is being increasingly described [4, 11]. Studies have indicated that beyond just an association between AKI and other organ failure, AKI itself may have a causative role in the failure of other organs. For example, models have described a lung-focused inflammatory process driven, in part, by cytokines that are produced with AKI [4]. Neonatal AKI has also been shown to be an independent risk factor for neurologic complications (intraventricular hemorrhage, poor neurocognitive outcomes) in infants [4]. Although this concept has not been examined in foals, if true, it would further support the need for focus to prevent, recognize, and treat AKI as quickly as possible.

While data in neonatal foals is less robust compared to humans, AKI has been repeatedly shown to be an independent risk factor for mortality in human neonates, even after correcting for multiple confounders [4, 12]. Specifically, neonates with AKI had an odds ratio for death that was 4.6 times higher than neonates without AKI after accounting for other factors [12]. In one study evaluating a relatively large group of neonatal foals admitted for ICU care, over 50% of the foals in the study would have met the criteria for AKI used in human neonates [13]. Similar to human neonates, the diagnosis, prevention, and treatment of AKI should be the overwhelming focus for equine neonatologists.

Sepsis-Associated Acute Kidney Injury

Sepsis-associated acute kidney injury (S-AKI) is a well-recognized concept; however, the mechanisms contributing to the renal injury that occurs with sepsis are complex, incompletely understood, and controversial [14]. It appears that direct cell death and hypoperfusion might not be the key (or only) events during this type of injury (Figure 26.1). S-AKI was formerly considered to be a disease of the renal macrocirculation resulting from global renal ischemia, cellular damage, and acute tubular necrosis [15, 16]. However, experimental and clinical studies have challenged this paradigm by showing that AKI can develop despite maintained, and in some cases increased, global renal blood flow [15, 16]. This notion is further supported by a large systemic review of 160 studies of experimental sepsis in which renal blood flow was shown to be either preserved or elevated in animal models and was characterized as hyperdynamic circulation (e.g. increased cardiac output) [17]. Moreover, microscopic examination of kidneys from patients that have succumbed to disease document patchy, heterogeneous tubular injury with apical vacuolization, but in the absence of tubular necrosis and minimal apoptosis. Thus, one theory suggests that renal defects associated with S-AKI may be functional rather than structural in nature [15]. However, an increase in global renal blood flow during sepsis does not preclude the possibility of redistribution of intra-renal microcirculatory blood flow

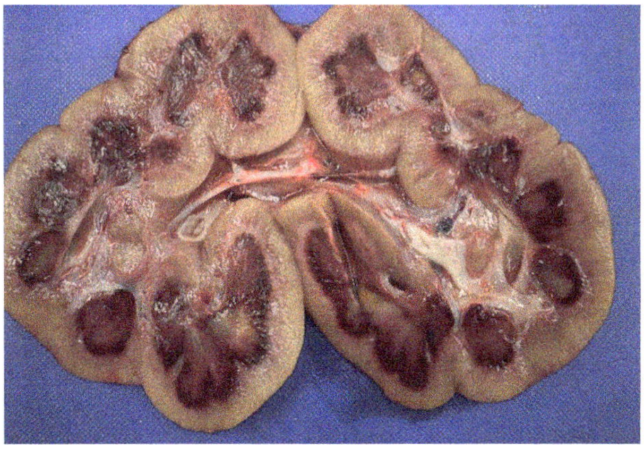

Figure 26.1 Kidney from a 7-day-old Thoroughbred foal that presented for septic shock and renal failure following dystocia. The foal was euthanized for continued deterioration despite intensive therapy. The medulla is diffusely hemorrhagic with pale streaking corresponding to areas of necrosis and early fibrosis, respectively. *Source:* Image courtesy of Dr. Rebecca Ruby, University of Kentucky.

resulting in some areas of the kidney receiving adequate perfusion at the expense of other regions exposed to local tissue ischemia and hypoxia [15]. Possible mechanisms that contribute to redistribution of intra-renal perfusion include excessive release of inflammatory cytokines, regional deficits in nitric oxide (vasodilation), generation of reactive oxygen and nitrogen species, damage to the glycocalyx, and/or disruption of the endothelial barrier.

Another pathophysiologic theory to explain S-AKI is that cells (in this case, kidney cells) may modulate their metabolism in order to survive during sepsis, and this modulation may result in the observed damage [14]. While these changes in metabolism help prevent the death of the cells, they lead to organ dysfunction – specifically, the S-AKI that is observed. This overall concept recognizes that disease resistance, as well as disease tolerance, are critical to survival for cells and that the latter may be a significant factor in the development of AKI [18]. Thus, the cellular changes that occur in order to survive a pathogen attack might be the more important cause of AKI rather than the direct effects of the pathogen or secondary cardiovascular dysfunction.

Recognition is a significant problem with sepsis and S-AKI in neonatal foals. While specific criteria have been proposed for the systemic inflammatory response syndrome (SIRS) and sepsis in horses, clinicians continue to struggle with reliable ways to recognize affected patients [19]. Biomarkers, clinical examination findings, and risk factors are all variables that can aid in sepsis-recognition in foals [20, 21]. Differentiation between sepsis and neonatal maladjustment syndrome (NMS) is particularly challenging. However, given that both sepsis and NMS can be associated with AKI, it may be more important to acknowledge that one or more risk factors is present in a patient and then to focus on the early recognition of AKI.

Again, it must be emphasized that the pathophysiologic mechanisms contributing to S-AKI are complex and not fully understood. This is exemplified by *in vitro* studies using cell cultures, where hemodynamic status is no longer a factor, but yet many cardinal features of S-AKI were reproduced in human epithelial tubular cells that were exposed to plasma from septic patients [8]. While ischemia and hypoxia may contribute to S-AKI, other mechanisms may also contribute or be involved. Other potential mechanisms involved with S-AKI include inflammation, heterogeneous distortion of microvascular flow at the peritubular and glomerular levels, and/or stimulation of mitochondrial control processes and cell cycle arrest [15, 16].

Toxin-Associated Acute Kidney Injury

Toxin-associated acute kidney injury (ToxAKI) can be associated with a variety of toxins, including medications, envenomation, and pesticides. However, for equine neonatologists, non-steroidal anti-inflammatory drugs (NSAIDs) and antimicrobials are frequently administered to foals and are the most discussed medications associated with AKI (Table 26.3). In one study in human patients, the administration of aminoglycosides for >3 days or the administration of >2 nephrotoxic medications in one day warranted an increased monitoring protocol to screen for the early development of AKI [22].

Table 26.3 Medications associated with AKI in horses or foals.

Medication	Mechanism of renal toxicity
Non-steroidal anti-inflammatory drugs	Inhibition of renal prostaglandins
Aminoglycosides	Acute tubular necrosis
Oxytetracycline	Acute tubular necrosis
Polymyxin-B	Acute tubular necrosis and dilation

NSAIDs can alter prostaglandin production. Many of these prostaglandins play an important role in modulating renal blood flow and filtration particularly in the presence of decreased perfusion [23]. It is interesting to note, however, that there are few reports of NSAID induced AKI in neonatal foals. In fact, flunixin meglumine was evaluated at a variety of dosages and showed minimal change in crude markers of renal function such as serum creatinine [24]. It is possible that with stricter monitoring protocols (such as those used in human neonates), early signs of AKI might have been recognized in these studies. Additionally, foals in these studies were typically healthy and therefore may have a much higher tolerance for NSAIDs than a neonate with ischemic injury or sepsis.

Nephrotoxicity with antibiotics such as aminoglycosides is also a concern in foals, however like NSAIDs, there are few reports of toxicity. In several studies, administration of gentamicin and amikacin to healthy foals did not create significant changes in renal function [25, 26]. Oxytetracycline has also been described as a cause for ToxAKI in foals; however, the medication was administered to treat flexural limb deformities in both reports with a different (higher) dose than what is used for antimicrobial purposes [27, 28]. Polymyxin B is another potentially nephrotoxic medication described for the treatment of endotoxemia in foals, but at an appropriate dosage there was no gross evidence of renal injury [29].

Similar to S-AKI, there is a continued focus on early recognition of ToxAKI using risk factors, traditional clinicopathology, and new biomarkers [30]. Important risk factors may include the use of multiple nephrotoxic drugs and the presence of hypotension. In many cases, antibiotics are being administered for the treatment of sepsis, however, recognizing that multiple risk factors for AKI are present may help the clinician to modify the choice of antibiotics. As discussed later, early recognition of AKI with toxic medications has the potential to significantly improve outcomes [22].

Myoglobin released during an episode of rhabdomyolysis can also be toxic to the kidneys. Mechanisms of toxicity associated with myoglobin include renal vasoconstriction, formation of tubular casts, and direct toxicity to the renal tubular cells. Rhabdomyolysis and subsequent renal injury have been described in neonatal foals associated with selenium/vitamin E deficiency [31]. AKI was identified in two foals with rhabdomyolysis that developed following oxytetracycline administration [28]. However, the renal injury could have been related to the oxytetracycline and not necessarily the toxic effects of myoglobin. Foals with hypoxic ischemic encephalopathy may also have elevations in muscle enzymes, but AKI in these foals may be more likely to be ischemic in origin rather than related to myoglobin. Polysaccharide storage myopathy and glycogen branching enzyme deficiency are infrequently described as causes of rhabdomyolysis in neonatal foals, but they theoretically could lead to this condition and associated renal injury. Compared to other causes of AKI (sepsis, medication toxicities, ischemia), rhabdomyolysis is an uncommon but recognized factor.

Ischemic Acute Kidney Injury

Ischemic acute kidney injury (I-AKI) is the third subcategory of AKI and involves changes to perfusion and/or oxygen delivery to all or parts of the kidney. The more classic division of "prerenal" and "renal" acknowledges that decreased perfusion begins with an appropriate "prerenal" response of compensatory mechanisms and modulation of blood flow. There is then progression to reversible and then irreversible renal cell injury as the degree of hypoperfusion advances. This localized or generalized reduction in blood flow represents a common pathway into AKI, but there are many factors contributing to this change [32]. For example, renal ischemia and subsequent reperfusion injury initiates a variety of signaling cascades that mediate renal cell necrosis, apoptosis, and inflammation, resulting in AKI [33]. The fate of the renal tubular cells exposed to ischemia depends on the extent of the injury. A mild, sublethal, injury results in disruption of the cytoskeletal integrity of the kidney; these cells can recover if the ischemic insult is brief. However, with more severe (lethal) injury, irreversible renal tubular cell death occurs via apoptosis or necrosis, resulting in renal dysfunction observed in AKI [33]. The inflammatory reaction associated with this process may also induce renal damage as inflammatory cascades are initiated by endothelial cell injury and activation and interaction of leukocytes via adhesion molecules. Neutrophils subsequently induce further damage through release of reactive oxygen species (ROS), proteinases, elastases, and myeloperoxidase [33].

In neonatal foals, I-AKI may be due to a variety of causes including hypoxemia during or shortly after birth, hypoperfusion due to hypothermia, or a number of factors causing hypotension. Similar to other subcategories of AKI, early recognition of I-AKI is based on risk factors, laboratory data, and specifically oxygenation and blood pressure monitoring.

Recognition of AKI

Chapter 24 discusses many of the diagnostics and laboratory testing used to diagnose renal disease in foals including creatine, serum symmetric dimethylarginine (SDMA), electrolytes, and urine output. Given the significant morbidity and mortality associated with AKI, early recognition cannot be overemphasized. There is a continuous search for new biomarkers for AKI and some of these are now being used for human neonates for earlier recognition of AKI (Table 26.4). Cystatin C (CysC) is a cysteine protease inhibitor that has been shown in serum to be potentially better than serum creatinine for evaluating glomerular filtration rate (GFR) [11]. CysC also appears to be a leading indicator for rises in creatine and may predict changes 1–4 days prior [34]. Neutrophil gelatinase-associated lipocalin (NGAL) is filtered by the glomerulus

Table 26.4 Newer biomarkers that have been described for the diagnosis and/or early recognition of AKI.

Biomarker	Brief description
Serum symmetric dimethylarginine (SDMA)	Released into circulation during protein catabolism – accumulates during renal dysfunction
Serum cystatin C (CysC)	Protein produced by all nucleated cells – better correlation with GFR than creatinine
Neutrophil gelatinase-associated lipocalin (NGAL)	One of the earliest induced proteins in the kidney after ischemic or nephrotoxic damage
Urinary tissue inhibitor of metalloproteinase 2 (TIMP-2)	Involved in G1 cell cycle arrest during the earliest phases of kidney injury
Insulinlike growth factor binding protein 7 (IGFBP-7)	Involved in G1 cell cycle arrest during the earliest phases of kidney injury

and reabsorbed in the proximal tubules [11]. It is a protein that is bound to neutrophil granules but is very sensitive and specific for AKI in perinatal asphyxia [35]. Perhaps more practical for equine neonatologists, a more recent study in human neonates showed the extraordinary benefit of daily serum creatine monitoring on patients receiving nephrotoxic medications [22]. This simple protocol change was credited with preventing 100 incidences of AKI in the study group. These results further emphasize the importance of early recognition of AKI in high-risk groups.

Increased serum creatinine concentrations are not uncommon at birth in neonatal foals particularly those that have undergone fetal stress [36]. Many foals may have serum creatinine concentrations two to three times the normal range or higher. A general guideline that has been proposed is that with normal renal function, creatinine concentrations should decrease by approximately 50% every 24 hours. However, given the high "baseline" value in these foals, detecting minor increases in creatinine may not be feasible in the face of an overall daily decline in concentration. A solution to this problem has been evaluated in humans, and a similar protocol is used practically by many equine clinicians [37]. Neonatal AKI could be defined not by an absolute serum creatinine concentration, or even a small rise in serum creatinine concentration, but instead by a failure of a normal reduction in creatinine. Serum creatinine concentrations that fall by a rate that is less than a "normal" 50% decrease over a 24-hour period could potentially be diagnosed with AKI based on these criteria, particularly if it is in combination with decreasing urine output. Similar to the neonatal KDIGO guidelines for humans, an increase in creatinine >0.3 g/dl should also be scrutinized and monitored closely.

Treatment of AKI

Treatment for AKI is also discussed in Chapter 24, but a few additional comments are presented here. For all categories of AKI, careful normalization of perfusion is warranted, but fluid administration should be monitored carefully to avoid fluid overload. The risk of fluid overload in neonates cannot be overemphasized due to their size and different physiology. Fluid overload in conjunction with AKI has been shown to increase the risk of mortality so careful attention should be paid to monitoring body weight, urine output, and overall fluid balance. Additional information on fluid therapy for neonatal foals is in Chapter 62.

If perfusion cannot be normalized with IV fluids alone, inotropes and vasopressors may be needed. This is especially important as the risk for fluid overload increases. In all cases of AKI, but particularly ToxAKI, nephrotoxic medications should be stopped if possible. In cases of S-AKI, treatments for sepsis (source control, antimicrobials, supportive care) are necessary in conjunction with specific treatments for AKI. If AKI is caught early and managed carefully, the renal damage is often reversible.

New treatments on the horizon for AKI include both theophylline and caffeine. These drugs are adenosine receptor antagonists that may be renoprotective by inhibiting adenosine-induced renal vasoconstriction. In studies that came out of the cohort from the AWAKEN database, both medications were associated with a decreased incidence of AKI [11]. Larger randomized clinical trials are needed. The use of caffeine in equine neonates with hypoxic–ischemic encephalopathy has been described, but unfortunately, this study did not report any data on the differences in renal function in the group of foals that received caffeine [38].

Renal replacement therapy (RRT) remains the ideal treatment for neonates with severe AKI and particularly when fluid overload is becoming life threatening. In humans, advancements in the available RRT machines and technology for neonates continue to improve outcomes. In equine neonates, a single report from the 1990s first described RRT in foals [27]. However, there have been more recent reports of RRT in foals in the last few years suggesting that the use of this treatment may become more readily available [39, 40]. As this treatment becomes more practical and available, the outcome of foals with severe AKI is likely to improve.

Renal Disorders Other than AKI

Renal Infection

Sepsis-associated AKI has been described previously, but S-AKI focuses on the renal effects from the systemic response to infection in locations other than the kidney. Conversely, the kidneys may be the source of the infection where the causative agent directly causes renal damage. *Actinobacillus equuli* is the most commonly described organism for this type of infection in foals, though Leptospira could also theoretically be associated with this disease.

Actinobacillus

A. equuli is often associated with severe septicemia of newborn foals and may result in decreased mentation. Thus, foals with *Actinobacillus* infection have been referred to having *sleepy foal disease* [41, 42]. A characteristic of neonatal septicemic actinobacillosis is severe multifocal embolic nephritis [43]. Disease severity is often greater with *Actinobacillosis* as compared to other bacteria [42]. Diagnosis can be made with blood and sometimes urine culture. *Actinobaccillus* sp. are usually susceptible to ceftiofur and doses of 5 mg/kg IV BID in neonatal foals should be effective.

Leptospirosis

Leptospirosis has been described as a cause of renal disease in foals (Figure 26.2). Animals 2 months of age and older are more often described while neonates do not appear to be commonly affected [40, 44]. Fever and azotemia are common findings, and the diagnosis is typically confirmed using real-time PCR on urine samples to detect Leptospira. Serology is often used to determine the serovar and other animals (including the dam) are often tested. *Leptospira interrogans* serogroup *australis* serovar Bratislava and *L. interrogans* serogroup *australis* serovar Australis were identified in one report from Europe as causative agents [40]. In North America, *L. interrogans* serovar Pomona is more commonly reported as causing disease [45]. Foals are often treated with doxycycline (10 mg/kg PO BID) but penicillins and cephalosporins are also likely to be effective. In one report, the severity of disease required RRT [40].

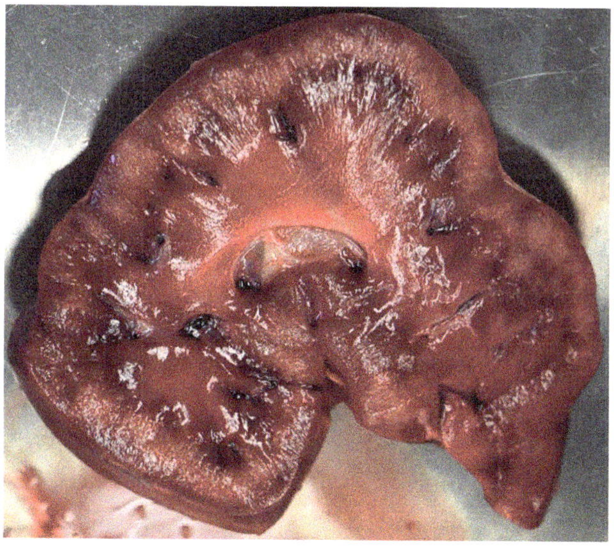

Figure 26.2 Kidney from a 10-month gestation thoroughbred fetus aborted due to leptospirosis. Pale, raised tan-white streaks extend throughout the cortex and medulla, corresponding with microscopic areas of suppurative tubulointerstitial nephritis. PCR performed on fetal kidney and placenta was positive as well as fetal heart blood titers for *L. Pomona*. *Source:* Image courtesy of Dr. Rebecca Ruby, University of Kentucky.

Congenital Abnormalities

Multiple congenital renal anomalies have been described either in isolation or in conjunction with other defects. Dysplasia of one or more kidneys has been reported multiple times, with complete absence of one or both kidneys being described less commonly [46]. If only one kidney is affected, clinical or laboratory abnormalities may be absent; however, if both kidneys are involved, the prognosis is poor. If the remaining kidney becomes diseased, clinical signs of renal failure can develop. Cystic disease affecting both kidneys [47] and uteropelvic polyps associated with hydronephrosis have also been reported [48].

As a general approach, neonatal foals with biochemical evidence of renal disease should have an ultrasound of the urogenital system to evaluate the kidney, bladder, and urachus. If the architecture of one or both kidneys is abnormal, additional testing may be required, but the possibility of a congenital renal abnormality should be considered. Other diagnostic modalities include biopsy and computed tomography. Depending on the congenital abnormality, some foals may have normal renal function and the abnormality may be found during imaging for other reasons.

Trauma

Trauma can be a cause for renal damage in animals of any age. A case of hemoperitoneum caused by capsular rupture and hemorrhage of the left kidney of a neonatal foal has been reported [49]. In this case, nephrectomy and stabilization of the foal was successful. Unilateral renal trauma may not generate abnormal renal makers on a biochemistry panel and clinical signs are unlikely to be specific for renal disease. External evidence of abdominal trauma may be apparent, but otherwise a foal with a painful or distended abdomen should undergo abdominal ultrasound evaluation as a routine part of the diagnostic workup. Ultrasonic evaluation of the kidneys may reveal evidence of a renal hematoma and possibly the presence of hemoperitoneum. The diagnosis of hemoperitoneum may be suspected from ultrasound alone, but in some cases a sample of abdominal fluid may need to be obtained for confirmation. Treatment consists of stabilization if blood loss has been severe. Nephrectomy may be required if hemorrhage is ongoing or significant renal damage has occurred.

Conclusions

AKI is the most important cause of renal dysfunction in neonatal foals and may be related to sepsis, nephrotoxic medications, or ischemia. Early detection of AKI is a current focus of research, and frequent monitoring for even very small changes in creatinine is likely to be extremely important. New biomarkers that identify renal injury are being explored in human neonates and may be more readily available for foals in the future. Standard treatment for AKI includes IV fluids, supportive care, and cessation of nephrotoxic medications. New research with caffeine and aminophylline may provide support for these medications for foals at risk for AKI. Renal replacement therapies also are now being used more frequently. Other renal disorders in foals include infection, congenital abnormalities, and trauma.

References

1 Makris, K. and Spanou, L. (2016). Acute kidney injury: definition, pathophysiology and clinical phenotypes. *Clin. Biochem. Rev.* 37: 85–98.

2 Kellum, J.A., Lameire, N., and For the KDIGO AKI Guideline Work Group (2013). Diagnosis, evaluation, and management of acute kidney injury: a KDIGO summary (part 1). *Crit. Care* 17: 204.

3 Jetton, J.G., Boohaker, L.J., Sethi, S.K. et al. (2017). Incidence and outcomes of neonatal acute kidney injury (AWAKEN): a multicentre, multinational, observational cohort study. *Lancet Child. Adolesc. Health* 1: 184–194.

4 Basu, R.K. and Wheeler, D.S. (2013). Kidney-lung cross-talk and acute kidney injury. *Pediatr. Nephrol.* 28: 2239–2248.

5 Askenazi, D., Abitbol, C., Boohaker, L. et al. (2019). Optimizing the AKI definition during first postnatal week using Assessment of Worldwide Acute Kidney Injury Epidemiology in Neonates (AWAKEN) cohort. *Pediatr. Res.* 85: 329–338.

6 Lameire, N., Van Biesen, W., and Vanholder, R. (2005). Acute renal failure. *Lancet* 365 (9457): 417–430.

7 Edwards, D.J., Brownlow, M.A., and Hutchins, D.R. (1990). Indices of renal function: values in eight normal foals from birth to 56 days. *Aust. Vet. J.* 67: 251–254.

8 Brewer, B.D., Clement, S.F., Lotz, W.S. et al. (1991). Renal clearance, urinary excretion of endogenous substances, and urinary diagnostic indices in healthy neonatal foals. *J. Vet. Int. Med.* 5: 28–33.

9 Holdstock, N.B., Ousey, J.C., and Rossdale, P.D. (1998). Glomerular filtration rate, effective renal plasma flow, blood pressure and pulse rate in the equine neonate during the first 10 days post partum. *Equine Vet. J.* 30: 335–343.

10 Buchanan, B.R., Sommardahl, C.S., Rohrbach, B.W. et al. (2005). Effect of a 24-hour infusion of an isotonic electrolyte replacement fluid on the renal clearance of electrolytes in healthy neonatal foals. *J. Am. Vet. Med. Assoc.* 227: 1123–1129.

11 Starr, M.C., Charlton, J.R., Guillet, R. et al. (2021). Advances in neonatal acute kidney injury. *Pediatrics* 148 (5): e2021051220.

12 Askenazi, D.J. (2020). AWAKEN-Ing a new frontier in neonatal nephrology. *Front. Pediatr.* 8: 21.

13 Rohrbach, B.W., Buchanan, B.R., Drake, J.M. et al. (2006). Use of a multivariable model to estimate the probability of discharge in hospitalized foals that are 7 days of age or less. *J. Am. Vet. Med. Assoc.* 228: 1748–1756.

14 Toro, J., Manrique-Caballero, C.L., and Gómez, H. (2021). Metabolic reprogramming and host tolerance: a novel concept to understand sepsis-associated AKI. *J. Clin. Med.* 10: 4184.

15 Ma, S., Evans, R.G., Iguchi, N. et al. (2019). Sepsis-induced acute kidney injury: a disease of the microcirculation. *Microcirculation* 26: e12483.

16 Gomez, H., Ince, C., De Backer, D. et al. (2014). A unified theory of sepsis-induced acute kidney injury: inflammation, microcirculatory dysfunction, bioenergetics and the tubular cell adaptation to injury. *Shock* 41: 3–11.

17 Langenberg, C., Bellomo, R., May, C. et al. (2005). Renal blood flow in sepsis. *Crit. Care* 9: R363–R374.

18 Huen, S.C. (2022). Metabolism as disease tolerance: implications for sepsis-associated acute kidney injury. *Nephron* 146: 291–294.

19 Taylor, S. (2015). A review of equine sepsis. *Equine Vet. Educ.* 27: 99–109.

20 Barr, B. and Nieman, N.M. (2022). Serum amyloid A as an aid in diagnosing sepsis in equine neonates. *Equine Vet. J.* 54: 922–926.

21 Wong, D.M., Ruby, R.E., Dembek, K.A. et al. (2018). Evaluation of updated sepsis scoring systems and systemic inflammatory response syndrome criteria and their association with sepsis in equine neonates. *J. Vet. Intern. Med.* 32: 1185–1193.

22 Stoops, C., Stone, S., Evans, E. et al. (2019). Baby NINJA (Nephrotoxic Injury Negated by Just-in-Time Action): reduction of nephrotoxic medication-associated acute kidney injury in the neonatal intensive care unit. *J. Pediatr.* 215: 223–228.e6.

23 Drożdżal, S., Lechowicz, K., Szostak, B. et al. (2021). Kidney damage from nonsteroidal anti-inflammatory drugs-Myth or truth? Review of selected literature. *Pharmacol. Res. Perspect.* 9 (4): e00817. https://doi.org/10.1002/prp2.817.

24 Carrick, J.B., Papich, M.G., Middleton, D.M. et al. (1989). Clinical and pathological effects of flunixin meglumine administration to neonatal foals. *Can. J. Vet. Res.* 53: 195–201.

25 Magdesian, K.G., Wilson, W.D., and Milhalyi, M. (1997). Pharmacokinetics and nephrotoxicity of high dose, once daily administered amikacin in neonatal foals. *AAEP Proc.* 396–397.

26 Burton, A.J., Giguère, S., and Arnold, R.D. (2015). Pharmacokinetics, pulmonary disposition and tolerability of liposomal gentamicin and free gentamicin in foals. *Equine Vet. J.* 47: 467–472.

27 Vivrette, S., Cowgill, L.D., Pascoe, J. et al. (1993). Hemodialysis for treatment of oxytetracycline-induced acute renal failure in a neonatal foal. *J. Am. Vet. Med. Assoc.* 203: 105–107.

28 Ellero, N., Freccero, F., Lanci, A. et al. (2020). Rhabdomyolysis and acute renal failure associated with Oxytetracycline Administration in two neonatal foals affected by flexural limb deformity. *Vet. Sci.* 7 (4): 160.

29 Wong, D.M., Sponseller, B.A., Alcott, C.J. et al. (2013). Effects of intravenous administration of polymyxin B in neonatal foals with experimental endotoxemia. *J. Am. Vet. Med. Assoc.* 243: 874–881.

30 Mussap, M., Noto, A., Fanos, V. et al. (2014). Emerging biomarkers and metabolomics for assessing toxic nephropathy and acute kidney injury (AKI) in neonatology. *Biomed. Res. Int.* 2014: 602526.

31 Perkins, G., Valberg, S.J., Madigan, J.M. et al. (1998). Electrolyte disturbances in foals with severe rhabdomyolysis. *J. Vet. Intern. Med.* 12: 173–177.

32 Kanagasundaram, N.S. (2015). Pathophysiology of ischaemic acute kidney injury. *Ann. Clin. Biochem.* 52 (Pt 2): 193–205.

33 Han, S.J. and Lee, H.T. (2019). Mechanisms and therapeutic targets of ischemic acute kidney injury. *Kidney Res. Clin. Pract.* 38: 427–440.

34 Nakashima, T., Inoue, H., Fujiyoshi, J. et al. (2016). Longitudinal analysis of serum cystatin C for estimating the glomerular filtration rate in preterm infants. *Pediatr. Nephrol.* 31: 983–989.

35 Tanigasalam, V., Bhat, V., Adhisivam, B. et al. (2016). Does therapeutic hypothermia reduce acute kidney injury among term neonates with perinatal asphyxia?--a randomized controlled trial. *J. Matern. Fetal. Neonatal Med.* 29: 2545–2548.

36 Chaney, K.P., Holcombe, S.J., Schott, H.C. 2nd et al. (2010). Spurious hypercreatininemia: 28 neonatal foals (2000–2008). *J. Vet. Emerg. Crit. Care (San Antonio)* 20: 244–249.

37 Gupta, C., Massaro, A.N., and Ray, P.E. (2016). A new approach to define acute kidney injury in term newborns with hypoxic ischemic encephalopathy. *Pediatr. Nephrol.* 31: 1167–1178.

38 Giguère, S., Slade, J.K., and Sanchez, L.C. (2008). Retrospective comparison of caffeine and doxapram for the treatment of hypercapnia in foals with hypoxic-ischemic encephalopathy. *J. Vet. Intern. Med.* 22: 401–405.

39 Wong, D.M., Ruby, R.E., Eatroff, A. et al. (2017). Use of renal replacement therapy in a neonatal foal with postresuscitation acute renal failure. *J. Vet. Intern. Med.* 31: 593–597.

40 Fouché, N., Graubner, C., Lanz, S. et al. (2020). Acute kidney injury due to *Leptospira interrogans* in 4 foals and use of renal replacement therapy with intermittent hemodiafiltration in 1 foal. *J. Vet. Intern. Med.* 34: 1007–1012.

41 Corley, K.T., Pearce, G., Magdesian, K.G. et al. (2007). Bacteraemia in neonatal foals: clinicopathological differences between Gram-positive and Gram-negative infections, and single organism and mixed infections. *Equine Vet. J.* 39: 84–89.

42 Stewart, A.J., Hinchcliff, K.W., Saville, W.J. et al. (2002). Actinobacillus sp. bacteremia in foals: clinical signs and prognosis. *J. Vet. Intern. Med.* 16: 464–471.

43 Layman, Q.D., Rezabek, G.B., Ramachandran, A. et al. (2014). A retrospective study of equine actinobacillosis cases: 1999–2011. *J. Vet. Diagn. Invest.* 26: 365–375.

44 van den Ingh, T.S., Hartman, E.G., and Bercovich, Z. (1989). Clinical *Leptospira interrogans* serogroup Australis serovar lora infection in a stud farm in The Netherlands. *Vet. Q.* 11: 175–182.

45 Divers, T.J., Chang, Y.F., Irby, N.L. et al. (2019). Leptospirosis: an important infectious disease in North American horses. *Equine Vet. J.* 51: 287–292.

46 Gilday, R.A., Wojnarowicz, C., Tryon, K.A. et al. (2015). Bilateral renal dysplasia, hydronephrosis, and hydroureter in a septic neonatal foal. *Can. Vet. J.* 56: 257–260.

47 Medina-Torres, C.E., Hewson, J., Stämpfli, S. et al. (2014). Bilateral diffuse cystic renal dysplasia in a 9-day-old Thoroughbred filly. *Can. Vet. J.* 55: 141–146.

48 Jones, S.L., Langer, D.L., Sterner-Kock, A. et al. (1994). Renal dysplasia and benign ureteropelvic polyps associated with hydronephrosis in a foal. *J. Am. Vet. Med. Assoc.* 204: 1230–1234.

49 Mitchell, K.J., Dowling, B.A., Hughes, K.J. et al. (2004). Unilateral nephrectomy as a treatment for renal trauma in a foal. *Aust. Vet. J.* 82: 753–755.

Chapter 27 Urinary Tract Disorders

David Wong, Annette M. McCoy, and Pamela A. Wilkins

Disorders involving the urinary tract occur with variable frequency with uroperitoneum and patent urachus being observed commonly in clinical practice. Other disorders such as ectopic ureters and megavesica occur rarely, but knowledge of these processes is important to the practitioner. This chapter discusses a variety of disorders that can occur involving the urinary tract in the neonatal foal.

Uroperitoneum

Uroperitoneum is a common clinical disorder in neonatal foals with a reported incidence of 0.2–2.5% [1]. This condition is most commonly associated with a tear or defect in the urinary bladder (53–81% of reported cases) or the urachus (19–47% of reported cases) [1–4]. Less common causes include urine leakage from the urethra or rarely, a defect in one or both of the ureters [1–4]. Occasionally there can be two sources of uroperitoneum, so evaluation of all possible causes of uroperitoneum during diagnostic evaluation is prudent [5, 6]. Possible underlying mechanisms of uroperitoneum include congenital defects within the bladder or ureters, parturient or external trauma, strenuous exercise, excessive pressure applied to a full bladder (during parturition or iatrogenic), focal necrotic cystitis, and urachal infections [1]. Additionally, critically ill foals can experience ruptured bladder from sepsis or urinary tract infections that can cause focal ischemia and necrosis from the infectious process, or iatrogenic bladder rupture from caretakers lifting and repositioning obtunded foals (e.g. foal with full bladder is lifted by the abdomen to move or reposition patient) [1, 2, 4, 6].

Regardless of the path by which urine enters the abdomen, specific physiologic and biochemical changes occur due to accumulation of urine within the abdominal cavity and exchange of electrolytes, fluid, and other molecules between the peritoneum and blood [7–10]. The peritoneum is an extensive serous membrane that lines the abdominal cavity, part of the pelvic inlet, and almost all the abdominal viscera, less a small portion of the liver that is attached directly to the diaphragm (area nuda hepatis) [7, 11]. Because the peritoneum is a semipermeable membrane, the components (e.g. creatinine, urea, potassium) within the free fluid (e.g. urine) in the abdomen exchange with the blood and eventually reach an equilibrium [1]. This "autodialysis" phenomenon is caused by a shift of water and solutes due to differences in relative osmolarity and concentration gradients between the two compartments—that is, the peritoneal cavity and intravascular space [7–10]. High urine osmolarity (Table 27.1) causes water to move from the intravascular space into the peritoneal cavity. Of note, urine osmolality varies considerably with age in the foal (e.g. mean of 544 mOsm/kg at 12 hours of age, decreasing to a mean of 138 mOsm/kg at 96 hours old, progressively increasing to a mean of 999 mOsm/kg as an adult). Therefore, movement of water between the intravascular and peritoneal spaces will vary [13]. Sodium and chloride concentrations are relatively low in the urine, resulting in these electrolytes in the blood to move down a concentration gradient and into the peritoneal cavity, subsequently resulting in hyponatremia and hypochloremia, respectively. Hyponatremia activates the renin-angiotensin-aldosterone system that acts at the distal tubule and collecting duct of the kidney nephron, resulting in increased reabsorption of sodium and water into the serum and secretion of potassium into the urine [7, 10]. In theory, urine that continues to leak into the peritoneal cavity will have declining sodium and increasing potassium concentrations [9]. Over time, the high solute concentration gradients of potassium, urea, and creatinine within the abdominal fluid/urine promote movement from the peritoneal cavity into the intravascular space, thereby causing elevated serum concentrations of these molecules (hyperkalemia, azotemia) [10].

Equine Neonatal Medicine, First Edition. Edited by David M. Wong and Pamela A. Wilkins.

Table 27.1 Urine and serum variables from healthy four-day-old foals expressed as least square means (range) [12].

	Urine	Serum
Sodium (mEq/l)	10 (7–13)	137 (136–138)
Potassium (mEq/l)	79.6 (24–212)	4.1 (3.9–4.2)
Chloride (mEq/l)	37 (16–72)	96 (92–100)
Creatine (mg/dl)	65.6 (15–183)	1.0 (0.8–1.3)
Osmolality (mOsm/kg)	210 (63–513)	267 (261–272)

Signalment and Clinical Findings

Foals that present with uroperitoneum typically range in age between 1 and 7 days old (reported range 0–42 days) [1, 2, 4, 14, 15]. In one study of 45 foals with uroperitoneum, the mean age at presentation was 2.5 days of age (range 1–6 days); in that study male foals presented earlier (mean 2 days, range 1–5 days) compared to female foals (mean 3.5 days, range 2–6 days) [16]. In other studies involving 18 and 31 foals with uroperitoneum, the mean age at the time of surgery was 4.6 and 4.8 days, respectively [1, 4]. In broad terms, foals with uroperitoneum secondary to bladder rupture typically present at 1–3 days of age, while foals with other causes such as urachal infection or ureteral rupture present with uroabdomen at a slightly older (7–10 days) age [17]. Historically, colts were believed to have a higher incidence of uroperitoneum because of parturient trauma and the inability of the colt to express a full bladder when compressed during parturition [1, 4]. However, this gender predilection has not always held true in studies. In one of the aforementioned studies, 17/18 foals were males, whereas another study no gender predilection was detected [1, 2]. Tears in the dorsal aspect of the bladder wall have been reported to be more common, although ventral tears are also possible [2]. Interestingly, in foals that had experimentally induced rupture of the neonatal bladder, rupture was exclusively characterized as a longitudinal tear of the dorsal surface of the cranial to mid-third of the urinary bladder with minimal bleeding, suggesting that the dorsal surface of the bladder is the weakest region [18].

A few studies have linked a history of dystocia with uroperitoneum and presentation of the foal to a hospital at a very young (<48 hours) age [4, 5]. In one study, 6/12 hospitalized foals that developed uroperitoneum had a history of dystocia [4]. The thin structure of the urachus and exposure to tearing forces during rupture of the umbilical cord make the urachus a more logical candidate for traumatic rupture in foals that experience dystocia, rather than the healthy, muscular, elastic urinary bladder wall [4].

Another cohort of foals with uroperitoneum are those that originally present for another medical concern (e.g. sepsis, neonatal encephalopathy) and develop uroperitoneum during hospitalization. These foals have more variation in age when they develop uroperitoneum with some studies suggesting that septic foals with uroperitoneum are older. For example, in one study of 31 foals, the average age of the septic foal with uroperitoneum was 7.1 days as compared to 3.1 days in nonseptic foals [1]. Conversely, in another study, foals that were hospitalized and developed uroperitoneum were significantly younger (mean 0.46 ± 0.52 days) compared to foals presenting for uroperitoneum as a primary compliant (mean 9.5 ± 10.8 days) [4].

Clinical signs associated with uroperitoneum are variable, but the foal may appear healthy for the first 24–48 hours of life followed by clinical signs of lethargy, lack of nursing, stranguria, urine dribbling, lateral recumbency, abdominal distension (Figure 27.1), tachycardia, and irregular heart rhythm [2, 4, 14, 16, 19]. Respiratory character can be altered and manifest as one or more of the following: tachypnea, labored and/or shallow breathing, flared nostrils, and respiratory distress [2, 4, 14, 16, 19]. Respiratory distress may be attributed to compression of the thorax by excessive free fluid in the abdomen and/or pleural fluid in thoracic cavity secondary to uroperitoneum. In some cases, the volume of free fluid within the abdomen increases intra-abdominal pressure to such an extent that pulmonary compliance and venous return to the heart is decreased. This situation, referred to as **intra-abdominal hypertension/abdominal compartment syndrome (ACS)**, has occasionally been reported in foals with uroperitoneum [19].

History of micturition varies, but affected foals typically appear healthy and have a history of passing urine

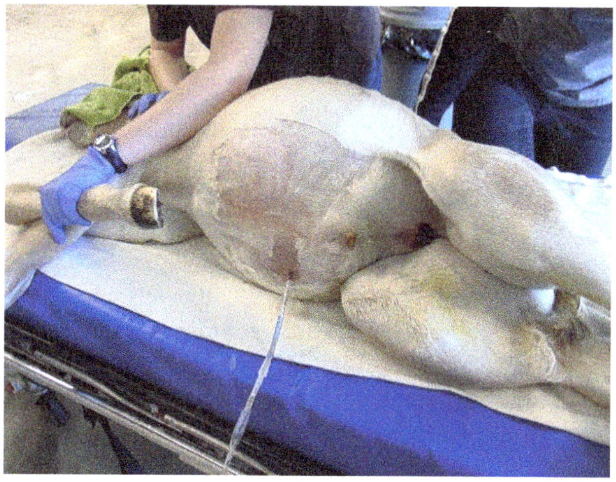

Figure 27.1 Neonatal foal with uroperitoneum. Note the abdominal distension as well as the abdominal drain placed to facilitate drainage of fluid from the abdominal cavity.

normally. At presentation for veterinary care, the foal may posture to urinate frequently and void small amounts of urine. Other signs that may be associated with uroperitoneum include weakness, injected mucous membranes, colic, ventral edema, fever, diarrhea, tenesmus associated with constipation, gastric reflux, neurologic signs, and intermittent focal seizures [1, 4, 14, 16]. These latter signs could also be related to comorbidities. Foals with urethral defects or defects of the subcutaneous portion of the urachus can develop edema and swelling of the perineum, inguinal region, and prepuce [5, 17].

On rare occasions, uroperitoneum can be associated with pleural effusion [2, 20, 21]. In such cases, ultrasonographic examination of the thorax can identify fluid and, if present, thoracocentesis and drainage of the pleural fluid improves ventilation [2]. One route by which fluid might pass from the abdomen to the thorax is the diaphragmatic lymphatics. The muscular portion of the diaphragm has a high concentration of lymphatic stomata that facilitates peritoneal drainage to the mediastinal lymph nodes [11, 21–23]. The relatively porous nature of the diaphragm may be one explanation of the clinical finding of secondary pleural effusion in foals with primary effusive diseases of the abdominal cavity, as reported in foals with uroperitoenum [2, 3, 24, 25]. Anatomic defects of the diaphragm or reno-pleural fistulas are other possible routes by which free abdominal fluid reaches the thorax [20]. The composition of the pleural effusion can also vary. In one case report, a 4-day-old filly presented originally for diarrhea developed uroperitoneum during hospitalization [20]. A rent in the urinary bladder was identified and repaired, but postoperatively, the foal was hypoxemic and pleural fluid was documented via ultrasonography. Subsequently, 350 mLs of clear yellow fluid was removed via thoracocentesis of the right hemithorax. Analysis of the pleural fluid revealed an elevated creatinine concentration of 2.8 mg/dL (serum creatinine 1.5 mg/dL), total protein of 7 g/L, and a total nucleated cell counts of <1000 cells/μL (60% nondegenerate neutrophils, 3% small lymphocytes, 37% mononuclear cells) [20]. The pleural fluid to serum creatinine ratio was 1.87, which was consistent with urinothorax (defined as a ratio> 1) [26]. In another report, a 2-day-old filly was diagnosed with a tear of urinary bladder resulting in uroperitoneum [21]. Uneventful surgical repair of the bladder was performed but 6 hours after anesthetic recovery, the filly was hypoxemic, tachycardic, and tachypneic. Thoracic ultrasound revealed a large amount of anechoic pleural fluid. Serosanguinous fluid (protein <25 g/L, total nucleated cell count 2090 cells/μL, 28 ,000 erythrocytes/μL) was drained from the right (700 mLs) and left (50 mLs) hemithorax. In this case, the creatinine concentration of the pleural fluid was 1.3 mg/dL suggesting that the pleural fluid was not urinothorax [21]. Possible causes of pleural effusion in this case included re-expansion pulmonary edema, acute lung injury or both processes [27].

Clinicopathologic changes occur because of urine collecting in the abdomen. The composition of neonatal foal urine includes high concentrations of creatinine and potassium and low concentrations of sodium and chloride when compared to serum (Table 27.1) [12]. Over time, as the electrolytes and creatinine reach an equilibrium across the peritoneal cavity, serum concentrations of these analytes are altered, often resulting in the classic biochemical profile of hyponatremia, hypochloremia, hyperkalemia, elevated creatinine concentrations, and decreased serum osmolality [2, 3, 5, 14, 24, 28, 29]. Serum urea nitrogen may be elevated but can be normal [3, 24]. However, the clinician must be cognizant of the fact that these electrolyte alterations do not always occur in foals with uroperitoneum. In one study involving 18 foals with uroperitoneum, 40% were hyponatremic, 43% were hypochloremic, 38% were hyperkalemic, and 88% were azotemic, thus highlighting the fact that electrolyte/creatinine changes, while common, are not consistent [2]. Electrolyte changes in foals that are hospitalized or receiving IV fluids that subsequently develop uroperitoneum can be normal or only slightly altered, likely due to the fact that these foals are receiving IV fluids that contain balanced electrolytes [1, 2].

Interestingly, in a study that induced ruptured bladder in adult mares, the abdominal fluid creatinine increased rapidly and dramatically. Within 2 hours post-bladder rupture, peritoneal fluid creatinine concentration increased by 33-fold from baseline and 97-fold within 16 hours. Concurrently, serum creatinine concentration increased by a factor of three in the first 20 hours [28]. In this study, the peritoneal: serum creatinine concentrations were greater than 2:1 within 2 hours of urinary bladder rupture [28]. Other clinicopathologic changes that may be associated with uroperitoneum include hyperglycemia and metabolic acidosis [1, 14, 15]. The hemogram can be normal, but leukocytosis or leukopenia can be observed and can also be altered if other disease processes such as sepsis are present [2, 4, 29].

Diagnosis

Prior to ultrasound, methods to support a diagnosis of uroperitoneum included contrast abdominal radiography or dye (sterile methylene blue or fluorescein) studies [30]. These studies are performed by injecting sterile contrast or dye through a urethral catheter and observing if the contrast material diffuses outside the urinary bladder on a subsequent abdominal radiograph (Figure 27.2) or dye within a sample of peritoneal fluid, respectively [2, 31]. Contrast studies may also be necessary to identify urethral tears or ruptures that have been reported in neonatal foals [5].

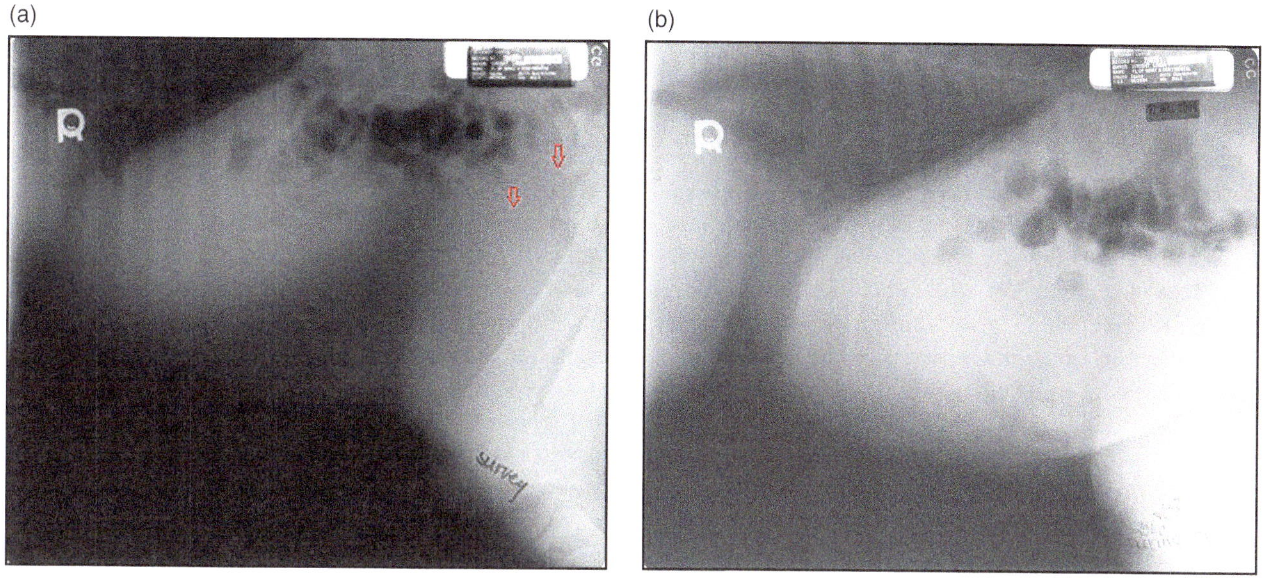

Figure 27.2 Pre- and post-contrast administration lateral radiographs in a foal with a ruptured bladder. Note the urinary catheter in the pre-contrast image (a; red arrows) and (b) the diffuse distribution of the contrast material throughout the abdomen in the post-contrast image.

Currently, ultrasonography of the abdomen plays a key role in identifying uroperitoneum. In healthy 1- and 7-day-old foals, the reported maximum bladder size when distended is 9 and 10 cm, respectively [32]. Foals with uroperitoneum demonstrate variable amounts of anechoic free fluid within the abdominal cavity; depending on the size and location of the defect, the bladder may contain anechoic urine or be collapsed and folded on itself (Figure 27.3) [1, 6]. In some instances, the defect in the bladder or urachus can be detected via ultrasound. A bubblegram can also be used to help identify a defect in the bladder and is performed by instilling sterile saline, that is shaken to produce air bubbles within the solution, into the bladder via urethral catheter and subsequently identifying the saline solution traversing the defect via ultrasound of the bladder [5, 33]. If a urethral defect is suspected, contrast radiography or urethral endoscopy should be considered [17]. If present, the classic clinicopathologic changes of hyponatremia, hypochloremia, hyperkalemia, and azotemia are highly suggestive of uroperitoneum. However, the clinician should be cognizant that these clinicopathologic alterations are present in approximately 50% of cases diagnosed with uroperitoneum [1]. Moreover, foals hospitalized for other conditions and/or those receiving IV fluid therapy may have either minimal changes or normal electrolyte concentrations [1, 2, 4]. Because creatinine diffuses relatively poorly across the peritoneal lining, a disparity between the peritoneal: serum fluid creatinine ratio develops during uroperitoneum with a ratio of at least 2 : 1 being highly suggestive of uroperitoneum [1]. Of note, serum creatinine and peritoneal: serum creatinine ratio are not significantly affected by IV fluid therapy [1, 4].

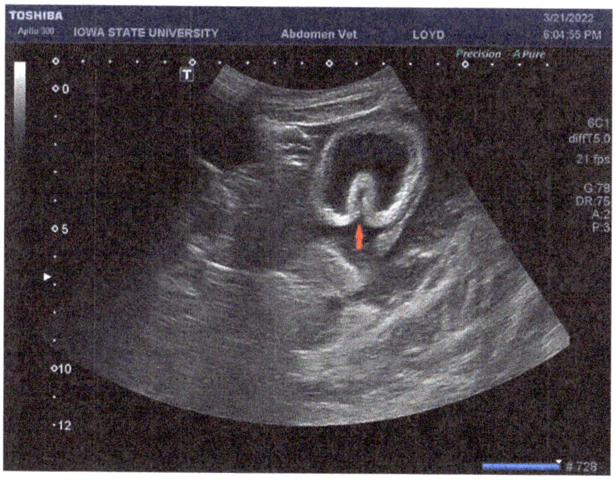

Figure 27.3 Abdominal ultrasound of a foal with a ruptured bladder. Note that the urinary bladder is folded in on itself (red arrow) and the anechoic free fluid within the abdomen.

Treatment

The initial treatment goals in a foal with uroperitoneum are to improve cardiovascular and respiratory function and correct electrolyte imbalances. Excess free fluid in the abdomen causes intra-abdominal hypertension and places pressure on the diaphragm which impacts the foal's ability to ventilate by decreasing the tidal volume, total lung capacity, and functional residual capacity and increases the work of breathing. As urine continues to fill the abdomen, the abdominal wall will distend to a point of reaching the limits of compliance; once this point is reached, intra-abdominal pressure increases. Thus, abdominal drainage is commonly indicated with uroperitoneum and can be performed using an abdominal drain (e.g. chest tube with one-way valve; Figure 27.1) for continuous drainage or a teat canula for intermittent drainage. In some cases, the drainage device can continually be blocked by omentum, making adequate drainage of free fluid from the abdomen difficult to impossible [19, 29]. The cardiovascular status should be closely monitored during and after drainage of large amounts of free fluid within the abdomen as hypotension can subsequently develop [29]. Although there is a reduction in intrathoracic and intraabdominal pressure after removing excess free fluid that facilitates improved cardiac output, there can also be expansion of the abdominal vasculature that consequently reduces systemic vascular resistance, thereby contributing to relative hypovolemia with a sum effect of a drop in blood pressure and development of hypotension [19, 29]. This situation can be particularly treacherous in neonatal foals as they are less able to compensate for hypotension since they maintain cardiac output primarily by altering their heart rate and because they have an immature sympathetic nervous system that has less vasomotor tone and therefore less capacity to control vasoconstriction [34, 35].

Hyperkalemia is corrected with IV administration of potassium poor fluids such as 0.9% saline. Dextrose can be added to IV fluids to help decrease hyperkalemia by inducing endogenous insulin release, which drives potassium from the serum into cells. Exogenous insulin has been administered to treat hyperkalemia but is used cautiously as hypoglycemia can consequently occur. Sodium bicarbonate (1–2 mEq/Kg slow IV over 15 minutes) can also be combined with IV fluids to help lower potassium concentrations by increasing the serum pH, which thereby liberates intracellular hydrogen ions [29]. As hydrogen ions exit the cells, potassium ions from the serum enter the cells in exchange to maintain electroneutrality. Of note, sodium bicarbonate should not be combined with calcium containing fluids as the two compounds are not compatible and may form precipitation in the solution. Calcium gluconate (4 mg/kg slow IV over 10–20 minutes) is sometimes administered to antagonize the effects of potassium on cardiomyocyte membranes (cardioprotective) [29]. Calcium administration does not lower potassium concentrations, but rather, increases extracellular free calcium which causes an increase in the threshold potential of excitable cells and counteracts the increased excitability that accompanies hyperkalemia (Figure 27.4) [14, 29]. For added safety, the dose of calcium can be added to a volume (e.g. 100 mL) of 5% dextrose in water. Administration of β_2-adrenergic agonists have also been used to treat hyperkalemia through activation of cyclic adenosine monophosphate (cAMP) and stimulation of the sodium–potassium ATPase pump, which shifts potassium into cells [35]. Table 27.2 provides a summary of methods used to treat hyperkalemia.

Because bacterial infections and sepsis are common in neonatal foals, broad-spectrum antimicrobials are frequently administered to hospitalized foals, including those with uroperitoneum. Sepsis can also directly impact the urinary bladder as demonstrated by foals that have concurrent cystitis and ruptured bladders [2]. In one report, foals had bacterial or fungal growth from bladder tissue and were hospitalized for sepsis, respiratory distress, or prematurity when uroperitoneum developed. Ischemia, necrosis, and infection have also been demonstrated microscopically on tissue samples of affected bladder tissue and one can

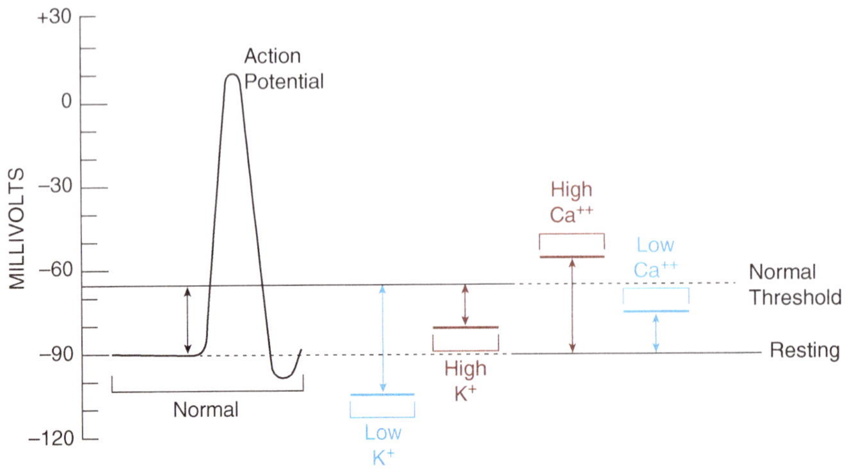

Figure 27.4 Effects of serum calcium and potassium on membrane potentials of excitable tissues. The concentration of potassium in extracellular fluids affects the resting potential, as compared to calcium concentrations that alter the threshold potential.

Table 27.2 Management of acute hyperkalemia [36, 37].

Medication	Response type	Onset of action	Duration of action	Mechanism of action	Dose
Ca gluconate	Rapid	1–2 min	30–60 min	Protects cardiomyocytes	4 mg/kg, slow IV over 10–20 min
Beta-agonists	Intermediate	3–5 min	1–4 h	Shift K^+ intracellularly	Salbutamol 0.5 µg/kg inhaled, q6–12h Albuterol 1–2 µg/kg inhaled q8–12h
Dextrose	Intermediate	10–20 min	2–6 h	Shift K^+ intracellularly	1–3% Dextrose IV
Dextrose + Insulin	Intermediate	10–20 min	2–6 h	Shift K^+ intracellularly	1–3% Dextrose IV Insulin (regular) 0.005–0.01 IU/kg/h
$NaHCO_3$	Intermediate	30–60 min	2–6 h	Shift K^+ intracellularly	1–2 mEq/kg, slow IV over 15–30 min
Furosemide	Delayed	5–30 min	2–6 h	Elimination of K^+ from body	1–2 mg/kg, IV, q6h

speculate that infection, sepsis, and associated local malperfusion might predispose the foal to focal lesions of the lower urinary tract and subsequent development of urinary leakage [4]. Thus, the clinician should consider submitting surgical tissue specimens for histologic examination and bacterial culture of bladder tissue [1, 4]. Rarely, postoperative bladder atony has been noted in foals and in these cases, bethanecol (0.4 mg/kg, PO, q8h, tapered [same dose] to q12h, then q24 hours over 10 days), a parasympathomimetic, can be considered to facilitate bladder contraction [37, 38].

Abdominal compartment syndrome (ACS) occurs when intraabdominal hypertension is sustained above 20 mmHg and new onset end organ dysfunction is present [39]. Increased intraabdominal pressure can result from increased intrabdominal volume, decreased abdominal compliance, or both [40]. The abdomen is a closed anatomic space where the compliance is largely determined by the elastic recoil of the abdominal wall and the diaphragm [39]. Abdominal compliance can be reduced by external constraints (e.g. abdominal bandage) or previous abdominal surgery [40]. Once the compliance limits are reached, an increase in intraabdominal volume causes a proportional increase in intrabdominal pressure [35]. Increased intraabdominal pressures and ACS can result in a number of negative physiologic effects on various organs [34, 39]. ACS has a direct effect on the pulmonary system as the pressure from excessive free abdominal fluid progressively decreases pulmonary compliance and reduces total lung capacity, functional residual capacity, and residual volume, all contributing to reduced capillary blood flow, increased dead-space, and ventilation-perfusion mismatch [39–41]. These changes impair gas exchange, resulting in hypoxemia, hypercapnia, and respiratory acidosis [42]. Movement of the diaphragm cranially can also result in atelectasis [35, 39]. Increased intraabdominal pressure also restricts movement of the diaphragm leading to hypoventilation which can contribute to development of hypoxemia [35].

Decreased cardiac output can also occur from increased intra-abdominal pressure due to reduced venous return from direct compression of the caudal vena cava and portal vein [41]. Increased intrathoracic pressure, secondary to excess abdominal fluid, results in reduced blood flow through the cranial vena cava, which further decreases venous return to the heart. Increased intrathoracic pressure (thoracic tamponade) also causes cardiac compression and a reduction in end diastolic volume, reduced ventricular compliance and contractility [39]. Concomitantly, increased systemic vascular resistance results from the combined effect of arterial vasoconstriction and increased intraabdominal pressure [41]. Collectively, these derangements result in reduced stroke volume. The effect of intraabdominal hypertension on systemic blood pressure is variable as both arterial hypertension and hypotension have been reported [42].

The renal, gastrointestinal, and hepatobiliary system can also be impacted by intraabdominal hypertension and ACS. With intraabdominal hypertension there is significant reduction in urine output because of reduced renal blood flow and function [39]. The elevated pressure also compresses mesenteric veins and reduces mesenteric blood flow resulting in intestinal edema; if severe this can result in worsening perfusion, bowel ischemia, and feeding intolerance and increases the likelihood of bacterial translocation [39, 42]. Likewise, intraabdominal hypertension can impair liver perfusion, and hepatic cell function.

Intra-abdominal pressure can be measured by direct (invasive, peritoneal puncture coupled to manometry) or indirect (noninvasive, insertion of a balloon monometer into visceral lumen such as the stomach, bladder, or rectum) methods [42]. Measurement of intra-abdominal pressure has not been extensively examined in horses but has been measured in healthy anesthetized recumbent adult horses (<7.4 mmHg), healthy standing horses using direct puncture of the right flank (mean ± SD, −5 ± 3 mmHg), healthy standing sedated horses using bladder catheterization and a water monometer (<5 mmHg), via gastric monometery, and in ill horses using direct abdominal needle puncture and a pressure transducer [43–47]. Measurement and evaluation of intraabdominal pressure has not been published in foals but use of an intra-bladder catheter seems relatively practical. Detailed description of techniques to measure intraabdominal pressure in horses are available [42, 44–46].

Drainage of abdominal fluid in patients with ACS results in nearly immediate reversal of the negative respiratory and cardiovascular effects [41]. However, decompression of the abdominal cavity should be performed at a controlled fashion, as too rapid a rate of drainage can cause significant hypotension as the sudden decrease in systemic vascular resistance results in a significant drop in blood pressure which may be compounded by preexisting hypovolemia. Cardiac arrhythmias and asystole have also been reported in foals and people [19, 29, 35, 41, 48, 49] after rapid removal of excess abdominal fluid and may be associated with a release of products of anaerobic metabolism such as potassium, lactic acid, and adenosine that have accumulated from previously ischemic tissues [34, 35, 41].

The sudden incorporation of these substances into the systemic circulation can cause arrhythmias, myocardial depression, and vasodilation. Additionally, bradycardia has been associated with rapid removal of intra-abdominal fluid as exemplified by a decrease in heart rate from 80 to 40 beats/min in a 5-day-old Thoroughbred filly that had 12 L of abdominal fluid (urine) removed over 30 seconds during celiotomy to repair a tear in the urinary bladder [35]. Pulmonary edema can develop after decompression (re-expansion pulmonary edema) likely secondary to increased pulmonary vascular permeability that occurs from hypoxic damage to capillary endothelium and mechanical damage to blood vessels from over stretching during the process of re-expansion [27]. Thus, frequent assessment of the heart rate, pulse pressure, and blood pressure is prudent during and after correction of ACS.

Surgical Repair

Primary surgical repair of a bladder tear should not be attempted prior to medical stabilization of the foal. Individual surgeons have personal preferences on repairing bladder tears, but a basic outline of the surgical technique is described herein. A caudoventral midline celiotomy is performed by way of a fusiform incision centered on ventral midline and extended lateral to the umbilicus through the skin and subcutaneous tissue. In male foals, the skin incision is directed paramedian to avoid the prepuce and penis, which are then retracted to expose the midline. The linea alba is then sharply incised to enter the abdomen and to release the urachus from the abdominal wall; alternatively, some surgeons prefer to initially enter the abdomen abaxial to the umbilicus to reduce the risk of damaging the umbilical vessels. Free abdominal fluid is removed via suction once the abdomen is entered. The bladder is isolated and elevated, and the tear or defect is identified (Figure 27.5). Placement of stay sutures to stabilize the bladder during primary repair is recommended. Some surgeons choose to debride the tear margins, especially if the tissue appears devitalized. A two-layer closure is used to repair the defect (e.g. simple continuous followed by an inverting [Cushing or Lembert] oversew) [14]. The suture should not penetrate the mucosa, to reduce the risk of formation of cystic calculi [50]. After the repair of the bladder is complete, an omphalectomy is performed, and the umbilical vessels are ligated with suture followed by transection. The urachus is then resected, taking care that the apex of the bladder remains intact. The integrity of the bladder repair is tested by distending the bladder with sterile saline (±sterile methylene blue) administered via urethral catheter [14]. Urachal tears are managed by omphalectomy and cystoplasty. Once the surgeon is satisfied with the repair, the abdomen should be copiously lavaged with 0.9% saline and the celiotomy incision closed in routine fashion.

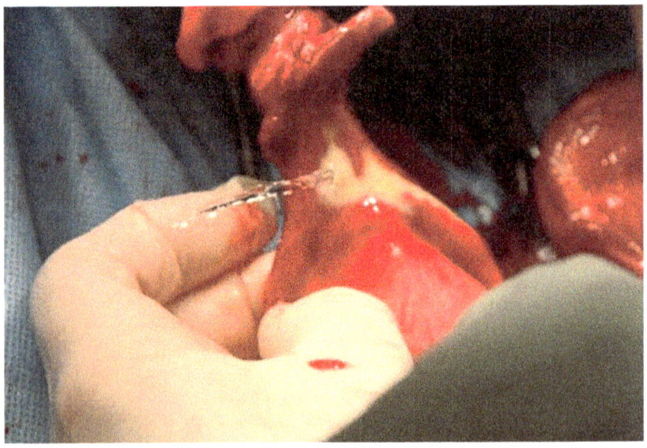

Figure 27.5 Intra-operative image demonstrating urine leakage from a small hole in the urachus along with a devitalized area of the bladder/urachus.

Antimicrobials, anti-inflammatory medications, and general supportive care (i.e. correction of serum electrolytes derangements and azotemia, provision of nutrition) are continued postoperatively [16]. Some clinicians suggest placement of a urinary catheter postoperatively whereas others avoid catheterization in attempts to avoid ascending infections. The use of a urinary catheter will vary based on individual case features, but clinicians should strongly consider maintaining a urinary catheter for at least 3 days postoperatively to allow the bladder tear to heal and avoid excessive bladder pressure in the immediate post-operative period. Although uroperitoneum is typically treated with surgical correction, a few reports of small urinary bladder defects have been managed successfully without surgery by use of an indwelling urinary catheter [4, 51, 52].

Postoperative complications following bladder repair are relatively uncommon, although one retrospective study involving 45 foals that had surgery for uroperitoneum noted that 9/45 foals (20%) had recurrence of uroperitoneum after primary closure while other reports noted recurrence rates of 12–27% [1, 3, 4, 16]. Recurrence of uroperitoneum can be related to surgical failure (e.g. dehiscence and leakage at original site of repair), latent tissue necrosis, overpressurization of the bladder causing leakage around suture tracts, or an additional urinary tract defect [16]. Recurrence was identified on average 48 hours (range 12–264 hours) after initial repair either by free abdominal fluid on postoperative ultrasound, observation of abdominal distension, and/or drainage from the abdominal incision postoperatively [16]. Of the nine foals with recurrence, four were treated with medical therapy, three underwent a second celiotomy, and two were euthanized [16]. Medical therapy was successful in the four foals with recurrence of uroperitoneum and consisted of continuous urine decompression with an indwelling urinary catheter and supportive care for 3–7 days [16]. Of the three foals that had a second celiotomy, bladder leakage was noted adjacent to or at the site of previous repair. In the two foals that were euthanized, focal bladder necrosis adjacent to the repair or leakage of urine from multiple suture tract sites were observed at necropsy [16]. Other comorbidities include persistent azotemia, peritonitis, pleural effusion, bladder atony, renal failure, intestinal adhesions, joint sepsis, abdominal dehiscence, and sepsis [16]. In one case, cystic calculi were noted 14 months after surgical repair of uroperitoneum [16].

Urethral defects are a much less common cause of uroperitoneum, but when present, treatment can be approached medically or surgically. Medical therapy involves allowing the defect to heal via second intention which is facilitated by catheterization of the bladder. This allows urine to bypass the urethra until granulation tissue surrounds the urethral defect and prevents subcutaneous urine accumulation [17]. The uroepithelium can bridge a defect within 3–21 days when urine is diverted away from the site of injury. Urethral stricture following second intention healing is rare [5]. If necrotic skin and extensive subcutaneous urine accumulation is present, these areas can be opened to allow drainage. If the skin is still intact over the identified site of urethral rupture, an incision can be made directly over the site, thereby allowing urine to drain and prevent further accumulation of subcutaneous urine [17]. This is an important because one factor that impacts urethral healing is urine extravasation [5]. Urine that contacts the periurethral tissues delays wound healing and can result in periurethral fibrosis [5]. Alternatively, primary closure of the urethral defect can be attempted surgically to facilitate primary healing of the urethral mucosa [5, 17]. This approach is appropriate following sharp transection or surgical incision into the urethra, but not following traumatic urethral rupture or necrosis. Urethral rupture that is secondary to necrosis/infection and managed with primary closure typically ends with dehiscence [5, 17].

Anesthesia

Anesthetic complications have been reported in foals with uroperitoneum that are undergoing a celiotomy to identify and repair the site of urine leakage [3, 19, 25, 52–54]. Historically, anesthetic complications were believed to be related to hyperkalemia and that anesthetic risks are minimized by decreasing serum potassium concentrations to <5.5 mEq/L prior to anesthetic induction [34]. Hyperkalemia reduces the resting potential across the cell membrane thereby moving the membrane potential closer to threshold potential and increasing the irritability of the myocardium (Figure 27.4) [35]. An initial increase in tissue excitability is typically observed with mild hyperkalemia and is followed by decreased excitability as plasma potassium concentrations continue to rise [29]. Hyperkalemia also reduces conduction velocity at the sinus and atrioventricular (AV) nodes potentially contributing to AV block or cardiac arrest [55]. Purkinje fibers seem to be more sensitive to hyperkalemia than the AV or sinus node, therefore precipitating the occurrence of AV block [29].

In one study, 9/18 foals developed life-threatening arrhythmias (most commonly third-degree AV block or cardiac arrest) under halothane anesthesia [3]. However, a more recent study noted anesthetic complications in only 16% of foals (4 foals) that received surgical correction of the defect; in this study, hyperkalemia was only present in half of the foals with anesthetic complications [4]. Two foals developed AV block and two foals developed conduction blocks. The reduced incidence of anesthetic complications may be related to less-severe electrolyte abnormalities because of earlier detection, improved peri-operative stabilization, and/or the routine use of isoflurane during general anesthesia. Other reports have noted second-degree AV block, third-degree AV

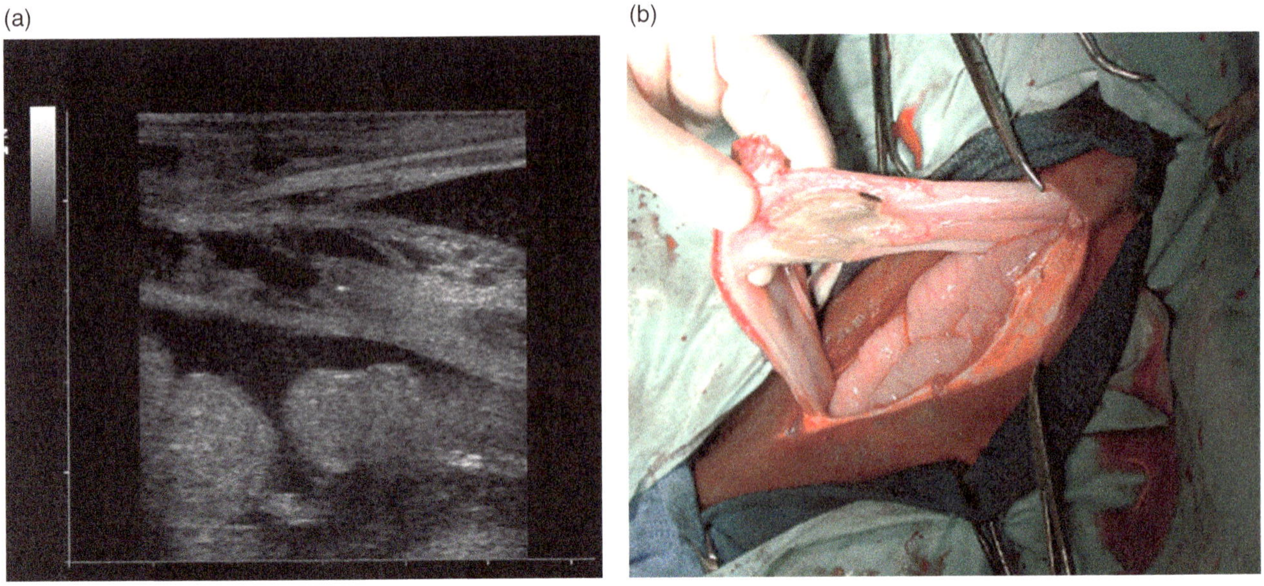

Figure 27.6 (a) Ultrasound and (b) intra-operative image of an infected urachus that resulted in septic peritonitis in a foal.

block, ventricular asystole, and bradycardia during anesthesia of foals with uroperiotneum [2, 19, 29, 56].

An inconspicuous but important variable that may contribute to anesthetic complications in the neonatal foal is movement of the anesthetized patient. Turning of the foal during anesthesia should be performed with care and heightened monitoring, as anecdotal reports of deaths have been associated with turning of the anesthetized patient [34, 57]. This may, in part, result from significant decrease in blood pressure when body position is changed in the foal [34, 58].

Prognosis of uroperitoneum is generally good following surgical repair, with short-term survival rates varying between 50% and 100% in various studies [1–4, 59]. If concurrent disease is present, especially sepsis or other severe illness, the prognosis is less favorable [1]. In one study, 8 of 14 foals with a positive sepsis score and uroabodmen survived [1]. In another study, only 9/18 foals were alive six months after surgical repair, and seven of the nine nonsurvivors were euthanized due to systemic fungal or bacterial infection [2].

Septic peritonitis has less commonly been reported in association with uroperitoneum [2, 30, 60–63]. In these cases, a septic focus typically involving the urachus or bladder is present, subsequently resulting in necrotic area(s) and loss of integrity of the structure causing leakage of urine (and bacteria) into the abdomen (Figure 27.6) [2, 30, 60–63]. In such cases, foals may be lethargic, tachycardic, tachypneic, and have evidence of generalized infection such as fever, ileus, and injected mucous membranes and sclerae. Examination of an abdominal fluid sample may reveal a turbid sample with a serosanguineous color along with increased red blood cells, total nucleated cell count (primarily nondegenerative and degenerative neutrophils), and total protein concentration [30, 61, 63]. Bacteria may also be visualized upon cytologic examination of abdominal fluid samples [30, 61]. Abdominal ultrasonography reveals increased amounts of hyperechogenic fluid with variable fibrin strands floating within the fluid [6, 63]. Celiotomy, surgical removal of infected tissue, and abdominal lavage is necessary in these cases, along with general supportive care. Urachal remnants and peritoneal fluid should be submitted for bacterial culture to potentially identify the causative organism(s) and guide antimicrobial therapy, which should be administered for at least 10–14 days. Septic peritonitis may increase the probability of adhesion formation and should be considered when establishing prognosis [60].

Subcutaneous Rupture of the Urachus

Occasionally, the urachus can rupture subcutaneously rather than intra-abdominally, resulting in a different clinical presentation than uroperitoneum, typically manifesting as subcutaneous swelling of the ventral abdomen. In one case series, foals with subcutaneous rupture of the urachus were relatively young (8–30 hours old) and presented for non-painful diffuse swelling of the umbilical region; the subcutaneous swelling increased in size over a short period of time to extend from the scrotum to the sternum [31]. Measurement of the creatinine or urea concentration from fluid aspirated from the subcutaneous swellings were elevated (urea, 135–420 mg/dL; creatinine

Table 27.3 Ultrasonographic measurements and images of various umbilical structures in the healthy foal at different ages. Umbilical vein (UV), umbilical artery (UA).

Age of foal (transverse)	UV cranial to umbilicus	UV midway to liver	UA at bladder apex	UA at mid-bladder	Urachus (transverse)
0–3 d	5–12 mm	4–10 mm	4–9 mm	3–8 mm	7–13 mm
4–7 d	4–10 mm	3–9 mm	3–7 mm	2–7 mm	5–13 mm
8–21 d	3–9 mm	3–7 mm	2–6 mm	2–6 mm	4–10 mm
1 mo	2–5 mm	2–5 mm	2–4 mm	2-5 mm	2–7 mm
	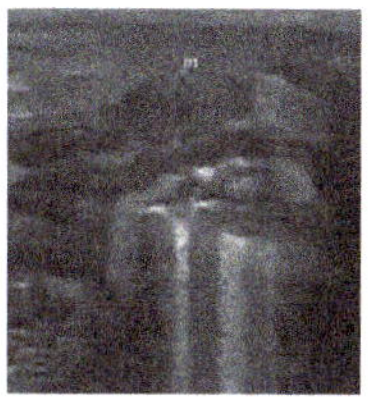	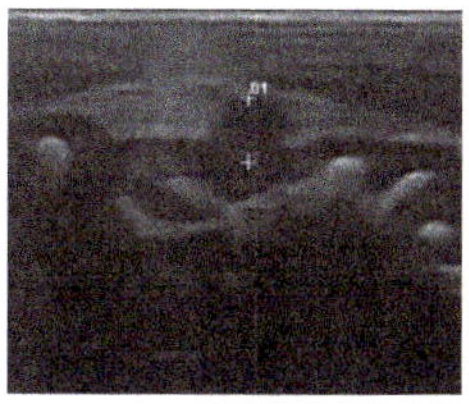	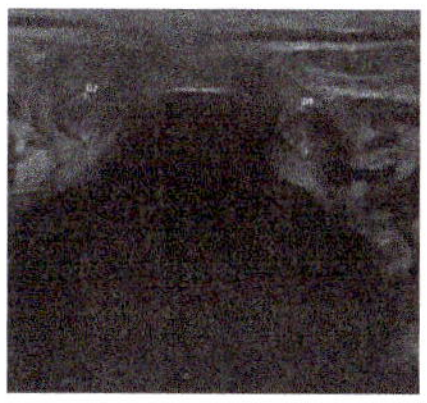	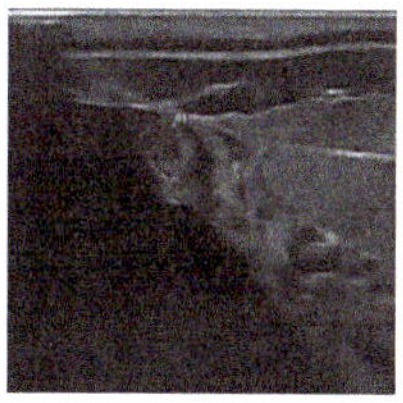	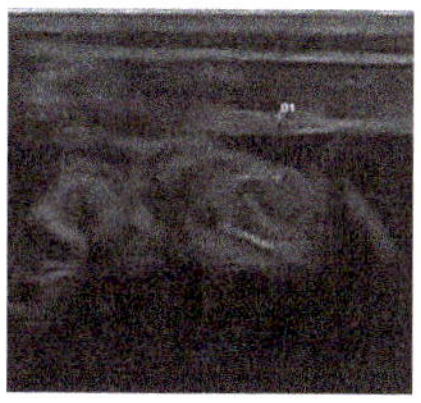
	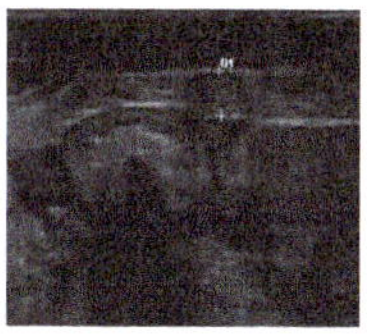	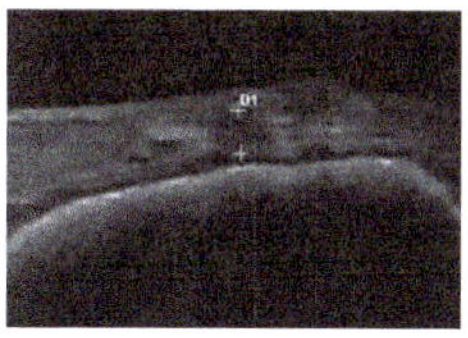	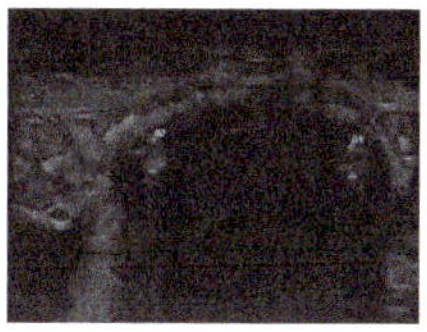	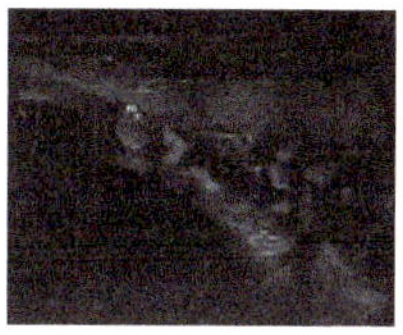	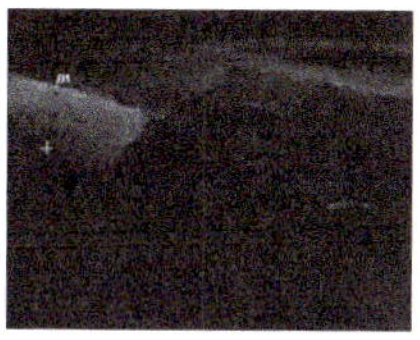
	Umbilical vein just cranial to the external umbilicus Top, 1-wk-old (5.9 mm) Bottom, 3-wk-old (4 mm)	Umbilical vein midway between the external umbilicus and liver: Top, 1-wk-old (4.3 mm) Bottom, 3-wk-old (2.9 mm)	Umbilical arteries at the apex of the bladder: Top, 1-wk-old (4.7/4.6 mm) Bottom, 3-wk-old (3.4/3.6 mm)	Umbilical artery (R) at mid-bladder: Top, 1-wk-old (5.7 mm) Bottom, 3-wk-old (3.7 mm)	Urachus in transverse view: Top, 1-wk-old with fluid Bottom, 3-wk-old with the space filled with tissue

3.2 mg/dL) when compared to serum concentrations. In one case, a defect was identified in the urachus that allowed urine to flow directly into the peritoneal cavity (uroperitoneum) and the subcutaneous tissue. Upon surgical exploration in these foals, defects (6–20 mm) of the subcutaneous portion of the urachi were identified, with corrective treatment involving resection of the urachus and cranial end of the bladder (cystoplasty). Subcutaneous or extraperitoneal rupture should be considered when a fluctuant swelling develops in the umbilical region of a neonatal foal with differential diagnoses including extraperitoneal rupture of the penile urethra or uroperitoneum due to rupture of the urachus or bladder and leakage of fluid into the subcutaneous tissue through the inguinal canals [31].

External infections may be detected clinically by the presence of heat, pain, swelling or enlargement, and/or purulent discharge from the umbilical stump; ultrasonographic examination of infected external umbilical remnants can reveal enlarged and thickened external umbilical structures along with hypoechoic to echogenic fluid within affected structures [6, 64, 65]. Internal infections are detected via ultrasonography of the umbilical remnants and appear as enlargement of one or more umbilical structure(s), intraluminal fluid, and possibly hyperechoic echoes representing gas formation due to anaerobic infection [6]. More than one umbilical remnant structure can be infected simultaneously with infection of the urachus and umbilical arteries being most common [6]. Maximum diameters of umbilical remnants in light horse foals are noted in Table 27.3, but variation in diameter size in healthy foals exists between breeds [66–68]. As the umbilical structures normally regress rapidly within the first few weeks of life, it is important to account for age when interpreting ultrasonographic findings [66]. Neutrophilic leukocytosis and hyperfibrinogenemia can be observed with infection of the umbilical remnants, but minimal changes are typically observed on serum biochemistry profile unless other disease processes are present [69, 70].

Discussing the individual umbilical remnants, the urachus retracts after birth and becomes the median ligament of the bladder; in health, it does not contain any fluid past a few days of age [66]. A common urachal disorder in neonatal foals is **patent urachus** in which a variable-sized conduit between the bladder and external urachus is present, resulting in urine dribbling, ranging from an intermittent dribble from the external umbilicus to near continuous flow of urine. Congenital (noninfectious) patent urachus can act as a portal for bacterial invasion, but infection within the urachus itself can result in an acquired patent urachus [70]. Umbilical remnant infections should be considered in any foal with a patent urachus because localized inflammation and necrosis in the arteries or veins can result in the urachus losing its seal [70]. Patent urachus appears as anechoic fluid within the urachus that is continuous with the bladder apex and the external umbilicus on ultrasound examination. Other defects or infection of the urachus can cause dissection of fluid resulting in subcutaneous ventral edema (noted above; subcutaneous portion of the urachus), uroperitoneum, or septic peritonitis. When the urachus is involved in cases of uroperitoneum, the bladder usually is round and fluid-filled as defects are generally small and result in slower leakage of urine into the peritoneal cavity [6]. Uncommonly, a urachal diverticulum can be present, which appears as a fluid-filled structure in the caudal urachal region continuous with the bladder apex [71, 72].

Disorders of the Umbilical Remnants

The umbilical remnants, including the umbilical vein, umbilical arteries, and urachus, can become infected. Common bacteria include Gram-negative enterobacteria and coccoid Gram-positive bacteria [64]. The average age at the time of diagnosis of umbilical infection ranges from 1 day to 3 months with a reported incidence of 17% (65 foals required omphalectomy of 378 admitted foals) in one referral hospital [65]. Umbilical remnant infections can occur externally, internally, or both and have been frequently incriminated as a port of bacterial entry potentially leading to bacteremia, sepsis, septic osteoarthritis, physitis, or peritonitis, uroperitoneum, and/or intra-abdominal adhesions [64, 65]. In one study evaluating 40 foals with confirmed umbilical infection, fever was noted in 47.5%, joint infection in 35.5%, and gastrointestinal disorders in 15% of foals [64].

The paired umbilical arteries course caudally from the external umbilicus and flank the urachus and urinary bladder. These arteries form the round ligaments of the bladder and are thick walled with a diameter ranging from approximately ≤5 mm at 24 hours of age to ≤2 mm at 5 weeks of age; an echogenic clot in the center is frequently observed [66]. Infection of the umbilical artery manifests as enlargement of the umbilical artery along with a thickened wall that contains anechoic to echoic fluid. The most common region to be enlarged occurs just caudal to the external umbilical remnant or at the apex of the bladder, although any area along the length of the artery can be affected [6, 73, 74]. Rarely, aortic aneurysms have been reported in foals in association with presumed umbilical artery infections in foals [75, 76]. Colic, pollakiuria, fever, and hematuria have been reported in these cases, which were identified via computed tomography or during surgical exploration. No foals survived this condition [75, 76].

The umbilical vein is located on midline extending from the external umbilicus to the liver and becomes the round ligament of the liver. The umbilical vein is small in healthy foals with an approximate diameter ranging from ≤7.5 mm at 24 hours of age to ≤2.5 mm at 6 weeks of age; the vein is oval to elliptical in shape with a thin echogenic wall and an anechoic center [6, 66]. Enlargement and thickening of the walls of the umbilical vein are suggestive of chronic infection, with some infections extending cranial into the liver (Figure 27.7). Occasionally this can result in formation of a hepatic abscess or suppurative hepatitis [6].

In one study, 78% (35/45) of foals were diagnosed with a combined urachal and arterial bundle enlargement, 53% (24/45) had right arterial enlargement, 40% (18/44) had left

(a) (b)

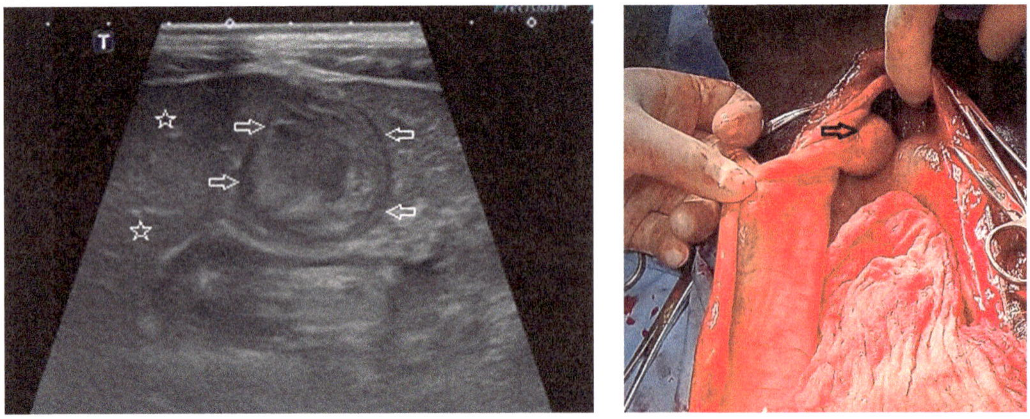

Figure 27.7 Umbilical vein abscess in a 9-day-old Percheron colt. (a) Ultrasonographic appearance of umbilical vein abscess (arrows) located adjacent to the liver (stars). Abscess measured 25 × 30 mm. (b) Appearance of umbilical vein abscess (arrow) intra-operatively. *Source:* Images courtesy of Dr. Avery Loyd, Iowa State University.

Table 27.4 Frequency of bacterial isolates obtained from 40 foals with confirmed umbilical remnant infections [64].

Bacterial isolate	Percentage (%)	Bacterial isolate	Percentage (%)
Streptococcus zooepidemicus	32.5% (13/40)	*Staphylococcus xilosus*	2.5 (1/40)
Escherichia coli	27.5% (11/40)	*Staphylococcus sciuri*	2.5 (1/40)
Staphylococcus faecalis	17.5% (7/40)	*Enterobacter aerogenes*	2.5 (1/40)
Enterococcus faecalis	7.5% (3/40)	*Pantoea agglomerans*	2.5 (1/40)
Klebsiella pneumonia	7.5 (3/40)	*Serratia marcescens*	2.5 (1/40)
Staphylococcus lentus	5 (2/40)	*Trueperella pyogenes*	2.5 (1/40)
Proteus mirabilis	5 (2/40)	*Salmonella enterica*	2.5 (1/40)

arterial enlargement, and 40% (18/45) had umbilical vein enlargement [65]. Bacterial culture of resected umbilical remnants was performed in 18 foals of which 14 (78%) were positive. Bacterial isolates included *Escherichia coli* (4), *Streptrococcus* (3), *Salmonella* spp. (2), *Klebsiella* spp. (1), *Bacillus* spp. (1), *Rhodococcus equi* (1), *Proteus* spp. (1), and mixed culture (1) [65]. In another study of 40 confirmed umbilical remnant infections, enlargement of the umbilical arteries were noted via ultrasonographic exam in 83%, umbilical vein in 55%, and 75% had an increased dimensions of the external umbilicus [64]. In this study, a single bacterial isolate was identified in 72.5%, while 22.5% had two or more isolates (Table 27.4). Additionally, 11/19 foals in which blood culture was obtained were also positive and 9/11 of these isolates were the same pathogen as that identified from culture of the umbilicus [64].

Rarely, hemorrhage from the umbilical cord at parturition can result in swelling of the internal umbilical vessels or perivascular tissues [6]. Hemoabdomen can result from rupture of the umbilical vein or artery during the postpartum period, which may appear as echogenic swirling fluid on ultrasound examination.

Treatment

Two approaches, medical and surgical, have generally been recommended to treat infection of one or more of the umbilical remnants and patent urachus. Medical treatment of mild cases, in which the foal is otherwise healthy and ultrasound examination does not reveal a discrete abscess, involves administration of broad-spectrum antimicrobials to directly treat infection within the umbilical remnants as well as decrease the chances of systemic dissemination of the infection [70]. Medical therapy might also be pursued in foals that are poor surgical candidates. In mild cases, oral antibiotics are frequently used because the treatment period ranges from 10–14 days or longer; thus, parenteral administration is not ideal for prolonged treatment unless the foal has an IV catheter for another medical reason. Ideally antimicrobial selection is based on culture and sensitivity results, but this is not always feasible. Oral medications that can be considered include chloramphenicol, macrolides ± rifampin, and trimethoprim-sulfamethoxazole, among others noted in Table 27.5. If parenteral antimicrobials are an option, the combination of an aminoglycoside and β-lactam typically is efficacious [64]. Medical management should

Table 27.5 Oral antibiotics available for medical management of umbilical remnant infections in neonatal foals [77, 78].

Medication	Dose	Comment
Amoxicillin	13–30 mg/kg, PO, q8h	Resistance may exist among enteric microbes
Azithromycin	10 mg/kg, PO, q24h; every 48 h after 5 d	Keep foal out of sunlight/heat
Cefadroxil	20–40 mg/kg, PO, q8–12h	First-generation cephalosporin
Cefalexin	25 mg/kg, PO, q6h or 30 mg/kg PO, q8h	First-generation cephalosporin
Cefpodoxime	10 mg/kg, PO, q6–8–12h	Third-generation cephalosporin; use q6h dosing for *Escherichia coli*
Clarithromycin	7.5 mg/kg, PO, q12h	Keep foal out of sunlight/heat
Chloramphenicol	50 mg/kg, PO, q12h days 1–2 of age; q8h days of age 3–5	Use gloves when administering drug
Doxycycline	10 mg/kg, PO, q12h	May cause tendon laxity
Minocycline	4 mg/kg, PO, q 12h	
Rifampin	5–7.5 mg/kg, PO, q12h	Use in combination with other antimicrobials to avoid bacterial resistance
Metronidazole	10 mg/kg, PO, q8–12h for first 2 wk of life	Use when culture reveals *Clostridial* infection [63]
Trimethoprim-sulfonamide	25–30 mg/kg, PO, q12h	

include serial ultrasound examinations and monitoring of the hemogram. If deterioration of either of these diagnostic tests is noted, surgical intervention should be considered.

Surgical excision may be necessary when medical therapy alone has failed to resolve the infection, more severe cases in which the foal shows systemic signs of sepsis or infection (fever, lethargy, tachycardia), changes on the hemogram (leukocytosis, hyperfibrinogenemia) are present, a discrete abscess is located, when multiple vascular structures are enlarged and contain purulent material, or when multiple sites of infection are present (e.g. septic arthritis) [64, 70]. Some small studies have reported improved survival rates with surgical excision (67%) compared to antimicrobial therapy alone (43%); surgical excision can also reduce the length of time that the foal requires treatment with antimicrobials [79, 80]. Surgery is most commonly performed via midline celiotomy, although a laparoscopic-assisted approach has been reported [81].

An infected umbilical vein is treated similarly to other infected umbilical structures (medical and/or surgical), however, in instances where complete excision of the vein is not possible because the infection is adjacent to or communicating with the liver parenchyma, marsupialization of the umbilical vein is suggested. This is accomplished by securing the vein in the cranial aspect of the incision (or a separate paramedian incision) in layers such that the external rectus sheath and subcutaneous tissue are sutured to the connective tissues and the vein wall in two layers, and the skin is sutured to the vein wall with nonabsorbable suture material. Postoperative treatment includes parenteral (3–5 days) followed by oral (7–10 days or longer) antimicrobials based on the clinical status of the foal and return of the white blood cell count and fibrinogen to normal reference intervals (if originally altered). The umbilical vein remnant is expected to close in 7–14 days; skin sutures are removed 14 days after the procedure [69].

Prognosis for survival of umbilical infections is favorable as long as appropriate therapy is provided with reported survival rates ranging from 56 to 91% [64, 65]. Combining results from four reports, 10 (91%) of 11 (laparoscopy) and 45 (86.5%) of 52 (routine celiotomy) foals undergoing surgical removal of the umbilical remnants survived as compared to 10 (59%) of 17 foals treated medically survived [53, 70, 74, 80, 81]. Prognosis is decreased if the foal has multiple concurrent disease processes [64, 65].

Prevention

Infection of the umbilical remnants may be thwarted by ensuring adequate passive transfer of immunity, daily cleaning of the external remnant, and maintaining a clean environment where the foal is housed. In one study, cultures were collected from the external umbilical stump from 139 healthy newborn foals within 10 minutes of birth [82]. In this study, coagulase-negative *Staphylococcus* was the most prevalent organism identified from the umbilical stump (59% of all foals), followed by *Diphtheroids* (40%), no growth (19%), *Bacillus* spp. (18%), *Acinetobacter* (14%), and various other isolates (<10% each isolate) [82]. Thus, the most common colonizers of the newborn's umbilical stump are skin and soil bacteria that are generally non-pathogenic in foals. In this study, cultures were repeated six hours after application of 1% povidone iodine, 2% iodine, 7% iodine tincture, 0.5% chlorhexidine, and no treatment. Application of 0.5% chlorhexidine and 7% iodine tincture was associated with a significant reduction in bacterial numbers, but application of the iodine tincture caused sloughing of adjacent skin, breaking off of the desiccated stump, and higher incidence of patent urachus. Due to the caustic nature of 7% iodine tincture and potential damaging effects on the skin, it is not an appropriate choice as a routine umbilical dip. Conversely, chlorhexidine suppresses the number of organisms colonizing the umbilicus, has sustained residual activity, is not inactivated by organic matter, and binds to the stratum corneum leaving a persistent residue. Therefore, chlorhexidine (q8–12h for the first 2–3 days of life) may be a better choice for dipping the foal's umbilical remnant [82].

Ureteral Tears and Defects

Ureteral tears and defects of one or both ureters are very uncommon but have been reported as a cause of either retroperitoneal accumulation of urine or uroperitoneum in neonatal foals [83–85]. Signalment of affected foals is variable, with age ranging from 4–11 days at the time of diagnosis [83–86]. Clinical signs are nonspecific and include lethargy and inappetence. Observation of an enlarged abdomen (commonly noted in uroperitoneum) may not be noted if the ureteral tear is only associated with retroperitoneal fluid accumulation; however, some ureteral tears eventually result in rupture of the retroperitoneal membrane and consequently a fluid filled abdomen [84].

Clinicopathologic changes tend to indicate disruption of the urogenital tract and include hyponatremia, hypochloremia, hyperkalemia, and azotemia, but these changes may be less evident compared to the classic changes associated with a ruptured bladder [83–85].

The diagnosis of ureteral tears/defects can be delayed due to the absence of the typical clinical and ultrasonographic findings or uroperitoneum, at least until rupture of the retroperitoneal membrane. The clinician should therefore assess the ureters as a source of uroperitoneum when defects of the urachus or urinary bladder are not identified.

Establishing a diagnosis of ureteral tears can be difficult, but ultrasound of the kidneys, urinary bladder, and urachus are appropriate first steps. In one case of a ureteral tear in the proximal left ureter, ultrasound findings included a large amount of anechoic fluid with some fluctuating particles surrounding the affected kidney in the retroperitoneal space (Figure 27.8). Multiphase computed tomography (CT) urography with contrast was used in one case to better characterize the ureteral defect [83]. Other reports used intravenous urography or retrograde ureteral infusion of methylene blue (via cystotomy and retrograde catheterization of the ureter) to identify the ureteral tear [84]. In one report, antegrade urography was performed by percutaneous injection of contrast medium through the kidney and into the renal pelvis [85]. This was accomplished by inserting a 22-gauge 3.5 in. spinal needle into the renal pelvis under ultrasonographic guidance followed by injection of contrast medium into the renal pelvis. Fluoroscopy was then used to determine the location of a urethral defect (nephropylocentesis and antegrade urography) [85].

(a)

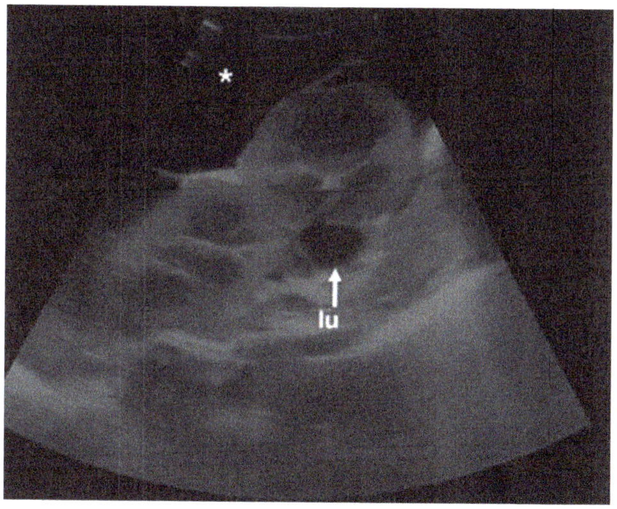

(b)

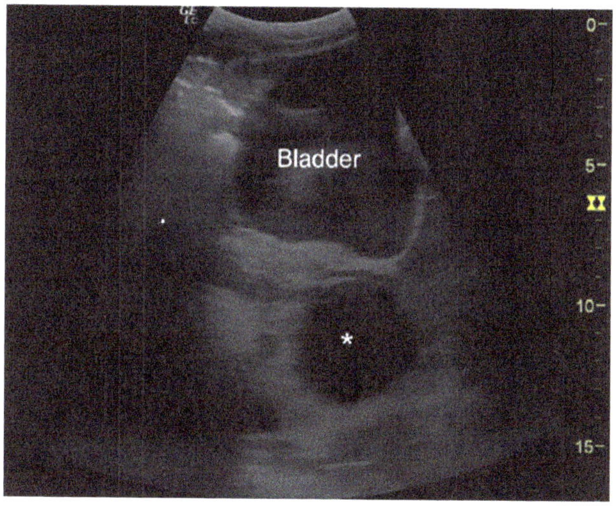

Figure 27.8 (a) Ultrasound image from left paralumbar fossa demonstrating fluid accumulation (*) around the left kidney in the retroperitoneal space and a mildly fluid-filled enlarged ureter (lu) exiting the renal pelvis (dorsal is left). (b) Transverse ultrasound image from the ventral window demonstrating a well- defined anechoic fluid filled structure (*) dorsal to the urinary bladder, later determined to be retroperitoneal accumulation of urine [83].

Ureteral tears can be repaired via primary closure [53, 87], however, a few cases of ureteral healing via secondary intention have been reported with small tears [87]. Administration of methylene blue through a ureteral catheter can help identify a ureteral defect intraoperatively, while minimizing extensive dissection of the entire length of the ureter to identify the defect. Aggressive dissection to expose the ureter has been associated with disruption of the ureteral blood supply in people [85]. Nephrectomy was used in one foal that had a tear in the proximal portion of the left ureter [84]. One of the most common complications observed after surgical repair of a ureteral defect is persistent or recurrent uroperitoneum, associated with leakage of urine at the repair site [84]. One method to potentially avoid this complication is placement of a ureteral catheter into the renal pelvis to divert urine flow and act as a stent to facilitate healing of the ureter [84].

Ectopic ureter is the most common congenital anomaly of the equine urinary tract and manifests as persistent urinary incontinence and urine scalding (dermatitis) of the perineum and hind legs (females) or ventral abdomen and hindlimbs (males) in an otherwise healthy animal [88]. This condition involves the terminal portion of one or both ureters in which the ureteral orifice is located caudal to the trigone of the urinary bladder [89]. Embryologically, this anomaly occurs due to failure of caudal migration of the metanephric duct in the developing fetus such that the ureter, which is eventually formed from this duct, opens caudal to the bladder and into the uterus, vagina, urethra, or part of the proximal reproductive tract [88, 90]. Foals with ectopic ureter are usually not diagnosed in the neonatal period, but rather later in life when foals present for veterinary care (incontinence, but otherwise healthy) with reported cases ranging in age between 3 weeks and 10 months of age or older [88, 89, 91–93]. Ectopic ureter is diagnosed with greater frequency in fillies, although the lower incidence in colts may reflect the absence of clinical signs and hence detection due to the gender-related anatomic differences (e.g. less frequent urine scalding in the colt) [90]. Normal urination may or may not be observed, along with incontinence, in reported cases [89, 92, 94].

Ectopic ureter can be suspected in foals/horses that have had urinary incontinence since birth but are otherwise healthy. Renal function is usually normal, but bilateral disease may manifest with abnormal kidney function [90]. Diagnosis is confirmed via retrograde or antegrade ureterography [88, 92], endoscopy of the vaginia [94] or bladder [95], contrast radiography [93, 94], ultrasonography [96], scintigraphy [97], or computed tomography [89]. Endoscopy and visualization of the aberrant ureteral opening(s) are facilitated by parenteral administration of dyes that discolor the urine such as phenolsulfonphthalein, methylene blue, indigo carmine, sodium flourescein (11 mg/kg, IV), azosulfamide (1.9 mg/kg, IM) or similar [90, 95]. Accurate imaging is required in order to determine the most appropriate surgical technique. The affected ureter is commonly markedly enlarged upon visualization of the urinary tract either via diagnostic imaging or intraoperatively [88].

Before attempting surgical correction of ectopic ureter(s), it is imperative to determine whether the disease is unilateral or bilateral, if urinary tract infection is present, if the detrusor muscle has normal function, and if the function of the renal system is appropriate [90]. Once the location of the ectopic ureter(s) is identified and the health of the contralateral kidney is confirmed, two procedures have been described to treat ectopic ureter in the horse. The first is unilateral ureteronephrectomy of the affected side, which can be performed as long as the other kidney has normal renal function [89]. Unilateral ureteronephrectomy may also be necessary when there is significant dilation of the distal ureter (ureterocele), as has been reported in some equine cases [89, 94]. The second treatment is ureterovesical anastomosis (ureteroneocystostomy, neoureterostomy) which involves re-implanting the affected ureter into the wall of the urinary bladder [94]. This procedure is indicated in the absence of ascending urinary tract infection or hydronephrosis, or in cases of bilateral ectopic ureters [88]. Ureterovesical anastamosis may be more difficult if the ectopic ureter is dilated [90]. Multiple different techniques have been described to perform a ureterovesical anastomosis as this procedure is frequently performed during renal transplantation in people [98]. End-to-side anastamosis with and without submucosal tunneling, as well as side-to-side anastomosis, have been reported in the limited cases available in the equine literature [88, 91, 93]. Of 11 cases of ectopic ureters across seven reports, ranging in age from 2.5 months to 3 years, 6 survived for greater than one year postoperatively. Of these, 3 were treated with unilateral nephrectomy (all survived), 6 with ureterovesical anastomosis (3 survived), and 2 were euthanized without treatment [88, 91, 93, 94, 99–101].

Other ureteral defects that have been infrequently reported include ureteral stenosis, ureteral agenesis, ureteritis, distal ureter stenosis, and ureteral atresia [3, 85, 86, 97]. In one case of ureteral atresia, uroperitoneum was present. Upon abdominal exploratory, the proximal portion of both ureters were enlarged (>2.5 cm) along its entire length except for the distal portion of the ureter, which was dense and fibrous [86]. Initial treatment involved bilateral resection of the distal fibrotic portions of the ureters and end-to-side anastomosis between the ureters and the bladder. In this case, uroperitoneum reoccurred 4 days after the original surgery due to disruption of the anastomosis site of the ureter; subsequently, unilateral nephrectomy was performed. The horse was reportedly healthy 4.5 years following the surgery [86]. In another unusual case where left ureteral stenosis and a right ureteral defect were diagnosed, treatment consisted of right ureterorrhaphy and left ureteroneocystostomy [85].

Megavesica is a rarely reported condition in which the foal's urinary bladder is greatly enlarged [38, 100, 102, 103]. The underlying cause of megavesica is unknown, but experimental ligation of the urachus and urethra in utero has resulted in megavesica in other species suggesting impediment of normal urine flow during gestation may be involved [38]. In one case, megavesica was described in a foal as an enlarged thin-walled urinary bladder in which a fibrous ligament was located instead of a normal urachus [102]. The foal was successfully treated by cutting the ligament that was suspected of impairing normal bladder emptying. In this case, it is possible that the fibrous band that adhered the bladder apex to the abdominal wall could have restricted bladder contraction and contributed to the development of megavesica [38, 102]. In another report, an enlarged thin-walled urinary bladder was identified in a newborn foal where part of the bladder wall and urachus were either ruptured or incompletely developed [100]. The authors speculated that an umbilical torsion may have caused the megavesica. The urinary bladder was partially resected and the foal recovered successfully [38, 100]. In a third case, a 1-day-old Warmblood colt was presented for lethargy, a distended abdomen, increased respiratory effort, an enlarged external umbilicus and urine dribbling from the penis [38]. A severely distended bladder was noted on ultrasonography in which the cranial margin of the bladder was cranial to the external umbilical remnant. The bladder was intermittently catheterized yielding 6, 4, and 4 L of urine over the next 2 days. Because of the consistently enlarged and malfunctioning bladder and abnormal umbilical structures, exploratory celiotomy was performed revealing a greatly enlarged and thickened bladder, a urinary diverticulum, and an abnormal umbilical remnant. The authors speculated that partial urachal obstruction secondary to malformation of the umbilical structure may have resulted in the enlarged bladder [38]. Overall, megavesica has rarely been reported in neonatal foals but should be considered if a greatly enlarged bladder is noted; identification of some form or urinary outflow obstruction may be a cause of the disorder.

Hematuria

Neonatal foal urine is usually a clear yellow color and maintains a low urine specific gravity (commonly <1.008) due to their milk diet [104]. Discolored urine can be caused by contamination with red blood cells (RBCs; hematuria) or hemoglobin or myoglobin (pigmenturia). Distinguishing hematuria from pigmenturia requires urinalysis and biochemical analysis. If urine discoloration is caused by RBCs, centrifugation of a urine sample results in a layer of RBCs at the bottom of the sample with clear urine above the red cells. Microscopic hematuria is generally defined as >5 RBCs/high powered field. Conversely, urine remains discolored after centrifugation with pigmenturia. Additionally, hematuria is likely if there is a large number of RBCs noted microscopically whereas absence of RBCs suggests pigmenturia. RBCs can rupture if urinalysis is delayed (for as little as 1–2 hours), especially if urine is dilute, resulting in false hemoglobinuria [105]. Hemoglobinuria can occur after systemic hemolysis (e.g. neonatal isoerythrolysis), resulting in pink to red discolored serum. If the foal has clinical signs of a myopathy as well as increased serum creatine kinase activity, myoglobinuria is likely the cause of urine discoloration; the serum of horses with myoglobinuria is typically clear because the pigment is rapidly cleared from the serum [105]. Hematuria, hemoglobinuria, and myoglobinuria all result in a positive reaction on urinalysis reagent strips.

Hematuria is not a common presenting problem in neonatal foals, but when it occurs, it can be caused by blood originating from the kidney, ureter, bladder, or urethra mixing with the urine. The timing of when urine discoloration is noted might provide a clue as to the source of hematuria. Blood at the beginning of the stream might indicate a urethral disorder as compared to the end or throughout the stream, which is suggestive origination from the bladder or kidney [105]. Potential causes of hematuria are noted in Table 27.6, with further description of some of these causes noted below.

Leptospirosis

Neonatal infection with Leptospira is uncommonly reported in foals, but clinical manifestations may include involvement of the kidney, liver, and lungs [106, 112]. In one case series involving five foals with Leptospirosis, all foals presented with severe respiratory distress; some foals had anemia, thrombocytopenia, azotemia, hyperbilirubinemia, hematuria, and pyuria [112]. Diagnosis was based on postmortem immunofluorescence of affected tissues or serologic microscopic agglutination tests (MAT). Leptospira was detected in the kidneys of four of five foals that did not survive or were euthanized with interstitial nephritis and glomerulonephritis documented on microscopic examination. Another case report described a 1-day old Thoroughbred foal presented for weakness and inability to stand or suckle. The foal was tachycardic,

Table 27.6 Causes of hematuria.

- Trauma to structure(s) of the urinary tract [106]
- Urinary tract infection/cystitis [107]
- Sepsis [106, 108]
- Cystic hematoma [110]
- Renal pseudoaneurysm [109]
- Renal infarct [108]
- Coagulopathy [114]
  - Thrombotic event (e.g. renal artery or vein thrombosis)
  - Vitamin K deficiency
  - Thrombocytopenia
- Congenital disorders
  - Renal arteriovenous malformation [115]
  - Renal dysplasia [116]
- Acute kidney injury (AKI)
  - Acute renal tubular necrosis [108]
  - Acute renal cortical necrosis [116]
  - Nephrotoxic medications (e.g. aminoglycosides, NSAIDs) [108]
  - Hypoxic–ischemic injury
- Residual blood from urachal bleeding from birth (<48 hr. old) [104]
- Iatrogenic (bladder catheterization, cystoscopy)
- Nephrolithiasis (reported in yearling) [117]
- Renal abscess [108, 111]
- Leptospirosis [106, 112]
- Hydronephrosis [113]

hypothermic and passed light red urine with some blood clots in the urine [106]. Leptospires were identified in the foal's urine and high serum titers were documented, suggesting that the hematuria was associated with Leptospirosis infection [106].

Renal Abscess

Abscesses involving the kidney have infrequently been reported in older (4.5–5 month) foals [108, 111]. In these cases, foals are presented for hematuria evident throughout micturition along with voiding of numerous large blood clots. Other clinicopathologic changes include anemia, leukocytosis, hematuria, pyuria, and proteinuria and bacteria may be identified on cytology of the urine. Cystoscopy aided diagnosis of the source of hematuria (e.g. ureter). In one foal, unilateral nephrectomy was performed and was curative, whereas another foal died due to severe hemorrhage secondary to the abscess eroding into the ureter and abdominal aorta [108, 111].

Cystic Hematomas

Hematomas in the bladder have been occasionally observed in foals and should be considered as a differential diagnosis for neonatal foals with hematuria [110]. In one case series involving three foals with cystic hematomas, foals ranged from 4 hours to 3 days of age and were of various breeds [110]. Two foals had a history of profuse bleeding from the umbilicus immediately after birth. Clinical signs consisted of tachycardia, stranguria, colic, and pigmenturia, with one foal passing a large blood clot via the urethra [110]. Clinicopathologic data was variable with no consistent findings among the three foals; however, gross hematuria was noted in all foals with microscopic examination of the urine, revealing RBCs that were too numerous to count. Diagnosis of cystic hematomas was established via ultrasound as homogenous echogenic masses within the ventral bladder, surrounded by urine (Figure 27.9). In addition, the urachus was larger than normal and was diffusely echogenic and heterogenous in two foals, while the third foal had a hematoma within the bladder, urachus, and umbilical arteries. Treatment included IV fluids to promote diuresis, prophylactic antimicrobials, careful handling of the abdomen (e.g. lifting the foal inappropriately could result in severe hemorrhage), general supportive care (adequate immunoglobulin G, nutrition), and treatment of other disease processes (if present). Foals passed the hematoma/blood via normal urination pattern, but some foals may require surgical correction if the urachus and/or umbilical arteries are involved [110]. The prognosis for foals with cystic hematomas is good, although concurrent disease processes must be considered.

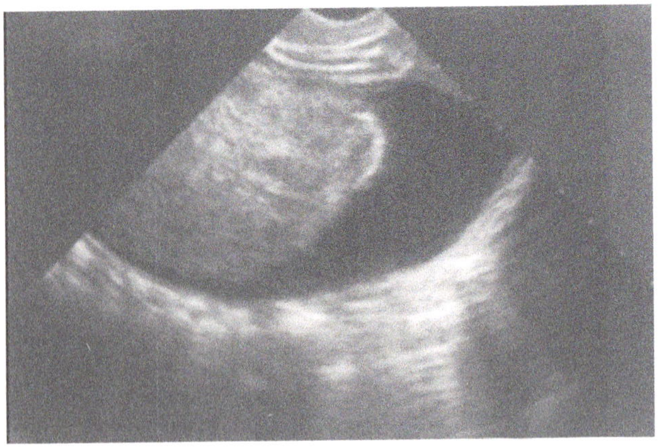

Figure 27.9 Ultrasonogram of the bladder of a Thoroughbred colt with pigmenturia and stranguria. Note the homogenous echogenic mass in the ventral aspect of the bladder presumed to be a cystic hematoma. From [110].

The exact cause of cystic hematomas in foals is not known, but it has been postulated that trauma to the umbilicus during the periparturient period can damage the umbilical vessels and urachal sheath, thereby resulting in retrograde bleeding into the proximal portion of the urachus, bladder, and umbilical arteries [110]. Foals with umbilical trauma might have gross hematuria or potentially, depending on the size of the cystic hematoma, some degree of urinary obstruction.

References

1 Kablack, K.A., Embertson, R.M., Bernard, W.V. et al. (2000). Uroperitoneum in the hospitalized equine neonate: retrospective study of 31 cases, 1988–1997. *Equine Vet. J.* 32: 505–508.

2 Adams, R., Koterba, A.M., Cudd, T.C., and Baker, W.A. (1988). Exploratory celiotomy for suspected urinary tract disruption in neonatal foals: a review of 18 cases. *Equine Vet. J.* 20: 13–17.

3 Richardson, D.W. and Kohn, C.W. (1983). Uroperitoneum in the foal. *J. Am. Vet. Med. Assoc.* 182: 267–270.

4 Dunkel, B., Palmer, J.E., Olson, K.N. et al. (2005). Uroperitoneum in 32 foals: influence of intravenous fluid therapy, infection, and sepsis. *J. Vet. Intern. Med.* 19: 889–893.

5 Castagnetti, C., Mariella, J., Pirrone, A. et al. (2010). Urethral and bladder rupture in a neonatal colt with uroperitoneum. *Equine Vet. Educ.* 22: 132–138.

6 McAuliffe, S.B. (2004). Abdominal ultrasonography of the foal. *Clin. Technol. Equine Pract.* 3: 308–316.

7 Clarke, H.S., Mills, M.E., Parres, J.A. et al. (1993). The hyponatremia of neonatal urinary ascites: clinical observations, experimental confirmation and proposed mechanisms. *J. Urol.* 150: 778–781.

8 Fleisher, D.S. and Gribetz, B. (1985). Autodialysis in neonatal urinary ascites. *Clin. Pediatr.* 24: 724–726.

9 Oei, J., Garvey, P.A., and Rosenberg, A.R. (2001). The diagnosis and management of neonatal urinary ascites. *J. Paediatr. Child Health* 37: 513–515.

10 Zani-ruttensock, E. and Zane, A. (2017). Neonatal ascites. In: *Pediatric Surgery*. Berlin, Heidelberg: Springer https://doi.org/10.1007/978-3-642-38482-0_73-1.

11 Capobianco, A., Cottone, L., Monno, A. et al. (2017). The peritoneum: healing, immunity, and diseases. *J. Pathol.* 243: 137–147.

12 Buchanan, B.R., Sommardahl, C.S., Rohrbach, B.W. et al. (2005). Effect of a 24-hour infusion of an isotonic electrolyte replacement fluid on the renal clearance of electrolytes in healthy neonatal foals. *J. Am. Vet. Med. Assoc.* 227: 1123–1129.

13 Edwards, D.J., Brownlow, M.A., and Dr, H. (1990). Indices of renal function: values in eight normal foals from birth to 56 days. *Aust. Vet. J.* 67: 251–254.

14 Butters, A. (2008). Medical and surgical management of uroperitoneum in a foal. *Can. Vet. J.* 49: 401–403.

15 Manning, M., Dubielzig, R., and McGuirk, S. (1995). Postoperative myositis in a neonatal foal: a case report. *Vet. Surg.* 24: 69–72.

16 Ford, M.G., Nelson, B.B., Ford, T.S. et al. (2022). Complications and comorbidities in foals undergoing surgical repair for uroperitoneum. *J. Equine Vet. Sci.* 110: 103852.

17 Hawkins, J.F. (2010). Evaluation and treatment of the foal with uroperitoneum. *Equine Vet. Educ.* 139–140.

18 Rooney, J.R. (1971). Rupture of the urinary bladder in the foal. *Vet. Pathol.* 8: 445–451.

19 Haga, H.A., Risberg, A., and Strand, E. (2011). Resuscitation of an anaesthetized foal with uroperitoneum and ventricular asystole. *Equine Vet. Educ.* 23: 502–507.

20 Vander Werf, K.A., Beard, L.A., and McMurphy, R.M. (2010). Urinothorax in a Quarter Horse filly. *Equine Vet. Educ.* 22: 239–243.

21 Wong, D.M., Leger, L.C., Scarratt, W.K. et al. (2004). Uroperitoneum and pleural effusion in an American paint filly. *Equine Vet. Educ.* 16: 290–293.

22 Kastelein, A.W., Vos, L.M.C., de Jong, K.H. et al. (2019). Embryology, anatomy, physiology and pathophysiology of the peritoneum and the peritoneal vasculature. *Semin. Cell Dev. Biol.* 92: 27–36.

23 Peroni, J.F. (2017). Diagnosis and treatment of peritonitis and hemoperitoneum. In: *The Equine Acute Abdomen* (ed. A.T. Blikslager, N.A. White, J.N. Moore, and T.S. Mair), 361–375. Wiley Blackwell.

24 Behr, M.J., Hackett, R.P., Bentinck-Smith, J. et al. (1981). Metabolic abnormalities associated with rupture of the urinary bladder in neonatal foals. *J. Am. Vet. Med. Assoc.* 178: 263–266.

25 Hackett, R.P. (1984). Rupture of the urinary bladder in neonatal foals. *Compend. Contin. Educ. Pract. Vet.* 6: S488–S494.

26 Garcia-Pachon, E. and Paddila-Navas, I. (2004). Urinothorax: case report and review of the literature with emphasis of biochemical diagnosis. *Respiration* 71: 533–536.

27 Wilkins, P.A. (2004). Respiratory distress in foals with uroperitoneum: possible mechanisms. *Equine Vet. Educ.* 16: 293–295.

28 Genetzky, R.M. and Hagemoser, W.A. (1985). Physical and clinical pathological findings associated with experimentally induced rupture of the equine urinary bladder. *Can. Vet. J.* 26: 391–395.

29 Marolf, V., Mirra, A., Fouche, N. et al. (2018). Advanced atrio-ventricular blocks in a foal undergoing surgical bladder repair: first step to cardiac arrest? *Front. Vet. Sci.* 5: 1–5.

30 Mendoza, F.J., Lopez, M., Diez, E. et al. (2010). Uroperitoneum secondary to rupture of the urachus associated with clostridium spp. infection in a foal: a case report. *Vet. Med.* 55: 399–404.

31 Lees, M.J., Easley, K.J., Sutherland, R.J. et al. (1989). Subcutaneous rupture of the urachus, its diagnosis and surgical management in three foals. *Equine Vet. J.* 21: 462–464.

32 Aleman, M., Gillis, C.L., Nieto, J.E. et al. (2002). Ultrasonographic anatomy and biometric analysis of the thoracic and abdominal organs in healthy foals from birth to age six months. *Equine Vet. J.* 34: 649–655.

33 Lillich, J.D. and Debowes, R.M. Urethra. In: *Equine Surgery*, 3e (ed. J.A. Auer and J.A. Stick), 877–887. St. Louis: Elsevier Saunders.

34 Love, E.J. (2011). Anaesthesia in foals with uroperitoneum. *Equine Vet. Educ.* 23: 508–511.

35 Petruccione, I., Levionnois, O., and Pawson, P. (2021). Hypoxaemia and bradyarrhythmia in a foal undergoing surgical bladder repair. *Vet. Rec. Case Rep.* 9: e35.

36 Magdesian, K.G. (2015). Foals are not just mini horses. In: *Equine Pharmacology* (ed. C. Cole, B. Bentz, and L. Maxwell), 99–117. Wiley Blackwell.

37 Booth, T.M., Howes, D.A., and Edwards, G.B. (2000). Bethanechol-responsive bladder atony in a colt foal after cystorrhaphy for cystorrhexis. *Vet. Rec.* 147: 306–308.

38 Toth, T., Liman, J., Larsdotter, S. et al. (2012). Megavesica in a neonatal foal. *Equine Vet. Educ.* 24: 396–403.

39 Rajasurya, V. and Surani, S. (2020). Abdominal compartment syndrome: often overlooked conditions in medical intensive care units. *World J. Gastroenterol.* 26: 266–278.

40 Padar, M., Blaser, A.R., Talving, P. et al. (2019). Abdominal compartment syndrome: improving outcomes with a multidisciplinary approach – a narrative review. *J. Multidiscip. Healthc.* 12: 1061–1074.

41 Wilkins, P.A. and Dunkel, B. Rupture of the urinary bladder. In: *Equine Neonatal medicine*, 1e (ed. M.R. Paradis), 237–245. Philadelphia: Elsevier Saunders.

42 Canola, P.A. and Johnson, P.J. (2013). Intra-abdominal hypertension in horses. *Equine Vet. Educ.* 25: 189–195.

43 Brosnahan, M.M., Holbrook, T.C., Gilliam, L.L. et al. (2009). Intra-abdominal hypertension in two adult horses. *J. Vet. Emerg. Crit. Care* 19: 174–180.

44 Hurcombe, S.D.A. and Scott, V.H.L. (2012). Direct intra-abdominal pressures and abdominal perfusion pressures in unsedated normal horses. *J. Vet. Emerg. Crit. Care* 22: 441–446.

45 Munstermann, A.S. and Hanson, R.R. (2009). Comparison of direct and indirect methods of intra-abdominal pressure measurement in normal horses. *J. Vet. Emerg. Crit. Care* 19: 545–553.

46 Munsterman, A.S. and Hanson, R.R. (2011). Evaluation of gastric pressures as an indirect method for measurement of intraabdominal pressures in the horse. *J. Vet. Emerg. Crit. Care* 21: 29–35.

47 Southwood, L.L. and Wilkins, P.A. (2005). Measurement of intra-abdominal pressure in normal horses. *J. Vet. Intern. Med.* 19: 488.

48 Eddy, V., Nunn, C., and Morris, J.A. (1997). Abdominal compartment syndrome. The Nashville experience. *Surg. Clin. N. Am.* 77: 801–812.

49 Cabrera, J., Falcon, L., Gorriz, E. et al. (2001). Abdominal decompression play a major role in early postparacentesis haemodynamic changes in cirrhotic patients with tense ascites. *Gut* 48: 384–389.

50 Kaminski, J.M., Katz, A.R., and Woodward, S.C. (1978). Urinary bladder calculus formation on sutures in rabbits, cats and dogs. *Surg. Gynecol. Obstet.* 146: 353.

51 Lavoie, J.P. and Harnagel, S.H. (1988). Nonsurgical management of a rupture urinary bladder in a critically ill foal. *J. Am. Vet. Med. Assoc.* 192: 1577–1580.

52 Kritchevsky, J.E., Stephens, D.L., Christopher, J. et al. (1984). Peritoneal dialysis for presurgical management of ruptured bladder in a foal. *J. Am. Vet. Med. Assoc.* 185: 81–82.

53 Robertson, J.T. and Embertson, R.M. (1988). Surgical management of congenital and perinatal abnormalities of the urogenital tract. *Vet. Clin. North Am. Equine Pract.* 4: 359–377.

54 Hardy, J. (1998). Uroabdomen in foals. *Equine Vet. Educ.* 10: 21–25.

55 Glazier, D.B., Littledike, E.T., and Evans, R.D. (1982). Electrocardiographic changes in induced hyperkalemia in ponies. *Am. J. Vet. Res.* 43: 1934–1937.

56 Keen, J.A. (2020). Bradyarrythnia in horses. *Vet. J.* 259: 105463.

57 Weichert, S.A., Di Concetto, S., Hepworth, K.L. et al. (2022). Successful cardiopulmonary cerebral resuscitation (CPCR) incorporating defibrillation in a filly with neonatal maladjustment syndrome following a routine anesthetic procedure. *Equine Vet. Educ.* 35: 77–85.

58 Braun, C., Trim, C.M., and Eggleston, R.B. (2009). Effects of changing body position on oxygenation and arterial blood pressure in foals anesthetized with guaifenesin, ketamine, and xylazine. *Vet. Anaesth. Analg.* 36: 18–24.

59 Bryant, J.E. and Gaughan, E.M. (2005). Abdominal surgery in neonatal foals. *Vet. Clin. North Am. Equine Pract.* 21: 511–535.

60 Cable, C.S., Fubini, S.L., Erb, H.N. et al. (1997). Abdominal surgery in foals: a review of 119 cases (1997–1994). *Equine Vet. J.* 29: 257–261.

61 Lores, M., Lofstedt, J., Martinson, S. et al. (2011). Septic peritonitis and uroperitoneum secondary to subclinical omphalitis and concurrent necrotizing cystitis in a bolt. *Can. Vet. J.* 52: 888–892.

62 Codina, L.R., Were, S.R., and Brown, J.A. (2019). Short-term outcome and risk factors for post-operative complications following umbilical resction in 82 foals (2004–2016). *Equine Vet. J.* 51: 323–328.

63 Hyman, S.S., Wilkins, P.A., Palmer, J.E. et al. (2002). Clostridium perfringens urachitis and uroperitoneum in neonatal foals. *J. Vet. Intern. Med.* 16: 489–493.

64 Rampacci, E., Passamonti, F., Bottinelli, M. et al. (2017). Umbilical infections in foals: microbiological investigation and management. *Vet. Rec.* 180: 1–5.

65 Oreff, G.L., Tatz, A.J., Dahan, R. et al. (2017). Surgical management and long-term outcome of umbilical infection in 65 foals (2010–2015). *Vet. Surg.* 46: 962–970.

66 McCoy, A.M., Lopp, C.T., Kooy, S. et al. (2020). Normal regression of the internal umbilical remnant structures in standardbred foals. *Equine Vet. J.* 52: 876–883.

67 Reef, V.B. and Collatos, C. (1988). Ultrasonography of umbilical structures in clinically normal foals. *Am. J. Vet. Res.* 49: 2143–2146.

68 Franklin, R.P. and Ferrell, E.A. (2002). How to perform umbilical sonograms in the neonate. *Proc. Am. Assoc. Equine Pract.* 48: 261–265.

69 Edwards, R.B. and Fubini, S.L. (1995). A one-stage marsupialization procedure for management of infected umbilical vein remnants in calves and foals. *Vet. Surg.* 24: 32–35.

70 Elce, Y.A. (2006). Infections in the equine abdomen and pelvis: perirectal abscesses, umbilical infections, and peritonitis. *Vet. Clin. Equine* 22: 419–436.

71 Reimer, J.M. (1998). The gastrointestinal tract: the foal. In: *Atlas of Equine Ultrasonography* (ed. J. Reimer), 200–211. St. Louis, MO: Mosby.

72 Dean, P.W. and Robertson, J.T. (1988). Urachal remnant as a cause of pollakiuria and dysuria in a filly. *J. Am. Vet. Med. Assoc.* 192: 375–376.

73 Reef, V.B. (1998). Pediatric abdominal ultrasound. In: *Equine Diagnostic Ultrasound* (ed. V. Reef), 364–403. Philadelphia, PA: Saunders.

74 Reef, V.B., Collatos, C., Spencer, P.A. et al. (1989). Clinical, ultrasonographic and surgical findings in foals with umbilical remnant infections. *J. Am. Vet. Med. Assoc.* 195: 69–72.

75 Archer, R.M., Gordon, S.J.G., Carslake, H.B. et al. (2012). Aortic Aneurysn presumed to be secondary to an infected umbilical artery in a foal. *N. Zeal. Vet. J.* 60: 65–68.

76 Nogradi, N., Magdesian, K.G., Whitcomb, M.B. et al. (2013). Imaging diagnosis – aortic aneurysm and ureteral obstruction secondary to umbilical artery abscessation in a 5-week-old foal. *Vet. Radiol. Ultrasound* 54: 384–389.

77 Magdesian, K.G. (2017). Antimicrobial pharmacology for the neonatal foal. *Vet. Clin. Equine* 33: 47–65.

78 Corley, K.T.T. and Hollis, A.R. (2009). Antimicrobial therapy in neonatal foals. *Equine Vet. Educ.* 21: 436–448.

79 Adams, R. (1990). Urinary tract disruption. In: *Equine Clinical Neonatology* (ed. A.M. Koterba, W.H. Drummond, and P.C. Kosch), 464–481. Philadelphia: Lea and Fibiger.

80 Adams, S.B. and Fessler, J.F. (1987). Umbilical core remnant infections in foals: 16 cases (1975–1985). *J. Am. Vet. Med. Assoc.* 190: 316–318.

81 Fischer, A.T. (1988). Laparoscopically assisted resection of umbilical structures in foals. *J. Am. Vet. Med. Assoc.* 214: 1813–1816.

82 Levan, R.P., Madigan, J.E., Walker, R. et al. (1995). Effects of disinfectant treatments on the bacterial flora of umbilicus of neonatal foals. *Biol. Reprod. Mono* 1: 77–85.

83 Beccati, F., Cercone, M., Angeli, G. et al. (2016). Use of multiphase computed tomographic urography in the diagnosis of ureteral tear in a 6-day-old foal. *Vet. Radiol. Ultrasound* 57: 10–15.

84 Cutler, T.J., Mackay, R.J., Johnson, C.M. et al. (1997). Bilateral ureteral tears in a foal. *Aust. Vet. J.* 75: 413–415.

85 Morisset, S., Hawkins, J.F., Franks, N. et al. (2002). Surgical management of a ureteral defect with ureterorrhaphy and of ureteritis with ureteroneocystostomy in a foal. *J. Am. Vet. Med. Assoc.* 220: 354–358.

86 Jean, D., Marcoux, M., and Louf, C.F. (1998). Congenital bilateral distal defect of the ureters in a foal. *Equine Vet. Educ.* 10: 17–20.

87 Divers, T.J., Byars, T.D., and Spirito, M. (1988). Correction of bilateral ureteral defects in a foal. *J. Am. Vet. Med. Assoc.* 192: 384.

88 Pringle, J.K., Ducharme, N.G., and Baird, J.D. (1990). Ectopic ureter in the horse: three cases and a review of the literature. *Can. Vet. J.* 31: 26–30.

89 Coleman, M.C., Chaffin, M.K., Arnold, C.E. et al. (2011). The use of computed tomography in the diagnosis of an ectopic ureter in a Quarter Horse filly. *Equine Vet. Educ.* 23: 597–602.

90 Chaney, K.P. (2007). Congenital anomalies of the equine urinary tract. *Vet. Clin. Equine* 23: 691–696.

91 Christie, B., Haywood, N., Hillbert, B. et al. (1981). Surgical correction of bilateral ureteral ectopia in a male appaloosa foal. *Aust. Vet. J.* 57: 336–340.

92 Tomlinson, J.E., Farnsworth, K., Sage, A.M. et al. (2001). Percutaneous ultrasound-guided pyelography aided diagnosis of ectopic ureter and hydronephrosis in a 3-week-old filly. *Vet. Radiol. Ultrasound* 42: 349–351.

93 Modransky, P.D., Wagner, P.C., Robinette, J.D. et al. (1983). Surgical correction of bilateral ectopic ureters in two foals. *Vet. Surg.* 12: 141–147.

94 Sullins, K.E., McIlwraith, C.W., Yovich, J.V. et al. (1988). Ectopic ureter managed by unilateral nephrectomy in two female horses. *Equine Vet. J.* 20: 463–466.

95 MacAllister, C.G. and Perdue, B.D. (1990). Endoscopic diagnosis of unilateral ectopic ureter in a yearling filly. *J. Am. Vet. Med. Assoc.* 197: 617–618.

96 Blikslager, A.T., Green, E.M., MacFadden, K. et al. (1992). Excretory urography and ultrasonography in the diagnosis of bilateral ectopic ureters in a foal. *Vet. Radiol. Ultrasound* 33: 41–47.

97 Getman, L.M., Ross, M.W., and Elce, Y.A. (2005). Bilateral ureterocystostomy to correct left ureteral atresia and right ureteral ectopia in an 8-month-old standardbred filly. *Vet. Surg.* 34: 657–661.

98 Alberts, V.P., Idu, M.M., Legemate, D.A. et al. (2014). Ureterovesical anastomotic techniques for kidney transplantation: a systemic review and meta-analysis. *Tranpl. Int.* 27: 593–605.

99 Ordidge, R.M. (1976). Urinary incontinence due to unilateral ureteral ectopica in a foal. *Vet. Rec.* 98: 384.

100 Rossdale, P.D. and Greet, T.R.C. (1989). Megavesica in a newborn foal. *ISVP News* 2: 10–13.

101 Houlton, J.E.F., Wright, I.M., Matic, S., and Herrtage, M.E. (1987). Urinary incontinence in a Shire foal due to ureteral ectopia. *Equine Vet. J.* 19: 244–247.

102 Dubs, B. (1976). Megavesica due to the absence of an urachus in a newborn foal. *Schweiz Arch. Tierheikd* 118: 393–395.

103 Rijkenhuizen, A. (2012). Megavesica and bladder rupture in foals. *Equine Vet. Educ.* 84: 404–407.

104 Axon, J.E. and Palmer, J.E. (2008). Clinical pathology of the foal. *Vet. Clin. Equine* 24: 357–385.

105 Schumacher, J. (2007). Hematuria and pigmenturia of horses. *Vet. Clin. Equine* 23: 655–675.

106 Bernard, W.V., Williams, D., Tuttle, P.A. et al. (1993). Hematuria and leptospiruria in a foal. *J. Am. Vet. Med. Assoc.* 203: 276–278.

107 Spiro, I. (2002). Hematuria and a complex congenital heart defect in a newborn foal. *Can. Vet. J.* 43: 375–377.

108 Johnston, J.K., Neely, D.P., and Latterman, S.A. (1987). Hematuria caused by abdominal abscessation in a foal. *J. Am. Vet. Med. Assoc.* 191: 971–972.

109 Larsdotter, S., Ley, C., and Pringle, J. (2009). Renal pseudoaneurysm as a cause of hematuria in a colt. *Can. Vet. J.* 50: 759–762.

110 Arnold, C.E., Chaffin, M.K., and Rush, B.R. (2005). Hematuria associated with cystic hematomas in three neonatal foals. *J. Am. Vet. Med. Assoc.* 227: 778–780.

111 Trotter, G.W., Brown, C.M., and Ainsworth, D.M. (1984). Unilateral nephrectomy for treatment of a renal abscess in a foal. *J. Am. Vet. Med. Assoc.* 11: 1392–1394.

112 Broux, B., Torfs, S., Wegge, B. et al. (2012). Acute respiratory failure caused by Leptospira spp. in 5 foals. *J. Vet. Intern. Med.* 26: 684–687.

113 Jones, S.L., Langer, D.L., Sterner-Kock, A. et al. (1994). Renal dysplasia and benign uteteropelvic polyps associated with hydroneprhosis in a foal. *J. Am. Vet. Med. Assoc.* 204: 1230–1234.

114 Jernigan, S.M. (2014). Hematuria in the newborn. *Clin. Perinatol.* 41: 591–603.

115 Schott, H.C., Barbee, D.D., Hines, M.T. et al. (1996). Renal arteriovenous malformation in a Quarter Horse foal. *J. Vet. Intern. Med.* 10: 204–206.

116 Gilday, R.A., Wojnarowicz, C., Tryon, K.A. et al. Bilateral renal dysplasia, hydronephrosis, and hydroureter in a septic neonatal foal. *Can. Vet. J.* 201;56: 257–260.

117 Juzwiak, J.S., Bain, F.T., Slone, D.E. et al. (1988). Unilateral nephrectomy for treatment of chronic hematuria due to nephrolithiasis in a colt. *Can. Vet. J.* 29: 931–933.

Neonatal Nervous System

Chapter 28 Embryology and Anatomy of the Neonatal Nervous System

Yvette Nout-Lomas and Rafael Alzola-Domingo

Embryology

In the mare, fertilization of the ovum occurs in the oviduct where initial symmetrical cleavages form a morula followed by a blastocyst (Figure 28.1). By the time the embryo enters the uterus (Day 6–7 post-ovulation), development has progressed to the late morula or early blastocyst stage. Around Day 9, the blastocyst contains an inner cell mass covered by a sheet of trophoblast that disappears by Day 14 and at Day 12 endoderm has enveloped the blastocyst cavity completely to form the yolk sac. In other species the yolk sac quickly becomes nonfunctional, but in the horse, it is a predominant structure for the first 3–4 weeks of pregnancy and is thought to play an important, if not critical, role in early embryonic nutritional supply [2]. Beginning around Day 14, mesoderm from the embryonic disc begins developing between the endodermal and ectodermal layers. This three-layered structure develops spherically from the region of the inner cell mass toward the abembryonic pole. In contrast to most domestic species in which the chorioallantois expands and elongates tremendously within the first 2 weeks of gestation, the equine conceptus remains essentially spherical throughout the first 6–8 weeks of gestation. Furthermore, the equine conceptus is extremely mobile and moves freely through the uterus until approximately Day 16, which is integral to maternal recognition of pregnancy in mares [3, 4]. Using transrectal ultrasonography, an equine embryonic vesicle is typically first identified around Day 10–11 following ovulation and mobility of the conceptus can be observed as early as Day 9 after ovulation, with a marked increase in mobility on Day 10, and maximum mobility between Days 11–14 [3, 5, 6].

The preimplantation period is a critical time during which the developing embryo responds to the maternal environment by permanently modifying its functional genome. It is during this stage that the gestational environment can have marked effects not only on birth weight and initial postnatal growth but also on neonatal adrenal and pancreatic functions and adult size. During this very early developmental stage (up to the blastocyst stage), the equine embryo is considered to be very sensitive to potential developmental advantages, as well as to disadvantageous developmental programming in response to adverse maternal metabolic status, health, or exposure to environmental toxins or pharmaceuticals [7].

Fixation of the embryo occurs around Day 15–16, and successful implantation requires a normally developing embryo, an appropriately primed uterus, and carefully coordinated communication between embryonic trophectoderm and maternal endometrium. This is necessary so that the endometrial surface is further modified to permit attachment and stimulate trophectoderm cells to proliferate, attach, and subsequently either invade into, or interdigitate, with the endometrium [7].

By Day 16, mesoderm begins to grow out from the embryo, envelopes half the yolk sac, and splits into somatic and splanchnic layers separated by the coelomic cavity. Folds of amnion begin to develop also and by Day 20 envelop the embryo. The allantois is visible at Day 21 as a bulge from the hind-gut region of the developing embryo and enlarges and spreads over the amnion and downward into the extraembryonic coelomic cavity so that by Day 25 it occupies one quarter of the embryo. At this stage, by Day 22, a fetal heart rate can be recognized [6]. Fusion of the allantois and chorion at the embryonic pole of the conceptus results in the allantochorion, consisting of inner allantoic endoderm, middle mesoderm, and thin layer of trophoblast overlying uterine epithelium. At the junction of the regressing yolk sac and advancing allantois, in a specific portion of the chorion, the outer trophoblast cells hypertrophy and proliferate to form an annulate band called the chorionic girdle. The trophoblast cells are arranged very closely to the underlying endometrium, and between Days 36 and 38 become separated entirely from

Equine Neonatal Medicine, First Edition. Edited by David M. Wong and Pamela A. Wilkins.

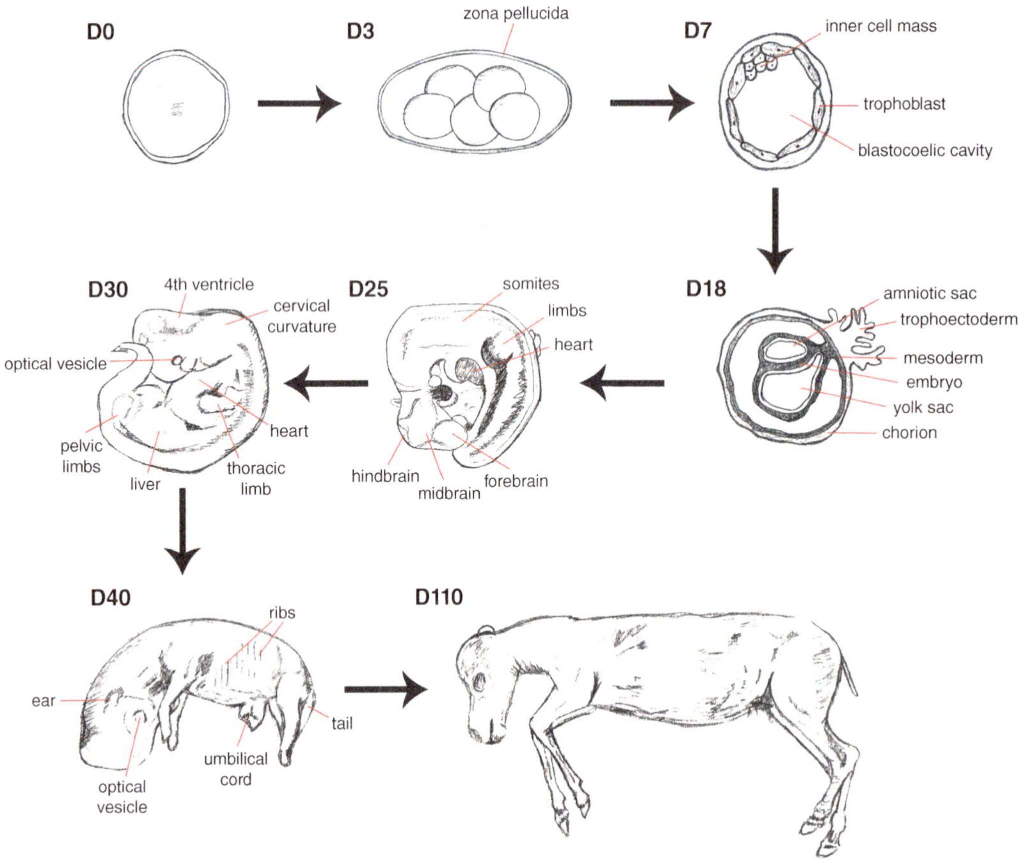

Figure 28.1 Stages of equine embryology. A Day 0 conceptus, a Day 3 morula, a Day 7 blastocyst, four stages of embryos (Day 18, 25, 30, and 40), and a Day 110 fetus are shown with annotations to specific developmental structures and organs [1].

the fetal membranes and actively invade maternal endometrium. These fetal cells form the endometrial cups and enlarge, become binucleate and secrete chorionic gonadotrophin. After Day 39 the first spontaneous movements have been shown to occur [6].

Fetal growth is not a uniform progression of cell replication, but a series of fundamentally different anabolic processes, which are integrated precisely. Development of the embryo before placental implantation involves rapid hyperplasia and pattern formation, which becomes apparent when primitive germ layers separate and presumptive organs can first be identified (Table 28.1). Metabolism at this time is anaerobic, and cells communicate by cell–cell contacts and by release of autocrine paracrine factors. The implantation of the placenta allows aerobic respiration and development of energy-expensive enzyme systems necessary for differentiated cell function. The appearance of the feto-placental circulation improves the delivery of nutrients to the tissues and, consequently, the rate of cell multiplication rises [8]. The equine fetus grows linearly during the second half of gestation and gains 75% of its final birth weight between mid and late gestation [9]. Therefore, fetal demand for nutrients to support this substantial tissue

Table 28.1 Embryonic age at which a first sign of organ system development is visible.

System	Age (Day after ovulation)	Identified characteristic
Musculoskeletal	15	Cartilaginous and mesenchymal tissues
Nervous	15	Discrete primordial vesicles
Senses: vison	15	Rudimentary optical vesicles
Appendices	15	Shape of ear; day 19: tail and limb buds
Dermatological	19	Translucent skin
Circulatory	19	Cardiac prominence
Digestive	21	Voluminous liver
Reproductive	25	Genital tubercle
Respiratory	35	Nasal area delimited
Urinary	37	Kidneys
Senses: auditory	37	Otic vesicles
Senses: olfactory	38	Olfactory epithelium
Senses: tactile	96	Tactile hairs on lips

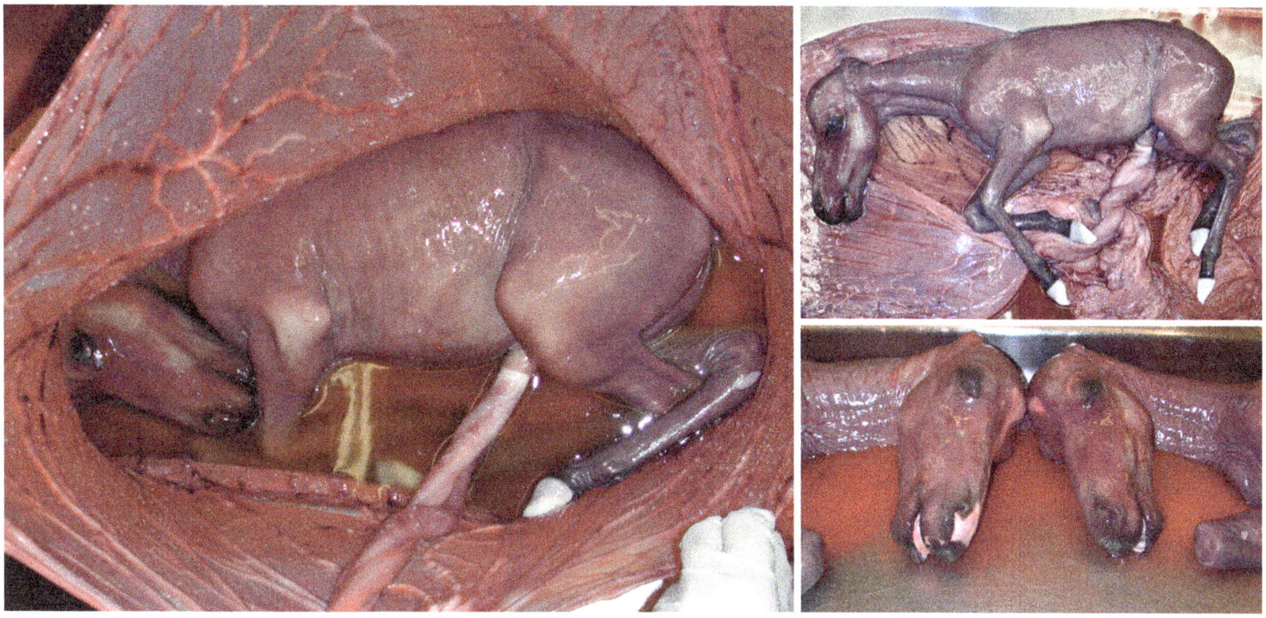

Figure 28.2 Twin pregnancy equine fetus aborted at 7 months' gestation.

accretion and oxidative metabolism increases rapidly during this time [10]. Figure 28.2 shows the appearance of an equine fetus at 7 months' gestation.

Development and Anatomy of the Nervous System

The field of neural development draws on studies of embryology, developmental biology, and neuroscience to describe and provide insight into the cellular and molecular mechanisms by which complex nervous systems form, develop during prenatal development, and continue to develop postnatally. The development of the nervous system includes the processes that generate, shape, and reshape the nervous system, from the earliest stages of embryonic development to adulthood. Landmarks of neural development in the embryo include neurogenesis, or the differentiation of neurons from stem cell precursors, migration of immature neurons to their final locations, outgrowth of axons from neurons and guidance of the motile growth cone through the embryo toward appropriate postsynaptic partners, generation of synapses between these axons and their postsynaptic partners, synaptic pruning, and changes in synapses, which underlie learning and memory. Neurodevelopmental processes occur through activity-independent and activity-dependent mechanisms. Activity-independent mechanisms are considered to be hardwired processes determined by genetic programs that occur within individual neurons. These processes occur independent of neural activity and sensory experience; examples include differentiation, migration, and axon guidance to the initial target areas. Once axons reach their target areas, activity-dependent mechanisms become important in further development. Neural activity and sensory experience mediate formation of new synapses, as well as synaptic plasticity, which is responsible for refinement of the nascent neural circuits. Many of these neurodevelopmental processes also are important in neural repair mechanisms following injury.

The nervous system has its origin in the neural plate that lies within the ectoderm of the embryonic disc. The margins of the plate become ridges or folds that grow toward each other and unite to form the neural tube (Figures 28.3 and 28.4). The neural tube first closes in its central portion, which corresponds to the future brainstem region. The cranial end of the neural tube segments into the three brain vesicles, namely the prosencephalon (forebrain), mesencephalon (midbrain), and rhombencephalon (hindbrain). The prosencephalon divides into the telencephalon and diencephalon, and the rhombencephalon divides into the metencephalon and myelencephalon. The cerebral hemispheres arise from the telencephalon. The cerebellum arises from the caudal section of the metencephalon. Neuroblasts proliferate from symmetric alar plates and form paired rhombic lips that thicken, project into the fourth ventricle, and extend progressively toward midline. The rhombic lips on the two sides fuse at midline, starting rostrally, to form the cerebellar vermis primordium [11]. From the ventral aspect of the telencephalon olfactory bulbs develop, which advance toward the developing nasal region. Neural crest cells migrate from the summits of the

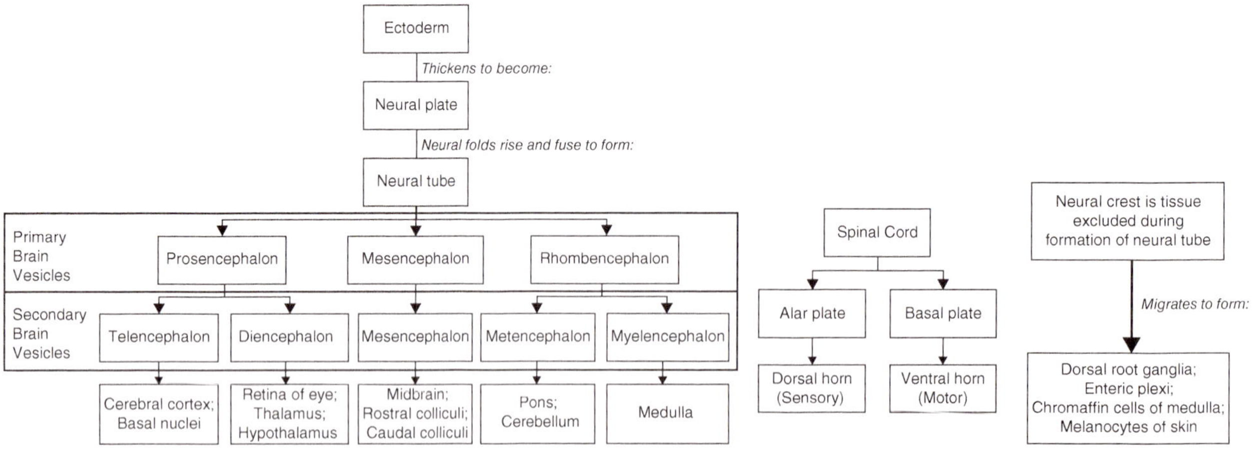

Figure 28.3 Schematic of nervous system development.

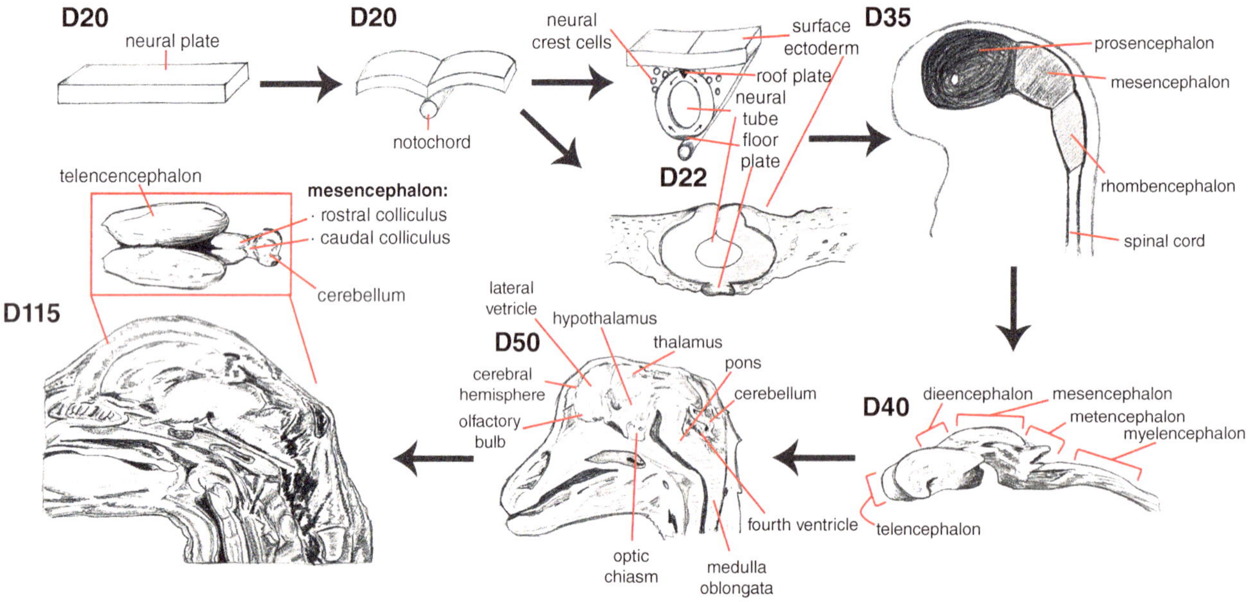

Figure 28.4 Equine embryonic and fetal neural development. Shown are stages of neural development from Day 0 to Day 115 gestation. Cells within the ectoderm germinal layer give rise to the neural plate, which folds and forms into the neural tube, surface ectoderm, and neural crest cells. The primary encephalic vesicles and spinal cord develop from the neural tube. Further development of secondary encephalic vesicles and formation of specific regions of the brain are indicated.

neural folds prior to closure and give rise to peripheral and autonomic ganglia, adrenal medulla, and a variety of other structures. The optic vesicles arise from the diencephalon and form the optic cups, which induce lens placodes in the overlying ectoderm. The inner layer of the optic cup becomes the retina, and axons from its nerve cells gradually extend as optic nerve fibers along the optic stalk to the brain. The otic vesicle that forms the inner ear is derived from ectoderm and eventually develops in a ductus endolymphaticus, cochlea, and three outpouchings, which become the semicircular canals.

In the equine embryo, one of the first organ systems of which development can be recognized by eye is the central nervous system (CNS) [1, 12, 13]. Mesenchymal tissue can be seen in the mesoderm cell layer using microscopy in embryos as early as Day 15 (Figure 28.1; Table 28.1). Table 28.2 shows at which embryonic or fetal age nervous system and sensory structures first become apparent microscopically. The spinal cord can be recognized in the thoracic cavity from Day 19 onward. Rudimentary optical vesicles on the cephalic region and primitive vesicles of the CNS can be seen that early as well. The three encephalic vesicles, the forebrain, midbrain, and hindbrain, can be recognized up to Day 39. The olfactory lobe is evident by Day 30. A weakly pigmented optical placodium can be seen by Day 25 and pigmentation of the retina by Day 38.

Table 28.2 Age in days postovulation at which development of specific nervous (bold) and sensory system structures become visible.

Age embryo (Day)	Structure
15–19	**Discrete primordial vesicles**
15–19	Rudimentary optical vesicles
19–40	**Development of encephalic vesicles and spinal cord**
19–26	Pigmented optical vesicles
24–40	Development and formation of tongue
26–38	Optical placodium weakly pigmented
35–47	Development of otic vesicles
37–40	**Pituitary, cerebellum, encephalic fourth ventricle, and choroid plexus**
38–47	Pigmentation of retina
40–107	**Formation of brainstem, spinal cord, and transition of brain vesicles to brain**
47–71	Eyes almost closed
47–107	Formation of external auricle
38–107	Development of olfactory epithelium
71–107	Orbit vesicle present
96–107	Tactile hairs on the lips

The spinal cord originates from the caudal part of the neural tube and appears as a thick neuroepithelium. Just beneath this neuroepithelium, a layer of smooth connective tissue is present that will form the primitive meninges. The pituitary gland has been seen as early as Day 38 and at that stage is bound to the hypothalamus by a pedicle. The cerebellum and the choroid plexus can be recognized with scanning microscopy at that stage also. After Day 40, the developing foal is referred to as a fetus, and at this stage the secondary embryonic brain vesicles (telencephalon, diencephalon, mesencephalon, metencephalon) and spinal cord can be recognized. Also, the thoracic limbs, pelvic limbs, and optic vesicles that are already pigmented can then be seen. Microscopically, other structures such as the fourth ventricle and its choroid plexus, dorsal root ganglia, primordial cartilage of the ribs and the sternum, tongue, heart, liver, cervical vertebrae, thoracic vertebrae, and caudal vertebrae are also seen.

The viable (>300 days gestation) newborn foal has a relatively well-developed neuraxis. Evidence of this is the presence of functional behavior at birth necessary for survival in a precocious species. In addition, foals are born with fully functional hearing and vision. Brainstem auditory evoked response testing in five healthy neonatal foals noted a functional auditory system comparable to that of adult horses when tested at 90 dB hearing level [14]. Further evidence that foals have a well-developed nervous system at birth is the presence of a gyral pattern similar to that seen in adults and mature myelin. Unlike pre- and full-term human infants that have somewhat primitive gyral development, the foal has a gyral pattern much like the adult horse [15]. Also, during conceptual ages 9–12 months, myelin in fetal foals matures, and there is evidence that, at birth, the spinal cord in foals is neurochemically more mature than in calves, lambs, and piglets [16].

Although the neonatal foal has a well-developed neuraxis, several factors indicate that cerebellar function lags behind that of the somatosensory, motor, vestibular and autonomic systems. Clinically, signs of incomplete cerebellar development include a deficient menace response, jerky head movements, a stiff, bouncy gait, prominent extensor tone and spinal hyperreflexia [15]. Furthermore, a state of deficient cerebellar function is corroborated by measurements of cerebellar and whole brain weights, the ratio of which rises during the conceptual ages of 9–12 months [15]. However, the cerebellum of the horse differentiates early on during embryonic development and is quite mature at birth. Moreover, the neonatal foal cerebellum is considered more mature than, for example the chick cerebellum, despite both species ambulating within hours after birth or hatching [11]. Relative to the chick, the cerebellar cortex of the newborn foal is more differentiated. In the foal the Purkinje cells are larger with well-formed, highly branched apical dendrites, the myelinated fibers in the white matter are more numerous and stained heavily with silver, the mossy and climbing fibers can be well-stained and can be seen coursing through the inner granule cell and Purkinje cell layers, and the external granule cell layer is 1–2 cells thick, which indicates that most of these cells have already migrated into the inner granule cell layer. The chick has 6–8 cell layers in the external granule layer, which is indicative of a less mature state at hatching than that exhibited by the equine fetus near birth.

Autonomic Nervous System Development

The autonomic nervous system is comprised of the sympathetic, parasympathetic, and enteric nervous systems. These systems develop in a stereotyped manner from the migration of the neural crest cells from specific rostrocaudal levels of the spinal cord to the growth of axons to their peripheral targets (Figure 28.3). Migration of the neural crest cells proceeds in two main streams: dorsolateral to the somites and ventromedially through the rostral portion of the somites. The latter stream produces neurons and non-neuronal cells of the autonomic nervous system, while the former stream produces pigment cells or melanocytes [17].

The enteric nervous system is thus derived from neural crest cells and receives innervation from the autonomic nervous system via the vagus nerve and prevertebral ganglia. Although the enteric nervous system receives considerable innervation from the autonomic nervous system, it can and does operate independently from the brain and spinal cord.

Similar to the remainder of the nervous system, in foals, the enteric nervous system is also well-developed. However, there are a number of differences that have been shown to be present between the neonatal and adult horse enteric nervous system. In foals, the density of myenteric plexuses and neurons is greater than healthy adult horses, which might be accounted for by spread with growth and neuron loss through cell death with aging [18]. In addition, in 1-day-old foals the myenteric plexus and neuron density in the right ventral, left ventral, and right dorsal colons is similar whereas in adult horses the density varies between different segments within the large colon. This might be explained by differences in growth of different segments of the colon [18]. Furthermore, in foals, neurons are localized within the edge of the myenteric plexus compared to a more central location in adults. Finally, the morphology of the myenteric plexus in foals differs from adult horses. The elongated bilobed myenteric plexuses present in foals is not seen in the large colon of adults and may represent the initial separation or expansion of plexuses which is completed with maturation [18].

Interstitial cells of Cajal generate pacemaker activity throughout the gastrointestinal (GI) tract by initiating the slow wave activity that is integral to the coordination of GI motility. In addition, interstitial cells of Cajal are thought to be involved in mediating neurotransmission via the autonomic nervous system and facilitating active propagation of electrical events. Interstitial cells of Cajal are a type of interstitial cell and are not derived from the neurocrest but are derived from the mesoderm. Developmental studies in other species have demonstrated that interstitial cells of Cajal start to colonize the GI tract about one-third to halfway through gestation. If this is the same for the equine fetus, interstitial cells of Cajal would likely be colonizing the GI tract around the fourth to sixth month of gestation [19]. In the equine fetus interstitial cells of Cajal have been found during the latter half of gestation and in the neonate. Furthermore, the distribution and density of interstitial cells of Cajal in the small intestine in the full-term fetus is similar to that of the neonatal animal. Similar to what has been shown for myenteric plexuses, it does appear that development of the interstitial cells of Cajal continues after birth. For example, interstitial cells of Cajal in the distal large intestine continue to further colonize the inner aspect of the circular muscle region after birth [19].

Fetal Movement

Fetal movement (motion of fetus caused by its own muscle activity) begins during the late embryonic stage and occurs as soon as muscles are innervated. The presence or absence of fetal movement reflects CNS function, with depressed CNS function resulting in decreased activity. Movement is required to ensure satisfactory muscular development and proper function of skeletal joints and the equine neonate is particularly dependent on the high level of development of these structures to ensure successful postnatal adaptation. Lack of fetal movement has been associated with a negative outcome [20]. Fetal motility can be classified as either elicited or spontaneous with spontaneous movements triggered by either the brain or spinal cord. The first movements are not reflexive but originate from action potentials generated within the spinal cord and as the nervous system matures, muscles can move in response to stimuli. In foals, first spontaneous movements have been recorded as early as day 34–39 after ovulation [5, 6]. Furthermore, videoendoscopic hysteroscopy has shown movement of fetal appendages as early as day 44 with movements appearing strong and coordinated by day 57 [5]. These simple and singular movements occur at an average rate of 2 every 10 minutes [21]. At these early stages of development, video-hysteroscopy has demonstrated that the fetus can also respond to both light and tactile stimuli [5].

Between 6 and 11 months of gestation, fetal movements consisting of fine-tuned activity as well as major movements. Fine-tuned activity includes fetal head nods, flexion and extension of extremities, suckling motion, lip movements, blinking, nostril flaring, auricular pinnae motion, opening and closure of the glottis and tail movements, whereas major movements are considered whole body advancements within the uterus in cranio-caudal and/or ventro-dorsal directions and vice versa, as well as rotation along the short and long axis. Additionally, fetal breathing movements can occasionally be seen as excursions of the diaphragm between thorax and abdomen and expansion of the ribcage. These have been shown to occur from 8 months gestation to term [20, 22].

In studies that have quantified fetal movements to assess fetal well-being, an increase in rate of movements from 4 to 9 months of gestation has been shown, with a peak of about 16 movements every 10 minutes [21]. In mares evaluated after 7 months of gestation, on average one to two fetal movements over the course of a 2-minute ultrasonographic evaluation can be detected [23], and major movements can be seen 3–5 times per hour [22]. There is considerable variation in major fetal movements with a reported range of occurrence of 1–84 per hour, and during the last 3 days prepartum, major movements increase in frequency to form a continuum of active periods of 10 minutes or greater duration [21]. These movements likely are related to final postural adjustments in anticipation of parturition.

Frequent changes in fetal presentation have been observed in studies investigating mobility of the equine fetus, and during the first 5 months of gestation, there is an equal likelihood of the equine fetus being in anterior or posterior presentation. After 5 months of gestation, variability of fetal presentation decreases as gestation advances, with an increased likelihood of the fetus being in anterior presentation [22, 24]. Dormant or inactive phases are observed in fetuses of all ages but are more common in late gestation and usually last <10 minutes, but longer phases, up to 60 minutes, have been detected. Long periods of true inactivity should be regarded as concerning, and lack of fetal movement has been associated with a negative outcome [20, 25].

References

1. Franciolli, A.L., Cordeiro, B.M., da Fonseca, E.T. et al. (2011). Characteristics of the equine embryo and fetus from days 15 to 107 of pregnancy. *Theriogenology* 76: 819–832.
2. Sharp, D.C. (2000). The early fetal life of the equine conceptus. *Anim. Reprod. Sci.* 60–61: 679–689.
3. Ginther, O.J. (1983). Mobility of the early equine conceptus. *Theriogenology* 19: 603–611.
4. McKinnon, A.O., Squires, E.L., Vaala, W.E. et al. (2011). *Equine Reproduction*, 2e. Wiley-Blackwell.
5. Allen, W.R. and Bracher, V. (1992). Videoendoscopic evaluation of the mare's uterus: III. Findings in the pregnant mare. *Equine Vet. J.* 24: 285–291.
6. Allen, W.E. and Goddard, P.J. (1984). Serial investigations of early pregnancy in pony mares using real time ultrasound scanning. *Equine Vet. J.* 16: 509–514.
7. Stout, T.A. (2016). Embryo-maternal communication during the first 4 weeks of equine pregnancy. *Theriogenology* 86: 349–354.
8. Han, V.K. (1993). Pathophysiology, cellular and molecular mechanisms of foetal growth retardation. *Equine Vet. J. Suppl.* 25: 12–16.
9. Platt, H. (1984). Growth of the equine foetus. *Equine Vet. J.* 16: 247–252.
10. Fowden, A.L., Giussani, D.A., and Forhead, A.J. (2020). Physiological development of the equine fetus during late gestation. *Equine Vet. J.* 52: 165–173.
11. Sisken, B.F., Zwick, M., Hyde, J.F. et al. (1993). Maturation of the central nervous system: comparison of equine and other species. *Equine Vet. J. Suppl.* 25: 31–34.
12. Rigoglio, N.N., Barreto, R.S.N., Favaron, P.O. et al. (2017). Central nervous system and vertebrae development in horses: a chronological study with differential temporal expression of nestin and GFAP. *J. Mol. Neurosci.* 61: 61–78.
13. Rigoglio, N.N., Smith, O.E., Matias, G.S.S. et al. (2019). Development of the central nervous system in equine twin fetuses derived by somatic cell nuclear transfer. *Reprod. Fertil. Dev.* 31: 941–952.
14. Aleman, M., Madigan, J.E., Williams, D.C. et al. (2014). Brainstem auditory evoked responses in an equine patient population. Part II: foals. *J. Vet. Intern. Med.* 28: 1318–1324.
15. Mayhew, I.G. (1988). Neurological and neuropathological observations on the equine neonate. *Equine Vet. J. Suppl.* 20: 28–33.
16. Sweasey, D., Patterson, D.S., and Leadon, D.P. (1982). Chemical composition of the spinal cord in the normal developing fetus and in the premature foal. *J. Reprod. Fertil. Suppl.* 32: 563–567.
17. Hill, C.E. (2004). Development of the autonomic nervous system. In: *Primer on the Autonomic Nervous System*, 2e (ed. D. Robertson, I. Biaggioni, G. Burnstock, et al.), 3–5. Elsevier.
18. Schusser, G.F. and White, N.A. (1994). Density of myenteric plexuses and neurons in the large and transverse colon of one-day-old foals. *Equine Vet. J.* 26: 337–339.
19. Fintl, C., Pearson, G.T., Ricketts, S.W. et al. (2004). The development and distribution of the interstitial cells of Cajal in the intestine of the equine fetus and neonate. *J. Anat.* 205: 35–44.
20. Reef, V.B., Vaala, W.E., Worth, L.T. et al. (1996). Ultrasonographic assessment of fetal well-being during late gestation: development of an equine biophysical profile. *Equine Vet. J.* 28: 200–208.
21. Fraser, A.F., Hastie, H., Callicott, R.B. et al. (1975). An exploratory ultrasonic study on quantitative foetal kinesis in the horse. *Appl. Anim. Ethol.* 1: 395–404.
22. Bucca, S., Fogarty, U., Collins, A. et al. (2005). Assessment of feto-placental well-being in the mare from mid-gestation to term: transrectal and transabdominal ultrasonographic features. *Theriogenology* 64: 542–557.
23. Luukkanen, L., Katila, T., and Koskinen, E. (1997). Some effects of multiple administration of detomidine during the last trimester of equine pregnancy. *Equine Vet. J.* 29: 400–402.
24. Ginther, O.J. and Griffin, P.G. (1993). Equine fetal kinetics: presentation and location. *Theriogenology* 40: 1–11.
25. Fraser, A.F. (1977). Fetal kinesis and a condition of fetal inertia in equine and bovine subjects. *Appl. Anim. Ethol.* 3: 89–90.

Chapter 29 Physiology of the Neonatal Nervous System

Yvette Nout-Lomas

Horses are a precocious species and are born with a more functionally developed brain than altricial species to enable survival as a prey animal [1]. For successful transition from the intrauterine to extrauterine environment, most structures and organ systems of the foal are therefore mature enough to be competent at birth. Rarely are congenital structural nervous system abnormalities noted in foals [2]; however, foal mortality is not uncommon, reported at 5.8% of live births in the first month of life in the USA (2015), of which 3.3% of deaths occurred within the first 2 days of life [3]. Abnormal periparturient and postpartum foal behavior is recognized as a consequence of disease, but also contributes or causes neonatal disease and subsequent death. This chapter briefly discusses physiological processes relevant to the periparturient period [4–7], and describes normal neonatal behavior.

Consciousness and Arousal after Birth

Activation of the fetal hypothalamic–pituitary–adrenal axis in the period before birth is important for many of the maturational processes essential for neonatal survival [5]. This activation results in a prepartum rise in cortisol concentrations in the fetal circulation, which induces functional and structural changes in a wide range of fetal tissues that must be functional at birth for survival. The prepartum endocrine changes in the fetus activate many physiological systems and homeostatic mechanisms that have little or no function in utero but are essential for survival in the newborn foal including glucoregulation, thermoregulation, maintenance of blood pressure and partial pressure of oxygen (PO_2), and perfusion of key tissues such as the brain.

Before birth, ungulate fetuses are actively maintained in a sleeplike unconscious state, even though their brains have the capacity for conscious perception and are neurologically mature at birth [6, 8]. Maintenance of this unconscious state is apparently due to combined neuroinhibitory effects of high circulating and cerebral concentrations of adenosine, allopregnanolone, pregnanolone, and prostaglandin D2, acting together with a placental neuroinhibitory peptide, warmth, buoyancy and cushioned tactile stimulation [6]. In precocial young, conscious perception does not occur until shortly after birth, when behaviors associated with survival become possible because the neurological apparatus has developed sufficiently to process sensory inputs from the environment, allowing them to find the dam and teat, or even seek shelter in cold conditions [9]. Factors that might contribute to the postnatal onset of consciousness and result in reduction of cerebral cortical inhibition include increased oxygenation through onset of breathing and loss of placental supply of adenosine and neuroactive steroids. Moreover, activators of arousal play a role in this process and include 17β-estradiol (primarily placental origin), stimulation of the locus coeruleus-noradrenaline system by strong intrapartum tactile stimulation and hypoxia, and postpartum exposure to cold ambient conditions (Table 29.1) [6].

Neurosteroids are steroids synthesized de novo in the nervous system as compared to neuroactive steroids, which are products of peripheral steroid hormones metabolized by nervous tissue. Both neurosteroids and neuroactive steroids modulate neuronal activity predominantly through agonistic effects at the gamma-aminobutyric acid (GABA) Type A receptor, typically leading to decreased neuronal excitability. Allopregnanolone, pregnanolone, and progesterone are examples of potent GABA Type A receptor agonists [10]. Furthermore, during acute fetal stress, concentrations of allopregnanolone, for example, increases to support trophic development (myelinogenesis, synaptogenesis, apoptosis) whereas in chronic fetal stress (e.g. restricted intrauterine growth), neuroactive steroids are inappropriately low (in part, due to high

Equine Neonatal Medicine, First Edition. Edited by David M. Wong and Pamela A. Wilkins.

Table 29.1 Summary of neuroinhibitory factors involved in maintaining late-term fetuses in unconscious sleeplike states and activators involved in arousal and onset of consciousness after birth [6].

Late-term fetus	After birth	
Inhibitors of movement	**Withdrawal of inhibition**	**Activators**
Adenosine	Onset of breathing and oxygenation	17β-esotradiol
Allopregnanolone	Loss of placental supply of inhibitors	Noradrenaline
Pregnanolone		Barrage of sensory impulses stimulating the locus coeruleus-noradrenergic system
Prostaglandin D_2		
Placental peptide inhibitor		
Warmth		
Low tactile stimulation through cushioning and buoyancy		

glucocorticoids), thereby altering neuronal and glial cell differentiation, brain development, and impairing the stress response, ultimately resulting in a multitude of postnatal complications [11]. In healthy foals, allopregnanolone concentrations were below the level of detection within 30 minutes of birth [12], although allopregnanolone concentrations are very high in term pregnant mares [13]. When a healthy 6-hour-old foal was administered allopregnanolone IV, the foal first appeared sedated, had decreased responsiveness to the environment, and became recumbent; higher IV doses resulted in stupor and unresponsiveness to the mare, environment, and sound and tactile stimulation [14]. In healthy foals, pregnenolone, a N-methyl-D-aspartate (NMDA)-receptor agonist, and progesterone concentrations were shown to rapidly decrease by 24 hours of age and remained subsequently low [12]. Neurosteroids and neuroactive steroids play an important role in the transition from intrauterine to extrauterine life in foals, and increased glucocorticoid [15] and progestogen concentrations [15–17], that are noted in critically ill foals suggest an imbalance in these compounds plays a role in development of abnormal neonatal behavior and disease. Moreover, in people, imbalances in neurosteroids and neuroactive steroids have been associated with psychiatric, behavioral, cognitive, and sleep disorders [18]. In foals, corticosteroids may interfere indirectly with the protective actions of neurosteroids and neuroactive steroids, favoring neurologic disease; it is also possible that foals have increased progestogen concentrations as a neuroprotective mechanism [7].

In addition to peripartum hormonal changes, there is significant change in tactile stimulation of the foal as it passes through the birth canal. Touch is the first sense to emerge in utero and is the most strongly developed at birth [1]. Neonatal foals are very sensitive to squeeze pressure; a rope-squeeze restraining technique can result in a state of somnolence in otherwise healthy foals [19]. Undoubtedly, the transition of foals from an unconscious sleeplike state in utero to a state of consciousness after birth is a coordinated process that requires changes in physical, hormonal, and other factors to act in concert.

Immediate Postpartum Behavior (0–3 hours)

Table 29.2 and Figure 29.1 illustrate postpartum behavior at 0–3 hours. Foals are minimally responsive during transit through the birth canal (Figure 29.1a and b). Dr.

Table 29.2 Time frame for normal post-parturient events and behavior in foals. For ponies, these time frames are typically shorter than for horses [20–23].

Parameter	Typical onset	Comments
Responsive to stimuli	Immediate	>5 min is concerning
Respiratory rhythm	Seconds	within 1 min
Sternal	Seconds – few minutes	>15 min is concerning
Severance umbilical cord	6–8 min (0–30 min)	
Vocalize	within 30 min	response to dam
Suckling reflex	1–30 min	>30 min is concerning
Stand	30–60 min (15 min – 2 h)	>2 h is concerning
Suckling	1–2 h (35 min – 3 h)	>3 h is concerning
Pass meconium	2–3 h (45 min – 4 h)	soon after standing or first meal
Urinate	6 h (colts) – 11 h (fillies)	
Pupillary light reflex	Present at birth	
Hyperreflexive spinal reflexes	Present at birth	
Crossed extensor reflex	Present at birth	lasts up to 3 wk
Menace	2 wk	

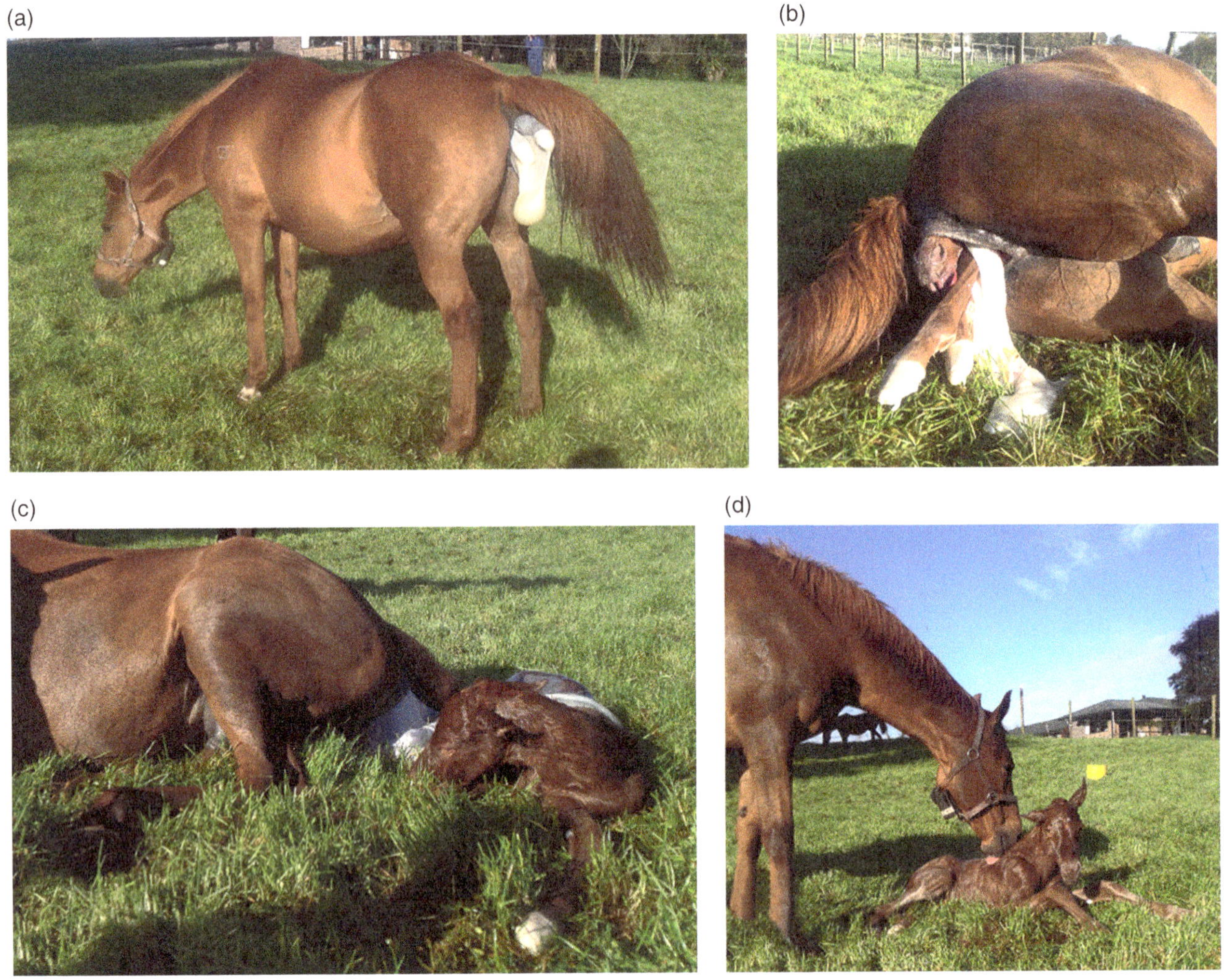

Figure 29.1 Normal foaling process. (a) Mare in stage two of labor. The chorioallantoic membrane has ruptured and the allantoic fluid has been released. The front feet are visible through the thin, transparent, whitish amniotic sack that encases the foal. (b) The mare has laid down and the amniotic sack has ruptured. (c) The newborn is actively positioning itself into sternal recumbency while its pelvic limbs remain the mare's reproductive tract. (d) The mare has stood up, the umbilical cord has ruptured, and the mare is licking the foal's thoracolumbar area. The foal has extended its thoracic limbs and is ready to start standing. *Source:* Photos courtesy Dr. Angela Hawker.

Rossdale [20], a pioneer of equine perinatology, noted that a noxious stimulus using a hypodermic needle around the nose did not elicit a response in foals before delivery of the hips. This is clinically significant because it suggests that it is nearly impossible to determine fetal/foal viability using reflex testing at this stage of birth, although a suckle reflex in some foals is present during parturition. Amazingly, foals are precocial, relatively mature, and mobile from the moment of birth, and within 5 minutes of birth should appear bright and alert and responsive to tactile, visual, and auditory stimuli. All senses are functional in the newborn foal, and they are capable of learning immediately after birth. In general, parturition in ponies is similar to larger breeds of horses, although the duration is shorter and pony foals stand and suckle sooner [21].

The foal frees itself from fetal membranes by raising its head and establishes a respiratory rhythm within 60 seconds of birth [24]. A foal is expected to be able to right itself into sternal recumbency within 5 minutes of birth, and this action is often completed while the pelvic limbs are still in the mare's reproductive tract (Figure 29.1c).

Most foals are in sternal recumbency, with the head up, before the umbilical cord breaks, and they assume this position within 15 minutes after birth (Figure 29.1d). Under natural circumstances, the umbilical cord remains intact until after the foal has established a respiratory rhythm. Horses have a long umbilical cord and, if the cord remains intact, approximately 1.5 l of blood can be transferred to the foal during the period when blood flow through the placenta decreases after birth [25]. Thus, leaving the umbilical cord attached when mare and foal remain recumbent is beneficial to optimize oxygenation, blood volume, and umbilical stump healing. On average, the umbilical cord is severed 8 minutes after foaling and typically occurs within 30 minutes of foaling through movements made by the foal or when the mare stands up [20].

Mares display maternal instincts such as nickering, looking at her flanks, and licking objects or her own body before a foal is delivered, during first and second stage labor. After foaling, the stimuli of smell and taste appear to be most important in promoting maternal behavior. Sight might be a less important stimulus, since mares give equal attention to foals that cannot stand or move normally as compared to healthy foals [24]; moreover, the mare's use of vision to recognize her foal develops once olfactory tags are in place [26]. Under normal circumstances, the dam shows interest in the foal immediately after expulsion and will look at and start nickering to the newborn. Mares show olfactory investigation including Flehmen responses toward the fetal membranes, the area where allantoic fluid has fallen, and occasionally the placenta and amnion. Mares vigorously lick the foal's haircoat and fetal fluids are likely important in stimulating the mare's maternal instincts as well as stimulating the foal's respiratory efforts, blood flow, and attempts to stand (Figure 29.1d). Within 30 minutes, the foal should vocalize, usually in response to the dam's nickering. In addition, the foal should make several attempts to stand within 30 minutes of birth [20]. The dam licks the foal along the lumbar paravertebral region and the foal (Figure 29.1d), in response to this stimulus, extends its forelimbs rigidly and simultaneously throws its head and neck dorsally while flexing and pushing up with both hindlimbs. This motion is similar to when the foal withdraws its hindlimbs from the vagina of the mare after her expulsive efforts cease on delivery of the hips [20].

Initially there is a base-wide swaying posture, and the foal staggers or rocks from side to side or back and forth. The foal may fall several times before getting solidly to its feet. After the standing position has been achieved for the first time, the foal is able to rise quickly and without difficulty from the recumbent position on subsequent efforts. By the time the foal stands, the head should follow movements of the mare around the stall. In the free-ranging state, the mare and foal leave the site of foaling soon after the placenta is discharged, about an hour after foaling [22].

The suckle reflex is often present during and immediately after parturition and should be present within 30 minutes after birth. The foal begins to search for the dam's udder once it stands solidly (within 30–60 minutes after birth) [20, 21]. Foals are innately driven to locate the teat and suckle, a response refined by learning. Coarse bobbing of the head and rocking of the body at this stage is normal. Before the foal suckles successfully, it will open and close the mouth in a slow-motion form of snapping with its head and neck in an extended position. During this time, the foal will often investigate the mare's pectoral region by sniffing or sucking around the front legs (Figure 29.2a), followed by exploration of the mare's mammary region often with initial attempts at sucking the dam's tail, inside of the back legs and stifle, and the sides of the udder, as well as making attempts to get to the udder through the mare's back legs. The mare can help the foal find the teats by standing still, stepping forward to bring the udder to the foal's head, flexing the back leg on the side away from the foal to angle the

(a) (b)

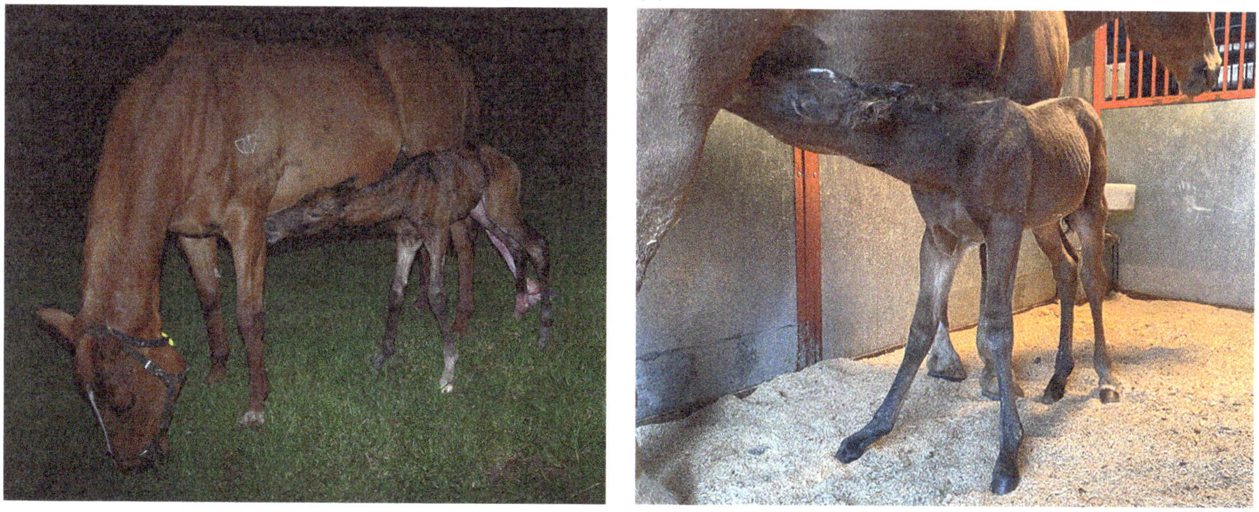

Figure 29.2 Newborn suckling behavior. (a) Within 30–60 minutes after birth, a newborn foal begins to search for the dam's udder, which often includes exploration of the mare's pectoral region. *Source:* Photo courtesy Dr. Angela Hawker. (b) Wide-based stance during suckling in a 24-hour-old foal.

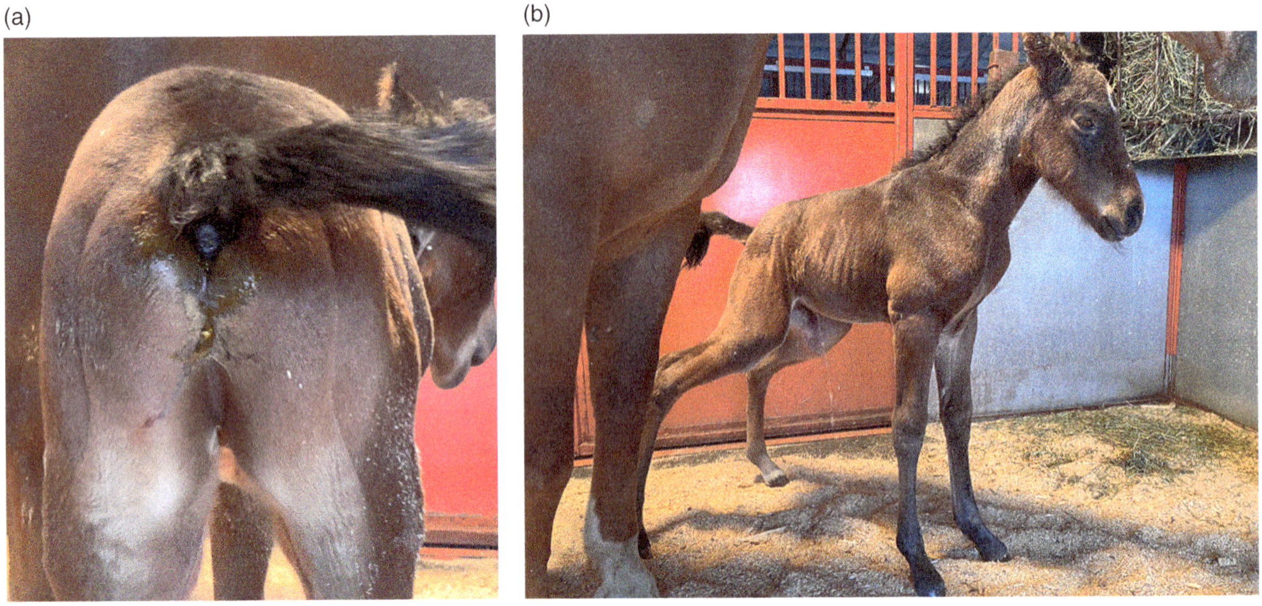

Figure 29.3 Neonatal eliminative behavior. (a) A 24-hour-old foal has passed all meconium and should start to pass yellow feces. (b) A neonatal colt's urinating posture is already similar to what is seen in male adult horses.

teats toward the foal's mouth, and occasionally pushing the foal toward the udder. When the foal finds the udder, its posture is base-wide and it takes hold of a teat and pushes its nose firmly into the udder before and sometimes during sucking (Figure 29.2b). Once the foal has successfully sucked from the teat, the maternal bond becomes increasingly established. After 1–2 hours, the foal should begin suckling for periods of 1–5 minutes [20, 21, 23]. The first suckling is considered crucial in the development of secure mare–foal attachment, similar to other species [27]. Successful suckling behavior within 2–3 hours after birth suggests that the relationship between foal and dam is firmly established. One study noted the mean interval from birth to standing and to suckling was shorter for fillies compared to colts [28]. Furthermore, some foals, and especially heavier ones take longer (~3 hours) to suckle naturally.

Suckling is often followed by a period of drowsiness characterized by the foal's head dropping repeatedly and the foal at times collapsing to the ground. The foal may sleep in lateral recumbency before standing to suckle again a few minutes later. The brown, green, or black pellets of meconium are passed within minutes of birth, and most foals pass meconium within 2–3 hours of birth.

Neonatal Behavior

In the first day of life, foals and their dams spend 96% of their time within 1 m of each other [29]. The foal's gait is noticeably exaggerated and hypermetric; usually within a day the foal is capable of trotting and galloping. Over the first day of life, foals develop a pattern of sleeping, standing, urinating, suckling, and exploring, which is then repeated. All meconium should be passed and replaced by yellow feces within 4 days of birth [30]. Meconium is only passed pre- or intrapartum when the fetus is distressed. First urination occurs about 6 hours after birth in colts and about 11 hours after birth in filly foals (Figure 29.3) [21].

Suckling and Feeding

Suckling commonly occurs after resting or after a disturbance, which has caused the foal to approach the dam. The frequency and duration of suckling is greatest in the first week of life [31]; however, not all suckling episodes are successful. Depending on the definition used for a suckling bout, foals have been shown to suckle four to seven times per hour in their first week of life [30, 32]. These bouts last an average of 2.5 minutes with individual foals having consistent patterns of short or long bouts, regardless of age [31, 33]. Udder-pushing, or bunting, stimulates release of oxytocin from the neurohypophysis, which in turn controls milk ejection in the udder. In foals, bunting is most frequent during the second week of life and declines rapidly thereafter [32]. Bunting can be uncomfortable to dams and elicit aversive or aggressive avoidance behavior by the dam. Maternal aggression during suckling is least frequent when the foal is very young and peaks when the foal is 4 to 5 months old [31, 33]. Foals react to normal maternal aggression during suckling by cessation of bunting and beginning of suckling, pauses in attempts to suckle, kicking the mare or threatening to, shifting body position while keeping the head at the udder, or ceasing attempts to suckle [31]. Suckling is usually terminated by the foal, but

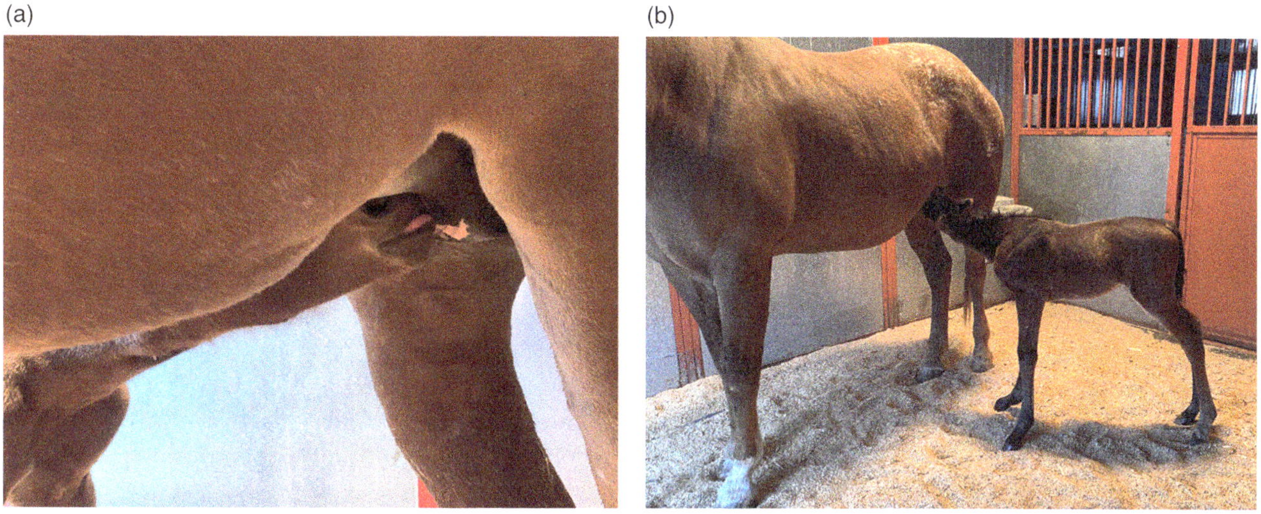

Figure 29.4 Neonatal suckling behavior. (a) The foal's head position during suckling is shown with its tongue surrounding the teat. (b) An alternative position during suckling is shown whereby the foal is positioned perpendicular to the dam rather than parallel to the dam.

mares are most likely to terminate suckling during the first week of the foal's life, when they are responsible for about half of terminations [31].

When suckling, the foal usually stands alongside the dam, facing the opposite direction of the mare. However, some foals occasionally suckle from behind the dam, facing in the same direction, but with the head bent round the dam's back leg. All variations between these two positions can be seen (Figure 29.4) [32]. Approximately one third of foals have an individual suckling preference either to the left or right, which further strengthens with age. This lateralized behavior is thought to develop and change during ontogeny and might be related to conformation [34]. In addition to providing nutrition, suckling provides comfort, since foals may suck on other objects (teats of others, sheaths of geldings) or suck the teats of their dam for long periods after they have emptied the udder of milk [31, 33].

Foals may be noted to eat other foodstuffs at a day old, and as they grow older, they spend progressively more time feeding in addition to suckling. By 3 weeks of age, foals spend 47% of their time eating [35], compared to adult horses that spend 50–60% of their time eating [36]. Almost all feeding by foals is done while their dams eat. Foals eat primarily during the early morning and evening. Suckling decreases with age, and by 3 to 4 months of age foals suckle on average once per hour, lasting a little more than a minute [32]. Of note, foals rarely drink water. The youngest age at which a foal was observed to drink water in one study was 3 weeks. In the same study, 8 of 15 foals were never observed to drink water before weaning [35].

Foals typically eat feces from their dam [37]. Coprophagia has been seen in foals as young as 5 days of age and occurs approximately once every 4 hours during the first 2 months of life, decreasing to once every 10–15 hours until 5months of age. After that, the incidence of coprophagia further decreases. The stimulus for coprophagia remains unclear, however, it could be a response to pheromones present in the manure. Possible benefits of coprophagia include introduction of normal gut flora, promotion of absorption of nutrients, vitamins, enzymes, proteins, and specific substances such as deoxycholic acid that possibly enhance gut immunocompetence and play a protective role against enterocolitis [37].

Sleeping and Resting

Neonates spend a considerable amount of time sleeping, but lying behavior is dependent on breed, age, weather, and time at pasture (Figure 29.5) [38]. In general, foals spend less time lying down and lie down less frequently as they age; moreover, foals spend less time lying down in wet, when compared to dry, conditions. Foals also lie down longer and more frequently when they are stalled compared to pasture. During the first week of life, a foal spends 32% of its time in recumbent rest [39], of which 15% in lateral recumbency, compared to 2% after weaning [40]. The time spent standing and alert decreases from 31% to 5% in the same period, while foraging increases from 13% to 62%. The milk supply from the dam may allow the foal to invest time in sleep and in exploration of their physical and social environment [40]. Time spent in lateral recumbency decreases from 15% in newborns to 3% in preweaning foals. When foals sleep, periods of limb extension and restlessness in sternal recumbency alternate with periods of sleep in lateral recumbency (Figure 29.6). When in lateral recumbency, foals may move their legs in running motions, and may also nicker and twitch their ears. A syndrome

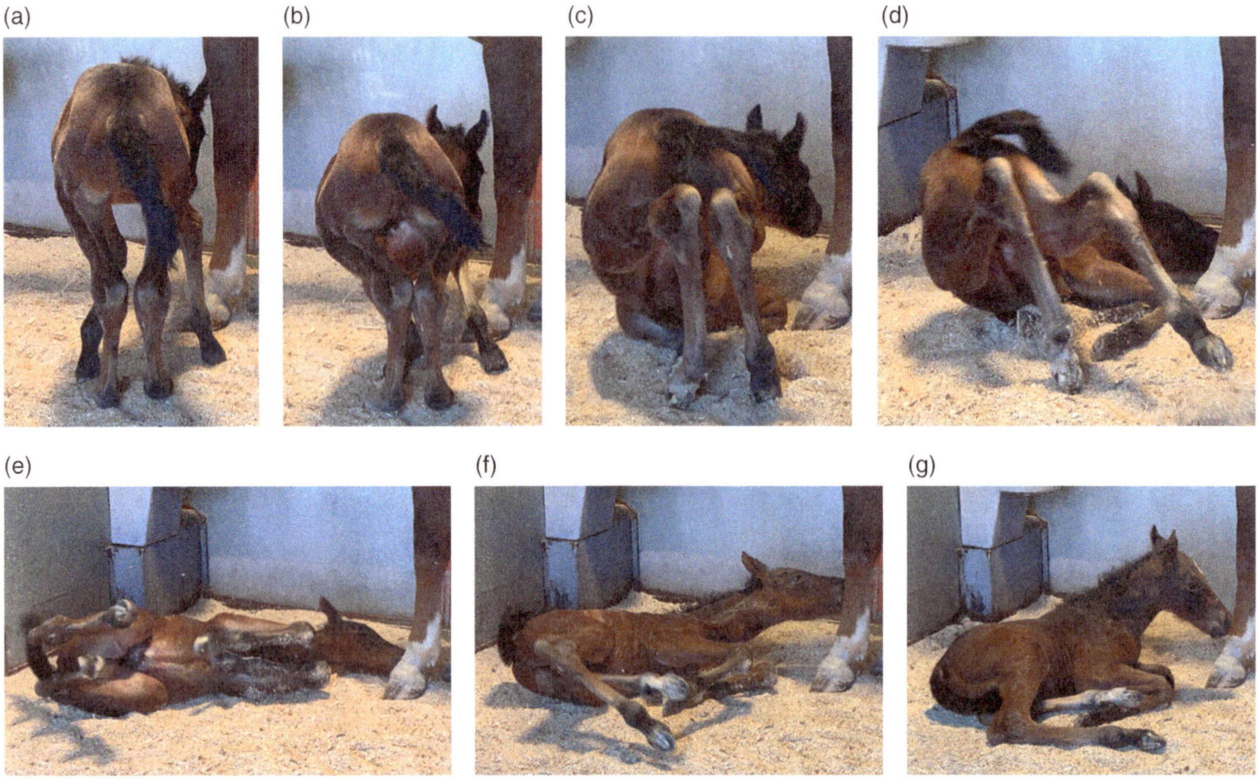

Figure 29.5 Sequence of a 24-hour-old foal lying down (a)–(f) into sternal recumbency (g). Similar to the adult horse the neonate flexes both thoracic and pelvic limbs and lowers the neck and thorax to the ground first (c); however, the neonate displays less strength and fine motor control resulting in a rough landing (d), (e). Occasionally foals are seen to collapse to the ground when they lie down.

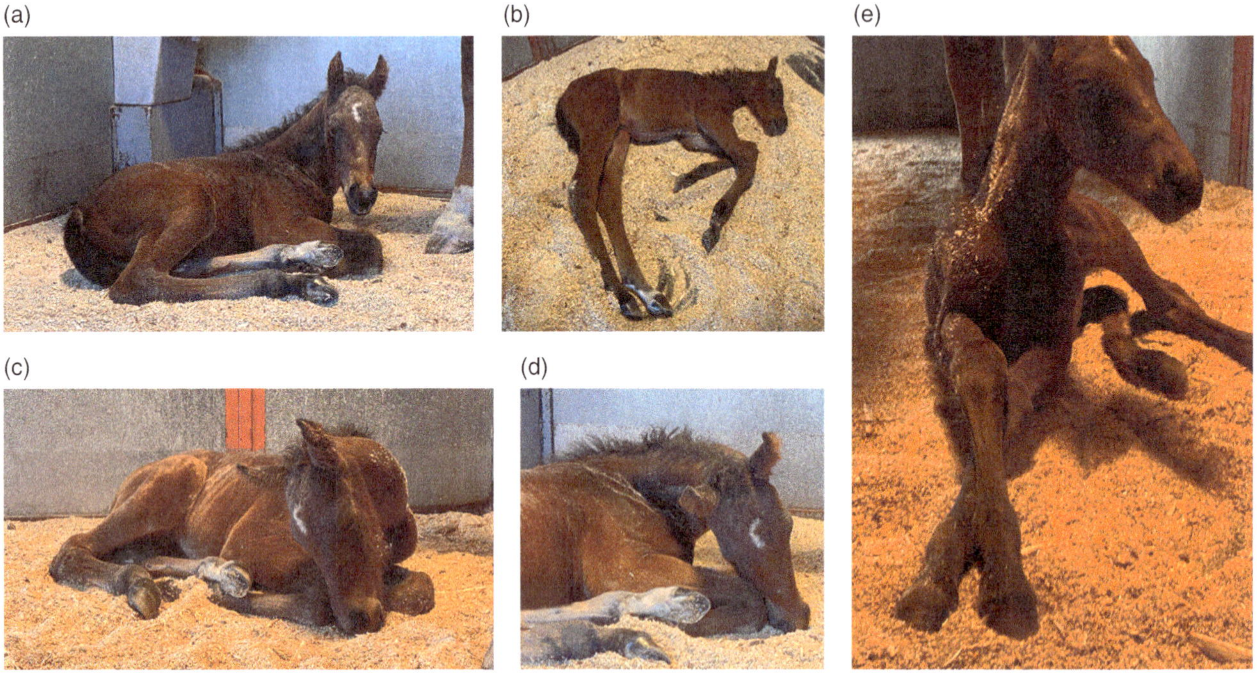

Figure 29.6 Neonatal resting behavior. Foals spend much time sleeping in sternal (a), (c), (d) or lateral recumbency (b). When foals sleep in lateral recumbency the thoracic limbs are commonly folded up (b). (e) A 24-hour-old foal is shown that is ready to stand up. Its thoracic limbs are positioned in rigid extension in front of itself; however, they are still crossed.

seen occasionally in healthy neonatal foals involves spontaneous, intermittent narcolepsy (sleep attacks), and cataplexy (sudden immobility), with areflexia (absent reflexes), from which foals seem to recover. This might be related to persistence of a fetal protective mechanism [41].

Mare–Foal Bond

Primary socialization is established within 2 hours of birth and separation of the mare and foal after this period results in disorientation of the foal and extreme excitement by the mare [30]. However, in free-ranging horses, bonding takes up to 2 weeks of close proximity and frequent interactions for the foal and mare to consolidate their bond [42]. During the first 3 days of life, the foal becomes increasingly confident and coordinated and, although it usually stays close to the mare, the foal develops a growing interest in the environment. During the first week of life, a foal spends over 90% of the time within 5 m of its dam and more than 80% of the time within 1 m [33, 43]. A mare spends a greater amount of time near her foal when it is recumbent and uses that time to rest upright, whereas when the foal is up she will be more relaxed and forage [22]. When foals encounter a novel or aversive stimulus, they will return to their dam. Dams use the unique calls of their foals to locate them when the pair is separated [22], and foals recognizes their dams through use of vision and olfaction [44].

Communication between mare and foal includes use of different sounds such as snorting, nickering, and whinnying. In general, mares initiate communication at closer mare–foal distances and preferentially use snorts, while foals initiate communication at farther distances using whinnies and nickers, the louder forms of communication [45]. When mares initiate communication, there is typically no change in animal distance or activity, whereas when foals initiate communication, suckling and a decrease in mare–foal distance are likely outcomes. With increasing age, foals are more likely to use snorts in lieu of whinnies, and suckling or decreases in the mare–foal distance are less likely outcomes of communication. Moreover, as foals age, the probability that mares initiate communication increases, but mares remain more or less constant in their signal choice.

In feral horses, foals that initiate communication at higher rates with their dams during the first 10 weeks of age survive longer than foals that initiate communication at lower rates [45]. This indicates the importance of maternal "style" to offspring survival and suggests that, in feral horses, communication may provide a mechanism by which dams facilitate both offspring independence and protection. Mares might assess risks and use snorts to signal both their position and that it is "safe" for their foals to continue current activities. Offspring allowed to play with conspecifics, interact with elders, and explore their environment are more likely to survive, and it may be that more communicative mares are facilitating these experiences for their foals, contributing to their future survival. It appears that the function of mother–offspring communication changes with increasing foal independence and mares may modulate risk to their foals and ensure safety while also encouraging independence [45].

Mutual grooming is uncommon in foals during the first month of life [30], but foals self-groom 5–12 times more often as their dams [30]. Foals use various self-grooming techniques in different proportions to adults. Foals usually scratch their head and neck with their back feet and bite and scratch the trunk and back legs with their teeth (Figure 29.7a). Flehmen is exhibited as early as 1 day of life, and colts have been seen to do this more than fillies (Figure 29.7b). Flehmen occurs frequently in response to mare urine, and it is possible that exposure to urinary pheromones is important for normal growth and sexual maturation in horses, similar to other species [30]. Play is a behavior that is important in development of appropriate horse behavior patterns and relationships. Fillies and colts engage in paly at the same rate; however, colts engage more in interactive play, whereas fillies engage more in general motor play. It is possible that increased interactive play displayed by colts is important in the development of dominance and mating behaviors [30].

Learning

Although imprinting is a general form of learning in which subjects become familiar with a stimulus as a result of being exposed to it, imprinting is unique since, before learning, no previous visual experience has affected brain development [46]. Typically during the imprinting phase, young animals undergo a process by which they establish social preferences shortly after birth [47]. Patterns of behavior, such as reduced fear to handling, established during such temporally sensitive periods for adaptive learning have been demonstrated in many species; however, the time frame for this period varies between species.

In horses, a time frame for imprinting has not been recognized but likely occurs much earlier than in predator species [48, 49]. Shortly after birth, imprinting of the mare with the foal occurs through licking, touching, and vocalizing. Foals learn immediately after birth, and foals that have been handled immediately after birth may be less fractious and easier to handle than foals that lacked immediate postnatal human contact [50]. Learning during this early time can include strategies such as desensitization, socialization, and sensitization, similar to those used to train adult horses, and can result in improved bonding with humans, desensitization to certain stimuli,

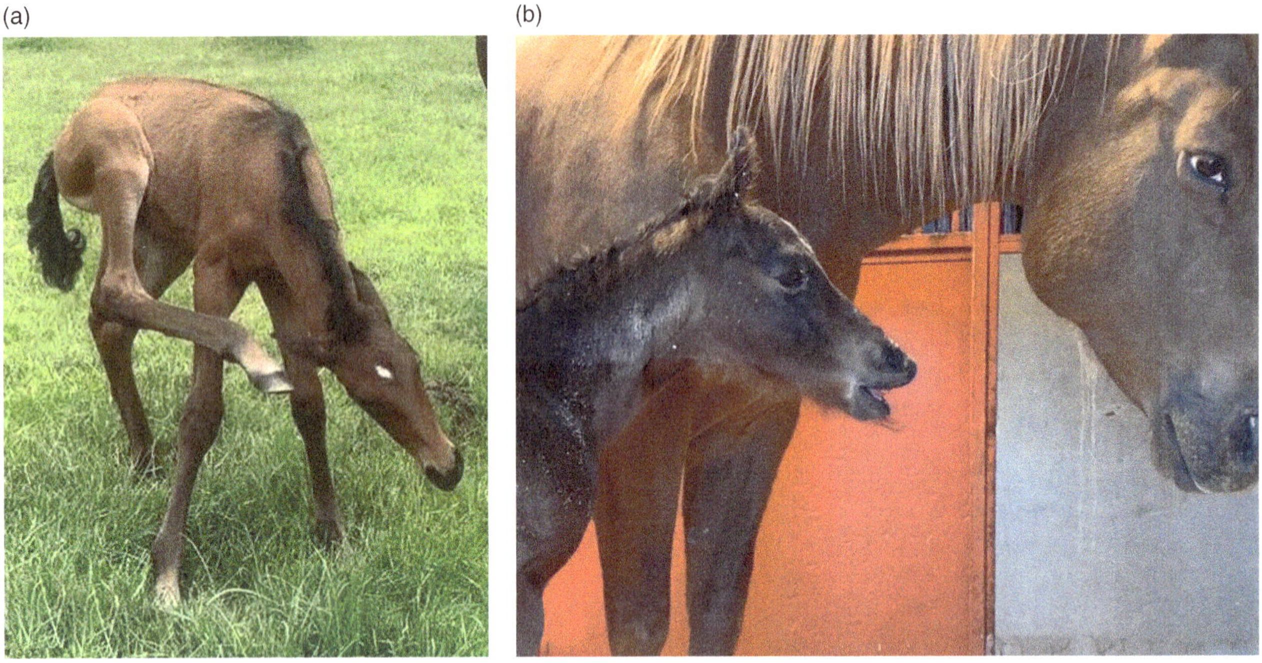

Figure 29.7 Neonatal behaviors. (a) Self-grooming. *Source:* Photo courtesy Dr. Angela Hawker. (b) Flehmen in a 24-hour-old colt.

sensitization to other stimuli such as yielding to pressure, and decreasing the fear response [49]. There are few studies of early learning in foals and much remains unknown with regards to critical periods of biological development and periods during which adult behavior is shaped. Although in one study, no effect of number of training sessions or timing of training sessions was found on foal behavior at 6 months of age [48]; another study showed reduced resistance to touching limbs and picking up feet in foals that received early handling [49].

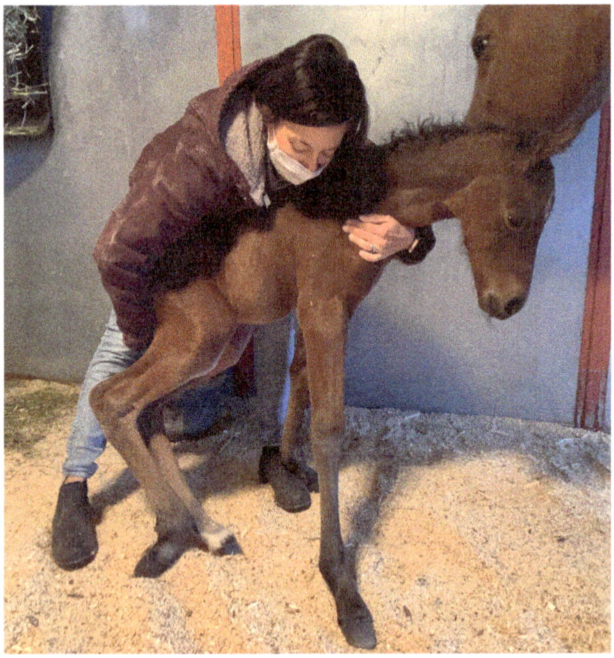

Figure 29.8 This foal is collapsing during restraint. Once pressure from the handler is reduced, the foal will jump back up again.

Restraint

Neonatal foals are very sensitive to squeeze pressure. When a handler firmly restrains a foal by placing one arm around the chest and the other one around the foal's hind quarters, the foal may collapse (Figure 29.8). Foals alternately struggle actively and collapse passively during this type of restraint. The evolutionary value of immobilization when squeezed might be related to potential benefits of reducing movement of the foal while it passes through the birth canal. This response to squeezing restraint in foals may represent a delayed loss of a protective intrauterine mechanism where there is suppression of motor activity during uterine confinement. Moreover, physical restriction has been hypothesized to reduce sympathetic stimulation to the ascending reticular activating system and decrease the level of arousal in human infants [51]. Restraint of animals may also influence the ascending reticular activating system, having a profound effect on consciousness and physical tone. During restraint, a foal may snap its teeth vigorously and urinate. Teeth snapping must be distinguished from grinding of the teeth (odontoprisis), continual ineffectual chewing, and teeth clenching (bruxism), and may represent normal submissive behavior [52].

In cattle and adult horses, rope-casting techniques are used to enable management and veterinary procedures to be performed [53]. As previously noted, a similar casting technique, termed *rope squeeze,* results in a state of somnolence when applied to neonatal foals [19]. The technique involves using a bowline knot to secure a rope around the foal's neck and under the shoulder. Then two half-hitch knots are used to loop the rope around the thorax and abdomen 5–25 cm from each other and perpendicular to the vertebral column. The half-hitch knots are positioned directly on the dorsal thoracolumbar area. One person stands behind the foal and pulls on the rope, which results in a generalized squeezing of the foal, and a second person assists the foal as it lies down [19]. When the rope squeeze is applied to healthy neonatal foals, a rapid onset of recumbency, somnolence, and slow wave sleep occurs, then quickly regain alertness when the rope is removed. Furthermore, after 20 minutes of squeeze pressure, an increase in adrenocorticotropic hormone, dehydroepiandrosterone sulfate, and androstenedione was measured in foals. The foals' tolerance to noxious stimuli significantly increased during restraint and was shown to be independent of the concentration of circulating β-endorphin [19].

Postnatal Central Nervous System Maturation

The angular head position, base wide stance, intention movements, hypermetric gait, and absent menace response in newborn foals is characteristic of cerebellar disease if observed in an adult. Other factors are likely involved in this as well, and final development of upper motor neuron inhibiting influences on reflex activity depend on many factors, including maturation of peripheral proprioceptors and inhibitory neurotransmitters, myelinization, as well as completion of anatomical pathways in the cerebellum.

The degree of differentiation of the major types of neurons and glia at birth appears to be correlated with the neonate's ability to function. The cerebellum of precocious newborn animals that can walk within the first few hours is more developed at birth than altricious newborn animals that may take months to perform such functions [54, 55]. Although maturation of the equine neonatal cerebellum is incomplete, it is one of the most mature seen in vertebrates. For example, the equine cerebellum at the time of birth is more mature than the chick cerebellum at the time of hatching, which is also a species that is up and moving immediately. Both the chick and equine cerebellum are more mature when compared to the human and rodent cerebellum at the time of birth [55].

References

1. Mellor, D.J. and Lentle, R.G. (2015). Survival implications of the development of behavioural responsiveness and awareness in different groups of mammalian young. *N. Z. Vet. J.* 63: 131–140.
2. Furr, M. (2015). Congenital malformation of the nervous system. In: *Equine Neurology*, 2e (ed. M. Furr and S. Reed), 401–405. Ames, Iowa: Wiley.
3. NAHMS (2015). Equine mortality in the United States, 2015. *Equine Mortality.* 4: 1–2.
4. Fowden, A.L., Forhead, A.J., and Ousey, J.C. (2012). Endocrine adaptations in the foal over the perinatal period. *Equine Vet. J. Suppl.* 130–139.
5. Fowden, A.L., Giussani, D.A., and Forhead, A.J. (2020). Physiological development of the equine fetus during late gestation. *Equine Vet. J.* 52: 165–173.
6. Diesch, T.J. and Mellor, D.J. (2013). Birth transitions: pathophysiology, the onset of consciousness and possible implications for neonatal maladjustment syndrome in the foal. *Equine Vet. J.* 45: 656–660.
7. Toribio, R.E. (2019). Equine neonatal encephalopathy: facts, evidence, and opinions. *Vet. Clin. North Am. Equine Pract.* 35: 363–378.
8. Mellor, D.J., Diesch, T.J., Gunn, A.J. et al. (2005). The importance of "awareness" for understanding fetal pain. *Brain Res. Brain Res. Rev.* 49: 455–471.
9. Mellor, D.J. and Gregory, N.G. (2003). Responsiveness, behavioural arousal and awareness in fetal and newborn lambs: experimental, practical and therapeutic implications. *N. Z. Vet. J.* 51: 2–13.
10. Olsen, R.W. (2018). GABAA receptor: positive and negative allosteric modulators. *Neuropharmacology* 136: 10–22.
11. Brunton, P.J. (2015). Programming the brain and behaviour by early-life stress: a focus on neuroactive steroids. *J. Neuroendocrinol.* 27: 468–480.
12. Aleman, M., McCue, P.M., Chigerwe, M. et al. (2019). Plasma concentrations of steroid precursors, steroids, neuroactive steroids, and neurosteroids in healthy neonatal foals from birth to 7 days of age. *J. Vet. Intern. Med.* 33: 2286–2293.
13. Ousey, J.C., Forhead, A.J., Rossdale, P.D. et al. (2003). Ontogeny of uteroplacental progestagen production in pregnant mares during the second half of gestation. *Biol. Reprod.* 69: 540–548.
14. Madigan, J.E., Haggettt, E.F., Pickles, K.J. et al. (2012). Allopregnanolone infusion induced neurobehavioural alterations in a neonatal foal: is this a clue to the pathogenesis of neonatal maladjustment syndrome? *Equine Vet. J. Suppl.* 109–112.
15. Dembek, K.A., Timko, K.J., Johnson, L.M. et al. (2017). Steroids, steroid precursors, and neuroactive steroids in critically ill equine neonates. *Vet. J.* 225: 42–49.

16 Aleman, M., Pickles, K.J., Conley, A.J. et al. (2013). Abnormal plasma neuroactive progestagen derivatives in ill, neonatal foals presented to the neonatal intensive care unit. *Equine Vet. J.* 45: 661–665.
17 Rossdale, P.D., Ousey, J.C., McGladdery, A.J. et al. (1995). A retrospective study of increased plasma progestagen concentrations in compromised neonatal foals. *Reprod. Fertil. Dev.* 7: 567–575.
18 Reddy, D.S. and Estes, W.A. (2016). Clinical potential of neurosteroids for CNS disorders. *Trends Pharmacol. Sci.* 37: 543–561.
19 Toth, B., Aleman, M., Brosnan, R.J. et al. (2012). Evaluation of squeeze-induced somnolence in neonatal foals. *Am. J. Vet. Res.* 73: 1881–1889.
20 Rossdale, P.D. (1967). Clinical studies on the newborn thoroughbred foal. I. Perinatal behaviour. *Br. Vet. J.* 123: 470–481.
21 Jeffcott, L.B. (1972). Observations on parturition in crossbred pony mares. *Equine Vet. J.* 4: 209–214.
22 McGreevy, P. (2012). *Equine Behavior a Guide for Veterinarians and Equine Scientists*, 2e. Saunders Elsevier.
23 MacKay, R.J. (2005). Neurologic disorders of neonatal foals. *Vet. Clin. North Am. Equine Pract.* 21 (387–406): vii.
24 Rossdale, P.D. (1968). Abnormal perinatal behaviour in the Thoroughbred horse. *Br. Vet. J.* 124: 540–553.
25 Rossdale, P. and Mahaffey, L.W. Parturition in the Thoroughbred mare with particular reference to blood deprivation in the new-born. *Vet. Rec.* 70: 142–152.
26 Leblanc, M.A. and Boissou, M.F. (1981). Development of a test to study material recognition of young in horses. *Biol. Behav.* 6: 283–290.
27 Hausberger, M., Henry, S., Larose, C. et al. (2007). First suckling: a crucial event for mother-young attachment? An experimental study in horses (*Equus caballus*). *J. Comp. Psychol.* 121: 109–112.
28 Rosales, C., Krekeler, N., Tennent-Brown, B. et al. (2017). Periparturient characteristics of mares and their foals on a New Zealand Thoroughbred stud farm. *N. Z. Vet. J.* 65: 24–29.
29 Barber, J.A. and Crowell-Davis, S.L. (1994). Maternal behavior of Belgian mares. *Appl. Anim. Behav. Sci.* 41: 161–189.
30 Crowell-Davis, S.L. (1986). Developmental behavior. *Vet. Clin. North Am. Equine Pract.* 2: 573–590.
31 Crowell-Davis, S.L. (1985). Nursing behaviour and maternal aggression among Welshponies (*Equus caballus*). *Appl. Anim. Behav. Sci.* 14: 11–25.
32 Carson, K. and Wood-Gush, D.G. (1983). Behaviour of Thoroughbred foals during nursing. *Equine Vet. J.* 15: 257–262.
33 Tyler, S.J. (1972). The behaviour and social organization of the New Forest ponies. *Anim. Behav. Monogr.* 5: 85–196.
34 Komarkova, M. and Bartosova, J. (2013). Lateralized suckling in domestic horses (*Equus caballus*). *Anim. Cogn.* 16: 343–349.
35 Crowell-Davis, S.L., Houpt, K.A., and Carnevale, J. (1985). Feeding and drinking behavior of mares and foals with free access to pasture and water. *J. Anim. Sci.* 60: 883–889.
36 Ralston, S.L. (1986). Feeding behavior. *Vet. Clin. North Am. Equine Pract.* 2: 609–621.
37 Crowell-Davis, S.L. and Houpt, K.A. (1985). Coprophagy by foals: effect of age and possible functions. *Equine Vet. J.* 17: 17–19.
38 Murase, H., Matsui, A., Endo, Y. et al. (2018). Changes of lying behavior in Thoroughbred foals influenced by age, pasturing time, and weather conditions. *J. Equine Sci.* 29: 61–66.
39 Crowell-Davis, S.L. (1994). Daytime and rest behaviour of the Welsh Pony (*Equus caballus*) mare and foal. *Appl. Anim. Behav. Sci.* 40: 197–210.
40 Boy, V. and Duncan, P. (1979). Time-budget of Camargue horses. 1. Developmental change in the time-budget of foals. *Behaviour* 71, 20: 188–202.
41 Mayhew, I.G. (1988). Neurological and neuropathological observations on the equine neonate. *Equine Vet. J. Suppl.* 28–33.
42 Houpt, K.A. (2002). Formation and dissolutiom of the mare foal bond. *Appl. Anim. Behav. Sci.* 78: 325–334.
43 Crowell-Davis, S.L. (1986). Spatial relations between mares and foals of the Welsh pony (*Equus caballus*). *Anim. Behav.* 34: 1007–1015.
44 Wolski, T.R., Houpt, K.A., and Aronson, R. (1980). The role of the senses in mare-foal recognition. *Appl. Anim. Ethol.* 6: 121–138.
45 Nunez, C.M.V. and Rubenstein, D.I. (2020). Communication is key: mother-offspring signaling can affect behavioral responses and offspring survival in feral horses (Equus caballus). *PLoS One* 15: e0231343.
46 Horn, G. (2004). Pathways of the past: the imprint of memory. *Nat. Rev. Neurosci.* 5: 108–120.
47 Bateson, P.P. (1966). The characteristics and context of imprinting. *Biol. Rev. Camb. Philos. Soc.* 41: 177–211.
48 Williams, J.L., Friend, T.H., Collins, M.N. et al. (2003). Effects of imprint training procedure at birth on the reactions of foals at age six months. *Equine Vet. J.* 35: 127–132.
49 Spier, S.J., Berger Pusterla, J., Villarroel, A. et al. (2004). Outcome of tactile conditioning of neonates, or "imprint training" on selected handling measures in foals. *Vet. J.* 168: 252–258.
50 Miller, R. (1991). *Imprint Training of the Newborn Foal.* Colorado, USA: Western Horseman Inc. Colorado Springs.

51 Giacoman, S.L. (1971). Hunger and motor restraint on arousal and visual attention in the infant. *Child Dev.* 42: 605–614.

52 Adams, R. and Mayhew, I.G. (1984). Neurological examination of newborn foals. *Equine Vet. J.* 16: 306–312.

53 Leahy, J.R. and Barrow, P. (1953). *Restraint of Animals*, 2e. Ithaca, NY: Cornell Campus Store.

54 DeLahunta, A., Glass, E.N., and Kent, M. (2014). *Veterinary Neuroanatomy and Clinical Neurology*, 4e. St. Louis, MO: Elsevier Saunders.

55 Sisken, B.F., Zwick, M., Hyde, J.F. et al. (1993). Maturation of the central nervous system: comparison of equine and other species. *Equine Vet. J. Suppl.* 31–34.

Chapter 30 Examination, Therapeutics, and Monitoring of the Nervous System

Section I Neurologic Examination of the Neonatal Foal

Cody Alcott and Yvette Nout-Lomas

The neonatal foal's nervous system has major similarities to the adult counterpart; however, examination techniques are unique. Neonates are prone to generalized encephalopathies (neonatal encephalopathy, infectious meningoencephalitis, kernicterus) that can challenge lesion localization, but this remains the goal of examination. Neurolocalization within the peripheral and central nervous systems (CNS) of the neonate requires careful consideration of clinical abnormalities. Concomitant disease and metabolic disturbances can further challenge a diagnosis of neurological disease as well as the neurological examination.

The equine neonate undergoes rapid maturation of its nervous system immediately following parturition. The ability of the neonate to right itself and stand shortly after birth is an amazing phenomenon and important measure of nervous system function, most importantly the cerebellum and vestibular system. Delays in the righting process, or achieving sternal recumbency, can suggest hypoxic events during parturition, maladaptation to the extrauterine environments post parturition, musculoskeletal disease, or developmental anomalies within the CNS. The recumbent neonate presents a unique opportunity to examine both the central and peripheral nervous systems, however this should not be performed at the sacrifice of mare-foal bonding, which is a critical part of neonatal survival.

The neurologic examination begins with observation of the foal's behavior, mentation, posture, and movement in its environment keeping in mind that behavior of healthy newborn foals changes rapidly within the first few hours of birth. Nonspecific bonding to objects or other horses can occur in neonates but does not necessarily suggest an abnormality is present. Dull mentation, wandering away from the dam, standing in corners of the stall, or circling suggest serious forebrain disturbances with sequalae of poor colostrum intake, dehydration, and sepsis. Neonatal encephalopathy is one of the most commonly recognized causes of forebrain dysfunction in the neonate [1].

Newborn foals are cognizant of their surroundings soon after birth and are responsive to the slightest disturbance in their environment. A foal usually stands within 2 hours of birth and locates its dam and suckles soon after. Healthy foals spend a considerable amount of time resting in recumbency, but are easily aroused, and this usually initiates suckling behavior. An alert neonatal foal carries its head with a noticeably more flexed angle at the atlantooccipital joint compared to adults (Figure 30.I.1), and movement of the head in response to visual, tactile, or auditory stimuli is jerky and exaggerated [2, 3]. Very young foals show rhythmic bobbing movements of the head while making sucking motions with the lips and tongue, in search of the udder. These findings are reminiscent of abnormal head movement seen in cerebellar disorders in older foals and horses [2].

The motor system of foals is well-developed, and the characteristic upright posture and slightly stiff, bouncy gait may represent a relative delay in maturation of cerebellar function [3]. Gait evaluation is best achieved by watching the free movement of the foal as it follows its dam. Intention movements of the head are often associated with the initiation of several steps. Forward movement is made with extremely exaggerated steps of short stride length that slap on the ground. In general, the foal's stride is short, rapid, and dysmetric [3]. With time and exercise, a gait that resembles the adult develops, and the foal learns to suckle and eat with one leg flexed rather than with base wide extension of the forelimbs. Foals that are confined to their stall or those that spend long periods recumbent are slower to develop the adult type stance and gait [3].

The newborn foal is extremely reactive to tactile stimuli along the neck and trunk. In addition to local subcuticular muscular contractions, foals flex their bodies away from the stimulus, shake their heads, and attempt to escape.

Equine Neonatal Medicine, First Edition. Edited by David M. Wong and Pamela A. Wilkins.

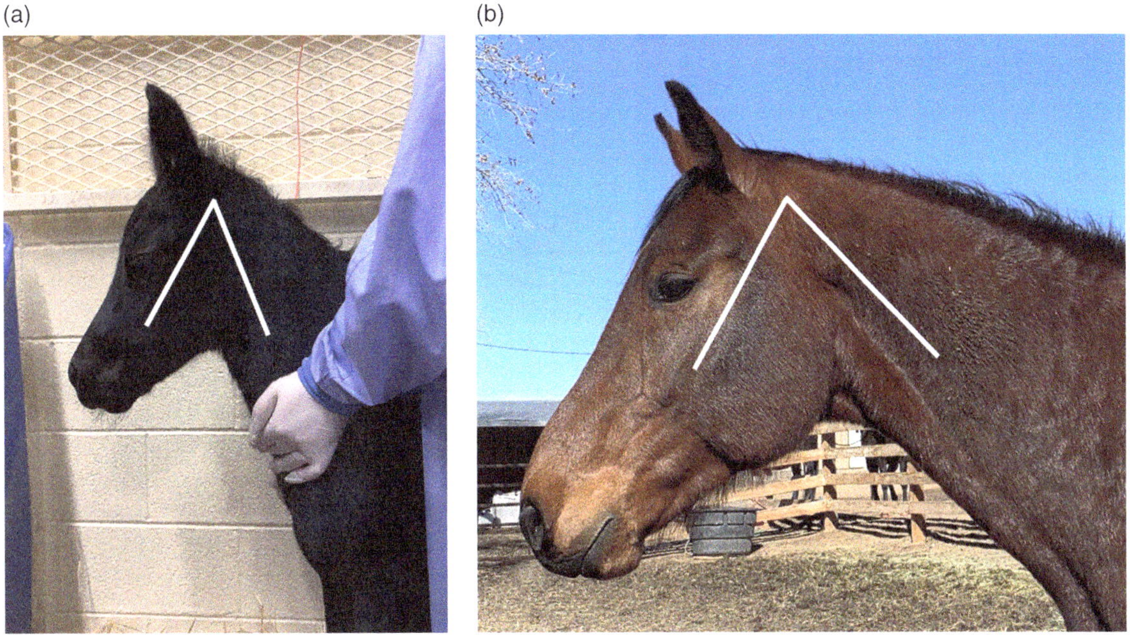

Figure 30.I.1 Head angle of the foal compared to the adult horse. A neonatal foal (a) carries its head with a noticeably more flexed angle at the atlantooccipital joint than in the adult horse (b).

Tactile stimuli along the cervical vertebrae cause a local muscle contraction as well as movement of the ipsilateral ear, eyelid, and lip. The foal's lip response is not as marked as the response in the adult. Foals are also very responsive to sensory stimuli along the trunk, flank, and hindlimbs. In very young foals, a dorsal head bob and forward movement can be elicited by pressure along the lumbar region, and a panniculus response can be elicited in the trunk and flank region similar to adults.

To evaluate the limbs more closely, the foal should be placed in lateral recumbency. Foals exhibit hyperreflexive spinal reflexes compared to adults. In lateral recumbency, the forelimbs of the newborn foal have substantial extensor tone. The tone in the foal's forelegs may be relaxed by repeated attempts to flex the leg. The triceps tendon reflex and extensor carpi radialis tendon reflex (radial nerve and C7-T1 spinal cord segments) are easily and consistently elicited in the foal. The withdrawal flexor reflex (musculocutaneous, median, and ulnar nerves, and C7 to T1 spinal cord segments) is also hyperreflexic compared to the adult. A marked reflex extension of the contralateral limb accompanies this forelimb flexion, and this prominent crossed extensor reflex can be present until 3 weeks of age [3]. In lateral recumbency the hindlimbs of foals have been observed to have less resting extensor tone than the forelimbs, but still more than the adult. In the newborn foal the patellar reflex (femoral nerve, L4–L5 spinal cord segments) is hyperreflexic, and can even exhibit clonus [3]. The gastrocnemius tendon reflex (tibial nerve) and the cranial tibial reflex (peroneal nerve) can be elicited consistently. The withdrawal flexor reflex in the hindlimb (sciatic nerve and L6-S2 spinal cord segments) is hyperreflexic and accompanied by crossed extension of the contralateral limb as seen in the forelimb. The recumbent extensor thrust reflex is present during the first 18 hours of life in both fore- and hindlimbs [3]; this reflex is evaluated by stabilizing the fetlock in extension, and then the toe is rapidly extended dorsally so sudden tension on the deep digital flexor tendon is placed. In response, the limb is thrust forcefully into rapid extension. This reflex is very prominent in the hindlimbs, and more difficult to elicit in the forelimbs, possibly because of the increased resting extensor tone of the forelimbs [3].

Locomotor examination is best performed from a distance given minimal acceptance of restraint by the neonate and proximity of the mare. Standing requires normal function of the entire nervous system. The normal neonate positions the thoracic limbs for standing first, a single thoracic limb is abducted for stabilization and the pelvic limbs are quickly extended after the head and neck are thrusted cranially. Appropriate proprioceptive positioning of all limbs relative to the body should be observed upon standing. Scuffing of the hooves while walking is typical, especially until the deciduate hoof capsule wears off. A "bunny hopping" gait of the pelvic limbs when running is common in the first week with neonates assuming a diagonal gait thereafter. Postural reaction testing, which is an assessment of proprioception, can be performed by holding a limb in flexion and observing the contralateral limb reaction time when pushing the trunk off midline. A brisk hop should be observed in the contralateral limb. The neonate affords a chance for examination of spinal nerve function not typically performed in the adult. Withdrawal reflexes can be assessed with hoof testers and a crossed extensor response will be observed in both thoracic and pelvic limbs.

Disturbances of the gait should be localized to intracranial (encephalitides), spinal cord (myelopathy-cervical, thoracolumbar or lumbosacral), or peripheral nervous system (neuropathy, neuromuscular junctionopathy, myopathy). Forebrain disturbances from a primary encephalopathy or secondary to systemic disease causes lethargy and ataxia in the neonate that are challenging to neurolocalize since metabolic perturbations simultaneously depress neuromuscular function. Cranial nerve deficits with ataxia are strong indicators of intracranial disease. Exercised induced weakness with appropriate mentation and cranial nerve examination suggest a peripheral nervous system disorder.

As already noted, the equine neonate normally has a hypermetric gait in all limbs, which is gradually refined after the first few weeks of life. Although the neonatal gait is exaggeratedly hypermetric, intention tremors at rest or with movement should not be observed. Disorders of the cerebellum (abiotrophy, dystrophy, hypoplasia, aplasia) might be evident early in life, although some variants can show progressive disease with common clinical signs of intention tremors, inconsistent menace response with appropriate vision, and ataxia [4–6]. Myelopathies within the cranial neck (spinal cord segments C1–C5) demonstrate tetraparesis and general proprioceptive ataxia in all four limbs with a spastic quality and delayed postural reactions in all limbs. Lateralized spinal cord lesions will result in hemiparesis with delayed postural reaction on the ipsilateral side as opposed to vestibular ataxia, which causes lateralized extensor hypertonus on the contralateral side with normal postural reactions. Malformations of C1 to C3 leading to vertebral canal stenosis and spinal cord compression are common causes of developmental myelopathy in the older foal; however, the neonate might not show clinical evidence of disease. Caudal neck myelopathies (C5–T2) can be differentiated from C1–5 if lower motor neuron weakness is observed in the thoracic limbs. The gait changes from cranial or caudal cervical myelopathy cannot always be differentiated. Horner's syndrome can manifest with spinal cord disease from C1 to T2.

Paraparesis and pelvic general proprioceptive ataxia are hallmarks of thoracolumbar spinal cord dysfunction (spinal cord segments T3–L3). Postural reaction deficits, pelvic limb circumduction and truncal sway when walking can be observed as part of general proprioceptive dysfunction. Lower motor neuron weakness due to myelopathies of the lumbar intumescence or sacral segments show absent or weak weight bearing in the pelvic limbs and varying degrees of urinary and fecal incontinence. Femoral nerve deficits can result in knuckling or walking on the dorsum of the distal metatarsus but is not typical with lesions cranial to the L3 spinal cord segment in the horse unlike other species. Sensory disturbances may occur circumferential to the tail head. Coccygeal segment dysfunction results in loss of anal tone, absent sensation surrounding the tail head and flaccid tail carriage, but thoracic and pelvic limb gait is normal.

A cranial nerve examination (Table 30.I.1) should be performed when assessing the neurologic function of the neonatal foal as cranial nerves, in general, are fully functional within hours of birth. Olfaction is likely significantly developed in the equine neonate based on evidence in other mammals [7]. Examination of olfaction is often limited to waving noxious substances (alcohol-soaked gauze) in front of the nares while monitoring for behavioral withdrawal of the head and is interpreted with caution. Several cranial nerves facilitate vision and position of the eye. In the foal, the angle of the pupil is often ventromedial to the palpebral fissure (Figure 30.I.2a). By 1 month old, the foal's pupil is similar to the adult (Figure 30.I.2b). Foals respond dramatically to visual and auditory cues and particularly to noxious stimuli to the face (cranial nerves II, V, VIII). Foals are visual, demonstrated by avoidance behavior to threatening movements; visual impairment can be assessed by watching environmental engagement of the foal. Within moments of birth, foals blink in response to a flash of bright light, but a functional visual cortex is not necessary for the latter [2, 3]. However, the menace response (e.g. closure of palpebral fissure in response to a sudden menacing gesture aimed toward the eye), is incomplete until 2 weeks of age [2]. The menace response is a measure of the entire visual pathway including the cerebrum (learning and motor response), brainstem (rostral colliculi, facial nucleus), and cerebellum (controlled motor response integrated with vestibular system). Unilateral loss of the menace response can be extracranial and result from intraocular (hyphema, retinal hemorrhage, uveitis, corneal ulcers) or retrobulbar (abscess, hematoma) diseases. Intracranial causes of unilateral loss of menace are typically contralateral diseases within the optic tract, brainstem, cerebrum, or rarely cerebellum due to 80–90% of optic nerve decussation at the chiasm. Bilateral loss of menace response without intraocular disease suggests a disturbance of the CNS from the optic chiasm centrally. Optic, oculomotor, and facial nerve examination via pupillary light and dazzle reflexes, both direct and indirect, are a measure of extracranial and intracranial visual pathways, however the cerebrum is not involved in these reflexes. A pupillary light reflex (PLR) is present at birth, but it is important to evaluate the size of the pupil before the PLR is tested because stress or excitement may cause sympathetic stimulation, which inhibits constriction of the dilated pupils when a

Table 30.I.1 Evaluation of reflexes and cranial nerves in the foal.

Observation	Localization	Result				
Mentation	Forebrain	BAR QR Dull/Lethargic	Stuporous	comatose		
		Nasal septum sensation		Present/Absent		
Head and neck position	Vestibular, spinal accessory	Appropriate				
		Tilt		Left	Right	
		Torticollis		Left	Right	
Menace response	Optic, facial, brainstem, cortex, cerebellum	Appropriate		OU	OD	OS
		Absent		OU	OD	OS
Pupillary light reflex	Optic, oculomotor brainstem	Appropriate (direct/indirect)				
		Absent	Direct	OU	OD	OS
			Indirect	OU	OD	OS
Palpebral and ariculo-palpebral responses	Trigeminal, facial, trochlear, brainstem	Appropriate	Bilateral	OU	OD	OS
	Facial	Ptosis		OU	OD	OS
	Trigeminal	Corneal sensation		OU	OD	OS
Vestibuloocular	Vestibular, oculomotor, trochlear, abducens, brainstem	Conjugate		OU		
		Ophthalmoplegia		OU	OD	OS
Nystagmus	Vestibular, brainstem, cerebellum	Physiologic		OU		
		Horizontal		OU	OD	OS
		Fast phase		Left	Right	
		Vertical		OU	OD	OS
		Rotary		OU	OD	OS
Strabismus	Vestibular, oculomotor Trochlear, abducens Brainstem, cerebellum	Appropriate		OU	OD	OS
	Oculomotor	Ventrolateral		OU	OD	OS
	Trochlear	Extorsion		OU	OD	OS
	Abducens	Medial		OU	OD	OS
Facial symmetry	Facial	Appropriate Paresis/deviation		Left	Right	
Lingual tone	Hypoglossal	Appropriate Paresis/deviation/atrophy		Left	Right	
Jaw tone	Trigeminal	Appropriate Masseter muscle weakness or atrophy		Left	Right	

BAR, bright, alert, responsive; QR, quiet, responsive to stimuli.

bright light is applied into the eye [2]. A slow PLR can be observed in young neonates but should resolve to a normal response time as the foal ages [8]. Vision requires a functional thalamus and occipital (visual) cerebral lobes, whereas the PLR and blink to bright light response requires a functional midbrain, pons, and medulla oblongata. Cortical blindness, specifically occipital lobe impairment, can result in an absent menace response, intact or incomplete PLRs, and resting mydriasis. Mydriasis with an intact PLR and absent menace response are common signs associated with cortical blindness. A complete fundic examination should be performed in any neonate with a visual disturbance.

Vestibuloocular reflexes integrate oculomotor, abducens, and trochlear nerve function with the vestibular system and cerebellum. In this reflex, conjugate eye movement should be observed, without dependence on vision, when the head and neck are moved from side to side. A slow-phase is observed away from the direction of lateral head movement with an intermittent fast-phase toward the direction of movement to correct globe position. Extension of the neck causes a physiologic bilateral ventrolateral strabismus.

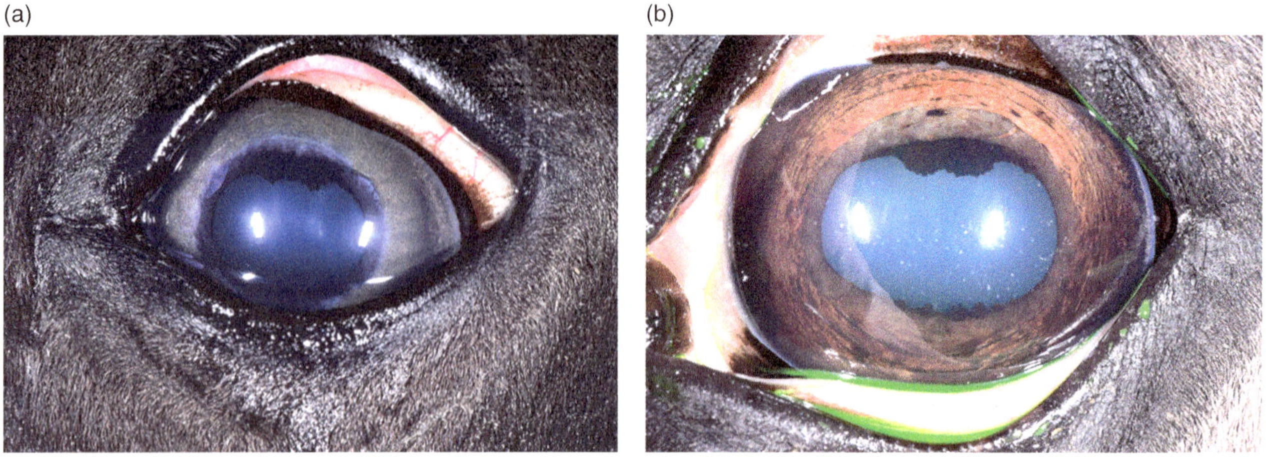

Figure 30.I.2 Position of the pupil within the eye. In a 4-day-old foal, the pupil is positioned ventromedial to the palpebral fissure (a) when compared to the adult horse (b). Note that medial is on the left side in these images.

Horizontal, vertical, or rotary pathologic nystagmus can be induced depending on head position and supports a disturbance of vestibular dysfunction (peripheral/central vestibular or cerebellar). Tilting of the head and abnormal oculocephalic reflexes can accompany vestibular dysfunction, with the head typically tilting ipsilateral to disease location. Differentiation of central from peripheral vestibular dysfunction is supported by centralizing clinical signs of other cranial nerve deficits, tight circling not influenced by size of confinement, and mentation disturbances.

Palpebral reflexes and behavioral responses to noxious stimuli are assessments of the mixed (sensory and motor) facial and trigeminal nerves function along with cortical integration. A blink reflex should be triggered by periocular touch. Trigeminal nerve dysfunction (sensory) results in absence of a blink or behavioral response to touch on the ipsilateral lesion side, whereas facial nerve dysfunction (motor) will show an absent blink, normal eye retraction, and behavior response to touch ipsilateral to the lesion. The muzzle and tongue deviate contralaterally with unilateral facial nerve deficit. Facial nerve deficits can lead to disturbances of lacrimation, desiccating the cornea and increased risk of corneal ulcer along with the risk of traumatic injury to the eye from lack of blink. Tear film production should be measured with suspected facial neuropathy. Ptosis can be observed with both facial nerve dysfunction and loss of sympathetic tone (Horner's syndrome), although facial nerve dysfunction tends to show a more severe palpebral droop. Horner's syndrome or oculosympathetic paresis in neonates can show varying degrees of ipsilateral ptosis, miosis, enophthalmos, protrusion of the nictitans, and sweating around the ear and eye [9]. Protrusion of the nictitans and ptosis is often mild in the neonate with Horner's syndrome. Sympathetic innervation of the eye begins in the brainstem, descending the spinal cord within the neck to the brachial plexus from where it ascends within the jugular groove to the eye [10]. Injuries to the spinal cord of the neck, brachial plexus, guttural pouch, petrosal temporal bone, or retrobulbar space can result in Horner's syndrome.

Amenable neonatal foals can be placed in dorsal recumbency to screen for induced pathologic nystagmus if vestibular dysfunction is suspected. However, this is not typically necessary since cranial nerve and gait evaluation often shows evidence of vestibular disease. Glossopharyngeal, vagal, and hypoglossal nerve function is orchestrated in the nucleus ambiguus of the brainstem. Foals should be evaluated for the presence of milk in their nostrils after suckling. This is occasionally the result of neurologic disease, pharyngeal paralysis, or congenital cleft palate, but is more commonly associated with weakness from generalized illness. Some healthy foals, particularly those that have not been allowed to suckle, hang their tongues out and suck on them, yet are able to pull their tongue into their mouth normally (Figure 30.I.3) [2].

Sounds made by the newborn foal should be carefully evaluated. A normal whinny or nicker made in response to another horse or following an attempt to stand is considered a sign of an alert foal. Ill foals may develop abnormal vocalizations. Diseases of these nerves manifest as disorders of prehension, dysphagia, weak tongue tone, or abnormalities of phonation. Developmental anomalies of the pharyngeal arch or soft palate should also be considered if the above symptoms are observed [11]. Guttural pouch tympany, empyema, or, rarely, mycosis (more common in the adult) can cause various disturbances of cranial nerves VII–XI along with Horner's syndrome [12]. Spinal accessory nerve influences head and neck position. Head tilt or torticollis without other evidence of vestibular dysfunction or cranial nerve deficits is observed with spinal cord disease affecting the cell bodies of the spinal accessory nerve or spinovestibular tracts.

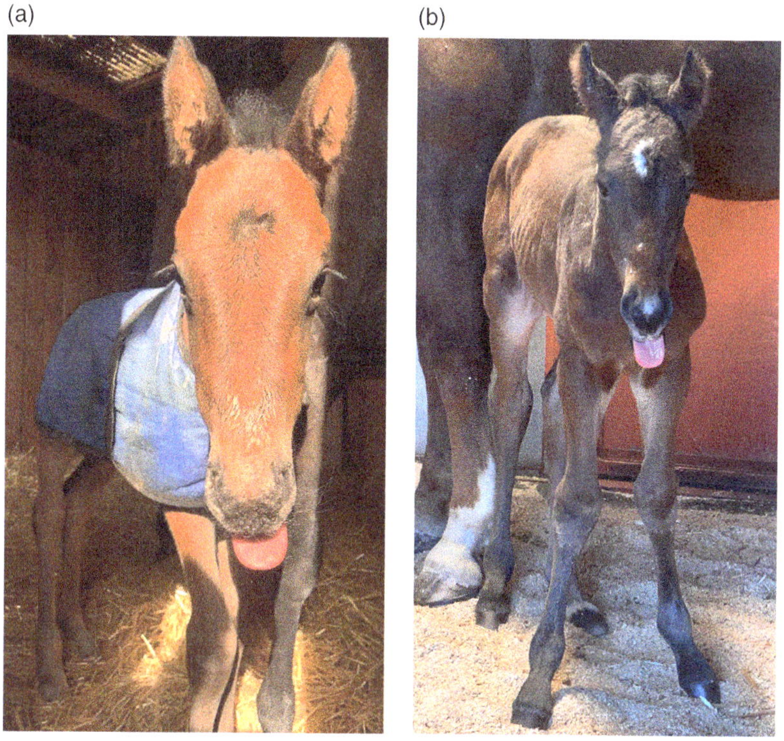

Figure 30.I.3 Examples of (a) two healthy neonates (b) that demonstrate tongue hanging from their mouths. Both foals suckled normally and did not display any signs of disease.

References

1 Wong, D., Wilkins, P.A., Bain, F.T. et al. (2011). Neonatal encephalopathy in foals. *Compend. Contin. Educ. Pract. Vet.* 33: E1–E10.

2 Mayhew, I.G. (1988). Neurological and neuropathological observations on the equine neonate. *Equine Vet. J. Suppl.* 5: 28–33.

3 Adams, R. and Mayhew, I.G. (1984). Neurological examination of newborn foals. *Equine Vet. J.* 16: 306–312.

4 Dungworth, D.L. and Fowler, M.E. (1966). Cerebellar hypoplasia and degeneration in a foal. *Cornell Vet.* 56: 17–24.

5 Cudd, T.A., Mayhew, I.G., and Cottrill, C.M. (1989). Agenesis of the corpus callosum with cerebellar vermian hypoplasia in a foal resembling the Dandy-Walker syndrome: pre-mortem diagnosis by clinical evaluation and CT scanning. *Equine Vet. J.* 21: 378–381.

6 Wong, D., Winter, M., Haynes, J. et al. (2007). Dandy-Walker-like syndrome in a quarter horse colt. *J. Vet. Intern. Med.* 21: 1130–1134.

7 Bloomfield, F.H., Alexander, T., Muelbert, M. et al. (2017). Smell and taste in the preterm infant. *Early Hum. Dev.* 114: 31–34.

8 Enzerink, E. (1998). The menace response and pupillary light reflex in neonatal foals. *Equine Vet. J.* 30: 546–548.

9 Smith, J.S. and Mayhew, I.G. (1977). Horner's syndrome in large animals. *Cornell Vet.* 67: 529–542.

10 DeLahunta, A. and Glass, E. (2009). *Veterinary Neuroanatomy and Clinical Neurology*, 3e. St. Louis, MO: Saunders Elsevier.

11 Holcombe, S.J., Hurcombe, S.D., Barr, B.S. et al. (2012). Dysphagia associated with presumed pharyngeal dysfunction in 16 neonatal foals. *Equine Vet. J.* 44: 105–108.

12 Borges, A.S. and Watanabe, M.J. (2011). Guttural pouch diseases causing neurologic dysfunction in the horse. *Vet. Clin. North Am. Equine Pract.* 27: 545–572.

Section II Cerebrospinal Fluid Collection and Analysis

David Wong

Cerebrospinal fluid (CSF) is an ultrafiltrate of plasma that bathes the entire central nervous system (CNS). The CSF functions to protect the brain from trauma, serves as a physiologic medium to transport compounds (e.g. neurotransmitters), and regulates and maintains the chemical environment of the CNS [1]. Just as in adult horses, evaluation of CSF samples from neonatal foals can help in the diagnostic evaluation of neurologic disease. CSF in the foal is typically collected from the atlanto-occipital (AO) space (Figure 30.II.1), although the lumbosacral space (LS) can also be used. Collection between the first and second cervical vertebrae (C1–C2) is another method reported in standing (sedated) adult horses but has not been described in foals [2]. A brief period of general anesthesia is necessary to collect CSF in foals as the patient needs to be completely immobilized.

A variety of methods can be used to induce anesthesia; one approach is to use diazepam (0.1 mg/kg, IV) and xylazine (0.25 mg/kg, IV) as a premedication followed by ketamine (1.5 mg/kg, IV) to induce anesthesia [3]. Alternatively, foals can be premedicated with xylazine (0.46 mg/kg, IV) and butorphanol (0.02 mg/kg, IV) and anesthesia induced with propofol (2.0 mg/kg, IV) [4]. After induction of anesthesia, the foal should be placed in lateral recumbency and the long axis of the cervical spine and head placed horizontal and parallel with the ground. The haircoat at the collection site (along midline from the poll and moving caudal) should be clipped with a #40 blade and the skin sterilely prepared with antiseptic. The foal's head should be flexed (to open the AO space) so that the median axis of the head is at a right angle to the median axis of the cervical vertebrae (Figure 30.II.2a) [5].

After donning sterile gloves, an 18- or 20-gauge 3.5 in. spinal needle is inserted at the intersection of imaginary lines drawn between the cranial borders of the atlas (C1) and along dorsal midline (Figure 30.II.2b) [5]. The needle is held parallel to the ground and aimed at the lower jaw or lips (perpendicular to the cervical vertebrae) and advanced slowly until the dorsal AO membrane and cervical dura mater are penetrated (Figure 30.II.2c,d). The clinician may feel a "pop" or change in resistance as it penetrates the membrane; the stylet should be withdrawn whenever a perceived change in resistance is felt to check for the presence of CSF. If no CSF is noted, the stylet should be replaced and the needle advanced at 1 mm intervals, checking for the presence of CSF after each advancement. Once the needle is correctly positioned, CSF should flow freely and collect in EDTA and plain tubes (Figure 30.II.2e,f) for cytology, biochemistry analysis, and/or culture. In the neonate, collection of 1–2 ml of CSF should be adequate; this volume minimizes the risk of tentorial hernation [1].

Once CSF is collected, the sample should be analyzed cytologically within 30 minutes of collection as the cells will undergo rapid degeneration because CSF has low concentrations of proteins and lipids (Table 30.II.1). The color of CSF is normally light yellow and clear although xanthochromia and slight turbidity can be a normal finding in newborn foals [6]. Normal CSF has <5 leukocytes/μl and the cell population should consist of monocytes and lymphocytes; neutrophils should not be present. In health, CSF does not contain red blood cells, but is commonly noted in samples due to iatrogenic blood contamination during sample collection [7]; one source suggests a red cell count in CSF in healthy foals of <500 cells/μl [8]. In healthy foals the normal CSF creatine kinase (CK) activity and glucose concentration should be 15 ± 9 U/l, and 80% of the blood glucose concentration, respectively [7]. Of note, the CSF glucose concentration peaks at birth, then decreases over the next 21 days [6]. CSF total protein and creatine

Equine Neonatal Medicine, First Edition. Edited by David M. Wong and Pamela A. Wilkins.

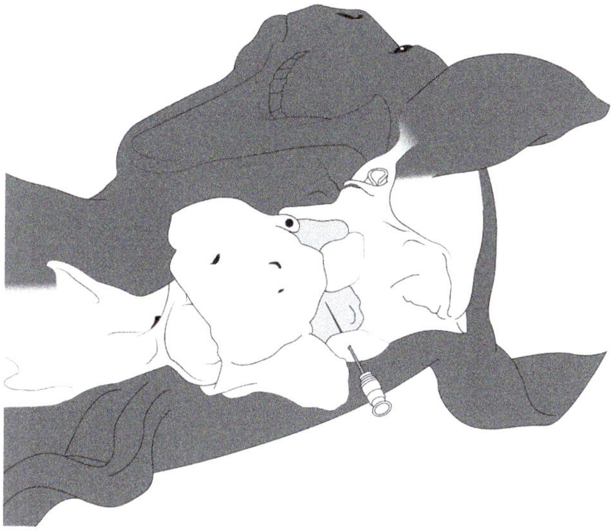

Figure 30.II.1 Drawing illustrating the placement of spinal needle into the AO space. Note cranial edge of the first cervical vertebrae (black dot).

kinase (CK) concentrations are also higher in foals <2 days of age; these higher values may reflect increased permeability in the blood-brain barrier (BBB) of neonatal foals [6, 7]. In one study in foals, no difference was detected in CSF protein when collected from the AO (82.8 ± 19.2 mg/dl) and lumbosacral (83.6 ± 16.1 mg/dl) space [9].

Other reported parameters in CSF from healthy pony foals (21 foals; <40 hours old) include aspartate aminotransferase (mean ± SD 16.1 ± 7.6 iu/l [range 6–26 iu/l]), lactate dehydrogenase (23.2 ± 10.7 iu/l [10–40 iu/l]), gamma glutamyl transferase (1.50 ± 1.5 iu/l [0.9–2.3 iu/l]) and chloride (109 ± 3.4 mmol/l [104–113 mmol/l]) [10]. Acid–base parameters in the CSF have also been evaluated in anesthetized foals (10 foals; <12 days of age) and include: pH 7.389 ± 0.009, PCO_2 37.8 ± 0.97 mmHg, PO_2 141.8 ± 6.79 mmHg, HCO_3 23.1 ± 0.19 mEq/l and TCO_2 24.3 ± 0.20 mEq/l [11].

Pathologic causes of elevated CSF protein include intrathecal hemorrhage, increased local synthesis of immunoglobulins, degeneration of neural tissue, and obstruction of CSF circulation (e.g. cervical vertebral malformations, abscess, tumor) [8]. Additionally, neurologic disease can alter the permeability of the BBB resulting in transudation of serum proteins into the CSF. The integrity of the BBB can be clinically evaluated using the albumin quotient (AQ = CSF albumin/serum albumin × 100). The ratio of albumin concentration in CSF and serum (AQ) is useful to evaluate CSF sample quality as albumin is the most abundant serum protein but is not produced in the CSF and must leak into the CSF from the systemic circulation [12]. Therefore, the total albumin concentration in CSF and the AQ can be compared to assess the integrity of the BBB with elevations in these parameters suggestive of increased BBB permeability or accidental blood contamination of the sample during the collection process [12].

Elevated concentrations of CSF IgG can also indicate abnormal BBB permeability or increased intrathecal synthesis by inflammatory cells [8]. The CSF IgG index is the ratio of total IgG concentration in CSF and serum (CSF IgG/serum IgG ÷ CSF albumin/serum albumin) and can be used to evaluate for intrathecal production of IgG and to further evaluate the BBB [12]. The CSF albumin and IgG concentration along with the AQ and IgG index from healthy foals is reported in Table 30.II.2 [9]. Of note, a statistical difference was not reported between the CSF values calculated when compared between the AO and LS space [9]. A CSF albumin concentration >85.2 mg/dl or an albumin quotient >2.4 may indicate increased BBB permeability, whereas an IgG index value of >1.0 suggests intrathecal IgG production [9].

Some disease processes that alter CSF composition include CNS trauma and septic meningitis. Trauma to the CNS can yield a xanthochromic or serosanguinous CSF with an increased concentration of protein and cell count. Erythrophagocytosis may also be observed. Septic meningitis, while uncommon in foals, can produce a turbid, serosanguineous CSF with increased protein concentration and WBC count (with presence of neutrophils). In one study evaluating septic meningitis in 10 foals, the mean CSF total nucleated cell count was 1215 cells/μl (range 13–5810) and the mean CSF total protein was 395 mg/dl (76–769 mg/dl) [13]. Low CSF glucose concentration may also be noted; an IgG index ≥1 suggests intrathecal IgG production. An increase in CSF CK activity can be observed with neural necrosis or degeneration and has been noted in foals with cerebellar abiotrophy [14].

Complications associated with CSF collection are rare but include alterations in intracranial pressure (ICP), herniation of the cerebrum or cerebellum, introduction of pathogens into the CNS, aseptic meningitis (from hemorrhage and swelling at site of needle entry), and spinal cord or brainstem injury [1]. In one report, cardiovascular sequela was observed after CSF was collected from the AO space. In that case, severe bradycardia (21 beats/min) and unconducted P waves were noted in a 3-month-old colt. Cardiopulmonary resuscitation was performed and was initially successful, but ultimately the foal was euthanized [15].

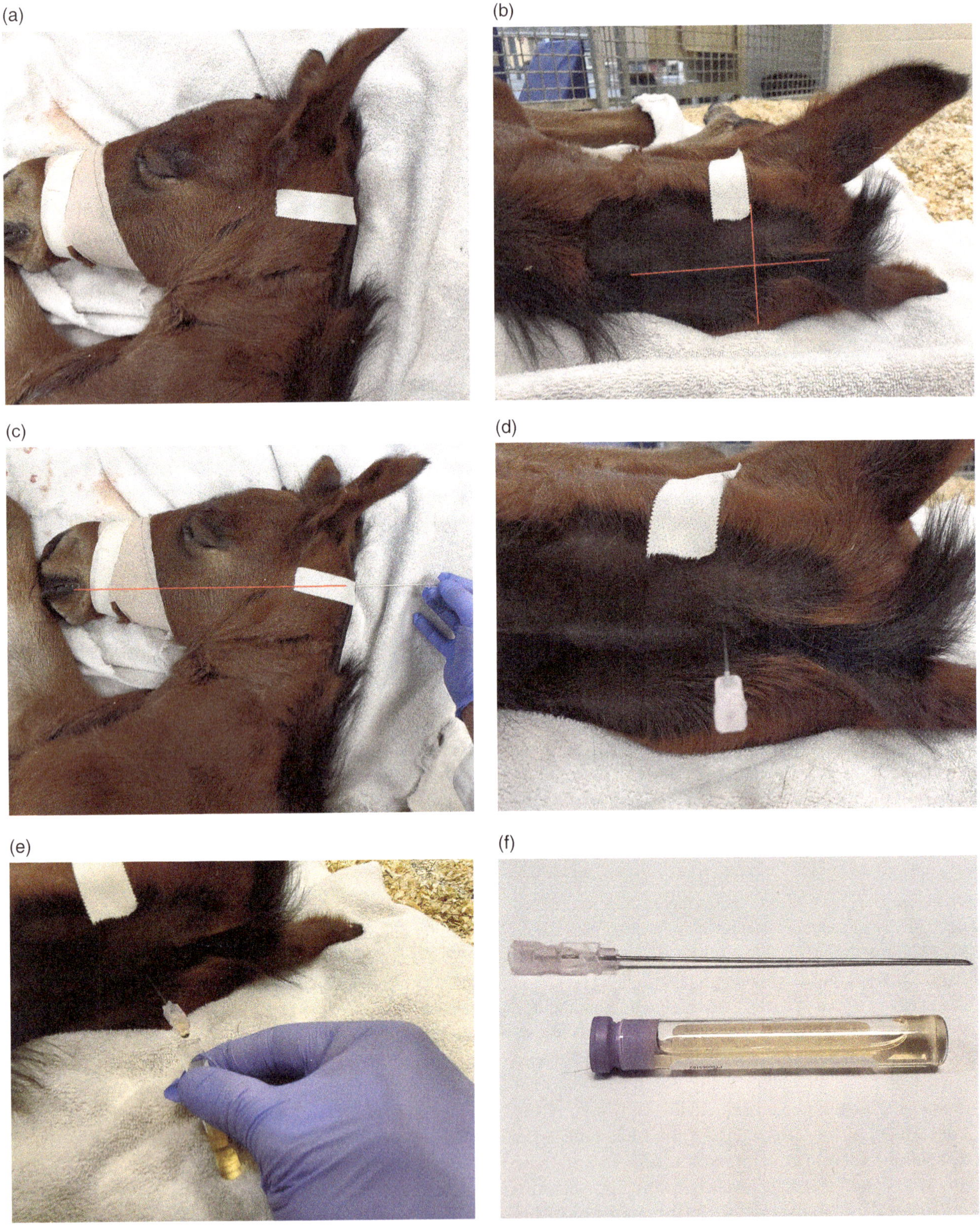

Figure 30.II.2 Technique to collect cerebrospinal fluid (CSF) from an anesthetized foal. (a) Foal is placed in lateral recumbency, the haircoat is clipped, and the skin undergoes sterile preparation. The foal's head should be flexed to open the atlantoaxial space. (b) The needle is inserted at the intersection of lines drawn between the cranial borders of the first cervical vertebra (C1; marked by white tape in image) and along the dorsal midline (red lines). (c) The needle is held parallel to the ground and aimed at the lower jaw/lip (red line) and advanced slowly. (d) The needle is advanced until a slight change in resistance is felt during insertion; the stylet is then withdrawn to see if free flow of CSF occurs. (e) If no CSF is noted, the stylet is replaced and the needle advanced in 1 mm intervals, checking for the presence of CSF after each advancement. (f) Once in the correct position, CSF should flow freely and collected into appropriate sterile tubes. In this case, the CSF has slight xanthochromia.

Table 30.II.1 Cerebrospinal fluid reference values in foals [6].

Age (d)	Glucose (mg/dl)	Protein (mg/dl)	Magnesium (mg/dl)	Sodium (mmol/l)	Potassium (mmol/l)
1.1 ± 0.4	98.8 ± 12.0	109.0 ± 9.7	2.43 ± 0.16	148.0 ± 7.2	3.01 ± 0.17
11.7 ± 1.5	76.3 ± 12.0	81.0 ± 22.8	2.51 ± 0.08	152.2 ± 1.2	3.60 ± 1.12
21.0 ± 0.0	65.3 ± 4.5	60.5 ± 22.4	2.65 ± 0.05	153.8 ± 2.5	3.06 ± 0.08
36.5 ± 6.3	70.0 ± 5.4	58.5 ± 17.0	2.55 ± 0.09	151.7 ± 1.5	2.96 ± 0.08
Adult	51.1 ± 2.5	60.3 ± 10.8	2.35 ± 0.09	152.3 ± 4.2	3.02 ± 0.08

Table 30.II.2 Cerebrospinal fluid albumin, albumin quotient (AQ), IgG, and IgG index from healthy foals; CSF collected from the AO and LS space [9].

	CSF albumin (mg/dl)	Albumin quotient	CSF IgG	IgG index
AO space	52.0 ± 8.6	1.86 ± 0.29	10.2 ± 5.5	0.519 ± 0.284
LS space	53.8 ± 15.7	1.85 ± 0.51	9.9 ± 5.7	0.482 ± 0.270
Interpretation of blood brain barrier permeability patterns:				
• Normal blood-CSF permeability			Normal CSF albumin, AQ, and IgG Index	
• Intrathecal IgG production, normal blood-CSF permeability:			Normal CSF albumin, AQ, increased IgG Index	
• Increased blood-CSF permeability w/o intrathecal IgG production:			Increased CSF albumin and AQ, normal IgG Index	
• Increased blood-CSF permeability with intrathecal production of IgG			Increased CSF albumin, AQ, and IgG index	

References

1 Furr, M. (2015). Cerebrospinal fluid and the blood-brain barrier. In: *Equine Neurology* (ed. M. Furr and S. Reed), 21–35. Ames Iowa: Wiley Blackwell.

2 Pease, A., Behan, A., and Bohart, G. (2012). Ultrasound-guided cervical centesis to obtain cerebrospinal fluid in the standing horse. *Vet. Radiol. Ultrasound* 53: 92–95.

3 Finno, C.J., Estell, K.E., Katzman, S. et al. (2015). Blood and cerebrospinal fluid α-tocopherol and selenium concentrations in neonatal foals with neuroaxonal dystrophy. *J. Vet. Intern. Med.* 29: 1667–1675.

4 Cook, A.G., Maxwell, V.B., Donaldson, L.L. et al. (2002). Detection of antibodies against Sarcocystis neurona in cerebrospinal fluid from clinically normal neonatal foals. *J. Am. Vet. Med. Assoc.* 220: 208–2011.

5 Mayhew, I.G. (1975). Collection of cerebrospinal fluid from the horse. *Cornell Vet.* 65: 500–511.

6 Furr, M.O. and Bender, H. (1994). Cerebrospinal fluid variables in clinically normal foals from birth to 42 days of age. *Am. J. Vet. Res.* 55: 781–784.

7 Axon, J.E. and Palmer, J.E. (2008). Clinical pathology of the foal. *Vet Clin Equine* 24: 357–385.

8 Siegel, A. (2020). Cerebrospinal fluid. In: *Equine Hematology, Cytology, and Clinical Chemistry*, 2e (ed. R.M. Walton, R.L. Cowell, and A.C. Valenciano), 293–303. Wiley Blackwell.

9 Andrews, F.M., Geiser, D.R., Sommardahl, C.S. et al. (1994). Albumin quotient, IgG concentration, and IgG index determinations in cerebrospinal fluid of neonatal foals. *Am. J. Vet. Res.* 55: 741–745.

10 Rossdale, P.D., Cash, R.S.G., Leadon, D.P. et al. (1982). Biochemical constituents of cerebrospinal fluid in premature and full term foals. *Equine Vet. J.* 14: 134–138.

11 Geiser, D.R., Andrews, F.M., Rohrbach, B.W. et al. (1996). Cerebrospinal fluid acid-base status during normocapnia and acute hypercapnia in equine neonates. *Am. J. Vet. Res.* 57: 1483–1487.

12 Dubey, J.P., Lindsay, D.S., Saville, W.J.A. et al. (2001). A review of Sarcocystis neurona and equine protozoal myeloencephalitis (EPM). *Vet. Parasitol.* 95: 89–131.

13 Viu, J., Jose-Cunilleras, E., Cesarini, C. et al. (2012). Clinical findings in 10 foals with bacterial meningoencephalitis. *Equine Vet. J.* 44: 100–104.

14 Turner-Beatty, M.T., Leipold, H.W., Cash, W. et al. (1985). Cerebellar disease in Arabian horses. *Proceedings of the 31st Annual Convention of American Association Equine Practitioner*, Toronto, 241. AAEP, Toronto.

15 Bennell, A.J. and Bardell, D. (2020). Asystole associated with cerebrospinal fluid collection in a 3-month-old foal under general anaesthesia. *Equine Vet Educ* early view on line.

Section III Electrodiagnostics in the Neonatal Foal

Monica Aleman

Neuroelectrodiagnostic testing is essential for the full investigation of disorders affecting the neurologic, neuromuscular, and muscular systems [1]. Neuroelectrodiagnostics will assist with identification, localization, severity, and follow-up assessment of neurologic abnormalities [1]. Although neuroelectrodiagnostics might not provide a definitive diagnosis in every case; it can provide direction or support of a clinical diagnosis [2]. Depending on diagnostic technique, patient cooperation, and state of health or disease, some techniques can be performed without sedation while others require sedation or general anesthesia [2]. Caution must be practiced when considering sedation and, more importantly, general anesthesia in the compromised ill neonatal foal. Foals with compromised cardiovascular, respiratory, or neuromuscular function or with hypoxic ischemic encephalopathy are not ideal candidates for sedation or anesthesia. Thus, risks and benefits of electrodiagnostic testing in the ill foal must be considered.

Most foals require some level of sedation (light sedation is usually adequate) for instrumentation (e.g. placement of subcutaneous needle electrodes) of specific electrodiagnostic techniques. The diagnostic value of various techniques will not be affected by general anesthesia except for electroencephalography (EEG). On the other end of the spectrum, certain techniques will require general anesthesia because of the application of a painful stimulus such as repetitive nerve stimulation (RNS) and motor and sensory nerve conduction studies (MNC, SNC; respectively) [1]. Examples of techniques that can be performed under sedation include: EEG, brainstem auditory evoked responses (BAER), visual evoked potentials (VEP, helpful for the study of central blindness), blink reflex, electroretinography (ERG, helpful for the study of blindness due to retinal disease), and electromyography (EMG) [2–11]. Single-fiber EMG (SF-EMG) can be done in the sedated animal but is preferred to be performed under anesthesia to avoid movement interfering with the performance and interpretation of results [2]. A variety of specific electrodiagnostic techniques used in foals is discussed below.

Electroencephalography

EEG is the recording of spontaneous electrical activity of the cortical neurons within the cerebral cortex with input from the brainstem, reticular activating system, and thalamus. The electrical activity represents ion changes (mainly sodium and chloride) that occur between the intracellular and extracellular spaces resulting in excitation or inhibition, termed excitatory postsynaptic potentials (EPSP) and inhibitory postsynaptic potentials (IPSP). The extracellular current is what gives rise to the recorded EEG, which is a valuable diagnostic technique for the study of seizures, sleep and sleep disorders, alterations in behavior, and distinguishing abnormal activity such as seizure-like episodes, tremors, myoclonic activity versus seizures, and collapse from cortical origin [12–15]. It is important to mention that a normal EEG study does not rule out seizures or other disorders; it just indicates that the events were not occurring at the time of recording and a second EEG might be necessary. The clinician should attempt to avoid performing an EEG under general anesthesia in the compromised foal; additionally, certain drugs and anesthetics can suppress or alter EEG recordings [16].

Seizures and Epilepsy

EEG along with clinical observations is helpful in the characterization and refinement of epileptic disorders in human medicine. Juvenile idiopathic epilepsy (JIE) of Egyptian Arabian foals is the only phenotypically characterized epileptic disorder in large animal species [12].

Equine Neonatal Medicine, First Edition. Edited by David M. Wong and Pamela A. Wilkins.

The disorder is suspected to be inherited as a dominant trait and affects foals from 2 days to 6 months of age, with a median age at onset of first seizures of 2 months [12]. Preictal events are rare with this disorder and usually spontaneous epileptic events are characterized by flipping backward and generalized tonic–clonic seizures with loss of consciousness occur [12]. Uncommonly, foals might start with a focal facial manifestation (e.g. twitch) but invariably will become generalized with loss of consciousness. Electroencephalographic studies showed epileptiform activity consisting of spikes (70 ms), sharp waves (70–200 ms), and spikes and waves. In most foals, paroxysmal activity is concentrated in the central cortical region before it spreads to other cortical areas of the brain (Figure 30.III.1) [12]. Voltage maximum frequently occurs at midline but at times on either side supporting the multifocal nature of paroxysmal activity. Photic stimulation has been used to induce or increase the number and duration of paroxysmal activity; however, no epileptic activity was seen in foals with JIE [12]. Postictally, foals appear disoriented with some becoming transiently ataxic. Cortical blindness occurs in all cases and lasts from a few seconds to 2–3 weeks, with the majority lasting a few minutes to hours. In all cases, blindness resolves. Interictally, foals appear neurologically normal. The frequency of seizures is variable. This self-limiting disorder apparently subsides by 1 year of age in most cases with a few horses up to 18 months old. Foals are clinically healthy provided no complications occur from seizures. Complications such as corneal ulceration from trauma and aspiration pneumonia from transient dysphagia following seizures can occur. Antiepileptic drugs such as diazepam or midazolam can be used in emergent situations (e.g. onset of seizure) or to manage seizures short-term. Most foals are managed long-term successfully with oral phenobarbital sodium, potassium bromide, or levetiracetam. Successful management must be discussed with the owner since success does not equal resolution. Rather, it means decreasing the frequency and severity of seizures while the foal outgrows epilepsy. However, in some cases seizures might not occur while on therapy. Striking similarities in phenotype including early onset and mode of inheritance to human neonatal and familial epileptic disorders caused by gene mutations exist; this raises the possibility that JIE might also be a familial, inherited disorder.

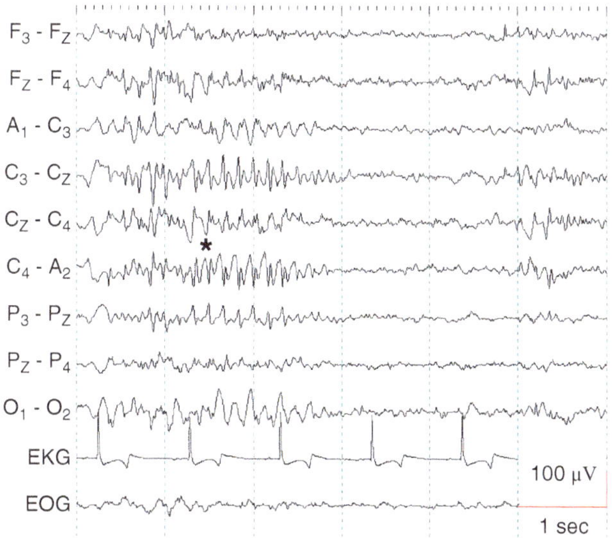

Figure 30.III.1 Paroxysmal activity in a 4-week-old colt. *Source:* Figure from Aleman et al. with permission [12].

Other disorder that can manifest with seizures includes lavender foal syndrome in Egyptian Arabian foals [17, 18]. This syndrome is a lethal inherited disorder caused by a frameshift mutation in exon 30 of the myosin Va gene (*MYO5A*) resulting in premature termination of transcription of the myosin Va protein [19]. This protein is part of a complex of proteins involved in the trafficking of melanosomes to keratinocytes, transportation of secretory granules, glutamate receptors, and mRNA in neurons. Foals are born with a dilute coat color and profound neurologic dysfunction such as lateral recumbency with inability to rise or assume sternal recumbency, opisthotonos, intermittent paddling, extensor rigidity, intermittent nystagmus, and ventral strabismus [17, 18].

Seizures can also be observed in foals with neonatal encephalopathy due to hypoxic ischemic injury or persistent elevation of neurosteroids [20, 21]. Seizures have been reported in 22% of foals with neonatal encephalopathy [20]. Septic foals with involvement of the central nervous system or foals with congenital anomalies can also present with seizures [15, 22]. Extracranial causes of seizures such as metabolic and liver disease must be ruled out [15]. Any disorder that might impair the ability of the neonatal foal to nurse will result in hypoglycemia, which, if left untreated, will invariably end up in alterations in mentation and seizures [23]. The effects of antiseizure medication in the patient can also be evaluated through EEG evaluation.

Sleep, Sleep Deprivation, and Sleep Disorders

Sleep disorders occur in the foal. The most common cause of altered sleep is neonatal maladjustment syndrome [24]. Neonatal foals do all their sleep in lateral recumbency (slow wave sleep, rapid eye movement sleep) including preceding drowsy states [24]. Sleeping while standing in neonatal foals is abnormal and will result in a cycle of disturbed sleep. Clinical observations of sleep and EEG in foals aid in the investigation of possible disorders. Sleep deprivation and sleep disorders are not the same [24]. Sleep deprivation is lack of sleep (e.g. constant disruption of sleep by hospital personnel, inability to lay down due to pain); whereas sleep disorders are characterized by primary alterations in sleep (e.g. hypersomnia, narcolepsy, altered rapid eye movement sleep) [24].

Evoked Potentials

Evoked potentials consist of a sequence of peaks (waves) characterized by polarity (negative or positive), latency, amplitude, shape, and distribution; and numbered in sequence (I, II, III, IV, V). These potentials are elicited by visual (visual EP = VEP), auditory (auditory EP = AEP), or electrical stimulation of sensory nerves (somatosensory EP = SEP). The most-used clinical EP in veterinary medicine is flash VEP, brainstem auditory evoked potentials (BAEP) to clicks, and SEP to electric stimulation of nerves. Evoked potentials are so sensitive that they aid in the detection of lesions not identified by clinical or laboratory techniques. Lesions in the three major sensory systems can be detected by delays, decreases of amplitude, or absence of peaks of VEP, AEP, and SEP. Evoked potentials abnormalities are detected by comparison with reference values from age-matched healthy individuals.

Visual Evoked Potentials

VEP evaluate the visual pathway from the retina to the visual cortex with each peak representing the different areas within this pathway. VEP vary with type of visual stimulus such as checkboard versus flash VEP. Transient flash VEP is used in patients who cannot focus on a patterned stimulus such as infants, small children, comatose patients, individuals with poor visual acuity, and animals. Therefore, this is the most commonly used technique in veterinary medicine [25]. VEP studies have been performed in foals demonstrating that they are visual at the time of birth with ongoing refining of the visual pathway continuing during early life [26]. This procedure can be done under light sedation. VEP and retinography aid in the differentiation of cortical (central) versus retinal blindness. Cortical blindness is the most common postictal alteration in Egyptian Arabian foals with JIE [12]. Postictal cortical blindness is also common in other types of epileptic activity [15].

Brainstem Auditory Evoked Response

Brainstem auditory evoked response (BAER) testing evaluates the integrity of the auditory pathway [11]. Five distinct peaks are recognized and represent an area within the auditory pathway such as the cochlear nerve (peak I), cochlear nucleus in the medulla (peak II), olivary nucleus in the medulla (peak III), lateral lemniscus at the pons (peak IV), and caudal colliculus in the midbrain (peak V). Neonatal foals, as prey animals, are born with fully developed hearing and peak latencies (Figure 30.III.2) comparable to adult horses [4, 11]. BAER testing is useful for the detection of complete, partial, uni- or bilateral auditory loss [11]. BAER studies can be performed relatively easy under sedation in foals but can also be performed under general anesthesia without significant alterations in results. Causes of hearing loss in foals include neonatal encephalopathy, sepsis, metabolic derangements such as marked hyperbilirubinemia causing kernicterus, prematurity, congenital, or inherited disorders such as those associated with multiple malformations and coat color patterns (e.g. lethal white foal syndrome), brainstem disease, trauma, and otitis among others [11]. Potential ototoxic drugs such as aminoglycosides commonly used in equine neonatal medicine must be considered [11].

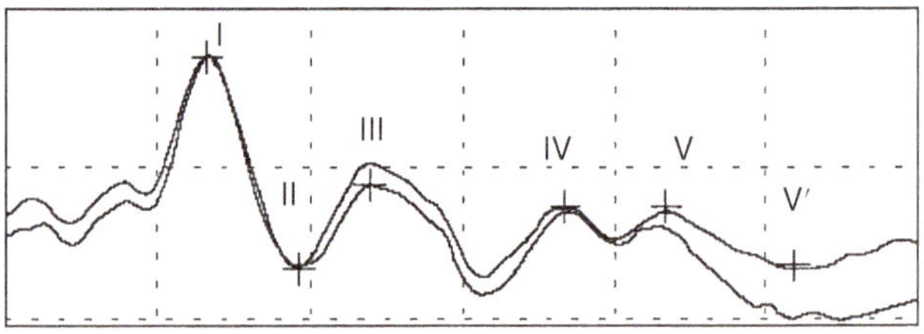

Figure 30.III.2 Normal brainstem auditory evoked response (BAER) from a neonatal foal. Note the various peaks.

Nerve Conduction Velocity

Nerve conduction velocity (NCV) studies evaluate multiple parameters (e.g. amplitude, latency, velocity) of motor and sensory evoked responses to stimulation of nerves [27]. NCV studies of the facial, radial, median, ulnar, lateral and medial palmar and plantar, sural, superficial, and deep peroneal nerves have been reported in adult horses and ponies [6, 28–36]. Because NCV studies are painful, the patient requires general anesthesia, which for the compromised foal might not be ideal.

Repetitive Nerve Stimulation

RNS is one of the most useful diagnostic techniques for the study of neuromuscular disease such as those characterized by myasthenia (muscle weakness) [5]. RNS testing has been used successfully to support botulism as a clinical diagnosis in neonatal foals [5]. Although the technique can be done under sedation, it is considered painful so general anesthesia is preferred. However, risks and benefits must be considered in the foal with compromised cardiovascular, respiratory, or generalized neuromuscular disease.

Electromyography

EMG is the study of the electrical activity of the muscle; the distribution of EMG abnormalities might aid in the localization of spinal cord segments, nerves, or muscles [37]. In acute neuropathic disorders, EMG abnormalities might not be evident immediately [37]. It might take up to 2 weeks to detect EMG alterations [37]. Although EMG usually does not provide a definitive diagnosis, it can support or refute a clinical diagnosis. For example, myotonic discharges are a hallmark feature of myotonic disorders but do not determine a specific myotonic disorder (e.g. myotonia congenita versus myotonia dystrophica or others) [2]. Abnormal activity such as complex repetitive discharges are seen in foals with hyperkalemic periodic paralysis (HYPP) [38]. EMG can be done under light sedation. It is important that the area of muscle to be studied is clean since a needle will be inserted into the muscle and redirected multiple times. Although risk of infection at the EMG site is very low, caution must be practiced in the immunocompromised or septic foal.

References

1 Dumitru, D. and Zwarts, M.J. (2002). The electrodiagnostic medicine consultation: approach and report generation. In: *Electrodiagnostic Medicine*, 2e (ed. D. Dumitru, A.A. Amato, and M.J. Zwarts), 515–540. Philadelphia: Hanley & Belfus, Inc.

2 Aleman, M. (2011). Miscellaneous neurologic or neuromuscular disorders in horses. *Vet. Clin. North Am. Equine Pract.* 27: 481–506.

3 Williams, D.C., Aleman, M., Tharp, B. et al. (2012). Qualitative and quantitative characteristics of the electroencephalogram in normal horses after sedation. *J. Vet. Intern. Med.* 26: 645–653.

4 Aleman, M., Holliday, T.A., Nieto, J.E. et al. (2014). Brainstem auditory evoked responses in an equine patient population: part I--adult horses. *J. Vet. Intern. Med.* 28: 1310–1317.

5 Aleman, M., Williams, D.C., Nieto, J.E. et al. (2011). Repetitive stimulation of the common peroneal nerve as a diagnostic aid for botulism in foals. *J. Vet. Intern. Med.* 25: 365–372.

6 Anor, S., Espadaler, J.M., Monreal, L. et al. (1999). Electrically elicited blink reflex in horses with trigeminal and facial nerve blocks. *Am. J. Vet. Res.* 60: 1287–1291.

7 Wijnberg, I.D. (2005). A review of the use of electromyography (EMG) in equine neurological diseases. *Equine Vet. Educ.* 17: 123–127.

8 Wijnberg, I.D., van der Kolk, J.H., Franssen, H. et al. (2003). Needle electromyography in the horse compared with its principles in man: a review. *Equine Vet. J.* 35: 9–17.

9 Finno, C.J., Aleman, M., Ofri, R. et al. (2012). Electrophysiological studies in American Quarter Horses with neuroaxonal dystrophy. *Vet. Ophthalmol.* 15 (Suppl. 2): 3–7.

10 Strom, L. and Ekesten, B. (2016). Visual evoked potentials in the horse. *BMC Vet. Res.* 12: 120.

11 Aleman, M., Madigan, J.E., Williams, D.C. et al. (2014). Brainstem auditory evoked responses in an equine patient population. Part II: foals. *J. Vet. Intern. Med.* 28: 1318–1324.

12 Aleman, M., Gray, L.C., Williams, D.C. et al. (2006). Juvenile idiopathic epilepsy in Egyptian Arabian foals: 22 cases (1985–2005). *J. Vet. Intern. Med.* 20: 1443–1449.

13 Wijnberg, I.D., van der Ree, M., and van Someren, P. (2013). The applicability of ambulatory electroencephalography (AEEG) in healthy horses and horses with abnormal behaviour or clinical signs of epilepsy. *Vet. Q.* 33: 121–131.

14 Lacombe, V.A., Podell, M., Furr, M. et al. (2001). Diagnostic validity of electroencephalography in equine intracranial disorders. *J. Vet. Intern. Med.* 15: 385–393.

15 Kube, S.A., Aleman, M., Williams, C.D. et al. (2004). How to work up a horse with seizures. *Am. Assoc. Equine Pract.* 418–424.

16 Williams, D.C., Brosnan, R.J., Fletcher, D.J. et al. (2016). Qualitative and quantitative characteristics of the electroencephalogram in normal horses during Administration of Inhaled Anesthesia. *J. Vet. Intern. Med.* 30: 289–303.

17 Page, P., Parker, R., Harper, C. et al. (2006). Clinical, clinicopathologic, postmortem examination findings and familial history of 3 Arabians with lavender foal syndrome. *J. Vet. Intern. Med.* 20: 1491–1494.

18 Fanelli, H.H. (2005). Coat colour dilution lethal ("lavender foal syndrome"): a tetany syndrome of Arabian foals. *Equine Vet. Educ.* 17: 260–263.

19 Brooks, S.A., Gabreski, N., Miller, D. et al. (2010). Whole-genome SNP association in the horse: identification of a deletion in myosin Va responsible for lavender foal syndrome. *PLos Genet.* 6: e1000909.

20 Lyle-Dugas, J., Giguère, S., Mallicote, M.F. et al. (2017). Factors associated with outcome in 94 hospitalised foals

diagnosed with neonatal encephalopathy. *Equine Vet. J.* 49: 207–210.

21 Aleman, M., Pickles, K.J., Conley, A.J. et al. (2013). Abnormal plasma neuroactive progestagen derivatives in ill, neonatal foals presented to the neonatal intensive care unit. *Equine Vet. J.* 45: 661–665.

22 Viu, J., Monreal, L., Jose-Cunilleras, E. et al. (2012). Clinical findings in 10 foals with bacterial meningoencephalitis. *Equine Vet. J. Suppl.* 100–104.

23 Aleman, M., Costa, L.R.R., Crowe, C. et al. (2018). Presumed neuroglycopenia caused by severe hypoglycemia in horses. *J. Vet. Intern. Med.* 32: 1731–1739.

24 Aleman, M., Williams, C.D., and Holliday, T.A. (2008). Sleep and sleep disorders in horses. *Am. Assoc. Equine Pract.* 180–185.

25 Ström, L., Bröjer, J., and Ekesten, B. (2020). Variability, repeatability and test-retest reliability of equine flash visual evoked potentials (FVEPs). *BMC Vet. Res.* 16: 261.

26 Ström, L., Michanek, M., and Ekesten, B. (2019). Age-associated changes in the equine flash visual evoked potential. *Vet. Ophthalmol.* 22: 388–397.

27 Daube, J.R. (1999). Nerve conduction studies. In: *Electrodiagnosis in Clinical Neurology*, 4e (ed. M.J. Aminoff), 253–289. Philadelphia: Churchill Livingstone.

28 Whalen, L.R., Wheeler, D.W., LeCouteur, R.A. et al. (1994). Sensory nerve conduction velocity of the caudal cutaneous sural and medial cutaneous antebrachial nerves of adult horses. *Am. J. Vet. Res.* 55: 892–897.

29 Wheeler, S.J. (1990). Effect of age on sensory nerve conduction velocity in the horse. *Res. Vet. Sci.* 48: 141–144.

30 Wheeler, S.J. (1989). Influence of limb temperature on sensory nerve conduction velocity in horses. *Am. J. Vet. Res.* 50: 1817–1819.

31 Huntington, P.J., Jeffcott, L.B., Friend, S.C. et al. (1989). Australian stringhalt--epidemiological, clinical and neurological investigations. *Equine Vet. J.* 21: 266–273.

32 Zarucco, L., Driessen, B., Scandella, M. et al. (2010). Sensory nerve conduction and nociception in the equine lower forelimb during perineural bupivacaine infusion along the palmar nerves. *Can. J. Vet. Res.* 74: 305–313.

33 Blythe, L.L., Kitchell, R.L., Holliday, T.A. et al. (1983). Sensory nerve conduction velocities in forelimb of ponies. *Am. J. Vet. Res.* 44: 1419–1426.

34 Blythe, L.L., Engel, H.N., and Rowe, K.E. (1988). Comparison of sensory nerve conduction velocities in horses versus ponies. *Am. J. Vet. Res.* 49: 2138–2142.

35 Henry, R.W. and Diesem, C.D. (1981). Proximal equine radial and median motor nerve conduction velocity. *Am. J. Vet. Res.* 42: 1819–1822.

36 Henry, R.W., Diesem, C.D., and Wiechers, D.O. (1979). Evaluation of equine radial and median nerve conduction velocities. *Am. J. Vet. Res.* 40: 1406–1410.

37 Dumitru, D. and Zwarts, M.J. (2002). Needle electromyography. In: *Electrodiagnostics in Diseases of Nerve and Muscle: Principles and Practice* (ed. D. Dumitru, A.A. Amato, and M.J. Zwarts), 257–291. Philadelphia: Hanley & Belfus, Inc.

38 Spier, S.J., Carlson, G.P., Holliday, T.A. et al. (1990). Hyperkalemic periodic paralysis in horses. *J. Am. Vet. Med. Assoc.* 197: 1009–1017.

Section IV Intracranial Pressure Monitoring

David Wong and Cody Alcott

Intracranial pressure (ICP) refers to the pressure exerted by the intracranial contents against the inelastic cranial vault [1]. Cerebral blood flow (CBF) is obviously critical for normal brain function and is impacted by increases in ICP and mean arterial pressure (MAP). CBF can be expressed by the formula for cerebral perfusion pressure (CPP) as CPP = MAP–ICP [1]. In infants, intracranial hypertension is generally defined as ICP >20 mmHg [2]. ICP monitoring is not routinely indicated in infants and children with mild or moderate head injury, based on the Glasgow Coma Score, but various pediatric studies have demonstrated an association between intracranial hypertension and poor neurologic outcome and/or increased mortality rate in more severe cases, thus supporting monitoring and treatment of intracranial hypertension in some instances [3]. Treatment and control of ICP within the reference range is intended to maintain adequate CPP, oxygenation, and metabolic substrate delivery to the brain and avoid cerebral herniation [3].

In comparison to neonatal infants with open fontanelles, the skull of the equine neonate is less forgiving because of the inelastic characteristics of the two main dural processes, the falx cerebri and membranous tentorium, and the complete nature of the skull [4, 5]. Therefore, increases in ICP are not well tolerated in the neonatal foal [5]. Currently, ICP monitoring is not a routine diagnostic performed in foals but the technique might be of benefit in certain clinical scenarios in which intracranial volume is increased such as head trauma, cerebral edema (noted on imaging), congenital anomalies of the central nervous system (CNS), meningitis or other acquired CNS disorders in the neonatal foal [5–7]. Such disorders of the CNS can manifest as seizures, ataxia, decreased ability to suckle, head-pressing, abnormal mentation, and motor dysfunction [5–8]. Cerebral edema and cerebellar herniation are other situations in which ICP monitoring may be indicated. One case series described four neonatal foals with confirmed or suspected sepsis that had clinical signs of altered mental status (e.g. comatose), seizures, abnormal respiratory pattern/respiratory arrest, and dilated unresponsive pupils that were noted to have cerebellar herniation of the cerebellum or cerebellar vermis in extremis [5]. Postmortem examination revealed herniation of the cerebellum or cerebellar vermis through the foramen magnum and cerebral edema.

A protocol to measure ICP has been documented in neonatal foals in which a subdural catheter was placed in healthy 3- to 4-hour-old newborn foals by sedating the foals and placing them in right lateral recumbency [4]. As described, the hair over the center of the coronal skull suture is clipped and the skin is surgically prepared. Local anesthetic is infiltrated into the subcutaneous and periosteal tissues and a 6-cm skin incision is made, centered over the coronal suture line, 2 cm left of midline. A small burr hole is subsequently created in the skull using an electric Dremel drill or pneumatic drill (Surgairtome, Linvated Inc., Key Largo, Florida) and 4-mm round cutting burr followed by perforation of the dura mater. A 2.7 mm Holter intraventricular catheter (e.g. Codman MicroSensor ICP transducer) or an 8 French, 2.7 mm Sovereign soft catheter is inserted into the subdural space so that the distal perforations are covered by dura mater (distance of 2–6 cm) [1, 4]. The distal end of the catheter is then tunneled out through a separate stab incision 1 cm distal to the surgical incision and an 18-gauge blunt needle is placed at the end of the catheter with the end of the needle fitted with an infusion plug (Figure 30.IV.1). The subdural catheter is then filled with sterile saline; patency and position can be verified by the observation of increased ICP when the jugular vein is occluded and a return to baseline values when the jugular is released. The skin incision is apposed with suture material and a sterile bandage is placed over the catheter and incision. To measure ICP, the foal is placed in right lateral recumbency with the head and neck in a neutral position. The subdural catheter is attached to a transducer system with the right external acoustic meatus used as the zero-reference level for ICP measurements.

Equine Neonatal Medicine, First Edition. Edited by David M. Wong and Pamela A. Wilkins.

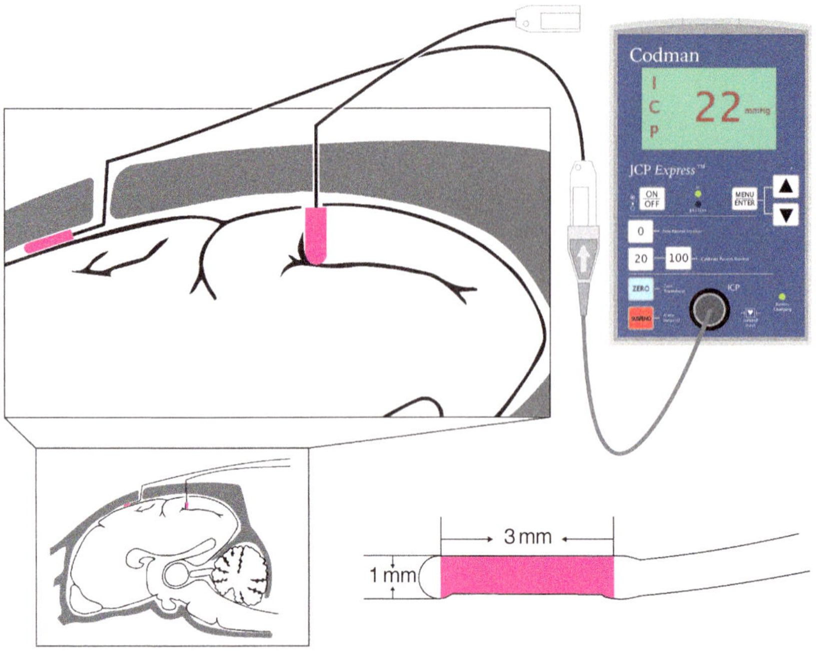

Figure 30.IV.1 Schematic drawing illustrating the subdural and intraparenchymal placement of Codman MicroSensor transducers. The cable interfaces with and intracranial pressure (ICP) monitoring to display ICP measurement.

ICP measurements in the eight healthy foals were recorded every 24 hours, starting at approximately 6 hours of age, for three readings [4]. Over this time, the mean ± standard deviation ICP was 5.83 ± 1.82, 8.81 ± 2.06, and 9.55 ± 1.55 mmHg for each 24-hour period, respectively. The CPP was calculated at 80.19 ± 10.34, 75.30 ± 10.86, and 76.80 ± 12.59 mmHg for each of the 24-hour periods, respectively. Of note, the clinical and neurologic examinations of the eight foals in this study were normal during and after the procedure and none of the foals had any side effects to the procedure. However, one foal developed generalized seizures at 21 days of age and was subsequently euthanized. Postmortem examination revealed that the dura mater was fused to the surface of the left occipital lobe with microscopic examination noting focal fibrosis of the dura mater of the left occipital lobe and a thin layer of granulation tissue adhered to the underlying subpial neuropil [4]. Interestingly, ICP was measured in adult horses in another study and noted a general trend of lower ICP values (2 ± 4, range −3 to 7 mmHg) and higher CPP measurements (101 ± 22, 78–152 mmHg) [9]. The practicality and usefulness of ICP in neonatal foals remains to be determined.

References

1 Sturges, B.K., Dickson, P.J., Tripp, L.D. et al. (2019). Intracranial pressure monitoring in normal dogs using subdural and intraparenchymal miniature strain-gauge transducers. *J. Vet. Intern. Med.* 33: 708–716.

2 Citerio, G., Prisco, L., Oddo, M. et al. (2019). International prospective observational study on intracranial pressure in intensive care (ICU): the SYNAPSE-ICU study protocol. *BMJ* 9: e026552.

3 Adelson, P.D., Bratton, S.L., Carney, N.A. et al. (2003). Guidelines for the acute medical management of severe traumatic brain injury in infants, children, and adolescents. Chapter 5. Indications for intracranial pressure monitoring in pediatric patients with severe traumatic brain injury. *Pediatr. Crit. Care Med.* 4 (3 Suppl): S19–S24.

4 Kortz, G.D., Madigan, J.E., Goetzman, B.W. et al. (1995). Intracranial pressure and cerebral perfusion pressure in clinically normal equine neonates. *Am. J. Vet. Res.* 56: 1351–1355.

5 Kortz, G.D., Madigan, J.E., Lakritz, J. et al. (1992). Cerebral edema and cerebellar herniation in four equine neonates. *Equine Vet. J.* 24: 63–66.

6 Anderson, J.M., Hecht, S., and Kalck, K.A. (2012). What is your diagnosis? Skull fracture in a foal. *J. Am. Vet. Med. Assoc.* 241: 181–183.

7 Hardefeldt, L.Y. (2014). Hyponatraemic encephalopathy in azotaemic neonatal foals: four cases. *Aust. Vet. J.* 92: 488–491.

8 Feary, D.J., Magdesian, K.G., Aleman, M.A. et al. (2007). Traumatic brain injury in horses: 34 cases (1994–2004). *J. Am. Vet. Med. Assoc.* 231: 259–266.

9 Brosnan, R.J., LeCouteur, R.A., Steffy, E.P. et al. (2002). Direct measurement of intracranial pressure in adult horses. *Am. J. Vet. Res.* 63: 1252–1256.

Section V Medications Acting on the Neonatal Nervous System

Edwina Wilkes

Diseases affecting the central nervous system (CNS) in foals are often encountered in equine practice. When considering treatment of CNS diseases, some unique features must be considered for appropriate pharmacological management. Neonatal encephalopathy is the most common neurologic condition affecting equine neonates with similarities to perinatal asphyxia syndrome (PAS) in human infants (Chapter 32). Other conditions that affect the neonatal CNS include trauma, bacterial meningitis/meningoencephalitis and less commonly, cerebellar abiotrophy, juvenile idiopathic epilepsy (Egyptian Arabian foals), equine degenerative myeloencephalopathy (EDM), and hydrocephalus. This chapter discusses important pharmacologic principles with reference to the neonatal CNS, specific drugs targeting the CNS, antimicrobial and anti-inflammatory therapy, drugs for the treatment of cerebral edema and other medications including antioxidants and free radical scavengers. These treatments are not necessarily specific for a particular disease as there is often overlap in treatment regimens for different diseases (Table 30.V.1).

Principles of Pharmacology (with Special Reference to the Neonatal CNS)

The blood-brain barrier (BBB) has the important function of maintaining the specific microenvironment required for brain homeostasis and providing protection from neurotoxic compounds that may be present in the systemic circulation [1]. The BBB is structured as a layer of endothelial cells surrounding the cerebral microvasculature, forming a tight barrier which directly influences the entry of pharmaceuticals into the brain (Figure 30.V.1) [1–3]. The BBB can be a major barrier in the effective delivery of therapeutic substances to the brain with more than 95% of drug candidates intended for the CNS restricted by the BBB [4, 5]. Other potential drug delivery routes to the brain used in people include intranasal and intrathecal (cerebrospinal fluid [CSF]) delivery [5], but these methods are not practical for routine use in horses.

Key features in the structure of the BBB include the interstitial cell space and tight junctions, providing a selective barrier between the brain parenchyma and blood [5]. Molecular weight, lipid solubility, ionization, and degree of plasma protein binding are important physicochemical properties of a drug, which determine its ability to penetrate the brain and CSF [6]. Only small, lipophilic compounds including oxygen or steroid hormones readily diffuse across the BBB [1]. Highly protein bound drugs have reduced capacity to cross the BBB [7, 8]. Some drugs with properties that would normally permit passive movement through the BBB capillary endothelium are actively transported from the endothelium back into the blood by carrier-mediated transport that has an affinity for some of these drugs [9]. The BBB of neonatal foals has increased permeability compared to adult horses [10]. Moreover, certain pathological states such as meningeal inflammation, infection, or damage to the BBB can compromise the integrity of the BBB, which can subsequently result in higher concentrations of drugs crossing the BBB; the significance of this varies between individual cases [6, 9, 11].

Other important pharmacological considerations associated with the unique physiology of the neonatal foal include absorption, distribution, metabolism, and/or elimination of drugs, which can differ significantly between foals and adult horses. Hence, caution is required when extrapolating doses from adult horses or other species. The volume of distribution for some drugs may vary with the age of the horse due to the high body water (and low fat) content of foals [12]. Polar drugs have larger volumes of distribution in foals and therefore, higher doses are required to attain the same plasma and tissue concentration as adults [13]. Additionally, foals have a lower serum

Equine Neonatal Medicine, First Edition. Edited by David M. Wong and Pamela A. Wilkins.

Table 30.V.1 Diseases affecting the central nervous system of foals and recommended treatment regimens.

Diagnosis	Anti-convulsants	Systemic antimicrobials	NSAIDs	Systemic corticosteroids	Anti-oxidants	Hyper-osmolar agents	Comments
Bacterial meningitis	•	•	•	•			
NE	•	•		Consider single adjunctive dose	•		
Cerebellar abiotrophy	•	•	•	•	•	•	Euthanasia typically recommended
Juvenile idiopathic epilepsy	•						Deep bedding, pad stall, and headgear to avoid trauma
EDM							Unlikely to be cured
Hydrocephalus							Euthanasia typically recommended

NE-neonatal encephalopathy; EDM-equine degenerative myelopathy constant rate infusion; NE, neonatal encephalopathy.
These treatments are in addition to general supportive and nursing care which is important in the management of critically ill neonates.

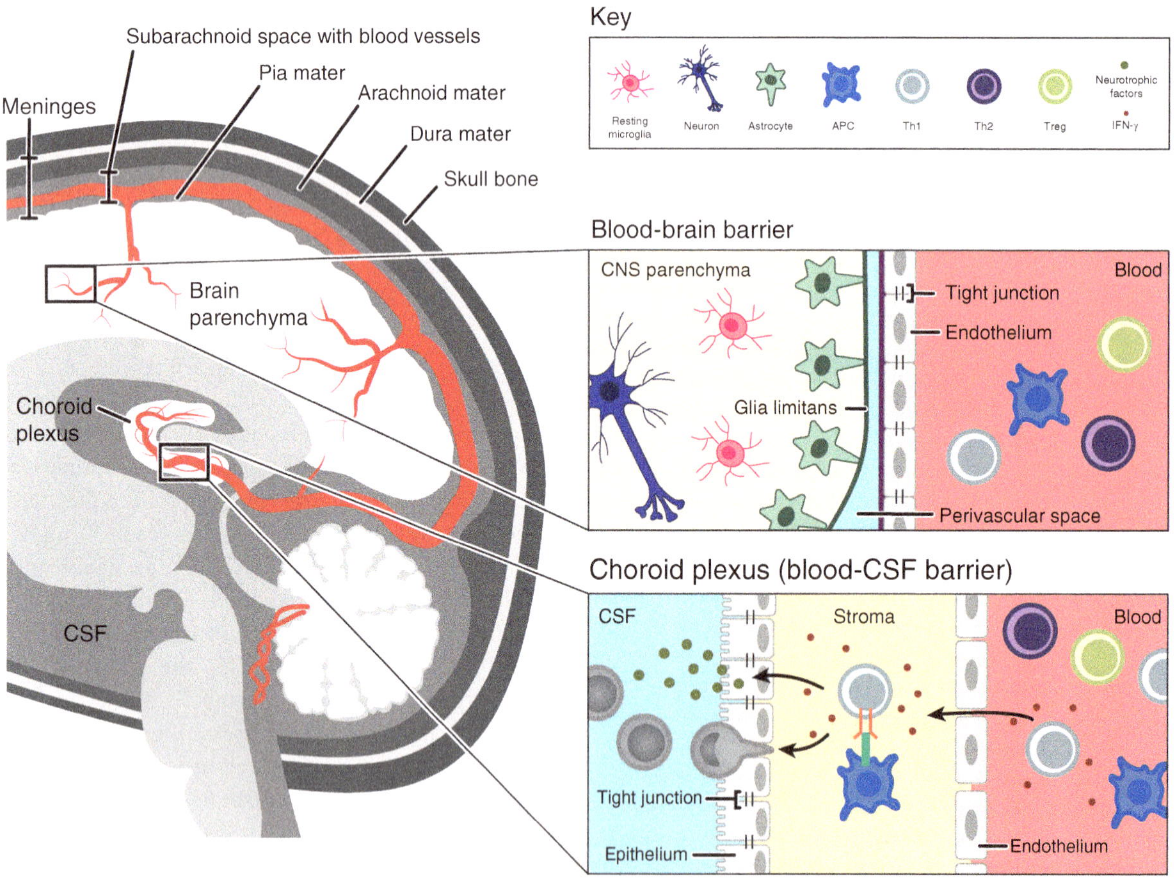

Figure 30.V.1 Central nervous system (CNS) borders. The blood–brain barrier (BBB) at the parenchymal vasculature and the meninges consists of a layer of endothelial cells (interconnected by tight junctions) and glia limitans (a surface made of astrocyte foot processes). The blood–CSF barrier (BCSFB) at the choroid plexus (CP) is a structure located in brain ventricles and comprises an endothelial wall of fenestrated blood capillaries and a monolayer of tight junction-connected epithelial cells. Whereas the BBB remains impermeable to immune cells under physiological conditions, the CP is viewed as a site of constant brain–immune dialogue, which supports CNS function by controlling leukocyte trafficking to the CNS territory and maintains the production of neurotropic factors from the CP epithelium. Abbreviations: APC, antigen presenting cell; IFN, interferon; Th1/2, type 1/2 T helper cell; Treg, regulatory T cell.

total protein concentration compared to adult horses [14] and when using highly protein bound drugs there may be a higher concentration of unbound/free drug in the serum compared to adult horses. The unbound fraction is active, and particular caution is required when using drugs with a narrow therapeutic index as this could result in toxicity [13]. Other pharmacologic considerations include longer elimination half-lives and decreased rates of clearance for some drugs when administered to foals, compared to adult horses. This is a result of overall decreased metabolic and excretory capacity in foals associated with gradual maturation of hepatic and renal function [13].

The pathophysiology and diagnosis of diseases affecting the neonatal CNS are discussed elsewhere in the text. For a number of these diseases, the treatment principles are consistent with some common goals of therapy for each disease. These include general supportive care, control of seizures, systemic antimicrobial therapy for the prevention/treatment of sepsis, and treatment of cerebral edema (Table 30.V.1) [15].

Specific Drugs Targeting the CNS

Anticonvulsant Drugs

Seizures are a common manifestation of neurological disease in the neonatal foal. Foals with neonatal encephalopathy often present with seizure activity of varying severity resulting from brain hypoxia. Hence, seizure control is an important feature of the treatment regimen for these foals. Prolonged, inadequately controlled seizure activity increases cerebral oxygen requirements and results in permanent neurologic injury [16]. The rationale behind the use of anticonvulsant drugs is to reduce the incidence, duration, and severity of seizures. Anticonvulsants can prevent spread of the seizure focus, increase the seizure threshold and decrease electrical excitement of abnormal neurons while maintaining normal function [17]. Table 30.V.2 lists anticonvulsants recommended for seizure control and prevention in foals. Additionally, accumulation of the excitatory neurotransmitter glutamate appears to contribute to the pathogenesis of neonatal encephalopathy and several agents used for seizure control in foals inhibit the release of glutamate (e.g. magnesium sulphate, potassium bromide, gabapentin, phenytoin).

Benzodiazepines

Benzodiazepines are recommended as first line drugs for the treatment of seizures, regardless of severity. High lipid solubility ensures rapid transport across the BBB [3]. Benzodiazepines potentiate the activity of endogenous gamma-aminobutyric acid (GABA), the major inhibitory neurotransmitter of the CNS. Benzodiazepines bind to a specific GABA binding site and activate GABA-gated chloride channels to increase chloride conductance resulting in hyperpolarization of the neuron and suppression of neuronal activity [3, 17]. Adverse effects such as respiratory depression or arrest might occur with prolonged use (multiple repeated doses) of benzodiazepines in foals [20].

Diazepam

Diazepam is used preferentially over other benzodiazepines for treatment of seizures as there is rapid distribution to the CNS following IV administration [17]. The limbic, thalamic, and hypothalamic regions of the CNS are depressed by diazepam producing anxiolytic, sedative, skeletal muscle relaxant, and anticonvulsant effects. Diazepam is highly lipophilic, has a large volume of distribution, rapid onset of action and is 99% protein bound [17, 21]. Once present in the systemic circulation, it undergoes rapid and extensive hepatic metabolism (first-pass-effect) to several pharmacologically active metabolites and is eliminated in the urine [22]. There are slight variations in the pharmacokinetic disposition of diazepam during the foal's first 21 days of life associated with changes in body composition and hepatic enzyme activity [20]. The volume of disposition is lower and clearance of diazepam is slower at 4 days of age compared to 21 days but the terminal half-life is not affected by age [20]. The dose ranges from 0.05–0.4 mg/kg, IV; repeated doses may be necessary to achieve adequate seizure control.

Midazolam

Midazolam is a water-soluble benzodiazepine with pharmacological and chemical structure properties similar to diazepam [21]. Midazolam has greater lipid solubility than diazepam, resulting in more rapid onset of action. It is also approximately three to four times more potent than diazepam and is 95% protein bound. Midazolam is shorter acting than diazepam with regard to metabolism and plasma clearance [21]; this characteristic allows reassessment of neurologic function shortly (1–2 hours) after discontinuation of the drug. The dose ranges from 0.05–0.2 mg/kg IV; a constant rate infusion (CRI) of 0.02–0.12 mg/kg/h (3–6 mg/h for 50 kg foal) can also be used. The lowest effective dose should be used and given slowly to avoid hypotension and respiratory depression. A CRI is recommended when there is inadequate response to single bolus doses or if more than two seizure episodes occur. The duration of the CRI required varies between individuals, but most foals respond within 72 hours; thus, the negative effects associated with long-term sedation that have been reported in human neonates are less likely in neonatal foals.

Phenobarbital

Phenobarbital is the most frequently used first-line antiepileptic agent in human neonates [23]. It is the most commonly used anticonvulsant in adult horses and used as maintenance therapy as well as occasionally for the initial

Table 30.V.2 Recommended anticonvulsant therapy for control and/or prevention of seizures in foals.

Drug	Indication	Dose	Adverse effects	Comments
Diazepam	Initial therapy for seizure control	0.05–0.4 mg/kg, IV	Respiratory depression or arrest after multiple repeated doses	Rapid onset of action. Repeated doses may be necessary to achieve adequate control
Midazolam	Initial therapy for seizure control; use CRI for recurrent seizures	0.05–0.2 mg/kg, IV 0.02–0.12 mg/kg/h (CRI)	Respiratory depression or arrest, hypotension	Rapid onset of action CRI used if inadequate response to single bolus doses or if >2 seizure episodes
Phenobarbital	Maintenance therapy for prevention of seizures	Loading dose: 16–20 mg/kg, IV diluted in 30 ml saline over 30 min Maintenance: 2–10 mg/kg, IV slowly over 20 min q8–12h or 4–10 mg/kg PO q12h	Sedation up to 8 h after administration; respiratory depression; bradycardia; hypotension; hypothermia	Bioavailability close to 100%; causes induction of hepatic cytochrome P450 complex; therapeutic monitoring recommended; dosage adjustments may be required after long-term therapy
Levetiracetam	Limited use in foals; used in other species for control of recurrent seizures	32 mg/kg, IV or PO q12h	Not yet reported in foals; sedation reported in dogs with initial dosing	Therapeutic range and target plasma concentration not established in foals
Potassium bromide	Maintenance therapy for prevention of seizures	25 mg/kg, PO q24h; 20% increase or decrease dose as required q2wk	Profound sedation, ataxia, proprioceptive deficits	May be more useful than phenobarbital for long-term maintenance of epilepsy
Magnesium sulphate ($MgSO_4$)	May decrease seizure incidence in foals with NE; Reduce CNS inflammation; inhibit free radical production	250 mg/kg over 1 h, q24h for 3 doses	Muscle tremors, hypotension with high doses	Dose is from human neonatal studies; dose unknown for foals [18, 19]
Gabapentin	Potential therapeutic agent in foals with NE to provide neuroprotection from ischemia	10–15 mg/kg/d PO divided equally given 3–4 times per day	Mild sedation with very high doses	Minimal information regarding clinical efficacy in foals with recurrent seizures
Phenytoin	Initial therapy for seizure control; maintenance therapy for prevention of seizures	1–5 mg/kg, IV or PO q4h up to 6 doses; then 1–5 mg/kg, PO q12h	Obtunded mentation, mild AV block, decreased blood pressure	Low therapeutic index and narrow therapeutic range
Sodium Pentobarbital	Initial therapy for seizure control; short term management (1–3 d) for recurrent seizures	2–10 mg/kg IV to effect	Profound respiratory depression with repeated doses	Control of seizure activity arises from anesthetic effects

AV, atrioventricular; CRI, constant rate infusion; NE, neonatal encephalopathy.

control of seizure activity in neonatal foals. The primary mechanism of action is facilitating neuronal stabilization via GABA receptors in postsynaptic neurons of inhibitory nerve terminals and increasing intracellular chloride conductance [24]. It also inhibits postsynaptic potentials produced by glutamate and voltage-gated calcium channels at excitatory nerve terminals, resulting in an increased seizure threshold [3]. Phenobarbital is well absorbed after oral administration, and the bioavailability in horses is near 100% [25]. The drug undergoes hepatic metabolism with induction of the hepatic cyctochrome P450 enzyme complex, which can result in rapid metabolism of concurrently administered drugs. Dosage adjustments may be required after long-term therapy to maintain serum concentrations within a therapeutic range [24]. The half-life is approximately 12 hours in foals after IV administration. A smaller proportion of the drug is protein bound in foals compared to adults and hence, the half-life is slightly shorter [25–28]. The dose of phenobarbital consists of a loading dose of 20 mg/kg IV diluted in 30 ml saline, administered slowly over 30 minutes followed by a maintenance dose of 2–10 mg/kg IV administered slowly over 20 minutes every 8–12 hours or 4–10 mg/kg PO every 12 hours. The half-life of phenobarbital is unknown after oral maintenance therapy in foals [24].

Therapeutic monitoring of serum concentrations is recommended to ensure adequate anticonvulsant concentrations are reached and to avoid toxicity. This is particularly important due to the variability in half-life, clearance, and metabolism of phenobarbital [24]. It is also important in foals due to alterations in distribution and elimination characteristics of drugs and the effects of hepatic induction and changes in body weight associated with growth [24]. The peak (approximately 2 ± 1.5 hours after oral dose administration) and trough concentration (prior to next dose) should be determined 3 days after initiation of treatment [26]. The therapeutic serum concentration in adult horses is 15–45 μg/ml which has been extrapolated from studies in humans and dogs [29]. An effective nontoxic therapeutic range of 5–30 μg/ml has been reported in foals [30]. Adverse effects in neonatal foals include sedation for up to 8 hours after administration, respiratory depression, bradycardia, hypotension, and hypothermia, particularly with larger doses [24, 28]. Foals should have their body temperature, blood pressure, and respiratory rate monitored during treatment.

Levetiracetam

Levetiracetam is a novel anticonvulsant drug with a nonconventional mechanism of action and has been well studied as an adjunctive therapy for partial epilepsy in human neonates [31]. While phenobarbital remains the most commonly used first-line agent in human neonates, levetiracetam is used as a second-line agent and is thought to be a safer treatment option with similar efficacy to other agents [31]. It has been shown to be safe and efficacious in dogs and is recommended as a second-line agent for seizures in this species. Although the clinical efficacy of levetiracetam for the treatment of seizure activity in neonatal foals requires further investigation, it likely provides a more favorable safety and tolerability profile over other traditional anticonvulsants [32].

Levetiracetam is the S-enantiomer of the ethyl analogue of piracetam and acts through synaptic vesicle glycoprotein 2A (SV2A), a protein thought to be involved in the release of neurotransmitters [33, 34]. The pharmacokinetics of levetiracetam in neonatal foals and adult horses have been investigated, however the therapeutic range and target plasma concentration have not been fully established [35]. Consequently, the accepted therapeutic range in human patients (5–45 mg/l) is currently proposed for veterinary species and a target plasma concentration of 35 mg/l has been used in adult horses [35]. The pharmacokinetics in foals are similar to those reported in adult horses [36] with minor differences in elimination half-life and volume of distribution and clearance, assumed to be attributed to age-related differences in these mechanisms [35].

Levetiracetam is metabolized by beta-esterases in the blood. Characteristics of the drug including minimal protein binding, lack of hepatic metabolism, and few reported drug–drug interactions are responsible for its optimal safety profile in people and are also desirable in foals [35, 36]. Levetiracetam can be administered IV or PO at a dose of 32 mg/kg every 12 hours in neonatal foals and has excellent intragastric bioavailability [35]. Adverse effects in horses have not been reported, but in dogs, sedation is the most common adverse effect with initial dosing [34]. Close monitoring in dogs with impaired renal function is recommended as a result of reduced drug clearance [34], and similar recommendations may be warranted in equine neonates.

Potassium Bromide

Potassium bromide has been used as an anticonvulsant in people since the 1800s, including management of refractory epilepsy in children [37]. It has also been used in the management of epilepsy in dogs. The exact mechanism of action is unknown, but it is believed to cause hyperpolarization of the neuronal membrane through the action of potassium bromide on chloride channels [3]. Electrical activity in the CNS is inhibited as concentrations of bromide increase and hence, seizure initiation is inhibited [37]. Potassium bromide has a synergistic effect with barbiturates and benzodiazepines [3]. There are limited reports on the pharmacokinetics of potassium bromide in horses [37, 38] and the target therapeutic range (700–2400 μg/l) has been extrapolated from other species. Potassium bromide has a shorter half-life in horses compared to other species, therefore dosing regimens for treatment of seizure disorders in horses are different from other species [38].

Few reports document the use of potassium bromide in foals; however, it has been used in the management of juvenile idiopathic epilepsy in three Egyptian Arabian foals when seizures were multiple, frequent, and ineffectively managed with phenobarbital [39]. Potassium bromide may also be more useful than phenobarbital for long-term maintenance of epilepsy as it has fewer side effects [40]. Metabolism of potassium bromide does not involve the liver, therefore it is a safe option for patients with a hepatopathy [39]. Gloves must be worn during administration as it is absorbed readily through intact skin [39]. The dose is 25 mg/kg PO every 24 hours with 20% increases or decreases as required every 2 weeks [39]. Adverse effects in horses include profound sedation, ataxia, and proprioceptive deficits [37] while side effects in other species include various CNS (drowsiness, sedation, stupor, recumbency, ataxia, paresis) and gastrointestinal tract effects (inappetence, weight loss, pancreatitis), along with increased water consumption and urination, muscle pain, and skin disorders [37].

Magnesium Sulphate

Magnesium sulphate is an N-methyl-D-aspartate (NMDA) receptor antagonist. NMDA receptors are a subtype of glutamate receptors, and their activation has been implicated in hypoxic–ischemic encephalopathy (HIE) [41]. A reduction of voltage-dependent magnesium blockade of NMDA current in mechanically injured neurons can be partially restored by increasing extracellular magnesium concentrations. Treatment with magnesium sulphate may decrease the incidence of seizures in foals with HIE, reduce secondary CNS inflammation and associated injury, stabilize cell membranes, and inhibit free radical production [42]. Increasing evidence in human medicine suggests the use of magnesium sulphate for treatment of traumatic brain injury may be associated with worse outcomes [43]. Hyperactivity of the glutamate NMDA receptor occurs within the first hour after brain injury, and the rationale behind the use of a CRI of magnesium during this time is to attenuate this stimulation. It has now been documented that NMDA receptor stimulation at 24 and 48 hours after injury may improve outcome, hence negating the potential beneficial effects of a magnesium infusion [43]. In addition, preclinical studies of magnesium sulphate for near-term HIE in human infants have concluded highly inconsistent histopathological impact of treatment both before and after the insult [42]. The inconsistencies might be related to a lack of temperature control during and after hypoxic ischemia (HI). Although there may be benefit in using magnesium sulphate as an adjunct therapy with hypothermia, further testing in translational animal models is needed [42]. In infants, magnesium sulfate is administered as a dose of 250 mg/kg over 1 hour, IV once daily for three doses. Adverse effects may include muscle tremors and hypotension, however this is usually only seen with very high doses [41].

Gabapentin

Gabapentin is used as an anti-epileptic medication in human medicine, but minimal information is known regarding the clinical efficacy in horses with epilepsy. Currently, the most common use for gabapentin in horses is in the management of neuropathic pain (e.g. severe laminitis). Gabapentin is a synthetic GABA analog that crosses the BBB. The primary mechanism of action is inhibition of excitatory neurotransmitter release (e.g. glutamate) via inhibition of voltage-dependent calcium channels [3]. Gabapentin is a potential therapeutic agent in foals with neonatal encephalopathy based on evidence demonstrating neuroprotection when used in ischemia, both as a sole agent as well as in combination with NMDA antagonists such as magnesium [41]. Pharmacokinetic studies in adult horses have demonstrated its safety at a variety of doses and it is rapidly absorbed after oral administration. Further studies are required to determine the efficacy and most appropriate dose in foals. As elimination of gabapentin occurs via the kidneys, ensuring adequate renal function prior to its use in neonatal foals is recommended. A dose of 10–15 mg/kg/day PO divided equally and given three to four times per day has been extrapolated from the human pediatric dose [41]. Side effects noted in horses include mild sedation after doses of 120 and 160 mg/kg were administered [44]. Gabapentin-related hepatotoxicity and chronic kidney disease has been reported in people [45, 46].

Phenytoin

Phenytoin is a hydantoin derivative that is not commonly used in horses, but has been suggested for anticonvulsant use in foals [3, 40]. Phenytoin reduces the release of the excitatory neurotransmitter glutamate by inactivating voltage-dependent neuronal sodium channels, thus preventing depolarization of the presynaptic neuronal membrane at the excitatory nerve terminal [47]. It also prevents opening of potassium channels leading to an increase in action potential duration and refractory period [3]. Phenytoin has a low therapeutic index and a narrow therapeutic range. Drug interactions leading to alterations in plasma concentrations may alter clearance of phenytoin and therefore should be avoided if possible [48]. In people, phenytoin is a potent inducer of cytochrome P450 microsomal enzyme activity, which can alter the pharmacokinetics of a number of drugs. Although not specifically studied in horses, it is likely that enzyme induction may lead to increased clearance of drugs that are metabolized by the cytochrome P450 pathway [48]. The dose of phenytoin ranges from 1 to 5 mg/kg IV or PO every 4 hours up to 6 doses, then 1–5 mg/kg PO every 12 hours. The bioavailability in horses can be variable; therefore, serum phenytoin concentrations should be determined during treatment [49]. Based on human studies, a steady-state concentration of 5–20 μg/ml is sufficient for effective seizure control [49]. Adverse effects include prolonged obtunded mentation in foals, mild atrioventricular block and decreased blood pressure [24].

Sodium Pentobarbital

Although not recommended for the management of seizure activity in adult horses, sodium pentobarbital has been used for short-term management (1–3 days) of seizures in neonatal foals, particularly in cases where there is poor response to other treatments [24]. Seizure control arises from the anesthetic effects of the drug. A dose of 2–10 mg/kg IV to effect can be used but profound respiratory depression can occur with repeated doses.

Antimicrobial Therapy for CNS Diseases

Infectious disease of the CNS is uncommon in foals, but includes meningitis, abscess formation, osteomyelitis of the vertebral column, infectious discospondylitis, and meningoencephalitis (Figure 30.V.2). Bacterial meningitis is more common in foals <6 months of age than in adults and is a reported complication of sepsis [10, 50]. The incidence of foals with septicemia that develop meningitis/meningoencephalitis is variable and likely a reflection of differences in management of septic foals and the ability to recognize and diagnose infectious disease of the CNS [50]. Diagnosis can be challenging and requires thorough evaluation of the CNS, thus the incidence of infectious disease of the CNS may be underreported.

In contrast to infectious disease in other peripheral sites, bacterial infection of the CNS initially requires disruption of the integrity of the BBB and blood-CSF barrier. Bacterial invasion is enhanced by the lack of immunoglobulins, complement, and leukocytes in the normal composition of the CSF, however, inflammatory cells and mediators are able to penetrate via the disrupted BBB [17]. A severe inflammatory response is initiated via bacterial cell walls of Gram-positive bacteria and endotoxin released from Gram-negative bacteria.

Risk factors for the development of infectious CNS disease in foals include increased permeability of the neonatal BBB and failure of transfer of passive immunity [10, 11, 51]. CNS infections in neonates are most commonly associated with bacteria causing generalized sepsis [50] with a predominance of Gram-negative organisms, particularly enteric bacteria such as *Escherichia coli, Enterobacter,* and *Klebsiella*. This is in contrast to adult horses in which

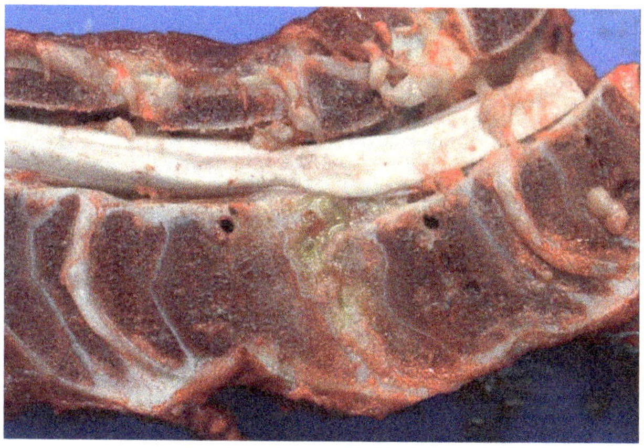

Figure 30.V.2 Postmortem specimen from a 2-week-old Thoroughbred filly presented for acute onset of neurological signs. The filly was unable to stand but was alert and responsive. Infectious discospondylitis and subsequent collapse of the vertebral joint space was note at C6–C7. Septic omphalophlebitis was also present and the likely source of hematogenous infection.

Gram-positive species are more commonly isolated in CNS infections [10]. Other commonly isolated organisms in septic foals include Gram-negative nonenteric bacteria such as *Actinobacillus* and *Pasteurella*. Mixed infections with Gram-negative and Gram-positive bacteria can also occur and include *Streptococci*, *Enterococci,* or *Staphylococci* [13].

Selection of an antimicrobial agent that can readily achieve appropriate concentrations in the CNS or CSF can be challenging [3]. Few antibiotics successfully cross the BBB, and antimicrobials commonly used in neonates for the treatment of sepsis are not adequate to treat bacterial CNS infections due to their lack of adequate CNS penetration [10]. Antimicrobials recommended for the treatment of bacterial CNS infections are summarized in Table 30.V.3. Ideally, antimicrobial selection should be based on culture and sensitivity testing of samples, including blood and CSF. However, empiric broad-spectrum treatment should begin prior to receiving final culture results.

In people, intrathecal injection into the lumbar CSF is a consideration as a more effective method of establishing high drug concentrations within the CNS, particularly if antimicrobials with poor CNS penetration are used [58]. It may also be useful with antimicrobials with high systemic toxicity, which can preclude increasing the systemic dose [58]. This method of delivery is very invasive and unlikely to be a practical in foals.

Determining the most appropriate duration of antimicrobial treatment in foals with bacterial meningitis or other CNS infections is difficult. Although specific guidelines do not exist, a minimum duration of 3 weeks is recommended and/or extending the treatment up to 10 days after resolution of clinical signs [50]. Ideally, repeat CSF analysis following discontinuation of antimicrobial treatment allows for accurate assessment of the response to treatment and helps determine if continued treatment is required. Treatment of a cerebral abscess may require prolonged antimicrobial administration and follow-up imaging (CT or MRI) to confirm resolution of the infection [50]. In addition to antimicrobial treatment, treatment of CNS infections must also address the immune response in the CNS, which can be particularly destructive and can significantly impair successful resolution of disease. Specifically, this involves inhibiting the activation of host inflammatory mediators using steroidal and nonsteroidal anti-inflammatory drugs. These drugs can modulate CSF leukocytosis and chemical abnormalities, and may limit intracranial pressure changes and the development of cerebral edema [17, 59].

Beta Lactams

Penicillin

The penicillins are bactericidal agents with activity against Gram-positive and some Gram-negative organisms, alone or in combination with a β-lactamase inhibitor. Differences

Table 30.V.3 Potential antimicrobials for the treatment of bacterial infections of the CNS in foals.[a]

Drug	Dose	Spectrum	CNS penetration	Comments
Ampicillin	22–30 mg/kg, IV or PO q6–8h	Gram+, some Gram−	Good	Achieves higher CNS concentration than penicillin when meningeal inflammation present
Cefepime	11 mg/kg, IV q8h	Broad-spectrum; Gram+ and Gram−, not effective against methicillin-resistant *Staphylococci* and *Enterococci*	Good	Routine empirical use not recommended; reserve for Gram− bacteria resistant to third-generation cephalosporins
Cefotaxime	40–50 mg/kg, IV q6h CRI 6.7 mg/kg/h (after initial loading dose of 40 mg/kg, IV)	Gram+, good activity against Gram− enteric organisms; many *Pseudomonas*, MRSA and some *E. coli* isolates may be resistant	Good	Slow infusion; CRI dosing protocol allows higher concentrations in other tissues. Compatible with 0.9% saline as diluent. Diluted formulation stable for at least 24 h (protect from light)
Ceftazidime	20–50 mg/kg, IV q12h	Good activity against multi-drug resistant Gram− bacteria	Good	Slow infusion
Ceftriaxone	25–50 mg/kg, IV q12h	Broad spectrum	Good	Use judiciously; use only when susceptibility data indicates that other options are limited
Chloramphenicol	40–50 mg/kg, PO q12h (1–2 d age) q8h (>3 d age)	Broad spectrum	Good	Risk of aplastic anemia in people; handlers should wear gloves. High oral bioavailability in foals
Doxycycline	10 mg/kg, PO q12h	Broad spectrum, limited activity against *Staphylococci*, *Enterococci* not susceptible	Poor	
Enrofloxacin	5.5 mg/kg, IV q12h 7.5 mg/kg, PO q12h	Broad spectrum, particularly Gram−	Good	Risk of arthropathy limits use in young foals
Metronidazole	10 mg/kg, PO q12h (neonates) 15 mg/kg, PO q12h (>10 d age)	Excellent anaerobic activity	Good	Anaerobic infections not reported in CNS, therefore use is limited
Minocycline	4 mg/kg, PO q12h		Intermediate	
Penicillin (potassium or sodium)	22 000–44 000 IU/kg, IV q6h	Gram+, especially beta-hemolytic *Streptococci*; some Gram− nonenteric microbes. Not effective against *Bacteroides fragilis*	Poor	Slow infusion
Rifampin	5–10 mg/kg, PO q12h	Primarily Gram+ aerobes	Good	Must be used in combination with other antimicrobial due to resistance; stains urine red
Trimethoprim-Sulfonamide	25–30 mg/kg, PO q12h	Broad spectrum; *Pseudomonas* spp., *Bacteroides* spp., and *Enterococci* usually resistant	Intermediate	Use based on susceptibility results

CRI, constant rate infusion.
[a] References Dowling [17], Furr [50], Gardner and Papich [52], Hewson et al. [53], Magdesian [13, 54], Morris et al. [55], Ringger et al. [56], Swain et al. [57].

in their naturally occurring side chains convey differences in antibacterial activity within this class. This also contributes to differences in their ability to penetrate the CSF [60]. Penicillin achieves concentrations in the CSF at approximately 10% of corresponding serum concentrations, although this may be variably increased in the presence of meningeal inflammation [3]. There are inconsistent reports suggesting that administration of aqueous penicillin G achieves higher CNS concentrations than intramuscularly administered procaine penicillin G. Of note, penicillin concentrations have been shown to remain detectable in the CSF for 12–24 hours following an intramuscular dose [60]. Ampicillin has good CNS penetration and achieves higher CSF concentrations than penicillin when meningeal inflammation is present [61].

Cephalosporins

Variability in the physicochemical properties of different cephalosporins exists consequently resulting in variation in their pharmacokinetic and bacteriologic profiles [60]. There is also variability in the ability to cross the BBB [60], with the variability being more pronounced in the presence of meningeal inflammation [3]. First- and second-generation cephalosporins do not achieve or sustain CNS concentrations as a result of their limited lipophilicity and hence, they are usually ineffective for the treatment of CNS infections [60]. Third- and fourth-generation cephalosporins have broad-spectrum activity and higher CSF:serum ratios than first- and second-generation cephalosporins. Third-generation cephalosporins demonstrate considerable activity against Gram-negative organisms and easily penetrate the BBB [55]. There have been limited studies on the pharmacokinetics of these drugs in horses and foals and hence, dosages are often extrapolated from human medicine. Spectrum of activity and recommended doses for third- and fourth-generation cephalosporins for the treatment of CNS infections in foals are listed in Table 30.V.3.

The third-generation cephalosporins that penetrate the BBB well include ceftriaxone, cefotaxime, and ceftazidime [54]. It is imperative that these antimicrobials are used judiciously as they are usually reserved for treatment of serious infections in people [54]. Ideally, use should be directed by antimicrobial sensitivity data. Ceftriaxone, another third-generation cephalosporin, is indicated for treatment of CNS infections in neonatal infants; CSF concentrations are 1.5 to 4 times greater in children with confirmed bacterial meningitis than in children with no evidence of meningeal inflammation [60]. In people, disease status is a better predictor of ceftriaxone CNS penetration than age or dose [60]. In horses, ceftriaxone has excellent penetration into many body tissues and is able to cross both the inflamed and healthy blood-CSF barrier [56]. Of the third-generation cephalosporins reported to cross the BBB well, ceftriaxone achieves the highest concentration within the CSF [54]. CSF concentrations exceed the minimal inhibitory concentration (MIC) for many pathogens and has therefore been recommended for the treatment of bacterial meningitis in horses. Similarly to people, the CSF concentrations may vary significantly between individual horses in the presence of CNS inflammation [3].

Cefotaxime has been used for the treatment of bacterial meningitis in foals, although specific CSF concentrations achieved have not been investigated [3]. In humans, cefotaxime is particularly effective for the treatment of bacterial meningitis, especially involving Gram-negative enteric organisms as it attains a bactericidal concentration for most Gram-negative organisms within CSF [55]. In children, cefotaxime and its microbiologically active desacetyl metabolite demonstrate excellent penetration into the CNS [60]. Ceftazidime (third-generation cephalosporin) has proven to be effective for the treatment of bacterial meningitis caused by multi-drug resistant Gram-negative bacteria in people [62]. In comparison to ceftriaxone and cefotaxime, ceftazidime is more active against *Pseudomonas aeruginosa* and *Acinetobacter* spp. *in vitro* and *in vivo* [62]. Ceftiofur (third-generation cephalosporin) does not achieve adequate concentrations in the CNS and is therefore not recommended for the treatment of CNS infections [3].

Cefepime (fourth-generation cephalosporin) has broad spectrum activity against Gram-positive and Gram-negative bacteria and is active against many Gram-negative bacteria that are resistant to third-generation cephalosporins [52]. Routine empiric treatment with cefepime is not recommended, however treatment may be indicated in Gram-negative infections caused by bacteria resistant to other routinely used antimicrobials or when fluoroquinolones are the only other alternative, as their use can result in cartilage injury in foals [52]. Treatment may also be considered in foals with confirmed Gram-negative infections and renal insufficiency, where the use of aminoglycosides is not recommended.

Aminoglycosides

The use of aminoglycosides is not recommended in the treatment of bacterial CNS disease because of limited penetration of the BBB [17].

Chloramphenicol

Chloramphenicol is bacteriostatic with broad-spectrum activity against Gram-positive and Gram-negative organisms as well as anaerobic bacteria. Enteric microbes have limited susceptibility, which may reduce its use in neonatal sepsis. However, it has high activity against *Enterococcus* isolates, which are common in neonatal sepsis and are often multidrug resistant [54]. Chloramphenicol is lipid soluble with low protein binding and is widely distributed throughout the body. It has good tissue penetration and enters intracellular fluids, bone, and the CNS [54]. CSF concentrations up to 50% of plasma concentrations have been reported with higher concentrations if meningeal inflammation is present [17]. The elimination half-life is age-dependent in foals due to hepatic metabolism through glucuronyl transferase activity. It has high oral bioavailability (83%) in foals 1–9 days of age and dosing should therefore be based on age [54, 63].

Potentiated Sulfonamides

Potentiated sulfonamides have broad spectrum of activity, although *Pseudomonas* spp., *Bacteroides* spp., and *Enterococci* are usually resistant. Frequent use of trimethoprim-sulfonamide combinations in horses has led to high rates of antimicrobial resistance, often in bacteria commonly isolated from septic neonatal foals. Thus, use is based on culture and sensitivity results [17]. They also have variable penetration of the CNS depending on the degree of protein binding and pK_a values. Meningeal inflammation does not improve their distribution in the CSF, thus their use in bacterial CNS infections may be limited [17].

Tetracyclines

Tetracyclines are broad-spectrum bacteriostatic antimicrobials but have limited activity against *Staphylococci* and *Enterococci*. In addition, *Pseudomonas* spp., *E. coli, Klebsiella* spp. and *Proteus* spp. are usually resistant. Although tetracyclines are lipid soluble, with distribution to many tissues, penetration intracellularly, and into the CSF is variable and therapeutic concentrations are often not reached in the CSF [17, 54]. Minocycline has the greatest degree of CSF penetration, followed by doxycycline [54].

Fluoroquinolones

Fluoroquinolones are bactericidal and have broad-spectrum activity, particularly against Gram-negative organisms, but have minimal activity against *Streptococci*. They are highly lipid-soluble and tissue penetration is very good, with high concentrations reaching the CNS following parenteral administration [64]. Bactericidal effects are concentration-dependent with a prolonged post-antibiotic effect. Fluoroquinolones are highly effective for the treatment of bacterial meningitis but use in foals is limited due to the high risk of arthropathy and effects on cartilage maturation.

Rifampin

Rifampin is a macrocyclic antimicrobial and is highly lipophilic, achieving high concentrations in the CSF. Rifampin is primarily effective against Gram-positive aerobes, including *Staphylococcus* spp., *Mycobacterium, Mycoplasma,* and *Chlamydia* and can be bactericidal or bacteriostatic, depending on the sensitivity of the organism [65]. Rifampin is primarily used in combination with other antimicrobials due to the rapid development of resistance if used as a monotherapy [54]. Rifampin is commonly used in foals in combination with macrolides or azalides for the treatment of *Rhodococcus equi* infection and occasionally used in combination with other antimicrobials including potentiated sulfonamides or aminoglycosides for susceptible infections that require higher levels of penetration (e.g. omphalophlebitis).

Metronidazole

Metronidazole is a nitroimidazole antimicrobial with excellent anaerobic activity. It is highly lipophilic and although it effectively achieves high concentrations in the CSF, anaerobic infections have not been reported in this location in the horse and hence, its value in treatment of CNS infections is limited [3]. Pharmacokinetic studies indicate that a range of dosages over the first 2 weeks of life are required due to age-dependent kinetics [57].

Anti-inflammatory Medications

The use of anti-inflammatories is an important consideration in the management of diseases affecting the neonatal CNS. Prostaglandin and thromboxane production occurs in the CNS in response to various clinical conditions, including seizures, traumatic brain injury, cerebral vascular disease, and hypoxic brain injury [3]. Inflammation plays an essential role in the pathogenesis of perinatal brain injury and neonatal encephalopathy [66, 67] and has been recognized as a major cause of long-term injury in neonatal infants [67]. Microglial cells within the CNS can be activated by excitatory amino acids and leukocyte migration in a hypoxic–ischemic insult. Microglia express inflammatory mediators and pro-inflammatory cytokines, which enhances the initial injury [67]. Cytokine-activated cells release toxic substances, including reactive oxygen species (ROS) and toxic granules such as proteolytic enzymes and myeloperoxidase. Pro-inflammatory cytokines (e.g. interleukin [IL]-1β, IL-6, IL-18, and tumor necrosis factor α [TNF-α]), can activate cytotoxic T cells, natural killer cells, and lymphokine-activated killer cells that can subsequently enhance excessive cellular and tissue damage, ultimately resulting in brain injury and cytotoxic oedema [67].

In infants, perinatal brain damage is a leading cause of life-long disability, cerebral palsy, seizure disorders, sensory impairment, and cognitive limitations. The initial insult may be hypoxic–ischemic, hemorrhagic, inflammatory, or a combination of insults [67]. Although the consequences of perinatal brain damage have different prognostic implications in foals, the role of CNS inflammation must still be considered when developing a therapeutic plan for foals with CNS disease in order to potentially reduce morbidity and mortality. Intuitively, the blockade of inflammatory cytokines should contribute to prevention of early brain damage in neonates, but use of anti-inflammatory medications remains controversial. The cytokines responsible for the unfavorable effects in the neonatal brain have also been associated with beneficial effects [67] as they contribute to tissue recovery through their role in elimination of cellular debris and in growth and repair. The activation of glial cells triggers the release of various factors, including colony-stimulating factor-1, which are vital for neuronal survival [67]. This can complicate the development of targeted therapeutic interventions to reduce the inflammatory response. In the treatment of CNS infections, control of inflammation is also important and in people with bacterial meningitis, outcomes are improved if there is adequate control of CNS inflammation [3].

Corticosteroids

Corticosteroids act on both the mineralocorticoid (MR) and glucocorticoid (GR) receptors and modulate inflammation and apoptosis in the brain. Corticosteroids have the potential to stabilize microvascular permeability, reduce edema formation, reduce intracranial pressure, decrease oxygen-derived free radicals and reduce damage to nervous tissue that may occur in the posttraumatic period [17]. Despite these beneficial effects, their use in neurologic disease remains controversial with few specific recommended dosing regimens. The use of corticosteroids in foals is usually reserved for cases of overwhelming localized or systemic inflammation [40]. Clinical use in neurological disease in equine neonates may include adjunctive treatment of neonatal encephalopathy, brain and spinal cord trauma and meningitis. The use of corticosteroids in the treatment of neonatal HI brain injury in people is controversial in that they can be both neuroprotective and neurotoxic when administered in the post-HI period [68]. The ability of corticosteroids to suppress neuroinflammation appears to be dependent on timing, dosing, and duration of exposure after the initial injury [68]. Administration of a single-dose of corticosteroids has been proposed as an adjunct treatment with hypothermia in human neonates with potential brain injury as the synergistic effects may minimize ongoing brain injury and improve patient outcome [68]. The use of corticosteroids in foals with HI encephalopathy is currently not recommended, but further research into use of single dose therapy as an adjunctive treatment is warranted. In the treatment of bacterial meningitis, corticosteroids decrease the risk of death and various neurological sequelae in people [3]. Supportive research in horses is lacking; however, it is likely that a similar benefit from reducing the degree of cerebral inflammation would result. The concern of corticosteroid induced immunosuppression and/or a delay in sterilization of the CSF in cases of meningitis has not been supported in human medicine [3, 17].

The dose of corticosteroids is variable and dependent on the drug selected. Dexamethasone is administered at a dose range of 0.05–0.2 mg/kg IV or IM every 12–24 hours, whereas hydrocortisone is administered at a range of 0.17–0.67 mg/kg IV every 4–6 hours (total dose 1–4 mg/kg/d). Prednisolone sodium succinate, a very short-acting corticosteroid, is administered at a dose of 1–2 mg/kg IV. With spinal cord trauma, prednisolone sodium succinate can be administered as an initial bolus of 30 mg/kg IV, followed by a CRI of 5 mg/kg/h for 8 hours. Prednisolone at a dose of 1 mg/kg PO every 12–24 hours can also be considered.

Nonsteroidal Anti-inflammatory Drugs (NSAIDS)

NSAIDS are common anti-inflammatory agents used to treat a range of conditions. Their use in neurological disease may be warranted for generalized systemic inflammation as well as specifically to target inflammatory processes in CNS tissues. NSAIDs are also used to regulate fever and patient discomfort. NSAIDS inhibit arachidonic acid synthesis via cyclooxygenase (COX) inhibition and include nonspecific COX inhibitors (phenylbutazone, flunixin meglumine), more selective COX-2 inhibitors (ketoprofen), and COX-2-specific drugs (meloxicam, firocoxib). The use of nonspecific COX inhibitors has been associated with adverse effects including gastrointestinal ulceration and renal injury [40]. Phenylbutazone is less commonly used in foals compared to adults due to the potential for toxicity. The use of COX-2-specific NSAIDS is recommended in foals with severe systemic inflammation, hypovolemia, or those at higher risk of gastrointestinal ulceration [40]. When using NSAIDS in neonatal foals, regular monitoring of serum creatinine concentration and urinalysis is recommended due to the risk of nephrotoxicity associated with these drugs. The doses of NSAIDs include: meloxicam at 0.6 mg/kg IV or PO every 12 hours (foals <6 weeks of age), flunixin meglumine at 0.25–1.1 mg/kg IV or PO every 12–24 hours, ketoprofen at 1.1–2.2 mg/kg IV every 24 hours, and firocoxib at 0.1 mg/kg PO or 0.09 mg/kg IV every 24 hours.

Dimethyl Sulfoxide

Dimethyl sulfoxide (DMSO) is an organic solvent used to treat a variety of inflammatory disorders in horses and foals, including neuroinflammation. Limited evidence supports its clinical use, and its pharmacological properties are incompletely understood [69]. For topical use only, 90% DMSO gel or liquid has been approved in veterinary medicine to reduce acute swelling [17, 69]. However in practice, IV administration of a 10% DMSO solution (diluted in saline) has been used to treat neuroinflammation [3]. If given at greater than a 20% solution, hemolysis may occur along with other signs of toxicity, including muscle trembling, loose feces, and colic [3]. Pharmacokinetic studies in horses demonstrate rapid distribution following IV administration, with an absence of plasma protein binding. Similarly, there is rapid absorption following oral administration, although this can be variable in the absence of food restriction [69].

Effects of DMSO in neurologic disease in laboratory animals have demonstrated reduction in excitotoxic neuronal cell death and enhancement of drug-induced blockade of calcium channels [70, 71]. In people with head trauma, DMSO has been shown to rapidly decrease intracranial pressure and improve cerebral perfusion pressure, thereby improving overall neurologic outcome [72]; a similar response might be noted in equine patients. DMSO has been used IV in other animal species to reduce intracranial pressure and volume [69] and in foals with HIE to decrease cerebral edema. The dose range for DMSO is 0.5-1 g/kg as (10% solution) IV every 12 hours.

Pentoxifylline

Pentoxifylline is a phosphodiesterase inhibitor that has multiple anti-inflammatory effects. It is used in adult horses for a variety of conditions associated with systemic inflammation and can be considered in neonatal encephalopathy to reduce cerebral inflammation. Pharmacokinetic studies have not been performed in foals; thus, the dosage is extrapolated from adult horses at 10 mg/kg, PO every 12 hours [40].

Medications for Cerebral Edema

Cerebral edema and increased intracranial pressure are important causes of morbidity and mortality in people with intracranial tumors, cerebral hematomas, traumatic brain injuries, cerebral infarcts, and intracranial hemorrhage [73]. Similarly, in other species including equine neonates, intracranial hypertension may develop secondary to a variety of intracranial disease processes, including traumatic brain injury, meningoencephalitis, hemorrhage, and status epilepticus, and can be life-threatening [74]. Targeted treatment of cerebral edema is often considered in foals presenting with traumatic brain injury or signs of CNS dysfunction. Mannitol and hypertonic saline are used primarily for their hyperosmolar effects [3] and both have similar effects on hemodynamics [73]. Hypertonic fluids contain a higher concentration of solute compared to plasma and interstitial fluid creating an osmotic gradient when administered, thereby drawing fluid from the interstitial space into the intravascular space [73]. In people, hyperosmolar therapy is a mainstay of conservative treatment for cerebral edema and increased ICP [75]. In foals with neonatal encephalopathy, cerebral edema is not typically present. Hence, the use of these medications is likely not warranted. However, foals presenting with acute traumatic brain injury, other metabolic derangements, or conditions that result in cerebral edema and increased ICP (e.g. hyponatremia) may be candidates for this treatment. In people with traumatic brain injury, edema is an important target for clinical intervention [76].

Mannitol

Mannitol is a crystalloid hyperosmolar solution that reduces intracranial pressure via osmotically driven movement of fluid from the tissue into the vascular compartment. This ultimately results in a reduction in tissue water content [3] which may be an important treatment goal if brain tissue is involved. Mannitol also induces changes in blood rheology and increases cardiac output resulting in improved cerebral oxygenation and perfusion pressure [77]. With improved cerebral oxygenation, subsequent cerebral artery vasoconstriction and reduction in cerebral blood volume and intracranial pressure occurs [77]. CSF production is also decreased by up to 50%, which can result in a prolonged decrease in intracranial pressure [78]. Adverse effects include renal and CNS effects as a result of persistent hyperosmolality. The administration of multiple doses of mannitol can induce diuresis and subsequent hypovolemia, hypotension, and reduction in cerebral blood flow [77]. The dose of mannitol ranges from 0.25–2.0 g/kg IV over 20 minutes as a 20% solution.

Hypertonic Saline

Hypertonic saline is an IV crystalloid composed of sodium chloride dissolved in water and has a higher concentration of sodium than plasma [73]. Administration of hypertonic saline causes an increase in blood osmolarity, with subsequent fluid shifts from the extravascular space into the intravascular space. In patients with increased ICP, this results in a decrease in brain edema, improved cerebral blood flow and decreased CSF production [73]. Volume resuscitation is augmented by a temporary increase in circulating blood volume and increased mean arterial blood pressure and cerebral perfusion pressure [77]. Hypertonic saline is associated with significant decreases in intracranial pressure and cerebral water content compared to treatment with isotonic fluids [77]. Following administration of hypertonic saline, isotonic fluids should be used for maintenance. Recent research has focused on establishing superiority between hypertonic saline and mannitol for the management of increased ICP. Hypertonic saline has been shown to provide a more robust and durable effect in lowering ICP and a tendency toward lower mortality rates in patients treated with hypertonic saline [79, 80]. It has also been suggested that hypertonic saline might be superior in the treatment of intracranial hypertension and in improving cerebral perfusion in dogs [74].

Adverse effects include excessive intravascular volume (particularly if active hemorrhage is still present), electrolyte abnormalities and coagulopathies [77]. Hypertonic saline causes significant increases in plasma sodium and chloride concentrations that can result in hyperchloremic metabolic acidosis. Hypertonic saline must be used judiciously in patients with renal dysfunction or pre-existing electrolyte derangements. The dose range for hypertonic saline is 4–6 ml/kg over 15 minutes for treatment of head trauma. Hypertonic saline can be administered intravenously as 3%, 5%, or 7% solutions. Contraindications include hypernatremia, renal failure, or ongoing intracerebral hemorrhage.

Other

Other treatments to consider in neonates with signs of CNS disease include antioxidants and neuroprotectants including allopurinol, thiamine, Vitamin E, and Vitamin C.

Thiamine

Thiamine has a neuroprotective role in supporting metabolic processes including mitochondrial metabolism and membrane Na^+/K^+/ATPases involved in maintaining cellular fluid balance. Thiamine is an essential coenzyme in glucose utilization by the brain and further provides metabolic support [47]. Thiamine can be administered at a rate of 10–20 mg/kg IV every 24 hrs, diluted in IV fluids.

Free Radical Scavengers

Allopurinol

The production of nitric oxide (NO), a free radical, is increased during cerebral hypoxia-ischemia in human neonates [81]. Both serum and CSF concentrations of NO have been correlated with the degree of HIE, supporting the role of NO in the pathophysiology following asphyxia. Xanthine oxidase catalyzes the reduction of nitrite and nitrate back to NO with enhancement of NO generation in ischemic or hypoxic tissues. For this reason, the use of xanthine oxidase-inhibiting compounds such as allopurinol has been investigated to decrease cerebral injury of asphyxiated human neonates [81]. In one study, serum NO levels were significantly decreased in asphyxiated neonates treated with allopurinol and this was associated with a better neurologic outcome [81]. No adverse effects were reported after administration of a single oral dose of allopurinol 6 hours after birth in foals born from mares with placentitis [82]. Treated foals also maintained normal glucose concentrations which potentially could be a result of treatment with allopurinol and its role in reducing cellular damage. Treatment with allopurinol also stabilized calcium concentrations, specifically within the first 6–12 hours after birth [82]. Hypocalcemia occurs commonly in foals suffering from perinatal asphyxia, most likely as a result of renal insufficiency from inadequate renal perfusion [82]. The dose of allopurinol is 44 mg/kg PO within 4 hours of birth.

Antioxidants

Equine immune function is decreased if the concentration of antioxidant molecules is depleted; supplementation may restore improved immune responses [83], justifying the use of antioxidants in adult horses for the treatment of a variety of conditions. In foals, it has been reported that oxidative stress does not increase among sick foals compared to healthy foals [83]. However, in neonatal foals presenting to the intensive care unit, the use of antioxidants following HI brain injury may have some merit. In premature infants, neonatal anoxia is one of the major causes of brain injury [84]. Restoration of oxygen equilibrium after hypoxia-ischemia results in a burst of free radical production that causes damage to tissues via lipid peroxidation within cellular membranes [85]. Hypoxic–ischemic brain injury involves increased oxidative stress and in asphyxiated newborns, iron deposited in the brain catalyzes formation of ROS [86]. In addition, newborns have lower levels of antioxidant enzymes and low-molecular antioxidants, making them particularly vulnerable to damage from free radicals [87].

Vitamin E

Vitamin E is an important lipophilic radical scavenging antioxidant [88] that protects the brain against excessive lipid oxidation. It reacts with ROS that have already been formed, resulting in their removal or inhibition [87]. Vitamin E can be given at a dose of 10–20 IU/kg SC or PO every 24 hours.

Vitamin C

The antioxidant effects of vitamin C (ascorbic acid) include scavenging of ROS and activation of other scavengers, including α-tocopherol [89, 90]. In people, vitamin C is used to treat sepsis or after ischemia/reperfusion injury to reduce oxidative damage to endothelial and other cells. This is thought to improve tissue perfusion and oxygenation and mitigate subsequent organ dysfunction [91]. Vitamin C is also reported to have NMDA receptor blockage properties [24] and similar beneficial effects as seen in humans may occur in foals with neonatal encephalopathy. The pharmacokinetics of vitamin C in horses has been investigated and although it is well absorbed following SC and IM injections, marked local irritation can occur. After oral administration, gastrointestinal absorption is very poor which is in contrast to humans and other species [92]. Therefore, IV administration is the only satisfactory means for appropriate supplementation of ascorbic acid in horses at a dose of 100 mg/kg every 24 hours [92].

Nonpharmacological Treatments

Hypothermia

Therapeutic hypothermia is standard of care for human neonatal HIE [93]. Evidence in neonatal infants suggests that hypothermia should be initiated within 6 hours of birth and continued for 72 hours, with a target temperature of 92.3 °F (33.5 °C) [94]. The underlying mechanisms of neuroprotection with hypothermia include modification of apoptosis, interruption of early necrosis, reduction of cerebral metabolic rate and reduction in release of excitotoxins and oxygen and nitrogen-free radicals [95, 96]. Hypothermia can be induced via two methods: whole body cooling and selective head cooling with mild systemic hypothermia. The rationale for selective head cooling is that the newborn infant's brain produces 70% of the total body heat along with concerns that systemic hypothermia may be physiologically harmful to ill neonates [93]. However, a significant reduction in deep brain temperature can only be achieved when core body temperature is lowered to 93.2 °F (34 °C), implying that a reduction in systemic temperature is required to achieve deep brain cooling [97].

Selective head cooling in equine neonates has not been investigated, however the use of a cooling collar, as has been trialed for racehorses with exertional heat illness as an adjunct to whole-body targeted cooling, may have merit [98]. Although the specific mechanism of action of the cooling collar is yet to be determined, proposed mechanisms include cooling of blood in the carotid arteries leading to cooling of the brain or induction of general body cooling with secondary cooling of the brain [98].

Physical Compression Squeeze Procedure

In the healthy foal, the transition of consciousness from intra- to extrauterine life includes a period where arousal stimulation is overridden by thoracic pressure while the fetus is in the birth canal. Thoracic pressure induces squeeze-induced somnolence and immobility [99]. Upon exit from the birth canal, the physical pressure is released and full stimulation occurs as the foal transitions to full consciousness and mobility. Maintenance of in utero unconsciousness involves neuromodulating hormones (neurosteroids) [99] and an association between neonatal maladjustment syndrome with the persistence of high concentrations of neruosteroids in the postnatal period has been proposed [100].

The physical compression squeeze procedure involves a rope compression system. When applied, the squeeze procedure produces a state of somnolence and immobility, termed "squeeze-induced somnolence" [99]. Applying the thoracic squeeze procedure to neonatal foals with neonatal encephalopathy for 20 minutes has been proposed to simultaneously elicit two responses mediated by different neural pathways. The first response is reflexive inhibition of physical movement and electrocortical activity leading to immobility and somnolence. The second response is locus coeruleus release of neuroactivating noradrenaline [99]. The squeeze procedure has been evaluated in healthy foals and foals with signs consistent with neonatal encephalopathy. In healthy foals, application of the rope-restraint device appeared to activate the hypothalamic–pituitary–adrenal (HPA) axis, decrease heart and respiratory rates, and cause dormancy in neonatal foals [101]. In another study, when the squeeze procedure was applied for 20 minutes, there was faster full recovery in some foals diagnosed with neonatal encephalopathy compared to foals treated medically [99]. Instructions on application of the squeeze procedure is available at: http://www.mdpi.com/2076-2615/7/9/69/s1, supplementary file title: Step-by-Step Written Instructions.

References

1 Tam, V.H., Sosa, C., Liu, R. et al. (2016). Nanomedicine as a non-invasive strategy for drug delivery across the blood brain barrier. *Int. J. Pharm.* 515: 331–342.

2 Patel, M.M., Goyal, B.R., Bhadada, S.V. et al. (2009). Getting into the brain: approaches to enhance brain drug delivery. *CNS Drugs* 23: 35–58.

3 Lacombe, V.A. and Furr, M. (2015). Pharmaceutical considerations for treatment of central nervous system disease. In: *Equine Neurology*, 2e (ed. M. Furr and S. Reed), 46–57. Wiley.

4 Pardridge, W.M. (1999). Non-invasive drug delivery to the human brain using endogenous blood-brain barrier transport systems. *Pharm. Sci. Technol. Today* 2: 49–59.

5 Copeland, C. and Stabenfeldt, S.E. (2020). Leveraging the dynamic blood-brain barrier for central nervous system nanoparticle-based drug delivery applications. *Curr. Opin. Biomed. Eng.* 14: 1–8.

6 Cole, C.A. and Bentz, B. (2015). Treatment of equine nervous system disorders. In: *Equine Pharmacology*, 1e (ed. C.A. Cole, B. Bentz, and L. Maxwell), 197–217. Wiley.

7 de Vries, H.E., Kooij, G., Frenkel, D. et al. (2012). Inflammatory events at blood-brain barrier in

neuroinflammatory and neurodegenerative disorders: implications for clinical disease. *Epilepsia* 53 (Suppl 6): 45–52.
8 Nau, R., Sörgel, F., and Prange, H.W. (1998). Pharmacokinetic optimisation of the treatment of bacterial central nervous system infections. *Clin. Pharmacokinet.* 35: 223–246.
9 Klein, B.G. (2012). Cerebrospinal fluid and the blood-brain barrier. In: *Cunningham's Textbook of Veterinary Physiology*, 5e (ed. B.G. Klein), 138–144. Saunders.
10 Viu, J., Monreal, L., Jose-Cunilleras, E. et al. (2012). Clinical findings in 10 foals with bacterial meningoencephalitis. *Equine Vet. J.* 44: 100–104.
11 Mayhew, I. (2009). *Large Animal Neurology*, 2e. Wiley.
12 Fielding, C.L., Magdesian, K.G., and Edman, J.E. (2011). Determination of body water compartments in neonatal foals by use of indicator dilution techniques and multifrequency bioelectrical impedance analysis. *Am. J. Vet. Res.* 72: 1390–1396.
13 Magdesian, K.G. (2015). Foals are not just mini horses. In: *Equine Pharmacology* (ed. C.A. Cole, B. Bentz, and L. Maxwell), 99–117. Wiley.
14 Runk, D.T., Madigan, J.E., Rahal, C.J. et al. (2000). Measurement of plasma colloid osmotic pressure in normal thoroughbred neonatal foals. *J. Vet. Intern. Med.* 14: 475–478.
15 MacKay, R.J. (2005). Neurologic disorders of neonatal foals. *Vet. Clin. North Am. Equine Pract.* 21 (387–406): vii.
16 Perlman, J.M. (2006). Intervention strategies for neonatal hypoxic-ischemic cerebral injury. *Clin. Ther.* 28: 1353–1365.
17 Dowling, P.M. (1999). Clinical pharmacology of nervous system diseases. *Vet. Clin. North Am. Equine Pract.* 15: 575–588.
18 Bhat, M.A., Charoo, B.A., Bhat, J.I. et al. (2009). Magnesium sulfate in severe perinatal asphyxia: a randomized, placebo-controlled trial. *Pediatrics* 123: Le764–Le769.
19 Rahman, S.U., Canpolat, F.E., Oncel, M.Y. et al. (2015). Multicenter randomized controlled trial of therapeutic hypothermia plus magnesium sulfate verses therapeutic hypothermica place placebo in the management of term and near-term infants with hypoxic ischemic encephalopathy: a pilot study. *J. Clin. Neonatal.* 4: 158–163.
20 Norman, W.M., Court, M.H., and Greenblatt, D.J. (1997). Age-related changes in the pharmacokinetic disposition of diazepam in foals. *Am. J. Vet. Res.* 58: 878–880.
21 Mason, D.E. (2004). Anesthetics, tranquilizers and opioid analgesics. In: *Equine Clinical Pharmacology*, 1e (ed. J.J. Bertone and L.J.I. Horspool), 267–309. Saunders.
22 Shini, S. (2000). A review of diazepam and its use in the horse. *J. Equine Vet. Sci.* 20: 443–449.
23 Martin, M., Jyes, Q., Hagen, E. et al. (2020). Evaluation of the neonate with seizures. *Pediatr. Ann.* 49: e292–e298.
24 Lacombe, V.A. and Furr, M. (2015). Differential diagnosis and management of horses with seizures or alterations in consciousness. In: *Equine Neurology*, 2e (ed. M. Furr and S. Reed), 79–92. Wiley.
25 Ravis, W.R., Duran, S.H., Pedersoli, W.M. et al. (1987). A pharmacokinetic study of phenobarbital in mature horses after oral dosing. *J. Vet. Pharmacol. Ther.* 10: 283–289.
26 Knox, D.A., Ravis, W.R., Pedersoli, W.M. et al. (1992). Pharmacokinetics of phenobarbital in horses after single and repeated oral administration of the drug. *Am. J. Vet. Res.* 53: 706–710.
27 Duran, S.H., Ravis, W.R., Pedersoli, W.M. et al. (1987). Pharmacokinetics of phenobarbital in the horse. *Am. J. Vet. Res.* 48: 807–810.
28 Spehar, A.M., Hill, M.R., Mayhew, I.G. et al. (1984). Preliminary study on the pharmacokinetics of phenobarbital in the neonatal foal. *Equine Vet. J.* 16: 368–371.
29 Dowling, P.M. (2004). Drugs acting on the neurological system and behaviour modification. In: *Equine Clinical Pharmacology*, 1e (ed. J.J. Bertone and L.J.I. Horspool), 145–154. Philadelphia: W.B. Saunders.
30 Hubbell, J.A.E., Kelly, E.M., Aarnes, T.K. et al. (2013). Pharmacokinetics of midazolam after intravenous administration to horses. *Equine Vet. J.* 45: 721–725.
31 Ramantani, G., Ikonomidou, C., Walter, B. et al. (2011). Levetiracetam: safety and efficacy in neonatal seizures. *Eur. J. Paediatr. Neurol.* 15: 1–7.
32 Costa, J., Fareleira, F., Ascenção, R. et al. (2011). Clinical comparability of the new antiepileptic drugs in refractory partial epilepsy: a systematic review and meta-analysis. *Epilepsia* 52: 1280–1291.
33 Talos, D.M., Chang, M., Kosaras, B. et al. (2013). Antiepileptic effects of levetiracetam in a rodent neonatal seizure model. *Pediatr. Res.* 73: 24–30.
34 Podell, M. (2013). Antiepileptic drug therapy and monitoring. *Top. Companion Anim. Med.* 28: 59–66.
35 MacDonald, K.D., Hart, K.A., Davis, J.L. et al. (2018). Pharmacokinetics of the anticonvulsant levetiracetam in neonatal foals. *Equine Vet. J.* 50: 532–536.
36 Cesar, F.B., Stewart, A.J., Boothe, D.M. et al. (2018). Disposition of levetiracetam in healthy adult horses. *J. Vet. Pharmacol. Ther.* 41: 92–97.
37 Raidal, S. and Edwards, S. (2008). Pharmacokinetics of potassium bromide in adult horses. *Aust. Vet. J.* 86: 187–193.
38 Fielding, C.L., Magdesian, K.G., Elliott, D.A. et al. (2003). Pharmacokinetics and clinical utility of sodium bromide (NaBr) as an estimator of extracellular fluid volume in horses. *J. Vet. Intern. Med.* 17: 213–217.

39 Aleman, M., Gray, L.C., Williams, D.C. et al. (2006). Juvenile idiopathic epilepsy in Egyptian Arabian foals: 22 cases (1985–2005). *J. Vet. Intern. Med.* 20: 1443–1449.

40 McKenzie, H.C. III (2018). Disorders of foals. In: *Equine Internal Medicine*, 4e (ed. S. Reed, W. Bayly, and D. Sellon), 1365–1459. St Louis, Missouri: Elsevier.

41 Wilkins, P.A. (2015). Perinatal asphyxia syndrome. In: *Current Therapy in Equine Medicine*, 7e (ed. K.A. Sprayberry and N.E. Robinson), 732–736. St. Louis, MO: Elsevier.

42 Galinsky, R., Bennet, L., Groenendaal, F. et al. (2014). Magnesium is not consistently neuroprotective for perinatal hypoxia-ischemia in term-equivalent models in preclinical studies: a systematic review. *Dev. Neurosci.* 36: 73–82.

43 Temkin, N.R., Anderson, G.D., Winn, H.R. et al. (2007). Magnesium sulfate for neuroprotection after traumatic brain injury: a randomised controlled trial. *Lancet Neurol.* 6: 29–38.

44 Gold, J.R., Grubb, T.L., Green, S. et al. (2020). Plasma disposition of gabapentin after the intragastric administration of escalating doses to adult horses. *J. Vet. Intern. Med.* 34: 933–940.

45 Zand, L., McKian, K.P., and Qian, Q. (2010). Gabapentin toxicity in patients with chronic kidney disease: a preventable cause of morbidity. *Am. J. Med.* 123: 367–373.

46 Jackson, C.D., Clanahan, M.J., Joglekar, K. et al. (2018). Hold the Gaba: a case of gabapentin-induced hepatotoxicity. *Cureus* 10: e2269.

47 Podell, M. (1998). Antiepileptic drug therapy. *Clin. Tech. Small Anim. Pract.* 13: 185–192.

48 Soma, L.R., Uboh, C.E., Guan, F. et al. (2001). Disposition, elimination, and bioavailability of phenytoin and its major metabolite in horses. *Am. J. Vet. Res.* 62: 483–489.

49 Kowalczyk, D.F. and Beech, J. (1983). Pharmacokinetics of phenytoin (diphenylhydantoin) in horses. *J. Vet. Pharmacol. Ther.* 6: 133–140.

50 Furr, M. (2015). Bacterial infections of the central nervous system. In: *Equine Neurology*, 2e (ed. M. Furr and S. Reed), 273–284. Wiley.

51 Pellegrini-Masini, A. and Livesey, L.C. (2006). Meningitis and encephalomyelitis in horses. *Vet. Clin. North Am. Equine Pract.* 22 (553–589): x.

52 Gardner, S.Y. and Papich, M.G. (2001). Comparison of cefepime pharmacokinetics in neonatal foals and adult dogs. *J. Vet. Pharmacol. Ther.* 24: 187–192.

53 Hewson, J., Johnson, R., Arroyo, L.G. et al. (2013). Comparison of continuous infusion with intermittent bolus administration of cefotaxime on blood and cavity fluid drug concentrations in neonatal foals. *J Vet Pharm Therap* 36: 68–77.

54 Magdesian, K.G. (2017). Antimicrobial pharmacology for the neonatal foal. *Vet. Clin. North Am. Equine Pract.* 33: 47–65.

55 Morris, D.D., Rutkowski, J.A., and Lloyd, K.C.K. (1987). Therapy in two cases of neonatal foal septicaemia and meningitis with cefotaxime sodium. *Equine Vet. J.* 19: 151–154.

56 Ringger, N.C., Brown, M.P., Kohlepp, S.J. et al. (1998). Pharmacokinetics of ceftriaxone in neonatal foals. *Equine Vet. J.* 30: 163–165.

57 Swain, E.A., Magdesian, K.G., Kass, P.H. et al. (2015). Pharmacokinetics of metronidazole in foals: influence of age within the neonatal period. *J. Vet. Pharmacol. Ther.* 38: 227–234.

58 Nau, R., Sörgel, F., and Eiffert, H. (2010). Penetration of drugs through the blood-cerebrospinal fluid/blood-brain barrier for treatment of central nervous system infections. *Clin. Microbiol. Rev.* 23: 858–883.

59 Tuomanen, E., Hengstler, B., Rich, R. et al. (1987). Nonsteroidal anti-inflammatory agents in the therapy for experimental pneumococcal meningitis. *J Infect Dis* 155: 985–990.

60 Sullins, A.K. and Abdel-Rahman, S.M. (2013). Pharmacokinetics of antibacterial agents in the CSF of children and adolescents. *Paediatr. Drugs* 15: 93–117.

61 Thea, D. and Barza, M. (1989). Use of antibacterial agents in infections of the central nervous system. *Infect. Dis. Clin. North Am.* 3: 553–570.

62 Nau, R., Prange, H.W., Kinzig, M. et al. (1996). Cerebrospinal fluid ceftazidime kinetics in patients with external ventriculostomies. *Antimicrob. Agents Chemother.* 40: 763–766.

63 Brumbaugh, G.W., Martens, R.J., Knight, H.D. et al. (1983). Pharmacokinetics of chloramphenicol in the neonatal horse. *J. Vet. Pharmacol. Ther.* 6: 219–227.

64 Cottagnoud, P. and Tauber, M.G. (2003). Fluoroquinolones in the treatment of meningitis. *Curr. Infect. Dis. Rep.* 5: 329–336.

65 Cole, C.A. (2015). Basics of antimicrobial therapy for the horse. In: *Equine Pharmacology* (ed. C.A. Cole, B. Bentz, and L. Maxwell), 16–43. Amers, IA: Wiley Blackwell.

66 Wong, D., Wilkins, P.A., Bain, F.T. et al. (2011). Neonatal encephalopathy in foals. *Compend. Contin. Educ. Vet.* 33: E5.

67 Ofek-Shlomai, N. and Berger, I. (2014). Inflammatory injury to the neonatal brain – what can we do? *Front. Pediatr.* 2: 30–30.

68 Concepcion, K.R. and Zhang, L. (2018). Corticosteroids and perinatal hypoxic-ischemic brain injury. *Drug Discov. Today* 23: 1718–1732.

69 Soma, L.R., Robinson, M.A., You, Y. et al. (2018). Pharmacokinetics, disposition, and plasma

concentrations of dimethyl sulfoxide (DMSO) in the horse following topical, oral, and intravenous administration. *J. Vet. Pharmacol. Ther.* 41: 384–392.

70 Lu, C. and Mattson, M.P. (2001). Dimethyl sulfoxide suppresses NMDA- and AMPA-induced ion currents and calcium influx and protects against excitotoxic death in hippocampal neurons. *Exp. Neurol.* 170: 180–185.

71 Wu, L., Karpinski, E., Wang, R. et al. (1992). Modification by solvents of the action of nifedipine on calcium channel currents in neuroblastoma cells. *Naunyn Schmiedebergs Arch. Pharmacol.* 345: 478–484.

72 Karaca, M., Bilgin, U.Y., Akar, M. et al. (1991). Dimethly sulphoxide lowers ICP after closed head trauma. *Eur. J. Clin. Pharmacol.* 40: 113–114.

73 Mason, A.K., Malik, A., and Ginglen, J.G. (2020). *Hypertonic Fluids*. Treasure Island, FL: StatPearls Publishing.

74 Hoehne, S.N., Yozova, I.D., Vidondo, B. et al. (2021). Comparison of the effects of 7.2% hypertonic saline and 20% mannitol on electrolyte and acid-base variables in dogs with suspected intracranial hypertension. *J. Vet. Intern. Med.* 35: 341–351.

75 Wang, J., Ren, Y., Wang, S.F. et al. (2021). Comparative efficacy and safety of glycerol versus mannitol in patients with cerebral oedema and elevated intracranial pressure: a systematic review and meta-analysis. *J. Clin. Pharm. Ther.* 46: 504–514.

76 Sawant-Pokam, P.A., Vail, T.J., Metcalf, C.S. et al. (2020). Preventing neuronal edema increases network excitability after traumatic brain injury. *J. Clin. Invest.* 130: 6005–6020.

77 Nout-Lomas, Y.S. (2015). Fluid therapy during neurologic disease. In: *Equine Fluid Therapy* (ed. C.L. Fielding and K.G. Magdesian), 228–238. Wiley.

78 White, H., Cook, D., and Venkatesh, B. (2006). The use of hypertonic saline for treating intracranial hypertension after traumatic brain injury. *Anesth. Analg.* 102: 1836–1846.

79 Mangat, H.S. (2018). Hypertonic saline infusion for treating intracranial hypertension after severe traumatic brain injury. *Crit. Care* 22: 37.

80 Mangat, H.S., Chiu, Y.L., Gerber, L.M. et al. (2015). Hypertonic saline reduces cumulative and daily intracranial pressure burdens after severe traumatic brain injury. *J. Neurosurg.* 122: 202–210.

81 Gunes, T., Ozturk, M.A., Koklu, E. et al. (2007). Effect of allopurinol supplementation on nitric oxide levels in asphyxiated newborns. *Pediatr. Neurol.* 36: 17–24.

82 Araujo, L.O., Nogueira, C.E.W., Pazinato, F.M. et al. (2016). Oral single dose of allopurinol in thoroughbred foals born from mares with placentitis. *Cienc. Rural* 46: 1119–1125.

83 Furr, M., Frellstedt, L., and Geor, R. (2012). Sick neonatal foals do not demonstrate evidence of oxidative stress. *J. Equine Vet. Sci.* 32: 297–299.

84 Barrett, R.D., Bennet, L., Davidson, J. et al. (2007). Destruction and reconstruction: hypoxia and the developing brain. *Birth Defects Res. C Embryo Today* 81: 163–176.

85 Blomgren, K. and Hagberg, H. (2006). Free radicals, mitochondria, and hypoxia-ischemia in the developing brain. *Free Radic. Biol. Med.* 40: 388–397.

86 Kletkiewicz, H., Nowakowska, A., Siejka, A. et al. (2016). Deferoxamine prevents cerebral glutathione and vitamin E depletions in asphyxiated neonatal rats: role of body temperature. *Int. J. Hyperthermia* 32: 211–220.

87 Kletkiewicz, H., Klimiuk, M., Woźniak, A. et al. (2020). How to improve the antioxidant defense in asphyxiated newborns –lessons from animal models. *Antioxidants (Basel)* 9 (9): 898.

88 Niki, E. (2014). Role of vitamin E as a lipid-soluble peroxyl radical scavenger: in vitro and in vivo evidence. *Free Radic. Biol. Med.* 66: 3–12.

89 Anderson, M.J., Ibrahim, A.S., Cooper, B.R. et al. (2020). Effects of administration of ascorbic acid and low-dose hydrocortisone after infusion of sublethal doses of lipopolysaccharide to horses. *J. Vet. Intern. Med.* 34: 2710–2718.

90 Berger, M.M. and Oudemans-van Straaten, H.M. (2015). Vitamin C supplementation in the critically ill patient. *Curr. Opin. Clin. Nutr. Metab. Care* 18: 193–201.

91 Oudemans-van Straaten, H.M., Spoelstra-de Man, A.M., and de Waard, M.C. (2014). Vitamin C revisited. *Crit. Care* 18: 460–460.

92 Löscher, W., Jaeschke, G., and Keller, H. (1984). Pharmacokinetics of ascorbic acid in horses. *Equine Vet. J.* 16: 59–65.

93 Jacobs, S.E., Berg, M., Hunt, R. et al. (2013). Cooling for newborns with hypoxic ischaemic encephalopathy. *Cochrane Database Syst. Rev.* 2013: Cd003311.

94 Gonzalez, F.F. (2019). Neuroprotection strategies for term encephalopathy. *Semin. Pediatr. Neurol.* 32: 100773.

95 Edwards, A.D., Yue, X., Squier, M.V. et al. (1995). Specific inhibition of apoptosis after cerebral hypoxia-ischemia by moderate post-insult hypothermia. *Biochem. Biophys. Res. Commun.* 217: 1193–1199.

96 Globus, M.Y., Alonso, O., Dietrich, W.D. et al. (1995). Glutamate release and free radical production following brain injury: effects of posttraumatic hypothermia. *J. Neurochem.* 65: 1704–1711.

97 Van Leeuwen, G.M., Hand, J.W., Lagendijk, J.J. et al. (2000). Numerical modeling of temperature distributions within the neonatal head. *Pediatr. Res.* 48: 351–356.

98 Brownlow, M.A. (2018). Alleviation of thermal strain after racing in the thoroughbred racehorse with the use

of a cooling collar. In: *CVE Control & Therapy Series*, 33–37. Sydney, NSW Australia: Centre of Veterinary Education.

99 Aleman, M., Weich, K.M., and Madigan, J.E. (2017). Survey of veterinarians using a novel physical compression squeeze procedure in the Management of Neonatal Maladjustment Syndrome in foals. *Animals (Basel)* 7.

100 Aleman, M., Pickles, K.J., Conley, A.J. et al. (2013). Abnormal plasma neuroactive progestagen derivatives in ill, neonatal foals presented to the neonatal intensive care unit. *Equine Vet. J.* 45: 661–665.

101 Toth, B., Aleman, M., Brosnan, R.J. et al. (2012). Evaluation of squeeze-induced somnolence in neonatal foals. *Am. J. Vet. Res.* 73: 1881–1889.

Chapter 31 Congenital Nervous System Disorders

Section I Juvenile Idiopathic Epilepsy

Diane Rhodes

Epilepsy is a disease of the brain defined by having two or more unprovoked seizures more than 24 hours apart and/or a confirmed diagnosis of an epilepsy syndrome [1, 2]. "Unprovoked" indicates that there is no reversible or precipitating factor at the time of the seizure [1–3]. The definition in people has been expanded to include individuals having one unprovoked seizure and who are at high risk of recurrence because of a persistently lowered seizure threshold [2]. Epileptic seizures are generally brief, lasting only 1–3 minutes, and may have multiple etiologies classified as idiopathic (proven or suspected genetic background), structural (known cerebral pathology), or unknown [1–3].

Juvenile idiopathic epilepsy (JIE) is a heritable epileptic disorder affecting Egyptian Arabian foals with pedigree analysis indicating an autosomal dominant mode of inheritance [3–6]. There is no sex predilection and the age of onset is reported to range from 2 days to 6 months of age (median 2 months) [3]. Equine JIE is self-limiting with seizure resolution achieved by 1–2 years of age [3, 5]. In the neonate, JIE must be differentiated from other intra- and extracranial causes of seizures including neonatal encephalopathy, trauma, central nervous system infections, sepsis, metabolic disturbances, and other developmental or genetic conditions such as lavender foal syndrome.

Clinical Signs

Foals with JIE are clinically normal at birth, which helps differentiate this disease from other genetic causes of seizures, primarily lavender foal syndrome, which also occurs in Egyptian Arabian foals [3, 4]. Foals with JIE present with recurring focal or generalized seizures typically lasting a few minutes. Although stress from handling can occasionally precipitate a seizure, many occur spontaneously without any external environmental stimuli (e.g. photosensitization). A focal or partial seizure involves one cerebral hemisphere, and in foals may be characterized by head or muzzle twitches [3, 7]. In people, the definition of a focal seizure is further divided into those with impaired or retained awareness, which is more difficult to ascertain in equine patients. Focal seizures may progress to generalized seizures or generalized seizures may occur spontaneously. Generalized seizures involve increased abnormal neuronal activity in both cerebral hemispheres and a loss of consciousness. Foals with JIE may present with generalized tonic (stiffness) seizures with clonic (twitching or jerking) motor activity or generalized tonic seizures followed by clonic seizures.

During the preictal phase, some foals will demonstrate abnormal behavior, hyperesthesia, ptyalism, and/or abnormal chewing behavior [3, 8]. The occurrence of preictal signs is inconsistent and may be missed by lay owners, particularly with respect to behavioral changes. During the postictal phase, the most common clinicals signs reported are blindness, ataxia, decreased suckle, obtundation, and disorientation [3, 8]. Foals are clinically normal between seizure events.

Complications following seizures include trauma and aspiration pneumonia. Organisms isolated from tracheal washes in foals with aspiration pneumonia are generally commensals of the nasopharynx and oral cavity [3]. Barring complications from seizures, long-term outcome and performance does not appear to be affected, however, reports are limited [4]. Reports of juvenile seizure disorders in people suggest that there are long-term neurobehavioral comorbidities associated with epilepsy [9, 10]. Jokinen et al. noted that Lagotto Romagnolo dogs with benign familial juvenile epilepsy (BFJE) exhibit behavior abnormalities resembling attention deficit disorder (ADHD) in people [11]. Further research is required to determine if there are similar findings in horses.

Equine Neonatal Medicine, First Edition. Edited by David M. Wong and Pamela A. Wilkins.

Pathogenesis

JIE is a genetic disease with a presumed autosomal dominant mode of inheritance. To date, the genetic cause is unknown and is being actively investigated. Two human neonatal epilepsy syndromes, benign familial neonatal epilepsy and benign neonatal-infantile seizures, are the result of mutations in genes coding for ion channels [12–14]. Benign familial neonatal epilepsy is caused by a mutation in either the KCNQ2 or KCNQ3 gene; these code for subunits that comprise a potassium channel for the muscarinic-regulated potassium current (M-current), which moderates neuronal excitability [14, 15]. Neonatal-infantile seizures result from a mutation in the gene SCN2A, which codes for the sodium voltage-gated channel alpha subunit 2 [12]. BFJE in Lagotto Romagnolo is caused by a mutation in the gene that codes for a protein called leucine-rich glioma-inactivated protein (LGI2) [16]. This protein has numerous functions, including modulating presynaptic voltage-gated potassium channels, interacting with scaffolding proteins, and a disintegrin and metalloprotease family of protein [16]. While these juvenile epilepsy syndromes may share phenotypic qualities with JIE, a specific mutation in equine KCNQ2, KCNQ3, SCN2A, and LGI2 has not been identified. Recent work suggests that JIE might result from a mutation in Tripartitis Motif-Containing 39-Ribonucleasep/mrp 21 kDa Subunit (TRIM39-RPP21); however, a follow-up study disproved this theory using EEG-confirmed JIE cases [14, 17, 18].

Diagnosis

JIE should be suspected in foals of Egyptian Arabian lineage presenting for recurrent seizures. Definitive diagnosis requires confirmation of epileptic seizures using electroenchephalography (EEG) and ruling out other possible causes. Abnormalities on the EEG include spikes, sharp waves, and spike and wave discharges (Figures 31.I.1, 31.I.2) [3, 5, 19]. While epileptiform changes on an EEG support the diagnosis of JIE, a normal EEG does not rule out epilepsy [5].

There are no specific hematologic or serum biochemical changes associated with JIE, however, foals may present with a stress leukogram, elevated muscle enzymes, and hyperglycemia [3]. Cerebral spinal fluid (CSF) may be xanthrochromic or normal [3]. In dogs with epilepsy, inflammatory, or neoplastic etiologies generally have higher CSF lactate concentrations than idiopathic or unknown causes, and focal seizures resulted in slightly higher lactate concentrations when compared to generalized seizures [20]. Another recent study in dogs suggested that high-mobility group box 1 (HMGB1), a nuclear protein that is released in response to neural inflammation by glial cells and neurons, may serve as a biomarker for idiopathic epilepsy [21].

Additional diagnostics, including ultrasound and radiography, may be indicated if there are comorbidities such as trauma or aspiration pneumonia. Advanced imaging, including computed tomography (CT) and magnetic resonance imaging (MRI), is unremarkable in foals with JIE just as it is in humans and dogs with heritable neonatal epilepsy syndromes [3, 22, 23].

Treatment

The treatment of JIE focuses on management of seizures and secondary complications, including aspiration pneumonia, and trauma. Early treatment of seizures can involve benzodiazepines (midazolam 0.1–0.2 mg/kg, IV or CRI 0.06–0.12 mg/kg/h, or diazepam 0.1–0.2 mg/kg, IV) followed by the use of barbiturates (phenobarbital), potassium bromide, or levetiracetam (Chapter 30) [3, 24].

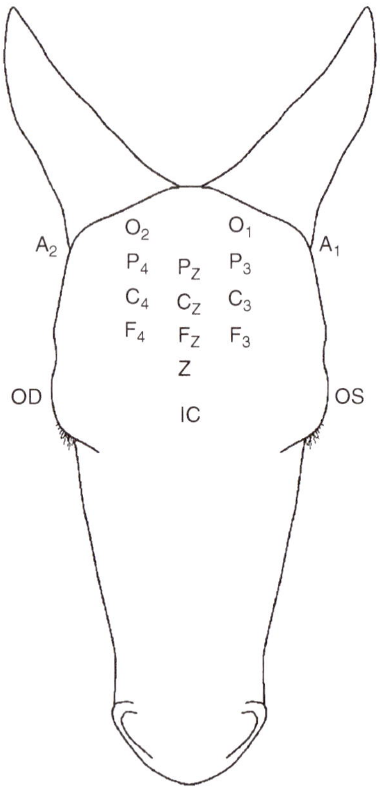

Figure 31.I.1 University of California–Davis–Veterinary Medical Teaching Hospital electrode placement protocol for electroencephalography in foals. Even numbers 5 right side, odd numbers 5 left side, z 5 midline, O 5 occipital, A 5 temporal, P 5 parietal, C 5 central, F 5 frontal, Z 5 ground, IC 5 intercanthus, OD 5 right eye, OS 5 left eye. *Source:* Image courtesy of Dr. Monica Aleman, University of California–Davis [3].

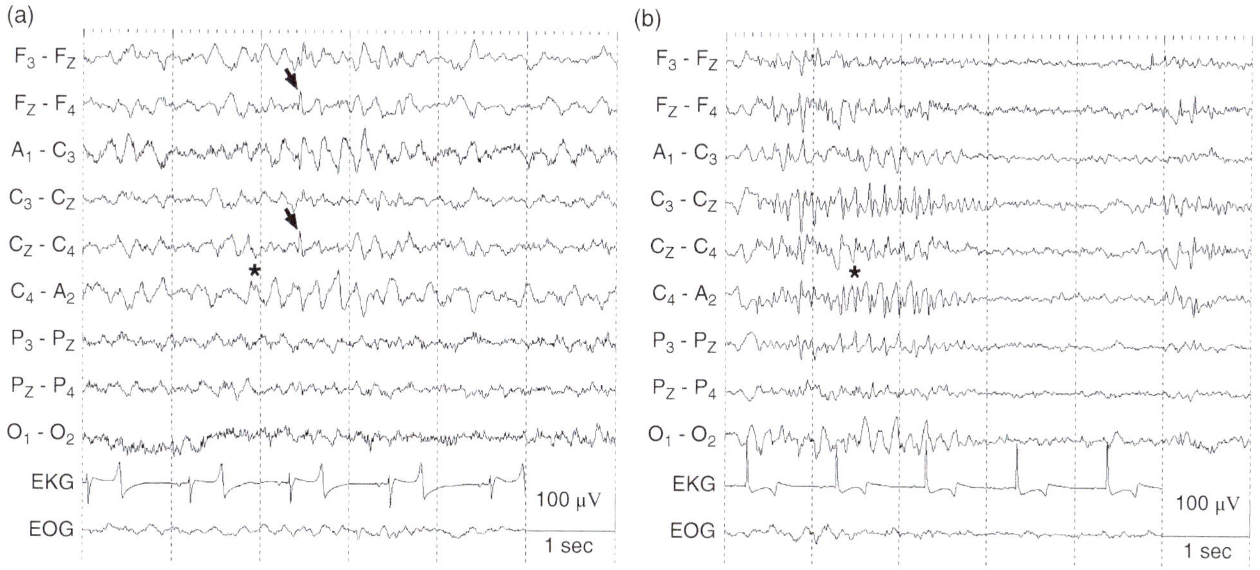

Figure 31.I.2 Electroencephalogram from a 3.5-week-old colt. (a) Frontocentral spike (arrow) and central theta burst (asterisk). (b) A burst of 6 Hz spike-and-wave discharges at C_Z/C_4 (asterisk) in a 4-week-old-colt. *Source:* Images courtesy of Dr. Monica Aleman, University of California–Davis [3].

Treatment is necessary until 1–2 years of age, which corresponds with cessation of seizure activity.

Additional therapies depend on concurrent conditions and may include fluid therapy, antimicrobials, and anti-inflammatories. Early work in people suggests that the gastrointestinal microbiome may play a role in epilepsy and may lead to the development of novel management strategies [25].

While long-term prognosis for foals with JIE is good, due to its suspected mode of inheritance, caution should be taken when deciding to keep these horses as breeding stock.

References

1 Berendt, M., Farquhar, R.G., Mandigers, P.J.J. et al. (2015). International veterinary epilepsy task force consensus report on epilepsy definition, classification and terminology in companion animals. *BMC Vet. Res.* 11 (1): 182.

2 Fisher, R.S., Acevedo, C., Arzimanoglou, A. et al. (2014). ILAE official report: a practical clinical definition of epilepsy. *Epilepsia* 55 (4): 475–482.

3 Aleman, M., Gray, L.C., Williams, D.C. et al. (2006). Juvenile idiopathic epilepsy in Egyptian Arabian foals: 22 cases (1985–2005). *J. Vet. Intern. Med.* 20: 1443–1449.

4 Aleman, M., Finno, C.J., Weich, K. et al. (2018). Investigation of known genetic mutations of Arabian horses in Egyptian Arabian foals with juvenile idiopathic epilepsy. *J. Vet. Intern. Med.* 32: 465–468.

5 Lacombe, V.A., Mayes, M., Mosseri, S. et al. (2012). Epilepsy in horses: Aetiological classification and predictive factors: epilepsy in horses. *Equine Vet. J.* 44 (6): 646–651.

6 Lichter-Peled, A., Polani, S., Stanyon, R. et al. (2013). Role of KCNQ2 and KCNQ3 genes in juvenile idiopathic epilepsy in Arabian foals. *Vet. J.* 196 (1): 57–63.

7 Fisher, R.S. (2017). The new classification of seizures by the international league against epilepsy 2017. *Curr. Neurol. Neurosci. Rep.* 17 (6): 48.

8 Mittel, L. (1987). Seizures in the horse. *Neurol Dis.* 3 (2): 323–332.

9 Baykan, B. and Wolf, P. (2017). Juvenile myoclonic epilepsy as a spectrum disorder: a focused review. *Seizure* 49: 36–41.

10 Wolf, P., Yacubian, E.M.T., Avanzini, G. et al. (2015). Juvenile myoclonic epilepsy: a system disorder of the brain. *Epilepsy Res.* 114: 2–12.

11 Jokinen, T.S., Tiira, K., Metsähonkala, L. et al. (2015). Behavioral abnormalities in Lagotto Romagnolo dogs with a history of benign familial juvenile epilepsy: a long-term follow-up study. *J. Vet. Intern. Med.* 29 (4): 1081–1087.

12 Melikishvili, G., Dulac, O., and Gataullina, S. (2020). Neonatal SCN2A encephalopathy: a peculiar recognizable electroclinical sequence. *Epilepsy Behav.* 111: 107187.

13 Maghera, J., Li, J., Lamothe, S.M. et al. (2020). Familial neonatal seizures caused by the Kv7.3 selectivity filter mutation T313I. *Epilepsia Open* 5: 562–573.

14 Edwards, L. and Finno, C.J. (2020). Genetics of equine neurologic disease. *Vet. Clin. North Am. Equine Pract.* 36 (2): 255–272.

15 Castaldo, P., del Giudice, E.M., Coppola, G. et al. (2002). Benign familial neonatal convulsions caused by altered gating of KCNQ2/KCNQ3 potassium channels. *J. Neurosci.* 22 (2): RC199–RC199.

16 Pakozdy, A., Patzl, M., Zimmermann, L. et al. (2015). LGI proteins and epilepsy in human and animals. *J. Vet. Intern. Med.* 29 (4): 997–1005.

17 Rivas, V.N., Aleman, M., Peterson, J.A. et al. (2019). TRIM39-RPP21 variants (Δ19InsCCC) are not associated with juvenile idiopathic epilepsy in Egyptian Arabian horses. *Genes* 10 (10): 816.

18 Polani, S., Dean, M., Lichter-Peled, A. et al. (2018). Sequence variant in the TRIM39-RPP21 gene readthrough is shared across a cohort of Arabian foals diagnosed with juvenile idiopathic epilepsy. *J. Gene Mutat.* 1: 103.

19 Lacombe, V.A., Podell, M., Furr, M. et al. (2001). Diagnostic validity of electroencephalography in equine intracranial disorders. *J. Vet. Intern. Med.* 15: 385–393.

20 Mariani, C.L., Nye, C.J., Ruterbories, L. et al. (2020). Cerebrospinal fluid lactate concentrations in dogs with seizure disorders. *J. Vet. Intern. Med.* 34 (6): 2562–2570.

21 Walker, L., Tse, K., Ricci, E. et al. (2014). High mobility group box 1 in the inflammatory pathogenesis of epilepsy: profiling circulating levels after experimental and clinical seizures. *The Lancet* 383: S105.

22 Pascual, F.T., Wierenga, K.J., and Ng, Y.-T. (2013). Contiguous deletion of KCNQ2 and CHRNA4 may cause a different disorder from benign familial neonatal seizures. *Epilepsy Behav. Case Rep.* 1: 35–38.

23 Erlen, A., Potschka, H., Volk, H.A. et al. (2020). Seizures in dogs under primary veterinary care in the United Kingdom: etiology, diagnostic testing, and clinical management. *J. Vet. Intern. Med.* 34 (6): 2525–2535.

24 MacDonald, K.D., Hart, K.A., Davis, J.L. et al. (2018). Pharmacokinetics of the anticonvulsant levetiracetam in neonatal foals. *Equine Vet. J.* 50 (4): 532–536.

25 Lum, G.R., Olson, C.A., and Hsiao, E.Y. (2020). Emerging roles for the intestinal microbiome in epilepsy. *Neurobiol. Dis.* 135: 104576.

Section II Lavender Foal Syndrome

Diane Rhodes

Lavender Foal Syndrome (LFS), also referred to as Coat Color Dilution Lethal (CCDL) or lethal dilute, is a fatal congenital disease affecting Arabian foals, particularly of Egyptian Arabian descent [1, 2]. The name stems from a coat color dilution that classically imparts a lavender hue to the hair coat, however, pale gray, pewter, and light chestnut (pink) have also been reported (Figure 31.II.1) [2]. The disorder is inherited in an autosomal recessive manner, following Mendelian genetics, with asymptomatic carriers. The carrier frequency in Egyptian Arabians is estimated to be 9.6–11.7%, depending on the region [4–6]. Other Arabian lineages may be affected; however, the estimated carrier frequency is significantly lower (1.8%) [4]. Investigation into LFS carrier frequency in breeds with Arabian influences, including the Thoroughbred, Standardbred, Quarter Horse, Morgan, and Percheron, did not identify any carriers, suggesting the mutation arose after their establishment [7].

Clinical Signs

Affected foals are neurologically abnormal at birth. Commonly reported clinical signs include seizures, nystagmus, ventral strabismus, paddling, opisthotonos, and failure to obtain sternal recumbency or stand [2, 3]. Paddling may be due to partial seizures or uncoordinated attempts to rise in the face of extensor rigidity [2, 3]; further study with additional diagnostics (i.e. electroencephalogram) is needed to identify the precise causes of these clinical signs [8, 9]. The suckle reflex may be strong or weak, and affected foals are able to swallow and vocalize [2, 3]. Withdrawal, cervicofacial, cutaneous trunci, and perineal reflexes are present, but interpretation may be complicated by exaggerated responses [3]. Pupillary light responses, both direct and indirect, are also normal [3].

Pathophysiology

LFS is caused by a single base-pair deletion in the mysoin Va gene (MYO5A), resulting in a frameshift mutation and premature stop codon in exon 30 [4]. In people, mutations in this gene cause Griscelli syndrome type-1 (GS1) and may be involved with a possible rare variant of GS1 called neuroectodermal melanolysosomal disease (Elejalde disease) [10]. Common clinical signs in people with GS1 include seizures, cerebellar signs, hemiparesis, spasticity, hypotonia, facial palsy, and psychomotor retardation. Additionally, affected individuals have hypopigmentation of the hair and skin [10]. Myosin Va interacts with proteins produced by the MLPH and RAB27A genes to form complexes that enable short-range organelle and macromolecule movement within cells [11]. In melanocytes, myosin Va facilitates transport of melanosomes to the periphery of the cell, allowing for transfer of melanin to tissues including the skin, hair, and eyes [12]. MYO5a is highly expressed in nervous tissue and is essential for the development and myelination of neurons, as well as transport of dendritic vesicles [12]. Dysfunction of myosin Va thus explains the impaired pigment delivery function and dilute coat color characteristic of affected foals as well as the multiple neurologic signs. To date, there is no evidence to suggest that LFS is related to juvenile idiopathic epilepsy (JIE), another heritable neurologic disorder seen in Egyptian Arabian foals [13].

Diagnosis and Treatment

The clinical signs associated with LFS may be similar to those for a variety of conditions, including sepsis, congenital malformations, and neonatal maladjustment syndrome [9]. The CBC and serum biochemistry profile is often unremarkable; however, hypoproteinemia and

Equine Neonatal Medicine, First Edition. Edited by David M. Wong and Pamela A. Wilkins.

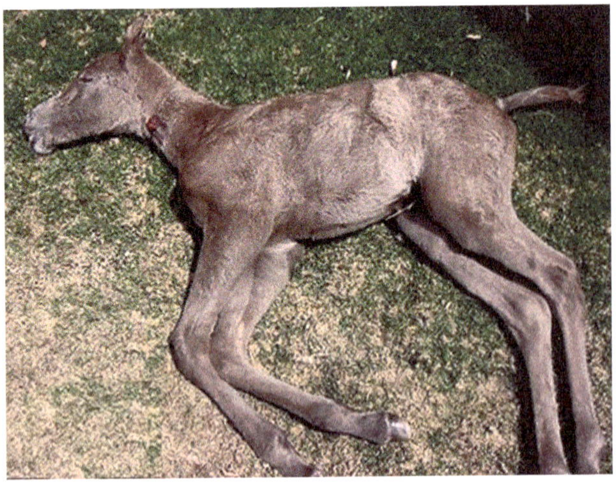

Figure 31.II.1 Typical appearance of a foal with lavender foal syndrome; note the dilute coat color [3].

hypoglycemia may be observed due to the foal's inability to stand and nurse. Further clinicopathologic abnormalities may be expected with other co-morbidities [2, 3]. There are no gross postmortem findings, but neuronal degeneration, vacuolization, and perivascular plasma cell infiltration may be seen on microscopic examination of neural tissue [9, 14]. A genetic test is commercially available and may be used to obtain a definitive diagnosis or determine a carrier state prior to breeding (sample type: 20–30 hairs with roots; test type: genotyping; test lab: UC Davis Veterinary Genetics Laboratory [http://vgl.ucdavis.edu/test/lfs]). There is no effective treatment for LFS. Anticonvulsive agents may provide short-term relief of symptoms, but lack of response to treatment and the overall grave prognosis of the disease typically necessitate euthanasia within the first few days of life [9].

References

1 Bowling, A.T. (1996). Medical genetics. In: *Horse Genetics* (ed. A.T. Bowling and A. Ruvinsky), 105–106. Wallingford: CAB International.

2 Fanelli, H.H. (2005). Coat colour dilution lethal ('lavender foal syndrome'): a tetany syndrome of Arabian foals. *Equine Vet. Educ.* 17: 260–263.

3 Page, P., Parker, R., Harper, C. et al. (2006). Clinical, clinicopathologic, postmortem examination findings and familial history of 3 Arabians with lavender foal syndrome. *J. Vet. Intern. Med.* 20: 1491–1494.

4 Brooks, B.A., Gabreski, N., Miller, D. et al. (2010). Whole-genome SNP association in the horse: identification of a deletion in myosin Va responsible for lavender foal syndrome. *PLos Genet.* 6: 1–7.

5 Efendić, M., Maćešić, N., Samardžija, M. et al. (2017). Determination of sublethal mutation causing lavender foal syndrome in Arabian horses from Croatia. *J. Equine Vet. Sci.* 61: 72–75.

6 Tarr, C.J., Thompson, P.N., Guthrie, A.J. et al. (2014). The carrier prevalence of severe combined immunodeficiency, lavender foal syndrome and cerebellar abiotrophy in Arabian horses in South Africa. *Equine Vet. J.* 46: 512–514.

7 Gabreski, N.A., Haase, B., Armstrong, C.D. et al. (2012). Investigation of allele frequencies for lavender foal syndrome in the horse. *Anim. Genet.* 43: 650.

8 Finno, C.J. and Aleman, A. (2013). Genetics of equine neurologic disease. In: *Equine Genomics* (ed. B.P. Chowdhary), 219–220. Germany: Wiley.

9 Edwards, L. and Finno, C.J. (2020). Genetics of equine neurologic disease. *Vet. Clin. Equine* 36: 255–272.

10 Gironi, L.C., Zottarelli, F., Savoldi, G. et al. (2019). Congenital hypopigmentary disorders with multiorgan impairment: a case report and an overview on gray hair syndromes. *Medicina (Kaunas, Lithuania)* 55: 78.

11 Hammer, J.A. and Wagner, W. (2013). Functions of class V myosins in neurons. *J. Biol. Chem.* 288: 28428–28434.

12 Eichler, T.W., Kögel, T., Bukoreshtliev, N.V. et al. (2006). The role of myosin Va in secretory granule trafficking and exocytosis. *Biochem. Soc. Trans.* 34: 671–674.

13 Aleman, M., Finno, C.J., Weich, K. et al. (2018). Investigation of known genetic mutations of Arabian horses in Egyptian Arabian foals with juvenile idiopathic epilepsy. *J. Vet. Intern. Med.* 32: 465–468.

14 Alkalamawy, N., Amin, D., Alkalamawy, I. et al. (2018). Lavender foal syndrome in Egyptian Arabian horses: molecular and pathological studies. *SVU-Int. J. Vet. Sci.* 1: 55–65.

Section III Cerebellar Abiotrophy

Kate L. Hepworth-Warren

Cerebellar abiotrophy (CA) is an inherited neurodegenerative condition described in horses, humans, sheep, goats, cattle, pigs, chickens, mice, cats, and dogs [1–4]. In equids, it occurs primarily in Arabian horses, but has been reported in other breeds of horse and one mule [5–8]. Foals with CA are often normal at birth but begin to show signs within the first year of life [9, 10].

Pathophysiology

Abiotrophy is described as premature degeneration of cells due to an innate defect in metabolism [11]. The key difference between abiotrophy and atrophy is that the degeneration results from an inborn error in the cells as opposed to external damage. In most instances, abiotrophy occurs as an inherited condition [11]. In cerebellar abiotrophy in the horse, there is degeneration of Purkinje cells that begins either at birth or within the first year of life [4, 11]. Apoptosis of the Purkinje cells has been suggested as a mechanism for this premature loss [12].

Epidemiology and Genetics

CA occurs primarily in Arabian horses, but has been reported in the Oldenburg, Gotland pony, Eriskay pony, and a mule [5, 8, 13]. An early case series of CA identified a gender predilection and noted that males were more likely to be affected; however, this has not been a consistent finding [10]. Unlike juvenile idiopathic epilepsy and lavender foal syndrome, which affects primarily Egyptian Arabians, CA does not appear to be specific to one type of Arabian horse [14–16].

In 2011, the putative mutation that leads to CA was identified on the ECA2 gene [1, 13]. This mutation is located approximately 1200 base pairs from MUTYH, which is involved in DNA repair. It has been proposed that the expression of MUTYH differed in affected horses when compared to normal horses, but its role in CA remains the focus of ongoing research [10, 13]. There have not been documented associations or co-mutations of CA and other known genetic diseases of Arabian horses, including lavender foal syndrome, severe combined immunodeficiency, occipitoatlantoaxial malformation and juvenile idiopathic epilepsy [15, 16].

The mode of inheritance for CA is autosomal recessive, therefore a mating between two carriers of the mutation will have a 25% risk of producing an affected foal, and a 50% risk of producing an unaffected carrier foal [17, 18]. Carriers of the mutation have been identified in Danish Sport Horses, Bashkir Curly horses, Trakehners, and Welsh ponies, all of known Arabian descent [6, 7]. A large study evaluating 808 Arabian horses and the mode of inheritance of CA identified a carrier frequency of 26.9%; however, the authors cautioned that this was a biased population with many related animals and could not be extrapolated to the breed [17]. More realistic carrier frequencies were identified in groups of Arabian horses in South Africa and Poland of 5.1% and 9.4%, respectively [14, 15].

Clinical Signs

Clinical signs of CA consist of cerebellar ataxia, intention tremors of the head, and an absent menace response that appear over the first year of life. Many foals with CA appear normal at birth, and signs develop within the first 6 weeks to 6 months of life, although it has been noted as early as birth, and diagnosed as late as 6 years of age [9, 10, 13, 19]. Fine head tremors are often the first sign observed, and may be exacerbated with intentional head movements, such as nursing. Head tremors can occur in either the lateral or vertical planes, although the latter is more common [9, 10].

Equine Neonatal Medicine, First Edition. Edited by David M. Wong and Pamela A. Wilkins.

The gait is hypermetric or dysmetric, with more pronounced dysmetria often noted in the thoracic limbs and truncal sway is often present in motion and at rest [9, 13]. The degree of ataxia ranges from mild stumbling to complete recumbency and inability to stand; gait deficits can be exacerbated when horses are walked over a curb, in small circles, or down a hill [9]. At rest affected horses display a wide-based stance. Menace response is often absent although the animal is visual, and nystagmus has not been reported [4, 9, 10, 20]. It is important to recall that normal foals do not have a consistent menace response until approximately 1--2 weeks of age. Affected animals can be hyperreactive and prone to falling when startled [9, 10].

Diagnosis

Clinical diagnosis of CA is based on the identification of cerebellar dysfunction in conjunction with the appropriate signalment, generally young Arabian horses. Differential diagnoses include other congenital diseases of the cerebellum (hypoplasia or aplasia), equine protozoal myeloencephalitis, viral encephalitides, neuroaxonal dystrophy, neoplasia, trauma, and vascular incidents [21]. Until recently, definitive diagnosis could only be obtained from histology of the cerebellum at postmortem examination thus exclusion of other differential diagnoses was crucial. However, genetic testing is now available through the University of California Davis, which can be performed antemortem on hair samples [18]. Genotypes reported as N/N genotypes will not have CA and are not carriers of the mutation, whereas heterozygotes N/CA are carriers but will not be affected by the condition. Horses with the CA/CA genotype will have cerebellar abiotrophy [18].

Clinicopathologic data from animals with CA, including hematology, serum biochemical profiles, and cerebrospinal fluid (CSF) analysis are generally unremarkable. Slight increases in activity of creatine kinase in CSF have been reported in horses with CA, but this is not a consistent finding [9]. Advanced imaging of the brain may be beneficial in excluding CA as a diagnosis, as macroscopic changes are often absent [22]. However, morphometric analysis of magnetic resonance imaging (MRI) of five horses with CA identified a significantly lower relative cerebellar size and increased CSF space in affected horses as compared to controls, although two of five affected horses did not show the latter [23]. An additional case report documented a reduction in cerebellar size via MRI performed on a foal with CA [24].

On postmortem examination, cerebellar hypoplasia has been described, but is not always evident on gross examination [9, 10, 20, 24, 25]. Histology of the cerebellar cortex of affected animals shows diffuse reduction in the number of normal Purkinje cells and the presence of swollen or shrunken degenerate Purkinje cells. Basket cells, or completely degenerate cells, can also be present in conjunction with gliosis and thinning of the granular and molecular layers of the cerebellum [9–11]. Mineralization within the thalamus of affected animals has been reported [9].

Prognosis

While CA is not fatal, there is no treatment. Thus, the majority of animals are euthanized as they are not safe to handle or ride. As signs are generally not progressive once present, some animals may learn to compensate for ataxia and be stable enough to be kept as a pasture animal [10]. However, owners should be educated as to the safety risks of keeping horses affected with CA and these animals should not be bred.

References

1 Brault, L.S., Cooper, C.A., Famula, T.R. et al. (2011). Mapping of equine cerebellar abiotrophy to ECA2 and identification of a potential causative mutation affecting expression of MUTYH. *Genomics* 97: 121–129.

2 de Lahunta, A. (1980). Comparative cerebellar disease in domestic animals. *Compend. Contin. Educ. Vet.* 11: 8–18.

3 Scaratt, W.K. (2004). Cerebellar disease and disease characterized by dysmetria or tremors. *Vet. Clin. Food Anim.* 20: 275–286.

4 Scott, E.Y., Woolard, K.D., Finno, C.J. et al. (2018). Cerebellar abiotrophy across domestic species. *Cerebellum* 17: 372–379.

5 Björck, G., Everz, K.E., Hansen, H.J. et al. (1973). Congenital cerebellar ataxia in the Gotland pony breed. *Zentralbl. Vet. Med. A* 20: 341–354.

6 Brault, L.S. and Penedo, M.C.T. (2011). The frequency of the equine cerebellar abiotrophy mutation in non-Arabian horse breeds. *Equine Vet. J.* 43: 727–731.

7 Fraser, H. (1966). Two dissimilar types of cerebellar disorders in the horse. *Vet. Rec.* 78: 608–612.

8 Suñol, A., Sanmarti Fierri, J., Foiani, G. et al. (2018). Cerebellar Purkinje cell degeneration in a mule foal (*Equus mulus mulus*). *Vet. Rec. Case Rep.* 6: e000560.

9 DeBowes, R.M., Leipold, H.W., and Turner-Beatty, M. (1987). Cerebellar Abiotrophy. *Vet. Clin. Equine* 3: 345–352.

10 Sponseller, M. (1967). Equine cerebellar hypoplasia and degeneration. In: *Proceedings of the Annual Convention of American Association of Equine Practitioners*, 123–126. AAEP.

11 de Lahunta, A. (1990). Abiotrophy in domestic animals: a review. *Can. J. Vet. Res.* 54: 65–76.

12 Blanco, A., Moyano, R., Vivo, J. et al. (2006). Purkinje cell apoptosis in Arabian horses with cerebellar abiotrophy. *J. Vet. Med.* 53: 286–287.

13 Edwards, L. and Finno, C.J. (2020). Genetics of equine neurologic disease. *Vet. Clin. Equine* 36: 255–272.

14 Bugno-Poniewierska, M., Stefaniuk-Szmukier, M., Piestrzynska-Kajtoch, A. et al. (2019). Genetic screening for cerebellar abiotrophy, severe combined immunodeficiency and lavender foal syndrome in Arabian horses in Poland. *Vet. J.* 248: 71–73.

15 Tarr, C.J., Thompson, P.N., Guthrie, A.J. et al. (2014). The carrier prevalence of severe combined immunodeficiency, lavender foal syndrome and cerebellar abiotrophy in Arabian horses in South Africa. *Equine Vet. J.* 46: 512–514.

16 Aleman, M., Finno, C.J., Weich, K. et al. (2018). Investigation of known genetic mutations of Arabian horses in Egyptian Arabian foals with juvenile idiopathic epilepsy. *J. Vet. Intern. Med.* 32: 465–468.

17 Brault, L.S., Famula, T.R., and Pineda, C.T. (2011). Inheritance of cerebellar abiotrophy in Arabians. *Am. J. Vet. Res.* 72: 940–944.

18 Veterinary Genetics Laboratory. Cerebellar abiotrophy. UC Davis Veterinary Medicine. https://vgl.ucdavis.edu/cerebellar-abiotrophy. Accessed April 14, 2021.

19 Foley, A., Grady, J., Almes, K. et al. (2011). Cerebellar abiotrophy in a 6-year-old Arabian mare. *Equine Vet. Educ.* 23: 130–134.

20 Palmer, A.C., Blakemore, W.F., Cook, W.R. et al. (1973). Cerebellar hypoplasia and degeneration in the young Arab horse: clinical and neuropathological features. *Vet. Rec.* 93: 62–66.

21 Johnson, A.L. (2011). Equine cerebellar abiotrophy: searching the genome for an explanation. *Equine Vet. Educ.* 23: 135–137.

22 Ferrell, E.A., Gavin, P.R., Tucker, R.L. et al. (2002). Magnetic resonance evaluation of neurologic disease in 12 horses. *Vet. Radiol. Ultrasound* 43: 510–516.

23 Cavelleri, J.M.N., Metzger, J., Hellige, M. et al. (2013). Morphometric magnetic resonance imaging and genetic testing in cerebellar abiotrophy in Arabian horses. *BMC Vet. Res.* 9: 1–9.

24 Pongratz, M.C., Kircher, P., Lang, J. et al. (2010). Diagnostic evaluation of a foal with cerebellar abiotrophy using magnetic resonance imaging. *Pferdeheilkunde* 4: 559–662.

25 Dungworth, D.L. and Fowler, M.E. (1966). Cerebellar hypoplasia and degeneration in a foal. *Cornell Vet.* 56: 17–24.

Section IV Deafness in Foals

Jamie Kopper

Hearing Loss

Hearing loss is an underrecognized clinical condition in horses, including foals, due to low sensitivity of identifying deafness or hearing loss based on history and physical examination as well as limited availability of advanced diagnostic testing (i.e. brainstem auditory evoked response, BAER) [1]. Hearing loss may result from trauma, inflammation, or infection of the peripheral auditory pathway, use of ototoxic medications (i.e. systemic administration of aminoglycosides and loop diuretics) and congenital sensorineural deafness [2–4].

Given the challenges of diagnosing hearing loss or deafness in animals, it remains underdiagnosed as compared to people. Although rarely reported in horses and not a congenital disorder per se, hearing loss secondary to systemic administration of aminoglycosides is of significant concern in people and may warrant consideration in neonatal foals, although this has yet to be evaluated in foals [2]. In humans, approximately 20% of individuals receiving aminoglycosides suffer from permanent hearing loss [5]. Aminoglycosides damage sensory hair cells, and they are not replaced when damaged, thus resulting in hearing loss. A single case report of aminoglycoside-related hearing loss exists in an adult horse [2], and a more recent prospective study evaluated 10 adult horses that were administered an IV dose (6.6 mg/kg) of gentamicin once daily for 7 days [6]. In this study, sensorineural auditory loss was documented in 7 of 10 healthy adult horses via BAER testing. Auditory loss developed during administration of gentamicin in six horses whereas loss was noted after discontinuation of gentamicin treatment in one horse. Dysfunction was partial [4] or complete [3], unilateral [6] or bilateral [1], and reversible [4] in some horses and irreversible in others [3]. The authors concluded that sensorineural auditory loss is a potential risk of gentamicin administration in horses, but studies in foals have not been conducted [6].

Congenital sensorineural deafness is associated with pigment alterations of the skin and/or irises in people and horses [1, 7, 8]. The exact role of these melanocytes is unknown. However, the presence of melanocytes within the inner ear is essential for hearing [9]. Magdesian and colleagues demonstrated similar associations between pigment alterations and deafness in American Paint Horses [1]. In many horses in this study, deafness was associated with the endothelin receptor B (EDNBR) genetic mutation [1]. Mutation of the ENDBR gene is best known for its association with overo lethal white foal syndrome [10].

Clinical Signs

Clinical signs vary. Owners report that some horses are calmer than their hearing counterparts, while others report an increased incidence of affected horses being startled [1]. This is likely even more challenging to assess clinically in neonatal foals. Failure of a foal to respond to sudden external noise outside of the foal's range of site may increase index of suspicion for complete bilateral deafness, but such examinations are subjective in nature. Otoscopic examinations of the external ear canal and ear are normal. In Paint Horses affected by congenital sensori-neural deafness, all 11 horses in one study had extensive white facial markers, with overo or tovero coat patterns and one or more blue irises with at least partially nonpigmented palpebral skin [1]. However, there was a wide variety of white

Equine Neonatal Medicine, First Edition. Edited by David M. Wong and Pamela A. Wilkins.

spotting within those coat patterns. Of the affected horses, many, but not all, had endothelin receptor B (EDNBR) genetic mutation. In the same study, all foals affected by overo lethal white syndrome were also deaf. Testing for EDNBR is commercially available (University of California Davis Equine Genetics Laboratory).

Ultimately, deafness is best diagnosed by brainstem auditory-evoked response (BAER) testing, which is described in detail elsewhere [1, 3], including the use in foals [1].

Treatment and Prognosis

There is no treatment for deafness in foals. Prognosis is generally good, as most horses compensate quite well for hearing loss, although variable clinical signs associated with deafness in horses have been reported [1]. In neonates, careful use of systemic ototoxic medications in critically ill foals – particularly those with comorbidities including prematurity and hypoxemia – may be warranted.

References

1 Magdesian, K.G., Williams, D.C., Aleman, M. et al. (2009). Evaluation of deafness in American Paint horses by phenotype, brainstem auditory-evoked responses and endothelin receptor B genotype. *J. Am. Vet. Med. Assoc.* 235: 1204–1211.
2 Dacre, K.J.P., Pirie, S., and Pince, D.P. (2013). Choke, pleuropneumonia, and suspected gentamicin vestibulotoxicity in a horse. *Equine Vet. Educ.* 15: 27–33.
3 Aleman, M., Puchalski, S.M., Williams, D.C. et al. (2008). Brainstem-auditory-evoked responses in horses with temporohyoid osteoarthropathy. *J. Vet. Intern. Med.* 22: 1196–1202.
4 Strain, G.M. (1996). Aetiology, prevalence and diagnosis of deafness in dogs and cats. *Br. Vet. J.* 152: 17–36.
5 Hudson, A.M., Lockard, G.M., Namjoshi, O.A. et al. (2020). Berbamine analogs exhibit differential protective effects from aminoglycoside-induced hair cell death. *Front. Cell. Neurosci.* 14 (234): eCollection2020.
6 Aleman, M.R., True, A., Scalco, R. et al. (2021). Gentamicin-induced sensorineural auditory loss in healthy adult horses. *J. Vet. Intern. Med.* 35: 3486–2494.
7 Giegy, C.A., Heid, S., Steffen, F. et al. (2007). Does a pleiotropic gene explain deafness and blue irises in white cats? *Vet. J.* 173: 548–553.
8 Matsushima, Y., Shinkai, Y., Kobayashi, Y. et al. (2002). A mouse model of Waardenburg syndrome type 4 with a new spontaneous mutation of the endothelin-B receptor gene. *Mamm Genome* 13 (1): 30–35.
9 Price, E.R. and Fisher, D.E. (2001). Sensorineural deafness and pigmentation genes: melanocytes and the *Mitf* transcriptional network. *Neuron* 30: 15–18.
10 Santschi, E.M., Purdy, A.K., Valberg, S.J. et al. (1988). Endothelin receptor B polymorphism associated with lethal white foal syndrome in horses. *Mamm Genome* 9: 306–309.

Section V Occipitoatlantoaxial Malformation (OAAM) in Foals

Jamie Kopper

Congenital malformations of the cervical vertebral column are rare in domestic animals [1–3], but of the domestic animals, they are most frequently described in horses [1, 2, 4–8]. Abnormalities associated with congenital occipitaoatlantoaxial malformations (OAAM) in horses can involve the occiput, atlas (first cervical vertebra, C1) and/or axis (second cervical vertebra, C2). In animals with OAAM, developmental errors occur during embryogenesis [1–3]. Originally, OAAMs were divided into three classifications [2] but have expanded to include up to six classifications [7–9] (Table 31.V.1).

Clinical Signs

Foals with OAAM have variable clinical signs including sudden death at birth, tetraparesis, ataxia, proprioceptive deficits, cervical sclerosis, head tilt, and other neurologic deficits [2, 10, 11]. These clinical abnormalities may be present at birth or develop over the first weeks to years of life [2, 10, 11]. Neurologic examination of clinically affected foals reveals a normal age-appropriate cranial nerve exam, normal mentation, and gait deficits due to vertebral stenosis affecting all four limbs. Additional clinical signs may include abnormal head position, extended neck posture, visible and/or palpable irregularities along the cervical spine, and/or a "clicking sound," which is thought to be due to luxation and replacement of a hypoplastic dens [12]. Although rare, in one Andalusian foal with cranioencephalic malformation with atlanto-occipital luxation, the foal displayed changes in mention, asymmetric decreased pupillary light reflexes, and apneic periods during cervical manipulation [7].

Diagnostics

Diagnosis of OAAM is typically made based on age and neurological exam with appropriate neurolocalization (i.e. cervical spinal cord) and confirmed with diagnostic imaging (i.e. radiographs [Figures 31.V.1 and 31.V.2a], computed tomography [Figure 31.V.2b]). Based on abnormalities identified in a neurological examination, other differentials for affected foals include trauma, osteomyelitis secondary to neonatal sepsis, equine degenerative myelopathy (EDM), equine protozoal myeloencephalitis (EPM), and cervical vertebral stenotic malformation (CVSM). Cerebral spinal fluid analysis typically reveals a normal fluid protein and normal-to-mild leukocytosis characterized by an increased number of macrophages [13]. To further characterize the lesion and confirm spinal cord compression a myelogram can be pursued.

OAAM in Arabian horses is inherited in an autosomal recessive manner without sex predilection [5, 14]. Investigations by Borbari and colleagues identified a 2.7 kb deletion of a conserved sequence within the HOXD 3/4 region in a clinically affected Arabian mare [12]. Genetic testing for OAAM is now available for Arabian horses and Arabian crosses (University of California Davis Veterinary Genetics Laboratory).

Equine Neonatal Medicine, First Edition. Edited by David M. Wong and Pamela A. Wilkins.

Table 31.V.1 OAAM classification schemes.

	Mayhew et al. [2]	Viu et al. [7]	Chowdhary [9]	BrÜnisholz et al. [8]
1	(A) Familial occipitalization of the atlas with atlantalization of the axis in Arabian horses	Occipitalization (occipital bone-like modification) of the atlas and atlantization (atlas bone-like modification) of the axis (familial in Arabian horses)	Occipitalization of the atlas with atlantalization of the axis; inherited in Arabian horses	(A) Atlanto-occipital fusion with hypoplasia and malformation of C2 including the dens and modification of atlanto-axial joint
2	(B) Congenital asymmetrical occipitoatlantoaxial malformation	Asymmetric malformations	Subluxation of the atlantooccipital joint and fusion of the atlas and axis with lateral deviation of the atlantoaxial joint and 20° rotation of the atlas	(B) Asymmetrical atlanto-occipital fusion; cervical sclerosis; presence of wedge-shaped bone caudally at C2
3	(C) Asymmetrical atlantooccipital fusion	Asymmetric atlanto-axial fusion	Congenital asymmetrical OAAM	(C) Asymmetrical atlanto-occipital fusion with aplasia of occipital condyles and cervical sclerosis
4		Duplication of C1	Asymmetric atlanto-occipital fusion	(D) Duplication of C1
5		Abnormalities similar to familial Arabian forms in non-Arabian individuals	Duplication of axis or atlas	
6			Symmetrical OAAM in non-Arabian horses	

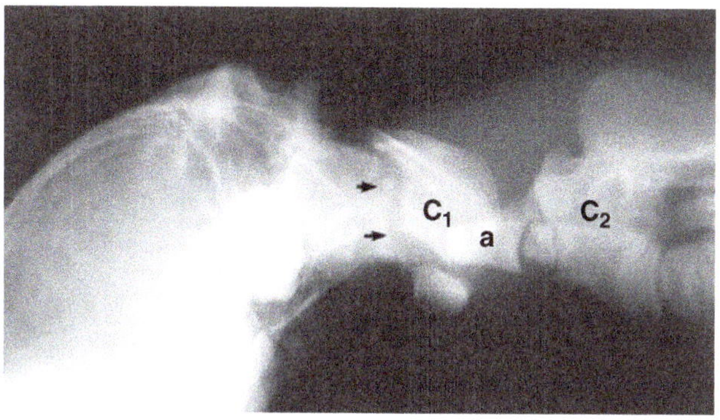

Figure 31.V.1 Lateral radiograph of a foal with OAAM. The foal's cervical vertebrae demonstrate fusion of a malformed C1 and occipital condyles (arrows) along with a hypoplastic dens (a) [13].

(a)

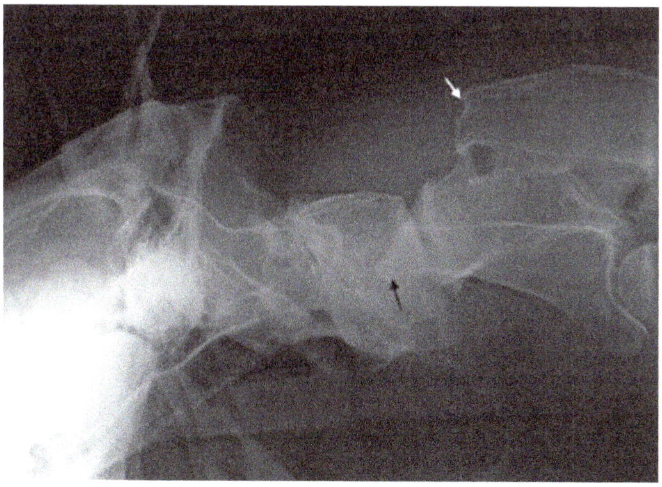

(b)

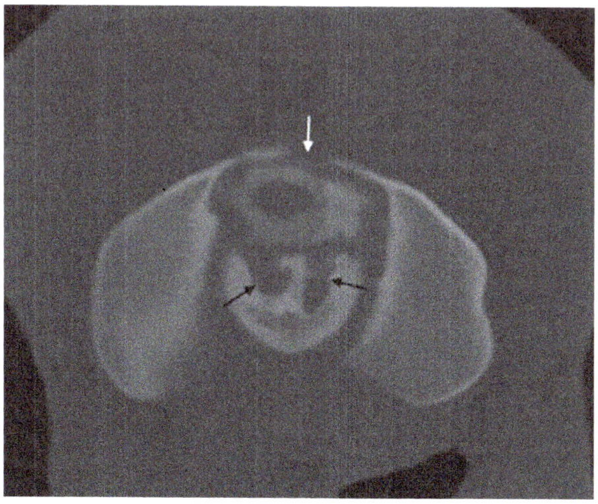

Figure 31.V.2 Imaging from a 3-year-old Warmblood mare with spinal ataxia secondary to congenital occipitoatlantoaxial malformation. (a) Lateral radiograph of the cranial neck. Note that the dorsal arch of C_1 is shortened and the dens of C_2 (black arrow) and cranial portion of the spinous process of C_2 (white arrow) are shortened and blunted. (b) Transverse computed tomography myelogram at the level of the atlanto-axial joint. Note the longitudinal defect within the dorsal arch (white arrow) of C_1 and the surface of the dens of C_2 (black arrows) is irregular [8].

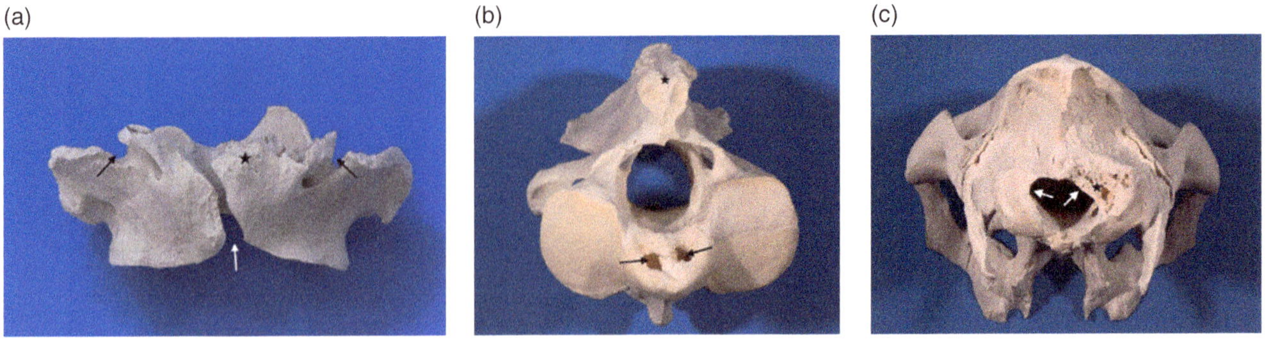

Figure 31.V.3 Postmortem samples from same horse as Figure 31.V.2. (a) Dorsal view of C_1. Note longitudinal split in the dorsal arch (white arrow) and presence of an incisura alare (black arrows) instead of a foramen alare. Also note the bony proliferations and rough appearance of the dorsal arch of C_1 (black star). (b) Cranial view of C_2. Note irregular shortened shape and surface of the dens containing several cavities (black arrows) and the irregularity of the spinous process of C_2 (black star). (c) Caudal view of occiput. Note the asymmetry of the foramen magnum (white arrows) and bony proliferations on the right occipital condyle (black star).

Treatment

Unfortunately, euthanasia is recommended for affected foals (Figure 31.V.3) due to a combination of bone fusion, spinal cord compression and vertebral instability caused by the defect(s) [13]. Surgical treatment has been suggested to correct atlantoaxial subluxation and scoliosis [15], but to date successful reports are not available. Given the autosomal recessive heritable nature in Arabian horses, genetic testing of related animals is recommended to inform future breeding decisions.

References

1 Wilson, W.B., Hughes, S.J., Ghoshal Ghoshal, N.G., and McNeel, S.V. (1985). Occipitoatlantoaxial malformation in two non-Arabian horses. *J. Am. Vet. Med. Assoc.* 187 (1): 36–40.

2 Mayhew, I.G., Watson, A.G., and Heissan, J.A. (1978). Congenital occipitoatlantoaxial malformations in the horse. *Equine Vet. J.* 10 (2): 103–113.

3 Watson, A.G., Wilson, J.H., Cooley, A.J. et al. (1985). Occipito-atlanto-axial malformation with atlanto-axial subluxation in an ataxic calf. *J. Am. Vet. Med. Assoc.* 187 (7): 740–742.

4 Leipold, H.W., Brandt, G.W., Guffy, M., and Blanch, B. (1974). Congenital atlantooccipital fusion in a foal. *Vet. Med. Small Anim. Clin.* 62: 646–653.

5 Watson, A.G. and Mayhew, I.G. (1986). Familial congenital occipitoatlantoaxial malformation (OAAM) in the Arabian horse. *Spine* 11: 334–339.

6 deLahunta, A., Hatfield, C., and Dietz, A. (1989). Occipitoatlantoaxial malformation with duplication of the atlas and axis in a half Arabian foal. *Cornell Vet.* 79: 185–193.

7 Viu, J., Armengou, L., Jose-Cunilleras, E. et al. (2010). Cranioencephalic malformation with atlanto-occipital luxation in an Andalusian neonatal foal. *J. Vet. Intern. Med.* 24: 639–642.

8 BrÜnisholz, H.P., Wildhaber, N., Hoey, S. et al. (2019). Congenital occipitoatlantoaxial malformation in a Warmblood mare. *Equine Vet. Educ.* 31 (5): 242–247.

9 Chowdhary, B.P. (2013). Genetics of equine neurologic disease. In: *Equine Genomics* (ed. B.P. Chowdhary), 229–231. Ames IA: Wiley.

10 Blikslager, A.T., Wilson, D.A., Constantinescue, G.M. et al. (1991). Atlantoaxial malformation in a half-Arabian colt. *Cornell Vet.* 81 (1): 67–75.

11 Mayhew, I.G. (1989). Tetraparesis, paraparesis, and ataxia of the limbs, and episodic weakness. In: *Large Animal Neurology: A Handbook for Veterinary Clinicians* (ed. I.G. Mayhew), 258–260. Philadelphia PA: Lea & Febiger.

12 Bordbari, M.H., Penedo, M.C.T., Aleman, M. et al. (2016). Deletion of 2.7 kb near HOXD3 in an Arabian horse with occipitoatlantoaxial malformation. *Anim. Genet.* 48: 287–294.

13 Gonda, C., Crisman, M., and Moon, N. (2001). Occipitoatlantoaxial malformation in a quarter horse foal. *Equine Vet. Educ.* 13 (6): 289–291.

14 Noden, D. and de Lahunta, A. (1985). Limb development. In: *The Embryology of Domestic Animals* (ed. G. Stamathis), 206–207. Baltimore: Williams and Wilkins.

15 Rush, B.R. (2012). Developmental vertebral abnormalities. In: *Equine Surgery*, 4e (ed. J.A. Auer and J.A. Stick), 693–699. St Louis MO: Elsevier Saunders.

Section VI Miscellaneous Congenital Disorders of the Nervous System

Kate L. Hepworth-Warren

Congenital defects of the equine neurologic system are rare and are often identified either on postmortem examination or by advanced imaging when foals fail to respond to therapy for more common neurologic conditions, such as neonatal maladjustment syndrome [1]. The majority of defects described here have only been identified in isolated cases. It is important to note that defects of the central nervous system (CNS) rarely occur alone, and many have other associated anomalies within the nervous system or other body systems [2–4]. Prognosis for the defects described in this chapter are generally grave [1–9].

Defects of the Brain and Cranial Nerves

Hydranencephaly

Hydranencephaly is a cerebral abnormality in which the neopallium (cerebral hemispheres) is reduced to a thin, nearly transparent pial/glial membrane with no associated parenchyma other than a thin layer of ependyma lining the expanded ventricle; the latter representing compensatory hydrocephalus secondary to the absence of cerebral parenchyma. It occurs when the developing cerebral hemispheres are destroyed in utero due to vascular compromise or viral infections [6, 10]. There have been three reported cases in the horse to date, one of which was identified in an aborted fetus. The most detailed report described a Welsh foal that was born 1 week premature and developed seizure activity at 12 hours of age [6]. The foal was able to hold itself in sternal recumbency and was alert, but never stood and was euthanized at four days of age when seizure activity became uncontrollable. Postmortem examination revealed severe collapse of both cerebral hemispheres, more severe on the right side (Figure 31.VI.1). The right cerebral hemisphere consisted of only a thin layer of neural tissue that ruptured during handling. The left hemisphere was significantly smaller than normal but had identifiable sulci and gyri. Both cerebral hemispheres had ventriculomegaly or dilated ventricles (compensatory hydrocephalus), but the brainstem and cerebellum were normally formed [6]. Hydranencephaly was also identified in an intentionally aborted Haflinger fetus and in one foal in a retrospective study [10–12]. In the aborted Haflinger fetus, hydranencephaly was identified in addition to cerebellar aplasia and severe scoliosis. The mare in this case was in the seventh month of gestation and abortion was induced after hydrops was diagnosed [11].

Hydrocephalus

Hydrocephalus develops when there is an interruption or obstruction to the normal flow or absorption of cerebrospinal fluid (CSF). It is classified as internal hydrocephalus when CSF accumulates within the ventricular system, or external hydrocephalus (also known as hydrocephalus ex vacuo) when the subarachnoid space becomes dilated with an excessive volume of CSF (Figure 31.VI.2) [13]. It is the most common congenital brain malformation in foals and was identified in 0.6 of every 1000 foals with congenital defects [14]. Hydrocephalus can occur spontaneously, or be acquired, and is associated with a specific mutation in Friesian horses [1, 13–15]. Hydrocephalus in Friesians (Figure 31.VI.3) has an autosomal recessive mode of inheritance and is associated with a mutation in the B3GALNT gene, which has also been identified in an aborted Belgian fetus with hydrocephalus [15, 17]. While Friesians appear to have a higher incidence of hydrocephalus than other breeds, it has also been reported in Standardbreds, Orlov Trotters, Thoroughbreds, Miniature Horses, Finnish Horses, Belgians, and Quarter Horses [12, 13, 15–20].

Foals with hydrocephalus often have a domed head/skull and display variable neurologic deficits at birth [12, 13, 18, 21, 22]. Due to the external abnormalities, hydrocephalus has been identified in 1–5% of foals born from dystocia and

Equine Neonatal Medicine, First Edition. Edited by David M. Wong and Pamela A. Wilkins.

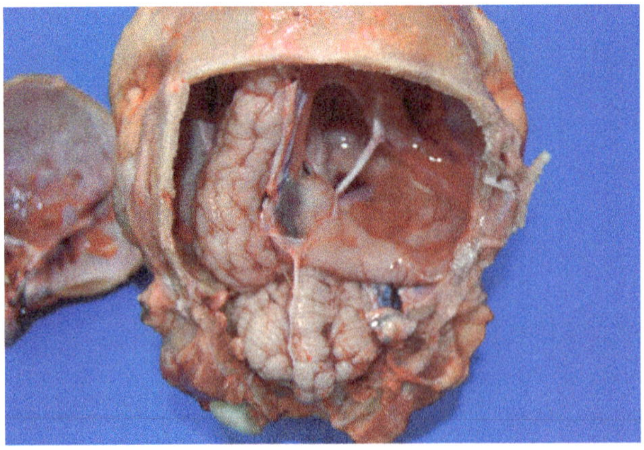

Figure 31.VI.1 Severely abnormal cerebral hemispheres in situ, which collapsed after escape of cerebrospinal fluid. While small, the left hemisphere is better preserved with a narrow cortex but retained gyri and sulci. The right cerebral hemisphere consists mostly of a thin, transparent, and congested membrane that has torn. *Source:* Image from [6].

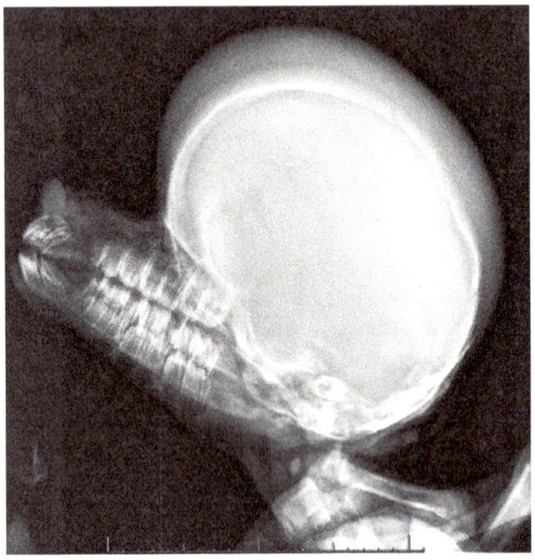

Figure 31.VI.2 Radiograph of a foal with severe cranial deformation. Note the ground glass appearance of the fluid within the skull consistent with hydrocephalic fluid [12].

is identified as a cause of stillbirth [15, 23, 24]. Affected foals may initially appear neurologically normal [13]. Clinical signs of hydrocephalus are consistent with forebrain and brainstem involvement and include obtundation, head pressing, seizure activity, compulsive walking, ventrolateral strabismus ("sunset eyes"), nystagmus, weakness, and ataxia [1, 10, 13, 18, 21, 25]. The menace response may not develop in affected foals [13, 22]. Affected foals that do not display the visible skull abnormalities may initially be diagnosed as having neonatal maladjustment syndrome based on an inability to stand, inappropriate behavior, and absent or decreased suckle [16, 18, 21, 22]. Prognosis for foals with hydrocephalus is grave and most are either euthanized or die shortly after birth [1, 13, 16].

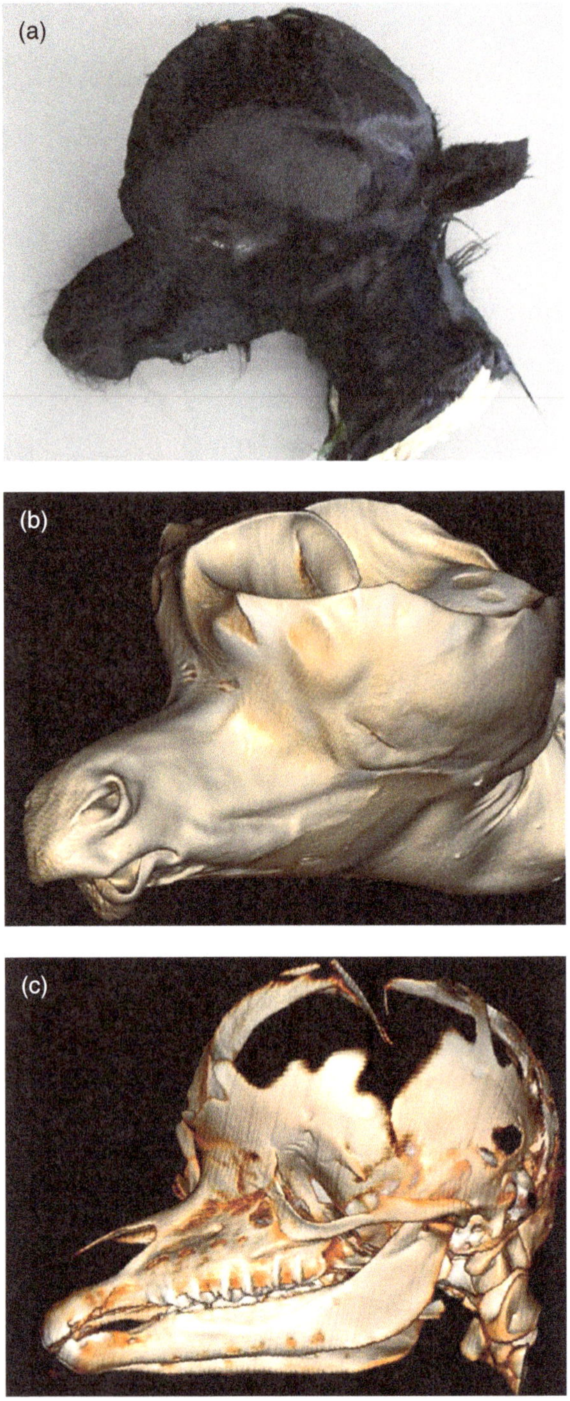

Figure 31.VI.3 Skull from a stillborn Friesian foal: (a) lateral view of a typical example of hydrocephalus; (b) middle-computed tomographic left lateral view of the skull of a Friesian foal; (c) three-dimensional reconstruction showing that ossification at the rostral part of the cranium is incomplete in hydrocephalus. *Source:* Image from [16].

While surgical treatment by placement of a ventriculoperitoneal shunt has been well-documented in other species, the procedure has only been reported once in the horse (Figure 31.VI.4) [21, 26]. In that report, hydrocephalus

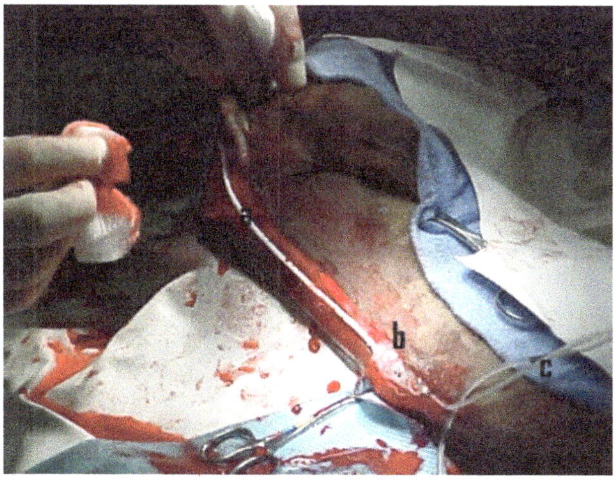

Figure 31.VI.4 Surgical implantation of a ventricular catheter (a) subcutaneously. The ventricular catheter is connected to the valve (b), which is subsequently connected to the peritoneal catheter (c) [21].

was diagnosed in a Quarter Horse filly and surgery performed at 30 days of age. The filly initially improved postoperatively but was euthanized 12 days after the procedure due to development of severe bacterial meningitis and peritonitis [21].

Dandy-Walker Malformation

Dandy-Walker malformation or syndrome is a cerebellar malformation that describes hypoplasia or complete agenesis of the cerebellar vermis that occurs in conjunction with cystic dilation of the fourth ventricle and may cause enlargement of the posterior (caudal) fossa (Figure 31.VI.5) [10, 27]. It has been associated with other malformations of the brain and congenital defects in other body systems in other species, though associated malformations outside of the nervous system have not been identified in horses [4, 27, 28]. Clinical signs that have been reported in horses include seizure activity, ataxia, nystagmus, absent suckle, apneic breathing, mental obtundation, aggression, inability to right themselves, truncal sway, intention tremors, and wide-based stance [4, 7, 27]. Consistent with Dandy-Walker malformations in other species, affected foals have had concurrent hydrocephalus, agenesis of the corpus collosum, and meningocele. It is important to note that without concurrent malformations, Dandy-Walker malformation alone would not lead to seizures and behavioral changes. Of the three foals described in the literature, two were euthanized within the first 3 days of life, and the third was euthanized at 6 months of age [4, 7, 27]. Computed tomography was utilized to make an ante-mortem diagnosis in one foal; advanced imaging should be considered when brain malformations are suspected [4].

Holoprosencephaly

Holoprosencephaly is characterized by the incomplete or entirely absent division of the cerebral hemispheres during embryonic development (Figures 31.VI.6 and 31.VI.7). It can develop from many causes in people, including drug, alcohol and tobacco use, toxic substances, diabetes mellitus, and can also be inherited [10, 29–31]. Holoprosencephaly has also been called arrhinencephaly because development of the olfactory system fails to occur [10]. Little is known about the cause in animals, but the condition has been reported in lambs, pigs, dogs,

(a) (b)

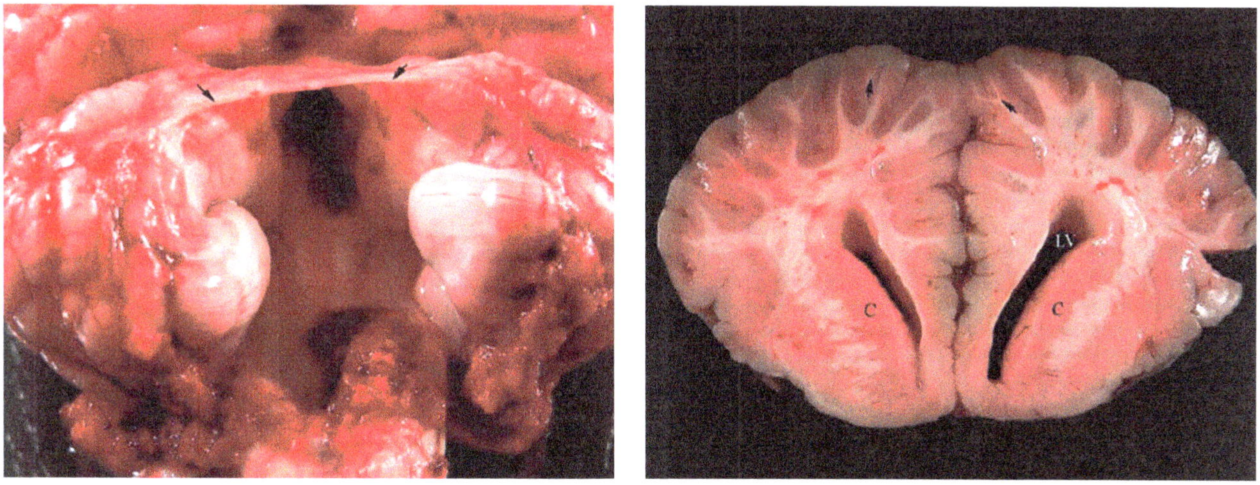

Figure 31.VI.5 Dandy-Walker malformation in a neonatal foal. (a) The fourth ventricle is evident because of complete lack of the cerebral vermis. There is a fibrous membrane covering the roof of the fourth ventricle (arrowheads); this was fused with the meninges forming a meningocele. (b) Cross-section of the brain at the level of the caudate nuclei (c) revealing a lack of the corpus callosum, mild dilation of the lateral ventricle (LV) and polymicrogyria (arrowheads) [4].

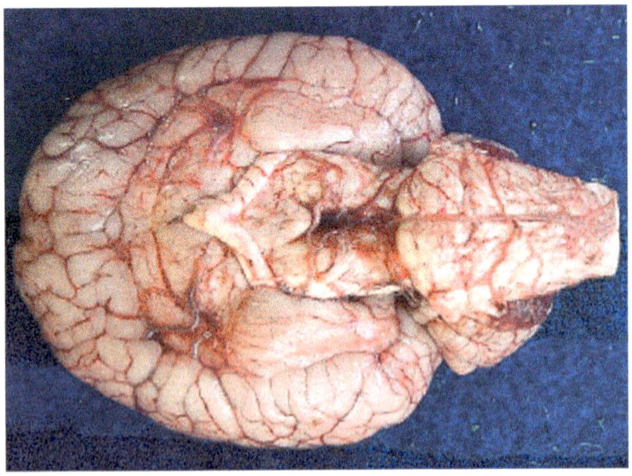

Figure 31.VI.6 Ventral view of the brain of a six-month-old Morgan with partial holoprosencephaly. Note the absence of any longitudinal cerebral fissure rostral to the optic chiasm and absence of olfactory bulbs and peduncles [10].

macaques, and three horses [29–31]. It is the most common congenital abnormality of forebrain development in people and is broken down into four subtypes classified by the degree of cleavage of the forebrain. These include alobar, semilobar, lobar, and a middle inter-hemispheric fusion variant. The most severe form is alobar, where the hemispheres completely fail to separate and only one cerebral ventricle develops with an absent corpus collosum and absent olfactory bulb [30, 31]. Alobar holoprosencephaly was identified in an aborted Quarter Horse fetus at nine months of gestation [30]. Semilobar holoprosencephaly is characterized by an interhemispheric fissure that is only visible in the caudal part of the cerebrum, and the olfactory bulbs and corpus collosum are absent [31]. It has been reported in a Morgan filly and a neonatal Quarter Horse colt [29, 31]. The Morgan filly had appropriate mentation but sporadically displayed abnormal behavior including persistent chewing of the dam's mane and tail, slow chewing without coordinated swallowing, and bruxism from a young age. Seizures developed around 6.5 months of age, and the filly was subjected to humane euthanasia [29]. On postmortem examination, there was also the absence of olfactory bulbs and peduncles, absence of cribriform plates, and absence of septum pellucidum.

Vascular Hamartoma

Vascular hamartomas are developmental anomalies of vessels that are present at birth and grow with the animal. There is a sole report in the literature in which a vascular hamartoma was identified in a Frieberger colt. The colt began showing signs of intermittent respiratory distress, laryngeal paralysis and dysphagia at birth that persisted until euthanasia at 4 weeks of age. Postmortem examination identified a dark red, well-demarcated mass in the obex of the white matter of the brain that was histopathologically identified as a vascular hamartoma [32].

Meningocele/Meningoencephalocele

A meningocele is a protrusion of the meninges through the cranium or vertebral canal (Figure 31.VI.8). Grossly, they appear as soft, fluctuant swellings located on midline and in multiple cases have not led to detectable neurological deficits [5, 8]. Meningoceles have been documented in live and stillborn foals and aborted fetuses in association with the brain and spinal cord [5, 8, 33]. Meningoencephaloceles are similar but also contain brain tissue and are more common in most species (Figure 31.VI.9) [10]. Meningoencepholoceles are due to ventricular dilation [10]. Surgical correction was

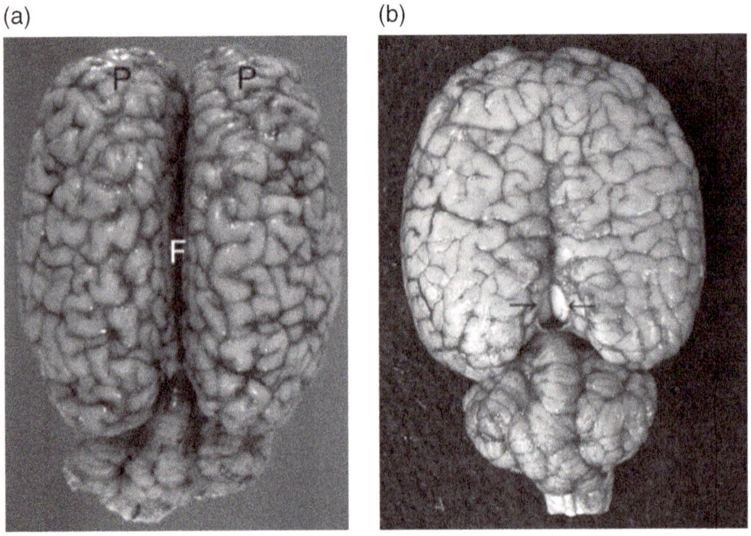

Figure 31.VI.7 Dorsal aspect of the brain from a healthy horse (a) and a horse with semilobar holoprosencephaly (b). (a) shows the longitudinal cerebral fissure (F), rostral poles of the cerebral hemispheres (P). In (b), there is no separation of the rostral components of the cerebrum, which forms a single, noncleaved structure. The longitudinal cerebral fissure is absent on the rostral third of the brain and inconspicuous along the middle third of the brain. An interhemispheric cleft is on the caudal part of the brain at the level of the rostral colliculi (arrows), which are readily visible through this small space. There is also diffuse flattening of the cerebral gyri [29].

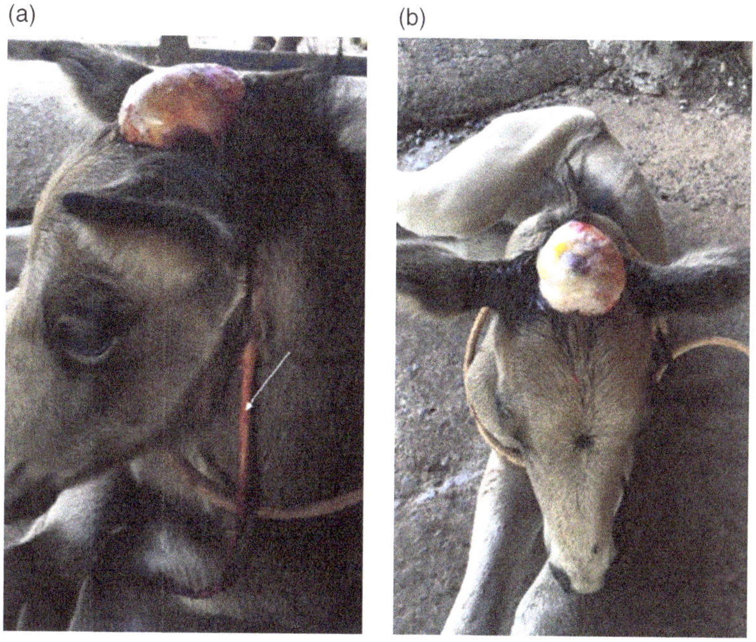

Figure 31.VI.8 Meningocele at birth. (a) Left lateral view. (b) Front view. *Source:* Image from Alonso [5].

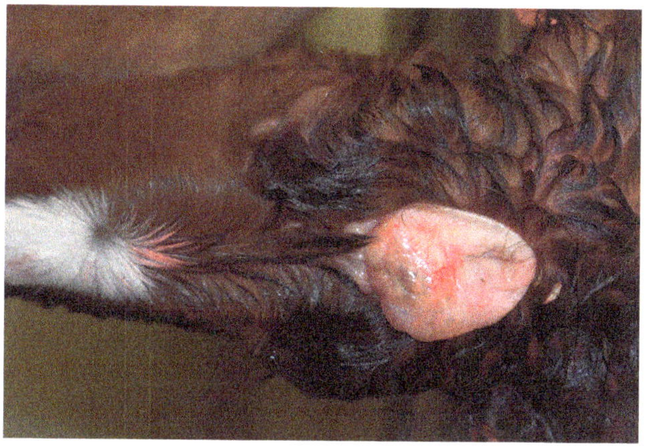

Figure 31.VI.9 A term foal born with a meningoencephalocele and incomplete brain formation. The foal displayed seizure activity and was euthanized due to cranial defects. *Source:* Image courtesy of Dr. Rebecca Ruby, University of Kentucky.

attempted in a 1-day-old Quarter Horse colt that was presented for evaluation of a cranial mass ultimately diagnosed as an occipital meningocele. Leakage of CSF was identified from the mass, but the foal was neurologically appropriate at presentation. Surgical closure of the defect was performed, and the foal was clinically normal for 48 hours following the procedure, but ultimately was euthanized after bacterial meningitis developed 14 days postoperatively [5]. Correction of a cervical and thoracic meningocele has also been attempted. In the former, the foal died within one week of discharge from the hospital, but in the latter case, the filly continued to do well until 6 months postoperatively, at which point the patient was lost to follow-up [8].

Congenital Facial Nerve Paralysis

Congenital facial nerve paralysis was identified in a 17-month-old Warmblood filly that presented for evaluation of facial asymmetry since birth. Neurologic examination identified a drooping right ear, ptosis of the right eye, mild mandibular lymphadenomegaly, deviation of the muzzle to the left, drooping of the right lower lip, right-sided green nasal discharge, and absent menace on the right side. The right masseter muscle was mildly atrophied in comparison to the left, which was attributed to disuse. Magnetic resonance imagining identified that the intracranial portion of the right facial nerve was significantly thinner than the left. The patient was euthanized, and histopathology identified atrophic neurons that contained a decreased number of smaller Nissl bodies than the left facial nerve. The extracranial portion of the nerve was completely aplastic and histopathologically was identified as connective tissue [34].

Epidermoid Cyst of the Brain

Epidermoid cysts develop from the sequestration of ectopic non-neural ectoderm in the brain at the time of neural tube closure. They grow gradually via keratin desquamation but may not induce clinical signs for many years [35, 36]. These cysts have been reported in two adult horses, a 15-year-old Connemara mare and a 12 -year-old Haflinger gelding [35, 36]. In both instances, the horses were neurologically normal until middle age at which time they developed episodic changes in mentation in between which they appeared normal. Both animals were humanely euthanized and large intracranial epidermoid cysts were identified at postmortem exam reaching up to 9 cm × 8 cm × 5 cm. In the Haflinger, the cyst was located in the region of the tentorium cerebelli and compressed the cerebellum and brainstem [36]. In the Connemara, the cyst was identified at the dorsolateral aspect of the left occipital lobe and compressed but did not invade the underlying tissue [35]. Histologically, the cysts were comprised of stratified squamous epithelium surrounded by a thick fibrous capsule [34, 35].

Chiari and Chiari-Like Malformation

Chiari malformation is a term used to describe a human anomaly that involves malformation of the occipital bone/skull, crowding of the caudal fossa, and cerebellar herniation through the foramen magnum [37, 38]. In people, four subtypes have been described and a fifth has been proposed [37, 38]. Defects similar to Chiari malformation have been well-documented in calves and dogs and are presumed to be heritable [39]. Affected calves are unable to make coordinated limb movements to stand after birth and frequently also show opisthotonus and nystagmus, although they are alert and visual [10]. The cerebellum is elongated, compressed, and displaced caudally in association with the brainstem. In addition to the cerebellar malformations, affected calves also have accompanying sacrocaudal spina bifida, meningomyelocele, and malformed tails [10]. To date, there have been two documented cases of Chiari or Chiari-like malformations in an Andalusian and a Thoroughbred foal [40, 41]. In both cases, malformations were most consistent with Type II Chiari malformation. The Andalusian colt was presented at 12 hours of age for evaluation of weakness and inability to stand. The foal showed visible signs of immaturity (domed forehead and flexor tendon laxity) and the skull had a prominent occipital crest. Relevant neurologic abnormalities included abnormal mentation, apnea induced by cervical manipulation, and an absent suckle reflex. Atlanto-occipital subluxation and a malformation of the skull was noted on radiographs. The foal was euthanized and postmortem exam demonstrated caudal displacement of the hindbrain and a misshapen cerebellar vermis due to compression from adjacent boney structures and accompanying hydrocephalus [40]. The Thoroughbred filly was presented at a few hours of age for evaluation of inability to stand and a soft swelling over the lumbar vertebral column. Neurologic evaluation identified paroxysmal movement of the thoracic limbs and total lack of coordinated movement, absent withdrawal reflex and absent nociception in the pelvic limbs. Lateral displacement of the thoracic vertebral column was noted in addition to a fluctuant swelling that was 4 × 5 cm protruding from the foal's lumbar region and was painful on palpation. Radiography identified severe scoliosis of the thoracolumbar vertebral column and the foal was humanely euthanized. Computed tomography and magnetic resonance imaging were performed postmortem. Postmortem examination identified scoliosis of the thoracolumbar vertebral column, spina bifida aperta from the fourth to sixth lumbar vertebrae, and meningomyelocele at this site. The foal also had herniation of the cerebellar vermis through the foramen magnum – consistent with a Type II Chiari malformation [41].

Defects of the Vertebral Column and Spinal Cord

Miscellaneous Vertebral Malformations

Vertebral and spinal cord malformations are classified according to their etiology, namely defects in neural tube development, inappropriate segmentation of the vertebrae, and defects of formation [42]. Aside from the well-described atlantoaxial malformations and malformations of the cervical vertebrae resulting in cervical vertebral stenotic myelopathy (CVSM, wobbler syndrome), vertebral malformations in the horse are rare [43]. While vertebral malformation in the cervical region frequently leads to spinal cord dysfunction, malformations have been identified without accompanying neurologic deficits [42]. Malformations are often identified on postmortem in aborted or stillborn fetuses, or shortly after birth. In animals that survive the immediate postpartum period, signs that have been identified in association with vertebral malformations include ataxia, paresis, kyphosis, and scoliosis [2, 43]. Many breeds have been affected, including Friesians, Clydesdales, Quarter Horses, Warmbloods, and Arabians [43–45].

Malformations that have been documented in the horse include hypoplasia of the fifth lumbar vertebra, fusion of thoracic vertebrae, a cleft of the fifth and sixth thoracic vertebrae, hemivertebrae, and interruption of normal fusion of the sixth and seventh thoracic vertebral bodies leading to butterfly vertebrae [3, 43, 45–47]. A subset of affected foals also had congenital defects outside of the nervous system, including cardiac ventricular septal defects, rib malformations, umbilical hernias, hydroureter/hydronephrosis, incomplete diaphragm development and subsequent hernia, rib deformities, joint contracture, skull deformities, and extraspinal cysts [44].

Cervical Vertebral Stenotic Myelopathy

The development of CVSM (wobbler syndrome) is multifactorial and can involve nutrition, familial influence, osteochondrosis dissecans, growth rate, gender, and trauma [48, 49]. While malformations or malarticulations may be present from birth, clinical signs consistent with spinal cord dysfunction often do not develop until later in life. In a retrospective study evaluating 807 horses with CVSM, only 6% were diagnosed at <6 months of age and horses from 6 to 11 months of age were 7.9 times more likely to be diagnosed than horses >11 years of age [50]. Males, Thoroughbreds, Tennessee Walking Horses, and Warmbloods are consistently overrepresented [48, 50].

Three types of CVSM have been described. Of those, Type I is the most likely to be present from birth, and the rarest. In Type I CVSM, there is a fixed malformation or malarticulation of two vertebral bodies, most commonly C2 and C3. Types II and III are generally a result of abnormal growth of the articular processes and thus are identified later in life [49]. More recently, the classification scheme has been altered and categorizes lesions as either dynamic or static [51]. Clinical signs of CVSM are reflective of a compressive spinal cord lesion, with Type I typically between C1 and C6. Affected animals display symmetric proprioceptive ataxia, hypermetria, spasticity, and upper motor neuron tetraparesis. Signs are often more prominent in the pelvic limbs [49]. Definitive diagnosis is best achieved via postmortem examination [49] but lateral and oblique radiographic projections can identify sites suspicious for compression of the spinal cord. Myelography via radiographs or computed tomography improves diagnosis [47, 51, 52]. Conservative management of young horses with CVSM consists of a restricted diet, anti-inflammatory therapy, and stall rest. Supplementation with vitamin E and selenium has been advocated and surgical correction via ventral stabilization is possible in certain cases [51].

Congenital Scoliosis/Kyphoscoliosis/Kyphosis

Scoliosis and kyphosis have been reported as singular defects but are also a component of contracted foal syndrome. Scoliosis is a lateral displacement of the vertebral column, whereas kyphosis is a dorsal deviation of the vertebral column. Kyphoscoliosis describes the defect when both anomalies are present and typically involves rotation of the vertebral bodies (Figure 31.VI.10) [53]. Contracted foal syndrome describes congenital, bilateral contraction of joints of either the thoracic limbs, pelvic limbs, or both, and occurs in conjunction with malformations of the vertebral column, including kyphosis and scoliosis, cranial deformation, and thinning of the ventral abdominal wall [2, 3, 54, 55]. Contracted foal syndrome was identified as the most frequent congenital defect in a study of 608 deformed foals and fetuses with congenital defects, accounting for 34.2% of the identified defects [14]. Another study identified contracted foal syndrome as the most common congenital defect in a group of 3,515 foals that

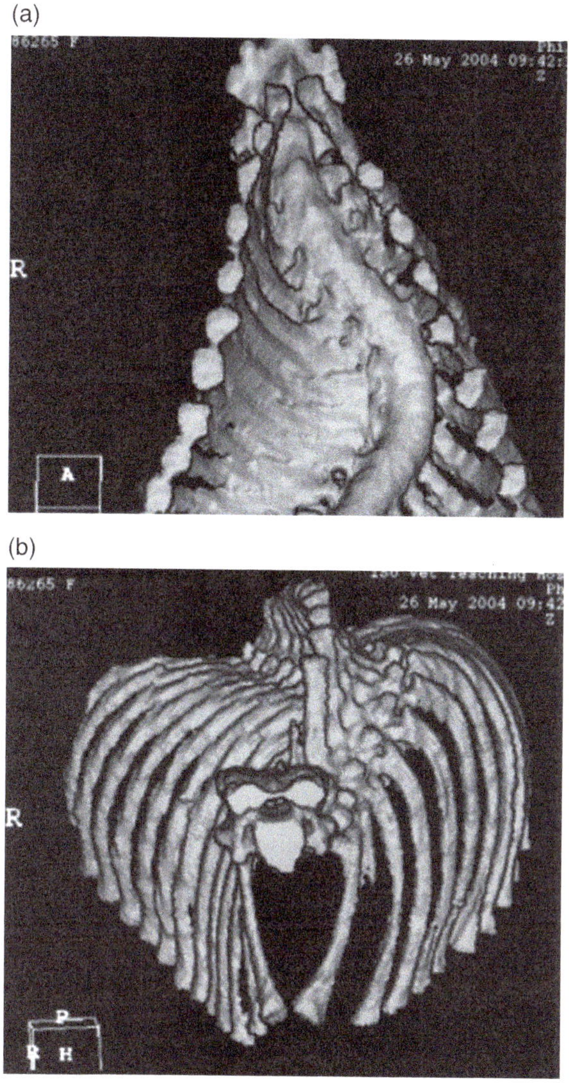

Figure 31.VI.10 Three-dimensional reformatted CT image of the thoracic spine of a neonatal foal with scoliosis (a). Abnormal alignment of the cranial thoracic vertebrae results in a curve of the spinous processes and ventral and dorsal displacement of the right and left hemithoraces, respectively (b) [9].

were either aborted, stillborn, or died within 24 hours of birth. The majority of foals with contracted foal syndrome cannot be delivered normally and require fetotomy or Caesarian section [54–56].

Scoliosis and kyphosis of the fetus can both lead to dystocia during parturition [57]. They are generally detectable visually and presenting complaints may include firm swellings over the dorsal or lateral aspects of the vertebral column, but imaging is required to characterize the anomaly. The visible swellings are not painful, and foals may or may not have neurologic deficits. Scoliosis and kyphosis can lead to spinal cord compression and associated neurological deficits, although foals with thoracolumbar lesions are often neurologically normal [47, 58]. Scoliosis can be congenital due to malformations of the vertebral column or acquired due to spinal cord lesions and denervation of surrounding musculature or afferent Ia fibers responsible for maintaining normal muscle tone. Congenital scoliosis in people is identified in approximately 1 out of 1000 live births but is far less common in horses [59]. Vertebral malformations and subsequent asymmetric growth of the vertebral column lead to scoliosis. Vertebrae may be abnormally small and asymmetric, which ultimately can lead to rotation of the vertebral column. The majority of reports in horses document cervical scoliosis, but thoracic lesions have also been reported [9, 47, 53, 57]. Radiography and computed tomography have been utilized to achieve final diagnosis [2, 9]. In human medicine, correction is often attempted with braces or surgical intervention. Affected foals may be identified shortly after birth, or the deformities can predispose them to dystocia during parturition [14, 33].

Spina Bifida

Spina bifida has been well-described in other species and is a specific vertebral malformation characterized by failure of the closure of the dorsal vertebral foramen of one or more vertebrae and is often associated with a meningocele or meningomyelocele. Fecal and urinary incontinence occur frequently in affected animals of other species in which the lumbar vertebrae and associated spinal cord and nerves are affected, and gait abnormalities and hypalgesia may or may not be present. The thoracolumbar and lumbar regions of the vertebral column are the most common sites of spina bifida [16].

Despite being reported with relative frequency in dogs, cats, and people, there are only a few reports of this defect in horses, including a Miniature Horse fetus, an aborted Thoroughbred fetus, and a live Thoroughbred foal [10, 16, 41, 60]. The Miniature Horse had hydrocephalus and a cervical meningomyelocele and the Thoroughbred had concurrent perosmus elumbis and cerebral aplasia [60]. The live foal was born prematurely at 320 days of gestation and was evaluated within hours of birth due to inability to stand and a prominent swelling over the lumbar vertebral column. The foal was euthanized after radiography identified severe scoliosis. In addition to spina bifida, postmortem exam also identified a meningomyelocele and a type II Chiari malformation [41].

Defects of the Spinal Cord

Meningomyelocele

Meningoceles, as described above, can occur in the spinal cord as well as the brain. A meningomyelocele is protrusion of nervous tissue in addition to the meninges through the vertebral canal, and typically occurs concurrently with spina bifida [10]. Grossly, meningomyeloceles may present as soft, fluctuant masses present along the dorsal midline although there is one report of a ventral meningomyelocele in an Arabian filly in the C7-T2 region identified on postmortem examination [61]. Clinical signs of meningomyelocele are consistent with a spinal cord lesion at the site of the defect [8, 16, 61, 62].

Syringomyelia/Syringohydromyelia

Syringomyelia is a congenital or acquired malformation where cavities develop within the spinal cord that are filled with fluid similar to normal CSF [63, 64]. It is reported with relative frequency in dogs but is less common in horses [65]. Signs are consistent with a spinal cord lesion at the affected site, and syringomyelia has been identified in the cervical, thoracic, and lumbar spinal cord [63, 64, 66]. Reported signs include lameness, spastic gait, stiffness, tremors, "bunny hopping," and scoliosis [63, 64, 66]. Clinical signs are often present shortly after birth, but in the acquired form, may develop later in life. Syringomyelia and syringohydromyelia have also been identified secondary to other congenital defects including Schwannosis and hamartomatous myelodysplasia of the spinal cord [67, 68].

Split Cord Malformation

Split cord malformation is a well-described malformation in people and leads to development of two separate hemicords, either within one dural sac (diplomyelia) or with two separate dural sacs (diastematomyelia). This has been described in a 9-year-old Thoroughbred that acutely developed inappetence, yawning, trembling, sweating, tachycardia, intermittent lateral recumbency, weakness, and lameness of the right forelimb after work that ultimately progressed to a narrow-based stance, cataplexy, ataxia, and recumbency. The horse was euthanized when signs failed to improve, and postmortem examination identified cerebellar asymmetry with mild hypoplasia of the right cerebellar hemisphere. A 7-cm-long segment of cervical spinal cord showed duplication of the cord with both portions having identifiable gray matter, although only the largest section was described as grossly having the typical "butterfly" appearance (Figure 31.VI.11). Findings were confirmed on histopathology. The delayed onset of clinical signs was considered most likely due to spinal cord tethering [62].

Perosmus Elumbis

Perosmus elumbis is a congenital defect characterized by agenesis of the lumbosacral spinal cord. The spinal cord defect then leads to failure of normal development of the associated vertebrae so affected animals may have absent lumbar, sacral, or coccygeal vertebrae. Anomalies of the urogenital tract and distal gastrointestinal tract can also develop. Perosmus elumbis has also been associated with

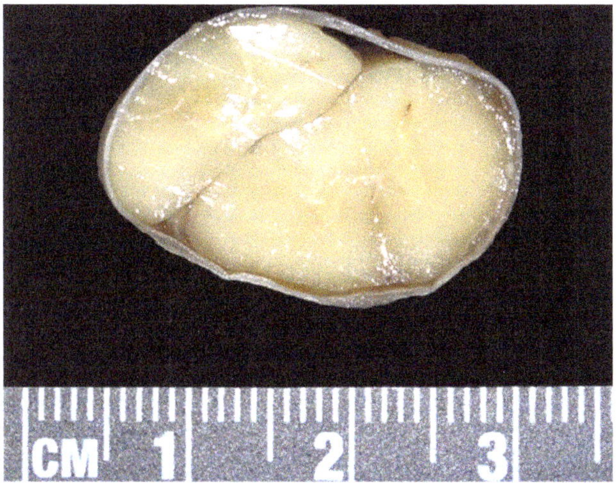

Figure 31.VI.11 Split cord malformation in a horse. Transverse section of asymmetrically duplicated cervical spinal cord covered with dura [62].

spina bifida and cerebral aplasia [60] and has been reported in many species, including cattle, dogs, human beings, pigs, camelids, and sheep [69]. There has been one report in a horse, where the defect was observed in an aborted female Thoroughbred fetus. Postmortem examination identified cranioschisis with a meningocele, absent cerebrum and cerebellum, and severe arthrogryposis. Thoracic ribs were malformed, the three most caudal thoracic vertebrae were fused, and the sacral and coccygeal vertebrae were absent. There were only four lumbar vertebrae present, all of which were also fused. Cervical spina bifida was present and there was no spinal cord or vertebral canal past the thoracic vertebrae [60].

Spinal Cord Hamartomatous Myelodysplasia

Hamartomatous myelodysplasia of the spinal cord is the term used to describe lesions characterized by disorganized spinal cord tissue and sometimes meningeal tissue forming a mass in the nervous system [68]. The term was proposed after identification of these changes in two horses that were presented at 5 weeks and 3 years of age with neurologic deficits. In the former case, a 5-week-old Holsteiner colt was presented for progressive muscle rigidity and spasms that had progressed since birth. The foal's mentation was appropriate, but electroencephalogram suggested abnormal discharges. Electromyography was normal. The foal was euthanized due to the progression of clinical signs, and a fluctuant dilation of the spinal cord filled with CSF was identified at the level of the fifth cervical vertebra and a mass was identified at the caudal end of the dilation. Histopathologically, the mass was comprised of streams and bundles of spindle-shaped and stellate cells mixed haphazardly with gray and white matter. The second case was a 3-year-old Thoroughbred colt presented for evaluation of pelvic and left thoracic limb ataxia. Ataxia progressed and the colt was euthanized. Post-mortem examination identified a multi-nodular tan mass at the level of the first lumbar vertebrae that was protruding from the surface of the spinal cord. Histopathologically, the mass was composed of gray and white matter with interspersed neurons and glial cells. There was no elaboration as to the suspected cause of the ataxia noted in the left thoracic limb. While similar lesions have been described, this was the first report using the term hamartomatous myelodysplasia to describe these lesions [68].

Miscellaneous

Schwannosis

Schwannosis is an anomaly characterized by invasion and proliferation of Schwann cells within the CNS in addition to myelination of central axons within the CNS. This condition is similar to, but not to be confused with, schwannomatosis, which is a type of neurofibromatosis in people. The cause of Schwannosis has not been elucidated, but it is most likely a dysplastic, maldevelopmental, or hamartomatous process. It has been reported in three foals, including two unrelated Quarter Horses and one Holsteiner. In all three animals, clinical signs consistent with spinal cord dysfunction were present from birth until the time of exam, which ranged from 5 to 11 weeks of age. Postmortem examinations on all cases identified Schwannosis. In two cases, Schwannosis was localized to a focal segment of the cord; one foal had Schwannosis at C4–C5 with lesions arising from the dorsal nerve roots and another had Schwannosis at T6–T8 with lesions in the ventral nerve roots. The third case had Schwannosis noted in all segments of the spinal cord arising from the dorsal and ventral nerve roots. Two of the three foals also had syringohydromyelia, one had scoliosis, and another had widespread neuronal dysplasia and small, asymmetric gyri in the cerebrum and folia within the cerebellum [67].

References

1 Johnson, A.L. (2010). Congenital malformations – uncommon but important causes of neurological signs in neonates. *Equine Vet. Educ.* 22: 599–601.

2 Binanti, D., Zani, D.D., De Zani, D. et al. (2014). Contracted foal syndrome associated with multiple malformations in two foals. *Anatom. Histol. Embryol.* 43: 71–74.

3 Boyd, J.S. (1976). Congenital deformities in two Clydesdale foals. *Equine Vet. J.* 8: 161–164.
4 Wong, D., Winter, M., Haynes, J. et al. (2007). Dandy-Walker-like syndrome in a quarter horse colt. *J. Vet. Intern. Med.* 21: 1130–1134.
5 Alonso, J.M., Filho, P.T.H., Ávila, A.R. et al. (2019). Surgical repair of an occipital meningocele in a foal. *J. Equine Vet. Sci.* 81: 102771.
6 Baiker, K., Saunders, N., Summers, B.A. et al. (2010). Hydranencephaly in a foal. *Equine Vet. Educ.* 22: 593–598.
7 Moreira, M., Kassem, I.G., and Palhares, M.S. (2015). Congenital cerebellar vermis aplasia associated with hydrocephalus in a foal. *Braz. J. Vet. Pathol.* 8: 6–9.
8 Van Hoogmoed, L., Yarbrough, T.B., Lecouteur, R.A. et al. (1999). Surgical repair of a thoracic meningocele in a foal. *Vet. Surg.* 28: 496–500.
9 Wong, D., Miles, K., and Sponseller, B. (2006). Congenital scoliosis in a quarter horse filly. *Vet. Radiol. Ultrasound* 47: 279–282.
10 de Lahunta, A., Glass, E., and Kent, M. (2020). *de Lahunta's Veterinary Neuroanatomy and Clinical Neurology*, 5e. Philadelphia: Saunders.
11 Waelchli, R.O. and Ehrensperger, F. (1988). Two related cases of cerebellar abnormality in equine fetuses associated with hydrops of fetal membranes. *Vet. Rec.* 123: 513–514.
12 Ferris, R.A., Sonnis, J., Webb, B. et al. (2011). Hydrocephalus in an American miniature horse foal: a case report and review. *J. Equine Vet. Sci.* 31: 611–614.
13 Foreman, J.H., Reed, S.M., Rantanen, N.W. et al. (1983). Congenital internal hydrocephalus in a quarter horse foal. *J. Equine Vet. Sci.* 3: 154–164.
14 Crowe, M.W. and Swerczek, T.W. (1985). Equine congenital defects. *Am. J. Vet. Res.* 46: 353–358.
15 Ducro, B.J., Schurink, A., Bastiaansen, J.W.M. et al. (2015). A nonsense mutation in B3GALNT2 is concordant with hydrocephalus in Friesian horses. *BMC Genom.* 16: 761.
16 Rivas, L.J., Hinchcliff, K.W., and Robertson, J.T. (1996). Cervical meningomyelocele associated with spina bifida in a hydrocephalic miniature colt. *J. Am. Vet. Med. Assoc.* 209: 950–953.
17 Kolb, D.S. and Klein, C. (2019). Congenital hydrocephalus in a Belgian draft horse associated with a nonsense mutation in B3GALNT2. *Can Vet. J.* 60: 197–198.
18 Marques, F.J., Semrad, S., and Peek, S. (2006). Congenital hydrocephalus in a neonatal foal. *Comp. Equine* 1: 105–110.
19 Ojala, M. and Ala-Huikki, J. (1992). Inheritance of hydrocephalus in horses. *Equine Vet. J.* 24: 140–143.
20 Sipma, K.D., Cornillie, P., Saulez, M.N. et al. (2013). Phenotypic characteristics of hydrocephalus in stillborn Friesian foals. *Vet. Pathol.* 50: 1037–1042.
21 Bentz, B.G. and Moll, H.D. (2008). Treatment of congenital hydrocephalus in a foal using a ventriculoperitoneal shunt. *J. Vet. Emerg. Crit. Care* 18: 170–176.
22 Schmidt, M. and Ondreka, N. (2019). Hydrocephalus in animals. In: *Pediatric Hydrocephalus* (ed. G. Cinallia, W.J. Maixner, and C. Sainte-Rose), 53–95. Cham: Springer International Publishing.
23 Frazer, G.S., Perkins, N.R., Blanchard, T.L. et al. (1997). Prevalence of fetal maldispositions in equine referral hospital Dystocias. *Equine Vet. J.* 29: 111–116.
24 Maaskant, A., De Bruijn, C.M., Schutrups, A.H. et al. (2010). Dystocia in Friesian mares: prevalence, causes and outcome following caesarean section. *Equine Vet. Educ.* 22: 190–195.
25 MacKay, R.J. (2005). Neurologic disorders of neonatal foals. *Vet. Clin. North Am. Equine* 21: 387–406.
26 Gillespie, S., Gilbert, Z., and De Decker, S. (2019). Results of oral prednisolone administration or ventriculoperitoneal shunt placement in dogs with congenital hydrocephalus: 40 cases (2005–2016). *J. Am. Vet. Med. Assoc.* 254: 835–842.
27 Cudd, T.A., Mayhew, I.G., and Cottrill, C.M. (1989). Agenesis of the corpus callosum with cerebellar Vermian hypoplasia in a foal resembling the Dandy-Walker syndrome: pre-mortem diagnosis by clinical evaluation and CT scanning. *Equine Vet. J.* 21: 378–381.
28 Parisi, M.A. and Dobyns, W.B. (2003). Human malformations of the midbrain and hindbrain: review and proposed classification scheme. *Mol. Genet. Metab.* 80: 36–53.
29 Koch, T., Loretti, A., Lahunta, A. et al. (2005). Semilobar holoprosencephaly in a Morgan horse. *J. Vet. Intern. Med.* 19: 367–372.
30 Henker, L.C., Invenstigation, M., Piva, M.M. et al. (2022). Alobar holoprosencephaly in an aborted American quarter horse fetus. *J. Equine Vet. Sci.* 112: 103898.
31 Pintore, M.D. and Cantile, C. (2016). Semilobar holoprosencephaly associated with multiple malformations in a foal. *Anatom. Histol. Embryol.* 45: 148–153.
32 Borel, N., Grest, P., Junge, H. et al. (2014). Vascular hamartoma in the central nervous system of a foal. *J. Vet. Diagn.* 26: 805–809.
33 Hong, C.B., Donahue, J.M., Giles, R.C.J. et al. (1993). Equine abortion and stillbirth in Central Kentucky during 1988 and 1989 foaling seasons. *J. Vet. Diagn. Invest.* 5: 560–566.
34 Schön, S., Wehrli Eser, M., Kircher, P.R. et al. (2019). Congenital unilateral facial nerve paralysis in a warmblood filly. *Equine Vet. Educ.* 31: 80–87.
35 Kelly, D.F. and Watson, W. (1976). Epidermoid cyst of the brain in the horse. *Equine Vet. J.* 8: 110–112.

36 Peters, M., Brandt, K., and Wohlsein, P. (2003). Intracranial epidermoid cyst in a horse. *J. Comp. Pathol.* 129: 89–92.

37 Holly, L.T. and Batzdorf, U. (2019). Chiari malformation and syringomyelia. *J. Neurosurg. Spine* 31: 619–628.

38 Tubbs, R.S., Muhleman, M., Loukas, M. et al. (2011). A new form of herniation: the Chiari V malformation. *Childs Nerv. Syst.* 28: 305–307.

39 Testoni, S., Dalla Pria, A., and Gentile, A. (2010). Imaging diagnosis-cerebellar displacement and spina bifida in a calf. *Vet. Radiol. Ultrasound* 51: 162–164.

40 Viu, J., Armengou, L., Jose-Cunilleras, E. et al. (2010). Cranioencephalic malformation with atlanto-occipital luxation in an Andalusian neonate foal. *J. Vet. Intern. Med.* 24: 639–642.

41 Lempe, A., Heine, M., Bosch, B. et al. (2012). Imaging diagnosis and clinical presentation of a Chiari malformation in a thoroughbred foal. *Equine Vet. Educ.* 24: 618–623.

42 Unt, V.E. and Piercy, R.J. (2009). Vertebral embryology and equine congenital vertebral anomalies. *Equine Vet. Educ.* 21: 212–214.

43 de Heer, N. and Nout, Y.S. (2011). Congenital kyphosis secondary to lumbar vertebral hypoplasia causing Paraparesis in a Friesian foal. *Equine Vet. Educ.* 23: 231–234.

44 Crochik, S.S., Barton, M.H., Eggleston, R.B. et al. (2009). Cervical vertebral anomaly and ventricular septal defect in an Arabian foal. *Equine Vet. Educ.* 21: 207–211.

45 Rendle, D.I., Durham, A.E., Bestbier, M. et al. (2008). Neurenteric cyst with associated butterfly vertebrae in a seven-month-old colt. *Vet. Rec.* 162: 558–561.

46 Doige, C.E. (1996). Congenital cleft vertebral centrum and intra- and extraspinal cyst in a foal. *Vet. Pathol.* 33: 87–89.

47 Wong, D.M., Scarratt, W.K., and Rohleder, J. (2005). Hindlimb paresis associated with kyphosis, hemivertebrae and multiple thoracic vertebral malformations in a quarter horse gelding. *Equine Vet. Educ.* 17: 187–194.

48 Levine, J.M. (2010). Multicenter case-control study of signalment, diagnostic features, and outcome associated with cervical vertebral malformation-malarticulation in horses. *J. Am. Vet. Med. Assoc.* 237: 812–822.

49 Reed, R., Grant, B., and Nout, Y. (2008). Cervical vertebral stenotic myelopathy. In: *Equine Neurology* (ed. M. Furr and S. Reed), 283–298. Ames, Iowa: Blackwell Publishing.

50 Levine, J.M., Nghei, P.P., Levine, G. et al. (2008). Associations of sex, breed, and age with cervical vertebral compressive myelopathy in horses 811 cases (1974–2007). *J. Am. Vet. Med. Assoc.* 233: 1453–1458.

51 Nout, Y.S. and Reed, S.M. (2003). Cervical vertebral stenotic myelopathy. *Equine Vet. Educ.* 15: 212–223.

52 Rovel, T., Zimmerman, M., Duchateau, L. et al. (2021). Computed tomographic myelography for assessment of the cervical spinal cord in ataxic warmblood horses 26 cases (2015–2017). *J. Am. Vet. Med. Assoc.* 259: 1188–1195.

53 Lerner, D.J. and Riley, G. (1978). Congenital kyphoscoliosis in a foal. *J. Am. Vet. Med. Assoc.* 172: 274–276.

54 Rooney, J.R. (1966). Contracted foals. *Cornell Vet.* 56: 172–187.

55 Finocchio, E.J. (1973). A case of contracted foal syndrome. *Vet. Med. Small Anim. Clin.* 68: 1254–1255.

56 Giles, R.C., Donahue, J.M., Hong, C.B. et al. (1993). Causes of abortion, stillbirth, and perinatal death in horses: 3,527 cases (1986–1991). *J. Am. Vet. Med. Assoc.* 203: 1170–1175.

57 Vandeplassche, M., Simoens, P., Bouters, R. et al. (1984). Aetiology and pathogenesis of congenital torticollis and head scoliosis in the equine foetus. *Equine Vet. J.* 16: 419–424.

58 Denoix, J.M. (2005). Thoracolumbar malformations or injuries and neurological manifestations. *Equine Vet. Educ.* 17: 191–194.

59 Hedequist, D. and Emans, J. (2007). Congenital scoliosis: a review and update. *J. Pediatr. Orthop.* 27: 106–116.

60 Gerhauser, I., Geburerk, F., and Wohlsein, P. (2012). Perosomus elumbis, cerebral aplasia, and spina bifida in an aborted thoroughbred foal. *Vet. Sci. Res. J.* 92: 266–268.

61 Harmelin, A., Egozi, O., Nyska, A. et al. (1993). Ventral meningomyelocele in a filly. *J. Comp. Pathol.* 109: 93–97.

62 De Jonge, B., Dufourni, A., Oosterlinck, M. et al. (2021). Split cord malformation in a thoroughbred horse. *J. Comp. Pathol.* 187: 68–74.

63 Kurz, J.P., Schoenhals, K., Hullinger, G. et al. (2018). Syringomyelia in an adult American paint horse. *Vet. Sci.* 5: 39.

64 Sponseller, B., Sponseller, B., Alcott, C.J. et al. (2011). Syringohydromyelia in horses: 3 cases. *Can Vet. J.* 52: 147–152.

65 Rusbridge, C., Greitz, D., and Iskandar, B.J. (2006). Syringomyelia: current concepts in pathogenesis, diagnosis, and treatment. *J. Vet. Intern. Med.* 20: 469–479.

66 Cho, D.Y. and Leipold, H.W. (1977). Syringomyelia in a thoroughbred foal. *Equine Vet. J.* 9: 195–197.

67 Miranda, I.C., Taylor, K.R., Castleman, W. et al. (2019). Schwannosis in three foals and a calf. *Vet. Pathol.* 56: 783–788.

68 Taylor, K.R., MacKay, R.J., Nelson, E.A. et al. (2016). Spinal cord Hamartomatous myelodysplasia in 2 horses with clinical neurologic deficits. *Vet. Pathol.* 53: 844–846.

69 Amaral, C.B., Romao, M., and Ferreira, A. (2012). Perosomus elumbis in a puppy. *J. Comp. Pathol.* 147: 495–498.

70 Tyler, C., Davis, R.E., Begg, A.P. et al. (1993). A survey of neurological diseases in horses. *Aust. Vet. J.* 70: 445–449.

Chapter 32 Nervous System Disorders

Section I Infectious and Inflammatory – Bacterial Meningoencephalomyelitis

Emil Olsen

Bacterial infection of the central nervous system is an uncommon condition in horses but appears to be more frequent in foals [1]. Bacterial meningoencephalomyelitis (MEM) is a possible complication of neonatal sepsis in up to 8–10% of septic foals and has a high mortality rate [1]. Risk factors such as the increased permeability of the neonatal blood-brain barrier (BBB) and the high incidence of failure of transfer of passive immunity may contribute to the higher incidence in foals. This section reviews MEM in the neonatal foal.

Pathophysiology

The brain and spinal cord are protected from invasion of microorganisms by the BBB and the lack of lymphatics. Predisposing mechanisms for BBB penetration include the systemic inflammatory response syndrome (SIRS), disseminated intravascular coagulation (DIC), and septicemia. However, once bacteria have crossed the BBB, the lack of immunocompetence makes the rapid bacterial invasion of meninges and neuroparenchyma possible. Bacteria cross the BBB transcellularly at either the choroid plexus epithelium or the cerebral microvascular endothelium. In foals, infections are most commonly hematogenous, spread from primary disease sites such as pneumonia, omphalophlebitis, omphaloarteritis, cystitis, liver abscess, osteomyelitis, or extension of infections from vertebrae, vertebral joints, eyes, ears, or the nasal cavity. For hospitalized foals, secondary spread from venous or arterial catheters, endotracheal tubes, and urinary catheters are also possible. Inflammation occurs in the meninges (dura, arachnoid, and pia mater) and neuroparenchyma (forebrain, brainstem, cerebellum, spinal cord) and is, therefore, most correctly called MEM. The neuroinflammation associated with MEM is extensive, and although needed for elimination of bacteria, is also a main cause of injury to the neuroparenchyma. The immune system can also encapsulate the bacteria to form an abscess, which may function as a space occupying lesion in the neuroparenchyma.

Clinical Signs

Neurolocalization of MEM is often multifocal due to the presence of infection in multiple areas of the brain or diffuse expansion across the meninges. Bacterial MEM often presents acutely with changes in mentation. The most common clinical sign reported in one report of 10 foals with MEM was altered mentation such as obtundation [1]. Other commonly noted signs were recumbency, tetraparesis, abnormal pupillary light reflexes (PLR), seizures, and nystagmus. Clinical signs in adult horses are similar to those of foals [2], whereas in dogs, the most common presenting clinical signs are cranial nerve abnormalities, paresis, ataxia, and seizures [3]. In one foal with MEM caused by *Streptococcus equi*, recumbency, and multiple cranial nerve abnormalities were described as well as neck pain [4]. Foals with abscess formation in the neuroparenchyma may present as described or with signs of increased intracranial pressure such as miotic pupils, bradycardia and hypertension (Cushing Reflex), altered mentation, and occasional opisthotonos. Abscess formation is most commonly due to Rhodococcus infection in older foals [5, 6] but has also been described with *S. equi* [7, 8].

Diagnostics

The diagnostic evaluation of a foal suspected of MEM includes careful neuroanatomical localisation and aggressive and rapid attempts to find the origin of the infection, including abdominal, thoracic, and umbilical ultrasound, thoracic and spinal radiographs or, if available and

Equine Neonatal Medicine, First Edition. Edited by David M. Wong and Pamela A. Wilkins.

clinically feasible, thoracic, abdominal, and/or spinal computed tomography (CT). CT can be performed under sedation or IV anesthesia with IV contrast to facilitate abscess detection. Sampling of possibly infected sites for fluid analysis and cultures (including blood and cerebrospinal fluid [CSF] culture) along with hematologic and serum biochemistry analysis can help divulge further information. In one study, the mean (range) values for various blood parameters from 10 foals with MEM included leukocytosis (10.67×10^3 cells/μl [0.68–27.18]), neutrophilia (8.11×10^3 cells/μl [0.4–19.57]), hyperfibrinogenemia (590 mg/dl [300–1000]), and hyperlactatemia (5 mmol/l [2.1–9.3 mmol/l]) [1]. For imaging of the brain, magnetic resonance imaging (MRI) is superior to CT for detection of edema, contrast enhancement, and inflammation as well as smaller abscesses. However, the clinician must ensure that the foal has a stable cardiovascular status for safe anesthesia. MRI also aids in diagnosis of elevated intracranial pressure, which increases the chance of herniation of cerebellum at the caudal fossa due to increased intracranial pressure associated with brain edema and infection or mass-effect from an intraparenchymal abscess. Once it has been determined that there is no increased intracranial pressure, CSF should be obtained as close to the affected site as possible, most commonly from the cerebello-medullary cistern. CSF should ideally be analyzed within 30 minutes for accurate cell count, cytology, total protein, lactate, and glucose and a second aliquot should be submitted for culture in pediatric blood culture medium or transport medium. In human medicine, a maximum of 50% of patients with bacterial MEM have positive CSF culture. Commonly, a neutrophilic pleocytosis with over 10% neutrophils and elevated total protein is documented upon CSF analysis in foals with MEM [1]. In CSF culture negative patients, intracellular bacteria on cytology of the CSF are also diagnostic, and Gram stains and blood cultures may aid the choice of antibiotics.

Etiologies

It is assumed that bacteria involved in neonatal sepsis are equally prevalent in central nervous system infections with *Escherichia coli* being the most commonly reported cultured bacteria in one case report of 10 foals with septic MEM. Other bacteria cultured included *Klebsiella* and *Salmonella*, but several foals did not have the CSF cultured [1]. One case report from Brazil found *Salmonella typhimurum* as the etiology in a foal with MEM [9]. In reports of abscess formation in foals, *S. Equi* and *Rhodococcus equi* have been identified [5–8]. In dogs, the most prevalent bacteria involved in MEM were *E. Coli, Streptococcus,* and *Klebsiella* [3]. Fungal MEM is prevalent in human neonatal MEM [10] and is notoriously difficult to treat, but appears uncommon in the foal.

Treatment

Commonly used antimicrobials administered to septic neonatal foals include penicillin and aminoglycosides, however, these antimicrobials are inadequate for bacterial MEM due to poor penetration of the BBB. A standard switch of antimicrobials from penicillin to ampicillin as well as addition of metronidazole can improve BBB penetration and is indicated until culture and sensitivity results are reported. Third-generation cephalosporins penetrate the BBB well and include ceftriaxone (best BBB penetration), cefotaxime, and ceftazidime; however, to maintain proper antimicrobial stewardship, empirical treatment with these antimicrobials should be limited, especially without evidence of CNS involvement and preferably with the support of culture and sensitivity results. Of note, cefpodoxime does not penetrate the BBB well. Chloramphenicol, can be used, when supported by culture and sensitivity results, for better BBB penetration [11]. For foals with *Rhodococcus equi* MEM, the combination of a macrolide and rifampin provides good penetration across the BBB. Anti-inflammatory doses of corticosteroids are often helpful initially to reduce the neuroinflammation in bacterial MEM. An initial IV dose of 0.15 mg/kg of dexamethasone followed by prednisolone 24 hours later (0.5 mg/kg PO q12h) for 10–14 days followed by a tapering dose over 2–3 weeks may be used to reduce inflammation. In the case of abscess formation, repeat CT or MRI should be performed before discontinuation of antimicrobials. If an abscess is well encapsulated and in a feasible location, surgical removal of an abscess or granulomatous infection could be attempted by an experienced neurosurgeon [8].

Prognosis

The prognosis is guarded to poor, nearing 20% survival in foals in one study [1]. Foals that recover have a risk of persistent neurologic deficits. In comparison, a mortality rate of 96% is reported in adult horses [2] and 43% in dogs with 20% lost to follow-up [3].

References

1 Viu, J., Monreal, L., Jose-Cunilleras, E. et al. (2012). Clinical findings in 10 foals with bacterial meningoencephalitis. *Equine Vet. J. Suppl.* 41: 100–104.

2 Toth, B., Aleman, M., Nogradi, N. et al. (2012). Meningitis and meningoencephalomyelitis in horses: 28 cases (1985–2010). *J. Am. Vet. Med. Assoc.* 240: 580–587.

3 Radaelli, S.T. and Platt, S.R. (2002). Bacterial meningoencephalomyelitis in dogs: a retrospective study of 23 cases (1990–1999). *J. Vet. Intern. Med.* 16: 159–163.

4 Finno, C., Pusterla, N., Aleman, M. et al. (2006). *Streptococcus equi* meningoencephalomyelitis in a foal. *J. Am. Vet. Med. Assoc.* 229: 721–724.

5 Janicek, J.C., Kramer, J., Coates, J.R. et al. (2006). Intracranial abscess caused by Rhodococcus equi infection in a foal. *J. Am. Vet. Med. Assoc.* 228: 251–253.

6 Morresey, P.R., Garrett, K.S., and Carter, D. Rhodococcus equi occipital bone osteomyelitis, septic arthritis and meningitis in a neurological foal. *Equine. Vet. Educ.* 23: 398–402.

7 Henderson, B. (2011). Cerebellar peduncle abscess secondary to disseminated strangles in a six-week-old miniature foal. *Vet. Sci. Dev.* 1: e12–e12.

8 Broux, B., van Bergen, T., Schauvliege, S. et al. (2019. http://dx.doi.org/10.1111/eve.12995). Successful surgical debridement of a cerebral *Streptococcus equi* equi abscess by parietal bone flap craniotomy in a 2-month-old Warmblood foal. *Equine. Vet. Educ.* 31 (10): 58–62.

9 de Oliveira, J.G., de Oliveira, J.G., Ramos, C.P. et al. (2019). Salmonella Typhimurium - associated meningoencephalomyelitis in a foal [Internet]. *Ciência Rural.* 49: http://dx.doi.org/10.1590/0103-847 8cr20190008.

10 McCarthy, M.W., Kalasauskas, D., Petraitis, V. et al. (2017). Fungal Infections of the Central Nervous System in Children. *J. Pediatric. Infect. Dis. Soc.* 6: e123–e133.

11 Magdesian, K.G. (2017). Antimicrobial Pharmacology for the Neonatal Foal. *Vet. Clin. North Am. Equine Pract.* 33: 47–65.

Section II Infectious and Inflammatory – *Sarcocystis* and *Neospora* in the Mare and Foal

Sharon Witonsky

Pregnant mares that develop neurologic disease or abortion should be assessed to identify the underlying cause. While not common, equine protozoal myeloencephalitis (EPM) caused by *Sarcocystis neurona* or *Neospora hughesi* should be considered, particularly if the mare has previously been diagnosed with EPM. Pregnancy is a risk factor for EPM due to *S. neurona*, in part because of altered immune responses associated with pregnancy, making the mare more susceptible to disease. While *Neospora* has similar clinical manifestations of disease as *S. neurona,* increased risk for EPM due to *Neospora* during pregnancy has not been documented, but likely exists. While uncommon, fetuses can be transplacentally infected by *N. hughesi;* transplacental infection with *S. neurona* is also suspected as neonates as young as 2 days of age have been documented to have clinical signs, antemortem diagnosis, and response to treatment of *S. neurona* [1, 2]. Knowledge of the transmission of antibodies against *S. neurona* and *N. hughesi* in the colostrum to the neonate is critical for diagnosing if a foal is infected or if anti-protozoal antibodies have been acquired via colostrum.

Clinical Signs

EPM is most commonly due to *S. neurona*, with *N. hughesi* being much less frequent. The definitive host of *S. neurona* is the opossum, with horses becoming infected by ingestion of contaminated feed or water [3, 4]. While the mechanism by which *S. neurona* enters the central nervous system (CNS) is unknown, *S. neurona* undergoes at least one replication in the gastrointestinal tract. The most likely pathways by which *S. neurona* enters the CNS is through leukocytes or endothelial cells [5–8]. Once *S. neurona* enters the CNS, it can localize anywhere, thus producing varied clinical signs which can be focal or multifocal and localize to the white or gray matter or both. Common clinical signs include asymmetric muscle atrophy and ataxia, but other signs include dysphagia, abnormal upper airway function, lameness, facial nerve dysfunction, and difficulty walking and standing. Ataxia is a sign of white matter involvement whereas weakness and atrophy are associated with damage to gray matter [4, 9–12]. Clinical signs can progress quickly or be subtle, progressing over months to years. In a minority of cases, signs are static. The time between exposure and development of clinical signs is unknown. In addition, stress factors such as pregnancy, illness, shipping, and performance can make horses susceptible to disease. The mechanism by which these factors increase the incidence of disease is unknown, but stress can alter the immune response [3, 4, 10]. The predicted protective immune response to *S. neurona* is a cell-mediated immune (CMI) response, based on equine and murine data, and CMI is necessary to prevent disease due to intracellular infection [4, 8, 13]. While most concerns regarding clinical disease of *N. hughesi* have been related to its role in neurologic disease, abortion likely due to *N. hughesi* has been reported [14].

Role of the Immune System in Disease

Pregnancy alters the immune response contributing to increased susceptibility to EPM in pregnant mares [3, 15, 16]. Before discussing how pregnancy alters the immune response, one must understand the different immune pathways involved. Four basic major pathways direct the immune response against allergens, intracellular and extracellular pathogens, and parasites. The T-helper cell 1 (CD4 Th1) and T-cytotoxic (CD8) pathways are cell mediated, with cells producing the cytokine IFN-gamma (IFN-γ). This pathway is needed for protection against

Equine Neonatal Medicine, First Edition. Edited by David M. Wong and Pamela A. Wilkins.

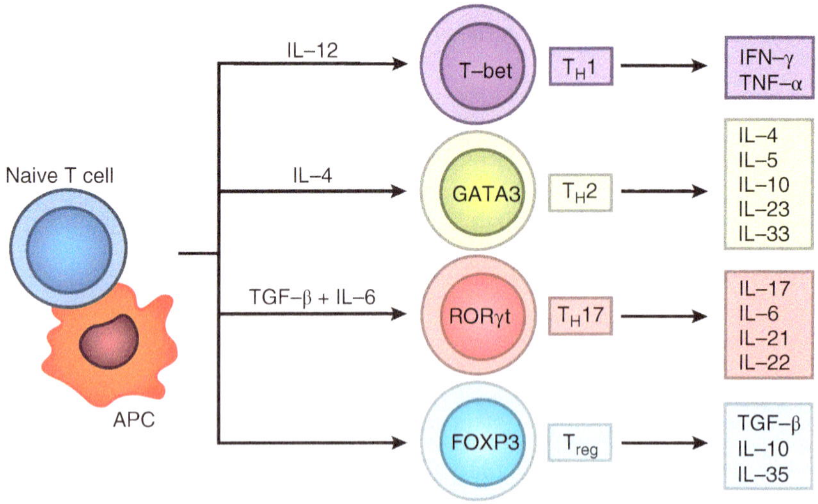

Figure 32.II.1 Differentiation of naïve T cells into T-cell subpopulations. In response to stimulation with antigens or cytokines, naïve T cells can differentiate into distinct subpopulations including T_H1, T_H2, T_H17, and T_{REG} cells. APC, antigen presenting cell; FOXP3, forkhead box P3; GATA3, trans-acting T-cell specific transcription factor; IFN, interferon; RORγ_t, RAR-related orphan receptor gamma; TGF, transforming growth factor, T_{REG} cell, regulatory T cell; TNF, tumor necrosis factor.

intracellular infections, such as *S. neurona* and *N. hughesi*. The T-helper-2 (CD4 Th2) pathway produces interleukin-4 (IL-4) and is needed to combat parasites (i.e. strongyles). The T-helper-17 (Th17) pathway helps control infection in response to some pathogens, but can also be involved in allergic conditions by contributing to the inflammatory component of the disease (i.e. asthma) [17]. The fourth pathway is the T-regulatory pathway (T-reg) that helps regulate the immune response and prevent dysfunction (Figure 32.II.1).

The mechanisms and extent of pregnancy-associated immunosuppression are still being elucidated, but studies support the theory that the immune response in the fetus, endometrium, and placenta, as well as overall peripheral immune response, are altered during pregnancy [18]. One reason for maternal immunosuppression is to dampen and prevent recognition of major histocompatibility class I (MHC class I) expression of paternal antigens in the fetus, but it is unclear if this unintentionally limits the protective immune response to pathogens including *S. neurona* and *N. hughesi* [18]. One pathway by which the immune response is limited is through the fetal production of a > 100 000 kd protein that inhibits interleukin-2 receptor (IL-2R) expression, thus inhibiting lymphocyte proliferation. Additionally, local factors from the endometrium, including prostaglandins, suppress lymphocyte proliferation *in vitro* [18]. The immune response is also altered due to increased expression of CD4 T-cells (CD4 T-reg), which express a regulatory molecule, fox p3, identified in endometrial cup folds. Systemically, some mares have increased IL-4 expression and CD4 Th2 type cells, which support a decreased CD4 Th1 CD8 immune response needed against some pathogens, including *S. neurona* and *N. hughesi*. Additionally, peripheral blood leukocytes from pregnant mares have decreased cytotoxic T-lymphocyte activity (CTL activity) against target cells from the stallion [18, 19].

Diagnosis

Diagnostic testing is warranted if a pregnant mare develops clinical signs consistent with EPM. When considering diagnostic tests for EPM in the pregnant mare, the clinician must balance the risks and stress of sedating the mare and collecting cerebrospinal fluid (CSF) compared to reliance on serologic results or clinical signs alone. A gold standard antemortem diagnostic test for EPM is yet to be identified but is currently based on clinical signs consistent with EPM along with intrathecal antibody production against the specific pathogen. For *S. neurona* and *N. hughesi*, commercial laboratories perform commercial testing such as the indirect fluorescent antibody test (IFAT), surface antigen (SAG 2 4/3, SAG 1,5,6), and polymerize chain reaction (PCR). Table 32.II.1 summarize commercially available diagnostic tests, cutoffs for positive/interpretation, and sensitivities and specificities for *S. neurona* and *N. hughesi* [4]. In some EPM cases due to *S. neurona*, a diagnosis is unclear based on diagnostic testing, and the Goldman Witmer co-efficient (C value) and antigen antibody specific index aid in diagnostic intrpretation [29].

$$\text{C value} = \text{CSF titer} \times \text{serum IgG} / \text{CSF IgG} \times \text{serum titer}$$

$$\text{AI}(\text{antibody index}) = \text{Qab}(\text{specific antibody quotient}) / \text{Qalbe}(\text{equine albumin quotient})$$

$$\text{Qalbe}(\text{equine albumin quotient}) = (\text{CSF albumin/serum albumin}) \times 1000$$

$$\text{Qab}(\text{specific antibody quotient}) = S.neurona \text{ titer}(\text{CSF}) \times 1000 / \text{serum albumin titer}$$

Another consideration in the mare is potential exposure over her lifetime, which is based on age, geographic location (i.e. Canada vs. Virginia), and housing (i.e. pasture vs. stall). Even mares that predominantly live in stalls can potentially be exposed to *S. neurona* through contaminated

Table 32.II.1 Performance of commercially available immunologic tests for antibodies against Sarcocystis neurona.

			Reported performance		
Test	Laboratory	Interpretation	Sample	Sensitivity	Specificity
WB	*EDS*	Band pattern read and interpreted visually (subjective)	Serum	89 [20], 80 [21], 89 [22]	71 [20], 38 [21], 87 [22]
	UC Davis IDEXX	Results usually reported as negative, weak positive, low positive, or positive	CSF	89 [20], 87 [21]	89 [20], 44 [21]
mWB	*Michigan*	Similar to standard WB (above)	Serum	100 [23], 89 [5]	98 [23], 69 [22]
IFAT	*UC Davis*	Serum positive at ≥1 : 80 has ≥55% probability[a] of EPM	Serum	89 [22], 83 [24], 94 [25], 59 [26]	100 [22], 97 [24], 85 [25], 71 [26]
		Serum negative at ≤1 : 40 has ≤33% probability[a] of EPM	CSF	100 [24], 92 [25], 65 [26]	99 [24], 90 [25], 98 [26]
		CSF positive at ≥1 : 5 has 92% probability[a] of EPM	S:C ratio	65 [26]	98 [26]
SAG 1 ELISA	*Antech*	Serum positive at ≥1 : 16 but recommended cutoff ≥1 : 32	Serum	68 [27], 13 [25]	71 [27], 97 [25]
SAG2,4/3 ELISA	*EDS*	Serum positive for exposure at ≥1 : 250	Serum	30–86[b] [28], 71 [26]	37–88[b] [28], 50 [26]
		CSF correlates well with EPM if ≥1:40	CSF	77–96[b] [28], 88 [26]	58–96[b] [28], 86 [26]
		Serum:CSF titer ratio very predictive of EPM if ≤100	S : C ratio	86 (cutoff ≤50), 93 (cutoff ≤100) [28], 88 [26]	96 (cutoff ≤50), 83 (cutoff ≤100) [28], 100 [26]
SAG1,5,6 ELISA	*Patho-genes*	Serum positive at ≥1 : 8, indicating infection	Serum	N/A	N/A

WB, Western blot; mWB, modified Western blot; IFAT, indirect fluorescent antibody test; SAG, surface antigen; ELISA, enzyme-linked immunosorbent assay; EDS, Equine Diagnostic Solutions (Lexington, KY); UC Davis, University of California at Davis; EPM, equine protozoal myeloencephalitis; CSF, cerebrospinal fluid; S : C, Serum : CSF titer.
[a] Based on pretest probability of 10%; see reference 85;
[b] Depending on cutoff.
Source: Adapted from Reed et al. [4].

hay. Because of these factors, older horses tend to have a higher serum and potentially CSF titer than younger horses; this factor should be considered in assessing serum and CSF titers. If serum and CSF are obtained, a serum : CSF ratio <100 based on SAG 2 4/3 (Equine Diagnostic Solutions), or ratio to support intrathecal antibody production supports a diagnosis of EPM. In many cases, the risks of CSF collection is too great, thereby necessitating diagnosis based on serology [4, 9, 10, 12].

Transplacental Infection of Neospora

Transplacental infection of *Neospora* likely occurs during the last trimester of pregnancy based on the following: (i) most affected mares do not abort; (ii) mares do not mount an antibody response, suggesting that infection occurs in late pregnancy; and (iii) neonates can develop high titers, which can occur if exposure occurs after the development of the fetal immune system (day 200 of gestation) [16, 30]. In cows, the probability of high antibody titers and transplacental infection on successive pregnancies is high [16, 31]. Although unknown, mares might behave similar to cows with persistent infections infecting subsequent fetuses. Diagnosis of transplacental infection is based on presuckle serum titers from newborn foals, which will likely be high in infected foals [16, 32]. If pre-suckle titers are not obtained and the foal consumes colostrum, the amount of *N. hughesi* antibodies in colostrum impacts the foal's serum titers [16]. Maternally derived antibodies decline as the foal ages; if a foal is suspected of being infected via transplacental infection, antibody titers can be measured serially to determine if they persist with time, supporting the possibility that the foal is still infected. Because there are so few reported cases of transplacental infection there is sparse information of the long-term outcome of infected foals. In one study in foals, one-third of foals developed neurologic disease [16, 33]. It was proposed that the transplacentally infected foal that later developed neurologic disease could have then had horizontal exposure in the environment. This may have overwhelmed the immune system, leading to neurologic signs [16, 33, 34].

S. Neurona Infection in Mares and Neonates

Infection with *S. neurona* is rare in foals, but foals between 2 days and 2 months of age have been identified with clinical signs due to *S. neurona* [1, 2]. Transplacental infection has not been demonstrated with *S. neurona* but could be possible based on the fact that a 2-day-old foal had compatible neurologic signs of EPM, coupled with a positive western blot against *S. neurona* and response to anti-protozoal treatment. Foals with clinical signs of EPM at <2 months of age raise the possibility of transplacental infection in a minority of cases [1, 2].

When performing diagnostic testing for *S. neurona* in neurologic foals, knowledge of the persistence of maternal antibodies in the foal's serum and CSF after colostrum ingestion is important. In one study, 33 neonatal foals were seronegative (western blot) prior to ingesting colostrum; post-colostrum, all 33 foals were seropositive [35]. By 9 months of age, 31 of 33 foals were seronegative with a mean seroconversion rate of 4.2 months. Thus, foals from seropositive mares that ingest colostrum will likely be seropositive for extended periods of time [35]. In a subsequent study, *S. neurona* antibodies in CSF were evaluated; in this study, 13 foals from 13 seropositive mares were seropositive to *S. neurona* (western blot) and 12 of 13 foals were CSF positive for antibodies to *S. neurona* [36]. CSF samples were collected periodically over subsequent weeks and demonstrated declining titers. However, three foals were weak positive (western blot) at 62–90 days of age and two were negative at 83–84 days [36]. Based on these studies, foals from seropositive mares will likely be serum and CSF positive for a period, regardless of the diagnostic test used. Thus, diagnostic testing for EPM in foals is complicated by maternal antibodies, but nonetheless should ideally include serum and CSF evaluation for *S. neurona* and *N. hughesi*. As noted, previous studies in foals for *S. neurona* were performed using western blot, but other tests (i.e. surface antigen testing [SAG 2 4/3], IFA) would have likely yielded similar results based on the high correlation between western blot and SAG 2 4/3 testing [37].

Treatment

Anti-protozoal medications for horses include ponazuril (Marquis), diclazuril (Protazil), and sulfadiazine pyrimethamine (Rebalance). Decoquinate and levamisole have also been used as an anti-protozoal and immune modulator [38]. Diclazuril and ponazuril are benzene acetonitrile drugs that act on the chloroplast like particles of the apicomplexan; therefore, they do not impact mammalian systems. Both are well-absorbed orally with relatively long half-lives (48–96 hours). Steady state concentrations are achieved after 7 days with both drugs if administered at labeled doses (ponazuril 5 mg/kg PO q24h; diclazuril 5 mg/kg PO q24h) [4, 9, 38]. Minimal toxicity has been reported when used at therapeutic drug levels [39]. Safety studies performed with up to 6 times the labeled dose of ponazuril (30 mg/kg PO q24h) noted few side effects but use in pregnant mares is extra-label. The Marquis label has reported histopathological findings included moderate edema in the uterine epithelium in three of four mares in the six times labeled dose group; two mares treated for 28 days and one treated for 56 days. A loading dose of 15 mg/kg ponazuril can be used to obtain steady state conditions in the CSF by day 2 [4, 40]. Safety studies with diclazuril have demonstrated safety at 5, 10, 25, and 50 times the therapeutic dose. At five times the labeled dose, horses failed to gain weight, but no other abnormalities were noted [38, 41]. Inflammation within the CNS after administration of anti-protozoal medications can result from death of pathogens subsequently leading to worsening neurological signs of up to one neurologic grade in this author's opinion, when using the labeled dose of ponazuril. Other factors to consider when using a loading dose include the severity of the affected mare and how acute the onset of signs is observed. Administration of a ½ cup of vegetable oil increases absorption of ponazuril up to 15% [42]. Horses treated with benzene acetonitrile drugs reported a 62–67% improvement (one neurologic grade) with treatment [4, 43]

Marquis and Protazil are labeled for 28 days of treatment. Initially it was proposed that 28 days of treatment would be effective with an estimated improvement of approximately 60% [9]. However, horses frequently do not obtain normal neurologic status after 28 days. Additionally, CSF testing noted that many horses were still positive for antibodies against *S. neurona* in the CSF. Therefore, treatment is often extended to 60 days or more; alternatively, ponazuril or diclazuril treatment is followed by an extended period of time with sulfadiazine (20 mg/kg)-pyrimethamine (1 mg/kg) PO q24h. This prolonged treatment may also reduce the incidence of neurologic relapse from EPM [4, 38].

The first FDA approved medication used for treating EPM was sulfadiazine pyrimethamine. This combination inhibits tetrahydrofolate synthesis, and as a result, purine and pyrimidine nucleic acid synthesis. When sulfadiazine is combined with pyrimethamine, their actions are synergistic. Potential adverse reactions include anemia, bone marrow depression, neutropenia, thrombocytopenia, urticaria, and intestinal disturbances [4, 38, 44]. Folate inhibition can result in anemia and pyrimethamine can be teratogenic; thus, it should not be used in pregnant mares. Folic acid supplementation does not help horses with side effects, and it can exacerbate adverse reactions in some cases [4, 9, 45, 46]. Improvement of two neurologic grades in 60–70% of the horses with 10% chance of relapse has been reported with sulfadiazine pyrimethamine. When used, this combination should be given either two hours before or after hay to maximize absorption [38, 47]. The ideal time between nursing for maximal absorption is not known in foals in regard to sulfadiazine/pyrimethamine.

Decoquinate/levamisole is another commercially available anti-protozoal/immune modulatory drug combination but is not FDA approved for treatment of EPM [48, 49]. There are no published data of its use in pregnant mares or foals. Decoquinate is a quinolone anti-coccidial drug, and thought to act on the *S. neurona* mitochondria [49]. Decoquinate has been shown to be effective in other diseases, such as *Toxoplasma gondii* in sheep, *Eimeria* in calves and kids, and *Cryptosporidium* in calves [50, 51]. Levamisole is an immunomodulatory drug used in many species [52–55]; however, little information is available in horses to better understand the mechanism of action and side effects [53, 54, 56, 57]. Levamisole is used to limit inflammation and control or prevent disease in a number of conditions ranging from inflammatory mediated diseases to neoplasia, as well as upregulate protective immune responses. However, lack of published data in horses has restricted its use. Ellison and Lindsay performed a study supporting its efficacy in the treatment of EPM based on improvement of affected horses (improved clinical signs, changes in serum titer) [48]. The concern for using decoquinate and levamisole in pregnant mares are the potential effect on the fetus/foal. Little is known in regard to the effect of decoquinate in the pregnant mare nor the residual products in mare's milk [58]. Similarly, limited information of the effects of levamisole on the systemic immune response in pregnant mares and how it affects susceptibility or resistance to other pathogens or parasites is known [19]. Data from other species suggest that the dam may be able to clear other parasitic pathogens [19, 59–62]. However, concerns of whether levamisole's effect on the overall immune status of the mare, specifically the placenta, and the ability to maintain immune tolerance to support pregnancy has not been assessed. Thus, the safety of decoquinate and levamisole in the pregnant mare is unknown.

In nonpregnant mares treated for EPM, one reason for using decoquinate and levamisole or sulfadiazine-pyrimethamine, based on *in vitro* studies, is that both are cidal drugs against *S. neurona*. Therefore, *S. neurona* does not have to be replicating for these anti-protozoals to eliminate *S. neurona in vitro*. In contrast, based on *in vitro* studies, both ponazuril and diclazuril are static drugs; therefore, *S. neurona* may have to be replicating to be eliminated. Recently, in an immune-deficient mouse model, *S. neurona* persisted and likely replicated after diclazuril therapy was discontinued [63]. Therefore, decoquinate and sulfadiazine/pyrimethamine are cidal drugs for *S. neurona* but ponazuril and diclazuril may have lower risks for complications. The concern with static medications is that these drugs may not eliminate persistent/latent infection. If the mare or foal becomes immunocompromised, recrudescence of clinical signs may occur. Little has been published on anti-protozoal treatment for *N. hughesi*; affected horses are therefore treated similar to *S. neurona* infected horses.

Treatment with anti-protozoal medications is aimed at resolution of clinical signs. With the intent to reduce risk of relapse, horses are often treated for prolonged periods of time (3–6 months). If an EPM-affected horse still has neurologic deficits after prolonged treatment, there is no way to reliably determine if the horse still has active infection or residual neurologic deficits, the latter of which requires more time to recover. Other treatments for affected mares and foals include nonsteroidal anti-inflammatory drugs (NSAIDs) along with agents such as DMSO and/or Vitamin E. Steroids should be avoided in pregnant mares. Based on the severity of signs and rate of improvement, NSAIDs may only be necessary for a few days. In nonpregnant horses with EPM, immune modulators are considered. Because of the regulation of the mare's immune system and the concern for how immunomodulators could affect the placenta and health of the fetus/foal, immunotherapy has an unknown risk/benefit. Exercise and turnout are focused on minimizing the mare's stress. In the author's opinion, if horses have neurologic deficits that are grade 2 or greater, they should be limited to stall rest or a small paddock.

Anti-Protozoal Treatment of Foals

Minimal information is available in regard to anti-protozoal treatment of foals with EPM. In one case, a 2-month-old Appaloosa colt was administered trimethoprim sulfadiazine (30 mg/kg q12h PO) and pyrimethamine (1 mg/kg PO q24h) to treat EPM [2]. The foal's cranial nerve deficits improved after 16 days. The owners were instructed to treat the colt for 6 months, but treatment was discontinued after 2 months. The foal presented 6 months after discharge for umbilical hernia repair; at that time the foal had mild residual neurological deficits with slight muzzle deviation and slight, though improved, bilateral dorsomedial strabismus. Other neurologic signs resolved. Foals receiving trimethoprim sulfadiazine should be monitored for anemia, bone marrow depression, neutropenia, and thrombocytopenia. For foals administered ponazuril, transferring the medication into a 6- or 12-ml syringe facilitate proper dosing and avoid overdose.

Nonempiric Treatment for Relapsing Horses

If a mare or foal is treated for EPM, and then develops recurrent signs during or after successful treatment, the animal should be reassessed. Differentials should be reviewed and diagnostic testing considered. If clinical signs are likely attributed to EPM, the mare/foal should be started on anti-protozoal medications. If the mare/foal demonstrates no improvement, the patient should be reassessed to identify other existing or coexisting diseases. If a mare/foal relapses more than twice from EPM, the author's opinion is that immune dysfunction is present and the mare/foal will likely need long-term treatment.

Summary

If a pregnant mare presents with neurologic signs consistent with EPM or abortion, *S. neurona* and *N. hughesi* should be considered as differentials. While ideal diagnostic testing of affected mares or foals includes serum and CSF testing for antibodies against *S. neurona* and *N. hughesi*, anti-protozoal medications should commence. Supportive therapies should be administered, including NSAIDS, vitamin E, and DMSO, based on severity of signs. Patients should be monitored closely for response to treatment and reassessed if not responding at the predicted rate.

References

1. Fayer, R., Mayhew, I., Baird, J. et al. (1990). Epidemiology of equine protozoal myeloencephalitis in North America based on histologically confirmed cases. *J. Vet. Intern. Med.* 4: 54–57.
2. Gray, L., Magedesian, K.G., Sturges, B. et al. (2001). Suspected protozoal myeloencephalitis in a two-month-old colt. *Vet. Rec.* 149: 269–273.
3. Saville, W., Reed, S., Morley, P. et al. (2000). Analysis of risk factors for the development of equine protozoal myeloencephalitis in horses. *J. Am. Vet. Med. Assoc.* 217: 1174–1180.
4. Reed, S., Furr, M., and Howe, D. (2016). Equine protozoal myeloencephalitis: an updated consensus statement with a focus on parasite biology, diagnosis, treatment, and prevention. *J. Vet. Intern. Med.* 30: 491–502.
5. Speer, C.A., Dubey, J.P., and Mattson, D.E. (2000). Comparative development and merozoite production of two isolates of *Sarcocystis neurona* and *Sarcocystis falcatula* in cultured cells. *J. Parasitol.* 86: 25–32.
6. Ellison, S., Greiner, E., Brown, K. et al. (2004). Experimental infection of horses with culture-derived *Sarcocystis neurona* merozoites as a model for equine protozoal myeloencephalitis. *Intern. J. Appl. Res. Vet. Med.* 2: 79–89.
7. Lindsay, D., Mitchell, S., Yang, J. et al. (2006). Penetration of equine leukocytes by merozoites of *Sarcocystis neurona*. *Vet. Parasitol.* 138: 371–376.
8. Witonsky, S.G., Ellison, S., Yang, J. et al. (2008). Horses experimentally infected with *Sarcocystis neurona* develop altered immune responses in vitro. *J. Parasitol.* 94: 1047–1054.
9. Furr, M. (2010). Equine protozoal myeloencephalitis. In: *Equine Internal Medicine*, 2e. St. Louis, MO: Saunders, Elsevier.
10. Dubey, J., Howe, D., Furr, M. et al. (2015). An update on *Sarcocystis neurona* infections in animals and equine protozoal myeloencephalitis (EPM). *Vet. Parasitol.* 209: 1–42.
11. James, K., Smith, W., Conrad, P. et al. (2017). Seroprevalences of anti–Sarcocystis neurona and anti–Neospora hughesi antibodies among healthy equids in the United States. *J. Am. Vet. Med. Assoc.* 250: 1291–1301.
12. Johnson, A. (2018). *Sarcocystis neurona* and *Neospora hughesi*. In: *Interpretation of Equine Laboratory Diagnostics*, 1e (ed. N. Pusterla and J. Higgins). Wiley.
13. Witonsky, S.G., Gogal, R.M., Duncan, R.B. et al. (2005). Prevention of meningo/encephalomyelitis due to *Sarcocystis neurona* infection in mice is mediated by CD8 cells. *Int. J. Parasitol.* 35: 113–123.
14. Anderson, J., Alves, D., and Cerqueira-Cézar, C. (2019). et al, Histologically, immunohistochemically, ultrastructurally, and molecularly confirmed neosporosis abortion in an aborted equine fetus. *Vet. Parasitol.* 270: 20–24.
15. Dubey, J., Schares, G., and Ortega-Mora, L. (2007). Epidemiology and control of neosporosis and Neospora caninum. *Clin. Microbiol. Rev.* 20: 323–367.
16. Pusterla, N., Conrad, P., Packham, A. et al. (2011). Endogenous transplacental transmission of Neospora hughesi in naturally infected horses. *J. Parasitol.* 97: 281–285.
17. Bettelli, E., Korn, T., and Kuchroo, V. (2007). Th17: the third member of the effector T cell trilogy. *Curr. Opin. Immunol.* 19: 652–657.
18. Noronha, L. and Antczak, D. (2010). Maternal immune responses to trophoblast: the contribution of the horse to

pregnancy. *Immunology. Am. J. Reprod. Immunol.* 64: 231–244.

19 Krakowski, L., Krzyzanowski, J., Wrona, Z. et al. (1999). The effect of nonspecific immunostimulation of pregnant mares with 1,3/1,6 glucan and levamisole on the immunoglobulins levels in colostrum, selected indices of nonspecific cellular and humoral immunity in foals in neonatal and postnatal period. *Vet. Immunol. Immunopathol.* 68: 1–11.

20 Granstrom, D. (1997). Equine protozoal myeloencephalitis: Parasite biology, experimental disease, and laboratory diagnosis. *International Equine Neurology Conference*, Ithaca NY, March 1997.

21 Daft, B.M., Barr, B.C., Gardner, I.A. et al. (2002). Sensitivity and specificity of western blot testing of cerebrospinal fluid and serum for diagnosis of equine protozoal myeloencephalitis in horses with and without neurologic abnormalities. *J. Am. Vet. Med. Assoc.* 221: 1007–1013.

22 Duarte, P.C., Daft, B.M., Conrad, P.A. et al. (2004). Comparison of serum indirect fluorescent antibody test with two Western blot tests for the diagnosis of equine protozoal myeloencephalitis. *J. Vet. Diagn. Invest.* 15: 8–13.

23 Rassano, M.G., Mansfield, L.S., Kaneene, J.B. et al. (2000). Improvement of western blot test specificity for detecting equine serum antibodies to *Sarcocystis neurona*. *J. Vet. Diagn. Invest.* 12: 28–32.

24 Duarte, P.C., Daft, B.M., Conrad, P.A. et al. (2004). Evaluation and comparison of an indirect fluorescent antibody test for detection of antibodies to *Sarcocystis neurona*, using serum and cerebrospinal fluid of naturally and experimentally infected, and vaccinated horses. *J. Parasitol.* 90: 379–386.

25 Johnson, A.L., Burton, A.J., and Sweeney, R.W. (2010). Utility of 2 immunological tests for antemortem diagnosis of equine protozoal myeloencephalitis (*Sarcocystis neurona* infection) in naturally occurring cases. *J. Vet. Intern. Med.* 24: 1184–1189.

26 Johnson, A.L., Morrow, J.K., and Sweeney, R.W. (2013). Indirect fluorescent antibody test and surface antigen ELISAs for antemortem diagnosis of equine protozoal myeloencephalitis. *J. Vet. Intern. Med.* 27: 596–599.

27 Hoane, J.S., Morrow, J.K., Saville, W.J. et al. (2005). Enzyme-linked immunosorbent assays for the detection of equine antibodies specific to *Sarcocystis neurona* surface antigens. *Clin. Diagn. Lab. Immunol.* 12: 1050–1056.

28 Reed, S.M., Howe, D.K., Morrow, J.K. et al. (2013). Accurate antemortem diagnosis of equine protozoal myeloencephalitis (EPM) based on detecting intrathecal antibodies against Sarcocystis neurona using the SnSAG2 and SnSAG4/3 ELISAs. *J. Vet. Intern. Med.* 27: 1193–1200.

29 Furr, M., Howe, D., Reed, S. et al. (2011). Antibody coefficients for the diagnosis of equine protozoal myeloencephalitis. *J. Vet. Intern. Med.* 25: 138–142.

30 Perryman, L., McGuire, T., and Torbeck, R. (1980). Ontogeny of lymphocyte function in the equine fetus. *Am. J. Vet. Res.* 41: 1197–1200.

31 Davison, H., Otter, A., and Trees, A. (1999). Estimation of vertical and horizontal transmission parameters of Neospora caninum infections in dairy cattle. *Int. J. Parasitol.* 29: 1683–1689.

32 Antonello, A., Pivotoa, F., Camilloa, G. et al. (2012). The importance of vertical transmission of *Neospora* sp. in naturally infected horses. *Vet. Parasitol.* 187: 367–370.

33 Finno, C., Aleman, M., and Pusterla, N. (2007). Equine protozoal myeloencephalitis associated with neosporosis in 3 horses. *J. Vet. Intern. Med.* 21: 1405–1408.

34 Dubey, J. and Schares, G. (2006). Diagnosis of bovine neosporosis. *Vet. Parasitol.* 140: 1–34.

35 Cook, A., Buechner-Maxwell, V., Morrow, J. et al. (2001). Interpretation of the detection of *Sarcocystis neurona* antibodies in the serum of young horses. *Vet. Parasitol.* 95: 187–195.

36 Cook, A., Buechner Maxwell, V., Donaldson, L. et al. (2002). Detection of antibodies against *Sarcocystis neurona* in cerebrospinal fluid from clinically normal neonatal foals. *J. Am. Vet. Med. Assoc.* 220: 208–211.

37 Hoane, J., Morrow, J., and Saville, W. (2005). Enzyme-linked immunosorbent assays for detection of equine antibodies specific to *Sarcocystis neurona* surface antigens. *Clin. Diagn. Lab. Immunol.* 12: 1050–1056.

38 Pusterla, N. and Tobin, T. (2017). Therapeutics for equine protozoal myeloencephalitis. *Vet. Clin. Equine* 33: 87–97.

39 Bentz, B., Dirikolu, L., Carter, W. et al. (2000). Equine protozoal myeloencephalitis (EPM): a clinical report. *Equine Vet. Educ.* 16: 258–263.

40 Reed, S., Wendel, M. and King, S. (2012). Pharmacokinetics of ponazuril in horses. *58th Annual Convention of the American Association of Equine Practitioners*, December 5th, Anaheim, CA, 572.

41 US FDA (2007). Protazil antiprotozoal pellets. 1.56% diclazuril. Freedom of Information Summary. Original new animal drug application. NADA 141–268. Available 96 Pusterla & Tobin https://animaldrugsatfda.fda.gov/adafda/app/search/public/document/downloadFoi/829 (accessed 7 July 2016).

42 Furr, M. and Kennedy, T. (2020). Effects of coadministration of corn oil and ponazuril on serum and cerebrospinal fluid concentrations of ponazuril in horses. *J. Vet. Intern. Med.* 34: 1321–1324.

43 Furr, M., Kennedy, T., MacKay, R. et al. (2001). Efficacy of ponazuril 15% oral paste as a treatment for equine protozoal myeloencephalitis. *Vet. Ther.* 2: 215–222.

44 Welsch, B.B. (1991). Treatment of equine protozoal myeloencephalitis. *Compend. Contin. Educ. Pract. Vet.* 13: 1599–1602.

45 Toribio, R., Bain, F., Mrad, D. et al. (1998). Congenital defects in newborn foals of mares treated for equine protozoal myeloencephalitis during pregnancy. *J. Am. Vet. Med. Assoc.* 12: 697–701.

46 Piercy, R., Hinchcliff, S., and Reed, S. (2002). Folate deficiency during treatment with orally administered folic acid, sulphadiazine and pyrimethamine in a horse with suspected equine protozoal myeloencephalitis (EPM). *Equine Vet. J.* 34: 311–316.

47 Reed, S.M. and Saville, W.J. (1996). Equine protozoal encephalomyelitis. *Proceedings of 1996 Veterinary Symposium*, (8–11 December). American Association of Equine Practitioners. Denver.

48 Ellison, S. and Lindsay, D. (2012). Decoquinate combined with levamisole reduce the clinical signs and serum SAG 1, 5, 6 antibodies in horses with suspected equine protozoal myeloencephalitis. *Intern. J. Appl. Res. Vet. Med.* 10: 1–7.

49 Lindsay, D., Nazir, M., and Maqbool, A. (2013). Efficacy of decoquinate against Sarcocystis neurona in cell cultures. *Vet. Parasitol.* 196: 21–23.

50 Taylor, M. and Bartram, D. (2012). The history of decoquinate in the control of coccidial infections in ruminants. *J. Vet. Pharmacol. Therap.* 35: 417–427.

51 Li, Q., Xie, L., Caridha, D. et al. (2017). Long-term prophylaxis and pharmacokinetic evaluation of intramuscular nano- and microparticle Decoquinate in mice infected with *P. berghei* sporozoites. *Malar. Res. Treat.* 7508291. 1–10.

52 Hanson, K. and Heidrick, M. (1991). Immunomodulatory action of levamisole— II. Enhancement of concanavalin a response by levamisole is associated with an oxidation degradation product of levamisole formed during lymphocyte culture. *Int. J. Immunopharmacol.* 13: 669–676.

53 Hanson, K., Nagel, D., and Heidrick, M. (1991). Immunomodulatory action of levamisole—I. structural analysis and immunomodulating activity of levamisole degradation products. *Int. J. Immunopharmacol.* 13 (6): 655–668.

54 Chen, L., Lin, Y., and Chiang, B. (2008). Levamisole enhances immune response by affecting the activation and maturation of human monocytederived dendritic cells. *Clin. Exp. Immunol.* 151: 174–181.

55 Chandy, M., Soman, C., Kumar, S. et al. (2016). Understanding molecular mechanisms of levamisole as an anti-helminthic, anti-inflammatory, antioxidant, anti-neoplastic and immunomodulatory drug. *J. Oral Maxillofac. Surg. Med. Pathol.* 28: 354–357.

56 Krakowski, L., Bartoszek, P., Krakowska, I. et al. (2017). Changes in blood lymphocyte subpopulations and expression of MHC-II molecules in wild mares before and after parturition. *J. Vet. Res.* 61: 217–221.

57 Witonsky, S., Buechner-Maxwell, V., Santonastasto, A. et al. (2019). Can levamisole upregulate the equine cell-mediated macrophage (M1) dendritic cell (DC1) T-helper 1 (CD4 Th1) T-cytotoxic (CD8) immune response in vitro? *J. Vet. Intern. Med.* 33: 889–896.

58 Clarke, L., Moloney, M., O'Mahony, J. et al. (2013). Determination of 20 coccidiostats in milk, duck muscle and non-avian muscle tissue using UHPLC-MS/MS. *Food Addit. Contam. Part A Chem. Anal. Control Expo. Risk Assess.* 30 (6): 958–969.

59 Oakley, G.A. (1982). Comparison of protection against lungworm infection between levamisole-treated and vaccinated calves. *Vet. Rec.* 111: 28–31.

60 Herd, R.P., Streital, R.H., McClure, K.E. et al. (1984). Control of hypobiotic and benzimidazole-resistant nematodes of sheep. *J. Am. Vet. Med. Assoc.* 184: 726–730.

61 Sun, X.M., Zou, J., Saeed, E. et al. (2011). DNA vaccination with a gene encoding toxoplasma gondii GRA6 induces partial protection against toxoplasmosis in BALB/c mice. *Parasit. Vectors* 213: https://doi.org/10.1186/1756-3305-4-213.

62 Zeynep, S.K., Yankik, K., Bilgin, K. et al. (2016). In vivo efficacy of drugs against *Toxoplasma gondii* combined with immunomodulators. *Jpn. J. Infect. Dis.* 69: 113–117.

63 Hay, A., Witonsky, S., Lindsay, D. et al. (2019). *Sarcocystis neurona*-induced Myeloencephalitis relapse following anticoccidial treatment. *J. Parasitol.* 105: 371–378.

Section III Infectious and Inflammatory – Tetanus in the Neonatal Foal

David Wong and Gaby van Galen

Tetanus is caused by *Clostridium tetani*, a Gram-positive anaerobic bacterium that is present in sporulated form in the environment, typically in the soil and manure. *C. tetani* is a commensal of the gastrointestinal tract and has been isolated from feces from a variety of animals, including horses, cows, sheep and dogs [1, 2]. Tetanus affects all mammals with each species having varying susceptibility to disease, but horses have been suggested to be the most susceptible [2–5]. *C. tetani* spores can enter the foal's body through the umbilicus, wounds, or minor abrasions, and under appropriate anaerobic conditions, the spores germinate to form vegetative bacteria that produce neurotoxin [3]. The two main toxins associated with *C. tetani* are tetanolysin and tetanospasmin, although a third less commonly noted toxin, non-spasmogenic toxin, has also been described [2, 5, 6].

Tetanolysin is a cytolytic toxin that damages viable host tissue by causing permeability changes in biological membranes, resulting in cell lysis and tissue necrosis. This consequently lowers the local redox potential creating a more favorable environment for expansion of the anaerobic infection [7]. Tetanospasmin, simply stated, inhibits the pre-synaptic release of glycine and gamma-aminobutyric acid (GABA) [8]. More specifically, tetanospasmin is a highly potent, zinc-dependent neurotoxin whose release is regulated by a complex system involving environmental signals and intrinsic regulatory factors [9]. After production by proliferating organisms, tetanospasmin diffuses locally and circulates in the blood to neuromuscular junctions throughout the body. The toxin then binds to presynaptic membranes at neuromuscular junctions causing initial clinical signs of localized tetanus, characterized by localized flaccid paralysis, resulting from interference with vesicular release of acetylcholine at the neuromuscular junction, similar to what occurs with botulinum toxin [9]. However, paralysis is typically overridden by spasmogenic effects at the inhibitory interneuron. Unlike botulinum toxin, tetanospasmin is internalized in the axons of the lower motor neuron and undergoes extensive retrograde transport, at a rate of 75–250 mm/day, through endogenous microtubule-based axonal pathways to reach the spinal cord and brainstem [9–11]. After 1 to 14 days, the toxin reaches the neuronal cell body within the central nervous system, is transported across synapses, and irreversibly binds presynaptic inhibitory interneurons [3, 9, 10]. These nerve endings are inhibitory GABAergic and/or glycinergic neurons that control the activity of the lower motor neuron [12, 13]. The substrate of tetanospasmin is vesicle-associated membrane protein 2 (VAMP2), also known as synaptobrevin-2, which is part of the complex that is normally needed for synaptic vesicle docking and neurotransmitter release [14]. Once inside inhibitory nerve terminals, tetanospasmin stops the formation of this complex by cleavage of VAMP2, thus preventing release of the inhibitory neurotransmitters GABA and glycine. This results in a reduction of motor nerve inhibition, increased muscle stimulation and the clinically characteristic spasms and rigidity noted with the disease [3, 9]. Since neuronal binding by the toxin is believed to be irreversible, recovery requires sprouting and growth of new nerve terminals; this process can take several weeks to months [2, 11]. Autonomic dysregulation can also be observed with tetanus and primarily affects the sympathetic nervous system with clinical signs arising from tetanospasmin's activity at central excitatory synapses binding to sympathetic adrenergic neurons [8, 14, 15].

Clinical Features

In the equine neonate, the umbilicus is the usual suspected site of entry [4, 16–18], but skin lacerations, wounds, burns, intramuscular injection, or abrasions can also serve as ports of entry [3, 9, 19]. The mean time between

Equine Neonatal Medicine, First Edition. Edited by David M. Wong and Pamela A. Wilkins.

inoculation to first clinical signs (incubation period) was 6 days with the mean period of onset (time of first signs to spasms) of 0.3 days, as reported in 21 foals with tetanus [18]. Disease severity is related to the speed of symptom evolution, with more rapid development of clinical signs associated with more severe disease [3, 20]. Stiffness and recumbency are typically the first clinical signs noted by the owner (Figure 32.III.1a). Although protrusion of the nictitating membrane and trismus are typical signs of tetanus, it is not unusual for foals to show these signs later in the course of disease, particularly trismus [18]. Other clinical signs reported carly in the course of disease in foals include: recumbency, muscle spasms, extended neck, and abnormal (decreased or absent) defecation and urination (Tables 32.III.1 and 32.III.2) [16–18, 21, 22]. In addition, signs of altered mental status such as lethargy, agitation, or anxiousness or common. Consciousness is usually not affected and clinical signs may be exacerbated by auditory, tactile or visual stimuli. Muscle stiffness may manifest as an abnormal stiff or difficult gait, wide-based stance, and a "saw-horse" or "rocking-horse" stance (e.g. tail extension, rigid and extended head and neck; Figure 32.III.1b) [4, 18]. Difficulty with prehension and mastication along with trismus (lockjaw), retracted lips and dysphagia can be observed and result from facial spasms [3, 16, 18, 23]. Tail extension, caudally placed or erect ears, and sweating along with dilated external nares, tachypnea, and dyspnea have been described. Pharyngeal, laryngeal, diaphragmatic, and intercostal muscle spasms can lead to dyspnea, respiratory stridor and dysfunction, pulmonary edema and aspiration [3, 4, 16–18, 22]. Generalized effects of tetanus can result in seizures, inability to stand or rise without assistance, and truncal rigidity (opistotonus). Death in equine tetanus is usually attributed to spasms of the laryngeal and respiratory muscles that cause respiratory failure [9, 16, 18–20]. Gastrointestinal impactions, diarrhea, dysuria, tachycardia or bradycardia, tachypnea, and hypo- or hyperthermia have also been reported [18].

Clinical manifestations associated with autonomic nervous system disturbances are well described in humans and dogs [24–26]. These signs can include hypertension, tachycardia, and sweating, but rapid changes in blood pressure or bradycardia also can occur [3]. These clinical signs are paralleled by increases in circulating adrenaline and noradrenaline [27, 28]. Other autonomic effects include abnormal bowel (gastric stasis, diarrhea) and bladder function, fever, and increased respiratory secretions, possibly reflecting the impact of tetanospasmin on the brainstem [19, 27]. Autonomic disturbances have been poorly described in horses but in one report, 3 of 21 foals had violent autonomic disturbances of the cardiovascular system (very severe tetanus score), while other foals demonstrated relative bradycardia in the face of painful muscle cramps, excessive sweating, fever, gastrointestinal impaction, diarrhea, and abnormal bladder function, all suggestive of tetanus-induced autonomic dysfunction [18]. Sensory

(a) (b)

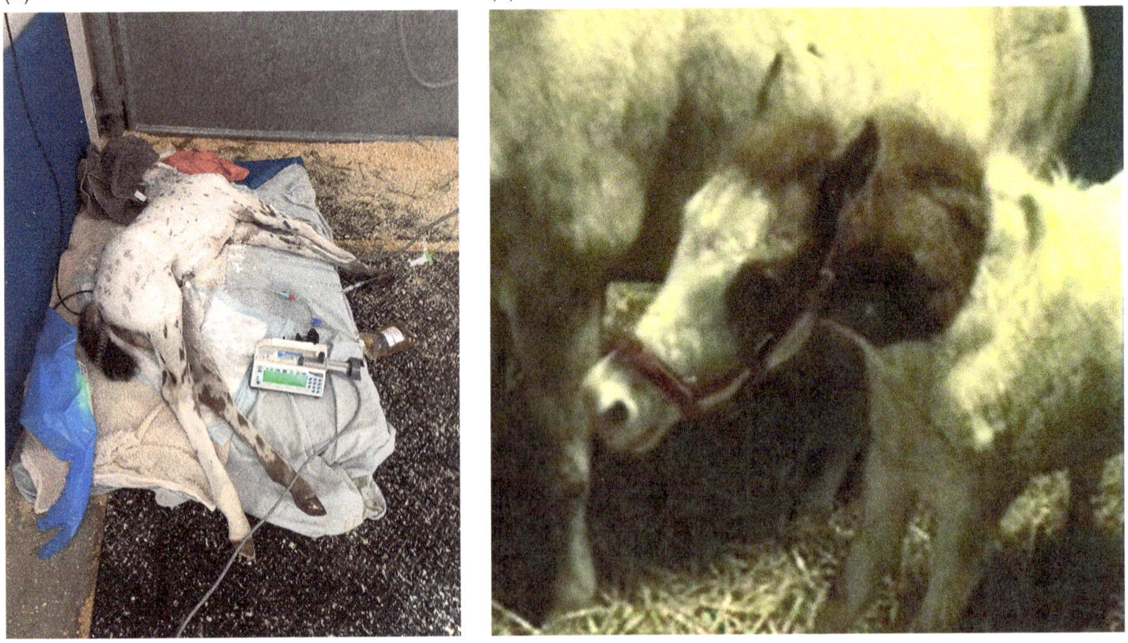

Figure 32.III.1 (a) Neonatal foal showing rigidity of the hindlimb muscles and recumbency secondary to tetanus. Photo courtesy of Dr. Kathryn Johnson, Iowa State University; (b) Foal with tetanus showing dilated nares, retracted ears, tense facial expression, extended neck, and wide-based stance.

Table 32.III.1 Clinical parameters reported on admission in 21 foals with tetanus (Median age 5.2 weeks; range 6 days to 6 months) [18].

Clinical Sign	Number foals observed	%	Clinical Sign	Number foals observed	%
Stiffness	21/21	100	Other neurologic signs		
Prolapse nictitating membrane	15/21	71.4	Recumbency	13/21	61.9
Trismus	8/21	38.1	Involuntary muscle spasms	12/20	60.0
Mentation			Wide-based stance	2/19	10.5
Normal	3/21	14.3	Retracted lips	2/20	10.0
Depressed	8/21	38.1	Pulled down ears	3/18	16.7
Generalized Seizures	6/20	30.0	Extended neck	11/20	55.0
Agitated	7/20	35.0	Elevated tail	5/19	26.3
Anxious	5/20	25.0	Dysphagia	4/18	22.2
Dyspnea	9/20	45.0			
Normal intestinal sounds	6/10	60.0	Clinical examination	Mean ± SD	Range
Normal defecation	3/10	30.0	Heart rate	97 ± 26	60–148
Anorexia	8/19	42.1	Respiratory rate	70 ± 38	20–160
Normal urination	4/8	50.0	Rectal temp Celsius	38.6 ± 0.8	36.2–39.6
Sweating	6/19	31.6	Fahrenheit	100.8 ± 1.4	97.2–103.2

Table 32.III.2 Complications and clinical signs that developed during hospitalization reported in 21 foals with tetanus (Median age 5.2 weeks; range 6 days to 6 months) [18, 20].

Clinical sign	Number foals observed	%
Dysphagia	9/19	47.4%
Recumbency	13/19	68.4%
Dyspnea	8/19	42.1%
Increased rectal temperature (>38.5°C)	13/19	68.4%
Seizures	6/19	31.6%
Gastrointestinal impaction	3/17	17.6%
Dysuria	2/19	10.5%
Laryngeal spasms and/or stridor	2/19	10.5%
Thrombophlebitis	1/19	5.3%
Diarrhea	1/19	5.3%
Aspiration pneumonia	2/18	11.1%

nerves may also be impacted by tetanospasmin, resulting in clinical signs of altered sensation such as pain and allodynia [29]. Interestingly, generalized nonpruritic asymmetric alopecia has been rarely reported in horses that have recovered from tetanus [2].

Clinical features of tetanus in foals are similar to adult horses, yet with clear differences. Wounds are more frequently identified in adult horses, as is protrusion of the nictitating membrane, trismus, wide-based stance, elevated tailhead, dysphagia, and normal urination compared to foals. In contrast, clinical signs of generalized seizures and recumbency are more commonly noted in foals along with development of increased rectal temperature during hospitalization [18]. Overall, adult horses tend to be moderately affected by tetanus, whereas foals have severe signs [18]. In addition, local forms of tetanus have been described in people, but not in foals [24]. Based on these differences, and the broader opportunities in intensive care opportunities in foals over adult horses (i.e., inherent size and weight limitations), tetanus in foals and adult horses are considered distinct syndromes, in line with human medicine [18].

A grading scale for foals with tetanus has been developed (Table 32.III.3) with one report involving 21 foals noting 29% mild, 19% moderate, 38% severe, and 13% very severe clinical signs, with the latter group including the previously noted cardiovascular autonomic signs [2, 18].

Diagnosis

Nearly always, tetanus in the neonatal foal is a diagnosis based on clinical signs and exclusion of other causes. Absence of maternal vaccination against tetanus, lack of administration of prophylactic tetanus antitoxin (TAT)

Table 32.III.3 Clinical Scoring System for foals with tetanus [18, 24].

Mild clinical signs	Mild-moderate trismus, generalized stiffness, no respiratory problems, no spasms, little or no dysphagia.
Moderate clinical signs	Moderate trismus, marked stiffness, mild-moderate short spasms, moderate respiratory embarrassment, mild dysphagia.
Severe clinical signs	Severe trismus, generalized stiffness, reflex prolonged spasms, respiratory embarrassment (tachypnea, apneic periods), severe dysphagia, tachycardia.
Very severe clinical signs	Similar criteria as severe grading plus violent autonomic disturbances of cardiovascular system (severe hypertension and tachycardia alternating with hypotension and bradycardia).

after birth, or failure of passive transfer of immunity may be reported [18]. Attempts can be made to culture *C. tetani* from infected wounds, identify the organism via Gram stains or detect the neurotoxic gene via PCR [30–32]. Despite frequent false negative results, these tests are currently considered the most sensitive test to diagnose tetanus in people [30–32]. However, the organism can be identified in patients without tetanus, so the presence of the bacteria is only supportive, not confirmatory [33]. Apart from diagnostic aid for tetanus, culture provides knowledge on the bacterial flora and antimicrobial susceptibility patterns of infected entry wounds and can be helpful to optimize wound care and direct antimicrobial therapy.

Tetanospasmin can be detected in serum by bioassay, but a negative bioassay result does not exclude tetanus [2, 34]. As *C. tetani* bacteremia has been described in people, albeit without signs of tetanus [35, 36], coupled with the fact that sepsis is a common occurrence in foals, it is recommended to perform blood cultures in foals with suspect tetanus. Affected foals may have nonspecific changes on CBC and serum biochemistry profile, including leukocytosis (mean ± SD; $16.5 \pm 5.6 \times 10^3/\mu l$), neutrophilia, moderately elevated creatine kinase (1247 ± 1186 U/l), hyperlactatemia (5.5 ± 2.5 mmol/l), and hyperfibrinogenemia [17, 18]. Other clinicopathologic changes include alterations in blood triglycerides, glucose, bilirubin, and urea if the foal is anorexic, and acid-base disturbances if seizure activity and/or respiratory compromise develops. Electromyography (EMG), although not examined in equids with tetanus, has been used in people with changes in the EMG related to reduced release of inhibitory neurotransmitters (continuous involuntary spontaneous motor activity, prolonged motor activity during attempted relaxation after voluntary contraction, increased F-wave amplitude, and absence of the silent period normally present after peripheral stimulation) [37–39].

Treatment

Treatment of foals with generalized tetanus, especially those that are recumbent, requires a dedicated owner committed to a potentially prolonged recovery and availability of sufficient veterinary staffing [16, 17, 40]. One report in foals that survived tetanus documented a mean ± SD hospitalization length of 10.1 ± 13.5 days with the total length of disease being 21 ± 17.2 days [18]. Overarching treatment goals include: elimination of *Clostridium tetani* (source of toxin), neutralization of unbound toxin, muscle relaxation and relief of pain, supportive care and physical therapy.

Eliminating Toxin Sources

Elimination of the source of the toxin involves thorough cleaning, debridement and lavage of any wounds, lacerations and/or the umbilical remnant and administration of antimicrobials, with the presumption that antimicrobials will eliminate and prevent local proliferation of *C. tetani*. Both penicillin and metronidazole have been used in people and foals with tetanus as first-line antimicrobials, but the development of resistance to these medications is possible [2, 17, 18, 31, 41]. Some controversy exists over the use of penicillin in cases of tetanus [31, 42]. The argument against the use of penicillin rests on the fact that penicillin is a GABA antagonist and thus produces a noncompetitive inhibition of GABA receptors, thereby obtunding postsynaptic inhibitory potentials [24, 42]. At high doses, penicillin can cause CNS hyperexcitability and convulsions and may theoretically potentiate the action of tetanospasmin and synergistically block GABA neuronal activity [19, 42]. However, this theory is not supported by some studies in people which did not note any difference in outcome when comparing penicillin and metronidazole [43]. Additionally, tetanus in foals has been successfully treated with penicillin [4, 16–18, 23]. Other references in people strongly recommend the use of metronidazole in the treatment of tetanus, as this drug is rapidly bactericidal against obligate anaerobes and its pharmacokinetic characteristics allows for distribution at effective therapeutic concentrations into anaerobic tissue environments [24]. Furthermore, a report in people described two cases where despite treatment with high doses of penicillin, *C. tetani* was still isolated from the wound after 16 days of intravenous therapy, suggesting penicillin may be inadequate for clearing infection in some cases and that local wound debridement is essential [31]. Additionally, penicillin can be inactivated by beta-lactamases produced by co-infecting bacteria. If possible, the intravenous route is recommended initially as to reduce any stimulation that may be caused by oral or intramuscular administration of medications [44]. Other suggested antibiotics include erythromycin, vancomycin, tetracycline, doxycycline, and chloramphenicol. However, considering antimicrobial stewardship, macrolides, and vancomycin should be avoided [19, 45]. Broad-spectrum antimicrobial coverage should be considered if the foal has leucopenia or partial or complete failure of transfer of immunity or signs of infection.

Neutralizing Unbound Toxins

Neutralization of unbound toxin is an established practice in the treatment of tetanus, but individual cases have been reported to survive tetanus without TAT [2, 18, 23]. Since tetanospasmin that has entered the nervous system is irreversible, efforts are placed on neutralizing circulating toxin before it enters the nervous system. Equine tetanus antitoxin has been administered to foals with tetanus at various dosages, ranging from a single administration of 1,000–2,500,000 iu given IV or IM, followed by lower doses over subsequent days [5, 18, 46]. Doses of 5,000–12,000 iu of TAT IV or IM, daily for 5–7 days is a good starting point as this dose and frequency has been reported in foals that have recovered from tetanus [4, 16–18]. Interestingly, 10 nonsurviving foals from one report had less frequent doses administered (1, 2, or 3 doses) compared to surviving foals [18], and showed a trend toward increasing survival rates with increased total TAT dose [18]. In comparison, the dose of TAT administered IV did not have an influence on survival rate in some equine studies [2, 16, 20, 45]. Administration of TAT via the intrathecal route during the early stages of disease has also been implemented in both people and foals, but the clinical benefit of this route of administration is unknown and the efficacy is skewed because this route is often attempted in more severe cases [4, 23, 46, 47]. The intrathecal route bypasses the blood-brain barrier and increases the concentration of TAT in the subarachnoid space, to a greater degree than that which is achieved with IM administration alone, and provides a means to neutralize tetanus toxin during its trans-synaptic transport within the nervous system [42]. Intrathecally administered TAT may even neutralize toxin that has already attached to the gray matter of the spinal cord [23]. In one study, 30 mLs of cerebrospinal fluid was withdrawn from the atlanto-occipital (AO) space and 30 mLs (30,000 iu) of TAT was administered to 6 foals; all 6 foals died [23]. In another report 6,000 iu of TAT was administered via the atlanto-occipital space in a 3-week-old foal coupled with IV administration of 5,000 iu of TAT, whereas 20,000 iu of TAT was administered via the lumbosacral space and 20,000 iu TAT IV in a yearling filly, both of which survived [4]. Seizures and collapse are rare reported complications of intrathecal administration of TAT [18, 46]. The clinician should consider the need to place the foal under general anesthesia when using the AO space for intrathecal administration, which may be a detriment, as compared to the lumbosacral space, which was the preferred route of intrathecal administration of TAT in one case series [4]. Conversely, it is unknown whether TAT will reach the cranial portions of the CNS due to the caudal flow of cerebrospinal fluid. Therefore, the clinician should consider the lumbosacral space only in cases of caudally located wounds. Tetanus infection does not impart immunity; therefore, active immunization with tetanus toxoid is also recommended and should be administered at a separate site from TAT administration to avoid interaction [19, 42].

Muscle Relaxation

Muscle relaxation is another therapeutic goal in foals with tetanus along with providing analgesia (Table 32.III.4). Benzodiazepines augment the effect of GABA on $GABA_A$ receptors of lower motor neurons and is standard therapy for tetanus in people as they not only provide muscle relaxation but also have anticonvulsant, sedative, and anxiolytic properties [9, 42]. Other medications administered to people to facilitate muscle relaxation include baclofen (acts on $GABA_B$ receptors), propofol ($GABA_A$ receptor modulator), nondepolarizing muscle relaxants such as pancuronium or pipecuronium (acts directly on muscle motor end plates by competing for acetylcholine binding site), and dantrolene (binds ryanodine receptor in muscle and reduces calcium mobilization thereby reducing muscle contraction) [9, 42]. Local muscle injection of botulism toxin has also been used to provide muscle relaxation in people [9].

Magnesium has multiple potential useful actions that may benefit a foal with muscle spasms and autonomic dysfunction. Magnesium blocks neuromuscular transmission, interferes with catecholamine release from nerves and the adrenal medulla, reduces receptor responsiveness to circulating catecholamines, is an anticonvulsant, and acts as a physiologic calcium antagonist that reduces acetylcholine release and reduces muscle response to acetylcholine [9, 11, 42].

Many of the medications used in people have been, or could be, used in foals with tetanus. Foals present with various severity of disease and have individual responses to medications used for muscle relaxation; therefore the clinician must titrate these medications appropriately. Phenothiazine tranquiller such as acepromazine or chlorpromazine have been used in foals, but hypotension has been associated with the phenothiazines [21, 48]. Other

Table 32.III.4 Medications available to provide muscle relaxation in foals with tetanus.

Drug	Dose	Route	Frequency	Effects	Side effects
Acepromazine	0.05–0.1 mg/kg	IV or IM	Repeated as needed	Muscle relaxant, anxiolytic	Hypotension [48]
Chlorpromazine	0.4–0.8 mg/kg	IV or IM	Repeated as needed	Muscle relaxant, anxiolytic	Hypotension
Xylazine	0.5–1 mg/kg	IV or IM	Repeated as needed	Muscle relaxant, analgesia	
Detomidine	5–20 μg/kg	IV	Repeated as needed	Muscle relaxant, analgesia (strong analgesia)	Duration of action 30–200 min. Bradycardia, arrhythmias, hyperglycemia, diuresis
Romifidine	30–80 μg/kg	IV	Repeated as needed	Muscle relaxant, analgesia (questionable analgesia)	Duration of action 30–200 min. Associated with bradycardia and arrhythmias of all α2 agonists, atropine could be co-administered to counter act these effects. Hyperglycemia, diuresis
Medetomidine	5–7 μg/kg	IV	Repeated as needed	Muscle relaxant, analgesia (analgesia similar or greater than detomidine)	Duration shorter than detomidine. Bradycardia, arrhythmias, hyperglycemia, diuresis
Diazepam	0.01–0.4 mg/kg	IV	Repeated as needed	Muscle relaxant, anticonvulsant	
Midazolam	0.04–0.1 mg/kg	IV	Repeated as needed	Muscle relaxant, anticonvulsant	Hypotension and apnea when rapid IV injection
	0.02–0.06 mg/kg/H	CRI using 50 mg midazolam added to 100 ml 0.9% saline			
Phenobarbital	2–5 mg/kg	IV slow over 15-20min		Muscle relaxant, anticonvulsant	Cardiovascular and respiratory depression, bradycardia, hypotension, hypothermia
5% sodium pentobarbitol				Muscle relaxant, anticonvulsant	Cardiovascular and respiratory depression, bradycardia, hypotension, hypothermia
Guaifenesin	50–100 mg/kg	IV to effect	Repeated as needed	Muscle relaxant, anticonvulsant	Hemolysis when administered in high concentration
Triple drip – 4% glycerol guiaicolate, 0.5 mg/ml xylazine, 1 mg/ml ketamine	1 ml/kg	IV		General anesthesia	General anesthesia
Methocarbamol	15–20 mg/kg	IV, PO		Muscle relaxant	Renal insufficiency
Magnesium	loading dose 0.05 mg/kg/hr, followed by maintenance dose of 0.025 mg/kg/hr	IV		Muscle relaxant	Hypermagnesemia can cause sweating, muscle weakness, recumbency, agitation, tachycardia, tachypnea, cardiovascular shock. Suggested target serum magnesium in people with tetanus is 2 to 4 mmol/l. [42]
Dantrolene	2–4 mg/kg	IV, PO, per rectum		Muscle relaxant	Hepatic toxicity

sedatives such as the α2 agonists xylazine, detomidine, romifidine, or medetomidine, alone or in combination with diazepam, can also provide muscle relaxation [2, 46]. The benzodiazepine midazolam has also been administered as a bolus or CRI for the treatment of seizures and provision of muscle relaxation [18, 20, 49]. In one report, tetany in a 2-week-old foal could not be completely controlled with diazepam (doses of 0.1 mg/kg every 30 minutes); therefore two doses of phenobarbital (5 mg/kg, IV × 2 [10mg/kg total]) were administered IV followed by continued oral dosing (10 mg/kg q 8 hr), which provided adequate relaxation [17]. Guaifenesin, methocarbamol, and chloral hydrate have also been attempted to control tetanic muscle spasms in foals [17, 18, 46, 50]. The use of IV magnesium to treat foals with tetanus has not been reported, but has been suggested for foals with neonatal encephalopathy [51]. A suggested target serum magnesium in people with tetanus is 2–4 mmol/l [42]. Muscle relaxation will provide some analgesia, but further analgesia may be necessary. Nonsteroidal anti-inflammatory medications such as meloxicam and flunixin meglumine can be used judiciously as an analgesic whereas opioids should be avoided as this class of drug can cause respiratory depression [5, 16–18].

Treatment of Autonomic Hyperactivity

Specific treatments to control autonomic hyperactivity have not been reported in equids, but epidural blockade with bupivacaine or sufentanil [52], intravenous α2-adrenoreceptor agonists clonidine [53] and dexmedetomidine [54], CRI of atropine [55], β-blockers such as labetolol [56] and esmolol [57], and morphine [58] have been used successfully in people with tetanus [42].

Supportive Care

A quiet, dim area is needed to reduce unnecessary stimuli that can exacerbate clinical signs. Auditory stimuli can be blocked by placing cotton or wool in the ears, although close observation should be made to ensure that the foal does not become distressed or irritated from foreign material in the ear. Intranasal oxygen can be administered if the foal has respiratory compromise or evidence of hypoxemia as reflected on arterial blood gas analysis. Mechanical ventilation following central muscle relaxation has improved outcome in people but has not been described in foals with tetanus [59, 60]. However, mechanical ventilation is an option if hypoxemia and hypercapnia become severe [61]. Nutrition and hydration can be facilitated by nasogastric tube feeding, if the foal is incapable of suckling, along with maintenance IV fluid therapy. If the foal is recumbent, provision of a thick mattress, fleece blankets and maintenance of a clean, dry environment will help prevent decubital skin ulcers. Urinary catheterization and the use of a closed urinary collection system may facilitate a clean and dry environment for the recumbent foal, and bandaging the distal limbs, head protection, and corneal lubrication help prevent self-induced injury. Foals should be placed in pain-free positions to avoid exacerbating discomfort of the disease process. Prolonged hospitalization may be necessary in foals with tetanus. For example, a 4-week-old Shetland foal demonstrated reduced signs of tetanus on day 6 of hospitalization while a 2-week-old draft foal required 3 weeks of hospitalization before being able to maintain a standing position, requiring assistance to rise [16, 17]. Because of the prolonged recumbency and slow recovery, physiotherapy, such as passive and active range of motion exercises, along with stretching and weight-bearing protocols can be used in foals to promote recovery (after the initial phases of disease) [17]. As the tetanic muscle spasms abate over days to weeks, the foal can be assisted to a weight-bearing position and encouraged to stand and/or walk; this activity may be facilitated by a large animal sling or walking frame (Figure 32.III.2). However, it is not recommended to use a sling if the foal does not put forth effort to voluntarily stand. This will result in the foal hanging in the sling, which consequently compromises breathing and increases discomfort and potential spasms. Attention to the mare is also needed with regular (every 2–4 hour) milking of the udder and provision of sedation if necessary to maintain a calm environment.

Outcome

Overall survival rates in horses of various ages has ranged between 24% and 75% [2, 18, 22, 23, 45, 46]. Throughout the literature, several reports of foals with tetanus are available (Table 32.III.5). Overall, foals with tetanus up to 1 year of age had a survival rate of 31%, but this may overestimate the success rate as most as these foals were admitted to a referral hospital for intensive care [2, 4, 16, 17, 20, 22, 23, 45, 46]. A poor outcome was reported in foals with tetanus younger than 2 months of age [20].

Prognostic factors have been identified in horses and foals with tetanus. Only one study compared surviving (n = 7) and nonsurviving foals (n = 10) and identified standing, voluntary eating soft food and drinking on admission to be associated to survival. Survivors also had a significantly older age and longer hospitalization delay compared to nonsurviving foals [20]. In another report, all five foals with an umbilical infection died and having an umbilical infection was therefore suggested to be a negative prognostic indicator. However, all of these foals were

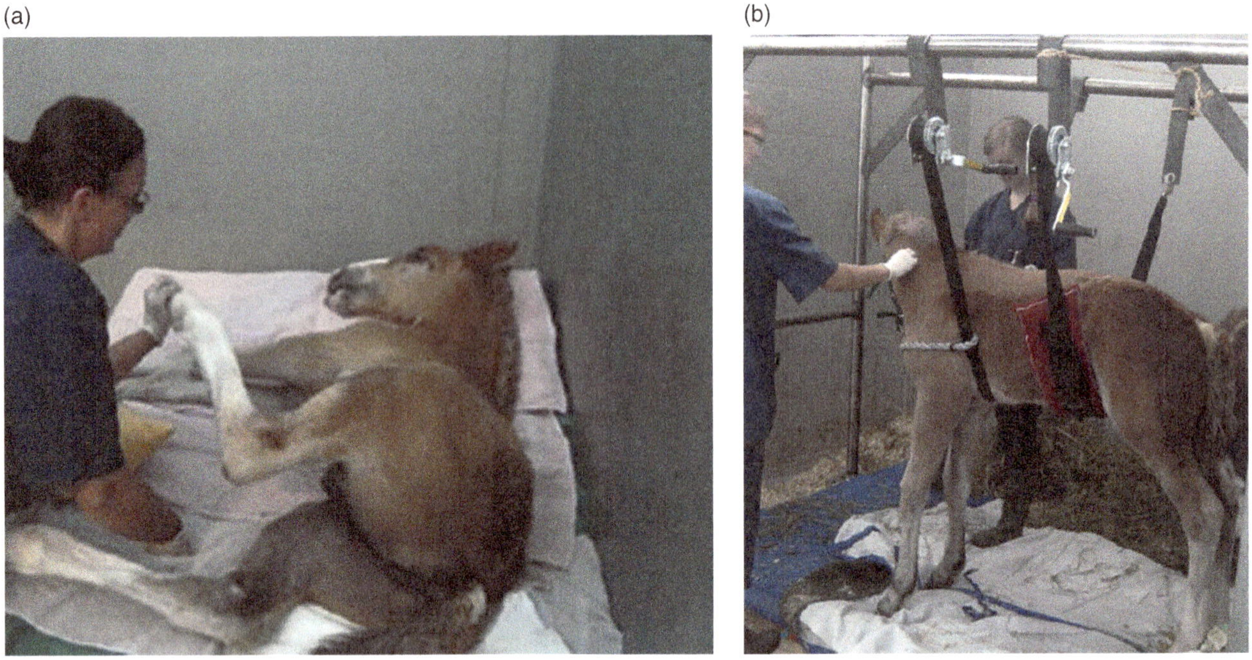

Figure 32.III.2 (a) Administration of physiotherapy in a foal recovering from tetanus; and (b) undergoing assisted standing exercise using a walking frame and sling [17].

Table 32.III.5 Summary of survival rate in reported cases of tetanus in foals

Reference	Country	Total number of horses	Number of foals	Age of foals	Survival (Foals)	Survival rate (%)
5	Brazil	70	5	< 1 month	0/5	0
			7	< 12 months	1/7	14
19	Europe	176	21	< 6 months	7/21	33.3
	Europe	176	17	< 2 months	3/17	17.6
19	Europe	176	47	< 12 months	16/47	34
17	Finland	1	1	2 weeks	1/1	100
22	Belgium	31	1	3.5 months	0/1	0
45	Brazil	76	4	< 12 months	0/4	0
2	Morocco	56	5	< 12 months	3/4	75
4	Israel	3	1	3 weeks	1/1	100
46	United States	20	4	< 12 months	0/4	4
23	Belgium	108	6	not indicated	0/6	0
16	Finland	1	1	4 weeks	1/1	100
Total				**< 12 months**	**23/75**	**31**
				<2 months	**6/24**	**25**

also <1 month of age, so age could have been a confounding factor [62]. Unless mechanical ventilation is a possibility, a worsening hypoxemia and increasing hypercapnia has previously been considered a poor prognostic indicator in foals or adult horses with compromised respiration of neuromuscular origin and can therefore be suggested as a poor prognostic indicator in foals with respiratory failure due to tetanus [63–65].

Poor prognostic indicators in adult horses with tetanus include: younger age [22], nonvaccination [46], rapid progression or short time of onset of disease/diagnosis [20, 45, 46], perforating lesions of the hoof sole [45], facial wounds [62], severe clinical signs [2, 20], recumbency [22, 45, 46, 55], sweating [62], dysphagia/aphagia/anorexia [20, 45, 55], tachycardia [2, 20], tachypnea [20], dyspnea [20, 22], the combination of recumbency, dysphagia and dyspnea [22], and seizures [22]. Many of these prognostic factors directly or indirectly relate to the severity of muscle spasms, or to the ability to eat and drink, highlighting the importance of a normally functioning gastrointestinal tract in horses with tetanus [22].

Postmortem findings in horses with tetanus are nonspecific and include pulmonary edema, atelectasis, pulmonary congestion, and bronchiolitis, likely related to increased respiratory effort and aspiration pneumonia [20, 46]. Traumatic lesions may be identified due to violent spasms or seizures [18].

Vaccination

Tetanus can be prevented by appropriate vaccination of the pregnant mare with tetanus toxoid within the last trimester of pregnancy and appropriate umbilical care in the neonatal foal (disinfective umbilical dips). If the mare is unvaccinated, TAT should be administered to the newborn foal or as soon as possible after a wound or umbilical infection is identified. Although rare, tetanus has been reported in horses that have been vaccinated with tetanus toxoid within 1 year of disease presentation [20, 46]. Additionally, clinical cases of neonatal tetanus have been reported in foals that were administered TAT at birth [18, 20]. Tetanus infection does not confer immunity; thus, patients should be vaccinated as part of the treatment [3, 9]. Of note, TAT has been associated with acute hepatic necrosis in horses [66].

Foals from vaccinated mares should receive tetanus toxoid three times at 4-week intervals at 4–6 months of age with a second dose 4–6 weeks later and the third dose at 11–12 months. Foals from nonvaccinated mares should be vaccinated three times at intervals beginning at 1–4 months of age [11]. The use of TAT given to healthy foals at birth is unnecessary in foals that receive adequate colostrum from a properly vaccinated mare. Doses of 1500–6000 iu of TAT have been given to foals born from unvaccinated mares [11, 50].

References

1 Ebisawa, I., Takayanagi, M., Kurata, M. et al. (1986). Density and distribution of Clostridium tetani in the soil. *Jpn J Exp Med* 56: 69–72.

2 Kay, G. and Knottenbelt, D.C. (2007). Tetanus in equids: A report of 56 cases. *Equine Vet Educ* 19: 107–112.

3 Yen, L.M. and Thwaites, C.L. (2019). Tetanus. *Lancet* 393: 1657–1668.

4 Steinman, A., Haik, R., Elad, D. et al. (2000). Intrathecal administration of tetanus antitoxin to three cases of tetanus in horses. *Equine Vet Educ* 12: 237–240.

5 Ansari, M.M. and Matros, L.E. (1982). Tetanus. *Compend Contin Educ Pract Vet* 4: S473–S479.

6 Cullinane, A.A., Bernard, W., Duncan, J.L. et al. (1999). Infectious diseases. In: *The Equine Manual* (ed. A.J. Higgins and I.M. Wright), 65–70. London: W.B. Saunders, 979–980.

7 Blumenthal, R. and Habig, W.H. (1984). Mechanism of tetanolysin-induced membrane damage: studies with black lipid membranes. *J Bacteriol* 157: 321–323.

8 Hilz, M.J., Liu, M., Sankanika, R. et al. (2019). Autonomic dysfunction in the neurological intensive care unit. *Clin Auton Res* 29: 301–311.

9 Hassel, B. (2013). Tetanus: Pathophysiology, treatment, and the possibility of using botulinum toxin against tetanus-induced rigidity and spasms. *Toxins* 5: 73–83.

10 Surana, S., Tosolini, A.P., Meyer, I.F.G. et al. (2018). The travel diaries of tetanus and botulinum neurotoxins. *Toxicon* 147: 58–67.

11 MacKay, R. (2014). Tetanus. In: *Equine Infectious Diseases*, 2e (ed. D. Sellon and M. Long), 368–372. St. Louis, MO: Saunders.

12 Gonzalez-Forero, D., Morcuende, S., Alvarez, F.J. et al. (2005). Transynaptic effects of tetanus neurotoxin in the oculomotor system. *Brain* 128: 2175–2188.

13 Schwab, M.E. and Thoenen, H. (1976). Electron microscopic evidence for a transsynaptic migration of tetanus toxin in spinal cord motoneurons: an autoradiographic and morphometric study. *Brain Res* 105: 213–227.

14 Schiavo, G., Matteoli, M., and Montecucco, C. (2000). Neurotoxins affecting neuroexocytosis. *Physiol Rev* 80: 717–766.

15 Shin, M.C., Nonaka, K., Wakita, M. et al. (2012). Effects of tetanus toxin on spontaneous and evoked transmitter release at inhibitory and excitatory synapses in the rat SDCN neurons. *Toxicon* 59: 385–339.

16 Finocchio, E.J. and Clement, J. (1974). Tetanus in a 4-week-old Shetland pony. *Vet Med Small Anim Clin* 69: 153–154.

17 Mykkanen, A.K., Hyytiainen, H.K., and McGowan, C.M. (2011). Generalized tetanus in a 2-week-old foal: use of physiotherapy to aid recovery. *Aust Vet J* 89: 447–451.

18 van Galen, G., Saegerman, C., Rijckaert, J. et al. (2017). Retrospective evaluation of 155 adult equids and 21 foals

with tetanus in Western, Northern, and Central Europe (2000–2014). Part 1: Description of history and clinical evolution. *J Vet Emerg Crit Care* 27: 684–696.

19 Goonetilleke, A. and Harris, J.B. (2004). Clostridial neurotoxins. *J Neurol Neurosurg Psychiatry* 75(Suppl III): iii45–iii39.

20 van Galen, G., Rijckaert, J., Mair, T. et al. (2017). Retrospective evaluation of 155 adult equids and 21 foals with tetanus from Western, Northern, and Central Europe (2000–2014). Part 2: Prognostic assessment. *J Vet Emerg Crit Care* 27: 697–706.

21 Berzo, G.A. (1980). Tetanus in a horse. *J Am Vet Med Assoc* 177: 1152–1154.

22 van Galen, G., Delguste, C., Sandersen, C. et al. (2008). Tetanus in the equine species: a retrospective study of 31 cases. *Tijdschr Diergeneeskd* 133: 512–517.

23 Muylle, E., Oyaert, W., Ooms, L. et al. (1975). Treatment of tetanus in the horse by injections of tetanus antitoxin into the subarachnoid space. *J Am Vet Med Assoc* 167: 47–48.

24 Attygalle, D. and Rodrigo, N. (2004). New trends in the management of tetanus. *Expert Rev Anti Infect Ther* 2: 73–84.

25 Bandt, C., Rozanski, E.A., Steinberg, T. et al. (2007). Retrospective study of tetanus in 20 dogs: 1988–2004. *J Am Anim Hosp Assoc* 43: 143–148.

26 Burkitt, J.M., Sturges, B.K., Jandrey, K.E. et al. (2007). Risk factors associated with outcome in dogs with tetanus: 38 cases (1987–2005). *J Am Vet Med Assoc* 230: 76–83.

27 Freshwater-Turner, D., Udy, A., Lipman, J. et al. (2007). Autonomic dysfunction in tetanus-what lessons can be learnt with specific reference to α-2 agonists? *Anaesthesia* 62: 1066–1070.

28 Kerr, J.H., Corbett, J.L., Prys-Roberts, C. et al. (1968). Involvement of the sympathetic nervous system in tetanus. Studies on 82 cases. *Lancet* 2: 236–241.

29 Burgess, J.A., Wambaugh, G.W., and Koczarski, M.J. (1992). Report of case: Reviewing cephalic tetanus. *J Am Dent Assoc* 123: 67–70.

30 Akbulut, D., Grant, K.A., and McLauchlin, J. (2005). Improvement in laboratory diagnosis of wound botulism and tetanus among injecting illicit-drug users by use of real-time PCR assays for neurotoxin gene fragments. *J Clin Microbiol* 43: 4342–4348.

31 Campbell, J.I., Lam, T.M., Huynh, T.L. et al. (2009). Microbiologic characterization and antimicrobial susceptibility of Clostridium tetani isolated from wounds of patients with clinically diagnosed tetanus. *Am J Trop Med Hyg* 80: 827–831.

32 Onuki, T., Nihonyanagi, S., Nakamura, M. et al. (2013). Clostridium tetani isolated from patients with systemic tetanus. *Kansenshogaku Zasshi* 87: 33–38.

33 Levy, P., Fournier, P.E., Lotte, L. et al. (2014). Clostridium tetani osteitis without tetanus. *Emerg Infect Dis* 20: 1571–1573.

34 Public Health England (2018). Tetanus: guidance for health professionals. https://www.gov.uk/government/publications/tetanus-advice-for-health-professionals (accessed 23 March 2023).

35 Lai, C.C., Chen, C.C., Hsu, H.J. et al. (2018). Clostridium tetani bacteremia in a patient with cirrhosis following transarterial chemoembolization treatment for hepatocellular carcinoma. *J Microbiol Immunol Infect* 51: 155–156.

36 Hallit, R.R., Afridi, M., Sison, R. et al. (2013). Clostridium tetani bacteraemia. *J Med Microbiol* 62 (Pt 1): 155–156.

37 Auger, R.G. (1994). AAEM mini-monograph #44: diseases associated with excess motor unit activity. *Muscle Nerve* 17: 1250–1263.

38 Risk, W.S., Bosch, E.P., Kimura, J. et al. (1981). Chronic tetanus: clinical report and histochemistry of muscle. *Muscle Nerve* 4: 363–366.

39 Struppler, A., Struppler, E., and Adams, R.D. (1963). Local tetanus in man. Its clinical and neurophysiological characteristics. *Arch Neurol* 8: 162–178.

40 Simonen, T. and Jarvimaa, T.A. (2001). Foals recovery from tetanus. *Finnish Vet J* 12: 696–700.

41 Hanif, H., Anjum, A., Ali, N. et al. (2015). Isolation and antibiogram of Clostridium tetani from clinically diagnosed tetanus patients. *Am J Trop Med Hyg* 93: 752–756.

42 Rodrigo, C., Fernado, D., and Rajapakse, S. (2014). Pharmacological management of tetanus: an evidence-based review. *Critical Care* 18: 217.

43 Ganesh Kumar, A.V., Kothari, V.M., Krishnan, A. et al. (2004). Benzathine penicillin, metronidazole and benzyl penicillin in the treatment of tetanus: A randomized, controlled trial. *Ann Trop Med Parasitol* 98: 59–63.

44 Thwaites, C.L., Beeching, N.J., and Newton, C.R. (2015). Maternal and neonatal tetanus. *Lancet* 385: 362–370.

45 Reichmann, P., Lisboa, J.A.N., and Araujo, R.G. (2008). Tetanus in equids: A review of 76 cases. *J Eq Vet Sci* 28: 518–523.

46 Green, S.L., Little, C.B., Baird, J.D. et al. (1970–1990). Tetanus in the horse: A review of 20 cases. *J Vet Intern Med* 8: 128–132.

47 White, S.S. and Christie, M.P. (1985). Acupuncture used as an adjunct in the treatment of a horse with tetanus. *Aust Vet J* 62: 25–26.

48 Pequito, M., Amory, H., de Moffarts, B. et al. (2013). Evaluation of acepromazine-induced hemodynamic alterations and reversal with norepinephrine infusion in standing horses. *Can Vet J* 54: 150–156.

49 Wilkins, P.A. (2005). How to use midazolam to control equine neonatal seizures. In: *AAEP Annual Convention*. Seattle: American Association of Equine Practitioners

https://www.ivis.org/library/aaep/aaep-annual-convention-seattle-2005/how-to-use-midazolam-to-control-equine-neonatal-seizures.
50 Knottenbelt, D.C. (2004). Chapter 6: Neonatal Conditions. In: *Equine Neonatalogy Medicine and Surgery* (ed. D.C. Knottenbelt, N. Holdstock, and J. Madigan), 155–364. Edinburgh: Saunders.
51 Wilkins, P.A. (2004). Disorders in Foals. In: *Equine Internal Medicine*, 2e (ed. S.M. Reed, W.M. Bayly, and D.C. Sellon), 1381–1431. St. Louis Missouri: Saunders.
52 Bhagwanjee, S., Basenberg, A.T., and Muckart, D.J. (1999). Management of sympathetic overactivity in tetanus with epidural bupivacaine and sufentanil: Experience with 11 patients. *Crit Care Med* 27L: 1721–1725.
53 Gregorakos, L., Kerezoudi, E., Dimopoulos, G. et al. (1997). Management of blood pressure instability in severe tetanus: the use of clonidine. *Inten Care Med* 23: 893–895.
54 Girgin, N.K., Iscimen, R., Gurbet, A. et al. (2007). Dexmedetomidine sedation for the treatment of tetanus in the intensive care unit. *Brit J Anaesth* 99: 599–600.
55 Dolar, D. (1992). The use of continuous atropine infusion in the management of severe tetanus. *Inten Care Med* 18: 26–31.
56 Dundee, J.W. and Morrow, W.F. (1979). Labetalol in severe tetanus. *Br Med J* 1: 1121–1122.
57 Beards, S.C., Lipman, J., Bothma, P.A. et al. (1994). Esmolol in a case of severe tetanus. Adequate haemodynamic control achieved despite markedly elevated catecholamine levels. *S Afr J Surg* 32 (33–35): 57.
58 Rocke, D.A., Wesley, A.G., Pather, M. et al. (1986). Morphine in tetanus – the management of sympathetic nervous system overactivity. *S Afr Med J* 70: 666–668.
59 Trujillo, M.H., Castillo, A., Espana, J. et al. (1987). Impact of intensive care management on the prognosis of tetanus. Analysis of 641 cases. *Chest* 92: 63–65.
60 Edmondson, R.S. and Flowers, M.S. (1970). Intensive care in tetanus: management, complications, and mortality in 100 cases. *Br Med J* 1: 1401–1404.
61 Palmer, J.E. (2005). Ventilatory support of the critically ill foal. *Vet Clin North Am Equine Pract* 21: 457–486.
62 Ribeiro, M.G., de Nardi, G., Megid, J. et al. (2018). Tetanus in horses: an overview of 70 cases. *Pesquisa Veterinaria Brasileira* 38: 285–293.
63 van Galen, G., Cerri, S., Porter, S. et al. (2013). Traditional and quantitative assessment of acid-base and shock variables in horses with atypical myopathy. *J Vet Intern Med* 27: 186–193.
64 Votion, D.M., Linden, A., Saegerman, C. et al. (2007). History and clinical features of atypical myopathy in horses in Belgium (2000–2005). *J Vet Intern Med* 21: 1380–1391.
65 Wilkins, P.A. and Palmer, J.E. (2003). Mechanical ventilation in foals with botulism: 9 cases (1989–2002). *J Vet Intern Med* 17: 708–712.
66 Tomlinson, J.E., Van de Walle, G.R., and Divers, T.J. (2019). What do we know about hepatitis viruses in horses? *Vet Clin Equine* 35: 351–362.

Section IV Toxicities – Neurotoxicities

Gaby van Galen

Published reports of toxicities targeting the nervous system are uncommon in foals. Yet, horses can be more sensitive to many toxins than other species (e.g. tetanus, ionophores) or uniquely affected by some (e.g. fumonisin mycotoxins) [1]. Neurotoxicity is more common than believed since almost every compound can become toxic if the dose is large enough [1]. In one review, over 200 industrial compounds were listed as known neurotoxins and linked to neurodevelopmental disorders in people and studies have incriminated over 1000 substances [2]. These lists represent a small fraction of all neurotoxic substances [3]. Most compounds are toxic across species as demonstrated by laboratory animal testing [3], therefore also likely to affect foals.

The Blood-Brain Barrier (BBB)

To understand how neurotoxicity can develop, knowledge of the protective barriers for the foal's brain is critical. There are two barriers that separate the central nervous system (CNS) from the systemic circulation: the blood-brain barrier (BBB) and blood-cerebrospinal barrier (Figure 32.IV.1). These are independent membrane barriers with separate functions (Table 32.IV.1) [3–8]. The literature often cites these barriers as the "BBB" without distinguishing between the two. A third barrier between blood and the brain parenchyma and the cerebrospinal fluid (CSF) is formed by the three layers of the meninges: the dura, arachnoid, and pia mater (arachnoid barrier) [4]. Due to these barriers, and because of compartmentalization, brain tissue and CSF concentrations of a drug or toxin may not be the same [9]. For ease, no distinction will be made between the barriers in the remainder of this chapter.

The BBB has the following barrier mechanisms:

1) *Tight junctions.* Restricting entry of water-soluble compounds into the CNS.
2) *Influx transport systems.* Responsible for passage of mainly water-soluble molecules such as glucose, amino acids, water, and ions into the CNS.
3) *Detoxifying and efflux transport systems.* Restricting entry of lipid soluble compounds into the CNS [3]. P-glycoprotein is a BBB efflux transporter that is central to neurotoxicity and linked with protection against toxicity from a number of drugs (e.g. ivermectin, digoxin, dexamethasone) [3]. Although P-glycoprotein is detectable very early in the fetus and shows efflux activity mid-gestation [10], it is incompletely expressed in the neonate [11]. Another BBB efflux transporter that limits entry of drugs into the CNS is Breast Cancer Related Protein (BCRP) [3]. BCRP is detectable early in development and remains the same throughout development [12]. Little information is available regarding these proteins in foals.

The ability of a compound to cross the BBB depends on its lipid solubility, molecular weight, and electrical charge (ionization) [9]. Many drugs are lipid soluble and easily penetrate, unless they are substrates of efflux proteins. The BBB excludes approximately 95% of drugs from entering the brain from the blood [13]. The historical belief amongst neurotoxicologists that the BBB in embryos and neonates is immature, leaky, or even absent has been argued to be incorrect as there is substantial evidence supporting a well-developed and functionally effective barrier [3, 14]. Most aspects of the adult BBB already exist and are functional in the fetus, including influx and efflux mechanisms and tight junctions. Some barrier mechanisms work to a lesser

Equine Neonatal Medicine, First Edition. Edited by David M. Wong and Pamela A. Wilkins.

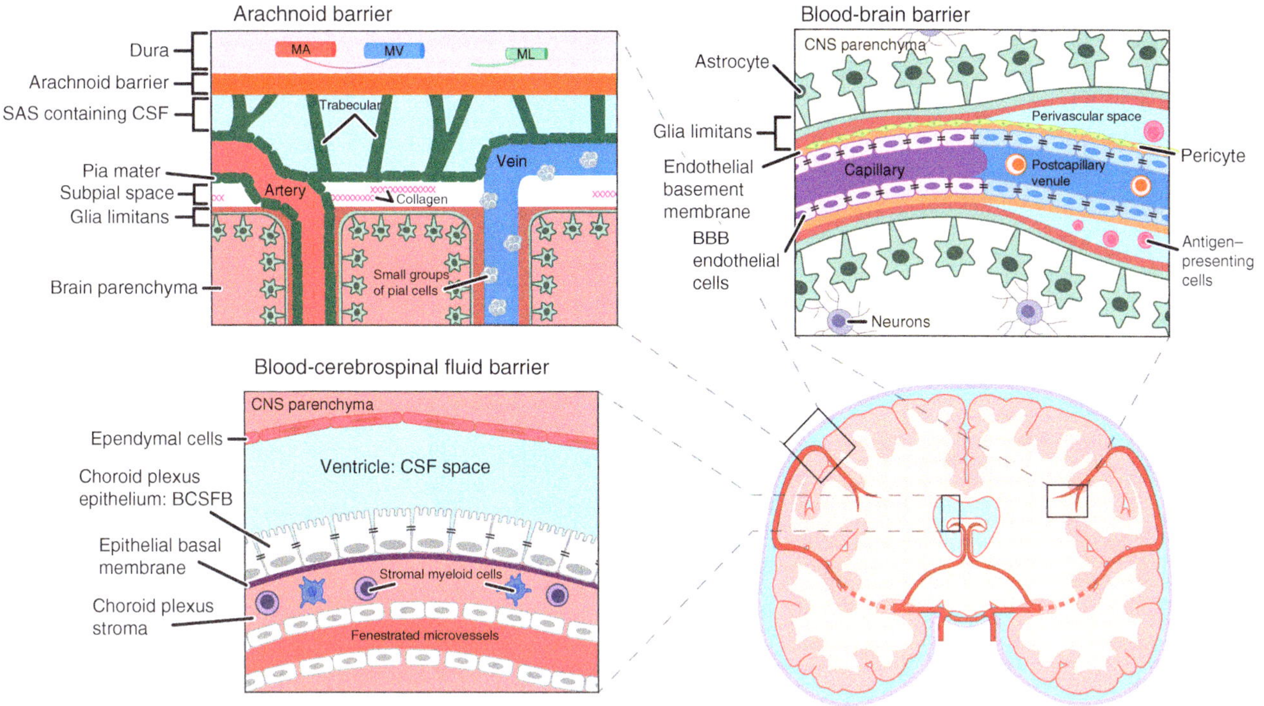

Figure 32.IV.1 Barriers of the CNS. The three main barriers of the CNS include the arachnoid barrier (upper left), the blood-brain barrier (upper right), and the blood-cerbrospinal-fluid barrier (lower left), all of which are identified in a schematic coronal brain section (lower right). Of the three barriers, the BBB maintains the closest proximity to the brain parenchyma [4]. BBB, blood-brain barrier; BCSFB-blood-cerbrospinal fluid barrier; CNS, central nervous system; CSF, cerbrospinal fluid; MA, meningeal artery; ML, meningeal lymphatics; MV, meningeal vein; SAS, subarachnoid space.

Table 32.IV.1 Characteristics of the barriers that separate the central nervous system from the general circulation.

	Blood-brain barrier	Blood cerbrospinal barrier
Function	Separates brain interstitial fluid from general circulation	Separates cerebrospinal fluid from the general circulation
Composition	Capillary endothelium, basal laminae, pericytes, astroglia, perivascular macrophages	Capillary endothelium, loose connective tissue, basal lamina, ependymal cells
Area	Large surface area; certain small areas do not have a BBB (hypothalamus, area presterma, subcommissural regions)	Much smaller area; choroid plexus and other small areas in the ventricles
Composition fluid determined by	Active tranport	Secretory processes

degree in developing animals, but others have a higher rate of function and some systems only exist in the fetus. However, *in utero* some toxins and drugs use these barrier mechanisms to enter the CNS and render the developing brain more vulnerable than the adult brain. For example, influx amino acid transporters are upregulated in the developing brain because of growth requirements and have the ability to co-transport various compounds and are relevant for neurotoxicity, especially in the developing brain [3]. Thus, barrier mechanisms and transport systems are related to stage of brain development and growth, in contrast to an adult brain that is optimized for maintenance [3, 14]. The concern about involvement of the BBB in the vulnerability of the brain to toxins and drugs in neonates is justified. Yet, its vulnerability is due to differences in essential physiological mechanisms, and not related to an absence of barrier mechanisms [3].

The Blood-Placental Barrier (BPB)

Toxin exposure can occur *in utero*. The placenta provides the fetus with oxygen and nutrients and removes waste products but also protects the fetus from harmful compounds in maternal blood, such as drugs and toxins [3]. Transplacental transport includes passive diffusion, pinocytosis and facilitated and active transport via transporters [15]. Similar to the BBB, P-glycoprotein and BCRP are major contributors to placental detoxification [3, 15]. In contrast to progressively increasing P-glycoprotein levels in the BBB, placental P-glycoprotein is higher early in gestation in human fetuses [15], representing an interplay between the two barriers to optimize fetal brain protection [3]. Also phase I and phase II metabolism occur in the placenta, suggested to remove toxins and metabolites from maternal blood [3]. Care is needed when extrapolating human placental drug passage studies, as horses have a diffuse epitheliochorial placentation with more tissue layers and higher levels of separation between fetal and maternal blood [16]. Consequently, a drug's ability to diffuse into fetal blood is likely more restricted, and active transfer of substances may be slower. Despite enhanced separation between fetal and maternal blood, the overall possibility to allow passage of substances is suggested not to be influenced [16].

Risk of Exposure

Risk of toxicities and response to toxins is different in neonatal foals compared to adult horses. Multiple factors create these differences such as toxin exposure, neonatal pharmacokinetics, toxin access to the CNS, and CNS susceptibility. Dependent on the toxin involved, these factors place neonatal foals at a higher or lower risk.

Exposure

Foals are less likely to ingest solid food in the neonatal period making neurotoxicities caused by toxic plants or contaminated foods uncommon. However, as the foal grows older, consumption of solid food and exposure risk soon match adult horses. Despite the fact that voluntary ingestion is lower in neonatal foals, they have greater exposure to drugs or toxins through the placenta, colostrum, and milk. Age-specific conditions, such as parasitic and bacterial infections, increase exposure to potential toxicities through iatrogenic drug administration. Incorrect dosing can also occur as owners and veterinarians are accustomed to adult volumes.

Pharmacokinetics

The safety margin of a drug is based on differences between the therapeutic and toxic dose. The toxic dose varies between drugs; many drugs are considered safe in adult horses with the toxic dose reached at 10-fold or more. Yet, an overdose of less than 10-fold can induce signs of neurotoxicity in foals because they are physiologically different than adults, which affects the pharmacokinetics of a drug or toxin. Foals absorb compounds more rapidly from the gastrointestinal tract (GI), have less plasma protein binding (increases active free plasma form of drug or toxin), have a larger volume of distribution, and have slower clearance compared to adult horses [17, 18]. These factors render them more susceptible to overdoses or toxicities. Their urine is acidic, which can increase renal clearance of weak bases [18] and decrease risk for toxicity compared to adult horses. Other pharmacokinetic differences in neonatal foals can be found in Chapter 60.

Loss of Integrity of Barriers

The BPB and BBB play vital roles in protecting the fetal and neonatal CNS but the integrity and functionality of these barriers can be affected by pathological conditions, causing drugs or toxins to cross the barrier where they would normally not. Examples include traumatic brain injury, cerebral hypoxia-ischemia, seizures, meningitis, and other inflammatory insults that affect BBB integrity in people [19–21], and systemic conditions such as sepsis and endotoxemia cause morphological and functional modifications and increased vulnerability of the BBB [22, 23]. Many ill foals suffer from hypoxic, septic, or inflammatory processes, systemically or locally in the CNS, and potentially have altered BBB integrity. The BPB can also loose integrity with chorioamnionitis and endotoxemia [15]. Thus, it is possible that fetuses of mares with placentitis or endotoxemia are at higher risk for toxicities following drug administration to the pregnant mare. The toxin itself may directly damage the barriers or barrier mechanisms [3]. For example, psychostimulants such as methamphetamine, cocaine, and nicotine produce BBB dysfunction and increased permeability [21, 24].

The BBB integrity can be assessed by the CSF total protein concentrations, albumin quotient ($Q_{Albumin} = albumin_{csf}/albumin_{serum} \times 100$), immunoglobin G index (IgG Index $= [IgG_{CSF}/IgG_{serum}]/[Alb_{CSF}/Alb_{serum}]$) and comparison of the electrophoretogram between serum and CSF [8, 25]. In pediatric medicine, physiologically based pharmacokinetic models are used to predict CSF drug concentrations following meningitis and sepsis, and guide therapeutic dosing [19] but are currently unavailable in equine medicine.

Susceptibility of the Developing Nervous System

Over all species, little is known about how much of a drug or toxin reaches the CNS or how it affects development [3]. Most likely, the developing brain is more susceptible and vulnerable than the adult brain, and effects of drugs on fetal development are dependent on gestational age [26].

Developing neurons undergo a maturation process during which neurons migrate and form complex neural networks. Disturbance of this maturation process can cause long-term effects on brain function [3, 23].

Mechanisms of Neurotoxicity: Toxidromes

Clinical signs are rarely pathognomic for a particular neurotoxin and merely indicate the involved mechanism – usually in an inhibitory or excitatory manner. These clusters of clinical signs are called **toxidromes.** Neurotoxins can act through one clearly identified mechanism or multiple mechanisms. Table 32.IV.2 summarizes the most common mechanisms.

Adverse Drug Reactions

Many neurotoxicities are iatrogenic in origin and develop following administration of medical drugs, either due to overdose or as adverse drug reactions.

Definitions and Terminology

An adverse drug reaction is "An appreciably harmful or unpleasant reaction, resulting from an intervention related to the use of a medicinal product, which predicts hazard from future administration and warrants prevention or specific treatment, or alteration of the dosage regimen, or withdrawal of the product" [27]. Adverse drug reactions are categorized into pharmacological and intrinsic toxicities. Both are dose-dependent and somewhat predictable. Pharmacological toxicities are exaggerated, and harmful effects associated with the pharmacological activity of a drug. Intrinsic toxicities are related to the drugs chemical property. A third category, idiosyncratic toxicities, are often unpredictable, difficult to reproduce and frequently described as drug hypersensitivity reactions [28].

Adverse Drug Reaction Database and Literature Searches

If suspicious of a neurotoxic adverse drug effect, a literature search can expose information to strengthen or weaken the suspicion, and should be extended to include small animal, livestock, and human literature. Searches can reveal previously described adverse drug reactions or a link between the mechanism of the particular drug and observed clinical signs. If the drug has anticholinergic properties and the patient has signs of increased anticholinergic activity, this reinforces the suspicion of a causal relation. The drug manufacturer should be contacted to discuss observed signs and if other concerns have been reported around toxicity of a specific product. Where previously described, adverse drug reactions or links between drug mechanism and clinical signs will strengthen your suspicion, but a lack of these does not negate a causal relationship. It is important to report adverse effects to national reporting centers.

Adverse Drug Reaction Probability Algorithms

In people, algorithms exist to determine the likelihood that a clinical reaction could be an adverse drug reaction. Examples are the Jones, the Naranjo (Table 32.IV.3), the Yale, the Karch, the Begaud, the ADRAC, and the WHO-UMC algorithms. These algorithms have better reproducibility than clinical judgment in rating adverse drug reactions and are useful in assessing causality. The algorithms depend on yes/no questions and can therefore lack specificity. Considering that there is no gold standard to test these algorithms, they cannot prove (or disprove) causality [30]. These scores are regularly used in literature to support and validate the conclusion on adverse drug reactions [28, 30].

Adverse Drug Reactions and Cytochrome P450

Cytochrome P450 (CYP) is a key enzyme in drug detoxification reactions widespread throughout the body. Drugs have no CYP activity, but are CYP inhibitors, or CYP inducers. Induction or inhibition of CYP is a main mechanism that underlies drug–drug interactions [31]. Drugs that inhibit an enzymatic pathway of CYP may cause increased concentrations of other drugs metabolized by the same pathway, resulting in drug toxicity or adverse drug reactions [32].

Neurotoxins

For this chapter, neurotoxicity is only considered when a toxin directly targets the nervous system. There are toxins that induce neurological signs as a consequence of targeting other organ systems (e.g. hepato-encephalopathy, electrolyte disturbances, severe cardiovascular impairment) but are not reviewed as neurotoxic in this chapter, but rather as differential diagnosis. Toxins that only cause neurotoxicity in adult horses through voluntary ingestion of contaminated food will not be listed, unless specifically reported to occur in foals.

Toxins that trigger neurological signs in foals include but are not limited to:

1) Most common neurotoxicities in equids that affect all ages
2) Neurotoxins that have been described specifically in foals
3) Toxicities supported by anecdotal reports in foals that are well supported by human literature

Table 32.IV.2 Common mechanisms through which neurotoxins can affect the neurologic system [1, 33–36].

Mechanism	Clinical signs	Toxins	Antidote/treatment	Drugs that enhance toxicity
Muscarinic Cholinergic Stimulation	▪ Profuse salivation ▪ Severe GI disturbances due to hypermotility, severe pain, abdominal cramps, increased defecation, diarrhea ▪ Excessive lacrimation ▪ Miosis ▪ Sweating ▪ Respiratory signs including cough, nasal discharge, dyspnea, cyanosis due to excessive respiratory tract secretions, bronchoconstriction ▪ Increased urination ▪ Bradycardia	▪ Cyanobacteria ▪ Cholinesterase-inhibiting carbamate insecticies ▪ Organophosphates	▪ Atropine sulfate 0.1–0.5 mg/kg ▪ Administer ¼ dose IV and remainder of dose IM or SC until control of autonomic signs; monitor for GI stasis ▪ Glycopyrrolate can also be used (has slower onset of action but longer duration than atropine)	▪ Drugs that target acetylcholinesterases: succinylcholine, phenothiazine, procaine, aminoglycosides
Nicotinic Cholinergic Stimulation	▪ Excessive stimulation of skeletal muscles: Muscle fasciculations, tremors, twitching, spasms, stiff/rigid gait, weakness, paresis/paralysis	▪ Cholinesterase-inhibiting carbamate	▪ Neuromuscular relaxants or blockers	▪ Inhalant anesthetics, magnesium, depolarizing and nondepolarizing neuro muscular blocking agents
Dopaminergic stimulation	▪ Decrease of prolactin in anterior pituitary ▪ Neurologic clinical signs: Depression, extrapyramidal signs	▪ Ergot alkaloids	▪ Dopamine D_2 receptor antagonists: ▪ Domperidone 1.1 mg/kg PO, q12h (does not cross BBB) ▪ Perphenazine, sulpride, acepromazine, metoclopramide ▪ Decreases brain dopamine: reserpine	▪ Dopamine agnoists
GABA and/or glycine stimulation	▪ Inhibition of skeletal muscle stimulation: ▪ Stupor or coma ▪ Decreased muscle tone ▪ Absent or decreased reflexes ▪ Involuntary temors	▪ Benzodiazepines ▪ Macrocyclic lactones (ivermectin and moxidectin)	▪ Sarmazenil 0.04 mg/kg, IV q2h ▪ Picrotoxin	
General CNS stimulation	▪ Anxiety, restlessness, hyperactivity, hypersensitivity, seizures	▪ Cholinesterase-inhibiting carbamate insecticides ▪ Organophosphates ▪ Chlorinated hydrocarbons		

Inhibition muscarinic cholinergic inhibition	▪ Abdominal discomfort due to hypomotility, decreased salivation, urinary retention, mydriasis, ptosis, restlessness, tachycardia	▪ Botulism ▪ Atropine overdose		
Nicotinic cholinergic Inhibition	▪ Inhibition of skeletal muscle function: ▪ Poor muscle tone (including tail tone), loss of muscle strength causing fasciculations, low head carriage ▪ Flaccid paralysis leading to recumbency ▪ Dysphagia and dyspnea due to affection of muscles involved with eating, swallowing, and respiration			▪ Drugs that can potentiate neuromuscular blockage: aminoglycosides, tetracyclines, procaine penicillin
GABA and/or glycine inhibition	▪ Continued stimulation of skeletal muscle: muscle contraction, muscle spasm, hyperesthesia, dysphagia, and dysphagia due to affection of muscles involved with eating, swallowing, and respiration, seizures	▪ Tetanus ▪ Cholinated hydrocarbons (some) ▪ Enrofloxacin	▪ Benzodiazepines (glycine and GABA-mimetic effects) such as diazepam, midazolam ▪ Other relaxing drugs: phenothiazines, α2-agonists, barbiturates, methocarbamol, guaifenesin	▪ Sarmazenil
Dopaminergic inhibition	▪ Vasoconstriction, extrapyramidal signs	▪ Carbon disulfide ▪ Ergot alkaloids ▪ Domperidone overdose ▪ Metoclopramide overdose		▪ Domperidone ▪ Metoclopramide

Table 32.IV.3 The Naranjo algorithm [29].

To assess the adverse drug reaction, please answer the following questionnaire and give the pertinent score

		Yes	No	Do not know or not done	Score patient for this question
1	Are there previous conclusive reports of this reaction?	+1	0	0	………
2	Did the adverse effect appear after the suspected drug was given?	+2	−1	0	………
3	Did the adverse reaction improve when the drug was discontinued, or a specific antagonist was given?	+1	0	0	………
4	Did the adverse reaction appear when the drug was re-administered?	+2	−2	0	………
5	Are there alternative causes that could have caused the reaction?	−1	+2	0	………
6	Did the reaction reappear when a placebo was given?	−1	+1	0	………
7	Was the drug detected in any body fluid in toxic concentrations?	+1	0	0	………
8	Was the reaction more severe when the dose was increased or less severe when the dose was decreased?	+1	0	0	………
9	Did the patient have a similar reaction to the same or similar drugs in any previous exposure?	+1	0	0	………
10	Was the adverse event confirmed by any objective evidence?	+1	0	0	………
TOTAL SCORE PATIENT					………

Total score:
9–10 = definite ADR[a]
5–8 = probably ADR
1–4 = possible ADR
0 = doubtful

[a] The original paper claimed that a score was a definite ADR because they used cases from published reports of adverse drug reactions. In reality the score cannot provide certainty.

Iatrogenic Toxicity

For most iatrogenic toxicities, foals are administered adult drug doses and are typically overdosed by at least tenfold. Toxicity can also occur following correct dosing because of the above described age-specific barrier mechanisms and brain vulnerability or because of adverse drug reactions. Furthermore, synergy between neurotoxic drugs and environmental toxins has been described in human and animal studies (and suggested in adult horses), leading to neurotoxicity at lower drug concentrations [41–43].

Anthelminthics

Ivermectin and **moxidectin** are anthelminthics commonly causing neurotoxicities in foals and belong to the group of **macrocyclic lactones (MLs)** used in equine deworming strategies. Because of their exclusion from the CNS in mammals, they have a wide margin of safety with clinical signs of toxicosis in horses being provoked at >10 times the recommended therapeutic dose [43, 44]. Although highly lipophilic molecules such as MLs readily diffuse across biological membranes, their penetration into the CNS is counteracted by the P-glycoprotein pump at the BBB [45, 46]. With lower expression of P-glycoprotein in neonatal infants [11], and presumably neonatal foals, accumulation of MLs in the brain is more likely to develop, making the safety margin lower. Literature mainly reports ML toxicosis caused by accidental overdose in which the foal receives the full syringe of the standard adult dose [43, 46–50]. Prefilled commercial oral syringes of wormer paste dose a 500–600 kg horse; thus, the smaller the foal the larger the potential for overdose and risk of clinical neurotoxicity [47, 50–51]. Based on information from the animal poison control center in the USA [44], and the fact that most affected horses reported in literature are <4 months old [47, 48, 50], it is suggested that horses are more susceptible when younger than 4 months of age. Alternatively, saturation of P-glycoprotein can occur by massive ML overdoses in older, healthy animals as demonstrated by a 11-month old foal that received >25-fold overdosing [46] and several adult horses that experimentally were overdosed at 10- to 60-fold for a safety trial [43].

Saturation of P-glycoprotein or damage to the BBB can develop secondary to co-exposure to other toxins. The latter has been described in two herds of adult horses after appropriate ivermectin dosing but following consumption of plants of the Solanum family (nightshade) [42, 51]. One report of three horses noted signs of toxicity in unrelated healthy horses that were not overdosed with possible concomitant exposure to toxic plants or other environmental toxins [41]. Moreover, genetic mutations in the encoding gene can lead to a lack of functional P-glycoprotein and a higher risk of adverse effects when exposed [52]. Such genetic defects have not been described in horses. ML toxicosis has also been described in a Miniature mule foal [47] and a zebra foal [53]. MLs are safe to administer to pregnant mares and have not been reported to cause neurotoxicity in the unborn foal, which is explained by high levels of P-glycoprotein at the BPB.

Clinical Signs

MLs trigger opening of gamma-aminobutyric acid (GABA)-gated chloride channels leading to hyperpolarization and blockade of neuronal impulses. MLs also affects the glycine inhibitory neurotransmitter system [54], which causes inhibition of skeletal muscle stimulation. ML toxicosis also can affect cranial nerves resulting in: blindness [43, 47, 53], mydriasis [41, 43, 47, 50], absent menace reflex [41, 47, 50], absent or decreased pupillary light reflexes [41, 47, 50], slow palpebral reflexes [47], absent or weak dazzle response [47, 50], decreased sensation of head and tongue [46], poor tone in tongue, jaw, lip, nose, and ear [40, 46], negative slap test [47], hypersalivation [41], and hypersensitivity to touch and sound [41]. Mentation can range from depression to obtundation [41, 43, 44, 47, 48, 53], with some foals progressing into coma or unconsciousness [44, 46, 49, 55]. Other clinical signs include head pressing, seizures, ataxia, tremors/fasciculations, weakness, and recumbency [41, 43, 44, 46, 47, 50, 53, 55]. Foals can develop systemic involvement with cardiovascular impairment, hypothermia, dyspnea, or hypoventilation [41, 43, 44, 46–48, 55]. One foal was also reported to suffer from a ruptured bladder and paralytic ileus [48].

Diagnosis is based on presence of neurologic signs following recent ML administration. Plasma levels of MLs are not helpful as they only confirm administration of the product but provide no information on how much crossed the BBB. Postmortem brain tissue concentrations in nonsurviving animals are considered more informative. These should be negligible in animals with an intact BBB [41, 54, 56].

Prognosis

Moxidectin is excreted slower and persists longer in plasma than ivermectin, potentially causing longer recovery times than ivermectin [41]. Clinical signs of ML toxicosis develop within 6–22 hours and last for 36–168 hours [41, 42, 44, 47, 50, 53, 55]. Most foals survive ML toxicity with supportive care [41, 44, 46, 47, 49, 50, 53, 55] although two foals [48, 49] and one adult horse [41] died from toxicosis and complications.

Treatment

Treatment consists of supportive care such as maintaining hydration (IV fluids), supplemental feedings/nutrition, ±urinary catheterization and maintaining a clean, dry, and well-padded environment. Several drugs may aid in reversing signs of ML neurotoxicity:

- *Sarmazenil* is a partial inverse benzodiazepine receptor agonist. One report (dose of 0.04 mg/kg, IV q2h) noted rapid regression of clinical signs of moxidectin toxicity without adverse effects [55]. It is unclear whether the reversal of clinical signs was aided by sarmazenil or if the foal would have shown reversal without, as described in other cases [49]. In another foal, sarmazenil did not reverse signs [46].
- *Picrotoxin* is a GABA-receptor antagonist used successfully in dogs with ML toxicity [57] but has a narrow safety margin and can cause seizures. In calves it was not useful in reversing clinical signs of ivermectin toxicity [54]. To the author's knowledge, picrotoxin has not been tested in foals with ML toxicity.
- *Physostigmine* is an anticholinesterase agent used in dogs, but effects are short-lasting (30–90 minutes) [58]. In cats, *neostigmine* has been used [59]. There are concerns about toxicity of these anticholinesterase drugs [41, 56]. These drugs may not be the best choice for ML toxicity since they stimulate skeletal muscle activity through the cholinergic system in order to override the GABA-induced inhibition of skeletal muscle activity, instead of directly acting on the GABA system. To the

author's knowledge, these drugs have not been used in horses with ML toxicity.
- Administration of *lipid emulsions* led to dramatic improvement in two foals [46, 50].

Other Anthelminthic Drugs

Bilateral laryngeal paralysis and a stiff gait was reported in five foals (23–35 days old) after use of haloxon as an anthelminthic (1–2 g at fortnightly intervals) starting at 2 days of age [60, 61]. Toxicity with an organic phosphate anthelminthic (Shell SD 15803) has been described in 2-month-old pony foals following excessive dosing [62] and the organic phosphate anthelminthic dichlorvos caused transient neurotoxicity in adult horses at 10–20 times the therapeutic dose [63]. Other anthelminthic drugs can cause neurotoxicity in adult horses with potential for toxicity in foals. The following are documented in literature:

- *Levamisole*: overdose causes hyperexcitability, muscle tremors, hyperactivity, excessive sweating, lacrimation, and death [60, 64].
- *Phenothiazine*: use has resulted in acute and unpredictable adverse effects such as hemolytic anemia, anorexia, weakness, CNS disturbances, and photosensitization [1].
- *Piperazine salts*: overdose causes a neuromuscular blockade "curare effect" with incoordination, depression, hyperesthesia, mydriasis, muscle tremors, constipation, and anorexia [1].
- *Topical application of amitraz*: old solutions can break down into components with increased toxicity and cause depression, ataxia, impaction colic, subcutaneous facial edema, diarrhea, dehydration, and acidosis [65].

Antimicrobials

Metronidazole

Metronidazole is usually well tolerated with no published reports describing neurotoxicity in horses. However, anecdotally suspected neurotoxicity in neonatal foals has been clinically witnessed (personal communication of G. van Galen, S. Hyldahl Laursen and D. Feary) and manifested as extra-pyramidal signs or ataxia that resolved within 24 hours after discontinuation of the metronidazole treatment. Literature supports the theory of metronidazole neurotoxicity but the pathophysiology is unknown. Metronidazole-induced encephalopathy in people is expressed by peripheral neuropathy, cerebellar dysfunction, visual impairment, vestibulotoxicity, cochleotoxicity, ataxic gait, dysarthria, seizures, and encephalopathy. The condition does not seem dose-dependent and affected individuals show MRI changes in the cerebellar dentate nuclei [66, 67]. Discontinuation of metronidazole results in rapid improvement and resolution of clinical signs, but long-lasting sequellae and fatality have been reported [66, 68]. Metronidazole-induced neurotoxicity has also been described in dogs [69, 70].

Fluoroquinolones

Fluoroquinolones cause seizures as a rare side effect in people, especially patients with a seizure history, electrolyte imbalances, receiving a dose not adjusted for renal insufficiency, or concurrent treatment with agents that lower the seizure threshold [71]. Despite the low risk, children are more frequently affected than adults [72]. Very high doses of enrofloxacin (25 mg/kg IV) as a bolus resulted in seizures of short duration in adult horses [73] and is assumed to result from transient high concentrations in the CSF binding to GABA receptors. To the author's knowledge, neurological signs after fluoroquinolone administration have not been reported in foals but could develop in foals that receive an overdose or have elevated risk. Supportive treatment and benzodiazepines would be useful.

Penicillins/Beta-Lactams

Benzylpenicillin is combined with procaine to provide longer therapeutic antimicrobial concentrations. Procaine is slowly absorbed from the intramuscular injection site, and plasma esterase hydrolyzes it to nontoxic para-aminobenzoic-acid (PABA). However, a sudden large bolus can overwhelm plasma esterases, leading to direct toxic effects on the CNS [74]. Analyses of plasma esterases from reacting horses demonstrate lower activity than nonreacting control horses, and low esterase activity was suggested to increase the possibility of procaine toxicity [75]. Accidental IV injection of penicillin procaine injection can result in neurologic signs [76] and is described in horses as young as 8 months [75]. Repeated intramuscular injections can increase the risk for accidental intravascular injection [75]. Patients show compulsive forward or backward movements, staggering, moving in a crazed manner or falling with muscle rigidity and spasms [76]; fatality has been reported [75]. Signs usually last for a few minutes, but can last several hours or days and up to 2 weeks [75]. There is no antidote or specific treatment; supportive treatment with sedative drugs can be attempted if signs are prolonged or severe.

Reports in people describe neurotoxicity related to beta-lactams (penicillins and cephalosporins) with reactions linked to the beta-lactam ring that shares structural similarities with GABA; this causes inhibition of GABA neurotransmission [77, 78]. Ampicillin in particular is noted to cause neurologic signs in neonates, primarily very low birth weight infants [79]. Therefore, if foals have a low birth weight (premature, dysmature), clinicians should be attentive to potential neurologic signs when receiving penicillins and cephalosporins.

Aminoglycosides

When aminoglycosides are administered concurrently with anesthetic agents, neuromuscular blockade of acetylcholine at nicotinic cholinergic receptors can occur [78]. This is a rare effect in adult horses, but potentially can occur in foals. Edrophonium (0.5 mg/kg IV) or calcium infusions (calcium gluconate 30–60 mg/kg IV or calcium chloride 10–20 mg/kg IV) reverse this effect [80, 81]. In addition, as a result of excitotoxic activation of NMDA receptors within the cochlea and subsequent formation of oxidative radicals, aminoglycosides can also cause ototoxicity [78]. This is a well-described side effect in people but is poorly documented in horses. Gentamicin administered at 5 mg/kg q8h did not result in ototoxicity in healthy ponies assessed by brain stem auditory-evoked responses [82]. One report suspected gentamicin induced vestibulotoxicity in an adult horse [83]. No reports describe aminoglycoside-induced ototoxicity or vestibulotoxicity in foals. Aminoglycoside-induced peripheral neuropathy and encephalopathy have also been described in people. Histological changes show lysosomal abnormalities similarly to aminoglycoside-induced nephrotoxicity [78]. There are no similar reports in horses.

Trimethoprim-Sulfonamides

Neurologic reactions have been described in four horses administered trimethoprim-sulfamethoxazole at normal dosages. Clinical signs include hypermetric gait, agitation, and erratic behavior with signs resolving after withdrawal of the medication; no residual effects were noted [28]. The same report included a suspected case of neurotoxicity in a 7-day-old foal following administration of an adult dose of pyrimethamine sulphadiazine. The foal developed acute onset of inability to nurse, recumbency, circling, facial grimace, manic chewing, biting the stable wall, and mild hypermetric gait. Administration of diazepam had little effect. Supportive care was provided and mentation improved and was considered normal within 3 days [28]. Dose-dependent headaches, psychoses, tremors, and aseptic meningitis are reported in people but are infrequent [84]. In horses, cardiovascular collapse also can occur following rapid IV administration or when combined with α2-agonists. Even though mentation can be severely altered when this happens, it is not caused by neurotoxicity.

Other Antimicrobials

Although rare in people, antimicrobial-induced neurotoxicity has been linked to erythromycin, clarithromycin, azithromycin, and tetracyclines [77, 78]. No neurotoxic effects have been reported following use of these drugs in horses.

Other Iatrogenic Neurotoxins

Lidocaine

Lidocaine neurotoxicity is caused by compromise of cortical inhibitory pathways from blockade of sodium channels, and consecutive excitatory features of sensory, visual, and muscular activation and seizure activity. Eventually a depressive phase with unconsciousness, coma, cardiovascular compromise, and respiratory arrest can follow in severe cases [85]. In adult horses, neurotoxicity following lidocaine constant rate infusion (CRI) is not uncommon and muscle fasciculations, dullness and ataxia have been described. Clinical signs are dose-dependent and resolve rapidly, often within minutes, following discontinuation of infusion [86–89].

Lidocaine toxicity has been reported in an 8-month-old foal during general anesthesia [90]. In awake patients neurologic effects are more pronounced than cardiovascular changes [89]. Because this incident occurred under general anesthesia, the classic neurologic signs could not be appreciated; instead signs of cardiovascular collapse became apparent (hypotension, drop-in end tidal CO_2 following asystole). The toxicity was successfully reversed during anesthesia with supportive treatments and administration of a lipid emulsion (see below) [90]. After recovery the foal was neurologically normal with the exception of visual impairment. In awake foals, neurological signs are likely associated with lidocaine toxicity and has anecdotally been observed (personal communication D. Feary). Neonatal infants are at greater risk than adults because of reduced plasma concentrations of the binding protein α1-acid glycoprotein and immature hepatic enzyme systems that increase the free plasma fraction of lidocaine. Reduced dosing by 15% is recommended in infants <4 months old [85]. As there are significant differences between species with regards to sensitivity to lidocaine [90], it is not known whether a similar dose reduction is warranted in foals. The risk for lidocaine toxicity also increases with concurrent administration of drugs that inhibit cytochrome P450 (e.g. ciprofloxacin [91], cimetidine [89]).

Sedatives and Opioids

Benzodiazepines, α2-agonists, and opioid-agonists induce sedation and cause drowsiness, ataxia, low head carriage, and occasionally recumbency and hypoventilation in foals. Overdoses can induce more severe neurologic signs. In addition to expected neurologic effects, opioids can cause seizures when administered in very large doses and intracarotid injection can cause agitation, collapse, or seizures [92]. The antidote for opioids is naloxone (0.01–0.05 mg/kg IV); α2-antagonists that reverse α2-agonists include yohimbine (0.04–0.15 mg/kg IV), tolazoline (2.0–6.0 mg/kg IV), or atipamezole (0.05–0.2 mg/kg IV) [92].

Neurotoxin Transmission from Mare to Foal

As it is unethical to place the unborn or newborn infant at risk, there is a lack of information about which drugs are safe to use during pregnancy and lactation [3, 37–39]. Similar gaps in knowledge occur in equine medicine. Yet, epidemiological studies demonstrate associations between drug use during pregnancy in women and birth defects [40]. Therefore, in women and horses, it is safest to avoid drugs during pregnancy or lactation, or restrict exposure by using the lowest effective dose and duration. Potential effects of drugs on fetal development are dependent on gestational age, dose, dosing frequency, route of administration and drug clearance. Furthermore, maternal active plasma drug concentrations can be different in pregnant versus non-pregnant mares because of altered pharmacokinetics that result from pregnancy-induced increase in blood volume, decrease in serum albumin, increase in glomerular filtration rates, and potential decrease in oral bioavailability [26]. Dependent on the drug administered, this can consequently place the fetus or neonate at increased or decreased risk.

Neurotoxin Transmission Through the Placenta

There are few reports on neurotoxins passing the placenta and causing clinical effects in newborn foals. Most are associated with anesthetic drugs.

Anesthetic Drugs

Anesthetics administered to periparturient mares cross the placenta and can induce effects in the fetus or newborn foal. Barbiturates produce fetal respiratory depression and arrest, with pentobarbital having more prominent effects than thiopental [93]. Ketamine can produce neurologic effects and respiratory depression in the newborn foal [93] and chloral hydrate can cause fetal depression [93, 94]. Although not reported, fetal depression should be considered if diazepam [89] and gas inhalants are administered to the mare just prior to parturition. Prudent use of anesthetic drugs in mares presented for dystocia or c-section is warranted and the foal delivered as soon as possible (ideally <20 minutes after start of general anesthesia) [95]. A separate team should be prepared for neonatal support or resuscitation. There are no antidotes available and treatment is based on general supportive care.

Sorghum

Ingestion of Sorghum spp. grasses by pregnant mares may cause arthrogryposis in the foal [73, 96].

Metals

Dietary lead can cross the BPB and BBB through amino acid transporters [3], with chronically exposed pregnant mares delivering potentially premature or small and weak foals [36]. Details of lead toxicity are described in environmental neurotoxins. In humans and animal studies, maternal exposure to other metals such as mercury, manganese, cadmium, iron, and arsenic are highly neurotoxic [3]. No reports of these heavy metal neurotoxicities in foals are available.

Pesticides/Organophosphates

Many pesticides are lipid soluble and likely cross the BPB and the BBB [3]. However, the BPB and the BBB afford protection to the fetus against some pesticides that are P-glycoprotein substrates [3]. Exposure to organophosphates caused degrees of cerebellar hypoplasia and ataxia and death in newborn piglets [97] and calves *in utero* [76]. To the author's knowledge, maternal exposure to pesticides has not been reported to cause neurotoxicity in foals.

Neurotoxin Transmission Through Colostrum and Milk

Drugs or toxins will transfer into milk to a certain degree but there can be a higher degree of excretion based on the lactation period and the concentration of casein in the milk [91]. Casein concentration is highest in colostrum and drops during the course of lactation; therefore, toxins or drugs strongly bound to casein, such as benzodiazepines, are present in higher concentrations in milk during the first days postpartum than later phases of lactation [98]. Toxin absorption through colostrum or milk rarely causes signs of neurotoxicity in the foal.

Accidental Administration of Domperidone Destined for the Mare

Accidental intoxication with domperidone intended for the mare to stimulate lactation has been witnessed in two neonatal foals (personal communication G. van Galen, I. Durie, D. De Clercq). One foal became comatose and died within 24 hours of administration. The second foal became comatose but woke up after 24–36 hours following IV fluid therapy and lipids, gastric emptying, and administration of paraffin oil and charcoal. Domperidone is a peripherally acting dopamine2-receptor antagonist [99]. Because it does not or only minimally cross the BBB in adult horses, CNS function is not altered [100, 101]. Symptoms of overdosage in people include restlessness, drowsiness, insomnia, headache, confusion, dizziness, acute dystonic reactions, and akathisia [102]. As reported by the Motilium® datasheet, depression, anxiety, headache, somnolence, agitation, nervousness, dizziness, disorientation, extrapyramidal disorders, and convulsions can occur [103]. Extrapyramidal manifestations are primarily reported in neonates and convulsion and agitation primarily in infants and children [103]. A specific antidote does not exist, but treatment with anticholinergics and anti-parkinsonian agents is suggested [103].

Pesticides/Insecticides

As toxin ingestion in neonatal foals is rare, only pesticides or insecticides that cause toxicity through inhalation or topical administration are listed (Table 32.IV.4). Despite this, the most common route of exposure to cause neurotoxicity for listed molecules is still oral exposure. Pesticide and insecticide toxicities are rare in horses, but younger animals might be more susceptible [76, 97].

Environmental Neurotoxins

Snake Envenomation

Not all snakes are venomous, and not all venomous snakes have neurotoxic venom. Most snake venom contains a mix of enzymes (e.g. digestive hydrolases), cytotoxins, neurotoxins, myotoxins, cardiotoxins, and hemotoxins. Neurotoxins are mostly found in elapids and hemotoxins in viperids. Exceptions occur as some elapids (e.g. black necked spitting cobra) do not carry neurotoxins and some viperids carry neurotoxins (e.g. Mojave rattlesnake) [114]. The following types of snake neurotoxins are commonly seen:

- *Fasciculins*. Toxins destroy acetylcholinesterase; acetylcholine cannot be broken down and remains in the receptor resulting in fasciculations and tetany.
- *Dendrotoxins*. Toxins block polarization/depolarization of nerves and cause nerve paralysis.
- *Alpha-neurotoxins*. Large group of toxins that act as acetylcholine mimetics, blocking the postsynaptic acetylcholine receptors and causing paralysis.

Suspected snake bite sites can be found around the muzzle, jaw, or distal limb, showing mild local swelling, erythema, and wheal formation. Occasionally, fresh blood or a pair of fang marks are visible [1, 115]. Systemic signs vary with the type of snake and type and dose of injected venom. Even if the snake venom does not carry neurotoxins, local peripheral nerve damage can occur because of tissue destruction and inflammation. Treatment is supportive; if available, snake antivenom can be administered.

Elapid Snakes

Elapid snakes include black, brown, and tiger snakes commonly encountered in Australia. Elapid venom typically contains potent neurotoxins. Nine Australian horses <1 year old were reported with elapid snake envenomation; eight survived [115]. Outside the local signs, others include unilateral facial nerve paralysis, neuromuscular weakness, unsteady or stiff gait, muscle fasciculations, dullness, inappetence, recumbency, colic, agitation, absent or slow pupillary light reflex, mydriasis, tongue paresis, dysphagia, pigmenturia, sweating, hyper- or hypothermia, tachycardia, and tachypnea. One of these cases was a 2-month-old colt presented in a comatose state. Prolonged clotting times, elevated CK, and elevated cardiac troponin are commonly encountered.

Treatment is supportive. If available, 1–5 vials of snake antivenom is administered slowly over 15–30 minutes; preferably each vial is diluted in 200–1000 ml of isotonic crystalloids [115] to allow controlled administration or discontinuation of infusions in case of an allergic reaction. Often premedication with dexamethasone, chlorpheniramine, flunixin meglumine, or a combination of these, is administered to avoid or reduce allergic reactions [115]. Antivenom should not be injected intramuscularly or into the bite or bite area [1]. Veterinary care is typically needed for 1–14 days for elapid snake bites [115].

Rattlesnakes

In the western USA, horses are primarily bit by rattlesnakes. Although rattlesnakes typically do not carry neurotoxins, some do. Rattlesnake bites can cause cardiac arrhythmia, hemolysis, and thrombocytopenia in horses [116–118]. They do not typically result in neurologic signs, although pharyngeal paralysis can develop as a chronic sign [117] and one horse has been described to develop bilateral facial nerve paralysis [116]. Of the 58 equine rattlesnake bite cases that were described, the youngest was 1 month old [116].

European Adder

European adder (Vipera berus) venom is a complex mixture of enzymes that contains, amongst others, a neurotoxic phospholipase A2 that blocks transmission of presynaptic nerve impulses. Clinical signs reported in seven affected horses from Sweden included local swelling, muscle fasciculations, depression, recumbency, and tachycardia. One of these horses was a 2-month-old Warmblood filly bitten in the plantar proximal metatarsus. The filly was severely depressed, recumbent, nonresponsive, had diffuse extensive swelling at the bite location, and developed extensive tissue necrosis in the flexor tendons; the filly was eventually euthanized [119].

Other Vipers

Several hundreds of horses every year are bitten by pit vipers, with 99% of all snake bites to animals due to pit vipers [1]. These bites produce dermomyonecrosis, hemorrhages, acute kidney injury, and death [120]. Palestine vipers (or true vipers) also envenomate horses, with the youngest being 3 days old [121]. Clinical signs include local swelling, tachycardia, tachypnea, and depression. The Palestine viper bite was fatal in 25/123 horses [121]; in this study, young age was not associated with fatality, but low body weight was [121], placing foals potentially at a higher

Table 32.IV.4 Pesticides and insecticides that can cause neurotoxicity [1, 36].

Toxin	Exposure/source	Mechanism of toxicity	Clinical signs	Diagnosis
Cholinesterase inhibiting carbamate insecticides (methiocarb, methomyl)[a, b] [35, 104–108]	Absorbed through GI tract, lungs, and skin	Reversible inhibition of acetylcholinesterase leading to muscarinic and nicotinic cholinergic overstimulation	Table 32.IV.3	Atropine test dose, acetylcholinesterase activity, residue analysis on biological samples
Treatment: Atropine sulfate 0.1–0.5 mg/kg, ¼ of the dose given IV, the remainder IM or SC (an initial low dose trial is recommended to assess the clinical response, but high doses are generally required to treat intoxications)				
Organophosphates[a, b, c] [35, 59, 60, 108, 109]	Absorbed through ingestion, topical exposure, or inhalation	Irreversible inhibition of acetylcholinesterase leading to muscarinic and nicotinic cholinergic overstimulation	Table 32.IV.3	Atropine test dose, acetyl cholinesterase activity, residue analysis, on biological samples
Treatment: Atropine sulfate 0.1–0.5 mg/kg, ¼ of the dose given IV, the remainder IM or SC (an initial low dose trial is recommended to assess the clinical response, but high doses are generally required to treat intoxications), Pralidoxime chloride (2-PAM) 20–50 mg/kg q4–12h, IM, SC or slow IV				
Metal phosphides[b] [110, 111]	Absorbed through ingestion, topical exposure or inhalation	Inhibition of cytochrome C leading to disruption of cellular aerobic metabolism	Sweating, tachycardia, tachypnea, pyrexia, ataxia, seizures, muscle	Residue analysis on biological samples
Treatment: None				
Chlorinated hydrocarbons (DDT and lindane)[a, b] [112]	Absorbed through ingestion, topical exposure or inhalation	Nonspecific stimulant of CNS, depolarizing effect on peripheral motor nerve and cholinergic stimulation, GABA inhibition	Table 32.IV.3, death	Residue analysis on biological samples
Treatment: No antidote				
Carbon disulfide[a, b] [113]	Absorbed through ingestion, topical exposure of inhalation	Potent fat solvent causing skin lesions; blocks enzymatic processes leading to neurologic Signs and hepatic necrosis	Burns, respiratory irritation, aggitation, lethargy, seizures, muscle spasms, coma	Iodine-azide test to find metabolites in urine (used in people)
Treatment: No antidote				
Nicotine[b]	Absorbed through ingestion, or topical exposure	Nicotinic cholinergic stimulation followed by blockade; caustic action on mucosa	Table 32.IV.3	Residue analysis on biological samples
Treatment: No antidote				

[a] Reported in adult horses; can occur at any age.
[b] Described in other species.
[c] Reported in foals.

risk. Neurologic signs are not induced by pit and Palestine vipers, however, if a foal were to be envenomated, severely altered mentation or a state of coma can be expected.

Ticks

Tick Paralysis

Tick paralysis is caused by soft (*Dermacentor variabilis*, *Dermacenter andersoni*) and hard ticks (Ixodes species, *Ornithodros lahorensis*). Tick toxins reduce acetylcholine release at neuromuscular junctions (Table 32.IV.3). Consequently, over hours to days, clinical signs develop and intensify from paresis to paraparesis, tetraparesis, recumbency, dysphagia, respiratory paralysis, and eventually death [73]. A presumptive diagnosis has been described in adult horses from Australia [122, 123] and North America [124] and a number of foals in Australia (55 foals <6 months old and 24 foals between 6 and 12 months old) [123, 125]. One report noted that 73% (75/103 cases) had a body weight <100 kg, suggesting low body weight is a risk factor for developing clinical signs of tick paralysis. Of these 75 cases <100 kg of body weight, 59 survived (78%). However, 28 horses that weighed >100 kg were more likely to die with a survival rate of only 60% [123]. The number of ticks present on affected horses at the time of diagnosis ranged from 1 to 100, with the majority having 1 or 2 ticks found on the head, neck, torso, axilla, and inguinal area [123]. Most Australian cases are presented between June and December [123]. Clinical signs can resolve after tick removal or application of topical or systemic acaricides [76, 122–124]. Treatment is supportive. Administration of >0.5 ml/kg of hyperimmune canine derived tick antiserum may reduce the odds of death [123].

Ear Ticks

Ear ticks have been reported to induce muscle spasm and seizures in horses [76, 126].

Neurotoxic Spider Bites

Some spiders have neurotoxic venom that cause neurological signs in people. Little evidence exists that spider bites cause neurologic signs in horses, likely because development of signs is linked to body weight. However, foals have a similar body weight as people, and in endemic areas of neurotoxic spiders, bites could be considered as a cause of neurologic signs:

- *Black widow spider*. Its neurotoxin, alpha-latrotoxin, binds presynaptic receptors causing increased release of acetylcholine leading to muscle cramping. Signs from systemic toxicity are referred to as lactrodectism [127]. Anecdotal bites causing local skin reactions, colic signs, muscle contractions and paralysis, respiratory distress and death are mentioned in websites and discussion forums [128].
- *Australian funnel web spider*. Its neurotoxin, atracotoxin, opens sodium channels, causing excessive neural activity leading to paresthesia, muscle contraction, unstable blood pressure, pulmonary edema, and potentially death. Some animal species are unaffected by its bite with no known reports in horses.
- *Brazilian wandering spider*. Its neurotoxin affects multiple types of ion channels, leading to severe pain, autonomic effects, cardiorespiratory failure, and possibly death.

Bee Mass Envenomation

Bee venom contains a mixture of toxic compounds including mellitins, phospholipase A2, hyaluronidases, mast cell degranulating peptides, and neurotoxin [129]. A mare and her 24-hour old foal suffered toxic envenomation by a swarm of bees with both developing urticaria, tachycardia, swelling of the head and muzzle, intermittent agitation and dullness, failure to pass urine and feces, and coagulopathy. The mare also demonstrated rolling, profuse sweating, maniacal repetitive circling, bucking, myoglobinuria, rhabdomyolysis, facial nerve paralysis, inspiratory stridor, anorexia, bruxism, and intravascular hemolytic anemia. The foal stopped nursing and developed swelling and subsequent necrosis of the eartips [129]. Bee stings have been described to be fatal in horses [130, 131]. Neurologic signs following bee mass envenomation have been described in dogs [132] and people [133]. Treatment is supportive.

Plants with Neurotoxins

Nettles

Ataxia, distress, muscle weakness, and urticaria following contact with stinging nettle (Urtica dioica) has been reported in three thin-coated horses. Spontaneous recovery occurred within 4 hours [134]. A presumptive nettle reaction has also been reported in a 4-hour-old Suffolk punch filly foal. Gestation and delivery were normal and the foal was healthy the first 3 hours of life. After pasture turnout and witnessed nettle exposure, the foal developed sudden onset recumbency, inability to rise or lift the head, drooping of the upper eyelids and flexion of head and neck to one side and periodical dorsiflexion. Skin changes were not noted. The foal recovered spontaneously over 4 hours [135]. There are no antidotes available and treatment is supportive. Skin decontamination is perhaps useful.

Blue Green Algae (Cyanobacteria)

Ingestion of blue green algae through contaminated water is not uncommon in livestock and horses are also susceptible [36]. Toxicosis can occur year-round, but is most likely during warm weather and when water is contaminated with fertilizer runoff or organic waste. The algae causes cholinergic stimulation or inhibition (Table 32.IV.3), sodium conductance blockage through excitable membranes, and hepatocellular necrosis. Clinical signs include colic, diarrhea, muscle tremors, seizures, recumbency, dyspnea, cyanosis, signs of liver damage, and death. Neurotoxic blooms can cause clinical signs within minutes including neurologic signs and death. Diagnosis is based on identification of cyanobacteria in gastric contents, liver, or suspect water. No antidote is available and treatment usually is not possible because of rapid death [36]. Literature does not report on affected foals.

Lead

Lead toxicity is one of the most commonly reported toxicities but is more rare in modern times [36]. Toxicity is linked to chronic ingestion following environmental contamination of habitat by industrial mining and smelting operations, lead based paints, oil, gasoline, and greases [1, 36, 136, 137]. Lead toxicity causes inhibition of sulfhydryl groups of essential metabolic enzymes, inhibition of heme synthesis, decreasing concentrations of essential trace metals, alterations of neurotransmitter release and interference with mitochondrial metabolism resulting in peripheral neuropathy through segmental demyelination, damaging the BBB and endothelial cells, and interference with humoral and cell-mediated immune responses. Clinical signs in horses include depression, weakness, weight loss, laryngeal and pharyngeal dysfunction, proprioceptive deficits, muscle tremors, seizures, and death [1, 36, 76, 138]. Signs usually progress slowly over several weeks [138] with diagnosis established by residue analysis on biological samples, blood lead concentrations [1, 36] and zinc protoporphyrin analysis [139]. Removing access to lead halts the outbreak and slowly reverses mild signs [76]. Supportive treatment may be needed, and lead chelation can be achieved by administration of $CaNa_2$-EDTA (75 mg/kg/day, slow IV infusion divided into two daily doses, diluted in normal saline or 5% dextrose as a 6.6% solution) or succimer (10 mg/kg PO q8h for 10 days) while monitoring whole blood lead concentrations [1]. Young and malnourished animals are more susceptible than older animals [36]. Lead poisoning has been described in foals [139], and chronically exposed mares can deliver premature or small and weak foals [36].

Clostridial Neurotoxins

Botulism and tetanus are described in detail elsewhere. Tetanus is caused by toxins of *Clostridium tetani* that prevent release of the inhibitory neurotransmitters GABA and glycine resulting in signs of increased muscle contraction and spasms (Table 32.IV.3). Botulism results from toxins of *Clostridium botulinum* that inhibit acetylcholine release at peripheral nerve terminals from skeletal and cholinergic nerves. Clinical signs include muscle weakness and similar to cholinergic inhibition (see Table 32.IV.3).

Clinical Approach in Cases of Suspected Toxicity

Differential Diagnosis for Neurotoxicities in Foals

Recognition of a possible neurotoxicity and identification of the toxin is challenging [1]. The nervous system has limited ways of responding to toxic insults; therefore, clinical signs are rarely pathognomic for a particular neurotoxin and are merely indicative of disturbed physiological mechanisms (Table 32.IV.3).

Nontoxic differentials should be considered when assessing foals with neurologic signs (Table 32.IV.6). Signs of neurotoxicities can easily be misinterpreted or missed because foals commonly develop neurologic signs following a variety of systemic diseases. Repeated seizures for example are more commonly associated with neonatal encephalopathy [77]. The foal's homeostatic processes that maintain body function within normal physiological ranges are less developed than adult horses, explaining why a wider severity range of changes such as electrolyte disturbances or cardiovascular/respiratory compromise impact the CNS more readily and result in secondary neurologic signs. Although the cause remains many times undetermined, exposure to teratogenic and neurotoxic chemicals or plants has also been suggested [142].

Stabilization of Vital Parameters

If suspicious of neurotoxicity in a foal, consider if any of the three major body systems (respiratory, cardiovascular, neurological) are compromised. Quick assessment of these systems allows for early recognition of abnormal vital parameters and rapid initiation of stabilization. Numerous neurotoxins affect the respiratory system by abnormal ventilation or ventilatory patterns, obstructed airways and/or failure of neuromuscular control of breathing. For example, snake bites cause localized swelling and edema [115], organophosphates induce increased bronchial secretions [1], and hypoventilation and respiratory failure occur with botulism [143], tetanus [144], tick paralysis [123], exposure to barbiturates or ketamine [93], or ivermectin/moxidectin toxicity [45, 51]. The cardiovascular system can also be severely affected by certain neurotoxins. For example, snake envenomation can induce cardiotoxicity, and cardiovascular impairment can be induced by lidocaine [88] or ivermectin/moxidectin toxicities [44, 51]. Neurologic dysfunction such as seizures and other neurological behaviors that can cause self-trauma to the foal or exacerbation of the neurologic lesions can be observed. Stabilization of vital parameters includes:

- Respiratory support by ensuring patency of the airways and ventilation
- Cardiovascular support through correction of hypovolemia, inotropic and vasopressor support, and antiarrhythmic drugs
- Neurological support by seizure control, muscle relaxants, and/or sedation

History, Clinical Assessment, and Diagnostic Tests

After stabilization, signalment and a thorough history should be obtained, including questioning about clinical signs, duration and evolution of signs, and exposure to potential drugs or environmental toxins. The presence of a toxin in the foal's environment does not assume exposure. If possible, an exposure assessment should be performed [1, 141, 145], which includes: (i) identification of toxin to which foal may have been exposed, (ii) confirmation of exposure (or highly suggested), (iii) amount of exposure or dose (including minimum and maximum amount foal could have been exposed to) and/or duration, (iv) date and time of exposure, (v) measures of the toxins toxicity (minimal lethal dose or lethal dose resulting in death of 50% of exposed individuals [LD50]), (vi) administration of medication that potentially worsen or improve toxicity, and (vii) body weight. Exposure assessment may not be able to be performed because of lack of information but when possible, suggests whether a patient has been exposed to a toxic amount of neurotoxin and assists in diagnostic and therapeutic decisions [1]. Close examination of pasture, feed, stable, and feed storage provide important clues. Local, regional, or national factors such as occurrence of toxic plants, snakes, ticks, heavy-metal exposure, or use of pesticides contribute to an increased suspicion of intoxications [1]. Furthermore, an adverse drug reaction algorithm (Table 32.IV.2) assesses the likelihood that the foal is displaying an adverse drug reaction. The foal should undergo clinical and neurologic examinations to attempt to localize the neurological lesions and if possible, identify the mechanism(s) of the toxin (Table 32.IV.1).

Complementary tests such as blood analysis (hematology, serum biochemistry, blood gas analysis), urinalysis, CSF analysis, and residue analysis in body fluids and gastric reflux can be used to investigate other causes of clinical signs (Table 32.IV.5). In certain cases, magnetic resonance imaging (MRI), electromyography (EMG), brainstem auditory evoked response testing (BAER), or electroencephalography (EEG) are useful. In fatal toxicities, postmortem examination is recommended, and gastric contents, brain, and liver can be sampled.

Toxin Detection

Tests are available to detect toxins including therapeutic drug monitoring (e.g. phenytoin), drug abuse tests (e.g. ketamine, barbiturates, benzodiazepines, and opioids), food contaminant tests (e.g. heavy metals), and food residue tests (e.g. antimicrobials, anthelminthic drugs, pesticides). These tests are performed on environmental, food or gastric content, and biological samples (CSF, saliva, urine, blood, tissues). In people, sweat analysis is used to monitor bioaccumulation of toxic elements, as many toxic elements are preferentially excreted through sweat. Moreover, some toxins readily identified in human sweat are not found in the serum of the same person [147]. The use of sweat for diagnostic purposes in ill foals would be challenging but might be useful in the future detection of certain toxins or drugs. Of note, blood concentrations of toxins do not necessary correlate with clinical features of toxicity; therefore, the main concern should be treatment of the patient and not of blood toxin concentrations [141].

Diagnostic Tests for Autonomic Involvement

A low-dose atropine test (0.02 mg/kg IV) can help differentiate the cause of autonomic signs. If the heart rate decreases and mydriasis occurs after administration, it is unlikely that signs were caused by organophosphates or carbamates as it takes a higher dose (0.1–0.5 mg/kg; ¼ of the dose given IV, the remainder SC or IM) to resolve autonomic signs caused by these pesticides [1, 35]. Serum cholinesterase levels can be measured to aid in the diagnosis of anticholinesterase drugs [141].

General Therapeutic Guidelines

Most foals require treatment in the absence of a diagnosis, because toxin detection and laboratory test results may only be available after several days.

Stop Exposure

Decontamination starts by preventing ongoing exposure. This is achieved by ceasing drug therapy, providing different food sources, or removing the foal from the environment. Following that, decontamination can include multiple systems.

Table 32.IV.5 Nontoxic differentials for foals with CNS signs [73, 142, 146].

Type of condition	Examples		
Infectious	■ Sepsis ■ Spinal or brain abscess	■ Meningitis (bacterial or fungal) ■ Botulism	■ Tetanus
Congenital, genetic or developemental	■ Idiopathic sizures (Arabian) ■ Meningoencephalocele ■ Cerebellar hypoplasia ■ Cervical spina bifida ■ Hemivertebrae ■ Dandy-Walker malformation	■ Cerebral agenesis ■ Hydrocephalus ■ Cerebral hypoplasia ■ Cervical compressive myelopathy ■ Block vertebrae	■ Spinal dysraphism ■ Lavender Foal Syndrome ■ Myelodysplasia ■ Butterfly vertebrae ■ Occipito-atlanto-axial malformation
Traumatic	■ Head trauma	■ Spinal cord trauma	
Metabolic	■ Severe acidosis ■ Severe azotemia ■ Severe electrolyte derangement (sodium, chloride, calcium, magnesium) ■ Rapid correction of sodium imbalances	■ Hepatoencephalopathy ■ Severe hypoglycemia	■ Kernicterus
Muscular	■ Atypical myopathy ■ Hyperkalemic periodic paralysis (HYPP) ■ Glycogen branching enzyme deficiency (GBED)	■ Nutritional myopathy (white muscle disease)	
Brain hypoxia due to Systemic conditions	■ Respiratory disease (hypoventilation, upper respiratory tract obstruction, pulmonary disease, pulmonary hypertension) ■ Cardiovascular compromise (shock, hypovolemia, anaphylaxis) ■ Cardiac disease (congenital abnormalities, arrhythmias) ■ Anemia (hemorrhage, neonatal isoerythrolysis) ■ Rapid injection of drugs that cause hypotension (trimethoprim sulphonamides, tetracyclines)		
Others	■ Neonatal encephalopathy ■ Sleep disorders	■ Intracarotid drug injection	■ Air embolism

Avoiding Further Uptake and Enhancing Toxin Removal from the Body

Treatment of toxicities in people have moved away from decontamination (i.e. emesis induction, gastric lavage, activated charcoal administration) but decontamination in equids is still warranted. The ability to treat toxicities is more limited due to financial restrictions and less readily available therapeutic modalities such as antidotes, plasmapheresis, hemodialysis, and mechanical ventilation [145]. The method of decontamination depends on the route of exposure and known responses of the toxic agent to the decontaminants. The selected method should be implemented aggressively to limit toxic effects [141]. Decontamination must be performed in a narrow window of time for most substances (generally <1 to 2 hours) [145].

Addressing the Gastrointestinal (GI) System

Following oral intake of a toxin, gastric lavage should be performed as soon as possible [145]. The first lavage sample should be used for toxicological analysis [1]. It is difficult to estimate the fraction that has already been taken up into the GI tract, therefore dilution and clearance from the GI tract should be promoted after gastric lavage. Dilution with water is useful because it reduces GI irritation by the toxin [141] and dilating the stomach increases defecation through the gastro-colic reflex. Laxatives repeatedly administered via nasogastric tube (tap water, electrolyte solutions or sodium or magnesium sulfate solutions) dilute and enhance clearance by decreasing transit time. Paraffin oil is not recommended in cases of toxicity as it is not successful in binding toxins [148] or decreasing systemic absorption from the GI tract in horses and can decrease the adsorptive ability of activated charcoal if administered together [1]. Furthermore, oil may carry certain toxins across cell barriers (e.g. carbamate compounds) [36]. Prokinetics are typically not used to enhance clearance, but if motility is reduced by the toxicity, use of metoclopramide or neostigmine can be attempted. Both can influence the nervous system, so before administration, verify that drug-toxin interactions do not enhance neurotoxic signs.

Milk is used in some toxicities in people as it acts as a diluent and has beneficial properties in cases of ingestion of caustic or irritant substances [141]. Milk is considered a natural laxative and contains hormones and peptides that are cytoprotective against toxins [149]. Secretory immunoglobin A in human milk has been shown to bind botulism toxin and inhibits toxin binding to intestinal epithelial cells [150]. Although milk content varies amongst species, similar effects can be expected from mare's milk. Ongoing nursing by the foal should be encouraged unless toxicity originates from exposure through the mare's milk or presence of reflux or ileus. In the absence of a suckle reflex, milk can be administered to the foal by nasogastric intubation. Milk may, however, reduce the efficacy of activated charcoal [141].

Addressing the Urinary System

For toxins primarily eliminated via the urine, excretion can be enhanced by forced diuresis through fluid therapy and diuretics. Many drugs are partially reabsorbed in the renal tubules, reducing the amount of toxin excreted despite increasing urinary output [141]. Ion trapping through manipulation of urinary pH is a means of forced diuresis; acidic molecules tend to remain ionized in alkaline urine, and basic molecules tend to remain ionized in acidic urine [141]. A foal's urine is slightly acidic and thus increases renal clearance of weak bases [18]. Forced alkaline diuresis can be helpful for barbiturate intoxication while forced acidic diuresis is dangerous in people and is rarely utilized [141]. Forced diuresis should be carefully controlled as to not worsen the clinical status of the foal, especially when the foal has CNS edema, pulmonary edema, renal or cardiac compromise, or electrolyte and acid base disturbances. In people, forced diuresis is recommended when the toxins or its active metabolites are excreted in urine, there is a high plasma concentration of the toxin and there is high likelihood that supportive therapy alone will not be sufficient, but there is no evidence that forced diuresis methods affect outcome [1, 141]. Peritoneal dialysis, hemodialysis, hemofiltration, charcoal hemoperfusion, or plasma or blood exchange can be considered [151]. Peritoneal dialysis can be of use following barbiturate toxicity and can be relatively easily implemented in foals (Chapter 24), but is less effective than hemodialysis [141].

Decontamination of the Skin

In cases of topical exposure to toxins (pesticides, topical anthelminthics), the skin is decontaminated by washing the foal with warm water or saline for at least 15 minutes [141]. Mild soap solutions [141] or liquid dishwashing detergent [35] can be used, especially for oily or greasy contaminants. The decontamination team should avoid self-contamination by wearing protective equipment. Nitrile gloves are recommended as latex gloves are not as chemical-resistant. Human (and likely equine) skin excretes drugs and toxins from the body through sweat, and sweating is a method for elimination of many toxic elements from the human body [147]. However, induced sweating is difficult in foals.

Clearing the Respiratory and Ophthalmic System

Following inhalational exposure, provision of fresh air is recommended [1] and humidified oxygen and hyperbaric oxygen have been suggested [141]. If uptake of the toxin has occurred through the eyes, they should be flushed with copious amounts of saline or tap water [1] for at least 15 minutes [141].

Inactivation of the Toxin

Antidote

Complete antidotes fully reverse toxicities leading to full resolution, typically almost immediately after administration. Partial antidotes counteract one of the toxic mechanisms, resulting in partial resolution. For most toxins, antidotes are either unavailable or not readily obtainable (Table 32.IV.3) [1].

Activated Charcoal

Activated charcoal absorbs many noxious substances onto its surface, preventing their absorption from the GI tract (Table 32.IV.6). The capacity to bind a substance depends on particle size, solubility, ionization, and pH of the substance and stomach contents [140]. Administration is not helpful if the toxin is known not to be adsorbed. However, in the event that the toxin is undetermined, administration of activated charcoal is recommended [140].

In horses, activated charcoal is given at a dose of 1–4 g/kg PO suspended in water (approx. 1 g/5 ml) via nasogastric intubation, repeated every 4–6 hours [1]. In human medicine, dosing is based on the amount of ingested toxin or patient's body weight [140]. When the amount of toxin absorbed is known, 10–40 times more activated charcoal is given. This is achievable for toxin intakes in the milligram range; otherwise dosages are calculated by body weight. There are many forms of activated charcoal, including powder and tablet form with or without cathartics (usually sorbitol). Activated charcoal should be given as soon as possible after ingestion of the toxin (ideally within 5 minutes) to be most effective [145]. When testing activated charcoal for 43 different toxins or drugs, a single-dose treatment in people effectively decreased toxin bioavailability by an average of 69% if the charcoal was given within 30 minutes and 34% if given within 1 hour of toxin ingestion [140]. Delayed administration, up to 6 hours post ingestion, may still be efficient for intoxications with (i) slow-release preparations, (ii) substances that inhibit GI motility (opiates, anticholinergics), or (iii) not readily digested materials such as toxic plants [140, 145].

Multidose treatment is beneficial in human intoxications for toxins that undergo enterohepatic or entero-enteric circulation, have high serum levels and long half-lives, or rapid elimination benefits the patient [140, 141, 145]. Therefore, multiple doses are likely beneficial in foals. Activated charcoal interrupts the enterohepatic and/or entero-enteric circulation and enhances excretion of the toxin from the body [140]. In the case of entero-enteric circulation, the intestinal wall functions as a semipermeable membrane and toxins diffuse out of the blood from serosa to mucosa onto the charcoal in the intestinal lumen (gastrointestinal dialysis) [140]. This multiple-dose approach is as efficacious as hemodialysis in people [141]. Multidose activated charcoal should not contain a cathartic because of risk for dehydration and secondary hypernatremia or hypermagnesemia.

Contraindications to activated charcoal are GI bleeding, impaired GI passage or reflux. Simultaneous administration of a laxative is not recommended [140] and simultaneous use of paraffin oil [1] or access to milk [141] decreases the adsorptive ability of charcoal. Moreover, oral medication and some antidotes bind to activated charcoal and negatively impact the efficacy of potentially life-saving treatment [141]. Side effects in people include: vomiting, constipation, diarrhea, nausea, urge to defecate, anal irritation, and rarely, aspiration pneumonia, small intestinal occlusion, and charcoal stercoliths [140, 141]. In horses activated charcoal likely has its maximal effect in the fore or mid-gut [152]. An *in vitro* analysis on microbial communities from horse's hindguts noted that if charcoal reaches the hindgut, it is unlikely to impact the flora significantly with no detrimental effect on hindgut fermentation [152].

Other adsorbents such as bentonite clay, aluminum silicates (kaolin), and di-tri-octahedral smectite (Biosponge®) are less efficient in binding toxins than activated charcoal [1]. An *in vitro* study tested different adsorbents for hypoglycin A binding and suggested that charcoal was the most suitable adsorbent to prevent atypical myopathy in horses [148].

Intravenous Lipid Emulsions (ILE)

ILE is a potential antidote for lipophilic drug toxicosis such as local anesthetics and MLs. ILE sequestrates the lipophilic toxin into the newly created intravascular lipid compartment, acting as a "lipid sink" thereby decreasing free toxin available to tissues [145]. It also provides the patient with energy substrates that support cardiac performance and skeletal muscle through free fatty acids in the circulation [145].

Dosages for foals are extrapolated from other species. Initially a 20% ILE bolus is administered at 1.5–4 ml/kg (between 0.3 and 0.8 g/kg), followed by a CRI of 0.25 ml/kg/min (0.05 g/kg/min) over 30–60 minutes. In non-responsive patients, intermittent bolusing at 1.5 ml/kg q4–6h for 24 hours can be attempted. Follow-up CRI doses (0.5 ml/kg/h) can be continued until signs improve (not to exceed 24 hours) or lipemia develops [145, 153]. Response to ILE varies from mild improvement to complete resolution of clinical signs [153]. In people, ILE is reserved for late stage treatment (once cardiopulmonary arrest has occurred) because of ILE's risk to interact with drugs [145, 153]. Use of ILE is therefore recommended in life-threatening intoxications, patients with severe symptoms or those that fail to respond to other therapies [145]. Adverse effects of ILE include anaphylactoid-like signs, hypertriglyceridemia, fat embolism, fat overload syndrome, worsening acute respiratory distress, pyrogenic reactions, coagulopathy, and infection following microbial contamination of ILE.

Table 32.IV.6 Neurotoxic substances that are known to be adsorbed or not to be adsorbed onto activated charcoal [140].

Neurotoxic substances that are absorbed		Neurotoxic substances absorbed insufficiently or not at all
Antidepressants	Antiepileptics	Alcohols (e.g. ethanol, methanol, glycols)
Barbiturates	Benzodiazepines	Anorganic salts (e.g. sodium chloride)
Neuroleptics	Tetracyclines	Metals and their anorganic compounds
Opiates	Nicotine	Organic solvents (e.g. acetone, dimethylsulfoxide)
Theophylline		Acids and bases
Strychnine		Cyanides

Complete list available in: [140, 141].

Administration of ILE has been described in two foals. Epinephrine, atropine and ILE rapidly reversed clinical signs of cardiopulmonary collapse following an overdose of lidocaine in an 8-month-old anesthetized foal weighing 140 kg. ILE was administered at a low dose of 100 ml 20% lipid emulsion followed by a CRI of 0.5 ml/kg BWT/h for 2 hours until recovery from anesthesia. Eight hours after collapse, the foal had mild hypertriglyceridemia (1.55 mmol/l) [37]. The second case was a 2-day-old 45 kg Arabian filly with accidental ivermectin toxicity. Twelve hours after admission the foal was not responsive to supportive treatment and was administered a 20% ILE solution at a dose of 1.5 ml/kg over 5 minutes and then 0.25 ml/kg/min for 30 minutes. Immediate clinical improvement was observed but another 12 hours passed before standing and 3 days to fully recover. A second ILE was not administered because of persistent hypertriglyceridemia (>346 mg/dl) [55].

Cytochrome P450 (CYP)

In patients with adverse drug reactions or pesticide intoxications, the clinician should avoid administration of drugs that inhibit CYP to allow for optimal metabolization and inactivation of the drug or pesticide. Commonly used CYP inhibitors include trimethoprim sulfonamides, phenylbutazone, omeprazole, macrolides, and antifungal drugs [154].

Symptomatic and Supportive Care

Symptomatic and supportive care has a greater influence on case outcome than any other factor [1]. In addition to the aforementioned treatments, the following aspects should be considered:

- Ongoing neurological support:
  - Controlling ongoing seizures and muscle tremors
  - Prevention of trauma: self-inflicted or on others or due to recumbency by use of sedation, well-bedded/padded stalls, maintaining the foal in sternal recumbency (to facilitate adequate ventilation), head and eye protection, and wound care.
- Ongoing cardiovascular support
  - Correction of fluid, acid-base, and electrolyte abnormalities
- Ongoing respiratory support
- Nutritional and GI support
- Renal and hepatic support

Recovery and Monitoring for Ongoing Damage

Swift decontamination, inactivation, increased excretion, and ceasing exposure will in some cases allow for rapid amelioration and normalization of toxin exposure. For others, recovery can take more time or damage can be irreversible or ongoing. The speed of which the return to normal neurologic function occurs is dependent on exposure dose, half-life of the drug or toxin, rate of metabolization into nontoxic metabolites, rate of excretion, amount of accumulation, time that toxins remain active, and/or attached to site of action, time the CNS requires to heal, and/or response to antidotes if available. Delayed effects can also occur. Based on clinical experience, an expectation can be set around the recovery time for each toxin when there is no ongoing exposure, although predictions do not always match real-life recoveries, which can be lengthy [75]. In general, rapid normalization (minutes to hours) occur with lidocaine toxicity [86], procaine penicillin reactions [75], and stinging nettles [134, 135], even without use of antidotes or any form of treatment. Recovery in one to several days is expected following ivermectin or moxidectin [44], metronidazole and trimethoprim sulfonamides toxicity [28]. Longer recoveries are encountered for lead toxicity, botulism [143], and tetanus [144], with acute death expected with blue green algae [36]. Ultimately recoveries can be uneventful for certain toxicities, but for others short-term and long-term sequellae can develop. Affected foals need to be monitored for potential ongoing damage that can involve the neurologic system or other body systems.

Other Potentially Exposed Animals

When neurotoxicity is suspected and believed to be of noniatrogenic origin, all in-contact animals should be examined because of potential co-exposure. Clinical examination, blood analyses, and close monitoring is indicated. Exposure should be restricted or stopped by ceasing administration of the same food or moving the horse out of the environment. Treatment should be initiated as soon as possible in cases that are suspected to have had significant exposure based on an exposure assessment and clinical indicators.

References

1 Poppenga, R.H. (2015). Toxicology. In: *Equine Emergency and Critical Care Medicine*, 1e (ed. L.L. Southwood and P.A. Wilkins), 555–620. Boca Raton: CRC Press.

2 Grandjean, P. and Landrigan, P.J. (2006). Developmental neurotoxicity of industrial chemicals. *Lancet* 368: 2167–2178.

3 Ek, C.J., Dziegielewska, K.M., Habgood, M.D. et al. (2012). Barriers in the developing brain and neurotoxicology. *Neurotoxicology* 33: 586–604.

4 Engelhardt, B., Vajkoczy, P., and Weller, R.O. (2017). The movers and shapers in immune privilege of the CNS. *Nat. Immunol.* 18: 123–131.

5 Brightman, M.W. (1977). Morphology of blood–brain interfaces. *Exp. Eye Res.* 25 (Suppl): 1–25.
6 Pardridge, W.M., Oldendorf, W.H., Cancilla, P. et al. (1986). Blood-brain barrier: interface between internal medicine and the brain. *Ann. Intern. Med.* 105: 82–95.
7 Gross, P.M. and Weindl, A. (1987). Peering through the windows of the brain. *J. Cereb. Blood Flow Metab.* 7: 663–672.
8 Furr, F. (2008). Cerebrospinal fluid and the blood brain barrier. In: *Equine Neurology*, 1e (ed. M. Furr and S. Reed), 33–46. Hoboken, NJ: Wiley.
9 Furr, F. (2008). Pharmaceutical considerations for treatment of central nervous system disease. In: *Equine Neurology*, 1e (ed. M. Furr and S.M. Reed), 55–63. Hoboken, NJ: Wiley.
10 Virgintino, D., Errede, M., Girolamo, F. et al. (2008). Fetal blood-brain barrier P-glycoprotein contributes to brain protection during human development. *J. Neuropathol. Exp. Neurol.* 67: 50–61.
11 Watchko, J.F., Daood, M.J., Mahmood, B. et al. (2001). P-glycoprotein and bilirubin disposition. *J. Perinatol.* 21 (Suppl 1): S43–S47.; discussion S59–S62.
12 Ek, C.J., Wong, A., Liddelow, S.A. et al. (2010). Efflux mechanisms at the developing brain barriers: ABC-transporters in the fetal and postnatal rat. *Toxicol. Lett.* 197: 51–59.
13 Pardridge, W.M. (1999). Non-invasive drug delivery to the human brain using endogenous blood-brain barrier transport systems. *Pharm. Sci. Technol. Today* 2: 49–59.
14 Saunders, N.R., Dreifuss, J.J., Dziegielewska, K.M. et al. (2014). The rights and wrongs of blood-brain barrier permeability studies: a walk through 100 years of history. *Front. Neurosci.* 8: 404.
15 Liu, L. and Liu, X. (2019). Contributions of drug transporters to blood-placental barrier. *Adv. Exp. Med. Biol.* 1141: 505–548.
16 Furukawa, S., Kuroda, Y., and Sugiyama, A. (2014). A comparison of the histological structure of the placenta in experimental animals. *J. Toxicol. Pathol.* 27: 11–18.
17 Baggot, J.D. and Short, C.R. (1984). Drug disposition in the neonatal animal, with particular reference to the foal. *Equine Vet. J.* 16: 364–367.
18 Sams, R.A. and Muir, W.W. (2009). principles of drug disposition and drug interaction in horses. In: *Equine Anesthesia, Monitoring and Emergency Therapy* (ed. W.W. Muir and J.A.E. Hubbell), 171–184. St. Louis, MO: Saunders Elsevier.
19 Verscheijden, L.F.M., Koenderink, J.B., de Wildt, S.N. et al. (2019). Development of a physiologically based pharmacokinetic pediatric brain model for prediction of cerebrospinal fluid drug concentrations and the influence of meningitis. *PLoS Comput. Biol.* 15: e1007117.
20 Loscher, W. and Friedman, A. (2020). Structural, molecular, and functional alterations of the blood-brain barrier during epileptogenesis and epilepsy: a cause, consequence, or both? *Int. J. Mol. Sci.* 21.
21 Hawkins, B.T. and Davis, T.P. (2005). The blood-brain barrier/neurovascular unit in health and disease. *Pharmacol. Rev.* 57: 173–185.
22 Kuperberg, S.J. and Wadgaonkar, R. (2017). Sepsis-associated encephalopathy: the blood-brain barrier and the sphingolipid rheostat. *Front. Immunol.* 8: 597.
23 Stolp, H.B., Johansson, P.A., Habgood, M.D. et al. (2011). Effects of neonatal systemic inflammation on blood-brain barrier permeability and behaviour in juvenile and adult rats. *Cardiovasc. Psychiatry Neurol.* 469046.
24 Kousik, S.M., Napier, T.C., and Carvey, P.M. (2012). The effects of psychostimulant drugs on blood brain barrier function and neuroinflammation. *Front. Pharmacol.* 3: 121.
25 Hacohen, Y., Singh, R., Forsyth, V. et al. (2014). CSF albumin and immunoglobulin analyses in childhood neurologic disorders. *Neurol. Neuroimmunol. Neuroinflamm.* 1: e10.
26 Al-Enazy, S., Ali, S., Albekairi, N. et al. (2017). Placental control of drug delivery. *Adv. Drug Deliv. Rev.* 116: 63–72.
27 Edwards, I.R. and Aronson, J.K. (2000). Adverse drug reactions: definitions, diagnosis, and management. *Lancet* 356: 1255–1259.
28 Stack, A. and Schott, H.C. 2nd (2011). Suspect novel adverse drug reactions to trimethoprim-sulphonamide combinations in horses: a case series. *Equine Vet. J.* 43: 117–120.
29 Naranjo, C.A., Busto, U., Sellers, E.M. et al. (1981). A method for estimating the probability of adverse drug reactions. *Clin. Pharmacol. Ther.* 30: 239–245.
30 Doherty, M.J. (2009). Algorithms for assessing the probablility of an adverse drug reaction. *Respir. Med. CME* 2: 63–67.
31 Manikandan, P. and Nagini, S. (2018). Cytochrome P450 structure, function and clinical significance: a review. *Curr. Drug Targets* 19: 38–54.
32 McDonnell, A.M. and Dang, C.H. (2013). Basic review of the cytochrome p450 system. *J. Adv. Pract. Oncol.* 4: 263–268.
33 Nout-Lomas, Y. (2018). Tetanus. In: *Equine Internal Medicine*, 4e (ed. S.M. Reed, W.M. Bayly, and D.C. Sellon), 668–672. Saunders.
34 Nout-Lomas, Y. (2018). Botulism. In: *Equine Internal Medicine*, 4e (ed. S.M. Reed, W.M. Bayly, and D.C. Sellon), 672–674. Saunders.
35 Plumlee, K.H. (2001). Pesticide toxicosis in the horse. *Vet. Clin. North Am. Equine Pract.* 17 (vii): 491–500.
36 Talcott, P. (2018). Toxicologic problems. In: *Equine Internal Medicine*, 4e (ed. S.M. Reed, W.M. Bayly, and D.C. Sellon), 1468–1484. Saunders.

37 Eyal, S. (2018). Use of therapeutics in pregnancy and lactation. *Pharm. Res.* 35: 107.

38 Verstegen, R.H.J. and Ito, S. (2019). Drugs in lactation. *J. Obstet. Gynaecol. Res.* 45: 522–531.

39 Anderson, P.O. (2018). Drugs in lactation. *Pharm. Res.* 35: 45.

40 Bracken, M.B. and Holford, T.R. (1981). Exposure to prescribed drugs in pregnancy and association with congenital malformations. *Obstet. Gynecol.* 58: 336–344.

41 Swor, T.M., Whittenburg, J.L., and Chaffin, M.K. (2009). Ivermectin toxicosis in three adult horses. *J. Am. Vet. Med. Assoc.* 235: 558–562.

42 Norman, T.E., Chaffin, M.K., Norton, P.L. et al. (2012). Concurrent ivermectin and Solanum spp. toxicosis in a herd of horses. *J. Vet. Intern. Med.* 26: 1439–1442.

43 Campbell, W.C. and Benz, G.W. (1984). Ivermectin: a review of efficacy and safety. *J. Vet. Pharmacol. Ther.* 7: 1–16.

44 Khan, S.A., Kuster, D.A., and Hansen, S.R. (2002). A review of moxidectin overdose cases in equines from 1998 through 2000. *Vet. Hum. Toxicol.* 44: 232–235.

45 Fardel, O., Lecureur, V., and Guillouzo, A. (1996). The P-glycoprotein multidrug transporter. *Gen. Pharmacol.* 27: 1283–1291.

46 Bruenisholz, H., Kupper, J., Muentener, C.R. et al. (2012). Treatment of ivermectin overdose in a miniature Shetland Pony using intravenous administration of a lipid emulsion. *J. Vet. Intern. Med.* 26: 407–411.

47 Plummer, C.E., Kallberg, M.E., Ollivier, F.J. et al. (2006). Suspected ivermectin toxicosis in a Miniature mule foal causing blindness. *Vet. Ophthalmol.* 9: 29–32.

48 Goehring, L.S. and Sloet van Oldruitenborgh-Oosterbaan, M.M. (1999). Moxidectin poisoning in a foal? *Tijdschr. Diergeneeskd.* 124: 412–414.

49 Johnson, P.J., Mrad, D.R., Schwartz, A.J. et al. (1999). Presumed moxidectin toxicosis in three foals. *J. Am. Vet. Med. Assoc.* 214: 678–680.

50 Pollio, D., Michau, T.M., Weaver, E. et al. (2018). Electroretinographic changes after intravenous lipid emulsion therapy in a dog and a foal with ivermectin toxicosis. *Vet. Ophthalmol.* 21: 82–87.

51 Mendell, C. (2006 (May 1)). Four horses dead, one ill; dewormer questioned. *The Horse* 24.

52 Merola, V.M. and Eubig, P.A. (2012). Toxicology of avermectins and milbemycins (macrocylic lactones) and the role of P-glycoprotein in dogs and cats. *Vet. Clin. North Am. Small Anim. Pract.* 42: 313–333, vii.

53 Hautekeete, L.A., Khan, S.A., and Hales, W.S. (1998). Ivermectin toxicosis in a zebra. *Vet. Hum. Toxicol.* 40: 29–31.

54 Button, C., Barton, R., Honey, P. et al. (1988). Avermectin toxicity in calves and an evaluation of picrotoxin as an antidote. *Aust. Vet. J.* 65: 157–158.

55 Muller, J.M., Feige, K., Kastner, S.B. et al. (2005). The use of sarmazenil in the treatment of a moxidectin intoxication in a foal. *J. Vet. Intern. Med.* 19: 348–349.

56 Hopper, K., Aldrich, J., and Haskins, S.C. (2002). Ivermectin toxicity in 17 collies. *J. Vet. Intern. Med.* 16: 89–94.

57 Sivine, F., Plume, C., and Ansay, M. (1985). Picrotoxin, the antidote to ivermectin in dogs? *Vet. Rec.* 116: 195–196.

58 Tranquilli, W.J., Paul, A.J., Seward, R.L. et al. (1987). Response to physostigmine administration in collie dogs exhibiting ivermectin toxicosis. *J. Vet. Pharmacol. Ther.* 10: 96–100.

59 Muhammad, G., Abdul, J., Khan, M.Z. et al. (2004). Use of neostigmine in massive ivermectin toxicity in cats. *Vet. Hum. Toxicol.* 46: 28–29.

60 Furr, M. (2008). Equine neurotoxic agents and conditions. In: *Equine Neurology*, 1e (ed. M. Furr and S.M. Reed), 337–356. Iowa: Blackwell Publishing.

61 Rose, R.J., Hartley, W.J., and Baker, W. (1981). Laryngeal paralysis in Arabian foals associated with oral haloxon administration. *Equine Vet. J.* 13: 171–176.

62 Bello, T.R. and Torbert, B.J. (1972). Toxicity of an organic phosphate anthelmintic (Shell SD 15803) at excessive dosages in two-month-old pony foals. *Am. J. Vet. Res.* 33: 329–334.

63 Reinecke, R.K., Loots, L.J., and Reinecke, P.M. (1980). The anthelmintic activity and toxicity of 2,2-dichlorovinyl dimethyl phosphate (dichlorvos) in equines. *J. S. Afr. Vet. Assoc.* 51: 21–24.

64 Drudge, J.H., Lyons, E.T., and Swerczek, T.W. (1974). Critical tests and safety studies on a levamisole-piperazine mixture as an anthelmintic in the horse. *Am. J. Vet. Res.* 35: 67–72.

65 Auer, D.E., Seawright, A.A., Pollitt, C.C. et al. (1984). Illness in horses following spraying with amitraz. *Aust. Vet. J.* 61: 257–259.

66 Ricci, L., Motolese, F., Tombini, M. et al. (2020). Metronidazole encephalopathy EEG features: a case report with systematic review of the literature. *Brain Sci.* 10: 227.

67 Agarwal, A., Kanekar, S., Sabat, S. et al. (2016). Metronidazole-induced cerebellar toxicity. *Neurol. Int.* 8: 6365.

68 Groothoff, M.V., Hofmeijer, J., Sikma, M.A. et al. (2010). Irreversible encephalopathy after treatment with high-dose intravenous metronidazole. *Clin. Ther.* 32: 60–64.

69 Tauro, A., Beltran, E., Cherubini, G.B. et al. (2018). Metronidazole-induced neurotoxicity in 26 dogs. *Aust. Vet. J.* 96: 495–501.

70 Dow, S.W., LeCouteur, R.A., Poss, M.L. et al. (1989). Central nervous system toxicosis associated with metronidazole treatment of dogs: five cases (1984–1987). *J. Am. Vet. Med. Assoc.* 195: 365–368.

71 Kushner, J.M., Peckman, H.J., and Snyder, C.R. (2001). Seizures associated with fluoroquinolones. *Ann. Pharmacother.* 35: 1194–1198.

72 Neame, M., King, C., Riordan, A. et al. (2020). Seizures and quinolone antibiotics in children: a systematic review of adverse events. *Eur. J. Hosp. Pharm.* 27: 60–64.

73 Bertone, A.L., Tremaine, W.H., Macoris, D.G. et al. (2000). Effect of long-term administration of an injectable enrofloxacin solution on physical and musculoskeletal variables in adult horses. *J. Am. Vet. Med. Assoc.* 217: 1514–1521.

74 Dawson, D.R. (2011). Toxins and adverse drug reactions affecting the equine nervous system. *Vet. Clin. North Am. Equine Pract.* 27: 507–526.

75 Olsen, L., Ingvast-Larsson, C., Brostrom, H. et al. (2007). Clinical signs and etiology of adverse reactions to procaine benzylpenicillin and sodium/potassium benzylpenicillin in horses. *J. Vet. Pharmacol. Ther.* 30: 201–207.

76 Mayhew, I.G.J. (2008). *Large Animal Neurology*. Wiley Blackwell.

77 Mattappalil, A. and Mergenhagen, K.A. (2014). Neurotoxicity with antimicrobials in the elderly: a review. *Clin. Ther.* 36: 1489, e1484–1511.

78 Grill, M.F. and Maganti, R.K. (2011). Neurotoxic effects associated with antibiotic use: management considerations. *Br. J. Clin. Pharmacol.* 72: 381–393.

79 Shaffer, C.L., Davey, A.M., Ransom, J.L. et al. (1998). Ampicillin-induced neurotoxicity in very-low-birth-weight neonates. *Ann. Pharmacother.* 32: 482–484.

80 Paradelis, A.G., Triantaphyllidis, C., and Giala, M.M. (1980). Neuromuscular blocking activity of aminoglycoside antibiotics. *Methods Find. Exp. Clin. Pharmacol.* 2: 45–51.

81 Hildebrand, S.V. and Hill, T. 3rd. (1994). Interaction of gentamycin and atracurium in anaesthetised horses. *Equine Vet. J.* 26: 209–211.

82 Nostrandt, A.C., Pedersoli, W.M., Marshall, A.E. et al. (1991). Ototoxic potential of gentamicin in ponies. *Am. J. Vet. Res.* 52: 494–498.

83 Dacre, K.J.P., Pirie, S., and Prince, D.P. (2003). Choke, pleuropneumonia and suspected gentamicin vestibulotoxicity in a horse. *Equine Vet. Educ.* 15: 27–30.

84 Cribb, A.E., Lee, B.L., Trepanier, L.A. et al. (1996). Adverse reactions to sulphonamide and sulphonamide-trimethoprim antimicrobials: clinical syndromes and pathogenesis. *Adverse Drug React. Toxicol. Rev.* 15: 9–50.

85 El-Boghdadly, K., Pawa, A., and Chin, K.J. (2018). Local anesthetic systemic toxicity: current perspectives. *Local Reg. Anesth.* 11: 35–44.

86 Dart, A.J. and Hodgson, D.R. (1998). Role of prokinetic drugs for treatment of postoperative ileus in the horse. *Aust. Vet. J.* 76: 25–31.

87 Brianceau, P., Chevalier, H., Karas, A. et al. (2002). Intravenous lidocaine and small-intestinal size, abdominal fluid, and outcome after colic surgery in horses. *J. Vet. Intern. Med.* 16: 736–741.

88 Seahorn, J. (2015). Sedation and analgesia. In: *Equine Emergency and Critical Care Medicine*, 1e (ed. L.L. Southwood and P.A. Wilkins), 685–696. Boca Raton, FL: CRC Press.

89 Rowe, E. (2008). Management of horses with gastrointestinal disorders. In: *The Equine Hospital Manual*, 1e (ed. K. Corley and J. Stephen), 499–515. Oxford: Blackwell Publishing.

90 Vieitez, V., Gomez de Segura, I.A., Martin-Cuervo, M. et al. (2017). Successful use of lipid emulsion to resuscitate a foal after intravenous lidocaine induced cardiovascular collapse. *Equine Vet. J.* 49: 767–769.

91 Isohanni, M.H., Ahonen, J., Neuvonen, P.J. et al. (2005). Effect of ciprofloxin on the pharmacokinetics of intravenous lidocaine. *Eur. J. Anaesthesiol.* 22: 795–799.

92 Muir, W.W. (2009). Anxiolytics, nonopioid sedative – analgesics, and opioid analgesics. In: *Equine Anesthesia, Monitoring and Emergency Therapy* (ed. W.W. Muir and J.A.E. Hubbell), 185–209. Missouri: Saunders Elsevier.

93 Muir, W.W. (2009). Intravenous anesthetic drugs. In: *Equine Anesthesia, Monitoring and Emergency Therapy* (ed. W.W. Muir and J.A.E. Hubbell), 243–259. Missouri: Saunders Elsevier.

94 Allen, W.E. (1986). Equine abortion and chloral hydrate. *Vet. Rec.* 118: 407.

95 Woodie, J.B. (2019). Uterus and ovaries. In: *Equine Surgery*, 5e (ed. J.A. Auer, J.A. Stick, J.M. Kummerle, and T. Prange), 1091. Missouri: Elsevier.

96 Prichard, J.T. and Voss, J.L. (1967). Fetal ankylosis in horses associated with hybrid Sudan pasture. *J. Am. Vet. Med. Assoc.* 150: 871–873.

97 Scheidt, A.B., Long, G.G., Knox, K. et al. (1987). Toxicosis in newborn pigs associated with cutaneous application of an aerosol spray containing chlorpyrifos. *J. Am. Vet. Med. Assoc.* 191: 1410–1412.

98 Stebler, T. and Guentert, T.W. (1990). Binding of drugs in milk: the role of casein in milk protein binding. *Pharm. Res.* 7: 633–637.

99 Barone, J.A. (1999). Domperidone: a peripherally acting dopamine2-receptor antagonist. *Ann. Pharmacother.* 33: 429–440.

100 Blodgett, D.J. (2001). Fescue toxicosis. *Vet. Clin. North Am. Equine Pract.* 17: 567–577.

101 Redmond, L.M., Cross, D.L., Strickland, J.R. et al. (1994). Efficacy of domperidone and sulpiride as treatments for fescue toxicosis in horses. *Am. J. Vet. Res.* 55: 722–729.

102 von During, S., Challet, C., and Christin, L. (2019). Endoscopic removal of a gastric pharmacobezoar

induced by clomipramine, lorazepam, and domperidone overdose: a case report. *J Med Case Reports* 13: 45.
103 Janssen (2018). Motilium (R) Domperidone Datasheet. edsafe.govt.nz motiliumtab.pdf (medsafe.govt.nz) (accessed 23 March 2023).
104 Edwards, H.G. (1986). Methiocarb poisoning in a horse. *Vet. Rec.* 119: 556.
105 Alexander, K.A. (1987). Methiocarb poisoning in a horse. *Vet. Rec.* 120: 47.
106 Kaye, B.M., Elliott, C.R., and Jalim, S.L. (2012). Methiocarb poisoning of a horse in Australia. *Aust. Vet. J.* 90: 221–224.
107 Krieger, R.I., South, P., Mendez Trigo, A. et al. (1998). Toxicity of methomyl following intravenous administration in the horse. *Vet. Hum. Toxicol.* 40: 267–269.
108 Wang, Y., Kruzik, P., Helsberg, A. et al. (2007). Pesticide poisoning in domestic animals and livestock in Austria: a 6 years retrospective study. *Forensic Sci. Int.* 169: 157–160.
109 Duncan, I.D. and Brook, D. (1985). Bilateral laryngeal paralysis in the horse. *Equine Vet. J.* 17: 228–233.
110 Easterwood, L., Chaffin, M.K., Marsh, P.S. et al. (2010). Phosphine intoxication following oral exposure of horses to aluminum phosphide-treated feed. *J. Am. Vet. Med. Assoc.* 236: 446–450.
111 Fox, J.H., Porter, B.F., Easterwood, L. et al. (2018). Acute hepatic steatosis: a helpful diagnostic feature in metallic phosphide-poisoned horses. *J. Vet. Diagn. Invest.* 30: 280–285.
112 St Omer, V.V. (1970). Chronic and acute toxicity of the chlorinated hydrocarbon insecticides in mammals and birds. *Can. Vet. J.* 11: 215–226.
113 Glenn, M.W. and Burr, W.M. (1972). Toxicity of a piperazine-carbon disulfide-phenothiazine preparation in the horse. *J. Am. Vet. Med. Assoc.* 160: 988–992.
114 Wikipedia (2020). Snake venom. Wikipedia.
115 Bamford, N.J., Sprinkle, S.B., Cudmore, L.A. et al. (2018). Elapid snake envenomation in horses: 52 cases (2006–2016). *Equine Vet. J.* 50: 196–201.
116 Fielding, C.L., Pusterla, N., Magdesian, K.G. et al. (2011). Rattlesnake envenomation in horses: 58 cases (1992–2009). *J. Am. Vet. Med. Assoc.* 238: 631–635.
117 Dickinson, C.E., Traub-Dargatz, J.L., Dargatz, D.A. et al. (1996). Rattlesnake venom poisoning in horses: 32 cases (1973–1993). *J. Am. Vet. Med. Assoc.* 208: 1866–1871.
118 Gilliam, L.L., Holbrook, T.C., Ownby, C.L. et al. (2012). Cardiotoxicity, inflammation, and immune response after rattlesnake envenomation in the horse. *J. Vet. Intern. Med.* 26: 1457–1463.
119 Anlen, K.G. (2008). Effects of bites by the European adder (*Vipera berus*) in seven Swedish horses. *Vet. Rec.* 162: 652–656.
120 Machado, M., Wilson, T.M., Ribeiro de Sousa, D.E. et al. (2019). Fatal lancehead pit viper (Bothrops spp.) envenomation in horses. *Toxicon* 170: 41–50.
121 Tirosh-Levy, S., Solomovich, R., Comte, J. et al. (2017). Daboia (Vipera) palaestinae envenomation in horses: clinical and hematological signs, risk factors for mortality and construction of a novel severity scoring system. *Toxicon* 137: 58–64.
122 Tee, S.Y. and Feary, D.J. (2012). Suspected tick paralysis (*Ixodes holocyclus*) in a Miniature Horse. *Aust. Vet. J.* 90: 181–185.
123 Ruppin, M., Sullivan, S., Condon, F. et al. (2012). Retrospective study of 103 presumed cases of tick (*Ixodes holocyclus*) envenomation in the horse. *Aust. Vet. J.* 90: 175–180.
124 Trumpp, K.M., Parsley, A.L., Lewis, M.J. et al. (2019). Presumptive tick paralysis in 2 American Miniature Horses in the United States. *J. Vet. Intern. Med.* 33: 1784–1788.
125 Bootes, B.W. (1962). A fatal paralysis in foals from ixodes holocyclus neumann infestation. *Aust. Vet. J.* 68–69.
126 Madigan, J.E., Valberg, S.J., Ragle, C. et al. (1995). Muscle spasms associated with ear tick (*Otobius megnini*) infestations in five horses. *J. Am. Vet. Med. Assoc.* 207: 74–76.
127 Camp, N.E. (2014). Black widow spider envenomation. *J. Emerg. Nurs.* 40: 193–194.
128 Wag (2023). Black widow spider bites in horses. https://wagwalking.com/horse/condition/black-widow-spider-bite (accessed 23 March 2023).
129 Lewis, N. and Racklyeft, D.J. (2014). Mass envenomation of a mare and foal by bees. *Aust. Vet. J.* 92: 141–148.
130 Cote, F.J. (1941). Death of a horse due to bee stinging. *Can. J. Comp. Med. Vet. Sci.* 5: 270.
131 Staempfli, H.R., Wollenebrg, G., and Jewell, G. (1993). Acute fatal reaction to bee stings in a mare. *Equine Vet. Educ.* 5: 250–252.
132 Wysoke, J.M., Bland van-den Berg, P., and Marshall, C. (1990). Bee sting-induced haemolysis, spherocytosis and neural dysfunction in three dogs. *J. S. Afr. Vet. Assoc.* 61: 29–32.
133 Daher, E.D., de Oliveira, R.A., da Silva, L.S.V. et al. (2009). Acute renal failure following bee stings: case reports. *Rev. Soc. Bras. Med. Trop.* 42: 209–212.
134 Bathe, A.P. (1994). An unusual manifestation of nettle rash in three horses. *Vet. Rec.* 134: 11–12.
135 Leaman, T.R. (2008). Nettle reaction in a foal. *Vet. Rec.* 162: 164.
136 Egan, D.A. and O'Cuill, T. (1970). Cumulative lead poisoning in horses in a mining area contaminated with galena. *Vet. Rec.* 86: 736–738.

137 Aronson, A.L. (1972). Lead poisoning in cattle and horses following long-term exposure to lead. *Am. J. Vet. Res.* 33: 627–629.

138 Dollahite, J.W., Younger, R.L., Crookshank, H.R. et al. (1978). Chronic lead poisoning in horses. *Am. J. Vet. Res.* 39: 961–964.

139 Kowalczyk, D.F., Naylor, J.M., and Gunson, D. (1981). The value of zinc protoporphyrin in equine lead poisoning: a case report. *Vet. Hum. Toxicol.* 23: 12–15.

140 Zellner, T., Prasa, D., Farber, E. et al. (2019). The use of activated charcoal to treat intoxications. *Dtsch. Arztebl. Int.* 116: 311–317.

141 Ju, C.A. (2000). Management of drug overdose and poisoning. *Nat. Pharm. Admin.* 3–89.

142 Furr, M. (2008). Congenital malformation of the nervous system. In: *Equine Neurology*, 1e (ed. M. Furr and S.M. Reed), 299–303. Hoboken, NJ: Wiley.

143 Wilkins, P.A. and Palmer, J.E. (2003). Mechanical ventilation in foals with botulism: 9 cases (1989–2002). *J. Vet. Intern. Med.* 17: 708–712.

144 van Galen, G., Saegerman, C., Rijckaert, J. et al. (2017). Retrospective evaluation of 155 adult equids and 21 foals with tetanus in Western, Northern, and Central Europe (2000–2014). Part 1: Description of history and clinical evolution. *J. Vet. Emerg. Crit. Care (San Antonio)* 27: 684–696.

145 Lee, J.A. (2015). Approach to drug overdose. In: *Small Animal Critical Care Medicine*, 2e (ed. D.C. Silverstein and K. Hopper), 385–389. Canada: Elsevier.

146 Lacombe, V. and Furr, F. (2008). Differential diagnosis and management of horses with seizures or alterations in consciousness. In: *Equine Neurology*, 1e (ed. M. Furr and S. Reed), 77–93.

147 Genuis, S.J., Birkholz, D., Rodushkin, I. et al. (2011). Blood, urine, and sweat (BUS) study: monitoring and elimination of bioaccumulated toxic elements. *Arch. Environ. Contam. Toxicol.* 61: 344–357.

148 Krageloh, T., Cavalleri, J.M.V., Ziegler, J. et al. (2018). Identification of hypoglycin A binding adsorbents as potential preventive measures in co-grazers of atypical myopathy affected horses. *Equine Vet. J.* 50: 220–227.

149 Buts, J.P. (1998). Bioactive factors in milk. *Arch. Pediatr.* 5: 298–306.

150 Matsumura, T., Fujinaga, Y., Jin, Y. et al. (2007). Human milk SIgA binds to botulinum type B 16S toxin and limits toxin adherence on T84 cells. *Biochem. Biophys. Res. Commun.* 352: 867–872.

151 Palm, C.A. and Kanakubo, K. (2015). Blood purification for intoxications and drug overdose. In: *Small Animal Critical Care Medicine*, 2e (ed. D.C. Silverstein and K. Hopper), 390–393. Canada: Elsevier.

152 Edmunds, J.L., Worgan, H.J., Dougal, K. et al. (2016). In vitro analysis of the effect of supplementation with activated charcoal on the equine hindgut. *J. Equine Sci.* 27: 49–55.

153 Fernandez, A.L., Lee, J.A., Rahilly, L. et al. (2011). The use of intravenous lipid emulsion as an antidote in veterinary toxicology. *J. Vet. Emerg. Crit. Care (San Antonio)* 21: 309–320.

154 Wikipedia (2020). List of cytochrome P450 modulators. https://en.wikipedia.org/wiki/List_of_cytochrome_P450_modulators (accessed 23 March 2023).

Section V Pathophysiology and Treatment of Central Nervous System Trauma in the Foal

Darien Feary and Gustavo Ferlini Agne

In the absence of clinical research evaluating treatments of traumatic central nervous system (CNS) injury in foals, clinicians must rely on overarching concepts extrapolated from people and small animal medicine to guide management. Some large human clinical trials have clear relevance and application to equids (prompt hemodynamic and respiratory support, seizure control, analgesia), while other recommendations are inconclusive (high-dose corticosteroids for acute spinal cord injury [SCI]; glucose supplementation) or difficult to achieve without advanced neuromonitoring and imaging (hyperosmolar therapy, decompressive surgery). Furthermore, some guidelines are not applied to foals because of reluctance to abandon traditional management approaches (use of DMSO and high-dose corticosteroids) when clinical impression suggests some benefit. Until more evidence of clinically effective therapies is available, acute management is driven by pathophysiologic principles and emphasis on interventions that attenuate secondary neurologic injury [1]. Priorities include prompt patient control to prevent further injury, early hemodynamic and respiratory support, seizure control, analgesia, nonsteroidal anti-inflammatory drug (NSAID) therapy, and hyperosmolar therapy when indicated. While clinical trials of many promising neuroprotective pharmacologic agents have yielded disappointing results, our understanding of the pathophysiology of CNS injury and repair is still evolving.

In many horses, long-term outcomes can be quite good following traumatic brain injury (TBI), even with substantial cortical loss, if the injury does not involve critical areas (e.g. visual cortex) [2–4]. Hence clinicians should be cautious about prognostication based on severity of clinical signs at initial presentation, particularly in young foals that are more amenable to intensive care than adult horses due to their smaller size. Each case should be evaluated individually with therapeutic decisions based on clinical and diagnostic information and provision for intensive care if required.

Pathophysiology of Traumatic CNS Injury

Traumatic CNS injury is conceptually divided into two phases: *primary* and *secondary* injury (Table 32.V.1). Current understanding of these mechanisms of injury in veterinary patients is based on literature addressing the complex and evolving understanding of traumatic CNS injury in experimental and clinical studies. It is reasonable to assume that similar pathophysiologic processes occur in foals. Reviews of the pathophysiology of traumatic CNS injury is found in the veterinary literature [3–7]. This section summarizes central pathophysiologic processes relevant to therapeutic and monitoring priorities.

Primary CNS Injury

Primary Injury refers to the physical damage to the brain or spinal cord parenchyma and blood vessels as a direct result of impact forces occurring immediately at the time of traumatic insult. Common types of primary TBI in foals include: (i) *coup* and *contracoup* contusions (Figure 32.V.1) or lacerations of the cerebral cortex resulting from acceleratory and deceleratory forces of impact to the frontal and parietal region (collisions, kicks, falls); and (ii) brainstem injury due to basioccipital, basisphenoid, or petrous bone fractures resulting from poll impact (flipping over backward). Associated vascular damage resulting in intracranial hemorrhage is an important effect of primary injury, potentially leading to progressive increases in intracranial pressure (ICP) and ischemia. Excessive traction of the optic nerve and pathway because of head trauma is an important type of primary brain injury,

Equine Neonatal Medicine, First Edition. Edited by David M. Wong and Pamela A. Wilkins.

Table 32.V.1 Primary injury and central secondary injury mechanisms involved in the pathophysiology of brain and spinal cord trauma.

	Secondary injury	
Primary injury	**Central nervous system**	**Systemic insults**
• Mechanical trauma	• Vascular damage	• Hypoxemia
	• Impaired pressure autoregulation	
	• BBB and BSCB breakdown	
• Hemorrhage	• Edema formation	• Hypotension
	• Vasogenic edema	
	• Cytotoxic edema	
	• Tissue hypoxia and Ischemia	• Hyper/hypoglycemia
	• Excitotoxicity	• Seizures
	• Increased extracellular glutamate	
	• NMDA receptor activation	
	• ATP-pump failure	
	• Na^{+} and Ca^{++} influx	
	• Intracellular Ca^{++} Accumulation	• Fever
	• Oxidative damage	
	• Reactive oxygen species	
	• Lipid peroxidation	
	• Pro-inflammatory and anti-inflammatory responses	
	• Cell death	
	• Necrosis	
	• Apoptosis	

Secondary injury may be exacerbated by systemic insults.
BBB, blood-brain barrier; BSCB, blood spinal cord barrier; NMDA, *N*-methyl-D-aspartate

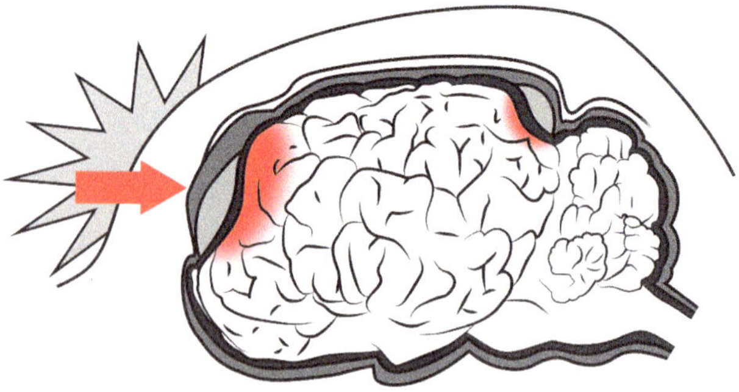

Figure 32.V.1 Coup-contrecoup injury describes the type of closed brain injury caused by rapid acceleration of the brain against the skull both at the site of impact (coup)[arrow], and also at the opposite side of the skull (contrecoup).

resulting in irreversible blindness in many cases. Specific types of brain and spinal injuries in foals are discussed elsewhere in this text.

Primary SCI in foals occurs from many of the same traumatic accidents that cause TBI, or from somersaulting and falls on a flexed neck [8]. These incidents likely result in compression and contusion type neuronal injury. Compression compromises spinal cord perfusion and causes direct mechanical damage to neurons. Although uncommon in equids, a displaced vertebral fracture can cause transection of the spinal cord. Foals appear to have a higher incidence of cranial cervical injuries associated with fractures and subluxations of the occipital or atlanto-axial bones. Pathologic vertebral fractures associated with osteomyelitis caused by bacterial pathogens (*Rhodococcus equi*, *Streptococcus equi*) are less common causes of spinal cord trauma. Unlike primary brain injury, traumatic vertebral fractures and luxations cause vertebral instability and repetitive spinal cord trauma. Prompt stabilization of unstable vertebra is necessary to prevent compounded primary injury.

Secondary CNS Injury

Damage caused by primary mechanical injury causes neuronal and vascular damage, which activates a complex cascade of biochemical pathways, referred to as *secondary injury,* that progresses minutes to weeks following trauma, and perpetuates further CNS injury. Although primary injury is irreversible and often dictates outcome following traumatic CNS injury, there is a window of opportunity post-trauma to prevent and treat secondary processes. Acute secondary CNS injury is characterized by several mechanisms common to both TBI and SCI including vascular changes and loss of pressure autoregulation, cellular ion dysregulation, ATP depletion, excitotoxity, intracellular calcium accumulation, oxidative damage, neuronal apoptosis, and initiation of proinflammatory and immune responses [9]. These mechanisms are conceptually illustrated as distinct biochemical pathways that have complex interactions (Figure 32.V.2).

Secondary injury is not easily measured but is clinically significant because secondary mechanisms are exacerbated by systemic variables such as hypotension, hypoxia, hyperthermia, and systemic inflammation. Understanding these mechanisms, along with prompt recognition and treatment of systemic insults, form the basis of a multimodal therapeutic approach to CNS injury in foals. The cellular and biochemical mechanisms of secondary injury

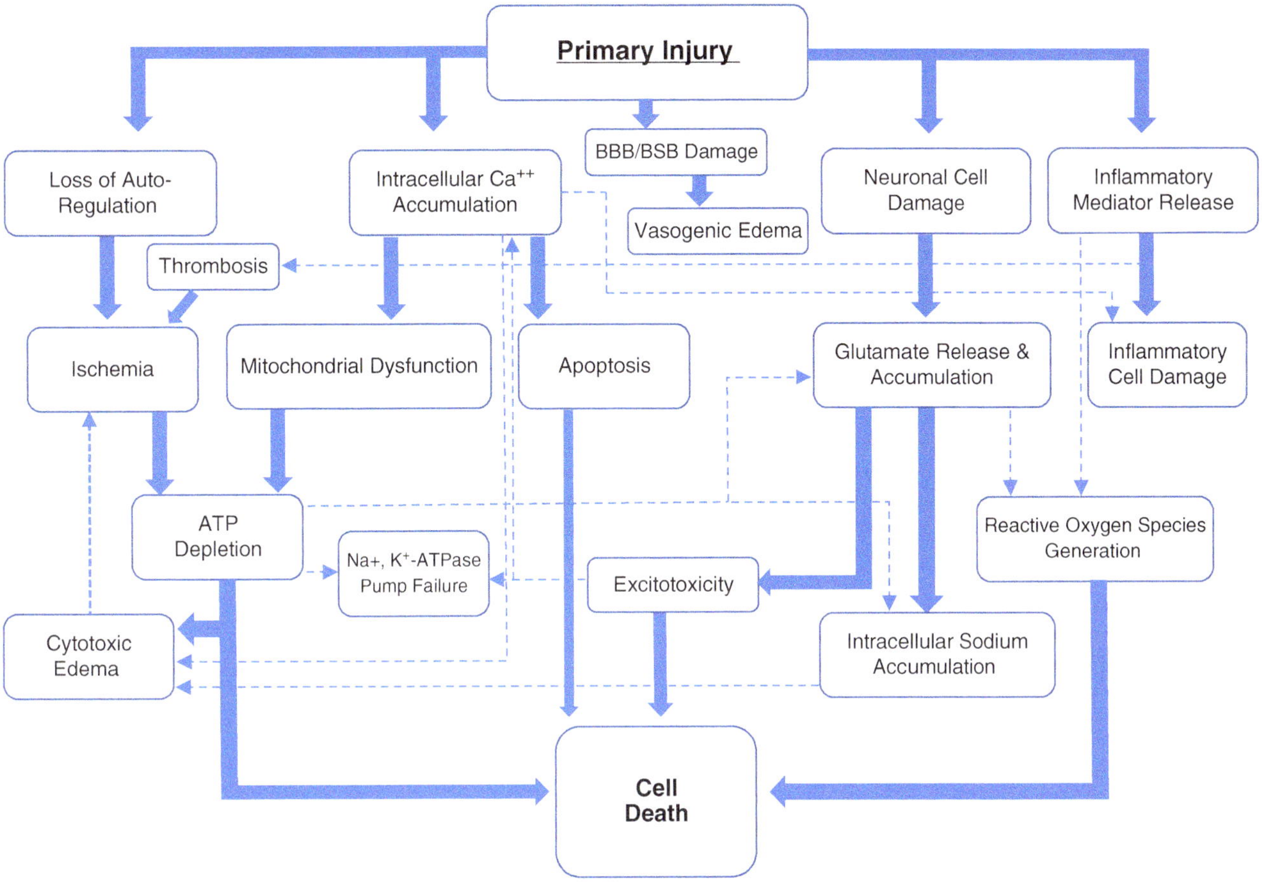

Figure 32.V.2 Overview of interrelated vascular and biochemical changes associated with secondary injury in central nervous system trauma; the secondary mechanisms involved have been targets of therapeutic interventions to improve patient outcome. BBB, blood-brain barrier; BSB, blood-spinal barrier. *Source:* modified from Park [6].

are similar for both TBI and SCI, however, there are significant anatomical differences that influence the development of ischemia in brain and SCI. These processes include ICP dynamics, types of edema, and spinal cord ischemia.

Intracranial Pressure Dynamics

ICP is central to the pathophysiology and management of TBI as progressive increases in ICP can overwhelm compensatory mechanisms, leading to decreased cerebral perfusion and subsequent brain ischemia. ICP is the combined pressure exerted by brain parenchyma, blood, and CSF within the rigid cranial vault. Under normal circumstances, the pressure-volume relationship between these three components remains constant, so that ICP is maintained within a normal range. Intracranial hemorrhage and brain edema increase intracranial volume, stimulating compensatory fluid shifts from the vascular and CSF compartments to protect the brain from increased ICP (*intracranial compliance*) [10]. If intracranial volume overwhelms the compensatory mechanism, ICP rises dramatically, leading to compromised cerebral perfusion pressure (CPP) and brain ischemia. The focus of therapy for TBI in people is reduction and management of ICP.

CPP is the main determinant of cerebral blood flow, and thus brain oxygenation and energy supply. CPP is related to ICP and mean arterial pressure (MAP) according to the formula: CPP = MAP − ICP. *Autoregulation* is the ability of blood vessels in the brain and spinal cord to constrict or dilate to maintain constant blood flow. In people and animals, autoregulation maintains a normal perfusion pressure between 50 and 140 mmHg [11]. According to this relationship in the brain, increased ICP or decreased MAP results in reduced CPP. Conversely, if MAP increases then CPP increases. A CPP <50 mmHg can result in cerebral hypoxia and ischemia, while a CPP >150 mmHg can result in cerebral edema [12]. *Systemic hypotension* is critically important because of potential loss of CPP autoregulation if CNS injury is severe. With loss of pressure autoregulation, cerebral and spinal cord blood flow becomes proportional to systemic blood pressure. Hence the importance of maintaining MAP when managing traumatic CNS injury. The autoregulatory system was believed to be similar in the brain and spinal cord [13]. However, experimental research notes that spinal cord autoregulation is not as robust as cerebral autoregulation and that oxygenation in the spinal cord is more pressure-dependent. This implies that avoiding hypotension is more important for maintaining the oxygenation level in the spinal cord compared to the brain [14].

Brain and Spinal Cord Edema

Two types of edema are recognized in traumatic CNS injury: vasogenic and cytotoxic (or cellular) edema. *Vasogenic edema* is characterized by *extracellular* fluid accumulation caused by disruption of the blood brain barrier (BBB) or blood spinal barrier (BSB) and increased permeability of capillary endothelial cells, allowing protein-rich fluid to accumulate and increasing extracellular fluid volume [15]. Vasogenic edema displaces CNS tissue and increases ICP or spinal interstitial pressure, reducing blood flow. Vasogenic edema was previously thought to be the predominant type of traumatic brain edema, hence the therapeutic use of hyperosmolar solutions to treat increased ICP. However, evidence suggests cytotoxic edema also plays a major role [16], and both types occur at different stages of the secondary brain injury cascade in experimental models. *Cytotoxic/cellular edema* is characterized by sustained *intracellular* fluid accumulation of astrocytes, neurons, and endothelial cells and develops through cellular energy failure due to local hypoxia, dysfunction of cell membrane Na^+, K^+-ATPase pumps, and subsequent intracellular sodium (Na^+) and calcium (Ca^{++}) influx and passive water accumulation. Cytotoxic edema occurs independently of BBB or BSB integrity, is not associated with increased capillary permeability, and results in decreased extracellular fluid volume.

Spinal Cord Hemorrhage and Ischemia

Primary injury to the CNS causes rapid local damage to microvessels and neuronal cells, acute and progressive hemorrhage, vasospasm, and ischemia that mainly affects the central gray matter of the spinal cord at the point of mechanical impact; this lesion represents central hemorrhagic necrosis and extends cranial and caudal to the site of injury [17, 18]. Progressive, small hemorrhages and vasoconstriction during the acute phase is a main causes of initial damage to the spinal cord [17]. Secondary injury mechanisms extend the central area of cell damage and death outward through necrosis and apoptosis, and eventually demyelination of axons in the white matter. Early endothelial cell death and BSB breakdown contributes to vasogenic edema and additional spinal cord compression. Spinal cord ischemia develops within several hours. Loss of pressure autoregulation in the spinal cord contributes to further hypoperfusion as blood flow becomes dependant on systemic blood pressure. Furthermore, systemic hypotension from hypovolemia or neurogenic shock (hypotension, bradycardia) contributes to ischemia and subsequent outcome in human patients [19].

Cellular and Biochemical Mechanisms of Secondary Injury

Excitotoxicity

Neuronal cell damage alters membrane permeability, allowing Na^+ and chloride (Cl^-) influx, potassium (K^+) efflux and release and extracellular accumulation of excitatory neurotransmitters. Excitotoxicity refers to overactivation of excitatory amino acid receptors because of excessive release of excitatory neurotransmitters, primarily glutamate. Excessive extracellular glutamate is an important mechanism in TBI and SCI [18, 20]. Glutamate is directly excitotoxic but also stimulates numerous receptors, notably *N*-methyl-D-aspartate (NMDA), kainic, and α-amino-3-hydroxy-5-methyl-4-isoxazolepropionic acid (AMPA) receptors and voltage-dependent Ca^{++} and Na^+ channels, producing rapid influx of Na^+ and slower influx of Ca^{++}. Low ATP concentrations from local tissue hypoxia result in failure of energy-dependant Na^+, K^+-ATPase pumps to actively remove Na^+ from neuronal cells. Uncontrolled Na^+ influx causes passive movement of water into neurons and glia resulting in cytotoxic edema. Intracellular Ca^{++} ion accumulation triggers numerous destructive processes that lead to cellular and vascular membrane degradation and ultimately necrotic or apoptotic cell death [6].

Intracellular Ca^{++} Accumulation

Sustained elevation of intracellular Ca^{++} is postulated as the final common pathway for cellular dysfunction and death in multiple tissues. Increased concentrations of cytosolic and mitochondrial Ca^{++} activate multiple pathways that destroy cell membranes, inhibit mitochondrial function, and bind phosphates to cause further ATP depletion. Calcium activates the arachidonic acid cascade (by binding phospholipase A_2), leading to production of inflammatory mediators that perpetuate secondary CNS injury. Excessive Ca^{++} also leads to formation of reactive oxygen species

(ROS) and lipid peroxidation. Calcium is also a major player in initiating cellular necrosis and apoptosis through activation of calpain and caspase enzymes [21].

Oxidative Damage

Neuronal cell membranes contain high concentrations of polyunsaturated fatty acids and cholesterol and are particularly susceptible to lipid peroxidation by ROS [10]. Post-traumatic oxidative damage is a significant and widely researched mechanism of secondary brain and SCI in experimental models [20, 22, 23]. ROS are produced early in the secondary injury cascade by Ca^{++}-dependent activation, ischemic conditions, arachidonic acid metabolites, activated neutrophils, and in the presence of iron and copper complexes within areas of hemorrhage [20]. Secondary hemorrhage occurs as petechial hemorrhages and continue to form during the first 24 hours following SCI injury [24]. Blood products are directly toxic to CNS cells through iron-dependant mechanisms and also catalyze lipid peroxidation and damage to neuronal cell membranes [25]. Lipid peroxidation initiates a cycle of ongoing oxidative damage to cell membrane pumps, cellular proteins and DNA and inhibits mitochondrial respiration [26].

Inflammatory and Immunological Responses

The CNS was previously considered to be an immune privileged site and therefore the inflammatory response to trauma and infection was believed to be less robust than other tissues [27]. Further understanding of posttraumatic neuroinflammation demonstrates that CNS inflammation is proportional to injury severity [28]. It is also well recognized that trauma activates both pro- and anti-inflammatory cytokines, and therefore has detrimental and beneficial effects [29]. Posttraumatic CNS inflammation is characterized by a rapid, robust production of pro-inflammatory cytokines and chemokines by local cells (microglia, astrocytes, oligodendrocytes, neurons, endothelial cells) at the injury site [11]. Pro-inflammatory cytokines are produced within minutes by locally activated microglial cells, perpetuating the inflammatory response, and cause further neuronal damage as well as recruit peripheral leukocytes that infiltrate the site of injury. Accumulation of peripheral leukocytes in the injured tissue is facilitated by increased vascular permeability and disruption of the BBB or BSB. These mediators promote metabolism of arachidonic acid and elaboration of proinflammatory prostanoids and kinins and activate complement and the coagulation cascade [7, 10]. These complex secondary injury reactions cause extensive neuronal damage and death and affect surrounding viable tissue. Thus, CNS injury can potentially be greater than the initial insult [11].

Although early inflammatory processes are detrimental, a subset of cells produced by the inflammatory response are important for neuronal regeneration and survival. The benefits of posttraumatic neuroinflammation include the ability of activated microglia to remove dying cell debris and produce neurotropic factors essential for repair [28]. Many cytokines themselves are also capable of anti-inflammatory action, reducing excitotoxicity, and promoting neurogenesis [29]. This evolving understanding of the complex effects of inflammatory response provides a possible explanation for the failure of initially promising interventions with single anti-inflammatory agents to improve outcomes in clinical trials (e.g. high-dose corticosteroids).

Systemic Contributions to Secondary Brain Injury

Systemic derangements in homeostasis contribute to secondary CNS injury and are critical to monitor and manage early in post-TBI and SCI. Addressing systemic hypotension and hypoxemia is critically important because they are independently associated with poor outcomes in adult and pediatric human patients with traumatic CNS injury [30–32]. Other important systemic derangements to address include hyperthermia, hyper- or hypoglycemia, hyper- or hypocapnia and abnormalities in electrolytes and acid–base balance.

Neurogenic Shock

Neurogenic shock is a form of distributive shock recognized in some patients following severe traumatic CNS injury, primarily involving the cervical and upper thoracic spinal cord, but also TBI. Circulatory changes result from dysfunction of descending sympathetic pathways and unopposed vagal tone, causing decreased systemic vascular resistance and vasodilation [19]. Neurogenic shock is clinically characterized by relative bradycardia in the setting of profound hypotension, although this represents a simplified definition. In reality, the hemodynamic derangements can be quite varied [33]. Hypothermia may develop readily in neonatal patients because of profound vasodilation and heat loss. Definitive diagnosis of neurogenic shock is problematic because of possible confounding hypovolemia and/or hemorrhage. Hypotension places patients at risk of secondary CNS injury due to loss of autoregulation. Neurogenic shock occurs almost immediately and persists for variable periods of time. Early management of neurogenic shock, typically in the field/prehospital setting, is important and can contribute to outcome [34, 35].

Treatment of Traumatic Brain and Spinal Cord Injury in Foals

General Considerations

Despite research identifying therapies that inhibit mediators of secondary CNS injury showing promise in experimental models, all have failed to demonstrate significant benefit in human trials. The mechanisms of CNS injury are extremely complex, and no single agent provides sufficient neuroprotection alone. A therapeutic approach that targets multiple aspects of injury is therefore logical. Previous recommendations for treatment of acute CNS injury in equids focused on aggressive reduction of inflammation [36–39]. Thus, anti-inflammatory therapy has been the mainstay of treatment of CNS trauma in horses, as was the case in people before publication of the landmark clinical trial (MRC CRASH trial) in 2004 [40]. Use of high doses of corticosteroids (dexamethasone, prednisolone sodium succinate, methylprednisolone) are routinely administered in horses, along with NSAIDs and DMSO [38, 39, 41–43]. There is scant literature on clinical management of traumatic CNS injury in foals with most case reports focused on the utility of advanced diagnostic imaging techniques [43–45].

As large-scale clinical trials regarding treatment of CNS injury in people have become available, treatment has focused on prehospital emergency management of trauma. Significantly improved outcomes have been achieved before patients reach the hospital by rapid recognition of hypoperfusion and hypoxemia, resuscitation, and direct transport to specialist facilities. In the hospital, advanced monitoring of ICP and optimizing CPP improve outcomes by minimizing secondary injury with early intervention [46, 47]. Equine practitioners are the first responders to traumatic CNS injury in foals and play a critical role in influencing outcome when the primary injury is not obviously incompatible with recovery. The following treatment recommendations suggest a prioritized approach to treatment of CNS injury in foals, emphasizing therapies with clear evidence-based justification for use. *Priority One* therapies focus on initial stabilization with consideration of optimal fluid therapy, airway and oxygenation, and seizure control (Table 32.V.2). *Priority Two* therapies include provision of anti-inflammatory, analgesic, nutrition, and antimicrobial therapies where indicated. Additional unproven therapies may be beneficial based on experimental research. Of note, in these recommendations:

- Medical management of elevated ICP using hyperosmolar therapy in foals is best performed when monitoring of fluid balance and blood biochemistry parameters are available.
- Neuromonitoring and advanced diagnostic imaging may not be readily available for foals. Instead, clinicians must interpret the patient's response to treatment based on frequent reassessment of neurologic examination. This is challenging when the foal's neurologic status is altered by co-morbidities or a requirement for continuous sedation.
- Use of corticosteroids is no longer standard-of-care for acute TBI or SCI in human or veterinary medicine. While anti-inflammatory therapy remains important in overall management of neurologic trauma, routine use of high-dose corticosteroids in equine CNS trauma should be reconsidered, and probably avoided altogether in foals with CNS injury.

Management Priorities and Initial Assessment

Triage of acute TBI includes an initial assessment, safety of personnel and the patient, and prioritized management until the patient receives systemic support and seizures are treated. More detailed diagnostic assessment can proceed following initial stabilization. Initial diagnostic assessment focuses on circulatory volume, perfusion parameters and respiratory pattern. Neurologic status is assessed based on level of consciousness, posture, motor activity, and pupillary responsiveness, prior to sedation (if required). Assessment of hematocrit, total solids, lactate, glucose, electrolytes, and blood gas analysis is indicated, and pulse oximetry and indirect blood pressure monitored, if available, during initial stabilization. Foals with TBI typically present with clinical signs consistent with the injured region of the cerebrum or brainstem. The most common injury in foals occurs to the brainstem from flipping over backward and striking the poll; common clinical signs include depressed mentation or stupor, head tilt, facial nerve paralysis, nystagmus, ataxia, circling, blindness, and possible hemorrhage from the nose and ear (Figure 32.V.3). Hemorrhage from the nose and/or ear indicates the possibility of an unstable basilar bone fracture and risk of asphyxia from hemorrhage into the guttural pouches and compression of the pharyngeal area. Establishing a patent airway may be urgently required in this scenario. A prioritized approach to acute and ongoing management is suggested (Table 32.V.2 for summary and drug dosages).

Priority One Treatments: Airway, Oxygen, and Ventilation

Airway

Indications for intubation (nasotracheal or endotracheal) in foals with brain or spinal cord trauma are listed in Table 32.V.3. The upper airway can become obstructed, particularly with poll injury secondary to flipping over

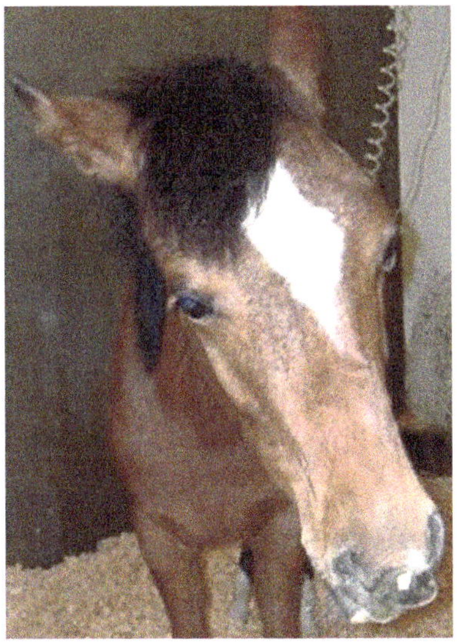

Figure 32.V.3 Weanling demonstrating head tilt toward the right after traumatic injury to the poll.

backward, as this type of injury can result in significant tissue disruption, hemorrhage, and swelling of the guttural pouches; this consequently results in pharyngeal compression and subsequent asphyxia. Foals with fresh blood from the nares and/or ear canal are at higher risk of asphyxia due to hemorrhage. In these cases, a patent airway should be established promptly (e.g. tracheostomy). Nasotracheal or endotracheal tube placement can be considered but requires head and neck extension that could potentially exacerbate further trauma in the presence of displaced basilar skull fractures. A significant amount of blood in the upper respiratory tract and risk of lower airway contamination must also be considered. Prehospital rapid endotracheal intubation improved neurologic outcomes and is recommended in pediatric patients with severe TBI for airway protection and ICP management [48, 49]. This recommendation should be considered in foals with clinical judgment used to determine if intubation is required.

Oxygen

Nasal oxygen insufflation is recommended with cerebral trauma if the foal tolerates administration without struggling or coughing. Decreased oxygen delivery to the brain is a main contributor to secondary brain injury and hypoxia following TBI and is an independent predictor of nonsurvival in adult and pediatric patients, as well as dogs [30, 50, 51]. Nasal oxygen is administered at 10–15 l/min during initial evaluation and stabilization of foals with cerebral trauma. If pulse oximetry and arterial blood gas analysis are available, oxygenation status can be directly assessed. The goal is to achieve normal oxygenation ($SpO_2 > 95\%$ and $P_aO_2 > 80\,mmHg$), although a $P_aO_2 > 60\,mmHg$ is recommended in human pediatric patients [52, 53]. The distal tip of the nasal cannula should not extend past the medial canthus to avoid communication with the cranial vault through a fracture site. Although uncommon, pneumocephalus has been reported in horses with head trauma and can complicate interpretation of neurologic status [54]. Some foals may require intubation and manual or mechanical ventilation to maintain normal oxygenation.

Ventilation

Carbon dioxide serves as a powerful determinant of cerebral blood flow by regulating vessel tone and diameter [53]. Hyperventilation lowers ICP by vasoconstriction and reduced cerebral blood flow and thereby cerebral blood volume in regions with intact CO_2 reactivity. The common practice of prophylactic hyperventilation ($P_aCO_2 < 30\,mmHg$) in older goal-directed neurocritical care is no longer recommended as it may cause excessive cerebral vasoconstriction, reduce global cerebral blood flow, and perpetuate hypoperfusion [55]. Short-term hyperventilation is reserved for patients with refractory intracranial hypertension and impending brain herniation [52]. Hypoventilation and subsequent increased P_aCO_2 may occur more readily in young foals because of their compliant chest, poor respiratory muscle tone, and low end-expiratory volume [56]. Hypoventilation could reasonably occur in foals with recent TBI due to traumatic injury to the brain's respiratory center, oversedation, mechanical airway obstruction, or thoracic pain and respiratory muscle fatigue. Ventilation should be assessed via arterial or venous blood gas analysis (venous CO_2 levels are typically 5 mmHg higher than corresponding P_aCO_2). If hypoventilation is identified ($P_aCO_2 > 60\,mmHg$ or $P_vCO_2 > 65\,mmHg$), then manual ventilation with a nasotracheal tube and ambubag can be performed in recumbent foals to maintain normocarbia (P_aCO_2 35–40 mmHg). Mechanical ventilation is indicated in foals with severe hypoxemia ($P_aO_2 < 60\,mmHg$) despite oxygen insufflation, severe hypoventilation ($P_aCO_2 > 65\,mmHg$), and when the ability to ventilate is impaired due to thoracic trauma, respiratory muscle failure, or fatigue.

Sedation, Analgesia, and Patient Positioning

Sedation and Analgesia

Control of clinical signs that contribute to further injury is important; sedation should be administered as necessary to avoid further trauma or implement treatment. Although neonatal foals are easily restrained, any cause of anxiety, pain, or fractious behavior will increase cerebral metabolic rate and ICP, which must be avoided [53]. Some foals with TBI present in an obtunded or comatose state and show no obvious signs of pain, but a traumatic insult requires

Table 32.V.2 Treatment summary of priority one, two, and adjunctive therapies for central nervous system injury.

Priority One

- Oxygen, airway, and ventilation
  - Ensure airway is patent
  - Nasal oxygen supplementation (if needed) at 10–15 l/min
  - Goal: $SpO_2 > 95\%$ and $P_aO_2 > 80$ mmHg
  - Manual or mechanical ventilation if hypoxemic ($P_aO_2 < 60$ mmHg) despite O_2 supplementation or severe hypoventilation ($PaCO_2 > 65$ mmHg)
- Sedation and analgesia
  - Benzodiazepine: Midazolam (0.02–0.2 mg/kg, IV or IM) or diazepam (0.02–0.2 mg/kg, IV) given alone or with
  - Opioid: Butorphanol (0.05–0.1 mg/kg, IV or IM)
  - Avoid alpha-2 agonists and acepromazine if possible (negative cardiovascular effects)
- Patient positioning
  - If foal recumbent, elevate head slightly (15–30° angle) from horizontal to optimize arterial and venous blood flow and reduce ICP
- Fluid therapy
  - Prevent or treat hypovolemia to avoid hypotension and decreased blood perfusion to brain; avoid overhydration
  - 10–20 ml/kg fluid boluses with frequent clinical reassessment
  - Normasol-R or Plasmalyte-148 preferred choice as they have more physiologic electrolyte concentrations
  - Normal (0.9%) saline may also be beneficial for initial resuscitation
- Maintain Homeostasis
  - Maintain mean arterial pressure: Target MAP of ≥75 mmHg for first few days following CNS injury; may need inotrope or vasopressor if MAP remains low despite adequate volume replacement
  - Glucose: maintain euglycemia (70–110 mg/dl); 1–5% dextrose in isotonic fluids if needed
  - Thiamine (Vitamin B_1) supplementation
- Seizure control
  - First-line: Midazolam (0.02–0.2 mg/kg, IV or IM;) or diazepam (0.02–0.2 mg/kg, IV)
  - Second-line: Phenobarbital (2–3 mg/kg, IV slow bolus to effect over 15 min), Levetiracetam (32 mg/kg, PO or IV, q12h), or midazolam CRI (0.02–0.06 mg/kg/h, IV)
  - Intractable seizures: Propofol (2 mg/kg, IV slow), pentobarbital (2–10 mg/kg, IV titrate to effect)
- Temperature control
  - Avoid fever/hyperthermia – favor permissive hypothermia (35–37 °C); If needed, active cooling with cold (4 °C) IV fluids, ice packs, fans, NSAIDs

Priority Two

- Hyperosmolar therapy
  - Use to decrease ICP or signs of brain herniation; only effective in management of vasogenic edema
  - Mannitol (20%; 0.25–1.0 g/kg, slow IV bolus over 10–20 min, every 4–8 h for maximum of 3 doses/24 h)
- Anti-inflammatory therapy
  - Corticosteroid therapy controversial in CNS trauma; not universally accepted
  - Dexamethasone sodium phosphate (0.1–0.25 mg/kg, IV), methylprednisolone sodium succinate (10–30 mg/kg, IV)
  - Flunixine meglumine (1.1 mg/kg, IV, q12h), ketoprofen (2.2 mg/kg, IV or IM, q24h), meloxicam (0.6 mg/kg, IV or IM, q24h), firocoxib (0.1 mg/kg, IV or PO, q12 -24 h following loading dose 0.3 mg/kg)
- Antimicrobial therapy
  - Broad-spectrum antimicrobials indicated with traumatic head injuries, cranial or vertebral fractures
  - Consider 3rd or 4th generation cephalosporins (Ceftriaxone, Cefotaxime), Chloramphenicol
- Nutritional support
  - Early enteral nutritional support; use IV dextrose supplementation if necessary

Adjunctive Therapies

- Antioxidant therapy
  - DMSO (0.5–1.0 g/kg, IV diluted to 10–20% in isotonic fluids); α-Tocopherol (Vitamin E; 1000–2000 U/day, PO), Thiamine (0.02 mg/kg IV or IM q 24hr) Vitamin C; (50–100 mg/kg IV q 6–12 hr, PO or 25 mg/kg, IV), Allopurinol (30–44 mg/kg, PO [poor bioavailability in foals, requires further study])
- Magnesium Sulfate: blocks NMDA receptors; 50 mg/kg, IV (diluted in IV fluids to ≤10%), then 15–20 mg/kg/h for 24 h
- Therapeutic hypothermia (see text)
- Tetracyclines – possible anti-inflammatory effects
  - Minocycline (4 mg/kg, PO, q12h) or Doxycycline (10 mg/kg, PO, q12h)

Table 32.V.3 Suggested indications for endotracheal/nasotracheal intubation in foals with traumatic brain or spinal cord injury.

- Upper respiratory tract obstruction: Basilar skull fracture and retropharyngeal hemorrhage (tracheostomy preferred)
- Comatose state
- $P_aO_2 < 60$ mmHg (despite oxygen therapy)
- $P_{a/v}CO_2 > 60–65$ mmHg
- Thoracic trauma/increased work of breathing

provision of analgesia and should be considered during initial stabilization. A combination of benzodiazepines and butorphanol is an excellent choice for sedation and analgesia of neonatal foals. Both provide good sedation and anxiolysis with minimal cardiovascular or intracranial effects; benzodiazepines cause muscle relaxation that can result in temporary recumbency [56]. Both agents have mild depressive effects on respiration but are manageable and reversible if hypoventilation occurs. Nasal insufflation of oxygen during sedation and recumbency is warranted. Midazolam (0.02–0.2 mg/kg IV or IM) or diazepam (0.02–0.2 mg/kg IV) can be given alone, or in combination with butorphanol (0.05–0.1 mg/kg IV or IM) and provide sedation for approximately 30 minutes in young foals. Benzodiazepines do not provide analgesia, so are best combined with an opioid in the management of traumatic CNS injury. The benzodiazepine–opioid combination should be attempted first but may not provide adequate sedation in juvenile foals 1–6 months of age [56]. Alpha-2 agonists and acepromazine should be avoided in foals with TBI due to negative cardiovascular effects. However, if safety dictates further restraint, small doses of xylazine (0.2–1.0 mg/kg IV or IM) combined with butorphanol should be considered in foals >2 weeks of age.

Patient Positioning for Traumatic Brain Injury

Head elevation is recommended as a simple method to minimize increases in ICP during initial evaluation of standing or recumbent foals. If the foal is horizontally recumbent, slight head elevation at a 15–30° angle from horizontal is recommended to optimize arterial and venous blood flow and reduce elevated ICP following TBI [4, 48, 53, 57]. The use of a board or firm padding to elevate the entire neck and head is useful to prevent bending of the neck and obstruction of jugular venous drainage, which results in elevated ICP (Figure 32.V.4) [3, 53]. For sternally recumbent or standing foals, the head should be supported in a neutral position using towels, hay bales, or other support (Figure 32.V.5). Bandaging around the neck for securing IV catheters must not be constrictive.

(a)
(b)

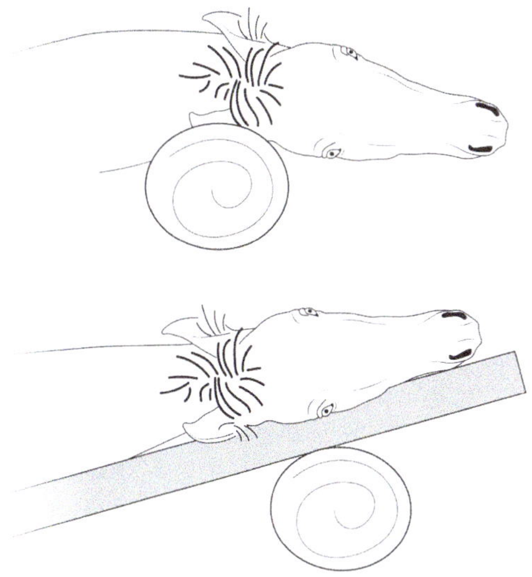

Figure 32.V.4 Elevated head position of up to 30° is recommended to reduce intracranial pressure and increase cerebral perfusion pressure. (a) Incorrect head elevation with a rolled-up towel leading to possible kinking of the neck and compression of jugular venous drainage. (b) Correct application of a rigid board or padding allowing head and neck elevation while avoiding obstruction of jugular venous drainage.

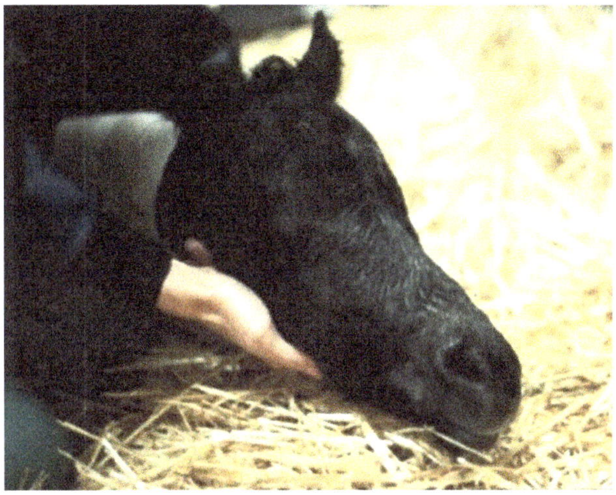

Figure 32.V.5 Position of obtunded foal in sternal recumbency with head elevated above shoulder level to prevent increased ICP following TBI. *Source:* Image courtesy of Dr. K.G. Magdesian, UC Davis.

Immobilization for traumatic SCI may be required in foals with suspected cervical vertebral fractures to prevent further primary injury. External stabilization is often not required in adult horses with suspected vertebral fractures because of the muscle mass surrounding the cervical and thoracolumbar vertebrae. Foals have much less muscle mass to stabilize the cervical spine, and consideration should be given to immobilize the spine with a supportive neck bandage or on a backboard during initial evaluation.

Fluid Therapy in CNS Trauma

General Principles

Early hemodynamic support is a priority in acute management of TBI and SCI (Table 32.V.4). Consistent evidence in people with TBI demonstrates the negative effect that even a single episode of hypotension can have on short and long-term outcome. Hemodynamic resuscitation (within 30 minutes of documented hypotension) during prehospital settings improves outcomes in pediatric TBI [58]. Therefore, prevention or treatment of hypovolemia and hypotension cannot be overemphasized in the initial and ongoing management of foals with CNS injury. A distinct difference in people with TBI is that the primary cause of hypotension is often associated with hemorrhage due to multiple extracranial injuries, rather than the head injury itself [59].

Hence the role of fluid resuscitation becomes critical to address the effects of hypotension from extracranial injuries on cerebral hemodynamics. Foals that experience significant hemorrhage secondary to basilar bone fractures are at highest risk for negative effects of hypotension on cerebral perfusion. The goal of fluid therapy in foals with CNS injury is normovolemia, while avoiding overhydration. Foals may not be hypovolemic if the injury is not associated with significant hemorrhage and are presented shortly after traumatic insult, although hypotension secondary to shock may be present. Neurogenic shock causing profound vasodilation and bradycardia is more common with traumatic SCI but may also occur in TBI.

Table 32.V.4 Summary of fluid therapy principles in foals with traumatic brain injury.

- Primary goal is to prevent or treat hypovolemia and hypotension to optimize cerebral perfusion and avoid overhydration.
- Isotonic crystalloid fluids are recommended for initial fluid therapy for foals with acute CNS injury. Isotonic fluid types that are iso-osmolar compared with equine plasma (Normasol-R/Plasmalyte 148) are preferred because of their more physiologic electrolyte components.
- Normal (0.9%) saline is a slightly hyperosmolar solution that can be beneficial for initial fluid resuscitation in foals with signs of elevated ICP to assist in maintaining adequate cerebral perfusion while minimizing cerebral edema. Use of 0.9% NaCl should be judicious and limited in foals because of its hyperchloremic acidifying effect and associated sodium load.
- Mannitol (20%) should remain the first choice for hyperosmolar therapy in young foals because of the risk of inducing sodium overload with hypertonic solutions.
- Administration of 3% hypertonic saline solutions as bolus or CRI may be considered for use in foals with persistent signs of elevated ICP refractory to treatment with mannitol, and in foals >2 wk with normal renal function.
- Provide IV dextrose supplementation during acute and ongoing management of TBI in foals to maintain euglycemia. Avoid inducing hyperglycemia and manage iatrogenic hyperglycemia with insulin therapy if needed.
- Avoid IV calcium supplementation during acute management of TBI in foals unless ionized hypocalcaemia is documented ($Ca^{++} < 1.0$ mmol/l).

Resuscitation

Isotonic fluids are the most appropriate fluid type for resuscitation and maintenance in foals with TBI and SCI. Balanced polyionic fluids such as Lactated Ringer's/Hartmanns, Normasol-R, and Plasmalyte-148 are readily available for resuscitation of critically ill foals, but the Na^+ concentration (130 mEq/l) in Lactated Ringers/Hartmann's solution is less than foals' normal plasma Na^+ concentration, as is the osmolality (272 mOsm/kg); these factors make Lactate Ringer's/Hartmann's solution less ideal in patients with cerebral edema. Normasol-R and Plasmalyte-148 have more physiologic Na^+ concentrations (140 mEq/l) and osmolality (295 mOsm/kg) and are better choices in patients with CNS injury. Normal (0.9%) saline (Na^+ 154 mEq/l; osmolality 308 mOsm/kg) is recommended by some authors for initial resuscitation of equine [41, 60] and human patients with TBI [52]. Normal saline is a reasonable choice as the higher osmolarity of 0.9% NaCl solution may be beneficial for initial resuscitation of foals with suspected elevated ICP, but given the acidifying effect (low strong ion difference), it is not recommended for ongoing fluid therapy. The choice of isotonic fluid for resuscitation is best made based on individual patient status and available fluid products.

Hypertonic saline is a reasonable resuscitative fluid in hypotensive adult horses following TBI due to its ability to simultaneously expand plasma volume and reduce ICP and cerebral edema. However, use of hypertonic (3–7.2%) saline is avoided in critically ill foals during the neonatal period for two reasons: (i) neonatal foals are prone to iatrogenic Na^+ overload because of their natural Na^+-conserving physiology and (ii) the negative effect of critical illness on renal Na^+-handling ability [61]. Careful use of small volumes of lower concentration hypertonic saline (3%) for osmotherapy may be considered, specifically for the management of suspected elevated ICP in older foals (>1 month) with TBI (discussed below). At this time, hypertonic saline is not recommended for fluid resuscitation in neonatal foals with TBI.

Colloids in TBI

Synthetic colloids have dose-related side effects, including coagulopathy, renal failure, anaphylaxis, and tissue storage in people. Given these concerns and risk of altered hemostasis in severe brain injury, synthetic colloids are avoided in foals with TBI. There is strong agreement in the human literature against the use of 4% albumin solution for patients with TBI due to higher mortality rates compared to 0.9% saline administration [62, 63]. It has been suggested that the hypotonic nature of the 4% albumin solution contributed to the higher mortality in this study.

Equine plasma may be necessary for the treatment of failure of passive transfer or significant blood loss during ongoing management of foals with TBI. The benefits of equine plasma for neonatal foals outweighs any yet-undetermined possible negative effects of albumin infusion. Furthermore, experimental models have shown that fresh-frozen plasma infusion is superior to both artificial colloid and normal saline solutions in reducing brain edema and lesion size [64]. Blood transfusion may be indicated in situations of significant blood loss according to the published blood transfusion recommendations in critically ill foals.

Fluid rates during resuscitation in foals with traumatic CNS injury should be approached judiciously, using small serial challenge doses of 10–20 ml/kg with frequent reassessment of clinical and neurologic parameters. Achieving hemodynamic stability is a priority for both TBI and SIC; however, overzealous fluid resuscitation should be strictly avoided in foals with TBI, as this contributes to worsening cerebral edema and increased ICP. Maintenance fluid rates should follow guidelines for fluid therapy in critically ill foals.

Mean Arterial Pressure (MAP) Goals

Traumatic Brain Injury

Guidelines in human medicine target CPP based on direct measurement of ICP and MAP according to the following relationship: CPP = MAP − ICP. In the absence of ICP monitoring, systemic MAP should be maintained within the normal age-specific range [65]. There are age-related differences in MAP and cerebral blood flow in people, with pediatric values lower than adults. The goal is to maintain MAP >90 mmHg for adults, and systolic blood pressure (SBP) >70 mmHg for children. A target MAP of ≥75 mmHg is recommended for neonatal foals with TBI.

Traumatic SCI

Neurogenic shock causing vasodilation, with concurrent hypotension and bradycardia, is more common with SCI than TBI, often necessitating treatment with pressor therapy and positive inotropes. The goal for hemodynamic management of SCI in people is a MAP to >85 mmHg to increase blood flow to the spinal cord for 7 days post-injury [66]. However, these guidelines assume that spinal cord perfusion pressure (SCPP)= MAP – cerebrospinal fluid pressure (CSFP). This concept is extrapolated from the TBI literature, even though the spinal cord is not contained in a rigid bony structure like the brain. Direct evidence of correlation between SCPP and MAP requires further research in which SCPP is measured directly at the injury site to determine an optimal pressure range and MAP goal [67].

The target MAP of >85 mmHg is likely to be unachievable in veterinary patients for 7 days, as even high-volume human trauma centers are unable to comply with this recommendation [67]. Nonetheless, a MAP of ≥75 mmHg in foals for the first few days following traumatic SCI with the use of fluid therapy and inotropes and/or pressor therapy is a reasonable goal. There is no consensus on a preferred vasopressor to achieve MAP recommendations for brain and SCI; however, norepinephrine is one common vasopressor used to support low peripheral vascular resistance while increasing heart rate and cardiac output with its positive chronotropic and inotropic effects [67, 68].

Glucose Supplementation

Continuous supply of glucose from the systemic circulation provides the main energy source for the brain. Therefore, adequate glucose supply is crucial to maintain brain function [69]. TBI induces increased energy demand; thus, endogenous levels of metabolic fuels may not be sufficient to meet increased demands in the injured brain. Experimental animal models of TBI demonstrate that provision of metabolic fuels (glucose, sodium pyruvate, ethyl pyruvate) early post-brain injury can be beneficial and improves outcome [70, 71]. Therefore a supplemental energy source may be needed to match the increased cerebral metabolic demands to avoid energy crisis after TBI in foals.

Conversely, adverse effects of hyperglycemia on ischemic brain injury have been well established. Early and persistent hyperglycemia (serum glucose >198 mg/dl [11 mmol/l]) following TBI is associated with increased risk of mortality and poor neurologic outcome in adults and children [72]. Hyperglycemia has also been associated with severity of head trauma in dogs and cats, but not with outcome [73]. Hyperglycemia is a secondary insult to the injured brain, resulting in increased glycolysis, increased lactate/pyruvate ratio, metabolic acidosis within brain parenchyma, overproduction of ROS, and ultimately neuronal cell death [74]. Detrimental effects of hyperglycemia in human and veterinary patients with TBI has led to recommendations in equine patients to avoid glucose supplementation during acute management of TBI, except if hypoglycemia is documented [5, 75, 76]. Iatrogenic hyperglycemia can also occur with high-dose corticosteroid administration and should be avoided. Both prolonged hyper- and hypoglycemia are detrimental in patients with brain injury. Insulin therapy that targets tight glucose control is no longer supported in caring of pediatric patients with TBI [66, 77]. Currently, a liberal glycemic-control strategy (maintain blood glucose concentrations of 144–180 mg/dl [8–10 mmol/l]) is recommended for adults following TBI [69]. However, there are variable practices for when glucose supplementation should be initiated and how hyperglycemia should be controlled in critically ill pediatric patients with TBI [78]. Recommendations for pediatric patients with TBI suggests withholding glucose containing fluids unless the serum glucose is <70 mg/dl (<4 mmol).

Neonatal foals are susceptible to hypoglycemia associated with illness and inability to nurse. Maintaining euglycemia (70–110 mg/dl) in foals with TBI and SCI is a priority, even if it requires IV glucose supplementation during initial management. If hypoglycemia is present (<70 mg/dl), dextrose can be added to IV fluids during resuscitation (20 ml/kg bolus) using a 1% dextrose (20 ml of 50% dextrose in 1 l isotonic crystalloid fluid) solution to avoid inducing hyperglycemia. Given the potential impact of both hyper- and hypoglycemia, optimal glycemic control in foals requires frequent monitoring of blood glucose concentrations and insulin therapy. If the foal is not receiving enteral nutrition, dextrose supplementation at 4–8 mg/kg/min is indicated [79].

Calcium Supplementation

Calcium plays a central role in secondary brain injury, contributing to excitotoxic neuronal cell damage and apoptotic cell death. Thus, calcium supplementation should be avoided in acute management of CNS injury unless ionized hypocalcemia is documented (Ca^{++} < 1.0 mmol/l) [80, 81]. Research has focused on investigating therapies that antagonize intracellular calcium influx following TBI [82, 83].

Thiamine (Vitamin B_1) Supplementation

Thiamine plays an important role as an enzyme cofactor in various pathways central to glucose metabolism and energy production. Thiamine deficiency has been associated with neuronal cell death due to glutamate-induced excitotoxicity and compromised mitochondrial function [84]. Whether supplementation of thiamine is indicated in acute CNS injury is not currently supported by published evidence. However, given the increased susceptibility of injured neuronal tissue to inadequate energy production and supply and the safety of its use, the common practice of thiamine supplementation for neurologic injury in large animals appears justified.

Seizure Management

Seizures are a common manifestation of neurological disease in neonatal foals. Early recognition and immediate control of seizures is a priority following head trauma as it increases cerebral metabolic rate and ICP and contributes to secondary brain injury by causing fluctuations in systemic blood pressure and arterial oxygenation [52, 85]. Infants and children are at greater risk of posttraumatic seizures compared with adults because of increased excitability of the developing brain [86]. In addition, development of posttraumatic seizures is correlated with severity of brain injury and younger age and is a poor prognostic indicator for recovery in pediatric patients [87]. Although not a direct comparison, foals with neonatal encephalopathy that show early onset, prolonged, and uncontrolled seizures have a poorer prognosis for survival compared with hospitalized foals without seizures [88, 89].

Benzodiazepines are first-line medications used for seizure control; either diazepam or midazolam are indicated for short-term (immediate) control of seizures due to their rapid onset of action and reliable efficacy in foals. Because of the short half-life, repeated doses may be necessary. Caution should be used as rapid IV injection and frequent, repeated, bolus administration may cause respiratory depression in foals requiring close monitoring and provision of nasal oxygen insufflation if available [90]. An advantage of midazolam is that it can be administered IV, IM, or as a CRI to foals with seizures. In healthy newborn foals, a bolus of 0.2 mg/kg midazolam IV has a rapid onset of effect (≤5 minutes), high plasma clearance (11.2 ml/min/kg bwt), and short half-life (2.2 hours; Feary, unpublished data). At this dose, midazolam does not produce detectable negative effects on cardiorespiratory status, but can produce muscle weakness, ataxia, and prolonged recumbency. Administration of more than three to four bolus doses of a benzodiazepine to treat ongoing seizures should be avoided and indicates the need for second-line or maintenance medications for seizures.

Second-line maintenance anticonvulsant therapy is indicated when seizures persist despite administration of first-line medications. Phenobarbital can be used for persistent seizures in adult horses and foals, with the dose in foals (2–3 mg/kg IV, slow bolus to effect over 15 minutes) being lower than adults [91]. The use of phenobarbital in critically ill foals can be problematic because of its slow onset of action, need to closely monitor and titrate to effect, and significant side effects. In addition, the prolonged half-life of phenobarbital can delay useful neurologic evaluation for several days once discontinued. Phenobarbital also complicates the care of already compromised neonatal foals due to respiratory depression, hypothermia, hypotension, and potential pharyngeal paralysis [92]. These safety concerns have stimulated clinical investigation of alternative safe and effective anticonvulsant drugs to manage equine neonatal seizures such as midazolam CRI and levetiracetam.

Midazolam CRI provides an alternative to phenobarbital for persistent seizures in equine neonates. Although the pharmacokinetics have not been investigated in foals, it is frequently administered to ill foals for seizure management at a dose ranging from 0.02–0.06 mg/kg/h [93]. Midazolam CRI is a reasonable choice for seizure management as it improves the ability to reassess neurologic status shortly after discontinuation and results in fewer side effects compared with phenobarbital [92].

Levetiracetam is a novel antiepileptic drug with promise as an effective and safe alternative to phenobarbital for controlling neonatal seizures in other species [94]. Levetiracetam is widely used in humans, dogs and cats and is safe and well tolerated in healthy adult horses [95] and foals [96]. Levetiracetam is a common add-on antiepileptic drug in dogs due to its rapid effect, minimal sedation, and efficacy for up to 8 hours for refractory seizures [97] and is recommended as a first-line drug for management of seizures in dogs with TBI [53]. The pharmacokinetics of levetiracetam have been studied in healthy neonatal foals; twice-daily administration of 32 mg/kg (IV or orally) maintains plasma concentrations within a proposed target concentration in people of 5–45 mg/l throughout the dosing interval [96]. The clinical efficacy and therapeutic dose range of levetiracetam requires further investigation in foals, thus individual adjustment of dose and frequency of administration may be required in a clinical setting for adequate seizure control [96]. At this time, the clinical efficacy of levetiracetam for seizure control in foals is based on anecdotal evidence. While reports are favorable, they suggest use of a higher loading dose of 60 mg/kg IV and report that foals may experience seizures through the loading dose and first 32 mg/kg maintenance dose, in which case midazolam CRI is administered, as needed, during that period (R. Bozorgmanesh; personnel communication). Current guidelines for TBI in pediatric patients recommend prophylactic anticonvulsant therapy for 7 days following severe TBI [66]. The use of prophylactic antiepileptic drugs in foals following TBI may not be indicated but considered in individual cases. Levetiracetam may be the prophylactic antiepileptic drug of choice based on twice daily IV or oral dosing and minimal sedative effects.

Emergency control of intractable seizures may necessitate immobilization by IV anesthesia using propfol. Propofol may be neuroprotective via modulation of GABA receptors and antioxidant effects, but also causes hypotension and hypoventilation [53]. Careful titration, meticulous monitoring, and supportive care are essential if IV anesthesia is used for seizure control. A suggested dose is 2 mg/kg slow IV [76]. Alternatively, infusion of pentobarbital for induction of a barbiturate coma can be considered as a last resort in foals refractory to other therapies. Pentobarbital is not a true anticonvulsant; seizure control results from its anesthetic effects. Pentobarbital causes profound respiratory depression with repeated doses. Initial doses of 2–15 mg/kg IV to effect are recommended in veterinary patients; the dose is carefully titrated to effect using small incremental boluses over 20 minutes. If seizure activity persists, barbiturate coma can be maintained using a CRI titrated to effect. Anecdotal reports suggest a starting dose of 7–8 mg/kg/h of pentobarbital diluted in isotonic saline and reduced slowly to minimize side effects (Bozorgmanesh, personal communication). Cardiovascular and respiratory depression leading to cardiac arrhythmias, hypotension, and hypoventilation are potential complications, thus intensive monitoring and assisted ventilation should be ensured prior to pentobarbital infusion to prevent adverse effects on cerebral perfusion [3, 53].

Targeted Temperature Control

Fever following acute neurologic injury is detrimental and associated with worse outcomes in pediatric patients. Therefore, prevention of hyperthermia following TBI in children is recommended [98]. The standard of care in pediatric TBI is controlled normothermia for the prevention of fever [66]. As such, controlled temperature management is recommended to avoid hyperthermia in foals with TBI. This recommendation translates to a clinical approach of permissive hypothermia (i.e. avoiding active warming of mildly hypothermic foals [35–37.0 °C (95–98.6 °F)] following TBI). Active cooling is indicated in foals with rectal temperature of >38.0 °C (100.4 °F) using cold (refrigerated 4 °C [39.2 °F]) IV fluids, ice packs, and fans. The use of NSAIDs is also indicated for the management of hyperthermia in foals with acute CNS injury. Therapeutic hypothermia for treating refractory increased ICP following TBI remains controversial in human critical care due to a lack of consistent benefits and possible harm (discussed below).

Priority Two

Once the foal is positioned to prevent further injury, IV fluid therapy has been initiated, oxygenation and ventilation stabilized, and seizures controlled, the foal should be assessed for other injuries. A neurologic examination should be performed but may be impeded by sedation and antiseizure medication. At this point, specific medical therapy for brain and SCI can be initiated as indicated.

Hyperosmolar Therapy for TBI

Evidence for use of hyperosmolar therapies for treatment if increased ICP is among the strongest within TBI management guidelines in human medicine. The principle of hyperosmolar therapy is establishing an osmotic gradient between the plasma and parenchymal brain tissue, thereby reducing brain water content and thus ICP. An intact BBB is necessary for this to be effective. Osmolar therapy is also only effective in the management of vasogenic edema, and not cytotoxic edema or oxidative processes involved in secondary brain injury. Given the lack of a consistent benefit of hyperosmolar agents over normal saline for initial resuscitation of patients with TBI, hyperosmolar therapy is only indicated in patients with clinical evidence of increased ICP and/or signs of brain herniation. Since direct ICP monitoring is not routinely performed in foals, clinicians do not have a quantitative ICP target to guide hyperosmolar therapy. Therefore, repeated neurologic examination is an indirect indicator of elevated ICP in foals. Examination focuses on level of consciousness, pupillary size and responsiveness, and motor activity. Clinical signs of elevated ICP include progressive reduction in level of consciousness and response to noxious stimuli, minimally responsive miotic or mydriatic pupils and development of paresis [5]. The foal's level of consciousness must also consider the influence of concurrent illness. Bilaterally miotic pupils and/or progression to unresponsive mydriasis or anisocoria indicates impending brain herniation and a grave prognosis [76]. Of note, the presence of seizures does not necessarily indicate elevated ICP.

Mannitol and hypertonic saline are commonly used hyperosmolar agents. Both solutions effectively lower ICP in patients with TBI. Mannitol has historically been the most widely used agent in people and animals with TBI and increased ICP [3, 99]. Despite promising evidence favoring use of hypertonic saline, studies do not suggest clear superiority for one treatment over another for lowering ICP in TBI [66, 100, 101]. Both mannitol and hypertonic saline are recommended for management of TBI in adult horses [8, 76, 102, 103]. Hyperosmolar therapy in foals should be considered carefully and guided by the principle of *primum non nocere*. Although mannitol and hypertonic saline are likely to be equally effective in reducing brain edema in foals, both solutions are associated with side effects that necessitate close attention to circulating fluid volume, electrolytes, acid–base status, and renal function. Hypertonic saline, particularly higher concentrations (7.2%), can be associated with more side effects in very young foals because of their reduced ability to accommodate large Na^{++} loads. If the BBB is compromised, infusion of hyperosmolar solutions could be detrimental because they may increase the size of cerebral contusions [104]. Since BBB integrity cannot be easily evaluated in the clinical setting, clinicians must use caution and clinical judgment when contemplating administration of hyperosmolar solutions. Optimum management of foals receiving more than a single dose of either hyperosmolar solution should include measurement of the following parameters prior to and every 4–8 hours during therapy: Na^{++}, Cl^{-}, osmolality, pH, lactate, and MAP. Renal parameters and urine output should be monitored daily. The therapeutic goal is to maintain serum osmolality ≤320 mOsm/l, and serum electrolytes within normal limits. If serum osmolality cannot be measured directly it can be estimated using the simplified equation based on serum Na^{++} and Cl^{-} concentrations: Serum osmolality = 2(Na+) + Glucose (mg/dl)/18 + Blood urea nitrogen (mg/dl)/2.8.

Hyperosmolar Therapy for Traumatic SCI

Hyperosmolar therapy is optimally guided by ICP monitoring in human patients, but measurement of spinal cord perfusion is not routinely performed. Studies demonstrate beneficial effects of serial bolus administration of 5% hypertonic saline for reducing spinal cord edema and hemorrhage in acute spinal cord trauma in a rodent model [105, 106]. Mannitol is not an effective treatment of SCI in small animals, and may potentially be harmful [10]. At this time, administration of hyperosmolar therapy for traumatic SCI is not indicated in foals, unless hypertonic saline (≤5%) is chosen as part of fluid resuscitation in hypovolemic older (>1 month) foals.

Mannitol

Mannitol should only be considered when the patient is hemodynamically stable and persistent clinical indications of increased ICP are noted. Mannitol reduces ICP by two mechanisms that have an additive effect on reducing ICP. Initially (first few minutes), reflex vasoconstriction of cerebral vasculature in response to transient reduction in blood viscosity occurs, followed by a slower onset osmotic effect that results in gradual movement of water out of the brain parenchyma and into the systemic circulation. This osmotic effect persists 5–6 hours but requires an intact BBB to be effective [66]. Mannitol also has free-radical scavenging effects. Adverse effects associated with multiple boluses are related to potent diuretic effects, making use contraindicated in hypovolemic patients. A concern that weighs against the use of mannitol in patients with intracranial hemorrhage is based on the theoretical risk of exacerbating active intracranial hemorrhage by its osmotic effect. Despite this widely cited contraindication, no clinical evidence supports this theory with the benefits of mannitol's ability to reduce ICP far outweighing this theoretical risk [3, 10, 57, 97]. Another theoretical disadvantage is a reverse osmotic shift, leading to brain edema and increase in ICP; however, reverse osmotic shift is unlikely with appropriate bolus use of mannitol [10].

Mannitol (20%) infusion has historically been part of the management of neonatal encephalopathy in foals based on a superseded understanding that the pathophysiology involves cerebral edema. The reported dose rate of mannitol (20%) administrated to neonatal foals is 0.25–1.0 g/kg slow IV bolus over 10–20 minutes [84]. This dose is the same as used for treatment of increased ICP in pediatric patients with TBI and is appropriate for foals with TBI [101]. Mannitol infusion can be repeated at 4–8 hour intervals (maximum three doses in 24 hours). Mannitol infusion is suggested by the author as the initial hyperosmolar therapy of choice in euvolemic neonatal foals with TBI and evidence of increased ICP. Hypertonic (3%) saline may be an appropriate first choice for older foals (>1 month). For comparison purposes, 0.5 g/kg of mannitol delivers the same osmolar dose as approximately 2.5 ml/kg of 3% hypertonic saline [66].

Hypertonic Saline

Hypertonic saline has additional beneficial effects that make it an attractive alternative to mannitol for treating increased ICP, particularly in hemodynamically unstable patients. In addition to augmenting plasma volume expansion and cerebral perfusion temporarily, hypertonic saline theoretically restores normal cellular resting membrane potential and cell volume and modulates the inflammatory response. These effects are maintained during concurrent infusion of isotonic crystalloids [27]. Furthermore, studies in both adult and pediatric populations have demonstrated the efficacy of hypertonic saline in treating refractory increases in ICP that have failed to respond to conventional therapy, including mannitol [99].

Hypertonic saline is commonly administered as a 3% solution to control ICP in pediatric patients at a dose of 1–3 ml/kg IV bolus infusion over 10 minutes [66, 101]. The recommended dose of 2 ml/kg of 7.2% hypertonic saline IV bolus every 4 hours for up to five infusions in adult horses with TBI is not, in the author's opinion, appropriate for foals [103]. Rather, a more cautious approach is recommended using a lower concentration (3%) compared to adults (7.2%). Continuous infusion of 3% hypertonic saline (0.1–1.0 ml/kg/h) is also recommended to maintain ICP <20 mmHg in pediatric patients [66]. The goal of a hypertonic saline CRI is to maintain plasma osmolality ≤320 mmol/l, decrease cerebral edema, and maintain cerebral perfusion [76]. Hypernatremia and hyperchloremia are likely with repeated doses, particularly in foals <2–4 weeks of age. While transient, mild elevations in Na^{++} and Cl^- are acceptable, sustained increases ($Na^+ > 150$ mEq/l; $Cl^- > 110$ mEq/l) for more than 12–24 hours may be detrimental to renal function and result in acidemia.

The incidence of hyperchloremia ($Cl^- > 110$ mEq/l) and acute kidney injury (AKI) is higher in people receiving hypertonic saline for treatment of severe neurologic injuries [106]. Given mounting evidence that hyperchloremia is associated with adverse outcomes including AKI and metabolic acidosis in people, close monitoring of serum electrolytes, osmolality, acid–base status, and renal function is prudent when administering repeated bolus or CRI of hypertonic saline to foals. As equine neonates are prone to Na^{++} overload [61], combined with the tendency of critically ill foals to retain Na^{++} and water [107], dictates that the use of hypertonic saline solutions in neonatal foals be carefully considered in light of potential side-effects of fluid overload and AKI.

Because of the risks of hypertonic saline use in neonatal foals, mannitol (20%) remains the first choice for hyperosmolar therapy in foals with TBI and increased ICP. However, administration of 3% hypertonic saline solutions as bolus or CRI may be considered in foals >2 weeks that are otherwise healthy or in foals with elevated ICP refractory to treatment with mannitol. Historically, furosemide was administered concurrently or immediately prior to hyperosmolar solutions based on the belief that it reduced CSF production and was synergistic with mannitol to reduce brain edema. Lack of evidence and risk of worsening hypovolemia has negated the use of furosemide in TBI [3, 46].

Anti-inflammatory Therapy in CNS Trauma

General Considerations

The inflammatory response to TBI is robust and proportional to the severity of injury [28]. Anti-inflammatory drugs are effective at reducing inflammation when administered before or soon after TBI in experimental models [108]. Consequently, conventional treatment of TBI focuses on negating the acute, deleterious effects of the neuroinflammatory response to injury. The traditional role of glucocorticoids for treatment of acute traumatic CNS in human medicine has been questioned and is no longer standard of care. The results of a large clinical trial of corticosteroid randomization after significant head injury (CRASH) demonstrated no benefit and increased risk of short- and long-term mortality in adults administered high doses of corticosteroids [40]. Thus, use of corticosteroids in TBI and head trauma patients has fallen out of favor [109].

Like most critical illness, the pro-inflammatory response to TBI is harmful, but the anti-inflammatory response has an important role that needs to be preserved to facilitate favorable outcomes. The disappointing findings of several experimental and clinical trials targeting complete inhibition of neuroinflammation using high dose glucocorticoids have led to the conclusion that nonspecific immunosuppression is detrimental to the injured brain [28, 40, 110]. Furthermore, the therapeutic window for efficacy of anti-inflammatory therapy is likely quite short (4–6 hours following injury). There are limited options for pharmacologic anti-inflammatory agents in neonatal foals. The most potent anti-inflammatory drugs (corticosteroids) are associated with the highest risk of adverse effects. The use of corticosteroids in foals with TBI or SCI is highly debated. In contrast, NSAIDs are indicated for their multiple effects to reduce neuroinflammation, provide analgesia, and reduce fever [111].

Corticosteroids in Foals with TBI

The rationale for corticosteroid administration for treatment of traumatic CNS injury is compelling based on their potent anti-inflammatory and antioxidant effects; moreover, use in traumatic CNS injury in horses is common and well-established [41, 76]. The apparent success of corticosteroid use in horses is suggested by numerous published case reports and widespread anecdotal evidence. While such evidence is the lowest quality, it is the only currently available evidence in the equine literature. Published case reports of horses administered corticosteroids have survived without complications [81], even with a prolonged course and concurrent bacterial meningitis [112].

The role of corticosteroids in acute TBI in people suggests some benefit, but also clearly no significant advantage or efficacy in the management of TBI [113]. Evidence in the pediatric population suggests that corticosteroids do not improve outcome or reduce ICP in children with TBI [114]. Furthermore, steroid treatment suppresses endogenous cortisol production for days and predisposes the patient to bacterial pneumonia [66]. In addition to not improving outcome, corticosteroids also cause hyperglycemia, immunosuppression, delayed wound healing, gastric ulceration, and exacerbate a catabolic state. These adverse effects, combined with increased mortality when used in people, has led to a lack of support for the use of corticosteroids when treating head trauma in small animal patients [3]. As mechanisms of the effects of corticosteroids and the pathophysiology of CNS trauma have become elucidated, it is understood that corticosteroids are most efficacious against inflammation related to vasogenic edema, but not cytotoxic edema (cytotoxic edema is predominate type in traumatic CNS injury in people) [48, 115]. Whether this is true for TBI and SCI in foals is unknown. In fact, the application of conclusions from these studies regarding corticosteroid use in people to equine CNS injury is controversial. The population of patients with TBI studied involved people with severe TBI that were administered a high-dose, tapering protocol of methylprednisolone, dexamethasone, or triamcinolone for multiple days [40, 116–119]. Primary endpoints in these studies focused on survival, long-term cognitive function, and fine motor skills. These outcomes are not relevant to horses as equine patients with moderate to severe brain injury generally require euthanasia because of poor prognosis. The types of traumatic CNS injuries to be managed in foals are therefore probably less severe and use of corticosteroids in the management of mild to moderate TBI may not be associated with worse outcomes.

The equine clinician is left with the dilemma of whether or not to administer corticosteroids in cases of TBI as has historically been widely accepted. The author adopts the position that routine use of corticosteroids for the management of TBI in foals should be reconsidered. Foals are likely to be particularly susceptible to adverse effects of corticosteroids and should therefore be avoided. Conversely, the potent anti-inflammatory effects of a single dose of corticosteroid administered within the first few hours following trauma is advocated for its potentially lifesaving effects in equine patients with rapid progression of signs or acute recumbency [76]; however, this notion may occur only because the potential benefit outweighs risk when death/euthanasia is the only other option.

There is limited data on corticosteroid pharmacokinetics and pharmacodynamics in foals, thus, dosages are extrapolated from adult horses [120]. Judicious use of corticosteroids within the acute setting and only when necessary, implies use of a single dose of rapidly acting corticosteroid administered IV. Recommended doses in adult horses include dexamethasone sodium phosphate (0.1–0.2 mg/kg IV), methylprednisolone sodium succinate (10–30 mg/kg IV), and prednisolone sodium succinate (1.0–2.5 mg/kg IV) [38, 76]. Given the number and severity of potential side effects, the decision to institute therapy with corticosteroids requires careful consideration of risks and benefits, especially in critically ill foals.

Corticosteroids in Traumatic SCI

The use of corticosteroids is also controversial in acute SCI. Methylprednisolone has more potent free-radical scavenging effect than other corticosteroids and is suggested to be superior for management of SCI for this reason [121, 122]. Both dexamethasone and prednisolone are not reported to be effective in the treatment of acute SCI in dogs and may be associated with a higher incidence of adverse effects [123, 124]. In people, the widespread adoption of high-dose methylprednisolone for patients treated within 8 hours of acute traumatic SCI was based on results in animal models [125], and supported by large clinical trials [126–128]. However, multiple reviews of these studies question the validity of the conclusions and novel evidence against the use of methylprednisolone has been accumulating over the past decade [129]. Current consensus statements do not recommend high dose methylprednisolone based on current available evidence [121]. However, because there is limited evidence to support alternative treatments, it remains a therapeutic option [129]. If therapy is elected, high-dose methylprednisolone protocols in people prescribe an initial dose of 30 mg/kg bolus over 15 minutes, followed by a 23–47 hour maintenance infusion of 5.4 mg/kg/h; this therapy is only indicated if given within 8 hours of injury [130]. A similar dose of 30 mg/kg slow IV bolus followed by repeated bolus doses of 15 mg/kg at 2 and 6 hours, then every 8 hours up to 48 hours following trauma is recommended in veterinary patients [131]. Use of corticosteroids for the treatment of acute SCI in foals should be carefully considered in light of the risks and benefits, especially in critically ill foals. If therapy is elected, methylprednisolone must be administered within 8 hours of injury at 15–30 mg/kg slow IV bolus followed by 1-2 additional doses of 15 mg/kg IV at 2 and 6 hours following the initial dose [10].

Nonsteroidal Anti-Inflammatory Drugs (NSAIDs)

Based on the importance of arachidonic acid metabolism in the pathogenesis of CNS injury, use of anti-inflammatory therapy with NSAIDs in foals with TBI is indicated, particularly in light of recommendations against the use of corticosteroids in veterinary patients [3, 53]. NSAIDs are also indicated for their analgesic and anti-pyretic effects. Specific NSAIDs that can be considered for the management of traumatic CNS injury in foals include flunixin meglumine, ketoprofen, meloxicam, and firocoxib [120]. Phenylbutazone should be avoided in compromised foals.

Antimicrobial Therapy

Broad-spectrum antimicrobial therapy is indicated in neonatal foals with traumatic head injuries, and in any foal in which cranium or vertebral fractures are suspected or confirmed due to the risk of septic meningitis. Bleeding from the nose or ears indicates a possible fracture of the basisphenoid, basioccipital, or petrous temporal bone from poll impact. Frontal injury may result in palpable fractures of the frontal or parietal bones. Bloody CSF suggests a fracture [76]. Antibiotic choice is based on culture and sensitivity testing, but culture samples are not always available. Thus, empirical antimicrobials to combat possible meningitis include third- and fourth generation cephalosporins (ceftriaxone, cefotaxime). Other options include chloramphenicol and rifampin. Poor antibiotic choices for CNS infection include penicillin, ampicillin, aminoglycosides, ceftiofur, and doxycycline as these compounds do not uniformly cross the BBB. Although meningeal inflammation increases penetration of many drugs into the CSF, therapeutic concentrations may still not be achieved [27]. Trimethoprim-sulfamethoxazole may not be an ideal choice for meningitis due to inadequate CSF concentrations for efficacy against a number of equine pathogens [27, 132].

Nutritional Support

Nutritional support is important in the management of all critically ill foals. Initiation of enteral nutritional support (within 36–72 hours from injury) is suggested to decrease mortality and improve outcome in human TBI [133]. Enteral feeding is preferred for its many beneficial effects, but intolerance to enteral feeding secondary to ileus, delayed gastric emptying, abdominal distension and diarrhea is documented in humans with TBI [134]. Enteral feeding with concurrent prokinetic therapy is recommended in human and veterinary patients with severe TBI due to the high incidence of delayed gastric emptying [3]. While early enteral nutrition is indicated in the management of foals with traumatic CNS injury, the author does not recommend use of prokinetics to facilitate enteral feeding. Rather, enteral feeding can be encouraged by allowing foals to nurse for short intervals, if able. If the foal is recumbent or unable to nurse, enteral nutrition is provided with conservative volumes (≤5% body weight/day) of mare's milk via an indwelling nasogastric tube. Additional caloric support can be provided with IV dextrose or partial parenteral nutrition as required. Foals that are unable to tolerate enteral feeding due to hypothermia, ileus, or inability to safely place a nasogastric tube without the risk of further injury, are candidates for parenteral nutrition. Parenteral nutrition should be initiated within the first 48 hours in neonatal foals and within 72–96 hours in older foals that are unable to nurse.

Adjunctive Therapies

Dimethylsulfoxide (DMSO)

DMSO has historically been used for treatment of traumatic CNS injury in horses for its anti-inflammatory and antioxidant effects [27, 60, 76]. DMSO might attenuate several mechanisms involved in secondary CNS injury, at least experimentally [135]. Specifically, DMSO has neuroprotective and stabilizing effects on cell membranes and has anti-inflammatory and ROS scavenging actions [136, 137].

DMSO also crosses the BBB and has potent diuretic effects. DMSO causes a transient reduction in ICP and brain edema when administered IV in experimental studies of TBI [22, 136, 138]. The beneficial effects of DMSO noted in experimental models have been challenged by other research that identified neurotoxic effects and evidence of damage from DMSO on brain development [139, 140]. Furthermore, several systemic side effects in people have been reported [138]. As a result, DMSO has not been extended into large clinical trials in people for TBI. Use of DMSO appears to be safe in horses, but studies determining efficacy in traumatic CNS injury do not exist.

DMSO is recommended (off-label) at a dose of 0.5–1.0 g/kg IV diluted to 10–20% in isotonic fluids given IV or via nasogastric tube once daily for three days in the acute management of traumatic CNS injury [27]. The pharmacokinetic parameters following a single 15-minute IV infusion of a 6% DMSO solution at a dose of 0.1 g/kg has been studied in healthy adult horses [141]. The changes in the plasma concentration–time curves are described by a two-compartment model with a rapid distribution half-life ($t_{1/2}\alpha$) of 29 minutes and elimination half-life ($t_{1/2}\beta$) of 14.1 hours. Use of DMSO for a variety of equine conditions in tertiary care settings has declined due to safety concerns, the unpleasant nature of handling DMSO, and lack of evidence-based data supporting its use. Nonetheless, some clinicians use DMSO for acute CNS injury in foals.

Antioxidants

The brain is particularly vulnerable to oxidative stress following injury, thus much research has focused on arresting or reversing free radical damage after a TBI [135]. Other antioxidant medications, outside of DMSO, used for acute CNS injury in adults and foals include alpha-tocopherol (vitamin E) and ascorbic acid (vitamin C). High doses of vitamin E are recommended (20,000 IU/adult) for horses with brain trauma, although clinical efficacy is unproven. A dose of 1000–2000 U/d is reasonable for a foal with CNS injury.

Ascorbic acid has reemerged as a potential antioxidant agent for further investigation due to promising findings in small cohort of people with septic shock [142]. Ascorbic acid depletion in critical illness, including CNS trauma, has been well documented and ascorbic acid has an excellent safety profile and is inexpensive [143, 144]. Ascorbic acid is believed to act as a neuromodulator that inhibits neurotransmitter binding to NMDA receptors. Plasma ascorbic acid concentrations have been measured in normal 7-day-old pony foals and found to be higher than in the dam [145]. The mares' ascorbic acid status had a large influence on the foals' ascorbic acid status at 7 days of age in this study, with ascorbic acid concentrations in colostrum and milk approximately 10 times higher than in foals' plasma. Foals that have failure of passive transfer or are not nursing may have reduced plasma ascorbic acid. Whether supplementation benefits foals with acute CNS injury is unknown and a suggested dose for neuroprotection has not been determined. However, a high dose of 200 mg/kg/d (administered as 50 mg/kg IV every 6 hours) has been a suggested in the management of TBI in people [146]. Based on pharmacokinetics of ascorbic acid in horses [147], an IV dose of 25 mg/kg has been reported to attenuate LPS-induced neutrophil depletion in an experimental study in adult horses [148]. Reported oral doses for foals vary from 50 to 100 mg/kg/d [84].

Allopurinol, a xanthine oxidase inhibitor, potentially protects against reperfusion-induced brain injury by reducing free-radical formation and has been investigated for its neuroprotective effects in human neonates with hypoxic-ischemic encephalopathy [149]. Anecdotal reports of its use in equine neonates with hypoxic-ischemic encephalopathy and adult horses with brain injury after head trauma exist, but clinical efficiency is unknown. The pharmacokinetics of IV allopurinol (5 mg/kg) administered to healthy horses demonstrated that allopurinol is rapidly metabolized with a short half-life ($t_{1/2}\beta = 0.09$H) suggesting that much of the activity of allopurinol may result from its metabolic conversion to oxypurinol which has a slightly longer $t_{1/2}\beta$ of 1.09 hours [150]. Oral bioavailability of allopurinol (30 mg/kg PO) in horses is low (14.3%). These findings suggest potential for use of allopurinol as a CRI in foals for antioxidant treatment for acute CNS injury, but further studies are warranted.

Magnesium sulfate ($MgSO_4$) infusion has potential benefit in re-establishing homeostatic regulation of pathways involved in secondary brain injury. Magnesium is a noncompetitive inhibitor of NMDA receptors and regulates calcium influx. Disruption of magnesium homeostasis and depletion of ionized magnesium has been observed in pathophysiological events after TBI in humans. Deficits in intracellular magnesium concentration following TBI and SCI are associated with poor neurological outcome in experimental studies and normalizing magnesium concentrations has resulted in improved neurological recoveries in preclinical studies [151]. In contrast, a metanalysis of $MgSO_4$ treatment after TBI failed to show consistent beneficial effects in mortality of TBI patients, but demonstrated a tendency to improved neurologic scores [152]. At this time $MgSO_4$ infusion is not considered standard of care for the management of TBI in humans.

Ongoing research of $MgSO_4$ for TBI includes coadministration of $MgSO_4$ with other agents in preclinical models of brain injury. Combined use of $MgSO_4$ with mannitol as a method of increasing brain bioavailability of magnesium is suggested to allow for a low and safe dose of magnesium to be administered and may improve clinical outcome in TBI patients. Safety data regarding the use of $MgSO_4$ for pediatric TBI concluded that $MgSO_4$ administration did not decrease MAP or CPP or adversely affect cardiac conduction [153]. Considering available evidence that $MgSO_4$ therapy helps attenuate neurodegeneration in several animal models of brain injury, it is reasonable to consider $MgSO_4$ infusion as part of multimodal therapy targeting various components of the secondary injury cascade in foals with TBI. Clinical efficacy of $MgSO_4$ for foals with TBI has not been established, but it has been used as a CRI in foals for its potential benefit in blocking cellular calcium influx and glutamate release [91]. Magnesium sulfate has been recommended either as a single dose of 50 mg/kg given slow IV (dilute in initial IV fluids), and as a CRI at a loading dose of 50 mg/kg IV following by 15–30 mg/kg/h for 24–48 hours [76, 91, 102, 154]. These dose rates are probably derived from recommendations in human medicine and although IV $MgSO_4$ appears to have a wide safety margin, it is important to monitor serum magnesium concentrations and for clinical signs of toxicity (neuromuscular weakness, flaccid paralysis, and hypocalcemia). $MgSO_4$ infusion is contraindicated in foals with renal failure, undiagnosed cardiac arrythmia, or elevated serum Mg concentrations [76].

Therapeutic Hypothermia

Use of therapeutic hypothermia (TH) in foals has not been reported but there is growing interest in this modality which can be considered as an adjunctive therapy in selected cases. Considering evidence in pediatric TBI, there are many potential benefits of TH for the management of TBI [155]. Experimental studies demonstrate that TH reduces secondary brain injury, cerebral metabolic rate, oxygen demand, and ICP via multiple mechanism and TH has proven to be an effective intervention to improve neurodevelopmental outcomes following perinatal HIE in infants [98]. However, favorable experimental findings have not translated into significant clinical benefits in randomized clinical trials with severe head injury. This may be because TH is associated with numerous complications. As such, the use of TH for neuroprotection following TBI remains controversial in human critical care due to a lack of consistent benefits and possible harm. Results of a landmark multicenter phase 3 randomized controlled trial compared TH and normothermia after severe TBI and noted that hypothermia (32–33 °C [89.6–91.4 °F]) for 48–72 hours with slow rewarming did not reduce mortality or improve outcome [156], despite promising phase 2 trial results in which hypothermia decreased mortality rate. The relevance of these clinical trials in neonatal foals is unknown.

Current recommendations do not support prophylactic use of TH in children following TBI [66, 157]. However, evidence suggests that moderate (32–34 °C [89.6–93.2 °F]) hypothermia has a role in patients with refractory intracranial hypertension (i.e. unresponsive to hyperosmolar therapy, continuous sedation or barbiturate coma), with a cautious rewarming rate of 0.5–1.0 °C (1.1–1.8 °F) every 12–24 hours to avoid complications and rebound intracranial hypertension. TH targeting body temperature of 34–35 °C [93.2–95 °F] could be considered in foals as an option for refractory cases (i.e. deterioration of neurologic status, persistent generalized seizures despite medical management) if intensive monitoring and continuous sedation and analgesia is available for 24–48 hours. An example of such a scenario might be foals that require more time while consideration is given for advanced diagnostic imaging procedures to make an informed decision about prognosis. TH would require considerable cost investment, owner dedication, and provision for management of complications. The application of TH in veterinary patients has been reviewed [158].

Application of TH

The sooner TH is initiated following TBI the better chance of success. Selective head cooling combined with mild systemic hypothermia (34.4–35 °C [93.9–95 °F]) is a well-tolerated method of reducing cerebral temperature in newborn infants after perinatal asphyxia [159]. The most readily available method of whole-body cooling in foals include surface application of ice packs around the head, neck, and axillary region, and evaporative cooling using fans, cool air conditioners, surface water misting, and administration of cold (4 °C [39.2 °F]) IV fluids. A rectal temperature of 35 °C (95 °F) was achieved in approximately 90 minutes using evaporative and surface cooling techniques in a 25 kg dog following TBI; intermittent hypothermia and high dose barbiturate therapy was maintained for 24 hours and credited for controlling post-traumatic seizures [160]. Use of the equine Cooling Collar (Figure 32.V.6) may be practical method of applying continuous surface

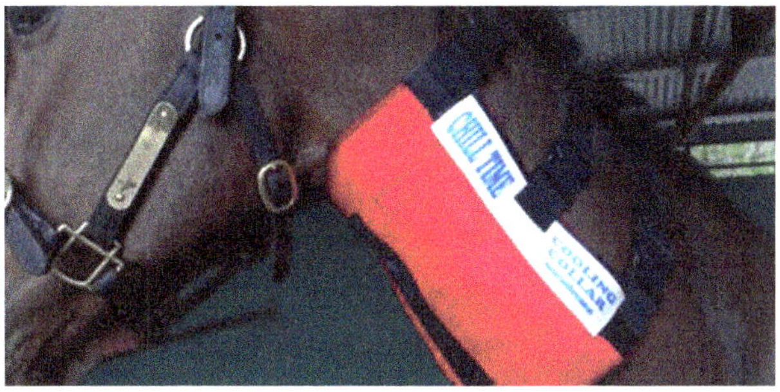

Figure 32.V.6 Application of the Cooling Collar in a racehorse. *Source:* Photo courtesy of Dr. Meg Brownlow. The cooling collar referred to is manufactured by Markey Saddlery, Australia.

cooling to the ventral neck of the foal as a possible means of cooling arterial blood to the brain. The Cooling Collar assists in prevention and management of exertional heat illness (EHI) in racehorses which is a syndrome characterized by neurologic dysfunction [161]. The basis for applying constant contact with crushed ice around the carotid artery and vein is that it creates a "heat sink" effect thus cooling blood flowing to the brain. In human athletes, application of ice packs to the lateral surface of the neck can reduce brain temperatures 0.2 °C–0.5 °C (0.3–0.9 °F) [162]. Although the exact mechanism by which the Cooling Collar assists in alleviation of neurologic signs of EHI in racehorses is unknown, application in foals with brain injury as a potentially selective head cooling technique is appealing. The cooling collar is designed for adult horses but has been custom made for racing greyhounds and could be adapted for foals.

Complications of TH

Numerous complications are associated with the cooling and rewarming phases of TH including bradycardia, arrhythmias, hypotension, decreased serum potassium, phosphorus, and magnesium, and increased blood glucose concentrations. Respiratory depression may require manual ventilation and cold diuresis can result from increased vascular resistance and associated suppression of ADH. Coagulopathy and increased risk of infection is also possible. TH also affects the pharmacokinetics and pharmacodynamics of many medications used in neonatal critical care, most notably benzodiazepines, opiates, and anti-epileptic drugs including barbituates [163]. These complications are manageable and reversible with rewarming but require intensive monitoring to facilitate prompt recognition and treatment, particularly during the rewarming phase to prevent rapid temperature increases.

Rewarming needs to be as slow as possible to prevent rewarming shock due to rapid peripheral vasodilation and blood pooling. This phenomenon is evident when surface rewarming is focused on the extremities rather than the core. A logical approach to rewarming in foals involves gradual cessation of active cooling and allowing the core body temperature to return to normal using tepid IV fluids, but it is important to avoid "overshooting" and causing hyperthermia with active warming techniques. Shivering is a frequent complication that requires prompt management to enable effective cooling, and to avoid associated increases in metabolic demand and cerebral energy consumption. Furthermore, feeling cold is an unpleasant, noxious stimulus. Shivering can be managed with continuous sedation and analgesia using opioids, benzodiazepines, and/or propofol. Gastrointestinal motility is reduced in hypothermic foals, thus enteral feeding should be avoided or limited to small, trophic feeds.

Other Therapies

Due to the controversial nature of corticosteroids in acute CNS injury, additional research involves development of therapies that address secondary brain and SCI; some are discussed briefly below.

Minocycline

Minocycline has beneficial neuroprotective effects in experimental and clinical trials for the management of TBI and SCI [164]. Minocycline and doxycycline are widely used antibiotics with anti-inflammatory effects. Minocycline appears to be more promising than other neuroprotective compounds studied because it targets multiple secondary injury mechanisms [165]. Minocycline also has lipophilic properties enabling superior BBB penetration, a wide safety margin, and sustained therapeutic efficacy (>3 hours) in experimental models [166]. Evidence of efficacy has not been investigated in large scale trials. However, minocycline and doxycycline have been recommended at therapeutic antimicrobial doses for traumatic CNS injury in horses based on their neuroprotective effects (minocycline, 4 mg/kg PO q12h; doxycycline, 10 mg/kg PO q12h) [76]. Until further evidence, use of tetracyclines in foals with TBI and SCI remain optional and open to clinical judgment.

Progesterone, erythropoietin, polyethylene glycol, calcium channel antagonists, and 21-aminosteroids are other compounds demonstrating promising neuroprotective effects in experimental models of CNS injury [28]. Clearly no single agent is likely to be effective, with current research focusing on multipotential drugs that modulate multiple secondary injury pathways. Until further clinical evidence becomes available, TBI and SCI in foals should focus on prioritizing acute stabilization and management and therapies that have clear indications for their use (Table 32.V.2). Management should also focus on diagnostic imaging and frequent re-assessment of response to therapy. Prognostic decisions are made based on anticipated future use of the foal and the owners wishes, recognizing that non-life-threatening neurologic improvement may require time.

Prognosis

Published reports of traumatic CNS injury in adult horses suggest a guarded prognosis for complete neurologic recovery [36, 42, 43, 167, 168]. Although prognosis is often dictated by severity of the primary injury, early and aggressive therapy targeting secondary injury can improve outcome. There is considerable variation in the types of neurologic injury and case presentations; hence, prognosis should be determined on an individual basis, with the foal's welfare held paramount. Foals 0–3 months of age have more opportunities for treatment success because of their small size, making them practically and financially more manageable for longer periods if recumbency compared to adult horses. The ability to perform advanced diagnostic imaging using MRI and CT is also an advantage in foals.

Initial neurologic improvement in response to medical management remains the best indicator of prognosis following CNS trauma. Diagnostic imaging provides valuable prognostic information to aid decision-making and whether to pursue treatment. Recumbent horses that receive prompt and appropriate intervention and respond by regaining the ability to stand with minimal assistance within 12–24 hours of initiating treatment have a reasonable prognosis for survival [102]. Foals with seizures and/or require continuous sedation should be afforded at least 48–72 hours to evaluate neurologic improvement. Residual deficits associated with vestibular and facial nerve injury may persist for long periods of time or permanently [154].

Some particular neurologic injuries carry a poorer prognosis for neurologic recovery than others. Traumatic optic neuropathy causing blindness and displaced basilar skull fractures have high morbidity and mortality and respond poorly to medical management due to the severity of the primary injury. Traumatic optic neuropathy is characterized by sudden onset of unilateral or bilateral blindness following blunt head trauma. Bilateral mydriasis with non-responsive pupils and a lack of menace response may be the only neurologic abnormality evident acutely. Over subsequent weeks following injury, ophthalmic examination reveals paling of the optic disc, marked reduction in retinal vasculature, and variable peripapillary pigment disruption [169]. Prognosis for return of vision is guarded to hopeless [169–171]. Displaced fractures of the basisphenoid bone from poll impact is also associated with a poor prognosis due to significant complications such as fracture fragments that can cause direct injury to brain tissue, life-threatening hemorrhage, risk of asphyxia from laceration of major vessels and development of bacterial meningitis [42, 81, 112, 172, 173] Despite a poorer prognosis, survival is possible in individual reported cases of basilar bone fracture if there is minimal injury to the brain parenchyma and major vessels and early and appropriate management [18, 112, 173]. For humane reasons, foals that survive traumatic CNS injury require a minimum level of neurologic function that enables them to independently maintain a good quality of life and ability to avoid further injury to themselves or their handlers. Equine athletes require near-normal neurologic and motor function and acceptable vision.

References

1 Stevens, R.D., Bhardwaj, A., Kirsch, J.R. et al. (2003). Critical care and perioperative management in traumatic spinal cord injury. *J. Neurosurg. Anesthesiol.* 15: 215–229.

2 Scrivani, P.V. (2011). Advanced imaging of the nervous system in the horse. *Vet. Clin. North Am. Equine Pract.* 27: 439–453.

3 Sande, A. and West, C. (2010). Traumatic brain injury: a review of pathophysiology and management. *J. Vet. Emerg. Crit. Care* 20: 177–190.

4 Mackay, R.J. (2004). Brain injury after head trauma: pathophysiology, diagnosis, and treatment. *Vet. Clin. North Am. Equine Pract.* 20: 199–216.

5 Nout-Lomas, Y.S. (2015). Fluid therapy during neurologic disease. In: *Equine Fluid Therapy* (ed. C.L. Fielding and K.G. Magdesian). Iowa: Wiley.

6 Park, E.H., White, G.A., and Tieber, L.M. (2012). Mechanisms of injury and emergency care of acute spinal cord injury in dogs and cats. *J. Vet. Emerg. Crit. Care* 22: 160–178.

7 Tennent-Brown, B.S. (2007). Trauma with neurologic sequelae. *Vet. Clin. North Am. Equine Pract.* 23: 81–101.

8 Matthews, H.K. and Nout, Y.S. (2004). Spinal cord, vertebral and intracranial trauma. In: *Equine Internal Medicine*, 2e (ed. S.M. Reed, W.M. Bayley, and D.C. Sellon). Missouri: Elsevier.

9 Kinoshita, K. (2016). Traumatic brain injury: pathophysiology for neurocritical care. *J. Intensive Care* 4: 29–29.

10 Dewey, C.W. (2002). Brain injury. In: *The Veterinary ICU Book* (ed. W.W. Wiingfield and M.R. Raffe). Wyoming: Teton New Media.

11 Mortazavi, M.M., Verma, K., Harmon, O.A. et al. (2015). The microanatomy of spinal cord injury: a review. *Clin. Anat.* 28: 27–36.

12 Josephson, L. (2004). Management of increased intracranial pressure: a primer for the non-neuro critical care nurse. *Dimens. Crit. Care Nurs.* 23: 194–207.

13 Hickey, R., Albin, M.S., Bunegin, L. et al. (1986). Autoregulation of spinal cord blood flow: is the cord a microcosm of the brain? *Stroke* 17: 1183–1189.

14 Kurita, T., Kawashima, S., Morita, K. et al. (2020). Spinal cord autoregulation using near-infrared spectroscopy under normal, hypovolemic, and post-fluid resuscitation conditions in a swine model: a comparison with cerebral autoregulation. *J. Intensive Care* 8: 1–10.

15 Nag, S., Manias, J.L., and Stewart, D.J. (2009). Pathology and new players in the pathogenesis of brain edema. *Acta Neuropathol.* 118: 197–217.

16 Unterberg, A.W., Stover, J., Kress, B. et al. (2004). Edema and brain trauma. *Neuroscience* 129: 1019–1027.

17 Hagg, T. (2013). Vascular mechanisms in spinal cord injury. In: *Vascular Mechanisms in CNS Trauma*, Springer Series in Translational Stroke Research, vol. 5 (ed. E. Lo, J. Lok, M. Ning, and M. Whalen). New York: Springer.
18 Hayta, E. and Elden, H. (2018). Acute spinal cord injury: a review of pathophysiology and potential of non-steroidal anti-inflammatory drugs for pharmacological intervention. *J. Chem. Neuroanat.* 87: 25–31.
19 Ruiz, I.A., Squair, J.W., Phillips, A.A. et al. (2018). Incidence and natural progression of neurogenic shock after traumatic spinal cord injury. *J. Neurotrauma* 35: 461–466.
20 Olby, N. (2010). The pathogenesis and treatment of acute spinal cord injuries in dogs. *Vet. Clin. North Am. Small Anim. Pract.* 40: 791–807.
21 Loane, D.J. and Faden, A.I. (2010). Neuroprotection for traumatic brain injury: translational challenges and emerging therapeutic strategies. *Trends Pharmacol. Sci.* 31: 596–604.
22 Ikeda, Y. and Long, D.M. (1990). Comparative effects of direct and indirect hydroxyl radical scavengers on traumatic brain oedema. *Acta Neurochir.* Suppl.51: 74–76.
23 Genovese, T. and Cuzzocrea, S. (2008). Role of free radicals and poly (ADP-ribose) polymerase-1 in the development of spinal cord injury: new potential therapeutic targets. *Curr. Med. Chem.* 15: 477–487.
24 Tator, C.H. and Fehlings, M.G. (1991). Review of the secondary injury theory of acute spinal cord trauma with emphasis on vascular mechanisms. *J. Neurosurg.* 75: 15–26.
25 Sadrzadeh, S.M. and Eaton, J.W. (1988). Hemoglobin-mediated oxidant damage to the central nervous system requires endogenous ascorbate. *J. Clin. Invest.* 82: 1510–1515.
26 Xiong, Y. and Hall, E.D. (2009). Pharmacological evidence for a role of peroxynitrite in the pathophysiology of spinal cord injury. *Exp. Neurol.* 216: 105–114.
27 Furr, M. (2008). Pharmaceutical considerations for treatment of central nervous system disease. In: *Equine Neurology* (ed. M. Furr and S. Reed). Wiley ProQuest Ebook Central.
28 Hellewell, S., Semple, B.D., and Morganti-Kossmann, M.C. (2016). Therapies negating neuroinflammation after brain trauma. *Brain Res.* 1640 (Part A): 36–56.
29 Ziebell, J.M. and Morganti-Kossmann, M.C. (2010). Involvement of pro- and anti-inflammatory cytokines and chemokines in the pathophysiology of traumatic brain injury. *Neurotherapeut. Neurotherapeut.* 7: 22–30.
30 Chesnut, R.M., Marshall, L.F., Klauber, M.R. et al. (1993). The role of secondary brain injury in determining outcome from severe head injury. *J. Trauma* 34: 216–222.
31 Spaite, D.W., Hu, C., Bobrow, B.J. et al. (2017). The effect of combined out-of-hospital hypotension and hypoxia on mortality in major traumatic brain injury. *Ann. Emerg. Med.* 69: 62–72.
32 Pigula, F.A., Wlad, S.L., Shackford, S.R. et al. (1993). The effects of hypotension and hypoxia on children with severe head injuries. *J. Pediatr. Surg.* 28: 310–316.
33 Summers, R.L., Baker, S.D., Sterling, S.A. et al. (2013). Characterization of the spectrum of hemodynamic profiles in trauma patients with acute neurogenic shock. *J. Crit. Care* 28: 531.e1–531.e5.
34 Levi, L., Wolf, A., and Belzberg, H. (1993). Hemodynamic parameters in patients with acute cervical cord trauma: description, intervention, and prediction of outcome. *Neurosurgery* 33: 1007–1016.
35 Furlan, J.C. and Fehlings, M.G. (2008). Cardiovascular complications after acute spinal cord injury: pathophysiology, diagnosis, and management. *Neurosurg. Focus* 25: E13.
36 DeBowes, M.R. and Gift, L. (1993). Trauma of the brain and spinal cord. In: *Current Therapy in Equine Medicine*, 3e (ed. N.E. Robinson), 535–539. Philadelphia: W.B. Saunders Co.
37 Moore, R.B. (1997). Central nervous system trauma. In: *Current Therapy in Equine Medicine*, 4e (ed. N.E. Robinson), 301–305. Philadelphia: Saunders.
38 Bernard, W. (2011). Neurologic disorders. In: *Equine Pediatric Medicine: Covering the Aetiology, Pathophysiology, Clinical Presentation, Differential Diagnosis, Diagnosis and Management* (ed. B. William and B.S. Barr). Manson Publishing, Limited.
39 Reed, S.M. (1993). Management of head trauma in horses. *Compend. Contin. Ed. Pract. Vet.* 15: 270–273.
40 Roberts, I., Yates, D., Sandercock, P. et al. (2004). CRASH trial collaborators. Effect of intravenous corticosteroids on death within 14 days in 10008 adults with clinically significant head injury (MRC CRASH trial): randomised placebo-controlled trial. *Lancet* 364 (9442): 1321–1328.
41 Reed, S.M. (2007). Clinical commentary head trauma: a neurological emergency. *Equine Vet. Educ.* 19: 365–367.
42 Feige, K., Fürst, A., Kaser-Hotz, B. et al. (2000). Traumatic injury to the central nervous system in horses: occurrence, diagnosis and outcome. *Equine Vet. Educ.* 12: 220–224.
43 De Zani, D., Zani, D., Binanti, P. et al. (2013). Magnetic resonance features of closed head trauma in two foals. *Equine Vet. Educ.* 25: 493–498.
44 Ragle, C.A., Koblik, P.D., Pascoe, J.R., and Honnas, C.M. (1988). Computed tomographic evaluation of head trauma in a foal. *Vet. Radiol.* 29: 206–208.
45 Barba, M. and Lepage, O.M. (2013). 2013 diagnostic utility of computed tomography imaging in foals: 10 cases (2008–2010). *Equine Vet. Educ.* 25: 29–38.
46 Brain Trauma Foundation; American Association of Neurological Surgeons; Congress of Neurological Surgeons; Joint Section on Neurotrauma and Critical

Care, AANS/CNS, Bratton, S.L. et al. (2007). Guidelines for the management of severe traumatic brain injury. VI. Indications for intracranial pressure monitoring. *J. Neurotrauma* 24 (Suppl 1): S37–S44.
47 Brain Trauma Foundation; American Association of Neurological Surgeons; Congress of Neurological Surgeons; Joint Section on Neurotrauma and Critical Care, AANS/CNS, Bratton, S.L., Chestnut, R.M. et al. (2007). Guidelines for the management of severe traumatic brain injury. IX. Cerebral perfusion thresholds. *J. Neurotrauma* 24 (Suppl 1): S59–S64.
48 Meyer, M.J., Megyesi, J., Meythaler, J. et al. (2010). Acute management of acquired brain injury part I: an evidence-based review of non-pharmacological interventions. *Brain Inj.* 24: 694–705.
49 Davis, D.P., Peay, J., Sise, M.J. et al. (2010). Prehospital airway and ventilation management: a trauma score and injury severity score-based analysis. *J. Trauma* 69: 294–301.
50 Sharma, D. and Holowaychuk, M. (2015). Retrospective evaluation of prognostic indicators in dogs with head trauma: 72 cases (January–March 2011). *J. Vet. Emerg. Crit. Care* 25: 631–639.
51 Ramaiah, V.K., Sharma, D., Ma, L. et al. (2013). Admission oxygenation and ventilation parameters associated with discharge survival in severe pediatric traumatic brain injury. *Childs Nerv. Syst.* 29: 629–634.
52 Bhalla, T., Dewhirst, E., Sawardekar, A. et al. (2012). Perioperative management of pediatric patient with traumatic brain injury. *Pediatr. Anesth.* 22: 627–664.
53 Kuo, K.W. and Taylor AR, B.L.M. (2018). Head trauma. *Vet. Clin. North Am. Small Anim. Pract.* 48: 111–128.
54 Dunkel, B., Corley, K.T.T., Johnson, A.L. et al. (2013). Pneumocephalus in five horses. *Equine Vet. J.* 45: 367–371.
55 Davis, D., Dunford, J., Poste, J. et al. (2004). The impact of hypoxia and hyperventilation on outcome after paramedic rapid sequence intubation of severely head-injured patients. *J. Trauma* 57: 1–8.
56 Sinclair, M. (2015). Chapter 182. Sedation and anesthetic management of foals. In: *Robinson's Current Therapy in Equine Medicine*, 7e (ed. K.A. Sprayberry and N.E. Robinson), 766–771. Elsevier Saunders.
57 Dewey, C.W. (2000). Emergency management of the head trauma patient: principles and practice. *Vet. Clin. North Am. Small Anim. Pract.* 30: 207–225.
58 Kannan, N., Wang, J., Mink, R.B. et al. (2018). The PEGASUS (pediatric guideline adherence and outcomes) study. Timely hemodynamic resuscitation and outcomes in severe pediatric traumatic brain injury: preliminary findings. *Pediatr. Emerg. Care* 34: 325–329.
59 Huang, M.S., Shih, H.C., Wu, J.K. et al. (1995). Urgent laparotomy versus emergency craniotomy for multiple trauma with head injury patients. *J. Trauma* 38: 154–157.
60 Reed, S.M. (2020). Medical aspects of traumatic brain injury in horses. In: *Equine Fracture Repair*, 2e (ed. A.J. Nixon). Wiley.
61 Palmer, J.E. (2004). Fluid therapy in the neonate: not your mother's fluid space. *Vet. Clin. North Am. Equine Pract.* 20: 63–75.
62 Finfer, S., Bellomo, R., Boyce, N. et al. (2004). A comparison of albumin and saline for fluid resuscitation in the intensive care unit. *N. Engl. J. Med.* 350: 2247–2256.
63 Reinhart, K., Perner, A., Sprung, C.L. et al. (2012). Consensus statement of the ESICM task force on colloid volume therapy in critically ill patients. *Intensive Care Med.* 38: 368–383.
64 Jin, G., DeMoya, M.A., Duggan, M. et al. (2012). Traumatic brain injury and hemorrhagic shock: evaluation of different resuscitation strategies in a large animal model of combined insults. *Shock* 38: 49–56.
65 Vavilala, M.S., Bowen, A., Lam, A.M. et al. (2003). Blood pressure and outcome after severe pediatric traumatic brain injury. *J. Trauma* 55: 1039–1044.
66 Kochanek et al. (2019). Guidelines for the Management of Pediatric Severe TBI, 3rd ed. update of the BTF guidelines. *Pediatr. Crit. Care Med.* 20 (3SSuppl 1): S1–S82.
67 Menacho, S.T. and Floyd, C. (2021). Current practices and goals for mean arterial pressure and spinal cord perfusion pressure in acute traumatic spinal cord injury: defining the gaps in knowledge. *J. Spinal Cord Med.* 44: 350–356.
68 Gao, X. and Dong, X. (2020). A retrospective study of hemodynamic management in traumatic spinal cord injury (abstract). *Crit. Care Med.* 48: 362.
69 Bouzat, P., Sala, N., Payen, J.F. et al. (2013). Beyond intracranial pressure: optimization of cerebral blood flow, oxygen, and substrate delivery after traumatic brain injury. *Ann. Intensive Care* 3: 1–9.
70 Moro, N., Ghavim, S., Harris, N.G. et al. (2013). Glucose administration after traumatic brain injury improves cerebral metabolism and reduces secondary neuronal injury. *Brain Res.* 1535: 124–136.
71 Shijo, K., Sutton, R.L., Ghavim, S.S. et al. (2017). Metabolic fate of glucose in rats with traumatic brain injury and pyruvate or glucose treatments: a NMR spectroscopy study. *Neurochem. Int.* 102: 66–78.
72 Elkon, B., Cambrin, J.R., Hirshberg, E.L. et al. (2014). An independent risk factor for poor outcome in children with traumatic brain injury. *Pediatr. Crit. Care Med.* 15: 623–631.
73 Syring, R.S., Otto, C.M., and Drobatz, K.J. (2001). Hyperglycemia in dogs and cats with head trauma: 122 cases (1997–1999). *J. Am. Vet. Med. Assoc.* 218: 1124–1129.
74 Rovlias, A. and Kotsou, S. (2000). The influence of hyperglycemia on neurological outcome in patients with severe head injury. *Neurosurgery* 46: 335–342.

75 Cole, C. and Bentz, B. (2015). Treatment of equine nervous system disorders. In: *Equine Pharmacology*, 1e (ed. C. Cole, B. Bentz, and L. Maxwell). Wiley.

76 Johnson, A.L. and Divers, T.J. (2014). Neurologic emergencies. In: *Equine Emergencies: Treatment and Procedures*, 4e (ed. J.A. Orsini and T.J. Divers). St. Louis, MO: Elsevier/Saunders.

77 Green, D., O'Phelan, K., Bassin, S. et al. (2010). Intensive versus conventional insulin therapy in critically ill neurologic patients. *Neurocrit. Care* 13: 299–306.

78 Mtaweh, H. and Bell, M.J. (2015). Management of pediatric traumatic brain injury. *Curr. Treat. Options. Neurol.* 17: 1–13.

79 Magdesian, K.G. (2015). Fluid therapy for neonatal foals. In: *Equine Fluid Therapy* (ed. C.L. Fielding and K.G. Magdesian). Iowa: Wiley.

80 Johnson, A.L. and Divers, T.J. (2008). Neurologic emergencies. In: *Equine Emergencies: Treatment and Procedures*, 3e (ed. J.A. Orsini and T.J. Divers). St. Louis, MO: Elsevier/Saunders.

81 Feary, D.J., Magdesian, K.G., Aleman, M.A. et al. (2007). Traumatic brain injury in horses: 34 cases (1994–2004). *J. Am. Vet. Med. Assoc.* 231: 259–266.

82 Xu, G.Z., Wang, M.D., Liu, K.G. et al. (2013). A meta-analysis of treating acute traumatic brain injury with calcium channel blockers. *Brain Res. Bull.* 99: 41–47.

83 Zhang, L., Wang, H., Zhou, X. et al. (2019). Role of mitochondrial calcium uniporter-mediated Ca2+ and iron accumulation in traumatic brain injury. *J. Cell. Mol. Med.* 23: 2995–3009.

84 Vaala, W.E. (2009). Supportive care of the abnormal newborn. In: *Large Animal Internal Medicine*, 4e (ed. B.P. Smith), 325–332. St Louis: Mosby.

85 Lacombe, V. and Furr, M. (2015). Differential diagnosis and management of horses with seizures or alterations in consciousness. In: *Equine Neurology*, 2e (ed. M. Furr and S. Reed). Wiley.

86 Liesemer, K., Bratton, S.L., Zebrack, C.M. et al. (2011). Early post-traumatic seizures in moderate to severe pediatric traumatic brain injury: rates, risk factors, and clinical features. *J. Neurotrauma* 28: 755–762.

87 Lewis, R.J., Yee, L., Inkelis, S.H. et al. (1993). Clinical predictors of post-traumatic seizures in children with head trauma. *Ann. Emerg. Med.* 22: 1114–1118.

88 Gold, J., Chaffin, M.K., Burgess, B.A. et al. (2016). Factors associated with non-survival in foals diagnosed with perinatal asphyxia syndrome. *J. Equine Vet. Sci.* 38: 82–86.

89 Savage, V.L., Collins, N.M., Axon, J.E. et al. (2015). The effect of generalised seizures on outcome in foals with neonatal encephalopathy: 246 cases. In: *Bain Fallon Memorial Lectures*, 11. Australia: Australian Equine Veterinary Association.

90 Norman, W.M., Court, M.H., and Greenblatt, D.J. (1997). Age-related changes in the pharmacokinetic disposition of diazepam in foals. *Am. J. Vet. Res.* 58: 878–880.

91 Wilkins, P.A. (2003). Hypoxic ischemic encephalopathy: neonatal encephalopathy. Recent advances in equine neonatal care. In: *International Veterinary Information Service (www.ivis.org)* (ed. P.A. Wilkins and J.E. Palmer). Ithaca, New York.

92 Wilkins, P. (2005). How to use midazolam to control equine neonatal seizures. *Proc. Am. Assoc. Equine Pract.* 51: 279–280.

93 Wong, D.M., Wikins, P.A., Bain, F.T. et al. (2011). Neonatal encephalopathy in foals. *Compend. Contin. Educ. Vet.* 33: E5.

94 Favrais, G., Ursino, M., Mouchel, C. et al. (2019). Levetiracetam optimal dose-finding as first-line treatment for neonatal seizures occurring in the context of hypoxic ischaemic encephalopathy (LEVNEONAT-1): study protocol of a phase II trial. *BMJ* 9: e022739.

95 Cesar, F.B., Stewart, A.J., Boothe, D.M. et al. (2017). Disposition of levetiracetam in healthy adult horses. *J. Vet. Pharmacol. Ther.* 41: 92–97.

96 Macdonald, K.D., Hart, K.A., Davis, J.L. et al. (2018). Pharmacokinetics of the anticonvulsant levetiracetam in neonatal foals. *Equine Vet. J.* 50: 532–536.

97 Platt, S., Freeman, C., and Beltran, E. (2016). Canine head trauma: an update. *In Pract.* 38: 3–8.

98 Jacobs, S.E., Berg, M., Hunt, R. et al. (2013). Cooling for newborns with hypoxic ischaemic encephalopathy. *Cochrane Database Syst. Rev.* (3): Available at EBM Reviews-Cochrane Database: http://ovidsp.ovid.com/ovidweb.cgi.

99 Vats, A., Chambliss, C.R., Anand, K.J.S. et al. (1999). Is hypertonic saline an effective alternative to mannitol in the treatment of elevated intracranial pressure in pediatric patients? *J. Intensive Care Med.* 14: 184–188.

100 Rickard, A.C., Smith, J.E., Newell, P. et al. (2014). Salt or sugar for your injured brain? A meta-analysis of randomised controlled trials of mannitol versus hypertonic sodium solutions to manage raised intracranial pressure in traumatic brain injury (review). *Emerg. Med. J.* 31: 679–683.

101 Stopa, B.M., Dolmans, R.G., Broekman, M.L. et al. (2019). Hyperosmolar therapy in pediatric severe traumatic brain injury – a systematic review. *Crit. Care Med.* 47: e1022–e1031.

102 Hurcombe, S.D.A. (2015). Acute neurologic injury. In: *Robinson's Current Therapy in Equine Medicine*, 7e (ed. K.A. Sprayberry and N.E. Robinson). St Louis, Missouri: Elsevier Inc.

103 Magdesian, K.G. (2009). Chapter 44. Critical care fluid therapy for horses. In: *Large Animal Internal Medicine*,

4e (ed. B.P. Smith), 1498–1501. St Louis Missouri: Mosby Elsevier.

104 Lescot, T., Degos, V., Zouaoui, A. et al. (2006). Opposed effects of hypertonic saline on contusions and noncontused brain tissue in patients with severe traumatic brain injury. *Crit. Care Med.* 34: 3029–3033.

105 Nout, Y.S., Mihai, G., Tovar, C.A. et al. (2009). Hypertonic saline attenuates cord swelling and edema in experimental spinal cord injury: a study utilizing magnetic resonance imaging. *Crit. Care Med.* 37: 2160–2166.

106 Erdman, M.J., Riha, H., Bode, L. et al. (2017). Predictors of acute kidney injury in neurocritical care patients receiving continuous hypertonic saline. *Neurohospitalist* 7: 9–14.

107 Fielding, C.L. (2015). Sodium and water homeostasis and derangements. In: *Equine Fluid Therapy* (ed. C.L. Fielding and K.G. Magdesian). Iowa: Wiley.

108 Bergold, P.J. (2016). Treatment of traumatic brain injury with anti-inflammatory drugs. *Exp. Neurol.* 275: 367–380.

109 Carney, N., Totten, A.M., O'Reilly, C. et al. (2017). Guidelines for the Management of Severe Traumatic Brain Injury, Fourth Edition. *Neurosurgery* 80: 6–15.

110 Browne, K., Iwata, A., Putt, M.E. et al. (2006). Chronic ibuprofen administration worsens cognitive outcome following traumatic brain injury in rats. *Exp. Neurol.* 201: 301–307.

111 Furr, M. (1996). Managing seizure disorders in neonatal foals. *Vet. Med.* 91: 772–778.

112 Atherton, R.P., Mitchell, E.V., McKenzie, K.C. et al. (2007). Traumatic fracture of the basisphenoid and secondary bacterial meningitis in a thoroughbred gelding. *Equine Vet. Educ.* 19: 359–364.

113 Akhigbe, T., Tope, A.D., and Anakwenze, A. (2018). Role of corticosteroids in the management of acute traumatic brain injury: literature review and critical appraisal of evidence. *Intern. J. Med. Rev. Case Rep.* 2: 22–28.

114 Fanconi, S., Kloti, J., Meuli, M. et al. (1988). Dexamethasone therapy and endogenous cortisol production in severe pediatric head injury. *Intensive Care Med.* 14: 163–166.

115 Hoshide, R., Cheung, V., Marshall, L. et al. (2016). Do corticosteroids play a role in the management of traumatic brain injury? *Surg. Neurol. Int.* 7: 84.

116 Braakman, R., Schouten, H.J., Blaauw-van Dishoeck, M. et al. (1983). Megadose steroids in severe head injury. Results of a prospective double-blind clinical trial. *J. Neurosurg.* 58: 326–330.

117 Grumme, T., Baethmann, A., Kolodziejczyk, D. et al. (1995). Treatment of patients with severe head injury by triamcinolone: a prospective, controlled multicenter clinical trial of 396 cases. *Res. Exp. Med.* 195: 217–229.

118 Saul, T.G., Ducker, T.B., Salcman, M. et al. (1981). Steroids in severe head injury: a prospective randomized clinical trial. *J. Neurosurg.* 54: 596–600.

119 Gaab, M.R., Trost, H.A., Alcantara, A. et al. (1994). "Ultrahigh" dexamethasone in acute brain injury. Results from a prospective randomized double-blind multicenter trial (GUDHIS). German Ultrahigh Dexamethasone Head Injury Study Group. *Zentralbl Neurochir* 55: 135–143.

120 Castagnetti, C. and Mariella, J. (2015). Anti-inflammatory drugs in equine neonatal medicine. Part II: corticosteroids. *J. Equine Vet. Sci.* 35: 547–554.

121 Breslin, K. and Agrawal, D. (2012). The use of methylprednisolone in acute spinal cord injury a review of the evidence, controversies, and recommendation. *Pediatr. Emerg. Care* 28: 1238–1248.

122 Hall, E.D. and Springer, J.E. (2004). Neuroprotection and acute spinal cord injury: a reappraisal. *NeuroRx* 1: 80–100.

123 Levine, J.M., Levine, G.J., Boozer, L. et al. (2008). Adverse effects and outcome associated with dexamethasone administration in dogs with acute thoracolumbar intervertebral disk herniation: 161 cases (2000–2006). *J. Am. Vet. Med. Assoc.* 232: 411–417.

124 Ruddle, T.L., Allen, D.A., Schertel, E.R. et al. (2006). Outcome and prognostic factors in nonambulatory Hansen type I intervertebral disc extrusions: 308 cases. *Vet. Comp. Orthop. Traumatol.* 19: 29–34.

125 Bracken, M.B., Collins, W.F., Freeman, D.F. et al. (1984). Efficacy of methylprednisolone in acute spinal cord injury. *JAMA* 251: 45–52.

126 Bracken, M.B., Shepard, M.J., Hellenbrand, K.G. et al. (1985). Methylprednisolone and neurological function 1 year after spinal cord injury. Results of the National Acute Spinal Cord Injury Study. *J. Neurosurg.* 63: 704–713.

127 Bracken, M.B., Shepard, M.J., Collins, W.F. et al. (1990). A randomized, controlled trial of methylprednisolone or naloxone in the treatment of acute spinal-cord injury. Results of the Second National Acute Spinal Cord Injury Study. *N. Engl. J. Med.* 322: 1405–1411.

128 Bracken, M.B., Shepard, M.J., Holford, T.R. et al. (1997). Administration of methylprednisolone for 24 or 48 hours or tirilazad mesylate for 48 hours in the treatment of acute spinal cord injury. Results of the third National Acute Spinal Cord Injury Randomized Controlled Trial. National Acute Spinal Cord Injury Study. *JAMA* 277: 1597–1604.

129 Bydon, M., Lin, J., Macki, M. et al. (2014). The current role of steroids in acute spinal cord injury. *World Neurosurg.* 82 (5): 848–854.

130 Kwon, B.K., Tetzlaff, W., Grauer, J.N. et al. (2004). Pathophysiology and pharmacologic treatment of acute spinal cord injury. *Spine J.* 4: 451–464.

131 Platt, S., Abramson, C., and Garosi, L. (2005). Administering corticosteroids in neurologic disease. *Compend. Contin. Educ. Pract. Vet.* 210–220.

132 Brown, M.P., Gronwall, R., and Castro, L. (1988). Pharmacokinetics and body fluid and endometrial concentrations of trimethoprim–sulfamethoxazole in mares. *Am. J. Vet. Res.* 1988 (49): 918–922.

133 Vavilala, M.S., Lujan, S.B., Qiu, Q. et al. (2017). Intensive care treatments associated with favorable discharge outcomes in Argentine children with severe traumatic brain injury: for the south American guideline adherence group. *PLoS One* 12: e0189296.

134 Kao, C.H., ChangLai, S., Cheing, P. et al. (1998). Gastric emptying in head injured patients. *Am. J. Gastroenterol.* 93: 1108–1112.

135 Jacob, S.W. and de la Torre, J.C. (2015). *Dimethyl Sulfoxide (DMSO) in Trauma and Disease*. NW: CRC Press, Taylor & Francis Group.

136 Jacob, S.W. and de la Torre, J.C. (2009). Pharmacology of dimethyl sulfoxide in cardiac and CNS damage. *Pharmacol. Rep.* 61: 225–235.

137 Di Giorgio, A.M., Hou, Y., Zhao, X. et al. (2008). Dimethyl sulfoxide provides neuroprotection in a traumatic brain injury model. *Restor. Neurol. Neurosci.* 26: 501–507.

138 Santos, N.C., Figueira-Coelho, J., Martins-Silva, J. et al. (2003). Multidisciplinary utilization of dimethyl sulfoxide: pharmacological, cellular, and molecular aspects. *Biochem. Pharmacol.* 65: 1035–1041.

139 Hanslick, J.L., Lau, K., Noguchi, K.K. et al. (2009). Dimethylsulfoxide (DMS0) produces widespread apoptosis in the developing nervous system. *Neurobiol. Dis.* 34: 1–10.

140 Yuan, C., Gao, J., Guo, J. et al. (2014). Dimethyl sulfoxide damages mitochondrial integrity and membrane potential in cultured astrocytes. *PLoS One* 9: e107447.

141 Soma, L.R., Robinson, M.A., You, Y. et al. (2018). Pharmacokinetics, disposition, and plasma concentrations of dimethyl sulfoxide (DMSO) in the horse following topical, oral, and intravenous administration. *J. Vet. Pharmacol. Ther.* 41: 384–392.

142 Fowler, A.A., Syed, A.A., Knowlson, S. et al. (2014). Phase I safety trial of intravenous ascorbic acid in patients with severe sepsis. *J. Transl. Med.* 12: 32.

143 Carr, A.C., Rosengrave, P.C., Bayer, S. et al. (2017). Hypovitaminosis C and vitamin C deficiency in critically ill patients despite recommended enteral and parenteral intakes. *Crit. Care* 21: 300.

144 Polidori, M.C., Mecocci, P., and Frei, B. (2001). Plasma vitamin C levels are decreased and correlated with brain damage in patients with intracranial hemorrhage or head trauma. *Stroke* 32: 898–902.

145 Marlin, D.J. and Allen, W.R. (2017). Ascorbic acid status in pony mares and young pony foals. *J. Equine Vet. Sci.* 76: 36–129.

146 Leichtle, S.W., Sarma, A.K., Strein, M. et al. (2020). High-dose intravenous ascorbic acid: ready for prime time in traumatic brain injury? *Neurocrit. Care* 32: 333–339.

147 Löscher, W., Jaeschke, G., and Keller, H. (1984). Pharmacokinetics of ascorbic acid in horses. *Equine Vet. J.* 16: 59–65.

148 Anderson, M.J., Ibrahim, A.S., Cooper, B.R. et al. (2020). Effects of administration of ascorbic acid and low-dose hydrocortisone after infusion of sublethal doses of lipopolysaccharide to horses. *J. Vet. Intern. Med.* 34: 2710–2718.

149 Annink, K.V., Franz, A.R., Derks, J.B. et al. (2017). Allopurinol: old drug, new indication in neonates? *Curr. Pharm. Des.* 23: 5935–5942.

150 Mills, P.C., Dunnett, M., and Smith, N.C. (1995). The pharmacokinetics of oral and intravenous allopurinol and intravenous oxypurinol in the horse. *J. Vet. Pharmacol. Ther.* 18: 451–456.

151 Sen, A.P. and Gulati, A. (2010). Use of magnesium in traumatic brain injury. *Neurotherapeutics* 7: 91–99.

152 Wen, L., Yin-An, B., Ya-Jun, L. et al. (2015). Magnesium sulfate for acute traumatic brain injury. *J. Craniofac. Surg.* 26: 393–398.

153 Natale, J.E., Guerguerian, A., Joseph, J. et al. (2007). Pilot study to determine the hemodynamic safety and feasibility of magnesium sulfate infusion in children with severe traumatic brain injury. *Pediatr. Crit. Care Med.* 8: 85.

154 Mackay, R. (2015). Trauma to the brain and cranial nerves. In: *Large Animal Internal Medicine*, 5e (ed. B.P. Smith), 927–931. St Louis: Mosby.

155 Li, H., Lu, G., Shi, W. et al. (2009). Protective effect of moderate hypothermia on severe traumatic brain injury in children. *J. Neurotrauma* 26: 1905–1909.

156 Cooper, D.J., Nichol, A.D., Bailey, M. et al. (2018). POLAR trial investigators and ANZICS clinical trials group. Effect of early sustained prophylactic hypothermia on neurologic outcomes among patients with severe traumatic brain injury: the POLAR randomized clinical trial. *JAMA* 320: 2211–2220.

157 Adelson, P.D., Wisniewski, S.R., Beca, J. et al. (2013). Comparison of hypothermia and normothermia after severe traumatic brain injury in children (cool kids): a phase 3, randomised controlled trial. *Lancet Neurol.* 12: 546–553.

158 Brodeur, A., Wright, A., and Cortes, Y. (2017). Hypothermia and targeted temperature management in cats and dogs. *J. Vet. Emerg. Crit. Care* 27: 151–163.

159 Battin, M.R., Penrice, J., Gunn, T.R. et al. (2003). Treatment of term infants with head cooling and mild systemic hypothermia (35.0 °C and 34.5 °C) after perinatal asphyxia. *Pediatrics* 111: 244–251.

160 Hayes, G.M. (2009). Severe seizures associated with traumatic brain injury managed by controlled hypothermia, pharmacologic coma, and mechanical ventilation in a dog. *J. Vet. Emerg. Crit. Care* 19: 629–634.

161 Brownlow, M. (2018). Alleviation of thermal strain after racing in the thoroughbred racehorse with the use of a cooling collar. *CVE Control Therapy Ser.* 293: 33–37.

162 Gordon, N.F., Bogdanffy, G.M., and Wilkinson, J. (1990). Effect of a practical neck cooling device on core temperature during exercise. *Med. Sci. Sports Exerc.* 22: 245–249.

163 Polderman, K.H. (2009). Mechanisms of action, physiological effects, and complications of hypothermia. *Crit. Care Med.* 37 (7 Suppl): S186–S202.

164 Meythaler, J., Fath, J., Fuerst, D. et al. (2019). Safety and feasibility of minocycline in treatment of acute traumatic brain injury. *Brain Inj.* 33: 679–689.

165 Shultz, R.B. and Zhong, Y. (2017). Minocycline targets multiple secondary injury mechanisms in traumatic spinal cord injury. *Neural Regen. Res.* 12: 702–713.

166 Elewa, H.F., Hilali, H., Hess, D.C. et al. (2006). Minocycline for short-term neuroprotection. *Pharmacotherapy* 26: 515–521.

167 Ramirez, O., Jorgensen, J.S., and Thrall, D.E. (1998). Imaging basilar skull fractures in the horse: a review. *Vet. Radiol. Ultrasound* 39: 391–395.

168 Reppas, G.P., Hodgson, D.R., McClintock, S.A. et al. (1995). Trauma-induced blindness in two horses. *Aust. Vet. J.* 72: 270–272.

169 Martin, L., Kaswan, R., and Chapman, W. (1986). Four cases of traumatic optic nerve blindness in the horse. *Equine Vet. J.* 18: 133–137.

170 Brooks, D.E., Plummer, C.E., Craft, S.L.M. et al. (2014). Optic neuropathy in the horse. *Equine Vet. Educ.* 26: 527–531.

171 Kullmann, A., Marteniuk, J.V., Williams, M.R. et al. (2014). Optic nerve avulsion. *Equine Vet. Educ.* 26: 523–526.

172 Stick, J.A., Wilson, T., and Kunze, D. (1980). Basilar skull fractures in three horses. *J. Am. Vet. Med. Assoc.* 176: 228–231.

173 Sweeney, C.R., Freeman, D.E., Sweeney, R.W. et al. (1993). Hemorrhage into the guttural pouch (auditory tube diverticulum) associated with rupture of the longus capitis muscle in three horses. *J. Am. Vet. Med. Assoc.* 202: 1129–1131.

Section VI Traumatic Brain and Spinal Cord Injury in the Foal

Gustavo Ferlini Agne and Darien Feary

Neurologic disease secondary to trauma to the central nervous system (CNS) occurs more frequently in foals compared to adult horses. However, information regarding this topic in foals is not readily available and is often extrapolated from adult horses and people. Traumatic events leading to neurologic deficits may occur at any stage of the foal's development. Perinatal neurologic disease secondary to trauma to the CNS has been reported in 6/28 foals in a study investigating neurologic disease in horses. From those foals, 5/6 had a history of dystocia and were diagnosed at necropsy to have brain, spinal cord, and subdural hemorrhage [1]. Most of the traumatic injuries related to the CNS occur while foals are being handled or restrained at the farm. Therefore, the attending veterinarian is essential in providing initial evaluation of the patient until referral to a hospital is possible. A thorough systematic neurological examination allows for initial neuroanatomical localization and determination of the extent of the initial insult, which will facilitate establishing a prognosis and treatment plan.

Neurologic examination can be challenging given the differences in response to stimuli in foals compared to adult horses. Furthermore, newborn foal's neurologic examination findings vary between different life stages [2]. In a study evaluating 49 foals within their first two weeks of life, a variety of singularities was displayed by newborn foals in contrast to adults. Foals have a flexed head–neck positioning and are often observed to walk with a rhythmic head bobbing movement, especially at the trot or when seeking the udder [3]. These are viewed as normal behavior and well documented during clinical investigation in order to allow differentiation from pathological conditions. The authors recommend performing neurological assessments with every physical examination, as neurologic deficits might change rapidly overtime.

Following strict protocols during examination is important, as there is high inter-observer variation often noted with the subjective nature of a neurologic evaluation [4]. An examination form aids in consistency between examiner and maintains accuracy of medical records during sequential examinations. A description of the neurologic examination is described elsewhere (Chapter 30) with the following focusing on examination associated with CNS pathology related to traumatic events.

Neurological Examination of the Neonatal Foal after CNS Trauma

Foals suspected of CNS trauma should be evaluated with caution. The environment should be conducive to safe observation from a distance and if the foal is not recumbent, allow for free interaction with the dam and for any abnormal behavior, posture, or gait deficits to be displayed. As with other clinical investigations, signalment and a detailed history are essential to guide neurologic assessment, as some breeds have higher predisposition for specific neurologic conditions that can lead to ataxia and seizure-induced trauma [5, 6]. Furthermore, history of specific traumatic events such as a foal falling while restrained or being stepped on or kicked by the dam can provide crucial information. Neuroanatomic localization of a specific lesion is extremely important and is facilitated by a thorough neurologic assessment with observation of the foal's level of consciousness, mental status, general behavior, head and body posture at rest, cranial nerve function, coordination, and gait [7].

Mental Status and Behavior

Normal neonate foals are aware of their surroundings shortly after birth and actively respond to different stimuli. Altered mental status and behavior is seen in cases of traumatic events localized to the cerebrum and brainstem. Impaired consciousness is a common clinical finding following traumatic brain injury (TBI) and is related to

Equine Neonatal Medicine, First Edition. Edited by David M. Wong and Pamela A. Wilkins.

Table 32.VI.1 Description of a modified Glasgow Coma Scale score used as a prognostic tool.

	Modified Glasgow Coma (mGCS) Scale	mGCS score
Level of consciousness	Occasional periods of alertness and responsiveness to the environment	6
	Depression or delirium, capable to responding but response may be inappropriated	5
	Semicomatose, responsive to visual stimuli	4
	Semicomatose, responsive to auditory stimuli	3
	Semicomatose, responsive only to repeated noxious stimuli	2
	Comatose, unresponsive to repeated noxious stimuli	1
Brainstem reflexes	Normal pupillary light reflexes (PLR) and physiological nystagmus	6
	Slow PLR and normal to reduced physiological nystagmus	5
	Bilateral unresponsive miosis with normal to reduced physiological nystagmus	4
	Bilateral unresponsive miosis with reduced to absent physiological nystagmus	3
	Unilateral unresponsive mydriasis with reduced to absent physiological nystagmus	2
	Bilateral unresponsive mydriasis with reduced to absent physiological nystagmus	1
Motor activity	Normal gait and spinal reflexes	6
	Hemiparesis, tetraparesis or decerebrate activity	5
	Recumbent with intermittent extensor rigidity	4
	Recumbent with constant extensor rigidity	3
	Recumbent with constant extensor rigidity and opisthotonos	2
	Recumbent, muscle hypotonia, depressed or absent spinal reflexes	1
	Overall suggested prognosis associated with final mGCS	**Final mGCS score**
Prognosis	Grave	3–8
	Guarded	9–14
	Good	15–18

Source: adapted from Platt et al. [8].

damage to the ascending reticular activating system (ARAS), a complex neural structure responsible for consciousness, which is located within the brainstem and cerebral cortex. Foals with CNS trauma/TBI may demonstrate altered consciousness with signs of dementia related to forebrain or midbrain injury leading to various degrees of awareness. Foals with mild TBI might present with lack of affinity for the mare's udder and unwillingness to nurse. With more significant trauma, foals may be obtunded and show signs of depression, unaware of surroundings, or unresponsive to tactile stimuli, or they may present, or progress quickly into, a comatose state. Foals that present or that progress into a comatose state may carry a worse prognosis for survival. Serial monitoring and assessment of the degree of coma is important and may be achieved by implementation of a modified Glasgow Coma Scale (mGCS) during examination, which allows for classification of the coma severity into mild, moderate, or severe based on level of consciousness (Table 32.VI.1) [8, 9].

Although studies evaluating this score system are lacking in equine neonates, it has been used successfully in humans, dogs, and cats with TBI. The mGCS demonstrated to be an objective tool to monitor severity and progression of neurologic deficits, effectiveness of therapeutic intervention, and was strongly correlated with survival, which aided in prognosis determination [8, 9].

During the first few days of life, the foal spends most of the time sleeping; these periods of rest are easily interrupted when aroused and followed by seeking the mare's udder and suckling. Foals are particularly prone to TBI when flipping over backward or when stepped on or kicked by the dam or other pasture mates. Foals with TBI may also present with clinical signs similar to neonatal encephalopathy (unable to latch on udder, seeking udder elsewhere on the mare instead of the inguinal region, attempting to nurse inanimate objects). Similar to foals with neonatal encephalopathy, foals with mild TBI may yawn repeatedly and not respond to training as expected [10]. Foals with moderate to severe TBI may demonstrate signs of dementia such as walking compulsively in circles, which can be a sign of cerebral damage with the foal usually circling toward the side of the lesion [10]. Other behavioral manifestations of TBI with trauma to the cerebrum include head pressing (Figure 32.VI.1), star gazing, hyperexcitability, or less commonly, aggression [10–12]. Foals with TBI can also present with different degrees of seizure activity, from pre-ictal to grand mal seizures with the latter usually followed by nystagmus, convulsions, and complete loss of consciousness. Neonatal foals with TBI are more prone to seizure development than adults, and seizure activity is also more frequent than what is observed in mature horses. In contrast to adult horses, where significant damage from TBI is already in place when seizure occurs, foals have a lower seizure threshold and might develop seizure activity even with minimal brain injury [13].

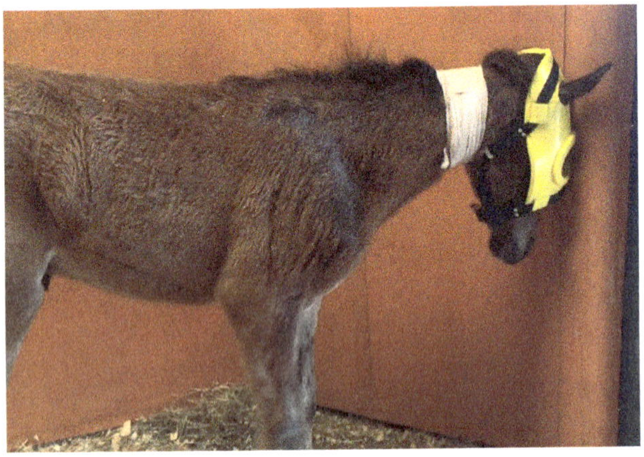

Figure 32.VI.1 Image of a 2-month-old Arabian foal with acute and severe traumatic brain injury after running into a fence post. Note the abnormal body posture with evidence of head pressing indicating possible damage to the cerebrum.

Head Posture

Equine neonates maintain their heads in an upright position with a somewhat flexed head–neck (Figure 32.VI.2a). Foals should be able to flex their neck to both sides and can be observed performing this maneuver with the intent of scratching their flanks or tail (Figure 32.VI.2b). Foals should be able to extend their neck and head without difficulties and maintain that position while suckling without losing balance (Figure 32.VI.2c). Unpredictable and bouncing movements of the head and neck resemble intention tremors, but are considered normal in foals and should not be confused with signs of cerebellar disease as seen in adult horses with trauma to the cerebellum or Arabian foals with cerebellar abiotrophy [14, 15]. Although the cerebellar layers are already histologically distinct at birth in prey animals such as horses, cerebellar development and myelination continues after birth, which might explain the rhythmic movements of the head resembling intention tremors [16]. Foals with abnormal head position such as a persistently stiff and extended neck should prompt further investigation, as cases of atlantoaxial subluxation or cranial cervical fractures might present with or without any signs of ataxia, and may only be characterized

(a) (b) (c)

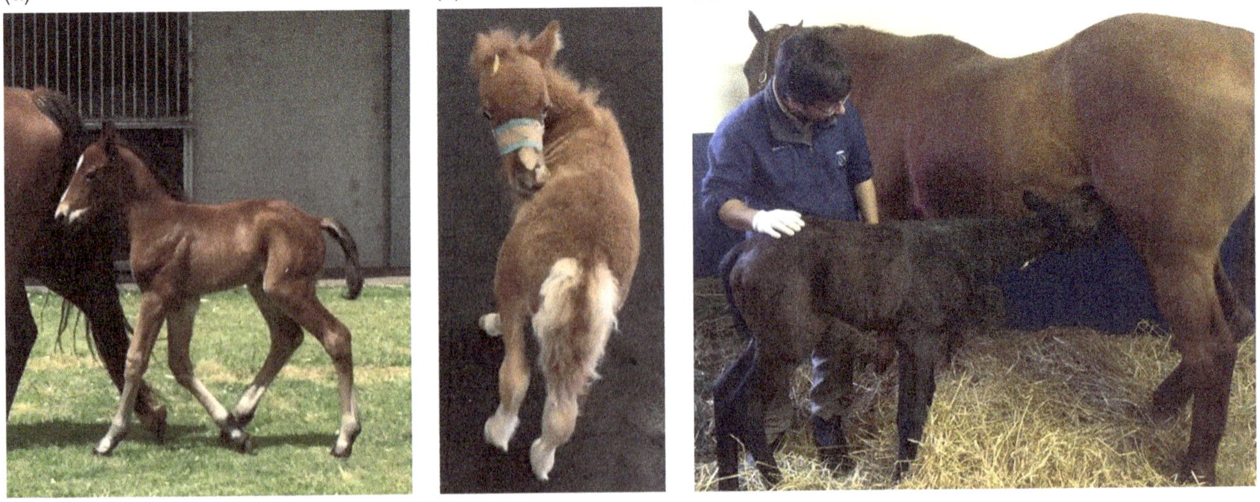

Figure 32.VI.2 Normal head and neck posture of a 2-week-old foal at the walk (a); normal neck and head lateral flexion of a 10-day-old foal while flank scratching (b); close observation of a foal nursing while maintaining the neck and head in extension (c).

by a stiff and painful cervical neck. Foals with altered mentation and a lower head carriage with a history of trauma are more likely enduring some degree of TBI localized to either the cerebral cortex or brainstem.

Cranial Nerve (CN) Examination in Equine Neonates with Trauma to the CNS

The foal's cranial nerve examination is similar to the adult horse, with cranial nerves being completely functional from birth [3].

CN I – Olfactory

CN I is difficult to assess especially in newborn foals but can be subjectively evaluated by exposing the foal to different scents (i.e. alcohol-infused gauze, gauze infused with milk). This might induce sneezing in foals with appropriate olfactory function when exposed to alcohol versus a curiosity behavior toward mare's milk, which might also lead to induction of a suckle reflex. It is important to compare the reaction of both pleasant and unpleasant scents since irritating substances such as alcohol and ammonia may stimulate nociceptors within the nasal mucosa, which will reflect in trigeminal nerve dendrites stimulation rather than olfactory nerve stimulation [17]. The olfactory nerve exits the cranium thorough the cribiform plate; therefore, traumatic lesions to this area could affect olfactory function [18]. Furthermore, lesions involving the frontal bone and calvarium with TBI to the olfactory bulbs can lead to loss of olfactory function but the extent of sequela based on clinical evaluation is difficult to impossible to determine.

CN II – Optic

In a study evaluating 52 full-term healthy equine neonates, a variety of biological anomalies were noted upon neuro-ophthalmic examination; the incidence of the abnormalities was inversely related to age [19]. Vision is present at birth as evidenced by the ability to move away from obstacles as well as compensate and guide movement. It is paramount to evaluate response to visual cues in conjunction with the remaining clinical presentation as foals with trauma to the cerebrum might be obtunded and wander into objects even with an intact visual pathway. Despite mature vision function at birth, a menace response is not present until 2 weeks of age as it is a learned response [2]. In the aforementioned study, dazzle reflex was observed in all foals ($n = 52$) whereas a menace response was absent in all foals <16 days of age ($n = 35$) [19]. Although not fully known if the menace pathway passes through the cerebellum, it is known that the ipsilateral cerebellar cortex is required for an intact menace response [17]. Therefore, lack of a blinking reflex after a menace test is likely related to a delay of complete development of the cerebellum. This hypothesis is supported by the wide-base stance in early stages of life, as well as a slightly rigid and bouncy gait due to relatively immature cerebellar function [2]. In foals >2–3 weeks of age, a menace response should be present and reflects the integrity of the entire visual pathway (i.e. retina, optic nerves and chiasm, thalamus, internal capsule, and occipital cortex). An abnormal menace response in older foals can indicate damage within the afferent pathway as it passes from the retina through the optic nerve and internal capsule, following toward the occipital lobe in the cerebrum. Abnormal menace response also can be due to trauma within the efferent pathway as it passes through the motor cortex via the pons toward the nucleus of CN VII within the medulla oblongata, and subsequently via the facial nerve toward the orbicularis oculi muscle inducing a blinking reflex [17]. Facial nerve paralysis leads to an inability to blink but an avoidance reflex of the head away from the menacing movement should still be present with a normal menace response. To test the menace response, separate hand movements toward the eye must be made from the nasal and temporal aspects to cover the entire visual arc. Traumatic lesions leading to optic nerve damage with partial or complete vision loss should be differentiated from TBI with cerebral damage related to the occipital cortex. Lesions to the cortical aspect of the brain might be followed by temporary or permanent cortical blindness and usually does not involve the optic nerve. Permanent or prolonged cortical blindness is related to extensive lesions to the cerebral cortex with pronounced edema or hemorrhage leading to ischemia of the occipital lobe cortex [20].

The foal's optic nerve arises from the retina and approximately 17% of its fibers cross the midline into the chiasm [20]. The fibers continue as the optic tract to form the lateral geniculate body. The collection of fibers from the lateral geniculate body and visual cortex within the occipital lobe form the optic radiation [20]. Differentiation of blindness secondary to lesions involving the retina or optic nerve from blindness due to occipital cortex damage is required and easily defined by the presence of a normal pupillary light reflex (PLR; direct and indirect) in cases of cortical blindness. A dazzle reflex, which is characterized by blinking in the presence of a bright light directed toward the eye is present moments after birth, and like the PLR, does not require a functional intact cortex to be elicited. Therefore, cases of traumatic events within the optic nerve tract will present without normal PLR and dazzle reflexes (Table 32.VI.2).

The equine neonate has symmetrical pupil sizes; evidence of anisocoria should prompt further investigation as it can indicate traumatic lesions to the cornea leading to miosis, or injury to neuro-ophthalmic structures such as the retina, optic nerve, optic chiasm, pretectal, and oculomotor nerve nuclei in the midbrain, CN III, ciliary

Table 32.VI.2 Neuro-ophthalmic lesion localization and its correlation with pupil size, vision, and PLR.

Lesion site	Pupil dilation		Vision status		PLR (direct)		PLR (indirect)	
Eye	**Left**	**Right**	**Left**	**Right**	**Left**	**Right**	**Left**	**Right**
Left CN II	Normal	Normal	ø	Normal	ø	Normal	Normal	ø
Left retina	Normal	Normal	ø	Normal	ø	Normal	Normal	ø
Optic chiasm	Dilated	Dilated	ø	ø	ø	ø	ø	ø
Occipital cortex	Normal	Normal	Normal	ø	Normal	Normal	Normal	Normal
Left CN III	Dilated	Normal	Normal	Normal	ø	Normal	ø	Normal
Left retrobulbar (CN II and CN III)	Dilated	Normal	ø	Normal	ø	Normal	ø	ø

PLR, pupillary light reflex; ø, Absent.

ganglia, and constrictor pupillae muscle. Anisocoria can also develop in the face of cervical sympathetic trunk lesions, such as seen in Horner's syndrome, as well as cervical fractures leading to spinal cord injuries [2]. Similar to adults, foals have a diphasic PLR and both direct and indirect PLR should be evaluated. Relying on PLR responses in foals that are excited or stressed can be deceiving, since overwhelming sympathetic stimulation may lead to midriasis and mask or change PLR test results.

Despite some challenges in assessing PLR in foals with neurologic disease, the authors recommend focused neuro-ophthalmic examination, as abnormalities can vary from subtle to pronounced. Equine neonates that present with bilateral miosis, which progress to bilateral midriasis that is unresponsive to light stimulation, are more likely to be affected by significant brain injury with possible brain herniation and therefore carry a more guarded prognosis [7]. TBI in one side of the forebrain will often lead to blindness in the eye opposite to the side of the lesion and usually does not affect the PLR. In cases of severe forebrain trauma with an increase in intracranial pressures due to edema or hemorrhage, other structures such as the CN III nucleus within the midbrain or CN III itself might be compressed, leading to an abnormal PLR with midriasis ipsilateral to the lesion site.

CN III (Oculomotor), CN IV (Trochlear), and CN VI (Abducens)

CN III, IV, and VI are evaluated together as they are responsible for innervation of the extraocular muscles responsible for positioning of the globe. To evaluate the position of the eyeball within the orbit, the foal's head should be at a horizontal position and the pupillary angle observed in comparison to the palpebral fissure in order to classify and determine the presence of abnormal positioning of the eye. Foals can move their eyes in all directions and have normal physiological nystagmus at birth. The presence of ocular asymmetry with unilateral or bilateral strabismus is abnormal and could be a consequence of TBI localized to the brainstem. In contrast to adult horses, which normally display a dorsomedial pupil angle to the palpebral fissure, newborn foals have ventromedial positioning of the pupil in relation to the palpebral fissure. This is normal until approximately one month of age when the pupillary angle shifts to a dorsomedial position [2]. Another study reported 57% of 1-day-old foals (8/14) presenting ventromedial strabismus with the incidence decreasing with age as only 4/21 foals (19%) between 2 to 5 days of age had a ventromedial pupillary angle. In foals <1 month old, a change in eye position with a dorsomedial pupillary angle can be related to TBI; this change is usually transitory as it returns to a ventromedial presentation with clinical improvement [2].

Foals are able to move their eyes in all directions due to a mature brainstem and extraocular muscles at birth: the medial rectus, inferior rectus, and superior rectus ocular muscles are innervated by the oculomotor; the lateral rectus muscle by the abducens nuclei; and the superior oblique muscle by the trochlear nucleus. TBI localized to the midbrain can lead to oculomotor nuclei damage and subsequent ventrolateral strabismus, whereas brainstem lesions with damage to the trochlear and abducens nuclei often result in a dorsomedial and medial strabismus, respectively (Figure 32.VI.3). It is important to note that strabismus related to CN III, IV, and VI deficits should be present even when maneuvering the head to different positions. A ventral or medial strabismus that disappears when moving the head in different directions may be a result of vestibular disease, with strabismus often being ipsilateral to the lesion. The oculomotor nerve exits the midbrain ventrally, traveling in rostral direction through the orbital fissure; therefore, TBI with lesions to the brainstem or traumatic events leading to hemorrhage and fracture within the retrobulbar space can affect CN III functionality [21].

CN V – Trigeminal

Sensory function of the trigeminal nerve is assessed by evaluating the nostril, face, corneal, and ear reflexes, as this nerve provides sensory innervation to the face,

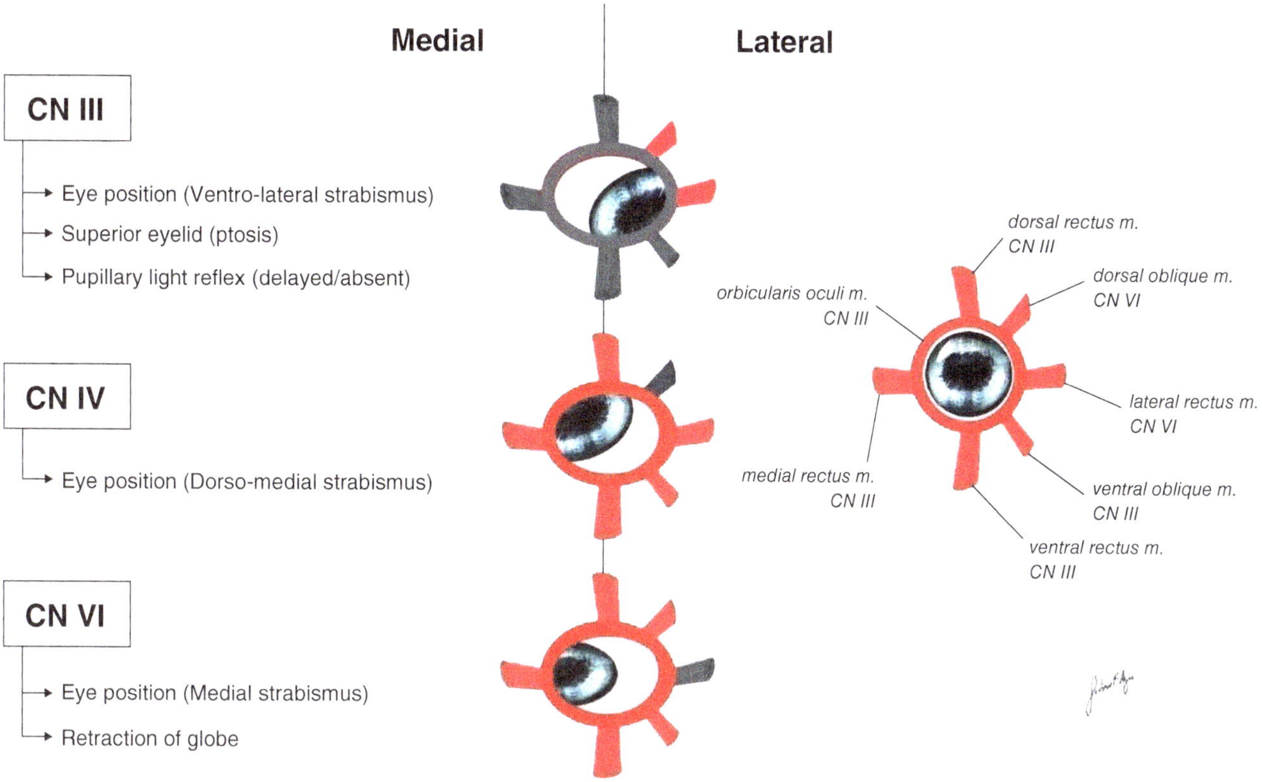

Figure 32.VI.3 Cranial nerves (III, IV, and VI) function and respective innervation of ocular muscles (CN III: medial rectus, inferior rectus, and superior rectus; CN IV: superior oblique; CN VI: lateral rectus). Ocular muscles in red represent muscles with normal function and innervation. Ocular muscles in gray represent abnormal muscle functionality secondary to cranial nerve deficits leading to ventro-lateral (CN III), dorso-medial (CN IV), and medial strabismus (CN VI).

medial aspect of the nasal mucosa, and cornea. Foals are hypersensitive to touch and often have an exacerbated reaction with an abrupt tossing of the head upon palpation of the face. The cornea can be gently stimulated with a cotton tip swab while restraining the foal's head, which elicits immediate closure of the eyelids, indicating normal innervation from the ophthalmic branch of CN V. Similarly, the nasal mucosa can be stimulated with the handler's finger or a cotton tip swab, which elicits a withdraw reaction with tossing of the head and might also induce sneezing (Figure 32.VI.4). The trigeminal nerve also provides motor function to the masseter, temporalis, and digastricus muscles; however, evaluation for loss of motor function is challenging due to the lower muscle mass foals have in this region compared to adults [2]. Nerveless, foals with trauma to the brainstem region with chronic lesions can have asymmetric masseter muscles and inappropriate mastication. Traumatic lesions to the ventrolateral aspect of the pons may induce both sensory and motor deficits as both components of CN V emerge as separate roots from this region [21]. Injury to the lateral surface of the medulla oblongata may also lead to CN V deficits, as the bulk of afferent fibers run toward the trigeminal spinal tract situated in the lateral surface of the medulla. Trauma to the lateral medulla oblongata might damage the sensory nucleus of CN V, leading to

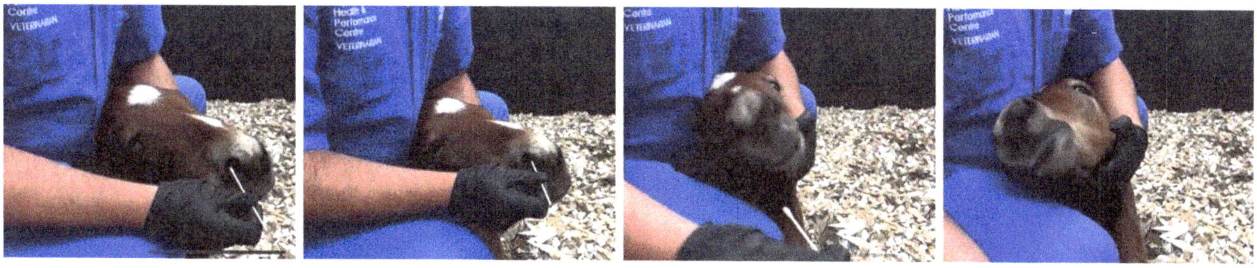

Figure 32.VI.4 Sequential images of a trigeminal nerve reaction in a foal with tossing of the head after stimulation of the nasal mucosa with a cotton tip swab.

hypalgesia and delayed reflexes of the face without changes in mandibular tone; this hypalgesia is different than the decrease in sensation caused by cerebral or thalamic injury, which leads to contralateral hypalgesia without evidence of hyporeflexia [22]. Bilateral lesions to the mid-pons may affect the trigeminal nerve motor nucleus, leading to complete loss of motor function of the mandibular nerve and an inability to masticate due to a flaccid jaw tone.

CN VII – Facial

Although facial nerve paralysis is common in adult horses, with trauma being the most common cause, traumatic facial nerve paralysis is not well documented in foals [1, 23]. The facial nerve arises within the skull from the brainstem, exits through the stylomastoid foramen, and divides into five different branches (auricular, auriculopalpebral, buccal, cervical, and digastricus branches). Therefore, TBI leading to brainstem damage can lead to facial nerve deficits (deviated muzzle to opposite site of the lesion, ear droop, ptosis, both ipsilateral to the lesion), as well as trauma to any of the specific branches as they exit the skull will lead to neurologic deficits secluded to the area innervated (e.g. auricopalpapebral nerve trauma causes ptosis and ear droop ipsilateral to the lesion). In addition to motor innervation, muscles responsible for facial expression and digastricus muscles, CN VII provides innervation to the pinnae and eyelids, supplies preganglionic parasympathetic fibers to several ganglia within the head and neck such as the lacrimal and salivary glands, and provides sensory input to approximately 67% of the rostral aspect of the tongue and oral cavity [23, 24]. While facial and nostril reflexes can be tested to assess sensory function of CN V, the same tests will provide information regarding facial nerve motor function. It is important to note that ear and lip tonicity are less pronounced in the newborn foal and even more so in dysmature foals. Therefore, bilateral ear droop and flaccid lower lip can be considered a normal finding that can be noted for a few hours after birth in a full-term foals and for a longer period in dysmature foals [2].

CN VIII – Vestibulocochlear

The vestibular apparatus is fully developed at birth with normal physiological nystagmus elicited when moving the head on a horizontal axis. The auditory component is also fully functional with evidence of hearing by exacerbated movements of the head or being startled when exposed to sudden sounds. A more objective assessment of hearing can be achieved via brainstem auditory-evoked response (Chapter 30) [25]. Trauma to the inner ear, medulla oblongata, or brainstem may lead to CN VIII deficits as the nerve fibers pass through the internal acoustic meatus within the petrosal bone, transitions to the lateral medulla oblongata, and terminates in the vestibular nuclei within the brainstem [22]. Evidence of horizontal nystagmus while the head is in a stationary/neutral position may indicate signs of peripheral vestibular disease with the fast phase away from the site of the lesion and away from the direction of the head tilt as seen in temporohyoid osteoarthropathy (THO). Vertical nystagmus or involuntary abnormal movement of the eye in multiple directions can be associated to central vestibular disease as a consequence of brainstem trauma. Although not commonly seen in foals, cases of THO secondary to trauma can occur if foals flip backward while restrained or halter trained and is often accompanied by vestibulocochlear and facial nerve deficits. A ventral or medial strabismus that disappears when moving the head in different directions may be a result of loss of normal vestibular function and deficits of the tonic mechanism controlling eye position. In these cases, the strabismus is ipsilateral to the vestibular lesion. Blindfolding the animal can exacerbate signs of CN VIII deficits, as visual compensation is required for appropriated accommodation to vestibular deficits.

CN IX – Glossopharyngeal, CN X – Vagus, and CN XI – Accessory

Foals with TBI might demonstrate difficulty in swallowing due to CN deficits, which can be detected by the presence or history of milk in the nostrils and secondary aspiration pneumonia. Assessment of function of CN IX to XI is challenging but can accomplished by observing the foal nursing while checking for appropriate swallowing. This is achieved by placing the examiner's hand over the esophageal groove while the foal is nursing to determine if esophageal peristalsis and milk passage through the esophagus is present. Alternatively, visualization of the swallowing reflex can be achieved with passage of a nasoesophageal tube or by endoscopic examination of the pharynx while instilling water through the endoscope, which normally elicits a swallowing reflex. The peripheral component of cranial nerves IX, X, and XI passes through each guttural pouch, thereby making foals with traumatic events associated with substantial hemorrhage and trauma to the guttural pouches more at risk for deficits related to these CNs. While injury to CN IX to XI can lead to inappropriate swallowing reflex, it is important to note that the feeding process is complex and involves other cranial nerves that control movement of the lips (CN VII), appropriate jaw tone (CN V), and ability to move and curl the tongue (CN XII) [2]. Also, inappropriate feeding behavior may be observed with TBI and lesions to the optic nerve or cerebrum leading to an inability to identify the mare's udder.

CN XII – Hypoglossal

The hypoglossal nerve is responsible for motor function of the tongue with deficits of CN XII function identified by inspection of tongue tone and muscle symmetry. Unilateral lesions will lead to unilateral muscle fasciculation or tongue atrophy with deficits being ipsilateral to the lesion side, but the foal should still be able to withdraw the tongue back into the mouth. TBI to the brainstem with bilateral damage to CN XII leads to inability or difficulty to withdraw the tongue back into the mouth once protruded. This can also be observed in cases of significant forebrain injury with pronounced weakness and signs of somnolence without specific damage to the hypoglossal nuclei or nerves [22]. The hypoglossal nerve exits the skull at the caudal aspect from the hypoglossal foramen and can be severely damaged with cranial cervical fractures caused by caudal compression of the skull through the atlantal ring, which often results in fragments of the atlas shearing off the hypoglossal nerve [7].

It is important to note the neuroanatomical location of the cranial nerves, as CN I and II are located within the forebrain whereas CN III to XII are closely located within the brainstem. Therefore, TBI with multiple CN involved likely occurs in cases of trauma with secondary injury to the brainstem. This is often observed in cases of basosphenoid fractures, which are most commonly caused when foals flip over their back while being restrained or halter trained [26].

Postural and Gait Evaluation in Neonatal Foals with Nervous System Trauma

Abnormalities of posture and gait can occur in foals with trauma to the brainstem, spinal cord, or peripheral nerves. Neurologic assessment is similar to adult horses with the extra challenge of not being able to lead a newborn foal in different directions for gait assessment. Postural reactions should be noted with the foal at rest and walking, as well as while being restrained and handled. In adult horses, evaluation of posture is performed while stationary, but this may not be possible in foals because of their inquisitive nature and infrequent tendency to stand still and quietly. Similarly, gait evaluation in adult horses is performed by walking the animal in a straight line, circling to both directions in wide and tight circles, walking in a serpentine direction, going up and down a curb and a slope, as well as walking backward. These are maneuvers that are not easily replicated in the foal and are better assessed by walking the mare in the desired directions while letting the foal follow without any sort of restraint (Figure 32.VI.5).

(a) (b)

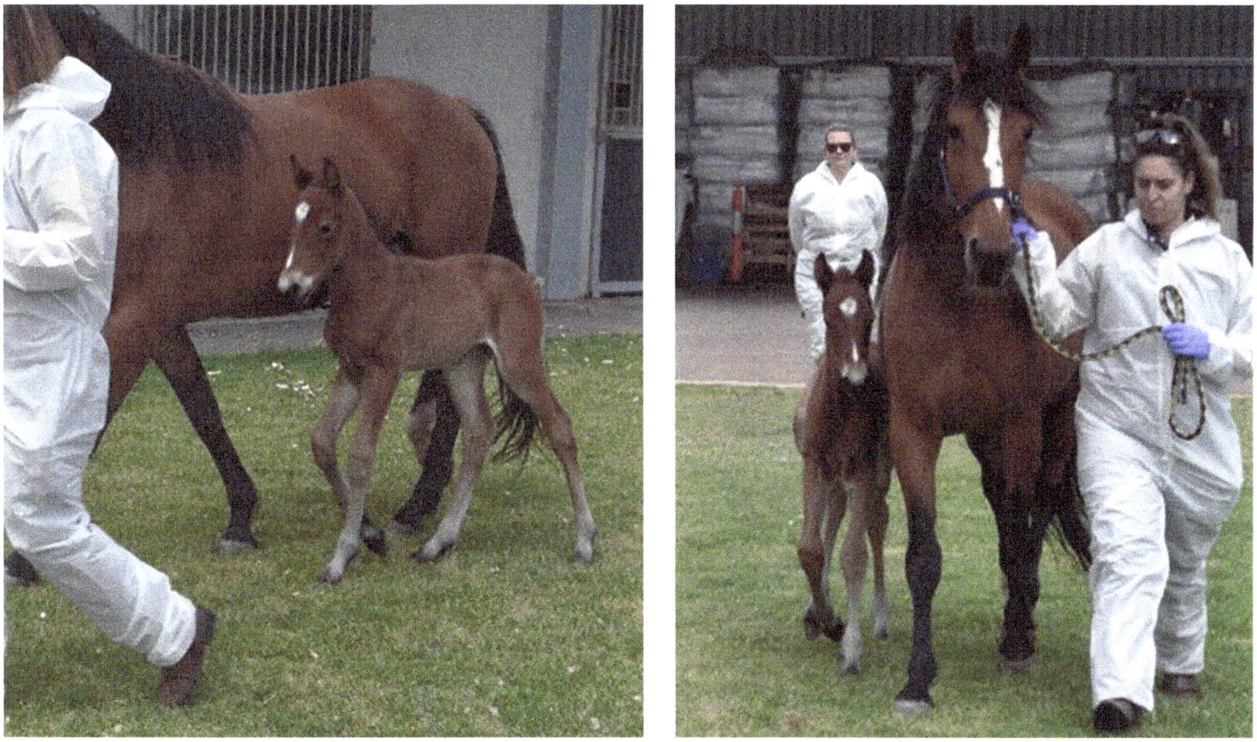

Figure 32.VI.5 Gait assessment during neurological examination in a 1-month-old foal. (a) observation from the side (b) observation from behind.

Postural Reactions

Newborn foals have well-developed brains and assume normal postural reactions readily after birth. The neonatal foal has enough muscle tone to assume sternal recumbency 1–2 minutes after birth and stand within 15–30 minutes. Once standing, foals initially assume a wide-base stance, especially within the thoracic limbs and is considered a normal stance in the first few days of life [16]. Neonatal foals display some differences regarding gait and postural reactions compared to older horses; therefore, close observation identifies age-related differences. Additionally, in the face of an abnormality, clinical examination will help differentiate between a musculoskeletal and a neurologic disorder. Restraining the foal by pulling toward the handler with one arm under and around the neck, while the other around the hamstring area or with the hand holding the tail, will lead to a common response of the foal pulling away from the handler. Also, foals usually attempt to lay down if firmly restrained while been held by the chest and hamstring. This postural reaction of collapsing toward the ground when firmly restrained should not be confused with weakness but rather a normal cataleptic reaction in foals [2]. Nevertheless, weakness can be observed in cases of spinal cord injury (SCI) with damage to the lower motor neuron (LMN) or upper motor neuron (UMN) pathways with interruption of the spinal reflex arc. The extent to which limbs are affected (thoracic, pelvic, or both) depends on the site of the lesion within the vertebral column.

Foals with trauma caudal to the second thoracic vertebrae (T2) with damage to the respective spinal cord segment are usually able to lift the thoracic limbs from the ground but are unable to use the pelvic limbs and therefore assume a dog-sitting position [27]. On the other hand, recumbent foals with an inability to stand on either the thoracic or pelvic limbs are likely to have a traumatic event leading to SCI at the level of the cervical vertebrae. SCI with lesions within the cervical spinal cord segments are also characterized by paresis in all four limbs, and foals may be unable to assume and maintain sternal recumbency. Postural deficits affecting the ability to raise the head and neck off the ground can be characteristic of severe cranial cervical SCI. Severe caudal cervical lesions may be characterized by a normal ability to lift the neck from the ground even though sternal recumbent posture might not be achievable.

Severe SCI with damage to the UMN pathway leads to abnormal voluntary effort with a decreased or even absent voluntary limb activity but with normal to increased muscle tone due to compensation from an intact LMN pathway. Foals with lesions to the LMN tract will present with a flaccid limb that trembles when bearing weight and an obvious decrease in muscle tone, which can be caused by lesions to the anterior horn cells, spinal nerve roots, or a peripheral nerve injury [27]. Muscle tone of the limbs is easily examined in healthy foals and foals with traumatic lesions to the CNS. The foal is placed in lateral recumbency, and the procedure is performed by repetitive manipulation while flexing and extending each limb. Evidence of limb spasticity that suddenly disappears (i.e. clasp-knife response) is indicative of an UMN lesion to the spinal cord [27]. In general, lesions to the UMN are characterized by normal muscle mass, normal to increased tonicity, hyperreflexia, and rhythmic muscle spasms (clonus); whereas lesions to the LMN are characterized by muscle wasting and fasciculation, decreased muscle tonicity, and hyporeflexia [27].

Proprioception and Gait Assessment in the Foal with CNS Trauma

Evaluation of proprioceptive function and gait assessment in neonatal foals with underlying CNS trauma involves assessment for the presence of weakness and ataxia. Foals with paresis or weakness have a shortened swing phase of the stride and may drag the limbs while walking, which can lead to abnormal hoof wear. Paresis can also manifest as muscle fasciculations and trembling of the affected limb(s) during weight bearing. Other signs of weakness include knuckling of the fetlocks or stumbling.

After neurologic assessment, the authors recommend video recording the foal's gait, which allows for further analysis of more subtle changes. Certain aspects of proprioception and gait assessment should be performed with caution in foals with suspected CNS trauma, such as walking up and down hills and walking while blindfolded; hopping should be done with caution to prevent falling and further injury. While hopping can be challenging in adult horses due to excessive body weight, foals can be easily hopped in one leg; however, if the foal resists such manipulation, it might elicit the foal to rear up or flip backward, increasing the chances for further CNS injury. Thus, use of hopping to evaluate proprioception should be limited to cases of mild to moderate ataxia. Although cerebral lesions do not affect gait or posture, a delayed hopping response may be elicited in foals with TBI involving the cerebrum [10]. This is most noticeable when the hopping test is performed with the foal blindfolded (again, note increased risk of further injury when blindfolding an untrained and hyperactive foal). In general, cerebral lesions elicit a delayed hopping response on the limb opposite to the lesion.

The sway test can be performed with the foal moving on a straight line while being held by the examiner with one arm around the neck and the other around the hamstring or holding the tail. While moving forward, the examiner applies force, pulling the foal by the tail or hamstring away and toward the examiner to assess for proprioceptive deficits and weakness within the pelvic limbs. In a similar manner, pressure should be placed in the scapular or withers area while pulling the foal away and toward the examiner to evaluate the thoracic limbs. Foals demonstrate an abnormal sway test with weakness that is characterized by exaggerated limb abduction and crossing while moving forward in cases of TBI or SCI, with lesions to the descending UMN pathway or ventral horn gray matter at the level of the limb tested (thoracic versus pelvic) [27]. The sway test should also be performed with the foal stationary, during which, in cases of profound weakness, the foal can be easily displaced from its original position, indicating a potential LMN lesion with a disrupted spinal reflex arc. The sway test at rest should not elicit signs of proprioceptive deficits and weakness in the face of UMN lesions without LMN pathways being affected. This exacerbated weakness at rest can also be observed in cases of peripheral nerve or musculoskeletal pathologies.

Foals with trauma to the cerebral cortex, internal capsule, or brainstem may present with signs of hemiparesis or hemiplegia as well as decreased conscious proprioception. With TBI localized to the brainstem, the hemiplegia is on the limb opposite to the side of the lesion, known as crossed hemiplegia. Neonatal foals with severe trauma to the pole region with TBI affecting the cerebellum will develop intention tremors, wide base stance, and signs of unconscious proprioceptive deficits as the information regarding limb position will pass through the general sensory pathways toward the cerebellum. One must understand the normal variations of gait in foals to differentiate a normal gait from ataxia. Foals are slightly dysmetric and have a noticeable head bob at the walk and trot, which is considered normal and not a sign of cerebellar ataxia [3]. Ataxia in newborn foals is similar to ataxia in adult horses, which can be divided in proprioceptive, cerebellar, and vestibular ataxia.

Proprioceptive Ataxia in Foals with CNS Trauma

Proprioceptive ataxia is mostly seen in cases of SCI and is characterized by abnormal limb stance and gait. Foals present with unconscious proprioceptive deficits such as exaggerated limb movements including abduction, adduction, or circumduction during the swing phase, as well as abnormal foot placement with exaggerated crossing of the limbs or stepping on the opposite foot. Proprioceptive ataxia can be presented with truncal sway, which can be observed on either the thoracic or pelvic limbs, or, in severe cases, the entire body can be swaying to one or both sides while walking. Signs of conscious proprioceptive deficits such as abnormal limb placement and knuckling may or may not be present with SCI leading to proprioceptive ataxia. Although most cases of proprioceptive ataxia are secondary to SCI, foals with TBI with lesions to the brainstem, thalamus, cortex, or basal nuclei can also develop proprioceptive ataxia, which is usually not as severe as seen in SCI. Furthermore, TBI leading to proprioceptive ataxia is often accompanied by cranial nerve deficits with or without other clinical signs such as behavioral changes, somnolence, compulsive walking/circling, and seizure activity. TBI with lesions secluded to the cerebrum do not cause changes in posture or gait.

Cerebellar Ataxia in Foals with CNS Trauma

Cerebellar ataxia is mostly seen as a congenital abnormality in purebred horses such as Arabian foals with cerebellar abiotrophy, rather than secondary to trauma. Cerebellar ataxia is characterized by an inability to control the range and frequency of steps resulting in dysmetria. This lack of fine control is represented by a prolonged protraction of the limb and should be differentiated from spasticity seen in cervical vertebral trauma with UMN damage. Foals with cerebellar ataxia alone do not have weakness nor show signs of unconscious or conscious proprioceptive deficits. Foals with trauma to the cerebellum leading to cerebellar ataxia present with exaggerated tremors of the head and neck (i.e. intention tremors), and wide base stance most noticeable in the pelvic limbs. Clinicians should use caution when handling foals with suspect trauma to the cerebellum as cases of cerebellar ataxia have a tendency to rear [28].

Vestibular Ataxia in Foals with CNS Trauma

Signs of vestibular ataxia vary if the lesion is unilateral or bilateral (symmetric), and if the central or peripheral portion of the vestibular system is affected. Symmetric or bilateral lesions are characterized by a hypometric and staggering gait, wide base stance, truncal sway or walking sideways, leaning, and sometimes losing balance to the point of falling. Similar signs are seen with unilateral lesions, although staggering, and abnormal posture is asymmetric with leaning and circling, with the head tilted toward the side of the lesion. Peripheral vestibular ataxia is frequently observed after head trauma and although central vestibular ataxia is not as common in foals with CNS trauma, it might occur in the face of brainstem lesions affecting the vestibular nuclei within the medulla oblongata or injury to the flocculonodular lobes and fastigial nuclei of the cerebellum. Peripheral vestibular disease occurs with trauma to the petrosal portion of the temporal bone affecting the membranous labyrinth of the inner ear, the vestibular ganglion, or the peripheral branch of CN VIII. Traumatic events leading to cranial cervical injuries may also elicit signs of vestibular ataxia as afferent input from the cranial cervical ligaments and muscles related to the C1–C3 dorsal spinal nerve roots arise from the spinal cord toward the vestibular nuclei [3, 22].

Central and peripheral vestibular signs in foals include head tilt and leaning or circling toward the side of the lesion. Normally, unilateral stimulation of the vestibular system leads to ipsilateral extensor tonus and contralateral flexor tonus of the limbs, which facilitates ipsilateral support against gravity. Therefore, in the face of a unilateral lesion, leaning and circling toward the lesion occurs due to an increase in ipsilateral flexor tonus and contralateral extensor tonus [22]. Central lesions are characterized by vertical or positional nystagmus and are usually seen along with additional CN deficits and changes in mentation (e.g. somnolence). Central vestibular disease is characterized by proprioceptive deficits that are ipsilateral to the lesion whereas peripheral vestibular disease does not cause proprioceptive deficits leading to weakness. Peripheral vestibular ataxia is characterized by a horizontal nystagmus (fast phase away from lesion) and no changes in mentation are observed unless in the face of concurrent TBI. Recumbency occurs with severe lesions and foals can have a preference to lie on the affected side [28].

Spinal Reflexes in Foals with CNS Trauma

In adult horses, assessment of peripheral nerve reflexes is usually only performed in recumbent patients. In contrast, spinal reflexes are easily evaluated in foals and is a part of every neurologic examination especially with potential CNS trauma. Sensory perception can be assessed with forceps by gently pricking the skin, which elicits a painful stimulus and subsequent local and cerebral response [22]. The local response is characterized by twitching of the skin and associated subcutaneous musculature. The consequence of the sensory response to noxious stimulus is the flexor and withdrawal reflex, whereas the cerebral response is characterized by vocalization, movement of the head toward the noxious stimulus, as well as changes in facial expression. The motor response of spinal reflexes of each nerve can also be elicited with the use of percussion reflex hammer (e.g. plexor).

Spinal Reflexes of the Cervical Spine and Thoracic Limbs

Foals have an exaggerated response to tactile stimuli with hyper-reflexive spinal reflexes compared to adult horses. This can make evaluation of reflexes difficult. This exaggerated response may be related to incomplete presence of UMN calming influences on reflex activity, which could be secondary to a combination of factors such as immature myelination, incomplete anatomical pathways in the cerebellum, and ongoing maturation of inhibitory neurotransmitter systems [2].

The *cervicofacial reflex* is evaluated in foals by gently striking the skin over the brachiocephalicus muscle on both sides. The normal reaction is movement of the ears and lip, as well as contraction of the brachiocephalicus and cutaneous colli muscles with associated twitching of the skin over the cervical region. The cervicofacial reflex is slightly different in neonatal foals, as movement of the lips in response to tactile stimulation is not as pronounced as compared to adults [2]. This difference in response might be related to tension in the facial musculature that foals develop when restrained. The response is ipsilateral to the tactile stimuli, and an abnormal reflex can be seen in foals with trauma to CN VII, damage to the sensory or motor fibers of the cervical nerves or nerve roots, or trauma to the cervical spinal cord (C1–C7). This reflex is usually decreased or absent at the level of the lesion albeit normal cranial and caudal to the lesion site.

Evaluation of the thoracic limb spinal reflexes is best performed while maintaining the foal in lateral recumbency. Reliable reflexes in foals include the flexor, triceps, and extensor carpi radialis reflexes [2]. *Flexor reflex* (withdrawal reflex) is stimulated after gently pricking the skin over the distal limb, which causes flexion of the fetlock, carpal, cubital, and scapulohumeral joints [22]. As with any other spinal reflex, a sensory and motor component is present, with the sensory aspect being provided by the musculocutaneous, median, and ulnar nerves, as well as spinal cord segments C7–T1 [2]. The motor portion of the flexor reflex is provided by motor fibers from a combination of the axillary, musculocutaneous, median, and ulnar nerves. Presence of conscious perception of the pain stimulus leading to the flexor reflex requires an intact afferent pathway of the median and ulnar nerves, an intact dorsal gray horn of the spinal cord segment C7–T1, as well as an undamaged sensory pathway of the spinal cord and brainstem [22]. This reflex is normally exaggerated in foals compared to adult horses, but foals with suspected CNS trauma that are presented with abrupt flexion of the limb due to an exaggerated flexor reflex may have a lesion cranial to C7 [29]. In this case, the limb may remain flexed for a prolonged period after elicitation by noxious stimuli. In cases of cerebral damage, a flexor reflex may be normal, although no evidence of perception of the noxious stimulus is present which may indicate a cerebral lesion. The flexor reflex is accompanied by a contralateral limb extension (i.e. crossed extensor reflex), which may be present in foals up to three weeks of age (Figure 32.VI.6a) [2]. The *triceps and extensor carpi radialis reflexes* are easily and consistently elicited in foals, and an abnormal response can be observed in cases of trauma to the radial nerve or damage to spinal cord segments C7–T1.

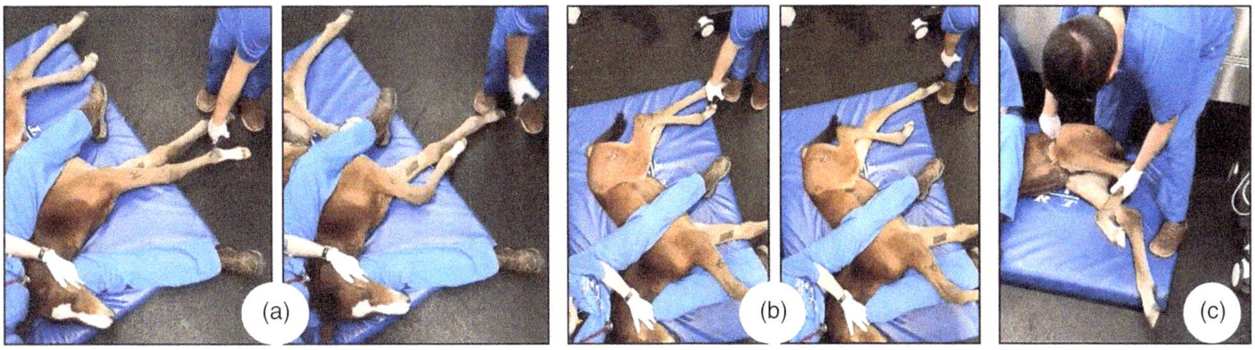

Figure 32.VI.6 Sequential images of thoracic limbs (a) and pelvic limbs (b) flexor reflexes: Note the flexion of the left thoracic limb (flexor reflex) and mild extension of the contralateral limb (crossed extensor reflex) on (a). Demonstration of the patellar reflex (c) being elicited with the use of a plexor hammer for tapping the middle patellar ligament.

Spinal Reflexes of the Trunk and Pelvic Limbs

Normal reflexes of the thoracic limbs but abnormal reflexes within the thoracolumbar area indicates a lesion between spinal cord segments T2–S2. Evaluation of spinal reflexes within the thoracolumbar area include assessment of the cutaneous trunci, pelvic limbs flexor reflex, and patellar reflex. The *cutaneous trunci reflex* is elicited by stimulation of the skin over the body wall of the thoracic and thoracolumbar area. This reflex leads to contraction of the cutaneous trunci muscle. In cases of severe traumatic lesions, the motor and sensory responses of this reflex are absent caudal to the site of the lesion. Evaluation of the *flexor reflex* of the pelvic limbs is performed similar to the thoracic limb flexor reflex where the local and cerebral response is observed after pricking the skin on the distal aspect of the limb. The pelvic limbs flexor reflex results in flexion of the fetlock, tarsocrural, femorotibial, and coxofemoral joints (Figure 32.VI.6b). Peripheral nerve damage to the sciatic nerve as well as spinal cord lesions between L5 and S3 results in abnormal pelvic limb flexor reflex due to damaged afferent or efferent pathways. The *patellar reflex* is assessed by tapping the middle patellar ligament with a percussion reflex hammer while maintaining the foal in lateral recumbency with the limb slightly flexed (Figure 32.VI.6c). A normal patellar reflex elicits extension of the femorotibial joint. A study evaluating neurologic particularities in newborn foals revealed they have an exaggerated response to spinal reflexes. Additionally, the gastrocnemius and cranial tibial reflexes are not consistent between animals and are therefore unreliable in clinical cases [2]. Evaluation of the sensory response to stimulation of the skin of the pelvic limb region can also facilitate neurolocalization: Trauma to the femoral nerve leads to loss of skin sensation in the medial aspect of the thigh; damage to the tibial nerve leads to hypalgesia or complete loss of sensory response to the plantar surface of the metatarsus; and a lesion to the peroneal nerve causes loss of skin sensation in the dorsal aspect of both the tarsus and metatarsus region [22].

Tail Tone and Perineal Reflex

Lesions of the sacrococcygeal spinal cord segments or sacrococcygeal innervation results in a flaccid tail without voluntary movement and decreased or absent tail tone. Tail tone can also be observed while evaluating the perineal reflex, which can be assessed by gently pricking the skin around the perineal area. This reflex should be evaluated with the foal laying down to avoid a kicking response, which poses risk to the examiner. The perineal reflex is easily evaluated by observing clamping the tail and contraction of the anal sphincter. Trauma to sacral spinal cord segment S1–S3 with damage to the caudal rectal branch of the pudendal nerve causes lack of anal sphincter contraction, whereas a lesion to the sacral and coccygeal nerves and spinal cord segments from S1 to the coccyx leads to an inability to flex the tail [22]. It is important to observe urination and defecation as cases of neuritis of the cauda equina present with flaccid paralysis and hypalgesia to analgesia of the bladder, rectum, anus, perineum, and tail. Neonatal foals with trauma to the lumbosacral segment also develop paresis, or in severe cases paralysis of the pelvic limbs, which is not observed in cases of neuritis of the cauda equina alone [22].

Neurolocalization of Traumatic Lesions to the CNS in Foals

Neurolocalization of the lesion is based on clinical signs and abnormalities noted during the neurologic examination; this will guide diagnostic intervention and development of differential diagnosis. Neurolocalization in equine neonates is the same as in adult horses (Table 32.VI.3). TBI is usually detected when evaluating mental status and CN

Table 32.VI.3 Description of lesion neurolocalization with respective clinical signs and regional functional deficits.

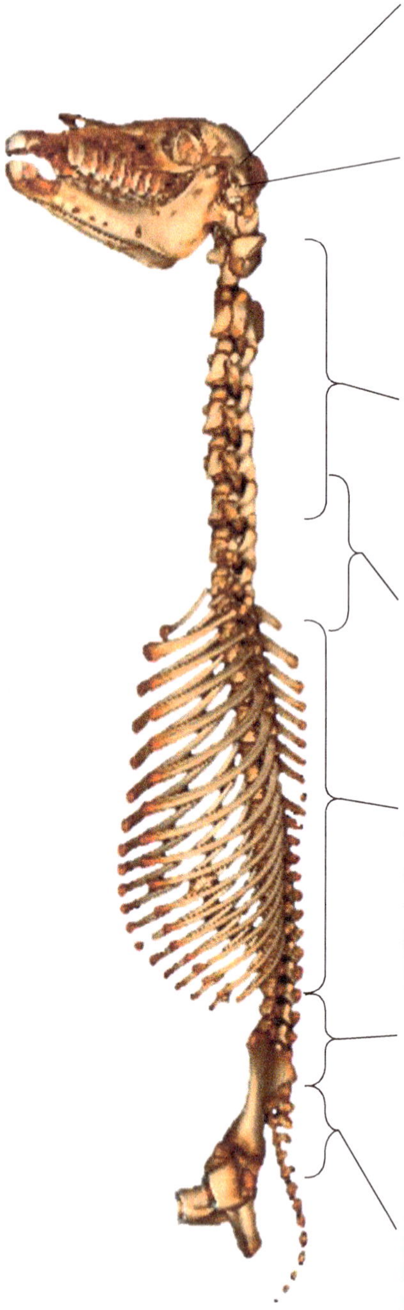

Lesion site	Limbs affected	Functional systems deficits
Cerebellum	Bilateral lesion: all 4 limbs Unilateral lesion: 2 limbs ipsilateral to lesion (1 thoracic and 1 pelvic)	**Motor:** • Normal strength. Dysmetric gait with loss of fine control; wide base stance, normal strength, head tremors. Tendency to rear when handled **Sensory:** • GP: normal • GSA: normal
Vestibular apparatus and C1–C3 (sensory dorsal nerve roots)	Peripheral: No proprioceptive deficits Central: 2 limbs ipsilateral to lesion (1 thoracic and 1 pelvic)	**Motor:** • Normal strength. Inappropriate posture and balance; hypometric gait, leaning; drifting, loss of balance/falling over, truncal sway, nystagmus and head tilt. Vestibular ataxia is exacerbated when blindfolded. Foals prefer to lie on affected side Central: vertical or positional nystagmus ± multiple cranial nerves involved along with changes in mentation Peripheral: horizontal nystagmus with fast phase away from lesion. No changes in mentation **Sensory:** • GP: normal • GSA: normal
C1–C6	Bilateral lesion: all 4 limbs* Unilateral lesion: 2 limbs ipsilateral to lesion 1 (thoracic and 1 pelvic) *More pronounced on pelvic limbs	**Motor:** • Tetraparesis to tetraplegia • UMN deficits on all limbs **Sensory:** • GP: Proprioceptive ataxia on all limbs with knuckling, abnormal foot placement (exaggerated crossing or stepping on opposite foot), abduction, adduction, or circumduction. Spastic and elongated stride • GSA: hypalgesia in all limbs
C6–T2	Bilateral lesion: all 4 limbs* Unilateral lesion: 2 limbs ipsilateral to lesion (1 thoracic and 1 pelvic) *More pronounced on thoracic limbs	**Motor:** • Tetraparesis to tetraplegia • LMN deficits on thoracic limbs and UMN deficits on pelvic limbs **Sensory:** • GP: Proprioceptive ataxia on all limbs with knuckling, abnormal foot placement (exaggerated crossing or stepping on opposite foot), abduction, adduction, or circumduction. Spastic and elongated stride • GSA: hypalgesia in all limbs
T3–L3	Bilateral lesion: both pelvic limbs Unilateral lesion: 1 pelvic limb ipsilateral to lesion	**Motor:** • Paraparesis to paraplegia • UMN deficits on pelvic limbs • Focal sweating and urinary incontinence **Sensory:** • GP: Proprioceptive ataxia on pelvic limbs with knuckling, abnormal foot placement (exaggerated crossing or stepping on opposite foot), abduction, adduction or circumduction. Spastic and elongated stride • GSA deficits: hypalgesia to analgesia of trunk and pelvic limbs caudal to the lesion site
L4–S1	Bilateral lesion: both pelvic limbs Unilateral lesion: 1 pelvic limb ipsilateral to lesion	**Motor:** • Paraparesis to paraplegia • LMN deficits on pelvic limbs • Urinary incontinence and obstipation **Sensory:** • GP: Proprioceptive ataxia on pelvic limbs with short stride due to decrease ability to support weight secondary to paraplegia • GSA deficits: hypalgesia to pelvic limbs caudal to the lesion site, tail and anus
S1-Coccigeal		**Motor:** • LMN to tail, anus, perineum, bladder, and rectum. • Urinary incontinence and obstipation **Sensory:** • GP: Normal • GSA deficits: hypalgesia to analgesia of tail, anus, perineum, bladder, and rectum

UMN, upper motor neuron; LMN, lower motor neuron; GP, general proprioception; GSA, general somatic afferent.
Source: Adapted from "Veterinary Neuroanatomy and Clinical Neurology" by A. De Lahunta, 2014 and Johnson [28].

deficits with multiple CN abnormalities localizing the lesion to the brainstem; significant changes in mental status indicate lesions within the forebrain or brainstem. Peripheral CN trauma can also alter CN function and, if lesions are isolated to peripheral nerves, clinical signs are not accompanied by altered mental status. Neonatal foals can present with ataxia secondary to trauma to the cerebellum, brainstem, and spinal cord. Trauma to the cerebellum is characterized by intention tremors, dysmetria, and a wide base stance without paresis. Unilateral trauma to the cerebellum will elicit signs of ataxia of the thoracic and pelvic limbs that are ipsilateral to the lesion, whereas bilateral cerebellar trauma will affect all four limbs [28]. Trauma to the cervical spinal cord or caudal brainstem elicits neurologic signs in all four limbs, with more pronounced deficits in the pelvic than thoracic limbs. This is often observed with compressive lesions as the spinocerebellar tract, which provides proprioceptive information to the hindlimbs, is localized toward the outside of the spinal cord and is the first portion of the spinal cord to be compressed and damaged upon trauma. Lesions affecting the white matter of the caudal brainstem are usually accompanied by CN deficits whereas cervical spinal cord lesions alone will infrequently be accompanied by CN abnormalities. Mild to moderate brainstem lesions or cervical spine lesions affect all four limbs with the pelvic limbs showing severe deficits, typically one grade worse than the thoracic limbs. Mild SCI within the cervical spine (C1–C6) may elicit no abnormalities within the thoracic limbs but noticeable mild changes within the pelvic limbs. Moderate to severe abnormalities within the pelvic limbs with no changes to the thoracic limbs can indicate SCI within the thoracolumbar segment of the spinal cord [22]. Neonatal foals that with all four limbs affected with neurologic deficits such that mild signs are observed in the thoracic limbs and severe signs involving the pelvic limbs (i.e. two grades worse in pelvic limbs compared to thoracic limbs), might be affected by multifocal traumatic lesions with a severe SCI in the thoracolumbar region and mild cervical (C1–C6) lesion. Foals presented with moderate to severe ataxia and weakness in the thoracic limbs and mild to no changes in the pelvic limbs are likely to have trauma with subsequent SCI and damage to the gray matter and lower motor pathways between spinal cord segments C6–T2 (brachial intumescence). Gait abnormalities to the thoracic limbs with normal pelvic limb function, can also be caused by peripheral nerve damage to the thoracic limbs. Bilateral SCI from C1–C6 as well as C6–T2 leads to clinical signs in all four limbs whereas unilateral lesions affect the thoracic and pelvic limbs ipsilateral to the lesion. Bilateral SCI localized to T3–L3 and L4–S1 spinal cord segments results in both pelvic limbs being affected whereas unilateral SCI (T3–L3 and L5–S1) causes clinical signs in the pelvic limb ipsilateral to the lesion.

Types of CNS Lesions Secondary to Trauma

Equine neonates are predisposed to CNS trauma as they are easily startled and have unexpected reactions when handled; they also have an inquisitive nature, putting them at risk for trauma from pasture mates. Among injuries to the CNS, head trauma is often observed because of a thinner calvarium providing less protection to the brain compared to adult horses [7]. Similarly, CNS trauma related to SCI is often observed in foals of all ages with trauma to the cervical spine most commonly presented to referral centers. Nervous system trauma can be divided into TBI, SCI, and peripheral nerve trauma.

Traumatic Brain Injury in the Foal

TBI in neonatal foals can progress rapidly with abrupt changes in demeanor and mental status [7]. Breathing pattern, respiratory and heart rate, pupil dilation, and response to light stimulation can change within hours of onset of trauma and warrant constant monitoring in order to determine clinical progression and prognosis. Foals are prone to trauma to the skull and calvarium with subsequent brain damage with insults such as flipping over backward and landing on the poll, being kicked by the dam, or being struck in the head by running into a fixed object such as a stall wall or fencepost.

Foals that flip over backward and land on the poll region experience tremendous impact toward the occiput, which can fracture at its thicker portion, with or without nuchal crest avulsion fractures. This impact can also fracture the occipital condyles and paramastoid processes. The impact that propagates through the occipital bone might disperse toward its base leading to basioccipital fractures, which often carry a worse prognosis [30]. Basilar skull fractures (e.g. basioccipital and basosphenoid bones) are facilitated by forces imposed by the rectus capitis ventralis muscles, which are the major muscles for flexion of the head that connect the basilar bones to the cervical vertebrae [10]. Although TBI with subsequent neurologic deficits in foals is most commonly associated with fractures to the skull, some foals may present with significant neurologic damage with an intact calvarium as seen in some adult horses with severe brain injury [10]. The neurologic damage may occur readily after trauma, although more frequently, the injury exacerbates hours to even days after the initial insult [7]. The signalment and history is paramount to establish the appropriate medical intervention as certain breeds are predisposed to neurologic diseases that might lead to trauma of the CNS. For example, Arabian foals with idiopathic epilepsy may present with TBI secondary to skull fractures due to striking the head on the ground during an epileptic episode.

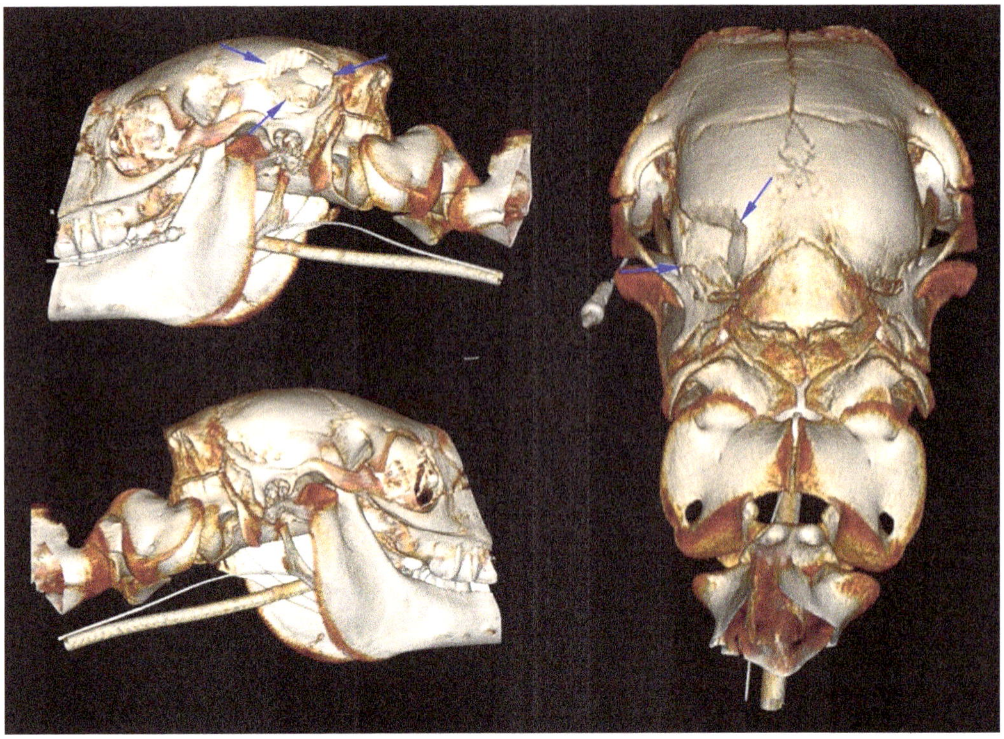

Figure 32.VI.7 Computed tomography three-dimensional skull reconstruction of a foal with depression fractures (blue arrows) of the left caudal aspect of the parietal and temporal bones. *Source:* Image courtesy of Dr. Emily Haggett, Rossdales Equine Hospital.

Types of Traumatic Brain Injury

TBI injury occurs due to primary forces imposed to the brain either at the point of contact of the skull with the impact source (coup lesion) or at the region opposite the site of impact (countercoup injury). The latter is a result of forces within the intracranial cavity that cause the brain to rebound in the opposite direction from the original site of impact. TBI with or without CN damage is more pronounced when foals are subjected to severe impact in the frontal and parietal skull region or when flipping over backward with the maximum forces of impact at the poll. Although TBI usually occurs due to primary forces with an impact directly to the head, TBI secondary to "whiplash" movements due to acceleration–deceleration of the head may also occur [10].

For classification purposes, TBI can occur due to primary or secondary injuries: primary injuries occur as a direct result from trauma and secondary injuries occur as an indirect result from the initial insult. Secondary injuries are discussed in section V of Chapter 32. Primary injuries are traumatic in origin and include skull fractures, contusions, concussions, lacerations, hemorrhages, and diffuse axonal injury. All of these can be a consequence of open or closed head injuries. Open head injuries are typically caused when a foal is kicked by another horse or strikes its head against a stationary object; this results in primary injuries such as skull fractures with disruption of the meninges and subsequent brain laceration and hemorrhage. Closed head injuries may occur with any primary injury but without penetrating the meninges. Closed injuries lead to TBI with focal brain damage and occur due to acceleration–deceleration injuries (whiplash) with abrupt movement of the brain within skull; this action results in a contusion (coup lesion) at the site of impact and a contusion (counter-coup lesion) on the area opposite from the impact site. Furthermore, close injuries may occur without a whiplash effect where the brain sustains a blow impact (e.g. stepped by the dam or pasture mate) without acceleration–deceleration forces but instead leading to a depression within the skull and subsequent brain tissue damage (Figure 32.VI.7).

Traumatic Brain Injury Related to Skull Fractures

Skull fractures leading to TBI can be divided into fractures of the roof or base of the skull. Compared to adult horses, where fractures of the roof of the skull are more common, foals are often presented with both types of fractures [26]. Fractures of the skull may be of different configuration with linear, compound, comminuted, stellate, and depressed being most commonly reported [10].

Foals can have explosive reactions when restrained and one common reaction during halter training is rearing,

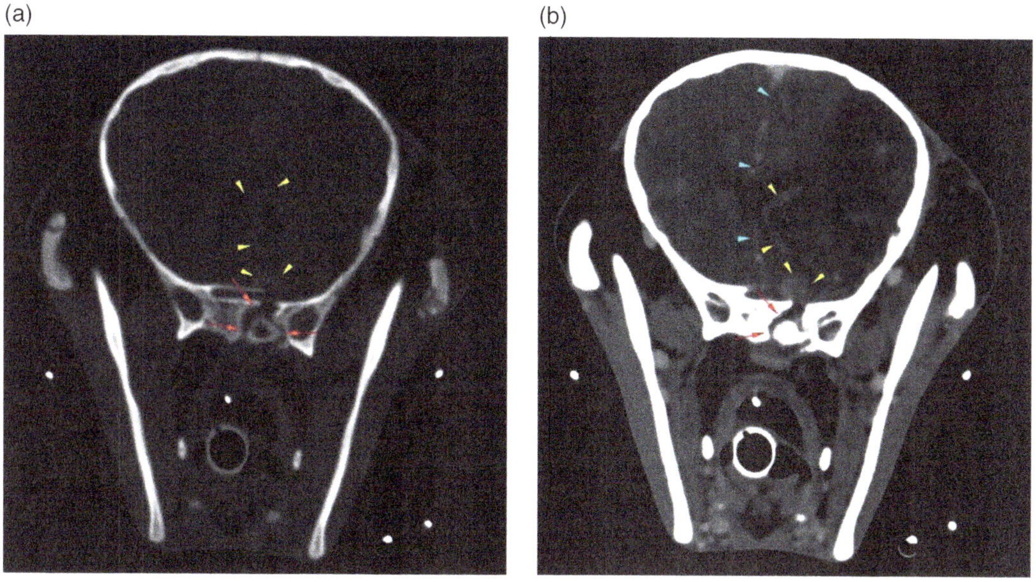

Figure 32.VI.8 Transverse pre- (a) and post-contrast (b) CT images of a 2-day-old miniature foal with multiple skulls fractures after being kicked by the damn. Red arrows indicate fractures. Intracranial hemorrhage is evidenced by hyperdense material within the cranial vault and left lateral ventricle (yellow arrowheads) with subsequent midline shift to the right (cyan arrowheads). *Source:* Image courtesy of Dr. Surita du Preez and Dr. Gustavo Ferlini Agne, University of Adelaide.

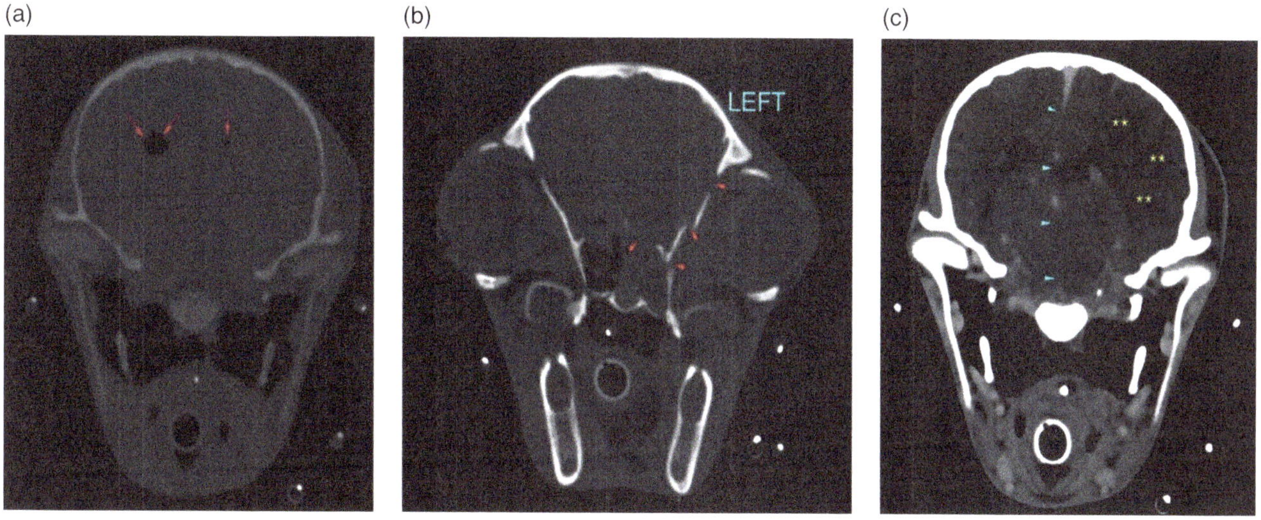

Figure 32.VI.9 Transverse pre- (a and b) and post-contrast (c) CT images of a 2-day-old miniature foal (same case as Figure 32.VI.8). Red arrows indicate gas within the lateral ventricles (a). Red arrowheads indicate lateral cranial vault and cribriform plate disruption (b). There is evidence of midline shift of the brain to the right (cyan arrowheads – c) and diffuse decreased attenuation of the left cerebral hemisphere affecting mostly the white matter tracts (yellow stars – c). *Source:* Image courtesy of Dr. Surita du Preez and Dr. Gustavo Ferlini Agne, University of Adelaide.

which can be followed by the foal flipping completely backward and hitting the poll of the skull on the ground. The primary impact site when flipping over backward is frequently the occipital bone protuberance, which creates a point of rotation axis for the head to extend backward, distributing the forces cranially toward the forebrain as well as stretching CNs, specifically the optic nerve. TBI secondary to a direct impact of the poll region after flipping over backward appears to be more severe when compared to flipping over backward and landing on an oblique direction striking the temporal region on the ground rather than the occipital region. Furthermore, neurologic deficits secondary to TBI can occur with fractures of the cerebral skull as a result of increase in intracranial pressure from the presence of hemorrhage and edema (Figures 32.VI.8 and 32.VI.9). The severity of neurologic deficits are directly related to the extent of the trauma, and the neurologic signs are defined by affected areas of the brain.

Trauma to the Frontal and Parietal Bone Region

Frontal and parietal fractures can cause direct damage to the cerebral cortex, especially if displaced fractures resulting in brain lacerations and hemorrhage to the underlying cortex are involved. Given the close proximity between bone and underlying surface of the cerebral cortex, impact between the supraorbital processes and the poll carry the highest risk for increase in TBI severity [31]. Decreased awareness and response to touch is observed in the contralateral side in cases of injury to the parietal (sensory) cortex. Similarly, in cases of direct impact to the frontal or parietal regions, a countercoup lesion to the occipital area may occur, which affects the occipital cortex leading to abnormal or absent vision and menace reflexes (cortical blindness) on the opposite side of the lesion (normal PLR still present). Therefore, a thorough neuro-ophthalmic examination should be performed to identify possible lesions to the occipital cortex. Evaluation of trauma to the parietal cortex with a decrease in sensation can be performed by evaluating the avoidance reflex after probing the nasal septal mucosa with a cotton-tip swab on both sides [10]. Commonly, neonatal foals present with transient epistaxis after trauma to the frontal and parietal bone region, which can indicate trauma to the nasal passage, paranasal sinus, or ethmoid turbinate. This temporary nasal hemorrhage is often bilateral and dark in color, suggesting an increased likelihood of being venous in origin, and of a small volume [10].

Forebrain Syndrome

Neurologic signs related to trauma to the frontal and parietal bone regions vary in severity and are often related to forebrain syndrome signs. Mild to moderate cases of forebrain syndrome have signs of concussion with temporary loss of conscious and a prolonged recovery period of depression and sternal recumbency. Severe signs of forebrain syndrome include persistent dementia with altered behavior, such as loss of affinity for the dam, yawning repeatedly, walking compulsively with or without circling (usually circling toward the lesion), and head pressing [10].

Midbrain Syndrome

Clinical signs of midbrain syndrome are uncommonly seen and are most often associated with trauma to the frontal and parietal regions. Injury to these regions can occur due to increase in intracranial pressure and subtentorial herniation of portions of the forebrain. Intracranial hemorrhage may also lead to signs of midbrain syndrome as well as trauma to the poll and rostral herniation of the cerebellum. Foals with midbrain syndrome are often comatose or depressed due to severe lesions affecting the ARAS. Vision is often intact, although severe cases may vary from bilateral miosis that progresses to bilateral pupillary dilation. In cases where the oculomotor nucleus is affected, the initial miosis is not observed and strabismus is seen along with bilateral dilation unresponsive to light stimulation. Midbrain syndrome without coma can be observed and is usually accompanied by bilateral weakness and ataxia with diffuse midbrain lesions. Unilateral midbrain lesions can occur with the neurologic deficits seen in the opposite site of the lesion [10]. TBI involving the midbrain and pons can result in deficits involving the oculomotor, trochlear, and abducens nerves, as their respective nuclei are located in this region. These nerves are also affected in skull fractures involving the orbital fissure as they exit the cranial cavity through the orbital foramen [21]. Although clinical signs of midbrain syndrome are more often observed after trauma to the frontal or parietal regions, it may also occur after traumatic events to the poll region.

Trauma to the Occiput (Poll) Region

Foals are predisposed to trauma to the poll specially when flipping backward while being handled or halter trained and are more prone to displaced fractures of the basilar bones due to incomplete ossification of the basioccipital-basisphenoidal suture (Figures 32.VI.10–32.VI.12). This suture line fuses, at the earliest, at 2 years of age, although it can take up to 4 years for complete fusion. Thus, not only foals but also young horses are susceptible to fracture and avulsion of the basilar bones [32]. Development of displaced basisphenoid fractures are facilitated by additional fractures of surrounding supporting bones such as the occipital, temporal, and parietal bone fractures [10]. Without the support of these surrounding bones, the basisphenoid fracture is more likely to displace ventrally from the basioccipital bone which will further increase the trauma and associated vasculature and brain tissue. Profuse epistaxis may be observed if the occipital vasculature is severed by bone fragments. The bleeding initially occurs into the retropharyngeal space and guttural pouches and later evidenced by epistaxis [10]. This epistaxis is sometimes arterial in origin with a bright red color, and often more profuse when compared to venous bleeding seen from the nasal passages after a frontal or parietal impact. Furthermore, basisphenoid fractures often lead to significant trauma to the brainstem region.

Hindbrain Syndrome

Although less often observed, signs of hindbrain syndrome can occur after significant trauma to the poll region. The cerebellum can be subjected to excessive acceleration–deceleration forces, leading to clinical signs of cerebellar ataxia (wide base stance, intention tremors). Severe cases can develop abnormal breathing pattern with shallow and rapid breathing observed.

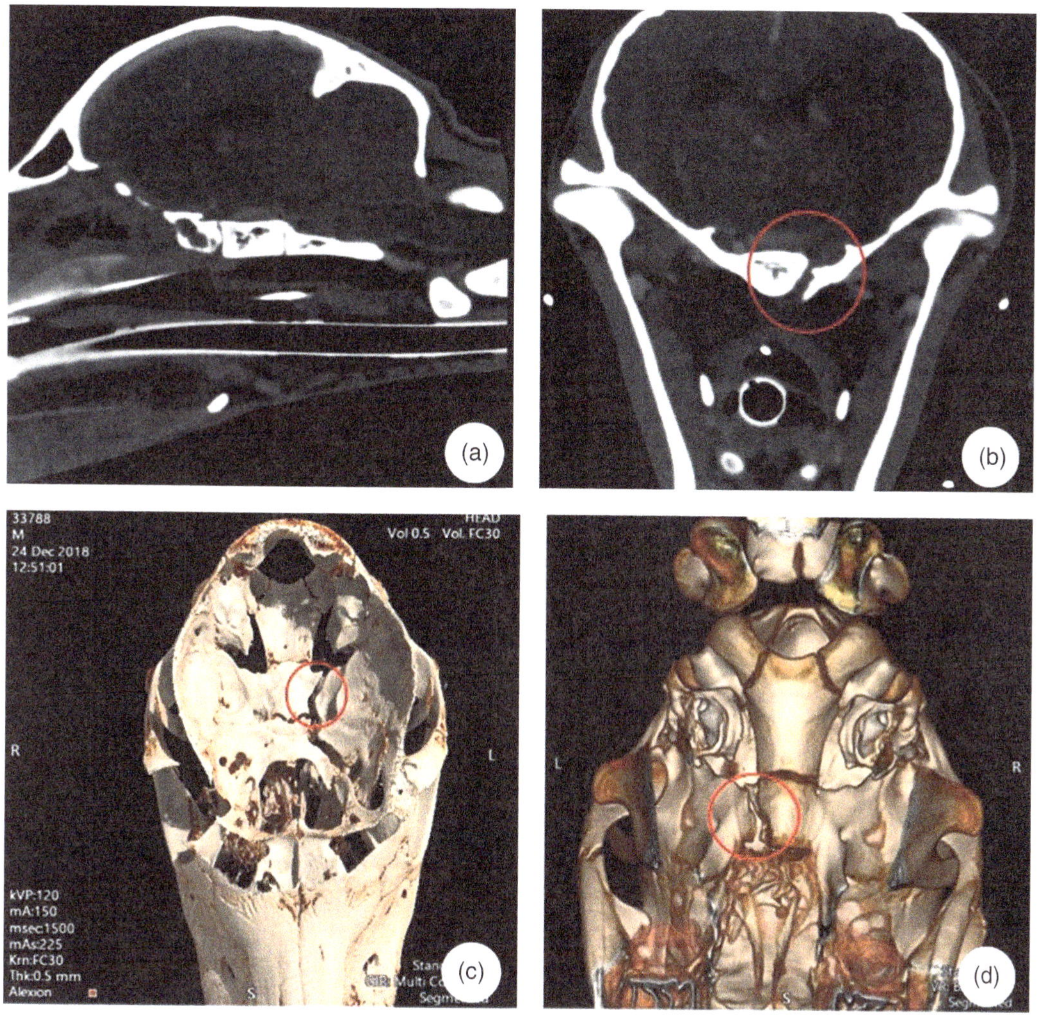

Figure 32.VI.10 Multiplanar post-contrast CT images (longitudinal [a], transverse [b]) and 3D reconstruction of the head (dorsal view [c], ventral view [d]) of a miniature foal with traumatic brain injury. Red circles demonstrate a regional fracture on the left aspect of the basisphenoid bone. *Source:* Image courtesy of Dr. Gustavo Ferlini Agne and Dr. Surita du Preez, University of Adelaide.

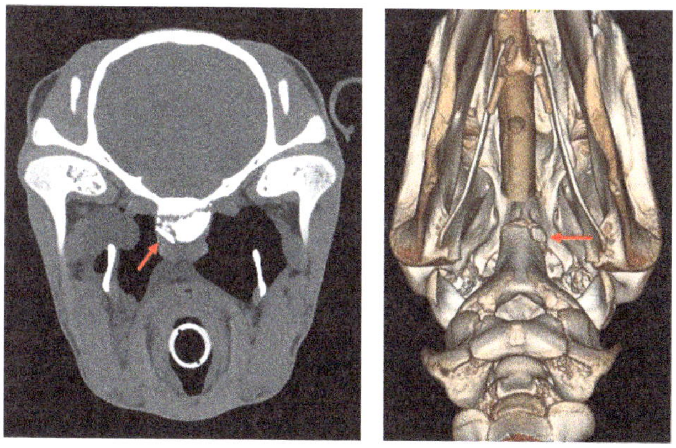

Figure 32.VI.11 Transverse and 3D head CT images of a 3-month-old Quarter Horse colt with acute neurologic signs after flipping backward. Evidence of a minimally displaced fracture of the rostral aspect of the basioccipital bone is seen (red arrow). *Source:* Image courtesy of Dr. Erin Groover, Auburn University.

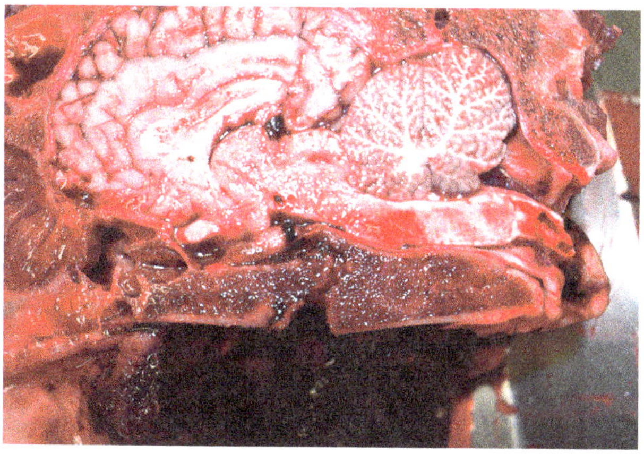

Figure 32.VI.12 Postmortem example of a basisphenoid bone fracture in a foal that struck its poll on the ground while flipped over backward. *Source:* Image courtesy of Dr. Rebecca Ruby, University of Kentucky.

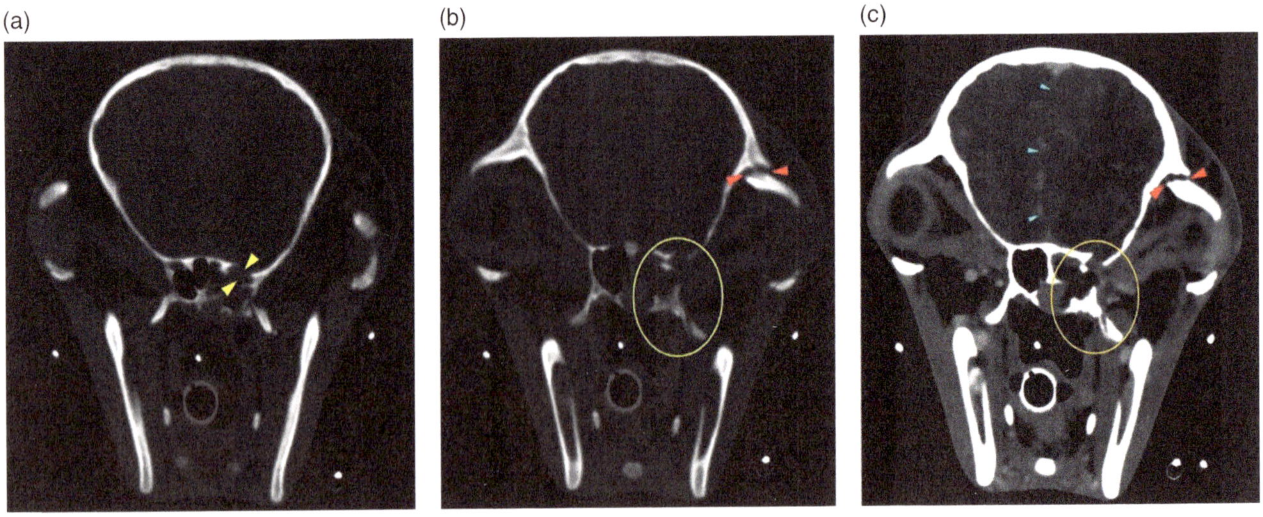

Figure 32.VI.13 Transverse pre- (a and b) and post-contrast (c) CT head slices of a miniature foal with traumatic brain injury with signs of unilateral blindness. This foal endured multiple skull lesions including optic canal fracture (yellow arrowheads – a), orbital fracture (red arrowheads b and c) and disruption of the left aspect of the base of the brain (yellow circle – b and c). Unilateral blindness was still present at a 12-month re-examination. *Source:* Image courtesy of Dr. Surita du Preez and Dr. Gustavo Ferlini Agne, University of Adelaide.

Optic Nerve Syndrome

Neonatal foals are at risk of permanent blindness due to stretching or complete resection of the optic nerves after a severe impact to the poll (Figure 32.VI.13). The strenuous forces of which the poll impacts the ground followed by the abrupt extension of the neck lead to acceleration–deceleration forces causing significant damage to the cerebral parenchyma and optic nerves. After the trauma, foals can develop bilateral midriasis that is unresponsive to light stimulation and partially or completely impaired vision. The prognosis for vision improvement is poor, as most commonly the secondary phase of the TBI continues and further aggravates the optic nerves damage.

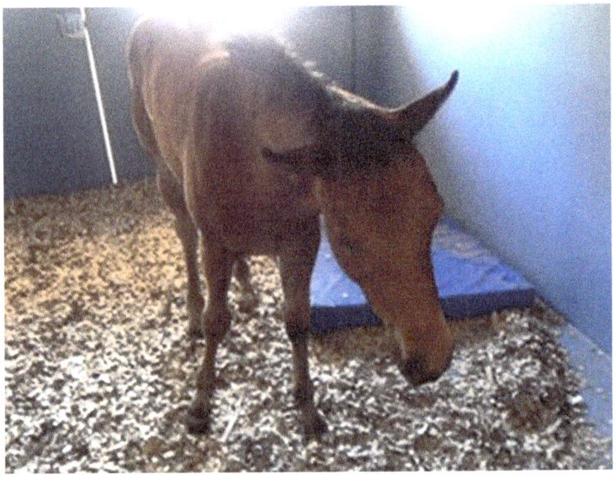

Figure 32.VI.14 Foal with a right-sided head tilt after a traumatic event to the lateral aspect of the poll with subsequent clinical signs of peripheral vestibular ataxia. *Source:* Image courtesy of Dr. Lidwien Verdegaal, University of Adelaide.

Vestibular Syndrome

Clinical signs of vestibular syndrome can be observed with trauma to the poll as tremendous forces to the occiput or temporal bone region (e.g. foal lands on head at an oblique angle toward the ground) lead to fracture of the petrous portion of the temporal bone, subsequently damaging the vestibular apparatus; this results in clinical signs of vestibular syndrome characterized by peripheral vestibular ataxia (Figure 32.VI.14). Lesions at the base of the skull might affect the nuclei of CN VIII within the brainstem and elicit signs of vestibular syndrome characterized by central vestibular ataxia. Examination of the neck/cervical spine is also warranted as afferent fibers pass through the C1–C3 dorsal spinal nerve roots and ascend from the spinal cord to the caudal vestibular nuclei. These nerves provide proprioceptive input from the cranial cervical vertebrae, ligaments, and muscles. Therefore, trauma to the cranial cervical neck could also elicit similar signs as trauma to the vestibular apparatus or damage to the CN VIII.

Multifocal Syndrome

Signs of multifocal disease often occur in foals with TBI given that secondary injury may develop and involve areas of the brain other than those directly involved in the original impact and trauma. Furthermore, foals that flip over while rapidly moving forward or backward are predisposed to endure traumatic events within their spinal cord segments.

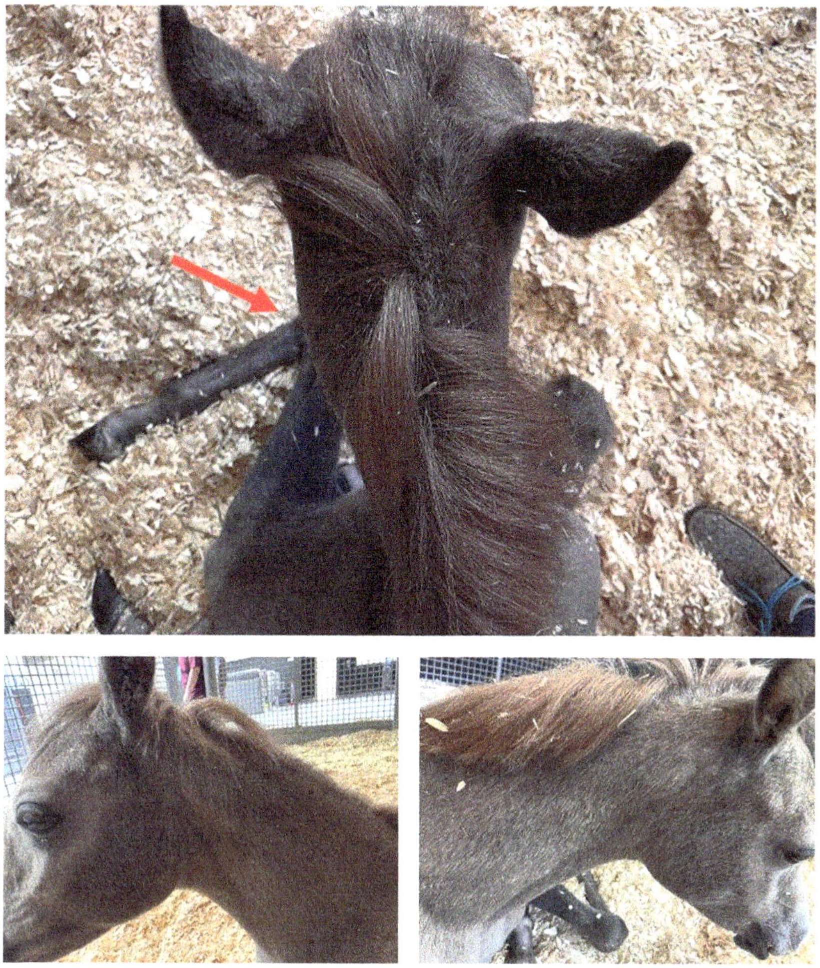

Figure 32.VI.15 Unilateral focal swelling within the cranial neck over the atlantoaxial region in a five-months-old Arabian filly. The foal had normal mentation, normal cranial nerve examination, and evidence of gross asymmetry of the left cranial neck (arrow) over the atlantoaxial region, although with no obvious pain or crepitus upon palpation. *Source:* Image courtesy of Dr. Camilla Jamieson, Equine Veterinary Medical Center.

Traumatic Spinal Cord Injury in the Foal

Traumatic events to the spinal cord are often related to vertebral fractures, with the cervical vertebrae being more commonly affected as they are less protected by soft tissue compared to other spinal cord segments. Similar to TBI, SCI can occur as a primary insult (e.g. trauma to the underlying spinal cord from compression or laceration due to a vertebral fracture or impact) or secondary injury that occurs within hours to days from the time of initial trauma. Clinical signs related to vertebral fractures vary according to the severity of the trauma and include neurologic deficits, obvious swelling within the area of the trauma (Figure 32.I.15), focal sweating (Figure 32.VI.16), hyper- or hypalgesia, and pruritus within the associated dermatome [33]. Mechanisms of spinal trauma include excessive flexion or extension, rotation, or strenuous shearing forces imposed to the spinal cord. SCI due to fractures can be divided into cervical, thoraco-lumbar, and caudal vertebral fractures.

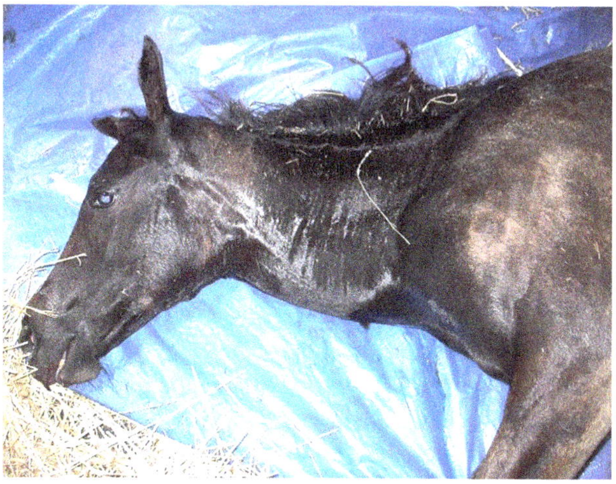

Figure 32.VI.16 Cervical focal sweating in a 6-month-old Thoroughbred foal with a C4–C5 fracture and spinal cord injury. The foal was quadriplegic on presentation. Note the moderate vertebral hyperextension and mydriatic pupil. *Source:* Image courtesy of Dr. Nathan Slovis, Hagyard Equine Medical Institute.

Cranial Cervical Vertebral Fractures (Atlantooccipital, Atlantoaxial, and C2–C3 Fractures)

Atlantooccipital and Atlantal Fractures

Head trauma can lead to skull fractures and TBI, but fractures to the occipital bone or the cranial cervical vertebrae can occur when foals hit their head into the ground or into a fixed object while traveling at high speeds. Upon impact, the forces are broadly distributed caudally from the front aspect of the skull toward the occipital condyles and subsequently toward the atlas [10]. Occipital condyle fractures are rare, with clinical signs including severe neck pain and inability or reluctance to move the head and usually occur without neurologic deficits [26]. Fractures to the atlas may occur more frequently than occipital condyle fractures, although less commonly seen compared to axial fractures.

In neonatal foals, the atlantal arches and wings are common sites for atlantal fractures but clinical signs often cannot be differentiated from atlantooccipital fractures. In cases of atlantooccipital fractures, fragments from the atlas may be displaced cranially with the impact and may lacerate the hypoglossal nerve as it exits the hypoglossal foramen, leading to difficulty in nursing and retracting the tongue. Spinal cord compression is a rare complication from atlantooccipital fractures and ataxia may or may not be present. Instead, foals often present with signs of swelling over the fractured area, a rigid and painful neck, and possibly a head tilt [26].

Diagnosis can be established via radiography using lateral, oblique, and ventrodorsal projections to evaluate atlantooccipital fractures (Figures 32.VI.17 and 32.VI.18). The dorsal aspect of the atlas has a distinct symphysis that should not be confused with fractures lines. Although radiographs may allow for a diagnosis, CT is useful in accurately defining comminuted fractures and developing a treatment plan. Surgical repair of atlantooccipital fractures are rarely reported, as many of these lesions are better managed with conservative medical therapy consisted of fiberglass splints placed on the ventral aspect of the cranial neck until healing and ossification of the fracture area occurs with appropriated alignment and stabilization of the atlantooccipital junction [26]. In cases of severe neurologic signs, callus formation with spinal cord compression may be present; this situation may necessitate myelography to confirm spinal cord compression. If confirmed, dorsal laminectomy of the caudal two-thirds of the dorsal lamina of the atlas can be performed with neurologic signs improving within 14 months postsurgical intervention [34].

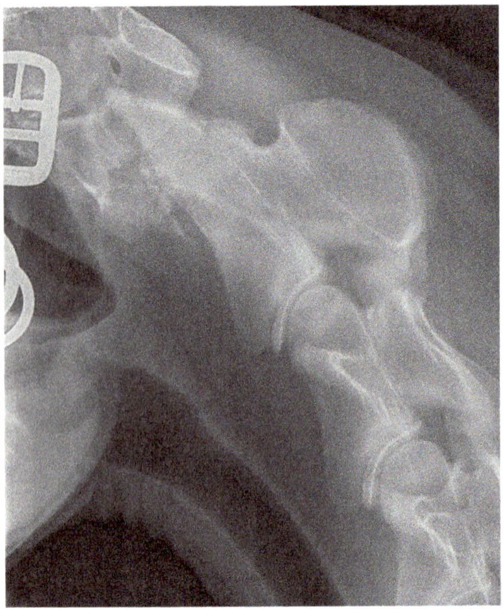

Figure 32.VI.17 Standing lateral radiograph of the cranial neck demonstrating a C1 fracture with rostral displacement of the dens and bone fragments near the ventral arch of the atlas. Ventrodorsal as well as oblique projections are required to better classify the lesion. *Source:* Image courtesy of Dr. Nicole Finazzo.

Axial Fractures

Fractures of the axis are not uncommon in foals with partial (Figure 32.VI.19) or complete fracture and separation of the dens (also known as odontoid process or odontoid peg) being most commonly reported [35, 36]. Note that the axis in foals, similar to other species, have ossification centers for the dens, the arch, as well as for the body and caudal epiphysis (Figure 32.VI.20) [37, 38]. The synchondrosis of the odontoid process and the body of the axis complete ossification at 7–8 months of age [39]. This area of synchondrosis should not be confused with fracture lines; however, these lines might be involved in fractures since they are weak points that do not tolerate excessive forces, making them more prone to injury, particularly during the initial months of life [26, 40]. Common types of axial fractures have been described in humans and a similar classification adapted to horses (Table 32.VI.4) [37, 41].

Clinical presentation is based on severity of the fracture and potential for spinal cord compression. Foals that are presented with unilateral swelling of the cranial neck, head tilt, and lateralization of the head may have endured a crush injury to the cranial articular process of the axis. This type of lesion is usually unilateral, affecting either the left or right cranial articular process of the second cervical vertebrae causing head positioning asymmetry and tilt. Axial fractures most commonly occur at the level of the dens with or without displacement of the axis body. Mild to moderate trauma without significant displacement of the

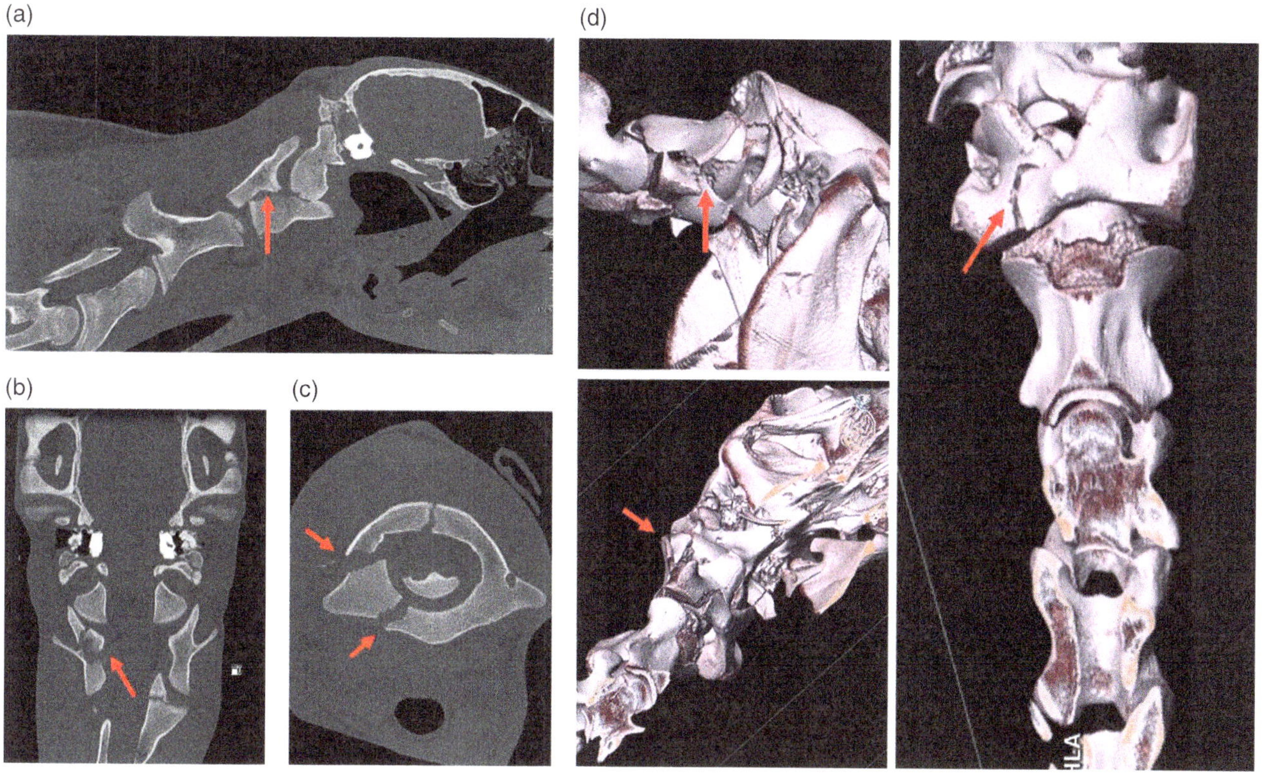

Figure 32.VI.18 Head and neck CT images from a foal with acute neurologic signs after a fall, which resulted in a comminuted fracture of the Atlas (same foal as in Figure 32.VI.15). Clinical signs of upper motor neuron paresis were evident in all four limbs (grade 3/5 on hind limbs and grade 2/5 on front limbs). Longitudinal CT lateral (a), longitudinal CT ventrodorsal (b), transverse CT slice of C1 (c), 3D reconstruction (d); This foal underwent conservative therapy consistent of prolonged stall rest and at recheck examination, evidence of upper motor neuron paresis, and proprioceptive deficits was still present, although with significant clinical improvement from presentation (grade 1/5 on hind limbs and normal on front limbs). Red arrows indicate fracture sites. *Source:* Image courtesy of Dr. Camilla Jamieson, Equine Veterinary Medical Center.

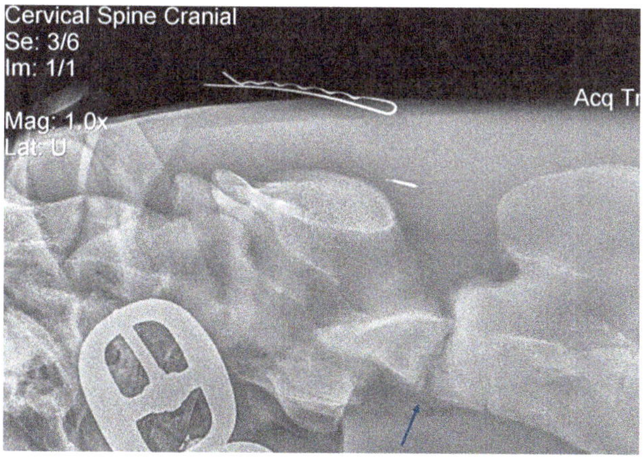

Figure 32.VI.19 Standing lateral radiograph of the cranial neck of a 2-month-old Quarter Horse foal with a type II fracture of dens (blue arrow) with no obvious fragments seen. *Source:* Image courtesy of Dr. Stacy Potter.

axis body usually does not result in spinal cord compression because of the large space between the caudal aspect of the atlas and cranial aspect of the axis; this allows for lateralization of the spinal cord from the fractured portion of the dens, subsequently lessening neurologic deficits [26]. In cases of severe impact and trauma, the fractured portion of the dens can remain attached to the ventral arch of the atlas by the dens ligament, whereas the body of the axis luxates ventrally in relation to the fractured dens due to tension from the nuchal ligament [26].

A variety of surgical techniques for spinal cord decompression and atlantoaxial joint stabilization have been described in foals and young horses [35, 42–44] with some success using a ventral stabilization and cancellous and cortical screws along with dynamic compression plates [45]. Evidence of arthrodesis and healing of the atlantoaxial joint was noted 2–3 months after surgical intervention, and no evidence of ataxia or proprioceptive deficits was present at long-term follow-up [42, 45]. The ventral surgical approach allows for decompression, alignment, and stabilization of the atlantoaxial joint. This technique seems to be superior to Steinmann pin fixation, although it does carry the risk for laryngeal paralysis [42]. Although surgical correction is possible, conservative therapy with splinting of the cranial neck for 4–6 weeks and stall rest (2 months) has also been reported, with successful

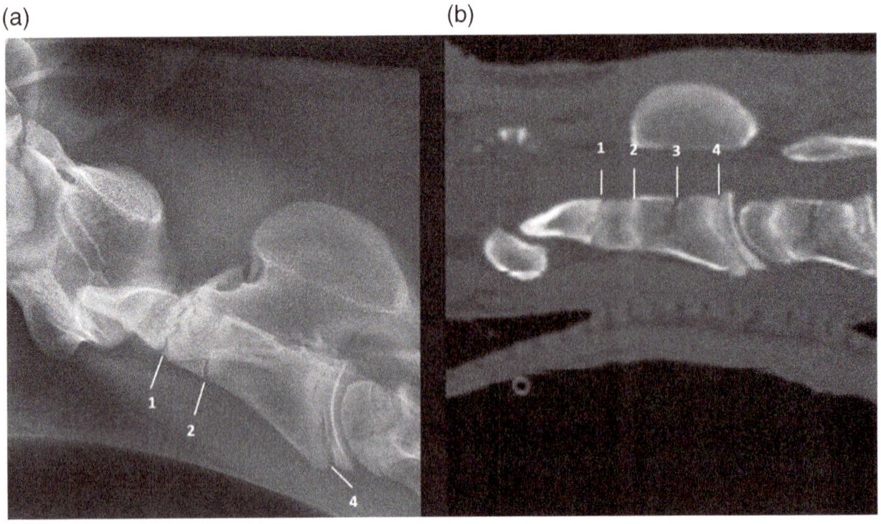

Figure 32.VI.20 Standing lateral radiograph (a) and longitudinal CT slice (b) of the cranial neck demonstrating the normal ossification centers of the dens [1], arch [2], body [3] and caudal physis of the axis [4].

Table 32.VI.4 Modified classification of fractures of the odontoid process of the axis.

Type of fracture		Fracture characteristic
Type I	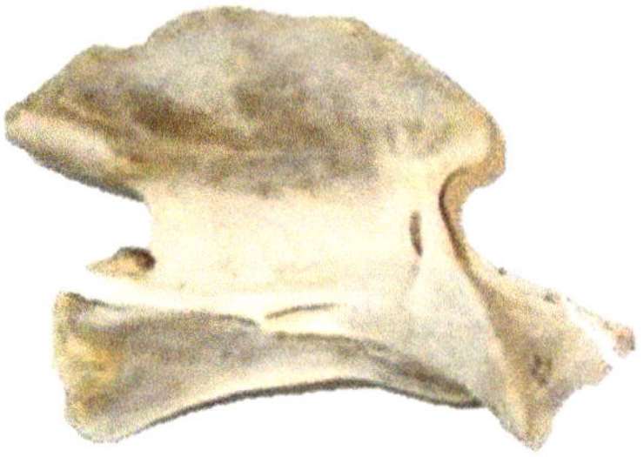	Oblique fracture line with avulsion of the upper portion of the odontoid process
Type II	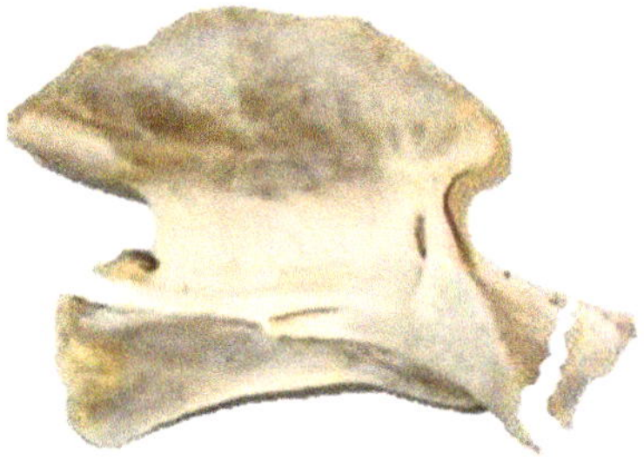	Fracture line at the synchondrosis of the odontoid process and the body of the axis
Type IIa	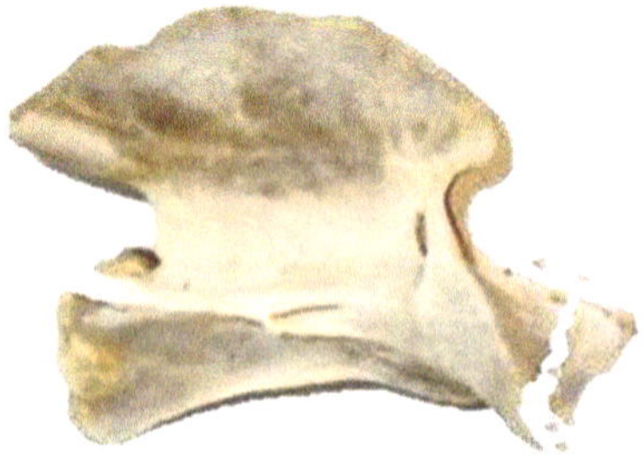	Fracture line at the synchondrosis of the odontoid process and the body of the axis with obvious bone fragments at the fracture site
Type III	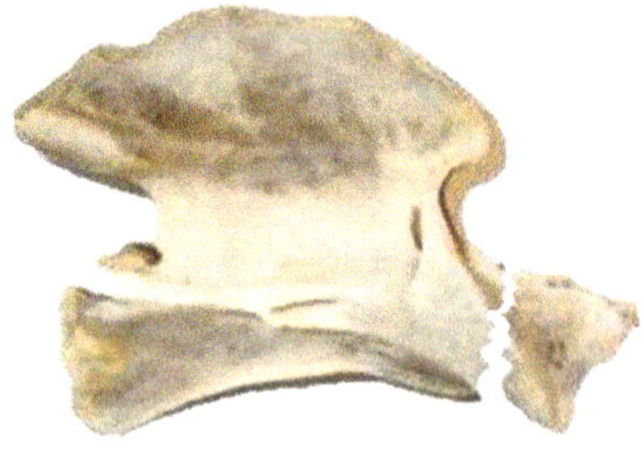	Fracture of the of axial body, which extends down into the cancellous bone

Source: Adapted from Vos et al. [37] and "Fractures of the odontoid process of the axis" by Anderson, *The Journal of Bone and Joint Surgery*, 1974.

results in adult horses. Conservative management may be an alternative for foals with less severe lesions (e.g. without compression of the spinal cord and significant neurologic deficits) or for cases without a surgical option due to financial constraints [35, 37]. Prognosis and decision for surgical intervention is related to the severity of neurologic deficits, with evidence of callus formation and spinal cord compression serving as indicators for surgical intervention and worse prognosis. Myelogram can be performed in cases with suspected spinal cord compression and subtotal dorsal laminectomy of the caudal two-thirds of the atlas can be attempt in order to achieve decompression [34].

Occiptoatlantoxial and Atlantoaxial Subluxation/Luxation

Traumatic events leading to atlantoaxial subluxation or luxation can occur in foals with or without fracture of the axis, although complete atlantoaxial luxation without vertebral fracture is rare [46]. Trauma with hyperflexion of the neck may result in soft tissue injury with disruption of the paired longitudinal ligaments of the dens, which offer the main source of stability for the odontoid peg within the atlas and occipital bone. Traumatic soft tissue injury with decreased stability of the dens within the atlas may appear as an increase in distance between the dens and the ventral arch of the atlas on radiographic assessment, indicating dorsal displacement of the dens [26]. Congenital malformations in foals such as blunting of the dens may predispose to this type of injury and has been reported in a Quarter Horse foal [47]. Similarly, congenital occipitoatlantoaxial malformation (OAAM) in foals can predispose to instability of the occipitoatlantoaxial junction, thereby facilitating subluxation. Arabian foals that present with a stiff, painful, and asymmetric cranial cervical neck, with or without signs of ataxia, warrant neurologic examination, diagnostic imaging, and genetic investigation, as deleterious mutations within the Homeobox D3 (HOXD3) gene has been related to OAAM [48]. Surgical and nonsurgical treatment for reduction and stabilization of occipitoatlantoaxial and atlantoaxial (sub)luxation have been described in foals with successful results [46]. Nonsurgical reduction of an occipitoatlantoaxial dislocation in a foal with notable ataxia has been successfully achieved after manipulation; the foal gradually improved within 5 days after the procedure. At the 14-month recheck examination, the foal had persistent but mild head tilt but no neurologic deficits; radiographs demonstrated evidence of ankylosing of the atlantoaxial joint [46]. Definite diagnosis for the presence and severity of spinal cord compression requires myelography, which in cases of atlantoaxial subluxation demonstrate exacerbation of spinal cord compression during extension and relief during flexion [26]. Cases of severe luxation of the atlantoaxial joint with complete ventral displacement and separation of the axis from the atlas frequently lead to tetraplegia, which ultimately requires euthanasia.

Mid (C3–C5) and Caudal (C5–C7) Cervical Vertebral Fractures

Neonate foals can sustain fractures of the mid and caudal cervical neck with subsequent SCI in the face of impact lesions with excessive hyperextension, hyperflexion, or excessive lateralization of the neck. Information identifying which vertebrae are most commonly affected in foals is not available, although a study in mature race horses indicated that C3 and C4 might be more susceptible to fractures [49]. Clinical presentation of foals with fractures of the mid and caudal cervical vertebrae can range from a painful and rigid neck without neurologic deficits to ataxia of varying severity, tetraplegia, recumbency or even sudden death [50]. Traumatic events with hyperextension of the neck may lead to distraction fractures of the caudal epiphysis of the mid cervical vertebrae (Figure 32.VI.21). These types of fractures are more likely to occur in foals up to 2 years of age due to the immature ossification within this area, although the caudal epiphysis (particularly the ventral aspect), has radiographic evidence of incomplete ossification for up to 4–5 years of age [51]. Severe hyperextension of the neck may also lead to fracture of the pedicles of the caudal articular processes as well as the lateral arches of the vertebral canal, resulting in deroofing lesions [52]. Deroofing lesions have noticeable malalignment of the vertebral bodies seen on lateral radiographs but do not seem to elicit substantial neurologic deficits initially; instead, a cascade of instability through the adjacent vertebrae may occur throughout the healing process. Therefore, cases with deroofing lesions of the spinal canal may present initially with minimal neurologic deficits that likely worsen over time [26, 51, 52]. Nevertheless, deroofing lesions with complete separation of the dorsal lamina and caudal pedicles may lead to compression of the spinal cord from the adjacent vertebrae leading to substantial spinal cord trauma and neurologic deficits.

Traumatic events with excessive lateral flexion of the neck may lead to unilateral or bilateral fractures of the articular processes with or without fractures of the associated vertebral pedicles (Figure 32.VI.22). Injury to the neck with strenuous forces during lateral flexion may also lead to tearing of the synovial joint capsule, which will further predispose to subluxation of the articular processes [53]. Fractures of the caudal cervical vertebrae occur less frequently when compared to cranial and mid-cervical fractures but the biomechanics for insult to the

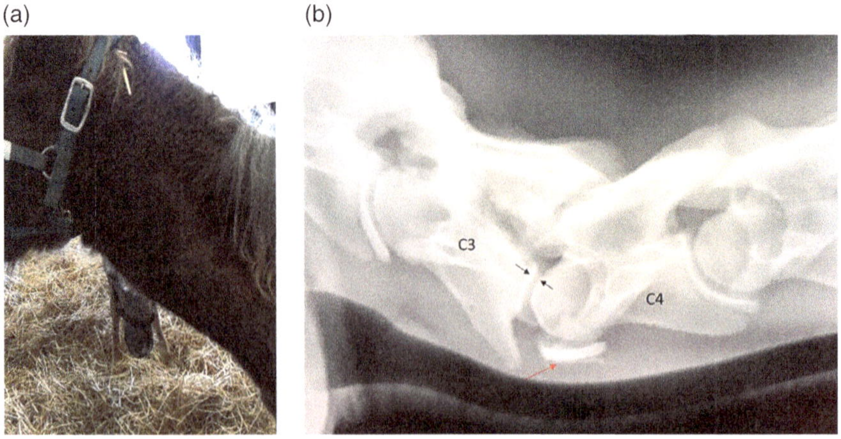

Figure 32.VI.21 Lateral view of the cranial cervical neck of a 3-month-old Thoroughbred foal with moderate to severe comminuted fracture of C3–C4. The foal was ambulatory on presentation with moderate swelling and mild hyperextension of C3–C4 region (a). Standing lateral radiograph demonstrates multiple fractures of C3, including a distraction fracture of the caudal epiphysis (red arrow) and an incomplete deroofing lesion with partial displacement of the dorsal laminae from the vertebral body (b). Evidence of bone remodeling around the fractures with poor definition of the caudal articular process of C3 as well as narrowing of craniodorsal aspect of C3–C4 intervertebral disk space (black arrows) is visible. Note the mild vertebral hyperextension of C3–C4 with associated tracheal compression. *Source:* Image courtesy of Dr. Nathan Slovis, Hagyard Equine Medical Institute.

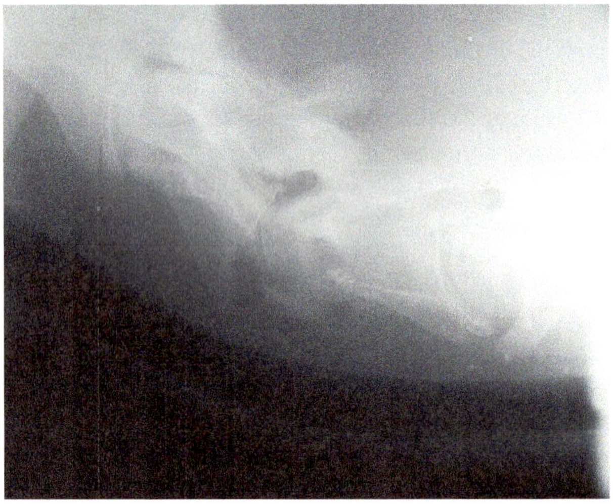

Figure 32.VI.22 Lateral radiograph of the mid cervical vertebrae from a 3-month-old Thoroughbred foal with severe comminuted fracture of C5–C6. Fracture of the articular processes is present and likely associated with exaggerated lateral flexion of neck during the fall. Distraction fracture of the caudal epiphysis of C5 is also visible. *Source:* Image courtesy of Dr. Nathan Slovis, Hagyard Equine Medical Institute.

spinal cord within this region are similar to those of mid cervical fractures. Different than cranial and mid cervical fractures where foals may present postural deficits affecting the ability to raise the head and neck off the ground, caudal cervical lesions may be associated with a normal ability to lift the neck from the ground, although sternal recumbency might not be achievable. Foals with ataxia and focal sweating along with signs of radial nerve paralysis may have abaxial fractures to C6–C7, as reported in adult horses. In those cases, lateral displacement of the fracture may cause SCI with damage to the descending sympathetic tracts causing ataxia and focal sweating. At the same time, damage to the dorsal nerve roots of the spinal nerves of C7 may also occur and contribute to deficits in the radial and musculocutaneous nerves [54]. Therefore, foals with a sudden history of radial nerve paralysis warrant a complete neurologic examination, including radiographic assessment of the caudal cervical neck.

Despite the site of fracture within the cervical neck, the severity of clinical signs is directly related to the degree of spinal cord trauma and compression. Comminuted fractures and fractures involving shattering of one or more vertebrae elicit the worst neurologic deficits and prognosis. Although cervical vertebral surgery is less challenging in foals because of their size, the softer bone density of the foal may lead to higher chances of implant failure compared to yearlings or adult horses that have denser vertebrae. Therefore, in cases of significant bone disruption such as severe comminuted fractures of the vertebral bodies, implant fixation may not be feasible, making conservative therapy with casting of the cervical neck an alternative [26, 41]. In cases of ventral fixation of the cervical vertebrae, neurologic deficits pre- and postoperatively are similar but are expected to improve within the initial 48 hours postoperatively [26]. Plate removal after ventral fixation of the cervical vertebrae has not been reported with the degree of recovery after surgical intervention being variable and dependent on the severity of the lesion as well as implant stability. Periods of up to 18 months are expected for complete recovery in older horses [26].

Spinal Cord Injury Secondary to Thoracolumbar Fractures

Trauma to the thoracolumbar vertebrae leading to SCI is uncommon in foals, making extrapolation of information from traumatic events in adult horses necessary. Clinical signs include neurologic deficits related to the specific spinal cord segment affected (see Neurolocalization section). Foals that flip over backward can fracture the thoracic spinous processes over the withers, although neurologic sequela might be absent unless the impact and forces imparted to the spinal cord are sufficient to cause primary or secondary SCI. Fractures to the body of the thoracic vertebrae usually result in significant neurologic deficits given the narrow space between the vertebral canal wall and the spinal cord at the thoracic level [26]. In adult horses, T1–T3, T12, T18–L6, and L5 are the most commonly fractured vertebrae [55]. It is unknown which sections of the thoracolumbar spine that foals are more likely to fracture, although areas of incomplete ossification such as the cranial and caudal vertebral body epiphyses of the thoracolumbar spine (do not have complete physeal closure until 3.5 years age) might be more easily injured and fractured [56]. Although vertebral end plate fractures related to trauma are more commonly reported in foals, vertebral body compression fractures have also been described, particularly within the thoracolumbar lesion.

Radiographic diagnosis of vertebral body compression fractures of the thoracolumbar region is possible in foals although it may be difficult to differentiate from congenital abnormalities such as hemivertebra [57]. Clinical signs of Schiff-Sherrington syndrome, characterized by extensor hypertonia of the thoracic limbs along with hypotonic paralysis of the hind limbs, was described in a 7-month-old foal with a compression fracture of the T15 vertebral body [57]. This clinical syndrome is rare in foals with such lesions demonstrating normal neck movement (unless a concurrent lesion within the cervical vertebrae), normal withdraw and patellar reflexes, and an absent or abnormal cutaneous trunci reflex at and caudal to the lesion site [57]. Compression fractures have also been described affecting the L2 vertebral body in a 3-week-old Thoroughbred colt with clinical sign of flaccid paralysis of the pelvic limbs, absent cutaneous trunci reflex and a subjectively conscious insensitivity to pin pricking [58]. Signs of both UMN and LMN deficits may develop in cases of compression fractures of the thoracolumbar spine due to compression of spinal vessels leading to ischemic SCI and neural degeneration of both upper and LMN pathways [58]. Foals with no history of trauma may have pathological fractures secondary to sepsis as reported in a 1-month-old Quarter Horse filly with hind limb paresis and diagnosed with a comminuted fracture of the L6 vertebral body and pedicle caused by *Rhodococcus equi* osteomyelitis [59].

Spinal Cord Injury Secondary to Lumbosacral Fractures

Fractures of the lumbosacral region are uncommon in foals with only one report of a sacral fracture described in a Thoroughbred foal with a history of dystocia [60]. The foal's vertebral column undergoes significant rotation (approximately 180°) during the second stage of parturition with the cervical and thoracic spine within the birth canal in a sternal position while the lumbosacral spine lying in a dorsal position [61]. This extreme rotation, in combination with malpresentation of the fetus, with or without feto-pelvic disproportion, can predispose the newborn to trauma of the spine, particularly at the cranial or caudal physis of the vertebral bodies. Therefore, foals that develop neurologic deficits such as hindlimb paralysis after assisted vaginal delivery warrant radiographic and, if available, CT evaluation of the vertebral column with a focus on the lumbosacral region.

References

1 Tyler, C., Davis, R., Begg, A. et al. (1993). A survey of neurological diseases in horses. *Aust. Vet. J.* 70: 445–449.

2 Adams, R. and Mayhew, I. (1984). Neurological examination of newborn foals. *Equine Vet. J.* 16: 306–312.

3 Mayhew, L. (1988). Neurological and neuropathological observations on the equine neonate. *Equine Vet. J.* 20: 28–33.

4 Olsen, E., Dunkel, B., Barker, W. et al. (2014). Rater agreement on gait assessment during neurologic examination of horses. *J. Vet. Intern. Med.* 28: 630–638.

5 Aleman, M., Gray, L.C., Williams, D.C. et al. (2006). Juvenile idiopathic epilepsy in Egyptian Arabian foals: 22 cases (1985–2005). *J. Vet. Intern. Med.* 20: 1443–1449.

6 Gonda, C., Crisman, M., and Moon, M. (2001). Occipitoatlantoaxial malformation in a Quarter Horse foal. *Equine Vet. Educ.* 13: 289–291.

7 Reed, S.M. (2019). Medical aspects of traumatic brain injury in horses. *Equine Fract. Repair* 800–803.

8 Platt, S.R., Radaelli, S.T., and McDonnell, J.J. (2001). The prognostic value of the modified Glasgow Coma Scale in head trauma in dogs. *J. Vet. Intern. Med.* 15: 581–584.

9 Platt, S. (2005). Evaluation and treatment of the head trauma patient. *In Practice* 27: 31–35.

10 MacKay, R.J. (2004). Brain injury after head trauma: pathophysiology, diagnosis, and treatment. *Vet. Clin. North Am. Equine* 20: 199–216.
11 Reed, S. (1993). Management of head trauma in horses. *Compend. Cont. Educ. Pract. Vet.* 15: 270–273.
12 Mayhew, I. (1996). Equine neurology and nutrition. *Proceedings of the 18th Australian Equine Veterinary Association Bain-Fallon Memorial Lectures,* 22nd–26th July 1996, Stamford Grand Hotel Glenelg, South Australia, Australia. Australian Equine Veterinary Association, 1–73.
13 Feary, D.J., Magdesian, K.G., Aleman, M.A. et al. (2007). Traumatic brain injury in horses: 34 cases (1994–2004). *J. Vet. Intern. Med.* 231: 259–266.
14 DeBowes, R.M., Leipold, H.W., and Turner-Beatty, M. (1987). Cerebellar abiotrophy. *Vet. Clin. North Am. Equine* 3: 345–352.
15 Brault, L.S., Cooper, C.A., Famula, T.R. et al. (2011). Mapping of equine cerebellar abiotrophy to ECA2 and identification of a potential causative mutation affecting expression of MUTYH. *Genomics* 97: 121–129.
16 Aleman, M. (2015). Neurologic examination in foals. *Proceedings of the 2015 WEVA – International Congress 2015* 10th October 2015, Guadalajara, Mexico. World Equine Veterinary Association.
17 Smith, B.P. (2014). *Large Animal Internal Medicine-E-Book*. Elsevier Health Sciences.
18 Scrivani, P.V. (2011). Advanced imaging of the nervous system in the horse. *Vet. Clin. Equine* 27: 439–453.
19 Leiva, M., Peña, T., and Monreal, L. (2011). Ocular findings in healthy newborn foals according to age. *Equine Vet. Educ.* 23: 40–45.
20 Saliou, G., d'Ablon, X., Théaudin, M. et al. (2020). Cerebral computed tomography scan demonstrating ischemic stroke in a filly after intravenous antibiotic administration. *J. Equine Vet. Sci.* 88: 102953.
21 Schmidt, M.J., Knemeyer, C., and Heinsen, H. (2019). Neuroanatomy of the equine brain as revealed by high-field (3Tesla) magnetic-resonance-imaging. *PLoS One* 14: e0213814.
22 Mayhew, I.G. (2009). *Large Animal Neurology*. Phildelphia: Lea & Febiger.
23 Boorman, S., Scherrer, N.M., Stefanovski, D. et al. (2020). Facial nerve paralysis in 64 equids: clinical variables, diagnosis, and outcome. *J. Vet. Intern. Med.* 34: 1308–1320.
24 Russell, C., Aboellail, T., and Nout-Lomas, Y. (2019). Congenital facial nerve dysfunction. *Equine Vet. Educ.* 31: 88–92.
25 Lecoq, L., Gains, M., Blond, L. et al. (2015). Brainstem auditory evoked responses in foals: reference values, effect of age, rate of acoustic stimulation, and neurologic deficits. *J. Vet. Intern. Med.* 29: 362–367.
26 Nixon, A.J. (2020). *Equine Fracture Repair*. Wiley.
27 Constable, P.D., Hinchcliff, K.W., Done, S.H. et al. (2016). *Veterinary Medicine-e-Book: A Textbook of the Diseases of Cattle, Horses, Sheep, Pigs and Goats*. Elsevier Health Sciences.
28 Johnson, A.L. (2010). How to perform a complete neurologic examination in the field and identify abnormalities. *AAEP Proceedings of the 56th Annual Convention of the American Association of Equine Practitioners*. Baltimore, Maryland, December 4–8, 2010. American Association of Equine Practitioners, 331–337.
29 Furr, M. and Reed, S. (2015). *Examination of the Nervous System. Equine Neurology*, 67–78. Ames, Iowa: Wiley Blakwell.
30 Avella, C. and Perkins, J. (2011). Computed tomography in the investigation of trauma to the ventral cranium. *Equine Vet. Educ.* 23: 333–338.
31 Sinha, A., Hendrickson, D., and Kannegieter, N. (1991). Head trauma in two horses. *Vet. Rec.* 128: 518–521.
32 Ramirez, O. III, Jorgensen, J.S., and Thrall, D.E. (1998). Imaging basilar skull fractures in the horse: a review. *Vet. Radiol. Ultrasound* 39: 391–395.
33 Scheffer, C.J., Blaauw, G., Dik, K.J. et al. (2001). Ataxia and pruritus in a pony due to a cervical vertebral fracture. *Tijdschrift voor diergeneeskunde* 126: 419–422.
34 Nixon, A. and Stashak, T. (1988). Laminectomy for relief of atlantoaxial subluxation in four horses. *J. Am. Vet. Med. Assoc.* 193: 677–682.
35 Owen, R. and Maxie, L. (1978). Repair of fractured dens of the axis in a foal. *J. Am. Vet. Med. Assoc.* 173: 854–856.
36 Jansson, N., Thoefner, M., and Bruun, H. (1998). Treatment of fractured odontoid process (dens of the axis) in a foal by coaptation casting: case report. *Dansk Veterinaertidsskrift (Denmark)* 81: 79–81.
37 Vos, N., Pollock, P., Harty, M. et al. (2008). Fractures of the cervical vertebral odontoid in four horses and one pony. *Vet. Rec.* 162: 116–119.
38 Butler, J.A., Colles, C.M., Dyson, S.J. et al. (2017). *Clinical Radiology of the Horse*. Wiley.
39 Maierl, J., Zechmeister, R., Schill, W. et al. (1998). Radiologic description of the growth plates of the atlas and axis in foals. *Tierarztliche Praxis Ausgabe G, Grosstiere/Nutztiere* 26: 341–345.
40 Hülsmeyer, V.-I., Flatz, K., Putschbach, K. et al. (2015). Traumatic odontoid process synchondrosis fracture with atlantoaxial instability in a calf: clinical presentation and imaging findings. *Irish Vet. J.* 68: 1–6.
41 Vos, N. (2008). Conservative treatment of a comminuted cervical fracture in a racehorse. *Irish Vet. J.* 61: 1–4.
42 McCoy, D., Shires, P., and Beadle, R. (1984). Ventral approach for stabilization of atlantoaxial subluxation

secondary to odontoid fracture in a foal. *J. Am. Vet. Med. Assoc.* 185: 545–549.

43 Barnes, H., Tucker, R., Grant, B. et al. (1995). Lag screw stabilization of a cervical vertebral fracture by use of computed tomography in a horse. *J. Am. Vet. Med. Assoc.* 206: 221–223.

44 Slone, D., Bergfeld, W., and Walker, T. (1979). Surgical decompression for traumatic atlantoaxial subluxation in a weanling filly. *J. Am. Vet. Med. Assoc.* 174: 1234–1236.

45 Smyth, G. (1992). Spinal cord decompression and stabilization of a comminuted axis fracture complicated by intraoperative malignant hyperthermia like reaction in a filly. *Aust. Equine Vet.* 10: 133–136.

46 Licka, T. (2002). Closed reduction of an atlanto-occipital and atlantoaxial dislocation in a foal. *Vet. Rec.* 151: 356.

47 Witte, S., Alexander, K., Bucellato, M. et al. (2005). Congenital atlantoaxial luxation associated with malformation of the dens axis in a Quarter Horse foal. *Equine Vet. Educ.* 17: 175–178.

48 Bordbari, M., Penedo, M., Aleman, M. et al. (2017). Deletion of 2.7 kb near HOXD 3 in an Arabian horse with occipitoatlantoaxial malformation. *Animal Genet.* 48: 287–294.

49 Vaughan, L and Mason B. (1975). A clinico-pathological study of racing accidents in horses. A report of a study on equine fatal accidents on racecourses financed by the Horserace Betting Levy Board.

50 Pinchbeck, G. and Murphy, D. (2001). Cervical vertebral fracture in three foals. *Equine Vet. Educ.* 13: 8–12.

51 Muno, J., Samii, V., Gallatin, L. et al. (2009). Cervical vertebral fracture in a Thoroughbred filly with minimal neurological dysfunction. *Equine Vet. Educ.* 21: 527–531.

52 Robertson, J.T. and Samii, V.F. (2012). Traumatic disorders of the spinal column. In: *Equine Surgery* (ed. J.A. Auer and A.A. Stick), 711–720. Elsevier.

53 Robinson, P. and Currall, J. (1981). Surgical repair of a cervical fracture/dislocation in a mature horse. *N. Z. Vet. J.* 29: 28–28.

54 Lopez, M.J., Nordberg, C., and Trostle, S. (1997). Fracture of the 7th cervical and 1st thoracic vertebrae presenting as radial nerve paralysis in a horse. *Can. Vet. J.* 38: 112.

55 Jeffcott, L. and Whitwell, K. (1977). Fractures of the thoracolumbar spine of the horse. *Proceedings Annual Convention of the American Association of Equine Practitioners*. December of 1976, Dallas, Texas, USA. American Association of Equine Practitioners.

56 Jeffcott, L. (1979). Radiographic features of the normal equine thoracolumbar spine. *Vet. Radiol.* 20: 140–147.

57 Chiapetta, J., Baker, J., and Feeney, D. (1985). Vertebral fracture, extensor hypertonia of thoracic limbs, and paralysis of pelvic limbs (Schiff–Sherrington syndrome) in an Arabian foal. *J. Am. Vet. Med. Assoc.* 186: 387–388.

58 Mason, B. (1971). A case of spinal cord compression causing paraplegia of a foal. *Equine Vet. J.* 3: 155–157.

59 Stewart, A., Salazar, P., Waldridge, B. et al. (2007). Computed tomographic diagnosis of a pathological fracture due to rhodococcal osteomyelitis and spinal abscess in a foal. *Equine Vet. Educ.* 19: 231–236.

60 Mackenzie, C., Haggett, E., Powell, S. et al. (2018). Traumatic sacral fracture following dystocia in a Thoroughbred foal. *Equine Vet. Educ.* 30: 518–521.

61 Jeffcott, L. and Rossdale, P. (1979). A radiographic study of the fetus in late pregnancy and during foaling. *J. Reprod. Fertil. Suppl.* 563–569.

Section VII Metabolic Causes of Neurologic Dysfunction

Emil Olsen

Multiple metabolic derangements can cause altered nervous system function in ill foals. Clinical signs associated with these metabolic derangements can be subtle (decreased mental awareness, generalized weakness, lethargy) to severe (ataxia, blindness, seizures). This section discusses various metabolic derangements that can impact nervous system function including hypoglycemia, hypo- and hypernatremia, osmotic demyelination syndrome, hypocalcemia, and hypomagnesemia.

Hypoglycemia

Hypoglycemia, defined as a blood glucose <80 mg/dl (<4.4 mmol/l), is very common in ill foals. In one study of 515 foals in a referral population, 34% were hypoglycemic; furthermore, strong evidence suggests that hypoglycemic foals have increased risk of bloodstream infection [1] with one study noting an adjusted odds ratio of 13.5 [2]. Moreover, decreased chance of survival was noted when severe hypoglycemia (blood glucose concentration <50 mg/dl [<2.8 mmol/l]) is measured at admission to an equine hospital [1]. Hypoglycemia can result from either decrease in glucose supply or increased glucose consumption. Decrease in glucose supply originates from a lack of nursing (e.g. due to limb deformity, systemic disease, separation from the mare), prematurity, metabolic disorders of glucose and lipids [3, 4], or hepatic dysfunction (portosystemic shunt). Increased use of glucose by the foal is most commonly associated with neonatal encephalopathy and sepsis where the systemic inflammatory response syndrome (SIRS) appears to reduce the availability of glucose systemically.

The brain utilizes glucose differently compared to other tissues where insulin is needed to facilitate glucose entrance into the cell. Glucose is the main energy substrate for the brain and crosses the blood-brain barrier (BBB) by passive diffusion from the blood and, as such, insulin is not needed [5]. Initially postpartum foals are dependent on existing circulating blood glucose and have a very low supply of glycogen in the liver, making foals entirely dependent on quickly getting up to nurse [6].

The brain's initial response to hypoglycemia is increased cerebral blood flow; however, this is unlikely to improve glucose availability without an increase in blood glucose concentration. As a result of persistent hypoglycemia, the brain reverts to altered amino acid metabolism for energy and production of the excitatory neurotransmitter glutamate. The effect of increased cerebral glutamate is activation of the N-methyl-D-aspartate (NMDA) receptors resulting in increased intracellular concentrations of sodium and calcium; this, in turn, alters the excitatory thresholds and cell membrane stability. Hypoglycemia also leads to depletion of adenosine triphosphate (ATP) and secondarily increases free radical damage to the mitochondria, which may result in apoptosis and necrosis. Hypoglycemia likely potentiates the effect of hypoxia with subsequent cytotoxic edema and neuronal apoptosis [5] and has been speculated to be involved in the pathogenesis of hypoxic ischemic encephalopathy in infants [7]. The state of persistent and/or profound hypoglycemia results in clinicals signs collectively termed *neuroglycopenia*, which is more common in foals compared to adult horses [8]. This term refers to altered neuronal function from persistent shortage of glucose (<70 mg/dl [<3.9 mmol/l]) in the brain, however clinical signs are more likely in foals with blood glucose concentrations <50 mg/dl (<2.8 mmol/l). Neurogenic symptoms result from the physiologic response to hypoglycemia by the autonomous nervous system. Common underlying causes of hypoglycemia in foals include sepsis, endotoxemia, neonatal encephalopathy, and SIRS with less common causes, including starvation and liver failure [8].

Equine Neonatal Medicine, First Edition. Edited by David M. Wong and Pamela A. Wilkins.

Clinical Signs

Clinical signs associated with hypoglycemia worsen based on the degree of hypoglycemia. Initial clinical signs in people with mild to moderate hypoglycemia (50–79 mg/dl [2.8–4.4 mmol/l]) include decreased cognition and cortical function which can manifest as disorientation, tremors, sweating, tachycardia and tachypnea. With moderate to severe altered mentation, clinical signs range from lethargy to coma with or without seizures [5, 9]. In foals, the most common clinical signs associated with neuroglycopenia are altered state of consciousness, disorientation, intermittent blindness and intermittent deafness [8]. A blood glucose cut-off for when foals and adult horses in a referral population displayed more severe mentation changes such as stupor and coma was <41 mg/dl (<2.3 mmol/l). The same study found an inverse relationship between high blood glucose concentrations and a decrease in risk of seizures [8].

Diagnosis

Diagnosis of hypoglycemia simply requires assessment of blood glucose concentration, preferably on-site via glucometer or serum biochemistry analysis. Blood glucose should be measured prior to administration of medication(s) for seizure control and if hypoglycemia is present, should be monitored every 2–4 hours. Magnetic resonance imaging is the diagnostic imaging modality of choice for foals with neurohypoglycemia and might show changes in the thalamus and basal ganglia with a high metabolic rate.

Treatment

Treatment of hypoglycemia involves administration of dextrose infusions; if the blood glucose is ≤50 mg/dl (≤2.8 mmol/l), a bolus of 2 ml/kg of 10% dextrose followed by a constant rate infusion (CRI) of 10% dextrose at maintenance- or correction rate (see Chapter 62 Fluid Therapy in the Neonatal Foal) is indicated. If seizures are associated with hypoglycemia, the primary disease process should be addressed, and dextrose supplementation administered. If the foal does not respond to glucose infusion within 5 minutes, therapy for seizures should be instituted, preferably with levetiracetam at a loading dose of 60 mg/kg followed by 32 mg/kg IV or PO q12h.

Prognosis

In a recent study looking at neuroglycopenia in foals, the mortality was 51% when generalized across foals and adults; the survival for horses with mild hypoglycemia (blood glucose <75 mg/dl [<4.2mmol/l]) was 34% and 58% for horses with severe hypoglycemia (blood glucose <50 mg/dl [<2.8mmol/l]) [8]. The prognosis in foals with hypoglycemia is usually associated with the primary disease process causing hypoglycemia. In one study, mild and severe hypoglycemia in neonatal foals on admission was associated with a poorer prognosis for survival to discharge [1], but this result was not repeated in a subsequent study [10].

Hyponatremia

Sodium (Na^+) is the main extracellular contributor to plasma osmolality, which in turn affects cell volume. At equilibrium, the extracellular and intracellular osmolality are equal with no net movement of water across cell membranes. Thus, changes in Na^+ concentration significantly contribute to intravascular (and intracellular) volume. Osmolality can be calculated (formula below) or measured whereas volume assessment is based on a less clear assessment of the clinical examination in combination with blood pressure, central venous pressure and urinalysis [38].

$$\text{Osmolality}_{\text{Europe}} = 2 \times \text{Serum Na}^+ + \text{Serum K}^+ + \text{Glucose} + \text{Urea}\ (\text{all in mmol / L})$$

$$\text{Osmolality}_{\text{North America}} = 2 \times \text{Serum Na}^+ + \text{Serum K}^+ + \text{BUN}/2.8 + \text{Glucose}/18\ (\text{Na}^+ \text{ and K}^+ \text{ in mEq/l, glucose and BUN in mg/dl})$$

Antidiuretic hormone (ADH) helps retain water in the kidneys and is secreted in the hypothalamus and transported to the neurohypophysis. Control of ADH release from the neurohypophysis is determined by osmoreceptors in the hypothalamus and baroreceptors in the vessel wall that sense changes in extracellular fluid osmolality. Thirst and ADH release are stimulated through small increases in osmolality (1%) and/or decrease in free water [38]. Short-term fluid regulation and hydration are a response to fluctuations in Na^+ and water balance. Longer-term fluid dynamics involve a complex interaction between ADH, aldosterone, the autonomic nervous system, other hormones and the kidneys. The kidneys regulate Na^+ reabsorption to maintain volume homeostasis as a response to decrease in intravascular volume, but the kidneys do not respond to the levels of Na^+ in the blood. Hypovolemia also leads to a response from the baroreceptors consequently releasing ADH and activation of the renin-angiotensin-aldosterone system (RAAS) and an increase in cardiac output, primarily by increasing heart rate and vasoconstriction. The RAAS helps maintain volume and blood pressure as well as electrolyte reabsorption in the kidneys. Serum tonicity is the concentration of particles and is often used for practical understanding of fluid dynamics [38].

In disease states where ill foals experience hyponatremia, the concomitant hypoosmolality promotes water to move from the extracellular space into the intracellular component, ultimately resulting in cell swelling. *In vitro* studies have demonstrated up to a doubling of intracellular fluid volume of cerebellar neurons in cell culture with rapid changes in tonicity [39]. Because the brain is constrained within the rigid skull, cell swelling can cause compression of the brain parenchyma. Conversely, hypernatremia results in hypertonicity, water movement out of the cell and cell shrinkage. The CNS is very sensitive to even minor changes in tonicity which can lead to notable clinical signs. The most dramatic effects of hyponatremia on the brain occur when there is a very rapid decrease in serum Na^+, as there is little time to allow for adaptation (Figure 32.VII.1). Of note, the clinical distinction between acute and chronic hyponatremia is a bit arbitrary hours duration, as it is believed that this is the time frame, after which complete mechanisms of brain adaption are in place, thereby making correction of hyponatremia potentially more harmful for the brain [14]. Interestingly, studies have demonstrated that brain water content does not increase as predicted after either chronic or acute hyponatremia. For example, after 6 hours of hyponatremia in an experimental model in rats, the brain water increased 40% of what was predicted and after 4 days of hyponatremia, there was only a 0.6% increase in brain water content [15]. This suggests that the brain can adapt to hypoosmolality using several mechanisms to counteract the negative effect of extracellular hypotonicity on cell volume. These counteractive mechanisms are collectively called regulatory volume decrease (RVD) as the aim is to restore the initial volume after swelling induced by hypotonicity [14].

The understanding of the RVD mechanism is incomplete but a variety of cells inside the BBB have osmoreceptors that activate intracellular bidirectional volume sensitive channels that may be activated during hypo- and hyper-tonicity. These volume sensitive channels have been identified throughout neurons inside the BBB and can utilize organic osmolytes such as ɣ-aminobutyric acid, taurine, glutamine, myoinositol, and betaine to regulate the impact of intracellular changes in tonicity [14]. In an experimental dilutional model in rats with intraperitoneal free water injection under general anesthesia, brain edema occurred with a maximum water increase between 6% and 9% after 3 hours [15, 16]. After 4 days of experimentally induced hyponatremia, the adaptation improved to a net water increase of the brain by 0.6% [12]. Further time allows the brain to normalize by reducing the intracellular osmolytes towards 0% net water increase and thus no edema after 14–28 days of hypoosmolality [14, 16, 17]. Hyponatremic encephalopathy is thus more likely to occur with acute changes in Na^+ and rapid correction in serum Na^+ greater than 1mEq/l/h [18].

Both early and late mechanisms of brain adaptation to hyponatremia exists. One of the first mechanisms against hypotonicity is water flow from the brain parenchyma into the cerebrospinal fluid, and later into the systemic circulation. Within minutes of hyponatremia, increased pressure inside the brain drives hydrostatic water movement into the CSF and then into the systemic circulation, thus helping guard against development of rapid brain edema. Another early mechanism of adaptation is movement of electrolytes from the intracellular to extracellular compartment. Within hours of hyponatremia, a significant decrease in intracellular Na^+, Cl^-, and K^+ occurs [14]. If hyponatremia persist (chronic situation), other osmotically active substances, termed organic osmolytes, balance brain water changes. This adaptation mechanisms were exemplified in a rat study in which, after 4 days of hyponatremia, the brain electrolyte concentration was reduced by 33%, 11%, and 17% for intracellular Cl^-, Na^+, and K^+, respectively, but the brain water content only increased by 0.6% [17]. Thus, the loss of electrolytes in chronic hyponatremia does not account for the magnitude of brain water changes suggesting that other osmotically active substances (organic osmolytes) help balance the osmolality and thereby minimize brain water changes [14].

Hyponatremia is one of the most common electrolyte abnormalities in foals and can be classified as mild (125–130 mEq/l), moderate (<125 but >122 mEq/l) or severe (<122 mEq/l), requiring attention and correction when present [13 and 19]. Hyponatremia is commonly split into a hyper-osmolar hyponatremia, hypo-osmolar hyponatremia and normo-osmolar pseudohyponatremia [38]. Further to this, a cerebral/renal salt wasting syndrome can also be responsible for a hyponatremic state. The most common type of hyponatremia in foals is *hypo-osmolar hypovolemic hyponatremia,* often caused by extrarenal losses of salt noted in cases of colitis, large volume gastric reflux, hemorrhage, peritonitis, urinary tract obstruction, and uroperitoneum [19]. Renal salt wasting may give a similar syndrome due to a nephropathy or diuretic excess. *Euvolemic hypo-osmolar hyponatremia* is less common in foals and is caused by hypothyroidism or the syndrome of inappropriate antidiuretic hormone secretion (SIADH) that may follow meningoencephalomyelitis or encephalopathy. *Hypervolemic hypo-osmolar hyponatremia* is caused by acute and chronic kidney disease as well as heart failure [38].

Hypertriglyceridemia, hypercholesterolemia, and hyperproteinemia result in a reduction in plasma water and a lower measurement of Na^+ in a so-called pseudohyponatremia or *isotonic hyponatremia*. Finally, *iatrogenic hyponatremia* is less common in foals but possible with inappropriate use of hypotonic fluids such as 5% dextrose. The most common causes of hyponatremia in foals include colitis, renal disease, uroperitoneum, pneumonia, and SIRS [19]. Less common causes include neonatal encephalopathy, congenital coagulopathy, neonatal isoerythrolysis, rhabdomyolysis, head trauma, meningoencephalomyelitis, and cerebral salt-wasting [19–21].

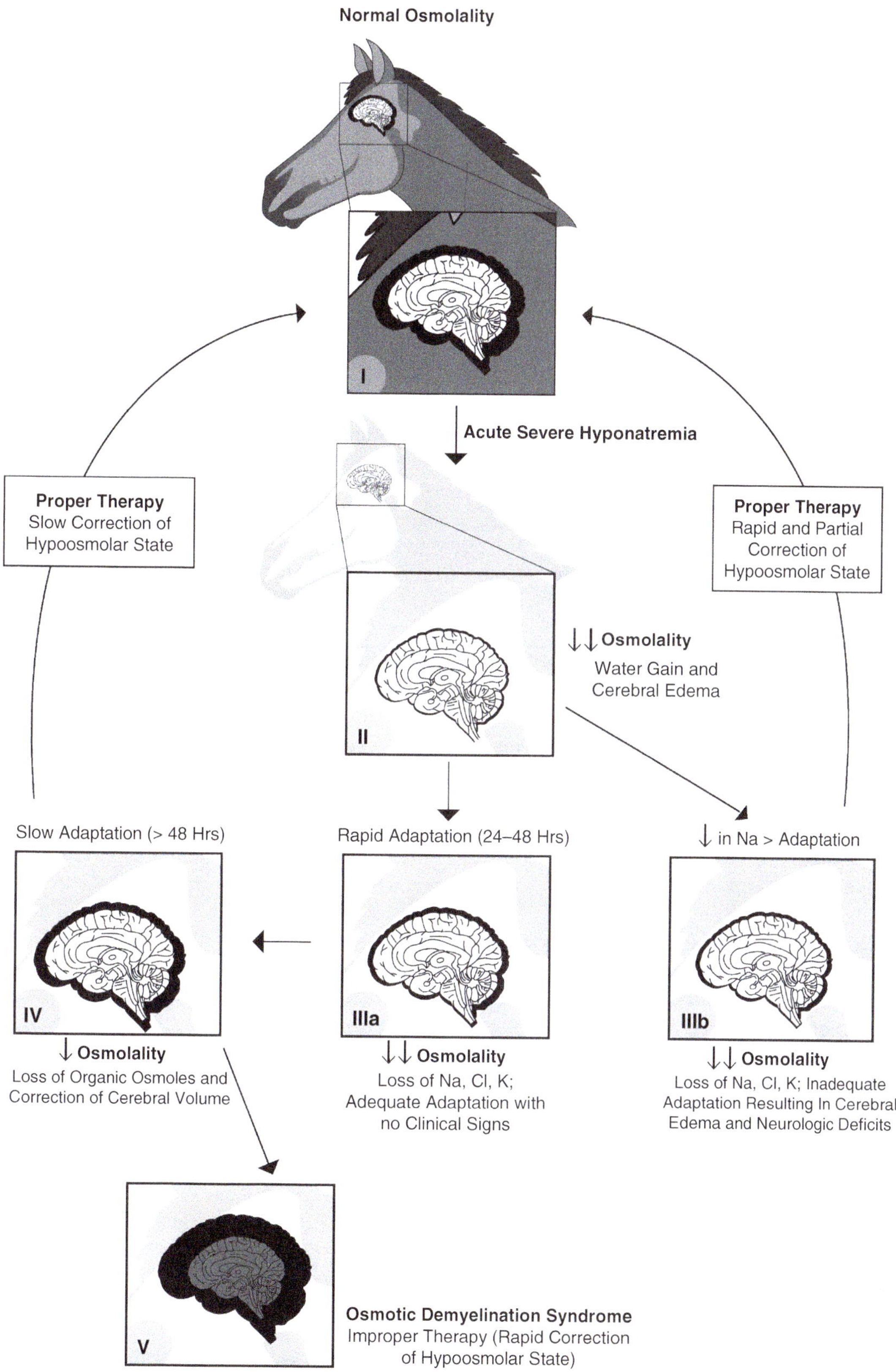

Figure 32.VII.1 Effects of hyponatremia on the brain, water balance and adaptive responses. (I) In health, the body maintains normal osmolality and tightly regulates cell volume. (II) Shortly after an acute decrease in serum osmolality (i.e. hyponatremia), intracellular water accumulates leading to cerebral edema and decreased osmolality in the brain. (IIIa) Rapid adaptation occurs within hours by loss of cellular electrolytes resulting in reduction of cerebral edema with no neurologic deficits. (IIIb) If decrease in cellular osmolality exceeds body's adaptive response to rapid loss or electrolytes, cerebral edema persists resulting in acute neurologic deficits. Proper therapy with rapid administration of sodium increases serum osmolality to subnormal level resulting in decreased cerebral edema and elimination or reduction in neurologic deficits. (IV) Slow (>48 hours) loss of organic osmoles further compensates for hypo-osmotic state. Low cellular osmolality persists despite normalization of brain volume. Proper therapy with slow correction of sodium results in a gradual return to normal osmolality. (V) Improper therapy associated with rapid sodium supplementation in chronic hyponatremia results in rapid cell dehydration and potential to develop osmotic demyelination syndrome [13].

The clinical signs of hyponatremic encephalopathy are associated with brain edema and in severe acute cases, herniation through foramen magnum, seizures, coma and death [14]. In people, the signs can be divided into early, advanced, and far advanced with early clinical signs including headache, muscular cramps, and weakness. Advanced clinical signs in people include lethargy, restlessness, disorientation, depressed reflexes, and seizures progressing to far advanced signs such as coma and respiratory arrest [22]. In foals, common clinical signs of hyponatremia include altered mentation and seizures (generalized or focal), with less common signs such as head pressing, ataxia, apparent blindness, and hyperesthesia also reported [13, 19]. The presence and severity of neurologic signs in foals are significantly associated with sodium concentrations [14] and likely the duration of hyponatremia. Diagnosis of hyponatremia is straightforward via assessment of serum electrolytes; other diagnostic tests such as a CBC, serum biochemistry analysis, blood gas analysis, and diagnostic imaging may be necessary to evaluate the primary cause of hyponatremia.

As the brain reaches relative homeostasis regarding the hypo-osmolar state, the clinician must be cognizant of the fact that rapid increases in osmolarity can significantly impact cellular fluid balance. If Na^+ correction occurs too rapidly, water can move out of the cells and into the extracellular fluid resulting in cell dehydration [13]. Therefore, treatment of hyponatremia involves addressing the primary disease process and deciphering whether the hyponatremia is acute or chronic. As noted above, the discrimination between acute and chronic hyponatremia is arbitrarily set at 24–48 hours due to the osmolar adaptation of the brain via the regulatory volume decrease mechanism. If acute hyponatremia has occurred, rapid correction will likely have minimal consequences; however, most patients rarely have clear evidence of acute hyponatremia, and as such, it is safer to assume a chronic situation. Patients with chronic Na^+ deficiencies may be more predisposed to osmotic injury after rapid Na^+ supplementation as cells in these patients have had a longer time to adapt to the hypo-osmolar condition with adequate time for organic osmoles to be removed from the cells [13]. However, complications of Na^+ correction, such as osmotic demyelination syndrome, are relatively rare in adults and even more rare in neonates. For example, in a retrospective study of 1490 people presenting to a hospital with a Na^+ <120 mEq/l, 0.5% ($n = 8$) of patients had evidence of osmotic demyelination on MRI, and of these, 7 (88%) had a documented Na^+ correction >8 mEq/l during any 24-hour period prior to MRI [23]. In the same study, 41% (606) of patients with severe hyponatremia had rapid correction of Na^+ (defined as >8 mEq/l) over a 24-hour period; of these patients with rapid correction, 1.3% (8 of 606) developed osmotic demyelination [23]. This may explain the lack of reports of osmotic demyelination syndrome in veterinary medicine although three case reports exist in dogs [24, 25]. The regulatory volume decrease mechanism is likely the cause of slow adaptation to correction of Na^+ levels in chronic hyponatremia and therefore, an increase in serum Na^+ concentrations at a rate of 8–10 mEq/l per 24 hours is recommended as this will significantly reduce the intracranial pressure and thus relieve clinical signs.

The clinician must balance Na^+ administration to avoid both over- and under-correction. If the Na^+ concentration is corrected too rapidly, a study in rats with hyponatremia noted that reinduction of hyponatremia with hypotonic fluids (e.g. 5% dextrose in water) reduced the risk of mortality and demyelination [26]. Conversely, under correction of Na^+ concentration was associated with longer ICU hospital stay in another study [27]. In human medicine, desmopressin (synthetic vasopressin analogue) has recently gained popularity to reduce the risk of overcorrection of Na^+. In a recent study, the mortality was lower when desmopressin was used [28]. The Adrogué-Madias formula [12] is commonly used to predict changes in serum Na^+ with administration of hypertonic saline solutions (Table 32.VII.1).

For practical use, a spreadsheet with the Na^+ concentration of available fluids (e.g. 5% dextrose, 0.45% NaCl, 3% NaCl, 7.2% NaCl, Ringer's acetate, Lactated Ringer's, etc.) is used to choose the maintenance fluid; ideally this fluid has a Na^+ concentration closest to and slightly above the patients serum Na^+; attach one or two additional constant rate infusions (CRIs) containing hypertonic NaCl; 7.2% NaCl is more readily available, but 3% NaCl is preferred. Although formulas help guide corrective therapy, they are only

Table 32.VII.1 Formulas for estimating sodium correction in hyponatremic patient.

- Effect of 1 liter of infusate on serum Na^+ = (Infusate Na^+ – serum Na^+)/total body water + 1 [12]. (Total body water in healthy neonatal foal = 0.74 l/kg) [29].
- Formula tends to underestimate correction because it does not account for K^+, ingestion of hypotonic fluids (water, milk), nor loss of Na^+ in the urine.
- Example: 50 kg foal with serum Na^+ of 115 mEq/l, administered 1 liter of Normosol (Na^+ content = 140 mEq/l); Effect of 1 liter of Normasol on foal's serum Na^+ = (140 mEq/l – 115 mEq/L)/(0.74 l/kg × 50 kg) + 1; = 25/37 + 1 = 0.66 increase in serum Na^+.

- Total amount of Na^+ needed to correct foal's serum Na^+ to 125 mEq/l (approximate concentration not associated with neurologic deficits) [13].
- Na^+ required (mEq/l) = 125 – measured Na^+ [mEq/l] × 0.74 × Body weight (kg) [13].
- Example: 50 kg foal with serum Na+ of 115 mEq/l: Na^+ required (mEq/l) = 125 – 115 mEq/l × 0.74 × 50 kg = approximately 370 mEq of Na^+ needed to correct Na^+ deficit to 125 mEq/l.

estimates that need to be compared to measured serum Na^+ concentrations; thus, the estimated correction is compared with the actual serum Na+ concentrations every 2–4 hours and CRIs are adjusted individually so that custom mixed maintenance fluids are avoided every time a change in correction rate is needed. Of note, many hyponatremic foals with enterocolitis also have metabolic acidemia and some clinicians administered sodium bicarbonate as a treatment for acidemia; the clinician should account for the sodium present in sodium bicarbonate solutions (1 mEq Na^+/ml of 8.4% solution; 0.6 mEq Na^+/ml in 5% solution; 0.156 mEq Na^+/ml in 1.3% solution).

As described above, if the correction of hyponatremia is too rapid, it may lead to demyelination of cells in the central nervous system, specifically in the area of the pons but also other areas of the brain. This phenomenon, termed *osmotic demyelination syndrome,* was previously known as pontine and extrapontine myelinolysis. Risk factors for developing osmotic demyelination syndrome in people are chronic severe hyponatremia and correction of Na^+ >8 mEq/l per 24 hours. Demyelination is preceded by protein aggregation in astrocytes and endoplasmic reticulum that leads to astrocyte death and subsequent decrease in nutritional support of oligodendrocytes responsible for myelin maintenance and subsequent demyelination [14]. In a canine model of hyponatremia, MRI of the brain in seven dogs revealed early changes were visible 2–3 days after rapid correction only on diffusion weighted imaging, prior to changes on other sequences such as gadolinium (contrast) enhancement, flair sequences and T_2 weighted sequences. The dogs rarely showed changes in the pons but more commonly in the thalamus, caudate nucleus and midbrain; affected areas varied between dogs [30]. MRI of the brain is standard practice in human medicine and may aid in early diagnosis of osmotic demyelination syndrome and possibly reversal of too rapid correction of hyponatremia.

The prognosis for foals with neurologic signs associated with hyponatremia is good, ranging from 67% to 76% in published reports [19, 20], but the underlying cause must be accounted for and treated and careful correction with frequent monitoring is warranted.

Hypernatremia

Hypernatremia in the neonatal foal is defined as a serum Na^+ >140 mEq/l [11] as compared to foals older than 7 days in which hypernatremia is defined as a serum Na^+ concentration >154 mEq/l. Hypernatremia in the foal is less commonly encountered as compared to hyponatremia but can occur with free water loss, overadministration of sodium containing fluids (iatrogenic), inappropriate mixing of milk replacer, or lack of access to free water in foals being fed milk replacer. Diseases processes that are associated with hypernatremia include neonatal encephalopathy, enterocolitis, and uncommonly, atresia coli, renal disease, excessive sodium ingestion, diabetes insipidus, the absence of a corpus callosum, and ependymoma of the hypophysis [11]. Iatrogenic hypernatremia is the most common cause of hypernatremia in foals because of a poor tolerance of isotonic fluids associated with a higher level of aldosterone in sick neonatal foals compared to adult horses [31, 32]. In a study using an isotonic electrolyte solution with 140 mEq/l of Na^+ administered at rate of 3.3 ml/kg/h, 4-day-old foals, but not adult mares, became hypernatremic [32]. To avoid hypernatremia in foals, a safe choice for maintenance IV fluids are solutions isotonic to somewhat hypotonic compared to the foal's serum Na^+ such as Lactated Ringer's (Na^+ concentration 130 mEq/l) or half strength saline 0.45% (Na^+ concentration 77 mEq/l). For field resuscitation in foals with moderate to severe dehydration, Lactated Ringer's solution is an appropriate fluid choice; if absolutely necessary, isotonic NaCl can be used when followed by fluids with a lower Na^+ content.

Diagnosis

Diagnosis of hypernatremia is established via measurement of serum Na^+ concentration in combination with assessment of dehydration level, but other diagnostics may be necessary to evaluate the primary disease as mentioned above. Treatment of hypernatremia involves addressing the primary disease, along with decreasing the serum Na^+ concentration at a maximum of 0.5 mEq/l of Na^+ per hour [11]. A human study of critically ill patients [33] did not demonstrate any adverse effects of rapid correction of Na^+ and indeed none have been described in veterinary medicine. Correction of hypernatremia can be guided by calculating the expected change per hour with the same formula described under hyponatremia (Table 32.VII.2) [12].

Monitoring of electrolytes every 2–4 hours during correction is essential to be able to change the rate of correction dynamically with enteral fluid intake and renal reabsorption affecting serum Na^+ concentration. A targeted decrease in serum Na^+ of 0.5 mEq/l/h allows brain adaption via the

Table 32.VII.2 Formula for estimating sodium correction in hypernatremic patient.

- Effect of 1 liter of any infusate on patient serum Na^+ = (infusate Na^+ – serum Na^+)/total body water + 1. (Total body water in the healthy neonatal foals = 0.74 l/kg) [30].
- Example: 50 kg foal with a serum Na^+ = 175 mEq/l, administered 1 liter of Plasma-Lyte (Na^+ content = 140 mEq/l): Effect of 1 liter of Plasma-Lyte on foal's serum Na^+ = (140 mEq/l – 175 mEq/l)/ (0.74 l/kg × 50 kg) + 1 = –35/37+1 = 0.9 mEq/l (0.9 mEq/l decrease in serum Na^+).

regulatory volume decrease mechanism [14] described under hyponatremia. For correction of hypernatremia, using a fluid with a Na^+ concentration slightly below the foals initial Na^+ or at the end target and a combination of multiple CRIs of 5% dextrose (markedly hypotonic) and a hypertonic solution such as 3% NaCl to help bridge the gap for too rapid correction. Overzealous rapid correction of hypernatremia has less of an adverse effect compared to overzealous correction of hyponatremia; this fact makes a convincing case for the use of half strength saline or even 5% dextrose to address the free water deficit. In particular, in foals with severely hypernatremia (Na^+ >170 mEq/l), the author recommends careful correction, targeting a lower rate of Na^+ decrease to a maximum of 0.5 mEq/l/h for safety.

Prognosis

66% of foals with hypernatremia survived to discharge; of these 81% were able to be registered for a race of which 62% raced. Foals with hypernatremia have increased mortality (OR 2.3) compared to foals with a normal Na^+ concentration [11].

Hypomagnesemia

Magnesium is essential microelement required for cellular energy-dependent reactions involving ATP (ion pump function, glycolysis, oxidative phosphorylation, protein synthesis) and plays an important role in regulation of calcium channel function and neurotransmitter release. Because of the vital role magnesium plays, its intracellular and extracellular concentrations are maintained within narrow limits. A number of diseases are associated with hypomagnesemia of varying severity and include enterocolitis, renal disease, sepsis, or SIRS. Decreased magnesium may increase the threshold in neurons leading to seizures [34] and result in tetany through delayed degradation of acetylcholinesterase and increased acetylcholine release from the neuromuscular junction [35]. Hypomagnesemia has been theorized to play a role in the pathogenesis or be a result of hypoxic ischemic encephalopathy in human neonates and foals. Indeed, magnesium has been suggested as a treatment for foals with neonatal encepahalopathy [36]. Clinical signs of hypomagnesemia are rare and primarily described in the adult horse where it includes weakness, muscle fasciculations, ventricular arrhythmias, seizures, ataxia, and coma [35]. Subclinical hypomagnesemia also increases the severity of SIRS, worsens the response to endotoxins, and can result in ileus, cardiac arrhythmias, refractory hypokalemia, and hypocalcemia [35]. Magnesium can be estimated via total magnesium (if there are no acid-base disturbances), but ionized magnesium can be measured by certain instruments not widely available in equine medicine. In one study, critically ill foals had a higher plasma magnesium compared to nonsurviving foals [37]. Treatment of foals with hypomagnesemia is recommended using a magnesium sulfate ($MgSO_4$) bolus of 8–32 mg/kg, IV over 10 minutes, or 50 mg/kg/hour for 1 hour followed by a CRI of 25 mg/kg/h [35].

Hypocalcemia

Calcium facilitates muscle contraction via actin-myosin activation in striated muscle and phosphorylation of myosin in smooth muscle. Hypocalcemia is defined as an ionized calcium <1.5 mmol/l with mechanisms leading to hypocalcemia related to dysfunction of the parathyroid gland, systemic illness, gastrointestinal disease, and tissue sequestration. Common causes of hypocalcemia in the neonatal foal include sepsis and SIRS, with less common causes including hypoparathyroidism, increased phosphate load, vitamin D deficiency, renal failure, hypomagnesemia, rhabdomyolysis, malignant hyperthermia, and heat stroke.

Clinical signs of hypocalcemia include ileus, tremors, muscle fasciculations, tetraparesis, seizures, and cardiac arrest [40]. Diagnosis requires measurement of serum total and ionized calcium concentrations, but clinicians should consider measurement of other serum analytes (magnesium, creatine kinase, aspartate, aminotransferase) and parathyroid hormone in cases that are either refractory to treatment or reoccur with discontinuation of calcium supplementation. Treatment of hypocalcemia involves addressing the primary disease process and correcting the calcium deficit based on concentration of ionized calcium (measured every 6–12 hours). Forms of parenterally administered calcium include calcium gluconate 23% (0.2–1 ml/kg over 2–3 hours) or calcium borogluconate 40% (0.1–0.5 ml/kg over 2–4 hours). Hyperparathyroidism causing hypocalcemia but not sepsis decreased survival in neonatal foals with hypocalcemia [41].

References

1 Hollis, A.R., Furr, M.O., and Magdesian, K.G. (2008). Blood glucose concentrations in critically ill neonatal foals. *Journal of veterinary [Internet].* https://onlinelibrary.wiley.com/doi/abs/10.1111/j.1939-1676.2008.0174.x.

2 Furr, M. and McKenzie, H. 3rd. (2020 Nov). Factors associated with the risk of positive blood culture in neonatal foals presented to a referral center (2000–2014). *J Vet Intern Med* 34: 2738–2750.

3 Valberg, S.J., Ward, T.L., Rush, B. et al. (2001). Glycogen branching enzyme deficiency in quarter horse foals. *J Vet Intern Med.* 15: 572–580.

4 Pinn, T.L., Divers, T.J., and Southard, T. (2018). Persistent hypoglycemia associated with lipid storage myopathy in a paint foal. *J Vet Intern Med* 32: 1442–1446.

5 Amendoeira, S., McNair, C., Saini, J. et al. (2020). Glucose homeostasis and the neonatal brain: A sweet relationship. *Neonatal Netw* 39: 137–146.

6 Barsnick, R.J. and Toribio, R.E. (2011). Endocrinology of the equine neonate energy metabolism in health and critical illness. *Vet Clin North Am Equine Pract* 27: 49–58.

7 Basu, S.K., Ottolini, K., Govindan, V. et al. (2018). Early glycemic profile is associated with brain injury patterns on magnetic resonance imaging in hypoxic ischemic encephalopathy. *J Pediat.* 203: 137–143.

8 Aleman, M., Costa, L.R.R., Crowe, C. et al. (2018). Presumed neuroglycopenia caused by severe hypoglycemia in horses. *J Vet Intern Med.* 32: 1731–1739.

9 Alsaleem, M., Lina, S., and Deepak, K. (2019). "Neonatal Hypoglycemia: A Review." *Clinical Pediatrics.* https://.doi: 10.1177/0009922819875540.

10 Armengou, L., Jose-Cunilleras, E., Ríos, J. et al. (2013). Metabolic and endocrine profiles in sick neonatal foals are related to survival. *J Vet Intern Med* 27: 567–575.

11 Collins, N.M., Carrick, J.B., Russell, C.M. et al. (2018). Hypernatraemia in 39 hospitalised foals: clinical findings, primary diagnosis and outcome. *Aust Vet J* 96: 385–389.

12 Adrogué, H.J. and Madias, N.E. (2000). Hypernatremia. *N Engl J Med* 342: 1493–1499.

13 Wong, D.M., Sponseller, B.T., Brockus, C. et al. (2007). Neurologic deficits associated with severe hyponatremia in 2 foals. *J Vet Emerg Crit Care* 17: 275–285.

14 Gankam Kengne, F. and Decaux, G. (2018). Hyponatremia and the Brain. *Kidney Int Rep* 3: 24–35.

15 Melton, J., Patlak, C., Pettigrew, K. et al. (1987). Volume regulatory loss of Na, Cl, and K from rat brain during acute hyponatremia. *Am J Physiol Renal Physiol* 252: F661–F669.

16 Verbalis, J.G. (2010). Brain volume regulation in response to changes in osmolality. *Neuroscience.* 168: 862–870.

17 Verbalis, J.G. and Drutarosky, M.D. (1988). Adaptation to chronic hypoosmolality in rats. *Kidney Int* 34: 351–360.

18 Sterns, R.H. (2018). Treatment of Severe Hyponatremia. *Clin J Am Soc Nephrol* 13: 641–649. https://doi.org/10.2215/CJN.10440917.

19 Dunkel, B., Dodson, F., Chang, Y.M. et al. (2020). Retrospective evaluation of the association between hyponatremia and neurologic dysfunction in hospitalized foals (2012–2016):109 cases. *J Vet Emerg Crit Care* 30: 66–73.

20 Collins, N.M., Axon, J.E., Carrick, J.B. et al. (2016). Severe hyponatremia in foals: clinical findings, primary diagnosis and outcome. *Aust Vet J* 94: 186–191.

21 Perkins, G., Valberg, S.J., Madigan, J.M. et al. (1998). Electrolyte disturbances in foals with severe rhabdomyolysis. *J Vet Intern Med* 12: 173–177.

22 Giuliani, C. and Peri, A. (2014). Effects of hyponatremia on the brain. *J Clin Med Res* 28: 1163–1177.

23 George, J.C., Zafar, W., Bucaloiu, I.D. et al. (2018). Risk factors and outcomes of rapid correction of severe hyponatremia. *Clin J Am Soc Nephrol* 6: 984–992.

24 Churcher, R.K., Watson, A.D., and Eaton, A. (1999). Suspected myelinolysis following rapid correction of hyponatremia in a dog. *J Am Anim Hosp Assoc* 35: 493–497.

25 O'Brien, D.P., Kroll, R.A., Johnson, G.C. et al. (1994). Myelinolysis after correction of hyponatremia in two dogs. *J Vet Intern Med* 8: 40–48.

26 Gankam Kengne, F., Soupart, A., Pochet, R. et al. (2009). Re-induction of hyponatremia after rapid overcorrection of hyponatremia reduces mortality in rats. *Kidney Int* 76: 614–621.

27 Pillai, K.S., Trivedi, T.H., and Moulick, N.D. (2018). Hyponatremia in ICU. *J Assoc Physicians India* 66: 48–52.

28 MacMillan, T.E. and Cavalcanti, R.B. (2018). Outcomes in severe hyponatremia treated with and without desmopressin. *Am J Med* 131: 317.e1–317.e10.

29 Fielding, C.L., Magdesian, K.G., and Edman, J.E. (2011). Determination of body water compoartments in neonatal foals by use of indicator dilution techniques and multifrequency bioelectrical impedance analtysis. *Am J Ve Res* 72: 1390–1396.

30 Laureno, R., Lamotte, G., and Mark, A.S. (2018). Sequential MRI in pontine and extrapontine myelinolysis following rapid correction of hyponatremia. *BMC Res Notes* 5: 707.

31 Hollis, A.R., Boston, R.C., and Corley, K.T.T. (2008). Plasma aldosterone, vasopressin and atrial natriuretic peptide in hypovolaemia: a preliminary comparative study of neonatal and mature horses. *Equine Vet J.* 40: 64–69.

32 Buchanan, B.R., Sommardahl, C.S., Rohrbach, B.W. et al. (2005). Effect of a 24-hour infusion of an isotonic electrolyte replacement fluid on the renal clearance of electrolytes in healthy neonatal foals. *J Am Vet Med Assoc.* 227: 1123–1129.

33 Chauhan, K., Pattharanitima, P., Patel, N. et al. (2019). Rate of correction of hypernatremia and health outcomes in critically ill patients. *Clin J Am Soc Nephrol.* 14: 656–663.

34 Chen, B.B., Prasad, C., Kobrzynski, M. et al. (2016). Seizures related to hypomagnesemia: A case series and review of the literature. *Child Neurol Open.* 3: 2329048X16674834.

35 Stewart, A.J. (2011). Magnesium disorders in horses. *Vet Clin North Am Equine Pract.* 27: 149–163.

36 Wilkins, P.A. (2001). Magnesium infusion in hypoxic ischaemic encephalopathy. *Proceedings of the Annual Veterinary Medical Forum, American College of Veterinary Internal Medicine*. 242–244.

37 Mariella, J., Isani, G., Andreani, G. et al. (2016). Total plasma magnesium in healthy and critically ill foals. *Theriogenology.* 85: 180–185.

38 Zieg, J. (2017). Pathophysiology of Hyponatremia in Children. *Front Pediatr*. Oct 16;5:213. doi: 10.3389/fped.2017.00213. PMID: 29085814; PMCID: PMC5650627.

39 Pasantes-Morales, H., Maar, T.E., Morán, J. (1993). Cell volume regulation in cultured cerebellar granule neurons. *J Neurosci Res*. Feb 1;34(2):219–24. doi: 10.1002/jnr.490340209. PMID: 8450565.

40 Toribio, R.E. (2011). Disorders of calcium and phosphate metabolism in horses. *Vet Clin North Am Equine Pract.* Apr;27(1):129–47. doi: 10.1016/j.cveq.2010.12.010. PMID: 21392658

41 Hurcombe, S.D., Toribio R.E., Slovis N.M., Saville W.J., Mudge, M.C., Macgillivray, K., Frazer, M.L. (2009). Calcium regulating hormones and serum calcium and magnesium concentrations in septic and critically ill foals and their association with survival. *J Vet Intern Med*. Mar-Apr;23(2):335–43. doi: 10.1111/j.1939-1676.2009.0275.x. Epub 2009 Feb 4. PMID: 19210311.

Section VIII Idiopathic – Neonatal Encephalopathy

Jenifer Gold and David Wong

Neonatal encephalopathy (NE) is one of the most common neurologic diseases affecting neonatal foals with a reported incidence of 1–2% of all equine births [1]. This disease has been documented in foals for over 90 years and has since acquired a variety of alternative names to describe this multi-systemic, noninfectious process. Descriptive names such as barker, wanderer, or dummy foal have been used, as well as hypoxic–ischemic encephalopathy (HIE), neonatal maladjustment syndrome (NMS), and perinatal asphyxia syndrome (PAS). The later names are more encompassing of a syndrome that has varying degrees of multi-systemic effects, as compared to solely neurologic disease. Reynolds first described NE in Thoroughbred foals in 1930 [2]. Since that time, multiple reports and reviews have been written [3–21] with Rossdale describing this syndrome as NMS (1968) with specific reference to behavioral dysfunction and disruption of normal adaptive responses needed for survival [12–16, 18]. Rossdale also suggested a classification of disorders of neonatal foals into various groups [14, 16, 18].

Out of these groups, one group included foals with abnormal behavior with a noninfectious cause [16]. These foals were further broken down into two categories based on gestation, foaling history, and time frame of when clinical signs developed. Category 1 foals were classified as having a normal gestation, parturition, and post-foaling behavior with clinical signs developing within 6–24 hours post-parturition; these foals maintained a good prognosis [19, 21]. Category 2 foals were those born to mares with placental disease but were subject to normal gestation and parturition; abnormal behavior was noted at birth and often accompanied by sepsis; these foals had a poor prognosis [19, 21]. Rossdale suggested that NMS was a disorder of the nervous and cardiovascular system around parturition [16]. This opinion remains relevant based on current theories and neonatal brain function. With the knowledge that foals with NE experience varying degrees of multisystemic effects due to a variety of potential underlying etiologies, NMS or NE have become preferred terms.

Mechanisms of Neonatal Encephalopathy in Foals

The exact pathophysiologic process(es) associated with NE in the foal are unknown, with most theories based on studies in other species. However, underlying clinical scenarios associated with NE in the foal can be broadly divided into potential events during the pre-, peri- and/or postpartum period (Table 32.VIII.1) [22].

As noted, some foals with NE do not have a history of peri-partum compromise, but other scenarios could contribute to the pathophysiologic processes involved in NE and can be divided into two different overarching mechanisms. The first mechanistic pathway involves hypoxic–ischemic (HI) damage, resulting from deprivation of energy substrates and subsequent reperfusion injury, hemorrhage, edema, and inflammation [22]. Foals with NE that are known to have adverse peripartum HI events likely follow the pathogenesis of other species with HI damage. This type of injury not only impacts the central nervous system (CNS), but can involve other organs with high metabolic and oxygen demands such as the gastrointestinal, renal, and cardiovascular systems. The second mechanistic pathway does not involve HI damage, but rather, is due to endocrine or neurotransmitter dysregulation [22]. Endocrine pathways potentially associated with NE include imbalances between systemic and neuroactive steroids and delayed decreases in endogenous progestogens in the postpartum period [23, 24]. Either of these possibilities could be associated with hypothalamic–pituitary–adrenal dysfunction. Another theory involved in the pathogenesis is

Equine Neonatal Medicine, First Edition. Edited by David M. Wong and Pamela A. Wilkins.

Table 32.VIII.1 Potential underlying scenarios that can contribute to development of NE.

Clinical scenario	Prepartum	Peripartum	Postpartum
Hypoxic–Ischemic Event	Systemic illness of dam	Dystocia cesarean section	Umbilical tear or hemorrhage Umbilical compression Neonatal isoerythrolysis
Placental disease	Placentitis Premature placental separation	Premature placental separation	
Healthy mare	Normal gestation	Normal parturition	Abnormal concentrations of neurosteroids

modifications in neurotransmitters, opioids, and cannabinoids, although scientific evidence is lacking [22]. Because so little research has been conducted in foals with NE, the true pathophysiologic processes are unknown, and may involve a combination of mechanisms.

Hypoxic-Ischemic (HI) Damage and Hypoxic–Ischemic Encephalopathy (HIE)

Because peri-partum HI injury occurs somewhat commonly in infants (2–3/1000 live births), a significant amount of research has investigated the pathophysiologic processes and treatment of HIE [25]. Much of this knowledge arises from animal models, but yet, a great deal remains to be explored [26–34]. HI injury is not a single event, but an ongoing process that causes neuronal death over hours to days after the initial HI event [35]. At an elementary level, brain damage caused by HI injury occurs due to decreased cerebral blood flow and associated decrease in energy substrates to the brain, subsequently resulting in a cascade of deleterious physiologic and biochemical events early within the postpartum period (hours to days). After a reversible HI event, neuronal injury/death occurs in two phases associated with primary and secondary energy failure [30–35]. The primary or immediate phase (primary neuronal death) is caused by energy failure, resulting from failure of oxidative metabolism, cytotoxic edema and accumulation of excitotoxins. After restoration of cerebral blood flow, the second phase (6–15+ hours after initial HI insult) is associated with excitotoxicity, apoptosis, and microglial activation (Figure 32.VIII.1) [35].

Primary energy failure results from the initial decrease in cerebral blood flow and associated decrease in oxygen and glucose delivery. This results in a drastic decline in available energy, including adenosine triphosphate (ATP), to the brain and increased lactate production [34, 36]. The lack of ATP has multiple consequences, but in particular, impacts the ability to maintain the normally low intracellular Ca^{++} concentrations and failure of Na^{+}/K^{+} pumps. Failure of Na^{+}/K^{+} pumps results in an influx of Na^{+} and concomitant movement of water, resulting in cell swelling and edema formation. Moreover, excessive Na^{+} causes depolarization of neurons, which precipitates release of the excitatory neurotransmitter glutamate. Glutamate binds to glutamate receptors, which further increases intracellular Na^{+} and Ca^{++}. Increased intracellular Ca^{++} has significant negative effects including cerebral edema, ischemia, and microvascular damage resulting in cell death by necrosis and apoptosis (see below). Ultimately, most of the cell death caused by primary energy failure is cellular necrosis through weakened cellular integrity and disruption of cytoskeleton and cell membrane.

Cellular necrosis occurs in conditions of extreme HI and results in cell swelling and rupture [33, 34]. Subsequently, cellular contents are released (damage-associated molecular patterns; DAMPS) and contribute to the inflammatory process [33, 34, 37]. In addition, microglia migrate to sites of inflammation and release additional inflammatory mediators [38]. The increase in inflammatory mediators results in damage to white matter, leading to scar tissue formation [38]. If the insult is less severe, cells can recover or become apoptotic [39]. The benefit of apoptosis, which can occur days following initial insult, is preservation of cell membranes, and therefore makes no further contribution to additional inflammation [33, 34].

The extent of primary energy failure plays a role in further damage during secondary energy failure [34]. When cerebral blood flow returns, recovery occurs for a short time [34]. The brief recovery/latent period is distinguished by normal cerebral metabolism. The length of the latent period depends on the severity of the initial HI event [40]. It is unclear when primary energy failure, the latent period and the secondary energy failure each begin, but secondary energy failure is believed to occur between 6 and 48 hours after initial injury [41]. The exact cause of secondary energy failure is unknown, but appears to be correlated to oxidative stress, excitotoxicity, and inflammation [41].

Oxidative Stress and Reperfusion Injury

Reperfusion injury is one of the main processes associated with CNS disorders such as stroke and traumatic brain injury and occurs when blood perfusion is re-established to

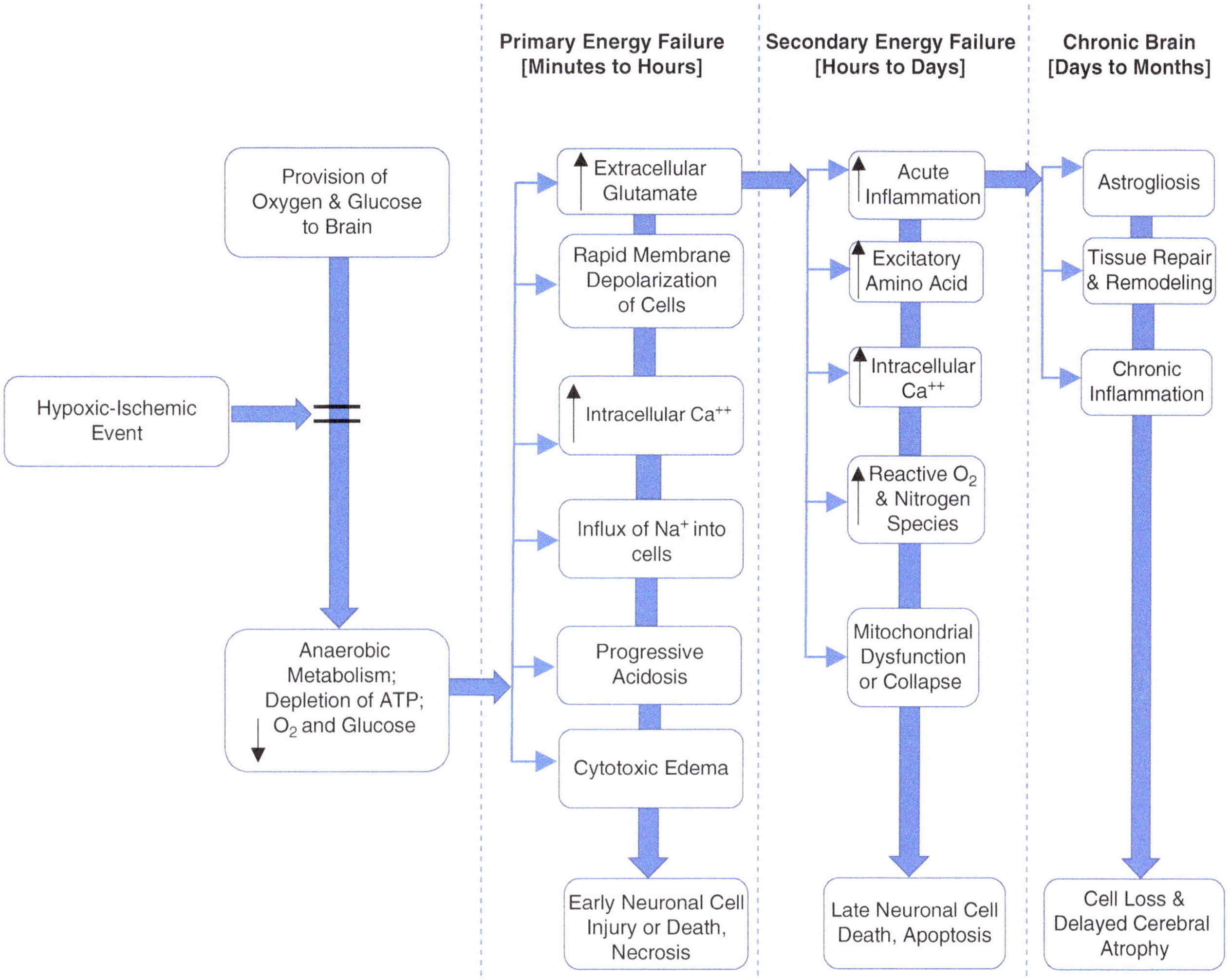

Figure 32.VIII.1 Overview of cascade of events associated with a peri-partum hypoxic-ischemic episode.

tissues after a HI event. When oxygen delivery returns to tissues, it can cause oxidative stress and damage, cellular dysfunction, and cell death via apoptosis or necrosis. Under healthy conditions, reactive oxygen species (ROS) are primarily generated in the mitochondria and are cleared by superoxide dismutase and glutathione peroxidase (Figure 32.VIII.2). During HI, ROS cannot be immediately eliminated by these antioxidant enzymes because metabolism is interrupted. Moreover, excessive ROS are generated from the mitochondrial electron transport chain, NADPH oxidases, xanthine oxidase, arachidonic acid, and nitric oxide (NO) synthase [35]. NO produced during hypoxia can result in lipid peroxidation, protein oxidation, nitration of nuclear membranes, DNA damage, apoptosis, and increased intracellular Ca^{++} [35]. Additionally, in response to ischemia, hypoxanthine is produced by xanthine dehydrogenase (Figure 32.VIII.3) and oxygen is converted to superoxide and hydroxyl radicals; NO reacts with superoxide to produce peroxynitrite, a highly toxic free radical. Free radicals, NO, and ROS react with cellular components (lipids, proteins, glycosaminoglycans) and alter cell function. Endothelial cells and leukocytes also produce ROS and contribute to additional damage.

The extensive production of free radicals causes damage to neuronal cell membranes and leads to apoptosis or necrosis from oxidative stress. Oxidative damage is particularly harmful to the neonatal brain because it has low concentrations of antioxidants and consumes a large amount of oxygen when transitioning from fetal to neonatal life. The neonatal brain also has a high concentration of unsaturated fatty acids, which break down to form more oxygen-free radicals [36]. Another damaging mechanism that occurs with HI is the release of protein-bound iron, allowing free iron to react with peroxides to form more free radicals [43]. Globally, the neonatal brain does not have the capacity to eliminate excessive free radicals and thus these free radicals cause damage to neuronal tissue [43].

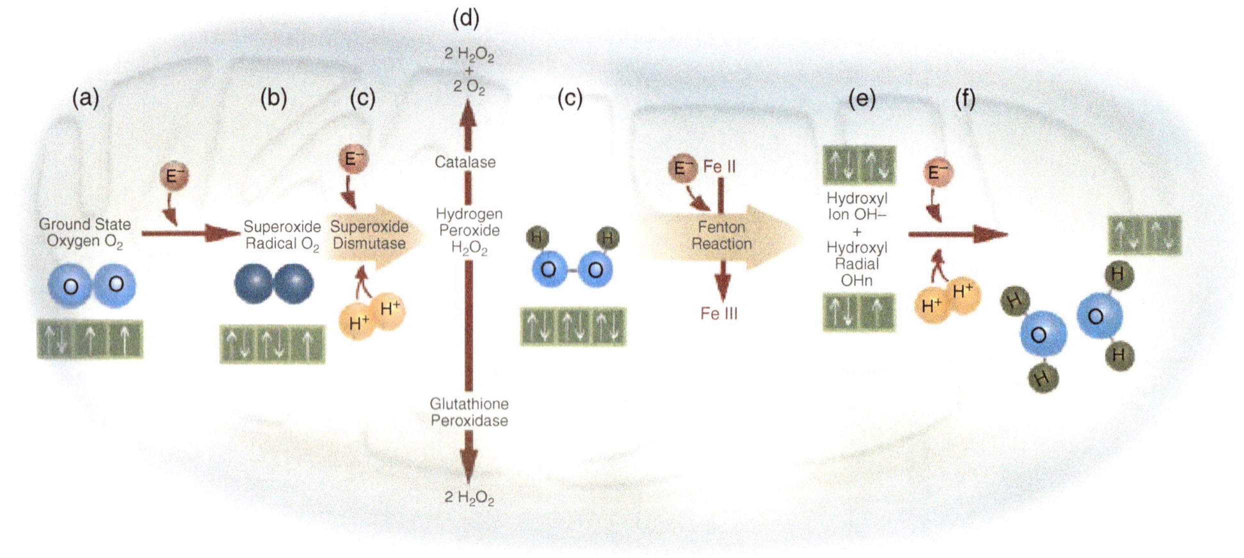

Figure 32.VIII.2 Reduction of molecular oxygen (O_2) to water in the mitochondria. Orbital diagrams demonstrate the electron configuration (green boxes and arrows) of each reactant. (a) Molecular O_2 has an outer shell occupied by two electrons spinning in opposite directions, whereas the other orbitals each contain a single electron, both of which spin in the same direction. (b) *First reaction*: an electron is added to O_2 forming superoxide radical ($O_2^{\bullet}$). (c) Subsequently, another electron is added along with two protons (H^+) forming hydrogen peroxide (H_2O_2). (d) Endogenous antioxidants metabolize H_2O_2 into H_2O via the catalase enzyme (within peroxisomes) or glutathione peroxidase (in the cytosol). (e) Remaining H_2O_2 forms two hydroxyl radicals. In this reaction (Fenton reaction), an electron is donated by ferrous iron (FeII) to form a hydroxyl ion (OH^-) and hydroxyl radical ($OH^{\bullet}$). (f) The fourth reaction involves addition of an electron and two protons (H+) to the hydroxyl radical, yielding two molecules of water [42].

Excitotoxicity

Excitotoxicity refers to cell death mediated by excessive stimulation of extracellular excitatory amino acid receptors [44]. This occurs during HI when large concentrations of extracellular neurotransmitters overstimulate excitatory receptors, thereby resulting in membrane depolarization and inappropriate opening of ion channels into the neuron [35]. Glutamate is the primary excitatory amino acid neurotransmitter in the brain and initiates biochemical changes via interaction with various receptors. These include ionotropic receptors, named because they are linked to ion channels, and include the N-methyl-D-Aspartate (NMDA) receptor (linked to Ca^{++} channels) and the α-amino-3-hydroxy-5-methyl-4-isoxazole propionic acid (AMPA) and kainite (KA) receptors (linked to Na^+ channels). In health, glutamate is continuously released from presynaptic nerve terminals when signaled by neuronal depolarization and is subsequently rapidly removed from the synaptic cleft by glutamate transporters in astrocytes and converted to glutamine, which in turn is returned to nerve terminals for reuse. This process is disrupted with HI and associated decrease in ATP and glucose to the brain. This situation lends to excess accumulation of extracellular glutamate and ensuing opening of ion channel, which, in turn, results in excess intracellular Ca^{++} influx into neurons, triggering Ca^{++}-dependent proteases, lipases, and endonucleases, as well as cytotoxic edema, mitochondrial dysfunction, and stimulation of pro-apoptotic pathways [35]. A variety of neuronal pathways utilize glutamate, including those associated with hearing, vision, somatosensory function, learning, and memory, which may explain some of the disruptive effects associated with NE on ensuing development [31].

Intracellular Calcium Accumulation

Increased intracellular Ca^{++} concentrations play a pivotal role in HI brain injury. In health, intracellular Ca^{++} concentrations are very low. The NMDA receptor is a main pathway of increased intracellular Ca^{++} in HI conditions. During a HI event, deprivation of oxygen and glucose triggers overstimulation of glutamate release; increased glutamate stimulates opening of the NMDA receptor channel, thereby allowing Ca^{++} to flow into neurons. Voltage-gated Ca^{++} channels further contribute to increased intracellular Ca^{++} concentrations [25]. High intracellular Ca^{++} activates lipases, proteases, endonucleases, and NO synthase resulting in neurotoxic cascades. Furthermore, increased Ca^{++}

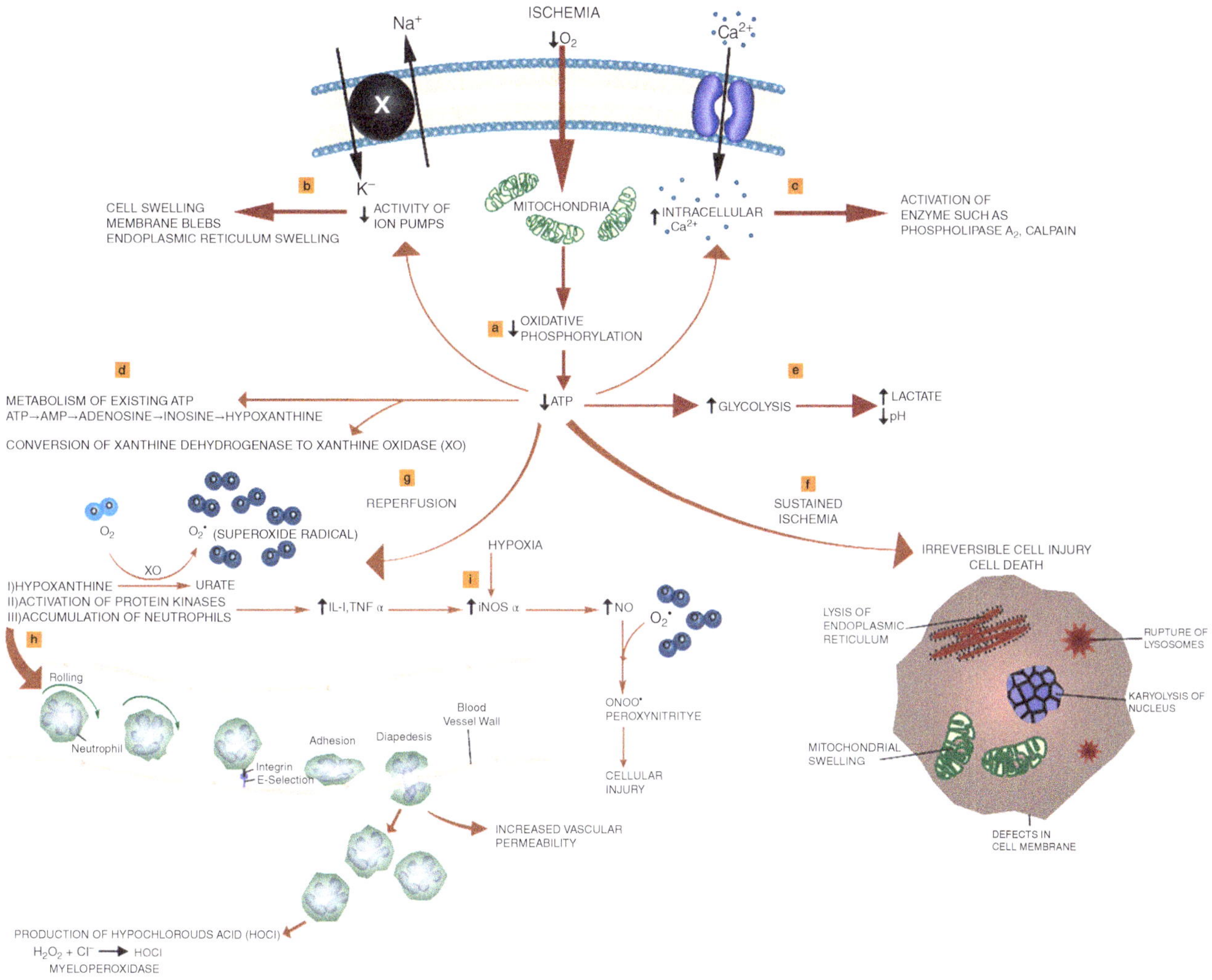

Figure 32.VIII.3 Mechanisms of ischemia–reperfusion injury. (a) During ischemic event, oxidative phosphorylation becomes uncoupled, resulting in decreased ATP production. (b) Decreased energy production results in decreased activity of membrane ion pumps and cell swelling. (c) Deceased energy production results in increased movement of Ca^{++} into the cell and activation of enzymes (e.g. phospholipase A2, calpain). (d) Concurrently, remaining ATP is metabolized, resulting in accumulation of hypoxanthine. Xanthine dehydrogenase is converted to xanthine oxidase as a result of increased intracellular Ca^{++} and calpain. (e) Anaerobic metabolism results in increased glycolysis, increased lactate, and decreased pH, further reducing ATP production. (f) Sustained ischemia results in cell death. (g) Alternatively, during reperfusion, accumulated hypoxanthine is metabolized to xanthine and urate, producing superoxide radicals. (h) Neutrophils migrate to previously ischemic tissue, releasing products that cause further damage. (i) activation of inducible nitric oxide synthase (iNOS) by inflammatory cytokines and/or hypoxia results in generation of large amounts of nitric oxide (NO). NO reacts with superoxide radical ($O_2^\bullet$) and produces highly toxic peroxynitrite ($ONOO^\bullet$) molecule, resulting in further cell injury [42].

induces mitochondrial dysfunction and mediates irreversible death of immature neurons via activation of Ca^{++}-dependent proteins (Figures 32.VIII.4 and 32.VIII.5) [22, 25].

Inflammation

In infants, inflammatory cells and mediators are believed to play an important role in the cascade of events resulting in neonatal brain injury [26, 27, 45]. Microglia, neutrophils, lymphocytes, cytokines, and immunoglobulins have a role in the inflammatory process activated by hypoxia [35]. When microglia are activated by an HI event, they release inflammatory and anti-inflammatory mediators, glutamate, NO, and ROS and also develop macrophage-like abilities such as phagocytosis, antigen presentation and production and release of matrix metalloproteinases (MMPs) [25, 35]. This activity subsequently causes dysfunction of neuronal, glial, and endothelium cells, and breaks down the blood-brain barrier (BBB) [28, 35, 46]. Consequently, peripheral leukocytes have access to the normally immunologically privileged area and the brain is

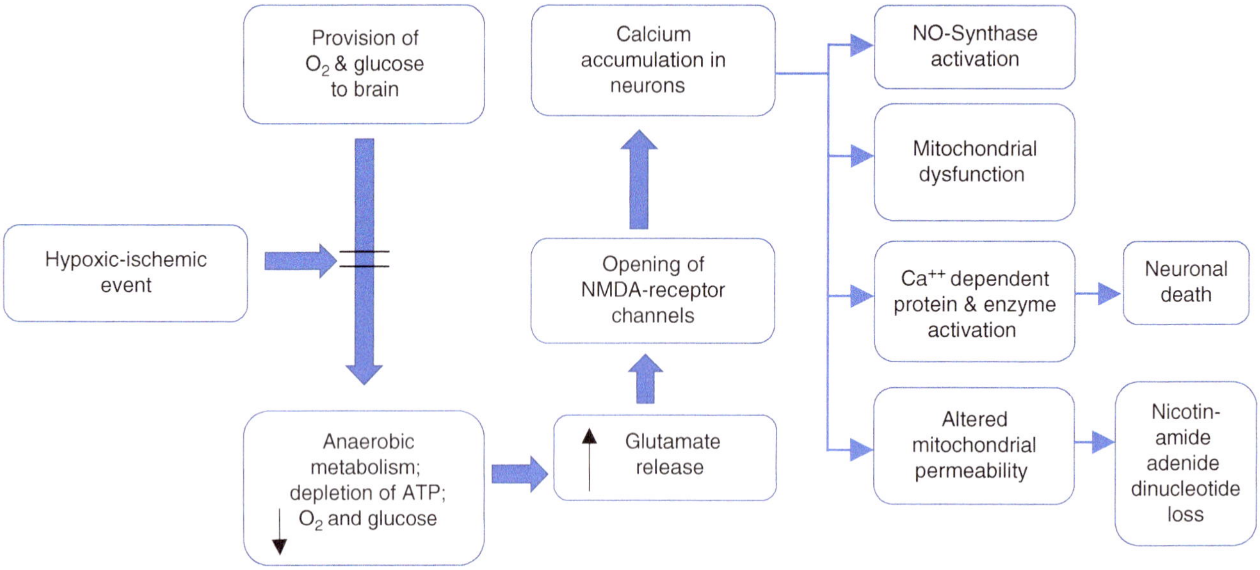

Figure 32.VIII.4 Association of hypoxic–ischemic events, increased intracellular calcium (Ca^{++}) and activation of several down-stream events.

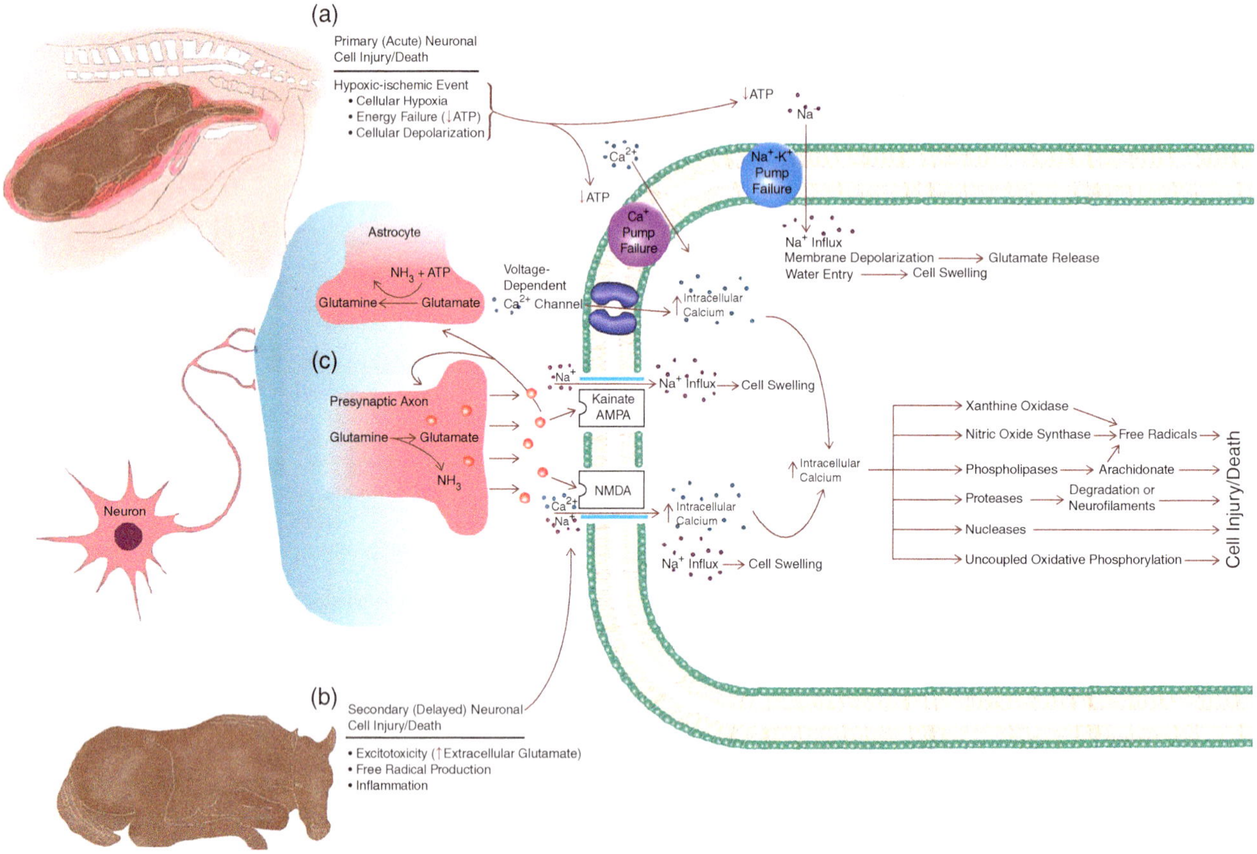

Figure 32.VIII.5 Potential phases of neuronal injury and death in foals with HIE. (a) HIE is associated with primary (acute) neuronal injury and death resulting from cellular hypoxia, energy failure and cellular depolarization. A hypoxic–ischemic event results in decreased ATP, failure of membrane pumps (Na^+-K^+, Ca^{++}) and influx of Na^+ and Ca^+ into neurons and other cells. Increased intracellular Na^{++} causes cell swelling, while membrane depolarization contributes to glutamate release. (b) Secondary neuronal death results from excess extracellular glutamate, oxidative damage and inflammation. (c) Presynaptic nerve ending and glutamate receptors within the neuronal cell membrane. Activation of these receptors results in influx of Na^+ (NMDA, AMPA, Kainate) and Ca^{++} (NMDA) into the cell. Increased intracellular Ca^{++} causes activation of numerous pathways that can contribute to cell injury and death [17].

subject to systemic responses. Studies in animal models indicate that infiltration of neutrophils into cerebral tissue occurs in the early stages (4–8 hours) of injury and worsen brain injury and cerebral edema via ROS production, release of cytotoxic agents and MMPs, and decreased microvascular flow due to neutrophil accumulation within the vessels [28, 35, 47]. Ultimately, neuroinflammation in the infant brain damages glial cells and neurons ultimately resulting in neurologic deficits [28].

Brain Injury and Astrocytes

As discussed above, energy depletion plays a large role in HI neuronal damage, but dysfunction of astrocytes also contributes to neuronal failure [48]. Astrocytes depend upon glycolysis and lactate production for energy whereas neurons depend on the tricarboxylic acid (TCA) cycle and pentose phosphate pathway to produce energy and maintain antioxidant capacity [46, 49]. Under normal conditions, the metabolism of astrocytes and neurons are coupled, despite having distinctly different metabolic processes. Most glucose in neurons goes into the pentose phosphate pathway and the use of 3-carbon glycolysis products such as pyruvate and lactate produced by the astrocytes (astrocyte-neuron lactate shuttle) are shuttled to the TCA cycle for oxidative phosphorylation to generate ATP [46, 49–51]. Within the neurons, ion pumps utilize ATP to maintain electrochemical gradients along with synaptic and action potentials.

Traumatic brain injury and ischemia cause glutamate accumulation which increases uptake of glucose and production of lactate by astrocytes [46]. Glutamate is co-transported with Na^+ into astrocytes, which stimulates Na^+ K^+-ATPase and consequently increases ATP utilization. Excess glutamate is converted to glutamine (GABA-glutamate-glutamine cycle) that requires 1 ATP/glutamate. When oxygen and energy supply are limited in astrocytes, the excess glutamate puts strain on astrocytes, which in turn can have negative effects on neuron function and survival. One of the key functions of astrocytes is water homeostasis; thus, dysfunction of astrocytes leads to brain edema and neuronal death. Astrocytes are also capable of producing neurosteroids when oxygen and energy are lacking [52].

Neuroactive Steroids, Progestogens, and Neonatal Encephalopathy

Clearly not every foal with NE has historic or microscopic evidence of a HI episode; thus, alternative pathophysiologic processes must be considered. One theory is that a subset of foals has altered concentrations of neurosteroids, resulting in clinical signs of NE. In particular, postnatal persistence of elevated pregnane (and/or other neuroactive steroids) concentrations may impact the onset of consciousness in the foal [6, 53]. Neuroactive steroids are synthesized from cholesterol in the peripheral and CNS by neurons and glial cells and are also synthesized as metabolites of steroid hormones from the peripheral tissues such as the adrenal glands, gonads, and placenta [54–62]. The terms *neuroactive steroid* and *neurosteroid* are used interchangeably, but by strict definition, neuroactive steroids are products of peripheral steroid hormones metabolized by nervous tissue whereas neurosteroids are produced de novo in the nervous system [54–62]. Steroids in the peripheral circulation can cross the BBB and be converted by neurons and glial cell into neuroactive steroids [63]. In other words, neurosteroids are synthetized in the brain and modulate neuronal activity whereas neuroactive steroids are steroids that modify neural activity independent of their tissue of origin [53]. Placental progesterone is the main substrate for steroids produced in the brain in primates; in horses, other pregnanes and androstanes are likely metabolized [22]. Neurosteroids are classified as pregnane, androstane, and sulfated neurosteroids with their production regulated by expression of 5α-reductase and 3α-hydroxysteroid dehydrogenase [55, 58–60].

Certain steroidal compounds, predominantly 5α-reductase pregnanes, have neuromodulatory effects and are potent allosteric modulators of $GABA_A$ receptors and, to a lesser extent, glutamate (NMDA, AMPA, kainite), glycine, serotonin, and sigma1 (σ1) receptors [23, 58–60]. The main target for neuroactive steroids is the $GABA_A$ receptor, which, when activated, facilitates chloride entry and hyperpolarization of the cell membrane, thereby decreasing neuronal excitability and modifying glial cell function [55, 58–60]. Sedative and anesthetic properties of progestogens were first described in rodents with the discovery leading to the development of commercial steroid anesthetics (benzodiazepines, barbiturates, propofol, etomidate) [22, 64–67]. Similarly, some pregnanes have comparable effects in foals [23, 24, 54, 68]. Other functions of neurosteroids include stimulation of neurogenesis and neuronal plasticity, organization of neuronal circuits (e.g. fetal brain programming, maternal behavior), and modulation of the stress response of the hypothalamic–pituitary–adrenal axis (HPAA), among many others [55, 56].

In utero, the equine fetus maintains a quiescent state compared to the precocious and active newborn foal that is observed within hours of birth. Maintenance of this sleep-like state in utero is believed to be due to neuroinhibitory effects of high circulating concentrations of adenosine, allopregnanolone, pregnanolone, and prostaglandin D_2 [6]. These compounds suppress brain activity and keep the fetus in a somnolent state while neurons and glial cells develop and differentiate [56]. The impact of allopregnanolone on the neonatal foal was experimentally demonstrated by IV administration to a healthy newborn foal. During IV infusion of allopregnanolone, sedation and decreased responsiveness were noted and, at higher doses, more dramatic effects such as recumbency, stupor, and unresponsiveness were observed [68]. Clinical signs persisted during infusion of allopregnanolone but diminished over 15 minutes after stopping the infusion and normal behavior was observed 30 minutes post-infusion. Other studies have documented increased concentrations of pregnenolone, progesterone, 17α-hydroxyprogesterone, allopregnanolone, androstenedione, and dehydroepiandrosterone (DHEA) sulfate in foals that were critically ill or premature or had NE [23, 24, 54, 69]. Mechanisms therefore exist to inhibit excessive fetal movement at the end of pregnancy and require precise timing during parturition to transition from fetal life to post-natal consciousness, rapid ambulation, and ability to nurse soon after birth: neurosteroids are thought to have a key role in this transition [23, 24, 54, 69, 70]. This transition may be regulated by a fetal-neural reflex that is triggered during parturition by the compression or squeeze that the fetus undergoes through the birth canal. Based on this information, some foals may have persistence of fetal HPAA axis (e.g. adrenal origin) activity and increased pregnanes (pregnenolone, progesterone, and metabolites) contributing to clinical signs of NE [23]. A pathophysiologic theory thus speculates that some nonhypoxic foals with NE lack the normal transition of the HPAA from synthesis to inhibition of specific neurosteroids associated with readiness for birth (failure to switch from fetal to neonatal neurosteroid profile). This theory may explain why some foals with NE do not have a peri-partum HI event and have a relatively rapid recovery without residual neurologic deficits [23].

Fetal Inflammatory Response Syndrome

Yet another theory, outside the framework of HI injury, that might be involved in the pathophysiology of NE in foals is the fetal inflammatory response to maternal chorioamnionitis (placentitis) and its impact on the fetus/neonate. Maternal inflammation (placenitis) is a common clinical syndrome in the pregnant mare. Chorio-amnionitis can be associated with the fetal inflammatory response syndrome (FIRS), with this inflammatory signal being transmitted across the BBB and inducing a neuroinflammatory response [71]. FIRS is a condition characterized by systemic activation of the fetal innate immune system and production of proinflammatory cytokines (interleukin [IL]-1, -6, -8, TNF-α) by monocytes-macrophages [71]. In infants, FIRS is defined by a fetal plasma IL-6 concentration greater than 11 pg/ml [71]. Intra-amniotic exposure to microorganisms (or experimental intra-amniotic injection of endotoxin) induces production of inflammatory mediators in the amniotic cavity and can initiate FIRS [72]. Consequently, FIRS affects multiple organs, including a detrimental neuroinflammatory response, mediated by microglia and peripheral immune effector cells [71, 72]. In infants, this cerebral inflammatory response is a risk factor for brain injury and neurodevelopmental conditions including cognitive, behavioral, and motor dysfunction [72]. The exact mechanism by which perinatal proinflammatory cytokines cause brain injury is not fully understood but proposed mechanisms include: increased permeability of the BBB to cytotoxic proteins, activation of microglia, dysmaturation of the oligodendrocyte lineage and hypomyelination, neuronal injury and cell death, modification of the endogenous stem cell populations, generation of reactive oxygen and nitrogen species, sensitization of the brain to subsequent HI insults and activation of the coagulation cascade [73]. Of note, perinatal CNS inflammation is also associated with HI injury (noted above) and may share common pathways as perinatal inflammation associated with FIRS: that is, placentitis or HI injury might initiate a common pathway of inflammatory injury to the perinatal brain, but much has to be learned in equine neonatology [74].

The clinician can clearly recognize that although multiple theories have been put forth in regard to the pathophysiologic mechanism(s) involved in the development of NE in the foal, the true cause is often unknown. It is likely that equine NE is a manifestation of a variety of disease processes and that multiple different mechanisms can result in clinical signs of NE. These different mechanisms contribute to the wide spectrum of clinical signs and severities observed in foals with NE. Regardless of the pedantic discussion of etiology, NE is one of the most common neurologic diseases noted in neonatal foals and fortunately maintains an overall promising prognosis.

Risk Factor for Neonatal Encephalopathy

The placenta, fetus, and mare can each contribute to risk factors for development of NE in the foal. Severe systemic maternal illness or inflammation can disrupt perfusion to the uteroplacental unit and serve as risk factors. Moreover, maternal hypotension secondary to endotoxemia, hemorrhage, anemia, severe respiratory disease or general anesthesia can also be involved [75–78]. Placentitis and premature placental separation could potentially cause NE by limiting oxygen and nutrients to the fetus. Fetal factors such as infection, twins, prematurity, dysmaturity, umbilical cord compression or accidents, congenital malformations, and meconium aspiration can also be involved [75–78]. Factors related to parturition such as dystocia, induced parturition, cesarean section, or post-term pregnancy (Fescue toxicity) can also be risk factors. In one study in 79 neonatal foals with a primary diagnosis of NE, placental abnormalities (55% of foals), gestational problems (21%), premature placental separation (34%), and dystocia (30%) were reported [1]. Alternatively, foals with NE may have no reported problems during gestation or parturition.

Clinical Signs

Foals with NE have a wide spectrum of clinical signs with varying severities. The median age at admission in 94 foals with NE was 12 hours (range 0–96 hours), therefore, the age of onset of clinical signs may vary within a relatively specific temporal window [9]. Some foals can demonstrate clinical signs of NE shortly after birth, whereas others may appear healthy for the first 12–24 hours (or less frequently >24 hours) and then develop clinical signs. In theory, the delayed onset of clinical signs may be attributed to the biphasic nature of neuronal damage (primary and secondary), but this remains speculative. Clinical signs include alterations of consciousness (hyperexcitability, lethargy, stupor, disorientation, somnolence, difficult to arouse, comatose), behavior (lack of affinity for the dam, abnormal to no udder seeking, lack of suckle reflex, wandering, inability to lie down, abnormal vocalization), neurologic function (ataxia, tremors, dysphagia, head pressing, abnormal respiratory rate and patterns, central blindness, proprioceptive deficits, localized or generalized seizures), muscle tone (weakness, hypotonia, arched neck, recumbency) along with other signs such as protrusion of the tongue, expiratory noise, hemorrhagic retinas, and inability to thermoregulate [2–22]. In a retrospective study involving 94 foals with NE, the most frequent clinical signs included abnormal udder seeking (59%), abnormal suckle (55%), inability to stand (42%), abnormal gastrointestinal motility (37%), abnormal consciousness (34%), and seizure activity (22%) [9]. Other organs such as the gastrointestinal (meconium impaction, ileus, colitis/enteritis), cardiac (arrythmias), renal (oliguric or anuria acute renal injury), and hepatic (elevated liver enzyme activity) systems can concurrently be affected [8, 9, 17–21]. Sepsis is a common secondary complication of NE due to failure of passive transfer of immunity and/or bacterial translocation, and other concurrent conditions such as prematurity, dysmaturity, patent urachus, omphalitis, limb deformities, colic, and uroperitoneium may also be observed [9].

Clinicopathologic Findings

Reported clinicopathologic abnormalities in foals with NE include hypoxemia, hypercapnia, acidosis, hyperlactatemia, hypoglycemia, hypocalcemia, hypomagnesemia, hypermagnesemia, and decreased thyroid concentrations [8, 9, 12, 17, 22, 54, 79–83]. These abnormalities are typically secondary to systemic disease and organ dysfunction and are not specific to NE. In a retrospective study, 32% of foals with NE had increased serum creatinine concentration and 61% of foals with NE had increased serum creatine kinase activity [1]. Another retrospective study evaluating spurious hypercreatininemia in 28 foals (mean creatinine concentration 13.6 mg/dl) noted that 20 foals (71%) had a clinical diagnosis of NE [84]. Increased concentrations of serum creatinine (>3.5 mg/dl) and/or low presuckle blood glucose concentrations (<35 to 40 mg/dl) have been associated with placental insufficiency in the foal [78]. Thus, elevations in serum creatinine and creatine kinase can be associated with a number of other disease processes in neonatal foals, but in the absence of compatible clinical signs (e.g. renal or muscle disorder), NE should be considered. Cerebrospinal fluid collection and examination is not typical performed in foals with NE, but it can be normal, xanthochromic or hemorrhagic [22].

Diagnosis

There is not a definitive antemortem diagnostic test for NE in foals. Currently, diagnosis is based on the veterinarian's clinical impression of clinical signs and neurologic examination of the foal coupled with historical information of the mare, maternal disease and parturition, and exclusion of other disease processes, and congenital abnormalities [9, 75–78]. Clinicopathologic findings are more demonstrative of other disease process rather than specific for NE. Biomarkers for brain injury have been reported in foals with NE [29]; more specifically, plasma concentrations of ubiquitin C-terminal hydrolase 1 (biomarker for brain injury) was significantly higher in foals with NE (mean 6.57 ng/ml; range 2.35–11.90 ng/ml) when compared with healthy foals (median 2.53 ng/ml; range 1.4–4.01 ng/ml). However, these markers are not readily measured, making them of limited clinical use.

Magnetic resonance imaging (MRI) is a mainstay in diagnosis of HIE in human infants; however, MRI is not used routinely in foals with suspected NE [5, 85]. MRI has been used to examine the healthy neonatal foal brain as well as other neurologic diseases in foals, but very few reports have described MRI findings in foals with presumptive NE [85–87]. In one report, MRI imaging revealed symmetrical, poorly delineated areas of high signal intensity (compared with gray matter regions elsewhere) involving the basal nuclei, ventral thalamic nuclei, and rostral aspect of the ventral midbrain (in the region of the substantia nigra) on T1-weighted (T1-W) images (Figure 32.VIII.6) [85]. Hyperintensity associated with the margins of the lateral ventricles were noted on T2-weighted (T2-W) and T2-W fluid attenuated inversion recovery (FLAIR) images [85]. The lesions noted in this foal were similar to those described in infants with HIE [88, 89]. The associated risks of general anesthesia and added client expense may preclude the use of MRI for the diagnosis of NE, but imaging studies might help elucidate the pathophysiology of NE in foals.

Cranial ultrasound has been used in infants to help identify neonates with HIE as well as other causes of fetal brain injury [90]. Changes in ventricular size, periventricular echogenicity, increased echogenicity in the thalamus, extra-axial fluid collection and intracranial hemorrhage have been observed with cranial ultrasound of infants with HIE [90]. In one study, cranial ultrasound was able to identify infants with a poor outcome, but MRI was better at identifying changes associated with HIE [91]. One study in foals examined ultrasonographic measurements of a number of variables viewed from the atlanto-occipital (AO) space in healthy foals and foals with NE using a 8 MHz micro-convex transducer at a depth of 6–8 cm [92]. In the described technique, the transducer is placed immediately cranial to the wings of the atlas to obtain a transverse image and then rotated 90° to obtain a longitudinal image [92]. The height of the spinal cord, depth of the dorsal sub-arachnoid space (mid-AO space), maximal depth of the dorsal sub-arachnoid space (cranial-AO space) and dorsoventral diameter of the ventral spinal artery are measured from longitudinal images. The height, width, and cross-sectional area of the spinal cord and spinal canal along with the depth of the dorsal sub-arachnoid space are measured from transverse images (Figure 32.VIII.7). In addition, ratios of the spinal canal to spinal cord height, spinal canal to cord width and spinal canal to cord cross sectional area measurements are calculated from transverse images. In foals with NE, the dorsoventral diameter of the ventral spinal artery (longitudinal images) and absolute measurements of the spinal cord height, width, and cross-sectional area (transverse images) were all significantly smaller when compared to healthy foals [92]. Ratios of spinal canal to spinal cord width and cross-sectional area were significantly larger in foals with NE when compared to healthy foals. Elevated intracranial pressure related to NE might explain the reduced spinal cord dimensions in foals with NE. The clinical application, utility, and reliability of ultrasonographic examination of the AO region in foals suspected to have NE is requires further study [92].

Treatment

Core therapies for NE revolve around supportive and nursing care, treatment or prevention of infection, along with targeted therapy for other organ systems that may be affected. This entails maintenance of adequate hydration and caloric needs, facilitation of gas exchange, maintenance of adequate blood pressure, treatment and/or prevention of infections, control of seizures (if present), antioxidants, neuroprotectants, and exceptional nursing care (keeping foal clean, dry, and comfortable). Diagnostic tests such as a complete blood count (CBC), serum biochemistry profile, arterial blood gas analysis, blood culture, urinalysis, and evaluation of passive transfer of maternal antibodies should be considered to provide a comprehensive assessment of the foal's condition and will help guide therapy. Table 32.VIII.2 provides an overview of various

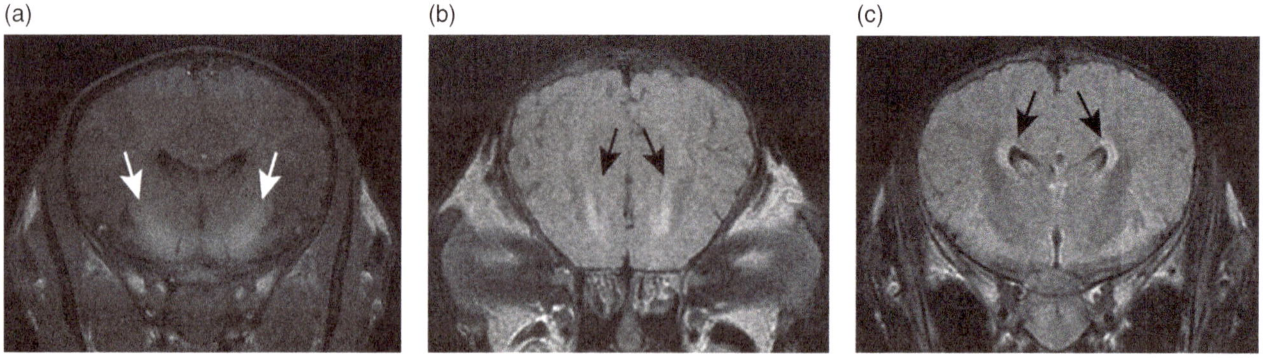

Figure 32.VIII.6 MRI scans of the brain of the foal, illustrating symmetrical abnormalities in the cerebrum. (a) T1W transverse image through the cerebral hemispheres immediately rostral to the pituitary. Arrows indicate regions of hyperintensity in the basal nuclei. (b) T2W FLAIR transverse image through the rostral limit of the lateral hemispheres. Arrows indicate areas of hyperintensity associated with the rostral poles of the hemispheres. (c) T2W FLAIR image through the cerebral hemispheres immediately rostral to the pituitary (same level as image in [a]). Arrows indicate regions of hyperintensity adjacent to the lateral ventricles [85].

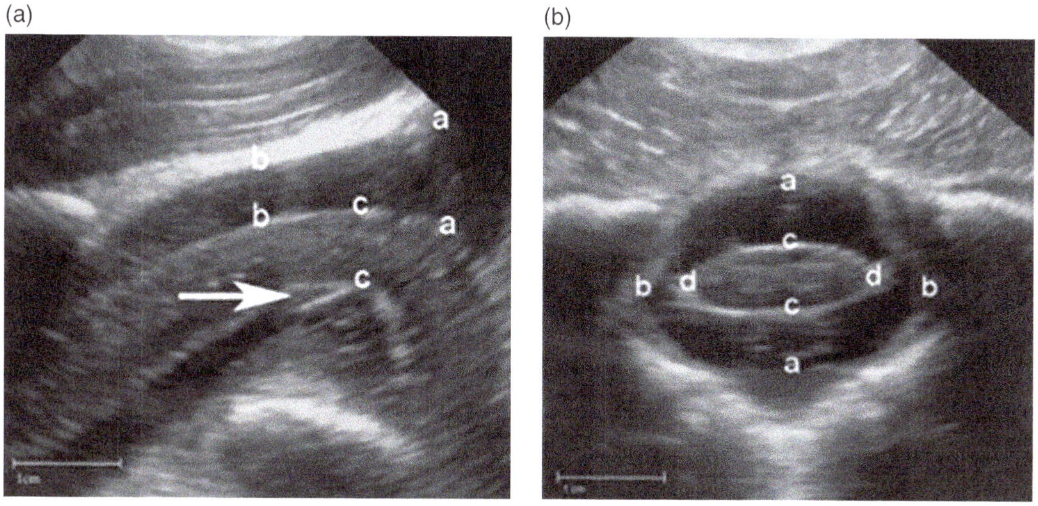

Figure 32.VIII.7 Ultrasonographic images of the atlanto-occipital region in a 1-day-old Thoroughbred foal with NE. (a) Longitudinal ultrasound image (cranial to right of image). Measurements of the maximal depth of the dorsal subarachnoid space (cranial atlanto-occipital space) (a to a), dorsal sub-arachnoid space (mid atlanto-occipital space) (b to b), height of the spinal cord (c to c) and dorsoventral diameter of the ventral spinal artery (arrow). (b) Transverse ultrasound image (right side of foal to right of image). Measurements of the spinal canal height (a to a) and width (b to b), spinal cord height (c to c) and width (d to d) and dorsal subarachnoid space (dorsal a to dorsal c). From Mackenzie et al. Ultrasonographic assessment of the atlanto-occipital space in healthy Thoroughbred foals and Thoroughbred foals with neonatal maladjustment syndrome [92].

supportive care techniques with detailed discussion on topics, such as nutritional support and fluid therapy, discussed in other chapters.

Based on the theory that NE might be caused by deficiencies in energy substrates, maintenance of adequate blood pressure, oxygen content, and glucose concentrations is a sensible goal. Adequate blood perfusion is needed to support cerebral perfusion and avoid further ischemic injury; therefore, IV fluid therapy (boluses, CRI) can be used to provide intravascular volume support; judicious use of inopressors can be implemented if fluid therapy is insufficient to maintain adequate perfusion. Since neonatal foals have limited energy reserves, supplemental nutrition in the form of dextrose or parenteral nutrition formulations is also prudent [106]. An arterial blood gas analysis should be performed as some foals with NE have poor oxygenation from a variety of underlying reasons; use of intranasal humidified oxygen may help raise the partial pressure of oxygen (P_aO_2) in hypoxemic foals. If seizures are observed in the foal, immediate therapy should be instituted as ongoing seizure activity greatly increases cerebral oxygen consumption and can further contribute to neuronal damage. Diazepam typically controls seizures in the neonatal foal and can be given intermittently if seizures are infrequent. Midazolam can also be used as a single IV dose or CRI to control seizures [99]. If seizure activity persists, phenobarbital may be necessary, but side effects such as sedation, ataxia and hypothermia may occur. Induction of anesthesia with propofol can be required for several hours to manage intractable cases of status epilepticus [20].

The pharmacokinetics of levetiracetam, a newer anticonvulsant, have been investigated in neonatal foals and may serve as an oral anticonvulsant administered once a day, but its efficacy in foals with seizures remains to be deteremined [100].

Another method used to reduce cerebral metabolic rate and energy consumption in infants is therapeutic hypothermia. Hypothermia also inhibits glutamate release from synaptic nerve endings, improves uptake of glutamate by astrocytes, inhibits microglial activation, reduces free radical production and NO synthesis, decreases cytotoxic edema, and acts as an immunosuppressant [37, 107, 108]. Hypothermia is the only treatment shown to decrease mortality, disabilities, and brain injury in infants with HIE and is considered standard of care [84]. In infants, hypothermia is started as early as possible, ideally within the first 6 hours of life (e.g. within the latent phase of injury), with a target brain temperature between 91.4–93.2 °F (33–34 °C) and continued for 72 hours [37, 109]. These guidelines are strictly adhered to as deviations (e.g. lower temperature, longer duration) can result in neuronal injury [109]. Therapeutic hypothermia has not been evaluated in foals with NE [37]. Mannitol is perhaps an outdated therapy for NE in foals, but has been used to counteract potential cerebral edema in both infants and foals with NE. Improved outcome with mannitol administration has not been identified in infant or animal models and no studies have evaluated its effect on foals with NE. Therefore, its use has become decreased by many veterinarians and obsolete in human neonatology [110–112]. Of note, cerebral edema is

Table 32.VIII.2 Summary of supportive therapy and potential treatments for foals with NE.

Body system	Treatment
Nutritional support	▪ Enteral nutrition, mare's milk at 5–25% foal's body weight via nasoesophageal tube, divided into every 2–4 h feedings ▪ Dextrose infusion, 4–8 mg/kg/min, IV, CRI [93] ▪ Parenteral Nutrition, IV, CRI
Fluid therapy	▪ If dehydrated: fluid boluses at 20 mg/kg, IV over 20 min; repeat up to 2–3 boluses [93] ▪ Maintenance fluid rate 80–120 ml/kg/d, IV CRI [94] ▪ Correct electrolyte derangements via oral or IV supplementation ▪ Correct acid–base abnormalities, if necessary, based on blood gas analysis
Blood pressure support	▪ Inopressor therapy if hypotension persists despite adequate rehydration Dobutamine, 1–3 µg/kg/min, IV, CRI [95] Dopamine, 2–5 µg/kg/min, IV, CRI (inotrope); 5–10 µg/kg/min, IV, CRI (vasopressor) [95] Norepinephrine, 0.1–1.5 µg/kg/min, IV, CRI [95] ▪ Colloid therapy Equine plasma 20–40 ml/kg, IV [94] Hetastarch 3–5 ml/kg, IV bolus; 0.5–1 ml/kg/h (up to 10 ml/kg/d) for hypooncotic foal [94] Tetrastarch 20 ml/kg, IV bolus (higher doses not investigated in foals) [96]
Blood pressure support	▪ Inopressor therapy if hypotension persists despite adequate rehydration Dobutamine, 1–3 µg/kg/min, IV, CRI [95] Dopamine, 2–5 µg/kg/min, IV, CRI (inotrope); 5–10 µg/kg/min, IV, CRI (vasopressor) [95] Norepinephrine, 0.1–1.5 µg/kg/min, IV, CRI [95] ▪ Colloid therapy Equine plasma 20–40 ml/kg, IV [94] Hetastarch 3–5 ml/kg, IV bolus; 0.5–1 ml/kg/h (up to 10 ml/kg/d) for hypooncotic foal [94] Tetrastarch 20 ml/kg, IV bolus (higher doses not investigated in foals) [96]
Respiratory support	▪ Oxygen therapy (uni- or bilateral nasal oxygen administration) if hypoxemic ($P_aO_2 \leq 90$ mmHg) 3–10 l/min humidified oxygen, maintain foal in sternal recumbency [97] ▪ Respiratory stimulant if hypoventilation present and $P_aCO_2 > 50$ mmHg Doxapram, 0.02–0.05 mg/kg/h, IV, CRI [98] Caffeine, loading dose 10 mg/kg; maintenance dose 2.5–5 mg/kg, PO [98] ▪ Persistent or severe hypoxemia and/or hypercapnia Mechanical ventilation Surfactant replacement
Infection control	▪ Specific antimicrobial(s) if blood culture results available ▪ Broad-spectrum antimicrobials if blood culture results unavailable or prophylactic infection control ▪ Plasma therapy, 20–40 ml/kg, IV; use serum IgG concentrations as guide
Seizure control	▪ Diazepam, 0.1–0.2 mg/kg, IV, PRN [78] ▪ Midazolam, 0.04–0.1 mg/kg, IV, PRN or 0.02–0.06 mg/kg/h, IV, CRI [99] ▪ Phenobarbital, 2–10 mg/kg, IV over 15 min, then 5 mg/kg, PO, q 12h [78] ▪ Pentobarbital, 2–10 mg/kg, IV [78] ▪ Levetiracetam, 32 mg/kg, PO, q 12h (unknown efficacy in foals with seizures) [100] ▪ Propofol (sedate with xylazine 0.5 mg/kg), then 2–3 mg/kg, IV over 1 min, then 0.3 mg/kg/min, IV, CRI [101] ▪ Ketamine 10–50 mcg/kg/min CRI
Antioxidants	▪ Vitamin C (ascorbic acid), 100 mg/kg, IV, q 24h [17] ▪ Vitamin E (α-tocopherol), 20 IU/kg, SC or PO, q 24h [17] ▪ Vitamin B (thiamine), 5–10 mg/kg, IV or SC, q 24h [17] ▪ Allopurinol, 40 mg/kg, PO given within 4 h of insult in infants with HIE [102]
Reduce CNS edema	▪ Dimethyl sulfoxide (DMSO), 0.5–1 g/kg as 10% solution over 20 min, IV, q 12–24h [17] ▪ Mannitol, 0.25–1.0 g/kg, warmed, as a 20% solution over 20 min, IV, q 12–24h [78] ▪ 7.5% hypertonic saline (4 mL/kg) has been used to reduce cerebral edema

Table 32.VIII.2 (Continued)

Body system	Treatment
Excitotoxicity (block NMDA receptor)	▪ Magnesium sulfate, 0.05 g/kg/h for first hour, then 0.025 g/kg/h, IV, CRI [103] ▪ Ketamine, dose unknown (unknown efficacy in foals with NE)
Gastrointestinal support	▪ Omeprazole, 4 mg/kg, PO, q 24h ▪ Sucralfate, 20–40 mg/kg, PO, q 6h ▪ Bismuth subsalicylate, 0.5–4.0 ml/kg, PO, q6–24h ▪ Prokinetic therapy Lidocaine, 1.3 mg/kg slow IV over 10 min, then 0.05 mg/kg/min, IV, CRI Bethanechol, 0.025 mg/kg, SC once, then 0.35 mg/kg, PO, q 8h; or 0.22–0.45 mg/kg, PO, q 6–8h Metoclopramide, 0.1–0.3 mg/kg, IV over 30 min, q 6h or 0.04 mg/kg/h, IV, CRI 0.1–0.25 mg/kg, PO, q 6h
Renal support	▪ Furosemide, 1 mg/kg, IV q 12–24h, or 0.12 mg/kg IV, loading dose then 0.12 mg/kg/h CRI ▪ Fenoldopam, 0.04 µg/kg/min, IV, CRI ▪ Mannitol, 0.5–1.0 g/kg, IV as a 20% solution over 20 min ▪ Consider closed urinary catheter and collection system if foal is recumbent
Miscellaneous	▪ Pentoxyfilline, 10 mg/kg, PO, q 12h as an anti-inflammatory ▪ Rope restraint/squeeze procedure [104, 105]

not a consistent finding on microscopic examination of foals with NE [9, 26, 113]. Dimethyl sulfoxide (DMSO) has been used ubiquitously in equine practice for its purported ability to scavenge free-radicals, reduce edema and act as an anti-inflammatory, but its efficacy unsubstantiated. Interestingly, a retrospective study in 94 foals with NE reported no significant difference in surviving and non-surviving foals that were administered mannitol, magnesium sulfate, vitamin E or DMSO [9]. While providing supportive care, attempts should be made to maintain recumbent foals in sternal recumbency to facilitate ventilation of both lung fields. The use of a "V"-pad is helpful for this purpose (Figure 32.VIII.8). Recumbent foals are also prone to skin abrasions/ulcers, especially if the skin is moist from urine pooling around the recumbent foal. Provision of soft bedding with clean dry blankets along and placement of a closed urinary catheter collection system helps prevent skin trauma and ulceration. Assessment of passive transfer of maternal antibodies should be evaluated as many NE foals fail to ingest enough colostrum and IV administration of equine plasma can be necessary.

Expanding on the theory that some foals have clinical signs of NE due to altered levels of consciousness as a result of abnormal neurosteroid concentrations, several studies have evaluated the rope restraint/squeeze procedure to evaluate if this procedure alters the foal's behavior and neurosteroid concentrations. The basis of this technique is that it mimics the fetal-neural reflex that occurs during parturition (e.g. labor-induced physical compression or squeezing of the fetus), thus activating the HPAA, modifying the neurosteroid profile and signaling the transition from in utero unconsciousness to extrauterine activity. The physical compression that occurs during parturition might be associated with changes in neurosteroid concentrations and consequent activity level [104, 105].

Part of this concept was tested in eight healthy neonatal foals in which a soft linen rope was secured around each foal's neck and under the shoulder and then looped around the thorax and abdomen using half-hitch knots positioned directly on the dorsal thoracolumbar area (Figure 32.VIII.9) [104]. Gentle pulling on the rope from behind the foal produced a generalized squeezing of the foal and the tension on the rope was maintained for 15–20 minutes [104, 105]. During the restraint, foals assumed lateral recumbency with relaxed, somnolent behavior in conjunction with a significant decrease in heart and respiratory rate and rectal temperature. Electroencephalographic recordings revealed patterns suggestive of slow wave sleep and plasma ACTH, β-endorphin, dehydroepiandrosterone sulfate and androstenedione concentrations significantly increased during restraint, compared to prerestraint values [104]. In a follow-up study, surveys were completed by equine clinicians who provided observational data in foals with NE that were treated with standard medical treatment only (nonsqueezed group) compared to the squeeze procedure with or without medical therapy (squeezed group) [105]. Respondents (51 clinicians) provided information on 195 foals with

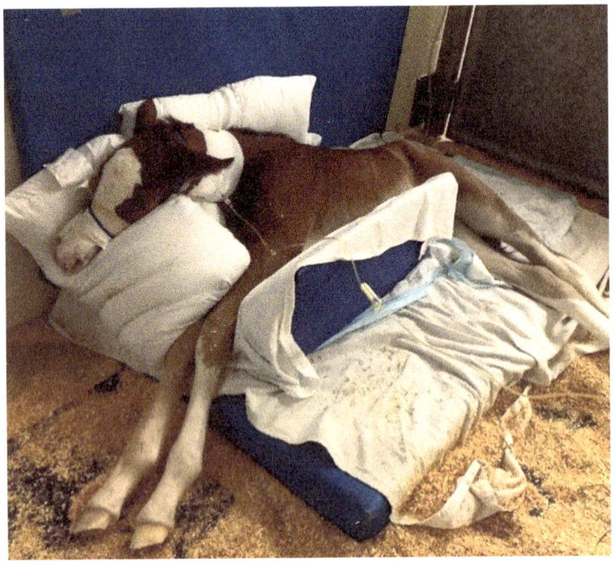

Figure 32.VIII.8 Neonatal foal with NE placed in a V-trough padded mat to help facilitate sternal recumbency. *Source:* Photo courtesy of Dr. Kathryn Johnson, Iowa State University.

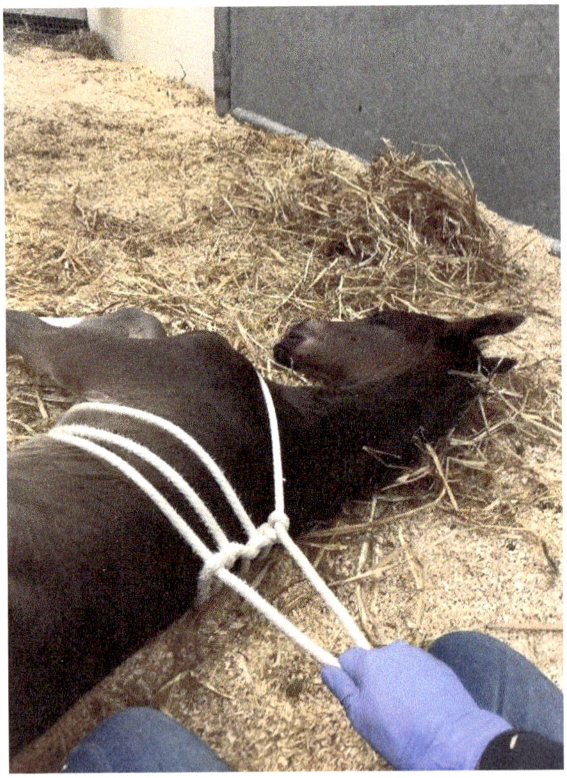

Figure 32.VIII.9 Neonatal foal demonstrating placement of a rope around the thorax to perform the rope restraint/squeeze technique. *Source:* Photo courtesy of Dr. Kathryn Johnson, Iowa State University.

NE (108 nonsqueezed; 87 squeezed). Based on the survey, foals that received the squeeze procedure with or without medical therapy had significantly faster recovery rates, were 3.7 times more likely to recover faster and 15 times more likely to recover in less than 1 hour compared to foals that were not squeezed [105]. The study suggested that foals that were squeezed for 20 minutes had significantly faster and higher recovery rates than foals that did not receive the procedure. However, several limitations were noted in this study, including nonblinded evaluations and variable medical treatments, but the authors proposed that the pressure from the birth canal that the fetus is exposed to during stage 2 of labor might influence the balance of neurosteroids and play a role in the neonatal transition from neuroinhibition to neuroactivation. Thus, simulation of stage 2 labor with the rope restraint may reset the balance of these neurosteroids and expedite recovery from NE thus facilitating normal behavior in the neonatal foal. Variable success has been seen with this technique however it is a safe procedure to consider for foals without evidence of perinatal ischemia [104, 105]. Further understanding of neurosteroid physiology may lead to other therapeutic options for NE foals.

Many foals with NE will respond to the aforementioned treatment suggestions within 3–5 days and have a complete recovery. However, other therapies can be considered with more complicated or severe cases of NE. Numerous medications have been suggested, mainly for infants with NE, that target specific pathophysiologic mechanisms that may be involved with the development of NE. As excitotoxicity has been implicated in the pathogenesis of NE, medications that block glutamate release or glutamate receptors have been examined. As calcium influx is necessary for glutamate release at presynaptic nerve endings, calcium channel blockers (flunarizine, nimodipine) have been administered to inhibit glutamate release in infants [106]. Magnesium is a more readily available calcium channel blocker that inhibits the NMDA receptor in infants with NE/HIE, but positive results have been inconsistent [61]. Magnesium sulfate has been used in neonatal foals with NE, however, no data is available as to its impact in either retrospective or prospective studies [17, 22]. Interestingly, one study found that NE foals with PAS actually had higher total magnesium concentrations then healthy or septic foals [114]. Ketamine, typically used as a dissociative anesthetic, also acts as a noncompetitive NMDA receptor antagonist that crosses the BBB and binds with the NMDA receptor-ion channel, thus blocking calcium conductance through the receptor channel [115]. In an experimental HI model in rats, ketamine administration provided partial protection to the brain [115]. Ketamine has been used anecdotally in foals with NE in attempts to halt seizures and block NMDA receptors but the benefit of this therapy is unknown. Another drug being investigated in people is xenon, which is used as a general anesthetic and has a high infinity for NMDA receptors. Clinical trials are ongoing with promising findings as it is protective against ischemia and not neurotoxic [116, 117].

Reducing or neutralizing ROS with medications such as allopurinol (xanthaine oxidase inhibitor), desferrioxamine (iron chelator), superoxide reductase, DMSO, and antioxidants (vitamin E, vitamin C, melatonin) have also been considered for treatment of NE [17, 21, 106, 108, 118–120]. A small study noted no adverse effects in foals administered a single oral dose of allopurinol (40 mg/kg), but pharmacokinetic data and effect on ROS was not examined [102]. Conversely, some studies have examined the neuroprotective effects of hyperbaric oxygen therapy in the treatment of NE and have shown that it reduces apoptosis, promotes neuronal stem cells, and enhances oxygen-free radical scavengers and delivery of oxygen to the brain [121, 122]. Hyperbaric oxygen therapy in infants decreases concentrations of malondialdehyde and NO and increases superoxide dismutase, all of which lead to improvement of neurologic assessment [123]. Hyperbaric oxygen therapy in NE foals has been documented to a limited extent with positive results [124].

Other medications evaluated in infants and animal models of NE include erythropoietin (anti-inflammatory, anti-apoptotic factors, angiongenesis, neurogenesis), melatonin (anti-inflammatory, anti-apoptotic, antioxidant), topiramate (glutamate receptor [AMPA, kainite] inhibition, blocks Na^+ channels and activates Ca^{++} currents), N-acetylcysteine (clears free radicals, restores glutathione levels, anti-inflammatory, reduces NO activity), edaravone (free radical scavenger), insulin-like growth factor-1 (anti-apoptotic), stem cells (modulate inflammation), azithromycin (neuroprotectant), monosialoganglioside (protect against apoptotic injury), docosahexaenoic acid (neuroprotectant), argon (neuroprotectant), and cannabinoids (decreased excitotoxicity), but remain to be evaluated in foals [125–128].

Unfortunately, there are no studies investigating the impact of majority of the medications noted above on the outcome of NE in foals. The clinician must realize that these have theoretical benefits, but their use is speculative and anecdotal. Therapeutic objectives of good supportive care, correction of clinicopathologic alterations, provision of nursing care, and medications that support or target abnormalities in other organ systems have remained the cornerstones of treatment over the years.

Prognosis

The prognosis for survival and athletic function in foals with a primary diagnosis of NE is typically good (range 70–80%), but also depends upon whether they are Category 1 (later onset) or Category 2 (signs present from birth) along with the presence or absence of complications [9, 75–79, 113]. The prognosis is poorer in foals that demonstrate clinical signs at the time of birth, have evidence of brain stem or spinal cord involvement, have multiple organs affected by HI injury, have complicating factors such as sepsis, remain comatose or are difficult to arouse, show no improvement in neurologic function in the first 5 days or have severe recurrent seizures [17, 75, 76]. The APGAR score is used in human infants to determine the severity of brain injury and has been modified to evaluate mentation and prognosis of neonatal foals, although is not commonly used [79, 80]. Recumbency was significantly associated with non-survival in one retrospective study (94 foals with NE) [9] and a different retrospective study (78 foals with NE) noted that neurologic signs lasted 1 day in 29 foals (29/59 foals that survived; 49%), 2 days in 17 foals (17/59; 29%), 3 days in 8 foals (13.5%), 4 days in 4 foals (6.8%), and 5 days in 1 foal (1/59; 1.7%); 19/78 foals (24%) did not survive [1]. A study by Lyle-Dugas et al., showed that high total serum calcium and low alkaline phosphatase activity were positively associated with survival in foals with NE, while foals treated with inotropes (indication of generalized hypoperfusion) was associated with mortality [9]. Rare long-term neurologic deficits including the inability to suckle from the mare, prolonged visual impairment, residual spasticity, recurrent seizures, and docility as adults have been reported [1, 77].

Necropsy

Gross necropsy findings of foals with NE have shown congestion, edema, hemorrhage, and necrosis of different areas of the brain. Microscopically, swelling, edema, necrosis, and malacia, along with neuronal and glial cell necrosis and apoptosis have been documented. In a retrospective study of foals with NE in which necropsy was performed, 10/11 foals had histological evidence of neuronal necrosis and/or degermation within the CNS consistent with ischemia [9]. In another study involving 18 foals with NE, necrosis of the cerebral cortex and local hemorrhage was noted in 9/18 foals [29], whereas neuronal necrosis of the gray matter of the cerebral cortex, caudate nuclei, thalamus, hippocampus, cerebellar cortex, and medulla oblongata was reported in 3 foals with NE in another report [113]. These lesions are similar to findings in experimental models of HIE in other animals, but the clinician must note that a selection bias toward the most severe cases of NE are typically examined microscopically, as many of the less-severe cases survive [22]. Neuronal and glial necrosis does not necessarily mean the pathophysiology is solely HI, but can also be caused by excitotoxicity or inflammation [22]. Not all foals that show signs of NE have lesions on postmortem examination [81]. In one study, many foals were reported to have a normal parturition, which suggests that other mechanisms may have triggered the findings at postmortem examination [18]. Lesions seen in other organs are variable and depend on the duration of clinical signs and comorbidities [81].

Prevention

Some risk factors for NE have been identified in the foal, but preventative measures need to focus on the health of the mare. Prevention of placentitis, and if present, treatment, decreasing inflammatory mediators during pregnancy, observation of parturition, and assistance if needed, are all actions that can help prevent NE. Preventive actions for the foal revolve around recognition of distress and initiating appropriate therapy such as oxygen supplementation, nutritional support, and fluid therapy. Neurosteroids may in the future become a preventative treatment for neonatal foals suffering from NE, but further research is needed before this therapy can be instituted.

Summary

Equine NE is one of the most common noninfectious neurologic conditions of neonatal foals. The diagnosis is based on history and clinical signs. Hypoxia-ischemia and endocrine imbalances (progestogens, neurosteroids) are likely major contributors to equine NE, but much research is still needed to help elucidate the pathophysiology. Lack of evidence and controversy surrounds specific treatments for NE; however, there is consensus that treatment should be directed at clinical signs. Clinicians should also be aware of the potential for damage to body systems outside the CNS because organs with high metabolic demands are often damaged in association with NE. Maintenance of the health of the mare, recognizing equine neonatal distress, along with supportive care are all key to management of NE.

References

1 Bernard, W., Reimer, J., and Cudd, T. (1995). Historical features, clinicopathologic findings, clinical features and outcome of equine neonates presenting with or developing signs of central nervous system disease. *Proc. Am. Assoc. Equine Pract.* 41: 222–224.
2 Reynolds, E.B. (1930). Clinical notes on some conditions met within the mare following parturition and in the newly born foal. *Vet. Rec.* 10: 277–280.
3 Baird, J.D. (1973). Neonatal maladjustment syndrome in a thoroughbred foal. *Aust. Vet. J.* 49: 530–534.
4 Cosgrove, J.S.M. (1955). The veterinary surgeon and the newborn foal. *Vet. Rec.* 97: 967.
5 Dickey, E.J., Long, S.N., and Hunt, R.W. (2011). Hypoxic ischemic encephalopathy–what can we learn from humans? *J. Vet. Intern. Med.* 25: 1231–1240.
6 Diesch, T.J. and Mellor, D.J. (2013). Birth transitions: pathophysiology, the onset of consciousness and possible implications for neonatal maladjustment syndrome in the foal. *Equine Vet. J.* 45: 656–660.
7 Galvin, N. and Collins, D. (2004). Perinatal asphyxia syndrome in the foal: review and a case report. *Ir. Vet. J.* 57: 707–714.
8 Gold, J.R. (2017). Perinatal asphyxia syndrome. *Equine Vet. Educ.* 29: 158–164.
9 Lyle-Dugas, J., Giguere, S., Mallicote, M.F. et al. (2017). Factors associated with outcome in 94 hospitalized foals diagnosed with neonatal encephalopathy. *Equine Vet. J.* 49: 207–210.
10 Estell, K.E., Aleman, M., Pickles, K.J. et al. (2013). Clinical signs, neurobehavioral score and electroencephalography recordings associated with infusion of pregnenolone derivative to induce neonatal maladjustment syndrome. *J. Vet. Intern. Med.* 27: 663–664.
11 Mahaffey, L.W. and Rossdale, P.D. (1957). Convulsive and allied syndrome in newborn foals. *Vet. Rec.* 69: 1277–1289.
12 Rossdale, P.D. (1967). Clinical studies on the newborn thoroughbred foal. Perinatal behaviour. *Br. Vet. J.* 123: 470–481.
13 Rossdale, P.D. (1968). Abnormal perinatal behaviour in the thoroughbred horse. *Br. Vet. J.* 124: 540–553.
14 Rossdale, P.D. (1969). Clinical studies on 4 newborn Thoroughbred foals suffering from convulsions with special reference to blood gas chemistry and pulmonary ventilation. *Res. Vet. Sci.* 10: 279–291.
15 Rossdale, P.D. (1970). The adaptive processes of the newborn foal. *Vet. Rec.* 87: 37–38.
16 Rossdale, P.D. (1972). Modern concepts of neonatal disease in foals. *Equine Vet. J.* 4: 117–128.
17 Wong, D., Wilkins, P.A., Bain, F.T. et al. (2011). Neonatal encephalopathy in foals. *Compend. Contin. Educ. Vet.* 33: E5.
18 Palmer, A.C. and Rossdale, P.D. (1975). Neuropathology of the convulsive foal syndrome. *J. Reprod. Fertil Suppl.* 23: 691–694.
19 Clement, S.F. (1987). Convulsive and allied syndromes of the neonatal foal. *Vet. Clin. North Am. Equine Pract.* 3: 333–344.
20 MacKay, R.J. (2005). Neurologic disorders of neonatal foals. *Vet. Clin. North Am. Equine Pract.* 21: 387–406.

21 Hess-Dudan, F. and Rossdale, P.D. (1996). Neonatal maladjustment syndrome and other neurological signs in the newborn foal: part 1. *Equine Vet. Educ.* 8: 24–32.

22 Toribio, R.E. (2019). Equine neonatal encephalopathy facts, evidence and opinions. *Vet. Clin. North Am. Equine Pract.* 35: 363–378.

23 Aleman, M., Pickles, K.J., Conley, A.J. et al. (2013). Abnormal plasma neuroactive progestogen derivatives in ill, neonatal foals presented to the neonatal intensive care unit. *Equine Vet. J.* 45: 661–665.

24 Rossdale, P.D., Ousey, J.C., McGladdery, A.J. et al. (1995). A retrospective study of increased plasma progestagen concentrations in compromised neonatal foals. *Reprod. Fertil. Dev.* 7: 567–575.

25 Yildez, E.P., Ekici, B., and Tatli, B. (2017). Neonatal hypoxic ischemic encephalopathy: an update on disease pathogenesis and treatment. *Expert Rev. Neurother.* 17: 449–459.

26 Badawi, N., Kurinczyk, J.J., Keogh, J.M. et al. (1988). Intrapartum risk factors for newborn encephalopathy: the Western Australian case-control study. *Br. Med. J.* 317: 1554–1558.

27 Shalak, L.F., Laptook, A.R., Jafri, H.S. et al. (2003). Clinical chorioamnionitis, elevated cytokines, and brain injury in term infants. *Pediatrics* 110: 673–680.

28 Liu, F. and McCullough, L.D. (2013). Inflammatory response in hypoxic ischemic encephalopathy. *Acta Phramacol. Sin.* 34: 1120–1130.

29 Ringer, N.C., Giguere, S., Morresey, P.R. et al. (2011). Biomarkers of brain injury in foals with hypoxic-ischemic encephalopathy. *J. Vet. Intern. Med.* 25: 132–137.

30 Allen, K.A. and Brandon, D.H. (2011). Hypoxic ischemic encephalopathy: pathophysiology and experimental treatments. *Newborn Infant Nurs. Rev.* 11: 125–133.

31 Fatemi, A., Wilson, M., and Johnston, M.V. (2009). Hypoxic ischemic encephalopathy in the term infant. *Clin. Pernatol.* 36: 835–838.

32 Periman, J.M. (2006). Summary proceedings from the neurology group on hypoxic-ischemic encephalopathy. *Pediatrics* 117: 28–33.

33 Volpe, J.J. (2001). Perinatal brain injury: from pathogenesis to neuroprotection. *Mental Retard. Dev. Disabil. Res. Rev.* 7: 56–64.

34 Cotton, C.M. and Shankaran, F.M. (2010). Hypothermia for hypoxic-ischemic encephalopathy. *Expert Rev. Obstet. Gynaecol.* 5: 227–239.

35 Greco, P., Nencini, G., Piva, I. et al. (2020). Pathophysiology of hypoxic-ischemic encephalopathy: a review of the past and a view of the future. *Acta Neurol. Belg.* 120: 277–288.

36 Shalak, L. and Perman, J.M. (2004). Hypoxic-ischemic brain injury in the term infant-current concepts. *Early Hum. Dev.* 80: 125–141.

37 Cho, K.H.T., Davidson, J.O., Dean, J.M. et al. (2020). Cooling and immunomodulation for treating hypoxic-ischemic brain injury. *Pediatr. Int.* 62: 770–778.

38 Alvarez-Diaz, A., Hilario, E., de Cerio, F.G. et al. (2007). Hypoxic-ischemic injury in the immature brain—key vascular and cellular players. *Neonatology* 92: 227–235.

39 Johnson, M.V., Ishida, A., Ishida, W.N. et al. (2009). Plasticity and injury in the developing brain. *Brain Dev.* 31: 1–10.

40 Iwata, O., Iwata, S., Thorton, J.S. et al. (2007). "Therapeutic time window" duration decreases with increasing severity of cerebral hypoxic-ischemia under normothermia and delayed hypothermia in newborn piglets. *Brain Res.* 1154: 173–180.

41 Laptook, A.R. (2009). Use of therapeutic hypothermia for term infants with hypoxic-ischemic encephalopathy. *Pediatr. Clin. North Am.* 56: 601–616.

42 Wong, D.M., Moore, R.M., and Brockus, C.W. (2012). Mechanisms of oxidative injury in equine diseases. *Compend. Contin. Educ. Equine* 34: E1–E8.

43 Buonocore, G. and Borenendaal, F. (2007). Anti-oxidant strategies. *Semin. Fetal Neonatal Med.* 79: 180–186.

44 Choi, D. and Rothman, S.M. (1990). The role of glutamate neurotoxicity in hypoxic ischemic neuronal death. *Ann. Rev. Neurosci.* 13: 171–182.

45 Ferriero, D.M. (2004). Neonatal brain injury. *N. Engl. J. Med.* 351: 1985–1995.

46 Magistretti, P.J. and Alleman, I. (2015). A cellular perspective on brain energy metabolism and functional imaging. *Neuron* 86: 883–901.

47 Palmer, C., Roberts, R.L., and Young, P.I. (2004). Timing of neutrophil depletion influences long-term neuroprotection in neonatal rat hypoxic-ischemic brain injury. *Pediatr. Res.* 55: 549–556.

48 Pasantes-Morales, H. and Vazquez-Juarez, E. (2012). Transporters and channels in cytotoxic astrocyte swelling. *Neurochem. Res.* 37: 2379–2387.

49 Stobart, J.L. and Anderson, C.M. (2013). Multifunctional role of astrocytes as gatekeepers of neuronal energy supply. *Front. Cell. Neurosci.* 7: 38.

50 Jakakumar, A.R. and Norenberg, M.D. (2010). The Na-K-Cl co-transporter in astrocyte swelling. *Metab. Brain Dis.* 25: 31–38.

51 Belanger, M., Allaman, I., and Magistretti, P.J. (2011). Brain energy metabolism: focus on the astrocyte-neuron metabolic cooperation. *Cell Metab.* 14: 724–738.

52 Brunton, P.J., Russell, J.A., and Hirst, J.J. (2014). Allopregnanolone in the brain: protecting pregnancy and birth outcomes. *Prog. Neurobiol.* 113: 106–136.

53 Aleman, M., McCue, P.M., Chigerwe, M. et al. (2019). Plasma concentrations of steroid precursors, steroids, neuroactive steroids, and neurosteroids in healthy

neonatal foals from birth to 7 days of age. *J. Vet. Intern. Med.* 33: 2286–2293.
54 Dembek, K.A., Timko, K.J., Johnson, L.M. et al. (2017). Steroids, steroid precursors, and neuroactive steroids in critically ill equine neonates. *Vet. J.* 225: 42–49.
55 Brunton, P.J. (2015). Programming the brain and behaviour by early-life stress: a focus on neuroactive steroids. *J. Neuroendocrinol.* 27: 468–480.
56 Hist, J.J., Kelleher, M.A., Walker, D.W. et al. (2014). Neuroactive steroids in pregnancy: key regulatory and protective roles in the foetal brain. *J. Steroid Biochem. Mol. Biol.* 139: 144–153.
57 Melcangi, R.C., Giatti, S., Pesaresi, M. et al. (2011). Role of neuroactive steroids in the peripheral nervous system. *Front. Endocrinol.* 2: 104.
58 Tuern, K.B. and Atey, T.M. (2017). Neuroactive steroids: receptor interactions and responses. *Front. Neurol.* 8: 422.
59 Reddy, D.S. and Estes, W.A. (2016). Clinical potential of neurosteroids for CNS disorders. *Trends Pharmacol. Sci.* 37: 543–561.
60 Longone, P., di Michele, F., D'Agati, E. et al. (2011). Neurosteroids as neuromodulators in the treatment of anxiety disorders. *Front. Endocrinol.* 2: 55.
61 Olsen, R.W. (2018). $GABA_A$ receptor: positive and negative allosteric modulators. *Neuropharmacology* 136: 10–22.
62 Wang, M. (2011). Neurosteroids and GABA-A receptor function. *Front. Endocrinol.* 2: 44.
63 Delelli, D. and Lambert, J.J. (2005). Neurosteroids: endogenous regulators of the GABA(A) receptor. *Nat. Rev. Neurosci.* 6: 565–575.
64 Selye, H. (1942). Studies concerning the correlation between anesthetic potency, hormonal activity and chemical structure among steroid compounds. *Curr. Res. Anesth. Analg.* 21: 41–47.
65 Merryman, W., Boiman, R., Barnes, L. et al. (1954). Progesterone anesthesia in human subjects. *J. Clin. Endocrinol. Metab.* 14: 1567–1569.
66 P'An, S.Y., Gardocki, J.F., Hutcheon, D.E. et al. (1955). General anesthetic and other pharmacological properties of a soluable steroid, 21-hydroxypregnanedione sodium succinate. *J. Pharmcol. Exp. Ther.* 115: 432–441.
67 Laubach, G.D., P'An, S.Y., and Rudel, H.W. (1955). Steroid anesthetic agent. *Science* 122: 78.
68 Madigan, J.E., Haggett, E.F., Pickles, K.J. et al. (2012). Allopregnanolone infusion induced neurobehavioural alterations in a neonatal foal: is this a clue to the pathogenesis of neonatal maladjustment syndrome? *Equine Vet. J. Suppl.* 41: 109–112.
69 Houghten, E., Holtan, D., Grainger, L. et al. (1991). Plasma progestagen concentrations in the normal and dysmature newborn foal. *J. Reprod. Fertil. Suppl.* 44: 609–617.
70 Mellor, D.J. (2010). Galloping colts, fetal feelings, and reassuring regulations: putting animal-welfare science into practice. *J. Vet. Med. Educ.* 37: 94–100.
71 Lu, H.Y., Zhang, Q., Wang, Q. et al. (2016). Contribution of histologic chorioamnionitis and fetal inflammatory response syndrome to increased risk of brain injury in infants with preterm premature rupture of membranes. *Pediatr. Neurol.* 61: 94–98.
72 Gussenhoven, R., Westerlaken, R.J.J., Ophelders, D.R.M.G. et al. (2018). Chorioamnionitis, neuroinflammation, and injury: timing is key in the preterm ovine fetus. *J. Neuroinflammation* 15: 113.
73 Anblagan, D., Pataky, R., Evans, M.J. et al. (2016). Association between preterm brain injury and exposure to chorioamnionitis during fetal life. *Sci. Rep.* 1: 37932.
74 Yellowhair, T.R., Noor, S., Maxwell, J.R. et al. (2018). Preclinical chorioamnionitis dysregulates CXCL1/CXCR2 signaling throughout the placental-fetal-brain axis. *Exp. Neurol.* 301: 110–119.
75 Furr, M. (1996). Perinatal asphyxia in foals. *Compend. Contin. Educ. Pract. Vet.* 18: 1342–1351.
76 Green, S. (1993). Current perspectives on equine neonatal maladjustment syndrome. *Compend. Contin. Educ. Vet.* 15: 1550–1552.
77 Valla, W. (1994). Peripartum asphyxia. *Vet. Clin. North Am. Equine Pract.* 10: 187–218.
78 Valla, W. (1999). Peripartum asphyxia syndrome in foals. *Proc. AAEP* 247–253.
79 Veronesi, M.C., Riccaboni, P., Faustini, M. et al. (2005). Potential association between placental features and Apgar scores after normal parturition in the Thoroughbred horse. *J. Am. Vet. Adv.* 4: 965–970.
80 Vaala, W.E. (2009). Perinatal asphyxia syndrome in foals. *Compend. Contin. Educ. Equine* 4: 134–140.
81 Gold, J.R., Chaffin, K., Burgess, B.A. et al. (2016). Factors associated with nonsurvival in foals diagnosed with perinatal asphyxia syndrome. *J. Equine Vet. Sci.* 38: 82–86.
82 Rossdale, P.D. (1993). Clinical view of disturbances in equine foetal maturation. *Equine Vet. J. Suppl.* 14: 3–7.
83 Pirrone, A., Panzani, S., Govoni, N. et al. (2013). Thyroid hormone concentrations in foals affected by perinatal asphyxia syndrome. *Theriogenology* 80: 624–629.
84 Chaney, K.P., Holcombe, S.J., Schott, H.C. et al. (2010). Spurious hypercreatininemia: 28 neonatal foals (2000–2008). *J. Vet. Emerg. Crit. Care* 20: 244–249.
85 Wong, D.M., Jeffery, N., Hepworth-Warren, K.L. et al. (2017). Magnetic resonance imaging of presumptive neonatal encephalopathy in a foal. *Equine Vet. Educ.* 29: 534–538.
86 Chaffin, M.K., Walker, M.A., McArthur, N.H. et al. (1997). Magnetic resonance imaging of the brain of normal neonatal foals. *Vet. Radiol. Ultrasound* 38: 102–111.

87 Ferrell, E.A., Gavin, P.R., Tucker, R.L. et al. (2002). Magnetic resonance for evaluation of neurologic disease in 12 horses. *Vet. Radiol. Ultrasound* 43: 510–516.

88 Barkovich, A.J., Westmark, K., Partridge, C. et al. (1995). Perinatal asphyxia: MR findings in the first 10 days. *Am. J. Neuroradiol.* 16: 427–438.

89 Massaro, A.N. (2015). MRI for neurodevelopmental prognostication in high-risk term infant. *Semin. Perinatol.* 39: 159–167.

90 Groenendaal, F. and de Vries, L.S. (2017). Fifty years of brain imaging in neonatal encephalopathy following perinatal asphyxia. *Pediatr. Res.* 81: 150–155.

91 Rutherford, M.A., Pennock, J.M., and Dubowitz, L.M. (1994). Cranial ultrasound and magnetic resonance imaging in hypoxic-ischaemic encephalopathy: a comparison with outcome. *Dev. Med. Child Neurol.* 36: 813–825.

92 Mackenzie, C.J., Haggett, E.F., Pinchbeck, G.L., and Marr, C.M. (2017). Ultrasonographic assessment of the atlanto-occipital space in healthy Thoroughbred foals and Thoroughbred foals with neonatal maladjustment syndrome. *Vet. J.* 223: 55–59.

93 Palmer, J.E. (2004). Fluid therapy in the neonate: not your mother's fluid space. *Vet. Clin. North Am. Equine Pract.* 20: 63–75.

94 Magdesian, K.G. and Madigan, J.E. (2003). Volume replacement in the neonatal ICU: crystalloids and colloids. *Clin. Tech. Equine Pract.* 2: 20–30.

95 Corley, K.T.T. (2004). Inotropes and vasopressors in adults and foals. *Vet. Clin. Equine* 20: 77–106.

96 Hepworth-Warren, K.L., Wong, D.M., Hay-Kraus, B.L. et al. (2015). Effects of administration of a synthetic low molecular weight/low molar substitution hydroxyethyl starch solution in healthy neonatal foals. *Can. Vet. J.* 56: 1069–1074.

97 Wong, D.M., Alcott, C.J., Wang, C. et al. (2010). Physiologic effects of nasopharyngeal administration of supplemental oxygen at various flow rates in healthy neonatal foals. *Am. J. Vet. Res.* 71: 1081–1088.

98 Giguere, S., Slade, J.K., and Sanchez, L.C. (2008). Retrospective comparison of caffeine and doxapram for the treatment of hypercapnia in foals with hypoxic–ischemic encephalopathy. *J. Vet. Intern. Med.* 22: 401–405.

99 Wilkins, P.A. (2005). How to use midazolam to control equine neonatal seizures. *Proc. Am. Assoc. Equine Pract.* 51: 279.

100 MacDonald, K.D., Hart, K.A., Davis, J.L. et al. (2018). Pharamacokinetics of the anticonvulsant levetiracetam in neonatal foals. *Equine Vet. J.* 50: 532–536.

101 Robertson, S.A. (1997). Sedation and general anaesthesia of the foal. *Equine Vet. Educ.* 9: 37–44.

102 de Araujo, L.O., Nogueira, C.E.W., Pazinato, F.M. et al. (2016). Oral single dose of allopurinol in Thoroughbred foals born from mares with placentitis. *Cienc. Rural* 46: 1119–1125.

103 Wilkins, P.A. (2004). Disorders in foals. In: *Equine Internal Medicine*, 2e (ed. S.M. Reed, W.M. Bayly, and D.C. Sellon), 1381–1440. St. Louis, MO: Saunders.

104 Toth, B., Aleman, M., Brosnan, R.J. et al. (2012). Evaluation of squeeze-induced somnolence in neonatal foals. *Am. J. Vet. Res.* 73: 1881–1889.

105 Aleman, M., Weich, K., and Madigan, J.E. (2017). Survey of veterinarians using a novel physical compression squeeze procedure in the management of neonatal maladjustment syndrome in foals. *Animals (Basel)* 7: 69.

106 Perlman, J.M. (2006). Intervention strategies for neonatal hypoxic-ischemic cerebral injury. *Clin. Ther.* 28: 1353–1356.

107 Calvert, J.W. and Zhang, J.H. (2005). Pathophysiology of a hypoxic-ischemic insult during the perinatal period. *Neurol. Res.* 27: 246–260.

108 Volpe, J.J. (2001). Perinatal brain injury: from pathogenesis to neuroprotection. *Mental Retard. Dev. Disabil. Res. Rev.* 7: 246–260.

109 Davies, A., Wassink, G., Bennet, L. et al. (2019). Can we further optimize therapeutic hypothermia for hypoxic-ischemic encephalopathy? *Neural Regener. Res.* 14: 1678–1683.

110 Vannucci, R.C. (1990). Current and potential new management strategies for perinatal hypoxic-ischemic encephalopathy. *Pediatrics* 85: 961–968.

111 Whitelaw, A. (2000). Systematic review of therapy after hypoxic-ischaemic brain injury in the perinatal period. *Semin. Neonatal* 5: 33–40.

112 Mujsce, D.J., Stern, D.R., Vannuccii, R.C. et al. (1988). Mannitol therapy in perinatal hypoxic-ischemic brain damage. *Ann. Nuerol.* 24: 338A.

113 Axon, J., Palmer, J.E., and Wilkins, P. (1999). Short- and long-term athletic outcome of neonatal intensive care unit survivors. *Proc. AAEP* 224–225.

114 Mariella, J., Isani, G., Andreani, G. et al. (2016). Total plasma magnesium in healthy and critically ill foals. *Theriogenology* 85: 180–185.

115 Spandou, E., Karkavelas, G., Soubasi, V. et al. (1999). Effect of ketamine on hypoxic-ischemic brain damage in newborn rats. *Brain Res.* 810: 1–7.

116 Ruegger, C.M., Davis, P.G., and Cheong, J.L. (2018). Xenon as an adjuvant to therapeutic hypothermia in near-term and term newborns with hypoxic-ischaemic encephalopathy. *Cochrane Database Syst. Rev.* (8): CD012753. https://doi.org/10.1002/14651858.CD012753.pub2.

117 Amer, A.R. and Oorschot, D.E. (2018). Xenon combined with hypothermia in perinatal hypoxic-ischemic encephalopathy: a noble gas a noble mission. *Pediatr. Neurol.* 84: 5–10.

118 Palmer, C., Roberts, R.L., and Bero, C. (1994). Deferoxamine posttreatment reduced ischaemic brain injury in neonatal rats. *Stroke* 25: 1039–1045.

119 Shahid, M., Beuoncore, G., Groenendaal, F. et al. (1998). Effect of deferoxamine and allopurinol on non-protein bound iron concentrations in plasma and cortical brain tissue of newborn lambs following hypoxia ischaemia. *Neurosci. Lett.* 22: 5–8.

120 Fan, X., Kaveklaars, A., Heijnen, C.J. et al. (2010). Pharmacological neuroprotection after perinatal hypoxic-ischaemic brain injury. *Curr. Neuropharmacol.* 8: 324–334.

121 Calvert, J.W., Yin, W., Patel, M. et al. (2002). Hyperbaric oxygenation prevented brain injury induced by hypoxia-ischemia in a neonatal rat model. *Brain Res.* 951: 1–8.

122 Liu, Z., Xiong, T., and Meads, C. (2006). Clinical effectiveness of treatment with hyperbaric oxygen for neonatal hypoxic-ischemic encephalopathy: systemic review of Chinese literature. *BMJ* 333: 374.

123 Zhou, B.Y., Ju, G.J., Huang, Y.Q. et al. (2008). Hyperbaric oxygen therapy under different pressures on neonatal hypoxic ischemic encephalopathy. *Zhonnguo Dang Dai Er Ke Za Zhi* 10: 133–135.

124 Slovis, N. (2008). Hyperbaric oxygen therapy in horses. *Proc. ACVIM* 150–152.

125 Greenwood, A., Evans, J., and Smit, E. (2018). New brain protection strategies for infants with hypoxic-ischaemic encephalopathy. *Paediatr. Child Health* 28: 405–411.

126 Nair, J. and Kumar, V.H.S. (2018). Current and emerging therapies in the management of hypoxic ischemic encephalopathy in neonates. *Children (Basel)* 5: 99.

127 Martinello, K., Hart, A.R., Yap, S. et al. (2017). Management and investigation of neonatal encephalopathy: 2017 update. *Arch. Dis. Child Fetal Neonatal Ed.* 102: F346–F358.

128 Barks, J.D.E., Liu, Y., Wang, L. et al. (2019). Repurposing azithromycin for neonatal neuroprotection. *Pediatr. Res.* 86: 444–451.

Section IX Idiopathic – Neonatal Epileptic Seizures

Emil Olsen

Epileptic seizures are common in the sick neonatal foal. If not successfully controlled, repeated, or constant seizure activity can lead to hyperthermia, permanent neuronal injury, acute kidney injury, rhabdomyolysis, and in the worst case, cardiac arrest.

Definitions

Established veterinary definitions for seizure classification and the various stages of a seizure are well described in companion animals by the International Veterinary Epilepsy Task Force with terminology adapted from the human International League Against Epilepsy (ILAE) [1–7]. This section seeks to implement these definitions in horses, with the objective of improving the consensus in equine internal medicine and neurology as well as standardize scientific reporting for seizures and epilepsy in horses.

Epilepsy is a pathologic state of the brain with a predisposition to generate epileptic seizures. In a more practical definition, the horse or foal needs to have at least two epileptic seizures more than 24 hours apart for it to be epilepsy. An epileptic seizure is a sudden onset transient and episodic clinical event representing abnormal forebrain electrical transmission as demonstrated via electroencephalogram (EEG). Epileptic seizures are brief and often last 15 seconds to 2–3 minutes. Neonatal seizures can be associated with a variety of disease processes, including vascular (hemorrhage, ischemic infarct), infectious/inflammatory (sepsis, bacterial, viral, fungal, or verminous meningoencephalomyelitis), traumatic (skull trauma, basisphenoid fracture), anatomic (porencephaly, hydrocephalus, lissencephaly), metabolic (kernicterus, hypoglycemia, hypocalcemia, hypernatremia, hypomagnesemia, transient hypoparathyroidism, portosystemic shunt), idiopathic (idiopathic epilepsy, neonatal encephalopathy, juvenile idiopathic epilepsy in Egyptian Arabian foals), neoplastic (teratoma), and degenerative (storage) disorders. Of these, more common causes of seizures in foals are neonatal encephalopathy, sepsis, and hypoglycemia. However, in many foals, the cause is not identified despite extensive diagnostic investigations. The epileptic seizure is characterized by synchronous rhythmic convulsions or focal motor, autonomic, or behavioral manifestations. Reactive or provoked seizures are: (i) a response to a transient disturbance of function by abnormal metabolic states or from a toxin [1], or (ii) provoked by an action such as approaching the foal or loud noises that causes the abnormal brain to react with abnormal electrical activity.

Idiopathic Epilepsy

Idiopathic epilepsy is an umbrella-term for three main etiologic subgroups: (i) *Idiopathic epilepsy* (genetic epilepsy) is a term used only when a gene for epilepsy has been identified; (ii) *idiopathic epilepsy* (suspected genetic epilepsy) can be utilized with increased breed prevalence (>2%) or familial accumulation of epileptic pets; and (iii) *idiopathic epilepsy* (epilepsy of unknown cause) [1], which is the most common in horses. Another etiologic subtype of epilepsy in companion animals is *structural epilepsy*. Structural epilepsy is more common in foals and is characterized by a primary cause such as vascular, infectious/inflammatory, traumatic, anomalous, neoplastic, or degenerative [1], all of which can be confirmed by diagnostic investigation, as described below.

Types of Epileptic Seizures

The two main types of epileptic seizures are *focal epileptic seizures* and *generalized epileptic seizures*. *Focal epileptic seizures* are characterized by lateralized clinical signs such as motor (facial twitches, repeated jerking of the head, repeated jerking of one extremity), autonomic

Equine Neonatal Medicine, First Edition. Edited by David M. Wong and Pamela A. Wilkins.

(hypersalivation, dilated pupils) and behavioral (restlessness, unexplainable fear reactions) changes. These focal epileptic seizures are a result of abnormal neuroelectric activity in a group of neurons within one hemisphere. In comparison, *generalized epileptic seizures* can evolve from a focal epileptic seizure or arise from both hemispheres with predominantly tonic, clonic, or tonic–clonic activity. An animal always loses consciousness during a generalized seizure, but this can be difficult to assess in the neonate. Salivation, urination, and/or defecation may occur during a generalized seizure [1]. Guidelines for definitions of epileptic seizures in human neonates [8] suggest modifications to the above described guidelines for classification because seizures in human neonates are different from adults. In one recent review, the most common causes of seizures in human infants were vascular events (stroke or hemorrhage), occurring in 45% of patients, and hypoxic ischemic encephalopathy, occurring in 25%. The drafted proposal of standardized terminology for human neonatal seizures suggests that there is no differentiation of focal or generalized seizures as most neonatal epileptic seizures in humans arise with focal manifestations. It is therefore proposed to establish a framework with three main seizure types in neonates: *motor* (automatisms, clonic activity, epileptic spasms, myoclonic jerks, sequential activity or tonic), *nonmotor* (autonomous nervous system, behavioral arrest), and *electrographic* (EEG confirmed). A different classification scheme has also been proposed to classify etiologies into hypoxic (neonatal maladjustment, hypoxic ischemic encephalopathy), structural (infarct, hemorrhage, trauma, malformations), infectious, metabolic, genetic, and unknown [8]. With seizures commonly seen in foals, a similar adaptation to equine neonates is reasonable.

Clinical Signs

Phases of an epileptic seizure are commonly described as *prodrome*, lasting from days to hours leading up to the seizure (with aggression, withdrawal, attention-seeking behavior), followed by the ictus (seizure activity) after which a post-ictal phase occurs (restoration of normal brain function), lasting minutes to days and commonly involve sleepiness, restlessness, hunger, thirst, blindness, confusion, or vocalization [1].

Clinical signs of seizures can be quite variable in foals; however, seizures can always be neurolocalized to the forebrain (cerebrum). Focal seizures in foals manifest as repeated jerking-head movements, rhythmic blinking, twitching of facial musculature, or repeated rhythmic jerking of one extremity. Focal seizures can progress to generalized seizures which have bilateral hemispheric involvement of the brain. Tonic, clonic, or tonic–clonic motor activity of all four legs, loss of consciousness, salivation, urination, and defecation can be observed with generalized seizures in foals and often evolve from focal seizure activity. In human neonates, subtle seizures are more common than generalized seizures and consist of: (i) ocular movements including rolling and nystagmus, (ii) oral-buccal and lingual movements such as sucking, smacking, chewing, or protruding of the tongue, and/or (iii) progressive movements, such as pedaling or thrashing, and long pauses in breathing [9]. In neonatal foals, it has been hypothesized that excessive stretching and repeated increases in extensor tone may be associated with subtle seizure activity, but this is poorly documented with EEG and appears to respond poorly to anti-epileptic drug therapy (AED).

Diagnostic Testing

Diagnostic testing to evaluate foals displaying epileptic seizures include assessment for primary etiologies noted above. Additional diagnostic tests are recommended soon after seizures are recognized to avoid missing any structural causes. Initial evaluation should include measurement of blood glucose, evaluation of the CBC, serum biochemistry profile (electrolytes, bile acids, liver enzymes, kidney parameters, muscle enzymes), venous or arterial blood gas analysis (pH, ionized calcium) and blood lactate, to aid in detection of any underlying infections or metabolic causes of seizures. Ideally EEG should be performed to document seizure activity. Behavior that can be confused with seizure activity include vestibular events with nystagmus and loss of balance, sometimes leading to the foal falling over. Vestibular events are commonly caused by vascular (infarct or hemorrhage) or infectious aetiologies. MRI and cerebrospinal fluid (CSF) analysis (total nucleated cell count, total protein, lactate, glucose) can help document anatomic causes or bacterial meningoencephalomyelitis, respectively. It is uncommon to obtain a positive bacterial culture from a CSF sample in foals with bacterial meningoencephalomyelitis; however, 1–3 ml of CSF may be added to a pediatric blood culture bottle to increase the odds of positive culture. In the author's opinion, a foal with multiple seizures over 24–48 hours with controlled systemic infection or no apparent cause should be anesthetized and an MRI of the brain with contrast should be performed; analysis of CSF should be collected while the foal is anesthetized for subsequent fluid analysis. Once a seizure focus is created in the brain, it may be more difficult to control with anti-epileptic medications, which lends to a poorer prognosis.

Treatment

Treatment of neonatal epileptic seizures target the cessation of seizure activity. For ease of implementation, this section is split into emergency and long-term management of foals with epileptic seizures. The objective of *emergency treatment* is stopping the seizure with sequential escalation in the drugs utilized. If the above diagnostic protocol is used and metabolic causes are demonstrated, it is imperative to address the primary cause, such as electrolyte abnormalities and hypoglycaemia first. If this does not resolve the seizure within 5 minutes of initiating treatment, the emergency protocol should be initiated. The question of when a foal should be treated for an epileptic seizure is often discussed. Treatment of a single seizure is initiated if it lasts over 2 minutes or the foal is seen after entering status epilepticus (≥5 minutes of ictal activity). First-line treatment includes midazolam or diazepam (Table 32.IX.1). Midazolam IV (or intranasally if no IV access exists) has been shown to shorten the seizure duration and reduce risk of a second in dogs compared to rectal administration of diazepam [10]. Administration of midazolam starts at a dose of 0.1 mg/kg and can be repeated several times with up to 0.2 mg/kg, IV or intranasally. The dose of diazepam starts at 0.1 mg/kg and can be increased with repeated dosing up to 0.5 mg/kg IV. If there is no effect, levetiracetam can be given as a single dose at 32 mg/kg or at a loading dose of 60 mg/kg IV or PO and thereafter repeated every 12 hours until at least 24 hours has evolved without seizures and the primary cause is under control. If the seizure activity is not controlled with these medications, or if seizures recur, the use of phenobarbital is appropriate and can be given as a single IV dose of 6.6 mg/kg or loaded using 4 mg/kg every 4 hours to effect up to a maximum of 12–16 mg/kg followed by a maintenance IV dose of 6.6 mg/kg every 12 hours [11]. A study in dogs suggests that if this does not resolve seizure activity, a constant rate infusion of midazolam may aid in seizure control at a dose of 0.2–0.3 mg/kg/h [12]. A propofol CRI at 0.15 mg/kg/min may be used for cases refractory to treatment with the above medications.

Once the seizure is controlled, consideration should be made whether AED therapy should be initiated for constant control. Recommendations for AED therapy in dogs and cats are: (i) seizures with identifiable structural lesion or prior history of brain disease or injury; (ii) status epilepticus with ictus lasting ≥5 minutes or ≥3 epileptic seizures occurring within a 24 hour period (so-called cluster); (iii) ≥2 or more epileptic seizure events within a 6-month period; or (iv) severe postictal signs [13]. For treatment beyond the emergency epileptic seizure, a first-choice treatment in neonatal foals is levetiracetam 32 mg/kg IV or PO q12h [14]. Levetiracetam is metabolized faster over time and as such, the effect may decrease and seizure frequency or severity may increase. Another option is phenobarbital, loaded to a total dose of 12–16 mg/kg over 24 hours, using 4 mg/kg every 4 hours until the loading dose is achieved. Thereafter 6.6 mg/kg IV is administered every 12 hours. When transitioning to oral therapy, a dose of 2–13 mg/kg has been described every 12 hours, preferably starting at the same dosage as used IV. Monitoring of therapeutic levels is essential after completion of loading and when it reaches steady state at 2 weeks, to adjust dosage and to control seizure activity. Therapeutic levels should be measured every 6 months to monitor drug concentrations and adjust dosage to a recommended blood concentration similar to that in dogs and cats (15–35 μg/ml) [13]. It is imperative to monitor for side effects, described in dogs but rarely in cats and poorly reported in

Table 32.IX.1 Treatment of epileptic seizures in foals, emergency treatment to stop a single seizure with the ictal phase lasting over 2 minutes or bring a foal out of status epilepticus (≥5 minutes of ictal activity).

Medication	Order[a]	Administration route	Dosage mg/kg	Max dosage mg/kg	Can be repeated # times	Dosage for loading	Frequency during load	Frequency after loading
Midazolam	1	IV	0.1	0.2	2	–	–	–
Midazolam	1	IN[b]	0.1	0.2	2	–	–	–
Diazepam	1	IV	0.1	0.5	2	–	–	–
Levetiracetam	2	IV/PO	32	60	2	60	once	Q12h
Phenobarbital	3	IV	6.6	12	3	4 mg/kg	Q4h	Q12h
Midazolam	4	IV	0.15[c]	1.0[c]	–	None	–	
Propofol	5	IV	0.15[d]	0.3[d]	–	–	CRI[d]	

References for the dosages can be found in the text above.

[a] Order of choice for emergency management. All order 1 medications have equal weight or priority. If a particular order 1 medication does not work, it can be swapped for another order 1 medication. If no effect, order 2 medications can be tried, and so forth.

[b] Intranasal (IN) administration, preferably with an atomizer.

[c] mg/kg/h.

[d] mg/kg/min as a Constant Rate Infusion (CRI).

horses, such as bone marrow depression, idiosyncratic anemia, and dose-dependent liver toxicity. A substantial sedative effect is expected in the first 10–14 days of therapy with phenobarbital [13].

There are no available protocols that outline discontinuation of AED therapy in equids; however, treatment is very costly and should be adjusted after evaluation of serum concentrations and as the foal increases in weight. If the primary cause of seizures is cured or controlled, the author recommends treating the foal for a seizure-free period of at least 4 weeks. Levetiracetam can be discontinued without a tapering dose whereas a 25% reduction in the phenobarbital dose is recommended every 2 weeks. The prognosis for survival is good to excellent with juvenile idiopathic epilepsy in Egyptian Arabic foals [15], but prognosis for other seizure conditions in foals are poorly described. In foals with neonatal encephalopathy, a seizure in the first 24 hours of life increases the likelihood of nonsurvival by 21 times [16].

References

1 Berendt, M., Farquhar, R.G., Mandigers, P.J.J. et al. (2015). International veterinary epilepsy task force consensus report on epilepsy definition, classification and terminology in companion animals. *BMC Vet. Res.* 11: 182.

2 Rusbridge, C., Long, S., Jovanovik, J. et al. (2015). International veterinary epilepsy task force recommendations for a veterinary epilepsy-specific MRI protocol. *BMC Vet. Res.* 11: 194.

3 Bhatti, S.F.M., De Risio, L., Muñana, K. et al. (2015). International veterinary epilepsy task force consensus proposal: medical treatment of canine epilepsy in Europe. *BMC Vet. Res.* 11: 176.

4 Volk, H.A. (2015). International veterinary epilepsy task force consensus reports on epilepsy definition, classification and terminology, affected dog breeds, diagnosis, treatment, outcome measures of therapeutic trials, neuroimaging and neuropathology in companion animals. *BMC Vet. Res.* 11: 174.

5 Potschka, H., Fischer, A., Löscher, W. et al. (2015). International veterinary epilepsy task force consensus proposal: outcome of therapeutic interventions in canine and feline epilepsy. *BMC Vet. Res.* 11: 177.

6 Matiasek, K., Pumarola, I., Batlle, M. et al. (2015). International veterinary epilepsy task force recommendations for systematic sampling and processing of brains from epileptic dogs and cats. *BMC Vet. Res.* 11: 216.

7 De Risio, L., Bhatti, S., Muñana, K. et al. (2015). International veterinary epilepsy task force consensus proposal: diagnostic approach to epilepsy in dogs. *BMC Vet. Res.* 11: 148.

8 Pressler, R.M., Cilio, M.R., Mizrahi, E.M. et al.(2018). The ILAE classification of seizures & the epilepsies: modification for seizures in the neonate. Proposal from the ILAE task force on neonatal seizures. http://www.saludinfantil.org/SubespecialidadesPediatricas/neurologia/Clasificacion%20Ilae.pdf (accessed 22 February 2023).

9 Martin, M., Querubin, J., Hagen, E. et al. (2020). Evaluation of the neonate with seizures. *Pediatr. Ann.* 49: e292–e298.

10 Charalambous, M., Bhatti, S.F.M., Van Ham, L. et al. (2017). Intranasal midazolam versus rectal diazepam for the management of canine status epilepticus: a multicenter randomized parallel-group clinical trial. *J. Vet. Intern. Med.* 31: 1149–1158.

11 Ravis, W.R., Duran, S.H., Pedersoli, W.M. et al. (1987). A pharmacokinetic study of phenobarbital in mature horses after oral dosing. *J. Vet. Pharmacol. Ther.* 10: 283–299.

12 Bray, K.Y., Mariani, C.L., Early, P.J. et al. (2020). Continuous rate infusion of midazolam as emergent treatment for seizures in dogs. *J. Vet. Intern. Med.* 35: 388–396.

13 Podell, M., Volk, H.A., Berendt, M. et al. (2016). 2015 ACVIM small animal consensus statement on seizure management in dogs. *J. Vet. Intern. Med.* 30: 477–490.

14 MacDonald, K.D., Hart, K.A., Davis, J.L. et al. (2018). Pharmacokinetics of the anticonvulsant levetiracetam in neonatal foals. *Equine Vet. J.* 50: 532–536.

15 Aleman, M., Gray, L.C., Williams, D.C. et al. (2006 Nov). Juvenile idiopathic epilepsy in Egyptian Arabian foals: 22 cases (1985–2005). *J. Vet. Intern. Med.* 20: 1443–1449.

16 Gold, J.R., Chaffin, K., Burgess, B.A. et al. (2016). Factors associated with nonsurvival in foals diagnosed with perinatal asphyxia syndrome. *J. Equine Vet. Sci.* 38: 82–86.

Section X Idiopathic – Narcolepsy in Foals

Jamie Kopper

Narcolepsy presents as excessive daytime sleepiness. In humans, narcolepsy typically occurs in conjunction with cataplexy (a brief and sudden loss of muscle tone that may result in collapse or partial paresis and is usually followed by a strong emotional response), sleep paralysis, and/or hypnagogic hallucinations [1]. However, some of these signs are difficult to assess in the horse. Narcolepsy with and without cataplexy has been described in several species in addition to people, including dogs, cattle, and horses with what appear to be both familial tendencies and sporadic cases.

The pathophysiology of narcolepsy remains unknown but is believed to be due to dysfunction of the brainstem, hypothalamus, limbic system, and/or striatum cortex [2, 3]. Hypocretin-1 levels play a role in some cases of human and canine narcolepsy, particularly those that are inherited, but a consistent role of hypocretin-1 has not been demonstrated in the horse. In one case report, elevated levels of a metabolite of norepinephrine and adrenergic neurons (MHPG) were found in an affected foal compared to normal foals and were hypothesized to play a role in clinical signs of disease [4]. However, a single unifying cause or abnormality has not been reported.

Clinical Signs

Onset of clinical signs can occur at any time from birth to the first several months of life in affected foals. Apparent familial tendencies have been reported in miniature foals [5], Lipizzaners [6] and sporadically in foals of other breeds [4, 7]. The exact mode of inheritance in horses is unknown. Foals with narcolepsy display excessive daytime sleepiness. This can present as paroxysmal sleep attacks with retention of muscle tone and reflexes [4]. Affected foals are often described as appearing in a "trance-like state" with a staggering gait [4]. Some affected foals also display apparent cataplexy in response to events interpreted as evoking an emotional response (i.e. resistance to handling, leaving the barn) [4–6].

Diagnostic Testing

Ultimately, a diagnosis of narcolepsy is made based on clinical signs and confirmation with provocative pharmacological testing [7, 8, 9]. As part of the examination, evidence of true sleep deprivation should be ruled out, including observation for overmothering by the mare, clinical examination for evidence of pain, and evaluation of the environment to ensure that environmental factors are not preventing the foal from getting appropriate sleep. Additionally, a thorough neurological examination to confirm appropriate neurolocalization and hematological evaluation (CBC, serum chemistry) should be performed to rule out any underlying disease. If collected, cerebral spinal fluid should be normal on cytological evaluation for foals with narcolepsy.

Pharmacological testing can be performed to confirm suspicions of narcolepsy after confirming that there is no evidence of underlying disease or sleep deprivation. Episodes or aggravation of narcolepsy can be induced with intravenous administration of physiostigmine (0.06 mg/kg IV) [4–6] and abated with intravenous administration of atropine sulfate (0.07 mg/kg) for up to 24 hours [4, 5]. Administering neostigmine, an anti-cholinesterase that does not cross the blood-brain barrier, with no effect rules out the possibility of peripheral neuromuscular dysfunction such as myasthenia gravis [5].

Equine Neonatal Medicine, First Edition. Edited by David M. Wong and Pamela A. Wilkins.

Treatment and Prognosis

Daily administration of imipramine hydrochloride has improved clinical signs of narcolepsy but did not appear to have an effect on cataplexy [5]. Of affected foals reported in the literature, many showed decreased frequency and severity of narcoleptic and cataplexic episodes with age, with improvement beginning around 6 months of age [5, 6] and/or with regular exercise [6].

References

1 Kales, A., Bueno, A.V., and Kales, J.D. (1987). Sleep disorders: sleep apnea and narcolepsy. *Ann. Intern. Med.* 106: 434–443.

2 Smith, K.M. and Cohen, F.L. (1988). Compound narcolepsy: development of biochemical imbalance. *Int. J. Neurosci.* 42: 229–252.

3 Strittmatter, M., Isenberg, E., Grauer, M.T. et al. (1996). CSF substance P stomatostatin and monoaminergic transmitter metabolites in patients with narcolepsy. *Neurosci. Lett.* 218: 99–102.

4 Bathen-Nothen, A., Heider, C., Fernandez, A.J. et al. (2009). Hypocretin measurement in an Icelandic foal with narcolepsy. *J. Vet. Intern. Med.* 23: 1299–1302.

5 Lunn, D.P., Cuddon, P.A., Shaftoe, S. et al. (1993). Familial occurrence of narcolepsy in miniature horses. *Equine Vet. J.* 25: 483–487.

6 Ludvikova, E., Nishino, S., Sakai, N. et al. (2012). Familial narcolepsy in the Lipizzaner horse: a report of three fillies born to the same sire. *Vet. Q.* 32: 99–102.

7 Sweeney, C.R., Hendricks, J.C., Beech, J. et al. (1983). Narcolepsy in a horse. *J. Am. Vet. Med. Assoc.* 183: 126–128.

8 Sweeney, C.R. and Hansen, T.O. (1987). Narcolepsy and epilepsy. In: *Current Equine Therapy* (ed. N.E. Robinson and W.B. Saunders), 349–353. Philadelphia PA: Saunders.

9 Mayhew, I.G. (1989). *Large Animal Neurology*, 137–139. Philadelphia PA: Lea and Febiger.

Section XI Autoimmune – Kernicterus

Rudy Madrigal

Kernicterus, or bilirubin encephalopathy, is an extremely rare condition in foals caused by the neurotoxic effects of unconjugated bilirubin (UB) on the central nervous system. The condition is characterized by elevated total bilirubin (hyperbilirubinemia), neurological deficits, and jaundice. Hyperbilirubinemia has been described in horses due to liver disease, glucose-6-phoshate dehydrogenase deficiency, intravascular hemolysis, and most commonly in foals, neonatal isoerythrolysis [1–3].

Bilirubin is formed by the breakdown of hemoglobin in senescent or hemolyzed red blood cells (RBCs). Degradation of heme leads to formation of biliverdin and carbon monoxide and release of iron. The biliverdin is reduced to water-insoluble unconjugated bilirubin (UB), primarily in macrophages, and subsequently transported in the blood ionically bound to albumin to the liver. Within the liver, UB is conjugated to glucuronic acid to form a nontoxic water-soluble molecule that is released in the bile into the small intestinal lumen [4]. Hyperbilirubinemia can be caused by increased production, deficiency of hepatic uptake, impaired hepatic conjugation of bilirubin or obstructive cholestasis [2, 5]. The most common cause of hyperbilirubinemia in foals is presumed increased production of bilirubin due to destruction of RBCs, as seen in neonatal isoerythrolysis (NI) [2].

Increased concentrations of circulating UB can enter different cell types and cross the more permeable neonatal blood–brain barrier (BBB). Albumin conjugated bilirubin is unable to cross the BBB; therefore, hypoalbuminemia increases the risk of kernicterus [6]. Unconjugated bilirubin is a substrate for an ATP-dependent plasma-membrane protein, P-glycoprotein, which is abundant in the BBB and normally limits influx into the central nervous system. With increased concentrations of UB, P-glycoprotein is overwhelmed, resulting in influx of bilirubin [4, 6, 7]. Other conditions including infection, acidosis, hyperoxia, sepsis, prematurity, and hyperosmolarity may also alter entry through the BBB. Bilirubin can lead to cellular injury and neurotoxic effects, with UB being more important than total bilirubin for cytotoxic effects. The duration of brain tissue exposure to increased concentrations of bilirubin is also an important determinant of neurotoxic effects [4]. A previous study noted that foals with total bilirubin of ≥27.0 mg/dl were 17 times more likely to develop neurologic problems compared to foals with lower total bilirubin concentrations [2]. The total bilirubin (TB) to albumin ratio (TB:A) and serum concentration of UB have been evaluated in order to better predict neurotoxicity prior to clinical signs; the protein binding of UB has been evaluated as a treatment to prevent or decrease clinical signs [8–10]. These parameters have currently not been evaluated in neonatal foals. The concentration of TB in which a foal may develop neurotoxicity is variable, as it is in infants, although both the concentration of TB and length of time of the elevation are also important variables [11].

Neurotoxicity is due to bilirubin's affinity for membrane phospholipids and inhibition of uptake of tyrosine (a marker of synaptic transmission) and inhibition of *N*-methyl-D-aspartate (NMDA) receptor ion channels, which may lead to interference with neuroexcitatory signals and impaired nerve conduction [4]. This occurs in selective regions of the brain, with studies showing primarily brainstem nuclei, the auditory, oculomotor, and vestibular region; motor control in the basal ganglia; and Purkinje cells. Rodent models have shown that these areas appear to be more commonly affected due to greater and longer-lasting accumulations of UB [12]. Further mechanisms by which bilirubin exerts damaging effects include inhibition of mitochondrial enzymes and functions, interference with DNA synthesis, induction of DNA-strand breakage and inhibition of protein synthesis and phosphorylation [4, 6]. Macroscopic pathologic changes of kernicterus in infants include brain edema, severe jaundice, yellow staining of the basal nuclei, hepatomegaly and splenomegaly; some of

Equine Neonatal Medicine, First Edition. Edited by David M. Wong and Pamela A. Wilkins.

these changes have been noted in the few reports of kernicterus in foals [13, 14]. Histopathologic changes such as necrosis of cerebral neurons, Purkinje cell necrosis and loss, yellow pigment in the cerebellar granular cell layer, and deposition of variable amounts of yellow pigment in other organ systems have been noted in infants and foals. Figures 32.XI.1–32.XI.5. show histopathologic abnormalities in a 5-day-old foal with kernicterus [13, 14].

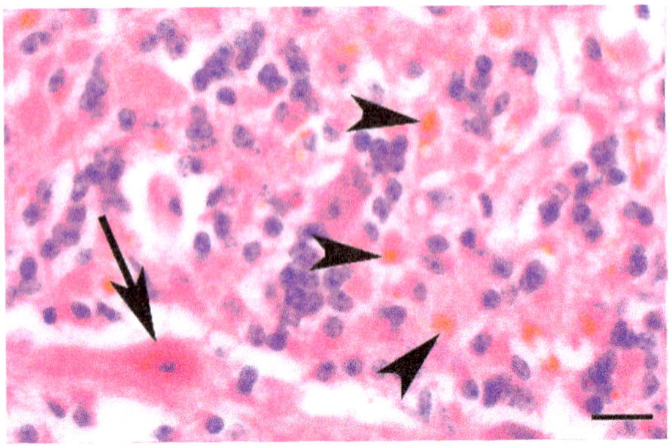

Figure 32.XI.1 Cerebellum, Purkinje, and granular cell layers. Purkinje cell necrosis (arrow) and granular cell layer contains yellow pigment (arrowheads). Bar = 20 μm.

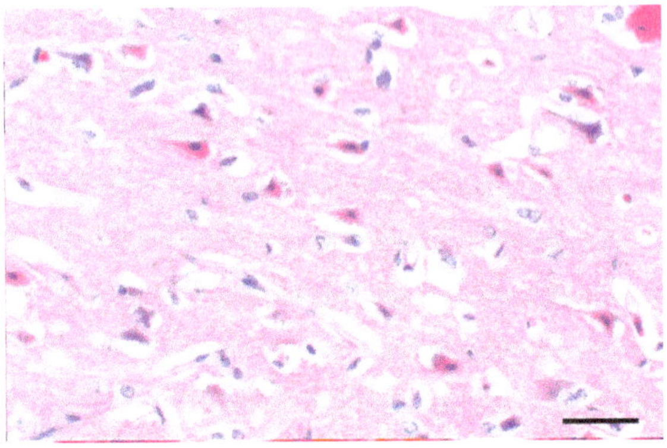

Figure 32.XI.2 Cerebrum, moderate numbers of necrotic neurons. Bar = 40 μm.

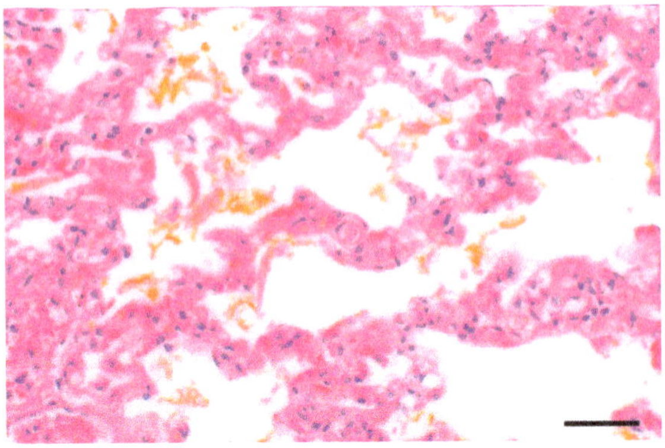

Figure 32.XI.3 Lung, amorphous strands of yellow pigment within alveolar spaces, often lining alveolar septa. Bar = 40 μm.

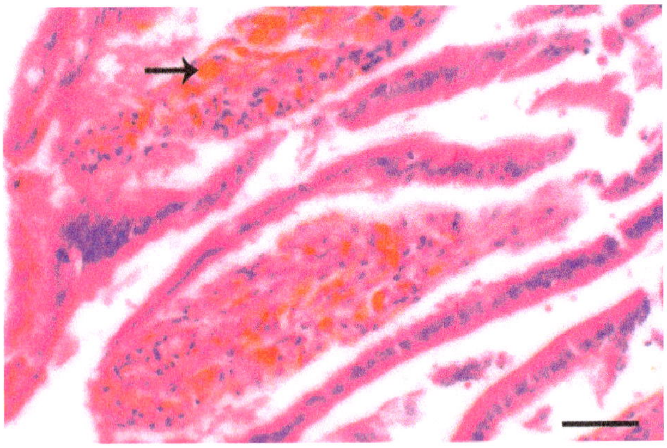

Figure 32.XI.4 Small intestine, yellow pigment throughout extracellular lamina propria and within macrophages (arrow). Bar = 40 μm. *Source:* Images from Loynachan et al. [13].

Clinical signs associated with the acute phase of hyperbilirubinemia in infants include neurologic deficits such as seizures, hypotonia, hypertonia, opisthotonos, setting-sun gaze (paresis of upward gaze) with eyelid retraction, and facial dystonia, making them appear stunned or scared [13]. Apnea has also been reported. Long-term, infants may experience motor dysfunction, auditory deficits with or without hearing loss, oculomotor impairments, and dysplasia of the enamel of deciduous teeth [15]. Bilateral absent brainstem auditory evoked response (BAER) testing has been reported in a foal with NI (with suspected kernicterus) and subsequent death in the foal [16]. Other clinical findings and signs in foals with kernicterus include those associated with NI (lethargy, weakness, decreased suckling, anemia, icterus, hyperbilirubinemia) along with marked seizure activity and possibly opisthotonus [13, 14]. Anemia is commonly reported in foals with hyperbilirubinemia ranging up to 45 mg/dl [13]. In one case report, cerebrospinal fluid (CSF) was collected from a foal with kernicterus immediately after death; the CSF was bright yellow and had increased white blood cells (28 cells/μl; normal, 0–8 cells/μl) and RBCs (65 cells/μl, normal 0 cells/μl). The majority of these cells were mononuclear cells, with a few containing yellow granules presumed to be bilirubin [14].

The primary treatment of kernicterus in infants is phototherapy during the acute phase and supportive care [1]. Rodent models using albumin administration have shown a neuroprotective role in acute hyperbilirubinemia [17]. Other novel treatments being investigated include hypothermia, caffeine, and minocycline [18–23]. Because foals with kernicterus likely have concurrent NI, whole blood transfusion should be considered to improve perfusion and oxygen-carrying capacity to organs [24]. Other therapies such as antioxidants (vitamins C, B_1, and E), plasma

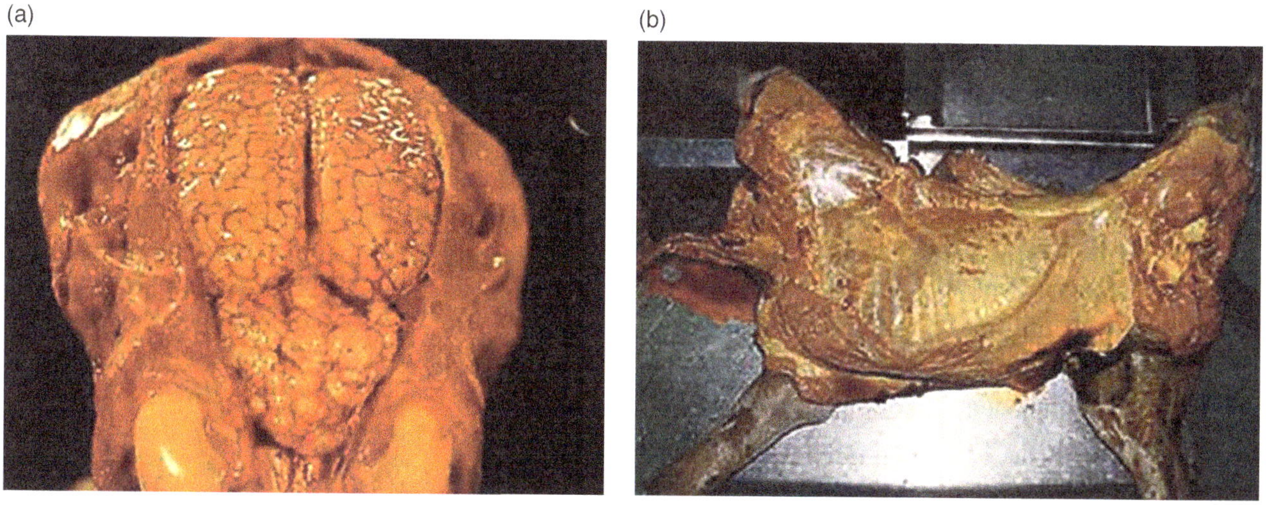

Figure 32.XI.5 Severe icterus of the leptomeningeal surface of the brain (a) and generalized icterus throughout the soft tissues (b) of a 4-day old foal with neonatal isoerythrolysis and kernicterus. *Source:* Images from J.B. David and T. Byars [14].

transfusion to increase protein binding, and supportive care may be attempted [24, 25]. Although not widely available, plasma exchange has been successfully reported in two neurologically normal foals for the treatment of hyperbilirubinemia [24]. In these two cases, plasma exchange was performed with a commercial plasmapheresis device, which withdraws blood from the foal, automatically separates plasma from RBCs by filtration, and subsequently returns RBCs to the patient, along with replacement plasma (3 l) from an equine donor [24]. While most therapies have been shown successful in rodent models, in-vitro studies, and limited peer review data in infants, the efficacy of any of these therapies is unknown in foals. The overall prognosis of kernicterus in foals appears to be guarded to poor, but few reported cases are available to formulate an accurate assessment of prognosis [13, 14, 25].

References

1 Riordan, S.M. and Shapiro, S.M. (2020). Review of bilirubin neurotoxicity I: molecular biology and neuropathology of disease. *Pediatr. Res.* 87: 327–331.

2 Polkes, A.C., Giguère, S., Lester, G.D. et al. (2008). Factors associated with outcome in foals with neonatal isoerythrolysis (72 cases, 1988–2003). *J. Vet. Intern. Med.* 22: 1216–1222.

3 Stockham, S.L., Harvey, J.W., and Kinden, D.A. (1994). Equine glucose-6-phosphate dehydrogenase deficiency. *Vet. Pathol.* 31: 518–527.

4 Dennery, P.A., Seidman, D.S., and Stevenson, D.K. (2001). Neonatal hyperbilirubinemia. *N. Engl. J. Med.* 344: 581–590.

5 Watchko, J.F. (2006). Neonatal hyperbilirubinemia – what are the risks? *N. Engl. J. Med.* 354: 1947–1949.

6 Calligaris, S.D., Bellarosa, C., Giraudi, P. et al. (2007). Cytotoxicity is predicted by unbound and not total bilirubin concentration. *Pediatr. Res.* 62: 576–580.

7 Watchko, J.F., Daood, M.J., and Hansen, T.W. (1998). Brain bilirubin content is increased in P-glycoprotein-deficient transgenic null mutant mice. *Pediatr. Res.* 44: 763–766.

8 Hulzebos, C.V., Van Imhoff, D.E., Bos, A.F. et al. (2008). Usefulness of the bilirubin/albumin ratio for predicting bilirubin-induced neurotoxicity in premature infants. *Arch. Dis. Child. Fetal Neonatal Ed.* 93: 384–388.

9 Hulzebos, C.V. and Dijk, P.H. (2014). Bilirubin-albumin binding, bilirubin/albumin ratios, and free bilirubin levels: where do we stand? *Semin. Perinatol.* 38: 412–421.

10 Amin, S.B. and Wang, H. (2018). Bilirubin albumin binding and unbound unconjugated hyperbilirubinemia in premature infants. *J. Pediatr.* 192: 47–52.

11 Zhang, F., Chen, L., Shang, S. et al. (2020). A clinical prediction rule for acute bilirubin encephalopathy in neonates with extreme hyperbilirubinemia: a retrospective cohort study. *Medicine (United States)* 99: 1–5.

12 Gazzin, S., Zelenka, J., Zdrahalova, L. et al. (2012). Bilirubin accumulation and Cyp mRNA expression in selected brain regions of jaundiced Gunn rat pups. *Pediatr. Res.* 71: 653–660.

13 Loynachan, A.T., Williams, N.M., and Freestone, J.F. (2007). Kernicterus in a neonatal foal. *J. Vet. Diagn. Invest.* 19: 209–212.

14 David, J.B. and Byars, T. (1988). Kernicterus in a foal with neonatal isoerythrolysis. *The Compendium* 20: 517–520.
15 Das, S. and van Landeghem, F.K.H. (2019). Clinicopathological spectrum of bilirubin encephalopathy/kernicterus. *Diagnostics* 9: 1–12.
16 Aleman, M., Madigan, J.E., Williams, D.C. et al. (2014). Brainstem auditory evoked responses in an equine patient population. Part II: foals. *J. Vet. Intern. Med.* 28: 1318–1324.
17 Schreuder, A.B., Rice, A.C., Vanikova, J. et al. (2013). Albumin administration protects against bilirubin-induced auditory brainstem dysfunction in Gunn rat pups. *Liver Int.* 33: 1557–1565.
18 Rice, A.C., Chiou, V.L., Zuckoff, S.B. et al. (2011). Profile of minocycline neuroprotection in bilirubin-induced auditory system dysfunction. *Brain Res.* 1368: 290–298.
19 Lin, S., Wei, X., Bales, K.R. et al. (2005). Minocycline blocks bilirubin neurotoxicity and prevents hyperbilirubinemia-induced cerebellar hypoplasia in the Gunn rat. *Eur. J. Neurosci.* 22: 21–27.
20 Geiger, A.S., Rice, A.C., and Shapiro, S.M. (2007). Minocycline blocks acute bilirubin-induced neurological dysfunction in jaundiced Gunn rats. *Neonatology* 92: 219–226.
21 Park, W.S., Chang, Y.S., Chung, S.H. et al. (2001). Effect of hypothermia on bilirubin-induced alterations in brain cell membrane function and energy metabolism in newborn piglets. *Brain Res.* 922: 276–281.
22 Kuter, N., Aysit-Altuncu, N., Ozturk, G. et al. (2018). The neuroprotective effects of hypothermia on bilirubin-induced neurotoxicity in vitro. *Neonatology* 113: 360–365.
23 Deliktaş, M., Ergin, H., Demiray, A. et al. (2019). Caffeine prevents bilirubin-induced cytotoxicity in cultured newborn rat astrocytes. *J. Matern. Neonatal. Med.* 32: 1813–1819.
24 Broux, B., Lefere, L., Deprex, P. et al. (2015). Plasma exchange as a treatment for hyperbilirubinemia in 2 foals with neonatal isoerythrolysis. *J. Vet. Intern. Med.* 29: 736–738.
25 Divers, T.J. (2011). Metabolic causes of encephalopathy in horses. *Vet. Clin. Equine* 27: 589–596.

Section XII Nervous System Neoplasia

Rebecca Ruby

Primary neoplastic conditions of the central nervous system (CNS) of horses are rare with the exception of pituitary adenomas frequently noted in adult horses. Neoplasia of the CNS in foals is considered even more uncommon. Reports of both primary neoplasia and metastatic involvement of the nervous system are limited to case reports or laboratory necropsy records.

A markedly enlarged, neoplastic pituitary gland resulting in mentation abnormalities and recumbency occurred in an 11-month-old Thoroughbred colt submitted for necropsy to the University of Kentucky Diagnostic Laboratory (UKVDL). The histologic features were consistent with a pituitary carcinoma. Placental germ cell tumors have been reported to metastasize in foals and fetuses and result in neurologic signs when metastatic spread involves the spinal column or brain [1–3]. Hepatoblastoma is a malignant neoplasm occurring in children and young animals with multiple reports in horses. A 2-hour-old foal was found to have metastatic hepatoblastoma within the cerebellum and meninges to the stylohyoid bone (Figure 32.XII.1) [4].

Vascular proliferations are most commonly recognized in the skin of foals, with occasional reports of these growths also occurring within the CNS. Vascular hamartomas are non-neoplastic anomalies of vessels, which may result in neurologic dysfunction as a space occupying mass or through bleeding. A 4-week-old Freiberger foal was diagnosed at necropsy with a vascular hamartoma in the obex region of the brain. The foal displayed multiple cranial nerve deficits from birth until euthanasia [5]. Leptomeningeal hemangiomatosis was reported in a 3-year-old horse with a history of intermittent seizures over the prior 2 months. This case had many pathologic similarities with Sturge–Weber syndrome in man and the changes were proposed to represent a form of neuroectodermal dysplasia [6]. A case submitted to the UKVDL of metastatic hemangiosarcoma in a 4-day old Thoroughbred involved widespread metastasis, which included the cerebral cortex.

Schwannosis, the proliferation of ectopic Schwann cells within the CNS, was reported in three foals ranging from 5 to 11 weeks old. All foals demonstrated clinical signs consistent with a spinal cord disorder from birth and were euthanized. Histopathologic findings demonstrated disorganized, dysplastic, hamartomatous, and heterotopic tissue with proliferative lesions consistent with Schwann cell proliferation [7].

Equine Neonatal Medicine, First Edition. Edited by David M. Wong and Pamela A. Wilkins.

(a)

(b)

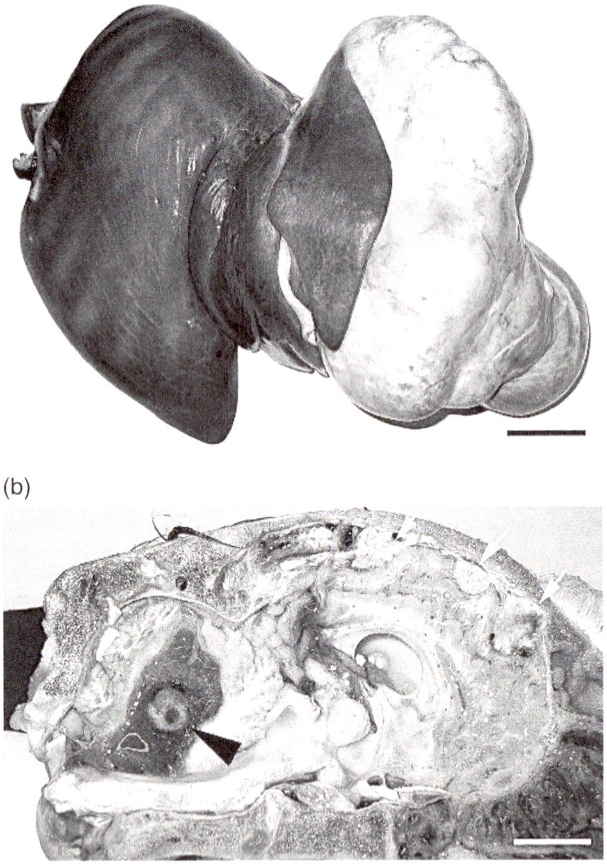

Figure 32.XII.1 Multilobulated, well-demarcated (20 × 16 × 11 cm) tan hepatic mass: (a) that extends from the left liver lobe in a Thoroughbred neonate (Bar = 5 cm) [4]; (b) Cerebellar and meningeal metastases and a Thoroughbred foal. The cerebellum is cavitated and contains a 1 cm in diameter well-demarcated pink mass (arrowhead) that is surrounded by yellow gelatinous material. Additional 0.3–1.25 cm in diameter reddish-tan mottled masses (arrows) are evident in the cerebral meninges. Bar = 2 cm.

References

1 Allison, N., Moeller, R.B. Jr., and Duncan, R. (2004). Placental teratocarcinoma in a mare with possible metastasis to the foal. *J. Vet. Diagn. Invest.* 16: 160–163.

2 Bockenstedt, M.M., Fales-Williams, A., and Haynes, J.S. (2015). Equine placental mixed germ cell tumor with metastasis to the foal. *Vet. Pathol.* 52: 360–363.

3 Hepworth-Warren, K.L., Wong, D.M., Galow-Kersh, N.L. et al. (2014). Metastatic tumor in pregnancy: placental germ cell tumor with metastasis to the foal. *J. Equine Vet. Sci.* 34: 1134–1139.

4 Loynachan, A.T., Bolin, D.C., Hong, C.B. et al. (2007). Three equine cases of mixed hepatoblastoma with teratoid features. *Vet. Pathol.* 2: 211–214.

5 Borel, N., Grest, P., Junge, H. et al. (2014). Vascular hamartoma in the central nervous system of a foal. *J. Vet. Diagn. Invest.* 26: 805–809.

6 McEntee, M., Summers, B.A., de Lahunta, A. et al. (1987). Meningocerebral hemangiomatosis resembling Sturge-Weber disease in a horse. *Acta Neuropathol.* 74: 405–410.

7 Miranda, I.C., Taylor, K.R., Castleman, W. et al. (2019). Schwannosis in three foals and a calf. *Vet. Pathol.* 56: 783–788.

Section XIII Peripheral Nerve Disorders – Nerve Injury Secondary to Dystocia

Steve Reed

Neurologic conditions of foals have been recognized for many years with seeming continuous changes as our understanding of neonatal physiology and neurologic conditions of neonates expands. Most of the literature focuses on the common condition of neonatal maladjustment syndrome. The focus of this chapter is to address peripheral nerve injuries secondary to dystocia and pulling injuries (i.e. injury to nerve(s) associated with the extraction/pulling of the fetus during a dystocia).

In human infants, conditions such as Erb's palsy, brachial plexus, and lumbosacral plexus injuries sometimes occur secondary to traction devices used in delivery of the infant [1–3]. Trauma to the peripheral nervous system is not uncommon in horses and foals; however, the incidence of these problems secondary to dystocia or pulling injuries appears very rare in the author's large primary and referral practice (Rood and Riddle Equine Hospital, Lexington, Kentucky). Some typical nerve injuries include Sweeney, brachial plexus avulsion and/or compression, radial nerve paralysis, and femoral and peroneal nerve paralysis [4–8]. However, in review of similar injuries related to dystocia occurring in our large private practice over the past 35 years, it appears very rare, about 1 per 1000 deliveries (Tom Riddle, personal communication).

Peripheral nerve injuries are often accompanied by loss of sensation over specific areas of the skin. Examples include the dorsal pastern region of the thoracic limbs for the median nerve, the medial and lateral regions of the forearm just below the elbow for the ulnar nerve, and the dorsum of the cannon bone region on the thoracic limbs for the musculocutaneous nerve and for the femoral nerve the medial aspect of the thigh. With tibial nerve paralysis sensory loss occurs on the medial and lateral aspects of the cannon bone region of the pelvic limbs, and with peroneal nerve injury loss of sensation occurs on the dorsal region of the cannon bone of the pelvic limbs [1, 9].

Examples of typical clinical signs for specific syndromes include Sweeney, which results from damage to the suprascapular nerve often caused by collisions between horses or with an inanimate object striking near the point of the shoulder. This syndrome has also been observed in draft horses due to a tight-fitting harness. As a result of the nerve injury, horses develop atrophy of the supraspinatus and infraspinatus muscles with subsequent outward rotation of the shoulder joint while walking [4]. Another commonly injured peripheral nerve in horses is the radial nerve [7, 10, 11]. This injury is observed approximately five to six times annually in our practice and is often seen secondary to horses running into each other at full gallop or when colliding with an immovable object. When observed in foals or adults, signs are quite dramatic as this appears to be a very painful injury. Signs include a dropped elbow along with knuckling of the fetlock and carpus. Radial nerve paralysis is sometimes seen post-anesthesia and may be observed in either the up or down leg of horses, which have been in prolonged lateral recumbency.

If faced with signs of multiple nerve injuries to the thoracic limb, one should suspect damage to the brachial plexus. In some foals where traction has been applied during parturition, especially when straps or chains have been applied to the thoracic limbs to aid with extraction of the foal, injury of the brachial plexus can occur. The most prominent signs often involve the radial nerve, which arises from nerve segments C7 and C8 [6]. Along with this, signs of Sweeney are often noted as well. Injury to the nerve root segments of C8 to T1 results in damage to the pectoral nerve and atrophy of one pectoral muscle will develop over time. Brachial plexus and radial nerve injuries are often very painful and foals or adult horses suffering brachial plexus injury appear as painful as a fracture of the humerus or other long bone of the thoracic limbs.

Equine Neonatal Medicine, First Edition. Edited by David M. Wong and Pamela A. Wilkins.

When the injury is severe enough, there can sometimes be avulsion of the brachial plexus from the spinal cord nerve roots resulting in permanent damage to the foal and a strong indication for euthanasia. Paralysis of the musculocutaneous nerve is rare but if injured the foal will show atrophy of the biceps and brachialis muscles over time but may not show a significant alteration of gait. Injury to the median and ulnar nerves results in a stiff and often "goose-stepping" gait with intermittent signs of weakness noted as toe dragging [9, 12].

In some foals injured during parturition there can be damage to the femoral nerve of one or both pelvic limbs. Damage to the femoral nerve results in inability to support weight along with inability to extend the stifle [13, 14]. When attempting to walk, the limb will buckle as the foal attempts to bear weight on it. When both femoral nerves have been injured, the foal will stand with a crouched posture and when attempting to walk will remain in this posture. Over a 2- to 3-week period, the foal will demonstrate signs of quadricep muscle atrophy and the patellar reflex can be depressed or absent.

Although rare, mares can sustain damage to the obturator nerve during parturition, which will result in loss of adductor function in the muscles of the pelvic limb. More typically, injury to the sciatic nerve and its branches can occur, leading to poor limb flexion with the stifle and hock extended while the fetlock remains in flexion. Bilateral sciatic nerve paralysis has occasionally been observed in foals receiving intramuscular injections of antibiotics or other medications. When the sciatic nerve or its branches are affected, clinical signs include unilateral or bilateral poor joint flexion, extension of the stifle and hock and flexion of the fetlock. When weight is applied to the limb (without extending the digit) the weight will be supported on the dorsum of the fetlock. Tibial nerve paralysis is uncommon in horses. When present, it results in a hypermetric "stringhalt-like" gait, with flexion of the hock and extension of the stifle while standing at rest and excessive hock flexion while walking.

Often times when the sciatic nerve is damaged the peroneal nerve is also involved. The nerve is most easily damaged following trauma to the lateral region of the stifle joint but is also sometimes seen following prolonged lateral recumbency during foaling or following a long period of general anesthesia. Injury to this nerve results in an inability to flex the hock and extend the digits, with the dorsum of the foot being dragged along the ground. If the foot is placed properly, the horse can bear weight until it attempts to walk.

Damage to the cranial gluteal nerve is most often associated with an injury to the fifth to sixth lumbar region of the lumbar spinal cord and thus can be seen in diseases like equine protozoal myeloencephalitis (EPM). The nerve may also be injured when a horse sustains a fracture of its pelvis.

Trauma to the dorsal sacrococcygeal vertebral region sometimes results in fracture of the S2 region, as this site is vulnerable due to anatomic constraints of the well-fixed sacrum and S1. Fractures in this region result in damage to the cauda equina from S2 caudally. Signs include paresis to paralysis of the tail and perineal region, decreased or loss of sensation in this region, a dilated rectum with fecal retention, and often a paralyzed bladder with urine overflow.

Injury to the facial nerve is not uncommon [15]. Horses can damage this nerve if a halter has a tight fit, pulling back on a restraint rope with pressure on the halter, prolonged lateral recumbency, or trauma to the side of the face. It is also a common feature in horses suffering from temperohyoid osteopathy (THO). Injury to this nerve may result in muzzle deviation, ptosis of the eyelid, and drooping of the ear. Sometimes all three signs are seen, depending on the site of injury to the nerve. In addition, the lacrimal branch of this nerve provides approximately one-third of tear production, such that if injured the horse may also develop severe keratitis and a partially dry eye.

Postpartum paralysis in the mare occurs most often when a small mare delivers a large foal. Signs are quite variable and may be as mild as pelvic limb stiffness to paraplegia following foaling. Signs can begin quite slowly and progress, sometimes rapidly, to weakness, ataxia, and paralysis. In some mares, hemorrhage in the region of the femoral nerves occurs, resulting in extensor weakness, patellar hyporeflexia, and loss of sensation on the medial side of the thigh. Horses with femoral nerve paralysis lose the ability to extend the stifle, resulting in difficulty to advance the limb and an inability to support weight on the limb, resulting in collapse. Following femoral nerve paralysis, the horse will rest with all joints of the affected limb in flexion. Over the next 2–3 weeks after injury, the quadriceps muscles begin to atrophy and the patellar reflex is lost or severely depressed. Patellar reflexes are most easily evaluated in foals rather than in adult horses. Femoral nerve injury appears to be the most common peripheral nerve injury in foals during parturition, usually secondary to hip or stifle lock. This injury is often associated with pelvic limb muscle rupture. Bilateral femoral nerve paralysis is sometimes seen secondary to dystocia or following general anesthesia, and occasionally following sacroiliac luxation with hemorrhage in the perineural region.

A muscle group that is sometimes ruptured at or near the time of foaling is the peroneus tertius. The function of the peroneus tertius is important to the normal reciprocal action of tarsal flexion with stifle flexion. It is the sole cranial component of the reciprocal mechanism and part of the passive stay apparatus, assisting the horse in standing with minimal effort. The peroneus tertius stretches during extension of the hock, centering the weight on the tarsus and recoiling elastically following breakover. This release of stored elastic energy during the terminal phase of the stride assists with efficient flexion of the hock. Therefore, an intact peroneus tertius is important to the normal combined movement of hock and stifle flexion.

Management of peripheral nerve injuries, regardless of cause is similar and is somewhat dependent on the severity of the injury. Classification of nerve injuries are divided into three categories. The least severe is neuropraxia and usually involves concussion of the nerve with minimal injury to the nerve fibers; it is therefore not associated with permanent damage to the nerve. Following this type of injury, the foal or mare may have loss of nerve function for 1–2 weeks followed by rapid return to full function over a few days. The second nerve injury is axonotmesis where delicate axons are injured while sparing the sturdy Schwann cell derived myelin sheaths. This loss of myelin will slow conduction down the nerve, which can sometimes be fully restored as long as the axon has a pathway to follow during remyelination. The third syndrome is neurotmesis and is defined by loss of structural integrity of both axons and the myelin sheaths and is often associated with permanent loss of function caused by inability of axonal regrowth rapid enough to avoid irreversible muscular fibrosis. Nerve regeneration occurs at approximately 1 mm per day or between 20 and 30 mm per month and can occur over a distance of about 300 mm, if regeneration does not occur within 6–12 months fibrosis is likely to stop further nerve healing.

Evaluation of nerve damage can be assisted by use of electromyography (EMG) [10]. This diagnostic technique is especially important when evaluating peripheral nerve injuries in horses. The EMG helps determine whether only one or more than one nerve has been injured. In addition, EMG can help determine the extent of nerve damage and whether reinnervation is occurring. The best time to perform EMG is 2–3 weeks following injury [16, 17]. By that time some degree of muscle atrophy is likely to be evident and sufficient time has passed for spontaneous denervation potentials to develop.

Following peripheral nerve injury, nerve regeneration is generally achieved by two fundamental responses: (i) myelin de-differentiation, and (ii) phenotype alteration in Schwann cells, along with activation of innate immune responses [7]. There are substantial changes in differentiation status of Schwann cells and damaged neurons in the distal position of injury so that there is a switch from myelin maintenance to that of axonal regrowth/repair. The process of peripheral nerve regeneration is profoundly dependent on regenerative capacity of Schwann cells and inherent competence of peripheral neurons for outgrowth [16]. Schwann cells, because of their plasticity for various ranges of activities such as myelination, regeneration, and myelinophagia, are major contributors in peripheral nerve regeneration [17]. Post-injury, cross talk between Schwann cells, extracellular molecules (ECM) and other nearby neurons is orchestrated and favors rebuilding damaged myelin sheaths; Schwann cells are reprogrammed into a proliferative feature and secrete plentiful healing factors for renovating disturbed nerves at a yield of 1–2 mm/d [18, 19].

Treatment of peripheral nerve injuries often relies on supportive care, facilitating ambulation with splints (if needed), physical therapy, anti-inflammatory medications, and enough time to allow nerve function to improve. In neonatal foals that are unable to suckle due to gait abnormalities secondary to nerve injury, provision of colostrum, supplemental feeding, and maintenance of hydration are needed. A well-crafted and padded splint should be fashioned if this will allow the foal to ambulate and suckle voluntarily. Splints should be removed periodically (every 8–12 hours) to evaluate the soft tissue under the splint as well as allow the skin to dry out from moisture/sweat that may develop under the splint. Other supportive care (e.g. antimicrobials, treatment of concurrent diseases) should also be provided. Physical therapy is needed to maintain range of motion and avoid contracture of the affected limb. Passive and active range of motion exercises should be implemented to facilitate long-term use of the affected limb.

References

1 Okafor, U.A., Akinbo, S.R.A., Sokunbi, O.G. et al. (2008). Comparison of electrical stimulation and conventional physiotherapy in functional rehabilitation in Erb's palsy. *Nig. Q. J. Hosp. Med.* 18: 202–205.

2 Kleinod, G. (1971). Prognosis of Erbs' obsteric paralysis. *Beitr. Orthop. Traumatol.* 18: 452–454.

3 Olugbile, A. and Mascarenhas, L. (2000). Review of shoulder dystocia at the Birmingham Women's hospital. *J. Obstet. Gynaecol.* 20: 267–270.

4 Emond, A.L., Bertoni, L., Seignour, M. et al. (2016). Peripheral neuropathy of a forelimb in horses: 27 cases (2000–2013). *J. Am. Vet. Med. Assoc.* 249: 1187–1195.

5 Dutton, D.M., Honnas, C.M., and Watkins, J.P. (1999). Nonsurgical treatment of suprascapular nerve injury in horses: 8 cases (1988-1998). *J. Am. Vet. Med. Assoc.* 214: 1657–1659.

6 Lopez, M.J., Nordberg, C., and Trostle, S. (1997). Fracture of the 7th cervical and 1st thoracic vertebrae

presenting as radial nerve paralysis in a horse. *Can. Vet. J.* 38: 112.
7 Rooney, J.R. (1963). Radial paralysis in the horse. *Cornell Vet.* 53: 328–337.
8 Schneider, J.E. (1985). Scapular notch resection for suprascapular nerve decompression in 12 horses. *J. Am. Vet. Med. Assoc.* 187: 1019–1020.
9 Blythe, L.L. and Kitchell, R.L. (1982). Electrophysiologic studies of the thoracic limb of the horse. *Am. J. Vet. Res.* 43: 1511–1524.
10 Henry, R.W. and Diesem, C.D. (1981). Proximal equine radial and median motor nerve conduction velocity. *Am. J. Vet. Res.* 42: 1819–1882.
11 Rijkenhuizen, A. (1996). True or false radial nerve paralysis in the horse. *Vet. Annual* 34: 126–133.
12 Henry, R.W., Diesem, C.D., and Wiechers, D.O. (1979). Evaluation of equine radial and median nerve conduction velocities. *Am. J. Vet. Res.* 40: 1406–1410.
13 Marolt, J., Bego, U., Zobundzija, M. et al. (1982). Dysfunction of femoral and tibial nerves in the horse in the light of clinical and anatomical experiments (author's transl). *Dtsch. Tierarztl. Wochenschr.* 89: 189–192.
14 Dyson, S., Taylor, P., and Whitwell, K. (1988). Femoral nerve paralysis after general anaesthesia. *Equine Vet. J.* 20: 376–380.
15 Boorman, S., Scherrer, M.N., Stefanovski, D. et al. (2020). Facial nerve paralysis in 64 equids: clinical variables, diagnosis, and outcome. *J. Vet. Intern. Med.* 34: 1308–1320.
16 Takahashi, Y., Mukai, K., Matsui, A. et al. (2018). Electromyographic changes in hind limbs of thoroughbreds with fatigue induced by treadmill exercise. *Am. J. Vet. Res.* 79: 828–835.
17 Graubner, C. (2020). Quantitative motor unit action potential analysis of paraspinal muscles, diagnostic imaging and necropsy findings in 36 horses suspected of cervical impairment. *Schweiz. Arch. Tierheilkd.* 162: 213–221.
18 Szabo, E.A., Pemberton, J.M., Gibson, A.M. et al. (1994). Application of PCR to a clinical and environmental investigation of a case of equine botulism. *J. Clin. Microbiol.* 32: 1986–1991.
19 Whitlock, R.H. and Buckley, C. (1997). Botulism. *Vet. Clin. North Am. Equine Pract.* 13: 107–128.

Section XIV Peripheral Nerve Disorders – Botulism

Sarah Colmer, Michelle Abraham, and Amy L. Johnson

Botulism is a disease of people and animals exposed to the neurotoxin of *Clostridium botulinum* (BoNT), which causes progressive flaccid paresis and cranial nerve deficits [1]. *C. botulinum* is a spore-forming, obligate anaerobic, Gram-positive bacterium found in soil with seven different serotypes (A-G, with C-α and C-β subgroups), each of which is distinguished by the unique properties of its toxin [2], though it has been theorized that toxic factors may be transferrable between different *Clostridia* [3]. The toxins are antigenically different and act specifically on various parts of the synaptic vesicle docking and fusion apparatus at the motor end plate to prevent release of acetylcholine (Ach). All vertebrates are susceptible to the development of botulism [4], and BoNT is widely regarded as the most potent and lethal toxin known to humankind in which end-stage disease leads to death by paralysis of the muscles of respiration [5]. Botulism was first recognized as a clinical disease in foals in the 1960s, most commonly identified in the mid-Atlantic United States and Kentucky. Botulism can be rapidly fatal without intervention, however with proper treatment, affected foals can survive. This chapter strives to outline epidemiological information, pathophysiology, diagnosis, treatment, prognosis, and prevention strategies for botulism in the equine neonate.

Epidemiology

C. botulinum spores are principally found in soil [5] and can be mobilized by heavy rains and wind. Spores are metabolically dormant and can resist extreme heat, radiation, acidic and basic environments as well as desiccation and many commercial disinfectants. Spores are ubiquitous in many regions of North America [6] where up to 18.5% of soil specimens evaluated were positive for the organism in one study [7]. Global understanding of the epidemiology of *C. botulinum* relies on a very limited number of reports [8], and unpredicted outbreaks have occurred worldwide [9]. Serotypes often vary based on geographic region. Botulism is prevalent in birds and cattle yielding global economic losses in agriculture, although it tends to be more sporadic in other species [5]. Despite its ubiquitous existence, *C. botulinum* spores may not always be toxic, which may explain the sporadic nature of both outbreaks and disease in individual people and animals [10].

Botulism in horses can be categorized in two ways, either by the *C. botulinum* serotype involved or by the route of acquisition of disease [11]. There are four predominant types of BoNT encountered in animal species – A, B, C, and D (Table 32.XIV.1). Both type A and type B are associated with soil, while type C and type D are associated with carrion. In the United States, type B is endemic in the mid-Atlantic states and Kentucky and is estimated to account for over 85% of equine cases diagnosed in the United States [12]. Type A is reported primarily in the western United States (California, Idaho, Montana, Oregon, Nebraska, Washington, and Wyoming) [12, 13]. Type C is seen sporadically across the country, though it is more commonly reported in Europe [13]. Confirmed cases of types D-G have not been reported in horses [13]. Horses with botulism almost always acquire the disease in one of three ways: ingestion of preformed toxin with feedstuffs (foodborne botulism in adults), ingestion of *C. botulinum* spores that subsequently germinate in the gastrointestinal tract and release toxin ("toxicoinfectious" botulism in foals), or through the contamination of wounds with *C. botulinum* yielding bacterial growth with toxin release ("wound" botulism) [13]. Foodborne botulism in adults and toxicoinfectious botulism in foals are more common than wound botulism [13].

Considering both serotype and route of acquisition, several trends are evident: toxicoinfectious botulism due to type B is common in foals in the mid-Atlantic region and Kentucky, foodborne botulism in adult horses most commonly results from spoiled forage contaminated with type B (in the eastern part of the country), or type A (in the western

Equine Neonatal Medicine, First Edition. Edited by David M. Wong and Pamela A. Wilkins.

Table 32.XIV.1 Botulism neurotoxin (BoNT) types, their predominant origin and endemic regions.

BoNT type	Predominant origin	Endemic region
A	Soil	Western United States
B	Soil	Mid-Atlantic United States, Kentucky
C	Carrion	Sporadic reports in the United States and Europe
D	Carrion	Not reported in the horse

part), and foodborne botulism due to type C is occasionally seen when carrion contaminates forage. Being aware of the most likely serotype present in one's region can inform treatment and prevention strategies, although diagnostic laboratory methods (see below) are still recommended to confirm serotype, which allows identification of unusual cases and new epidemiologic trends [11]. Clinical signs might vary slightly between types, but not reliably enough to allow distinction of serotype based on clinical signs. Although toxicoinfectious botulism is most common in foals, wound botulism has been suspected in some foal cases [14]. Toxicoinfectious botulism in foals is similar to "infant botulism" in humans, which **has been** the most diagnosed form of botulism in the United States since the late 1970s [15].

Pathophysiology

Foals ingest *C. botulinum* spores while nursing or nosing around on the ground, given that spores are commonly found in the soil of endemic regions as previously mentioned. Interestingly, **it does not seem possible** to induce the disease in young, healthy foals via oral inoculation with live organism [16]. Reported incubation periods in various species range from 2 hours to 2 weeks, though many toxicoinfectious cases exhibit signs between 12 and 48 hours after ingestion [14]. *C. botulinum* can establish itself in the gastrointestinal tract and outcompete normal intestinal bacteria [17]. Germination of *C. botulinum is* triggered by anaerobic conditions, a pH >4, and by host- or pathogen-specific "germinants" which can consist of amino acids, sugars, ribosides, or various ions [18]. Once spores germinate within the digestive tract, the vegetative form immediately produces toxin (BoNT), which is subsequently absorbed into the bloodstream across the intestinal epithelium via transcytosis [19]. Other routes of infection occur by way of ingestion of preformed toxin, which is similarly absorbed in the context of foodborne botulism, or via germination of spores in devitalized tissue (such as an infected umbilicus) and with absorption into the bloodstream as is the case with wound botulism [20].

Regardless of route of entry, the toxin ultimately binds to polysialogangliosides, which are large, negatively charged molecules on the nerve terminals of both autonomic and voluntary motor neuromuscular junctions (NMJs) [21]. The ganglioside/toxin complex then binds to a specific protein receptor on the terminal end plate of the motor neuron and is internalized. Botulinum neurotoxin cleaves proteins that are responsible for release (exocytosis) of acetylcholine (Ach). Botulinum toxin types A and E cleave SNAP-25, types B, D, F, and G cleave VAMP (synaptobrevin), and type C cleaves syntaxin [21]. Protein cleavage results in either the interruption of voltage-gated calcium channel activation at the nerve terminus preventing Ach release, or prevention of exocytosis of synaptic vehicles by inhibiting fusion of vesicles with the presynaptic membrane; both outcomes ultimately result in neuromuscular paralysis.

Clinical Diagnosis

The gold standard of botulism diagnosis is identification of BoNT in serum samples from patients with compatible signs by using the mouse bioassay test [22]. However, **clinical diagnosis is most often** based on compatible history and clinical signs, since laboratory confirmation with the mouse bioassay can be difficult. Historical details that increase suspicion of botulism include **the foal residing in an endemic region, particularly the mid-Atlantic states** and Kentucky, an unvaccinated dam, and, less commonly, recent wounds or infections. Consumption of fermented forages or large-bale hay is an important historical factor to determine in adult horses, but is less consequential in foals, since foals are usually exposed through soil contamination. Historical information may help identify the type of BoNT involved, and there may be differences in the potency between types of toxins; type A has been theorized to be more toxic than types B or C [11].

Regardless of botulinum toxin type, the clinical signs of botulism intoxication are the same: progressive flaccid paresis or paralysis and cranial nerve deficits including, but not limited to; dysphagia, weak tongue tone (Figure 32.XIV.1), weak eyelid tone, and mydriasis with slow pupillary light reflexes. Of note, neurological deficits are generally symmetrical, which can help differentiate botulism from other neurologic conditions in horses. The most common clinical syndrome in foals specifically is referred to as *shaker foal syndrome* because the predominant clinical signs are muscle fasciculations and excessive recumbency. It was first identified in foals in the 1960s [23]. Some owners and clinicians first notice milk coming from the foal's nose or mouth, while others do not identify overt dysphagia. In one retrospective

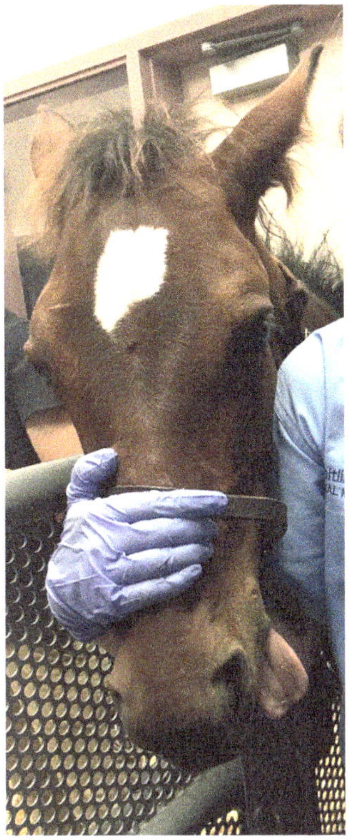

Figure 32.XIV.1 Demonstration of poor tongue tone in a foal with toxicoinfectious botulism during a tongue stress test. *Source:* Image courtesy of Dr. Caitlin Moore, University of Pennsylvania.

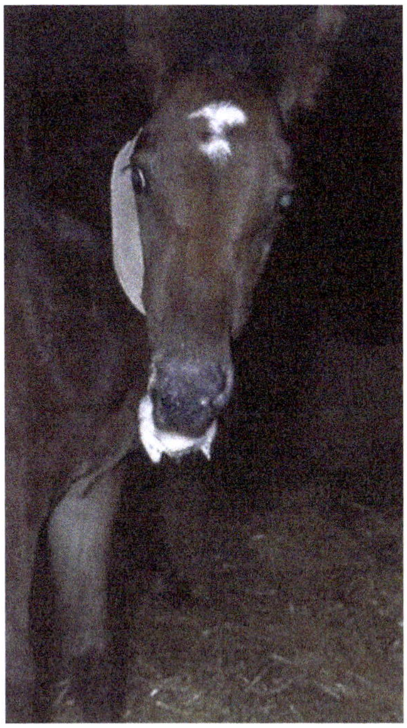

Figure 32.XIV.2 A foal exhibiting frothy saliva as a consequence of its dysphagia. *Source:* Image courtesy of Dr. Corinne Sweeney, University of Pennsylvania.

report out of a tertiary care facility, the most common clinical complaints were weakness and recumbency, though some cases presented for colic signs and others for pneumonia or respiratory distress [17]. Most foals present without fever and with mild tachycardia and tachypnea. Mentation is usually appropriate, although dehydration secondary to dysphagia may be present in some cases, causing dullness. Frothy saliva may be present at the mouth of dysphagic foals (Figure 32.XIV.2). Weak tail and anal tone **may also be observed**, and in some cases, urine dribbling or bladder distension is possible. Although weakness is observed in affected animals, ataxia is not typically seen as part of this disease.

More mildly affected foals can often stand, initially appearing relatively healthy before beginning to fatigue. Number and duration of episodes of recumbency will often increase in foals. Fine muscle fasciculations progress to coarser trembling as weakness increases, and soon the foal is forced to lie down again. After being recumbent for a period of time, muscle tremors and fasciculations subside and the foal may appear normal. This cycle might occur repeatedly, or more severely affected foals rapidly progress to complete recumbency. As mentioned, toxin dose and time since intoxication are strongly associated with severity of clinical signs, though these details may not be known in many cases. Botulism usually has an acute onset and short clinical course in accordance with the severity of intoxication. Death is most often the result of respiratory failure.

Two clinical tests have been described that may increase suspicion for a botulism diagnosis in the horse, though their diagnostic accuracy has not been clearly established in clinical cases [24]. The first is known as the tongue tone or tongue stress test in which the examiner gently withdraws the tongue from the foal's mouth and assesses the ability of the foal to pull it back while gently holding the jaw closed (Figure 32.XIV.1). Another test more frequently utilized for adult horses is known as the grain test and involves feeding the horse 8 oz of grain in a bucket while timing how long it takes for the horse to consume the feed. Normal horses finish in less than 2 minutes, whereas horses with dysphagia do not. This test in less useful in nursing foals that might not be interested in grain, however. In foals where aspiration of milk is suspected, auscultation of the trachea during nursing may yield a tracheal gurgle or rattle during swallowing to provide further convincing evidence of dysphagia.

Laboratory Diagnosis

Routine hematology and biochemical tests are often largely within normal limits. However, dysphagic foals can develop secondary aspiration pneumonia, which might lead to changes in the leukogram and increases in acute phase protein concentrations. Some foals have evidence of hemoconcentration secondary to dehydration, particularly if dysphagic. Others may have mildly increased muscle enzyme activities such as serum creatinine phosphokinase (CPK) or aspartate aminotransferase (AST) due to increased recumbency. Foals with wound botulism might also have clinicopathologic abnormalities related to infection. Importantly, cerebrospinal fluid cytologic analysis is normal in foals with botulism but might assist in ruling out other neurologic conditions that cause tremors and weakness, such as bacterial meningitis. Arterial blood gas analysis in foals with botulism might be normal in mildly affected foals but is likely to show abnormalities consistent with progressive hypoventilation in more severely affected, recumbent foals. Typical findings include acidemia, hypercapnia, hypoxemia, and desaturation of hemoglobin [11].

Although clinical diagnosis by experienced practitioners is reasonably accurate in predicting botulism, and serotype may be predicted based on known serotype prevalence in a geographic region and likely means of exposure, confirmation of serotype must be made in the diagnostic laboratory. For suspected equine cases or outbreaks, the most appropriate samples to submit include forage, gastrointestinal contents, and feces. As noted, the gold standard for laboratory diagnosis is the mouse bioassay, which detects BoNT. Unfortunately, detection of BoNT in equine samples is difficult. When compared to other species, horses are highly sensitive to BoNT and develop clinical signs after exposure to smaller amounts of toxin. Any circulating toxin is quickly bound to receptors and internalized in motor end plates, becoming undetectable. Furthermore, toxin remaining in the gastrointestinal tract is degraded by microbial organisms and their enzymes. Although preformed toxin may be detected by the mouse bioassay in a small number of foal cases (approximately 20%) [11], it is rarely detected in adult cases. Therefore, toxin testing is generally performed or repeated after culture enrichment, which allows any spores in the original sample to germinate and elaborate toxin, thus increasing the diagnostic yield of the assay. These culture-enriched samples are positive in approximately 53% of suspected foal cases and 32% of suspected adult cases [25]. The identification of *C. botulinum* spores in the original sample is considered presumptive evidence of botulism in animals with compatible clinical signs, as this organism is not part of the normal gastrointestinal flora.

Regarding the mouse bioassay, effective samples (pre- or post-culture enrichment) from a suspect case are injected into mice, which are observed for signs consistent with botulism, while additional mice pretreated with antiserum are observed for the same signs. If the latter group of mice is protected, botulism is confirmed and serotype can be determined. As can be intuited, the mouse bioassay has a high positive predictive value (100% for foals and 89% for adults) but lower negative predictive value (51% for foals and 67% for adults) [25]. Additionally, it requires live animal use, is performed at a limited number of facilities, and has an extended lag time for results, limiting its practicality in many clinical scenarios.

Due to the limitations of the mouse bioassay, PCR technology has been investigated to improve diagnostic accuracy and speed while reducing live animal use. This modality is particularly appropriate for equine samples, which more commonly contain *C. botulinum* spores than preformed toxin. A validated, quantitative real-time PCR assay for the detection of the neurotoxin gene of *C. botulinum* type B in equine diagnostic samples was optimized; this assay was faster, more sensitive, and more economical than the mouse bioassay [26]. Subsequently, PCR capabilities were expanded to a multiplex assay for types A and B as well as a singleplex assay for type C [27]. Results indicate that both the A/B multiplex assay and the C singleplex assay are highly specific and more sensitive than the mouse bioassay for detecting *C. botulinum* in equine samples. Lastly, an ELISA has been developed to detect type C and D botulinum toxins in various fluids; however, cross-reactivity with *Clostridium novyi* yields decreased specificity compared to the mouse bioassay, and it was not commercially available at the time of this publication [28].

Ancillary Diagnostic Techniques

Aspiration pneumonia may result from pharyngeal dysfunction in foals with botulism. In the foal population, aspiration pneumonia may or may not be symptomatic, depending on the chronicity and how widespread the lesions are. Although clinicopathologic changes consistent with infection may be useful, imaging techniques (ultrasonography and radiology) are an important tool in diagnosing and monitoring aspiration pneumonia. Radiographs in cases of aspiration pneumonia most often exhibit alveolar and mixed bronchointerstitial patterns [29]. Ultrasonographic findings may include ventral lung field consolidation and pleural irregularities ("comet tails"). Lesion distribution is typically in the lung overlying the caudal heart, however in recumbent foals with botulism, atypical distributions can be seen.

Electrodiagnostic testing has been described for foals with botulism utilizing repetitive nerve stimulation (RNS) of the peroneal nerve [30]. The main finding consistent with a botulism diagnosis is facilitation, which is identified with incremental responses in both amplitude and area under the curve when stimulus rate is high. Availability of equipment for performing RNS may be limited in many clinical scenarios, however. One differential for the described RNS findings is hypomagnesemia and

Table 32.XIV.2 Differential diagnoses for clinical signs seen in foals with botulism.

Dysphagia	Neurologic	Systemic	Musculoskeletal
▪ Guttural pouch disease	▪ Bacterial meningitis	▪ Sepsis/SIRS	▪ Hyperkalemic periodic paralysis
▪ Cleft palate	▪ Discospondylitis	▪ Enterocolitis	▪ Polysaccharide storage myopathy
▪ Soft palate mass	▪ Rabies	▪ Hypothermia	▪ Nutritional myodegeneration
▪ Megaesophagus	▪ Tick paralysis	▪ Anemia	▪ Pain associated with orthopedic condition (fracture, osteomyelitis, synovial sepsis)
▪ Esophageal stricture	▪ Toxicity (lead, organophosphate)	▪ Cachexia	
▪ Equine neonatal dysphagia associated with polycyclic aromatic hydrocarbons		▪ Electrolyte derangements	

identifying normal serum ionized magnesium concentrations may be helpful to rule this out.

Although late-stage botulism in the foal is fairly characteristic for the syndrome, early signs are broad and can be attributable to various disease processes. Appropriate mentation and lack of dramatic clinical pathology alterations may help rule out a variety of infectious, metabolic, or toxic causes in the foal. Dysphagia in foals can have multiple causes (Table 32.XIV.2), and neonatal foals with dysphagia should be assessed for guttural pouch disease or congenital anomalies such as cleft palate, soft palate masses, megaesophagus and esophageal stricture, many of which can be identified by endoscopic evaluation. Of note, recent literature has cited the potential for the influence of environmental exposure to unconventional gas development activity on the occurrence of equine neonatal dysphagia [31]. In this study, the dysphagic period was transient with a median duration of 11 days. Additionally, neurologic conditions resulting in dysphagia include Rabies virus as well as some toxicities.

Muscle tremors and weakness as well as other commonly observed signs in horses with botulism can have multiple etiologies (Table 32.XIV.2), including neurologic disease, systemic illness, and musculoskeletal problems. When assessing the weak, trembling foal, the clinician must determine whether a neuromuscular or non-neuromuscular problem is the cause. Eliminating non-neurologic causes can be easier than confirming a diagnosis of neuromuscular disease in many cases. Thorough anamnesis and physical examination should be performed to assess whether systemic disease or a painful condition is the likely cause of tremors and weakness. Systemic problems that are common in the foal and that can induce tremors and weakness include sepsis, systemic inflammatory response syndrome (SIRS), shock, enterocolitis, hypothermia, electrolyte abnormalities such as hypocalcemia, severe anemia, or severe cachexia. Various drug reactions or intoxications – such those associated with white snakeroot, ionophores, organophosphates or lead – are additional appropriate differential diagnoses. Finally, visceral or musculoskeletal pain can cause tremors and weakness. Abdominal pain can cause tremors and frequent recumbency that mimics neuromuscular weakness, as can painful orthopedic problems such as multiple limb lameness or pelvic fracture.

Botulism is a diffuse neuromuscular disease that causes a characteristic narrow-based stance and short-strided gait, with frequent weight-shifting and recumbency. An important differential diagnosis in adult horses is equine motor neuron disease (EMND), which develops after a prolonged period of vitamin E deficiency. However, this condition has not been reported in foals. Nutritional myodegeneration (white muscle disease) can occur in regions where dietary deficiency of selenium and vitamin E is common; foals with nutritional myodegeneration have marked increases in muscle enzyme activities which would be detectable on serum biochemistry. Although they do not frequently manifest in young foals, genetic myopathies such as HYPP and PSSM should be considered in affected breeds, such as Quarter Horse foals. Tick paralysis can occur in certain geographic regions, such as Australia.

Treatment

Antitoxin administration is considered a mainstay of therapy for botulism and should be administered as soon as possible, as it greatly increases odds of foal survival and minimizes the severity of clinical signs [17, 32, 33]. Prior to antitoxin use in foals, the disease was nearly uniformly fatal within 12–72 hours after the onset of clinical signs beyond those very mildly affected [17, 34]. Antitoxin can be difficult to obtain – often, veterinary teaching hospitals are the best resource. Currently there are two commercially available antitoxins: a trivalent antitoxin against types A, B, and C (Lake Immunogenics, Ontario, NY) and a monovalent antitoxin against type B (Plasvacc, Templeton, CA).

Antitoxin will only bind circulating toxin, not toxin bound at motor end plates or internalized, so clinical signs can continue to progress for 12–24 hours after administration. Since toxin is irreversibly bound and regrowth of motor end plates is required for recovery, administration of antitoxin will not reverse clinical signs. The authors' experience is such that one treatment of antitoxin tends to be adequate, with no change in outcome seen when repeated treatments are administered.

In the case of wound botulism, tissue debridement is recommended and may include fasciotomy as needed to disturb the anaerobic environment in which the spores are germinating to effectively eliminate the organism. In addition to debridement, antimicrobial administration is recommended in cases of wound botulism. Importantly, aminoglycosides [35], tetracyclines, and procaine penicillin [36] are known to potentiate neuromuscular weakness and should thus be avoided, while potassium penicillin is considered appropriate. Antimicrobials are not essential in cases of gastrointestinal botulism, as antimicrobials have not been proven to clear the bacterium from the intestine.

Despite the lack of antimicrobial efficacy in treating *Clostridium* infections themselves, the incorporation of antimicrobials in a botulism foal's therapeutic plan can be useful to prevent or reduce the consequences of aspiration pneumonia when appropriate. When dysphagia is marked and/or aspiration pneumonia is identified on previously described imaging modalities, broad-spectrum IV antimicrobial therapy is recommended. A retrospective study at a veterinary teaching hospital found that ceftiofur sodium was the most commonly used antimicrobial, with trimethoprim sulfa drugs utilized in those that required additional treatment after hospitalization [17]. Potassium penicillin was also used in some cases. Of note, metronidazole is not only ineffective in treating botulism in foals but might potentiate colonization of the intestinal tract by *C. botulinum*, as has been shown in adult laboratory mice [37].

Nutritional management is an essential component of supportive therapy. Dysphagic foals require their hydration and nutritional requirements to be met through enteral (preferred) or parenteral administration. The administration of milk or milk replacer through an indwelling nasogastric or nasoesophageal tube is tolerated in many cases with small, intermittent meals every few hours. Due to their total or increased recumbency, as well as BoNT's tendency to cause gastrointestinal ileus, foals with botulism often do best when fed a smaller percentage of their body weight (BW) in milk (10% of their BW as opposed to 20–25% BW), at least initially, until one can determine that they can tolerate increased feedings. Parenteral administration may be more appropriate for those foals with a component of ileus who do not tolerate enteral feedings, in which case partial or total parenteral nutrition may be necessary. Diarrhea is not uncommon in the general foal population nor in those with botulism and should be treated as needed symptomatically. Disturbances in gastrointestinal function are theorized to be either primarily associated with botulism via alterations at cholinergic motor synapses or secondary in the face of ileus or altered gastrointestinal microbiota.

Although historic postulates of colonization of gastroduodenal ulcers by *C. botulinum* were published, this has not been proven to be a component of toxicoinfectious clinical botulism [16]. In a retrospective study, 17 foals were treated with ulcer medications (sucralfate, ranitidine, cimetidine) while 13 foals were not treated, with no significant difference in case outcome, nor any clinically apparent gastroduodenal ulceration [17]. As such, prophylactic gastric ulcer treatment in foals is not recommended.

Horses with moderate-to-severe botulism require thick bedding and/or padding to prevent complications associated with excessive recumbency such as decubital ulceration. Even horses receiving high-quality nursing care will develop necrosis of skin and underlying muscle over pressure points if recumbency is prolonged. Topical antimicrobials such as silver sulfadiazine can be used for local treatment. Additionally, corneal ulceration can result from prolonged recumbency even in well-bedded situations. Protecting the "down" eye with a towel or other soft surface (i.e. if foal is on a mattress) may be recommended and daily ocular examinations should be performed. Preventative ocular lubricant ointment is recommended to decrease the development of keratitis and ulceration.

Foals should not be forced to rise frequently or stand for prolonged periods, as depletion of acetylcholine stores will increase weakness and lead to progression of signs. Along these lines, keeping foals in quiet locations is recommended. The use of sling support is generally not suggested for use during initial treatment (first 1–3 days). In addition to exhaustion, maintaining foals in slings can result in compression of the chest and worsen respiratory ability. However, after antitoxin treatment and stabilization of signs, some severely affected foals may benefit from the use of a sling to assist them to rise and remain standing. Due to their size, recumbent foals can be more readily turned every 2 hours compared to their adult counterparts, and physical therapy (such as passive range of motion exercises isolated at each joint) should be performed frequently to prevent the development of flexural deformities. Splinting may also be beneficial to prevent or improve flexural deformities when needed.

Additional elements of nursing supportive care that may be necessary include evacuation of the bladder and rectum in some cases. While foals are recumbent, it is best to monitor urine and fecal output and identify when manual intervention may be needed. Additional complications in foals with

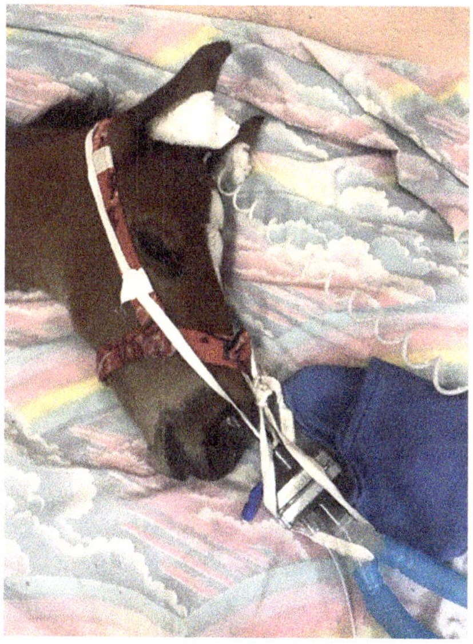

Figure 32.XIV.3 Thoroughbred colt that presented for botulism, intubated and on a ventilator.

botulism include cellulitis, myositis, colic, cystitis, pneumonia, and salmonellosis, however, development of complications has not been associated with nonsurvival [17].

In foals that exhibit respiratory weakness, monitoring of arterial blood gas measurements may prove helpful in identifying those that require respiratory support. Intranasal oxygen insufflation can be implemented with relative ease if infrastructure allows. Mechanical ventilation (Chapter 6) can be utilized in foals with botulism exhibiting respiratory failure (Figure 32.XIV.3). In these foals, mechanical ventilation can provide the opportunity of additional time for recovery of affected NMJs (particularly those in which the intercostal muscles and diaphragm are affected). Choosing cases for which mechanical ventilation is appropriate generally involves **selecting those which become** progressively acidemic and hypercapnic on blood gas analysis [33]. A retrospective study described **a survival rate of 87.5%** of mechanically ventilated foals with botulism [33].

Importantly, although the use of neurostimulants such as neostigmine or 4-aminopyridine may be tempting to help maintain foals in standing positions for nursing and give them temporary periods of strength via increased Ach release at the NMJ, these medications are not recommended. Such compounds often only hasten the depletion of Ach, and the resultant periods of increased neuromuscular strength are short-lived, further exhausting the Ach supply.

In foals with botulism, it is important to establish early client communications and establish realistic timeline for intensive care needs and return of neuromuscular function. If the foal is recumbent, it is likely to remain so for 7–10 days, which can be cost- or manpower-prohibitive for some. Ventilated foals will often have longer hospital stays, with the previously mentioned retrospective study noting an average of an additional 7 days of hospitalization when mechanical ventilation is implemented [33]. Regarding muscle strength, recovery can take up to 10 days to regenerate docking proteins at the NMJ, and full muscle strength recovery can take up to 1 month [38]. If the foal experienced more severe generalized weakness, this recovery may take even longer.

Prognosis

Prognosis is determined by the amount of toxin present in the affected foal, which unfortunately is often unknown, restricting extrapolations on survival in most cases. Type of botulism toxin can be helpful in determining prognosis. Limited reports in both adults and foals make prognosticating difficult. However, a dataset of 30 foals treated for botulism at New Bolton Center revealed an overall 96% survival rate among treated foals, with an 88% survival rate among the 8 treated foals requiring mechanical ventilation [17, 33]. Based on laboratory confirmation (when available) and characteristics of the referral area, these foals likely all had type B botulism. In published literature, a mean combined case-fatality rate of about 70% was seen in several outbreaks (horses of all ages) involving type-B toxin [39–41].

Survival rates in foals are substantially higher than in adult horses. A retrospective study of adult horses treated for botulism at New Bolton Center showed an overall survival rate of 48% [41]. This survival rate was substantially higher than that reported in outbreak situations, which had survival rates of 10–30%. Horses that maintained the ability to rise without assistance were more likely to survive than those that could not rise unassisted. Survival rate for horses that arrived at the hospital with the ability to rise was 67%, and if they maintained the ability to rise throughout hospitalization, their survival rate was 95%. Conversely, horses that could not rise had a survival rate of only 18%, even with aggressive hospital treatment [42].

Prevention

Only one USDA-approved vaccine against equine botulism is available in the United States (BotVax® B, Neogen Corporation;http://animalsafety.neogen.com/en/neogenvet-botvax-b). This product is a killed (toxoid) vaccine directed against *C. botulinum* type B. The initial series consists of three doses administered at 4-week intervals, with subsequent yearly boosters. Pregnant mares should receive their primary series and then be revaccinated 4–6 weeks prior to foaling. Passively acquired maternal antibodies do not appear to interfere with the foal's serologic response, so foals can have their primary series started as early as 2 weeks of age, although it is more commonly started at 1–3 months of age. It is important to note that in endemic areas, early vaccination (2 weeks) of foals is often recommended since botulism can be seen in foals born to vaccinated dams, even with adequate transfer of passive immunity (IgG > 800 mg/dl).

Unfortunately, there are no licensed vaccines available for preventing types A or C botulism, and there is no cross-protection between types. Horses affected by botulism may not develop protective immunity, as the amount of toxin required for intoxication is less than that required to stimulate an immune response. Therefore, affected horses and foals should be vaccinated during or after recovery, assuming that *C. botulinum* type B is the serotype of concern.

Regarding prevention of wound botulism, appropriate care of penetrating wounds or umbilical infections in foals is imperative. Other preventative measures for botulism in the foal and adult include fastidious feeding practices involving fresh, good-quality grain and forages where applicable.

References

1 Rocke, T.E. (1993). Clostridium botulinum. In: *Pathogenesis of Bacterial Infections*, 2e (ed. C.L. Gyles and C.O. Thoen), 86–96. Ames, IA: Iowa State University Press.
2 Rings, D.M. (1987). Bacterial meningitis and diseases caused by bacterial toxins. *Vet. Clin. North Am. Equine Pract.* 3: 85–97.
3 Zhou, Y., Sugiyamam, H., and Johnson, E.A. (1993). Transfer of neurotoxigenicity from clostridium butyricum to a nontoxigenic clostridium botulinum type E-like strain. *Appl. Environ. Micribiol.* 59: 3825–3831.
4 Lamanna, C. (1959). The most poisonous poison. *Science* 130: 763–772.
5 Christine, R.E., Lemichez, E., and Popoff, M.R. (2020). Public health risk associated with botulism as foodborne zoonoses. *Toxins* 12 (1): 17.
6 Smith, L.D.S. (1979). Clostridium botulinum: characteristics and occurrence. *Rev. Infect. Dis.* 1: 637–641.
7 Smith, L.D.S. (1978). The occurrence of clostridium botulinum and clostridium tetani in the soil of the United States. *Health Lab. Sci.* 15: 74–80.
8 Fleck-Derderian, S., Shankar, M., Rao, A.K. et al. (2017). The epidemiology of foodborne botulism outbreaks: a systematic review. *Clin. Infect. Dis.* 66 (suppl1): S73–S81.
9 Espelund, M. and Klaveness, D. (2014). Botulism outbreaks in natural environments – an update. *Front. Microbiol.* 5: 287.
10 Galey, F.D.G. (2001). Botulism in the horse. *Toxicology* 17: 579–588.
11 Johnson, A.L., McAdams, S.C., and Whitlock, R.H. (2010). Type a botulism in horses in the United States: a review of the past ten years (1998–2008). *J. Vet. Diagn. Invest.* 22: 165–173.
12 Semrad, S. and Peek, S. (2002). Equine botulism. *Compend. Contin. Educ. Pract.* 24: 169–172.
13 Whitlock, R.H. and McAdams, S. (2006). Equine botulism. *Clin. Tech. Equine Pract.* 5: 37–42.
14 Spickler, AR. (2018). Botulism. http://www.cfsph.iastate.edu/DiseaseInfo/factsheets.php (accessed 21 March 2023).
15 Shapiro, R.L., Hatheway, C.L., and Swerdlow, D.L. (1998). Botulism in the United States: a clinical and epidemiological review. *Ann. Intern. Med.* 129: 221–228.
16 Swerczek, T.W. (1980). Toxicoinfectious botulism in foals and adult horses. *J. Am. Vet. Med. Assoc.* 176: 217–220.
17 Wilkins, P.A. and Palmer, J.E. (2003). Botulism in foals less than 6 months of age: 30 cases (1989–2002). *J. Vet. Intern. Med.* 17: 702–707.
18 Böhnel, H. and Gessler, F. (1999). Clostridia and clostridioses. *Immunol. Med. Microbiol.* 24: 4.
19 Rosow, L.K. and Strober, J.B. (2015). Infant botulism: review and clinical update. *Pediatr. Neurol.* 52: 487–492.
20 Jeffery, I.A. and Karim, S. (2021). Botulism. In: *StatPearls*. Treasure Island (FL): StatPearls Publishing https://pubmed.ncbi.nlm.nih.gov/29083673/.
21 Peng, L., Liu, H., Ruan, H. et al. (2013). Cytotoxicity of botulinum neurotoxins reveals a direct role of Syntaxin 1 and SNAP-25 in neuron survival. *Nat. Commun.* 4: 1472.
22 Lindstrom, M. and Korkeala, H. (2006). Laboratory diagnostics of botulism. *Microbiol. Rev.* 298–314.
23 Rooney, J.R. (1967). Shaker foal syndrome. *Mod. Vet. Pract.* 48: 44–47.
24 Whitlock, R.H. (1994). Botulism type C experimental and field cases in the horse. *Proc. Annu. Meet. Am. College Vet. Int. Med.* 13: 720–723.
25 Johnson, A.L., McAdams-Gallagher, S.C., and Aceto, H. (2016). Accuracy of a mouse bioassay for the diagnosis of botulism in horses. *J. Vet. Intern. Med.* 30: 1293–1299.
26 Johnson, A.L., Sweeney, R.W., McAdams, S.C. et al. (2012). Quantitative real-time PCR for detection of the neurotoxin gene of clostridium botulinum type B in equine and bovine samples. *Vet. J.* 194: 118–120.

27 Johnson, A.L., McAdams-Gallagher, S.C., and Sweeney, R.W. (2014). Quantitative real-time PCR for detection of neurotoxin genes of *Clostridium botulinum* types A, B, and C in equine samples. *Vet. J.* 199: 157–161.

28 Thomas, R.J. (1991). Detection of *Clostridium botulinum* types C and D toxin by ELISA. *Aust. Vet. J.* 68: 111–113.

29 Holcombe, S.J., Hurcombe, S.D., Barr, B.S. et al. (2011). Dysphagia associated with presumed pharyngeal dysfunction in 16 neonatal foals. *Equine Vet. J.* 44: 105–108.

30 Aleman, M., Williams, D.C., Jorge, N.E. et al. (2011). Repetitive stimulation of the common peroneal nerve as a diagnostic aid for botulism in foals. *J. Vet. Intern. Med.* 25: 365–372.

31 Mullen, K.R., Rivera, B., Tidwell, L.G. et al. (2020). Environmental surveillance and adverse neonatal health outcomes in foals born near unconventional natural gas development activity. *Sci. Total Environ.* 731: 138497.

32 Vaala, W.E. (1991). Diagnosis and treatment of *Clostridium botulinum* infection in foals: A review of fifty-three cases. In: *Proceedings of the 9th Annual Veterinary Medical Forum*. New Orleans, LA: American College of Veterinary Internal Medicine.

33 Wilkins, P.A. and Palmer, J.E. (2003). Mechanical ventilation in foals with botulism: 9 cases (1989–2002). *J. Vet. Intern. Med.* 17: 708–712.

34 Johnson, J.K. and Whitlock, R.W. (1987). Botulism. In: *Current Therapies in Equine Medicine and Surgery*, 2e (ed. N.E. Robinson), 367–370. Philadelphia, PA: WB Saunders.

35 Paradelis, A.G., Triantaphyllidis, C., and Giala, M.M. (1980). Neuromuscular blocking activity of aminoglycoside antibiotics. *Methods Find. Exp. Clin. Pharmacol.* 2: 45–51.

36 Cook, D. and Simons, D.J. (2021). *Neuromuscular Blockade*. Treasure Island (FL): StatPearls Publishing PMID: 30855885.

37 Whitlock, R.H. and Buckley, C. (1997). Botulism. *Vet. Clin. North Am. Equine Pract.* 13: 107–128.

38 Wang, Y. and Sugiyama, H. (1984). Botulism in metronidazole-treated conventional adult mice challenged orogastrically with spores of clostridium botulinum type A or B. *Infect. Immun.* 46: 715–719.

39 Witchell, J.J. and Whitlock, R.H. (1991). Botulism associated with feeding alfalfa hay to horses. *J. Am. Vet. Med. Assoc.* 199: 471–474.

40 Ricketts, S.W., Greet, T.C.R., Glyn, P.J. et al. (1984). Thirteen cases of botulism in horses fed big bale silage. *Equine Vet. J.* 16: 515–518.

41 Bernard, W., Divers, T.J., Whitlock, R.H. et al. (1987). Botulism as a sequel to open castration in a horse. *J. Am. Vet. Med. Assoc.* 191: 73–74.

42 Johnson, A.L., McAdams-Gallgher, S.C., and Aceto, H. (2015). Outcome of adult horses with botulism treated at a veterinary hospital: 92 cases (1989–2013). *J. Vet. Intern. Med.* 5: 311–319.

Neonatal Musculoskeletal System

Chapter 33 Embryology and Anatomy of the Neonatal Musculoskeletal System

Emma Adam

The horse is a species that gives birth to precocious young. Within hours of birth a foal can run with its dam over some distance and at speed if necessary (Figure 33.1). This breathtaking feat of evolutionary success is even more astounding considering that a foal's skeleton is immature. The scope for growth within the neonatal skeleton is extensive and part of an incredible continuum of musculoskeletal embryological development. Postnatally, the advantages and synergy of the vertebrate musculoskeletal system are obvious to the observer. These include bony protection of the brain, a pliable vertebral column, synovial joints that endow flexibility, and long tendons and sesamoids that confer mechanical advantage, to name but a few. In the embryo developing *in utero*, the genesis of these complex structures is part of an utterly magnificent, orchestrated program.

The musculoskeletal system is composed of tissues with diverse biomechanical properties that confer huge evolutionary advantages. The body plan of tetrapods is highly conserved, and its development is tightly regulated by patterning and differentiating factors that govern the number, size, and shape of musculoskeletal elements, as well as the fate of the cells comprising these structures.

Soon after fertilization, the process of cell division occurs to first generate a ball of cells, the morula, followed by the generation of a fluid-filled ball, called the blastula, that clearly distinguishes cells that will form the fetal membranes from the embryo proper. The three germ layers – ectoderm, mesoderm, and endoderm – are formed during the next process, gastrulation, when anterior–posterior polarity is also established. During the next stage of embryogenesis, neurulation occurs. This critical step heralds the start of organogenesis from germ layer tissues. Once organogenesis is complete, the embryo is referred to as a fetus. The rearrangement of the germ layer components results in the formation of different regions of mesoderm tissue. The mesoderm contributes massively to the formation of the musculoskeletal system. Figure 33.2 shows the contributions of the mesoderm to morphogenesis, which include:

- Chordamesoderm: forming the notochord.
- Paraxial mesoderm: (also called the somitic mesoderm) forming muscle, connective tissue of the back, vertebrae, and ribs.
- Intermediate mesoderm: forming the kidneys, gonads, adrenal cortex.
- Lateral plate mesoderm: forming the heart, circulatory system, pelvic, and limb skeleton.

Germ Layer Contributions

Somites are bilaterally paired blocks of paraxial mesoderm tissue that form simultaneously on both sides of the neural tube (Figure 33.2). Somites are specified according to their anterior–posterior position in the paraxial mesoderm. This is under the control of highly conserved expression of *Hox* genes. Thirty-nine Hox genes are found in humans as four paralogous clusters *(Hoxa, Hoxb, Hoxc, Hoxd)*. The position of the cluster corresponds to the expression pattern along the anterior–posterior axis of the developing embryo's head, trunk, and limbs [2]. While the structures that the somites go on to develop is determined, the differentiation fate of the cells within each somite is still subject to influences from cell–cell interaction, cell signaling molecules, and the expression of key transcription factors. The first portion of the somite to differentiate is the ventromedial portion which becomes the sclerotome. The transcription factor, Sonic hedgehog (Shh), and the bone morphogenetic protein (BMP) antagonist signaling protein, Noggin, are secreted by the notochord to induce sclerotome formation. The sclerotome forms the vertebrae and proximal portions of the ribs, trunk muscle tendons, and the vertebral joints [3]. The remaining portion of the somite becomes the

Equine Neonatal Medicine, First Edition. Edited by David M. Wong and Pamela A. Wilkins.

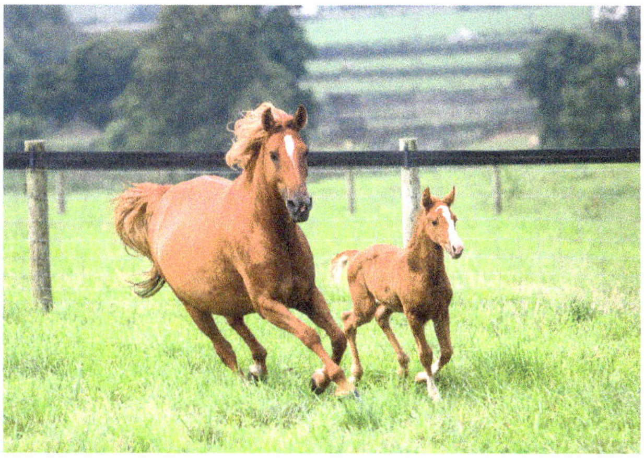

Figure 33.1 Mare with neonatal foal at foot. The foal is a few days old. *Source:* Image courtesy of University of Kentucky, College of Agriculture, Food and Environment.

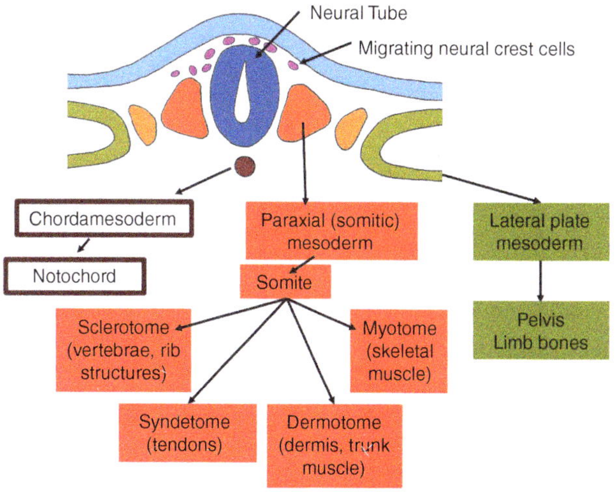

Figure 33.2 Schematic representation of the three embryologic germ layers in a cross section of a neurula stage embryo showing their contribution to various musculoskeletal body structures. (Note: Not all derivatives shown). *Source:* Diagram drawn by Grace Adam, adapted from Gilbert [1].

dermomyotome. The skeletal muscles of the trunk and limbs are all generated from this compartment of cells. Cells of the dermomyotome are multipotent. They become committed to their cell fate through a host of extracellular signaling pathways such as Wnt/β-catenin signaling and BMP family proteins and transcription factors such as Shh. Development of the vertebral column will not be covered in this chapter; the reader is referred to an excellent review by Scaal [4].

Cells within the dermomyotome under the influence of Wnt1, Wnt 3a, and Shh become determined for a myogenic fate at this stage, developing into the myotome. The fourth compartment of the somite is the syndetome, which forms later as the cells between the dermatome and myotome are influenced by Fgf8 produced by the adjacent myotome [1]. The syndetome is the source of tendon progenitor cells in the trunk and limbs.

Limb Development

The appendicular skeleton arises from limb buds that form in set positions on both sides of the early embryo. In mice, with a gestation of 19–20 days as a frame of reference, this occurs around E9 in the forelimb with the hindlimb lagging behind by ~0.5 days (E9 is 9 days of embryonic development counted from the morning after coitus). These early limb buds consist of loose undifferentiated lateral plate mesoderm derived mesenchyme surrounded by ectoderm origin epithelium. Seminal *in ovo* chick studies performed in the 1940s recognized that the apical ectoderm of the limbs bud, termed the apical ectodermal ridge (AER), was a critical signaling center [1]. Subsequent studies in chicks and mammalian species revealed it to be responsible for continued outgrowth of the limb bud and maintenance of plasticity of the underlying mesenchyme. A positive feedback loop of Fgf8 from the ectoderm and Fgf10 from the mesenchyme is critical for continued growth of the limb bud. Hox gene interactions, along with gradients of signaling molecules, such as retinoic acid, interact to specify forelimb and hindlimb designation [5, 6]. Hox genes associated with murine forelimbs and hindlimbs are *Tbx4* and *Tbx5/Pitx1,* respectively [7]. In addition to the AER, the Zone of Polarizing Activity and "positional information" gradients generate the anterior–posterior and dorsal-ventral pattern orientation of the tetrapod limb pattern (Figure 33.3) [8]. The sequential formation of a single element stylopod, double-element zeugopod, and multiple rays of the autopod is a conserved theme in the tetrapod limb across multiple species. The chemical-mathematical model for limb element patterning was proposed by Alan Turing in 1952 [9]. Since that time, it has received much attention and supporting research data.

In horses, only the central rays of the autopod are maintained. These develop into metacarpals/metatarsals II, III, and IV, and phalanges of the central digit. Little is known about this stage of equine embryological limb development. However, as seen in Figure 33.4a, the tissue in the limb bud at this stage is as yet ill-defined. Comparing the images in Figure 33.4 with Figure 33.3, the advanced limb patterning and skeletal tissue development that has taken place in the intervening 10 days is truly remarkable.

Development of Cartilaginous Primordia

Mesenchymal cells in the developing limb bud transiently stop proliferating and express adhesion molecules such as N-cadherin and tenascin-C. They form precartilaginous condensations in a proximal to distal order in the limb via

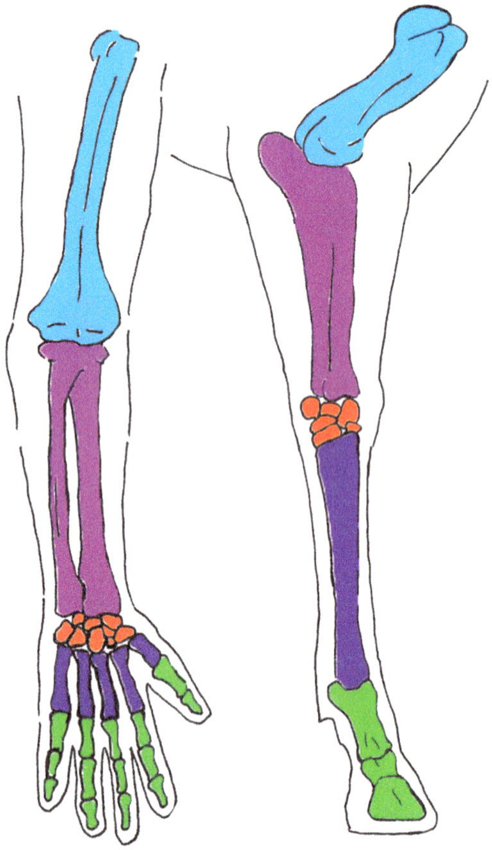

Figure 33.3 The tetrapod limb. Homologous elements of the tetrapod limb are compared between the human (*left*) and equine (*right*) forelimb. In the forelimb the stylopod develops as the humerus, the zeugopod consists of the radius and ulna, and the autopod consists of the metacarpals and digit(s). In the hindlimb the stylopod develops as the femur, the zeugopod consists of the tibia and fibula, and the autopod consists of the metatarsals and digit(s). *Source:* Diagram by Grace Adam.

poorly understood mechanisms. Most peripheral cells of these condensed cell aggregates differentiate into chondrocytes. Once formed, chondrocytes in these cartilaginous primordia, or anlagen (anlage singular), start proliferating again and produce cartilage extracellular matrix driven largely by the Sox triad of transcription factors, Sox5, Sox6, and Sox9, under BMP signaling [10]. Part of a small anlage may be seen in the forelimb bud of the equine fetus at 35 days postovulation (Figure 33.4). The most peripheral cells of the anlage remain skeletogenic and become the perichondrium (Figure 33.5). At this stage of development, the as-yet unpatterned vascular growth entering the developing limb undergoes spatial rearrangement in response to the developing skeleton. Vessels regress from the more central area of the limb tissue as mesenchyme condenses in this position as the anlagen form [11]. Unlike the developing musculature, it is the anlagen that are prerequisite for the development of limb vasculature [12].

Skeletogenesis

Skeletogenic cells are multipotent mesenchymal cells that migrate to specific body locations and commit to a skeletal fate. The primary skeleton is cartilaginous and able to grow rapidly. The majority of this cartilage is replaced by bone through endochondral ossification (Figures 33.6 and 33.7). The bony skeleton confers locomotor mechanical advantage while also participating in mineral homeostasis. Endochondral ossification is one mechanism of bone formation. A second process, intramembranous ossification, also contributes to the skeleton but will not be discussed in detail here. In brief, in flat bones, such as those of the skull,

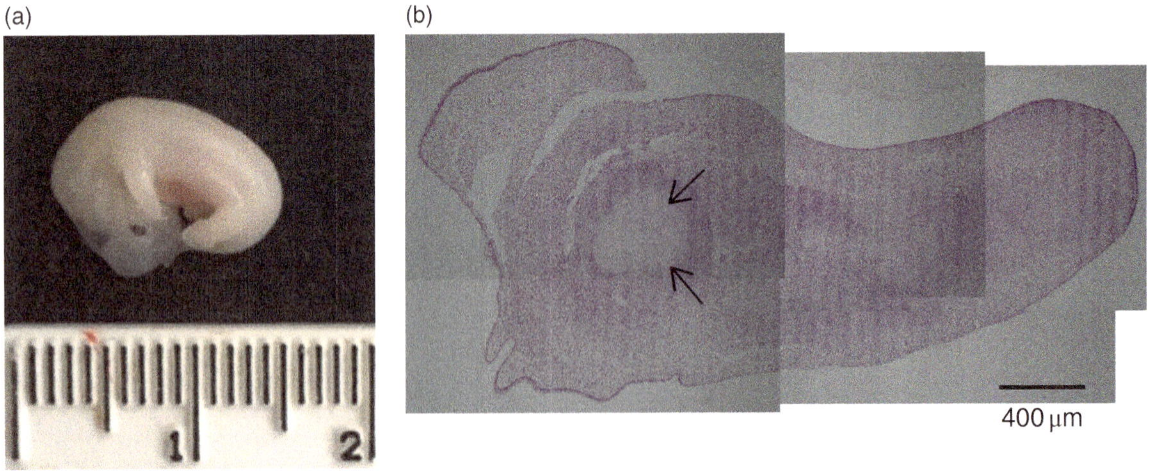

Figure 33.4 (a) Photograph of an equine embryo 35 days postovulation. The forelimb and hindlimb buds are clearly visible but shorter than the tail. The scale bar is in centimeters. (b) Composite photomicrographs of the forelimb of this embryo stained with hemotoxylin and eosin in sagittal section. The tip of the limb bud is on the right of the image. In the left part of the image, corresponding to the proximal part of the limb bud, an area of cartilaginous tissue is visible (black arrows). *Source:* Image courtesy of Emma Adam, James MacLeod Laboratory, Gluck Equine Research Center.

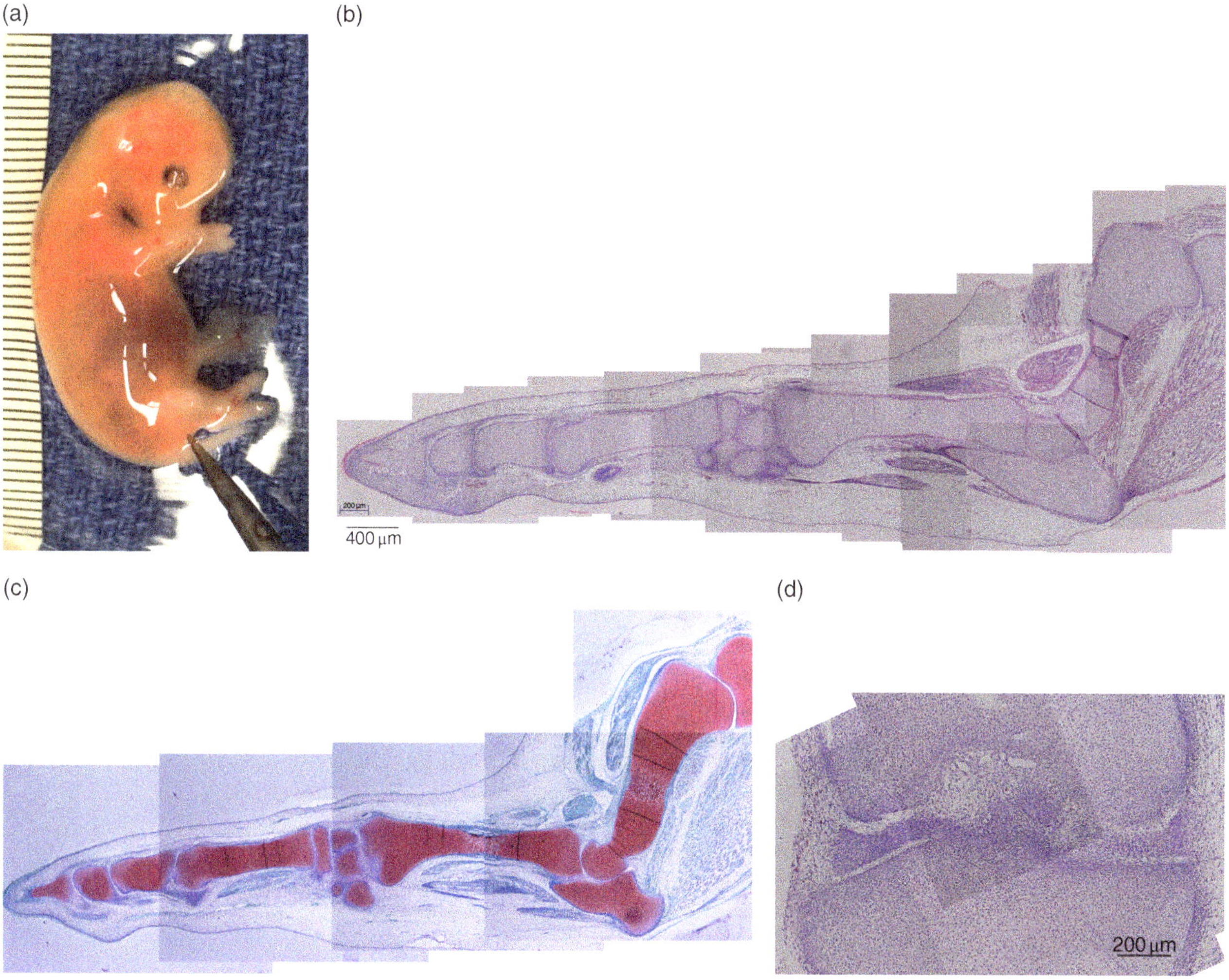

Figure 33.5 (a) Photograph of an equine embryo 46 days postovulation. The limbs are slightly longer than the tail. The scale bar to the left is in millimeters. (b) and (c) Composite photomicrographs of the forelimb of this embryo in sagittal view stained with hemotoxylin and eosin (b) and safranin-O and fast green (c). In both images nascent centers of ossification are visible in the humerus and just distinguishable in mid radius (there are transverse artefactual lines from tissue section folding in both humeri). Safranin-O stains proteoglycans in cartilage matrix red. In image (c) the proximal sesamoid bone is visible. All joints in the forelimb of this age of embryo appear to be cavitated. (d) Shows the stifle of this embryo cut in the frontal plane. The menisci are clearly visible between the femoral condyles and proximal tibia. The nascent cruciate ligaments are also evident. In this section it is unclear as to whether the joint is completely cavitated. *Source:* Image courtesy of Emma Adam, James MacLeod Laboratory, Gluck Equine Research Center.

skeletogenic cells condense into compact nodules and form bone directly without a cartilage primordia intermediary. By definition, skeletogenic cells are undifferentiated. Lineages are largely established by the expression of master transcription factors such as Sox9 for chondroprogenitor cells and Runx2 for osteoprogenitor cells. However, multiple mechanisms are in place to keep them under proper control.

Development of Synovial Joints

The synovial joint is a remarkable structure composed of opposing articular cartilage surfaces on the ends of bone, within a fibrous capsule. The capsule is lined by synovial cells that synthesize synovial fluid in the synovial cavity. Some synovial joints have intra-articular structures such as ligaments and menisci, but what they all have in common is their remarkable embryological origins. Like other areas of embryology and morphogenesis, our understanding of joint formation has progressed tremendously by leveraging techniques such as cell lineage tracing, selective, and inducible knock in/knock out genetic models and elegant imaging techniques.

Each putative joint site is initially seen as a region of flattened, condensed cells at a specific point in the as-yet uninterrupted cartilaginous anlage in the developing limb [14]. This region is termed the interzone. Removal of, or damage to, interzone tissue results in incomplete

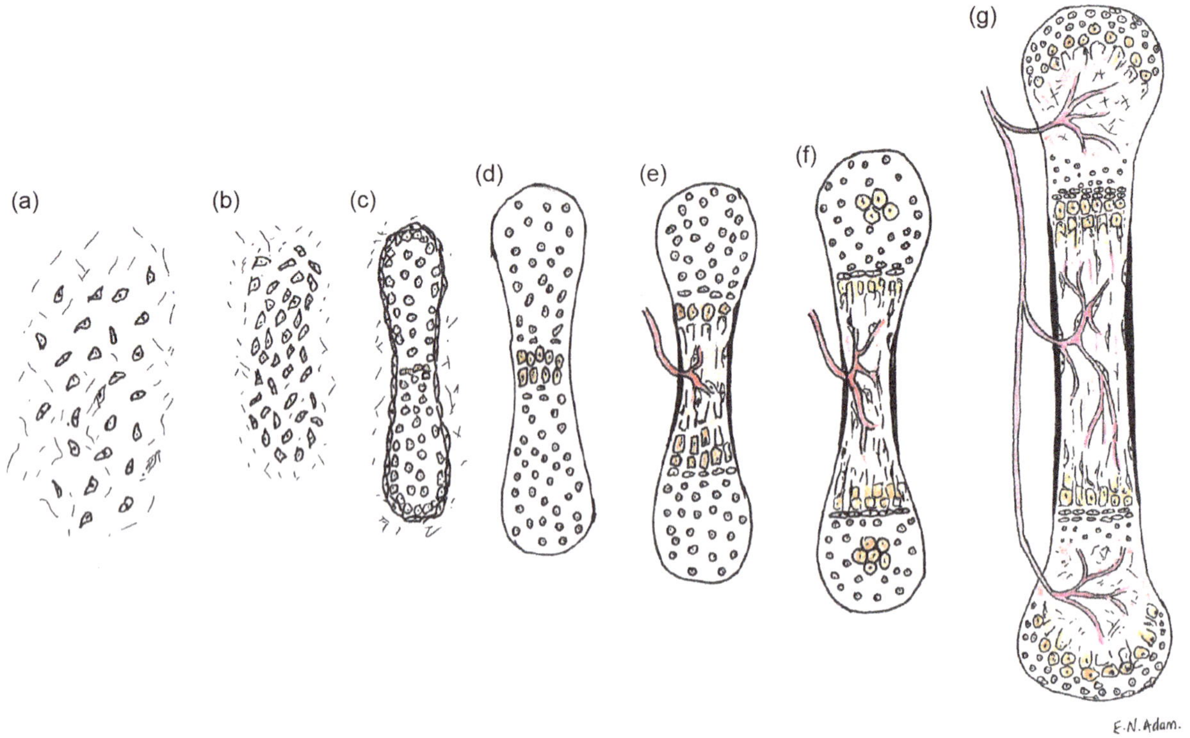

Figure 33.6 Schematic diagram of the process of endochondral ossification from the stages of precondensation mesenchyme to the immature long bone with active primary and secondary centers of ossification: (a) precondensation mesenchyme cells in the limb bud; (b) condensed mesenchyme forming an anlage; (c) anlage showing the chondrocytes surrounded by perichondrium; (d) hypertrophy of the chondrocytes in the central portion of the anlage; (e) invasion of blood vessels in the region of chondrocyte hypertrophy and maturation. Emergence of a bone collar in the central area of the diaphysis; (f) establishment of bone marrow and further development of cortical bone around the mid-diaphyseal region; (g) establishment of secondary centers of ossification in the epiphyses at each end of the developing bone, with bone developing in these locations (perichondrium not depicted in images (d), (e), (f), and (g)). Adapted and drawn by Emma Adam from W. A. Horton [13].

formation or failure of the joint to form [15–17]. Joint formation takes place in a proximal to distal direction within the limb, starting with the appearance of the cellular interzone, which then forms a cavitated synovial joint. The initially cellular joint becomes cavitated through the synthesis of hyaluronic acid, which hydrostatically forms an acellular space within the interzone [16]. The process of joint formation takes a matter of days in the embryo of mice and in the equine embryo likely occurs between 35 and 50 days of gestation counted from ovulation (E.N. Adam and J.N. MacLeod personal communication). One published study examining the equine stifle supports this time frame with the observation of the presence of an interzone at day 37 and well-formed intra-articular structures by day 50 [18]. Images of a fetal forelimb and the stifle at day 46 postovulation (Figure 33.5) show that joint formation appears to be more advanced in the proximal joints compared to the distal joints, as well as showcasing the remarkable detail of limb formation already present at this age.

Soon after formation, the interzone develops a tri-layer appearance with two outer compacted cell layers and a more loosely packed cell layer centrally [15, 19]. Interzone cells express *Gdf5*, which is considered a hallmark gene, although gene expression patterns between the outer and inner layers are different [20, 21]. Studies suggest that the compacted outer layer goes on to form the articular cartilage [20]. Remarkable tracing studies have shown this cell population is responsible for all of the intra-articular structures of the joint: articular cartilage, intra-articular menisci and ligaments, and the synovial membrane [22–25]. More recent work suggests that there is a continuous influx of *Gdf5*$^{-}$/*Sox9*$^{+}$/*Col2a1*$^{-}$ cells that migrate to the interzone and then start to express *Gdf5* [26]. These fascinating studies suggest that the tissues of the synovial joint arise from a broad, heterogeneous interzone progenitor cell population found within the developing anlagen with contributions from progenitor cells flanking the prospective joint sites [26, 27]. As the fetus grows, the articular cartilage continues to develop. At term, the neonatal articular

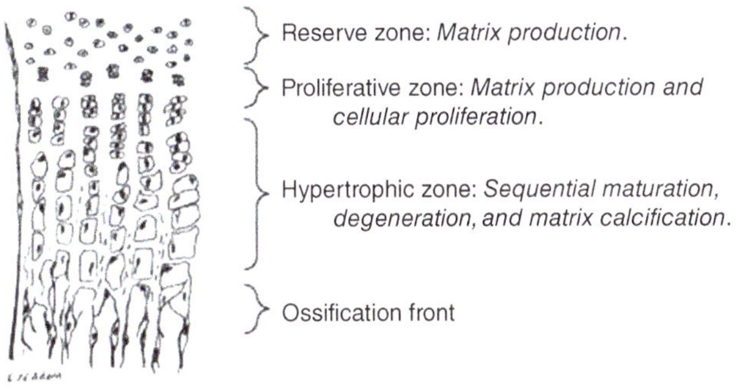

Figure 33.7 Schematic representation of the epiphyseal growth plate depicting the sequence of cellular events of endochondral ossification. *Source:* Drawing by Emma Adam.

cartilage is much more cellular than adult articular cartilage and exhibits differences in gene expression and extracellular matrix composition [28, 29].

Endochondral Ossification

Chondrocyte proliferation and hypertrophy are the drivers of cartilaginous primordia elongation. Chondrocytes in all but the very ends of the bones, where articular cartilage exists, are destined to be replaced by bone through the process of endochondral ossification. The cellular sequence of events is such that anlagen chondrocytes stop proliferating, become pre-hypertrophic, hypertrophic, and then, after calcification of the matrix around them by synthesis of alkaline phosphatase, undergo apoptosis as terminal chondrocytes [30]. The majority of lengthening of the developing bone primordia is a attributed to chondrocyte hypertrophy in the growth plate (Figures 33.6 and 33.7) [31]. It is believed that all hypertrophic chondrocytes undergo apoptosis at this stage, but definitive proof is lacking [31].

Almost concordant to chondrocyte apoptosis, lacunae of the dead cells and calcified cartilage matrix are invaded by osteoblast progenitors differentiating from mesenchymal tissue and translocating with the invasion of blood vessels [32]. Locally acting factors such as Indian Hedgehog (Ihh) from prehypertrophic chondrocytes and the expression of *Runx2* induce the perichondrium to form osteoblast progenitor cells [32, 33]. This leads to the formation of a bone collar in the outer layer of the perichondrium through intramembranous ossification, and the perichondrium in this region becomes a periosteum. The production of vascular endothelial growth factor (VEGF) by prehypertrophic chondrocytes promotes an initial vascular invasion that brings osteoclasts and endothelial cells, as well as translocating osteoblast precursor cells to the center of the cartilage primordia [32]. This heralds the formation of the primary ossification center in the bone [34].

Critical transcription factors related to osteogenesis include Runx2, which is required for full osteoblastic differentiation, as well as osterix (Osx), which is required for osteoblast formation and differentiation into mature osteocytes. As osteoblasts differentiate, they produce matrix proteins, including the main bone constituent, type I collagen (Col1). Mature osteoblasts that become embedded in the bone matrix differentiate into resident osteocytes [35].

Local and systemic factors regulate proliferation, differentiation, and apoptosis of growth plate chondrocytes. As previously mentioned, Ihh is produced by prehypertrophic chondrocytes. In addition to promoting proliferation of chondrocytes in the proliferative zone and hypertrophy, it also stimulates osteoblast differentiation and synthesis of parathyroid hormone-related peptide (PTHrP) in the perichondrium. PTHrP inhibits the transition of proliferative chondrocytes to prehypertrophic cells, thus establishing a negative feedback loop that controls the size and activity of the proliferative zone in the growth plate. This is critical to the coupling of cortical bone formation and the longitudinal growth of the bone. This has been investigated somewhat in foals and lambs with angular limb deformities where this mechanism may play a part in disproportionate bone length [36]. The perichondrium has a bigger role in bone growth than previously thought. It synthesizes fibroblast growth factor 18 (Fgf18), which acts to negatively regulate chondrocyte proliferation, and through Ext1- and Ext2 glycosyltransferases exerts a boundary function regulating growth and differentiation of the growth plate [37].

As the fetus grows and the primary ossification center expands, secondary ossification centers form in one or both ends of the developing bone (Figure 33.6). The images in Figure 33.8 show three early equine fetuses and the extent of ossification of their skeleton as seen by digital radiographs.

Development of Skeletal Muscle

Skeletal muscle is derived from the dermomyotome. The major transcription factors for muscle formation are the myogenic regulatory factors (MRFs), of which MyoD, Myf5, myogenin, and MRF4 are the most influential. Myf5, MRF4, and MyoD are myogenic determination factors and myogenin is a differentiation factor. These myogenic factors function with positive feedback loops tempered by factors such as myostatin. Myostatin (*Mstn* gene symbol) is released by myocytes to inhibit myogenesis.

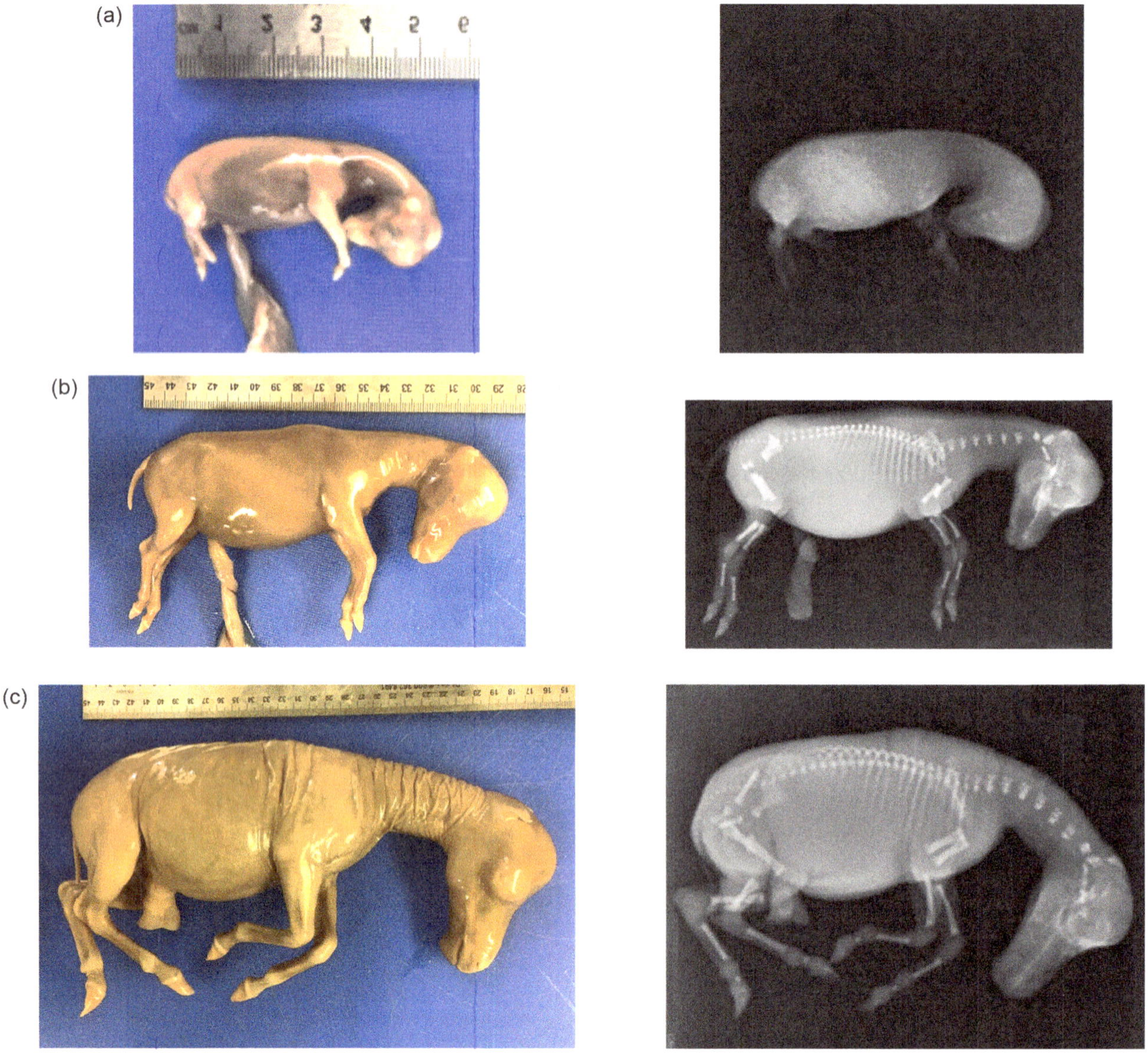

Figure 33.8 Three equine fetuses collected from pregnant mares that presented to a veterinary diagnostic laboratory for necropsy following death from other causes. The approximate ages of the fetuses are (a) 60 days, (b) 95 days, and (c) 140 days. Images on the right show the level of ossification as imaged by routine digital radiography. Vertebral body ossification is just visible in image (a). *Source:* Fetuses graciously loaned by Sara Welch, UKVDL, and radiographs kindly performed by Hagyard Equine Medical Institute.

The initial cascade of differentiation into committed muscle progenitor cells, called myoblasts, commences with *Pax3*$^+$ cells being activated to express *Myf5* by Wnt signaling in the presence of Shh and the absence of BMPs. Hepatocyte Growth Factor secreted by limb mesenchyme acts as a paracrine signal for the migration of myogenic precursor cells into the limb bud [3]. In a proximal to distal developmental progression myoblasts differentiate and fuse together to form myofibers. To achieve this, myoblasts exit the cell cycle, alter cell adhesion molecule expression, such as the cadherins, and fuse their membranes. Membrane fusion is mediated by metalloproteinases called meltrins.

Muscle retains the ability to hypertrophy and repair damage into adulthood as a function of the retention of unfused muscle progenitor cells, called satellite cells. Satellite cells contain both stem cells and progenitor cells demonstrated by different anti-apototic and myogenic genes [38]. Stem cells are *Pax7*$^+$/*Myf5*$^-$ and make up an estimated 10% of the population, while satellite progenitor cells are *Pax7*$^+$/*Myf5*$^+$, which make up the majority of the satellite cell population and differentiate into muscle [38]. The signaling cascade that regulates muscle repair is analogous to that which acts on muscle formation in embryogenesis [3].

Development of Tendons

Tendon progenitor cells (TPC) arise from the syndetome compartment of the somite. In the developing limb they are found in the subectodermal mesenchyme in a proximal to distal direction as the limb bud extends and develops [39]. The tendon's specific transcription factor, Scleraxis (*Scx*) is expressed in these cells, but also in muscle progenitor cells that are found in a similar location, but the two populations are considered different [40]. Cartilage primordia (anlagen) and muscle differentiation generally precede that of tendons. In the mouse, for example, cartilage, muscle, and tendon differentiation and basic patterning are in place by E10.5, E11.5, and E13.5, respectively [40]. Tendon progenitors, following induction, become organized in parallel bundles along the axis of where the tendon will form [41]. The initial induction of tendon progenitor cells occurs in locations that are dorsal and ventral to the more central cartilage analgen. In the mouse, distinct tendon patterns are present by day E12.5 and by E13.5 they have condensed to form tendon structures, concurrently expressing critically important tendon related and tendon specific genes including tenomodulin (*Tnmd*), *Mkx*, *Egr1*, *Egr2*, and Collagen type 1 (*Col1a1*). Primary tendon patterning is complete 1 day later, but the splitting and coalescing of certain tendons to generate the final pattern may not be complete at this time. Mechanical stimulation is important in tendon formation even at these early stages of development [42, 43].

In the images of the equine fetal limb (Figure 33.5), the tendon structures are clearly present and appear to be patterned. The flexor tendons and extensor tendons at this stage of fetal development are already different in size (author's personal observation). Little is known about the development of fetal tendons in the horse, but one equine study corroborates findings in other species that the immature digital tendon in term fetuses is more cellular than adult tendon [44].

The requirement of movement and the presence of muscle tissue for tendon development has been investigated in other organisms with some interesting results [40]. In spite of earlier studies suggesting muscle and tendon can develop autonomously, further work has shown that while the presence of muscle may not be required for development, it is required for the later differentiation and maintenance of tendon [40]. Little is known about tendon development in the autopod, although it is independent of muscle formation [43]. Likewise, autopod cartilage is known to play a critical role in tendon formation, but exactly how is unknown. A study in mice demonstrated that the position of the origin of the superficial digital flexor musculotendinous unit actually translocates from the paw to the forearm [45]. This concept has not been explored in the equine limb where long digital tendons are common.

The origin of the enthesis, the tendon-bone attachment, is considered to be different from that of the tendon proper [46]. Indeed, tracing studies show that these bony eminences do not arise from chondroprogenitor cells as once thought, but from a separate population of $Scx^{+}/Sox9^{+}/Col2a1^{-}$ cells under the regulation of TGFβ/BMP4 signaling. These findings may have bearings on studies examining the origins of sesamoids.

Sesamoids

Sesamoids are small auxiliary bones near joints and are typically embedded in tendons. They contribute to the stability and function of the joint. In other species they can be highly variable in size and number, but in the horse their size and position are stable. Sesamoids of the equine skeleton include the navicular bone (distal sesamoid bone), proximal sesamoid bones adjacent to the metacarpo/metatarsophalangeal joints, and the patella. The development of sesamoids in the horse is poorly understood but is the subject of ongoing study. A few case reports discuss bipartite navicular bones that may be the result of aberrations in bone development [47]. In Figure 33.5 a nascent proximal sesamoid bone is clearly visible adjacent to the fetlock joint.

Original theories regarding the formation of sesamoid bones include: (i) they are induced within tendons under mechanical forces generated during embryonic movement; or (ii) they detach from the cartilage anlage during joint development [10]. Recent studies have demonstrated that both theories have merit. The patella has been shown in mice to arise as part of the femur and separate during femoropatellar joint formation under stimuli from mechanical load [48]. Furthermore, similar to bone eminences, these cells are from $Sox9^{+}/Scx^{+}$ progenitor cells (cartilage forming chondroprogenitor cells are typically $Sox9^{+}/Scx^{-}$) that require TGFβ for specification, BMP2 signaling for growth, and BMP2 and/or BMP4 for differentiation [46]. The development of digital sesamoids (and that of the fabella) differs from that of the patella. Again, in mice, they originate from $Scx^{+}/Sox9^{+}$ progenitor cells but independent of mechanical stimulation, and the formation of their fibrocartilaginous articulating surface is not Gdf5 dependent [49]. Taken together, the distinct cohorts of progenitor cells that form different sesamoids under different stimuli may be of note when considering repair processes in postnatal musculoskeletal injuries.

The embryological processes that generate the musculoskeletal system are both fascinating and impressive. It is remarkable that patterning and structure layout are complete by approximately 50 days postovulation in a gestation lasting approximately 340 days. The continued growth of the musculoskeletal system and the progressive ossification of bony structures is a process that continues postnatally. These processes, and the remarkable adaption they are capable of for athletic function, are of intense interest to equine veterinarians and equestrians alike. Investing in a better understanding of these developmental processes may enable us to overcome the frustrations and difficulties that relate to tissue injury, repair, and regeneration in the adult horse.

References

1 Gilbert, S. (2014). *Developmental Biology*, 10e. Sunderland, MA: Sinauer Associates, Inc.
2 Wellik, D.M. (2007). Hox patterning of the vertebrate axial skeleton. *Dev. Dyn.* 236: 2454–2463.
3 Endo, T. (2015). Molecular mechanisms of skeletal muscle development, regeneration, and osteogenic conversion. *Bone* 80: 2–13.
4 Scaal, M. (2016). Early development of the vertebral column. *Semin. Cell Dev. Biol.* 49: 83–91.
5 Taher, L., Collette, N.M., Murugesh, D. et al. (2011). Global gene expression analysis of murine limb development. *PLoS One* 6: e28358.
6 Butterfield, N.C., McGlinn, E., and Wicking, C. (2010). The molecular regulation of vertebrate limb patterning. *Curr Topics Develop Biol* 90: 319–341.
7 Tickle, C. (2015). How the embryo makes a limb: determination, polarity and identity. *J. Anat.* 227: 418–430.
8 Young, J.J. and Tabin, C.J. (2017). Saunders's framework for understanding limb development as a platform for investigating limb evolution. *Dev. Biol.* 429: 401–408.
9 Turing, A.M. (1952). The chemical basis of morphogenesis. *Philos. Trans. R. Soc. Lond. Ser. B Biol. Sci.* 237: 37–72.
10 Hall, B.K. and Miyake, T. (2000). All for one and one for all: condensations and the initiation of skeletal development. *Bioessays* 22: 138–147.
11 Eshkar-Oren, I., Viukov, S.V., Salameh, S. et al. (2009). The forming limb skeleton serves as a signaling center for limb vasculature patterning via regulation of Vegf. *Development* 136: 1263–1272.
12 De Angelis, L., Berghella, L., Coletta, M. et al. (1999). Skeletal myogenic progenitors originating from embryonic dorsal aorta coexpress endothelial and myogenic markers and contribute to postnatal muscle growth and regeneration. *J. Cell Biol.* 147: 869–878.
13 Horton, W.A. (1990). The biology of bone growth. *Growth Genet. Hormones* 6 (1): 1–3.
14 Fell, H. (1925). The histogenesis of cartilage and bone in the long bones of the embryonic fowl. *J. Morphol.* 40: 417–459.
15 Decker, R.S., Koyama, E., and Pacifici, M. (2014). Genesis and morphogenesis of limb synovial joints and articular cartilage. *Matrix Biol.* 39C: 5–10.
16 Khan, I.M., Redman, S.N., Williams, R. et al. (2007). The development of synovial joints. In: *Current Topics in Developmental Biology* (ed. P.S. Gerald), 1–36. Academic Press.
17 Pacifici, M., Koyama, E., Shibukawa, Y. et al. (2006). Cellular and molecular mechanisms of synovial joint and articular cartilage formation. *Ann. N. Y. Acad. Sci.* 1068: 74–86.
18 Jenner, F., van Osch, G.J., Weninger, W. et al. (2015). The embryogenesis of the equine femorotibial joint: the equine interzone. *Equine Vet. J.* 47: 620–622.
19 Rux, D., Decker, R.S., Koyama, E. et al. (2019). Joints in the appendicular skeleton: developmental mechanisms and evolutionary influences. *Curr. Top. Dev. Biol.* 133: 119–151.
20 Jenner, F., Cleary, M., Heijsman, D. et al. (2014). Differential gene expression of the intermediate and outer interzone layers of developing articular cartilage in murine embryos. *Stem Cells Dev.* 23: 1883–1898.
21 Storm, E. and Kingsley, D.M. (1999). GDF5 coordinates bone and joint formation during digit development. *Dev. Biol.* 209: 11–27.
22 Koyama, E., Ochiai, T., Rountree, R.B. et al. (2007). Synovial joint formation during mouse limb Skeletogenesis. *Ann. N. Y. Acad. Sci.* 1116: 100–112.
23 Koyama, E., Shibukawa, Y., Nagayama, M. et al. (2008). A distinct cohort of progenitor cells participates in synovial joint and articular cartilage formation during mouse limb skeletogenesis. *Dev. Biol.* 316: 62–73.
24 Hyde, G., Boot-Handford, R.P., and Wallis, G.A. (2008). Col2a1 lineage tracing reveals that the meniscus of the knee joint has a complex cellular origin. *J. Anat.* 213: 531–538.
25 Hyde, G., Dover, S., Aszodi, A. et al. (2007). Lineage tracing using matrilin-1 gene expression reveals that articular chondrocytes exist as the joint interzone forms. *Dev. Biol.* 304: 825–833.
26 Shwartz, Y., Viukov, S., Krief, S. et al. (2016). Joint development involves a continuous influx of Gdf5-positive cells. *Cell Rep.* 15: 2577–2587.
27 Rountree, R.B., Schoor, M., Chen, H. et al. (2004). BMP receptor signalling is required for postnatal maintenance of articular cartilage. *PLoS Biol.* 2: 1815–1827.
28 Mienaltowski, M., Huang, L., Bathke, A. et al. (2010). Transcriptional comparisons between equine articular

repair tissue, neonatal cartilage, cultured chondrocytes and mesenchymal stromal cells. *Brief. Funct. Genomics* 9: 238–250.

29 Mienaltowski, M., Huang, L., Stromberg, A. et al. (2008). Differential gene expression associated with postnatal equine articular cartilage maturation. *BMC Musculoskelet. Disord.* 9: 149.

30 St-Jacques, B., Hammerschmidt, M., and McMahon, A.P. (1999). Indian hedgehog signaling regulates proliferation and differentiation of chondrocytes and is essential for bone formation. *Genes Dev.* 16: 2072–2086.

31 Lefebvre, V. and Bhattaram, P. (2010). Vertebrate skeletogenesis. *Curr. Top. Dev. Biol.* 90: 291–317.

32 Maes, C., Kobayashi, T., Selig, M.K. et al. (2010). Osteoblast precursors, but not mature osteoblasts, move into developing and fractured bones along with invading blood vessels. *Dev. Cell* 19: 329–344.

33 Berendsen, A.D. and Olsen, B.R. (2015). Bone development. *Bone* 80: 14–18.

34 Karsenty, G. and Wagner, F. (2002). Reaching a genetic and molecular understanding of skeletal development. *Dev. Cell* 2: 389–406.

35 Wagner, E.F. and Karsenty, G. (2001). Genetic control of skeletal development. *Curr. Opin. Genet. Dev.* 11: 527–532.

36 Liesegang, A., Giezendanner, R., Tanner, S. et al. (2010). Systemic and local effects of disproportional longitudinal growth of bones in foals and lambs and the impact on bone mineral density and content. *Pferdeheilkunde* 26: 495–502.

37 Huegel, J., Mundy, C., Sgariglia, F. et al. (2013). Perichondrium phenotype and border function are regulated by Ext1 and heparan sulfate in developing long bones: a mechanism likely deranged in hereditary multiple exostoses. *Dev. Biol.* 377: 100–112.

38 Kuang, S., Kuroda, K., Le Grand, F. et al. (2007). Asymmetric self-renewal and commitment of satellite stem cells in muscle. *Cell* 129: 999–1010.

39 Arvind, V. and Huang, A.H. (2017). Mechanobiology of limb musculoskeletal development. *Ann. N. Y. Acad. Sci.* 1409: 18–32.

40 Huang, A.H. (2017). Coordinated development of the limb musculoskeletal system: tendon and muscle patterning and integration with the skeleton. *Dev. Biol.* 429: 420–428.

41 Connizzo, B.K., Yannascoli, S.M., and Soslowsky, L.J. (2013). Structure-function relationships of postnatal tendon development: a parallel to healing. *Matrix Biol.* 32: 106–116.

42 Benjamin, M. and Ralphs, J.R. (2000). The cell and developmental biology of tendons and ligaments. *Int. Rev. Cytol.* 196: 85–130.

43 Huang, A.H., Lu, H.H., and Schweitzer, R. (2015). Molecular regulation of tendon cell fate during development. *J. Orthop. Res.* 33: 800–812.

44 Stanley, R.L., Fleck, R.A., Becker, D.L. et al. (2007). Gap junction protein expression and cellularity: comparison of immature and adult equine digital tendons. *J. Anat.* 211: 325–334.

45 Huang, A.H., Riordan, T.J., Wang, L. et al. (2013). Repositioning forelimb superficialis muscles: tendon attachment and muscle activity enable active relocation of functional myofibers. *Dev. Cell* 26: 544–551.

46 Blitz, E., Sharir, A., Akiyama, H. et al. (2013). Tendon-bone attachment unit is formed modularly by a distinct pool of Scx- and Sox9-positive progenitors. *Development* 140: 2680–2690.

47 Dyson, S.J. (2010). Fracture of the navicular bone and congenital bipartite navicular bone. In: *Diagnoses and Management of Lameness in the Horse*, 2e (ed. M.W. Ross and S.J. Dyson), 243–344. St. Louis: Elsevier.

48 Eyal, S., Blitz, E., Shwartz, Y. et al. (2015). On the development of the patella. *Development* 142: 1831–1839.

49 Eyal, S., Rubin, S., Krief, S. et al. (2019). Common cellular origin and diverging developmental programs for different sesamoid bones. *Development* 146: dev167452.

Chapter 34 Clinical Neonatal Musculoskeletal Physiology

Ashlee Watts

The healthy foal is born responsive to stimulation, is sternal within a few minutes, and will be circling the mare in short bursts of running within 2–3 hours of birth. To support this degree of movement, the musculoskeletal system must be well developed at birth and continue to develop rapidly in the early postnatal period. The normal physiology of musculoskeletal system in the neonatal period will be discussed in this chapter.

Bone

In accordance with Wolff's law, bone is an intensely dynamic tissue that models and remodels throughout life dependent on the loads placed on it. In short, low strain leads to osteocyte apoptosis and bone resorption whereas high strain results in deposition of bone and an increase in bone mass with targeted remodeling of damaged bone. Prenatal bone development occurs independent of the load it experiences, and this is termed *anticipative bone modeling*. Anticipative bone modeling is particularly important in a precocial species that will be running within hours of birth [1]. The effect of anticipative bone modeling is in both bone composition/quantity and bone architecture/quality (bone is anisotropic at birth), and it appears to be genetically programed to prepare the bone for a dramatic increase in load in the postnatal period [1–3].

Another precocial characteristic is that the foal is born with only small amounts of unossified growth cartilage in the epiphyses and short bones. These areas in the articular-epiphyseal-complex will ossify to form subchondral bone starting in patches that are related to the amount of load experienced. These patches of subchondral bone development and differences in trabecular bone architecture at birth may dictate predilection sites for osteochondrosis lesions or possibly even common areas of bone fracture in adults [1, 2].

In the early postnatal period, bone continues to respond in accordance with Wolff's law (i.e. bone adapts to loads under which they are placed). The importance of play behavior in foals and its optimization of strain applied to bone has been shown [4]. When pasture-kept foals exhibiting normal play behavior were additionally exercised in canter, there was a significant increase in size and strength of the first phalanx and the cannon bone compared to non-exercised foals, and these differences may persist into adulthood [5–7].

Cartilage

Articular cartilage in the newborn foal is a "blank slate" in that there is no heterogeneity in the proteoglycan content, collagen content or collagen cross-linking, and no anisotropy, like there is in the adult. This blank slate rapidly develops into the heterogeneous phenotype of mature cartilage in response to normal locomotion of the foal [8]. The high metabolism of articular cartilage in the neonatal foal is reflected by high synovial fluid concentrations of hydroxyproline and glycosaminoglycans (GAG) that decline rapidly in the first months of life [9]. When box-rested foals were compared to pastured and exercised foals, there were significant differences in GAG, DNA, collagen, and hydroxylysine content at 5 months of age [10]. This was termed a delay in *functional adaptation* of the box-rested foals. This delay of functional adaptation of articular cartilage may translate to increased risk for osteochondral injury. Additionally, if functional adaptation does not occur in the postnatal period, subsequent adaptation may be delayed or incomplete, especially for the collagen characteristics of articular cartilage [10, 11].

The articular cartilage is also part of the articular-epiphyseal complex (AEC), which is the growth cartilage responsible for the formation of the secondary ossification

Equine Neonatal Medicine, First Edition. Edited by David M. Wong and Pamela A. Wilkins.

center in the postnatal period. This occurs via calcification of growth cartilage, invasion by blood vessels, chondrification, chondroclastic removal of calcified cartilage, and bone production by osteoblasts. Prior to and during this process of ossification, the blood supply is provided by cartilage canals throughout the AEC. Cartilage canals with their vessels run transversely to the articular surface superficially within the AEC and perpendicularly at the osteochondral junction. The anastomosis between the transverse and perpendicular cartilage canal might be a site for premature vessel failure. Failure of the blood supply due to occlusion by thrombi, bacteria, or trauma results in chondronecrosis that can lead to osteochondrosis lesions [3, 8, 12, 13]. Bacterial adhesion may be predisposed at this site because cartilage canals are surrounded by collagen type I rather than cells [3]. Osteochondrosis is less common in pony breeds, and this may be because pony foals have fewer cartilage canals and thinner growth cartilage than horse foals [14].

The physis is also a vascularized growth cartilage that undergoes endochondral ossification with calcification of cartilage, invasion by blood vessels, chondrification, chondroclastic removal of calcified cartilage, and bone production by osteoblasts. The blood supply to the physis changes with age. The foal is born with metaphyseal-origin arteries to the physis. In 1- to 10-day-old foals, the physis has both metaphyseal- and epiphyseal-origin arteries. After 15 days of age, the physis has epiphyseal-origin arteries only. Vessels in the cartilage have a monopodial branching pattern, and vessels in epiphyseal and metaphyseal bone have a monopodial and dichotomous branching pattern [15].

Tendon and Ligament

Neonatal tendon and ligament is highly cellular and has a larger and more uniform fibril size compared to tendon in the adult horse [16, 17]. Unlike adult tendon, foal tendon is highly adaptable [18, 19] and exercise is critical for normal tendon development [20]. When foals were pastured, kept in stalls, or kept in stalls with forced exercise, the pastured foals had stronger, more elastic superficial digital flexor tendons (SDFTs) with a large cross-sectional area and a trend toward increased hysroxylysine and hydroxypuridonline cross-links as well as higher cellularity, polysulfated glycosaminoglycan (PSGAG), hyaluronic acid (HA), and cartilage oligomeric matrix protein (COMP) content [21–23]. While size and mechanical characteristics of tendons [24] change with exercise of foals, cellularity does not. These data support that at-will exercise and normal play behavior of foals is critical for normal tendon and ligament development, and it is possible that additional forced exercise in pasture-kept foals could be beneficial [4, 20, 23].

Muscle

Like the other musculoskeletal tissues, the muscle of postnatal foals is highly developed and fully functional at birth. However, major changes still occur in the postnatal period. The distribution of myosin heavy-chain type 1 (slow), type 2a (fast oxidative), and type 2d (fast glycolytic) fiber types changes with a decrease in fast fibers and an increase in slow fibers in the first 5 months of age and loss of developmental myosin heavy chain fibers by 2 months of age [25]. The effect of training on postnatal muscle composition has been studied. The concentration of Na^+, K^+-ATPase increased in gluteus medius and semitendinosus muscle, but not in masseter muscle, in 5-month-old foals that were exercised compared to stalled foals, which suggests a benefit of improved performance by training [26, 27]. There are several inherited congenital muscle abnormalities reported in horses that result in abnormal metabolism and/or neuroconduction (Chapter 36).

References

1 Gorissen, B.M.C., Wolschrijn, C.F., van Vilsteren, A.A.M. et al. (2016). Trabecular bone of precocials at birth; are they prepared to run for the wolf? *J. Morphol.* 277: 948–956.
2 Anne-Archard, N., Martel, G., Fogarty, U. et al. (2019). Differences in third metacarpal trabecular microarchitecture between the parasagittal groove and condyle at birth and in adult racehorses. *Equine Vet. J.* 51: 115–122.
3 Hellings, I.R., Dolvik, N.I., Ekman, S. et al. (2017). Cartilage canals in the distal intermediate ridge of the tibia of fetuses and foals are surrounded by different types of collagen. *J. Anat.* 231: 615–625.
4 Rogers, C.W. and Dittmer, K.E. (2019). Does juvenile play programme the equine musculoskeletal system? *Animals (Basel)* 9: 646.
5 Firth, E.C., Rogers, C.W., van Weeren, P.R. et al. (2011). Mild exercise early in life produces changes in bone size and strength but not density in proximal phalangeal, third metacarpal and third carpal bones of foals. *Vet. J.* 190: 383–389.
6 Firth, E.C., Rogers, C.W., van Weeren, P.R. et al. (2012). The effect of previous conditioning exercise on diaphyseal and metaphyseal bone to imposition and withdrawal of training in young thoroughbred horses. *Vet. J.* 192: 34–40.

7 Rogers, C.W., Firth, E.C., McIlwraith, C.W. et al. (2008). Evaluation of a new strategy to modulate skeletal development in thoroughbred performance horses by imposing track-based exercise during growth. *Equine Vet. J.* 40: 111–118.

8 Lecocq, M., Girard, C.A., Fogarty, U. et al. (2008). Cartilage matrix changes in the developing epiphysis: arly events on the pathway to equine osteochondrosis? *Equine Vet. J.* 40: 442–454.

9 van den Boom, R., PAJ, B., Kiers, G.H. et al. (2004). Assessment of the effects of age and joint disease on hydroxyproline and glycosaminoglycan concentrations in synovial fluid from the metacarpophalangeal joint of horses. *Am. J. Vet. Res.* 65: 296–302.

10 PaJ, B., TeKoppele, J.M., Bank, R.A. et al. (2002). Development of biochemical heterogeneity of articular cartilage: influences of age and exercise. *Equine Vet. J.* 34: 265–269.

11 Brama, P.A., Tekoppele, J.M., Bank RA et al. (2000). Functional adaptation of equine articular cartilage: the formation of regional biochemical characteristics up to age one year. *Equine Vet. J.* 32: 217–221.

12 Olstad, K., Hendrickson, E.H.S., Carlson, C.S. et al. (2013). Transection of vessels in epiphyseal cartilage canals leads to osteochondrosis and osteochondrosis dissecans in the femoro-patellar joint of foals; a potential model of juvenile osteochondritis dissecans. *Osteoarthr. Cartil.* 21: 730–738.

13 Olstad, K., Ytrehus, B., Ekman, S. et al. (2008). Epiphyseal cartilage canal blood supply to the distal femur of foals. *Equine Vet. J.* 40: 433–439.

14 Hendrickson, E.H.S., Olstad, K., Nødtvedt, A. et al. (2015). Comparison of the blood supply to the articular-epiphyseal growth complex in horse vs. pony foals. *Equine Vet. J.* 47: 326–332.

15 Wormstrand, B.H., Fjordbakk, C.T., Griffiths, D.J. et al. (2021). Development of the blood supply to the growth cartilage of the medial femoral condyle of foals. *Equine Vet. J.* 53: 134–142.

16 Crevier-Denoix, N., Collobert, C., Sanaa, M. et al. (1998). Mechanical correlations derived from segmental histologic study of the equine superficial digital flexor tendon, from foal to adult. *Am. J. Vet. Res.* 59: 969–977.

17 Parry, D., Craig, A.S., and Barnes, G. (1978). Tendon and ligament form the horse: An ultrastructural study of collegen fibrils. *Proceedings of Royal Society* 203 (1152): 293–303.

18 Young, N.J., Becker, D.L., Fleck, R.A. et al. (2009). Maturational alterations in gap junction expression and associated collagen synthesis in response to tendon function. *Matrix Biol.* 28: 311–323.

19 Dowling, B.A. and Dart, A.J. (2005). Mechanical and functional properties of the equine superficial digital flexor tendon. *Vet. J.* 170: 184–192.

20 Smith, R.K., Birch, H., Patterson-Kane, J. et al. (1999). Should equine athletes commence training during skeletal development?: changes in tendon matrix associated with development, ageing, function and exercise. *Equine Vet. J. Suppl.* 30: 201–209.

21 Cherdchutham, W., Becker, C., Smith, R.K. et al. (1999). Age-related changes and effect of exercise on the molecular composition of immature equine superficial digital flexor tendons. *Equine Vet. J. Suppl.* 31: 86–94.

22 Cherdchutham, W., Becker, C.K., Spek, E.R. et al. (2001). Effects of exercise on the diameter of collagen fibrils in the central core and periphery of the superficial digital flexor tendon in foals. *Am. J. Vet. Res.* 62: 1563–1570.

23 Cherdchutham, W., Meershoek, L.S., van Weeren, P.R. et al. (2001). Effects of exercise on biomechanical properties of the superficial digital flexor tendon in foals. *Am. J. Vet. Res.* 62: 1859–1864.

24 Stanley, R.L., Goodship, A.E., Edwards, B. et al. (2008). Effects of exercise on tenocyte cellularity and tenocyte nuclear morphology in immature and mature equine digital tendons. *Equine Vet. J.* 40: 141–146.

25 Dingboom, E.G., Dijkstra, G., Enzerink, E. et al. (1999). Postnatal muscle fibre composition of the gluteus medius muscle of dutch warmblood foals; maturation and the influence of exercise. *Equine Vet. J. Suppl.* 31: 95–100.

26 Suwannachot, P., Verkleij, C.B., Kocsis, S. et al. (2001). Specificity and reversibility of the training effects on the concentration of Na+, K+-atpase in foal skeletal muscle. *Equine Vet. J.* 33: 250–255.

27 Suwannachot, P., Verkleij, C.B., Weijs, W.A. et al. (1999). Effects of training on the concentration of Na+, K+-ATPase in foal muscle. *Equine Vet. J. Suppl.* 31: 101–105.

Chapter 35 Examination, Therapeutics, and Monitoring of the Neonatal Musculoskeletal System

Section I Diagnostic Tests

Dustin Major

Submission of blood for assessment of a CBC and serum biochemistry profile in the neonatal foal is an invaluable tool to aid in diagnosis of disease and monitoring response to treatment. Given the concern for sepsis in neonatal foals, particularly those presenting in a hospital setting, blood culture is also often indicated. Alterations in the CBC or biochemistry profile are not typically observed in foals with noninfectious orthopedic disease such as angular or flexural limb deformities or congenital musculoskeletal anomalies; however, clinicopathologic changes can occur secondary to noninfectious orthopedic disease. For example, a foal with a severe flexural limb deformity may be unable to stand/suckle, thereby resulting in failure of passive transfer of immunity and sepsis. Conversely, foals with infectious orthopedic disease frequently have alterations in the CBC and elevation of serum fibrinogen concentration; these parameters can be serially monitored throughout treatment as a reflection of response to therapy, or lack thereof. Moreover, elevations in muscle enzymes may suggest myopathy in the neonatal foal. Evaluation of the neonate's CBC and biochemistry analysis is provided elsewhere in this text; the purpose of this section is to provide specific alterations that occur with musculoskeletal disease.

Complete Blood Count and Serum Biochemistry

White blood cell (WBC) counts and cell differentials in neonatal foals are comparable to adult horses and, from a clinical perspective, can be interpreted similarly when evaluating for disease processes. For example, neutropenia with or without degenerative and/or toxic changes is a hallmark of sepsis just as it is for systemic inflammatory response syndrome (SIRS) in the adult. However, changes to the WBC in foals immediately after birth are reflective of conditions experienced in utero. Infections under these circumstances often result in leukocytosis, with or without true infection of the foal itself [1].

When considering localized infections such as omphalophlebitis, enteritis, or septic arthritis, WBC parameters can be variable, and even normal, depending on severity and presence or absence of systemic sepsis [2]. In one study foals with septic arthritis had significantly greater leukocytosis (mean 16,000 cells/μl) compared to adults with the same condition [3]. Additionally, it is prudent to consider whether or not these localized infections are a result of sepsis (i.e. seeding of a joint in a foal with bacteremia), contributing to active sepsis, or an isolated problem not resulting in systemic disease. Another retrospective study noted that 61.8% of foals with septic arthritis in addition to osteomyelitis demonstrated leukogram abnormalities, most commonly a mild-to-marked leukocytosis (12,400–33,900 cells/μl; reference range 5200–12,000 cells/μl). A small portion of foals had normal total WBC counts with elevated band neutrophils (430–1340 bands/μl). The vast majority of foals in this study (86.8%) also demonstrated hyperfibrinogenemia (500–1100 g/dl; reference range 200–400 g/dl) [1].

Normal reference intervals of packed cell volume (PCV) and platelets are established (Chapter 42) [1, 4, 5]. The PCV is slightly higher at birth and drops rapidly with colostrum/milk intake. Increased PCV may indicate dehydration, which, in turn, can be an indication of inadequate nursing for any reason. Decreases in PCV may result from blood loss, red blood cell destruction (i.e. hemolysis), or decreased production, the latter being rare. Platelet numbers in normal neonates are similar to those of adults. Platelet counts in some septic foals are within reference limits (110,000–300,000/μl) from admission through 48 hours of hospitalization; in one study, there were no differences in platelet count between survivors and nonsurvivors [3]. It has been the author's experience that this is largely true for foals with septic arthritis as well, and the literature

Equine Neonatal Medicine, First Edition. Edited by David M. Wong and Pamela A. Wilkins.

examining leukogram and hemogram changes in these foals make no mention of changes in platelet numbers [3–6]. Thrombocytopenia can be due to lab error (platelet clumping in EDTA), increased platelet use (septic foal with coagulopathy), destruction of platelets by infectious agents (equine herpes virus-1, equine viral arteritis), or allo- or autoimmune reactions. Interpretation of thrombocytopenia in foals should be made in light of the clinical picture as absolute number of platelets does not always correlate with clinical signs [4, 6].

Total serum and plasma protein values in healthy foals are reported in Chapter 44 but these parameters increase with colostrum ingestion, though albumin levels are relatively static. Total protein levels will also increase with dehydration and chronic disease, particularly the globulin component in the latter. Hypertriglyceridemia in foals will falsely elevate total protein concentrations as measured by refractometer as the triglyceride molecules are also refractile. Acute phase proteins, namely fibrinogen and serum amyloid A (SAA), are useful in tracking progression of inflammatory/infectious diseases, both localized and systemic, as well as response to treatment. Fibrinogen concentrations are low at birth (117 ± 39 mg/dl) [7], with elevated values (i.e. >400 mg/dl) in the newborn suggestive of an abnormal intra-uterine environment. Expected SAA ranges have been published for healthy foals (median 0.9 μg/ml; 1 day old) [8–11] as well as for those with bronchopneumonia (median for *Rhodococcus equi* cases 212 μg/ml vs 27 μg/ml for other bacteria) [12], LPS-induced (between 150 and 200 μg/ml in serum and 100–150 μg/ml in synovial fluid) and naturally occurring septic arthritis (median 195 μg/ml) [8, 13], diarrhea, sepsis, localized abscesses, viral infection, GI disease, various noninfectious neonatal diseases, and abortion [8]. One study demonstrated higher SAA in obese foals at 90 and 180 days, which were also at higher risk of osteochondrosis. However, there was no difference between normal and obese foals at birth [14], and the relationship between these factors is uncertain. Clinically, both fibrinogen and SAA are most useful when performed as serial measurements, taken every 24 hours or more, with trends in SAA facilitating evaluation of progression of disease and treatment.

Serum creatine kinase (CK) and aspartate aminotransferase (AST) are used to evaluate muscle injury or disease. CK activity may increase for reasons unrelated to myonecrosis/muscle injury. In adult horses, moderate exercise can result in elevations up to 500 IU/l; and recumbent horses can have elevations up to 3000 IU/l. Baseline activity, on the other hand, is considered to be <250 IU/l with peak activity typically observed 4–6 hours postinjury. Rhabdomyolysis generally results in very high elevations (>100,000 IU/l). The half-life of CK is short in comparison to AST, with AST peaking 24 hours postinjury. This dichotomy allows the clinician to interpret the progression of muscle insult. If CK is still rising with little or no change in AST, injury is ongoing and very recent while concurrent increases in CK and AST indicates ongoing injury that is somewhat older in onset. If CK is decreasing but AST is rising or static, injury is in the early stages of resolving. If the activity of one or both of the enzymes remains elevated, the injury is ongoing [15].

Electromyography (EMG) aids in differentiating between neurogenic, neuromuscular, or myopathic disease as well as assisting in more accurate neurologic lesion localization. This procedure involves insertion of small needles into skeletal muscle to measure motor unit action potentials and is usually reserved for referral hospitals rather than field settings [16, 17]. EMG can be useful in foals with abnormal neurologic signs in the absence of other localizing signs or diagnostic findings. This is particularly true in cases where overlapping disease processes makes accurate assessment of the inciting cause difficult (e.g. foal with botulism that did not nurse, developed failure of passive transfer and subsequent sepsis, and is also catatonic and experiencing seizure activity due to hypoglycemia).

EMG does not provide a diagnosis, but rather provides further insight into interpretation of other physical/neurologic examination and diagnostic tests. In the neonatal foal, EMG can be used to assist in the diagnosis of organophosphate toxicity [17], HYPP [18], equine motor neuron disease (EMND) [19], congenital myotonia [20], botulism [21], and congenital centronuclear myopathy [22]. The combination of standard (radiography and ultrasound) and advanced (computed tomography [CT] and magnetic resonance imaging [MRI]) imaging as well as serum biochemistry analysis (CK, AST) aid in facilitating a diagnosis. Additional diagnostics such as muscle biopsy may be necessary. The gluteus medius muscle and semimembranosus muscles are commonly used sites for biopsy [22, 23] although the sacrocaudalis dorsalis muscle is preferred for the diagnosis of EMND [19].

Radiographic evaluation of the musculoskeletal system in the neonatal foal is commonly utilized to assess congenital anomalies of the appendicular or axial skeleton, assess injuries for osseous involvement/fracture, examine painful or enlarged physes, and characterize the extent of septic arthritis. Images taken to assess the thorax for detection of fractured rib(s) are typically performed in lateral recumbency with or without sedation based on the activity level and disease state of the foal; however, ultrasonography has been shown to be more sensitive [24, 25]. Every foal should be examined closely for the presence of rib fractures and any suspects should be imaged as thoracic trauma and lung laceration from fracture fragments can have life threatening consequences. Radiographic assessment of the head and spine is also typically performed in lateral recumbency in the neonate. Assessment of the neonatal spine can be

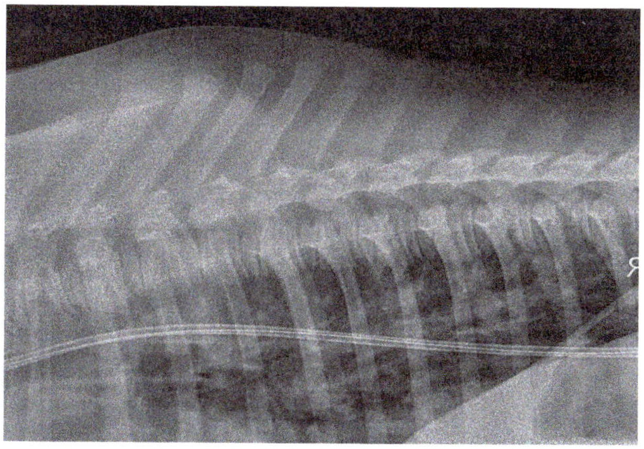

Figure 35.I.1 Neonatal Paint Horse colt presented for meconium impaction. Note the open endplate physes at the cranial and caudal aspects of each vertebral body.

difficult due to the presence of multiple physes in each vertebra. Normal vertebrae will have two endplate physes with their corresponding epiphyses, centers of ossification of the two arches, and the main body (Figure 35.I.1). Congenital malformations of the skull such as wry nose, as well as any injuries, typically require multiple views and/or advanced imaging.

The appendicular skeleton can be imaged either standing or in lateral recumbency depending on the status of the foal. Congenital abnormalities such as angular limb deformities and incomplete ossification of the cuboidal bones are assessed with the foal standing, if possible (Figure 35.I.2a) as this allows better appreciation for the angulation of the limb(s) during weight bearing. While it is often possible to obtain radiographs of both limbs in the same image (Figure 35.I.2b), significant rotation often accompanies angular limb deformities. Separate images of each affected limb from directly dorsopalmar are recommended in order to obtain more accurate measurements of angulation. This also allows for better evaluation of the physes for signs of infection or inflammation (physitis). Conversely, incomplete ossification can be assessed with both limbs in the same image. The best images for assessment are obtained in a dorsopalmar view for the carpi and a lateromedial view of the tarsi. A grading system has been created for this condition, with Grade 4 foals considered normal and Grade 1 having one or more carpal or tarsal bones with no radiographic evidence of ossification [26]. Radiographs should be obtained in a serial fashion throughout the management of the foal in order to guide treatment decisions and inform prognosis.

(a) (b)

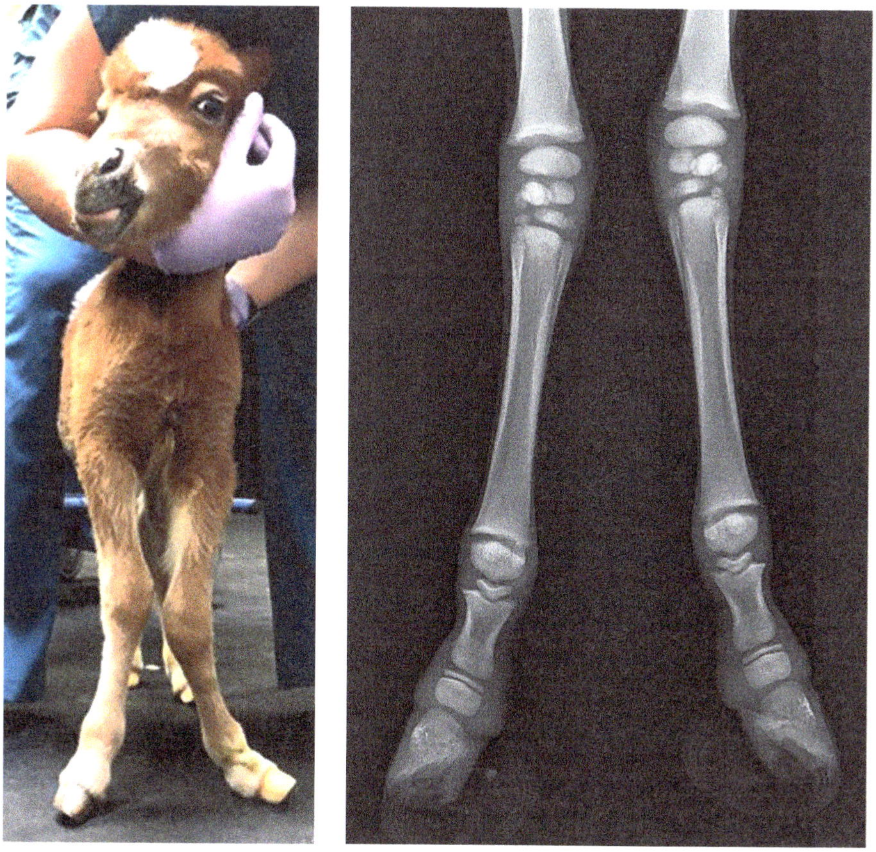

Figure 35.I.2 (a) Three-week-old miniature horse colt born with severe incomplete ossification of the cuboidal bones along with severe carpal and fetlock valgus. Note the coronary band contacts the ground, which results in painful sores.
(b) Dorsopalmer radiograph of same foal with corrective shoes in place.

Radiographs are less useful in cases of contracture or laxity in the absence of evidence of trauma and/or lameness. Lameness in the neonatal foal should be approached diligently as they can rapidly develop contracture in the affected limb and varus angular limb deformity of the contralateral limb. Radiographic examination of a joint that is swollen, painful and/or has heat is always indicated. Joint sepsis in foals is classified as S- (synovial), E- (epiphyseal), P- (physeal), or C-type (cuboidal) with the S-type being the most common in the neonate [27]. However, it is possible for the primary site of infection to spread to affect the adjacent tissues given enough time; and radiography provides a means of assessing for this possibility (Figure 35.I.3).

Radiographs are also indicated if any instability, crepitus, or other evidence of a fracture is noted on orthopedic evaluation. Fractures are rare in the neonate and prognosis for recovery is better than that of adults due to decreased biomechanical forces and increased healing capacity of foals. Diagnosis of fractures can be complicated by the presence of multiple physes; comparison with the same anatomy in similarly aged foal or contralateral side of the same animal can help aid in differentiating normal from abnormal images. Interestingly, a study noted that 74% of 19 normal foals >2 months of age had fractures of the palmar process, none of which demonstrated any lameness [28, 29].

Advanced imaging has become more widely used in the hospital setting. Computed tomography (CT) is a rapid imaging modality that utilizes an X-ray generator and its detectors mounted on a circular gantry to obtain images of slices of anatomy as thin as 1 mm at a time. As the generator and detectors spin around the circle within the gantry tube, the patient is moved into this space within the gantry on the CT table, which is synchronized with the machine. The X-ray detectors continually measure the degree of attenuation of the X-ray beam as it passes through the intervening anatomy, and a computer creates transverse plane images. Images in the dorsal and sagittal planes are extrapolated; in addition, three-dimensional models can be created of the examined anatomy. Description of CT images differs from standard radiographic terminology in that regions of anatomy are described as hyper- or hypoattenuating when they are brighter or darker, respectively. However, the same principles of X-ray beam attenuation by air, soft tissue, mineral, and metal apply. Metallic objects will create a significant artifact on CT examination.

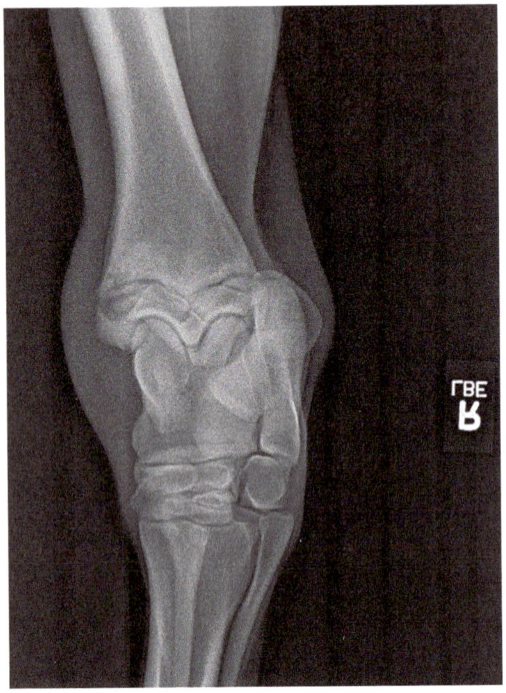

Figure 35.I.3 DLPMO radiograph of a septic physitis (P-type) in a 4-month-old Quarter Horse colt. Note the irregular, asymmetrical lysis, and associated metaphyseal sclerosis in addition to the soft tissue swelling over the affected bone.

Fortuitously, neonatal foals are small enough to allow full body imaging in large bore gantry machines. Image acquisition is significantly faster than MRI and has excellent spatial resolution. A lack of contrast resolution makes evaluation of low contrast regions of anatomy (abdomen, muscle) difficult. However, inherently high contrast anatomic regions such as the head, distal limbs, and lungs/thorax are ideal for CT imaging. The modality has been used not only to evaluate foals for distal limb disease such as septic arthritis [30, 31] and physitis [30, 32], but is recognized as the gold standard for fracture imaging. Studies describe CT use in evaluation, description, diagnosis, and/or treatment of persistent right aortic arch [33], ureteral tearing [34], fracture of the palmar process of P3 [28, 29], normal head and lungs of foals [35, 36], normal paranasal sinuses [37], head trauma [38], temporohyoid osteoarthropathy [39], cervical cord compression with myelography [40], and cardiac tamponade [41].

MRI has also provided an increasingly accurate evaluation of various portions of equine anatomy as this technology has become more advanced and increasingly available. Image acquisition is similar to CT in that there is a circular gantry into which the area of interest is placed. However, the patient is on a stationary table, and only limited regions of anatomy can be imaged before having to move the patient to allow imaging of another region, in contrast to the continuous motion of the CT table into and out of the gantry. Within the gantry the region of anatomy to be imaged is placed within a gradient coil; the size of the bore within the gantry and coil limit the anatomy that can be introduced and imaged. Both standing and recumbent MRI units are available, but only low-field magnets (<1 Tesla [T] of magnetic field strength) are used in standing units. The relatively low power of the magnet, coupled with micro-motion from the standing horse, limits the anatomy that can be imaged to the foot and distal pastern and results in extremely low spatial and contrast resolution. The only logistically viable option for MRI imaging in the neonate is a recumbent unit with the foal under general anesthesia using either a low- or high-field magnet.

Image acquisition using MRI involves alignment of hydrogen proton spinning by application of the magnetic field, followed by excitation of these hydrogen protons by a radio frequency pulse that is then removed. The fall-out of energy of the protons as they return to their native state is measured and converted to a computer-generated image. The different sequences used to obtain images (e.g. STIR, PD, T2-weighted) differ in their measurement and interpretation of the fall-out energy from removal of the radio frequency pulse, and each must be obtained by a separate scan for every plane in which they are obtained (i.e. transverse, dorsal, or sagittal). This results in a much longer total image acquisition time compared to CT. However, high-field magnets have excellent spatial resolution and improved contrast resolution compared to CT, allowing much better soft tissue imaging and identification of fluid (edema, hemorrhage, necrosis) within bone and soft tissue. Additionally, rapid, computed, gradient echo sequences have been engineered allowing more rapid image acquisition with very small (i.e. 1 mm) slice thickness.

In the neonate, soft tissue injuries to the distal limb are relatively uncommon and CT evaluation is arguably better and certainly faster when assessing bony abnormalities as stated above. Evaluation of the thorax and abdomen with MRI is often not possible due to the limitations of gantry and coil size. Therefore, MRI is clinically utilized to evaluate the head and rostral/cranial central nervous system in young foals. MRI descriptions of the brain anatomy in healthy neonatal foals [42] as well foals with neonatal encephalopathy [43], closed head trauma [44], bacterial meningoencephalitis [45], cerebellar abiotrophy [46], hydrocephalus [47], Chiari malformation [48], and mandibular ossifying fibroma have been reported [49].

Muscle Biopsy

Myogenic disorders in neonatal foals are diagnosed through physical and neurologic exam, as well as evaluation of serum muscle enzyme activity (CK, AST), urinalysis, EMG, and muscle biopsy. CK and AST can be difficult to interpret as they can be mildly elevated in recumbent foals, but are typically severely elevated in cases of myopathies.

Histopathology of muscle biopsy samples, in conjunction with other diagnostic tests, has been used to diagnose EMND [19], selenium/vitamin E deficiency (white muscle disease or nutritional muscular dystrophy) [50, 51], polysaccharide storage myopathies (PSSM) [22], glycogen-branching enzyme deficiency (GBED) [52], and congenital centronuclear myopathy [22]. The gluteus medius muscle and semimembranosus muscles are common sites for biopsy [22, 23] with the sacrocaudalis dorsalis muscle preferred for diagnosis of EMND [19]. Ultrasonography can be useful to evaluate the proposed biopsy site not only for any abnormalities associated with the architecture and/or echogenicity of the musculature but also to determine the depth necessary to obtain a sample when using a Bergstrom needle. Biopsy of the gluteus medius muscle is performed along a straight line between the point of the tuber coxa and the tail head at a depth of as little as 1 cm [23]. Alternatively, a small linear incision can be made over the muscle to be biopsied, and a 1 cm biopsy can be obtained with direct visualization of the muscle sampled. Light sedation and a local anesthesia are sufficient to obtain muscle biopsies by either method.

Synoviocentesis and Cytologic Evaluation

Septic arthritis is common in neonatal foals. Wounds involving articular communication also occur with relative frequency, but diagnosis of articular involvement does not differ significantly from that of adult horses. Bacteremia can distribute organisms hematogenously, resulting in localized disease such as septic arthritis. Bacteria can settle in end capillary beds within the physes and joint capsule, resulting in localized infection. Affected foals are typically severely lame and maintain recumbeny more often. This behavior is difficult for inexperienced owners to detect since healthy newborn foals spend a large portion of time sleeping [26]. Owners also frequently attribute severe lameness to trauma from being stepped on by the dam, even though this type of injury rarely occurs. The affected joint(s) are typically severely effusive and warm with periarticular edema. This differentiates them from foals with sterile (immune-mediated) polysynovitis or clinically insignificant physeal enlargement. One retrospective study of foals <60 days of age with hematogenous septic arthritis revealed that a single synovial structure was most commonly affected (77% of cases) with the tarsocrural joint most commonly affected, followed by the femoropatellar and femorotibial joints [53]. It is worth noting that immune-mediated polysynovitis is relatively common in foals with *R. equi* pneumonia and most commonly affects the tarsi and stifle joints [54].

A thorough physical exam, CBC, and diagnostic imaging are standard for evaluation of foals with suspected septic arthritis. Survey radiographs are sufficient for most cases, but ultrasound and advanced imaging may be necessary for persistent or complicated cases. Synoviocentesis is a critical tool in the diagnosis and treatment of septic arthritis and should be performed in any foal suspected to have S-,

E-, or P-type infections. Due to severe joint effusion, fluid is easily obtained. Collection of fluid can be performed with a sterile 3 ml syringe with the sample transferred into EDTA tubes for cytology, total protein, and lactate measurement. Serum clot tubes are used to collect samples for total protein, lactate measurements and bacterial culture.

Although culture can provide important information, it is not always successful, even in confirmed cases of synovial infection. In a clinical study of foals <60 days old, bacterial culture was only positive in 39% of samples submitted. Of the 22 isolates, 12 were Gram-negative and 10 Gram-positive. The most common isolates were *Streptococcus* spp.(6), followed by *Actinobacillus spp* (4), *Pasteurella* spp. (4), *Escherichia coli* (3), and *Staphylococcus* spp. (2) [53]. A similar distribution of Gram stain and culture results were identified in foals with septic osteomyelitis with and without joint sepsis in another retrospective study in Australia [53]. In order to increase the likelihood of isolating the offending organism(s), synovial fluid samples should be placed in blood culture vials with antimicrobial binding agents since most foals have received antimicrobials prior to synoviocentesis. These samples are submitted for aerobic and anaerobic culture and sensitivity testing. Aggressive management using broad-spectrum systemic antimicrobials and active lavage of the joint (needle lavage, arthroscopy, physeal debridement) should be considered.

Normal synovial fluid should be transparent, straw colored, and highly viscous with a total nucleated cell count (TNCC) of <1500 cells/μl and a total protein <1.5 g/dl. Lymphocytes should comprise >90% of the nucleated cells on a differential count. Joint sepsis results in serosanguineous synovial fluid with decreased viscosity, a TNCC of >30,000 cells/μl with >90% neutrophils, typically degenerate, and >4 g/dl protein. However, blood contamination of the sample and sympathetic ("bystander") inflammation from periarticular trauma and/or infection (i.e. periarticular soft tissue and/or E- or P-type infections) can result in mildly increased TNCC, neutrophil percentages of 30–80%, and significantly increased protein levels [30].

L-lactate can be useful when measured on repeated synovial samples taken over the course of treatment, but single measurements can be difficult to interpret as the value is typically higher than systemic values and highly variable between individuals. While a synovial L-lactate concentration >4.9 mmol/l is consistent with sepsis in adult horses [55, 56], the author's clinical experience suggests that values higher than this can be seen in joints that are not septic. SAA values also increase in the synovial fluid of horses experimentally injected with LPS [13] as well as those with synovial sepsis [11, 57]. Interestingly, SAA has been reported not to increase significantly in cases of repeated synoviocentesis, intra-articular amikacin administration, and joint lavage, unlike TNCC and total protein values [58–60]. Finally, synovial pH (<6.9) and serum-synovial glucose difference (>39.6 mg/dl) have been examined and can also be used as indicators of synovial sepsis [56]. These parameters are less clinically useful in the author's experience.

References

1 Axon, J.E. (2020). Laboratory data. In: *Large Animal Internal Medicine*, 6e (ed. B. Smith, D.C. Van Metre, and N. Pusterla), 260–261. St. Louis, MO: Mosby Elsevier.

2 Koterba, A.M., Brewer, B.D., and Tarplee, F.A. (1984). Clinical and clinicopathological characteristics of the septicaemic neonatal foal: review of 38 cases. *Equine Vet. J.* 16: 376–382.

3 Schneider, R.K., Bramlage, L.R., Moore, R.M. et al. (1992). A retrospective study of 192 horses affected with septic arthritis/tenosynovitis. *Equine Vet. J.* 24: 436–442.

4 Hance, S.R. (1998). Hematogenous infections of the musculoskeletal system in foals. *AAEP Proc.* 44: 159–166.

5 Schaer, B.L.D., Bentz, A.I., Boston, R.C. et al. (2009). Comparison of viscoelastic coagulation analysis and standard coagulation profiles in critically ill neonatal foals to outcome. *J. Vet. Emerg. Crit. Care* 19: 88–95.

6 Neil, K.M., Axon, J.E., Begg, A.P. et al. (2010). Retrospective study of 108 foals with septic osteomyelitis. *Aust. Vet. J.* 88: 4–12.

7 Barton, M.H., Morris, D.D., Crowe, N. et al. (1995). Hemostatic indices in healthy foals from birth to one month of age. *J. Vet. Diagn. Invest.* 7: 380–385.

8 Hultèn, C. and Demmers, S. (2010). Serum amyloid A (SAA) as an aid in the management of infectious disease in the foal: comparison with total leucocyte count, neutrophil count and fibrinogen. *Equine Vet. J.* 34: 693–698.

9 Jacobsen, S., Kjelgaard-Hansen, M., Hagbard Petersen, H. et al. (2006). Evaluation of a commercially available human serum amyloid A (SAA) turbidometric immunoassay for determination of equine SAA concentrations. *Vet. J.* 172: 315–319.

10 Stoneham, S.J., Palmer, L., Cash, R. et al. (2010). Measurement of serum amyloid a in the neonatal foal using a latex agglutination immunoturbidimetric assay: determination of the normal range, variation with age and response to disease. *Equine Vet. J.* 33: 599–603.

11 Jacobsen, S., Thomsen, M.H., and Nanni, S. (2006). Concentrations of serum amyloid a in serum and

synovial fluid from healthy horses and horses with joint disease. *Am. J. Vet. Res.* 67: 1738–1742.

12 Giguère, S., Berghaus, L.J., and Miller, C.D. (2016). Clinical assessment of a point-of-care serum amyloid A assay in foals with bronchopneumonia. *J. Vet. Intern. Med.* 30: 1338–1343.

13 Jacobsen, S., Niewold, T.A., Halling-Thomsen, M. et al. (2006). Serum amyloid A isoforms in serum and synovial fluid in horses with lipopolysaccharide-induced arthritis. *Vet. Immunol. Immunopathol.* 110: 325–330.

14 Robles, M., Nouveau, E., Gautier, C. et al. (2018). Maternal obesity increases insulin resistance, low-grade inflammation and osteochondrosis lesions in foals and yearlings until 18 months of age. *PLoS One* 13: 1–25.

15 Valberg, S.J., Spier, S.J., Parish, S.M. et al. (2020). Diseases of muscle. In: *Large Animal Internal Medicine*, 6e (ed. B.P. Smith, D.C. Van Metre, and N. Pusterla), 1422. St. Louis, MO: Mosby Elsevier.

16 Winjnberg, I.D., Back, W., Jong, M. et al. (2010). The role of electromyography in clinical diagnosis of neuromuscular locomotor problems in the horse. *Equine Vet. J.* 36: 718–722.

17 Aleman, M. (2020). Electromyography. In: *Large Animal Internal Medicine*, 6e (ed. B.P. Smith, D.C. Van Metre, and N. Pusterla), 1012. St. Louis, MO: Mosby Elsevier.

18 Traub-Dargatz, J.L., Ingram, J.T., Stashak, T.S. et al. (1992). Respiratory stridor associated with polymyopathy suspected to be hyperkalemic periodic paralysis in 4 Quarter Horse foals. *J. Am. Vet. Med. Assoc.* 201: 85–89.

19 Divers, T.J., Mohammed, H.O., and Cummings, J.F. (1997). Equine motor neuron disease. *Vet. Clin. North Am. Equine Pract.* 13: 97–105.

20 Wijnberg, I.D., Owczarek-Lipska, M., Sacchetto, R. et al. (2012). A missense mutation in the skeletal muscle chloride channel 1 (CLCN1) as candidate causal mutation for congenital myotonia in a New Forest pony. *Neuromuscul. Disord.* 22: 361–367.

21 Aleman, M., Williams, D.C., Jorge, N.E. et al. (2011). Repetitive stimulation of the common peroneal nerve as a diagnostic aid for botulism in foals. *J. Vet. Intern. Med.* 25: 365–372.

22 Polle, F., Andrews, F.M., Gillon, T. et al. (2014). Suspected congenital centronuclear myopathy in an Arabian-cross foal. *J. Vet. Intern. Med.* 28: 1886–1891.

23 De La Corte, F.D., Valberg, S.J., and MacLeay, J.R.M. (2002). Developmental onset of polysaccharide storage myopathy in 4 quarter horse foals. *JVIM* 16: 581–587.

24 Jean, D., Picandet, V., Macieira, S. et al. (2007). Detection of rib trauma in newborn foals in an equine critical care unit: a comparison of ultrasonography, radiography and physical examination. *Equine Vet. J.* 39: 158–163.

25 Lugo, J. and Carr, E.A. (2019). Thoracic disorders. In: *Equine Surgery*, 5e (ed. J.A. Auer, J.A. Stick, J.M. Kummerle, et al.), 812. Louis, MO.

26 Coleman, M.C. and Whitfield-Cargile, C. (2017). Orthopedic conditions of the premature and dysmature foal. *Vet. Clin. North Am. Equine Pract.* 1–9.

27 Firth, E.C. (1983). Current concepts of infectious polyarthritis in foals. *Equine Vet. J.* 15: 5–9.

28 Faramarzi, B., McMicking, H., Halland, S. et al. (2015). Incidence of palmar process fractures of the distal phalanx and association with front hoof conformation in foals. *Equine Vet. J.* 47: 675–679.

29 Faramarzi, B. and Dobson, H. (2017). Palmar process fractures of the distal phalanx in foals: a review. *Equine Vet. Educ.* 29: 577–580.

30 Glass, K. and Watts, A.E. (2017). Septic arthritis, physitis, and osteomyelitis in foals. *Vet. Clin. North Am. Equine Pract.* 33: 299–314.

31 Barba, M. and Lepage, O.M. (2013). Diagnostic utility of computed tomography imaging in foals: 10 cases (2008–2010). *Equine Vet. Educ.* 25: 29–38.

32 Munsterman, A.S., Alexander, K., Samii, V.F. et al. (2007). Computed tomography in the diagnosis of septic physitis in two foals. *Equine Vet. Educ.* 19: 200–206.

33 Bauer, S., Livesey, M.A., Bjorling, D.E. et al. (2010). Computed tomography assisted surgical correction of persistent right aortic arch in a neonatal foal. *Equine Vet. Educ.* 18: 32–36.

34 Beccati, F., Cercone, M., Angeli, G. et al. IMAGING DIAGNOSIS – use of multiphase computed tomographic urography in the diagnosis of ureteral tear in a 6-day-old foal. *Vet. Radiol. Ultrasound* 57: E10–E15.

35 Smallwood, J.E., Wood, B.C., Eric Taylor, W. et al. (2002). Anatomic reference for computed tomography of the head of the foal. *Vet. Radiol. Ultrasound* 43: 99–117.

36 Schliewert, E.C., Lascola, K.M., O'Brien, R.T. et al. (2015). Comparison of radiographic and computed tomographic images of the lungs in healthy neonatal foals. *Am. J. Vet. Res.* 76: 42–52.

37 Bahar, S., Bolat, D., Dayan, M.O. et al. (2014). Two- and three-dimensional anatomy of paranasal sinuses in Arabian foals. *J. Vet. Med. Sci.* 76: 37–44.

38 Ragle, C.A., Koblik, P.D., Pascoe, J.R. et al. (1988). Computed tomographic evaluation of head trauma in a foal. *Vet. Radiol.* 29: 206–208.

39 Inui, T., Yamada, K., Itoh, M. et al. (2017). Computed tomography and magnetic resonance imaging findings for the initial stage of equine temporohyoid osteoarthropathy in a thoroughbred foal. *J. Equine Sci.* 28: 117–121.

40 Yamada, K., Sato, F., Hada, T. et al. (2016). Quantitative evaluation of cervical cord compression by computed

tomographic myelography in thoroughbred foals. *J. Equine Sci.* 27: 143–148.
41 Yamada, K., Sato, F., Horiuchi, N. et al. (2016). Autopsy imaging for cardiac tamponade in a thoroughbred foal. *J. Equine Sci.* 27: 115–118.
42 Chaffin, M.K., Walker, M.A., Mcarthur, N.H. et al. (1997). Magnetic resonance imaging of the brain of normal neonatal foals. *Vet. Radiol. Ultrasound* 38: 102–111.
43 Wong, D.M., Jeffery, N., Hepworth-Warren, K.L. et al. (2017). Magnetic resonance imaging of presumptive neonatal encephalopathy in a foal. *Equine Vet. Educ.* 29: 534–538.
44 De Zani, D., Zani, D.D., Binanti, D. et al. (2013). Magnetic resonance features of closed head trauma in two foals. *Equine Vet. Educ.* 25: 493–498.
45 Viu, J., Armengou, L., De La Fuente, C. et al. (2012). Magnetic resonance imaging of bacterial meningoencephalitis in a foal. *Case Rep. Vet. Med.* 1–4.
46 Pongratz, M.C., Kircher, P., Lang, J. et al. (2010). Diagnostic evaluation of a foal with cerebellar abiotrophy using magnetic resonance imaging (MRI). *Pferdeheilkunde* 26: 559–562.
47 Oey, L., Müller, J.M.V., Klopmann, T.V. et al. (2011). Diagnosis of internal and external hydrocephalus in a warmblood foal using magnetic resonance imaging. *Tierarztl Prax Ausgabe G Grosstiere – Nutztiere* 39: 41–45.
48 Lempe, A., Heine, M., Bosch, B. et al. (2012). Imaging diagnosis and clinical presentation of a Chiari malformation in a thoroughbred foal. *Equine Vet. Educ.* 24: 618–623.
49 Van Thielen, B., Busoni, V., Chiers, K. et al. (2013). MRI and CT features of an equine juvenile mandibular ossifying fibroma. *J. Equine Vet. Sci.* 33: 658–662.
50 Löfstedt, J. (1997). White muscle disease of foals. *Vet. Clin. North Am. Equine Pract.* 13: 169–185.
51 Roneus, B. and Craig, J. (1984). Muscular dystrophy in foals. *Trans. R. Acad. Med. Ireland* 30: 95–103.
52 Valberg, S.J., Ward, T.L., Rush, B. et al. (2001). Glycogen branching enzyme deficiency in quarter horse foals. *J. Vet. Intern. Med.* 15: 572–580.
53 Wright, L., Ekstrøm, C.T., Kristoffersen, M. et al. (2017). Haematogenous septic arthritis in foals: short- and long- term outcome and analysis of factors affecting prognosis. *Equine Vet. Educ.* 29: 328–336.
54 Giguère, S. and Prescott, J.F. (1997). Clinical manifestations, diagnosis, treatment, and prevention of *Rhodococcus equi* infections in foals. *Vet. Microbiol.* 56: 313–334.
55 Nieto, J.E., Dechant, J.E., le Jeune, S.S. et al. (2015). Evaluation of 3 handheld portable analyzers for measurement of L-lactate concentrations in blood and peritoneal fluid of horses with colic. *Vet. Surg.* 44: 366–372.
56 Dechant, J.E., Symm, W.A., and Nieto, J.E. (2011). Comparison of pH, lactate, and glucose analysis of equine synovial fluid using a portable clinical analyzer with a bench-top blood gas analyzer. *Vet. Surg.* 40: 811–816.
57 Robinson, C.S., Singer, E.R., Piviani, M. et al. (2017). Are serum amyloid A or D-lactate useful to diagnose synovial contamination or sepsis in horses? *Vet. Rec.* 181: 425.
58 Sanchez-Teran, A.F., Bracamonte, J.L., Hendrick, S. et al. (2016). Effect of arthroscopic lavage on systemic and synovial fluid serum amyloid A in healthy horses. *Vet. Surg.* 45: 223–230.
59 Sanchez Teran, A.F., Rubio-Martinez, L.M., Villarino, N.F. et al. (2012). Effects of repeated intra-articular administration of amikacin on serum amyloid A, total protein and nucleated cell count in synovial fluid from healthy horses. *Equine Vet. J.* 44: 12–16.
60 Sanchez-Teran, A.F., Bracamonte, J.L., Hendrick, S. et al. (2016). Effect of repeated through-and-through joint lavage on serum amyloid A in synovial fluid from healthy horses. *Vet. J.* 210: 30–33.

Section II Medications for Intra-articular and Musculoskeletal Use in the Neonatal Foal

Christopher Byron

Septic processes require urgent care in neonatal foals. These infections can manifest as systemic disease, local organ disease, or both. Musculoskeletal infections can be particularly difficult to treat because of challenging anatomic considerations, difficulty in achieving effective antimicrobial drug concentrations, and potential for life-long debilitation resulting from bone and cartilage damage. Common locations of musculoskeletal sepsis in neonates include joints, physes, and bones. Septic arthritis, physitis, and osteomyelitis in foals typically results from hematogenous spread of bacteria but other possible causes include lacerations, penetrating wounds, and periarticular infections that result in direct ingress of bacteria to a joint [1, 2]. Because hematogenous spread is usually responsible for musculoskeletal sepsis, infection in multiple joints and concurrent septic osteomyelitis and arthritis are common findings [3]. Infection in these structures can be accompanied by infection in other tissues. It is therefore important to identify all areas of sepsis early and institute aggressive treatment. Treatments are commonly multi-modal and include systemic antimicrobials, local or regional antimicrobial administration, pain management, mechanical lavage, and possibly surgical debridement. Because multiple medications are commonly administered simultaneously and via various routes, clinicians must be cognizant of the additive effects of these drugs on organ systems and monitor for development of adverse effects. This section discusses local and regional use of medications for neonatal foals with musculoskeletal sepsis, including considerations for selection of drugs, routes, and methods for administration, and adverse effects.

Considerations for Local and Regional Treatment of Musculoskeletal Sepsis

Medications for treatment of musculoskeletal conditions in horses are employed to treat a variety of conditions including soft tissue injuries, osteoarthritis, and septic arthritis. Such treatments often involve systemic, local, and/or regional administration of drugs. Treatment of musculoskeletal sepsis in neonates can be complicated by failure of transfer of passive immunity [4]. Importantly, musculoskeletal infection in foals is associated with reduced survival [5] and future athletic performance [6]. Considering this, antimicrobial drug selection and knowledge of pharmacologic properties are critical. The overall treatment goal is eliminating infection and minimizing permanent damage of structures from actions of bacteria and local cellular responses. For instance, high concentrations of matrix metalloproteinases and other degradative enzymes may cause loss of critical cartilage extracellular matrix components in the face of infection; together with mechanical loading, permanent cartilage damage, and subsequent osteoarthritis can develop.

When selecting medications and routes of administration for neonates with musculoskeletal infections, it is important to identify all anatomic sites and tissue types affected. Standard diagnostics include musculoskeletal palpation, radiography, ultrasonography, and peripheral blood and synovial fluid analyses. Use of three-dimensional imaging adds useful information and more accurately reveals the extent of involvement. Modalities such as computed tomography and magnetic resonance imaging (MRI)

Equine Neonatal Medicine, First Edition. Edited by David M. Wong and Pamela A. Wilkins.

can uncover changes in bone density not detected with radiographs [7]. In a retrospective study of foals with suspected infectious arthritis, 19 osteomyelitis lesions were identified on MRI images, only 4 of which were detected on radiographs [8].

Treatment of neonatal foals follows similar principles as for adult horses and it is important to recognize that much of the clinical and scientific knowledge regarding local and regional use of antimicrobials in equids relates to adult animals; thus, techniques for foals are usually inferred. Early initiation of treatment is all the more important in light of the fact that neonates often have septicemia and a compromised immune system. Therefore, systemic and local/regional antimicrobial treatment should be started before results of other diagnostic tests (e.g. aspirate, synovial, and blood sample culture and sensitivity) are known. Broad-spectrum coverage is desired, typically including a combination of beta-lactam (penicillin, cephalosporins) and aminoglycoside (gentamicin, amikacin) drugs. Because neonates have a greater extracellular fluid compartment than adult horses, antimicrobials administered at adult doses may not achieve desired concentrations. For example, the dose of an aminoglycoside may need to be increased to achieve target plasma concentrations, and administration of part of the systemic dose via regional limb perfusion can help avoid toxicity [9]. Development of bacterial antimicrobial resistance further complicates treatment selection [10, 11].

Overview of Antimicrobial Selection for Local and Regional Administration

Antimicrobial selection, dosage, route of administration, target organism(s), and anatomic location of infection are important considerations when designing a therapeutic protocol. Antimicrobial effectiveness is dependent on both pharmacokinetics (distribution and clearance of drugs within the patient) and pharmacodynamics (mechanisms of action and effects of drugs on target organisms). Area under the concentration time curve from 0 to 24 hours (AUC_{0-24}), minimum inhibitory concentration (MIC), maximum plasma concentration (C_{max}), and time plasma concentrations exceed MIC all contribute to effects [12]. Antimicrobials can be classified as concentration- or time-dependent drugs: concentration-dependent antimicrobials rely on maximal drug concentrations for bacterial killing (regardless of time above MIC) whereas time-dependent drugs require local concentrations to exceed MIC for a prolonged period of the inter-dosing interval. For concentration-dependent drugs, an AUC_{0-24} : MIC ratio of 125 : 1 and a C_{max} : MIC of 10 : 1 are recommended to achieve high efficacy. Time-dependent drug concentrations should exceed MIC by one to five times for 40–100% of the inter-dosing interval [12]. The most commonly used antimicrobials for local and regional administration are aminoglycosides (concentration-dependent) and beta-lactams (time-dependent). Of these, aminoglycosides (amikacin, gentamicin) are most used because regional drug administration at frequent intervals is not clinically practical and use of concentration-dependent drugs allows a prolonged inter-dosing interval while maintaining efficacy. An additional advantage is that it is easier to achieve very high AUC_{0-24} : MIC and C_{max} : MIC ratios via regional administration than by systemic administration. Despite advantages of concentration-dependent drugs for local and regional use, time-dependent drugs may be selected when results of bacterial sensitivity profiles indicate they are a better choice. Of note, fluoroquinolones should be avoided as they are associated with development of musculoskeletal abnormalities in young growing animals [13–16].

Aminoglycosides have rapid bactericidal activity via irreversible binding the 30S subunit of bacterial ribosomes resulting in interference with mRNA translation. A post-antibiotic effect whereby efficacy is maintained after environmental drug concentrations fall below MIC also contributes to concentration-dependent activity. They are effective against a wide variety of Gram-negative organisms and *Staphylococci*; *Streptococci*, and *Enterococci* are generally resistant. Concurrent treatment with beta-lactam antimicrobials is recommended to prevent development of resistance in *Staphylococci* and improve efficacy against resistant microbes [17]. Anaerobic bacteria are naturally resistant because oxygen is required for transport of aminoglycosides into bacteria. Amikacin typically has greater activity against Gram-negative bacteria than other aminoglycosides because it is more resistant to degradation by bacterial enzymes. The activity of aminoglycosides is reduced by low pH and cellular debris (e.g. abscesses) and are inactivated by beta-lactams when physically combined; therefore, these medications should be administered separately. A high peak concentration relative to MIC is a major factor in success of aminoglycoside treatment [18]. For aminoglycosides, the maximum plasma drug concentration should be >8 times the MIC of the bacteria [19] and trough concentration should be ≤2 μg/ml [20]. This allows maximal efficacy while minimizing risk of side effects such as nephrotoxicity, ototoxicity (vestibular and auditory), and, rarely, neuromuscular blockade and hypersensitivity reactions [21]. Local and regional delivery methods such as intraarticular (IA) and intravenous regional limb perfusion (IVRLP) routes allow high concentrations with reduced risk of systemic adverse effects. The total body dose of aminoglycosides via IV, IVRLP, and IA routes should not exceed the total body dose unless peak/trough testing is performed.

Cephalosporins are beta-lactam class antimicrobials that are commonly used via local and regional routes of administration when indicated. These drugs have bactericidal activity by disruption and prevention of synthesis of bacterial cell walls. They bind to and interfere with cell wall synthesis enzymes (penicillin-binding proteins); this activity is slow, thus beta-lactam drugs are slowly bactericidal. This results in a time-dependent manner of bacterial killing. Therefore, beta-lactams are best used with more frequent dosing than aminoglycosides. Highly susceptible Gram-positive bacterial infections may require less frequent dosing. Also, third-generation cephalosporins (e.g. ceftiofur) that have activity against Gram-positive and Gram-negative bacteria have longer half-life and may require less frequent dosing [22]. As with other beta-lactam drugs, the critical pharmacokinetic-pharmacodynamic parameter is time above MIC. Despite belonging to a time-dependent antimicrobial class, ceftiofur can be effective when administered regionally or locally. The choice of a cephalosporin over an aminoglycoside is based on culture and sensitivity results, and consideration should be made for more frequent administration to maximize efficacy.

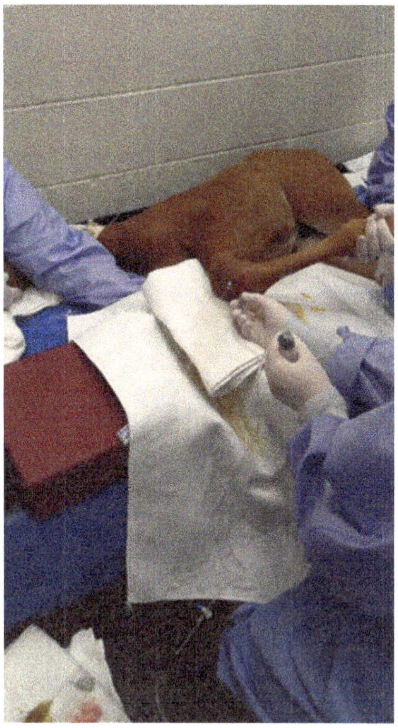

Figure 35.II.1 Septic joint lavage and intraarticular injection performed with needles under a short injectable general anesthesia episode in lateral recumbency. Intraarticular administration of antimicrobials should be performed immediately after lavage. After lavage the egress needle should be removed then antimicrobials injected through the ingress needle.

Septic Arthritis in Equine Neonates

The most common organisms causing septic arthritis in equine neonates are *Actinobacillus* spp., *Escherichia coli*, *Klebsiella* spp., *Pseudomonas* spp., and *Salmonella* spp. [2] However, Gram-positive organisms such as *Streptococcus* spp., *Staphylococcus* spp., and *Clostridium* spp. can also be involved [23]. Approximately 60% of bacterial isolates from synovial structures are Gram-positive and 40% are Gram-negative [24]. Therefore, broad-spectrum antimicrobial coverage is important, at least until results of culture and sensitivity testing are known. Initial systemic antimicrobial selection is based on the assumption that septic arthritis may be caused by Gram-positive and/or Gram-negative bacteria. Results of culture and sensitivity testing for peripheral blood, synovial fluid, and tissue samples or aspirates can be used to subsequently modify treatments. Use of regional and local delivery methods in addition to systemic administration should be considered standard of care for foals with septic arthritis. Local and regional delivery of antimicrobials is often not practical more than once daily because they require more preparation and restraint than systemic administration. In addition, these procedures usually require sedation or general anesthesia in foals. Therefore, concentration-dependent antibiotics such as aminoglycosides are typically chosen. However, ceftiofur concentrations remain above MIC for prolonged periods after IA administration [25], making this a good alternate in appropriate cases. Antimicrobials may be administered via IVRLP or IA injection. High-volume lavage with sterile isotonic fluids is typically required on multiple days; IVRLP can be performed at the same time as lavage. Alternately, antimicrobials can be administered IA after completion of lavage (Figure 35.II.1). In general, IVRLP is a better choice when multiple tissue types are infected, such as cellulitis or septic osteitis concurrent with septic arthritis. IA administration is faster and more convenient when infection is isolated to a synovial cavity. Details regarding these procedures are discussed below. The prognosis for life for foals with septic arthritis is fair to good, with 57–78% surviving to hospital discharge [24, 26]. The prognosis for athletic use for surviving foals is similar to horses that did not have neonatal septic arthritis [26].

Septic Physitis and Osteomyelitis

Septic physitis or osteomyelitis can occur in isolation or concurrent with septic arthritis. Up to 70% of foals with septic osteomyelitis have concurrent septic arthritis [3]. Clinical signs are nonspecific and include lameness and local heat, pain, and edema. Diagnosis is established via detection of osseous changes in imaging, although it can be difficult to detect subtle changes, particularly early in the course of disease. A plasma fibrinogen concentration ≥900 mg/dl is suggestive of physeal or epiphyseal osteomyelitis [27], which can be helpful in detecting cases. Septic physitis and osteomyelitis should be treated with systemic and local antimicrobial delivery in addition to surgical curettage when indicated. The most common organisms isolated from septic physes are *Salmonella* spp. and *Rhodococcus equi* [28]. Antimicrobials that reach effective concentrations in bone include rifampin (in combination with another antimicrobial), tetracyclines, chloramphenicol, fluoroquinolones, and cephalosporins. In addition to systemic antimicrobial administration, foals should be treated via intraosseous (IO), IA, and/or IVRLP routes. Interestingly, there is no significant difference between IVRLP and IA routes in periarticular bone concentrations of gentamicin, and both routes result in levels >MIC for 8 hours [29]; thus, the choice is made based on lesion location, local musculoskeletal anatomy, presence of other lesions, technical expertise, available equipment, and clinician preference. For *R. equi* infections, systemic treatment with a macrolide and rifampin along with erythromycin IVRLP may be used [30].

Treatment of septic physitis and osteomyelitis can be challenging but the prognosis can be good. In a report of 17 foals with septic physitis, 15 survived to 9-month follow-up with good musculoskeletal function [31]. In another report, 87 of 108 (81%) foals with septic osteomyelitis were discharged from the hospital. Six of 8 foals with septic osteomyelitis of the patella survived long term [32]. Multimodal treatment including systemic and local antimicrobials in addition to surgical removal of infected tissue can result in quite favorable outcomes.

Intrasynovial Antimicrobial Injection

Intrasynovial injection of antimicrobials is a rapid and efficient method of achieving very high drug concentrations in joints and other synovial cavities. The technique is most useful for simple synovial sepsis but can also benefit patients with concurrent periarticular septic osteitis. IA injection is used after synovial lavage as it is generally accepted that antimicrobials should not be used in lavage fluid because the primary function of lavage is to physically remove bacteria and debris, fluid is not in contact with the joint tissues for an appreciable amount of time, and such use may increase bacterial resistance to drugs. IA injection can be performed directly after arthroscopic or needle lavage and repeated as needed (Figure 35.II.1). IA injection allows use of low drug doses and volumes with decreased risk of systemic side effects with several antimicrobials appropriate for IA use in horses (Table 35.II.1).

Table 35.II.1 Selected references for intra-articular antimicrobial drugs in horses and foals.

Drug	Dose	Reference
Amikacin sulfate	150 mg	[3]
Amikacin sulfate	500 mg	[32]
Amikacin sulfate	125–500 mg	[33]
Ceftiofur sodium	150 mg	[25]
Ceftiofur sodium	150 mg	[3]
Ceftiofur sodium	250–1000 mg	[33]
Gentamicin sulfate	1 g	[29]
Gentamicin sulfate	150 mg	[3]
Gentamicin sulfate	1 g	[32]
Imipenem-cilastatin	125–250 mg	[32]
Tobramycin sulfate	240 mg	[34]

Aminoglycosides and ceftiofur are good choices for IA treatment because they maintain concentrations above MIC for 24 hours after injection [25, 35]. Amikacin is typically used as a first-choice antimicrobial until results of culture and sensitivity testing is available and is bactericidal in a concentration-dependent manner. Neonates should be sedated or anesthetized for IA injection. Hair is clipped over the synovial structure to facilitate arthroscopy or needle lavage. The injection site chosen should be away from areas of trauma or dermatitis and prepared in a sterile manner with antimicrobials injected using sterile technique. A 1.5-in. 22- or 20-gauge needle is sufficient for administration. Joints of the proximal limb may require a longer spinal needle. Successful needle placement should be confirmed by observing synovial fluid in the needle hub, and a sample collected for analysis at this time, prior to antimicrobial injection. If joints are to be lavaged before IA antimicrobial administration, larger gauge needles (14- to 16-g) are used; drugs are injected after removal of the egress needle and through the ingress needle.

IA administration of antimicrobials results in much greater concentrations what can be achieved after systemic administration. Gentamicin levels are >700-fold higher after IA administration (150 mg) versus IV administration (2.2 mg/kg) in healthy adult horses, and simultaneous IA and IV administration increases IA concentrations further while limiting systemic levels [35]. Although IVRLP and IA administration both result in gentamicin levels >MIC for 24 hours, synovial fluid concentrations are >700 times higher 1 hour after IA injection and 17 times higher 24 hours later [29]. Synovial fluid ceftiofur sodium concentrations are >700 times higher after IA injection (150 mg) than after IV injection (2.2 mg/kg;) and synovial concentrations remain > MIC_{90} for >24 hours after IA injection versus only 8 hours after IV administration [25].

Typical doses of IA antimicrobials are 125–250 mg of amikacin, 500 mg of gentamicin, and 500 mg of cefazolin. Frequency of IA administration is typically q24h initially; dose intervals may be extended depending on clinical course of infection and response to treatment. Increased IA aminoglycoside dosing intervals may decrease adaptive resistance of microorganisms [36] as well decrease chemical synovitis [34]. IA ceftiofur sodium or amikacin every 48 hours after arthroscopic lavage and debridement results in decreased nucleated cell counts in septic joints [33]. This data supports use of a 48-hour inter-dose interval. Synovial fluid analysis is often repeated as a monitoring tool for response to treatment; however, nucleated cell count may have limited utility as a monitoring tool to determine response to treatment [33]. This is complicated by the fact that IA amikacin causes changes in synovial fluid clinical pathologic parameters that can be mistaken as evidence of sepsis [37, 38]. Decisions regarding duration of IA antimicrobial administration should therefore be made considering all clinical parameters including laboratory analysis, physical examination, and imaging.

There is some concern over the effects of antimicrobials on articular tissues, particularly effects of aminoglycosides. Most research has focused on experimental effects in healthy adult horses. There is scant information regarding effects of IA antimicrobials on foal cartilage, but available data from adult horses should be considered when designing a treatment plan. For example, IA gentamicin administration results in substantially increased synovial fluid nucleated cell counts [35, 39]. However, IA gentamicin via CRI did not cause significant changes in histologic appearance of cartilage or synovium [40], suggesting prolonged administration of lower amounts is less likely to induce reaction. In one study, IA amikacin (500 mg) did not induce significant chemical synovitis or increased cell counts [41], but clinically relevant concentrations rapidly induced toxic changes and apoptotic cell death in chondrocytes [42, 43]. Amikacin-induced chondrocyte toxicity is concerning because it can lead to joint tissue degeneration and eventual functional compromise, although this has not been documented in clinical cases. Particularly in foals, consequences could compromise joint function and athletic performance. Interestingly, low dose IV amikacin may be effective against Gram-negative infections in horses [44], so lower single administration concentrations or use of CRI may alleviate potential adverse effects. IA aminoglycosides have been used to treat septic arthritis for many years but there is still question as to effective dose with minimal effects on joint tissues. In comparison, IA ceftiofur sodium (150 mg) has minimal effects on synovial nucleated cell counts, total protein, and gross or microscopic appearance of cartilage and synovium in adult horses [25] and may be a good choice for susceptible infections. IA tobramycin (240 mg) results in transient chemical synovitis but appears safe for use in joints [34] and serves as an alternative to other aminoglycosides (based on susceptibility testing), particularly *Psudomonas* spp. infections [21]. IA injection of antimicrobials may impact clearance of systemically administered drugs and potentially contribute to drug toxicity, however in practice this is not common. Amounts injected IA are typically small and do not alter aminoglycoside pharmacokinetics when concurrently administered IV [34, 35]. Despite the risks, the benefits of IA antimicrobial injection outweigh potential adverse effects for treatment of septic joints in foals.

Intravenous Regional Limb Perfusion

IVRLP has revolutionized treatment of musculoskeletal wounds and infections in distal limbs of horses and foals. Advantages include maximizing efficacy of antimicrobials by allowing local tissue concentrations to greatly exceed the MIC for organisms and potentially reducing systemic adverse effects. Many antimicrobials have been investigated for IVRLP (Table 35.II.2) but aminoglycosides are preferred because they are concentration-dependent antimicrobials. Synovial inflammation dramatically increases maximal concentration (C_{max}) and decreases time to maximal concentration (T_{max}) of aminoglycosides in synovial fluid [45], potentiating the benefits. Beta-lactam antimicrobials such as penicillins and cephalosporins can also be used when indicated. Since these are time-dependent antimicrobials, administration may need to be more frequent. Use of an indwelling RLP catheter can make repeated administration more convenient. Because of the need for frequent dosing with beta-lactams, aminoglycosides are usually chosen unless results of culture and susceptibility testing indicate another choice would be better. Enrofloxacin has been studied for RLP in adult horses [56] but should be avoided in foals because it causes vasculitis and potentially cartilage damage [13–16].

In adult horses, IVRLP is usually performed with the patient standing [73] whereas this procedure is more practically performed in sedated neonatal foals placed on a clean mattress/pad (Figure 35.II.2). A minimum of 3 people (1 restraining the head and administering sedation as needed, 1 assistant, and 1 performing the IVRLP) helps the procedure proceed smoothly. IVRLP may be performed with moderate to heavy sedation in foals that are unlikely to move because of depressed mentation secondary to concurrent systemic disease. General anesthesia is strongly advised for foals with normal mentation and when restraint under sedation is anticipated to be difficult. For foals that

Table 35.II.2 Selected references for doses of IV regional limb perfusion antimicrobial drugs in horses and foals. Where available, dose is reported as total amount, amount/kg, or both.

Drug	Dose	Notes	Reference
Amikacin sulfate	5 mg/kg		[45]
Amikacin sulfate	500 mg		[46]
Amikacin sulfate	1 g (1.5–2.4 mg/kg)		[47]
Amikacin sulfate	1 g (2.7–3.1 mg/kg)		[48]
Amikacin sulfate	5 mg/kg	1/3 systemic dose	[49]
Amikacin sulfate	2 g (3.3–3.8 mg/kg) 3 g (4.9–5.7 mg/kg)		[50]
Amikacin sulfate	2 g (3.6–4.9 mg/kg) 1 g (1.8–2.4 mg/kg)	2 g in cephalic or saphenous vein 1 g in palmar digital vein	[51]
Amikacin sulfate	2 g (3.4–3.9 mg/kg)		[52]
Amikacin sulfate	2.5 g (5.0–6.0 mg/kg)		[53]
Amikacin sulfate	2 g (3.6–4.3 mg/kg)		[54]
Amikacin sulfate	2 g (4.6–7.9 mg/kg)		[55]
Amikacin sulfate	250 mg	Therapeutic concentrations not attained	[56]
Amikacin sulfate	2 g (3.5–4.1 mg/kg)		[57]
Amikacin sulfate	1 g (1.9–2.1 mg/kg)		[58]
Amikacin sulfate	250–500 mg	Foals; in 40 ml 0.9% NaCl	[23]
Amphotericin B	50 mg (0.12–0.5 mg/kg)	In 10% DMSO	[59]
Ceftiofur sodium	2 g (mean, 4.6 mg/kg)		[60]
Ceftiofur sodium	500 mg	Foals	[23]
Ceftiofur Sodium	2 g (approx. 4.4 mg/kg)		[61]
Chloramphenicol	2 g (3.6–5.3 mg/kg)		[62]
Enrofloxacin	1.5 mg/kg		[56]
Erythromicin lactobionate	1 g	In 40 ml saline	[30]
Erythromicin lactobionate	1 g (1.8–2.4 mg/kg) 2 g (3.6–4.9 mg/kg)	1 g in palmar digital veins (not therapeutic) 2 g in cephalic or saphenous vein	[63]
Gentamicin sulfate	400–600 mg		[3]
Gentamicin sulfate	2.0 mg/kg	Foals	[31]
Gentamicin sulfate	500 mg (0.9–1.2 mg/kg)		[64]
Gentamicin sulfate	1 g (1.5–2.6 mg/kg)		[29]
Gentamicin sulfate	500 mg	Foals; in 40 ml 0.9% NaCl	[23]
Imipenem	500 mg (1.0–1.3 mg/kg)		[65]
Marbofloxacin	0.67 mg/kg		[66]
Meropenem	500 mg (0.8–1.25 mg/kg)	Therapeutic concentrations not attained	[67]
Penicillin G sodium	10 million International Units	Administered w/amikacin; Penicillin G concentration > MIC for only 6 h	[68]
Penicillin (benzylpenicillin sodium)	10 million International Units (20,000–31 250 IU mg/kg)	Administered with amikacin	[69]
Polymyxin B	25–300 mg (0.05–0.62 mg/kg)		[70]
Ticarcillin/Clavulanate	7 g	Combined with amikacin (2.5 g); combination not recommended	[71]
Vancomycin	300 mg (0.7–0.9 mg/kg)		[72]

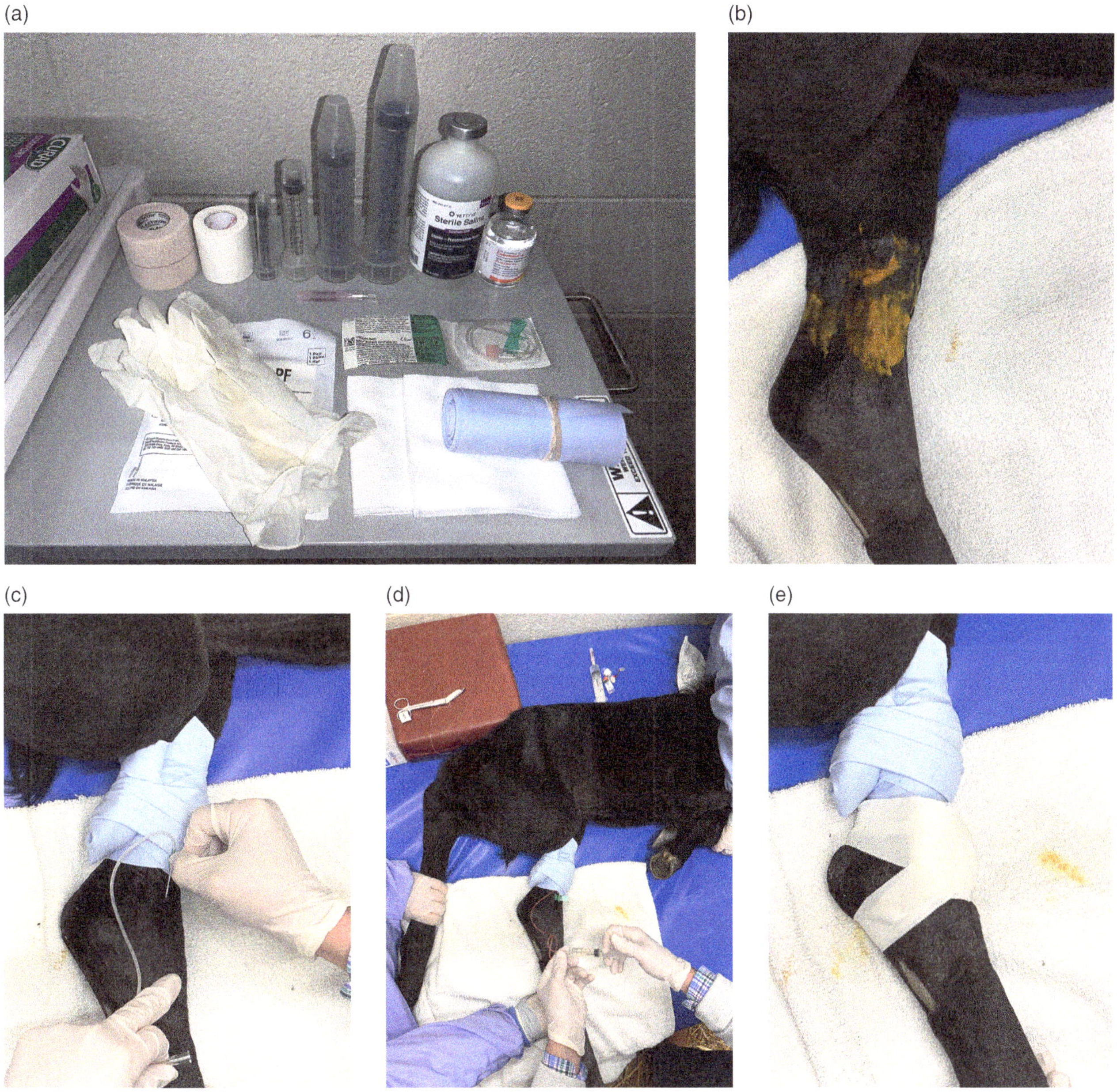

Figure 35.II.2 Steps in performing regional limb perfusion. (a) Materials should be gathered prior to patient sedation of the patient and aseptic preparation of the injection site. (b) The injection site is clipped and aseptically prepared with the foal sedated in lateral recumbency. (c) If necessary, the foal is anesthetized. Then, the pneumatic or Esmarch (pictured) tourniquet is applied tightly proximal to the injection site and butterfly catheter placed. Alternately, an indwelling catheter may be placed before the tourniquet. A second tourniquet may be placed distally for proximal infection sites. (d) Blood is allowed to flow into the catheter tubing to confirm placement in the vein and then the perfusate is injected. (e) A temporary pressure bandage of gauze squares and medical tape is placed when the butterfly catheter is removed to prevent hematoma formation while the tourniquet is in place.

will be anesthetized, it can be helpful to prepare the limb for IVRLP under sedation and induce general anesthesia immediately before the RLP procedure to decrease anesthesia time and reduce the risk of a light anesthetic plane while the tourniquet is applied. Inhalant or IV injectable general anesthesia may be used. For distal limb infections and when using palmar digital veins for IVRLP, foals can be placed in lateral recumbency. When saphenous or cephalic veins are to be used the procedure is easier in lateral recumbency with the affected limb down. Once the foal is sedated and restrained in lateral recumbency the IVRLP injection site is identified, clipped, and prepared aseptically. A small injection of local anesthetic over the IVRLP site or a ring block just proximal to the site can minimize the reaction to injection. Keeping the limb motionless during the procedure is important to ensure complete injection of medication and prevent hematoma formation, which can hinder subsequent IVRLP attempts.

The antimicrobial should be prepared prior to placement of a tourniquet and catheter. In foals, IA administration of 1/3 the systemic amikacin dose is typically used; the remaining two-thirds of the total calculated dose is administered IV on those days. If higher doses are used, the systemic dose should be further reduced to prevent nephrotoxicity. Alternately, the entire calculated systemic dose may be administered via IVRLP without additional IV administration on those days. In general, the total dose (IV + IVRLP) should not exceed the calculated daily dose; if susceptible infections are not responding to treatment, determination of peak and trough concentrations may be indicated to help adjust dosing. As with IA injection, other antimicrobial classes may be used when appropriate. Ceftiofur sodium IVRLP (dose of 4.4–4.6 mg/kg) results in concentrations above MIC in synovial fluid for >24 hours, plasma for 12 hours, and soft tissue for 24 hours [60]; however, effective concentrations in bone are only maintained while the tourniquet is in place [61]. Some individual antimicrobial peculiarities do exist. For example, ceftazidime is unsuitable for once-daily RLP because concentrations rapidly decrease after tourniquet removal [74]. Imipenem IVRLP achieves therapeutic concentrations in distal limbs of horses [65]. Use of the beta-lactam antimicrobial meropenem in IVRLP does not reliably reach tissue concentrations above MIC, which may lead to development of bacterial resistance [67]. Chloramphenicol RLP has been experimentally investigated [62] and IVRLP of erythromycin has been used to treat *R. equi* septic arthritis and physitis in a foal [30]. Amphotericin B in 10% DMSO has been used to treat pythiosis in foals and adult horses [59]. Other antimicrobials investigated for IVRLP include marbofloxacin [66] and polymyxin B [70].

Antimicrobial combinations can expand the spectrum of activity of treatments for orthopedic disorders. Aminoglycosides are often combined with beta-lactam antimicrobials for systemic administration to treat mixed infections or offer broad coverage when the causative agent is unknown. IVRLP with a combination of 2 g amikacin and 10 million units penicillin maintains therapeutic concentrations of both drugs in synovial fluid of adult horses for >24 hours [69], although other studies noted that the same combination resulted in therapeutic penicillin concentrations of only 6 hours [68]. The combination of amikacin and ticarcillin/clavulanate results in lowered synovial amikacin concentrations and antimicrobial activity than amikacin alone [71]. Therefore, caution should be used when selecting antimicrobial combinations for IVRLP as drug interactions may decrease efficacy.

Antimicrobials are diluted in sterile saline solution prior to injection. Perfusate volume should be high enough to increase intravascular pressure and drive diffusion into tissues but not so high that substantial leakage of drug past the tourniquet occurs [75]. Typical total perfusate volumes in adult horses range up to 60 ml, although higher volumes are occasionally employed. Perfusate volumes of 20–40 ml are used in foals but there is conflicting information regarding effect of perfusate volume on tissue concentrations of antimicrobials. Volumes between 10 and 120 ml do not affect synovial fluid gentamicin or amikacin concentrations in some studies [58, 64], but increasing perfusate volumes up to 100 ml did increase amikacin concentrations in synovial fluid samples in another study [55].

A butterfly (20–25 g) or short over-the-needle (20 g) catheter is used if a longer-term indwelling catheter is not elected. Alternately, a longer IV catheter may be placed if repeat injections are anticipated (particularly if a time-dependent antimicrobial is used), if the catheter can be adequately protected, and there is adequate staffing to monitor and maintain the catheter. For indwelling catheters, an extension set for access outside the protective bandage should be attached to skin via cyanoacrylate glue or sutures. Polytetrafluoroethylene catheters are less likely to kink than polyurethane catheters and may be maintained up to 7 days [76].

Tourniquets are placed proximal to the injection site. Single-use catheters should be placed immediately after tourniquet placement while indwelling catheters should be placed beforehand. Traditionally, an Esmarch bandage is applied in a spiral fashion from the coronary band to the proposed tourniquet site to force intravascular fluid and blood out of the target region. However, limb exsanguination via this method seems to be unnecessary [54, 77]. Either a pneumatic tourniquet or wide elastic Esmarch bandage is then placed to restrict arterial inflow and venous outflow from the limb, allowing accumulation of high concentrations of drug in local tissues. Pneumatic tourniquet cuff pressures used in adult horses range from 400 to 420 mmHg, but lower pressures of 200–300 mmHg are recommended in foals [78]; the effect of lower pressures on antimicrobial tissue concentrations is unknown. Other types of tubing (e.g. narrow rubber tubing) or bandage materials are not suitable because they do not adequately restrict venous outflow [53]. There is some disagreement whether an Esmarch bandage or pneumatic tourniquet is most effective at isolating the limb [46, 53], but either is sufficient to achieve antimicrobial concentrations >MIC. The tourniquet should be circumferentially secured with medical tape or tied to itself. At this point the distal spiral Esmarch (if placed) is removed. A second tourniquet may be placed below the targeted treatment site provided there are no other septic sites distal and the injection site is far enough proximal in the limb. Use of a second tourniquet effectively increases drug concentrations in the target tissue which is important when using lower doses of amikacin and volumes of perfusate [77]. Palmar digital, cephalic, or saphenous veins are typically used for RLP. When palmar digital veins are used, the tourniquet is placed in the mid-metacarpal/metatarsal region; when cephalic or saphenous veins are used, the tourniquet is placed in the mid-radius or mid-tibia. Placement of tourniquets proximally still achieves adequate concentrations of antimicrobial in distal joints and use of cephalic/saphenous veins is preferred, although higher drug doses may be needed because of greater tissue volume [63], particularly when using only one proximal tourniquet [58]. Because some joints achieve higher amikacin concentrations when RLP is performed standing [47], it is important to ensure tourniquets are applied tightly and limb movement is minimized when the procedure is performed in recumbent foals.

Antimicrobial injection commences immediately after the tourniquet and catheter are in place. Blood is allowed to flow into the indwelling catheter extension or butterfly catheter tubing to confirm placement. Traditionally, the volume of blood equal to the IVRLP volume is aspirated or allowed to freely flow from the tubing to reduce intravenous pressure. This may be unnecessary, particularly when perfusing larger tissue volumes. Injection of diluted antimicrobial is performed slowly over 60–120 seconds. During injection the catheter site should be closely observed; injection should cease, and catheter placement rechecked if the injection becomes more difficult, subcutaneous extravasation of fluids is observed, or a hematoma develops. It is helpful to frequently stop injection and allow a small amount of blood to flow back into the catheter extension tubing to ensure intravascular placement; blood should be allowed to backflow by intravascular pressure and should not be forcibly aspirated. Once injection is complete, indwelling catheters are lightly bandaged or temporary catheters removed. During removal of temporary catheters, pressure should be applied to the injection site with gauze and temporarily taped in place to maintain pressure on the site while the tourniquet is applied to prevent hematoma formation. Septic joints can be lavaged simultaneously if necessary; this does not reduce the effectiveness of amikacin IVRLP [46]. The tourniquet can be left in place for up to 30 minutes, however, 20 minutes [47], or even 10 minutes [52] may be sufficient if the full 30-minute tourniquet application is unattainable. This is supported by the fact that T_{max} for amikacin in the distal interphalangeal joint is 15 minutes, and C_{max} does not increase beyond that time [57]. IVRLP for 30 minutes is recommended when using time-dependent antimicrobials. When the IVRLP period is finished, the tourniquet and gauze pad over the injection site (if present) are removed. Topical application of 1% diclofenac liposomal cream over the injection site helps decrease inflammation and edema, preserving the vein for subsequent IVRLP procedures [79].

Table 35.II.3 Selected references for regional limb perfusion analgesics in horses.

Drug	Dose	Reference
Butorphanol tartrate	10 mg (0.02 mg/kg)	[80]
Lidocaine hydrochloride	1.3 mg/kg	[81]
Mepivacaine hydrochloride	500 mg (1.3–1.6 mg/kg)	[48]
Mepivacaine hydrochloride	1.3 mg/kg	[81]
Morphine sulfate	0.1 mg/kg	[82]

Analgesics may also be administered via IVRLP (Table 35.II.3). Inclusion of mepivacaine hydrochloride in the IVRLP can provide analgesia during and after the procedure without decreasing amikacin concentrations or antimicrobial efficacy [48]. Butorphanol tartrate (0.02 mg/kg) results in measurable concentrations in joints and increases mechanical nociceptive threshold for 1 hour [80]; it remains unknown whether higher doses result in longer duration of analgesia. IVRLP with morphine (0.1 mg/kg) results in measurable synovial concentrations in healthy horses [82]; importantly, inclusion of gentamicin in the perfusate does not alter regional distribution of morphine and could be a useful analgesic adjunct to antimicrobial IVRLP.

Regional limb perfusion is only suitable for infections at or distal to the distal radial and tibial physes. Therefore, sepsis of more proximal joints (shoulder, elbow, coxofemoral, stifle joints) must be treated via other methods, such as repeated lavage, arthroscopic debridement, and IA antimicrobial injection. Complications of IVRLP include vasculitis, hematoma, and thrombosis [73], which can be prevented with meticulous technique and proper injection site care. Severe cellulitis, non-weight-bearing lameness, neurologic dysfunction, and dehydration were reported in one horse after erythromycin IVRLP [63], but these adverse effects are uncommon. The primary complication associated with indwelling catheters for IVRLP is phlebitis [76]. IVRLP with amikacin does not negatively affect wound healing [49], so the technique can be safely used in the face of soft tissue damage.

Intraosseous Antimicrobial Administration

IO administration may be preferable when osteomyelitis is the primary or only orthopedic infection. Antimicrobials are delivered through a cannula, needle, or cannulated screw placed into the bone. The technique is more time-consuming than other local or regional delivery techniques and is not as effective against infections in other tissues. IO antimicrobial treatment has a higher complication rate than IVRLP [73], and osteonecrosis has been reported in an adult horse after IO gentamicin administration [83]. Nonetheless, IO delivery of antimicrobials is an option for foals without reliable IV access for IVRLP, since the medullary cavity of bone is noncollapsible. The injection site should allow access to a long bone with an accessible medullary cavity through a percutaneous approach with minimal soft tissue coverage and the site should be as close as practical to the septic tissue. It is important to avoid synovial structures, tendons, ligaments, veins, arteries, and nerves. Suitable locations with minimal soft tissue coverage include the medial tibia and radius and medial or lateral metacarpus/metatarsus. Gentamicin (2.2 mg/kg in 0.1 ml/kg sterile saline solution) administered IO in the metacarpus results in bone and synovial fluid concentrations exceeding MIC in the distal limb [84]. IO vancomycin has been evaluated at a dose of 300 mg in 60 ml saline [72]. A combination of 500 mg amikacin and 1 million units of potassium G penicillin was used via IO delivery in a third metacarpal bone to treat a 2-week-old foal with septic distal radial physitis [85].

IO delivery of antimicrobials should be performed under general anesthesia in neonates unless depressed mentation allows completion of the procedure under sedation. As with IVRLP, foals can be sedated and restrained in lateral recumbency for preparation of the injection site, with anesthetic induction occurring immediately before the procedure. The injection site is clipped, aseptically prepared, and desensitized with local anesthetic. Using sterile technique, a stab incision is made through skin, subcutaneous tissue, and periosteum. There are several options for gaining access to the medullary cavity. If a temporary injection cannula or needle will be used, a Steinmann pin, Jamshidi needle, or hypodermic needle (in premature neonates) can be used to penetrate the cis (near) cortex of bone. The trans (far) cortex should not be penetrated. Alternately, an indwelling cannulated cortical screw may be placed using the appropriate drill and tap for the screw. A tourniquet should be placed just proximal to the port. A second tourniquet can be applied distally for more proximal injection sites. Antimicrobial selection and dilution volumes are similar to those for IVRLP. Injection of 2 ml of local anesthetic into the medullary cavity prior to antimicrobial administration decreases pressure-induced discomfort and helps maintain an adequate plane of anesthesia. The tourniquets should be removed after 20–30 minutes and the injection site bandaged. Indwelling cannulated screws should be capped and protected with a bandage. Complications include screw loosening or breakage, local exudate, and difficulty with injection [73]. Other adverse effects include infection, hemorrhage, and periosteal or endosteal damage with subsequent ossifying reaction.

Intraarticular Catheters and CRI Bulb Infusion

Catheters may be placed IA to allow repeated bolus dosing or CRI of antimicrobials via administration bulbs. This circumvents repeated introduction of needles into joints. IV catheters or commercially available synovial catheters may be placed IA; the advantage of the latter is that the catheter wall is thicker than IV catheters and is less prone to kinking and collapse. Catheters are best placed under arthroscopic guidance but may also be placed blindly or under ultrasonographic guidance. Catheters should be placed in a synovial pouch that allows location of the catheter away from weight-bearing joint surfaces. Catheters are introduced over guide stylets or wires, depending on the system, but use of a J-wire is easiest. Catheters should be trimmed so that 2–5 cm (depending on anatomic location) remains within the synovial cavity with the hub flush against the skin, then sutured or glued in place and maintained under a sterile bandage and monitored daily. Meticulous maintenance of IA catheters is imperative including being covered with a sterile dressing and cleaned with sterile 1% betadine solution daily. Catheters are removed 24–48 hours after resolution of infection, usually within 7 days. However, use of IA catheters under a cast for longer periods can be successful when necessary; maintenance of an IA catheter under a cast up to 18 days has been reported [86].

Elastomeric/balloon pumps may be used for CRI of antimicrobials into joints. The walls of the pump exert pressure on the liquid antimicrobial solution inside the pump, creating a constant flow of drug. A flow restrictor is included in the pump design to maintain flow within a specified range. Positive pressure within a septic joint can slow flow below that specified by the manufacturer. This method may be particularly advantageous when administering time-dependent antimicrobials IA as it allows continuous infusion of drug allowing concentrations to remain above MIC for prolonged periods. Pumps are refilled as needed (typically q24h) for continued drug delivery. This is also advantageous for proximal joints not amenable to IVRLP [87]. Continuous rate IA infusion of gentamicin (approx. 0.1 mg/kg/h) results in significantly higher drug concentrations in synovial fluid, synovial membrane, and joint capsule versus IV administration [88], and synovial fluid concentrations are >100 times the MIC for common pathogens [89].

Use of intrasynovial CRI of antimicrobials resulted in resolution of infection and hospital discharge in 28 of 31 horses, including 8 foals [90]. In this study, drug choice was guided by results of bacterial culture and sensitivity testing with one-third of the systemic dose given via CRI in the joint (antimicrobials may be diluted with sterile saline) and two-thirds administered IV. Gentamicin was used in infusion systems in metacarpophalangeal/metatarsophalangeal and midcarpal/radiocarpal joints of five foals with septic osteomyelitis and concurrent septic arthritis [3]. CRI of gentamicin appears to be safe, having no significant effect on articular cartilage or synovial membrane [40]. Clinical complications include catheter obstruction and synovial fistula formation [86].

Antimicrobial-Impregnated Slow-Release Vehicles

Implantation of antimicrobial-impregnated slow-release vehicles into tissues is an alternative method of achieving high tissue concentrations. These include nonbiodegradable (polymethylmethacrylate [PMMA]) and biodegradable (inorganic salts [plaster of Paris, hydroxyapatite, tricalcium phosphate], collagen sponges, and other biocompatible materials) products [91]. The advantage is that controlled release of drugs over the course of several days to weeks obviates the need for repeated IVRLP procedures. Disadvantages include variable or nonideal drug release profiles, mechanical inflexibility of the vehicle, and lack of absorption necessitating removal at a later date. PMMA beads implanted into joints cause synovitis and cartilage erosion [92], so they are best used in soft tissue and periosseous locations. Plaster of Paris beads are also unsuitable for intraarticular use because they degrade quickly in liquid media and cause synovitis. Antimicrobials used in slow-release formulations should be stable in the carrier, be compatible with target tissues, and have activity against infectious organisms. Typically, antimicrobials will have an initial burst release followed by prolonged slower release [91]. Between 1 and 4 g of antimicrobial are mixed with 20 g of vehicle (e.g. PMMA, plaster of Paris) and the appropriate liquid for the vehicle is added in a 2 : 1 liquid-to-powder ratio and mixed thoroughly for one minute. The mixture is then formed by hand into small (5–6 mm) spherical or cylindrical beads or placed into bead molds (Figure 35.II.3). Smaller beads have a larger surface area-to-volume ratio, which increases the rate of drug elution. Beads may be formed over a strand of suture to allow ease of application and bead retrieval from tissues. If beads are made in a sterile manner, they may be used immediately.

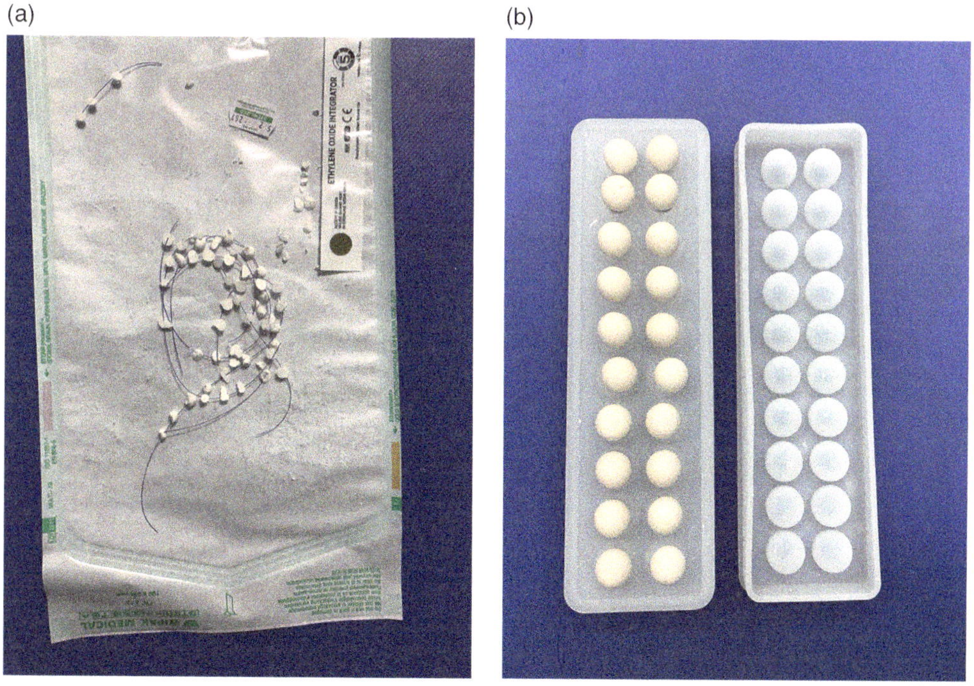

Figure 35.II.3 PMMA and Plaster-of-Paris beads may be formed by hand (a) or in a mold (b). Forming beads around a strand of suture makes application and removal easier. Beads can be aseptically prepared for immediate use or gas-sterilized for later use.

If sterilization is required, steam sterilization should be avoided as the antimicrobial may be inactivated. The number of beads used is determined by the volume of septic tissue to be treated. They may be temporarily sutured in place or held with a bandage. Plaster of Paris beads biodegrade and do not require removal. PMMA beads may be left in place in deeper tissues or retrieved and, if necessary, exchanged for new beads 7–10 days after implantation. PMMA beads with gentamicin sulfate (100 mg in 2 g PMMA), and ceftiofur sodium (100 mg in 2 g PMMA) have been used in foals with septic osteitis [3].

Collagen sponges have also been investigated as an IA antimicrobial delivery vehicle. Collagen sponges impregnated with 130 mg of gentamicin placed in tarsocrural joints of horses resulted in concentrations >20 times the MIC for common pathogens and did not cause significant inflammation or joint trauma [93]. A rapid release of antimicrobial is observed followed by quickly declining synovial concentrations. Therefore, this method may not have any advantage over direct injection.

Intraarticular Sodium Hyaluronate for Synovial Sepsis

Under certain conditions, IA use of other adjunctive medications may be beneficial. Hyaluronic acid may be a useful adjunct IA treatment for foals with septic arthritis. In a study of adult horses with experimentally induced *Staphylococcus aureus* tarsocrural infection, joints treated with 10 mg sodium hyaluronate had significantly less inflammation than contralateral control joints, as indicated by decreased total protein concentration, WBC counts, cellular infiltrate, and granulation tissue formation as well as more normal synovial villus structure. Treated joints also had significantly less lameness and smaller joint circumference [94]. In another study IA sodium hyaluronate (20 mg) and IM polysulfated glycosaminoglycan (500 mg q7d for four to seven treatments) was used in foals after resolution of septic osteomyelitis and arthritis [32]. Although the mechanism of action is unknown, beneficial effects may be attributable to reduced inflammation.

References

1 Cohen, N.D. (1994). Causes of and farm management factors associated with disease and death in foals. *J. Am. Vet. Med. Assoc.* 204: 1644–1651.

2 Hardy, J. (2006). Etiology, diagnosis, and treatment of septic arthritis, osteitis, and osteomyelitis in foals. *Clin. Tech. Equine Pract.* 5: 309–317.

3 Neil, K.M., Axon, J.E., Begg, A.P. et al. (2010). Retrospective study of 108 foals with septic osteomyelitis. *Aust. Vet. J.* 88: 4–12.

4 Robinson, J.A., Allen, G.K., Green, E.M. et al. (1993). A prospective study of septicaemia in colostrum-deprived foals. *Equine Vet. J.* 25 (3): 214–219.

5 Giguère, S., Weber, E.J., and Sanchez, L.C. (2017). Factors associated with outcome and gradual improvement in survival over time in 1065 equine neonates admitted to an intensive care unit. *Equine Vet. J.* 49 (1): 45–50.

6 Chidlow, H., Giguère, S., and Sanchez, L.C. (2019). Factors associated with long-term athletic outcome in thoroughbred neonates admitted to an intensive care unit. *Equine Vet. J.* 51 (6): 716–719.

7 Haggett, E.F., Foote, A.K., Head, M.J. et al. (2012). Necrosis of the femoral condyles in a four-week-old foal: clinical, imaging and histopathological features. *Equine Vet. J. Suppl.* 41: 91–95.

8 Gaschen, L., LeRoux, A., Trichel, J. et al. (2011). Magnetic resonance imaging in foals with infectious arthritis. *Vet. Radiol. Ultrasound* 52: 627–633.

9 Axon, J.E., Russell, C.M., and Wilkins, P.A. (2014). Chapter 9: neonatology. In: *Equine Emergency and Critical Care Medicine* (ed. L.L. Southwood and P.A. Wilkins), 511–554. Boca Raton, FL: CRC Press.

10 Theelen, M.J.P., Wilson, W.D., Edman, J.M. et al. (2014). Temporal trends in *in vitro* antimicrobial susceptibility patterns of bacteria isolated from foals with sepsis: 1979–2010. *Equine Vet. J.* 46: 161–168.

11 Gilbertie, J.M., Schnabel, L.V., Stefanovski, D. et al. (2018). Gram-negative multi-drug resistant bacteria influence survival to discharge for horses with septic synovial structures: 206 cases (2010–2015). *Vet. Microbiol.* 226: 64–73.

12 McKellar, Q.A., Sanchez Bruni, S.F., and Jones, D.G. (2004). Pharmacokinetic/pharmacodynamic relationships of antimicrobial drugs used in veterinary medicine. *J. Vet. Pharm. Ther.* 27: 503–514.

13 Stahlmann, R., Kuhner, S., Shakibaei, M. et al. (2000). Chondrotoxicity of ciprofloxacin in immature beagle dogs: immunohistochemistry, electron microscopy and drug plasma concentrations. *Arch. Toxicol.* 73: 564–572.

14 Davenport, C.L.M., Boston, R.C., and Richardson, D.W. (2001). Effects of enrofloxacin and magnesium deficiency on matrix metabolism in equine articular cartilage. *Am. J. Vet. Res.* 62: 160–166.

15 Vivrette, S.L., Bostian, A., Bermingham, E. et al. (2001). Quinolone-induced arthropathy in neonatal foals. *AAEP Proc.* 47: 376–377.

16 Khazaeil, K., Mazaheri, Y., Hashemitabar, M. et al. (2012). Enrofloxacin effect on histomorphologic and histomorphometric structure of lamb cartilage. *Global Vet.* 9: 447–453.

17 Papich, M.G. and Riviere, J.A. (2018). Chapter 35: aminoglycoside antibiotics. In: *Veterinary Pharmacology*

and Therapeutics, 10e (ed. J.E. Riviere and M.G. Papich), 877–902. Hoboken, NJ: Wiley Blackwell.

18 Moore, R.D., Lietman, P.S., and Smith, C.R. (1987). Clinical response to aminoglycoside therapy: importance of the ratio of peak concentration to minimal inhibitory concentration. *J Infect Dis* 155: 93–99.

19 Deziel-Evans, L.M., Murphy, J.E., and Job, M.L. (1986). Correlation of pharmacokinetic with therapeutic outcome in patients receiving aminoglycosides. *Clin. Pharm.* 5: 319–324.

20 Sanchez-Alcaraz, A., Vargas, A., Quintana, M.B. et al. (1998). Therapeutic drug monitoring of tobramycin: once-daily versus twice-daily dosage schedules. *J. Clin. Pharm. Ther.* 23: 367–373.

21 Gonzalez, U.S. and Spencer, J.P. (1998). Aminoglycosides: a practical review. *Am. Fam. Physician* 58 (8): 1811–1820.

22 Papich, M.G. (2018). Chapter 33: β-lactam antibiotics: penicillins, cephalosporins, and related drugs. In: *Veterinary Pharmacology and Therapeutics*, 10e (ed. J.E. Riviere and M.G. Papich), 826–857. Hoboken, NJ: Wiley Blackwell.

23 Annear, M.J., Furr, M.O., and White, N.A. (2011). Septic arthritis in foals. *Equine Vet. Educ.* 23 (8): 422–431.

24 Hepworth-Warren, K.L., Wong, D.M., Fulkerson, C.V. et al. (2015). Bacterial isolates, antimicrobial susceptibility patterns, and factors associated with infection and outcome in foals with septic arthritis: 83 cases (1998–2013). *J. Am. Vet. Med. Assoc.* 246: 785–793.

25 Mills, M.L., Rush, B.R., St Jean, G. et al. (2000). Determination of synovial fluid and serum concentrations, and morphologic effects of intraarticular ceftiofur sodium in horses. *Vet. Surg.* 29 (5): 398–406.

26 O'Brien, T.J., Rosanowski, S.M., Mitchell, K.D. et al. (2021). Factors associated with survival and racing performance of 114 thoroughbred foals with septic arthritis compared with maternal siblings (2009–2015). *Equine Vet. J.* 53: 935–943.

27 Newquist, J.M. and Baxter, G.M. (2009). Evaluation of plasma fibrinogen concentration as an indicator of physeal or epiphyseal osteomyelitis in foals: 17 cases (2002–2007). *J. Am. Vet. Med. Assoc.* 235: 415–419.

28 Baird, A.N., Taylor, J.R., and Watkins, J.P. (1990). Debridement of septic physeal lesions in 3 foals. *Cornell Vet.* 80 (1): 85–95.

29 Werner, L.A., Hardy, J., and Bertone, A.L. (2003). Bone gentamicin concentration after intra-articular injection or regional intravenous perfusion in the horse. *Vet. Surg.* 32: 559–565.

30 Kelmer, G. and Hayes, M.E. (2009). Regional limb perfusion with erythromycin for treatment of septic physitis and arthritis caused by *Rhodococcus equi*. *Vet. Rec.* 165: 291–292.

31 Hall, M.S., Pollock, P.J., and Russell, T. (2012). Surgical treatment of septic physitis in 17 foals. *Aust. Vet. J.* 90: 479–484.

32 Kay, A.T., Hunt, R.J., Rodgerson, D.H. et al. (2012). Osteomyelitis of the patella in eight foals. *Vet. Surg.* 41 (41): 307–315.

33 Cousty, M., Stack, J.D., Tricaud, C. et al. (2017). Effect of arthroscopic lavage and repeated intra-articular administrations of antibiotic in adult horses and foals with septic arthritis. *Vet. Surg.* 46: 1008–1016.

34 Newman, J.C., Prange, T., Jennings, S. et al. (2013). Pharmacokinetics of tobramycin following intravenous, intramuscular, and intra-articular administration in healthy horses. *Vet. Pharm. Ther.* 36: 532–541.

35 Lloyd, K.C., Stover, S.M., Pascoe, J.R. et al. (1988). Plasma and synovial fluid concentrations of gentamicin in horses after intra-articular administration of buffered and unbuffered gentamicin. *Am. J. Vet. Res.* 49 (5): 644–649.

36 Gilleland, L.B., Gilleland, H.E., Gibson, J.A. et al. (1989). Adaptive resistance to aminoglycoside antibiotics in *Pseudomonas aeruginosa*. *J. Med. Microbiol.* 29: 41–50.

37 Sanchez Tieran, A.F., Rubio-Martinez, L.M., Villarino, N.F. et al. (2012). Effects of repeated intra-articular administration of amikacin on serum amyloid A, total protein and nucleated cell count in synovial fluid from healthy horses. *Equine Vet. J. Suppl.* 43: 12–16.

38 Dykgraaf, S., Dechant, J.E., Johns, J.L. et al. (2007). Effect of intrathecal amikacin administration and repeated centesis on digital flexor tendon sheath synovial fluid in horses. *Vet. Surg.* 36: 57–63.

39 Stover, S.M. and Pool, R.R. (1985). Effect of intra-articular gentamicin sulfate on normal equine synovial membrane. *Am. J. Vet. Res.* 46 (12): 2485–2491.

40 Lescun, T.B., Adams, S.B., Ching, C. et al. (2002). Effects of continuous intra-articular infusion of gentamicin on synovial membrane and articular cartilage in the tarsocrural joint of horses. *Am. J. Vet. Res.* 63: 683–687.

41 Taintor, J., Schumacher, J., and DeGraves, F. (2006). Comparison of amikacin concentrations in normal and inflamed joints of horses following intra-articular administration. *Equine Vet. J.* 38 (2): 189–191.

42 Bolt, D.M., Ishihara, A., Weisbrode, S.E. et al. (2008). Effects of triamcinolone acetonide, sodium hyaluronate, amikacin sulfate, and mepivacaine hydrochloride, alone and in combination, on morphology and matrix composition of lipopolysaccharide-challenged and unchallenged equine articular cartilage explants. *Am. J. Vet. Res.* 69 (7): 861–867.

43 Pezzanite, L., Chow, L., Soontararak, L. et al. (2020). Amikacin induces rapid dose-dependent apoptotic cell death in equine chondrocytes and synovial cells in vitro. *Equine Vet. J.* 52 (5): 715–724.

44 Pinto, N., Schumacher, J., Taintor, J. et al. (2011). Pharmacokinetics of amikacin in plasma and selected body fluids of healthy horses after a single intravenous dose. *Equine Vet. J.* 43 (1): 112–116.

45 Am, B.-V., Epstein, K.L., and White, C.L. (2011). Effect of experimentally induced synovitis on amikacin

concentrations after intravenous regional limb perfusion. *Vet. Surg.* 40 (7): 891–897.

46 Alkabes, S.B., Adams, S.B., Moore, G.E. et al. (2011). Comparison of two tourniquets and determination of amikacin sulfate concentrations after metacarpophalangeal joint lavage performed simultaneously with intravenous regional limb perfusion in horses. *Am. J. Vet. Res.* 72 (5): 613–619.

47 Aristizabel, F.A., Nieto, J.E., Guedes, A.G. et al. (2016). Comparison of two tourniquet application times for regional intravenous limb perfusions with amikacin in sedated or anesthetized horses. *Vet. J.* 208: 50–54.

48 Colbath, A.C., Wittenburg, L.A., Gold, J.R. et al. (2016). The effects of mepivacaine hydrochloride on antimicrobial activity and mechanical nociceptive threshold during amikacin sulfate regional limb perfusion in the horse. *Vet. Surg.* 45: 798–803.

49 Edwards-Milewski, M.L., Morello, S.L., Zhao, Q. et al. (2016). The effect of intravenous regional perfusion of the distal limb with amikacin sulfate on wounds healing by second intention in horses. *Vet. Surg.* 45: 125–132.

50 Harvey, A., Kilcoyne, I., Byrne, B.A. et al. (2016). Effect of dose on intra-articular amikacin sulfate concentrations following intravenous regional limb perfusion in horses. *Vet. Surg.* 45: 1077–1082.

51 Kelmer, G., Bell, G.C., Martin-Jimenez, T. et al. (2012). Evaluation of regional limb perfusion with amikacin using the saphenous, cephalic, and palmar digital veins in standing horses. *Vet. Pharm. Ther.* 36: 236–240.

52 Kilcoyne, I., Dechant, J.E., and Nieto, J.E. (2016). Evaluation of 10-minute versus 30-minute tourniquet time for intravenous regional limb perfusion with amikacin sulfate in standing sedated horses. *Vet. Rec.* 23: 585.

53 Levine, D.G., Epstein, K.L., Ahern, B.J. et al. (2010). Efficacy of three tourniquet types for intravenous antimicrobial regional limb perfusion in standing horses. *Vet. Surg.* 39: 1021–1024.

54 Sole, A., Nieto, J.E., Aristizabal, F.A. et al. (2016). Effect of emptying the vasculature before performing regional limb perfusion with amikacin in horses. *Equine Vet. J.* 48: 737–740.

55 Oreff, G.L., Dahan, R., Tatz, A.J. et al. (2016). The effect of perfusate volume on amikacin concentration in the metacarpophalangeal joint following cephalic regional limb perfusion in standing horses. *Vet. Surg.* 45: 625–630.

56 Parra-Sanchez, A., Lugo, J., Boothe, D.M. et al. (2006). Pharmacokinetics and pharmacodynamics of enrofloxacin and a low dose of amikacin administered via regional intravenous limb perfusion in standing horses. *Am. J. Vet. Res.* 67: 1687–1695.

57 Kilcoyne, I., Nieto, J.E., Knych, H.K. et al. (2018). Time required to achieve maximum concentration of amikacin in synovial fluid of the distal interphalangeal joint after intravenous regional limb perfusion in horses. *Am. J. Vet. Res.* 79: 282–286.

58 Moser, D.K., Schoonover, M., Holbrook, T.C. et al. (2016). Effect of regional intravenous limb perfusate volume on synovial fluid concentration of amikacin and local venous blood pressure in the horse. *Vet. Surg.* 45: 851–858.

59 Dória, R.G.S., Carvalho, M.B., Freitas, S.H. et al. (2015). Evaluation of intravenous regional perfusion with amphotericin B and dimethylsulfoxide to treat horses for pythiosis of a limb. *BMC Vet. Res.* 11: 152.

60 Pille, F., De Baere, S., Ceelen, L. et al. (2005). Synovial fluid and plasma concentrations of ceftiofur after regional intravenous perfusion in the horse. *Vet. Surg.* 34: 610–617.

61 Cox, K.S., Nelson, B.B., Wittenburg, L. et al. (2017). Plasma, subcutaneous tissue and bone concentrations of ceftiofur sodium after regional limb perfusion in horses. *Equine Vet. J.* 49: 341–344.

62 Kelmer, G., Tatz, A.J., Famini, S. et al. (2014). Evaluation of regional limb perfusion with chloramphenicol using the saphenous or cephalic vein in standing horses. *J. Vet. Pharm. Ther.* 38: 35–40.

63 Kelmer, G., Martin-Jimenez, T., Saxton, A.M. et al. (2012). Evaluation of regional limb perfusion with erythromycin using the saphenous, cephalic, or palmar digital veins in standing horses. *J. Vet. Pharm. Ther.* 36: 434–440.

64 Hyde, R.M., Lynch, T.M., Clark, C.K. et al. (2013). The influence of perfusate volume on antimicrobial concentration in synovial fluid following intravenous regional limb perfusion in the standing horse. *Can. Vet. J.* 54: 363–367.

65 Kelmer, G., Tatz, A.J., Britzi, M. et al. (2017). Evaluation of the pharmacokinetics of imipenem following regional limb perfusion using the saphenous and the cephalic veins in standing horses. *Res. Vet. Sci.* 114: 64–68.

66 Lallemand, E., Trencart, P., Tahier, C. et al. (2013). Pharmacokinetics, pharmacodynamics and local tolerance at injection site of marbofloxacin administered by regional intravenous limb perfusion in standing horses. *Vet. Surg.* 42: 649–657.

67 Fontenot, R.L., Langston, V.C., Zimmerman, J.A. et al. (2018). Meropenem synovial fluid concentrations after intravenous regional limb perfusion in standing horses. *Vet. Surg.* 47: 852–860.

68 Nieto, J.E., Trela, J., Stanley, S.D. et al. (2016). Pharmacokinetics of a combination of amikacin sulfate and penicillin G sodium for intravenous regional limb perfusion in adult horses. *Can. J. Vet. Res.* 80: 230–235.

69 Dahan, R., Oreff, G.L., Tatz, A.J. et al. (2019). Pharmacokinetics of regional limb perfusion using a combination of amikacin and penicillin in standing horses. *Can. Vet. J.* 60: 294–299.

70 Snowden, R.T., Schumacher, J., Blackford, J.T. et al. (2019). Tarsocrural joint polymyxin B concentrations achieved following intravenous regional limb perfusion of the drug via a saphenous vein to healthy standing horses. *Am. J. Vet. Res.* 80 (12): 1099–1106.
71 Zantingh, A.J., Schwark, W.S., Fubini, S.L. et al. (2014). Accumulation of amikacin in synovial fluid after regional limb perfusion of amikacin sulfate alone and in combination with ticarcillin/clavulanate in horses. *Vet. Surg.* 43: 282–288.
72 Rubio-Martínez, L., López-Sanromán, J., Cruz, A.M. et al. (2005). Medullary plasma pharmacokinetics of vancomycin after intravenous and intraosseous perfusion of the proximal phalanx in horses. *Vet. Surg.* 34: 618–624.
73 Rubio-Martínez, L.M., Elmas, C.R., Black, B. et al. (2012). Clinical use of antimicrobial regional limb perfusion in horses: 174 cases (1999–2009). *J. Am. Vet. Med. Assoc.* 241: 1650–1658.
74 Oreff, G.L., Tatz, A.J., Dahan, R. et al. (2017). Pharmacokinetics of ceftazidime after regional limb perfusion in standing horses. *Vet. Surg.* 46: 1120–1125.
75 Rubio-Martínez, L.M. and Cruz, A.M. (2006). Antimicrobial regional limb perfusion in horses. *J. Am. Vet. Med. Assoc.* 228: 706–712.
76 Kelmer, G., Catasus, C.T., Saxton, A.M. et al. (2009). Evaluation of indwelling intravenous catheters for the regional perfusion of the limbs of horses. *Vet. Rec.* 165: 496–501.
77 Schoonover, M.J., Moser, D.K., Young, J.M. et al. (2017). Effects of tourniquet number and exsanguination on amikacin concentrations in the radiocarpal and distal interphalangeal joints after low volume intravenous regional limb perfusion in horses. *Vet. Surg.* 46: 675–682.
78 Paradis, M.R. (2018). Regional limb perfusion in the neonatal foal. In: *Manual of Clinical Procedures in the Horse* (ed. L.R.R. Costa and M.R. Paradis). Hoboken NJ: Wiley Blackwell.
79 Levine, D.G., Epstein, K.L., Neelis, D.A. et al. (2009). Effect of topical application of 1% diclofenac sodium liposomal cream on inflammation in healthy horses undergoing intravenous regional limb perfusion with amikacin sulfate. *Am. J. Vet. Res.* 70: 1323–1325.
80 Crabtree, N.E., Mochal-King, C.A., Sloan, P.B. et al. (2019). Synovial butorphanol concentrations and mechanical nociceptive thresholds after intravenous regional limb perfusion in standing sedated horses. *Vet. Surg.* 48: 1473–1482.
81 Mendez-Angulo, J.L., Granados, M.M., Modesto, R. et al. (2020). Systemic and local effects of lidocaine or mepivacaine when used for intravenous regional anaesthesia of the distal limb in standing sedated horses. *Equine Vet. J.* 52: 743–751.
82 Hunter, B.G., Parker, J.E., Wehrman, R. et al. (2015). Morphine synovial concentrations after intravenous regional limb perfusion in standing horses. *Vet. Surg.* 44: 679–686.
83 Parker, R.A., Bladon, B.M., McGovern, K. et al. (2010). Osteomyelitis and osteonecrosis after intraosseous perfusion with gentamicin. *Vet. Surg.* 39: 644–648.
84 Mattson, S., Bouré, L., Pearce, S. et al. (2004). Intraosseous gentamicin perfusion of the distal metacarpus in standing horses. *Vet. Surg.* 33: 180–186.
85 Kettner, N.U., Parker, J.E., and Watrous, B.J. (2003). Intraosseous regional perfusion for treatment of septic physitis in a two-week-old foal. *J. Am. Vet. Med. Assoc.* 222: 346–350.
86 Stewart, A.A., Goodrich, L.R., Byron, C.R. et al. (2010). Antimicrobial delivery by intrasynovial catheterization with systemic administration for equine synovial trauma and sepsis. *Aust. Vet. J.* 88: 115–123.
87 Glass, K. and Watts, A.E. (2017). Septic arthritis, physitis, and osteomyelitis in foals. *Vet. Clin. Equine* 33: 299–314.
88 Lescun, T.B., Ward, M.P., and Adams, S.B. (2006). Gentamicin concentrations in synovial fluid and joint tissues during intravenous administration or continuous intra-articular infusion of the tarsocrural joint of clinically normal horses. *Am. J. Vet. Res.* 67: 409–416.
89 Lescun, T.B., Adams, S.B., Ching, C. et al. (2000). Continuous infusion of gentamicin into the tarsocrural joint of horses. *Am. J. Vet. Res.* 61: 407–412.
90 Lescun, T.B., Vasey, J.R., Ward, M.P. et al. (2006). Treatment with continuous intrasynovial antimicrobial infusion for septic synovitis in horses: 31 cases (2000–2003). *J. Am. Vet. Med. Assoc.* 228: 1922–1929.
91 Haerdi-Landerer, M.C., Habermacher, J., Wenger, B. et al. (2010). Slow release antibiotics for treatment of septic arthritis in large animals. *Vet. J.* 184: 14–20.
92 Farnsworth, K.D., White, N.A., and Robertson, J. (2001). The effects of implanting gentamicin-impregnated polymethylmethacrylate beads in the tarsocrural joint of the horse. *Vet. Surg.* 30: 126–131.
93 Ivester, K.M., Adams, S.B., Moore, G.E. et al. (2006). Gentamicin concentrations in synovial fluid obtained from the tarsocrural joints of horses after implantation of gentamicin-impregnated collagen sponges. *Am. J. Vet. Res.* 67 (9): 1519–1526.
94 Brusie, R.W., Sullins, K.E., White, N.A. et al. (1992). Evaluation of sodium hyaluronate therapy in induced septic arthritis in the horse. *Equine Vet. J. Suppl.* 11: 18–23.

Chapter 36 Congenital and Acquired Musculoskeletal Disorders in the Neonatal Foal

Annette M. McCoy and Rebecca Bishop

Abnormalities of the Appendicular Skeleton

Conformational deviations of the limb are common in neonatal foals and can be divided into flexural limb deformities (deviation of limb in sagittal plane) and angular limb deformities (deviation of limb in frontal plane). Both flexural and angular limb deformities can be classified based on etiology as congenital or acquired. Less common conditions affecting the neonatal appendicular skeleton include patellar luxation, polydactyly, and phalangeal hypoplasia.

Flexural Limb Deformities

Flexural limb deformities refer to a joint or joints that are held in an abnormally flexed or extended position. Although commonly referred to as contracted tendons, in most cases deformation arises from incongruent growth, resulting in flexor tendon units, which are functionally shortened relative to the osseous structures. Conversely, laxity of flexor tendons results in hyperextension deformities. By convention, the deformity is named by the involved joint(s). More commonly, a single joint is affected in a given limb with forelimbs more commonly affected than hindlimbs. Congenital abnormalities are present at birth, and prognosis is generally related to the amount of mobility on manual manipulation of the affected joint. Severe deformities that are not manually correctable may be refractory to any treatment. Acquired flexural deformities most often occur during periods of rapid growth (1–4 months of age; around 1 year of age) or may be secondary to any painful condition that limits weight-bearing. Contracture of the palmar/plantar joint capsule can occur with chronic flexural deformity, underscoring the importance of early diagnosis and treatment.

Congenital Flexural Deformities

Flexural limb deformities are considered congenital when present at birth. Severe flexural deformities may cause dystocia or prevent the foal from standing after birth (Figure 36.1). Severe (typically bilateral) deformities are often combined with axial skeletal deformities; this combination is referred to as contracted foal syndrome. Contracted foal syndrome and other congenital anomalies were reported to cause 8.5% and 9.9% of abortions, stillbirths, and perinatal deaths in two large surveys [1, 2].

Even mild deformities are readily recognized on visual examination. The foal should be evaluated while standing on a level surface, free of deep bedding or grass that may mask deformities involving the lower limb. The limb(s) should be manipulated to assess the range of motion and determine the degree to which manual straightening is possible. Flexural deformities may be overlooked in recumbent foals; thorough orthopedic examination is warranted in foals presented for recumbency so that appropriate treatment can be instituted. Radiography or other imaging is typically not required. Many factors may play a role in disease etiology, including exposure of the mare to teratogens or disease during pregnancy (locoweed, hybrid Sudan grass, equine goiter, influenza, abnormal intrauterine positioning, large size of foal relative to size of mare), and genetic predisposition (neuromuscular disorders, dominant gene mutation in the sire, and lathyrism). The metacarpophalangeal joint and carpus are most commonly affected, with the tarsus, metatarsophalangeal, distal, and proximal interphalangeal joints less commonly involved.

Treatment Early identification of affected foals is critical, as most flexural deformities require immediate conservative treatment and continued monitoring for the best outcome:

- **Exercise** is critical to stretch and lengthen the involved palmar/plantar soft tissues (musculotendinous units, ligaments, and joint capsule) and may be the only treatment necessary in young foals that are able to stand and ambulate. Moderate, controlled exercise should be

Equine Neonatal Medicine, First Edition. Edited by David M. Wong and Pamela A. Wilkins.

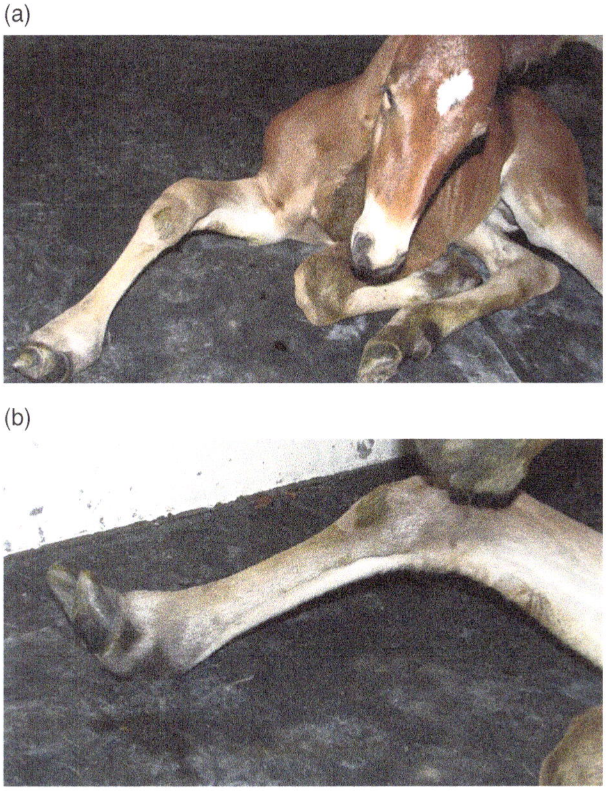

Figure 36.1 (a, b) Foal with a moderate to severe flexural deformity of the right carpus that made it difficult to rise without assistance. The left carpus was more mildly affected (not shown in this image). This foal also had a concurrent congenital skeletal anomaly, polydactyly, affecting both forelimbs.

encouraged, but overexertion can worsen the deformity and cause lameness.

- **Farriery** for flexural limb deformities focuses on protecting the toe and increasing tensile forces on the deep digital flexor tendon (DDFT) during ambulation. Application of a dorsal hoof wall extension protects the toe from excess wear, facilitates a delay in breakover, and compensates for lack of extension in the phalangeal region.
- **Oxytetracycline** makes tendons and ligaments of young foals more susceptible to elongation and is used to augment stretching of tendons and ligaments during exercise. The mechanism of oxytetracycline-mediated tendon and ligament relaxation is inhibition of tractional structuring of collagen fibrils by myofibroblasts, including dose-dependent inhibition of collagen gel contraction and decreases in matrix metalloproteinase-1 mRNA expression by equine myofibroblasts [3]. A single dose of oxytetracycline (2–3 g in 250–500 mL of saline, slow IV) results in correction or improvement of deformity within 24–48 hours. This dose may be repeated one to two times within the first few weeks of life if needed. Caution should be used in systemically compromised foals as oxtetracycline can be nephrotoxic. Serum biochemical monitoring is important; while no effect was seen on renal biochemical parameters following a single dose of oxytetracycline [4], acute renal failure has been reported in one foal [5].
- **External coaptation** with splints or casts can be effective for many flexural deformities, including the metacarpo-phalangeal/metatarsophalangeal joints, carpus, and tarsus. Splints can be made from PVC pipe, wood, fiberglass, or thermoplastic and are cost-effective options (Figure 36.2). Splints can be removed regularly and easily reapplied, allowing for repeated examination of the flexural deformity and monitoring for development of pressure sores. Pressure sores must be evaluated diligently as they can progress to septic arthritis or osteomyelitis. Splints should be placed over adequate padding to protect the skin, but sparse enough to prevent displacement of the splint when padding compresses. Sedation and analgesia facilitate splint placement and allows maximal extension of the limb.
- **Analgesics**, specifically nonsteroidal anti-inflammatory drugs (NSAIDs), are often warranted to encourage ambulation, as both the primary deformity and treatments may be painful.
- **Surgical intervention** is not usually required for treatment of congenital flexural deformities and is reserved for severe cases or those refractory to medical therapies (see "Acquired flexural limb deformities" section for site-specific surgical interventions).

Acquired Flexural Deformities

Acquired flexural deformities can occur in horses of any age but are most common in rapidly growing foals. Proposed etiologies are divided into contraction of the musculotendinous unit in response to pain or disparity in bone and tendon/ligament growth. As with congenital flexural deformities, acquired deformities can be readily diagnosed on visual exam. Deformities of the distal limb may be hidden by grass if the foal is on pasture, thus regular examination on hard, level ground facilitates early diagnosis.

Treatment Early diagnosis and treatment greatly improve prognosis. Underlying causes of pain should be addressed first. Surgical intervention should be considered if initial conservative management is unsuccessful unless the deformity is severe. Specific surgical interventions are discussed below.

- **Nutrition** plays a significant role in growth rate of foals. Overfeeding, either excessive concentrates or by heavily lactating mares, can increase growth as can an abrupt

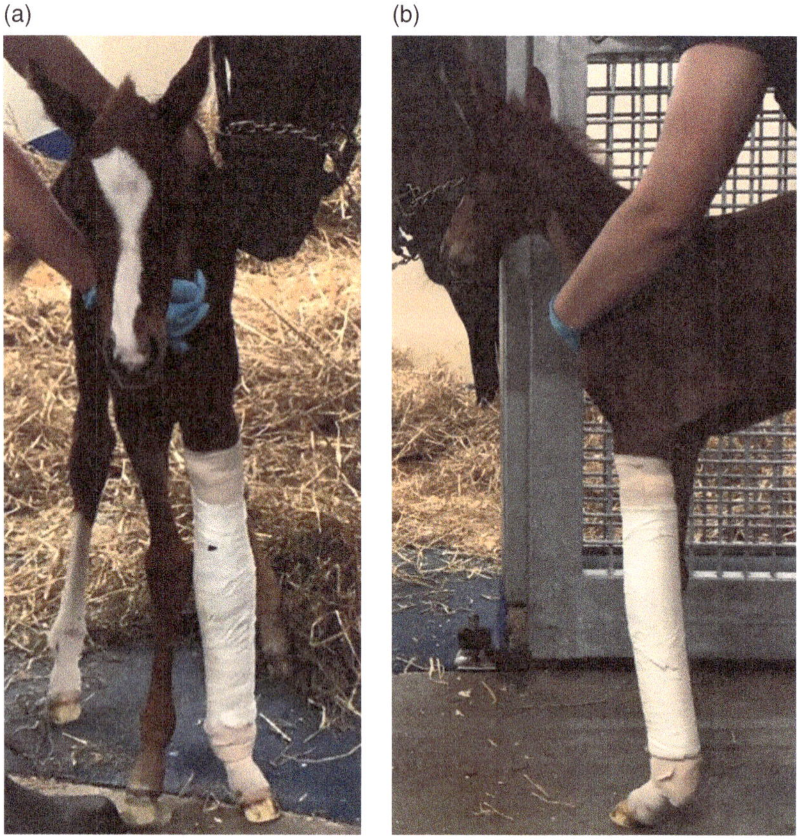

Figure 36.2 (a, b) Filly with external coaptation (splint) on the left forelimb. Note that the foot has been left out, as is typical for deformities involving the carpus and metacarpophalangeal joint. This foal also exhibits a mild carpus valgus of the right forelimb. *Source:* Images courtesy of Dr. Alessandro Migliorisi.

increase in the plane of nutrition. When a flexural deformity is identified, the foal should be weaned (if not already) or the mare's concentrate ration decreased. Weanlings or yearlings should be fed minimal concentrate with a hay and mineral supplement. Dietary mineral balance, especially calcium and phosphorous, also plays a role in developmental orthopedic disease. Mineral composition of diet, soil, and drinking water should be evaluated and supplemented as needed.

- **Physiotherapy** for treatment of acquired flexural deformities is controversial. If the deformity is secondary to a painful condition, exercise restriction is indicated to decrease pain and limit overloading of the contralateral limb. If the deformity is not secondary to pain, then regular exercise is recommended. In all cases, passive range of motion exercises can be used to help stretch the tendons.
- **Analgesics** should be considered for pain resulting from both the inciting cause and treatment of flexural deformity.

Distal Interphalangeal Joint (DIPJ)

Flexural deformities of the DIPJ almost always affect the forelimbs, primarily in foals 1–4 months of age and are often bilateral. A functional shortening of the DDFT results in excessive tension on the third phalanx, resulting in palmar rotation of the foot. The accessory ligament of the DDFT (ALDDFT or inferior check ligament) limits passive elongation of the DDFT, contributing to the deformity. Changes in the external appearance of the hoof (clubbed foot) occur secondary to abnormal position of the third phalanx. Initially, the hoof wall appears more vertical, and in acute cases the heel may not even contact the ground. With time, the heels overgrow and the foot develops a box-like appearance. Increased stress and wear of the toe results in widening of the white line and flaring of the dorsodistal hoof wall. DIPJ flexural deformities are classified as Stage I or Stage II based on the external appearance of the foot. In Stage I (Figure 36.3a), the dorsal hoof wall is upright but has not passed the vertical plane (angle between dorsal hoof wall and sole is $>60°$ and $<90°$). In Stage II, the dorsal hoof wall is beyond the vertical plane (angle between wall and sole is $>90°$). Radiographs may show secondary changes, including remodeling of the dorsodistal aspect of P3, rotation of P3 within the hoof capsule and osteoarthritis of the DIP joint (Figure 36.3b).

Conservative treatment of DIPJ flexural deformities focuses on stretching the DDFT, minimizing pain, and protecting the toe from excessive wear. Analgesics help reduce pain and encourage exercise. Farriery should address the boxy foot conformation by gradually rasping back the heels to realign the hoof-pastern axis, so long as the heel is

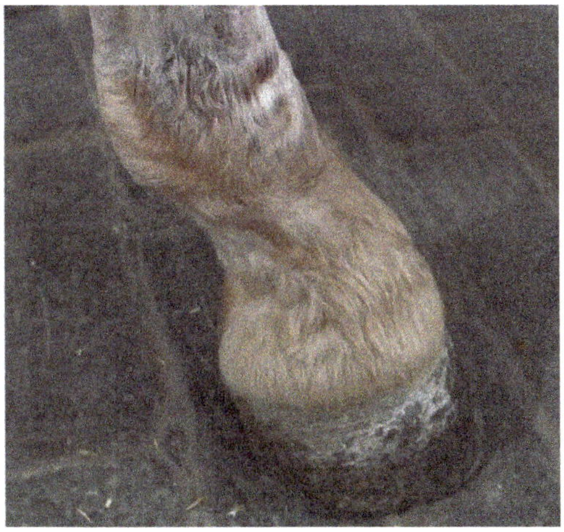

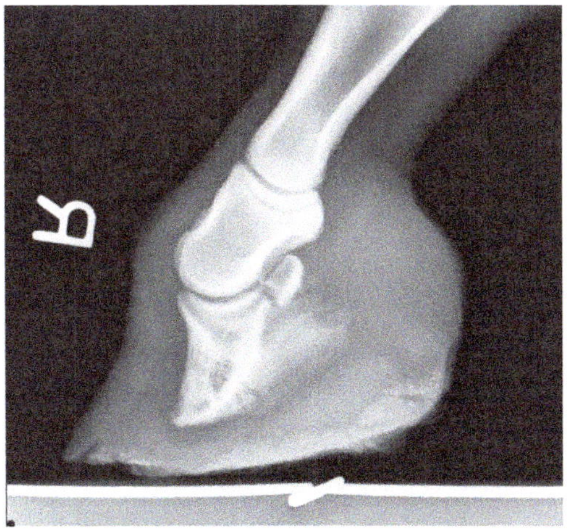

Figure 36.3 (a) Stage I flexural deformity of the right distal interphalangeal joint (DIPJ) of a foal ("club foot"). Note the characteristic boxy appearance of the hoof with an upright dorsal hoof wall. This foal was treated with an inferior check ligament desmotomy. (b) Radiograph of a more severe (nearly Stage II) flexural limb deformity of the right DIPJ. Note radiographic changes indicative of chronicity including rotation of P3 relative to the hoof capsule and osseous remodeling of P3. This foal was treated with a deep digital flexor tenotomy.

touching the ground. If necessary, desomotomy of the ALDDFT is the surgical treatment of choice for Stage I deformity. Immediate correction or improvement of the deformity is expected, although toe protection/extension is often required for the best outcome. Postoperative management includes regular hoof trims with rasping of the heel and controlled exercise. DDFT tenotomy is indicated for Stage II deformities that do not correct after desmotomy of the ALDDFT. Postoperative correction is immediate but can be associated with significant pain, and the deformity can reappear within months of surgery [6]. Historically viewed as a salvage procedure, some horses are sound for riding following tenotomy of the DDFT [7]. Nevertheless, the prognosis for full athletic function is guarded [8].

Prognosis following ALDDFT desmotomy is good for athletic function. Eighty six percent of pleasure/show horses treated before 1 year of age were used for their intended purpose (78% after 1 year of age) [9]. In Standardbreds, the prognosis was better for foals treated <8 months of age [10]. Prognosis is worse for Stage II compared to Stage I and worsens with radiographic changes or increased time before treatment. Over time, abnormal forces within the foot result in permanent changes to the soft tissue structures and bones. Distraction of the dorsodistal hoof wall can result in seedy toe or subsolar abscesses. However, even mature horses may return to athletic use following ALDDFT desmotomy for flexural deformity of the distal interphalangeal joint [11, 12].

Proximal Interphalangeal Joint (PIPJ)

Acquired flexural deformities of the PIPJ are primarily diagnosed in the hind limbs of rapidly growing weanlings between 10 and 18 months old. Foals with straight hind limb conformation are more commonly affected and the condition is typically bilateral. Deformity of the PIPJ is caused by shortening of the DDFT, with concurrent laxity in the superficial digital flexor tendon (SDFT). Diagnosis is based on dorsal subluxation of the PIPJ, and an audible click may be noted during walking. The click may resolve with rest due to periarticular fibrosis; joint deformity usually persists, and secondary osteoarthritis is likely. Surgical management, consisting of ALDDFT desmotomy and tenotomy of the medial head of the DDFT resolved subluxation in a small case series [13]. Arthrodesis of the PIPJ may be required with persistent subluxation and osteoarthritis.

Metacarpophalangeal or Metatarsophalangeal Joint (MCPJ/MTPJ)

This deformity is more common in the forelimb (Figure 36.4) than the hindlimb and most often develops around 1 year of age. Functional shortening of the SDFT, DDFT, and less commonly the suspensory ligament may contribute to the deformity. Three grades of MCPJ/MTPJ deformity have been described:

- **Mild**: Straight joint that rarely flexes more than 180° but remains caudal to the foot at all times.
- **Moderate**: >180° joint angle when standing, such that the joint is dorsal to the foot, but the fetlock extends to a caudal position when walking.
- **Severe**: Joint maintains >180° flexion at all time, with laxity in the flexor tendons and suspensory ligament; prominent, taut extensor tendons preventing further flexion of the joint.

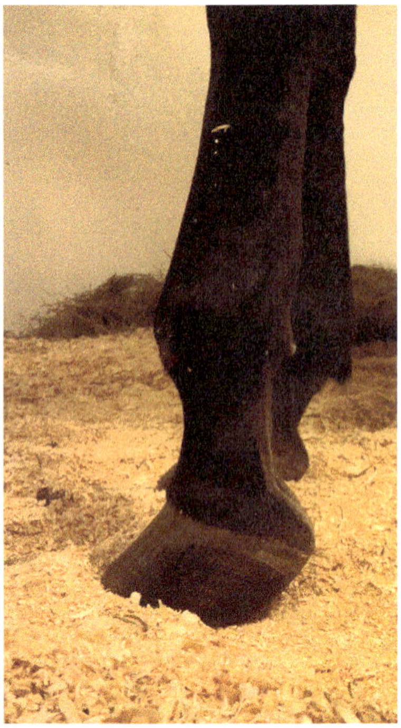

Figure 36.4 Flexural limb deformity affecting the left metacarpophalangeal joint.

Conservative management relies on correction of nutritional excesses, corrective farriery, and physiotherapy. Significant pain is associated with correction; thus, analgesics are always indicated. Surgical intervention should be considered if unresponsive to conservative management or if the fetlock joint angle is >180°. As both the SDFT and DDFT can contribute to deformity, desmotomies of the ALDDFT and accessory ligament of the superficial digital flexor tendon (ALSDFT), singly or together, may be used. The primarily affected tendinous structure is determined by palpation of the limb. Application of pressure to the dorsal joint surface creates tension in the flexor tendons; the tightest structure is the first to be released surgically. Prognosis is good with conservative treatment if the deformity is diagnosed and treated early. If surgical intervention is required, the prognosis is guarded to poor. Severe and chronic deformities respond poorly to any treatment, including surgery.

Carpal Flexural Deformities

Acquired flexural deformities of the carpus are commonly secondary to another injury that prevents weightbearing and develops suddenly following a prolonged period of non-weightbearing lameness. To prevent development of carpal flexural deformities, application of splints should be considered early in convalescence for foals with long-term injuries that prevent normal weightbearing. Passive stretching and controlled exercise (as permitted by original injury) are combined with splinting to prevent contracture and maintain normal range of motion. Splints must be monitored for development of pressure sores. Tenotomy of the ulnaris lateralis and flexor carpi ulnaris tendons can have good outcomes in cases resistant to conservative treatment. Carpal splints and controlled exercise are important during the postoperative period.

Congenital Digital Hyperextension Deformities (Flexor Tendon Laxity)

Digital hyperextension of varying severity is commonly seen in newborn foals. Affected foals have a more acute angle to the MCPJ or MTPJ when standing and/or are unable to maintain the toe on the ground (Figure 36.5). In severe cases, foals may stand and walk on the palmar/plantar aspect of the phalanges. Diagnostic imaging is unnecessary as imaging abnormalities are not expected. Digital hyperextension is attributable to flaccidity of the flexor muscles and often improves or resolves without specific treatment over the initial few weeks of life. Resolution is due to increased muscle tone and negative allometric growth of the tendons relative to the bones of the distal limb.

Conservative therapy is typically sufficient to address this condition:

- **Moderate exercise** to strengthen the musculotendinous unit is recommended; excessive exercise should be avoided as fatigue worsens hyperextension. If hyperextension worsens, exercise restriction should be increased.

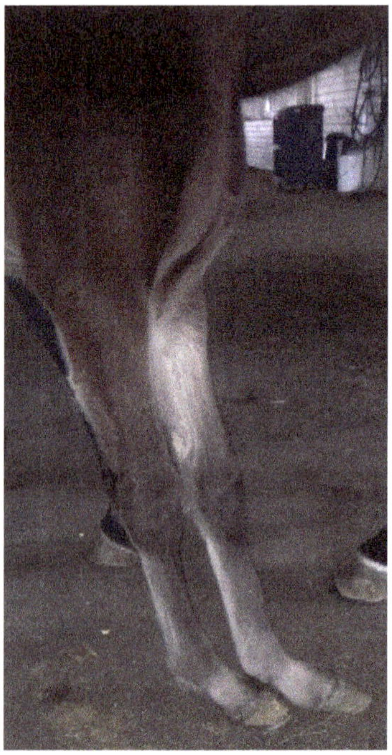

Figure 36.5 Foal with severe congenital tendon laxity of both forelimbs. This image was taken after several weeks of conservative therapy, including heel extensions and limited exercise.

- **Farriery** includes light rasping to shorten the toe and reduce the palmar/plantar hoof to increase contact with the ground. Heel extensions are indicated to maintain contact between the sole and ground in severely affected foals where the toe is lifting off the ground or weight-bearing is occurring on the pastern.
- **Light bandages** should be applied to protect the skin of the distal limb from trauma. Foals that bear weight on the palmar/plantar pastern are at risk of excoriation and necrosis of the skin in that region. Likewise, padding applied over heel extension devices protects the skin of the phalanges from injury and may prevent the mare or foal from prematurely dislodging the devices. Heavy bandages, splints, or casts that incorporate the foot are contraindicated.

Angular Limb Deformities

Angular limb deformity (ALD) is defined as a conformational deviation of the limb in the frontal plane. The deformity is described by the direction of deviation of the limb distal to the point of origin. Valgus describes lateral deviation while varus describes medial deviation (Figure 36.6). Axial rotation of the limb is commonly identified in conjunction with ALD: outward rotation with valgus deformity (splay foot) and inward rotation with varus deformity (pigeon toed). "Windswept" describes a foal with a varus deformity in one limb and a valgus deformity

(a) (b)

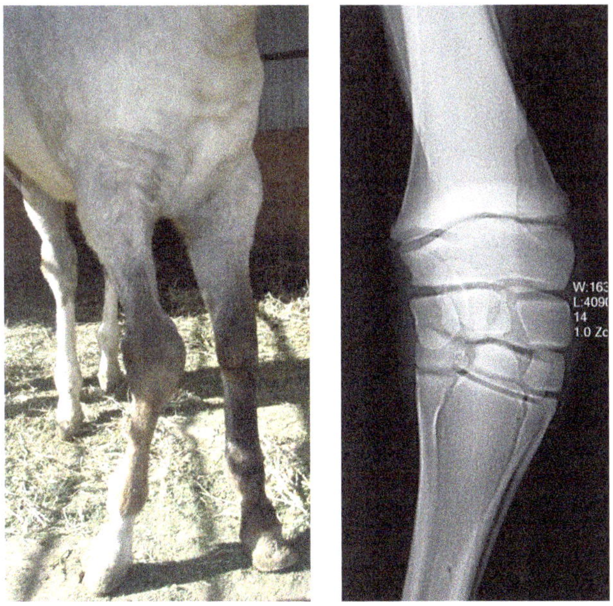

Figure 36.6 Foal with severe carpus valgus of the right forelimb. (a) Gross appearance of the limb; (b) radiograph of the affected limb. This foal also had compensatory fetlock varus of the affected limb, diagnosed radiographically.

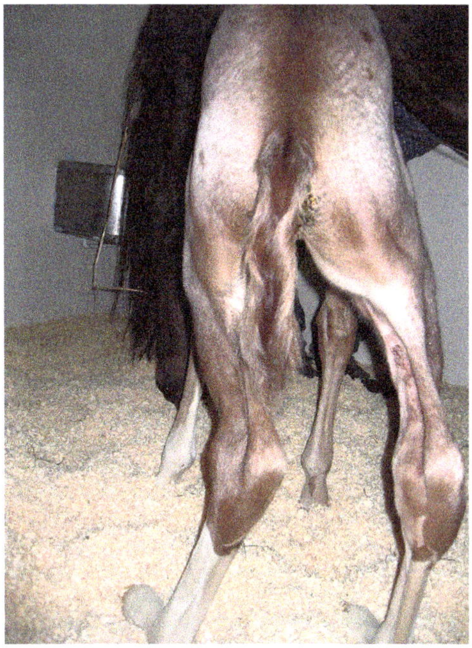

Figure 36.7 Neonatal foal with windswept hindlimbs. *Source:* Photo courtesy of Dr. David Wong, Iowa State University.

in the contralateral limb (Figure 36.7). "Bench knees" describes a limb with a straight appearance, but knees that are offset from the limb. This is the result of two opposing ALDs: valgus of the distal radius and varus at proximal MCIII.

ALD may be perinatal or acquired. While disproportionate growth at the metaphyseal growth plate is the most common cause of ALD, abnormalities of the cuboidal bones of the carpus or tarsus or the diaphysial or epiphyseal region of long bones can also contribute. Congenital laxity of the periarticular structures leads to joint instability and should be suspected if multiple severe ALDs are present, in windswept foals, and if oscillation between varus and valgus deformities are noted. Laxity initially results in ALD when weightbearing, but can lead to severe permanent ALD, especially in cases with concurrent incomplete ossification of cuboidal bones (**Chapter 37**). Prolonged disproportionate loading of the growth plate distal to the origin of primary ALD can result in a compensatory ALD. This compensatory deformity may appear to straighten the limb axis, but the joint will not be perpendicular to the axis of the limb, resulting in abnormal rotation of the joint during motion. Incidence of ALD has been reported in 36–94% of foals at birth, decreasing to 16–34% by 6 months of age [14, 15].

Factors suggested to contribute to uneven bone development include genetic predisposition, dietary imbalances, trauma, excessive exercise, physeal dysplasia, heavy birth weight, and physeal overload [14, 16]. Hypotheses for the underlying etiology for periarticular laxity include aberrant development of the long bones relative to soft tissues, gestational hormonal imbalance or abnormal intrauterine positioning [17]. The limb should be evaluated with the clinician oriented perpendicular to the frontal plane of the limb. If outward rotation of the limb is present (common in neonates), evaluation should be performed from a craniolateral position.

The foal should be examined while standing and while moving. Thorough palpation and assessment of passive range of motion in all planes should be performed. If the deformity is caused by laxity of the periarticular structures, the limb should be easily straightened by manual pressure. If the limb cannot be manually straightened, underlying osseous abnormality should be suspected. Radiography is the only method to identify the exact location and objectively determine the degree of angular deformity and is useful to identify concurrent osseous abnormalities such as abnormally shaped, fractured, or incompletely ossified cuboidal bones, congenital abnormalities, atavisms, or physitis.

Treatment

Periarticular laxity is usually self-limiting and resolves with growth. Controlled exercise to strengthen muscles and associated soft tissues is beneficial. Treatment of ALD of physeal origin depends on age of the foal, location and severity of deformity, and progression of condition. Young foals with a mild deformity that is not progressive may be managed conservatively with restricted exercise ± corrective farriery (trimming and/or foot extensions). Timing of growth plate closure dictates earlier surgical intervention in the fetlock than in the carpus or tarsus. Surgical interventions can be broadly divided into procedures for growth acceleration or growth retardation and may be used in combination:

- **Hemi-circumferential periosteal transection and elevation (HCPTE or periosteal stripping)** has historically been described to encourage growth acceleration on the concave side of the limb with ALD. The mechanism through which HCPTE mediates correction of deformity is thought to be a decrease in static compression at the physis, resulting in accelerated growth of physeal cells. Although a good prognosis following HCPTE has been described [18, 19], some studies have called its utility into question [20].
- **Methods of surgical growth retardation include stapling, screws and cerclage wire, single transphyseal screw, or application of a small bone plate**. The principle of growth retardation procedures is to increase static compression on the cells of the physis to a supraphysiologic level. Implants are applied to the convex aspect of the bone across the physis, allowing the shorter aspect of the bone (concave side) to continue growing. For all surgical growth retardation techniques, the timing of implant removal is determined by response to treatment as judged by frequent re-evaluation and monthly radiographs. The goal is to remove the implant before complete correction, as minor correction of ALD will continue for a short time after implant removal. Ideally, 85–95% of the desired correction should occur at the time of implant removal [21]. Prognosis for athletic use following surgical growth retardation techniques is good in foals without concurrent incomplete ossification of cuboidal bones, although Thoroughbred racehorses treated as foals had lower performance indices compared to untreated siblings [21–23].
- **Corrective osteotomy and ostectomy** may be considered for correction of diaphyseal and metaphyseal/epiphyseal ALDs in foals with closed growth plates. Prognosis for future athletic use is guarded to fair following these procedures [24].
- **Nonsurgical local growth retardation** has been described by application of a radial shockwave generator to the convex aspect of the limb with ALD [25]. In the reported study, weekly application was tolerated by sedated foals, and straightening of limbs occurred between 15 and 76 days.

Other Appendicular Skeleton Abnormalities

Other less common congenital abnormalities of the appendicular skeleton include patellar luxation, polydactyly, and congenital phalangeal hypoplasia. Patellar luxation is most commonly reported in Miniature Horses, while only sporadic reports of the other conditions exist.

Patellar Luxation

Lateral luxation of the patella is a rare condition in horses, most commonly observed as a congenital condition in foals and Miniature Horses. The etiology is unknown but it is believed to be heritable [26]. Traumatic lateral patellar luxation has also been reported but is less common [27]. The condition may be unilateral or bilateral with varying clinical signs, depending on the severity of displacement. With complete luxation, the quadriceps muscle acts as a flexor instead of an extensor of the stifle. Affected foals assume a classic crouched position and may be unable to stand (Figure 36.8). Incomplete lateral patellar luxation is typified by limb stiffness and variable degrees of lameness, femoropatellar joint effusion, and crepitus. Luxation can typically be reduced manually, thus confirming the diagnosis, but the position of the patella can be assessed radiographically in both caudocranial and lateromedial views. Radiographs should be evaluated for the degree of joint

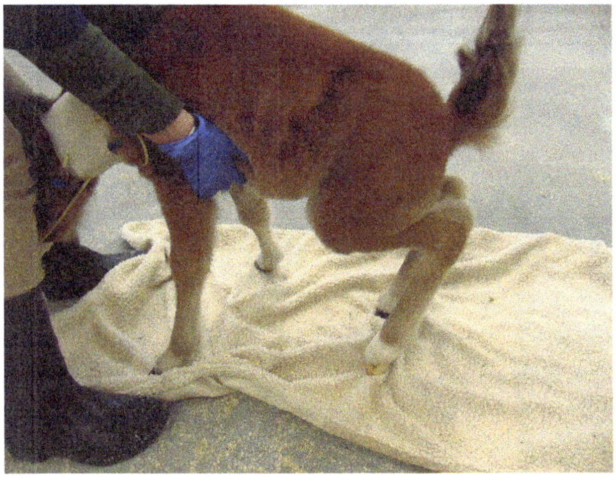

Figure 36.8 Neonatal Miniature Horse foal with bilateral lateral luxation of the patella. Foal was unable to stand on its own and assumed a crouched position. *Source:* Photo courtesy of Dr. David Wong, Iowa State University.

degeneration, the depth of the trochlear groove, and the shape and degree of ossification of the patellar and trochlear ridges.

Surgical correction of lateral patellar luxation involves release of tension from lateral soft tissue structures (lateral release) and reinforcement of the medial supporting structures (medial imbrication). Sulcoplasty has been described to address instability of the patella within the trochlear groove or lateral ridge hypoplasia, in combination with the other procedures [28]. Successful outcomes have been reported in foals, resulting in a functional femorpatellar joint and minimal to no lameness in some cases [27–29]. Positioning of the patella should be confirmed with intra- or postoperative radiographs.

Polydactyly

Polydactyly varies in phenotype from a small vestigial hoof at the fetlock to a full extra digit that articulates at the carpus (Figure 36.1). The forelimb is affected in 80% of cases, and the supernumerary digit is more often on the medial aspect of the limb. Unlike cattle, there is no evidence of a genetic etiology in horses. Polydactyly is associated with other congenital musculoskeletal malformations, including adactylia, congenital arthrogryposis, and jaw abnormalities [30, 31]. Diagnosis of polydactly is made based on the distinctive gross appearance. However, radiographs of the affected limb(s) should be obtained to evaluate the bony anatomy prior to surgical intervention, as the anatomy may be more complex internally than external appearance reveals.

Surgical removal of the supernumerary digit(s) is indicated to improve cosmetic appearance and prevent ongoing trauma to the digit but should be delayed until the foal is older to decrease anesthetic risk. The supernumerary digit will have extensor and flexor tendons, a suspensory ligament, sesamoid bones, and nerves and vessels like other digits. The digit is removed by osteotomy at the middle of the metacarpal bone or disarticulation, depending on the individual anatomy. Destabilization of the carpal joint should be avoided to prevent development of osteoarthritis or ALD. Incomplete removal of the digit increases risk of future lameness and poor cosmetic outcome [32].

Congenital Phalangeal Hypoplasia

Sporadic cases of osseous hypo- or aplasia of the appendicular skeleton have been described, including one case of patellar agenesis, agenesis of a forelimb distal to the radius, and four cases involving the phalanges and/or navicular bone [30, 33]. There is no documented etiology for phalangeal hypoplasia. Inherited transmission as a single recessive trait has been suggested, but no pattern of heritability has been documented in reported cases. Environmental teratogen exposure or random defects during embryogenesis are other plausible explanations. Radiographic examination of the affected limb should be performed to document the presence and severity of osseous hypoplasia. In a series of three foals, all had severe hypoplasia of the distal phalanx, two had concurrent hypoplasia of the middle phalanx, and two had hypo- or aplasia of the navicular bone [33]. No specific treatment has been described; rather, treatment aims to support the biomechanics of the affected limb. Of the few described cases, most have been lost to follow up. Based on the resultant severe hoof wall deformation, future athletic potential is unlikely.

Abnormalities of the Axial Skeleton

Developmental abnormalities of the vertebral column result in a variety of clinical presentations. While congenital abnormalities of the axial skeleton are, by definition, present at birth, defects may not become apparent until later in life. Cervical vertebral stenotic myelopathy (CVSM) and occipitoatlantoaxial malformation (OAAM) are the most common developmental abnormalities of the vertebral column in horses.

Less commonly, deviations of the thoracic vertebral column resulting from some form of vertebral malformation (e.g., hemivertebrae) are often, but not always, readily appreciated on physical exam at birth and may occur in the vertical (kyphosis, lordosis) and/or horizontal (scoliosis) planes. Hemivertebrae result from failure of formation of part of a vertebra, typically a part of the vertebral body [34]. Depending on the portion of the vertebra that fails to form, hemivertebra can be wedge-shaped with the base oriented dorsally, ventrally, or medially [34]. If the central portion of the vertebra does not form, two hemivertebrae may be noted within the same segment (termed butterfly vertebra). Hemivertebra can be incidental findings on diagnostic imaging studies or necropsy but can also result in neurologic disease from stenosis of the vertebral canal, progressive deformity of spinal angulation with growth, or instability [34].

Of note, deformation of vertebral bodies resulting from alteration in the shape or structure of a vertebra that was initially normally differentiated is not considered a true congenital abnormality. Multiple vertebral abnormalities may be present simultaneously. For example, OAAM may be associated with congenital cervical scoliosis [35]. Thus, recognition of one axial abnormality should prompt a search for associated lesions.

Cervical Vertebral Stenotic Myelopathy

CVSM is a common, multifactorial disease characterized by stenosis of the vertebral canal and spinal cord compression resulting in spinal ataxia in young horses. Genetic predisposition and nutritional factors are thought to be the most significant causes of postnatal vertebral deformation in CVSM. Affected animals demonstrate rapid growth and are more likely to be affected by developmental orthopedic disease of the appendicular skeleton. CVSM presents as proprioceptive neurologic deficits that are more severe in the pelvic limbs. Type I CVSM commonly occurs between 6 months and 3 years of age and is defined by dynamic instability resulting from malformation and malarticulation. Type II CVSM, caused by static compression, results from cervical osteoarthropathy in older horses, and is beyond the scope of this chapter.

Pathophysiology

Vertebral malformations associated with CVSM include flaring of caudal epiphyses of vertebral bodies, abnormal ossification of the articular processes, malalignment between adjacent vertebrae, ligamentous hypertrophy, synovial cysts, disc herniation, epidural hematomas, osteoarthritis of the articular processes, and extension of the dorsal laminae. Spinal cord lesions include focal loss of white matter neurons and Wallerian degeneration of ascending fibers cranial to the lesion and descending fibers caudal to the lesion. Clinical signs result from focal compression of the cervical spinal cord at single or multiple intervertebral articulations. Ataxia is often worse in the hindlimbs than in the forelimbs as descending tracts to the hindlimb tracts are located superficially within the spinal cord and are therefore more affected by external compression. Compression of the cervical intumescence at the C6–C7 articulation may result in more severe forelimb signs. Clinical signs are consistent with upper motor neuron deficits and include symmetric weakness, stumbling, toe dragging, delayed proprioceptive positioning, truncal sway, circumduction and pivoting of hind limbs when circling, and spastic or stiff-legged gait.

Diagnosis

Imaging modalities are most useful for diagnosing CVSM, although further tests can rule out other neurological diseases. Analysis of cerebrospinal fluid (CSF) is unremarkable although horses with acute compression may have mild xanthochromia or increased protein concentration.

- **Plain radiography** can diagnose CVSM with 50% sensitivity and 70% specificity [36]. High-quality, precise lateromedial radiographs facilitate determination of spinal canal diameter. Subjective evaluation of vertebral deformation (vertebral subluxation, flared caudal epiphysis, extension of dorsal laminae, abnormal ossification or osteoarthritis of articular facets) is not reliable for the diagnosis of CVSM [36]. Measurements of minimal sagittal diameter and vertebral body width are obtained to calculate intra- and intervertebral sagittal ratios. Intravertebral sagittal ratios should exceed 52% for C2–C4 and 56% at C7 in horses weighing more than 320 kg [37, 38]. Intervertebral sagittal ratio of 0.485 or less indicates CVSM [39].
- **Myelography**, including neutral and stressed views, provides more accurate lesion localization and allows for differentiation between dynamic (type I) and static (type II) spinal cord compression. Compression is evaluated based on the height of the myelographic dye column, defined as at least a 20% reduction of minimal intervertebral dural diameter compared to maximum intravertebral dural diameter or a 50% reduction of the dorsal myelographic dye column at the minimum intervertebral height compared to maximum intravertebral height [40]. Dural or dye column ratios are more reliable than absolute measurements of column height. Agreement between myelographic findings and necropsy ranges from 50 to 80%.
- **Computed tomographic (CT)** and post-myelographic CT provides the most reliable antemortem diagnosis of spinal cord compression and can confirm the results of radiographic studies. However, like radiography, CT cannot provide information regarding the integrity of the spinal cord.

Treatment

Nutritional management may be effective in foals <1 year of age with radiographic evidence of CVSM with or without clinical signs [41]. The goal is to allow cervical vertebral sagittal diameter to enlarge by slowing bone growth and increasing bone metabolism. Dietary management consists of restricted energy and protein intake. The diet should be balanced in vitamins and minerals, with supplemental selenium and vitamins A and E. Affected foals should be stall confined to minimize repetitive spinal cord compression caused by dynamic instability. Administration of anti-inflammatory medications may reduce edema, resulting in transient improvement in neurologic signs.

The goal of surgical treatment is to reduce spinal cord impingement by stabilization of affected intervertebral articulations. Surgical options include vertebral interbody fusion and subtotal dorsal decompression laminectomy, although the latter is not widely performed due to surgical difficulty and high frequency of postoperative complications [42, 43]. Vertebral interbody fusion can be performed with a Kerf-cut cylinder (Seattle Slew implant) or by ventral cervical vertebral fusion with a locking compression plate. Complications of interbody fusion include fracture of adjacent vertebral body, seroma formation, failure or migration of implants, laryngeal hemiplegia, Horner's syndrome, esophageal rupture, and laryngospasm.

Case selection for surgical intervention is critical to satisfactory outcome. Factors related to successful outcomes include number of sites of spinal cord compression, type of compression (static or dynamic), severity and duration of clinical signs, and temperament, age, and intended use of the horse. Expected improvement following surgical intervention is 1–2 neurological grades on a five-point scale. Therefore, severely affected horses may improve but remain unable to return to athletic use following surgical treatment. Horses should be evaluated for concurrent appendicular developmental orthopedic disease prior to surgical intervention and the implication of concurrent lesions on outcome and intended use carefully considered.

Scoliosis, Kyphosis, and Lordosis

Deformation of the vertebral column is described by the deviation from normal alignment. Dorsal and ventral bending is referred to as *kyphosis* and *lordosis*, respectively. Bending to either side is called scoliosis, and combinations of these conditions may occur (i.e. kyphoscoliosis) (Figure 36.9). Torticollis, or wry neck, specifically refers to deformation in the cervical spinal column resulting in an uncorrectable deviation of the neck to one side. Reports of these congenital abnormalities are rare, with most affected foals exhibiting a combination of abnormalities in both the axial and appendicular skeleton (i.e. contracted foal syndrome) [44–47]. Severely affected foals may be stillborn or die or are euthanized in the perinatal period. However, some foals that are born via cesarean section with deformities restricted to the neck and limbs that can stand and are otherwise healthy have been reported to recover [48].

Congenital scoliosis, kyphosis, and lordosis are typically the result of malformation of one or more cervical and/or thoracic vertebrae. The etiology of this condition is debated, but toxin exposure, genetic factors, and restricted intrauterine environment have been proposed as possible causes [35, 44, 48]. Mild deviations of the vertebral column may not be appreciated clinically, and in these cases radiography or CT may be useful for diagnosis and characterization of the abnormality [45]. These mild disorders may not preclude an athletic career, as a large survey of horses

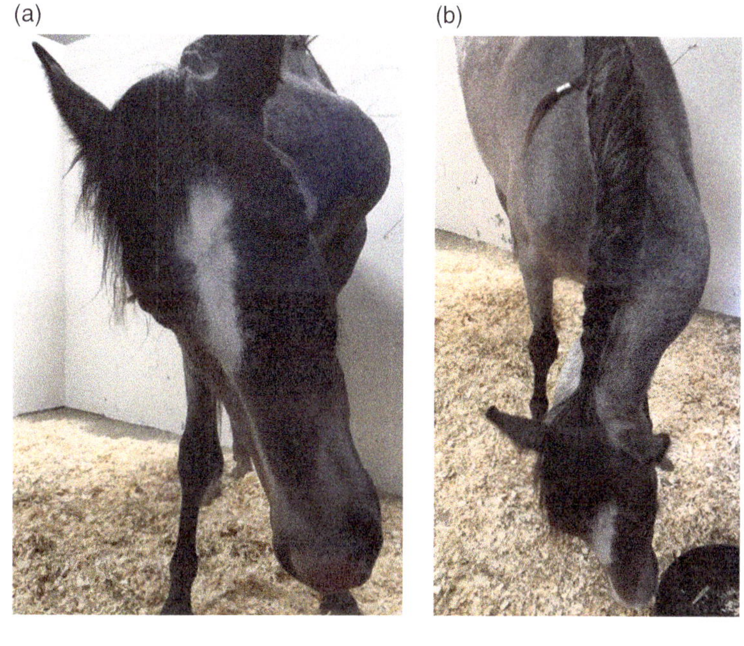

Figure 36.9 (a, b) Filly with chronic congenital lordoscoliosis affecting the cervical spine. The filly could not raise her head above the level of her shoulders. Necropsy examination revealed asymmetrical cervical vertebrae.

6 months to 18 years of age presenting for evaluation of thoracolumbar pain revealed vertebral malformations (scoliosis, lordosis, kyphosis) in 2.9% of this clinical population [49]. Kyphosis, or "roach back," may also occur secondarily to painful conditions of the back or abdomen; in this case, no underlying vertebral malformation exists.

Other Axial Skeleton Abnormalities

Other less common congenital abnormalities of the axial skeleton include hereditary multiple exostoses and osteopetrosis.

Hereditary Multiple Exostoses

Also referred to as multiple cartilaginous exostoses or osteochondroma, hereditary multiple exostoses is a rare heritable congenital condition. This condition manifests as multiple abnormal bony projections or solitary osteochondromas arising from the long bones, ribs, and pelvis. These benign growths typically do not continue to grow beyond skeletal maturity, and single lesions may be amenable to surgical removal.

Osteopetrosis

Osteopetrosis is an inherited disorder of osteoclasts with a wide range of phenotypic expression, related to an imbalance between bone apposition and resorption. The disease has been described in five foals and a donkey [50–53].

Affected equids present for failure to thrive, inability/reluctance to stand, and failure of passive transfer. Marked brachygnathia is an additional common feature. Of the six cases reported, the Peruvian Paso breed (4/6) and males (4/6) were overrepresented [50–53]. Radiographs reveal increased opacity of medullary bone throughout the axial and appendicular skeleton. Parallel linear columns of bone originating from the physis toward the diaphysis create an hourglass appearance in long bones. Osteosclerosis is also apparent in the cervical vertebrae, as well as abnormal development and malpositioning of incoming premolar and molar dentition. Pathologic fractures of the ribs, radius, tibia, and spinous or transverse processes have been reported, reflecting abnormally stiff and brittle bones. Multiple rib fractures with various degrees of callous formation suggests that fractures occur in utero as well as peripartum. Affected individuals have normal serum calcium and phosphorus levels, but increased serum alkaline phosphatase. Treatment consists of supportive care and symptomatic management for complications. All reported cases were euthanized by 8 days of age due to various systemic complications.

Complex Congenital Musculoskeletal Disorders

Arthrogryposis

Congenital arthrogryposis (also called congenital articular rigidity or arthrogryposis multiplex congenita) is a syndrome resulting from rigid fixation of joints. Typically, multiple joints are involved, with affected joints fixed in flexion. The etiology in foals is unknown, although a relation to autosomal trisomy has been proposed [54]. In cattle and swine, arthrogryposis has been associated with in utero infection with akabane virus and ingestion of toxic plants, in addition to hereditary forms. Few reports of arthrogyposis in horses exist as the condition is often conflated with flexural limb deformities or contracted foal syndrome. In one report of an affected Thoroughbred foal, hypoplasia of muscles, nerves, and bones were described in the affected limb [55]. Affected animals are unlikely to improve and are often euthanized [6]. Aggressive intervention, such as arthrodesis or wedge osteotomy, may be attempted as a salvage procedure [56].

Schistosoma Reflexus

Schistosoma reflexus is a rare type of fetal deformity, more often observed in cattle than horses. Schistosomus refers to exposure of viscera due to failure of the thoracic and abdominal cavities to close appropriately. Reflexus describes the characteristic extreme lordosis of the vertebral column, with the tail and head in close proximity. Facial deformity may also be present in affected animals. As with other deformities, abnormal fetal posture may result in dystocia, requiring fetotomy or cesarean section for resolution.

Schistocoelia

Schistocoelia is the eventration of viscera through a closure defect of the body wall without severe lordosis and is more often reported in equids than schistosoma reflexus [57–59]. Schistocoelia may present as a component of contracted foal syndrome, along with kyphoscoliosis and arthrogryposis.

Functional Musculoskeletal Abnormalities

Several functional musculoskeletal abnormalities are reported in horses, including glycogen branching enzyme deficiency (GBED), hyperkalemic periodic paralysis (HYPP), myotonia congenital and dystrophica, and polysaccharide storage myopathy (PSSM). These are primary muscle diseases and have a known or suspected inherited etiology. Testing and breeding strategies are in place in certain breeds to reduce the incidence of these diseases.

Glycogen Branching Enzyme Deficiency

GBED is a hereditary glycogen storage disease inherited as an autosomal recessive trait, primarily in Quarter Horses and American Paint Horses. The disease is caused by a point mutation in the *GBE1* gene that prevents normal synthesis of glycogen storage enzyme and thus disrupts glycogen metabolism [60]. Frequency of the causative allele in the affected breeds is reported to range between 2.0 and 5.4% [61, 62], although it is more common in the cutting subtype of Quarter Horses. A commercial genetic test is available for the GBED mutation and is required under certain circumstances by both the American Quarter Horse and American Paint Horse Associations. GBED is a fatal disorder, with many affected fetuses aborted or stillborn. Foals that are born alive demonstrate progressive clinical signs including hypoglycemic seizures, muscle weakness, respiratory failure, and death. One study reported that 2.5% of fetal and early neonatal foal deaths from cases presented to two diagnostic laboratories were affected with GBED [62]. Typical histopathologic changes include globular deposits of abnormal polysaccharide in cardiac and skeletal muscle tissue, as well as inclusion bodies in cardiac muscle, particularly Purkinje fibers [62].

Hyperkalemic Periodic Paralysis

HYPP is a hereditary myotonia inherited in an autosomal dominant fashion in Quarter Horses and related breeds. The causative point mutation is located within the voltage-dependent skeletal muscle sodium channel alpha subunit [63]. This changes one amino acid in one type of voltage dependent sodium channel, thereby allowing muscle to be more permeable to sodium. Normally, sodium channels open to allow rapid membrane depolarization in the first phase of an action potential and then close once the membrane is depolarized. In HYPP, the channel remains open, resulting in the membrane potential being more depolarized and closer to threshold, making muscle more likely to contract spontaneously. This mutation is traced to the American Quarter Horse sire "Impressive" with an overall estimated frequency in the general Quarter Horse and Paint populations of 1.0–2.5% [61]. However, breeding practices in halter and pleasure horse groups that favor maintenance of the heterozygote state due to a heavily muscled phenotype have resulted in a much higher allele frequency in these subpopulations [61]. A genetic test is commercially available for the HYPP mutation and is required under certain circumstances by both the American Quarter Horse and Paint Horse associations. Horses that are homozygous for the defect have been barred from registration by the American Quarter Horse Association since January 1, 2007.

Clinical signs vary widely between affected individuals, ranging from intermittent muscle fasciculations and weakness to sudden death. Homozygous individuals usually have more severe clinical signs than heterozygotes. Dysphagia is a particular clinical sign that can be observed in nursing foals with HYPP [64]. Muscle fasciculations generally begin locally in the face, flanks, neck, or shoulders, but may progress to generalized tremors and weakness with dog-sitting or collapse. Once the episode is over (up to an hour in severe cases) horses generally have a normal gait, and mentation should remain normal throughout. Although the widespread use of the genetic test allows owners to know their horse's HYPP status before they ever see clinical signs, owners of unregistered Quarter Horses may not recognize the clinical signs and therefore miss mild episodes. Hyperkalemia (6–9 mEq/L) during or immediately after an episode is highly suggestive of the disease but not definitive. Triggers for HYPP episodes include diets high in potassium, sudden diet changes, fasting, anesthesia, or any other kind of stress. Exercise is not a triggering factor in of itself, and in fact, mild exercise may help abrogate clinical signs in mild cases. Prognosis for athletic use is generally good, particularly heterozygotes, that are appropriately managed.

Treatment and Prevention

Many horses recover from mild HYPP episodes without intervention. Prevention includes avoidance of high-potassium feeds such as alfalfa and molasses, feeding multiple small meals throughout the day, and regular exercise and turnout. More severe episodes may require intervention:

- **Feeding grain or corn syrup** stimulates insulin-mediated intracellular movement of potassium.
- **IV fluids with calcium gluconate** (0.2–0.4 ml/kg of 23% solution) **or dextrose** (6 ml/kg of 5% dextrose solution) promotes uptake of potassium and has a more immediate effect than feeding grain or giving corn syrup. Sodium bicarbonate (1–2 mEq/kg) may be administered IV to alkalinize the serum and indirectly drives potassium intracellularly via hydrogen/potassium exchange.
- **Acetazolamide** (2–4 mg/kg PO q8–12h) is used as a daily preventative for horses prone to HYPP episodes, despite dietary management, or as a short-term medication administered around planned stressful events (e.g. anesthesia and surgery). There is inadequate evidence to suggest how far in advance of a stressful event acetazolamide should be given for optimal effect or duration of administration. An alternative medication to consider is hydrochlorothiazide (0.5–1 mg/kg PO q12h).
- Emergency tracheotomy may be required in severe episodes resulting in respiratory obstruction.

Myotonia Congenita and Dystrophica

Myotonia congenita and myotonia dystrophica are myotonic muscle disorders. They share similar features with HYPP but are less common, with only a few isolated cases reported [65–68]. Affected foals are generally well-muscled and exhibit a stiff-legged gait, particularly in the hind end. Dimpling of the muscles of the upper hind limb and gluteal region is exacerbated by percussion, which results in a large area of sustained (1–2 minutes) tight contraction, followed by slow relaxation. Foals with myotonia congenita typically do not exhibit progression of clinical signs after 6–12 months of age and may improve with exercise. In contrast, clinical signs in foals with myotonica dystrophica progress to include muscle atrophy and fibrosis over the first 1–2 years of life. Muscle stiffness in these cases worsens with exercise. The etiology of these conditions is unknown; a genetic cause is suspected and at least one presumptive causal mutation has been reported [69].

Presumptive diagnosis is based on physical exam findings, but definitive diagnosis requires electromyography. Presence of crescendo-decrescendo, high-frequency repetitive bursts of activity with a characteristic "dive-bomber" sound is considered pathognomonic for the condition [66]. Dystrophic changes with or without muscle fiber atrophy are appreciated on histopathologic examination of muscle biopsies from horses with myotonia dystrophica, but not myotonia congenita. No specific treatment exits for these conditions, although mild exercise can provide some clinical improvement due to decreased muscle stiffness. Concurrent abnormalities include retinal dysplasia and testicular atrophy [67, 68]. Euthanasia is often elected due to the progression of clinical signs. Prognosis for athletic potential is poor.

Polysaccharide Storage Myopathy (PSSM)

Two types of PSSM have been described. Type 1 PSSM is caused by a mutation in the gene encoding the skeletal muscle glycogen synthase enzyme (*GYS1*), whereas Type 2 PSSM is a term used to describe any horse that has clinical signs of exercise intolerance and abnormal aggregates of polysaccharide in muscle fibers that does not possess the *GYS1* mutation [70]. Clinical signs are not commonly observed in neonatal foals although severe rhabdomyolysis has been reported in foals with PSSM, exacerbated by concurrent conditions including strangles [71] and pneumonia [72, 73]. More commonly PSSM is diagnosed when affected individuals begin training. Genetic tests are available to confirm a diagnosis of type 1 PSSM but not type 2 PSSM [70]. Type 1 PSSM affects many breeds, but has an especially high prevalence in Belgians and Quarter Horses [73–77]. Muscle biopsy is required for a diagnosis of type 2 PSSM in adults; however, biopsies may not be diagnostic in foals [78]. Long-term management of PSSM includes minimal stall confinement, regular exercise, and a low-starch, high-fat diet [79]. Many horses with PSSM can be successfully managed with appropriate exercise and diet; however, recurrent episodes of rhabdomyolysis with intense exercise is possible.

References

1 Hong, C.B., Donahue, J.M., Giles, R.C. et al. (1993). Equine abortion and stillbirth in central Kentucky during 1988 and 1989 foaling seasons. *J. Vet. Diagn. Invest.* 5: 560–566.

2 Giles, R.C., Donahue, J.M., Hong, C.B. et al. (1993). Causes of abortion, stillbirth, and perinatal death in horses: 3,527 cases (1986–1991). *J. Am. Vet. Med. Assoc.* 203: 1170–1175.

3 Arnoczky, S.P., Lavagnino, M., Gardner, K.L. et al. (2004). In vitro effects of oxytetracycline on matrix metalloproteinase-1 mRNA expression and on collagen gel contraction by cultured myofibroblasts obtained from the accessory ligament of foals. *Am. J. Vet. Res.* 65: 491–496.

4 Madison, J.B., Garber, J.L., Rice, B. et al. (1992). Oxytetracycline decreases fetlock joint angle in newborn foals. *Proc. Am. Assoc. Equine Pract.* 38: 745–746.

5 Vivrette, S., Cowgill, L., Pascoe, J. et al. (1993). Hemodialysis for treatment of oxytetracycline-induced acute renal failure in a neonatal foal. *J. Am. Vet. Med. Assoc.* 203: 105–107.

6 Adams, S.B. and Santschi, E.M. (2000). Management of congenital and acquired flexural limb deformities. *Proc. Am. Assoc. Equine Pract.* 46: 117–125.

7 Caldwell, F.J. (2017). Flexural deformity of the distal interphalangeal joint. *Vet. Clin. Equine Pract.* 33: 315–330.

8 Greet, T.R.C. (2000). Managing flexural and angular limb deformities: the Newmarket perspective. *Proc. Am. Assoc. Equine Pract.* 46: 130–136.

9 Blackwell, R.M. (1980). Response of acquired flexural deformity of the metacarpophalangeal joint to desmotomy of the inferior check ligament. *Proc. Am. Assoc. Equine Pract.* 26: 107–111.

10 Stick, J.A., Nickels, F.A., and Williams, M.A. (1992). Long-term effects of desmotomy of the accessory ligament of the deep digital flexor muscle in standardbreds: 23 cases (1979–1989). *J. Am. Vet. Med. Assoc.* 200: 1131–1132.

11 Yiannikouris, S., Schneider, R.K., Sampson, S.N. et al. (2011). Desmotomy of the accessory ligament of the deep digital flexor tendon in the forelimb of 24 horses 2 years and older. *Vet. Surg.* 40: 272–276.

12 Tracey, A. and McClure, S.R. (2018). Retrospective analysis of distal limb conformation and lameness in

mature horses after desmotomy of the accessory ligament of the deep digital flexor tendon for management of a flexural deformity. *Equine Vet. Educ.* 30: 53–56.

13 Shiroma, J.T., Engel, H.N., Wagner, P.C. et al. (1989). Dorsal subluxation of the proximal interphalangeal joint in the pelvic limb of three horses. *J. Am. Vet. Med. Assoc.* 195: 777–780.

14 Santschi, E.M., Leibsle, S.R., Morehead, J.P. et al. (2006). Carpal and fetlock conformation of the juvenile Thoroughbred from birth to yearling auction age. *Equine Vet. J.* 38: 604–609.

15 Robert, C., Valette, J.P., and Denoix, J.M. (2013). Longitudinal development of equine forelimb conformation from birth to weaning in three different horse breeds. *Vet. J. (London, England: 1997)* 198 (Suppl 1): e75–e80.

16 Bridges, C.H. and Harris, E.D. (1988). Experimentally induced cartilaginous fractures (osteochondritis dissecans) in foals fed low-copper diets. *J. Am. Vet. Med. Assoc.* 193: 215–221.

17 Shaver, J.R., Fretz, P.B., Doige, C.E. et al. (1979). Skeletal manifestations of suspected hypothyroidism in two foals. *J. Equine Med. Surg.* 3: 269–275.

18 Auer, J.A. and Martens, R.J. (1982). Periosteal transection and periosteal stripping for correction of angular limb deformities in foals. *Am. J. Vet. Res.* 43: 1530–1534.

19 Auer, J.A., Martens, R.J., and Williams, E.H. (1982). Periosteal transection for correction of angular limb deformities in foals. *J. Am. Vet. Med. Assoc.* 181: 459–466.

20 Baker, W.T., Slone, D.E., Ramos, J.A. et al. (2015). Improvement in bilateral carpal valgus deviation in 9 foals after unilateral distolateral radial periosteal transection and elevation. *Vet. Surg.* 44: 547–550.

21 Baker, W.T., Slone, D.E., Lynch, T.M. et al. (2011). Racing and sales performance after unilateral or bilateral single transphyseal screw insertion for varus angular limb deformities of the carpus in 53 thoroughbreds. *Vet. Surg.* 40: 124–128.

22 Dutton, D.M., Watkins, J.P., Honnas, C.M. et al. (1999). Treatment response and athletic outcome of foals with tarsal valgus deformities: 39 cases (1988–1997). *J. Am. Vet. Med. Assoc.* 215: 1481–1484.

23 Mitten, L.A., Bramlage, L.R., and Embertson, R.M. (1995). Racing performance after hemicircumferential periosteal transection for angular limb deformities in thoroughbreds: 199 cases (1987–1989). *J. Am. Vet. Med. Assoc.* 207: 746–750.

24 Epp, T.L. (2007). Step ostectomy as a treatment for varus deformity of a metatarsophalangeal joint in a 4.5-month-old colt. *Can. Vet. J.* 48: 519–521.

25 Bathe, A.P., Rowlands, D.S., and Boening, K.J. (2006). Treatment of angular limb deformities using radial extracorporeal shock wave therapy: a prospective clinical trial. *Proc. World Equine Vet. Assoc.* 9: 167–168.

26 Hermans, W.A., Kersjes, A.W., Mey, G.J.W. et al. (1987). Investigation into the heredity of congenital lateral patellar (sub) luxation in the Shetland pony. *Vet. Q.* 9: 1–8.

27 Ogden, N., Doyle, C., Fraser, B. et al. (2019). Clinical presentation and surgical repair of traumatic lateral patellar luxation associated with a complete tear of the vastus medialis muscle in a neonatal cob foal. *Equine Vet. Educ.* 31: 472–477.

28 Kobluk, C.N. (1993). Correction of patellar luxation by recession Sulcoplasty in three foals. *Vet. Surg.* 22: 298–300.

29 Engelbert, T.A., Tate, L.P., Richardson, D.C. et al. (1993). Lateral patellar luxation in Miniature Horses. *Vet. Surg.* 22: 293–297.

30 Leipold, H.W. and Macdonald, K.R. (1971). Adactylia and polydactylia in a Welsh foal. *Vet. Med. Small Anim. Clin. VM, SAC* 66: 928–930.

31 Nes, N., Lomo, O.M., and Bjerkas, I. (1982). Hereditary lethal arthrogryposis ("muscle contracture") in horses. – Abstract – Europe PMC. *Nord. Vet. Med.* 34: 425–430.

32 McGavin, M.D. and Leipold, H.W. (1975). Attempted surgical correction of equine polydactylism. *J. Am. Vet. Med. Assoc.* 166: 63–64.

33 Bertone, A.L. and Aanes, W.A. (1984). Congenital phalangeal hypoplasia in Equidae. – Abstract – Europe PMC. *J. Am. Vet. Med. Assoc.* 185: 554–556.

34 Wong, D.M., Scaratt, W.K., and Rohleder, J. (2005). Hindlimb paresis associated with hyphosis, hemivertebrae and multiple thoracic vertebral malformations in a Quarter Horse gelding. *Equine Vet. Educ.* 17: 187–194.

35 Mayhew, I.G., Watson, A.G., and Heissan, J.A. (1978). Congenital occipitoatlantoaxial malformations in the horse. *Equine Vet. J.* 10: 103–113.

36 Levine, J.M., Scrivani, P.V., Divers, T.J. et al. (2010). Multicenter case-control study of signalment, diagnostic features, and outcome associated with cervical vertebral malformation-malarticulation in horses. *J. Am. Vet. Med. Assoc.* 237: 812–822.

37 Moore, B.R., Reed, S.M., Biller, D.S. et al. (1994). Assessment of vertebral canal diameter and bony malformations of the cervical part of the spine in horses with cervical stenotic myelopathy. *Am. J. Vet. Res.* 55: 5–13.

38 Hughes, K.J., Laidlaw, E.H., Reed, S.M. et al. (2014). Repeatability and intra- and inter-observer agreement of cervical vertebral sagittal diameter ratios in horses with neurological disease. *J. Vet. Intern. Med.* 28: 1860–1870.

39 Hahn, C.N., Handel, I., Green, S.L. et al. (2008). Assessment of the utility of using intra- and intervertebral minimum sagittal diameter ratios in the

diagnosis of cervical vertebral malformation in horses. *Vet. Radiol. Ultrasound* 49: 1–6.
40 Papageorges, M., Gavin, P.R., Sande, R.D. et al. (1987). Radiographic and myelographic examination of the cervical vertebral column in 306 ataxic horses. *Vet. Radiol.* 28: 53–59.
41 Donawick, W.J., Mayhew, I.G., Galligan, D.T. et al. (1989). Early diagnosis of cervical vertebral malformation in young thoroughbred horses and successful treatment with restricted, paced diet and confinement. *Proc. Am. Assoc. Equine Pract. (USA)* 35: 525–528.
42 Nixon, A.J. and Stashak, T.S. (1985). Surgical therapy for spinal cord disease in the horse. *Proc. Am. Assoc. Equine Pract. (USA)* 31: 61–74.
43 Grant, B.D., Barbee, D.D., Wagner, P.C. et al. (1985). Long-term results of surgery for equine cervical vertebral malformation. *Proc. Am. Assoc. Equine Pract. (USA)* 91–96.
44 Binanti, D., Zani, D.D., De Zani, D. et al. (2014). Contracted foal syndrome associated with multiple malformations in two foals. *Anat. Histol. Embryol.* 43: 71–74.
45 Wong, D., Miles, K., and Sponseller, B. (2006). Congenital scoliosis in a Quarter Horse filly. *Vet. Radiol. Ultrasound* 47: 279–282.
46 Boyd, J.S. (1976). Congenital deformities in two Clydesdale foals. *Equine Vet. J.* 8: 161–164.
47 Kirberger, R.M. and Gottschalk, R.D. (1989). Developmental kyphoscoliosis in a foal. *J. S. Afr. Vet. Assoc.* 60: 146–148.
48 Vandeplassche, M., Simoens, P., Bouters, R. et al. (1984). Aetiology and pathogenesis of congenital torticollis and head scoliosis in the equine foetus. *Equine Vet. J.* 16: 419–424.
49 Jeffcott, L.B. (1980). Disorders of the thoracolumbar spine of the horse – a survey of 443 cases. *Equine Vet. J.* 12: 197–210.
50 Berry, C.R., House, J.K., Poulos, P.P. et al. (1994). Radiographic and pathologic features of osteopetrosis in two Peruvian paso foals. *Vet. Radiol. Ultrasound* 35: 355–361.
51 Sanger, V.I. and Whitenack, D.I. (1981). Osteopetrosis in a foal [skeletal diseases]. *Equine Pract.* 3: 30–36.
52 Nation, P.N. and Klavano, G.G. (1986). Osteopetrosis in two foals. *Can. Vet. J.* 27: 74–77.
53 Williamson, A.J., Stent, A.W., Milne, M. et al. (2016). Osteopetrosis in a neonatal donkey. *Aust. Vet. J.* 94: 358–361.
54 Buoen, L.C., Zhang, T.Q., Weber, A.F. et al. (1997). Arthrogryposis in the foal and its possible relation to autosomal trisomy. *Equine Vet. J.* 29: 60–62.
55 Mayhew, I.G. (1984). Neuromuscular arthrogryposis multiplex congenita in a Thoroughbred foal. *Vet. Pathol.* 21: 187–192.
56 Whitehair, K.J., Adams, S.B., Toombs, J.P. et al. (1992). Arthrodesis for congenital flexural deformity of the metacarpophalangeal and metatarsophalangeal joints. *Vet. Surg.* 21: 228–233.
57 Addo, P.B., Cook, J.E., and Dennis, S.M. (1984). Schistocoelia in a twin foal. *Equine Vet. J.* 16: 69–71.
58 Johnstone, R. (1981). Equine schistosomus fetus. *Vet. Record* 109: 125–125.
59 Proctor, P.T. (1982). Foetal monstrosity in a Thoroughbred mare resembling shistosomus reflexus. *Equine Vet. J.* 14: 340–340.
60 Ward, T.L., Valberg, S.J., Adelson, D.L. et al. (2004). Glycogen branching enzyme (GBE1) mutation causing equine glycogen storage disease IV. *Mamm. Genome* 15: 570–577.
61 Tryon, R.C., Penedo, M.C., McCue, M.E. et al. (2009). Evaluation of allele frequencies of inherited disease genes in subgroups of American Quarter Horses. *J. Am. Vet. Med. Assoc.* 234: 120–125.
62 Wagner, M.L., Valberg, S.J., Ames, E.G. et al. (2006). Allele frequency and likely impact of the glycogen branching enzyme deficiency gene in Quarter Horse and Paint Horse populations. *J. Vet. Intern. Med.* 20:1207–1211.
63 Rudolph, J.A., Spier, S.J., Byrns, G. et al. (1992). Periodic paralysis in Quarter Horses: a sodium channel mutation disseminated by selective breeding. *Nat. Genet.* 2: 144–147.
64 Traub-Dargatz, J.L., Ingram, J.T., Stashak, T.S. et al. (1992). Respiratory stridor associated with polymyopathy suspected to be hyperkalemic periodic paralysis in four Quarter Horse foals. *J. Am. Vet. Med. Assoc.* 201: 85–59.
65 Jamison, J.M., Baird, J.D., Smith-Maxie, L.L. et al. (1987). A congenital form of myotonia with dystrophic changes in a Quarter Horse. *Equine Vet. J.* 19: 353–358.
66 Reed, S.M., Hegreberg, G.A., Bayly, W.M. et al. (1988). Progressive myotonia in foals resembling human dystrophia myotonica. *Muscle Nerve* 11: 291–296.
67 Montagna, P., Liguori, R., Monari, L. et al. (2001). Equine muscular dystrophy with myotonia. *Clin. Neurophysiol.* 112: 294–299.
68 Hegreberg, G.A. and Reed, S.M. (1990). Skeletal muscle changes associated with equine myotonic dystrophy. *Acta Neuropathol.* 80: 426–431.
69 Wijnberg, I.D., Owczarek-Lipska, M., Sacchetto, R. et al. (2012). A missense mutation in the skeletal muscle chloride channel 1 (CLCN1) as candidate causal mutation for congenital myotonia in a New Forest pony. *Neuromuscul. Disord.* 22: 361–367.
70 Valberg, S.J., Finno, C.J., Henry, M.L. et al. (2021). Commercial genetic testing for type 2 polysaccharide storage myopathy and myofibrillar myopathy does not correspond to a histopathological diagnosis. *Equine Vet. J.* 53: 690–700.

71 De La Corte, F.D., Valberg, S.J., JM, M.L., and Mickelson, J.R. (2002). Developmental onset of polysaccharide storage myopathy in Quarter Horse foals. *J. Vet. Intern. Med.* 16: 581–587.

72 Byrne, E., Cohen, N., Jones, S.L. et al. (2000). Rhabdomyolysis in two foals with polysaccharide storage myopathy. *Compend. Contin. Educ. Pract. Vet.* 22: 503–510.

73 McCue, M.E., Valberg, S.J., Miller, M.B. et al. (2008). Glycogen synthase (GYS1) mutation causes a novel skeletal muscle glycogenosis. *Genomics* 91: 458–466.

74 Baird, J.D., Valberg, S.J., Anderson, S.M. et al. (2010). Presence of the glycogen synthase 1 (GYS1) mutation causing type polysaccharide storage myopathy in continental European draught horse breeds. *Vet. Rec.* 167: 781–784.

75 McCoy, A.M., Schaefer, R., Petersen, J.L. et al. (2014). Evidence of positive selection for a glycogen synthase (gys1) mutation in domestic horse populations. *J. Hered.* 105: 163–172.

76 McCue, M.E., Anderson, S.M., Valberg, S.J. et al. (2010). Estimated prevalence of the type 1 polysaccharide storage myopathy mutation in selected North American and European breeds. *Anim. Genet.* 41: 145–149.

77 Stanley, R.L., McCue, M.E., Valberg, S.J. et al. (2009). A glycogen synthase 1 mutation associated with equine polysaccharide storage myopathy and exertional rhabdomyolysis occurs in a variety of UK breeds. *Equine Vet. J.* 41: 597–601.

78 McKenzie, E. and MacLeay, J. (2011). Muscle disorders. In: *Equine Reproduction*, 2e (ed. A. McKinnon, E. Squires, W. Vaala, and D. Varner), 463–468. West Sussex, UK: Wiley Blackwell.

79 Valberg, S.J. (2002). A review of the diagnosis and treatment of rhabdomyolysis in foals. *Proc. 48th Annu. Conven. Am. Assoc. Equine Pract.* 48: 117–121.

Chapter 37 Musculoskeletal Disorders

Section I Infectious Neonatal Musculoskeletal Disorders

Kira Epstein and Jarred Williams

Sepsis is a leading cause of morbidity and mortality in neonatal foals. Prompt administration of empirical broad-spectrum antimicrobials is a key component to treatment of all foals with a clinical diagnosis of sepsis. Although positive blood cultures confirm the diagnosis and are used to refine antimicrobial choice, negative blood cultures do not rule out sepsis. As such, treatment with antimicrobials should not be delayed or forgone in order to obtain blood culture samples or results. Despite rapid implementation of appropriate antimicrobial therapy, complications of sepsis still occur. One complication is hematogenous spread of bacteria to joints or bone. Hematogenous spread of bacteria can also occur in foals that do not have generalized signs of sepsis during transient bacteremia. One of the more common causes of transient bacteremia in foals is translocation of microorganisms from the gastrointestinal tract; for this reason, the authors also recommend treatment with antimicrobials in foals with diarrhea. This chapter discusses the types of orthopedic infections that can occur secondary to sepsis or bacteremia in foals, diagnostic tests that aid in identification of the disease process, treatment options, complications, and prognosis for athletic outcome.

Overview and Classification

Orthopedic infections of the neonate most commonly involve joints (septic arthritis) and/or bones (septic osteomyelitis) with concurrent infections being fairly common. Bone involvement has been reported in 26%–80% of septic arthritis [1–9]. Historically, infectious arthritis was described as "joint ill," and although any joint can become infected, the tarsus is reportedly the most common [8]. Joint ill, while generic, does accurately describe septic arthritis or synovitis, but fails to describe infection involving the bone, primarily or secondarily as a result of spreading from the joint. Early reports described infections, of presumed hematogenous origin, to the metaphysis, epiphysis, and physis of bone leading to osteomyelitis [6, 10, 11]. Other routes of joint infection include periarticular wound infection or inoculation of the joint by a puncture wound. On the basis of clinical, radiological, and pathological findings, orthopedic infections can be classified as described by Firth (Table 37.I.1) [12]. The presence of a serofibrinous or fibrinopurulent arthritis in one or more joint is classified as an S-type infection; osteomyelitis of the epiphysis at the subchondral bone and cartilage junction is classified as an E-type infection; osteomyelitis directly adjacent to the physis is classified as P-type infection [12]. In addition to these original three types, osteomyelitis of the central tarsal bone, T-type infection, was added and is a separate classification that has now been expanded to include other cuboidal bones of the tarsus and carpus [13].

S-Type Infections

S-type infections, in which septic synovitis occurs without bone involvement, are the most common type of infectious orthopedic disease in the foal. Affected foals are usually <2 weeks old, and concurrently, systemically ill. Though S-type infections can occur in foals that seem otherwise healthy, a nidus of infection can often be identified on further examination (i.e. infected umbilical vein or artery) or historically (i.e. diarrhea or placentitis). Foals may present with acute, obvious lameness. However, lameness may be challenging to observe if the orthopedic infection is less severe or if the foal is recumbent and/or has abnormal mentation due to severity of systemic disease or neonatal encephalopathy. Additionally, multiple joints may be affected with varying degrees of severity and associated lameness. Therefore, diagnosis often relies on careful palpation of joints for periarticular swelling, effusion, heat, or

Equine Neonatal Medicine, First Edition. Edited by David M. Wong and Pamela A. Wilkins.

Table 37.I.1 Septic arthritis and osteomyelitis syndromes in the neonatal foal [12–15].

	S type	E type	P type	T type
Characteristics	Synovial infection Resulting in joint swelling accompanied by periarticular swelling; may have more than one joint involved; may have concurrent or historical infection/illness	Infection of joint and adjacent epiphysis; may have more than one joint involved; may have concurrent or historical infection/illness	Infection initially restricted to physis; nonseptic effusion of adjacent joint may occur rarely	Infection of small cuboidal bones of carpus and/or tarsus
Age of foal	Few days old to 2 wk	3–4 wk	1–12 wk	<1 mo
History	Acute onset lameness, systemically ill	Acute onset lameness (may be severe), may appear only to have orthopedic problem, ±previous illness	Variable degree of lameness, past history of diarrhea or pneumonia	Previous history of systemic disease, twin birth, premature, dysmature
Common sites	Tarsus, stifle, fetlock carpus	Medial and lateral femoral condyles, tibial tarsal condyles, lateral styloid process of distal radius, distal tibia and patella	Distal radial physis, distal tibial physis, metacarpal/tarsal physis	Small tarsal or carpal bones
Clinical signs	One or several joints distended, warm, painful; lameness of varying severity	Joint distension, warm, painful in two or more joints	Swelling over physis, painful on palpation, ±joint distention, variable lameness	Multiple joints affected; moderate to severe lameness, tibial tarsal and small tarsal joint capsule distended
Radiographic changes	Soft tissue swelling, joint distension	Lucencies in epiphysis, cuboidal bones may be involved	Lucencies in metaphysis, physis, epiphysis, possible sequestra	Lucencies in third and central tarsal bones and proximal metatarsus
Synovial fluid analysis	Purulent, increased protein and WBC count; Gram stain positive	Purulent, increased protein and WBC count; Gram stain positive	±Increased protein; ±Increased WBC, ±Gram stain positive	Abnormal in small tarsal or carpal joints, ±tibial tarsal joint abnormal
Commonly cultured bacteria	*Escherishia coli, Klebsiella, Actinobacillus, Streptococcal* spp.	*E. coli, Streptococcus, Salmonella* spp.	*Salmonella* spp., *Klebsiella* spp., *Streptococcal* spp., *Rhodococcus equi*	*E. coli, Salmonella*
Necropsy lesions	Primarily synovial membrane, superficial cartilage loss; subchondral bone usually not affected	Fibrinopurulent arthritis; purulent bone lesions corresponding to radiographic lucencies	Osteomyelitis of physis, metaphysis, epiphysis; infectious arthritis, ±subcutaneous abscess	Fibrinopurulent arthritis; cartilage may be cracked and bone shape irregular or fractured
Prognosis to involved even if controlled	May die early in life due to critical illness	Often poor prognosis because of widespread osteomyelitis and septic	Aggressive surgical curettage may help well-localized lesions; poor prognosis due to physeal damage and bone destruction	Poor prognosis due multiple joints and degenerative arthritis in tarsus infection is

pain and should be part of the routine physical examination in any foal with suspected sepsis, or presenting with an infected umbilicus, colitis, or pneumonia. Affected joints are most likely swollen and effusive. Synoviocentesis should be performed in any joint under suspicion and the joint fluid analyzed for color, clarity, viscosity, total protein concentration, white blood cell (WBC) count, and cytologic assessment. Additionally, the fluid should be microscopically evaluated for the presence of intra- and extracellular bacteria and submitted for bacterial culture. Note that many infected joints can be bacterial culture negative, despite being infected. Nonetheless, isolation of the pathogen and results of an antimicrobial susceptibility pattern justify attempting bacterial culture.

Radiography of the affected joints may only demonstrate soft tissue swelling and effusion; however, due to the risk

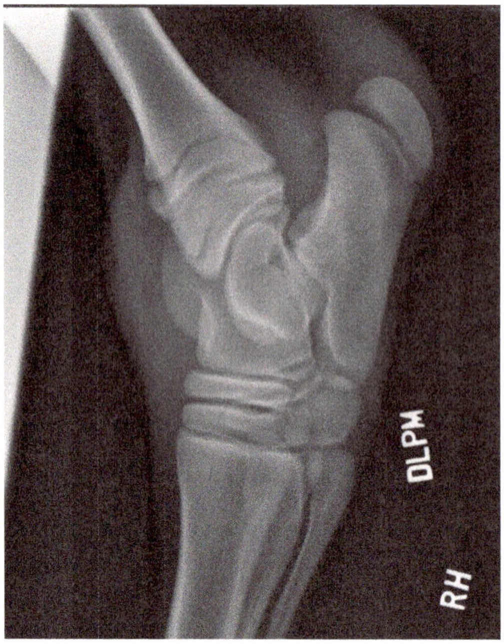

Figure 37.I.1 Dorsolateral plantaromedial oblique radiograph of the right hind tarsus of foal with tarsocrural effusion. Note the marked soft tissue opacity throughout the dorsal and plantar aspects of the joint. Additionally, note the gas shadowing throughout the soft tissue swelling. This joint was filled with fibrin, increased volumes of synovial fluid, and proliferation of the synovium.

of osteomyelitis and associated impact on treatment and prognosis, diagnostic imaging is recommended (Figure 37.I.1). The tarsus, stifle, and fetlock are the most commonly affected joints; however, all joints are at risk. The coffin joint, elbow, and hip are uncommon sites to become infected, but can be challenging to identify and treat when involved.

E-Type Infection

E-type infections involving the joint and adjacent epiphysis tend to present for veterinary care later in the neonatal period (i.e., 3–4 weeks of age) and are typically more severe than S-type infections. Given the similar hematogenous pathogenesis to S-type infections, foals with E-type infections also commonly present with concurrent or historical infections/illness and often involve multiple joints. As a result of the more severe pathology, foals with E-type infection are likely to have severe lameness, spending much of their time recumbent, and have significant abnormalities on palpation of the affected joint(s). Arthrocentesis and synovial fluid analysis with cytology and culture of suspected joints is recommended. Because the history, clinical signs, and synovial fluid analysis findings of E-type infections resemble that of S-type infections, imaging is necessary to discern between the two types of infections.

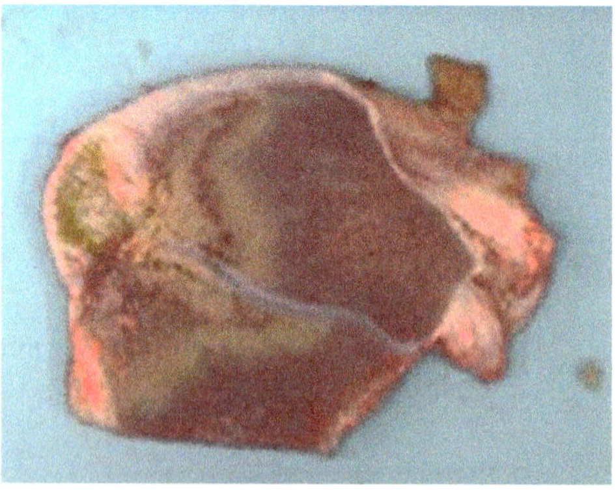

Figure 37.I.2 Well-demarcated area of osteomyelitis with areas of necrosis and hemorrhage affecting the epiphysis and diaphysis with destruction of the growth plate. *Source:* Image courtesy of Dr. Rebecca Ruby, University of Kentucky.

Radiographs of the affected joint should be performed. The presence of radiolucent lesions of variable size in the epiphysis are diagnostic for E-type infections. Of note, radiographic evidence of osteomyelitis often underestimates, and has a temporal lag behind, the damage to the bone. Therefore, in foals in which the lesions of the epiphysis are ill-defined, or involvement of the epiphysis is suspected but not confirmed with radiography, advanced imaging via computed tomography (CT) or magnetic resonance (MRI) is recommended.

Although foals with E-type infections have infection of the joint and epiphyseal/subchondral bone (Figure 37.I.2), the cartilage that separates the two is variably affected. Thus, arthroscopy or necropsy of the affected joint will reveal serofibrinous or fibrinopurulent arthritis. However, there may or may not be a visible defect in the surface of the articular cartilage or even change in contour of the joint surface at the site of osteomyelitis. As a result, arthroscopy, like radiography, often fails to accurately identify the severity of bone involvement. Probing of the cartilage overlying the abnormal subchondral bone during arthroscopy, or bone sectioning during necropsy, can provide a better estimate of the extent of pathology. Specifically, upon histopathology, subchondral bone lesions consisting of purulent osteomyelitis and necrosis may be present.

The shortcomings of radiographs, and even arthroscopy, for accurately identifying and quantifying the degree of bony involvement should be carefully considered when deliberating on response to treatment, advanced imaging, and prognosis. Importantly, some S-type lesions unresponsive to treatment may in fact be misdiagnosed E-type lesion. Thus, additional diagnostic results that more definitively define the problem should be considered promptly in these cases. Commonly affected sites are the medial and lateral femoral condyles, talus, distal radius, and distal tibia, though any epiphysis is at risk.

P-Type Infections

P-type infections occur when bone infections are adjacent to the metaphyseal growth plate and more commonly affect older foals (9–90 days of age). In one report the mean age of foals presenting with P-type infections was 38 days of age [6]. Foals may present with a continuation of a prior lameness or a new, acute lameness. P-type infections most commonly affect one physis and the foal may exhibit heat and pain upon palpation of the affected physis. The nearest joint may or may not be affected by secondary inflammation or spread of infection. Severity of swelling and other clinical signs and joint fluid analysis will be related to degree of involvement. With severe cases of P-type infections, or moderate cases that progress, subcutaneous edema and pain may worsen, with or without the presence of cellulitis or abscessation. As infection spreads through the physis and accompanying bone, the ability to bear weight worsens; ultimately, pathologic fracture can occur.

Depending on the duration and severity of the infection, P-type infections can be diagnosed based on radiographic abnormalities. Common radiographic abnormalities include osteolysis, bone resorption, and cavitation with the physis and adjacent epiphysis and metaphysis (Figure 37.I.3). As with E-type infections, radiographic abnormalities may lag behind and underestimate the degree of bony damage compared to three-dimensional imaging and histopathology. Histopathologic examination may reveal osteomyelitis in all areas of radiographic suspicion, as well as infection extending into affiliated diaphysis, metaphysis, physis, epiphysis, periosteum, joint capsule, articular cartilage, synovium, and adjacent soft tissue structures such as subcutaneous tissue, tendons and ligaments. The most commonly affected regions include the distal radius, distal tibia, and distal metacarpus/metatarsus.

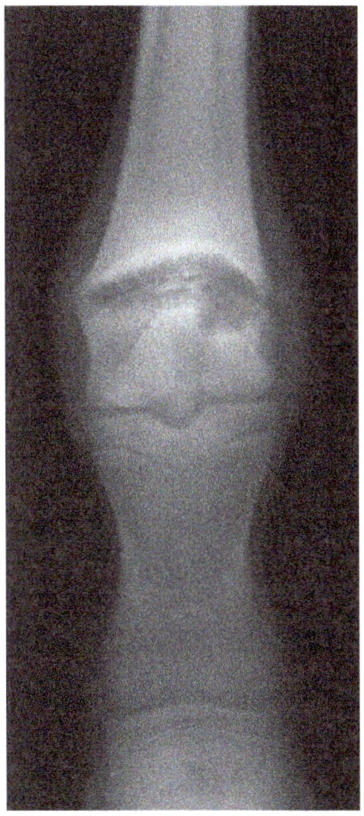

Figure 37.I.3 Dorsopalmar radiograph of the distal metacarpus of a foal. There is marked lysis of the distal metacarpal physis, with gas shadowing overlying the physis and periphyseal sclerosis. Additionally, there is soft-tissue swelling and mineralization adjacent to the physis.

T-Type Infections

Infection of the cuboidal bones of the carpus or tarsus are called T-type infections. These infections are most commonly identified in premature or dysmature foals. Noticeable effusion of the radiocarpal, middle carpal, or tibiotarsal joints can be expected. These foals tend to spend much of the time in a recumbent position and can be quite lame. Clinical examination, joint fluid analysis, and imaging (radiology, CT, or MRI) aid in a complete diagnosis. Sequela of T-type infections are crushing, disfigurement, or osteolysis of the cuboidal bones leading to significant arthritis if the infection resolves and survives the infection [13].

Pathogenesis

While not exclusively, orthopedic infections in foals are hematogenous in origin, unless proven otherwise [13, 14, 16, 17]. The synovium, epiphysis, and physis are highly vascular making exposure of these structures to pathogens during bacteremia or septicemia high. Moreover, the neonatal foal's immature bones and joints are in a rapid growth phase that requires increased blood flow through these capillaries. These areas have dense capillary beds that form hairpin bends that end in wide venous sinusoids, which may lead to infection by "trapping" the bacteria as they pass through these areas of decreased blood flow, low pressure (i.e. pooling in sinusoids), and lower oxygen tension [14, 17–19]. More specifically, the articular blood supply is provided via a main arteriole that branches to the synovial membrane and epiphysis (Figure 37.I.4). Blood supply to the metaphysis is supplied by the nutrient artery, but in neonatal foals, transphyseal vessels exit and connect the metaphyseal and epiphyseal blood supply. In young foals, these functional transphyseal vessels allow communication of the metaphysis and epiphysis such that bacteria can localize preferentially to the synovial membrane and subchondral bone. This is part of the reason why young foals are more prone to types S and E infections [20]. In contrast closure of transphyseal vessels starts to occur at approximately 7–10 days of age, localizing infection more

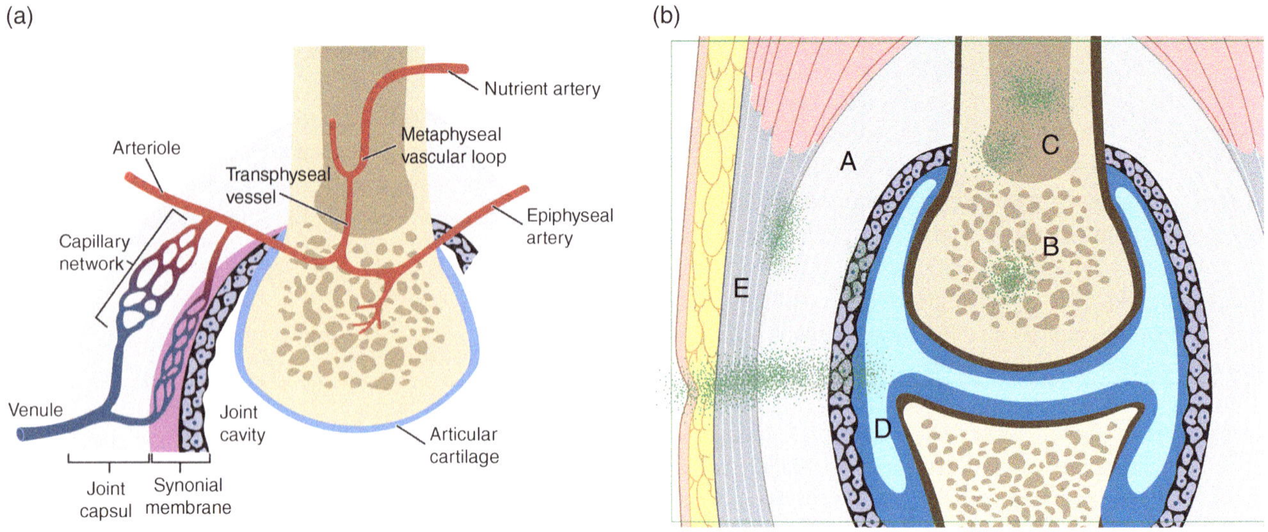

Figure 37.I.4 (a) Illustration of the arterial blood supply to an equine neonatal joint demonstrating the relationship between the nutrient artery, synovial capillary network and epiphyseal vessels. (b) Possible routes of bacterial inoculation of a joint: A, B, and C are hematogenous, resulting in synovial membrane infection (A), epiphyseal infection (B), and physeal infection (C). In C, the joint capsule attachment includes the physis; therefore, inoculation of the physis will also result in septic arthritis. If the physis is extra-articular, septic arthritis does not always occur concurrently with septic physitis. Joint inoculation via puncture wound (D) or from contiguous soft tissue infection (E) [20].

commonly to the metaphyseal vessel loops in older foals. Therefore, physeal infections are more commonly noted in foals older than 7 days of age.

Failure of passive transfer of colostral IgG is one of the most important risk factors for bacteremia and sepsis [21, 22] and is common in foals with septic arthritis and osteomyelitis [1, 2, 6, 23, 24]. In retrospective studies of foals with septic arthritis, 50%–88% of affected foals had partial or complete failure of passive transfer [1, 2]. Additionally, studies in foals with confirmed sepsis, 26% and 28% of foals had concurrent septic arthritis or osteomyelitis, respectively [3, 7]. The gastrointestinal and respiratory tract as well as the umbilicus are likely entry points for bacteria and sites of concurrent infection in foals with orthopedic infection [1, 22]. Thus, foals with enteritis, colitis, or pneumonia should be treated with antimicrobials to prevent bacteremia and monitored closely for development of orthopedic infections. Every foal should have their umbilicus evaluated and monitored frequently, even if initially normal.

Tissue damage and pain associated with orthopedic infections are not solely the result of toxins produced by bacteria. The inflammatory response of the host, including increases in inflammatory cytokines, arachadonic acid metabolites, reactive oxygen species, matrix metalloproteinases (MMPs), and procoagulant activity interfere with normal function and promote damage of surrounding tissues, including cartilage [25, 26]. More specifically, bacterial colonization of the periarticular vessels can result in thrombosis and ischemic necrosis of the physeal region along with thrombosis of the vessels of the synovial membrane [18]. This, in turn, results in impaired synovial fluid production and exchange due to increased vascular permeability [27]. Premature and dysmature foals can maintain this vascular pattern for prolonged periods, predisposing these foals to orthopedic infections [28]. Consequently, normal production and drainage of synovial fluid is impaired, thus impacting cartilage metabolism as the cartilage derives its nutrients from synovial fluid [18]. An increase influx of serum proteins, WBCs and proteolytic enzymes in the synovial fluid occurs and disrupts the reparative nature of chondrocytes, eventually causing degradation of the articular cartilage if left untreated [18]. In addition, fibrin deposition on articular cartilage and reduced joint mobility (secondary to pain) results in impaired delivery of nutrients to articular cartilage. Proinflammatory cytokines act directly on synoviocytes and chondrocytes to increase the release of MMPs that contribute to articular cartilage destruction [14]. With chronicity, normal synoviocyte function is continually impaired, decreased hyaluronic acid, is secreted and increased inflammatory mediators are released further contributing to joint pathology [14].

The pathogen(s) causing an orthopedic infection is likely to be the one causing septicemia, therefore, the list of commonly isolated bacterial species isolated from orthopedic infections are similar and include *Escherishia coli*, *Salmonella* spp., *Actinobacillus* spp., *Klebsiella* spp., *Enterobacter* spp., *Pseudomonas* spp., *Staphalococcus* spp., *Streptococcus* spp., *Clostridia* spp., and *Bacteroides* spp. [8, 14, 23, 29] Common organisms isolated from septic physitis include *Salmonella* spp. and *Rhodococcus equi* [20].

Clinical Signs and Diagnosis

Lameness, moderate to severe synovial swelling, and pain on palpation or from passive movement of the affected joint are common clinical signs and presenting complaints for foals with orthopedic sepsis [23, 29]. Physical examination should include careful palpation of all limbs and the spine and a thorough lameness examination. However, lameness may be subtle despite the severity of infection and may be difficult to detect in foals with concurrent systemic illnesses that limit their mobility and coordination. Swelling associated with septic arthritis is typically manifested as joint effusion though periarticular edema may be present, whereas foals with osteomyelitis typically have more diffuse periarticular swelling and edema and variable joint effusion. With physeal infection, the presence of concurrent synovial effusion is dependent on whether the growth plate is intra- or extra-articular [20]. Osteomyelitis also frequently results in increased lameness, heat, and pain. Multiple sites of infection can be present and careful evaluation of all limbs should be performed, even if an obvious abnormality is identified [1, 17, 23]. Additional diagnostics aimed at locating and identifying the bacterial source from the primary site should be performed as needed (Figure 37.I.5).

A CBC and serum fibrinogen concentration might identify evidence of inflammation. Although leukocytosis is expected, WBC counts and differentials in foals with orthopedic infections can vary depending on concurrent disease and duration of infection. Elevated serum fibrinogen concentration is common and expected in orthopedic infections [1, 30]. Leukocytosis, neutrophilia, and hyperfibrinogenemia were more pronounced in osteomyelitis compared to septic arthritis in one study [30]. In that study, serum fibrinogen concentration between 900 and 1500 mg/dl had good positive and negative predictive value for septic osteomyelitis [30]. Plasma biochemistry analysis should also be performed to evaluate for concurrent disease and when deciding on antimicrobial and anti-inflammatory therapy (e.g. kidney function).

Sterile arthrocentesis (18- or 20-gauge needle) to collect synovial fluid for cytologic and biochemical analysis should be performed prior to initiating treatment on any joint with effusion. Synovial fluid analysis are important and useful diagnostic tests for septic arthritis (Figure 37.I.6). Normal joint fluid has a total protein of <2.0 g/dl, <200 cells/μl and <10% neutrophils [25, 31–34]. Gram staining of synovial fluid is a rapid and simple method to detect bacteria and used as a screening test to guide initial therapy while awaiting culture results. In one study, Gram stain identified the etiologic agent in up to 25% of cases in which bacterial culture results were negative [35]. The pH of the synovial fluid can be used as evidence of infection as normal synovial fluid pH is 7.3 whereas the pH of septic synovial fluid is usually acidic with a pH as low as 6.2 [33]. The presence of inflammation within the joint results in an increase in vascular permeability of the synovial membrane; alterations in the total protein concentration occurs first in response to inflammation, followed by increases in WBC count 12–24 hours after initiation of infection [33]. Therefore, changes consistent with sepsis include increased total protein concentration and nucleated cell count and increased percentage of neutrophils with a decreased percentage of mononuclear cells (Figure 37.I.7). Neutrophils may also exhibit toxic changes. Nucleated cell counts are typically markedly elevated (>30,000 cells/μl), with neutrophil counts >90%; WBC counts >100,000 cells/μl being pathognomonic for infection [25, 31]. However, even mild changes (>10,000 cells/μl) may be indicative of disease; particularly, periarticular infection and sympathetic inflammation as may occur with P- and E-type infections. If the foal has a separate physeal infection, in which the physis is extraarticular, there may only be a moderate increase in WBC count with <90% neutrophils [20]. Alternatively, falsely low synovial fluid WBC counts may be noted when cells aggregate within fibrin clots [18]. While joint fluid should be evaluated for bacteria, treatment should be based on physical examination and cytology [8, 25]. Synovial fluid analysis is also valuable for monitoring response to treatment, with declining synovial fluid WBC counts suggestive of clearance of bacteria and inflammatory mediators and improved joint health.

Although culture results are unlikely to be available to guide initial antimicrobial therapy, obtaining appropriate samples for culture and sensitivity is important to allow modification of antimicrobial therapy, if indicated, by sensitivity results and clinical response. Ideally, samples should be obtained prior to initiating antimicrobials, but samples should be collected even if this is not possible. In foals already receiving antimicrobials, timing collection of culture samples to coincide with trough antimicrobial blood concentrations (i.e. just prior to the next dose) can be considered. Additionally, the use of culture media containing resin beads to bind and decrease the effect of antimicrobials may increase the chances of obtaining a positive culture [34].

In cases with suspected joint sepsis, synovial fluid samples for culture and sensitivity can be obtained at the same time as samples for cytology. Using blood culture bottles/media (thioglycolate broth) to incubate synovial fluid (ideally 5–10 ml) may increase the likelihood of a positive culture result [16, 28]. Between 63% and 89% of infected synovial structures are reported to have positive

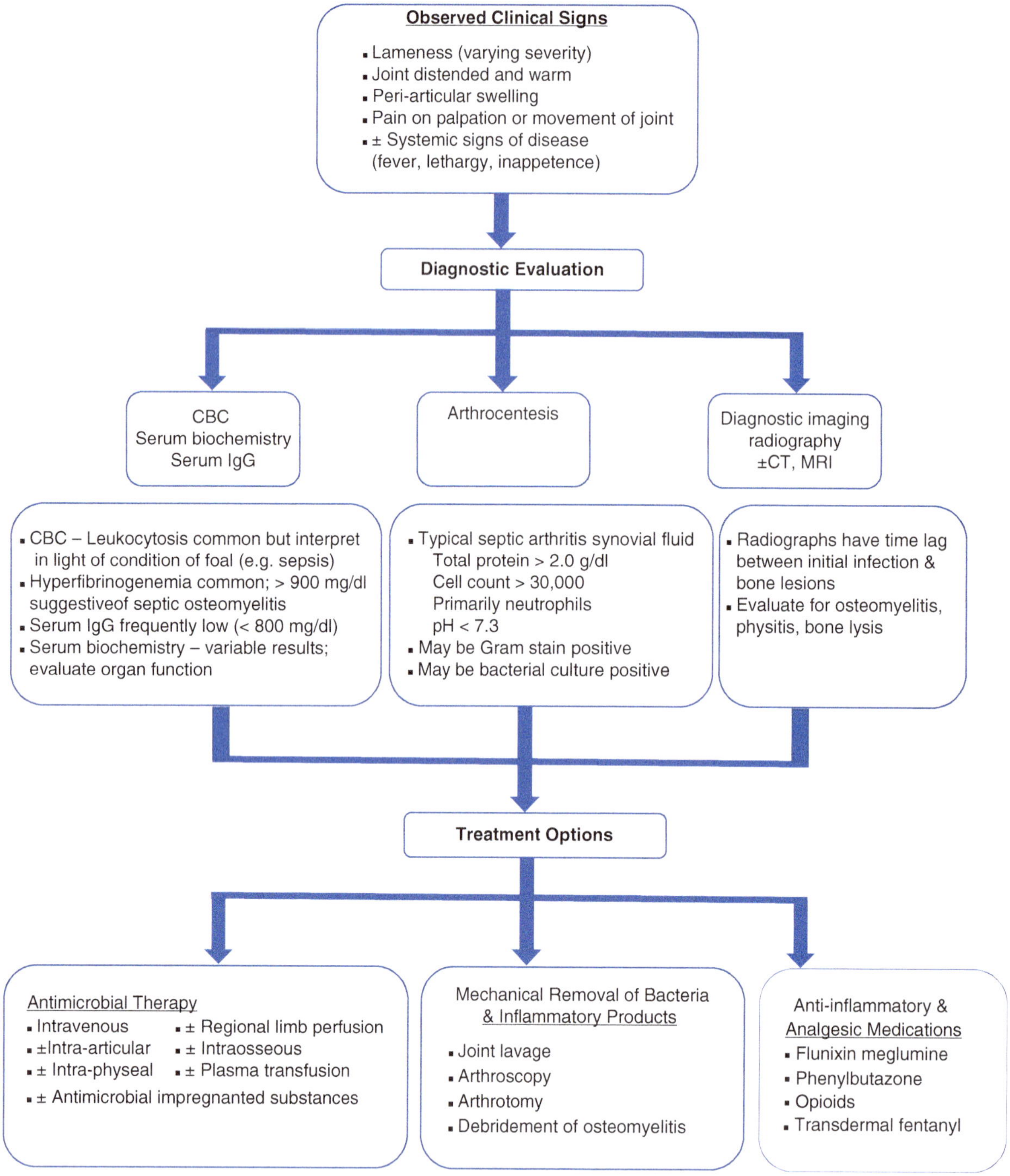

Figure 37.I.5 Overview of examination and treatment of septic orthopedic disease in the foal.

cultures [1, 2, 8, 35–37]. One report showed that of 70 synovial fluid samples submitted for culture, 60 (85.7%) yielded growth of 72 bacterial isolates. Of the 72 isolates, 45 (62.5%) were Gram negative and 27 (37.5%) were Gram positive [37]. Other samples to consider for bacterial culture include synovium and/or fibrin clots removed from the joint during therapy [18]. It is unclear if culturing these additional samples improves the likelihood of success [1, 13, 35, 38].

In cases of osteomyelitis, samples from the suspected region should be submitted for bacterial culture if possible. If the physis is suspected to be the site of infection, a needle can be placed into the physis and an aspirate can be collected. Synovial samples from adjacent joints may also yield positive culture results and should be submitted [23].

Radiographs are indicated in cases of suspected infectious lameness and should be carefully evaluated for

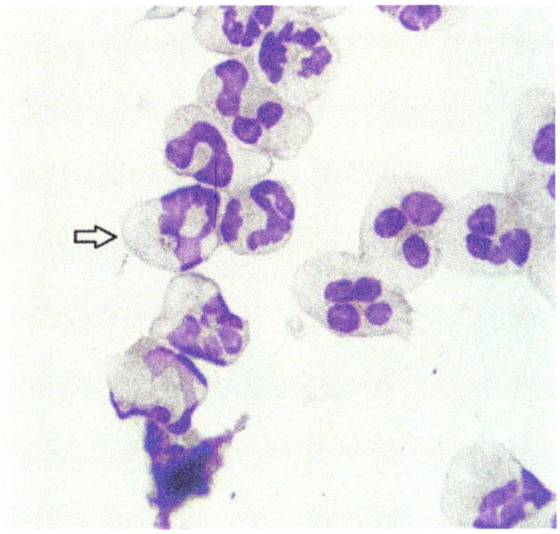

Figure 37.I.6 Synovial fluid sample from a 3-day-old Thoroughbred with septic arthritis of the tarsus. Note the abundant neutrophils and intracellular bacteria (arrow). *Source:* Photo courtesy of Dr. Wong, Iowa State University.

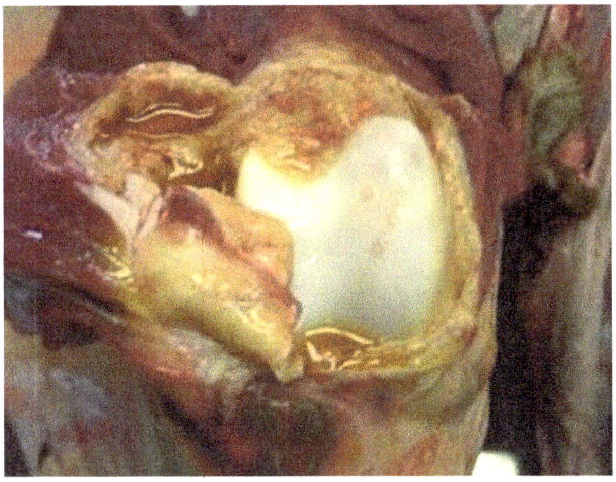

Figure 37.I.7 Joint space from a neonatal foal with septic arthritis. Note the increased amount of thin orange-red fluid; the synovium is discolored yellow and modestly thickened, and the surrounding connective tissue is mildly edematous. *Source:* Image courtesy of Dr. Rebecca Ruby, University of Kentucky.

evidence of bony involvement. Radiographic changes including osteomyelitis, physitis, or osteoarthritis have been reported in 38–80% of foals with septic arthritis [1–4]. The clinician must be cognizant of the fact that most joints in foals appear quite different compared to adults and identifying normal versus abnormal structures can be challenging. Additionally, it is often difficult to distinguish incomplete ossification associated with skeletal immaturity from bone lysis as a result of infection, and both can be present simultaneously. If uncertain, radiographs of the opposite, presumably unaffected joint, can provide a reference. Unfortunately, radiographic evidence of bony involvement is frequently not apparent initially and can take weeks or longer to appear [25]. Therefore, serial monitoring of radiographs or pursuing more advanced imaging, particularly in cases not responding to therapy as expected, is recommended.

Additional diagnostic imaging may include ultrasound, nuclear scintigraphy, or three-dimensional imaging (CT/MRI) (Figures 37.I.8 and 37.I.9). Ultrasound evaluation of the joint and periarticular soft tissue may be helpful to identify the extent of fibrin clot formation and compartmentalization of the joint (Figure 37.I.9). Ultrasound can also identify thickening of the joint capsule and increased echogenicity of synovial fluid and may also be useful for evaluation of osteomyelitis [39]. Fluid accumulation adjacent to the area of infection and irregularities in the bony surface may be observed. Traditional nuclear scintigraphy or nuclear scintigraphy using radiolabeled WBCs can be performed [18, 31]. However, the use of nuclear scintigraphy in foals with septic orthopedic disease is limited and the high level of bone activity in foals should be kept in mind during interpretation [40]. Although less widely available, the images provided by CT and MRI provides higher sensitivity and improved detail and may be useful in defining the extent of disease, particularly in early cases with ambiguous diagnostic findings [14, 18, 31]. As the use of and experience with these techniques in horses expands, these modalities might have an increasing role in evaluation of foals with orthopedic infections.

Treatment

Treatment of septic arthritis in the neonatal foal is considered an emergency, requiring immediate assessment and treatment. These cases are challenging due to the potential for simultaneous multisystemic diseases, some of which can be critical. Early and aggressive treatment of septic arthritis is indicated, but one form of treatment is not necessarily superior to others, and in reality, a combination of multiple therapies will result in the best chance of treatment success. The economic situation also dictates therapy as treatment of septic arthritis can be costly. The goals of treatment include elimination of the causative organism(s), resolution of inflammation, removal of inflammatory products, reduction of joint effusion, and reestablishment of normal synoviocyte and cartilage function [14]. With these goals in mind, the cornerstones of therapy involve antimicrobial therapy and drainage and lavage of the affected joint(s).

Appropriate antimicrobials are important in treatment of any infectious disease. Ideally, antimicrobial therapy is based on bacterial culture and sensitivity results. However, culture results are not available at the time of initial therapy, with the exception of blood culture results from foals with a history of sepsis. Therefore, antimicrobials are

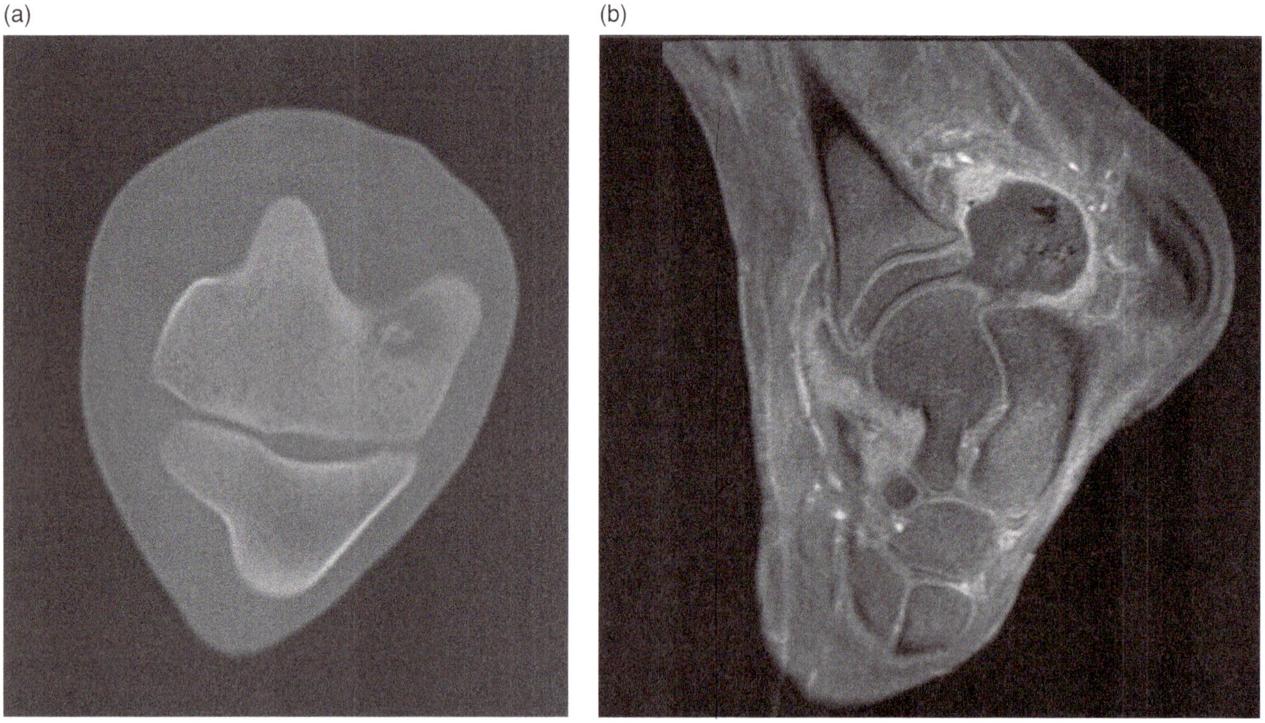

Figure 37.I.8 (a) Left image – transactional slice from CT of a tarsocrural joint of a foal with septic osteomyelitis of the talus. Note the area of osteolysis with within the trochlear ridge. Within the region of osteolysis is a focal area of increased signaling. Additionally, note the increased signaling surrounding the lesion, consistent with sclerosis. (b) Right image – longitudinal slice from an MR of the tarsocrural joint of a different foal with septic arthritis. Note the significant amount of fibrin with fluid pockets within the joint space, particularly in the plantar pouch planar to the distal tibia and proximal to the calcaneus. This image is from the tarsus of the same foal radiographed in Figure 37.I.1. The difference in detail obtained between the MR and radiography of this joint is evident and should be considered in cases that are not responding to treatment as expected.

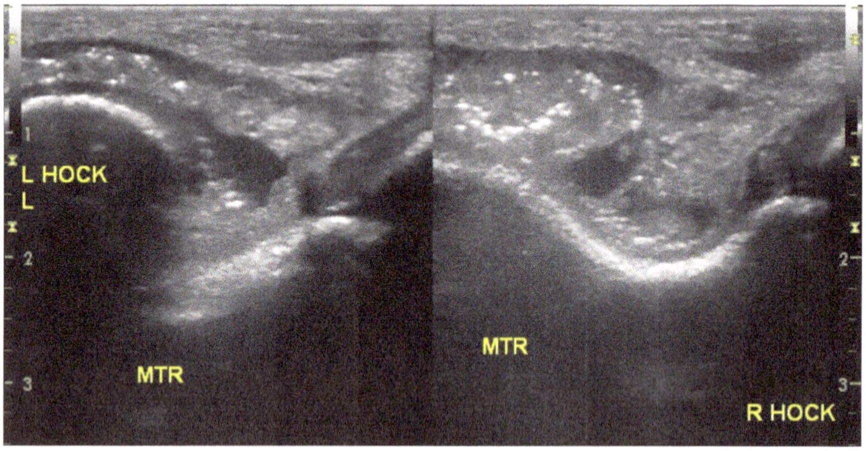

Figure 37.I.9 Ultrasound images obtained from the left and right tarsocrural joints of a foal with a septic arthritis. Note the pronounced fibrin accumulation with gas shadowing, pockets of effusion, and thickened joint capsule.

chosen empirically and modified based on culture and sensitivity and/or lack of response to treatment. In cases of orthopedic sepsis, systemic antimicrobials are frequently combined with local administration of antimicrobials to increase tissue concentrations in areas of concern. Systemic antimicrobial therapy should be initiated as soon as possible and is most commonly administered IV to foals with orthopedic infections because of the reliability of administration and types and number of antimicrobials available.

When choosing antimicrobials, they should ideally be bactericidal, have minimal adverse effects (e.g. nephrotoxicity), and achieve adequate concentrations in the bone and synovia. A combination of antimicrobials that will collectively provide activity against Gram-positive and Gram-negative organisms is recommended. The most common antimicrobials with strong Gram-positive spectrum are β-lactams (penicillins, cephalosporins) combined with antimicrobials with strong Gram-negative spectrum, such as the aminoglycocides (amikacin, gentamicin). Amikacin is used more frequently in foals because bacterial resistance is less common along with the suggestion that nephrotoxicity may be reduced compared to gentamicin [41, 42]. However, the acidic environment of septic synovial fluid along with the presence of purulent material can decrease the efficacy of aminoglycosides [43]. In foals with concern of impaired renal function (azotemia, abnormalities on urinalysis), alternative antimicrobials with strong Gram-negative spectrum include late generation and extended spectrum β-lactams (ceftiofur, cefotaxime, imipenem, timentin). Systemic antimicrobial therapy is continued well after resolution of clinical and clinicopathologic signs (2–3 weeks for septic arthritis, 2–3 months for septic osteomyelitis) [14, 16, 18]. Based on clinician preference, culture and sensitivity results, and duration, IV antimicrobials can be continued or a switch to oral antimicrobials can be made. An important factor to emphasize is that the duration of antimicrobials is very important in these cases. Discontinuing antimicrobials too early can result in incomplete resolution of the disease process despite improved clinical signs.

A variety of methods for local delivery of antimicrobials exist including regional limb perfusion (RLP), intra-articular (IA) injection, injection into an infected region of the physis, and placement of antimicrobial impregnated substances such as polymethylmethacrylate, plaster of paris, and collagen. The most commonly used methods are RLP and IA injection. When performing these methods, the antimicrobial used should be a concentration dependent and nonirritating. Of note, high concentrations of antimicrobials may be damaging to local tissues, but likely to a lesser extent than the effects of infection [44–46]. RLP can be used as a local therapy for septic arthritis or osteomyelitis. Performing IV RLP in foals that are recumbent (appropriate sedation required) daily or every other day will provide the greatest opportunity for the success of the perfusion. If the antimicrobial chosen is the same as one of the systemic antimicrobials, the clinician should consider timing RLP with the systemic administration and administering two-thirds the dose systemically and one-third locally. Intraosseous perfusion (Chapter 59), where drugs are administered through the medullary cavity, is another route to achieve high regional concentrations of antimicrobial.

IA injection involves intermittent or continuous infusion of antimicrobials into the affected joint through a needle or indwelling catheter. IA injections are typically used for cases of septic arthritis. However, IA injection of gentamicin resulted in higher synovial fluid concentrations and similar concentrations in bone adjacent to the injected joint when compared with RLP in experimental horses [47]. Therefore, IA injection may be useful in cases of orthopedic sepsis involving the joint or periarticular bone. Several studies have reported the use of IA antimicrobials for treatment of septic arthritis with and without associated osteomyelitis in horses and foals with good success [48–50]. If the clinician choses to perform intermittent injection through a needle, sedation will be required and injections are generally performed at the time other procedures are being done (i.e. collection of synovial fluid samples or joint lavage); these injections will likely be daily or every other day. The clinician should be aware of the fact that inflammation appears to increase clearance of the antimicrobial from the joint and daily injection may be required to keep concentrations above the minimal inhibitory concentration for the bacteria [50]. Doses of antimicrobials used for IA injection are not well defined, but 125–250 mg of amikacin, 500 mg of gentamicin, and 500 mg of cefazolin have been suggested [14]. Indwelling catheter systems allow administration without sedation multiple times per day or continuously [49]. This method allows the use of time-dependent antimicrobials more effectively.

Mechanical removal of bacteria and inflammatory products (fibrin), cells, and mediators (cytokines, arachadonic acid metabolites, MMPs) is an important aspect of treatment of orthopedic infections [51]. This is particularly true for cases of septic arthritis, where accumulated fibrin can harbor bacteria, making resolution of infection difficult or impossible; moreover, inflammatory mediators can cause irreversible damage to the joint. Thus, joint lavage should be performed in all cases of confirmed or suspected septic arthritis. In cases of osteomyelitis, debridement should be performed in all cases where the lesion communicates with the joint and in cases without joint involvement based on clinical judgment and response to treatment. If osteomyelitis does not involve the joint, debridement should be avoided when the lesion is too close to an unaffected joint as this may introduce bacteria into a sterile joint. Additionally, debridement can result in instability of the respective bone [6, 52, 53]. Successful treatment with and without debridement has been reported [23, 54].

Joint lavage can be performed with needles (14–16 gauge), arthroscopy, or arthrotomy. A thorough lavage should access all regions of the joint – biaxial, proximal, and distal, dorsal (cranial) and palmar/plantar (caudal). A large volume of polyionic, isotonic fluid (at least 1–2 l minimum) should be used for each joint with the foal heavily sedated or anesthetized. Two techniques can be used to perform joint lavage: distension-irrigation and through-and-through lavage. In the first method, a large-gauge needle (14–18 gauge) is placed into the joint; the joint is then alternately infused with sterile fluid to distend the joint and then aspirated. In the second method, which is more commonly used, two or more large-gauge needles (14–18 gauge) are placed at distant sites from each other within the joint;

one needle then serves as the ingress of sterile lavage fluids and the other(s) serves as the egress. Use of a fluid pressure bag or pump facilitates expedient lavage of the joint. IA administration of a selected antimicrobial is typically performed through the ingress needle after the joint lavage is completed, just prior to removal of the needle; of note, the systemic dose of aminoglycoside should be adjusted if IA aminoglycosides are utilized concurrently. Repeated lavage every 24–48 hours is frequently indicated and should be based on clinical judgment and response to therapy. In one study, the average number of lavage procedures was 3.3 (range 2–11) [2].

Needle lavage may be insufficient if large amounts of fibrin have accumulated or there is cartilage/bone involvement. Once fibrin accumulates within the joint, which can occur as fast as 48 hours postbacterial inoculation, bacteria can become trapped within the fibrin making it difficult to adequately decrease the organisms within the joint until the fibrin is removed. Arthroscopy allows large volumes of fluid to be used rapidly, assessment of damage to the joint, visual guidance to remove fibrin, performance of synovectomy, and debriding cartilage/bone. In contrast, arthrotomy allows large volumes of fluid for lavage along with visual inspection of the joint and debridement of fibrin [14]. Arthroscopy portals and arthrotomy sites can be left open for drainage or repeat lavage, but ascending infection should be considered an important complication [55]. The relative importance of volume of lavage and location and size of needle/portal placement is not well documented. One experimental study examined recovery of microspheres, similar to the size of a WBC, from tarsocrural joints in adult horses and noted no benefit of volumes greater than 1 l; however, improved microsphere recovery was noted when two egress needles (one dorsal, one plantar) were used as compared to a single egress arthroscopy portal (dorsal) [56]. As a general guideline, needle lavage is recommended for foals without evidence of concurrent osteomyelitis and a short (<2 days) history of clinical signs whereas arthroscopy is recommended if there is evidence of concurrent osteomyelitis, longer history of clinical signs, or failure to respond to needle lavage.

The technique for debridement of osteomyelitis lesions depends on the location. As noted, if the lesion communicates with the joint, arthroscopy is used to guide debridement. If the lesion does not communicate with the joint, imaging such as fluoroscopy or radiography, can be used to guide drilling and/or curettage. If the lesion is close to the surface of the bone, curettage can be performed alone. However, if the lesion is further from the cortex, a drill and 5 mm drill bit may be necessary to create a path from the surface of the bone to the lesion to allow removal of infected and/or necrotic bone via curettage and rongeurs. The bone cavity is then flushed with sterile electrolyte solution and left open to drain under a sterile bandage. In a retrospective study of 108 foals with osteomyelitis, 42 foals received surgical debridement [23].

The articular cartilage itself is devoid of nerve endings, but the joint capsule contains many nociceptors that extend into the synovial membrane [14]. In cases of septic arthritis, joint effusion distends the joint capsule and is an important source of pain. Additionally, prostaglandin E2 is released as part of the inflammatory cascade and enhances pain perception [14]. Because inflammation within the joint is damaging and painful, nonsteroidal anti-inflammatory (NSAIDs) drugs, specifically cyclooxygenase (COX) inhibitors, are frequently administered to foals with septic arthritis. The combination of analgesia and decreased inflammation can promote better antibiotic penetration into synovial membranes by allowing better clearance of pro-inflammatory mediators and degradative enzymes within the synovial fluid through the lymphatic system [57]. Careful monitoring for renal and gastrointestinal side effects is important when using NSAIDs and gastroprotectants (e.g. omeprazole, ranitidine, sucralfate) may be considered based on clinician preference. Flunixin meglumine and phenylbutazone are the most common NSAIDs used in foals.

Pain associated with infectious orthopedic disease can have a significant impact on the systemic health of the foal as well as orthopedic consequences. Foals that are painful are less likely to nurse appropriately and can become dehydrated and lose or fail to gain appropriate amounts of weight. Decreased weight bearing in the affected limb can result in contracture while increased weight bearing in the contralateral limb can result in fetlock hyperextension and/or angular limb deformity. Additionally, foals that are down for extended periods of time can become weak and have tendon laxity. Thus, it is important to control pain with the most important analgesic being resolution of the infection and associated inflammation.

NSAIDs remain the primary analgesic used. However, if NSAIDs cannot be used or are not controlling the pain, other analgesics should be considered. Opioids, such as butorphanol and morphine are options and transdermal fentanyl patches have been evaluated in foals [58, 59]. With any opioid there is the potential for gastrointestinal ileus and sedation and these effects should be balanced against the benefits of analgesia and increased nursing behavior [58].

While not universally implemented, IA administration of sodium hyaluronate has been suggested as an adjunctive therapy in septic arthritis in foals [14, 60]. Hyaluronic acid is synthesized by synoviocytes and is an important component of synovial fluid and articular cartilage but can become depleted in septic arthritis. In one study of induced septic arthritis in adult horses, 10 mg of sodium hyaluronate was administered into the tarsal joint after standard joint lavage, with the contralateral joint serving as the control [60]. The sodium hyaluronate treated joints demonstrated significant reductions in lameness, tarsal circumference, synovial fluid protein concentration, and WBC counts. Additionally, treated joints contained less cellular infiltrate and less granulation tissue formation and retained more normal villous structure compared to control joints. The reason for the improved outcome is unknown, but in horses with noninfectious inflammatory and degenerative arthropathy, sodium hyaluronate improves lubrication of soft tissues, decreases loss of cartilage matrix by binding of surface proteoglycans, and decreases permeability of the synovial membrane [60]. The authors of that study suggested that IA sodium hyaluronate may be a useful treatment in septic arthritis in horses when used in conjunction with other standard therapies (e.g. joint lavage, antimicrobials). Alternatively, IV or IA administration of hyaluronic acid has been suggested only after the infection has been completely eliminated from the joint to provide lubrication and aid in repair of the synovial membrane [18].

In addition to resolving the infection, limited exercise is indicated to allow restoration of normal joint health and attempt to preserve future athletic function. Low range of motion exercise is suggested in foals with septic arthritis to help maintain and restore joint function without contributing to further damage. As the infection resolves, the foal may ambulate more readily and enthusiastically, but excessive exercise should be avoided as the joint cartilage is vulnerable to traumatic damage for some time after severe inflammatory disease [14]. This predisposition for articular damage from septic arthritis is a result of depleted proteoglycan matrix and disrupted collagen framework, both of which make the cartilage less resistant to compressive forces. Thus, a prolonged period (e.g. 3–4 weeks) of stall rest and controlled hand-walking after resolution of septic arthritis is suggested as to avoid excessive exercise and induction of further joint injury [14].

Prognosis

The prognosis for athleticism in a foal with an orthopedic infection should be interpreted in light of the fact that the orthopedic infection is likely secondary to systemic disease. Therefore, prognosis for athleticism in ill neonates in general is useful information. A study evaluating 454 Thoroughbred foals admitted to a neonatal intensive care unit between 1982 and 2008 reported that 269 of the foals (59%) raced [61]. When evaluating those that were registered and hospitalized and also had registered siblings that were not hospitalized, 68% of the hospitalized foals raced compared to 79% of their healthy siblings [61]. Foals with dysmaturity/prematurity were significantly less likely to race compared to their siblings, and for those that did race, they had significantly fewer starts, wins, and lower earnings [60]. Finally, foals with orthopedic disease were significantly less likely to race than their siblings, and those that did had a lower percentage of wins compared to their siblings [61].

Many foals with septic arthritis may also have umbilical remnant infections. A study on foals undergoing resection of the umbilical remnant reported an 89% (73/82) survival rate to discharge [62]. Concurrent diseases were present in approximately 61% of the foals prior to surgery, with diarrhea and septic arthritis as the two most common diseases [62]. The presence of septic arthritis and/or physitis were significantly associated with nonsurvival [62]. Failure of passive transfer and longer surgery times were associated with increased odds for a postoperative complication [62].

Septic arthritis has reported survival rates of 42–84% [1, 2, 8, 17]. Prognosis for athletic performance appears to be worse with only 37–48% of Thoroughbred foals with septic arthritis starting more than one race [1, 17, 19]. Thoroughbred foals were also older at the first race start and less likely to start than control siblings [17]. Several factors have been associated with decreased prognosis: delay of treatment (>2 days after clinical signs) [1], multiple affected joints [1, 3, 6], concurrent osteomyelitis [5], multisystemic disease [17], and isolation of *Salmonella* spp. [1] Another study reported that 47/83 (56.6%) foals with septic joints survived to discharge [37]. In that study, the median number of joints affected per foal was 2 (range 1–10 joints) [36]. The survival rate was positively associated with serum fibrinogen concentration and negatively associated with the number of affected joints [37].

Foals with osteomyelitis have a reported survival rate of 80.6% and a prognosis for starting a race of 48% (65.8% of short-term survivors that reached racing age) [23]. This study found a significant decrease in prognosis associated with foals <30 days of age, foals with critical illness, and foals with multiple sites of osteomyelitis; a worse prognosis was also associated with concurrent arthritis and osteomyelitis caused by *E. coli*, *Salmonella* spp., and *Klebsiella* spp. [23]

Septic arthritis and osteomyelitis have been described as a plausible cause of some osteochondral lesions in horses [63]. In that report, samples of infected orthopedic lesions were histologically examined from seven foals that were euthanized with septic arthritis or osteomyelitis. The anatomic sites evaluated included the third metacarpal bone (2), ilium (1), femur (6), tibia (5), talus (2), and third metatarsal bone (2). Bacteria were present in the cartilage canals, thus deeming them septic cartilage canals. Septic cartilage canals that were necrotic and contained neutrophils were termed acute, while septic canals with granulation tissue and neutrophils were termed chronic. Acute and chronic septic canals were associated with ischemic chondronecrosis in the articular-epiphyseal cartilage complex of five cases and in the physis of two cases. In five of those cases, endochondral ossification was focally delayed. These findings shed light on possibility of septic orthopedic conditions as another factor in the development of osteochondral lesions [63].

References

1 Steel, C.M., Hunt, A.R., Adams, P.L. et al. (1999). Factors associated with prognosis for survival and athletic use in foals with septic arthritis: 93 cases (1987–1994). *J. Am. Vet. Med. Assoc.* 215: 973–977.

2 Meijer, M.C., van Weeren, P.R., and Rijkenhuizen, A.B. (2000). Clinical experiences of treating septic arthritis in the equine by repeated joint lavage: a series of 39 cases. *J. Vet. Med. A Physiol. Pathol. Clin. Med.* 47: 351–365.

3 Raisis, A.L., Hodgson, J.L., and Hodgson, D.R. (1996). Equine neonatal septicaemia: 24 cases. *Aust. Vet. J.* 73: 137–140.

4 Firth, E.C. and Goedegebuure, S.A. (1988). The site of focal osteomyelitis lesions in foals. *Vet. Q.* 10: 99–108.

5 Paradis, M.R. (1992). Septic arthritis in the equine neonate: A retrospective study. *Proceedings of the 10th American College Veterinary Medicine Forum*, 458–459. May 1992, San Diego, Ca, American College of Veterinary Internal Medicine.

6 Martens, R.J. and Auer, J.A. (1980). Haematogenous septic arthritis and osteomyelitis in the foal. *Proc. Am. Assoc. Equine Pract.* 26: 47–63. December 2–5, 1979, Miami Beach, Fl, American Association of Equine Practitioners

7 Koterba, A.M., Brewer, B.D., and Tarplee, F.A. (1984). Clinical and clinicopathological characteristics of the septicaemic neonatal foal: review of 38 cases. *Equine Vet. J.* 16: 376–382.

8 Schneider, R.K., Bramlage, L.R., Moore, R.M. et al. (1992). A retrospective study of 192 horses affected with septic arthritis/tenosynovitis. *Equine Vet. J.* 24: 436–442.

9 Gayle, J.M., Cohen, N.D., and Chaffin, M.K. (1998). Factors associated with survival in septicemic foals: 65 cases (1988–1995). *J. Vet. Intern. Med.* 12: 140–146.

10 Van Pelt, R.W. and Riley, W.F. (1969). Clinicopathologic findings and therapy in septic arthritis in foals. *J. Am. Vet. Med. Assoc.* 155: 1467–1480.

11 Bennett, D. (1978). Pathological features of multiple bone infection in the foal. *Vet. Rec.* 103: 482–485.

12 Firth, E.C., Goedegebuure, S.A., Dik, K.J. et al. (1985). Tarsal osteomyelitis in foals. *Vet. Rec.* 116: 261–266.

13 Firth, E.C. (1983). Current concepts of infectious polyarthritis in foals. *Equine Vet. J.* 15 (1): 5–9.

14 Annear, M.J., Furr, M.O., and White, N.A. (2011). Septic arthritis in foals. *Equine Vet. Educ.* 23: 422–431.10.

15 Adams, R. (1990). Polyarthritis and osteomyelitis. In: *Equine Clinical Neonatology* (ed. A.M. Koterba, W.H. Drummond, and P.C. Kosch), 317–330. Philadelphia: Lea & Febiger.

16 Martens, R.J., Auer, J.A., and Carter, G.K. (1986). Equine pediatrics: septic arthritis and osteomyelitis. *J. Am. Vet. Med. Assoc.* 188: 582–585.

17 Smith, L.J., Marr, C.M., Payne, R.J. et al. (2004). What is the likelihood that thoroughbred foals treated for septic arthritis will race? *Equine Vet. J.* 36: 452–456.

18 Trumble, T.N. (2005). Orthopedic disorders in neonatal foals. *Vet. Clin. North Am. Equine* 21: 357–385.

19 Firth, E.C. (1992). Specific orthopedic infections. In: *Equine Surgery* (ed. J.A. Auer), 932–946. Philadelphia: WB Saunders.

20 Hardy, J. (2006). Etiology, diagnosis, and treatment of septic arthritis, osteitis, and osteomyelitis in foals. *Clin. Tech. Equine Pract.* 5: 309–317.

21 Robinson, J.A., Allen, G.K., Green, E.M. et al. (1993). A prospective study of septicaemia in colostrum-deprived foals. *Equine Vet. J.* 25: 214–219.

22 McGuire, T.C., Crawford, T.B., Hallowell, A.L. et al. (1977). Failure of colostral immunoglobulin transfer as an explanation for most infections and deaths of neonatal foals. *J. Am. Vet. Med. Assoc.* 170: 1302–1304.

23 Neil, K.M., Axon, J.E., Begg, A.P. et al. (2010). Retrospective study of 108 foals with septic osteomyelitis. *Aust. Vet. J.* 88: 4–12.

24 Platt, H. (1977). Joint-ill and other bacterial infections on thoroughbred studs. *Equine Vet. J.* 9: 141–145.

25 Bertone, A. (1996). Infectious arthritis. In: *Joint Disease in the Horse*, 1e (ed. C. McIlwraith and G. Trotter), 397–409. Philidelphia: WB Saunders.

26 Palmer, J.L. and Bertone, A.L. (1994). Joint structure, biochemistry and biochemical disequilibrium in synovitis and equine joint disease. *Equine Vet. J.* 26: 263–277.

27 Curtiss, P.H. (1973). The pathophysiology of joint infections. *Clin. Orthop.* 96: 129.

28 Stoneham, S.J. (1997). Septic arthritis in the foal: practical considerations on diagnosis and treatment. *Equine Vet. Educ.* 9: 25.

29 Neil, K.M., Axon, J.E., Todhunter, P.G. et al. (2007). Septic osteitis of the distal phalanx in foals: 22 cases (1995–2002). *J. Am. Vet. Med. Assoc.* 230: 1683–1690.

30 Newquist, J.M. and Baxter, G.M. (2009). Evaluation of plasma fibrinogen concentration as an indicator of physeal or epiphyseal osteomyelitis in foals: 17 cases (2002–2007). *J. Am. Vet. Med. Assoc.* 235: 415–419.

31 Morton, A.J. (2005). Diagnosis and treatment of septic arthritis. *Vet. Clin. North Am. Equine Pract.* 21: 627–649.

32 Van Pelt, R. (1974). Interpretation of synovial fluid findings in the horse. *J. Am. Vet. Med. Assoc.* 165: 91–95.

33 Tulamo, R.M., Bramlage, L.R., and Gabel, A.A. (1989). Sequential clinical and synovial fluid changes associated with acute infectious arthritis in the horse. *Equine Vet. J.* 21: 325–331.

34 Spaargaren, J., van Boven, C.P., and Voorn, G.P. (1998). Effectiveness of resins in neutralizing antibiotic activities in bactec plus aerobic/F culture medium. *J. Clin. Microbiol.* 36: 3731–3733.

35 Madison, J.B., Sommer, M., and Spencer, P.A. (1991). Relations among synovial membrane histopathologic findings, synovial fluid cytologic findings, and bacterial culture results in horses with suspected infectious arthritis: 64 cases (1979–1987). *J. Am. Vet. Med. Assoc.* 198: 1655–1661.

36 Ross, M.W., Orsini, J.A., Richardson, D.W. et al. (1991). Closed suction drainage in the treatment of infectious arthritis of the equine tarsocrural joint. *Vet. Surg.* 20: 21–29.

37 Hepworth-Warren, K.L., Wong, D.M., Fulkerson, C.V. et al. (2015). Bacterial isolates, antimicrobial susceptibility patterns, and factors associated with infection and outcome in foals with septic arthritis: 83 cases (1998–2013). *J. Am. Vet. Med. Assoc.* 246 (7): 785–793.

38 Bertone, A.L., McIlwraith, C.W., Jones, R.L. et al. (1987). Comparison of various treatments for experimentally induced equine infectious arthritis. *Am. J. Vet. Res.* 48: 519–529.

39 Reef, V.B., Reimer, J.M., Reid, C.F. (1992). Ultrasonographic findings in horses with osteomyelitis. *Proceedings of the 37th Annual Convention of the American Association of Equine Practitioners*, 381–391. December 1–4, 1991, San Francisco, CA. American Association of Equine Practitioners.

40 Hardy, J. (1999). Septic arthritis in the foal. *Large Animal Proceedings of the Ninth Annual Symposium of the American College of Veterinary Surgeons*, 63–66. September 30–October 3, 1998, San Francisco, CA, Wiley.

41 Lerner, S.A., Schmitt, B.A., Seligsohn, R. et al. (1986). Comparative study of ototoxicity and nephrotoxicity in patients randomly assigned to treatment with amikacin or gentamicin. *Am. J. Med.* 80: 98–104.

42 Lerner, S.A., Seligsohn, R., and Matz, G.J. (1977). Comparative clinical studies of ototoxicity and nephrotoxicity of amikacin and gentamicin. *Am. J. Med.* 62: 919–923.

43 Wichtel, M.E., Buys, E., DeLuca, J. et al. (1999). Pharmacologic considerations in the treatment of neonatal septicemia and its complications. *Vet. Clin. North Am. Equine Pract.* 15: 725–746.

44 Lloyd, K.C., Stover, S.M., Pascoe, J.R. et al. (1988). Effect of gentamicin sulfate and sodium bicarbonate on the synovium of clinically normal equine antebrachiocarpal joints. *Am. J. Vet. Res.* 49: 650–657.

45 Stover, S.M. and Pool, R.R. (1985). Effect of intra-articular gentamicin sulfate on normal equine synovial membrane. *Am. J. Vet. Res.* 46: 2485–2491.

46 Lloyd, K.C., Stover, S.M., Pascoe, J.R. et al. (1990). Synovial fluid pH, cytologic characteristics, and gentamicin concentration after intra-articular administration of the drug in an experimental model of infectious arthritis in horses. *Am. J. Vet. Res.* 51: 1363–1369.

47 Werner, L.A., Hardy, J., and Bertone, A.L. (2003). Bone gentamicin concentration after intra-articular injection or regional intravenous perfusion in the horse. *Vet. Surg.* 32: 559–565.

48 Lescun, T.B., Vasey, J.R., Ward, M.P. et al. (2006). Treatment with continuous intrasynovial antimicrobial infusion for septic synovitis in horses: 31 cases (2000–2003). *J. Am. Vet. Med. Assoc.* 228: 1922–1929.

49 Stewart, A.A., Goodrich, L.R., Byron, C.R. et al. (2010). Antimicrobial delivery by intrasynovial catheterisation with systemic administration for equine synovial trauma and sepsis. *Aust. Vet. J.* 88: 115–123.

50 Schneider, R.K., Bramlage, L.R., Mecklenburg, L.M. et al. (1992). Open drainage, intra-articular and systemic antibiotics in the treatment of septic arthritis/tenosynovitis in horses. *Equine Vet. J.* 24: 443–449.

51 Taintor, J., Schumacher, J., and DeGraves, F. (2006). Comparison of amikacin concentrations in normal and inflamed joints of horses following intra-articular administration. *Equine Vet. J.* 38: 189–191.

52 Baird, A.N., Taylor, J.R., and Watkins, J.P. (1990). Debridement of septic physeal lesions in three foals. *Cornell Vet.* 80: 85–95.

53 Desjardins, M.R. and Vachon, A.M. (1990). Surgical management of *Rhodococcus equi* metaphysitis in a foal. *J. Am. Vet. Med. Assoc.* 197: 608–612.

54 Hall, M.S., Pollock, P.J., and Russell, T. (2012). Surgical treatment of septic physitis in 17 foals. *Aust. Vet. J.* 90: 12.

55 Bertone, A.L., Davis, D.M., Cox, H.U. et al. (1992). Arthrotomy versus arthroscopy and partial synovectomy for treatment of experimentally induced infectious arthritis in horses. *Am. J. Vet. Res.* 53: 585–591.

56 Loftin, P.G., Beard, W.L., Guyan, M.E. et al. (2016). Comparison of arthroscopic lavage and needle lavage techniques, and lavage volume on the recovery of colored microspheres for the tarsocrural joints of cadaver horses. *Vet. Surg.* 45: 240–245.

57 Palmer, J.L. and Bertone, A.L. (1996). Joint biomechanics in the pathogenesis of traumatic arthritis. In: *Joint Disease in the Horse* (ed. C.W. McIlwraith and G.W. Trotter), 104–119. Philadelphia: WB Saunders.

58 Arguedas, M.G., Hines, M.T., Papich, M.G. et al. (2008). Pharmacokinetics of butorphanol and evaluation of physiologic and behavioral effects after intravenous and intramuscular administration to neonatal foals. *J. Vet. Intern. Med.* 22: 1417–1426.

59 Eberspacher, E., Stanley, S.D., Rezende, M. et al. (2008). Pharmacokinetics and tolerance of transdermal fentanyl administration in foals. *Vet. Anaesth. Analg.* 35: 249–255.

60 Bruise, R.W., Sullins, K.E., White, N.A. et al. (1992). Evaluation of sodium hyaluronate therapy in induced septic arthritis in the horse. *Equine Vet. J.* 24: 18–23.

61 Chidlow, H., Giguere, S., and Sanchez, L.C. (2019). Factors associated with long-term athletic outcome in Thoroughbred neonates admistted to an intensive care unit. *Equine Vet. J.* 51: 716–719.

62 Reig Codina, L., Were, S.R., and Brown, J.A. (2019). Short-term outcome and risk factors for postoperative complications following umbilical resection in 82 foals (2004–2016). *Equine Vet. J.* 51: 323–328.

63 Wormstrand, B., Ostevik, L., Ekman, S. et al. (2018). Septic arthritis/osteomyelitis may lead to osteochondrosis-like lesions in foals. *Vet. Pathol.* 55 (5): 693–702.

Section II Noninfectious Neonatal Musculoskeletal Disorders

Heidi Reesink

Incomplete Ossification/Cuboidal Bone Collapse

Pathophysiology

In the healthy equine fetus, the calcaneus is first radiographically apparent by 125 days gestation, the talus by 220–260 days gestation and the central, second, third, and fourth tarsal bones by day 280–320 gestation [1]. The first tarsal bone is normally partially ossified at birth while the second tarsal bone is nearly fully ossified. Incomplete ossification of the carpal and tarsal cuboidal bones is commonly observed in premature, dysmature, and newborn twin foals [2] as normal cuboidal bone ossification occurs in the final 2–3 weeks of gestation [3]. Incomplete ossification is typically bilateral, though one limb may be more severely affected. The cuboidal bones of the carpi and tarsi in affected foals commonly have radiographically small centers of calcification surrounded by a thick layer of cartilage when observed postmortem [1]. Incomplete ossification of the navicular bone has also been reported in combination with the carpal and tarsal bones in a dysmature foal [4] as the navicular bone typically ossifies after the cuboidal bones [3].

Clinical Presentation

Premature and dysmature foals may present with more immediate clinical signs secondary to more nefarious underlying processes (sepsis, neonatal encephalopathy), but all premature/dysmature foals should be evaluated for incomplete ossification once initial stabilization is complete. The degree of incomplete ossification, if present, can have substantial impact on the long-term prognosis. Alternatively, some foals with incomplete ossification of the carpal bones can present with a carpal valgus angular limb deformity (ALD) while foals in which the tarsal bones are affected commonly present with hyperextension and a broken distal tarsal axis (sickle-hocked) conformation [5]. It is not uncommon for both the carpal and tarsal bones to be involved at varying severities. Lameness is uncommon in the forelimbs; however, carpal valgus may enable earlier detection of the condition in the forelimbs. An altered hindlimb gait or sickle-hocked conformation may not be readily clinically apparent in the newborn/neonatal foal, resulting in failure to recognize the condition until later in life [6], though some foals will present with a characteristic "bunny hopping" gait. If left untreated, incomplete ossification can result in juvenile "spavin" caused by osteoarthritis of the distal hock joints, with the distal intertarsal joint more severely affected than the tarsometatarsal joint [6].

Diagnosis

Diagnosis of incomplete ossification can be confirmed with standard radiographic views, which is recommended in any premature or dysmature foal or foals that are small for gestational age [7]. Although orthogonal films are always recommended, the dorsopalmar projection is most useful for evaluating cuboidal bone ossification of the carpus and lateromedial projections of the tarsus (Figure 37.II.1). These radiographic views also enable assessment of carpal ALD in the frontal plane and tarsal hyperextension or a sickle-hocked conformation in the sagittal plane, respectively.

A skeletal ossification index (SOI) has been established to standardize radiographic interpretation of carpal and tarsal regions in neonatal foals (Table 37.II.1), ranging from Grade 1 (least ossified) to Grade 4 (most ossified) [7]. More recently, a modified SOI was used to differentiate foals with cuboidal bones with rounded edges from unaffected, fully ossified cuboidal bones with square edges [1]. Premature Thoroughbred foals (gestation length of

Equine Neonatal Medicine, First Edition. Edited by David M. Wong and Pamela A. Wilkins.

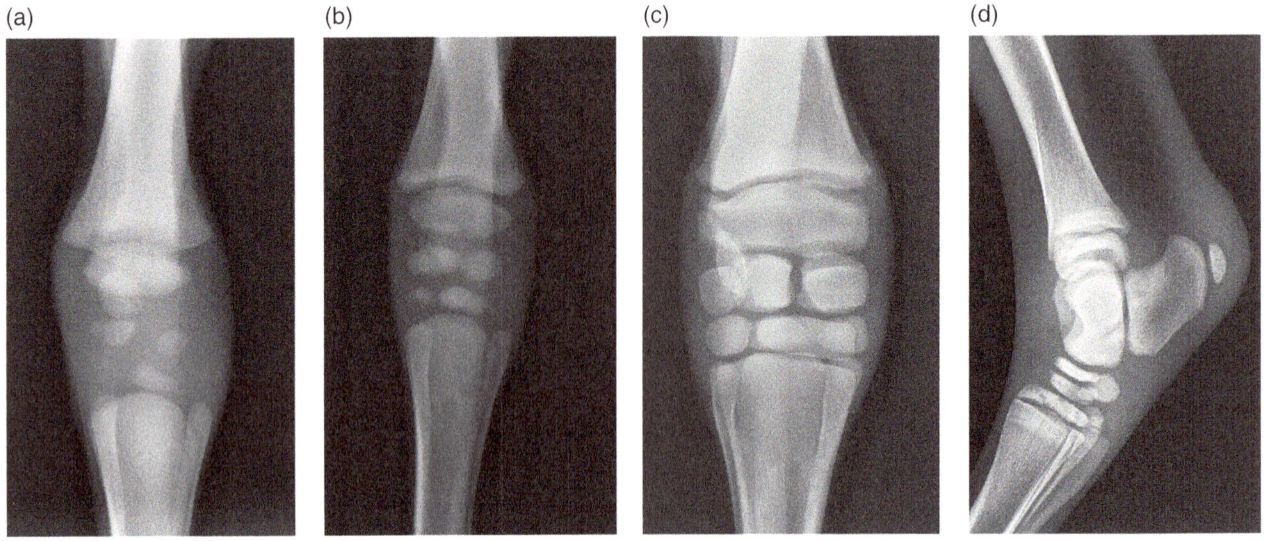

Figure 37.II.1 (a)–(c) Incomplete ossification of the carpi from a Thoroughbred colt born 28 days prematurely. Progression of ossification was assessed using dorsopalmar radiographic views, revealing (a) grade 1 ossification at 7 days of age, (b) grade 2 ossification at 32 days of age, and (c) grade 4 ossification at 51 days of age. (d) Lateromedial radiograph of the right tarsus of a 2-day-old Standardbred filly delivered prematurely, demonstrating grade 2–3 ossification of the tarsal cuboidal bones.

Table 37.II.1 Skeletal ossification indices for classification of incompletely ossified cuboidal bones in neonatal foals.

Grade	Skeletal ossification index [7]	Modified skeletal ossification index [1]
1	Some cuboidal bones without ossification	Some cuboidal bones without ossification
2	All cuboidal bones have radiographic evidence of some ossification	All cuboidal bones have radiographic evidence of some ossification
3	Small and round cuboidal bones	Small and round cuboidal bones
4	Cuboidal bones shaped like mature bones	Cuboidal bones with rounded edges
5	–	Fully ossified cuboidal bones with square edges

<325 days) commonly have Grades 1 and 2 ossification while term foals typically had Grades 3 and 4 [1].

Treatment

Treatment depends upon the severity of incomplete ossification, age of the foal, ambulatory status and the limbs affected. Exercise restriction is indicated until ossification is complete. Application of sleeve casts, which extend from the elbow to the fetlock in the forelimb or from the stifle to the fetlock in the hindlimb, changed at 2-week intervals (or sooner as dictated by growth of the foal), are frequently used to align the limb and protect the cartilaginous templates of the cuboidal bones from crush injury (Figure 37.II.2). Bandage casts or bandages and splints have also been used. Stall confinement is recommended for foals with rigid coaptation. For nonambulatory foals, bandaging may be sufficient while the foal is recumbent, transitioning to more rigid external coaptation once the foal becomes ambulatory. Foals with bilateral sleeve casts or bandages may have difficulty rising and need assistance to nurse. Ossification should be assessed using serial radiographs, and foals may transition to less rigid forms of coaptation as ossification progresses.

Prognosis

Prognosis depends on the degree of normal cuboidal ossification and absence of osteochondrosis (OC) or osteoarthritic lesions [5]. If not diagnosed early and treated appropriately, incomplete ossification can lead to carpal ALD and juvenile spavin, wedging or collapse of cuboidal bones and chronic lameness. The tarsal bones, especially the central and third tarsal bones, are more likely to be affected by crush injury than the carpal bones [5]. In one study, foals with minor tarsal bone collapse, defined as <30% of the affected bones (type I), were able to perform athletically whereas more severe tarsal bone collapse and fragmentation (type II) precluded animals from being used for their intended purposes [8].

The prognosis for becoming a high-performance athlete is guarded, especially with incomplete ossification of the tarsal bones [4]. A retrospective study of 115 Thoroughbred

(a) (b)

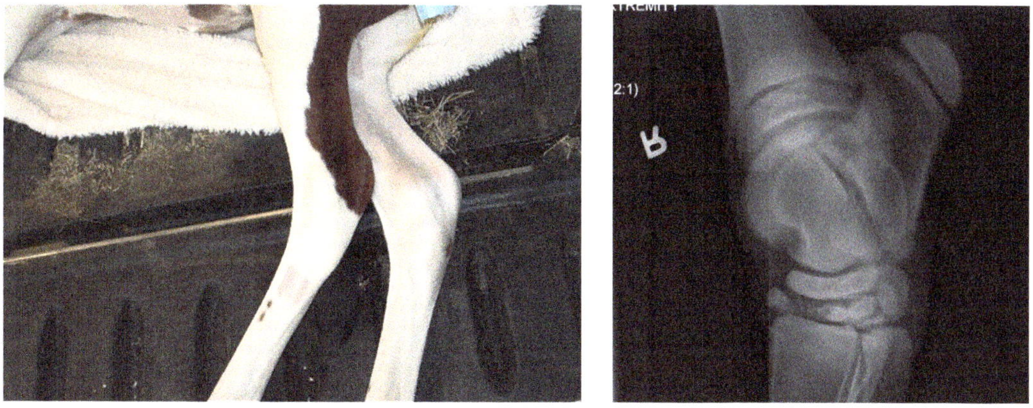

Figure 37.II.2 (a) Foal with sickle hock appearance of the hindlimbs. (b) Radiograph of the right hind tarsus demonstrating crushing and displacement of the tarsal bones. *Source:* Images courtesy of Dr. David Wong, Iowa State University.

foals revealed that foals with Grades 2 and 3 incomplete ossification of the tarsal bones were less likely to race than their maternal siblings, and foals with Grades 1–4 incomplete ossification earned less money [1]. If significant cuboidal bone wedging, fragmentation or collapse has already occurred at the time of presentation, the prognosis is guarded regardless of any treatment, and osteoarthritis and joint abnormalities are likely to be performance limiting.

White Muscle Disease (Nutritional Myodegeneration)

Pathophysiology

White muscle disease (WMD), also referred to as nutritional myodegeneration (NMD), is most commonly observed in foals <30 days of age in regions with selenium-deficient soils and forages, including the northeast, northwest, mid-Atlantic and Great Lakes regions of the United States, in addition to regions in Japan [9] and the Netherlands [10]. Foals are born with low serum selenium and low-to-normal serum vitamin E concentrations [9–11] as a result of deficiency in the mare. The underlying pathology is believed to result from free-radical mediated rhabdomyolysis with the disease acquiring its name from the characteristic pale discoloration of muscles observed at necropsy, which demonstrate bilaterally symmetrical dry myodegeneration. Since muscular exercise results in increased production of free radicals and reactive oxygen species, muscles with high physiological motion, including the diaphragm, intercostal muscles, gluteal muscles, tongue, muscles of mastication, and myocardium are most severely affected. Selenium is an important redox-sensitive element and constituent of glutathione peroxidase, which is essential for neutralizing reactive oxygen species while vitamin E serves as an antioxidant be combating formation of reactive oxygen species during lipid peroxidation. Depending on the severity of the selenium deficiency, foals may either present with an acute or subacute form of the disease.

Clinical Presentation

WMD affects both skeletal and cardiac muscle. Foals with acute disease demonstrate significant muscular weakness, which may quickly progress to recumbency and death (sometimes within hours) as a result of myocardial and respiratory muscle failure [12]. Foals with subacute disease may be able to stand at birth but develop progressive musculoskeletal pathology, including muscle atrophy, weakness, fasciculations, trismus, or other orthopedic abnormalities along with recumbency, tachypnea, dyspnea, and dysphagia [11]. In some foals, dysphagia may be the only presenting sign [10]. Myoglobinuria, malaise, weight loss/poor weight gain, neurologic signs, gastrointestinal symptoms, and immune dysfunction may also be present [11], in addition to distal limb edema associated with myonecrosis (Figures 37.II.3 and 37.II.4).

Diagnosis

WMD is suspected based on clinical signs of rapidly progressive muscular weakness and confirmed via presence of increased serum muscle enzymes (creatine kinase [CK], aspartate aminotransferase [AST]), decreased blood selenium (frequently <1.26 microm/l or 10 μg/dl in one study) [11], and decreased glutathione peroxidase activity. Serum CK activity ranged from 710 to 172 800 IU/l (reference interval 0–269 IU/l) in one report of 8 foals with WMD [10]. Foals can develop profound electrolyte abnormalities (hyperkalemia, hyponatremia, hypocalcemia, hypochloremia) with

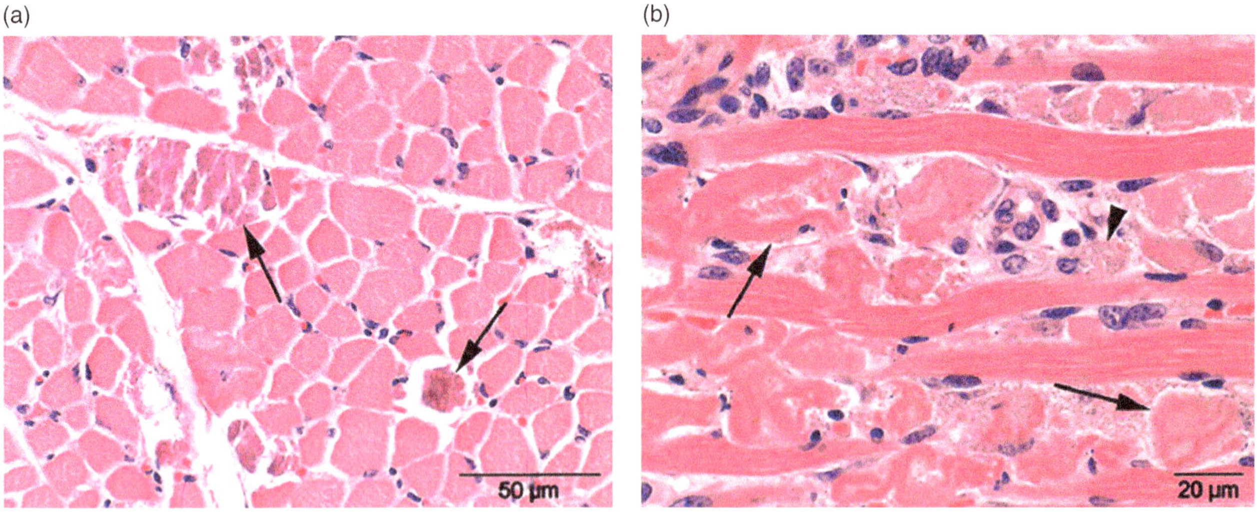

Figure 37.II.3 Histologic image of cross-section of affected skeletal muscle in a foal with WMD. (a) Multifocal mineralization of muscle fibers (arrows) H&E stain. (b) Longitudinal section of severely affected skeletal muscle demonstrating hyalinization and fragmentation of muscle fibers (arrows) and influx of macrophages phagocytizing myofiber remnants (arrowhead) H&E stain. *Source:* Image from Deleselle [10].

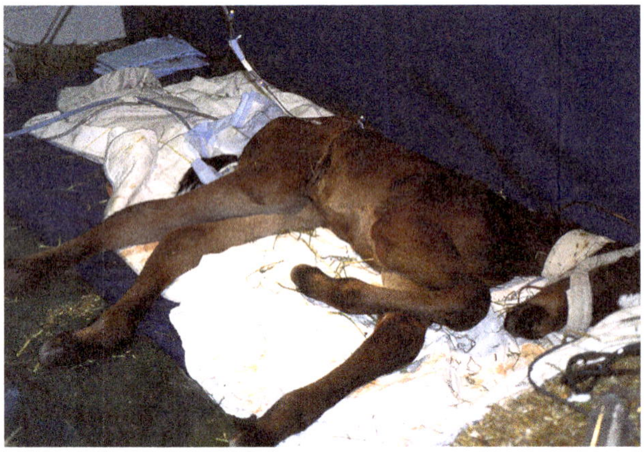

Figure 37.II.4 Recumbent 3-day-old foal presenting for subacute WMD with severe distal limb edema and myoglobinuria. *Source:* Image courtesy of Dr. Thomas Divers, Cornell University.

secondary cardiac arrhythmias, and renal failure may be a sequela of pigment nephropathy secondary to myoglobinuria [10, 13].

Treatment

Treatment of WMD predominantly consists of supportive care, including IV fluid therapy, diuresis, nutritional support and selenium and vitamin E supplementation. Selenium is given intramuscularly at a dose of 0.06 mg/kg; treatment can be repeated at 3 and 8–10 days after initial dose (do not exceed product label dose to avoid selenium toxicity). Vitamin E, given in the form of DL-α-tocopheryl acetate can be administered at a dose of 2–6 IU/kg, by mouth every 24 hours [10, 12]. Nasogastric feeding or parenteral nutrition may be necessary to provide appropriate nutritional requirements for dysphagic foals. In addition, it is important to treat any concurrent diseases (sepsis, hypoxia/reperfusion injury) which may be present in dysmature foals [13].

Prognosis and Necropsy Findings

The prognosis is guarded initially, ranging from 30% to 45% [10]; however, foals that regain the ability to stand have a more favorable prognosis [10]. If the myocardium is affected, the muscle is usually extensively affected and invariably fatal [10]. The disease can be prevented by ensuring that mares have adequate vitamin E and selenium intake throughout pregnancy [9, 14]. In endemic areas, prophylactic parenteral administration of vitamin E (2–6 IU/kg, PO, q24h) and selenium (0.055–0.067 mg/kg, IM) to newborn foals can be helpful [10, 12].

Acute Rhabdomyolysis

Pathophysiology

Causes of rhabdomyolysis in foals include hypoxia, polysaccharide storage myopathy (PSSM) and glycogen branching enzyme deficiency (GBED) [10]. PSSM and GBED are both heritable diseases. Type 1 PSSM is caused by a mutation in the gene encoding the skeletal muscle glycogen synthase enzyme (*GYS1*) whereas GBED is caused by a mutation in the glycogen branching enzyme (*GBE1*) gene. Rarely reported causes of rhabdomyolysis in foals include atypical myotonia congenita [15], atypical myopathy [16], lipid storage myopathy [17], white snake root toxicity [18], and toxic envenomation by bees *(Hymenoptera)* [19]. This section focuses on general treatment strategies for acute rhabdomyolysis in foals, including the more common genetic causes of rhabdomyolysis, PSSM, and GBED.

Clinical Presentation

Foals with acute rhabdomyolysis present with clinical signs similar to those described for WMD including weakness, muscle stiffness, elevated serum muscle enzyme activity, electrolyte abnormalities (hyperkalemia, hyponatremia, hypocalcemia, hyperphosphatemia, hypochloremia) and myoglobinuria [10]. Though PSSM is not typically diagnosed until affected individuals begin training, severe rhabdomyolysis has been reported in foals with PSSM, exacerbated by concurrent conditions including strangles [20] and pneumonia [21]. Conversely, GBED is an important cause of stillbirth and early neonatal death [22, 23], with foals presenting with weakness, hypothermia, intermittent hypoglycemia, seizures, and other nonspecific clinical signs that may be difficult to differentiate from neonatal sepsis [10, 24]. Respiratory failure and sudden death may occur secondary to exercise [10].

Diagnosis

Increased muscle enzymes, including serum CK and AST, electrolyte abnormalities and myoglobinuria support a diagnosis of acute rhabdomyolysis [10]. Genetic tests are available to confirm a diagnosis of type 1 PSSM and GBED but not type 2 PSSM. Type 1 PSSM affects many breeds, but has an especially high prevalence in Belgians and Quarter Horses [25–29]. GBED occurs in Quarter Horse and Paint breeds [22, 23, 30]. Muscle biopsy is required for a diagnosis of type 2 PSSM in adults; however, biopsies may not be diagnostic in foals [23].

Treatment

Treatment for rhabdomyolysis is focused on pain management, restoring fluid and electrolyte balance, preventing renal failure secondary to myoglobinuria and, if possible, eliminating the inciting cause [10]. Supportive care and treatment should also be directed at concurrent conditions. Long-term management of PSSM includes minimal stall confinement, regular exercise, and a low-starch, high-fat diet [10]. There is no treatment available for GBED.

Prognosis

The prognosis for acute rhabdomyolysis depends on inciting cause and comorbidities. Many horses with PSSM can be successfully managed with appropriate exercise and diet; however, recurrent episodes of rhabdomyolysis with intense exercise is possible. GBED is a fatal genetic disorder, with most foals dying/euthanized in the first weeks of life, with no reports of survival beyond 18 weeks of age [10, 23].

Rib Fractures

Pathophysiology

Fractured ribs are common in newborn foals, with 9% of 760 necropsied foals diagnosed with thoracic trauma in one report [31]. Rib fractures occur during parturition, especially in primiparous mares or secondary to dystocia [32], with an increased incidence in Thoroughbred foals [33]. The shape of the Thoroughbred foal's thorax, retention of a flexed elbow during parturition, a narrow maternal pelvic canal and excessive manipulation during foaling have been proposed as contributing factors [32]. Ribs 3–8 are most commonly affected, occurring either at the costochondral junction or just proximal to the costochondral junction [31]; however, fractures have been documented in ribs 1–17 [34].

Clinical Presentation

Foals with rib fractures present with clinical signs of lethargy, recumbency, groaning or grunting, subcutaneous edema over the ribs or ventral thorax, crepitus, and pain on palpation of the thorax [35].

Diagnosis

Rib fracture is an important differential diagnosis for foals presented with respiratory signs such as tachypnea, dyspnea, and shallow breathing [33, 34]. When in lateral recumbency, a depression may be observed or palpated near the costochondral junction and palpation of affected ribs may elicit crepitus and pain. Ultrasonography is the most sensitive modality to confirm diagnosis of rib fracture and can also reveal associated lung and internal organ pathology [34]. In addition, ultrasonography can differentiate whether displaced distal fracture fragments are axially deviated toward the heart or are simply overriding. Although some rib fractures can be detected radiographically, this form of imaging is much less sensitive for diagnosing rib fractures than ultrasound and provides little information about the orientation of the fracture extremities [32–34].

Treatment

Many rib fractures can be managed conservatively with stall rest and supportive therapy including supplemental intranasal oxygen and non-steroidal anti-inflammatory drugs. However, displaced rib fractures can cause pulmonary contusion, collapse, pneumothorax, and hemothorax; diaphragmatic hernia; hemopericardium; and myocardial laceration, all of which can be life-threatening (Figure 37.II.5) [33, 35]. Surgical repair of rib fractures is indicated when severe internal thoracic injury is present or the potential for severe internal injury is possible, especially myocardial laceration [33]. Axial displacement of fracture fragment extremities of ribs 3–5 of the left hemithorax place the foal at highest risk for cardiac injury, and the distal fracture fragment is typically the fragment deviated toward the heart with potential for myocardial laceration (Figure 37.II.6) [35]. Surgical treatment is also indicated for treatment of flail chest, an uncommon condition in which two or more consecutive ribs are fractured in at least two sites, resulting in a free-floating segment of chest wall and paradoxical respiration [33, 35]. Several techniques have been described to repair rib fractures in foals, including internal fixation with 2.7 mm reconstruction plates and screws ± cerclage wire [33], 2.7 mm reconstruction plates and cerclage wires without screws, stainless steel wire in a figure-of-eight pattern, nylon strand suture (Securos Cranial Cruciate Ligament Repair System) in a figure-of-eight pattern [36], and commercially available nylon cable ties, both with [37] and without fracture reduction (Figure 37.II.7) [38]. Surgical treatment is typically recommended within the first 24–72 hours after birth, but it is not typically necessary to repair every fractured rib when multiple rib fractures are present.

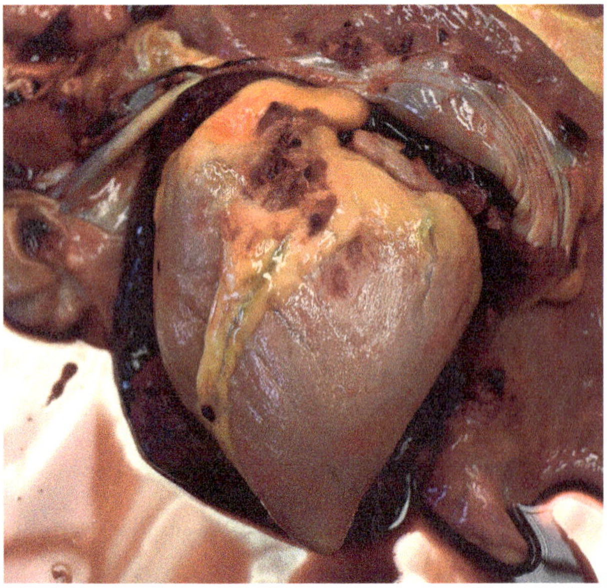

Figure 37.II.5 Postmortem image of a neonatal foal that died from a laceration to the coronary artery secondary to a rib fracture. *Source:* Image courtesy of Dr. Rebecca Ruby, University of Kentucky.

Prognosis

The prognosis for foals with rib fractures depends upon the number and location; displacement and orientation of fracture fragment extremities; extent of internal injury; and presence of comorbidities (e.g. sepsis) [35]. Sudden death from myocardial laceration can occur with axially displaced fractures affecting ribs 3–5 of the left hemithorax; therefore, surgical intervention is recommended for these cases [32, 35]. Other causes of death attributable to complications associated with rib fractures include pulmonary contusion, hemothorax, pneumothorax, diaphragmatic hernia, hemoabdomen, and hemopericardium [35]. The prognosis for foals with non-displaced rib fractures or displaced rib fractures in locations unlikely to result in myocardial trauma is fair-to-good with conservative management, in the absence of comorbid conditions [32], however, there are no studies directly comparing conservative versus surgical management.

Common Neonatal Physeal and Long Bone Fractures

Pathophysiology

Long bone fractures in foals can occur due to external trauma, such as a kick from another horse, being stepped on by the dam or having a limb pinned under the body, or as a result of internal trauma due to misloading or falling. Additional considerations relevant to neonates include involvement of the growth plate, or physeal fractures, which account for approximately 20% of long bone fractures in foals [39, 40]. Physeal fractures are described using the Salter-Harris classification system (Table 37.II.2), with type 1 and 2 Salter-Harris fractures most common in foals. Common fracture locations include the proximal and distal femur, proximal tibia, proximal radius, distal humerus, and, rarely, the distal third metacarpus/metatarsus or proximal phalanx [41–43]. Fractures of other physes, including the distal radius, proximal humerus, distal tibia, and distal scapula are not common in foals [39, 43].

Other fracture locations include the proximal sesamoid bones and distal phalanx. Foals are susceptible to most proximal sesamoid bone fracture configurations that adults are; however, apical and basilar fractures are most common [44, 45]. Biaxial midbody proximal sesamoid bone fractures can be seen in young foals galloping to keep up with their dams, as the tensile forces of the suspensory apparatus overwhelm the bone yield strength once the muscles fatigue [46]. Most distal phalanx (P3) fracture types are uncommon in foals (Table 37.II.3), with the exception of type 7 and type 4 (extensor process) fractures [44, 47, 48]. Type 7 fractures – also called palmar

(a) (b) (c) (d)

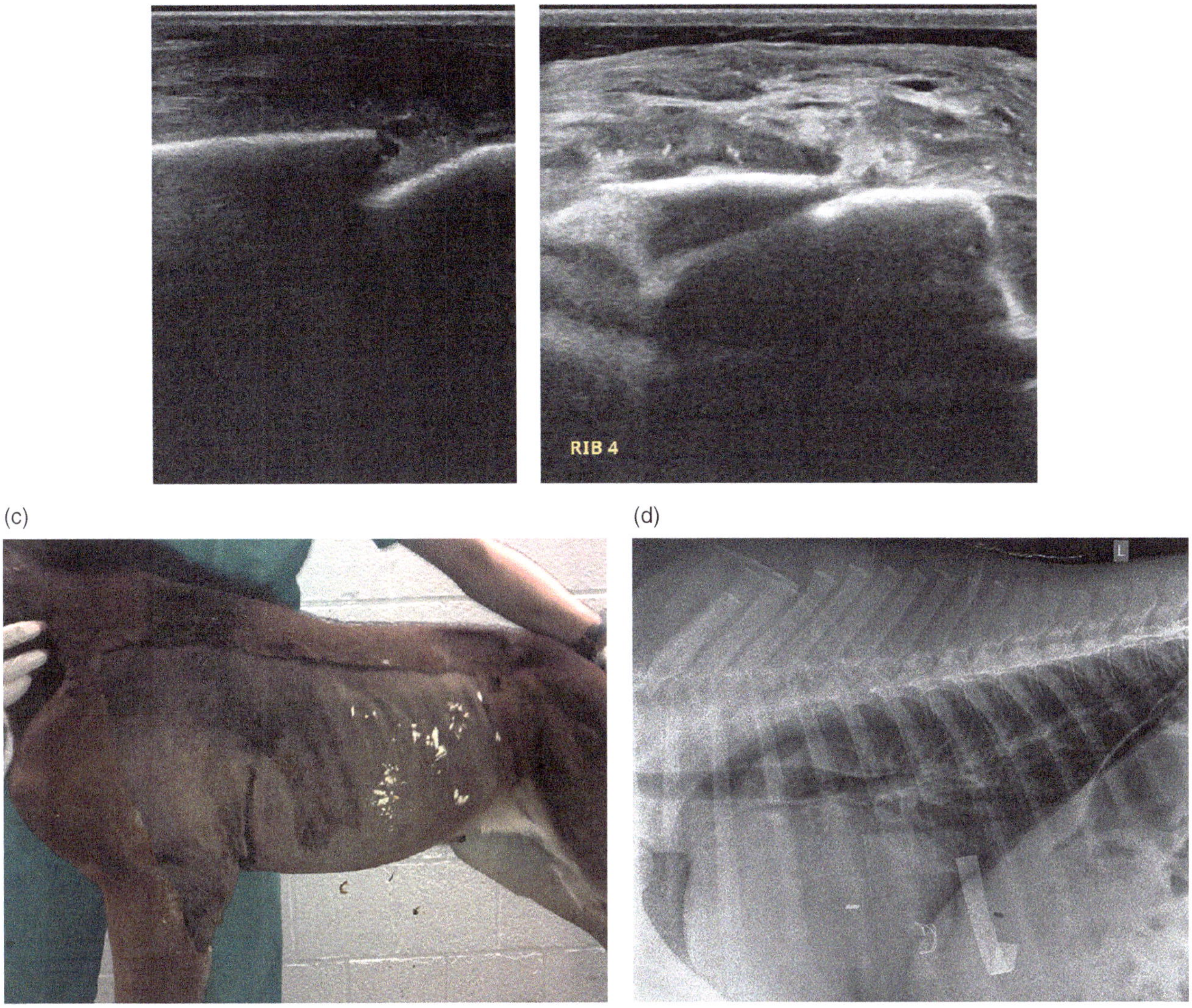

Figure 37.II.6 (a) and (b) Ultrasonographic images of (a) mildly overriding and (b) axially displaced ventral fracture fragments of rib 4 on the left side of the thorax in a Standardbred filly at 2 days and 1 week after birth, respectively (dorsal is to the left). Left-sided rib fractures involving ribs 3–8; only ribs 4 and 5 were significantly displaced with axial deviation. Ribs 4 and 5 were surgically repaired using a combination of nylon strand suture and stainless-steel wire, with (c) images of the incision and (d) radiographs of the thorax post-operatively.

(a) (b)

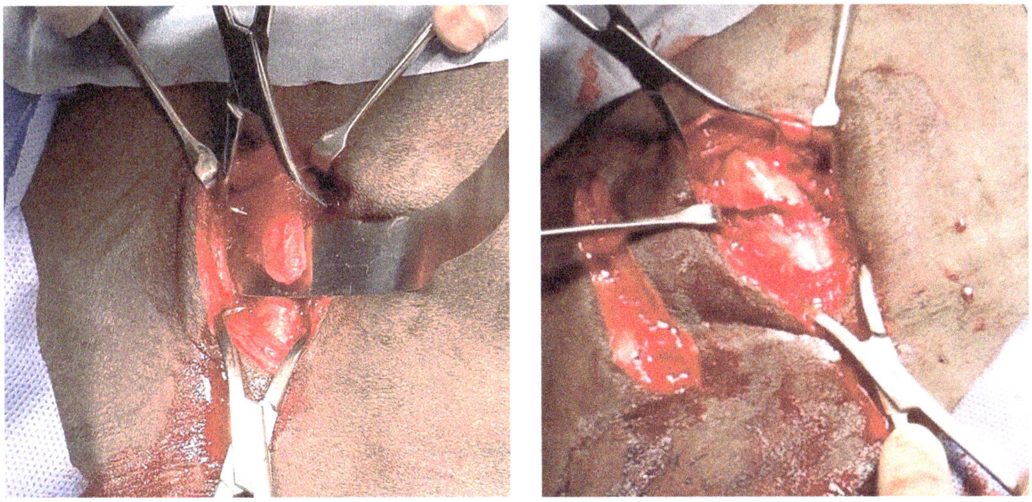

Figure 37.II.7 Three-day-old Quarter Horse foal with four fractured ribs of the left hemithorax. (a) Isolation of rib fracture, and (b) alignment of fracture site prior to fixation. *Source:* Images courtesy of Dr. Annette McCoy.

Table 37.II.2 Salter-Harris classification system for physeal fractures.

Type	Description
I	Fracture through the physis only
II	Fracture through the physis and metaphysis
III	Fracture through the physis and epiphysis, entering the joint
IV	Fracture involving epiphysis, physis, and metaphysis
V	Crush/compression injury to the physis with minimal to no displacement
VI	Periosteal bridge between metaphysis and epiphysis

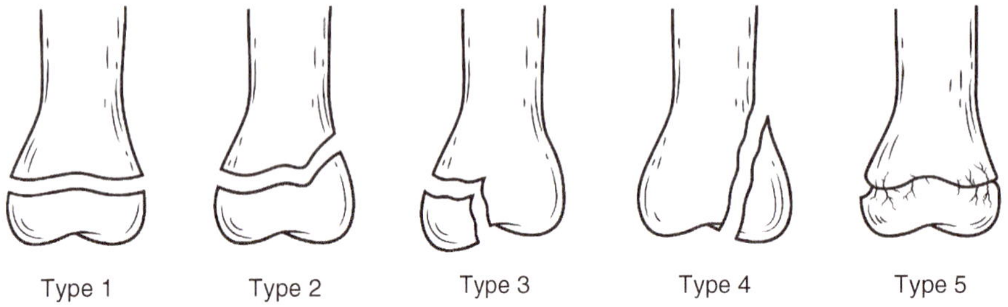

Table 37.II.3 Classification system for distal phalanx fractures.

Type	Description
1	Nonarticular fractures of palmar/plantar processes
2	Oblique, articular fractures of palmar/plantar processes
3	Articular, midsagittal fractures
4	Extensor process fractures
5	Comminuted fractures
6	Nonarticular, solar margin fractures
7[a]	Nonarticular, solar margin fractures dorsal to palmer/ plantar process[a]

[a] Foal specific distal phalanx fracture

process fractures [48], osseous bodies, or ossicles [47] – are unique to foals with proposed etiologies including acute trauma [47, 49], separate centers of ossification, and developmental orthopedic disease [47]. There is a higher prevalence of type 7 fractures in Thoroughbred foals, possibly associated with hoof conformation [48]. Type 4 fractures are thought to be either traumatic, due to hyperextension or avulsion injury, or developmental, with bilateral fragments thought to be a result of a separate center of ossification or OC [50].

Clinical Presentation

Foals with long-bone and physeal fractures typically present with severe weightbearing to non-weightbearing lameness. Crepitus can be appreciated with physeal and long-bone fractures that are still moderately aligned. In severely displaced and overriding long-bone fractures, crepitus may not be appreciated, but limb malalignment and significant swelling associated with hematoma formation may be appreciable.

Diagnosis

Radiography can be used to confirm/characterize a suspected fracture and provides information about the severity of injury. As with adults, fractures in foals are described as either open or closed, complete or incomplete, and displaced or nondisplaced; also reported are the bones and joints involved and whether the fracture is comminuted. The Salter-Harris classification system is commonly used to describe fractures of compression physes (Table 37.II.2), whereas simple anatomic description of fractures involving tension physes, such as the olecranon tuberosity or calcaneal tuber, is appropriate [43].

Treatment

Treatment of neonatal physeal and long-bone fractures depends on the site and configuration of the fracture; however, the same principles of accurate anatomic reduction and stabilization through interfragmentary compression are recommended to return the foal to early weightbearing and prevent complications, including angular and flexural limb deformities of both the fractured and contralateral limb. Detailed descriptions of fracture repair techniques for physeal and long-bone fractures are beyond the scope of this chapter and readers are directed to other references [43, 51–53].

Internal fixation is commonly indicated for most long bone fractures in foals. Some Salter-Harris physeal fractures can be adequately stabilized with screw fixation and coaptation alone, whereas the majority of diaphyseal long bone fractures require repair with open reduction and internal fixation [43]. Locking compression plate or dynamic compression plate fixation is indicated for most metacarpal/metatarsal, radial and tibial fractures, whereas stack pinning, bone plating, and intramedullary interlocking nail fixation have all been successful for humeral and femoral fractures [41, 53]. Where possible, the surgeon should avoid placing constructs that bridge the physis to prevent limb shortening or angular limb deformities due to premature physeal closure [41, 43]. A subset of minimally displaced, stable fractures are candidates for healing with stall confinement alone, but most fractures are best repaired with internal fixation to minimize the likelihood of support limb complications such as varus deformity, carpal contracture of the affected limb or, rarely, support limb laminitis [53]. Treatment with external coaptation alone of minimally displaced physeal fractures, including proximal phalangeal and distal metacarpal/metatarsal fractures may be appropriate in neonatal foals [43]. A critical aspect of emergency care and triage for neonatal foals with long bone or physeal fractures is appropriate coaptation and transport, with some differences from the adult given the likelihood of recumbency during transport. Although discussed in detail elsewhere [43, 53], brief considerations specific for bandaging and external coaptation for foal fractures are listed below (Table 37.II.4).

Prognosis

Open fractures are associated with a reduced prognosis due to bacterial contamination and likelihood of surgical site infection [41]. Rarely are surgical site infections eradicated in the presence of orthopedic implants and, if a fracture is able to heal despite the presence of infection, implant removal is nearly always indicated. In general, the prognosis for foals with long bone fractures is better than adults due to their smaller size, rapid healing, and reduced risk for development of contralateral limb laminitis [41, 53]. However, it is still ideal to obtain rigid fixation in order to return foals to comfortable weightbearing due to the potential for rapid development of contralateral limb varus deformity and other support limb complications. Similar to adults, more highly comminuted fractures, fractures with articular components and more proximal fractures have a worse prognosis. Nonetheless, fractures of the pelvis, femur, humerus, radius, ulna, and tibia have been successfully repaired in foals. Radial, ulnar, and tibial fractures are more amenable to surgical repair than femoral and humeral fractures [45]; however, diaphyseal femoral and humeral fractures can be repaired successfully in foals as they are more likely to involve simple, oblique fracture configurations as compared to fractures in adults [53–57].

Physeal fractures can be associated with more complications than diaphyseal fractures due to risks of disturbed limb growth and articular involvement [39, 40, 42, 43]. Whereas the prognosis for some physeal fractures, including proximal phalangeal, distal metacarpal/metatarsal, and ulnar fractures is good, the prognosis for proximal and distal humeral and femoral physeal fractures is guarded to poor [43]. Radial physeal fractures and proximal tibial physeal fractures have a good prognosis with appropriate anatomic reduction and sparing of the physis, with more uncertainty or a less favorable prognosis for distal tibial fractures and distal scapular fractures [43].

Table 37.II.4 Recommended coaptation for long-bone fractures of the forelimb and hind limb in the neonatal foal.

Location	Coaptation
Scapula	None
Humerus	None
Ulna	None for displaced fracture; fixing the carpus in extension may reduce likelihood of a nondisplaced fracture becoming displaced
Radius	Caudal splint to level of elbow, lateral splint to shoulder
Femur	None
Tibia	Caudal splint to level of stifle, lateral splint to the croup
Metacarpus/metatarsus	Lateral splint to level of elbow/stifle; caudal splint to elbow/point of hock
Phalangeal	Dorsal (fore) or caudal (hind) splint to level of carpus/tarsus with the dorsal cortices of the phalanges aligned

Proximal Sesamoid Bone and Distal Phalanx Fractures

Clinical Presentation

Foals with small or minimally displaced fractures of the proximal sesamoid bones may only display mild or transient lameness [46]. In contrast, larger displaced uniaxial proximal sesamoid bone fractures often result in fetlock effusion, moderate lameness, and pain on palpation and fetlock joint flexion [44]. Biaxial proximal sesamoid bone fractures result in non-weightbearing lameness and fetlock hyperextension. Foals with distal phalanx fractures may present with variable clinical presentations, with some type 7 distal phalanx fractures resulting in mild-to-moderate lameness while other type 7 fractures do not have localizing signs and are incidental radiographic findings [44, 47, 48]. Lameness associated with type 4 fractures ranges from mild–moderate [58], whereas other distal phalanx fractures with significant articular involvement, though rare in foals, are associated with more severe lameness [49].

Diagnosis

Radiography is the primary imaging modality utilized for diagnosis of proximal sesamoid and distal phalangeal fractures. Computed tomography (CT) can be useful for complex or occult phalangeal fracture configurations. Proximal sesamoid bone fractures are described based on the region of the bone affected: apical, basilar, mid-body, abaxial, axial, and comminuted. In foals, apical, basilar, and mid-body proximal sesamoid bone fractures are most common [44, 45]. Distal phalanx fractures are described with the grading system used for adult fractures, which consists of 7 fracture types (Table 37.II.3). Type 7 fractures involve the abaxial wings of the third phalanx and are unique to foals [44, 47].

Treatment

Most simple, uniaxial proximal sesamoid bone fractures in neonatal foals will heal adequately with conservative treatment, even when mild fracture displacement is present [44, 46]. Conservative treatment includes stall rest for 4–8 weeks, followed by gradual turnout [45]. Arthroscopic removal of apical proximal sesamoid bone fractures is commonly performed in weanlings and yearlings [59, 60], but there are few reports of surgical treatment of proximal sesamoid bone fractures in young foals [46]. Biaxial proximal sesamoid bone fractures that result in complete suspensory apparatus disruption and fetlock instability can be treated with exercise restriction and external coaptation with splinting alone [61] or with fetlock arthrodesis if metacarpophalangeal joint subluxation or luxation is present [44, 45]. Because mid-body proximal sesamoid bone fractures commonly occur in foals galloping to keep up with their dams or paddock-mates [46, 61], it is important to incrementally introduce exercise to allow the proximal sesamoid bones to adapt to loading, especially for foals that have been stall confined for any reason related to mare or foal health.

Similar to proximal sesamoid bone fractures, the majority of distal phalanx fractures observed in foals heal via bony union with conservative treatment [44]. Nonarticular distal phalanx fractures, including type 1, 6, and 7 fractures can be treated with exercise restriction and soft footing alone. Some type 7 fractures are incidental radiographic findings and do not require specific treatment. Small, non- or minimally displaced type 4 fractures in foals may not require treatment, but arthroscopic removal may be performed when the foal is older. There is one report of screw fixation of a type 4 fracture in a foal [58]; however, the majority of type 4 fractures will heal with exercise restriction alone. Unlike adults, long-term placement of a shoe is contraindicated in foal distal phalanx fractures due to the potential for significant contracture of the hoof [44, 49].

Prognosis

The prognosis for neonatal foals with small apical and basilar proximal sesamoid bone fractures is good [46]. In a study of 151 Thoroughbred weanlings and yearlings that underwent arthroscopic removal of apical proximal sesamoid bone fractures, the prognosis for racing was excellent for hindlimb fractures and good for forelimb fractures, with medial fractures of the forelimb associated with the worst prognosis [59]. Biaxial proximal sesamoid bone fractures typically preclude any high level of athleticism; however, these animals can be salvaged for breeding or pasture soundness. The prognosis for type 7 distal phalanx fractures in foals is excellent, and the prognosis for most other common distal phalanx fractures is good [44, 47, 48]. Most distal phalanx fractures treated conservatively in foals will heal with a bony union.

Common Digital Extensor Tendon Rupture

Pathophysiology

Rupture of the common digital extensor tendon is most frequently observed in combination with flexural (contractual) deformities of the carpus and/or metacarpophalangeal joints [62–64], but can also be observed independently [63]. Extensor tendon rupture can be unilateral or bilateral and may also accompany incomplete ossification and, in older foals, ALD [65]. The condition has been described as a congenital disorder [65] as well as a occurring within the first few days of life [66]. The cause of the tendon rupture is unknown but hypothesized to occur from contraction of the flexor musculotendinous unit in foals with carpal or forelimb fetlock flexural deformities with excessive strain [62, 67].

Clinical Presentation and Diagnosis

Foals present differently depending on the severity of the underlying condition; however, a common feature is the pathognomonic tendon sheath swelling at the dorsolateral aspect of the carpus, both proximal and distal to the carpus (Figure 37.II.8) [65]. The ruptured ends of the common digital extensor tendon or myotendinous junction can be palpated within the distended tendon sheath. Some foals also have an "over-at-the-knee" or bowlegged appearance due to the tendon sheath swelling and buckling at the carpus or knuckling over at the metacarpophlangeal joint [65]. Additional

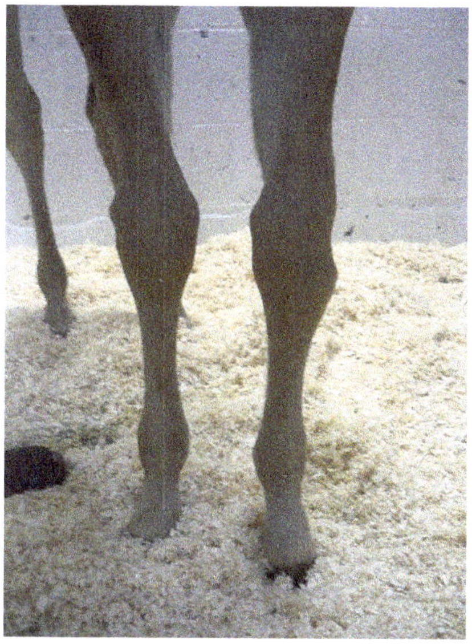

Figure 37.II.8 Unilateral common digital extensor tendon sheath swelling on the dorsolateral aspect of the left carpus, both proximal and distal to the carpus, pathognomonic for common digital extensor tendon rupture, in a 4-week-old Quarter Horse filly.

diagnostics are usually not necessary for diagnosis; however, ultrasonography can identify the torn ends of the tendon within the effusive tendon sheath and radiographs can be used to determine if incomplete ossification is present.

Treatment

When occurring in combination with forelimb flexural deformities, treatment of common digital extensor tendon rupture should focus on resolution of underlying contracture, often through external coaptation in combination with analgesia, controlled exercise and oxytetracycline or, in severe cases, surgical intervention [67]. Flexural limb deformities are described elsewhere in the textbook. Surgical intervention for common digital extensor tendon rupture is not necessary, and bandaging and coaptation is typically only needed for as long as the underlying flexural deformity is present, but may speed healing of the torn common digital extensor tendon. Box stall confinement is indicated initially to prevent knuckling and associated trauma. The torn ends of the common digital extensor tendon typically fibrose and re-appose within 6 months with minimal swelling [63, 64].

Prognosis

The prognosis for common digital extensor tendon rupture is favorable, provided that concurrent underlying conditions, including flexural deformities, incomplete ossification, or angular limb deformities are not performance limiting.

Rupture of the Origin of the Peroneus Tertius and Long Digital Extensor Muscles

Pathophysiology

The peroneus (fibularis) tertius originates from the common tendon of origin of the peroneus tertius and long digital extensor muscles within the extensor fossa on the lateral aspect of the distal femur and inserts on the dorsoproximal aspect of metatarsal III, the calcaneus, and the third and fourth tarsal bones. The tendon is part of the cranial hindlimb reciprocal apparatus, coordinating simultaneous flexion of the stifle and tarsus.

Clinical Presentation

Peroneus tertius rupture is uncommonly reported in neonates and typically involves traumatic rupture near the origin of the peroneus tertius and long digital extensor muscles coupled with avulsion fracture or fragmentation of the femur [68–71]. Unlike mid-body peroneus tertius tears in adult horses, the pathognomonic signs of tarsal extension combined with stifle flexion are less commonly reported with avulsion fractures of the peroneus tertius origin in foals, possibly because the avulsed bone is constrained by the joint capsule [69], though disruption of the cranial reciprocal apparatus may be detected upon manipulation of the limb [71]. Instead, foals commonly present with unilateral hindlimb lameness and painful swelling over the lateral aspect of the stifle joint, along with effusion of the femoropatellar and femorotibial joints [69].

Diagnosis

Diagnosis is made via physical examination and stifle radiography; however, ultrasonography may be beneficial in some cases to define the location of fragmentation. The caudocranial and caudolateral-craniomedial oblique views of the stifle are usually diagnostic, revealing single or multiple distally displaced avulsion fractures of the common tendon of origin involving the lateral condyle and/or lateral trochlear ridge of the femur (Figure 37.II.9) [68, 69].

Treatment

Depending on the number, size, and location of avulsion fragments, stifle arthroscopy or an open surgical approach can be performed for fragment removal. If the fragments are intra-articular, arthroscopy will enable assessment of concurrent stifle pathology, even if the size of the fragments necessitates conversion to an open approach. Removal of small bone fragments is recommended, but some authors have suggested that large fragments embedded in the joint capsule are better left in place [69].

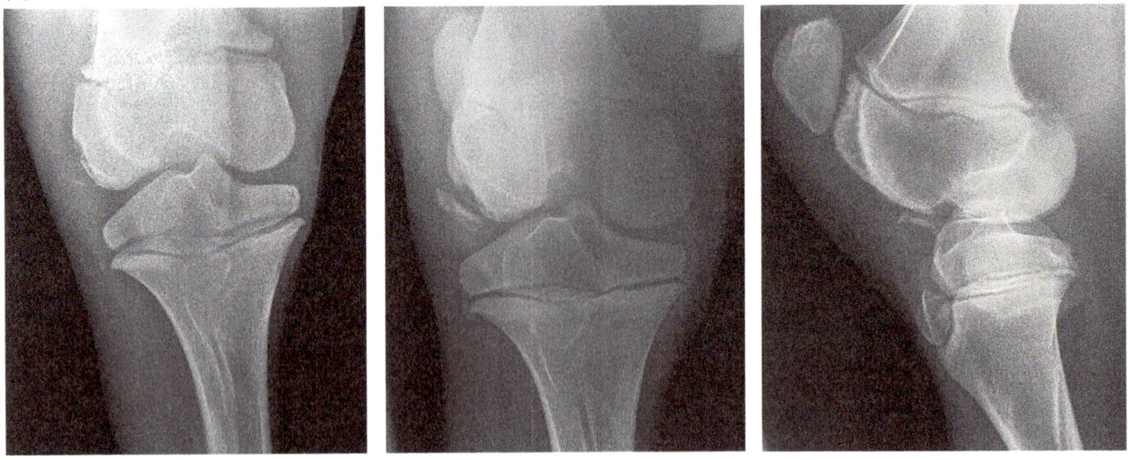

Figure 37.II.9 Avulsion injury of the origin of the peroneus tertius and long digital extensor tendons in a 1-month-old Thoroughbred colt. (a) Caudocranial stifle radiograph on the day of injury, revealing a minimally displaced fracture fragment. (b) and (c) Caudocranial and lateromedial stifle radiographs obtained 2 weeks post-injury, revealing additional ossification and distolateral displacement of the fracture fragments into the lateral femorotibial joint. Arthroscopic fragment removal was recommended. *Source:* Images courtesy of Dr. Alanna Zantingh, Cambridge Equine Hospital, NZ.

Prognosis

The prognosis for athleticism and return to full soundness following avulsion injury is guarded [68, 70]; however, resolution of lameness has been reported 6 months and 1 year postoperatively in two cases [69, 72].

Gastrocnemius Muscle Rupture

Pathophysiology

The gastrocnemius muscle originates on the supracondylar tuberosities on the caudal surface of the femur and inserts as the common calcanean tendon on the calcaneal tuber, functioning as a flexor of the stifle and primary extensor of the tarsus. In concert with the peroneus tertius on the cranial aspect of the limb, the gastrocnemius muscle is the primary caudal component of the reciprocal apparatus, coordinating concurrent flexion-extension of the stifle and tarsus. Partial disruption or complete rupture of the gastrocnemius muscle in foals has been associated with uncoordinated attempts to stand *postpartum* [73], dystocia, and assisted delivery, with hip lock being the most commonly reported cause of dystocia in one case series [74]. Gastrocnemius rupture has also been reported in foals with normal parturition and in foals delivered by caesarian section [75]. Unilateral disruption is most common, though bilateral injury can occur due to manual attempts to straighten the hindlimbs of foals with bilateral contracture of the tarsocrural joints [73]. In neonates, disruption of the gastrocnemius muscle most commonly occurs near its origin on the caudal surface of the femur [73, 75]; however, rupture of the tendon has been reported adjacent to the insertion of the gastrocnemius in a 3-month-old foal [76].

Clinical Presentation

More severely affected foals present with inability to rise or stand without assistance at birth, while foals with less severe tears or partial disruption can stand but have a dropped tarsus with extension of the stifle due to disruption of the caudal reciprocal apparatus (Figure 37.II.10 a, b). Mild to severe swelling may be present in the caudal thigh in addition to hematoma formation as a result of tearing of both gastrocnemius muscle fibers and the caudal femoral artery or its branches [73].

Diagnosis

Complete rupture of the gastrocnemius muscle is diagnosed via the pathognomonic appearance of caudal reciprocal apparatus disruption with an extended stifle and flexed, dropped tarsus. Additional localizing signs include the presence of swelling caudal to the stifle, instability of the stifle joint, and stifle joint effusion [74]. Ultrasonography is most useful to confirm the location and extent of the gastrocnemius muscle fiber disruption and to characterize the swelling (Figure 37.II.11) [74, 75]. Both radiography and ultrasonography are useful in identifying the presence of avulsion fragments associated with distal femoral avulsion fracture [74, 75]. Though avulsion fracture was uncommon in one report (1/28 foals) [75], avulsion fractures were detected in 2/6 foals in another report [74], and heterotopic ossification or ossification consistent with a

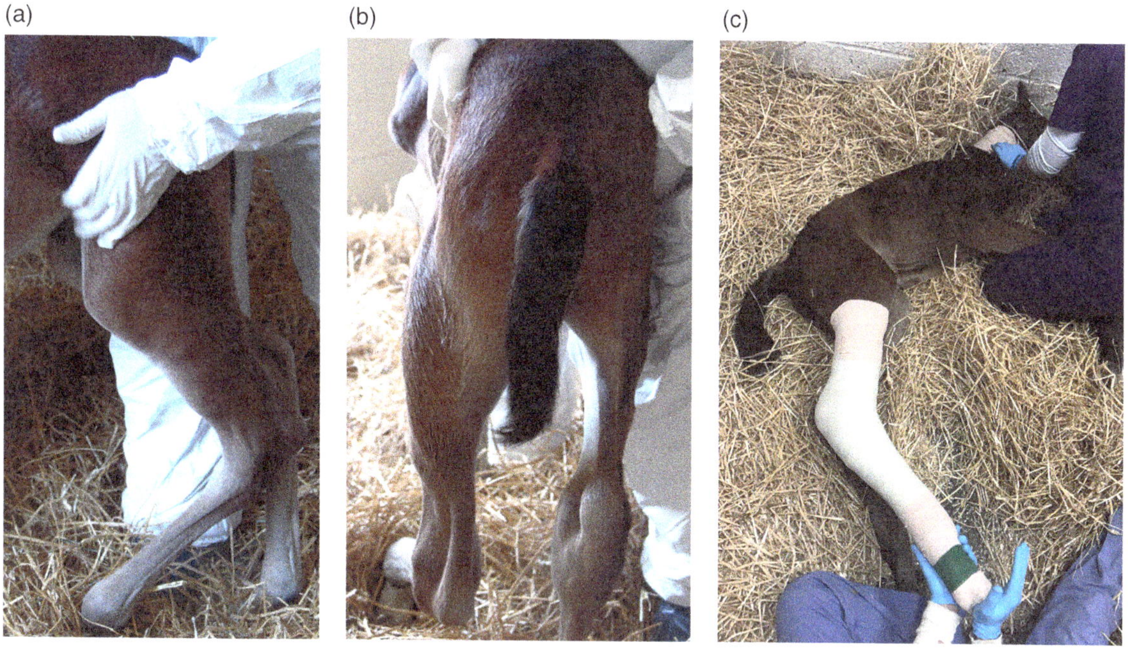

Figure 37.II.10 (a), (b) Gastrocnemius rupture of the left hindlimb in a neonatal Thoroughbred colt demonstrating the characteristic disruption of the caudal reciprocal apparatus with a flexed tarsus and extended stifle. (c) Application of a sleeve cast from the proximal tibia to the distal metatarsal 3 in the right hindlimb of a foal with gastrocnemius disruption. *Source:* Images courtesy of Dr. Travis Tull, Ocala Equine Hospital.

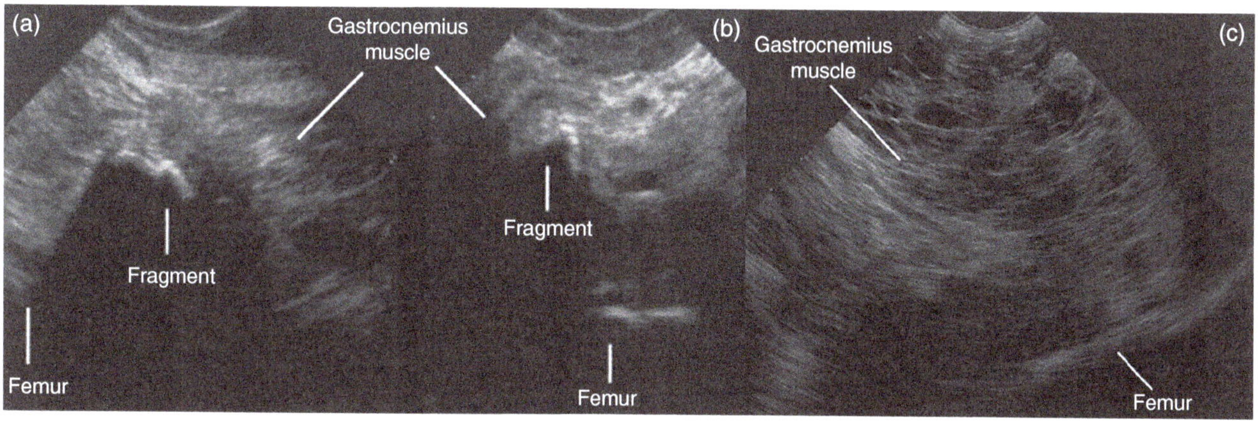

Figure 37.II.11 Ultrasonographic images of the left hind limb (a), (b) of a foal with gastrocnemius rupture. (a) Note avulsion fragments distracted from caudal aspect of distal portion of the femur; bone fragments are hyperechoic and cast clean acoustic shadows. Image from proximodistal plane, with proximal to right of image. (b) Same view as (a), from mediolateral plane. Lateral is to the right. (c) Ultrasonographic image of right hind limb of a 13-day-old Standardbred foal with tear in the gastrocnemius muscle sustained at birth. Note the loculated pattern of fluid among muscle and fibrin strands in the body of the gastrocnemius muscle. Image from proximodistal plane, proximal to the right. Images from Jesty et al. [74].

possible avulsion fragment were identified at necropsy in 2/3 foals in a third series [77].

Treatment

Treatment includes stall rest alone or in combination with coaptation, depending on the degree of caudal reciprocal apparatus dysfunction and systemic status of the foal [75]. Stall rest may be sufficient for foals with incomplete rupture and minimal disruption of the caudal reciprocal apparatus, whereas external coaptation in the form of a sleeve cast or a hemi-circumferential dorsal splint is indicated with more significant disruption [75]. Coaptation should extend from the proximal tibia to the distal aspect of the third metatarsus in a weightbearing position (Figure 37.II.10c), unless digital flexor tendon laxity requires incorporation of the hoof [75]. Successful repair of gastrocnemius tendon rupture near the insertion on the tuber calcanei in a 3-month-old filly has been reported using carbon fiber suture [76].

Prognosis

While gastrocnemius rupture can lead to life-threatening hemorrhage or hypovolemic shock secondary to injury [74, 75, 78], a recent case report in 28 Thoroughbred foals suggests that athletic prognosis is favorable, with 82% of survivors of racing age (13/16) entering race training or starting a race [75]. Historically, a poor to guarded prognosis for athleticism was reported, but many foals in those case studies were afflicted by significant concurrent diseases or were euthanized due to economic constraints and perceived poor prognoses [73, 74]. Factors associated with reduced prognosis for athleticism include concurrent systemic disease processes and abscess formation in the gastrocnemius muscle injury site [75].

Physitis/Physeal Dysplasia

Pathophysiology

Physitis or physeal dysplasia, characterized by inflammation and firm enlargement of the physeal region of long bones, is common in growing horses. Although physitis is most commonly bilaterally symmetrical and diagnosed in weanlings from 4 to 8 months of age, it can occasionally be noted in neonates. Nutritional, genetic and/or exercise-induced physitis should be suspected when multiple limbs are involved, whereas trauma or overloading can explain single-site involvement.

Clinical Presentation

Physitis most commonly affects the distal physes of the third metacarpal/metatarsal bones, the radius and the tibia. Young foals may present with a stiff gait, increased recumbency, trembling when standing or buckling at the carpus or fetlock [42, 79]. In neonates <2 weeks old, physitis is more likely secondary to trauma or excessive compression of the affected physis due to severe ALD or compensatory overloading.

Diagnosis

Diagnosis of physitis is made via clinical presentation, presence of enlarged physes (painful to deep palpation) and radiographic evidence of physeal changes, including paraphyseal new bone production (physeal lipping or metaphyseal flaring) [79], physeal radiolucency/widening, metaphyseal asymmetry, epiphyseal wedging, metaphyseal sclerosis adjacent to the physis, and asymmetric cortical thickness [42].

Treatment

Treatment in neonatal foals is directed at resolving the underlying cause of physitis, including bandaging or coaptation to help align limbs with moderate-to-severe ALD and addressing the underlying cause of lameness that is resulting in compensatory overloading. Severe angular limb deformities may require surgical growth retardation to prevent physeal crush injury and premature closure of the overloaded portion of the physis.

Prognosis

The prognosis depends on the underlying cause of physitis. Most cases of symmetrical, multi-limb physitis are mild and self-limiting. Cases of severe physitis resulting in angular or flexural limb deformities or premature physeal closure may limit athleticism [79, 80].

Developmental Orthopedic Disease (DOD)

Developmental orthopedic disease is a broad term that encompasses several conditions including: incomplete ossification, physitis/physeal dysplasia and subsequent ALD, OC, subchondral cystic lesions, flexural limb deformities, and cervical vertebral malformations [42, 81]. The pathophysiology of DOD is complex, with genetics, nutrition, cartilage vascularization, biomechanics, exercise, and trauma all potentially contributing to disease. Incomplete ossification and physitis/physeal dysplasia are discussed earlier in this chapter, and angular and flexural limb deformities are discussed in Chapter 37 Section I. Although OC, subchondral cystic lesions and cervical vertebral malformation are common causes of lameness in weanlings and yearlings, they are uncommonly diagnosed as a clinical problem in foals <2–4 months old [81] and rarely in neonates.

References

1 Haywood, L., Spike-Pierce, D.L., Barr, B. et al. (2018). Gestation length and racing performance in 115 thoroughbred foals with incomplete tarsal ossification. *Equine Vet. J.* 50: 29–33.

2 Coleman, M.C. and Whitfield-Cargile, C. (2017). Orthopedic conditions of the premature and dysmature foal. *Vet. Clin. North Am. Equine Pract.* 33: 289–297.

3 Guffy, M.M., Bergin, W.C., and Gier, H.T. (1970). Radiographic fetometry of the horse. *Cornell Vet.* 60: 359–371.
4 Wong, D.M., Scarratt, W.K., Maxwell, V. et al. (2010). Incomplete ossification of the carpal, tarsal and navicular bones in a dysmature foal. *Equine Vet. Educ.* 15: 72–81.
5 McIlwraith, C.W. (2010). Incomplete ossification of carpal and tarsal bones in foals. *Equine Vet. Educ.* 15: 79–81.
6 Ernst, N.S., Trumble, T.N., and Baxter, G.M. (2020). Lameness in the young horse: angular limb deformities (ALDs) and cuboidal bone malformations. In: *Adams and Stashak's Lameness in Horses*, 7e (ed. G.M. Baxter), 1048–1058. Wiley.
7 Adams, R. and Poulos, P. (1988). A skeletal ossification index for neonatal foals. *Vet. Radiol.* Wiley 29 (5): 217–222.
8 Dutton, D.M., Watkins, J.P., Walker, M.A., and Honnas, C.M. (1998). Incomplete ossification of the tarsal bones in foals: 22 cases (1988–1996). *J. Am. Vet. Med. Assoc.* 213: 1590–1594.
9 Higuchi, T., Ichijo, S., Osame, S. et al. (1989). Studies on serum selenium and tocopherol in white muscle disease of foal. *Nippon juigaku zasshi Jpn. J. Vet. Sci.* 51: 52–59.
10 Delesalle, C., de Bruijn, M., Wilmink, S. et al. (2017). White muscle disease in foals: focus on selenium soil content. A case series. *BMC Vet. Res.* 13: 121.
11 Streeter, R.M., Divers, T.J., Mittel, L. et al. (2012). Selenium deficiency associations with gender, breed, serum vitamin E and creatine kinase, clinical signs and diagnoses in horses of different age groups: a retrospective examination 1996–2011. *Equine Vet. J. Suppl.* 43: 31–35.
12 McKenzie, H.C. III (2018). Disorders of foals. In: *Equine Internal Medicine*, 4e (ed. S.M. Reed, W.M. Bayly, and D.C. Sellon), 1365–1459. St. Louis: Elsevier.
13 Perkins, G., Valberg, S.J., Madigan, J.M. et al. (1998). Electrolyte disturbances in foals with severe rhabdomyolysis. *J. Vet. Intern. Med.* 12: 173–177.
14 Karren, B.J., Thorson, J.F., Cavinder, C.A. et al. (2010). Effect of selenium supplementation and plane of nutrition on mares and their foals: selenium concentrations and glutathione peroxidase. *J. Anim. Sci.* 88: 991–997.
15 Schooley, E.K., MacLeay, J.M., Cuddon, P. et al. (2004). Atypical myotonia congenita in a foal. *J. Equine Vet. Sci.* 24: 483–488.
16 Karlíková, R., Široká, J., Mech, M. et al. (2018). Newborn foal with atypical myopathy. *J. Vet. Intern. Med.* 32: 1768–1772.
17 Pinn, T.L., Divers, T.J., Southard, T. et al. (2018). Persistent hypoglycemia associated with lipid storage myopathy in a paint foal. *J. Vet. Intern. Med.* 32: 1442–1446.
18 Sanders, M. (1983). White snakeroot poisoning in a foal: a case report. *J. Equine Vet. Sci.* 3: 128–129.
19 Lewis, N. and Racklyeft, D.J. (2014). Mass envenomation of a mare and foal by bees. *Aust. Vet. J.* 92: 141–148.
20 De La Corte, F.D., Valberg, S.J., MacLeay, J.M. et al. (2002). Developmental onset of polysaccharide storage myopathy in 4 quarter horse foals. *J. Vet. Intern. Med.* 16:581–587.
21 Byrne, E., Cohen, N., Jones, S.L. et al. (2000). Rhabdomyolysis in two foals with polysaccharide storage myopathy. *Compend. Contin. Educ. Pract. Vet.* 22: 503–510.
22 Valberg, S.J., Ward, T.L., Rush, B. et al. (2001). Glycogen branching enzyme deficiency in quarter horse foals. *J. Vet. Intern. Med.* 15: 572–580.
23 McKenzie, E. and MacLeay, J. (2011). Muscle disorders. In: *Equine Reproduction*, 2e (ed. A. McKinnon, E. Squires, W. Vaala, and D. Varner), 463–468. West Sussex, UK: Wiley Blackwell.
24 Sponseller, B.T., Valberg, S.J., Ward, T.L. et al. (2003). Muscular weakness and recumbency in a quarter horse colt due to glycogen branching enzyme deficiency. *Equine Vet. Educ.* 15: 182–188.
25 McCue, M.E., Valberg, S.J., Miller, M.B. et al. (2008). Glycogen synthase (GYS1) mutation causes a novel skeletal muscle glycogenosis. *Genomics* 91: 458–466.
26 Baird, J.D., Valberg, S.J., Anderson, S.M. et al. (2010). Presence of the glycogen synthase 1 (GYS1) mutation causing type 1 polysaccharide storage myopathy in continental European draught horse breeds. *Vet. Rec.* 167: 781–784.
27 McCoy, A.M., Schaefer, R., Petersen, J.L. et al. (2014). Evidence of positive selection for a glycogen synthase (gys1) mutation in domestic horse populations. *J. Hered.* 105: 163–172.
28 McCue, M.E., Anderson, S.M., Valberg, S.J. et al. (2010). Estimated prevalence of the type 1 polysaccharide storage myopathy mutation in selected north American and European breeds. *Anim. Genet.* 41: 145–149.
29 Stanley, R.L., McCue, M.E., Valberg, S.J. et al. (2009). A glycogen synthase 1 mutation associated with equine polysaccharide storage myopathy and exertional rhabdomyolysis occurs in a variety of UK breeds. *Equine Vet. J.* 41: 597–601.
30 Wagner, M.L., Valberg, S.J., Ames, E.G. et al. (2006). Allele frequency and likely impact of the glycogen branching enzyme deficiency gene in quarter horse and paint horse populations. *J. Vet. Intern. Med.* 20: 1207–1211.
31 Schambourg, M.A., Laverty, S., Mullim, S. et al. (2003). Thoracic trauma in foals: post mortem findings. *Equine Vet. J.* 35: 78–81.
32 Jean, D., Laverty, S., Halley, J. et al. (1999). Thoracic trauma in newborn foals. *Equine Vet. J. Br. Equine Vet. Assoc.* 31: 149–152.

33 Bellezzo, F., Hunt, R.J., Provost, P. et al. (2004). Surgical repair of rib fractures in 14 neonatal foals: case selection, surgical technique and results. *Equine Vet. J.* 36: 557–562.

34 Jean, D., Picandet, V., Macieira, S. et al. (2007). Detection of rib trauma in newborn foals in an equine critical care unit: a comparison of ultrasonography, radiography and physical examination. *Equine Vet. J.* 39: 158–163.

35 Sprayberry, K.A., Bain, F.T., Seahorn, T.L. et al. (2001). Cases of rib fractures in neonatal foals hospitalized in a referral center intensive care unit from 1997–2001. *Proc. Am. Assoc. Equine Pract.* 56: 395–399.

36 Kraus, B.M., Ross, M.W., and Boston, R.C. (2005). Surgical and nonsurgical management of sagittal slab fractures of the third carpal bone in racehorses: 32 cases (1991–2001). *J. Am. Vet. Med. Assoc.* 226: 945–950.

37 Downs, C. and Rodgerson, D. (2011). The use of nylon cable ties to repair rib fractures in neonatal foals. *Can. Vet. J.* 52: 307–309.

38 Williams, T.B., Williams, J.M., and Rodgerson, D.H. (2017). Internal fixation of fractured ribs in neonatal foals with nylon cable tie using a modified technique. *Can. Vet. J.* 58: 579–581.

39 Embertson, R.M., Bramlage, L.R., Herring, D.S., and Gabel, A.A. (1986). Physeal fractures in the horse: I. Classification and Incidence. *Vet. Surg.* 15: 223–229.

40 Embertson, R.M., Bramlage, L.R., and Gabel, A.A. (1986). Physeal fractures in the horse II. Management and outcome. *Vet. Surg.* 15: 230–236.

41 Watkins, J.P. (2006). Etiology, diagnosis, and treatment of long bone fractures in foals. *Clin. Tech. Equine Pract.* 5: 296–308.

42 Tartarniuk, D.M., Trumble, T.N., and Baxter, G.M. (2020). The physis/physeal fractures/physitis. In: *Adams and Stashak's Lameness in Horses*, 7e (ed. G.M. Baxter), 1033–1047. Wiley.

43 Levine, D.G. and Aitken, M.R. (2017). Physeal fractures in foals. *Vet. Clin. North Am. Equine Pract.* 33: 417–430.

44 Reesink, H.L. (2017). Foal fractures: osteochondral fragmentation, proximal sesamoid bone fractures/sesamoiditis, and distal phalanx fractures. *Vet. Clin. North Am. Equine Pract.* 33: 397–416.

45 Hunt, R.J. (2020). Lameness in foals. In: *Adams and Stashak's Lameness in Horses*, 7e (ed. G.J. Baxter), 1081–1089. Chichester, West Sussex: Wiley.

46 Ellis, D.R. (1979). Fractures of the proximal sesamoid bones in thoroughbred foals. *Equine Vet. J.* 11: 48–52.

47 Kaneps, A.J., O'Brien, T.R., Redden, R.F. et al. (1993). Characterisation of osseous bodies of the distal phalanx of foals. *Equine Vet. J.* 25: 285–292.

48 Faramarzi, B., Mcmicking, H., Halland, S. et al. (2015). Incidence of palmar process fractures of the distal phalanx and association with front hoof conformation in foals. *Equine Vet. J.* 47: 675–679.

49 Yovich, J.V., Stashak, T.S., DeBowes, R.M., and Ducharme, N.G. (1986). Fractures of the distal phalanx of the forelimb in eight foals. *J. Am. Vet. Med. Assoc.* 189: 550–554.

50 Furst, A.E. and Lischer, C.J. (2020). Foot. In: *Equine Surg*, 5e (ed. J.A. Auer, J.A. Stick, J.M. Kummerle, and T. Prange), 1543–1587. St. Louis: Elsevier.

51 Nixon, A.J. (2020). *Equine Fracture Repair*, 2e (ed. A.J. Nixon). Hoboken, NJ: Wiley Blackwell.

52 Auer, J.A. and Kummerle, J.M. (2019). Musculoskeletal System. In: *Equine Surgery*, 5e (ed. J.A. Auer, J.A. Stick, J.M. Kummerle, and T. Prange), 1220–1835. St. Louis: Elsevier.

53 Glass, K. and Watts, A.E. (2017). Diagnosis and treatment considerations for nonphyseal long bone fractures in the foal. *Vet. Clin. North Am. Equine Pract.*. W.B. Saunders 33 (2): 431–438.

54 Orsini, J.A., Buonanno, A.M., Richardson, D.W., and Nunamaker, D.N. (1990). Condylar buttress plate fixation of femoral fracture in a colt. *J. Am. Vet. Med. Assoc.* 197: 1184–1186.

55 Carter, B.G., Schneider, R.K., Hardy, J. et al. (1993). Assessment and treatment of equine humeral fractures: retrospective study of 54 cases (1972–1990). *Equine Vet. J.* 25: 203–207.

56 Rakestraw, P.C., Nixon, A.J., Kaderly, R.E., and Ducharme, N.G. (1991). Cranial approach to the humerus for repair of fractures in horses and cattle. *Vet. Surg.* 20: 1–8.

57 Hance, S.R., Bramlage, L.R., Schneider, R.K., and Embertson, R.M. (1992). Retrospective study of 38 cases of femur fractures in horses less than one year of age. *Equine Vet. J.* 24: 357–363.

58 MacLellan, K.N.M., MacDonald, D.G., and Crawford, W.H. (1997). Lag screw fixation of an extensor process fracture in a foal with flexural deformity. *Can. Vet. J.* 38: 226–228.

59 Schnabel, L.V., Bramlage, L.R., Mohammed, H.O. et al. (2007). Racing performance after arthroscopic removal of apical sesamoid fracture fragments in Thoroughbred horses age <2 years: 151 cases (1989–2002). *Equine Vet. J.* 39: 64–68.

60 Kamm, J.L., Bramlage, L.R., Schnabel, L.V. et al. (2011). Size and geometry of apical sesamoid fracture fragments as a determinant of prognosis in Thoroughbred racehorses. *Equine Vet. J.* 43: 412–417.

61 Honnas, C.M., Snyder, J.R., Meagher, D.M., and Ragle, C.A. (1990). Traumatic disruption of the suspensory apparatus in foals. *Cornell Vet.* 80: 123–133.

62 Yovich, J., Stashak, T., and McIlwraith, C. (1984). Rupture of the common digital extensor tendon in foals. *Compend. Contin. Educ. Pract. Vet.* 6: 373–378.

63 Myers, V. and Gordon, G. (1976). Ruptured common digital extensor tendons associated with contracted flexor

tendons in foals. *Proc. 21st Ann Conv Am Assoc. Equine Prat* 67–74.

64 Fackelman, G. (1981). Equine flexural deformities of developmental origin. *Proc. 26th Ann Conv Am Assoc. Equine Prat.* 97–105.

65 Auer, J.A. (2006). Diagnosis and treatment of flexural deformities in foals. *Clin. Tech. Equine Pract.* 5: 282–295.

66 Stevenson, W.L. and Stevenson, W.G. (1942). Rupture of the common digital extensor. *Can. J. Comp. Med. Vet. Sci.* 6: 197–203.

67 Trumble, T.N. (2005). Orthopedic disorders in neonatal foals. *Vet. Clin. North Am. Equine Pract.* 21: 357–385.

68 Blikslager, A.T. and Bristol, D.G.D. (1994). Avulsion of the origin of the peroneus tertius tendon in a foal. *J. Am. Vet. Med. Assoc.* 204: 1483–1485.

69 Holcombe, S.J. and Bertone, A.L. (1994). Avulsion fracture of the origin of the extensor digitorum longus muscle in a foal. *J. Am. Vet. Med. Assoc.* 204: 1652–1654.

70 Szabuniewicz, M. and Titus, R.S. (1967). Rupture of the peroneus tertius in the horse. *Vet. Med. Small Anim. Clin.* 62: 993–995.

71 Koch, C., Brounts, S., and Foerner, J. (2009). What is your diagnosis? *J. Am. Vet. Med. Assoc.* 234: 1389–1390.

72 Beccati, F., Pepe, M., Dante, S. et al. (2013). Avulsion fracture of the origin of the peroneus tertius in a foal. *Ipplogia* 24: 15–20.

73 Sprinkle, F., Swerczek, T., and Crowe, M. (1985). Gastrocnemius muscle rupture and hemorrhage in foals. *Equine Pract.* 7: 10–17.

74 Jesty, S.A., Palmer, J.E., Parente, E.J. et al. (2005). Rupture of the gastrocnemius muscle in six foals. *J. Am. Vet. Med. Assoc.* 227: 1965–1968.

75 Tull, T.M., Woodie, J.B., Ruggles, A.J. et al. (2009). Management and assessment of prognosis after gastrocnemius disruption in thoroughbred foals: 28 cases (1993–2007). *Equine Vet. J.* 41: 541–546.

76 Valdez, H., Coy, C.H., and Swanson, T. (1982). Flexible carbon fiber for repair of gastrocnemius and superficial digital flexor tendons in a heifer and gastrocnemius tendon in a foal. *J. Am. Vet. Med. Assoc.* 181: 154–157.

77 Sato, F., Shibata, R., Shikichi, M. et al. (2014). Rupture of the gastrocnemius muscle in neonatal thoroughbred foals: a report of three cases. *J. Equine Sci.* 25: 61–64.

78 Pascoe, R.R. (1975). Letter: death due to rupture of the origin of the gastrocnemius muscles in a filly. *Aust. Vet. J.* 51: 107.

79 Bramlage, L. (1993). Identification, examination, and treament of physitis in the foal. *Proc. 39th Ann Conv Am Assoc. Equine Prat* 39: 57–62.

80 Bramlage, L.R. (2011). Physitis in the horse. *Equine Vet. Educ.* 23: 548–552.

81 Hunt, R. (2011). Lameness in foals. In: *Diagnosis and Management of Lameness in the Horse*, 2e (ed. M. Ross and S.J. Dyson), 1242–1252. St. Louis: Saunders.

Neonatal Integumentary System

Chapter 38 Embryology and Anatomy of the Integument

Rebecca Ruby

Anatomy of the integument is based on the major function of this organ, which is to serve as a boundary between the environment and the remainder of the body. Additionally, the skin acts as a sensory organ, allows for movement, assists with thermoregulation, and aids immune function. To this effect, the outermost layer of the integument is the stratum corneum, which helps decrease water loss and is composed of terminally differentiated keratin squames. This layer is constantly renewed and shed which results in physical removal of potential pathogens. Additionally, this layer contains antimicrobial peptides and lipids to provide additional layers of defense. The integument is composed of the epidermis, dermis, subcutis, adnexal glands, and hooves (Figure 38.1). Adnexal units include hair follicles, epithrichial apocrine glands, eccrine glands, sebaceous glands, and arrector pilli muscles.

The epidermis has four distinct layers, the stratum basale, stratum spinosum, stratum granulosum, and stratum corneum. Stem cells within the basal layer proliferate into amplifying cells which then detach from the basement membrane and differentiate into keratinocytes. The stratum basale is a single layer of cells that rests on the basement membrane zone and is attached the basement membrane by hemidesmosomes. Basal cells are attached to each other and the overlying keratinocytes by desmosomes, adhesion molecules that are the target of several dermal autoimmune diseases. The stratum spinosum and stratum granulosum are thicker in areas of nonhaired skin. The outer stratum corneum is composed of anucleate cells, which create a hydrophobic barrier.

Cells in the epidermis that are not keratinocytes include melanocytes, which provide melanin pigment to keratinocytes. In addition, Langerhans cells are antigen-presenting cells found in the stratum basale and stratum spinosum. The junction between the epidermis and dermis is the basement membrane zone, which anchors the epidermis to the dermis. Abnormalities in the basement membrane zone are associated with severe bullous diseases. Underlying the basement membrane zone is the dermis which is responsible for the strength and elasticity of the skin. Within the dermis are collagen, elastin, blood vessels, nerves, lymphatics, and low numbers of lymphoid cells, predominantly T helper cells.

Hair begins to form in the developing fetus at approximately 9.5 months of gestation. In the full-term fetus, the normal hair coat density should be present. The hair follicle of horses is a simple follicle in which a single hair emerges from the follicular opening. The hair bulb is composed of proliferating matrix cells and melanocytes. The outer root sheath is an extension of the epidermis while the inner root sheath arises from the matrix cells.

The integument system includes the skin, hair, hooves, and skin glands. Embryologically, the integument is formed from the endoderm, ectoderm, and neural crest [1]. The epidermis is derived from the ectoderm while the dermis is derived from the mesoderm. The epidermis is derived from a single layer of cuboidal cells that divide into multiple layers, beginning with the periderm and basal layer or stratum germinativum. The periderm undergoes apoptosis at the time when epidermal and amniotic exchange of water and electrolytes ends. The basal layer is retained and continues to divide to form the epidermis and differentiates into hair germs, which will become hair follicles, sebaceous glands, and sweat glands. Melanoblasts migrate from the neural crest to the basal layer of the epithelium where they differentiate into melanocytes, which synthesize melanin pigment [1]. Langerhans cells migrate from bone marrow to the stratum spinosum and other layers; here they function as antigen presenting cells for T lymphocytes.

Beneath the epidermis is the dermis which is derived from dermatomal cells and somatopleural mesoderm and forms collagenous and elastin fibers [1]. In most of the body, the layer underneath the dermis is the hypodermis, also referred to as the subcutaneous connective tissue or

Equine Neonatal Medicine, First Edition. Edited by David M. Wong and Pamela A. Wilkins.

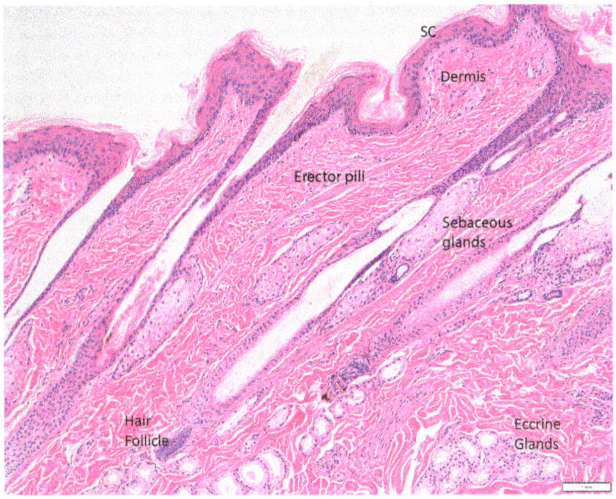

Figure 38.1 Histopathological section of integument contains epidermis (stratum corneum that is a hydrophobic barrier) (SC), dermis, hair follicle, erector pili muscle, sebaceous glands, and eccrine glands. Image courtesy of Dr. Amanda Fales-Williams, Iowa State University.

superficial fascia. This layer of tissue anchors the skin to the structures beneath it. Horses have a relatively thin hypodermis, which results in the skin having low mobility and clearly outlines the underlying bone and muscle.

Hair follicle formation requires interactions between the epidermis and mesoderm to stimulate local development while inhibiting development in adjacent tissue, resulting in appropriate spacing. Proliferation of the basal layer of the epidermis into the mesoderm forms hair buds. As the hair bud extends into the dermis, the hair papilla projects into the tip. The epidermal ingrowth and papilla are called the hair follicle and the inner epidermal layer gives rise to the hair shaft and epithelial root sheaths. Three bulges are formed in this process: the lowest is the attachment for the arrector pili muscle; the middle differentiates into the sebaceous gland; and the upper buldge forms the epitrichial sweat gland. Arrector pili muscles are derived from mesenchymal cells surrounding the developing follicle, and sebaceous glands form from outgrowths of the basal layer. Sweat glands develop from more superficial portions of the follicular wall. Horses only have primary hair follicles, distributed evenly in rows that are simple follicles (only one hair shaft emerges from one follicular infundibulum) [1].

Hair growth is cyclical with the active growing stage (anagen) followed by a transitional (catagen) and resting stage (telogen). The hair's cycle is independent of neighboring hairs, and length is related to rate of growth and duration of the anagen phase. Horses have well-developed sebaceous glands that secrete a combination of lipid, keratin, and keratinohylaline granules. The content of these granules combine with the high protein content from sweat glands to create the thick, white lather seen when horses sweat heavily. The apocine or epitrichial sweat glands are developed from the primary hair germ and function in thermoregulation.

Underlying the dermis is the subcutis formed by lipocytes, collagen, and blood vessels. This layer is of mesenchymal origin and is typically the thickest layer of the skin. It functions as an energy reserve, insulation, and support, and is involved in steroid metabolism, acting as a reservoir and site of metabolism and production. The thickness of the skin decreases from dorsal to ventral on the trunk and proximally to distally on the limbs.

The hoof is developed from the epidermis on the dorsal and lateral portions of the terminal region of the third digit. In the first 2 months of gestation the epidermis thickens and covers a thin dermis. In the third month the cornium and hypodermis increase in growth and the frog and heal bulbs increase in depth leading to features and shape of the adult hoof. The hoof is anchored to the underlying connective tissue by secondary laminae, which are derived from both the coronary cushion and hoof wall; these interdigitate with each other.

Peripheral nerves are comprised of connective tissue and conducting fibers [2]. The area of the skin supplied by branches of one spinal nerve is the dermatome. The sensory innervation to the skin is a precise process in which axons from each dorsal root ganglion extend along a predetermined pathway to the appropriate dermatome. The connective tissue structures of the peripheral nerves consist of three distinct sheaths: endoneurium, perineurium, and epineurium, from innermost to outermost, respectively [2]. All peripheral nerves, myelinated or unmyelinated, are surrounded by Schwann cells. The embryonic origin of non-neuronal components (perineurial cells, endoneurial fibroblasts, and pericytes) of the peripheral nerve connective tissue is poorly understood. It is suggested that multipotent neural crest stem cells generate neurons, Schwann cells, and myofibroblasts [2]. Peripheral nerve development is a complicated and integrated process. Axons grow toward their target organs with variation in chemical difference between axons directing targeted growth. The axon is led on its route by a growth cone that depends on both attraction and repulsion through contact and chemical signals.

References

1 Som, P.M., Laitman, J.T., and Mak, K. (2017). Embryology and anatomy of the skin, its appendages, and physiologic changes in the head and neck. *Neurographics* 7 (5): 390–415.

2 Onger, M.E., Türkmen, A.P., Elibol, E. et al. (2015). Embryology of the peripheral nerves. *Nerves and Nerve Injuries* 1: 37–40.

Chapter 39 Diagnostics, Therapeutics, and Monitoring of Skin Diseases in the Foal

Darren Berger

During the neonatal period in horses there are a limited number of dermatologic conditions that occur. These cutaneous processes can be broken down to inherited or congenital diseases such as junctional epidermolysis bullosa and fragile foal syndrome or acquired skin disorders including lacerations, secondary infections, or parasitic conditions. Although the number of diseases is limited given the general timeframe under discussion, the diagnostic and therapeutic options available are similar in horses at any age. The following is an overview of dermatologic diagnostics and basic dermatologic therapies.

Skin Scraping, Acetate Tape Impression, and Combing

Skin scraping is primarily used to identify ectoparasites, which may be causing cutaneous lesions. The procedure is inexpensive and easy to perform but is limited in the neonatal foal given the lack of parasitic infestations that are recognized during this time frame. To perform a skin scrape, the hair can be lightly clipped from an affected site to facilitate sample collection. Mineral oil should then be placed directly on the skin and on a clean glass slide. A clean #10 scalpel blade or a small medical metal spatula (Figure 39.1) is used to scrape the affected site. The area scraped and procedure varies slightly with the suspected ectoparasite. In the case of superficial parasites that reside outside of the hair follicle (*Chorioptes* spp. or lice), a large area roughly the size of a monetary bill should be scrapped. In instances where the parasite causes a folliculitis (*Pelodera* dermatitis), the skin should be pinched or massaged prior and then a deeper scraping performed over a surface area about the size of a large coin. The collected material is then placed on a glass slide with mineral oil to distribute the sample evenly. A glass coverslip is placed over the sample to decrease the depth of field and enhance refractility along with protecting the microscope. The sample is scanned with the microscope condenser closed under 4x to 10x magnification. Lower magnification increases speed but should only be used by the experienced practitioner.

Acetate tape impression is a simple alternative to skin scraping but requires practice and is only beneficial for superficial parasites in outer surface debris (*Dermanyssus gallinae, Trombicula* spp., or *Oxyuris equi*). The tape is firmly pressed over affected areas and then placed on a glass slide with mineral oil between the glass and adhesive side of the tape. A drop or two of mineral oil and a glass cover slip may also be placed over the back side of the tape. The tape sample is then scanned in a similar manner to a skin scrape, with the observer using the fine focus of their microscope to view the different planes. Although quicker and easier than scraping, this technique is limited and requires time to view all the planes in the sample.

In cases of suspected lice infestation, a fine-toothed comb such as a flea comb can be used to collect and comb surface debris into a collection vessel. The debris is then grossly examined or transferred to mineral oil on a glass slide, similar to a skin scrape, and observed under low magnification.

Direct Examination of Hair (Trichogram)

Direct examination of hair can provide useful information but is limited in that it is highly sensitive and can be similar to finding the proverbial "needle in a haystack." To perform this procedure, hairs are plucked by pulling in the direction of hair growth to minimize trauma to the hairs and acquire whole hairs. The hairs are then positioned in a similar orientation on a glass slide with mineral oil and a cover slip placed over the sample to decrease the number of focal

Equine Neonatal Medicine, First Edition. Edited by David M. Wong and Pamela A. Wilkins.

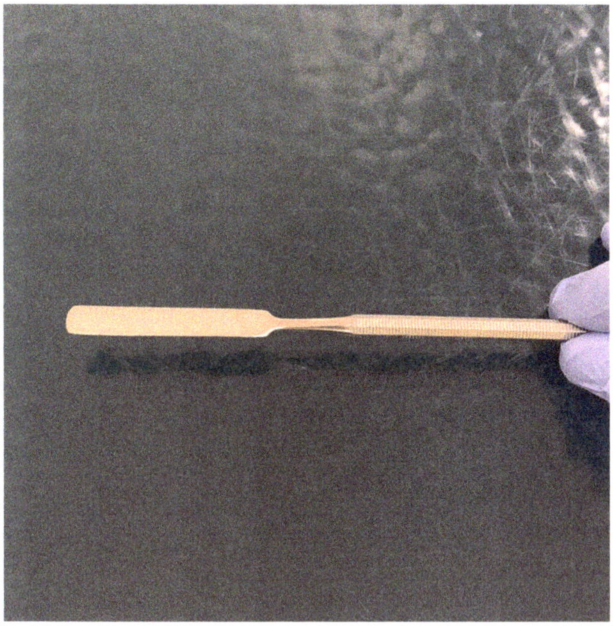

Figure 39.1 Medical metal spatula used as an alternative to scalpel blades for acquiring skin scrape samples.

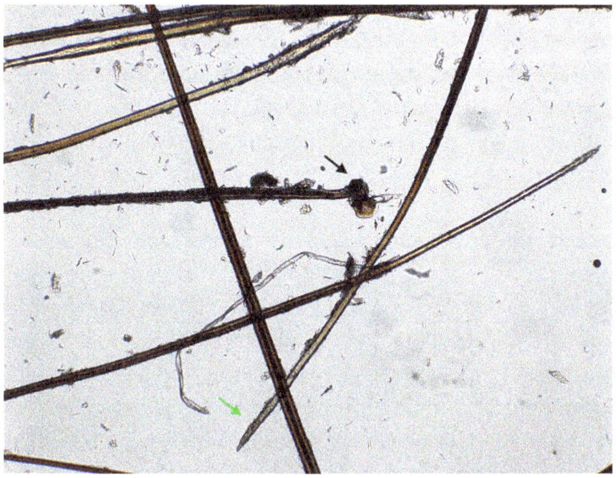

Figure 39.2 Trichogram from a horse. Black arrow denotes a bent or curled root end seen with anagen hairs, while the green arrow identifies a spear-like appearance observed with telogen hairs.

planes and protect the microscope. An adequate sample should contain roughly 20 hairs. The growth phase (anagen vs. telogen) of the hairs is determined by examining the roots. Anagen hairs have a rounded and bent-over root while telogen hairs have a more pointed or irregular root (Figure 39.2). Plucked hairs should be a mixture of anagen and telogen. Examination of the hair shaft is also performed. Irregular or twisted hairs might indicate nutritional disorders, while fractured or split hairs are suggestive of self-trauma associated with pruritus. Swollen and misshapen hair shafts are observed with dermatophytosis (Figure 39.3).

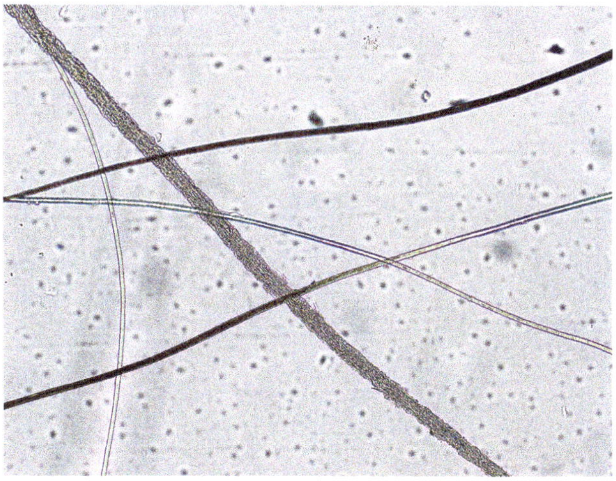

Figure 39.3 Trichogram from a horse showing a swollen hair affected by a dermatophyte species, causing loss of hair definition and "ball-like" ectothrix spores lining the outside of the hair shaft.

Cytology

Cytology is the most common dermatologic technique performed when evaluating any horse presenting for cutaneous disease. There are several different techniques for acquiring samples, which depend on the lesion and individual procuring the sample. Two of the more common methods are the use of acetate tape and a simple impression smear. Acetate tape is helpful for dry, scaly, or hard-to-sample areas such as around the head. This sample requires some practice reading, as the technique tends to yield a large amount of material on the sample to look through. Impression smears are more useful for exudative lesions and is collected by pressing a clean glass slide directly to the lesion or using the edge of the slide to rupture a pustule or lift a crust up prior to directly pressing the slide onto the exudate. Again, these are two of many described methods for sample acquisition, with the purpose of any cytologic technique being to get a sample on a slide to stain and examine. Special consideration for dermatophilosis (rain rot of scald) is worth mentioning. When suspected, early exudative crusted lesions may be removed, and the exudative surface pressed to the glass slide. If older dry lesions are present, the crusts can be removed and placed in a small amount of sterile saline and then macerated prior to placing a drop of the mixture on a glass slide to subsequently air dry and then stain. Most cytologic samples are stained with a Romanowsky stain variant such as Diff-Quik. It is important to note that if an adhesive cytology technique such as acetate tape is utilized, that these samples are not placed through the fixative (first stain) as it will cloud the sample and make it incredibly difficult to review. Additionally, Gram stain is a simple and

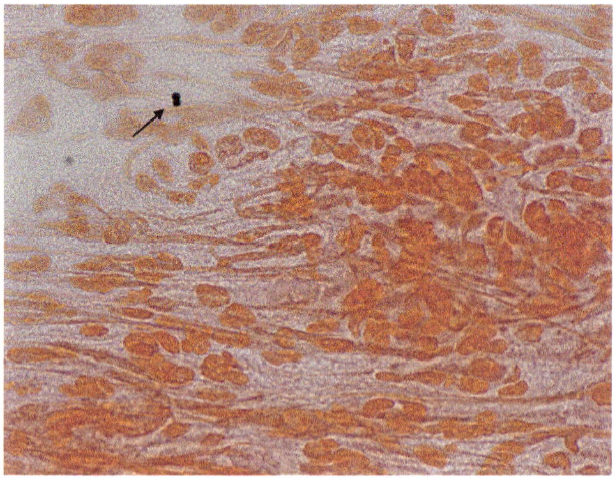

Figure 39.4 Gram stain of an impression smear from an ulcerated lesion in a horse. The black arrow identifies a pair of Gram-positive coccoid bacteria consistent with *Staphylococcus* spp., which are easily seen against the pink background of white blood cells.

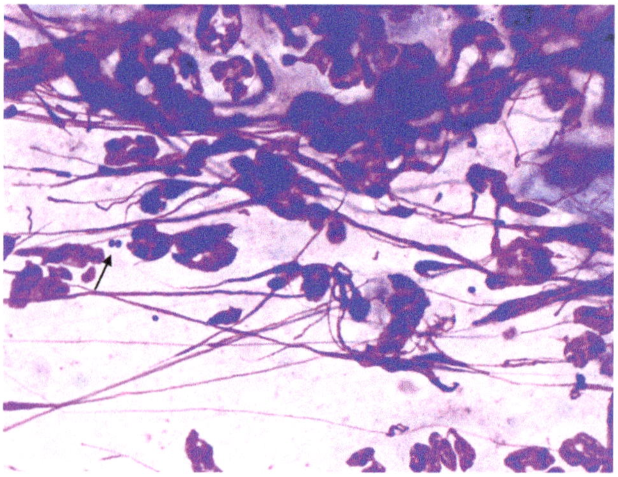

Figure 39.5 Diff-Quik stain of an impression smear from the same ulcerated lesion as Figure 39.4. The black arrow indicates a pair of extracellular coccoid-shaped bacteria that is commonly observed with staphylococcal infections.

inexpensive stain, which can be helpful to highlight bacteria and provide further information regarding bacterial populations present (Figure 39.4).

Following staining, samples are microscopically reviewed. When examining a slide, the clinician should first view the slide under a low power objective to find areas of interest (presence of leukocytes) and to gain a general impression of what is present on the sample. Once scanned, the sample should then be reviewed under a high dry or oil immersion lens. The presence and type of inflammatory cells may provide information regarding the underlying disease process and chronicity. When examining a slide to determine if potential secondary infections are present, it is helpful to consider the type of lesion that was sampled. It is common for nonintact or covered lesions to reveal a mixed bacterial population or the presence of environmental molds. The presence of intracellular bacteria is ideal to facilitate a diagnosis of bacterial infection, but many bacteria such as *Staphylococcus* spp. are also commonly found extracellularly (Figure 39.5). Clinical judgment is always warranted when interpreting cytology samples from horses as no predetermined number, type, or shape of bacteria or yeast will determine if treatment should be instituted.

Fine-Needle Aspiration

Fine-needle aspiration is not commonly used in equine dermatology but may be helpful for nodular or vesicular lesions. A small-gauge needle (22 g) is attached to a 6 ml syringe and inserted into the lesion. Once the needle is in the lesion, a small amount of negative pressure is maintained on the syringe, while the needle is redirected. Once complete, the negative pressure is released prior to removing the needle from the lesion. The needle is then removed from the syringe, the syringe is filled with air before the needle is reattached, and then the contents are blown or expelled onto a clean sample slide; the sample is then smeared using a second glass slide into a monolayer for examination. Smaller or larger syringes may be used, which will either create less or more negative pressure, respectively, during aspiration. An alternative method known as fenestration can also be performed where a small-gauge needle is held between the clinician's fingers while the hub of the needle is covered. The needle is then repeatedly inserted and redirected in the lesion to collect the sample. The needle is then attached to an air-filled syringe to expel the collected material onto a slide. Slides can either be stained, similar to cytology samples, or submitted to reference laboratories.

Culture and PCR

Bacterial culture and antimicrobial susceptibility testing are helpful for proper identification of organisms and guiding appropriate antimicrobial decision-making when disease is severe, rapidly progressive, or initial empiric therapy has failed. A knowledge of the clinical relevance of various bacterial agents and the degree of care when sampling is highly imperative with obtaining and interpreting bacterial culture results from foals. Isolation of a coagulase-positive *Staphylococcal* spp. should be seen as a significant finding with the incidence of encountering methicillin-resistant strains rates growing [1]. Coagulase-negative *Staphylococci* are common commensals on the skin of healthy horses and are common contaminants. These strains are also frequently methicillin-resistant in isolation [2]. When isolated, coagulase-negative species should be considered a contaminate and the diagnosis re-evaluated unless it is the only organism isolated and cytologic evidence was consistent with the presence of *Staphylococcus* spp. [3].

Dermatophytosis is not common in immunocompetent horses but is seen more frequently in foals. It should be suspected in any case where patchy alopecia and crusting are encountered. Cultures for dermatophytes are acquired either by collecting hairs from the margin of new lesions or via toothbrush sampling. To obtain a toothbrush sample, a sterile toothbrush is used to brush the hairs in the affected region until the bristles visibly contain scales and hairs. Submission of samples to veterinary diagnostic laboratories that have experience with dermatophyte isolation and identification from horses is preferred to in-hospital commercial media preparations due to rapid overgrowth of the plates with commensal and environmental fungi. Wiping suspected lesions with alcohol and allowing it to air dry prior to sampling has been a proposed strategy to avoid issues with contaminant overgrowth. When performing in-house cultures, it is important to realize that dermatophytes do not yield pigmented colony growth on culture plates and that many things may cause color changes with selective media. All suspect growth should be examined microscopically for pathogen identification.

Recently, PCR-based diagnostic tests for identification of dermatophyte species have become commercially available. These tests offer a rapid alternative to traditional culture-based techniques and can be helpful to prevent disease outbreaks and environmental contamination. Samples are often collected and submitted in a similar fashion to those for traditional dermatophyte culture. Exact submission criteria should always be checked with the diagnostic laboratory prior to sample submission as variations in criteria exist. Although these tests offer expedited results, they should be combined with traditional culture to improve the overall accuracy and clinical utility and to avoid false negative and positive results [4].

Biopsy

Biopsy with histopathologic interpretation is an underutilized diagnostic in equine dermatology. Biopsy, in many instances, is the only diagnostic test that provides a definitive diagnosis of conditions that afflict the horse, especially foals. Most samples can be acquired with local anesthesia (i.e. lidocaine) or mild sedation combined with local anesthesia. Samples should be acquired with no surgical preparation as preparing the skin may remove scales or crusts or damage fragile lesions that are needed for diagnosis. Clipping of hair should also be avoided for similar reasons. When punch biopsies are used, samples should be acquired with the largest punch (6 or 8 mm) from the center of the primary lesions and multiple samples should be obtained. If 1 cm or larger samples are indicated, incisional biopsies with a scalpel blade are preferred. Similarly, to using a punch biopsy, the transitional zone of normal to affected skin should be avoided as once the sample is place in formalin the two areas cannot be differentiated. As a result, lesions may be missed when samples are sectioned during sample processing at the diagnostic laboratory. Two other considerations are that if nodules are present, samples should be taken from unruptured lesions, and if the sample is being submitted for tissue culture, the surface should be surgically prepped, rinsed with sterile saline, and the epidermis removed from the sample to increase the chances of culturing a primary deep pathogen.

Dermatologic Therapy

Therapeutic intervention in neonatal foals is usually a combination of topical and systemic medications. In many cases topical interventions are preferred given the possible complications associated with many systemic medications in the equine species. However, knowledge of the lesion type and purpose of therapy is needed to determine which route or if combination therapy are needed to provide a successful outcome. Topical therapy is preferred when superficial and focal lesions are present while diffuse and deep lesions require systemic therapy. When deep lesions (draining tracts, cellulitis) are present, topical medications are unlikely to penetrate the entire lesion depth and should not be used as monotherapy.

Topical therapy has many advantages including decreased requirement or therapeutic course of systemic medications, physical removal of crusts and pathogens, delivery of high concentrations of medication to the affected site, and improving overall cutaneous health. Historically, many topical formulations used were products marketed for small animals that also were labeled for horses. Recently, newer topical products have been directly produced for horses and prepared in a variety of formulations that are more suited to the horse and include shampoos, sprays, and salves that are more intuitive and size appropriate for horse owners. Regardless of the topical product selected, contact time is an essential element of successful therapy. With sprays, leave-on lotions, and shampoos, many dermatologists prefer a contact time of 10 minutes before the product is rinsed away.

The most common reason topical therapy is instituted in a neonatal foal is the treatment of secondary bacterial infections. Although many products have been advocated for this purpose, there is a lack of well-designed controlled trials that provide evidence to guide medical decisions. As a result, extrapolation from other species where similar infections arise is commonly used, along with expert opinion. The active ingredients that are commonly suggested based on these criteria are chlorhexidine (2–4%), benzoyl peroxide, and silver sulfadiazine. Benzoyl peroxide is also beneficial for removing crusts and for greasy lesions, but it can be drying, irritating, and disrupt the epidermal barrier if overused. Silver sulfadiazine cream may be occlusive and need to be avoided in overly exudative lesions. Chlorhexidine is consistently effective for *Staphylococcal* pyoderma and in many instances can be used as a sole therapy when applied frequently. Chlorhexidine is also very effective in the treatment of dermatophilosis.

Systemic therapy for dermatologic conditions should be used with caution in horses due to many adverse events that have been encountered, specifically those that are gastrointestinal in nature. The most commonly utilized medications administered systemically include glucocorticoids and antimicrobials. Glucocorticoids are predominantly used for immune-mediated and inflammatory conditions. Dexamethasone tends to be the most commonly prescribed while prednisolone is also routinely used. It is worth noting that prednisone cannot be substituted for prednisolone during therapy due to a lack of hepatic metabolism in the horse. Doses and protocols for treatment with glucocorticoids vary widely based on the condition and formulation being utilized. The reader is advised to consult other drug reference books for specific doses and protocols for the specific condition being treated. With regards to systemic antimicrobials, oral potentiated sulfonamides are preferred given their distribution to the skin and microbial organisms commonly associated with skin infections (*Staphylococcus* spp. and *Dermatophilus congolensis*).

Monitoring

Monitoring of dermatologic care in the neonatal foal should be daily to weekly, depending on the severity of the specific condition being treated. Skin infections should show noticeable improvement within 5–7 days with appropriate medical intervention. If clinical worsening or a lack of improvement is seen over 7 days, the therapeutic intervention should be reevaluated and likely changed. If a foal is placed on a systemic antimicrobial, particular attention for any signs of lameness and GI motility disturbances should be monitored. When glucocorticoids are required for therapy, it is important to ensure they are continued daily until full clinical resolution is appreciated prior tapering. Early tapering prior to complete resolution of clinical symptoms can result in disease flare-ups that may be more recalcitrant to therapeutic intervention.

References

1. Boyen, F., Smet, A., Hermans, K. et al. (2013). Methicillin resistant staphylococci and broad-spectrum B-lactamse producing *Enterbacteriaceae* in horses. *Vet. Microbiol.* 167: 67–77.
2. Vengust, M., Anderson, M.E., Rousseau, J. et al. (2006). Methicillin-resistant staphylococcal colonization in clinically normal dogs and horses in the community. *Lett. Appl. Microbiol.* 43: 602–606.
3. Rook, K.A., Brown, D.C., Ranken, S.C. et al. (2012). Case-control study of *Staphylococcus lugdunensis* infection isolates from small companion animals. *Vet. Dermatol.* 23: 476–e90.
4. Tartor, Y.H., El Damaty, H.M., and Mahmmod, Y.S. (2016). Diagnostic performance of molecular and conventional methods for identification of dermatophyte species from clinically infected Arabian horses in Egypt. *Vet. Dermatol.* 27: 401–e102.

Chapter 40 Congenital and Inherited Skin Disorders

Rebecca Ruby

Numerous congenital and inherited disorders involving the dermis and mucous membranes are recognized in foals. The majority of these conditions were first identified as a spectrum of clinical and/or pathologic findings, often within one or two specific breeds. Significant advances in the last several decades have resulted in identification of the genetic basis for many of these conditions.

Lavender Foal Syndrome (LFS)

Lavender foal syndrome (LFS) is a lethal inherited disease primarily seen in foals with Egyptian Arabian breeding and is inherited in an autosomal recessive pattern. Lavender foal syndrome is clinically recognized by the combination of a dilute hair color and multiple neurologic abnormalities, including seizure-like activity, opisthotonos, and paddling. Foals fail to stand and nurse and may be misdiagnosed with neonatal enceophalopathy. Despite the name, affected foals are often not lavender or silver but rather light gray or pale chestnut, depending on the color coat dilution [1]. Affected foals are homozygous for a mutation in the MYO5A gene, which was identified as responsible for this condition [2]. This gene is involved in organelle transport and membrane trafficking, along with axonal and dendrite transport in neurons [3]. Diagnosis is based on signalment and characteristic coat color dilution, with definitive diagnosis made via DNA testing to demonstrate the presence of the mutated MYO5A gene (see Chapter 31).

Epitheliogenesis Imperfecta and Junctional Epidermolysis Bullosa

Epitheliogenesis imperfecta and junctional epidermolysis bullosa are reported in the literature as rare, hereditary mechanobullous diseases. Epitheliogenesis imperfecta is a mechanobullous disease characterized by segmental absence of the epidermis and epithelial derived structures of the skin. Epidermolysis bullosa includes a number of epidermal disorders manifesting as blistering and fragility of the skin and mucosa. In people, different forms of epidermolysis bullosa are recognized and differ genotypically, phenotypically, and by anatomic site of epidermal disruption. The junctional form of epidermolysis bullosa referred to as junctional epidermolysis bullosa involves blistering within the lamina lucida of the basement membrane zone and is associated with mutations in genes that encode the polypeptide subunits that comprise the laminin 5 molecule. Laminin 5 is involved in cell adhesion, motility, and proliferation.

Epitheliogenesis imperfecta was historically diagnosed in American Saddlebred and Belgian foals; however, histopathologic features and identification of the causative genetic mutation indicate these are actually cases of junctional epidermolysis bullosa (Figures 40.1 and 40.2) [4]. Clinically, foals present at birth or within 48 hours with vesicles and bullae progressing to ulceration with marked crusting and exudate. The most severely affected areas are the mucocutaneous junctions and sites over bony prominences. These skin defects may be variable in size; foals often do not nurse well because of oral lesions. The teeth of affected foals may also be pitted and irregular (Figure 40.1) [6]. No treatment is available so affected foals are often euthanized or die from complications if significant amounts of skin are affected. American Saddlebred foals with these lesions were identified to have a mutation in the LAMA3 gene, which codes for the α-3 glycoprotein subunit of laminin 5 (Figure 40.2). The frequency of the mutation in American Saddlebreds is estimated at 0.026 [5].

Belgian draft horses with junctional epidermolysis bullosa have a mutation causing a cytosine insertion in the LAMC2 gene, which results in abnormal laminin 5 [7]. Junctional epidermolysis bullosa in Belgian draft horses is

Equine Neonatal Medicine, First Edition. Edited by David M. Wong and Pamela A. Wilkins.

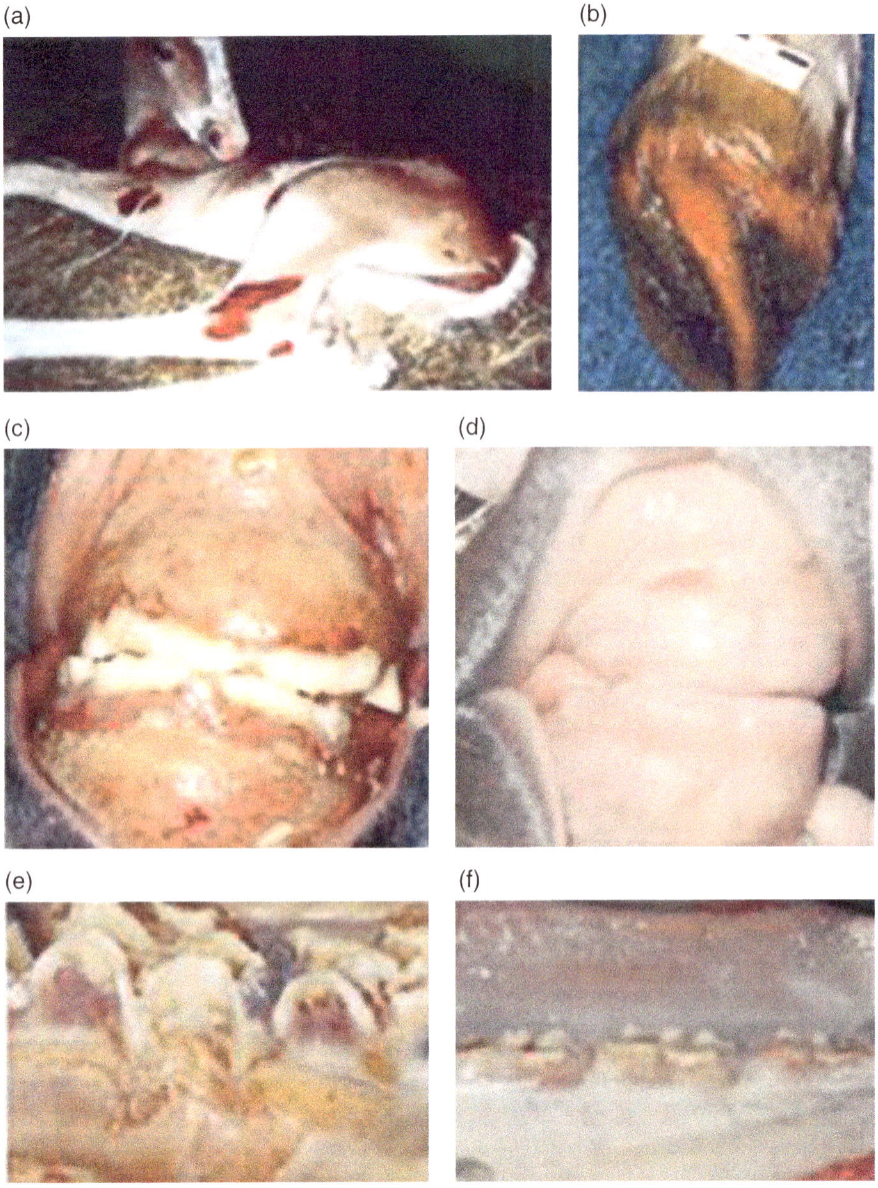

Figure 40.1 (a)–(f) Belgian foal with junctional epidermolysis bullosa demonstrating extensive erosions over the pressure points of carpal, tarsal, and femorotibial joints (a) and exungulation of the hoofs (b). Extensive loss of buccal mucous membrane around junction of teeth and gums, detected at bith (c), Erosions are associated with eruption of deciduous incisor (c) and premolar teeth (e), which are irregularly shaped, with serrated edges and pitted enamel. Normal mucous membranes and premolars for comparison (d), (f) [4].

an autosomal recessive trait for which a DNA test is available to identify carriers. In North America, 17% of Belgian horses were carriers of the mutation and in Europe 8–27% were carriers [8]. Over 100 American Saddlebred horses, including the dam and sire of a foal with junctional epidermolysis bullosa, were tested for this mutation, and there was no evidence that the LAMC2 mutation was responsible for cases of junctional epidermolysis bullosa in American Saddlebreds [9].

The gross appearance is nearly pathognomonic for junctional epidermolysis bullosa; however, vesiculobullous diseases from autoimmune or drug reactions are differentials. Subepidermal bullous disease was identified in a 1-day-old Appaloosa foal that presented with vesicles and bullae over the oral, anal, and genital mucosal surfaces. Ulcers and petechial hemorrhages were also evident on the oral mucosa. Biopsies of affected skin were consistent with a subepidermal vesiculobullous disease with neutrophilic infiltrates. The foal was treated with ceftiofur sodium therapy for 1 week. All skin lesions resolved 2 weeks following discharge and the foal was reported to be normal at 9 months. The presumptive diagnosis was bullous drug eruption secondary to topical iodine exposure at birth [10].

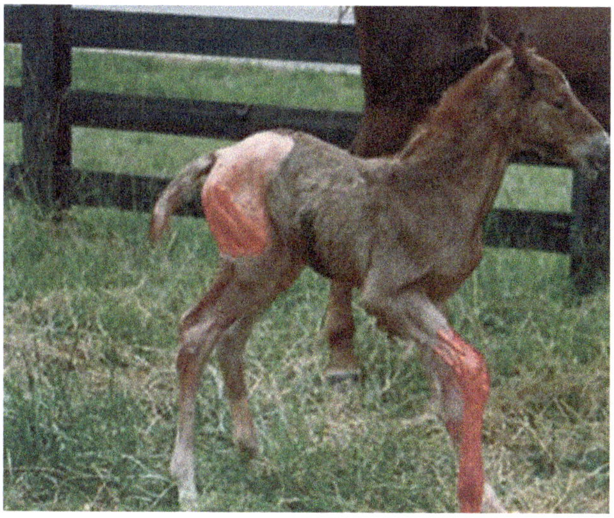

Figure 40.2 Saddlebred foal with epitheliogenesis imperfecta, more currently defined as junctional epidermolysis bullosa [5].

Hereditary Equine Regional Dermal Asthenia (HERDA)

Hereditary Equine Regional Dermal Asthenia (HERDA) occurs due to a genetic mutation affecting collagen of the skin and connective tissues of Quarter Horses and horses with Quarter Horse lineage (Appaloosas, American Paint Horses). The disease has an autosomal recessive mode of inheritance and is a form of Ehlers-Danlos Syndrome. Prior to identification of the causative genetic mutation, HERDA was referred to as hyperelastosis cutis, dermatosparaxis, and cutaneous asthenia. Males and females are equally affected with clinical signs typically recognized by 1.5 years of age. These signs include hematomas, seromas, slow-healing wounds, and loosely tented skin [8]. A wrinkled-skin appearance of the whole body may also be evident. The genetic defect is a G to A substitution at codon 115 in equine cycophilin B (PPIB), which plays a role in protein folding of collagens [11]. Genetic testing is the diagnostic method of choice, as skin biopsies are only abnormal from affected areas of skin and may have subtle, nondiagnostic findings. There is no cure for this condition, and the majority of homozygous animals are humanely destroyed. Dedicated owners have successfully managed horses for a normal lifespan through a combination of environmental and dietary management [12]. Due to the success of heterozygous horses in competition, the incidence of the carrier state of this disease is increasing [11]. Dermal lesions are most commonly identified; however abnormal connective tissue has been demonstrated within the cornea, musculoskeletal system, and cardiac valves [12].

Cutaneous Asthenia/Hyperelastosis Cutis

Cutaneous asthenia/hyperelastosis cutis is a defect in dermal collagen resulting in loose, easily tented skin. This condition has been referred to as cutaneous asthenia, Ehlers-Danlos syndrome, and HERDA. Rarely, similar clinical findings to HERDA have been reported in horses, which do not have the inherited cyclophilin B gene mutation [13]. A 7-year-old Quarter Horse gelding presented for signs similar to those seen with HERDA but had negative testing for mutations in the PPIB gene. [13] The horse in another case report was 9 years old at the time of euthanasia, with clinical signs first noted at 6 years of age, suggesting a variable phenotype of hyperelastosis cutis. Similar signs were described in a 3.5-year-old cross mare with no mutations identified in the RRIB or PLOD1 genes [14].

In one case example, a 6-week-old Warmblood colt presented with multiple hematomas and failure of wound healing. The foal was seen in the first 3 weeks of life for numerous lacerations, hematomas, and wound dehiscence (Figure 40.3). On examination, the skin was noted to be hyperextensible, and seromas formed at the sites of extension. Histopathology was generally unremarkable with subjective variation in dermal collagen bundle thickness and orientation. The diagnosis of cutaneous asthenia is primarily based on clinical signs, which include fragile and loose skin, slow healing, and development of seromas and hematomas. While there is some overlap with the skin fragility seen in HERDA, the age when clinical signs are noted and location of lesions is different [15].

Albinism

The lack of pigment in the skin, hair, and iris is known as albinism. Melanocytes are present but fail to produce melanin. This is an autosomal dominant trait with homozygotes being nonviable. True albinism has not been recognized in horses. Horses that appear white may have one or two copies of the dominant white gene or in some cases may not be true white in color and rather represent a dilution coat color pattern [16]. A full discussion of coat color genetics is beyond the scope of this chapter. In contrast, lethal white foal syndrome produces white foals due to a lack of melanocytes, rather than a lack of pigment.

Curly Coat

Foals with curly coat syndrome have abnormally long, curly hair coats, a curly mane and tail associated with hypotrichosis, and alopecia due to follicular dysplasia

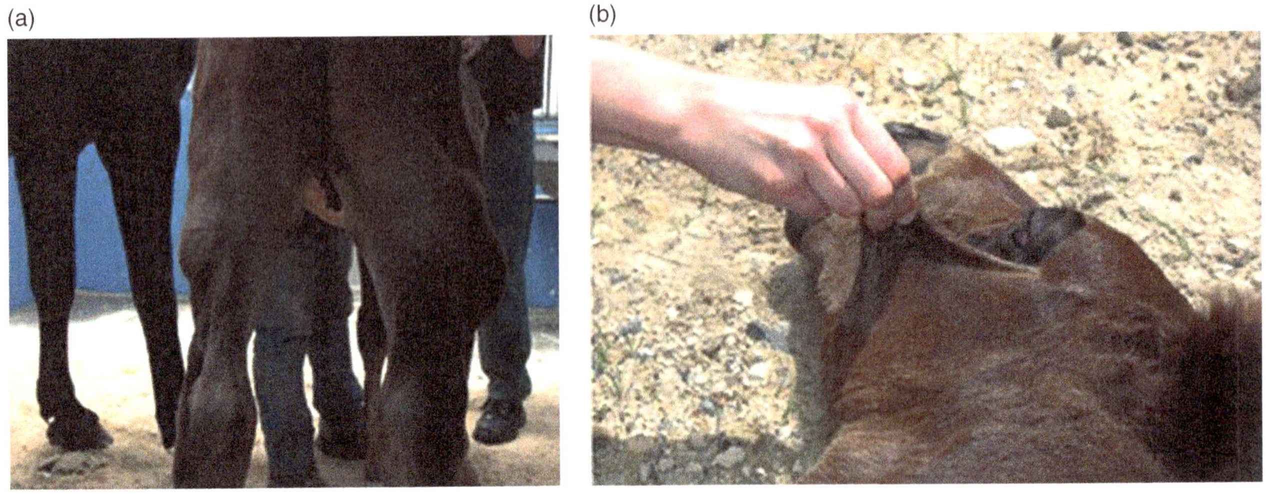

Figure 40.3 Cutaneous asthenia in a 6-week-old Warmblood colt. (a) Large hematoma over right stifle. (b) Hyperextensible skin of the left cheek [15].

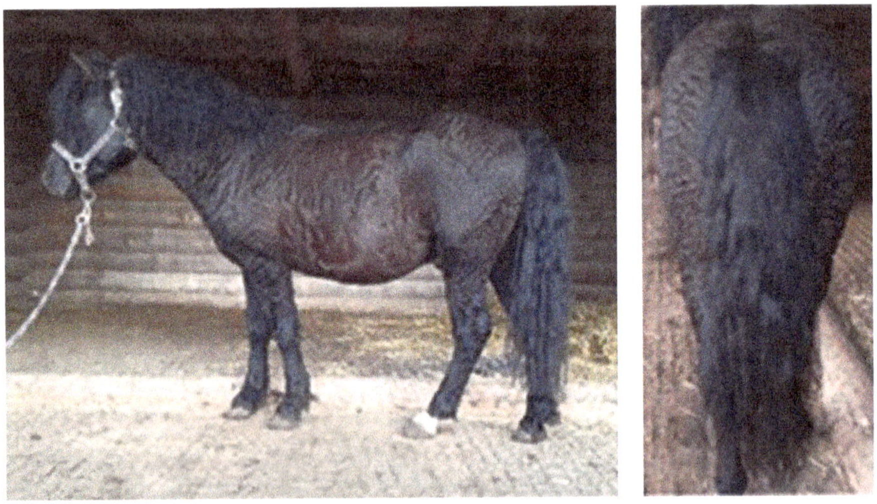

Figure 40.4 Example of curly coat syndrome in an adult horse; not the abnormally long curly hair coat, including the main and tail [17].

(Figure 40.4). Curly coat syndrome is most common in Bashkir Curly Horses and Missouri Foxtrotters, although it has been described in many other breeds [16]. There is no systemic illness, and this condition is considered a cosmetic disease with variation in the degree of curly coat length. Molecular investigation suggests at least two different genes with missense variants may act independently on development of curly coat [17].

Warmblood Fragile Foal Syndrome

Warmblood Fragile Foal Syndrome is a monogenetic defect with autosomal recessive inheritance characterized by a point mutation of the gene coding for the procollagen-lysine, 2-oxoglutarate 5-dioxygenase 1 (Plod-1) [18]. Mutations in this gene in people cause Ehlers Danlos-syndrome, which is characterized by hyperelasticity of the skin and joints along with defects in vessels and the cardiac and ocular systems (Figures 40.5 and 40.6). In Germany, 10–15% of Warmblood horses are heterozygous for this mutation.

No homozygous adult horses have been identified, confirming that homozygous animals do not survive extrauterine life. Heterozygous animals have been identified in Germany, Brazil, and the United States. Testing of 7343 horses of variable breeds demonstrated a carrier frequency of 0.12–0.58% across a variety of breeds including Draft horses, Quarter Horses and Paint Horses [20]. One clinical report of a foal with Warmblood Fragile Foal Syndrome noted dermal lesions, incomplete closure of the abdominal wall and a think dermis with insufficient interlinking of collagen fibers observed histologically [18]. Cutaneous lesions were present in most, but not all, homozygous positive foals. Findings included abnormal flexibility of the digital joints and contracted forelimbs, intracranial hemorrhage [19].

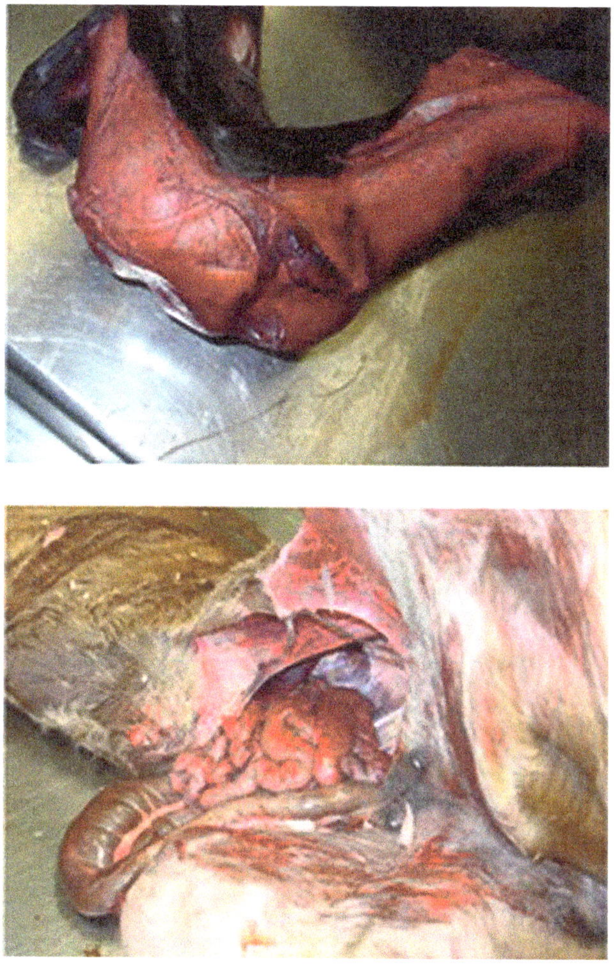

Figure 40.5 Clinical presentation of a foal with Warmblood Fragile Foal Syndrome demonstrating severe ablation of skin on the right forelimb (top image) and open abdomen and eventration of small intestines (bottom image) [18].

Naked Foal Syndrome

Naked foal syndrome is a genodermatosis in the Akhal-Teke horse breed, a breed with its origin in central Asia known for endurance and a metallic shine to the hair coat. Affected foals are born hairless and die within days to years of birth. Histopathologic evaluation shows change consistent with follicular dysplasia in affected foals. The underlying genetic defect is suspected to be a mutation in the ST14 gene, which is involved in epidermal development [21].

Hypotrichosis/Alopecia

Congenital alopecia, also referred to as hypotrichosis, is extremely rare in horses and is characterized by a decreased amount of hair. Many reports are anecdotal without histopathologic correlation. Congenital hypotrichosis has been described in a Percheron foal; the foal was born with patchy alopecia of the trunk and legs that was progressive and nearly complete by 1 year of age (Figure 40.7). Histopathological evaluation of the skin was consistent with severe follicular hypoplasia [22]. Animals with congenital hypotrichosis may be born with variable degrees of alopecia and progress over months to years until hair loss is diffuse. No known treatment exists, and the condition is

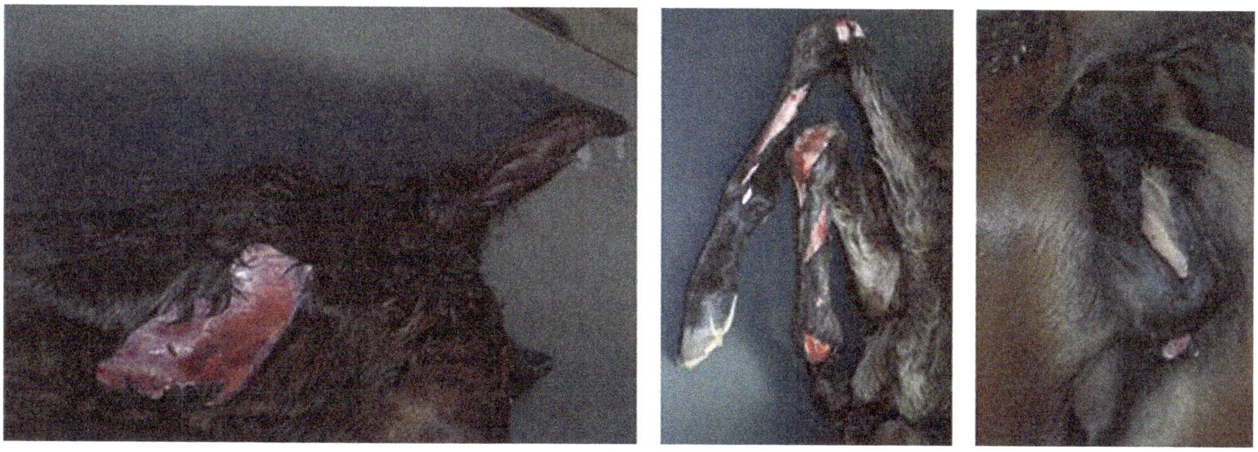

Figure 40.6 Skin defects on the head (left), forelimbs (middle) and ventral to the vulval (right image) in a foal [19].

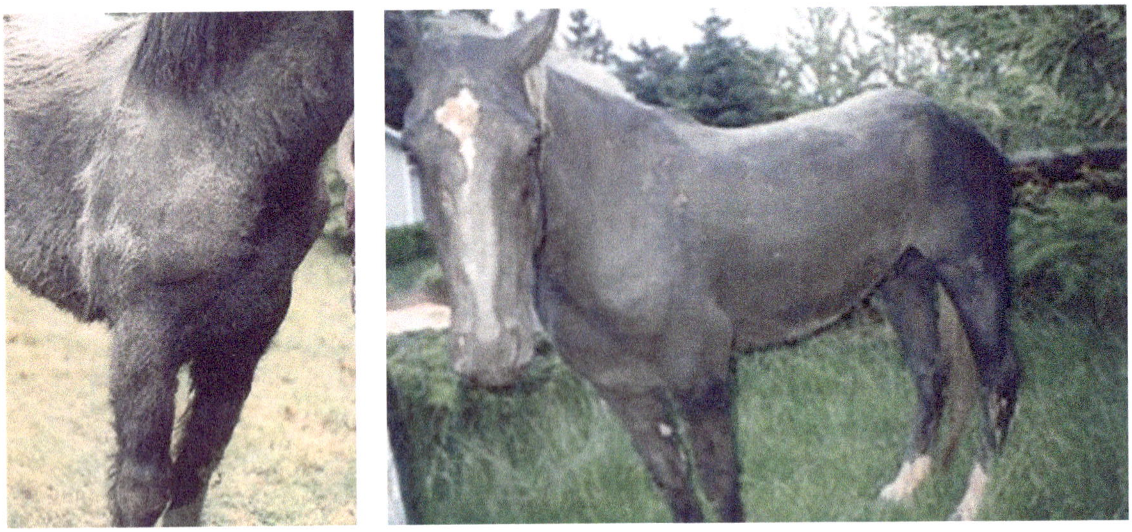

Figure 40.7 Five-month-old Percheron foal with hypotrichosis; the mane was full, but body hair was sparse and consisted of long coarse hairs (left). Same horse at 5 years of age; there is near complete absence of body hair with sparse mane and tail (right). Raised erythematous plaques are present due to solar damage on nonpigmented areas of skin [22].

primarily cosmetic; however, due to the potential for heritability, breeding of these animals should be discouraged. Hypotrichosis has been described in the Arabian horse breed as hair thinning, primarily around the eyes and toward the muzzle; the skin may feel thin or scaly. Other causes of alopecia, such as alopecia areata or defluxion, should be considered with biopsy necessary for definitive diagnosis.

Insect Bite Hypersensitivity

Hypersensitivity to insect bites is the most common allergic skin disease of the horse, commonly caused by hypersensitivity to the salivary antigens of the *Culicoides* sp. These insects are known by many names with approximately 1000 species throughout the world. Prevalence of insect bite hypersensitivity in horses varies by country and region, with a range from 3% in Great Britain to 60% in Queensland Australia [23]. Insect bite hypersensitivity is a type I and type IV hypersensitivity with strong support for a genetic and familial predisposition [24]. Clinically any breed, sex, or coat color may be affected. Most affected horses present with clinical signs between 2 and 3 years of age, but some studies report 3% of cases occurring in horses <1 year of age [23]. Certain breed predispositions exist, and familial involvement has been documented. Signs of insect bite hypersensitivity are seasonal coinciding with the presence of *Culicoides*, which varies geographically. Early in the course of the disease the mane and tail may be the initial sites affected, resulting in hair damage in these areas. Distribution of lesions may be dorsal, ventral, or a combination, and is characterized by pruritus and in some cases crusted papules. As the condition progresses and self-trauma occurs, the lesions of erosive or ulcerative disease, hair loss, lichenification, and hyperpigmentation may occur. Behavior changes are often observed and range from aggressiveness to irritation. The degree of self-trauma and behavior changes can decrease the horse's welfare and performance. Secondary bacterial infections may occur along with weight loss; euthanasia might be elected in severe cases. Diagnosis requires clinical history, eliminating other causes and response to insect control. The management of insect-bite hypersensitivity includes insect control and pharmaceutical control of pruritus. Significant research is ongoing at multiple institutions to determine the genetic basis, as well as the development of new management or vaccination therapies [24].

Dermoids

Dermoids, also called choristomas, are collections of normal tissue found in aberrant locations. They are congenital in nature and histologically represent normal skin and skin appendages. The occurrence is most common along the dorsal midline in horses <18 months of age and may be recognized at birth (Figure 40.8). They occur singly or in clusters and are typically covered with haired skin. Surgical excision is diagnostic and curative.

(a) (b)

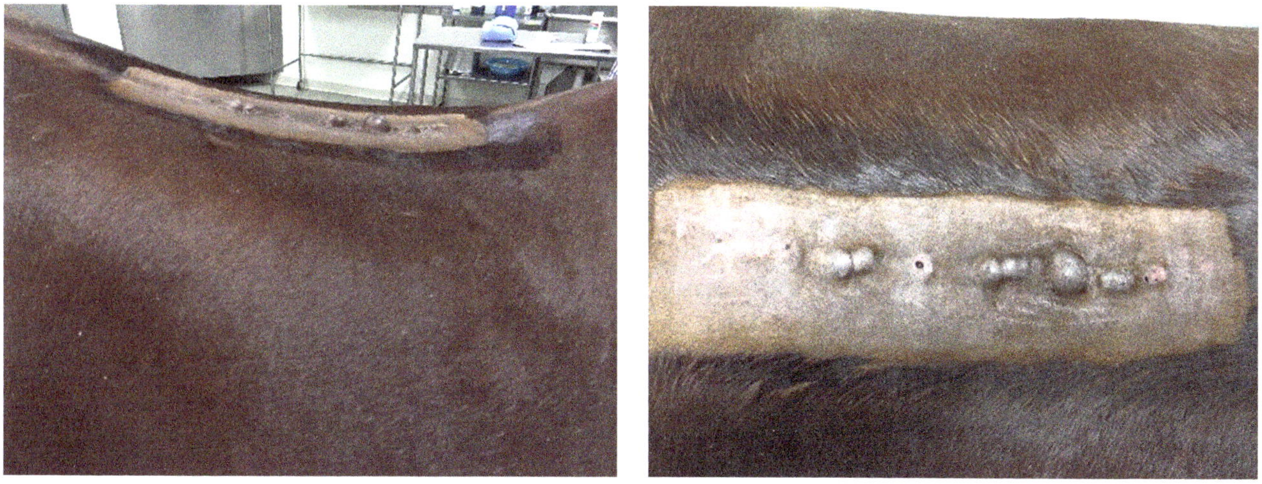

Figure 40.8 Dermoids on the dorsal midline of an adult horse as viewed from the right side of the horse (a) and the dorsal aspect of the horse (b). *Source:* Images courtesy of Dr. Stephanie Caston, Iowa State University.

Epidermoid Cysts

Epidermoid cysts (atheroma) are developmental cystic structures of the epidermis, with the most common site being the false nostril; other sites include the limbs and head. These are freely movable, well circumscribed, firm growths that contain fluid with no adnexal structures. Growth is usually slow or static and, in many cases, removal is not required. Aspiration of the fluid from these cysts yields squamous cells, with occasional cholesterol crystals and an oily consistency.

Dentigerous Cysts

These cysts are characterized by a swelling in the temporal region and arise from tooth germ cell tissue. Clear, opaque, or sticky drainage may be associated with the site and biopsy reveals dental tissue and stratified squamous epithelium (Figure 40.9 a and b). These cysts are most commonly found attached to the temporal bone; rarely these growths may be identified within the sinuses or cranial vault. Surgical removal is curative; however, care should be taken to avoid fracture of attachment of the tooth to bone [25–27].

(a) (b)

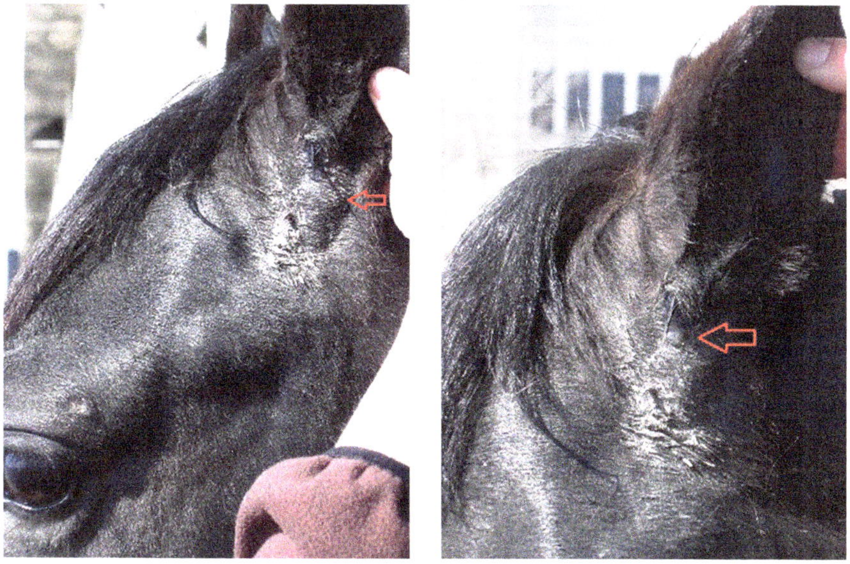

Figure 40.9 Dentigerous cysts located at the base of the ear (a and b), note the opaque (arrow) drainage. *Source:* Images courtesy of Dr. Kevin Kersh.

(a) (b)

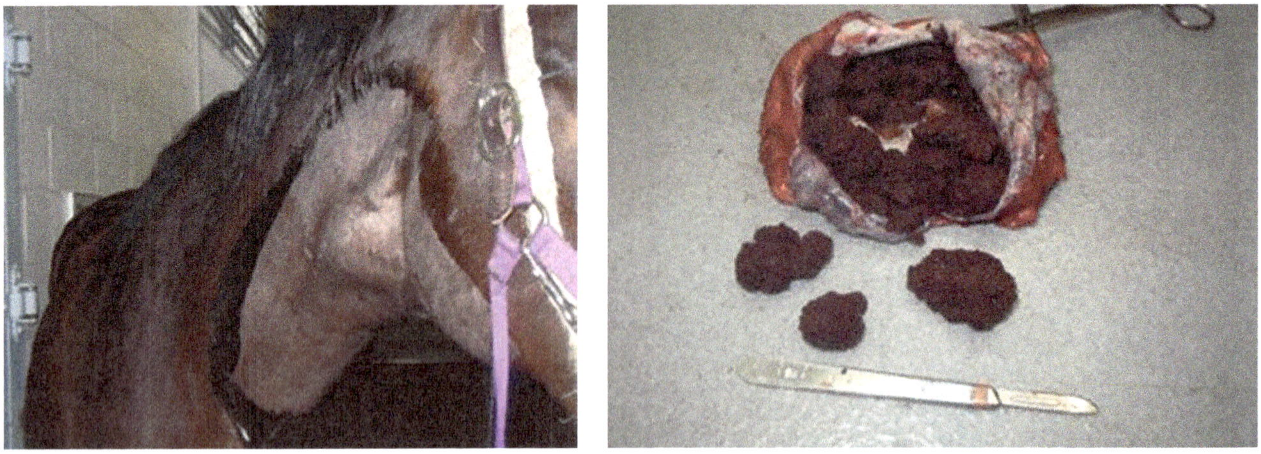

Figure 40.10 Branchial remnant cyst in a mature horse. A firm mass is noted near the region of the thyroid glands (a). Branchial remnant cysts after surgical excision; cysts typically had a fibrous capsule that contained material consistent with previous hemorrhage (b) [28].

Branchial Cysts

Brachial cysts are clinically identified as masses associated with a brachial arch remnant. These cysts vary in the presence of internal or external openings. In a retrospective study, two of seven horses with branchial remnant cysts were <6 months of age. Foals presented for respiratory distress or stridor, and a mass was identified caudal to the pharynx using ultrasonography and radiographs. Laryngeal cartilage anomalies were often diagnosed or suspected. Surgical removal of the cyst is typically curative with postoperative complications common (Figure 40.10 a and b) [28].

Cutaneous Hemangioma

Cutaneous hemangioma also known as vascular hamartoma, vascular nevus, hemangioendotheliomas, or proliferative angioma, has been reported in foals ranging from birth to several months of age [29]. These structures are benign tumors of vascular endothelial cells. Their appearance is variable and may be hyperpigmented, alopecic, hyperkeratotic, or firm-flocculent nodules with variable alopecia, ulceration, or normal haired skin.

The clinical course is inconsistent, with some neoplasms showing no growth, while others increase rapidly in size, necessitating surgical removal [30]. Complete removal of these masses is considered curative, but regrowth may occur after incomplete excision. The most common location is on the distal limb, which may inhibit surgical removal (Figure 40.11) [32]. One report successfully used brachytherapy for treatment of a nonresectable vascular hamartoma, indicating that this modality may be an option for growths on the distal limb [31]. Other locations where these tumors may be observed include the distal limb, base of the ear, and the flank (Figure 40.12) [33]. Metastatic hemangiosarcoma has also been described in neonates with both dermal and visceral involvement noted in some cases; prognosis is considered grave due to the generalized involvement of the dermis and potential for internal metastasis at the time of diagnosis [34].

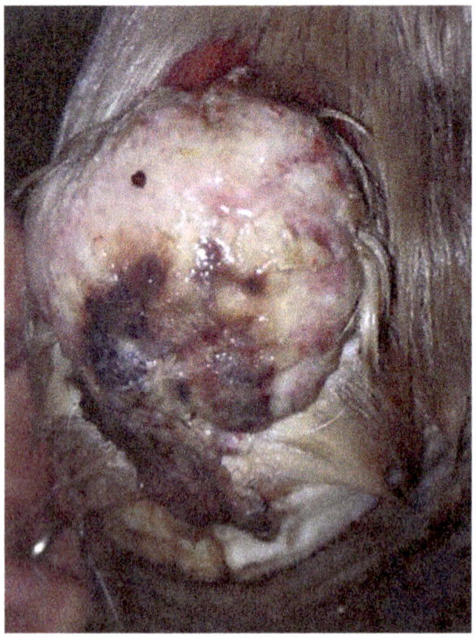

Figure 40.11 Nonresectable dermal vascular hamartoma localized on the hoof coronary band in a colt [31].

Congenital Papillomas

Congenital papillomas have been recognized in adult horses, neonatal foals, and fetuses. In adult horses, papillomas are typically acquired, viral-induced neoplasms.

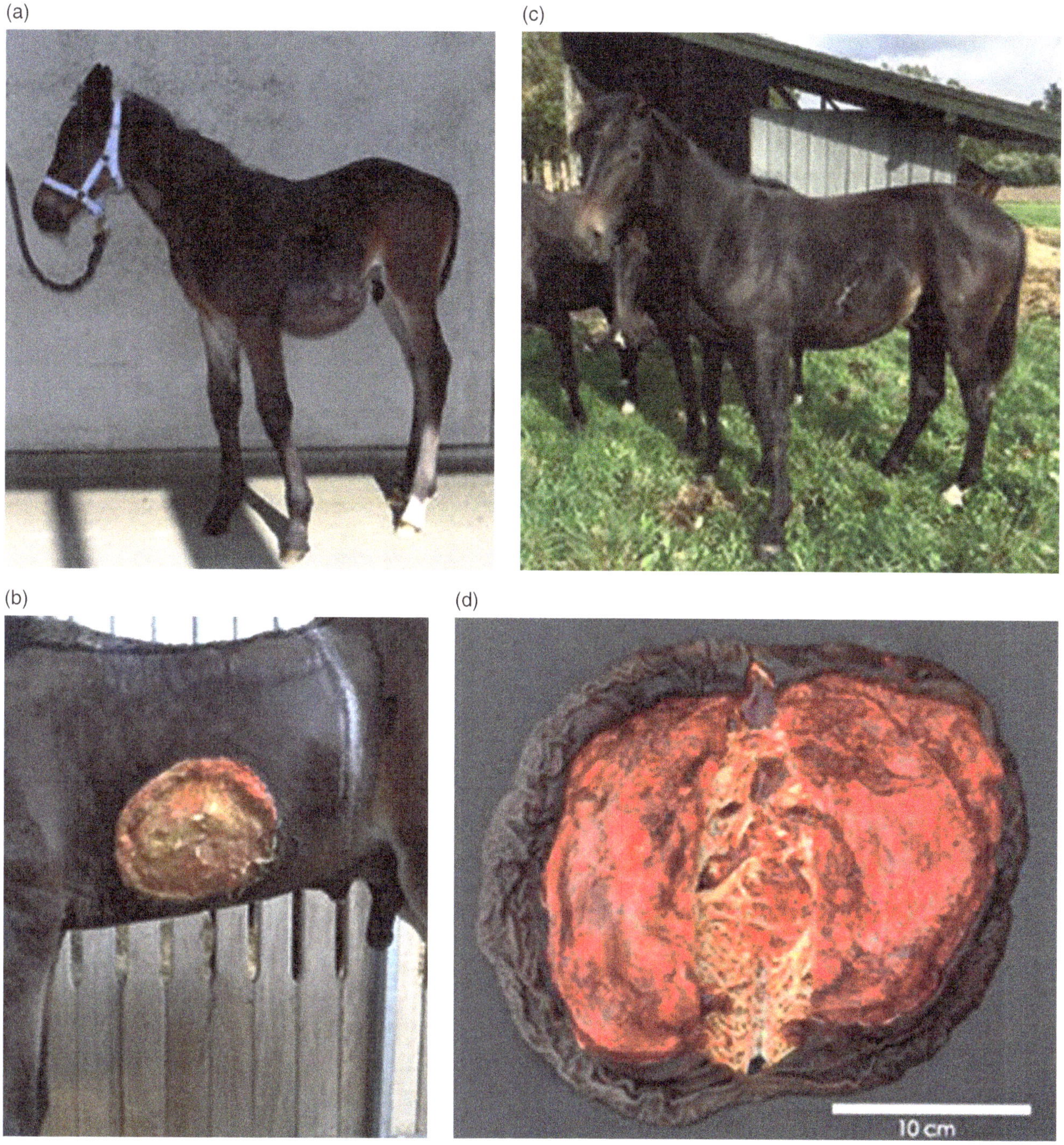

Figure 40.12 Hemangioma on the lateral thorax in a 2.5-week-old Oldenburg colt prior to surgery (a), 4 days postoperatively (b) and 1.5 years after surgery (c) [30]. Cut surface of hemangioma (d) after extirpation; surface was covered by smooth soft tissue. Incision of the mass revealed cystic structure with meshwork of intermingling connective tissue bands and abundant amounts of serosanguinous fluid.

Congenital papilloma in foals lack immunohistochemical or histologic evidence of papillomavirus and therefore it is suggested that congenital papillomas are a form of epidermal nevus or hamartoma [35]. The gross appearance is a pedunculated mass with a wart-like to cauliflower-like surface with variable pigmentation (Figure 40.13). These growths have been reported in fetuses and newborn foals with multiple locations on the head, and less commonly on the thorax or limb [33]. Excision is curative and spontaneous regression has not been reported.

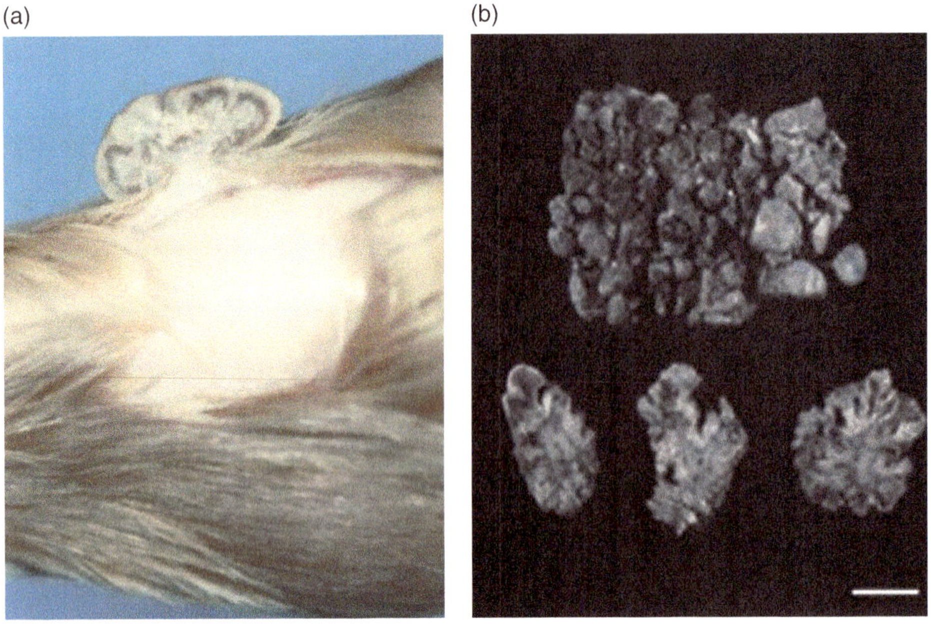

Figure 40.13 Congenital papilloma (a) in the skin of a full-term stillborn Thoroughbred filly; (b) mass is pedunculated with a cauliflower-like surface. Mass has been hemisected. Multiple congenital papillomas, fixed in formalin, from a 2-day-old Paint foal. Masses are pedunculated with a verrucous surface [35].

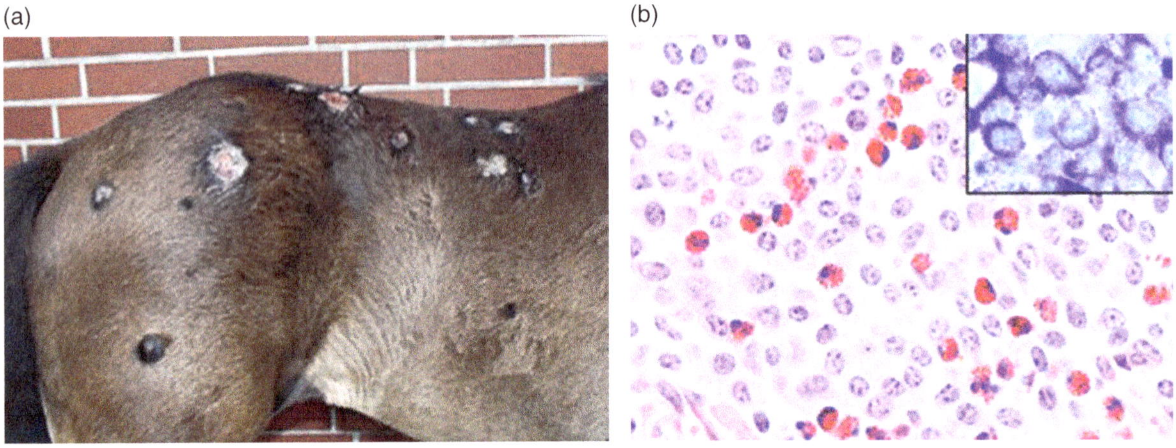

Figure 40.14 A 2.5 month old Warmblood filly with neonatal equine mastocytosis; (a) the skin has multiple nodular masses, some of which were ulcerated. (b) Histopathology of mast cells which are well differentiated with moderate amounts of light, bsophilically stippled cytoplasm containing metachromatic granules (inset), unremarkable nuclei and few mitosis. Hematoxylin and eosin stain; inset toluidine blue stain, bot 600× magnification [39].

Lymphoma

Lymphoma has been reported in foals and aborted fetuses. These animals may have cutaneous and visceral involvement of multiple sites and organs [36–38].

Cutaneous Maculopapular Mastocytosis

Cutaneous maculopapular mastocytosis has been rarely described in foals, with one report documenting two of three foals with systemic mast cell infiltration of multiple organs. Mastocytosis restricted to the skin was described in a 2.5-month Warmblood foal with multiple skin nodules present since birth (Figure 40.14). Long-term prognosis is unknown as most foals are euthanized. In one newborn foal, spontaneous regression of most of the nodules occurred by one year of age [33]. In people and dogs, this condition is reported to be a self-limiting, spontaneously resolving condition. Lesions are typically sharply demarcated and raised with histopathologic examination demonstrating sheets of mast cells with minimal features of cellular atypia [39].

One foal with cutaneous mastocytosis was extensively studied over a period of a year. In this foal dermal lesions developed throughout the first month of life with numbers decreasing over the following year. Examination of the lymph nodes, spleen, and bone marrow revealed large numbers of mast cells. The lesions regressed spontaneously with only residual lesions noted at necropsy at a year of age when euthanasia was elected [40]. It is proposed that this condition will spontaneously regress but documentation of animals reaching adulthood is lacking due to elective euthanasia and the rarity of this condition.

References

1 Fanelli, H.H. (2005). Coat colour dilution lethal ('lavender foal a'): syndrome tetany syndrome of Arabian foals. *Equine Vet. Educ.* 17: 260–263.
2 Brooks, S.A., Gabreski, N., Miller, D. et al. (2010). Whole-genome SNP association in the horse: identification of a deletion in myosin Va responsible for Lavender Foal Syndrome. *PLoS Genet.* 6.
3 Bierman, A., Guthrie, A.J., and Harper, C.K. (2010). Lavender foal syndrome in Arabian horses is caused by a single-base deletion in the MYO5A gene. *Anim. Genet.* 41: 199–201.
4 Spirito, F., Charlesworth, A., Ortonne, J.P. et al. (2002). Animal models for skin blistering conditions: absence of laminin 5 causes hereditary junctional mechanobullous disease in the Belgian horse. *J. Invest. Dermatol.* 119: 684–691.
5 Graves, K.T., Henney, P.J., and Ennis, R.B. (2009). Partial deletion of the LAMA3 gene is responsible for hereditary junctional epidermolysis bullosa in the American Saddlebred Horse. *Anim. Genet.* 40: 35–41.
6 Lieto, L.D., Swerczek, T.W., and Cothran, E.G. (2002). Equine epitheliogenesis imperfecta in two American Saddlebred foals is a lamina lucida defect. *Vet. Pathol.* 39: 576–580.
7 Milenkovic, D., Chaffaux, S., Taourit, S. et al. (2003). A mutation in the LAMC2 gene causes the Herlitz junctional epidermolysis bullosa (H-JEB) in two French draft horse breeds. *Genet. Select.* 35: 1–8.
8 Finno, C.J., Spier, S.J., and Valberg, S.J. (2009). Equine diseases caused by known genetic mutations. *Vet. J.* 179: 336–347.
9 Baird, J.D., Millon, L.V., Dileanis, S. et al. (2003). Junctional epidermolysis bullosa in Belgian draft horses. *Proc. Am. Assoc. Equine Pract.* 49: 122–126.
10 Ginn, P.E., Hillier, A., and Lester, G.D. (1998). Self-limiting subepidermal bullous disease in a neonatal foal. *Vet. Dermatol.* 9: 249–256.
11 Tryon, R.C., White, S.D., and Bannasch, D.L. (2007). Homozygosity mapping approach identifies a missense mutation in equine cyclophilin B (PPIB) associated with HERDA in the American Quarter Horse. *Genomics* 90: 93–102.
12 Rashmir-Raven, A.M. and Spier, S.J. (2015). Hereditary equine regional dermal asthenia (HERDA) in quarter horses: a review of clinical signs, genetics and research. *Equine Vet. Educ.* 27: 604–611.
13 Steelman, S.M., Jackson, N.D., Conant, E. et al. (2014). Ehlers-Danlos syndrome in a quarter horse gelding: a case report of PPIB-independent hereditary equine regional dermal asthenia. *J. Equine Vet. Sci.* 34: 565–568.
14 Oliveira-Filho, J.P., Badial, P.R., Liboreiro, R.M. et al. (2017). Ehlers-Danlos syndrome in a Mangalarga-Campolina Crossbreed Mare. *J. Equine Vet. Sci.* 57: 95–99.
15 Marshall, V.L., Secombe, C., and Nicholls, P.K. (2011). Cutaneous asthenia in a Warmblood foal. *Aust. Vet. J.* 89: 77–81.
16 Sponenberg, D.P. (1990). Dominant curly coat in horses. *Genet. Select.* 22: 257–260.
17 Thomer, A., Gottschalk, M., Christmann, A. et al. (2018). An epistatic effect of KRT25 on SP6 is involved in curly coat in horses. *Sci. Rep.* 8: 1–2.
18 Monthoux, C., de Brot, S., Jackson, M. et al. (2015). Skin malformations in neonatal foal tested homozygous positive for Warmblood Fragile Foal Syndrome. *BMC Vet. Res.* 11: 12.
19 Aurich, C., Müller-Herbst, S., Reineking, W. et al. (2019). Characterization of abortion, stillbirth and non-viable foals homozygous for the Warmblood Fragile Foal Syndrome. *Anim. Reprod. Sci.* 211: 106.
20 Martin, K., Brooks, S., Vierra, M. et al. (2020). Fragile foal syndrome (PLOD1 c. 2032G> A) occurs across diverse horse populations. *Anim. Genet.* 52: 178–138.
21 Bauer, A., Hiemesch, T., Jagannathan, V. et al. (2017). A nonsense variant in the ST14 gene in Akhal-Teke horses with naked foal syndrome. *G3* 7: 1315–1321.
22 Valentine, B.A., Hedstrom, O.R., Miller, J.R. et al. (2001). Congenital hypotrichosis in a Percheron draught horse. *Vet. Dermatol.* 12: 215–217.
23 Schaffartzik, A., Hamza, E., Janda, J. et al. (2012). Equine insect bite hypersensitivity: what do we know? *Vet. Immunol. Immunopathol.* 147: 113–126.
24 Jonsdottir, S., Cvitas, I., Svansson, V. et al. (2019). New strategies for prevention and treatment of insect bite hypersensitivity in horses. *Curr. Dermatol. Rep.* 8: 303–312.
25 Hunt, R.J., Allen, D., and Mueller, P.O. (1991). Intracranial trauma associated with extraction of a temporal ear tooth (dentigerous cyst) in a horse. *Cornell Vet.* 81: 103–108.

26 McClure, S.R., Schumacher, J., and Morris, E.L. (1993). Dentigerous cyst in the ventral Conchal sinus of a horse. *Vet. Radiol. Ultrasound* 34: 334–335.

27 Smith, L.C., Zedler, S.T., Gestier, S. et al. (2012). Bilateral dentigerous cysts (heterotopic polyodontia) in a yearling standardbred colt. *Equine Vet. Educ.* 24: 573–578.

28 Nolen-Walston, R.D., Parente, E.J., Madigan, J.E. et al. (2009). Branchial remnant cysts of mature and juvenile horses. *Equine Vet. J.* 41: 918–923.

29 Platt, H. (1987). Vascular malformations and angiomatous lesions in horses: a review of 10 cases. *Equine Vet. J.* 19: 500–504.

30 Jacobsen, S., Christophersen, M.T., Tnibar, A. et al. (2018). Surgical treatment of a large congenital cavernous haemangioma on the thorax of a foal. *Equine Vet. Educ.* 30: 289–294.

31 Contia, F., Poujetb, L., Lallemandc, E. et al. (2021). High dose rate (HDR) interstitial 192--Ir brachytherapy for the treatment of a recurrent dermal vascular hamartoma in a horse: a case report. ESVONC

32 Sartin, E.A. and Hodge, T.G. (1982). Congenital dermal hemangioendothelioma in two foals. *Vet. Pathol.* 19: 569–571.

33 Misdorp, W. (2003). Congenital tumors and tumor-like lesions in domestic animals. 3. Horses. A review. *Vet. Q.* 25: 61–71.

34 Dunkel, B.M., Piero, F.D., Kraus, B.M. et al. (2004). Congenital cutaneous, oral, and periarticular hemangiosarcoma in a 9-day-old Rocky Mountain Horse. *J. Vet. Intern. Med.* 18: 252–255.

35 White, K.S., Fuji, R.N., Valentine, B.A. et al. (2004). Equine congenital papilloma: pathological findings and results of papillomavirus immunohistochemistry in five cases. *Vet. Dermatol.* 15: 240–244.

36 Tomlinson, M.J., Doster, A.R., and Wright, E.R. (1979). Lymphosarcoma with virus-like particles in a neonatal foal. *Vet. Pathol.* 16: 629–631.

37 Haley, P.J. and Spraker, T. (1983). Lymphosarcoma in an aborted equine fetus. *Vet. Pathol.* 20: 647–649.

38 Seahorn, T.L., Carter, G.K., Morris, E.L. et al. (1988). Lymphosarcoma in a foal: a case report. *J. Equine Vet. Sci.* 8: 317–319.

39 Junginger, J., Geburek, F., Khan, M.A. et al. (2016). Cutaneous form of maculopapular mastocytosis in a foal. *Vet. Dermatol.* 27: 202–e51.

40 Cheville, N.F., Prasse, K., Van Der Maaten, M. et al. (1972). Generalized equine cutaneous mastocytosis. *Vet. Pathol.* 9: 394–407.

Chapter 41 Skin Disorders in the Neonatal Foal

Rebecca Ruby and David Wong

Overall, neonatal foals are not often afflicted with skin disorders except for decubitus ulcers in recumbent neonatal foals, which occurs somewhat frequently. This section briefly highlights some of the reported skin disorders in foals with a slightly longer discussion of decubitus ulcers.

Pemphigus Foliaceous

Pemphigus foliaceous is an autoimmune disease characterized by vesicles and pustules with prominent acantholysis. It has been recognized in foals as young as 2 months of age [1]. Horses often develop lesions on the head and limbs with progression of lesions over several months to the remainder of the body. Due to the fragility of the primary vesicles and pustules, lesions rapidly progress to erosions, crusts, alopecia, and scaling. Foals with pemphigus foliaceous may be depressed and febrile and present with skin crusting, oozing serum, distal edema, and variable clinicopathologic findings. Horses under 1 year of age have a better prognosis compared to older horses, with younger horses reported to spontaneously regress, despite having severe clinical disease [2]. Diagnosis is based on cytological and/or histopathologic findings from affected skin. As with adult horses, dermatophytosis should be ruled out as a differential diagnosis by a combination of fungal culture and examination of skin biopsies for fungal elements.

Ulcerative Dermatitis, Thrombocytopenia, and Neutropenia

Ulcerative dermatitis, thrombocytopenia, and neutropenia in neonatal foals has been described in foals <4 days of age [3]. These foals present with ulceration of the oral cavity along with crusting and erythema of the skin. Common clinicopathologic abnormalities included severe thrombocytopenia, mild leukopenia, and mild neutropenia. Some foals display evidence of coagulopathy characterized by petechiae, ecchymosis, and increased bleeding (Figure 41.1). Subepidermal clefting with vascular dilation, dermal hemorrhage, and superficial papillary necrosis may be noted on histopathologic exam of the skin. Reported cases have recovered with a variety of medical treatments and were healthy as yearlings. Mares are known to have multiple affected foals unless an alternate source of colostrum is used [3, 4]. The mechanism to explain the occurrence of these skin lesions and thrombocytopenia is not understood, and the dermal lesions alone are suggestive of a transient epidermal bullous dermatosis.

Neutrophilic Dermatitis

Neutrophilic dermatitis has been reported in a 3-day-old Morgan filly. This disorder is similar to Sweet's syndrome in people. This foal was reported to have crusted papules and plaques over the entire body (Figure 41.2) but remained bright and actively nursing. A hemogram and serum biochemistry profile were unremarkable, and histopathology of the lesions showed a severe suppurative superficial perivascular to diffuse dermatitis with mural and necrotizing folliculitis. Bacterial and fungal culture was negative. The filly responded well to a tapering dose of dexamethasone sodium phosphate treatment and was reportedly normal during a 3-month follow-up [5].

Linear keratosis is characterized by one or more vertically oriented linear areas of alopecia, which may range from a few centimeters to a meter and most observed on the neck and lateral thorax. There is no associated pruritus and crusting and scaling are variable. Despite the linear orientation, these lesions do not follow vasculature or dermatomes. Biopsy samples have revealed lymphocytic mural folliculitis that can progress to epithelioid cells and giant cells infiltrating the outer root sheath. The end stage of this condition is a permanent, nonreversible alopecia [6].

Equine Neonatal Medicine, First Edition. Edited by David M. Wong and Pamela A. Wilkins.

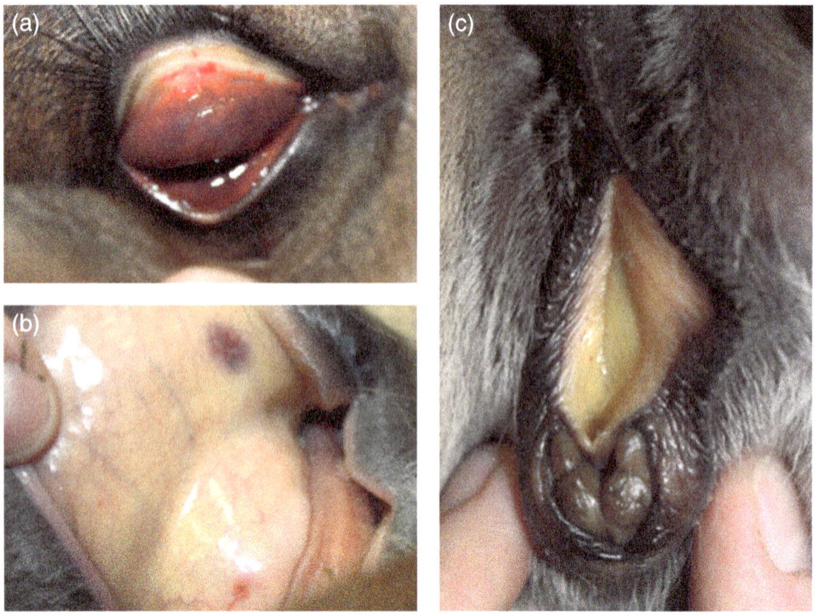

Figure 41.1 Three-day-old Standardbred filly with thrombocytopenia, neutropenia, and ulcerative dermatitis. Note the multifocal petechial and coalescing ecchymotic hemorrhages of the (a) conjunctiva; (b), buccal; and (c) vulval mucosa [4].

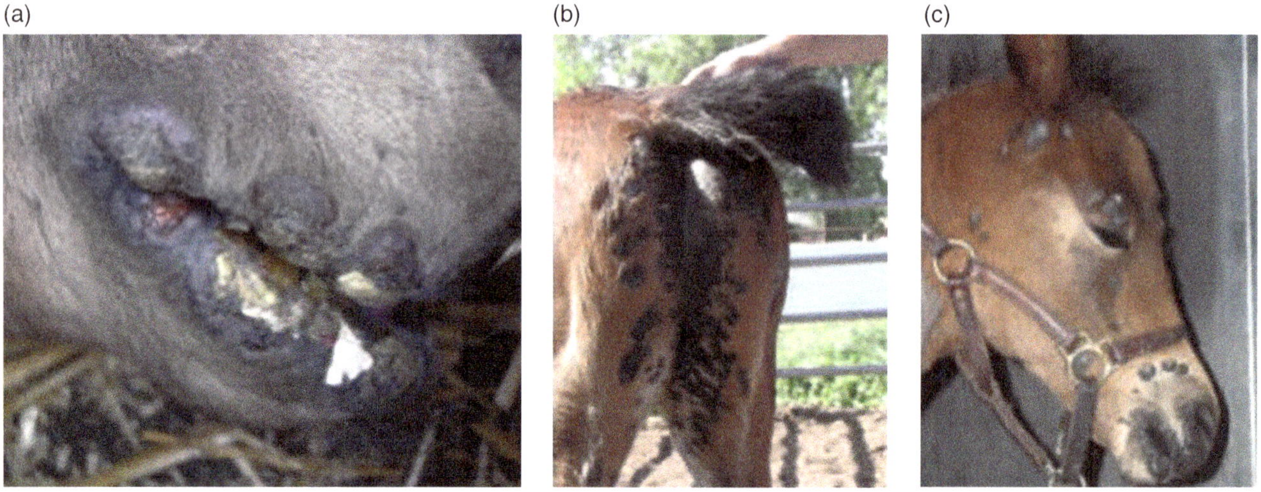

Figure 41.2 Morgan foal with neutrophilic dermatosis. (a) Crusted plaques on the lips of foal. Resolving lesions from same foal involving the perineal area (b) and lips (c) one week after hospital discharge [5].

Melanoma

Melanocytic tumors are typically classified as benign (melanocytoma or melanocytic nevus), malignant or metastatic. Congenital melanocytic neoplasms typically have a low mitotic rate and may occur in multiple coat colors. The location of melanocytic tumors is variable but commonly affect cutaneous tissue. Melanomas have been reported in foals with a generally good prognosis if complete surgical excision is achieved. Melanoma is considered a malignancy; however, congenital metastatic melanoma has only been reported in one foal. The remaining reported cases of congenital malignant melanoma have been cured when complete surgical excision is possible [7].

Melanoma of noncutaneous tissue or those with an invasive nature carry a more guarded prognosis, likely due to the inability to achieve surgical control. A malignant epibulbar melanoma was reported in a 6-month-old Hanoverian foal. The mass was completely excised with enucleation and the animal was reported to have no recurrence at 14 months following surgery [8]. In another case, a primary malignant melanoma was found within the esophagus of a 2-month-old filly who presented for colic surgery and subsequent euthanasia for a ruptured stomach [9].

Skin Disease Related to Treatment of Equine Protozoal Myeloencephalitis

Three foals born to mares receiving treatment for EPM including sulfadiazine or sulfamethozazole-trimethoprim, pyrimethamine, folic acid, and vitamin E were reported to have associated side effects involving the skin. Affected foals had anemia, leukopenia, azotemia, hyponatremia, and hyperkalemia. Skin lesions included a thin wooly coat and histologically apparent epidermal necrosis without inflammation [10].

Telogen defluxion/effluvium results in a temporary, nonpruritic alopecia, which occurs when a large number of telogen hairs are shed when anagen follicles enter catagen and telogen. The normal hair cycle growth includes the anagen (growth), catagen (transition), and telogen (resting) phases. During telogen, hair growth ceases and the hair is not shed until another cycle of anagen occurs; the new hair then displaces the old hair. Many triggers for telogen defluxion have been proposed including stress, starvation, pregnancy, lactation, shock, fever, surgery, and anesthesia [11]. These events typically occur 1–4 months prior to the clinical appearance of alopecia. Histopathology may reveal that the majority of follicles appear normal due to the time lag in clinical signs. Diagnosis is best achieved by plucked hair examination, which shows nonpigmented telogen roots.

Anagen Defluxion

With anagen defluxion, severe disease may cause anagen arrest in hair follicles. This is due to a factor inhibiting synthesis in the hair bulb during the anagen phase and the defective portion of the hair shaft then breaking. Anagen defluxion is most associated with severe stress or chemical compounds such as antimitotic agents. There are often only a few days to weeks before the inciting event and recognition of alopecia [11]. Diagnosis is by plucked hair examination, which shows fragmented hair shafts and absence of root.

Acquired Alopecia

Acquired alopecia is divided into cicatricial and noncicatricial types. With noncicatricial alopecia, future hair growth has the potential to occur while cicatricial alopecia is characterized by permanent destruction of hair follicles and in which growth will not recur. Causes of cicatricial alopecia include direct injury to the skin (physical, chemical, or thermal), severe infection, or neoplasia. Causes of noncicatricial alopecia include trauma, telogen and anagen defluxion, follicle dystrophies, and inflammation or infection of the hair shaft. A diagnosis is achieved with a combination of clinical history, dermal biopsy, and evaluation of hair shafts microscopically [11].

Ioderma eruption was suspected in a 1-day-old Appaloosa colt that developed subepidermal vesiculobullous lesions (Figure 41.3). The foal presented with ptyalism, depression, and problems suckling. Mucosal surfaces were covered by vesicles and bullae. Ulcers were present in the oral mucosa and tongue. Vesicles were also present on the muzzle and eyelids. The distal limbs were swollen and painful on palpation and oozed serum as did the stifles and ventral abdomen. The primary differential was a drug eruption, with the foal having had its umbilicus dipped in 7% iodine at birth. All lesions resolved within 2 weeks of presentation and no concerns were noted at 1- and 9-months postdischarge. Based on the histopathologic findings, clinical history, and resolution of signs, an iododerma eruption was suspected. These have been described in humans [12].

Decubitus ulcers, also referred to as pressure ulcers, pressure sores, or bedsores, are by far the most common type of skin disorder observed in the care of ill neonatal foals that are recumbent for prolonged periods. The word *decubitus* arises from the Latin *decumbere*, meaning "to lie down," referring to the constant pressure that can occur from prolonged recumbency [13, 14]. Pressure sores can be a serious complication in foals and can substantially delay

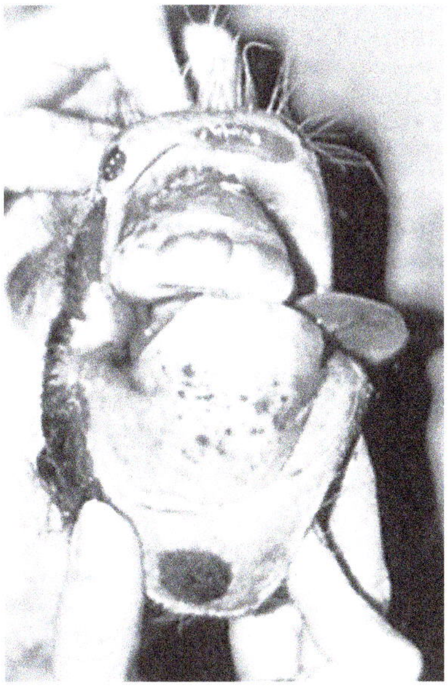

Figure 41.3 One-day-old Appaloosa colt with subepidermal bullous disease. Note the petechia of the buccal surface and a large intact bullae of the upper lip margin. An ulcer is also present on the upper lip [12].

hospital discharge of otherwise recovered/healthy foals. Decubitus ulcers manifest as wounds that develop in the upper layers of the skin as a result of sustained, externally applied pressure; these wounds then enlarge both radially (outward) and into the deeper tissue layers [13]. Decubitus ulcers are frequently accompanied by inflammation and local bacterial colonization [13]. In people, decubitus ulcers are classified according to the depth of extension into the skin and underlying tissues (Table 41.1) by the National Pressure Ulcer Advisory Panel [14].

Decubitus ulcers are commonly observed in foals that cannot move for a protracted length of time because of an underlying medical condition (severe sepsis, neonatal encephalopathy); this sustained recumbency results in impaired blood supply and tissue malnutrition. During prolonged recumbency, externally applied pressure on prominent body surfaces (Figure 41.4) may exceed the capillary pressure within the tissue, which thereby interferes with normal circulation, causing hypoxic tissue damage and necrosis [13, 14]. Areas of the body where bony or cartilaginous prominences have minimal soft tissue overlying (hips, stifles, elbows) are particularly prone to pressure injury. The exact duration of ischemia that causes pressure injury varies between individuals and specific regions of the body, but in people, a duration of 30–240 minutes is enough time to cause tissue injury [13]. Increase susceptibility to decubitus ulcers can arise from external (pressure, friction, shear force, moisture) and internal (fever, malnutrition, anemia, endothelial dysfunction) factors. Other factors such as poor vascular perfusion/vasoconstriction and nutritional deficiencies (cachexia, inadequate fluid replacement) can impair oxygen and nutrient delivery to peripheral tissues contributing to development of decubitus ulcers [13].

Table 41.1 Classification of decubitus ulcers in people [14].

Stage 1	Intact skin with signs of impending ulceration such as blanching and/or non-blanching erythema, warmth, and induration. This stage results from hypoperfusion and pressure injury of the upper layers of the skin and results in a circumscribed area of erythema and induration. Damage can be reversed by removing excessive pressure that is causing the ulcer.
Stage 2	Shallow ulcer (including epidermis and possibly dermis) with pigmentation changes. Lesion may present as an abrasion, blister, or superficial ulcer. This stage results when cells of the basal layer die and become detached and necrosis progresses beyond the basal membrane into deeper layers. An open wound is now present and thus, the normal barrier function of the intact skin is lost.
Stage 3	Full-thickness loss of skin with extension through subcutaneous tissue, but not underlying fascia. Lesions present as necrotic, foul-smelling crater. Stage 3 represents the "typical" decubitus ulcer.
Stage 4	Full-thickness skin and subcutaneous tissue loss, with ulcer penetration into the deep fascia, resulting in involvement of muscle, bone, tendon, or joint capsule. Osteomyelitis may be present along with sinus tracts and severe undermining of adjacent tissue.

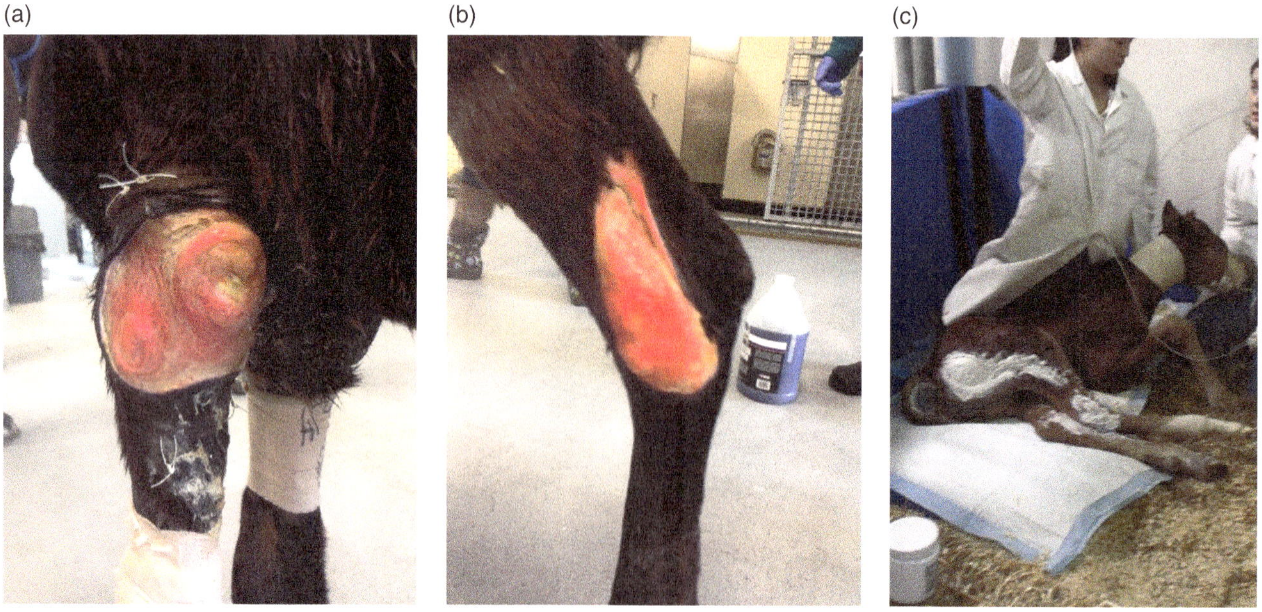

Figure 41.4 Decubitus ulcers in foals. Severe deep decubitus ulcers of the elbow (a) and lateral aspect of the tarsus (b) in a neonatal foal. This foal was recumbent and managed at the owner's facility on a poorly bedded concrete surface for several days prior to presentation for veterinary care. (c) Superficial decubitus ulcers of the lateral aspect of the pelvis and tarsus in a foal that was lying in urine for prolonged period prior to presentation for veterinary care. Note, the wounds are covered with silver sulfadiazine (white cream) in this case.

Outside prolonged recumbency, specific contributing factors that occur in ill foals that predispose the foal to the development of decubitus ulcers include moisture, dysfunction of autonomic regulatory mechanisms of local flood flow, and hypotension. With regard to moisture, foals with prolonged recumbency frequently urinate while lying down, thereby contaminating the area they are laying in with urine. The skin then becomes urine soaked. Moisture does not cause pressure injury per se, but it promotes skin injury by softening the upper layers of skin (maceration) and changes the cutaneous chemical environment (alters pH) [13]. Over time, the moisture causes the skin to become weakened and friable and predisposes areas to the development of decubitus ulcers. A common scenario is a recumbent foal that is laying in urine resulting in moist skin, especially of the hindlimbs and hips; the foal then makes attempts to stand (pushing off with the back legs), resulting in further abrasion (friction, shear forces) and damage to the skin (Figure 41.4). Therefore, critically ill foals that are unable to stand need to be kept dry and should have a urinary catheter placed and a closed urinary collection system implemented to retain urine in a confined bag. If foals become wet from urine, they should be toweled dry; some clinicians also use hair dryers on a low heat or cool setting to help dry the hair coat. Other less common factors that can cause moist skin in the foal include diarrheic feces or constant contact with chemicals such as chlorhexidine or povidone iodine. Loss of regulatory mechanisms of local blood flow and hypotension can also impair oxygen and nutrient delivery to tissues. These conditions (loss of control of blood flow, hypotension) are not uncommon in foals with sepsis and the systemic inflammatory response syndrome and can contribute to formation of pressure sores [15]. Moreover, use of vasopressors in septic patients can also potentially limit nutrient delivery to peripheral tissues and the skin in foals and has been associated with increased risk of pressure ulcers in people treated for shock [16].

Treatment of decubitus ulcers in people involve multiple modalities, including: (i) pressure reduction and prevention of additional ulcers, (ii) wound management, (iii) surgical intervention, and (iv) nutrition. The cornerstone of treatment of decubitus ulcers is reduction or elimination of pressure on vulnerable or affected areas of the body. This is accomplished through adequate support surfaces, regular turning, appropriate positioning and padding, and, if possible, mobilization of the patient [14]. Use of pressure relief devices such as pillows, foam cushions, and mattresses help reduce pressure, while regular (every 2 hours) turning/moving of the patient reduces continuous pressure on vulnerable areas. The skin of high-risk areas (little fat or muscle) such as bony prominences should be carefully monitored. In the foal, these areas include the elbow and lateral aspect of the stifle, pelvis, and tarsus.

Once an ulcer develops, wound management is vital. The wound should be kept clean and effective drainage and absorption should be facilitated to ensure effective healing. Fleece-type blankets allow for fluid to drain away from the surface and diaper drapes provide an absorbent surface to wick away moisture. Necrotic tissue should be debrided and the skin adjacent to the ulcer should also be protected to prevent enlargement of the wound. Various dressings and bandages are available to facilitate healing of wounds based on wound location and clinician preference. Infection control is important for wound healing and can be managed via clean dressings and bandages, and removal of any debris from the ulcer. Infection plays various roles in the etiology, healing, and complications of pressure ulcers. Therefore, treatment of infection is another aspect to consider. In people with ulcers that are cultured and produce $>1 \times 10$ [6] CFU of bacteria/g of tissue or any tissue level of beta hemolytic streptococci, topical antimicrobials are used until the bacterial balance is restored [17]. The use of antibacterial ointments such as silver containing compounds can be valuable in treating pressure ulcers in foals. Other management strategies include provision of adequate nutrition to promote growth of granulation tissue and healing (malnourished patients have higher susceptibility for ulcer formation), blood transfusions if the patient is anemic, IV fluids if the patient is dehydrated, and placement of a urinary catheter and closed urinary collection system to avoid moisture to the skin. Although not readily available, one case series utilized mesenchymal stem cells to treat pressure sores in seven hospitalized neonatal foals. In this brief report, foals treated with mesenchymal stem cells had a statistically improved mean sore regression rate compared to the control group [18]. In people with severe (stage III or IV ulcers) decubitus ulcers, surgical flaps are sometimes implemented to facilitate healing, but this type of therapy has not been reported in foals [14]. Serial photographic documentation with a ruler included for scale in pictures facilitates monitoring of the progression and healing of the ulcer. Of note, persistent exudation from large, damaged skin areas can also result in fluid and protein loss [14].

Prevention of decubitus ulcers is always preferred and measures such as facilitating patient movement/ambulation, protection of pressure areas using positioning, pressure removal from high-risk areas through frequent position changes, use of well-padded mats, pillows, and/or beds for recumbent foals, and treatment of malnutrition, impaired perfusion, and any underlying disease(s) that restrict mobility. Although some decubitus ulcers can be severe, with proper (and potentially prolonged) care, ulcers can heal.

References

1 Laing, J.A., Rothwell, T.L., and Penhale, W.J. (1992). Pemphigus foliaceus in a 2-month-old foal. *Equine Vet. J.* 24: 490–491.

2 Vandanbeele, S.I.J., White, S.D., Affolter, V.K. et al. (2004). Pemphigus foliaceus in the horse: a retrospective study of 20 cases. *Vet. Dermatol.* 15: 381–388.

3 Perkins, G.A., Miller, W.H., Divers, T.J. et al. (2005). Ulcerative dermatitis, thrombocytopenia, and neutropenia in neonatal foals. *J. Vet. Intern. Med.* 19: 211–216.

4 Du Preez, S. and Hughes, K.J. (2018). Thrombocytopenia, neutropenia, ulcerative dermatitis and haemarthrosis in a neonatal foal. *Equine Vet. Educ.* 30: 647–653.

5 Rodeheaver, R.M., Tillotson, K., Traub-Dargatz, J. et al. (2007). Neutrophilic dermatitis in a neonatal Morgan foal. *Equine Vet. Educ.* 19: 375–379.

6 Fadok, V.A. (1995). Update on four unusual equine dermatoses. *Vet. Clin. N. Am. Equine Pract.* 11: 105–110.

7 Foley, G.L., Valentine, B.A., and Kincaid, A.L. (1991). Congenital and acquired melanocytomas (benign melanomas) in eighteen young horses. *Vet. Pathol.* 28: 363–369.

8 McMullen, R.J., Clode, A.B., Pandiri, A.K. et al. (2008). Epibulbar melanoma in a foal. *Vet. Ophthalmol.* 11: 44–50.

9 Caston, S.S. and Fales-Williams, A. (2010). Primary malignant melanoma in the oesophagus of a foal. *Equine Vet. Educ.* 22: 387–390.

10 Toribio, R.E., Bain, F.T., Mrad, D.R. et al. (1998). Congenital defects in newborn foals of mares treated for equine protozoal myeloencephalitis during pregnancy. *J. Am. Vet. Med. Assoc.* 212: 697–701.

11 Rosychuk, R.A. (2013). Noninflammatory, nonpruritic alopecia of horses. *Vet. Clin. N. Am. Equine Pract.* 29: 629–641.

12 Ginn, P.E., Hillier, A., and Lester, G.D. (1998). Self-limiting subepidermal bullous disease in a neonatal foal. *Vet. Dermatol.* 9: 249–256.

13 Anders, J., Heinemann, A., Leffmann, C. et al. (2010). Decubitus ulcers: pathophysiology and primary prevention. *Dtsch. Arztebl. Int.* 107: 371–382.

14 Bansal, C., Scott, R., Stewart, D. et al. (2005). Decubitus ulcers: a review of the literature. *Int. J. Dermatol.* 44: 805–810.

15 Eachempati, S.R., Hydo, L.J., and Barie, P.S. (2001). Factors influencing the development of decubitus ulcers in critically ill surgical patients. *Crit. Care Med.* 29: 1678–1682.

16 Cox, J. and Roche, S. (2015). Vasopressors and development of pressure ulcers in adult critical care patients. *Am. J. Crit. Care* 24: 501–510.

17 Whitney, J., Phillps, L., Aslam, R. et al. (2006). Guidelines for the treatment of pressure ulcers. *Wound Repair Regen.* 14: 663–679.

18 Iacono, E., Lanci, A., Merlo, B. et al. (2016). Effects of amniotic fluid mesenchymal stem cells in carboxymethyl cellulose gel on healing of spontaneous pressure sores: clinical outcome in seven hospitalized neonatal foals. *Turk. J. Biol.* 40: 484–492.

Neonatal Hematology and Clinical Chemistry

Chapter 42 Development of Hemopoiesis in the Foal

Charles Brockus

Introduction

Hematopoiesis or hemopoiesis is defined as the formation and development of blood cells and cell components (*Hemo* or *hemato* meaning *blood* and *poiesis* meaning *to make*). Bone marrow is the major organ for production of blood cells (erythrocytes, leukocytes) and cell components (platelets) and is primarily found throughout the long bones but other bones are also involved. In times of extreme demand for blood cells extramedullary hematopoiesis can occur through other tissues that supplement cell production. The bone marrow microenvironment provides substratum, growth factors, and nutrients necessary for blood cell production. Turnover of cells within the hematopoietic system of an adult human is approximately 1.5×10^6 cells/second[1]. This rapid turnover is due to the different limited life spans of mature blood cells and replacement of senescent cells that have been removed from circulation or response to signals for increasing proliferation of these cells. Red cells (erythrocytes) in circulation are anuclear but have the longest circulating lifespan of approximately 145 days in horses. Peripheral circulating cells originate from a hematopoietic stem cell (HSC), which produces all marrow cells for eventual release into the circulating peripheral blood. How HSCs either self-renew or differentiate is unknown. At any given moment, a relatively small portion of the total stem cell pool is composed of cells beginning to differentiate along one of several pathways of hematopoietic development through an extremely complex process, ultimately giving rise to the wide variety of cells within the circulation that perform numerous functions within the peripheral blood and tissues. The first step in hematopoietic differentiation involves commitment of the stem cell to progenitor cells (myeloid, lymphoid, and megakaryocytic-erythrocytic progenitor cells). Subsequently, progeny of cells committed to each pathway become obligated to a specific sub-pathway of development. After becoming committed to a specific pathway, or lineage, these cells are referred to as committed progenitor cells.

Major pathways followed by the myelocytic progenitor cell is the myelocytic pathway, lymphoid progenitor cell is the lymphocytic pathway, and the megakaryocytic-erythroid progenitor cell (MEP) are the erythrocytic and megakaryocytic pathways (Figure 42.1). The erythrocytic cell line does not go through additional subdivisions but gives rise specifically to red blood cells (RBCs, erythrocytes) used for oxygen transfer from the lungs to peripheral tissues. The megakaryocytic line also does not go through additional subdivisions but provides blood platelets (components of megakaryocyte cytoplasm) that protect against hemorrhage and play a major role in maintaining and repairing vascular endothelium. The myelocytic pathway undergoes numerous complex subdivisions with eventual maturation and release of numerous cell types into circulation. Leukocytes are divided into granulocytic and mononuclear cells and follow an orderly synchronous proliferation and maturation process, provided adequate nutrients, blood flow, and necessary activity factors are available. Granulocytes are divided into neutrophils, eosinophils, and basophils while monocytes and lymphocytes comprise the mononuclear cell population. The granulocyte pathway divides into neutrophilic, eosinophilic, and basophilic pathways. Neutrophils are the body's main defense against bacterial infections and are the most common circulating nucleated cells in healthy horses followed by lymphocytes, monocytes, eosinophils, and basophils, respectively. Circulating monocytes exit the blood and mature within tissues to various classes of macrophages that are derived from the monocytic pathway. Eosinophils play an important role in allergic states and in combating various parasitic infestations. Although there is a lymphocytic pathway for lymphocyte production, the bone marrow is not the major producer of lymphocytes; rather, this

Equine Neonatal Medicine, First Edition. Edited by David M. Wong and Pamela A. Wilkins.

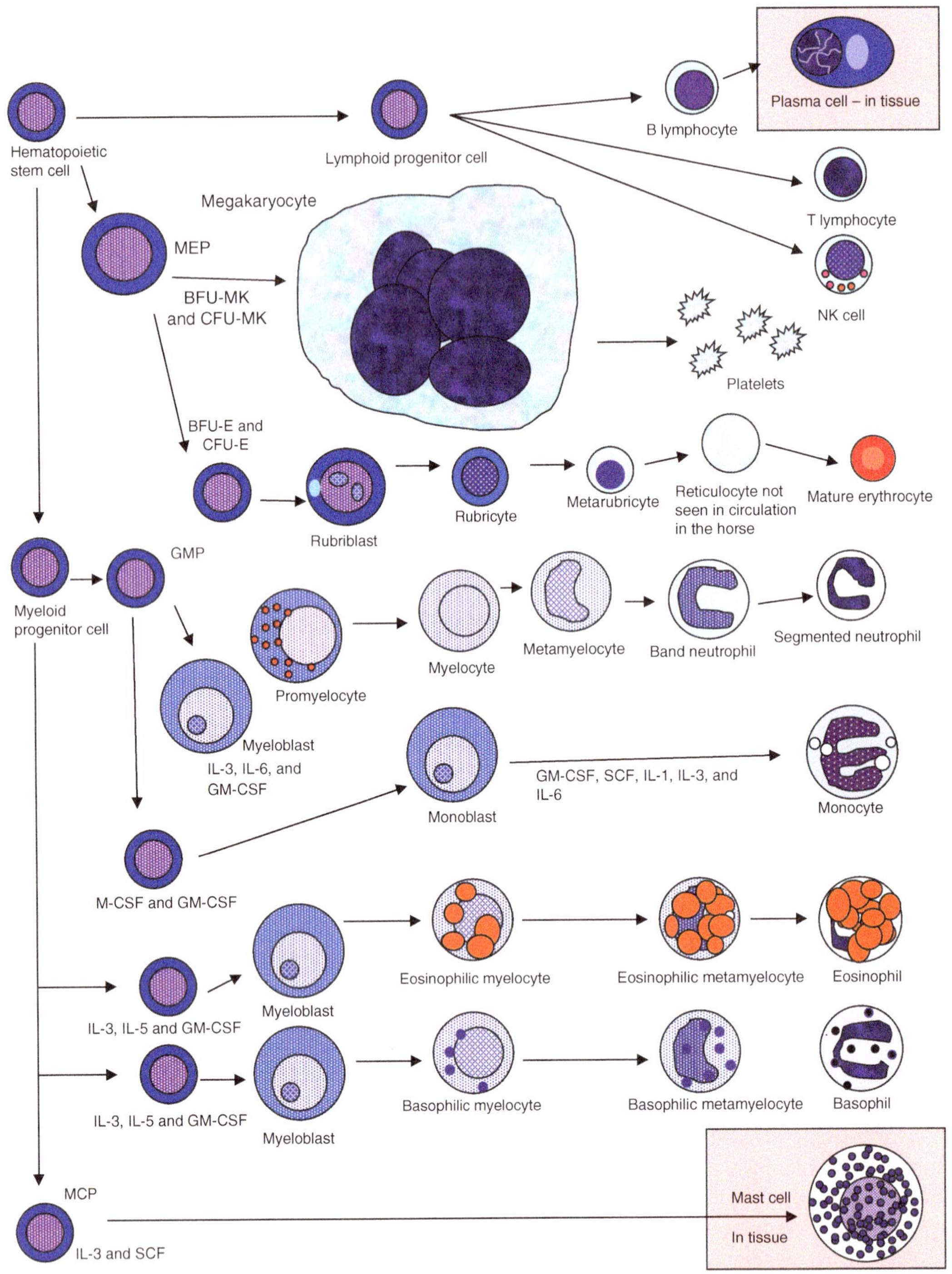

Figure 42.1 Generalized bone marrow proliferation sequence. Hematopoietic stem cell (HSC), megakaryocyte-erythrocyte progenitor (MEP), blast forming unit-megakaryocyte (BFU-MK), BFU-E (blast forming unit-erythrocyte), CFU-E (colony forming unit-erythrocyte), granulocyte monocyte progenitor (GMP), mast cell progenitor (MCP), granulocyte/monocyte-colony stimulating factor (GM-CSF), granulocyte-colony stimulating factor (G-CSF), monocyte-colony stimulating factor (M-CSF), interleukin-1 (IL-1), interleukin-3 (IL-3), interleukin-5 (IL-5), interleukin-6 (IL-6), and stem cell factor (SCF).

is attributed to extramedullary tissues (i.e. thymus, spleen, lymph nodes, etc.).

Hematopoiesis is the collective result of extremely complex regulated signaling pathways facilitated by numerous growth factors and cytokines and their receptors. Many activity factors are released to affect the proliferation and differentiation of the HSC into the required cells. Both soluble and membrane bound factors exist. Soluble factors reach the area of activity through the bloodstream and tend to act on more differentiated cells affecting growth,

Table 42.1 Main hematopoietic growth factors, cytokines, and nutrients involved in hemopoiesis [1–5].

Nutrients	Iron, vitamin B_{12}, and folic acid
Growth factors supporting proliferation of multipotential progenitors, cellular lineages, differentiation, and cell kinetics	Erythropoietin (EPO) Granulocyte Colony Stimulating Factor (G-CSF) Thrombopoietin (TPO) Granulocyte-Macrophage Colony Stimulating Factor (GM-CSF) Insulin-like growth factor-1 (IGF-1) Stem cell factor (SCF) Flt-3 ligand
Cytokines supporting proliferation of multipotential progenitors, cellular lineages, differentiation, and cell kinetics	Interleukin-1 (IL-1) Interleukin-3 (IL-3) Interleukin-5 (IL-5) Interleukin-6 (IL-6) Interleukin-7 (IL-7)

differentiation, and maturation [1–5]. Many have been extensively studied and are in clinical use, including erythropoietin (Epogen®, Eprex®, Retacrit®, Procrit®) and granulocyte-colony stimulating factor (G-CSF; Neupogen®, Granix®, Zarxio®). Using the human recombinant form is effective; however, there is a risk of developing neutralizing antibodies with chronic administration. The main factors promoting hemopoiesis are listed in Table 42.1. Some late-acting factors have synergistic activity with early-acting factors to activate dormant stem cells into the cell cycle.

Lymphocyte Production

Development of the adaptive equine immune system occurs during fetal life, with the thymus being the first lymphoid organ to develop. In the equine fetus, thymic corticomedullary organization of lymphocytes and antigen-responsive lymphocytes are present by day 80 of gestation [6, 7]. Lymphocytes are present within fetal peripheral blood by day 120 and proliferate in response to mitogens by day 140 of gestation [7]. Periarteriolar lymphatic sheaths, well-developed germinal centers, and significant responses to mitogens are present within the fetal spleen by day 200 [7]. Peripheral lymph nodes and intestinal lamina propria are populated with lymphocytes around fetal day 90, and response to mitogens can be detected within the mesenteric lymph node by day 200 [6, 7]. Immunoglobulin production is detectable in the serum of fetuses older than 185 days, and presuckle newborn foals have IgM concentrations of approximately 16 mg/dl [7]. Concentration of IgG is typically low and likely reflects the degree of in utero antigenic stimulation. Functional T lymphocytes appear to be present in the equine fetus by day 100 of gestation and functional B lymphocytes are present by day 200.

Foals are born with circulating lymphocytes with counts similar to the low reference value of adult horses; however, they rapidly increase over subsequent months. Increase in peripheral blood lymphocytes results from an increase in both T and B lymphocytes and is concurrent with an increase in serum IgG and IgM concentrations. This indicates activation/stimulation of the humoral immune system. The percentage of T and B lymphocytes remains constant from birth to 6 months of age with the absolute count and percentage of circulating B lymphocytes being higher in foals than in adult horses [8]. Proliferation of peripheral blood lymphocytes in response to mitogens is slightly reduced at birth but rapidly increases to adult counts. Neonatal foals have significantly fewer T lymphocytes expressing major histocompatibility (MHC) class II antigens on their surface. Expression of MHC class II molecules increases progressively during growth, reaching adult totals by approximately 4 months of age [9]. This indicates progressive development of the adaptive immune system and numbers of antigen-activated memory T lymphocytes. Collectively, neonatal foals are immunocompetent at birth but immunologically naïve. In addition, foals do not have organized lymphoid tissue within their lungs at birth, and lymphocytes and plasma cells are virtually absent from the lungs in the first week of life. Plasma cells producing IgG, IgA, or IgM are present by 8 weeks of age, and foals exhibit well-developed bronchus- and bronchiole-associated lymphoid tissue (BALT) by 12 weeks of age [10].

Hematology of Foals

When interpreting hematological changes associated with a disease process, age related data is best. The neonatal foal's hematology parameters over the first 30 days of life are in rapid flux in specific patterns. Generally, all hematologic values for foals (Table 42.2) are within the much wider reference intervals for the adult horse [2, 11]. As noted, using data within the same approximate age is best, but also, data from the same breed and gender are often even more exact. One report discussed the need for extensive reference intervals for the neonatal foal since their hematology and clinical chemistry parameters are in constant flux; [15] however, the practicality of establishing nearly hourly reference intervals is unlikely due to this process being a very costly and extensive procedure. Therefore, reference intervals covering numerous breeds, ages, and

Table 42.2 Hematology reference intervals for foals at 1, 2, 7, 14, 30, and 90 days of age [11–14].

Parameter	Day 1	Day 2	Day 7	Day 14	Day 30	Day 90	Adult
WBC ($\times 10^3/\mu l$)	6.2–13.0	6.8–8.1	9.5–10.9	8.8–10.4	8.4–9.8	11.6–13.1	5.4–14.3
Neutrophil ($\times 10^3/\mu l$)	4.1–9.6	5–6.4	6.6–7.8	5.5–6.5	5.1–5.9	5.4–7.1	2.3–8.6
Lymphocyte ($\times 10^3/\mu l$)	1.3–3.1	1.6–1.9	2.3–2.7	2.7–3.2	2.5–3.3	4.8–5.7	1.5–7.7
Monocyte ($\times 10^3/\mu l$)	0.4–0.8	0.1–0.2	0.3–0.4	0.3–0.4	0.3–0.3	0.4–0.5	0–1.0
Eosinophil ($\times 10^3/\mu l$)	0	0–0.1	0–0.1	0.1–0.1	0.1–0.1	0.1–0.2	0–1.0
Basophil ($\times 10^3/\mu l$)	0–0.9	0–0	0–0.1	0–0.1	0–0	0–0.1	0–0.29
RBC ($\times 10^6/\mu l$)	9.1–11.9	9.3–10.3	8.9–9.9	9.1–10	9.3–9.9	10.1–11.1	6.8–12.9
Hemoglobin (mg/dl)	12.9–15.5	13.3–14.8	12.3–13.8	12.2–13.3	11.4–12.5	12.2–13.2	11.9–19.0
Packed cell volume (%)	38.4–45.6	34.2–39.8	34.2–39.8	31.3–38.7	34.7–41.3	39.9–42.1	0–0.43
MCV (fL)	36–44	41–43	41–42	40–41	36–38	34–36	42.6–47.4
MCH (pg)	13–15	14–14.6	14–14.3	13.3–14	12.4–12.9	12–12.3	15.7–17.5
MCHC (%)	32–36	33–35	34–35	33–34	34–35	34–35	25.2–49.2
Platelet ($\times 10^3/\mu l$)	163–369	189–213	162–195	217–243	233–274	177–210	95–183

WBC, white blood cell count; RBC, red blood cell count; MCV, mean corpuscular volume; MCH, mean corpuscular hemoglobin; MCHC, mean corpuscular hemoglobin concentration.

genders may not be available. Other factors have also been known to affect blood chemistry and hematology in horses, including stress, altitude, and handling of samples.

The equine neonate from birth to 30 days has red and white cell parameter variability. Narrowing the data field specifically for foals of a specific age can be of significant benefit when interpreting hematology data. The foal's RBC mass parameters (hemoglobin concentration [Hgb], packed cell volume [PCV]) are initially high in the newborn. However, after 12–24 hours after birth, these values begin to decrease, reaching a nadir at approximately 2–3 weeks of age. The rapid decline in RBC, Hgb, and PCV during this time frame have previously been reported [16–18]. The initial higher RBC mass is associated with significant placental blood transfer from the placenta to the foal that occurs immediately after birth and may account for the transient initial increase in PCV reported at 30–45 minutes postpartum [19, 20]. Many reasons have been suggested for the physiological decline in RBC mass, including catecholamine release with fluid balance from colostral proteins (hemodilution), decreased RBC production, decreased iron delivery to bone marrow, increased erythrocyte destruction (shorter RBC half-life than adults), and decreased 2,3-diphosphoglycerate concentrations [11, 14, 21]. However, these theories have not been proven. The rapid decrease in RBC production over the first 2–3 weeks and subsequent decrease in PCV is potentially attributed to an increase in oxygenation, as the source of oxygen switches to normal respiration of the lungs. Alternate theories resulting in decreased RBC mass is erythrocyte destruction during the first week postpartum [16], but this has not been determined and other indicators of hemolysis are not documented. Lastly, hemodilution associated with the effects of expanding plasma volume attributed with growth and the osmotic effects of absorbed colostral proteins potentially accounts for the decrease in PCV observed 24 hours after birth [20]. Colostral absorption ceases after 24 hours with most colostral protein absorption occurring before 12 hours of age [21]. However, caution is needed in interpreting changes in RBC mass in horses because of the large splenic erythrocyte pool [18, 22]. Changes may occur as a result of contraction or relaxation of the spleen resulting in changes of RBC mass. Red cell indices parameters, including mean corpuscular volume (MCV), mean corpuscular hemoglobin (MCH), and mean corpuscular hemoglobin concentration (MCHC), also vary with age. MCV is high at birth and then decreases, reaching a nadir at 3–5 months. It remains lower until nearly a year of age, when it reaches adult values [11, 14]; MCH and MCHC remain relatively stable over the first 30 days of life. Interestingly, horses do not have circulating reticulocytes during a regenerative response, except in rare cases [2, 5].

The total white blood cell count varies little during the first 30 days of life of the equine neonate, but the individual types of leukocytes, including neutrophils, lymphocytes, monocytes, eosinophils, and basophils fluctuate (Table 42.2). Neutrophils and lymphocytes are the primary leukocytes that contribute to the total white cell count with fewer monocytes and even fewer eosinophils and only occasional basophils. Over the first 30 days of life, neutrophil counts decrease slightly with a general pattern of lower counts, while lymphocyte counts increase and nearly double. Increases in peripheral lymphocyte counts during the first month of life have been theorized to increase because of continued development and maturation of the lymphoid system after birth [2, 23]. Monocytes increase minimally, to just under twofold higher. Eosinophils were not reported at <12 hours postpartum, with counts gradually and continuously increasing through Day 30. Basophils transiently increased over the first week, then decreased until Day 30. Eosinophils and basophils are usually easily identified if increased dramatically. More emphasis is usually placed on neutrophil, lymphocyte, monocyte, and eosinophil counts when considering interpretive information. As noted, the reference intervals for adult horses generally straddle the foal's hematological changes during the first 30 days, indicating the importance of age-related reference intervals. In addition, variability in reporting hematological measurements may be present when considering different hematology analyzers used for these measurements. Use of point of care hematology analyzers may result in different results when compared with a laboratory analyzer that goes through many different quality-control measures during the day. However, hematological parameter results are relatively stable, and they may not vary enough to alter interpretation.

Serum Iron (SI) and related parameters total iron binding capacity [TIBC], unbound iron binding capacity [UIBC], and transferrin saturation percent (Sat%, ferritin) are infrequenlty requested laboratory measurements, but are documented for the first year of life (Table 42.3). Measurements vary noticeably during this time frame. Serum iron and Sat% measurements are initially high the first 12 hours of life, then decrease markedly, with SI reaching a nadir after approximately 3 days and Sat% reaching a nadir at approximately 2–4 weeks of age [18]. TIBC is initially high the first 12 hours of life, then decrease incrementally during the first 3 days to 1-week, and then increase to a peak value at 1 month of age. Unsaturated iron binding capacity (UIBC) is quite low post-partum but then increases to a peak value at one month of age.

Table 42.3 Serum iron (SI) and unbound (UIBC) and total (TIBC) iron binding capacity from healthy foals from birth through 1 year of age [18, 22].

Age	SI (mg/l)	UIBC (mg/l)	TIBC (mg/l)	Sat%
<12 h	3.82 ± 0.68 (2.62–4.88)	0.55 ± 0.39 (0.10–1.62)	4.37 ± 0.49 (3.40–5.30)	87 ± 9 (63–98)
1 d	2.14 ± 0.78 (0.68–3.67)	1.45 ± 1.00 (0.22–4.65)	3.59 ± 0.77 (2.17–5.93)	60 ± 22 (22–93)
3 d	0.95 ± 0.51 (0.28–2.17)	2.29 ± 0.90 (0.92–4.16)	3.24 ± 0.77 (1.91–4.81)	30 ± 16 (10–62)
1 wk	1.74 ± 0.77 (0.66–3.15)	2.10 ± 0.99 (0.26–4.29)	3.84 ± 0.82 (2.14–5.71)	46 ± 20 (16–92)
2 wk	1.11 ± 0.44 (0.22–2.01)	3.87 ± 0.85 (2.35–4.99)	4.99 ± 0.55 (3.88–5.71)	23 ± 11 (4–44)
3 wk	1.28 ± 0.50 (0.51–2.13)	4.18 ± 0.78 (2.42–4.99)	5.46 ± 0.56 (4.00–6.46)	24 ± 10 (10–41)
1 mo	1.38 ± 0.64 (0.49–2.60)	4.27 ± 0.85 (2.33–4.99)	5.65 ± 0.65 (4.11–6.60)	25 ± 12 (9–50)
2 mo	1.81 ± 0.57 (1.10–3.26)	3.68 ± 0.80 (2.15–4.91)	5.49 ± 0.60 (4.27–6.44)	33 ± 11 (19–60)
3 mo	1.75 ± 0.56 (0.61–2.83)	3.32 ± 0.92 (1.27–4.70)	5.07 ± 0.49 (4.10–5.95)	35 ± 14 (12–69)
4 mo	1.46 ± 0.47 (0.54–2.19)	3.13 ± 0.63 (1.61–4.24)	4.59 ± 0.51 (3.47–5.31)	32 ± 11 (14–58)
5 mo	1.29 ± 0.45 (0.44–2.22)	3.09 ± 0.74 (1.91–4.84)	4.38 ± 0.68 (3.22–5.40)	30 ± 10 (8–45)
6 mo	1.69 ± 0.38 (0.86–2.33)	3.05 ± 0.66 (1.85–4.37)	4.74 ± 0.58 (3.61–5.82)	36 ± 8 (17–53)
9 mo	1.97 ± 0.51 (0.49–3.06)	2.72 ± 0.67 (1.50–4.25)	4.68 ± 0.56 (3.74–5.56)	42 ± 11 (10–60)
12 mo	1.84 ± 0.38 (1.11–2.57)	2.83 ± 0.54 (1.85–3.88)	4.68 ± 0.61 (3.76–5.79)	40 ± 7 (24–53)

Values are mean ± standard deviation. Limits in parentheses are minimum and maximum values in 22 foals.

References

1 Car, B.D. (2010). The hematopoietic system. In: *Schalm's Veterinary Hematology*, 6e, vol. 5 (ed. D.K. Weiss and K.J. Wardrop), 27–35. Iowa: Wiley Blackwell.

2 Schalm, O.W., Jain, N.C., and Carroll, E.J. (1975). *Veterinary Hematology*, 3e. Philadelphia: Lea & Febiger.

3 Radin, J.M. and Wellman, M.L. (2010). Granulopoiesis. In: *Schalm's Veterinary Hematology*, 6e, vol. 7 (ed. Feldman, Zinkl, and Jain), 43–49. Lippincott, Williams, and Wilkins.

4 Boudreaux, M.K. (2010). Thrombopoiesis. In: *Schalm's Veterinary Hematology*, 6e, vol. 9 (ed. D.K. Weiss and K.J. Wardrop), 56–60. Iowa: Wiley Blackwell.

5 Olver, C.S. (2010). Erythropoiesis. In: *Schalm's Veterinary Hematology*, 6e, vol. 6 (ed. D.K. Weiss and K.J. Wardrop), 36–42. Iowa: Wiley Blackwell.

6 Mackenzie, C.D. (1975). Histological development of the thymic and intestinal lymphoid tissue of the horse. *J. S. Afr. Vet. Assoc.* 46: 47–55.

7 Perryman, L.E., McGuire, T.C., and Torbeck, R.L. (1980). Ontogeny of lymphocyte function in the equine fetus. *Am. J. Vet. Res.* 41: 1197–1200.
8 Flaminio, M.J., Rush, B.R., and Shuman, W. (1999). Peripheral blood lymphocyte subpopulations and immunoglobulin concentrations in healthy foals and foals with *Rhodococcus equi* pneumonia. *J. Vet. Intern. Med.* 13: 206–212.
9 Flaminio, M.J., Rush, B.R., Davis, E.G. et al. (2000). Characterization of peripheral blood and pulmonary leukocyte function in healthy foals. *Vet. Immunol. Immunopathol.* 73: 267–285.
10 Giguère, S. and Polkes, A.C. (2005). Immunologic disorders in neonatal foals. *Vet. Clin. Equine* 21: 241–272.
11 Grondin, T.M. and DeWitt, S.F. (2010). Normal hematology of the horse and donkey. In: *Schalm's Veterinary Hematology*, 6e, vol. 109 (ed. D.K. Weiss and K.J. Wardrop), 821–828. Iowa: Wiley Blackwell.
12 Faramarzi, B. and Rich, L. (2019). Haematological profile in foals during the first year of life. *Vet. Rec.* 184: 503–507.
13 Jain, N.C. (1986). *Schalm's Veterinary Hematology*, 4e. Philadelphia: Lea & Febiger.
14 Grondin, T.M. and Dewitt, S.F. (2010). Normal hematology of the horse and donkey. In: *Schalm's Veterinary Hematology*, 6e, vol. 109 (ed. D.J. Weiss and K.J. Wardrop), 821–828. Ames, IA: Wiley-Blackwell.
15 Duncan, N.B., Johnson, P.J., Crosby, M.J. et al. (2019). Serum chemistry and hematology changes in neonatal stock-type foals during the first 72 hours of life. *J. Equine Vet. Sci.* 84: 102855.
16 Medeiros, L.O., Ferri, S., Barcelos, S.R. et al. (1971). Hematologic standards for healthy newborn Thoroughbred foals. *Biol. Neonate* 17: 351–360.
17 Sato, T., Oda, K., and Kubo, M. (1979). Hematological and biochemical values of Thoroughbred foals in the first six months of life. *Cornell Vet.* 69: 3–19.
18 Harvey, J.W., Asquith, R.L., McNulty, P.K. et al. (1984). Haemotology of foals up to one year old. *Equine Vet. J.* 16: 347–353.
19 Kitchen, H. and Rossdale, P.D. (1975). Metabolic profiles of newborn foals. *J. Reprod. Fertil. Suppl.* 23: 705–707.
20 Rossdale, P.D. and Ricketts, S.W. (1980). *Equine Stud Farm Medicine*, 2e. Philadelphia: Lea & Febiger.
21 Jeffcott, L.B. (1975). The transfer of passive immunity to the foal and its relation to immune status after birth. *J. Reprod. Fertil. Suppl.* 23: 727–733.
22 Harvey, J.W. (1990). Normal Hematologic Values. In: *Equine Clinical Neonatology* (ed. A.M. Koterba, W.H. Drummond, and P.C. Kosch), 561–570. Philadelphia: Lea & Febiger.
23 Jeffcott, L.B. (1977). Clinical haematology of the horse. In: *Comparative Clinical Haematology* (ed. R.K. Archer and L.B. Jeffcott), 161–213. Oxford: Blackwell Scientific Publications.

Chapter 43 Evaluation of the Hematopoietic System – Flow Cytometry

M. Julia B. Felippe

Flow Cytometric Testing

Flow cytometry is a cell-flow laser-based technique that characterizes individual cells and cell populations based on their size, granularity, and *expression* of molecules or metabolites detected with fluorescent monoclonal antibodies or dyes. The clinical application of flow cytometry is expanding for the equine species as more reagents become available, and with a better understanding of physiologic development and pathophysiologic mechanisms of diseases. Flow cytometry has been used for the diagnosis of human prenatal and neonatal hematological and immunological disorders, including measuring immune cell distribution and activation, genetic carrier analysis, sepsis biomarkers, and immune and hematopoietic reconstitution after bone marrow transplantation [1, 2].

Flow Cytometric Assays for the Diagnosis of Immunodeficiencies

Immunodeficiency can be defined as a failure to build protection against pathogens. In primary immunodeficiencies, a genetic mutation impairs immune cell development and/or function, and the effect may be specific to that cell or include other components of the immune system. Such conditions can be congenital, inheritable, and permanent. When available, a genetic test provides the definitive diagnosis at a young age. In human medicine, infants are screened at birth for hundreds of genetic mutations routinely or when there is familial predisposition [3]. Currently, two commercial genetic tests are available for the diagnosis of severe combined immunodeficiency in Arabian and cross-Arabian horses, and foal immunodeficiency syndrome in Fell Pony, Dales, and crossbred horses [4–7].

In the absence of a genetic test, the diagnosis of an underlying immunodeficiency in foals is challenging, but starts at clinical recognition. The diagnosis of a primary versus a transient or delayed developmental immune disorder is particularly difficult. Equine neonates commonly present with infections due to prenatal exposure to placentitis; failure of transfer of immunoglobulins through colostrum; respiratory, gastrointestinal and umbilical infections; and the physiologic transition from an immunologic naïve state to a developing pathogen-specific immunity [8–12]. Nevertheless, infections caused by opportunistic pathogens (e.g. *Pneumocystis jiroveci*, *Cryptosporidium parvum*, adenovirus) should raise the suspicion of a suspected immunodeficiency.

Peripheral blood lymphocyte immunophenotyping using flow cytometry aids in the diagnosis of immunodeficiencies. Results need to be interpreted in the context of clinical history; risk factors; presence of fever and signs of infection; type of pathogens involved; absolute lymphocyte counts; serum IgM and IgG concentrations; and laboratory reference intervals. Repeated immunologic testing in the initial 2–24 months of age may be necessary to observe either improvement, which characterizes a transient condition, or no improvement, which indicates a permanent condition of known or unknown pathologic mechanism.

Both absolute counts and subpopulation distributions of peripheral blood lymphocytes reflect lymphoid tissue activity, as lymphocytes constantly circulate throughout the body. An increase in peripheral blood absolute lymphocyte count with age (values two to three times greater than at birth), as well as in the distribution of CD4 T cells, CD8 T cells, and B cells is an important sign of normal immunologic development with population expansion in the young foal [11, 12].

A recognizable immunodeficiency in the foal is the failure to increase the peripheral blood CD4 T-cell

Equine Neonatal Medicine, First Edition. Edited by David M. Wong and Pamela A. Wilkins.

population with age, when compared with age-matched (and potentially breed-matched) healthy foals. Low CD4 T-cell distribution or failure to expand this population with time may have implications on cytotoxic and/or humoral functions, depending on the underlying mechanism [13, 14]. This condition is often transient in the foal, and normalizes by 12 months of age, but can take a longer period in rare cases. Occasionally transient hypogammaglobulinemia is diagnosed concomitantly, but it is uncertain if both conditions (i.e. transient CD4 T-cell lymphopenia and delayed hypogammaglobulinemia) involve the same disorder background because they can also present independently (Felippe, personal observation). Therefore, serum IgM and IgG concentrations should be measured at the same time points to evaluate overall immunocompetence. In foals with transient hypogammaglobulinemia, serum IgG concentration is below protective levels (<500 mg/dl), and IgM concentration is often <50 mg/dl. The transient hypogammaglobulinemia may last for a few months (e.g. 5–10 months of age) or longer (e.g. 18–24 months of age).

Lymphocyte function can be further characterized using flow cytometry based on the expression of molecules with a specific developmental profile. Foal lymphocytes show an age-dependent expression of cell surface major histocompatibility (MHC) class II and intracellular interferon-gamma (IFNg) production from birth to 12 months of age. Physiological increase in the expression of these molecules seems to reflect maturation and activation of the immune system secondary to antigen exposure, and they can be used as markers of immune maturation [12, 15–17]. Foals may have delayed expression of these markers in their first or second year of age.

Flow cytometry can also be used for lymphocyte proliferation assays that test for cell dysfunction. By labeling lymphocytes with carboxyfluorescein succinimidyl ester (CSFE) and stimulating the cells *in vitro* with mitogens or cell signaling stimulants (e.g. phytohemagglutinin; pokeweed; concanavalin A; phorbol 12-myristate 13-acetate plus ionomycin), rounds of cell division can be measured based on the decrease of cell fluorescence in the daughter cells. Results that suggest intrinsic cell dysfunction with impaired cell proliferation are rarely observed in foals, with the exception of primary immunodeficiencies (Felippe, personal observation) [12]. However, this assay adds information about the foal's lymphocyte competence when combined with the expression of MHC class II and IFNg upon stimulation, particularly when there is minimal change in their expression with age in blood samples.

Immunologic testing requires fresh samples that are chilled at all times with an ice pack or in the refrigerator, and shipped overnight to specialized laboratories in order to preserve their integrity and cellular function. Prolonged storage and hemolysis affect cell viability and profile. For lymphocyte immunophenotyping (CD4 T cell, CD8 T cell, and B cell distributions), molecular expression (MHC class II, IFNg), and proliferation, whole blood samples preserved in anticoagulant preservative ethylenediaminetetraacetic acid (EDTA) or sodium heparin (preferably) can be submitted to specialized laboratories for immunophenotyping. Along with serum IgM and IgG concentrations, these tests can be repeated every two months to determine progress in immunologic competence, and guidance for the need of antibiotic therapy (i.e. when immunologic parameters reach reference intervals for the age, antibiotic therapy may be discontinued).

In addition to lymphocyte evaluation, phagocyte activity can be tested using flow cytometry. Although inherited forms of neutrophil dysfunction have not been described in the horse to date (e.g. granulomatous disease, lack of integrin molecules), phagocytic dysfunction may be investigated in cases of recurrent infection (dermatitis, cutaneous or intracavitary abscesses, cellulitis, periodontal diseases) not associated with humoral immunodeficiency (normal serum IgG concentration), and caused by *Staphylococcus*, *Pseudomonas*, *Serratia*, *Klebsiella*, or fungi (*Aspergillus, Candida*). Phagocytosis and oxidative burst activity can be measured *in vitro* using opsonized inactivated fluorescence-conjugated bacteria (e.g. *Staphylococcus aureus, Escherichia coli*) and a fluorescent indicator of production of reactive oxygen species (e.g. oxidation of 123 dihydrorhodamine into fluorescent 123 rhodamine) [18, 19]. These assays require whole blood samples preserved in sodium heparin (not in EDTA).

Flow Cytometric Assays for the Diagnosis of Neonatal Isoerythrolysis

Neonatal isoerythrolysis (NI) is an acquired form of immune-mediated hemolytic anemia in the foal that develops within hours to a few days of life, and involves alloantibodies absorbed through the colostrum produced by the mare against paternally inherited, incompatible surface molecules expressed on the foal's red cells [20]. The absorbed anti-erythrocyte antibodies cause red cell agglutination, removal by the mononuclear phagocyte system (extravascular hemolysis), and/or destruction via complement activation (intravascular hemolysis) [21, 22].

The use of flow cytometry to detect the percentage of antibody-bound red cells has been successfully applied for the diagnosis of equine NI [23–25]. Whole blood samples should be carefully collected into tubes with EDTA anticoagulant as this prevents complement fixation to red cells *in vitro*. Direct immunofluorescence flow cytometry consists of incubating washed red cells from the patient with fluorescence-conjugated monospecific antibody against immunoglobulins of different isotypes (e.g. anti-IgG, IgM, or IgA), and measuring positive fluorescence (i.e. antibody-coated red cell) using a flow cytometer. Background levels of antibody binding are measured using washed red cells from a healthy control horse. In one study, flow cytometric tests on equine whole blood samples were compared to direct antiglobulin test (Coombs test); the flow cytometric test showed a sensitivity of 100% and a specificity of 87.5%, with positive and negative predictive values of 92% and 100%, respectively [26]. Importantly, this assay measures antibody-bound red cells of different isotypes (i.e. IgG, IgM, and IgA), and can be used to reevaluate direct antiglobulin test-negative results [27, 28].

Flow Cytometric Assays for the Diagnosis of Neonatal Alloimmune Thrombocytopenia or Neutropenia

Neonatal alloimmune thrombocytopenia or neutropenia involves alloantibodies absorbed through the colostrum produced by the mare against paternally inherited, incompatible surface molecules expressed on the foal's platelets or neutrophils, respectively. The alloantibodies bind to platelets or neutrophils of the foal, and accelerate their removal and destruction.

Direct immunofluorescence flow cytometry is used to test for the presence of IgG-, IgM-, and IgA-bound platelet in whole blood samples [23, 29–31]. The test consists of first washing platelets to remove unbound-antibodies present in the blood, adding a fluorescence-conjugated anti-IgG, anti-IgM or anti-IgA, and running the sample in a flow cytometer. Approximately 10 000 platelets are screened, and a positive result is indicated by >8% fluorescent positive (antibody-bound) platelets. The test should always include negative control blood from a healthy horse, which has normally <4% fluorescent positive platelets.

The flow cytometric test has the potential for false-positive results because not every detected antibody on a platelet is an anti-platelet antibody [32]. Platelets naturally express fragment crystallizable (Fc) antibody receptors on the surface, and these receptors can bind to: (i) the constant region of fluorescence-conjugated antibody reagent (e.g. anti-horse IgG); and (ii) the constant region of any circulating antibodies, which then become targets for the antibody reagent. In addition, platelet alpha-granules contain IgG acquired by fluid phase endocytosis from plasma, also becoming a target for the antibody reagent [33, 34]. False negative results may occur when there are low numbers of antibody-coated platelets in the sample due to their removal (thrombocytopenia) or bound-antibodies are removed from platelets during the washing process. The addition of epitope specific (e.g. CD41a and CD42 glycoproteins) anti-platelet antibodies improve the sensitivity and specificity of the test in human samples, but these reagents are not currently available for horses [31]. Similar implications of false positive and negative results occur, but perhaps in greater magnitude, when attempting to diagnose antibody-bound neutrophils, for they express high levels of functional Fc receptors. The use of an antigen-binding fragment F(ab')2 reagent that lacks the constant region improves the specificity of the test. Severe neutropenia can also affect results. In cases such as alloimmune neonatal neutropenia, a flow cytometric assay that relies on antibody-reagents requires careful controls, including individually testing foal and mare's neutrophils treated with their serum in a cross design [35, 36, 37]. In any condition, flow cytometric results should be corroborated by agglutination tests. Nevertheless, when carefully interpreted in the clinical context, this relatively simple and rapid test can be useful in the early diagnosis of alloimmune thrombocytopenia or neutropenia, for immediate treatment decisions and clinical monitoring.

Megakaryocytic hyperplasia is an expected response to platelet destruction in the peripheral circulation, and its absence may indicate immune-mediated destruction of megakaryocytes (or myelophthisic disease). Thrombopoiesis can be assessed by a blood smear and flow cytometry. In the latter, platelets from the patient are treated with thiazole orange, which dyes ribonucleic acid (RNA). The fluorescent RNA is then quantified using flow cytometry: young platelets have greater mRNA content than older cells, and their presence characterizes thrombopoiesis, while their absence or paucity suggests inadequate platelet production in the bone marrow [32, 33].

Flow Cytometric Assays for the Diagnosis of Sepsis

The early diagnosis of human and equine neonatal sepsis can be difficult and delayed. Therefore, blood markers for sepsis have been studied, but data are conflicting and show insufficient sensitivity and specificity [19, 38–40]. One of the reasons for such difficulty is the dynamic expression of inflammatory markers, which is dependent on the age of the neonate (including pre-term or full-term), disease process, and the variable temporal and quantitative influence of inflammatory cytokines on the expression of cell markers [2]. To date, flow cytometric blood cell markers have not been determined for the diagnosis of sepsis in equine neonates.

References

1 Curtis, M.G., Walker, B., and Denny, T.N. (2011). Flow cytometric methods for prenatal and neonatal diagnosis. *J. Immunol. Methods* 5: 198–209.

2 Umlauf, V.N., Dreschers, S., and Orlikowsky, T.W. (2013). Flow cytometry in the detection of neonatal sepsis. *Int. J. Pediatr.* 763191.

3 Yu, J.E., Orange, J.S., and Demirdag, Y.Y. (2018). New primary immunodeficiency diseases: context and future. *Curr. Opin. Pediatr.* 30: 806–820.

4 Shin, E.K., Perryman, L.E., and Meek, K. (1997). Evaluation of a test for identification of Arabian horses heterozygous for the severe combined immunodeficiency trait. *J. Am. Vet. Med. Assoc.* 211: 1268–1270.

5 Wiler, R., Leber, R., Moore, B.B. et al. (1995). Equine severe combined immunodeficiency: a defect in V(D)J recombination and DNA-dependent protein kinase activity. *Proc. Natl. Acad. Sci.* 92: 11485–11489.

6 Fox-Clipsham, L.Y., Brown, E.E., Carter, S.D. et al. (2011). Identification of a mutation associated with fatal foal immunodeficiency syndrome in the fell and dales pony. *PLoS Genet.* 7: e1002133.

7 Fox-Clipsham, L.Y., Carter, S.D., Goodhead, I. et al. (2011). Population screening of endangered horse breeds for the foal immunodeficiency syndrome mutation. *Vet. Rec.* 169: 655–658.

8 Perryman, L.E. and McGuire, T.C. (1980). Evaluation for immune system failures in horses and ponies. *J. Am. Vet. Med. Assoc.* 176: 1374–1377.

9 Perryman, L.E., McGuire, T.C., and Torbeck, R.L. (1980). Ontogeny of lymphocyte function in the equine fetus. *Am. J. Vet. Res.* 41: 1197–1200.

10 LeBlanc, M.M., Tran, T., Baldwin, J.L. et al. (1992). Factors that influence passive transfer of immunoglobulins in foals. *J. Am. Vet. Med. Assoc.* 200: 179–183.

11 Flaminio, M.J., Rush, B.R., and Shuman, W. (1999). Peripheral blood lymphocyte subpopulations and immunoglobulin concentrations in healthy foals and foals with *Rhodococcus equi* pneumonia. *J. Vet. Intern. Med.* 13: 206–212.

12 Flaminio, M.J., Rush, B.R., and Shuman, W. (2000). Characterization of peripheral blood and pulmonary leukocyte function in healthy foals. *Vet. Immunol. Immunopathol.* 73: 267–285.

13 Tanaka, S., Kaji, Y., Taniyama, H. et al. (1994). *Pneumocystis carinii* pneumonia in a thoroughbred foal. *J. Vet. Med. Sci.* 56: 135–137.

14 Flaminio, M.J., Rush, B.R., Cox, J.H. et al. (1998). CD4+ and CD8+ T-lymphocytopenia in a filly with *Pneumocystis carinii* pneumonia. *Aust. Vet. J.* 76: 399–402.

15 Lunn, D., Holmes, M., and Duffus, W. (1993). Equine T-lymphocyte MHC II expression: variation with age and subset. *Vet. Immunol. Immunopathol.* 35: 225–238.

16 de Jager, W., Velthuis, H.T., Prakken, B.J. et al. (2003). Simultaneous detection of 15 human cytokines in a single sample of stimulated peripheral blood mononuclear cells. *Clin. Diagn. Lab. Immunol.* 10: 133–139.

17 Breathnach, C.C., Sturgill-Wright, T., Stiltner, J.L. et al. (2006). Foals are interferon gamma-deficient at birth. *Vet. Immunol. Immunopathol.* 112: 199–209.

18 Flaminio, M.J., Rush, B.R., Davis, E.G. et al. (2002). Simultaneous flow cytometric analysis of phagocytosis and oxidative burst activity in equine leukocytes. *Vet. Res. Commun.* 26: 85–92.

19 Gardner, R.B., Nydam, D.V., Luna, J.A. et al. (2007). Serum opsonization capacity, phagocytosis, and oxidative burst activity in neonatal foals in the intensive care unit. *J. Vet. Intern. Med.* 21: 797–805.

20 Boyle, A.G., Magdesian, K.G., and Ruby, R.E. (2005). Neonatal isoerythrolysis in horse foals and a mule foal: 18 cases (1988–2003). *J. Am. Vet. Med. Assoc.* 227: 1276–1283.

21 Becht, J.L., Page, E.H., Morter, R.L. et al. (1983). Evaluation of a series of testing procedures to predict neonatal isoerythrolysis in the foal. *Cornell Vet.* 73: 390–402.

22 Becht, J.L. (1983). Neonatal isoerythrolysis in the foal, part I. background, blood group antigens, and pathogenesis. *Compend. Contin. Educ. Dent.* 5: S5591.

23 Davis, E.G., Wilkerson, M.J., and Rush, B.R. (2002). Flow cytometry: clinical applications in equine medicine. *J. Vet. Intern. Med.* 16: 404–410.

24 Roback, J.D., Barclay, S., and Hillyer, C.D. (2004). Improved method for fluorescence cytometric immunohematology testing. *Transfusion* 44: 187–196.

25 Alzate, M.A., Manrique, L.G., Bolaños, N.I. et al. (2015). Simultaneous detection of IgG, IgM, IgA complexes and C3d attached to erythrocytes by flow cytometry. *Int. J. Lab. Hematol.* 37: 382–389.

26 Wilkerson, M.J., Davis, E., Shuman, W. et al. (2000). Iso-type specific antibodies in horses and dogs with immune-mediated hemolytic anemia. *J. Vet. Intern. Med.* 14: 190–196.

27 Thedsawad, A., Taka, O., and Wanachiwanawin, W. (2001). Development of flow cytometry for detection and quantitation of red cell bound immunoglobulin G in autoimmune hemolytic anemia with negative direct Coombs test. *Asian Pac. J. Allergy Immunol.* 29: 364–367.

28 Chaudhary, R., Das, S.S., Gupta, R. et al. (2006). Application of flow cytometry in detection of red-cell-bound IgG in Coombs-negative AIHA. An automatable

format for accurate immunohematology testing by flow cytometry. *Hematology* 11: 295–300.

29 Nunez, R., Gomes-Keller, M.A., Schwarzwald, C. et al. (2001). Assessment of equine autoimmune thrombocytopenia (EAT) by flow cytometry. *BMC Blood Disord.* 1: 1.

30 McGurrin, M.K., Arroyo, L.G., and Bienzle, D. (2004). Flow cytometric detection of platelet-bound antibody in three horses with immune-mediated thrombocytopenia. *J. Am. Vet. Med. Assoc.* 224: 83–87.

31 Tomer, A. (2006). Autoimmune thrombocytopenia: determination of platelet-specific autoantibodies by flow cytometry. *Pediatr. Blood Cancer* 47: 697–700.

32 Neunert, C., Lim, W., Crowther, M. et al. (2011). The American Society of Hematology 2011 evidence-based practice guideline for immune thrombocytopenia. *Blood* 117: 4190–4207.

33 George, J.N. (1991). Platelet IgG: measurement, interpretation, and clinical significance. *Prog. Hemost. Thromb.* 10: 97–126.

34 Harrison, P. and Cramer, E.M. (1993). Platelet alpha-granules. *Blood Rev.* 7: 52–62.

35 Wong, D.M., Alcott, C.J., Clark, S.K. et al. (2012). Alloimmune neonatal neutropenia and neonatal isoerythrolysis in a thoroughbred colt. *J. Vet. Diagn. Invest.* 24: 219–226.

36 Davis, E.G., Rush, B., Bain, F. et al. (2003). Neonatal neutropenia in an Arabian foal. *Equine Vet. J.* 35: 517–520.

37 Jiménez, M.M., Guedán, M.J., Martín, L.M. et al. (2006). Measurement of reticulated platelets by simple flow cytometry: an indirect thrombocytopoietic marker. *Eur. J. Intern. Med.* 17: 541–544.

38 Aydin, M., Barut, S., Akbulut, H.H. et al. (2017). Application of flow cytometry in the early diagnosis of neonatal sepsis. *Ann. Clin. Lab. Sci.* 47: 184–190.

39 Zabrecky, K.A., Slovis, N.M., Constable, P.D. et al. (2015). Plasma C-reactive protein and haptoglobin concentrations in critically ill neonatal foals. *J. Vet. Intern. Med.* 29: 673–677.

40 Borba, L.A., Nogueira, C.E.W., Bruhn, F.R.P. et al. (2020). Peripheral blood markers of sepsis in foals born from mares with experimentally ascending placentitis. *Vet. Rec.* 187: 29–29.

Chapter 44 Clinical Chemistry in the Foal

Jenifer Gold

Foals undergo dynamic physiologic changes during the neonatal period that cause unique differences in clinicopathologic parameters compared to adult horses. Changes are noted in all clinicopathologic facets from hematology to serum biochemistry profiles and electrolytes. Placental abnormalities may also influence clinicopathologic results in the newborn in the first several days of life [1]. Additionally, serum biochemistry values change, particularly during the first 4 weeks of life; therefore, age-specific parameters should be used when evaluating ill foals.

Hepatic Indices

The liver has multiple roles in homeostasis, including protein, lipid and carbohydrate metabolism, vitamin storage, production of coagulation factors, detoxification of blood, and excretion of metabolic waste products. Total bilirubin concentration, which is primarily unconjugated (indirect) bilirubin, is considerably higher in neonatal foals compared to adult horses, peaking in the first week of life (up to 5 mg/dl), and remain increased over the first 2 weeks of life [2–4]. Unconjugated bilirubin concentrations are often two to four times higher than adult values during this period and are even higher in premature foals compared to foals of appropriate gestational length [5].

In neonatal infants, unconjugated bilirubin is physiologically elevated due to shorter life span of red blood cells (RBC), reduced hepatocellular uptake of bilirubin, reduced activity of UDP-glucoronosyltransferase (enzyme responsible for conjugation), and increased intestinal uptake of bilirubin by an unidentified component in breast milk [6]. Physiologic hyperbilirubinemia in neonatal foals can be exacerbated by anorexia. Foals tend to have smaller RBCs and less hemoglobin per cell; thus, they have a "physiologic anemia" [7]. The physiologic hyperbilirubinemia and anemia during the neonatal period can be misinterpreted as evidence of hemolytic anemia [7]. A variety of hepatic and nonhepatic causes of hyperbilirubinemia occur in foals (Table 44.1). In comparison, donkey foals do not have elevated bilirubin values as seen in horse foals and are often within adult donkey reference intervals [8, 9].

Foals have less stored glycogen compared to adult horses and have not developed a hindgut. Because of these factors, blood glucose concentrations in foals vary greatly, depending on stress, nursing frequency, and demand. Blood glucose values in foals tend to be higher than adult concentrations during the first month of life, many times up to two times the upper reference range of adults (Table 44.2) [7]. Moreover, healthy foals can also have elevated serum triglyceride concentrations, as high as 340 mg/dl, in the first months of life compared to that of adult horses, which rarely go above 50 mg/dl [2, 3, 7, 9].

The neonatal foal's liver-associated enzyme activity is generally higher and have greater variability between individuals when compared to adult horses (Table 44.3) [7, 12]. Serum gamma-glutamyl transferase (GGT) activity increases in the first 2 weeks of life and returns to, and remains within, the adult reference range thereafter [3, 4, 13]. Elevations of serum GGT activity may be due to induction of hepatic enzymes seen with hepatocellular maturation after birth. Equine colostrum contains very little GGT, therefore neonatal foals have no correlation between transfer of passive immunity and serum GGT concentrations, unlike ruminant neonates. Premature foals can have significantly increased serum GGT concentrations [5]. Interestingly, a retrospective study in 147 foals examined the clinical implications of elevated liver enzyme activity in hospitalized foals <30 days of age [14]. Foals in the study had increased sorbital dehydrogenase (SDH) and GGT concentrations, with septic foals more likely to have higher liver enzyme activity and less likely to survive than foals without sepsis [13]. However, elevated liver enzyme activity alone was not useful as a negative prognostic indicator [14].

Equine Neonatal Medicine, First Edition. Edited by David M. Wong and Pamela A. Wilkins.

Table 44.1 Potential causes of hyperbilirubinemia in the foal [1].

- RBC hemolysis
  - Neonatal isoerythrolysis
  - Sepsis
- Absorption from internal hemorrhage
  - Fractured ribs and hemothorax
  - Internal umbilical remnant hemorrhage
- Neonatal hyperbilirubinemia
- Meconium impaction
- Hepatotoxicity
- Iron toxicity
- Decreased hepatic function
  - Hypoxic–ischemic injury
  - Sepsis/SIRS
- Congenital liver disease
  - Biliary atresia
  - Congenital hepatic fibrosis and cystic bile duct formation in Swiss Freiberger
- Cholangiohepatitis secondary to:
  - Gastroduodenal ulcer syndrome
  - Ileus
  - Enteritis
- Infectious hepatitis
  - Bacterial (*Actinobacillus equuli, Clostridium piliforme* [Tyzzer's disease], secondary to sepsis)
  - Viral (EHV-1)

During the first 2 weeks of life, the liver specific enzyme SDH is comparable to adult concentrations, and then increases between week 1–4 of life [3, 7, 12]. Elevations in GGT and SDH may be seen in foals with sepsis, neonatal encephalopathy, systemic inflammatory response syndrome, or other liver diseases. GGT may also increase in foals with ascending infections of the biliary ducts from gastroduodenal ulcers [1]. Alkaline phosphatase (ALP) activity is very high in the first week of life in foals due to increased osteoblastic activity in growing bones and intestinal activity, development, and pinocytosis during the first 24 hours of life [3, 11, 15–17]. ALP can increase up to 3000 U/l in the first week of life and remain in the upper reference limit for adult horses for the first year of life [2, 3, 18].

Despite the fact that foals ingest an exclusively milk diet, ammonia produced by the colonic microbiota is less than adult horses. Therefore, ammonia concentrations are lower in the neonatal period, which may make its accuracy as an indicator of hepatic function skewed [1]. Ammonia concentrations in adult horses range between 19 and 94 μg/dl whereas measurements in foals (neonate to 1 month of age) is low [1]. However, hyperammonemia of Morgan foals and congenital portosystemic shunts may cause hyperammonemia and causes neurologic signs in foals from 6 to 12 weeks of age [19].

Bile acids are also used commonly as an indicator of liver function [4], but are significantly higher in foals during the first 6 weeks of life compared to adult concentrations, with radioimmunoassay values exceeding enzymatically determined concentrations [4]. Elevated bile acid concentrations during the neonatal period may be due to upregulation of hepatic production, reduced excretion into bile, distinctive effects of intestinal microflora on bile acid composition of the neonate, or heightened intestinal absorption or uptake from the portal circulation [7]. Thus foals may be mistakenly diagnosed with liver disease during the neonatal time frame due to normal elevations in bile acids, bilirubin, GGT, SDH, and ALP [7].

Renal Indices

In the first 24–36 hours of life, newborn foals often have increased serum creatinine concentrations (2.5 ± 0.6 mg/dl) compared to adult horses [2]. Substantial increases in serum creatinine concentrations in newborn foals can be associated with placental pathology and fetal stress [1, 5, 20, 21]. Elevated fetal concentrations are a result of compensatory redistribution of fluid secondary to an insult (e.g. placentitis) to the fetus, which in turn leads to increased ingestion of allantoic fluid and thus creatinine by the fetus [22]. In cases in which the serum creatinine concentration is caused by fetal stress, the creatinine values decrease substantially in the first few days of life. Alternatively, if serum creatinine concentrations remain elevated or decrease slowly, renal injury or other causes of azotemia should be considered (Table 44.4).

In a retrospective study, elevated serum creatinine concentrations were evaluated in 28 foals less than 2 days of age [20]. The purpose of the study was to examine spurious hypercreatininemia (13.6 ± 7.5 mg/dl) at admission to the hospital, assess resolution of the hypercreatininemia, and determine its association with survival in neonatal foals [20]. Of the 28 foals with spurious hypercreatininemia, 5 foals had acute renal failure [20]. Twenty of 28 foals

Table 44.2 Blood glucose concentrations (mg/dl) in healthy foals [10].

Birth	1 h	6 h	12 h	24 h	7 d	30 d
82.3 ± 6.27	107.0 ± 9.7	126.4 ± 7.3	145.5 ± 4.9	169.8 ± 5.1	163.7 ± 3.4	148.6 ± 4.7

Table 44.3 Foal serum enzyme activity and organic molecules related to the liver at various ages [2–4, 11].

Age	ALP	GGT	SDH	AST	ALT	Total bilirubin	Conj. bilirubin	Unconj. bilirubin	Cholesteol	Triglyceride	Bile acids
<12 h	152–2835	13–39	0.2–4.8	97–315	0–47	0.9–2.8	0.3–0.6	0.8–2.5	111–432	24–88	21.7–81.7
Days											
1	861–2671	18–43	0.6–4.6	146–340	0–49	1.3–4.5	0.3–0.7	1.0–3.8	110–562	30–193	26.0–74.3
3	283–1462	9–40	0.6–3.7	80–580	0–52	0.5–3.9	0.2–0.8	0.2–3.3	142–350	63–342	
5	156–1294	8–89	0.8–5.3	—	—	1.2–3.6	0.1–0.7	0.8–2.8	127–361	52–340	
7	137–1169	237–620	4–50	0.8–3.0	0.3–0.7	0.8–3.0	0.3–0.7	0.5–2.3	139–445		16.7–29.4
14	182–859	16–169	0.6–4.3	240–540	1–9	0.7–2.2	0.3–0.6	0.5–1.6	164–287	39–200	11.3–30.6
21	146–752	16–132	1.0–8.4	226–540	0–45	0.5–1.6	0.2–0.5	0.2–1.1	74–276	34–124	7.2–18.4
28	210–866	17–99	1.2–5.9	252–440	5–47	0.5–1.7	0.1–0.6	0.4–1.2	83–233	45–155	9.0–17.1
Months											
2	201–741	8–38	1.1–4.6	282–484	7–57	0.5–2.0	0.2–0.5	0.3–1.5	98–242	10–148	
3	206–458	0–27	1.1–3.9	282–480	8–65	0.4–2.0	0.1–0.7	0.4–1.4	110–226	28–151	
4	124–222	0–27	1.5–4.4	280–520	8–65	0.3–1.0	0.1–0.6	0.2–0.4	91–207	14–148	
5	105–239	0–30	1.3–4.8	225–420	0–65	0.3–1.8	0.1–0.7	0.1–1.1	51–137	14–57	
6	155–226	0–26	0.3–3.3	300–620	7–20	0.3–1.3	0.1–0.7	0.1–0.6	83–173	35–76	
9	158–232	0–26	0.3–3.3	246–728	4–27	0.3–1.1	0.1–0.7	0.2–0.6	11–187	38–86	
12	—	—	—	283–720	5–20	0.4–1.4	0.1–1.0	0.2–0.6	—	—	
Adult	64–214	5–28	0.5–3.0	149–267	4–10	0.5–1.8	0.2–0.7	0.3–1.0	58–109	6–44	4–11.5
Units	IU/l	IU/l	IU/l	IU/l	IU/l	mg/dl	mg/dl	mg/dl	mg/dl	mg/dl	μmol/l

ALP, alkaline phosphatase; GGT, gamma-glutamyl transferase; SDH, sorbital dehydrogenase; AST, aspartate aminotransferase; ALT, alanine aminotransferase; Conj, conjugated; Unconj, unconjugated.

in the study had neonatal encephalopathy [20]. Serum creatinine concentrations decreased by 50% within the first 24 hours of standard neonatal care and were in the reference intervals in all but one foal within 72 hours of hospitalization [20]. Blood urea nitrogen (BUN) concentrations in foals are similar to adult values at birth and then drop to below the lowest limit of the adult reference range (~12 mg/dl) from the first few days of life, up to 5 months of age [2]. However, BUN can also increase in foals due to tissue breakdown for energy production with negative energy balance. This is a common finding in critically ill or newborn foals that had in utero stress and catabolism [1].

Muscle Indices

Aspartate aminotransferase (AST) is primarily associated with muscle in foals, although some AST is also produced by the liver (Tables 44.5 and 44.8). During the first week of life, AST concentrations tend to be equal to or slightly lower than adult horse values and become within adult reference ranges as they continue to exercise and grow [2, 12]. Premature foals have been reported to have elevated AST concentrations [8].

Creatine kinase (CK) activity is similar to adult reference range, although some foal's values may decrease below adult values in the first few months of life [2]. Other circumstances that might increase CK concentrations include neonatal encephalopathy [21], which is likely due to placentitis, perinatal asphyxia, dystocia, trauma at birth, prolonged recumbency, and/or seizures that can occur secondary to neonatal asphyxia; CK values can be increased up to 10 times the adult reference range values [1]. "Sick cell syndrome," which occurs from reduced functioning of the cellular Na^+/K^+ pump and causes loss of homeostasis due to global insult, may also contribute to the increase in CK [24, 25].

Electrolyte Indices

Foals typically maintain serum electrolyte concentrations within a narrow range for the first 6 months of life, similar to adult reference ranges (Table 44.4) [15]. Sodium concentrations may transiently be at the lower end of adult reference ranges in the first 24–48 hours of life. This mild hyponatremia is likely due to hemodilution following osmotic fluid expansion secondary to absorption of

Table 44.4 Organic molecules related to the kidney and electrolyte concentrations (mean ± SD) at various ages in the foal.

Age	BUN	Creatinine	Na^+	K^+	Cl^-	CO_2	HPO_4^-	Ca^{++}	Mg^{++}	Anion Gap
<12 h	12–27	1.7–4.2	148 ± 15	4.4 ± 1.0	105 ± 12	25 ± 5	4.7 ± 1.6	12.8 ± 2.0	1.5 ± 0.8	21 ± 12
Days										
1	9–40	1.2–4.3	141 ± 18	4.6 ± 10	102 ± 12	27 ± 6	5.6 ± 1.8	11.7 ± 2.0	2.4 ± 1.8	16 ± 8
3	2–29	0.4–2.1	142 ± 19	4.8 ± 1.4	101 ± 11	28 ± 12	6.4 ± 2.6	12.1 ± 4.4	2.1 ± 0.9	23 ± 4
5	—	—							2.2 ± 2.0	—
7	4–20	1.0–1.7	142 ± 12	4.8 ± 1.0	102 ± 8	28 ± 4	7.4 ± 2.0	12.5 ± 1.2	2.0 ± 0.6	17 ± 8
14	6–13	0.9–1.8	143 ± 8	4.6 ± 0.8	103 ± 6	26 ± 7	7.8 ± 1.8	12.4 ± 1.2	2.1 ± 1.1	18 ± 6
21	6–14	0.6–2.0	144 ± 8	4.3 ± 1.0	104 ± 11	27 ± 6	7.6 ± 0.8	12.3 ± 1.0	2.3 ± 3.0	18 ± 8
28	6–21	1.1–1.8	145 ± 9	4.6 ± 0.8	103 ± 6	27 ± 5	7.1 ± 2.2	12.2 ± 1.2	2.0 ± 1.1	19 ± 6
Months										
2	6–11	1.1–2.1	148 ± 12	4.8 ± 1.0	105 ± 12	27 ± 5	7.4 ± 1.4	12.3 ± 0.6	2.0 ± 0.8	21 ± 10
3	7–20	0.7–2.2	148 ± 8	4.6 ± 1.2	106 ± 4	27 ± 3	7.3 ± 1.0	12.2 ± 1.0	2.2 ± 0.6	20 ± 8
4	9–25	1.3–2.1	147 ± 12	4.8 ± 1.0	105 ± 11	27 ± 4	6.7 ± 1.8	12.3 ± 1.6	2.4 ± 0.7	21 ± 8
5	11–33	1.2–2.1	145 ± 12	4.5 ± 1.4	107 ± 7	27 ± 5	6.3 ± 1.6	11.8 ± 1.4	2.4 ± 0.6	16 ± 10
6	15–30	1.2–2.1	143 ± 10	4.2 ± 1.4	105 ± 7	26 ± 4	6.2 ± 1.4	11.8 ± 1.6	2.4 ± 0.7	17 ± 8
9	16–26	1.1–2.2	143 ± 5	3.7 ± 1.0	102 ± 6	28 ± 4	6.0 ± 1.4	12.0 ± 1.2	2.3 ± 0.4	16 ± 8
12	15–24	1.3–2.1	146 ± 12	3.8 ± 1.6	104 ± 5	29 ± 2	6.0 ± 0.8	12.7 ± 1.4	—	17 ± 12
Adult	12–24	0.9–2.0	139 ± 8	4.2 ± 1.0	101 ± 6	26 ± 4	4.5 ± 1.4	12.0 ± 1.2	2.2 ± 0.6	18 ± 8
Units	mg/dl	mg/Dl	mEq/l	mEq/l	mEq/l	mEq/l	mg/dl	mg/dl	mg/dl	mEq/l

BUN, blood urea nitrogen; Na^+, sodium, K^+, potassium; Cl^-, chloride; CO_2, carbon dioxide; HPO_4^{2-}, phosphorus; Ca^{++}, calcium.

Table 44.5 AST parameters in neonatal foals [5].

	Healthy foal		Premature foal		Reference value	
	Birth	24 h	Birth	24 h	Birth	24 h
AST (U/l)	96 ± 10	196 ± 17	139 ± 15	185 ± 15	49–111	113–275

colostrum. The healthy neonatal and growing foal's sodium, potassium, chloride, bicarbonate, and magnesium concentrations remain within adult reference ranges.

When newborn foals have abnormal electrolyte concentrations, it is usually due to placental dysfunction and an altered in utero environment. Hyponatremia, hypochloremia, hypo/hyperkalemia, hypo/hypercalcemia, and hyperphosphatemia in the newborn are caused by severe placental disease. Foals can have classic electrolyte disturbances of hyperkalemia, hyperphosphatemia, hyponatremia, hypochloridemia, and hypocalcemia with uroperitoneum and renal insufficiency, but this can be masked if the foal is hospitalized and concurrently receiving IV polyionic fluids [26]. Foals have also been reported to have the same electrolyte abnormalities as above with nutritional myodegeneration [27]. Healthy newborn foals will have ionized and total calcium concentrations 25–30% higher than adult reference ranges, which is likely due to active placental transport [28]. The calcium concentrations begin to decrease soon after birth, become approximately 20% lower than adult reference range, and progressively return to the adult reference range over the first few days of life and remain within this range [2].

Critically ill foals with neonatal encephalopathy or sepsis may create a global insult to cellular membranes that can result in leakage of many cellular constituents. This may lead to clinicopathologic abnormalities such as hypercalcemia, hyperkalemia, hypochloremia, hyponatremia and increases in creatinine kinase. Many of these foals also have an osmolar gap (i.e. difference between measured and calculated plasma osmolality), which supports the concept of sick cell syndrome [2, 24, 25]. Potential causes of neonatal electrolyte derangements are noted in Table 44.6.

Lactate

Blood L-lactate concentrations are frequently evaluated in the critical care setting because it is an affordable, rapid, and readily available (point-of-care lactometers) parameter to measure (Table 44.7). L-lactate has been historically viewed as a marker of global perfusion and tissue hypoxia [23, 29–35]. However, lactate can also serve as an

Table 44.6 Potential causes of increased or decreased serum/plasma electrolyte concentrations in the foal [1].

Parameter	Increased	Decreased

Sodium	▪ Placental dysfunction
	▪ Excessive water loss
	  ▪ Increased insensible losses
	    ▪ Increased respiratory rate
	    ▪ Fever
	    ▪ Large skin defects
		▪ Placental dysfunction
		▪ Renal loss
		  ▪ Renal tubular disorders ephrotoxic drugs, SIRS)
		  ▪ Diuretic therapy
		  ▪ Congenital abnormalities
		  ▪ Hypoxic–ischemic injury
		▪ Gastrointestinal loss
		▪ Uroperitoneum
		▪ Increased osmotic agents (unidentified osmoles, lipids)
		▪ Inappropriate antidiuretic hormone secretion
		▪ Excessive intravenous fluid administration
		▪ Severe rhabdomyolysis

Potassium	▪ Renal failure
	▪ Uroperitoneum
	▪ Sick cell syndrome
	▪ Metabolic acidosis
	▪ Severe rhabdomyolysis
	▪ Prolonged sample storage
		▪ Anorexia
		▪ Renal loss
		  ▪ Renal tubular disorders (nephrotoxic drugs, SIRS)
		  ▪ Diuretic therapy
		  ▪ Congenital abnormalities
		  ▪ Hypoxic–ischemic injury
		▪ Metabolic alkalosis
		▪ GI loss

Chloride	▪ Placental dysfunction
	▪ Metabolic compensation for acidosis
	▪ Metabolic compensation for in utero respiratory acidosis
		▪ Placental dysfunction
		▪ GI loss
		▪ Renal loss
		  ▪ Renal tubular disorders (hypoxic–ischemic injury, nephrotoxic drugs, SIRS)
		  ▪ Diuretic therapy
		  ▪ Congenital abnormalities
		▪ Severe rhabdomyolysis

Calcium	▪ Sick cell syndrome ▪ Severe placentitis	▪ Hypoalbuminemia ▪ Severe rhabdomyolysis ▪ Uroperitoneum
Phosphorus	▪ Uroperitoneum ▪ Renal disease ▪ Severe rhabdomyolysis ▪ Severe placentitis ▪ Excessive use of phosphate containing enemas	

important carbohydrate intermediate shuttled between tissues. Energy production is an extensive biochemical discussion; thus, only a brief review will follow (Figure 44.1). Adenosine 5′-triphosphate (ATP) is the primary source of energy for the cell and is generated by two sequential pathways: glycolysis (anaerobic process) and the citric acid cycle (aerobic process). Intermediates produced by the citric acid cycle enter the electron transport chain for oxidative phosphorylation, where most ATP is generated. In the presence of oxygen, pyruvate is converted to acetyl coenzyme A (acetyl CoA) via enzyme pyruvate dehydrogenase for subsequent metabolism in the citric acid cycle. Alternatively, under anaerobic conditions, pyruvate is preferentially converted into lactate. This conversion regenerates the nicotinamide adenine dinucleotide (NAD) that is needed for continued glycolysis and ATP production. In health, the liver converts 50–70% of plasma lactate to pyruvate and can increase this rate if required [29]. Most pyruvate derived from hepatic lactate metabolism is processed to the citric acid cycle for oxidation or the Cori cycle for gluconeogenesis. The kidney and skeletal muscle are responsible for the remainder of plasma lactate metabolism.

Various studies have shown blood or plasma lactate values measured at birth or shortly postpartum to be as high

Table 44.7 Some causes of type A and B hyperlactatemia [29].

Type A	Type B
Decreased oxygen delivery	*B_1: Hyperlactatemia associated with underlying disease*
■ Hypotension	■ Sepsis/systemic inflammatory response syndrome
■ Hypovolemia	
■ Blood loss	■ Liver disease
■ Cardiogenic shock	■ Parenteral nutrition
■ Septic shock	■ Diabetes mellitus
■ Severe anemia	■ Malignancy
■ Severe hypoxemia	■ Thiamine deficiency
■ Carbon monoxide poisoning	*B_2: Hyperlactatemia associated with drugs or toxins*
Increased oxygen demand	■ Propylene glycol
■ Exercise	■ Bicarbonate
■ Seizures	■ Catecholamines
■ Shivering	*B_3: Hyperlactatemia associated with mitochondrial dysfunction*
	■ Congenital metabolic defects

as 4.9 ± 1.0 mmol/l in healthy foals and may remain higher than adult concentrations for at least 3 days after birth [23, 29–35]. The reason for this is not known but may be related to a combination of peripartum events and immature hepatic function in the newborn, as fetal lactate concentrations are close to adult values [29]. Lactate is also an important carbohydrate substrate for the fetus, and this might contribute to normal periparturient hyperlactatemia [29]. Foals between 1 and 6 months of age have lactate concentrations the same as adult reference ranges [29].

Hyperlactatemia can be categorized as type A or type B. Type A hyperlactatemia occurs with relative or absolute tissue oxygen deficit; in comparison, type B occurs when tissue oxygenation is maintained. Type B hyperlactatemia is divided into three further subcategories: B_1 is associated with underlying disease process, B_2 is associated with drugs or toxins, and B_3 is associated with congenital metabolic defects [29]. Clinically, type B typically causes modest elevations in blood L-lactate (2–3 mmol/l) concentrations whereas moderate to severe hyperlactatemia (>6 mmol/l) is associated with global oxygen deficiency. Furthermore, type A and B may occur concurrently in some ill foals. In the ill neonatal foal, common causes of hyperlactatemia include decreased oxygen perfusion to tissues or increased metabolic demand, which can occur with the systemic inflammatory response syndrome, sepsis, shivering, or seizures [2]. One study demonstrated the median admission lactate was significantly higher in foals with bacteremia (7.65 mmol/l) and neonatal encephalopathy (8.5 mmol/l) compared to foals with local bacterial infection (2.0 mmol/l) and colitis (1.7 mmol/l) [31]. Potential causes of hyperlactatemia are noted in Table 44.7. Additionally, lactate concentrations have been studied as prognostic indicators in critically ill neonates with the sensitivity and specificity in predicting outcome in the range of 60–75% [23, 30–35]. Intuitively, higher lactate concentrations at hospital admission is associated with more severe disease and nonsurvival in equine neonates, compared to survivors [23, 31–35]. However, defining a specific blood lactate concentration cutoff between survivors and nonsurvivors is difficult. In one study, overall foal survival to discharge was 67%; if the arterial lactate concentration was <3.9 mmol/l the survival rate was 80% whereas if the lactate was >6.0 mmol/l the survival rate decreased to <40% [31, 33]. Serial lactate concentrations over the first few days of life may be more valuable than a single point measurement. Prognosis tends to be worse if blood lactate concentrations remain high despite adequate fluid resuscitation and therapy. As noted, although some blood lactate

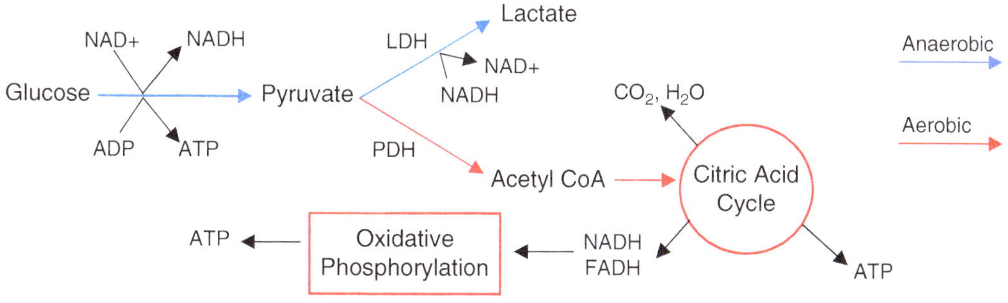

Figure 44.1 General principles of energy production. Glycolysis occurs in cytoplasm of cell and converts glucose to pyruvate (anaerobic process). During glycolysis, adenosine triphosphate (ATP) is produced from adenosine diphosphate (ADP) and reduced nicotinamide adenine dinucleotide (NADH) is generated from oxidized NAD (NAD^+). The final step in glycolysis is conversion of pyruvate to lactate via the enzyme lactate dehydrogenase (LDH); during this process, NAD^+ is created and is essential for glycolysis to proceed. In well-oxygenated tissues, pyruvate is preferentially converted to acetyl CoA via pyruvate dehydrogenase (PDH), at which point acetyl CoA enters the citric acid cycle and oxidative phosphorylation to produce ATP. Flavin adenine dinucleotide (FAD).

concentration cutoff points have been suggested, the author recommends that serial blood lactate concentrations be used to help direct therapy and prognostication in combination with other variables such as trends in vital parameters, blood pressure, clinicopathologic variables and the patient's mentation.

Serum Amyloid A

Acute phase proteins increase with infectious disease and inflammation. They are not specific for disease but are indications of systemic inflammation and infection. Serum amyloid A (SAA) correlates well with systemic inflammatory response syndrome (SIRS) and infection (Table 44.8). The SAA concentration in healthy foals <3 days of age ranges from 0 to 27.1 mg/dl (95% confidence interval), within the reference range reported for healthy adult horses [36]. The highest concentrations in healthy foals appeared to be around 2 days of age [36]. Values of SAA >100 mg/l are suggestive of infection in foals [36].

Arterial Blood Gas Analysis

Arterial oxygen tension (P_aO_2) in the adult horse ranges from 90 ± 2.2 to 101.7 ± 1.6 mmHg with concentrations <80 mmHg indicating hypoxemia [37]. When a foal is first born, inflation of the lungs and closing of vascular and cardiac shunts used during fetal circulation result in rapid changes in arterial blood gas analysis postpartum (Table 44.9). It is important to note that significant changes can occur in P_aO_2 in foals depending on their position (standing or recumbent). The P_aO_2 can be significantly decreased, up to 14 mmHg, when the sample is obtained when the foal is in lateral recumbency [1]. Foals are normally hypoxemic after birth with normal P_aO_2 concentrations as low as 40–50 mmHg when in lateral recumbency [7]. Arterial oxygen tension obtained from foals in lateral recumbency tends to stay ≤80 mmHg for the first 24 hours of life and approach the lower limit of adult reference range between 1 and 3 days of life [39]. The neonatal foal has a carbon dioxide tension that is only slightly higher than the adult mean range in the first 24 hours of life and then decreases to the adult reference range of 40–44 mmHg [39].

Table 44.8 Miscellaneous organic molecules at various ages in the foal [2, 3, 11, 23].

Age	Glucose	CK	AST	Venous L-Lactate	SAA	Total protein	Albumin	Total globulin
Birth				1.9–5.7				
<12 h	108–190	65–380	97–315	1.5–4.1		4.0–7.9	2.7–3.9	1.1–4.8
Days								
1	121–233	40–909	146–340	1.3–2.9	12.3[a]	4.3–8.1	2.5–3.6	1.5–4.6
2				1.1–2.3	36.6[a]			
3	101–226	21–97	80–580	1.2–2.6	27.1[a]	4.4–7.6	2.8–3.7	1.6–4.5
5	—	29–208						
7	121–192	52–143	237–620			4.4–6.8	2.7–3.4	1.6–3.9
14	137–205	46–208	240–540			4.8–6.7	2.6–3.3	2.0–3.5
21	130–240	44–210	226–540			4.7–6.5	2.6–3.2	1.7–3.6
28	130–216	81–585	252–440			5.0–6.7	2.7–3.4	1.8–3.7
Months								
2	119–204	50–170	282–484			5.2–6.5	2.7–3.5	1.9–3.8
3	88–170	57–204	282–480			5.5–7.0	2.8–3.5	2.6–4.1
4	113–196	60–266	280–520			5.7–7.3	2.8–3.7	2.7–3.9
5	95–210	60–125	225–420			6.0–6.9	2.9–3.4	2.7–4.0
6	110–210	97–396	300–620			6.0–6.9	3.0–3.5	2.8–3.7
9	104–207	97–396	246–728			5.6–6.7	3.0–3.6	2.2–3.1
12	106–165	—	283–720			5.8–6.6	3.1–3.8	2.2–3.5
Adult	57–96	69–272	149–267	< 2.5	0.5–20	5.5–7.9	2.8–4.8	1.9–3.8
Units	mg/dl	mg/dl		mmol/l	mg/l	g/dl	g/dl	g/dl

[a] 95% percentile.

Table 44.9 Arterial blood gas values and ventilation parameters at various ages in the foal [38].

Age	pH	P_aCO_2	P_aO_2	HCO_3	V_E	V_T	VO_2	Breaths	Weight
Minutes of age									
Birth	7.41 ± 0.02	60.7 ± 1.5	32.7 ± 2.5	24.0 ± 0.8	418 ± 32	6.1 ± 0.50	7.8 ± 0.8	71 ± 6	44 ± 2.7
2	7.31 ± 0.02	54.1 ± 2.0	56.4 ± 2.3	24.0 ± 1.2					
15	7.32 ± 0.03	50.4 ± 2.7	57.5 ± 3.6	24.4 ± 1.6	463 ± 65	8.1 ± 0.76	10.5 ± 1.7	58 ± 5	44 ± 2.7
30	7.35 ± 0.01	51.5 ± 1.5	57.0 ± 1.8	25.3 ± 0.7	376 ± 37	7.1 ± 0.72	7.7 ± 1.0	53 ± 4	44 ± 2.7
60	7.36 ± 0.01	47.3 ± 2.2	60.9 ± 2.7	25.3 ± 1.0	349 ± 38	8.9 ± 0.95	7.4 ± 1.0	40 ± 3	44 ± 2.7
Hours of age									
2	7.36 ± 0.01	47.7 ± 1.7	66.5 ± 2.3	25.0 ± 0.9					
4	7.35 ± 0.02	45.0 ± 1.9	75.7 ± 4.9	23.6 ± 1.1	380 ± 46	6.7 ± 0.57	6.6 ± 0.9	57 ± 6	44 ± 2.7
12	7.36 ± 0.02	44.3 ± 1.2	73.5 ± 3.0	23.2 ± 1.6	245 ± 37	6.8 ± 0.52	5.2 ± 1.1	32 ± 5	25 ± 2.9
24	7.39 ± 0.01	45.5 ± 1.5	67.6 ± 4.4	26.2 ± 1.1	260 ± 22	6.4 ± 0.46	4.8 ± 0.6	42 ± 4	46 ± 2.9
Days									
2	7.37 ± 0.01	46.1 ± 1.1	74.9 ± 3.3	25.7 ± 0.6	271 ± 56	6.0 ± 0.45	4.6 ± 0.6	44 ± 7	47 ± 3.1
4	7.40 ± 0.01	45.8 ± 1.1	81.2 ± 3.1	23.2 ± 2.1	284 ± 31	6.1 ± 0.40	5.7 ± 0.8	46 ± 4	50 ± 2.9
7	7.37 ± 0.01	46.7 ± 1.1	86.9 ± 2.2	25.6 ± 0.8	320 ± 28	8.1 ± 1.21	7.0 ± 0.6	42 ± 5	54 ± 3.1
Units	—	mmHg	mmHg	mEq/l	ml/kg/min	ml/kg	ml/kg/min	per min	kg

P_aCO_2, partial pressure of carbon dioxide in arterial blood; P_aO_2, partial pressure of oxygen in arterial blood; HCO_3, bicarbonate; V_E, minute respiratory volume; V_T, tidal volume, VO_2, oxygen consumption.

Colloid Oncotic Pressure

Colloid oncotic pressure (COP) associates indirectly to circulating volume and perfusion. It helps to cater treatment to maintain intravascular volume and can help indicate the inclination to develop edema [40]. Monitoring COP may be useful in management of critically ill patients by prioritizing the need for colloids versus crystalloid fluid therapy. Foals commonly have hypo-oncotic diseases with various critical illnesses such as SIRS, endothelial integrity compromise, protein consumption, renal and gastrointestinal loss of proteins, hepatic dysfunction, and failure of passive transfer of immunity.

Oncotic pressure can be measured by direct or indirect means. Direct colloid osmometry is performed via a colloid osmometer, which utilizes a semipermeable membrane to separate saline from a test chamber where the test sample (blood, plasma or serum) is injected [40, 41]. A pressure transducer senses the pressure gradient created by movement of water from the saline side in response to the oncotic pressure exerted by the test sample. Alternatively, indirect assessment of COP can be calculated using numerous different equations. In a study performed by Magdesian et al. [42], the most accurate equation was the Landis-Pappenheimer (L-P) equation, which is used to estimate COP in people: $COP = 2.1TP + (0.16TP^2) + (0.009TP^3)$, where TP is the serum total protein [40–50]. When compared with measured COP, the L-P equation had a mean error of -0.8 ± 3.8 mmHg [42]. Values for COP were obtained from critically ill hospitalized and control foals in this study in which COP values were not significantly different between groups [51]. Interestingly critically ill foals with a blood lactate of ≥3 mmol/l had lower COP values than foals with a lactate ≤3 mmol/l. [51] Despite the close approximation of COP in healthy and ill foals, when measuring COP in critically ill foals, direct measurement should be utilized (if available), particularly with the relationship of COP and lactate concentrations. Measured COP values in healthy and critically ill foals was 17.7 ± 2.4 and 17.1 ± 2.4 mmHg, respectively [42].

Coagulation

Hemostasis is a dynamic physiologic process that starts in utero and develops into the adult system in the postnatal period [52]. However, placental transfer of coagulation or fibrinolytic factors does not occur, and the neonate's coagulation system must develop independently (Tables 44.10 and 44.11). The hemostatic system plays an important role in survival of the neonate and is influenced by age. Thus, the clinician should be aware that concentrations of many hemostatic proteins are dependent on gestational and postnatal stages [61]. Hemostatic mechanisms do not complete maturation until the first week of life, which facilitates the adaptation to extrauterine life [62]. Of interest, coagulopathy is a common occurrence in critically ill foals, with a study finding

Table 44.10 Summary of coagulation tests used to evaluate coagulopathies.

Parameter	Abbreviation	Comment
Activated clot time	ACT	Assesses secondary hemostasis and intrinsic clotting cascade, quantity and function of platelets, and concentration of fibrinogen. Reference interval (seconds): 124–333 (1 d); 130–288 (1 wk); 158–281 (>1 wk).
Prothrombin time	PT	Assesses extrinsic and common clotting cascade, activation of factor X by factor VII, and factors VI, X, V, II, and I (fibrinogen).
Activated partial thrombo-plastin time	APTT	Assesses intrinsic and common clotting cascade, activation of factor X by factors XII, XI, IX and VIII:C, and factors V, II, and I
Antithrombin	AT	Serine protease inhibitor that targets proteases of coagulation pathway such as activated forms of factors IXa, Xa, XIa, XIIa, IIa, and VIIa
Platelet count	PLT	Quantification of platelet numbers; key cell component in primary hemostasis and formation of platelet plug
Fibrinogen	Factor I	Quantification of fibrinogen; elevated in infection or decreased with consumption or liver disease
Template bleeding time	TBT	Measures number and function of platelets, level of von Willebrand's protein and vascular integrity; reference interval (minute): 6.8–12.8 (1 d); 1.7–8.1 (1 wk); 2.5–5.8 (>1 wk)
Fibrin degradation products	FDP	Measures presence of fibrin from action of plasmin on fibrin and fibrinogen
D-dimer	None	Specific evaluation for plasmin degradation of cross-linked fibrin
Thrombin time	None	Evaluates conversion time of fibrinogen to fibrin

Table 44.11 Coagulation parameters reported from healthy foals expressed as mean ± standard deviation except for D-dimers, which is expressed as the median (25th–75th range) [53–60].

Diagnostic test	<7 h	<24 h	48 h	4–7 d	10–14 d	25–30 d	Adult
PT (s)	10.4 ± 0.4	10.9 ± 0.6	11.1 ± 1.8	9.6 ± 0.6	9.5 ± 0.4	9.4 ± 0.4	9.5 ± 0.3
aPTT (s)	52.8 ± 8.1	56.8 ± 6.3	55.6 ± 10.4	39.8 ± 4.0	39.9 ± 4.8	40.8 ± 6.0	42.0 ± 8.9
Fibrinogen (mg/dl)	226.4 ± 57.3	116.8 ± 39.1	316.8 ± 42.8	196.8 ± 26.6	199.6 ± 50.0	221.1 ± 48.0	195 ± 54
Platelets ($\times 10^3/\mu l$)	381.6 ± 58.9	243 ± 170	222.2 ± 60.6	181 ± 60	218 ± 57	245 ± 59	153 ± 49
FDPs $(\mu g/ml + 1)^{1/2}$	—	8.2 ± 2.7	—	5.6 ± 3.4	4.5 ± 3.1	3.5 ± 2.6	1.8 ± 0.6
Antithrombin (%)	147.6 ± 15.0	107 ± 41	133.0 ± 20.7	164 ± 35	170.9 ± 40.9	166.5 ± 40.6	202 ± 82
D-dimers (ng/ml)	—	101 (36–270)	220 (140–472)	—	453 (304–716)	—	677 ± 119
TBT (min)	—	4 ± 2	—	4 ± 2	4 ± 2	4 ± 2	4 ± 2
ACT (min)	—	5.8 ± 1.3	—	5.8 ± 1.3	5.8 ± 1.3	5.8 ± 1.3	2.6 ± 0.5
Thrombin time (s)	—	—	—	—	—	—	13.5 ± 5.5
Protein C antigen (%)	—	63.5 ± 11.9	—	—	93.4 ± 10.6	—	98.9 ± 9.0
Protein C activity (%)	—	113 ± 23	—	—	84.6 ± 12.0	—	86.5 ± 17.6
Plasminogen (%)	—	82.3 ± 15.8	—	99.2 ± 16.1	98.1 ± 14.4	102 ± 14.4	114 ± 14
α-2 antiplasmin (%)	—	197 ± 40	—	207 ± 47.8	175 ± 55.5	174 ± 50.7	209 ± 43.6
TPA (U/ml)	—	2.2 ± 1.3	—	—	5.4 ± 4.6	8.9 ± 5.5	2.8 ± 1.9
PAI (U/ml)	—	39.0 ± 25.8	—	—	22.0 ± 10.3	10.0 ± 12.2	8.2 ± 2.5

TBT, template bleeding time; ACT, activated clotting time; TPA, tissue plasminogen activator; PAI, plasminogen activator inhibitor.

at least one abnormal coagulation test result in 64% of foals with septic shock [53].

The method in which these tests are performed impacts the reference intervals, particularly for coagulation testing. Collection of blood in citrate tubes assures accurate platelet counts [51, 63–65]. Platelet counts are equal or slightly higher in foals during the first few days of life, and then become analogous to adult concentrations [51, 54, 66, 67]. Although platelet counts are comparable, platelet function is impaired in the first week of life, being less responsive to factors that initiate aggregation [54]. PT and APTT are similar or longer and fibrinogen values are lower in the foal's first days of life when compared to adult horses [51, 52, 54, 66, 67]. Fibrin degradation products (FDP) are significantly higher in foals compared to adult horse for the first 2 weeks of life [66, 67]. D-dimer concentrations are lowest at birth and increase during the first week to a month of life [54], but were not different between foals 1–6 months of age compared to adult horses [68]. At this time, no studies exist comparing D-dimer concentrations between healthy neonatal foals and adult horses.

Miscellaneous Biochemical Markers

Biomarkers of myocardial injury in foals include measurement of serum cardiac troponin I (cTnI), cardiac troponin T (cTnT), and myocardial isoenzyme of creatine kinase (CKMB). In one study of 52 healthy foals between 12 and 48 hours of age, the 95th percentiles for cTnI was 0.49 ng/ml (range 0.01–0.51), cTnT was 0.03 (range 0.009–0.041), and CKMB was 7.4 ng/ml (range 0.40–9.3) [69]. Higher concentrations of cTnT and CKMB were noted in septic foals, as compared to healthy foals, but there was no differences among septic foals in regards to survival.

Several acute phase proteins (APP) produced by the liver have also been examined as a biomarker of the acute phase response to sepsis and include C-reactive protein (CRP) and haptoglobin. The median CRP and haptoglobin concentrations from 39 healthy, 24-hour-old foals was 39 mg/ml (range 0–240) and 1627 mg/ml (range 601–3224). Both of these markers are elevated in response to inflammation, but in one study neither CRP or haptoglobin was significantly higher in septic or ill neonatal foals when compared to healthy foals [70].

A variety of cytokines and other biomarkers have also been examined in foals, particularly in efforts to identify septic foals or predict survival and include interleukin (IL)-1β, IL-6, IL-8, IL-10, interferon-γ [71, 72], procalcitonin (PCT) [73], transforming growth factor-β [73], vasopressin [74, 75], adrenocorticotropin hormone [75], endothelin 1 [76], and adrenomedullin [77], among many others. Mixed results were reported in these studies, and the reader is encouraged to review them individually based on interest.

References

1 Axon, J.E. and Palmer, J.F. (2008). Clinical pathology of the foal. *Vet. Clin. Equine* 24: 357–385.
2 Bauer, J.E. (1990). Normal blood chemistry. In: *Equine Clinical Neonatalogy* (ed. A. Koterba, W. Drummond, and P. Kosch), 602–614. Philidephia: Lea and Febiger.
3 Bauer, J.E., Asquith, R.L., and Kivipelo, J. (1989). Serum biochemical indicators of liver function in neonatal foals. *Am. J. Vet. Res.* 50: 2037–2041.
4 Barton, M.H. and LeRoy, B.E. (2007). Serum bile acid concentrations in healthy and clinically ill neonatal foals. *J. Vet. Intern. Med.* 21: 508–513.
5 Feijo, L.S., Curcio, B.R., Pazinato, F.M. et al. (2018). Hematological and biochemical indicators of maturity in foals and their relation to the placental features. *Pesqui. Vet. Bras.* 38: 1232–1238.
6 Anderson, N.B. and Calkins, K.L. (2020). Neonatal indirect hyperbilirubinemia. *Neoreviews.* 21: 749–760.
7 Barton, M.H. and Hart, K.A. (2020). Clinical pathology in the foal. *Vet. Clin. Equine* 36: 73–85.
8 D'Allesandro, A.G., Casamassima, D., Palazzo, M. et al. (2012). Values of energetic proteic and hepatic serum profiles in neonatal foals of the Martina Franca donkey breed. *Maced. J Anim Sci.* 2: 213–217.
9 Berryhill, E.H., Magdesian, K.G., Kass, P.H., and Edman, J.E. (2017). Triglyceride concentrations in neonatal foals: serial measurements and effects of age and illness. *Vet. J.* 227: 23–29.
10 Boakari, Y.L., Alonso, M.A., Riccio, A.V. et al. (2021). Evaluation of blood glucose and lactate concentrations in mule and equine foals. *J. Equine Vet. Sci.* 101: 103369.
11 Bauer, J.E., Harvey, J.W., Asquith, R.L. et al. (1984). Clinical chemistry reference values of foals during the first year of life. *Equine Vet J.* 16 (4): 361–363.
12 Gosset, K.A. and French, D.D. (1984). Effect of age on liver enzyme activities in serum of healthy Quarter Horses. *Am. J. Vet. Res.* 45: 354–356.
13 Patterson, W.H. and Brown, C.M. (1986). Increases of serum gamma-glutamyltransferase in neonatal Standardbred foals. *Am. J. Vet. Res.* 47 (11): 2461–2463.
14 Haggett, E.F., Magdesian, K.G., and Kass, P.H. (2011). Clinical impllications of high liver enzyme activities in

hospitalized neonatal foals. *J. Am. Vet. Med. Assoc.* 239: 661–667.
15 Rumbaugh, G.E. and Adamson, P.J.W. (1983). Automated serum chemistry analysis in the foal. *J. Am. Vet. Med. Assoc.* 183: 768–772.
16 Kitchen, H. and Rossdale, P.D. (1975). Metabolic profiles of newborn foals. *J. Reprod. Fertil. Suppl.* 23: 705–707.
17 Rose, R.J., Backhouse, W., and Chan, W. (1979). Plasma biochemistry changes in Thoroughbred foals during the first 4 weeks of life. *J. Reprod. Fertil. Suppl.* 27: 601–605.
18 Hank, A.M., Hoffmann, W.E., Sanecki, R.K. et al. (1993). Quantitative determination of equine alkaline phosphatase isoenzymes in foal and adult serum. *J. Vet. Intern. Med.* 7: 20–24.
19 Divers, T.J. and Perkins, G.A. (2003). Urinary and hepatic disorders in neonatal foals. *Clinical Tech. Equine Pract.* 2 (1): 67–78.
20 Chaney, K.P., Holcombe, S.J., Schott, H.C. et al. (2010). Spurious hypercreatininemia: 28 neonatal foals (2000–2008). *J. Vet. Emerg. Crit. Care* 20 (2): 244–249.
21 Bernard, W.V., Hewlett, L., Cudd, T. et al. (1995). Historical factors, clinicopathologic findings, clinical features, and outcome of equine neonates presenting or developing signs of central nervous system disease. *Am. Assoc. Equine Pract. Proc. Annu. Convent.* 41: 222–224.
22 Palmer, J. (2006). Recognition and resuscitation of the critically ill foal. In: *Equine Neonatal Medicine: A Case-Based Approach* (ed. M.R. Paradis), 135–148. Philadelphia: Elseveir Saunders.
23 Castagnetti, C., Pirrone, A., Mariella, J. et al. (2010). Venous blood lactate evaluation in equine neonatal intensive care. *Theriogenology* 73: 343–357.
24 Guglielminotti, J., Pernet, P., Maury, E. et al. (2002). Osmolar gap hyponatremia in critically ill patients: evidence of sick cell syndrome? *Crit. Care Med.* 30: 1051–1055.
25 Gilla, G.V., Osypiwb, J.C., Shearere, E. et al. (2005). Critical illness with hyponatremia and impaired cell membrane integrity the "sick cell syndrome" revisited. *Clin. Biochem.* 38: 1045–1048.
26 Dunkel, B., Palmer, J.E., Olson, K.N. et al. (2005). Uroperitoneum in 32 foals: influences of intravenous fluid therapy, infection and sepsis. *J. Vet. Intern. Med.* 19 (6): 889–893.
27 Perkins, G.A., Valberg, S.J., Madigan, J.E. et al. (1998). Electrolyte disturbances in foals with severe rhabdomyolysis. *J. Vet. Intern. Med.* 12: 173–177.
28 Wooding, F.B., Morgan, G., Fowden, A.L. et al. (2000). Separate sites and mechanisms for placental transport of calcium, iron, and glucose in the equine placenta. *Placenta* 21 (7): 635–645.
29 Tennent-Brown, B. (2014). Blood lactate measurement and interpretation in critically ill equine adults and neonates. *Vet. Clin. North Am. Equine Pract.* 30: 399–413.
30 Sheahan, B.J., Wilkins, P.A., Lascola, K.M. et al. (2016). The area under the curve of L-latate in neonatal foals from birth to 14 days of age. *J. Vet. Emerg. Crit. Care* 26: 305–309.
31 Corley, K.T.T., Donaldson, L.L., and Furr, M.O. (2005). Arterial lactate concentration, hospital survival, sepsis and SIRS in critically ill neonatal foals. *Equine Vet. J.* 37 (1): 51–59.
32 Wotman, K., Palmer, J.E., Boston, R.C. et al. (2005). Lactate concentrations in foals presenting to a neonatal intensive care unit: association with outcome. *J. Vet. Intern. Med.* 19 (3): 409.
33 Borchers, A., Wilkins, P.A., Marsh, P.M. et al. (2012). Association of admission L-lactate concentration in hospitalized equine neonates with presenting complaint, periparturient events, clinical diagnosis and outcome: a prospective multicenter study. *Equine Vet. J. Suppl.* 41: 57–63.
34 Borchers, A., Wilkins, P.A., Marsh, P.M. et al. (2013). Sequential L-lactate concentration in hospitalized equine neonates: a prospective multicenter study. *Equine Vet. J.* 45: 2–7.
35 Dunkel, B., Kapff, J.E., Naylor, R.J. et al. (2013). Blood lactate concentrations in ponies and miniature horses with gastrointestinal disease. *Equine Vet. J.* 45: 666–670.
36 Stoneham, S.J., Palmer, L., Cash, R. et al. (2001). Measurement of serum amyloid A in the neonatal foal using latex agglutination immunoturbidimetric assay: determination of the normal range, variation with age, and response to disease. *Equine Vet. J.* 33: 599–603.
37 Magdesian, K.G. (1992). Monitoring the critically ill equine patient. *Vet. Clin. North Am. Equine Pract.* 24: 399–401.
38 Stewart, J.H., Rose, R.J., and Barko, A.M. (1984). Respiratory studies in foals from birth to seven days old. *Equine Vet. J.* 16: 323–328.
39 Madigan, J.E., Thomas, W.P., and Backus, K.Q. (1992). Mixed venous blood gases in recumbent and upright positions in foals from birth to 14 days of age. *Equine Vet. J.* 24: 399–401.
40 Niki, K., Thoh, T., Nose, H. et al. (1987). Estimation of plasma volume from hematocrit and plasma oncotic pressure during volume expansion in dog. *Jpn. J. Physiol.* 37 (4): 687–698.
41 Brewer, B.D. (1990). Neonatal infection. In: *Equine Clinical Neonatalogy* (ed. A.M. Koterba, W.H. Drummond, and P.C. Kosch), 295–316. Philiadelphia, PA: Lee and Febiger.
42 Madgedesian, K.G., Fielding, C.L., and Madigan, J.E. (2004). Measurement of plasma colloid oncotic pressure in neonatal foals under intensive care: comparison of direct and indirect methods and the

association of COP with selected clinical and clinicopathologic variables. *J. Vet. Emerg. Crit. Care* 14 (2): 108–114.

43 Landis, E.M. and Pappenheimer, J.R. (1963). Exchange of substance through capillary walls. In: *Handbook of Physiology* (ed. W.F. Hamilton), 961–984. Washington, DC: The American Physiological Society, Circulation.

44 Thomas, L.A. and Brown, S.A. (1992). Relationship between colloid oncotic pressure and plasma protein concentrations in cattle, horses, dogs and cats. *Am. J. Vet. Res.* 53 (12): 2241–2244.

45 Brown, S.A., Dusza, K., and Boehmer, J. (1994). Comparison of measured and calculated values for colloid oncotic pressure in hospitalized animals. *Am. J. Vet. Res.* 55 (7): 910–915.

46 Runk, D.T., Madigan, J.E., Rahal, C.J. et al. (2000). Measurement of plasma colloid oncotic pressure in normal Thoroughbred neonatal foals. *J. Vet. Intern. Med.* 14: 475–478.

47 Jones, P.A., Bain, F.T., Byers, T.D. et al. (2001). Effect of hydroxyethyl starch solutions in hypoproteinemic horses. *J. Am. Vet. Med. Assoc.* 218 (7): 1130–1135.

48 Jones, P.A., Tomasic, M., and Gentry, P.A. (1997). Oncotic hemodilutional, and hemostatic effects of isotonic saline and hydroxethyl starch solutions on clinically normal ponies. *Am. J. Vet. Res.* 58 (8): 541–548.

49 McFarland, D. (1999). Hetastarch: a synthetic colloid with potential in equine patients. *Compend. Contin. Educ. Pract. Vet.* 21: 867–873.

50 Mullins, R.E., Pappas, A.A., and Gadsen, R.H. (1983). Correlation of standardized serum protein determinations with calculated and measured colloid osmotic pressure. *Am. J. Clin. Pathol.* 80: 170–175.

51 Barton, M.H., Morris, D.D., Crowe, N. et al. (1995). Hemostatic indices in healthy foals from birth to 1 month of age. *J. Vet. Diagn. Invest.* 7: 380–385.

52 Diaz-Miron, J., Miller, J., and Vogel, A.M. (2013). Neonatal hematology. *Semin. Pediatr. Surg.* 22: 199–204.

53 Benz, A.I., Wilkins, P.A., Boston, R.C. et al. (2009). Prospective evaluation of coagulation in critically ill neonatal foals. *J. Vet. Intern. Med.* 23: 161–167.

54 Armengou, L., Monreal, L., Taracon, I. et al. (2008). Plasma D-dimer concentration in sick newborn foals. *J. Vet. Intern. Med.* 22: 411–417.

55 Barton, M.H., Morris, D.D., Crowe, N. et al. (1995). Hemostatic indices in healthy foals from birth to one month of age. *J. Vet. Diagn. Invest.* 7: 380–385.

56 Monreal, L., Angles, A., Espada, Y. et al. (2000). Hypercoagulation and hypofibrinolysis in horses with colic and DIC. *Equine Vet. J. Suppl.* 32: 19–25.

57 Hinchcliff, K.W., Kociba, G.J., and Mitten, L.A. (1993). Diagnosis of EDTA-dependent pseudothrombocytopenia in a horse. *J. Am. Vet. Med. Assoc.* 203: 1715–1716.

58 Knottenbelt, D., Holdstock, N., and Madigan, J. (2004). *Equine Neonatology Medicine and Surgery*. Philadelphia: Elsevier Science.

59 Lassen, E.D. and Swardson, C.J. (1995). Hematology and hemostasis in the horse: normal functions and common abnormalities. *Vet. Clin. North Am. Equine Pract.* 11: 351–389.

60 Feige, K., Ehrat, F.B., Kastner, S.B.R. et al. (2004). The effects of automated plasmapheresis on clinical, haematological, biochemical and coagulation variables in horses. *Vet. J.* 169: 102–107.

61 Chalmers, E.A. (2004). Neonatal coagulation problem. *Arch. Dis. Child. Fetal Neonatal Ed.* 89: F475–F478.

62 Rossdale, P.D. (2004). The maladjusted foal influence of intrauterine growth retardation and birth trauma. In: *Proceedings of the 50th Annual Convention of the American Association of Equine Practitioners*, 75–76. Denver, CO: AAEP.

63 Ehhrmann, C. (2015). An overview of equine hematology. *Pract. Tierazt* 96: 480–486.

64 Hinchcliff, K.W., Kociba, G.J., and Mittle, L.A. (1993). Diagnosis of EDTA-dependent pseudo-thrombocytopenia in a horse. *J. Am. Vet. Assoc.* 203: 1715–1716.

65 Williams, T.L. and Archer, J. (2016). Effect of prewarming EDTA blood samples to 37 degrees C on platelet count measured by Sysmex XT-2000iV in dogs, cats and horses. *Vet. Clin. Pathol.* 45: 444–449.

66 Darien, B.J., Carleton, C., Kurdowska, A. et al. (1991). Hemostasis and antithrombin III in the full-term newborn foal. *Comp. Haemtol. Int.* 1: 161–165.

67 Piccion, G., Arfuso, F., Quartucci, M. et al. (2015). Age-related developmental clotting profile and platelet aggregation in foals over the first month of life. *J. Equine Vet. Sci.* 35: 89–94.

68 Watts, A.E., Fubini, S.L., Todhunter, R.J. et al. (2011). Comparison of plasma and peritoneal indices of fibrinolysis between foals and adult horses with and without colic. *Am. J. Vet. Res.* 72: 1535–1540.

69 Slack, J.A., McGuirk, S.M., Erb, H.N. et al. (2005). Biochemical markers of cardiac injury in normal, surviving septic, or nonsurviving septic neonatal foals. *J. Vet. Intern. Med.* 19: 577–580.

70 Zabrecky, K.A., Slovis, N.M., Constable, P.D. et al. (2015). Plasma C-reactive protein and haptoglobin concentrations in critically ill neonatal foals. *J. Vet. Intern. Med.* 29: 673–677.

71 Castagnetti, C., Mariella, J., Pirrone, A. et al. (2012). Expression of interleukin-1β, interleukin-8, and interferon-γ in blood samples obtained from healthy and sick neonatal foals. *Am. J. Vet. Res.* 73: 1418–21427.

72 Burton, A.B., Wagner, B., Erb, H.N. et al. (2009). Serum interleukin-6 (IL-6) and IL-10 concentrations in normal and septic neonatal foals. *Vet. Immunol. Immunopathol.* 132: 122–128.

73 Pusterla, N., Magdesian, K.G., Mapes, S. et al. (2006). Expression of molecular markers in blood of neonatal foals with sepsis. *Am. J. Vet. Res.* 67: 1045–1049.

74 Borchers, A., Magdesian, K.G., Schenck, P.A. et al. (2014). Serial plasma vasopressin concentration in healthy and hospitalized neonatal foals. *Equine Vet. J.* 46: 306–310.

75 Hurcombe, S.D., Toribio, R.E., Slovis, N. et al. (2008). Blood arginine vasopressin, adrenocorticotropin hormone, and cortisol concentrations at admission in septic and critically ill foals and their association with survival. *J. Vet. Intern. Med.* 22: 639–647.

76 Giordano, A., Castagnettic, C., Panzani, S. et al. (2015). Endothelin 1 in healthy foals and in foals affected by neonatal diseases. *Theriogenology* 15: 667–673.

77 Toth, B., Slovis, N.M., Constable, P.D. et al. (2014). Plasma adrenomedullin concentrations in critically ill neonatal foals. *J. Vet. Intern. Med.* 28: 1294–1300.

Chapter 45 Hematologic Disorders

Bettina Dunkel

Hematologic disorders are not uncommon in neonatal foals and can be a primary problem or develop secondary to other disease processes such as sepsis. A brief physiology review involving various hematology parameters is presented here, with this section placing more emphasis on hematologic disorders.

Anemia

Physiologic Anemia of the Foal

Plasma volume, red blood cell volume, and blood volume have been determined in foals <24 hours and 2 days old in three studies using different methods [1–3]. Both methods and all studies reported comparable results: the plasma volume in the neonatal foal is 93–96 ml/kg, the red blood cell volume 59 ml/kg, and blood volume approximately 150 ml/kg [1–3].

Red blood cell variables change significantly during the first days and weeks of life in foals. Immediately after birth, packed cell volume (PCV) and hematocrit (Hct) are high, likely due to placental transfer of blood to the foal and splenic contraction of the foal during parturition. The difference can be substantial with immediate postpartum PCV ranging from 45% to 50% decreasing to 35–40% within the first days of life due to hemodilution after colostrum absorption followed by a further decrease [4]. Values should remain within the normal to low normal reference ranges for adult horses. The subsequent continuous slow decrease in PCV, Hct, and hemoglobin (Hgb) concentration in the first weeks of life can be accompanied by a decrease in mean corpuscular volume (MCV) and mean corpuscular hemoglobin (MCH) [5], which indicates that red blood cell numbers remain the same but become smaller and contain less Hgb over time. Mean corpuscular hemoglobin concentration (MCHC) remains normal to slightly low compared to adult values. Other studies documented no change in MCV, which might be due to the concurrent presence of micro- and macrocytes [6]. Thus, after an initial increase immediately after birth, foals develop a slight, often microcytic anemia during the first months of life, which is considered physiologic [4, 7]. Another difference in foals (1–18 days of age) is a higher erythrocyte osmotic fragility compared to mares [6]. The reasons for this finding and clinical relevance remain currently speculative.

Parameters relating to iron metabolism are also slightly different in foals compared to adult horses. The ferritin concentration is high in colostrum (354 ± 42 ng/ml), but low in milk (25 ± 2 ng/ml) [8]. Serum ferritin concentrations therefore increase after ingestion of colostrum and are briefly above adult reference ranges before rapidly decreasing during or after the first 24 hours of life [7, 8]. Thereafter, ferritin concentration decrease gradually to a minimum of 61 ± 6 ng/ml at 3 weeks of age followed by an increase to adult values at 6 months of age. The decrease and then increase in serum ferritin concentration occurs concomitantly with opposite changes in serum total iron-binding capacity [8].

Anemia of Chronic Disease

Inflammatory diseases result in release of acute phase proteins. Hepcidin is an acute-phase reactant that is predominately expressed in the liver in horses [9]. Plasma concentration increase in response to inflammation and after exposure to lipopolysaccharide [10]. Hepcidin binds to ferroportin-1 and induces degradation of the hepcidin-ferroportin complex, particularly in duodenal enterocytes and macrophages. As a result, iron absorption is reduced and storage in macrophages increases. This deprives rapidly dividing cells and invading microbes of iron. Serum iron concentrations are decreased despite an increase in ferritin due to intracellular iron sequestration.

Equine Neonatal Medicine, First Edition. Edited by David M. Wong and Pamela A. Wilkins.

Anemia develops when there is insufficient iron for red cell production. Anemia of chronic disease initially presents as mild to moderate normocytic normochromic anemia but can progress to microcytic and hypochromic if the inflammatory conditions remain [10]. The PCV usually remains greater than 20% [11]. Treatment is directed against the primary disease process; iron supplementation is usually not beneficial, as iron is not available rather than being deficient.

Anemia Secondary to Blood Loss or Hemolysis

Blood Loss Anemia

Foals might suffer from internal or external blood loss in the neonatal period. External blood loss is usually due to trauma and easily diagnosed. Internal blood loss into the thoracic or abdominal cavity might be associated with trauma sustained during parturition such as rib fractures, other external trauma or secondary to acquired or congenital coagulopathies. Blood transfusions might be necessary to stabilize foals with substantial blood loss. The half-life of the foal's own red blood cells (RBCs) after an autologous transfusion is approximately 12 days compared to 4–6 days for erythrocytes from the dam or a donor [12]. With internal bleeding into body cavities, an autotransfusion, although so far not reported in foals, could be considered. However, it is unknown if the increased life span also applies to autologous blood recovered from a body cavity. Autotransfusions are either performed by collecting blood aseptically from the affected body cavity using no anticoagulant or a reduced amount. This is due to the depletion of coagulation factors and platelets when blood comes in contact with serosal surfaces [13]. A ratio of 1:15 of 3.8% citrate to blood has been recommended [14]. The blood is then transfused back into the patient following routine procedures, ideally using a transfusion set with a filter.

Hemothorax

Thoracic trauma, particularly rib fractures, sustained during parturition is common in foals [15]. Physical evidence of rib fractures or chostochondral dislocation can be identified in up to 20% of foals <3 days old [16]. Considering the low sensitivity and specificity of physical examination, the true number of rib fractures in foals is likely much higher as ultrasonography identified rib fractures in 65% of hospitalized foals [15]. The injury is often clinically insignificant, particularly if nondisplaced and if only individual ribs are affected [15, 16]. However, displaced rib fractures can lead to hemothorax, hemoabdomen, and hemopericardium as well as pulmonary contusion, pneumothorax, diaphragmatic herniation, and myocardial laceration. In cases with internal thoracic injury, or a high likelihood of such an injury occurring, surgical stabilization is indicated, with several techniques described [17–19]. In cases with multiple rib fractures, fixation of one or two ribs might be sufficient to achieve stability in adjacent ribs [17].

Hematuria

Foals can experience cystic and urachal hematomas, which might manifest as stranguria, pigmenturia, or hematuria. This is often seen secondary to prolonged bleeding from the umbilicus with presumed retrograde blood flow into the urachus, umbilical arteries, and bladder [20]. Anemia is usually not reported with these cases but surgical removal of large cystic hematomas causing urinary tract obstruction might be necessary.

Leptospira Infection

Leptospira infection has been reported as cause of hematuria in a newborn foal and as a cause of fever, microcytic anemia, and thrombocytopenia along with azotemia, hyponatremia, and hypochloremia secondary to acute renal injury in foals 2 months of age [21, 22]. All foals survived although one required renal replacement therapy. In Europe, infection has also been associated with icterus, anemia, thrombocytopenia, azotemia, hematuria, or pyuria, and acute respiratory distress secondary to intrapulmonary hemorrhage in foals 3–20 weeks of age [23].

Only one of five foals survived in this case series suggesting a guarded prognosis. Diagnosis is achieved by PCR testing of tissue, fluids, and urine or the microscopic agglutination test (MAT) [24]. Paired serology can also be performed but is clinically less useful due to the time delay in confirming a titer increase [24]. Treatment with penicillin, ampicillin, ticarcillin, cephalosporins, macrolides, tetracyclines, and fluroquinolones has been reported together with supportive therapy [24].

Neonatal Icterus and Hyperbilirubiemia

In infants, neonatal icterus is caused by hyperbilirubinemia. Total bilirubin concentrations, predominately composed of indirect bilirubin, are higher in neonatal foals during the first days of life before gradually decreasing to adult concentrations within the next 2 weeks [4, 25]. Reported values range 2.1–3.6 mg/dl in newborn foals but clinically noticeable icterus is rarely present [25, 26]. Premature foals might even have higher concentrations with total and indirect bilirubin concentrations of up to 8.8 ± 0.9 and 6.8 ± 0.9 mg/dl, respectively [26]. Other causes of icterus in neonatal foals include hemolytic anemia, most frequently caused by neonatal isoerythrolysis, hepatic disease, neonatal piroplasmosis, and neonatal equine herpes virus 1 infection [27, 28].

Neonatal Piroplasmosis

A rarely reported causes of icterus, mild anemia, hemoglobinuria, and thrombocytopenia at birth is transplacental *Theileria equi* infection [29, 30]. Parasitemia might be evident on a blood smear and clinically affected foals reportedly die quickly. Foals can also be born apparently healthy following transplacental transmission and act as carriers [31, 32] although overall, transplacental admission appears to be rare [33]. Suspected transplacental transmission has also been reported for *Babesia caballi* [34].

Neonatal Isoerythrolysis

Neonatal isoerythrolysis (NI) is an immune-mediated hemolytic anemia (IMHA) caused by antibodies contained in the mare's plasma that react with the foal's RBC antigens. It is the most common cause of hemolytic anemia and icterus in neonatal foals. Most foals present within the first 3 days of life, but NI has been reported up to 12 days old [35, 36]. The prerequisites for development of NI are that the stallion has RBC antigens different from the mare's, and the foal has inherited the antigens from the stallion. In addition, the dam must have developed antibodies against the stallion's RBC antigens and transferred those to the foal via colostrum in sufficient quantities to cause clinical hemolysis. Exposure to RBC antigens that the mare does not have may occur from previous blood transfusions or prior foaling(s) as NI is most common in multiparous mares; however, NI has been reported in foals from maiden mares [37].

Historically, the RBC antigens Qa and Aa have been predominately associated with NI, largely because of their relatively high frequency in the horse population, the likelihood of a foal inheriting the factors, and their high degree of antigenicity. However, in one study these antigens only accounted for 55% of the cases suggesting that approximately half of all cases are caused by other antigens [36]. Other reported antigens include Ab, Ac, Qrs, Qb, Qc, Dc, Da, Db, Dg, Ka, Pa, and Ua [38–40]. Nonspecific hemolytic alloantibodies reacting with all tested equine blood types except the dam's own have been identified in Friesian mares with NI foals [39]. The anti-Ca alloantibody may protect against NI but extensive information is lacking [41]. Due to a donkey-specific antigen (donkey factor) on donkey RBCs, which is a xenoantigen to horses, all mule pregnancies (donkey sire × horse dam) are incompatible and are therefore at increased risk of NI (prevalence of NI in mule foals is up to 10%) [42, 43]. Most foals with NI will have adequate transfer of passive immunity but the condition has also been reported in foals with failure of passive transfer [36].

Common clinical signs of NI relate to hemolytic anemia including weakness, lethargy, tachypnea, icterus (Figure 45.1), fever, and tachycardia [35, 36] with the most pertinent clinicopathologic findings, including anemia (although the true degree can be masked by hemoconcentration) that is sometimes accompanied by thrombocytopenia, which might be more common in mule foals. The white cell count can be normal, low, or high. Other common abnormalities include hyperbilirubinemia, hemoglobinemia, hemoglobinuria, increased lactate concentrations, and acidosis.

(a) (b)

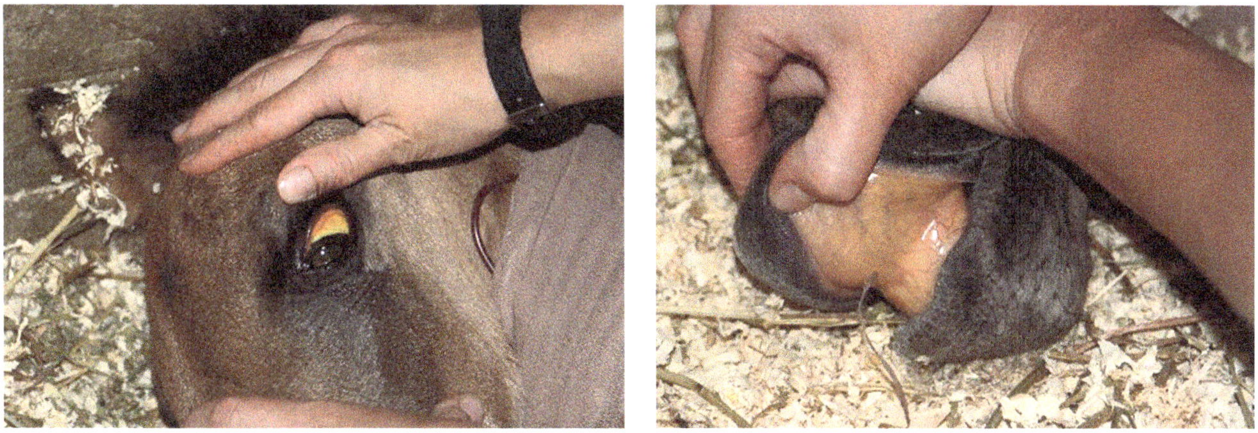

Figure 45.1 (a) Foal with neonatal isoerythrolysis; note the icteric sclera and (b) mucous membranes. *Source:* Images courtesy of David Wong, Iowa State University.

Diagnosis of NI is usually based on the age of the foal (typically <3 days of age) combined with clinical signs and physical examination abnormalities (lethargy, weakness, tachycardia, icterus) and laboratory results (anemia, hyperbilirubinemia). Definitive diagnosis is achieved by demonstrating antibodies in the mare's serum or colostrum that react with the foal's RBCs. A hemolytic cross match, rather than just agglutination, is recommended but requires the addition of exogenous complement. A direct Coombs test demonstrating antibodies bound to the foal's RBC surface can also be used but is considered less sensitive.

The Jaundiced Foal Agglutination (JFA) test assesses agglutination when the mare's colostrum is mixed with the foal's RBCs. The test can be used diagnostically but might be more useful when performed preventively in at risk mares before the foal is allowed to nurse. To perform the test, the dams colostrum is diluted with saline (1 ml of colostrum: saline dilutions at 1:2; 1:4; 1:8; 1:16, and 1:32) and each dilution is mixed with a drop of the foal's blood, which should be obtained before suckling. Following ingestion of colostrum, the foal's cells may become antibody-coated and auto-agglutinate in the JFA, even if colostral or milk antibodies are no longer present in significant amounts [44]. Pure saline and the mare's blood serve as negative control. The presence of agglutination can be observed after centrifugation for 2–3 minutes at medium speed and inversion of the tubes, best performed under a microscope. Alternatively, the test can be performed on glass slides. Rouleaux formation can resemble agglutination, which makes interpretation of the test more difficult and less reliable. Agglutination seen at dilutions of 1:16 or greater indicate a high risk for NI and the foal should not be allowed to ingest the colostrum or nurse from the mare in the first 36–48 hours.

Treatment depends on the severity of anemia and presence of concurrent disease processes. In mild cases, observation and supportive care might be sufficient. If the anemia is severe or if the Hct drops rapidly (e.g. over 6–12 hours), a blood transfusion will be necessary. Theoretically, washed RBCs from the mare are ideal. However, no differences between the use of whole blood from an unrelated donor or washed maternal RBCs and survival, total number of transfusion required, or total volume of blood administered during hospitalization have been noted [35]. As washing of maternal RBCs offers no clear advantage, using a compatible donor identified by cross match is more convenient. However, washing of RBCs should be considered if a suitable donor cannot be identified. If facilities for centrifugation of the mare's RBCs are not available, serial gravity sedimentation with isotonic saline and removal of the supernatant is a viable but time-consuming option. The half-life of transfused RBCs is 4–6 days and not different between RBCs from the dam or an unrelated gelding [12]. A different study found longer half-lives for transfused RBC in healthy foals, ranging from 9 to 21 days (median 14.6 days) [45]. For mule foals that require a blood transfusion a horse blood donor, ideally a gelding, should be chosen; the mare's washed RBCs would also be suitable if effective washing can be performed.

The need for a transfusion should be carefully considered, as with each additional administration of blood products the odds of nonsurvival increase 8.4 times. Hepatic injury secondary to hypoxia or, more commonly, administration of blood products and secondary iron overload can occur [35]. Histologically, lesions in foals with NI are similar to those reported after oral administration of ferrous fumarate to newborn foals [35, 46]. Due to the low tolerance of foals to iron (16 mg/kg of ferrous fumarate is often fatal) [47] more than 2–3 l of blood products can induce toxicity in a 50 kg foal (each liter of blood transfused delivers approximately 400–500 mg of iron) [35, 45]. Deferoxamine mesylate is a drug that chelates intra- and extracellular iron from ferritin and hemosiderin by forming a stable complex and is excreted in the urine or bile, thereby preventing iron from entering into further chemical reactions [45, 48]. In a randomized controlled study, administration of deferoxamine (20 mg/kg, SC q12h) for 14 days to neonatal foals that received a 3 l transfusion of packed washed maternal RBCs was associated with significantly lower liver iron concentrations and significantly higher urine iron concentrations and fractional excretion of iron in treated foals as compared to control foals. This study suggested that deferoxamine enhances urinary iron elimination and decreases hepatic iron accumulation after blood transfusion and may be a valuable adjunct therapy in foals with NI that require numerous blood transfusions. Its use has been reported as beneficial in preventing iron toxicity in one clinical case of NI in a foal [45, 49].

Kernicterus is another complication of excessively high bilirubin concentrations (Chapter 32) with a total bilirubin concentration >27 mg/dl increasing the odds of developing kernicterus 17 times [35]. Plasma exchange with a commercial plasmapheresis device has been used in foals with hyperbilirubinemia to decrease the risk of kernicterus, achieving a decrease in bilirubin concentrations between 44% and 57% [50]. Renal function should also be monitored closely. In one report, 67% of nonsurvivors showed histological evidence of renal damage and pigment nephropathy leading to acute kidney injury is a risk.

The prognosis for survival of hospitalized foals with NI is 75–88% [35, 36]. Considering that more severe cases are usually referred for hospital treatment, the overall prognosis is good. The only factor influencing nonsurvival in the largest study of NI in foals was the number of transfusions with blood products. While the need for repeated transfusions signifies more severe disease, it is likely that the additional iron load contributes to hepatic compromise and ultimately nonsurvival. The main reasons for nonsurvival in hospitalized foals were hepatic failure and neurological signs, often secondary to kernicterus or hepatic encephalopathy [35, 36]. The odds of liver failure increased by 2.1 with each liter of blood product administered, and the total volume of blood products administered was the only significant factor influencing development of liver failure [35]. The main factor for development of kernicterus was the total bilirubin concentration. Complications from sepsis also contributed to nonsurvival in both studies, highlighting that affected foals should be carefully evaluated for concomitant disease processes [35, 36].

Prevention can be divided into pre- and postbreeding strategies. Prebreeding, mares at risk can be determined by the fact that a previous foal has suffered from NI or by her blood type [44]. Mares negative for the blood types Aa or Qa or both have traditionally been considered at risk if bred to stallions positive for these antigens as they are likely to form antibodies against these factors if exposed. Estimates of the percentage of mares at risk because they are Aa-negative are 2% for Thoroughbreds, 3% for Arabians, 3% for Standardbred trotters, 22% for Standardbred pacers, and 25% for Quarter Horses. Estimates of the percentage of mares at risk because they are Qa-negative are 16% for Thoroughbreds, 72% for Arabians, 68% for Quarter Horses, and 100% for Standardbreds [44]. Prebreeding prevention would therefore include breeding to a compatible stallion; however, such a match might not always be desired or a suitable stallion might be hard to find. If an incompatibility is known or if a mare has produced NI foals in the past, postbreeding strategies should be implemented. As donkeys' RBCs carry an additional antigen (donkey factor), all mule pregnancies are considered high-risk. Postbreeding strategies can include testing the mare for presence of anti-RBC antibodies 14 days before the due date. This should be repeated every 14 days if the mare carries the foal longer than expected. Testing is usually performed for antibodies to Aa, Qa, Qc, and Ua. Alternatively, the colostrum can be tested for antibodies using the JFA test. If the mare is determined to be at increased risk for producing NI in a newborn foal or if the JFA test is positive, the foal should be muzzled for 36–48 hours to prevent further colostrum intake and the foal should receive mare's milk from a NI negative mare, goat's milk, or milk replacer. The dam should be thoroughly milked out at regular intervals and the colostrum discarded. Adequate passive transfer of immunity can be achieved by providing another source of colostrum or performing a plasma transfusion. The JFA test can be used to repeatedly test the dam's milk to determine when it is safe to allow the foal to nurse.

Other Causes of Hemolysis

A congenital enzyme defect causing severe deficiency of glucose-6-phosphate dehydrogenase resulted in persistent hemolytic anemia, hyperbilirubinemia, and Howell-jolly bodies in a Saddlebred colt and his dam [51]. NI was initially suspected and appeared to initially resolve until the foal represented at 6 months of age for persistent anemia secondary to increased RBC destruction.

Nonregenerative Anemia

Iron Deficiency Anemia

While iron deficiency is a rare cause of anemia in adult horses as iron intake via forage is usually more than sufficient, iron deficiency anemia develops more rapidly in neonatal foals due to their milk-based diet and absent or low forage consumption. Deficiency can be due to limited storage of body iron, increased iron demand during growth, and low concentration of iron in the dam's milk [52]. The first indications of iron deficiency are low serum ferritin concentration and decreased stainable iron stores in the bone marrow. Once iron concentrations have decreased to a level that affects erythropoiesis, a decreased percentage of plasma transferrin saturation, increased total iron binding capacity (TIBC), hypochromic RBCs (decreased MCHC), and release of small cells (microcytosis; decreased MCV) are noted.

Iron-deficiency anemia has been reported in foals without access to pasture and in a hospitalized foal treated for presumed sepsis [52, 53]. In the latter, microcytosis and hypochromasia were absent but multiple RBC abnormalities – including echinocytosis, keratocytosis, and schistocytosis – were noted [52]. In neonatal foals with confirmed iron-deficiency anemia, treatment with ferric sulfate (2 mg/kg PO q 12h) should be implemented. Prophylactic iron supplementation in healthy foals is not recommended, and acute and fatal hepatic failure has been reported following administration of products containing ferric fumarate (16 mg/kg of ferric fumarate) to neonatal foals ≤48 hours of age; foals with low levels of vitamin E and selenium are thought to be at particular risk. Colostrum provides large quantities of vitamin E, making administration of iron preparations before colostrum intake particularly perilous [47, 54–56].

Foal Immunodeficiency Syndrome/Fell Pony Syndrome

Foal immunodeficiency syndrome, previously known as Fell pony syndrome, is a fatal autosomal recessive disorder of foals of the Fell pony and Dales pony breed caused by a genetic mutation [57, 58]. The disease is characterized by severe nonregenerative anemia and B-cell lymphopenia [57, 59]. Foals are born healthy but clinical signs of pneumonia, diarrhea, and opportunistic infections begin to manifest within the first month of life. Foals rarely survive longer than 3 months of age [59]. Genetic testing on hair samples to identify carriers has significantly reduced the incidence of the disease [58].

Leukocyte Physiology in Foals

Foals are particularly vulnerable to infections and are affected by pathogens that normally do not cause disease in adult horses. This suggests a degree of immaturity and decreased effectiveness of the immune system during the first months of life [60]. The function and regulation of the foal's immune system and its gradual change over time toward adult immunocompetence are incompletely understood and investigations are ongoing.

Differences in immune functions described in foals including reduced antibody and T-cell responses and modified cytokine profiles to stimulation by pathogens [60]. The normal white cell and differential count in mature foals are largely comparable to adult values with few, clinically insignificant changes occurring during the first months of life (Chapter 42) [5]. The most common cause of either leukopenia and neutropenia or leukocytosis and neutrophilia in foals is sepsis or other severe, often infectious, systemic diseases. An increased presence of band neutrophils and toxic changes are also suggestive of sepsis. Less commonly, premature foals with incomplete adrenal maturation have a low total white blood cell and neutrophil counts and a neutrophil: lymphocyte ratio <1 : 1 [61, 62]. Anecdotally, failure to increase the total white cell and neutrophil counts over the initial 24–48 hours of treatment might indicate a poor prognosis for premature foals [62].

Leukocyte Disorders

Alloimmune Neonatal Neutropenia

Immune-mediated destruction of neutrophils in foals has been reported in a Thoroughbred and an Arabian colt [40, 63]. Both mares were primiparous; one had received a blood transfusion during gestation but in the other mare no inciting cause could be established. A further report describes neutropenia in three foals of varying breeds but sepsis was not convincingly ruled out [64]. Clinical signs attributed to the disease might be minimal, and the disease could go unrecognized if the foal doesn't experience secondary infections or blood samples are evaluated for other reasons. Leukocyte counts on presentations were 1200 and 3500/μl but neutropenia was severe, 620 and 950/μl, respectively. In one foal, a nadir of 8 neutrophils/μl was reached [63]. A granulocyte agglutination test and flow cytometry were used diagnostically to confirm the clinical suspicion. The pathophysiology is presumed to be similar to NI but the disease appears to be comparatively rare or rarely recognized. Administration of a single injection of granulocyte-colony stimulating factor (G-CSF; 3.5–6 μg/kg SC) resulted in a considerable increase in peripheral neutrophils, but one foal required repeated injections every 3 to 4 days (four injections total). Studies on G-CSF doses in adult horses investigated a range of 5–10 μg/kg and concluded that 7.5 μg/kg administered once subcutaneously achieved the best results (L. Riddell et al.; unpublished data). Both foals recovered completely.

Hemostasis

Repair of microvascular and macrovascular injury is essential for survival, particularly at times of disease or injury. Effective hemostasis is tightly controlled and relies on the interaction of the vascular wall, particularly the endothelium, platelets, and soluble plasma proteins. Spontaneous coagulation is prevented by several anticoagulant mechanisms. The healthy endothelium is covered by a glycocalyx, a complex network of negatively charged macromolecules formed by cell-bound proteoglycans, glycosaminoglycan side chains, and sialoproteins. Attached to these macromolecules are soluble molecules including albumin, hyaluronic acid, heparan sulphate, thrombomodulin, and antithrombin [65]. The glycocalyx plays a key role in regulating microvascular tone and endothelial permeability, maintaining an oncotic gradient, regulating adhesion and extravasation of leukocytes, and inhibiting intravascular thrombosis [65].

The quiescent state of circulating platelets and presence of the circulating coagulation factors in an inactive zymogen form also prevent spontaneous clot formation. Many coagulation factors have pro- or anti-inflammatory properties. Due to the extensive crosstalk between the inflammatory and coagulation systems, activation of the coagulation system and coagulopathies should be expected in patients with signs of systemic inflammation. Dysregulation of hemostasis is a major source of morbidity and mortality in foals and both increased bleeding and inappropriate clot formation can occur.

Primary and Secondary Hemostasis

Plasma-based factors broadly serve four different functions: coagulation, anticoagulation, fibrinolysis, and antifibrinolysis. However, functions of individual factors are not strictly separated, and one factor might have several roles, depending on circumstances and effects of negative and positive feedback loops. Inappropriate clot formation (hypercoagulability) is favored by a procoagulant environment, decreased anticoagulant activity, and inhibition of clot lysis (antifibrinolysis). Increased bleeding (hypocoagulation) occurs with high antithrombotic and fibrinolytic activities, decreased activity of coagulation factors and decreased platelet numbers or function. Two main components, primary and secondary hemostasis, initiate closure and repair of any defect. Primary hemostasis refers to platelet aggregation to form an initial platelet plug. Activated platelets adhere to the site of injury and to each other, thereby forming a platelet plug. Secondary hemostasis refers to the conversion of fibrinogen into an insoluble fibrin mesh that stabilizes the platelet plug. Defects of primary hemostasis are characterized by petechiae, ecchymosis, spontaneous bleeding from mucosal surfaces (including epistaxis and gingival bleeding), hyphema, hematuria, and melena. Defects of secondary hemostasis present as hematoma formation and bleeding into subcutaneous tissues, body cavities, muscles, or joints.

Overlap exists and particularly in acquired disorders, such as disseminated intravascular coagulation (DIC), multiple hemostatic defects cause clinical signs compatible with dysfunction of primary and secondary hemostasis. Similarly, mild von Willebrand disease might resemble a primary hemostatic defect, but in severe cases signs of a secondary hemostatic disorder are also present. Available hemostasis and coagulation tests and interpretation of the results in horses have been reviewed [66].

Coagulation

Earlier cascade or waterfall models that divided the coagulation process into intrinsic and extrinsic pathways have been replaced by cell-based models [67]. A key event in coagulation is the activation of prothrombin to thrombin, triggering the subsequent conversion of fibrinogen into fibrin. In the new models, tissue factor (TF) is the most important activator of coagulation. TF is highly expressed in extravascular tissue and becomes exposed with vascular damage. Platelets then adhere to the damaged site, mediated by von Willebrand factor, and aggregate through interactions of platelet receptors with extracellular ligands and soluble proteins. Trace amounts of thrombin formed during this process have multiple effects on other coagulation factors and platelets. This process and its progression can be divided into three phases: initiation, amplification, and propagation.

In the initiation phase (extrinsic pathway in cascade model), exposed TF binds and activates factor VII (FVII). The TF/FVIIa complex activates FIX and FX (FIXa and FXa). FXa and cofactor FVa build a prothrombinase complex on TF-expressing cells and convert prothrombin (FII) into thrombin [67]. The small amounts of thrombin generated in the initiation activate further platelets at the injury site (amplification phase). The propagation phase (intrinsic pathway in cascade model) takes place on phospholipid-containing cell surfaces, predominantly activated platelets. Activated FXIa converts FIX into FIXa, which then associates with thrombin-cleaved FVIII. On phosphatidylserine-exposing cell membranes, the FIXa/FVIIIa complex catalyzes the conversion of FX to FXa, which complexes with FVa to form enough thrombin to procedure fibrin fibers. As a final step, the thrombin-activated FXIIIa catalyzes covalent crosslinking between adjacent fibrin fibers, generating a fibrin clot [67]. Via multiple enforcement loops, large amounts of fibrin are formed, stabilizing the earlier-generated platelet plug [67].

Vitamin K is an essential coenzyme for factors II, VII, IX, and X and is necessary for their synthesis in the liver. Vitamin K deficiency can cause severe and even fatal hemostatic dysfunctions, which has been reported in foals [68]. Vitamin K catalyzes post-transcriptional carboxylation of glutamic acid residues on factors II, VII, IX, and X. In the absence of carboxylation, vitamin K–dependent factors cannot bind to platelets leading to hemostatic dysfunctions. Deficits of vitamin K can occur quickly due to the short half-life of the vitamin K-dependent coagulation factors. Vitamin K is lipid soluble and present in two types: K_1 (phylloquinone) is found in greens and oils, and K_2 (menaquinone) is produced by the intestinal microflora. Absorption occurs in the intestine in the presence of bile salts.

Anticoagulation

Mechanisms of anticoagulation prevent spread of coagulation to unaffected areas and retain clot formation at sites of injury. The three main pathways include the protease inhibitors antithrombin with its cofactor heparin, tissue factor pathway inhibitor (TFPI) and the protein C/protein S pathway [69]. Antithrombin is one of the most important inhibitors of thrombin generation because of its high affinity for FIXa, FXa, and thrombin. In the presence of its cofactor heparin, activity is increased up to 1000-fold. TFPI directly inhibits FXa and interacts with TF/FVIIa/FXa complex. Thrombin itself initiates anticoagulation by binding to thrombomodulin, which enables activation of endothelial-bound protein C. The complex of activated protein C (APC) and its cofactor protein S inactivate FVIIIa and FVa.

Fibrinolysis and Antifibrinolysis

The final step in the process of fibrinolysis is conversion of the circulating zymogen plasminogen into active plasmin. This is achieved by tissue-type plasminogen activator (t-PA) and, to a lesser degree, urokinase. In the presence of fibrin, binding of both plasminogen and t-PA to fibrin increases plasmin generation more than twofold [65]. The co-localization of both factors on fibrin aims to minimize indiscriminate fibrinolysis. Plasma inhibitors (α_2-antiplasmin and plasminogen activator inhibitor [PAI]-1 and PAI-2) also limit plasmin activity locally and its generation in the circulation. The recently described thrombin activatable fibrinolysis inhibitor (TAFI), which is activated by thrombin concentrations near recently formed clots, appears to inhibit premature clot lysis by preventing docking of t-PA and plasminogen to fibrin [65].

Coagulation and Inflammation

In the past decade, intricate connections between innate immunity, platelet activation, and coagulation have emerged. Part of this interplay between innate immunity and coagulation is termed *immunothrombosis* and represents an important host defense mechanism aiming to immobilize and fixate pathogens to limit systemic distribution through the circulation [70]. However, excessive activation or systemic spread of immunothrombosis can lead to widespread formation of thromboembolisms and secondary organ damage. The main contributors to immunothrombosis are leukocytes, platelets, the complement system, and activated endothelial cells. Platelets can migrate within the vasculature and function as scavengers that collect bacteria on their surface and present them to neutrophils [70]. The contact between neutrophils and platelets or exposure of neutrophils to soluble signals released by activated platelets trigger neutrophil activation and formation of neutrophil extracellular traps (NETs), a process called NETosis. NETs are three-dimensional structures consisting of nuclear DNA, histones and neutrophil granular proteins including myeloperoxidase, matrix metalloprotease-9 and neutrophil elastase, that are released by neutrophils following contact with infectious and noninfectious stimuli [69, 70]. NETs are recognized as major contributors to the development of DIC (discussed below) [69]. Another key mediator in immunothrombosis is tissue factor (TF), a strongly prothrombotic activator of coagulation. TF is not only expressed in the extravascular tissue but also by activated intravascular cells including endothelial cells, monocytes, platelets, and is contained within microparticles released from macrophages [71]. Thrombosis, in turn, can also trigger and exacerbate inflammation. Thrombin stimulates the release of proinflammatory cytokines and chemokines from immune cells and endothelial cells, providing another direct link between coagulation and inflammation [70, 72]. Many aspects of immunothrombosis and its role in critical illness are yet to be discovered, and a full review is beyond the scope of this chapter.

Neonatal Coagulopathies

Hemostatic and fibrinolytic indices for healthy foals are slightly different from adult values (Chapter 44). When investigating coagulation parameters in foals, inclusion of an age matched control is ideal but often not available. In their absence, published values offer guidance. Healthy neonatal foals have lower antithrombin, plasminogen, and tissue plasminogen activator (t-PA) activities, protein C antigen, and fibrinogen concentrations than adult horses. Protein C and PAI-1 activities and fibrin degradation products are significantly higher [73, 74]. D-dimer concentrations have been determined in healthy foals <24 hours of age up to 8–21 days of age and increased during this time from 101 ng/ml (36–270 ng/ml) to 453 ng/ml (304–716 ng/ml) [75]. This is slightly higher than values in healthy adult horses (164 ± 68 ng/ml) [76]. Prothrombin (PT) and activated partial thromboplastin (aPTT) times are slightly prolonged in foals [73, 74].

Mean platelet component (MPC), a variable measured by many hematology analyzers that indicates platelet activation, is also higher in neonates <21 days old compared to adult horses [77]. With the exceptions of antithrombin and t-PA activities, all hemostatic indices measured in foals at 1 month of age are equivalent to adult values; MPC has not been investigated in different age groups [73, 74]. Coagulopathies are common in ill neonatal foals and in most cases secondary to sepsis or other severe systemic diseases [75, 78–80]. While earlier studies predominately identified evidence of hypocoagulation in the form of bleeding [78, 79], fibrin deposits were detected in the microvasculature of 88% of septic nonsurviving foals consistent with a postmortem diagnosis of DIC and the presence of hypercoagulation [81]. Clinically, signs of hypocoagulation such as petechiae, ecchymosis, or bleeding from venipuncture sites are more frequently noticed than clinically noticeable thrombosis but both hypo- and hypercoagulation can occur [78, 79].

Hypercoagulation and Vascular Thrombosis

Hypercoagulation can lead to microthrombi in the microcirculation or thrombus formation in larger veins and arteries [81–86]. Confirmation of hypercoagulation states with commonly used laboratory tests is difficult as plasma-based coagulation tests including D-dimers and viscoelastographic methods have so far failed to reliably identify patients at risk of thrombus formation [75]. Thromboelastography demonstrated hypercoagulation in a small number of septic foals compared to healthy and sick nonseptic foals [87]. However, viscoelastography is affected by large intra- and inter-individual differences and intra- and inter-operator variability depending on the personnel performing the test [76, 88, 89]. Whether the method is sensitive and specific enough to tailor therapy in foals according to test results remains to be demonstrated in a larger population before it can be recommended to guide therapy. With sensitive microscopic detection methods, microthrombi can frequently be visualized in the tissues of euthanized foals with sepsis. The lungs are the most commonly affected organ, but a statistical association between organ failure and fibrin deposition could not be established [81].

Clinical signs associated with thrombus formation in larger vessels depends on the location and extend of the thrombus and associated vascular obstruction. Thrombi have been reported in the right ventricle, saphenous vein [83], portal vein [85], brachial artery [84, 90], distal aorta and ileac arteries [82, 91], and distal limb and digital arteries [86, 92, 93]. Lameness, cold distal limbs, absence of a peripheral pulse, skin discoloration, edema and separation of the hoof capsule from the coronary band might be observed with thrombosis of the limb arteries. The affected areas can be painful to palpation or show a decreased or absent pain sensation [86]. Diagnosis depends on the location of the suspected thrombus. Doppler ultrasonography might be able to confirm presence of an intraluminal thrombus and absence of blood flow. Contrast radiography and nuclear angiography have also been described [82, 84, 92].

Treatment of established thrombi is difficult. IV administration of t-PA (0.038 mg/kg) resulted in bleeding diathesis in one foal and subsequent euthanasia [82]. However, one intra-cardiac thrombus resolved spontaneously within one month [83] suggesting that intrinsic fibrinolysis can be highly effective if the foal survives long enough. This foal received anticoagulant medications in the form of warfarin, heparin, and acetylsalicylic acid but these only limit propagation of the existing thrombus and should not be expected to contribute to thrombus resolution [83]. Initiation of anti-coagulant therapy in at-risk patients before thrombosis occurs is ideal. As mentioned, identification of hypercoagulation is difficult as readily available plasma-based coagulation tests are not designed to detect hypercoagulation. Thromboelastography might be useful in the future as a tool to monitor and tailor therapy [87]. Routine anticoagulant treatment in septic foals might enhance the risk of bleeding and is so far not widely recommended. A low molecular weight heparin (dalteparin) dose of 100 IU/kg subcutaneously once daily has been recommended for neonatal foals to achieve adequate antifactor-Xa activity [94]. Fresh or fresh frozen plasma, with or without the addition of heparin (1000–1500 u/l used anecdotally) might be helpful in hypercoagulation as antithrombin concentrations, one of the main anticoagulants, are frequently low in septic foals [78, 79]. Disappointingly, administration of plasma had no effect on coagulation parameters and viscoelastography, and thereby indirectly outcome, in one study [80] but further investigations are necessary. Other treatments aimed at modifying platelet function such as clopidogrel have no or only limited effects on equine platelets and coagulation [95, 96]; clinical effects in ill foals need to be established.

Disseminated Intravascular Coagulation (DIC)

DIC is an acquired dysregulation of the coagulo-fibrinolytic system that occurs secondary to severe systemic disease processes. DIC is characterized by systemic intravascular activation of coagulation and suppressed fibrinolysis [72]. In people, the major conditions associated with DIC are sepsis, trauma, and whole body ischemia–reperfusion as it occurs following cardiac arrest and resuscitation [69]. Platelet activation and NET formation are recognized as major contributors to the development of DIC [69]. In addition, tissue factor (TF)-mediated activation of coagulation and thrombin generation is also seen as principal initiator of DIC. The procoagulant environment is further exacerbated by impairment of the three major anticoagulation pathways. Antithrombin, TFPI and activated protein C activities are decreased due to reduced synthesis, increased consumption and extravasation secondary to glycocalyx degradation and increased vascular permeability [69]. In addition, fibrinolysis is suppressed by inactivation of t-PA by PAI, which is produced by endothelial cells [72].

The diagnosis of DIC is based on the presence of a predisposing disease process and clinical or laboratory evidence of coagulopathy. Most cases of DIC in adult horses are subclinical, but particularly in septic foals, clinical signs such as thrombosis or bleeding diathesis can be observed [78, 86, 97]. Laboratory abnormalities classically associated with DIC include prolonged coagulation times (PT, aPTT), evidence of increased coagulation (increased fibrinogen/fibrin degradation products [FDP] and D-dimer concentrations and decreased fibrinogen concentrations), decreased platelet count and decreased antithrombin activity [97, 98]. However, these abnormalities best describe the consumptive coagulopathy observed late in the disease process [72] and the correlation between laboratory abnormalities and postmortem findings of DIC in horses is poor [99]. Recently, it has been suggested that the combination of biomarkers for thrombin generation such as thrombin-antithrombin complex (TAT) and fibrinolytic suppression, such as PAI, increase the predictive value for DIC and mortality in human patients [72]. Unfortunately, both are not routinely measured in horses.

No universally effective treatment for DIC has been identified. Treatment of the underlying disease process, supportive treatment and, in bleeding patients, platelet and fresh plasma transfusions are still the main stem of therapy [100]. Use of anticoagulants has not been universally beneficial in people and an increased risk of bleeding has been identified [72]. The presence and severity of coagulopathies secondary to a systemic disease process has repeatedly been linked to a worse prognosis in adult horses but findings in foals are less consistent [78, 80, 97, 98].

Upon stimulation with infectious and noninfectious insults, neutrophils release NETs presenting matrix DNA and histones with neutrophil components, such as neutrophil elastase and matrix metalloprotease 9, extracellular histones, cell-free DNA, and NETs formation are now recognized as major contributors to the development of DIC extracellular histones, cell-free DNA and NETs formation are now recognized as major contributors to the development of DIC Extracellular histones, cell-free DNA and NETs formation are now recognized as major contributors to the development of DIC Extracellular histones, cell-free DNA, and NETs formation are now recognized as major contributors to the development of DIC.

Vitamin K Deficiency Bleeding in Neonatal Foals

Vitamin K deficiency bleeding (VKDB), formerly known as hemorrhagic disease of the newborn, is a bleeding disorder caused by low levels of vitamin K-dependent clotting factors. Acquired VKDB is more common in human neonates. Neonates are very susceptible to vitamin K deficiency because of low stores at birth, poor placental transfer, low concentrations in milk and lack of production by an immature intestinal microflora [101]. Routine prophylactic administration of vitamin K has made human VKDB a rarity in most developed countries. In mares, transfer of vitamin K across the placenta is limited and foals are dependent on vitamin K intake from the mare's milk. While supplementation of mares during pregnancy increased vitamin K concentrations in milk, no differences in foals' plasma concentrations were detected [102]. VKDB has been suspected in a 4-week-old Standardbred colt presenting with hemarthrosis, spontaneous bleeding from the gingiva, blood covering of feces, and hematoma formation after venipuncture [68]. Activities of vitamin K-dependent factors II, VII, IX, and X were markedly decreased and improved following supplementation with vitamin K_1 (2 mg/kg SC q12h for 2 days, then 0.5 mg/kg PO q 12h for 17 days). Subcutaneous administration is preferred to avoid hematoma formation and risk of anaphylactoid reactions after intramuscular and IV administration, respectively. The condition was also suspected in a half-sibling colt but not further investigated. It is therefore unclear whether the condition was inherited or acquired.

Hemophilia A (Factor VIII Deficiency) and Multiple Clotting Factor Deficiency

Hereditary hemophilia A has been reported in Thoroughbreds, Standardbreds, Quarter Horses, a Tennessee Walking Horse, and in an Arabian colt with multiple clotting defects including factors VIII, IX, and X and to a lesser degree factor VII and prothrombin [103–107]. The disorder is caused by a mutation in the F8 gene, located on the X-chromosome; the mode of inheritance is X-linked recessive [108]. Carriers show no clinical signs despite often low factor VIII concentrations. Affected females have two nonfunctional copies and males have one nonfunctional copy of the F8 gene, making hemophilia A much more common in males [108].

In horses, the disease has only been reported in colts. Clinical signs can occur within the first days to months of life and relate to prolonged bleeding from the umbilical cord, repeated bleeding episodes, hematoma formation, epistaxis, hemarthrosis, and bleeding into body cavities [104, 107, 109]. Depending on the severity of the bleeding, moderate to severe anemia might be observed [107]. Coagulation tests reveal a normal platelet count and PT but prolonged aPTT. Fibrinogen concentrations might be decreased if inflammatory stimulation is absent. Treatment is supportive, and most animals that show clinical signs at a young age eventually die or are euthanized due to the poor long-term prognosis [104, 105].

Von Willebrand Disease

Von Willebrand disease is caused by quantitative and/or qualitative defects of von Willebrand factor (vWF), a multimeric glycoprotein synthesized by endothelial cells and megakaryocytes. The factor mediates platelet adhesion and aggregation and stabilizes factor VIII in circulation [110]. Without vWF platelet binding to collagen is reduced and primary hemostasis disrupted. Von Willebrand's disease can be congenital or acquired and in people, six different types (1, 3, 2A, 2B, 2M, 2N) have been described [110]. Von Willebrand's disease is rare in horses; so far, only congenital deficiencies corresponding to human type 2A and one suspected case of type 1 in an 8-day-old Quarter Horse colt have been reported [111–113]. Clinical signs in horses include bleeding from mucosal surfaces, epistaxis, hematoma formation, hemarthrosis, and prolonged bleeding from venipuncture sites, injuries, or after surgery. Bleeding times are prolonged whereas platelet count and PT are normal; aPTT can be normal or increased if factor VIII is deficient. A definitive diagnosis can be achieved by measuring plasma von Willebrand antigen using an enzyme-linked immunosorbent assay (ELISA); results will be low or normal, depending on type. Treatment in other species includes plasma transfusion or administration of desmopressin [114]. Desmopressin is a synthetic vasopressin analogue that increases release of vWF from endothelial cells and is particularly effective in type 1 cases. The prognosis depends on the age at presentation and severity of clinical signs. The neonatal foal was euthanized; another filly that presented at 3 days of age and animals that were older at the time of diagnosis survived [111–113].

Prekallikrein Deficiency

Without functional prekallikrein, activation of factor XII is less efficient, which might result in abnormal bleeding. However, the phenotype can be subtle, and severe bleeding is rare in people [108]. Prekallikrein deficiency causes prolonged aPTT with normal PT and fibrinogen levels. Prekallikrein deficiency has been diagnosed in a family of Belgian and Miniature Horses [115, 116]. Excessive hemorrhage and a markedly prolonged aPTT prompted further investigation, which led to diagnosis. It was presumed that animals with low prekallikrein activity might be homozygous for prekallikrein deficiency, whereas close relatives with values closer to normal might be heterozygous for the genetic defect. Platelet function and von Willebrand factor testing was not carried out, raising suspicion that other abnormalities could have remained undetected [108].

Platelet Disorders

Neonatal foals have similar to slightly higher platelet counts compared to adult horses [5, 73, 117], but platelet aggregation in response to some stimuli such as ADP and collagen is reduced in the first days of life [74, 117]. All values approach adult levels within the first weeks of life. Congenital platelet disorders are recognized in horses, including Glanzmann thrombasthenia and atypical equine thrombasthenia, but clinical signs are usually first noticed in young adult or adult horses and have not been reported in foals [118–121].

Thrombocytopenia

Thrombocytopenia has been reported in foals with sepsis but is an inconsistent finding and most studies have not found an association with sepsis or survival [78, 80, 122–124].

Neonatal Alloimmune Thrombocytopenia

Immune-mediated thrombocytopenia following ingestion of preformed antiplatelet antibodies in colostrum has been reported in horse and mule foals and is suspected to be more common in the latter [36, 125]. Thrombocytopenia can occur alone or in combination with NI. In mule foals, platelet destruction is suspected to be IgG mediated targeting the collagen receptor (GP I/IIa). Platelet dysfunction secondary to adhering antibodies has been described in these foals, highlighting the fact that risk of bleeding is not only determined by platelet numbers but also by their functional state [126]. The risk of hemorrhage depends on platelet numbers, platelet function, the activation state of the coagulation and fibrinolysis system and integrity of the endothelium and vascular wall. In adult horses, a platelet count <30,000 to 50,000/μl is likely to be associated with clinical signs such as petechiae or epistaxis and a platelet count <10,000/μl often manifests as active bleeding after venipuncture or hematoma formation [125, 127]. A platelet or whole blood transfusion is indicated if prolonged bleeding is observed or suspected due to a progressively decreasing hematocrit. Administration of whole blood might be the easiest option. Alternatively, platelet-rich plasma can be prepared in house. Citrate-based anticoagulant solutions are recommended and it is important not to underfill containers as platelet function is affected by increasing citrate concentrations [128]. Glass bottles are not suitable as glass surfaces activate platelets. RBCs are allowed to sediment by gravity, leaving the smaller platelets suspended in the plasma, which can be used as a platelet transfusion. If not administered immediately, the platelet-rich plasma should be stored at room temperature (72 °F [22 °C]) as exposure to temperatures below 59 °F (15 °C) induces irreversible changes and significantly decreases platelet function. In dogs, a fresh whole-blood transfusion of 10 ml/kg of body weight is expected to increase the recipient's platelet count by a maximum of 10,000/μl [129]. No guidelines are available for horses but similar to slightly lower increases might be expected, depending on the donor's platelet count. Drugs that negatively affect platelet function (acetylsalicylic acid, clopidogrel, heparin) should be avoided. Other nonsteroidal anti-inflammatory drugs such as flunixin meglumine and phenylbutazone have minimal effects on *in vitro* platelet function and can be used if necessary [130]. Administration of G-CSF to foals increases not only the neutrophil count but also platelets [63, 131]. The increase might be caused by G-CSF receptors on platelets [63] and in people, not only increased platelet numbers but also increased platelet activation and aggregation has been noticed [132], which could be beneficial in foals at risk of bleeding. Doses of 3.5–6 μg/kg administered subcutaneously have been used in foals [40, 63] and

7.5 μg/kg might be ideal as shown in adult horses (L. Riddell et al., unpublished data).

Thrombocytopenia, Neutropenia, Ulcerative Dermatitis

A syndrome of ulcerative dermatitis, thrombocytopenia, and neutropenia has been described in neonatal foals of varying breeds (Figure 45.2) [131, 133]. All mares of affected foals were multiparous and foals had adequate transfer of passive immunity. Two mares had two affected foals each in subsequent years [131]. Most foals had petechiae or ecchymosis and prolonged bleeding from venipuncture sites with one foal presenting with hemarthrosis, subcutaneous hematomas, and hematuria [133]. Platelet counts ranged from 0 to 30,000/μl, leukocyte counts from 1,900 to 3,200/μl, neutrophil counts from 500 to 1,900/μl and anemia with a PCV of 17% was reported in one foal [133]. Prothrombin time and aPTT were prolonged in one and two foals, respectively. Histology of the skin lesions identified multifocal ulcerations in the epidermis with abnormalities at the dermoepidermal junction adjacent to the ulceration. Early changes were characterized by subepidermal vesicular change, superficial dermal edema, vascular congestion, and superficial dermal hemorrhage, while more developed lesions showed dermoepidermal separation with fibrin, cellular debris, and RBCs filling the cleft [131]. Treatment included antimicrobials in all but one foal and corticosteroids in some foals; in two foals the thrombocytopenia appeared to be responsive to corticosteroid administration.

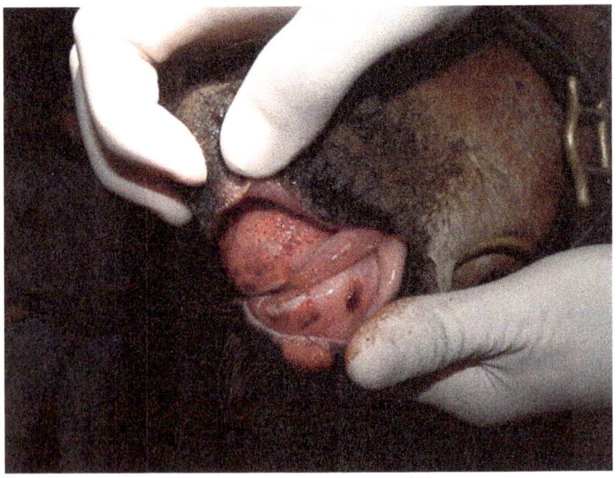

Figure 45.2 Petechiae and ecchymosis of the oral mucous membranes in a foal with thrombocytopenia, neutropenia, and ulcerative dermatitis. *Source:* Image courtesy of Kim Sprayberry, Hagyard Equine Medical Institute.

Whole blood or platelet rich plasma transfusions were also administered and G-CSF was used in one foal. This foal experienced a marked increase in neutrophil and platelet count [131]. The increase in platelet count has been observed in another foal before and might be caused by G-CSF receptors on platelets [63]. In people, not only increased platelet numbers but also increased platelet activation and aggregation has been noticed after G-CSF administration [132]. Although the exact etiology for the syndrome was not established, acquisition of antibodies or other factors via the colostrum was strongly suspected in all cases and is corroborated by the fact that two mares had affected foals in subsequent years [131, 133].

References

1 Persson, S.G. and Ullberg, L.E. (1981). Blood volume and rate of growth in Standardbred foals. *Equine Vet. J.* 13: 254–258.
2 Spensley, M.S., Carlson, G.P., and Harrold, D. (1987). Plasma, red blood cell, total blood, and extracellular fluid volumes in healthy horse foals during growth. *Am. J. Vet. Res.* 48: 1703–1707.
3 Fielding, C.L., Magdesian, K.G., and Edman, J.E. (2011). Determination of body water compartments in neonatal foals by use of indicator dilution techniques and multifrequency bioelectrical impedance analysis. *Am. J. Vet. Res.* 72: 1390–1396.
4 Barton, M.H. and Hart, K.A. (2020). Clinical pathology in the foal. *Vet. Clin. North Am. Equine Pract.* 36: 73–85.
5 Faramarzi, B. and Rich, L. (2019). Haematological profile in foals during the first year of life. *Vet. Rec.* 184: 503.
6 Arfuso, F., Quartuccio, M., Bazzano, M. et al. (2016). Erythrocyte osmotic fragility and select hematologic variables in postparturient mares and their foals. *Vet. Clin. Pathol.* 45: 260–270.
7 Kohn, C.W., Jacobs, R.M., Knight, D. et al. (1990). Microcytosis, hypoferremia, hypoferritemia, and hypertransferrinemia in Standardbred foals from birth to 4 months of age. *Am. J. Vet. Res.* 51: 1198–1205.
8 Harvey, J.W., Asquith, R.L., Sussman, W.A. et al. (1987). Serum ferritin, serum iron, and erythrocyte values in foals. *Am. J. Vet. Res.* 48: 1348–1352.
9 Oliveira-Filho, J.P., Badial, P.R., Cunha, P.H. et al. (2012). Lipopolysaccharide infusion up-regulates hepcidin mRNA expression in equine liver. *Innate Immun.* 18: 438–446.
10 Chambers, K., Ashraf, M.A., and Sharma, S. (2021). *Physiology, Hepcidin*. Treasure Island (FL): StatPearls.

11 Chervier, C., Cadore, J.L., Rodriguez-Pineiro, M.I. et al. (2012). Causes of anaemia other than acute blood loss and their clinical significance in dogs. *J. Small Anim. Pract.* 53: 223–227.

12 Smith, J.E., Dever, M., Smith, J. et al. (1992). Post-transfusion survival of 50Cr-labeled erythrocytes in neonatal foals. *J. Vet. Intern. Med.* 6: 183–185.

13 Fouche, N., Cornelisse, K., Gerber, V. et al. (2014). Noncitrated blood transfusions used as adjunctive treatment in a 7-year-old Shetland pony with haemoperitoneum due to a ruptured corpus haemorrhagicum. *Equine Vet. Educ.* 26: 250–254.

14 Finding, E.J.T., Eliashar, E., Johns, I.C. et al. (2011). Autologous blood transfusion following an allogenic transfusion reaction in a case of acute anaemia due to intra-abdominal bleeding. *Equine Vet. Educ.* 23: 339–342.

15 Jean, D., Picandet, V., Macieira, S. et al. (2007). Detection of rib trauma in newborn foals in an equine critical care unit: a comparison of ultrasonography, radiography and physical examination. *Equine Vet. J.* 39: 158–163.

16 Jean, D., Laverty, S., Halley, J. et al. (1999). Thoracic trauma in newborn foals. *Equine Vet. J.* 31: 149–152.

17 Bellezzo, F., Hunt, R.J., Provost, R. et al. (2004). Surgical repair of rib fractures in 14 neonatal foals: case selection, surgical technique and results. *Equine Vet. J.* 36: 557–562.

18 Williams, T.B., Williams, J.M., and Rodgerson, D.H. (2017). Internal fixation of fractured ribs in neonatal foals with nylon cable tie using a modified technique. *Can. Vet. J.* 58: 579–581.

19 Kraus, B.M., Richardson, D.W., Sheridan, G. et al. (2005). Multiple rib fracture in a neonatal foal using a nylon strand suture repair technique. *Vet. Surg.* 34: 399–404.

20 Arnold, C.E., Chaffin, M.K., and Rush, B.R. (2005). Hematuria associated with cystic hematomas in three neonatal foals. *J. Am. Vet. Med. Assoc.* 227 (778–780): 741.

21 Fouche, N., Graubner, C., Lanz, S. et al. (2020). Acute kidney injury due to Leptospira interrogans in 4 foals and use of renal replacement therapy with intermittent hemodiafiltration in 1 foal. *J. Vet. Intern. Med.* 34: 1007–1012.

22 Bernard, W.V., Williams, D., Tuttle, P.A. et al. (1993). Hematuria and leptospiruria in a foal. *J. Am. Vet. Med. Assoc.* 203: 276–278.

23 Broux, B., Torfs, S., Wegge, B. et al. (2012). Acute respiratory failure caused by Leptospira spp. in 5 foals. *J. Vet. Intern. Med.* 26: 684–687.

24 Divers, T.J., Chang, Y.F., Irby, N.L. et al. (2019). Leptospirosis: an important infectious disease in North American horses. *Equine Vet. J.* 51: 287–292.

25 Barton, M.H. and LeRoy, B.E. (2007). Serum bile acids concentrations in healthy and clinically ill neonatal foals. *J. Vet. Intern. Med.* 21: 508–513.

26 Feijo, L.S., Curcio, B.R., Pazinato, F.M. et al. (2018). Hematological and biochemical indicators of maturity in foals and their relation to placental features. *Pesq. Vet. Bras.* 38: 1232–1238.

27 Murray, M.J., del Piero, F., Jeffrey, S.C. et al. (1998). Neonatal equine herpesvirus type 1 infection on a thoroughbred breeding farm. *J. Vet. Intern. Med.* 12: 36–41.

28 Hess-Dudan, F. (1994). Four possible causes of hepatic failure and/or icterus in the newborn foal. *Equine Vet. Educ.* 6: 310–315.

29 Georges, K.C., Ezeokoli, C.D., Sparagano, O. et al. (2011). A case of transplacental transmission of *Theileria equi* in a foal in Trinidad. *Vet. Parasitol.* 175: 363–366.

30 Chhabra, S., Ranjan, R., Uppal, S.K. et al. (2012). Transplacental transmission of *Babesia equi* (*Theileria equi*) from carrier mares to foals. *J. Parasit. Dis.* 36: 31–33.

31 Allsopp, M.T., Lewis, B.D., and Penzhorn, B.L. (2007). Molecular evidence for transplacental transmission of *Theileria equi* from carrier mares to their apparently healthy foals. *Vet. Parasitol.* 148: 130–136.

32 Phipps, L.P. and Otter, A. (2004). Transplacental transmission of *Theileria equi* in two foals born and reared in the United Kingdom. *Vet. Rec.* 154: 406–408.

33 Tirosh-Levy, S., Gottlieb, Y., Mimoun, L. et al. (2020). Transplacental transmission of *Theileria equi* is not a common cause of abortions and infection of foals in Israel. *Animals (Basel)* 10: 341.

34 Santos, T.M., Santos, H.A., and Massard, C.L. (2008). Molecular diagnostic of congenital babesiosis in neonates foals from state of Rio de Janeiro, Brazil. *Rev. Bras. Parasitol. Vet.* 17 (Suppl 1): 348–350.

35 Polkes, A.C., Giguere, S., Lester, G.D. et al. (2008). Factors associated with outcome in foals with neonatal isoerythrolysis (72 cases, 1988–2003). *J. Vet. Intern. Med.* 22: 1216–1222.

36 Boyle, A.G., Magdesian, K.G., and Ruby, R.E. (2005). Neonatal isoerythrolysis in horse foals and a mule foal: 18 cases (1988–2003). *J. Am. Vet. Med. Assoc.* 227: 1276–1283.

37 Jalali, S.M., Razi-Jalali, M., Ghadrdan-Mashhadi, A. et al. (2018). Occurrence, hematologic and serum biochemical characteristics of neonatal isoerythrolysis in Arabian horses of Iran. *Iranian J. Vet. Sci. Technol.* 10: 39–45.

38 MacLeay, J.M. (2001). Neonatal isoerythrolysis involving the Qc and Db antigens in a foal. *J. Am. Vet. Med. Assoc.* 219 (79–81): 50.

39 de Graaf-Roelfsema, E., van der Kolk, J.H., Boerma, S. et al. (2007). Non-specific haemolytic alloantibody causing equine neonatal isoerythrolysis. *Vet. Rec.* 161: 202–204.

40 Wong, D.M., Alcott, C.J., Clark, S.K. et al. (2012). Alloimmune neonatal neutropenia and neonatal isoerythrolysis in a thoroughbred colt. *J. Vet. Diagn. Invest.* 24: 219–226.

41 Bailey, E., Albright, D.G., and Henney, P.J. (1988). Equine neonatal isoerythrolysis: evidence for prevention by

maternal antibodies to the ca blood group antigen. *Am. J. Vet. Res.* 49: 1218–1222.
42 McClure, J.J., Koch, C., and Traub-Dargatz, J. (1994). Characterization of a red blood cell antigen in donkeys and mules associated with neonatal isoerythrolysis. *Anim. Genet.* 25: 119–120.
43 Traub-Dargatz, J.L., McClure, J.J., Koch, C. et al. (1995). Neonatal isoerythrolysis in mule foals. *J. Am. Vet. Med. Assoc.* 206: 67–70.
44 McClure, B.J. (2003). Strategies to prevent neonatal isoerythrolysis in horses and mules. *Equine Vet. Educ.* Manual 6: 6–10.
45 Elfenbein, J.R., Giguere, S., Meyer, S.K. et al. (2010). The effects of deferoxamine mesylate on iron elimination after blood transfusion in neonatal foals. *J. Vet. Intern. Med.* 24: 1475–1482.
46 Acland, H.M., Mann, P.C., Robertson, J.L. et al. (1984). Toxic hepatopathy in neonatal foals. *Vet. Pathol.* 21: 3–9.
47 Mullaney, T.P. and Brown, C.M. (1988). Iron toxicity in neonatal foals. *Equine Vet. J.* 20: 119–124.
48 Gummery, L., Johnston, P.E.J., Sutton, D.G.M. et al. (2019). Two cases of hepatopathy and hyperferraemia managed with deferoxamine and phlebotomy. *Equine Vet. Educ.* 31: 575–581.
49 Wilkes E, Feary D, Raidal S, et al. (2018). The use of deferoxamine mesylate for the management of iron overload in a foal with neonatal isoerythrolysis. Poster presented at 40th Bain Fallon Memorial Lectures, Sydney, Australia.
50 Broux, B., Lefere, L., Deprez, P. et al. (2015). Plasma exchange as a treatment for hyperbilirubinemia in 2 foals with neonatal isoerythrolysis. *J. Vet. Intern. Med.* 29: 736–738.
51 Stockham, S.L., Harvey, J.W., and Kinden, D.A. (1994). Equine glucose-6-phosphate dehydrogenase deficiency. *Vet. Pathol.* 31: 518–527.
52 Fleming, K.A., Barton, M.H., and Latimer, K.S. (2006). Iron deficiency anemia in a neonatal foal. *J. Vet. Intern. Med.* 20: 1495–1498.
53 Brommer, H. and Sloet van Oldruitenborgh-Oosterbaan, M.M. (2001). Iron deficiency in stabled Dutch Warmblood foals. *J. Vet. Intern. Med.* 15: 482–485.
54 Divers, T.J., Warner, A., Vaala, W.E. et al. (1983). Toxic hepatic failure in newborn foals. *J. Am. Vet. Med. Assoc.* 183: 1407–1413.
55 Swerczek, T.W. and Crowe, M.W. (1983). Hepatotoxicosis in neonatal foals. *J. Am. Vet. Med. Assoc.* 183: 388.
56 Mullaney, T.P., Brown, C.M., Watson, G.L. et al. (1984). Suspected hepatotoxicity in neonatal foals: preliminary report of an emerging syndrome. *Vet. Rec.* 114: 115–117.
57 Fox-Clipsham, L.Y., Carter, S.D., Goodhead, I. et al. (2011). Identification of a mutation associated with fatal foal immunodeficiency syndrome in the Fell and Dales pony. *PLoS Genet.* 7: e1002133.
58 Carter, S.D., Fox-Clipsham, L.Y., Christley, R. et al. (2013). Foal immunodeficiency syndrome: carrier testing has markedly reduced disease incidence. *Vet. Rec.* 172: 398.
59 Tallmadge, R.L., Stokol, T., Gould-Earley, M.J. et al. (2012). Fell pony syndrome: characterization of developmental hematopoiesis failure and associated gene expression profiles. *Clin. Vaccine Immunol.* 19: 1054–1064.
60 Perkins, G.A. and Wagner, B. (2015). The development of equine immunity: current knowledge on immunology in the young horse. *Equine Vet. J.* 47: 267–274.
61 Jeffcott, L.B., Rossdale, P.D., and Leadon, D.P. (1982). Haematological changes in the neonatal period of normal and induced premature foals. *J. Reprod. Fertil. Suppl.* 32: 537–544.
62 Lester, G.D. (2005). Maturity of the neonatal foal. *Vet. Clin. North Am. Equine Pract.* 21: 333–355.
63 Davis, E.G., Rush, B., Bain, F. et al. (2003). Neonatal neutropenia in an Arabian foal. *Equine Vet. J.* 35: 517–520.
64 Leidl, W., Cwik, S., and Schmid, D.O. (1980). Neonatal isoimmune leukopenia in foals. *Berl. Munch. Tierarztl. Wochenschr.* 93: 141–144.
65 Draxler, D.F. and Medcalf, R.L. (2015). The fibrinolytic system-more than fibrinolysis? *Transfus. Med. Rev.* 29: 102–109.
66 DeNotta, S.L. and Brooks, M.B. (2020). Coagulation assessment in the equine patient. *Vet. Clin. North Am. Equine Pract.* 36: 53–71.
67 Versteeg, H.H., Heemskerk, J.W., Levi, M. et al. (2013). New fundamentals in hemostasis. *Physiol. Rev.* 93: 327–358.
68 McGorum, B.C., Henderson, I.S., Stirling, D. et al. (2009). Vitamin K deficiency bleeding in a Standardbred colt. *J. Vet. Intern. Med.* 23: 1307–1310.
69 Gando, S. and Wada, T. (2019). Disseminated intravascular coagulation in cardiac arrest and resuscitation. *J. Thromb. Haemost.* 17: 1205–1216.
70 Stark, K. and Massberg, S. (2021). Interplay between inflammation and thrombosis in cardiovascular pathology. *Nat. Rev. Cardiol.*.
71 Ito, T., Kakuuchi, M., and Maruyama, I. (2021). Endotheliopathy in septic conditions: mechanistic insight into intravascular coagulation. *Crit. Care* 25: 95.
72 Iba, T., Connors, J.M., Nagaoka, I. et al. (2021). Recent advances in the research and management of sepsis-associated DIC. *Int. J. Hematol.* 113: 24–33.
73 Barton, M.H., Morris, D.D., Crowe, N. et al. (1995). Hemostatic indices in healthy foals from birth to one month of age. *J. Vet. Diagn. Invest.* 7: 380–385.

74 Piccione, G., Arfuso, F., Quartuccio, M. et al. (2015). Age-related developmental clotting profile and platelet aggregation in foals over the first month of life. *J. Equine Vet. Sci.* 35: 89–94.

75 Armengou, L., Monreal, L., Tarancon, I. et al. (2008). Plasma D-dimer concentration in sick newborn foals. *J. Vet. Intern. Med.* 22: 411–417.

76 Dunkel, B., Chan, D.L., Boston, R. et al. (2010). Association between hypercoagulability and decreased survival in horses with ischemic or inflammatory gastrointestinal disease. *J. Vet. Intern. Med.* 24: 1467–1474.

77 Segura, D., Monreal, L., Armengou, L. et al. (2007). Mean platelet component as an indicator of platelet activation in foals and adult horses. *J. Vet. Intern. Med.* 21: 1076–1082.

78 Barton, M.H., Morris, D.D., Norton, N. et al. (1998). Hemostatic and fibrinolytic indices in neonatal foals with presumed septicemia. *J. Vet. Intern. Med.* 12: 26–35.

79 Bentz, A.I., Palmer, J.E., Dallap, B.L. et al. (2009). Prospective evaluation of coagulation in critically ill neonatal foals. *J. Vet. Intern. Med.* 23: 161–167.

80 Dallap Schaer, B.L., Bentz, A.I., Boston, R.C. et al. (2009). Comparison of viscoelastic coagulation analysis and standard coagulation profiles in critically ill neonatal foals to outcome. *J. Vet. Emerg. Crit. Care (San Antonio)* 19: 88–95.

81 Cotovio, M., Monreal, L., Armengou, L. et al. (2008). Fibrin deposits and organ failure in newborn foals with severe septicemia. *J. Vet. Intern. Med.* 22: 1403–1410.

82 Duggan, V.E., Holbrook, T.C., Dechant, J.E. et al. (2004). Diagnosis of aorto-iliac thrombosis in a Quarter Horse foal using Doppler ultrasound and nuclear scintigraphy. *J. Vet. Intern. Med.* 18: 753–756.

83 Banse, H., Holbrook, T.C., Gilliam, L. et al. (2012). Right ventricular and saphenous vein thrombi associated with sepsis in a Quarter Horse foal. *J. Vet. Intern. Med.* 26: 178–182.

84 Triplett, E.A., O'Brien, R.T., Wilson, D.G. et al. (1996). Thrombosis of the brachial artery in a foal. *J. Vet. Intern. Med.* 10: 330–332.

85 Ness, S.L., Kennedy, L.A., and Slovis, N.M. (2013). Hyperammonemic encephalopathy associated with portal vein thrombosis in a thoroughbred foal. *J. Vet. Intern. Med.* 27: 382–386.

86 Brianceau, P. and Divers, T.J. (2001). Acute thrombosis of limb arteries in horses with sepsis: five cases (1988–1998). *Equine Vet. J.* 33: 105–109.

87 Mendez-Angulo, J.L., Mudge, M., Zaldivar-Lopez, S. et al. (2011). Thromboelastography in healthy, sick non-septic and septic neonatal foals. *Aust. Vet. J.* 89: 500–505.

88 Thane, K., Bedenice, D., and Pacheco, A. (2017). Operator-based variability of equine thromboelastography. *J. Vet. Emerg. Crit. Care (San Antonio)* 27: 419–424.

89 Epstein, K.L., Brainard, B.M., Lopes, M.A. et al. (2009). Thrombelastography in 26 healthy horses with and without activation by recombinant human tissue factor. *J. Vet. Emerg. Crit. Care (San Antonio)* 19: 96–101.

90 Spier, S. (1985). Arterial thrombosis as the cause of lameness in a foal. *J. Am. Vet. Med. Assoc.* 187: 164–165.

91 Moore, L.A., Johnson, P.J., and Bailey, K.L. (1998). Aorto-iliac thrombosis in a foal. *Vet. Rec.* 142: 459–462.

92 Forrest, L.J., Cooley, A.J., and Darien, B.J. (1999). Digital arterial thrombosis in a septicemic foal. *J. Vet. Intern. Med.* 13: 382–385.

93 Lawhon, S.D., Lopez, F.R., Joswig, A. et al. (2014). Weissella confusa septicemia in a foal. *J. Vet. Diagn. Invest.* 26: 150–153.

94 Armengou, L., Monreal, L., Delgado, M.A. et al. (2010). Low-molecular-weight heparin dosage in newborn foals. *J. Vet. Intern. Med.* 24: 1190–1195.

95 Norris, J.W., Watson, J.L., Tablin, F. et al. (2019). Pharmacokinetics and competitive pharmacodynamics of ADP-induced platelet activation after oral administration of clopidogrel to horses. *Am. J. Vet. Res.* 80: 505–512.

96 Brooks, M.B., Divers, T.J., Watts, A.E. et al. (2013). Effects of clopidogrel on the platelet activation response in horses. *Am. J. Vet. Res.* 74: 1212–1222.

97 Dolente, B.A., Wilkins, P.A., and Boston, R.C. (2002). Clinicopathologic evidence of disseminated intravascular coagulation in horses with acute colitis. *J. Am. Vet. Med. Assoc.* 220: 1034–1038.

98 Dallap, B.L., Dolente, B., and Boston, R.C. (2003). Coagulation profiles in 27 horses with large colon volvulus. *J. Vet. Emerg. Crit. Care* 13: 215–225.

99 Cesarini, C., Cotovio, M., Rios, J. et al. (2016). Association between necropsy evidence of disseminated intravascular coagulation and hemostatic variables before death in horses with colic. *J. Vet. Intern. Med.* 30: 269–275.

100 Smith, L. (2021). Disseminated intravascular coagulation. *Semin. Oncol. Nurs.* 37: 151135.

101 Lembo, C., Buonocore, G., and Perrone, S. (2021). The challenge to define the optimal prophylactic regimen for vitamin K deficiency bleeding in infants. *Acta Paediatr.* 110: 1113–1118.

102 Fischer, T.J., Coyle, M.P., Regtop, H.L. et al. (2017). Placental transfer of vitamin K in the horse. *J. Equine Vet. Sci.* 52: 57.

103 Archer, R.K. and Allen, B.V. (1972). True haemophilia in horses. *Vet. Rec.* 91: 655–656.

104 Littlewood, J.D., Bevan, S.A., and Corke, M.J. (1991). Haemophilia A (classic haemophilia, factor VIII deficiency) in a Thoroughbred colt foal. *Equine Vet. J.* 23: 70–72.

105 Henninger, R.W. (1988). Hemophilia A in two related Quarter Horse colts. *J. Am. Vet. Med. Assoc.* 193: 91–94.

106 Sanger, V.L., Mairs, R.E., and Trapp, A.L. (1964). Hemophilia in a foal. *J. Am. Vet. Med. Assoc.* 144: 259–264.

107 Norton, E.M., Wooldridge, A.A., Stewart, A.J. et al. (2016). Abnormal coagulation factor VIII transcript in a Tennessee Walking Horse colt with hemophilia A. *Vet. Clin. Pathol.* 45: 96–102.

108 Dahlgren, A.R., Tablin, F., and Finno, C.J. (2021). Genetics of equine bleeding disorders. *Equine Vet. J.* 53: 30–37.

109 Hinton, M., Jones, D.R., Lewis, I.M. et al. (1977). A clotting defect in an Arab colt foal. *Equine Vet. J.* 9: 1–3.

110 Bykowska, K. and Ceglarek, B. (2020). Clinical significance of slightly reduced von Willebrand factor activity. *Pol. Arch. Intern. Med.* 130: 225–231.

111 Brooks, M., Leith, G.S., Allen, A.K. et al. (1991). Bleeding disorder (von Willebrand disease) in a Quarter Horse. *J. Am. Vet. Med. Assoc.* 198: 114–116.

112 Rathgeber, R.A., Brooks, M.B., Bain, F.T. et al. (2001). Clinical vignette. Von Willebrand disease in a Thoroughbred mare and foal. *J. Vet. Intern. Med.* 15: 63–66.

113 Laan, T.T., Goehring, L.S., and Sloet van Oldruitenborgh-Oosterbaan, M.M. (2005). Von Willebrand's disease in an eight-day-old Quarter Horse foal. *Vet. Rec.* 157: 322–324.

114 Keeshen, T.P., Case, J.B., Runge, J.J. et al. (2017). Outcome of laparoscopic ovariohysterectomy or ovariectomy in dogs with von Willebrand disease or factor VII deficiency: 20 cases (2012–2014). *J. Am. Vet. Med. Assoc.* 251: 1053–1058.

115 Geor, R.J., Jackson, M.L., Lewis, K.D. et al. (1990). Prekallikrein deficiency in a family of Belgian horses. *J. Am. Vet. Med. Assoc.* 197: 741–745.

116 Turrentine, M.A., Sculley, P.W., Green, E.M. et al. (1986). Prekallikrein deficiency in a family of Miniature Horses. *Am. J. Vet. Res.* 47: 2464–2467.

117 Clemmons, R.M., Dorsey-Lee, M.R., Gorman, N.T. et al. (1984). Haemostatic mechanisms of the newborn foal: reduced platelet responsiveness. *Equine Vet. J.* 16: 353–356.

118 Macieira, S., Rivard, G.E., Champagne, J. et al. (2007). Glanzmann thrombasthenia in an Oldenbourg filly. *Vet. Clin. Pathol.* 36: 204–208.

119 Norris, J.W., Pratt, S.M., Auh, J.H. et al. (2006). Investigation of a novel, heritable bleeding diathesis of Thoroughbred horses and development of a screening assay. *J. Vet. Intern. Med.* 20: 1450–1456.

120 Norris, J.W., Pratt, S.M., Hunter, J.F. et al. (2007). Prevalence of reduced fibrinogen binding to platelets in a population of Thoroughbreds. *Am. J. Vet. Res.* 68: 716–721.

121 Christopherson, P.W., Insalaco, T.A., van Santen, V.L. et al. (2006). Characterization of the cDNA encoding alphaIIb and beta3 in normal horses and two horses with Glanzmann thrombasthenia. *Vet. Pathol.* 43: 78–82.

122 Sellon, D.C., Levine, J., Millikin, E. et al. (1996). Thrombocytopenia in horses: 35 cases (1989–1994). *J. Vet. Intern. Med.* 10: 127–132.

123 Giguere, S., Weber, E.J., and Sanchez, L.C. (2017). Factors associated with outcome and gradual improvement in survival over time in 1065 equine neonates admitted to an intensive care unit. *Equine Vet. J.* 49: 45–50.

124 Weber, E.J., Sanchez, L.C., and Giguere, S. (2015). Re-evaluation of the sepsis score in equine neonates. *Equine Vet. J.* 47: 275–278.

125 Buechner-Maxwell, V., Scott, M.A., Godber, L. et al. (1997). Neonatal alloimmune thrombocytopenia in a Quarter Horse foal. *J. Vet. Intern. Med.* 11: 304–308.

126 Ramirez, S., Gaunt, S.D., McClure, J.J. et al. (1999). Detection and effects on platelet function of anti-platelet antibody in mule foals with experimentally induced neonatal alloimmune thrombocytopenia. *J. Vet. Intern. Med.* 13: 534–539.

127 McGurrin, M.K., Arroyo, L.G., and Bienzle, D. (2004). Flow cytometric detection of platelet-bound antibody in three horses with immune-mediated thrombocytopenia. *J. Am. Vet. Med. Assoc.* 224 (83–87): 53.

128 Dunkel, B., Chan, D., and Monreal, L. (2009). Influence of citrate concentration and material of blood tubes on thromboelastographic parameters in horses. *J. Vet. Emerg. Crit. Care* 19: A14.

129 Ohto, H. and Nollet, K.E. (2011). Overview on platelet preservation: better controls over storage lesion. *Transfus. Apher. Sci.* 44: 321–325.

130 Johnstone, I.B. (1983). Comparative effects of phenylbutazone, naproxen and flunixin meglumine on equine platelet aggregation and platelet factor 3 availability in vitro. *Can. J. Comp. Med.* 47: 172–179.

131 Perkins, G.A., Miller, W.H., Divers, T.J. et al. (2005). Ulcerative dermatitis, thrombocytopenia, and neutropenia in neonatal foals. *J. Vet. Intern. Med.* 19: 211–216.

132 Spiel, A.O., Bartko, J., Schwameis, M. et al. (2011). Increased platelet aggregation and in vivo platelet activation after granulocyte colony-stimulating factor administration. A randomised controlled trial. *Thromb. Haemostat.* 105: 655–662.

133 du Preez, S. and Hughes, K.J. (2018). Thrombocytopenia, neutripenia, ulcerative dermatitis and haemathrosis in a neonatal foal. *Equine Vet. Educ.* 30: 647–653.

Neonatal Immunology & Infection

Chapter 46 Innate Immunity in the Foal

Lindsay M.W. Piel and Kelsey A. Hart

Overview of the Innate Immune System

The innate immune system is responsible for the initial host response to tissue damage or infection. Both acellular and cellular factors play key roles in the innate immune response. The noncellular, or humoral, portion of the innate immune system is fast and nonspecific and is vitally important in the initial response to a potential pathogen. The humoral innate immune system is composed of soluble or fixed macromolecules, including immunoglobulins, C-reactive proteins, complement, LPS binding protein, collectins, pentraxins, and defensins [1, 2]. The cellular portion of the innate immune system includes epithelial and immune cells. Epithelial cells comprise important barriers between the internal and external environments, which is critically important in limiting direct host-pathogen interactions [2–4]. In addition to their barrier function, however, some epithelial cells also have direct immune effects. A good example of this are the Paneth cells in the intestinal crypts, which release humoral immune molecules like lysozyme, α-defensins, and angiogenins [4]. Immune cells are also obviously vital players in the innate immune response, with key cellular players including neutrophils, macrophages, dendritic cells, natural killer cells (NK cells), mast cells, eosinophils, and γδ T-lymphocytes [2].

The ability to generate a rapid innate immune response to a potential pathogen is even more important in neonates compared to adults, as they are coming from a predominantly sterile in utero environment and being exposed to both beneficial and pathogenic organisms [1, 5–7]. Unfortunately, the adaptive immune response is naïve in the neonatal foal and takes upwards of 8–12 weeks to generate a targeted attack [2, 5, 6, 8]. This leaves transfer of maternal immunity and the innate immune system at the foundation of the neonatal foal's initial defenses against infection [9]. However, there are also factors within the neonatal foal's innate immune system that are not mature in their ability to protect the host. These shortcomings will be discussed herein and compared to the capacities of the adult horse.

Humoral (Acellular) Components of the Innate Immune System

Complement

While complement comprises a portion of the humoral innate immune system, it works closely with innate immune cells. Complement contains a multitude of both soluble and surface associated proteins that monitor for pathogens, cellular damage, and apoptosis. Upon recognizing any one of these components, the complement system activates to promote clearance of debris or to engage in an immune system attack [10]. There are three mechanisms of complement activation: the classic pathway, the lectin pathway, and the alternative pathway. Each pathway overlaps in the use of complement components as depicted in Figure 46.1 [10, 11].

Both the classical and lectin complement pathways are activated through recognition of a substrate [10, 11]. The most well-known stimulant of the classical pathway is an antigen–antibody complex; however, stimulation may also occur by apoptotic cells, necrotic cells, or C-reactive protein [10]. Activation occurs when one of the aforementioned compounds interacts with the collagen-like tail present on C1q. C1q is present in a soluble protein complex made up of six C1q molecules, two C1r molecules, and two C1s molecules. When C1q is bound, a conformational change occurs that leads to the activation of the serine proteases C1r and C1s. Together C1r and C1s work to cleave C4 and C2 into C4a, C4b, C2a, and C2b [10, 12]. The active portion of this reaction is known as C3

Equine Neonatal Medicine, First Edition. Edited by David M. Wong and Pamela A. Wilkins.

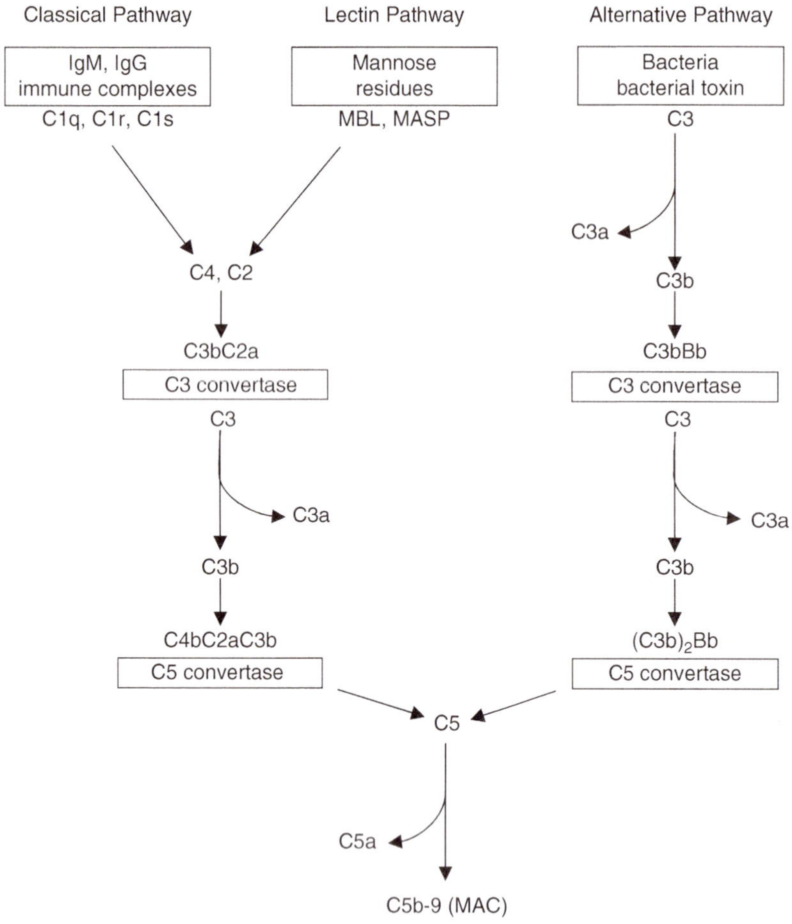

Figure 46.1 Overview of the complement pathways and their components. See text for further description. MBL, Mannose-binding lectin; MASP, Mannose-associated serine protease; MAC, membrane attack complex.

convertase and is comprised of C4b and C2a held together by a noncovalent bond.

Activation of the lectin pathway also leads to formation of C3 convertase. However, instead of antigen–antibody complex activation, the lectin pathway is encouraged by the presence of pathogenic carbohydrates. Recognition of these foreign carbohydrates occurs via mannose-binding lectin (MBL). When MBL contacts foreign carbohydrates on pathogen surfaces it causes activation of MBL-associated serine proteases, which also cleave C4 and C2. In contrast to the lectin and classical pathways, the alternative pathway is constantly undergoing random activation by means of spontaneous thioester bond hydrolysis. This hydrolysis allows the formation of C3(H_2O) that can bind complement factor B (CFB). After CFB interaction with C3(H_2O), another serine protease, known as complement factor D (CFD), can cleave CFB to generate an alternate form of C3 convertase (C3(H_2O)Bb) [10].

Generation of either C3 convertase allows further cleavage of C3 into C3a and C3b, where incorporation of C3b into this enzyme complex generates C5 convertase. Cleavage of C5 by C5 convertase produces C5a and C5b. Thereafter, C5b will interact with C6–C9 to form the membrane attack complex (MAC), a vital effector molecule of the complement system. The function of MAC is to incorporate into cellular membranes to cause destruction of or substantial damage to the abnormal/foreign cell [10].

Along with MAC generation, the complement system functions by producing anaphylatoxins and opsonization [1, 10]. C3a and C5a yielded earlier are the anaphylatoxins that cause alterations in hemodynamics and immune cell reactivity. Within the vasculature, C5a and C3a cause vasodilation and increase permeability, allowing for chemotaxis of immune cells through endothelial cells. Furthermore, C5a and C3a act as chemoattractants for macrophages, neutrophils, basophils, mast cells, B cells, and T cells, helping to deliver immune cells to the site of infection or tissue damage. Lastly C5a and C3a will mediate a respiratory burst from macrophages, neutrophils, and eosinophils, where basophils will be stimulated to release histamine.

C3b and C4b also serve to help opsonize pathogens by covalently bonding to foreign material [1, 10, 13]. This allows for easier recognition of this material by immune cells to facilitate phagocytosis and killing of pathogens by macrophages, neutrophils, and dendritic cells [2, 10]. This process uses the CR3 receptor present on myeloid cells and the CR4 receptor present on myeloid and lymphoid cells to permit better interaction with pathogenic material. Furthermore, the inactive version of C3b (iC3b) will still interact with CR3 and CR4 providing additional means of opsonization [10, 14, 15].

Regulation of the complement cascade is essential, since activation leads to an intensive proinflammatory state [10]. Plasma enzymes work rapidly to metabolize C5a and C3a to prohibit excessive signaling and inflammation. Complement factor H (CFH) will cleave either C3b or C4b to cause complement inactivation. Other means of deactivating complement include decay-accelerating factor (DAF) and C1 inhibitor (C1INH), where DAF works to dissociate either of the C3 convertase complexes and C1INH irreversibly binds C1r, C1s, and MASPs [10, 12].

Other Soluble Factors

Many other soluble factors, including lactoferrin, C-reactive protein, and pentraxins, defensins, and collectins play critical roles in the innate immune response. These factors are generally produced by innate immune cells, and thus are discussed in relation to those cells below.

Innate Immunity at Mucosal Surfaces

Infectious diseases in neonates are often introduced through either the respiratory or gastrointestinal tracts [3, 16]. Therefore, understanding the innate immune defenses present at these mucosal surfaces is critical. M-cells, or microfold-cells, are a modified epithelial cell type that has the capacity to sample antigen from the adjacent lumen. M-cells then deliver this antigen to dendritic cells in the lamina propria by completing a process known as transcytosis, which is similar to the absorption of antibodies from colostrum and milk [16]. Alternatively, dendritic cells adjacent to epithelial surfaces can also directly sample for antigen by extending a dendrite into the lumen [4].

Lymphoid tissue commonly known as mucosa-associated lymphoid tissue (MALT) is located in association with epithelial regions containing M-cells [16]. MALT consists of both B cells and T cells that interact directly with antigen presenting cells like M-cells and dendritic cells. MALT can be further named depending on its anatomical region, including nose-associated lymphoid tissue (NALT), larynx- and trachea-associated lymphoid tissue (LTALT), bronchus-associated lymphoid tissue (BALT), and gut-associated lymphoid tissue (GALT) [17].

Within the gut, the neonatal immune system develops with the exposure to the gastrointestinal microbiome. Experiments with germ-free mice have shown that depletion of the microbiome prohibits immune system development, wherein immune system stimulation occurs when microbial species are added back [4]. The Treg phenotype is predominantly present, which results in IL-10 and TGF-β production [4, 7, 17–19]. These cytokines will suppress dendritic cell activity and cause the production of inhibitory molecules for T-cell differentiation [18]. The other less predominant T-cell phenotype within the gastrointestinal tract is Th17. It is believed, that the Th17 polarization may help with IgA production and therefore prevent the colonization with pathogenic microbes, where IgA is also being attained through ingested milk [4, 19]. Further work to better understand microbiome-host immune interactions in foals and horses is needed.

Cellular Components of the Innate Immune System

Humoral and mucosal components of the innate immune system can function to prevent infection or directly kill invading pathogens, but are usually not effective at fully eliminating substantial infections in the absence of a cellular immune response. Key functions of innate immune cells include uptake and removal of pathogens by phagocytosis, release of antimicrobial compounds such as lactoferrin and reactive oxygen species (ROS), and antigen presentation to stimulate the more targeted adaptive immune response. Several cell types play vital roles in these innate immune processes, including neutrophils, macrophages/monocytes, dendritic cells, and NK cells. Activation of the innate immune cells in general and specific cellular functions are discussed in more detail below.

Specific Functions of Innate Immune Cells

Phagocytosis and Clearance of Infected Cells

Cells take up extracellular components, or sample their environment, through either pinocytosis, micropinocytosis, endocytosis, or phagocytosis [14, 20]. Phagocytosis is important when cells are ingesting particles >0.5 μm in size [14, 21]. Therefore, this represents the main means by which immune cells engulf invading pathogens. Of the innate immune system cells, the macrophage and neutrophil are considered professional phagocytes. Many cells have the capability to complete phagocytosis, but these respective cell types have an increased repertoire of receptors available for use and are able to phagocytose at a faster rate to help clear infections [14].

Overall, phagocytosis is the encapsulation of external particles using the cellular plasma membrane and remodeling of the actin cytoskeleton. Closing of the membrane around the particle of interest generates the nascent phagosome, which then undergoes a series of maturation steps to become a phagolysosome. During maturation, a number of vesicles fuse to share compounds with the phagosome to generate an inhospitable environment that prohibits growth or destroys the phagocytosed organism or material [14]. Key factors in this process include ROS, reactive nitrogen species, an acidic environment, nutrient deprivation, and hydrolytic enzymes [14, 15, 21]. Neutrophils also contain azurophilic granules, discussed below, which deliver additional hydrolytic enzymes [22].

There are multiple receptors available for the initial recognition of pathogenic organisms, which work together to mediate phagocytosis. These include the Fcγ receptor, complement receptors, scavenger receptors, and the mannose receptor [14]. While each of these receptors helps in the recognition of extracellular particles that should be phagocytosed, some of the receptors are better at mediating phagocytosis than others. It is important to note that the phagocytosis process is most efficient if the particles have been opsonized by complement or by immunoglobulins from the humoral immune response.

In general, opsonization with immunoglobulins results in the most efficient phagocytosis. The Fcγ receptor (FcγR) recognizes the Fc portion of IgG immunoglobulins [14, 15]. Receptor activation results in a tightly adhered phagosomal membrane around the ingested particle and generation of ROS [14, 15]. In contrast, complement receptors CR3 and CR4 cause phagocytosis to occur in a sinking fashion, where the phagosomal membrane is only attached to the ingested particle in focal areas [14, 15]. Release of ROS to damage pathogens due to complement receptor ligation occurs only in neutrophils, not macrophages [14, 15]. Another complement receptor, CR1, only plays a part in recognition of an opsonized particle when a secondary activating signal helps stimulate phagocytosis [14]. CR1 also binds the mannose binding protein (MBP) and C1q of the complement system [12, 15, 23]. This mannose binding protein is important for monocyte binding of pathogens containing the mannose sugar on their surface, because monocytes (but not macrophages) lack a cell surface mannose receptor that can directly interact with pathogen-associated mannose or fucose [14, 23]. The innate immune system's ability to recognize mannose is particularly important for recognizing lipopolysaccharide (LPS, endotoxin) in Gram-negative bacteria [23]. Lastly, scavenger receptors are important in the clearance of apoptotic, or senescent, host cells, particularly by macrophages [5]. Dying host cells alter their surface molecules by increasing phosphatidyl serine, altering surface charge, and altering glycosylation, which signals to macrophages that they are ready to be cleared [14].

Release of Immune Effector and Antimicrobial Compounds

Neutrophils contain vesicles known as granules that carry an assortment of different immune effector proteins. These aid in extravasation for circulating neutrophils and support the initial immune response at sites of infection. Three separate granule types have been defined: (i) primary/azurophilic; (ii) secondary/specific, and (iii) tertiary/gelatinase granules [21]. These granules have different propensities for release after neutrophil stimulation, with tertiary granules released first and primary granules released last [21, 22]. This step-wise granule release is important as early release of primary granules can cause significant tissue damage.

The initial step in granule release is activation of secretory vesicles in the neutrophil. These secretory vesicles are essential because they contain receptors important for the neutrophil adhesion cascade and secretion of cytokines for immune system polarization [21, 22]. One important membrane receptor present in the secretory vesicle is the integrin receptor, which binds vessel endothelium [22]. Once the secretory vesicle is attached to the endothelium, the tertiary granules are released. Tertiary/gelatinase granules carry gelatinase, arginase 1, matrix metalloproteinase-9, and lysozyme, which help the neutrophil generate a pathway through the basement membrane of vasculature endothelium [21, 22]. Once in the interstitium, neutrophils release secondary granules, which contain more metalloproteinases, lactoferrin, cathelicidin, and lipocalin 2 [21]. These proteins again help the neutrophil move through the connective tissue of the host, and some, like lactoferrin, also inhibit bacterial growth by sequestering iron away from bacteria [5].

The last, and most potent, granule released are the primary, or azurophilic, granules, which contain potent hydrolases like neutrophil elastase, myeloperoxidase, azuracidin, and defensins [21]. Primary/azurophilic granules may be released into the extracellular environment or delivered to the maturing phagolysosome [22]. The function of these primary granules is to kill and digest foreign microorganisms [21]. In summary, granules are important both for neutrophil transmigration and bactericidal capacity, during the early cellular innate response.

Activated neutrophils, and to a lesser degree macrophages, also produce and release ROS. These highly reactive molecules contain oxygen (ROS) and are produced during many cellular processes, including phagocytosis. Specifically, reactive oxygen molecules are produced on the phagosomal endosomal membranes via nicotinamide adenine dinucleotide phosphate (NADPH) oxidase [24]. This process is triggered by many foreign antigens, including bacterial lipopolysaccharide and by inflammatory cytokines produced by host cells. Key ROS produced during immune responses include superoxide, hydrogen peroxide, hydroxyl radicals, singlet oxygen, peroxynitrite, and hypochlorous acid. ROS can damage invading pathogens by damaging bacterial and function cell membranes and microbial DNA. Additionally, ROS can work through receptor-mediated pathways to play a key role in antiviral defenses and can activate other immune cells like macrophages and T cells to support both innate and adaptive responses. However, it is important to note that ROS can also directly damage host cells.

Natural Killer Cells

Natural killer (NK) cells are a subgroup of lymphocytes that lack antigen-specific cell surface receptors, and thus are generally considered part of the innate immune response. They play a key role in early antiviral defenses, in addition to tumor recognition. NK cells directly lyse host cells expressing stress or damage signals, but they also appear to have a vital effector function in production of cytokines that activate and direct both innate and adaptive immune responses [24]. Specifically, NK cells are a key producer of IFN-γ, as well as a myriad of other pro- and anti-inflammatory cytokines; this allows them to both stimulate and regulate immune responses and play roles in both pathogen clearance and immune tolerance [24].

Activation of the Adaptive Immune Response

In addition to NK cells, other innate immune responses directly work to stimulate a more targeted adaptive immune response after sensing a potential threat. This occurs via two specific mechanisms: (i) releasing specific cytokines that activate other leukocytes to target particular types of microbes; or (ii) by directly presenting antigen to adaptive immune cells to activate their specific response to that antigen. Both these mechanisms are discussed below.

Damage to an epithelial lining causes the release of constitutively expressed inflammatory cytokine mediators such as IL-1α [25, 26]. This pro-inflammatory cytokine response causes fever, increases leukocyte adhesion molecule presentation, increases migration of leukocytes, alters the endocrine stress response, and increases the lifespan of innate immune cells. Leukocytes themselves can also detect the presence of tissue damage or foreign antigen through pathogen recognition receptors (PRR) or damage receptors. These well-conserved host receptors recognize common pathogen associated molecular patterns (PAMPs) and damage associated molecular patterns (DAMPs), respectively [2, 4, 5, 27]. Interactions between host leukocyte PRRs such as toll-like receptors (TLRs) with common microbial PAMPs such as lipopolysaccharide, flagellin, and peptidoglycans, among many others, play a key role in stimulating the initial cellular innate immune response. Global stimulation of these receptors is integral to the pathogenesis of the systemic inflammatory response syndrome (SIRS) and sepsis (Chapter 50).

Cytokines released from damaged tissues or from activated innate immune cells after PRR stimulation work together to coordinate an appropriate adaptive immune response. Table 46.1 summarizes cytokines and their general function in the immune system. Specific combinations of these cytokines can polarize the adaptive immune response toward a particular type of adaptive response. To date, there have been three well characterized adaptive immune cell responses, comprised of T-helper cells 1, 2, and 17 (Th1, Th2, and Th17). Additionally, T cells can be polarized to a T-regulatory cell population, which mediates tolerance of the immune system to certain constitutive stimulants like the gut microbiome. Each of these T-cell polarized phenotypes is known to be most effective against certain pathogen types. Table 46.2 details these T-helper cell polarizations and the cytokine environment that elicits each polarization; these responses are discussed in more detail below.

Direct presentation of antigen by innate immune cells to adaptive immune cells is also vital for generation of an

Table 46.1 General functions of many important cytokines (not an exhaustive list) [28–31].

Cytokine	Function
IFNα/β	Exerts antiviral properties
IFNγ	Activates macrophages and NK cells, defense against intracellular pathogens and viruses
IL-1	Increase adhesion molecules for leukocyte migration, produces fever, and alters lifespan of macrophages and neutrophils
IL-6	Release of acute phase proteins, differentiate B and T cells, decrease serum iron, angiogenesis, keratinocyte proliferation
IL-8	Neutrophil chemotactic protein
IL-10	Anti-inflammatory cytokine with multiple pleiotropic effects in immunoregulation and inflammation. Downregulates expression of Th1 cytokines and MHCII antigens and enhances B-cell survival, proliferation, and antibody production
IL-12	Development of naïve T cells
IL-15	Activate NK cells and CD8+ T cells
IL-18	Increase epithelial tight junctions, upregulate adhesion molecules, help activate macrophages
IL-23	Promote endothelial adhesion of leukocytes by upregulation of ICAM-1 and VCAM-1; activate memory T cells
IL-27	Initially promotes Th1 response; long-term presence causes anti-inflammatory Treg response
IL-33	M2 macrophage phenotype
TNFα	Immune cell differentiation, proliferation, and survival

IFN, Interferon; NK, Natural killer; IL, Interleukin; TNF, Tumor necrosis factor; ICAM-1, Intracellular adhesion molecule 1; VCAM-1, Vascular cell adhesion molecule-1.

Table 46.2 T-helper cell polarization functions and the cytokines that stimulate their production [18, 32].

T-helper cell polarization	Key helper cell phenotype	Cytokines driving polarization	Main effector cytokines
Th1	Kill intracellular bacteria and antiviral state	IL-12, IFN α/β, IFNγ IL-15, IL-18	IFN-γ, IL-2
Th2	Antibody production and parasitic response	IL-33, IL-25	IL-4, IL-13, IL-5
Th17	Kill extracellular bacteria	IL-23, IL-1β, IL-6, TGF-β	IL-17, IL-22
Treg	Wound healing and antigen tolerance	TGF-β, IL-10	TGF-β, IL-10, IL-35

IL, Interleukin; IFN, Interferon; TGF, Transforming growth factor.

effective and directed adaptive immune response. The main mediators of antigen presentation to the adaptive immune system are dendritic cells, macrophages, and B cells, which are all considered professional antigen presenting cells [21]. Once a pathogen of interest has been phagocytosed and destroyed, a portion of the agent will be loaded into major histocompatibility complex II (MHCII) molecules on the cell surface [18]. MHCII is only expressed in these professional antigen presenting cells, while MHCI is expressed in all cells and is key for the ability of the host to distinguish self-antigens [2]. The antigen-MHCII complex then interacts with T-cell receptors until an appropriate "matching" counterpart is found [7, 18]. This interaction between the antigen presenting cell expressing antigen on its surface MHCII molecules with a T-cell receptor specific for that antigen results in activation of the T cell. Dendritic cells are the only antigen presenting cells capable of activating naïve T cells and are of exceptional importance in the neonate [33].

Response of the T cell to antigen presentation will depend on multiple factors, including affinity of the TCR-MHCII complex, the co-receptors present, and the local cytokine environment [18]. Co-receptors serve to either augment or inhibit T-cell responses to presented MHCII-antigen complexes [7, 18]. The co-stimulating receptor pair most recognized is CD80 or CD86 on the antigen presenting cell, and CD28 on the T cell [18]. Interaction of all these receptors on the antigen presenting cell and the T cell ultimate result in downstream signaling that supports T-cell proliferation and cytokine secretion. Inhibiting co-receptors, such as cytotoxic T-lymphocyte antigen-4 or programmed death-1 ligands, may also be expressed on the antigen presenting cell or T cell, and work to prevent generation of an adaptive immune response [18].

Once the T cell is activated by the antigen presenting cell through this complex process, the predominant cytokine milieu will determine the specific type of T-cell response (Tables 46.1 and 46.2). There are a variety of different cytokines that the immune system uses in order to generate an organized response to varied types of invading pathogens. In addition to functioning in the described paracrine manner, cytokines are also able to stimulate or inhibit the cell of origin in an autocrine manner; some circulating cytokines can even impact cells and tissues far away from the inflamed site in an endocrine fashion. In sum, the innate and adaptive immune systems must function in concert to complete the common goal of maintaining health and homeostasis.

Innate Immune Responses and Limitations in the Foal

Transcriptome analysis of peripheral blood leukocyte populations in foals reveals gradual development of adaptive immune functions during foal maturation. This includes increase in mRNA responsible for homologous DNA recombination, T-cell co-stimulation molecules, and antibody production [7]. This means that the newborn foal is very much dependent on innate immune responses (and transfer of maternal immunity) for protection during the neonatal period. Unfortunately, in addition to the general limitations of the innate immune response such as lack of specificity and potential for substantial host tissue damage, the foal has inherent and specific age-related limitations in multiple aspects of the innate immune system.

Complement and Other Humoral Innate Immune Factors in the Foal

Limitations in complement function in the neonate has been described for several species, including cattle, sheep, pigs, mice, humans, and foals. The hemolytic activity of complement, representing formation of the MAC, is approximately 40% of the adult capability in neonates that have not received colostrum. These results may need to be analyzed cautiously as the hemolytic assay uses red blood cells, which only require one molecule of C9 for lysis, where bacteria require a multimeric structure of C9 for destruction [5]. Even so, C9 represents the lowest complement factor present in human neonates and this alternate capacity for RBCs would only serve to falsely heighten the ability of the neonate to form an active MAC [5]. Levels of C3 in piglets and calves are lower than their adult counterparts, suggesting a decreased ability to opsonize present microorganisms. Furthermore, it has been demonstrated that C3 activity is diminished in the neonate due to the inability of the thioester bond to spontaneously hydrolyze, thereby directly affecting the function of the alternate complement pathway [5].

Studies specific to the foal have shown that complement activity is roughly 15% at birth as compared to an adult horse [1, 9]. The ability of complement to function within neonates steadily increases over the following months, reaching about 85% activity at 5 months of age [1]. Many studies have suggested that complement activity is heightened in the neonate once colostrum has been ingested [5, 34]. Gardner et al. demonstrated this phenomenon by isolating presuckle foal serum and incubating it with adult horse phagocytes to determine opsonization capacity [8]. There was an approximately twofold increase in fluorescent capacity of cells following incubation with prelabeled *Staphylococcus aureus* between one and two days of age, wherein the first day of sampling the foal had not yet suckled. Additionally, foal serum in this study had a steady increase in C3 concentration from 1 day to roughly 2 weeks in age. Notably, this expansion of C3 was not due to acquisition from colostrum, as serum levels surpassed the C3 concentration measured in colostrum [8]. Ironically, measurement of MAC capacity in foal serum suggested that healthy foals not receiving colostrum had a higher ability to lyse RBCs and had higher C3 serum concentrations [8]. Therefore, there is conflicting evidence as to what signals complement development, whether it be from components in colostrum, epigenetic remodeling, or environmental regulation. It is known that complement and maternal antibodies together help mediate opsonization of invading pathogens for foal phagocytes [1, 23, 35].

Mucosal Immunity in the Foal

In equine neonates, it has been determined that NALT, LTALT, and GALT start to organize during gestation, but that BALT formation doesn't begin until approximately one week of age [17, 36]. When BALT does develop in foals, a predominance of IgA production is seen. This is in contrast to adult horses, which chiefly generate IgG in their lower airways and IgA in their upper airways [36].

Bronchoalveolar lavage of neonatal foals has shown that the immune cell makeup matures over the first three months of life [1]. Initially, alveolar macrophages make up approximately 85% of the immune cells present in the respiratory tissue [1, 37]. As these foals aged, the percentage of alveolar macrophages present dropped to roughly 50% of the population [1]. Thus, the initial relative preponderance of macrophages and relative paucity of lymphocytes in the respiratory tract may play a role in the development of respiratory infections in young foal. This idea is further supported from the failure of neonatal alveolar macrophages to undergo chemotaxis in the presence of appropriate stimuli and the decreased ability to phagocytose *Streptococcus aureus*. Each of these discrepancies from adult horses was alleviated by 2 months of age [1, 37].

Innate Immune Cells in the Foal

Neutrophils

Functional limitations in neonatal neutrophils in comparison to adult neutrophils has long been accepted in a variety of species, including foals, calves, piglets, kittens, and human infants [5]. Key neutrophil functions include chemotaxis to sites of inflammation/infection, phagocytosis, and oxidative burst activity. Foal neutrophils exhibit some degree of limitations in all these functions during the neonatal period. Specifically, foal neutrophils are not fully mature in their capacity to complete chemotaxis at birth, but a plasma component confounds this issue. Neonatal foal neutrophils exhibit decreased capacity to migrate toward endotoxin-activated plasma before ingestion of colostrum [1, 34, 37]. This resolves by 4–21 days after birth, when foal neutrophils exhibit similar chemotaxis to adult neutrophils [34]. This functional change coincides with the alteration of histone methylation in genes important in neutrophil signaling and trafficking but may also be impacted by soluble factors in foal plasma [9]. Foal neutrophils obtained prior to colostral ingestion can more readily migrate when incubated with plasma from an adult horse than with foal plasma [34]. It is not clear if this is due to an inhibitory factor in foal plasma or a stimulatory factor in adult horse plasma.

Foal neutrophils also exhibit limitations in phagocytic function and bactericidal capacity, some of which also may be due to availability of specific soluble plasma factors. Foal neutrophils collected prior to colostral ingestion exhibit highly deficient phagocytosis of yeast or bacterial agents [34, 35]. However, this ability is restored to adult-like levels when yeast is phagocytosed in the presence of adult plasma [1, 34], suggesting soluble opsonins present only in adult plasma may be key for ideal neutrophil function. Over the first 2 weeks of life, phagocytic capacity of foal neutrophils increases even in the presence of autologous foal plasma; adult functional capacity is not yet reached, but function is not substantially impaired [13, 34, 35]. Neonatal foal neutrophils exhibit phagocytic function almost identical to adult horse neutrophils by approximately 2 months of age [13, 34].

CD18 is expressed in higher levels on foal neutrophils as compared to adult neutrophils [1, 5, 13]. This surface marker is important for the interaction of neutrophils with C3b or iC3b [1, 13]. As noted previously, C3b and iC3b are components of the complement system that help with opsonization of invading pathogens [10]. Spontaneous activation of C3 is depreciated in neonatal neutrophils as the thioester bond does not function appropriately, leaving complement deficient in its ability to covalently bond pathogens for immune system recognition [5]. Furthermore, foal complement opsonization and C3 concentration steadily increases over the first few weeks of life [8]. Therefore, this may explain the depreciation in phagocytosis when serum is heat inactivated.

Bactericidal capacity of the neutrophil is also very important [9, 38–40]. In the presence of adult serum, foal neutrophils show an adult-like capacity to destroy *S. aureus*. This ability trends downward from 4 to 113 days following birth and thereafter starts to increase again [38]. When neutrophils obtained from foals between 1 and 56 days of age were stimulated with a TLR9 activator, CpG-oligodeoxynucleotide, there was no difference in the secretion of the azurophilic granule marker β-D-glucouronidase [40]. Together, these results suggest that neutrophils are fully capable of destroying foreign agents.

Confounding these results are the outcomes of studies looking at ROS production. McTaggart et al. showed that neutrophils from 7-day-old foals were competent in their ability to produce ROS [39]. Importantly, while ROS production from neonatal neutrophils is possible, it was completely obliterated when foal neutrophils were incubated with either adult or foal serum. This contrasts the outcome when adult neutrophils are tested, as addition of serum generates an earlier ROS burst compared to antigen stimulation alone [39]. Therefore, while neonatal neutrophils are able to generate ROS *in vitro*, it may be that their *in vivo* capability has not been accurately represented.

Lastly, neutrophils are important in their ability to polarize the immune response through cytokine signaling [41]. Neonatal neutrophils that have not been stimulated still produce a baseline amount of cytokine mRNA, or transcript signal [40, 41]. The greatest basal cytokine transcription levels were noted for IL-8, TNF-α, IL-6, and IL-23p19 [40]. These cytokines support neutrophil migration and activation of the acute-phase response [42, 43]. Cytokines that increased in basal mRNA expression from 2 to 56 days of age were IFN-γ, IL-4, IL-6, IL-17, and TNF-α, which are all generally considered pro-inflammatory cytokines [40]. This basal cytokine profile from foal neutrophils supports the foal's dependency on the innate immune response early in life, and their propensity toward pro-inflammatory bias when an immune response is required, which plays a key role in the pathogenesis of SIRS and sepsis in foals.

Monocytes and Antigen Presentation

Macrophages and monocyte-derived dendritic cells (MoDC) represent the main population of cells that have been studied to determine foal antigen presentation capabilities [7, 20, 44]. As mentioned previously, antigen presenting cells require MHC II expression, co-stimulatory surface markers, and cytokine expression profiles to mediate an adaptive immune response. While it is accepted that MHCII expression is lower in foals as compared to adult horses, it is controversial as to whether the percentage of cells expressing the protein is decreased or if the amount of MHCII on each cell is inadequate [8, 20, 28]. One study that isolated stimulated dendritic cells through flow cytometry determined that dendritic cell populations express MHCII in similar levels as compared to adult DCs, but that less of the cellular population has MHCII on their surface [20]. This decreased propensity of foal MoDCs to express MHCII does not appear to be due to a lack of proficiency in foreign particle uptake, as foal MoDCs perform adequately at micropinocytosis [20].

While low expression of specific MHCII genes decreases the ability to present certain antigens, inhibitory and co-stimulatory surface marker expression is required for stimulation of T-cell proliferation and effector function. CD86 on MoDC or monocyte-derived macrophages (MoMc) from foals is expressed in appropriate levels as compared to adult cells [28, 44]. While not significant, the intensity of CD86 on MoMc increased when exposed to virulent *Rhodococcus equi*, but not an avirulent strain. This expression was incrementally gained in association with maturation from 1 to 3 months of age [44]. This may show an increased disposition of macrophages to become activated in the coming months following birth. While MoDC in the prior study did not show an elevation in CD86 following virulent *R. equi* infection, they did show an increase in the CD40 co-stimulation receptor at 2 months of age [44]. Importantly, the percentage of MoDC expressing CD86 was depressed in foals sampled on day 1 and 7 of life compared to day 30 and adult horse cells; this first week of life represents a major time in which foals are more susceptible to infection [20]. In sum, these studies suggest that foal dendritic cells may have limited ability to stimulate an effective adaptive response during the first week of life, but antigen presentation may mature by 1–2 months of age.

The ability of monocyte-derived macrophages and dendritic cells to respond to specific TLR agonists or whole bacteria has been assessed through cytokine expression profiles, TLR transcript quantities, and NF-κβ activation [20, 28]. TLR9 transcript levels are comparable to adult horses and are stimulated by incubation with cytosine-phosphate-guanosine oligodeoxynucleotide (CpG), which is reminiscent of bacterial DNA structure [28]. With this stimulant, foal MoDC, and macrophages up to 3 months in age were not able to produce inflammatory cytokine transcripts for IL-12p35, IL-12p40, or IFNα as compared to adult horses, where TLR9 stimulation should lead to a strong Th1 mediated response [27, 28]. Similarly, stimulation of MoDC with a Gram-positive bacterium (*S. aureus*) was not able to induce proinflammatory cytokines (IL-4, IL-17, or IFN-γ) for the first 30 days of life [20]. Importantly, stimulation with CpG specifically targets TLR9 responses, while stimulation with whole bacteria functionally ligates multiple TLRs at the same time. During MoDC incubation with a Gram-negative bacterium (*Escherichia coli*) the ability to produce cytokines was seen when foals were 7 or 30 days old, where IL-17 was produced above basal levels at 7 days of age and IFN-γ and IL-4 were produced above basal levels at 30 days of age [20]. This indicates that certain pathogens may produce different immune responses early in life and that the foal might be more capable of generating inflammatory responses to *E. coli* as compared to *S. aureus*. This concept is further supported during assays using the major foal pathogen *R. equi*. While mRNA expression levels of IL-12p40 or IL-12p35 were not significantly lowered from adult levels, MoMc and MoDC began to increase their IL-12p40 transcript numbers between 1 and 3 months of age after bacterial exposure [44]. For MoDC specifically, IL-12p35 mRNA levels increased by 3 months of age when incubated with both virulent and avirulent *R. equi* [44]. It is important to note that studies investigating cytokine profiles after *R. equi* incubation measured alterations in mRNA levels, while studies using *E. coli* and *S. aureus* stimulation quantified cytokine protein secretion [20, 44]. It is possible, that the increase in mRNA profiles after *R. equi* exposure did not lead to mature protein release.

Furthermore, foal MoDC were able to produce the predominantly anti-inflammatory cytokine IL-10 from day 1 to 30 in a fashion similar to adult horses [20]. Interestingly, the transcription factor responsible for production of many pro-inflammatory cytokines, NF-κβ, was not altered in its activation in foals as compared to adults [44]. Therefore, the inability to make certain cytokines during the neonatal life stage may be due to epigenetic modification of certain histones related to proinflammatory cytokine promoters or from some unknown inhibitory signal. Histone modifications were also found in association with neutrophil immune response promoters [9]. Alterations in gene expression at these promoters was seen at 30 days of life and therefore may represent a mass alteration in immune system regulation.

Summary

The innate immune system is integral in the initial recognition of invading pathogens in adults and neonates. It is also responsible for initiating and coordinating an appropriate adaptive immune response to obtain a more precise attack on the invading organism. Foals are very dependent on their innate immune response during the neonatal period as the adaptive immune response is not fully mature. However, the foal's innate immune response also exhibits functional limitations during the neonatal period. While macrophage and dendritic cells require 1–2 months to reach functional maturity, neutrophils can generate an inflammatory phenotype more rapidly after birth and reach adult levels of activity by roughly a week in age. Foal neutrophil maturation may be driven by increases in availability of complement and other soluble factors that start to increase in concentration shortly after birth. Thus, limitations in innate immune function in newborn foals result from inherent cellular immaturity and altered plasma factors that govern leukocyte function. Further study to increase understanding of specific cellular defects and key circulating factors that regulate immune function may permit the development of specific preventative approaches or immunomodulatory therapies for neonatal foals.

References

1 Giguere, S. and Polkes, A. (2005). Immunologic disorders in neonatal foals. *Vet. Clin. Equine* 21: 241–272.

2 Turvey, S.E. and Broide, D.H. (2010). Innate immunity. *J. Allergy Clin. Immunol.* 125 (2 Suppl. 2): S24–S532.

3 Martin, T.R. and Frevert, C.W. (2005). Innate immunity in the lungs. *Proc. Am. Thorac. Soc.* 2: 403–411.

4 Salzman, N.H. (2014). The role of the microbiome in immune cell development. *Ann. Allergy Asthma Immunol.* 113: 593–598.

5 Firth, M.A., Shewen, P.E., and Hodgins, D.C. (2005). Passive and active components of neonatal innate immune defenses. *Anim. Health Res. Rev.* 6: 143–158.

6 Perkins, G.A. and Wagner, B. (2015). The development of equine immunity: current knowledge on immunology in the young horse. *Equine Vet. J.* 47: 267–274.

7 Tallmadge, R.L., Wang, M., Sun, Q. et al. (2018). Transcriptome analysis of immune genes in peripheral blood mononuclear cells of young foals and adult horses. *PLoS One* 13: e0202646.

8 Gardner, R.B., Nydam, D.V., Luna, J.A. et al. (2007). Serum opsonization capacity, phagocytosis, and oxidative burst activity in neonatal foals in the intensive care unit. *J. Vet. Intern. Med.* 21: 797–805.

9 Dindot, S.V., Doan, R.N., Kuskie, K.R. et al. (2018). Postnatal changes in epigenetic modifications of neutrophils of foals are associated with increased ROS function and regulation of neutrophil function. *Dev. Comp. Immunol.* 87: 182–187.

10 Noris, M. and Remuzzi, G. (2013). Overview of complement activation and regulation. *Semin. Nephrol.* 33: 479–492.

11 MacKay, R.J. (2000). Inflammation in horses. *Vet. Clin. North Am. Equine Pract.* 16: 15–27.

12 Tenner, A.J., Robinson, S.L., and Ezekowitz, R.A. (1995). Mannose binding protein (MBP) enhances mononuclear phagocyte function via a receptor that contains the 126,000 M(r) component of the C1q receptor. *Immunity* 3: 485–493.

13 Grondahl, G., Johannisson, A., Demmers, S. et al. (1999). Influence of age and plasma treatment on neutrophil phagocytosis and CD18 expression in foals. *Vet. Microbiol.* 65: 241–254.

14 Aderem, A. and Underhill, D.M. (1999). Mechanisms of phagocytosis in macrophages. *Annu. Rev. Immunol.* 17: 593–623.

15 Underhill, D.M. and Ozinsky, A. (2002). Phagocytosis of microbes: complexity in action. *Annu. Rev. Immunol.* 20: 825–852.

16 Jonsdottir, I. (2007). Maturation of mucosal immune responses and influence of maternal antibodies. *J. Comp. Pathol.* 137 (Suppl. 1): S20–S26.

17 Liebler-Tenorio, E.M. and Pabst, R. (2006). MALT structure and function in farm animals. *Vet. Res.* 37 (3): 257–280.

18 Kaiko, G.E., Horvat, J.C., Beagley, K.W. et al. (2008). Immunological decision-making: how does the immune system decide to mount a helper T-cell response? *Immunology* 123: 326–338.

19 Kumar, S.K. and Bhat, B.V. (2016). Distinct mechanisms of the newborn innate immunity. *Immunol. Lett.* 173: 42–54.

20 Lopez, B.S., Hurley, D.J., Giancola, S. et al. (2019). The effect of age on foal monocyte-derived dendritic cell (MoDC) maturation and function after exposure to killed bacteria. *Vet. Immunol. Immunopathol.* 210: 38–45.

21 Rosales, C. (2020). Neutrophils at the crossroads of innate and adaptive immunity. *J. Leukoc. Biol.* 108: 377–396.

22 Hager, M., Cowland, J.B., and Borregaard, N. (2010). Neutrophil granules in health and disease. *J. Intern. Med.* 268: 25–34.

23 Kuhlman, M., Joiner, K., and Ezekowitz, R.A. (1989). The human mannose-binding protein functions as an opsonin. *J. Exp. Med.* 169: 1733–1745.

24 Vivier, E., Raulet, D.H., Moretta, A. et al. (2011). Innate or adaptive immunity? The example of natural killer cells. *Science* 331: 44–49.

25 Garlanda, C., Dinarello, C.A., and Mantovani, A. (2013). The interleukin-1 family: back to the future. *Immunity* 39: 1003–1018.

26 Palomo, J., Dietrich, D., Martin, P. et al. (2015). The interleukin (IL)-1 cytokine family–balance between agonists and antagonists in inflammatory diseases. *Cytokine* 76: 25–37.

27 Kawai, T. and Akira, S. (2010). The role of pattern-recognition receptors in innate immunity: update on toll-like receptors. *Nat. Immunol.* 11: 373–384.

28 Flaminio, M.J., Borges, A.S., Nydam, D.V. et al. (2007). The effect of CpG-ODN on antigen presenting cells of the foal. *J. Immune Based Ther. Vaccines* 5: 1.

29 Stetson, D.B. and Medzhitov, R. (2006). Type I interferons in host defense. *Immunity* 25: 373–381.

30 Hunter, C.A. and Kastelein, R. (2012). Interleukin-27: balancing protective and pathological immunity. *Immunity* 37: 960–969.

31 Parameswaran, N. and Patial, S. (2010). Tumor necrosis factor-alpha signaling in macrophages. *Crit. Rev. Eukaryot. Gene Expr.* 20: 87–103.

32 Zhu, J. (2018). T helper cell differentiation, heterogeneity, and plasticity. *Cold Spring Harb. Perspect. Biol.* 10: 10.

33 Sallusto, F. and Lanzavecchia, A. (2002). The instructive role of dendritic cells on T-cell responses. *Arthritis Res.* 4 (Suppl. 3): S127–S132.

34 Bernoco, M., Liu, I.K., Wuest-Ehlert, C.J. et al. (1987). Chemotactic and phagocytic function of peripheral blood polymorphonuclear leucocytes in newborn foals. *J. Reprod. Fertil. Suppl.* 35: 599–605.

35 Grondahl, G., Sternberg, S., Jensen-Waern, M. et al. (2001). Opsonic capacity of foal serum for the two neonatal pathogens *Escherichia coli* and *Actinobacillus equuli*. *Equine Vet. J.* 33: 670–675.

36 Blunden, A.S. and Gower, S.M. (1999). A histological and immunohistochemical study of the humoral immune system of the lungs in young Thoroughbred horses. *J. Comp. Pathol.* 120: 347–356.

37 Fogarty, U. and Leadon, D.P. (1987). Comparison of systemic and local respiratory tract cellular immunity in the neonatal foal. *J. Reprod. Fertil. Suppl.* 35: 593–598.

38 Wichtel, M.G., Anderson, K.L., Johnson, T.V. et al. (1991). Influence of age on neutrophil function in foals. *Equine Vet. J.* 23: 466–469.

39 McTaggart, C., Yovich, J.V., Penhale, J. et al. (2001). A comparison of foal and adult horse neutrophil function using flow cytometric techniques. *Res. Vet. Sci.* 71: 73–79.

40 Bordin, A.I., Liu, M., Nerren, J.R. et al. (2012). Neutrophil function of neonatal foals is enhanced in vitro by CpG oligodeoxynucleotide stimulation. *Vet. Immunol. Immunopathol.* 145: 290–297.

41 Tecchio, C., Micheletti, A., and Cassatella, M.A. (2014). Neutrophil-derived cytokines: facts beyond expression. *Front. Immunol.* 5: 508.

42 Tanaka, T., Narazaki, M., and Kishimoto, T. (2014). IL-6 in inflammation, immunity, and disease. *Cold Spring Harb. Perspect. Biol.* 6: a016295.

43 Espigol-Frigole, G., Planas-Rigol, E., Ohnuki, H. et al. (2016). Identification of IL-23p19 as an endothelial proinflammatory peptide that promotes gp130-STAT3 signaling. *Sci. Signal.* 9: ra28.

44 Flaminio, M.J., Nydam, D.V., Marquis, H. et al. (2009). Foal monocyte-derived dendritic cells become activated upon *Rhodococcus equi* infection. *Clin. Vaccine Immunol.* 16: 176–183.

Chapter 47 Humoral Immunity & Transfer of Maternal Immunity

Kelsey A. Hart and David Wong

Overview of Humoral Immunity

Humoral immunity encompasses the immune responses that are mediated by macromolecules in extracellular fluids, primarily in plasma and at mucosal surfaces. Key components in the humoral immune response include secreted antibodies produced by B lymphocytes, complement proteins, and antimicrobial peptides. Complement and antimicrobial peptides play a role in microbial destruction and are components of the innate immune system. Antibodies, also known as immunoglobulins or gamma globulins, are circulating proteins that are produced in all vertebrates in response to foreign antigens and are vital parts of the adaptive immune response. Adaptive immunity is stimulated by exposure to foreign antigen and infectious agents and is characterized by increasing magnitude and efficacy of defensive response with each serial exposure to a specific microbe or antigen. This chapter focuses primarily on the humoral aspects of the adaptive immune response and provides a general description of antibody availability and production in the foal.

B lymphocytes (and activated plasma cells) are the only cells that synthesize antibodies. Antibodies can be either bound to the surface of B lymphocyte antigen receptors or secreted into the plasma, tissues, or at mucosal surfaces. Either way, all antibody molecules function to bind antigens and all share the same basic structure that includes two heavy chains and two light chains, that come together in a "Y" shape (Figure 47.1). Each heavy chain and light chain has a variable region at the amino-terminus and a constant region at the carboxy-terminus. While the general structure is conserved across antibody molecules, the antigen-binding sites necessarily exhibit great variety to permit the immune system to recognize an enormous capacity of structurally diverse molecules as foreign and initiate an immune response. This unique antigen-specificity is provided by the variable regions at the amino-terminal ends, which form the antigen-binding site. In contrast, the constant regions at the carboxy-terminal ends are responsible for the effector functions of the antibody molecule.

Membrane-bound antibodies function as antigen-receptors to alert and activate B cells to the presence of foreign antigens and are discussed in more detail in relation to cell-mediated immunity (Chapter 48). Secreted antibodies, however, play a vital role in humoral immunity by binding to foreign antigen to trigger a variety of effector mechanisms that ultimately help the host eliminate the invading microbe. These effector mechanisms generally involve interaction with other components of the immune system such as phagocytes, natural killer (NK) cells, mast cells, and complement that eventual work to destroy the invader.

There are five major antibody isotypes that differ to a degree in both structure and function: IgM, IgG, IgA, IgE, and IgD. The constant region of the heavy chain of each of these isotypes is encoded by a different gene (mu, gamma, alpha, epsilon, and delta, respectively). Characteristics and functions of these isotypes are detailed in Table 47.1.

Transfer of Maternal Humoral Immunity to the Foal

Humoral immunity in neonatal mammals is initially provided via transfer of passive immunity from the dam. Passive immunity is defined as short term immunity resulting from the introduction or administration of antibodies from another individual. In contrast, active immunity is induced by exposure to foreign antigen, as the immune system of that individual plays an active role in the process of generating the immunity. Passive immunity in the neonate can be provided by administration of plasma or serum containing antibodies from an individual immunized against a specific antigen, or via transfer of naturally occurring

Equine Neonatal Medicine, First Edition. Edited by David M. Wong and Pamela A. Wilkins.

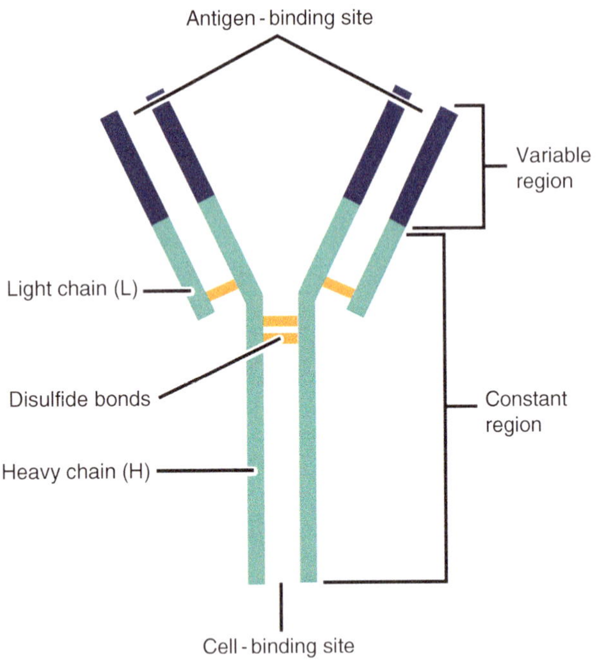

Figure 47.1 Diagram demonstrating the structure of an antibody. Note the "Y" shape along with the heavy and light chain regions and antigen binding sights.

Table 47.1 Specific characteristics and key functions of the five general antibody isotypes.

Antibody isotype	Characteristics and function
IgA	• Produced at mucosal surfaces • Directly neutralizes microbes and prevents binding to host cells • Opsonization for phagocytosis • Integral for mucosal immunity
IgD	• Naïve B cell antigen receptor, usually expressed on cell-surface in conjunction with IgM • Important for activation of naïve B lymphocytes • Very low concentrations in serum
IgE	• Degranulates mast cells • Important for allergy and in defense against parasites • Found in blood and tissues (skin, mucosa) in low concentrations
IgG	• Directly neutralizes microbes and prevents binding to host cells • Opsonization for phagocytosis • Activates complement • Important in antibody-mediated cell-mediated cytotoxicity • Produced slightly later in infection than IgM, especially after first exposure to an antigen • The most prevalent circulating immunoglobulin, with a half-life 4–5 times longer than other isotypes
IgM	• Naïve B cell antigen receptor also expressed on cell-surface • Secreted from activated B cells early in infection • Directly neutralizes microbes and prevents binding to host cells • Activates complement

antibodies from the dam to a fetus or neonate across the placenta and/or via ingestion of colostrum after birth. In many mammalian species, trans-placental transfer of maternal antibodies occurs throughout part or most of gestation. In the horse, however, the unique epitheliochorial placentation prevents any in utero transfer of circulating maternal antibodies to the foal. Thus, the foal is completely dependent on ingestion of good quality colostrum for provision of adequate passive immunity during the immediate postnatal period.

This process of transfer of maternal immunity to the newborn is often referred to as "passive transfer" of immunity, but this is a bit of a misnomer for the foal. In the foal, reception of maternal immunity is an incredibly active process that requires active contributions from both the foal and the dam. The dam must produce sufficient volume and good-quality colostrum and retain that colostrum without leaking milk prior to foaling. Then, within hours of birth, the foal must stand without assistance, locate the udder, and coordinate a strong suckle to repeatedly nurse and consume a large quantity of colostrum prior to closure of the intestinal mucosal barrier. Consumed colostral immunoglobulins are absorbed by specialized epithelial cells of the small intestine through the process of pinocytosis [1].

Through this process, microglobules of protein pass to the back of the epithelial cells and merge to form one or more large globulues [2]. Subsequently, these protein-containing globules are discharged at the base of the cell into the intracellular space, pass into the local lymphatics, and finally reach the systemic circulation [3]. If a foal nurses within 1–3 hours of birth, immunoglobulins can be detected in the serum by 6 hours [1]. Of note, the absorptive cells are non-selective in their uptake and any large molecules present within the intestine are absorbed. These specialized intestinal cells have a rapid turnover rate and are replaced by more mature cells within 38 hours of life [3]. Thus, maximum efficacy of intestinal absorption of immunoglobulins from colostrum occurs at birth, and falls to approximately 25% by 3 hours of age and further decreases to <1% at 20 hours of life [1, 3, 4]. In fact, by 12 hours of age, many of the cells of the small intestine are no longer able to absorb colostral immunoglobulins due to gut closure [2, 3, 5].

Of note, withholding consumption or administration of macromolecules does not delay closure of the equine neonatal small intestine to immunoglobulin absorption but foals that suckle large quantities of colostrum by the first 1–2 hours of age experience gut closure sooner than foals that are weak/ill, orphaned at birth, or consume colostrum with low IgG content [5] (Table 47.2). In these foals, absorption of macromolecules ceases by 24 hours of age [1]. Therefore, if either the mare (e.g. poor colostrum quality/quantity, premature lactation) or foal (e.g. missing, reduced, or delayed colostrum intake, insufficient absorption) fail on their active contribution to this process, veterinary intervention is needed to provide adequate passive immunity to the foal. Thus, it is more appropriate to refer to this process as "transfer of passive immunity" than "passive transfer of immunity" when referring to the foal.

Colostrum is produced as the mammary gland concentrates immunoglobulins from the blood into the mammary secretions during the last few weeks of pregnancy under the influence of estrogen and progesterone with the average mare producing 2–3 l of colostrum [1, 6]. Colostrum not only contains immunoglobulins, but cytokines, complement proteins, growth factors, lactoferrin, ferritin, hormones, enzymes, and cells (lymphocytes, macrophages, neutrophils, epithelial cells) that are likely important in the development of local gastrointestinal immunity and modulation of the newborn foal's response to antigens [1]. The principal immunoglobulin in equine colostrum is IgG (1,500–5,000 mg/dl) with lesser amounts of IgA (500–1,500 mg/dl), IgM (100–350 mg/dl), and IgG(T) (500–2,500 mg/dl) [6]. In very good-quality colostrum, IgG concentration exceeds 8000 mg/dl, whereas 5,000–8,000 mg/dl is considered good quality, 2,800–5,000 mg/dl as fair quality, and <2,800 mg/dl considered poor-quality colostrum [7, 8]. Protein concentrations within colostrum decline rapidly in the first 8 hours post-parturition as the foal suckles, and immunoglobulin concentrations become negligible by 12 hours with regular suckling [6]. It is important to reiterate that antibodies specific to important potential pathogens in the foal's immediate environment are a critical component of colostrum. Specifically, antibodies against *Clostridium* spp., *Actinobacillus* spp., *Streptococcus equi*, *Rhodococcus equi*, and common equine viral diseases have been demonstrated in equine colostrum [9].

Table 47.2 Concentrations (mean ± SD) of IgG, IgM, and IgA in the colostrum, milk, and serum of horses [5].

		Immunoglobulin (mg/dl)		
Sample	*n*	IgG	IgA	IgM
Colostrum	36	8912 ± 6200	957 ± 1098	123 ± 77
	6	16 583 ± 3618	NM	104 ± 35
	5	26 800 ± 5814	900 ± 300	NM
Milk	5	50 ± 22	70 ± 20	NM
Serum (birth)	35	5 ± 5	NM	16 ± 6
	5	3 ± 0.3	ND	NM
Serum (24 h)	36	1953 ± 1635	58 ± 42	34 ± 30
	10	1600 ± 280	NM	50 ± 6
	5	3900 ± 412	40 ± 10	NM
Serum (30 d)	10	1180 ± 280	NM	41 ± 8
	5	1770 ± 454	6 ± 4	NM
Serum (120 d)	10	1360 ± 320	NM	46 ± 8
Serum (adult)	35	2464 ± 1337	305 ± 337	136 ± 218
	6	2233 ± 262	ND	104 ± 25
	25	1955 ± 413	NM	103 ± 40

NM, not measured; ND, not done.

In sum, all of these components play a vital role in the foal's humoral immunity in the neonatal period and beyond. In fact, colostral-derived antibodies provide protection for the foal for the first 2–4 months of life until their endogenous antibody production is sufficient to offer protection.

The importance of transfer of passive immunity cannot be overstated. Several studies have demonstrated a high correlation between foals with failure of transfer of passive immunity (FTPI) and the development of sepsis or other infections in foals within the first few weeks of life, especially those foals with IgG concentrations <200–400 mg/dl [10–13]. In one particular study involving 8 colostrum-deprived foals with complete FTPI, 7 foals demonstrated signs of sepsis, of which 5/7 were blood culture positive [14]. In a much larger study investigating FTPI, the mortality rate in 597 foals with complete FTPI, partial FTPI, and adequate transfer of passive immunity was 29% (57/198), 23% (39/167), and 7% (17/232), respectively [15]. Of note, foals with partial FTPI (i.e. IgG concentrations of 400–800 mg/dl) do not always have increased prevalence of disease or death, suggesting that the amount of transfer of passive immunity is not the only factor that impacts outcome; other factors such as environmental conditions, stress, concurrent disease, and management practices also contribute to development of disease [1, 6].

Evaluation and Management of Transfer of Passive Immunity in the Foal

Incidence of FTPI in Foals

The exact serum IgG concentration that constitutes adequate transfer of passive immunity in foals is not known and is likely variable, depending on environmental factors, management conditions, comorbidities (e.g. perinatal disease such as neonatal encephalopathy), pathogen virulence, and number of invading microorganisms [13, 16, 17]. In most healthy foals, serum IgG concentrations are higher than the 800 mg/dl breakpoint that is often used to define transfer of passive immunity. In one study involving six healthy neonatal foals, the mean serum IgG concentration was 1,508 mg/dl [14]. The IgG concentration at which infections are more common is debatable, but one study did recently validate the commonly used cutoff values indicating adequate transfer of passive immunity (>800 mg/dl) [15]. In this study involving hospitalized foals, foals with complete or partial FTPI (IgG concentration of <400 and <800 mg/dl, respectively) had increased risk of dying compared to foals with an IgG >800 mg/dl [15].

The incidence of FTPI has been reported in a number of studies and has ranged from 2.9–24% and up to 30–42% in hospitalized foals [13, 17–19]. Some inherent variability in the reported incidence could be related to the different tests used to measure IgG concentrations, different reference ranges, and the age at which the foal was tested [13, 17, 19]. In a large study of 323 Thoroughbred foals from a single breeding farm, the incidence of FTPI (IgG <800 mg/dl) was 9.6% (31/323) [16]. In this study, factors associated with FPTI included male foals, time of birth (foals born late in the foaling season), and the need for human assistance at parturition. In addition, IgG concentration <800 mg/dl at 12–24 hours was significantly associated with increased incidence of septic conditions (septicemia, osteomyelitis, respiratory infection). In another study, foals that took longer than 6 hours postpartum to consume colostrum had a higher risk (odds ratio 5.39) of FTPI, whereas foals that were born on pasture had a lower risk (odds ratio 0.23) of FTPI when compared to foals born in stables [16].

Methods for Assessing Transfer of Passive Immunity in Foals

Because adequate transfer of passive immunity is so imperative for preventing infection in the neonatal foal, screening individual foals for FTPI is extremely important. Estimation of serum IgG concentrations based on serum total solids, total protein, or total globulin measurements are not adequately sensitive or specific for FTPI diagnosis in foals but can provide some preliminary information [18, 20–24]. For example, in one study involving 88 newborn foals, the mean total protein in foals with FTPI was 4.26 ± 0.42 g/dl (range 3.5–4.9 g/dl) compared to 5.89 ± 0.55 g/dl (range 4.7–7.0 g/dl) in foals with adequate transfer of passive immunity [17]. The authors of that study suggested that a foal (>18 hours of age) with a total protein <4.7 g/dl is likely to have complete or partial FTPI [17]. In another study involving 65 foals, the authors proposed that a serum total protein concentration of ≤4.5 g/dl suggested FTPI, whereas values ≥6.0 g/dl suggested adequate IgG concentrations [18]. In a third study, a total protein concentrations of 5.4 g/dl (sensitivity 67%, specificity 84%) and 5.1 g/dl (sensitivity 65%, specificity 77%) suggested sufficient serum IgG concentrations for levels of 800 and 400 mg/dl, respectively [25]. In that same study, total globulins of 2.7 g/dl (sensitivity 75%, specificity 82%) and 2.4 g/dl (sensitivity 76%, specificity 78%) suggested IgG concentrations for levels of 800 and 400 mg/dl, respectively [25]. While serum total protein or globulin concentrations might serve as a preliminary guide, the clinician must be cognizant of the fact that these values are impacted by the foal's hydration status and are less reliable; therefore, assessment of transfer of passive immunity should be confirmed with a more accurate test.

A number of quantitative and semi-quantitative methods for diagnosis of FTPI in foals have been described, but radial immunodiffusion (RID) is considered the gold standard method. Unfortunately, both RID and another similarly accurate method, serum protein electrophoresis, are expensive and require specialized laboratory equipment and training to perform and interpret. These tests also take longer to report results if performed in hospital and even longer if they are mailed to outside testing laboratories. Several other, more rapid, less-expensive, semi-quantitative methods for diagnosis of FTPI in foals have been evaluated in attempts to provide clinicians a rapid screening test for foals in a farm or hospital setting. Some of these tests include the point-of-care ELISA, glutaraldehyde coagulation, and zinc sulfate turbidity methods; these tests are acceptably accurate for detecting FTPI [20, 26–28], but do not provide a quantitative IgG measurement (Table 47.3). Turbidometric immunoassay methodology that permits quantitative IgG assessment in foals has been developed and offers acceptable sensitivity and specificity [24, 31, 32], but a validated point-of-care system employing this methodology is not universally available to date. Newer tests to evaluate IgG concentrations such as the immunocrit test (ammonium sulphate precipitation) have been evaluated but widespread use has not occurred [33].

An important component to consider when testing for FTPI is the sensitivity and specificity of the test. A test that produces few false positive results has a high specificity whereas a test that produces few false negative results has a high sensitivity. Regarding testing for FTPI, a false positive test (test reports FTPI when foal's IgG is truly adequate) and false negative test (test reports adequate IgG when foal's IgG is truly inadequate) are both concerns. Ideally, a test would be both highly sensitive and specific, such as radioimmunodiffusion. However, most tests for evaluating serum IgG concentrations are typically not both sensitive and specific. Considering the complications associate with FTPI, a test with high sensitivity is desired to minimize the number of foals with FTPI misclassified as having adequate passive transfer (false negative). Table 47.4 reports the sensitivity and specificity of a variety of tests used for detection of FTPI.

Table 47.3 Various methods of testing for transfer of passive immunity in the neonatal foal.

Enzyme-Linked Immune-Sorbent Assay (ELISA)	Monoclonal antibodies that react specifically with an antigen (e.g. equine IgG) are firmly fixed in a strip (situated in windows) within a nitrocellulose base. Free moving antibodies that are specific to the antigen are initially found in the well receiving the test sample. The second group of antibodies contain an enzyme that converts a colorless reagent into a dark color. The intensity of the color change (dependent on foal's serum IgG concentration) corresponds to predetermined IgG concentrations (>800 mg/dl, 400–800 mg/dl, <400 mg/dl).
Glutaraldehyde Coagulation	Glutaraldehyde is an aldehyde that reacts primarily with uncharged amino groups of lysine residues to form intermolecular cross-linkages and is more specific for basic proteins. Gammaglobulin proteins in serum react with glutaraldehyde to form insoluble complexes. The test is performed by mixing 1 volume of reagent with 10 volumes of serum and observing the coagulation time (time to form a solid gel). The required glutaraldehyde concentration was established for various threshold levels of IgG as determined by radial immunodiffusion [29].
Zine Sulfate Turbidity Test	Semiquantitative assay in which a solution of zinc sulfate precipitates with the globulin fraction in serum samples at certain serum IgG levels (e.g. 400 mg/dl) [30].
Turbidimetric Immunoassay	Immunologic agglutination and light scattering of the agglutination products. Sample is mixed with solution containing high concentration of antibody (anti-equine IgG); antigen–antibody complexes form large aggregates that scatter light; this results in turbidity proportional to the immunoglobulin concentration of the sample. The nonscattered light is measured by spectrophotometry at 700 nm, a wavelength that is not absorbed by either the sample or immunoprecipitate. The nonscattered light from the sample is compared to a standard curve prepared from the instrument [31].

Table 47.4 Accuracy and diagnostic performance (95% confidence interval) of some commercially available assays for the detection of serum IgG at concentrations of <400 or <800 mg/dl in neonatal foals [5, 18, 34].

	Performance of assay for detection of IgG ≤ 400 mg/dl		
Assay	**Accuracy**	**Sensitivity**	**Specificity**
DVM Stat (Colorimetric immunoassay)[A]	97.0 (91.5–99.4)	100 (89.5–100)	96.0 (88.5–99.1) [18]
Equi Z Equine FPT Test Kit (Zinc sulfate turbidity)[B]	82.0 (73.1–89.0)	88.9 (70.8–97.7)	79.4 (68.4–88.0) [18]
Plasma Foal IgG quick Test Kit (Immunoturbudimetric)[C]	81.0 (71.9–88.2)	88.9 (70.8–97.7)	78.1 (66.9–86.9) [18]
Snap Foal IgG (Semi-quantitative ELISA)[D]	93.4 (87.3–97.7)	88.9 (70.8–97.7)	95.8 (88.3–99.1) [18]
Snap Foal IgG (Semi-quantitative ELISA)[D]	Not available	90.0 (71.0–98)	79.0 (71.0–82.0) [22]
Glutaraldehyde coagulation	Not available	95.0 (92.0–98.0)	80.0 (74.0–85.0) [34]
	Performance of assay for detection of IgG ≤ 800 mg/dl		
	Accuracy	**Sensitivity**	**Specificity**
DVM Stat (Colorimetric immunoassay)[A]	89.0 (81.2–94.4)	97.6 (87.4–99.9)	82.8 (70.6–91.4) [18]
Equi Z Equine FPT Test Kit (Zinc sulfate turbidity)[B]	67.0 (56.9–76.1)	81.0 (65.9–91.4)	56.9 (43.2–69.8) [18]
Plasma Foal IgG quick Test Kit (Immunoturbudimetric)[E]	80.0 (70.8–87.3)	52.4 (36.4–68.0)	100 (95.0–100) [18]
Snap Foal IgG (Semi-quantitative ELISA)[D]	88.9 (81.0–94.3)	81.0 (65.9–91.4)	94.7 (85.4–98.9) [18]
Snap Foal IgG (Semi-quantitative ELISA)[D]	Not available	95.0 (71.0–98.0)	52.0 (39.0–57.0) [22]
Gamma-Check-E (Glutaraldehyde coagulation)[D]	73.0 (63.2–81.4)	92.9 (80.5–98.5)	58.6 (44.9–71.4) [18]
Glutaraldehyde coagulation	Not available	100 (100)	58.0 (52.0–65.0) [34]

A – VDx Inc., Belgium, WI; B – VMRD Inc., Pullman, WA; C – Midland BioProducts, Boone, IA; D – Snap ELISA, IDEXX Labs, Westbrook ME; E – Midland Bioproducts, Boone, IA (800).

Timing of assessment of transfer of passive immunity in newborn foals is also important. Absorption of colostral immunoglobulins occurs most efficiently in the first 12 hours of life, but complete gut closure does not occur until 12–24 hours of age [35]. Thus, screening for FTPI can be done as early as 8–12 hours of age. Testing serum IgG concentrations at 12 hours may permit remediation of FTPI with oral administration of another source of colostrum or commercial colostrum replacer, while documentation of FTPI closer to 18–24 hours of age or after requires intravenous administration of plasma to ensure adequate immunoglobulin levels. In sick foals, even if adequate transfer of passive immunity was documented on the first day of life, repeat screening is recommended as immunoglobulin consumption in illness can result in serum IgG falling below protective levels early in life [9].

FTPI can be partial (generally described as IgG concentration of 400–800 mg/dl) or complete (IgG <400 mg/dl) [9]. Some, but not all, semi-quantitative methods for assessment allow the clinician to distinguish between these immunoglobulin concentrations. Foals with partial FTPI may have adequate immunity, but there is little data to suggest their specific risk of illness. In general, treatment for FTPI with plasma transfusion to provide IgG supplementation is recommend for both partial and complete FTPI.

Prevention and Management of FTPI in Foals

Prevention of FTPI in foals is centered on ensuring that a healthy newborn foal receives an appropriate amount of good-quality colostrum before the gastrointestinal mucosal barrier begins to close. Good farm management strategies are an important first step. Mares with a previous history of having had a foal with FTPI should have their colostral quality assessed in subsequent foalings. Digital or optical refractometry are simple methods for assessing equine colostral quality with values ≥23% suggestive of good quality colostrum (IgG >60 g/l) [1, 36–38]. Alternatively, colostral IgG concentration is directly related to its specific gravity; therefore a modified hydrometer that measures the specific gravity of colostrum (colostrometer) can be used to evaluated colostral quality (Figure 47.2). Colostrum with a specific gravity of ≥1.060 is considered good quality colostrum [1] as exemplified in one study in which a colostral specific gravity value <1.060 was associated with an increased likelihood of FTPI [17, 39]. The clinician should also be mindful that colostral IgG content drops by 60–75% by eight hours after foaling [1]. The foal should be supplemented with colostrum from another source or plasma if colostral quality is deemed inadequate. If available, 1–2 liters of high-quality colostrum is recommended for a 45 kg foal with feedings beginning at 1–2 hours of age in volumes of 200–300 ml/feeding [6]. Similar actions should be taken if the mare is observed to drip/stream milk for a substantial period before parturition, or if the mare has inadequate udder development. Of note, if colostrum is to be harvested and banked for future use, it should be collected immediately after the foal first suckles. It is safe to collect up to 250 ml of colostrum from a mare without harming her foal [1].

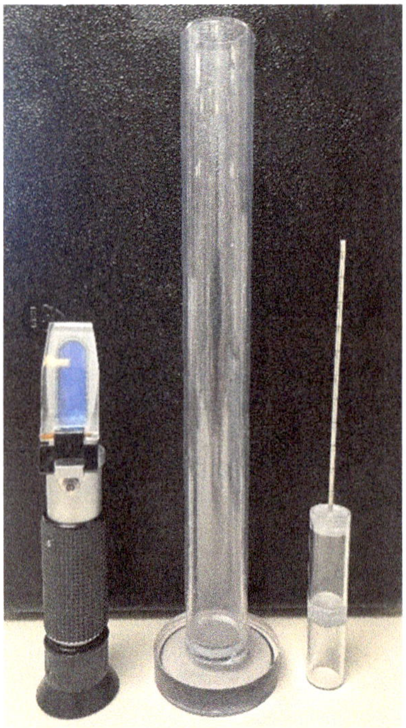

Figure 47.2 Devices used to evaluate the quality of colostrum include the Brix refractometer (left) and colostrometer (right).

Colostrum or plasma administration, as discussed above, should be considered for newborn foals that are not able to stand or suckle normally to attempt to prevent FTPI. The mare's own colostrum, frozen colostrum from another mare, or commercial equine colostrum replacer can be administered via nasogastric intubation to ensure adequate delivery. Alternatively, plasma can be given intravenously to ensure a rapid increase in serum IgG – this is the only option for foals >18–24 hours of age, and the required treatment in most cases of FTPI which is typically diagnosed at this age or beyond. The volume of plasma necessary to raise the serum IgG concentration to adequate concentrations (i.e. >800 mg/dl) cannot be predicted accurately because the response to exogenously administered plasma depends on a number of variables, including the severity of FTPI, the quantity of IgG contained in the plasma, the weight of the foal, and possible ongoing infections [4]. Commercially available equine plasma typically has an IgG concentration of ≥2000 mg/dl and is available in one-liter units. In general, one liter of plasma containing 1500–1700 mg/dl of IgG increases the recipient's IgG by approximately 200–300 mg/dl [1].

Therefore, on average, 1–2 units are needed to reach adequate IgG levels >800 mg/dl, but some foals with complete FTPI or ill foals with ongoing immunoglobulin consumption due to neonatal illness may require additional plasma supplementation. Reassessment of IgG concentration 24–48 hours after plasma transfusion is ideal [38]. Foals with sepsis should have their serum IgG concentrations reassessed as these foals may differ in catabolism and distribution of immunoglobulins and thus may require additional and repeated administration of plasma throughout the course of their disease to achieve and maintain adequate serum IgG concentrations [5].

Ideally, IgG concentrations of >800 mg/dl should be achieved in newborn foals. However, plasma administration may be declined due to financial constraints by some owners. Interestingly, studies of FTPI suggest that otherwise heathy foals with no other known risk factors for sepsis (e.g. dystocia, prematurity/dysmaturity, neonatal encephalopathy, endemic farm pathogens, etc.) and a serum IgG concentration of 400–800 mg/dl may not require a plasma transfusion to provide adequate immune protection for the first weeks of life [40, 41]. However, owners should be advised of the risks of declining IgG supplementation in foals with serum IgG concentrations in this range and foals should be closely monitored for evidence of infection and maintained in a clean environment with minimal exposure to potential pathogens.

Frozen plasma should be thawed and warmed to body temperature slowly before administration. A whole-blood filter should be used to administer plasma and other blood products. A slow rate of administration is initiated for the first 50–100 ml to observe for potential adverse reactions (tachypnea, tachycardia, hyperthermia, urticaria, behavior change). If no reactions are noted within the first 15–20 minutes of slow administration, the remainder of the transfusion can be administered at 20–30 ml/kg/h, although some manufacturers recommend much faster rates [5]. Rapid administration rates of multiple units of plasma to normovolemic foals are discouraged to avoid volume overload. If minor reactions are noted, the infusion rate should be decreased until signs abate. However, if adverse reactions occur, even with a slower rate, the process should be discontinued.

Development of Endogenous Humoral Immunity in the Foal

The foal's immune organs and immune cells develop during fetal life, and essentially, the foal is born immunocompetent but immunologically naïve. Thus, the newborn foal is initially heavily dependent on innate immune responses as the adaptive immune system is less robust and rapid than in adult animals, due to the fact that the foal's immune system has not been exposed to foreign antigens to develop important immunological memory. Humoral immunity in the neonatal foal is initially centered on innate humoral factors such as complement, and on maternal antibodies and other factors transferred via colostrum as described above.

It is important to note, however, that the newborn foal is capable of generating an antigen-specific humoral immune response. The foal's lymphoid organs develop during early to mid-gestation, with the thymus detectable at approximately 80 days of gestation and circulating lymphocytes apparent by approximately 120 days gestation [9]. These cells are capable of making antibodies, as healthy, full-term foals are born with detectable but low serum concentrations of IgM and IgG and foals exposed to pathogens in utero, such as foals born to mares with *Neospora hughesi* placentitis, have high levels of specific antibodies even prior to suckling [9].

Clearly, the foal's humoral immune system demonstrates some degree of antigen-independent activity during gestation and is capable of responding to foreign antigens and pathogens in late gestation, if present, by producing specific antigens in multiple different isotypes [9]. However, it is not until shortly after birth, upon exposure to a massive number of diverse environmental and commensal organisms, that an enormous expansion of antigen-specific lymphocyte subpopulations is induced. Specifically, an approximately twofold increase in circulating lymphocyte numbers is observed by 2–3 months of age, which is coupled with substantial increase in the mass of secondary lymphoid tissues [9, 42]. This increase in lymphoid mass is especially apparent in the gastrointestinal-associated lymphoid tissue and is likely driven by constant exposure to microbial antigens as the gut is colonized by commensal flora. Interestingly, this process is much slower in the respiratory tract, with bronchial-associated lymphoid tissue not observed until 12 weeks of age [9].

Circulating lymphocyte numbers (both B and T cells) increase steadily until about 4–5 months of age until stabilizing at higher levels than noted in adult horses. Lymphocyte numbers then taper to adult levels by 7–9 months of age [9, 43, 44]. The ability of foal lymphocytes to proliferate in response to mitogens *in vitro* is comparable to adult responses [42].

Endogenous antibody production increases steadily over the first several months of life in the foal upon exposure to environmental, commensal, and pathogenic organisms, but specific timing varies among isotypes. IgA is not present in the foal's respiratory tract until approximately 4 weeks of age, but the foal is still protected by initial mucosal immunity provided by maternal antibodies. In fact, IgG, presumably of maternal origin, is detectable in the foal's respiratory tract shortly after colostral ingestion.

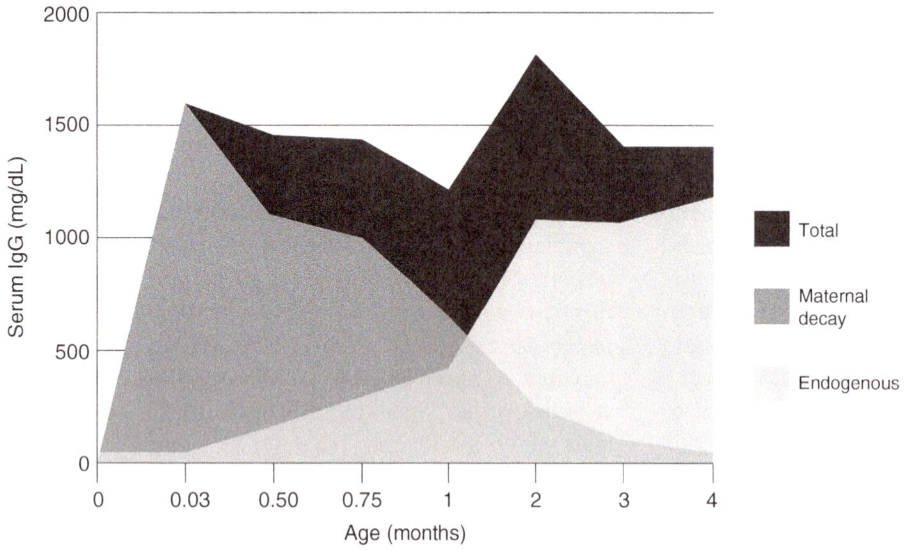

Figure 47.3 Serum immunoglobulin concentrations of young foals ranging from the newborn-neonatal period to several months of age. The total serum IgG concentration is initially composed of colostrum-derived antibodies that slowly wane over 3–4 months (half-life 28–32 days). Endogenously produced immunoglobulins begin in the neonatal period and gradually increase over time.

Colostral IgA also plays a vital protective role in neutralizing and opsonizing potential pathogens in the gut during early life. IgE production is also quite limited in the newborn foal, for a much longer period of time; maternally-derived IgE is undetectable by 4 months, but endogenous IgE production does not begin in earnest until 6–11 months of age [45].

Endogenous production of IgM and IgG steadily increases over the first months of life, but maternally derived antibodies are simultaneously decreasing during this time (half-life of immunoglobulins is approximately 30 days). Thus, the foal's serum immunoglobulin concentration reaches a nadir at 1–3 months of age when maternal antibody concentrations are waning and endogenous production has not yet reached substantial levels (Figure 47.3) [9, 46]. Considering the 30-day half-life, it may be more prudent to consider an IgG of ≥1,000–1,200 mg/dl rather than ≥800 mg/dl as adequate transfer of passive of immunity after birth, to ensure that the foal continue to have protective levels of circulating immunoglobulins (≥500 mg/dl) at this nadir before the foal's endogenous immunoglobulin production is enough to reach this threshold for protection [9, 46].

The presence of maternal antibodies has been described to interfere with the foal's own humoral immune responses, potentially by clearing pathogens prior to immune activation or inhibition of B-cell activation [9, 47]. However, a number of studies have demonstrated that foals can generate antigen-specific immune responses from an early age, even in the presence of circulating maternal antibodies [48–52]. In sum, the foal's humoral immune system is present and competent at birth, though months of diverse antigen exposure are needed until it functions at a robust level adequate for production of a protective antibody response. In the meantime, the newborn foal depends heavily on maternally derived humoral immune components and the innate immune system for protection from infection.

References

1 LeBLanc, M.M. (2001). Update on passive transfer of immunoglobulins in the foal. *Pferdeheilkunde* 17: 662–665.

2 Jeffcott, L.B. (1974). Some practical aspects of the transfer of passive immunity to newborn foals. *Equine Vet. J.* 6: 109–115.

3 Jeffcott, L.B. (1974). Studies on passive immunity in the foals. II the absorption of 1241-labelled PVP (polyvinyl pyrrolidone) by the neonatal intestine. *J. Comp. Pathol.* 84: 279–289.

4 Francesca, F., Jole, M., Aliai, L. et al. (2017). Efficacy and safety of a commercial fresh-frozen hyperimmune plasma in foals with failure of passive transfer of immunity. *J. Equine Vet. Sci.* 48: 174–181.

5 Giguere, S. and Polkes, A.C. (2005). Immunologic disorders of neonatal foals. *Vet. Clin. North Am. Equine Pract.* 21: 241–272.

6 Sellon, D.C. (2000). Secondary immunedeficiences of horses. *Vet. Clin. North Am. Equine* 16: 117–130.

7 Pearson, R.C., Hallowell, A.L., Bayly, W.M. et al. (1984). Times of appearance and disappearance of colostral IgG in the mare. *Am. J. Vet. Res.* 45: 186–190.
8 Turini, L., Nocera, I., Bonelli, F. et al. (2020). Evaluation of brix refractometry for the estimation of colostrum quality in Jennies. *J. Equine Vet. Sci.* 92: 103172.
9 Tallmadge, R. (2016). The immune system of the young horse. In: *Equine Clinical Immunology* (ed. M.J. Felippe), 11–22. Ames, IA: Wiley.
10 Mcguire, T.C., Crawford, T.B., Hallowell, A.L. et al. (1977). Failure of colostral immunoglobulin transfer as an explanation for most infections and deaths of neonatal foals. *J. Am. Vet. Med. Assoc.* 170: 1302–1304.
11 Mcguire, T.C., Poppie, M.J., and Banks, K.L. (1975). Hypogammaglobulinemia predisposing to infection in foals. *J. Am. Vet. Med. Assoc.* 166: 71–75.
12 Bublitz, U., Gerhards, H., and Deegen, E. (1991). Incidence of failure of passive transfer of colostral immunoglobulins to neonatal foals: a field study. *Pferdeheikunde* 7: 155–165.
13 Raidal, S.L. (1996). The incidence and consequences of failure of passive transfer of immunity on a Thoroughbred breeding farm. *Aust. Vet. J.* 73: 201–206.
14 Robinson, J.A., Allen, G.K., Green, E.M. et al. (1993). A prospective study of septicaemia in colostrum-deprived foals. *Equine Vet. J.* 25: 214–219.
15 Liepman, R.S., Dembek, K.A., Slovis, N.M. et al. (2015). Validation of IgG cut-off values and their association with survival in neonatal foals. *Equine Vet. J.* 47: 526–530.
16 Ayala, M.S.F. and Oliver-Espinosa, O.J. (2016). Risk factors associated with failure of passive transfer of colostral immunoglobulins in neonatal Paso Fino foals. *J. Equine Vet. Sci.* 44: 100–104.
17 Tyler-McGowan, C.M., Hodgson, J.L., and Hodgson, D.R. (1997). Failure of passive transfer in foals: incidence and outcome on four studs in New South Wales. *Aust. Vet. J.* 75: 56–59.
18 Davis, R. and Giguere, S. (2005). Evaluation of five commercially available assays and measurement of serum total protein concentration via refractometry for the diagnosis of failure of passive transfer of immunity in foals. *J. Am. Vet. Med. Assoc.* 227: 1640–1645.
19 Morris, D.D., Meirs, D.A., and Merryman, B.S. (1985). Passive transfer failure in horses: incidence and causative factors on a breeding farm. *Am. J. Vet. Res.* 46: 2294–2299.
20 Fouché, N., Graubner, C., and Howard, J. (2014). Correlation between serum total globulins and gamma globulins and their use to diagnose failure of passive transfer in foals. *Vet. J.* 202: 384–386.
21 Hurcombe, S.D., Matthews, A.L., Scott, V.H. et al. (2012). Serum protein concentrations as predictors of serum immunoglobulin G concentration in neonatal foals. *J. Vet. Emerg. Crit. Care. (San Antonio)* 22: 573–579.
22 Metzger, N., Hardy, J., Schwarzwald, C.C., and Wittum, T. (2006). Usefulness of a commercial equine IgG test and serum protein concentration as indicators of failure of transfer of passive immunity in hospitalized foals. *J. Vet. Intern. Med.* 20: 382–387.
23 Rumbaugh, G.E., Ardans, A.A., Ginno, D. et al. (1978). Measurement of neonatal equine immunoglobulins for assessment of colostral immunoglobulin transfer: comparison of single radial immunodiffusion with the zinc sulfate turbidity test, serum electrophoresis, refractometry for total serum protein, and the sodium sulfite precipitation test. *J. Am. Vet. Med. Assoc.* 172: 321–325.
24 Wong, D.M., Giguère, S., and Wendel, M.A. (2013). Evaluation of a point-of-care portable analyzer for measurement of plasma immunoglobulin G, total protein, and albumin concentrations in ill neonatal foals. *J. Am. Vet. Med. Assoc.* 242: 812–819.
25 Sievert, M., Schuler, G., Buttner, K. et al. (2022). Comparison of different methods to determine the absorption of colostral IgG in newborn foals. *J. Equine Vet. Sci.* 114: 104008.
26 Bauer, J.E. and Brooks, T.P. (1990). Immunoturbidimetric quantification of serum immunoglobulin G concentration in foals. *Am. J. Vet. Res.* 51: 1211–1214.
27 Clabough, D.L., Conboy, H.S., and Roberts, M.C. (1989). Comparison of four screening techniques for the diagnosis of equine neonatal hypogammaglobulinemia. *J. Am. Vet. Med. Assoc.* 194: 1717–1720.
28 Kent, J.E. and Blackmore, D.J. (1985). Measurement of IgG in equine blood by immunoturbidimetry and latex agglutination. *Equine Vet. J.* 17: 125–129.
29 Beetson, S.A., Hilbert, B.J., and Mills, J.N. (1985). The use of the glutaraldehyde coagulation test for detection of hypogammaglobulinaemia in neonatal foals. *Aust. Vet. J.* 62: 279–281.
30 LeBlanc, M.M., Hurtgen, J.P., and Lyle, S. (1990). A modified zinc sulfate turbidity test for the detection of immune status in newly born foals. *J. Equine Vet. Sci.* 10: 36–39.
31 Davis, D.G., Schaefer, D.M., Hinchcliff, K.W. et al. (2005). Measurement of serum IgG in foals by radial immunodiffusion and automated turbidimetric immunoassay. *J. Vet. Intern. Med.* 19: 93–96.
32 Ujvari, S., Schwarzwald, C.C., Fouche, N. et al. (2017). Validation of a point-of-care quantitative equine IgG turbidimetric immunoassay and comparison of IgG concentrations measured with radial immunodiffusion and a point-of-care IgG ELISA. *J. Vet. Intern. Med.* 31: 1170–1177.
33 Mortola, E., Miceli, G., Alarcon, L. et al. (2020). Assessment of the immunocrit method to detect failure of passive immunity in newborn foals. *Equine Vet. J.* 52: 760–764.

34 McClure, J.T., Miller, J., and Deluca, J.L. (2003). Comparison of two ELISA screening tests and a non-commercial glutaraldehyde coagulation screening test for the detection of failure of passive transfer in neonatal foals. *AAEP Proc.* 49: 301–305.

35 Jeffcott, L.B. (1971). Duration of permeability of the intestine to macromolecules in the newly-born foal. *Vet. Rec.* 88: 340–341.

36 Rampacci, E., Mazzola, K., Beccati, F. et al. (2023). Diagnostic characteristics of refractometry cut-off points for the estimation of immunoglobulin G concentration in mare colostrum. *Equine Vet. J.* 55: 102–110.

37 Waelchli, R.O., Hässig, M., Eggenberger, E. et al. (1990). Relationships of total protein, specific gravity, viscosity, refractive index and latex agglutination to immunoglobulin G concentration in mare colostrum. *Equine Vet. J.* 22: 39–42.

38 Elsohaby, I., Riley, C.B., and McClure, J.T. (2019). Usefulness of digital and optical refractometers for the diagnosis of failure of transfer of passive immunity in neonatal foals. *Equine Vet. J.* 51: 451–457.

39 LeBlanc, M.M., McLaurin, B.I., and Bowsell, R. (1986). Relationships among serum immunoglobulin concentration in foals, colostral specific gravity, and colostral immunoglobulin concentration. *J. Am. Vet. Med. Assoc.* 189: 57–60.

40 Baldwin, J.L., Cooper, W.L., Vanderwall, D.K. et al. (1991). Prevalence (treatment days) and severity of illness in hypogammaglobulinemic foals. *J. Am. Vet. Med. Assoc.* 198: 423–428.

41 Clabough, D.L., Levine, J.F., Grang, G.L. et al. (1991). Factors associated with failure of passive transfer of colostral antibodies in Standardbred foals. *J. Vet. Intern. Med.* 5: 335–340.

42 Flaminio, M., Rush, B., Davis, E. et al. (2000). Characterization of peripheral blood and pulmonary leukocyte function in healthy foals. *Vet. Immunol. Immunopathol.* 73: 267–285.

43 Flaminio, M., Rush, B., and Shuman, W. (1999). Peripheral blood lymphocyte subpopulations and immunoglobulin concenrations in healthy foals and foals with *Rhodococcus equi* pneumonia. *J. Vet. Intern. Med.* 13: 206–212.

44 Smith, R., Chaffin, M., Cohen, N. et al. (2002). Age-related changes in lymphocyte subsets of Quarter Horse foals. *Am. J. Vet. Res.* 63: 531–537.

45 Wagner, B., Flaminio, J.B., Hillegas, J. et al. (2006). Occurrence of IgE in foals: evidence for transfer of maternal IgE by the colostrum and late onset of endogenous IgE production in the horse. *Vet. Immunol. Immunopathol.* 110: 269–278.

46 Felippe, M.J. (2016). Immunodeficiencies. In: *Equine Clinical Immunology* (ed. M.J. Felippe), 193–204. Ames, IA: Wiley.

47 Siegrist, C.A. and Aspinall, R. (2009). B-cell responses to vaccination at the extremes of age. *Nat. Rev. Immunol.* 9: 185–194.

48 Jacks, S., Giguere, S., Crawford, P. et al. (2007). Experimental infection of neonatal foals with *Rhodococcus equi* triggers adult-like gamma interferon induction. *Clin. Vaccine Immunol.* 14.

49 Ryan, C., Giguere, S., Hagen, J. et al. (2010). Effect of age and mitogen on the frequency of interleukin-4 and interferon gamma secreting cells in foals and adult horses as assessed by an equine-specific ELISPOT assay. *Vet. Immunol. Immunopathol.* 133: 66–71.

50 Chong, Y.C. and Duffus, W.P. (1992). Immune responses of specific pathogen free foals to EHV-1 infection. *Vet. Microbiol.* 32: 215–228.

51 Chong, Y.C., Duffus, W.P., and Hannant, D. (1992). Natural killer cells in normal horses and specific-pathogen-free foals infected with equine herpesvirus. *Vet. Immunol. Immunopathol.* 33: 103–113.

52 Harris, S.P., Hines, M.T., Mealey, R.H. et al. (2011). Early development of cytotoxic T lymphocytes in neonatal foals following oral inoculation with *Rhodococcus equi*. *Vet. Immunol. Immunopathol.* 141: 312–316.

Chapter 48 Cellular Immunity in the Neonatal Foal

Brett Sponseller

In general, cell-mediated immunity (CMI) refers to one of the arms of the adaptive immune system that does not involve the production of antibodies to protect the body against microbial invasion. CMI is further distinguished from innate immune responses, which include, among others, immune protective features such as skin, phagocytic white blood cells, activation of the complement cascade, cytokine induction of immune cells, and activation of adaptive immune responses by presentation of antigen. While immune functions may be easily categorized, there can be extensive overlap in the roles and functions that cells play in immune responses. The clinical significance of differential CMI responses in neonatal foals compared to adult horses is exemplified by "foalhood" diseases, such as rotaviral enteritis and Rhodococcal pneumonia, that rarely cause clinical disease in adult horses. At birth, foals lack B- and T-cell memory and fully functional effector cells, which contribute to adult protection from these same diseases.

The acquisition and development of CMI entails the activation of phagocytes, antigen-specific cytotoxic T-lymphocytes (CTLs) and release of cytokines in response to antigen. Upon exposure to potential pathogens or to vaccine antigen, different subsets of helper T cells produce a distinct profile of cytokines (Table 48.1, Figure 48.1) that bias regulation of adaptive immune responses. It is apparent that the cytokine profile elicited by exposure to antigen, whether a microbial pathogen or vaccine derived, differs between adult horses and foals throughout the first year of life [1–3]. Foals have a T_h1-biased cytokine response but at a level that is much lower than that of the adult horse. Importantly, T_h2 cytokine responses are barely detectable for weeks to months after birth [1, 4, 5]. The T_h1-response predominates in the foal for several months, resulting in concurrently lower CMI responses compared to the adult horse. As a result, despite the predominance of a T_h1 response, which generally is effective at eliminating intracellular pathogens, the neonatal foal is much more susceptible to intracellular pathogens than the adult.

Helper T cells (T_h cells), also designated as CD4+ cells, play an important role in adaptive immunity, primarily through the release of cytokines which are small cell-signaling molecules. From the standpoint of CMI, helper T cells help promote the activation of cytotoxic T cells and enhance the phagocytic activity of macrophages. Macrophages are important antigen presenting cells and when antigen is expressed by a macrophage on MHC class II, T_h cells interface directly with the macrophage through specific proteins, CD40 on the surface of the macrophage and CD154 (or CD40 ligand) on the surface of the T_h cell [6]. Macrophages and T_h cells also communicate in a noncontact dependent way via cytokines. T_h cells also play a central role in activation of antigen-specific cytotoxic T cells, which, in turn, can induce apoptosis of other cells that display epitopes of foreign antigen on the cellular surface, including virally infected cells, cells harboring intracellular bacteria, and cancer cells expressing tumor antigens. Regarding neonatal foals, their particular vulnerability to viral and bacterial pathogens emphasizes the importance of T_h cells in the activation of CTLs.

T-Cell Immunity

Cytokines elaborated by T_h cells play important roles in regulating CMI responses. In spite of the reduced and delayed cytokine responses of young foals vis-à-vis adult horses, young foals' CMI responses are T_h1 biased with T_h2 responses developing much later [1, 7]. Indeed, IFN-γ produced by T_h1 cells and CTLs is detected shortly after birth and increases with age. However, IL-4 producing T_h2 cells are virtually absent for the first several months of life in foals [1]. RNA and protein expression changes are highly dynamic and frequently discordant, especially in states of disease [8]. Consequently, measurement of protein levels of cytokines of interest directly from target cells versus RNA has been proposed to provide the best representation of elaboration of cytokines from T_h cells.

Equine Neonatal Medicine, First Edition. Edited by David M. Wong and Pamela A. Wilkins.

Table 48.1 Cytokine profiles produced by T-Helper cell subtypes.

T-Helper cell subtype	Secreted factors	Signature cytokine	Response involved with
T_h1	IFN-γ, IL-2, IL-10, TNF-α, TNF-β	IFN-γ	• Cell mediated immunity • Inflammation • Intracellular pathogens (viruses and bacteria) • Autoimmunity
T_h2	IL-4, IL-5, IL-9, IL-10, IL-13, IL-21, IL-31	IL-4	• Humoral immune response and antibody-mediated immunity • Extracellular parasites • Allergy

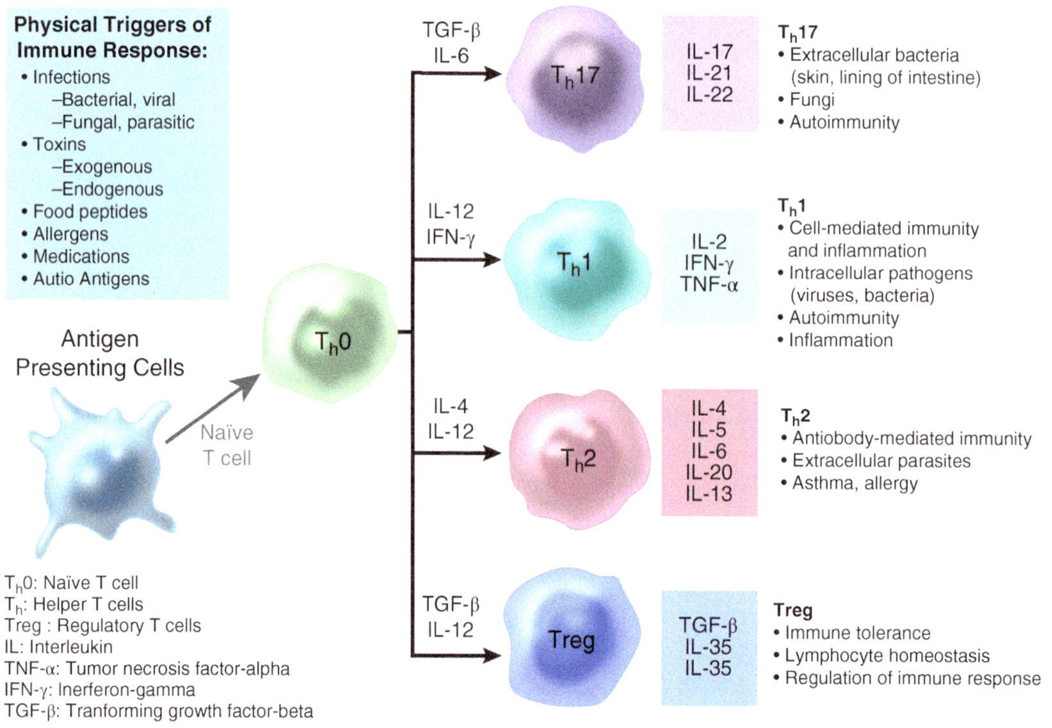

Figure 48.1 Overview of the various cell types and associated cytokines and functions involved in the immune response.

Wagner et al. evaluated intracellular IFN-γ and IL-4 in T cell subsets [1]. These investigators demonstrated that young foals have a T_h1 bias, produce IFN-γ by T_h1 and CD8+ CTLs, and that IL-10, a regulatory cytokine, is effectively produced as well [1]. In contrast, foal T cells produce comparatively less IL-4, indicating an impaired T_h2 response. In a separate study of foals less than 3 weeks of age, Liu et al. studied peripheral blood mononuclear cell (PBMC) cytokine responses to *in vitro Rhodococcus equi* antigen by mRNA expression and demonstrated rapid increases in IL-4 and, most notably, IL-17 [7]. IL-17 is the signature cytokine of T_h17 cells, a distinct subcategory of T cells that assists development of robust T_h1 responses and elaboration of IL-8 by macrophages and epithelial cells [7]. A subcategory of T regulatory cells (T_{Reg}) are easily detectable at 6 weeks of age, but not during the neonatal period. T_{regs} help maintain peripheral tolerance, limit inflammation in the case of autoimmunity and play important roles in immunoregulation [1]. Despite having a full complement of responsive T_h cells, foals are clearly more predisposed to certain pathogens than adult horses, and their immature immune system is one plausible explanation that accounts for an apparent susceptibility to particular infections, including *R. equi*, equine herpesvirus-1, and rotavirus. Indeed, despite a T_h1 bias, foals do not produce as much IFN-γ as adults, which may contribute to susceptibility to these foalhood diseases as early as the neonatal period [4, 9–11].

Plasmacytoid Dendritic Cells and Natural Killer Cells

In addition to T_h cells, plasmacytoid dentritic cells (PDC) and natural killer cells (NK) play an important role in cellular immunity during the initial innate response to intracellular infections. PDC produce large amounts of IFN-α, but also contribute to adaptive immunity by cross-presentation of antigen to autologous T cells (CD8+ T cells). NK cells play important roles in mitigating viral infections (generally) by (i) directly killing infected cells and (ii) by producing IFN-γ, which promotes polarization of a T_h1 adaptive response. NK are activated by dendritic cells (DC), by direct contact, and by DC elaborated cytokines. IFN-α enhances NK cytolytic activity; reciprocally, NK cells augment DC T-cell responses and have been demonstrated to present antigen to T cells under experimental conditions.

Previous studies demonstrated that weanlings' responses to *in vitro* recall EHV-1 infection yielded increased IFN-γ and IL-4 in CD2+ CD4− CD8− PBMC (NK cells) [12] indicating that NK cells play a role in immune protection in young horses to infection with EHV-1. While NK cells appear to play an important role in young horses, specific studies in neonatal foals are lacking. Within the past decade it has also been appreciated that NK cells have features often attributed to T cells [13]. NK cells go through a pathogen-specific expansion phase upon encounter of a cognate ligand, a memory maintenance phase, where a stable population of long-lived memory cells resides in lymphoid and nonlymphoid tissues, and a so-called secondary or recall response phase [14, 15]. The implication of such findings is not only that NK cells may play a role in defense of intracellular infections, but that they can be primed by vaccination. This aspect of NK cell biology has not been extensively studied in the horse; however, many of the same cytokines, including inteferons, are implicated in functional NK and DC T-cell responses.

In a broad context, CMI is directed primarily at intracellular pathogens, including virally infected cells, fungal and protozoal organisms, as well as intracellular bacteria and neoplastic processes. While the distinct vulnerability of neonatal foals to intracellular pathogens is well described, interferon-γ production by T_h1 and cytotoxic T cells is detectable a few days after birth in neonatal foals and increases gradually with age [1, 4]. In contrast, IL-4 production by T_h2 cells is nearly absent for the first several months of life [1]. While CMI is but one aspect of adaptive immunity, our current understanding of CMI responses that do not compare favorably to adult levels points to plausible deficits that likely contribute to the susceptibility of neonatal foals to infectious agents.

References

1 Wagner, B., Burton, A., and Ainsworth, D. (2010). Interferon-gamma, interleukin-4 and interleukin-10 production by T helper cells reveals intact Th1 and regulatory TR1 cell activation and a delay of the Th2 cell response in equine neonates and foals. *Vet. Res.* 41: 47.

2 Wagner, B., Stokol, T., and Ainsworth, D.M. (2010). Induction of interleukin-4 production in neonatal IgE+ cells after crosslinking of maternal IgE. *Dev. Comp. Immunol.* 34: 436–444.

3 Lopez, A.M., Hines, M.T., Palmer, G.H. et al. (2003). Analysis of anamnestic immune responses in adult horses and priming in neonates induced by a DNA vaccine expressing the vapA gene of *Rhodococcus equi*. *Vaccine* 21: 3815–3825.

4 Breathnach, C.C., Sturgill-Wright, T., Stiltner, J.L. et al. (2006). Foals are interferon gamma-deficient at birth. *Vet. Immunol. Immunopathol.* 112: 199–209.

5 Paillot, R., Daly, J.M., Luce, R. et al. (2007). Frequency and phenotype of EHV-1 specific, IFN-gamma synthesising lymphocytes in ponies: the effects of age, pregnancy and infection. *Dev. Comp. Immunol.* 31: 202–214.

6 Sponseller, B.A., Clark, S.K., Gilbertie, J. et al. (2016). Macrophage effector responses of horses are influenced by expression of CD154. *Vet. Immunol. Immunopathol.* 180: 40–44.

7 Liu, M., Bordin, A., Liu, T. et al. (2011). Gene expression of innate Th1-, Th2-, and Th17-type cytokines during early life of neonatal foals in response to *Rhodococcus equi*. *Cytokine* 56: 356–364.

8 Cheng, Z., Teo, G., Krueger, S. et al. (2016). Differential dynamics of the mammalian mRNA and protein expression response to misfolding stress. *Mol. Syst. Biol.* 12: 855.

9 Boyd, N.K., Cohen, N.D., Lim, W.S. et al. (2003). Temporal changes in cytokine expression of foals during the first month of life. *Vet. Immunol. Immunopathol.* 92: 75–85.

10 Dawson, T., Horohov, D.W., Meijer, W.G. et al. (2010). Current understanding of the equine immune response to *Rhodococcus equi*. An immunological review of *R. equi* pneumonia. *Vet. Immunol. Immunopathol.* 135: 1–11.

11 Liu, T., Nerren, J., Liu, M. et al. (2009). Basal and stimulus-induced cytokine expression is selectively

impaired in peripheral blood mononuclear cells of newborn foals. *Vaccine* 27: 674–683.

12 Platt, R., Sponseller, B.A., Chiang, Y.W. et al. (2010). Cell-mediated immunity evaluation in foals infected with virulent equine herpesvirus-1 by multi-parameter flow cytometry. *Vet. Immunol. Immunopathol.* 135: 275–281.

13 Vivier, E., Raulet, D.H., Moretta, A. et al. (2011). Innate or adaptive immunity? The example of natural killer cells. *Science* 331: 44–49.

14 Hou, X., Zhou, R., Wei, H. et al. (2009). NKG2D-retinoic acid early inducible-1 recognition between natural killer cells and Kupffer cells in a novel murine natural killer cell-dependent fulminant hepatitis. *Hepatology* 49: 940–949.

15 Sun, J.C., Beilke, J.N., and Lanier, L.L. (2009). Adaptive immune features of natural killer cells. *Nature* 457: 557–561.

Chapter 49 Congenital Disorders of Immunity

M. Julia B. Felippe

Immunodeficiency

Immunodeficiency is a rare condition of failure to build protection against pathogens. *Primary immunodeficiencies* are rare, congenital, often inheritable, and permanent disorders that may affect one of more components of the immune system. Examples in the equine species include Foal Immunodeficiency Syndrome (FIS) and Severe Combined Immunodeficiency Syndrome (SCID). Agammaglobulinemia in colts was described in the literature but a genetic disorder for this condition has not been identified. Although possible, the diagnosis of common variable immunodeficiency (CVID) has not been diagnosed in equine neonates or horses <2 years of age. More commonly diagnosed disorders in foals are age-dependent or developmental immune conditions, such as transient hypogammaglobulinemia of the young and selective IgM deficiency (Figure 49.1). *Secondary immunodeficiencies* are acquired disruptions of the immune function that reduce the ability to combat opportunistic and/or pathogenic organisms and include failure of transfer of passive immunity (FTPI) through colostrum, viral infections, endocrine disorders, nutritional deficiencies, immunosuppressive treatments, and lymphoma/lymphosarcoma. The effect of these conditions on the immune system is variable. Neonatal immunodeficiency may manifest with severe bacterial infections and/or septicemia (e.g. pneumonia, diarrhea, osteomyelitis, meningitis) and, more obviously, infections with opportunistic organisms (e.g. adenovirus, *Cryptosporidium*, *Pneumocystis jiroveci*). In addition, affected foals may fail to gain weight and grow properly.

Clinical recognition and diagnosis of an underlying immunodeficiency in the equine neonate can be difficult because of the common presentation of infections at this age, often associated with placentitis (prenatal infection) or FTPI through colostrum (postnatal infection). In addition, the physiologic, age-dependent development of the immune system results in natural functional limitations of both innate and acquired immune responses [1–4]. Therefore, in the absence of a genetic test, definitive diagnosis of a primary immunodeficiency requires periodic immunologic testing in the initial 6–24 months of age, and beyond the confounding presence of colostrum- or plasma transfusion-derived circulating immunoglobulins. When available, genetic tests are diagnostic and definitive for primary immunodeficiencies.

Age-Dependent Immune Development: Immune Preparedness and Immune Priming

The immune system of the equine *fetus* develops physiologically in the absence of foreign antigens and produces the pre-immune repertoire of cells. Initially the yolk sac, then the liver, and, subsequently, the bone marrow produce lymphoid and myeloid cells that populate the primary and secondary lymphoid organs, tissue parenchyma, and circulation during gestation [5]. Functional organization of B and T cells in primary and secondary lymphoid organs starts at 80–100 days of gestation and, by 200 days, the equine fetus is equipped to respond to intrauterine vaccination with the production of antigen-specific IgM and IgG [2, 6–8]. Under physiological conditions, serum IgM concentration of 10-22 mg/dl may be measured in fetuses older than 185 days of gestation, and values around 25 mg/dl in the pre-suckle serum of healthy foals, in comparison to minimal IgG concentration (0.2-17 mg/dl) at birth [2, 9]. Yet, the very presence of IgG indicates that recombination of immunoglobulin genes for isotype switching occurs during fetal life [5, 9–11]. In addition, in an antigen-independent manner, the fetal pre-immune immunoglobulin repertoire undergoes expansion and limited-diversity between 100 days of gestation and birth, preparing the foal

Equine Neonatal Medicine, First Edition. Edited by David M. Wong and Pamela A. Wilkins.

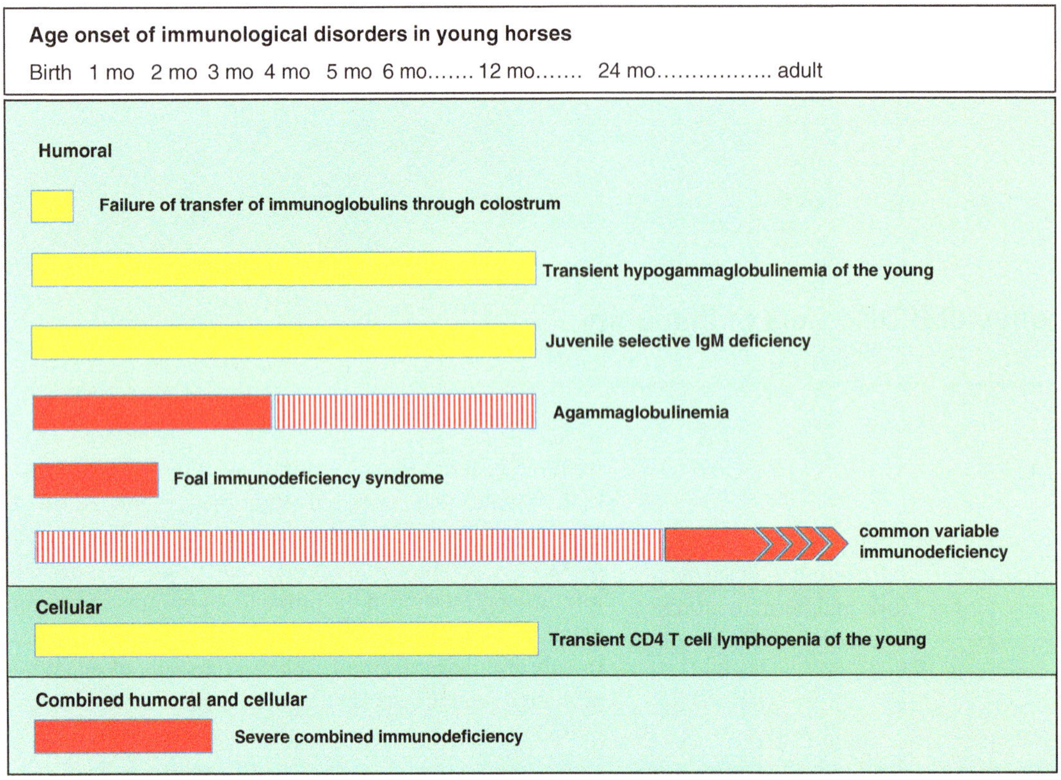

Figure 49.1 Age onset of clinical recognition of immunological disorders in horses. Humoral, cellular and combined immunodeficiencies described in foals are shown in yellow (transient conditions) and red (permanent conditions) bars according to the age of clinical signs; red hashed bars indicate rare diagnosis at this age (mo; months).

to respond to pathogens encountered immediately after delivery and throughout life.

The epitheliochorial placenta of the horse prevents transfer of maternal immunoglobulins to the fetus in utero. Colostrum, therefore, fills the gap between immunologic preparedness during fetal life in the naive uterine environment and immunity during neonatal life in the pathogen-challenging environment. High amounts of IgG, and small amounts of IgM, IgA, and IgE immunoglobulins, plus complement, serum amyloid A, inflammatory cytokines (tumor necrosis factor alpha, interleukin-4, interleukin-6), lysozyme, ferritin, and maternal lymphocytes, neutrophils, macrophages, and epithelial cells in colostrum are readily absorbed in the small intestine of the healthy equine neonate during the first 8 hours of life, and with decreasing efficiency of absorption up to 24–36 hours after birth [8, 12–23]. The equine neonate is critically dependent on this precious colostral formula to fight infections and survive. Albeit in a small scale, healthy foals start producing antigen-specific immunoglobulins immediately after birth, when exposed to environmental organisms, but endogenous protective levels take at least 3 months to be achieved. Meanwhile, colostrum-derived IgG circulates with a half-life of 28–32 days, and milk provides high concentrations of IgA that act with neutralizing properties for bacterial, viral and toxin at the intestinal surface [24].

Phagocytic function in the healthy equine neonate is quite reliable: in response to infections, the bone marrow efficiently releases neutrophils and band neutrophils that express high levels of immunoglobulin, complement, and toll-like receptors to identify opsonized and non-opsonized pathogens; integrins and inflammatory cytokines that allow diapedesis, chemotaxis, and amplification of immune responses; and provide cell degranulation, and strong pathogen phagocytic and killing activities [25–29]. Undeniably, the equine neonate relies on its phagocytes for protection against pathogens but efficient phagocytic function is remarkably dependent on the synergism of different opsonins [17, 30–32]. For instance, phagocytosis and killing of encapsulated bacteria is more efficiently accomplished when pathogens are opsonized by both complement and immunoglobulins. The foal is born with low serum complement activity, colostrum offers low levels of complement, and serum complement is rapidly consumed during sepsis [17, 28, 33]. Therefore, foals rely on the other types of opsonins in colostrum (or transfused plasma) and on their endogenous production of complement and immunoglobulins after birth [28, 29]. In fact, opsonic capacity in foals becomes comparable to that of adult horses only by 5 months of age [17, 28]. Therefore, the protective role of colostrum applies to the period immediately after birth but is required to last months, particularly its immunoglobulin component.

Antigen presenting cells of foals also show age-dependent development and response to stimulus after birth. For instance, *in vitro* dendritic cells and macrophages from equine neonates express 11 to 12 times, respectively, less expression of major histocompatibility complex (MHC) class II molecules than adult horse cells; and lower cytokine production upon bacterial exposure, perhaps limiting their potential for antigen presentation to and activation of T cells for certain organisms [34–37]. Those differences progressively subside by 3 months of age. Nevertheless, the exposure to an abundant and diverse population of pathogens in early life induces a massive expansion of antigen-specific, primed lymphocyte populations, reflected by an increase in mass of secondary lymphoid tissues and, consequently, two to four times increase in the number of circulating lymphocytes notably by 3–6 months of age [3, 4, 38, 39]. In addition, age-dependent increase in CD4 and CD8 T cells occurs naturally from birth through the first 12 months of age [4, 40]. In addition, foal lymphocytes also show an age-dependent interferon-gamma (IFNg) production and MHC class II expression from birth to 12 months of age, upon pathogen antigen exposure, and these can be used as markers of immune maturation [4, 41–43]. Importantly, individual variability and timeline in the expansion and distribution of different lymphocyte subpopulations and functional markers are possible, and many foals may take longer to achieve such immune structure, perhaps delaying their immunocompetence.

The development of intestinal lymphoid tissue is marked after birth, and Payer's patches and mesenteric lymph nodes become grossly obvious beyond 3 weeks of age [38]. The gut-associated lymphoid tissue's protective function requires microbial stimulation provided by the initial bacterial colonization after birth, and energy substrate present in the milk [44]. Nondigestible milk carbohydrates create the appropriate acidic environment for proliferation of probiotic/ commensal bacteria, which subsequently promote the development of the mucosal immunity via the expression of pathogen-associated molecular patterns (PAMPs).

The respiratory tract is a common route of infection in the neonate. Remarkably, foals do not present organized lymphoid tissue in the lungs at birth. T lymphocytes and plasma cells are virtually absent in lung tissues in the first week of life, and bronchus-associated lymphoid tissue is only observed by 12 weeks of age [38]. The concentration of leukocytes in bronchoalveolar lavage fluid (BALF) in foals <3 weeks of life is one-half the values of adult horses [4]. While CD4 T cells in BALF increase markedly in the first 3 weeks of age, B cells are almost undetectable in the first 4 weeks, and only reach values comparable to adult horses by 8 weeks of age [45]. Around this same time, higher levels of IgA, IgG, and IgM are detected in BALF. Therefore, the respiratory tract of the foal seems poorly protected in the first 8 weeks of age and, together with decreasing levels of colostrum-derived immunoglobulins, may explain the high incidence of respiratory conditions during this period.

Failure of Transfer of Passive Immunity

FTPI occurs when the foal does not suckle adequate amounts of colostrum soon after birth, the foal cannot absorb immunoglobulin efficiently through the intestinal epithelium (e.g. ischemic hypoxia, immaturity/dysmaturity), and/or the colostrum does not contain adequate amounts of immunoglobulin (e.g. colostral specific gravity <1.060, mares with systemic illness late in gestation, prepartum loss of colostrum) [46]. This topic is further covered in Chapter 47. In brief, FTPI results in hypogammaglobulinemic foals that are susceptible to infections and sepsis with environmental pathogens [47–49]. FTPI through colostrum is classically defined based on serum or blood IgG concentration <800 mg/dl by 24 hours of life [16, 46, 50–53]. Evaluation of foal serum or blood IgG concentration at 12–14 hours post-suckling allows remediation with colostrum supplementation or, with more certainty, IV plasma transfusion.

Foals with total or partial FTPI are more likely to present with pulmonary and/or gastrointestinal infections, and sepsis within the first week of life. Nevertheless, foals with adequate passive transfer may also become septic, or foals may be born septic when there is intrauterine infection [48, 49]. Moreover, foals that did not have FTPI at birth, as classically defined, but had marginal transfer of immunoglobulins through colostrum (around 800 mg/dl) may not have adequate humoral protection when circulating colostrum-derived immunoglobulins drop to levels below protection before 3 months of age, and while endogenous production is still rising. These foals tend to present with recurrent fevers and pneumonia 1–4 months of age, or until endogenous serum IgG concentration reaches protective levels (>800 mg/dl); these foals may require antibiotic therapy during this transition period to treat infections.

Therefore, passive transfer of IgG through colostrum or plasma transfusion plays a major role in humoral protection not only around birth but also in the initial few months of life. Given the IgG half-life of 28–32 days, a post-suckle value >1,000 mg/dl would be more certain of protection in the first few months of life [13]. Indeed, passive transfer of immunoglobulins occurs naturally at levels >1,100 mg/dl, often reaching values >2,000 mg/dl [4]. The use of a quantitative (rather than a semi-quantitative) assay, such as the immunoturbidimetric or radial immunodiffusion assay, provides the actual blood immunoglobulin concentration achieved after passive transfer at birth, which could be used for predicting immunoglobulin coverage and clinical monitoring of foals at risk of developing infections in the first few months of age. Also, testing serum IgG concentration in foals with pneumonia or diarrhea would inform if a low IgG concentration was contributing to susceptibility to infection.

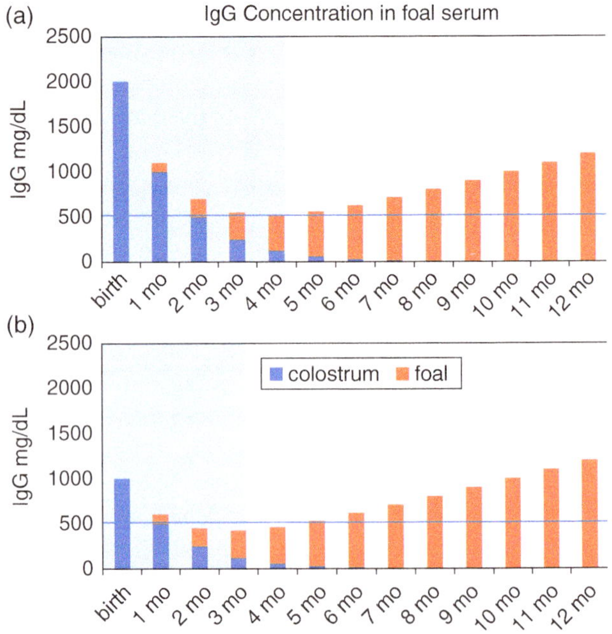

Figure 49.2 Hypothetical serum IgG concentration in foals during their first year. Circulating colostrum-derived immune-globulins in the foal serum are shown in blue bars, and their decay was calculated with a half-life of 30 days. Serum endogenous IgG is shown in orange bars, calculated at 100 mg/dl production by the foal per month (mo). Passive transfer of immunoglobulins after birth are depicted at 2,000 mg/dl (a) and 1,000 mg/dl (b). There is a physiologic window of susceptibility around 2–4 months of age that is dependent on the amount of IgG transferred through colostrum (compare the values in A and B at 500 g/dl, which is typically measured in foals between 3mo and 5mo). Lower colostrum-derived immune-globulin levels after birth and/or a delay in endogenous antibody production creates a greater susceptibility to infections. Blue shaded area indicates the age in which the diagnosis of humoral immunodeficiencies is challenged by the presence of circulating colostrum-derived antibodies.

Humoral Immunodeficiencies

Immunoglobulin deficiency may be caused by intrinsic failure of B-cell development or dysfunction, or inadequate co-stimulation for B-cell differentiation in the lymphoid tissues, such as the critical interactions with CD4 helper T cells. The consequence of the lack of B cells or dysfunctional B cells is inadequate production of immunoglobulins, affecting IgG and other isotypes (e.g., IgM, IgA, IgE). In general, lack of IgG is the most significant humoral deficiency because its major role in antigen neutralization, opsonization, and complement activation. Other isotype-selective deficiencies (e.g. selective IgM deficiency with normal IgG production) may be asymptomatic or transitory in the young. The lack of IgG leads to susceptibility to bacterial infections, particularly encapsulate bacteria (e.g. *Streptococcus* spp, *Staphylococcus* spp, *Klebsiella* spp, *Actinobacillus equuli, Escherichia coli*) because effective phagocytosis and killing of these organisms by neutrophils require opsonization with both immunoglobulin and complement.

Transient Hypogammaglobulinemia of the Young Foal

Transient hypogammaglobulinemia results from a delay or inadequate endogenous immunoglobulin production during early life [47]. In heathy foals, a brief physiologic hypogammaglobulinemia may occur around 2 and 5 months of age when circulating colostrum-derived IgG concentration drops – or earlier; if transfer of passive immunoglobulins at birth was partial (Figure 49.2). In most cases, this physiologic response has no clinical impact when the foal has normal endogenous immunoglobulin production. However, in foals with delayed production of immunoglobulins, the hypogammaglobulinemia persists for a longer period, predisposing to infections. In affected foals, the challenging pathogens are often encapsulated bacteria, as they require both immunoglobulin and complement for effective opsonization and phagocytic function. Appropriate antibiotic therapy often protects foals during the period of abnormal immunoglobulin production; plasma transfusions can also be used if the infection is severe or refractory to antibiotic therapy; in this case, treatment confounds monitoring of endogenous IgG production.

In these foals, serum IgG concentration is below protective levels (<500 mg/dl), and IgM concentration is often <50 mg/dl. The transient hypogammaglobulinemia may last for a few months (e.g. 5–10 months of age) or potentially longer (e.g. 18–24 months of age; Felippe, personal observation). In most cases, the peripheral blood B- and T-lymphocyte counts and distributions are normal; however, some cases have decreased CD4 T-cell population distribution, with a low CD4:CD8 ratio for the age, and decreased expression of MHC class II in lymphocytes when compared to age-matched healthy foals. In addition, there is a delay in the physiologic, age-dependent increase in these values (Felippe, personal observation). T-cell proliferation response to mitogen *in vivo* (skin) and *in vitro* has been reported to be normal, perhaps discarding intrinsic or lasting lymphocyte dysfunction [47].

Affected foals are managed with continuous or intermittent antibiotic therapy, and routine physical examination and serial complete blood counts to monitor for infections. Immunologic testing based on serum IgG and IgM concentrations and peripheral blood lymphocyte immunophenotyping (distribution of CD4 and CD8 T cells, B cells, and expression of MHC class II in lymphocytes) every 2 months can be used to determine positive progression of immunologic competence, and guidance for the need of antibiotic therapy. Serum IgM concentration more clearly reflects endogenous humoral function, and improvement in this condition is revealed when levels become >50 mg/dl. When serum IgG concentration reach values >800–1,000 mg/dl, infections are typically controlled by the foal, and antibiotic therapy may no longer be needed.

It is still not common practice to measure serum IgG and IgM concentrations in foals beyond the first week of age, and rarely beyond 2 months of age; therefore, this condition may be more frequent than reported. Despite recurrent infections, commonly respiratory, most foals maintain normal development when intermittently treated with antibiotic therapy. As indicated above, it may take up to 24 months before normal immunoglobulin production establishes. If B-cell distribution is low or there are no signs of immunoglobulin production during this period, other types of immunodeficiency should be considered (e.g. CVID, lymphoma/lymphosarcoma).

In affected foals, the response to vaccines is unknown; at this time, a full vaccination program with boosters based on current guidelines (e.g. starting at 3 months of life) would be recommended to promote development of immunologic memory to vaccine antigens. This same program could be repeated when serum IgG concentrations become normal, a sign of humoral competency, to ensure long-lasting protection.

Juvenile Selective IgM Deficiency

In *selective* immunoglobulin deficiencies, serum immunoglobulin concentration for only *one* immunoglobulin isotype is two standard deviations below the normal mean reference interval, while all other immunoglobulin isotype concentrations are within normal reference intervals for the age. *Selective IgM deficiency* has been reported in foals with chronic infections when serum IgM concentrations were two standard deviations below the normal mean reference, and IgG and IgA were within normal reference intervals for the age group [54, 55]. The onset of infections occurred between 2–10 months of age, and involved both male and female foals of different breeds. Clinical sings included recurrent fevers, bronchopneumonia, arthritis, enteritis, dermatitis, and lymph node pyogranulomatous response, caused by encapsulated bacteria [56–58].

This condition did not seem to involve an intrinsic B- or T-cell impaired development or dysfunction because peripheral blood lymphocyte counts, B- and T-cell distributions, and proliferation responses *in vitro* were normal, and most reported foals recovered, with normal IgM production as yearlings [1, 59]. The definition and pathogenesis of selective IgM deficiency are unclear and intriguing. All naive B cells must express IgM on the cell surface during development in the bone marrow, and IgM is produced readily in response to foreign antigens after a brief interaction of B and CD4 T helper cells; in contrast, the production of other immunoglobulin isotypes requires multiple rounds of interaction with CD4 T helper cells and antigen for immunoglobulin receptor selection before isotype switching (IgG, IgA, IgE) in the germinal centers.

It is uncertain if the published selective IgM deficiency was an independent condition diagnosed based on a particular reference range interval or reflective of transient hypogammaglobulinemia of the young, given that most cases were reported at a time when serum IgG concentrations could also include colostrum-derived immunoglobulins. Nevertheless, serum IgM concentration can be used to more readily evaluate B-cell function and endogenous immunoglobulin production capacity during the first 3 months of age because IgM production already occurs in utero, and colostrum-derived IgM has a short half-life of 5–16 days [9, 24]. When values <50 mg/dl are measured, both serum IgM and IgG concentrations should be monitored to evaluate for persistence or change in values with age.

Common Variable Immunodeficiency

CVID is a *late-onset* immunologic disorder of B cell depletion and inadequate immunoglobulin production due to impaired B-cell differentiation in the bone marrow [60–63]. Clinical signs manifest more commonly in adult horses (average age 10 years, range 2–27 years). Although this disease can potentially present and progress in young foals, the diagnosis would require repeated immunologic testing in the first several months of age to monitor the progress and rule out other humoral conditions. Affected patients are unrelated, of both sexes, different breeds, and living in distinct geographic areas. To date, only isolated cases in a herd have been diagnosed. The intrinsic impaired B-cell production in the bone marrow involves epigenetic gene silencing of signature lineage transcriptional factors [64, 65].

Although patients are likely born with B cells and can produce immunoglobulins during a period of their lives, the late-onset B-cell depletion leads to inadequate immunoglobulin production. By the time clinical signs such as recurrent infection and sometimes septicemia with encapsulated bacteria develop, serum IgG (<800 mg/dl) and IgM (<25 mg/dl) concentrations are no longer protective [62, 63, 66, 67]. Antibiotic therapy may help with controlling infections for a period, but organ failure due to chronic infections makes this condition fatal. The distribution of T-lymphocyte population in blood and lymphoid tissues is normal, and these cells respond to mitogenic stimulation *in vitro*. In some cases, there is a relative increase in the percentage of circulating CD8 T cells and CD4 T cells [63].

Diagnosis is based on clinical history of recurrent infections, persistent B-cell depletion from blood, and unresolved hypogammaglobulinemia. In some cases, B-cell distribution in blood is at the low normal reference interval (~5–7%), but immunoglobulin production is not sustained. Gross pathology and histopathology confirm the paucity of B cells in the bone marrow, lack of germinal cells, lymphoid hypoplasia, and paucity of plasma cells in various lymphoid and mucosal tissues [62, 63].

Agammaglobulinemia

Agammaglobulinemia is a very rare, congenital, and fatal immunodeficiency caused by intrinsic failure of B-cell differentiation and function, with subsequent inability to produce immunoglobulins. This condition was described only in colts of young age and of different breeds in the late 1970s and early 1980s, but there have been no recent reports in the literature [68, 69]. Although a congenital disorder of B-cell depletion, clinical signs of recurrent infections manifest around 3 months of age, when circulating colostrum-derived IgG concentration decreases below protective levels (<500 mg/dl). Serum IgM and IgA concentrations are undetectable, and serum IgG values do not increase with age; affected foals fail to produce immunoglobulins upon vaccination [70]. These foals are born with depletion of B cells and plasma cells, and lymphoid follicles. T lymphocytes are present in normal counts, and they proliferate in response to mitogenic stimulation *in vitro* and *in vivo* [1].

Colts with this condition develop fevers, bacterial infections of the respiratory and/or gastrointestinal systems and skin; peripheral lymphadenopathy is common; and foals appear unthrifty and with poor development. Infections are temporarily responsive to antibiotic and plasma therapies, but complications lead to death or euthanasia before 18 months of age [68, 70, 71].

Foal Immunodeficiency Syndrome

FIS is an autosomal recessive, congenital, hereditary condition characterized by profound anemia and septicemia described in the Fell Pony, Dales, and, potentially, other breeds that include their common ancestors [72-76]. Affected foals are born apparently healthy, but illness develops within 1 month of age, and death occurs generally soon after. The foals present with weight loss and dullness along with signs of infection, including enterocolitis, bronchopneumonia, and glossal hyperkeratosis often caused by opportunistic organisms (e.g. *E. coli*, *Cryptosporidium* spp., and adenovirus) [77–79]. Management of infections and subsequent septicemia may be temporarily treated with antibiotic and supportive therapy, but the severe progressive anemia is fatal.

At birth, hemoglobin and hematocrit values may be within the low normal reference interval, and peripheral blood B cell distribution may be equivalent to healthy foals [80, 81]. Within the first few weeks of life, however, profound anemia and B cell lymphopenia develop. The severe, progressive anemia results from lack of erythrocyte production in the bone marrow. Bone marrow cytology in samples collected prospectively from Fell Pony neonates showed that affected foals were born with erythroid precursors, but rapidly evolved to erythrocyte hypoplasia, with rare and binucleated proerythroblasts [81]. During this period, myeloid precursors and megakaryocytes were present, but myeloid dysplasia puts into question broader bone marrow dysfunction.

Absolute lymphopenia in affected foals likely reflects poor lymphocyte development in primary and secondary lymphoid tissues, and failure of lymphocyte population expansion with age [81]. The B lymphopenia limits the ability of affected foals to produce immunoglobulins; nevertheless, serum IgG concentration is often normal when clinical signs are detected within the first month of life due to the presence of circulating colostrum-derived immunoglobulins. Septicemia may develop despite normal serum IgG concentrations. Serum IgM concentration (a parameter not confounded by colostrum-derived immunoglobulins at this age) is low (<25 mg/dl) in affected foals, and strongly suggest impaired primary humoral immune responses. The CD4 and CD8 T-cell distributions are reported normal in affected foals; however, T-cell dysfunction is possible due to the small thymus, and opportunistic infections with *Cryptosporidium* and adenovirus [82]. In addition, the expression of MHC class II molecule in peripheral blood lymphocytes is decreased and/or fail to increase with age in affected foals when compared to healthy foals, also supporting abnormal lymphocyte development [80, 81].

In the postmortem, abnormal gross findings include generalized tissue pallor, thymic hypoplasia, inflammation, and lymphadenopathy associated with infections of multiple organs (e.g. necrotizing enteritis, pyogranulomatous bronchopneumonia, pancreatitis, myocarditis). The medullary cavities of bones often do not contain red marrow and, instead, are filled with pale or tan fatty tissue, with severe erythroid hypoplasia. Despite lymphadenopathy, there is severe lymphocytic hypoplasia and lack of secondary lymphoid follicles in the lymphoid organs; in addition, plasma cells are absent. Immunohistochemical staining detects no B lymphocytes in bone marrow, and rare or few B cells in the lymph nodes and spleen, dispersed in the tissues without forming germinal centers. In addition, peripheral ganglionopathy characterized by neuronal chromatolysis involving trigeminal, cranial mesenteric and dorsal root ganglia has been reported [77, 79].

A genome-wide study identified a mutation in the gene SLC5A3 on chromosome ECA26 associated with the syndrome [83, 84]. The mechanistic implications of this mutation have not been fully resolved. The gene must be disrupted in both chromosome alleles in the affected foal; hence, the mutation must be present in one allele of each parent. Carrier horses are heterozygous for the defective gene and are immunocompetent. The breeding of two affected horses will produce an affected foal in 25% of the offspring [78, 85]. The Fell Pony breed experienced loss of genetic diversity due to the small numbers of animals and overuse of prominent stallions. The DNA-based test was developed by the Animal Health Trust, Newmarket, UK, and offers herd management planning to avoid mating of two carriers with the genetic defect. The test, therefore, should be performed in all Fell Pony, Dales, and crossbred horses used in reproduction. The appropriate planning of breeding of carriers prevents the outcome of affected foals and decreases the incidence of the mutant gene in the population.

Combined Immunodeficiency

Combined immunodeficiency involves both the humoral (immunoglobulin production) and cellular (cytotoxicity) arms of the acquired immune system.

Severe Combined Immunodeficiency

Severe combined immunodeficiency (SCID) is an autosomal recessive, congenital, hereditary condition that impairs the development of B and T cells in affected Arabian foals or breeds with Arabian ancestors [1, 86, 87]. Both humoral and cellular immunity are impaired in these patients and, consequently, SCID foals are susceptible to organisms that require B- and T-cell function [88]. This condition manifests clinically in both male and female foals around 2 months of age, when colostrum-derived immunoglobulin concentrations drop below protective levels. Foals may show clinical signs of bacterial bronchopneumonia or *P. jiroveci* pneumonia and adenovirus inclusions in the lungs and pancreas can be observed. Diarrhea associated with *Cryptosporidium parvum* and coronavirus is present in some cases [89, 90].

Affected foals present with severe peripheral blood lymphopenia (<1,000 cells/ul), and IgM (<25 mg/dl) and IgA deficiency; although the production is completely impaired, serum IgG concentration is often low and reflects colostrum-derived immunoglobulins [91, 92]. Affected foals also fail to respond to vaccination. The lymphoid tissues in SCID foals are hypoplastic for both B and T cells, and the thymus is depleted of lymphocytes and is infiltrated with adipose tissue instead. The secondary lymphoid tissues lack germinal centers and periarteriolar lymphocytic sheaths. The few recognized lymphocytes do not respond to mitogenic stimulation *in vitro*, and one-way mixed lymphocyte cultures revealed failure of SCID mononuclear cells to respond to allogenic stimulation.

Treatment of affected foals is challenging and palliative [93, 94]. Antibiotic therapy and IV plasma transfusion provide limited control of infections, and death occurs before 5 months of age. Successful experimental replacement of functional B and T cells in SCID foals has been accomplished with bone marrow and thymus transplantation from compatible donors [1, 95, 96].

The defective development of B and T cells is caused by a faulty V(D)J recombination during B- and T-cell receptor formation. A frame-shift mutation in the gene encoding DNA-dependent protein kinase catalytic subunit (DNA-PKc) results in complete absence of this protein in affected foals [97, 98]. Therefore, DNA repair during gene recombination of the variable region of the receptors is not achieved, B- and T-cell receptors do not develop, and B and T-cell lymphopoiesis is blocked. The gene must be disrupted in both chromosome alleles in the affected foal; hence, the mutation must be present in one allele of each parent. Carrier horses are heterozygous for the defective gene and are immunocompetent. The breeding of two affected horses will produce disease in 25% of the offspring. The definitive diagnosis of carriers and affected foals can be done by a DNA test (VetGen, Veterinary Genetic Services, Michigan, USA) of whole blood or cheek swab samples [98]. The test should be performed in all Arabian and Arabian-crossbred horses used in reproduction. The appropriate planning of breeding of carriers prevents the outcome of affected foals and decreases the incidence of the mutant gene in the population.

Cellular Immunodeficiencies

Cellular immunodeficiencies are more difficult to diagnose and, therefore, apparently less prevalent in equids. Peripheral blood lymphocyte counts and subpopulation distributions reflect lymphoid tissue activity, as lymphocytes constantly circulate throughout the body. Therefore, immunophenotyping of CD4 and CD8 T cells and B cells in peripheral blood using flow cytometry may show unbalanced or inadequate activity in lymphoid tissues (Chapter 43). In addition, the expression of MHC class II and IFNg in lymphocytes can be used as developmental markers of lymphocyte activity since these molecules have age-dependent expression in foals [41].

Transient CD4 T-Cell Lymphopenia

Cellular immune disorders may result from impaired CD4 T helper cell function, with implications to cytotoxic and/or humoral responses, depending on the underlying mechanism. Cellular dysfunction may also originate at upstream events, through inadequate antigen presentation and signaling, and consequent failure to activate T lymphocytes.

Infections with opportunistic organisms in the foal (e.g., *P. jiroveci*, *C. parvum*, adenovirus) suggest the presence of a primary or transient/delayed cellular immunodeficiency. Primary conditions, such as FIS and severe combined immunodeficiency are described above. In transient or delayed conditions, peripheral blood immunophenotyping shows decreased CD4 T-cell distribution and, consequently, decreased CD4:CD8 ratio when compared to age-matched healthy foals (Felippe, personal observation) [3, 99, 100]. This finding is often accompanied by a decrease in distribution of lymphocytes expressing the MHC class II molecule. Affected foals also show a delay in the physiologic increase of CD4 T-cell distribution, and expression of MHC class II in lymphocytes with age (Flaminio, personal observation) [3, 4, 100]. Yet, lymphocyte proliferation response *in vitro* upon mitogenic stimulation is normal, discarding intrinsic or lasting lymphocyte dysfunction. The expression of IFNg has not been systematically studied in these patients.

B-cell distribution and age-dependent changes are normal and serum IgG concentrations may be comparable to values in healthy foals. Occasionally, serum IgG concentration is also decreased for the age, indicating a delay in humoral function; in this case, both CD4 T-cell distribution and IgG immunoglobulin production tend to reach normal values at the same age, suggesting a connection between both conditions.

Long-term antibiotic therapy (e.g. trimethoprim-sulfadiazine to treat infection with *P. jiroveci*) may be necessary during this transition period. Periodic leukograms, thoracic ultrasound and radiographs, and immunologic testing (CD4+ and CD8+ T cells, B cells, MHC class II, and IFNg expression) along with serum IgG and IgM concentrations measured every 2 months may help with determining the need of treatment, and document improvement of immunologic function. Diagnostic assays for other potential etiologies of impaired cellular immunity in the foal (e.g. co-stimulatory molecule CD40 ligand expression) are under development.

Phagocytic Deficiencies

Inherited forms of neutrophil dysfunction have not been described in the horse but should be suspected in cases of recurrent infection (dermatitis, cutaneous, or intracavitary abscesses, cellulitis) not associated with humoral immunodeficiency (normal serum IgG concentration), and caused by *Staphylococcus*, *Pseudomonas*, *Serratia*, *Klebsiella*, or fungi (*Aspergillus, Candida*).

Septicemia in foals <1 week of age is a life-threatening systemic condition that may arise from prenatal intrauterine placentitis, or postnatal respiratory, oral, and umbilical routes of infection [101, 102]. Sepsis involves a systemic inflammatory response during infection, and foals respond effectively with neutrophilia and a left shift, unless they present with prematurity or immaturity. Although healthy foals are born with competent neutrophil function, septic foals demonstrate a transient decrease in phagocytosis and oxidative burst activity that improves once infection is controlled with antibiotics [17, 103]. In addition, opsonins are highly consumed during sepsis and, if not replaced with plasma transfusion, their shortage can further affect phagocytic function [17, 104]. However, primary complement deficiency has not been described in the horse.

Pelger-Huët anomaly of neutrophils, which present as dumbbell-shaped bilobed nuclei, has been identified in the horse but their phagocytic function is normal (Felippe, unpublished data; Wilkerson, personal communication). Some of the diseases associated with phagocytic disorders described in other species, but not in horses to date, include leukocyte adhesion deficiency (failure to express the CD18 integrin), chronic granulomatous disease (inability to produce oxygen reactive species), cyclic neutrophil hematopoiesis (cyclic changes in blood neutrophil), and Chediak-Higashi syndrome (giant granules in neutrophils).

Immunostimulants and Immunomodulators

Immunostimulants promote nonspecific activation of immune cells and amplify different areas of immune defense with variable effect according to their structure, including phagocytosis and killing of pathogens, antigen presentation, cytotoxic and antiviral activity, and cytokine expression. They can be fragments of inactivated whole organisms that preserve their PAMP for recognition by toll-like receptors on immune cells. Their interaction leads to a short-term cell activation with cytokine release and inflammatory response, and they are used as adjunctive therapy or prophylaxis. The brief effect prevents exacerbation of inflammation to deleterious levels. Repeated use, though, may lead to the development of neutralizing antibodies and decreased effect. Immunostimulants may help with temporary and developmental conditions in foals, such as sepsis, transient hypogammaglobulinemia of the young, and transient CD4 T-cell lymphopenia, but will not change permanent conditions caused by intrinsic cell defects.

Examples of such immunostimulants used in foals to increase immune response to pathogens are inactivated *Propionibacterium acnes*, parapoxvirus ovis, and short single-stranded synthetic DNA molecules (unmethylated CpG oligodeoxynucleotides) [31, 32, 105–108]. In addition, granulocyte-colony stimulating factor promotes the production of neutrophils in the bone marrow and may aid in immune protection of foals with alloimmune neutropenia, premature foals with neutropenia, and foals with sepsis [109, 110].

Immunomodulators are substances that normalize the immune system and aid in the control of inflammation [111]. Interferon alpha, a cytokine with antiviral property, and levamisole, a synthetic anthelmintic, have been shown to have immunomodulatory effects [112, 113]. Overall, more clinical studies are needed to better understand the application and outcomes of immunostimulants and immunomodulators in equine neonates.

References

1 Perryman, L.E. and McGuire, T.C. (1980). Evaluation for immune system failures in horses and ponies. *J. Am. Vet. Med. Assoc.* 176: 1374–1377.

2 Perryman, L.E., McGuire, T.C., and Torbeck, R.L. (1980). Ontogeny of lymphocyte function in the equine fetus. *Am. J. Vet. Res.* 41: 1197–1200.

3 Flaminio, M.J., Rush, B.R., and Shuman, W. (1999). Peripheral blood lymphocyte subpopulations and immunoglobulin concentrations in healthy foals and foals with *Rhodococcus equi* pneumonia. *J. Vet. Intern. Med.* 13: 206–212.

4 Flaminio, M.J., Rush, B.R., and Shuman, W. (2000). Characterization of peripheral blood and pulmonary leukocyte function in healthy foals. *Vet. Immunol. Immunopathol.* 73: 267–285.

5 Prieto, J.M.B., Tallmadge, R.L., and Felippe, M.J.B. (2017). Developmental expression of B cell molecules in equine lymphoid tissues. *Vet. Immunol. Immunopathol.* 183: 60–71.

6 Martin, B.R. and Larson, K.A. (1973). Immune response of equine fetus to coliphage T2. *Am. J. Vet. Res.* 34: 1363–1364.

7 Morgan, D.O., Bryans, J.T., and Mock, R.E. (1975). Immunoglobulins produced by the antigenized equine fetus. *J. Reprod. Fertil. Suppl.* 23: 735–738.

8 Mackenzie, C.D. (1975). Histological development of the thymic and intestinal lymphoid tissue of the horse. *J. S. Afr. Vet. Assoc.* 46: 47–55.

9 Tallmadge, R.L., McLaughlin, K., Secor, E. et al. (2009). Expression of essential B cell genes and immunoglobulin isotypes suggests active development and gene recombination during equine gestation. *Dev. Comp. Immunol.* 33: 1027–1038.

10 Tallmadge, R.L., Tseng, C.T., King, R.A. et al. (2013). Developmental progression of equine immunoglobulin heavy chain variable region diversity. *Dev. Comp. Immunol.* 41: 33–43.

11 Tallmadge, R.L., Tseng, C.T., and Felippe, M.J. (2014). Diversity of immunoglobulin lambda light chain gene usage over developmental stages in the horse. *Dev. Comp. Immunol.* 46: 171–179.

12 Jeffcott, L.B. (1974). Studies on passive immunity in the foal. Gamma-globulin and antibody variations associated with the maternal transfer of immunity and the onset of active immunity. *J. Comp. Pathol.* 84: 93–101.

13 Lavoie, J.P., Spensley, M.S., Smith, B.P. et al. (1989). Complement activity and selected hematologic variables in newborn foals fed bovine colostrum. *Am. J. Vet. Res.* 50: 1532–1536.

14 Kohn, C.W., Knight, D., Hueston, W. et al. (1989). Colostral and serum IgG, IgA, and IgM concentrations in Standardbred mares and their foals at parturition. *J. Am. Vet. Med. Assoc.* 195: 64–68.

15 Sheoran, A.S., Timoney, J.F., Holmes, M.A. et al. (2000). Immunoglobulin isotypes in sera and nasal mucosal secretions and their neonatal transfer and distribution in horses. *Am. J. Vet. Res.* 61: 1099–1105.

16 Stoneham, S.J., Digby, N.J., and Ricketts, S.W. (1991). Failure of passive transfer of colostral immunity in the foal: incidence, and the effect of stud management and plasma transfusions. *Vet. Rec.* 128: 416–419.

17 Gardner, R.B., Nydam, D.V., Luna, J.A. et al. (2007). Serum opsonization capacity, phagocytosis, and oxidative burst activity in neonatal foals in the intensive care unit. *J. Vet. Intern. Med.* 21: 797–805.

18 Wagner, B., Flaminio, J.B., Hillegas, J. et al. (2006). Occurrence of IgE in foals: evidence for transfer of maternal IgE by the colostrum and late onset of endogenous IgE production in the horse. *Vet. Immunol. Immunopathol.* 110: 269–278.

19 Burton, A.B., Wagner, B., Erb, H.N. et al. (2009). Serum interleukin-6 (IL-6) and IL-10 concentrations in normal

and septic neonatal foals. *Vet. Immunol. Immunopathol.* 132: 122–128.
20 Secor, E.J., Matychak, M.B., and Felippe, M.J. (2012). Transfer of tumour necrosis factor-α via colostrum to foals. *Vet. Rec.* 170: 51.
21 Numata, M., Kondo, T., Nambo, Y. et al. (2013). Change of antibody levels to ferritin in the sera of foals after birth: possible passive transfer of maternal anti-ferritin autoantibody via colostrum and age-related anti-ferritin autoantibody production. *Anim. Sci. J.* 84: 782–789.
22 Perkins, G.A., Goodman, L.B., Wimer, C. et al. (2014). Maternal T-lymphocytes in equine colostrum express a primarily inflammatory phenotype. *Vet. Immunol. Immunopathol.* 161: 141–150.
23 Mariella, J., Castagnetti, C., Prosperi, A. et al. (2017). Cytokine levels in colostrum and in foals' serum pre- and post-suckling. *Vet. Immunol. Immunopathol.* 185: 34–37.
24 Lavoie, J.P., Spensley, M.S., Smith, B.P. et al. (1989). Absorption of bovine colostral immunoglobulins G and M in newborn foals. *Am. J. Vet. Res.* 50: 1598–1603.
25 Bernoco, M., Liu, I.K., Wuest-Ehlert, C.J. et al. (1987). Chemotactic and phagocytic function of peripheral blood polymorphonuclear leucocytes in newborn foals. *J. Reprod. Fertil. Suppl.* 35: 599–605.
26 Wichtel, M.G., Anderson, K.L., Johnson, T.V. et al. (1991). Influence of age on neutrophil function in foals. *Equine Vet. J.* 23: 466–469.
27 Gröndahl, G., Johannisson, A., Demmers, S. et al. (1999). Influence of age and plasma treatment on neutrophil phagocytosis and CD18 expression in foals. *Vet. Microbiol.* 65: 241–254.
28 Gröndahl, G., Sternberg, S., Jensen-Waern, M. et al. (2001). Opsonic capacity of foal serum for the two neonatal pathogens *Escherichia coli* and *Actinobacillus equuli*. *Equine Vet. J.* 33: 670–675.
29 Flaminio, M.J., Rush, B.R., Davis, E.G. et al. (2002). Simultaneous flow cytometric analysis of phagocytosis and oxidative burst activity in equine leukocytes. *Vet. Res. Commun.* 26: 85–92.
30 Nerren, J.R., Martens, R.J., Payne, S. et al. (2009). Age-related changes in cytokine expression by neutrophils of foals stimulated with virulent *Rhodococcus equi* in vitro. *Vet. Immunol. Immunopathol.* 127: 212–219.
31 Liu, M., Liu, T., Bordin, A. et al. (2009). Activation of foal neutrophils at different ages by CpG oligodeoxynucleotides and *Rhodococcus equi*. *Cytokine* 48: 280–289.
32 Bordin, A.I., Liu, M., Nerren, J.R. et al. (2012). Neutrophil function of neonatal foals is enhanced in vitro by CpG oligodeoxynucleotide stimulation. *Vet. Immunol. Immunopathol.* 145: 290–297.
33 Leblanc, M.M. and Pritchard, E.L. (1988). Effects of bovine colostrum, foal serum immunoglobulin concentration and intravenous plasma transfusion on chemiluminescence response of foal neutrophils. *Anim. Genet.* 19: 435–445.
34 Flaminio, M.J., Borges, A.S., Nydam, D.V. et al. (2007). The effect of CpG-ODN on antigen presenting cells of the foal. *J. Immune Based Ther. Vaccines* 5: 1.
35 Flaminio, M.J., Nydam, D.V., Marquis, H. et al. (2009). Foal monocyte-derived dendritic cells become activated upon *Rhodococcus equi* infection. *Clin. Vaccine Immunol.* 16: 176–183.
36 Lopez, B.S., Hurley, D.J., Giancola, S. et al. (2019). The effect of age on foal monocyte-derived dendritic cell (MoDC) maturation and function after exposure to killed bacteria. *Vet. Immunol. Immunopathol.* 210: 38–45.
37 Sponseller, B.A., de Macedo, M.M., Clark, S.K. et al. (2009). Activation of peripheral blood monocytes results in more robust production of IL-10 in neonatal foals compared to adult horses. *Vet. Immunol. Immunopathol.* 127: 167–173.
38 Banks, E.M., Kyriakidou, M., Little, S. et al. (1999). Epithelial lymphocyte and macrophage distribution in the adult and fetal equine lung. *J. Comp. Pathol.* 120: 1–13.
39 Smith, R., Chaffin, M.K., Cohen, N.D. et al. (2002). Age-related changes in lymphocyte subsets of quarter horse foals. *Am. J. Vet. Res.* 63: 531–537.
40 Tallmadge, R.L., Wang, M., Sun, Q. et al. (2018). Transcriptome analysis of immune genes in peripheral blood mononuclear cells of young foals and adult horses. *PLoS One* 13: e0202646.
41 Lunn, D., Holmes, M., and Duffus, W. (1993). Equine T-lymphocyte MHC II expression: variation with age and subset. *Vet. Immunol. Immunopathol.* 35: 225–238.
42 Breathnach, C.C., Sturgill-Wright, T., Stiltner, J.L. et al. (2006). Foals are interferon gamma-deficient at birth. *Vet. Immunol. Immunopathol.* 112: 199–209.
43 Sun, L., Adams, A.A., Page, A.E. et al. (2011). The effect of environment on interferon-gamma production in neonatal foals. *Vet. Immunol. Immunopathol.* 143: 170–175.
44 Forchielli, M.L. and Walker, W.A. (2005). The role of gut-associated lymphoid tissues and mucosal defense. *Br. J. Nutr.* 93 (Suppl 1): S41–S48.
45 Balson, G.A., Smith, G.D., and Yager, J.A. (1997). Immunophenotypic analysis of foal bronchoalveolar lavage lymphocytes. *Vet. Microbial.* 56: 237–246.
46 LeBlanc, M.M., Tran, T., Baldwin, J.L. et al. (1992). Factors that influence passive transfer of immunoglobulins in foals. *J. Am. Vet. Med. Assoc.* 200: 179–183.
47 McGuire, T.C., Poppie, M.J., and Banks, K.L. (1975). Hypogammaglobulinemia predisposing to infection in foals. *J. Am. Vet. Med. Assoc.* 166: 71–75.

48 Raidal, S.L. (1996). The incidence and consequences of failure of passive transfer of immunity on a thoroughbred breeding farm. *Aust. Vet. J.* 73: 201–206.

49 Robinson, J.A., Allen, G.K., Green, E.M. et al. (1993). A prospective study of septicaemia in colostrum-deprived foals. *Equine Vet. J.* 25: 214–219.

50 Baldwin, J.L., Cooper, W.L., Vanderwall, D.K. et al. (1991). Prevalence (treatment days) and severity of illness in hypogammaglobulinemic and normogammaglobulinemic foals. *J. Am. Vet. Med. Assoc.* 198: 423–428.

51 Clabough, D.L., Levine, J.F., Grant, G.L. et al. (1991). Factors associated with failure of passive transfer of colostral antibodies in Standardbred foals. *J. Vet. Intern. Med.* 5: 335–340.

52 Tyler-McGowan, C.M., Hodgson, J.L., and Hodgson, D.R. (1997). Failure of passive transfer in foals: incidence and outcome on four studs in New South Wales. *Aust. Vet. J.* 75: 56–59.

53 Erhard, M.H., Luft, C., Remler, H.P. et al. (2001). Assessment of colostral transfer and systemic availability of immunoglobulin G in new-born foals using a newly developed enzyme-linked immunosorbent assay (ELISA) system. *J. Anim. Physiol. Anim. Nutr.* 85: 164–173.

54 Perryman, L.E., McGuire, T.C., and Hilbert, B.J. (1977). Selective immunoglobulin M deficiency in foals. *J. Am. Vet. Med. Assoc.* 170: 212–215.

55 Perkins, G.A., Nydam, D.V., Flaminio, M.J.B.F. et al. (2003). Serum IgM concentrations in normal, fit horses and horses with lymphoma or other medical conditions. *J. Vet. Intern. Med.* 17: 337–342.

56 Perryman, L.E. (2000). Primary immunodeficiencies of horses. *Vet. Clin. North Am. Equine* 16: 105–116.

57 McGuire, T.C., Perryman, L.E., and Davis, W.C. (1983). Analysis of serum and lymphocyte surface IgM of healthy and immunodeficient horses with monoclonal antibodies. *Am. J. Vet. Res.* 44: 1284–1288.

58 Boy, M.G., Zhang, C., Antczak, D.F. et al. (1992). Unusual selective immunoglobulin deficiency in an Arabian foal. *J. Vet. Intern. Med.* 6: 201–205.

59 Weldon, A.D., Zhang, C., Antczak, D.F. et al. (1992). Selective IgM deficiency and abnormal B-cell response in a foal. *J. Am. Vet. Med. Assoc.* 201: 1396–1398.

60 Freestone JF, Hietala S, Moulton SJ, et al. 1987. Acquired immunodeficiency in a seven-year-old horse. *J. Am. Vet. Med. Assoc.* 1987;190:689–691.

61 MacLeay, J.M., Ames, T.R., Hayden, D.W. et al. (1997). Acquired B lymphocyte deficiency and chronic enterocolitis in a 3-year-old quarter horse. *Vet. Immunol. Immunopathol.* 57: 49–57.

62 Flaminio, M.J., LaCombe, V., Kohn, C.W. et al. (2002). Common variable immunodeficiency in a horse. *J. Am. Vet. Med. Assoc.* 22: 1296–1302.

63 Flaminio, M.J.B.F., Tallmadge, R., Salles-Gomes, C.M. et al. (2009). Common variable immunodeficiency in horses is characterized by B cell depletion in primary and secondary lymphoid tissues. *J. Clin. Immunol.* 29: 107–116.

64 Tallmadge, R.L., Such, K.A., Miller, K.C. et al. (2012). Expression of essential B cell developmental genes in horses with common variable immunodeficiency. *Mol. Immunol.* 51: 169–176.

65 Tallmadge, R.L., Shen, L., Tseng, C.T. et al. (2015). Bone marrow transcriptome and epigenome profiles of equine common variable immunodeficiency patients unveil block of B lymphocyte differentiation. *Clin. Immunol.* 160: 261–276.

66 Pellegrini-Masini, A., Bentz, A.I., Johns, I.C. et al. (2005). Common variable immunodeficiency in three horses with presumptive bacterial meningitis. *J. Am. Vet. Med. Assoc.* 227: 114–122.

67 Tennent-Brown, B.S., Navas de Solis, C., Foreman, J.H. et al. (2010). Common variable immunodeficiency in a horse with chronic peritonitis. *Equine Vet. Educ.* 22: 393–399.

68 McGuire, T.C., Banks, K.L., Evans, D.R. et al. (1976). Agammaglobulinemia in a horse with evidence of functional T lymphocytes. *Am. J. Vet. Res.* 37: 41–46.

69 Perryman, L., McGuire, T.C., and Banks, K.L. (1983). Animal model of human disease. Infantile X-linked agammaglobulinemia. Agammaglobulinemia in horses. *Am. J. Pathol.* 111: 125–127.

70 Deem, D.A., Traver, D.S., Thacker, H.L. et al. (1979). Agammaglobulinemia in a horse. *J. Am. Vet. Med. Assoc.* 175: 469–472.

71 Banks, K.L., McGuire, T.C., and Jerrells, T.R. (1976). Absence of B lymphocytes in a horse with primary agammaglobulinemia. *Clin. Immunol. Immunopathol.* 5: 282–290.

72 Scholes, S.F., Holliman, A., May, P.D. et al. (1998). A syndrome of anaemia, immunodeficiency and peripheral ganglionopathy in Fell pony foals. *Vet. Rec.* 142: 128–134.

73 Jelinek, F., Faldyna, M., and Jasurkova-Mikutova, G. (2006). Severe combined immunodeficiency in a Fell pony foal. *J. Vet. Med. A Physiol. Pathol. Clin. Med.* 53: 69–73.

74 Dixon, J.B., Savage, M., Wattret, A. et al. (2000). Discriminant and multiple regression analysis of anemia and opportunistic infection in Fell pony foals. *Vet. Clin. Pathol.* 29: 84–86.

75 Richards, A.J., Kelly, D.F., Knottenbelt, D.C. et al. (2000). Anaemia, diarrhoea and opportunistic infections in Fell ponies. *Equine Vet. J.* 32: 386–391.

76 Fox-Clipsham, L.Y., Swinburne, J.E., Papoula-Pereira, R.I. et al. (2009). Immunodeficiency/anaemia syndrome in a Dales pony. *Vet. Rec.* 165: 289–290.

77 Bell, S.C., Savidge, C., Taylor, P. et al. (2001). An immunodeficiency in Fell ponies: a preliminary study into cellular responses. *Equine Vet. J.* 33: 687–692.

78 Butler, C.M., Westermann, C.M., Koeman, J.P. et al. (2006). The Fell pony immunodeficiency syndrome also occurs in the Netherlands: a review and six cases. *Tijdschr. Diergeneeskd.* 131: 114–118.

79 Thomas, G.W., Bell, S.C., Phythian, C. et al. (2003). Aid to the antemortem diagnosis of Fell pony foal syndrome by the analysis of B lymphocytes. *Vet. Rec.* 152: 618–621.

80 Gardner, R.B., Hart, K.A., Stokol, T. et al. (2006). Fell Pony syndrome in a pony in North America. *J. Vet. Intern. Med.* 20: 198–203.

81 Tallmadge, R.L., Stokol, T., Gould-Earley, M.J. et al. (2012). Fell Pony syndrome: characterization of developmental hematopoiesis failure and associated gene expression profiles. *Clin. Vaccine Immunol.* 19: 1054–1064.

82 McDonald, V., Robinson, H.A., Kelly, J.P. et al. (1994). Cryptosporidium muris in adult mice: adoptive transfer of immunity and protective roles of CD4 versus CD8 cells. *Infect. Immun.* 62: 2289–2294.

83 Fox-Clipsham, L.Y., Brown, E.E., Carter, S.D. et al. (2011). Identification of a mutation associated with fatal foal immunodeficiency syndrome in the Fell and Dales Pony. *PLoS Genet.* 7: e1002133.

84 Fox-Clipsham, L.Y., Carter, S.D., Goodhead, I. et al. (2011). Population screening of endangered horse breeds for the foal immunodeficiency syndrome mutation. *Vet. Rec.* 169: 655–658.

85 Thomas, G.W., Bell, S.C., and Carter, S.D. (2005). Immunoglobulin and peripheral B-lymphocyte concentrations in Fell pony foal syndrome. *Equine Vet. J.* 37: 48–52.

86 McGuire, T.C. and Poppie, M.J. (1973). Hypogammaglobulinemia and thymic hypoplasia in horses: a primary combined immunodeficiency disorder. *Infect. Immun.* 8: 272–277.

87 Perryman, L.E., Boreson, C.R., Conaway, M.W. et al. (1984). Combined immunodeficiency in an Appaloosa foal. *Vet. Pathol* 21: 547–548.

88 Lew, A.M., Hosking, C.S., and Studdert, M.J. (1980). Immunologic aspects of combined immunodeficiency disease in Arabian foals. *Am. J. Vet. Res.* 41: 1161–1166.

89 Clark, E.G., Turner, A.S., Boysen, B.G. et al. (1978). Listeriosis in an Arabian foal with combined immunodeficiency. *J. Am. Vet. Med. Assoc.* 172: 363–366.

90 Mair, T.S., Taylor, F.G., Harbour, D.A. et al. (1990). Concurrent cryptosporidium and coronavirus infections in an Arabian foal with combined immunodeficiency syndrome. *Vet. Rec.* 126: 127–130.

91 Wyatt, C.R., Magnuson, N.S., and Perryman, L.E. (1987). Defective thymocyte maturation in horses with severe combined immunodeficiency. *J. Immunol.* 139: 4072–4076.

92 Lunn, D.P., McClure, J.T., Schobert, C.S. et al. (1995). Abnormal patterns of equine leucocyte differentiation antigen expression in severe combined immunodeficiency foals suggests the phenotype of normal equine natural killer cells. *Immunology* 84: 495–499.

93 Thompson, D.B., Spradborw, P.B., and Studdert, M. (1976). Isolation of an adenovirus from an Arab foal with a combined immunodeficiency disease. *Aust. Vet. J.* 52: 435–437.

94 Perryman, L.E. and McGuire, T.C. (1978). Mixed lymphocyte culture responses in combined immunodeficiency of horses. *Transplantation* 25: 50–52.

95 Ardans, A.A., Trommershausen-Smith, A., Osburn, B.I. et al. (1977). Immunotherapy in two foals with combined immunodeficiency, resulting in graft versus host reaction. *J. Am. Vet. Med. Assoc.* 170: 167–175.

96 Bue, C.M., Davis, W.C., Magnuson, N.S. et al. (1986). Correction of equine severe combined immunodeficiency by bone marrow transplantation. *Transplantation* 42: 14–19.

97 Wiler, R., Leber, R., Moore, B.B. et al. (1995). Equine severe combined immunodeficiency: a defect in V(D)J recombination and DNA-dependent protein kinase activity. *Proc. Natl. Acad. Sci.* 92: 11485–11489.

98 Shin, E.K., Perryman, L.E., and Meek, K. (1997). Evaluation of a test for identification of Arabian horses heterozygous for the severe combined immunodeficiency trait. *J. Am. Vet. Med. Assoc.* 211: 1268–1270.

99 Tanaka, S., Kaji, Y., Taniyama, H. et al. (1994). *Pneumocystis carinii* pneumonia in a thoroughbred foal. *J. Vet. Med. Sci.* 56: 135–137.

100 Flaminio, M., Rush, B.R., Cox, J.H. et al. (1998). CD4+ and CD8+ T-lymphocytopenia in a filly with Pneumocystis carinii pneumonia. *Aust. Vet. J.* 76: 99–402.

101 Koterba, A.M., Brewer, B.D., and Tarplee, F.A. (1984). Clinical and clinicopathological characteristics of the septicaemic neonatal foal: review of 38 cases. *Equine Vet. J.* 16: 376–382.

102 Morris, D.D. and Whitlock, R.H. (1987). Therapy of suspected septicemia in neonatal foals using plasma-containing antibodies to core lipopolysaccharide (LPS). *J. Vet. Intern. Med.* 1: 175–182.

103 Hotchkiss, R.S. and Karl, I.E. (2003). The pathophysiology and treatment of sepsis. *N. Engl. J. Med.* 348: 138–150.

104 McTaggart, C., Penhale, J., and Raidala, S.L. (2005). Effect of plasma transfusion on neutrophil function in healthy and septic foals. *Aust. Vet. J.* 83: 499–505.

105 Flaminio, M.J., Rush, B.R., and Shuman, W. (1989). Immunologic function in horses after non-specific immunostimulant administration. *Vet. Immunol. Immunopathol.* 63: 303–315.

106 Ryan, C., Giguère, S., Fultz, L. et al. (2010). Effects of two commercially available immunostimulants on leukocyte function of foals following ex vivo exposure to *Rhodococcus equi*. *Vet. Immunol. Immunopathol.* 138: 198–205.

107 Sturgill, T.L., Strong, D., Rashid, C. et al. (2011). Effect of *Propionibacterium acnes*-containing immunostimulant on interferon-gamma production in the neonatal foal. *Vet. Immunol. Immunopathol.* 141: 124–127.

108 Cohen, N.D., Bourquin, J.R., Bordin, A.I. et al. (2014). Intramuscular administration of a synthetic CpG-oligodeoxynucleotide modulates functional responses of neutrophils of neonatal foals. *PLoS One* 9: e109865.

109 Davis, E.G., Rush, B., Bain, F. et al. (2003). Neonatal neutropenia in an Arabian foal. *Equine Vet. J.* 35: 517–520.

110 Wong, D.M., Alcott, C.J., Clark, S.K. et al. (2012). Alloimmune neonatal neutropenia and neonatal isoerythrolysis in a Thoroughbred colt. *J. Vet. Diagn. Invest.* 24: 219–226.

111 Rush, B.R. and Flaminio, M.J. (2000). Immunomodulation in horses. *Vet. Clin. North Am. Equine Pract.* 16: 183–188.

112 Moore, B.R. (1996). Clinical application of interferons in large animal medicine. *J. Am. Vet. Med. Assoc.* 208: 1711–1715.

113 Moore, I., Horney, B., Day, K. et al. (2004). Treatment of inflammatory airway disease in young standardbreds with interferon alpha. *Can. Vet. J.* 45: 594–601.

Chapter 50 Neonatal Infection

Section I Bacterial Sepsis

David Wong and Pamela A. Wilkins

Sepsis and the Systemic Inflammatory Response Syndrome

Pathophysiology of Sepsis

Documentation of sepsis in the neonatal foal is well established and is a clinically relevant disease entity. Sepsis in foals is a common cause of morbidity and mortality in the early neonatal period and is also an important comorbidity of other neonatal diseases such as neonatal encephalopathy and prematurity. Over the last several decades, a main research focus surrounding sepsis in people has been describing the basic cellular and molecular biology of the body's response to infection and why, in some cases, the body reacts with a hyper-reactive inflammatory response and in other cases, this does not occur. In 1991, a consensus conference proposed updated definitions for sepsis and organ failure in people and it was at this point that the systemic inflammatory response syndrome (SIRS) was defined [1]. In this document, sepsis was defined as the systemic response to infection, with the systemic response described as fulfilling two or more SIRS criteria (SIRS criteria: fever or hypothermia, tachycardia, tachypnea, leukocytosis or leucopenia, or >10% immature band neutrophils) [1]. This definition of sepsis has dominated clinical practice and the literature over the last several decades. A subsequent 2001 consensus conference reviewed the definitions and noted that the SIRS concept was valid in the sense that systemic inflammation can be elicited by a variety of infectious and noninfectious conditions, but the definition of SIRS was overly sensitive and nonspecific to be useful in diagnosing a cause of the syndrome or identifying a distinct pattern of host response [2]. Subsequently, the International Pediatric Sepsis Consensus Conference recognized that physiologic parameters change as a child ages, and thus clinical variables used to define SIRS and organ dysfunction were age-adjusted and based on age-specific vital parameters and laboratory data [3]. In the more recent 2016 consensus sepsis definition in people (Sepsis-3), sepsis was defined as life-threatening organ dysfunction due to a dysregulated host response to infection [4]. The SIRS concept was removed from the definition of sepsis (SIRS considered unhelpful in identifying sepsis) and organ dysfunction was determined by an increase in a predefined grading scale, known as the Sequential Organ Failure Assessment (SOFA) score [4]. Moreover, the task force recommended eliminating the terms sepsis syndrome, septicemia, and severe sepsis.

The definition of sepsis and the usefulness of the SIRS concept has evolved over the years, but a large amount of information describing the underlying host response to injury is now available. The body's response to infection or cell damage involves tightly regulated relationships between pro- and anti-inflammatory mediators in concert with the immune, hemostatic, cardiovascular, nervous, and endocrine systems. There is an obvious benefit of the host response to microbial invasion (i.e. containment and elimination of microbes) and these complex interactions participate in a fine balance involving the host's protective response to infection or injury and activation of the immune system. However, the host response can play a dichotomous role: when activation of the inflammatory response is exaggerated, inadequate, chronic, or directed against normal tissue, the hyper-activation of pro-inflammatory responses can be detrimental to the host [5–7]. Sepsis is one such situation in which a misguided innate immune response occurs and an over abundant inflammatory response results in organ injury and potentially death, a sentiment that is captured in the Sepsis-3 definition [4].

PAMPs and DAMPs

The early innate and inflammatory response associated with microbial infection or tissue damage is regulated by an overlapping network of *pathogen associated molecular*

Equine Neonatal Medicine, First Edition. Edited by David M. Wong and Pamela A. Wilkins.

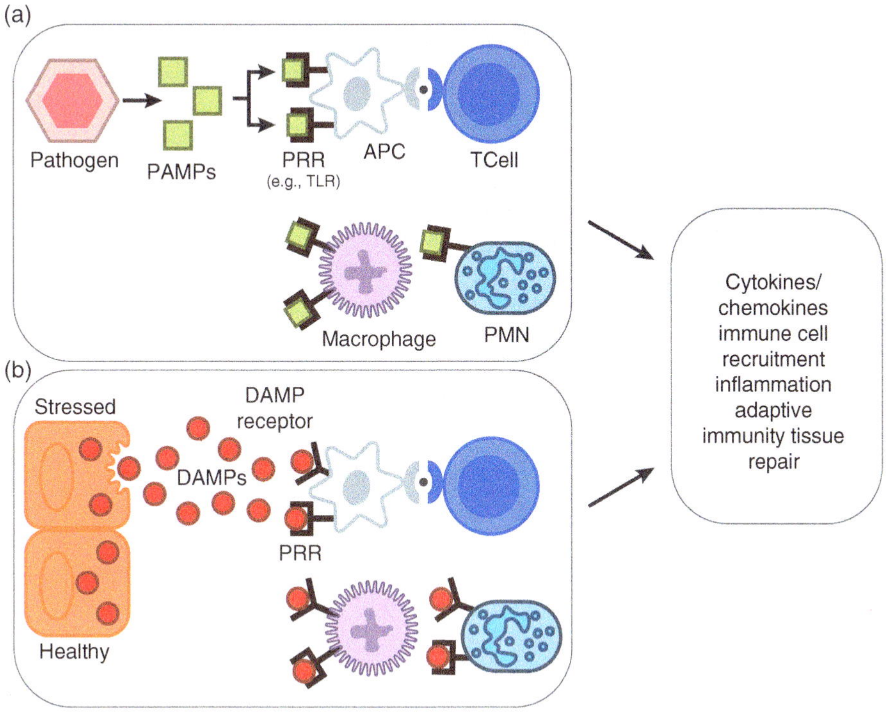

Figure 50.I.1 DAMPs and PAMPs – (a) Pathogenic bacteria or viruses cause release of pathogen associated molecular patterns (PAMPs) that bind to pathogen recognition receptors (PRR), such as toll-like receptors (TLR), on immune cells and stimulate an innate immune response accompanied by inflammation and activation of adaptive immunity. They eventually acts to resolve infection and promote tissue repair. (b) Danger associated molecular patterns (DAMPs), normally hidden in the cell, are released from stressed, injured, or necrotic cells. Extracellularly, DAMPs bind to TLRs or other specialized DAMP receptors to elicit an immune response by promoting release of proinflammatory mediators and recruiting immune cells to infiltrate the tissue. Immune cells that participate in these processes include antigen presenting cell (e.g. APC; dendritic cells, macrophages), T cells, and polymorphonuclear (PMN) cells. *Source:* Copyright Sara Anais Gonzalez, 2022.

patterns (PAMPs) and *damage-associated molecular patterns* (DAMPs; Figure 50.I.1). A multitude of PAMPs and DAMPs have been identified and are recognized by the host's cell surface and cytosolic *pathogen recognition receptors* (PRR). Classes of PRRs include toll-like receptors (TLRs), C-type lectin receptors, nucleotide-binding domain leucine-rich repeat containing proteins (NLRs) and retinoic acid-inducible gene-1-like receptors (RLRs) [6, 8, 9]. These PRRs can reside on the cell surface, in the endoplasmic reticulum, in the cytosol, or in endosomes, lysosomes, or endolysosomes [9]. Subsequent activation of PRRs leads to a more limited number of signaling pathways such as activation of the nuclear factor kappa-light-chain-enhancer of activated B cells (NF-ĸB), mitogen-activated protein kinase (MAPK), or interferon regulatory factor (IRF) which control expression of cytokines, chemokines, and interferons [6–8]. A comprehensive review of equine PRRs and ligands has been published [9].

Recognition of PAMPs is the first step in mounting the early innate immune response. The most intensely studied PAMPs include lipopolysaccharide (LPS; endotoxin), lipoproteins, peptidoglycans, lipoteichoic acid, and nucleic acids [7, 10]. Perhaps the most infamous PAMP recognized by equine veterinarians and human physicians alike is endotoxin (LPS). Detailed descriptions of the molecular pathways of LPS and its role in activation of the inflammatory response are available elsewhere [11]. For the purposes of this text, suffice it to say Gram-negative bacteria possess large quantities of LPS which bind to the TLR 4 complex on primarily macrophages and monocytes ultimately culminating in the production of potent inflammatory mediators such as interleukin (IL)-1 and tumor necrosis factor (TNF)-α [11]. Another PAMP is lipoprotein, which is a component of all bacteria and shares a common chemical motif; lipoproteins induce the inflammatory response via TLR2 signaling [12]. Gram-positive bacteria contain peptidoglycan (PGN) which serves as a PAMP and is recognized through several peptidoglycan molecules such as cluster of differentiation (CD) 14 and TLR2 [7]. Lipoteichoic acid (LTA) is an additional PAMP that is bound to cell membranes and projects through the peptidoglycan layer of most Gram-positive bacteria. Lysozyme and cationic peptides from leukocytes cause bacteriolysis and release LTA which subsequently induces NF-ĸB, MAPK, and phosphoinositide 3-kinase activation via TLR2-CD14 [13]. Pathogen-derived nucleic acids are yet another group of PAMPs that are primarily recognized intracellularly during bacterial phagocytosis, viral replication or reverse transcriptase and are recognized via TLR9 resulting in a potent inflammatory response [7, 14, 15].

Host cells can also activate the immune system through endogenous DAMPs that are released from damaged cells, cell death that occurs during sepsis or trauma, or actively released molecules in response to cell stress [7]. Well-described DAMPs include high mobility group box (HMGB) nuclear proteins, S100 proteins, host mitochondrial and nuclear DNA and advanced glycosylated end products (AGEs) [7]. Endogenous DAMPs can also be actively secreted as alarm signals (alarmins) that notify the host of danger by activating the innate immune system [16]. Alarmins are normal nuclear proteins that are produced from necrotic and physiologically stressed cells [17, 18]. Once in the local and systemic circulation these endogenous molecules activate the innate immune and inflammatory responses [19]. If a cell is under stress or dying, HBGB nuclear proteins are released and act as an alarmin and pro-inflammatory mediator. In addition, HMGB nuclear proteins are actively secreted by monocytes and macrophages during the early inflammatory response [20, 21]. Elevated concentrations of HMGB have been demonstrated in conditions such as septic shock and severe trauma [22, 23]. S100 proteins are calcium-binding homodimeric proteins within the cytoplasm of phagocytes that are released or secreted during cell stress or cell damage [24, 25]. Upon release, S100 proteins act as endogenous ligands of TLR4 and subsequently induce TNFα production [26]. Endogenous nuclear and mitochondrial DNA can also act as DAMPs when they are released into the circulation after cell damage and necrosis and produce an inflammatory response [27].

Stimulation of PRR results in downstream signaling that produces both a common, non-specific response and a pathogen-specific host cellular response [7]. Early non-specific responses target suppressing microbial replication, tissue invasion, and propagation of microbes from the original site of infection [28]. In the prototypical response, the innate immune system is the first line of defense and is coupled with disruption of cells and the extracellular matrix which results in activation of a number of endogenous host mechanisms and release or exposure of a multitude of mediators. These mediators promote the vasoactive and phagocytic phases of inflammation. In the *vasoactive phase of inflammation*, a local environment within the infected or traumatized tissues is infiltrated by phagocytic cells. Vasodilation occurs from vasoactive mediators including bradykinin, histamine, inducible nitric oxide synthase (iNOS), and cyclooxygenase 2 (COX-2) that consequently increase blood flow while simultaneously slowing blood flow velocity to affected areas [28, 29]. In addition, activation of the coagulation cascade by inflammatory cytokines and exposure of tissue factor (thromboplastin) on endothelial cells paired with inhibition of the anti-coagulant protein C results in a hyper-coagulable state which reduces microvascular perfusion and increases endothelial permeability, resulting in potential microvascular thrombosis and ischemia [30–32]. Increased endothelial permeability also allows formation of local edema, enabling a more aqueous environment for leukocyte migration through the normally condensed extracellular matrix [28]. These alterations in blood flow dynamics, along with increased expression of adhesion molecules, allow for margination and diapedesis of leukocytes to infected and injured areas with the intended goal of reducing blood loss and trapping microbes locally [7, 29, 33]. Furthermore, chemokines provide specific signals for leukocyte trafficking into inflamed tissue [34]. During the *phagocytic phase of inflammation*, up-regulation of selectin and adhesion molecules on endothelial cells facilitates adherence and margination of circulating neutrophils and monocytes under the guidance of chemoattractants [29, 33]. Pro-inflammatory cytokines such as TNF-α, IL-1β, IL-2, IL-6, IL-8, IL-12, and IFN, produced by monocytes and macrophages, help heighten the phagocytosis of pathogens, enhance cell-mediated immunity, upregulate acute phase protein synthesis and facilitate removal of degenerating and dead host cells [8, 35]. Other protective mediators released during infection include proteolytic enzymes, reactive oxygen species, and neutrophil extracellular traps (NETs), which are chromatin fiber structures extruded by activated neutrophils, that produce a physical barrier that prevents further spread of pathogens and provides a high local concentration of endogenous antimicrobial components that bind and kill microbes [36, 37]. This process in which cytokine and chemokine release attracts leukocytes to the local area can cause local tissue destruction (abscess) or cellular injury (pus) that are necessary by-products of an effective local inflammatory response aimed at healing of host tissues. Antigen presenting cells simultaneously process microbial antigens and deliver secondary signals at the site of infection along with draining lymph nodes. The secondary release of cytokines and other mediators modulate and recruit additional inflammatory cells that promote an environment for the adaptive immune response, which further enhances microbial elimination [7].

Offsetting the pro-inflammatory environment is the concurrent production of *anti-inflammatory mediators* that attempt to maintain immune homeostasis and balance the host's defenses against infection or cell trauma while minimizing self-induced tissue injury [38, 39]. Cytokine antagonists such as soluble TNF receptors and IL-1 receptor antagonist bind and inactivate TNF-α and IL-1, respectively [31]. Anti-inflammatory cytokines include IL-4, IL-5,

Table 50.I.1 Proposed equine neonatal SIRS criteria using age-specific parameters; SIRS is present when at least 3 of the following criteria must be present, one of which must be abnormal temperature or leukocyte count [46].

Parameter	Newborn foal (Birth to 3 d of age)	Neonatal foal (4–14 d of age)	Juvenile foal (15 d to 6 mo)	Weanling foal (7 mo to 1 yr)
Fever or hypothermia (rectal temperature)	>102.6 °F (39.2 °C) or <99.0 °F (37.2 °C)	>102.6 °F (39.2 °C) or <99.0 °F (37.2 °C)	>102.6 °F (39.2 °C) or <99.0 °F (37.2 °C)	>102.6 °F (39.2 °C) or <99.0 °F (37.2 °C)
Tachycardia (beats/min)	>115	>120	>96	>60
Tachypnea (breaths/min)	>56	>56	>44	>20
Leukocytosis ($\times 10^3$), Leukopenia ($\times 10^3$), or >5% band neutrophils	>14.4 or <6.9	>12.5 or <4.0	>12.5 or <4.0	>12.5 or <4.0
Venous blood lactate level (mmol/l)	>5.0	>2.5	>2.5	>2.5
Venous blood glucose level (mg/dl)	<50	<50	<50	<50

IL-10, IL-13, and transforming growth factor (TGF)-β. These cytokines inhibit expression of cytokines that contribute to sepsis and promote the humoral immune response by stimulating B-cell differentiation and antibody production while dampening pro-inflammatory mediators [31, 38, 40]. Another component of the immune response to sepsis is the neuro-immune reflex in which vagal nerve activity impacts the immune response via the cholinergic anti-inflammatory pathway. In this response, afferent nerve fibers are stimulated by immunogenic mediators resulting in efferent signaling to the spleen and other organs via the vagus nerve. The subsequent release of acetylcholine activates cholinergic receptors (7-nicotinic receptors) on macrophages, which then dampens the release of pro-inflammatory cytokines [37]. Just as the pro-inflammatory response can become dysregulated in sepsis, this compensatory response can also become dysregulated.

The *compensatory anti-inflammatory response syndrome* (CARS) can arise if over-activity of the anti-inflammatory pathway occurs resulting in immunosuppression and potentially enhanced susceptibility of the host to infection. Septic patients can demonstrate immunosuppressive trends such as leukocyte anergy, reduction and apoptosis of lymphocytes, decreased pro-inflammatory cytokine production, repression of T-cell, B-cell, and natural killer cell function, decreased antigen-presentation by monocytes and increased expression of immunosuppressive cytokines [31, 41, 42].

Sepsis in the Equine Neonate

In regard to the equine neonate, a specific definition of sepsis has not been universally agreed upon. In the recent task force on sepsis in people (Sepsis-3), sepsis was defined as life-threatening organ dysfunction due to a dysregulated host response to infection [4]. Likewise, septic shock in neonatal foals has not been defined, but has been defined in people as a subset of sepsis in which circulatory, cellular, and metabolic abnormalities are associated with a greater risk of mortality than sepsis alone. The clinical criteria in people representing septic shock were the need for vasopressor therapy to maintain a mean arterial pressure (MAP) ≥60mmHg and a serum lactate concentration >2 mmol/l, persisting after fluid therapy [4]. Most equine clinicians rely on clinical observations, blood culture, and/or the use of the modified sepsis score to identify septic foals. The SIRS concept has also been used to help categorize neonatal foals in a variety of research studies utilizing the original SIRS parameters proposed for people [43–45]. In addition, equine neonatal SIRS criteria, using age-specific parameters, have also been proposed (Table 50.I.1) [46]. A study evaluating both the original and equine neonatal SIRS criteria and their ability to predict sepsis in foals reported a sensitivity and specificity of 60% and 69%, respectively, when the original SIRS criteria were met and 42% and 76%, respectively, when the equine neonatal SIRS criteria were met [46]. Therefore, use of the original SIRS criteria may provide a rapid diagnostic screen in identifying foals at risk for sepsis, but should not be the sole method for determining sepsis in foals.

A few equine studies have examined and compared *molecular markers* and *cytokine profiles* between septic, sick nonseptic, and healthy neonatal foals [47, 48]. In a study by Pusterla et al., peripheral blood mononuclear cells (PBMC) from all foals had certain transcription levels for TNF-α, IL-1β, IL-6, IL-8, IL-10, procalcitonin (PCT), and TGF-β [47]. Interestingly, TNF-α, and TGF-β were significantly lower and IL-8 was significantly higher in sick-nonseptic and septic foals as compared to healthy foals [47]. No significant difference was noted in gene expression of IL-1β, IL-6, and PCT between groups [47]. These cytokine profiles were also observed in another study comparing septic and healthy foals [48]. IL-10, noted for suppressing macrophage, T-cell, and natural killer cell function, was significantly higher in foals that died suggesting possible immunosuppression in non-survivors [47]. In another small study involving 26 ill foals, no significant difference in mRNA expression of IL-1β, IL-6, or TNF-α was noted between septic and sick-nonseptic foals, but IL-8 expression was significantly lower in septic foals when compared to sick non-septic foals, a finding opposite to the study by Pusterla et al. [47, 49] Additionally, IL-4 gene expression was initially down-regulated and TLR4 expression up-regulated in PBMC from septic foals [50]. In a different study, median IL-6 serum concentrations were significantly lower in septic foals (491 ng/ml) when compared to healthy foals (3242 ng/ml) [40]. Interestingly, equine colostrum had notable amounts of IL-6 (≥215 ng/ml) and prior to ingestion of colostrum, serum IL-6 concentrations was undetectable in healthy foals [40]. Thus, passive transfer of maternally derived IL-6 to healthy foals may explain the higher IL-6 in this group as compared to septic foals that may have failure of transfer of passive immunity (FTPI) [40]. Investigations into molecular markers that could aid in the early detection of sepsis such as plasma concentrations of PCT, C-reactive protein, serum amyloid A (SAA), haptoglobin, and adrenomedullin have been evaluated in foals, but thus far no specific marker has proved to be reliable at identifying sepsis in the foal [47, 51–53]. The small study groups, different measurement methodologies, and large standard deviations in measured markers likely contributed to the lack of significant differences between groups and inconsistencies between studies [40, 43–49]. Further investigation characterizing the neonatal foal's molecular responses to infection is needed.

Risk Factors

Risk factors for development of sepsis can partly be founded on published information, but many proposed risk factors are based on anecdotal clinical experience [54–56]. Risk factors can be divided into peri-parturient history of the mare, pre-natal/maternal, and post-natal factors, although many of these are inter-related (Table 50.I.2). For example,

Table 50.I.2 Risk factors for the development of sepsis in the neonatal foal.

Prior peri-parturient history of the mare	Prenatal/maternal factors	Postnatal/newborn foal factors
* Previous abortions, stillbirths or twins * Previous premature, dysmature, or compromised foals * Previous foals with neonatal isoerythrolysis * Previous maternal aggression or nursing avoidance towards foal	<u>Environmental Factors</u> * Unsanitary foaling conditions * Endemic infectious diseases *Salmonella*, *Clostridium* * High density of horses or overcrowding <u>Maternal</u> * Serious illness * Poor nutritional status * Prolonged transport in last 30 d of gestation * Placental disease Placentitis Vaginal discharge Villus atrophy Placental edema * Premature placental separation * Mare with colic episode * Mare with endotoxemia * Clinical or subclinical Salmonellosis * Dystocia * Cesarean section * Early signs of parturition * Induction of parturition * Prolonged second stage of labor * Premature lactation * Poor colostral quality	* Premature/Dysmature foal * Failure of transfer of passive immunity * Neonatal encephalopathy * Meconium staining * Abnormal appearance of fetal membranes of fluids * Prolonged time to stand or nurse * Musculoskeletal disorder preventing normal ambulation Severe flexural limb deformities Severe angular limb deformities Myopathies [57] - Nutritional myodegeneration - Glycogen branching enzyme deficiency [58] - Lipid storage myopathy [59] - Atypical myopathy [60]

placentitis can be associated with prenatal clinical signs such as vaginal discharge, premature lactation, and early parturition along with post-natal risk factors such as abnormal appearance of fetal fluids and membranes, poor colostral quality and FTPI. In regard to prior maternal history, if a mare has had previous abortions, still-births, or premature/dysmature foals, careful attention to the mare's vaccination history (e.g. herpes abortion), diet (e.g. malnutrition, fescue toxicity, goitrogenic plants) and reproductive tract conformation (e.g. abnormalities that predispose mare to placentitis such as pneumovagina, vestibule-vaginal reflux or cervical fibrosis, tears, or adhesions) should be made. FTPI is a risk factor for the development of sepsis, but the amount of risk varies with the degree of FTPI as well as environmental and farm management conditions and virulence of invading microbes [61]. In one study, complete deprivation of colostrum in 8 neonatal foals resulted in development of sepsis in 7 foals [62]. Another study examined 50 ill foals and found a significantly larger proportion of foals with FTPI were diagnosed with sepsis (26/28; 93%) compared to septic foals with adequate TPI (10/22; 45%) [63]. Conversely, other studies have not documented a relationship between IgG concentration and blood culture status in hospitalized ill foals and in a well-managed Standardbred farm situation, there was not a greater risk of disease in foals with partial FTPI as compared to adequate transfer of passive immunity [44, 64, 65]. Thus it is likely that a combination of risk factors impact the incidence of sepsis. Despite the variable reports, certainly maternal antibodies infer a degree of protection to the immunologically naïve foal, thus situations that compromise the quality and quantity of colostrum or ability of the foal to consume colostrum serve as risk factors. Other situations, such as endemic infectious diseases (e.g. *Salmonella*), overcrowding, or unsanitary environmental conditions might increase the bacterial load presented to the neonate's gastrointestinal (GI) tract, particularly during initial phase of locating the udder, thus increasing the likelihood of sepsis [56].

Clinical Signs

Clinical signs of sepsis in the neonatal foal are quite variable and at times vague, ranging from no overt clinical signs to recumbency and unresponsiveness. Changes in mentation can range from depression and lack of awareness of the surrounding environment to thrashing, seizures, or a comatose state. Weakness may manifest as a reluctance to rise or inability to stand and ambulate. The mare's udder may appear full from abbreviated or absent suckling; the presence of dried milk might appear on the foal's forehead as ill foals often stand with their head underneath the mare's udder allowing streaming milk to collect on the foal's forehead and muzzle in the absence of regular suckling. Aberrations in blood components can result in icteric mucous membranes and sclera or petechia of the mucous membranes or skin of the inner pinnae [54, 66–68]. Changes in blood perfusion parameters such as hyperemic or dark red mucous membranes, coronitis, decreased pulse quality, cold extremities, pale mucous membranes, increased capillary refill time, prolonged jugular refill, decreased urine output, and variable tachycardia can also be observed (Figure 50.I.2 a,b,c) [54, 68]. Tachypnea or respiratory distress can be variably present in septic foals along with hypo- or normothermia during the early stages of sepsis followed by fever in other instances [66]. In one study of 85 septic foals, rectal temperature ranged from 90 to 105 °F (median 100.8 °F), heart rate ranged from 44 to 180 beats/minute (median 100 beats/min) and respiratory rate ranged from 12 to 88 breaths/minute (median 36 breaths/min) at hospital admission [68]. If left untreated, clinical signs can progress rapidly resulting in deterioration of the cardiovascular system, septic shock, and death. Organ specific or localizing clinical signs of infection include colic, diarrhea, respiratory distress, uveitis, joint effusion (with or without lameness), omphalitis, patent urachus, and subcutaneous abscessation [56, 65, 67].

Body Systems Involved in Sepsis

Hematologic System

Hematologic changes associated with sepsis include alterations in total white cell count and neutrophil count. Leukopenia, characterized by neutropenia and a toxic (Dohle bodies, toxic granulation, vacuolization) regenerative or degenerative left shift is the most common hematologic alteration associated with acute sepsis, especially in neonates <7 days of age [70]. In one study, 70% (19/27) of blood culture positive septic foals had neutropenia ($<4.0\times10^3$ cells/µl), 89% (24/27) had a left shift ($>0.2\times10^3$ band neutrophils/µl) and 89% (24/27) had toxic granulation observed [66]. In a larger study of 85 septic foals, lower mean peripheral white blood cell and lymphocyte counts and more toxic band neutrophils were observed in foals with Gram-negative bacteremia as compared to Gram-positive bacteremia, but 40% of septic foals had a white cell count within normal reference intervals [68]. Septic foals presented at an older age (8–14 days) can display leukocytosis, neutrophilia, and left shift [56, 66, 70]. Septic foals may also have significantly lower lymphocyte counts and higher monocyte counts when compared to age-matched healthy foals [70].

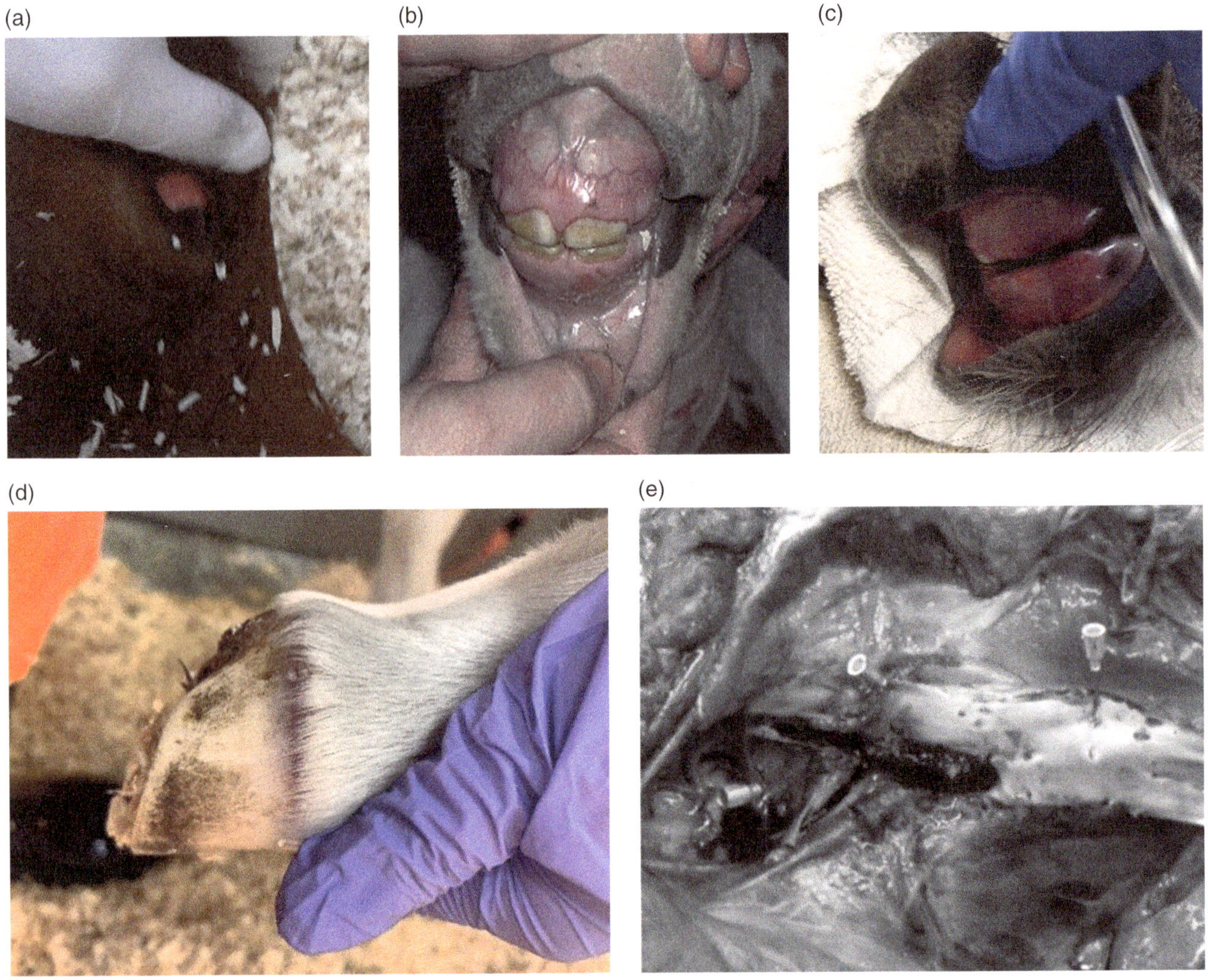

Figure 50.I.2 Clinical signs associated with sepsis in the neonatal foal. (a) Injection of vessels of the sclera. (b) Vasodilation of the oral vasculature. (c) Severe congestion of the oral mucous membranes in a septic foal. (d) Poor perfusion of the coronet in a septic foal with severe diarrhea (*Note:* All four feet were involved). (e) Thrombosis at the bifurcation of the abdominal aorta [69].

Coagulation System

In health, the coagulation system maintains a precise equilibrium between pro-coagulant, anti-coagulant, and fibrinolytic mechanisms to maintain homeostasis. However, coagulopathies are not infrequent in septic foals owing to the fact that inflammatory mediators alter normal hemostatic balance. Sepsis and ensuing production of inflammatory mediators such as IL-1 and TNF-α promote expression of tissue factor on endothelial cells, monocytes, and macrophages [30, 32]. Tissue factor (also called Factor III [FIII], thromboplastin, or CD142) initiates the coagulation pathway by binding and activating factor VII (FVII) on cell surfaces and forming tissue factor-FVIIa complex; this in turn results in activation and amplification of factor X (FX), factor V (FV) and conversion of prothrombin to thrombin [30, 32]. Pro-inflammatory cytokines also disrupt endogenous anti-inflammatory mediators such as antithrombin, tissue factor pathway inhibitor, and activated protein C [30, 71]. Collectively, these changes result in a pro-coagulant state in septic patients.

Clinical signs of coagulopathy in neonatal foals can range from subclinical laboratory abnormalities with no clinical evidence of coagulopathy to development of petechial hemorrhages to more significant changes such as thrombosis of blood vessels or disseminated intravascular coagulation (DIC) [16, 72]. Clinically detectable bleeding was reported in 47% of foals with sepsis or septic shock in one study [73] and a few case reports have documented thrombi within the heart or involving the central (aorta-iliac; Figure 50.I.2e) or peripheral arteries and veins. Reported clinical signs included cold limbs, limb edema, weak/absent peripheral pulses, and dark red/purple coronets (Figure 50.I.2d) [69, 74–79]. Foals with sepsis can have prolonged prothrombin time (PT), activated partial thromboplastin time (aPTT) and increased concentrations of fibrin degradation products (FDPs) and D-dimers along with decreased anti-coagulant factors such as anti-thrombin activity and protein C antigen [70, 80]. One prospective study identified coagulopathy, defined as 3 or more abnormal coagulation tests, in 25% of foals in septic shock and 16% of foals with sepsis [73] while another study noted that 50% of septic foals had clinicopathologic evidence of DIC, although none of those foals showed clinical signs of bleeding disorders [80]. Of note, unlike infants with sepsis, thrombocytopenia is inconsistently reported in septic foals [70, 73, 75, 81]. Collectively, sepsis-related inflammation can potentially cause coagulopathies contributing to bleeding disorders, micro- or gross vascular thrombosis, and possible organ dysfunction.

Organ Dysfunction

Organ dysfunction associated with sepsis results from local and systemic release of mediators that exert deleterious effects at both the site of infection and organs distant to the inciting infection. Organ dysfunction, sometimes referred to as multiple organ dysfunction syndrome (MODS), is a continuum with varying degrees of severity and physiologic derangements of individual organs and can be reflected in clinical signs and on serum biochemistry analysis. Common manifestations observed in septic foals include abnormalities in blood glucose regulation and alterations that reflect compromise of the renal, hepatic, respiratory, cardiovascular, GI, and endocrine systems. Septic foals can lose glycemic control and present with hyper-, normo-, or hypoglycemia. Hypoglycemia can be related to low fat and glycogen stores coupled with decreased or absent caloric intake and increased catabolism, or arise, in part, from endotoxemia which decreases hepatic gluconeogenesis and increases peripheral glucose uptake [11, 44, 82]. Septic foals that have a peri-parturient asphyxial or ischemic insult may also become hypoglycemic as asphyxia results in rapid metabolism of glucose by the brain and other tissues for energy [44]. In a retrospective study involving 515 neonatal foals, hypoglycemia (blood glucose <75.6 mg/dl) was significantly associated with sepsis, a positive blood culture, and SIRS [44]. Of the 515 foals, 37% were hyperglycemic (>131 mg/dl), 34% were hypoglycemic and 29% were normoglycemic. Moreover, hypoglycemia and severe hyperglycemia (blood glucose >180 mg/dl) were both significantly associated with a worse prognosis to hospital discharge [44]. In another study, septic foals had a significantly lower blood glucose (median 86.5 mg/dl, range 3–329 mg/dl) as compared to sick nonseptic (median 133 mg/dl, range 34–272 mg/dl) and healthy (median 144 mg/dl, range 110–182 mg/dl) foals [83, 84]. A possible link between abnormal glucose regulation and somatotropic axis (growth hormone, insulin-like growth factor-1) resistance might play a part in sepsis mediated blood glucose dynamics [83, 84].

Acute Kidney Injury (AKI)

There is little published information regarding sepsis-induced acute kidney injury (AKI) in the neonatal foal, although it undoubtedly occurs [31, 45]. AKI can be defined as a sudden decline in kidney function accompanied by an acute and reversible increase in serum creatinine concentration, derangements in fluid and electrolyte balance, and altered waste produce clearance; this condition may or may not be associated with a reduction in urine output [85]. The exact pathophysiology of sepsis-induced renal injury is unknown but various theories have been put forth. One theory suggests that pro-inflammatory cytokines and SIRS causes induction of nitric oxide synthase, which in turn results in arterial vasodilation, decreased systemic vascular resistance (SVR) and hypotension; this contributes to renal hypoperfusion and acute tubular necrosis [31, 86]. Another theory suggests that microvascular dysfunction occurs in the presence of normal or increased renal blood flow, and manifests with a decreased glomerular filtration rate resulting in tubular dysfunction [31]. Another possible explanation is that sepsis-induced expression of inflammatory cytokines and leukocyte activity cause capillary plugging and micro-thrombi. This, coupled with disturbances in microcirculatory oxygen delivery, production of reactive oxygen species, and induction of nitric oxide synthase can damage the kidney [85, 87].

Sepsis combined with perinatal asphyxia, a situation that frequently occurs in ill foals, can collectively contribute to renal injury as well [85]. Clinicopathologic changes that reflect renal compromise include elevated or rising serum creatinine concentrations, an atypically slow decrease in creatinine concentrations from birth values, elevation in blood urea nitrogen (BUN), and hyperkalemia [88]. Of note, these serum changes are not exclusive to sepsis-induced kidney injury. Moreover, the clinician must interpret serum creatinine concentrations in light of spurious hypercreatininemia, in which greatly elevated serum creatinine (mean ± SD: 13.5 ± 7.5 mg/dl) concentrations are noted in the first 1–2 days of life in neonatal foals with normal renal function [88]. In such cases, serum creatinine concentrations should decline by 50% within 24 hours of hospitalization [88]. A proposed cause of this phenomenon is placental dysfunction and redistribution of fluid and creatinine from the allantoic cavity, which normally has creatinine concentrations of 160–200 mg/dl, to the fetus [67, 89]. Uroabdomen should also be ruled out, as this can cause azotemia and electrolyte imbalances. Urinalysis and urine output can be monitored for evidence of renal injury as well.

Healthy foals produce approximately 148 ml/kg/d (6 ml/kg/h) of urine, with the mean specific gravity in 2-day-old foals of 1.009 (range 1.002–1.027) [90]. However, if the foal is being administered IV fluids, these parameters may not have as much relevance. Decreased to absent urine production, isosthenuria, and evidence of renal injury on urinalysis (hematuria, casts, bacteria, proteinuria, glucosuria) in the presence of suspected or confirmed sepsis may support sepsis-associated kidney injury. The urine GGT to creatinine ratio ($U_{GGT}/U_{Cr} \times 100$) has also been used as an indicator of renal injury in adult horses and can potentially serve as a marker of tubular injury in foals (mean ± SD ratio in healthy neonatal foals 8.16 ± 5.7) [90, 91].

Necropsy examination of septic neonatal foals with renal involvement can note discrete aggregates of bacteria present in glomerular tufts, tubules, and intertubular capillaries, microabscesses in the renal cortex and outer medulla, and renal cortical necrosis with hemorrhage [31, 45]. As previously noted, sepsis activates the coagulation system and inhibits fibrinolysis creating a hypercoagulable state responsible for acute thrombosis [45, 75]. In a study involving 32 nonsurviving septic neonatal foals, hypercoaguability was evaluated by the presence and degree of fibrin deposits in tissues where secondary organ injury (liver, lung, kidney) is commonly observed with sepsis [45]. In that study, fibrin deposits (Figure 50.I.3) were observed in 87.5% (28/32) of septic foals with renal fibrin deposits noted in 44% (14/32), suggesting sub-clinical or clinical renal involvement is not uncommon [45].

Acute Liver Injury

Elevated liver enzyme activity such as GGT and SDH along with hyperbilirubinemia are commonly observed in neonatal foals and can originate from primary hepatic diseases such as *Clostridium piliforme* infection (Tyzzer's disease), bacterial infection of the liver via direct hematogenous spread or ascending biliary ducts, or secondary to sepsis, perinatal asphyxia, or enteritis [31, 92, 93]. Bacteria, such as *Actinobacillus equuli* and *Salmonella typhimurium*, have been cultured from liver specimens from neonatal foals collected at necropsy [31, 92]. Other causes of neonatal liver disease include equine herpesvirus-1 infection, neonatal isoerythrolysis, toxic hepatopathy, and congenital abnormalities [94–98].

Hyperbilirubinemia is common in septic infants and neonatal foals and is attributed to rapid hemolysis caused by bacteria or endotoxin [66, 99]. In one retrospective study, high liver enzyme activity characterized by elevations in GGT (median 49, range 9–505 [reference range 20–45 U/l]) and SDH (median 20, range 0–495 U/l [reference interval 2–11 U/l]), were identified in 36% (147/410) of hospitalized foals <30 days of age [92]. Septic foals were significantly more likely to have high liver enzymes activity (51%, [66/130]) compared to nonseptic foals (27%, [70/255]) [92]. However, an association between magnitude of increase in GGT or SDH activity and disease severity was not observed. Furthermore, septic foals with high liver enzyme activity were no less likely to survive than septic foals without elevated activity [92]. Neutrophilic hepatitis, hepatic congestion, hepatocellular necrosis, and hepatic fibrin deposits suggestive of activation of the

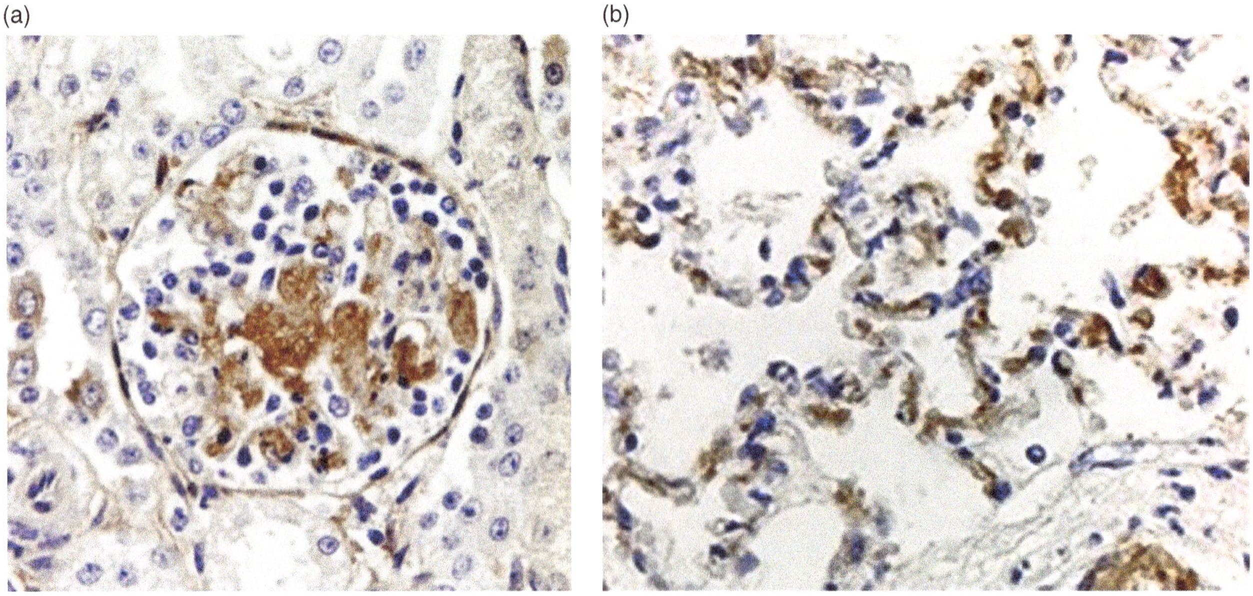

Figure 50.I.3 Fibrin deposits in the glomerular capillaries and lungs from foals with severe sepsis demonstrated by immunohistochemistry (brown). Fibrin deposits obliterate the glomerular capillaries (a) and occlude alveolar capillaries (b) [45].

coagulation cascade, can also be observed microscopically in foals with sepsis-related liver disease [45, 92].

Acute Lung Injury (ALI)

Hypoxemia and *tachypnea* are frequently documented in neonatal foals and arise from a number of pulmonary causes such as surfactant deficiency (neonatal equine respiratory distress syndrome [NERDS]), lung atelectasis (especially in recumbent foals), persistent pulmonary hypertension, airway obstruction, or non-pulmonary causes including congenital heart disease and, relevant to this chapter, sepsis [100]. Clinical evidence of septic pneumonia was documented in 19% (12/62) of septic foals in one study and can occur from bacteremia or secondary to aspiration [101].

In health, the alveolus is lined by a thin alveolar-capillary barrier that maintains an air-liquid interface. This barrier is comprised of the epithelial cell layer (Type I and II pneumocytes) and the microvascular endothelial cell layer; these two layers are separated by interstitial space with alveolar macrophages residing on top of the epithelia (Figure 50.I.4) [103]. Sepsis impacts the respiratory system via similar pathophysiologic processes seen in the rest of the body including activation of the innate immune system, production of inflammatory mediators, neutrophil infiltration, development of a pro-coagulant environment, and microthrombosis [104]. Sepsis-induced lung injury can vary in severity in neonatal foals ranging from mild to moderate injury to the respiratory microvascular endothelium and variable amounts of pulmonary edema, which is more commonly suspected clinically, to more severe degrees of acute lung injury (ALI), which is less commonly reported in neonatal foals.

In regard to ALI, injury to the lung can originate from the epithelial (direct lung injury) or endothelial (indirect injury) side leading to loss of alveolar-capillary barrier integrity, neutrophil recruitment, surfactant dysfunction, and alveolar edema [103]. Direct lung injury can occur from pneumonia, pulmonary contusion, or inhalation injury whereas indirect lung injury occurs from sepsis or severe trauma [100, 104]. Thus, it must be noted that ALI occurs with sepsis, but other inciting causes exist. Lung injury secondary to sepsis in foals may manifest clinically as hypoxemia, in some instances despite supplemental oxygen, and/or hypercapnia. Of note, respiratory rate and lung auscultation can be normal despite pulmonary involvement, thus thoracic radiography, ultrasonography, and

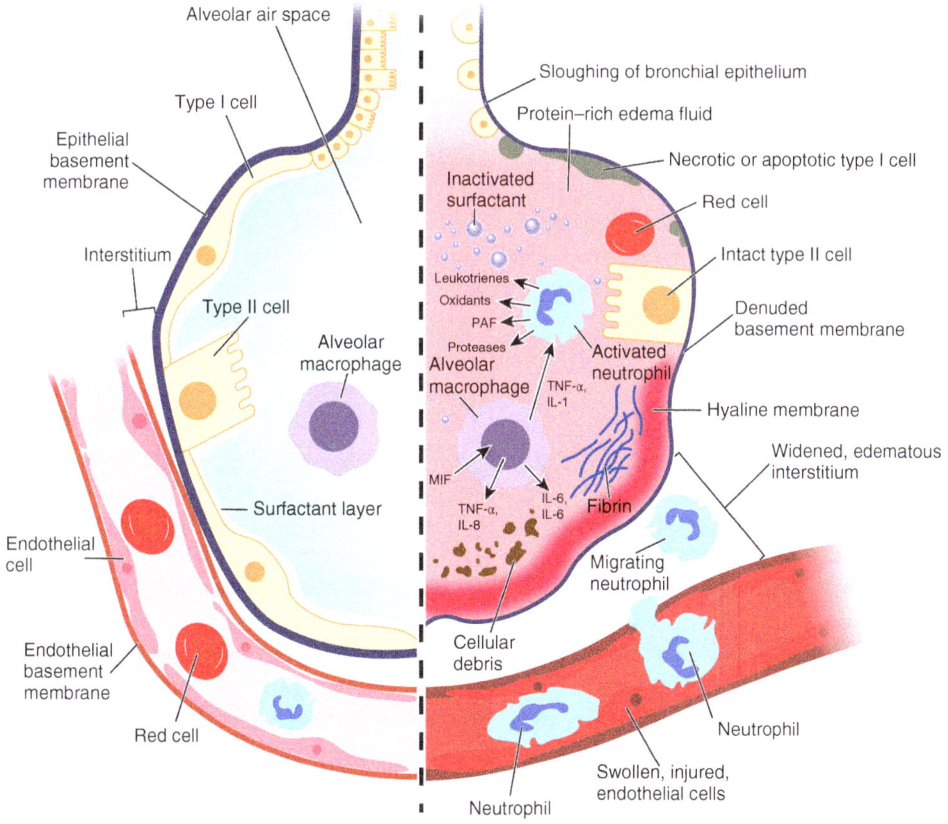

Figure 50.I.4 Schematic diagram of the healthy lung (left) and potential pathophysiologic mechanisms associated with the injured alveolus in the acute phase (right) of acute lung injury [102].

arterial blood gas analysis is needed to facilitate identification of lung pathology.

Acute Respiratory Distress Syndrome (ARDS)

Acute respiratory distress syndrome (ARDS) is the most severe form of ALI and is characterized by pulmonary inflammation causing diffuse alveolar damage and loss of the alveolar-capillary barrier leading to pulmonary edema, hypoxemia, and respiratory failure [104]. In people, ARDS is defined clinically by acute onset of hypoxemia accompanied by bilateral radiographic infiltrates consistent with pulmonary edema that cannot be explained by heart failure; a specific definition of ARDS has also been proposed in foals (Chapter 8) [100]. ALI and ARDS have been reported in older foals (1.5–8 months) presented for acute respiratory distress, tachycardia, tachypnea and radiographic findings consistent with ALI/ARDS definitions [105, 106]. However, neither syndrome has been well-documented in neonatal foals [107]. In regard to post-mortem findings of lung injury, in the aforementioned study involving 32 nonsurviving septic neonatal foals, 28% had thickened alveolar septae, 19% had patchy alveolar edema and hemorrhage, and 9% had intra-alveolar inflammatory cell infiltration [45]. Extensive diffuse fibrin deposition along the septae (16%), alveolar capillaries (60%), and alveolar fluid (16%) was also observed suggesting moderate frequency of pulmonary involvement in non-surviving septic foals [45].

Cardiovascular Injury

Hemodynamic alterations in the neonate occur in the context of incomplete myocardial and vascular development; therefore, cardiovascular responses targeted at restoring homeostasis are likely different than adult horses. Information regarding the neonatal cardiovascular system is still developing in infants, and even less is known in neonatal foals. Thus, much information regarding the foal's cardiovascular system is extrapolated from other species. In the neonate, basal contractility is near maximal levels with little contractile reserve, suggesting that the neonatal myocardium has nominal ability to respond to further cardiac demands [108]. Accordingly, in the euvolemic foal, heart rate (HR) is a primary determinant of cardiac output ($CO = SV \times HR$) as the neonate does not have the ability to significantly alter stroke volume (SV) [109]. Sepsis can impact the cardiovascular system in a number of ways including a pathologic decrease in vascular tone that contributes to circulatory compromise.

Decreased vascular tone is caused, at least in part, by cytokines that up-regulate the expression of iNOS in the vasculature [86]. Nitric oxide causes vascular smooth muscle relaxation via the secondary messenger cyclic guanosine monophosphate (cGMP) with dysregulated production of nitric oxide resulting in decreased SVR [86, 109, 110]. A concomitant decrease in perfusion pressure occurs resulting in hypotension despite normal or elevated cardiac output [110]. Concurrently, hypovolemia, which can arise from external or internal (edema formation) fluid losses, contributes to circulatory compromise [37]. In adult people, the hemodynamic hallmark of sepsis is generalized arterial vasodilation and decreased SVR, although two different manifestations of septic shock have been described: vasodilatory (warm) and vasoconstrictive (cold) shock [86, 110].

Warm (also called hyperdynamic) shock is characterized by high cardiac output and peripheral vasodilation whereas cold (also called hypodynamic) shock is typified by low cardiac output and peripheral vasoconstriction. Adult people with sepsis generally present with warm shock but up to 50% of pediatric patients present with cold shock [111]. Some pediatric patients do not benefit hemodynamically as much as adults from increased heart rate because their resting heart rates are higher than adults and tachycardia may not allow adequate diastolic filling; therefore, pediatric patients respond with vasoconstriction [111]. Both warm and cold shock can be seen in foals with sepsis. Differences in the type of shock exhibited may relate to different time points in which shock is clinically recognized, different hemodynamic responses to different pathogens, or age-related cardiovascular immaturity [110, 111].

Interestingly, an experimental sepsis model in healthy foals administered IV endotoxin reported increased mean values for SVR and peripheral vascular resistance (PVR) as well as increases in pulmonary artery pressure (PaP), pulmonary artery wedge pressure (PaW) and right atrial pressure (RaP) over baseline measurements [112]. The discordance between low SVR in people with septic shock as compared to high SVR in foals administered endotoxin may reflect the fact that experimental models do not completely mimic natural cases of sepsis. However, warm shock and hypotension have been described as a cause of inadequate tissue blood supply in septic foals with one particular case series describing the use of norepinephrine as a treatment for refractory hypotension in seven neonatal foals [43, 109, 113]. Septic foals likely have a continuum of changes in vascular tone and myocardial function depending on age, host response to various pathogens, genetic factors, as well as what time point veterinary intervention is first initiated [108]. Additionally, inflammatory cytokines such as TNF-α, IL-2, and IL-6 reduce the contractility of cardiac myocytes [109]. Myocardial evaluation of both systolic and diastolic echocardiographic parameters in people have demonstrated myocardial depression and dysfunction in septic patients that contribute to hypotension [109, 114]. As well, acute myocardial injury can be a component of sepsis in foals as demonstrated by higher cardiac troponin T (cTnT) and cardiac isoenzyme of creatine kinase (CKMB) concentrations in septic foals when compared to healthy counterparts along with anecdotal reports of mild to moderate ventricular dilation and hypo-contraction in septic foals [109, 115]. Many of the clinical findings of cardiovascular compromise in septic foals overlap with other organ dysfunction and disease processes but clinical observations include tachycardia, weak pulses, cold extremities, low blood pressure, decreased urine output and elevated blood L-lactate [113].

GI Tract Injury

The exact manner in which the GI tract is impacted by sepsis is incompletely understood and various hypotheses have been proposed on how the gut might be involved in sepsis-associated organ dysfunction. One theory suggests sepsis alters gut permeability and mucosal integrity allowing bacterial translocation through the gut wall and into the portal circulation whereas another theory proposes that toxic mediators are released from injured gut mucosa and are transported to the mesenteric lymph nodes and cause organ dysfunction [37, 116, 117]. A more recent theory suggests that the intestinal microbiome plays a role in critical illness. In health, the gut microbiome plays an important role in maintaining immune homeostasis in the systemic environment [118]. For example, gut commensals and their derived products (PAMPs, short-chain fatty acids) modulate the immune system at distant organs by priming the innate immune system, influencing the cytokine response to infection, and enhancing neutrophil function [86, 118]. In contrast, septic patients have profoundly altered intestinal microbiome (dysbiosis) due to hypoxic injury, inflammation, intestinal dysmotility, disrupted epithelial integrity, shifts in intraluminal pH values and secondary to treatment with antibiotics, vasopressors, parenteral feedings, proton-pump inhibitors, and opioids, among others [118]. This sepsis-induced dysbiosis may negatively impact patients through immunosuppression, altered immune responses and other undefined mechanisms. Minimal information is known regarding the neonatal foal's gut microbiome as it relates to critical illness. Clinically, diarrhea is a relatively common early localizing sign of GI involvement in foals with sepsis and no other evidence of enteric pathogens [11, 55]. In studies that mimic sepsis in foals (via IV administration of endotoxin), colic and diarrhea are consistently observed [112, 119] and in a clinical study of neonatal foals presented with a primary complaint of diarrhea, 49.6% (66/133) of foals were bacteremic with the most common blood culture isolate being *Enterococcus* spp. (29.3% of diarrheic foals) [44]. Other clinical signs in septic neonatal foals that point to GI involvement include GI dysmotility characterized by ileus, intestinal distension, gastric reflux or intolerance to feeding [44, 55, 67].

Experimental endotoxin studies in adult horses have documented dramatic cessation and altered function of intestinal smooth muscle which can manifest clinically as ileus and intestinal distention in septic foals [120]. Moreover, necropsy findings in experimental endotoxin studies in horses have shown edematous thickening of the intestine along with congestion, scattered petechiae and ecchymoses of the serosa and mucosa; these post-mortem findings have been observed in septic foals (Figure 50.I.5) [120]. Microscopic changes observed in experimental endotoxin studies include edematous degeneration and coagulation necrosis of smooth muscle cells in the intestinal muscularis with electron microscopy revealing disruption of intercellular gap junctions and nexuses in intestinal smooth muscle, implying decreased or absent electrical transmission of intestinal electrical impulses might contribute to intestinal dysmotility [120].

Hypothalamic-Pituitary-Adrenal Axis (HPAA)

The hypothalamic-pituitary-adrenal axis (HPAA) plays an important role in maintaining water homeostasis along with cardiovascular, immunologic, and metabolic functions and is the primary neuroendocrine pathway mediating host responses to the stress of infection [49, 121]. The prototypical endocrine response to stress (e.g. sepsis) and inflammatory cytokines is secretion of corticotropin-releasing hormone (CRH) from the hypothalamus which in turn stimulates the adenohypophysis to release adrenocorticotropic hormone (ACTH). ACTH stimulates the adrenal cortex to produce and release cortisol. In septic foals, inflammatory cytokines (IL-1, IL-6, TNF-α) are strong stimulators of the HPAA which initially acts to increase blood cortisol [49, 121, 122]. However, prolonged stimulation of the HPAA may blunt or exhaust the HPAA. Historically, investigations have focused on dysfunction of the HPAA along with inappropriately low secretion or activity of cortisol in septic infants and foals with terms such as relative adrenal insufficiency (RAI) and critical-illness related corticosteroid insufficiency (CIRCI) being used [48, 121–123]. Adrenal exhaustion may manifest grossly and microscopically as hemorrhagic adrenal glands in some foals that succumb to sepsis (Figure 50.I.6).

More recently, ACTH-cortisol dissociation (ACD; low ACTH and high cortisol) has been proposed, as impaired cortisol metabolism may raise peripheral cortisol concentrations and suppress ACTH secretion [124]. In addition, other HPAA-related hormones such as pregnenolone, progesterone, aldosterone, vasopressin, and dehyroepiandrosterone sulfate (DHEAS) have been measured in septic foals as these hormones are also released with HPAA activation [122]. In a study of 326 foals, septic foals ($n = 134$) had significantly higher median concentrations of ACTH, cortisol, aldosterone, 17α-OH-progesterone, and DHEAS when compared to

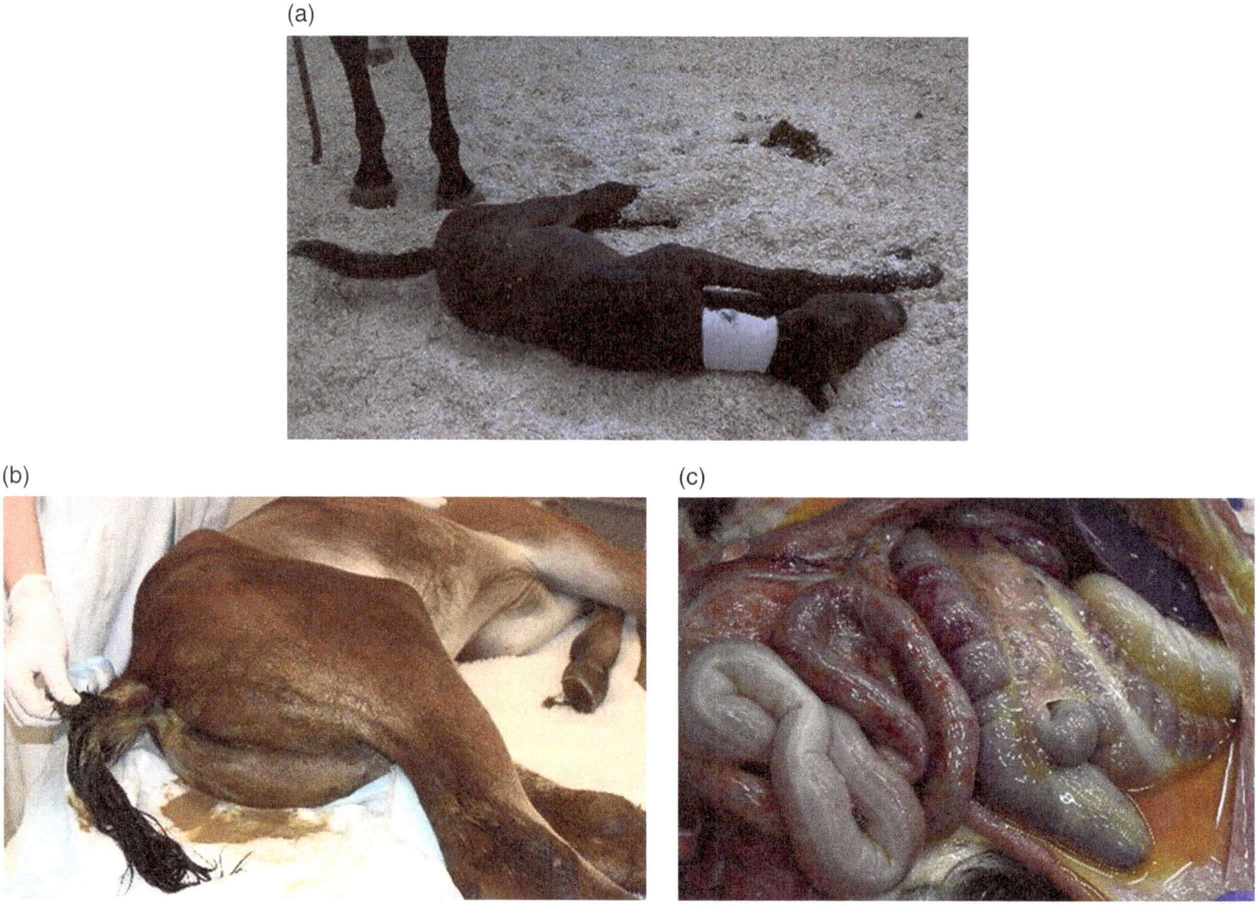

Figure 50.I.5 (a) Septic foal with intermittent colic. (b) Diarrhea secondary to sepsis in a neonatal foal. (c) Scattered petechiae and ecchymoses on the serosal surface of the intestinal tract in a foal with severe sepsis.

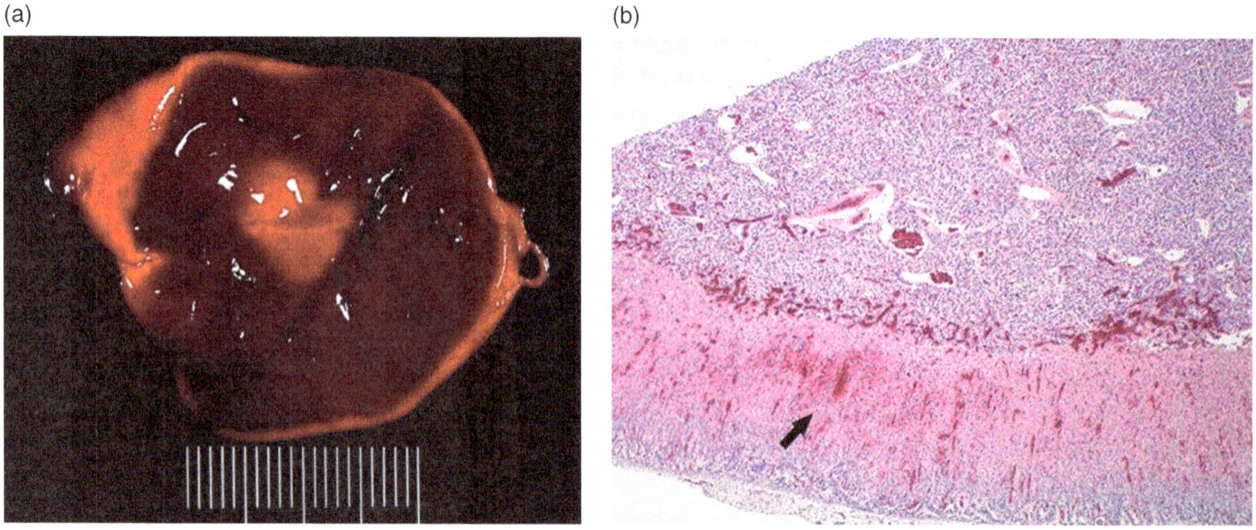

Figure 50.I.6 (a) Gross appearance of a hemorrhagic adrenal gland from a foal that died from severe sepsis. (b) Low-power microscopic image of an adrenal gland from a septic foal demonstrating hemorrhage within the adrenal cortex. *Source:* Images courtesy of Dr. Katarzyna A. Dembek (North Carolina State University) and Dr. Rebecca Ruby (University of Kentucky).

sick non-septic ($n = 128$) and healthy ($n = 64$) foals indicating an appropriate response to sepsis in the majority of septic foals [122]. However, 24 septic and sick-nonseptic foals had ACTH-cortisol imbalance consistent with reduced steroid synthesis suggesting that some foals have HPAA dysfunction and do not have appropriate hormonal stress responses to critical illness [122]. Similar findings were noted in another study in that ACTH and cortisol concentrations were significantly higher in septic foals (median cortisol 72.6 ng/ml) as compared to sick-nonseptic (36 ng/ml) and healthy (8.6 ng/ml) foals [125]. It is likely that most septic foals are able to mount a proper HPAA response with elevated concentrations of cortisol and other related hormones, but a small subset of septic foals have HPAA dysfunction that contributes to morbidity and mortality [122, 125, 126].

Another endocrine system impacted by sepsis in foals is related to energy metabolism and includes insulin, glucagon, and glucose. Insulin increases cellular glucose uptake, glycogenesis, and fatty acid synthesis and decreases proteolysis, lipolysis and gluconeogenesis whereas glucagon has the opposite actions including gluconeogenesis, glycogenolysis, and lipolysis [84]. In a study of 44 septic, 62 sick-nonseptic, and 19 healthy neonatal foals, ill (septic and sick-nonseptic) foals had significantly lower insulin and higher triglyceride concentrations when compared to healthy foals suggesting that ill foals have an appropriate metabolic response to decreased energy intake [84]. The only variable that was significantly higher in septic foals, compared to healthy and sick non-septic foals, was glucagon concentrations. This was interpreted as an appropriate physiologic response as glucagon is a catabolic hormone that stimulates gluconeogenesis [84]. Despite these investigations, a good degree of uncertainty remains regarding endocrine function in septic patients.

Diagnosis of Sepsis

Outside of clinical intuition, the main diagnostic tools available for identifying septic foals are blood cultures and the equine sepsis score. The diagnosis of sepsis has always been beset by the fact that the gold standard for identifying sepsis, positive blood culture, has questionable sensitivity. However, blood cultures have the advantage of isolating specific microorganisms and providing valuable information regarding invading organism's antimicrobial susceptibility.

Blood Culture

Factors that influence recovery of pathogens from blood include timing of blood collection, number of blood culture sets collected, and amount of blood sampled [127]. Historically, it was recommended to collect blood samples for culture at the time of a febrile episode, however, studies have not found a significant association between enhanced recovery of bacteria and collection of samples when the patient is febrile [127]. At least two sets of blood cultures (two bottles per set: one aerobic and one anaerobic) should be obtained, and when possible from different sites, as single set blood cultures are associated with a lower sensitivity to detect bacteremia [128]. More than one set of blood cultures may also help differentiate bacterial contaminants when only one bottle is positive, from clinically relevant pathogens. As an example, a large retrospective study in people evaluated 112,570 blood culture sets and noted a significantly higher number of culture positive results were obtained when two sets of samples were collected (10.9%) as compared to single sets (6.5%) [128]. Although not always practical in equine medicine, recovery of bacteria might be improved by collecting three to four blood culture sets over a 24-hour period based on studies in people [129, 130]. In a study in people in which ≥ 3 blood cultures were obtained, 73.1% of blood stream infections were detected with the first blood culture, 89.7% with the first two blood cultures, 98.2% with the first three blood cultures and 99.8% when evaluating four blood cultures [129]. Another finding in this study was that certain pathogens, in this case *Staphylococcus aureus*, was detected in the first blood culture in 90% of cases whereas *Pseudomonas aeruginosa* bacteremia was only detected 60% of the time on the first blood culture suggesting that some organisms may be more difficult to detect [129]. If multiple samples are collected, they are ideally collected one to several (6–36) hours apart, but it is appropriate to obtain blood from 2 separate sites within minutes of each other from patients who are acutely ill and have a high likelihood of continuous bacteremia [130]. It is best if blood culture samples are collected prior to antimicrobial administration, but antimicrobials should not be delayed more than 45 minutes just to obtain initial or additional samples [131]. Equine clinicians are typically not restricted by the amount of blood they can practically collect from neonatal foals and should follow the recommendation for adult people of 10 ml of blood for each blood culture bottle (20 ml per set) [130]. Antimicrobial administration to foals prior to blood culture collection can decrease the likelihood of identifying causative bacteria, as demonstrated in one retrospective study in which the proportion of foals with positive blood culture was significantly lower in foals treated with antimicrobials prior to admission (36.6% positive blood culture) compared to foals not treated with antimicrobials prior to admission (44.4%), but this should not deter clinicians from submitting blood cultures [132]. Antibiotic-neutralizing substances such as charcoal or antibiotic-binding resin beads are added to commercial blood culture bottles and a number of retrospective studies have noted positive growth despite antimicrobial administration prior to blood collection [63, 132, 133]. In another retrospective study, 36.6% (94 of 257) of foals treated with antimicrobials prior to admission had a positive blood culture which was significantly lower than foals that were not treated with antimicrobials prior to admission (44.4%; 359 of 808) [132]. Smaller studies have ranged from 43% (9/21) to 91% (10/11) of blood culture positive foals that received antimicrobials prior to referral [63, 133].

In a different equine study, blood cultures were collected from neonatal foals at the time of admission and after ≥48 hours of hospitalization and antimicrobial treatment. Of the 267 septic foals, 51 had positive cultures after ≥48 hours of hospitalization; 21/51 foals had positive cultures at admission and after ≥48 hours hospitalization whereas 30 foals hand negative cultures at admission, but positive cultures after ≥48 hours of hospitalization [134]. *Escherichia coli* was isolated most frequently from samples collected at hospital admission; in comparison, there were much higher odds of culturing *Acinetobacter, Enterococcus, Klebsiella, Psuedomonas*, and *Serratia* after ≥48 hours hospitalization. Bacterial isolates after ≥48 hours of hospitalization were less susceptible to antimicrobial drugs and combinations compared to those isolated at admission [134]. This study suggests that antimicrobial resistance can develop in small percentage of septic foals and that repeat bacterial blood culture may be indicated in ill/septic foals that do not appear to be recovering despite antimicrobial therapy.

The exact incidence of sepsis and sensitivity of blood culture is unknown in foals, but a few studies have examined this topic. In one study, sepsis was confirmed in foals by results of ante-mortem culture of blood or joint fluid samples or culture of necropsy specimens of internal organs [135]. In that study, 47 foals were confirmed to be septic where 38/47 (81%) had positive blood culture results with a false negative blood culture rate of 19%; another study reported 12% false-negative blood culture results [135, 136]. Other retrospective studies reveal an incidence of positive bacterial growth of blood samples in neonatal foals ranging from 25 to 50% of samples submitted from foals presented to various veterinary hospitals (Table 50.I.3). A wide variety of bacterial isolates have been identified in retrospective studies with *E. coli* being the most frequent pathogen isolated in a number of studies. In one analysis, the 6 most prevalent isolates identified from blood cultures from neonatal foals, in descending order, included *E. coli, Actinobacillus, Enterobacter, Enterococcus, Streptococcus*, and *Klebsiella* [145].

Sepsis Score

In contrast to blood cultures, the original equine *sepsis score* was developed in the 1980s as an adjunctive method to blood culture to provide clinicians a rapid tool to predict the likelihood of sepsis in foals [146, 147]. This scoring system utilizes subjective clinical criteria and objective clinicopathologic data and assigns a number for each criterion [146, 147]. Points are summated with the original cut-point to predict sepsis of >11 [146, 147]. Subsequently a modified sepsis score was proposed that eliminated some variables (e.g. metabolic acidosis, P_aO_2) to make the system more practical [92]. Retrospective analysis of the modified sepsis score demonstrated good sensitivity (94%) and specificity (86%), but more recent evaluations have yielded lower sensitivity (56–74%) and specificity (52–76%), suggesting that score cut-points might be hospital-dependent [138, 147–150]. An updated sepsis score was more recently evaluated and incorporated the SIRS criteria as well as commonly available blood parameters such as L-lactate, glucose, creatinine, and lymphocyte count; inclusion of these parameters did not significantly improve the scoring systems sensitivity or specificity [138].

Treatment of Sepsis

The therapeutic approach to septic foals is quite variable based on severity of illness, degree of sepsis-associated complications, clinician preference, and financial resources available. Baseline assessment of the foal includes measurement of heart rate, respiratory rate, rectal temperature, capillary refill time, evaluation of mucous membrane color, peripheral (limb) perfusion, umbilical structures, presence or absence of rib fractures and assessment of blood L-lactate, blood glucose, packed cell volume (PCV), total protein, serum IgG (if >12 hours old) and indirect blood pressure. A complete blood count and biochemistry profile is indicated and an arterial blood gas analysis and blood culture should be performed, if available. Clinical improvement and response to therapy is assessed by re-evaluation of aforementioned parameters. Cornerstones of treatment include elimination of infection, hemodynamic stabilization to ensure adequate microcirculatory perfusion, and supportive and nursing care.

Elimination of Infection

Several antimicrobials, alone or in combination, are used to target the diversity of bacteria encountered in equine neonatal sepsis. Foals have a wider availability of antimicrobials compared to adults as they are not yet hindgut fermenters and thus, antimicrobials that cause colitis in adult

Table 50.I.3 Incidence of positive bacterial growth in blood cultured from various studies examining sepsis in the foal.

Inclusion criteria for study	Blood culture positive	Median age at presentation (range)	Single organism isolated	Multiple organisms isolated	Gram negative isolates	Gram positive isolates	Most common bacterial isolate	Overall survival	Reference
All foals <14 d age admitted to hospital and blood culture done	143/429 (33%)	2.7 d (mean)	112/143 (78%)	31/143 (22%)	88/178 (49%)	90/178 (51%)	*Escherichia coli* (17%)	110/141 (78%) Septic foals only	Furr [137] 2020
All foals admitted to hospital with IV catheter	11/43 (25.6%)	9.4 d (mean) (1–146 d)	7/11 (64%)	4/11 (36%)	4/16 (25%)	12/16 (75%)	*Staphylococcus* spp. *(50%)*	30/43 (69.7%)	Fouche [134] 2018
All foals admitted to ICU <30 d age	112/273 (41%)	12 h (birth-22 d)	92/112 (82%)	20/112 (18%)	71/135 (53%)	63/135 (47%)	*E. coli* (11.2%)	217/273 (79.5%)	Wong [138] 2018
Foals <30 d age admitted with diagnosis of umbilical infection	11/19 (57.8%)	Not reported (1–30 d)	11/11 (100%)	0/11 (0%)	8/11 (73%)	3/11 (27%)	*E. coli* (45%)	31/40 (77.5%)	Rampacci [139] 2017
7 healthy Quarter Horse foals	4/7 (57%)	Not applicable (0–72 h)	8/9 (89%)	1/9 (11%)	0/9 (0%)	9/9 (100%)	*Bacillus* spp. *(67%)*	7/7 (100%)	Hackett [140] 2015
All medically compromised foals	22/50 (44%)	2 d (hours-42 d)	18/22 (82%)	4/22 (18%)	12/22 (54.5%)	6/22 (27.3%)	*E. coli* (33.3%)	26/50 (52%)	Hytychova [63] 2015
Neonates with diarrhea <30 d age	66/133 (49.6%)	4 d (0–30 d)	57/66 (86%)	9/66 (14%)	43/75 (57%)	32/75 (43%)	*Enterococcus* spp. (29.3%)	100/127 (78.7%)	Hollis [44] 2008
All foals admitted to ICU <7 d age	110/427 (25.8%)	Not reported	97/110 (88%)	13/110 (12%)	71/124 (57%)	50/124 (40%)	*E. coli* (31.4%)	344/427 (80.6%)	Russell [141] 2008
All foals presented to ICU with bacteremia	423/423 (100%)	Not reported	Not reported	Not reported	375/554 (68%)	145/554 (26%)	*E. coli* (31%)	254/423 (60%) Septic foals only	Sanchez [142] 2008
Only foals <10 d of age with positive blood culture	85/85 (100%)	40 h (birth-10 d)	66/85 (78%)	19/85 (22%)	81/109 (74%)	23/109 (21%)	*E. coli* (44%)	57/85(67%) Septic foals only	Corley [68] 2007
All foals with positive blood culture	101/101 (100%)	48 h (birth-113 d)	71/101 (70%)	30/101 (30%)	64/101 (64%)	30/101 (30%)	*E. coli* (39%)	56/101 (55%) Septic foals only	Stewart [65] 2002

(*Continued*)

Table 50.I.3 (Continued)

Inclusion criteria for study	Blood culture positive	Median age at presentation (range)	Single organism isolated	Multiple organisms isolated	Gram negative isolates	Gram positive isolates	Most common bacterial isolate	Overall survival	Reference
All foals admitted to neonatal ICU <30 d age	155/543 (28.5%)	Not reported	145/174 (83%)	26/174 (15%)	96/145 (66%)	49/145 (34%)	*E. coli* (6.6%)	Not reported	Marsh [143] 2001
All foals diagnosed with sepsis <4 wk of age	29/35 (82.8%)	Not reported (1–11 d)	16/29 (55%)	13/29 (45%)	24/29 (83%)	2/29 (7%)	*E. coli* (30%)	29/65 (45%)	Gayle [101] 1998
Only foals <14 d of age with positive blood culture	24/24 (100%)	3.2 d (0–7 d)	Not reported	Not reported	22/24 (92%)	2/24 (8%)	*E. coli* (50%)	17/24 (71%) Septic foals only	Raisis [144] 1996
Only foals ≤7 d of age with positive blood or tissue culture	27/105 (25.7%)	Not Reported (0–7 d)	25/27 (93%)	2/27 (7%)	25/27 (93%)	2/27 (7%)	*E. coli* (56%)	7/27 (26%) Septic foals only	Koterba [66] 1984

horses do not carry similar risk in foals. In addition, some antimicrobials are cost-prohibitive because of the size of adult horses, whereas foals do not have this limitation.

Of note, neonatal foals have a higher percentage of body mass comprised of water compared to adult horses, therefore dosages are typically higher [113, 151]. Ideally, first-choice antimicrobials should be bactericidal and broad spectrum as septic foals have a less robust immune system, are often neutropenic, and blood culture results are not immediately available or may have not been performed [145]. The IV route of administration is preferred as intestinal and muscle perfusion may be reduced thereby decreasing bioavailability of drugs administered orally or intramuscularly [145]. The combination of a beta-lactam antimicrobial (e.g. ampicillin, potassium penicillin, ceftiofur) and an aminoglycoside (e.g. amikacin or gentamicin) is commonly used with the combination of ampicillin and amikacin yielding the highest percentage (91.5%) of susceptible isolates in one study of 306 bacterial isolates cultured from the blood of 213 foals [152]. Other drug combinations with a high percentage of susceptible bacterial isolates included ceftiofur and amikacin (89.6%) and penicillin and amikacin (88.6%). The combination of penicillin and gentamicin, commonly used in adults, yielded an 82% susceptibility rate to bacterial isolates [152]. IV antimicrobials should be administered as soon as possible as each hour delay in administration has been associated with increased mortality in septic people [132]. Antimicrobials should be administered IV for the first 7–10 days with de-escalation of antimicrobials based on susceptibility testing, if possible. De-escalation involves evaluating if the empiric antibiotic(s) that were started initially can be reduced in number and/or narrowed in spectrum thus facilitating antimicrobial stewardship programs [132, 153]. Typically, oral or intramuscular antibiotics should be administered for another 7–10 days after IV antimicrobials are discontinued to lengthen the duration of antimicrobial therapy and lessen the chance of complications of sepsis (e.g. septic umbilical structure, septic arthritis). Some antimicrobials used in foals are noted in Table 50.I.4 and Chapter 61.

Hemodynamic Stabilization

Hemodynamic stabilization is another central tenet of treatment. Oxygen delivery (DO_2) to the vascular beds is dependent on cardiac output (CO) and arterial oxygen concentration (CaO_2), expressed as: $DO_2 = CO \times CaO_2$. In most clinical situations, IV fluid therapy is the first step in increasing blood flow and oxygen delivery to the body. Improving circulating blood volume increases the venous return to the heart thereby increasing stroke volume (SV) and consequently CO. Thus, an IV jugular catheter is vital to treat foals in need of fluid resuscitation and should be aseptically placed upon initial examination, if deemed necessary. IV boluses of isotonic fluids with a normal strong ion difference at a dose of 20 mg/kg (1 l in 50 kg foal) over 10–20 minutes is used in foals with hypovolemia from sepsis, high-volume diarrhea, or acute hemorrhage [154]. Administration of large volumes of fluids with no strong ion difference (e.g. saline) have an acidifying effect and should be avoided [154]. After each bolus, perfusion parameters should be reevaluated with warmer limbs and improved pulse quality, heart rate, mental status, urine production, blood L-lactate, and arterial blood pressure suggesting improved hemodynamics.

Measurement of indirect arterial blood pressure is readily available and is an important parameter used to monitor hemodynamic status of foals. MAP is the driving pressure of tissue perfusion; if MAP falls below 60 mmHg, tissue perfusion becomes linearly dependent on arterial pressure [132]. Indirect assessment of mean and diastolic blood pressure can be accurately measured in foals using the coccygeal or metatarsal artery and the oscillometric method with a targeted MAP for adequate tissue perfusion of ≥60–65 mmHg [113, 132, 155]. Indirect MAP is also correlated with blood L-lactate with one study noting that all foals with a MAP ≤60 mmHg had a L-lactate concentration of >7 mmol/l. [156] Repeat fluid boluses can be administered, if necessary, up to a total of 60–80 ml/kg; if perfusion parameters are still not improved, vasoactive medications are indicated [154]. To this point, sepsis can be a problem of vascular capacitance rather than true hypovolemia, thus restoring vascular tone with vasopressors in addition to fluid resuscitation may prove to be more effective at restoring circulating volume in some foals [67]. Once hemodynamic stability and adequate blood perfusion is achieved, maintenance fluid therapy can be instituted (Chapter 62).

If a hospitalized septic foal appears adequately hydrated while receiving maintenance IV fluids, yet develops hypotension during the course of treatment, administering an IV fluid bolus challenge with crystalloid fluids (2–3 ml/kg) can help determine if the foal is hypovolemic [113]. If MAP and other hemodynamic parameters improve after the bolus, the IV maintenance fluid rate may need to be increased; conversely, if hypotension persists despite the fluid challenge, vasoactive medications may be indicated. A number of vasoactive agents, indications for use, and mechanisms of action are described in Chapter 11. In brief, the main agents used are inotropes, such as dobutamine, dopamine, and epinephrine, which increase CO primarily by increasing stroke volume, and vasopressors such as norepinephrine, dopamine, and vasopressin, which increase blood pressure via direct arteriolar vasoconstriction [109].

The use of vasoactive medications must be tailored to individual foals, and frequent reassessment is necessary to gauge response. In general, vasopressors increase cardiac afterload and can therefore decrease CO; thus, it is safer to

Table 50.I.4 Antimicrobial doses and routes of administration used in neonatal foals. See also Chapter 61.

Drug	Dosage	Route/frequency	Comment
Penicillins			
Ampicillin	22–30 mg/kg	IV or PO, q6–8h	Oral pivampicillin 19.9 mg/kg
Amoxicillin	13–30 mg/kg	PO, q8h	
Amoxicillin-clavulanic acid	10–30 mg/kg	PO, q6–8h	
Penicillin (potassium or sodium)	22 000–44 000 IU/kg	IV q6h	Infuse slowly
Ticarcillin-clavulanic acid	50 mg/kg	IV, q6h	Slow and dilute infusion
Imipenem	15 mg/kg	IV, q6–8h	Use only when culture dictated
Meropenem	15 mg/kg	IV, q6h	Use only when culture dictated
First-generation cephalosporins			
Cefazolin	15–22 mg/kg	IV, q6–8h	
Cephalothin	10–20 mg/kg	IV, q6h	
Cefadroxil	20–40 mg/kg	PO, q8–12h	
Cephalexin	25 mg/kg 30 mg/kg	PO q6h PO q8h	
Second-generation cephalosporins			
Cefuroxime Na	16–33 mg/kg	IV, q8h	
Cefoxitin	20 mg/kg	IV q6h	
Third-generation cephalosporins			
Ceftazidime	20–50 mg/kg	IV q6h	Slow infusion; Crosses BBB
Cefoperazone	30 mg/kg	IV q8h	Slow infusion
Cefotaxime	40–50 mg/kg	IV q6h	Slow infusion, Crosses BBB
Cefotaxime CRI	40 mg/kg loading dose, then 6.7 mg/kg/h	IV, CRI	Can go up to 8.3 mg/kg/h
Ceftizoxime	20–50 mg/kg	IV, q6h	Slow infusion
Cefpodoxime proxetil	10 mg/kg	PO, q6–8–12h	q6h for *Escherichia coli*
Ceftriaxone	25–50 mg/kg	IV, q12h	Crosses BBB
Ceftiofur	5–10 mg/kg	IV, SC, IM q6–12h	High doses given slowly
Ceftiofur CRI	5 mg/kg loading dose, then 0.42 mg/kg/h	IV, CRI	Can double the dose depending on MIC
Fourth-generation cephalosporins			
Cefepime	11 mg/kg	IV, q8h	Crosses BBB
Cefquinome	1 mg/kg	IV or IM, q12h	2.5 mg/kg q6–8 has been used
Aminoglycosides			
Amikacin	25 mg/kg	IV, q 24 h	TDM recommended
Gentamicin	8–16 mg/kg	IV, q 24 h	TDM recommended
Other Antimicrobials for foals			
Erythromycin	20–30 mg/kg	PO, q6h	
Azithromycin	10 mg/kg	PO, q24h; q48h after 5 d	Keep foal out of sunlight/heat
Clarithromycin	7.5 mg/kg	PO, q12h	Keep foal out of sunlight/heat
Chloramphenicol	40–50 mg/kg	PO, q12h days 1–2 of age; q8h days 3–5 of age	
Doxycycline	10 mg/kg	PO, q12h	May cause tendon laxity
Minocycline	4 mg/kg	PO, q12h	
Rifampin	5 mg/kg	PO, q12h	
Metronidazole	10 mg/kg	PO or IV, q8–12h for 1st 2 wk	
Trimethoprim-sulfonamide	25–30 mg/kg	PO, q12h	

BBB, blood brain barrier; TDM, therapeutic drug monitoring.

start with inotropes unless the clinician has the ability to measure CO. [109] Dobutamine at a dose of 1–5 μg/kg/min (up to 20 g/kg/min) diluted in isotonic saline, 5% dextrose or Lactated Ringer's solution, is a good first-line inotrope for foals [67, 109]. If hypotension persists despite inotropes and appropriate fluid therapy, vasopressors such as norepinephrine can be titrated from a starting dose of 0.1 μg/kg/min, up to 1.5 μg/kg/min [43, 109]. Of note, sepsis may cause a reduced response to vasopressor therapy such as administration of norepinephrine due, in part to, the potent vasodilatory effects of nitric oxide [86].

Supportive and Nursing Care

Transfer of Passive Immunity (TPI)

Another therapeutic component of infection control is assurance of adequate transfer of passive immunity (TPI). If the foal is <18 hours old (preferably <12 hours old), oral administration of quality colostrum is ideal if the serum IgG is <800 mg/dl. A retrospective study reexamined the cut-off values of TPI and its relationship to foal survival and confirmed that foals with the time-honored value of >800 mg/dl had a higher likelihood of survival as compared to foals with IgG values <800 mg/dl [157]. Outside the obvious benefit of IgG antibodies, mare's colostrum contains cytokines such as IL-4, IL-6, IL-8, IFN-γ, and TNF-α as well as other growth factors that are passed to the foal and enhance the activity and efficiency of the neonatal immune system [40, 62, 158, 159]. If the foal is beyond the age in which colostrum can be absorbed via the intestine, IV administration of approximately 1–3 l of plasma is needed to sufficiently raise the serum IgG in a 50 kg foal. Plasma provides critical antibodies as well as complement and coagulation factors and also helps increase the oncotic pressure thereby facilitating improved circulating blood volume that may be compromised in septic foals.

An additional benefit of TPI, via colostrum or plasma administration, is the provision of opsonins (i.e. immunoglobulins, complement proteins, secreted PRR) that facilitate phagocytosis of pathogens. These opsonins are consumed in sepsis, with one study noting that foals with sepsis had lower phagocytic function compared to healthy foals, likely impacting the ability to kill pathogens [160]. Interestingly, IV administration of plasma to foals improved their opsonization capacity and in one study, administration of plasma to septic foals at admission increased probability of survival [101, 160, 161]. Therefore, IV plasma transfusions may play a role in treatment of septic foals, regardless of IgG concentration at admission [160].

Although IgG may be >800 mg/dl upon admission, serum IgG concentrations may decrease over a shorter than natural time frame in foals with sepsis due to opsonization of bacteria, protein (e.g. IgG) loss across compromised vasculature, and protein catabolism due to negative energy balance [162]. Consideration should be made to rechecking serum IgG concentrations during the course of treatment. The type of equine plasma to administer to foals is still debatable as the benefits of the use of commercial equine plasma that is rich in anti-endotoxin antibodies is not certain. One study documented greater survival in septic foals that received plasma rich in anti-endotoxin antibodies (survival rate 68%) as compared to standard hyperimmune equine plasma (survival rate 52%) [150], but a separate study did not identify any survival benefit with anti-endotoxin antibodies [163]. In generally, most clinicians use standard hyperimmune equine plasma in foals.

Prophylactic Treatment

Abnormal coagulation parameters are not uncommon in septic foals but specific treatment protocols for coagulopathies in foals with sepsis have not been established. Randomized controlled trials related to prophylactic fresh frozen plasma transfusion in septic people with coagulation abnormalities are not available and the current recommendation in people is to treat septic patients with abnormal coagulation tests with fresh frozen plasma only if active bleeding is present [132]. Based on this, continued clinical and hemostatic monitoring is suggested for septic foals that have alterations in coagulation parameters with no clinical evidence of bleeding. Interestingly, one study noted no significant differences in coagulation parameters between septic foals treated with isotonic fluids and those treated with plasma [73].

Likewise, no uniform recommendations are available for treatment of more severe coagulopathies such as DIC [73, 80]. The pathogenesis of DIC is reviewed elsewhere, but in brief, DIC can be described as widespread activation of the coagulation system, secondary to conditions such as sepsis, colitis or endotoxemia, resulting in a procoagulant state with subsequent production of fibrin and micro-thrombi formation of blood vessels [164, 165]. Spontaneous diffuse hemorrhage throughout the body may also occur, resulting from the consumption and depletion of platelets and coagulation factors. Consequently, DIC is a continuum between diffuse thrombosis and hemorrhage with clinical signs varying and dependent on which system, coagulation or fibrinolysis, dominates. Treatment of the primary disorder is indicated in DIC, but heparin has been used in some instances to help prevent microthrombi formation and resultant obstruction of microvasculature that can cause organ dysfunction or failure. The use of heparin is controversial in both human and veterinary medicine, but the rationale for its use during DIC stems from its ability to inactivate thrombin and factor Xa and XIa, which theoretically prevents further conversion of fibrinogen to fibrin, thus reducing microthrombus formation [166, 167].

Table 50.I.5 Mean ± SD arterial blood gas and tracheal variables in nine healthy neonatal foals breathing room air (baseline) and during administration of supplemental humidified oxygen at various flow rates from unilateral and bilateral nasal cannulae [171].

		Unilateral supplemental O_2 (ml/kg/min)				Bilateral supplemental O_2 (ml/kg/min)			
Variable	Baseline	50	100	150	200	50	100	150	200
FiO_2 (%)	18±0.7	23±1.4	30.9±2.1	44.2±5.8	52.6±8.3	30.9±2.6	48.7±6.2	56.5±3.4	74.6±4.2
P_aO_2 (mmHg)	92.5±8.2	135.9±13.2	175.2±14	219.6±31.9	269.7±40.8	174.3±26.8	261.2±38.3	307.8±41	374.2±58.2
P_aCO_2 (mmHg)	47.7±2.8	49.7±2.4	50.5±2.3	50.1±2.8	51.3±3.1	55.6±2.8	55.3±6.0	55.2±5.1	55.3±4.8

A specific directive in regard to when to administer (or if it should even be administered) heparin in septic foals cannot be recommended, but if the clinician chooses to use heparin, a dose of 100 IU/kg of low molecular weight heparin, administered once daily subcutaneously has been shown to reach therapeutic concentrations in healthy and septic neonatal foals [168]. Heparin therapy can also be considered to prevent the occurrence or progression of phlebitis or thrombophlebitis that can occur secondary to neonatal sepsis in foals, but it will not dissolve existing thrombi [78, 169, 170]. Systemic coagulopathies, injury to the vascular endothelium (i.e. IV catheterization, repeated venipuncture), type of catheter material, type(s) of IV medications administered and blood stasis help fulfill Virchow's triad and predispose septic foals to thrombophlebitis [169, 170]. Removal of IV catheters, avoidance of venipuncture and topical anti-inflammatory salves are other methods of treating thrombophlebitis [170]. Thrombosis of central and larger peripheral vessels is a particularly devastating complication of sepsis in foals and warrants a guarded to poor prognosis [75, 169]. Although thrombolytic agents such as tissue plasminogen activator have been used in foals with vessel thrombosis with variable success, aggressive treatment of the primary disease coupled with prophylactic administration of anticoagulants such as aspirin or heparin may help prevent vessel thrombosis, but identifying foals at high risk of thrombosis and defining specific criteria for when to administer anticoagulants is unknown in foals [75, 169].

Respiratory compromise is not infrequent in septic foals and arterial blood gas analysis helps identify and characterize pulmonary involvement. General principles of respiratory support in septic neonatal foals include maintaining recumbent foals in a sternal position to prevent atelectasis in the dependent lung and administration of intranasal oxygen if hypoxemia is detected (i.e. partial pressure of oxygen [P_aO_2] <80 mmHg). Intranasal oxygen will optimize gas transport and decrease the work of breathing by increasing the fraction of inspired oxygen (F_iO_2) of room air (18–20% oxygen content) up to a F_iO_2 of approximately 50–75% using unilateral or bilateral nasal insufflation of humidified oxygen, respectively (Table 50.I.5) [171]. Reassessment of P_aO_2 should be performed after instituting intranasal oxygen as prolonged hyperoxia should be avoided. If the foal is hypercapnic from hypoventilation, respiratory stimulants such as doxapram (0.02–0.05 mg/kg/h, IV CRI) or caffeine (loading dose 10 mg/kg PO, then 2.5–5 mg/kg PO, daily) can be administered [172]. Mechanical ventilation can be considered if these interventions fail to increase the P_aO_2 and/or decrease the P_aCO_2 (Chapter 6).

Serum biochemistry profile results may identify *compromised renal or hepatic function*. Renal function can be further assessed with urinalysis, and monitoring urine output. Placement of a urinary catheter and closed urinary collection system should be considered to monitor urine output and/or to keep recumbent foals clean and dry thereby facilitating nursing care and decreasing the risk of decubital ulceration. Abnormally increased daily body weight gain provides insight into fluid retention from decreased urine output or overzealous IV fluid administration. Elevations in liver enzyme activity may be detected in serum biochemistry analysis secondary to sepsis, but in general, broad-spectrum antimicrobials and concomitant supportive care will frequently facilitate liver recovery. Tyzzer's disease (*Clostridium piliforme*) should be ruled out and is discussed, along with other liver diseases (Chapter 19).

Another vital treatment component of septic foals is provision of *adequate nutritional support*. Some septic foals maintain their appetite and the adequacy of their nutritional needs can be monitored by measuring weight gain. Healthy neonatal foals suckle four to five times every hour and gain approximately 1.3–1.5 kg/d during the first 30 days of life [151]. The daily gross energy needs of a healthy neonatal foal is approximately 150–160 kcal/kg/d with ill foals having lower energy requirements of approximately 40–50 kcal/kg/d [151, 173, 174]. If the foal is not suckling voluntarily, nutritional support can be provided via the enteral or parenteral route. If the GI tract is functional (i.e. no evidence of gastric reflux, intestinal distension, or ileus), enteral nutrition is preferred because it allows delivery of a natural and physiologic diet, provides necessary nutrients to the intestinal mucosa and is less expensive. Mare's milk is an obvious first choice and if the foal is not suckling, the mare's udder should be stripped of milk every 2–4 hours to maintain milk production. This will promote adequate lactation and availability of sufficient amounts of milk upon the foal's recovery. If mare's milk is not available or production is inadequate, commercial mare's milk replacer or goat's milk can be used [151]. A nasoesophageal feeding tube can be placed with initial milk feedings consisting of 5–10% of the foal's body weight, divided into frequent feedings (e.g. 5% × 50 kg = 2.5 l ÷ 12 feedings/d = 200 ml every 2 hours). The amount of milk can slowly be increased over several days as a healthy foal normally consumes 20–27% of their body weight in milk (10–13.5 l/d in a 50 kg foal) [151]. If the GI tract is not a viable route to supply nutritional needs or if a supplemental energy source is needed while increasing the amount of enteral feeding, one can consider short-term caloric supplementation with IV dextrose. The placental glucose transfer rate in the fetal foal is 6.8 mg/kg/min and the provision of 4–8 mg/kg/min of dextrose to neonatal foals has been suggested [154, 175]. The caloric content of 50% dextrose solution is 1.7 kcal/ml and can be administered undiluted via an infusion pump, provided that additional isotonic (i.e. maintenance) fluids are being administered concurrently to avoid phlebitis caused by hypertonic solutions. An infusion rate of 1 ml/kg/h of 50% dextrose delivers approximately 40 kcal/kg/d (1.7 kcal/kg/h × 24 hours = 41 kcal/kg/d) or approximately 8 mg/kg/h of dextrose [176]. Blood glucose should be measured every 2–4 hours initially to check for hyperglycemia; if present, the dextrose rate can be decreased or regular insulin therapy added as a CRI of 0.00125 to 0.05 U/kg/h [67]. One method of instituting insulin therapy is an initial small dose of 0.0025 U/kg/h, then doubling the infusion rate every 4 hours until blood glucose is controlled or the infusion is >0.2 U/kg/h. [67] Solutions containing 5% dextrose (0.17 kcal/ml) can be used but require excessively high fluid volumes to deliver the same amount of kcal (10 ml/kg/h to deliver 41 kcal/kg/d) [176]. Nutritional support should be reevaluated at the end of 24 hours and partial parenteral nutrition should be considered if enteral feedings are still not feasible; this is necessary as dextrose-containing fluids are an incomplete nutritional source and should not be used alone for extended periods of time. Chapter 58 provides a review of enteral and parenteral nutrition.

The prophylactic use of gastroprotectants is debatable in septic people and neonatal foals. Part of the argument against prophylactic use of acid-suppressive medications such as omeprazole, ranitidine, and cimetidine in people include increased risk of *Salmonellosis*, *Clostridium difficile*-associated diarrhea and bacterial colonization of the usually sterile upper GI tract, as well as increased risk of bacterial sepsis in human neonates [177–180]. The incidence of gastric ulcers in the subcategory of neonatal foals with sepsis is unknown, but necropsy examinations documented gastric ulcers in 13% (11/85) to 15% (54/354) of ill neonatal foals of which 65% (230/354) of those foals had a diagnosis of sepsis in one study [181, 182]. Comparatively, 62% (38/61) of foals (1–85 days of age) with a variety of clinical disorders had one or more gastric ulcers noted on gastroscopy [183]. In the ill neonatal foal, administration of anti-ulcer medications has been associated with increased odds of developing diarrhea and was associated with sepsis in a retrospective study; moreover, the use of anti-ulcer medications has not been proven to decrease the incidence of gastric ulcers in ill neonatal foals [181, 182, 184]. The pathogenesis of gastric ulcers in neonatal foals is unclear but may be related to alterations in gastric mucosal perfusion, ileus, hypoxia, use of nonsteroidal anti-inflammatory drugs or feeding frequency and volume in hospitalized foals [181, 184]. Full-term neonatal foals can produce gastric acid by 2 days of age and maintain a mean gastric pH between 0.8 and 6 between feedings [56, 185]. However, critically ill neonatal foals have more variable gastric pH that is often alkaline [185]. Considering the lack of evidence to support the use of prophylactic acid-suppressive medications in septic foals, the prophylactic use of sucralfate (22 mg/kg, PO, q8h), a cytoprotective medication, might be considered unless gastroscopy confirms the presence of gastric ulcers at which time acid-suppressive drugs are indicated [186]. Chapter 17 reviews gastric ulceration syndrome.

Sepsis in foals results in changes in hormonal concentrations but the rapid and fluctuant alterations of these temporal hormone profiles is difficult to interpret or therapeutically manage. In recent years, focus on the subset of septic foals with HPAA dysfunction has occurred and is characterized by inappropriately low secretion or activity of cortisol, that might contribute to morbidity and mortality [122, 125, 126]. Investigations identifying foals with abnormal cortisol metabolism are still ongoing, thus recommendations that clearly identify septic foals in need of supplemental hydrocortisone cannot be made. However, in the surviving sepsis campaign, IV hydrocortisone is recommended in septic people only when adequate fluid resuscitation and vasopressor therapy is unable to restore hemodynamic stability [132]. A few anecdotal reports have used bolus doses of steroids such as dexamethasone or hydrocortisone in severe cases of septic hypotensive foals with the intent to maintain adequate blood pressure and/or decrease the requirement for vasopressors [109]. A specific hydrocortisone dose for septic foals is unknown, but in healthy neonatal foals, a 3.5 day tapering dose starting with 1.3 mg/kg/d for 48 hours, then 0.65 mg/kg day for 24 hours, then 0.33 mg/kg/d for 12 hours dampened the pro-inflammatory cytokine response to ex vivo endotoxin exposure without significantly suppressing neutrophil function; the total daily dose was divided into six doses and administered as an IV bolus every 4 hours [187]. Whether septic foals benefit from corticosteroid therapy remains uncertain, but side effects such as hyperglycemia, leukocytosis, neutrophilia, and hypernatremia can be relevant [109].

Anti-Inflammatory Therapy

Unlike adult horses with sepsis or endotoxemia that are frequently administered anti-inflammatory therapy (i.e. nonsteroidal anti-inflammatory drugs, NSAIDs), the use of these medications is controversial and less frequently used in septic neonatal foals. Although the goal of anti-mediator therapy is to suppress production of inflammatory mediators, those same mediators (cytokines, complement, coagulation factors) also have protective roles in defending the host [67]. Moreover, blocking a targeted signaling pathway may be insufficient in suppressing inflammation as many aspects of the inflammatory cascade have redundant activation pathways [67]. These reasons likely contribute to the failure to identify a medication that targets a signaling or response pathway in clinical trials in septic people. Despite this, some clinicians use anti-mediator therapy in the treatment of septic foals and include flunixin meglumine, polymyxin B, pentoxyifylline, and dimethyl sulfoxide (DMSO), among others. Caution must be exercised when using flunixin and polymyxin B as they are potentially nephrotoxic. Flunixin also has the potential for gastric ulceration. Little evidence supports use of any of these medications but administration of polymyxin B (6000 u/kg, IV, q8h) did lower blood L-lactate, TNF-α, and thromboxane B_2 concentrations and improved blood glucose and attitude scores in neonatal foals administered endotoxin [119]. In addition, meloxicam (0.6 mg/kg, PO, q12h) was well tolerated in healthy foals with no observed side effects. The clinical benefit of any of these medications in septic foals is unknown [188].

The preceding information serves as a starting point for developing a treatment plan for septic foal. Individual variations in the course of sepsis and response to treatment as well as the development of septic complications (e.g. septic arthritis) is anticipated and the clinician must observe, monitor, recheck, and adjust the treatment plan accordingly. Other body systems impacted by sepsis such as the musculoskeletal system (septic arthritis, osteomyelitis), central nervous system (meningoencephalitis) and umbilical remnants (septic omphalitis, omphalophlebitis) are reviewed in system specific chapters within this textbook.

Prognosis, Survival, and Prevention

The survival rate of hospitalized critically ill neonatal foals has improved over the past decades ranging from 58% survival rate in the 1980s to 69% in the 1990s and 81% in 2000s as reported from one institution [133, 142]. Table 50.I.3 provides information from previous studies that have examined survival rate in septic equine neonates and ranges from 26 to 71%. Other studies have documented a survival rate of septic foals in the range of 49% (25/51) to 68% (30/44) with larger retrospective studies ranging from 60% (254/423) to 76% (85/113) [84, 121, 133, 142, 150]. In general, an approximate survival rate of 60–70% would seem appropriate for septic foals, but individual factors and financial resources greatly influence outcome. Complications such as septic arthritis and meningoencephalitis decrease survival rate. In regard to long-term performance, no statistically significant differences were detected between 102 surviving septic foals compared to their healthy siblings when evaluating the percentage of starters, percentage of winners, or number of race starts. However surviving foals had significantly lower number of wins, total earnings, and standard start index values [142].

A number of studies have evaluated various historical, examination findings, and clinicopathologic data and their relationship with survival [133]. Septic foals infected with a single organism have a significantly higher likelihood of survival (62–74%) compared to foals with a polymicrobial infection (41–50%) [68, 152]. Foals with Gram-negative sepsis were less likely to survive (10%; 1/10) compared to Gram-positive sepsis (40%; 2/5) in a small study, but no significant difference in survival rate between Gram-positive (85%) and Gram-negative (68%) bacteremia was noted in a larger study of 85 foals [68, 70]. Moreover, an association between survival and different bacterial isolates in septic foals was not identified in 101 blood culture positive foals [65]. In one study in which initial empiric antimicrobial treatment administered to septic foals was known (186 foals), the likelihood of survival was 65.4% if the bacteria isolated from a foal was susceptible to initial treatment as compared to 41.7% if one or more bacteria were resistant [152]. However, 34.6% of foals that received the "correct" antimicrobials still died and 63.4% of foals that received the "incorrect" antimicrobials survived, thus emphasizing the influence of other factors on outcome [152]. A host of other clinical (e.g. standing at presentation, cold extremities, age at admission, others) and clinicopathologic variables (e.g. neutrophil count, band neutrophil count, serum creatinine concentration, arterial blood pH, others) have been linked to survival rates, but each individual variable will not be discussed here [133, 142].

No single strategy can prevent the occurrence of sepsis in neonatal foals, but a few guidelines can be discussed with horse owners to potentially decrease the incidence. Addressing risk factors for the development of sepsis (Table 50.I.1) as early as possible is one step to aid in prevention. Meticulous birth hygiene is also important and includes maintaining a clean environment where parturition will occur, thus reducing bacterial load within the environment. Additionally, after foaling but prior to suckling, thoroughly washing the mare's hindquarters, perineum and udder with soap and water followed by drying these areas might decrease the bacterial load that the foal is exposed to, but this activity is labor intensive and requires a degree of commitment on the part of the owner. Providing appropriate umbilical care (e.g. chlorhexidine dips or sprays), ensuring the consumption of quality colostrum within the first few hours of life and confirming adequate TPI are other factors that can be done with the hopes of decreasing the incidence of sepsis.

References

1 Bone, R.C., Balk, R.A., Cerra, F.B. et al. (1992). Definitions for sepsis and organ failure and guidelines for the use of innovative therapies in sepsis. The AACP/SCCM Consensus Conference Committee. American College of Chest Physicians/ Society of Critical Care Medicine. *Chest* 101: 1644–1655.

2 Levy, M.M., Fink, M.P., Marshall, J.C. et al. (2003). 2001 SCCM/ESICM/ACCP/ATS/SIS International sepsis definitions conference. *Intensive Care Med.* 29: 530–538.

3 Goldstein, B., Giroir, B., Randolph, A. et al. (2005). International Pediatric Sepsis Consensus Conference: definitions for sepsis and organ dysfunction in pediatrics. *Pediatr. Crit. Care Med.* 6: 2–8.

4 Singer, M., Deutschman, C.S., Seymour, C.W. et al. (2016). The third international consensus definitions for sepsis and septic shock (Sepsis-3). *JAMA* 801–810.

5 de Jong, H.K., van der Poll, T., and Wiersinga, W.J. (2010). The systemic pro-inflammatory response in sepsis. *J. Innate Immun.* 2: 422–430.

6 Angus, D.C. and van der Poll, T. (2013). Severe sepsis and septic shock. *N. Engl. J. Med.* 369: 840–851.

7 Raymond, S.L., Holden, D.C., Mira, J.C. et al. (2017). Microbial recognition and danger signals in sepsis and trauma. *Biochim. Biophys. Acta* 1863: 2564–2573.

8 Lewis, D.H., Chan, D.L., Pinheiro, D. et al. (2012). The immunopathology of sepsis: Pathogen recognition, systemic inflammation, the compensatory anti-inflammatory response, and regulatory T cells. *J. Vet. Intern. Med.* 26: 457–482.

9 Werners, A.H. and Bryant, C.E. (2012). Pattern recognition receptors in equine endotoxaemia and sepsis. *Equine Vet. J.* 44: 490–498.

10 Erridge, C. (2010). Endogenous ligands of TLR2 and TLR4: agonists or assistants? *J. Leukoc. Biol.* 87: 989–999.

11 Sanchez, L.C. (2018). Endotoxemia. In: *Equine Internal Medicine*, 4e (ed. S.M. Reed, W.M. Bayly, and D.C. Sellon), 723–738. St. Louis MO: Elsevier.

12 Janeway, C.A. and Medzhitov, R. (1999). Lipoproteins take their toll on the host. *Curr. Biol.* 9: R879–R882.

13 Schwandner, R., Dziarski, R., Wesche, H. et al. (1999). Peptidoglycan- and lipoteichoic acid-induced cell activation is mediated by toll-like receptor 2. *J. Biol. Chem.* 274: 17406–17409.

14 Diebold, S.S., Kaisho, T., Hemmi, H. et al. (2004). Innate antiviral responses by means of TLR7-mediated recognition of single-stranded RNA. *Science* 303: 1529–1531.

15 Hemmi, H., Takeuchi, O., Kawai, T. et al. (2000). A toll-like receptor recognizes bacterial DNA. *Nature* 408: 740–745.

16 Denk, S., Perl, M., and Huber-Lang, M. (2012). Damage- and pathogen-associated molecular patterns and alarmins: Keys to sepsis? *Eur. Surg. Res.* 48: 171–179.

17 Lord, J.M., Midwinter, M.J., Chen, Y.F. et al. (2014). The systemic immune response to trauma: an overview of pathophysiology and treatment. *Lancet* 384: 1455–1465.

18 Manson, J., Thiemermann, C., and Brohi, K. (2010). Trauma alarmins as activators of damage-induced inflammation. *Br. J. Surg.* 99 (Suppl 1): 12–20.

19 Matzinger, P. (1994). Tolerance, danger, and the extended family. *Annu. Rev. Immunol.* 12: 991–1045.

20 Degryse, B., Bonaldi, T., Scaffidi, P. et al. (2001). The high mobility group (HMG) boxes of the nuclear protein HMG1 induce chemotaxis and cytoskeleton reorganization in rat smooth muscle cells. *J. Cell Biol.* 152: 1197–1206.

21 Wang, H., Bloom, O., Zhang, M. et al. (1999). HMG-1 as a late mediator of endotoxin lethality in mice. *Science* 285: 248–251.

22 Cohen, M.J., Brohi, K., Calfee, C.S. et al. (2009). Early release of high mobility group box nuclear protein 1 after severe trauma in humans: role of injury severity and tissue hypoperfusion. *Crit. Care* 13: R174.

23 Gibot, S., Massin, F., Cravoisy, A. et al. (2007). High-mobility group box 1 protein plasma concentrations during septic shock. *Intensive Care Med.* 33: 1347–1353.

24 Steiner, J., Marquardt, N., Pauls, I. et al. (2011). Human CD8(+) T cells and NK cells express and secrete S100B upon stimulation. *Brain Behav. Immun.* 25: 1233–1241.

25 Rohde, D., Schon, C., Boerries, M. et al. (2014). S100A1 is released from ischemic cardiomyocytes and signals myocardial damage via Toll-like receptor 4. *EMBO Mol. Med.* 6: 778–794.

26 Vogl, T., Tenbrock, K., Ludwig, S. et al. (2007). Mrp8 and Mrp14 are endogenous activators of Toll-like receptor 4, promoting lethal endotoxin-induced shock. *Nat. Med.* 13: 1042–1049.

27 Zhang, Q., Raoof, M., Chen, Y. et al. (2010). Circulating mitochondrial DAMPs cause inflammatory responses to injury. *Nature* 464: 104–107.

28 Fry, D.E. (2012). Sepsis, systemic inflammatory response, and multiple organ dysfunction: the mystery continues. *Am. Surg.* 78: 1–8.

29 Khan, F.A. and Khan, M.F. (2010). Inflammation and acute phase response. *Int. J. Appl. Pharm. Tech.* 1: 312–321.

30 O'Brien, J.M., Ali, N.A., Aberegg, S.K. et al. (2007). Sepsis. *Am. J. Med.* 120: 1012–1022.

31 Blatt, N.B., Srinivasan, S., Mottes, T. et al. (2014). Biology of sepsis: Its relevance to pediatric nephrology. *Pediatr. Nephol.* 29: 2273–2287.

32 Chu, A.J. (2011). Tissue factor, blood coagulation, and beyond: an overview. *Int. J. Inflamm.* 2011: 367284.

33 Barkhausen, T., Krettek, C., and van Griensven, M. (2005). L-selectin: Adhesion, signaling and its importance in pathologic posttraumatic endotoxemia and non-septic inflammation. *Exp. Toxicol. Pathol.* 57: 39–52.

34 Charo, I.F. and Ransohoff, R.M. (2006). The many roles of chemokines and chemokine receptors in inflammation. *N. Engl. J. Med.* 354: 610–621.

35 Mackay, I. and Rosen, F.S. (2000). Advances in Immunology: Innate Immunity. *N. Engl. J. Med.* 343: 338–344.

36 Brinkmann, V., Reichard, U., Goosmann, C. et al. (2004). Neutrophil extracellular traps kill bacteria. *Science* 303: 1532–1535.

37 Lelubre, C. and Vincent, J.L. (2018). Mechanisms and treatment of organ failure in sepsis. *Nat. Rev. Nephrol.* 14: 417–427.

38 Adib-Conquy, M. and Cavaillon, J.M. (2009). Compensatory anti-inflammatory response syndrome. *Thromb. Haemost.* 101: 36–47.

39 Osuchowski, M.F., Welch, K., Siddiqui, J. et al. (2006). Circulating cytokine/inhibitor profiles reshape the understanding of the SIRS/CARS continuum in sepsis and predict mortality. *J. Immunol.* 177: 1967–1974.

40 Burton, A.B., Wagner, B., Erb, H.N. et al. (2009). Serum interleukin-6 (IL-6) and IL-10 concentrations in normal and septic neonatal foals. *Vet. Immunol. Immunopathol.* 132: 122–128.

41 Shubin, N.J., Monaghan, S.F., and Ayala, A. (2011). Anti-inflammatory mechanisms of sepsis. *Contrib. Microbiol.* 17: 108–124.

42 Ward, N.S., Casserly, B., and Ayala, A. (2008). The compensatory anti-inflammatory response syndrome (CARS) in critically ill patients. *Clin. Chest Med.* 29: 617–625.

43 Corley, K.T., McKenzie, H.C., Amoroso, L.M. et al. (2000). Initial experience with norepinephrine infusion in hypotensive critically ill foals. *J. Vet. Emerg. Crit. Care* 10: 267–276.

44 Hollis, A.R., Wilkins, P.A., and Palmer, J.E. (2008). Bacteremia in equine neonatal diarrhea: a retrospective study. *J. Vet. Intern. Med.* 22L: 1203–1209.

45 Cotovio, M., Monreal, L., Armengou, L. et al. (2008). Fibrin deposits and organ failure in newborn foals with severe septicemia. *J. Vet. Intern. Med.* 22: 1403–1410.

46 Wong, D.M. and Wilkins, P.A. (2015). Defining the systemic inflammatory response syndrome in equine neonates. *Vet. Clin. North Am. Equine* 31: 463–481.

47 Pusterla, N., Magdeisan, K.G., Mapes, S. et al. (2006). Expression of molecular markers in blood of neonatal foals with sepsis. *Am. J. Vet. Res.* 67: 1045–1049.

48 Gold, J.R., Divers, T.J., Barton, M.H. et al. (2007). Plasma adrenocorticotropin, cortisol, and adrenocorticotropin/cortisol ratios in septic and normal-term foals. *J. Vet. Intern. Med.* 21: 791–796.

49 Gold, J.R., Cohen, N.D., Welsh, J.R. et al. (2012). Association of adrenocorticotrophin and cortisol concentrations with peripheral blood leukocyte cytokine gene expression in septic and nonseptic neonatal foals. *J. Vet. Intern. Med.* 26: 654–661.

50 Gold, J.R., Perkins, G.A., Erb, H.N. et al. (2007). Cytokine profiles of peripheral blood mononuclear cells isolated from septic and healthy neonatal foals. *J. Vet. Intern. Med.* 21: 482–488.

51 Zabrecky, K.A., Slovis, N.M., Constable, P.D. et al. (2015). Plasma C-reactive protein and haptoglobin concentrations in critically ill neonatal foals. *J. Vet. Intern. Med.* 29: 673–677.

52 Toth, B., Slovis, N.M., Constable, P.D. et al. (2014). Plasma adrenomedullin concentrations in critically ill neonatal foals. *J. Vet. Intern. Med.* 28: 1294–1300.

53 Stoneham, S.J., Palmer, L., Cash, R. et al. (2001). Measurement of serum amyloid A in the neonatal foal using a latex agglutination immunoturbidimetric assay: determination of the normal range, variation with age and response to disease. *Equine Vet. J.* 33: 599–603.

54 Fielding, C.L. and Magdesian, K.G. (2015). Sepsis and septic shock in the equine neonate. *Vet. Clin. Equine* 31: 483–496.

55 Koterba, A.M., Drummond, W.H., and Kosch, P.C. (1990). Neonatal Infection. In: *Equine clinical Neonatoogy* (ed. A.M. Koterba), 295–316. Philadelphia: Lea & Febiger.

56 Sanchez, L.C. (2015). Equine neonatal sepsis. *Vet. Clin. Equine* 21: 273–293.

57 Aleman, M. (2008). A review of equine muscle disorders. *Neuromuscul. Disord.* 18: 277–287.

58 Valberg, S.J., Ward, T.L., Rush, B. et al. (2001). Glycogen branching enzyme deficiency in quarter horse foals. *J. Vet. Intern. Med.* 15: 572–580.

59 Pinn, T.L., Divers, T.J., Southard, T. et al. (2018). Persistent hypoglycemia associated with lipid storage myopathy in a paint foal. *J. Vet. Intern. Med.* 32: 1442–1446.

60 Karlikova, R., Siroka, J., Mech, M. et al. (2018). Newborn foal with atypical myopathy. *J. Vet. Intern. Med.* 32: 1768–1772.

61 Raidal, S.L. (1996). The incidence and consequences of failure or passive transfer of immunity on a Throughbred breeding farm. *Aust. Vet. J.* 73: 201–206.

62 Robinson, J.A., Allen, G.K., Green, E.M. et al. (1993). A prospective study of septicaemia in colostrum-deprived foals. *Equine Vet. J.* 25: 214–219.

63 Hytychova, T. and Bezdekova, B. (2015). Retrospective evaluation of blood culture isolates and sepsis survival rate in foals in the Czech Republic: 50 cases (2011–2013). *J. Vet. Emerg. Crit. Care* 25: 660–666.

64 Baldwin, J.L., Cooper, W.L., Vanderwall, D.K. et al. (1991). Prevalence (treatment days) and severity of illness in hypogammaglobulinemic and normogammaglobulinemic foals. *J. Am. Vet. Med. Assoc.* 198: 423–428.

65 Stewart, A.J., Hinchcliff, K.W., Saville, W.J.A. et al. (2002). Actinobacillus sp. Bacteremia in foals: clinical signs and prognosis. *J. Vet. Intern. Med.* 16: 464–471.

66 Koterba, A.M., Brewer, B.D., and Tarpless, F.A. (1984). Clinical and clinicopathological characteristics of the septicaemic neonatal foal: Review of 38 cases. *Equine Vet. J.* 16: 376–383.

67 Palmer, J.E. (2014). Update on the management of neonatal sepsis in horses. *Vet. Clin. Equine* 30: 317–336.

68 Corley, K.T.T., Pearce, G., Magdesian, K.G. et al. (2007). Bacteraemia in neonatal foals: clinicopathological differences between Gram-positive and Gram-negative infections, and single organisms and mixed infections. *Equine Vet. J.* 39: 84–89.

69 Duggan, V.E., Holbrook, T.C., Dechant, J.E. et al. (2004). Diagnosis of aorto-iliac thrombosis in a Quarter Horse foal using Doppler ultrasound and nuclear scintigraphy. *J. Vet. Intern. Med.* 18: 753–756.

70 Barton, M.H., Morris, D.D., Norton, N. et al. (1998). Hemostatic and fibinolytic indices in neonatal foals with presumed septicemia. *J. Vet. Intern. Med.* 12: 26–35.

71 Sarangi, P.P., Lee, H.W., and Kim, M. (2010). Activated protein C action in inflammation. *Br. J. Haematol.* 148: 817–833.

72 Frick, I.M., Bjorck, L., and Herwald, H. (2007). The dual rold of the contact system in bacterial infectious disease. *Thromb. Haemost.* 98: 497–502.

73 Bentz, A.I., Palmer, J.E., and Dallap, B.L. (2009). Prospective evaluation of coagulation in critically ill neonatal foals. *J. Vet. Intern. Med.* 23: 161–167.

74 Banse, H., Holbrook, T.C., Gilliam, L. et al. (2012). Right ventricular and saphenous vein thrombi associated with sepsis in a Quarter Horse foal. *J. Vet. Intern. Med.* 26: 178–182.

75 Brianceau, P. and Divers, T.J. (2001). Acute thrombosis of limb arteries in horses with sepsis: five cases (1988–1998). *Equine Vet. J.* 33: 105–109.

76 Moore, L.A., Johnson, P.J., and Bailey, K.C. (1998). Aorto-iliac thrombosis in a foal. *Vet. Rec.* 142: 459–462.

77 Forrests, L.J., Cooley, A.J., and Darien, B.J. (1999). Digital arterial thrombosis in a septicemic foal. *J. Vet. Intern. Med.* 13: 382–385.

78 Triplett, E.A., O'Brien, R.T., Wilson, D.G. et al. (1996). Thrombosis of the brachial artery in a foal. *J. Vet. Intern. Med.* 10: 330–332.

79 Spier, S. (1985). Arterial thrombosis as the cause of lameness in a foal. *J. Am. Vet. Med. Assoc.* 187: 164–165.

80 Armengou, L., Monreal, L., Tarancon, I. et al. (2008). Plasma D-dimer concentration in sick newborn foals. *J. Vet. Intern. Med.* 22: 411–417.

81 Sola-Visner, M., Sallmon, H., and Brown, R. (2009). New insights into the mechanisms of nonimmune thrombocytopenia in neonates. *Semin. Perinatol.* 33: 43–51.

82 Fowden, A.L., Mundy, L., Ousey, J.C. et al. (1991). Tissue glycogen and glucose 6-phosphate levels in fetal and newborn foals. *J. Reprod. Fertil.* 44 (Suppl): 537–542.

83 Barsnick, R.J.I.M., Hurcombe, S.D.A., Dembek, K. et al. (2014). Somatotropic axis resistance and ghrelin in critically ill foals. *Equine Vet. J.* 46: 45–49.

84 Barsnick, R.J.I.M., Hurcombe, S.D.A., Smith, P.A. et al. (2011). Insulin, glucagon, and leptin in critically ill foals. *J. Vet. Intern. Med.* 25: 123–131.

85 Sweetman, D.U. (2017). Neonatal acute kidney injury – severity and recovery prediction and the role of serum and urinary biomarkers. *Early Hum. Dev.* 105: 57–61.

86 Schrier, R.W. and Wang, W. (2004). Acute renal failure and sepsis. *N. Engl. J. Med.* 351: 159–169.

87 Poston, J.T. and Koyner, J.L. (2019). Sepsis associated acute kidney injury. *BMJ* 364: K4891.

88 Chaney, K.P., Holcomb, S.J., Schott, H.C. et al. (2010). Spurious hypercreatininemia: 28 neonatal foals (2000–2008). *J. Vet. Emerg. Crit. Care* 20: 244–249.

89 Pirrone, A., Antonelli, C., Mariella, J. et al. (2014). Gross placental morphology and foal serum biochemistry as predictors of foal health. *Theriogenology* 81: 1293–1299.

90 Brewer, B.D., Clement, S.F., Lotz, W.S. et al. (1991). Renal clearance, urinary excretion of endogenous substances, and urinary diagnostic indices in healthy neonatal foals. *J. Vet. Intern. Med.* 5: 28–33.

91 Bayly, W.M., Brobst, D.F., Elfers, R.S. et al. (1986). Serum and urinary biochemistry and enzyme changes in ponies with acute renal failure. *Cornell Vet.* 76: 306–316.

92 Haggett, E.F., Magdesian, K.G., and Kass, P.H. (2011). Clinical implications of high liver enzyme activities in hospitalized neonatal foals. *J. Am. Vet. Med. Assoc.* 239: 661–667.

93 Koterba, A.M., Drummond, W.H., and Kosch, P.C. (1990). Neonatal hyperbilirubinemia. In: *Equine Clinical Neonatoogy* (ed. A.M. Koterba), 589–601. Philadelphia: Lea & Febiger.

94 Murray, M.J., del Piero, F., Jeffrey, S.C. et al. (1998). Neonatal equine herpesvirus type 1 infection on a thoroughbred breeding farm. *J. Vet. Intern. Med.* 12: 36–41.

95 Acland, H.M., Mann, P.C., Rpbertson, J.L. et al. (1984). Toxic hepatopathy in neonatal foals. *Vet. Pathol.* 21: 3–9.

96 Bastianello, S.S. and Nesbit, J.W. (1986). The pathology of a case of biliary atresia in a foal. *J. S. Afr. Vet. Assoc.* 57: 117–120.

97 Boyle, A.G., Magdesian, K.G., and Ruby, R.E. (2005). Neonatal isoerythrolysis in horse foals and a mule foal: 18 cases (1988–2003). *J. Am. Vet. Med. Assoc.* 15: 1276–1283.

98 Haecheler, S., Van den Ingh, T.S., Rogivue, C. et al. (2000). Congenital hepatic fibrosis and cystic bile duct formation in Swiss Freiberger horses. *Vet. Pathol.* 37: 669–671.

99 Zhu, J., Xu, Y., Zhang, G. et al. (2012). Total serum bilirubin levels during the first 2 days of life and subsequent neonatal morbidity in very low birth weight infants: a retrospective review. *Eur. J. Pediatr.* 171: 669–674.

100 Wilkins, P.A., Otto, C.M., Baumgardner, J.E. et al. (2007). Acute lung injury and acute respiratory distress syndromes in veterinary medicine: consensus definitions: the Dorothy Russell Havemeyer working group on ALI and ARDS in veterinary medicine. *J. Vet. Emerg. Crit. Care* 4: 333–339.

101 Gayle, J.M., Cohen, N.D., and Chaffin, M.K. (1998). Factors associated with survival in septicemic foals: 65 cases. *J. Vet. Intern. Med.* 12: 140–146.

102 Bakowitz, M., Bruns, B., and McCunn, M. (2012). Acute lung injury and the actue respiratory distress syndrome in the injured patient. *Scand. J. Trauma Resusc. Emerg. Med.* 20: 54.

103 Englert, J.A., Bobba, C., and Baron, R.M. (2019). Integrating molecular pathogenesis and clinical translation in sepsis-induced acute respiratory distress syndrome. *JCI Insight* 4: e124061.

104 Ware, L.B. (2006). Pathophysiology of acute lung injury and the acute respiratory distress syndrome. *Semin. Respir. Crit. Care Med.* 27: 337–349.

105 Dunkel, B., Dolente, B., and Boston, R.C. (2005). Acute lung injury/acute respiratory distress syndrome in 15 foals. *Equine Vet. J.* 37: 435–440.

106 Lakritz, J., Wilson, W.D., Berry, C.R. et al. (1993). Bronchointerstitial pneumonia and respiratory distress in young horses: clinical, clinicopathologic, radiographic, and pathologic findings in 23 cases (1984–1989). *J. Vet. Intern. Med.* 7: 277–288.

107 Wilkins, P.A. and Seahorn, T. (2004). Acute respiratory distress syndrome. *Vet. Clin. Equine* 20: 253–273.

108 Barrington, K.J. (2013). Common hemodynamic problems in the neonate. *Neonatology* 103: 355–340.

109 Corley, K.T.T. (2004). Inotropes and vasopressors in adults and foals. *Vet. Clin. Equine* 20: 77–106.

110 Noori, S. and Seri, I. (2015). Evidence-based versus pathophysiology-based approach to diagnosis and treatment of neonatal cardiovascular compromise. *Semin. Fetal Neonatal Med.* 20: 238–245.

111 Emr, B.M., Alcamo, A.M., Carcillo, J.A. et al. (2018). Pediatric sepsis update: how are children different? *Surg. Infect. (Larchmt.)* 19: 176–183.

112 Lavoie, J.P., Madigan, J.E., Cullor, J.S. et al. (1990). Haemodynamic, pathological, haematological and behavioural changes during endotoxin infusion in equine neonates. *Equine Vet. J.* 22: 23–29.

113 Corley, K.T.T. (2002). Monitoring and treating haemodynamic disturbances in critically ill neonatal foals. Part 1: haemodynomic monitoring. *Equine Vet. Educ.* 14: 270–279.

114 Raj, S., Killinger, J.S., Gonzalez, J.A. et al. (2014). Myocardial dysfunction in pediatric septic shock. *J. Pediatr.* 164: 72.

115 Slack, J., McGuirk, S.M., Erb, H.N. et al. (2005). Biochemical markers of cardiac injury in normal, surviving septic, or nonsurviving septic neonatal foals. *J. Vet. Intern. Med.* 19: 577–580.

116 Mittal, R. and Coopersmith, C.M. (2014). Redefining the gut as the motor of critical illness. *Trends Mol. Med.* 20: 214–223.

117 Klingensmith, N.J. and Coopersmith, C.M. (2016). The gut as the motor of multiple organ dysfunction in critical illness. *Crit. Care Clin.* 32L: 203–212.

118 Haak, B.W. and Wiersinga, W.J. (2017). The rold of the gut microbiota in sepsis. *Lancet Gastroenterol. Hepatol.* 2: 135–143.

119 Wong, D.M., Sponseller, B.A., Alcott, C.J. et al. (2013). Effects of intravenous administration of polymyxin B in neonatal foals with experimental endotoxemia. *J. Am. Vet. Med. Assoc.* 243: 874–881.

120 Oikawa, M., Ohnami, Y., Koike, M. et al. (2007). Endotoxin–induced injury of the central, autonomic and enteric nervous systems and intestinal muscularis in Thoroughbred Horses. *J. Comp. Pathol.* 136: 127–132.

121 Hurcombe, S.D.A., Toribio, R.E., Slovis, N. et al. (2008). Blood arginine vasopressin, adrenocorticotropin hormone, and cortisol concentrations at admission in septic and critically ill foals and their association with survival. *J. Vet. Intern. Med.* 22: 639–647.
122 Dembek, K.A., Timko, K.J., Johnson, L.M. et al. (2017). Steroids, steroid precursors, and neuroactive steroids in critically ill equine neonates. *Vet. J.* 225: 42–49.
123 Hart, K.A., Slovis, N.M., and Barton, M.H. (2009). Hypothalamic-pituitary-adrenal axis dysfunction in hospitalized neonatal foals. *J. Vet. Intern. Med.* 23: 901–912.
124 Boonen, E., Bornstein, S.R., and Van Den, B.G. (2015). New insights into the controversy of adrenal function during critical illness. *Lancet Diabetes Endocrinol.* 3: 805–815.
125 Armengou, L., Cunilleras, E.J., Rios, J. et al. (2013). Metabolic and endocrine profiles in sick neonatal foals are related to survival. *J. Vet. Intern. Med.* 27: 567–575.
126 Wong, D.M., Vo, D.T., Alcott, C.J. et al. (2009). Baseline plasma cortisol and ACTH concentrations and response to low-dose ACTH stimulation testing in ill foals. *J. Am. Vet. Med. Assoc.* 234: 126–132.
127 Bard, J.D. and TeKippe, E.M. (2016). Diagnosis of bloodstream infections in children. *J. Clin. Microbiol.* 54: 1418–1424.
128 Tarai, B., Jain, D., Das, P. et al. (2018). Paired blood cultures increase the sensitivity for detecting pathogens in both inpatients and outpatients. *Eur. J. Clin. Microbiol. Infect. Dis.* 37: 435–441.
129 Lee, A., Mirrett, S., Reller, L.B. et al. (2007). Detection of bloodstream infection in adults: how many blood cultures are needed? *J. Clin. Microbiol.* 45: 3546–3548.
130 Ntusi, N., Aubin, L., Oliver, S. et al. (2010). Guideline for the optimal use of blood cultures. *S. Afr. Med. J.* 100: 839–843.
131 Rhodes, A., Evans, L.E., Alhazzani, W. et al. (2017). Surviving sepsis campaign: International guidelines for management of sepsis and septic shock: 2016. *Intensive Care Med.* 43: 304–377.
132 Giguere, S., Weber, E.J., and Sanchez, L.C. (2017). Factors associated with outcome and gradual improvement in survival over time in 1065 equine neonates admitted to an intensive care unit. *Equine Vet. J.* 49: 45–50.
133 Fouche, N., Gerber, V., Thomann, A. et al. (2018). Antimicrobial susceptibility patterns of blood culture isolates from foals in Switzerland. *Schweiz. Arch. Tierheilkd.* 160 (11): 665–671.
134 Theelen, M.J.P., Wilson, W.D., Byrne, B.A. et al. (2020). Differences in isolation rate and antimicrobial susceptibility of bacteria isolated from foals with sepsis at admission and after ≥48 hours of hospitalization. *J. Vet. Intern. Med.* 34: 955–963.
135 Wilson, W.D. and Madigan, J.E. (1989). Comparison of bacteriologic culture of blood and necropsy specimens for determining the cause of foal septicemia: 47 cases (1978–1987). *J. Am. Vet. Med. Assoc.* 195: 1759–1763.
136 Brewer, B.D. and Koterba, A.M. (1985). The diagnosis and treatment of equine neonatal septicemia. *Proc. Am. Assoc. Equine Pract.* 31: 127–135.
137 Furr, M. and McKenzie, H. (2020). Factors associated with the risk of positive blood culture in neonatal foals presented to a referral center (2000–2014). *J. Vet. Intern. Med.* 34: 2738–2750.
138 Wong, D.M., Ruby, R.E., Dembek, K.A. et al. (2018). Evaluation of updated sepsis scoring systems and systemic inflammatory response syndrome criteria and their association with sepsis in equine neonates. *J. Vet. Intern. Med.* 32: 1185–1193.
139 Rampacci, E., Passamonti, F., Bottinelli, M. et al. (2017). Umbilical infections in foals: microbial investigation and management. *Vet. Rec.* 180: 543–547.
140 Hackett, E.S., Lunn, D.P., Ferris, R.A. et al. (2015). Detection of bacteraemia and host response in healthy neonatal foals. *Equine Vet. J.* 47: 405–409.
141 Russell, C.M., Axon, J.E., Blishen, A. et al. (2008). Blood culture isolates and antimicrobial sensitivities from 427 critically ill neonatal foals. *Aust. Vet. J.* 86 (7): 266–271. 82/110 (74.5%) septic foals.
142 Sanchez, L.C., Giguere, S., and Lester, G.D. (2008). Factors associated with survival of neonatal foals with bacteremia and racing performance of surviving Thoroughbreds: 423 cases (1982–2007). *J. Am. Vet. Med. Assoc.* 233: 1446–1452.
143 Marsh, P.S. and Palmer, J.E. (2001). Bacterial isolates from blood and their susceptibility patters in critically ill foals: 543 cases (1991–1998). *J. Am. Vet. Med. Assoc.* 218: 1608–1610.
144 Raisis, A.L., Hodgson, J.L., and Hodgson, D.R. (1996). Equine neonatal septicaemia: 24 cases. *Aust. Vet. J.* 73: 137–140.
145 Magdesian, K.G. (2017). Antimicrobial pharmacology for the neonatal foal. *Vet. Clin. Equine* 33: 47–65.
146 Brewer, B.D. and Koterba, A.M. (1988). Development of a scoring system for the early diagnosis of equine neonatal sepsis. *Equine Vet. J.* 20: 18–22.
147 Brewer, B.D., Koterba, A.M., Carter, R.L. et al. (1988). Comparison of empirically developed sepsis score with a computer generated and weighted scoring system for the identification of sepsis in the equine neonate. *Equine Vet. J.* 20: 23–24.
148 Corley, K.T.T. and Furr, M.O. (2003). Evaluation of a score designed to predict sepsis in foals. *J. Vet. Emerg. Crit. Care* 13: 149–155.
149 Weber, E.J., Sanchez, L.C., and Giguere, S. (2015). Re-evaluation of the sepsis score in equine neonates. *Equine Vet. J.* 47: 275–278.

150 Peek, S.F., Semrad, S., McGuirk, S.M. et al. (2006). Prognostic value of clinicopathologic variables obtained at admission and effect of antiendotoxin plasma on survival in septic and critically ill foals. *J. Vet. Intern. Med.* 20: 569–574.

151 Buechner-Maxwell, V.A. (2005). Nutritional support for neonatal foals. *Vet. Clin. Equine* 21: 487–510.

152 Theelen, M.J.P., Wilson, W.E., Byrne, B.A. et al. (2019). Initial antimicrobial treatment of foals with sepsis: do our choices make a difference? *Vet. J.* 243: 74–76.

153 Masterton, R.G. (2011). Antibiotic de-escalation. *Crit. Care Clin.* 27: 149–162.

154 Palmer, J.E. (2004). Fluid therapy in the neonate: not your mother's fluid space. *Vet. Clin. Equine* 20: 63–75.

155 Nout, Y.S., Corlety, K.T.T., Donaldson, L.L. et al. (2002). Indirect oscillometric and direct blood pressure measurement in anesthetized and conscious neonatal foals. *J. Vet. Emerg. Crit. Care* 12: 75–80.

156 Corley, K.T.T., Donaldson, L.L., and Furr, M.O. (2005). Arterial lactate concentration, hospital survival, sepsis and SIRS in critically ill neonatal foals. *Equine Vet. J.* 37: 53–59.

157 Liepman, R.S., Dembek, K.A., Slovis, N.M. et al. (2015). Validation of IgG cut-off values and their association with survival in neonatal foals. *Equine Vet. J.* 47: 526–530.

158 Secor, E.J., Matychak, M.B., and Felippe, M.J. (2012). Transfer of tumour necrosis factor – via colostrum to foals. *Vet. Rec.* 170: 51.

159 Mariella, J., Castagnetti, C., Prosperi, A. et al. (2017). Cytokine levels in colostrum and in foals' serum pre- and post-suckling. *Vet. Immunol. Immunopathol.* 185: 34–37.

160 Gardner, R.B., Nydam, D.V., Luna, J.A. et al. (2007). Serum opsonization capacity, phagocytosis, and oxidative burst activity in neonatal foals in the intensive care unit. *J. Vet. Intern. Med.* 21: 797–805.

161 Grondahl, G., Johannisson, A., Demmers, J. et al. (1999). Influence of age and plasma treatment on neutrophil phagocytosis and CD18 expression in foals. *Vet. Microbiol.* 65: 241–254.

162 Tennent-Brown, B. (2011). Plasma therapy in foals and adult horses. *Compend. Contin. Educ. Vet.* 33: E1–E4.

163 Morris, D.D. and Whitlock, R.H. (1987). Therapy of suspected septicemia in neonatal foals using plasma-containing antibodies to core lipopolysaccharide (LPS). *J. Vet. Intern. Med.* 1: 175–182.

164 Levi, M. and Ten Cate, H. (1999). Disseminated intravascular coagulation. *N. Engl. J. Med.* 341: 586–592.

165 Morris, D.D. (1988). Recognition and management of disseminated intravascular coagulation in horses. *Vet. Clin. North Am. Equine Pract.* 4: 115–143.

166 Zhang, Y., Scandura, J.M., Van Nostrand, W.E. et al. (1997). The mechanism by which heparin promotes the inhibition of coagulation factor XIa by protease nexin-2. *J. Biol. Chem.* 272: 26139–26144.

167 Scarlatescu, E., Tomescu, D., and Arama, S. (2017). Anticoagulant therapy in sepsis. The importance of timing. *J. Crit. Care Med.* 3: 63–69.

168 Armengou, L., Monreal, L., Delgado, M.A. et al. (2010). Low-molecular-weight heparin dosage in newborn foals. *J. Vet. Intern. Med.* 24: 1190–1195.

169 Divers, T.J. (2003). Prevention and treatment of thrombosis, phlebitis, and laminitis in horses with gastrointestinal diseases. *Vet. Clin. North Am. Equine Pract.* 19: 779–790.

170 Morris, D. (1989). Thrombophlebitis in horses: The contribution of hemostatic dysfunction to pathogenesis. *Compend. Contin. Educ. Pract. Vet.* 11: 1386–1395.

171 Wong, D.M., Alcott, C.J., Wang, C. et al. (2010). Physiologic effects of nasopharyngeal administration of supplemental oxygen at various flow rates in healthy neonatal foals. *Am. J. Vet. Res.* 71: 1081–1088.

172 Giguere, S., Slade, J.K., and Sanchez, L.C. (2008). Retrospective comparison of caffeine and doxapram for the treatment of hypercapnia in foals with hypoxic-ischemic encephalopathy. *J. Vet. Intern. Med.* 22: 401–405.

173 Paradis, M.R. (2001). Nutrition and indirect calorimetry in neonatal foals. In: *Proceedings of the 19th American College of Veterinary Internal Medicine Forum*, 245–247. Lakewood, CO: American College of Veterinary Internal Medicine.

174 Jose-Cunilleras, E., Viu, J., Corradini, I. et al. (2012). Energy expenditure of critically ill neonatal foals. *Equine Vet. J.* Suppl 41: 48–51.

175 Silver, M. and Comline, R.S. (1976). Fetal and placental O2 consumption and the uptake of different metabolites in the ruminant and horse during late gestation. *Adv. Exp. Med. Biol.* 75: 731–736.

176 McKenzie, H.C. and Geor, R.J. (2009). Feeding management of sick neonatal foals. *Vet. Clin. Equine* 25: 109–119.

177 Graham, P.L., Begg, M.D., Larson, E. et al. (2006). Risk factors of late onset Gram-negative sepsis in low birthweight infants hospitalized in the neonatal intensive care unit. *Pediatr. Infect. Dis. J.* 25: 113–117.

178 Williams, C. (2001). Occurrence and significance of gastric colonization during acid inhibitory therapy. *Best Pract. Res. Clin. Gastroenterol.* 15: 511–521.

179 Thorens, J., Froehlich, F., Schwizer, W. et al. (1996). Bacterial overgrowth during treatment with omeprazole compared with cimetidine: a prospective randomized double blind study. *Gut* 39: 54–59.

180 Buendgens, L., Bruensing, J., Matthes, M. et al. (2014). Administration of proton pump inhibitors in critically ill medical patients is associated with increased risk of developing *Clostridium difficile*-associated diarrhea. *J. Crit. Care* 29: 696.

181 Elfenbein, J.R. and Sanchez, L.C. (2012). Prevalence of gastric and duodenal ulceration in 691 nonsurviving foals (1995–2006). *Equine Vet. J. Suppl.* 41: 76–69.

182 Barr, B.S., Wilkins, P.A., DelPiero, F., and Palmer, J.E. (2000). Is prophylaxis for gastric ulcers necessary in critically ill neonates? A retrospective study of necropsy cases 1989–1999. *J Vet Intern Med* 14 (3): 328.

183 Murray, M.J. (1989). Endoscopic appearance of gastric lesions in foals: 94 cases (1987–1988). *J. Am. Vet. Med. Assoc.* 195: 1135–1141.

184 Furr, M.O., Murray, M.J., and Ferguson, D.C. (1992). The effects of stress on gastric ulceration, T3, T4, reverse T3 and cortisol in neonatal foals. *Equine Vet. J.* 24: 37–40.

185 Sanchez, L.C., Lester, G.D., and Merrit, A.M. (2001). Intragastric pH in critically ill neonatal foals and the effect of ranitidine. *J. Am. Vet. Med. Assoc.* 218: 907–911.

186 Borne, A.T. and MacAllister, C.G. (1993). Effect of sucralfate on healing of subclinical gastric ulcers in foals. *J. Am. Vet. Med. Assoc.* 292: 1465–1468.

187 Hart, K.A., Barton, M.H., Vandenplas et al. (2011). Effects of low-dose hydrocortisone therapy on immune function in neonatal horses. *Pediatr. Res.* 70: 72–77.

188 Raidal, S.L., Edwards, S., Pippia, J. et al. (2013). Pharmacokinetics and safety of oral administration of meloxicam to foals. *J. Vet. Intern. Med.* 27: 300–307.

Section II Viral Infections

Gabriele Landolt

The equine neonate is exposed to a wide range of potential pathogens in the first months of life. Although colostrum-derived maternal antibodies protect foals from many systemic pathogens, viral infection at mucosal surfaces occurs with high frequency and can cause significant morbidity and mortality. Part of this elevated risk can be attributed to the functions of the neonatal immune system. Numerous qualitative differences between the neonatal and adult immune system have been described and may reflect a transitionary stage from the intrauterine environment. In utero, materno-fetal tolerance is of utmost importance and may require regulation of fetal cellular and innate immune functions, including differential expression of class I MHC molecules [1], altered natural killer (NK) cell activity [2], increased numbers of regulatory T cells, and myeloid-derived suppressor cells [3, 4], as well as differences in toll-like receptor (TLR) responses [5]. While these mechanisms may be critical in the intrauterine environment, some or all of these may contribute to the vulnerability to infection of neonates.

Even though the foal's immune system can respond to antigens and is immunocompetent at birth, the cellular branch of the immune system is thought to be immature at birth. While equine neonatal B cells can express most immunoglobulin isotypes by the time of birth, serum levels are markedly lower than in older animals. Despite this, following antigen administration, foals mount an antigen-specific immune response consisting of antigen-specific isotype-switched antibodies as well as cytotoxic T-cells [6], albeit of a lesser magnitude than in adult horses [7]. Similarly, human and murine neonatal humoral responses demonstrate a delayed onset of antibody production following challenge, with lower levels of antibodies produced, less efficient antibody affinity maturation, and higher levels of B-cell apoptosis compared to the adult humoral response [8, 9]. Moreover, in humans and mice, the neonatal T-cell response appears to be skewed toward a T helper (Th)2-type and Th17 response pattern [10], typified by the production of interleukin (IL)-4 and IL-13, following a microbial insult. While Th2-type responses are central in defending against helminths as well as driving allergic pathologies, Th1-type responses play a key role in combating challenges posed by intracellular pathogens, including viruses. While T-helper bias has not been conclusively demonstrated to exist in neonatal foals, studies suggest that newborn foals express relatively low levels of IFN-γ at birth [11] and are deficient in their ability to produce IFN-γ in response to stimulation [12]. Neonatal foals also fail to induce substantial IL-4 production in response to stimulation with mitogens [13, 14], which suggests that there is no clear bias toward a Th2 response in equine neonates [7].

Similar to the adaptive immune response, striking differences in neonatal innate immunity have also been characterized. Foal peripheral blood mononuclear cells (PBMCs) are comprised of fewer dendritic cells (DCs) and more B1-like $CD5^{hi}$ cells than adult horses [15–17]. As the name suggests, B1 cells are a B-cell subset, but they exhibit more innate immune functions than conventional B cells. Following stimulation with lipopolysaccharide (LPS), production of IL-12 (a key innate Th1 cytokine) by cord mononuclear cells was found to be far less than adult PBMCs [18]. As discussed in greater detail below, both cell surface and cytoplasmic pattern recognition receptors (PRR), including TLRs, nucleotide oligomerization domain (NOD)-like receptors, and retinoic acid induced gene I (RIG-I)-like receptors, play important roles in innate recognition of common microbial products (e.g. LPS, double-stranded RNA). They are central players in triggering immune responses in key innate effector cells such as monocytes and dendritic cells.

Studies have shown that neonatal responses of cord blood dendritic cells to several TLR ligands are both quantitatively and qualitatively different from adult responses. For example, human neonatal dendritic cells express low amounts of MHC II receptors, CD80, CD86, and

Equine Neonatal Medicine, First Edition. Edited by David M. Wong and Pamela A. Wilkins.

intracellular adhesion molecule-1 (ICAM1), thus impairing efficiency for antigen presentation and T-cell stimulation [19, 20]. In addition, following stimulation with several TLR agonists, neonatal monocytes and dendritic cells produced more IL-6, IL-23, and IL-1β, but less interferon-α (IFN), IFN-γ, and tumor-necrosis factor (TNF)-α [5]. While NK cells are present in higher numbers in peripheral blood of neonates compared to adults, the neonatal NK cells express more inhibitory receptors (e.g. CD94/NKG2A) and have lower overall functionality than adult counterparts, including reduced cytolytic activity [21]. Likewise, upon LPS stimulation, neonatal macrophages produce more IL-10 but less IL-1β, IL-12, and TNF-α compared to adult macrophages and are less responsive to IFN-γ activation [22, 23]. As the innate immune system is essential for initial detection of invading viruses and subsequent activation of adaptive immunity, these immature patterns of innate immunity might affect the outcome of viral infection of the neonate. Highlighting the importance of innate immunity in the foal's immune defense, a study comparing the transcriptome of neonates to older foals and adult horses found higher expression of innate immune genes, such as genes for antimicrobial proteins, PRRs, cytokines, and chemokines, early in life compared to a higher expression of adaptive immune genes (e.g. B- and T-cell receptor diversity genes, DNA replication enzymes, cell adhesion molecules etc.) in older animals [24].

Cellular Recognition of Virus Infection

Following attachment and invasion of virus into the host cell, the innate immune system is the first line of defense to prevent viral replication and dissemination, before protection by adaptive immune mechanisms can be achieved. As replicating viruses are obligate intracellular pathogens and utilize host cell protein and nucleic acid processing machinery, the critical discrimination of "self" versus "nonself" (i.e. virus) is usually achieved through recognition of virus-associated nucleic acid motifs [25]. Mammalian cells, under physiological conditions, possess a limited variety of nucleic acids, including double-stranded DNA with methylated CpG motifs and capped single-stranded RNAs (ssRNA). In contrast, the structure of viral nucleic acids is much more diverse and includes linear double-stranded DNA (dsDNA), circular dsDNA, single-stranded DNA (ssDNA), ssRNA, and double-stranded RNA (dsRNA) [25]. These viral nucleic acids often contain unique modifications and polarity that virus-infected cells can detect through PRRs. At least three classes of PRRs have been implicated in sensing virus-associated nucleic acids in infected cells: (i) TLRs; (ii) retinoid acid-inducible gene (RIG)-I-like receptors (RLRs); and (iii) NOD-like receptors (NLRs) [26]. A potential fourth group of viral nucleic acid-based sensors consists of a heterogenous family of cytoplasmic and possibly nuclear DNA sensors [27]. In addition to PRRs, recognition of cell damage or stress induced by viral host cell infection has also been suggested as a nucleic acid-independent mechanism for virus sensing [25]. While TLR and RLR activation results in the production of type I interferons (IFNs) and other cytokines, NLR signaling ultimately results in activation of caspase-1, which processes pre-IL-1β into mature IL-1β [25].

The TLRs are the best-studied family of PRRs and, to date, more than 10 distinct TLRs have been identified in mammalian cells (Table 50.II.1) [29]. Many viruses employ the host cells' endocytic pathways to gain entry or exit the cell, and these compartments are intensely surveyed by innate immune sensors. All endosomal TLRs, including TLR3, TLR7, TLR8, and TLR9, are activated by various viral nucleic acid moieties. For example, TLR3 is activated by dsRNA [30], TLR7 by ssRNA [31, 32], and TLR9 by unmethylated CpG DNA motifs [33]. In contrast to TLR3, that is expressed in many cell types including conventional dendritic cells, TLRs7 and 9 are predominantly found in plasmacytoid dendritic cells (pDCs) [34], which produce large amounts of type I interferons in response to virus infection. While all TLR activation ultimately culminates in the induction of type I interferon (IFN-I), as well as early response inflammatory cytokine genes, not every TLR capable of viral molecular pattern sensing is activated during viral infection. For instance, vesicular stomatitis virus RNA is recognized by TLR7 [35] and IFN-I production in response to adenovirus infection occurs in a TLR9-dependent manner [36].

Cytoplasmic detection of viral RNAs is mediated by the plasmin-receptor protein (PRL) family, which consists of RIG-I and the melanoma differentiation-associated gene 5 (MDA5). These cytoplasmic pattern recognition sensors play a key role in detection of many enveloped viruses that enter the cell without exposing their nucleic acids in the endosomal compartment (e.g. influenza A virus). Although both RIG-I and MDA5 activation results in IFN-I production, the pathogen-associated molecular patterns (PAMPs) resulting in their activation differ between them. Specifically, RIG-I activation is accomplished by either binding of short dsRNA or 5′-triphosphate-containing ssRNA, while MDA5 activation follows binding of long dsRNA species. Accordingly, the RIG-I-mediated antiviral response is elicited upon infection with paramyxoviruses, vesicular stomatitis virus, influenza virus, and Japanese encephalitis virus [37, 38], and an MDA5-mediated innate immune response is observed following reovirus and picornavirus infection [39, 40]. While PRL-mediate immune activation can generate a potent antiviral response, several

Table 50.II.1 Characteristics of human toll-like receptors (TLRs) [28].

TLR member	TLR expression	TLR coreceptor	Origin	Signaling adaptors
TLR1	Cell membrane	TLR2	Nonviral	BCAP, TIRAP, MyD88, SCIMP
TLR2	Cell membrane	TLR1, 2, 6 & 10 CD14, CD36, integrin, RP105, MBL, LBP	Nonviral	BCAP, TIRAP, MyD88, SCIMP
TLR3	Endoplasmic reticulum, Lysosomal membrane	CD14, Mex3B	Viral	SARM, SCIMP, TRIF, TICAM1
TLR4	Cell membrane, Endoplasmic reticulum, Lysosomal membrane	MD2, LY96, CD14, CD36, LBP, RP105	Nonviral TICAM1, TICAM2	BCAP, TIRAP, MyD88, SARM, SCIMP,
TLR5	Cell membrane		Nonviral	MyD88, TICAM1
TLR6	Cell membrane	TLR2, CD36, LBP	Nonviral	BCAP, TIRAP, MyD88, SCIMP
TLR7	Cell membrane Endoplasmic reticulum, Lysosomal membrane	CD14	Viral	MyD88
TLR8	Endoplasmic reticulum, Lysosomal membrane		Viral	MyD88
TLR9	Endoplasmic reticulum, Lysosomal membrane	CD14	Viral	TIRAP, MyD88, SCIMP
TLR10	Cell Membrane		Nonviral	MyD88

BCAP, B-cell adaptor for phosphoinositide; CD, cluster of differentiation; LPB, lipopolysaccharide binding protein; MBL, Mannan-binding lectin; MyD88, Myeloid differentiation primary response protein 88; SARM, Sterile α- and armadillo-motif-containing protein; SCIMP, SLP adaptor and CSK interacting membrane protein; TICAM, Toll-IL-1 receptor homology domain-containing adapter molecule; TIR, Toll-interleukin-1 receptor domain; TIRAP, TIR domain-containing adapter protein; TRIF, TIR-domain-containing adaptor protein that induces IFN-γ.

viruses have evolved mechanisms to counter viral nucleic acid recognition by the host's innate immune system. For example, the Ebolavirus-encoded VP35 binds to and caps the dsRNA blunt ends, therefore reducing RLR blunt-end dsRNA recognition, which results in reduced IFN induction [41, 42].

The members of the NLR family consist of a number of cytosolic sensors (e.g. in humans, 22 NLR homologs) that recognize various PAMPs (e.g. bacterial cell-wall derivates, microbial toxins, viral nucleic acid) and danger-associated molecular patterns (DAMPs), such as endogenous byproducts of tissue injury. NLR activation is translated through distinct signaling pathways, which may either initiate the formation of inflammasomes or activate nuclear factor κB (NF-κB), stress kinases, interferon response factors (IRFs), and inflammatory caspases as well as autophagy [43]. The term *inflammasome* describes a cytoplasmic multiprotein complex, which consists of a sensor (NLR), an adaptor protein (apoptosis-associated speck-like protein containing CARD [ASC]), and an effector molecule (pro-CASP1) [44]. These are essential components of the innate response and play an important role in clearance of bacteria, fungi, viruses, and damaged cells. Upon inflammasome activation, pro-caspase-1 is converted to its catalytically active form caspase-1, which mediates the enzymatic cleavage of pro-interleukin-1β (pro-IL-1β) and pro-interleukin-18 (pro-IL-18) into their functionally active forms [43] and subsequent release of these cytokines from the cell. Numerous studies have demonstrated the critical role of NLRs in the activation of innate immune responses to various microbial pathogens, including influenza A virus [45, 46].

Host Cell Interferon Response to Viral Infection and Induction of the Antiviral State

Detection of viral nucleic acid moieties by PRRs in infected or immune cells ultimately leads to the induction of genes that encode proteins with antiviral, antiproliferative, and immunomodulatory activities. These host cell responses eventually prevent viral spread and promote the onset of adaptive immunity. Genes that contribute to the generation of the antiviral state, and an intracellular environment that antagonizes virus replication, can be divided into early and delayed response genes. Expression of early genes is regulated by transcription factor families, including NF-κB, ATF-2/c-Jun, and interferon regulatory factors (IRFs). These transcription factors are present in the cell in an inactive state and are post-translationally activated by phosphorylation to regulate the expression of the early genes. Genes that fall into the early antiviral response category include genes encoding Type I (IFN-α and IFN-β) and Type III IFNs (IFN-λ), RANTES, IL-15, major histocompatibility class I, and inducible nitric oxide synthase. After secretion of IFNs, interferon-induced delayed response genes are activated, which encode hundreds of antiviral host effector proteins including protein kinase, RNA-activated (PKR), Mx protein GTPases, 2′-5′-oligoadenylate synthase (OAS), and ribonuclease L (RNase L) genes.

Type I IFNs can be produced and secreted by professional innate immune cells (dendritic cells, macrophages), but also by all nucleated nonprofessional cell types. Moreover, as the type I IFNα/β receptor (IFNAR) is expressed on virtually all cells, they all can generate antiviral responses. In contrast, IFN-λ binds to a distinct receptor, which is primarily found on epithelial cells that are present at mucosal barriers and some immune cells (e.g. neutrophils) [47] and consists of INF-λ receptor 1 and another subunit shared with the IL-10 receptor [48]. Even though type I and III IFNs share many functional similarities, due to its more restricted tissue tropism, IFN-λ is thought to represent an epithelial cytokine that protects mucosal surfaces without widespread activation of antiviral and pro-inflammatory responses. In contrast, with more ubiquitous expression of IFN-α, -β, and their receptor, type I IFNs represent a more general and potent system that is activated once the mucosal barrier is breached. In addition to epithelial innate immunity, IFN-λ serves immunomodulatory functions. These include modulation of NK and DC function and result in a more potent NK cell activation and skewing of T-cell activation toward an antiviral Th1-type responses [49, 50].

Binding of IFNs to their respective receptors activates transcription factor complex IFN-stimulated gene factor 3 (ISGF-3) [51]. Following its translocation into the nucleus, ISGF-3 binds to IFN-stimulated response elements (ISRE) and results in transcriptional activation of interferon-inducible genes [52]. These IFN-inducible genes are involved in eliminating viral components from infected cells (e.g. 2′-5′-oligoadenylate synthase), inducing apoptosis of infected cells (e.g. PKR, IRF-3) and conferring resistance to viral infection to adjacent, uninfected cells. Interestingly, many of the PRR and IRFs are encoded on interferon-inducible genes themselves, which allows for further amplification of viral sensing and antiviral immune responses.

Following dsRNA mediated autophosphorylation of PKR, the activated enzyme catalyzes phosphorylation of several other proteins including additional PKR molecules [53], the α-subunit of protein synthesis initiation factor 2 (eIF-2α) [54], and transcription inhibitory factor κB (IκB) [55]. In eukaryotic cells, eIF-2 plays a key role in mRNA translation by mediating the GTP-dependent transfer of Met-tRNAi to the 40S ribosomal subunit. The PKR-mediated phosphorylation of the α subunit of eIF-2 (eIF-2α) prevents formation of the eIF2.GTP.Met-tRNAi complex and thus, inhibits cellular protein synthesis. As viruses rely on the host cell's machinery for their own protein synthesis, phosphorylation of eIF-2α effectively blocks viral (as well as cellular) RNA translation and thus, viral replication. Many viruses have evolved mechanisms to evade the antiviral effects of PKR. For example, PKR activation is prevented by adenovirus-associated RNA [56] as well as the nonstructural protein (NS1) of influenza A virus [57].

Another potent, PKR-independent, antiviral mechanism triggered by IFN is the 2′,5′-linked oligoadenylates (2-5A) response, which results in degradation of intracellular RNA, including viral RNAs and all components of cellular protein translation machinery (e.g. mRNAs, tRNAs, and 28S/18S rRNAs) [58]. The 2-5A mediated arrest of protein translation is initiated by conserved small RNAs that contain 2-5A and requires action of two enzymes: OAS and RNase L [59]. Following the binding of viral (or cellular) dsRNA, OASs are activated and catalyze synthesis of oligoadenylates with a 2′,5′-phosphodiester bond linkage. 2-5A binds to RNase L resulting in its activation as well as dimerization, and subsequent cleavage of intracellular RNAs. In addition to viral protein synthesis, RNase L activity inhibits all cellular protein translation, including IFNs production.

Despite the efficacy of these IFN-induced innate immune pathways, virtually all viruses have evolved one or several mechanisms to, at least partially, counteract IFN-mediated innate immune functions. Viral interference with the type I IFN system is accomplished at several levels including disruption of intracellular IFN signaling pathways, interference with IFN production, as well as disruption of antiviral protein function [60]. For example, poxviruses encode a soluble interferon receptor homolog, which bind secreted IFN and thus prevents activation of cellular IFN-receptors [59]. The nonstructural protein 1 (NS1) of influenza A virus blocks interferon-dependent and independent antiviral responses by binding to dsRNA-binding region of PKR, thus blocking its activation, and inhibiting the activation of IRF-3 and NFκB [61–63]. The adenoviral E1A protein inhibits the DNA binding activity of ISGF-3, thus blocking transcriptional activation of interferon-inducible genes [64]. In addition to several other immunomodulatory strategies (e.g. interference with complement-mediated clearance and suppression of MHC-1 expression), equine herpesvirus-1 (EHV-1) has been found to suppress type I IFN production in endothelial cell cultures by down-regulating IRF-3 and inhibiting its nuclear translocation as well as by interfering with signaling pathways [65, 66]. In contrast to EHV-4, the EHV-1 envelope glycoprotein gG has also been found to bind and block activity of a broad range of chemokines and inhibit the migration of equine neutrophils in response to IL-8 [67, 68].

To counteract viral immune evasion strategies, infected cells transmit signals to adjacent uninfected cells by an IFN-independent mechanism, which is mediated by transfer of extracellular vesicles between neighboring cells [69]. A well-studied example of such extracellular vesicles is the exosome, which is formed in multivesicular bodies by inward budding of the endosomal membrane. Studies have shown that infected cells can encapsulate viral components, such as viral RNAs and proteins, within exosomes or exosome-like vesicles and transfer these vesicles to in-contact cells [69]. Similar to paracrine actions of IFN, the transfer of these components triggers a response in neighboring cells in the absence of viral infection. Moreover, *in vitro* data showed that such exosome-mediated transfer of material from infected cells plays a key role in activation of pDCs [70]. This alternative pathway for pDC activation has been demonstrated for various RNA viruses (e.g. *Flaviviridae*, *Arenaviridae*, *Retroviridae*, and *Picornaviridae*) [70–74] and has been hypothesized for some DNA viruses (e.g. herpes simplex virus) [75]. Interestingly, the exosomal pathway has also been employed by some viruses (e.g. hepatitis C virus) as a mode of viral transmission between cells [76].

Cellular Components of the Innate Immune Response and Their Role in Antiviral Immune Defense

Dendritic cells serve as immune sentinels that instruct both innate and adaptive immune responses. They are central in orchestrating pathogen-directed immunity and regulation of viral pathogenesis and also direct a myriad of immune responses, including activation of T cells, NK cells, and maturation of antigen-presenting cells. Different subsets of DCs respond in unique fashion to orchestrate antiviral responses. Among these, pDCs are crucial in the early antiviral response, as they can produce vast amounts of type I and type III IFNs [77, 78]. As discussed previously, pDC activation is primarily triggered by TLR7 and TLR9-mediated sensing of viral nucleic acid species and the cells' importance in the early stages of viral infection has been highlighted in several studies [79–82]. As outlined above, despite being permissive for many viral agents, pDCs preferentially sense viral infection via close cell-to-cell contact with infected cells. This restriction of pDC activation to the site of infection may serve a host-protective function, as abundant, systemic production of IFNs and other cytokines has detrimental effects on the host and has been correlated with immune dysfunction characterized by inhibition of DC differentiation and weakening of the $CD8^+$ T-cell response [83–85], tissue damage, and increased vascular permeability [86]. Interestingly, it has been suggested that some viruses induce an overwhelming IFN-α/β production causing profound immunosuppression as a means of viral immune evasion [84]. To further illustrate the importance of controlled IFN production, the pDC response is likely also modulated by the local environment, as studies note a heterogenous distribution in several organs of pDC subsets with varied abilities to produce IFNs [87].

NK cells are a distinct lineage of lymphoid cells defined by expression of CD56 and NKp46 and absence of CD3 [88]. These cells recognize virus infected cells without the need for prior sensitization. Cytokines and chemokines released by dendritic cells, macrophages, and infected cells activate NK cells. Activated NK cells in turn produce cytokines and chemokines important for control of viral infections as well as shaping the subsequent adaptive immune responses. They represent an early defense against viral infection and their importance as innate immune system effectors is highlighted by their rapid activation after viral infection [89]. NK cells can eliminate virus-infected (and tumor) cells via antibody-dependent cellular cytotoxicity (ADCC), release of perforin and granzyme B, and by TNF-related apoptosis-inducing ligand (TRAIL) and FasL-mediated apoptosis [90–92]. Through production of various cytokines (e.g. IL-5, IL-10, IFN-γ, GM-CSF, TNF-α, TGF-β) they have important immune regulatory functions, such as induction of Th1 responses and upregulation of MHC-1 expression [88]. Moreover, as NK cells interact with other immune cells (e.g. DCs, B, and T cells), they serve as a bridge between innate and adaptive immune responses [93].

NK cells express a variety of receptors including killer cell immunoglobulin-like receptor (KIR) and killer cell lectin-like receptors (KLR; e.g. CD94/NKG2, Ly49) through which cell recognition is mediated. Binding of ligand to these receptors is selective and requires presentation of peptides in association with an MHC I molecule, which allows distinction of "self" versus "nonself" [94]. Following interaction with a virus infected target cell, the NK cell releases perforin and granzymes [95]. Perforin binds to and polymerizes phospholipid head groups in the cell membrane, thus forming transmembrane channels. Cellular uptake of granzyme ultimately triggers cellular pathways that result in apoptosis [96]. As with other host cell immune defense strategies, several viruses have evolved mechanisms to downregulate expression of MHC I molecules to evade cytotoxic T-cell-mediated immunity. While these "missing-self" cells should thus become susceptible to NK cell-mediated lysis, certain viruses permit the selective expression of some forms of MHC-I heavy chain receptors (e.g. HLA-C and HLA-E) [89]. As these MHC-I ligands are preferentially recognized by human NK cell inhibitory receptors, NK-mediated cytotoxicity is inhibited. Similarly, several herpes viruses (e.g. murine and human cytomegalovirus) encode MHC class I analogues that bind to inhibitory NK cell receptors [97, 98]. Interestingly, infection of foals with EHV-1 did not result in suppression (or enhancement) of NK cell-mediated cytotoxicity [99]. Lastly, viruses may affect the ability of target cells to express adhesion and co-stimulatory molecules necessary to efficiently activate NK and other immune cells [100].

In newborn infants there is a higher percentage of circulating NK cells, particularly the less-mature $CD56^{-}CD16^{+}$ subset, compared to adults [101–103]. These cells have a lower level of cytotoxicity compared to NK cells in adults [91, 104], which potentially is due to a lower expression of cell-adhesion molecules (e.g. L-selectin, ICAM-1) [105], and increased expression of inhibitory receptors (e.g. CD94/NKG2A) [106]. Moreover, in humans, neonatal NK cells rarely express CD57, which is a marker of terminal differentiation [107]. While there are fewer TNF-α producing NK cells in neonates, they exhibit higher INF-γ production and CD69 (a transmembrane lectin protein) expression following stimulation with IL-12 and IL-18 than adult counterparts [108, 109]. Adult people have higher frequency of NK cells, expressing an inhibitory KIR receptor for self-MHC-I compared to infants [110]. As these cells show enhanced effector function (i.e. NK licensing), the reduced clonal frequency found in newborns might contribute to their greater infection susceptibility [111]. Additional phenotypic and functional differences of neonatal NK cells compared to adult counterparts may further compromise antiviral immune defenses. For example, in humans, influenza A virus can directly infect NK cells and induce their apoptosis [112]. This influenza-induced apoptosis was more pronounced in neonatal NK cells than adult cells, which may contribute to greater morbidity of infants following infection with influenza [113].

Viral Pathogens Affecting Foals

Several viral pathogens can impact equine neonates with infection occurring either vertically or horizontally following parturition (Table 50.II.2). Viral agents infecting the pregnant mare that can cause abortion include EHV-1/4, equine viral arteritis (EVA), and equine infectious anemia (EIA). However, infection of the dam does not always result in abortion and foals are sometimes born alive but infected. These foals may be clinically normal at birth but develop viral pneumonia within the first few days of life and die from severe respiratory disease shortly thereafter. Vertical transmission of nonprimate hepacivirus (NPHV) has also been described, although the clinical relevance of in utero fetal infection remains unclear [114, 115]. Lastly, viral pathogens can infect foals in the postnatal period and can cause disease ranging from mild to severe. Agents that fall into this last category include the equine herpesviruses, equine arteritis virus (EAV), equine adenovirus, equine rotavirus, equine influenza virus (EIV), equine rhinitis virus, equine coronavirus (ECoV), equine encephalosis virus (EEV), and cowpox virus.

Equine Herpesviruses

Members of the *Herpesviridae* family, equine herpesviruses 1 and 4 are classified as alphaherpesvirinae. They are large, enveloped viruses containing a linear, double-stranded DNA genome. The virus encodes 80 (with at least 76 distinct genes and four duplicates) and 79 (with 76 unique genes and 3 duplicates) open reading frames (ORFs), respectively, and encodes 77 proteins, which are classified as immediate early, early, and late [116]. Nucleotide homology of EHV-1 and EHV-4 ORFs ranges from 55% to 84% [117, 118]. Despite the genetic and antigenic similarities between these viruses, EHV-1 and EHV-4 demonstrate substantial differences in pathogenicity. While EHV-4 primarily infects and replicates in the respiratory tract, EHV-1 infection can be accompanied by a cell-associated viremia with subsequent systemic distribution of virus. While the pathogenic potential of EHV-1 clearly is greater than EHV-4, differences in pathogenicity have also been demonstrated between various EHV-1 strains particularly pertaining to their neuropathogenic potential.

Studies elucidating the neurovirulence of EHV-1 described a single nucleotide polymorphism (A/G) at location 2254 in ORF30, which encodes the viral DNA polymerase, resulting in substitution of asparagine (N) with aspartic acid (D) at position 752 [119, 120]. These studies noted that viruses recovered from horses with equine herpesvirus myeloencephalopathy (EHM) more frequently encoded D752 than N752 [119]. In contrast, historically abortion appeared to have been associated more closely with the N752 genotype, although in recent years abortions have increasingly been reported following infection with the D752 mutation [119, 120].

EHV-1 has a significant equine health impact through its potential to cause late term abortions, EHM, and chorioretinopathy; viral pathogenesis has been extensively reviewed [121, 122]. While EHV-4 occasionally causes secondary disease (e.g. abortion), this occurs much less

Table 50.II.2 Summary of clinical signs and diagnostic tests for common viral diseases in foals.

	Family	Clinical signs	Diagnosis
Equine herpesvirus	Herpesviridae Alphaherpesvirinae ■ Equine herpesvirus 1 ■ Equine herpesvirus 4	■ Late-term abortion (1 and 4) ■ Infected fetuses in which foal is born alive are weak, jaundiced and typically die from respiratory disease within first few days of life (1) ■ Infection typically self-limiting respiratory disease in older foals (1 and 4)	■ PCR ■ Paired serology ■ Virus isolation ■ IHC
	Gammaherpesviruses ■ Equine herpesvirus 2 ■ Equine herpesvirus 5	■ Keratoconjunctivitis, pharyngitis, respiratory disease, ocular disease ■ Unknown in foals	■ PCR ■ PCR
Equine arteritis virus	Arteriviridae	■ Abortion ■ Interstitial pneumonia; fever, weakness anorexia, limb edema, colic, diarrhea	■ Virus Isolation ■ PCR ■ IHC ■ Paired serology
Equine adenovirus	Adenoviridae ■ Equine adenovirus 1 ■ Equine adenovirus 2	■ Respiratory disease, diarrhea ■ Pyrexia, ocular & nasal discharge, cough tachypnea	■ PCR ■ Paired serology ■ Electron microscopy
Equine rotavirus	Reoviridae	■ Diarrhea, lethargy, fever, dehydration	■ Electron microscopy ■ Virus isolation ■ PCR ■ ELISA
Equine influenza virus	Orthomyxoviridae	■ Pyrexia, anorexia, lethargy, nasal discharge, cough	■ Virus isolation ■ PCR ■ IHC ■ Paired serology ■ Fluorescent antibody

IHC, Immunohistochemistry.

commonly then observed for EHV-1. For both viruses, primary infection occurs at the respiratory epithelium with subsequent viral spread to respiratory tract lymph nodes. Nasal virus shedding is typically observed for 4–7 days post infection but can persist up to 14 days. EHV-1 establishes a lymphocyte-associated viremia, which is how the virus reaches the pregnant uterus, central nervous system, and other tissues. Infection of endothelial cells at these sites results in vasculitis, hemorrhage, thrombosis, and ischemic tissue necrosis. In pregnant mares, vasculitis of the small arteriolar branches of the glandular layer of the endometrium and transplacental spread of the virus to the fetus can result in abortion, although fetal infection is not a prerequisite for abortion [123]. EHV-1 DNA has also been detected in sperm of infected stallions, but venereal transmission has not been demonstrated [124, 125]. Abortion commonly occurs in the last 4 months of pregnancy, but occasionally can occur as early as the second trimester [121].

Pathologic lesions in the fetus include multifocal areas of necrosis in the lungs, adrenal glands, and lymphoid tissues, as well as hepatic necrosis, evident as white spots on the liver capsule and cut surface (Figure 50.II.1) [126].

PCR analysis of tissues from aborted fetuses demonstrated presence of virus in the placenta, lung, liver, spleen, and thymus [127]. Some infected foals are born alive but are weak and jaundiced, and they die from respiratory failure within the first few days of life. Death is typically a consequence of primary viral pneumonia with or without secondary bacterial infection. The leukogram

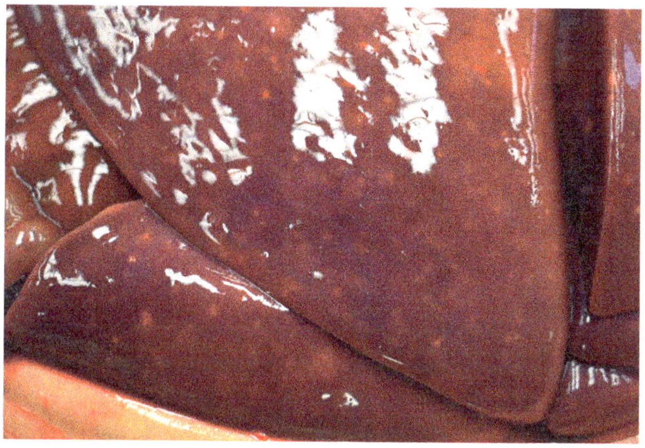

Figure 50.II.1 Liver from a foal with equine herpes virus infection; note the white spots on the surface of liver. *Source:* Image courtesy of Dr. Rebecca Ruby, University of Kentucky.

of EHV-1 infected neonates <24 hours old has significantly lower lymphocyte counts compared to foals that were deemed normal, premature, dysmature, and suffering from bacterial infection or neonatal encephalopathy [128]. In addition, extensive depletion of thymic and splenic lymphocytes has been described, which promotes the foal's susceptibility to secondary bacterial infections [129].

Analysis of bone marrow from foals succumbing to EHV-1 infection demonstrated severe myeloid depletion with toxic myeloid series cells, an increased left shift index, and high numbers of atypical lymphocytes with vacuolated cytoplasm and metamyelocytes with ring nuclei [128]. While damage to parenchymal and lymphoreticular organs is often severe, some neonatal foals survive infection [130]. Moreover, natural infection of young foals (7–11 days old) has been documented in several studies, with some infected foals remaining asymptomatic [131, 132]. Viral shedding was also detected in two premature foals born to mares experimentally infected with EHV-1. As virus shedding was detected starting on days 4 and 5 post-parturition, it was hypothesized that foals were infected during or immediately after parturition. Interestingly, despite detectable shedding of virus, neither foal displayed clinical signs of infection [127].

The establishment of latency is a key feature in the epidemiology of herpesviruses, including EHV-1 and EHV-4, and allows the virus to persist for lengthy periods, and likely life-long within its equine host. Latency is established in the lymphoreticular system and in the trigeminal ganglion [121]. Reactivation and subsequent nasal virus shedding can result in infection of new susceptible horses and possibly in disease in the latently infected horse itself. There is ample evidence that primary infection of most horses occurs early in life, with the likely source of infection being the dam. For instance, EHV-1 and EHV-4 DNA was identified in nasal secretions of foals born to EHV vaccinated mares as early as 22 days and 11 days postpartum, respectively [131]. Interestingly, many of the infected foals did not demonstrate overt signs of respiratory disease [131]. Experimental infection of specific pathogen-free foals lacking maternally derived antibodies resulted in a mild, self-limiting upper respiratory tract disease [133]. Another study demonstrated peak incidence of EHV-1 infection in weanling foals approximately 130 days of age, suggesting foal-to-foal spread of virus both prior and after weaning [134]. These findings support the presence of a silent cycle of virus spread, in which virus stemming from lactating mares spreads to their asymptomatic foals with subsequent subclinical spread of virus from these foals to other foals [131, 134, 135]. Thus, establishment of latency with subsequent viral reactivation resulting in viral shedding likely makes elimination of these viruses from the equine population impossible. Another critical feature for EHV-1 maintenance is its ability to evade both innate and acquired immunity. For example, the virus has evolved mechanisms to interfere with ADCC and cytotoxic T lymphocyte (CTL) -mediated lysis of infected cells and through the action of its envelope protein gG; the virus also blocks the activity of a broad range of host cell chemokines [67, 116]. Thus, protective immunity following natural infection or vaccination is typically brief, and control of EHV-1 by vaccination remains incomplete. While evidence supports the fact that vaccination can reduce viral nasal shedding and provide some protection from respiratory disease, there is little evidence that vaccination can prevent EHM. Conflicting information is available on the use of vaccination for prevention of abortion [136, 137].

Diagnosis of EHV-1/4 infection relies on demonstration of viral antigen, its genome, or virus isolation. Conventional and real-time EHV-1/4 PCR assays are offered by diagnostic laboratories. In addition, many commercially available PCR assays are capable of distinguishing between neuropathogenic and non-neuropathogenic EHV-1 strains. While serological assays are widely available and cost-effective, diagnosis of active infection relies on testing paired samples and demonstration of seroconversion between acute and convalescent samples. Except for a commercially available gG-specific enzyme-linked immunosorbent assay (ELISA), most serological assays cannot distinguish between EHV-1 and EHV-4 infection [138, 139].

As disease caused by EHV-1/4 is often mild and self-limiting in foals, treatment is typically symptomatic. Antiviral therapy, consisting of administration of acyclovir and valganciclovir, has been used in horses with EHM with varying results. Anecdotal reports suggest a potential benefit of acyclovir administration in neonatal foals with EHV-1 infection [130].

Equine herpesvirus 2 and 5, members of equine gammaherpesviruses, were historically named *equine cytomegaloviruses* because of their slow-developing cytopathic effect and high cell-association [140]. Also designated as an equine gammaherpesvirus, the donkey is the natural host of EHV-7 (also called asinine herpesvirus 2 [AHV-2]) [141]. Like the alphaherpesviruses, EHV-2 and EHV-5 contain a linear, double-stranded DNA genome. In conserved sequences, the viruses share approximately 60% sequence homology; this includes homology in genes encoding the DNA polymerase and glycoprotein B [142]. In contrast to alphaherpesviruses, gammaherpesviruses demonstrate substantial genomic diversity due to frequent deletion and insertional mutations [143–145]. Interestingly, studies note recombination events occur even in genomic regions previously characterized as stable [146]. This substantial genomic variability of EHV-2 and EHV-5 may explain why horses can be infected with multiple strains over their lifetime [147].

Both viruses appear to have a worldwide distribution and similar to alphaherpesviruses, primary infection likely occurs early in life, with subsequent establishment of latent infection and periodic reactivation. For EHV-2, latent infection occurs in B lymphocytes and the virus or its DNA can frequently be detected in nasopharyngeal swabs, either due to recrudescence of latent infection or as the result of reinfection with a different EHV-2 [147]. While foals as young as 25 days of age can shed virus in nasal secretion, primary EHV-5 infection appears to occur later in life [148]. Despite this, nasal virus shedding occurs in foals as young as 1 month of age [148, 149]. The source of primary infection of the foal is likely the dam, as viruses isolated from foals and their dams were found to share the same gB sequence [147, 148]. While the presence of colostrum-derived antibodies can delay onset of nasal virus shedding in the foal, the presence of EHV-2 specific antibodies does not protect from infection [147]. Following primary infection, virus can subsequently be transmitted horizontally among in-contact foals [150]. Likely due to the development of an adaptive immune response, viral load, and gB diversity was shown to decrease at 3–5 months of age [147, 151].

Infection of horses with EHV-2 and EHV-5 has been associated with a wide range of clinical signs, including respiratory disease, ocular disease, poor performance, pharyngitis, abortion, granulomatous dermatitis, oral and esophageal ulcers, and equine multinodular pulmonary fibrosis [152]. As viruses can be detected in horses with or without clinical disease, their clinical significance has remained debatable. In foals, EHV-2 has been isolated from animals suffering from keratoconjunctivitis, pharyngitis, and respiratory disease. Following experimental infection, foals developed mild to severe chronic pharyngitis and was also observed following natural infection [153]. Mild signs of upper respiratory tract disease with rhinitis, lymphadenopathy, and pyrexia have also been described [149, 151].

Detection of equine gammaherpesviruses is accomplished employing PCR-based methods, although the virus can also be isolated using cell culture techniques. As the viruses share close antigenic similarities, serological methods are not commonly employed in the routine diagnostic setting [154].

Equine Arteritis Virus

EAV, a member of the family *Arteriviridae*, is an enveloped positive-sense, single-stranded RNA virus. The virus was first identified in lung tissue of an aborted foal during a widespread outbreak of respiratory disease and abortion in Standardbred horses in 1953 [155, 156]. The virus has a polycistronic genome of approximately 12.7 kb, which contains at least 10 functional ORFs. The ORFs 1a and 1b encode two replicase proteins that are translated to produce two polyproteins (pp1a and pp1ab) that are extensively processed by viral proteases (nsp1, nsp2, and nsp4) to generate at least 13 nonstructural proteins. The remaining ORFs encode seven envelope proteins and viral nucleocapsid protein. The envelope protein GP5 serves as the major viral neutralization determinant, and four neutralization sites (A–D) have been identified. Based on genetic determinants, viruses fall into either a North American or European clade. Interestingly, while only a single EAV serotype has been identified, virus isolates display substantial differences in virulence [157]. Similar to other enveloped viruses, EAV is readily inactivated by lipid solvents and disinfectants. Of epidemiological importance, however, is the fact that the virus can remain infectious for extended periods of time at subfreezing temperatures.

Transmission of EAV occurs by respiratory and venereal routes, and persistently infected carrier stallions are central to maintenance and spread of virus throughout horse populations [158, 159]. The virus persists mainly in the ampulla of the vas deferens, and the carrier state has been shown to be testosterone dependent, as castration resolves infection [159]. Breeding of seronegative mares with EAV-contaminated semen can result in infection rates as high as 85–100% [159]. Following infection, virus can be spread to seronegative animals by respiratory droplets, contact with aborted fetuses and fetal membranes, contaminated fomites, and via embryo transfer [158–161]. The duration of nasal virus shedding is 7–14 days but can last up to 21 days [161]. Systemic dissemination of virus with further replication of virus in the adrenals, thyroid, liver, and testes is accomplished through viremia, which can last up to 21 days.

As the name suggests, the virus infects and replicates in endothelial cells and infection results in vasculitis characterized by fibrinoid necrosis of small muscular arteries, leukocyte infiltration, and perivascular hemorrhage and edema [162]. While most infections are asymptomatic or mild in adult horses, disease can be severe and fatal. Generally, the severity of EVA tends to be greater in very young and old horses. Clinical signs associated with infection of adult horses and weanlings include fever, lethargy, anorexia, ventral, and periorbital edema, conjunctivitis (pink eye), photophobia, epiphora, urticaria, nasal discharge, cough, submandibular lymphadenopathy, and petechial hemorrhage [156]. Depending on the infecting strain, abortion rates range between 10% and 70%, occur from 2 to 10 months of gestation, and may occur without premonitory signs in the mare. Abortion is thought to be a consequence of placental dysfunction because of vasculitis or necrotic myometritis, although transplacental transmission of virus to the fetus has also been documented [156, 163, 164]. The fetus is typically well-preserved, and if lesions are found, they are usually mild [162].

In contrast to adult horses, perinatal infection of foals often results in severe respiratory disease characterized by interstitial pneumonia and high mortality. Clinical signs observed in neonatal foals include fever, weakness, anorexia, limb edema, colic, and diarrhea [155, 156, 165]. One report described two distinct EAV outbreaks in neonatal foals at two Standardbred breeding farms and reported sudden death with no prior evidence of disease [166]. While gastrointestinal tract involvement has been documented in some affected foals [165], respiratory signs typically predominate [166]. Although not considered diagnostic, complete blood count abnormalities may include leukopenia and thrombocytopenia [166]. The most prominent lesions found at necropsy are congested and edematous lungs as well as pleural and pericardial effusion [165]. Histopathology demonstrates the presence of interstitial pneumonia, hypertrophy and hyperplasia of alveolar pneumocytes, alveolar infiltration with macrophages and neutrophils, and hyaline membrane formation [162]. Lymphocytic vasculitis affecting the small arteries and venules of the lungs and several other organs (kidneys, adrenals, spleen), can also be observed [162, 166].

Diagnosis of EVA infection relies on detection of virus via virus isolation, RT-PCR, or immunological methods (e.g. immunohistochemistry) [157]. Histopathology, in combination with immunohistochemistry, is also useful in the diagnosis of EAV-induced abortion and neonatal foal death [166]. Serological diagnosis is based on demonstration of seroconversion in paired samples. Despite the development of several ELISA-based assays, the virus neutralization (VN) test is still considered the principal serological assay for detection of EAV specific antibodies [157].

EVA control measures include identification of carrier stallions, isolation and testing of horses prior to introduction into resident horse populations, segregation of pregnant mares and newborn foals, and vaccination [167]. Serological testing should be performed in all stallions prior to the breeding season; if seropositivity is detected in a stallion with no known vaccination history, testing of the semen for presence of EAV should be conducted. Seronegative mares that are being bred to carrier stallions or with their semen should be vaccinated [167]. While both a modified live and a killed vaccine are commercially available in some countries, only the modified live virus (MLV) vaccine is licensed in the United States. Protection following vaccination is only partial – viral replication still occurs [167]. Moreover, antibodies raised following vaccination do not appear to neutralize all EAV strains with equal efficiency [168, 169]. The manufacturer does not recommend the use of this vaccine in foals <6 weeks of age and in pregnant mares. Vaccination of pregnant mares during the last 2 months of gestation has been associated with the risk of abortion [170].

Equine Adenovirus

Equine adenovirus is a member of the *Adenoviridae* family, which comprises a group of nonenveloped, icosahedral DNA viruses. Two equine adenoviruses have been identified: equine adenovirus 1 (EAdV1) and equine adenovirus 2 (EAdV2) [171]. The virus has a worldwide distribution [172], and serological studies performed in horse populations indicate widespread exposure [173–175]. Virus transmission is thought to occur by direct contact with virus-containing secretions or indirectly via fomites. The virus persists in the upper respiratory tract of adult horses that can serve as a virus reservoir. The virus is also stable and can remain infectious up to 1 year when stored at 4 °C.

Infection of the immunocompetent host often results in localized and mild disease, and the virus has been isolated from healthy adult horses and foals [176, 177]. Conversely, the virus has been implicated as being the cause of acute respiratory tract disease, intestinal infection, and diarrhea in immunocompetent foals [178–182]. It is also well-documented that the virus can cause progressive, fatal pneumonia, particularly in Arabian foals with severe combined immunodeficiency (SCID) [183, 184]. Following experimental infection of a yearling, clinical signs observed were mild and mostly consisted of serous nasal discharge [185]. In contrast, foals developed more significant clinical signs following experimental inoculation, such as intermittent pyrexia, ocular/nasal discharge, cough, and tachypnea [178]. In addition, a quarter of the foals developed transient diarrhea. Foals also developed mild lymphopenia in early infection followed by lymphocytosis.

Recovery occurred in all foals on day 10 postinoculation [178]. Postmortem examination of foals euthanized 14–21 days after infection revealed pulmonary atelectasis and suppurative bronchopneumonia. Histological findings included hyperplasia of airway epithelial cells and presence of intranuclear inclusion bodies [186]. In contrast to the milder disease observed in immunocompetent foals, disease in foals with SCID is progressive and fatal. Gross necropsy findings include conjunctivitis, rhinitis, tracheitis, and pneumonia. Acute pancreatitis and sialoadenitis with histological demonstration of inclusion bodies in acinus and ductal cells have also been described [185, 187]. While no vaccine is currently available, the virus appears to have limited clinical significance for the immunocompetent foal.

Equine Rotavirus

Equine rotaviruses belongs to the family *reoviridae* and are icosahedral, nonenveloped viruses with a segmented double-stranded RNA genome encoding 12 proteins [188]. Rotaviruses replicate in the cytoplasm of cells and encode six nonstructural proteins (NSP1–6) that aid in replication and morphogenesis. Except for NSP1, all nonstructural proteins are essential for virus replication. Like the influenza A virus NS1 protein, NSP1 is an RNA-binding protein that interacts with IRF-3 and antagonizes the host's type I IFN response [189]. The rotavirus virion consists of three layers of capsid proteins, including an inner capsid layer composed of viral protein (VP)1, 2, and 3, an intermediate capsid layer consisting of VP6, and an outer capsid formed by VP7 with spike proteins consisting of VP4 [188].

VP4 serves as the viral attachment; VP6 is used to classify rotaviruses into groups A-H, with equine rotavirus classified into group A. While VP7 is the major neutralizing antigen and used to classify the group A viruses in 27 G types (6 of which have been reported in horses), VP4 is a minor neutralizing antigen and determines the 35 viral G types (6 demonstrated in horses). Despite the vast genetic and antigenic diversity, the majority of circulating equine rotaviruses belong to two G and P types, namely G3P[12] and G14P[12]. Based on differences in three antigenic regions of VP7, G3 viruses are further subdivided into two subtypes – G3A and G3B – with G3A being the predominant subtype in several geographical areas. While other P and G types have been sporadically isolated from foals, they are thought to mainly originate from isolated cross-species transmission events of viruses stemming from other animals such as pigs and cattle [190, 191].

Rotavirus is a significant cause of diarrhea in foals with infection characterized by lethargy, fever, diarrhea, and dehydration [192]. Older foals can be infected, but clinical disease is typically more severe in young foals [193]. Rotavirus can sometimes be identified in feces of adult horses, including the dam [194], but the clinical significance of this is not known. Disease transmission occurs via fecal-oral route and studies in pigs note an infectious dose as low as 90 viral particles [195]. The virus replicates efficiently within the gastrointestinal tract and is shed in high virus titers in the feces. In fact, up to 10^{10} virus particles per gram of feces were found in the feces of infected pigs [195]. Fecal virus shedding might persist well past resolution of clinical signs, which results in substantial environmental contamination [194, 196]. In contrast to most enveloped viruses, rotaviruses can remain infectious for several months in feces at room temperature and are resistant to several disinfectants (e.g. quaternary ammonium compounds), making environmental contamination and fomite transmission major routes for disease spread [197].

The incubation period is short; clinical signs are apparent within 1–4 days post infection. The pathogenesis of equine rotavirus infection is thought to be similar to other species and involves infection of epithelial cells located at the tips of duodenal, jejunal, and ileal villi [192]. Viral replication results in enterocyte destruction, desquamation and inflammation of the mucosa, and subsequent loss in absorptive capacity [198]. In addition to malabsorption, viral NSP4 causes osmotic diarrhea by reducing sodium-glucose cotransport and disrupting Ca^{2+} homeostasis [199, 200]. It has also been speculated that enteric nervous system activation plays a role in rotaviral pathogenesis [201].

Diagnosis is accomplished by several methods, including detection of rotavirus particles in feces by electron microscopy (EM), cell culture-based virus isolation, ELISA and other immune-based assays, and by RT-PCR-based assays. In contrast to both ELISA and RT-PCR, the diagnostic sensitivity of EM and virus isolation is low [192, 202].

Prevention is based on management practices, including reduction of foal density and vaccination. While live attenuated orally delivered vaccines given to foals have been investigated, the mainstay of prevention is administration of an inactivated vaccine to the dam [192]. The vaccines include two monovalent products, which employ either the H-2 G3AP[12] or HO-5 G3BP[12] strain of virus and a trivalent product containing the equine H-2 strain, a simian G3P[2] strain, and a bovine G6P[1] strain [203–205]. Even though all three products substantially increase neutralizing antibodies in mares and their foals, prevention of infection of the foal was only partial following experimental infection and foals from vaccinated mares still developed disease [194, 196]. Results from studies investigating whether disease severity was lessened in foals from vaccinated compared to foals from unvaccinated mares are ambiguous [203–205]. Further information regarding equine rotavirus is found in Chapter 17.

Equine Influenza Virus

EIV is a member of the *Orthomyxoviridae* family and is classified as an influenza A virus. The virus is enveloped and contains a segmented, single-stranded, negative-sense RNA genome [206]. Based on antigenic properties of hemagglutinin (HA) and neuraminidase (NA) proteins, influenza A viruses are divided into subtypes and 18 HA and 11 NA subtypes have been described to date [206–208]. While two subtypes, H3N8 and H7N7, have been associated with equine infections, the H7N7 viruses have not been isolated since the 1970s [209]. Since the mid-1980s, the H3N8 viruses have evolved to form genetically distinct evolutionary lineages, namely Eurasian and American, with subsequent divergence of the American lineage into three antigenically distinct sublineages: South American, Kentucky, and Florida lineage [210]. Currently, viruses belonging to two clades (1 and 2) of the Florida sublineage are the predominant strains circulating in the equine population throughout most of the world [210, 211].

Clinical signs of influenza virus infection include pyrexia, anorexia, lethargy, nasal discharge, and cough. Complications associated with influenza infection include secondary bacterial pneumonia, myositis, myocarditis, and limb edema. Neurological disease due to a nonsuppurative encephalitis has also been described in rare cases [212]. While the disease can have a significant negative impact on the welfare of horses, it is seldom fatal in vaccinated animals. However, in unvaccinated horses and particularly donkeys, deaths have been reported during epidemics [213].

Horses of all ages can be infected following experimental inoculation but there is a lower incidence of disease in foals. Only one published report exists of a widespread outbreak of influenza in foals <6 months of age [214], although sporadic fatalities have been reported to occur in foals. Gross necropsy findings in these foals primarily reveals bronchointerstitial pneumonia [214, 215]. Histological changes in the lung include bronchiolar and alveolar septal necrosis, airway epithelial and alveolar type II pneumocyte hyperplasia, hyaline membrane formation, occasional syncytial cell formation, and infiltration and accumulation of neutrophils, fluid, and cellular debris in alveolar and bronchiolar spaces [215].

The lower incidence of disease in young foals is likely due to the presence of maternally derived antibodies. The duration of protection from colostrum derived antibodies is ill-defined but likely can be improved by vaccinating mares a few weeks prior to foaling [216]. As there is evidence of interference of maternally derived antibodies with inactivated, subunit and modified live vaccine efficacy, primary vaccination should occur after passive immunity has waned (around 6 months of age) [217–220]. In addition, the inefficient antigen presentation in young foals compared to mature horses may affect vaccine efficacy [221]. Induction of tolerance has also been reported to occur after administration of a subunit vaccine to 3-month-old foals [222].

Diagnosis of EIV infection is accomplished by demonstration of virus using virus isolation, its genome by RT-PCR, or viral antigens (e.g. fluorescent antibody testing, immunohistochemistry) in nasal secretion or lung tissue. Serological assays, such as the hemagglutination inhibition assay, are widely available but confirmation of active infection requires the demonstration of seroconversion.

Viral Pathogens of Lesser Clinical Importance in the Equine Neonate

Several viruses sporadically cause disease in foals and include equine rhinitis viruses, ECoV, EEV, and cowpox virus. For many of these viral agents, questions remain regarding their impact on foal health.

Equine Rhinitis Viruses

As the clinical illness was thought to resemble the common cold, equine rhinitis viruses historically were referred to as equine rhinoviruses and classified as members of the genus *Rhinovirus*. While they have remained part of the *Picornaviridae*, the equine rhinitis viruses have since been reclassified into the genus *Aphthovirus* (equine rhinitis A virus [ERAV]) and *Erbovirus* (equine rhinitis B virus [ERBV]), respectively. The genus *Erbovirus* includes three genetically related but serologically distinct viruses: ERBV1 (formerly equine rhinovirus 2), ERBV2 (formerly equine rhinovirus 3), and acid-stable equine picornavirus (ERBV3). The viruses are nonenveloped, single-stranded RNA viruses. The clinical significance of ERAV and ERBV remains ill-defined, as both viruses have been isolated from healthy animals and from horses with respiratory disease [223–227]. First described in 1962, ERAV is endemic in the horse population worldwide [228]. The ERAV seropositivity rate increases with age with only 16% of horses between the ages of 6–12 month found to be seropositive in one study [227]. Waning maternal antibodies, stress, season (i.e. late winter and spring), and increased contact with other horses may be predisposing factors for infection [229–231]. Virus transmission occurs via respiratory droplets. In addition, as ERAV has been found in urine and feces, environmental contamination and fomite transmission may contribute to spread of virus [232]. While recent seroprevalence studies indicate high frequency of exposure to ERBV1 and ERBV2, their clinical significance also remains unclear, as both of these viruses have been isolated from horses with and without signs of acute respiratory illness [229, 233, 234].

Equine Coronavirus

ECoV belongs to the *Coronaviridae* family, which consists of enveloped, positive-stranded RNA viruses that contain a large, polycistronic genome. Based on genetic characteristics, the subfamily *Coronavirinae* is divided into the genera *Alpha-*, *Beta-* and *Gammacoronavirus*. The *Alphavirus* group include human coronaviruses 229E, canine and feline coronavirus, porcine transmissible gastroenteritis virus, porcine and epidemic diarrhea virus. *Betacoronaviruses* are divided into groups A-D, with bovine and ECoVs falling into group A and SARS-CoV and MERS-CoV assigned to group B. Lastly, the *Gammacoronaviruses* include mostly avian coronaviruses [235]. While questions to clinical significance of ECoV remain, reported clinical signs of infection in adult horses include fever, anorexia, leukopenia, colic, and diarrhea [236, 237]. In support of ECoV's role as an enteric disease agent in adults, clinical signs were observed following experimental infection in draft horses [238]. In contrast, isolation of ECoV from a foal with diarrhea was first described in 2000 [239], but Bass and Sharpee first described electron microscopic detection of coronavirus-like particles in fecal samples from three foals with diarrhea [240]. As with many other infectious agents discussed here, the clinical significance of ECoV infection of neonatal foals remains ill-defined, mostly due to the ability to detect virus in foals with and without enteric disease [241]. However, the virus may have significance as a coinfecting agent in enteric disease in neonates, as presence of ECoV may facilitate secondary infection [241]. Surveillance studies suggest a higher prevalence of infection in the United States [242], although ECoV infection has also been detected in other countries [243–247]. While a study found age not to be a risk factor for ECoV seropositivity, the study population lacked horses <1 year of age [242].

Equine Encephalosis Virus

First isolated from horses in South Africa in 1967, EEV is an arthropod-borne virus belonging to the *Reoviridae* family [248]. The virus was considered endemic in South Africa, but recent reports have found a wider geographical distribution including Israel, Palestine, Jordan, and India [249–251]. The virus is transmitted by *Culicoides* midges, including *C. imicola* and *C. bolitinos* [251]. While most infections are subclinical, clinical signs can include anorexia, pyrexia, icterus, and edema. In geographic areas where African Horse Sickness (AHS) is seen, EEV is an important differential diagnosis, as clinical signs can resemble AHS [252]. While clinical disease is typically mild, foals in endemic areas may be susceptible to infection, even in the presence of colostrum derived maternal antibodies [253]. The mortality rate is <5% [252].

Cowpox Virus

Belonging to the genus *Orhopoxvirus* in the family *Poxviridae*, cowpox virus infection of horses occurs rarely [254–256]. Despite its name, the reservoir hosts of cowpox virus are rodents and voles. The virus can occasionally infect other species, including cats, rats, dogs, primates, cattle, elephants, cheetahs, and horses [257]. Infection of a 7-year-old horse resulted in generalized cutaneous pox lesions [256], while infection of a pregnant mare resulted in abortion, with multifocal papules covering the skin, mucocutaneous junctions, and oral cavity of the fetus [255]. Interestingly, perinatal infection of a foal, confirmed by transmission EM, virus isolation, and sequencing, did not result in development of cutaneous pox-like lesions, but virus was found to be present in ulcerative lesions in the buccal mucosa, tongue, esophagus, and stomach [254].

References

1 Hunt, J.S., Petroff, M.G., McIntire, R.H. et al. (2005). HLA-G and immune tolerance in pregnancy. *FASEB J.* 19: 681–693.

2 Szekeres-Bartho, J. (2008). Regulation of NK cell cytotoxicity during pregnancy. *Reprod. BioMed. Online* 16: 211–217.

3 Aluvihare, V.R., Kallikourdis, M., and Betz, A.G. (2004). Regulatory T cells mediate maternal tolerance to the fetus. *Nat. Immunol.* 5: 266–271.

4 Chabtini, L., Mfarrej, B., Mounayar, M. et al. (2013). TIM-3 regulates innate immune cells to induce fetomaternal tolerance. *J. Immunol.* 190: 88–96.

5 Kollmann, T.R., Crabtree, J., Rein-Weston, A. et al. (2009). Neonatal innate TLR-mediated responses are distinct from those of adults. *J. Immunol.* 183: 7150–7160.

6 Tallmadge, R.L., Miller, S.C., Parry, S.A. et al. (2017). Antigen-specific immunoglobulin variable region sequencing measures humoral immune response to vaccination in the equine neonate. *PLoS One* 12: e0177831.

7 Ryan, C. and Giguère, S. (2010). Equine neonates have attenuated humoral and cell-mediated immune responses to a killed adjuvanted vaccine compared to adult horses. *Clin. Vaccine Immunol.* 17: 1896–1902.

8 Adkins, B., Leclerc, C., and Marshall-Clarke, S. (2004). Neonatal adaptive immunity comes of age. *Nat. Rev. Immunol.* 4: 553–564.

9 Tian, C., Kron, G.K., Dischert, K.M. et al. (2006). Low expression of the interleukin (IL)-4 receptor alpha chain

and reduced signalling via the IL-4 receptor complex in human neonatal B cells. *Immunology* 119: 54–62.
10 Restori, K.H., Srinivasa, B.T., Ward, B.J. et al. (2018). Neonatal immunity, respiratory virus infections, and the development of asthma. *Front. Immunol.* 9: 1249.
11 Boyd, N.K., Cohen, N.D., Lim, W.S. et al. (2003). Temporal changes in cytokine expression of foals during the first month of life. *Vet. Immunol. Immunopathol.* 92: 75–85.
12 Breathnach, C.C., Sturgill-Wright, T., Stiltner, J.L. et al. (2006). Foals are interferon gamma-deficient at birth. *Vet. Immunol. Immunopathol.* 112: 199–209.
13 Ryan, C., Giguère, S., Hagen, J. et al. (2010). Effect of age and mitogen on the frequency of interleukin-4 and interferon gamma secreting cells in foals and adult horses as assessed by an equine-specific ELISPOT assay. *Vet. Immunol. Immunopathol.* 133: 66–71.
14 Wagner, B., Burton, A., and Ainsworth, D. (2010). Interferon-gamma, interleukin-4 and interleukin-10 production by T helper cells reveals intact Th1 and regulatory TR1 cell activation and a delay of the Th2 cell response in equine neonates and foals. *Vet. Res.* 41: 47.
15 Hamza, E., Mirkovitch, J., Steinbach, F. et al. (2015). Regulatory T cells in early life: comparative study of CD4+CD25 high T cells from foals and adult horses. *PLoS One* 10: e0120661.
16 Mérant, C., Breathnach, C.C., Kohler, K. et al. (2009). Young foal and adult horse monocyte-derived dendritic cells differ by their degree of phenotypic maturity. *Vet. Immunol. Immunopathol.* 131: 1–8.
17 Prieto, J.M.B., Tallmadge, R.L., and Felippe, M.J.B. (2017). Developmental expression of B cell molecules in equine lymphoid tissues. *Vet. Immunol. Immunopathol.* 183: 60–71.
18 Lee, S.M., Suen, Y., Chang, L. et al. (1996). Decreased interleukin-12 (IL-12) from activated cord versus adult peripheral blood mononuclear cells and upregulation of interferon-gamma, natural killer, and lymphokine-activated killer activity by IL-12 in cord blood mononuclear cells. *Blood* 88: 945–954.
19 Upham, J.W., Rate, A., Rowe, J. et al. (2006). Dendritic cell immaturity during infancy restricts the capacity to express vaccine-specific T-cell memory. *Infect. Immun.* 74: 1106–1112.
20 Willems, F., Vollstedt, S., and Suter, M. (2009). Phenotype and function of neonatal DC. *Eur. J. Immunol.* 39: 26–35.
21 Guilmot, A., Hermann, E., Braud, V.M. et al. (2011). Natural killer cell responses to infections in early life. *J. Innate Immun.* 3: 280–288.
22 Chelvarajan, R.L., Collins, S.M., Doubinskaia, I.E. et al. (2004). Defective macrophage function in neonates and its impact on unresponsiveness of neonates to polysaccharide antigens. *J. Leukocyte Biol.* 75: 982–994.
23 Maródi, L., Goda, K., Palicz, A. et al. (2001). Cytokine receptor signalling in neonatal macrophages: defective STAT-1 phosphorylation in response to stimulation with IFN-gamma. *Clin. Exp. Immunol.* 126: 456–460.
24 Tallmadge, R.L., Wang, M., Sun, Q. et al. (2018). Transcriptome analysis of immune genes in peripheral blood mononuclear cells of young foals and adult horses. *PLoS One* 13: e0202646.
25 Shayakhmetov, D.M., Di Paolo, N.C., and Mossman, K.L. (2010). Recognition of virus infection and innate host responses to viral gene therapy vectors. *Mol. Theory* 18: 1422–1429.
26 Takeuchi, O. and Akira, S. (2009). Innate immunity to virus infection. *Immunol. Rev.* 227: 75–86.
27 O'Neill, L.A.J. and Bowie, A.G. (2010). Sensing and signaling in antiviral innate immunity. *Curr. Biol.* 20: R328–R333.
28 Sameer, A.S. and Nissar, S. (2021). Toll-like receptors (TLRs): structure, functions, signaling, and role of their polymorphisms in colorectal cancer susceptibility. *BioMed. Res. Int.* 1157023.
29 Takeda, K. and Akira, S. (2005). Toll-like receptors in innate immunity. *Int. Immunol.* 17: 1–14.
30 Alexopoulou, L., Holt, A.C., Medzhitov, R. et al. (2001). Recognition of double-stranded RNA and activation of NF-kappaB by toll-like receptor 3. *Nature* 413: 732–738.
31 Diebold, S.S., Kaisho, T., Hemmi, H. et al. (2004). Innate antiviral responses by means of TLR7-mediated recognition of single-stranded RNA. *Science* 303: 1529–1531.
32 Heil, F., Hemmi, H., Hochrein, H. et al. (2004). Species-specific recognition of single-stranded RNA via toll-like receptor 7 and 8. *Science* 303: 1526–1529.
33 Hemmi, H., Takeuchi, O., Kawai, T. et al. (2000). A toll-like receptor recognizes bacterial DNA. *Nature* 408: 740–745.
34 Lund, J., Sato, A., Akira, S. et al. (2003). Toll-like receptor 9-mediated recognition of herpes simplex virus-2 by plasmacytoid dendritic cells. *J. Exp. Med.* 198: 513–520.
35 Lee, H.K., Lund, J.M., Ramanathan, B. et al. (2007). Autophagy-dependent viral recognition by plasmacytoid dendritic cells. *Science* 315: 1398–1401.
36 Iacobelli-Martinez, M. and Nemerow, G.R. (2007). Preferential activation of toll-like receptor nine by CD46-utilizing adenoviruses. *J. Virol.* 81: 1305–1312.
37 Kato, H., Sato, S., Yoneyama, M. et al. (2005). Cell type-specific involvement of RIG-I in antiviral response. *Immunity* 23: 19–28.
38 Melchjorsen, J., Jensen, S.B., Malmgaard, L. et al. (2005). Activation of innate defense against a paramyxovirus is mediated by RIG-I and TLR7 and TLR8 in a cell-type-specific manner. *J. Virol.* 79: 12944–12951.

39 Gitlin, L., Barchet, W., Gilfillan, S. et al. (2006). Essential role of mda-5 in type I IFN responses to polyriboinosinic: polyribocytidylic acid and encephalomyocarditis picornavirus. *Proc. Natl. Acad. Sci. U.S.A* 103: 8459–8464.

40 Kato, H., Takeuchi, O., Mikamo-Satoh, E. et al. (2008). Length-dependent recognition of double-stranded ribonucleic acids by retinoic acid-inducible gene-I and melanoma differentiation-associated gene 5. *J. Exp. Med.* 205: 1601–1610.

41 Leung, D.W., Prins, K.C., Borek, D.M. et al. (2010). Structural basis for dsRNA recognition and interferon antagonism by Ebola VP35. *Nat. Struct. Mol. Biol.* 17: 165–172.

42 Leung, D.W., Shabman, R.S., Farahbakhsh, M. et al. (2010). Structural and functional characterization of Reston Ebola virus VP35 interferon inhibitory domain. *J. Mol. Biol.* 399: 347–357.

43 Velloso, F.J., Trombetta-Lima, M., Anschau, V. et al. (2019). NOD-like receptors: major players (and targets) in the interface between innate immunity and cancer. *Biosci. Rep.* 39: BSR20181709.

44 Latz, E., Xiao, T.S., and Stutz, A. (2013). Activation and regulation of the inflammasomes. *Nat. Rev. Immunol.* 13: 397–411.

45 Allen, I.C., Scull, M.A., Moore, C.B. et al. (2009). The NLRP3 inflammasome mediates in vivo innate immunity to influenza a virus through recognition of viral RNA. *Immunity* 30: 556–565.

46 Thomas, P.G., Dash, P., Aldridge, J.R. et al. (2009). The intracellular sensor NLRP3 mediates key innate and healing responses to influenza a virus via the regulation of caspase-1. *Immunity* 30: 566–575.

47 Galani, I.E., Triantafyllia, V., Eleminiadou, E.-E. et al. (2017). Interferon-λ mediates non-redundant front-line antiviral protection against influenza virus infection without compromising host fitness. *Immunity* 46: 875–90.e6.

48 Sommereyns, C., Paul, S., Staeheli, P. et al. (2008). IFN-lambda (IFN-lambda) is expressed in a tissue-dependent fashion and primarily acts on epithelial cells in vivo. *PLoS Pathog.* 4: e1000017.

49 Koltsida, O., Hausding, M., Stavropoulos, A. et al. (2011). IL-28A (IFN-λ2) modulates lung DC function to promote Th1 immune skewing and suppress allergic airway disease. *EMBO Mol. Med.* 3: 348–361.

50 Lasfar, A., de laTorre, A., Abushahba, W. et al. (2016). Concerted action of IFN-α and IFN-λ induces local NK cell immunity and halts cancer growth. *Oncotarget* 7: 49259–49267.

51 Levy, D.E., Kessler, D.S., Pine, R. et al. (1988). Interferon-induced nuclear factors that bind a shared promoter element correlate with positive and negative transcriptional control. *Genes Dev.* 2: 383–393.

52 Levy, D.E., Marié, I.J., and Durbin, J.E. (2011). Induction and function of type I and III interferon in response to viral infection. *Curr. Opin. Virol.* 1: 476–486.

53 Ortega, L.G., McCotter, M.D., Henry, G.L. et al. (1996). Mechanism of interferon action. Biochemical and genetic evidence for the intermolecular association of the RNA-dependent protein kinase PKR from human cells. *Virology* 215: 31–39.

54 Kuhen, K.L. and Samuel, C.E. (1999). Mechanism of interferon action: functional characterization of positive and negative regulatory domains that modulate transcriptional activation of the human RNA-dependent protein kinase Pkr promoter. *Virology* 254: 182–195.

55 Kumar, A., Haque, J., Lacoste, J. et al. (1994). Double-stranded RNA-dependent protein kinase activates transcription factor NF-kappa B by phosphorylating I kappa B. *Proc. Natl. Acad. Sci. U.S.A.* 91: 6288–6292.

56 Mathews, M.B. and Shenk, T. (1991). Adenovirus virus-associated RNA and translation control. *J. Virol.* 65: 5657–5662.

57 Li, S., Min, J.Y., Krug, R.M. et al. (2006). Binding of the influenza A virus NS1 protein to PKR mediates the inhibition of its activation by either PACT or double-stranded RNA. *Virology* 349: 13–21.

58 Choi, U.Y., Kang, J.-S., Hwang, Y.S. et al. (2015). Oligoadenylate synthase-like (OASL) proteins: dual functions and associations with diseases. *Exp. Mol. Med.* 47: e144.

59 Samuel, C.E. (2001). Antiviral actions of interferons. *Clin. Microbiol. Rev.* 14: 778.

60 Grandvaux, N., tenOever, B.R., Servant, M.J. et al. (2002). The interferon antiviral response: from viral invasion to evasion. *Curr. Opin. Infect. Dis.* 15: 259–267.

61 Bergmann, M., Garcia-Sastre, A., Carnero, E. et al. (2000). Influenza virus NS1 protein counteracts PKR-mediated inhibition of replication. *J. Virol.* 74: 6203–6206.

62 Talon, J., Horvath, C.M., Polley, R. et al. (2000). Activation of interferon regulatory factor 3 is inhibited by the influenza A virus NS1 protein. *J. Virol.* 74: 7989–7996.

63 Krug, R.M., Yuan, W., Noah, D.L. et al. (2003). Intracellular warfare between human influenza viruses and human cells: the roles of the viral NS1 protein. *Virology* 309: 181–189.

64 Leonard, G.T. and Sen, G.C. (1997). Restoration of interferon responses of adenovirus E1A-expressing HT1080 cell lines by overexpression of p48 protein. *J. Virol.* 71: 5095–5101.

65 Sarkar, S., Balasuriya, U.B.R., Horohov, D.W. et al. (2016). Equine herpesvirus-1 infection disrupts interferon regulatory factor-3 (IRF-3) signaling pathways in equine endothelial cells. *Vet. Immunol. Immunopathol.* 173: 1–9.

66 Sarkar, S., Balasuriya, U.B.R., Horohov, D.W. et al. (2016). The neuropathogenic T953 strain of equine herpesvirus-1 inhibits type-I IFN mediated antiviral activity in equine endothelial cells. *Vet. Microbiol.* 183: 110–118.

67 Bryant, N.A., Davis-Poynter, N., Vanderplasschen, A. et al. (2003). Glycoprotein G isoforms from some alphaherpesviruses function as broad-spectrum chemokine binding proteins. *EMBO J.* 22: 833–846.

68 Van de Walle, G.R., May, M.L., Sukhumavasi, W. et al. (2007). Herpesvirus chemokine-binding glycoprotein G (gG) efficiently inhibits neutrophil chemotaxis in vitro and in vivo. *J. Immunol.* 179: 4161–4169.

69 Assil, S., Webster, B., and Dreux, M. (2015). Regulation of the host antiviral state by intercellular communications. *Viruses* 7: 4707–4733.

70 Dreux, M., Garaigorta, U., Boyd, B. et al. (2012). Short-range Exosomal transfer of viral RNA from infected cells to plasmacytoid dendritic cells triggers innate immunity. *Cell Host Microbe* 12: 558–570.

71 Décembre, E., Assil, S., Hillaire, M.L.B. et al. (2014). Sensing of immature particles produced by dengue virus infected cells induces an antiviral response by plasmacytoid dendritic cells. *PLoS Pathog.* 10: e1004434.

72 Feng, Z., Li, Y., McKnight, K.L. et al. (2015). Human pDCs preferentially sense enveloped hepatitis A virions. *J. Clin. Invest.* 125: 169–176.

73 Takahashi, K., Asabe, S., Wieland, S. et al. (2010). Plasmacytoid dendritic cells sense hepatitis C virus–infected cells, produce interferon, and inhibit infection. *Proc. Natl. Acad. Sci. U.S.A.* 107: 7431–7436.

74 Wieland, S.F., Takahashi, K., Boyd, B. et al. (2014). Human plasmacytoid dendritic cells sense lymphocytic choriomeningitis virus-infected cells. *J. Virol.* 88: 752–757.

75 Megjugorac, N.J., Jacobs, E.S., Izaguirre, A.G. et al. (2007). Image-based study of interferongenic interactions between plasmacytoid dendritic cells and HSV-infected monocyte-derived dendritic cells. *Immunol. Invest.* 36: 739–761.

76 Ramakrishnaiah, V., Thumann, C., Fofana, I. et al. (2013). Exosome-mediated transmission of hepatitis C virus between human hepatoma Huh7.5 cells. *Proc. Natl. Acad. Sci. U.S.A.* 110: 13109–13113.

77 Swiecki, M. and Colonna, M. (2015). The multifaceted biology of plasmacytoid dendritic cells. *Nat. Rev. Immunol.* 15: 471–485.

78 Webster, B., Assil, S., and Dreux, M. (2016). Cell-cell sensing of viral infection by plasmacytoid dendritic cells. *J. Virol.* 90: 10050–10053.

79 Machmach, K., Leal, M., Gras, C. et al. (2012). Plasmacytoid dendritic cells reduce HIV production in elite controllers. *J. Virol.* 86: 4245–4252.

80 Pichyangkul, S., Endy, T.P., Kalayanarooj, S. et al. (2003). A blunted blood plasmacytoid dendritic cell response to an acute systemic viral infection is associated with increased disease severity. *J. Immunol.* 171: 5571–5578.

81 Smit, J.J., Rudd, B.D., and Lukacs, N.W. (2006). Plasmacytoid dendritic cells inhibit pulmonary immunopathology and promote clearance of respiratory syncytial virus. *J. Exp. Med.* 203: 1153–1159.

82 Swiecki, M., Gilfillan, S., Vermi, W. et al. (2010). Plasmacytoid dendritic cell ablation impacts early interferon responses and antiviral NK and CD8+ T cell accrual. *Immunity* 33: 955–966.

83 Teijaro, J.R., Ng, C., Lee, A.M. et al. (2013). Persistent LCMV infection is controlled by blockade of type I interferon signaling. *Science* 340: 207–211.

84 Hahm, B., Trifilo, M.J., Zuniga, E.I. et al. (2005). Viruses evade the immune system through type I interferon-mediated STAT2-dependent, but STAT1-independent, signaling. *Immunity* 22: 247–257.

85 McNally, J.M., Zarozinski, C.C., Lin, M.-Y. et al. (2001). Attrition of bystander CD8 T cells during virus-induced T-cell and interferon responses. *J. Virol.* 75: 5965–5976.

86 Costa, V.V., Fagundes, C.T., Souza, D.G. et al. (2013). Inflammatory and innate immune responses in dengue infection: protection versus disease induction. *Am. J. Pathol.* 182: 1950–1961.

87 Zucchini, N., Bessou, G., Robbins, S.H. et al. (2007). Individual plasmacytoid dendritic cells are major contributors to the production of multiple innate cytokines in an organ-specific manner during viral infection. *Int. Immunol.* 20: 45–56.

88 Lee, Y.-C. and Lin, S.-J. (2013). Neonatal natural killer cell function: relevance to antiviral immune defense. *Clin. Dev. Immunol.* 2013: 427696.

89 French, A.R. and Yokoyama, W.M. (2003). Natural killer cells and viral infections. *Curr. Opin. Immunol.* 15: 45–51.

90 Fehniger, T.A., Cai, S.F., Cao, X. et al. (2007). Acquisition of murine NK cell cytotoxicity requires the translation of a pre-existing pool of granzyme B and perforin mRNAs. *Immunity* 26: 798–811.

91 Nguyen, Q.H., Roberts, R.L., Ank, B.J. et al. (1998). Interleukin (IL)-15 enhances antibody-dependent cellular cytotoxicity and natural killer activity in neonatal cells. *Cell. Immunol.* 185: 83–92.

92 Zhang, Y., Cheng, G., Xu, Z.-W. et al. (2013). Down regulation of TRAIL and FasL on NK cells by cyclosporin A in renal transplantation patients. *Immunol. Lett.* 152: 1–7.

93 Robbins, S.H., Bessou, G., Cornillon, A. et al. (2007). Natural killer cells promote early CD8 T cell responses against cytomegalovirus. *PLoS Pathog.* 3: e123.

94 Ljunggren, H.-G. and Kärre, K. (1990). In search of the missing self: MHC molecules and NK cell recognition. *Immunol. Today* 11: 237–244.

95 Kerr, J.F.R., Wyllie, A.H., and Currie, A.R. (1972). Apoptosis: a basic biological phenomenon with wideranging implications in tissue kinetics. *Br. J. Cancer* 26: 239–257.

96 Barber, G.N. (2001). Host defense, viruses and apoptosis. *Cell Death Differ.* 8: 113–126.

97 Farrell, H.E., Vally, H., Lynch, D.M. et al. (1997). Inhibition of natural killer cells by a cytomegalovirus MHC class I homologue in vivo. *Nature* 386: 510–514.

98 Kubota, A., Kubota, S., Farrell, H.E. et al. (1999). Inhibition of NK cells by murine CMV-encoded class I MHC homologue m144. *Cell. Immunol.* 191: 145–151.

99 Chong, Y.C., Duffus, W.P.H., and Hannant, D. (1992). Natural killer cells in normal horses and specific-pathogen-free foals infected with equine herpesvirus. *Vet. Immunol. Immunopathol.* 33: 103–113.

100 Coscoy, L. and Ganem, D. (2001). A viral protein that selectively downregulates ICAM-1 and B7-2 and modulates T cell costimulation. *J. Clin. Invest.* 107: 1599–1606.

101 Chin, T.W., Ank, B.J., Murakami, D. et al. (1986). Cytotoxic studies in human newborns: lessened allogeneic cell-induced (augmented) cytotoxicity but strong lymphokine-activated cytotoxicity of cord mononuclear cells. *Cell. Immunol.* 103: 241–251.

102 Gaddy, J. and Broxmeyer, H.E. (1997). Cord blood CD16+56−cells with low lytic activity are possible precursors of mature natural killer cells. *Cell. Immunol.* 180: 132–142.

103 López, M.C., Palmer, B.E., and Lawrence, D.A. (2009). Phenotypic differences between cord blood and adult peripheral blood. *Cytometry B Clin. Cytom.* 76B: 37–46.

104 Lin, S.-J., Yang, M.-H., Chao, H.-C. et al. (2000). Effect of interleukin-15 and Flt3-ligand on natural killer cell expansion and activation: umbilical cord vs. adult peripheral blood mononuclear cells. *Pediatr. Allergy Immunol.* 11: 168–174.

105 Lin, S.J. and Yan, D.-C. (2000). ICAM-1 (CD54) expression on T lymphocytes and natural killer cells from umbilical cord blood: regulation with Interleukin-12 and Interleukin-15. *Cytokine Cell. Mol. Ther.* 6: 161–164.

106 Wang, Y., Xu, H., Zheng, X. et al. (2007). High expression of NKG2A/CD94 and low expression of granzyme B are associated with reduced cord blood NK cell activity. *Cell. Mol. Immunol.* 4: 377–382.

107 Tanaka, H., Kai, S., Yamaguchi, M. et al. (2003). Analysis of natural killer (NK) cell activity and adhesion molecules on NK cells from umbilical cord blood. *Eur. J. Haematol.* 71: 29–38.

108 Krampera, M., Tavecchia, L., Benedetti, F. et al. (2000). Intracellular cytokine profile of cord blood T-, and NK- cells and monocytes. *Haematologica* 85: 675–679.

109 Nomura, A., Takada, H., Jin, C.-H. et al. (2001). Functional analyses of cord blood natural killer cells and T cells: a distinctive interleukin-18 response. *Exp. Hematol.* 29: 1169–1176.

110 Cooley, S., Xiao, F., Pitt, M. et al. (2007). A subpopulation of human peripheral blood NK cells that lacks inhibitory receptors for self-MHC is developmentally immature. *Blood* 110: 578–586.

111 Kim, S., Poursine-Laurent, J., Truscott, S.M. et al. (2005). Licensing of natural killer cells by host major histocompatibility complex class I molecules. *Nature* 436: 709–713.

112 Mao, H., Tu, W., Qin, G. et al. (2009). Influenza virus directly infects human natural killer cells and induces cell apoptosis. *J. Virol.* 83: 9215–9222.

113 Lin, S.-J., Cheng, P.-J., Lin, T.-Y. et al. (2012). Effect of influenza a infection on umbilical cord blood natural killer function regulation with Interleukin-15. *J. Infect. Dis.* 205: 745–756.

114 Gather, T., Walter, S., Todt, D. et al. (2016). Vertical transmission of hepatitis C virus-like non-primate hepacivirus in horses. *J. Gen. Virol.* 97: 2540–2551.

115 Pronost, S., Fortier, C., Marcillaud-Pitel, C. et al. (2019). Further evidence for in utero transmission of equine hepacivirus to foals. *Viruses* 11.

116 Ma, G., Azab, W., and Osterrieder, N. (2013). Equine herpesviruses type 1 (EHV-1) and 4 (EHV-4)—masters of co-evolution and a constant threat to equids and beyond. *Vet. Microbiol.* 167: 123–134.

117 Telford, E.A., Watson, M.S., Perry, J. et al. (1998). The DNA sequence of equine herpesvirus-4. *J. Gen. Virol.* 79: 1197–1203.

118 Telford, E.A.R., Watson, M.S., McBride, K. et al. (1992). The DNA sequence of equine herpesvirus-1. *Virology* 189: 304–316.

119 Nugent, J., Birch-Machin, I., Smith, K.C. et al. (2006). Analysis of equid herpesvirus 1 strain variation reveals a point mutation of the DNA polymerase strongly associated with neuropathogenic versus nonneuropathogenic disease outbreaks. *J. Virol.* 80: 4047–4060.

120 Goodman, L.B., Loregian, A., Perkins, G.A. et al. (2007). A point mutation in a herpesvirus polymerase determines neuropathogenicity. *PLoS Pathog.* 3: e160.

121 Allen, G., Kydd, J., Slater, J. et al. (2004). Equid herpesvirus 1 and equid herpesvirus 4 infections. *Infect. Dis. Livest.* 2: 829–859.

122 Kydd, J., Hannant, D., and Mumford, J. (1996). Residence and recruitment of leucocytes to the equine lung after EHV-1 infection. *Vet. Immunol. Immunopathol.* 52: 15–26.

123 Smith, K.C., Whitwell, K.E., Binns, M.M. et al. (1992). Abortion of virologically negative foetuses following

experimental challenge of pregnant pony mares with equid herpesvirus 1. *Equine Vet. J.* 24: 256–259.

124 Hebia-Fellah, I., Léauté, A., Fiéni, F. et al. (2009). Evaluation of the presence of equine viral herpesvirus 1 (EHV-1) and equine viral herpesvirus 4 (EHV-4) DNA in stallion semen using polymerase chain reaction (PCR). *Theriogenology* 71: 1381–1389.

125 Walter, J., Balzer, H.-J., Seeh, C. et al. (2012). Venereal shedding of equid herpesvirus-1 (EHV-1) in naturally infected stallions. *J. Vet. Intern. Med.* 26: 1500–1504.

126 Foote, A.K., Ricketts, S.W., and Whitwell, K.E. (2012). A racing start in life? The hurdles of equine feto-placental pathology. *Equine Vet. J.* 44: 120–129.

127 Gardiner, D.W., Lunn, D.P., Goehring, L.S. et al. (2012). Strain impact on equine herpesvirus type 1 (EHV-1) abortion models: viral loads in fetal and placental tissues and foals. *Vaccine* 30: 6564–6572.

128 Chavatte, P., Brown, G., Ousey, J.C. et al. (1991). Studies of bone marrow and leucocyte counts in peripheral blood in fetal and newborn foals. *J. Reprod. Fertil. Suppl.* 44: 603–608.

129 Bryans, J.T., Swerczek, T.W., Darlington, R.W. et al. (1977). Neonatal foal disease associated with perinatal infection by equine herpesvirus I. *J Eq Med Surg* 1: 20–26.

130 Murray, M.J., del Piero, F., Jeffrey, S.C. et al. (1998). Neonatal equine herpesvirus type 1 infection on a Thoroughbred breeding farm. *J. Vet. Intern. Med.* 12: 36–41.

131 Foote, C.E., Love, D.N., Gilkerson, J.R. et al. (2004). Detection of EHV-1 and EHV-4 DNA in unweaned Thoroughbred foals from vaccinated mares on a large stud farm. *Equine Vet. J.* 36: 341–345.

132 Mumford, J.A., Rossdale, P.D., Jessett, D.M. et al. (1987). Serological and virological investigations of an equid herpesvirus 1 (EHV-1) abortion storm on a stud farm in 1985. *J. Reprod. Fertil. Suppl.* 35: 509–518.

133 Gibson, J.S., Slater, J.D., Awan, A.R. et al. (1992). Pathogenesis of equine herpesvirus-1 in specific pathogen-free foals: primary and secondary infections and reactivation. *Arch. Virol* 123: 351–366.

134 Gilkerson, J.R., Whalley, J.M., Drummer, H.E. et al. (1999). Epidemiology of EHV-1 and EHV-4 in the mare and foal populations on a Hunter Valley stud farm: are mares the source of EHV-1 for unweaned foals. *Vet. Microbiol.* 68: 27–34.

135 Gilkerson, J.R., Whalley, J.M., Drummer, H.E. et al. (1999). Epidemiological studies of equine herpesvirus 1 (EHV-1) in Thoroughbred foals: a review of studies conducted in the Hunter Valley of New South Wales between 1995 and 1997. *Vet. Microbiol.* 68: 15–25.

136 Hannant, D., Jessett, D.M., O'Neill, T. et al. (1993). Responses of ponies to equid herpesvirus-1 Iscom vaccination and challenge with virus of the homologous strain. *Res. Vet. Sci.* 54: 299–305.

137 Kydd, J.H., Townsend, H.G.G., and Hannant, D. (2006). The equine immune response to equine herpesvirus-1: the virus and its vaccines. *Vet. Immunol. Immunopathol.* 111: 15–30.

138 Balasuriya, U.B., Crossley, B.M., and Timoney, P.J. (2015). A review of traditional and contemporary assays for direct and indirect detection of equid herpesvirus 1 in clinical samples. *J. Vet. Diagn. Invest.* 27: 673–687.

139 Fuentealba, N., Sguazza, G., Scrochi, M. et al. (2014). Production of equine herpesvirus 1 recombinant glycoprotein D and development of an agar gel immunodiffusion test for serological diagnosis. *J. Virol. Methods* 202: 15–18.

140 Gleeson, L.J. and Coggins, L. (1985). Equine herpesvirus type 2: cell-virus relationship during persistent cell-associated viremia. *Am. J. Vet. Res.* 46: 19–23.

141 Davison, A.J., Eberle, R., Ehlers, B. et al. (2009). The order Herpesvirales. *Arch. Virol* 154: 171–177.

142 Telford, E.A.R., Studdert, M.J., Agius, C.T. et al. (1993). Equine herpesviruses 2 and 5 are γ-herpesviruses. *Virology* 195: 492–499.

143 Franchini, M., Akens, M., Bracher, V. et al. (1997). Characterisation of gamma herpesviruses in the horse by PCR. *Virology* 238: 8–13.

144 Holloway, S., Lindquester, G., Studdert, M. et al. (2000). Analysis of equine herpesvirus 2 strain variation using monoclonal antibodies to glycoprotein B. *Arch. Virol* 145: 1699–1713.

145 Dunowska, M., Holloway, S., Wilks, C. et al. (2000). Genomic variability of equine herpesvirus-5. *Arch. Virol* 145: 1359–1371.

146 Sharp, E.L., Farrell, H.E., Borchers, K. et al. (2007). Sequence analysis of the equid herpesvirus 2 chemokine receptor homologues E1, ORF74 and E6 demonstrates high sequence divergence between field isolates. *J. Gen. Virol.* 88: 2450–2462.

147 Brault, S.A., Bird, B.H., Balasuriya, U.B. et al. (2011). Genetic heterogeneity and variation in viral load during equid herpesvirus-2 infection of foals. *Vet. Microbiol.* 147: 253–261.

148 Bell, S.A., Balasuriya, U.B.R., Gardner, I.A. et al. (2006). Temporal detection of equine herpesvirus infections of a cohort of mares and their foals. *Vet. Microbiol.* 116: 249–2557.

149 Dunowska, M., Wilks, C., Studdert, M. et al. (2002). Equine respiratory viruses in foals in New Zealand. *N. Z. Vet. J.* 50: 140–147.

150 Browning, G. and Studdert, M. (1987). Epidemiology of equine herpesvirus 2 (equine cytomegalovirus). *J. Clin. Microbiol.* 25: 13–16.

151 Fu, Z., Robinson, A., Horner, G. et al. (1986). Respiratory disease in foals and the epizootiology of equine herpesvirus type 2 infection. *N. Z. Vet. J.* 34: 152–155.
152 Hartley, C.A., Dynon, K.J., Mekuria, Z.H. et al. (2013). Equine gammaherpesviruses: perfect parasites? *Vet. Microbiol.* 167: 86–92.
153 Blakeslee, J.R. Jr., Olsen, R.G., McAllister, E.S. et al. (1975). Evidence of respiratory tract infection induced by equine herpesvirus, type 2, in the horse. *Can. J. Microbiol.* 21: 1940–1946.
154 Fortier, G., van Erck, E., Pronost, S. et al. (2010). Equine gammaherpesviruses: pathogenesis, epidemiology and diagnosis. *Vet. J.* 186: 148–156.
155 Bryans, J.T., Crowe, M.E., Doll, E.R. et al. (1957). Isolation of a filterable agent causing arteritis of horses and abortion by mares; its differentiation from the equine abortion (influenza) virus. *Cornell Vet.* 47: 3–41.
156 Bryans, J.T., Doll, E.R., and Knappenberger, R.E. (1957). An outbreak of abortion caused by the equine arteritis virus. *Cornell Vet.* 47: 69–75.
157 Balasuriya, U.B.R., Go, Y.Y., and MacLachlan, N.J. (2013). Equine arteritis virus. *Vet. Microbiol.* 167: 93–122.
158 Timoney, P.J., McCollum, W.H., Roberts, A.W. et al. (1986). Demonstration of the carrier state in naturally acquired equine arteritis virus infection in the stallion. *Res. Vet. Sci.* 41: 279–280.
159 Timoney, P.J., McCollum, W.H., Murphy, T.W. et al. (1987). The carrier state in equine arteritis virus infection in the stallion with specific emphasis on the venereal mode of virus transmission. *J. Reprod. Fertil. Suppl.* 35: 95–102.
160 Broaddus, C.C., Balasuriya, U.B.R., Timoney, P.J. et al. (2011). Infection of embryos following insemination of donor mares with equine arteritis virus infective semen. *Theriogenology* 76: 47–60.
161 McCollum, W.H., Prickett, M.E., and Bryans, J.T. (1971). Temporal distribution of equine arteritis virus in respiratory mucosa, tissues and body fluids of horses infected by inhalation. *Res. Vet. Sci.* 12: 459–464.
162 Del Piero, F. (2000). Equine viral arteritis. *Vet. Pathol.* 37: 287–296.
163 Coignoul, F.L. and Cheville, N.F. (1984). Pathology of maternal genital tract, placenta, and fetus in equine viral arteritis. *Vet. Pathol.* 21: 333–340.
164 Golnik, W. (1981). Natural equine viral arteritis in foals. *Schweiz. Arch. Tierheilk.* 123: 523–533.
165 Vaala, W.E., Hamir, A.N., Dubovi, E.J. et al. (1992). Fatal, congenitally acquired infection with equine arteritis virus in a neonatal Thoroughbred. *Equine Vet. J.* 24: 155–158.
166 Del Piero, F., Wilkins, P.A., Lopez, J.W. et al. (1997). Equine viral arteritis in newborn foals: clinical, pathological, serological, microbiological and immunohistochemical observations. *Equine Vet. J.* 29: 178–185.
167 Balasuriya, U.B.R., Carossino, M., and Timoney, P.J. (2018). Equine viral arteritis: a respiratory and reproductive disease of significant economic importance to the equine industry. *Equine Vet. Educ.* 30: 497–512.
168 Balasuriya, U.B.R., Zhang, J., Go, Y.Y. et al. (2014). Experiences with infectious cDNA clones of equine arteritis virus: lessons learned and insights gained. *Virology* 462–463: 388–403.
169 Zhang, J., Timoney, P.J., Shuck, K.M. et al. (2010). Molecular epidemiology and genetic characterization of equine arteritis virus isolates associated with the 2006–2007 multi-state disease occurrence in the USA. *J. Gen. Virol.* 91: 2286–2301.
170 Broaddus, C.C., Balasuriya, U.B.R., White, J.L.R. et al. (2011). Evaluation of the safety of vaccinating mares against equine viral arteritis during mid or late gestation or during the immediate postpartum period. *J. Am. Vet. Med. Assoc.* 238: 741–750.
171 Giles, C., Vanniasinkam, T., Barton, M. et al. (2015). Characterisation of the equine adenovirus 2 genome. *Vet. Microbiol.* 179: 184–189.
172 Studdert, M., Wilks, C., and Coggins, L. (1974). Antigenic comparisons and serologic survey of equine adenoviruses. *Am. J. Vet. Res.* 35: 693–699.
173 De Boer, G., Osterhaus, A., Van Oirschot, J. et al. (1979). Prevalence of antibodies to equine viruses in the Netherlands. *Vet. Q.* 1: 65–74.
174 Harden, T., Pascoe, R., Spradbrow, P. et al. (1974). The prevalence of antibodies to adenoviruses in horses from Queensland and New South Wales. *Aust. Vet. J.* 50: 477–482.
175 Obi, T. and Taylor, W. (1984). Serological survey of adenovirus antibodies in domestic animals in Nigeria. *Comp. Immunol. Microbiol. Infect. Dis.* 7: 63–68.
176 Harden, T. (1974). Characterization of an equine adenovirus. *Res. Vet. Sci.* 16: 24–250.
177 Wilks, C. and Studdert, M. (1972). Isolation of an equine adenovirus. *Aust. Vet. J.* 48: 580–581.
178 McChesney, A. and England, J. (1975). Adenoviral infection in foals. *J. Am. Vet. Med. Assoc.* 166: 83.
179 Dutta, S. (1975). Isolation and characterization of an adenovirus and isolation of its adenovirus-associated virus in cell culture from foals with respiratory tract disease. *Am. J. Vet. Res.* 36: 247.
180 Gleeson, L., Studdert, M., and Sullivan, N.D. (1978). Pathogenicity and immunologic studies of equine adenovirus in specific-pathogen-free foals. *Am. J. Vet. Res.* 39: 1636–1642.

181 Studdert, M. and Blackney, M. (1982). Isolation of an adenovirus antigenically distinct from equine adenovirus type 1 from diarrheic foal feces. *Am. J. Vet. Res.* 43: 543.

182 Picard, J.A. (2007). *Respiratory Pathogens in Thoroughbred Foals up to One Year of Age on a Stud Farm in South Africa*. University of Pretoria.

183 McGuire, T. (1974). Combined (B-and T-lymphocyte) immunodeficiency: a fetal genetic disease in Arabian foals. *J. Am. Vet. Med. Assoc.* 164: 70–76.

184 Thompson, D., Spradborw, P., and Studdert, M. (1976). Isolation of an adenovirus from an Arab foal with a combined immunode ficiency disease. *Aust. Vet. J.* 52: 435–437.

185 Pascoe, R., Harden, T., and Spradbrow, P. (1974). Experimental infection of a horse with an equine adenovirus. *Aust. Vet. J.* 50: 278.

186 McChesney, A.E., England, J.J., Whiteman, C.E. et al. (1974). Experimental transmission of equine adenovirus in Arabian and non-Arabian foals structure and assembly. *Am. J. Vet. Res.* 35: 1015–1023.

187 Whitlock, R., Dellers, R., and Shively, J. (1975). Adenoviral pneumonia in a foal. *Cornell Vet.* 65: 393–401.

188 Pesavento, J.B., Crawford, S.E., Estes, M.K. et al. (2006). Rotavirus proteins: structure and assembly. *Curr. Top. Microbiol. Immunol.* 309: 189–219.

189 Graff, J.W., Mitzel, D.N., Weisend, C.M. et al. (2002). Interferon regulatory factor 3 is a cellular partner of rotavirus NSP1. *J. Virol.* 76: 9545–9550.

190 Ciarlet, M., Isa, P., Conner, M.E. et al. (2001). Antigenic and molecular analyses reveal that the equine rotavirus strain H-1 is closely related to porcine, but not equine, rotaviruses: interspecies transmission from pigs to horses? *Virus Genes* 22: 5–20.

191 Gulati, B.R., Deepa, R., Singh, B.K. et al. (2007). Diversity in Indian equine rotaviruses: identification of genotype G10,P6[1] and G1 strains and a new VP7 genotype (G16) strain in specimens from diarrheic foals in India. *J. Clin. Microbiol.* 45: 972–978.

192 Bailey, K.E., Gilkerson, J.R., and Browning, G.F. (2013). Equine rotaviruses—current understanding and continuing challenges. *Vet. Microbiol.* 167: 135–144.

193 Dwyer, R., Powell, D., Roberts, W. et al. (1991). A study of the etiology and control of infectious diarrhea among foals in central Kentucky. *Proceedings of the Annual Convention of the American Association of Equine Practitioners* 36: 337–355.

194 Conner, M.E. and Darlington, R. (1980). Rotavirus infection in foals. *Am. J. Vet. Res.* 41: 1699–1703.

195 Payment, P. and Morin, E. (1990). Minimal infective dose of the OSU strain of porcine rotavirus. *Arch. Virol* 112: 277–282.

196 Higgins, W.P., Gillespie, J.H., Schiff, E.I. et al. (1988). Infectivity and immunity studies in foals with cell culture-propagated equine rotaviruses. In: *Equine Infectious Diseases V: Proceedings of the Fifth International Conference*, 241–247. Lexington: University of Kentucky Press.

197 Springthorpe, V.S., Grenier, J.L., Lloyd-Evans, N. et al. (1986). Chemical disinfection of human rotaviruses: efficacy of commercially available products in suspension tests. *Epidemiol. Infect.* 97: 139–161.

198 Woode, G. and Crouch, C. (1978). Naturally occurring and experimentally induced rotaviral infections of domestic and laboratory animals. *J. Am. Vet. Med. Assoc.*.

199 Beau, I., Cotte-Laffitte, J., Géniteau-Legendre, M. et al. (2007). An NSP4-dependant mechanism by which rotavirus impairs lactase enzymatic activity in brush border of human enterocyte-like Caco-2 cells. *Cell. Microbiol.* 9: 2254–2266.

200 Morris, A.P., Scott, J.K., Ball, J.M. et al. (1999). NSP4 elicits age-dependent diarrhea and Ca2+ mediated I− influx into intestinal crypts of CF mice. *Am. J. Physiol.* 277: G431–G444.

201 Lundgren, O., Peregrin, A.T., Persson, K. et al. (2000). Role of the enteric nervous system in the fluid and electrolyte secretion of rotavirus diarrhea. *Science* 287: 491–495.

202 Storch, G. (2007). Diagnostic virology. In: *Fields Virology* (ed. D.M. Knipe and P.M. Howle), 493–531. Philadelphia: Lippincott Williams & Wilkins.

203 Barrandeguy, M., Parreno, V., Lagos, M.M. et al. (1998). Prevention of rotavirus diarrhoea in foals by parenteral vaccination of the mares: field trial. *Dev. Biol. Stand.* 92: 253.

204 Imagawa, H., Kato, T., Tsunemitsu, H. et al. (2005). Field study of inactivated equine rotavirus vaccine. *J. Equine Sci.* 16: 35–44.

205 Powell, D., Dwyer, R., Traub-Dargatz, J. et al. (1997). Field study of the safety, immunogenicity, and efficacy of an inactivated equine rotavirus vaccine. *J. Am. Vet. Med. Assoc.* 211: 193.

206 Lamb, R. and Krug, R. (2001). Orthomyxoviruses: the viruses and their replication. In: *U: Fields Virology* (ed. D.M. Knipe and P.M. Howley). Philadelphia: Lippincott-Raven.

207 Tong, S., Zhu, X., Li, Y. et al. (2013). New world bats harbor diverse influenza A viruses. *PLoS Pathog.* 9: e1003657.

208 Zhu, X., Yu, W., McBride, R. et al. (2013). Hemagglutinin homologue from H17N10 bat influenza virus exhibits divergent receptor-binding and pH-dependent fusion activities. *Proc. Natl. Acad. Sci. U.S.A.* 110: 1458–1463.

209 Webster, R. (1993). Are equine 1 influenza viruses still present in horses? *Equine Vet. J.* 25: 537–538.

210 Lai, A., Chambers, T., Holland, R. Jr. et al. (2001). Diverged evolution of recent equine-2 influenza (H3N8) viruses in the Western Hemisphere. *Arch. Virol* 146: 1063–1074.

211 Bryant, N.A., Rash, A.S., Russell, C.A. et al. (2009). Antigenic and genetic variations in European and North American equine influenza virus strains (H3N8) isolated from 2006 to 2007. *Vet. Microbiol.* 138: 41–52.

212 Daly, J., Whitwell, K., Miller, J. et al. (2006). Investigation of equine influenza cases exhibiting neurological disease: coincidence or association? *J. Comp. Pathol.* 134: 231–255.

213 Powell, D., Watkins, K., Li, P. et al. (1995). Outbreak of equine influenza among horses in Hong Kong during 1992. *Vet. Rec.* 136: 531–536.

214 Peek, S.F., Landolt, G., Karasin, A.I. et al. (2004). Acute respiratory distress syndrome and fatal interstitial pneumonia associated with equine influenza in a neonatal foal. *J. Vet. Intern. Med.* 18: 132–134.

215 Patterson-Kane, J., Carrick, J., Axon, J. et al. (2008). The pathology of bronchointerstitial pneumonia in young foals associated with the first outbreak of equine influenza in Australia. *Equine Vet. J.* 40: 199–203.

216 Paillot, R., Hannant, D., Kydd, J.H. et al. (2006). Vaccination against equine influenza: Quid novi? *Vaccine* 24: 4047–4061.

217 Conboy, H.S., Berry, D., Fallon, E. et al. (1997). Failure of foal seroconversion following equine influenza vaccination. *Proceedings of the Annual Convention of the American Association of Equine Practitioners* 43: 22–23.

218 Holland, R., Conboy, H., Berry, D. et al. (1999). Age dependence of foal vaccination for equine influenza: new evidence from the USA. In: *Proceedings of the Eighth International Conference Quine Infect Dis.* (ed. U. Werney, J.F. Wade, U. Mumford, and O.R. Kaaden). Newmarket: RandW Publications.

219 Van Maanen, C., Bruin, G., de Boer-Luijtze, E. et al. (1992). Interference of maternal antibodies with the immune response of foals after vaccination against equine influenza. *Vet. Q.* 14: 13–13.

220 Wilson, W.D., Mihalyi, J., Hussey, S. et al. (2001). Passive transfer of maternal immunoglobulin isotype antibodies against tetanus and influenza and their effect on the response of foals to vaccination. *Equine Vet. J.* 33: 644–650.

221 Lopez, A.M., Hines, M.T., Palmer, G.H. et al. (2003). Analysis of anamnestic immune responses in adult horses and priming in neonates induced by a DNA vaccine expressing the vapA gene of Rhodococcus equi. *Vaccine* 21: 3815–3825.

222 Cullinane, A., Weld, J., Osborne, M. et al. (2001). Field studies on equine influenza vaccination regimes in Thoroughbred foals and yearlings. *Vet. J.* 161: 174–185.

223 Fukunaga, Y., Kumanomido, T., Kamada, M. et al. (1983). Equine Picornavirus. *Bull. Earthquake Res. Inst.* 1983: 103–109.

224 Flammini, C. and Allegri, G. (1970). Rhino-virus strain as a possible cause of equine respiratory infection. *Archivio Veterinario Italiano* 21: 309–316.

225 Li, F., Drummer, H.E., Ficorilli, N. et al. (1997). Identification of noncytopathic equine rhinovirus 1 as a cause of acute febrile respiratory disease in horses. *J. Clin. Microbiol.* 35: 937–943.

226 Plummer, G. and Kerry, J. (1962). Studies on an equine respiratory virus. *Vet. Rec.* 74: 967–970.

227 Studdert, M. and Gleeson, L. (1978). Isolation and characterisation of an equine rhinovirus. *Zentralbl. Vet. Reihe B* 25: 225–237.

228 Plummer, G. (1962). An equine respiratory virus with enterovirus properties. *Nature* 195: 519–520.

229 Black, W.D., Wilcox, R.S., Stevenson, R.A. et al. (2007). Prevalence of serum neutralising antibody to equine rhinitis A virus (ERAV), equine rhinitis B virus 1 (ERBV1) and ERBV2. *Vet. Microbiol.* 119: 65–71.

230 Holmes, D., Kemen, M., and Coggins, L. (1978). Equine rhinovirus infection: serologic evidence of infection in selected United States horse populations. *J. Equine Med. Surg. Suppl.*.

231 Klaey, M., Sanchez-Higgins, M., Leadon, D. et al. (1998). Field case study of equine rhinovirus 1 infection: clinical signs and clinicopathology. *Equine Vet. J.* 30: 267–269.

232 Horsington, J., Lynch, S.E., Gilkerson, J.R. et al. (2013). Equine picornaviruses: well known but poorly understood. *Vet. Microbiol.* 167: 78–85.

233 Burrell, M., Wood, J., Whitwell, K. et al. (1996). Respiratory disease in Thoroughbred horses in training: the relationships between disease and viruses, bacteria and environment. *Vet. Rec.* 139: 308–313.

234 Carman, S., Rosendal, S., Huber, L. et al. (1997). Infectious agents in acute respiratory disease in horses in Ontario. *J. Vet. Diagn. Invest.* 9: 17–23.

235 Zhang, J., Guy, J.S., Snijder, E.J. et al. (2007). Genomic characterization of equine coronavirus. *Virology* 369: 92–104.

236 Pusterla, N., Mapes, S., Wademan, C. et al. (2013). Emerging outbreaks associated with equine coronavirus in adult horses. *Vet. Microbiol.* 162: 228–231.

237 Pusterla, N., Vin, R., Leutenegger, C. et al. (2016). Equine coronavirus: an emerging enteric virus of adult horses. *Equine Vet. Educ.* 28: 216–223.

238 Nemoto, M., Oue, Y., Morita, Y. et al. (2014). Experimental inoculation of equine coronavirus into Japanese draft horses. *Arch. Virol* 159: 3329–3334.

239 Guy, J.S., Breslin, J.J., Breuhaus, B. et al. (2000). Characterization of a coronavirus isolated from a diarrheic foal. *J. Clin. Microbiol.* 38: 4523–4526.

240 Bass, E. and Sharpee, R. (1975). Coronavirus and gastroenteritis in foals. *Lancet* 306: 822.

241 Slovis, N.M., Elam, J., Estrada, M. et al. (2014). Infectious agents associated with diarrhoea in neonatal foals in Central Kentucky: a comprehensive molecular study. *Equine Vet. J.* 46: 311–316.

242 Kooijman, L., James, K., Mapes, S. et al. (2017). Seroprevalence and risk factors for infection with equine coronavirus in healthy horses in the USA. *Vet. J.* 220: 91–94.

243 Bryan, J., Marr, C.M., Mackenzie, C.J. et al. (2018). Detection of equine coronavirus in horses in the United Kingdom. *Vet. Rec.* 184: 123.

244 Hemida, M., Chu, D., Perera, R. et al. (2017). Coronavirus infections in horses in Saudi Arabia and Oman. *Trans. Emerg. Dis.* 64: 2093–2103.

245 Miszczak, F., Tesson, V., Kin, N. et al. (2014). First detection of equine coronavirus (ECoV) in Europe. *Vet. Microbiol.* 171: 206–209.

246 Nemoto, M., Oue, Y., Higuchi, T. et al. (2015). Low prevalence of equine coronavirus in foals in the largest thoroughbred horse breeding region of Japan, 2012–2014. *Acta Vet. Scand.* 57: 1–4.

247 Nemoto, M., Schofield, W., and Cullinane, A. (2019). The first detection of equine coronavirus in adult horses and foals in Ireland. *Viruses* 11: 946.

248 Erasmus, B., Adelaar, T., Smit, J. et al. (1970). The isolation and characterization of equine encephalosis virus. *Bull. Off. Int. Epizoot.* 74: 781–789.

249 Tirosh-Levy, S., Gelman, B., Zivotofsky, D. et al. (2017). Seroprevalence and risk factor analysis for exposure to equine encephalosis virus in Israel, Palestine and Jordan. *Vet. Med. Sci.* 3: 82–90.

250 Wescott, D.G., Mildenberg, Z., Bellaiche, M. et al. (2013). Evidence for the circulation of equine encephalosis virus in Israel since 2001. *PLoS One* 8: e70532.

251 Yadav, P.D., Albariño, C.G., Nyayanit, D.A. et al. (2018). Equine encephalosis virus in India, 2008. *Emerg. Infect. Dis.* 24: 898.

252 Howell, P., Guthrie, A., and Coetzer, J. (2004). *Equine Encephalosis. Infectious Diseases of Livestock*, 2e, 1247–1251. Cape Town, Southern Africa: Oxford University Press.

253 Grewar, J.D., Thompson, P.N., Lourens, C.W. et al. (2015). Equine encephalosis in Thoroughbred foals on a South African stud farm. *J. Vet. Res.* 82: 1–4.

254 Ellenberger, C., Schüppel, K.F., Möhring, M. et al. (2005). Cowpox virus infection associated with a streptococcal Septicaemia in a foal. *J. Comp. Pathol.* 132: 101–105.

255 Franke, A., Kershaw, O., Jenckel, M. et al. (2016). Fatal cowpox virus infection in an aborted foal. *Vector Borne Zoonotic Dis.* 16: 431–433.

256 Pfeffer, M., Burck, G., and Meyer, H. (1999). Cowpox viruses in Germany: an analysis of 5 cases in 1998. *Berl. Münch Tierärztl. Wochenschr.* 112: 334–338.

257 Marennikova, S., Shelukhina, E., and Efremova, E. (1984). New outlook on the biology of cowpox virus. *Acta Virol.* 28: 437–444.

Neonatal Ophthalmology

Chapter 51 Embryology and Anatomy of the Equine Eye

Bianca Martins and Paula Galera

Ocular Embryology

Understanding the development of the ocular structures is key to comprehending the normal ocular anatomy, physiology, and relationship of ocular structures. Furthermore, it is crucial for understanding how congenital abnormalities develop and the implications they bear to the individual. The ocular development is fairly similar among species, with the same sequence of events displayed, albeit with different timelines [1–3]. In the horse, nasolacrimal system atresia, congenital aniridia, iridial hypoplasia and coloboma, uveal cyst, and cataracts are among the most commonly reported ocular malformations; however, microphthalmos, dermoid (of the eyelids, nictitans, cornea, and conjunctiva), cornea globosa, retinal dysplasia, and optic disc colobomas have been reported, among others [4–12]. This chapter provides an overview of the normal development of the ocular structures and punctuates developmental aspects that may lead to ocular malformations.

Eye formation begins relatively early in development in the forebrain, after gastrulation and formation of the three classic germ layers: ectoderm, mesoderm, and endoderm [1–3]. The ectoderm is the most critical germ layer for ocular development and gives rise to three important embryonic tissues: surface ectoderm, neural crest, and neuroectoderm. As gastrulation proceeds, a portion of the surface ectoderm proliferates and forms two elevations (neural folds), which give rise to the neuroectoderm. As the neural folds approximate to each other, a specialized cell population called the neural crest is formed at the junction of the neuroectoderm and surface ectoderm. The neural crest produces the mesenchyme or embryonic connective tissue [1, 2].

A bilateral evagination is present in the forebrain neuroectoderm – the **optic sulcus** (or optic groove), which will then expand and form the **optic vesicle** (Figure 51.1). The optic vesicles are outward extensions of the forebrain lined by neuroectoderm that will eventually develop into the eyes. If the optic vesicle does not form properly, *microphthalmia* (small eye) develops [1–3]. The optic vesicle is connected to the forebrain by the **optic stalk**, a structure critical to the formation of the optic nerve (Figure 51.1). As the optic vesicle expands, its neuroectoderm contacts the surface ectoderm, triggering the induction of the **lens placode** (Figure 51.1a). The contact of the optic vesicle with the surface ectoderm (inducing the lens placode) is critical to determining the size of the palpebral fissure, and abnormalities on the development of the optic vesicle and its contact with the surface ectoderm (either area of contact or time of contact) lead to a combination of microphthalmia and microblepharon [1–3]. The lens placode then invaginates onto itself (Figure 51.1b), creating a double layer of neuroectoderm, the **optic cup** (Figure 51.1c), which remains connected to the forebrain via the optic stalk.

The outer layers of the optic cup will become the neurosensory retina and the inner layer will become the retinal pigmented epithelium (RPE) of the retina. As the neurosensory retina develops, it differentiates into distinct cell layers comprised of photoreceptor nuclei, an inner nuclear layer composed of multiple cell types, and the innermost ganglion cell layer [1–3, 13]. The anterior aspect of the optic cup extends forward to form the posterior aspect of the iris (posterior pigmented epithelium, iris sphincter, and iris dilator muscles), while neural crest mesenchyme will form the anterior aspect of the iris (stroma). The optic cup also originates the ciliary body. Folding of the double layers results in the formation of the ciliary processes. The inner, nonpigmented epithelium of the ciliary body is contiguous with the neurosensory retina, while the outer, pigmented epithelium of the ciliary body is contiguous with the RPE. Meanwhile, the neural crest mesenchyme originates the ciliary body stroma [1–3]. Failure of adhesion of the inner and outer layers of the optic cup result in uveal cysts,

Equine Neonatal Medicine, First Edition. Edited by David M. Wong and Pamela A. Wilkins.

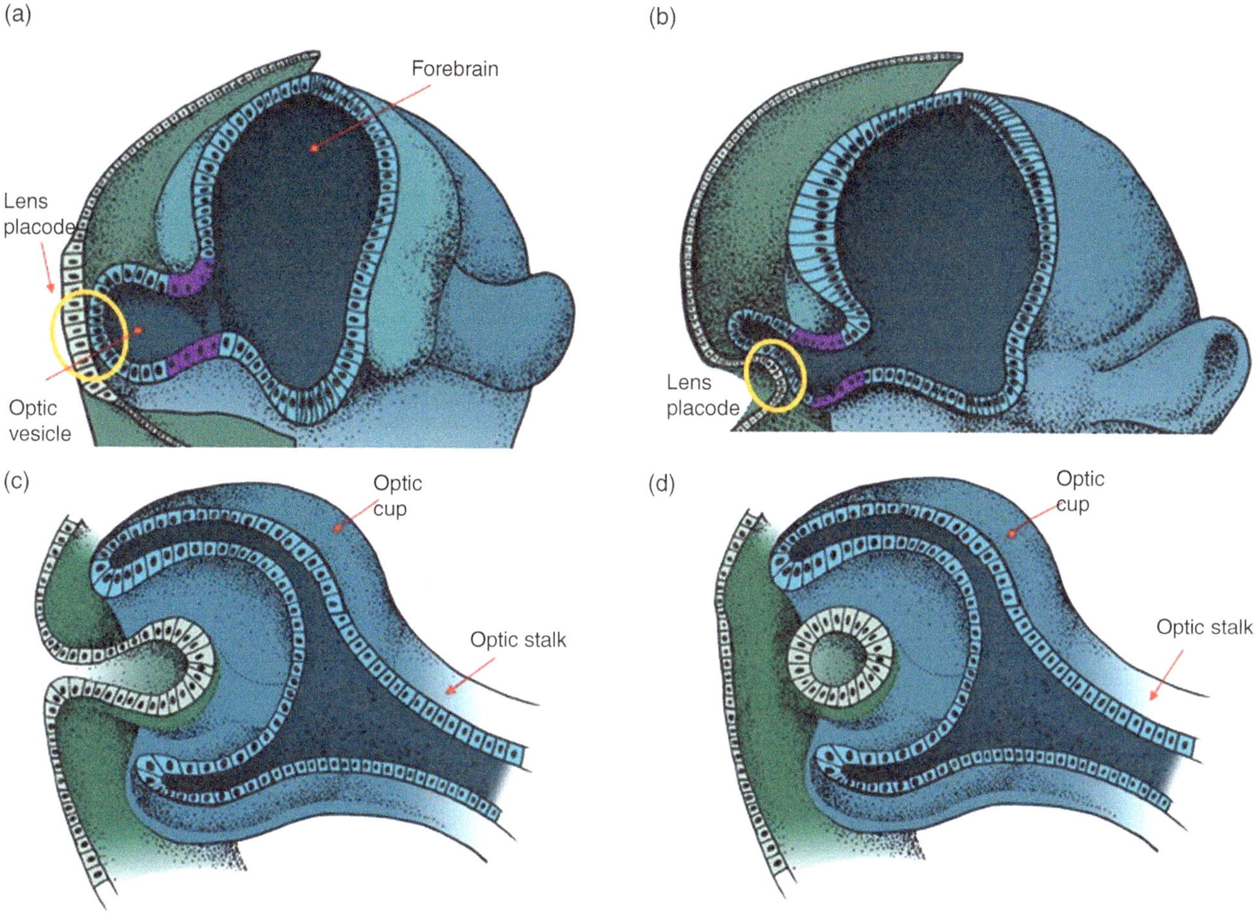

Figure 51.1 Formation of the optic cup (a–c) and lens vesicle (d). The three germinal layers are displayed: surface ectoderm (green), neuroectoderm (blue), and neural crest (magenta). The contact between the neuroectoderm and the surface ectoderm of the optic vesicle induces the lens placode (yellow circle) (a), which then invaginates (b) and forms the optic cup (c) and the lens vesicle (d).

commonly observed in horses. Of particular importance are cysts of the posterior iris, ciliary body, and peripheral retina observed in horses with multiple congenital ocular anomalies (MCOA), a generic inherited syndrome associated with a missense mutation of the PMEL17 gene, reported in Rocky Mountain horses, Kentucky Mountain Saddle Horses, Standardbred horses, American Miniature Horses, Morgans, Belgians and Icelandic Horses, among others [10–12, 14–18].

The invagination of the lens placode also leads to the formation of the *lens vesicle*, a hollow sphere surrounded by lens epithelial cells, which pinches off the surface ectoderm (Figure 51.1d).

Following separation of the lens placode/lens vesicle from the surface ectoderm, the lens fibers from the posterior aspect of the lens vesicle start to elongate and obliterate the lens cavity, forming the lens. Lens fibers will continue to proliferate throughout life. If the lens placode does not separate completely from the surface ectoderm, anterior segment dysgenesis occurs [19].

It is important to note also that lens abnormalities may be a result of abnormalities early in the development before the formation of the lens vesicle. For example, an abnormal orientation of the optic vesicle as it approaches the lens placode leads to a small lens vesicle, resulting in microphakia (small lens) [1–3].

While the optic cup and lens vesicle forms, the optic vesicle and optic stalks also invaginate dorsoventrally, forming the *choroidal fissure* inferiorly – a hollow canal that allows the hyaloid artery to enter the developing eye, thus providing vascular supply and nutrition to the primitive ocular structures. The hyaloid expands from the lens vesicle to the optic stalk and regresses later in development (after the ciliary body begins to produce aqueous humor) and should be completely regressed by the time the animal opens the eyelid [20]. The location where the hyaloid artery was attached to the lens vesicle can sometimes be observed clinically at the posterior lens capsule and is known as Mittendorf's dot. The previous attachment of the hyaloid artery to the optic nerve can also be clinically observed in some cases and is known as Bergmeister's papilla. Later in the development, the choroidal fissure should close completely [1–3, 21]. Failure of the complete closure of the choroidal fissure leads to the formation of typical colobomas (located ventrally) of the iris, choroid, or optic nerve. Complete closure of the choroidal fissure also allows intraocular pressure (IOP) to be established [1–3].

Following lens formation, the cornea starts to develop. The surface ectoderm will differentiate into corneal epithelium, while cells from the neural crest will originate the stroma, Descemet membrane, and endothelium. The anterior chamber forms as a space develops between the lens and the cornea. Neural crest also forms the pupillary membrane, a solid sheet of tissue continuous with the iris, covering the pupil aperture and the lens. The pupillary membrane provides nourishment to the developing lens and should regress later in development. Failure of the complete involution of the pupillary membrane is a common developmental abnormality known as *persistent pupillary membrane* [1–3]. They are commonly observed in horses, as complete regression of the pupillary membrane is rare.

The eyelids are comprised by surface ectoderm (epidermis, cilia, and conjunctival epithelium) and neural crest mesenchyme (dermis and tarsus). The eyelid and extraocular muscles (EOM) originate from *somitomeres* – condensations of mesoderm. The sclera, choroid, and tapetum are neural-crest derived tissues, and induced by the outer layer of the optic cup, meaning that normal RPE is necessary to the development of those structures. The primary vitreous forms between the primitive lens and the inner layer of the optic cup. It is composed of vessels of the hyaloid system, collagenous fibrillar material, and primitive hyalocytes, which produce collagen fibril that will expand the vitreous [1–3].

The Anatomy of Eye in the Neonatal Foal

The definition of the neonatal period can vary but as discussed here is considered from birth until before adulthood in foals [22]. Healthy term foals are considered a precocial species at birth, with mature eyes and vision and open eyelids [23]. The structures of foals' eyes are smaller than adult horses, although the anterior segment is thicker than 30- to 35-year-old horses. In foals, the anterior segment in foals constitutes 17% of the sagittal globe axis, while lens and vitreous make up 26% and 57% of its content, respectively [24]. The globe itself has a mild ventromedial orientation at birth, which resolves at 2–4 weeks of age [23].

The horse displays a complete orbit with an entirely bony orbital rim, which provides extra protection to the globe. The horse's orbit is positioned laterally, enhancing the monocular vision [25] and providing a panoramic field of vision, exceeding 340° [26]. The frontal, lacrimal, zygomatic, temporal, palatine, and sphenoid bones comprise the enclosed orbit, being the closure of the temporal side accomplished by the union of the zygomatic and the frontal bone (Figure 51.2). The palatine and sphenoid bones form the orbit's medial wall (Figure 51.3), and soft tissue by fat and pterygoid muscles form the orbit floor. Vessels and nerves pass from the cranial cavity and alar canal through foramina and fissures. The orbital space contains the globe, third eyelid, EOM, nerves, vessels, lacrimal gland, and fat [25–27].

The maxillary artery and nerve gain the orbit via the alar and rostral foramen, while the ethmoidal foramen permits passage of the ethmoidal vessels and nerve. The orbital foramen allows cranial nerves III (oculomotor), IV (trochlear), V (trigeminal – ophthalmic branch), and VI (abducens) to enter the orbit, while cranial nerve II (optic) and the internal ophthalmic artery enter the orbit via the optic foramen [25–27]. The orbital fascia envelopes all the structures within the orbit, being subdivided into periorbita, orbita bulbi (or Tenon's capsule), and fascial sheaths of the EOM [27].

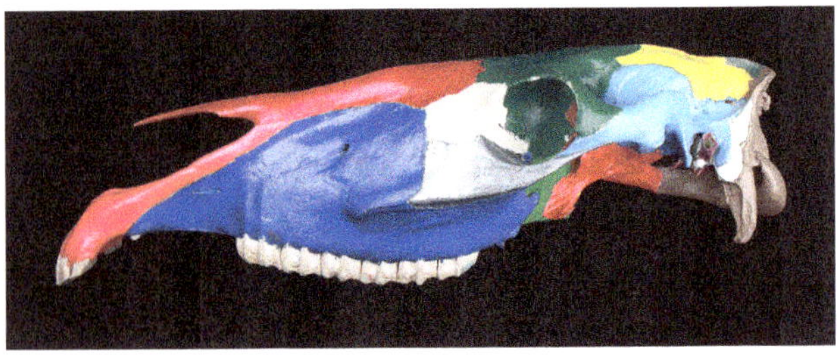

Figure 51.2 Side view of the equine cranium. Note the complete bony orbit laterally positioned on the head. The orbital rim is comprised by the frontal (dark green), lacrimal (white), zygomatic (silver), and temporal (light blue) bones. Other bones that comprise the interior portion of the orbit are the sphenoid (red) and palatine (light green) bones. *Source:* Courtesy: UC Davis Veterinary Ophthalmology Service.

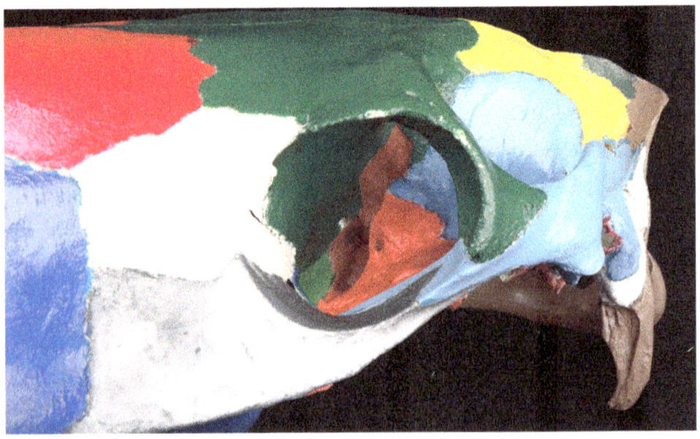

Figure 51.3 Close-up image of the equine orbit comprised by the frontal (dark green), lacrimal (white), zygomatic (silver), temporal (light blue), sphenoid (red), and palatine (light green) bones. *Source:* Courtesy: UC Davis Veterinary Ophthalmology Service.

Seven EOM are responsible for suspending the globe in the orbit and providing ocular motility [27]. The four rectus muscles (dorsal, ventral, lateral, and medial) move the eye in the direction that they are named. The superior oblique muscle attaches to the superior/lateral aspect of the globe, rotating the superior portion of the globe inferiorly and nasally. The inferior oblique muscle attaches to the inferior/lateral aspect of the globe, moving the globe superiorly and nasally. The retractor bulbi muscle consists of four muscle bellies that withdraw the globe posteriorly. The retractor bulbi muscle is one of the largest EOM, or at least it seems so when evaluating a horse with a painful eye. Origination of the muscle is from the posterior orbital wall, and insertion is to the posterior sclera. Innervation of the superior, inferior, medial rectus, and inferior oblique muscles is via the oculomotor nerve (cranial nerve III). The superior oblique muscle is innervated by the trochlear nerve (cranial nerve IV), and the lateral rectus and retractor bulbi muscles are innervated by the abducens nerve (cranial nerve VI) [27].

The eyelids have a crucial function on ocular surface health and protection through blink reflex, production of the lipidic layer of the tear film, and distribution of tears across the ocular surface [27, 28]. The upper (superior) and lower (inferior) eyelids are folds of skin and contain, from exterior to interior aspects, skin, subcutaneous tissue, the tarsal plate, the orbicularis oculi muscle, the levator palpebrae superioris muscle, Mueller's muscle, and the palpebral conjunctiva [25, 27]. The junction of the superior and inferior eyelids creates the lateral and medial canthus (canthi), and the opening of this structure forms the palpebral fissure. The tarsal plate, formed by dense connective tissue, contains Meibomian glands (around 40–50) that secrete the lipidic layer of the tear film. The orbicularis oculi muscle, innervated by the facial nerve, acts on the eyelids closure, and the levator palpebrae superioris muscle, innervated by the oculomotor nerve, is responsible for elevation of the superior lid [25].

In the horse, the eyelids fit the globe precisely, except in the medial canthus, where the caruncula (a protuberance of variable size) is found and may have a droopy aspect [23, 27]. The equine periocular skin contains vibrissae, cilia, and dermal hair [28]. The equine cilia are long and well developed in the upper eyelid and few or absent on the lower eyelid [27, 28]. Vibrissae are present on the base of the lower eyelid and on the medial aspect of the base of the upper eyelid, providing tactile stimuli via cranial nerve V, leading to eyelid closure if touched. Dermal hairs cover the eyelid surface [27].

The eyelids' interior region is the palpebral conjunctiva, a thin layer of loose connective tissue that continues through the bulbi (over the sclera), being called bulbar conjunctiva in this location [27]. Conjunctival hyperemia and hemorrhage are commonly observed at birth, with spontaneous resolution usually taking place by 10–14 days [23]. There conjunctiva carries goblet cells that are responsible for mucin secretion and lymphoid follicles, especially in the posterior aspect of the third eyelid [27].

The nasolacrimal system has a secretory and a drainage portion. The third eyelid, in the medial canthus, contains a T-shaped cartilage plate and a serous gland on its base (accessory lacrimal gland, third eyelid gland, or nictatans gland). The main lacrimal gland (a tubulo-acinar gland) is located on the dorsolateral aspect of the globe. The lacrimal and third eyelid gland are responsible for aqueous tears secretion [27].

The nasolacrimal system drains tears. After secretion, tears are drained through the upper and lower proximal lacrimal puncta, which are oval openings located 8–9 mm lateral to the medial canthus on the upper and lower eyelid margin. Each proximal puncta continues as upper and lower canaliculi, which are 3–4 mm diameter tubes, and join each other to form the lacrimal sac, which, in the horse, is much less developed than in other species. The nasolacrimal duct initiates at the lacrimal sac and runs distally 7–8 cm within the maxillary and lacrimal bones. The lacrimal duct ends at the distal nasolacrimal puncta on the ventral floor of the nasal vestibule (Figure 51.4) [28]. All these structures encompass the nasolacrimal drainage apparatus [27, 28].

Three layers (or tunics) form the globe itself: fibrous (extern), vascular (medium), and nervous (intern) tunics. The fibrous tunic is composed of the cornea and sclera, both formed mainly by collagen. This tunic is responsible

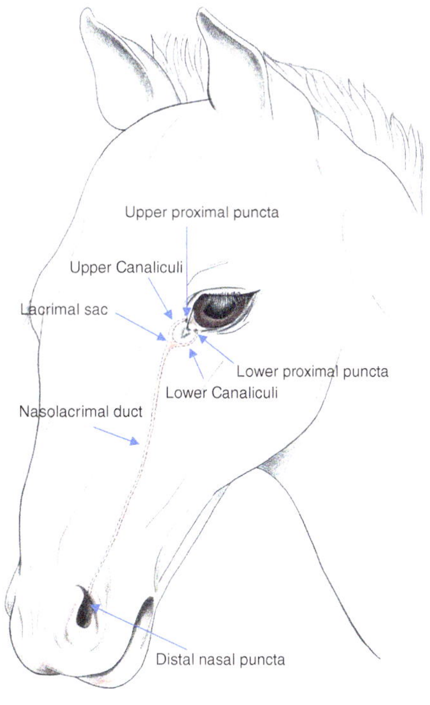

Figure 51.4 Equine drainage nasolacrimal apparatus.
Source: **Roselia Araujo**

for the eye shape and form, alongside refraction due to the cornea's transparency. The equine globe is flattened in the anteroposterior axis compared to other mammals [27–29]. The cornea is the most powerful refractive structure, which also supports the intraocular content and promotes the transmission of light [29]. Its transparency results from the lack of blood vessels, presence of a nonkeratinized epithelium, lack of pigmentation, and size and organization of the collagen fibrils [27]. Sensory nerves supply the cornea by the long ciliary nerves derived from the ophthalmic branch of the trigeminal nerve; it is important to note that newborn foals have reduced corneal sensitivity compared to mature animals [23–27].

In young horses, the cornea measures 20.5–26.6 mm horizontally and 19.5–24.0 mm vertically and is relatively flat compared to other mammals. The cornea is thicker dorsally and ventrally relative to centrally, medially, and laterally [29]. A bilateral perilimbal vascular ring associated with diffuse edema has been described in day-old foals, without ocular abnormalities [23].

The equine cornea has four layers: the epithelium (lipophilic), stroma (hydrophilic), Descemet's membrane (lipophilic), and endothelium (lipophilic). The corneal epithelium exhibits good regenerative capability and is composed of 8–12 layers of nonkeratinized, stratified squamous cells, wing cells, and basal cells, which are anchored by hemidesmosomes to its basement membrane [27–29]. The stroma comprises 90% of corneal thickness and is composed of water (75–80%), regularly arranged collagen fibers (mainly collagen I and V), and keratocytes [29]. The collagen fibrils run parallel in the cornea's diameter, an essential factor in maintaining the cornea's transparency; this arrangement permits light to enter without being scattered. Changes in this structural arrangement will result in the opacity of the cornea [27, 29]. The stroma is the only cornea layer with hydrophilic properties. Descemet membrane is a specialized basement membrane of the endothelium and becomes thicker with age due to its continuous secretion through life. Descemet membrane is acellular and composed of collagen; however, elastic properties are observed in the horse [27, 29]. The corneal endothelium is the innermost layer of the cornea and is organized as a single layer of hexagonal cells. The endothelium is responsible for maintaining the dehydrate status (deturgescence) of the cornea, as required for transparency. This layer works as a barrier (preventing aqueous humor from entering the stroma), as well as actively through the Na^{+}/K^{+} adenosine triphosphatase (ATPase) pump to move water out of the stroma. The endothelium's regenerative ability in young or immature animals is variable between species and, as the animal ages, the density of these cells decreases [27, 29].

The sclera comprises the remainder of the fibrous tunic and, together with the cornea, is responsible for support and protection to intraocular structures and providing shape to the globe. The scleral shelf (or overhang) is more prominent dorsally and ventrally, preventing the visualization of the iridocorneal angle in this location [27].

The second most important refractive structure of the eye is the lens, which helps focus the incoming light into the retina [23, 30]. This biconvex structure is transparent, since it has no vascular or innervation structures, and grows from embryologic development throughout life. The lens is anatomically divided into three regions: the nucleus (inner center), the cortex (surrounding the nucleus), and the lens capsule (externally) [27, 30]. The lenses in foals are thinner than the adult lenses and are placed more anteriorly with prominent suture lines [24]. The lens divides the globe into anterior segment (from cornea to lens) and posterior segment (from lens to retina) [27, 30].

The iris, ciliary body, and choroid compose the vascular tunic of the eye, also known as uveal tract. The iris divides the anterior segment into anterior and posterior chambers, which communicates through the pupil and is responsible for controlling the light entering the eye, resulting in miosis (constricted pupil) or mydriasis (dilated pupil) [27, 31]. The anterior surface of the iris lacks an epithelial layer and, instead, is composed of connective tissue and melanocytes. The iris stroma lays just beneath the anterior surface of the iris and is composed of collagen, fibroblasts, and a dense mesh of blood vessels. The stroma houses both iris muscles responsible for pupil shape and size: the parasympathetically innervated iris sphincter muscle (located at the pupillary margin) and the sympathetically innervated iris dilator muscle (oriented in a radial fashion). The inner aspect of the iris is composed of the posterior pigmented epithelium [27, 31]. The iris exhibits a slight gray coloration, with possible tan mottling in the periphery [23, 32]. The pupil has a round aspect at birth and acquires a horizontal oval shape by the first month of life (Figure 51.5) [23, 32]. Once dilated, the pupil becomes more round [31, 32]. The equine iris has a dorsal structure called the corpora nigra (or granula iridica), which is a cystic projection of the posterior pigmented epithelium of the iris. In some breeds (Thoroughbred, Standardbred, Saddlebred), this structure can also be prominent ventrally [31].

Posterior to the base of the iris is the ciliary body, a triangular structure divided into pars plicata (anteriorly) and pars plana (posteriorly). The pars plicata consists of a ring of around 100-folds called ciliary processes from which the lens zonules extend toward the equatorial lens region. The pars plana is smooth and relatively flat and extends from the pars plicata to the ora ciliaris retinae (the most peripheral aspect of the retina) [27, 31]. The inner surface of the ciliary body (in contact with the vitreous) is lined with a

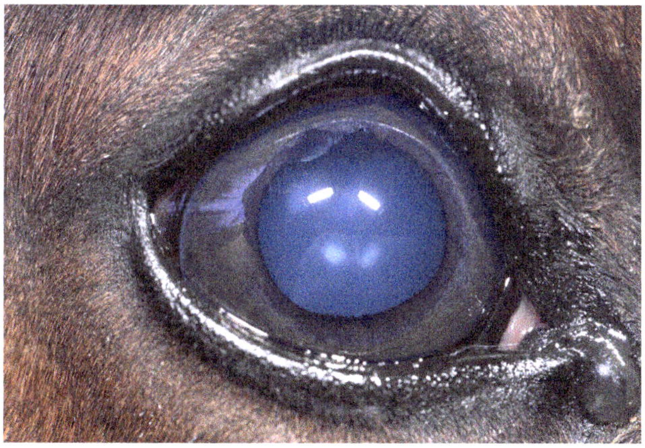

Figure 51.5 Photographic image of a foal's eye. Note the round pupil and slightly gray coloration of the iris, typical of equine neonates. *Source:* Courtesy: UC Davis Veterinary Ophthalmology Service.

double layer of epithelial cells: the nonpigmented epithelium (NPE) (inner) and the pigmented epithelium. It produces aqueous humor, the fluid responsible for nourishing the lens and cornea and maintaining IOP. The ciliary body is also responsible for lens accommodation once its contraction pulls the lens zonules, which alters the shape of the lens. The blood supply of the ciliary body derives from the two long posterior ciliary arteries and the anterior ciliary arteries [27, 31].

The choroid is the posterior component of the uveal tract and is composed of blood vessels and connective tissues. It is the principal source of nourishment of the outer layers of the retina. The dorsal portion of the choroid harbors the reflective tissue called tapetum lucidum, which reflects the light that passes through the retina and stimulates the retinal photoreceptor cells [27, 31]. In horses, the tapetal layer is composed of regularly arranged collagenous fibers, called *tapetal fibrosum,* and the color varies with breed, age, and amount of pigmentation. The horse is born with mature eyes, which give this species a well-developed tapetum at birth. However, in color-dilute horses, the tapetum may be hypoplastic or absent, allowing the observation of the choroidal vessels. Small blood vessels (capillaries) penetrate the tapetum and ophthalmoscopically are seen as multiple dark dots uniformly distributed, known as *Star of Winslow* [27, 31].

The nervous layer or retina is composed of the sensory retina (composed of nine layers) and the RPE [33]. The RPE is a continuation of the pigmented epithelial layer of the ciliary body, being the outermost layer of the retina. The RPE is formed by polygonal cells and transports nutrients from the choriocapillaris to the retina. These cells are pigmented, although the dorsal area overlying the tapetum lucidum (also called nontapetal area) is absent of melanin, permitting the light to pass through the RPE and reflect back to the photoreceptors [27, 33]. The photoreceptor cells (rods and cones) contain photopigments that change when exposed to the light-producing chemical energy, which is converted to electrical energy. This energy is then transmitted to the visual cortex of the brain. The rods (more dominant on the equine retina) are responsible for achromatic low-light vision, and the cones for vision in bright light and color vision [27, 33].

The horse has a paurangiotic retina, meaning that it is partially vascularized with 30–60 small vessels around the elliptical optic disk, less prominent dorsal, and ventral to the optic disk [31]. The remainder of the retina is avascular, and nutrition is supplied by the choroid vessels. A remnant of the hyaloid artery can usually be observed in foals up to 21 days [32]. The optic nerve and optic tracts connect the retina to the brain [23, 32]. The optic disc, located in the nontapetal fundus, is an oval, salmon-pink structure, although some foals may exhibit a round disc [23, 32, 33]. Mild to moderate optic nerve head congestion has been described in foals; however, this alteration disappears with age, and no treatment is required [23].

The vitreous is the largest structure in the eye and occupies almost two-thirds of the globe's volume functioning as a gelatinous support for the retina [27]. It is a transparent and uniform medium composed of type II collagen fibrils, hyaluronic acid, and water. It is divided into cortical, intermediate, and central zones [27, 33]. The functions of the vitreous include transmission of light, maintenance of the shape of the eye, and support for the position of the retina [27].

References

1 Cook, C.S. (2021). Ocular embryology and congenital malformations. In: *Veterinary Ophthalmology*, 6e (ed. K.N. Gelatt), 3–40. Hoboken: Wiley.

2 Stromland, K., Miller, M., and Cook, C. (1991). Ocular teratology. *Surv. Ophthalmol.* 35: 429–446.

3 Saraiva, I.Q. and Delgado, E. (2020). Congenial ocular malformations in dogs and cats: 123 cases. *Vet. Ophthalmol.* 23: 964–978.

4 Ewart, S.L., Ramsey, D.T., and Meyers, D. (2000). The horse homolog of congenital aniridia conforms to codominant inheritance. *J. Heredity* 91: 93–98.

5 Ueda, Y. (1990). Aniridia in a Thoroughbred horse. *Equine Vet. J.* 22 (s10): 9.

6 Joyce, J.R., Martin, J.E., Storts, R.W. et al. (1990). Iridial hypoplasia (aniridia) accompanied by limbic dermoid and

cataracts in a group of related Quarter Horses. *Equine. Vet. J.* 22 (s10): 26–28.
7 Schuh, J.C. (1989). Bilateral colobomas in a horse. *J. Comp. Pathol.* 100: 331–335.
8 Matthews, A.G. (2000). Lens opacities in the horse: a clinical classification. *Vet. Ophthalmol.* 3: 65–71.
9 Wheeler, C.A. and Collier, L.L. (1990). Bilateral colobomas involving the optic discs in a Quarter Horse. *Equine Vet. J.* 22: 39–41.
10 Dziezyc, J., Samuelson, D.A., and Merideth, R. (1990). Ciliary cysts in three ponies. *Equine Vet. J.* 22 (s10): 22–25.
11 Grahn, B.H., Pinard, C., Archer, S. et al. (2008). Congenial ocular anomalies in purebred and crossbred Rocky and Kentucky Mountain horses in Canada. *Can. Vet. J.* 49: 675–681.
12 Plummer, C.E. (2021). Equine ophthalmology. In: *Veterinary Ophthalmology*, 6e (ed. K.N. Gelatt), 1841–1982. Hoboken: Wiley.
13 Crispin, S.M., Matthews, A.G., and Parker, J. (1990). The equine fundus I: examination, embryology, structure and function. *Equine Vet. J.* 22: 42–49.
14 Komaromy, A.M., Rowlan, J.S., La Croix, N.C. et al. (2011). Equine multiple congenital ocular anomalies (MCOA) syndrome in PMEL17 (silver) mutant ponies: five cases. *Vet. Ophthalmol.* 14: 313–320.
15 Barsotti, G., Sgorbini, M., Marmorini, P. et al. (2013). Ocular abnormalities in healthy Standardbred foals. *Vet. Ophthalmol.* 16: 245–250.
16 Pinard, C.L. and Basrur, P.K. (2011). Ocular anomalies in a herd of exmoor ponies in Canada. *Vet. Ophthalmol.* 14: 100–108.
17 Plumer, C.E. and Ramsey, D.T. (2011). A survey of ocular abnormalities in miniature horses. *Vet. Ophthalmol.* 14: 239–243.
18 Ramsey, D.T., Ewart, S.L., Render, J.A. et al. (1999). Congenital ocular abnormalities of Rocky Mountain Horses. *Vet. Ophthalmol.* 2: 47–59.
19 Beebe, D.C. and Coats, J.M. (2000). The lens organizes the anterior segment: specification of neural crest cell differentiation in the avian eye. *Dev. Biol.* 220: 424–431.
20 Browning, J., Reichelt, M.E., Gole, G.A. et al. (2001). Proximal arterial vasoconstriction precedes regression of the hyaloid vasculature. *Curr. Eye Res.* 22: 405–411.
21 Ozeki, H., Ogura, Y., Hirabayashi, Y. et al. (2000). Apoptosis is associated with formation and persistence of the embryonic fissure. *Curr. Eye Res.* 20: 367–372.
22 Turner, A.G. (2004). Ocular conditions of neonatal foals. *Vet Clin Eq* 20: 429–440.
23 Leiva, M., Peña, T., and Monreal, L. (2011). Ocular findings in healthy newborn foals according to age. *Equine Vet. Educ.* 23: 40–45.
24 Svaldenienė, E., Paunksnienė, M., and Babrauskienė, V. (2004). Ultrasonographic study of equine eyes. *Ultragarsas* 4: 49–51.
25 Carastro, S.M. (2004). Equine ocular anatomy and ophthalmic examination. *Vet. Clin. Equine* 20: 285–299.
26 Hartley, C. and Grundon, R.A. (2017). Diseases and surgery of the globe and orbit. In: *Equine Ophthalmology*, 3e (ed. B.C. Gilger), 151–196. Ames: Wiley.
27 Meekins, J.M., Rankin, A.J., and Samuelson, D.A. (2021). Ophthalmic anatomy. In: *Veterinary Ophthalmology*, 6e (ed. K.N. Gelatt), 41–123. Hoboken: Wiley.
28 Giuliano, E.A. (2017). Diseases of the adnexa and nasolacrimal system. In: *Equine Ophthalmology*, 3e (ed. B.C. Gilger), 197–251. Ames: Wiley.
29 Brooks, D.E., Matthews, A., and Clode, A.B. (2017). Diseases and surgery of the cornea. In: *Equine Ophthalmology*, 3e (ed. B.C. Gilger), 253–368. Ames: Wiley.
30 McMullen, R.J. Jr. and Gilger, B.C. (2017). Diseases and surgery of the lens. In: *Equine Ophthalmology*, 3e (ed. B.C. Gilger), 416–452. Ames: Wiley.
31 Gilger, B.C. and Hollingsworth, S.R. (2017). Diseases of the uvea, uveitis, and recurrent uveitis. In: *Equine Ophthalmology*, 3e (ed. B.C. Gilger), 369–415. Ames: Wiley.
32 Latimer, C.A., Wyman, M., and Hamilton, J. (1983). An ophthalmic survey of the neonatal horse. *Equine Vet. J.* 15: 9–14.
33 Allbaugh, R.A., Townsend, W.M., and Wilkie, D. (2017). Diseases of the equine vitreous and retina. In: *Equine Ophthalmology*, 3e (ed. B.C. Gilger), 469–507. Ames: Wiley.

Chapter 52 Ocular Physiology and Vision in the Equine Neonate

Ralph Hamor and David Whitley

Introduction

The focus of this chapter is to highlight where ocular physiology in the neonatal foal has been specifically studied and/or compared to the adult horse. Knowledge of normal parameters, as well as normal variations in the foal allows the clinician to better evaluate the globe and vision in equine neonates. Additionally, this information allows identification of lesions that require intervention or referral to a veterinary ophthalmologist.

Birth

The globe of the neonatal foal is functionally and structurally different than the adult horse [1]. It is believed that neonatal foals have functional vision at birth. Although the neonatal foal may lack a menace response, most avoid objects in their environment and pull their head away from potential threats, indicating the presence of some degree of functional vision [2, 3]. In contrast to earlier studies [4–6], more recent investigations have determined that acquired ophthalmic disease is more common in neonatal foals than congenital disease [7, 8].

Anatomic Pathways for Vision

Conscious perception of vision requires a transparent or partial clarity of ocular media including the tear film, cornea, pupil, lens, and vitreous. The cell bodies in the retina convert light to electrical impulses, which are transmitted via the optic nerve to the visual cortex to be converted to images. The cell bodies within the retinal ganglion cell (RGC) layer are actually within the central nervous system (CNS). The axons of the RGCs form the "optic nerve." The optic nerve is actually a tract of the CNS and is myelinated by oligodendrocytes [9]. At the equine optic chiasm, approximately 80% of the RGC axons decussate and 20% remain ipsilateral [10, 11]. Beyond the optic chiasm, the RGC axons continue as the optic tract and course caudodorsally and laterally to synapse in the lateral geniculate nucleus (LGN). The axons from the cell bodies within the LGN project caudally as the optic radiation and terminate in the visual cortex of the occipital lobe of the brain to produce conscious visual perception (Figure 52.1) [9].

Visual perception is "seeing" or the image that the foal perceives; it is not a photographic image that captures every detail that the eyes transmit and visual cortex processes. The visual system of many species processes the received data or image and uses shortcuts to process the image more rapidly into useful information to guide or alter behaviors [12]. The eye can be compared to a camera with optical elements (cornea and lens) capable of altering focus, an adjustable light diaphragm (pupil) that assists in the control of the amount of light that passes through to the neurosensory layers (retina) and captures the image. Visual perception is a complex series of events as follows:

1) Light from the environment is focused on the retina.
2) The retina converts light energy into chemical energy and subsequently to electrical energy.
3) These impulses are separated into categories (e.g. motion, brightness, movement, velocity, direction, location, distance, size, shape, color, position) and this information is transmitted to the brain.
4) The brain processes the information to a useful format.
5) The relevant parts of the image are selected for priority and further action [13].

To facilitate the ability to identify an object (threat) from the surroundings environment, horses have a very large globe that allows more light to enter the globe in dim light. Dim light perception is also improved, when present, by a fibrous tapetum lucidum located in the dorsocentral

Equine Neonatal Medicine, First Edition. Edited by David M. Wong and Pamela A. Wilkins.

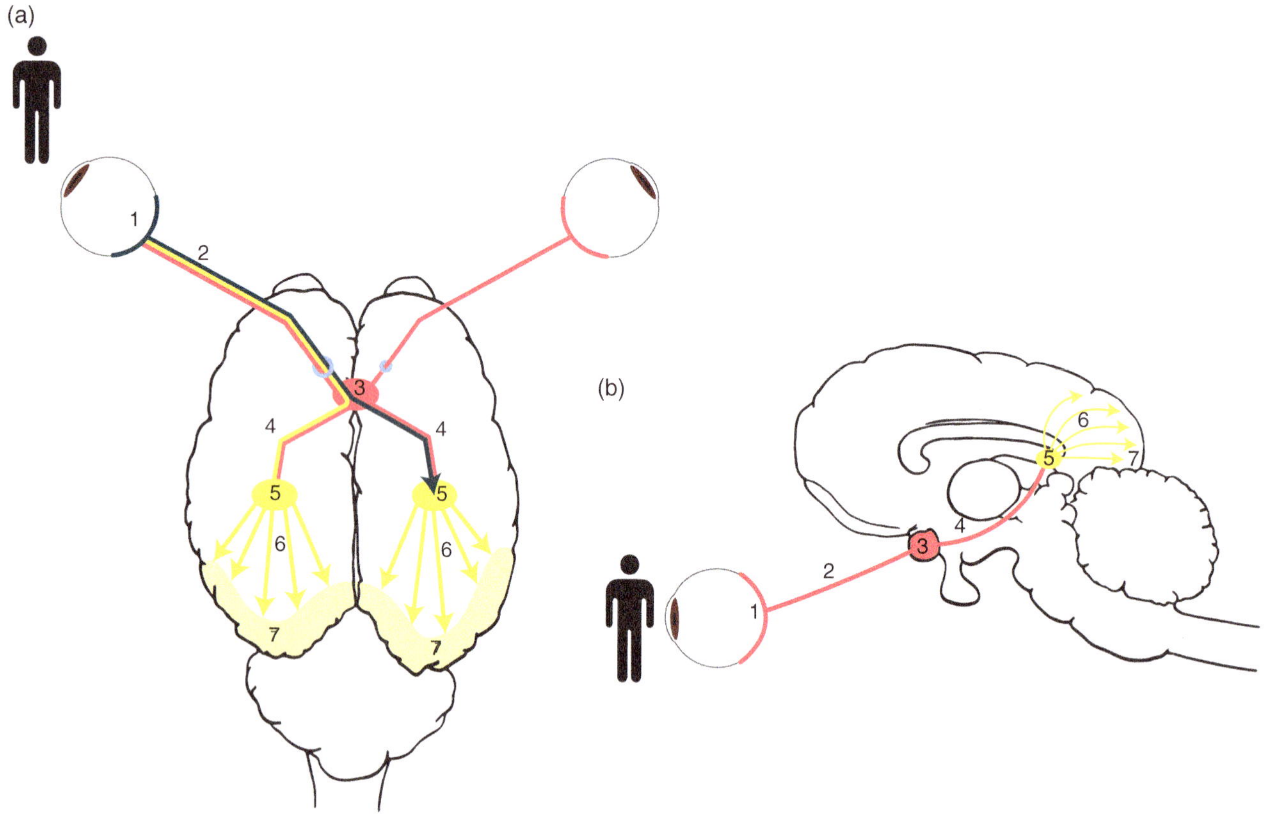

Figure 52.1 Schematic of the neuroanatomic pathway for conscious vision. (a) Dorsal and (b) Lateral views. 1. Retina, 2. Optic nerve, 3. Optic chiasm, 4. Optic tract, 5. Lateral geniculate nucleus (LGN), 6. Optic radiation, 7. Visual cortex of the occipital lobe.

portion of the fundus. This structure likely allows for light to be reflected back through the retina a second time. The horizontal pupil of the horse also allows more light to enter the back of the globe, even when the pupil is constricted.

Evaluation of vision relies on assessment of the foal in its surroundings, its response to visual stimuli, and an ophthalmic examination. It is best to examine the foal within the first 12–24 hours of life with examination performed in the presence of the mare with minimal restraint and in a quiet stall that can be darkened. Normal parameters of the ophthalmic examination are found here and in Chapter 53. While there are no specific reports evaluating visual acuity in neonatal foals, it is generally accepted that precocious species, including foals, are born with a mature visual system. The presence of a dazzle reflex, an intact pupillary light reflex (PLR), along with normal ambulation in its environment suggest normal vision in a neonatal foal. More details regarding vision in horses can be found elsewhere [12].

Menace Response

The menace response is elicited by the examiner making a threatening gesture toward the eye and observing for the closure of the eyelids. The afferent or sensory pathway includes the retina, optic nerve, optic chiasm, contralateral optic tract, contralateral LGN, contralateral optic radiation, and visual cortex. The efferent or motor pathway involves the occipital cortex, with impulses transmitted by association fibers to the motor cortex or frontal cortex. Axons from the pontine nucleus decussate and enter the cerebellum. The cerebellum then activates the facial nuclei in the rostral medulla oblongata [9]. The cerebellar interposital nucleus sends fibers via the red nuclei in the midbrain; the red nucleus then sends fibers to the facial nucleus [14]. The axons leave the medulla oblongata, and the facial nerve innervates the orbicularis oculi muscle in the eyelid, causing a blink response (Figure 52.2).

The menace response in neonatal foals is absent at birth but is usually present by 14 days of age [2, 3, 15–18]. In one report involving 52 healthy neonatal foals, the menace response was not identified consistently until 16–21 days of age [13]. While most reports were empiric, a longitudinal evaluation of the development of the menace response was performed in 26 neonatal foals [3]. In this study, only 1 foal had a menace response on day one. After day 1, most foals developed a menace response between days 5–8, with all having a menace response by day 9. Not all neonatal foals developed a symmetric menace response in both eyes. In 5 neonatal foals, one eye developed a menace response 1 day earlier than the other eye. Two other studies have documented that a partial menace

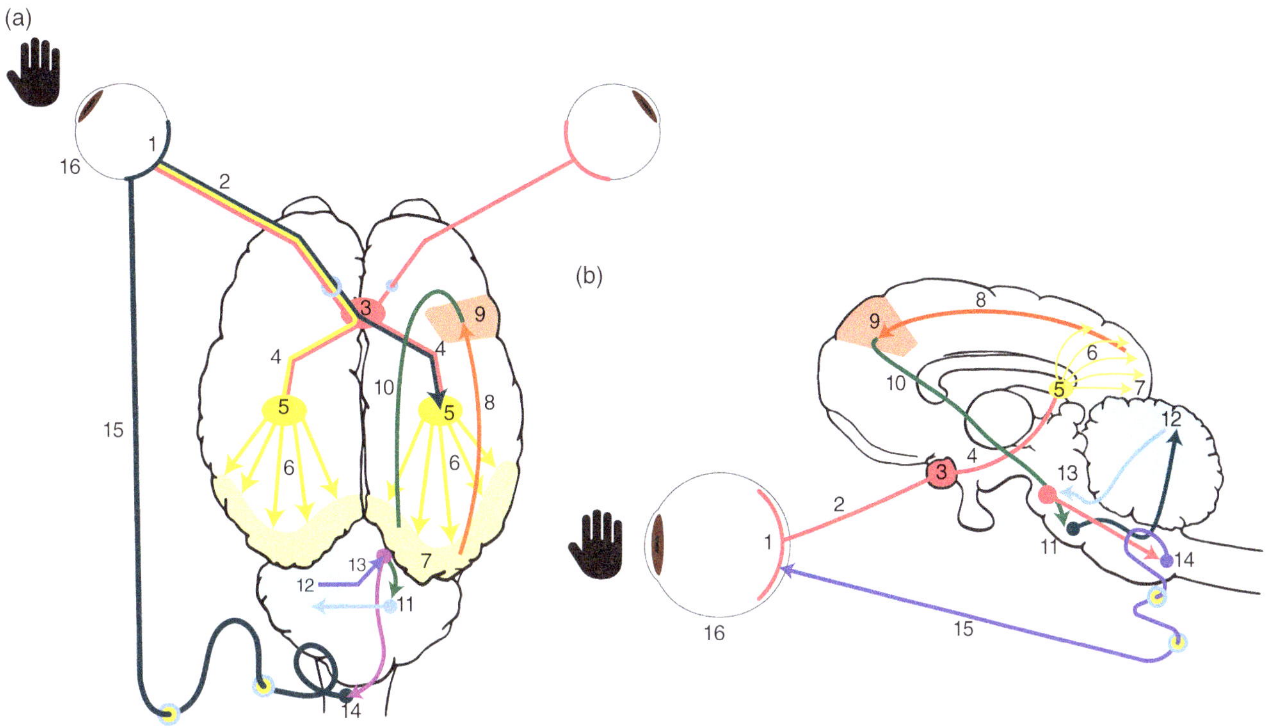

Figure 52.2 Schematic of the neuroanatomic pathway for the menace response. (a) Dorsal and (b) lateral views. 1. Retina; 2. Optic nerve; 3. Optic chiasm; 4. Optic tract; 5. Lateral geniculate nucleus; 6. Optic radiation; 7. Visual cortex of the occipital lobe; 8. Association fibers; 9. Frontal cortex; 10. Projection fibers; 11. Pontine nucleus; 12. Cerebellar cortex; 13. Red nucleus; 14. Facial nucleus; 15. Facial nerve; 16. Orbicularis oculi muscle.

response may be present 1 day prior to the presence of a complete menace response [2, 3]. While the menace response is generally present by 14–16 days after birth, it may be diminished until several weeks of age [3, 19].

Dazzle Reflex

The dazzle reflex (also called the photic blink reflex) is present from birth and is a subcortical reflex elicited by directing a very bright light into the eye, which causes the eyelid to blink [1]. The blink is usually bilateral but can be more complete in the tested eye. The afferent arm of the reflex is similar to the pupillary light response: however, the exact neuroanatomic pathways have not been elucidated. It is presumed that the efferent pathway is via the facial nerve. Optic tract axons synapse in the rostral colliculus and tectonuclear fibers course caudally to synapse in the facial nucleus in the medulla oblongata. The facial nerve then courses to innervate the orbicularis oculi muscle and causes a blink or palpebral reflex (Figure 52.3) [9].

Pupillary Light Reflex (PLR)

The PLR occurs in response to light stimulating the retina and is elicited by shining a bright, focal light into each pupil of the eye. The neuroanatomic pathway has been described in these steps:

1) Light stimulates the retina.
2) Light impulses travel via the retinal axons in the optic nerve to the optic chiasm, where approximately 80% decussate to the contralateral optic tract and 20% remain ipsilateral.
3) Axons synapse in the pretectal nucleus.
4) Fibers then travel to the parasympathetic components of the oculomotor or Edinger-Westphal nucleus [9].
5) The oculomotor nerve courses to the ciliary ganglion.
6) The short ciliary nerve innervates the sphincter muscle of the iris causing constriction (Figure 52.4).

The larger superior and smaller inferior corpora nigra of the equine iris may act as a shield to reduce glare and to augment constriction of the pupil.

The PLR is present in both eyes of newborn foals but may be sluggish and incomplete for the first few days of life [3, 18, 20]. Similar to adults, the PLR of neonatal foals is biphasic with an initial rapid but small reduction in pupil diameter, followed by a slower but more complete reduction in pupil size. The evaluation of a PLR in a neonatal foal is best performed in a quiet area with minimal stress or excitement. It is important to remember that the PLR is not an assessment of vision but a

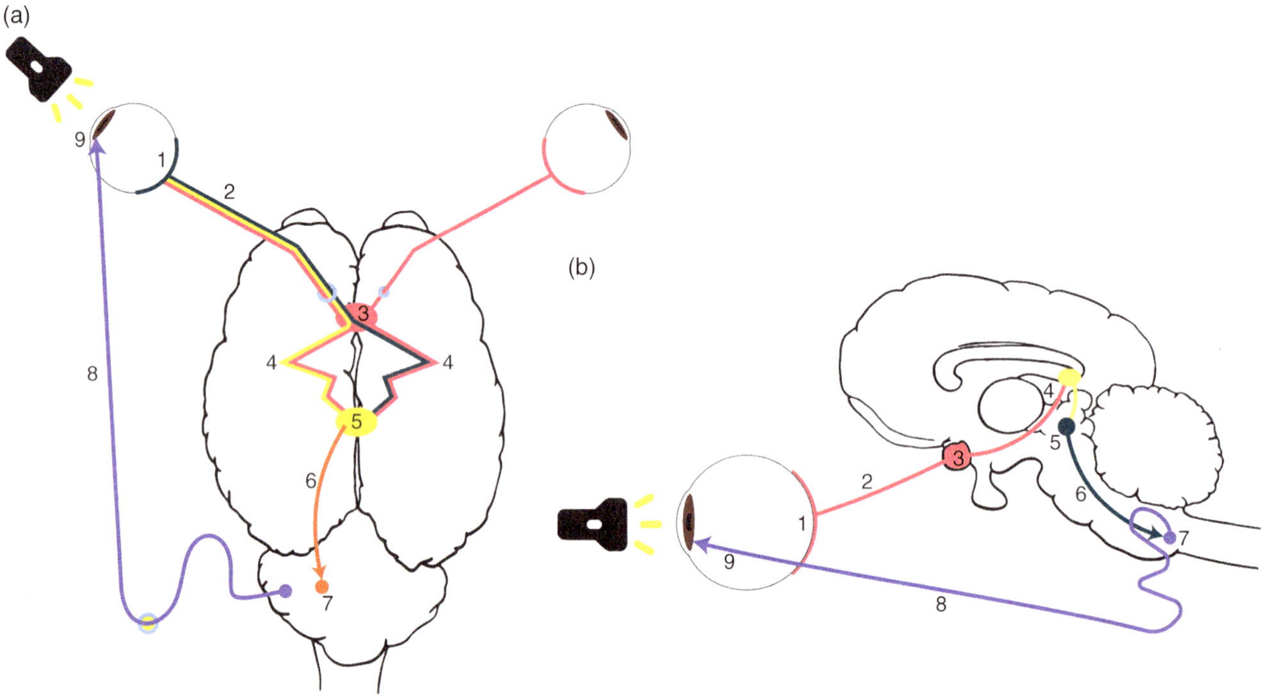

Figure 52.3 Proposed neuroanatomic pathway involved in the dazzle reflex. (a) Dorsal and (b) lateral views. 1. Retina; 2. Optic nerve; 3. Optic chiasm; 4. Optic tract; 5. Rostral colliculus; 6. Tectonuclear fibers; 7. Facial nucleus; 8. Facial nerve; 9 Orbicularis oculi muscle.

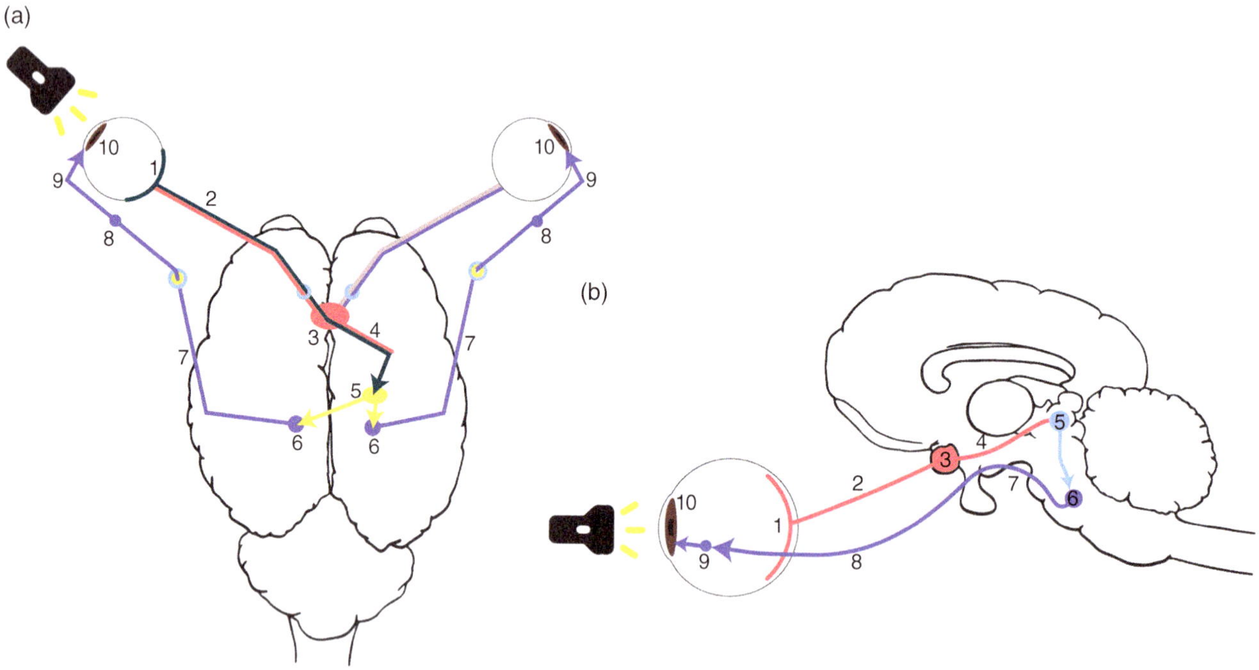

Figure 52.4 Schematic of the neuroanatomic pathway involved in the pupillary light reflex. (a) Dorsal and (b) lateral views. 1. Retina; 2. Optic nerve; 3. Optic chiasm; 4. Optic tract; 5. Pretectal nucleus; 6. Parasympathetic components of the oculomotor or Edinger-Westphal nucleus; 7. Oculomotor nerve; 8. Ciliary ganglion; 9. Short ciliary nerve; 10. Iris sphincter muscle.

reflex that involves only a portion of the entire visual pathway. The presence of a dazzle reflex, a menace response, and intact PLRs, along with appropriate visual behavior, are needed to assume normal vision in a neonatal foal.

Palpebral Reflex

This reflex is elicited by touching the medial and lateral canthus. The sensory innervation to the eyelids is through the trigeminal nerve (CN V) and efferent innervation via the facial nerve (CN VII). A recent study regarding the development of palpebral reflex in a large number of neonatal foals indicates that the reflex is similar to that of adult horses, and may even be hypersensitive in foals [2, 6]. This information is in contrast to an earlier study that reported a reduced palpebral reflex in neonatal foals [10].

Oculocardiac Reflex

The oculocardiac reflex results in slowing of the heart rate due to pressure on the globe, tension on extraocular muscles or the iris, or increased intraorbital pressure. The most common effect is bradycardia, but cardiac arrest and ventricular fibrillation can occur. Complications of the oculocardiac reflex have been reported in a foal [21]. The afferent arc of the oculocardiac reflex begins with the ciliary nerves to the ciliary ganglion. The ophthalmic branch of the trigeminal nerve (CN V) continues to the trigeminal nucleus and the afferent arc continues along fibers to connect with the efferent pathway in the motor nucleus of the vagus nerve (CN X) to the myocardium [22]. Sensory stimulation of the eye and orbit causes stimulation of the vagal nucleus in the brainstem, leading to a reflex bradycardia or other cardiac disorder.

Tear Film Physiology in the Foal

The preocular tear film (PTF) maintains an optically smooth and transparent corneal surface by filling in and smoothing out irregularities in the corneal epithelial surface, removing foreign material, providing nutrients to the avascular cornea, and lubricating the cornea and conjunctiva. Tear flow rates are difficult to measure but in the horse, it has been estimated to be 34 µl/min with a tear volume of 234 µl and a total tear volume turnover of 7 minutes [23]. The PTF is commonly divided into three layers (outer, middle, and deep layer) that intermix to some degree. The outer or surface layer is a very thin oily or lipid layer that stabilizes the air-tear interface, decreases PTF evaporation, and prevents overflow of tears onto the eyelids. This oily or lipid layer is produced by the Meibomian or tarsal glands of the eyelids. These sebaceous glands undergo holocrine secretion, with cell rupture releasing the entire cell contents. The primary component of the lipid layer is the Meibomian gland secretions of a lipid rich mixture. The main lipid classes found are long-chain cholesteryl esters, wax esters, and (O-acryl)-omega-hydroxy fatty acids (OAHFA) [24]. The middle or aqueous layer is the thickest of the three layers of the PTF and occupies >60% of the PTF thickness. This layer is approximately 98% water and 2% solids, predominantly proteins. The aqueous layer is produced by the orbital lacrimal gland and the gland of the nictitating membrane. The deep or mucin layer of the PTF is composed of mucins produced by the apocrine conjunctival goblet cells, as well as a glycocalyx associated with the corneal and conjunctival microvilli [22]. The distribution of goblet cells varies among species. In the horse, the conjunctival fornix has the highest concentration [25]. The glycocalyx is composed of polysaccharides produced by stratified squamous epithelium of the cornea and conjunctiva [26].

The nasolacrimal drainage system eliminates used PTF and excessive tears. The PTF accumulates along the eyelid margins and, with eyelid closure (blinking) from lateral to medial, is forced medially into the lacrimal puncta. When tears are in the lacrimal lake and puncta, and facial muscles relax, the tears flow into the canaliculi by capillary action. Normal breathing movements also increase flow into the canaliculi [22]. Blinking of the eyelids closes the lacrimal sac, which acts as a passive pump of tears into the nasolacrimal duct. Pseudoperistaltic motion of the nasolacrimal duct facilitates movement of tears into the nasal cavity [27].

Globe

At birth, the globe and adnexal tissues of the neonatal foal are fully developed [1]. The globe of the neonatal foal demonstrates a mild, ventromedial orientation at birth, which generally resolves slowly within a few days, however, it may take 2–4 weeks to completely resolve [2, 20].

Eyelids

Healthy neonatal foals may demonstrate droopy eyelids [20]. In a study of healthy, neonatal Standardbred foals, 3.9% (4/102) had entropion of the lower eyelid margin that was not associated with a corneal ulcer [8]. In 3/4 of these foals, entropion was associated with prematurity with no other systemic signs. Anatomic or primary entropion was present in 5.7% (4/70) of neonatal foals [7].

Cornea

The interface between the cornea and PTF is responsible for 70–80% of the refractive power of the eye. The cornea is composed of layers: epithelium, stroma, Descemet's membrane, and an endothelial cell layer. The epithelial layer consists of 8–12 layers of nonkeratinized squamous cells, wing cells, and basal cells. The stroma comprises 90% of the corneal thickness, and is composed of water, collagen fibrils, and a proteoglycan matrix made up of proteins linked to glycosaminoglycans (GAGS) [28]. Just posterior to the stroma is Descemet's membrane which is acellular and is composed primarily of collagen. Descemet's membrane is the basement membrane of the endothelial cells, and is formed throughout life (thickness increases with age). Beneath Descemet's membrane is a single layer of metabolically active hexagonal cells. In addition to producing Descemet's membrane, the endothelium serves a barrier function and is physiologically responsible for maintaining the osmotic gradient between the hydrophilic stroma and the aqueous humor (AH) required for corneal transparency.

Factors contributing to corneal transparency or clarity include the lack of pigment and blood vessels, absence of keratinization of the anterior surface epithelium, the barrier function of the anterior epithelium, nonmyelinated nerve fibers, hypocellularity and transparency of cells, small uniform diameter of stromal collagen fibrils, consistent interfibrillar spacing, the lattice-like organization of the stromal collagen fibrils, the active fluid pump in the endothelial cells, and the state of relative dehydration [29].

Various corneal proteinases (proteolytic enzymes), proteinase inhibitors, and growth factors in the PTF and aqueous humor play a role in the balance of natural turnover of corneal tissue [30]. Maintenance and repair of the stromal extracellualar matrix requires a highly regulated homeostasis of extracellualar matrix synthesis, degradation, and remodeling [31]. Proteinases perform physiological functions in the turnover and remodeling of corneal stroma. Excessive degradation of normal healthy tissue is prevented by naturally occurring proteinase inhibitors in the PTF and cornea [32, 33]. Pathologic degradation of the corneal stromal collagen and proteoglycans occurs when the homeostasis between proteinases and proteinases inhibitors is tilted toward the former [34]. The rapid degradation of the corneal stromal collagen occurring in some severe corneal ulcers is caused by proteinases and is referred to as *keratomalacia* or "corneal melting."

The cornea of a neonatal foal, similar to adults, is clear, oval and thinnest at its central axis [1]. The central corneal thickness in foals (0–180 days of age), as measured by high-frequency ultrasound and ultrasound biomicroscopy, was $802 \pm 36\,\mu m$ [35]. The cornea is primarily innervated by the terminal ciliary nerves from the ophthalmic branch of the trigeminal nerve (CN V). The anterior cornea is the most sensitive structure in the mammalian body. The corneal reflex is elicited by gently touching the unanesthetized central cornea with a wisp of cotton or a sterile cotton or Dacron-tipped swab, which results in closure of the eyelid and retraction of the globe. This subcortical reflex is in response to an uncomfortable stimulus to the cornea. The afferent pathway is through the ophthalmic branch of the trigeminal nerve (CN V) and the efferent arm for closure of the eyelid is via the facial nerve (CN VII) and the retraction is mediated by the abducens nerve (CN VI).

The corneal touch threshold is a measure of corneal sensitivity and can be quantified using an esthesiometer. The corneal touch threshold is the threshold of the stimulus that results in a corneal reflex. The Cochet-Bonet esthesiometer has been used in foals to evaluate corneal touch threshold. The device contains a small diameter nylon or platinum filament with an adjustable length of 0.5–6.0 cm. The filament is applied to the cornea at different lengths until a corneal reflex is attained and noted as the corneal touch threshold. The longer the filament required to elicit the corneal reflex, the more sensitive the cornea.

In healthy neonatal foals, the mean corneal touch threshold is 5.01 ± 0.61 cm [36]. The same study demonstrated that healthy foals had the most sensitive corneas, compared with sick neonatal foals and healthy adult horses. In addition, the cornea of sick, hospitalized neonatal foals was significantly less sensitive than both adult horses and healthy neonatal foals. The dorsal and temporal peripheral corneas of both healthy and sick neonatal foals were the least sensitive areas of the cornea, but these differences were not significant.

Bilateral perilimbal corneal vascularization has been reported in a 1-day-old foal [37] and physiologic corneal vascularization has been reported in another study of neonatal foals [20]. In each report, no treatment was prescribed, and the corneal vessels resolved by day 10. A proposed cause of the transient corneal vessels is an insult to the cornea from the amniotic or allantoic fluid in the last few days of gestation [20].

Iris

The iris of a neonatal foal may have a slight gray color [1] and the pupil is initially round and becomes horizontal and elliptical within the first week of life [16, 19, 20, 38, 39]. As in an adult horse, the presence of iris-to-iris persistent pupillary membranes is likely a normal variation [6, 39]. These appear as fine strands of pigmented tissue originating from the iris collarette and generally run along the iris (Figure 52.5). In more rare instances, they may project from the iris into the anterior chamber, to the cornea, or onto the lens capsule. If this occurs, a corneal or lenticular opacity may result.

Intraocular Pressure (IOP)

Aqueous humor is continually produced by the ciliary body processes in the pars plicata. The AH exits the equine eye by uveoscleral and conventional outflow pathways and provides nutrition and supplies the metabolic requirements of the avascular structures of the eye such as the

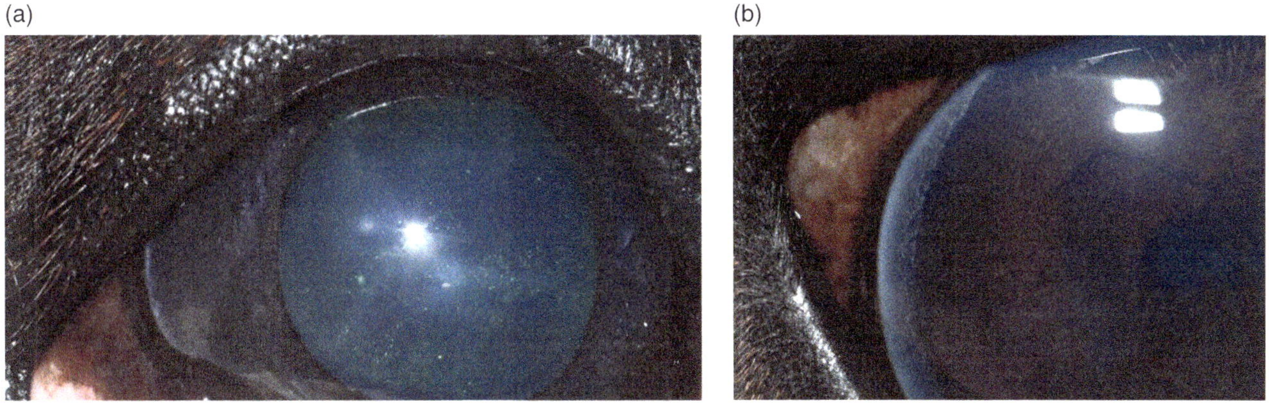

Figure 52.5 (a and b) Persistent pupillary membrane in an adult horse. These fine strands of pigmented tissue originate from the iris collarette and typically run along the iris. *Source:* Images courtesy of Caren Plummer, University of Florida.

cornea and lens. The inner surface of the ciliary body is lined by two layers of epithelial cells. The innermost layer (nearest the vitreous) is nonpigmented and called the nonpigmented epithelium (NPE). The NPE is continuous at the ora ciliaris retinae as the nine layers of the neurosensory retina (NSR). This layer is continuous anteriorly with the posterior iris epithelium. The second (outermost) layer of the ciliary body lies beneath the NPE and is pigmented with melanin and referred to as the pigmented epithelial layer of the ciliary body. Posteriorly, this layer is contiguous with the retinal pigmented epithelium (RPE), and, anteriorly, with the outer most layer of the posterior iris epithelium. Tight junctions between NPE represent the epithelial portion of the blood -aqueous barrier [40]. Deep to the two layers of ciliary body epithelium, each ciliary process has a central portion of vascular plexus, which is fenestrated, allowing leakage of plasma into the ciliary body stroma. The NPE portion of the blood-aqueous filters plasma, removing all cells and protein. This implies that AH is an ultrafiltrate of plasma. Additionally, the NPE contains the enzyme carbonic anhydrase, which catalyzes the active transport of AH [41].

The majority of AH is produced via active secretion by the ciliary body processes of the pars plicata, using energy and carbonic anhydrase. A lesser portion of AH is formed by passive diffusion and ultrafiltration of blood (plasma) in the ciliary body circulation. After formation, AH flows from the posterior chamber through the pupil into the anterior chamber. AH circulates by convection currents in the anterior chamber, providing nutrients and removing waste. Aqueous fluid exits the anterior chamber by way of the iridocorneal angle through the trabecular meshwork, the intrascleral plexus, and into the vortex veins. Aqueous humor flows into the iridocorneal angle between pectinate ligaments through the trabecular beams of the uveal trabecular meshwork, the corneoscleral trabecular meshwork, the angular aqueous plexus, and into the intrascleral plexus comprising the conventional aqueous outflow pathway. The AH then flows from the intrascleral plexus into vortex veins that empty into the choroid [42, 43]. The uveal trabecular meshwork composes 74.3% of the iridocorneal angle area [41–44]. The unconventional or uveoscleral AH outflow in the horse drains via the iris, ciliary body, and choroid [41, 44–46]. Ocular microsphere perfusion studies in horses have shown that suprachoroidal and supraciliary spaces allow an extensive unconventional outflow pathway to the sclera and choroid [43].

The aqueous dynamics of the neonatal foal have not been studied but are suspected to be similar to the adult horse. In one study the mean IOP in 102 neonatal Standardbred foals was 17.1 ± 2.6 mmHg [8] whereas another study measured a mean IOP of 17.6 ± 4.5 mmHg in neonatal foals [7] without uveitis (both measured by applanation tonometry).

Lens

The lens aids in properly focusing images onto the retina as well as accommodation. The ciliary body has circumferentially oriented smooth muscle innervated by the parasympathetic nervous system where contraction of ciliary body muscle allows accommodation, the process whereby the optical power changes to focus on an object. When these muscles contract, zonules attached to the lens relax, allowing the lens to passively thicken, allowing for near vision. When the ciliary body muscle is relaxed, the zonules tighten, and the lens thins, allowing for far vision. Most nonhuman primates possess poorly developed ciliary body muscles, and therefore have limited accommodative ability. Accommodation in the horse is believed to be only about two diopters [12].

As with most other species, a singular layer of lens epithelial cells is located immediately behind the anterior lens capsule and bend at the lens equator to form the lens bow. This layer of lens epithelial cells performs most of the metabolic functions of the lens to move products between the lens and the aqueous humor and to maintain transparency of the lens. Aside from the lens capsule and the anterior lens epithelial cells, the remainder of the lens is comprised of lens fibers. Lens fibers are originally created at the lens bow and mature into cells that have lost most of their metabolic functions to allow for clarity of the lens. At birth, the lens is primarily made up of the embryonic and fetal lens nucleus. As the horse matures, lens fibers are continually created throughout life, causing the lens to grow and the central nucleus to become denser, resulting in nuclear sclerosis. Loss of the precise arrangement of lens fibers and/or changes in metabolic function of the lens results in cataract formation. As with other highly diurnal species, the lens of the horse contains yellow pigments that filter out blue light that are believed to reduce glare and improve contrast [12]. Most horses are within 1.5 diopters of emmetropia and have a low incidence of astigmatism [12].

The lens of a neonatal foal is smaller than in an adult horse and increases in size and thickness into adulthood. The lens suture lines of neonatal foals are very prominent [7, 19, 20, 39] and should not be mistaken as a cataract. In a study of 102 healthy, neonatal Standardbred foals, 1% (1/102) had a congenital, unilateral, immature, nuclear cataract [8]. In another study of 70 neonatal foals, the most common nonpathological lesions of the lens were prominent Y-suture lines in 7.1% (5/70) and congenital cataracts noted in 8.6% (6/70) of neonatal foals [7].

Vitreous Humor or Hyaloid Apparatus System Functions

The vitreous body is the largest structure within the globe, occupying about 80% of the eye [47] and a volume of about 28 ml in the adult horse. The vitreous is a large hydrogel in the poster globe composed of >98% water. Collagen makes up the framework of the vitreous and provides its gel-like plasticity. The spaces between collagen fibrils are filled with hyaluronic acid. An increase in in the water or decrease in the collagen content makes the vitreous more fluid, thereby offering less support of the retina and other intraocular structures. The vitreous contributes to eye growth, optics, structure, physiology, and metabolism. Vitreal elongation lengthens the pathway for light to reach the retina, resulting in axial myopia. The vitreous body is also thought to contribute to accommodation [48]. The vitreous also plays a role in ocular metabolism and serves as a storage depot for retinal metabolites of glycogen, amino acids, and potassium [49–51]. The vitreous absorbs retinal and lenticular waste products helping to protect the lens and retina from toxic products [47, 52]. The vitreous also provides some structural and mechanical protection to the internal eye during eye movement and ocular trauma.

The vitreous body forms in three stages: primary, secondary, and tertiary (adult) vitreous. Primary vitreous forms between the primitive lens and the optic cup. It contains blood vessels, mesenchymal cells, collagen fibrillar material, and macrophages. Secondary vitreous forms as the fetal fissure closes and contains a matrix of fibrillar and cellular material including primitive monocytes, hyalocytes, and hyaluronic acid [53, 54]. The embryonic vitreous is quite dense and translucent. As an animal matures, the axial length of the vitreous increases, collagen content remains static, hyaluronic acid increases, and vitreous liquification increases. As the vitreous becomes more liquid, the posterior vitreous cortex separates from the retinal inner limiting membrane, which may predispose to retinal tears and detachment.

Numerous studies have documented that remnants of the hyaloid vascular system are expected in neonatal foals [7, 20, 39, 55]. These can appear as linear, white, or blood-filled structures surrounding the lens and/or present in the vitreous. The presence of these structures in a neonatal foal is considered normal and do not require treatment as most slowly fade away. In a study of 204 adult Thoroughbreds, only one foal had a persistent hyaloid artery [55].

Retina

The visual optics portion of the visual process ends when photons strike the outer segments of the photoreceptors of the retina. The neuronal part of the visual process begins when the photons are captured and absorption of their energy by the outer segments of the rods and cones occurs, where a chain of biochemical reactions begin. As in the adult, the retina of the foal consists of nine layers of the NSR and one layer of retinal pigment epithelium (RPE). Like other species, the NSR has both rods and cones. In the equine, the rods greatly outnumber the cones. The rods are responsible for low-light and motion detection vision, while cones account for color vision and bright-light vision. The horse lacks a macula and fovea but rather has a visual streak accompanied by the highest cell density and maximum visual acuity. The area centralis in the horse is located at the temporal end of the visual streak and has the highest cell density and is responsible for binocular vision [56–58]. The visual streak in the horse is a horizontal band 1 mm × 22 mm located about 3 mm dorsotemporal to the optic disc [59, 60]. Variation in the ganglion cell density has been shown in different areas of the retina and in the area centralis; variation also occurs among breeds of horse and skull confirmation [61]. The horse has a very large retinal surface area compared to humans.

The horse perceives color in a dichromatic pattern with a short (spectral peak 425 nm) and a medium (spectral peak of 540 nm) wavelength cone [62]. This likely means color vision of blue-gray and yellow-green spectrum. The horse has demonstrated color discrimination [63], but likely has trouble differentiating orange and blue [12]. Due to the temporal placement of the eyes, horses have a visual field of approximately 350° with a relatively narrow, 65–80° of binocular vision [12, 58, 64]. The inner nuclear layer of the retina contains the nuclei of the horizontal, bipolar, amacrine and Mueller cells.

Bipolar cells provide the radial connections between the photoreceptors and the ganglion cells whereas amacrine cells provide horizontal integration between bipolar cells, ganglion cells, and other amacrine cells. The RGCs receive information from both bipolar and amacrine cells. Vertical information pathways come from the photoreceptors to the bipolar cells and then to the ganglion cells. Horizontal information pathways come from photoreceptors to horizontal cells to bipolar cells to amacrine cells and then to ganglion cells [65]. The ganglion cells are collected into the optic nerve axons. Mueller cells are primarily the structural supporting cells of the retina but also function to provide some nutrients.

The fundus (retina and optic nerve head) of the neonatal foal is similar to that of an adult horse with a few differences [1]. The optic nerve head generally appears more rounded, can be pale to deep pink in color and may have axons appearing as light gray streaks in the peripapillary area [2, 4, 20]. The optic nerve head may also show mild to moderate congestion in neonatal foals between 1 and 16 days [20, 66] that resolves without treatment and leaves no visual deficits [20].

Retinal hemorrhage was noted in 18.6% (19/102) of healthy neonatal Standardbred foals [8]. These hemorrhages were always in the tapetum dorsal to the optic disc. There was no association between their presence and foal size, and all resolved with 7 days. In another study, retinal hemorrhage was noted in 16.2% (27/167) of healthy, neonatal Thoroughbred foals [66]. Bilateral hemorrhage was significantly more common, particularly in females. There was also a significant relationship between the size of the foal and the presence of retinal hemorrhage. There was no relationship between retinal hemorrhages and lack of vision, menace response or PLRs but there was an association between the presence of retinal hemorrhage and foaling difficulty. All retinal hemorrhages resolved within 10 days, were not associated with short- or long-term complications, and were not associated with any abnormal foal behavior. In another study, retinal hemorrhage was noted in 11.4% (8/70) of neonatal foals evaluated for nonophthalmic disease [7]. Only one affected foal was known to have been born to a dam with dystocia. In contrast, in a recent survey of neonatal foals no retinal hemorrhages were noted [20]. Historically retinal hemorrhage was thought to be associated with neonatal encephalopathy but these reports of retinal hemorrhage in foals without neonatal encephalopathy or known dystocia suggest that retinal hemorrhage is transient in the neonatal foal.

Choroid

The choroid is a highly vascular structure between the retina and the sclera. In most cases, choroidal vessels are obscured by the tapetum and the pigment of the RPE. However, in lightly pigmented animals, the choroidal vessels can be seen radiating across the fundus. As horses have a paurangiotic retinal vascular pattern with retinal vessels limited to the peripapillary retina, the choroid is responsible for supplying nutrition to most of the retina.

Imaging

Ultrasonographic imaging of 22 healthy neonatal foal eyes <7 days old showed a mean anterior chamber depth of 2.2 ± 0.5 mm, central lens thickness of 9.9 ± 0.8 mm, vitreous chamber depth of 15.5 ± 1.1 mm, an axial globe length of 27.6 ± 1.6 mm, a longitudinal globe length of 35.8 ± 1.2 mm, and a lens pole distance of 16.4 ± 1.0 mm [67]. In this study, intraocular measurements were not influenced by gender, laterality (right or left globe), or body weight. Two other ultrasonographic studies have evaluated the eyes of foals <180 days of age [35, 68]. These two studies (and other reports) noted that axial globe length was dependent on age rather than body size [69, 70]. Table 52.1 provides data from all three studies.

Table 52.1 Ultrasonographic measurements of the globe of neonatal or young foals. Values are expressed in mm and as mean value ± standard deviation.

Intraocular measurements	Foals 1–7 d-old (44 eyes) [67]	Foals 0–180 d-old (33 eyes) [28]	Foals 42–116 d-old (20 eyes) [70]
Anterior chamber depth	2.2 ± 0.5	2.9 ± 0.6	4.94 ± 0.49
Central lens thickness	9.9 ± 0.8	9.1 ± 0.4	9.38 ± 0.59
Vitreous chamber depth	15.5 ± 1.1	19.3 ± 1.0	18.96 ± 0.86
Axial globe length	27.6 ± 1.6	32 ± 1.4	33.32 ± 0.83

Electroretinography

Minimal research is available regarding electrodiagnostic evaluation of the retina and visual system in the neonatal foal. The visual evoked potential measures the integrity of the visual system, and the electroretinogram measures the function of the retina. Flash-generated visual-evoked potential (FVEP) and electroretinogram (FERG) data have been harvested in neonatal foals [71, 72]. The amplitudes for all FVEP peaks in neonatal foals were significantly larger than in adult horses, and some of the implicit times were significantly shorter in foals. There were no significant differences in the mean amplitudes or implicit times in the FERG of neonatal foals as compared to adult horses. The presence of an intact FVEP suggests that the visual pathway of neonatal foals is intact even though a menace reflex may not be present. The authors recommend using age-matched controls when harvesting FVEP data in horses <3 years of age.

Conclusions

Some studies regarding the specific ophthalmic parameters and physiology of neonatal foals have been accomplished. In certain instances, there are specific differences that must be noted when evaluating both healthy and sick neonatal foals. In the absence of specific data involving the neonatal foal, however, it is reasonable to assume that the ocular and adnexal physiology of the neonatal foal is similar to the adult horse.

References

1 Leiva, M. and Pena, T. (2017). Ophthalmic diseases in foals. In: *Equine Ophthalmology*, 3e (ed. B.C. Gilger), 112–150. Hoboken, NJ: John Wiley & Sons.

2 Adams, R. and Mayhew, I.G. (1984). Neurological examination of newborn foals. *Equine Vet. J.* 16: 306–312.

3 Enzering, E. (1998). The menace response and pupillary light reflex in neonatal foals. *Equine Vet. J.* 30 (6): 546–548.

4 Gelatt, K.N. (1993). Congenital and acquired ophthalmic diseases in the foal. *Anim. Eye. Res.* 12: 15–27.

5 Munroe, G.A. and Barnett, K.C. (1984). Congenital ocular disease in the foal. *Vet. Clin. North Am. Large Anim. Pract.* 6: 519–537.

6 Turner, A.G. (2004). Ocular conditions in neonatal foals. *Vet. Clin. North Am. Equine Pract.* 20: 429–440.

7 Labelle, A.L., Hamor, R.E., Townsend, W.M. et al. (2011). Ophthalmic lesions in neonatal foals evaluated for nonophthalmic disease at referral hospitals. *J. Am. Vet. Med. Assoc.* 239: 486–492.

8 Barsotti, G., Scorbini, M., Marmorini, P. et al. (2013). Ocular abnormalities in healthy Standardbred foals. *Vet. Ophthalmol.* 16: 245–250.

9 de Lahunta, A., Glass, E.G., and Kent, M. (2015). Visual system. In: *Veterinary Neuroanatomy and Clinical Neurology*, 4e (ed. A. de Lahunta, E.N. Glass, and M. Kent), 409–454. St. Louis: Elsevier Saunders.

10 Herron, M.A., Martin, J.E., and Joyce, J.R. (1978). Quantitative study of the decussating optic axons in the pony, cow, sheep, and pig. *Am. J. Vet. Res.* 39: 1137–1139.

11 Cummings, J.F. and de Lahunta, A. (1969). An experimental study of the retinal projections in the horse and sheep. *Ann. N.Y. Acad. Sci.* 167: 293–316.

12 Miller, P.E. and Murphy, C.J. (2017). Equine vision. In: *Equine Ophthalmology*, 3e (ed. B.C. Gilger), 508–544. Hoboken, NJ: John Wiley & Sons.

13 Galambos, R. and Johasz, G. (2001). How patterns of bleached rods and cones become visual perceptual experiences: a proposal. *Proc. Natl. Acad. Sci. U.S.A.* 98: 11702–11707.

14 Sun, L.W. (2012). Transynaptic tracing of conditioned eyeblink circuits in the mouse cerebellum. *Neuroscience* 203: 122–134.

15 Mayhew, I.G. (1989). Neurologic evaluation. In: *Large Animal Neurology: A Handbook for Veterinary Clinicians* (ed. I.G. Mayhew), 15–47. Philadelphia: Lea and Febiger.

16 Roberts, S.M. (1993). Ocular disorders. In: *Equine Reproduction* (ed. A.L. McKinnon and J.L. Voss), 1076–1087. Philadelphia: Lea and Febiger.

17 Mayhew, I.G. (1995). Neuro-ophthalmology. In: *Color Atlas and Text of Equine Ophthalmology* (ed. K.C. Barnett, S.M. Crispin, J.D. Lavach, and A.G. Matthews), 215–222. London: Mosby-Wolfe.

18 Whitley, R.D. (1990). Neonatal equine ophthalmology. In: *Equine Clinical Neonatology* (ed. A.M. Koterba, W.H. Drummond, and P.C. Kosch), 531–557. Philadelphia: Lea & Febiger.

19 Latimer, C.A. and Wyman, M. (1985). Neonatal ophthalmology. *Vet. Clin. North Am. Equine Pract.* 1: 235–259.

20 Leiva, M., Pena, T., and Monreal, I. (2011). Ocular findings in healthy newborn foals according to age. *Equine Vet. Educ.* 23: 40–45.

21 Short, C.E. and Rebhun, W.C. (1980). Complications caused by the oculocardiac reflex during anesthesia in a foal. *J. Am. Vet. Med. Assoc.* 176: 630–631.

22 Hendrix, D.V.H., Thomasy, S.M., and Gum, G.G. (2021). Physiology of the eye. In: *Veterinary Ophthalmology*, 6e, vol. 1 (ed. K.N. Gelatt, G. Ben-Shlomo, B.C. Gilger, et al.), 124–167. Wiley.

23 Chen, T. and Ward, D.A. (2010). Tear volume, turnover rate, and flow rate in ophthalmoscopically normal horses. *Am. J. Vet. Res.* 71: 671–676.

24 Butavich, I.A., Borowiak, A.M., and Eule, J.C. (2011). Comparative HPLC MSn analysis of canine and human Meibomian lipidomes: many similarities, a few differences. *Sci. Rep.* 1: 24 https://doi.org/10.1038/srep00024.

25 Bourges-Abella, N., Raymond-Letron, I., Diquelou, A. et al. (2007). Comparison of cytologic and histologic evaluations of the conjunctiva in the normal equine eye. *Vet. Ophthalmol.* 10: 12–18.

26 Dartt, D.A. (2011). Formation and function of the tear film. In: *Adler's Physiology of the Eye*, 11e (ed. L.A. Levin, S.F.E. Nilsson, J. Ver Hoeve, and S.M. Wu), 350–362. New York: Elsevier Saunders.

27 Francois, J. and Neetens, A. (1973). Tear flow in man. *Am. J. Ophthalmol.* 76: 351–358.

28 Hassell, J.R. and Birk, D.E. (2010). The molecular basis of corneal transparency. *Exp. Eye Res.* 91: 326–335.

29 Goldman, J.N., Benedek, G.B., Dohlman, C.H. et al. (1968). Structural alterations affecting transparency in swollen human corneas. *Invest. Ophthalmol. Vis. Sci.* 7: 501–519.

30 Sivak, J.M. and Fini, M.E. (2002). Emerging roles for matrix metalloproteinases in ocular physiology. *Rofrress Retinal Eye Res.* 21: 1–14.

31 Ollivier, F.J., Gilger, B.C., Barrie, K.P. et al. (2007). Proteinases of the cornea and preocular tear film. *Vet. Ophthalmol.* 10: 199–206.

32 Hibbets, K., Hines, B., and Williams, D. (1999). An overview of protease inhibitors. *J. Vet. Intern. Med.* 13: 302–308.

33 Twining, S.S., Fukuchi, T., Yue, B.Y. et al. (1994). Alpha 2-macroglobulin is present in and synthesized by the cornea. *Invest. Ophthalmol. Vis. Sci.* 35: 3226–3233.

34 Geerling, G., Joussen, A.M., Daniels, J.T. et al. (1999). Matrix metalloproteinases in sterile corneal melts. *Ann. N.Y. Acad. Sci.* 878: 571–574.

35 Herbig, L.E. and Eule, J.C. (2015). Central corneal thickness measurements and ultrasonographic study of the growing equine eye. *Vet. Ophthalmol.* 18: 462–471.

36 Brooks, D.E., Clark, C.K., and Lester, G.D. (2000). Cochet-Bonnet aesthesiometer-determined corneal sensitivity in neonatal foals and adult horses. *Vet. Ophthalmol.* 3: 133–137.

37 Munroe, G.A. (1995). Congenital corneal vascularisation in a neonatal Thoroughbred foal. *Equine Vet. J.* 27 (2): 156–157.

38 Barnett, K.C. (1975). The eye of the newborn foal. *J. Reprod. Fertil.* 23 (Suppl): 701–702.

39 Latimer, C.A., Wyman, M., and Hamilton, J. (1983). An ophthalmic survey of the neonatal horse. *Equine Vet. J. Suppl.* 2: 9–14.

40 Gilger, B.C. and Hollingsworth, S.R. (2017). Diseases of the uvea, uveitis, and recurrent uveitis. In: *Equine Ophthalmology*, 3e (ed. B.C. Gilger), 369–415. Ames, Iowa: Wiley.

41 Meekins, J.M., Rankin, A.J., and Samuelson, D.A. (2021). Ophthalmic anatomy. In: *Veterinary Ophthalmology*, 6e (ed. K.N. Gelatt, G. Ben-Shlomo, B.C. Gilger, et al.), 41–123. Hobokin: Wiley.

42 De Geest, J.P., Lauwers, H., Simoens, P. et al. (1990). The morphology of the equine iridocorneal angle: a light and scanning electron microscopic study. *Equine Vet. J. Suppl.* 22: 30–35.

43 Smith, P.J., Samuelson, D.A., Brooks, D.E. et al. (1986). Unconventional aqueous humor outflow of microspheres perfused into the equine eye. *Am. J. Vet. Res.* 47: 2445–2453.

44 Samuelson, D.A., Smith, P.J., and Brooks, D.E. (1989). Morphologic features of the aqueous humor drainage pathways in horses. *Am. J. Vet. Res.* 50: 720–727.

45 Miller, T.L., Willis, A.M., Wilke, D.A. et al. (2001). Description of ciliary body anatomy and identification of sites for transscleral photocoagulation in the equine eye. *Vet. Ophthalmol.* 4: 183–190.

46 Smith, P.J., Gum, G.G., and Whitley, R.D. (1990). Tonometric and tonographic studies in the normal pony eye. *Equine Vet. J. (Suppl.)* 10: 36–38.

47 Sebag, J. (1989). *The Vitreous: Structure, Function, and Pathology*. New York: Springer.

48 Croft, M.A., Nork, T.M., McDonald, J.P. et al. (2013). Accommodative movements of the vitreous membrane, choroid, and sclera in young presbyopic human and nonhuman primate eyes. *Invest. Ophthalmol. Vis. Sci.* 54: 5049–5058.

49 Newman, E.A. (1984). Regional specialization of retinal glial cell membrane. *Nature* 309: 155–157.

50 Reddy, V.N. (1979). Dynamics of transport systems in the eye. *Invest. Opthalmol. Vis. Sci.* 18: 1000–1008.

51 Weiss, H. (1972). The carbohydrate reservein the vitreous body and retina of the rabbit eye during and after pressure ischemia and insulin hypoglycemia. *Ophthalmic Res.* 3: 360–371.

52 Ueno, N., Sebag, J., Hirokawa, H. et al. (1987). Effects of visible light irradiation on vitreous structure in the presence of a photosensitizer. *Exp. Eye Res.* 44: 863–870.

53 Murthy, K.R., Goell, R., Subbannayya, Y. et al. (2014). Proteomic analysis of human vitreous humor. *Clin. Proteomics* 11: 29–40.

54 Akiya, S., Uemura, Y., Tsuchiya, S. et al. (1986). Electron microscopic study of the developing human vitreous collagen fibrils. *Ophthalmic Res.* 1986 (18): 199–202.

55 Munroe, G. (2000). Study of the hyaloid apparatus in the neonatal thoroughbred foal. *Vet. Rec.* 146: 579–584.

56 Hurn, S.D. and Turner, A.G. (2006). Ophthalmic examination findings of Thoroughbred racehorses in Australia. *Vet. Ophthalmol.* 9: 95–100.

57 Guo, X. and Sugita, S. (2000). Topography of ganglion cells in the retina of the horse. *J. Am. Vet. Med. Assoc.* 62: 1145–1150.

58 Harman, A.M., Moore, S., Hoskins, R. et al. (1999). Horse vision and an explanation for the visual behavior originally explained by the ramp retina. *Equine Vet. J.* 31: 384–390.

59 Hebel, R. (1976). Distribution of retinal ganglion-cells in 5 mammalian species (pig, sheep, ox, horse, dog). *Anat. Embryol.* 150: 45–51.

60 Brooks, D.E., Komaromy, A.M., and Kallberg, M.E. (1999). Comparative retinal ganglion cell and optic nerve morphology. *Vet. Ophthalmol.* 2: 3–11.

61 Evans, K.E. and McGreevey, P.D. (2007). The distribution of ganglion cells in the equine retina and its relationship to skull morphology. *Anat. Histol. Embryol.* 36: 151–156.

62 Carroll, J., Murphy, C.J., Neitz, M. et al. (2001). Photopigment basis for dichromatic color vision in the horse. *J. Visualization* 1: 80–87.

63 Hall, C.A., Cassaday, H.J., Vincent, C.J. et al. (2006). Cone excitation ratios correlate with color discrimination performance ion the horse (Equus caballus). *J. Comp. Psychol.* 120: 438–448.

64 Hughes, A. (1977). The topography of vision in mammals of contrasting life style: comparative optics and retinal organization. In: *Handbook of Sensory Physiology*, The Visual System in Vertebrates, vol. vii/5 (ed. F. Crescitelli), 613–756. Berlin: Springer.

65 Sigelman, J. and Ozanics, V. (1988). Retina. In: *Biomedical Foundations of Ophthalmology*, vol. 1 Chapter 19 (ed. T.D. Duane and E.A. Jaeger), 1–63. Philadelphia PA: JB Lippincott.

66 Munroe, G. (2000). Survey of retinal haemorrhages in neonatal Thoroughbred foals. *Vet. Rec.* 146: 95–101.

67 Valentini, S., Castagnetti, C., Musella, V. et al. (2014). Assessment of intraocular measurements in neonatal foals and association with gender, laterality, and body weight: a clinical study. *PLoS One* 9 (10): e109491.

68 Townsend, W.M., Wasserman, N., and Jacobi, S. (2012). A pilot study on the corneal curvature and ocular dimensions of horses less than one year of age. *Equine Vet. J.* 45: 256–258.

69 Plummer, C.E., Ramsey, D.T., and Hauptman, J.G. (2003). Assessment of corneal thickness, intraocular pressure, optical corneal diameter, and axial globe dimensions in Miniature Horses. *Am. J. Vet. Res.* 64: 661–665.

70 Mouney, M.C., Townsend, W.M., and Moore, G.E. (2012). Association of height, body weight, age, and corneal diameter with calculated intraocular lens strength of adult horses. *Am. J. Vet. Res.* 73: 1977–1982.

71 Strom, L., Michanek, M., and Ekeston, B. (2019). Age-associated changes in the equine flash visual evoked potential. *Vet. Ophthalmol.* 22: 388–397.

72 Strain, G.M., Graham, M.C., Claxton, M.S. et al. (1989). Postnatal development of brainstem auditory-evoked potentials, electroretinograms, and visual-evoked potentials in the calf. *J. Vet. Intern. Med.* 3: 231–237.

Chapter 53 Examination, Diagnostics and Therapeutics of the Neonatal Equine Eye

Elizabeth A. Giuliano

Ophthalmic disease is commonly encountered in neonatal foals, arising from a variety of reasons. As with any examination, it is important that a complete ocular examination is performed to the fullest extent possible when a foal presents with ocular disease. In this chapter, the minimum ophthalmic data base (MODB) using basic instrumentation and viewing techniques will be discussed. Other sections in this text detail specific ocular conditions and treatments. Exceptions to the MODB rules will be highlighted, as examination of the neonatal equine eye presents unique challenges.

As a general rule, the equine ocular examination includes obtaining a detailed history and signalment, inspecting the patient in a well-lit environment, examining the ocular structures in both light and darkened environments, facilitating the ophthalmic examination with restraint, sedation, and local nerve blocks as needed, and collecting relevant diagnostic samples or data [1-3]. In healthy foals, ocular examinations are typically performed without sedation or lid blocks, with an assistant restraining the foal as needed, and the examiner steadying the head. If very active, the foal can be backed into the stall corner to minimize motion and facilitate examination. Conversely, in recumbent foals, the examiner may need to examine one eye at a time while an assistant holds the head. Whenever possible, foals should be examined near their dams to minimize anxiety.

Examination Components

A thorough history is important to best interpret ophthalmic abnormalities in foals [4-17]. Common questions asked of owners/breeders/caretakers of the foal include:

- What first made you think your foal has an ocular problem? This question is of particular relevance, as many owners perceive neurologic problems as vision impairment.
- Date first noted, progression, and duration of the ocular problem.
- What medications have been administered and how did medical therapy alter the appearance of the ocular abnormality?
- Is vision perceived to be better in well-lit or dark environmental conditions?
- Is the abnormality unilateral or bilateral?
- Does the dam, stud, or any other equine relatives have any known ocular disease?

The essentials of a complete ophthalmic examination in any species are based on a systematic manner, referred to as the MODB. After overview of the foal from a distance, the components of the MODB, in order, are noted in Table 53.1. Advanced diagnostics include ocular ultrasonography, electroretinography (ERG), radiography, computed tomography (CT), or magnetic resonance imaging (MRI) [18-21]. Foals may need to be referred for specialist care if advanced diagnostic techniques are warranted. As we consider the MODB in more detail, consideration for foals specifically will be discussed.

Overall Patient Examination as Related to Normal Ocular Development and Vision

The initial examination of a foal should be performed prior to sedation or regional lid blocks in a well-lit, quiet environment. Examining the neonatal foal without the presence of the dam is not possible and, in most cases, not recommended. In contrast to performing complete ophthalmic examinations in adult horses where sedation and regional eyelid blocks are usually necessary, neither are routinely required in neonatal foals [1]. Of all possible regional eyelid blocks, the auriculopalpebral (AP) nerve block is most commonly used to facilitate examination of

Equine Neonatal Medicine, First Edition. Edited by David M. Wong and Pamela A. Wilkins.

Table 53.1 Components of the minimum ophthalmic data base (MODB), performed in sequential order.

1) Perform the menace response.
2) Check the palpebral reflex.
3) Evaluate direct and consensual pupillary light reflex (PLR).
4) Perform Schirmer tear test (STT).
5) Apply fluorescein staining to the cornea.
6) Measure the intraocular pressure measurement (IOP) of the globe.

Additional commonly performed diagnostics can then be obtained as needed including culture and cytology

the globe. The AP block results in akinesia of the superior eyelid and significantly aids in gently opening the eyelids. The AP block is warranted in cases where globe structural integrity is at risk due to a deep or perforated corneal wound, especially if the foal is noncompliant. The AP nerve can be palpated over the zygomatic arch in the region of the temporo-frontal suture. The sensation of this palpation is likened to "strumming a guitar string" when locating the nerve. Once located, approximately 1.5 mL of 2% lidocaine is injected using a 25-gauge, ⅝-inch needle over the zygomatic arch. Using a finger, rub the local anesthetic transcutaneously for approximately 10–15 seconds. Successful administration of the AP block results in a highly compliant, "loose" upper eyelid that can then be elevated to facilitate ocular examination with minimal to no pressure on the globe.

It is worth remembering that vision testing in animals, even in adult horses, is subjective at best and relies on assessing a foal's behavior in his/her environment, the menace response, dazzle reflex, and possibly maze testing (difficult to perform in very young foals). Evaluation of one or more of these tests may help the clinician to determine complete blindness but subtle deficits in vision can be easily missed. While advanced diagnostic testing such as ocular ultrasound and ERG testing can help determine retinal abnormalities specifically, it is important to remember that ERG testing is not a test of visual function. Many foals presenting for ocular problems may be depressed, ataxic, have vestibular disease, or are obtunded secondary to systemic disease. In this author's opinion, most consultations performed on foals, particularly in the first week of life, are often diagnosed with an ophthalmic abnormality secondary to systemic disease (e.g., bilateral uveitis).

Providing the neonatal foal can stand normally, the clinician is positioned in front of the foal to assess the head, bony orbit, position and health of the eyelids, and pupillary symmetry. Foals with unilateral ocular discomfort typically have a narrowed palpebral fissure with eyelashes directed ventrally, and if the affected globe is retracted, third eyelid elevation may be evident. Other reasons besides blepharospasm for ventral eyelash deviation include enophthalmos or ptosis. By contrast, enlargement of the interpalpebral fissure with upward eyelash deviation may be observed with exophthalmos (normal-sized globe protruding forward) or buphthalmos (enlarged globe). Once the overall assessment of the foal's head is complete, the examiner should proceed with the MODB. If a foal is recumbent due to systemic disease, assistants will be needed to assess both eyes. Care should be taken, as neonatal foals are kept with their dams. Protective mares can become dangerous to the foal, the examiners, and in some cases themselves, thus light sedation of the dam may be advisable prior to examination of the neonatal foal [2, 5, 22].

Menace Response and Palpebral Reflex

The neuro-ophthalmic portions of the MODB (menace response, palpebral, and PLR reflexes) should be performed prior to sedation or regional eyelid blocks. The menace response is learned and not reliably present in foals under two weeks of age; thus, this test of vision is frequently not reliable in neonatal foals. This neuro-ophthalmic test assesses the retina, cranial nerve II (afferent arm) and the orbicularis oculi muscle innervated by the palpebral branch of cranial nerve VII (efferent arm). When present and normal, a threatening movement, usually performed with the examiner's finger or hand, results in protective eyelid closure with or without retraction of the globe or an avoidance movement of the head. When performing this test, the clinician should avoid causing air currents or touching the vibrissae, lest cranial nerve V (trigeminal nerve) be stimulated. To try and best determine if vision is present in different visual fields of an eye, the finger or hand performing the menace response is independently directed towards both the nasal and temporal visual fields.

The palpebral reflex should be present in neonatal foals. By first touching the nasal and then the temporal aspect of the eyelid canthus (CN V), the foal should blink (CN VII) in response to these stimuli. Abnormalities in a foal's palpebral reflex may be due to facial nerve paralysis or secondary to severe chemosis, making the eyelids unable to close. It is often useful to combine the first two components of the MODB, the menace response and the palpebral reflex, in relatively rapid succession of one another to serve as a reminder to the patient that a threatening finger gestured toward the eye may make contact. This can be a helpful technique in depressed foals to ascertain both vision and functionality of eyelid movement, providing the foal is old enough to have learned a menace response. Again, the menace response is a crude test of functional vision and is often not present in very young or premature neonatal foals, especially those that are depressed from systemic illness, and thus an absent menace in such cases does not necessarily imply a visual deficit.

Pupillary Light Reflex

PLRs are most reliably elicited by a bright focal light source such as a transilluminator with the foal in a darkened examination area. A dark blanket may be placed over the examiner and assistant(s) to aid in the creation of a darkened environment, but care should be taken to avoid alarming the dam. From approximately an arm's distance away from a standing foal's head, with the transilluminator positioned at the examiners temple and pointing parallel to the examiner's line of sight, with slight side to side movement of the examiner, both pupils can be examined using retroillumination (light shines into the patient's eye and is reflected back toward the examiner). Retroillumination is an effective way to determine pupil symmetry or lack thereof. Direct ophthalmoscopy can also be used to assess pupil size by setting the instrument at 0 diopters and observing the tapetal reflections of both eyes while standing an arm's distance away from the front of the foal.

Foals with heterochromia iridis, especially when one iris is blue and the contralateral iris is brown, may demonstrate some degree of normal anisocoria, with the larger pupil on the same side as the blue iris. A normal PLR (both direct and consensual) is slower than what is observed in a small animal patient. Recall that an adult equid's pupil is horizontally ellipsoid and thus vertical movement is greater than horizontal movement when stimulated by bright light [1]. In foals, pupils are slightly rounder [5]. The PLR pathway involves the retina, CN II, midbrain, and CN III. When light is shown into one eye, the result should be constriction in the illuminated eye (direct reflex) and the contralateral eye (indirect or consensual reflex). Indirect PLRs are more difficult to examine in horses as a result of their weaker and slower response time; this is due to approximately 85% decussation of pupillomotor fibers at the optic nerve chiasm. In a recumbent foal, consensual PLRs are challenging to accurately determine [23].

If a very bright light is available, the foal's dazzle reflex can be evaluated. Unlike the cortically mediated menace response, the dazzle reflex is a subcortical reflex that is considered more of a "pain response" to very bright light. Clinically the dazzle reflex may be useful in a foal whose posterior segment cannot be evaluated due to ocular abnormalities such as hyphema, cataract, or severe corneal edema, to assess if any part of the retina is still functional. The bright light source is shown into the eye and the foal responds with blepharospasm and/or moving of the head in an avoidance maneuver. Importantly, neither positive PLRs nor dazzle reflexes indicate that the foal has functional vision.

MODB Diagnostics

Schirmer Tear Test (STT)

The STT is performed by placing a standardized commercially available paper strip, folded at its notch 5 mm from its end, in the lower middle conjunctival sac and millimeters of wetting in 60 seconds is recorded. More specifically, a STT I is performed with no topical anesthesia applied to the eye and measures the amount of basal and stimulated aqueous component of tears. By contrast, the STT II test is performed after the application of topical anesthesia and is purported to measure only the basal aqueous tear production. This is the first diagnostic test to be performed when conducting the MODB, as the test should be performed prior to significant manipulation of the eye and orbit during examination to minimize reflex tearing. Dry eye or keratoconjunctivitis sicca is much less common in horses than in dogs [1]. It is perhaps for this reason that STT are often not routinely performed in horses, coupled with the finding that there is wide variability in the STT I in normal horses and ponies (range of 11 to >30 mm wetting/60 seconds) [24]. There is a paucity of scientific reports on STT values in horses, especially in foals. STT I values for ill (14.2 $\pm$ 1 mm wetting/min) and healthy (12.8 $\pm$ 2.4 mm/min) neonatal foals were not significantly different in one report but were slightly lower than STT I values from healthy adult horses (18.3 $\pm$ 2.1 mm/min) [1, 25]. A recent study examined the effect of AP nerve block on STT I values in normal horses and found no difference [26].

Fluorescein Stain

In ill neonatal foals, low tear production, reduced blinking rate, increased corneal exposure, and in some cases eyelid abnormalities (e.g., entropion) render patients at increased risk of corneal disease [2]. There are various ophthalmic dyes available for use including sodium fluorescein, rose bengal, lissamine green, alcian blue, trypan blue, and methylene blue. The most commonly used stain in clinical practice is sodium fluorescein. Application of fluorescein stain to the cornea is indicated in all complete ocular examinations in neonatal foals. Uptake of fluorescein stain will occur in corneal ulceration where it binds to exposed hydrophilic stroma but does not adhere to healthy lipophilic corneal epithelium or to Descemet's membrane (Figures 53.1 and 53.2). This stain can also be used to assess tear film stability (e.g. Tear Film Break-up Time) and patency of the nasolacrimal outflow tract.

Fluorescein stain is commonly purchased in sterile impregnated paper strips. Due to the vertical position of the standing foal, in most cases application of topical fluorescein involves the use of a 1- or 3-mL syringe with a 25-gauge

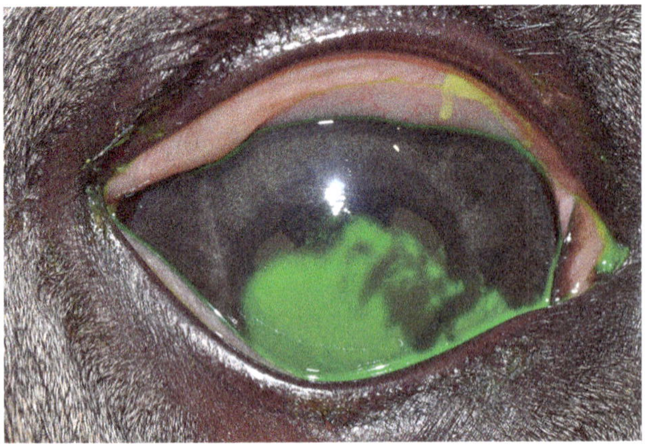

Figure 53.1 A 3-week-old foal with an irregular superficial corneal ulcer as denoted by the areas of green fluorescein stain uptake. *Source:* Photo courtesy of Dr. Caryn Plummer, University of Florida.

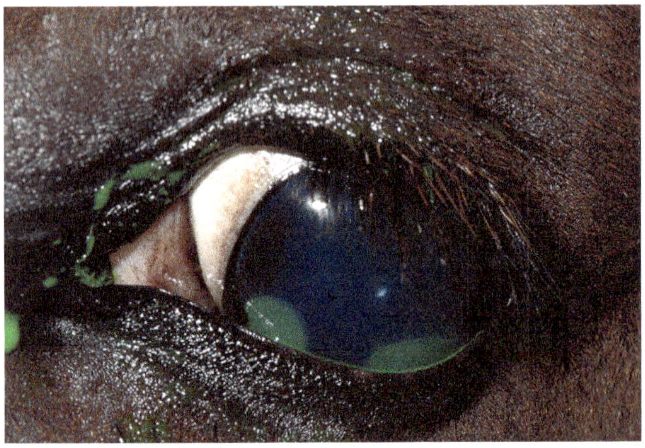

Figure 53.2 A 15-day-old foal with two ventral healing corneal ulcers resulting from entropion during the first week of life. Note the two areas of positive fluorescein staining.

needle and sterile eyewash solution. The impregnated dye end of the fluorescein strip is torn off and placed into a syringe, which is then filled with sterile eyewash; the plunger is replaced, and the needle is manually broken off leaving only the hub of the 25-gauge needle in place. The syringe is gently shaken to distribute the dye within the eyewash. The diluted fluorescein stain is then squirted onto the ocular surface and blinking of the eyelids distributes the stain evenly across the ocular surface. If the foal is recumbent, the moistened fluorescein tip may be touched to the dorsal sclera and the eyelids blinked to evenly distribute the stain. Excess fluorescein stain using either technique can be removed with gentle irrigation of sterile eyewash. Note that use of undiluted topical fluorescein stain may better highlight subtle lesions consistent with corneal and conjunctival erosions. In dim light conditions, blue light, typically available on a direct ophthalmoscope, will highlight areas of stain retention.

Fluorescein staining is useful for two other purposes: to detect leakage of aqueous humor through the cornea (i.e. Seidel test) and to test patency of the nasolacrimal outflow system (i.e. Jones test). The Seidel test, best performed using undiluted fluorescein stain, can detect full thickness, actively leaking corneal perforations. If a corneal wound (i.e. penetrating foreign body, deep ulcer, or corneal suture abnormalities) is leaking, the high concentration of fluorescein stain over the leak will result in diluted rivulets as the aqueous humor egresses out of the wound, thus a positive Seidel test diagnosis.

Fluorescein staining is useful in determining the patency of the nasolacrimal outflow track, which consists of a medial upper and lower eyelid lacrimal puncta, two canualiculi that meet to form a rudimentary nasolacrimal sac, the main nasolacrimal duct, and the exit to the nasal puncta located on the floor of the nasal vestibule. The nasolacrimal outflow tract can be obstructed for numerous reasons, both acquired (foreign body, calcification, dentition abnormalities, inflammation/infection, or neoplastic processes) or congenital abnormalities. The most common congenital defect of the nasolacrimal duct is atresia of the duct and/or an imperforate nasal punctum [27, 28]. Mild to moderate unilateral or bilateral epiphora is initially observed in neonatal foals (Figure 53.3), but by 4–6 months of age, foals often exhibit severe mucopurulent ocular discharge due to the development of secondary bacterial dacryocystitis (Figure 53.4). The Jones test evaluates nasolacrimal duct patency by instillation of fluorescein stain onto the corneal and conjunctival surfaces. After several minutes, stain should be visible running out of the nasal punctum (i.e. positive Jones test). An imperforate nasal punctum is diagnosed by a negative Jones test, an inability to locate the opening of the distal nasal opening in the vestibule, and an inability to irrigate the nasolacrimal outflow tract in a normograde direction. Swelling of the nasal epithelium distally, near the area of normal punctal opening,

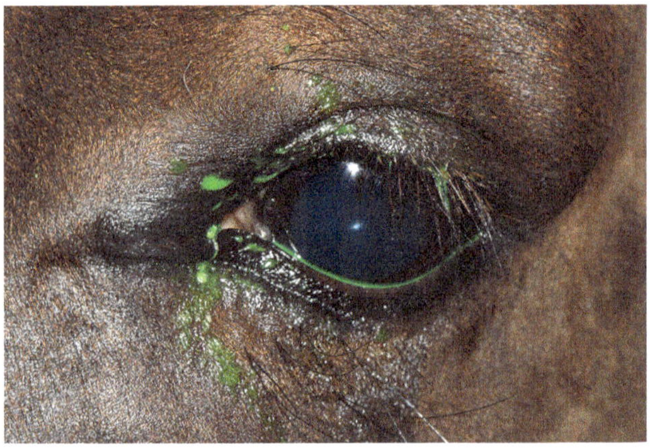

Figure 53.3 A 1-month-old foal exhibiting moderate epiphora.

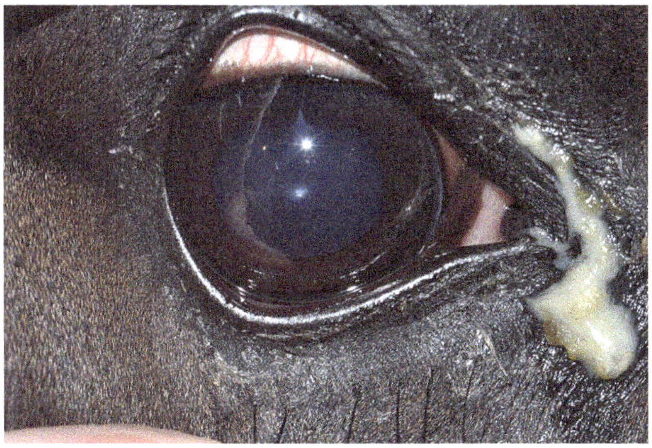

Figure 53.4 A 4-month-old foal with mucopurulent discharge predominantly at the medial canthus secondary to nasolacrimal duct atresia. *Source:* Photo courtesy of Dr. Caryn Plummer, University of Florida.

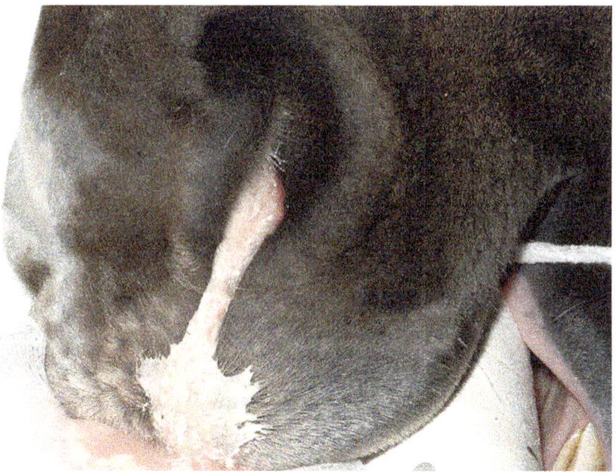

Figure 53.6 Same foal as shown in Figure 53.5. Note the copious mucopurulent discharge flowing from the surgical opening at the level of the imperforate nasal punctum as a result of the foal's dacryocystitis.

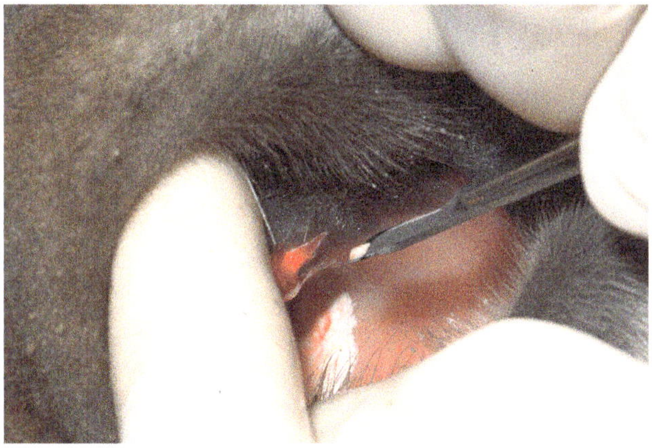

Figure 53.5 A 15 blade is being used to incise over the area of an imperforate nasal punctum in the nose of a 3.5-month-old Quarter Horse foal.

suggests atresia and can usually be digitally palpated as a focal flocculent area when normograde flushing is performed. If that is the case, a #15 blade can be used to create an opening overlying the swelling (Figure 53.5) at which point, if secondary infection is present, copious amounts of mucopurulent discharge will exude out the nose (Figure 53.6). If patency is surgically successful, a long piece of tubing (e.g. red rubber catheter) is kept in place for 4–6 weeks postoperatively until the nasal mucosa has healed (Figure 53.7).

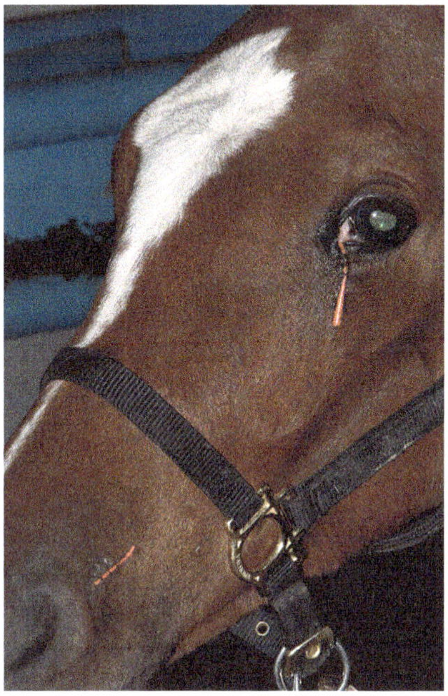

Figure 53.7 Once patency of an obstructed nasolacrimal system is surgically established, tubing (in this case a red rubber catheter) should be sutured into place for 4–6 weeks postoperatively until the nasal mucosa has healed, thereby helping to ensure a permanent functional nasolacrimal outflow tract.

Intraocular Pressure Measurement

Measurement of intraocular pressure (IOP) is warranted in "any red eye" in cases of corneal edema (Figure 53.8), blunt force trauma, or in an abnormal globe where structural integrity is intact. IOP should not be performed in foals with very deep ulcers at risk of rupture or if corneal rupture has already occurred. Tonometry in foals is performed by one of two methods: rebound tonometry (TonoVet® Icare Finland, Oy, Helsinki) or applanation tonometry (Tono-Pen Vet®, Reichert Inc., NY). In brief, applanation tonometers measure the force required to flatten, or applanate, a precise area of corneal surface and, using assumptions about physical features of the cornea (thickness, curvature), convert this force to an estimate of IOP [29]. Rebound tonometers use characteristics of the motion created when a probe is

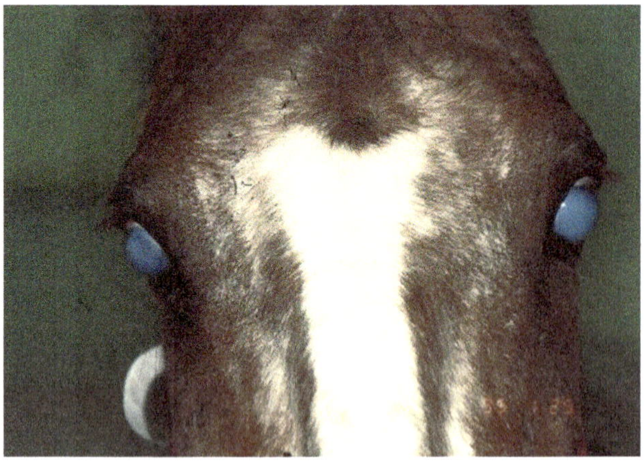

Figure 53.8 Congenital glaucoma in a 1-month-old foal. Note bilateral buphthalmos and diffuse corneal edema. *Source:* Photo courtesy of Dr. Caryn Plummer, University of Florida.

electromagnetically propelled to contact and then rebound from the corneal surface [3]. IOP measurement in foals can be challenging in healthy foals with ocular conditions. While topical anesthetic is recommended prior to use of applanation tonometry, the author uses anesthetic for either method as it improves patient compliance. By contrast, in systemically ill or severely depressed foals, IOP measurements can often be obtained without topical anesthetic. Rebound tonometry is generally preferred in standing healthy foals as the small disposable probe and reduced contact time results in greater patient compliance. However, in ill recumbent foals, use of the rebound tonometer is difficult as the probe should be maintained in a position parallel to the horizon and perpendicular to the cornea. In recumbent foals, applanation tonometry is often easier to use for IOP measurement. Reference ranges for IOP in healthy horses varies considerably, with values between 20–28 mmHg considered normal. Of note, IOP varies considerably depending on factors such as head position, exercise, drugs (systemic or topical) administered, time of day, and presence of corneal disease (e.g. fibrosis or significant corneal edema) [3, 30–37]. If the IOP measurements between eyes of the same foal vary by >5–10 mmHg, the clinician should repeat the technique, and if repeatable differences are detected, search for underlying causes of difference (i.e. glaucoma, uveitis, or both) [37].

Completion of Ocular Examination after MODB Diagnostics

After the MODB has been obtained, ocular examination should then make use of a combination of three forms of light: direct, retro-, and tangential illumination. Diffuse illumination simply uses a Finoff tansilluminator to broadly illuminate the eyelids, conjunctiva, cornea, and anterior segment to include the anterior chamber, iris, and lens. If a direct ophthalmoscope is available, using the smallest round aperture or the rectangular "slit" beam, when held close to the cornea in a darkened environment, the clinician should examine the foal for aqueous flair (pathognomonic for anterior uveitis). Since most clinicians do not have access to a slit-lamp biomicroscope, the author recommends holding the direct ophthalmoscope within 1 inch (2 cm) of the eye and then, while wearing a pair of magnifying loops, examine the anterior chamber from a side angle of 30–45° to the beam of light. The clarity and depth of the anterior chamber should be examined. In a healthy foal, no internal reflection of light from the aqueous will be present (no appearance of "fog in the headlights"); the anterior chamber should look clear. With uveitis, either primary or secondary, blood vessels in the uveal tract become inflamed and leak protein and cells into the aqueous humor. These solids reflect light (i.e. Tyndall effect). This turbidity results in visualization of the beam of light traversing the anterior chamber, referred to as aqueous flare. If the examiner only has diffuse direct illumination available, uveitis should be strongly suspected if the anterior chamber appears murky making it difficult to visualize the iris (Figure 53.9).

Tangential illumination is performed by holding the transilluminator to the side of the eye and aiming the beam of light tangentially across the anterior chamber. This is a useful form of illumination to better visualize abnormalities in the anterior chamber, iris, or a displaced lens. Recall that the dorsal aspect of the iris, and to a lesser extent the ventral aspect, possess protruding pigmented structures known as granula iridica or corpora nigra. These are part of a horse's normal iridal anatomy and believed to aid in decreasing glare in bright light conditions (Figures 53.10 and 53.11).

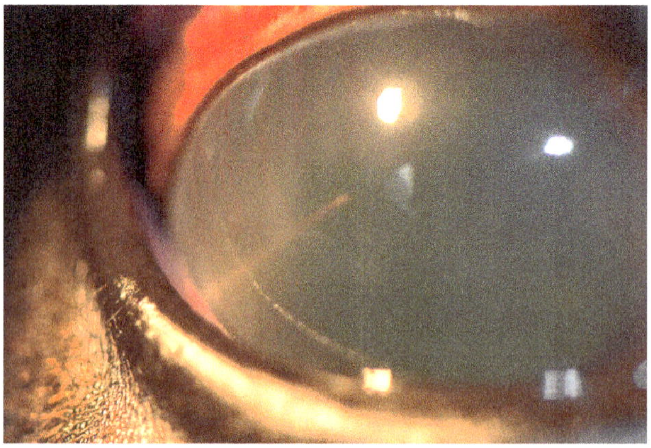

Figure 53.9 Three-week-old Saddlebred foal with linear foreign body in the anterior chamber surrounded by 3+ flare and fibrin in the anterior chamber. The pupil is pharmacologically dilated. There is mild diffuse corneal edema and conjunctival hyperemia evident in the superior temporal quadrant of the globe. Superficial corneal neovascularization is present.

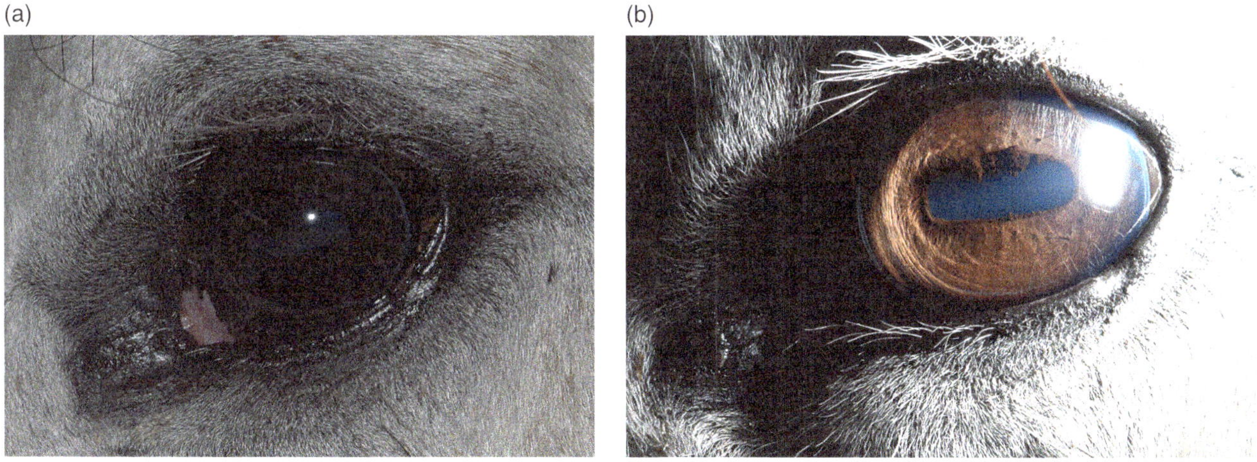

Figure 53.10 An adult Arabian mare's left eye and adnexa demonstrating direct diffuse illumination (a) and tangential illumination (b). Tangential illumination will "bleach" out eyelid structures but is useful in visualizing structures in the anterior chamber and iris.

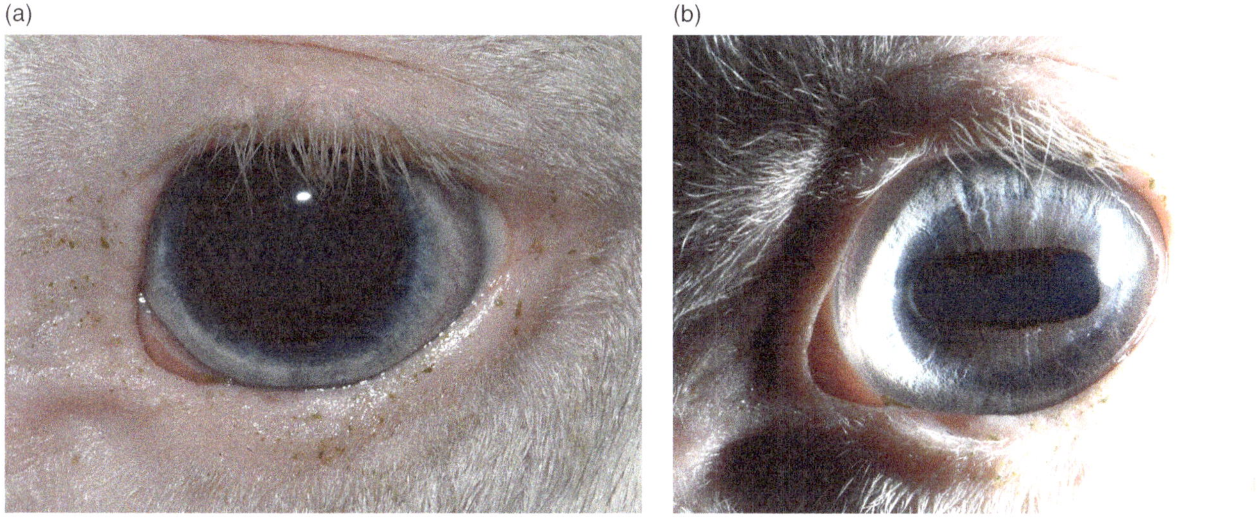

Figure 53.11 An adult American Paint gelding's left eye and adnexa demonstrating direct diffuse illumination (a) and tangential illumination (b). As with horses with dark brown irides, tangential illumination is not as helpful for adnexal evaluation but is useful in visualizing structures in the anterior chamber and iris of blue irises.

Retroillumination is an illumination technique whereby light is cast into the eye and allowed to be reflected back by the tapetum and posterior segment to the examiner, who is standing at least an arm's distance away from the globe. It is a useful technique to determine ocular abnormalities such as anisocoria, lesions affecting the cornea (Figure 53.12), anterior chamber, cataracts and vitreous, owing to the fact that opacities in these areas will reflect, refract, or obstruct returning light. Retroilluminated light will appear yellow to green and sometimes red depending on the skin color of the foal. Because the neonatal foal's tapetum is not fully developed, the reflected light can sometimes appear bluish-gray in color (Figure 53.13).

Unlike adult horses that typically require chemical restraint with regional nerve blocks to complete an ocular exam, neonatal foals, especially if depressed from systemic disease, do not. Neonatal foals are typically housed with their dam, making use of stocks irrelevant. The dam may need light sedation to quiet anxiety and the standing neonate restrained with the help of assistants. When possible, the heads of the foal and dam should be positioned near each other to decrease anxiety.

Now that the distance examination and the MODB is complete, examination of each eye at this juncture should include evaluation of the eyelids, third eyelid, and conjunctiva. Topical anesthetic can be applied if the posterior aspect of the third eyelid needs to be examined using small-toothed forceps to retract the third eyelid from the cornea in search of foreign body material. The cornea should be examined for loss of clarity including, but not limited to, ulceration (Figures 53.14) with careful attention to corneal malacia (Figure 53.15), blood vessels, and diffuse or focal

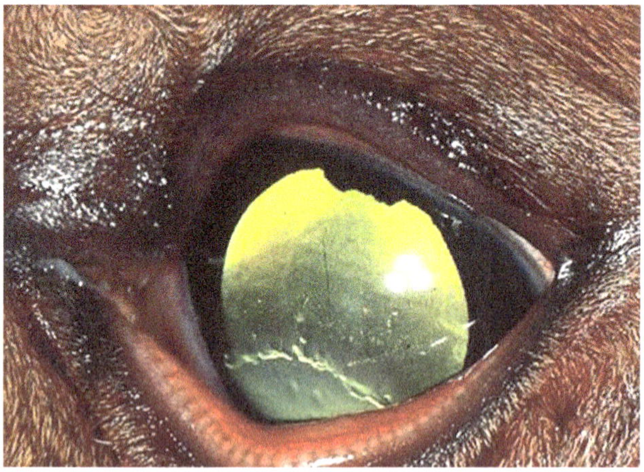

Figure 53.12 A 2-week-old Quarter Horse foal that is pharmacologically dilated, demonstrating retroillumination. The greenish-yellow tapetal reflection is "backlighting" the semi-circular margin of the ventral corneal ulcer in this extraocular photograph. *Source:* Photo courtesy of Dr. Caryn Plummer, University of Florida.

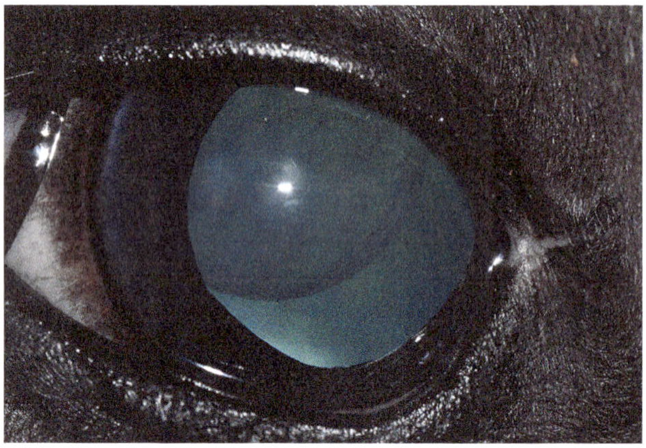

Figure 53.13 A 3-week-old black Andalusian foal with a posterior subluxated immature cataractous lens. Faint retroillumination demonstrates a blue-gray immature tapetal color captured in this image. *Source:* Photo courtesy of Dr. Caryn Plummer, University of Florida.

corneal edema (Figure 53.16). The three aforementioned illumination techniques should be used to assess the anterior chamber (Figure 53.17) and iris with regards to texture, contour, pupil shape, and mobility. Severity of corneal disease and/or anterior chamber opacities can preclude completion of examination into the foal's eye (Figure 53.18).

Deeper structures of the eye should be examined next; this is best performed using a short acting mydriatic such as tropicamide, providing IOP measurement is not elevated. If IOP measurement reveals glaucoma, pupillary dilation is contraindicated in most cases to prevent further escalation of IOP. Thorough lenticular, vitreal, and fundus examinations are best achieved once pupillary dilation is achieved. Topical tropicamide takes 15–20 minutes to reach full effect and lasts 4–6 hours in most horses. Lenticular and anterior vitreal examinations are best examined with a slit-lamp biomicroscope. As most clinicians do not possess this instrumentation, use of the three forms of

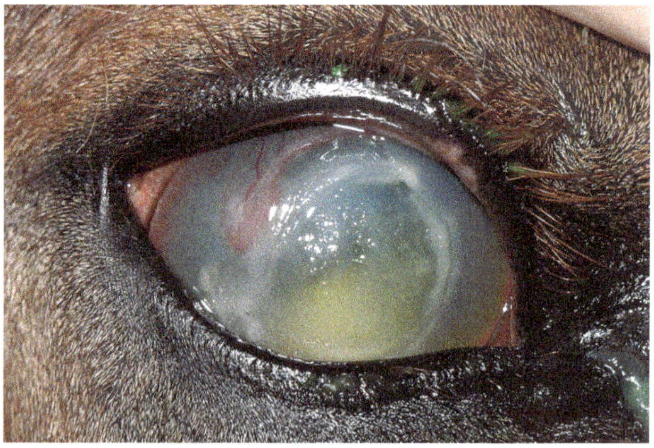

Figure 53.14 Severe equine ulcerative keratitis with approximately 50% stromal loss in the ulcer bed. Other typical hallmark features include diffuse corneal edema, superficial as well as deep corneal neovascularization, anterior uveitis with a fibrin clot seen in the anterior chamber.

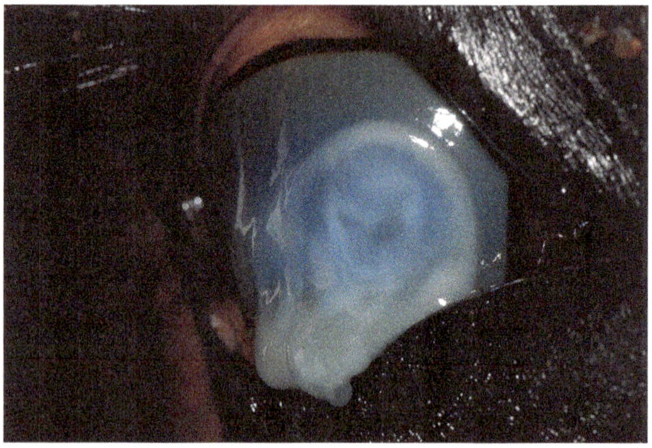

Figure 53.15 Severe equine corneal malacia. Note the creamy white appearance to the malacic stroma.

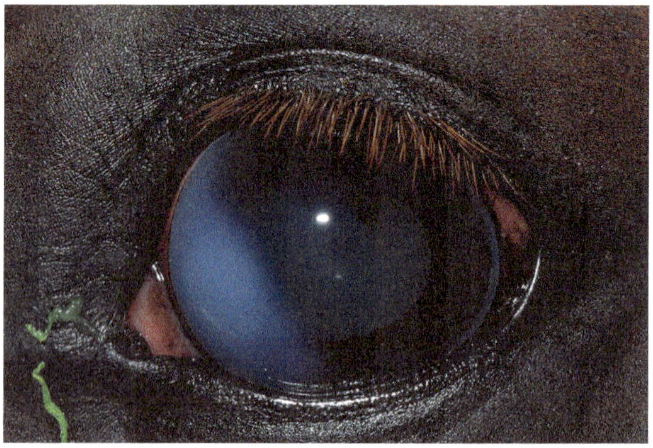

Figure 53.16 Focal medial corneal edema in a 3-week-old Saddlebred foal from blunt force trauma.

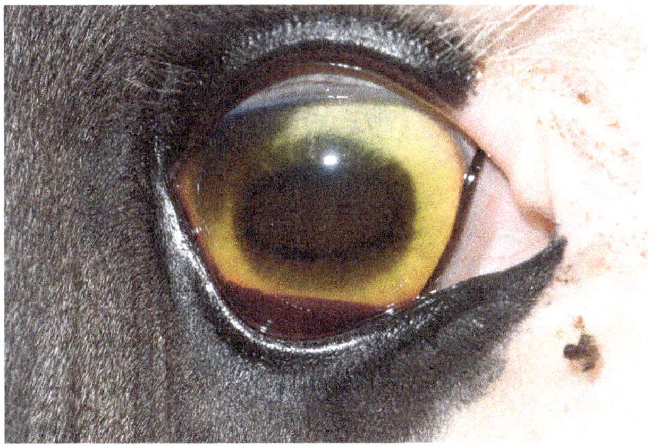

Figure 53.17 Severe anterior uveitis in a 2.5-week-old Paint foal. Note the hyphema settled in the ventral anterior chamber and the yellowish hue to the otherwise normally blue heterochromic iris due to the presence of fibrinous anterior uveitis.

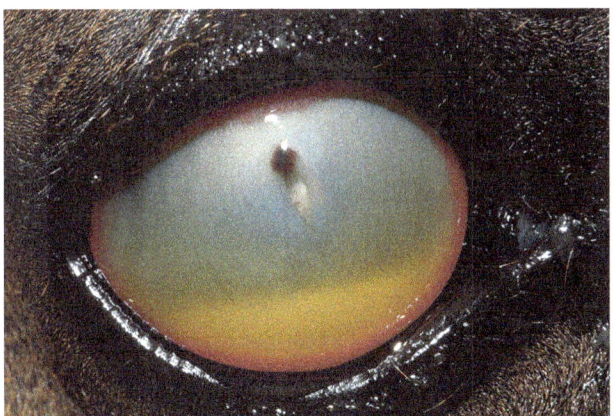

Figure 53.18 Dark brown penetrating foreign body is present in the superior axial corneal of this foal with accompanying diffuse corneal edema, ciliary flush, and hypopyon. All these clinical findings are consistent with severe anterior uveitis secondary to a penetrating full thickness corneal injury.

illumination previously discussed can help detect ocular abnormalities. For example, vitreous transillumination may reveal small posterior polar remnants of the hyaloid artery in foals and areas of light reflection between vitreous planes. Healthy horses possess a large tapetum fibrosum, which occupies the dorsal two-thirds of the fundus. End-on views of choroidal blood vessels are called Stars of Winslow. Tapetal color varies from green/yellow (most common) to a blue/purple and is often underdeveloped (pale orange to red color) in horses with albinotic or subalbinotic coat colors. The nontapetal fundus is usually dark brown due to melanin present in the retinal pigmented epithelium (RPE), which may be absent, depending on coat and anterior uveal tract (i.e., iris) coloration. In cases of poorly or absent pigment in the nontapetum, choroidal vessels are visualized and should not be mistaken for retinal hemorrhage. The junction of the tapetal and nontapetal areas of the equine fundus is well-delineated. The healthy optic disc is salmon-pink in color, horizontally oval, and located just temporal and ventral in the nontapetum. Retinal vessels radiate out only a short distance from the optic disc (i.e., paurangiotic retinal vasculature pattern) and are usually absent at the ventral optic disc border.

Posterior segment examination of the vitreous and fundus is achieved using either direct or indirect ophthalmoscopy techniques. Recall that the fundus is a "composite picture" of the neurosensory retina, superimposed on the choroid, which contains the tapetum fibrosum, superimposed on the sclera, and includes the optic nerve. In general, due to the ability to use both eyes and therefore maintain stereopsis (i.e. depth perception), the author advocates use of indirect over direct ophthalmoloscopy. Both techniques are discussed below.

Purported advantages of direct ophthalmoscopy include an upright image, availability of different viewing apertures such as slit and graticule, ability to alter the dioptric power of the ophthalmoscope, and high magnification. Disadvantages include shorter working distance to the foal's head, small field of view, lack of stereopsis, difficulty examining the peripheral fundus, and difficulty viewing the posterior segment when the visual axis is not clear. Importantly, when using direct ophthalmoscopy as the sole method for funduscopic viewing, it is difficult to interpret the "big picture" of the fundus compared to the larger field of view provided by indirect ophthalmoscopy. There are at least two dials on the direct ophthalmoscope head piece: one dial controls the size and shape of the light beam and a second dial controls the focal point of the light beam. When performing direct ophthalmoloscopy in a foal that has undergone pupillary dilation, set the horizontal dial to project a large circular white light beam while using the vertical dial to adjust the focus on the structure(s) of interest, (e.g. start at 0 for viewing the fundus). By adjusting the focusing distance of the direct ophthalmoscope, the examiner uses the instrument to examine all visible intraocular structures; however, its most common use is examination of the posterior portion of the globe. Green or black numbers represent convex or converging lenses, and red numbers represent concave or diverging lenses. Practically, when the vertical dial is set on 0, subtracting diopters (i.e. −1, −2, −3, etc.) moves the focal point away from the viewer. Conversely, when diopters are added (e.g., +1, +2, +3, etc.) the focal distance is brought closer to the viewer. Note, if the examiner wears corrective eyewear and removes his/her glasses when performing direct ophthalmoscopy, the refractive power of the examiner will need to be adjusted for (thus, the diopter power needed to achieve focus for various ocular structures may vary slightly from person to person).

Indirect ophthalmoscopy involves using a focused light (Finoff transilluminator or binocular headset) and a condensing lens (15-20-28 diopters) to view the fundus (Table 53.2). Advantages of indirect ophthalmoscopy include a wider field of view, safer working distance from the foal's head, stereopsis (i.e. depth perception), greater view of the peripheral fundus, an improved ability to view posterior segment structures through opacities in the anterior aspects of the viewing axis, and ability to alter the magnification by utilizing different diopter strength lenses.

Table 53.2 Key points regarding indirect ophthalmoscopy in foals.

- This technique is performed using a hand-held lens and bright focal light source; an indirect headset can also be used and provides stereopsis (binocular indirect ophthalmoscopy).
- Indirect ophthalmoscopy, depending in part on the dioptric power of the handheld lens used, renders an image
- Significantly less magnified than that seen with direct ophthalmoscopy, thus has a much larger field of view, and is overall a much better technique for routine screening of the eye.
- Indirect ophthalmoscopy provides the examiner with an inverted, reversed image.
- Indirect ophthalmoscopy is inexpensive and requires only of a bright focal light source and a 15 or 20/2.2 diopter lens. It is performed as follows:

  Step 1: Begin at arm's length from patient. An assistant is usually required to restrain the foal.

  Step 2: Darken the exam room or use a dark blanket to cover the head of both the foal and the examiner.

  Step 3: With a focal light source (transilluminator or penlight) held close to the lateral canthus of your dominant eye or at your cheek and standing at approximately arm's length from the patient, visualize the tapetal reflection (a red reflex will be seen in foals with poorly developed or no tapetum).

  Step 4: Hold a 20 or 15 diopter condensing lens in your other hand between the thumb and index finger and use your ring finger and pinky to elevate the upper lid. Initially, hold the lens to one side of the eye until the tapetal reflection is established, then rotate the lens such that the eye can be observed through it. Initially, hold your lens close to the corneal surface (~1/2 inch from eye) and slowly pull the lens toward you until the image of the fundus fills the lens (usually ~1–3 inches away from the foal's eye, depending on diopter power of condensing lens used). When the image is lost (usually because of movement), immediately rotate the lens away from the patient's eye (left ring finger and pinky continue to hold up the upper lid), reestablish the tapetal reflex, and again, rotate the lens back into place in front of the eye so the fundus comes into view.

  Step 5: Maintain alignment with your light source, lens, and patient's eye and move up, down, left, or right to examine all quadrants of the patient's fundus (remember that the image is inverted, so move in the opposite direction to the image). If the image is lost, move the lens out of the light beam and start again.

Disadvantages of indirect ophthalmoscopy include an inverted and reversed image and the expense of equipment. The author does not believe that indirect ophthalmoscopy requires a skill set that is any more difficult to master than correct usage of the direct ophthalmoscope. Using the indirect technique, the vitreous can also be examined for congenital remnants (retained hyaloid structures) and other opacities (degenerative materials, hemorrhage, or exudates).

Indirect ophthalmoscopy is relatively easy to master providing the skill set is practiced regularly. Various lenses are commercially available for indirect ophthalmology and provide varying magnification and field of view. The less the magnification, the greater the field of view. Because of the unique optical properties of the equine globe (i.e. the largest terrestrial animal eye), using a 20 D lens will actually "minify" the size of any pathology. For this reason, most ophthalmologist start by using a 20 or 2.2 diopter lens, but quickly move on to a 15 diopter lens to provide better magnification. A 5.5 MAC lens can be used for further magnification as well, although comfort with this size indirect lens takes some practice.

A final consideration when examining the posterior segment of foals involves a hybrid approach. Welch-Allyn produces a monocular indirect ophthalmoscope (PanOptic, Welch-Allyn, Skaneateles Falls, NY) that has five times greater magnification and a wider visual field than the direct ophthalmoscope. As with direct, the PanOptic view is an upright nonreversed fundus image. The author recommends a complete posterior segment exam in foals to be conducted first using indirect ophthalmoscopy to more easily detect posterior segment disease, followed by use of the PanOptic to better assess any specific lesions noted on indirect funduscopy (Figures 53.19 and 53.20). Regardless of the most effective method used for any one veterinarian, he/she should be sensitive to the patient's comfort level and avoid using illumination on its highest setting for protracted periods of time.

Additional Diagnostics

Once the MODB and a thorough eye exam has been completed, other routine diagnostics commonly performed include collection of conjunctival and/or corneal culture and cytology, flushing of the nasolacrimal system, and eyelid or conjunctival biopsy. Collection of these samples are warranted in various cases where ocular pathology is evident, including but not limited to, eyelid masses, conjunctival swellings, and ulcerative keratitis [38-42]. Procurement of samples does not vary widely from collection sites at other aspects of the body, although culture and cytology

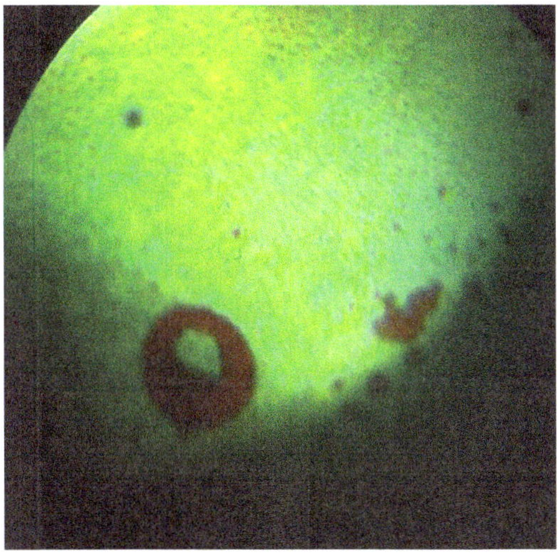

Figure 53.19 Dot-blot intra-retinal as well as larger preretinal hemorrhages are visible in the tapetal area of this foal's fundus. *Source:* Photo courtesy of Dr. Caryn Plummer, University of Florida.

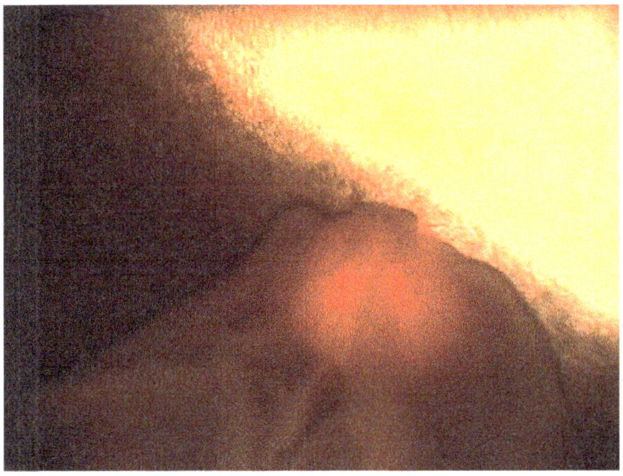

Figure 53.20 Complete retinal detachment. The neurosensory retina is only attached in the peri-papillary area with its remaining structure floating ventrally in the vitreous. *Source:* Photo courtesy of Dr. Caryn Plummer, University of Florida.

taken from a deep corneal ulcer should be done with great caution due to risk of globe rupture. Use of regional and local anesthesia via injectable (e.g. lidocaine, bupivacaine) and topical (e.g. proparacaine HCl 0.5%, oxibuprocaine cloridrate 0.4%, tetracaine) is strongly recommended prior to any biopsy of the eyelid/conjunctiva or corneal cytologic samples being taken. Once regional anesthesia is attained, biopsy of the eyelid can be performed using a combination of punch biopsy, Bishop harmon forceps, and Steven tenotomy scissors. Cytology samples can be acquired with cytology brushes or the back small end of a sterile #10 blade. Nasolacrimal flushing can be performed normograde or retrograde using a 5-French male silastic or plastic urinary catheter and flushed with a 10 ml syringe filled with sterile eyewash or saline.

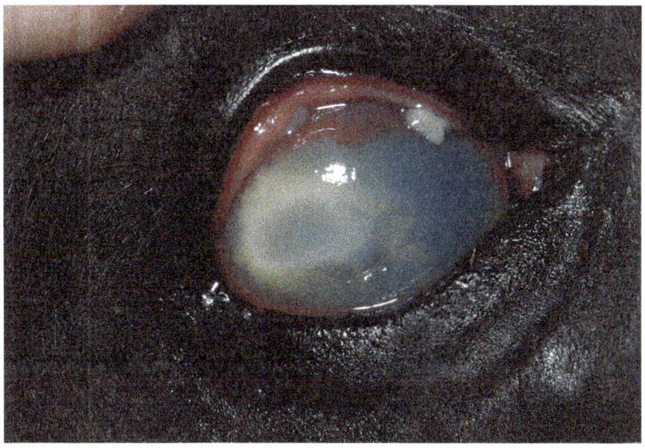

Figure 53.21 A 9-day-old Quarter Horse foal referred for an infected corneal ulcer. White cellular infiltrate is evident with ventral stromal loss, diffuse corneal edema, and perilimbal ciliary flush. The owners elected medical management only.

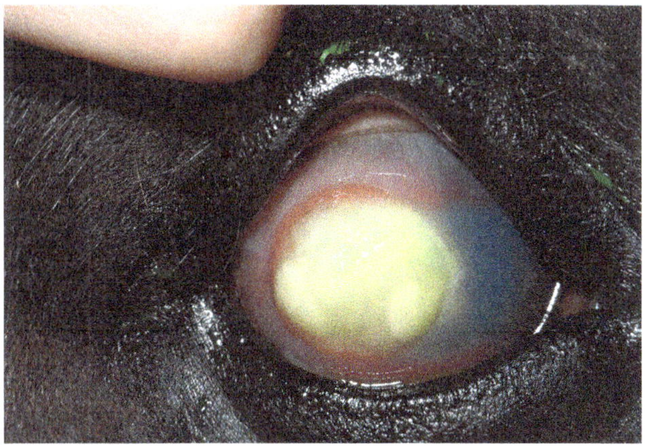

Figure 53.22 Same foal as shown in Figure 53.21, 10 days after initial presentation. The infectious keratitis has progressed to include a robust stromal abscess. Despite further ingrowth of corneal vessels into the area of abscessation, additional stromal loss was evident. Due to loss of vision and patient discomfort, the owners elected enucleation.

Referral to a specialist is recommended to aid in the diagnosis and treatment of complicated ophthalmic disease in foals. In many cases, neonatal foals are referred to multispecialty hospitals due to the patient's systemic illness and ophthalmologists are consulted to address systemic manifestations of ophthalmic disease. Alternatively, in systemically healthy foals, referral may be warranted in challenging primary ophthalmic cases that are worsening and/or vision is threatened (Figures 53.21 and 53.22). Advanced imaging such as contrast dacryocystorhinography (DCR) may help determine the exact location of obstruction in the nasolacrimal outflow tract. Other advanced imaging modalities include CT or MRI. A relatively common reason foals are referred to veterinary ophthalmologists is for the evaluation of cataracts (Figure 53.23) [43, 44]. In late immature or mature cataracts, where the posterior segment cannot be

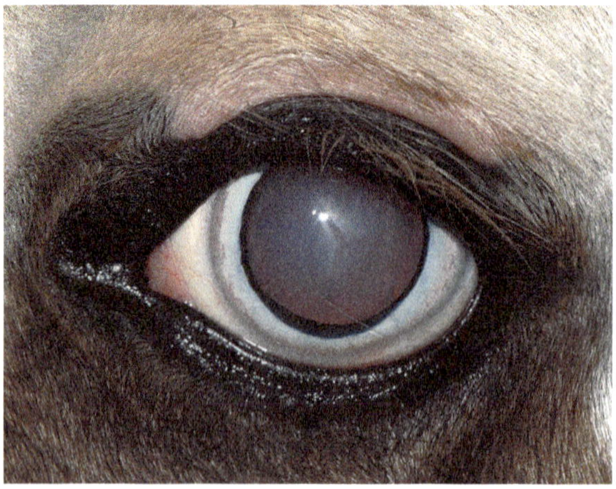

Figure 53.23 Late immature cataract in an American Paint foal.

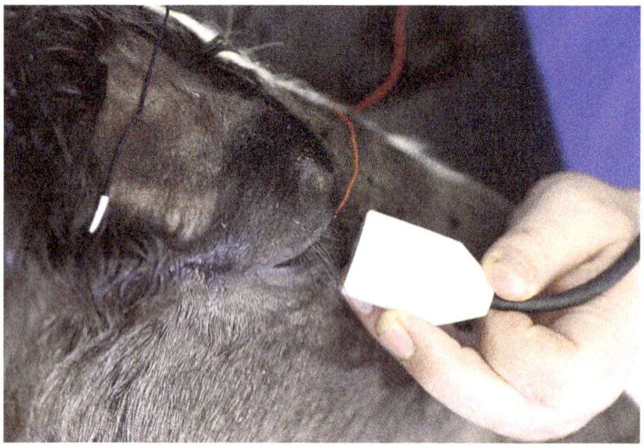

Figure 53.24 An electroretinogram is being performed in this 6-week-old Thoroughbred foal. *Source:* Photo courtesy of Dr. Tim Knott, Rowe Referrals, UK.

adequately visualized, ocular ultrasonography and ERG are performed to determine patient candidacy for surgery (Figure 53.24) [21]. In recent years, with the widespread use of smartphones, digital photography often plays a pivotal role in communication between the client, primary veterinarian, and ophthalmologist.

Therapeutics

A list of systemic and topical agents commonly used in equine ophthalmology is noted in Table 53.3. For additional details, refer to specific medical and surgical ocular conditions affecting foals in the other sections of this text. Uveitis in foals merits additional consideration beyond what is listed in Table 53.1, as uveitis is usually a result of sepsis in neonatal foals [17, 45-48]. Treatment of neonatal foals with sepsis is challenging and warrants use of appropriate antimicrobial drugs with careful deployment of anti-inflammatory drugs at this age in light of their propensity to interfere with maturation in addition to traditional toxic side effects (personal communication, Philip J. Johnson BVSc [Hons]). The physiology of neonates differs from that of adult horses; thus, drug doses tend to be different. At the author's institution (University of Missouri Veterinary Health Center), flunixin meglumine is dosed up to 1.1 mg/kg, PO/IV, q 12h in adult horses, but the high end of the dose in neonates is 1.5 mg/kg (Table 53.3). Depending on the underlying ocular condition and frequency of topical medications needs, subpalpebral lavage tubes greatly facilitate treatment [49].

Monitoring

As with treatment regimens, monitoring frequency is dependent on the ocular condition that is being treated. At times, frequent monitoring is not possible due to either accessibility to the foal (hospitalized or on a farm) and owner finances. Neonatal foals presenting to a specialist facility will benefit from a team approach to case management. For example, a systemically ill foal with jaundice secondary to systemic disease and concurrent entropion (with or without corneal ulceration) is primarily managed by equine internists while ophthalmologist place temporary tacking sutures to correct the entropion and perform regular ocular examinations (Figure 53.25). By contrast, an otherwise healthy foal that presents for cataract surgery is managed by the ophthalmology service with twice daily examinations of the eyes in the early postoperative period and daily examinations of the mare and foal by equine internists to ensure that both remain healthy while hospitalized (Figures 53.26 and 53.27). Foals that have undergone cataract surgery require regular follow-up ophthalmic examinations, especially for the first 3–6 months (Figure 53.28). Finally, the clinician may be presented with a foal that appears to have a severe ocular abnormality perceived as emergent but, when carefully examined, little to no treatment is required due to the end-stage nature of the disease process (e.g. phthisis bulbi; Figures 53.29 and 53.30).

Table 53.3 Common medications used in the ophthalmic examination or treatment of the horse.

Medication	Dosage	Comments
Anesthetics		
• Lidocaine	2% s/c	Local anesthesia and akinesia
• Mepivicaine	2% s/c	Local anesthesia and akinesia
• Proparacaine	0.5% topically	Topical anesthesia; may induce minor superficial corneal irregularities; may decrease tear production
• Tetracaine	0.5% topically	Topical anesthesia; may induce minor superficial corneal irregularities; may decrease tear production
Antibiotics		
• Bacitracin-neomycin-polymyxin B	o/o topically q2-8h	Broad-spectrum bactericidal
• Chloramphenicol	1% o/o topically q2-8h	Gram-positive spectrum
• Ciprofloxacin	0.3% o/s topically q2-8h	Broad-spectrum bactericidal fluoroquinolone; reserve for treatment of severe infections by sensitive organisms
• Gatifloxacin	0.3% topically q2-8h	Fourth generation fluoroquinolone
• Gentamicin	0.3% o/s topically q2-8h	Bactericidal aminoglycoside; Gram-negative spectrum, some Gram-positive aerobes,
• Moxifloxacin	0.5% topically q2-8h	Fourth-generation fluoroquinolone
• Ofloxacin	0.3% o/s topically q2-8h	Broad-spectrum antibiotic with better Gram-positive spectrum and less topical irritation than ciprofloxacin
• Tobramycin	0.3% o/s topically q2-8h	Gram-negative spectrum; restrict use to severe corneal infections, particularly *Pseudomonas aeruginosa*
Anticollagenolytics		
• Acetylcysteine	10% o/s topically q1-4h	
• EDTA	0.05% o/s topically	
• Serum	Topically q2-6h	Contains α-macroglobulins; inhibits matrix metallo-proteases, serine proteases; collect new autogenous sample every 7 days
Antifungals		
• Amphotericin B	1.5% o/s topically	Broad-spectrum polyene; poor intraocular penetration when given parenterally; poor corneal penetration topically
• Fluconazole	0.2% o/o topically q4-8h; 1 mg/kg PO, q12h	Imidazole
• Itraconazole	1% o/o topically q4-8h; 3 mg/kg PO, q12h	Imidazole; high corneal concentration; compounded in ointment with 30% dimethylsulfoxide
• Miconazole	1% o/s topically q4-8h	Imidazole; excellent corneal penetration; also active against Gram-positive cocci
• Natamycin	5% o/s topically q4-8h	Only commercially available antifungal
• Povidone-iodine	2% solution topically	Antibacterial, antiviral, antiprotozoal
• Voriconazole	1% o/s q4-8h	Triazole; effective against Aspergillus

(Continued)

Table 53.3 (Continued)

Medication	Dosage	Comments
Anti-inflammatories		
• Dexamethasone	0.05-0.1 mg/kg IV, q24h0.1% o/o or o/s topically	Corticosteroid
• Diclofenac	0.1% o/s topically	Non-steroidal anti-inflammatory
• Dimethylsulfoxide	30% o/o topically	Topical ointment compounded with itraconazole
• Flurbiprofen	0.03% o/s topically	Non-steroidal anti-inflammatory
• Prednisolone acetate	1% o/s topically	Corticosteroid
• Flunixine meglumine	1 mg/kg, IV or PO q12-24h	Non-steroidal anti-inflammatory; can cause GI ulceration
• Phenylbutazone	2.2-4.4 mg/kg, PO/IV,	Non-steroidal anti-inflammatory; can cause GI ulceration q12-48h
• Dipyrone	10-20 mg/kg, q12–24h, IV	Non-steroidal anti-inflammatory
• Firocoxib	0.1 mg/kg, PO, q 24h	Non-steroidal anti-inflammatory
• Ketoprofen	2 mg/kg, q12–24h, IV	Non-steroidal anti-inflammatory
• Methylprednisolone	1-3 mg/kg, q12–24h, IV	Steroid
• Prednisolone sodium succinate	1.0-2.5 mg/kg, q6-24h, IV	Steroid
• Pentoxifylline	7.5-10 mg/kg, PO/IV, q8-12h	Anti-tumor necrosis factor-α
Mydriatic/Cycloplegics		
• Atropine	1% o/o or o/s topically	Parasympatholytic mydriatic, cycloplegic; use q8-12h until pupil dilates, then according to clinical needs
• Tropicamide	1% o/s topically	Shorter duration than atropine

s/c, subcutaneous; o/o, ophthalmic oinment; o/s, ophthalmic solution; IV, intravenous; PO, per os

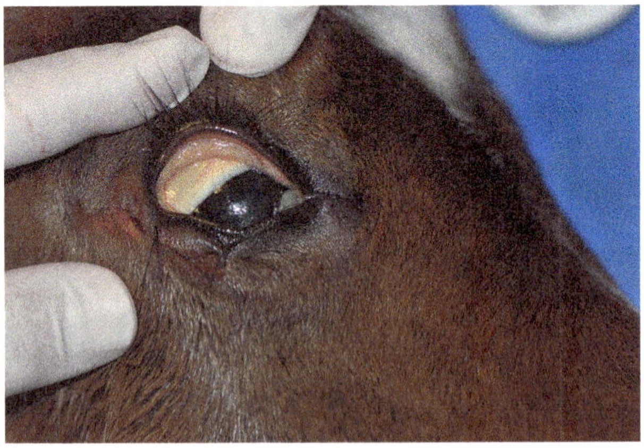

Figure 53.25 A 1-week-old systemically ill Quarter Horse foal with jaundice as seen in the sclera and two temporary eyelid tacking sutures in the lower eyelid due to entropion. *Source:* Photo courtesy Dr. Allison Fuchs, MU-Ophthalmology resident 2019–2022.

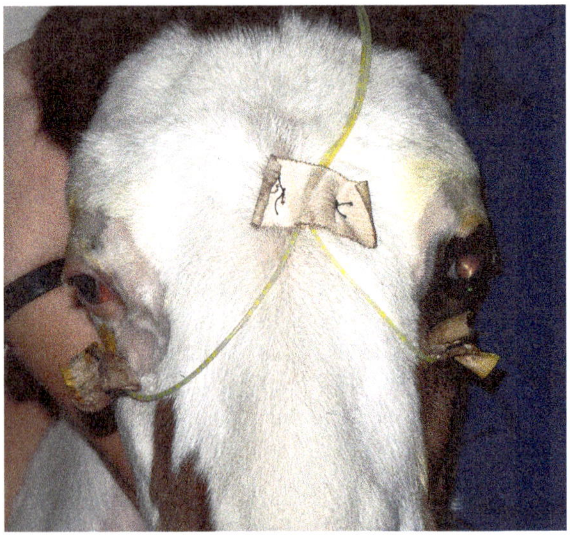

Figure 53.26 A 2-month-old American Paint foal 10 days post cataract surgery OU with bilateral inferonasal subpalpebral lavage tubes.

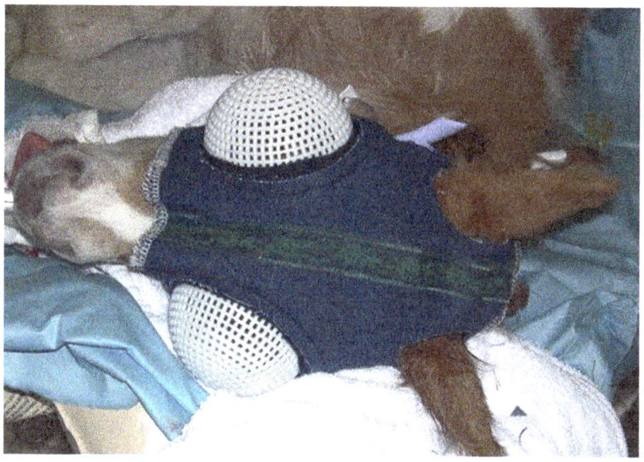

Figure 53.27 A 3-month-old Miniature Horse foal immediately after bilateral cataract surgery. Note that due to the small size of this foal, a protective "eye cup" was hand-made to adequately fit the foal's head and protect the eyes while healing.

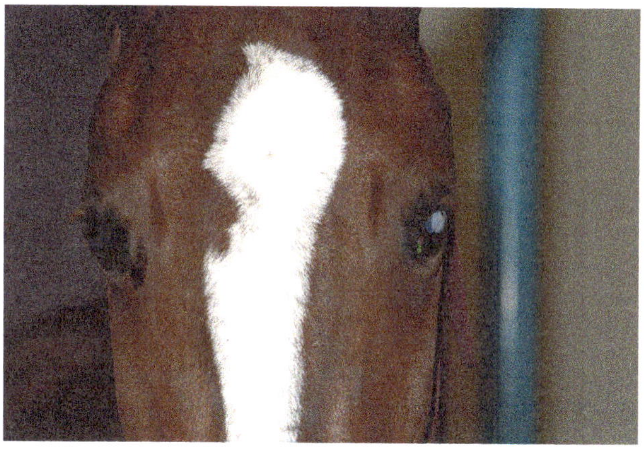

Figure 53.29 A 4-week-old Quarter Horse foal with phthisis bulbi OS secondary to severe trauma in the first week of life.

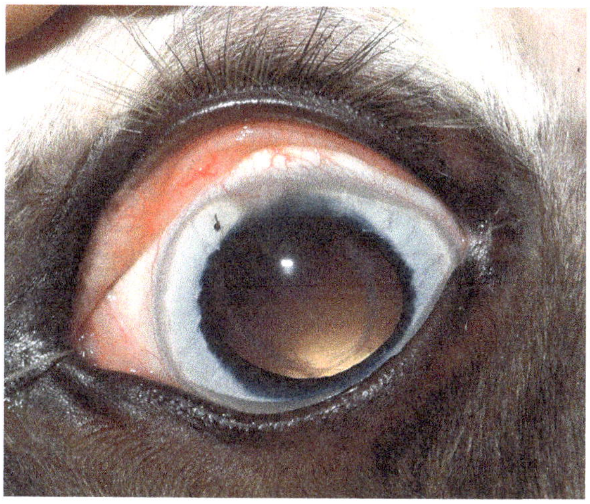

Figure 53.28 Same foal as shown in Figure 53.26, now 8 weeks after cataract surgery. The left eye's corneal incision is healed, the pupil is pharmacologically dilated, the anterior continuous curvilinear capsulorhexis is visible, there are no obvious signs of intraocular inflammation, and there is a clear visual axis. An intraocular lens was not placed in this eye.

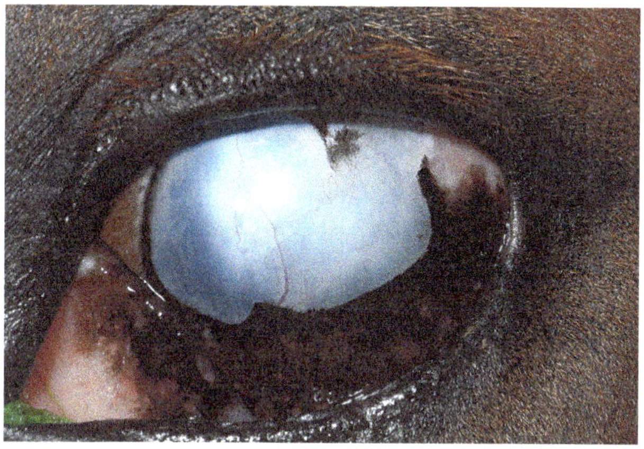

Figure 53.30 Same foal as Figure 53.29 in which the nonvisual left eye can be seen to have severe fibrosis, corneal neovascularization, ventral sympblepharon, and be too small in size resulting in elevation of the third eyelid.

References

1 Stoppini, R. and Gilger, B.C. (2017). Equine ocular examination basic techniques. In: *Equine Ophthalmology*, 3e (ed. B.C. Gilger), 1–39. Ames, Iowa: John Wiley & Sons, Inc.

2 Labelle, A.L., Hamor, R.E., Townsend, W.M. et al. (2011). Ophthalmic lesions in neonatal foals evaluated for nonophthalmic disease at referral hospitals. *J Am Vet Med Assoc* 239: 486–492.

3 Lassaline, M. and Latimer, C. (2018). Ophthalmic disorders. In: *Equine Pediatric Medicine*, 2e (ed. W.V. Bernard and B.S. Barr), 249–267. Boca Raton: CRC Press.

4 Sandmeyer, L.S. and Bellone, R. (2017). Inherited ocular disorders. In: *Equine Ophthalmology*, 3e (ed. B.C. Gilger), 545–566. Ames, Iowa: John Wiley & Sons, Inc.

5 Leiva, M. and Peña, T. (2017). Ophthalmic diseases of foals. In: *Equine Ophthalmology*, 3e (ed. B.C. Gilger), 112–150. Ames, Iowa: John Wiley & Sons, Inc.

6 Greenberg, S.M., Plummer, C.E., Sledge, D. et al. (2016). Bilateral microphthalmos with cyst in a neonatal foal. *Vet Ophthalmol* 19: 332–339.

7 Casteleyn, C., Cornillie, P., Tüllmann, V. et al. (2016). *Campylorrhinus lateralis*, Bilateral microphthalmia and odontoma temporalis in an Oldenburg Foal. *Reprod Domest Anim* 51: 330–334.

8 Depecker, M., Ségard, E., and Cadoré, J.L. (2013). Phenotypic description of multiple congenital ocular anomalies in Comtois horses. *Equine Vet Educ* 25: 511–516.

9 Barsotti, G., Sgorbini, M., Marmorini, P. et al. (2013). Ocular abnormalities in healthy Standardbred foals. *Vet Ophthalmol* 16: 245–250.

10 Leiva, M., Peña, T., and Monreal, L. (2011). Ocular findings in healthy newborn foals according to age. *Equine Vet Educ* 23: 40–45.

11 Baumgartner, W.A., Storey, E.S., and Paulsen, D.B. (2009). Bilateral intraocular glandular choristomas in a Thoroughbred foal. *Vet Ophthalmol* 12: 106–114.

12 Slovis, N.M. (2008). The eye and related structures. In: *Color Atlas of Diseases and Disorders of the Foal* (ed. S.B. McAuliffe and N.M. Slovis), 326–346. New York: Saunders/Elsevier.

13 Munroe, G. (2000). Survey of retinal haemorrhages in neonatal thoroughbred foals. *Vet Rec* 146: 95–101.

14 Munroe, G. (2000). Study of the hyaloid apparatus in the neonatal thoroughbred foal. *Vet Rec* 146: 579–584.

15 Cutler, T.J., Brooks, D.E., Andrew, S.E. et al. (2000). Disease of the equine posterior segment. *Vet Ophthalmol* 3: 73–82.

16 Munroe, G. (1999). Subconjunctival haemorrhages in neonatal thoroughbred foals. *Vet Rec* 144: 279–282.

17 Hendrix, D.V.H., Ward, D.A., and Guglick, M.A. (1997). Disseminated candidiasis in a neonatal foal with keratomycosis as the initial sign. *Veterinary & Comparative Ophthalmology* 7: 10–13.

18 Cooley, S.D., Scrivani, P.V., Thompson, M.S. et al. (2016). Correlations among ultrasonographic measurements of optic nerve sheath diameter, age, and body weight in clinically normal horses. *Vet Radiol Ultrasound* 57: 49–57.

19 Townsend, W.M., Wasserman, N., and Jacobi, S. (2013). A pilot study on the corneal curvatures and ocular dimensions of horses less than one year of age. *Equine Vet J* 45: 256–258.

20 Parikh, P.V., Jhala, S.K., and Mehraj u din D. (2011). Surgical management of soft cataract in a foal. *Intas Polivet* 12: 108–110.

21 Scotty, N.C., Cutler, T.J., Brooks, D.E. et al. (2004). Diagnostic ultrasonography of equine lens and posterior segment abnormalities. *Vet Ophthalmol* 7: 127–139.

22 Latimer, C.A. and Wyman, M. (1985). Neonatal ophthalmology. *Vet Clin North Am Equine Pract* 1: 235–259.

23 Enzerink, E. (1998). The menace response and pupillary light reflex in neonatal foals. *Equine Vet J* 30: 546–548.

24 Beech, J., Zappala, R.A., Smith, G. et al. (2003). Schirmer tear test results in normal horses and ponies: effect of age, season, environment, sex, time of day and placement of strips. *Vet Ophthalmol* 6: 251–254.

25 Brooks, D.E., Clark, C.K., and Lester, G.D. (2000). Cochet-Bonnet aesthesiometer-determined corneal sensitivity in neonatal foals and adult horses. *Vet Ophthalmol* 3: 133–137.

26 Visser, H.E., Diehl, K.A., Whitley, R.D. et al. (2017). Effect of auriculopalpebral nerve block on Schirmer tear test I values in normal horses. *Vet Ophthalmol* 20: 568–570.

27 Theoret, C.L., Grahn, B.H., and Fretz, P.B. (1997). Incomplete nasomaxillary dysplasia in a foal. *Can Vet J* 38: 445–447.

28 Turner, A.G. (2004). Ocular conditions of neonatal foals. *Vet Clin North Am Equine Pract* 20: 429–440, vii–viii.

29 Valentini, S., Castagnetti, C., Musella, V. et al. (2014). Assessment of intraocular measurements in neonatal foals and association with gender, laterality, and body weight: a clinical study. *PLoS One* 9: e109491.

30 Allbaugh, R.A., Keil, S.M., Ou, Z. et al. (2014). Intraocular pressure changes in equine athletes during endurance competitions. *Vet Ophthalmol* 17 (Suppl 1): 154–159.

31 Barnett, K.C., Cottrell, B.D., Paterson, B.W. et al. (1988). Buphthalmos in a Thoroughbred foal. *Equine Vet J* 20: 132–135.

32 Gelatt, K.N. (1973). Glaucoma and lens luxation in a foal. *Vet Med Small Anim Clin* 68: 261.

33 Komaromy, A.M., Garg, C.D., Ying, G.S. et al. (2006). Effect of head position on intraocular pressure in horses. *Am J Vet Res* 67: 1232–1235.

34 Monk, C.S., Brooks, D.E., Granone, T. et al. (2017). Measurement of intraocular pressure in healthy anesthetized horses during hoisting. *Vet Anaesth Analg* 44: 502–508.

35 Mughannam, A.J., Buyukmihci, N.C., and Kass, P.H. (1999). Effect of topical atropine on intraocular pressure and pupil diameter in the normal horse eye. *Vet Ophthalmol* 2: 213–215.

36 Stine, J.M., Michau, T.M., Williams, M.K. et al. (2014). The effects of intravenous romifidine on intraocular pressure in clinically normal horses and horses with incidental ophthalmic findings. *Vet Ophthalmol* 17 (Suppl 1): 134–139.

37 Wilkie, D.A. and Gilger, B.C. (2004). Equine glaucoma. *Vet Clin North Am Equine Pract* 20: 381–391. vii.

38 Kammergruber, E., Rahn, C., Nell, B. et al. (2019). Morphological and immunohistochemical characteristics of the equine corneal epithelium. *Vet Ophthalmol* 22: 778–790.

39 Bae, Y., Lee, E., Song, M. et al. (2019). Treatment of melting ulcer in a foal. *Journal of Veterinary Clinics* 36: 88–92.

40 Pigatto, J.A.T., Albuquerque, L., Bacchin, Â.B.O. et al. (2017). Diamond burr for the treatment of an indolent corneal ulcer in a foal. *Acta Scientiae Veterinariae* 45: 198.

41 Sgorbini, M., Barsotti, G., Nardoni, S. et al. (2008). Fungal Flora of Normal Eyes in Healthy Newborn Foals Living in the Same Stud Farm in Italy. *J Equine Vet Sci* 28: 540–543.

42 McMullen, R.J., Clode, A.B., Pandiri, A.K. et al. (2008). Epibulbar melanoma in a foal. *Vet Ophthalmol* 11 (Suppl 1): 44–50.

43 Brooks, D.E., Plummer, C.E., Carastro, S.M. et al. (2014). Visual outcomes of phacoemulsification cataract surgery in horses: 1990-2013. *Vet Ophthalmol* 17 (Suppl 1): 117–128.

44 Harrington, J.T., McMullen, R.J. Jr., Clode, A.B. et al. (2013). Phacoemulsification and +14 diopter intraocular lens placement in a Saddlebred foal. *Vet Ophthalmol* 16: 140–148.

45 Tarancón, I., Leiva, M., Jose-Cunilleras, E. et al. (2019). Ophthalmologic findings associated with *Rhodococcus equi* bronchopneumonia in foals. *Vet Ophthalmol* 22: 660–665.

46 Zak, A., Siwinska, N., Slowikowska, M. et al. (2018). Conjunctival aerobic bacterial flora in healthy Silesian foals and adult horses in Poland. *BMC Vet Res* 14: 1–6.

47 Borel, N., Grest, P., Junge, H. et al. (2014). Vascular hamartoma in the central nervous system of a foal. *J Vet Diagn Invest* 26: 805–809.

48 Leiva, M., Peña, T., Armengou, L. et al. (2010). Uveal inflammation in septic newborn foals. *J Vet Intern Med* 24: 391–397.

49 Giuliano, E.A., Maggs, D.J., Moore, C.P. et al. (2000). Inferomedial placement of a single-entry subpalpebral lavage tube for treatment of equine eye disease. *Vet Ophthalmol* 3: 153–156.

Chapter 54 Congenital Ocular Abnormalities in the Foal

Roxanne M. Rodriguez Galarza

In general, the incidence of congenital ophthalmic abnormalities is low in the foal, but when they occur, these abnormalities can be due to congenital or inherited disorders as well as acquired conditions secondary to systemic infection, inflammation, or toxicity [1, 2]. Following ophthalmic examination of the foal, if ocular abnormalities are observed, the mare and stallion should be further examined, as these conditions may be inherited.

Orbit and Globe

Microphthalmos and Anophthalmos

Microphthalmos is a congenital disorder that results in an abnormally small globe along with additional ophthalmic malformations. Microphthalmia has been reported in 7–14.7% of horses [1, 3]. Anophthalmia is a congenital disorder that leads to a complete absence of the globe. Anophthalmia is usually associated with other nonocular malformations that are not compatible with life [4]. In practice, most cases of suspected anophthalmia are incorrectly diagnosed, as the presence of ocular tissues in the orbit are typically noted upon histopathology.

Strabismus

Strabismus refers to abnormal deviation of the globe. A slight ventromedial strabismus has been described in foals of <1 month of age [5, 6]. Following 1 month of age, the strabismus resolves. Strabismus has also been reported in Appaloosa foals [7]; convergent, asymmetrical strabismus has been reported in mules [8].

Adnexa

Unlike most small animals, foal's eyelids are open at birth. Ankyloblepharon, or adhesion of the eyelids, has been reported in a Shetland-cross foal [9]. Eyelid agenesis, or eyelid coloboma, refers to a congenital defect of the eyelid in which the eyelid is not formed. Ankyloblepharon and eyelid agenesis are infrequently reported in the horse [5, 10–12]. Although still rare, dermoids of the third eyelid are the most common reported congenital disorder of the third eyelid [13, 14]. See cornea section for further information on dermoids.

Entropion

Entropion describes an inward rolling of the eyelid and results in secondary trichiasis of the haired skin contacting the ocular surface. Entropion is more commonly diagnosed in dehydrated or premature and dysmature foals with the lower eyelids more commonly affected [15]. Although less common, inherited congenital entropion has also been suspected and investigated in Thoroughbreds and Quarter Horses [11, 12]. Affected foals can experience blepharospasm, epiphora, conjunctivitis, keratitis, and corneal ulcers.

If the degree of entropion is mild (i.e. minimal to mild epiphora), topical lubrication may be sufficient to create a barrier between the hair (from the rolled-in eyelid) and ocular surface. If moderate to severe clinical signs are noted, permanent surgical correction to roll the eyelid outward is recommended. However, permanent surgical correction (e.g. Hotz-Celsus procedure) is discouraged until the foal is fully developed [16]. Early permanent surgical correction can result in overcorrection and ectropion (outward rolling of the eyelid), which can be more challenging to surgically correct. In these cases, a temporary eversion of the eyelids is recommended. The authors' preferred method includes the use of vertical mattress suture pattern placed with nonabsorbable suture (e.g. 4-0 nylon suture). Other techniques described include the use of subcutaneous injection of procaine penicillin G, liquid paraffin, silicone, or hyaluronic acid [11, 17, 18]. However, injection of these substances may lead to local eyelid inflammation. In addition to suture, temporary vascular staples/clips can also be used [15].

Equine Neonatal Medicine, First Edition. Edited by David M. Wong and Pamela A. Wilkins.

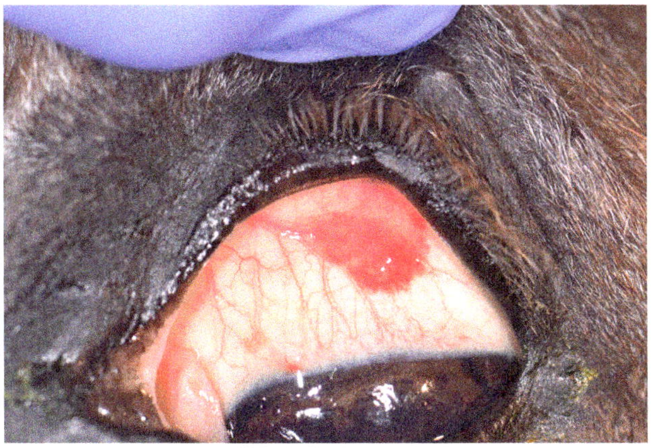

Figure 54.1 Representation of a large conjunctival hemorrhage in an adult Pony of the Americas. Also, note dorsonasally focal smaller conjunctival hemorrhage adjacent to the limbus.

Conjunctiva

Although not truly congenital, conjunctival hemorrhage has been reported in the neonatal foal, but is likely acquired during parturition [4]. Conjunctival hemorrhage has been reported in 8.3–36% of healthy neonatal foals [19–21]. Conjunctival hemorrhages typically resolve within 4–10 days of birth, depending on the severity (Figure 54.1) [10, 20]. Although reported in healthy foals, it is important to note that other potential underlying etiologies may cause conjunctival hemorrhage, such as neonatal encephalopathy, trauma, vasculitis, coagulopathy, and other underlying systemic conditions. These should be considered more likely, depending on the overall physical examination of the foal.

Nasolacrimal System

Nasolacrimal Duct Atresia

Nasolacrimal duct atresia is one of the most common congenital disorder in the horse and can occur as a unilateral or bilateral disorder [3, 22–24]. Although congenital, affected foals rarely show clinical signs at birth but, rather, present with epiphora at a young age that progresses to severe mucopurulent discharge, due to secondary dacryocystitis by 6 months of age [25].

Abnormalities anywhere along the nasolacrimal duct can occur, but imperforate nasal punctum is the most common presentation [25]. Diagnosis can be made by a lack of visualization of the nasal punctum or inability to flush the nasolacrimal duct normograde (from lacrimal puncta to nasal punctum). When normograde flushing is attempted, the nasal mucosa overlying the duct atresia can become distended. If the atresia has occurred at the level of the upper and lower eyelid punctum, when retrograde flushing (from nasal punctum to lacrimal puncta by the eye) is attempted, the conjunctival mucosa overlying becomes distended. In addition to examination and attempted flushing, advance imaging, such as dacryocystorhinography, can also be useful in determining the location of the atresia and surgical approach [26].

If the only abnormality of the nasolacrimal duct is present at the level of the nasal punctum, several surgical options exist. The goal of treatment is to create an opening that results in a stoma that restores passage. Following placement of a normograde urinary catheter, an incision with a number 11 scalpel blade over the distended nasal mucosa (or over an area where the catheter is palpated) can be made [5]. A urinary catheter should be left within the lumen and newly created opening for a few weeks to create a stoma. In order to secure the catheter within the lumen, the catheter can be sutured in place as it exits near the eyelid and nares. Systemic nonsteroidal anti-inflammatory drugs and topical antibiotics are recommended postoperatively. More recently, 980 nm diode laser has been described to ablate the nasal mucosa overlying the distal end of the nasolacrimal duct [27]. This technique was associated with decreased surgical time and hemorrhage.

Corneal Diseases

Congenital corneal diseases, such as microcornea, megalocornea, cornea globosa, dermoids, and leukoma are uncommon in the horse. Megalocornea and microcornea refer to an eye with a large or small corneal diameter, respectively. Sometimes confused as megalocornea, cornea globosa refers to a cornea with an increased corneal curvature and, thus a deepened anterior chamber. Cornea globosa is most commonly seen in horses with multiple congenital ocular anomalies (MCOA). See uvea section for further information on MCOA.

Dermoids

Periocular and ocular dermoids are classified as choriostomas and hamartomas. Choriostomas refer to congenital overgrowth of normal epithelial and dermis-like tissue that is found in an abnormal location, such as the cornea, limbus, and conjunctiva. Hamartomas refer to congenital overgrowth of disorganized tissue that is normal for the location it is found, such as an eyelid dermoid. Corneal dermoids have been documented as a single finding as well as in combination with other ophthalmic malformations in Standardbreds and related Quarter Horses [28, 29]. Clinically, they can appear as a raised pink island of tissue that has varying pigmentation and may be haired or nonhaired. Affected foals can have chronic epiphora or ocular discharge due to constant irritation of the associated hairs. Depending on the size of the dermoid, they can also obstruct vision. In those that are large or lead to irritation, surgical excision of the dermoid is recommended. Most corneal dermoids are superficial; thus, superficial keratectomy, sclerokeratectomy, and conjunctivectomy are all curative.

Linear Keratopathy

Linear keratopathy, due to congenital thinning of Descemet's membrane (basement membrane on innermost aspect of the cornea), is seen as mostly horizontal thin (1–2 mm) linear posterior refractive opacities or bands [30]. Clinically, the bands from linear keratopathy appear very similar to Haab's striae. However, the bands from Haab's striae occur due to breaks (not thinning) in Descemet's membrane from blunt trauma or glaucoma. As such, foals with horizontal linear corneal opacities should be further examined for findings that may be suggestive of glaucoma or blunt trauma (such as corneal edema, increased intraocular pressures, mydriasis from glaucoma, periocular swelling, corneal edema, hyphema, miosis, and lens instability).

Uvea

Aniridia and Iris Hypoplasia

Congenital abnormalities of the uvea are infrequently reported in horses. Aniridia describes complete lack of the iris that allows visualization of the lens equator and ciliary processes. This condition has been reported in the Belgian Draft Horse, Quarter Horse, Thoroughbred, Thoroughbred/Welsh cross, and Tennessee Walking Horse [31–34]. Iris hypoplasia, or incomplete development of the iris, is commonly reported in horses with blue or heterochromia irides [35]. Clinically, iris hypoplasia manifests as a dark, anterior bulging of the iris stroma, with the dorsal iris being most commonly affected (Figure 54.2). Iris hypoplasia is also in MCOA affected horses (see MCOA section for further details).

Persistent pupillary membranes (PPMs) are remnants from incomplete regression of the fetal pupillary membrane and are commonly noted incidentally in adult horses. The fetal pupillary membrane provides nutrition to the anterior segment and lens in utero and regresses toward the end of gestation. PPMs can be classified depending on what structure the strand is adherent to: iris to iris (can span the iris), iris to lens (can cause lens opacities), and iris to cornea (can cause corneal opacities). The PPM can also become detached leading to a small tag off of the iris collarette or a strand free floating in the anterior chamber. In one study, 100% of examined miniature horses had PPMs, most frequently extending from iris to iris [36].

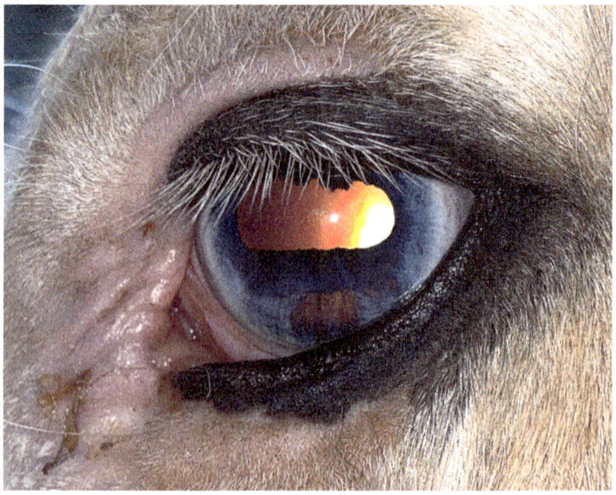

Figure 54.2 Ventral iris hypoplasia in a blue-eyed Paint horse gelding. It is important to note that, dorsal iris hypoplasia is more prevalent.

Iris Coloboma

Iris colobomas have also been reported in foals. Clinically, iris coloboma manifests as a focal notch or defect of the iris. Iris colobomas can be classified as typical and atypical depending on their location. Typical colobomas are described as defects located at the 6 o'clock position. Any other locations are defined as atypical coloboma. In horses, atypical colobomas are more common than typical colobomas [4].

Uveal Cysts

Uveal cysts may arise from the posterior pigmented epithelium of the iris or from ciliary body epithelium. Clinically, they can be apparent as adhered or free-floating thin-walled cysts on the corpora nigra (Figure 54.3a) in the anterior chamber, posterior to the iris and peripheral retina. If enlarged, especially those associated with the corpora nigra, they can lead to visual disturbances due to pupillary obstruction. This is most commonly reported when the horse is being worked in a well-lit environment that would lead to pupillary constriction. Uveal cysts can be deflated with needle aspiration or transcorneal laser or endolaser photocoagulation (Figure 54.3b) [37].

MCOA is a heritable syndrome that can affect horses with silver coating and has been described in the Rocky Mountain Horse, Icelandic Horse, Shetland Pony, Exmoor Pony, American Miniature Horse, Kentucky Mountain Saddle Horse, Mountain Pleasure Horse, Belgian Draft Horse, Morgan, and Comtois Horse [36, 38–44]. The pattern of inheritance is incomplete dominance, leading to homozygotes being more affected than heterozygotes. Ocular findings in affected horses can include cornea globosa (anterior bulging of cornea), iris hypoplasia (miosis

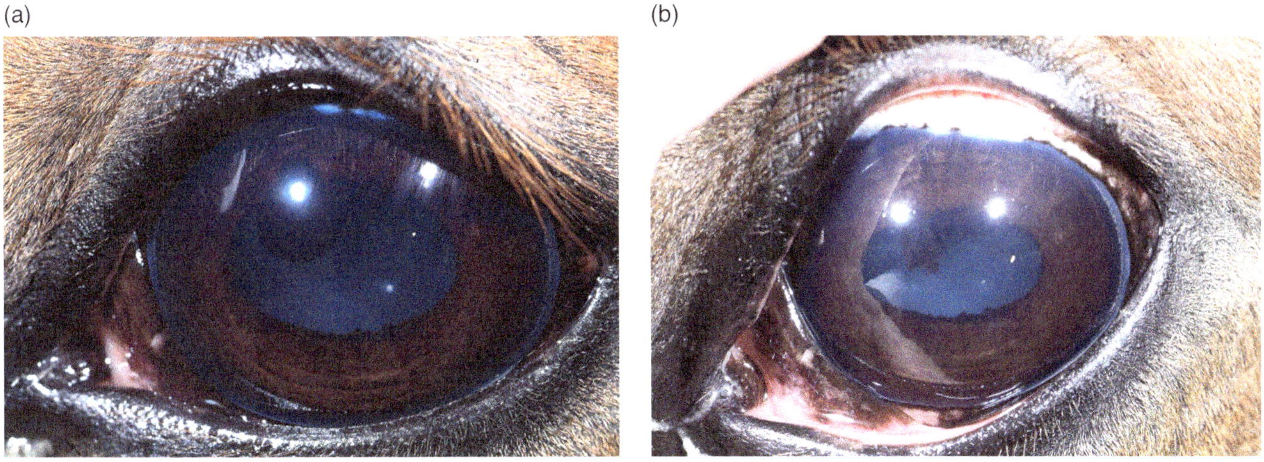

Figure 54.3 (a) Corpora nigra cyst noted along the dorsal pupillary margin. (b) Same eye following treatment with transcorneal diode laser. Note immediate deflation of cyst. *Source:* Photograph courtesy of Dr. Ian Herring.

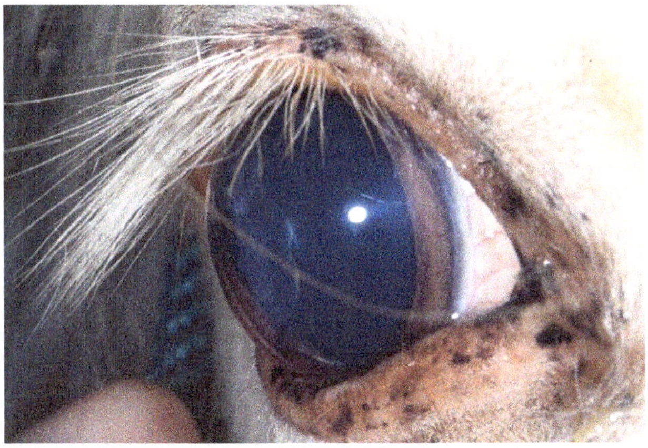

Figure 54.4 Visualization of temporal ciliary body cyst in a heterozygote affected horse. The pupil has been pharmacologically dilated. *Source:* Photograph courtesy of Dr. Ian Herring.

with incomplete response to pharmacologic dilation), uveal cysts (commonly found arising from temporal ciliary body and iris), abnormal pectinate ligaments, cataract, and retinal dysplasia [40, 45]. Heterozygote horses are typically only affected by the presence of cysts while homozygotes have the additional above-mentioned anomalies (Figure 54.4). On occasions, uveal cysts arising from the temporal ciliary body can sometimes extend into peripheral retina. This syndrome is not progressive; however, cataracts may progress leading to changes in their vision.

Lens

Cataracts

Cataracts, an opacification of the lens, can be inherited, infectious/inflammatory, traumatic, nutritional, or secondary to radiation. Congenital cataracts have been reported between 33.6% and 35.3% of congenital defects in foals, accounting for the most common congenital abnormality in one study [1, 3, 5]. Inherited cataracts have been reported in the Thoroughbred, Quarter Horse, Belgian Draft, and Morgan breeds [7, 32, 34, 40, 46, 47]. Although cataracts have been identified as a single ophthalmic finding, they have also been associated with other abnormalities, such as hyaloid remnants, PPMs, and aniridia [28, 34]. Cataracts have also been reported in horses with MCOA.

To determine an underlying etiology of a foal's cataract, a thorough physical examination, medical history, and examination of mare and stallion should be performed. However, an underlying etiology of cataracts in foals is frequently undetermined. Cataracts are classified as follows, depending on lens involvement: incipient (<1–15% of lens is affected), immature (in between incipient to mature), mature (near 100% of lens is affected), and hypermature (noted resorption). They can be further classified depending on their location: anterior and posterior capsular, anterior and posterior cortex, and nucleus (Figure 54.5). Depending on how much of the lens is involved, affected foals may or may not have visual deficits present.

Cataracts may remain unchanged or progress until the entirety of the lens is involved. Therefore, affected foals should be reexamined to document any cataract progression or if changes in vision are noted. Cataract surgery can be pursued in healthy foals and adult horses that have cataracts that result in visual deficits. It is important to note that foals with underlying systemic diseases or accompanying uveitis are associated with less postoperative success. Additionally, prior to pursuing surgery, foals should be weaned and be accustomed to handling as postoperative care is crucial.

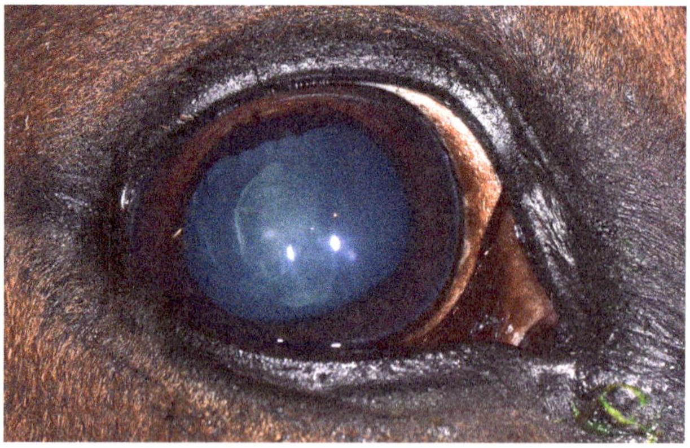

Figure 54.5 Nuclear cataract noted in in yearling Quarter Horse gelding. The pupil has been pharmacologically dilated.

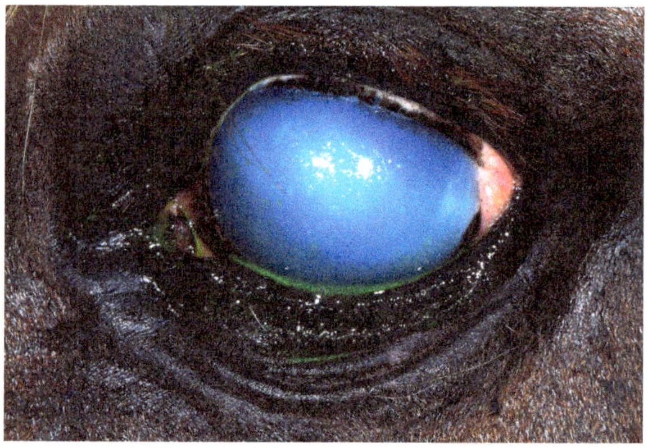

Figure 54.6 Representative image of glaucoma in a middle-aged Quarter Horse. Note diffuse corneal edema, deeper perilimbal vascularization, and multifocal bullae formation. This image was taken following fluorescein administration, allowing delineation of bullae. *Source:* Photograph courtesy of Dr. Ian Herring.

Glaucoma

Glaucoma is a progressive, blinding disease in which elevated intraocular pressures lead to damage to the optic nerve. Glaucoma can be classified as congenital, primary, or secondary. Primary glaucoma occurs due to an inherited anatomical abnormality of the iridocorneal angle. Secondary glaucoma occurs due to an identified underlying cause that leads to obstruction of the iridocorneal angle, such as uveitis, lens instability, or neoplasia. Congenital glaucoma occurs due to developmental abnormalities of the iridocorneal angle and is commonly found with anterior segment dysgenesis and lens luxation [48, 49]. Although uncommon, congenital glaucoma has been reported in Thoroughbred, Arabian, and Standardbred foals [50–53].

Glaucoma is diagnosed based on clinical signs and documentation of increased intraocular pressures (>25–30 mmHg) via tonometry. Clinical signs associated with glaucoma include: blepharospasm, tearing, episcleral injection, focal or diffuse corneal edema with or without bullae (blister) formation, Haab's striae, mydriasis, vision loss, retinal, optic nerve atrophy, and buphthalmos (enlargement of the globe due to sustained elevated intraocular pressures) (Figure 54.6).

Glaucoma treatment is aimed at decreasing intraocular pressures with both medical and surgical management. Medical management in horses is limited to the use of topical carbonic anhydrase inhibitors and beta blockers, as other topical medications (prostaglandin analogues) have shown limited response. The topical use of combination carbonic anhydrase inhibitor/beta blocker (dorzolamide 2%/timolol 0.5%) can reduce intraocular pressures by 13% in normal horses [54]. Surgical management of glaucoma in potential visual eyes includes trans-scleral or endo-laser cyclophotocoagulation and the use of gonioimplants. For end-stage eyes that are nonvisual, enucleation is recommended. In many cases of congenital glaucoma, the prognosis for vision is poor and enucleation is most commonly pursued.

Posterior Segment

Congenital abnormalities of the posterior segment in the horse are uncommon.

Retinal dysplasia is a congenital retinal malformation that results in disorganization and retinal folds (rosettes). Additional etiologies, across species, include inherited, viral infections, vitamin A deficiency, radiation, toxicities, and intrauterine trauma. In horses, retinal dysplasia can be seen as a sole abnormality but also as part as MCOA. In one study, retinal dysplasia comprised 3.5% of all congenital ocular abnormalities [1]. Clinically, retinal dysplasia can be visualized as focal, multifocal, or geographic lesions of altered tapetal reflectivity and pigmentation [4]. These lesions are nonprogressive and rarely cause visual disturbances.

Posterior Colobomas

Colobomas of the posterior segment have been reported and include of the optic nerve and retinal pigmented epithelium (RPE) [55–61]. In horses, atypical colobomas (those not at the 6 o'clock position) are more common than typical colobomas [4]. Posterior segment colobomas can be seen as a single abnormality but also with others, such as with MCOA. Colobomas of the posterior segment can be seen incidentally but can also affect vision, often leading to the reason for veterinary examination. Clinically, an optic disc coloboma manifests as a focal notch or defect of the optic disc and/or peripapillary retina. Colobomas of the RPE are visualized as "window defects," noted more commonly in the nontapetal retina, allowing direct visualization of the choroid and/or sclera [4].

Retinal Hemorrhage

Similar to conjunctival hemorrhage, retinal hemorrhage has been reported in the foal, but is likely acquired during parturition [4]. Retinal hemorrhage has been reported in 11.4–29% of healthy foals [11, 19, 21, 62], but it is important to note that other underlying etiologies may contribute to hemorrhage, such as vasculitis, coagulopathy, and other underlying systemic conditions. Just as with conjunctival hemorrhages, an underlying etiology should be considered more likely depending on the overall physical examination of the foal. Retinal hemorrhages can resolve spontaneously in 7–10 days, with punctate peripheral hemorrhages resolving quicker than larger or central hemorrhages [19, 21].

Persistent Hyaloid Artery

Persistent hyaloid artery (or tunica vasculosa lentis) results from an incomplete regression of the hyaloid artery. In utero, the hyaloid artery, a branch of the ophthalmic artery, supplies the lens as it extends from the optic disc. In the horse, regression of the hyaloid artery starts prior to parturition with complete resorption occurring by 3–9 months of age [1, 11, 19, 21]. Therefore, remnants of the posterior hyaloid artery should be considered a normal finding in foals up to the age of 9 months. Persistent hyaloid artery, in conjunction with other ophthalmic abnormalities, in horses has been rarely reported in the literature [8, 15].

Congenital Stationary Night Blindness

Congenital stationary night blindness manifests as nonprogressive scotopic (dark or dim-light) vision deficits. This condition has been described in humans, dogs, and horses [63–66]. It has been reported in the Appaloosa, Thoroughbred, Standardbred, Miniature Horse, and Paso Fino breeds [7, 67–70]. Congenital stationary night blindness has been associated with homozygosity of the leopard complex gene (Lp) [67, 69].

These horses present with a change in vision or apprehension during scotopic conditions (nyctalopia), but otherwise are visually normal. Affected horses may also exhibit dorsomedial strabismus, nystagmus, and "stargazing" (dorsal ocular deviation and head tilt/elevation). Severely affected horses may also exhibit a change in vision during photopic conditions (well-lit environment or daytime) [67, 71].

Although diagnosis can be made based off of signalment and clinical signs, congenital stationary night blindness can be confirmed with electroretinogram (ERG). Affected horses have a normal a-wave but a decreased photopic and absent scotopic b-wave, commonly referred as a negative ERG [57, 67, 68]. There is no treatment for affected horses, but the condition is otherwise nonprogressive. Because the condition is heritable, affected animals should not be bred [57]. A genetic test is available from the Veterinary Genetics Laboratory at UC Davis.

References

1 Roberts, S.M. (1992). Congenital ocular anomalies. *Vet. Clin. N. Am. Equine* 8: 459–478.

2 Latimer, C.A., Wyman, M., and Hamilton, J. (1983). An ophthalmic survey of the neonatal horse. *Equine Vet. J.* 15 (S2): 9–14.

3 Priester, W.A. (1972). Congenital ocular defects in cattle, horses, cats, and dogs. *J. Am. Vet. Med. Assoc.* 160: 1504–1511.

4 Leiva, M.P. and Peña, T. (2016). Ophthalmic diseases of foals. In: *Equine Ophthalmology* (ed. B.C. Gilger), 112–150. Hoboken, NJ: Wiley.

5 Turner, A.G. (2004). Ocular conditions of neonatal foals. *Vet. Clin. Equine* 20: 429–440.

6 Adams, R. and Mayhew, I.G. (1984). Neurological examination of newborn foals. *Equine Vet. J.* 16: 306–312.

7 Gelatt, K.N. (1993). Congenital and acquired ophthalmic disease in the foal. *Anim. Eye Res.* 1–2: 15–27.

8 Gelatt, K. (1982). The eye. In: *Equine Medicine and Surgery*, 3e (ed. R.A. Mansmann, E.S. McAllister, and P.W. Pratt). Santa Barbara, California: American Veterinary Publications.

9 Fox, L.T. (1969). Bilateral ankyloblepharon congenital in a newborn foal. *Vet. Med. Small Anim. Clin. VM, SAC* 64: 237–238.

10 Latimer, C.A. and Wyman, M. (1985). Neonatal ophthalmology. *Vet. Clin. N. Am. Equine Pract.* 1: 235–259.

11 Munroe, G.A. and Barnett, K.C. (1984). Congenital ocular disease in the foal. *Vet. Clin. N. Am. Large Anim. Pract.* 6: 519–539.

12 Barnett, K.C. (1975). The eye of the newborn foal. *J. Reprod. Fertil.* 23 (Suppl): 701–702.

13 Greenberg, S.M., Plummer, C.E., Brooks, D.E. et al. (2012). Third eyelid dermoid in a horse. *Vet. Ophthalmol.* 15: 351–354.

14 Gornik, K.R., Pirie, C.G., and Beamer, G.L. (2015). Unilateral choristoma of the nictitating membrane in a horse. *J. Am. Vet. Med. Assoc.* 246: 231–235.
15 Whitley, R.D. (1990). Neonatal equine ophthalmology. In: *Equine Clinical Neonatology* (ed. A.M. Koterba, W.H. Drumoond, and P.C. Kosch), 242. Philadelphia: Lea & Febiger.
16 Moore, C.P. (1992). Eyelid and nasolacrimal disease. *Vet. Clin. N. Am. Equine* 8: 499–519.
17 Craven, J.R. (1971). Significance of lesions of the cornea and lens in the examination of horses for soundness. *Equine Vet. J.* 3: 141–143.
18 Lavach, J.D. (1990). *Large Animal Ophthalmology*. CV. Mosby Co.
19 Leiva, M., Peña, T., and Monreal, L. (2011). Ocular findings in healthy newborn foals according to age. *Equine Vet. Educ.* 23: 40–45.
20 Munroe, G. (1999). Subconjunctival haemorrhages in neonatal Thoroughbred foals. *Vet. Rec.* 144: 279–282.
21 Barsotti, G., Sgorbini, M., Marmorini, P. et al. (2013). Ocular abnormalities in healthy Standardbred foals. *Vet. Ophthalmol.* 16: 245–250.
22 Latimer, C.A. and Wyman, M. (1984). Atresia of the nasolacrimal duct in three horses. *J. Am. Vet. Med. Assoc.* 184: 989–992.
23 Lundvall, R.L. and Carter, J.D. (1971). Atresia of the nasolacrimal meatus in the horse. *J. Am. Vet. Med. Assoc.* 159: 289–291.
24 Mason, T.A. (1979). Atresia of the nasolacrimal orifice in two Thoroughbreds. *Equine Vet. J.* 11: 19–20.
25 Giuliano, E. (2016). Diseases of the adnexa and nasolacrimal system. In: *Equine Ophthalmology*, 3e (ed. B.C. Gilger), 197–251. Hoboken, NJ: Wiley.
26 Sandmeyer, L.S., Bauer, B.S., Breaux, C.B. et al. (2011). Congenital nasolacrimal atresia in 4 alpacas. *Can. Vet. J.* 52: 313–317.
27 Stoppini, R., Tassan, S., and Barachetti, L. (2014). Diode laser photoablation to correct distal nasolacrimal duct atresia in an adult horse. *Vet. Ophthalmol.* 17 (Suppl 1): 174–178.
28 Joyce, J.R., Martin, J.E., Storts, R.W. et al. (1990). Iridial hypoplasia (aniridia) accompanied by limbic dermoids and cataracts in a group of related Quarterhorses. *Equine Vet. J.* 22 (S10): 26–26.
29 McLaughlin, S. and Brightman, A. (1983). Bilateral ocular dermoids in a colt. *Equine Practice* 5: 10–14.
30 Walde, I. (1983). Band opacities. *Equine Vet. J.* 15 (S2): 32.
31 Ueda, Y. (1990). Aniridia in a Thoroughbred horse. *Equine Vet. J.* 22 (S10): 29.
32 Joyce, J.R. (1983). Aniridia in a Quarterhorse. *Equine Vet. J.* S2: 21–22.
33 McCormick, K., Ward, D., and Newkirk, K. (2013). Aniridia in two related Tennessee Walking horses. Case reports. *Vet. Med.* 703732.
34 Eriksson, K. (1955). Hereditary aniridia with secondary cataract in horses. *Nord. Vet. Med.* 7: 773–779.
35 Crispin, S.M. (2000). Developmental anomalies and abnormalities of the equine iris. *Vet. Ophthalmol.* 3: 93–98.
36 Plummer, C.E. and Ramsey, D.T. (2011). A survey of ocular abnormalities in Miniature Horses. *Vet. Ophthalmol.* 14: 239–243.
37 Gemensky-Metzler, A.J., Wilkie, D.A., and Cook, C.S. (2004). The use of semiconductor diode laser for deflation and coagulation of anterior uveal cysts in dogs, cats and horses: a report of 20 cases. *Vet. Ophthalmol.* 7: 360–368.
38 Komáromy, A.M., Rowlan, J.S., La Croix, N.C. et al. (2011). Equine multiple congenital ocular anomalies (MCOA) syndrome in PMEL17 (silver) mutant ponies: five cases. *Vet. Ophthalmol.* 14: 313–320.
39 Andersson, L.S., Juras, R., Ramsey, D.T. et al. (2008). Equine multiple congenital ocular anomalies maps to a 4.9 megabase interval on horse chromosome 6. *BMC Genet.* 9: 88.
40 Ramsey, D.T., Ewart, S.L., Render, J.A. et al. (1999). Congenital ocular abnormalities of Rocky Mountain horses. *Vet. Ophthalmol.* 2: 47–59.
41 Grahn, B.H., Pinard, C., Archer, S. et al. (2008). Congenital ocular anomalies in purebred and crossbred Rocky and Kentucky Mountain horses in Canada. *Can. Vet. J.* 49: 675–681.
42 Andersson, L.S., Axelsson, J., Dubielzig, R.R. et al. (2011). Multiple congenital ocular anomalies in Icelandic horses. *BMC Vet. Res.* 7: 21.
43 Kaps, S.S. and Spiess, B.M. (2010). Multiple congenital ocular abnormalities (MCOA) in Rocky Mountain horses and Kentucky Mountain Saddle horses in Europe. *Pferdeheilkunde* 26 (4): 536–540.
44 Depecker, M., Ségard, E., and Cadoré, J.-L. (2013). Phenotypic description of multiple congenital ocular anomalies in Comtois horses. *Equine Vet. Educ.* 25: 511–516.
45 Ramsey, D.T., Hauptman, J.G., and Petersen-Jones, S.M. (1999). Corneal thickness, intraocular pressure, and optical corneal diameter in Rocky Mountain horses with cornea globosa or clinically normal corneas. *Am. J. Vet. Res.* 60: 1317–1321.
46 Beech, J., Aguirre, G., and Gross, S. (1984). Congenital nuclear cataracts in the Morgan horse. *J. Am. Vet. Med. Assoc.* 184: 1363–1365.
47 Beech, J. and Irby, N. (1985). Inherited nuclear cataracts in the Morgan horse. *J. Hered.* 76: 371–372.
48 Pickett, J. and Ryan, J. (1993). Equine glaucoma: a retrospective study of 11 cases from 1988 to 1993. *Vet. Med. (USA)* 88: 756–763.

49 Cullen, C.L. and Grahn, B.H. (2000). Equine glaucoma: a retrospective study of 13 cases presented at the Western College of Veterinary Medicine from 1992 to 1999. *Can. Vet. J.* 41: 470–480.

50 Gelatt, K.N. (1973). Glaucoma and lens luxation in a foal. *Vet. Med. Small Anim. Clin.* 68: 261.

51 Wilkie, D., Peckham, E.S., and Paulic, S. (2001). Equine glaucoma and diode laser transscleral cyclophotocoagulation: 27 cases. *Vet. Ophthalmol.* 4: 294.

52 Barnett, K.C., Cottrell, B.D., Paterson, B.W. et al. (1988). Buphthalmos in a Thoroughbred foal. *Equine Vet. J.* 20: 132–135.

53 Halenda, R.G., Sorden, S., and Collier, L. (1997). Congenital equine glaucoma: clinical and light microscopic findings in two cases. *Vet. Comp. Ophthalmol.* 7: 105–109.

54 Tofflemire, K.L., Whitley, E.M., Flinn, A.M. et al. (2015). Effect of topical ophthalmic dorzolamide(2%)-timolol(0.5%) solution and ointment on intraocular pressure in normal horses. *Vet. Ophthalmol.* 18: 457–461.

55 Pinard, C.L. and Basrur, P.K. (2011). Ocular anomalies in a herd of Exmoor ponies in Canada. *Vet. Ophthalmol.* 14: 100–108.

56 Williams, D. and Barnett, K. (1993). Bilateral optic disc colobomas and microphthalmos in a Thoroughbred horse. *Vet. Rec.* 132: 101–103.

57 Allbaugh, R.T. and Wilkie, D.A. (2016). Diseases of the equine vitreous and retina. In: *Equine Ophthalmology*, 3e (ed. B.C. Gilger), 469–507.

58 Schuh, J.C. (1989). Bilateral colobomas in a horse. *J. Comp. Pathol.* 100: 331–335.

59 Wheeler, C.A. and Collier, L.L. (1990). Bilateral colobomas involving the optic discs in a Quarter Horse. *Equine Vet. J. Suppl.* 10: 39–41.

60 Bildfell, R., Watrous, B., Maxwell, S. et al. (2003). Bilateral optic disc colobomas in a Quarter Horse filly. *Equine Vet. J.* 35: 325–327.

61 Martín-Suárez, E.M., Galán, A., Gallardo Galero, J.M. et al. (2009). Bilateral typical complete colobomas in a donkey: retinographic and fluorangiographic description. *Vet. Ophthalmol.* 12: 338–342.

62 Labelle, A.L., Hamor, R.E., Townsend, W.M. et al. (2011). Ophthalmic lesions in neonatal foals evaluated for nonophthalmic disease at referral hospitals. *J. Am. Vet. Med. Assoc.* 239: 486–492.

63 Carr, R.E., Ripps, H., Siegel, I.M. et al. (1966). Visual functions in congenital night blindness. *Invest. Ophthalmol.* 5: 508–551.

64 Narfström, K., Wrigstad, A., and Nilsson, S.E. (1989). The Briard dog: a new animal model of congenital stationary night blindness. *Br. J. Ophthalmol.* 73: 750–756.

65 Kondo, M., Das, G., Imai, R. et al. (2015). A naturally occurring canine model of autosomal recessive congenital stationary night blindness. *PLoS One* 10: e0137072.

66 Miraldi Utz, V., Pfeifer, W., Longmuir, S.Q. et al. (2018). Presentation of TRPM1-associated congenital stationary night blindness in children. *JAMA Ophthalmol.* 136: 389–398.

67 Sandmeyer, L.S., Breaux, C.B., Archer, S. et al. (2007). Clinical and electroretinographic characteristics of congenital stationary night blindness in the Appaloosa and the association with the leopard complex. *Vet. Ophthalmol.* 10: 368–375.

68 Nunnery, C., Pickett, J.P., and Zimmerman, K.L. (2005). Congenital stationary night blindness in a thoroughbred and a Paso Fino. *Vet. Ophthalmol.* 8: 415–419.

69 Sandmeyer, L.S., Bellone, R.R., Archer, S. et al. (2012). Congenital stationary night blindness is associated with the leopard complex in the Miniature Horse. *Vet. Ophthalmol.* 15: 18–22.

70 Rebhun, W.C. (1992). Retinal and optic nerve diseases. *Vet. Clin. North Am. Equine Pract.* 8: 587–608.

71 Witzel, D.A., Smith, E.L., Wilson, R.D. et al. (1978). Congenital stationary night blindness: an animal model. *Invest. Ophthalmol. Vis. Sci.* 17: 788–795.

Chapter 55 Inherited Ocular Disorders

David Whitley and Ralph Hamor

The genomes of many species, including the horse, have been sequenced and are available at http://www.ncbi.nlm.nih.gov/Genomes/index.html [1]. Wade et al. reported the equine genome sequence in 2009, which has enhanced the study of genetic disease, both simple and polygenetic traits in the horse [2]. Several inherited or presumed inherited ocular diseases in horses have been described [3] and several genetic tests are available for identifying horses with inherited ocular disease or those at risk for such disorders [4]. This chapter reviews the ocular conditions in the horse for which a genetic basis is known or suspected (Table 55.1) [5, 6]. Hereditary ocular disease and hereditary diseases with ophthalmic manifestations have also been described in horses [1, 3–5]. However, these have not been studied in the detail that hereditary diseases in humans, mice, and dogs have been.

Inheritance

The instructions for biological life are encoded in nucleotide sequences that are passed from one generation to the next in the form of deoxyribonucleic acid (DNA) that is organized into genes contained on chromosomes in each cell nucleus. The chromosomal position where a gene is located is called a locus and this term is often used colloquially to refer to the gene at that site. Information encoded within the components of the DNA is translated into structural proteins, enzymes, and other cellular components through a complex process. Briefly, a specific sequence of paired nucleotides comprising each DNA strand is consistently transcribed into messenger RNA, which is translated into a specific protein. These paired nucleotides are called a base pair (bp) and are the building blocks of the DNA double helix [7].

The genome of the horse is composed of approximately 2.4–2.7 billion base pairs and contains about 20 000 genes [3, 7]. The base pairs are divided among 32 chromosomes. A horse has two copies of every chromosome, one copy inherited from the sire and the other from the dam. One pair of chromosomes determines the sex of the animal (sex chromosomes); in mammals XX for females and XY for males. In females, one X chromosome is inactivated in each cell [7]. The inactivated X chromosome is seen as the Barr body. This process occurs during embryonic development and is referred to as random X chromosome inactivation [7].

The type of cell division that occurs in the ovaries and testes to produce gametes (eggs and spermatids, respectively) is called meiosis. During meiosis, one cell replicates its DNA, then divides twice to form four daughter cells, each with half of the normal amount of DNA and half the number of chromosomes, a condition called "haploid" [1, 3]. These haploid cells have one copy of all the chromosomes from the original cell. As the gametes form, there is exchange of genetic material among chromosomes, so that the original paternal chromosome may receive a section of maternal chromosome material, and likewise the maternal chromosome may receive genetic material from the paternal chromosome. This genetic recombination process results in new combinations of the genetic code on the gametes' chromosomes. Subsequent fusion of sperm and egg during fertilization results in a genetically unique diploid zygote that undergoes further development into an individual animal.

Genetic Variation

On occasion, when a cell replicates the DNA, a mistake in copying the order of nucleotides may occur. If the mistake is not repaired by DNA repair enzymes, the new strand of DNA becomes a permanent change in the sequence of bases (referred to as a mutation or polymorphism) [3]. If the mistake is a single base, it is termed a single nucleotide polymorphism (SNP). Mutation is the primary source of

Equine Neonatal Medicine, First Edition. Edited by David M. Wong and Pamela A. Wilkins.

Table 55.1 Inherited or suspected inherited eye diseases in different horse breeds.

	Mini	SBD	App	Arab	AusTB	Belg	Comtois	Exmoor	Fries	Half	Ice	Knub	Lip	Mor	Mount	Nor	Paso	POA	PPaso	QH	RMH	Shet	STB	TB	WB
Aniridia						X																			
Cataracts		X	X			X				X				X						X				X	
Coloboma (posterior segment)			X																	X					
Congenital Hypertropia			X																						
Corneal dystrophy									X																
CSNB	X		X									X				X	X	X		X			X	X	
Distichiasis									X																
Entropion																				X			X	X	
ERU			X																						X
Glaucoma congenital primary				X										X			X			X			X	X	X
Iris Hypoplasia			X																						
Iris pigmentation alteration“Tiger Eye”																			x	x					
Limbal dermoid						X														X					
Linear Keratopathy					X							X													
MCOA							X	X		X	X		X		X						X	X			
Melanoma												X													
Microphthalmos				X										X										X	
Progressive retinal degeneration																								X	
Retinal detachment																							X	X	
Sarcoid			X	X																X					
SCC										X															
Scleral Ectasia				X																					
Strabismus			X																						

CSNB, Congenital stationary night blindness; MCOA, Multiple congenital ocular anomalies syndrome; ERU. Equine recurrent uveitis; SCC, squamous cell carcinoma.
Mini, American Miniature Horse; SBD, Saddlebred; App, Appaloosa; Arab, Arabian; AusTB, Australian Thoroughbred; Belg, Belgian; Fries, Friesian; Half, Halflinger; Ice, Icelandic horse.
Knub, Knubstrupper; Lip, Lipizzaner; Mor, Morgan; Mount, Mountain Pleasure Horse; Nor, Noriker; Pas, Paso Fino; POA, Pony of the Americas; PPasa, Puerto Rican Paso Fino.
QH, Quarter Horse; RMH, Rocky Mountain Horse; Shet, Shetland Pony; STB, Standardbred; TB, Thoroughbred; WB, Warmblood.

genetic variation. Alternative forms of a gene that arise by mutation are called alleles. Within a species, there can be numerous alleles for a single gene. When there are two different alleles present for a single gene, the individual is defined as heterozygous for that allele. If the alleles are identical, the individual is homologous for the allele. Which alleles are inherited or the genetic makeup for a particular locus is termed the genotype [3, 7].

Phenotype, Expression, and Penetrance

The phenotype is the observable or clinical appearance of a trait such as coat color pigmentation, or status of an eye disease. The terms *affected* and *not affected* are used to describe the presence or absence of an individual trait. The phenotype is the result of the both the genotype and environmental influences. Expressivity is the degree or extent that a genotype exhibits its phenotype expression. Variable expressivity occurs when all animals carrying a gene express the trait but to variable degrees. Variable expressivity can occur if the characteristic is controlled by more than one gene (i.e. is polygenetic), or is due to a genotype-environment interaction. Equine recurrent uveitis (ERU) in the Appaloosa breed is an example of variable expression due to genotype-environment interaction. Appaloosas with ERU exhibit variable expression, with some horses more severely affected than others, and the expression of this trait is regulated by several loci (genes) and by environmental factors [8].

Penetrance is a measurement of the proportion of individuals in a population that carry the allele for a trait and express the phenotype. Incomplete penetrance is when all animals in a population are known to carry a particular allelic variation (i.e. a uniform genotype among the population), but only some of the animals exhibit the trait [3, 7]. The gene appears to penetrate and be expressed by some animals but not by others. Multiple congenital ocular anomalies syndrome (MCOA) is an example of a dominant trait with incomplete penetrance.

Modes of Inheritance

Pedigree analysis is used to investigate for the possibility of a genetic basis for a clinical trait.

Autosomal recessive – With autosomal inheritance, the causal gene is located on an autosomal chromosome (non-sex chromosome). The incidence of the phenotype is expected to be equal in males and females. Recessive traits are only expressed in individuals that are homologous (two mutant alleles) for the causative gene. Individuals with one mutant allele and one normal allele (e.g. heterozygous for the trait) do not express the disease phenotype and are carriers for the mutant allele. The offspring of two heterozygous (carrier) animals have a one in four chance of being homozygous for the gene and of expressing the phenotype [7].

Autosomal Dominant

In autosomal dominant inheritance, the causal genetic mutation lies on an autosomal chromosome and is likely to be inherited by both male and female animals in the group. Phenotypes caused by dominant alleles will be expressed in every offspring carrying the allele, regardless of if they have one or two copies of the mutation allele. Breeding between an affected individual (heterozygous for the defect) and an unaffected individual will result in a 50% chance of producing an affected offspring [1, 3].

X-linked Recessive

With X-linked recessive inheritance, the causal gene mutation lies on the X chromosome. An X-linked recessive mode of inheritance is implicated when there are more males with the disease than females. This is due to the one affected X chromosome result in the disease phenotype [3]. When both X chromosomes in a female are mutated, that female will exhibit the defect. All female offspring from an affected male will at least be carriers for the mutant allele.

X-linked Dominant

In X-linked dominant inheritance, the causal gene mutation lies on the X chromosome. All animals carrying the gene, male or female, will be affected. Therefore, each affected animal must have one affected parent. Affected males (XY) mated to normal females will not pass the gene to any of their male offspring, because they receive the Y chromosome from the sire. Affected males bred to normal females will pass the affected X chromosome to all female offspring. Both sons and daughters of a heterozygous female will have a 50% chance of being affected [1, 3]. Heterozygous females may exhibit a less severe phenotype of the disease than homozygous females or affected males. Since only one X chromosome is active in each cell and one X chromosome is inactive, a heterozygous female may have more cells with the normal allele on the active X chromosome, resulting in expression of some amount of the normal gene product [1, 7].

Mitochondrial Inheritance

Mitochondria within normal cells contain their own genomes. Mitochondria are only transmitted in the ova, not in the sperm, so each animal inherits mitochondria only from the dam [8]. Inherited diseases from mutations in mitochondrial DNA therefore are maternally inherited. At present, there are no known equine diseases caused by defects in the mitochondrial genome [8].

Ocular Disorders of the Horse with Known or Suspected Genetic Basis

Congenital stationary night blindness (CSNB) is reported in the Appaloosa breed [9, 10]. Horses with this condition are born with the inability to see in the dark. The condition is nonprogressive, and the retina is morphologically normal [10, 11]. The dark-adapted electroretinogram (ERG) has a characteristic "negative" waveform response, an absent b-wave, and a depolarizing a-wave [10–12]. The pathogenesis is defective neural transmission within the rod photoreceptor pathway – specifically, the inability of the retinal bipolar cells to respond after hyperpolarization of the rods [12, 13].

CSNB is a recessive autosomal defect in low-light vision in several horse breeds [14]. Horses homozygous for the characteristic Appaloosa pigmented oval spots known as "leopard spots" occur in the white-patterned areas. The white-spotted-patterns differ by the amount of white on the flank and range from horses that display only a few white flecks to those that are almost completely white. It is thought that modifier genes are responsible for determining the size of the white-pattern that is inherited [15, 16].

Leopard complex spotting is inherited by the incompletely dominant locus, *LP*, which also causes CSNB in homozygous horses [13, 17]. Archeological equine bones investigated for *TRMP1* gene, date back to Pleistocene time (17 000 YBP) and the genes in Turkey date back to 2700–2200 BCE. During the Iron Age, LP reappeared probably by introduction into the domestic gene pool from wild horses [17]. Leopard complex spotting in the Appaloosa is characterized by patches of white in the coat that vary in size and tend to be symmetrical and centered over the hips or flank. Other pigmentation traits include nonpigmented sclera, striped hooves, and mottled pigmentation around the muzzle, genitalia, and anus [18].

Horses that are homozygous *LP/LP* are affected by CSNB [12, 13]. The cause of both CSNB and LP is a defect in expression of the *TRPM1* gene [19]. Lack of expression of TRMP1 in CSNB-affected horses explains the "negative ERG" seen in affected horses. The rod photoreceptors hyperpolarize in response to light and cause the a-wave, but the ON bipolar cells cannot depolarize, leading to an absent b-wave [20, 21]. TRMP1 has also been demonstrated in the synaptic ribbons of rods and melanopsin-expressing photosensitive retinal ganglion cells, which may suggest other roles for this gene in the visual process [22, 23]. It is suggested that TRPM1 SNP can act independently and suggests a selective advantage for the apparently deleterious CSNB trait [16].

CSNB has been associated with specific coat color patterns in the Appaloosa breed [12]. The haircoat spotting patterns (referred to as the leopard complex spotting) are caused by a single incompletely dominant allele (LP). Leopard complex spotting also occurs in the Knabstrupper, Noriker, Pony of the Americas (POA), American Miniature horse, and British Spotted pony. CSNB probably occurs in all breeds with LP spotting but has been confirmed only in the Appaloosa, American Miniature Horse, and the Knabstrupper [13].

A genetic test is available for CSNB and LP [4]. Electroretinography and genetic testing are the best ways to confirm the diagnosis. The genotype cannot be accurately assessed based on the pigment spotting. The *LP* genotype is important from both breeding and management standpoints. Horses homozygous for LP (*LP/LP*) are important breeding animals to produce desired haircoat-patterns. However, since LP and CSNB are both caused by the same mutation, it is impossible to eliminate CSNB from the gene pool without eliminating the desired coat patterns. Most horses with CSNB function very well in the lighted environment and adapt well to their dim light visual deficits. Confirming the diagnosis of CSNB is worthwhile in that it allows adjusted management and handling of affected animals, to enhance the safety of the horse and interacting humans [1].

Multiple Congenital Ocular Anomalies Syndrome (MCOA)

A second ocular disease associated with coat pigmentation is MCOA Syndrome, which is a pleotropic effect of the silver coat color dilution gene in the horse [24]. The condition was originally described as anterior segment dysgenesis in Rocky Mountain horses in 1999 [24, 25]. More recently, the syndrome has been identified in the American Miniature Horse, Belgian Draft, Comtois, Kentucky Mountain Saddle Horse, Mountain Pleasure, and the Icelandic horse [26–31]. The silver coat-color is a dilution of black (eumelanin) pigment determined by a dominant gene, which phenotypically controls the color of the mane and tail, producing a silver or flaxen color. In a black base color, it reduces the pigment in the haircoat, lightening the dark black coat to a dark chocolate color [32]. The silver gene encodes for the premelanosome protein (PMEL). PMEL is a pigment cell-specific membrane protein located in the melanosomes, which synthesizes the black and brown pigment eumelanin [33–35].

Ocular signs of MCOA syndrome occur as two distinct phenotypes: (i) Temporal cysts originating from the ciliary body or peripheral retina (cyst phenotype), and (ii) Multiple congenital ocular anomalies (MCOA phenotype). These congenital anomalies include ciliary body or peripheral retinal cysts and iris hypoplasia. Ocular changes associated with iris hypoplasia include dyscoria, miosis, flattened granula iridica, absence of an iris collarette, a visible pupillary sphincter muscle, and incomplete pupillary dilation after instillation of mydriatic drugs [25]. In addition, some horses with MCOA have corneal globosa, an exaggerated abnormal corneal curvature or megalocornea, megaloblpharon, immature nuclear cataracts, retinal dysplasia, and iridocorneal angle hypoplasia or adhesions [25, 26, 36]. It is presumed that animals heterozygous for the mutant allele express the ciliary body or retinal cyst phenotype, and homozygous animals express the MCOA phenotype [24]. The mutation results in an incomplete dominant trait with homozygous animals demonstrating more serious ocular defects, while heterozygous animals have less severe defects [26, 37]. A study linking ocular lesions, age, and genotype identified a missense mutation in exon 11 of the *PMZEL* gene on the ECA6 chromosome as the cause of the silver coat coloration [38].

To avoid the risk of producing foals with MCOA, silver horses should not be bred to each other. In addition, since only bay- and black-based coat colors express the phenotype, it is strongly advised to have chestnut-based foals produced from silver breedings tested for PMEL mutation, along with strictly avoiding breeding those horses with the silver mutation to each other [1].

Equine Recurrent Uveitis (ERU)

ERU or immune-mediated anterior and/or posterior uveitis has a worldwide distribution and is likely the most common cause of blindness in horses [39]. It is characterized by chronic, recurring bouts of uveal inflammation. The condition is usually bilateral, but severity is not symmetrical. Three clinical forms of the disease are recognized: classic, insidious, and posterior. Classic ERU is most common and is characterized by bouts of active inflammation in the eye, followed by periods with minimal observable inflammation or quiescent periods. Insidious ERU is characterized by persistent low-grade uveal inflammation, with a gradual and progressive destructive pathology of the eye, instead of the typical or classical ERU with painful ocular episodes. The insidious type is commonly observed in Appaloosa and draft breeds. Posterior uveitis affects mainly the choroid, retina, and vitreous and is most common in Warmbloods, draft breeds, and horses imported from Europe to the United States [39].

The etiology and pathophysiology of ERU is multifaceted and not completely defined. It is most likely an autoimmune disease, but the etiology, inciting causes, and reasons for recurrent inflammatory episodes are not fully elucidated. The association of *Leptospira* spp. with ERU is well documented, but the true role is not completely known. It has been theorized that infection with *Leptospira* spp. is at least one of the inciting causes of ERU [40–49]. The inflammatory cells infiltrating the equine uveal tract in ERU are predominately $CD4^+$ T cells, supporting involvement of the adaptive immune system [49].

Consistent with an immune-mediated pathogenesis, it is plausible that the genetic make-up plays a substantial role in determining the susceptibility of the factors that incite the disorder along with development and severity of future inflammatory recurrences. Genetic associations for ERU have been identified in the Appaloosa and the German Warmblood breeds [8, 50]. In both breeds, associations with genes involved in immune function, specifically the major histocompatibility complex (MHC), have been determined [1, 51].

ERU in the Appaloosa

The incidence of ERU in the Appaloosa is much higher than in the general horse population, and the disease is more severe and more likely to be bilateral and cause blindness in this breed [43, 52]. In the Appaloosa breed, the insidious form of ERU is more common than other forms, resulting in a gradual, cumulative destruction of the uveal tract, lens, retina, and vitreous [53]. Investigations using a candidate gene approach identified three genetic markers significantly associated with insidious ERU in the Appaloosa [8]. The three included a SNP within intron 11 of the *TRMP1* gene (the gene causing the white coat spotting pattern typical of the breed), an MHC class I microsatellite, and an MHC class II microsatellite in intron 1 of the *DRA* gene [8].

In the Appaloosa, the risk of ERU is two to three times higher with each A allele for the *TRPM1* intron [8]. One supposition is that the link between the coat color patterns of the Appaloosa and the increased risk of insidious ERU may be an immune-mediated reaction to altered TRPM1 protein in uveal melanocytes. However, this has not been confirmed. Another possible pathogenetic mechanism is that TRPM1 plays a more primary role in immune function. The risk of ERU in other LP horse breeds should be investigated [1, 3, 4].

ERU in the German Warmblood

German Warmblood horses have a high risk of ERU, and heredity has a role in this breed as well [54]. In a serological study in the German Warmblood, an association between ERU and equine MHC class I haplotypes was demonstrated; at least one copy of the ELA-A9 haplotype appeared in 41% of ERU cases and in none of the normal, control animals [55]. Additionally, an association of SNP on ECA20 located near the candidate genes IL-17A and IL-17F has been posited [54]. IL-17 is a pro-inflammatory cytokine associated with cell damage in autoimmune diseases, including ERU. Similarly, a SNP near the crystalline gene cluster on ECA18 was strongly associated with the most severe cases of ERU [54]. These authors hypothesized that genetic variations in mutations in crystalline genes may contribute to cataract formation in ERU in the German Warmblood breed [54]. Further genetic studies should identify genes that will help explain the variability and severity of ERU and improve understanding of the cause and pathogenesis of ERU. The availability of DNA testing will help predict the risk of ERU in susceptible horse breeds and serve as a valuable tool to provide early diagnosis and a more accurate prognosis.

Squamous cell carcinoma (SCC) is the most common tumor type of the eye and eyelids of horses [56]. The third eyelid, limbus, and eyelids are the most common ocular sites affected [56–58]. In all breeds, the reported prevalence usually increases with age and is more common in geldings than mares [56]. SCC is more common in gray, paint (white-patterned), and dilute chestnut horses than in black, brown, or bay horses [57]. Horse breeds at increased risk include American Paint Horse, Appaloosas, draft breeds, Haflingers, and Thoroughbreds [56–62]. Haflingers are overrepresented for the development of limbal SCC [59, 61, 63]. Following pedigree evaluation, a recessive mode of inheritance is suspected [63]. A genome-wide association study identified a locus on ECA12 significantly associated with limbal SCC. Sequencing the most relevant gene from ECA12 identified a missense mutation on damage-specific DNA binding protein 2 (DDB2) [64]. This DDB2 variant is also present in the Belgian and Percheron breeds, suggesting that it may be a SCC risk factor for these breeds, as well [64]. The incidence of ocular and periocular SCC in horses increases with altitude and exposure to ultraviolet (UV) radiation [56, 65]. It is widely accepted in human medicine that COX-2 expression and the abundance of its enzymatic product PGE_2 have key roles in influencing the development, promoting tumor maintenance and progression of cancer in human beings [66]. Immunoreactivity for cyclo-oxygenase (COX)-1 and -2 is elevated in corneal SCC in horses, possibly indicating that the COX-prostaglandin inflammatory pathway plays a role in the pathogenesis of the tumor [62, 67].

Distichiasis in the Friesian Horse Breed

Distichiasis is an ocular disorder in which aberrant eyelashes (cilia, hairs) grow in the eyelid tissue and exit via the meibomian gland openings in the eyelid margin and has been reported in Friesian horses. A genome-wide association study was performed using an equine genotyping array to query genotypes of affected Friesian horses and nonaffected controls [68]. Only the locus on ECA13 reached genome-wide significance and provided evidence for a recessive mode of inheritance [68]. Hisey et al. identified a 16 kilobase deletion on ECA13 was associated with distichiasis in the Friesian breed [68].

Corneal Dystrophy in the Friesian Breed

A progressive, typically bilateral, and geographically symmetrical focal stromal thinning (in some cases leading to corneal perforation) has been reported in a group of related Friesian horses [69]. The condition has been termed a dystrophy since it is usually bilateral and symmetric and has an absence of inflammation. The breed predisposition and bilateral nature suggests a genetic component. A limited pedigree analysis revealed a common ancestor within six generations; thus, a genetic basis is suspected. The condition is more common in males, with the average age of the first eye diagnosis being 10.7 years [69].

Cataract

Congenital and developmental cataracts have been reported in several equine breeds; however, extensive genetic studies have not been performed. In foals with congenital cataracts, especially bilateral, suggests a disorder with a genetic basis. Familial occurrence of cataracts has been described in the Arabian, Quarter Horse, and Thoroughbred breeds [70–74]. The published reports are observations made by veterinary ophthalmologists and the true genetic behavior of these cataracts is unproven. Lavach reported cataracts in three successive foals from a Quarter Horse mare that were sired by three different stallions, suggestive of a dominant inheritance [70]. Whitley et al. reported cataracts in multiple foals from the same affected Quarter Horse mare with different unrelated sires [71, 72]. Millichamp and Dziezyc described two independent families of Arabians in which cataracts occurred in related members suggestive of a genetic transmission; however, no mode of inheritance was postulated [73]. Severin mentions congenital nuclear cataracts in Thoroughbreds as a dominant inheritance supported by test breeding, but pedigree analysis was not made available [74]. In the Morgan breed, congenital nuclear cataracts have been reported as an inherited trait [75, 76]. The cataracts are described as bilateral, finely reticulated, spherical translucencies, of the embryonal and fetal nucleus, that are not progressive. Occasionally the translucencies extend to the posterior "Y" suture. These cataracts in the Morgan horse are not associated with other ocular defects and do not impair sight. Pedigree analysis has shown that they are inherited as an autosomal dominant trait [76], but more females than males were affected.

Cataracts have been reported in a group of Exmoor ponies in Canada, as a suspected inherited trait [77]. The cataracts had a varied severity, most were punctate or intermediate, with the majority located anterior cortical or anterior capsular. Cataract progression was not reported. An inherited etiology is likely, but mode of inheritance was not definitely determined. In this study, inheritance did not appear to be autosomal recessive or dominant. However, more females were affected than males, similar to the cataracts reported in Morgan horses. These findings suggest a sex-linked or, at minimum, a sex-influenced inheritance [75–77].

Cataracts are also reported, in association with other inherited ocular anomalies in horses, including MCOA syndrome in horses with the silver mutation, and iridal hypoplasia in the Belgian and Quarter Horse breeds [24–31, 37, 78–80]. Worldwide, ERU is considered the most common cause of cataracts and of blindness in horses. Heredity has been demonstrated to play a role in the development of ERU in the Appaloosa and German Warmblood breeds [8, 50, 54]. As an aside, a genome-wide association study in German Warmbloods identified a significant SNP near the crystalline gene cluster on ECA18. The exact role of this mutation is not known, but it may be associated with cataract formation along with ERU [50].

Aniridia (Iris hypoplasia) describes partial or complete absence of iris tissue. Iris hypoplasia of varying extent is a more appropriate term, especially when some amount of iris tissue is present. This can be difficult to differentiate clinically without light microscopic examination. Aniridia or iris hypoplasia has been described in the Belgian, Quarter Horse, Swedish Warmblood, Tennessee Walking Horse, Welsh Thoroughbred cross, and Thoroughbred breeds [78–84].

In the Belgian and Quarter Horse breeds, aniridia or iridal hypoplasia has been reported. In 1955, Erickson reported inherited aniridia in the Belgian breed [78]. Bilateral aniridia and cataracts were diagnosed in a Belgian stallion and 65 of his descendants. Affected horses were photophobic with large unresponsive circular pupils. Cataracts were present in affected offspring after 2 months of age. Dermoids and a nonulcerative keratitis were diagnosed in several of the affected horses. Pedigree analysis supported an autosomal dominant mode of inheritance [78]. Affected animals were excluded from breeding stock of the Belgian breed and there have been no further reports.

Bilateral congenital aniridia (iris hypoplasia) was reported in a Quarter Horse and in some of his offspring; [79, 80] in addition, cataracts were observed in most of the offspring. Cataracts were not diagnosed clinically in the stallion at 18 months of age but were present and large on light microscopic examination postmortem. Histology of affected eyes did indicate the presence of some iris tissue, indicating iris hypoplasia instead of true aniridia, along with dermoids [80]. Limbal dermoids, along with nonulcerative, pigmented, and vascularized keratitis were seen in the dorsal limbus. Seven of eight of the Quarter Horse stallion's offspring, produced by unaffected and unrelated dams, were affected with iris hypoplasia and cataracts. An autosomal dominant mode of inheritance was hypothesized [80].

Iris hypoplasia, cataracts, and dermoids (nonulcerative keratitis) have been described in Swedish Warmbloods; it is suggested that the mode of inheritance is not a dominant trait [84]. Iris hypoplasia, cataract, and dorsal nonulcerative keratitis have been reported in two Tennessee Walking Horses, a Welsh Thoroughbred mixed breed filly, and one Thoroughbred colt, but the mode of inheritance has not been determined [81–83].

"Tiger Eye" in Puerto Rican Paso Fino Horses is a unique eye color and is characterized by a prominent yellow, amber, or orange iris [85]. Pedigree analysis identified a simple autosomal recessive mode of inheritance and a genome wide association study found a locus on ECA 1; this locus harbors the candidate gene SLC24A5 with roles in pigmentation in other species [84]. The "Tiger Eye" defect does not cause ocular anomalies or clinical alteration in coat color.

Ocular Manifestations of Equine Diseases Caused by Known Genetic Mutations

Hereditary Equine Regional Dermal Asthenia (HERDA), also called hyperelastosis cutis, is an autosomal recessive disorder of Quarter Horses [86, 87] and is characterized by loose, hyperextendable skin, and fragile skin that tears easily and heals poorly [86, 88, 89]. Temperature and UV radiation exposure play a role in clinical progression of the disease with the most noticeable lesions seen over the dorsal midline [90]. Horses with HERDA have an increased risk of infection and the occurrence of certain types of neoplasia, such as disseminated SCC, both related to a decreased immune surveillance due to T-cell malfunction [90]. Ophthalmic conditions seen with HERDA include thinner corneas and an increased incidence of corneal ulcers [91]. Affected animals also have a larger corneal curvature and corneal diameter than normal horses [92]. The pathogenesis of disease related to HERDA is defects in collagen biosynthesis and organization of collagen architecture [90, 92–95]. A missense mutation in the cyclphilin B gene (PPIB) has been identified as the most likely cause of the disorder [90].

Hyperkalemic periodic paralysis (HYPP) is an autosomal dominant trait affecting Quarter Horses. Clinical signs are variable, ranging from asymptomatic to frequent muscle fasciculations, weakness, and recumbency [96–99]. Ocular manifestations include third-eyelid protrusion secondary to globe retraction [96]. The genetic mutation has been traced back to a single Quarter Horse stallion [97–99]. The molecular genetic mutation for HYPP is a missense mutation in the alpha-subunit of the skeletal muscle sodium channel alpha-subunit [100].

Junctional epidermolysis bullosa (JEB) is an autosomal recessive trait in American Saddlebred horses, Belgian, Italian, Trait Breton, and Trait Comtois draft horse [101–104]. Clinical signs include mechanical stress-related blistering of the skin and mucous membranes. Blisters rapidly progress to erosions and ulcerations. These typically occur at sites of minor frictional irritation such as the oral mucosa, lips, distal extremities, and coronary bands [104, 105]. Ocular manifestations are most commonly seen as corneal ulceration [101, 105–107]. Histologically, the lesions are described as separation of the epidermis and dermis within the lamina lucida leaving the epidermis and dermis intact. The disorder is caused by a defective basement membrane zone in the skin [102, 103]. Genetic mutations involving two different genes coding for the laminin 332 protein complex have been associated with the disease in horses [108]. Laminin is a necessary basement membrane protein for the structure and function of the dermal-epidermal junction. In American Saddlebreds the genetic defect is a deletion in the LAMA3 gene [108]. The mutation in draft breeds (Belgian, Italian Toit Breton, and Trait Comtois) is a cytosine insertion creating a premature stop codon in the LAMC2 gene [103, 104], [108].

Summary

Genetic mutations have been described for a small number of ocular disorders in horses (CSNB, MCOA) and several systemic conditions with ocular manifestations (HERDA, HYPP, JEB). Genetic tests are available for these mutations. In other ocular conditions, a simple genetic basis is supported by pedigree analysis: limbal SCC in the Haflinger, corneal dystrophy in the Friesian, and cataract in the Quarter Horse, Arabian, Thoroughbred, Swedish Warmblood, Exmoor pony, and Tennessee Walking Horse. Additional ocular disorders may be more genetically complex involving several genes and genetic associations have been reported which include ERU in the Appaloosa and German Warmblood. For other ocular disorders, single-gene inheritance is highly suspected but specific mutations have not been determined; cataract in the Morgan, aniridia/iris hypoplasia in the Belgian and Quarter Horse.

The study of equine genetic disease has been limited until the equine genome sequence is published and advances are made in genetic and genomic technologies became available. When a mutation is found that causes or is associated or amplifies a disease and a DNA test is readily available, informed breeding decisions can be enhanced with the hope to lower the incidence or eliminate the disease from affected breeds.

When risk alleles are identified for inherited ocular disorders or associated disorders, veterinarians can use DNA testing to identify animals that should be examined more frequently, with earlier detection and therapy, and improved prognosis. Several laboratories offer genetic testing for coat color and for genetic diseases. The Veterinary Genetics laboratory at the University of California Davis offers testing for many of the equine disease listed in Table 55.1. New discoveries in DNA testing and in gene therapy will improve diagnosis and treatment of inherited ocular diseases in the equine industry.

References

1. Sandmeyer, L.S. and Bellone, R. (2017). Inherited ocular disorders. In: *Equine Ophthalmology*, 3e (ed. B.C. Gilger), 545–566. Ames, Iowa: Wiley Blackwell.
2. Wade, C.M., Giulotto, E., Sigurdsson, S. et al. (2009). Genome sequence, comparative analysis, and population genetics of the domestic horse. *Science* 326: 865–867.
3. Bellone, R.R. (2020). Genetics of equine ocular disease. *Vet. Clin. North Am. Equine Pract.* 36: 303–322.
4. Bellone, R.R. (2017). Genetic testing as a tool to identify horses with or at risk for ocular disorders. *Vet. Clin. North Am. Equine Pract.* 33: 627–645.
5. Whitley, R.D. and Vygantas, K.R. (2010). Presumed inherited ocular diseases. In: *Ophthalmic Diseases in Veterinary Medicine* (ed. C.L. Martin), 421–487. London: Manson Publishing/The Veterinary Press.
6. Boveland, S.D. (2019). Presumed inherited ocular diseases. In: *Ocular Diseases in Veterinary Medicine*, 2e (ed. C.L. Martin, J.P. Pickett, and B. Speiss), 651–696. Boca Raton, FL: CRC Press.
7. Peterson-Jones, S. and Ewart, S. (2011). Inherited ocular disorders. In: *Equine Ophthalmology*, 2e (ed. B.C. Gilger), 434–442. Missouri: Elsevier.
8. Fritz, K.L., Kaese, H.J., Valberg, S.J. et al. (2014). Genetic risk factors for insidious equine recurrent uveitis in Appaloosa horses. *Anim. Genet.* 45: 392–399.

9 Witzel, D.A., Riis, R.C., Rebhun, W.C. et al. (1977). Night blindness in the Appaloosa sibling occurrence. *J. Equine Med. Surg.* 1: 383–386.

10 Witzel, D.A., Smith, E.L., Wilson, R.D. et al. (1978). Congenital stationary night blindness: an animal model. *Invest. Ophthalmol. Vis. Sci.* 17: 788–795.

11 Rebhun, W.C., Loew, E.R., Riis, R.C. et al. (1984). Clinical manifestations of night blindness in the Appaloosa horse. *Compend. Contin. Educ. Pract. Vet.* 6: S103–S106.

12 Sandmeyer, L.S., Breaux, C.B., Archer, A. et al. (2007). Clinical and electroretinographic characteristics of congenital stationary night blindness in the Appaloosa and the association with the leopard complex. *Vet. Ophthalmol.* 10: 368–375.

13 Sandmeyer, L.S., Bellone, R.R., Archer, S. et al. (2012). Congenital stationary night blindness is associated with the leopard complex in the miniature horse. *Vet. Ophthalmol.* 15: 18–22.

14 Scott, M.L., John, E.E., Bellone, R.R. et al. (2016). Redundant contribution of a transient receptor potential cation channel member 1 exon 11 single nucleotide polymorphism to equine congenital stationary night blindness. *BMC Vet. Res.* 21: 121.

15 Bellone, R.R., Holl, H., Setaluri, V. et al. (2013). Evidence for a retroviral insertion in TRPM1 as the cause of congenital stationary night blindness and leopard complex spotting in the horse. *PLoS One* 8: e78280.

16 Holl, H.M., Brooks, S.A., Sandmeyer, L. et al. (2016). Differential gene expression with PATN1, a modifier of leopard complex spotting. *Anim. Genet.* 47: 91–101.

17 Ludwig, A., Reissmann, M., Benecke, N. et al. (2015). Twenty-five thousand years of fluctuating selection on leopard complex spotting and congenital night blindness in horses. *Philos. Trans. R. Soc. Lond. B Biol. Sci.* 370 (1660): 20130386.

18 Sponenberg, D.P., Carr, G., Simak, E. et al. (1990). The inheritance of the leopard complex of spotting patterns in horses. *J. Hered.* 81: 323–331.

19 Bellone, R.R., Brooks, S.A., Sandmeyer, L. et al. (2008). Differential gene expression of TRPM1, the potential cause of congenital stationary night blindness and coat spotting pattern (LP)in the Appaloosa horse (*Equus caballus*). *Genetics* 179: 1861–1870.

20 Morgans, C.W., Zhang, J., Jeffrey, B.G. et al. (2009). TRPM1 is required for the depolarizing light respone in retinal ON bipolar cells. *Proc. Natl. Acad. Sci. U. S. A.* 106: 19174–19178.

21 Morgans, C.W., Brown, R.L., Duvoisin, R.M. et al. (2010). TRPM1: the endpoint of the mFluR6signal transduction cascade in retinal ON-bipolar cells. *Bioessays* 32: 609–614.

22 Klooster, J., Blokker, J., Ten Brink, K.B. et al. (2011). Ultrastructural localization and expression of TRMP1 in the human retina. *Invest. Ophthalmol. Vis. Sci.* 52: 8356–8362.

23 Hughes, S., Pothecary, C.A., Jagannath, A. et al. (2012). Profound defects in pupillary responses to light in TRPM channel null mice: role for TRPM channels I non-image-forming photoreceptors. *Eur. J. Neurosci.* 3591: 34–43.

24 Anderson, L.S., Wilbe, M., Viluma, A. et al. (2013). Equine multiple congenital anomalies and silver coat color result from the pleiotropic effects of mutant PMEL. *PLoS One* 8 (9): e75639.

25 Ramsey, D.T., Sl, E., Render, J.A. et al. (1999). Congenital ocular abnormalities of Rocky Mountain horses. *Vet. Ophthalmol.* 2: 47–59.

26 Grahn, R.H., Pinard, C., Archer, S. et al. (2008). Congenital ocular anomalies in purebred and crossbred rocky and Kentucky Mountain horses in Canada. *Can. Vet. J.* 49: 675–681.

27 Anderson, L.S., Axelsson, J., Dubielzig, R.R. et al. (2011). Multiple congenital ocular anomalies in Icelandic horses. *BMC Vet. Res.* 7: 21.

28 Plummer, C.E. and Ramsey, D.T. (2011). A survey of ocular abnormalities in miniature horses. *Vet. Ophthalmol.* 14: 239–243.

29 Komaromy, A.M., Rowlan, J.S., La Croiz, N.C. et al. (2011). Equine multiple congenital ocular anomalies (MCOA) syndrome in PMEL17 (silver) mutant ponies: five cases. *Vet. Ophthalmol.* 14: 313–320.

30 Depecker, M., Segard, E., and cadore JL. (2013). Phenotypic description of multiple congenital ocular anomailies in Comtois horses. *Equine Vet. Educ.* 25: 511–516.

31 Kaps, S. and Spies, B.M. (2010). Multiple congenital ocular abnormalities (MCOA) in Rocky Mountain horses and Kentucky Mountain Saddle horses in Europe. *Pferdehdelkunde* 26: 536–540.

32 Sponenberg, D.P. (1996). Colors built from the basic colors. In: *Equine Color Genetics* (ed. D.P. Sponenberg), 41–42. Ames: Iowa State University Press.

33 Lee, Z.H., Hou, L., Moellmann, G. et al. (1996). Characterization and subcellular localization of human PMEL 17/silver, a110-kDa (pre)melanosomal membrane protein associated with 5,6-dihydroxyindole-2-caroxylic acid (DHICA) converting activity. *J. Invest. Dermatol.* 106: 605–610.

34 Theos, A.C., Truschel, S.T., Raposo, G. et al. (2006). The silver locus product PMEL 17/gp100/Silv/ME20: controversial in name and in function. *Pigment Cell Melanoma Res.* 18: 322–336.

35 Berson, J.F., Harper, D.C., Tenza, D. et al. (2001). PMEL17 initiates premelanosome morphogenesis within multivesicular bodies. *Mol. Biol. Cell* 12: 3451–3464.

36 Ramsey, D.T., Hauptman, J.G., and Peterson-Jones, S.M. (1999). Corneal thickness, intraocular pressure and optical corneal diameter in Rocky Mountain horses with cornea globosa or clinically normal corneas. *Am. J. Vet. Res.* 60: 1317–1321.

37 Ewart, S.L., Ramsey, D.T., Xu, J. et al. (2000). The horse homolog of congenital aniridia conforms to codominant inheritance. *J. Hered.* 91: 93–98.

38 Bromberg, E., Andersson, L., Cochran, G. et al. (2006). A missense mutation in PMEL17 is associated with the silver coat color in the horse. *Biomed. Central Genet.* 7: 46.

39 Gilger, B.C. (2010). Equine recurrent uveitis. The viewpoint from the USA. *Equine Vet. J. Suppl.* 37: 57–61.

40 Whitley, R.D. and Gelatt, K.N. (1981). Ocular manifestations of systemic disease in the horse. In: *Veterinary Ophthalmology* (ed. K.N. Gelatt), 724–741. Philadelphia: Lea & Febiger.

41 Dwyer, A.E., Crocett, R.S., and Klsow, C.M. (1995). Association of leptospiral seroreactivitiy and breed with uveitis and blindness in horses 372 cases (1986–1993). *J. Am. Vet. Med. Assoc.* 207: 1327–1331.

42 Wollanke, B., Gerhards, H., Brem, S. et al. (1998). Intraocular and serum antibody titers to Leptospira in 150 horses with equine recurrent uveitis (ERU) subjected to vitrectomy. *Berl. Munch. Tierarztl. Wochenschr.* 111: 134–139.

43 Wollanke, B., Rohrback, B.W., and Gerhards, H. (2001). Serum and vitreous humor antibody titers in and isolation of Leptospria interrogens from horses with recurrent uveitis. *J. Am. Vet. Med. Assoc.* 219: 795–800.

44 Brem, S., Gerhards, H., Wollanke, B. et al. (1999). 35 Leptospira isolated from the vitreous body of 32 horses with recurrent uveitis(ERU). *Berl. Munch Tierarztl WochenschrJ* 112: 390–393.

45 Faber, N.A., Crawford, M., LeFebvre, R.B. et al. (2000). Detection of Leptospira spp. in the aqueous humor of horses with naturally acquired recurrent uveitis. *J. Clin. Microbiol.* 38: 2731–2733.

46 Deeg, C.A., Ehrenhofer, M., Thurau, S.R. et al. (2002). Immunopathology of recurrent uveitis in spontaneously diseased horses. *Exp. Eye Res.* 75: 127–133.

47 Pearce, J.W., Galle, L.E., Kleiboeker, S.B. et al. (2007). Detection of Leptospira interrogans DNA and antigen in fixed equine eyes affected with end-stage equine recurrent uveitis. *J. Vet. Diagn. Invest.* 19: 686–690.

48 Gilger, B.C., Samon, J.H., Yi, N.Y. et al. (2008). Role of bacteria in the pathogenesis of recurrent uveitis in horses from the southeastern United States. *Am. J. Vet. Res.* 68: 1329–1335.

49 Gilger, B.C., Malok, E., Cutter, K.V. et al. (1999). Characterization of T-lymphocytes in the anterior uvea of eyes with chronic equine recurrent uveitis. *Vet. Immunol. Immunopathol.* 71: 17–28.

50 Kulbrock, M., Lehner, S., Metzger, J. et al. (2013). A genome-wide association study identifies risk loci to equine recurrent uveitis in German warmblood horses. *PLoS One* 8: e71619.

51 Janeway, C.A. Jr., Travers, P., Walort, M. et al. (2001). *Immunobiology: The Immune System in Health and Disease*, 5e. New York: Garland Science.

52 Angelos, J., Oppenheim, Y., Rebhun, W. et al. (1998). Evaluation of breed as a risk factor for sarcoid and uveitis in horses. *Anim. Genet.* 19: 417–425.

53 Gilger, B.C. and Hollingsworth, S.R. (2017). Diseases of the uvea, uveitis, and recurrent uveitis. In: *Equine Ophthalmology*, 3e (ed. B.C. Gilger), 369–415. Ames, Iowa: Wiley Blackwell.

54 Kulbrock, M., von Borstel, M., Rohn, K. et al. (2013). Occurrence and severity of equine recurrent uveitis in Warmblood horses –a comparative study. *Pferdcheilkunde* 29: 27–36.

55 Deeg, C.A., Marti, E., Gaillard, C. et al. (2004). Equine recurrent uveitis is strongly associated with the MHC class I haplotype ELA-A9. *Equine Vet. J.* 36: 73–75.

56 Dugan, S.J., Curtis, C.R., Roberts, S.M. et al. (1991). Epidemiologic study of ocular/adenexal squamous cell carcinoma in horses. *J. Am. Vet. Med. Assoc.* 198: 251–256.

57 Schwink, K. (1987). Factors influencing morbidity and outcome of equine ocular squamous cell carcinoma: a retrospective morphological description in 10 horses. *Equine Vet. J.* 19: 198–200.

58 Plummer, C.E., Smith, S., Andrew, S.E. et al. (2007). Combined keratectomy, strontium irradiation and permanent bulbar conjunctival grafts for corneolimbal squamous cell carcinoma in horses (1990–2002): 38 horses. *Vet. Ophthalmol.* 10: 37–42.

59 Michau, T.M., Davidson, M.G., and Gilger, B.C. (2012). Carbon dioxide laser photoablation adjunctive therapy following superficial lamellar keratectomy and bulbar conjunctivectomy for the treatment of corneolimbal squamous cell carcinoma in horses: a review of 24 cases. *Vet. Ophthalmol.* 15: 245–253.

60 Payne, R.I., Lean, M.S., and Greer, T.R. (2009). Third-eyelid resection as treatment for suspected squamous cell carcinoma in 24 horses. *Vet. Rec.* 165: 740–743.

61 Bosch, G. and Klein, W.R. (2005). Superficial keratectomy and cryosurgery as therapy for limbal neoplasms in 13 horses. *Vet. Ophthalmol.* 8: 241–246.

62 Smith, K.M., Scase, T.J., Miller, J.L. et al. (2008). Expression of cyclooxygenase-2 by equine ocular and adnexal squamous cell carcinoma. *Vet. Ophthalmol.* 11: 9–14.

63 Lassaline, M., Cranford, T.L., Latimer, C.A. et al. (2015). Limbal squamous cell carcinoma in Haflinger horses. *Vet. Ophthalmol.* 18 (5): 404–408.

64 Bellone, R.R., Liu, J., Petersen, J.L. et al. (2017). A missense mutation in damage-specific DNA binding protein 2 is a genetic risk factor for limbal squamous cell carcinoma in horses. *Int. J. Cancer* 141: 342–353.

65 Sironi, G., Riccaboni, P., Mertel, L. et al. (1999). p53 protein expression in conjunctival squamous cell carcinoma of domestic animals. *Vet. Ophthalmol.* 2: 227–231.

66 Greenbough, A., Smartt, H.J.M., Moore, A.M. et al. (2009). The COX-2PGE$_2$ pathway: key roles in the hallmarks of cancer and adaptation to the tumour microenvironment. *Cacinogenesis* 30: 377–386.

67 Elce, Y.A., Orsini, J.A., and Blikslager, A.T. (2007). Expression of cyclooxygenase and −2 in naturally occurring squamous cell carcinoma in horses. *Am. J. Vet. Res.* 68: 76–80.

68 Hisey, E.A., Hermans, H., Avila, F. et al. (2020). Whole genome sequencing identified a 16 kilobase deletion on ECA13 associated with distichiasis in Friesian horses. *BMC Genomics* 21: 848.

69 Lassaline-Utter, M., Gemensky-Metzler, G., Scherrer, N.M. et al. (2014). Corneal dystrophy in Friesian horses may represent a variant of pellucid marginal degeneration. *Vet. Ophthalmol.* 17: 186–194.

70 Lavach, J.D. (1990). Lens. In: *Large Animal Ophthalmology* (ed. J.D. Lavach), 185–201. St Louis: Mosby.

71 Whitley, R.D. (2005). Diseases and surgery of the lens. In: *Equine Ophthalmology* (ed. B.C. Gilger), 269–284. St Louis: Elsevier.

72 Whitley, R.D., Meek, L.A., Millichamp, N.J. et al. (1990). Cataract surgery in the horse: a review of six cases. *Equine Vet. J.* (Suppl): 85–90.

73 Millichamp, N.J. and Dziezyc, J. (2003). Cataract phacofragmentation in horses. *Vet. Ophthalmol.* 3: 157–164.

74 Severin, G.A. (1996). *Severin's Veterinary Ophthalmology Notes*, 3e, 379–406. Fort Collins: Colorado State University.

75 Beech, J., Aquirre, G., and Gross, S. (1984). Congenital nuclear cataracts in the Morgan horse. *J. Am. Vet. Med. Assoc.* 184: 1363–1365.

76 Beech, J. and Irby, N. (1985). Inherited nuclear cataracts in the Morgan horse. *J. Hered.* 76: 371–372.

77 Pinard, C.L. and Basrur, P.K. (2011). Ocular anomalies in a herd of Exmoor ponies in Canada. *Vet. Ophthalmol.* 14: 100–108.

78 Erikson, K. (1955). Hereditary aniridia with secondary cataracts in horses. *Nord. Vet. Med.* 7: 773–793.

79 Joyce, J.R., Martin, J.E., Storta, R.W. et al. (1990). Iridal hypoplasia (aniridia) accompanied by limbic dermoids and cataracts in a group of related quarter horses. *Equine Vet. J. Suppl.* 10: 26–28.

80 Joyce, J.R. (1983). Aniridia in a Quarter Horse. *Equine Vet. J. Suppl.* 2: 21–22.

81 Irby, N.L. and Aquirre, G.D. (1985). Congenital aniridia in a pony. *J. Am. Vet. Med. Assoc.* 186: 281–283.

82 McCormick, K.A., Ward, D., and Newkirk, K.M. (2013). Aniridia in two related Tennessee Walking Horses. *Case Rep. Vet. Med.* 703732.

83 Hakanson, N. (1993). Iris hypoplasi hos hast. *Svensk Veterinartidning* 45: 99–103.

84 Mack, M., Kowalski, E., Grahn, R. et al. (2017). Two variants in SLC24A5 are associated with "tiger-eye" iris pigmentation in Puerto Rican Paso Fino horses. *G3* 7: 2799–2806.

85 White, S.D., Affolter, V.K., Bannash, D.L. et al. (2004). Hereditary equine regional dermal asthenia ("hyperelastosis cutis") in 50 horses clinical histologic, immunohistologic and ultrastructural findings. *Vet. Dermatol.* 15: 207–217.

86 Tryon, R.C., White, S.D., and Bannash, D.L. (2007). Homozygousity mapping approach identifies a missense mutation in equine cyclophilin B (PPIB) associated with HERDA in the American Quarter Horse. *Genomics* 90: 93–102.

87 Brounts, S.H., Rashmir-Raven, A.M., and Black, S.S. (2001). Zonal dermal separation: a distinctive histopathological lesion associated with hyperelastosis cutis in a Quarter Horse. *Vet. Dermatol.* 12: 219–224.

88 Borges, A.S., Conceicao, L.G., Alves, A.L. et al. (2005). Hereditary equine regional dermal asthenia in three related quarter horses in Brazil. *Vet. Dermatol.* 16: 125–130.

89 Rashmir-Raven, A.M. (2013). Hereitable equine regional dermal asthenia. *Vet. Clin. North Am. Equine Pract.* 29: 689–702.

90 Mochal, C.A., Miller, W.W., Colley, J.A. et al. (2010). Ocular findings in Quarter Horses with hereditary equine regional dermal asthenia. *J. Am. Vet. Med. Assoc.* 237: 304–310.

91 Badial, P.R., Cisneros-Alvarez, L.E., Brandao, C.V.S. et al. (2015). Ocular dimensions, corneal thickness, and corneal curvature in Quarter horses with hereditary equine regional dermal asthenia. *Vet. Ophthalmol.* 18: 385–392.

92 Grady, J.G., Elder, S.H., Ryan, P.L. et al. (2009). Biomechanical and molecular characteristics of hereditary equine regional dermal asthenia in Quarter Horses. *Vet. Dermatol.* 20: 591–599.

93 Bachinger, H.P. (1987). The influence of peptidyl-prolyl cis-trans-isomerase on the in vitro folding of type III collagen. *J. Biol. Chem.* 262: 17144–17148.

94 Steinmann, B., Bruckner, P., and Superti-FurgaA. (1991). Cyclopsporine A slows collagen triple-helix formation in vivo: indirect evidence for a physiologic role of peptidyl-prolyl cis-trans-isomerase. *J. Biol. Chem.* 266: 1299–1303.

95 Cullen, C.L. and Webb, A.A. (2013). Ocular manifestations of systemic disease. Part 3: the horse. In: *Veterinary Ophthalmology*, 5e (ed. K.N. Gelatt, B.C. Gilger, and T.J. Kern), 2037–2070. Ames: Wiley.

96 Bowling, A.T., Byrns, G., and Spier, S. (1996). Evidence for a single pedigree source of the hyperkalemic periodic paralysis susceptibility gene in Quarter Horses. *Anim. Genet.* 27: 279–281.

97 Naylor, J.M. (1994). Selection of Quarter Horses affected with hyperkalemic periodic paralysis by show judges. *J. Am. Vet. Med. Assoc.* 204: 926–927.

98 Naylor, J.M. (1994). Equine hyperkalemic periodic paralysis: a review and implications. *Can. Vet. J.* 35: 279–285.

99 Rudolph, J.A., Spier, S., Byrns, G. et al. (1992). Periodic paralysis in Quarter Horses: a sodium channel mutation disseminated by selective breeding. *Nat. Genet.* 2: 144–147.

100 Kohn, C.W., Johnson, G.C., Garry, F.B. et al. (1989). Mechanobullous disese in two Belgian foals. *Equine Vet. J.* 21: 297–301.

101 Lieto, L.D., Swerczek, T.W., and Cothan, E.G. (2009). Equine epithliogenesis imperfect in two American Saddlebred foals is a lamina lucida defect. *Vet. Pathol.* 39: 575–580.

102 Milenkovic, D., Chaffauz, S., Taourit, S. et al. (2003). A mutation in the LAMC2 gene causes the Herlitz junction epidermolysis bullosa (H-JE) in two French draft horse breeds. *Genet. Sel. Evol.* 35: 249–256.

103 Cappelli, K., Brachelente, C., Passamonti, F. et al. (2015). First report of junctional epidermolysis bullosa (JEB) in the Italian draft horse. *BMC Vet. Res.* 11 (55): 1–4.

104 Johnson, G.C., Kohn, C.W., Johnson, C.W. et al. (1988). Ultrastructure of junctional epidermolysis bullosa in Belgian foals. *J. Comp. Pathol.* 98: 329–336.

105 Dubielzig, R., Wilson, J.W., Beck, K.A. et al. (1986). Dental dysplasia and epitheliogenesis imperfect in a foal. *Vet. Pathol.* 23: 325–327.

106 Shapiro, F. and McEwen, B. (1995). Mechanobullous disease in a Belgian foal in eastern Ontario. *Can. Vet. J.* 36: 572.

107 Graves, K.T., Henney, P.J., and Ennis, R.B. (2009). Partial deletion of the LAMA3 gene is responsible for hereditary junctional epidermolysis bullosa in the American Saddlebred horse. *Anim. Genet.* 40: 35–41.

108 Spirito, F., Charlesworth, A., Linder, K. et al. (2002). Animal models for skin blistering conditions: absence of laminin 5 causes hereditary junctional mechanbullous disese in the Belgian horse. *J. Invest. Dermatol.* 119: 684–691.

Chapter 56 Acquired Ocular Diseases in Neonatal Foals

Sara M. Smith and Brian C. Gilger

Ocular abnormalities recognized in neonatal foals are defined as congenital, inherited, or acquired. Congenital ocular defects, assumed to arise because of genetic abnormalities or various in utero insults, including infection, trauma, exposure to drugs or toxins, nutrient or vitamin deficiencies or excesses, ionizing radiation, and other unknown or idiopathic factors, are reviewed in Chapter 54. This chapter reviews ocular conditions in foals that develop in the neonatal period (≤30 days of age). To be able to assess the eyes of neonatal foals, clinicians must be able to differentiate between normal and abnormal ophthalmic examination findings. Therefore, a summary of normal ocular examination findings and diagnostics in equine neonates and how they differ from adult horses will be briefly reviewed with a full description discussed in Chapter 53. This is followed by a discussion of the diagnosis and treatment of ocular abnormalities associated with parturition followed by ocular conditions associated with neonatal encephalopathy including entropion and corneal ulceration. Uveal inflammatory conditions related to systemic disease such as those associated with septicemia and *Rhodococcus equi* infection will be discussed followed by traumatically acquired ocular conditions. For a comprehensive review of ocular abnormalities in foals, the reader is directed to additional specific references [1–4].

Ophthalmic Examination in Neonatal Foals

Normal ocular parameters of neonatal foals are listed in Table 56.1. The menace response in foals may not be present until 10–14 days after birth. In one study, a positive menace response was observed more frequently with increasing age, with most foals having a positive menace response at 5 days of age, and all foals exhibiting a positive menace by 9 days of age [5]. In another study, a menace response was not consistently observed until 16–21 days after birth [3]. Dazzle reflex and direct and consensual pupillary light reflexes (PLR) are present from birth, although PLR may be sluggish and possibly absent in excited foals [3, 5]. However, an abnormal PLR is a common clinical sign of bacterial meningoencephalitis in neonatal foals, so this condition should be considered if other neurologic abnormalities are present [8]. In healthy foals, during the first few days after birth, the pupils are oval to round in shape and assume the more adult shape (horizontal oval) by 3–5 days of age [1, 2]. Some foals also exhibit bilateral, ventromedial strabismus that resolves by 6–7 days after birth [3]. Regarding fundic examination findings, hyaloid artery remnants and optic disc hyperemia are present in nearly all neonatal foals [3, 4, 9, 10]. Standard ophthalmic diagnostic tests (i.e. intraocular pressure [IOP], tear production, fluorescein stain) can be performed in neonatal foals with proper restraint, many times without sedation. The mean IOP of foals is similar to adult horses, approximately 13.0 ± 5.0 mmHg (applanation tonometer) or 14.5 ± 4.0 mmHg (rebound tonometer) [4]. Corneal sensitivity, evaluated by use of the corneal touch threshold (CTT) with a Cochet-Bonnet aesthesiometer, was similar between foals and adult horses (CTT of approximately 5.0 cm). However, corneal sensitivity is decreased in ill neonatal foals and is hypothesized to be a factor in the frequent development of corneal ulcers [6]. Furthermore, in the same study, Schirmer tear test I values (STT, tear production) were significantly lower in healthy foals (12.8 ± 2.4 mm) compared to adult horses (18.3 ± 2.1 mm) [6]. Based on ocular ultrasound, the mean axial globe length (central cornea to retina) of neonatal foals measured 35.8 ± 1.2 mm (compared to 43.7 mm in an adult horse [11]) with no associations between gender, laterality (i.e. right vs left eyes), or body weight of the foal [7].

Equine Neonatal Medicine, First Edition. Edited by David M. Wong and Pamela A. Wilkins.

Table 56.1 Normal ocular parameters of healthy neonatal foals.

Ocular parameter	Age of onset	Comment/value	References
▪ Menace response	9, 16–21 d	—	[3, 5]
▪ Pupillary light reflex	At birth	Sluggish	[3, 5]
▪ Dazzle reflex	At birth	—	[3, 5]
▪ Pupil shape – round	1–5 d	Oval >5 d	[1, 2]
▪ Intraocular pressure	At birth	13–14 mmHg	[4]
▪ Schirmer tear test I	At birth	12.8 ± 2.4 mm	[6]
▪ Corneal touch threshold	At birth	5.0 cm	[6]
▪ Globe axial length	At birth	35.8 ± 1.2 mm	[7]

Ocular Abnormalities Associated with Parturition

Subconjunctival and retinal hemorrhages are commonly observed in foals during the early postnatal period (Table 56.2) [3, 4, 10, 12–14]. In a survey of Thoroughbred [12] and Standardbred [10] foals, 8.3% and 12.7%, respectively, had dorsal nasal bulbar subconjunctival hemorrhages (Figure 56.1), especially in the early neonatal period. Subconjunctival hemorrhages were also observed in some foals on the third eyelid [10]. Subconjunctival hemorrhages were not associated with other ocular or systemic disease and resolved spontaneously within 4–10 days [12]. In one study, 4/14 (35%) of 1-day-old foals had subconjunctival hemorrhages observed, but none were observed in foals 2–21 days of age, suggesting if present, the hemorrhages resolve rapidly [3].

Similarly, retinal hemorrhages are commonly observed in the early neonatal period, with reported incidences of 11.4% [4], 16% [13], and 18.6% [10]. Hemorrhages were most commonly observed in both eyes, were multifocal within the tapetal area, and located in the retinal or subretinal space (Figure 56.2) [3, 13, 14]. Retinal hemorrhages were not associated with other ocular or systemic disease and there was no discernable effect on vision [13]. Retinal hemorrhages spontaneously resolved within 10 days of birth [13]; however, one survey did not observe retinal hemorrhages after 1 day postpartum [3]. The cause of subconjunctival and retinal hemorrhages in neonatal foals is unknown, but trauma associated with parturition is suspected. It was suggested that larger foals (>51 kg), were at increased risk of retinal hemorrhages [13]; however, this was not supported in a later study where all foals with retinal hemorrhages were <45 kg. The clinician should note that these hemorrhages are common in foals, especially in the early neonatal period, and typically resolve spontaneously.

Other ocular conditions occur sporadically and have been suggested to be associated with parturition, especially with dystocia. These include eyelid injuries (blepharitis, hemorrhage, lacerations), conjunctival hyperemia, and ulcerative and nonulcerative keratitis [1–3, 14].

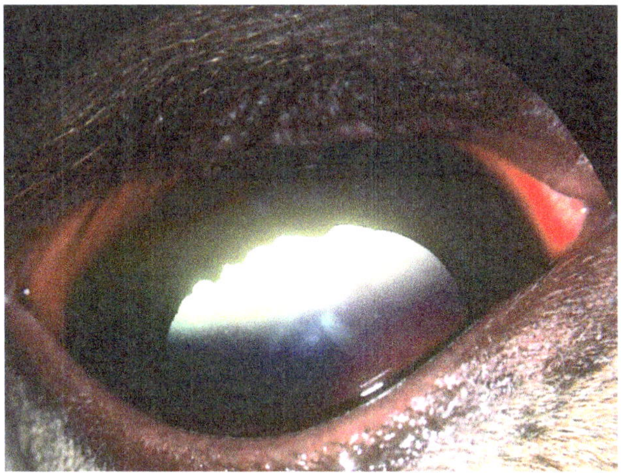

Figure 56.1 Bulbar subconjunctival hemorrhage in a neonatal foal. This is a common finding in foals and is thought to be associated with parturition trauma. Subconjunctival hemorrhage generally resolves spontaneously. *Source:* Image provided by Dr. Andy Matthews.

Table 56.2 Ocular abnormalities possibly associated with parturition in the early neonatal period in the foal.

Ocular abnormality	Resolution	Prevalence	References
▪ Subconjunctival hemorrhages	4–10 d	8.3–12.7%	[3, 10, 12]
▪ Retinal hemorrhages	<10 d	11.4–18.6%	[3, 4, 10, 13]
▪ Conjunctival hyperemia	<15 d	48%	[3]
▪ Blepharitis/lacerations	<7 d	—	[4]
▪ Ulcerative and nonulcerative keratitis	<7 d	—	[1, 3]

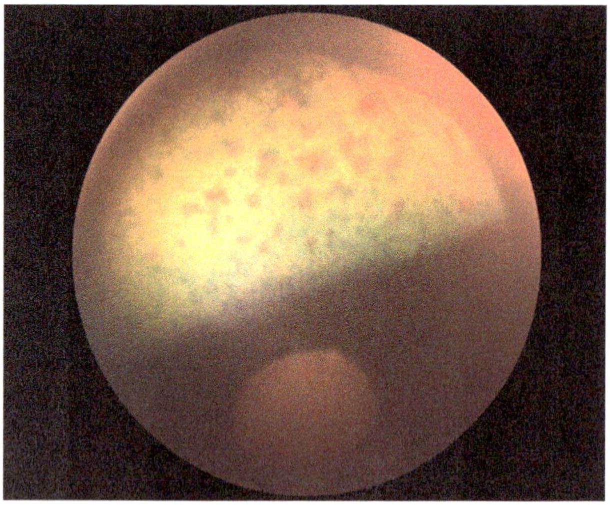

Figure 56.2 Retinal hemorrhages in the tapetal fundus of a newborn foal. *Source:* Image provided by Dr. Marta Leiva.

Ocular Disease Associated with Prematurity and Neonatal Encephalopathy

Prematurity and neonatal encephalopathy are common clinical entities in foals [15–17]. Ocular disease observed in foals that are premature or that have neonatal encephalopathy commonly fall into two categories: eyelid and corneal disease. The most common eyelid disease is entropion, which can be present in one or both eyelids; however, the lower lid is more commonly affected than the upper eyelid (Figure 56.3). Generally, entropion in foals is most often secondary to dehydration, where the globe becomes enophthalmic and the eyelids roll inward [14]. Corneal ulceration, also seen more commonly in ill dehydrated foals, can result in spastic contraction of the orbicularis oculi muscle because of corneal pain, aggravating the resultant spastic entropion, and subsequently inducing further irritation of the cornea. The treatment of entropion depends on the cause and severity. In dehydrated, premature, and encephalopathic foals, supportive care including IV fluids and frequent lubrication of the corneal surface with a protective ophthalmic ointment may be sufficient. If entropion does not resolve or if corneal ulceration is present, vertical mattress tacking sutures (4-0 or 5-0 nylon or silk nonabsorbable sutures) can be placed to evert the eyelid margin for 10–14 days (Figure 56.3). Rarely, a Hotz-Celsus entropion surgical procedure is necessary if entropion does not resolve or recurs after 10–14 days following suture removal. Hyaluronic dermal fillers, injected into the eyelid at the area of the entropion, may be a biocompatible and less scarring treatment for foal entropion [18], but additional study needs to be evaluated before routine use in foals is recommended.

Corneal Ulcers (Ulcerative Keratitis)

Corneal ulcers, with or without entropion, are common in ill foals (Figure 56.4). Corneal sensitivity is significantly lower in ill foals and those with neonatal encephalopathy compared with adult horses [6]. The combination of lower tear production and decreased corneal sensitivity in ill foals may explain the higher incidence of corneal disease seen when compared to adult horses [6, 14]. Superficial corneal ulcers develop when the epithelium has been removed, usually as a result of trauma or persistent irritation (i.e. entropion, cornea in direct contact with bedding), exposing the underlying corneal stroma (Figure 56.4). Diagnosis of corneal ulceration is made by application of topical

(a) (b)

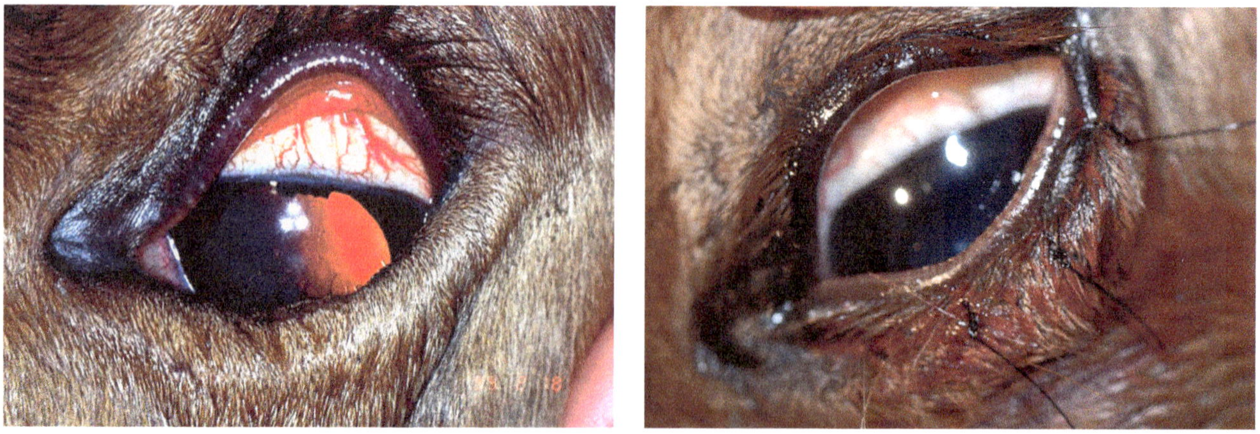

Figure 56.3 Entropion. (a) Lower eyelid entropion in a neonatal foal. (b) Correction of entropion after placement of three vertical mattress sutures.

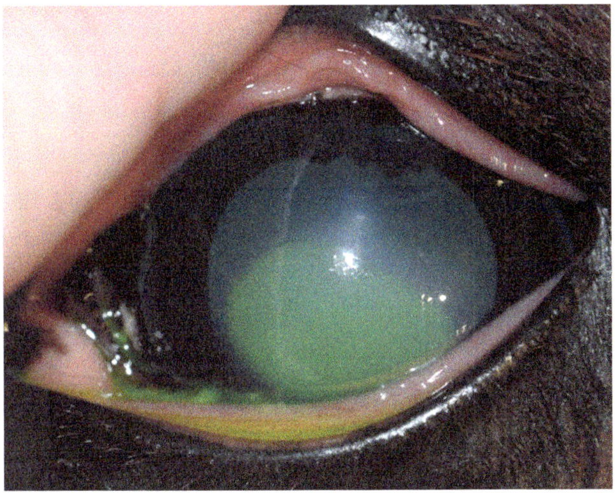

Figure 56.4 Superficial corneal ulcer in a foal following trauma. These superficial ulcers have epithelial loss but no corneal stromal involvement.

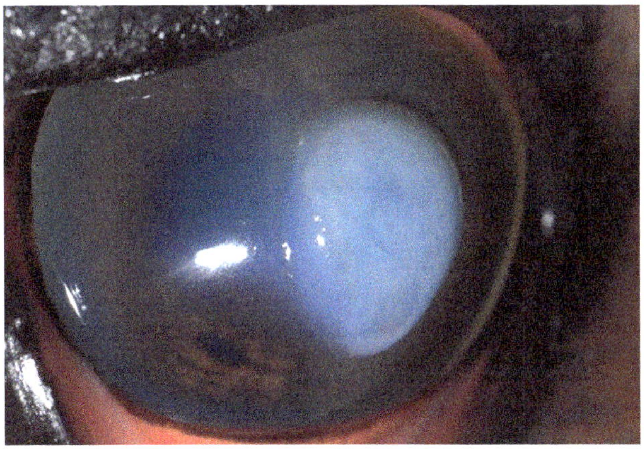

Figure 56.5 Complicated, malacic corneal ulcer in a foal. Culture, cytology, and aggressive medical therapy is warranted.

fluorescein dye to the corneal surface, which is retained by exposed corneal stroma, but not retained by intact corneal epithelium. As long as there is no persistent underlying irritation or presence of infection, superficial corneal ulcers heal rapidly, typically within 5–7 days. For superficial, uncomplicated corneal ulcers, treatment consists of topical prophylactic antibiotic (q 6–8h), such as neomycin-bacitracin-polymyxin (Table 56.3). However, if a visible stromal defect or corneal divot, white or yellow stromal cellular infiltrate, or extensive corneal edema is present, infection may be present and more aggressive diagnostics and treatment is warranted (Figure 56.5). For complicated stromal corneal ulcers, samples for bacterial and fungal culture should be collected followed by scraping of the cornea (i.e. periphery of the ulcer) for immediate cytologic examination to evaluate for presence of inflammatory cells and/or microorganisms. Aggressive therapy is needed for complicated corneal ulcers including a second-line topical antibiotic such as moxifloxacin or ofloxacin (q 3–4h). Topical antifungals, mydriatics, systemic nonsteroidal anti-inflammatory drugs (NSAIDs) and systemic antibiotics should also be considered depending on clinical and cytologic findings (Table 56.3). When medications are required more than four times a day, placement of a

Table 56.3 Common treatment regimens for uncomplicated versus complicated corneal ulceration.

Route of therapy	Treatment	Frequency	Duration
Superficial uncomplicated	▪ Topical antibiotic (triple antibiotic, oxytetracycline)	q6–8h	5–10 d
	▪ Topical mydriatic (atropine)	q24h	3–7 d
Stromal complicated	▪ Topical antibiotic[a] (moxifloxacin, ofloxacin)	q6–8h[b]	10–14 d[c]
	▪ Topical mydriatic (atropine)	q12–24h	7–14 d[c]
	▪ Topical antifungal (voriconazole)	q6–8h[b]	10–14 d[c]
Systemic	▪ Systemic nonsteroidal anti-inflammatory drug (NSAID)	q12h	Up to 7 d
	▪ Supportive care	—	—

[a] Choice of antibiotic or antifungal depends on cytologic and culture results.
[b] Recommend that a SPL be placed to deliver medications when required more frequently than every 6 hours.
[c] Duration of therapy depends on how quickly ulcer heals. In some cases, therapy may be required for 4–6 weeks.

subpalpebral lavage catheter (SPL) is recommended. A SPL catheter allows delivery of medication to the surface of the eye through the catheter without the caretaker having to touch the eye itself. This is not only more protective for the eye, but also less stressful and less painful for the foal. For more information on performing and interpreting corneal cytology and placing an SPL, please see this reference [19].

If there is progressive deepening of corneal ulceration, especially if the ulcer is estimated to be ≥50% of the corneal depth, or if the cornea becomes malacic (i.e. melting; Figure 56.5), then surgical repair should be considered. Surgical repair consists of debridement of the infected tissue followed by a conjunctival, amnion, or synthetic graft. Following surgery, medications to manage the infection and intraocular inflammation are continued for 4–8 weeks (Table 56.3).

Uveitis Associated with Systemic Disease

Uveitis is inflammation of the uveal tract, which includes the iris and ciliary body (anterior uveitis) or the choroid and retina (posterior uveitis). Uveitis can occur secondary to local ocular disease such a corneal ulceration, blunt or penetrating trauma, or can result from systemic disease. Any infectious or noninfectious inflammatory condition may compromise the blood ocular barrier leading to influx of inflammatory mediators and subsequent leakage of protein, fibrin, and inflammatory and/or red blood cells from uveal tissue into the aqueous and vitreous humor.

Reports of ocular manifestations of systemic disease in neonatal foals are primarily limited to those related to neonatal septicemia [4, 20] and *R. equi* infection [21–25] with individual reports involving adenoviral infection [26], equine herpesvirus-1 [27], and neonatal isoerythrolysis [28]. Other infectious diseases such as *Streptococcus equi* subsp. *equi* (strangles) [29, 30], *Borrelia burgdorferi* [31, 32], leptospirosis [33–36], and equine viral arteritis [37, 38] are also reported causes of uveitis, but are typically observed in adult horses.

Clinical Signs of Anterior Uveitis

Clinical signs of anterior uveitis are similar among etiologies with no pathognomonic finding for any specific disease. Ocular examination findings can range in severity with nonspecific signs of blepharospasm, conjunctival hyperemia, epiphora, blepharitis, and photophobia while miosis, aqueous flare, intraocular fibrin, and/or hypopyon formation are specific findings for anterior uveitis and indicative of blood aqueous barrier breakdown (Figure 56.6; Table 56.4). Posterior uveitis is associated with retinal hemorrhage, retinal detachment, chorioretinal infiltrates, and/or swelling or hemorrhage of the optic nerve head (optic neuritis). However, it is not uncommon for the extent of anterior inflammation to preclude examination of the ocular posterior segment (i.e. vitreous humor, retina, choroid, optic nerve). When associated with a systemic disease, clinical signs of uveitis are often bilateral and can be symmetrical or asymmetrical [20, 21]. The development of uveitis secondary to systemic disease has been linked to poorer outcomes

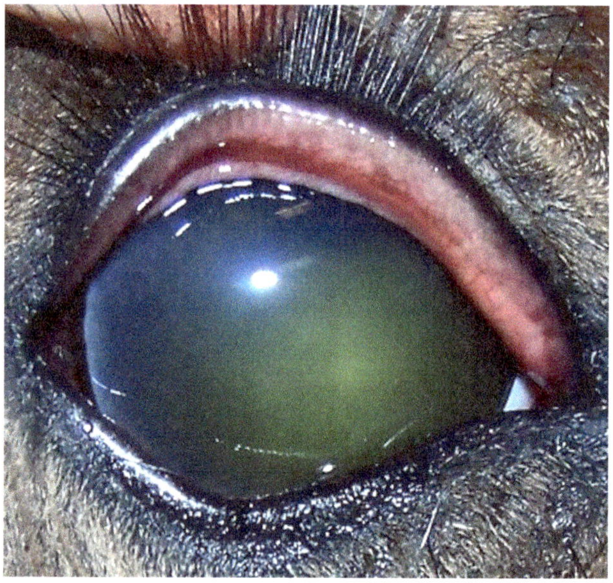

Figure 56.6 Uveitis in a neonatal foal with *Rhodoccocus* spp. The green-colored aqueous humor in foals is characteristic of uveitis secondary to *Rhodococcus* infections. *Source:* image provided by Dr. Ann Dwyer.

Table 56.4 Ocular findings with anterior uveitis.

■ Lacrimation	■ Blepharospasm	■ Photophobia
■ Conjunctival hyperemia	■ Ciliary injection	■ Corneal edema
■ Corneal vascularization	■ Changes in iris color	■ Miosis
■ Hypotony	■ Fibrin formation	■ Hypopyon
■ Hyphemia		

and decreased survival rates compared to systemically ill foals that do not develop uveitis [4, 20, 21].

Uveitis must be treated aggressively to rapidly minimize inflammation and prevent further damage to the ocular structures associated with anterior uveitis. Systemic treatment is aimed at treating the underlying disease process, and systemic anti-inflammatories are recommended in cases of uveitis, ensuring they can be safely tolerated by the foal. Whether or not systemic anti-inflammatories can be administered, topical corticosteroids or NSAIDs are the mainstay of treatment to decrease intraocular inflammation along with topical atropine to minimize intraocular pain and prevent adhesion formation (Table 56.5). Untreated or unresponsive uveitis can result in permanent ocular sequelae including corneal edema, iris fibrosis and hyperpigmentation, synechia formation, corpora nigra degeneration, permanent miosis, cataract formation, vitreous and retinal degeneration, and in an end-stage eye, blindness, and phthisis bulbi formation (small and shrunken eye).

The development or presence of corneal ulceration in eyes with uveitis will affect treatment regimens as topical corticosteroids are contraindicated in the presence of corneal ulceration. Topical corticosteroids can delay healing and are associated with the development and severity of fungal keratitis [39]. Therefore, the use of systemic anti-inflammatories is warranted in these cases, along with appropriate topical antimicrobials.

Table 56.5 Common treatment regimen for neonatal foals with uveitis.

Route of therapy	Treatment	Frequency	Duration
Systemic	▪ NSAID	q12h	up to 7 d
	▪ Treat underlying systemic disease process	—	—
	▪ Supportive care	—	—
Topical	▪ Anti-inflammatory (dexamethasone, prednisone, NSAID)	q6h	10–14 d (taper)
	▪ Antibiotic (triple antibiotic, oxytetracycline)	q6h	10–14 d[a]
	▪ Mydriatic (atropine)	q24h	Up to 7 d
	▪ Lubricant (ointment, hyaluronic acid)	q6h	10–14 d

[a] Duration of therapy depends on how quickly ulcer heals. In some cases, therapy may be required for 4–6 weeks.

Uveitis Associated with Neonatal Septicemia

Anterior uveitis is well documented in septic neonatal foals, especially those with failure of passive transfer or with other immunodeficiencies [4, 20]. Sepsis results in alterations of microcirculation, vascular insult, and subsequent disruption of endothelial barriers [40]. Both Gram-positive and Gram-negative bacteria have been associated with anterior uveitis in septic foals; however, Gram-negative organisms such as *Escherichia coli* are more frequently isolated [8, 20]. Additionally, studies in humans suggest that infections caused by Gram-positive organisms are associated with a lower inflammatory response than Gram-negative sepsis [41].

The incidence of uveitis in septic foals has been reported to be 25–26% and associated with a variety of underlying systemic diseases including enteritis, pneumonia, polyarthritis, meningoencephalitis, umbilical abscesses, failure of passive transfer, and neonatal encephalopathy [4, 20]. In septic foals, those with a positive blood culture had a higher incidence of uveitis (40%) compared to nonbacteremic septic foals (19%), suggesting an important role of bacteremia in triggering anterior uveitis. Foals with uveitis often display bilateral signs with varying degrees of asymmetry, while more severe clinical signs such as fibrin formation and posterior uveitis are typically observed in foals with bacteremia [20]. Additionally, significantly poorer outcomes and survival rates have been associated with septic foals with uveitis compared to septic foals without uveitis [4, 20].

The presence of anterior uveitis and optic neuritis along with various neuro-ophthalmic abnormalities including nystagmus, ventrolateral positional strabismus, and decreased to absent PLRs have been observed in foals diagnosed with bacterial meningoencephalitis secondary to sepsis [8]. As bacterial meningoencephalitis is a severe complication of sepsis, these foals had an even higher incidence of poorer outcomes, with only 20% of foals in one study surviving to discharge [8].

Uveitis Associated with *Rhodococcus equi*

R. equi, a Gram-positive coccobacillus, causes pyogranulomatous bronchopneumonia and is a well-described cause of morbidity and mortality in foals 3 weeks to 6 months of age. Extrapulmonary disorders (EPD) from direct or hematogenous extension of infection or from immunological response are frequently identified with a prevalence rate of at least one EPD in 54–76% of foals with *R. equi* pneumonia [24, 42, 43]. Reported EPD associated with *R. equi* include septic and nonseptic polysynovitis, immune-mediated hemolytic anemia, intrabdominal abscesses, peritonitis, nephritis, hepatitis, ulcerative enterocolitis and typhlitis, meningitis, and uveitis [21–23, 25, 44–47]. The incidence of uveitis ranges from 11% to 31% in foals with *R. equi* pneumonia [21, 24].

A recent report specifically characterizing ocular inflammatory findings in foals with *R. equi* bronchopneumonia observed anterior uveitis in 30.8% (12/39) of cases [21]. All foals exhibited bilateral, symmetrical anterior uveitis with 25% considered to have mild uveitis, while 75% (9/12) of affected foals were considered to have severe bilateral uveitis. Additionally, five of the severely affected uveitic foals had a green-colored aqueous flare (Figure 56.6), an ocular finding not previously described in the literature. No aqueous humor cytology nor histopathology was performed on these eyes, but acute ocular inflammation with high concentration of polymorphonuclear cells could cause this change in aqueous coloration, and green aqueous flare could be considered a suggestive sign of *R. equi* in foals with clinical signs of bronchopneumonia [21]. Despite aggressive systemic treatment, 23% of foals died with 44% of these nonsurviving foals having concurrent severe uveitis. The case fatality rate differed significantly between foals with and without uveitis, being 33.3% in uveitis-affected foals and 18.5% in foals without uveitis. Results from this study demonstrate that bilateral anterior uveitis is prevalent in about a third of foals with *R. equi* bronchopneumonia and severity of uveitis might be a nonsurvival prognostic factor [21].

As anterior uveitis is commonly associated with systemic disease, a complete ocular examination should be routinely performed in any ill foal with suspected sepsis, infectious disease, or immunocompromised immune status. Early identification of anterior uveitis in foals not only allows for appropriate treatment and prevention of permanent ocular sequela but can also provide additional diagnostic and prognostic information.

Traumatically Acquired Ocular Diseases

Acquired disease is common in foals because of their prominent laterally positioned eyes with common sources of trauma in their environment including bedding, hay, vegetation, stalls, and other horses. Eyelid lacerations, blunt trauma, abrasions, contusions, blepharitis, and blepharoedema are all possible injuries from trauma [1], especially foals with visual impairment (congenital cataracts, severe intraocular inflammation, severe corneal ulceration) or recumbency due to illness. Systemically ill foals not only have a lower reported corneal sensitivity compared to healthy foals [6] but are also typically recumbent with eyelids in direct contact with bedding, which pose and even higher risk of corneal disease and periocular skin irritation. Appropriate supportive care, bedding changes, and position changes are needed, along with frequent ocular monitoring, as these foals may not show typical outward clinical signs (blepharospasm, epiphora) of ocular discomfort compared to healthy foals. In ill foals with prolonged recumbency, corneal injury can be prevented/lessened through appropriate positioning, avoidance of bedding into the eye, correction of entropion (if present), frequent use of ocular lubricants, and routine (daily) fluorescein staining of the eye to check for the presence of early ulcers.

Eyelid Lacerations

Eyelid lacerations and blunt trauma resulting in orbital fractures are infrequently reported in foals, but treatment and surgical management of these conditions are similar to those in adult horses. The extent of eyelid injury can vary from involving only a portion of a single eyelid to affecting large sections of both the upper and lower eyelids, often seen with ripping of the eyelid along its orbito-palpebral sulcus (Figure 56.7).

Even with severe lacerations, the eyelids are highly vascularized and often heal well with primary closure [48]. In rare cases, when eyelid trauma is so severe that repair is not possible, such that the eyelids are completely severed and/or there is extensive concurrent ocular damage (globe rupture, large corneal laceration with iris prolapse), then exenteration is indicated and the wound is allowed to heal by second intention. During initial evaluation, a complete ocular examination should be performed to identify the extent of the trauma and identify any concurrent abnormalities, such as corneal ulceration or secondary uveitis that would require additional treatment [49].

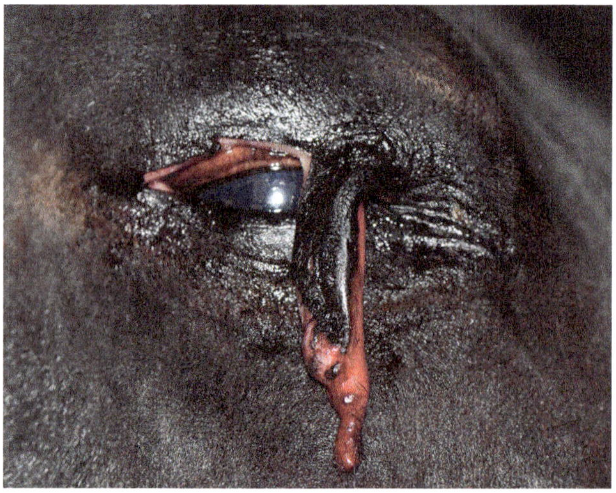

Figure 56.7 Eyelid laceration in the upper eyelid of a foal. Surgical correction of the eyelid was performed.

Eyelid lacerations should be repaired surgically and quickly, as unrepaired eyelid injuries can result in permanent defects that can lead to chronic keratitis, trichiasis (eyelid hairs contacting corneal surface), and recurrent corneal ulceration. Surgical repair can be performed under sedation with local anesthetic blocks with the foal in lateral recumbency or under general anesthesia. When repairing an eyelid laceration, the goal is to maintain integrity of the eyelid margin with as perfect apposition as possible. Gentle debridement of any necrotic tissue may be needed to obtain clean, fresh wound edges; however, it is imperative to take meticulous care to not cut or remove unnecessary amounts of tissue. Overly aggressive eyelid debridement or excision of too much eyelid margin can result in persistent exposure keratitis and discomfort. For more information on repair of eyelid lacerations in horses, the reader is directed to these references [49–51].

Postoperatively, the foal should wear a protective visor to prevent rubbing at the incision. Treatment consists of topical antimicrobials administered q6–8h, systemic anti-inflammatories for 3–5 days, and often systemic antibiotics. Topical treatment should be continued until skin sutures are removed in 10–14 days. Prognosis for eyelid lacerations is generally good as long as surgery was performed accurately.

Orbital Fractures

Fractures of the equine orbit and skull in foals (Figure 56.8) can result from trauma associated with direct kicks, collisions with stationary objects, and rearing in confined spaces. The equine orbit is formed from the frontal, lacrimal, zygomatic, and temporal bones to form a complete, bony orbital rim, while the internal wall of the orbit is formed form the sphenoid and palatine bones. The dorsal orbital rim, especially the zygomatic process of the frontal bone and zygomatic arch, are most prone to trauma. Orbital fractures can be diagnosed by digital palpation, radiographically, or by magnetic resonance imaging (MRI) or computed tomography (CT). Due to the complexity of the equine orbit and superimposition of bony structures on radiographs, advanced imaging such as CT is recommended to best guide treatment, surgical planning, and prognosis. Fractures of orbital bones can lead to impingement or damage of orbital structures including the globe, optic nerve, extraocular muscles, and nasolacrimal apparatus (Figure 56.8). Poll trauma, typically from rearing backward, can result in blindness due to damage of the sphenoid bones that form the optic canal and internal orbital wall.

Fractures can be treated medically or surgically, with the decision based on severity and displacement of the fractures and effects on ocular structures. Surgically, fractures can be repaired in a closed reduction or open exploration and reduction with the use of internal fixation implants [49, 52, 53]. Most reports on orbital and skull trauma occur in adult horses, however there are a few cases of orbital fractures in foals ranging from 2 weeks to 7 months of age. A 2.5-week-old Quarter Horse was diagnosed with left-sided sphenoid bone and palatine bone fractures secondary to head trauma from the mare rolling during a violent colic episode. The foal had concurrent left-sided facial swelling, corneal ulceration, and lack of vision. This foal was treated medically and improved neurologically, however vision in the left eye remained diminished at 15 months postinjury [54]. Open, surgical repair for displaced fractures of the zygomatic process of the frontal bone is described in foals between 3-7 months of age, which resulted in excellent postoperative cosmesis and good functional outcome [55, 56].

(a) (b)

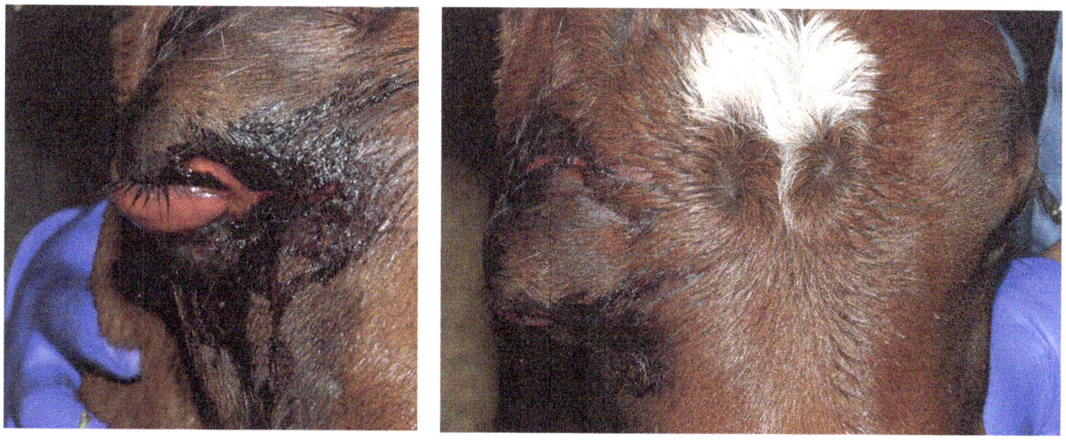

Figure 56.8 (a and b). Severe subconjunctival hemorrhage, periorbital swelling, and periocular lacerations in a foal that sustained direct trauma to the right globe and orbit. A scleral rupture was diagnosed via orbital ultrasound, and a fracture of the dorsal orbital rim was diagnosed on direct palpation. Due to the severity of the trauma, this right eye was enucleated.

Other Acquired Ocular Diseases

Various case reports on other acquired ocular findings in neonatal foals are few. In foals diagnosed with neonatal isoerythrolysis, in addition to systemic signs of icterus, pale mucous membranes, and progressive lethargy and tachycardia, ocular signs can include pale to icteric conjunctiva with scleral and conjunctival hemorrhages [57]. A recent case report described a 2-day-old Arabian filly presenting for neurologic impairment and blindness following accidental ingestion of an entire tube of 1.87% ivermectin paste. The foal was laterally recumbent on presentation, and ophthalmic examination revealed bilateral absent menace response, absent dazzle reflex and absent PLRs with pupils remaining fixed and dilated. Corneal sensation and palpebral reflexes were intact, and the remainder of the ophthalmic examination, including the retina and optic nerve, was normal. Treatment consisted of IV fluids, systemic antibiotics, and an IV 20% intralipid emulsion. Significant improvement was observed following 12 hours of lipid therapy, and the foal regained menace and PLRs at 72 hours following treatment [58].

Conclusions

Acquired ocular diseases in foals are very common, especially in premature foals and those with septicemia or neonatal encephalopathy. Daily ocular examinations of these foals are recommended, and preventative care, such as the use of frequent ocular lubricants, is recommended to minimize ocular irritation and trauma. Any evidence of ocular inflammation warrants an extensive systemic workup because of the common association between uveitis and systemic illness, such as septicemia. Furthermore, because of common ocular and periocular trauma in neonatal foals, caring for them in a safe, protective environment is needed.

We thank Erin Barr for photography and for acquiring images used in this chapter.

References

1 Latimer, C.A., Wyman, M., and Hamilton, J. (2010). An ophthalmic survey of the neonatal horse. *Equine Vet. J.* 15: 9–14.

2 Leiva, M. and Peña, T. (2016). Ophthalmic diseases of foals. In: *Equine Ophthalmology*, 3e (ed. B.C. Gilger), 112–150. Wiley Blackwell.

3 Leiva, M., Peña, T., and Monreal, L. (2011). Ocular findings in healthy newborn foals according to age. *Equine Vet. Educ.* 23: 40–45.

4 Labelle, A.L., Hamor, R.E., Townsend, W.M. et al. (2011). Ophthalmic lesions in neonatal foals evaluated for nonophthalmic disease at referral hospitals. *J. Am. Vet. Med. Assoc.* 239: 486–492.

5 Enzerink, E. (1998). The menace response and pupillary light reflex in neonatal foals. *Equine Vet. J.* 30: 546–548.

6 Brooks, D.E., Clark, C.K., and Lester, G.D. (2000). Cochet-Bonnet aesthesiometer-determined corneal sensitivity in neonatal foals and adult horses. *Vet. Ophthalmol.* 3: 133–137.

7 Valentini, S., Castagnetti, C., Musella, V. et al. (2014). Assessment of intraocular measurements in neonatal foals and association with gender, laterality, and body weight: a clinical study. *PLoS One* 9: e109491.

8 Viu, J., Monreal, L., Jose-Cunilleras, E. et al. (2012). Clinical findings in 10 foals with bacterial meningoencephalitis. *Equine Vet. J.* 44: 100–104.

9 Munroe, G. (2000). Study of the hyaloid apparatus in the neonatal Thoroughbred foal. *Vet. Rec.* 146 (20): 579–584.

10 Barsotti, G., Sgorbini, M., Marmorini, P. et al. (2013). Ocular abnormalities in healthy standardbred foals. *Vet. Ophthalmol.* 16: 245–250.

11 Visser, H.E., Diehl, K.A., Whitley, R.D. et al. (2017). Effect of auriculopalpebral nerve block on Schirmer tear test I values in normal horses. *Vet. Ophthalmol.* 20: 568–570.

12 Munroe, G. (1999). Subconjunctival haemorrhages in neonatal Thoroughbred foals. *Vet. Rec.* 144: 279–282.

13 Munroe, G. (2000). Survey of retinal haemorrhages in neonatal Thoroughbred foals. *Vet. Rec.* 146: 95–106.

14 Turner, A.G. (2004). Ocular conditions of neonatal foals. *Vet. Clin. North Am. Equine Pract.* 20: 429–440.

15 MacLeay, J.M. (2000). Neonatal maladjustment syndrome. *J. Equine Vet. Sci.* 20: 88–90.

16 Gold, J.R. (2017). Perinatal asphyxia syndrome. *Equine Vet. Educ.* 29: 158–164.

17 Vaala, W.E. (2003). Perinatal asphyxia syndrome in foals. In: *Current Therapy in Equine Medicine*, 5e (ed. N.E. Robinson). Elsevier https://doi.org/10.1016/B978-0-7216-9540-2.50182-1.

18 Beasley, K.L., Weiss, M.A., and Weiss, R.A. (2009). Hyaluronic acid fillers: a comprehensive review. *Facial Plast. Surg.* 25: 86–94.

19 Dwyer, A.E. (2016). Practical field ophthalmology. In: *Equine Ophthalmology*, 3e (ed. B.C. Gilger). Wiley Blackwell https://doi.org/10.1002/9781119047919.ch3.

20 Leiva, M., Peña, T., Armengou, L. et al. (2010). Uveal inflammation in septic newborn foals. *J. Vet. Intern. Med.* 24: 391–397.

21 Tarancón, I., Leiva, M., Jose-Cunilleras, E. et al. (2019). Ophthalmologic findings associated with *Rhodococcus equi* bronchopneumonia in foals. *Vet. Ophthalmol.* 22: 660–665.

22 Blogg, J.R., Barton, M.D., Graydon, R. et al. (2010). Blindness caused by *Rhodococcus equi* infection in a foal. *Equine Vet. J.* 15: 25–26.

23 Patterson-Kane, J., Buergelt, C., and Brown, C. (2001). *Rhodococcus equi* septicemia with pyogranulomatous hepatitis and panuveitis in an Arabian foal. *Eur. J. Vet. Pathol.* 7: 31–33.

24 Reuss, S.M., Keith Chaffin, M., and Cohen, N.D. (2009). Extrapulmonary disorders associated with *Rhodococcus equi* infection in foals: 150 cases (1987–2007). *J. Am. Vet. Med. Assoc.* 235: 855–863.

25 Huber, L., Giguère, S., Berghaus, L.J. et al. (2018). Development of septic polysynovitis and uveitis in foals experimentally infected with *Rhodococcus equi*. *PLoS One* 13 (2): e0192655.

26 McChesney, A.E., England, J.J., and Rich, L.J. (1973). Adenoviral infection in foals. *J. Am. Vet. Med. Assoc.* 162: 545–549.

27 McCartan, C.G., Russell, M.M., Wood, J.L. et al. (1995). Clinical, serological and virological characteristics of an outbreak of paresis and neonatal foal disease due to equine herpesvirus-1 on a stud farm. *Vet. Rec.* 136: 7–12.

28 Wotman, K.L. and Johnson, A.L. (2017). Ocular manifestations of systemic disease in the horse. *Vet. Clin. North Am. Equine Pract.* 33: 563–582.

29 Barratt-Boyes, S.M., Young, R.L., Canton, D.D. et al. (1991). *Streptococcus equi* infection as a cause of panophthalmitis in a horse. *J. Equine Vet. Sci.* 11: 229–231.

30 Roberts, S.R. (1971). Chorioretinitis in a band of horses. *J. Am. Vet. Med. Assoc.* 158: 2043–2046.

31 Priest, H.L., Irby, N.L., Schlafer, D.H. et al. (2012). Diagnosis of borrelia-associated uveitis in two horses. *Vet. Ophthalmol.* 15: 398–405.

32 Johnstone, L.K., Engiles, J.B., Aceto, H. et al. (2016). Retrospective evaluation of horses diagnosed with neuroborreliosis on postmortem examination: 16 cases (2004–2015). *J. Vet. Intern. Med.* 30: 1305–1312.

33 Gerding, J.C. and Gilger, B.C. (2016). Prognosis and impact of equine recurrent uveitis. *Equine Vet. J.* 48: 290–298.

34 Dwyer, A.E., Crockett, R.S., and Kalsow, C.M. (1995). Association of leptospiral seroreactivity and breed with uveitis and blindness in horses: 372 cases (1986–1993). *J. Am. Vet. Med. Assoc.* 207: 1327–1331.

35 Frazer, M.L. (1999). Acute renal failure from leptospirosis in a foal. *Aust. Vet. J.* 77: 499–500.

36 Divers, T.J., Chang, Y.F., Irby, N.L. et al. (2019). Leptospirosis: an important infectious disease in North American horses. *Equine Vet. J.* 51: 287–292.

37 Balasuriya, U.B.R. (2014). Equine viral arteritis. *Vet. Clin. North Am. Equine Pract.* 30: 543–560.

38 Cole, J.R., Hall, R.F., Gosser, H.S. et al. (1986). Transmissibility and abortogenic effect of equine viral arteritis in mares. *J. Am. Vet. Med. Assoc.* 189: 769–771.

39 Cho, C.H. and Lee, S.B. (2019). Clinical analysis of microbiologically proven fungal keratitis according to prior topical steroid use: a retrospective study in South Korea. *BMC Ophthalmol.* 19: 207.

40 Lundy, D.J. and Trzeciak, S. (2009). Microcirculatory dysfunction in sepsis. *Crit. Care Clin.* 25 (4): 721–731.

41 Laborada, G., Rego, M., Jain, A. et al. (2003). Diagnostic value of cytokines and C-reactive protein in the first 24 hours of neonatal sepsis. *Am. J. Perinatol.* 20: 491–501.

42 Zink, M.C., Yager, J.A., and Smart, N.L. (1986). *Corynebacterium equi* infections in horses, 1958–1984: a review of 131 cases. *Can. Vet. J.* 27: 213–217.

43 Takai, S., Higuchi, T., Matsukura, S. et al. (2000). Some epidemiological aspects of *Rhodococcus equi* infection in foals in Japan: a review of 108 cases in 1992–1998. *J. Equine Sci.* 11: 7–14.

44 Wilkes, E.J.A., Hughes, K.J., Kessell, A.E. et al. (2016). Successful management of multiple extrapulmonary complications associated with *Rhodococcus equi* pneumonia in a foal. *Equine Vet. Educ.* 28: 186–192.

45 Muscatello, G. (2012). *Rhodococcus equi* pneumonia in the foal – part 1: pathogenesis and epidemiology. *Vet. J.* 192: 20–26.

46 Johns, I.C., Desrochers, A., Wotman, K.L. et al. (2011). Presumed immune-mediated hemolytic anemia in two foals with *Rhodococcus equi* infection. *J. Vet. Emerg. Crit. Care* 21: 273–278.

47 Vázquez-Boland, J.A., Giguère, S., Hapeshi, A. et al. (2013). *Rhodococcus equi*: the many facets of a pathogenic actinomycete. *Vet. Microbiol.* 167: 9–33.

48 Anderson, B. and Wyman, M. (1979). Anatomy of the equine eye and orbit: histological structure and blood supply of the eyelids. *J. Equine Med. Surg.* 3: 4–14.

49 Schaer, B.D. (2007). Ophthalmic emergencies in horses. *Vet. Clin. North Am. Equine Pract.* 23: 49–65.

50 De Linde, H.M. and Brooks, D.E. (2014). Standing ophthalmic surgeries in horses. *Vet. Clin. North Am. Equine Pract.* 30: 91–110.

51 Giuliano, E.A. (2016). Diseases of the adnexa and nasolacrimal system. In: *Equine Ophthalmology*, 3e (ed. B.C. Gilger). Wiley Blackwell https://doi.org/10.1002/9781119047919.ch6.

52 Caron, J.P., Barber, S.M., Bailey, J.V. et al. (1986). Periorbital skull fractures in five horses. *J. Am. Vet. Med. Assoc.* 188: 280–284.

53 DeBowes, R. (1996). Fractures of the cranium. In: *Equine Fracture Repair*, 1e (ed. A. Nixon), 313–322. Philadelphia: Saunders.

54 Anderson, J.M., Hecht, S., and Kalck, K.A. (2012). What is your diagnosis? Skull fracture in a foal. *J. Am. Vet. Med. Assoc.* 241: 181–183.

55 Gerding, J.C., Clode, A., Gilger, B.C. et al. (2014). Equine orbital fractures: a review of 18 cases (2006–2013). *Vet. Ophthalmol.* 17: 97–106.

56 Derham, A.M., Johnson, J.P., Kearney, C.M. et al. (2019). Surgical repair of a depressed, comminuted fracture of the zygomatic process of the frontal bone using a locking compression plate in a Thoroughbred colt foal. *Clin. Case Rep.* 7: 110–114.

57 Boyle, A.G., Magdesian, K.G., and Ruby, R.E. (2005). Neonatal isoerythrolysis in horse foals and a mule foal: 18 cases (1988–2003). *J. Am. Vet. Med. Assoc.* 227: 1276–1283.

58 Pollio, D., Michau, T.M., Weaver, E. et al. (2018). Electroretinographic changes after intravenous lipid emulsion therapy in a dog and a foal with ivermectin toxicosis. *Vet. Ophthalmol.* 21: 82–87.

General Treatment Principles for the Equine Neonate

Chapter 57 Neonatal Care at the Farm

Scott Austin

Considerable advances have been made in equine neonatology over the last four decades, resulting in an increase in the level of care available at referral centers and a corresponding decrease in foal mortality. Veterinarians on the farm remain the first line for diagnosis and treatment of ill neonates with decisions on the farm greatly influencing subsequent mortality by early recognition of these conditions and prompt institution of therapy. If abnormalities are detected, it is paramount that field practitioners are able to assist owners with the decision whether the foal can be managed on the farm or should be referred to a specialty hospital for further care. The primary care clinician is in a unique position to evaluate historical, environmental, and management considerations that may impact the ability to successfully attend to the foal's needs on the farm and initiate appropriate therapeutics to improve odds for successful treatment. Other factors to consider include value and insurance status of the foal, prognosis related to suspected abnormalities, availability of referral centers, and availability of trained personnel to attend to the foal's needs [1].

Assessing the Newborn Foal

Timing of Examination

The timing of the initial foal examination depends on multiple factors but includes a recognition of increased risk secondary to perinatal factors. Perinatal risk factors affecting the mare include previous and concurrent disease, malnutrition, poor perineal conformation, placentitis, premature lactation, twinning, prolonged transport during pregnancy, and a history of delivering a previous ill foal [2]. Mares at high risk should be monitored during pregnancy, and a veterinarian should attend the foaling or examine the mare and foal as soon as possible after delivery. An immediate veterinary examination is recommended for foals that are premature (<320 days gestation), small for gestational age, dysmature, arrive during inclement weather, experience premature placental separation (red-bag) delivery, or are born after a period of dystocia [1, 2].

If perinatal risk factors are not identified, the timing of the first examination depends on whether the foal achieves predictable milestones that signify normal transition to extrauterine life: the foal should be sternal by 5 minutes after birth, have a normal suckle response within 10 minutes, successfully stand by 1 hour, and nurse within the first 2 hours after birth. Larger breed foals may take slightly long to stand and suckle. If the foal is slow in achieving these milestones, a veterinarian should be consulted, and an earlier examination is recommended. If the foal stands and nurses during the expected time frame, then the veterinary examination should occur during the first 12–24 hours of life [3]. Additionally, the placenta should be protected from predation, trauma, and freezing and saved for examination.

Examination of the Neonate

A complete history should be obtained at the time of the initial foal examination, especially if the veterinarian is not familiar with the mare or the client. The length of gestation, vaccination history, concurrent mare abnormalities during gestation, leaking of colostrum prior to foaling, dystocia, premature placental separation, and history of previous pregnancies, including gestational length, should be recorded. It is also important to inquire about the time and location of parturition and if the foaling was observed. Additionally, questions should be asked about foal behavior since birth to determine if it is nursing, urinating, and passing meconium. The examination should begin with observation of the foal from a distance to observe nursing behavior, assess ambulation and musculoskeletal abnormalities, and determine resting respiratory rate. This is an opportunity to assess the foal's interactions with the mare, environment, and handler, as well as evaluating the mare's

Equine Neonatal Medicine, First Edition. Edited by David M. Wong and Pamela A. Wilkins.

attitude to outside intervention before the veterinarian enters the stall. Alterations in foal behavior can be the earliest indication of sepsis or neurological dysfunction. Normal foals nurse in short bouts (90 seconds), at a frequency of up to 7–10 times per hour. Milk staining on the foal's forehead and muzzle suggests impaired nursing and onset of potential problems. The normal gait of the foal, as compared to an adult, is characterized by base-wide stance, mild hypermetria, and flexed head posture. Signs of prematurity should be noted and include short, soft hair coat, pliant lips and ears, laxity of the distal limbs (foot to withers test), and a domed forehead (Figure 57.1). Poor body condition typified by obvious appearance of ribs and bony prominences and a lower birthweight may be present with either prematurity or intrauterine growth restriction [3].

The order of the examination is not critical if a routine is established that ensures a comprehensive examination each time. Examinations usually begin with determination of vital parameters. The body temperature of a healthy foal is 37–39 °C (99–101.5 °F) (Table 57.1). Healthy foals can regulate body temperature at birth but are susceptible to hypothermia because of minimal energy reserves, minimal subcutaneous fat stores, and increased body surface area to body weight ratio that increases heat loss when the foal is exposed to low environmental temperatures. Ingestion of milk soon after birth and high activity are necessary for maintenance of normal body temperature, so a subnormal body temperature may indicate decreased suckling, reduced activity, and potential onset of illness [3]. Sepsis or the systemic inflammatory response syndrome (SIRS) may cause fever or hypothermia; altered body temperature is an indication for laboratory assessment of the foal.

Respiratory frequency is best determined by observation before entering the stall and handling the foal. Examination of the thorax should occur with the foal in sternal recumbency or standing while gently restrained. Auscultation of the lung sounds are typically louder than adults due to the thinner body wall. Careful observation of breathing effort is informative, as there is a poor correlation between the character of ausculted sounds and lung pathology. Typically, the respiratory rate is 60–80 breaths per minute soon after birth and decreases to 20–40 breath per minute within the first day of life (Table 57.1). A persistently elevated respiratory rate can be an early indicator of pulmonary disease. A gentle in-and-out motion is characteristic of normal respiration, while exaggerated intercostal movement with synchronous abdominal effort and an expiratory grunt typifies dyspnea. Paradoxical movement of the chest and abdomen signify that the foal is approaching respiratory failure [3]. With the foal standing, the thorax should be carefully palpated for rib fractures, which may click or grind during palpation and simultaneous auscultation and are often accompanied by subcutaneous swelling and edema. Fractures are most frequently observed at the level or slightly above of the costochondral junction over ribs 3–5 [4]. Fracture of ≥3 ribs is associated with increased risk of death because the fracture segment frequently lies over the heart [5]. When multiple ribs are fractured, the rib cage moves inward as the chest expands, and the identification of a "flail" chest signifies that surgical intervention is necessary. Such foals should be handled with care to limit further damage to underlying structures.

During the first 24–48 hours of life, a grade 1–4 holosystolic murmur can be detected over the left heart base. Additionally, transient irregularities in heart rhythm may be present immediately after birth secondary to high vagal tone and hypoxia associated with delivery [6]. Murmurs that are loud (>grade 4/6), pansystolic,

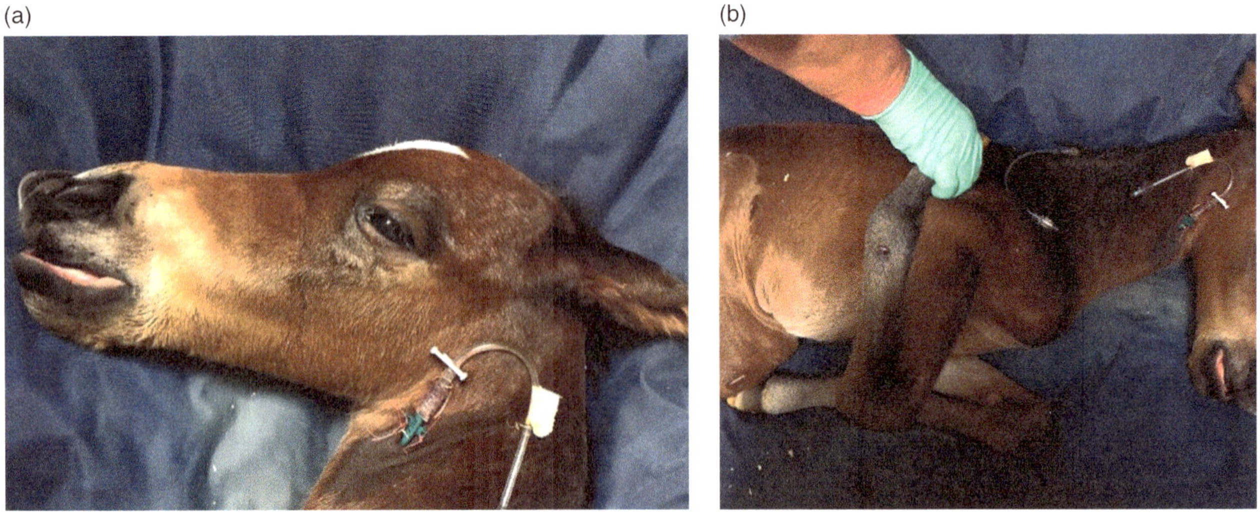

Figure 57.1 (a) Premature foal demonstrating the characteristic domed forehead and pliant lips and ears. (b) Premature foal exhibiting laxity of limbs as demonstrated by the "foot to withers" test.

Table 57.1 Normal vital parameters in the neonatal foal by age [4].

Age (h)	Temperature °F (°C)	Heart rate (beats/min)	Respiratory rate (breaths/min)
At birth	99.0–100.5 (37–39)	60–80	40–60
0–2	99.0–100.5 (37–39)	120–150	60–80
>2	99.0–101.5 (37–39)	90–120	20–40

bilateral, diastolic, or right-sided are more likely to be associated with pathological, rather than physiological, causes [7]. After 96 hours of age, persistent arrythmias and murmurs should be investigated further. At birth, the heart rate is usually 60–80 beats/minute but increases to 120–150 beats/minute when the foal first stands. The heart rate will remain increased (90–120) over the first 2 days of life followed by a decrease to 60–80 beat/minute [8].

Poor pulse quality, prolonged capillary refill time (>2 seconds), decreased jugular fill (>2 seconds) and cool ears and distal extremities indicate decreased peripheral perfusion and signify that further investigation and early intervention are warranted. Dehydration is suspected when mucous membranes are tacky, eyes appear sunken, skin tent is prolonged, and urination is decreased in frequency or amount. Tenting of the skin of the eyelids is a more reliable location to evaluate hydration status than the neck. Pale mucous membranes signify anemia or inadequate perfusion, while sepsis is associated with mucous membrane, sclera, ear, and coronary band hyperemia, and/or petechiation. Yellow mucous membranes occur with hyperbilirubinemia secondary to liver disease or hemolysis.

The eyes should be examined for cataracts, corneal ulcers, and entropion; abnormal injection or color of the cornea should be noted. The menace response is a learned behavior and is not reliably present until 2 weeks of age [9]. Superficial corneal ulcers should be treated with antimicrobial ophthalmic ointment every 4–6 hours, and corneas should be stained with fluorescein 1–2 times/day [10]. Entropion normally resolves upon correction of dehydration; however, entropion occasionally requires surgical or medical therapy. Entropion can be corrected with several vertical mattress sutures placed in the lower lid or temporary injection of the lower lid with procaine penicillin to roll the lid out. The benefit of penicillin is it gradually absorbs and may or may not need to be performed again.

Neonates should be observed as they ambulate around the stall, and the limbs, joints, and tendons should be examined to detect potential abnormalities. The external umbilicus should be examined while inspecting the abdominal wall for inguinal and umbilical hernias. To decrease the risk of bacterial contamination and possible internal migration, the umbilicus should be dipped in 0.5% chlorhexidine solution (1 part 2% chlorhexidine solution: 3 parts sterile water), and the client should be instructed to dip the navel three times daily for the first 3 days of life. Chlorhexidine has greater residual activity than betadine solution but may cause delay in the drying of the umbilical stump. The addition of surgical alcohol (60 ml of ethyl alcohol added to 440 ml of 0.5% chlorhexidine) to the navel dip will speed drying and help seal the umbilicus [11, 12]. Discarded syringe cases or small disposal cups may be used for navel dipping but should be discarded after single use to prevent contamination of the dipping solution.

The mare and placenta should be evaluated at the time of the foal inspection. Examination of the mare should include temperature, pulse, and respiratory rates, mucous membrane color, inspection of the udder, and evaluation of the perineum for foaling injuries. The placenta should be examined to ensure the entire placenta has been passed and to determine if there are abnormalities suggestive of placental infection. Heavy placentas (>11% of foal weight) [13] and overly long or short umbilical cords have been linked to increase likelihood of neonatal foal disease (normal umbilical length is 36–83 cm) [14, 15]. Signs of neonatal illness are usually nonspecific and include decreased activity, loss of suckle, loss of affinity for the mare, increased sleepiness, and alterations in body temperature (increased or decreased). Since the signs are frequently subtle, the owner may see streaming of milk from the udder of the mare or milk staining of the foal's head and muzzle before overt signs of illness in the foal are recognized.

Point of Care Diagnostic Testing

Evaluation of Passive Transfer

Foals are immunocompetent at birth but immunologically naïve and reliant upon ingestion and absorption of maternal antibodies as colostrum to provide protection from pathogens during the neonatal period. Approximately 3% to 38% of foals fail to absorb adequate amounts of colostrum [16]. Immunoglobulins in the colostrum are absorbed across specialized intestinal cells in the newborn's gut, with maximal absorption occurring during the first 3 hours after birth. Colostral antibody absorption decreases to 22% of initial rate by 3 hours after birth and is <1% by 24 hours of age [17, 18]. Therefore, if there is a delay in nursing, antibody absorption is negatively impacted and affected foals are at risk for failure of passive transfer of antibodies.

Complete failure of transfer is equated to a serum IgG <400 mg/dl and levels between 400 and 800 mg/dl are described as partial failure of antibody transfer [19–28]. Proposed causes include poor-quality colostrum, dripping of colostrum in the late peripartum period, failure to ingest adequate colostrum prior to gut closure, and insufficient absorption of colostral antibodies by the foal. During late gestation, mares produce between 1.8 and 2.8 l of colostrum [23]. Factors that decrease colostrum quality include mare illness during pregnancy, early season foaling, mares >10 years of age, and ingestion of endophyte-infected fescue [29, 30]. Normal colostrum is yellow, cloudy, and sticky, but physical characteristics alone do not ensure adequate colostrum antibody content. The quality of colostrum can be assessed using a colostrometer[1] or brix refractometer, with good-quality colostrum having a specific gravity of at least 1.060 or specific gravity of 25, respectively [31]. Premature or dysmature foals may fail to absorb antibodies across the intestinal tract despite ingestion of adequate amounts of good quality colostrum.

Sepsis is a leading causes of foal mortality [32]. Numerous studies have established the link between inadequate ingestion/absorption of maternal antibodies and risk of sepsis [19–21, 23–25, 27, 30, 33–35]; therefore, all foals should be evaluated for failure of passive transfer. Colostral antibodies peak in the foal at 18–24 hours after birth [36], so foals can be tested as early as 8–18 hours of age [37]. Numerous commercial tests are available to evaluate IgG levels in foal serum [38–41]. These tests are good at identifying foals with complete failure of passive antibody transfer but may underestimate IgG levels in some foals that have antibody levels between 400 and 800 mg/dl resulting in unnecessary treatment of some foals that have adequate serum antibody levels [41]. Determination of serum total protein as a surrogate for serum IgG, although simple, is not sensitive enough to identify foals with insufficient antibodies to protect against sepsis in the neonatal period [38, 41].

Laboratory Testing

A complete blood count (CBC) is recommended for any abnormal foal and may be required by insurance companies before issuance of foal insurance. Red blood cell (RBC) and packed cell volume (PCV) are influenced by transfer of placental blood prior to umbilical cord breakage, catecholamine release, and fluid balance. Premature rupture of the umbilical cord or neonatal isoerythrolysis may result in reduction in PCV and RBC counts. In the newborn foal, with normal adrenocortical function, the neutrophil: lymphocyte ratio should be higher than 2 : 1. Alterations in the white blood cell count (WBC), such as an increase or decrease in absolute number of neutrophils, band neutrophils, or degenerative neutrophils, are suggestive of a systemic inflammatory response and should prompt investigation and intervention [2, 42]. Platelet counts should be similar to adult values and decreased numbers may be seen with immune-mediated disease [43] or secondary to sepsis [44].

Stall-side testing is valuable to ambulatory practitioners since results that establish and monitor the status of foals are available at the point-of-care (POC) [1]. For example, serum amyloid A (SAA) is an acute inflammatory marker that increases significantly within 24–48 hours after an inflammatory insult (up to >100 mg/l; normal range 0–27 mg/l) and has the advantage of being available as a POC test (Stablelab).[2] Levels also decrease rapidly when therapeutic intervention is successful at ameliorating the inflammatory response [45].

The handheld lactate analyzer (Lactate Scout)[3] has proven utility as a POC test for determination of whole blood lactate in neonatal foals [46]. Elevations in serum lactate are not specific for any condition but typically indicate poor perfusion/oxygen delivery to tissues associated with conditions such as sepsis, hemorrhagic shock, prematurity, or complicated neonatal encephalopathy [46, 47]. Healthy newborn foals have modest increases in blood lactate at birth but values stabilize at 2.1 mmol/l (range 1.0–3.7 mmol/l) by 24 hours of age. Because of the variability in lactate levels in healthy foals at birth, lactate clearance is a more useful predictor of survival, and persistent hyperlactatemia in the face of appropriate therapy is associated with a poor outcome [47].

Foals that are not nursing or developing sepsis frequently develop life-threatening hypoglycemia that can be identified using a POC glucometer. Periodic monitoring of blood glucose can identify alterations in glucose metabolism and allow rapid corrections in the field. Monitoring of blood glucose is essential for any foal that is receiving IV glucose supplementation. Devices designed to measure blood glucose in humans may be highly variable when measuring equine blood glucose, so a glucometer designed for veterinary use is required [48, 49].

Imaging

The ability of the clinician to evaluate foals is improved with the availability of portable ultrasonography. Examination of the lungs and thoracic wall can greatly assist in identification of lung pathology and rib fractures. Ultrasound has proven to be more accurate than either physical examination or radiography in the detection of rib fractures, commonly overlying the heart in the cranioventral thorax [50, 51]. The identification of a “step” in rib contour in addition to swelling or edema at the fracture site are confirmatory. Examination of the umbilicus is recommended for foals that demonstrate lethargy and fever or

Table 57.2 Dimensions of umbilical remnants in newborn foals.

Structure	Location	Dimensions (cm) 0–24 hours old [52]	6 h to 4 wk old [53]
Umbilical vein	Immediately cranial to umbilicus	0.83 (0.77–1.09)[a]	0.61 ± 0.20[b]
	Midway between umbilicus and liver	0.70 (0.60–0.76)	0.52 ± 0.19
	At liver	0.76 (0.69–0.82)	0.60 ± 0.19
Umbilical arteries	Single artery	0.61 (0.56–0.70)	0.85 ± 0.21
	Urachus	1.07 (1.02–1.14)	–
	Both arteries and urachus	–	1.75 ± 0.37

[a] Median diameter (inter-quartile range).
[b] mean ± SD.

develop a patent urachus. Potential infection of the internal umbilical remnants is suspected when structures are increased in size (Table 57.2) [52–54]. In healthy foals, the umbilical remnants are largest at birth and regress linearly over time to 50% of original values by 1 month. The umbilical remnants continue to regress and are difficult to detect by 5–6 weeks of age [52].

Ultrasonography can also be used to assess intestinal motility, confirm retained meconium, identify intestinal intussusception, and determine if abdominal distention is the result of free fluid within the abdomen or from intestinal distention. The most common cause of increased abdominal free fluid is rupture of the urinary bladder or urachus. A bladder that is collapsed upon itself into a characteristic U-shape, often with a visible dorsal defect, is further evidence that a bladder rupture has occurred. In these instances, the foal requires immediate medical stabilization and referral to a surgical facility. Confirmation of uroperitoneum requires abdominocentesis and demonstration that peritoneal creatinine is at least twice that of serum creatinine [55, 56].

General Nursing Care

If referral of the foal is not necessary or unavailable, the ambulatory clinician is responsible for making recommendations regarding management of the foal's environment. A clean, draft-free stall with secure footing and adequate bedding is essential. Wet foals should be dried, as their large surface to mass ratio increases heat loss to their environment. The heat loss, coupled with limited energy reserves and low environmental temperatures, can result in healthy foals becoming hypothermic. Additionally, ill foals have impaired ability to regulate body temperature and are better cared for with supplemental heat [57, 58]. In unheated barns, heat lamps and space heaters may be used to improve the foal's environment (ensure heaters are kept clear of flammable materials). Heat lamps are less likely to be a fire risk but can inadvertently cause thermal damage if positioned too close to the foal. To avoid burns, keep lamps at least 5 feet away from the foal. Air blankets (Bair Hugger)[4] are safe and effective, provided that the warmer unit is kept clear of flammable materials.

Recumbent foals require a clean, dry, and well-padded environment. Large beanbags are relatively inexpensive and easily adapted to a foal bed. The surface may be mildly abrasive, so a padded blanket that can be changed once wet will help prevent sores. Pillows can be used to prop the foal into sternal position to aid pulmonary ventilation. If the foal will not maintain sternal position and attempts at repositioning result in a struggle that has a detrimental result on the foal, then the recumbent foal will need to be turned every 2 hours. Disposable incontinence pads may be used to absorb urine and changed as needed. Wet skin should be dried, and zinc oxide ointment may be used to protect the perineum and points of contact. Artificial tears may be applied every 6–12 hours, and corneas should be stained with fluorescein daily because of the increased risk of corneal ulcers in recumbent foals [1].

A significant challenge in caring for ill foals, on the farm or in a hospital, is the need for constant trained supervision to protect the foal and facilitate treatment. Instructions to caregivers should be in writing and include specific parameters that require further investigation by a veterinarian. It is important that the veterinarian and owner discuss limitations of on farm care and agree on the frequency of reevaluation provided by the veterinarian. POC lactate, glucose, IgG, and SAA tests are available, but hematology, blood gas, and biochemistry profiles are not usually immediately available, so emerging abnormalities as determined by laboratory values may necessitate additional veterinary visits [1].

Venous access for drug and fluid delivery is an essential part of foal care. The practitioner has a choice between Teflon or polyurethane catheters. Teflon (over-the-needle) catheters are more rigid and easier to insert but rarely can be maintained for a prolonged period because of increased risk for clotting and infection compared to polyurethane catheters (over-the-wire) [59, 60]. Polyurethane catheters are more flexible, are easier to maintain, and have fewer complications, so the added expense of over-the-wire catheters is justified. If long-term venous access is anticipated, then the longest catheter suited for the insertion site is recommended, especially if medications are potentially irritating to the vein [61]. If short-term fluids or a single bolus of fluid and/or plasma is the objective, then a shorter catheter should be chosen since flow rate is proportional to catheter length [61].

Nutrition

Since neonates are born with limited energy reserves, they depend on ingestion of colostrum for energy and passive transfer of antibodies. A healthy foal will nurse frequently (7–10 times/hour), in bouts of 90–120 minutes each. If the foal is slow to nurse, hypoglycemia, dehydration, hypothermia, and lethargy may ensue and contribute to poor suckle and udder seeking behavior in as little as 2–4 hours after birth. Common problems associated with failure of the foal to nurse include musculoskeletal disease, congenital defects, intrauterine (newborn) infections, and maternal behavior that precludes the foal from nursing (aggressive or nervous mares).

Tube-feeding foals in the field can be challenging and labor intensive. Recumbent foals and those demonstrating signs of colic should be checked for gastric reflux. Supplemental feeding should be withheld if the foal's temperature is <37.5 °C (99.5 °F), borborygmi are absent, or fluid resuscitation is required [62]. A foal that is slow to nurse or loosing sufficient strength to nurse effectively, will benefit from a single feeding of colostrum or milk through a nasogastric (NG) tube. If necessary and safe to provide supplemental nutrition in the field, a small-bore indwelling NG tube can be placed. Correct tube placement is confirmed by palpation of the tube dorsal to the trachea in the proximal portion of the neck. If correct tube position cannot be confirmed via palpation, radiography, or endoscopy should be utilized to confirm placement prior to use. Commercially available NG feeding tubes with stylet[5] are designed to remain in the stomach or retracted into the distal esophagus. When placed in the stomach, there is no need to reposition the tube to check for reflux prior to feeding; however, there is a risk of milk regurgitation around the tube when placed through the cardia, but the small diameter of commercially available tubes minimizes the risk of reflux [63]. The position of the tube relative to the nostril should be clearly marked to ensure that the tube has not retracted from the desired placement and is securely attached to the nostril. The tube should be secured in place either by direct suturing to the naris or taping of the tube to the rounded end of a tongue depressor as it exits the nostril. The clinician should be sure that the foal can open its mouth sufficiently to nurse once the tube is secured to muzzle of the foal [1].

Properly placed feeding tubes provide essential nutrition to weak foals and are easy to use by farm personnel with minimal training. It is important that explicit feeding instructions are left on the farm (Table 57.3). Tubes can become soiled, so it is important to emphasize cleaning of the tube end to minimize unnecessary bacterial burdens. Mares should be milked every 2–4 hours and the milk filtered through gauze to remove gross particulates prior to administration. Excess milk should be refrigerated or discarded if milk production greatly exceeds foal needs. Refrigerated milk should be warmed prior to administration, and all equipment should be cleaned between feedings. Decreased milk letdown is common in mares that are being milked. A warm cloth can be used to gently clean the udder and stimulate milk letdown. Also, milking can be facilitated with oxytocin (1–3 IU/450 kg body weight IV). Mares with insufficient milk production should be treated with domperidone (1.1 mg/kg body weight orally q24h) or sulpiride (0.5 mg/kg orally q12h) [1].

Table 57.3 Use of indwelling feeding tube.

1) **Check foal position.** The foal should be standing or in sternal position with the head position above stomach level.
2) **Check for abdominal distention.** Measure abdominal size at a consistent location. Do not feed if foal is demonstrating colic or the abdomen is enlarging over three consecutive feedings in absence of discomfort.
3) **Confirm tube location.** A mark is present on the tube at the naris. If the distance between the mark and the nostril has increased, do not administer milk, and call your veterinarian.
4) **Clean and clear the tube.** Wipe the end of the tube with alcohol, uncap tube, clear tube with a small amount of air.
5) **Check for reflux.** Apply gentle suction to the tube with a catheter tipped syringe. Delay next feeding by 2 h if >30 ml of reflux is obtained. Reflux at 2 consecutive feedings should prompt a call to your veterinarian.
6) **Flush the tube.** Flush tube with 20 ml water. If tube is patent and foal is comfortable, proceed with scheduled feeding.
7) **Feed the foal.** Use gravity flow only.
8) **Flush the tube.** Use 20 ml of water to flush milk from the tube.
9) **Clean and cap the tube.** Use an air bolus to clear water from tube, clean, and dry tube end, and secure the cap.

Overfeeding of foals may increase the risk of hyperglycemia, hypercapnia, and azotemia [64]. Healthy foals consume up to 25% of their body weight (50 kg foal × 0.25 = 12.5 l/day) as milk; however, requirements in sick neonates may be reduced by 50% [65]. Enteral feeding is the preferred method for providing nutrition to foals that are unable to nurse, and local nutrition (30–60 ml every 2 hours) is required for appropriate development of enterocytes, even in foals that do not tolerate significant amounts of enteral nutrition [66]. It is best to start nutritional supplementation by giving 5–7% of body weight the first day, divided into 12 equal feedings. Once the foal is more stable, the amount of milk is gradually increased. The energy needs of a sick foal can be met with 10% of the body weight of the foal administered as milk or milk replacer [63].

Impaired gastric and intestinal motility is common in ill foals; thus, caregivers should monitor for abdominal distention and ileus. Repeated measurement of the abdomen at a marked location provides objective evidence of abdominal distention and is used in conjunction with ultrasonographic assessment of intestinal motility to ascertain the degree of ileus. Clear communication to caregivers as to when veterinary reexamination is necessary is essential any time an ill neonate is managed on the farm. Foals with increasing abdominal distention accompanied by colic signs or reflux should be reassessed by a veterinarian and the indwelling feeding tube removed and replaced by a NG tube of sufficient diameter to remove accumulated reflux. Enteral feeding is halted until reflux and bloating are resolved. In addition to intestinal ileus, ill foals are prone to alterations in fecal consistency, especially when fed milk replacer. If constipation is evident, the fluid plan should be reevaluated to ensure that adequate fluid is being provided. Foal attendants should record frequency of defecation and urination and periodically catch urine to assess hydration status; urine specific gravity of adequately hydrated foals is <1.012. Diarrhea may indicate developing sepsis or concurrent infectious disease. Diarrhea can also be secondary to increased bacterial loads during enteral feeding or incorrect mixing of milk replacer resulting in an excessively concentrated replacer. The onset of diarrhea should prompt immediate reassessment of the foal. Most foals that require nutritional support in the field will resume suckling or can be transitioned to bucket feeding after 1–2 days. Foals that are not able to tolerate calculated amounts of nutrition are in danger of developing dehydration and hypoglycemia and will require IV fluid therapy. Foals that are too ill to resume nursing or are intolerant to enteral feeding require more intensive management that cannot easily be provided in the field.

Fluid Therapy

In neonates, dehydration is rarely a problem immediately at birth, but develops rapidly if nursing is delayed or ceases. Hypovolemia may be recognized by depression, decreased activity, poor pulse quality, prolonged capillary refill time and jugular fill, and cool extremities. Initial fluid therapy consists of IV boluses of 20 ml/kg body weight over 20–30 minutes and reevaluation. A positive clinical response is indicated with improved pulse quality, warming of distal extremities, improved attitude, increased activity, return of borborygmi, and increased urine production [67]. Fluid boluses may be repeated every 20 minutes until signs of volume depletion resolve or a total of 3-4 boluses have been administered. Failure to respond appropriately after repeated boluses indicates more intensive therapy is required and referral should be considered [67]. If dehydration is present after resuscitation, then additional fluid should be administered over time. Mild, moderate, and severe dehydration in foals is estimated at 5%, 10%, and 15% of body weight, respectively. Mild dehydration is recognized as a slight decrease in urine production and increased urine specific gravity. Moderate dehydration is characterized by tacky mucous membranes, mild increase in heart rate, minimal urine production, lethargy, sunken eyes, and loss of skin turgor. Severe dehydration is recognized by dry mucous membranes, tachycardia, absent urine production, lethargy, sunken eyes, loss of skin turgor and tachypnea, thready pulse, delayed capillary refill time, mottled mucous membranes and decreased activity or recumbency. Fluid deficits should be corrected over the first 12 hours of therapy followed by maintenance rate fluids [10]. Fluids used for resuscitation should have a strong ion difference, which helps restore normal anion gap and correct metabolic acidosis [62]. Following resuscitation, a biochemistry panel should be evaluated to identify disorders of organ function and establish the level of electrolyte derangement. Electrolyte abnormalities should be corrected slowly over time to prevent subsequent neurologic disorders.

In ill neonates, hypoglycemia is often observed concurrently with disorders of fluid homeostasis secondary to limited energy reserves and decreased nursing. Correction of hypoglycemia can be lifesaving, but glucose should not be administered as a bolus. After correction of hypovolemia, 5% glucose may be used to provide 4 mg/kg/min for the first 24 hours, then glucose concentration increased to 8 mg/kg/min if the foal tolerates the increasing glucose [67]. Blood glucose can be monitored using a POC glucometers with a blood glucose goal between 72 and 100 mg/dl (4.0 and 5.5 mmol/l) [1]. Glucose infusion is insufficient to meet caloric needs alone, but parenteral nutrition is rarely undertaken in the field. Maintenance fluids are administered at 2–4 ml/kg/h or calculated using the Holliday-Segar formula (Table 57.4) to calculate a "dry" rate based on the basal metabolic rate of the foal [62, 67].

Daily fluid requirements are formulated after adding the estimated ongoing loses to the maintenance fluid rate. Long-term use of replacement fluids for maintenance therapy can lead to water retention and interstitial edema secondary to the equine neonate's limited ability to excrete sodium. Therefore, except for neonates with diarrhea, maintenance fluids should have a lower sodium concentration. Suitable fluids for maintenance therapy include Normosol-M, 5% dextrose, and a combination of 5% dextrose with Lactated Ringer's solution [62]. Normal saline and other fluids with high chloride concentration should be avoided because they have significant acidifying effects. Ongoing fluid therapy

Table 57.4 Holliday-Segar formula for calculation of maintenance fluid rate.

Body weight (kg)	Fluid requirement (ml/kg/d)	50 kg foal (example)
1–10	100	First 10 kg × 100 ml/kg/d = 1000 ml/d
11–20	50	Second 10 kg × 50 ml/kg/d = 500 ml/d
Each additional kg >20	25	Remaining 30 kg × 25 ml/kg/d = 750 ml/d
		Total fluid requirement = 2250 ml/d

requires periodic laboratory monitoring to assess hydration status, organ function, and electrolyte levels. Foals that are not being fed and do not suffer from kidney disorders or ruptured bladder are prone to hypokalemia. However, IV potassium administration can be dangerous if the rate is not controlled by fluid pump and experienced personnel to monitor therapy. If the foal will tolerate enteral therapy, oral supplementation is safer.

Therapy of Specific Disease

Diseases of the Immune System

Failure of transfer of passive immunity (FTPI) is a commonly treated on the farm. Multiple tests are available and allow stall-side detection of FTPI, which should be evaluated at 8–24 hours of age. Failure of passive transfer can occur in otherwise healthy foals with the decision to treat influenced by the experience of the clinician, farm history, and wishes of the owner. Healthy foals with complete failure (IgG <400 mg/dl) and high-risk foals with partial (IgG 400–800 mg/dl) or complete failure of passive transfer should be treated to increase serum immunoglobulin to >800 mg/dl [68]. If foals are to be insured, the veterinarian and owner should check with the proposed insurer to ensure stipulations for coverage are met.

If IgG is recognized as suboptimal when the foal is <18 hours of age, oral colostrum can be supplemented. Normally 1–2 l of good quality colostrum is required and should be administers in 200–400 ml aliquots every 30 minutes. Concentrated equine serum and lyophilized immunoglobulin products can be used, but recommended doses frequently fail to increase immunoglobulin levels to >800 mg/dl [69]. If the foal is >24 hours of age, IV plasma is needed to correct deficiencies in passive transfer. Plasma should be thawed slowly and administered with a filtered administration set. Typically, equine plasma that contains 12 g/l of IgG will increase a 45 kg foal by 200 mg/dl while hyperimmune products that contain >25 g/l increase IgG levels about 400 mg/dl [68, 70]. IgG concentrations should be checked 12–24 hours after plasma administration to ensure adequate IgG concentrations have been achieved. Reactions are rare when commercial plasma is administered through a blood administration set that includes an inline filter. An initial flow rates of 0.5 ml/kg is used with the foal closely monitored for reactions (piloerection, fever, tachypnea, tachycardia). After the first 15 minutes, the rate of administration is increased to 40 ml/kg/h if adverse signs are not seen [71]. If adverse signs are observed, transfusion should be slowed or stopped. If signs recur when administration is resumed, further attempts to administer plasma should be abandoned [71]. Foals that develop respiratory distress should receive IV epinephrine (0.5 ml of 0.1%). IV plasma has been described to cause reactions in foals that have previously received milk replacer. Many milk replacers have bovine proteins and plasma that has anti-bovine antibodies may result in the formation of immune complexes. If plasma transfusion is considered likely, plasma should be administered before providing nutritional supplementation as milk replacer. The blood volume of a 50 kg foal is 5 l, so volume overload can easily occur when giving supplemental plasma. Signs of volume overload include hyperventilation, sweating, and increased heart rate. One liter of plasma can safely be administered in 15–20 minutes, but if 2 l are anticipated then the minimum time for administration is 2 hours. Any time signs of fluid overload occur, the rate of plasma administration must be slowed.

Neonatal isoerythrolysis (NI) is an immune disease that is occasionally encountered. This condition primarily affects multiparous mares that are negative for the Aa and Qa red cell antigens but were sensitized to Aa or Qa antigens during previous pregnancies or blood transfusions. Once sensitized, mares will concentrate antibodies against Aa and Qa red cell antigens in colostrum. Foals that inherited either Aa or Qa red cell antigens are susceptible to red cell agglutination or hemolysis after ingestion of colostrum containing antibodies against the Aa and Qa surface antigens. Other blood antigens can be involved to at a lesser frequency. NI also occurs in neonatal mules secondary to ingestion of colostrum containing a specific donkey factor [71].

Affected foals are normal at birth with clinical signs dependent on ingestion and absorption of colostrum. The severity of red cell hemolysis and resulting anemia is variable and clinical signs are typically observed between 5 hours to 7 days of age [10]. Depression, tachypnea, tachycardia, and pale or icteric mucous membranes are typically seen in mildly affected foals and may not be apparent for several days after birth. More severely affected foals may be febrile, stop nursing, become icteric and develop pigmenturia. Sudden death without premonitory signs may happen on occasion. NI is one of the most frequent causes of icterus in foals [71]. A decreased PCV is expected in affected foals, and severity of clinical signs correlates with speed and degree of PCV decrease. Serum biochemistry is recommended to evaluate for potential complications such as acute kidney injury, kernicterus, of hepatic damage.

Acutely affected foals should be muzzled or separated from the dam and alternative sources of nutrition provided. Nursing from the dam should be prevented (e.g. muzzle foal) until gut closure has occurred (about 24 hours of age). The dam should be milked, and the milk must be discarded. Foals with PCV <12–15% may require a blood transfusion, which can prove difficult in an ambulatory setting. In an emergency, blood from an unrelated gelding can be collected into acid-citrate dextrose (ACD) anticoagulant (9 parts blood:1 part ACD) and 1–3 l for a 50 kg foal may be administered over 2–4 hours [10]. The volume of donor blood required to raise the recipients PCV can be estimated via the formula:

$$\left(PCV_{\text{desired}} - PCV_{\text{recepient}}\right) \times 150\,ml/kg^{*} \times \text{body weight}\left(\text{kg}\right) \div PCV_{\text{donor}}\left({}^{*}\text{estimated blood volume 2} - \text{day old foal}\right)$$

Prevention of NI is preferable to treating clinically affected foals. Thus, at-risk mares can be screened during late pregnancy for presence of circulating alloantibodies. Mares with existing alloantibodies can be milked and colostrum discarded. For the first 24 hours, the foal should be provided with an alternative source of colostrum and milk [71].

Meconium Impaction

As a prevention or treatment of meconium impaction, an enema may be administered by farm personnel or at the time of first veterinary examination. While attempting to defecate, affected foals will often arch the back, stand with hind legs camped-under, and flag the tail. In contrast, urination is associated with a flat back and the hind legs stretch backward. Additional signs include colic and ineffective nursing. Abdominal distention and patent urachus can be seen in foals with longer duration impactions. Affected foals that develop patent urachus should receive antiseptic care of the umbilicus and prophylactic antibiotic therapy. Commercial sodium phosphate or warm, soapy water (2–3 ml of liquid detergent in 500 ml water delivered by gravity flow) may be used to assist in passage of the meconium. If straining continues after the first enema, the foal should be examined by a veterinarian before administration of additional enemas. Digital rectal examination, abdominal palpation, or abdominal ultrasonography can confirm retained meconium. Fluid therapy, NG administration of laxatives, and acetylcysteine enemas have been recommended to resolve persistent impactions. Mineral oil (100–200 ml) administered by NG tube has been used for its laxative effects. Flunixin meglumine (0.25–0.5 mg/kg IV q12h), hyoscine N-butylbromide (0.14 mg/kg IV), or a combination of diazepam (0.05–0.2 mg/kg IV) and butorphanol (0.01–0.04 mg/kg IV) have been recommended for pain control [10]. Acetylcysteine retention enemas are delivered through a 30 French Foley catheter that is inserted into the rectum and the balloon cuff inflated. Gravity flow is used to deliver 200 ml of a 4% acetylcysteine solution, and the catheter is clamped for 20 minutes. The retention enema can be repeated in 12 hours if the impaction is not resolved. Success rate is reported to be 93% using this technique, with 40% requiring more than one enema (Chapter 17) [72].

Sepsis

Early recognition of sepsis and prompt referral to a hospital is associated with improved outcome. Signs of sepsis are nonspecific and include decreased activity and nursing, lethargy progressing to recumbency, and injected mucous membranes. Petechia of the mucous membranes, sclera, and inside of the ears, along with uveitis and coronary band hyperemia, may be apparent with these changes representative of SIRS [73, 74]. Sepsis scoring systems aid the practitioner in recognizing sepsis, allowing appropriate referral as soon as possible [75–78]. Recumbent foals require appropriate cardiovascular and environmental support prior to referral. If antibiotics are deemed necessary prior to transport, aseptic collection and inoculation of blood culture media prior to administering antibiotics is ideal. Culture media should accompany the foal to the hospital and can be invaluable in directing subsequent antibiotic therapy. Initial antibiotic therapy should be broad-spectrum, as both Gram-negative and Gram-positive infections occur in neonates. Clinical experience dictates antimicrobials likely to be effective in a region [79, 80], but β-lactam drugs combined with an aminoglycoside or high-dose ceftiofur are acceptable empiric choices until culture and sensitivity testing are available. In some foals, localized infections (with limited signs of systemic disease) may be observed and include joint infection or omphalophlebitis. Initially, IV antibiotics are preferred in foals <7 days of age, but the intramuscular route may be used in a field setting if it is difficult/impossible to maintain an IV catheter. Foals with suspected bacteremia without localizing signs should be treated at least 10–14 days. Routine use of prophylactic antibiotics is not recommended, but in some instances such as high-risk environment and failure of transfer of passive antibodies, antibiotic therapy is prudent. Prophylactic antibiotics are usually administered for 3–5 days [62].

Neonatal Encephalopathy

Neonatal encephalopathy (NE) is one of the most common disorders of the equine neonate. Clinical signs manifest at any time between birth and 48 hours of age. Signs include any combination of lack of affinity for the dam, increased sleepiness, loss of suckle response, aimless wandering, abnormal vocalization, and decreased responsiveness to external stimulation. Careful observation may identify increased limb stiffness, intermittent nystagmus, or limb paddling before overt seizures are seen [62]. This condition is multifactorial and proposed causes include hypoxic–ischemic damage, reperfusion injury, dysregulation of neuropregnanes, and increased inflammatory mediators in the brain [81]. Management of NE is best accomplished in a hospital environment with trained personnel, immediate laboratory support, and ready access to continuous care. If referral is not an option, treatment goals include nutritional and fluid support, control of seizures, antioxidants, and prophylactic antibiotic therapy. In addition to alterations in brain function, affected foals may also have multisystemic involvement including renal, gastrointestinal, and respiratory dysfunction. It is imperative to assess passive transfer of antibodies as affected foals are prone to insufficient ingestion of colostrum. Despite alterations in multiple body systems, seizure activity, and altered mentation, the prognosis for future athletic function is good in surviving foals (Chapter 32) [81].

Musculoskeletal Abnormalities

Musculoskeletal abnormalities are encountered with some frequency in ambulatory practice and include angular limb deformities, tendon laxity and tendon contracture. Mild to moderate angular limb deformities should be monitored, as most will improve over the first 30 days of life. Fetlock deformities that persist beyond 10–14 days, and carpal/tarsal abnormalities that fail to correct or worsen beyond the first 60 days should be further evaluated for possible surgical correction. All premature foals should have carpal and tarsal radiographs to evaluate ossification of cuboidal bones. Stall rest and exercise restriction are necessary until the cuboidal bones have completely ossified or permanent limb angulation may result.

Flexural laxity is usually transient and rarely causes long-term issues. Affected foals should have reduced exercise initially to prevent trauma to the heel bulbs. Light bandages over the fetlock may be used to prevent trauma, but full leg bandages should be avoided as they will increase laxity. If tendon laxity fails to improve after the first few days, glue-on shoes with heel extensions can be applied to force the hoof plantigrade and aid in correction of the laxity.

Tendon contractures involving the carpus, fetlock, pastern, and distal interphalangeal joint are also encountered frequently. Specific therapy may not be required if the foal is able to stand and nurse without assistance. However, if contracture is not improving or worsening, a combination of full limb bandaging, analgesia, and IV oxytetracycline may be used to facilitate relaxation. Flunixin meglumine (0.5 mg/dl IV q12h) or ketoprofen (2.2 mg/kg IV q12–24h) may be used for 1–2 days to provide adequate pain relief to allow lengthening of tendons and improved ambulation. Oxytetracycline (40–60 mg/kg, IV diluted and given slowly) has been recommended daily for 1–3 treatments to facilitate tendon lengthening but should be used with caution in dehydrated foals as renal damage may occur [82]. More severe cases of contracture may require heavy bandaging and polyvinyl chloride splints. Affected foals should be confined and carefully monitored to assure they are able to stand and nurse effectively.

Referral of Critical Foals

At the time of first visitation, the field veterinarian must assess the foal, determine prognosis and treatment strategies for any abnormalities, and discuss optimal treatment plans. Minor abnormalities can be addressed on the farm, but severely ill foals often require referral to a hospital for intensive management. The client should be informed of identified problems, treatment requirements, cost of therapy, and prognosis for athletic use. If referral is necessary, then the clinician must make recommendations to ensure the foal arrives at its destination with the best possible chance for survival.

Temperature Regulation and Respiratory Support During Transport

In most instances, it is best to place the mare in the adjacent stall within sight and smell of the foal to avoid possible injury to the foal during transport. Sedation of the mare may be required to facilitate safe transport. Ambulatory foals may be protected from heat loss during transport by adding a sweatshirt or jacket, with the foal's front legs passed through the sleeves and the jacket fasted over the back [83]. Recumbent foals require special care as they are challenged to maintain body temperature and rapidly lose body heat if not adequately insulated. During extreme weather, the best option may be to transport the foal separately in a heated car or truck and bring the mare separately in a trailer. Under no circumstances should the foal be transported in the trunk of a car or the back of a pickup truck [83]. Blankets and sleeping bags can be added to insulate recumbent foals from the floor of the transport and to minimize heat loss. Leg bandages may be applied to foals that are thrashing to protect pressure points from trauma during transport. Recumbent foals are frequently energy depleted and hypoglycemic. If possible, blood glucose should be checked prior to transport. Foals with glucose <45 mg/dl (2.5 mmol/l) and a journey that will last more than 1–2 hours will require supplemental glucose administered as a 5% solution at a rate of 4 ml/kg/h. At no time should attendants travel in the trailer with a recumbent foal. Foals that are active but unable to nurse may be given 200–250 ml of milk by NG tube, provided reflux is not present. A bolus of highly concentrated glucose solution is not recommended, as this stimulates insulin release and may cause a profound rebound hypoglycemia. Fluids may be kept warm using a commercial fluid-warming device available from several commercial sources.

Foals with respiratory compromise present significant challenges [84]. While transporting, efforts are directed at ensuring that the nostrils remain free from bedding and other potential obstructions and keeping the foal in a sternal position. Sternal positioning provides rapid and consistent improvement in P_aO_2 and decreases the effort of breathing by alleviating dependent lung atelectasis. Pillows and blankets can be used to wedge the foal in sternal position, but some foals will manage to thwart all well-intentioned efforts to prop them in sternal. Inexpensive beanbags can be used to prop foals and a pillow over the extended carpi to rest the head upon will help maintain the nostrils free of debris. Foals that resist attempts to position sternal, should be turned at least every hour [84].

Foals with decreased (<30 per minute) or increased (>80 per minute) respiratory rates, labored respiration characterized by exaggerated intercostal and abdominal effort, cyanotic mucous membranes, or restlessness should be provided oxygen therapy if available [84]. Intranasal administration of supplemental oxygen is effective at increasing the P_aO_2 and oxygen saturation in neonatal foals [85] and may be required during transport in compromised foals. Small oxygen tanks (E size cylinder) can deliver flow rates of 5 l per minute for up to 1 hour [86], but the tanks must be firmly secured to the vehicle to prevent unintentional damage to the cylinder or valve. Conversely, the use of oxygen concentrators has been described in horses and could be adapted to proving supplemental oxygen to compromised foals via nasal insufflation [87]. If the foal has not nursed and the mare is dripping milk, collect the colostrum and send it with mare and foal to the referral hospital to prevent further wasting of the colostrum.

Notes

1 Lane Manufacturing Co., Denver, Colorado, USA.
2 Zoetis, Parsippany, N.J. USA.
3 SensLab, GmbH, Leipzig Germany.
4 3-M, St. Paul, Minnesota, USA.
5 Mila International, Inc., Florence, KY, USA.

References

1 Austin, S.M. (2013). Assessment of the equine neonate in ambulatory practice. *Equine Vet. Educ.* 25: 585–589.
2 LeBlanc, M.M. Immunological considerations. In: *Equine Clinical Neonatology* (ed. A.M. Koterba, W.H. Drummond, and P.C. Kosch), 55–70. Philadelphia: Lea and Febiger.
3 Stoneham, S.J. Assessing the newborn foal. In: *Equine Neonatal Medicine: A Case-Based Approach*, 1e (ed. M.R. Paradis), 1–13. Philadelphia: Elsevier Saunders.
4 Wilkins, P.A. and Dolente, B. Body wall tear in late gestational mare and birth resuscitation of a compromised foal. In: *Equine Neonatal Medicine: A Case-Based Approach*, 1e (ed. M.R. Paradis), 22–29. Philadelphia: Elsevier Saunders.
5 Schambourg, M.A., Laverty, S., Mullin, S. et al. (2003). Thoracic trauma in foals: postmortem findings. *Equine Vet. J.* 35: 78–81.
6 Yamamoto, K., Yasuda, J., and Too, K. (1992). Arrhythmias in newborn foals. *Equine Vet. J.* 24: 169–173.
7 Chope, K. Cardiac disorders. In: *Equine Neonatal Medicine: A Case-Based Approach*, 1e (ed. M.R. Paradis), 247–258. Philadelphia: Elsevier Saunders.
8 Rossdale, P.D. (1967). Clinical studies on the newborn Thoroughbred foal: II heart rate, auscultation, and electrocardiogram. *Br. Vet. J.* 123: 521–531.
9 Enzerink, E. (1998). The menace response and papillary light reflex in neonatal foals. *Equine Vet. J.* 30: 546–548.
10 Axon, J.E., Russell, C.M., and Wilkins, P.A. Neonatology. In: *Equine Emergency and Critical Care* (ed. L. Southwood and P. Wilkins), 511–554. Baca Raton: CRC Press.
11 Madigan, J.E. (1990). Management of the newborn foal. *Proc. Am. Assoc. Equine Pract.* 36: 99–116.
12 Kavan, R.P., Madigan, J.E., and Walker, R. (1994). Effect of disinfectant treatments on bacterial flora of the umbilicus of neonatal foals. *Proc. Am. Assoc. Equine Pract.* 40: 37–38.
13 Whitwell, K. and Jeffcott, L.B. (1975). Morphological studies on the fetal membranes of the normal singleton foal at birth. *Res. Vet. Sci.* 19: 44–55.

14 Cottril, C.M. (1991). Placental evaluation in the field. *Equine Vet. Educ.* 3: 204–207.
15 Cottril, C.M., Jeffers-Lo, J., Ousey, J.C. et al. (1991). The placenta as a determinant of fetal well-being in normal and abnormal pregnancies. *J. Reprod. Fertil. Suppl.* 44: 591–601.
16 McCue, P.M. (2007). Evaluation of a turbidometric immunoassay for measurement of plasma IgG concentrations in neonatal foals. *Am. J. Vet. Res.* 68: 1005–1009.
17 Jeffcott, L.B. (1971). Duration of permeability of the intestine to macromolecules in the newly-born foal. *Vet. Rec.* 8: 340–341.
18 Jeffcott, L.B. (1974). Studies on passive immunity in the foal II. The absorption of 125 – labeled pvp (polyvinyl pyrrolidone) by the neonatal intestine. *J. Comp. Pathol.* 84: 279–289.
19 McGuire, T.C., Crawford, T.B., Hallowell, A.L. et al. (1977). Failure of colostral immunoglobulin transfer as an explanation for most infections and deaths of neonatal foals. *J. Am. Vet. Med. Assoc.* 170: 1302–1304.
20 Perryman, L.E. and McGuire, T.C. (1980). Evaluation for immune system failures in horses and ponies. *J. Am. Vet. Med. Assoc.* 176: 1374–1377.
21 Koterba, A.M., Brewer, B.D., and Tarplee, R.L. (1984). Clinical and clinicopathological characteristics of the septicemic neonatal foal: review of 38 cases. *Equine Vet. J.* 16: 276–383.
22 Morris, D.D., Meirs, D.A., and Merryman, G.S. (1985). Passive transfer failure in horses: incidence and causative factors on a breeding farm. *Am. J. Vet. Res.* 46: 2294–2299.
23 Kohn, C.W., Knight, D., Hueston, W. et al. (1989). Colostral and serum IgG, IgA, and IgM concentrations in standardbred mares and their foals at parturition. *J. Am. Vet. Med. Assoc.* 195: 64–68.
24 Baldwin, J.L., Cooper, W.L., Vanderwall, D.K., and Erb, H.N. (1991). Prevalence (treatment days) and severity of illness in hypogammaglobulinemia and normogamma-globulinemia foals. *J. Am. Vet. Med. Assoc.* 198: 423–428.
25 Clabough, D.L., Levine, J.F., Grant, G.L., and Conboy, H.S. (1991). Factors associated with failure of passive transfer of colostral antibodies in Standardbred foals. *J. Vet. Intern. Med.* 5: 335–340.
26 Stoneham, S.J., Wingfield Digby, N.J., and Ricketts, S.W. (1991). Failure of passive transfer of colostral immunity in the foal: incidence, and the effect of stud management and plasma transfusions. *Vet. Rec.* 128: 416–419.
27 Raidal, S.L. (1996). The incidence and consequences of failure of passive transfer of immunity on a thoroughbred breeding farm. *Aust. Vet. J.* 73: 201–206.
28 McClure, J.T., Miller, J., and DeLuca, J.L. (2003). Comparison of two ELISA screening tests and a non-commercial gluteraldehyde coagulation screening test for the detection of failure of passive transfer in neonatal foals. *Proc. Am. Assoc. Equine Pract.* 49: 301–305.
29 Clabough, D.L. (1990). Factors associated with failure of passive transfer in Standardbred foals. *Proc. Am. Colloids Vet. Intern. Med.* 8: 555–558.
30 LeBlanc, M.M., Tran, T., Baldwin, J.L., and Pritchard, E.L. (1992). Factors that influence passive transfer of immunoglobulins in foals. *J. Am. Vet. Med. Assoc.* 200: 179–183.
31 LeBlanc, M.M., McLaurin, B.I., and Boswell, R. (1986). Relationships among serum immunoglobulin concentrations in foals, colostral specific gravity, and colostral immunoglobulin concentrations. *J. Am. Vet. Med. Assoc.* 189: 57–60.
32 Cohen, N.D. (1994). Causes of and farm management factors associated with disease and death in foals. *J. Am. Vet. Med. Assoc.* 204: 1644–1651.
33 Robinson, J.A., Allen, G.K., Green, E.M. et al. (1993). A retrospective study of septicaemia in colostrum-deprived foals. *Equine Vet. J.* 25: 214–219.
34 Raidal, S.L., McTaggart, C., and Penhale, J. (2005). Effect of withholding macromolecules on the duration of intestinal permeability to colostral IgG in foals. *Aust. Vet. J.* 83: 78–81.
35 Liepman, R.S., Dembek, K.A., Slovis, N.M. et al. (2015). Validation of IgG cut-off values and their association with survival in neonatal foals. *Equine Vet. J.* 47: 526–530.
36 Sheoran, A.S., Timoney, J.F., Holmes, M.A. et al. (2000). Immunoglobulin isotypes in sera and nasal mucosal secretions and their neonatal transfer and distribution in horses. *Am. J. Vet. Res.* 61: 1099–1105.
37 LeBlanc, M.M. (2001). Update on passive transfer of immunoglobulins in the foal. *Pferdheilkunde* 17: 662–665.
38 Rumbaugh, G.E., Ardans, A.A., Ginno, D. et al. (1978). Measurement of neonatal immunoglobulins for assessment of colostral immunoglobulin transfer: comparison of single radial immunodiffusion with zinc sulfate turbidity test, serum electrophoresis, refractometry of total serum protein, and the sodium sulfite precipitation test. *J. Am. Vet. Med. Assoc.* 172: 321–325.
39 Clabough, D.L., Conboy, H.S., and Roberts, M.C. (1989). Comparison of four screening techniques for the diagnosis of equine neonatal hypoglobulinemia. *J. Am. Vet. Med. Assoc.* 194: 1717–1720.
40 Pusterla, N., Pusterla, J.B., Spier, S.J. et al. (2002). Evaluation of the SNAP foal IgG test for the semiquantitative measurement of immunoglobulin G in foals. *Vet. Rec.* 151: 258–260.
41 Davis, R. and Giguere, S. (2005). Evaluation of five commercially available assays and measurement of

serum total protein concentration via refractometry for the diagnosis of failure of passive transfer of immunity in foals. *J. Am. Vet. Med. Assoc.* 227: 1640–1645.

42 Harvey, J.W., Asquith, R.L., McNulty, P.K. et al. (1984). Haematology of foals up to one year old. *Equine Vet. J.* 16: 347–353.

43 Buechner-Maxwell, V., Scott, M.A., Godber, L., and Kristensen, A. (1997). Neonatal alloimmune thrombocytopenia in a Quarter Horse foal. *J. Vet. Intern. Med.* 11: 304–308.

44 Bentz, A.I., Wilkins, P.A., MacGillivray, K.C. et al. (2002). *J. Vet. Intern. Med.* 16: 494–497.

45 Stoneham, S.J., Palmer, L., Cash, R., and Rossdale, P.D. (2001). Measurement of serum amyloid A in the neonatal foal using a latex agglutination immunoturbidimetric assay: determination of the normal range, variation with age and response to disease. *Equine Vet. J.* 33: 599–603.

46 Castagnetti, C., Pirrone, A., Mariella, J. et al. (2010). Venous blood lactate evaluation in equine neonatal intensive care. *Theriogenology* 73: 343–357.

47 Henderson, I.S.F., Franklin, R.P., Wilkins, P.A., and Boston, R.C. (2008). Association of hyperlactatemia with age, diagnosis, and survival in equine neonates. *J. Vet. Emerg. Crit. Care* 18: 496–502.

48 Hackett, E.S. and McCue, P.M. (2010). Evaluation of a veterinary glucometer for use in horses. *J. Vet. Intern. Med.* 24: 617–621.

49 Wilkins, P.A. (2011). The equine neonatal intensive care laboratory: point-of-care testing. *Clin. Lab. Med.* 31: 125–137.

50 Bellezzo, F., Hunt, R.J., Provost, P. et al. (2004). Surgical repair of rib fractures in 14 neonatal foals: case selection, surgical technique and results. *Equine Vet. J.* 36: 557–562.

51 Jean, D., Picandet, V., Maciera, S. et al. (2007). Detection of rib trauma in newborn foals in an equine critical care unit: a comparison of ultrasonography, radiography, and physical examination. *Equine Vet. J.* 39: 158–163.

52 McCoy, A.M., Lopp, C.T., Kooy, S. et al. (2020). Normal regression of the internal umbilical remnant structures in standardbred foals. *Equine Vet. J.* 52: 876–883.

53 Reef, V.B. and Collatos, C.A. (1989). Ultrasonography of umbilical structures in clinically normal foals. *Am. J. Vet. Res.* 49: 2143–2146.

54 Franklin, R.P. and Ferrell, E.A. (2002). How to perform umbilical sonograms in the neonate. *Proc. Am. Assoc. Equine Pract.* 48: 261–265.

55 Adams, R., Koterba, A.M., Cudd, T.C. et al. (1988). Exploratory celiotomy for suspected urinary tract disruption in neonatal foals: a review of 18 cases. *Equine Vet. J.* 20: 13–17.

56 Kablack, K.A., Embertson, R.M., Bernard, W.V. et al. (2000). Uroperitoneum in the hospitalized equine neonate: retrospective study of 31 cases, 1988–1997. *Equine Vet. J.* 32: 505–508.

57 Ousey, J.C., McArthur, A.J., Murgatroyd, P.R. et al. (1992). Thermoregulation and total body insulation in the neonatal foal. *J. Thermal Biol.* 17: 1–10.

58 Morresey, P.R. (2014). Assessing the weak foal. *Proc. Am. Assoc. Equine Pract. Focus on the First Year of Life* 60: 10–15.

59 Hunter, A.C. (1989). Practical intravenous fluid therapy. *Aust. Vet. Pract.* 19: 223–226.

60 Smith, B.P. (1996). Fluid delivery systems. In: *Large Animal Internal Medicine*, 2e (ed. B.P. Smith), 778–779. St Louis: Mosby.

61 Tan, R.H.H., Dart, A.J., and Dowling, B.A. (2003). Catheters: a review of the selection, utilization and complications of catheters for peripheral venous access. *Aust. Vet. J.* 81: 136–139.

62 Axon, J.E. and Wilkins, P.A. (2015). The neonate. In: *Equine Emergency and Critical Care Medicine* (ed. L. Southwood and P. Wilkins), 797–808. Boca Raton: CRC Press.

63 Buechner-Maxwell, V. (2012). Practical approach to nutritional support of the dysphagic foal. *Proc. Am. Assoc. Equine Pract.* 58: 412–424.

64 Klein, C.J., Stanek, G.S., and Wiles, C.E. III (1998). Overfeeding macronutrients to critically ill adults: metabolic complications. *J. Am. Diet. Assoc.* 98: 795–806.

65 Paradis, M.R. (2001). Nutrition and indirect calorimetry in neonatal foals. *Proc. Am. Colloids Vet. Int. Med.* 19: 245–247.

66 Rothman, D., Udall, J.N., Pang, K.Y. et al. (2004). The effect of short-term starvation on mucosal barrier function in the newborn rabbit. *Pediatr. Res.* 19: 727–731.

67 Palmer, J.E. (2004). Fluid therapy in the neonate: not your mother's fluid space. *Vet. Clin. North Am. Equine Pract.* 20: 63–75.

68 Korterba, A.M., Brewer, B., and Drummond, W.H. (1985). Prevention and control of infection. *Vet. Clin. North Am. Equine Pract.* 1: 41–50.

69 Vivrette, S.L. (2001). Colostrum and oral immunoglobulin therapy in newborn foals. *Compend. Contin. Educ. Pract. Vet.* 23: 286–291.

70 Wilkins, P.A. and Dewan-Mix, S. (1994). Efficacy of intravenous plasma therapy in newborn foals. *Cornell Vet.* 84: 7–14.

71 Sellon, D.C. (2006). Neonatal immunology. In: *Equine Neonatal Medicine* (ed. M.R. Paradis), 31–39. Philadelphia: Elsevier.

72 Pusterla, N., Magdesian, K.G., Maleski, K. et al. (2004). Retrospective evaluation of the use of acetylcysteine enemas in the treatment of meconium retention in foals: 44 cases (1987–2002). *Equine Vet. Educ.* 16: 133–136.

73 Fielding, C.L. and Magdesian, K.G. (2015). Sepsis and septic shock. In: The equine neonate. *Vet. Clin. North Am. Equine Pract.* 31: 483–496.

74 Wong, D.M. and Wilkins, P.A. (2015). Defining the systemic inflammatory response syndrome in equine neonates. *Vet. Clin. North Am. Equine Pract.* 31: 463–481.

75 Brewer, B.D. and Koterba, A.M. (1988). Development of a scoring system for the early diagnosis of equine neonatal sepsis. *Equine Vet. J.* 20: 18–22.

76 Brewer, B.D. Neonatal infection. In: *Equine Clinical Neonatology* (ed. A.M. Koterba, W. Drummond, and P. Kosch), 310. Philadelphia: Lea and Febiger.

77 Corley, K.T.T. and Furr, M.O. (2003). Evaluation of a score designed to predict sepsis in foals. *J. Vet. Emerg. Crit. Care* 13: 149–155.

78 Weber, E.J., Sanchez, L.C., and Giguere, S. (2015). Re-evaluation of the sepsis score in equine neonates. *Equine Vet. J.* 47: 275–278.

79 Sanchez, L.C. (2005). Equine neonatal sepsis. *Vet. Clin. North Am. Equine Pract.* 21: 273–293.

80 Russell, C.M., Aon, J.E., Bishen, A. et al. (2008). Blood culture results from 427 critically ill neonatal foals (1999 to 2004). *Aust. Vet. J.* 86: 266–271.

81 Gold, J.R. (2017). Perinatal asphyxia syndrome. *Equine Vet. Educ.* 29: 158–164.

82 Trumble, T.N. (2005). Orthopedic disorders in neonatal foals. *Vet. Clin. North Am. Equine Pract.* 21: 358–385.

83 DeBoer, S. (1992). Transporting ill or injured foals safely. *Equine Vet. Educ.* 4: 150–153.

84 Kosch, P.C. and Koterba, A.M. (1987). Respiratory support for the newborn foal. In: *Current Therapy in Equine Medicine*, 2e (ed. N.E. Robinson), 247–253. Philadelphia: WB Saunders.

85 Wong, D.M., Alcott, C.J., Wang, C. et al. (2010). Physiologic effects of nasopharyngeal administration of supplemental oxygen at various flow rates in healthy neonatal foals. *Am. J. Vet. Res.* 71: 1081–1088.

86 Knottenbelt Transport of the sick or injured foal. In: *Equine Neonatology* (ed. D.E. Knottenbelt, N. Holstock, and J.E. Madigan), 456–458. London: Elsevier Ltd.

87 Coutu, P., Caulkett, N., Pang, D., and Boysen, S. (2015). Efficacy of a portable oxygen concentrator with pulsed delivery for treatment of hypoxemia during equine field anesthesia. *Vet. Anaesth. Analg.* 42: 18–26.

Chapter 58 Feeding the Neonatal Foal

Harold McKenzie and Bettina Dunkel

Developing an appropriate nutritional plan for a foal can be challenging, as one needs to ensure that the foal has adequate nutrients not only for basal metabolism but also to support immune function and growth. This process can be straightforward for healthy orphan foals, but the situation for ill foals is more complex, as their energy requirements are less well understood and the ability of ill foals to appropriately utilize the nutrients provided is not guaranteed. The clinician must formulate the best plan possible with available information and ensure that the foal is closely monitored and the goals of the nutritional plan are met while minimizing complications.

Nutritional Requirements of the Foal

The caloric requirements of the healthy foal are substantial, due to the need to support high basal metabolic needs and maintain a rate of growth of as much as 2.5% of body weight per day. This equates to a caloric requirement as great as 150 kcal/kg body weight/d (kcal/kg/d), which decreases gradually to around 120 kcal/kg/d at three weeks of age and then 80–100 kcal/kg/d by 1–2 months of age [1, 2]. The initial energy source for the foal is mare's milk, which has considerably greater lactose content than cow's milk and lower milk fat content. On a dry-matter basis, mare's milk averages about 64%, 22%, and 13% sugar, protein, and fat, respectively, as compared to 38%, 26%, and 30% sugar, protein, and fat, respectively, for cow's milk. Mare's milk derives most of its energy content from carbohydrates, and appropriate endogenous production of insulin is required for the foal to metabolize and utilize these carbohydrates appropriately.

Maturation of pancreatic β-cell function occurs late in gestation. Following birth, there is a gradual maturation of the endocrine response to ingested carbohydrates. Studies in healthy newborn pony foals have demonstrated impaired glucose clearance following administration of exogenous glucose on the first day of life, suggesting a degree of insulin resistance [3]. By 10 days of age, foals demonstrate increased rates of glucose clearance, but this response remains lower than what is observed in healthy adult horses. This gradual maturation may be an appropriate response to changes in the composition of mare's milk, as colostrum contains little lactose, and in the volume of milk ingested, which is less on the first day of life than on subsequent days [1, 3].

When evaluating the ill neonatal foal, one must always keep in mind the possibility that the disease processes might have originated in utero. Maternal illness, malnutrition, or toxin exposure along with placentitis and placental insufficiency all have the potential to profoundly influence the development and maturation of fetal metabolism [4, 5]. This prenatal programming may affect the neonatal foal's ability to appropriately metabolize nutrients in the clinical setting, with some foals from compromised placental environments exhibiting insulin resistance and carbohydrate intolerance. Foals suffering from systemic inflammation (e.g. sepsis) may also exhibit hyperglycemia due to insulin resistance and carbohydrate intolerance [6]. Conversely, hypoglycemia, complicated by decreased endogenous energy reserves and impairment of nursing due to concurrent weakness, depression, and/or difficulty standing, is a common problem in ill neonatal foals, although this risk tends to decrease with advancing age [7].

Determining the caloric needs of the ill foal is one of the greatest challenges in designing a nutritional strategy. The energy requirements of ill foals are not as great as previously thought [8], as there is a reduction in the overall metabolic rate due to a decrease in activity in combination with a temporary reduction in growth rate. Indirect calorimetry testing of clinically ill neonatal foals demonstrated a resting energy requirement (RER) of only 45–50 kcal/kg/d, which is one-third of the energy requirement for growing,

Equine Neonatal Medicine, First Edition. Edited by David M. Wong and Pamela A. Wilkins.

active, healthy foals [9, 10]. As ill foals recover, their energy requirements gradually increase to approximately 65–70 kcal/kg/d, which is similar to the energy requirements of age-matched control foals [10].

In managing the critically ill neonatal foal, using a hypocaloric approach may be preferable, wherein one endeavors to prevent the foal from entering a severely catabolic state while accepting that all of the nutritional needs of the patient may not be met [11, 12]. This approach addresses the fact that aggressive nutritional support can result in overfeeding, the risks of which can outweigh the benefits of providing nutritional support. Excessive carbohydrate administration will lead to increased generation of carbon dioxide and can worsen hypercapnia in foals with compromised respiratory function. Excessive carbohydrate delivery will also cause hyperglycemia, which is considered a proinflammatory stimulus and associated with worsening of outcome in human critical illness [13, 14]. Overfeeding of protein will result in increased protein catabolism and can result in the potentiation and/or development of azotemia [14]. The excessive administration of lipids may result in hypertriglyceridemia [15]. In contrast to the risks of overfeeding, there is little evidence in people that short-term hypocaloric nutrition results in worsened outcomes as compared to regimens designed to meet the patient's metabolic needs [12, 16]. Some evidence suggests that this approach, especially in regards to maintaining appropriate control of blood glucose levels, is associated with decreased rates of complications and improved outcomes [13, 16].

Enteral Feeding

The first step in developing a nutritional plan is selection of the route of nutrient delivery. The enteral route is generally preferred for two reasons: (i) it is the most natural and physiologic means of nutrient delivery, and (ii) the intestinal mucosa is partially dependent on products of digestion for energy and nutrients. A thorough evaluation of gastrointestinal (GI) function is needed before institution of enteral nutritional, as foals with evidence of GI dysfunction such as gastric reflux, bowel distension, increased bowel wall thickness, and ileus are unlikely to tolerate enteral feeding. A conservative approach to enteral feeding is also indicated for premature or dysmature foals that may have incomplete development of the GI tract. Foals with perinatal asphyxia syndrome may also be intolerant of enteral feeding due to ileus and GI dysfunction from intestinal ischemic injury.

Mare's milk is the preferred substrate for enteral feeding, as it is highly digestible and obviously provides the correct balance of nutrients for normal growth and development. The caloric content of mare's milk varies by breed, diet, and other factors, but is approximately 480 kcal/l (0.48 kcal/ml) [17]. Commercial mare's milk replacers are commonly used, but these products are bovine in origin and have lower digestibility compared with mare's milk. This increases the risk of intestinal dysfunction associated with enteral feeding. When mixed according to label recommendations these products also are hyperosmolar and can cause electrolyte and GI disturbances in foals, but mixing them at a rate of 1 part solids to 10 parts water can minimize these risks [18]. Providing free access to fresh water can also help decrease the risk of electrolyte abnormalities, especially following transition to voluntary intake. Goat's milk or semi-skimmed (2% fat) cow's milk supplemented with 20 g/l dextrose (equivalent to 40 ml of 50% dextrose solution per liter) also can be used if mare's milk or mare's milk replacer is unavailable [18]. Foals that are unable to nurse the mare may be fed through a bottle, bowl, or nasogastric feeding tube. Many ill, recumbent foals have a weak and/or uncoordinated suckle reflex, however, and due to the risk of aspiration should be fed using a nasogastric tube.

Use of small-bore indwelling feeding tubes and provision of small volumes at frequent intervals is preferred over repeated passage of a feeding tube, as large-bolus feedings may overwhelm digestive capacity, and repeated passage of a feeding tube is traumatic and stressful. Small-bore indwelling tubes still allow voluntary intake of feed and water so the tube may be left in place as the foal is transitioned to feeding from the mare or a bucket. Prior to placement, the tube can be held along the foal's side to estimate the length needed for the tube to reach the distal esophagus. Placement in the distal esophagus is preferable to the stomach, as this allows for normal sealing of the cardiac sphincter and minimizes the likelihood of inadvertent milk reflux from the tube as well as aspiration of air. The feeding tube should be inserted with the foal standing or in sternal recumbency, and correct placement confirmed by palpation of the tube within the cervical esophagus, radiography, or endoscopy. The tube is then fastened to the external nares by sutures. At each feeding, it is important to check that the tube is still in place and that there is no reflux. The foal should be in sternal recumbency or standing when fed via tube, and milk should be administered by gravity flow followed by a small amount of clean water to flush the tube. The tube should be capped between feedings to prevent aspiration of air. Some clinicians replace feeding tubes every 3–4 days to reduce risk of GI tract infection.

A suggested initial rate of milk delivery is 2–3 ml/kg body weight/h or 100–150 ml/h for a 50-kg foal (Table 58.1). This provides 2.4–3.6 l of milk to a 50-kg foal during the first 24 hours of enteral support. Parenteral nutrition can

Table 58.1 Enteral feeding recommendations for neonatal and growing foals.

Foal age (days)	Energy requirement	Volume of mare's milk or milk replacer	Percentage of body weight fed
0–1	50–150 kcal/kg/d	2–3 ml/kg/h	5–7%
2–3	100–150 kcal/kg/d	4–5 ml/kg/h	10–12%
4–7	150 kcal/kg/d	6–8 ml/kg/h	14–20%
8–30	120 kcal/kg/d	9–10 ml/kg/h	22%
30 – weaning	80–100 kcal/kg/d	Gradual decreasing, replaced with solid feed	

be administered to provide additional nutrition during the transition to an adequate level of enteral feeding. The feeding rate can be gradually increased over the next 2–3 days (e.g. increase to 4–5 ml/kg/h on day 2, 6–8 ml/kg/h on day 3). Simultaneously, IV nutritional support may be gradually withdrawn. This feeding level (6–8 ml/kg/h) will likely meet the RER of hospitalized foals. Depending on degree of clinical improvement and length of hospitalization, it may be possible to increase the volume of feeding to 20–22% body weight/day, which approximates the milk intake of healthy neonatal foals. The frequency of feeding can be reduced as the foal demonstrates that is can tolerate enteral feedings, especially when consuming milk or milk replacer voluntarily. Clinical monitoring includes frequent assessment of GI function, as gastric reflux, bloating, colic, diarrhea, or constipation can indicate intolerance to enteral feeding and the need for adjustments to the feeding program such as a decrease in volume or frequency of enteral feedings. In some situations, the foal's GI tract may not be able to digest and absorb lactose, as in rotaviral infections where production of lactase by the enterocytes is likely impaired. In these cases, lactase enzyme (such as Lactaid®, McNeil Nutritionals, LLC, Ft. Washington, PA) can be added to the milk or milk replacer prior to feeding, at the rate of 9000 units (one tablet) per feeding. Additional volumes of enteral fluid may be required in foals with diarrhea, and a simple balanced isotonic enteral solution can be formulated by adding 5.6 g of table salt (NaCl), 0.6 g of Lite Salt® (50% NaCl, 50% KCl), and 3.4 g of baking soda ($NaHCO_3$) per liter of water [19].

Parenteral Nutrition (PN)

Enteral feedings are preferred to support foals [2, 20], but ill foals may have conditions that preclude enteral nutrition or inability to tolerate the volume of enteral nutrition required to support basal metabolism and growth. These range from the critically ill neonate with GI complications to the suckling foal with severe enterocolitis. The rapid institution of parenteral nutrition (PN) can help prevent the development of protein/calorie malnutrition and substantial energy deficits. Limitations of PN include the expense, the risk of secondary complications (e.g. hyperglycemia, hypertriglyceridemia, electrolyte disturbances, azotemia, thrombophlebitis), and an increased risk of bloodstream infections.

A reasonable goal for PN administration in foals is 30–40 kcal/kg/d, while human studies suggests that initial therapy may only need to target rates of 15 kcal/kg/d [21]. This hypocaloric approach does not completely meet the theoretical energy requirements of the healthy neonate but comes close to meeting the RER in hospitalized foals [1, 9]. In this situation, PN is used purely as temporary support to prevent the foal from entering a severely catabolic state, in which protein catabolism increases to utilize amino acids for energy production [1, 11, 22]. Failure to provide adequate nutritional support may also have a negative influence on the immune response [22–24].

PN Formulations and Administration

Short-term parenteral supplementation (<24 hours) may consist of IV carbohydrate solutions, but if prolonged PN is expected, a more complete formula should be utilized. Carbohydrate-containing solutions represent the simplest means of providing IV caloric support to foals. While fluids containing small amounts of dextrose (~1%) can be utilized for initial fluid bolus resuscitation, fluids containing 5% dextrose should not be used for this purpose, as this will almost certainly result in excessive amounts of dextrose to a foal with any degree of dehydration, resulting in profound hyperglycemia. Following initial fluid resuscitation, maintenance fluids containing electrolytes as well as dextrose (0.45% saline with 5% dextrose, Normosol-M with 5% dextrose, Plasmalyte-56 with 5% dextrose) may be used as primary fluids in foals with minimal ongoing fluid losses. Dextrose 5% in water is not a good choice as a maintenance solution due to the absence of electrolytes. Additional nutritional support is likely to be needed, using the enteral or parenteral route, as the caloric content of 5% dextrose solution is 0.17 kcal/ml. This means that an infusion rate of 10 ml/kg/h would be required to deliver approximately 40 kcal/kg/d (0.17 kcal/kg/h × 24 hours/d = 41 kcal/kg/d). This rate of infusion is excessive, as it is over twice the maintenance rate for a neonatal foal; if additional calories are needed, they should be provided in another way.

Alternatively, 50% dextrose solution can be delivered using an infusion pump, provided that additional isotonic fluids are administered concurrently to provide dilution of the hypertonic dextrose solution as it is being delivered to the foal. This reduces the risk of endothelial injury due to the hypertonic nature of this solution. Use of 50% dextrose solution should be avoided if an infusion pump is not available, as it is easy to inadvertently administer an excessive amount of dextrose, leading to hyperglycemia. The caloric content of 50% dextrose solution is 1.7 kcal/ml, so an infusion rate of 1 ml/kg/h of this solution will deliver approximately 40 kcal/kg/d (1.7 kcal/kg/h × 24 h/d = 41 kcal/kg/d). This low infusion rate warrants that primary fluid needs are met with dextrose-free electrolyte solutions in which the administration rate can be altered in response to changes in patient fluid status without concerns related to the nutritional plan. At the end of the first 24 hours of treatment, the fluid and nutritional plans should be revisited to determine if the foal can begin to rely on enteral fluid and nutritional intake or if continued parenteral therapy is required. Continued PN support requires formulation of a more complete solution that provides amino acids and possibly lipids.

One important aspect of providing PN beyond initial stabilization is inclusion of a protein source, as early provision of protein may improve clinical outcomes [25]. The metabolic response to injury and sepsis is increased protein degradation of muscle; this catabolic response can be reduced by increasing energy intake and/or by supplying a source of amino acids. Traditionally it has been recommended to provide PN with a ratio of 100–200 non-protein calories per gram of nitrogen [26]. In a 50 kg foal receiving 30 kcal/kg/d of PN, this would equate to 7.5–15 g of nitrogen per day, or 0.15–0.3 g nitrogen/kg/d. Current human recommendations, however, are to provide amino acids at a rate of 1.5 (1.2–2.5) grams nitrogen/kg/d [27], and there are suggestions that providing adequate amounts of protein may actually be more important than caloric adequacy [16, 28].

The inclusion of lipids in PN formulations provides a larger number of calories per unit volume compared with solutions containing only dextrose. Another advantage of lipid emulsions is that they are isotonic, thereby moderating the hypertonicity of PN and potentially decreasing the risk of thrombophlebitis. Formulating PN solutions with lipids substantially increases the daily costs associated with PN and increases the risk of complications [29]. Hyperlipidemia can occur in association with lipid administration to foals, but does not appear to result in adverse effects [15, 29]. Of greater concern, lipid-containing formulations are much more susceptible to contamination and promote bacterial growth, requiring formulation under controlled, sterile conditions to reduce risk of contamination. These conditions are typically only available in pharmacies associated with large veterinary hospitals or human hospitals. Due to the risk of contamination, IV lines through which lipid-containing solutions are administered must also be changed daily, substantially increasing client costs. While the use of lipid-containing PN solutions in one report allowed for the provision of 40–92 kcal/kg/d (mean = 63 kcal/kg/d) to foals, as opposed to only 25–66 kcal/kg/d (mean = 41 kcal/kg/d) with a dextrose based solution, in most situations such high levels of caloric support are not required [15].

There are two basic approaches to formulating PN to foals. The first involves exact determination of anticipated metabolic needs of the patient and development of a formulation that will meet all of these needs in a precise manner, using a mixture of dextrose, amino acids, and lipids (Table 58.2). This approach is complex and is best performed using a computerized spreadsheet to perform various calculations. The second approach is more practical and consists of using simple, basic parenteral nutrition formulas (Table 58.3). One of these solutions is intended for short-term use and consists of 50% dextrose and 8.5% amino acid solutions (Solution I). The second solution incorporates a lipid energy source and is preferred for long-term administration or for administration to foals that are poorly tolerant of infused dextrose (Solution II). Solution I is formulated using 2000 ml of 50% dextrose and 2000 ml of 8.5% amino acids, while Solution II is formulated with

Table 58.2 Useful conversions for the preparation of parenteral nutrition.

1 kcal = 4.184 kJ = 4184 J	1 g glucose = 3.4 kcal
1 g amino acids = 4.0 kcal	1 g lipids = 9.0 kcal
1 ml of 50% dextrose = 0.5 g/ml = 500 mg/ml dextrose	1 ml of 50% dextrose = 1.7 kcal
1 g protein = 0.16 g nitrogen	1 g nitrogen = 6.25 g protein
1 ml of 8.5% amino acid solution = 85 mg/ml AA = 13.6 g nitrogen = 0.32 kcal/ml	
1 ml of 10% amino acid solution = 100 mg/ml = 16 g nitrogen = 0.4 kcal/ml	
1 ml of 20% amino acid solution = 200 mg/ml = 32 g nitrogen = 0.8 kcal/ml	
1 ml 10% lipid solution = 100 mg/ml = 0.9 kcal/ml	
1 ml 20% lipid solution = 200 mg/ml = 1.8 kcal/ml	

Table 58.3 Formulation of parenteral nutrition solutions.

Formulation	Composition	Caloric density (kcal/ml)	Non-protein calories/g N	Osmolarity
Compounded solutions				
Formula 1	1500 ml 50% dextrose, 1500 ml 8.5% amino acids	1.02	125	1675
Formula 2	1500 ml 50% dextrose, 500 ml 20% lipids, 2000 ml 8.5% amino acids	1.08	131	1395
Premixed solutions				
Clinimix 4.25/20	4.25% amino acids, 25% dextrose	1.02	125	1675
Procalamine	3% amino acids, 3% glycerol Sodium 35 mEq/l; Potassium 24.5 mEq/l; Calcium 3 mEq/l; Magnesium 5 mEq/l; Chloride 41 mEq/l; Phosphate 7 mEq/l; Acetate 47 mEq/l	0.25	28	735
Clinimix E 2.75/5	2.75% amino acids, 5% dextrose Sodium 35 mEq/l; Potassium 30 mEq/l; Calcium 4.5 mEq/l; Magnesium 5 mEq/l; Chloride 39 mEq/l; Phosphate 15 mEq/l; Acetate 51 mEq/l	0.28	37	665

1500 ml of 50% dextrose, 500 ml of 20% lipids, and 2000 ml of 8.5% amino acids (e.g. Dextrose 50%, Travasol® 8.5%, Intralipid®, Baxter Healthcare Corp., Clintec Nutr. Div., Deerfield, IL, USA) [15]. The total caloric density of these solutions is 1.02 kcal/ml for Solution I and 1.08 kcal/ml for Solution II. If solution I is used in a foal to deliver 30 kcal/kg/d this will achieve delivery of 0.2 g nitrogen/kg.

Alternatively, a shelf-stable premixed multi-chamber bag preparation identical to Solution I is manufactured for human use (Table 58.3), and is cost-effective and practical for use in foals (e.g. Clinimix® 4.25/25 sulfite-free 4.25% Amino Acid in 25% Dextrose Injection, Baxter Healthcare Corp., Clintec Nutr. Div., Deerfield, IL, USA). The bag is separated into two compartments such that the dextrose and amino acid solutions are not intermixed until the barrier between compartments is manually released prior to administration to the patient. Eliminating the need for formulation in a fume hood greatly reduces the risk of contamination of the PN solution, and multichambered bag PN formulations have been shown to significantly reduce the risk of bloodstream infections in human patients as compared to compounded PN [30]. Premixed PN solutions are typically less expensive than compounded PN [31], and having a readily available PN solution also allows for more rapid institution of PN therapy in the veterinary setting, especially outside of normal business hours. Where one might normally institute dextrose supplementation alone, the use of this type of product allows for early administration of amino acids as well. While not currently available in the United States, similar three-chamber bag products are available in Europe that include dextrose, amino acids, and lipids.

Another premixed, shelf-stable option exists for PN administration (e.g. Procalamine®, Braun Medical Inc., Bethlehem, PA). In veterinary medicine, this product has primarily been used in dogs as a supplement to enteral nutrition and has similar utility in foals [32]. Procalamine is substantially different in formulation from other PN solutions, and is essentially a maintenance-type crystalloid fluid (Table 58.3) with moderate amounts of added carbohydrates (3% glycerol) and amino acids (3%). This solution is less hypertonic than PN solutions described above, and in humans is considered safe for peripheral, rather than central, vein administration [33]. The use of glycerol as the carbohydrate is potentially beneficial, as glycerol metabolism is insulin-independent [34]. Hyperglycemia is less likely to develop with glycerol infusion, and the need for exogenous insulin is less in human patients receiving glycerol-containing fluids compared to dextrose-containing fluids [34]. The total caloric content of Procalamine is 0.25 kcal/ml, which is less than a fourth of Solution I above, but the relative amount of protein to carbohydrates is nearly four times greater (28 nonprotein calories/g N). Olan et al. reported delivering an average of 33% of the RER in canine patients using Procalamine [32]. By using this product to meet the baseline maintenance fluid needs of the neonatal foal (at 4 ml/kg/h) one would achieve delivery of 24 kcal/kg/d and 0.7 g protein/kg. It is not recommended to exceed this rate of delivery in most patients, as this solution contains low concentrations of electrolytes and hyponatremia so hypochloremia may result. Additional isotonic polyionic fluid therapy may be required in patients with ongoing losses or electrolyte abnormalities. If a greater degree of caloric support is desired, Procalamine can be supplemented with additional administration of 50% dextrose, as previously described. A similar product formulated with dextrose rather than glycerol is also available in a shelf stable multi-chamber bag formulation (Table 58.3).

An electronic infusion pump should always be used when administering PN solutions, as the rate must be tightly controlled. Excessive rates of administration can induce profound hyperglycemia, which has been shown in other species to be associated with severe complications and increased risk of death [35]. The solutions used for PN are all hypertonic and can cause injury to the vascular endothelium, increasing the risk of thrombophlebitis. For this reason, it is recommended that PN solutions be administered through a 20 cm long polyurethane long-term catheter placed in the jugular vein, as this provides a "central" line in most foals. While not required, the use of a multiple lumen catheter allows for one lumen to be dedicated to infusion of the PN solution and other fluids, minimizing the risks of contamination. Catheter management is extremely important when foals are receiving PN, and the catheter site and vein should be monitored at least twice daily for heat, swelling, or exudation. Increased resistance to fluid flow in the catheter may be an indication of vessel thrombosis.

Clinical Application

Components of compounded PN solutions must be compounded in a sterile manner prior to administration (Table 58.4) and care should be taken when adding any medications to a PN solution. The bag containing the final PN composition should be protected from light (i.e. covered with a brown plastic bag) to avoid degradation of amino acids within the solution. The rate of infusion (in ml/h) is calculated based upon the desired kcal/kg/d to be administered. A reasonable initial goal is 30–40 kcal/kg/d.

Table 58.4 Instructions on how to prepare parenteral nutrition under sterile conditions.

- Clean inside of flow hood/ surface of working area thoroughly, as last step spray all surfaces with alcohol and allow alcohol to evaporate.
- Wear gown, mask, and sterile gloves when preparing the solution.
- Spray/wipe all injection ports with alcohol.
- Close all lines leading to compounding bag before connecting bottles to compounding bag.
- Connect lines of compounding bag with dextrose and amino acid containers; mix amino acids and dextrose first (to assess aqueous solution for any signs of precipitation).
- Allow solutions to run into compounding bag by gravity. Close lines to change dextrose/amino acid bottles and reopen once reconnected.
- Add lipids and additives (vitamins, KCL) last.
- Close lines, close mixing bag with clamp provided and note date of mixing on label.
- Keep refrigerated at 4–8 °C (or as indicated by manufacturer) and use within 48 h.

The initial infusion rate of PN solutions should be 25% of the calculated final rate, and gradually increased every 1–3 hours following monitoring of blood glucose concentration to ensure that hyperglycemia (blood glucose >150 mg/dl) is not present [36]. If the patient tolerates PN well and maintains blood glucose concentrations at or near normal concentrations, the PN administration rate can be increased to a maximum of 50–60 kcal/kg/d, but this is rarely required [37]. When discontinuing PN, it is recommended to gradually reduce the infusion rate in 25–50% increments every 4–6 hours while gradually introducing enteral feeding. It is important that blood glucose monitoring is continued during this weaning process, in order to detect or prevent the development of hypoglycemia.

Foals must be frequently monitored, especially during the initial phase of PN therapy. This includes a general physical examination, with close attention to neurological status, respiratory function, and monitoring of rectal temperature, as fever is a common early manifestation of systemic infection. Blood glucose concentrations should be frequently monitored, initially on an hourly basis, until the patient has stabilized with the appropriate rate of PN infusion, followed by monitoring every 3–6 hours for the first day of therapy. The frequency of blood glucose monitoring is dependent upon the stability of the patient, and may need to be more frequent in the very critically ill, but may not need to be monitored beyond every 12 hours in the stable patient. Continuous blood glucose monitoring holds promise for use in foals, although work continues to determine the most appropriate and accurate devices in foals [38]. Monitoring urine output and urine glucose concentration may also aid in detection of hyperglycemia-induced diuresis and glucosuria. The actual renal threshold for glucose is not well described in foals, but glucosuria and diuresis are typically seen when blood glucose levels exceed 180 mg/dl. Serum electrolytes should be monitored at least twice daily with particular attention paid to serum potassium and phosphorus concentrations as they can decrease rapidly, especially in foals receiving insulin therapy. Ideally, body weight should be assessed on a daily basis, to ensure that the foal is at least maintaining body weight while on PN. Foals receiving PN solutions containing lipids should be monitored for the development of hypertriglyceridemia [15, 39].

Insulin Therapy

Critically ill foals often demonstrate carbohydrate intolerance, making it difficult to achieve even a conservative rate of administration of IV nutrition. This situation can be addressed by lowering the rate of infusion or use of a lipid containing PN solution. If hyperglycemia persists, the only alternative is administration of exogenous insulin. The administration of insulin to the neonatal foal is not to be

Table 58.5 Setting up a continuous rate infusion of insulin.

Setting up an insulin infusion:

- Confirm that blood glucose concentration exceeds set limit on two consecutive readings (usually 1 h apart).
- Check regular insulin concentration: usually 100 U per ml.
- Set up insulin infusion by adding regular insulin to 0.9% sodium chloride.
  - 10 units to 100 ml sodium chloride 0.9% = 0.1 unit/ml.
  - 100 units to 100 ml sodium chloride 0.9% = 1 unit/ml.
  - 100 units to 500 ml sodium chloride 0.9% = 0.2 unit/ml.
- Start at rate of 0.01 U/kg/h = 0.5 U/h for 50 kg foal = 5 ml/h of a 0.1unit/ml solution.
- Monitor blood glucose concentration initially hourly until stable at the desired concentration.

Precautions:

- Insulin infusions must be accompanied with supportive parenteral glucose or parenteral nutrition supplementation.
- Insulin should be stored (e.g. refrigerated) and used as directed by the manufacturer (e.g. some insulin preparations require rolling or shaking before use).
- Insulin adsorbs to plastic tubing, decreasing the concentration in the solution. Current recommendations suggest flushing of the tubing with 20 ml of the infusion solution followed by starting the infusion. Leaving the solution in the tube for a longer dwell time is no longer recommended [42].

undertaken lightly as it places additional demands on the clinician and nursing staff to ensure that profound hypoglycemia does not occur. Intermittent dosing of subcutaneous insulin offers some advantages in terms of simplicity of administration, expense and moderation of effects, but does not allow for changes in dosage over the short term. One recommended dosage for subcutaneous insulin in foals is 0.1–0.5 IU of regular insulin every 12 hours [40]. A retrospective report of foal PN described subcutaneous insulin dosage rates 0.02–0.1 IU/kg given every 6–24 hours [39]. This approach may be associated with a greater risk of hypoglycemia or hyperglycemia as it is much more challenging to achieve homeostasis in terms of blood glucose concentrations when using intermittent bolus insulin therapy [41].

The use of continuous rate infusion (CRI) of insulin (Table 58.5) allows for a fairly rapid onset of action while facilitating rapid adjustment of dosage. Due to the gradual saturation of cellular insulin receptors, the maximal effect of CRI insulin is not typically seen until 60–90 minutes after initiation of the infusion. The response to alterations of infusion rates occurs over a similar time frame, so care must be taken to avoid altering the rate of infusion of PN solutions too soon after changing the rate of insulin infusion. An initial insulin infusion rate of 0.01–0.07 IU/kg/h of regular insulin has been reported to be well tolerated, and it represents a reasonable starting point in foals intolerant of PN [11, 43]. Starting at the low end of this dosage range is safe and may be sufficient, especially if using a hypocaloric approach and/or low carbohydrate concentration PN formulations, but may require a longer period of time before the dose is titrated to a high enough level to control refractory hyperglycemia.

When "fine-tuning" insulin therapy, it is best to avoid simultaneous alterations in both the insulin and PN infusion rates, as this leads to a "roller-coaster ride" wherein the blood glucose concentration is rising and falling wildly due to the delay in the body's response to these changes (Figure 58.1) [11]. Blood glucose monitoring should be

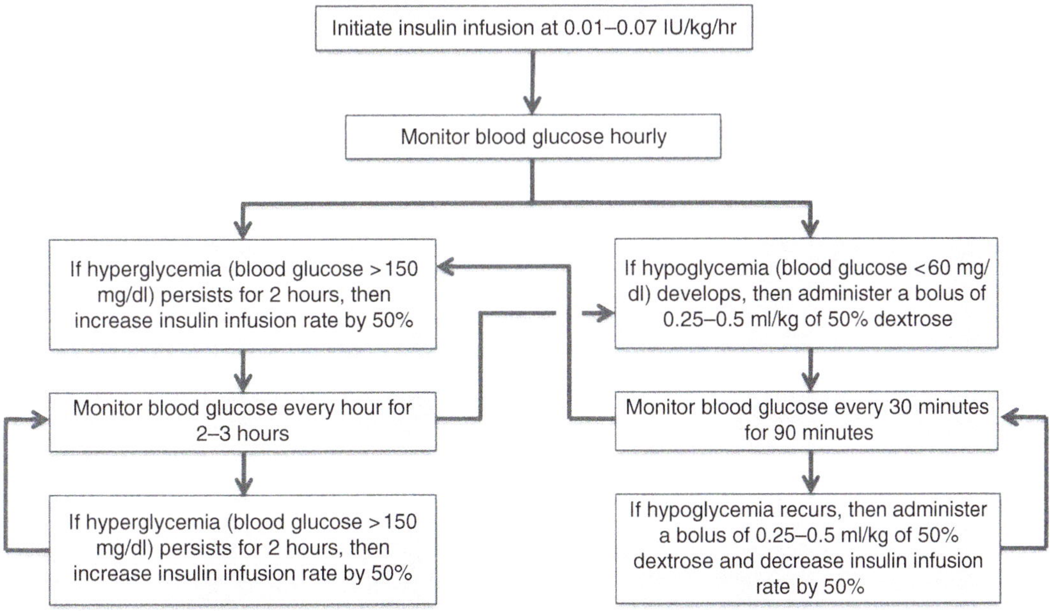

Figure 58.1 Protocol for the monitoring and regulation of insulin when administered as a continuous rate infusion to foals. *Source:* Adapted from: McKenzie and Geor [11].

performed at least hourly for the first 2–3 hours after initiation of the insulin CRI; if hyperglycemia (blood glucose >150 mg/dl) persists beyond the first 2 hours of insulin therapy, then the insulin infusion rate may be increased by 50%, followed by hourly blood glucose monitoring for a further 2–3 hours. This procedure for increasing the insulin infusion rate may be repeated if hyperglycemia persists. Conversely, if hypoglycemia (blood glucose <60 mg/dl) is noted then a bolus of 0.25–0.5 ml/kg of 50% dextrose solution should be administered intravenously over 3–5 minutes. The blood glucose level should then be reassessed every 30 minutes for at least 90 minutes to ensure that hypoglycemia does not recur. If hypoglycemia recurs, a second bolus of dextrose is administered and the insulin infusion rate is decreased by 50%. Close monitoring is required for a further 60–90 minutes to ensure that hypoglycemia does not recur and that hyperglycemia does not develop. Further changes to the insulin infusion rate are not usually necessary once a steady state is achieved. Patient reassessment is indicated if the foal becomes even more insulin resistant (requiring additional insulin administration in order to avoid hyperglycemia), as there may be an overall deterioration in the patient's condition accompanied by increasing systemic inflammation. When discontinuing insulin therapy, the insulin rate should be gradually titrated downward in parallel with the PN rate, but there can be a substantial lag between changes in the insulin infusion rate and the patient's response to this change. Importantly, foals being weaned from insulin CRIs should receive enteral nutrition during the transition period.

References

1 Ousey, J.C., Holdstock, N.B., Rossdale, P.D. et al. (1996). How much energy do sick neonatal foals require compared with healthy foals? *Pferdeheilkunde* 12: 231–237.

2 Ousey, J.C., Prandi, S., Zimmer, J. et al. (1997). Effects of various feeding regimens on the energy balance of equine neonates. *Am. J. Vet. Res.* 58: 1243–1251.

3 Holdstock, N.B., Allen, V.L., Bloomfield, M.R. et al. (2004). Development of insulin and proinsulin secretion in newborn pony foals. *J. Endocrinol.* 181: 469–476.

4 Robles, M., Nouveau, E., Gautier, C. et al. (2018). Maternal obesity increases insulin resistance, low-grade inflammation and osteochondrosis lesions in foals and yearlings until 18 months of age. *PLoS One* 13: e0190309.

5 Fowden, A.L., Giussani, D.A., and Forhead, A.J. (2020). Physiological development of the equine fetus during late gestation. *Equine Vet. J.* 52: 165–173.

6 Hollis, A.R., Furr, M.O., Magdesian, K.G. et al. (2008). Blood glucose concentrations in critically ill neonatal foals. *J. Vet. Intern. Med.* 22: 1223–1227.

7 Barr, B. (2018). Pediatric nutrition. In: *Equine Pediatric Medicine* (ed. W. Bernard and B. Barr), 311–319. London: Manson Publishing, Ltd.

8 Ousey, J. (1994). Total parenteral nutrition in the young foal. *Equine Vet. Educ.* 6: 316–317.

9 Paradis, M.R. (2001). Caloric needs of the sick foal: determined by the use of indirect calorimetry. *Dorothy Havemeyer Foundation Neonatal Septicemia Workshop (III)*, 1–5.

10 Jose-Cunilleras, E., Viu, J., Corradini, I. et al. (2012). Energy expenditure of critically ill neonatal foals. *Equine Vet. J. Suppl.* 48–51.

11 McKenzie, H.C. 3rd and Geor, R.J. (2009). Feeding management of sick neonatal foals. *Vet. Clin. North Am. Equine Pract.* 25: 109–119, vii.

12 Marik, P.E. and Hooper, M.H. (2016). Normocaloric versus hypocaloric feeding on the outcomes of ICU patients: a systematic review and meta-analysis. *Intensive Care Med.* 42: 316–323.

13 Dandona, P., Mohanty, P., Chaudhuri, A. et al. (2005). Insulin infusion in acute illness. *J. Clin. Invest.* 115: 2069–2072.

14 Klein, C.J., Stanek, G.S., and Wiles, C.E. 3rd. (1998). Overfeeding macronutrients to critically ill adults: metabolic complications. *J. Am. Diet. Assoc.* 98: 795–806.

15 Krause, J.B. and McKenzie, H.C. 3rd. (2007). Parenteral nutrition in foals: a retrospective study of 45 cases (2000–2004). *Equine Vet. J.* 39: 74–78.

16 Koekkoek, K.W. and van Zanten, A.R. (2017). Nutrition in the critically ill patient. *Curr. Opin. Anaesthesiol.* 30: 178–185.

17 Jastrzębska, E., Wadas, E., Daszkiewicz, T. et al. (2017). Nutritional value and health-promoting properties of mare's milk – a review. *Czeh J. Anim. Sci.* 62: 511–518.

18 Stoneham, S.J., Morresey, P., and Ousey, J. (2017). Nutritional management and practical feeding of the orphan foal. *Equine Vet. Educ.* 29: 165–173.

19 Lopes, M.A. (2003). Administration of enteral fluid therapy: methods, composition of fluids and complications. *Equine Vet. Educ.* 15: 107–112.

20 Settle, C.S. and Vaala, W.E. (1991). Management of the critically ill foal: initial respiratory, fluid and nutritional support. *Equine Vet. Educ.* 3: 49–54.

21 Rugeles, S.J., Ochoa Gautier, S.B., Dickerson, R.N. et al. (2017). How many nonprotein calories does a critically ill patient require? A case for hypocaloric nutrition in the critically ill patient. *Nutr. Clin. Pract.* 32: 72S–76S.

22 Furr, M.O. (2002). Intravenous nutrition in horses: clinical applications. *20th Annual ACVIM Forum*, 186–187.

23 Lopes, M.A. and White, N.A. (2002). Parenteral nutrition for horses with gastrointestinal disease: a retrospective study of 79 cases. *Equine Vet. J.* 34: 250–257.

24 Naylor, J.M. and Kenyon, S.J. (1981). Effect of total calorific deprivation on host defence in the horse. *Res. Vet. Sci.* 31: 367–372.

25 Mehta, N.M., Skillman, H.E., Irving, S.Y. et al. (2017). Guidelines for the Provision and Assessment of Nutrition Support Therapy in the Pediatric Critically Ill Patient: Society of Critical Care Medicine and American Society for Parenteral and Enteral Nutrition. *JPEN J. Parenter. Enteral. Nutr.* 41: 706–742.

26 Hansen TO (1990). Nutritional support: parenteral feeding. In: *Equine Clinical Neonatology* (ed. A.M. Koterba, W.H. Drummond, and P.C. Kosch), 747–762. Philadelphia: Lea and Febiger.

27 Hoffer, L.J. (2017). Parenteral nutrition: amino acids. *Nutrients* 9: 257.

28 McClave, S.A., Taylor, B.E., Martindale, R.G. et al. (2016). Guidelines for the Provision and Assessment of Nutrition Support Therapy in the Adult Critically Ill Patient: Society of Critical Care Medicine (SCCM) and American Society for Parenteral and Enteral Nutrition (A.S.P.E.N.). *JPEN. J. Parenter. Enteral Nutr.* 40: 159–211.

29 Hansen, T.O. (1986). Parenteral nutrition in foals. *32nd Annu Conv AAEP*, 153–156.

30 Pontes-Arruda, A., Zaloga, G., Wischmeyer, P. et al. (2012). Is there a difference in bloodstream infections in critically ill patients associated with ready-to-use versus compounded parenteral nutrition? *Clin. Nutr.* 31: 728–734.

31 Miller, S.J. (2009). Commercial premixed parenteral nutrition: is it right for your institution? *Nutr. Clin. Pract.* 24: 459–469.

32 Olan, N.V. and Prittie, J. (2015). Retrospective evaluation of ProcalAmine administration in a population of hospitalized ICU dogs: 36 cases (2010–2013). *J. Vet. Emerg. Crit. Care (San Antonio)* 25: 405–412.

33 Madsen, H. and Frankel, E.H. (2006). The Hitchhiker's guide to parenteral nutrition management for adult patients. *Pract. Gastroenterol.* 40: 46–68.

34 Sun, L.C., Shih, Y.L., Lu, C.Y. et al. (2006). Randomized controlled study of glycerol versus dextrose in postoperative hypocaloric peripheral parenteral nutrition. *J. Invest. Surg.* 19: 381–385.

35 Hays, S.P., Smith, E.O., and Sunehag, A.L. (2006). Hyperglycemia is a risk factor for early death and morbidity in extremely low birth-weight infants. *Pediatrics* 118: 1811–1818.

36 Jacobi, J., Bircher, N., Krinsley, J. et al. (2012). Guidelines for the use of an insulin infusion for the management of hyperglycemia in critically ill patients. *Crit. Care Med.* 40: 3251–3276.

37 Tillotson, K., Traub-Dargatz, J.L., and Morgan, P.K. (2002). Partial parenteral nutrtition in equine neonatal clostridial enterocolitis. *Compend. Contin. Educ. Pract. Vet.* 24: 964–969.

38 Hug, S.A., Riond, B., and Schwarzwald, C.C. (2013). Evaluation of a continuous glucose monitoring system compared with an in-house standard laboratory assay and a handheld point-of-care glucometer in critically ill neonatal foals. *J. Vet. Emerg. Crit. Care (San Antonio)* 23: 408–415.

39 Myers, C.J., Magdesian, K.G., Kass, P.H. et al. (2009). Parenteral nutrition in neonatal foals: clinical description, complications and outcome in 53 foals (1995–2005). *Vet. J.* 181: 137–144.

40 Stratton-Phelps, M. (2008). Nutritional management of the hospitalised horse. In: *The Equine Hospital Manual* (ed. K. Corley and J. Stephen), 261–311. Oxford: Blackwell Publishing.

41 Neff, K., Donegan, D., MacMahon, J. et al. (2014). Management of parenteral nutrition associated hyperglycaemia: a comparison of subcutaneous and intravenous insulin regimen. *Ir. Med. J.* 107: 141–143.

42 Thompson, C.D., Vital-Carona, J., and Faustino, E.V. (2012). The effect of tubing dwell time on insulin adsorption during intravenous insulin infusions. *Diabetes Technol. Ther.* 14: 912–916.

43 Han, J.H., McKenzie, H.C., McCutcheon, L.J. et al. (2011). Glucose and insulin dynamics associated with continuous rate infusion of dextrose solution or dextrose solution and insulin in healthy and endotoxin-exposed horses. *Am. J. Vet. Res.* 72: 522–529.

Chapter 59 Critical Care Techniques in the Neonatal Foal

Section I Foal Restraint and Handling

Bonny Millar

To reduce stressful situations in a newborn foal, especially in a veterinary setting, it is important to familiarize foals with human handling at the earliest opportunity. Appropriate restraint allows the veterinary team a safe means of assessing the neonate and can be of benefit when performing minor procedures without sedation.

The Standing Foal

A handler can restrain the newborn foal by placing one arm around the front of the foal's chest and another around its hindquarters. When the foal is cradled in this way, it will often exhibit what is known as the "floppy foal" response. This is a normal and natural reaction when pressure is applied around its chest and the tail head is held firmly (Figure 59.I.1). In many cases, this will cause the foal to relax, often sinking to the ground. When the handler lets go or releases some of the pressure, the foal instantly becomes alert, resulting in the foal springing up into a standing posture. This is an innate reaction, believed to be in response to being caught by a perceived predator. When that predator (i.e. the handler) releases the foal (i.e. the prey), it rises quickly and runs away. The handler should always be alert to the restrained and relaxed foal suddenly mobilizing unexpectedly in the middle of a procedure.

Leading Foals

Some neonates are fitted with a leather foal slip or leather halter in the first days of life. These must not be used for leading or restraint until the foal has acclimatized and been trained to these devices. Placing an arm or soft towel around the neck can help the handler guide the foal in a controlled manner (Figure 59.I.2). Additionally, a hand placed on the hindquarters or a soft rope draped around the hindquarters and pulled forward will encourage the foal to move onward. Foals are known to resist in the opposite direction to being lead and can flip over backward with inexperienced handlers. Staff should ensure that individuals assisting with handling do not position themselves between the mare and foal, as the mare might become anxious if her view of the foal is obscured. Once a foal is accustomed to its halter and shows compliance when led, a slip rope without a buckle can be used through the halter to further teach the foal about leading.

Lifting and Transportation

There are a number of ways a foal can be carried when it is unable to walk. One person can lift and carry a small neonate, supporting its whole body, as long as care is taken to prevent self-injury. One arm is wrapped around to support the hindquarters, while the other arm cradles the chest, distal to the humeral joint (Figure 59.I.3). This method prevents pressure being placed on the foal's abdomen or thorax thus preventing possible injury to the bladder or ribs. Alternatively, with enough assistance, a stretcher, padded mat with handles, or wheeled cart with padding can be used to safely transport foals of varying sizes.

It is often necessary to lay a foal down from the standing position to allow examination or other medical procedures such as venipuncture of the cephalic vein, IV catheter placement, application of limb splints or therapeutic shoes, and for other short, minimally invasive surgical procedures. A specific technique that allows neonates to be gently placed in lateral recumbency is called "folding" a foal. It is a safe, simple, and effective technique that enables these procedures to be carried out in controlled manner, while minimizing anxiety and harm (Figure 59.I.4).

Equine Neonatal Medicine, First Edition. Edited by David M. Wong and Pamela A. Wilkins.

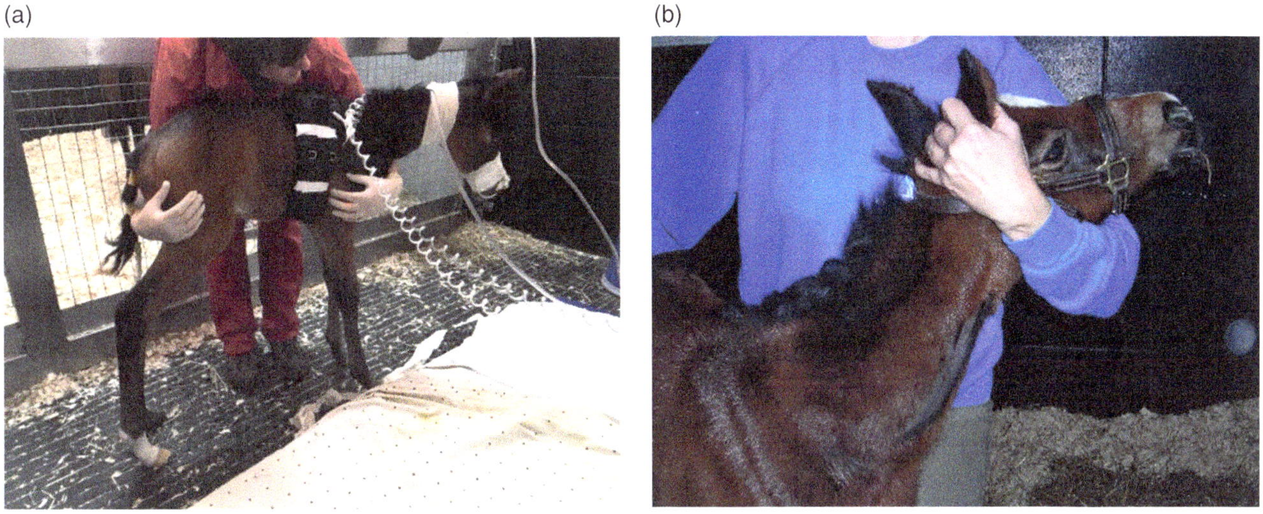

Figure 59.I.1 (a) Restraint of the neonatal foal can be accomplished by cradling one arm around the chest and the other arm around the hindquarters or tail head; (b) IV catheter placement in the standing foal. Note how the foal is restrained with an extended neck so the vein is visualized and remains prepped for catheter placement.

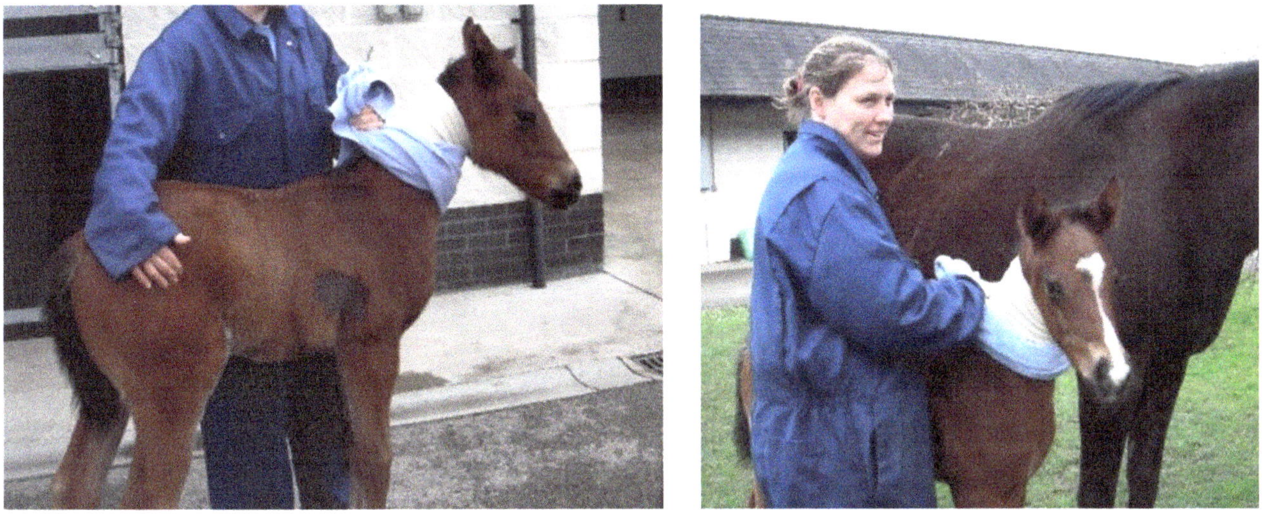

Figure 59.I.2 Foal being led with mare using a towel around the foal's neck.

Folding is only effective on young foals, typically those <4 weeks old and/or <80 kg in weight. Foals that are older are deceptively strong and can easily injure the handler or themselves if the handler attempts to lay it down unaided. It is worth mentioning that foals with neonatal encephalopathy find it harder to lie down compared to rising, so this method is useful in giving these foals assistance in getting down to rest:

- Both the handler and the foal should be positioned away from walls and other obstacles in the stable. It is easier and safer to "fold" the foal toward the handler so it is important to provide a deep layer of bedding or a mat behind the handler for the foal to fall back on.
- The handler cradles the foal around the base of the neck with one arm while holding the base of the tail or hindquarters with the other hand. Keep the foal close to the handler's body.
- The handler gently but firmly turns the foal's head and neck away toward its side, while curling the hindquarters closer to the head. The handler is effectively "folding" the foal while supporting it against their body. As

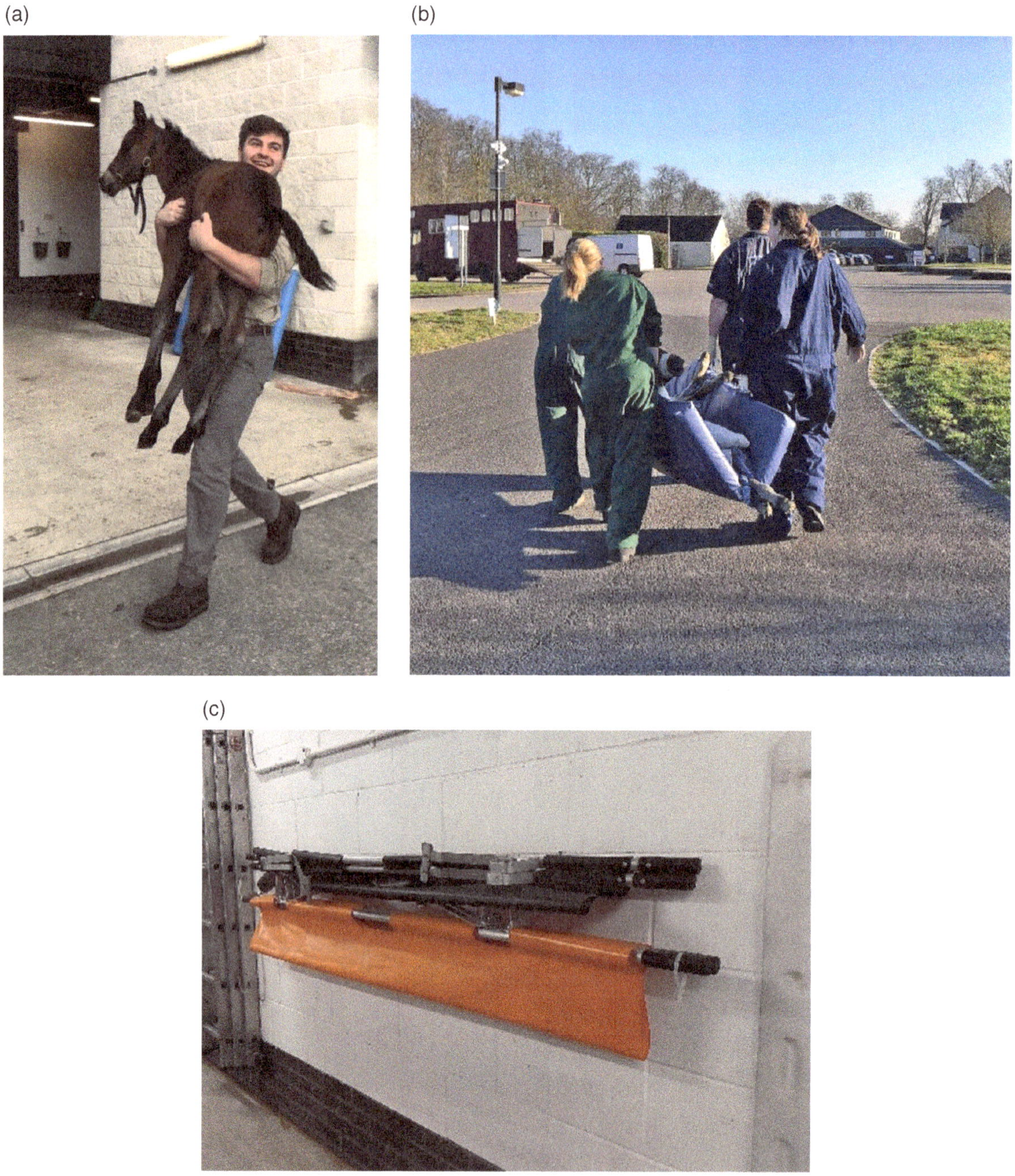

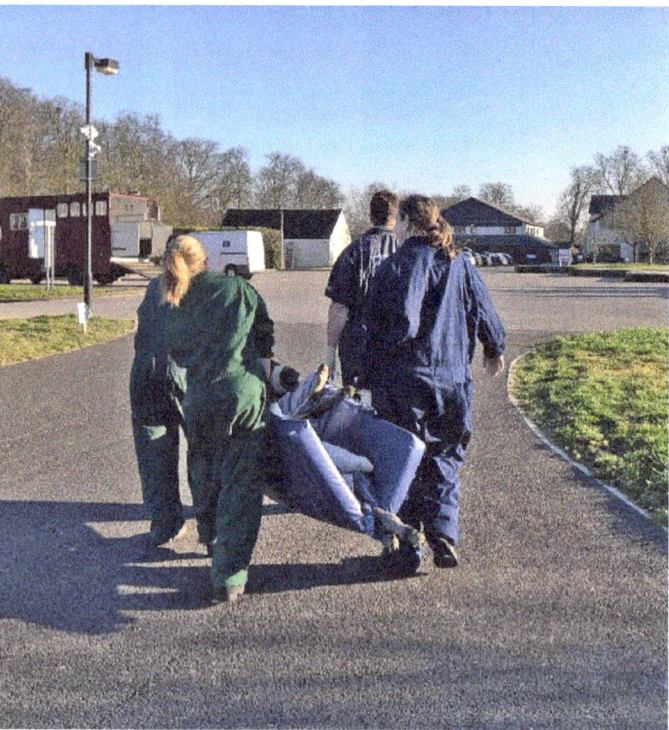

Figure 59.I.3 Examples of methods to carry a neonatal foal; (a) one person can carry smaller foals while (b, c) a padded mat or stretcher can be used but requires multiple individuals to assist.

the foal's head moves around to its side, the handler's arm moves up from its neck with the forearm exerting pressure against the foal's head.

- The foal should start to lean against the handler and relax. With larger foals, the handler may need to brace to maintain balance when the foal leans against them. As the handler takes a step backward, the foal will slide down the handler's body, with its legs positioned away from the handler. The handler should continue to bring the head and tail together. The head is supported as the foal sinks into lateral recumbency onto the mat or floor. The handler moves down to the floor with the foal.
- When the foal is in lateral recumbency, the handler remains kneeling behind its back. The foal can be maintained in this position by exerting light pressure

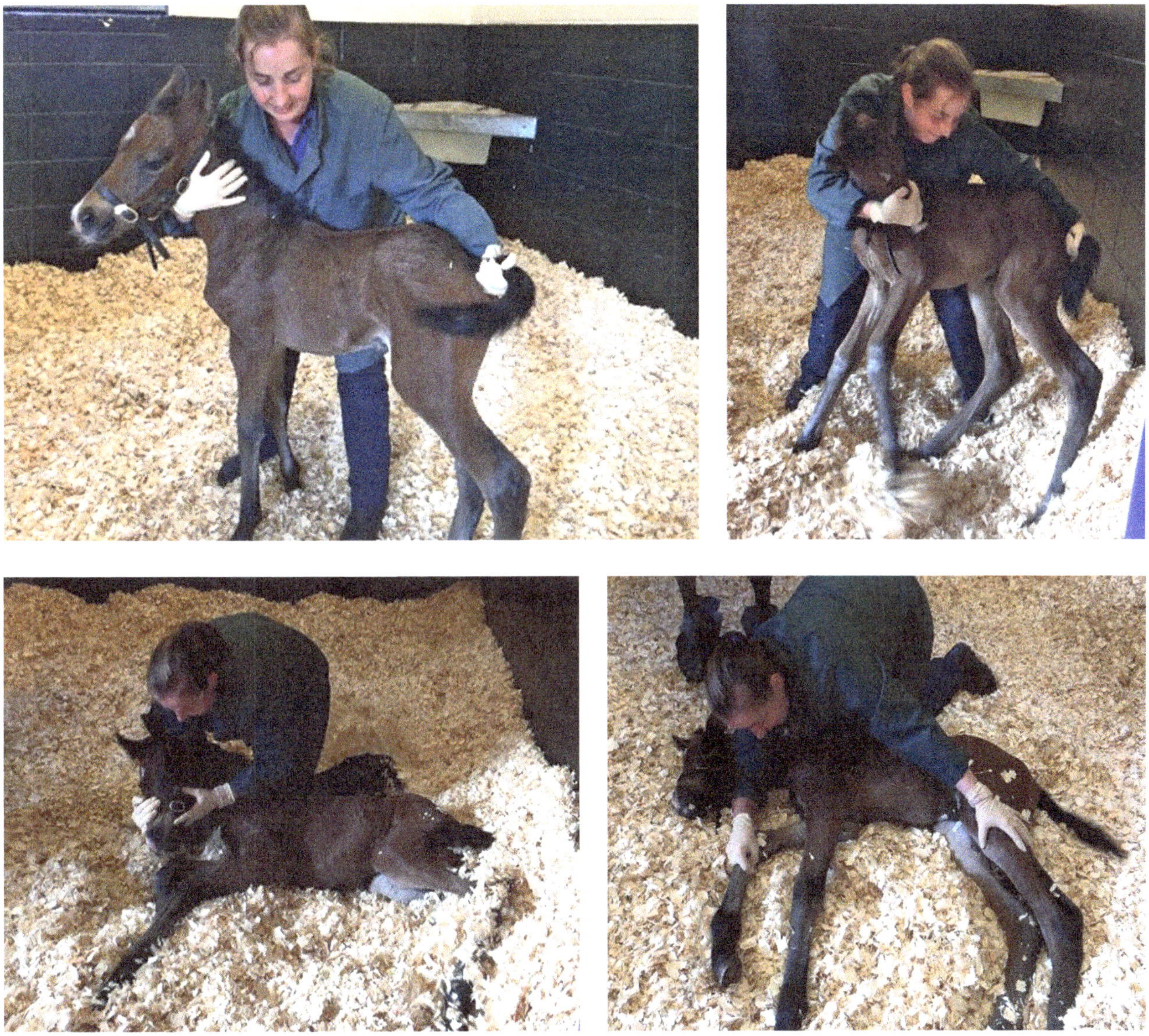

Figure 59.I.4 Technique for safely "folding" neonatal foals into lateral recumbency.

on the neck while holding the down foreleg at the carpus to prevent it from rising into sternal. The handler can use their other arm to steady the hind legs. With older and strong foals, an additional assistant may be needed to hold or straddle the foal's hind legs to prevent it from kicking out.

- Laying a towel across the foal's eyes will help it stay calm and relaxed. Sedation is not usually required prior to "folding" foals, but it may be needed if the subsequent procedure is stimulating or causes discomfort. It is not uncommon for the foal to go to sleep, especially if there is limited stimulus.

Section II Sedation of the Neonatal Foal

Bonnie Hay-Kraus

Sedation is sometimes needed in neonatal foals to accomplish minor procedures or diagnostics such as IV catheter placement, joint lavage/flush, regional limb perfusion, radiography, or ultrasonography. The type of sedation can be based on the age of the foal and the health status.

Foals <7 Days of Age and/or Sick Foals

Midazolam (0.1 mg/kg IV) + Butorphanol (0.05 mg/kg IV for sedation, 0.1 mg/kg IV for analgesia) typically provides moderate sedation and recumbency. Diazepam can be substituted for midazolam at a similar dose, depending on drug availability and cost. Alpha-2 agonists are generally avoided in young neonatal (<7 days) and/or sick foals because it can cause cardiovascular depression.

Foals >7 Days and Healthy

The above protocol may be used and typically provides mild–moderate sedation/recumbency depending on the physical status of the patient. Alpha-2 agonists can be added if the above protocol does not provide sufficient sedation/chemical restraint OR the alpha-2 agonist can be substituted for the benzodiazepine: (Xylazine 0.1–0.5 mg/kg IV or Detomidine 0.002–0.08 mg/kg IV) + Butorphanol (0.05 mg/kg IV for sedation, 0.1 mg/kg IV for analgesia).

If additional chemical restraint is needed, ketamine (0.5–2.0 mg/kg IV) can be administered in the sedated foal at small IV boluses to desired effect. Local anesthetic cream/gel (lidocaine gel or cream or EMLA cream) is recommended to decrease the foal's response to noxious stimuli such as IV catheters, arterial blood gas sampling and regional limb perfusion. Keep in mind the onset of action is ~30 minutes for lidocaine and 30–60 minutes for EMLA cream but will significantly decrease the need for parenteral drugs and physical restraint.

Foals should be administered nasal flow by oxygen 50–100 ml/kg/min if recumbent. Heart rate and respiratory rate should be monitored; pulse oximetry is helpful in monitoring pulse rate and oxygen saturation. Patients under short general anesthesia should also have indirect blood pressure monitoring with oscillometry or Doppler if the procedure lasts >10–15 minutes. Lubricant eye ointment should be applied in all recumbent/anesthetized foals.

Drug	<7 days	>7 days
Premedication/Sedation		
Benzodiazepines	Midazolam 0.02–0.1 mg/kg IV or IM (typical IV dose 0.1 mg/kg) Diazepam 0.02–0.1 mg/kg IV	Midazolam 0.05–0.2 mg/kg IV or IM (typical IV dose 0.1 mg/kg) Diazepam 0.05–0.2 mg/kg IV
Opioids	Butorphanol 0.05 mg/kg for sedation, 0.1 mg/kg for analgesia	Butorphanol 0.05 for sedation, 0.1 mg/kg for analgesia
α-2 agonists	Xylazine 0.1–0.2 mg/kg[a]	Xylazine 0.1–0.5 mg/kg[b] Detomidine 0.002–0.08 mg/kg[b]

[a] Use only for procedural sedation or if other sedatives are not effective, avoid in sick foals or as premedication for general anesthesia.
[b] Use higher end doses for IM administration.

Equine Neonatal Medicine, First Edition. Edited by David M. Wong and Pamela A. Wilkins.

Section III Nasotracheal and Orotracheal Intubation

David Wong

Intubation of the trachea via the nasal or oral route is a relatively straightforward procedure and might be required under controlled circumstances (e.g. induction of anesthesia) or under more dire situations (e.g. cardiopulmonary resuscitation). Familiarity with the procedure prior to an emergent situation is prudent. Orotracheal intubation is technically easier and allows for the passage of larger bore endotracheal tubes, but conscious foals can damage the endotracheal tube with their teeth. Nasotracheal intubation can also be performed in the conscious foal, without damage to the tube. In the emergent situation (cardiopulmonary arrest), either method is appropriate with bias toward the nasotracheal route followed by the orotracheal route if the former is unsuccessful after one or two attempts. A 55-cm cuffed endotracheal tube is typically used to intubate foals with the tube diameter size dependent on the foal's size/breed (Table 59.III.1) [1, 2]. Ideally, the largest diameter endotracheal tube that fits in the airway should be used to minimize airway resistance created by the endotracheal tube.

Nasotracheal Intubation

In general, nasotracheal intubation is preferred over orotracheal intubation because the tube is less likely to be damaged or become dislodged as the foal recovers. However, orotracheal intubation should be pursued if nasotracheal intubation is unsuccessful after one or two attempts. Proper patient positioning will facilitate passage of the nasotracheal tube in the neonatal foal. If the foal is conscious, sedation should be administered and the foal restrained in the standing position or placed in sternal recumbency. The head should be extended in-line with the neck (dorsiflexion), allowing an easy and relatively straight passage of the endotracheal tube into the trachea. Sterile lubricant should be applied to the endotracheal tube to facilitate passage. Once the tube reaches the level of the arytenoids, a twisting motion of the tube can facilitate passage by allowing the beveled end of the tube to spread the arytenoids. An assistant can also apply gentle external pressure over the left side of the pharynx near the throatlatch to occlude the esophagus. One technique to facilitate passage is holding the end of the mandible with the palm of the nondominant hand and extend the head and neck; the fingers of the same hand are used to direct the end of the nasotracheal tube ventromedially, into the ventral meatus [1]. If the foal is recumbent or unconscious, either due to sedation or primary disease process, the foal should be placed in lateral recumbency and the head extended so that the ventral neck is parallel to the lower jaw. The endotracheal tube can be passed as described above. There should be little resistance to endotracheal tube advancement once the end of the tube is in the trachea.

Orotracheal Intubation

The foal should be placed on the ground with the head extended so that the head and neck are in a straight line. The tongue is then grasped with the nondominant hand and gently pulled to the side to help stabilize the larynx. The endotracheal tube (with the natural curvature of the endotracheal tube pointing downward) is advanced over the tongue on midline. As the endotracheal tube reaches the oropharynx, rotation of the tube in either direction can facilitate passage through the larynx and into the trachea.

It is important to ensure that the endotracheal tube is placed into the trachea rather than the esophagus.

Equine Neonatal Medicine, First Edition. Edited by David M. Wong and Pamela A. Wilkins.

Table 59.III.1 Approximate endotracheal tube size (internal diameter) based on weight of the foal [1, 2].

Weight of foal	Typical breeds	Approximate sizes for nasotracheal intubation	Approximate sizes for orotracheal intubation
20–30 kg	Premature foal	7 mm	9 mm
	Pony foal	9 mm	10 mm
25–50 kg	Arab foal	8 mm	9 mm
	Large pony breed foal	9 mm	10 mm
45–60 kg	Thoroughbred foal	9 mm	10 mm
	Warmblood foal	10 mm	12 mm
60–80 kg	Draft breed foal	12 mm	12–14 mm

If the tube is placed in the esophagus it can typically be palpated externally; this is a simple means of detecting improper placement. Endotracheal placement also can be confirmed by gently compressing the thorax and simultaneously identifying expired air at the proximal end of the endotracheal tube. The thoracic wall should also rise and fall when mechanical respirations are provided by the clinician. Other methods of identifying proper placement include placement of an end-tidal carbon dioxide ($ETCO_2$) monitor on the proximal end of the tube to identify the presence of expired CO_2 if placed in the trachea ($ETCO_2$ levels may be variable with cardiopulmonary arrest) or endoscopy to visually confirm placement. Once placement is confirmed, the cuff of the endotracheal tube should be inflated.

References

1 Corley, K. (2008). Procedures in the neonatal foal. In: *The Equine Hospital Manual* (ed. K. Corley and J. Stephen), 120–146. Blackwell.

2 Palmer, J.E. (2007). Neonatal foal resuscitation. *Vet. Clin. Equine* 23: 159–182.

Section IV Placement of Nasal Insufflation Tube

David Wong

Ill neonatal foals frequently require intranasal oxygen for a variety of underlying causes to improve global oxygenation and treat hypoxemia (P_aO_2 <70–80 mmHg). Placement of nasal insufflation tube(s) can be performed in a unilateral or bilateral fashion, depending on the oxygen deficit. Various types of tubing can be used to provide supplemental oxygen. In general, a small diameter soft flexible tubing should be used (red rubber catheter, plastic feeding tube). Other equipment required includes a humidifier, oxygen source with flowmeter, adhesive tape, and suture material.

The distance that the tube should be inserted into the naris can be estimated externally by measuring the distance from the naris to the medial canthus of the eye; placement of adhesive tape at this location serves as a reference point for placement and an anchoring point for suturing the tube in place. With the foal in standing or sternal recumbency, pass the tube ventromedially into the ventral meatus to the level of the adhesive tape. Once the tube is in proper position, place two simple interrupted sutures through the adhesive tape and into the foal's nostril (Figure 59.IV.1).

Oxygen can then be administered at flow rates of 2–10 l/min, depending on patient needs. Oxygen should be humidified as it is delivered to the foal to prevent drying of the mucous membranes. In addition, the lowest flow rate that provides a P_aO_2 of 80–100 mmHg should be used as higher oxygen tensions can cause hyperoxemia and oxygen toxicity to the lungs. It is not uncommon for a small amount of nasal discharge to develop with prolonged treatment with nasal oxygen. Table 59.IV.1 provides an estimate of the expected fraction of inspired oxygen (F_iO_2) and partial pressure of oxygen (P_aO_2) and carbon dioxide (P_aCO_2) in healthy foals receiving unilateral and bilateral intranasal oxygen at different flow rates [1].

Equine Neonatal Medicine, First Edition. Edited by David M. Wong and Pamela A. Wilkins.

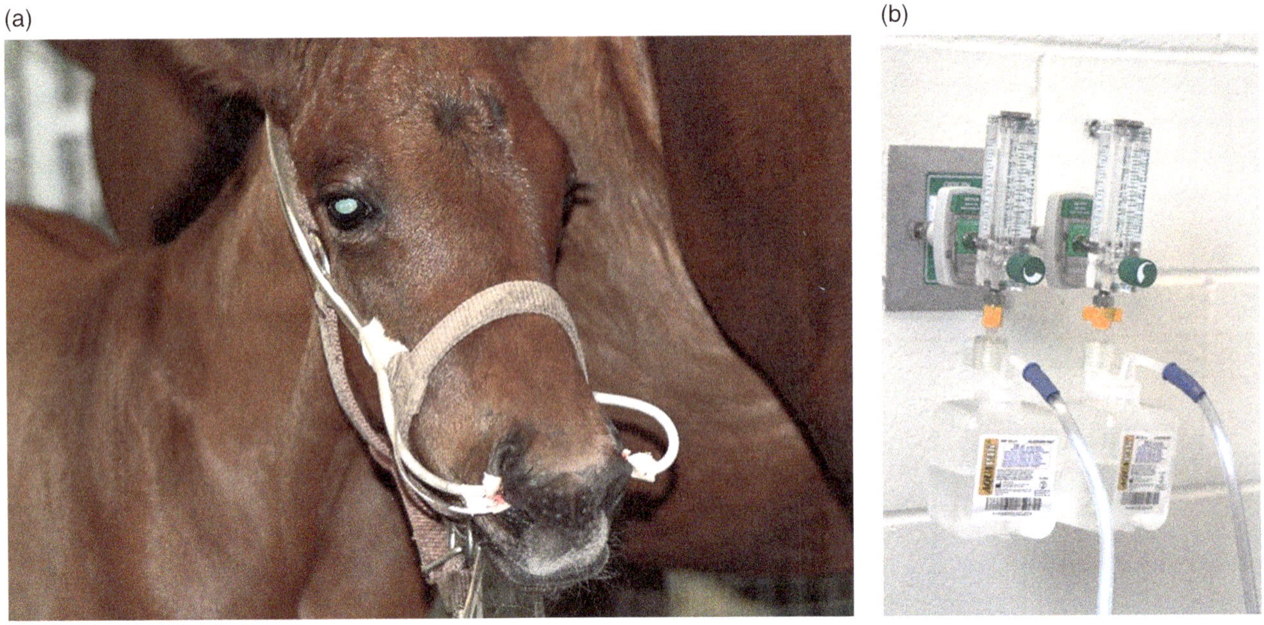

Figure 59.IV.1 (a) Neonatal foal receiving bilateral intranasal oxygen. (b) Oxygen is delivered through humidifiers and regulated by flow meters.

Table 59.IV.1 Mean ± SD tracheal and arterial blood gas variables in nine healthy neonatal foals before (baseline) and during administration of supplemental oxygen at various flow rates via 1 or 2 nasal cannulae [1].

		Oxygen delivery							
		Unilateral (ml/kg/min)				Bilateral (ml/kg/min)			
	Baseline	50	100	150	200	50	100	150	200
F_iO_2 (%)	18 ± 0.7	23 ± 1.4	31 ± 2.0	44 ± 6.0	53 ± 8.3	31 ± 2.6	49 ± 6.2	56 ± 3.4	75 ± 4.2
P_aO_2 (mmHg)	93 ± 8.2	136 ± 13	175 ± 15	220 ± 32	270 ± 41	174 ± 27	261 ± 38	308 ± 41	374 ± 52
P_aCO_2 (mmHg)	48 ± 2.8	50 ± 2.4	51 ± 2.3	50 ± 2.8	51 ± 3.1	50 ± 1.8	51 ± 2.2	50 ± 2.9	49 ± 3.6

Reference

1 Wong, D.M., Alcott, C.J., Wang, C. et al. (2010). Physiologic effects of nasopharyngeal administration of supplemental oxygen at various flow rates in healthy neonatal foals. *Am. J. Vet. Res.* 71: 1081–1088.

Section V Nasogastric Tube Placement

Bonny Millar

Placement of an indwelling nasogastric (NG) tube is frequently performed in ill neonates to allow for the administration of enteral nutrition or check for gastric reflux in foals with ileus or colic. Ill foals may have a weak or absent suckle reflex, abnormal swallowing, and/or decreased or absent nursing behavior. Indwelling NG tubes are also used to supplement nutrition to foals in which the mare is not producing adequate amounts of milk. Once the NG tube is placed, but prior to initiating enteral feedings, the clinician should ensure that there is no/minimal gastric reflux and that the intestinal tract is functional. A variety of commercially available, neonatal-specific, NG tubes are available, but larger tubes can be utilized if the smaller versions are not accessible (Figure 59.V.1). Table 59.V.1 provides the equipment needed and steps taken to place an NG tube in the neonatal foal (Figure 59.V.1).

Complications of NG tube placement include kinking of the NG tube. Significant resistance to injection of water into the NG tube may indicate improper placement despite appearing to be correctly placed. In this instance, it is possible that the NG tube has formed a hairpin loop and double-backed on itself within the esophagus. The stylet may be very difficult to remove as well. Another potential reason that an NG tube cannot be passed into the stomach is severe gastric distention (compresses esophageal opening into the stomach) or increased tone at the esophageal cardia. This should not be mistaken for lack of gastric reflux. In this instance, a small volume (3–5 ml) of lidocaine can be injected down the NG tube to relax the cardiac sphincter. Inadvertent placement of the NG tube within the trachea is another common possibility during placement; the clinician should be aware that the coughing reflex in neonatal foals is suppressed, and confirmation of correct NG tube placement should be based on palpation or endoscopy/radiography. Some clinicians/hospitals confirm placement by performing endoscopy of the upper airway or thoracic radiography to ensure that the NG tube is in correct position. Once the NG tube is in place, long-term indwelling NG tubes can cause irritation of pharynx (smaller tubes are less likely to cause pharyngitis) that can result in occasional cough and mild purulent material from the nares.

Equine Neonatal Medicine, First Edition. Edited by David M. Wong and Pamela A. Wilkins.

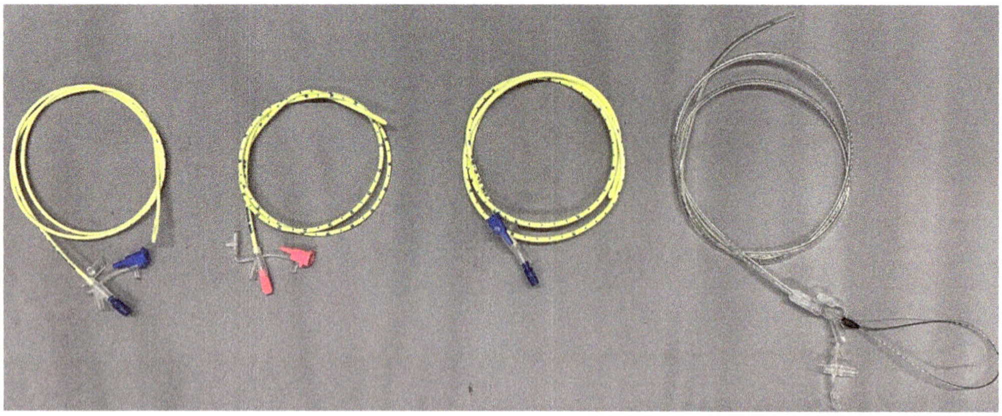

Figure 59.V.1 Various size NG tubes available for indwelling placement in the foal. Sizes, from L to R: 8, 10, 12, and 14 French.

Table 59.V.1 Technique for placement of an indwelling nasogastric (NG) tube.

Equipement needed for NG tube placement – Collect all equipment in an instrument tray to have readily available during placement

- 8–15 French indwelling polyurethane nasogastric (NG) feeding tube with stylet and multi-access ports
- Porous medical (white) tape
- Gauze swabs
- Sterile lubricant
- Monofilament suture with swaged-on straight needle
- Sterile or exam gloves
- Dose syringe (60 ml) and tap water

Determine distance/length of NG tube

- Estimate distance to the stomach by measuring length of NG tube on the outside of the foal, from the nostril to just behind the elbow, following the estimated path of the esophagus. Mark the distance to the stomach on the NG tube with indelible marker. Of note, some clinicians prefer to place the distal end of the NG tube at the level of the distal esophagus, as this allows normal sealing of the cardiac sphincter and minimizes the likelihood of inadvertent milk reflux from the tube or aspiration of air.
- It is helpful to measure and mark the distance from the nostril to the back of the oropharynx to provide a reference point of the approximate distance to the opening of the esophagaus.

Procedure for placement of NG tube

- A foal handler or assistant restrains foal in sternal recumbency if the foal is down. An NG tube may be placed in the standing foal, but sedation should be avoided, if possible, as sedation makes the swallow reflex sluggish.
- Clean nostrils of debris with gauze swabs.
- Lubricate tip of NG tube and insert it, with the inner stylet in the lumen, into a nostril, advancing ventrally and medially into the ventral conchal sinus. Ventroflex the head to divert NG tube from entering the trachea. Placing the NG tube in a refrigerator for several minutes prior to placement helps prevent softening and folding of NG tube when in the larynx.
- Stop advancing the NG tube when it enters the pharynx and rests against the epiglottis (approximately 15–17 cm in 50 kg foal), resulting in soft and pliable resistance. If the tip of the NG tube feels like it is against a hard structure (check indelible mark referencing back of oropharynx), it may have slipped dorsally into the ethmoid turbinates (approximately 8–12 cm in 50 kg foal). If this occurs, withdraw NG tube a few centimeters and advance from a different angle. "Tickling" the epiglottis with the tip of the NG tube will usually initiate a swallow reflex, as will blowing a small amount of air down the NG tube or sticking a gloved finger into the foal's mouth.
- As the foal swallows, gently advance the NG tube into the esophagus.
- Palpate the tip of the NG tube in the cranial esophagus as it advances caudally. It may be necessary to firmly squeeze both sides of the neck just behind the trachea to feel the tip of the NG tube.
- Stop advancing the NG tube when the indelible mark referencing the distal esophagus or stomach is just visible inside the nostril. On some occasions, it may be difficult to advance the tube through the cardiac sphincter.
- Place porous medical tape "wings" around the NG tube at the mark and suture to the upper caudal, medial nares. A Chinese finger-trap suture pattern around the NG tube will further prevent dislodging. Alternatively, the tube can be taped around the curvature of a tongue depressor and secured to the side of the face with elastic tape.

Table 59.V.1 (Continued)

- Remove stylet once the NG tube is fixed in place.
- Some clinicians prefer to confirm correct positioning by endoscopic exam or radiography.
- When correct placement has been confirmed, check for ease of flow and patency of the NG tube by administering a few milliliters of tap water (gravity fed). The flow of water should be unrestricted.
- Loop and fix the tube to the side of the face with loosely applied flexible bandage material around the muzzle. Ensure the end of the tube does not hit the eyes and that the foal can freely open its mouth.
- When not feeding the foal, keep the end of the NG tube plugged.
- Feeding via the NG tube must occur when the foal is either standing or in sternal recumbency.
- Foals can nurse well from the mare or bottles while the NG tube is in situ, providing it has a strong, coordinated suck and swallow reflex.

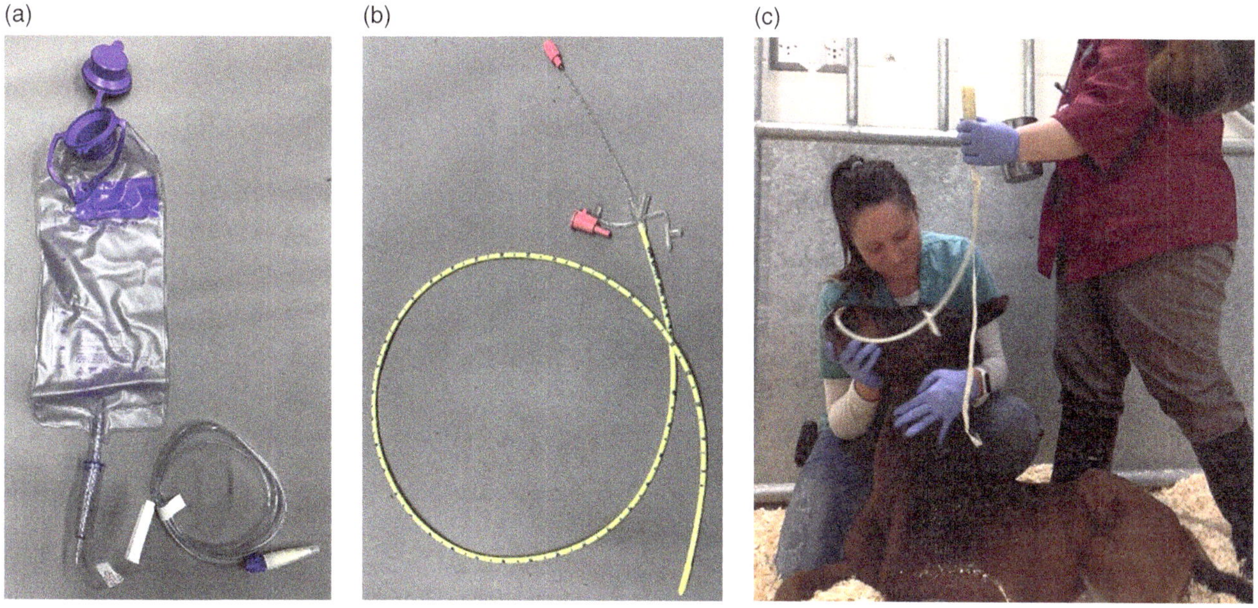

Figure 59.V.2 (a) Commercially available feeding bag to facilitate gravity fed milk feeding. (b) Feeding tube with metal stylet partially removed. (c) Feeding a foal colostrum.

Section VI Intravenous Catheter Selection, Placement, Maintenance, and Monitoring

Bonny Millar and David Wong

Intravenous catheters (IV) are essential for the treatment of ill neonatal foals as they allow for the easy administration of antimicrobials, supplementary medications, IV fluids, and total parental nutrition. They can also be used for blood sampling and central venous pressure monitoring. Long-term, polyurethane catheters are the standard for critical-care foal medicine with a variety of commercially available catheters with single, double, and triple lumens along with integrated extension sets available for neonatal use. As foals are prone to sepsis, a silver zirconium phosphate coating is added to some catheters to inhibit bacterial growth, alleviating some risk of bacterial contamination of the catheter while in situ. Over-the-needle catheters can also be used; however, they are easily dislodged in recumbent or active foals. When inserted, over-the-wire catheters afford less trauma to the vein and remain more secure in situ when sutured correctly (Figure 59.VI.1).

Common complications of IV catheterization include phlebitis, thrombophlebitis, localized cellulitis, and infection (Chapter 13). The vein should be examined and carefully palpated daily and whenever medications are given, or replacement fluid bags are attached. Signs of heat, venous thickening, generalized skin swelling, and pain may require immediate removal of the catheter. Remove the catheter using aseptic technique and consider submission of the catheter tip for bacterial culture if deemed necessary.

Additionally, the catheter, extension sets, and fluid administration sets should be examined whenever the catheter is heparinized. Leaks, breaks in sterility, or trauma from the patient require immediate change of fluid administration lines and extension sets. Inadvertent patient interference can lead to catheter damage as well. A rare but serious complication of IV catheter use in foals is dislodgement or fragmentation of the catheter while in situ, subsequently resulting in a fragment of the catheter becoming lodged within the cardiovascular system. In foals, catheter fragments can remain in the jugular vein or migrate to the vena cava, heart, or pulmonary artery and can be identified radiographically and/or ultrasonographically. The most common cause of catheter fragmentation and dislodgement is inadvertent cutting of the catheter at the level of the catheter hub during attempted catheter removal [1]. Other causes include breakage at the hub of the catheter, inappropriate insertion or removal of the catheter, or as a result of disruption or damage to the catheter by the foal [1, 2]. Retrieval of a guidewire used for over-the-wire catheter insertion has also been reported in an adult horse and could potentially occur in foals [3].

Although the long-term complications and outcome of leaving foreign bodies within the vascular system is unknown in foals, standard-of-care in people with lodged catheter fragments suggests removal [4]. Mortality and serious complication rates are quite high in people, depending on the site at which the fragment lodges [5]. Potential complications of retained catheter fragments in situ include sepsis, endocarditis, lung abscess, pulmonary embolism, dysrhythmias, cardiac perforation, pulmonary or caval thrombosis, and death [1]. Retrieval should be attempted as soon as feasible as reports in people indicate that early intervention reduces the number of complications and allows easier recovery due to the fact that a greater proportion of fragments lie proximal to the tricuspid valve and the fragment is less likely adhered to the vessel wall [4, 6]. In people, catheter fragments are most commonly located in the pulmonary artery or right ventricle; in experimental catheter fragmentation in six adult horses, five fragments were located in the pulmonary artery, and one was located in the cranial vena cava at necropsy (30 hours after fragmentation) [7, 8].

Removal of catheter fragments has been reported in a limited number of foals and adult horses [1, 2, 4, 7, 8]. Interventional radiologic techniques have simplified retrieval of fragments using relatively noninvasive

Equine Neonatal Medicine, First Edition. Edited by David M. Wong and Pamela A. Wilkins.

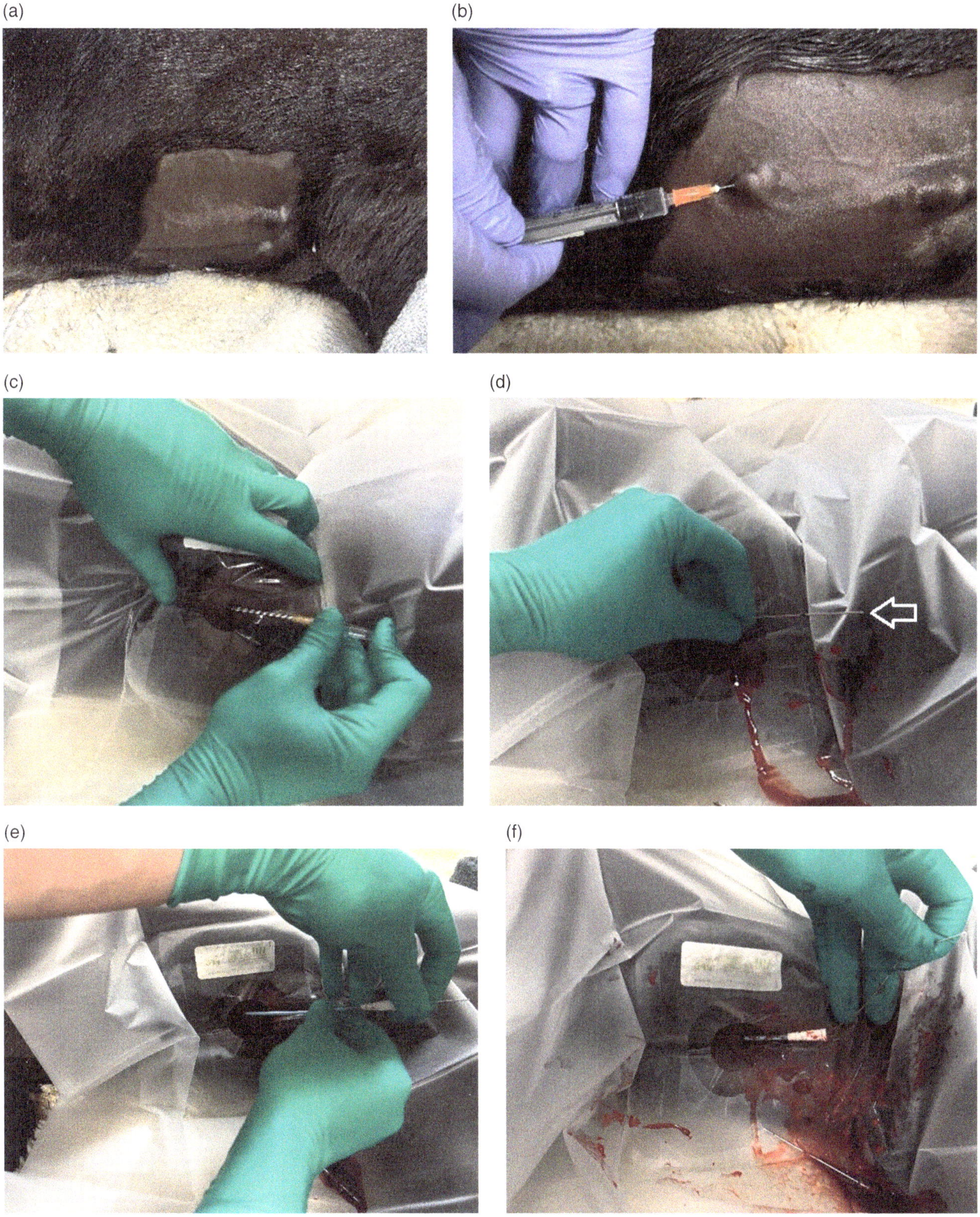

Figure 59.VI.1 Technique for placement of an over-the-wire IV catheter using the Seldinger technique. (See Table 59.VI.1 for legend).

(g) (h)

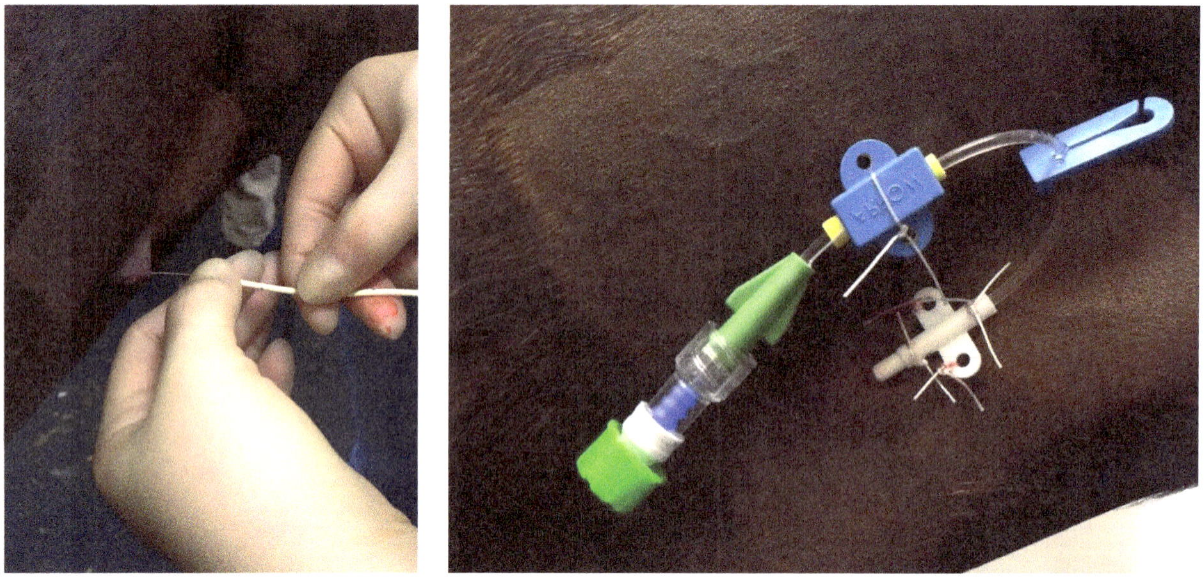

Figure 59.VI.1 (Continued)

Table 59.VI.1 Technique for placement of an intravenous catheter using the Seldinger technique.

Equipment needed for IV catheter placement – collect all equipment and have readily available during placement

- Clippers with # 40 blade
- Sterile surgical scrub materials
- Sterile gloves for catheter placement
- Heparinized saline flush
- Needle-free connectors[b]
- Nonsterile exam gloves
- Small sterile drapes
- 1.0 ml local anesthetic (e.g. mepivicaine) in syringe with 23 g needle
- Disinfecting caps[a]
- Four metric nonabsorbable nylon suture with swaged on needle
- Long-term IV catheter kit[c] (16-gauge single lumen or a 14g/18g double lumen is ideal for neonates)
- Dressing/adhesive bandaging or tubular neck covering (TUBIGRIP™ size J)
- Optional – blood collection tubes; whole blood samples can be aspirated from catheter at time of insertion, prior to flushing with heparinized saline.

Procedure for placement of IV catheter in the jugular vein

- Assistance will be needed to restrain the foal for either standing or recumbent placement.
- If the foal is weak, place foal in lateral recumbency on a clean padded surface. If the foal is standing, and likely to remain so, an assistant can hold the foal with one arm around the cranial neck holding the head against the assistant's body with the head slightly extended, enabling access to the jugular vein. With the foal's body braced against the assistant, the other hand holds the base of the tail or hindquarters. While it is possible to insert a catheter in this manner, there may be better control of the procedure with the foal in lateral recumbency. In most instances, chemical restraint is not needed in the neonate; if necessary, IV diazepam will facilitate placement in active foals.
- In recumbency, position the foal with the head and neck flat on a padded table or resting on the lap of an assistant sitting on the mat. The foal's nose and neck is extended, allowing the jugular vein to be easily visualized. Additionally, a rolled-up towel placed underneath the neck can assist in raising the jugular furrow.
- Check that the vein can be easily distended, without evidence of thickening or other abnormalities. Clip a large patch on the cranial half of the foal's neck, with the jugular furrow central in the clipped area. The clipped area should be large enough to ensure the catheter, extension set, and injection connectors sit completely within the clipped area.
- Remove loose hair from the area and dampen the surrounding hair on the neck to prevent flyaway hair from landing within the sterile field. Place a sterile drape cranial or caudal to the clipped site if it will mitigate inadvertent breaks in sterility.
- Don nonsterile gloves and begin the first aseptic preparation of the clipped site. Excessive scrubbing is contraindicated as it can lead to micro abrasions of the foal's delicate skin, potentially leading to the introduction of bacteria. Spray the prepared area or wipe with alcohol-soaked sterile swabs (Figure 59.VI.1a).

Table 59.VI.1 (Continued)

- Inject 0.5 ml of mepivacaine subcutaneously, using a 23 g needle, exactly over the catheter insertion site and where the extension set will be sutured (Figure 59.VI.1b). The insertion site should be located cranially to accommodate the length of the catheter without it entering the right atrium. If central venous pressure measurements are required, it is safe to have the distal tip located within the cranial vena cava.
- Don nonsterile gloves and perform a second aseptic preparation within the clipped area. Open the catheter pack, and while maintaining sterility of all materials, place inside an instrument tray. Keep the tray within easy reach. Remove nonsterile gloves and don sterile gloves. If preferred, additional sterile drapes can be placed around the site.
- Raise the vein, within the clipped area, by placing a finger or two deep into the jugular furrow. With the bevel of the introducer needle facing the operator, and positioned parallel to the jugular vein, insert it into the desensitized skin proximally, at a 45° angle. Some kits include an over-the-needle catheter, which can take the place of the introducer needle (preferred method by some clinicians). Continue steadily advancing the needle until the vein is punctured and blood is visible in the hub. Next, angle the needle slightly more parallel (flatter) to the vein and advance it slightly. The continued rise of blood in the needle hub confirms placement is within the lumen of the vein (Figure 59.VI.1c). If a short term catheter is used, the stylet is removed, leaving the catheter in situ.
- The guidewire, encased in a circular sleeve and straightener, fits into the needle hub. Thread the guidewire into the vein using the thumb notch on the straightener. The wire should advance freely, without resistance. Observe for the appearance of the black witness marks on the wire and stop advancing when three black marks are visible. At least 10 cm of guidewire will remain externally. Remove the circular wire sleeve and straightener, making sure the grip on the guidewire is sustained and sterility is maintained (Figure 59.VI.1d). **Always keep a secure hold on the wire!**
- Remove the introducer needle or catheter while keeping the wire fixed in place.
- Insert the tissue dilator over the guidewire and gently tunnel the beveled tip into the skin until the subcutaneous space is reached (Figure 59.VI.1e,f). Remove the dilator, once again keeping the wire in place. This step enables the catheter to advance freely through the skin without causing drag and puckering.
- Grasp the guidewire with the hand used to hold off the vein; using the other "clean" hand, insert the wire into the distal tip of the catheter (Figure 59.VI.1g). Advance the catheter over the wire, carefully bringing the wire up through the catheter until it appears at the end of the integrated extension set. Grasp the wire securely, and again, **do not let go of the wire!**
- The catheter can now be advanced smoothly and easily, without resistance, following the path of the wire down into the vein. Once the catheter is inserted up to the hub, the wire can safely be removed.
- If required, remove a whole-blood sample prior to heparinizing the catheter and attach a needle-free connector. Attach a disinfecting cap if not immediately using for fluid therapy. Note that long catheters with integrated extension sets will require additional volumes of heparinized saline flush to accommodate their extra length.
- Suture the catheter to the skin through the holes on the wings and in the groove of the hub closest to the catheter. Skillful suturing will fix the hub into the jugular furrow, preventing excess movement that could expose the white catheter, thus causing kinks (Figure 59.VI.1h). The additional wings are fitted over the extension tubing and sutured in place. A loop in the extension tubing is left to ensure there is no pull on the catheter insertion site when the tubing is handled. All sutures should be placed within the clipped area.
- Cover the neck and catheter site in the desired manner.

Maintenance: The catheter will need to be flushed with heparinized saline every 3–4 h to maintain patency, which is recommended even when administering fluid therapy. Needle-free connectors maintain a constantly closed system and only require replacing every 7 d. Disinfecting caps are also changed every 7 d.

[a] Curos™ disinfecting cap for needless connectors (3M™, 3M Center, St Paul, MN, USA).
[b] Bionector TKO® (Vygon, Lansdale, PA, USA).
[c] Long Term MILACATH™ (MILA International Inc., Florence, Kentucky, USA).

procedures. Prior to interventional radiology, surgical intervention was necessary (thoracotomy, sternotomy) and was associated with considerable morbidity [2, 4]. If fragmentation of the catheter is recognized instantly, immediate occlusion of the distal jugular vein with a rope tourniquet around the caudal cervical region is warranted, as one report involving two neonatal foals and one adult horse successfully retrieved catheter fragments by jugular venotomy along with the use of a caudal cervical tourniquet to prevent distal migration of the fragment [7, 8]. In another case, a catheter fragment was lodged in the jugular vein in a 4-month-old Thoroughbred filly, approximately 10 cm distal to the site of catheter entry [4]. In this case, an endovascular snare was used to retrieve the fragment under fluoroscopic guidance. The loop snare technique has been extensively evaluated and implemented in people and is the method of choice for interventional radiologist [4]. For successful use of the loop snare technique, a free end of the catheter fragment must be accessible; if the fragment is positioned such that both ends are lodged against the vessel walls, a hooked catheter, IV forceps, or pigtail catheter can be used to dislodge and expose a free end [4]. Typically, attempts at fragment removal are performed under general anesthesia with fluoroscopy essential to guide catheter location and retrieval. An ECG should be

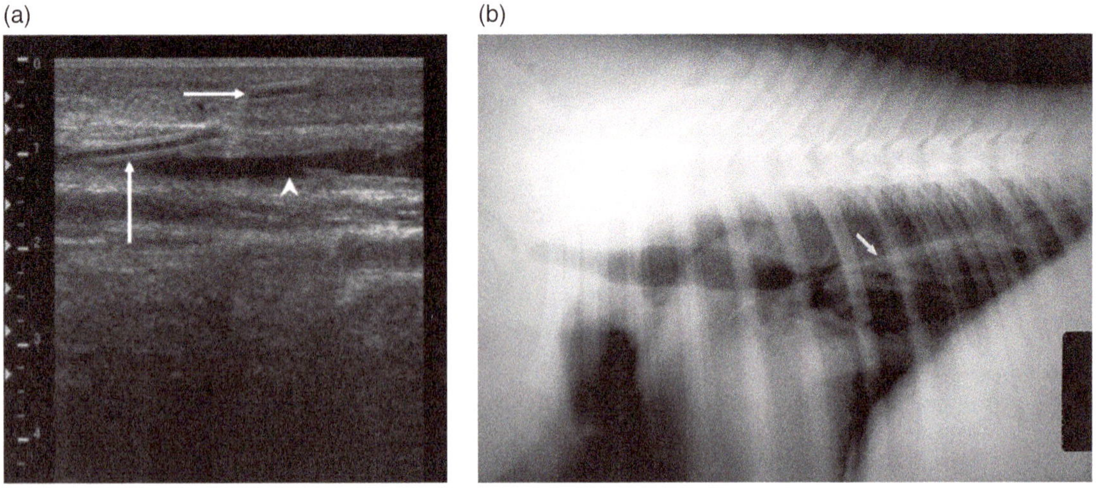

Figure 59.VI.2 (a) Ultrasonographic image of the left jugular vein in a 4-month-old foal with a large catheter fragment (white arrow) lodged in the wall of the jugular vein and a smaller fragment lodged in the subcutaneous tissues (horizontal white arrow). The jugular vein is identified by the white arrowhead. Scale on left is in centimeters. *Source:* From Culp et al. [4]. (b) Lateral thoracic radiograph of a foal with a fragmented catheter. Note the radiopaque catheter fragment in the dorsocaudal lung field extending from the base of the heart to the caudal aspect of the lung (arrow). *Source:* From Little et al. [1].

used during retrieval procedures as ventricular tachycardia and premature atrial contractions were reported during manipulation of the catheter fragment in foals [9, 10]. Transient tachycardia and cardiac murmurs (point of maximal intensity over pulmonic or tricuspid valve) have also been associated with catheter fragments lodged within the heart in foals, prior to removal [2, 10].

In one particular case involving a 7-day-old Arabian foal, the IV catheter fragment was located predominantly in the pulmonary artery with approximately 1 cm remaining in the right ventricle (Figure 59.VI.2). A 3-French microvascular snare (vascular retrieval forceps, Cook Inc., Bloomington, IN) was first used, under fluoroscopic guidance, but was unsuccessful at retrieving the fragment. Subsequently, an 8-French 65 cm catheter and 4-French helical stone basket (wire basket microvascular snare, Boston Scientific, Waterstown, MA) was passed under fluoroscopic guidance to the vicinity of the fragment. The basket was deployed and closed on the fragment and was subsequently removed; the foal was reportedly healthy 2 months after discharge [1]. Other reports in foals have noted catheter fragments in the right ventricle (removed via thoracotomy), cranial vena cava, and azygos vein and right ventricle and atrium (removed via percutaneous method) [2, 9, 10]. The percutaneous approach utilized a basket retrieval catheter and snare, but other instrumentation such as endoscopic forceps and ureteral stone baskets have also been used.

Another rare but important complication of IV catheters is vascular air embolus (VAE), which is the entrainment of air from a communication with the environment into the venous or arterial vasculature that produces systemic effects. Factors that determine the morbidity and mortality of VAE are directly related to the volume of air entrainment and the rate of accumulation. Lethal volumes of air entrained as an acute bolus have been experimentally determined to be approximately 0.5–0.75 ml/kg in rabbits, 7.5–15 ml/kg in dogs, and 3–5 ml/kg in adult people [11]. In one study conducted in 1934, rapid injection of 500 ml of air into the jugular was fatal in a horse, whereas 100 ml caused no clinical signs [12]. The rate of air entrainment is also a factor because the pulmonary circulation and alveolar interface provide a reservoir for dissipation of intravascular gas. Animal data suggests that the lung can act as a physiologic filter but becomes overwhelmed above 0.4 ml/kg/min of air [13]. If the air entrainment is slow, the patient is more apt to withstand large quantities of air over a prolonged period (e.g. dogs were able to withstand up to 1400 ml of air over several hours) [14]. Another proposed factor that impacts the degree of detrimental effects of VAE is the proximity of the vein to the right heart; the closer the vein to the right heart, the smaller amount of air is required to be lethal [11].

If the VAE is large ($\geq$5 ml/kg), a gas airlock can immediately occur, resulting in a complete outflow obstruction from the right ventricle. This is due to the inability of the heart to decompress the tension of the ventricular wall (Figure 59.VI.3). This subsequently results in heart failure and immediate cardiovascular collapse. More modest volumes of air can still result in significant right ventricular outflow obstruction, decreased cardiac output, hypotension, and myocardial and cerebral ischemia (and possibly death) [11]. Air entrainment in the pulmonary vasculature can lead to pulmonary vasoconstriction, release of

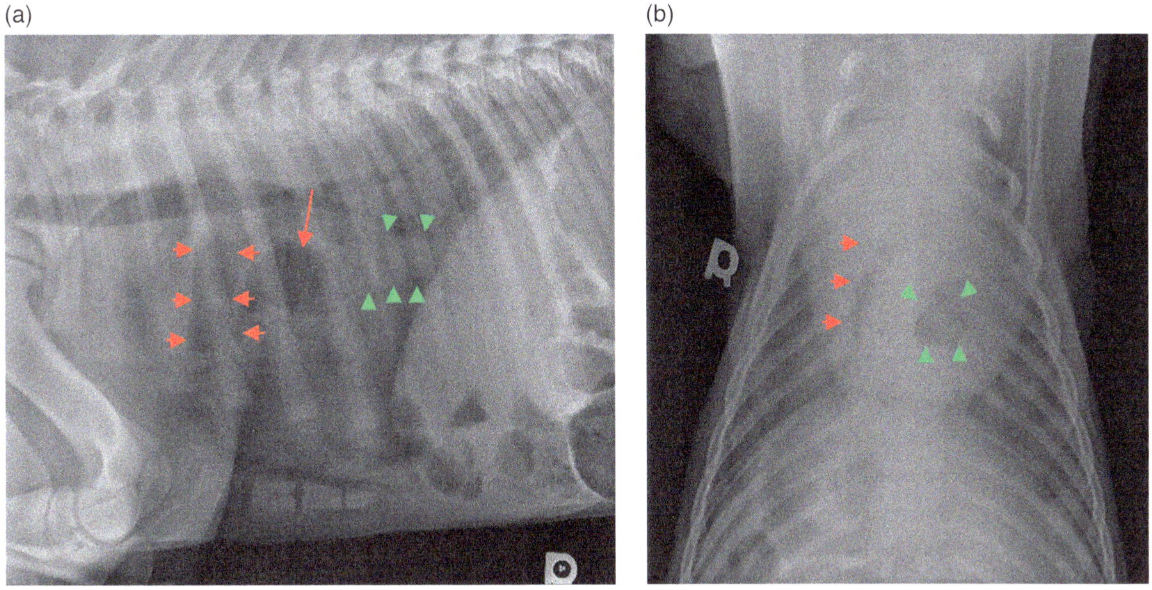

Figure 59.VI.3 (a) Right lateral radiograph in a foal that died after receiving a rapid infusion of an air bolus during fluid therapy with a pressure bag. Note the large amount of air in the right outflow tract, particularly the right atrium (large red arrow) and pulmonary artery (small red arrows) along with the dilated caudal vena cava (green arrows). (b) Dorsoventral radiograph of the same foal; note air within the right pulmonary artery (red arrows) and likely left ventricle (green arrows). Large air emboli can cause paradoxical arterial embolization by acutely increasing right atrial pressure, which facilitates right-to-left shunting through a patent foramen ovale or patent ductus arteriosus [16]. *Source:* Images courtesy of Dr. Jared Janke, Iowa State University.

inflammatory mediators, bronchoconstriction, and increased ventilation/perfusion mismatch – all contributing to hypoxemia [11]. If the volume of air received is not immediately lethal, VAE can have cardiovascular, pulmonary, and neurologic sequelae as a result of ischemia in the organ in which the air is trapped [15]. The impact on the cardiovascular system can manifest as tachyarrhythmias and myocardial ischemia, whereas pulmonary signs might include acute dypsnea, coughing, and chest pain [11, 16]. Neurologic signs can result from ischemia and cerebral hypoperfusion secondary to cardiovascular collapse and reduced cardiac output.

Reported clinical signs of VAE in 32 adult horses included tachypnea (80%), tachycardia (77%), muscle fasciculations (63%), transient recumbency (57%), agitation (57%), and colic (40%) [17]. Behavioral changes were also observed and included excitement (hyperreactivity, erratic behavior, compulsive circling, flank biting, kicking) with a small number of horses demonstrating lethargy or obtundation [17]. Neurologic signs such as seizures (23%), apparent central blindness (27%), and head tilt (10%) were also reported. Less common signs included hyperesthesia, pruritis, head pressing, decreased facial sensation, and delayed-onset dysphagia. Sudden death was reported in two horses with an overall mortality of 19%. Initial signs were observed either concurrently with or within minutes of detection of catheter disconnection in all but one case that developed seizures after 2 hours [17].

Situations that serve as risk factors for VAE include damage or detachment of catheter connections, failure to occlude the needle hub or catheter during insertion or removal, dysfunction of self-sealing valves, presence of a persistent catheter tract following removal, deep inspiration during insertion or removal (increases magnitude of negative pressure in thorax), and hypovolemia (reduces central venous pressure) [11]. In the retrospective review of 32 cases of air embolism in horses, the cause of air aspiration was disconnection of the extension set or injection cap from the hub of the catheter in the majority of cases [17].

General management strategies of VAE include prevention of further air entrainment, administration of high flow (100%) oxygen (maximize oxygenation during cardiovascular compromise), reduction of embolic obstruction (relieve air-lock in right side of heart by placing in left lateral recumbency), immediate initiation of cardiopulmonary resuscitation (CPR), aspiration of air from the right atrium using a properly placed catheter (low success rate), and hemodynamic support (inotropic drugs). In the retrospective study of VAE in horses, treatments included non-steroidal anti-inflammatory drugs, sedatives, dexamethasone, dimethyl sulfoxide, and oxygen insufflation [17].

Intravenous catheters are an essential component of critical care medicine and should be used without reservation but must be maintained and monitored carefully. Although rare, the clinician should be aware of catheter fragmentation and VAE as a serious complication of IV catheters.

References

1 Little, D., Keene, B.W., Bruton, C. et al. (2002). Percutaneous retrieval of a jugular catheter fragment from the pulmonary artery of a foal. *J. Am. Vet. Med. Assoc.* 220: 212–214.

2 Lees, M.J., Read, R.A., Klein, K.T. et al. (1989). Surgical retrieval of a broken jugular catheter from the right ventricle of a foal. *Equine Vet. J.* 21: 3840387.

3 Nannarone, S., Falchero, V., Gialletti, R. et al. (2013). Successful removal of a guidewire from the jugular vein of a mature horse. *Equine Vet. Educ.* 25: 173–176.

4 Culp, W.T.N., Weisse, C., Berent, A.C. et al. (2008). Percutaneous endovascular retrieval of an intravascular foreign body in five dogs, a goat, and a horse. *J. Am. Vet. Med. Assoc.* 232: 1850–1856.

5 Fisher, R.G. and Ferreyro, R. (1978). Evaluation of current techniques for nonsurgical removal of intravascular iatrogenic foreign bodies. *Am. J. Roentgenol.* 130: 541–548.

6 Rose, G.E. (1984). Intravenous catheter fragment irretrievable by radiographically-guided non-surgical techniques. *J. R. Soc. Med.* 77: 615–616.

7 Scarratt, W.K., Moll, H.D., and Pleasant, R.S. (1997). Fragmentation of intravenous catheters in three horses. *J. Equine Vet. Sci.* 17: 608–611.

8 Scaratt, W.K., Pyle, R.L., Buechner-Maxwell, V. et al. (1998). Transection of an intravenous catheter in six horses. *Proc. Annu. Meet. Am. Assoc. Equine Pract.* 44: 294–295.

9 Hoskinson, J., Wooten, P., and Evans, R. (1991). Nonsurgical removal of a catheter embolus from the heart of a foal. *J. Am. Vet. Med. Assoc.* 199: 233–235.

10 Ames, T.R., Hunter, D.W., and Caywood, D.D. (1991). Percutaneous transvenous removal of a broken jugular catheter from the right ventricle of a foal. *Equine Vet. J.* 23: 392–393.

11 Mirski, M.A., Lele, A.V., Fitzsimmons, L. et al. (2007). Diagnosis and treatment of vascular air embolism. *Anesthesiology* 106: 164–177.

12 Lapolla, L. (1934). Pathogenesis of air embolism. *Clin. Vet.* 57: 593–606.

13 Butler, B.D. and Hills, B.A. (1985). Transpulmonary passage of venous air emboli. *J. Appl. Physiol.* 59: 543–547.

14 Hybels, R.L. (1980). Venous air embolism in head and neck surgery. *Laryngoscope* 80: 946–954.

15 Van Hulst, R.A., Klein, J., and Lachmann, B. (2003). Gas embolism: pathophysiology and treatment. *Clin. Physiol. Funct. Imaging* 23: 237–246.

16 Palmon, S.C., Moore, L.E., Lundberg, J. et al. (1997). Venous air embolism: a review. *J. Clin. Anesth.* 9: 251–257.

17 Parkinson, N.J., McKenzie, H.C., Barton, M.H. et al. (2008). Catheter-associated air embolism in hospitalized horses: 32 cases. *J. Vet. Intern. Med.* 32: 805–814.

Section VII Intraosseous Infusion Technique

David Wong

Resuscitative and maintenance fluids as well as a variety of medications are most frequently administered to neonatal foals using the IV route. However, there are instances when venous access is not achievable or will be critically delayed (e.g. severe hypovolemia, circulatory collapse, hypotensive conditions, neonatal miniature horses, venous thrombosis), thereby necessitating an alternative route of fluid and/or medication administration. In such instances, intraosseous (IO) infusion may provide a bridge for therapy until IV access is available. Intraosseous infusion accesses the foal's central circulation through the intramedullary vessels within the bone marrow, which are not subject to collapse because of the rigid bony structure that maintains the vascular space. Substances injected into the marrow flow through sinusoids into large medullary venous channels, which subsequently travel through the nutrient and emissary veins into the central circualtion [1]. Once accessed, IO infusion allows abrosption of exogenously administered fluids or medications at a rate similar to the IV route [1].

Two main locations have been used for IO infusion in the foal, the proximal radius and the proximal tibia. Although either site can provide access to the medullary vessels, the proximal tibia was shown to be easier to access and allowed faster infusion rates in one study [1]. Advantages of the tibial site include rapid identification, lack of soft tissue structures over the bone, flat entry surface, and ease of penetrating the marrow. If the foal requires resuscitation, it is a site away from areas occupied by other clinicains performing resuscitation (Figure 59.VII.1) [2]. A more recent study examined the feasibilty of additional sites of IO infusion including the lateral diaphysis of the humerus, lateral diaphysis of the radius, dorsolateral diaphsyis of the third metacarpal bone, craniomedical diaphysis of the tibia, and the tuber coxae in weanling age foals (3–5 months of age) [3]. In that study, the tuber coxae proved to be an unacceptable site for IO needle placement; however, the other sites were acceptable and may provide alternative sites for IO infusion [3]. The equipment needed, locations, and procedure to place an IO needle is described in Table 59.VII.1.

In mature newborn foals, a standard IO needle designed for people is ideally used. Another type of IO infusion method is the cannulated screw [4]. These are placed at the same sites as previously mentioned, but a 3.2 mm hole is drilled through the cortex and then tapped with a 4.5 mm tap to allow placement of a 4.5 mm cannulated screw (Figure 59.VII.2). If a purpose-specific IO needle is not available, a bone marrow biospy or aspiration needle (e.g. Jamshidi needle) can also be placed into the tibia [5]. The same types of needles can be used in premaure/dysmature foals, twins, or foals with intrauterine growth restriction/incomplete ossification, but this group of foals may have a softer bone cortex allowing placement of a 14- to 18-gauge standard hypodermic needle [2, 5]. Once the needle is in the proper place, fluid should flow easily with minimal extravasation.

In the original study describing IO infusion technique in foals, mean time to needle placement in the tibia and radius was 33 and 63 seconds, respectively [1]. The fastest fluid flow rates achieved at these locations were 67 ml/min and 27 ml/min, respectively [1]. Bone pain has been reported in people receiving IO infusions that exceed a pressure of 35 mmHg [6]; the pressure was not measured in neonatal foals, but a pressure bag was utilized to facilitate infusion with no noted discomfort [1]. In contrast, in the study using weanling foals, a pressure of 300 mmHg was used to infuse fluids to which foals demontrated discomfort; administration of lidocaine prior to infusion appeared to eleviate the discomfort [3]. Complications associated with the IO procedure include subcutaenous and subperiosteal fluid leakage, malposition of the IO needle, IO

Equine Neonatal Medicine, First Edition. Edited by David M. Wong and Pamela A. Wilkins.

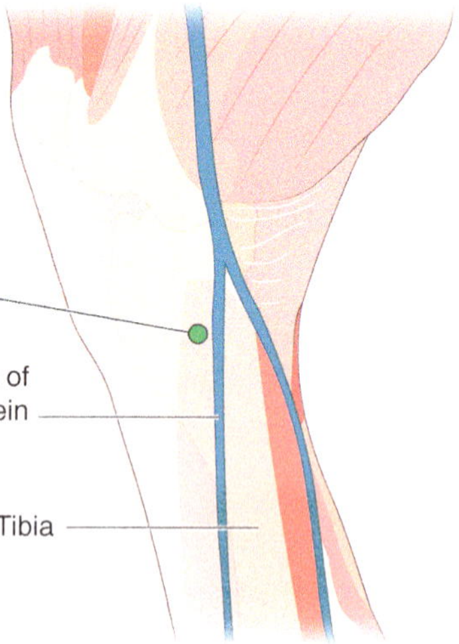

Figure 59.VII.1 Preferred site for placement of IO needle in the neonatal foal. The site is on the medial side of the proximal tibia, approximately 3 cm distal to the tendinous band from the semitendinosus muscle.

needle dislodgement, and partial occlusion of the IO needle. Following IO needle removal, localized soft tissue swelling and firm hard swelling occurred at the IO sites. These typically resolved within 1–4 weeks [1].

The pharmacodynamics of IO infused drugs are nearly the same as those for the IV route. In one study in healthy neonatal foals, plasma concentration-time profiles and pharamacokinetic parameters were identical when comparing IO and IV administered amikacin and suggested that medications and fluids administered IO nearly instantantly reached the central circulation and exerted effects equivalent to those achieved via IV administration [6, 7]. In the aforementioned study in weanling-age foals, the humeral site was comparable to jugular vein infusion in regard to delivery time of medications to the central circulation, but a 30–60 second delay was reported for the radius, tibia, and third metacarpal bones [3]. This brief delay was considered clinically negligible. Some drugs that can be administered via the IO route include replacement fluids, glucose, sodium bicarbonate, calcium choloride, blood, plasma, epinephrine, lidocaine, atropine, dopamine, dobutamine, vasopressin, antimicrobials, phenobarbital, diazepam, butorphenol, insulin, and mannitol, as well as other drugs that are formulated for intravenous administration [2].

Table 59.VII.1 Technique for placement of intraosseous (IO) needle.

Equipment needed for intraosseous infusion technique

- Clippers with #40 blade
- Supplies for aseptic preparation of site
- Sterile gloves
- Local anesthetic (2% lidocaine or similar)
- #15 scalpal blade
- Heparin-saline solution
- Sterile wrap
- 12- or 15-gauge IO needles or Sur-fast Cook IO needle (Cook Critical Care, Bloomington, Indiana)
- If purpose-specific IO needles are not available, a 14 to 18-gauge needle can be used but may require a #4 Steinmann pin and Jacobs chuck to facilitate insertion of needle into marrow.

Location of intraosseous infusion needle placement

Tibia	Radius
A flat area devoid of vessels is located at the proximal medial one-third of the tibia, approximately 3 cm distal to a tendinous band from the semitendinous muscle. Of note, a branch of the saphenous vein crosses tibia approximately 2 cm distal to IO infusion site.	A flat area is located in the proximal medial radius, cranial to the median vein, artery, and nerve. The site is approximately 1 cm distal to the mediocutaneous antebrachial nerve.

Procedure for placement of intraosseous infusion needle

- Sedate foal if necessary and position in lateral recumbency.
- Clip hair and aseptically prepare IO site.
- Desensitize skin, subcutaneous tissues, and periosteum over IO site with local anesthetic.
- Incise skin and subcutaneous tissues with #15 scalpel blade.
- Using an IO needle (with stylet) or large-gauge needle, apply firm pressure downward while using a twisting motion on bone until a loss or resistance is noted.
- If IO needle is not available and clinician is not able to apply enough pressure to insert a large-gauge needle, use #4 Steinmann pin and Jacobs chuck to penetrate cortex into the marrow cavity, remove Steinman pin, and insert large-gauge needle.
- The needle should stand without support, and placement into the medullary cavity can be confirmed by aspirating blood and/or marrow contents.
- Flush with 5–10 ml of sterile heparin-saline solution; needle should be flushed every 4–6 h until needle is removed.
- Remove IO needle after stabilzation of patient and IV access is obtained. Although infrequently needed, IO needle can be left in place for prolonged period (2–3 d) if necessary, but should be wrapped with sterile bandage.

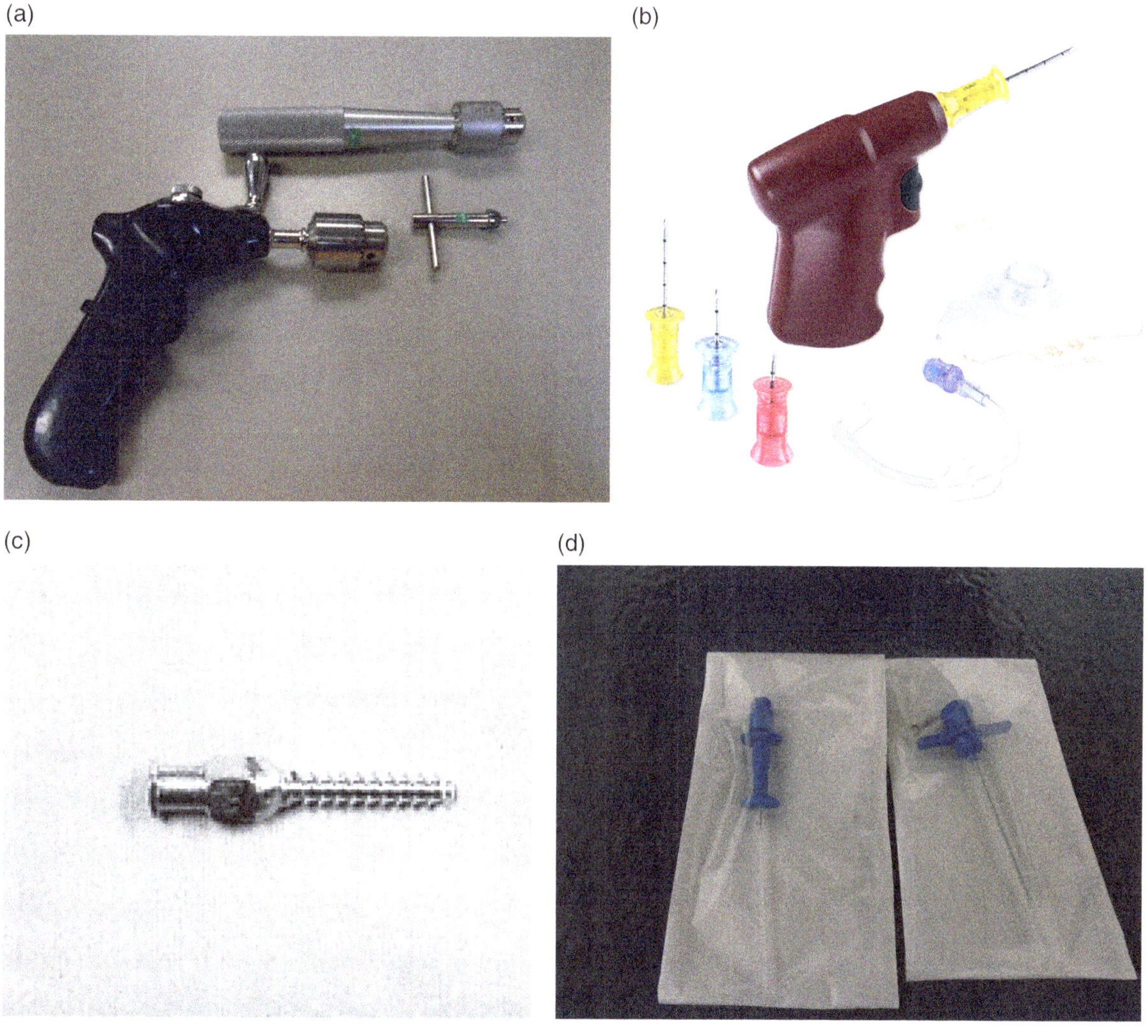

Figure 59.VII.2 Equipment used in placement of IO needle or screw. (a) Use of a Jacob chuck (top) or hand drill and a #4 Steinmann may be necessary to create a hole in the cortex and allow passage of a needle into the marrow. (b) Example of an IO catheter kit, including steel luer-lock catheters of various sizes (Arrow, Inc.). (c) Cannulated screw used for IO administration of fluids [4]. (d) Bone marrow needles used for IO infusion procedure. Pictured is an Illinois Bone Marrow Aspiration/Interosseous Infusion needle (left) and a Jamshidi needle (right) with luer-lock adapters to facilitate attachment of fluid administration set.

References

1 Golenz, M.R., Carlson, G.P., Madigan, J.E. et al. (1993). Preliminary report: the development of an intraosseous infusion technique for neonatal foals. *J. Vet. Intern. Med.* 7: 377–382.

2 Palmer, J.E. (2007). Neonatal Foal Resuscitation. *Vet. Clin. Equine* 23: 159–182.

3 Tate, L.P., Berry, C.R., and King, C. (2003). Comparison of peripheral-to-central cirulation delivery times between intravenous and intraosseious infusion in foals. *Equine Vet. Educ.* 15: 201–206.

4 Nils-Uwe, K., Parker, J.E., and Watrous, B.J. (2003). Intraosseous regional perfusion for treatment of septic physitis in a two-week-old foal. *J. Am. Vet. Med. Assoc.* 222: 346–350.

5 Nogaradi, N. and Magdesian, K.G. (2018). Intaosseous needle placement in the neonatal foal. In: *Manual of Clinical Procedures in the Horse* (ed. L.R.R. Costa and M.R. Paradis), 472–475. Wiley Blackwell.

6 Wilson, W.D. (1995). Intraosseous drug administration to foals. *Proc 17th Bain-Fallon Memoral Lectures*, 213–220.

7 Golenz, M.R., Wilson, W.D., Carlson, G.P. et al. (1994). Effect of route of administration and age on the pharmacokinetics of amikacin administered by the intravenous and intraosseous routes to 3 and 5-day-old foals. *Equine Vet. J.* 26: 367–373.

Section VIII Treatment of Hypothermia

David Wong

Accidental hypothermia, defined as an unintentional decline in the core body temperature because of exposure to ambient temperature less than core temperature, is a well-documented condition in people [1, 2]. Although little information specifically related to accidental hypothermia is available in foals, it remains a geographic and seasonal occurrence in newborn foals, particularly those born during cold environmental temperatures [2]. Although most horse owners monitor and plan for parturition to avoid accidental hypothermia, unexpected pregnancy or early delivery of a foal is not uncommon and can cause accidental hypothermia.

Body temperature is regulated by the hypothalamus, which receives input from thermoreceptors along the internal carotid artery, posterior hypothalamus, and peripheral skin receptors [1]. Core body temperature can be measured via the rectum or esophagus in the foal and is representative of the central body temperature away from the effects of vasoconstriction that might occur at the peripheral vasculature. Body temperature should range from 99 to 102 °F (37–39 °C) in newborn to 24-hour-old foals [3]. Normal heat loss occurs through four mechanisms: radiation (heat transfer in the form of infrared electromagnetic radiation), conduction (direct heat transfer to adjacent colder object or medium), convection (direct heat transfer to air or water currents), and evaporation (vaporization of water through insensible losses and perspiration) [4]. In people, approximately 55–65% of loss is through radiation whereas only 2–3% is lost via conduction [5]. In contrast, animals lose heat primarily from conduction and convection [6]. Moreover, conduction increases dramatically when wet, as might occur in the newborn foal. Homeothermic responses to cold include vasoconstriction, increased muscle tone, and shivering along with metabolic increases from release of catecholamines and thyroxine (Table 59.VIII.1) [1, 5]. Shivering is controlled by the posterior hypothalamus and spinal cord with thermogenesis via shivering causing a twofold to fivefold increase in basal metabolic rate and markedly increased oxygen consumption.

Several factors predispose the newborn foal to hypothermic episodes, with the ambient temperature being a major contributing component (e.g. average low temperature in January is 12 °F [−11 °C] in Ames, IA). With primary hypothermia, the foal has no underlying health condition but the compensatory responses to heat loss are overwhelmed by exposure [5]. Secondary hypothermia is low body temperature that can result from a variety of systemic diseases that lower the temperature set-point. Factors in the foal that predispose to hypothermia are noted in Table 59.VIII.2.

Hypothermia, depending on severity, can have various effects on the body including the cardiovascular, respiratory, neurologic, renal and coagulation systems [5]. Mild hypothermia, in patients with normal thermoregulation, causes an increase in oxygen consumption and cardiac output. However, the cardiovascular system is depressed with moderate to severe hypothermia, often manifesting as decreased inotropic function of the heart, decreased cardiac output and hypotension. Cardiac cycle prolongation occurs because the conduction system is more sensitive to cold than the myocardium. Bradycardia occurs as a result of decreased spontaneous depolarization of the pacemaker cells [5]. Arrhythmias can arise from cold-induced conduction abnormalities with atrial irritability a feature of early hypothermia. In addition, hypothermia causes a decrease in transmembrane resting potential that thereby decreases the threshold for ventricular dysrhythmias, which are common with moderate to severe hypothermia [5]. Reentrant dysrhythmias are caused by decreased conduction velocity along with increased myocardial conduction time and decreased absolute refractory periods [5].

In regard to the respiratory system, hypothermia initially stimulates respiration followed by progressive decrease in minute ventilation proportional to decreasing metabolism and depression of the brainstem respiratory center [1, 5].

Equine Neonatal Medicine, First Edition. Edited by David M. Wong and Pamela A. Wilkins.

Table 59.VIII.1 Classification and clinical signs associated with hypothermia in people [1, 4, 5].

	Mild	Moderate	Severe
Degree of hypothermia °F (°C)	89.6–95 [32–35]	82.4–89.6 [28–32]	68–82.4 [20–28]
General/Metabolic	Shivering, ↑ O_2 consumption	↑ O_2 Consumption	Acidosis
Cardiac	Vasoconstriction ↑ Blood pressure and cardiac output from catecholamines	Atrial arrythmias Bradycardia	Ventricular arrythmias, Decreased cardiac output
Respiratory/Neurologic	Tachypnea, bronchospasm Confusion, hyperreflexia	Decreased respiratory drive Depressed consciousness Hyporeflexia	Apnea, coma, Absent reflexes
Renal, GI, Coagulation	Decreased motility Platelet dysfunction, Impaired clotting enzyme function	Cold diuresis	
Endocrine	↑ Stress hormones (cortisol) catecholamines, thyroxin		

Table 59.VIII.2 Factors predisposing foal to hypothermia.

Decreased heat production	Increased heat loss	Miscellaneous
■ Lactic acidosis ■ Insufficient calories (hypoglycemia, malnutrition) ■ Inactivity	■ Environmental temperature ■ Immersion (wet when born)	■ Multisystem trauma ■ Infection ■ Shock

In people, carbon dioxide production decreases by 50% with a 8 °C fall in body temperature [1, 5]. With severe hypothermia, the normal stimuli for respiratory control is altered and carbon dioxide retention with respiratory acidosis can occur [5]. The central nervous system is also progressively depressed with hypothermia with cerebral blood flow highly sensitive to changes in core temperature [1]. For example, in people, a 1 °C decrease in core temperature can cause a drop in cerebral blood flow of 6–7% [1].

The kidney's response to simple cold exposure is diuresis, regardless of the individual's state of hydration [5]. With more severe hypothermia, renal blood flow is decreased and the kidneys excrete a large amount of dilute urine, termed cold diuresis. Cold diuresis is essentially glomerular filtrate that does not clear nitrogenous waste products [5]. This compensatory response might occur because of the initial relative central hypervolemia observed in severe hypothermia as a consequence of peripheral vasoconstriction; diuresis attempts to decrease overall blood volume [1, 5]. Hematologically, hypothermia increases coagulation, which may be a result of catecholamine or steroid release, simple circulatory collapse, or release of tissue thromboplastin from cold ischemic tissue [7]. Interestingly, the enzymatic nature of the activated clotting factors are depressed by the cold, but coagulation tests performed in the clinical pathology laboratory are typically completed at 37 °C. Therefore, there can be a disparity between the *in vivo*, clinically evident coagulopathy and the potentially normal prothrombin time and partial thromboplastin time [5, 8]. Cold-induced thrombocytopenia can also occur from direct bone marrow suppression or splenic and hepatic sequestration, and platelet function is decreased due to decreased production of thromboxane B_2 and expression of platelet surface molecules [5].

The term *core temperature afterdrop* is sometimes used in hypothermic patients to refer to the further decline in core temperature after removal from cold. This occurs as a result of circulatory changes and temperature equilibration across a gradient. In other words, a counter-current cooling of blood occurs when cold tissues receive more blood perfusion, resulting in a temperature decline until the gradient is eliminated [9, 10]. Core temperature afterdrop is clinically important in foals with a large temperature gradient between core and peripheral tissues [6].

Treatment and Rewarming Options

Severe hypothermia can often be overlooked because standard rectal thermometers only measure to approximately 93 °F (34 °C) [6]. Electronic thermistors can be used to measure core temperatures from the esophagus or rectum, with some instruments having the ability to provide continuous readings. Additional diagnostics include a standard minimum database, including a complete blood count and serum biochemistry profile to evaluate for leukopenia, thrombocytopenia, or elevated hematocrit (hematocrit increases 2% for every 1.8 °F decline in temperature) and other analyte (hypokalemia, hyper- or hypoglycemia) and organ (azotemia) anomalies [1, 5, 6].

Rewarming of the hypothermic patient can be approached using passive and/or active methods (Table 59.VIII.3). Passive rewarming optimizes environmental conditions while allowing the patient's endogenous heat-generating capabilities to correct decreased core temperature. Passive rewarming techniques include removing the foal from a cold environment, increasing the ambient room temperature, and providing blanket coverage, while endogenous heat production restores core temperature [1]. This type of therapy is simple and noninvasive but can result in significant anaerobic metabolism and lactic acidosis, and therefore is the treatment of choice for only mild cases of hypothermia [1].

Active rewarming (external or internal) utilizes direct transfer of exogenous heat to the foal and is indicated in cases with more severe hypothermia and clinical signs such as cardiovascular instability, poikilothermia (inability to regulate body temperature), inadequate rate or failure to rewarm, endocrinologic insufficiency, or presence of predisposing factors (Table 59.VIII.1) [5]. Active external rewarming techniques are implemented with moderate hypothermia (82–90 °F [28–43 °C]) and include use of hot-water bottles, heating blankets, convective air blankets, reflective blankets, and radiant heat shields [6]. Caution must be exercised with active external rewarming as externally heating the extremities may result in direct damage to the skin and contribute to a drop in core temperature by causing vasodilation in the peripheral extremities; this can be limited by applying external heat to the thorax only [2].

Table 59.VIII.3 Rewarming techniques.

Passive rewarming	Active external rewarming	Active internal rewarming
▪ Remove from cold environment ▪ Increase ambient room temperature ▪ Blanket coverage	▪ Forced-air warming ▪ Hot-water bottles ▪ Heating pads/blankets ▪ Reflective blankets ▪ Radiant heat sources	▪ Warmed IV fluids ▪ Airway rewarming ▪ Warm irrigation fluids into body cavities (gastric, colonic) ▪ Warm peritoneal dialysis

One of the simplest methods of active internal rewarming is administration of warmed IV fluids. Warmed IV fluids increase core temperature by conduction, which is the most effective method of heat transfer [1]. Crystalloid fluids can be warmed in a water bath to a temperature of 104 °F (40 °C) and administered to hypothermic patients. Administration of warmed IV fluids will also address dehydration, which is common in the hypothermic patient. If the foal requires administration of plasma, frozen products should be rewarmed to adequate temperatures. In addition to warming IV fluids prior to administration, the use of in-line fluid warmers can be implemented to facilitate heat transfer. Countercurrent fluid warmers are most effective at heating IV fluids as these devices pass fluid through a water bath contained in a length of thin aluminum tubing, which has much higher thermal conductivity than plastic tubing [1]. Airway rewarming (ventilation with warmed air) via mask or endotracheal tube is another method of active internal rewarming, as it limits the normal heat and water loss from respiration; however this method has low thermal conductivity and should not be used as a sole method of rewarming [1].

Body cavity lavage is another active internal method of rewarming and transfers a large amount of heat to patients suffering from moderate to severe hypothermia because water has a rate of heat transfer 32 times greater than air. Cavity lavage can be accomplished via peritoneal or pleural lavage, but is obviously a more invasive method of rewarming and should be reserved for more severe cases of hypothermia. Interestingly, intraperitoneal fluids have been used as both an alternative and an adjunct to intravenous fluid therapy in dehydrated human patients [11, 12]; however, the intraperitoneal route may not reliably replace fluid volume in dehydrated patients [12]. The peritoneal crystalloid dialysate can be heated to 104–113 °F (40–45 °C) and administered at a dose of 10–20 ml/kg [6]. Peritoneal lavage should be avoided with cases of hemoperitoneum, free air in the abdomen, or a foal with a prior laparotomy. Pleural lavage has been described in people and small animals and may provide an easier route of fluid return than peritoneal lavage, but it has not been described in the hypothermic neonatal foal [8, 13]. Appropriate volumes of warmed fluids can also be administered into the stomach or colon, but the surface area of these organs is limited.

References

1 Tsuei, B.J. and Kearney, P.A. (2004). Hypothermia in the trauma patient. *Inj. Int. J. Care Injured* 35: 7–15.

2 Stephen, J.O., Baptiste, K.E., and Townsend, H.G.G. (2000). Clinical and pathologic findings in donkeys with hypothermia: 10 cases (1988–1998). *J. Am. Vet. Med. Assoc.* 216: 725–729.

3 Carr, E.A. (2014). Field triage of the neonatal foal. *Vet. Clin. Equine* 30: 283–300.

4 Chavala, M.L.A., Gallardo, M.A., Marteinez, I.S. et al. (2019). Management of accidental hypothermia: a narrative review. *Med. Intensiva* 43: 556–568.

5 Danzl, D. (2002). Hypothermia. *Semin. Respir. Crit. Care Med.* 23: 57–68.

6 Wingfield, W.E. (2002). Accidental hypothermia. In: *The Veterinary ICU Book* (ed. W.E. Wingfield and M.R. Raffe), 1116–1129. Jackson Hole, Wyoming: Teton New Media.

7 Cosgriff, N., Moore, E.E., Sauaia, A. et al. (1997). Predicting life-threatening coagulopathy in the massively transfused trauma patient: hypothermia and acidoses revisited. *J. Trauma* 42: 857–861.

8 Eddy, V.A., Morris, J.A., and Cullinane, D.C. (2000). Hypothermia, coagulopathy, and acidosis. *Surg. Clin. North Am.* 80: 845–854.

9 Hayward, J.S., Eckerson, J.D., and Kemna, D. (1984). Thermal and cardiovascular changes during three methods of resuscitation from mild hypothermia. *Resuscitation* 11: 21–33.

10 Giesbrecht, G.G., Johnston, C.E., and Bristow, G.K. (1998). The convective afterdrop component during hypothermic exercise decreased with delayed exercise onset. *Aviat. Space Environ. Med.* 69: 17–22.

11 Asheim, P., Uggen, P.E., Aasarod, K. et al. (2006). Intraperitoneal fluid therapy: an alternative to intravenous treatment in a patient with limited vascular access. *Anesthesia* 61: 502–504.

12 Wenzel, R.P. and Phillips, R.A. (1971). Intraperitoneal infusion for initial therapy of cholera. *Lancet* 298: 494–495.

13 Peng, R.Y. and Bongard, F.S. (1999). Hypothermia in trauma patients. *J. Am. Coll. Surg.* 188: 685–696.

Section IX Direct and Indirect Blood Pressure Measurement

David Wong

Disturbances of the cardiovascular system are frequently encountered in ill neonatal foals, especially those afflicted with sepsis and neonatal encephalopathy. Although this section focuses on blood pressure measurement, assessment of mentation, heart rate, pulse pressure, mucous membranes, and capillary refill time provide a more comprehensive and accurate evaluation of the cardiovascular status of the foal. Moreover, measured values of blood lactate, urine output, and central venous pressure complement physical examine of the cardiovascular system.

Blood flow and blood pressure are distinct physical entities with global blood flow (e.g. cardiac output) rather than blood pressure being the critical determinant of tissue perfusion [1]. Measurement of cardiac output is not a commonly used modality in ill equine neonates; thus, arterial blood pressure is used as an indication for potential blood flow [1]. Blood pressure (BP) is the product of cardiac output (CO) and systemic vascular resistance (SVR), expressed as $BP = CO \times SVR$ [1]. The clinician should be cognizant of the fact that adequate organ perfusion is dependent on blood flow rather than directly on blood pressure. Because blood flow is difficult to quantify clinically, clinicians often use blood pressure as a marker of blood flow. Based on studies in other species and anecdotal evidence in foals [2], mean blood pressures <60 mmHg are likely to be deleterious as it is at this pressure at which autoregulatory control of blood flow to the heart, brain, and kidneys ceases and organ perfusion becomes pressure-dependent [2]. In regard to hemodynamic support, therapy should be titrated to the mean blood pressure, rather than systolic pressure, as mean pressure better predicts organ perfusion pressure [3]. The normal mean arterial blood pressure in the Thoroughbred foal is 69–111 mmHg [4].

Blood pressure can be measured using direct and indirect (oscillometric, Doppler) methods. Direct blood pressure is considered the gold standard and is accomplished by direct cannulation of a peripheral artery. In foals, a 20-gauge 1.5-in. (3.8 cm) catheter is commonly placed in the dorsal metatarsal artery for direct blood pressure measurement. Alternative sites include the facial, radial, and caudal auricular arteries [5, 6]. Once placed, the catheter is fixed in place via rapid drying adhesive glue and/or sutures. Both over-the-needle and over-the-wire catheters have been used to cannulate arteries in foals, but over-the-wire catheters may be easier to place in hypotensive foals or patients with peripheral edema. Once the catheter is secured in place, it is connected to an electronic pressure transducer at the level of the sternal manubrium; the transducer is placed and zeroed at this level [1, 2]. Arterial catheters require intermittent flushing every 3–4 hours using heparinized saline solution to maintain patency. Although direct arterial blood pressure monitoring provides an accurate and continuous display of blood pressure, direct cannulation is difficult to maintain, is not without risk, requires specific technical skill and equipment, and is not always indicated in noncritical cases.

Alternatively, noninvasive blood pressure (NIBP) techniques can be used because of their ease of use, availability and noninvasive nature. NIPB measurements are more clinically practical in foals and can be accomplished via oscillometric or Doppler techniques. The oscillometric technique detects pressure fluctuations produced in an air bladder within the occluding cuff resulting from the pressure pulse [7]. In foals, common sites to obtain oscillometric measurements include placement of the cuff around the base of the tail (coccygeal artery), at the proximal aspect of the metatarsus (dorsal metatarsal artery) or around the forelimb between the carpus and elbow (median artery); the posterior digital artery is another possible location [2]. Use of appropriately sized cuffs should be placed using careful and tight positioning to ensure the most accurate results. In dogs and cats, the recommended cuff width is 30–40% of the circumference of the appendage that the cuff is placed on; however, the ideal cuff bladder width is

Equine Neonatal Medicine, First Edition. Edited by David M. Wong and Pamela A. Wilkins.

not known in foals [7]. Reportedly, cuffs with bladder widths that are too wide relative to appendage circumference result in falsely low measurements and cuffs with bladders that are too small result in falsely high measurements [8]. Interestingly, in the limited studies in foals, no correlation was found between cuff ratios and bias [1, 9]. A cuff width of 52 mm was used in one foal study and provided acceptable results [9]. It is also recommended to collect four to six consecutive measurements over a 5–10 minute period and use the average of those measurements to provide a more representative measurement.

Oscillometry has been examined in anesthetized and conscious foals with the overall consensus that this technique provides acceptable estimates of mean arterial blood pressure when measured from the tail, when compared to direct mean arterial blood pressure measured from the metatarsal artery [1]. In one study, a significant interaction was noted between type of monitor used and site of cuff placement. In this study, significantly lower bias was noted when the cuff was placed over the coccygeal artery as compared to the median or metatarsal artery [1]. Collectively, the lowest mean arterial pressure bias was −1.07 mmHg and the narrowest limits of agreement were −9.39 to 7.25 [1, 9]. Of note, the degree of correlation between various oscillometric machines and direct blood pressure measurements will likely vary, along with different sites of cuff placement; thus, the global cardiovascular status should be assessed through both physical examination parameters and other measured blood variables (e.g. lactate).

Doppler measurements are made using a Doppler flowmeter that detects blood flow by emitting an ultrasound signal that produces an auditory signal generated by the change in emitted versus returning frequencies (frequency shift) reflected back to the transducer by underlying moving red blood cells [7]. Blood pressure is estimated by the operator using an aneroid manometer that is connected to an occluding cuff placed proximal to the Doppler transducer. When a good pulse wave is identified (e.g. audible sound when placed over artery), the cuff proximal to the transducer is inflated to a level that abolishes the pulse wave. The cuff pressure is slowly released and the point at which flow audibly returns approximates the systolic arterial pressure. The Doppler technique is less frequently used in clinical practice, but an older study successfully utilized the Doppler technique in 12 pony foals, although results were not compared to direct measurements (Table 59.IX.1) [10]. As with the oscillometric technique, an average of several measurements should be used with the Doppler technique.

Table 59.IX.1 Mean (± standard deviation) blood pressure measurements from 12 healthy pony foals using the Doppler technique (coccygeal artery) [10].

Age	Systolic (mmHg)	Diastolic (mmHg)	Mean[a] (mmHg)
1	81 ± 10	35 ± 7	50 ± 8
7	104 ± 21[b]	40 ± 14	61 ± 15
14	100 ± 16[b]	41 ± 7	61 ± 6[b]
21	107 ± 28[b]	48 ± 17[b]	68 ± 16[b]
30	114 ± 21[b]	54 ± 13[b]	74 ± 11[b]
60	103 ± 12[b]	53 ± 20[b]	70 ± 6[b]
90	111 ± 15[b]	57 ± 19[b]	75 ± 16[b]

[a] Calculated value.
[b] Significantly different than day 1 ($P < 0.05$).

References

1 Giguere, S., Knowles, H.A., Valverde, A. et al. (2005). Accuracy of indirect measurement of blood pressure in neonatal foals. *J. Vet. Intern. Med.* 19: 571–576.
2 Corley, K.T.T. (2002). Monitoring and treating haemodynamic disturbances in critically ill neonatal foals. Part 1: Haemodynamic monitoring. *Equine Vet. Educ.* 14: 279–279.
3 Hollenberg, S.M., Ahrens, T.S., Astiz, M.E. et al. (1999). Practice parameters for hemodynamic support of sepsis in adult patients in sepsis. *Crit. Care Med.* 27: 639–660.
4 Franco, R.M., Ousey, J.C., Cash, R.S. et al. (1986). Study of arterial blood pressure in newborn foals using an electronic sphygmomanometer. *Equine Vet. J.* 18: 475–478.
5 Vaala, W.E. and Webb, A.I. (1990). Cardiovascular monitoring of the critically ill foal. In: *Equine Clinical Neonatology* (ed. A.M. Koterba, W.H. Drummond, and P.C. Kosch), 262–272. Philadelphia: Lea and Fibiger.
6 Taylor, P.M. (1981). Techniques and clinical application of arterial blood pressure measurement in the horse. *Equine Vet. J.* 13: 271–275.
7 Henik, R.A., Dolson, M.K., and Wenholz, L.J. (2005). How to obtain a blood pressure measurement. *Clin. Tech. Small Anim. Pract.* 20: 144–150.
8 Magdesian, K.G. (2004). Monitoring the critically ill equine patient. *Vet. Clin. North Am. Equine Pract.* 20: 11–39.
9 Nout, Y.S., Corley, K.T.T., Donaldson, L.L. et al. (2002). Indirect oscillometric and direct blood pressure measurements in anesthetized and conscious neonatal foals. *J. Vet. Emerg. Crit. Care* 12: 75–80.
10 Lombard, C.W., Evans, M., Martin, L. et al. (1984). Blood pressure, electrocardiogram and echocardiogram measurements in the growing pony foal. *Equine Vet. J.* 16: 342–347.

Section X Urinary Catheter Placement

Bonny Millar

After birth, neonates urinate for the first time between 6 and 10 hours of age, with fillies taking marginally longer. Their first urination produces concentrated urine. The healthy neonate who is well hydrated and nurses frequently will yield large volumes (6–7 l/d/50 kg foal) of dilute urine, especially after nursing. Their high fluid intake results in acidic urine with a low specific gravity (1.001–1.008) [1]. The neonate will not have a fully mature and functional renal system for a few weeks. In the early neonatal period, a transient proteinuria exists and in some cases there is an elevated creatinine that gradually decreases to age-specific normal values. Blood urea concentrations are low and remain so for a few months due to the fast growth of the foal. Erythrocytes, leukocytes, hemoglobin, bilirubin, myoglobin, or casts should not be present in normal foal urine.

An indwelling urinary catheter is necessary in recumbent ill foals that cannot stand to urinate or are in the postoperative recovery period after repair of a ruptured urinary bladder (Table 59.X.1). Where hypoperfusion is suspected, accurate measurement of urine output is needed. Monitoring of ill neonatal foals can be accomplished by utilizing a closed urinary system to collect and monitor urine output. Sick neonates are also at risk of developing sepsis, often resulting in weakness and an inability to stand. These foals are more susceptible to a number of urinary associated complications. For example, if the foal continuously lays in a wet, urine-soaked stable or on a nonabsorbent mat, scalding can occur, especially in neonates that cannot stand and posture to void correctly (Figure 59.X.1). The placement of an indwelling urinary catheter can prevent the delicate ventral abdomen and perineal skin from urine scald.

Complications

- Catheter failure – If the balloon bursts or the valve on the balloon port malfunctions, the catheter will displace and need to be replaced.
- Catheter kinks and obstructions – Following aseptic technique, remove and replace with a new sterile catheter.
- Ascending urinary tract infections – Maintaining a closed collection system decreases the prevalence of urinary infections that enter via the catheter. Whenever a catheter is replaced, observe aseptic technique for the procedure.
- Patent urachus – In utero, the allantois and fetal bladder are connected by the urachus, which should close at birth. In the ill and recumbent neonate, there may be added pressure on the bladder that can delay or prevent the closure of the urachus. On rare occasions it is possible to inadvertently advance the urinary catheter into the bladder and through the length of the urachus (Figure 59.X.4). To reposition the catheter, clean the catheter and urachal stump, retract the catheter into the bladder, and remove completely. Replace with a new sterile catheter.

Equine Neonatal Medicine, First Edition. Edited by David M. Wong and Pamela A. Wilkins.

Table 59.X.1 Technique for placement of an indwelling urinary catheter.

Equipment needed for urinary catheter placement. Collect all equipment in an instrument tray and have readily available during placement.

- Dilute povidine – iodine solution soaked swabs
- Exam gloves
- Small sterile drape
- Sterile water soluble lubricant
- Sterile gloves
- Sterile silicone foley catheter with inflatable balloon[a]
- Sterile urine collection bag with emptying valve[b] (Figure 59.X.2)
- Porous medical (white) tape
- 10 ml syringe filled with sterile water (for filling the catheter balloon cuff)
- Sterile 50 ml catheter tip syringe

Determine required size of urinary cather

- Fillies – 12F to 14F, 30 cm (10F in very small fillies)
- Colts – 10F to 12F, 30 cm

The diameter of the catheter should fit the urethral opening well enough to prevent urine from leaking around the exterior of the catheter. Many catheters are also available in a 55 cm length. While these may be prefered in some foals, consider that when the foal is standing and mobile, they are more likely to catch and remove a long catheter.

Procedure for the placement of urinary catheters

Colts

- The foal will need to be placed in lateral recumbency with the uppermost leg lifted up and out of the way of the person inserting the catheter. Ensure there is sufficient restraint, as it is easy to be kicked during this procedure. With effective restraint, sedation is rarely required.
- Assistant dons gloves and exteriorizes the penis clear from the prepuce. This is done by holding the shaft and gently pushing the prepuce downward and the penis outward and clear of the sheath. They will be required to hold the penis in this manner to prevent it from retracting during the procedure. (Note: Some colts have a persistent frenulum, making it difficult to exteriorize the penis. If this is the case, do not force the penis up and out of the prepuce. It is still possible to visualize the urethral orifice when the prepuce is pushed down, thus enabling catheterization.)
- Clean the urethra and urethral fossa with dilute povidine-iodine or other appropriate antiseptic wash followed by a wipe with a swab soaked in sterile water. Avoid using cotton wool as small fibers can be left behind within the prepuce.
- Don sterile gloves and have assistant open up catheter and aseptically pass the catheter to the individual inserting it. Check for leaks by injecting sterile water into the catheter balloon. Withdraw the sterile water and lubricate the tip of the catheter. Attach a catheter tip syringe to the distal end to prevent air ingress into the bladder during insertion.
- Gently insert the tip of the catheter into the urethral opening and advance until it just enters the bladder. There may be some resistance when the catheter passes through the pelvic brim or if the penis is held too firmly. Urine is often seen entering the drainage port and the attached syringe. If urine is not present, gently aspirate the syringe to check for position and patency.

Fillies

- Catheterization of a filly's bladder is more challenging as the insertion requires a blind approach to the urethra. Experience is an advantage and supervision may be required. Sedation is rarely required as long as the foal is restrained correctly.
- Place the filly in lateral recumbency with an assistant restraining the hind legs.
- Clean the filly's perineum and vulval with dilute povidine-iodine or other appropriate anti-septic wash, followed by a wipe with a swab soaked in sterile water. Avoid using cotton wool as small fibers can be left behind within the vulva.
- Don sterile gloves and have an assistant open up the catheter and aseptically pass it to individual placing the catheter. Check for leaks by injecting sterile water into the catheter balloon. Withdraw the sterile water and lubricate the tip of the catheter. Attach a catheter tip syringe to the distal end to prevent air ingress into the bladder during insertion.
- Lubricate an index finger, inserting it into the vulva with the tip of the catheter positioned on the ventral surface of the finger, directing it toward the vestibular floor. The other hand advances the catheter, following the contour of the index finger, ventrally into the urethral opening.
- Urine should be visible at the drainage port once the catheter enters the bladder. Gentle aspiration with the syringe can confirm position of the catheter if the urine does not appear spontaneously.

Continuing (for both sexes)

- Inflate the catheter's balloon with the sterile water. The recommended amount is printed on the side of the balloon port. Slight underinflation is preferable to overinflation.

(*Continued*)

Table 59.X.1 (Continued)

• Attach the urine collection bag and tape securely to the catheter. Running the catheter between the hind legs, tape the catheter and bag connection to the foal's tail, leaving a loop when taped to the tail so it does not pull against the bladder. Care must be taken to ensure the tape is not wrapped around the tail too tightly. Foals are very tolerant of having this system attached to their tails even when they are mobile (Figure 59.X.3). • Urine can be removed for measurement of volume and specific gravity without disconnecting the bag by opening the exit valve and emptying the urine into a container.

[a] SurgiVet® Premium foley catheters, Smiths Medical, Upper Metro Place, Dublin, Ohio, U.S.A. and Eureka Park, Lower Pemberton, Ashford, Kent, UK.
[b] Uriplan® urine collection systems, Bard Medical, Tilgate Forest Business Park, Crawley, West Sussex, UK and Industrial Boulevard, Covington, GA, USA.

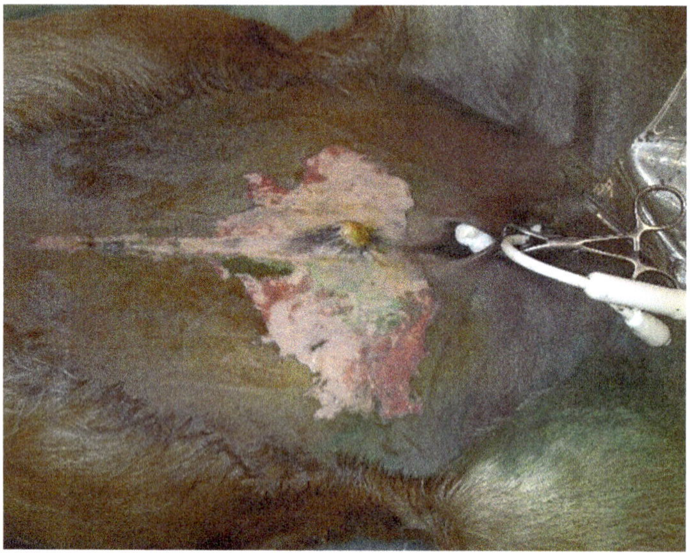

Figure 59.X.1 Urine scalding of the ventral abdominal skin secondary to continuous recumbency and exposure to urine-soaked environment in an ill neonatal foal.

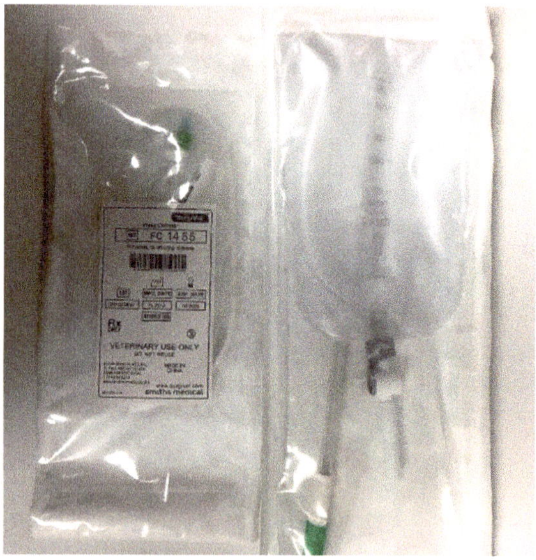

Figure 59.X.2 Sterile urine collection bag with emptying valve.

(a) (b)

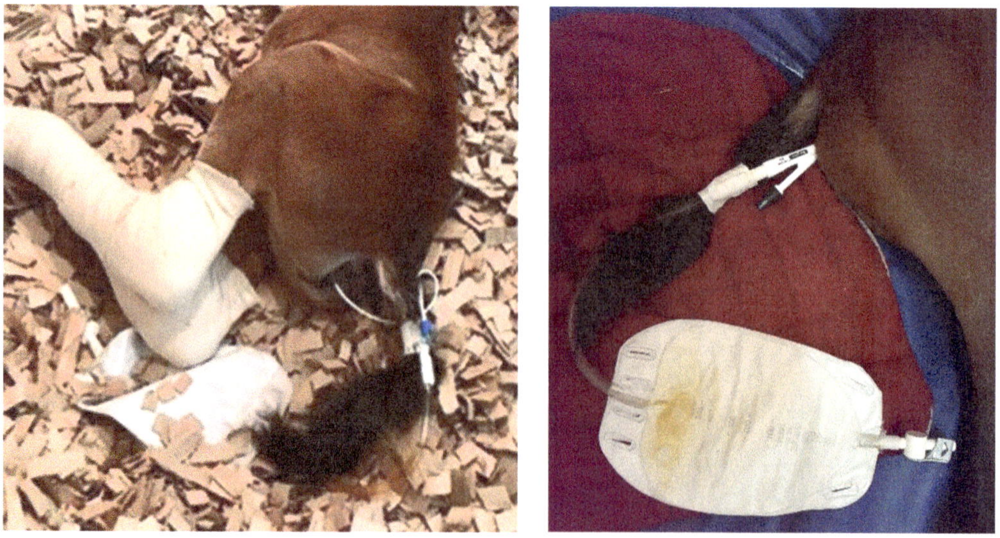

Figure 59.X.3 Fillies with urinary catheters and urine collection bags attached and affixed to tails.

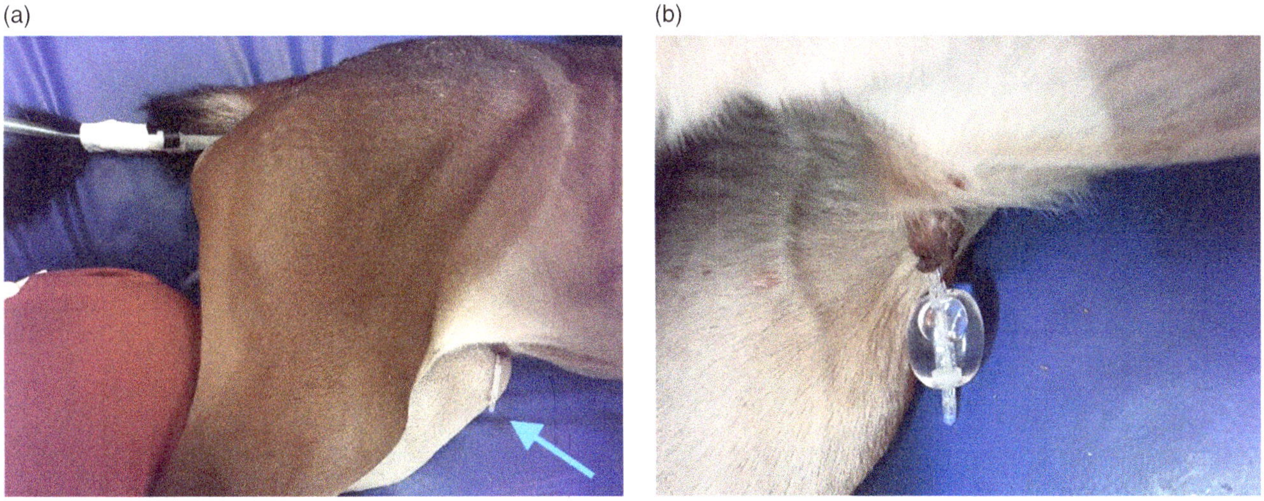

Figure 59.X.4 Filly with urinary catheter inserted, which passed through urinary bladder and urachus, and out urachal stump.

Reference

1 Orsini, J.A. and Divers, T.J. (2013). Neonatology. In: *Equine Emergencies: Treatment and Procedures*. Elsevier.

Section XI Arterial and Venous Blood Gas Collection

Bonny Millar

Arterial blood collection is commonly performed for blood gas analysis and has become a routine procedure in equine neonatology (Table 59.XI.1). Since the introduction of portable point-of-care analyzers (Figure 58.XI.1), with their improved accuracy and reliability, stall-side analysis has become more affordable for general practitioners as well as equine hospitals. Blood from arterial sampling is preferred to venous blood as it provides more accurate and current information on pulmonary function. The blood vessels of foals are easily accessible, such as the brachial artery, located on the medial aspect of the humerus, and the dorsal metatarsal artery, situated along the plantar lateral aspect of the third metatarsal (Figure 59.XI.2). Both sites allow for repeat sampling provided measures are taken to prevent hematomas. Arterial catheters can be placed in the dorsal metatarsal artery, but much care is needed to maintain patency as the active foal can dislodge them easily.

Although arterial sampling is preferred, venous blood gas (VBG) measurement can provide some useful information. Venous blood can be collected from the jugular, cephalic, or saphenous vein in the neonate. VBG analysis differs from arterial results, due to tissue metabolism. Arterial blood gas collection can be more difficult if hypotension and hypothermia are present, thus venous sampling may be the only option. Components analyzed in blood gas analysis include partial pressure of oxygen (PO_2) and carbon dioxide (PCO_2), total CO_2, pH, bicarbonate (HCO_3), base excess, and serum concentrations of electrolytes and ionized calcium.

Complications

Major complications are rare. Repeat sampling can lead to hematomas, localized cellulitis, pain, and phlebitis. Placing support bandages on the distal hindlimb, when not sampling, may decrease swelling. These conditions will eventually resolve when sampling has ceased.

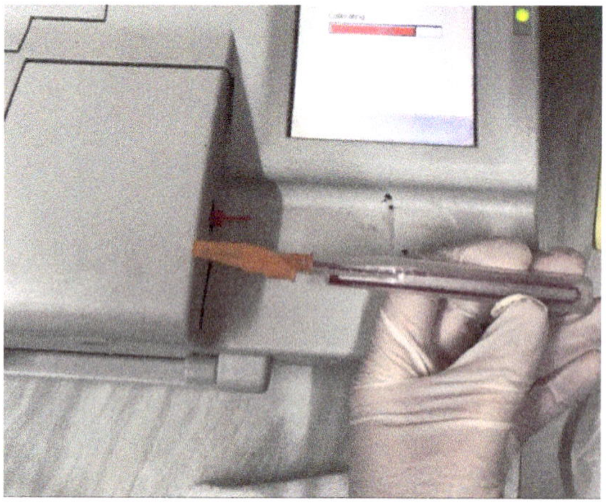

Figure 59.XI.1 Point of care blood gas analyzer and microsampler, testing an arterial sample from a neonatal foal.

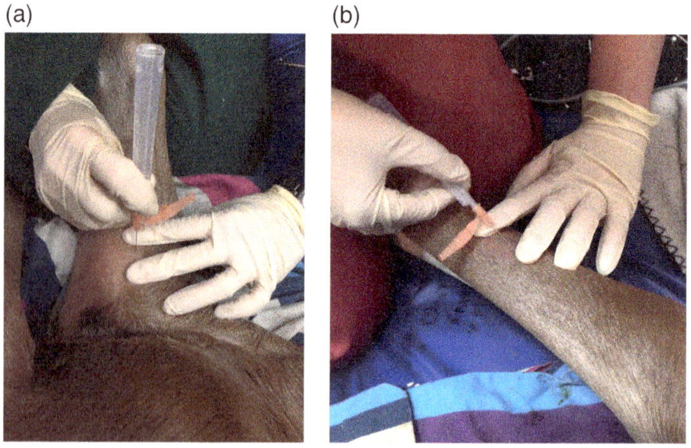

Figure 59.XI.2 (a) Arterial blood gas sample being collected from the brachial artery from the right forelimb in a neonatal foal. (b) Arterial blood gas sample being collected from the metatarsal artery from the left hindlimb in a neonatal foal.

Equine Neonatal Medicine, First Edition. Edited by David M. Wong and Pamela A. Wilkins.

Table 59.XI.1 Technique for collecting arterial blood gas samples.

Equipment needed for artierial blood collection – Collect all equipment in an instrument tray and have readily available during placement.

- Clippers with #40 blade
- Surgical prep materials or alcohol soaked gauze swabs
- Exam gloves
- Proprietary arterial blood gas syringe[a] (Figure 59.XI.3), or a 2 ml syringe internally coated with lithium heparin (1000 μ/ml)
- 23- or 25-gauge needle
- Ice pack and cool box
- Optional – local anesthetic gel, cream or spray[b] for desensitizing the puncture site

Procedure for collection of arterial blood samples in the neonate

- The foal should be standing or in sternal recumbency for a few minutes prior to collection to allow for normal ventilation of the lungs. The foal should then be placed in lateral recumbency and restrained for the procedure. The person taking the blood can kneel and straddle the fore or hind limb (depending on artery used) as a means of restricting movement.
- Clip a small patch of skin over the dorsal metatarsal and/or brachial artery. These vessels are most commonly used in the ill neonatal foal for arterial puncture. Increased pressure or vigorous disinfecting may cause the artery to spasm, thus losing the pulse sensation needed to determine the location of the vessel for needle placement. Applying a warm compress may help with arterial dilation and aid palpation.
- Desensitizing the skin might be advantageous in highly reactive foals. If indicated, apply a very small amount of topical anesthetic gel or cream, directly over the puncture site. Applying excess amounts may cause vasoconstriction, making palpation of the pulse difficult. Application should be at least 15–30 minutes prior to sampling.
- If not using a proprietary blood gas syringe, prepare a syringe and needle by aspirating a small amount of heparin to cover the inner surface of the syringe. To prevent sample dilution, discard all the heparin except that which remains in the hub.
- Don exam gloves and disinfect the area. Palpate for the arterial pulse, being aware that the sensation of the pulse may be diminished while wearing gloves.
  - Dorsal metatarsal approach – feel for the pulse proximal to the puncture site and insert the needle just distal to the operator's fingers, parallel to the vessel at a shallow angle. This is a superficial artery, so care must be taken to avoid puncturing through it. Be aware that limb retraction is common when arteriopuncture occurs; thus, the leg should be held firmly.
  - Brachial approach – when palpating the pulse, straddle the artery with two fingers, stabilizing it in place so the needle enters the artery from a 90° angle, perpendicular to the limb. Advance the needle at this angle until blood is seen in the hub.

  If using tubes that fill by capillary action, pulsing of the blood will be observed as it fills, indicating the presence of an arterial sample. In syringes with plungers, the blood may fill the hub rapidly before the syringe is attached. Care must be taken to not dislodge the placement of the needle when drawing back the plunger.
- When collection is complete, immediately remove any air bubbles and cap the needle with a rubber stopper. Proprietary blood gas syringes may have an integrated cap that will snap over the needle to prevent ingress of atmospheric air.
- Place the sealed sample in a cool environment (ice packs in a cool box) and immediately transport for analysis. Arterial samples left at room temperature must be analyzed within 30 minutes.
- Apply direct pressure with a gauze swab over the puncture site for several minutes to prevent hematoma formation.
- Arterial blood samples must not be exposed to room air or be allowed to clot. This results in increased PO_2 and pH, with a decrease of PCO_2, rendering the results nondiagnostic. Otherwise, the sample can be stored on ice up to 90 minutes without skewed results.

[a] Roche Microsampler Protect, F. Hoffmann-La Roche AG, Basel, Switzerland and Pro- Vent Arterial Sampling Kit, Smiths Medical ASD, Inc. Keene, NH, USA.
[b] EMLA™ lidocaine/prilocaine cream 5%, Aspen Pharma Ireland Limited, Maidenhead, UK.

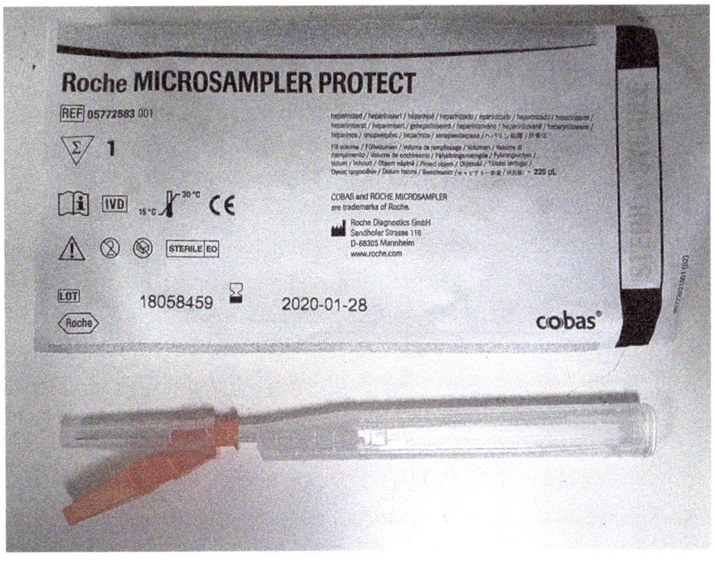

Figure 59.XI.3 Example of a commercially available blood gas syringe that is pre-filled with heparin to inhibit clotting of the sample.

Section XII Capnography

David Wong

Assessment of respiratory function is routinely performed in critically ill neonatal foals, with monitoring of oxygenation and ventilation being vital components of evaluation. These variables can be evaluated via arterial blood gas analysis, pulse oximetry, and capnography. Capnography is a noninvasive measurement that provides physiologic information on ventilation (effectiveness of carbon dioxide [CO_2] elimination), perfusion (CO_2 transportation in vasculature), and metabolism (production of CO_2 by cellular metabolism) and is a measurement of the CO_2 from the airway opening during inspiration and expiration [1]. Capnography can be measured by mainstream or side-stream devices. Mainstream devices measure CO_2 using in-line devices and are designed for intubated patients whereas side-stream units continuously aspirate gas through microtubing to a sensor remote from the patient's airway and can be used in the intubated and nonintubated patient.

A capnogram consists of two stages, inspiration and expiration, which is further divided into four different phases (Table 59.XII.1). The maximum partial pressure of CO_2 is measured at the end of exhalation and is referred to as end-tidal CO_2 ($EtCO_2$), and in the healthy patient is between 35 and 40 mmHg. In the foal with normal ventilation and lung function, the capnograph has a trapezoidal waveform. When exhalation begins, atmospheric air at the sensor has minimal CO_2 yielding a baseline reading of zero (I; inspiratory baseline). As exhalation progresses, air from anatomic dead space is cleared and alveolar air admixes with atmospheric air, resulting in a rapid raise in expired CO_2 (II; expiratory upstroke). During the latter part of exhalation, concentration of CO_2 stabilizes, reflecting primarily alveolar gas (III; alveolar plateau), with the highest CO_2 at end expiration representing the $EtCO_2$. With inspiration, atmospheric air devoid of CO_2 rushes by the sensor, resulting in a rapid decline back to baseline (0; inspiratory downstroke) [2, 3]. Variables that impact capnography include CO_2 production, CO_2 transport, ventilation, and ventilation to perfusion ratio changes [1].

When utilizing capnography, interpretation involves consideration of $EtCO_2$, shape of the capnogram, and the difference between partial pressure of arterial CO_2 (P_aCO_2) and $EtCO_2$ pressure (normally 2–5 mmHg) [1, 2]. The P_aCO_2-$PEtCO_2$ difference has been evaluated in healthy and ill foals with a mean ± SD gradient of 0.1 ± 5.0 mmHg [4]. When gas exchange in the lungs is impaired, $PEtCO_2$ decreases relative to $PaCO_2$ thereby increasing the P_aCO_2-$PEtCO_2$ gradient. Conditions that increase anatomic dead space (shallow breathing, open ventilator circuit) or increase physiologic dead space (low cardiac output, pulmonary embolism, obstructive lung disease) can be associated with a higher P_aCO_2-$PEtCO_2$ gradient.

There are a variety of factors that can alter the normal capnograph as well as a number of uses of capnography in the critical care of neonatal foals (Tables 59.XII.2 and 59.XII.3). Variables that alter the capnograph include sepsis, pulmonary embolism, and metabolic acidemia. Sepsis is associated with hyperlactatemia with $EtCO_2$ having an inverse relationship with blood lactate concentrations. Therefore, sepsis-induced hyperlactatemia is associated with decreased $EtCO_2$ and increased mortality. A pulmonary embolus is another variable that can alter the capnogram and is associated with decreased perfusion to a segment of lung while ventilation remains normal. Pulmonary embolism increases alveolar dead space and is associated with lower expired CO_2 and increases in the P_aCO_2-$EtCO_2$ gradient. $EtCO_2$ is also linearly correlated with serum bicarbonate; thus, in disease states that cause a metabolic acidemia (decreased bicarbonate and venous pH), respiratory compensation occurs, thereby decreasing $EtCO_2$ [1, 2].

Specific clinical situations in which capnography can be used to monitor respiratory function in foals include neonatal encephalopathy, verifying and monitoring endotracheal

Equine Neonatal Medicine, First Edition. Edited by David M. Wong and Pamela A. Wilkins.

Table 59.XII.1 Phases of capnography.

	Phase	Event
Inspiration	0	• Inspiration begins, clearing of CO_2
	β-angle	• Located between phase III and descending part of inspiration; normally 90°
Expiration	I	• Anatomical dead space; should not contain CO_2
	II	• Rapid rise in CO_2 concentration as breath reaches upper airway from alveoli; mixture of anatomical and alveolar dead space
	III	• Alveolar plateau; CO_2 reaches uniform level in airway; height of slope of the line provides information on ventilation and perfusion ratio; height related to cardiac output
	α-angle	• Located between phase II and III; normally 100°

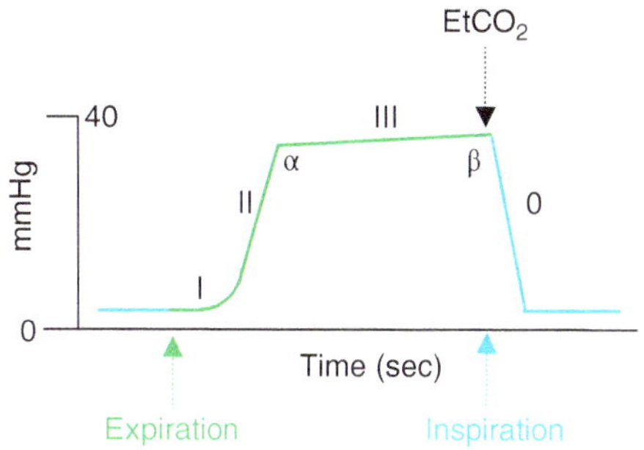

Table 59.XII.2 Conditions that alter $EtCO_2$ [1].

Etiology of abrnomality	$EtCO_2$ decrease	$EtCO_2$ increase
Metabolic	• Hypothermia • Metabolic acidemia	• Malignant hyperthermia
Respiratory	• Pulmonary edema • Intrapulmonary shunt • Hyperventilation	• Hypoventilation • Severe COPD/asthma
Circulatory	• Anesthesia induction • Pulmonary embolism • Hypovolemia • Hemorrhagic shock • Cardiogenic shock • Intracardiac shunt	• Release of tourniquet • Treatment of acidemia
Technical	• Equipment disconnection • Blocked/kink in tubing	• CO_2 absorber dysfunction • Monitor contamination

Table 59.XII.3 Capnography waveform interpretation and etiologies [1].

Waveform	Potential condition
• High $EtCO_2$ with normal respiratory rate	• Low minute volume with normal rate or rapidly rising body temperature
• High $EtCO_2$ with low rate	• Respiratory depression without compensation (e.g. neonatal encephaolpathy)
• Low $EtCO_2$ with normal rate	• Circulatory shock, low body temperature, high minute volume on ventilator, compensation of metabolic acidosis
• Low $EtCO_2$ with low rate	• Low body temperature, damage to central nervous system
• Low $EtCO_2$ with fast rate	• Pain, compensation of metabolic acidosis or hypoxia, severe shock, ventilator with high rate and minute volume
• Sudden decrease in $EtCO_2$ to 0	• Complete obstruction of airway or endotracheal tube, apnea, disconnection of ventilator ciruit
• Gradual decreasing $EtCO_2$ levels	• Hyperventilation (increased respiratory rate or tidal volume), decrease in metabolic rate or CO_2 production, fall in body temperature
• Sudden increase in $EtCO_2$	• Sudden increase in blood pressure (return of spontaneous circulation during CPR or administratin of vasopressor), injection of sodium bicaronate
• Elevation of baseline	• Rebreathing of expired air

tube placement, monitoring cardiac arrest, and monitoring sedation/anesthesia. Neonatal encephalopathy is a common neurologic disorder in foals with a portion of affected foals developing hypoventilation or periods of apnea, resulting in severe respiratory acidosis; these changes in respiratory pattern are presumably caused by loss of recognition of hypercapnia by the chemosensitive area in the respiratory center [4]. In a retrospective study involving 16 foals with hypercapnia secondary to neonatal encephalopathy, the mean P_aCO_2 ranged from 66 to 69 mmHg [5]. Arterial blood gas analysis is needed to evaluate foals with neonatal encephalopathy and hypoventilation. However, $EtCO_2$ is used as a surrogate for monitoring P_aCO_2 in infants and can also be used in foals for the same purpose by fashioning a modified nasal tube connected to a side-stream capnography and inserted into the naris of the foal [2, 4, 6]. One study noted strong and significant linear correlation between P_aCO_2 and $PEtCO_2$ in neonatal foals with the 95% limits of agreement of −9.9 to 10.1 mmHg [4].

Capnography can also be used to confirm endotracheal intubation in the neonatal foal and help distinguish between endotracheal and esophageal tube placement. With correct placement of the endotracheal tube, a normal capnogram waveform will be observed. Conversely, a flat capnogram suggests placement of the tube in the esophagus or, less commonly, obstruction in the endotracheal tube, prolonged cardiac arrest or complete airway obstruction distal to the tube [1].

Another use of capnography is to monitor the effectiveness of cardiopulmonary resuscitation (CPR). The level of $EtCO_2$ reflects cardiopulmonary blood flow with $EtCO_2$ measurements directly associated with chest compressions. Positive waveform tracing should be observed during effective chest compressions. In people, an $EtCO_2$ of >20 mmHg is targeted during CPR with levels <10 mmHg suggesting improved CPR technique or rotation of the individual performing compressions [1]. An abrupt increase in $EtCO_2$ is an early indicator of return of spontaneous circulation (ROSC) during CPR.

Capnography can also be used to monitor respiratory function during sedation or anesthesia of the neonatal foal. Capnography detects hypoventilation earlier than pulse oximetry and can also detect upper airway obstruction, laryngospasm, or bronchospasm [1]. Respiratory depression/hypoventilation will manifest as abnormally high $EtCO_2$.

References

1 Long, B., Koyfman, A., and Vivirito, M.A. (2017). Capnography in the emergency department: a review of uses, waveforms and limitations. *J. Emerg. Med.* 53: 829–842.

2 Nagler, J. and Krauss, B. (2008). Capnography: a valuable tool for airway management. *Emerg. Med. Clin. North Am.* 26: 881–897.

3 Anderson, C.T. and Breen, P.H. (2000). Carbon dioxide kinetics and capnography during critical care. *Crit. Care* 4: 207–215.

4 Wong, D.M., Alcott, C.J., and Wang, C. (2011). Agreement between arterial partial pressure of carbon dioxide and saturation of hemoglobin with oxygen values obtained by direct arterial blood measurements verses noninvasive methods in conscious healthy and ill foals. *J. Am. Vet. Med. Assoc.* 239: 1341–1347.

5 Giguere, S., Slade, J.K., and Sanchez, L.C. (2008). Retrospective comparison of caffeine and doxapram for the treatment of hypercapnia in foals with hypoxic-ischemic encephalopathy. *J. Vet. Intern. Med.* 22: 401–405.

6 Moses, J.M., Alexander, J.L., and Agus, M. (2009). The correlation and level of agreement between end-tidal and blood gas pCO_2 in children with respiratory distress: a retrospective analysis. *BMC Pediatr.* 9: 20.

Section XIII Neonatal Transfusion Therapy

Jamie Kopper

Plasma Transfusions

Indications

Primary indications for plasma transfusions in foals include of transfer of passive immunity (FTPI) due to decreased intake, absorption and/or increased consumption of immunoglobulins, and hypoalbuminemia contributing to decreased colloid oncotic pressure (COP). In some instances, hyperimmune plasma may be utilized with the intent to provide the foal with increased immunity to endemic infectious to on-farm agents (i.e. *Rhodoccus equi*).

Potential Beneficial Effects of Plasma

Plasma provides numerous potential benefits to critically ill neonatal foals, in addition to provision of immunoglobulins. Natural colloid solutions, particularly fresh frozen plasma, contain several components that benefit critically ill patients [1–4]. Albumin is the most abundant protein in plasma and is responsible for approximately 75% of COP [5]. In addition to the role albumin plays in maintaining COP, albumin also transports endogenous and exogenous compounds with low water solubility [6], contributes to the endothelial glycocalyx to maintain vascular barrier integrity [7], plays an important role in acid–base balance [8] and has anti-oxidant and anti-inflammatory properties [9]. Further, albumin can bind lipopolysaccharide and cytokines and, thereby, modulate inflammation [10, 11]. Plasma products may also provide clotting factors, anti-thrombin, protein C, and other endogenous anti-inflammatory compounds [9, 12]. All of these roles, in addition to assistance in improving and maintaining COP, may be beneficial to critically ill foals.

Equine Plasma Types

Equine plasma can be purchased from several commercial vendors as well as prepared in-house, as described by Wilson and colleagues [11]. Equine plasma is typically stored frozen; defrosting plasma should be performed gradually in a room temperature (22 °C) to slightly warm (37 °C) water bath as opposed to a warm water bath (57 °C) or microwave oven, as the later result in denaturation and loss of valuable immunoglobulins and clotting factors [13, 14].

Use of hyperoncotic colloids (i.e. 5% albumin) may be more practical and effective at improving COP, particularly in the face of ongoing losses [15]. The use of 5% equine albumin has been reported in adult horses with colic [16], however at this time does not appear to be commercially available. Lyophilized pooled canine albumin (Animal Blood Resources International, Dixon, CA) and pooled human albumin have been used in critically ill canine patients with beneficial effects including expansion of intravascular volume and increase in COP. Interestingly, naturally occurring antibodies against human albumin have been identified in dogs with no previous transfusion history although the rate of severe transfusion reactions is rare in critically ill dogs [17, 18]. At this time, the use of nonequine albumin products has only been reported in a small number of adult horses. In one case series, seven horses were treated with 25% human albumin; the total albumin of horses treated with human albumin was 3.2 ± 1.0 g/dl and 3.7 ± 0.9 g/dl, pre- and post-treatment, respectively, while the COP was 9.7 ± 2.3 mmHg and 16.6 ± 2.4 mmHg, pre- and post-treatment respectively. Furthermore, serum albumin was 1.5 ± 0.3 g/dl and 2.2 ± 0.3 g/dl, pre- and post-treatment. No changes were

Equine Neonatal Medicine, First Edition. Edited by David M. Wong and Pamela A. Wilkins.

noted in vital parameters during human albumin infusion but a wider safter study has not been conducted [19]. Hyperoncotic albumin-based products may be beneficial at improving COP and other albumin-specific roles but would not have a significant effect on immunoglobulin replacement or supplementation for foals with FTPI.

Plasma Transfusion Administration and Complications

Administration of any equine origin biologic product has the potential to result in one of several allergic reactions with clinical signs ranging from mild (i.e. fever, urticaria) to severe (i.e. anaphylaxis, death). Prior to initiating a plasma transfusion, the foal's pre-transfusion vital parameters (heart rate, respiratory rate, rectal temperature) and source of plasma (manufacturer and lot or donor horse) should be recorded. Plasma should initially be administered to the foal slowly with vital parameters monitored every 5 minutes. If the foal appears to be tolerating the transfusion well, the rate of administration is gradually increased with evaluation every 5 minutes. After 15–30 minutes, if the foal continues to maintain stable vital parameters, the remaining volume of plasma can be administered as a bolus, if indicated. However, particularly when being used to treat hypoalbuminemia and improve COP, administration of plasma as a continuous rate infusion (CRI, i.e. part of the maintenance fluid requirement) may be more efficacious at restoring and maintaining blood albumin levels [20]. If, at any point, the foal develops an increased rectal temperature, tachycardia, and/or tachypnea, the transfusion should be stopped and the foal carefully monitored. If clinical signs consistent with a transfusion reaction progress the foal can be administered a dose of non-steroidal anti-inflammatory medication, or short acting corticosteroid. In the rare event of severe anaphylaxis, epinephrine should be used. According to Wilson and colleagues [11], the development of clinical signs consistent with a plasma transfusion reaction was rare (<10%) in adult horses receiving in-hospital prepared plasma. Similar studies have not been reported, specifically in foals. See Table 59.XIII.1 for an example of plasma transfusion-recording sheet for neonates.

Administration of volumes of plasma >60 ml/kg per 24 hours should be avoided in otherwise euvolemic foals due to the risk of causing volume overload; if >60 ml/kg of colloid is required due to refractory FTPI, ongoing consumption of immunoglobulins or loss of albumin, administration should be divided among several days. Additionally, a study reported significant variations in the composition of commercial equine plasma with regards to electrolyte (sodium, chloride and potassium) and albumin composition [21]. Electrolyte values reported in this study ranged from sub to supraphysiologic values (i.e. sodium concentrations of 104–305 mEq/l). Although use of these products resulted in only minor transient changes in patient serum values, this study was performed in adult horses where the dose of product administered was

Table 59.XIII.1 Plasma transfusion monitoring worksheet.

Patient name:		Medical record number:		Date:
Patient weight:		Company, lot number:		
Clinician call parameters:				
Time (minutes)	**Temperature**	**Heart rate**	**Respiratory rate**	**Notes**
0				
5				
10				
15				
20				
25				
30				
Comments, notes:				
Emergency drug calculations:				
Drugs	**Dose**	**Concentration**	**mg (units) to be administered**	**Volume to be administered**
Epinephrine				
Dexamethasone				
Flunixin meglumine				

approximately 10 times less than that used in foals. Given this finding, when providing large volume plasma transfusions, monitoring of serum electrolytes may be warranted. Variations in pathogen specific IgG concentrations in commercial equine plasma have also been reported and may contribute to varied results when using these products for disease prevention [22].

Red Blood Cell Transfusions

Indications

Red blood cell (RBC) transfusions (whole blood or packed red blood cells [pRBCs]) are options for foals with significant anemia resulting in impaired oxygen delivery [23]. Clinical signs or hematological parameters consistent with impaired oxygen delivery are provided in Table 59.XIII.2. Using an absolute packed cell volume (PCV) to trigger a transfusion can be misleading, due to delayed reduction of the PCV in cases of whole blood loss; however, a foal with a PCV of <15% likely will need a blood transfusion to support adequate oxygen exchange. Other indicators that the patient may require a blood transfusion include tachycardia, tachypnea, increased systemic lactate concentration, increased oxygen extraction ratio, and lethargy. Table 59.XIII.2 provides general guidelines for clinical indicators in foals that a blood transfusion may be warranted. The goal, when providing a blood transfusion, is not necessarily to return the PCV to normal but rather to improve/normalize oxygen carrying and delivery capacity. If the anemia is severe enough to result in impaired oxygen delivery (DO_2), the oxygen extraction ratio (O_2ER) will increase [24, 25]. The oxygen extraction ratio (below) is calculated using information from arterial and mixed venous blood samples.

Table 59.XIII.2 Clinical signs and treatment guidelines for foals with anemia.

	Consider transfusion	Continue to monitor
Attitude	Dull, lethargic	Alert, interactive, nursing
Heart rate (beats per minute)	>120	<120
Respiratory rate (breaths per minute)	>32	<32
Source anemia	Uncontrolled	Controlled
Systemic lactate (mmol/l)	>2	<2
O_2 extraction ratio	>40%	<40%

Oxygen Delivery DO_2

$$DO_2 = CO \times \left(1.39 \times \left[Hb\right] \times SaO_2 + \left(0.003 \times PaO_2\right)\right) \quad (59.XIII.1)$$

DO_2 = Rate of oxygen delivery (ml per minute)
CO = Cardiac output (l per minute)
1.39 = Oxygen binding capacity of hemoglobin
Hb = Hemoglobin concentration (grams per liter)
SaO_2 = Hemoglobin oxygen saturation expressed as a fraction
$0.003 + PaO_2$ = Amount of dissolved oxygen in blood
PaO_2 = Oxygen pressure in arterial blood

Oxygen Consumption VO_2

$$VO_2 = CO \times \left(CaO_2 - CvO_2\right) \quad (59.XIII.2)$$

CaO_2 = arterial oxygen content = $(1.34 \times [Hb] \times SaO_2/100) + (0.0031 \times PaO_2)$
CvO_2 = mixed venous oxygen content = $(1.34 \times [Hb] \times SvO_2/100) + (0.0031 \times PvO_2)$

Oxygen Extraction Ratio O_2ER

$$O_2ER = VO_2 / DO_2 \text{ or } SaO_2 - SvO_2 / SaO_2 \quad (59.XIII.3)$$

The three most common overarching causes of significant anemia include (i) destruction of RBCs; (ii) loss of whole blood (i.e. hemorrhage); and (iii) failure to produce RBCs, with destruction of RBCs due to neonatal isoerthrolysis (NI) being the most common cause in neonates. Foals with NI can suffer a precipitous drop in PCV due to translocation of the mare's anti-RBC antibodies in colostrum consumed by the foal which target the foal's red blood cell antigens resulting in mass destruction.

Types of Blood Transfusions

Depending on the source of anemia (i.e. loss of whole blood versus hemolysis), administration of whole blood transfusions versus pRBCs may be considered. Whole blood transfusions are specifically indicated in animals with anemia and hypovolemia (i.e. blood loss) and have the potential benefit of also providing plasma, which contains additional beneficial components, whereas pRBCs supply a concentrated collection of RBCs without plasma. pRBCs are desirable in patients with hemolysis due to the ability to provide a larger number or RBCs, which improves PCV and oxygen carrying capacity, without risking volume overload. However, whole blood transfusions tend to be more common in equine medicine due to limited availability of the specialized equipment necessary to create aliquots of pRBCs. For foals with NI, the ideal transfusion substrate would be washed RBCs from the mare, but this is time consuming and requires specialized equipment, which may not be available or practical at every hospital.

Donor Selection and Crossmatching

Horses are recognized to have eight blood groups (A, C, D, K, P, Q, U, and T) and greater than 30 RBC antigens, which results in over 400,000 possible antigenic combinations [23, 26]. Given this, it is unlikely that a horse would receive a truly "type specific" blood transfusion. However, careful selection of donors and ideally performing major and minor crossmatching can significantly reduce or eliminate the probability of a clinically significant transfusion reaction.

Ideally, a typed donor horse would be used to ensure compatibility between donors and recipients prior to blood transfusions. Unfortunately, equine blood typing is limited to a few laboratories and is time consuming [27]. However, in the absence of horses with known blood types, a healthy gelding of the same breed should be used with a PCV >35% and free of known disease. In foals with NI, blood from the mare should not be administered to the foal unless it has first been washed free of alloantibodies.

Prior to performing a blood transfusion, a major crossmatch (and potentially minor) is recommended. In theory, animals should be able to receive one "free" blood transfusion because the majority of horses do not carry antibodies against other blood types unless they have been previously exposed to blood products [24]; sensitization typically occurs after the first exposure. However, many neonates receiving blood transfusions are suffering from NI, meaning that they in fact do carry anti-RBC antibodies acquired via ingestion of colostrum.

Major crossmatching evaluates the recipient's serum versus the donor's RBCs to ensure that the recipient does not possess antibodies targeted against the donor's RBCs that would result in hemolysis or agglutination. This test evaluates for the most severe and common blood transfusion reactions. Minor crossmatching evaluates the donor's serum, with the recipient's RBCs for hemolysis or agglutination. However, dilution of donor serum during transfusion makes it unlikely that a clinically significant transfusion reaction would occur.

Several methods exist for performing major crossmatching in horses. Traditionally, donor-recipient crossmatch procedures are available as a benchtop assay[27]; unfortunately, this method is relatively time consuming and requires training and expertise. Recently, several studies have evaluated the use of point-of-care methods including a gel column crossmatch [28, 29] and a Ca blood typing immunochormatographic strip [29]. Both studies found that the gel column methods for crossmatching were simple with varying accuracy – most discrepancies being low-grade agglutination, which may be of limited clinical significance. In adult horses, use of crossmatched blood has been demonstrated to significantly prolong the half-life of red blood cells in the recipient compared to use of non-crossmatched blood (~5 vs ~33 days) [30].

Collection and Administration of Red Blood Cell Transfusions

Several equations (Eqs. 59.XIII.4 or 59.XIII.5) aid in determining the volume of blood necessary to achieve a significant increase in PCV (and thus O_2 carrying capacity). An adult horse can safely donate up to 20% of its blood volume for transfusion, which is equivalent to approximately 16 ml/kg of lean body weight (Eq. 59.XIII.6). To collect blood, the donor should be restrained and an IV catheter placed in a jugular vein. Blood can be collected, via the IV catheter into commercially available blood collection kits, or by collecting blood into a sterile IV fluid bag with anticoagulant (ACD, CPD-A1 or 3.8% citrate) at a rate of 1 ml of anticoagulant per 9 ml of blood (i.e. 1 : 10 dilution).

$$\text{Volume}(\text{ml})\text{of} = 2\times(\%\ \text{desired increase in PCV}) \times \text{Bwt}(\text{kg})\ \text{blood needed} \tag{59.XIII.4}$$

Case example: A 50 kg foal with a PCV of 10%, which you desire to increase to 20%.

Volume of blood needed = 2×(10%)×50 kg = 1000 ml of blood needed.

$$\text{Volume of blood needed}(\text{l}) = \text{VDB}\times\text{BW}(\text{kg}) \times \frac{\text{Desired PCV}(\%) - \text{Recipient PCV}(\%)}{\text{Donor PCV}(\%)} \tag{59.XIII.5}$$

VDB = volume of distribution of blood (l/kg); typically assumed to be 8%.

Case example: A 50 kg foal with PCV of 10%, which you desire to increase to 20% and the donor PCV is 35%.

$$\text{Volume of blood needed} = 0.08\times 50\,\text{kg}\times\frac{20\% - 10\%}{35\%} = 1.11\ \text{of blood needed}$$

$$\text{Volume of blood to safely donate} = 16\,\text{ml}\times\text{Bwt}(\text{kg}) \tag{59.XIII.6}$$

Case example: For a 500 kg horse

Volume of blood to donate = 16×500 = 8000 ml, or 8 l.

If necessary, collected blood can be stored at 4 °C for up to several weeks [31]. However, storage without leukoreduction results in metabolic waste product accumulation, leading to a decrease in pH of the transfusion, accumulation of inflammatory cytokines, increase in free iron and changes in RBC membranes that result in hypercoagulability [31]. In humans and small animals, use of blood >2 weeks of storage is discouraged due to the accumulation of proinflammatory cytokines.

pRBCs (and platelet-rich plasma, see below) can be made via gravity sedimentation due to the high erythrocyte sedimentation rate of equine blood, or via centrifugation [32]. Using gravity sedimentation, blood is collected as described above, and subsequently the plasma is allowed to separate and is removed. When centrifugation is available, blood is collected and centrifuged by one of several protocols: 40 × g for 15 minutes [33], 250 × g for 3 minutes [34], or 1000 × g for 4 minutes [35]. The plasma is then gently pressed into a second collection bag.

Whole blood should be administered using a filter administration set. Similar to administering a plasma transfusion, an initial physical examination should be performed and recorded prior to initiating the transfusion and then repeated every 5 minutes. Throughout the transfusion the patient should be carefully monitored for evidence of a transfusion reaction including increase in rectal temperature, tachycardia, tachypnea, urticaria, and pruritus. The rate at which the transfusion is administered may be gradually increased every 5 minutes, and if the patient's exam parameters have remained unchanged at 30 minutes, the transfusion may be administered as rapidly as dictated by the patient's needs. Similar to plasma administration, total volumes of >60 ml/kg/d should be avoided due to risk for volume overload. If the patient requires a second transfusion 2 weeks or later after the first, crossmatching is strongly recommended as adequate time has passed for the foal to have become sensitized and produced antibodies against the initial transfusion blood type.

Common complications or reactions associated with blood product transfusions include immunologic reactions (febrile nonhemolytic transfusion reactions, urticaria, hemolytic reactions, immune suppression, and thrombocytopenia) and nonimmunologic reactions (disease transmission, citrate toxicity leading to hypocalcemia and circulatory overload). Febrile nonhemolytic reactions, the most commonly reported transfusion reactions, are associated with white blood cells in the transfused blood product. Unfortunately, prophylactic treatment with steroids or antihistamines is not advantageous as histamine release is not a component of febrile nonhemolytic transfusion reactions.

Massive transfusions (i.e. transfusion of a volume of whole blood that is greater than the patient's blood volume), replacement of half of the patient's blood volume in 3–4 hours, or administration of blood at a rate of ≥1.5 ml/kg/min over 20 minutes, are associated with several notable concerns, including electrolyte disturbances (specifically hypocalcemia, hypomagnesemia, and hyperkalemia), hemostatic defects, hypothermia, metabolic acidosis, immunosuppression, delayed wound healing, and acute lung injury. Patient's receiving massive transfusions should be monitored carefully for these potential complications.

Platelet Transfusions

In rare cases, foals with immune mediated thrombocytopenia may benefit from platelet transfusions. Platelet transfusions are not typically recommended unless platelet counts are <10,000–20,000/μl. If a patient has a concurrent need for whole blood and platelets, care should be taken with blood collection to preserve platelet function including avoiding the use of collection of administration equipment containing latex or glass bottle collection devices, as both will result in premature activation of platelets. Platelets can be collected and prepared from whole blood [32] as described above or via platelet apheresis [36]. Given the small size of platelets, relative to the size of red blood cells, freshly harvested plasma via gravity sedimentation contains the vast majority of blood platelets and can be used as a platelet transfusion [32, 37]. Storage of blood products at <15 °C results in irreversible changes in platelet function and should be avoided if administration of platelets is a goal of transfusion [37].

In summary, there are numerous instances in which critically ill foals may benefit from plasma or red blood cell transfusions. Care should be taken to choose the most appropriate product for each patient, based on clinical goals and patient needs and to reduce the risk of transfusion related reactions.

References

1 Dolente, B.A., Wilkins, P.A., and Boston, R.C. (2002). Clinicopathologic evidence of disseminated intravascular coagulation in horses with acute colitis. *J. Am. Vet. Med. Assoc.* 220: 1034–1038.

2 Collatos, C., Barton, M.H., Prasse, K.W., and Moore, J.N. (1995). Intravascular and peritoneal coagulation and fibrinolysis in horses with acute gastrointestinal tract diseases. *J. Am. Vet. Med. Assoc.* 207: 465–470.

3 Welch, R.D., Watkins, J.P., Taylor, T.S. et al. (1992). Disseminated intravascular coagulation associated with colic in 23 horses (1984–1989). *J. Vet. Intern. Med.* 6: 29–35.

4 Monreal, L., Angles, A., Espada, Y. et al. (2000). Hypercoagulation and hypofibrinolysis in horses with colic and DIC. *Equine Vet. J. Suppl.* 32: 19–25.

5 Artigas, A., Wernerman, J., Arroyo, V. et al. (2016). Role of albumin in diseases associated with severe systemic inflammation: pathophysiologic and clinical evidence in sepsis and in decompensated cirrhosis. *J. Crit. Care* 33: 62–70.

6 Vincent, J.L. (2009). Relevance of albumin in modern critical care medicine. *Best Pract. Res. Clin. Anaesthesiol.* 23: 183–191.

7 Fleck, A., Raines, G., Hawker, F. et al. (1985). Increased vascular permeability: a major cause of hypoalbuminaemia in disease and injury. *Lancet* 1: 781–784.

8 Reeves, R.B. (1976). Temperature-induced changes in blood acid-base status: Donnan rCl and red cell volume. *J. Appl. Physiol.* 40: 762–767.

9 Quinlan, G.J., Margarson, M.P., Mumby, S. et al. (1998). Administration of albumin to patients with sepsis syndrome: a possible beneficial role in plasma thiol repletion. *Clin. Sci.* 95: 459–465.

10 Jurgens, G., Muller, M., Garidel, P. et al. (2002). Investigation into the interaction of recombinant human serum albumin with Re-lipopolysaccharide and lipid A. *J. Endotoxin Res.* 8: 115–126.

11 King, T.P. (1961). On the sulfhydryl group of human plasma albumin. *J. Biol. Chem.* 236: Pc5.

12 Wilson, E.M., Holcombe, S.J., Lamar, A. et al. (2009). Incidence of transfusion reactions and retention of procoagulant and anticoagulant factor activities in equine plasma. *J. Vet. Intern. Med.* 23: 323–328.

13 O'Rielly, J.L. (1993). A comparison of the reduction in immunoglobulin (IgG) concentration of frozen equine plasma treated by three thawing techniques. *Aust. Vet. J.* 70: 442–444.

14 Isaacs, M.S., Scheuermaier, K.D., Levy, B.L. et al. (2004). In vitro effects of thawing fresh-frozen plasma at various temperatures. *Clin. Appl. Thromb. Hemost.* 10: 143–148.

15 Liu, D.T. and Silverstein, D.C. (2015). Chapter 58: crystalloids, colloids and hemoglobin-based oxygen carrying solutions. In: *Small Animal Critical Care Medicine*, 2e, 311–315. St. Louis, MO, USA: Elsevier.

16 Belli, C.G., Tavor, J.P.F., Ferreira, R.A. et al. (2013). Evaluation of equine albumin solution in fluid therapy of horses with colic. *J. Equine Vet. Sci.* 33: 509–514.

17 Martin, L.G., Luther, T.Y., Alperin, D.C. et al. (2008). Serum antibodies against human albumin in critically ill and healthy dogs. *J. Am. Vet. Med. Assoc.* 232: 1004–1009.

18 Mathews, K.A. and Barry, M. (2005). The use of 25% human serum albumin: outcome and efficacy in raising serum albumin and systemic blood pressure in critically ill dogs and cats. *J. Vet. Emerg. Crit. Care* 15: 110.

19 DeWitt, S.F. and Paradis, M.R. (2004). Use of human albumin as a colloidal therapy in the hypoproteinemic equine. *J. Vet. Intern. Med.* 18: 394.

20 Greissman, A., Silver, P., Minkoff, L., and Sagy, M. (1996). Albumin bolus administration versus continuous infusion in critically ill hypoalbuminemic pediatric patients. *Intensive Care Med.* 22: 495–499.

21 McKenzie, E.C., Johns, J., and Busby, M. (2019). Biochemical characteristics of a commercial plasma product and response to transfusion of clinically diseased horses. *J. Vet. Intern. Med.* 33: 2375–2547.

22 Sanz, M.G., Oliveira, A.F., Page, A. et al. (2014). Administration of commercial Rhodococcus equi specific hyperimmune plasma results in variable amounts of IgG against pathogenic bacteria in foals. *Vet. Rec.* 175: 485–485.

23 Sandberg, K. (July 1996). *Guidelines for the Interpretation of Blood Typing Tests in Horses*. Brisbane, Australia: International Society for Animal Genetics.

24 Weiss, S.L., Peters, M.J., Alhazzani, W. et al. (2020). Surviving sepsis campaign international guidelines for the management of septic shock and sepsis associated organ dysfunction in children. *Pediatr. Crit. Care Med.* 21: e52–e106.

25 Rhodes, A., Evans, L.E., Alhazzani, W. et al. (2017). Surviving sepsis campaign: international guidelines for Management of Sepsis and Septic Shock: 2016. *Crit. Care Med.* 45: 486–552.

26 Bowling, A. (2000). Red blood cell antigens and blood groups in the horse. In: *Schalm's Veterinary Hematology* (ed. B. Feldman, J. ZInkl, and N. Jan), 774–777. Baltimore, MD: Lippincott, Williams & Wilkins.

27 Weiss, D.J. and Wardrop, K.J. (2000). Clinical blood typing and crossmatching. In: *Schlam's Veterinary Hematology* (ed. B. Feldman, J. Zinkl, and N. Jain), 1101–1105. Baltimore, MD: Lippincott, Williams & Wilkins.

28 Casenave, P., Leclere, M., Beauchamp, G. et al. (2019). Modified stall-side crossmatch for transfusions in horses. *J. Vet. Intern. Med.* 33: 1775–1783.

29 Luethy, D., Owens, S.D., Stefanovski, D. et al. (2016). Comparison of tube, gel and immunochromatographic strip methods for evaluation of blood transfusion compatibility in horses. *J. Vet. Intern. Med.* 30: 1864–1871.

30 Tomlinson, J.E., Taberner, E., Boston, R.C. et al. (2015). Survival time of cross-match incompatible red blood cells in adult horses. *J. Vet. Intern. Med.* 29: 1683–1688.

31 Mudge, M.C., Macdonald, M.H., Owens, S.D. et al. (2004). Comparison of 4 blood storage methods in a protocol for equine pre-operative autologous donation. *Vet. Surg.* 33: 475–486.

32 Sprayberry, K.A. (2003). Neonatal transfusion medicine: the use of blood, plasma, oxygen-carrying solutions and

adjunctive therapies in foals. *Clin. Tech. Equine Pract.* 2: 31–41.

33 Ramirez, S., Gaunt, S.D., McClure, J.J. et al. (1999). Detection and effects on platelet function of anti-platelet antibody in mule foals with experimentally induced neonatal alloimmune thrombocytopenia. *J. Vet. Intern. Med.* 13: 534–539.

34 Ketcham, E.M. and Cairns, C.B. (1999). Hemoglobin-based oxygen carriers: development and clinical potential. *Ann. Emerg. Med.* 33: 326–337.

35 Buechner-Maxwell, V., Scott, M.A., Godber, L. et al. (1997). Neonatal alloimmune thrombocytopenia in a Quarter Horse foal. *J. Vet. Intern. Med.* 11: 304–308.

36 Dunkel, B. (2013). Platelet transfusion in thrombocytopenic horses. *Equine Vet. Educ.* 25: 359–362.

37 Ohto, H. and Nollet, K.E. (2011). Overview on platelet preservation: better controls over storage lesion. *Transfus. Apheresis Sci.* 44: 321–325.

Section XIV Umbilical Care

Bonny Millar

The neonate's umbilical cord should be allowed to break naturally, right after the birth of the foal, at the end of the second stage of labor. This initiates a recoil response, where the urachus and umbilical vessels are stimulated to retract internally and seal naturally. The cord breaks at its narrowest point, approximately 5 cm from the body wall, thus leaving a short protruding stump. Following an assisted delivery or cesarean, the cord will be clamped and ligated by the veterinary team. In the immediate postnatal period neonates should have their umbilicus examined and treated with a skin disinfectant to aid desiccation and prevent infection (Figure 59.XIV.1). Chlorhexidine gluconate is a recommended skin disinfectant as it is effective at reducing bacterial colonization and has a desirable residual effect (Table 59.XIV.1). The umbilicus is recognized as a primary portal for the introduction of pathogens. Appropriate umbilical care can lessen the likelihood of bacterial omphalitis occurring.

Complications

The use of harsh disinfectants or other caustic agents, e.g. highly concentrated tincture of iodine, should be avoided as they can encourage tissue necrosis of the ventral abdominal skin thus increasing the possibility of infection and a persistent patent urachus.

Equine Neonatal Medicine, First Edition. Edited by David M. Wong and Pamela A. Wilkins.

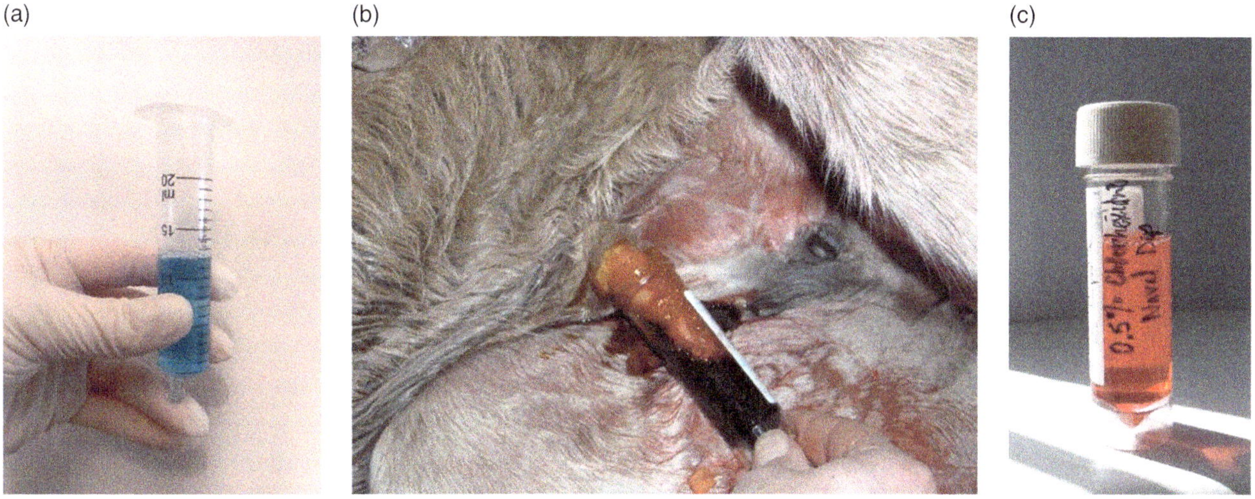

Figure 59.XIV.1 (a) Disinfectant placed in a 20 ml Syringe barrel. (b) Placement of disinfectant against the external umbilicus. (c) Disinfectant ready for applying from a narrow necked container.

Table 59.XIV.1 General principles for treatment of the neonatal umbilicus.

Equipment needed for umbilical care

- Exam gloves.
- Sterile specimen cup, preferably with a narrow opening or a 20/30 ml syringe barrel.
- Chlorhexidine gluconate solution[a] – dilute to make a 0.5% solution. (Calculating the dilutions will vary depending on the concentration of the original chlorhexidine preparation.)
- In the absence of the recommended chlorhexidine solution, a 1% povidone iodine solution may be substituted.
- Gauze swabs.

Procedure for treating the umbilicus

- With clean gloved hands, examine the umbilicus for heat, pain, swelling, and/or purulent discharge. Also important to note is the presence of wet hair surrounding the urachus or dripping urine. Either will indicate a patent urachus. Observations of the umbilicus must be carried out prior to each treatment with disinfectant.
- Fill the sterile specimen cup or syringe barrel about half full with dilute 0.5% chlorhexidine solution. It is important to avoid using chlorhexidine scrub as it contains a detergent that can cause chemical irritation. Using a narrow-necked specimen cup prevents the solution from coming in contact with large areas of the surrounding skin.
- With the foal restrained while standing or in lateral recumbency, advance the cup over the umbilicus, up close to the abdominal wall. Keep in place for a couple seconds, ensuring the solution saturates the umbilicus.
- Remove the cup and with the swabs wipe up any excess solution that spills onto the abdomen or legs. Soaking up excess moisture will prevent maceration and irritation of the surrounding skin.
- Alternatively, the umbilicus can be painted with the solution, thus providing targeted application.
- Either method may not be easy in the standing foal as they often react with a kick in protest.
- Repeat every 6 h until the umbilicus shrinks and dries up. In the healthy neonate, treatment rarely needs to continue past the first couple days postpartum. If there is evidence of a persistent patent urachus, then further investigations are warranted.

[a] Nolvason® 2% solution, Zoetis Inc., Kalamazoo, MI 49007. In the absence of the recommended chlorhexidine solution, a 1% povidone iodine solution may be substituted.

Section XV Point-of-Care Monitors in Neonatal Medicine

David Wong

Biomarkers are specific blood analytes that are used to monitor normal or disease processes in foals. These biomarkers help identify phases of diseases, monitor illness severity, evaluate response to therapy, and aid in predicting prognosis [1]. Point-of-care (POC) devices refer to benchtop diagnostic modalities that have been translated into portable, easy-to-use formats that allow measurement of a variety of blood analytes [2]. These small, typically handheld devices have a lower initial and maintenance expense compared with benchtop equipment and are intended to be performed patient-side, but quality control remains a concern with POC devices. Despite this, POC devices provide a rapid measurement of common blood analytes used to evaluate critically ill foals, thereby providing near immediate appraisal of blood parameters using a small sample volume from the patient.

Types of POC Monitors

The purpose of this section is to discuss types of POC monitors available for the diagnostic evaluation and treatment of neonatal foals with the goal of improving clinical or economic outcome; these include glucose, L-lactate, serum amyloid A (SAA), blood gas analysis, creatinine, and cardiac troponin.

Glucose Monitors

Glucose is possibly the most commonly assessed POC analyte measured in neonatal foals because of the vital role that glucose plays as an energy source for the body and the fact that the critically ill neonatal foal's blood glucose is frequently deranged due to low glycogen stores, decreased and absent nursing behavior, and elevated metabolic rate noted in disease states such as sepsis [3]. Critically ill neonatal foals may present with varying severities of hypo- or hyperglycemia, although some may maintain a normal blood glucose concentration despite being quite ill [3, 4]. In addition, glucose monitoring is needed in the critical care setting because many foals are administered drugs that alter glucose homeostasis (corticosteroids, insulin) or are receiving dextrose infusions or parenteral nutrition.

A number of POC glucometers have proved sufficiently accurate in neonatal foals including the Accu-Check Aviva and Alpha TRAK glucometers [3, 4]. These devices use enzymatic indirect approaches to measure blood glucose, but results can be affected by environmental (oxygen tension, electrochemical currents) and patient factors (azotemia, severe polycythemia) [5]. Another important variable that impacts the accuracy of the measurement is the fact that most benchtop analyzers use plasma or serum, rather than whole blood, to measure glucose; therefore, most POC devices use conversion algorithms to report plasma values despite being measured from whole blood [5].

In people, glucose equilibrates relatively equally between erythrocytes and plasma with a correction multiplier used to convert whole blood measurement to reported plasma value of 1.11 [5]. In contrast, in the neonatal foal, glucose is largely present in plasma (approximately 82 mg/dl) with less measurable glucose in erythrocytes (15 mg/dl) [6]. Because of this, many glucometers designed for people have poor correlation with biochemistry analyzers when using whole blood from horses, with more accurate results obtained when using plasma samples [3]. The Alpha TRAK veterinary glucometer accounts for the larger proportion of glucose in the plasma of veterinary species and in a study of healthy and ill adult horses and foals, glucose concentration measured in equine whole blood correlated well to a biochemistry analyzer that used plasma samples [4]. Because of the numerous glucometers commercially available, each ICU should evaluate its glucometry method by periodically comparing results to gold standard devices to ensure glucose results of POC devices are within an acceptable target range of the gold standard [5].

Equine Neonatal Medicine, First Edition. Edited by David M. Wong and Pamela A. Wilkins.

Continuous Glucose Monitoring Systems

Continuous glucose-monitoring systems (CGMS) are newer POC devices initially designed to monitor interstitial glucose concentrations in diabetic people, but have also been used in the critical care setting in people, companion animals, foals, and adult horses [7–13]. These devices use a small sensor to measure blood glucose concentrations within the interstitial space of the subcutaneous tissue via a reaction of glucose with the enzyme glucose oxidase (Figure 59.XV.1) [14]. This reaction converts glucose into gluconic acid and hydrogen peroxide and generates an electric signal proportional to the glucose concentration, which is then converted to a standard unit of measure (mg/dl); this signal is then transmitted via Bluetooth technology to a remote device reader [14]. Benefits of CGMS are the ability of these devices to measure and monitor patient glucose without entering the stall, elimination of frequent blood collections, and facilitation of continuous glucose monitoring, which aids in the detection of hypo- or hyperglycemic periods. Once set, the sensors can provide continuous glucose measurements for up to 10 days (Figure 59.XV.2). After calibration, CGMS allow user-selected high and low glucose values to be set; if the blood glucose value goes above or below these preset values, the device reader will set of an audible alarm. In one study, glucose concentrations were measured via a glucometer (AlphaTrak) and CGMS (Dexcom G6) and compared to a chemistry analyzer (gold standard) in healthy and ill neonatal foals; the CGMS was significantly correlated with ($r = 0.72$), and had a mean bias of 3.49 mg/dl, when compared with the chemistry analyzer [12]. In that study, the glucometer had a larger mean bias (22.73 mg/dl) and tended to overestimate blood glucose when compared to the chemistry analyzer [12]. The CGMS provided meaningful and immediate continuous glucose measurements in neonatal foals over a 5-day period and eliminated the need for repeated restraint for blood collection. This could translate clinically into continuous blood glucose information available in ill foals along with lower diagnostic test costs and decreased nursing demands in the ICU setting.

L-Lactate

L-lactate is routinely measured from blood samples in critically ill foals, but can also be measured from peritoneal, thoracic, or synovial fluid [15]. Hyperlactatemia is most

(a) (b)

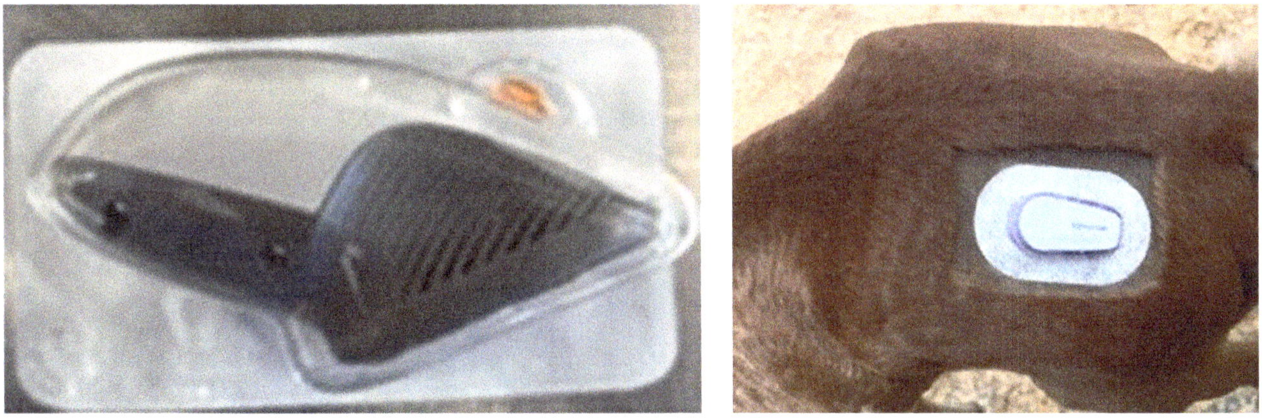

Figure 59.XV.1 (a) Continuous glucose monitoring system (Dexcom) prior to application. (b) Placement of the sensor and transmitter onto the dorsal aspect of the croup in a foal.

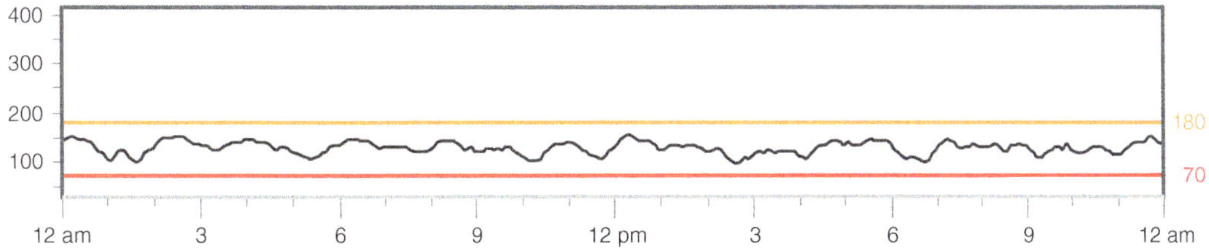

Figure 59.XV.2 Continuous glucose measurements (mg/dl) from a neonatal foal with pneumonia over a 24-hour time period (black line) using the Dexcom G6 CGMS. The yellow and red lines indicate preset glucose concentrations to which an alarm would sound if the foal were to become hyper- or hypoglycemic, respectively.

commonly attributed to abnormal or inadequate tissue perfusion and oxygen delivery, but other causes include mitochondrial dysfunction or decreased L-lactate clearance. Whole blood samples should be measured within 30 minutes of collection as L-lactate concentrations can increase with storage [16]. Elevated peritoneal fluid L-lactate concentrations are attributed to intestinal ischemia in horses and septic bacterial infections of closed cavities (abdomen, thorax) or joint fluid coupled with decreased glucose concentrations in the same fluid sample may help distinguish if a septic or nonseptic effusion is present [1].

Several POC devices are commercially available and measure L-lactate by placing a drop of sample fluid on a reagent pad; plasma is separated from erythrocytes within the test strip and L-lactate determined by reflectance photometry using an enzyme-mediated colorimetric reaction. Available devices include the Accutrend (formerly called Accusport; Roche Diagnostics, Mannheim, Germany), Lactate Pro (Arkray Global, Kyoto, Japan), Lactate Scout (SensLab GmbH, Leipzig, Germany), Lactate Plus (Nova Biomedical, Waltham, Massachusetts), and i-STAT (Abaxis, location). Details of these POC devices are detailed in Table 59.XV.1 [1, 15–24].

Immunoglobulin G

Immunoglobulin G (IgG) is another frequently evaluated parameter in which POC devices are used to evaluate neonatal foals. The single radial immunodiffusion (RID) is considered the most accurate method to quantify IgG, but testing requires performance in a laboratory, with results available 18–24 hours after receipt. Even if testing is done in-house, the duration of time needed to run the test is considered prolonged and can pose a serious delay in the treatment of foals with failure of transfer of passive immunity (FTPI). To expedite measurement of IgG, several stall-side diagnostic tests have been developed for use in foals. More commonly used tests include the enzyme immunoassay (SNAP Foal IgG test, IDEXX, Westbrook, Maine) and turbidimetric immunoassay (ARS Foal IgG, Animal Reproduction Systems, Ontario, CA) test, but older tests such as the glutaraldehyde coagulation test (GammaCheck-E, Plasvacc USA Inc., Templeton, CA), zinc sulfate turbidity test (Equi-Z Equine PFT Test Kit, WMRD Inc., Pullman, WA), and latex agglutination test (foal check, Centaur Animal Health, Olathe, KS) are also available. The SNAP test is perhaps the most commonly used semiquantitative enzyme immunoassay that provides quick, reliable, stall-side results in foals. In one study, the sensitivity of the SNAP test for detecting IgG concentrations ≤400 and ≤800 mg/dl was 90% and 95%, respectively, whereas the specificity was 79% and 52%, respectively [25]. This study implies that few foals with failure of transfer of passive immunity (FTPI) remain undetected, but the low specificity results in many foals with adequate transfer of passive immunity being diagnosed with FTPI [25, 26]. The immunoturbidimetric assay is an alternative method for measurement of serum/plasma IgG concentrations in which an antibody is directed at, and binds to, IgG and forms a complex that consequently causes a change in the turbidity of the sample. The change in turbidity reduces the amount of light transmitted through the sample, which in turn is measured via spectrophotometry and provides a measure of the analyte [27]. In one study, a POC turbidimetric assay (Rapid DVM test II, MAI Animal Health, Melksham, Wiltshire, UK) demonstrated fair to good agreement with the RID and had better sensitivity and specificity than the SNAP test [28, 29]. A full review of FTPI and testing methods is located in Chapter 47.

Table 59.XV.1 Various lactometers used in horses.

Lactometer	Characteristics
Accutrend	• Close agreement with NOVA benchtop blood gas analyzer (plasma samples); whole blood samples are less reliable [17]. • Underestimated blood lactate concentration when concentrations >10 mmol/l. [18–21]
Lactate Pro	• Linear relationship with radiometer benchtop analyzer (correlation r = 0.90) over range of lactate concentrations (1.0–18.6 mmol/l) [22, 23].
Lactate Scout	• High intra-analyzer variability at medium blood lactate concentrations [23].
Lactate Plus	• Good correlation ($r = 0.978$) with chromogenic benchtop analyzer; underestimated blood lactate concentration by 0.39 mmol/l [24].
i-Stat	• Measures blood lactate as a panel with other analytes; significant bias between i-STAT and automated analyzer [15].

Serum Amyloid A (SAA)

SAA is a small apoprotein and an acute phase protein. The acute phase response is a physiologic response to inflammation, infection, trauma or neoplasia and is a component of the innate immune system [1]. Activated tissue macrophages, blood monocytes and dendritic cells at the site of tissue damage release cytokines that are responsible for inducing hepatocellular production of acute phase proteins such as fibrinogen, C-reactive protein, haptoglobin, α-1 antitrypsin, complement components, coagulation proteins and SAA, among others [1]. SAA is degraded by the liver with a half-life of 30 minutes to 2 hours and has been studied in horses as a marker of inflammation as it has a low basal concentration in health, short half-life, and demonstrates an acute and pronounced increase in blood concentrations during acute phase responses (peaks 24–48 hours after stimulation) [30–32]. Serum concentrations of SAA in Thoroughbred foals 1–3 days of age was 27.1 mg/l (95th percentile; range 0–99 mg/l) using an immunoturbidimetric method [32]. In that study, elevations in SAA were noted in foals suffering from sepsis (279.9 mg/l) and focal infection (195 mg/l) with the authors suggesting SAA concentrations >100 mg/l are likely to be from infectious challenge [32]. In another study, SAA was significantly higher in eight foals with bacterial infections (mean 65 mg/l) compared to foals with nonbacterial disease processes (mean 1.6 mg/l) [33].

SAA can be measured by a variety of methods (single RID, ELISA, slide reversed passive agglutination, electroimmunoassay, immunoturbidometry) [30, 32, 34], but the commercially available POC analyzer (StableLab SAA, Zoetis, Parsippany, NJ) uses a proprietary lateral flow membrane-based immunoassay using either blood or serum, although the manufacturer reports serum provides more accurate results [1]. The POC analyzer provides values between 0 and 3000 μg/ml and demonstrated acceptable accuracy and precision for clinical diagnostic purposes in equine serum/plasma samples with SAA concentrations up to at least 1000 μg/ml [35, 36]. In one study, the POC analyzer had consistent negative bias (lower readings) when compared to an automated analyzer at SAA concentrations >500 ng/l [36].

Blood Gas Analysis

Blood gas analysis can provide valuable clinical information in regard to respiratory function, acid–base status (partial pressure of oxygen [PO_2] and carbon dioxide [PCO_2], saturation of hemoglobin [SO_2], pH, bicarbonate) and blood electrolytes concentrations (potassium, sodium, chloride, ionized calcium). Some POC devices also have the ability to measure creatinine and cardiac troponin. A number of POC analyzers are available including the IRMA Trupoint Blood Analysis System (LifeHealth, Roseville, MN) and i-STAT (Abbot Laboratories, Princeton, NJ). Other POC blood gas analyzers include the Element POC (Heska, Loveland, CO), EPOC (Siemens Medical, Malvern, PA), VetStat analyzer (IDEXX Laboratories, Westbrook, ME) and StatPal II (Unifet Inc. La Jolla, CA). Several studies have compared POC blood gas analyzers with benchtop analyzers using equine samples with results noted to be sufficient for diagnostic purposes [37–42].

Creatinine and Cardiac Troponin

Creatinine is a byproduct of muscle metabolism that is eliminated by the kidneys and is a commonly measured blood analyte used to evaluate kidney function via assessment of glomerular filtration. Azotemia is a relatively insensitive test for detection of early kidney disease because of the kidney's vast renal reserves, but elevations in creatinine are frequently observed in ill neonatal foals. Specific indications where POC measurement of creatinine may be informative include ischemic or toxic damage to the kidney or suspected cases of uroabodmen in the foal. Creatinine can be measured using the i-STAT as an individual test or in combination with other biochemistry analytes (CHEM8+ cartridge) [1].

Cardiac tropnin I (cTnI) is a sensitive and specific biomarker of myocardial injury and can be used to evaluate primary cardiac disease as well as the impact of other types of critical illness such as hypoxic injury, endotoxemia, inflammation, and sepsis and septic shock on cardiac health [43–47]. Septic foals were noted to have increased cTnI concentrations, but elevations did not have an association between myocardial injury and survival [47]. cTnI can be measured with the i-STAT POC analyzer using plasma, serum, or heparinized whole blood with concentrations in normal horses, ranging from 0.0–0.06 ng/ml using a POC device [46]. Cardiac troponin is measured via enzyme-linked immunosorbent assay (ELISA) with a sensitivity of 0.02 ng/ml and a reportable range of 0.0–50 ng/ml. The POC device provided similar cTnI concentrations in adult horses when compared to a benchtop immunoassay, but has not been specifically evaluated in foals [2, 46].

Summary

In summary, POC monitors serve an important function, as described in this chapter. In addition, a variety of other analytes can be measured via POC devices such as triglyceride, urea nitrogen, hematocrit, prothrombin time, as well as others, but many of these POC devices and analytes have not been validated in foals. Nonetheless, POC monitors aid in the diagnostic evaluation and monitoring of critically ill foals. As a general rule, trends in POC analytes may be more informative than a single-point measurement. Moreover, results of POC devices should be validated with a reliable gold-standard to ensure that accurate POC results are provided.

References

1 Radcliffe, R.M., Buchanan, B.R., Cook, V.L. et al. (2015). The clinical value of whole blood point-of-care biomarkers in large animal emergency and critical care medicine. *J. Vet. Emerg. Crit. Care* 25: 138–151.

2 Slovis, N.M., Browne, N., and Bozorgmanesh, R. (2020). Point-of-care diagnostics in equine practice. *Vet. Clin. Equine* 36: 161–171.

3 Hollis, A.R., Furr, M.O., Magdesian, K.G. et al. (2008). Blood glucose concentrations in critically ill neonatal foals. *J. Vet. Intern. Med.* 22: 1223–1227.

4 Hackett, E.S. and McCue, P.M. (2010). Evaluation of a veterinary glucometer for use in horses. *J. Vet. Intern. Med.* 24: 617–621.

5 Wilkins, P.A. (2011). The equine neonatal intensive care laboratory: point-of-care testing. *Clin. Lab. Med.* 31: 125–137.

6 Goodwin, R.F.W. (1956). The distribution of sugar between red cells and plasma: variations associated with age and species. *J. Physiol.* 134: 88–101.

7 Lheureux, O., Prevedollo, D., and Presier, J.C. (2019). Update on glucose in critical care. *Nutrition* 14–20.

8 Preiser, J.C., Lheureux, O., Thooft, A. et al. (2018). Near continuous glucose monitoring makes glycemic control safer in the ICU patients. *Crit. Care Med.* 46: 1224–1229.

9 Wernerman, J., Desaive, T., Finfer, S. et al. (2014). Continuous glucose control in the ICU: report of a 2013 round table meeting. *Crit. Care* 18: 226–236.

10 Brunner, R., Kitzberger, R., Miehsler, W. et al. (2011). Accuracy and reliability of a subcutaneous continuous glucose-monitoring system in critically ill patients. *Crit. Care Med.* 39: 659–664.

11 Shah, V.N., Laffel, L.M., Wadwa, R.P. et al. (2018). Performance of a factory-calibrated real-time continuous glucose monitoring system utilizing an automated sensor applicator. *Diabetes Technol. Ther.* 20: 428–433.

12 Wong, D.M., Malik, C., Dembek, K. et al. (2021). Evaluation of a continuous glucose monitoring system in neonatal foals. *J. Vet. Intern. Med.* 35: 1995–2001.

13 Malik, C., Wong, D.M., Dembek, K. et al. (2022). Comparison of two glucose monitoring systems for use in horses. *Am. J. Vet. Res.* 83: 222–228.

14 Wiedmeyer, C., Johnson, P.J., Cohn, L.A. et al. (2005). Evaluation of a continuous glucose monitoring system for use in veterinary medicine. *Diabetes Technol. Ther.* 7: 885–895.

15 Dechant, J.E., Symm, W.A., and Nieto, J.E. (2011). Comparison of pH, lactate, and glucose analysis of equine synovial fluid using a portable clinical analyzer with a bench-top blood gas analyzer. *Vet. Surg.* 40: 811–816.

16 Biedler, A., Schneider, S., Bach, F. et al. (2007). Methodological aspects of lactate measurement-evaluation of the accuracy of photometric and biosensor methods. *Open Anesthesiol. J.* 1: 1–5.

17 Tennent-Brown, B.S., Wilkins, P.A., Lindborg, S. et al. (2007). Assessment of a point-of-care lactate monitor in emergency admissions of adult horses to a referral hospital. *J. Vet. Intern. Med.* 21: 1090–1098.

18 Evans, D.L. and Golland, L.C. (1996). Accuracy of accusport for measurement of lactate concentrations in equine blood and plasma. *Equine Vet. J.* 28: 398–402.

19 Constable, P., Sulimai, N., Tinkler, S. et al. (2014). Accuracy of a point-of-care lactate analyzer for measuring blood and plasma L-lactate concentrations in exercising Standardbreds. *Equine Vet. J.* 46: 20.

20 Lindner, A. (1996). Measurement of plasma lactate concentration with accusport. *Equine Vet. J.* 28: 403–405.

21 Schulman, M.L., Nurton, J.P., and Guthrie, A.J. (2001). Use of accusport semi-automated analyzer to determine blood lactate as an aid in the clinical assessment of horses with colic. *J. S. Afr. Vet. Assoc.* 28: 398–402.

22 Van Oldruitenborgh-Oosterbaan, M.M.S., Van Den Broek, E.T.W., and Spierenburg, A.J. (2008). Evaluation of the usefulness of the portable device Lactate Pro for measurement of lactate concentrations in equine whole blood. *J. Vet. Diagn. Investig.* 20: 83–85.

23 Nieto, J.E., Dechant, J.E., le Jeune, S.S. et al. (2015). Evaluation of 3 handheld portable analyzers for measurement of L-lactate concentrations in blood and peritoneal fluid of horses with colic. *Vet. Surg.* 44: 366–372.

24 Hauss, A.A., Stablein, C.K., Fisher, A.L. et al. (2014). Validation of the lactate plus lactate meter in the horse and its use in a conditioning program. *J. Equine Vet. Sci.* 34: 1064–1068.

25 Metzger, N., Hinchcliff, K.W., Hardy, J. et al. (2006). Usefulness of a commercial equine IgG test and serum protein concentration as indicators of failure of transfer of passive immunity in hospitalized foals. *J. Vet. Intern. Med.* 20: 382–387.

26 Pusterla, N., Pusterla, J.B., Speir, S.J. et al. (2002). Evaluation of the SNAP foal IgG test for the semiquantitative measurement of immunoglobin G in foals. *Vet. Rec.* 151: 258–260.

27 Wong, D.M., Giguere, S., and Wendel, M.A. (2013). Evaluation of a point-of-care portable analyzer for measurement of plasma immunoglobulin G, total protein, and albumin concentrations in ill neonatal foals. *J. Am. Vet. Med. Assoc.* 242: 812–819.

28 Kent, J.E. and Blackmore, D.J. (1985). Measurement of IgG in equine blood by immunoturbidimetry and latex agglutination. *Equine Vet. J.* 17: 125–129.

29 Ujvari, S., Schwarzwald, C.C., Fouche, N. et al. (2017). Validation of a point-of-care quantitative equine IgG turbidimetric immunoassay and comparison of IgG concentrations measure with radial immunodiffusion and a point-of-care IgG ELSIA. *J. Vet. Intern. Med.* 31: 1170–1177.

30 Jacobsen, S., Kjelgaard-Hansen, M., Hagbard Petersen, H. et al. (2006). Evaluation of a commercially available human serum amyloid A (SAA) turbidometric immunoassay for determination of equine SAA concentrations. *Vet. J.* 172: 315–319.

31 Uhlar, C.M. and Whitehead, A.S. (1999). Serum amyloid A, the major vertebrate acute-phase reactant. *Eur. J. Biochem.* 265: 501–523.

32 Stoneham, S.J., Palmer, L., Cash, R. et al. (2010). Measurement of serum amyloid A in the neonatal foal using a latex immunoturbidimetric assay: determination of the normal range, variation with age and response to disease. *Equine Vet. J.* 33: 599–603.

33 Hulten, C. and Demmers, S. (2002). Serum amyloid A (SAA) as an aid in the management of infectious disease in the foal; comparison with total leucocyte count, neutrophil count and fibrinogen. *Equine Vet. J.* 34: 693–698.

34 Nunokawa, Y., Fujinaga, T., Taira, T. et al. (1993). Evalution of serum amyloid A protein as an acute-phase reactive protein in horses. *J. Vet. Med. Sci.* 55: 1011–1016.

35 Jacobsen, S. and Kjelgaard-Hansen, M. (2008). Evaluation of a commercially available apparatus for measuring the acute phase protein serum amyloid A in horses. *Vet. Rec.* 163: 327–330.

36 Schwartz, D., Pusterla, N., Jacobsen, S. et al. (2018). Analytical validation of a new point-of-care assay for serum amyloid A in horses. *Equine Vet. J.* 50: 678–683.

37 Mitten, L.A., Hinchcliff, K.W., and Sams, R. (1995). A portable blood gas analyzer for equine venous blood. *J. Vet. Intern. Med.* 9: 353–356.

38 Looney, A.L., Ludders, J., Erb, H.N. et al. (1998). Use of a handheld device for analysis of blood electrolyte concentrations and blood gas partial pressures in dogs and horses. *J. Am. Vet. Med. Assoc.* 213: 526–530.

39 Grosenbaugh, D.A., Gadawski, J.E., and Muir, W.W. (1998). Evaluation of a portable clinical analyzer in a veterinary hospital setting. *J. Am. Vet. Med. Assoc.* 213: 691–694.

40 Klein, L.V., Soma, L.R., and Nann, L.E. (1999). Accuracy and precision of the portable StatPal II and the laboratory-based NOVA stat proile 1 for measurement of pH, P(CO_2), and P(O_2) in equine blood. *Vet. Surg.* 28: 67–76.

41 Peiro, J.R., Borges, A.S., Goncalves, R.C. et al. (2010). Evaluation of a portable clinical analyzer for the determination of blood gas partial pressures, electrolyte concentrations, and hematocrit in venous blood samples from cattle, horses, and sheep. *Am. J. Vet. Res.* 71: 515–521.

42 Elmeshreghi, T.N., Grubb, T.L., Greene, S.A. et al. (2018). Comparison of enterprise point-of-care and nova biomedical critical care Xpress analyzers for determination of arterial pH, blood gas, and electrolyte values in canine and equine blood. *Vet. Clin. Pathol.* 47: 415–424.

43 Langhorn, R., Oyama, M.A., King, L.G. et al. (2013). Prognostic importance of myocardial injury in critically ill dogs with systemic inflammation. *J. Vet. Intern. Med.* 27: 895–903.

44 Kraus, M.S., Kaufer, B.B., Damiani, A. et al. (2013). Elimination half-life of intravenously administered equine cardiac troponin I in healthy ponies. *Equine Vet. J.* 45: 56–59.

45 Nath, L.C., Anderson, G.A., Hinchcliff, K.W. et al. (2012). Serum cardiac troponin I concentrations in horses with cardiac disease. *Aust. Vet. J.* 90: 351–357.

46 Kraus, M.S., Jesty, S.A., Gelzer, A.R. et al. (2014). Measurement of plasma cardiac troponin I concentration by use of a point-of-care analyzer in clinically normal horses and horses with experimentally induced cardiac disease. *J. Equine Vet. Sci.* 34: 1064–1068.

47 Slack, J., McGuirk, S.M., Erb, H.N. et al. (2005). Biochemical markers of cardiac injury in normal, surviving, septic, or nonsurviving septic neonatal foals. *J. Vet. Intern. Med.* 19: 577–580.

Chapter 60 Special Considerations in Pharmacology of the Neonatal Foal

Jennifer Davis

Foals, particularly neonatal foals, represent a treatment challenge for veterinarians for practical reasons, but also due to differences in drug pharmacokinetics and pharmacodynamics found between adult horses and foals of different ages [1–3]. Drug dosages and dosing regimens for adults may not be appropriate for neonatal foals. Additionally, dosages cannot always be extrapolated between neonatal foals and older foals up to weanling age. This chapter describes the differences between neonatal foals, older foals, and adult horses regarding pharmacology and treatment regimens. For definition purposes, a neonatal foal is regarded as <2 weeks of age.

Routes of Administration

One practical consideration for drug administration is the route by which the drug is to be administered. Oral administration of drugs is a common route in horses and can be used in foals as well, with a few considerations. The foal's suckle reflux should be strong and the medication should be administered relatively slowly and in as small a volume as possible. This is to prevent aspiration of the drug into the lungs with resultant pneumonitis. Similarly, the foal should be encouraged to drink, or the mouth should be rinsed after drug administration to ensure complete intake and prevent residual drug in the oral cavity/pharynx, which may induce local irritation. For extravascular parenteral administration, intramuscular (IM) or subcutaneous (SC) routes can be utilized. However, it is important to remember that foals have reduced muscle mass compared to adult horses and the IM route is limited to smaller volumes. The SC route, in contrast, is rarely utilized in adult horses, but may be more viable in foals. Injection site reactions for some drugs are minimized by this route in foals – for example, ceftiofur crystalline free acid [4, 5]. The SC route is more susceptible to changes in blood flow with dehydration; therefore, hydration status and continued fluid/milk intake of the foal should be considered when choosing this route.

The intravenous (IV) route is the preferred route for septic foals or those requiring resuscitation as it ensures complete drug administration, and the highest concentrations will be reached almost immediately after administration. However, it is also technically the most difficult route to achieve, particularly in the presence of severe hypotension. The jugular vein is used most frequently for drug administration; however, the cephalic or saphenous veins can be accessed relatively easily in recumbent animals. Foal veins are unforgiving to multiple injections compared to adults and therefore more prone to development of hematomas or thrombosis. Additionally, the proximity of the jugular vein to the carotid artery in the neck make intracarotid injections more of a possibility, especially in an uncooperative patient. Using smaller gauge, shorter needles (e.g. 22 g × 1 in.) is recommended.

Placement of an IV catheter can overcome the need for multiple needle injections but is difficult to maintain in the farm setting. Owners require education on proper hygiene and catheter etiquette, and the veterinarian should be called for catheter removal to prevent accidental loss of the catheter in the vein. If a catheter is left in place, it should be monitored multiple times per day for development of thrombi, which typically begin near the tip of the catheter, and insertion site reactions. The catheter should be removed promptly if either of these occur. If infection of the catheter is a concern, the tip of the catheter can be cultured if it is collected properly, with thorough cleansing of the skin and sterile gloves worn during removal. Foals may be more susceptible to sepsis with the development of septic thrombi and should be monitored for the development of fever, joint pain and swelling, and other signs of sepsis during and after catheter placement.

Equine Neonatal Medicine, First Edition. Edited by David M. Wong and Pamela A. Wilkins.

In severe shock cases, venous access via peripheral veins may be difficult to impossible to obtain due to severe hypotension. In those cases, temporary placement of an intraosseous (IO) needle or catheter can provide access to the venous system for fluid therapy or administration of IV medications (Chapter 59) [6]. This route is typically used only in emergency situations and, as these foals are usually recumbent and minimally responsive, can be performed with little to no restraint or sedation. Any accessible long bone can be used. The proximal tibia is the most common site used, particularly for administration of fluids or large volume medications. With proper needle or catheter placement, fluids and drugs should flow freely into the IO space.

Other routes of administration include topical, local, or transdermal, when applicable. Inhalation or nebulization therapy (Chapter 6) has been used in foals for administration of mucolytics or antibiotics directly to the respiratory system. When using these alternate routes, it is important to use nonirritating drugs designed specifically for the route in horses or other veterinary species.

Differences in Oral Drug Absorption

Oral drug absorption in the foal is frequently different from that in the adult horse. In general, foals have a slower absorption, but a higher bioavailability of many drugs, when compared to adults. Healthy neonatal foals have the highest bioavailability, with drug absorption decreasing with age. Older foals up to weanling age will demonstrate oral absorption similar to adults. This is especially true for β-lactam antibiotics. For example, a well-designed study looking at absorption of cefadroxil in foals over a range of 0.5–5 months showed that the oral absorption became faster with age, but bioavailability decreased from 99.6% at 0.5 months to 14.5% at 5 months [7].

The difference in oral drug absorption between foals and adult horses is likely multifactorial. One contributing factor may be increased intestinal permeability due to decreased mucosal integrity in young foals. This is supported by a study in foals that examined the absorption of xylose at varying ages, where xylose absorption following intragastric administration was higher in younger foals of 1 month of age, then decreased at 2 months and reached a similar level as adult horses by 3 months of age [8]. It is also evident in a neonatal foal's ability to absorb large molecules, including antibodies from colostrum, in the first 24 hours of life.

Another explanation for the differences in oral absorption in foals may be differences in gastric pH as the foal ages. Gastric pH in healthy foals is constantly changing, and is affected by milk consumption in varying ways. A high gastric pH tends to be acidified by milk, whereas a low pH tends to be neutralized by milk intake [9]. The influence of gastric pH on drug absorption varies, depending on the drug being administered. A high gastric pH favors absorption of weakly basic compounds and reduces absorption of weakly acidic compounds. The converse is also true for low pH and weakly acidic compounds. These effects contribute to varying drug absorption based on feeding schedules. As the foal ages and more roughage is added to the diet, the stomach acid should become neutralized for longer periods of time, making the difference in drug absorption based on feeding less distinct. However, neutralizing the gastric pH would also decrease the bioavailability of weakly acidic drugs as the foal ages, which has been seen with acidic drugs such as ampicillin [10]. In critically ill foals, gastric pH is highly variable and response to drugs that increase pH is often less pronounced [11]. Recumbency, lack of feed intake, and decreased mucosal blood flow due to hypotension are all variables that may affect gastric pH.

In human neonates, differences in gastric motility and gastrointestinal (GI) transit times have also been cited as causing differences in oral drug absorption. Human neonates have slower rates of gastric emptying than adults. Delayed gastric emptying increases the time for absorption, manifested as a longer time to reach maximum concentration (T_{max}) for most drugs, as absorption typically only occurs in the proximal small intestine. Delayed absorption has been seen in foals with several drugs, and alterations in gastric motility may be a contributing mechanism.

Oral absorption in foals may also be affected by differences in GI flora compared to adult horses. Some bacteria are able to metabolize drugs in the ileum or large colon, preventing absorption. The bacterial flora in the foal intestine is incomplete at birth and significant differences in fecal microbiota have been detected in foals as they transition from a milk diet to fibrous plant material [12]. As the foal ages and achieves a more typical adult gut microbiome, this may decrease absorption of some drugs if the bacterial population changes to contain flora capable of drug degradation/metabolism. The differences in bacterial flora may also be the reason that some drugs can be administered to foals without causing diarrhea as they do in adult horses. For instance, erythromycin can be safely administered to young foals, but can cause severe colitis in adult horses.

Increased oral absorption of some drugs in foals may also be due to decreased presence of metabolizing enzymes, such as cytochrome P450, in the small intestinal enterocyte or in the liver, resulting in a decreased first-pass effect. This has been studied in human neonates [13] and may apply to foals as well. Similarly, p-glycoprotein drug efflux pumps have been shown to have age-related development in the gut and liver of neonatal pigs and humans [14]. P-glycoprotein functions as a transmembrane efflux pump, pumping drugs and other substrates from inside to outside the cell. The result of these efflux pumps in the gut and liver is typically decreased drug absorption as drugs are pumped back into the gut lumen or the biliary ducts prior to reaching the systemic circulation. A combined lack of metabolizing enzymes and efflux transporters in the GI tract would therefore result in increased bioavailability of drugs that are substrates. However, this may have a negative effect on the absorption of drugs administered as prodrugs, which require metabolism for activation. Evidence supporting this was shown with administration of cefpodoxime proxetil to foals and horses. The appearance of cefpodoxime in the plasma after administration of oral cefpodoxime proxetil (10 mg/kg) was slower in neonates and 3- to 4-month-old foals, as expected. However, the maximum serum concentration (C_{max}) was significantly higher in adult horses compared to both neonatal and older foals [15]. This may indicate a greater ability of adult horses to metabolize the drug at the level of the gut or liver into its parent form through cleavage of the proxetil ester.

Differences in Drug Distribution

A horse's age affects drug distribution in a significant way. The extent of differences in distribution of a drug in neonates compared to adults depends to a great degree on the drug's solubility characteristics and its pharmacodynamics (e.g. concentration dependent versus time dependent antibiotics). This can be explained by a larger extracellular fluid compartment in young animals which results in a larger volume of distribution of water-soluble drugs [16]. A larger volume of distribution (V_d) for neonatal foals results in lower plasma concentrations, as related to in the equation:

$$V_d = D * C_{max}$$

where D is the dose administered and C_{max} is the maximum plasma concentration of the drug.

For drugs where the therapeutic effect relates to the C_{max} (e.g. aminoglycoside antibiotics), this necessitates a higher dose administered to neonates to achieve adequate plasma concentrations. For example, in adult horses an appropriate dose for amikacin is 10 mg/kg once daily [17]. However, because foals have a higher volume of distribution, a larger proportion of the administered dose is distributed to extracellular fluid and this results in a lower plasma C_{max}. The volume of distribution in neonatal foals has been measured at 0.5–0.7 l/kg, compared to adults at 0.17 and 0.26 l/kg. Therefore, the dose of amikacin for neonatal foals should be increased to 20–25 mg/kg once daily [18]. The effects of age on volume of distribution for time dependent drugs (e.g. beta-lactam antibiotics) and lipophilic drugs (e.g. macrolide antibiotics) are less well defined and changes in dosing typically relate more to alterations in metabolism or clearance than distribution. In fact, the lack of fat on neonatal animals may actually increase plasma concentrations of lipid soluble drugs since there is less of a fat layer into which drugs may distribute [19].

In neonatal animals, some drugs may distribute into protected sites they might not otherwise reach in adult animals due to immature barriers and a lack of drug efflux pumps. One example that can have significant clinical effects is the central nervous system. In foals <2 weeks of age, cerebrospinal fluid (CSF) protein concentrations and albumin quotients are elevated compared to adults, which may be attributed to a more permeable blood-brain barrier (BBB) [20, 21]. This effect may last for up to 2 months of age [22]. Because the BBB may not be fully mature at birth, drug penetration into the CSF might be increased, and may also explain the increased neurotoxicity of some drugs in neonates compared to adult horses, such as ivermectin and moxidectin. A lack of functional p-glycoprotein efflux pumps in the BBB may also account for the increased toxicity with these drugs in foals.

Drugs in the circulation bind to plasma proteins to a varying degree. The most common proteins that drugs bind to include albumin, which binds weak acids, and α_1-acid glycoprotein, which binds weak bases. Plasma protein binding has been shown to be a major determinant of drug distribution in horses, with those drugs that have high protein binding having limited diffusion into extracellular fluids. This likely occurs due to the fact that protein bound drugs are too large to translocate out of the vasculature by either the paracellular or transcellular route. Another important aspect of drug protein binding to consider is that protein bound drugs are not biologically active. Foals have lower total plasma protein concentrations for the first 4–6 weeks of life, compared to adult horses [22]. Hypoproteinemia may lead to an increase in free, active drug concentration and greater distribution into the interstitial fluid. However, in healthy neonates, this is primarily due to decreased globulin concentrations, which may have less of an effect on drug binding and activity.

Differences in Drug Metabolism

Drug metabolism, or biotransformation, may be impaired in young foals due to a deficiency in hepatic drug metabolizing capacity. Metabolism is divided into two general phases. Phase I metabolism is dependent on cytochrome P450 enzymes involved in reduction, oxidation and hydrolysis reactions. Phase II metabolism involves conjugation reactions of drugs through glucuronidation, sulfation or acetylation reactions, among others. The goal of drug metabolism is to prepare the drug for elimination by making it more polar and hydrophilic. Therefore, any changes of drug metabolism in the neonate can result in changes in drug elimination.

At this point, no quantitative research has been performed that specifically examines the development of phase I cytochrome (CYP) 450 metabolic pathways in the neonatal foal. In humans, some CYP450 enzymes are active in utero, however CYP enzymes in fetal liver are only 30–60% of adult values and full CYP activity does not develop until 2 years of age [23]. It is likely that a similar phenomenon occurs in foals where CYP activity is decreased in the early stages, but it is assumed that they develop more rapidly and are within a similar range as adult horses within the first 3–4 weeks of life [24].

Phase II metabolism likewise is decreased at birth but may develop rapidly in the foal. Glucuronide conjugation pathways, often important in drug metabolism, appear to develop later than other drug metabolizing pathways in neonates [25]. This has been demonstrated in foals administered chloramphenicol, where clearance and elimination half-life are age-dependent, although values approach normal adult values within 1 week of life [26]. Chloramphenicol is extensively metabolized in the liver via glucuronic acid conjugation and is mostly excreted through the biliary system into the feces. There are several other examples of drugs with slow or diminished metabolism in foals compared to adult horses. Salicylate shows decreasing elimination half-lives over the first 4 weeks of life [27]. Neonatal foals also had no detectable concentrations of ciprofloxacin after enrofloxacin administration, whereas in adult horses, ciprofloxacin concentrations are approximately 17% of the enrofloxacin concentrations [28].

The degree to which a drug's metabolism is affected by age is also dependent on the degree of metabolism of the specific drug administered and the natural capacity for metabolism in a healthy animal. For hepatic metabolism, drugs are often divided into high or low extraction ratio drugs. High extraction ratio drugs have a large innate metabolizing capacity (i.e. enzyme concentration) and therefore the rate limiting step to biotransformation is drug delivery to the liver in the blood stream. Low extraction ratio drugs have a lower enzyme concentration and the rate limiting step to biotransformation is enzyme production.

Differences in Drug Elimination

In most instances, the kidney is the major route of drug elimination from the body. This is particularly true for water-soluble drugs that are ionized at physiologic pH. Once a drug reaches the kidney, there are three possible consequences: glomerular filtration of protein unbound drugs, tubular secretion via carrier-mediated excretion of polar compounds, or passive reabsorption of nonionized lipid soluble drugs. Immature glomerular filtration is present in several species of neonatal animals. However, the foal and some ruminant species develop adult capacity within several days after birth [24]. Foals are reported to have glomerular filtration rates and renal plasma flow similar to adult horses as early as 2–4 days of age, based on inulin and para-aminohipurrate clearances [29]. Therefore, in healthy neonatal foals, the pharmacokinetics of drugs eliminated primarily by glomerular filtration are not likely to be greatly affected. In other species, tubular secretion capacity develops much more slowly than glomerular filtration. Although this has not been definitively studied in neonatal foals, assuming they follow a similar trend as other veterinary species, the capacity may take weeks to months to develop, resulting in delayed elimination and a longer elimination half-life for drugs excreted primarily by this route.

The final process a drug may undergo in the kidneys is passive reabsorption. As previously stated, this applies mainly to non-ionized, lipophilic drugs. The degree of ionization is affected by urinary pH and the acid/base status of the drug. Compared to adult horses, foal urine is acidic [22]. As "like is nonionized in like," weak acids will be less ionized in foal urine and therefore more available for reabsorption back into the blood stream. The ultimate effect is a delay in drug elimination. The converse would subsequently be true for weak bases, which may have a more rapid elimination in foals. Urine flow rate is another factor that affects drug reabsorption in the kidney and can be influenced by hydration status and administration of fluids.

Effects of Illness on Pharmacokinetics of Drugs in Foals

The above discussion primarily revolves around pharmacokinetic studies performed in healthy foals. However, foals receiving veterinary care are often critically ill. In particular, septic foals represent a therapeutic challenge, due to further alterations in drug pharmacokinetics and pharmacodynamics related to the physiologic effects of sepsis/septic shock on drug disposition (Table 60.1).

Sepsis is a heterogeneous syndrome associated with an uncontrolled body response to systemic infection which can ultimately result in dysregulated pro- and anti-inflammatory cascades. Septic shock is a continuum of these events leading to severe hypotension, circulatory failure and organ dysfunction. Pathophysiologic changes result in decreased blood flow to the organs responsible for drug absorption (e.g. gut, subcutaneous space), metabolism (e.g. liver) and elimination (e.g. kidneys). It is important to note that, although these changes most

Table 60.1 Summary of pharmacokinetic differences seen in healthy and septic foals, and potential mechanisms.

	Neonates		Septic neonates	
Phase	**Effect**	**Mechanism**	**Effect**	**Mechanism**
Absorption	Increased oral absorption Slower oral absorption	Increased intestinal permeability; slower gastric emptying rates; variability in gastric pH; decreased efflux pumps; decreased metabolizing enzymes; incomplete GI flora; esophageal groove (pre-ruminants)	Decreased oral absorption Slower oral absorption	Decreased perfusion of gut; mucosal edema; hypomotility
	Variable IM absorption	Decreased muscle mass and blood flow; increased water content (hydrophilic drugs)	Decreased IM and SC absorption	Decreased perfusion of muscles and skin
	Increased transdermal absorption	Thinner skin	Decreased transdermal absorption	Decreased perfusion of skin
	Decreased absorption/activation of prodrugs	Decreased metabolizing enzymes	Decreased absorption/activation of prodrugs	Decreased metabolizing enzymes
Distribution	Increased volume of distribution (hydrophilic drugs)	Larger extracellular fluid compartment and increased total body water; decreased protein binding; incomplete diffusion barriers	Increased volume of distribution (hydrophilic drugs)	Same as for normal neonates, but the extent may be altered due to changes in tissue perfusion; more severe hypoproteinemia; alterations in permeability of tissue membranes
	Decreased volume of distribution (lipophilic drugs)	Decreased fat stores	Decreased volume of distribution (lipophilic drugs)	Decreased fat stores; decreased perfusion of fat
Metabolism	Impaired hepatic metabolism (particularly glucuronidation)	Decreased hepatic metabolizing enzymes	Impaired hepatic metabolism	Hepatic blood flow is decreased; hepatocellular enzyme activity is reduced; endotoxin decreases CYP450 activity
Elimination	Decreased renal elimination	Impaired glomerular filtration (duration is species dependent); impaired tubular secretion (duration is species dependent); develops later than glomerular filtration rate (GFR)	Decreased renal elimination	Same as for normal neonates, but the extent may be greater due to pre-renal, renal and post-renal compromise
	Ion trapping due to acidic urine	Decreased elimination of acidic drugs; increased elimination of basic drugs	Ion trapping due to acidic urine	Same as for normal neonates, but the extent may be more or less if on acidifying or alkalinizing fluid therapy, or if urine output is decreased

likely result in differences in drug pharmacokinetics and pharmacodynamics, there are relatively few studies examining these processes and therefore there is little information available to inform dosing regimens in septic neonatal foals. However, certain assumptions can be made based on known effects of sepsis and the principles of pharmacokinetic drug distribution.

Drug Absorption in Disease

To bypass the effects of sepsis/septic shock on drug absorption, the IV or potentially IO (if vascular access is limited) route is preferred. Oral drug administration should be avoided in septic neonatal foals, unless a direct effect on the GI tract is desired. Numerous physiologic changes in the GI tract could result in decreased oral drug absorption, including decreased blood perfusion, splanchnic blood pooling, mucosal edema and hypomotility or ileus [30]. These effects will vary with severity of disease and are therefore difficult to predict. Gastric pH differences in horses and foals may also affect absorption. At birth, the foal gastric pH is >4.0 but decreases to <2.0 within 1 week [31]. With nursing, the pH rapidly increases. Septic or sick foals that are not nursing will have a consistently lower gastric pH, which may affect drug absorption as previously described.

Other parenteral routes, such as SC or IM, are also not recommended, due to decreased perfusion of the SC space and musculature. Of these, the SC route of administration would be the most affected, as it is already more susceptible to dehydration, which may occur in septic animals. Additionally, foals have reduced muscle mass compared to adult horses, therefore large volume IM injections are often not possible and may result in more muscle damage.

Drug Distribution in Disease

Sick or septic foals would still be expected to have a larger volume of extracellular fluid into which a drug may distribute compared to adult horses; however, the degree of change may differ from healthy neonatal foals in two ways. Sick foals may have significant volume contraction due to fluid loss (e.g. from diarrhea) and/or lack of fluid intake. The resulting dehydration decreases the volume of distribution for water soluble drugs. On the other hand, septic foals are often treated with fluids simultaneously with drug administration. This can normalize fluid volumes, or even increase them if the foal experiences fluid overload due to decreased excretory ability. Pleural effusion, peritoneal effusion and pulmonary edema, among others, may affect drug distribution. They may also result in the need to alter the dose of a drug, as they affect body weight. For water-soluble drugs, the excess water accumulation may result in lower plasma concentration (and potentially decreased efficacy). For lipid-soluble drugs that would not be expected to distribute into water, it may result in higher plasma concentrations (and increased risk for toxicity).

As previously stated, plasma protein binding affects drug distribution into the interstitial fluid. While healthy foals have decreased total protein, this is typically due to decreases in globulins, not in proteins associated with protein binding (albumin or α_1-acid glycoprotein). Sick or septic foals, on the other hand, often have exaggerated protein loss due to loss of albumin through the GI tract or kidneys, in addition to a potentially decreased globulin concentration from failure of passive transfer. Hypoalbuminemia may result in decreased protein binding of acidic drugs and subsequent increased distribution. In a foal with a functioning elimination pathway (e.g. adequate renal/hepatic function), this change may not result in differences in drug pharmacokinetics, as unbound drug is more available for elimination via glomerular filtration. However, in foals where renal or hepatic function is compromised, this may result in accumulation of free drugs in the animal and subsequent increased risk for toxicity.

Inflammation can also alter drug distribution into sites that otherwise achieve minimal drug concentrations. For example, systemic inflammation may result in a breakdown in the BBB (which is already less effective in foals), higher concentrations of drug in the central nervous system (CNS), and potentially increased efficacy in the early stages of treatment for meningitis, but also an increased risk for development of toxicity with neurotoxic drugs (e.g. metronidazole). Inflammation also induces increased α_1-acid glycoprotein, thus potentially increasing protein binding of weak bases.

Drug Metabolism and Elimination in Disease

In addition to the decreased drug metabolic capacity present in neonatal foals, drug metabolism in septic foals may be impaired in other ways. Decreased hepatic blood flow due to liver disease or general dehydration and poor tissue perfusion may occur. This decreases the biotransformation of high extraction ratio drugs. Furthermore, endotoxin is known to inhibit phase I metabolism by depressing CYP450 activity [32]. As many sick neonatal foals have Gram-negative sepsis and endotoxemia, this may affect drug metabolism in this population.

Drug elimination in sick neonatal foals may be affected by compromised renal function due to disease (renal), dehydration (prerenal), or physical factors such as a ruptured bladder (postrenal). This can result in severe drug accumulation if treatment is initiated prior to resolving any renal disturbances. Alternatively, if the foal is being administered fluids during drug treatment, this can affect elimination in multiple ways. Normalization of renal function should result in increased drug elimination. Fluid therapy also increases urine flow, which decreases time available for drug reabsorption at the level of the renal tubules, resulting in more rapid clearance. Finally, most fluid solutions administered have either an alkalinizing or acidifying effect and therefore alter urine pH, increasing or decreasing ion trapping and elimination based on whether the drug is a weak acid or weak base.

More studies on pharmacokinetics of commonly used drugs in sick and septic neonatal foals are necessary. Alterations in pharmacokinetics of drugs may result in subtherapeutic or toxic drug concentrations. Caution should be used, particularly with drugs that have a narrow therapeutic index or that are known to have toxic effects in neonates of other species. Additionally, all attempts should be made to normalize fluid volumes to allow for adequate tissue perfusion and renal function.

References

1 Baggot, J.D. (1994). Drug therapy in the neonatal foal. *Vet. Clin. North Am. Equine Pract.* 10: 87–107.

2 Vaala, W.E. (1985). Aspects of pharmacology in the neonatal foal. *Vet. Clin. North Am. Equine Pract.* 1: 51–75.

3 Caprile, K.A. and Short, C.R. (1987). Pharmacologic considerations in drug therapy in foals. *Vet. Clin. North Am. Equine Pract.* 3: 123–144.

4 Hall, T.L., Tell, L.A., Wetzlich, S.E. et al. (2011). Pharmacokinetics of ceftiofur sodium and ceftiofur crystalline free acid in neonatal foals. *J. Vet. Pharmacol. Ther.* 34: 403–409.

5 Fultz, L., Giguère, S., Berghaus, L.J. et al. (2013). Comparative pharmacokinetics of desfuroylceftiofur acetamide after intramuscular versus subcutaneous administration of ceftiofur crystalline free acid to adult horses. *J. Vet. Pharmacol. Ther.* 36: 309–312.

6 Costa, L.R.R. and Paradis, M.R. (ed.) (2017). Nogradi N, Magdeisan KG. Intraosseus needle placement in the neonatal foal. In: *Manual of Clinical Procedures in the Hors Eds. Costa LRR, Paradis MR*, 472–475. New Delhi, India: Wiley.

7 Duffee, N.E., Stang, B.E., and Schaeffer, D.J. (1997). The pharmacokinetics of cefadroxil over a range of oral doses and animal ages in the foal. *J. Vet. Pharmacol. Ther.* 20: 427–433.

8 Merritt, T., Mallonée, P.G., and Merritt, A.M. (1986). D-xylose absorption in the growing foal. *Equine Vet. J.* 18: 298–300.

9 Baker, S.J. and Gerring, E.L. (1993). Gastric pH monitoring in healthy, suckling pony foals. *Am. J. Vet. Res.* 54: 959–964.

10 Brown, M.P., Gronwall, R., Kroll, W.R. et al. (1984). Ampicillin trihydrate in foals: serum concentrations and clearance after a single oral dose. *Equine Vet. J.* 16: 371–373.

11 Javsicas, L.H. and Sanchez, L.C. (2008). The effect of omeprazole paste on intragastric pH in clinically ill neonatal foals. *Equine Vet. J.* 40: 41–44.

12 De La Torre, U., Henderson, J.D., Furtado, K.L. et al. (2019). Utilizing the fecal microbiota to understand foal gut transitions from birth to weaning. *PLoS One* 14: e0216211.

13 Brussee, J.M., Yu, H., Krekels, E.H.J. et al. (2018). First-pass CYP3A-mediated metabolism of midazolam in the Gut Wall and liver in preterm neonates. *CPT Pharmacometrics Syst. Pharmacol.* 7: 374–383.

14 Van Peer, E., Verbueken, E., Saad, M. et al. (2014). Ontogeny of CYP3A and P-glycoprotein in the liver and the small intestine of the Göttingen minipig: an immunohistochemical evaluation. *Basic Clin. Pharmacol. Toxicol.* 114: 387–394.

15 Carrillo, N.A., Giguère, S., Gronwall, R.R. et al. (2005). Disposition of orally administered cefpodoxime proxetil in foals and adult horses and minimum inhibitory concentration of the drug against common bacterial pathogens of horses. *Am. J. Vet. Res.* 66: 30–35.

16 Kami, G., Merritt, A.M., and Duelly, P. (1984). Preliminary studies of plasma and extracellular fluid volume in neonatal ponies. *Equine Vet. J.* 16: 356–358.

17 Pinto, N., Schumacher, J., Taintor, J. et al. (2011). Pharmacokinetics of amikacin in plasma and selected body fluids of healthy horses after a single intravenous dose. *Equine Vet. J.* 43: 112–116.

18 Magdesian, K.G., Wilson, W.D., and Mihalyi, J. (2004). Pharmacokinetics of a high dose of amikacin administered at extended intervals to neonatal foals. *Am. J. Vet. Res.* 65: 473–479.

19 Mzyk, D.A., Bublitz, C.M., Hobgood, G.D. et al. (2018). Effect of age on the pharmacokinetics and distribution of tulathromycin in interstitial and pulmonary epithelial lining fluid in healthy calves. *Am. J. Vet. Res.* 79: 1193–1203.

20 Furr, M.O. and Bender, H. (1994). Cerebrospinal fluid variables in clinically normal foals from birth to 42 days of age. *Am. J. Vet. Res.* 55: 781–784.

21 Andrews, F.M., Geiser, D.R., Sommardahl, C.S. et al. (1994). Albumin quotient, IgG concentration, and IgG index determinations in cerebrospinal fluid of neonatal foals. *Am. J. Vet. Res.* 55: 741–745.

22 Barton, M.H. and Hart, K.A. (2020). Clinical pathology in the foal. *Vet. Clin. North Am. Equine Pract.* 36: 73–85.

23 O'Hara, K., Wright, I.M., Schneider, J.J. et al. (2015). Pharmacokinetics in neonatal prescribing: evidence base, paradigms and the future. *Br. J. Clin. Pharmacol.* 80: 1281–1288.

24 Reiche, R. (1983). Drug disposition in the newborn. In: *Veterinary Pharmacology and Toxicology*

(ed. Y. Ruckebusch, P.-L. Toutain, and G.D. Koritz), 49–55. Dordrecht: Springer Netherlands.

25 Ecobichon, D.J., D'Ver, A.S., and Ehrhart, W. (1988). Drug disposition and biotransformation in the developing beagle dog. *Fundam. Appl. Toxicol.* 11: 29–37.

26 Adamson, P.J., Wilson, W.D., Baggot, J.D. et al. (1991). Influence of age on the disposition kinetics of chloramphenicol in equine neonates. *Am. J. Vet. Res.* 52: 426–431.

27 Davis, L.E., Westfall, B.A., and Short, C.R. (1973). Biotransformation and pharmacokinetics of salicylate in newborn animals. *Am. J. Vet. Res.* 34: 1105–1108.

28 Bermingham, E.C., Papich, M.G., and Vivrette, S.L. (2000). Pharmacokinetics of enrofloxacin administered intravenously and orally to foals. *Am. J. Vet. Res.* 61: 706–709.

29 Brewer, B.D., Clement, S.F., Lotz, W.S. et al. (1990). A comparison of inulin, Para-aminohippuric acid, and endogenous creatinine clearances as measures of renal function in neonatal foals. *J. Vet. Intern. Med.* 4: 301–305.

30 De Paepe, P., Belpaire, F.M., and Buylaert, W.A. (2002). Pharmacokinetic and pharmacodynamic considerations when treating patients with sepsis and septic shock. *Clin. Pharmacokinet.* 41: 1135–1151.

31 Murray, M.J. and Grodinsky, C. (1989). Regional gastric pH measurement in horses and foals. *Equine Vet. J. Suppl.* 21: 73–76.

32 Shedlofsky, S.I., Israel, B.C., McClain, C.J. et al. (1994). Endotoxin administration to humans inhibits hepatic cytochrome P450-mediated drug metabolism. *J. Clin. Invest.* 94: 2209–2214.

Chapter 61 Antimicrobial Therapy in the Neonatal Foal

Jennifer Davis

Principles of Therapy

Antibiotic therapy in horses has always been challenging due to potential adverse gastrointestinal (GI) effects and lack of approved products. Foals, in particular, present a therapeutic challenge as they often need highly active drugs due to potential immunocompromised status at the time of treatment, further limiting drug choices [1]. Additionally, differences in drug disposition in foals versus adults result in specific dosing regimens that are necessary to achieve microbial and clinical cures in foals. Differences in absorption, volume of distribution, metabolism, and clearance between foals and adults must be considered when selecting their antibacterial dosage regimens [2–4].

Pharmacokinetic-Pharmacodynamic Optimization of Doses

To achieve a microbial cure, the antibiotic concentration *at the site of the infection* must be above the minimum inhibitory concentration (MIC), or some multiple of the MIC, of the bacteria being treated for at least a portion of the dose interval. Antibacterial dosage regimens are designed around this concept, as long as the pharmacokinetics of the drug in the species and age group being treated are known. Pharmacokinetic-pharmacodynamic (PK-PD) relationships describe the interactions of plasma concentrations and MICs in order to predict microbial cures. These interactions take into account whether the antibiotic is cidal or static against a given bacterium. For a drug that is bactericidal, the PK-PD relationship is often classified as concentration or time dependent. Concentration-dependent antibiotics typically have maximum effect when doses used will optimize the maxiumum concentration (C_{max})/MIC ratio or the area under the curve (AUC_{24})/MIC ratio. For time-dependent antibiotics, the drug works best when concentrations are maintained above the MIC for a proportion of the dosage interval (T > MIC). The T > MIC may differ depending on immune status of the patient. For bacteriostatic drugs, the PK-PD relationships are less well described, however in general, dosage regimens are designed to keep drug concentrations above MIC at the site of action for as long as possible during the dosing interval.

PK-PD relationships are well defined for drug classes such as aminoglycosides and beta-lactam antibiotics. Aminoglycosides are concentration-dependent and reach optimal efficacy if the dose administered produces a maximum concentration 8–10 times the MIC. This is sufficient due to the rapid bactericidal effect and long post-antibiotic effect seen with these drugs. Beta-lactam antibiotics are time-dependent, and concentrations should be maintained above the MIC for at least 50% of the dosing interval in immunocompetent animals. In neutropenic or otherwise immunocompromised patients, maintaining concentrations >MIC for 90–100% of the dosing interval is required for maximal bactericidal action, sometimes necessitating a constant rate infusion for greatest effect [5, 6].

Drug Concentrations at the Site of Action

For most tissues, antibiotic drug concentrations in the serum or plasma predict drug concentration in the interstitial fluid, the site of most infections, as no physical barrier impedes drug diffusion from the vascular compartment to extracellular tissue fluid [7]. Pores in the capillary endothelium are typically large enough to allow protein unbound drug molecules to distribute from the vasculature into the interstitial fluid. Therefore, with most antimicrobial drugs, the plasma drug concentrations correlate to tissue fluid concentrations that are similar to steady-state plasma drug concentrations as the surface area of the capillaries is high relative to the volume into which the drug diffuses.

Equine Neonatal Medicine, First Edition. Edited by David M. Wong and Pamela A. Wilkins.

Exceptions to this include drugs with high protein binding, which may impair diffusion, or tissues with altered blood flow or anatomic barriers to drug distribution.

Drug diffusion into a granuloma, abscess, or cavitated lesion relies on simple drug diffusion from the plasma compartment, and is ultimately affected by the blood supply to the area. Diffusion is often delayed because the surface area of vessels supplying the abscess is much lower relative to the volume into which drug must diffuse. This results in a lower surface area to volume (SA/V) ratio, lower peak drug concentrations, and a slower equilibrium between plasma and tissue, all of which may result in lower antimicrobial efficacy.

Tissues that lack pores or channels may inhibit penetration of some drugs due to the presence of a barrier membrane caused by tight junctions between endothelial capillaries that represents a barrier to drug diffusion. In these cases, a drug must be sufficiently lipid soluble or have a mechanism for carrier-mediated transport across the membrane to reach effective concentrations in tissues. Tissues that have such barriers include the central nervous system (CNS), eye, alveoli, and prostate. Lipophilic antibiotic classes include macrolides, fluoroquinolones, phenicols, tetracyclines, trimethoprim, and metronidazole. Drugs in these classes may be more likely to diffuse through lipid membranes and produce a microbial cure with infections occurring in these tissues.

The role of inflammation in drug penetration across these barriers is debatable. In the early stages of infection, these barriers will be broken down and many drugs, regardless of solubility, will be able to diffuse freely into the affected area. However, this is not always the case. Therapeutic concentrations of amikacin in the CSF of adult horses were not reached when drug was administered to animals with either an intact or inflamed blood-brain barrier (BBB) [8]. Foals are considered to have an incomplete BBB for the first few months of life, as evidenced by increased protein concentrations and albumin quotients [9–11]. This may result in higher antibiotic drug concentrations in the CSF of foals, but also may present an increased risk for neurotoxicity with some drugs, such as metronidazole.

Some tissues once assumed to present a barrier to drug diffusion, including joints and other synovial structures, actually attain adequate drug penetration. Ampicillin and gentamicin achieve therapeutic concentrations [12], although equilibrium is often delayed because of the synovial volume (low SA/V). Once equilibrium is achieved, synovial fluid concentrations either parallel plasma drug concentrations or decline more slowly. These antibiotics penetrate acutely inflamed joints more rapidly and achieved higher concentrations compared to healthy joints [13], which is assumed to be a result of increased blood flow to the joint. However, chronic inflammation may result in purulent material and fibrosis, which may impede drug diffusion and decrease drug efficacy.

Most bacterial infections are located extracellularly, and a cure can be achieved with adequate drug concentrations in the extracellular (interstitial) space rather than intracellular space. Intracellular infections, however, present a different problem. For drugs to reach intracellular sites, they must be lipophilic enough to diffuse passively into the cell, or utilize a transport process. Several important pathogens affecting older foals reside intracellularly, and therefore may be resistent *in vivo* to antibiotics that show *in vitro* activity. For example, drugs traditionally used for treatment of *Rhodococcus equi* pneumonia in foals include macrolides and rifampin because of their known ability to achieve high concentrations intracellularly [14]. *Lawsonia intracellularis* is another pathogen of older foals that requires higher intracellular concentrations for efficacy. Staphylococci and *Salmonella* sp. may become resistant to treatment in some cases because of intracellular survival. Examples of drugs that accumulate in leukocytes, fibroblasts, macrophages, and other cells are fluoroquinolones, tetracyclines (doxycycline, minocycline), macrolides (erythromycin, clarithromycin), and the azalides (azithromycin) [15]. Beta-lactam antibiotics and aminoglycosides do not reach therapeutic concentrations within cells. Doxycycline, despite high protein binding in horses, achieves leukocyte concentrations 17 times greater than maximum plasma concentrations [16]. The erythromycin derivative azithromycin achieves particularly high concentrations of active drug intracellularly. Concentrations of azithromycin achieved in phagocytes are up to 200 times the corresponding plasma concentrations and persist for multiple days after administration of a single dose [17].

Local Factors That Affect Antibiotic Effectiveness

Local tissue factors may decrease antimicrobial effectiveness. Examples include purulent and necrotic debris present at the site of infection that may bind and inactivate vancomycin or aminoglycoside antibiotics. Cellular material also can decrease the activity of topical agents such as polymyxin B. Biofilm (glycocalyx) formation at the site of foreign material or surgically implants can protect bacteria from antibiotics and phagocytosis [18]. Cations at the site of infection (e.g. calcium in bone) may adversely affect the activity of antimicrobials by chelating some drug classes, notably fluoroquinolones and tetracyclines. These cations, including magnesium, iron, and aluminum and drugs containing those cations such as sucralfate, can also inhibit absorption of these drugs when co-administered orally.

Infected tissue may become acidic due to the presence of lactic acid producing bacteria. An acidic environment is known to decrease the effectiveness of macrolides, fluoroquinolones, and aminoglycosides. Hemoglobin at the site of infection will decrease the activity of penicillin and tetracycline. Aminoglycoside antibiotics require oxygen for bacterial uptake of the drug, therefore they are not effective in an anaerobic environment. Tissues, particularly abscesses or purulent infections, may contain thymidine and para-aminobenzoic acid (PABA), which inhibit the action of trimethoprim and sulfonamides, respectively. Because of this, these drugs alone or in combination are sometimes not effective in the patient despite *in vitro* susceptibility [19].

Effective antibacterial drug concentrations may not be attained in tissues that are poorly vascularized (e.g. extremities during shock, sequestered bone fragments, endocardial valves). An abscess rarely responds to antibiotic therapy alone because several factors hamper successful therapy: poor blood supply, material in tissue fluid and pus that inactivate drugs, and a small SA/V ratio of the infected site. In these instances, removal of necrotic tissue, drainage and lavage of abscess fluid, and maintenance of tissue perfusion through the use of fluid and pressor therapy is often required for microbial and clinical cures.

Specific Antibiotics Used in Foals (Table 61.1)

β-Lactam Antibiotics

Drugs in Class: Any antibiotic with a beta-lactam ring structure falls into this class and includes penicillins, cephalosporins, carbapenems, and monobactams. Procaine penicillin G, ampicillin sodium, ceftiofur, and cefquinome are all labeled for use in horses in some countries. Many other drugs in this class have been studied in foals.

Mechanism of Action: β-lactam antimicrobial drugs bind to penicillin binding proteins (PBP), a subgroup of transpeptidases which are essential for synthesis of the bacterial cell wall. By binding to PBPs, these drugs prevent cross-linking of cell wall precursors, resulting in pore formation in the cell wall, which allows fluid into the cell, resulting in cell swelling and death.

Mechanisms of Resistance: There are several well-established methods for development of resistance to beta-lactam antibiotics [20]. The most common is through production of β-lactamase enzymes that hydrolyze and inactivate the beta-lactam ring. Beta-lactamases are often produced by several strains of common bacteria, including staphylococci, Gram-negative Enterobacteriaceae and *Bacteroides fragilis*. Carbapenems are inherently more resistant to beta-lactamases, and the addition of a beta-lactamase inhibitor to a penicillin can result in bacterial susceptibility. Resistance to the anti-staphylococcal drugs methicillin and oxacillin is conferred through the mecA gene, resulting in alterations of PBPs and an inability to bind the beta-lactam ring. Presence of the mecA gene should be interpreted as producing resistance to all drugs in this class, even in the presence of *in vitro* susceptibility. Another common mechanism of resistance in Gram-negative bacteria is decreased permeability into the cell wall due to the presence of an outer cell membrane.

Spectrum of Activity: The spectrum of activity varies among the drugs. The penicillin subclasses consist of benzylpenicillins, aminopenicillins, anti-staphylococcal penicillins, and anti-pseudomonal penicillins. The benzylpencillins (i.e. penicillin G) are mostly active against streptococci and anaerobic bacteria. The aminopenicillins have slightly more activity against Gram-negative bacteria, although resistance has developed over the years and they are not routinely used for this purpose unless the infection is in the lower urinary tract.

The cephalosporin antibiotics are often classified according to generations. First-generation drugs have good Gram-positive spectrum. As the generation number increases, so does the activity against Gram-negative bacteria. Third- and fourth-generation cephalosporins are commonly used in human medicine to treat life-threatening Gram-negative sepsis; therefore, they should be considered reserved antibiotics in veterinary medicine. Carbapenems are also reserved antibiotics. They have an extended spectrum of activity against Gram-negative bacteria, including some *Pseudomonas* sp.

Pharmacokinetics: In general, beta-lactam antibiotics have low plasma protein binding and distribute well to the interstitial fluid; however, their hydrophilic nature prevents distribution across membranes and they remain confined to the extracellular space. Most drugs in this class have a short half-life, unless affected by formulation (e.g. ceftiofur crystalline free acid [CCFA]). Metabolism is considered minimal, except for ceftiofur, which is rapidly metabolized to an active metabolite, desfuroylceftiofur. They are eliminated almost exclusively through the kidneys via glomerular filtration and active tubular secretion, resulting in urine concentrations up to 1000 times higher than plasma concentrations.

Pharmacodynamics: All drugs in this class are time dependent; therapeutic success is associated with concentrations being greater than the bacterial MIC (T>MIC) for 50% of the dosing interval in immunocompetent patients with gram-positive infections.

Table 61.1 Antimicrobial formulary for neonatal foals.

Drug	Dosing information in foals	MIC[a, b]	Clinical comments
Amikacin	20–30 mg/kg, IM, IV, q24h.	≤2–4 μg/ml	Increased dose is required for foals due to the larger volume of distribution. Therapeutic drug monitoring and monitoring of urinalysis and creatinine during treatment are recommended.
Ampicillin sodium Ampicillin trihydrate	10–20 mg/kg IV, q6–8h. 6.6–22 mg/kg q12–q24h.	≤0.25 μg/ml	Doses at the higher end of the dose range should be used for anaerobic infections. Doses of 25–40 mg/kg every 6–8 h have been used for refractory infections. Resistance among gram-negative organisms is high, therefore ampicillin should be combined with an aminoglycoside for treatment of neonatal sepsis.
Amoxicillin	10–20 mg/kg IV or IM, q6h. 20–30 mg/kg PO, q4–6h.	≤0.25 μg/ml	Oral bioavailability decreases rapidly within the first few months of life and this route should not be used in older foals.
Azithromycin	10 mg/kg PO, q24h for 5–7 d, then q48h for 21 d.	≤1 μg/ml	Doses are based on treatment of predominantly intracellular organisms, including *Rhodococcus equi* and *Lawsonia intracellularis*.
Cefadroxil	20–40 mg/kg PO, q8–12h.	≤0.5 μg/ml	1st generation. Bioavailability decreases from 99.6% in 2 wk old foals to 14.5% in 5 mo old foals.
Cefazolin	10–22 mg/kg IV, q6–8 h.	≤2 μg/ml	1st generation. May have some efficacy against Gram-negative organisms involved in neonatal sepsis.
Cefepime	11 mg/kg IV, q8h.	≤8 μg/ml	4th generation. Crosses the blood–brain-barrier.
Cefoxitin	20 mg/kg IV or IM, q4–6h.	–	2nd generation. Often used for its increased anaerobic spectrum, including many strains of *Bacteroides fragilis*.
Cefotaxime	40 mg/kg IV q6h.	≤1 μg/ml	3rd generation. Crosses the blood–brain-barrier.
Cefpodoxime proxetil	10 mg/kg PO, q12h.	≤0.2 μg/ml	3rd generation. More frequent dosing (q8h) should be used for Salmonella or *E. coli* infections.
Cefquinome	1 mg/kg IV or IM q12h.	<0.125 μg/ml	4th generation. A higher dose of 4.5 mg/kg IV q12h is recommended for treatment of bacteria with MICs of 0.125–0.5 μg/ml.
Ceftiofur sodium	5–10 mg/kg IV or IM q6–12h.	≤0.5 μg/ml	3rd generation. For refractory infections with MIC ≤4 μg/ml, a loading dose of 2.2 mg/kg IV followed by a constant rate infusion of 12.5 μg/kg/min can be used.
Ceftiofur crystalline free acid	13.2 mg/kg SC.	≤0.5 μg/ml	3rd generation. The initial dose should be repeated at 48 h and then q72 h afterwards. Older foals can follow recommendations for adult dosing (6.6 mg/kg IM, repeated at 96 h). Consider a loading dose of ceftiofur sodium. This formulation is not recommended for severely ill foals.
Chloramphenicol	35–50 mg/kg PO, q6–8h; 25 mg/kg IV q6–8h.	≤4 μg/ml	Dosing interval should be increased to q12h in foals 1–2 d of age and q8h for foals 3–5 d of age. Prematurity may result in an even greater prolongation of half-life. Wear gloves when handling.
Clarithromycin	7.5 mg/kg PO, q12h.	≤0.12 μg/ml	Doses are based on treatment of predominantly intracellular organisms, including *R. equi*.

(Continued)

Table 61.1 (Continued)

Drug	Dosing information in foals	MIC[a, b]	Clinical comments
Doxycycline	10 mg/kg PO, q12h.	≤3 μg/ml	Do not administer IV. Combining with rifampin may result in anemia and liver disease.
Enrofloxacin	8 mg/kg PO or IV q24h.	≤0.12 μg/ml	Should only be used when culture dictates and no other options are available due to potential cartilage toxicity. If used, strict stall rest during and after treatment is recommended.
Erythromycin estolate	25 mg/kg PO, q6–8h.	≤0.25 μg/ml	Oral erythromycin must be administered as a salt as the erythromycin base degrade rapidly in gastric acid.
Erythromycin phosphate	37.5 mg/kg PO, q12h.		
Gamithromycin	6.6 mg/kg IV IM once a week.	≤1 μg/ml	Dosing presumed to be effective for *R. equi* and *Strep. zooepidemicus*. To avoid injection site reactions, drug can be diluted using 0.4 ml/kg qs to 50 ml in distilled water.
Gentamicin	12–14 mg/kg IV or IM, q24–36h.	≤2 μg/ml	Increased dose is required for foals due to the larger volume of distribution. Therapeutic drug monitoring and monitoring of urinalysis and creatinine during treatment are recommended.
Imipenem	15 mg/kg IV, q6–8h.	≤1 μg/ml	Should be combined with cilastatin to decrease risk of nephrotoxicity. Use only when indicated by culture.
Marbofloxacin	2–4 mg/kg PO q24h.	≤1 μg/ml	Should only be used when culture dictates and no other options are available due to potential cartilage toxicity. If used, strict stall rest during and after treatment is recommended.
Meropenem	15 mg/kg IV, q6h.	≤1 μg/ml	Use only when indicated by culture.
Metronidazole	10–15 mg/kg PO or IV q12h.	≤4 μg/ml	Due to alterations in drug clearance in 1- to 2.5-d old foals, the lower dose should be used. Intravenous dosing should be by slow IV bolus over at least 20 min to prevent neurotoxicity.
Oxytetracycline	50–70 mg/kg IV, 2 doses given 24 h apart.	N/A	This dose is used for treatment of contracted tendons. Antimicrobial doses have not been reported for neonates but are likely much lower.
Penicillin G	Sodium or potassium salts: 22 000–44 000 U/kg IV, q6h; Procaine: 22 000–44 000 U/kg IM, q12h.	≤0.5 μg/ml	Slow IV bolus for sodium or potassium salts. Avoid IV injection with procaine containing products.
Rifampin	5–10 mg/kg PO, q12h.	<1 μg/ml	Always used in combination with a macrolide; will alter the pharmacokinetics of the macrolide.
Trimethoprim-sulfonamide combinations	20–30 mg/kg PO, q12h.	≤0.25/4.75 μg/ml	Resistance among gram-negative organisms is high and this combination should be reserved for non-life-threatening infections. Efficacy *in vivo* is less than *in vitro* for anaerobic infections, and purulent infections or abscesses.

[a] The listed MIC represents the highest MIC that should be considered susceptible based on PK-PD interactions. Data are taken from specific studies where available.
[b] CLSI breakpoints for adult horses or dogs are used when this data is not available. Specific CLSI breakpoints for foals are only available for amikacin.

For immunosuppressed patients or for treatment of Gram-negative bacteria, it is recommended that the T > MIC be 80–90% of the dosing interval. Gram-negative bacteria inherently have higher MICs; therefore, dosing regimens for those infections may need to include higher doses and/or more frequent dosing. Some drugs in this class have a post-antibiotic effect, although this may only occur with specific drug-bacterial combinations. However, health status of the treated foal may also affect the duration of the PAE. In critically ill humans, when serum concentration of time dependent antibiotics falls below the bacterial MIC, bacterial multiplication occurs almost immediately [5].

Adverse Effects: These drugs are relatively safe in animals in general, and in neonates in particular. Due to their safety profile, they are frequently administered to foals and pregnant mares. Rare hypersensitivity reactions have been reported and high doses of some cephalosporins can result in thrombocytopenia. The procaine included in some penicillin formulations can cause severe CNS reactions if injected IV.

Drug Interactions: β-lactam antibiotics are commonly combined with aminoglycoside antibiotics. This combination results in an enhanced antibacterial spectrum, as well as a synergistic effect *in vivo*; *in vitro* inactivation can occur, however, and these drugs should not be mixed in the same syringe or catheter. They can also be combined with fluoroquinolone antibiotics for additive effects. Combination with bacteriostatic antibiotics (i.e. tetracyclines and sulfonamides) can result in a possible antagonistic effect, depending on the bacteria being treated [21, 22].

Use in Foals: Procaine penicillin and potassium penicillin are frequently used in foals, often combined with aminoglycosides, for treatment of neonatal sepsis and streptococcal infections. A report on the treatment of neonatal sepsis suggested that the combination of ampicillin and amikacin had the highest chance for treatment success, although the dose and formulation of ampicillin used was not listed [23]. Formulation will affect dose, frequency, and route of administration. Ampicillin trihydrate suspension (Polyflex®) is administered IM at a dose of 6.6–22 mg/kg q12 to q24h. Ampicillin sodium is administered IV at 10–20 mg/kg q6-8h or IM at 10–22 mg/kg q12h. Using the high end of the dose range, ampicillin reaches plasma concentrations that should be effective against bacteria with an MIC ≤2.0 μg/ml.

Ceftiofur sodium (Naxcel®) is a commonly used cephalosporin in neonatal foals, particularly in patients with renal compromise that cannot tolerate aminoglcoside antibiotics. It is unique among the beta-lactam antibiotics as it is rapidly and efficiently metabolized to an active metabolite, desfuroylceftiofur. Ceftiofur sodium is approved for use in horses for treatment of respiratory tract infections caused by *Streptococcus equi* subsp. *zooepidemicus* at a dose of 2.2–4.4 mg/kg q24h IM. Higher doses or more frequent intervals have been recommended for treating Gram-negative organisms. In septic neonatal foals, doses as high as 10 mg/kg IV q6h have been used, although lower doses (5 mg/kg IV, SC q12h) may be sufficient for bacteria with a MIC ≤0.5 μg/ml [24]. Constant rate infusion of ceftiofur has also been shown to be safe in foals at doses up to 20 mg/kg/day. This dose rate is adequate for the treatment of bacteria with MICs up to 4 μg/ml [24].

A newer formulation of ceftiofur has been approved for use in horses (CCFA, Excede®). This formulation is a sustained release formulation, providing therapeutic plasma concentrations for days after administration of a single dose. The main adverse effect associated with this formulation is injection site reactions, which can be minimized by splitting the dose into two different injection sites [25]. The pharmacokinetics differ in neonatal foals and age specific doses are required [25]. Current recommended doses are 13.2 mg/kg SC, repeated once at 48 hours, then every 72 hours after that [26]. This is much higher than the adult horse label dose of 6.6 mg/kg IM repeated once at 96 hours. Foals 4–6 months of age also exhibit different pharmacokinetics, however these differences were not significant enough to necessitate a difference in dosing regimen [27].

Cefquinome (Cobactan®) is a fourth-generation cephalosporin labeled for use in foals in some European countries for treatment of *Escherichia coli* sepsis at a dose of 1 mg/kg IV or IM q12h. This dose regimen should be effective against bacteria with an MIC ≤0.12 μg/ml; higher doses of 4.5 mg/kg IV q12h are recommended for bacteria with MICs up to 0.5 μg/ml [28].

The carbapenems are the newest class of β-lactam antimicrobials. Clinical use in foals should be limited to severe, life-threatening sepsis or cases where culture indicates no other treatment options. Imipenem (combined with cilastatin) has been used in foals at 15 mg/kg IV infused over 20 minutes q6–8h. Slow IV infusion is necessary to prevent potential seizures during administration. Meropenem has also been used IV as a frequent bolus, or constant rate infusion, as well as intra-articular or for regional limb perfusions.

Oral use of β-lactam drugs is often not possible in adult horses due to low bioavailability resulting in subtherpaeutic plasma concentrations. Foals have higher oral absorption of several β-lactam antibiotics, presumably due to a lack of degradation in the stomach by microbial flora or digestive enzymes. Bioavailability decreases rapidly with age, however, and is insufficient for treatment within 2–4 weeks of life. Conversely, examination of the pharmacokinetics of an ester prodrug formulation of cefpodoxime, cefpodoxime proxetil, showed lower concentrations of the active drug, cefpodoxime in foals compared to adults after oral administration [29]. This likely represents decreased metabolizing ability at the level of the gastrointestinal tract or liver; however, oral absorption was adequate and a dose of 10 mg/kg q6–12h produced plasma concentrations that would potentially treat infections in foals.

Aminoglycosides

Drugs in Class: Amikacin and gentamicin are the two drugs in this class most commonly used in foals.

Mechanism of Action: Aminoglycosides primarily bind to a specific receptor protein on the 30S ribosomal subunit and cause formation of nonfunctional proteins. These nonfunctional proteins also insert in the cell wall and lead to altered cell wall permeability and increased drug uptake. This binding is irreversible. There is also variable activity at the 50S ribosomal subunit.

Mechanisms of Resistance: Enzymes produced by both Gram-positive and Gram-negative bacteria can inactivate aminoglycosides. These include acetyltransferases, adenyltransferases, and nucleotidyltransferases [20]. Amikacin is the least susceptible to inactivation, and is therefore considered more active than gentamicin. Altered ribosomal binding may also be present and has a greater effect on drugs that do not have multiple ribosomal binding sites. Anaerobic bacteria and bacteria growing in an anaerobic environment are inherently resistant to aminoglycosides because transport into the bacterial cell requires oxygen. Activity of aminoglycosides is also reduced in the presence of cations, organic debris, and an acidic pH.

Spectrum of Activity: Aminoglycosides are commonly used for treatment of Gram-negative bacteria, including enteric bacteria (*E. coli, Klebsiella*) and *Pseudomonas*. Staphylococci, including methicillin resistant staphylococci, are potentially sensitive. Activity against streptococci is poor, although regional differences have been noted. They are inactive against enterococci and obligate anaerobic bacteria.

Pharmacokinetics: Aminoglycosides are not absorbed orally although they are occasionally administered orally to have a local effect on GI flora (e.g. neomycin and ammonia producing bacteria); systemic concentrations are not expected. Aminoglyocosides are administered IV or IM. Drugs in this class have low plasma protein binding, are hydrophilic and highly polar; therefore, they are confined to the extracellular space. They do not distribute intracellularly, into protected sites, or into abscesses. As neonates have a larger extracellular fluid volume, they have a larger volume of distribution of aminoglycosides compared to adult horses. This results in lower plasma concentrations and therefore higher doses are needed for efficacy. Aminoglycosides undergo minimal metabolism and are primarily eliminated by the kidneys via glomerular filtration. Despite a short half-life, these drugs are dosed once a day due to a rapid bactericidal effect and a long post-antibiotic effect.

Pharmacodynamics: Aminoglycosides are concentration dependent. Dose regimens are designed to produce drug concentrations 8–10 times the MIC of susceptible bacteria. Breakpoints for *E. coli* have been determined specifically for amikacin in neonatal foals. Using a dose of 20 mg/kg IV q24h, bacteria are considered to be susceptible at an MIC ≤2 μg/ml. Higher doses (25–30 mg/kg IV q24h) will likely be effective against bacteria with an MIC ≤4 μg/ml, which coincides with the breakpoint for adult horses [30]. The gentamicin breakpont MIC for horses is ≤2 μg/ml. As with amikacin, higher doses are necessary for similar efficacy in neonatal foals [31].

Adverse Effects: Nephrotoxicity is the most concerning clinical adverse effect associated with aminoglycoside antibiotics and this toxicity is increased in young horses [32]. There is also an increased risk for nephrotoxicity with multiple daily doses, or doses which result in trough concentrations that are ≥2–3 μg/ml. Foals that are dehydrated, febrile, on concurrent nephrotoxic drugs, or have preexisting renal disease are also at higher risk of nephrotoxicity. Impaired renal development in the fetus, ototoxicity, vestibular toxicity, and neuromuscular blockade are all rare effects.

Drug Interactions: β-lactam antibiotics are frequently coadministered with aminoglycosides due to *in vivo* synergism, although they should not be mixed *in vitro*. Coadministration with other nephrotoxic drugs increases the risk of nephrotoxicity. In cases of overdose, prompt administration of calcium can mitigate the nephrotoxic effects of aminoglycosides [33].

Use in Foals: Aminoglycosides, amikacin in particular, are frequently used for the treatment of foal sepsis combined with either ampicillin or potassium penicillin. Foal specific doses have been determined based on pharmacokinetic studies in neonates. Doses needed are much higher in animals <2 weeks of age due to a higher volume of distribution in foals, which results in a lower C_{max}. However, clearance may be decreased in foals with imparied renal function, therefore a longer dosing interval may be required. Whenever possible, therapeutic drug monitoring should be performed to personalize dosing to the individual animal. Plasma concentrations from the patient can be used to design a dose regimen that results in a C_{max} of 8–10 times the MIC (typically 20–40 μg/ml) and a trough concentration of less than 2–3 μg/ml.

Potentiated Sulfonamides

Drugs in Class: A potentiated sulfonamide is a combination of a sulfa drug with a dihydrofolate reductase (DHFR) inhibitor drug. There are several potentiated sulfonamide formulations approved for use in horses that are combinations of sulfadiazine and trimethoprim. Human generic formulations are also used in horses, which combine trimethoprim with sulfamethoxazole. A formulation containing pyrimethamine and sulfadiazine is also approved in horses for treatment of equine protozoal myelitis.

Mechanism of Action: These drugs work by inhibiting folic acid synthesis at two levels within the folic acid synthesis pathway. This results in differential toxicity to bacterial cells, as mammalian cells can use dietary folate for this pathway, whereas bacteria must synthesize their own. The sulfonamide component blocks dihydropteroate synthase, which is responsible for the conversion of PABA to dihydropteroic acid in the folic acid synthesis pathway. Trimethoprim and pyrimethamine work at a separate enzyme further down in the pathway, DHFR. This combined action at different sites in the folic acid sythesis pathway result in a bactericidal effect.

Mechanisms of Resistance: Bacteria may contain a second dihydropteroate synthase with low affinity for sulfonamides or they may synthesize one that is sulfa resistant. Increased synthesis of PABA, as occurs in abscesses or with co-administration of procaine, or increased synthesis of pteridine may also decrease efficacy of sulfonamides. Similarly, increased production of normal DHFR or production of DHFR that does not bind trimethoprim or pyrimethamine can result in decreased efficacy.

Spectrum of Activity: In theory, potentiated sulfonamides are broad-spectrum antibiotic combinations, however in practice, resistance is common and their efficacy *in vivo* may not relate to culture and susceptibility results. Gram-positive and Gram-negative aerobic bacteria may be susceptible. Anaerobic activity *in vitro* does not equate to activity *in vivo,* and these drugs are not recommended for treatment of anaerobic bacteria, even if culture results indicate susceptibility. Potentiated sulfonamides may also be used for treatment of protozoal infections. A susceptibility test should always measure inhibition of the combination, not the individual drugs.

Pharmacokinetics: Potentiated sulfonamides are readily absorbed orally, but bioavailability may be affected by feeding [34]. They have moderate protein binding and are moderately hydrophilic; however, they distribute well into peritoneal, cerebrospinal, and synovial fluid, as well as urine. These drugs are metabolized by the liver and primarily excreted in urine, although excretion through feces, bile, milk, sweat, and tears also occurs. Trimethoprim typically has a much shorter half-life than the sulfonamides, however tissue concentrations of both drug types persist long enough to allow twice-daily dosing. Studies have directly compared the pharmacokinetics of trimethoprim sulfa combinations in foals to those in adult horses. Following IV administration, trimethoprim pharmacokinetics are similar, regardless of age; however, clearance of sulfamethoxazole was slower and volume of distribution was larger in foals compared to adult horses [35]. Following oral administration of trimethoprim-sulfadiazine to foals, plasma concentrations are higher compared to adults, likely related to increased oral absorption.

Pharmacodynamics: Studies performed in cattle and horses support a T > MIC parameter as most important for clinical success [36, 37]. Therefore dosage regimens should be designed to produce plasma and tissue combinations above the MIC for the majority of the dosing interval. This requires twice daily drug administration. Most labratories use the human breakpoint MIC values for trimethoprim-sulfamethoxazole combinations of 0.5/9.5 μg/ml. Sensitivity to sulfamethoxazole typically equates to sensitivity to sulfadiazine. An FDA approval for oral trimethoprim-sulfadiazine suspension demonstrate an MIC_{90} for treatment successes for *Streptococcus zooepidemicus* of 0.25/4.75 μg/ml.

Adverse Effects: Potentiated sulfonamides are considered relatively safe for use in foals. The main adverse effects are the development of diarrhea and bone marrow suppression (long-term administration).

Drug Interactions: Co-administration of trimethoprim-sulfonamide combinations with the alpha-2 agonist drug detomidine may result in severe cardiac arrhythmias and death. This drug interaction may be more dangerous when the antibiotic is administered IV [38].

Use in Foals: Due to the relatively high prevalence of resistance, trimethoprim-sulfonamide combinations are not considered effective for empiric treatment of septicemia in foals. Use is typically reserved for minor infections or aerobic bacteria for which culture results document susceptibility. Despite the differences documented in pharmacokinetics between foals and adult horses, doses are typically similar in both age groups.

Tetracyclines

Drugs in Class: Oxytetracycline, doxycycline, and minocycline are used in horses although no formulations are approved for use in horses.

Mechanism of Action: Tetracyclines reversibly bind to the 30S ribosomal subunit and cause inhibition of protein synthesis. They are bacteriostatic at all concentrations.

Mechanisms of Resistance: Resistance is widespread and plasmid-mediated. The most common mechanism relates to a failure of active transport of drug into the bacterial cell.

Spectrum of Activity: Tetracyclines are considered broad spectrum and have activity against Gram-positive and Gram-negative bacteria, *Chlamydia*, rickettsia, spirochetes mycoplasma, L-form (cell wall deficient) bacteria, and some protozoa. Of this group, minocycline is the most active.

Pharmacokinetics: Oral absorption can be affected by other drugs and diet, due to chelation. Oral absorption is poor in adult horses; however, specific studies of doxycycline and minocycline in foals 6–9 weeks of age show increased oral bioavailability. A study examining the oral absorption of doxycycline in young foals (4–8 weeks of age) showed a maximum plasma concentration of 2.54 μg/ml following a single dose of 10 mg/kg [39]. This is in contrast to studies in adult horses that have reported a Cmax of 0.32 μg/ml after the same dose [40]. For minocycline, pharmacokinetic variables for IV administration to foals 6–9 weeks of age were not significantly different from those in adult horses. After oral administration of 4 mg/kg, however, bioavailability was significantly higher in foals (57.8%) compared to adult horses (32.0%) [41]. Doxycycline and minocycline are more lipophilic than oxytetracycline, therefore they distribute better to most tissues. This class of drugs does accumulate intracellularly. There are no significant active metabolites. Oxytetracycline is primarily eliminated through the kidneys, doxycycline elimination is both renal and hepatic, and minocycline is mainly hepatic.

Pharmacodynamics: For therapeutic success, concentrations in plasma should reach an AUC_{24h} : MIC >25. Other sources cite a T > MIC for the majority of the dosing interval. Based on T > MIC, suggested breakpoint MICs for foals with respiratory disease for doxycycline are ≤3 μg/ml and for minocycline, ≤1 μg/ml.

Adverse Effects: Tetracycline antibiotics can induce dental discoloration and inhibit long bone growth in neonates and fetuses exposed in utero [42]. Foals seem to be less susceptible to these effects as significant effects have not been reported. In humans, doxycycline and minocycline are less likely to cause these effects, possibly due to the fact that they are less potent chelators compared to other drugs in the class. IV administration of doxycycline results in fatal arrhythmias in horses [43]. IV use is not recommended in foals. Nephrotoxicity with high doses of oxytetracycline, such as those used for treatment of flexural deformities, can be seen [44].

Drug Interactions: Coadministration of doxycycline and rifampin produced hemolytic anemia and evidence of liver dysfunction in 2- to 3-month-old foals [45]. Coadministration of tetracyclines with beta-lactam antibiotics have the potential to cause antagonism due to the static vs cidal activity of these drugs. Although it has not been demonstrated specifically in foals, in other species, coadministration of sucralfate with doxycycline decreases oral absorption of doxycycline; oral dosing should be separated by at least 2 hours[46].

Use in Foals: Due to their bacteriostatic nature, these drugs are seldom used for treatment of neonatal sepsis but may be useful for minor bacterial infections, particularly umbilical abscesses caused by susceptible bacteria. Doxycycline has been studied as a possible treatment for macrolide resistant *R. equi* alone or in combination with azithromycin [47]. Drugs in this class are the treatment of choice for *L. intracellularis* in weanling age foals [48]. Oxytetracycline at supratherapeutic doses (2–3 g/foal) is used to treat contracted tendons in newborn foals.

Amphenicols

Drugs in Class: Chloramphenicol is the only drug in this class studied and used in neonatal foals. It is not labeled for use in horses and may be prohibited in horses in some countries due to residue concerns.

Mechanism of Action: Chloramphenicol reversibly binds to the 50S ribosomal subunit and causes inhibition of protein synthesis. It is considered bacteriostatic at most concentrations, although this may differ depending on the bacteria being treated.

Mechanism of Resistance: Inactivation can occur through bacterial enzyme production or decreased permeability into cell.

Spectrum of Activity: Chloramphenicol is a broad spectrum antibiotic, with activity against Gram-positive and Gram-negative aerobic and anaerobic bacteria, as well as *Rickettsia*, *Chlamydia*, and *Mycoplasma* spp. Activity against Enterobacteriaceae is unpredictable, and activity against *Pseudomonas* is poor.

Pharmacokinetics: Chloramphenicol is moderately well absorbed following oral administration with bioavailability reported up to 83% when administered as a sodium succinate suspension in neonatal foals [49]. Absorption percent may depend on formulation, however. Due to its highly lipophilic nature, chloramphenicol distributes widely intracellularly and into abscesses and the CNS. It is extensively metabolized by the liver via glucuronidation. This metabolism may be deficient in premature foals, or full-term foals 1–3 days old. Only a small percentage of parent drug is eliminated via the kidneys. The elimination half-life for chloramphenicol in foals decreased from 5.29 hours to 1.35 hours to 0.61 hours in 1-, 3-, and 7-day-old foals, respectively [50].

Pharmacodynamics: Plasma PK-PD relationships for therapeutic success are not well defined. At commonly administered doses, plasma concentrations rarely reach the canine breakpoint MIC of ≤4 μg/ml for canine skin and soft tissue infection. Efficacy may therefore be a result of drug accumulation and activity at the site of infection, including intracellularly and within abscesses.

Adverse Effects: The most clinically important adverse effect with chloramphenicol use is dose-dependent bone marrow suppression. This typically occurs with longer-term use and is reversible. Idiosyncratic aplastic anemia can occur in susceptible humans [51]. Client communication is important, including wearing gloves while handling the drug and patient, dissolving tablets instead of crushing or grinding, and cleaning residues on surfaces. Chloramphenicol may cause anorexia due to poor taste.

Drug Interactions: Hepatic microsomal enzyme inhibition by chloramphenicol may decrease clearance of some drugs, including phenylbutazone and barbiturates [52]. Coadministration of other drugs that work at the 50s ribosomal subunit (e.g. macrolides) may result in competitive inhibition for drug binding sites and antagonism.

Use in Foals: Chloramphenicol is typically used for the treatment of abscesses in foals, or for other minor infections where susceptibility is documented. It may be an option for treatment of *R. equi* in cases where macrolides are not effective or not tolerated.

Nitroimidazoles

Drugs in Class: Metronidazole is the only drug in this class used clinically in foals. It is not labeled for horses and may be prohibited from use in horses in some countries.

Mechanism of Action: Reduction of the nitro group on the antibiotic by nitroreductases from susceptible bacteria results in formation of highly reactive intermediates that disrupt bacterial DNA. Metronidazole is bactericidal.

Mechanisms of Resistance: Oxygen competes with the antibiotic for electrons necessary to perform the nitroreductase reaction. Therefore nitroimidazoles are only active in an anaerobic environment.

Spectrum of Activity: Gram-positive and Gram-negative anaerobic bacteria are typically susceptible to nitroimidazole antibiotics. Metronidazole is active against *B. fragilis*, a β-lactamase producing anaerobic bacteria that is often resistance to penicillin. In addition, they have some activity against protozoa.

Pharmacokinetics: Metronidazole is well absorbed following oral administration and bioavailability approaches 100% in neonatal and adult horses [53]. Different feeding regimens do not affect bioavailability. Metronidazole also has excellent distribution into tissues, including the CNS and abscesses. Clearance is decreased and the elimination half-life is longer in foals aged 1–2.5 days compared to 10–12 days of age [53]. Compared to adult horses, C_{max} was similar in foals, but the time to C_{max} after intragastric administration was longer in foals.

Pharmacodynamics: The appropriate PK-PD association for metronidazole is debated. Some sources recommended T > MIC for the entire dosing interval, whereas others recommend an AUC_{24h}:MIC of 25–30. Based on studies in healthy neonates, oral or IV administration of 10 mg/kg q 12h for newborn foals, and 15 mg/kg q12h for 10–12 day old foals would reach either PK-PD association for bacteria with MIC ≤4 μg/ml [53].

Adverse Effects: In general, metronidazole is a safe antibiotic. However, neurotoxicity may be seen with high plasma concentrations or rapid IV injection. For IV administration, drug is typically given via infusion pump over 20–30 minutes to prevent seizures and muscle fasciculations. Metronidazole has a metallic taste that causes decreased appetite in foals and aversion to medicating.

Drugs Interactions: Metronidazole is often combined with other antimicrobials to increase their anaerobic spectrum. Hepatic enzyme inducers, including phenobarbital and phenytoin, may increase the clearance of metronidazole, and therefore decrease efficacy [54].

Clinical Use: The most common use of metronidazole in foals is treatment of Clostridial enteritis. Metronidazole has anti-inflammatory effects in the GI tract of humans, and some clinicians add this drug to the antibiotic regimen in foals with colitis of unknown etiology for this reason.

Macrolides and Derivatives

Drugs in Class: Erythromycin, clarithromycin, azithromycin, tulathromycin, gamithromycin. There are no formulations labeled for use in the horse.

Mechanism of Action: Drugs in this class bind reversibly to the 50S ribosomal subunit and result in inhibition of protein synthesis. They are bacteriostatic against most bacteria at commonly achieved plasma concentrations.

Mechanisms of Resistance: Resistance may occur with decreased drug entry into (or increased efflux from) the bacterial cell, an inability to bind to the bacterial 50S ribosomal subunit, or plasmid-mediated production of esterases. Resistance to *R. equi* isolates is an emerging clinical problem. Estimated resistance rates are between 4% and 14%, although rates as high as 40% may be found on individual farms [55]. The mechanism of resistance in these isolates has been confirmed as a novel, transferable erythromycin-resistance methylase gene, *erm(46)*, which encodes for a methyltransferase targeting the 50S ribosomal subunit [56]. Extensive cross-resistance has been demonstrated between the macrolides and rifampin.

Spectrum of Activity: The predominant spectrum of macrolides is against Gram-positive aerobic bacteria. Susceptible bacteria include staphylococci, streptococci, and *R. equi*. Macrolides are not effective against Gram-negative bacteria, except some strains of *Pasteurella* and *Haemophilus*. Azithromycin has more activity against Gram-negative bacteria and anaerobes, although it is seldom used for this purpose in practice. *Mycoplasma* sp. may also be susceptible.

Pharmacokinetics: Pharmacokinetic data exists for multiple macrolide drugs in foals (2–3 months of age) [17, 57–60]. Large differences in plasma pharmacokinetics exist between drugs in this class. Erythromycin, azithromycin, and clarithromycin can be administered orally with moderate bioavailability. Absorption of erythromycin is highly formulation dependent; however, the pure base is degraded in gastric acid. Tulathromycin and gamithromycin are administered intramuscularly. Macrolides and their derivatives are known for their wide volume of distribution, particularly into the pulmonary compartment. Volumes of distribution (Vd/F) are typically >12 l/kg for drugs in this class. They also concentrate intracellularly, which makes them ideal for susceptible intracellular organisms. Concentrations of azithromycin and clarithromycin in bronchoalveolar lavage cells were significantly higher than erythromycin [61]. The significant pulmonary tropism noted with these drugs also make them well-suited for treatment of respiratory disease. Metabolism is via the liver, although only clarithromycin has an active metabolite thought to contribute significantly to its effect. Elimination is also primarily through the liver. The elimination half-life varies with each drug, with the shortest half-life belonging to erythromycin, followed by clarithromycin. Azithromycin, gamithromycin, and tulathromycin have prolonged plasma half-lives, as well as persistence in the pulmonary epithelial lining fluid and cells, resulting in extended dosing intervals for these drugs of every 48 hours, up to 7 days following administration.

Pharmacodynamics: The PK-PD interactions associated with therapeutic success for macrolides are not well defined. This is because plasma concentrations are often below the MIC of the bacteria for all or part of the dosing interval. Studies in cattle and swine suggest an AUC_{24h}:MIC >24 may be most predictive; however, there is currently no published threshold ratio for commonly treated bacteria in foals. It is assumed that the therapeutic success of these drugs is more closely related to pulmonary kinetics, than plasma concentrations. There are currently no CLSI breakpoints for macrolides in foals. For *R. equi* isolates, susceptibility for erythromycin is determined as a zone diameter >23 mm for disk diffusion or an MIC <0.5 μg/ml.

Adverse Effects: Macrolides are associated with diarrhea, particularly in adult horses and older foals. This may be because of the effects on the GI microbiome, but may also be due to a prokinetic effect in the GI tract through agonist actions at the motilin receptor. This limits their use in adult horses, and older foals administered macrolide antibiotics should be monitored closely for development of loose stool. Anecdotally, compounded formulations are more frequently associated with adverse effects in older foals and yearlings. Hyperthermia due to anhidrosis has also been documented in foals [62]. Sweating is decreased shortly after initiation of treatment and persists for several days after stopping treatment. This effect is greatest with erythromycin, but also occurs with clarithromycin and azithromycin [63]. Injection site reactions have been documented with tulathromycin and gamithromycin, some of which may be severe and require analgesic administration. For this reason, it is recommended to administer only small volumes of drug per injection site, deep IM in the semimembranosus/semitendinosus muscles. Tilmicosin is associated with cardiotoxicity in horses and humans.

Drug Interactions: Macrolides and derivatives are commonly coadministered with rifampin. These drugs are synergistic and result in a lowering of the MIC for *R. equi*. The combination is also thought to reduce development of resistance to rifampin. However, there are pharmacokinetic interactions with these drug combinations. Rifampin administration results in decreased plasma concentrations of clarithromycin and tulathromycin. Bioavailability of clarithromycin is decreased by up to 90% [64, 65]. Conversely, coadministration of rifampin with gamithromycin results in increased concentrations of gamithromycin and decreased concentrations of the rifampin [66]. Erythromycin is a microsomal enzyme inhibitor and may decrease elimination of drugs metabolized by the same cytochrome P450 enzyme system. Administration of erythromycin with theophylline doubles plasma theophylline concentrations and may result in seizures in foals.

Use in Foals: Macrolides, with or without rifampin, are considered the treatment of choice for *R. equi* infections in foals. Specific criteria for treatment of this disease have been recommended as many foals will recover from the disease without treatment and indiscriminate use of these drugs has been shown to directly correlate with development of macrolide (and rifampin) resistance [67]. Only foals with clinical signs of respiratory disease (fever >39.5 °C, dyspnea, tachypnea), in addition to abscesses totaling >8–15 cm should be treated. Using this criteria, morbidity/mortality rates are similar to prior treatment protocols that encouraged treatment of any foals with abscesses noted on ultrasound [68]. Treatment duration has historically been 2–8 weeks for pneumonic foals. Given the persistence of some of these drugs within the pulmonary macrophages there is some evidence that treatment periods as short as 2 weeks are adequate for drugs like azithromycin. These drugs are also effective therapy for equine proliferative enteropathy due to *L. intracellularis*, an uncommon disease in weanling age foals [69]. Due to the potential for anhidrosis and hyperthermia, during treatment of foals with macrolides and derivatives for any indication, foals should be kept inside during periods of high temperature with access to shade and potable water.

Rifamycins

Drugs in Class: Rifampin, also known as rifampicin, is the only drug used clinically in foals in this class.

Mechanism of Action: Rifampin inhibits bacterial DNA-dependent RNA synthesis by inhibiting bacterial DNA-dependent RNA polymerase. It can be bacteriostatic or bactericidal, depending on the bacteria being treated.

Mechanism of Resistance: Resistance to rifampin develops rapidly and is frequently due to a genetic change in the β subunit of bacterial RNA polymerase.

Spectrum of Activity: Rifampin is effective against a variety of mycobacterium species, which is its main use in human medicine. Staphylococci, including methicillin resistant staphylococci, are often susceptible. *R. equi* is also commonly susceptible to rifampin, however resistant strains have been increasing and are commonly cross-resistant with macrolides.

Pharmacokinetics: Bioavailability of rifampin in adult horses is approximately 70%. Although the absolute bioavailability in foals is not known, oral administration does lead to therapeutic plasma concentrations. Rifampin is highly lipophilic and penetrates most tissues including cells, abscesses, and the CNS. It is active at the acidic pH found in phagocytic cells, making it useful for treatment of intracellular pathogens. Metabolism and elimination is primarily hepatic. Due to immature hepatic metabolism, elimination of rifampin is delayed in very young foals [70]. Rifampin itself is an inducer of hepatic microsomal enzymes and, as such, can induce its own metabolism, resulting in a shorter elimination half-life following multiple doses.

Pharmacodynamics: The PK-PD interactions are not well described for rifampin. The high intracellular concentrations may make it difficult to predict *in vivo* therapy results based on *in vitro* sensitivity tests.

Adverse Effects: Co-administration of rifampin and doxycycline produced hemolytic anemia and evidence of liver dysfunction in 2- to 3-month-old foals [45]. Hepatotoxicity or increased hepatic enzymes have been reported in other species on rifampin alone. Rifampin turns urine, sweat, and tears a red or orange color.

Drugs Interactions: Microsomal enzyme induction from rifampin may shorten the elimination half-life and decrease plasma drug concentrations of chloramphenicol, corticosteroids, theophylline, itraconazole, ketoconazole, warfarin, and barbiturates. Drug interactions between rifampin and other macrolide antibiotics are described above.

Clinical Use: Rifampin is primarily used in the treatment of *R. equi* or *L. intracellularis* infections in foals in combination with a macrolide or a macrolide derivative.

Fluoroquinolones

Drugs in Class: Ciprofloxacin, enrofloxacin, danofloxacin, marbofloxacin, orbifloxacin, difloxacin, pradofloxacin. There are no formulations labeled for use in the horse. In some countries, their use is prohibited in horses intended for food production.

Mechanism of Action: This class of antibiotics works by inhibiting DNA gyrase (also called topoisomerase II). DNA gyrase is required for bacterial DNA replication, transcription, repair, and recombination. Some newer fluoroquinolone antibiotics also have activity against topoisomerase IV, which broadens their spectrum against Gram-positive bacteria. They are considered bactericidal against most pathogens with a moderate post-antibiotic effect.

Mechanisms of Resistance: Resistance is mediated through chromosomal mutations in DNA gyrase (gyrA), which confers cross-resistance to other fluoroquinolones.

Spectrum of Activity: Fluoroquinolones have a broad spectrum of activity and are often the treatment of choice for Gram-negative bacteria, including Enterobacteriaceae such as *E. coli* and *Klebsiella. Pseudomonas sp* have higher MICs, susceptibility is unpredictable, and resistance may develop during treatment. Activity is good against staphylococci, and these drugs may be an option for treatment of methicillin resistant *S. aureus* and *Staphylococcus epidermidis. Brucella, Legionella, Chlamydia, Leptospira,* and sometimes *Mycobacteria* will respond to treatment with fluoroquinolone antibiotics. Activity against streptococci is variable, and these drugs are not active against enterococci.

Pharmacokinetics: The pharmacokinetics of multiple fluoroquinolone antibiotics have been studied in adult horses [71–75]. In adults, these drugs are moderately well absorbed orally, with the exception of ciprofloxacin. Fluoroquinolones distribute well to tissues and penetrate intracellularly. Enrofloxacin is the most lipophilic and therefore reaches the highest concentration inside cells. Enrofloxacin is also the only drug with an active metabolite. It is metabolized *in vivo* to ciprofloxacin, but the degree of metabolism is species and age dependent. Elimination is typically via the kidney, and these drugs are often highly effective for treating resistant urinary tract infections. Enrofloxacin and pradofloxacin undergo varying degrees of hepatic elimination as well. These drugs have a moderate half-life and post-antibiotic effects, resulting in once-daily dosing for most drugs. Enrofloxacin is the only drug to be studied in foals [76]. IV administration resulted in slower clearance and longer half-life compared to adults. Oral absorption was lower in foals (42% compared to approximately 68% in adults), potentially due to cations present in the milk diet of foals.

Pharmacodynamics: Fluoroquinolones are considered most effective if the doses used result in an AUC_{24hr}:MIC of 100–125 for Gram-negative bacteria. Some sources cite a ratio of 55 for Gram-positive bacteria. For IV administration, a C_{max}:MIC of 8–10 is occasionally used, however these criteria are rarely met with extravascular drug administration. Based on an oral dose of 7.5 mg/kg PO in adult horses, CLSI has set a breakpoint for sensitivity for enrofloxacin in horses of ≤0.12 μg/ml, with intermediate sensitivity at 0.25 μg/ml and resistance at ≥0.5 μg/ml.

Adverse Effects: Age and dose dependent effects on joint cartilage and tendons limit the use of these drugs in young animals. Changes in cartilage have been noted using *in vitro* methods in horses up to 4 years of age [77]. These drugs are not recommended for empiric treatment of animals <2 years of age to prevent this adverse effect. While antibiotic associated colitis is considered rare with this groups of drugs, ciprofloxacin has resulted in fatal diarrhea and endotoxemia in adult horses, regardless of route of administration [73]. High doses or rapid IV administration of enrofloxacin can cause CNS excitement, confusion, or seizures.

Drugs Interactions: Fluoroquinolones are routinely combined with beta-lactam antibiotics to expand their spectrum against streptococci and anaerobic bacteria. The combination is considered additive. Coadministration with drugs containing cations, including sucralfate, may decreased oral drug absorption due to chelation. Fluoroquinolones are known to increase plasma concentrations of methylxanthine drugs, including theophylline and caffeine, potentially resulting in toxicity related to the methylxanthine drug [78].

Use in Foals: Although these drugs are commonly used for treatment of Gram-negative sepsis in adults, they should not be used routinely in foals due to the potential adverse effects on cartilage. When 2-week-old foals were administered enrofloxacin (10 mg/kg PO q24h), moderate to severe joint swelling and lameness, as well as histologic evidence of chondrocyte damage and loss of proteoglycans developed [79]. If used in any neonate, strict stall confinement to decrease weight bearing should be enacted to decrease adverse effects on cartilage. Several studies have been published examining the effects of enrofloxacin administration to pregnant mares on the development of cartilage in the fetus. Results of these studies indicate that a 2-week course of treatment to pregnant mares in early or late pregnancy did not result in cartilage lesions in the foals [79–81]. Some clinicians report fewer cartilage effects with marbofloxacin in foals, but this has not been confirmed experimentally, and pharmacokinetics in neonates and older foals is not known.

Dosing Antibiotics in Foals

Whenever possible, dosing regimens determined specifically in neonatal foals should be used for treatment. Table 61.1 includes doses for commonly used antibiotics in foals, with differences from adult doses described where possible.

References

1 Magdesian, K.G. (2017). Antimicrobial pharmacology for the neonatal foal. *Vet. Clin. North Am. Equine Pract.* 33: 47–65.

2 Vaala, W.E. (1985). Aspects of pharmacology in the neonatal foal. *Vet. Clin. North Am. Equine Pract.* 1: 51–75.

3 Baggot, J.D. (1994). Drug therapy in the neonatal foal. *Vet. Clin. North Am. Equine Pract.* 10: 87–107.

4 Caprile, K.A. and Short, C.R. (1987). Pharmacologic considerations in drug therapy in foals. *Vet. Clin. North Am. Equine Pract.* 3: 123–144.

5 Stewart, S.D. and Allen, S. (2019). Antibiotic use in critical illness. *J. Vet. Emerg. Crit. Care (San Antonio)* 29: 227–238.

6 Varghese, J.M., Roberts, J.A., and Lipman, J. (2011). Antimicrobial pharmacokinetic and pharmacodynamic issues in the critically ill with severe sepsis and septic shock. *Crit. Care Clin.* 27: 19–34.

7 Nix, D.E., Goodwin, S.D., Peloquin, C.A. et al. (1991). Antibiotic tissue penetration and its relevance: impact of tissue penetration on infection response. *Antimicrob. Agents Chemother.* 35: 1953–1959.

8 Brown, M.P., Embertson, R.M., Gronwall, R.R. et al. (1984). Amikacin sulfate in mares: pharmacokinetics and body fluid and endometrial concentrations after repeated intramuscular administration. *Am. J. Vet. Res.* 45: 1610–1613.

9 Furr, M.O. and Bender, H. (1994). Cerebrospinal fluid variables in clinically normal foals from birth to 42 days of age. *Am. J. Vet. Res.* 55: 781–784.

10 Andrews, F.M., Geiser, D.R., Sommardahl, C.S. et al. (1994). Albumin quotient, IgG concentration, and IgG index determinations in cerebrospinal fluid of neonatal foals. *Am. J. Vet. Res.* 55: 741–745.

11 Barton, M.H. and Hart, K.A. (2020). Clinical pathology in the foal. *Vet. Clin. North Am. Equine Pract.* 36: 73–85.

12 Bowman, K.F., Dix, L.P., Riond, J.L. et al. (1986). Prediction of pharmacokinetic profiles of ampicillin sodium, gentamicin sulfate, and combination ampicillin sodium-gentamicin sulfate in serum and synovia of healthy horses. *Am. J. Vet. Res.* 47: 1590–1596.

13 Firth, E.C., Klein, W.R., Nouws, J.F. et al. (1988). Effect of induced synovial inflammation on pharmacokinetics and synovial concentration of sodium ampicillin and kanamycin sulfate after systemic administration in ponies. *J. Vet. Pharmacol. Ther.* 11: 56–62.

14 Villarino, N. and Martín-Jiménez, T. (2013). Pharmacokinetics of macrolides in foals. *J. Vet. Pharmacol. Ther.* 36: 1–13.

15 Pascual, A. (1995). Uptake and intracellular activity of antimicrobial agents in phagocytic cells. *Rev. Med. Microbiol.* 6: 228–235.

16 Davis, J.L., Salmon, J.H., and Papich, M.G. (2006). Pharmacokinetics and tissue distribution of doxycycline after oral administration of single and multiple doses in horses. *Am. J. Vet. Res.* 67: 310–316.

17 Davis, J.L., Gardner, S.Y., Jones, S.L. et al. (2002). Pharmacokinetics of azithromycin in foals after i.v. and oral dose and disposition into phagocytes. *J. Vet. Pharmacol. Ther.* 25: 99–104.

18 Habash, M. and Reid, G. (1999). Microbial biofilms: their development and significance for medical device-related infections. *J. Clin. Pharmacol.* 39: 887–898.

19 Van Duijkeren, E., Vulto, A.G., and Van Miert, A.S. (1994). Trimethoprim/sulfonamide combinations in the horse: a review. *J. Vet. Pharmacol. Ther.* 17: 64–73.

20 Schwarz, S. and Chaslus-Dancla, E. (2001). Use of antimicrobials in veterinary medicine and mechanisms of resistance. *Vet. Res.* 32: 201–225.

21 Ocampo, P.S., Lázár, V., Papp, B. et al. (2014). Antagonism between bacteriostatic and bactericidal antibiotics is prevalent. *Antimicrob. Agents Chemother.* 58: 4573–4582.

22 Coetzee, J.F., Magstadt, D.R., Sidhu, P.K. et al. (2019). Association between antimicrobial drug class for treatment and retreatment of bovine respiratory disease (BRD) and frequency of resistant BRD pathogen isolation from veterinary diagnostic laboratory samples. *PLoS One* 14: e0219104.

23 Theelen, M.J.P., Wilson, W.D., Byrne, B.A. et al. (2019). Initial antimicrobial treatment of foals with sepsis: do our choices make a difference? *Vet. J.* 243: 74–76.

24 Meyer, G.A., Lin, H.C., Hanson, R.R. et al. (2001). Effects of intravenous lidocaine overdose on cardiac electrical activity and blood pressure in the horse. *Equine Vet. J.* 33: 434–437.

25 Hall, T.L., Tell, L.A., Wetzlich, S.E. et al. (2011). Pharmacokinetics of ceftiofur sodium and ceftiofur crystalline free acid in neonatal foals. *J. Vet. Pharmacol. Ther.* 34: 403–409.

26 Pusterla, N., Hall, T.L., Wetzlich, S.E. et al. (2017). Pharmacokinetic parameters for single- and multi-dose regimens for subcutaneous administration of a high-dose ceftiofur crystalline-free acid to neonatal foals. *J. Vet. Pharmacol. Ther.* 40: 88–91.

27 Credille, B.C., Giguère, S., Berghaus, L.J. et al. (2012). Plasma and pulmonary disposition of ceftiofur and its metabolites after intramuscular administration of ceftiofur crystalline free acid in weanling foals. *J. Vet. Pharmacol. Ther.* 35: 259–264.

28 Smiet, E., Haritova, A., Heil, B.A. et al. (2012). Comparing the pharmacokinetics of a fourth generation cephalosporin in three different age groups of new Forest ponies. *Equine Vet. J. Suppl.* 52–56.

29 Carrillo, N.A., Giguère, S., Gronwall, R.R. et al. (2005). Disposition of orally administered cefpodoxime proxetil in foals and adult horses and minimum inhibitory concentration of the drug against common bacterial pathogens of horses. *Am. J. Vet. Res.* 66: 30–35.

30 Magdesian, K.G., Wilson, W.D., and Mihalyi, J. (2004). Pharmacokinetics of a high dose of amikacin administered at extended intervals to neonatal foals. *Am. J. Vet. Res.* 65: 473–479.

31 Burton, A.J., Giguère, S., Warner, L. et al. (2013). Effect of age on the pharmacokinetics of a single daily dose of gentamicin sulfate in healthy foals. *Equine Vet. J.* 45: 507–511.

32 Riviere, J.E., Coppoc, G.L., Hinsman, E.J. et al. (1983). Species dependent gentamicin pharmacokinetics and nephrotoxicity in the young horse. *Fundam. Appl. Toxicol.* 3: 448–457.

33 Brashier, M.K., Geor, R.J., Ames, T.R. et al. (1998). Effect of intravenous calcium administration on gentamicin-induced nephrotoxicosis in ponies. *Am. J. Vet. Res.* 59: 1055–1062.

34 Bogan, J.A., Galbraith, A., Baxter, P. et al. (1984). Effect of feeding on the fate of orally administered phenylbutazone, trimethoprim and sulphadiazine in the horse. *Vet. Rec.* 115: 599–600.

35 Brown, M.P., McCartney, J.H., Gronwall, R. et al. (1990). Pharmacokinetics of trimethoprim-sulphamethoxazole in two-day-old foals after a single intravenous injection. *Equine Vet. J.* 22: 51–53.

36 Greko, C., Bengtsson, B., Franklin, A. et al. (2002). Efficacy of trimethoprim-sulfadoxine against Escherichia coli in a tissue cage model in calves. *J. Vet. Pharmacol. Ther.* 25: 413–423.

37 van Duijkeren, E., Ensink, J.M., and Meijer, L.A. (2002). Distribution of orally administered trimethoprim and sulfadiazine into noninfected subcutaneous tissue chambers in adult ponies. *J. Vet. Pharmacol. Ther.* 25: 273–277.

38 Taylor, P.M., Rest, R.J., Duckham, T.N. et al. (1988). Possible potentiated sulphonamide and detomidine interactions. *Vet. Rec.* 122: 143.

39 Womble, A., Giguère, S., and Lee, E.A. (2007). Pharmacokinetics of oral doxycycline and concentrations in body fluids and bronchoalveolar cells of foals. *J. Vet. Pharmacol. Ther.* 30: 187–193.

40 Bryant, J.E., Brown, M.P., Gronwall, R.R. et al. (2000). Study of intragastric administration of doxycycline: pharmacokinetics including body fluid, endometrial and minimum inhibitory concentrations. *Equine Vet. J.* 32: 233–238.

41 Giguère, S., Burton, A.J., Berghaus, L.J. et al. (2017). Comparative pharmacokinetics of minocycline in foals and adult horses. *J. Vet. Pharmacol. Ther.* 40: 335–341.

42 Cross, R., Ling, C., Day, N.P. et al. (2016). Revisiting doxycycline in pregnancy and early childhood – time to rebuild its reputation? *Expert Opin. Drug Saf.* 15: 367–382.

43 Riond, J.L., Riviere, J.E., Duckett, W.M. et al. (1992). Cardiovascular effects and fatalities associated with intravenous administration of doxycycline to horses and ponies. *Equine Vet. J.* 24: 41–45.

44 Vivrette, S., Cowgill, L.D., Pascoe, J. et al. (1993). Hemodialysis for treatment of oxytetracycline-induced acute renal failure in a neonatal foal. *J. Am. Vet. Med. Assoc.* 203: 105–107.

45 Venner, M., Astheimer, K., Lämmer, M. et al. (2013). Efficacy of mass antimicrobial treatment of foals with subclinical pulmonary abscesses associated with *Rhodococcus equi*. *J. Vet. Intern. Med.* 27: 171–176.

46 KuKanich, K. and KuKanich, B. (2015). The effect of sucralfate tablets vs. suspension on oral doxycycline absorption in dogs. *J. Vet. Pharmacol. Ther.* 38: 169–173.

47 Wetzig, M., Venner, M., and Giguère, S. (2020). Efficacy of the combination of doxycycline and azithromycin for the treatment of foals with mild to moderate bronchopneumonia. *Equine Vet. J.* 52: 613–619.

48 Sampieri, F., Hinchcliff, K.W., and Toribio, R.E. (2006). Tetracycline therapy of *Lawsonia intracellularis* enteropathy in foals. *Equine Vet. J.* 38: 89–92.

49 Brumbaugh, G.W., Martens, R.J., Knight, H.D. et al. (1983). Pharmacokinetics of chloramphenicol in the neonatal horse. *J. Vet. Pharmacol. Ther.* 6: 219–227.

50 Adamson, P.J., Wilson, W.D., Baggot, J.D. et al. (1991). Influence of age on the disposition kinetics of chloramphenicol in equine neonates. *Am. J. Vet. Res.* 52: 426–431.

51 Flach, A.J. (1982). Chloramphenicol and aplastic anemia. *Am. J. Ophthalmol.* 93: 664–666.

52 Burrows, G.E., MacAllister, C.G., Tripp, P. et al. (1989). Interactions between chloramphenicol, acepromazine, phenylbutazone, rifampin and thiamylal in the horse. *Equine Vet. J.* 21: 34–38.

53 Swain, E.A., Magdesian, K.G., Kass, P.H. et al. (2015). Pharmacokinetics of metronidazole in foals: influence of age within the neonatal period. *J. Vet. Pharmacol. Ther.* 38: 227–234.

54 Gupte, S. (1983). Phenobarbital and metabolism of metronidazole. *N. Engl. J. Med.* 308: 529.

55 Giguère, S., Berghaus, L.J., and Willingham-Lane, J.M. (2017). Antimicrobial Resistance in *Rhodococcus equi*. *Microbiol. Spectrom.* 5.

56 Anastasi, E., Giguère, S., Berghaus, L.J. et al. (2015). Novel transferable erm(46) determinant responsible for emerging macrolide resistance in *Rhodococcus equi*. *J. Antimicrob. Chemother.* 70: 3184–3190.

57 Berlin, S., Randow, T., Scheuch, E. et al. (2017). Pharmacokinetics and pulmonary distribution of gamithromycin after intravenous administration in foals. *J. Vet. Pharmacol. Ther.* 40: 406–410.

58 Womble, A.Y., Giguère, S., Lee, E.A. et al. (2006). Pharmacokinetics of clarithromycin and concentrations in body fluids and bronchoalveolar cells of foals. *Am. J. Vet. Res.* 67: 1681–1686.

59 Scheuch, E., Spieker, J., Venner, M. et al. (2007). Quantitative determination of the macrolide antibiotic tulathromycin in plasma and broncho-alveolar cells of foals using tandem mass spectrometry. *J. Chromatogr. B Analyt. Technol. Biomed. Life Sci.* 850: 464–470.

60 Lakritz, J., Wilson, W.D., Marsh, A.E. et al. (2000). Effects of prior feeding on pharmacokinetics and estimated bioavailability after oral administration of a single dose of microencapsulated erythromycin base in healthy foals. *Am. J. Vet. Res.* 61: 1011–1015.

61 Suarez-Mier, G., Giguère, S., and Lee, E.A. (2007). Pulmonary disposition of erythromycin, azithromycin, and clarithromycin in foals. *J. Vet. Pharmacol. Ther.* 30: 109–115.

62 Stieler, A.L., Sanchez, L.C., Mallicote, M.F. et al. (2016). Macrolide-induced hyperthermia in foals: role of impaired sweat responses. *Equine Vet. J.* 48: 590–594.

63 Stieler Stewart, A.L., Sanchez, L.C., Mallicote, M.F. et al. (2017). Effects of clarithromycin, azithromycin and rifampicin on terbutaline-induced sweating in foals. *Equine Vet. J.* 49: 624–628.

64 Berlin, S., Spieckermann, L., Oswald, S. et al. (2016). Pharmacokinetics and pulmonary distribution of clarithromycin and rifampicin after concomitant and consecutive administration in foals. *Mol. Pharm.* 13: 1089–1099.

65 Venner, M., Peters, J., Höhensteiger, N. et al. (2010). Concentration of the macrolide antibiotic tulathromycin in broncho-alveolar cells is influenced by comedication of rifampicin in foals. *Naunyn Schmiedebergs Arch. Pharmacol.* 381: 161–169.

66 Berlin, S., Wallstabe, S., Scheuch, E. et al. (2018). Intestinal and hepatic contributions to the pharmacokinetic interaction between gamithromycin and rifampicin after single-dose and multiple-dose administration in healthy foals. *Equine Vet. J.* 50: 525–531.

67 Huber, L., Giguère, S., Slovis, N.M. et al. (2019). Emergence of resistance to macrolides and rifampin in clinical isolates of *Rhodococcus equi* from foals in Central Kentucky, 1995 to 2017. *Antimicrob. Agents Chemother.* 63: e01714–e01718.

68 Arnold-Lehna, D., Venner, M., Berghaus, L.J. et al. (2020). Changing policy to treat foals with *Rhodococcus equi* pneumonia in the later course of disease decreases antimicrobial usage without increasing mortality rate. *Equine Vet. J.* 52: 531–537.

69 van den Wollenberg, L., Butler, C.M., Houwers, D.J. et al. (2011). Lawsonia intracellularis-associated proliferative enteritis in weanling foals in the Netherlands. *Tijdschr. Diergeneeskd.* 136: 565–570.

70 Burrows, G.E., MacAllister, C.G., Ewing, P. et al. (1992). Rifampin disposition in the horse: effects of age and method of oral administration. *J. Vet. Pharmacol. Ther.* 15: 124–132.

71 Haines, G.R., Brown, M.P., Gronwall, R.R. et al. (2000). Serum concentrations and pharmacokinetics of enrofloxacin after intravenous and intragastric administration to mares. *Can. J. Vet. Res.* 64: 171–177.

72 Lopez, B.S., Giguère, S., Berghaus, L.J. et al. (2015). Pharmacokinetics of danofloxacin and N-desmethyldanofloxacin in adult horses and their concentration in synovial fluid. *J. Vet. Pharmacol. Ther.* 38: 123–129.

73 Yamarik, T.A., Wilson, W.D., Wiebe, V.J. et al. (2010). Pharmacokinetics and toxicity of ciprofloxacin in adult horses. *J. Vet. Pharmacol. Ther.* 33: 587–594.

74 Carretero, M., Rodríguez, C., San Andrés, M.I. et al. (2002). Pharmacokinetics of marbofloxacin in mature horses after single intravenous and intramuscular administration. *Equine Vet. J.* 34: 360–365.

75 Davis, J.L., Papich, M.G., and Weingarten, A. (2006). The pharmacokinetics of orbifloxacin in the horse following oral and intravenous administration. *J. Vet. Pharmacol. Ther.* 29: 191–197.

76 Bermingham, E.C., Papich, M.G., and Vivrette, S.L. (2000). Pharmacokinetics of enrofloxacin administered intravenously and orally to foals. *Am. J. Vet. Res.* 61: 706–709.

77 Beluche, L.A., Bertone, A.L., Anderson, D.E. et al. (1999). In vitro dose-dependent effects of enrofloxacin on equine articular cartilage. *Am. J. Vet. Res.* 60: 577–582.

78 Intorre, L., Mengozzi, G., Maccheroni, M. et al. (1995). Enrofloxacin-theophylline interaction: influence of enrofloxacin on theophylline steady-state pharmacokinetics in the beagle dog. *J. Vet. Pharmacol. Ther.* 18: 352–356.

79 Ellerbrock, R.E., Canisso, I.F., Larsen, R.J. et al. (2020). Fluoroquinolone exposure in utero did not affect articular cartilage of resulting foals. *Equine Vet. J.* 53: 385–396.

80 Ellerbrock, R.E., Canisso, I.F., Podico, G. et al. (2019). Diffusion of fluoroquinolones into equine fetal fluids did not induce fetal lesions after enrofloxacin treatment in early gestation. *Vet. J.* 253: 105376.

81 Ellerbrock, R.E., Canisso, I.F., Roady, P.J. et al. (2020). Administration of enrofloxacin during late pregnancy failed to induce lesions in the resulting newborn foals. *Equine Vet. J.* 52: 136–143.

Chapter 62 Fluid Therapy in the Neonatal Foal

Langdon Fielding

Administration of intravenous (IV) fluids is a cornerstone of treatment of neonatal foals for a variety of medical conditions. The large size of an adult horse makes routine fluid administration relatively safe, but the unique physiology and small size of neonatal foals requires a much more careful approach to IV fluid administration [1, 2]. This chapter focuses on criteria used to determine if IV fluids are needed, to decide on the type of fluid, to delineate the rate the fluids should be administered, and define when the fluids can be discontinued.

Reasons for IV Fluid Therapy

There are four primary reasons to administer IV fluids to neonatal foals: (i) resuscitation due to inadequate perfusion; (ii) replacement of fluid deficits; (iii) provision of maintenance fluids when adequate enteral fluid therapy is not possible; and (iv) management of electrolyte or other metabolic derangements. In many cases, fluids are administered for more than one of these reasons or started for one reason and continued for a different reason. Regardless of the rationale for initiating fluids, throughout the course of treatment, the type and rate of fluids should be reconsidered. Discontinuing fluid therapy, as soon as it is no longer needed, is the goal.

Resuscitation

A common mistake in equine emergency medicine is to initiate aggressive resuscitation with IV fluids when the foal may only require maintenance fluids, dextrose supplementation, or electrolyte management. This increased/excessive fluid load may have detrimental physiologic effects and can frequently take days to properly distribute throughout various physiologic spaces (e.g., vascular space, intracellular, interstitium) and be excreted [2]. Determining if fluid resuscitation is truly needed is an important skill and can potentially contribute to the outcome of the case. The need for fluid resuscitation should be guided by a set of parameters (Table 62.1). No single clinical finding or laboratory test can be universally used to identify patients that require fluid resuscitation. However, when a combination (typically >2 parameters) of results indicate that resuscitation is indicated, fluid therapy is likely needed. The physiology behind these examination and laboratory variables is beyond the scope of this chapter with additional information found throughout this textbook.

Type of Resuscitation Fluid

The type of fluid used for resuscitation of neonatal foals is controversial and there is minimal research in foals or even human neonates to support a strong recommendation. The factors to consider include overall tonicity, electrolyte composition, and colloidal activity.

Tonicity

The general recommendation for IV fluid resuscitation is to avoid hypotonic fluids such as 5% dextrose in water or 0.45% sodium chloride. The choice between isotonic and hypertonic fluids is more complicated. Isotonic fluids should primarily affect the extracellular fluid space, but they quickly distribute between the vascular and interstitial spaces. Hypertonic fluid resuscitation should theoretically expand the extracellular fluid volume at the expense of the intracellular fluid volume. Additionally, hypertonic fluids may provide brief but significant expansion of the vascular space depending on other properties of the fluid. However, most hypertonic fluids add a significant amount of sodium, and often chloride, to a foal that is already struggling metabolically.

Equine Neonatal Medicine, First Edition. Edited by David M. Wong and Pamela A. Wilkins.

Table 62.1 Guide for assessing fluid needs in the foal.

<u>Clinical examination findings consistent with the need for IV fluid resuscitation</u>

- Increased heart rate (>100 beats/min) – variably present in foals
- Cold extremities
- Poor pulse quality
- Pale mucous membranes
- Capillary refill time >2 seconds
- Lethargy, dull mentation
- Prolonged jugular refill
- Decreased urine output (<0.5 ml/kg/hr)

<u>Laboratory findings supporting the need for IV fluid resuscitation</u>

- Blood lactate concentration >2.0 mmol/l
- Central venous oxygen (ScV_{O2}) <70%

<u>Hemodynamic variables consistent with the need for IV fluid resuscitation</u>

- Mean arterial blood pressure (cutoffs age dependent)
- Central venous pressure (CVP) <8 cmH_2O
- Pulse pressure variation >12%

Research on the use of hypertonic resuscitation fluids is limited in human and equine neonates, but more information is available from neonatal calves. Studies were primarily conducted on calves with diarrhea, with beneficial effects of hypertonic saline and hypertonic bicarbonate solutions described [3]. These fluids have historically been avoided for resuscitation in foals, but these practices may need to be revisited in light of this newer research. At this time, the author is not aware of many hospitals that are using hypertonic fluids for resuscitation of equine neonates.

Electrolyte Composition

If an isotonic crystalloid fluid is used for resuscitation, common choices include a balanced acetate containing fluid (e.g., Normosol R, Plasmalyte 148), Lactated Ringer's solution, Hartmann's solution, and 0.9% sodium chloride (Table 62.2). A balanced acetate containing fluid is used most commonly in equine neonatal medicine, but concerns with hypotension following the bolus of acetate have been raised in other species [4]. Lactated Ringer's solution is an acceptable alternative; however, if the foal has impaired lactate clearance (e.g., liver disease) this could be a less optimal fluid choice [5]. Additionally, Lactated Ringer's solution has a higher chloride concentration than acetated fluids, but most studies have focused on the higher chloride load of 0.9% saline and the increased risk of acute kidney injury (AKI) [6]. The use of 0.9% sodium chloride was very common with fluid resuscitation in humans, but the high chloride content has continued to raise concerns about renal injury. However, in some studies changing to a balanced electrolyte solution from saline did not identify clinically significant differences [7]. A 0.9% sodium chloride solution is also slightly hypertonic relative to foal plasma.

If hypertonic fluids are used, the most common option for resuscitation is hypertonic saline (commonly 7.2%), but hypertonic sodium bicarbonate solution (8.4%) could also theoretically be administered. Both fluids have effects on acid-base balance and represent a large amount of sodium that the foal must eventually excrete. In either case, a more balanced isotonic or slightly hypotonic crystalloid fluid should be used following infusion with one of these hypertonic fluids. Hypertonic saline may have a number of additional physiologic effects including improvements in cardiac contractility and vascular

Table 62.2 Common IV solutions used in foals.

Solution	Ringer's	Lactated Ringer's solution	Plasma-Lyte 56	Plasma-Lyte 148	Plasma-Lyte R	Normosol-R Plasma-Lyte A	Hartman's solution	0.9% Sodium chloride
Na^+ (mEq/l)	147	130	40	140	140	140	131	154
K^+ (mEq/l)	4	4	13	5	10	5	5.4	
Ca^{++} (mEq/l)	4	3			5		1.8	
Mg^{++}(mEq/l)			3	1.5	3	3		
Cl^- (mEq/l)	156	109	40	98	103	98	112	154
Gluconate (mEq/l)				23		23		
Lactate(mEq/l)		28			8		28	
Acetate (mEq/l)			16	27	47	27		
Osmolarity (mOsm/l)	310	272	111		312	295	277	310

tone [8]. Hypertonic bicarbonate has been associated with a variety of cardiovascular changes including an increase in contractility [9].

Colloids

Colloids can be natural (e.g. plasma) or artificial (e.g. hydroxyethyl starch). These substances have a high molecular weight and are better contained within the vascular space than crystalloids in healthy individuals [10]. Synthetic colloid solutions containing hydroxyethyl starch (HES) are readily available for use in foals, but improved survival in ill foals with these solutions remains to be proven. Hydroxyethyl starches are nonionic starch polymers derived from branched-chain glucose polymers obtained by hydrolysis of the maize or potato starch, amylopectin. Subsequent hydroxyethylation of glucose units provides water solubility and conservation from degredation [11]. Hydroxyethyl starch solutions are categorized by their mean molecular weight (kDa) as high, medium, or low molecular weight solutions, ranging from 70 to 670 kDa. Additionally, the molar substitution ratio, which is the number of hydroxyethyl groups per glucose molecule, further categorize solutions [12]. The physicochemical characteristics of HES solutions are determined by concentration (e.g., 6% or 10% solution), mean molecular weight, and degree of molar substitution [12]. Synthetic colloid solutions with lower molecular weights have more active molecules to contribute to oncotic pressure compared to higher molecular weight products with similar concentrations. Thus, more beneficial effects on colloid osmotic pressure (COP) and intravascular volume are conferred with lower molecular weight solutions [13]. The disadvantage of lower molecular weight solutions is that they are degraded more rapidly, as compared to higher molecular weight solutions, thereby decreasing the duration of clinical effect [13].

The use of synthetic colloids has been associated with coagulopathies and AKI in randomized clinical trials in human patients with sepsis [14, 15]. The mechanism by which synthetic colloids induce coagulopathy includes dilution of and interference with clotting factors, fibrinolysis, and platelet function [11, 16]. Reduced concentrations of von Willebrand factor (vWF) and factor VIII as well as prolongation of prothrombin time (PT) and activated partial thromboplastin time (aPTT) have been documented in horses administered 10 mL/kg body weight of 6% HES (600/0.75) [16–19]. Elevated plasma oncotic pressure, as observed with administration of hyper-oncotic colloid solutions, has the potential to produce kidney dysfunction or acute renal failure because colloids might decrease glomerular filtration [20, 21]. In one study, synthetic colloid solutions were associated with kidney dysfunction and a higher incidence of renal failure when 10% HES (200/0.5) was used, as compared to crystalloids [14]. Another proposed mechanism of renal dysfunction is induction of urine hyperviscosity by infusing a hyperoncotic agent to a dehydrated patient. In turn, glomerular filtration of hyperoncotic molecules results in hyperviscous urine and stasis of tubular flow [22]. In addition, accumulation of small molecules in the tubules may account for acute tubular toxicity [12]. These negative side effects are dose-related and are more common with colloid solutions that have higher molecular weight and molar substitution ratios [23–25]. In contrast, studies in people evaluating preparations of lower molecular weight and molar substitution ratios (130/0.38–0.45) have been noted to be safer and had fewer side effects [23].

A few studies regarding synthetic colloid solutions in horses have evaluated higher molecular weight/molar substitution ratio HES solutions ranging from 600 to 670 molecular weight and 0.75 molar substitution ratio [16]. More recently a lower molecular weight/molar substitution ratio solution (Vetstarch; 130/0.4 in 0.9% sodium chloride) has been examined in foals and was noted to be safe and significantly increased COP for 3 hours post-administration [26]. A study in adult horses documented more effective volume expansion and arterial blood pressure support as well as a more sustained effect on COP with the use of this low molecular weight synthetic colloid solution compared to 0.9% NaCl [17]. In addition, a shorter duration of adverse effects on platelet function was noted with Vetstarch, as compared to HES [17]. Furthermore, an *in vitro* study using equine blood suggested less impairment of coagulation when low molecular weight/low molar substitution solutions were used [16]. In summary, the use of artificial colloids has been described in foals and has shown improved vascular volume expansion and colloid osmotic pressure as compared to crystalloids [26]. However, in children, artificial colloids have not been consistently shown to be superior as a resuscitation fluid compared to crystalloids [27]. Therefore, the use of colloids during resuscitation in foals remains uncertain.

In contrast, the most common natural colloid used in neonatal foals is plasma. The beneficial effects of specific types of hyperimmune plasma have been documented in foals, but the trial did not compare the use of a colloid to a crystalloid for fluid resuscitation [28]. In practice, IV plasma transfusions are somewhat commonly used in neonatal foals to address failure of transfer of passive immunity or hypoalbuminemia in critically ill foals (e.g. enterocolitis and diarrhea). However, at this time, there is not sufficient evidence to recommend colloids as a superior resuscitation fluid compared to crystalloids in neonatal foals.

Rate of Fluid Resuscitation

The rate for administering shock resuscitative fluids is typically rapid with 20 ml/kg over 10–15 minutes. If there is a clear need for fluid resuscitation (based on clinical exam, clinicopathologic variables, point-of-care lactate), then the first bolus of fluids should be given immediately and quickly. If subsequent boluses are needed, some clinicians decrease the rate of the additional boluses to 20 ml/kg infusions administered over 1–2 hours. However, it is important to remember that isotonic crystalloids move out of the vascular space quickly and therefore the hemodynamic benefits may be more limited if administered slowly [29].

End Points for Fluid Resuscitation

One approach to determining the total amount of resuscitative fluids needed is to calculate the fluid deficit for the foal and aim to administer a percentage of this deficit (e.g. 75% of the fluid deficit) during the resuscitation period. The potential pitfall with this strategy is that it can be difficult to accurately estimate fluid deficits. Additionally, some foals may have a relative hypovolemia with poor perfusion, but not necessarily an absolute hypovolemia or the ability to tolerate large fluid volumes. The practice of administering a predetermined amount of fluid based on a calculated deficit can be risky and prone to fluid overload or under resuscitation.

A more finessed approach to fluid resuscitation is to administer a bolus of a resuscitative fluid and then reevaluate the parameters that were used to determine the need for fluids prior to resuscitation. If the majority of parameters are normalizing or significantly improving, then the resuscitative phase of fluid administration can be discontinued. Conversely, if there is no improvement or parameters are deteriorating, then an additional bolus of fluids should be administered and the reevaluation repeated. It is important to remember that laboratory values such as blood lactate may often increase with initial fluid expansion and then gradually improve over a period of days. Clinical experience with neonatal foals will help the clinician to combine the examination and laboratory parameters to determine if the overall clinical picture of the foal is improving.

Until more recently, the benefits of fluid resuscitation were considered to outweigh potential risks of fluid overload and many clinicians would err on the side of additional fluids. Fluid overload is discussed in more detail later in this chapter, but recognition of morbidity and mortality associated with fluid overload has caused a shift in the approach to resuscitation fluids in human neonates [30]. Due to their physiology and size, careful evaluation during the resuscitation phase is extremely important to avoid fluid overload. If a foal has received more than 40-60 ml/kg of rapidly administered IV isotonic fluids with no improvement in perfusion parameters, additional fluids should be carefully considered. Other treatments to improve perfusion in addition to IV fluids include inotropes or vasopressors. At the end of fluid resuscitation, all IV fluids can be stopped and the foal monitored carefully. However, it is more common to move into a maintenance phase of fluid administration depending on the foal's underlying condition and ability to tolerate oral feeding.

Maintenance Fluid Therapy

IV maintenance fluids are needed when a foal is unable to maintain normal fluid and electrolyte balance with enteral fluids alone. While many foals are hospitalized when they are unable to safely nurse or drink from a pan, a large number of these foals will tolerate fluids through a feeding tube. However, if the foal has large volumes of reflux or develops signs of colic with enteral fluid administration, then IV maintenance fluids are warranted.

Tonicity

The ideal tonicity of maintenance fluids for neonates has become more controversial in the last decade where numerous studies in human pediatric care identifying significant risks of hyponatremia with the use of hypotonic IV fluids [31]. While maintenance isotonic fluids have been evaluated in healthy foals, concerns have been raised about the large amount of sodium that is administered with these products [32]. When using isotonic fluids, the risk of hypernatremia exists, but appears to be less common than the risk of hyponatremia when using hypotonic fluids [31]. Many of the recommendations in human neonates have begun to change to incorporate isotonic fluids for maintenance fluid therapy.

It may not be possible to extrapolate human neonatal studies on the tonicity of maintenance fluids to neonatal foals, as both have unique physiologic aspects. However, careful monitoring of sodium concentration and/or osmolality is indicated for foals receiving relatively hypotonic fluids. Many clinicians use a 50/50 combination of 5% dextrose in water and a balanced electrolyte solution (Normosol-R, Lactated Ringer's, etc.) as maintenance fluids. In foals where the sodium concentration is decreasing, increasing the proportion of isotonic crystalloid and decreasing the amount of 5% dextrose in water may be prudent.

Rate

The rate of maintenance fluid administration is almost as controversial as the tonicity of the fluids. A complicating variable is that different breeds of foals can be dramatically

Table 62.3 Holliday-Segar method for calculating maintenance fluid rate [2, 33, 35].

First 10 kg body weight	100 ml/kg/day (4 ml/kg/hr)
Second 10 kg body weight	50 ml/kg/day (2 ml/kg/hr)
Additional 10 kg body weight	20 ml/kg/day (1 ml/kg/hr)

Example for a 50 kg foal:
First 10 kg = 100 ml × 10 kg/day = 1000 ml
Second 10 kg = 50 ml × 10 kg/day = 500 ml
Additional 10 kg (remaining 30 kg) = 20 ml × 30 kg/day = 600 ml
Total volume = 1000 ml + 500 ml + 600 ml = 2100 ml/day

Table 62.4 Fluid administration rates for neonatal foals.

Foal size	Fluid rate
10–20 kg	5 ml/kg/hr
20–60 kg	4 ml/kg/hr
>60 kg	3–4 ml/kg/hr

different in size from as little as 8–10 kg for a Miniature Horse foal to 10 times that size for a draft horse foal. In clinical practice, there are two primary approaches to calculating the maintenance fluid rate for neonates:

1) Holliday-Segar formula (or variation on this approach)
2) Flat rate (4–6 ml/kg/hr) depending on size of the foal

The Holliday-Segar method (Table 62.3) has been used for decades as a way to estimate maintenance fluid requirements for neonatal and pediatric patients [33]. Of the two approaches discussed here, it is the more conservative approach to maintenance fluid therapy and can result in administration rates that are potentially 50% less than alternative calculations. This approach is less likely to lead to volume overload. More recently, a single equation has been proposed to calculate maintenance fluid requirements for children, but the results are similar to values obtained using Holliday-Segar [34]; this equation is as follows:

$$\text{Daily maintenance fluid requirement}(\text{ml / day}) = 300 \times \text{BW}^{1/2} \text{ where BW} = \text{body weight of the foal}(\text{kg}) \quad (62.1)$$

This equation may be easier to use for equine neonatologists particularly considering that foals come in a very wide range of sizes and body weight can be easily inserted into the formula.

The major risks with the Holliday-Segar method are that inadequate fluid volume is administered or hyponatremia develops when using a lower sodium maintenance fluid. Neonatal foals have many reasons to develop AKI; inadequate intravascular fluid volume will only increase the risks. The Holliday-Segar calculation may result in a fluid rate that allows little room for error (e.g. malfunctioning fluid pump or catheter), thus monitoring of blood pressure and renal function is extremely important. A hypotonic fluid is often used with the Holliday-Segar calculation and development of hyponatremia is a common problem in human neonates [36]. Hyponatremia is also commonly reported in sick neonatal foals for a variety of reasons; however, many of these foals were not receiving this more conservative fluid plan [37].

The more aggressive maintenance fluid plan used in equine neonatal medicine is to administer fluids according to the general guidelines provided in Table 62.4.

These fluid rates can be as much as double the rate calculated under the Holliday-Segar method but may be less likely to result in volume underloading and AKI. However, fluid overload can be a problem, particularly in foals born from cesarean-sections or following a dystocia. Patients with sepsis may also be vulnerable to excess fluid administration. These fluid rates allow for a larger margin of error for problems with catheters and fluid pump malfunctions, but also require careful monitoring to avoid fluid overload. Similar to the discussion above, hypotonic fluids can be used, but foals need to be monitored carefully for hyponatremia.

End Point for IV Maintenance Fluids

When the neonatal foal tolerates enough enteral feeding to meet hydration requirements, IV fluids can be discontinued. This simple statement would suggest that foals that tolerate at least 8–10% of their body weight per day via enteral feeding should be stable enough to allow the discontinuation of IV fluids. However, many clinicians will slowly decrease maintenance fluids over 24–48 hours once the foal is tolerating this rate of enteral feeding. Another reason that maintenance fluids may be continued for an extended period is to manage electrolyte imbalances or provide additional dextrose. Additionally, some medications that are provided continuously (e.g. lidocaine, metoclopramide) are more easily administered when a constant rate of fluids are being given concurrently. While these foals technically do not require maintenance IV fluid therapy, practical considerations may prevail, and fluids will be continued for a longer period.

Management of Metabolic Derangements

IV fluids are frequently used to provide dextrose and manage electrolyte disorders. While the primary goal of these fluids may not be to provide fluid volume, the type of fluid and rate of fluid administration are still extremely important. The following is a summary of the approach to using IV fluids to manage common conditions in neonatal foals.

Hypoglycemia

Hypoglycemia has many causes in the neonatal foal, including inadequate nutrition, sepsis, liver failure, and some genetic disorders [38]. While the mechanisms for hypoglycemia may be very different, the options for providing dextrose supplementation are more uniform. When dextrose supplementation is required, foals typically receive 4–8 mg/kg/min of dextrose as a constant rate infusion (CRI) if no other form of nutrition (e.g. enteral) is being provided. However, in severe cases of liver failure, sepsis, and glycogen branching disorder, higher rates of dextrose may be needed (12 mg/kg/min or more). There are two general approaches to providing dextrose supplementation through IV fluids, and the decision is often a practical one.

A common approach is to use a 5% dextrose in water solution as half of the IV fluids for the foal and a balanced isotonic crystalloid for the other half – e.g. 100 ml per hour of 5% dextrose in water and 100 ml per hour of Normosol-R. The amount of dextrose in the water solution can be adjusted up to 10% or even 15% to reach the 4–8 mg/kg/min that is often needed. The challenge with this approach is that the fluid rate often needs to be adjusted based on the hydration needs of the foal. If the fluid rate needs to be increased but the dextrose rate needs to be decreased, new fluids will need to be made or the amount of dilution calculated.

Another approach is to "piggyback" a 50% dextrose solution onto the fluids that are being used and adjusting the rates of the dextrose solution and isotonic fluids independently. This allows the dextrose rate to be adjusted without affecting the overall fluid rate. With this approach, a separate fluid pump is needed; it is very important to consider how the 50% dextrose interacts with other fluids in the administration line and to be cognizant of whether this hypertonic fluid is being administered through a central vein.

Hyponatremia

Hyponatremia represents excess free water in relation to the total amount of sodium and is a condition well recognized in foals [37, 39]. A foal that is hyponatremic can be hypovolemic, normovolemic, or hypervolemic. While it is easiest to identify foals with extreme hypervolemia or hypovolemia, more subtle changes in volume status can be challenging. Alternatively, a short list of common differentials for hyponatremia in neonatal foals includes diarrhea, renal failure, uroperitoneum, excess free water administration/consumption, and syndrome of inappropriate antidiuretic hormone (ADH) secretion. As a general approach, the diagnosis of diarrhea/enteritis, renal failure, and ruptured bladder is relatively straightforward and covered in other chapters. Recognizing excess free water due to excessive administration or consumption can be more challenging and often requires a careful history and evaluation of the neurologic status of the foal. Finally, the syndrome of inappropriate ADH secretion (SIADH) is based on a specific set of criteria including euvolemia, inappropriate urinary concentration, decreased extracellular fluid volume (ECFV) osmolality, increase urinary sodium concentration, an absence of renal insufficiency or other endocrine disorder, and absence of diuretic administration [40].

As hyponatremia develops, there is a tendency for water to move from the ECFV into the cells. As water moves into cells in the brain, neurologic signs can develop. As the serum sodium concentration is corrected with fluid therapy, there is the potential for water to quickly move out of the cells, resulting in osmotic demyelination syndrome. The treatment of hyponatremia depends not only on the cause but also on the severity. Treatment for hyponatremia is also covered in Chapter 32, with the following providing basic guidelines for treatment of severe hyponatremia that may need to be addressed regardless of the cause.

Foals with serum sodium concentrations <125 mmol/l are candidates for specific treatment for hyponatremia, but foals often do not show clinical signs until concentrations ≤110 mmol/l. The speed at which the sodium concentration drops may affect the presence of clinical signs. Treatment of hyponatremia <120 mmol/l involves gradually raising the sodium concentration in the blood using a fluid with a higher sodium content. In people, 3% hypertonic saline can be used as either a bolus or CRI and both methods appear to be equally effective [41]. In foals, an isotonic crystalloid (Normosol-R or LRS) is often used; alternatively, the relatively hypertonic 0.9% saline can be administered. The goal of treatment is to increase sodium concentration by approximately 0.5 mmol/l/hr while not exceeding a change of >10–12 mmol/l in a 24-hour period. Frequent monitoring (every 2–6 hours) is required, and overcorrection is possible. If the serum sodium concentration is increased too rapidly, osmotic demyelination syndrome can occur [41].

Hypernatremia

Hypernatremia represents a free water deficit relative to the amount of total sodium in the foal. Similar to hyponatremia, the foal can be hypovolemic, euvolemic, or hypervolemic and still have significant hypernatremia. Thus, the sodium concentration only reflects the balance between sodium and water and not the absolute amount of sodium in the foal. Hypernatremia is observed less commonly in foals, but a case series has been reported where sepsis and neonatal maladjustment syndrome were the most common conditions associated with this disorder [42]. Other possible causes include water deprivation, improper mixing of milk replacers, iatrogenic administration of high sodium fluids, lack of thirst mechanism, and diuretic administration.

In general, foals with working kidneys, access to free water and/or milk with a low sodium concentration, and an intact thirst mechanism usually do not develop severe hypernatremia. In foals that are receiving milk replacer and do not have access to free water, mixing errors in the preparation of the milk replacer (e.g. too little water for the amount of powder) can lead to hypernatremia. If the foal has no other source of fluid intake, the hypernatremia can be severe. Similarly, hospitalized foals given IV fluids with a high concentration of sodium without access to free water (enteral or parenteral) will also develop hypernatremia depending on the sodium concentration of the fluid being administered. While diuretic administration would be unlikely to cause hypernatremia in most foals, it is possible with prolonged use of certain diuretics if the appropriate fluid is not being administered.

As hypernatremia develops and the osmolality of the ECFV increases, water will move out of the cells. To prevent this movement, idiogenic osmoles are generated by cells to help retain water within the cells and maintain a more normal cell volume. As the serum sodium concentration begins to drop with treatment, water will now move back into the cells due to these idiogenic osmoles. This increased influx of water can damage the cells and cause neurologic sequelae.

Similar to hyponatremia, correction of hypernatremia should occur at a slow rate that does not exceed approximately 0.5 mmol/hr. In mild to moderate cases of hypernatremia, this can be achieved with isotonic crystalloid fluids. However, in cases with severe hypernatremia (170 mmol/l), fluids with a sodium concentration approximately halfway between Normosol-R (140 mmol/l) and the patient's sodium concentration should be used (i.e. adding hypertonic saline to Normosol-R to increase sodium to specific mmol/l). As the sodium concentration decreases, the administered fluid will need to be adjusted.

Hypokalemia

The majority of potassium in animals is located intracellularly. As the newborn foal grows, there is a net retention of potassium over time to account for growth and the shift to a relatively larger intracellular fluid volume. Mare's milk and foal milk replacers are rich in potassium and are adequate in the foal that is nursing or drinking normal quantities. However, if foals are not receiving enteral nutrition, they may have a dramatically decreased intake of potassium. In addition to the potential for decreased potassium intake, many sick neonatal foals receive significant volumes of IV fluids that promote diuresis and leads to increased excretion of potassium in the urine. Additionally, dextrose and/or insulin administration (if part of the treatment plan) promotes movement of potassium out of the extracellular fluid space and into cells. Foals can also have a low serum magnesium concentration, which is yet another factor that can contribute to hypokalemia (Table 62.5) [43].

For these reasons, hypokalemia is often observed in sick neonatal foals undergoing treatment with IV fluids. Hypokalemia can contribute to clinical signs of weakness and cardiac arrhythmias, but most clinical signs in sick foals are attributable to the primary disease. Regardless, the correction of hypokalemia is usually recommended, and potassium chloride (KCl) is typically added to IV maintenance fluids. The general rule for potassium supplementation is that the rate of administration should not exceed 0.5 mEq/kg/hr of KCl. For an average foal that weighs 50 kg, this equates to 25mEq of KCl/hour. Mild cases of hypokalemia often resolve as foals begin enteral feeding.

Hyperkalemia

Potassium concentrations above the normal range in foals are most commonly related to abnormalities of the urogenital system including ruptured bladder and acute renal failure (Table 62.6) [44]. Excess potassium administration in fluids (parenteral or enteral) is a less common cause. Hyperkalemia can be a life-threatening emergency and

Table 62.5 Factors contributing to hypokalemia in neonatal foals.

Decreased intake if unable to tolerate enteral feeding
Intravenous fluid diuresis
Dextrose and insulin administration
Hypomagnesemia

Table 62.6 Common causes of hyperkalemia in foals.

Acute renal failure
Ruptured bladder
Excessive potassium administration in oral or IV fluids

therefore the cause should be identified quickly and treatment initiated as soon as possible.

There are five core treatment principles for hyperkalemia:

1) *Slow administration of IV calcium*. Calcium helps protect the heart from the effects of hyperkalemia. This treatment is often not used until the potassium concentrations exceeds 6–6.5 mmol/l. However, some clinicians may institute this treatment at lower concentrations of potassium if there are concerns that the level is rising rapidly. Calcium administration will not have a significant effect on the actual potassium concentration but can mitigate the electrocardiogram abnormalities. A common approach is to dilute 50 ml of 23% calcium gluconate in 1 l of IV fluids and administer over 30 minutes. If the foal is in acute renal failure, the fluid volume may need to be reduced to 500 ml or less to prevent fluid overload.
2) *Diuresis with IV fluid administration*. Fluid administration and increased urine production helps remove potassium from the extracellular fluid and decrease the concentration. While fluids that do not contain potassium (saline, bicarbonate) would theoretically be preferred compared to potassium-containing fluids, research from other species suggests that other properties of the fluid (e.g., acidity) are more important than the potassium concentration when treating hyperkalemia [45]. A balanced crystalloid such as Normosol-R may be appropriate at a rate of 20 ml/kg/hr over 1 hour.
3) *Fluids containing dextrose*. The rapid administration of fluids containing large amounts of dextrose can have adverse effects on fluid balance and metabolism. Administering dextrose at a rate of 8 mg/kg/min can help release endogenous insulin and move potassium into the intracellular space.
4) *Exogenous insulin administration*. While insulin administration has been shown to be an effective technique for lowering the potassium concentration, it is important to recognize that critically ill neonatal foals may already have deranged metabolism and insulin will need to be administered carefully. IV dextrose will almost always be administered concurrently, and blood glucose concentrations should be monitored to avoid hypoglycemia or hyperglycemia. An insulin infusion rate of 0.01 IU/kg/hr is a reasonable starting rate for insulin but may need to be increased if the glucose levels are stable and hyperkalemia is refractory.
5) *Other treatments* such as furosemide or beta-agonists can be used in addition to those outlined above [46]. Furosemide can be administered as a CRI at a rate of 0.12 mg/kg/hr and most clinicians use this same dose in foals [31]. There is minimal information on the safety and efficacy of using beta-agonists for the treatment of hyperkalemia in foals, but it has been shown to be effective in other species [47]. Bicarbonate administration has been evaluated for the treatment of hyperkalemia in calves, though evidence of its efficacy in humans has been equiovacal [48].

Hypochloremia

Similar to hyperchloremia, chloride concentrations can mirror sodium in cases of free water excess or present in the face of normal or increased sodium concentrations. Hypochloremia is present with hyponatremia in cases of ruptured bladder and excess free water administration but can also be present in septic foals [44, 49]. In many cases, treatment of the sodium disorder resolves the hypochloremia when balanced crystalloid solutions are used.

Hypochloremia with a normal or increased sodium concentration is not common in neonatal foals. This abnormality can be observed in foals being treated with isotonic bicarbonate solutions for maintenance fluid therapy or in foals that have metabolic compensation for an ongoing respiratory acidosis. As a general rule, hypochloremia rarely requires specific treatment in neonatal foals beyond that of the primary condition leading to the electrolyte abnormality.

Hyperchloremia

Hyperchloremia is not a commonly discussed electrolyte abnormality in neonatal foals, though in one study, ill foals had a significantly higher chloride concentration than control animals [50]. Hyperchloremia can be seen in conjunction with hypernatremia, particularly where free water is not available and milk replacer has not been prepared correctly. In foals with enteritis, hyperchloremia can be observed [50]. In some foals with diarrhea, a relative hyperchloremia is often seen where the chloride concentration can be normal in conjunction with a decreased sodium concentration. Hyperchloremia can also develop in foals receiving parenteral nutrition if the chloride content in the amino acid solutions is significantly increased [51]. In cases of free water deficits (where sodium and chloride have increased together), treatment of hyponatremia typically resolves the hyperchloremia as well. It is often unnecessary to make special adjustments to the fluid for chloride. In cases of hyperchloremia associated with enteritis, administration of isotonic sodium bicarbonate (often supplemented with other electrolytes such as potassium) may be needed to resolve the hyperchloremia (Table 62.7).

Calcium

Sepsis is one of the more common causes of hypocalcemia encountered in hospitalized equine neonates [52, 53]. Monitoring ionized calcium allows the clinician to identify hypocalcemia early in the course of disease. Calcium

Table 62.7 General tips for electrolyte disorders in foals.

1) Sodium disorders should be corrected slowly depending on the chronicity of the abnormality.
2) Hyperkalemia needs to be addressed as an emergency.
3) Hypokalemia usually results from a combination of decreased intake and renal losses.
4) Chloride abnormalities that parallel changes in sodium concentration are often resolved with the treatment of the dysnatremia.
5) Hypochloremia does not typically require treatment with fluids containing high concentrations of chloride.

supplementation is usually started when Ca^{++} falls below the normal range and a rate of 1 ml/kg/day of 23% calcium gluconate is often used IV when available. Calcium is diluted in a larger volume of IV fluids and given over hours and should not be combined with bicarbonate or incompatible medications. Thoroughbred foals that do not respond to calcium supplementation may be affected by a genetic refractory hypocalcemia [54, 55].

Magnesium

Total magnesium has been evaluated in healthy and sick newborn foals and shown to be increased in nonsurviving foals [56]. In one study, septic foals did not have significantly different ionized magnesium concentrations compared to healthy foals [53]. Magnesium supplementation has been described for the treatment of hypoxic ischemic encephalopathy in foals, as well as for the treatment of ventricular arrhythmias [57]. Foals with hypomagnesemia and consistent clinical signs may be candidates for treatment; however, maintenance fluids such as Normosol-R already contain magnesium. Infusions at rates of 25 mg/kg/h of magnesium have been described [57].

Fluid Overload

Fluid overload is usually described as an absolute gain in total body water with or without clinical signs, but overload can also be relative where clinical signs (e.g. edema) develop without an absolute excess in total body water. This might occur when a severely dehydrated patient with acute anuric renal failure is rapidly given a large volume of IV fluids. In this case, the animal may still have a total body water deficit, but the rapidly given fluids have overwhelmed the ECFV and the patient develops signs of fluid overload. Clinical signs of fluid overload typically occur when there is excess fluid in the ECFV that is accumulating outside of the vascular space. A detailed discussion of fluid balance is beyond the scope of this chapter, but the concepts are usually discussed using the Starling equation;

$$\text{Net filtration} = K_f\left[\left(P_{cap} - P_{int}\right) - \left(\pi_{plasma} - \pi_{int}\right)\right]$$

The factors affecting fluid movement between the vascular space and interstitium include capillary permeability (K_f), plasma oncotic pressure (π_{plasma}), interstitial oncotic pressure (π_{int}), interstitial hydrostatic pressure (P_{int}), and capillary hydrostatic pressure (P_{cap}). Newer research has elucidated the role of the glycocalyx in fluid balance and the changes that occur with inflammation leading to fluid movement into the interstitium. From a clinical standpoint, it is still easiest to consider factors that place the patient at risk for fluid overload (Table 62.8) and how best to manage these foals.

Dystocia/Cesarean section (C-section)

Foals born following a difficult dystocia, especially if a C-section is required, appear to be at high risk for developing fluid overload during hospitalization. While some of these foals develop sepsis and have other risk factors, in the author's experience the post-C-section foal is one of the most likely patients to develop fluid overload. From the beginning of treatment, the rate of fluid administration and total amount of fluids administered for the neonatal foal following dystocia and/or C-section should be considered very carefully. These foals should be intensively monitored for signs of excess fluid accumulation even if clinical signs have not yet developed.

Systemic Inflammatory Response Syndrome/Sepsis

The systemic inflammatory response syndrome (SIRS) can be associated with changes in the glycocalyx and capillary permeability as well as hypoproteinemia [58]. Additionally, these foals are often receiving large amounts of fluids for resuscitation, maintenance, as well as infusions of antibiotics and other medications. AKI can occur even if the creatinine values are still in the reported normal ranges. These factors contribute to creating a patient that is prone to fluid overload.

Table 62.8 List of common conditions associated with fluid overload in foals.

Foals born following prolonged dystocia and/or C-section
Systemmic inflammatory response syndrome – (with or without sepsis)
Hypoproteinemia
Anuric/oliguric renal failure
Heart failure
Blood product administration

Hypoproteinemia

Foals develop hypoproteinemia for many reasons, including failure of passive transfer, liver disease, malnutrition, and protein losing enteropathies [59]. While hypoproteinemia as an isolated laboratory result might not lead to fluid overload, this abnormality combined with aggressive fluid resuscitation or changes in capillary permeability creates a patient at risk for fluid gain.

Renal Failure

Acute kidney injury is common is neonatal foals treated at intensive care units and results from hypoxic injury, sepsis, nephrotoxic medications, and hypovolemia [39, 60]. Decreases in glomerular filtration rate and urine output can quickly result in fluid overload, particularly if IV fluids are administered at an aggressive rate. Patients with decreased urine output in the face of normovolemia should be watched carefully for fluid overload, particularly if kidney values are increasing or above the normal range. Renal failure is one of the most difficult factors to manage in the context of fluid overload because the options for improving renal function are limited in many settings.

Heart Failure

Heart failure is not a common cause of fluid overload in newborn foals. However, foals with altered myocardial function should be considered at risk for fluid overload and fluid administration should be carefully monitored.

Recognizing Fluid Overload

Identifying patients at risk for fluid overload and modifying the fluid therapy plan accordingly is an extremely important. In these high-risk patients (or any neonatal foal in the ICU), careful monitoring for early signs of fluid overload is essential. Clinical examination, body weight monitoring, monitoring fluid ins/outs, laboratory testing, and hemodynamic monitoring are all methods to recognize fluid overload, but these methods can have conflicting results [61].

Clinical examination findings including peripheral edema formation in the triceps region or distal limbs suggest that fluid overload may be occurring. Changes in respiratory effort/rate or auscultation of abnormal lung sounds are also potential indications of fluid overload. Frothy nasal discharge associated with fulminant pulmonary edema would be consistent with severe and life-threatening fluid overload.

Monitoring fluid ins/outs requires serial recording of fluid administration including IV crystalloids, colloids, and fluids used to administer medications (particularly continuous infusions). Additionally, some percentage of parenteral nutrition can also be counted as fluid intake. Enteral fluid administration should also be recorded. Fluid outs include urination that is ideally measured through a closed catheter system attached to the foal (Figure 62.1). Other "outs" include diarrhea and other losses, but these are difficult to quantify. Foals in which the "ins" far exceed the "outs" are likely to be experiencing some form of fluid overload even if clinical signs have not developed.

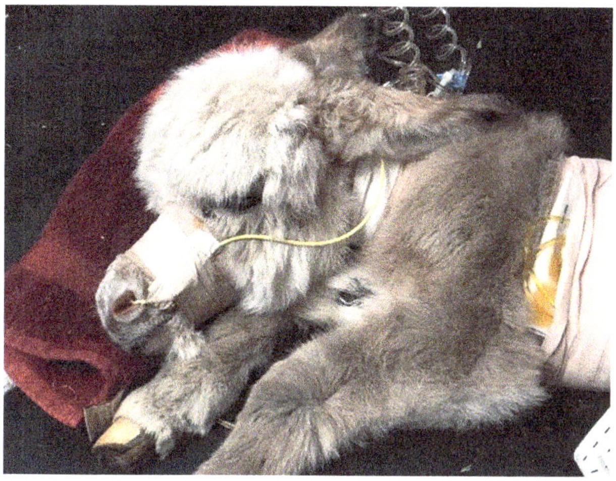

Figure 62.1 Miniature donkey foal with closed urinary system attached to the patient.

Perhaps the simplest and most effective way to monitor fluid overload is to record body weight multiple times per day. Many ICUs measure body weight daily in stable foals that are not at high risk of fluid overload but may record the weight two to three times per day in foals at higher risk. The temperament of the mare and the foal as well as available staffing are factors that make this challenging in some patients. Average weight gain of more than 1–2% per day would be a warning sign that fluid overload may occur.

Laboratory testing may help raise concerns for fluid overload, but it is often difficult to use in isolation. For example, a sudden drop in packed cell volume could occur with fluid overload, but also following neonatal isoerythrolysis or hemorrhage. Similarly, a drop in total protein might be from excessive fluid expansion of the vascular space but could also indicate worsening gastrointestinal disease with a protein losing enteropathy. Changes in the partial pressure of arterial oxygen could suggest fluid overload affecting oxygenation but might also be associated with developing or worsening lung disease. Ultimately, laboratory values can support a concern of fluid overload, but are difficult to use without other corroborating evidence.

Hemodynamic monitoring is often considered an important tool for monitoring fluid overload. Specifically, persistent increases in central venous pressure would be consistent with fluid overload and have been associated with increased mortality in children [62]. However, strong evidence is not available to suggest that CVP monitoring can help prevent fluid overload. Hemodynamic variables such as pulse pressure variation could be useful in ventilated patients to help gauge the need for fluids and are likely superior to CVP monitoring [63]. This technique would be limited to very sick foals that are quietly resting on ventilators.

In summary, monitoring changes in weight, computing fluid ins/outs, and frequently evaluating for peripheral edema may be some of the best ways to detect fluid overload early. Once fluid overload is recognized, specific steps can be taken to modify the treatment plan and prevent worsening of clinical signs.

Treatment of Fluid Overload

Foals with mild signs of fluid overload (e.g., minimal distal limb edema) may not require specific treatment particularly if the foal's clinical condition is improving and the foal is becoming stronger and more ambulatory. If the foal is early in the course of treatment (first 24 hours after C-section) or the clinical signs are moderate to severe, changes to the treatment plan are warranted.

Changing the rate of IV fluid administration is one of the simplest steps that helps modify fluid overload. If the rate of fluid administration is above normal and the foal is stable with good urine output and renal function, then decreasing the fluid rate by 30–50% is a very reasonable first step. Blood lactate values, renal function, and urine output should be monitored when this type of change is made. Foals that already have compromised renal function or signs of poor perfusion may be more difficult to manage on lower fluid rates. These challenging foals may require alternative support in the form of inotropes or vasopressors. Ideally, the lowest fluid rate should be used that does not result in hypoperfusion and detrimental changes in organ function. Unfortunately, that ideal rate is not clear a priori and sometimes an element of trial and error is necessary.

Changing the type of IV fluid is another strategy when signs of fluid overload occur. While the argument has been made that colloids could be used to treat patients with fluid overload to prevent worsening edema, there is little evidence that this strategy is successful. Decreasing the rate of fluid administration or increasing the rate of fluid excretion is likely to be more effective than changing the type of fluid administered.

In foals with anuric or oliguric renal failure, improving the rate of fluid removal should be considered a priority as fluid overload develops. The use of diuretics, specifically furosemide, is often a practical option with CRI being commonly used. A more detailed discussion of the treatments for renal failure is included in Chapter 26.

Renal replacement therapies (RRT) have been described in foals and are another means to facilitate fluid removal, but this treatment option is not widely available [64]. Even in foals without renal failure but signs of severe fluid overload (i.e. pulmonary edema), a combination of judicious fluid administration combined with diuretic administration may represent the best "rescue" option when fluid overload becomes a clinical problem. In all cases, treatment of the primary condition (sepsis, heart failure, etc.) should be a priority.

In summary, the art and science of fluid therapy in equine practice is required at the highest level with equine neonates. The choice to use fluid therapy, the type of fluid, the rate of fluid administration, and the stopping point are all critical. Core principles and controversies are noted involving this topic, but continued research and clinical practice improve our understanding of how to manage these challenging patients.

References

1 Magdesian, K.G. (2015). Chapter 22: Fluid therapy for neonatal foals. In: *Equine Fluid Therapy*, 1e (ed. C.L. Fielding and K.G. Magdesian), 279–298. Hoboken, NJ: Wiley.
2 Palmer, J.E. (2004). Fluid therapy in the neonate: not your mother's fluid space. *Vet. Clin. North Am. Equine Pract.* 20: 63–75.
3 Koch, A. and Kaske, M. (2008). Clinical efficacy of intravenous hypertonic saline solution or hypertonic bicarbonate solution in the treatment of inappetent calves with neonatal diarrhea. *J. Vet. Intern. Med.* 22: 202–211.
4 Holbert, R.D., Pearson, J.E., and Gonzalez, F.M. (1976). Effect of sodium acetate infusion on renal function in the dog. *Arch. Int. Pharmacodyn. Ther.* 219: 211–222.
5 Connor, H., Woods, H.F., Murray, J.D. et al. (1982). Utilization of L(+) lactate in patients with liver disease. *Ann. Nutr. Metab.* 26: 308–314.
6 Rein, J.L. and Coca, S.G. (2019). "I don't get no respect": the role of chloride in acute kidney injury. *Am. J. Physiol. Renal Physiol.* 316: F587–F605.
7 Barhight, M.F., Nelson, D., Moran, T. et al. (2021). Association between the use of balanced fluids and outcomes in critically ill children: a before and after study. *Crit. Care* 25: 266.
8 van Haren, F.M., Sleigh, J., Boerma, E.C. et al. (2012). Hypertonic fluid administration in patients with septic shock: a prospective randomized controlled pilot study. *Shock* 37: 268–275.

9 Berchtold, J.F., Constable, P.D., Smith, G.W. et al. (2005). Effects of intravenous hyperosmotic sodium bicarbonate on arterial and cerebrospinal fluid acid–base status and cardiovascular function in calves with experimentally induced respiratory and strong ion acidosis. *J. Vet. Intern. Med.* 19: 240–251.
10 Mitra, S. and Khandelwal, P. (2009). Are all colloids same? How to select the right colloid? *Indian J. Anaesth.* 53: 592–607.
11 Struden, M.S., Heckel, K., Goetz, A. et al. (2011). Perioperative fluid and volume management: physiological basis, tools and strategies. *Ann. Int. Care* 1: 2.
12 Niemi, T.T., Miyashita, R., and Yamakage, M. (2010). Colloid solutions: a clinical update. *J. Anesth.* 24: L913–L925.
13 Jungheinrich, C. and Neff, T.A. (2005). Pharmacokinetics of hydroxyethyl starch. *Clin. Pharmacokinet.* 44: 681–699.
14 Brunkhorst, F.M., Engel, C., Bloos, F. et al. (2008). Intensive insulin therapy and pentastarch resuscitation in severe sepsis. *N. Engl. J. Med.* 358: 125–139.
15 Schortgen, F., Lacherade, J.C., Bruneel, F. et al. (2001). Effects of hydroxyethylstarch and gelatin on renal function in severe sepsis: a multicenter randomized study. *Lancet* 357: 911–916.
16 Blong, A., Epstein, K., and Brainard, B. (2013). In vitro effect of three formulations of hydroxyethyl starch solutions on coagulation and platelet function in horses. *Am. J. Vet. Res.* 74: 712–720.
17 Epstien, K.L., Bergren, A., Giguere, S. et al. (2014). Cardiovascaular, colloid osmotic pressure, and hemostatic effects of 2 formulations of hydroxyethyl starch in healthy horses. *J. Vet. Intern. Med.* 28: 223–233.
18 Schusser, G.F., Rieckhoff, K., Ungemach, F.R. et al. (2007). Effect of hydroxyethyl starch solution in normal horses and horses with colic or acute colitis. *J. Vet. Med. A Physiol. Pathol. Clin. Med.* 54: 592–598.
19 Jones, P.A., Tomasic, M., and Gentry, P.A. (1997). Oncotic, hemodilutional, and hemostatic effects of isotonic saline and hydroxyethyl starch solutions in clinically normal ponies. *Am. J. Vet. Res.* 58: 541–548.
20 Nearman, H.S. and Herman, M.L. (1997). Toxic effects of colloids in the intensive care unit. *Crit. Care Clin.* 7: 713–723.
21 Moran, M. and Kapsner, C. (1987). Acute renal failure associated with elevated plasma oncotic pressure. *N. Engl. J. Med.* 317: 150–153.
22 Chinitz, J.L., Kim, K.E., Onesti, G. et al. (1971). Pathophysiology and prevention of dextran-40-induced anuria. *J. Lab. Clin. Med.* 77: 76–87.
23 Langeron, O., Doelberg, M., Ang, E.T. et al. (2001). Voluven, a substituted novel hydroxyethyl starch (HES 130/0.4), causes fewer effect on coagulation in major orthopedic surgery than HES 200/0.5. *Anesth. Analg.* 92: 855–862.
24 Konrad, C.J., Markl, T.J., Schuepfer, G.K. et al. (2000). In vitro effects of different medium molecular hydrocyethyl starch solutions and lactated Ringer's solution on coagulation using SONOCLOT. *Anesth. Analg.* 90: 274–279.
25 Westphal, M., James, M.F., Kozek-Langenecker, S. et al. (2009). Hydroxyethyl starches: Different products-different effects. *Anesthesiology* 111: 187–202.
26 Hepworth-Warren, K.L., Wong, D.M., Hay-Kraus, B.L. et al. (2015). Effects of administration of a synthetic low molecular weight/low molar substitution hydroxyethyl starch solution in healthy neonatal foals. *Can. Vet. J.* 56: 1069–1074.
27 Upadhyay, M., Singhi, S., Murlidharan, J. et al. (2005). Randomized evaluation of fluid resuscitation with crystalloid (saline) and colloid (polymer from degraded gelatin in saline) in pediatric septic shock. *Indian Pediatr.* 42: 223–231.
28 Peek, S.F., Semrad, S., McGuirk, S.M. et al. (2006). Prognostic value of clinicopathologic variables obtained at admission and effect of antiendotoxin plasma on survival in septic and critically ill foals. *J. Vet. Intern. Med.* 20: 569–574.
29 Drobin, D. and Hahn, R.G. (2002). Kinetics of isotonic and hypertonic plasma volume expanders. *Anesthesiology* 96: 1371–1380.
30 Matsushita, F.Y., Krebs, V.L.J., and de Carvalho, W.B. (2021 Nov 2). Association between fluid overload and mortality in newborns: a systematic review and meta-analysis. *Pediatr. Nephrol.* https://doi.org/10.1007/s00467-021-05281-8. Epub ahead of print. PMID: 34727245.
31 Tuzun, F., Akcura, Y., Duman, N. et al. (2020). Comparison of isotonic and hypotonic intravenous fluids in term newborns: is it time to quit hypotonic fluids. *J. Matern. Fetal Neonatal Med.* 29: 1–6.
32 Buchanan, B.R., Sommardahl, C.S., Rohrbach, B.W. et al. (2005). Effect of a 24-hour infusion of an isotonic electrolyte replacement fluid on the renal clearance of electrolytes in healthy neonatal foals. *J. Am. Vet. Med. Assoc.* 227: 1123–1129.
33 Holliday, M.A. and Segar, W.E. (1957). The maintenance need for water in parenteral fluid therapy. *Pediatrics* 19: 823–832.
34 Amano, Y. (2020). Estimated basal metabolic rate and maintenance fluid volume in children: A proposal for a new equation. *Pediatr. Int.* 62: 522–528.
35 Meyers, R.S. (2009). Pediatric fluid and electrolyte therapy. *J. Pediatr. Pharmacol. Ther.* 14: 204–211.
36 Fuchs, J., Adams, S.T., and Byerley, J. (2017). Current Issues in Intravenous Fluid Use in Hospitalized Children. *Rev. Recent Clin. Trials* 12: 284–289.
37 Dunkel, B., Dodson, F., Chang, Y.M. et al. (2020). Retrospective evaluation of the association between

hyponatremia and neurological dysfunction in hospitalized foals (2012–2016): 109 cases. *J. Vet. Emerg. Crit. Care* 30: 66–73.
38 Hollis, A.R., Furr, M.O., Magdesian, K.G. et al. (2008). Blood glucose concentrations in critically ill neonatal foals. *J. Vet. Intern. Med.* 22: 1223–1227.
39 Collins, N.M., Axon, J.E., Carrick, J.B. et al. (2016). Severe hyponatraemia in foals: clinical findings, primary diagnosis and outcome. *Aust. Vet. J.* 94: 186–191.
40 Yasir, M. and Mechanic, O.J. (2021). Syndrome of inappropriate antidiuretic hormone secretion. In: *StatPearls [Internet]*. Treasure Island, FL: StatPearls Publishing https://www.statpearls.com/articlelibrary/viewarticle/29810/.
41 Baek, S.H., Jo, Y.H., Ahn, S. et al. (2021). Risk of Overcorrection in Rapid Intermittent Bolus vs Slow Continuous Infusion Therapies of Hypertonic Saline for Patients With Symptomatic Hyponatremia: The SALSA Randomized Clinical Trial. *JAMA Intern. Med.* 181: 81–92.
42 Collins, N.M., Carrick, J.B., Russell, C.M. et al. (2018). Hypernatraemia in 39 hospitalised foals: clinical findings, primary diagnosis and outcome. *Aust. Vet. J.* 96: 385–389.
43 al-Ghamdi, S.M., Cameron, E.C., and Sutton, R.A. (1994). Magnesium deficiency: pathophysiologic and clinical overview. *Am. J. Kidney Dis.* 24: 737–752.
44 Dunkel, B., Palmer, J.E., Olson, K.N. et al. (2005). Uroperitoneum in 32 foals: influence of intravenous fluid therapy, infection, and sepsis. *J. Vet. Intern. Med.* 19: 889–893.
45 Cunha, M.G., Freitas, G.C., Carregaro, A.B. et al. (2010). Renal and cardiorespiratory effects of treatment with lactated Ringer's solution or physiologic saline (0.9% NaCl) solution in cats with experimentally induced urethral obstruction. *Am. J. Vet. Res.* 71: 840–846.
46 Johansson, A.M., Gardner, S.Y., Levine, J.F. et al. (2003). Furosemide continuous rate infusion in the horse: evaluation of enhanced efficacy and reduced side effects. *J. Vet. Intern. Med.* 17: 887–895.
47 Long, B., Warix, J.R., and Koyfman, A. (2018). Controversies in Management of Hyperkalemia. *J. Emerg. Med.* 55: 192–205.
48 Trefz, F.M., Constable, P.D., and Lorenz, I. (2017). Effect of Intravenous Small-Volume Hypertonic Sodium Bicarbonate, Sodium Chloride, and Glucose Solutions in Decreasing Plasma Potassium Concentration in Hyperkalemic Neonatal Calves with Diarrhea. *J. Vet. Intern. Med.* 31: 907–921.
49 Dembek, K.A., Onasch, K., Hurcombe, S.D. et al. (2013). Renin-Angiotensin-aldosterone system and hypothalamic-pituitary-adrenal axis in hospitalized newborn foals. *J. Vet. Intern. Med.* 27: 331–338.
50 Viu, J., Armengou, L., Ríos, J. et al. (2017). Acid base imbalances in ill neonatal foals and their association with survival. *Equine Vet. J.* 49: 51–57.
51 Gomez, D.E., Biermann, N.M., and Sanchez, L.C. (2015). Physicochemical Approach to Determine the Mechanism for acid–base Disorders in 793 Hospitalized Foals. *J. Vet. Intern. Med.* 29: 1395–1402.
52 Myers, C.J., Magdesian, K.G., Kass, P.H. et al. (2009). Parenteral nutrition in neonatal foals: clinical description, complications and outcome in 53 foals (1995–2005). *Vet. J.* 181: 137–144.
53 Aguilera-Tejero, E. (2015). Calcium homeostasis and derangements. Chapter 5. In: *Equine Fluid Therapy*, 1e (ed. C.L. Fielding and K.G. Magdesian), 55–75. Hoboken, NJ: Wiley.
54 Hurcombe, S.D., Toribio, R.E., Slovis, N.M. et al. (2009). Calcium regulating hormones and serum calcium and magnesium concentrations in septic and critically ill foals and their association with survival. *J. Vet. Intern. Med.* 23: 335–343.
55 Rivas, V.N., Magdesian, K.G., Fagan, S. et al. (2020). A nonsense variant in Rap Guanine Nucleotide Exchange Factor 5 (RAPGEF5) is associated with equine familial isolated hypoparathyroidism in Thoroughbred foals. *PLos Genet.* 16: e1009028.
56 Mariella, J., Isani, G., Andreani, G. et al. (2016). Total plasma magnesium in healthy and critically ill foals. *Theriogenology* 85 (2): 180–185.
57 Stewart, A.J. (2015). Magnesium homeostasis and derangements. In: *Equine Fluid Therapy*, 1e (ed. C.L. Fielding and K.G. Magdesian), 76–87. Hoboken, NJ: Wiley.
58 Juffermans, N.P., van den Brom, C.E., and Kleinveld, D.J.B. (2020). Targeting Endothelial Dysfunction in Acute Critical Illness to Reduce Organ Failure. *Anesth. Analg.* 131: 1708–1720.
59 Magdesian, K.G., Hirsh, D.C., Jang, S.S. et al. (2002). Characterization of *Clostridium difficile* isolates from foals with diarrhea: 28 cases (1993–1997). *J. Am. Vet. Med. Assoc.* 220: 67–73.
60 Ellero, N., Freccero, F., Lanci, A. et al. (2020). Rhabdomyolysis and Acute Renal Failure Associated with Oxytetracycline Administration in Two neonatal foals affected by Flexural Limb Deformity. *Vet. Sci.* 7: 160.
61 Schneider, A.G., Baldwin, I., Freitag, E. et al. (2012). Estimation of fluid status changes in critically ill patients: fluid balance chart or electronic bed weight? *J. Crit. Care* 27: 745.e7–745.e12.
62 Choi, S.J., Ha, E.J., Jhang, W.K. et al. (2018). Elevated central venous pressure is associated with increased mortality in pediatric septic shock patients. *BMC Pediatr.* 18: 58.

63 Kannan, G., Loganathan, S., Kajal, K. et al. (2021 https://doi.org/10.1007/s12630-021-02130-y). The effect of pulse pressure variation compared with central venous pressure on intraoperative fluid management during kidney transplant surgery: a randomized controlled trial. *Can. J. Anaesth.* 69: 62–71.

64 Wong, D.M., Ruby, R.E., Eatroff, A. et al. (2017). Use of Renal Replacement Therapy in a Neonatal Foal with postresuscitation Acute Renal Failure. *J. Vet. Intern. Med.* 31: 593–597.

Chapter 63 Nonsteroidal Anti-inflammatory Drugs and Analgesics in the Neonatal Foal

Jennifer Davis

Nonsteroidal Anti-inflammatory Drugs (NSAIDs)

Nonsteroidal anti-inflammatory drugs (NSAIDs) are the most commonly used drugs for treatment of mild to moderate pain, inflammation, and pyrexia in adult horses (Table 63.1). Use in foals is less widespread due to concerns over potential adverse effects, as well as known alterations in pharmacokinetics in neonates. This makes determining safe dosage regimens difficult as they cannot be extrapolated from adult doses. These drugs work through inhibition of cyclooxygenase (COX), the enzyme responsible for converting arachidonic acid into prostaglandins. Blocking prostaglandins results in anti-inflammatory, analgesic, antipyretic, and antithrombotic effects.

Two different, distinct forms of COX have been identified in the horse. In simplified terms, COX-1 is the constitutively expressed form necessary for normal homeostatic mechanisms in the body, whereas COX-2 is the inducible form produced in response to injury [1]. For this reason, some newer NSAIDs target only COX-2 in an effort to inhibit the inflammatory response without inhibiting normal physiologic processes. While these drugs present a safer option for treatment, adverse effects associated with non-selective NSAID inhibition may still occur with administration, therefore careful monitoring is required during treatment.

Adverse Effects of NSAIDs

NSAID administration is frequently associated with gastric ulceration in multiple species and is well documented to occur under experimental conditions in horses and foals [1]. NSAIDs decrease production of prostaglandin E_2 (PGE_2), which is responsible for maintaining mucosal blood flow throughout the gastrointestinal (GI) tract. It is also responsible for mucosal healing in cases of preexisting disease. In the stomach, inhibition of COX can also increase acid secretion, decrease output of mucus and bicarbonate, impair vasodilation, and diminish epithelial restitution, cell division, and angiogenesis. Clinical signs often include anorexia, bruxism, ptyalism, diarrhea, and mild colic, although colic signs in foals may be severe. Prognosis for full recovery is good as long as lesions are diagnosed, NSAID administration is discontinued, and appropriate treatment is instituted.

Right dorsal colitis (RDC) is an ulcerative condition of the GI tract unique to horses. Lesions associated with RDC include mucosal ulceration, edema, neutrophilic inflammation, and mural thickening of the right dorsal colon. The etiology is thought to be similar to gastric ulceration, but it is not known why this particular segment of the intestine is affected greater than other areas. This condition has been diagnosed primarily in adult horses given toxic doses of NSAIDs, in particular phenylbutazone, as well as those receiving label doses when dehydrated [2]. Horses will show varying signs of colic and diarrhea and often have a low plasma protein concentration with or without signs of endotoxemia. Prognosis in cases of RDC is usually guarded unless recognized and treated early. Complications include chronic colic, colonic rupture or stricture. Ulceration in other parts of the GI tract typically occurs concurrently.

The kidneys are the other major organ susceptible to adverse effects following NSAID administration [3]. Inhibition of PGE_2 and PGI_2 result in dysregulation of renal blood flow and vasoconstriction of renal blood vessels. These effects are enhanced in dehydrated patients or those with preexisting renal disease that may already have compromised renal blood flow [4]. The lesions are characterized by medullary crest or papillary necrosis, as the medulla normally receives less blood flow than the cortex, making it more vulnerable to insult. These areas also

Equine Neonatal Medicine, First Edition. Edited by David M. Wong and Pamela A. Wilkins.

Table 63.1 Nonsteroidal anti-inflammatory drugs and analgesics used in neonatal foals.

Drug	Dose	Comments
NSAIDS		
Flunixin meglumine	1.1–1.65 mg/kg IV or PO q24–36h	Doses were determined in healthy foals. Lower doses or longer dosing intervals may be needed for septic foals. Use with caution in foals that are anorexic or dehydrated.
Phenylbutazone	2.2 mg/kg IV or PO q24h	
Ketoprofen	2.2–3.6 mg/kg IV or IM q24h	
Meloxicam	0.6 mg/kg IV or IM q 12–24h	
Firocoxib	0.1–0.2 mg/kg IV or PO q 12–24h	
Diclofenac	7.3 mg (1.27 cm strip) topically q 12h	
Opioids		
Buprenorphine	0.01–0.02 mg/kg IV or oral transmucosal (OTM)	Lower doses may produce sedation while higher doses produce mild excitement and increased locomotor activity. Higher doses needed for antinociception.
Butorphanol	0.005–0.05 mg/kg IV	
Fentanyl	100 μg/h transdermal patch (change q 72h)	
Tramadol	3 mg/kg IV	
Alpha-2 agonists		
Xylazine	0.5–1.0 mg/kg IV	May cause excessive sedation, respiratory depression and arrhythmias. Use with extreme caution in sick or septic foals.
Romifidine	0.07 mg/kg IV	
Detomidine	0.01–0.04 mg/kg IV	
Anticholinergics		
N-butylscopolammonium bromide	0.3 mg/kg IV	Single dose only. Visceral pain only.
Sodium channel blockers		
Lidocaine	1.3 mg/kg, loading dose IV; 0.05 mg/kg/min constant rate infusion	Accumulation of the metabolite occurs in septic foals, which may increase risk for adverse effects such as CNS excitement and cardiovascular collapse.

contribute most to concentrating urine; therefore, the most consistent laboratory finding is decreased urine specific gravity. Azotemia may also be detected with more severe disease. In acute NSAID toxicosis, overt hematuria (or occult blood) and increased white blood cells in the urine may be noted. In chronic cases, other than decreased urine specific gravity, urinalysis results are typically normal. Prognosis is related to duration of renal compromise prior to diagnosis, as well as response to fluid therapy. Horses that remain oliguric or anuric after aggressive therapy have a guarded prognosis.

Another potentially dangerous adverse effect of NSAIDs in horses relates to the route of administration. Deliberate intramuscular injection or accidental perivascular injection can result in severe injection site reactions, particularly with flunixin meglumine and phenylbutazone. Despite a label claim for this route of administration in horses, flunixin meglumine is highly irritating with reports of abscessation and clostridial myositis secondary to IM administration [5]. Perivascular injection of phenylbutazone can result in severe tissue necrosis and sloughing, with potential damage to underlying structures, including the esophagus, recurrent laryngeal nerves, vago-sympathetic trunk, and great vessels of the neck. Ketoprofen has a label for IM administration in some countries (not the US) and, being more water soluble and less irritating, has been used safely for short term administration IM in foals. Neither meloxicam nor firocoxib injections are labeled for IM use in the horse.

There are numerous other adverse effects of NSAIDs reported, although they do not appear to be common in the horse. NSAIDs can alter hemostasis through effects on platelets as well as vascular epithelium. Inhibition of COX-1 prevents platelet aggregation, which is catalyzed by thromboxane A_2. Inhibition of COX-2 blocks the release of prostacyclin (PGI_2) from intact vascular endothelium, which allows for spread of the platelet plug and initiation of intravascular clotting. Therefore, selective inhibition of COX-1 may lead to bleeding tendencies, whereas selective inhibition of COX-2 may lead to hypercoagulation. Immune-mediated hemolytic anemia/thrombocytopenia has rarely been attributed to NSAIDs in horses. Clinical signs should diminish with proper treatment and removal of the drug. Blood dyscrasias, including a fatal pancytopenic bone marrow failure, have been reported in humans and dogs exposed to phenylbutazone. Dose-dependent and dose-independent hepatotoxicity has been reported in some animal species, but not horses.

Flunixin Meglumine

Flunixin meglumine is frequently used for treatment of colic and endotoxemia. It has historically been considered inferior to phenylbutazone for musculoskeletal pain. However, it is commonly used over phenylbutazone in septic neonatal foals with concurrent septic arthritis due to its superior efficacy against the cardiovascular effects of endotoxin [6].

Flunixin meglumine is absorbed well orally in adult horses. Its bioavailability in neonates and older foals is unknown. Area under the curve, clearance, and half-life of flunixin meglumine are significantly greater in newborn foals (<24 hours old) compared to adult horses. The half-life increases from 1–2 hours in adults to 6–8 hours in foals [7]. These differences are no longer significant at 10 days of age [8]. Despite the differences in pharmacokinetics, thromboxane suppression was similar in 24- to 28-hour-old foals compared to 10- to 11-day-old and 28-day-old foals for up to 12 hours after administration of the same dose, suggesting increases in dosing are not necessary. The slower clearance, however may indicate that the dosing intervals should be longer in very young foals to decrease risks for toxicity.

Administration of escalating doses (0.55–6.6 mg/kg) of flunixin meglumine IV to neonatal foals for five consecutive days resulted in an increased incidence of diarrhea which appeared to be independent of dose [9]. Pathological lesions included ulceration of the glandular stomach, petechiation or congestion of the cecum, and petechiation, congestion, or edema of the colon, although these lesions were seen in placebo-treated foals as well. Chronic administration of flunixin meglumine orally (1.1 mg/kg q12h) or intramuscularly (1.1 mg/kg q24h) for 30 days resulted in glandular ulceration/erosions by either route and oral ulceration by the oral route [10].

There are no studies examining the pharmacokinetics and safety of flunixin meglumine in sick or septic neonates and older foals, but it is assumed they are higher risk for drug-induced toxicity compared to healthy foals. Caution should be used when dosing.

Phenylbutazone

Phenylbutazone is another popular NSAID used in adult horses. This drug is an affordable and effective treatment of musculoskeletal conditions, including navicular disease, laminitis, and chronic osteoarthritis. It has also been shown to be effective in preventing prostanoid production after endotoxin challenge; however, it is not as effective as flunixin in preventing the cardiovascular changes associated with endotoxin. Phenylbutazone also has a beneficial effect on gut motility and gastric emptying in an endotoxin challenge model [11].

Oral bioavailability of phenylbutazone approaches 91% in adult horses. The time to peak plasma concentration is affected by feeding a hay diet, which may affect foals as they age. Bioavailability has not been reported in foals but pharmacokinetic data are available for foals <24 hours old. Volume of distribution was larger, clearance was slower, and half-life was longer in neonatal foals compared to adults [12]. The pharmacokinetics of phenylbutazone are dose-dependent, with longer-elimination half-lives reported with higher doses. This is likely due to saturation of metabolizing enzymes, which can be assumed to occur in neonates as well. Phenylbutazone has an active metabolite, oxyphenbutazone. Exposure of foals to phenylbutazone or its metabolite through milk is minimal [13]; however, in utero exposure can occur. Both phenylbutazone and oxyphenbutazone cross the placenta, and the elimination of both are significantly prolonged in newborn foals compared to elimination in the mares [14].

Phenylbutazone has a higher incidence of adverse effects in horses and foals when compared to flunixin and ketoprofen. When administered at 5 mg/kg PO q12h for 7 days in 7- to 10-day-old foals, morphologic, histologic, and ultrasonographic changes in the kidney were seen, particularly in the medulla and the corticomedullary junction [15]. Chronic administration (12–42 days) of the same dose to older foals 3–10 months of age resulted in a high incidence of GI lesions (erosions, ulcerations), as well as elevated blood urea nitrogen, decreased total plasma protein, inappetence, and diarrhea [16]. Phenylbutazone has a direct cytotoxic effect on oral and esophageal mucosa. Therefore, it should not be used via the oral route in animals with dysphagia or decreased suckle reflex. The toxic effects are greatly amplified in horses that are anorexic or dehydrated. Sucralfate administration appears partially protective against mucosal lesions and diarrhea in foals [17].

There are no studies examining the pharmacokinetics and safety of phenylbutazone in sick or septic neonates and older foals. Due to the high risk of toxicity, use in foals is not recommended. If used, careful monitoring for adverse effects is required. The lowest effective dose at the longest effective dosing interval should be used.

Ketoprofen

Ketoprofen is labeled for use in horses for similar indications as flunixin meglumine and phenylbutazone. Ketoprofen is not as effective in reducing lameness scores in animals with navicular disease. Clinical efficacy in lameness, endotoxemia, and other inflammatory syndromes is similar to other NSAIDs when higher than label doses are administered. Oral formulations are not commercially available, however oral absorption of the injectable formulation is relatively high in adult horses. The injectable formulation is less irritating than flunixin meglumine or phenylbutazone, therefore repeated intramuscular injections rarely cause problems. Ketoprofen is a racemic mixture of R(−) and S(+) enantiomers. The S(+) enantiomer is responsible for the anti-inflammatory activity, but also the toxic effects of the drug. Chiral inversion occurs in the adult horse, resulting in higher concentrations of the S(+) enantiomer. Pharmacokinetics in the neonatal foal (<24 hours old) showed a slower clearance and a larger volume of distribution compared to adult horses, although specific enantiomers weren't studied [18].

Ketoprofen has a higher therapeutic index than either flunixin or phenylbutazone, with fewer adverse effects noted when used at the label dose in adult horses and miniature donkeys [19, 20]. Anecdotally, it is effective for fevers that are not responsive to flunixin meglumine and can be used as an anti-pyretic in foals.

Meloxicam

Meloxicam is a COX-2 selective inhibitor labeled for use as an anti-inflammatory drug in the horse in some countries (not the US). Pharmacokinetic-pharmacodynamic analysis of meloxicam in adult horses has shown a therapeutic effect at plasma concentrations of approximately 0.2 μg/ml, which translates into a daily dose of 0.6 mg/kg [21]. This dose has proven effective in lameness models, as well as experimental models of colic and abdominal pain. Meloxicam is typically given as an injection, however oral bioavailability is nearly complete, and absorption is not affected by feeding. Bioavailability of meloxicam in foals is not known; however, it has been studied per os [22]. Following oral administration of 0.6 mg/kg PO to foals 2–23 days of age, maximum concentrations were similar to adult horses administered the same dose. Oral clearance, however, was faster and half-life was shorter (2.5 hours in foals vs. 10.2 hours in horses).

Meloxicam may be a safer option for use in foals. Repeated oral dosing at 0.6 mg/kg PO q12h for 14 days in foals 17–33 days of age (at the start of dosing) did not reveal any clinical or clinicopathologic changes and only mild (grade 1) ulcerations on endoscopy [22]. Doses of up to 1.8 mg/kg PO q12h were also considered safe when administered for up to 7 days in foals less than 1 week old.

Firocoxib

Firocoxib is the most recent NSAID licensed for use in the horse. Paste, tablet, and injectable formulations are available. Of the drugs studied in the horse, it has the highest COX-2 selectivity. In adult horses, oral bioavailability is high, although maximum concentrations are relatively low and therapeutic concentrations are not reached until adequate drug accumulation has occurred (five to seven doses) [23–25]. For this reason, as well as a prolonged half-life in adult horses, a loading dose of three times the label dose is recommended for faster effect [25]. The pharmacokinetics differ significantly in foals <2 weeks of age. Firocoxib is more rapidly absorbed following oral administration of the paste formulation and reaches a higher initial maximum concentration [26]. Firocoxib administration in foals has a shorter half-life, however, which results in less drug accumulation with multiple doses. Steady state is achieved after approximately three doses, and a loading dose is not currently recommended. Intravenous dosing shows a more rapid plasma clearance compared to adults, although volume of distribution is comparable [27].

In healthy foals, no clinically apparent adverse effects were noted after oral administration at 0.1 mg/kg q24h for 9 consecutive days or IV at 0.09 mg/kg q24h for 7 days. No significant clinicopathologic changes or lesions on endoscopy were noted. Firocoxib may be a safer alternative to use in foals, but further work is needed to find the most effective dose. Higher doses and/or shorter dosing intervals may be required in foals to produce results comparable to those in adult horses.

Diclofenac

Diclofenac is a nonspecific COX inhibitor that may also inhibit the lipoxygenase pathway by reducing arachidonic acid release from cells, as well as enhancing its reincorporation into triglycerides. There are no reports of the use of diclofenac as a systemic anti-inflammatory agent in neonates, however topical preparations are available. A 1% liposomal cream is available in the United States for topical treatment of joint inflammation. It has good effects on pain and lameness scores, with minimal systemic absorption, and therefore minimal adverse effects [28, 29].

Topical diclofenac has been studied in foals 2–14 days of age. Application of 7.3 mg (1.27-cm strip of liposomal cream) q12h for 7 days resulted in maximum plasma concentrations of <1 ng/ml, suggesting minimal systemic exposure [30]. No changes in physical exam parameters, clinicopathologic measurements, urinalysis, gastroscopy, or ultrasonographic examination of the kidneys or right dorsal colon were noted during the course of treatment.

Opioid Drugs

Opioids are classically used for treatment of moderate to severe pain but can be useful as sedatives in neonatal foals. Drugs studied in foals work at either the μ or κ receptors. The μ receptors are associated with a greater analgesic effect, but they also cause the most side effects. Adverse effects of μ receptor agonists include bradycardia, hypoventilation, and GI ileus. These effects may exacerbate preexisting conditions in septic neonatal foals. The partial μ agonists produce less respiratory effects, however, there is a ceiling effect, which limits their use in severe pain. Kappa opioid agonists produce less ventilatory depression and may cause more sedation in foals. Buprenorphine, butorphanol, fentanyl, and tramadol have all been studied in foals.

Buprenorphine is a partial μ agonist labeled for use in horses in some countries (not the US) for postoperative analgesia and potentiation of sedative effects of α-2 agonists. When given alone, it may cause central nervous system (CNS) excitement in horses, and also caused increased locomotor activity in foals [31, 32]. Buprenorphine is considered long-acting compared to many opioid medications, with an elimination half-life of approximately 4 hours in adult horses. Pharmacokinetics in foals show a larger volume of distribution, and a faster drug clearance with a half-life of <2 hours [32]. Buprenorphine is administered transmucosally rather than orally to avoid first-pass metabolism in the gut and liver. Following transmucosal administration to foals, maximum concentrations (0.61 ± 0.11 ng/ml) approached therapeutic concentrations in other species and bioavailability was approximately 25%. In horses <1 year of age, analgesic effects have been noted with transmucosal administration, with no signs of concurrent CNS excitement. Intramuscular administration of 0.01 mg/kg to neonatal foals (2–11 days old) resulted in an antinociceptive effect [33]. Sedation when left undisturbed, increased locomotion when handled, and tachypnea were also noted.

Butorphanol is an opioid drug with κ receptor agonist and μ receptor antagonist effects. It is labeled for use in horses and has been studied extensively in equine colic, as well as for standing sedation and as an anti-tussive. It has also been evaluated in neonatal foals. Administration at 0.05 mg/kg IV to foals <14 days of age resulted in a higher volume of distribution, faster clearance and shorter half-life compared to adult horses [34]. Bioavailability after IM administration was only 66%, and neither route produced concentrations considered to be antinociceptive in horses (20–30 ng/ml). Subsequent evaluation of 0.1 mg/kg showed a significant antinociceptive effect for up to 2.5 hours after administration to neonatal (1–2 weeks old) and older foals (4–8 weeks old) [35]. Treated foals exhibit sedation, decreased responsiveness, and decreased physical activity as well as increased suckling behavior and mild decreases in respiratory rate, body temperature, and GI sounds.

Fentanyl is a very potent μ receptor agonist that also decreases the release of neurotransmitters involved in pain perception (e.g. substance P). It is frequently used in small animal medicine for severe pain, with minimal cardiorespiratory effects. However, due to its short half-life, it is typically administered as a constant rate infusion. Pharmacokinetics in neonatal foals also demonstrate a short elimination half-life (<1 hour). Doses of 0.004 mg/kg produce sedation, whereas doses >0.008 mg/kg produce ataxia, increased locomotor activity, muscle rigidity, head pressing, and recumbency [36]. Constant rate infusion doses have not been evaluated in foals but may present a method of administration that produces analgesia without adverse effects. Transdermal administration is another method to provide a constant level of drug exposure without high peaks associated with adverse effects. Application of commercially available transdermal patches containing fentanyl released at 100 μg/h produced detectable drug concentrations in plasma within 20 minutes [37]. Peak concentrations varied between 0.1–28.7 ng/ml and were not reached until a mean of 14 hours after patch application; concentrations were undetectable 12 hours after patch removal which occurred at 72 hours. No adverse effects were noted in that study; however, the results indicate transdermal fentanyl should not be used as the sole analgesic medication in foals.

Tramadol is a weak μ receptor agonist that also has effects on norepinephrine and serotonin reuptake. Its metabolite (M1) has 200× the opioid binding affinity of the parent compound and is associated with a greater analgesic effect in humans and cats. It is considered a mild analgesic in horses but is sometimes used in combination with NSAIDs. Adult horses make the active M1 metabolite; however, it is rapidly glucuronidated and inactivated [38]. The ability to glucuronidate the M1 metabolite is age-dependent, with significantly less glucuronidation occurring in the first week of life (6–8 days) compared to foals 2–6 weeks of age when administered at 3 mg/kg IV as a single dose [39]. Inactivity, muscle fasciculations, and weight shifting were noted in some foals, which did not appear to be age related. Data on the use of oral tramadol in foals are not available.

Alpha-2 Agonist Drugs

The sympathomimetic drugs xylazine, detomidine and romifidine cause dose-dependent sedation, analgesia and muscle relaxation through agonist action at the α-2 adrenergic receptor. Unfortunately, significant cardiovascular and respiratory depression may occur with administration. These effects are of particular concern in sick or septic neonatal foals and limit their use. Foals with upper or lower airway compromise may be particularly susceptible as they may develop upper airway obstruction because of laryngeal and pharyngeal relaxation after administration. The pharmacokinetics of these drugs have not been reported in neonatal or older foals. There are several studies available examining their pharmacodynamic effects in healthy foals, however. These suggest that lower doses should be administered to avoid adverse effects compared to the label doses for adult horses. Administration of xylazine at typical pre-anesthetic doses used for adult horses (1.1 mg/kg) resulted in marked ataxia, recumbency, bradycardia without arrhythmia, hypotension, and decreased respiratory rate in 10- and 28-day-old foals [40]. Detomidine administration at doses of 0.01–0.04 mg/kg resulted in similar effects as xylazine, but also included arrhythmias, sweating, and frequent urination. A significant analgesic effect was only seen at the highest dose [41]. Romifidine at 0.07 mg/kg IV likewise produced similar clinical signs, but also produced a better level of sedation compared to xylazine (1 mg/kg), allowing for easier examination and nasogastric tube passage with less physical restraint [42].

In some instances, the sedation observed with α-2 agonists may be too severe or may result in excessive cardiovascular compromise. In these cases, the drugs can be reversed using several reversal agents, including atipamezole and yohimbine. The affinity of atipamezole for α −2 receptors is 100 times higher than other antagonists. These drugs have not specifically been studies in foals. Anecdotally, 0.05 mg/kg IM atipamezole and 0.1–0.2 mg/kg IM yohimbine have been used in foals.

Anticholinergic Drugs

N-butylscopolammonium bromide has recently been approved by the FDA as a spasmolytic drug for the treatment of abdominal pain in horses caused by spasmodic colic, flatulent colic and simple impactions. It is available in several other countries combined with metamizole (also known as dipyrone). It works via an anticholinergic effect resulting from competitive inhibition of muscarinic receptors on intestinal smooth muscle cells. It has been shown to improve pain scores and attitude in treated horses with colic. It has also been shown to facilitate rectal examinations in horses by decreasing rectal pressure and reducing straining during examination. It is only labeled for use as a single injection. This drug has not been studied as an analgesic in foals, but it has been used at doses of 0.3 mg/kg IV to facilitate colonoscopy in a case of atresia coli in a foal [43]. It may have use as an antispasmodic in foals with colic or meconium impactions, although careful diagnosis should be made prior to use.

Local Anesthetic Drugs

Local anesthetics, such as lidocaine, block sodium channels resulting in decreased nerve conduction and pain sensation. Lidocaine has also been shown to have anti-inflammatory effects in the gut wall, and is used to treat arrhythmias such as ventricular tachycardia. Local infiltration along surgical incisions, catheter insertion sites, or centesis sites is often used in foals to facilitate procedures. IV administration can be accomplished using a constant rate infusion as lidocaine has a half-life <30 minutes in adult horses. This also allows for rapid titration of plasma concentrations as lidocaine has a narrow therapeutic index. Adverse effects include CNS excitement and cardiovascular collapse. In adult horses, plasma concentrations between 1 and 2 μg/ml are considered therapeutic, but toxicity has been seen at concentrations of 1.85–4.53 μg/ml [44]. Toxicity has also been noted in a foal receiving a constant rate infusion of lidocaine that was successfully treated with IV lipid emulsion [45].

The plasma pharmacokinetics of lidocaine and its active metabolite monoethylglycylxylidide (MEGX) in healthy foals <3 months of age have been investigated using the adult loading dose of 1.3 mg/kg IV over 15 minutes, followed by 0.05 mg/kg/min for 6 hours. At this dose rate, plasma concentrations were lower than reported for adult horses and below the presumed therapeutic concentrations of 1–2 μg/ml [46]. Additionally, healthy foals had a larger volume of distribution at steady state, faster clearance, and a shorter half-life ($t_{1/2}$) compared to healthy adult horses. In sick neonatal foals, lidocaine elimination was similar to healthy foals, however accumulation of MEGX occurred to a greater extent in sick foals [46]. Adverse effects attributed to lidocaine were not noted in the sick foals, although evaluation was more difficult in these patients due to their underlying conditions.

Multimodal Therapy

Combination drug therapy can be performed, which utilizes drugs with different modes of action to block multiple areas of the pain pathway. The above-mentioned drug classes may be combined to improve analgesia, as well as decrease the dose of individual drugs, which would likely decrease the risk of toxicity. Care should be taken with combinations of anticholinergic drugs and α-2 agonist drugs, as they can potentiate severe arrhythmias, especially in patients with systemic cardiovascular compromise [47]. Additionally, different NSAIDs should not be administered in combination, including nonselective and COX-2 selective drug combinations. Combination NSAID therapy increases the risk for adverse effects above the risk for each drug administered alone [48].

References

1 Little, D., Jones, S.L., and Blikslager, A.T. (2007). Cyclooxygenase (COX) inhibitors and the intestine. *J. Vet. Intern. Med.* 21: 367–377.

2 Davis, J.L. (2015). Nonsteroidal anti-inflammatory drug associated right dorsal colitis in the horse. *Equine Vet. Educ.* 29: 104–113.

3 Gunson, D.E. (1983). Renal papillary necrosis in horses. *J. Am. Vet. Med. Assoc.* 182: 263–266.

4 Gunson, D.E. and Soma, L.R. (1983). Renal papillary necrosis in horses after phenylbutazone and water deprivation. *Vet. Pathol.* 20: 603–610.

5 Peek, S.F., Semrad, S.D., and Perkins, G.A. (2003). Clostridial myonecrosis in horses (37 cases 1985–2000). *Equine Vet. J.* 35: 86–92.

6 King, J.N. and Gerring, E.L. (1989). Antagonism of endotoxin-induced disruption of equine bowel motility by flunixin and phenylbutazone. *Equine Vet. J. Suppl.* 21: 38–42.

7 Crisman, M.V., Wilcke, J.R., and Sams, R.A. (1996). Pharmacokinetics of flunixin meglumine in healthy foals less than twenty-four hours old. *Am. J. Vet. Res.* 57: 1759–1761.

8 Semrad, S.D., Sams, R.A., and Ashcraft, S.M. (1993). Pharmacokinetics of serum thromboxane suppression by flunixin meglumine in healthy foals during the first month of life. *Am. J. Vet. Res.* 54: 2083–2087.

9 Carrick, J.B., Papich, M.G., Middleton, D.M. et al. (1989). Clinical and pathological effects of flunixin meglumine administration to neonatal foals. *Can. J. Vet. Res.* 53: 195–201.

10 Traub-Dargatz, J.L., Bertone, J.J., Gould, D.H. et al. (1988). Chronic flunixin meglumine therapy in foals. *Am. J. Vet. Res.* 49: 7–12.

11 Valk, N., Doherty, T.J., Blackford, J.T. et al. (1998). Phenylbutazone prevents the endotoxin-induced delay in gastric emptying in horses. *Can. J. Vet. Res.* 62: 214–217.

12 Wilcke, J.R., Crisman, M.V., Sams, R.A. et al. (1993). Pharmacokinetics of phenylbutazone in neonatal foals. *Am. J. Vet. Res.* 54: 2064–2067.

13 Crisman, M.V., Sams, R.A., and Irby, M.H. (1989). The disposition of phenylbutazone in lactating mares and its effect on nursing foals. In: *Proceedings of the Annual Meeting American Association of Equine Practitioners*, vol. 35, 127–131.

14 Crisman, M.V., Wilcke, J.R., Sams, R.A. et al. (1991). Concentrations of phenylbutazone and oxyphenbutazone in post-parturient mares and their neonatal foals. *J. Vet. Pharmacol. Ther.* 14: 330–334.

15 Léveillé, R., Miyabayashi, T., Weisbrode, S.E. et al. (1996). Ultrasonographic renal changes associated with phenylbutazone administration in three foals. *Can. Vet. J.* 37: 235–236.

16 Traub, J.L., Gallina, A.M., Grant, B.D. et al. (1983). Phenylbutazone toxicosis in the foal. *Am. J. Vet. Res.* 44: 1410–1418.

17 Geor, R.J., Petrie, L., Papich, M.G. et al. (1989). The protective effects of sucralfate and ranitidine in foals experimentally intoxicated with phenylbutazone. *Can. J. Vet. Res.* 53: 231–238.

18 Wilcke, J.R., Crisman, M.V., Scarratt, W.K. et al. (1998). Pharmacokinetics of ketoprofen in healthy foals less than twenty-four hours old. *Am. J. Vet. Res.* 59: 290–292.

19 MacAllister, C.G., Morgan, S.J., Borne, A.T. et al. (1993). Comparison of adverse effects of phenylbutazone, flunixin meglumine, and ketoprofen in horses. *J. Am. Vet. Med. Assoc.* 202: 71–77.

20 Mozaffari, A.A., Derakhshanfar, A., Alinejad, A. et al. (2010). A comparative study on the adverse effects of flunixin, ketoprofen and phenylbutazone in miniature donkeys: haematological, biochemical and pathological findings. *N. Z. Vet. J.* 58: 224–228.

21 Toutain, P.L. and Cester, C.C. (2004). Pharmacokinetic-pharmacodynamic relationships and dose response to meloxicam in horses with induced arthritis in the right carpal joint. *Am. J. Vet. Res.* 65: 1533–1541.

22 Raidal, S., Edwards, S., Pippia, J. et al. (2013). Pharmacokinetics and Safety of Oral Administration of Meloxicam to foals. *J. Vet. Intern. Med.* 27: 300–307.

23 Letendre, L.T., Tessman, R.K., McClure, S.R. et al. (2008). Pharmacokinetics of firocoxib after administration of multiple consecutive daily doses to horses. *Am. J. Vet. Res.* 69: 1399–1405.

24 Holland, B., Fogle, C., Blikslager, A.T. et al. (2015). Pharmacokinetics and pharmacodynamics of three formulations of firocoxib in healthy horses. *J. Vet. Pharmacol. Ther.* 38: 249–256.

25 Cox, S., Villarino, N., Sommardahl, C. et al. (2013). Disposition of firocoxib in equine plasma after an oral loading dose and a multiple dose regimen. *Vet. J.* 198: 382–385.

26 Hovanessian, N., Davis, J.L., McKenzie, H.C. 3rd et al. (2014). Pharmacokinetics and safety of firocoxib after oral administration of repeated consecutive doses to neonatal foals. *J. Vet. Pharmacol. Ther.* 37: 243–251.

27 Wilson, K.E., Davis, J.L., Crisman, M.V. et al. (2017). Pharmacokinetics of firocoxib after intravenous administration of multiple consecutive doses in neonatal foals. *J. Vet. Pharmacol. Ther.* 40: e23–e29.

28 Schleining, J.A., McClure, S.R., Evans, R.B. et al. (2008). Liposome-based diclofenac for the treatment of inflammation in an acute synovitis model in horses. *J. Vet. Pharmacol. Ther.* 31: 554–561.

29 Frisbie, D.D., McIlwraith, C.W., Kawcak, C.E. et al. (2009). Evaluation of topically administered diclofenac

liposomal cream for treatment of horses with experimentally induced osteoarthritis. *Am. J. Vet. Res.* 70: 210–215.

30 Barnett, S.E., Sellon, D.C., Hines, M.T. et al. (2017). Randomized, controlled clinical trial of safety and plasma concentrations of diclofenac in healthy neonatal foals after repeated topical application of 1% diclofenac sodium cream. *Am. J. Vet. Res.* 78: 405–411.

31 Davis, J.L., Messenger, K.M., LaFevers, D.H. et al. (2012). Pharmacokinetics of intravenous and intramuscular buprenorphine in the horse. *J. Vet. Pharmacol. Ther.* 35: 52–58.

32 Grubb, T.L., Kurkowski, D., Sellon, D.C. et al. (2019). Pharmacokinetics and physiologic/behavioral effects of buprenorphine administered sublingually and intravenously to neonatal foals. *J. Vet. Pharmacol. Ther.* 42: 26–36.

33 Risberg, Å.I., Spadavecchia, C., Ranheim, B. et al. (2015). Antinociceptive effect of buprenorphine and evaluation of the nociceptive withdrawal reflex in foals. *Vet. Anaesth. Analg.* 42: 329–338.

34 Arguedas, M.G., Hines, M.T., Papich, M.G. et al. (2008). Pharmacokinetics of butorphanol and evaluation of physiologic and behavioral effects after intravenous and intramuscular administration to neonatal foals. *J. Vet. Intern. Med.* 22: 1417–1426.

35 McGowan, K.T., Elfenbein, J.R., Robertson, S.A. et al. (2013). Effect of butorphanol on thermal nociceptive threshold in healthy pony foals. *Equine Vet. J.* 45: 503–506.

36 Knych, H.K., Steffey, E.P., Casbeer, H.C. et al. (2015). Disposition, behavioural and physiological effects of escalating doses of intravenously administered fentanyl to young foals. *Equine Vet. J.* 47: 592–598.

37 Eberspächer, E., Stanley, S.D., Rezende, M. et al. (2008). Pharmacokinetics and tolerance of transdermal fentanyl administration in foals. *Vet. Anaesth. Analg.* 35: 249–255.

38 Knych, H.K., Corado, C.R., McKemie, D.S. et al. (2013). Pharmacokinetics and selected pharmacodynamic effects of tramadol following intravenous administration to the horse. *Equine Vet. J.* 45: 490–496.

39 Knych, H.K., Steffey, E.P., White, A.M. et al. (2016). Effects of age on the pharmacokinetics of tramadol and its active metabolite, O-desmethyltramadol following intravenous administration to foals. *Equine Vet. J.* 48: 65–71.

40 Carter, S.W., Robertson, S.A., Steel, C.J. et al. (1990). Cardiopulmonary effects of xylazine sedation in the foal. *Equine Vet. J.* 22: 384–388.

41 Oijala, M. and Katila, T. (1988). Detomidine (Domosedan) in foals: sedative and analgesic effects. *Equine Vet. J.* 20: 327–330.

42 Naylor, J.M., Garven, E., and Fraser, L. (2005). A comparison of romifidine and xylazine in foals: the effects on sedation and analgesia. *Equine Vet. Educ.* 7: 89–94.

43 Hunter, B. and Belgrave, R.L. (2010). Atresia coli in a foal: diagnosis made with colonoscopy aided by N-butylscopolammonium bromide. *Equine Vet. Educ.* 22: 429–433.

44 Meyer, G.A., Lin, H.C., Hanson, R.R. et al. (2001). Effects of intravenous lidocaine overdose on cardiac electrical activity and blood pressure in the horse. *Equine Vet. J.* 33: 434–437.

45 Vieitez, V., Gómez de Segura, I., Martin-Cuervo, M. et al. (2017). Successful use of lipid emulsion to resuscitate a foal after intravenous lidocaine induced cardiovascular collapse. *Equine Vet. J.* 49: 767–769.

46 Ohmes, C. (2014). *The Disposition of Lidocaine During a 6-Hour Intravenous Infusion to Young Foals*, 67. Manhattan, KS: Department of Clinical Sciences, College of Veterinary Medicine Kansas State University.

47 Morton, A.J., Varney, C.R., Ekiri, A.B. et al. (2011). Cardiovascular effects of N-butylscopolammonium bromide and xylazine in horses. *Equine Vet. J.* 43: 117–122.

48 Reed, S.K., Messer, N.T., Tessman, R.K. et al. (2006). Effects of phenylbutazone alone or in combination with flunixin meglumine on blood protein concentrations in horses. *Am. J. Vet. Res.* 67: 398–402.

Chapter 64 Anesthesia of the Neonatal Foal

Bonnie Hay-Kraus

Introduction

Foals are precocious at birth compared to other veterinary species. A healthy full-term foal is born after 11 months of gestation (approximately 335–342 days) [1]. Foals up to 1 month of age are considered neonates, pediatric at 1–3 months, and juvenile when they are 3–4 months of age. By 3–5 months, foals may be treated similar to young adult horses from an anesthesia standpoint [2]. Neonatal foals (<7–10 days old) are given special consideration because mortality is approximately seven times higher than adult horses. This section focuses on sedation and anesthesia of the neonatal foal; information regarding anesthesia of pediatric and juvenile foals can be found elsewhere [2]. Common reasons for anesthesia in the first 4 weeks of life include treatment of ruptured urinary bladder, patent urachus, umbilical remnant resection, colic, musculoskeletal trauma, and septic arthritis. Perhaps more common than general anesthesia is the need for sedation and/or analgesia to facilitate a variety of procedures in foals such as IV catheter placement, abdominocentesis, arthrocentesis, cast application, or cerebrospinal fluid (CSF) collection [3]. The transition from the uterine environment and the changes in physiology, especially with respect to the cardiovascular and respiratory systems and metabolic pathways, make neonatal foals particularly vulnerable during anesthesia since they are less able to compensate for changes in homeostasis.

Morbidity and Mortality

The Confidential Enquiry into Perioperative Fatalities (CEPEF) has indicated that foals <1 month of age have the greatest anesthetic risk. Overall, neonatal foals have a mortality rate of ~1.5%, whereas foals aged 1–5 months have a mortality rate on par with noncolic adult horses <14 years of age [4]. Foals <1 week of age that are anesthetized for reasons other than colic are approximately seven times more likely to die than adult horses anesthetized for elective procedures. Foals 1–4 weeks old have a mortality risk approximately two times adult horses. By age 1–5 months, mortality is on par with the adult horses. The original CEPEF (February 1991–March 1994) indicated that foals <7 days of age had the highest mortality rate (up to 21%); the mortality rate decreased but was still elevated in foals aged 1–4 weeks compared to adult horses aged 2–4 years [5].

Although many neonatal foals requiring anesthesia are systemically ill and require emergent anesthesia and surgery (e.g. ruptured urinary bladder), even healthy foals have a higher risk of death. Postulated reasons for this higher mortality include physiologic differences between neonatal foals and adult horses. Additionally, the very short time frame of foaling season makes it difficult for anesthetists to gain and maintain proficiency in managing foal anesthesia, including familiarity with differences in anesthetic equipment.

The CEPEF indicated that anesthetic agents and protocols can also influence mortality. Protocols consisting of total inhalational anesthesia (including induction) that lack any premedication were associated with the highest risk of mortality. Total inhalational anesthesia, which was used in 510 foals <1 year of age in the study, was associated with a markedly increased risk of dying (15/510; 2.9%) [4]. CEPEF Phase 1 studied cases from February 1991–March 1994 and Phase 2 from April 1994–February 1997. The use of total inhalational anesthesia in neonatal foals reflects common practice at that time likely due to concern over metabolic capacity for barbiturates and as well as other drugs [3, 6, 7]. CEPEF-4 was launched in 2012 and will hopefully evaluate if newer, shorter-acting induction

Equine Neonatal Medicine, First Edition. Edited by David M. Wong and Pamela A. Wilkins.

anesthetics such as propofol and alphaxalone influence the mortality rate in neonatal foals. There are numerous physiological differences between neonatal foals and adult horses that may account for an increase in anesthetic risk; it is important that the anesthetist be aware and have a plan for intervention.

Physiology

The foal transitions from intra- to extrauterine life during the first few days and weeks after birth. The time frame of this transition varies by body system, with that of the cardiopulmonary system the most critical at the time of birth. Major physiologic changes also occur in the peripheral and central nervous system (CNS), liver and renal function, metabolism and tissue composition, as well as thermoregulation. These adaptations are also critical but occur over a longer period of time following birth. Understanding physiologic changes and differences from adult horses allows the anesthetist to better prepare and tailor a plan for the special needs of the neonatal foal (Tables 64.1 and 64.2).

Cardiovascular System

One of the most dramatic changes that occur at birth is the adaptation from fetal to neonatal circulation. During gestation, the gas exchange "organ" is the placenta. Oxygenated blood is delivered from the dam to the fetus via the umbilical vein which travels to the right atrium via the caudal vena cava. The fetal circulation functionally bypasses the pulmonary circulation and noninflated lungs by shunting through the foramen ovale (FA) and ductus arteriorsus (DA); a process dependent on high pulmonary arterial resistance. Most of the blood entering the right atrium is diverted to the left atrium through the FA. A smaller portion of blood from the right atrium enters the right ventricle and pulmonary artery. This blood bypasses the lung through the DA, which connects the pulmonary

Table 64.1 Cardiorespiratory variables in neonatal foals compared to adult horses [2, 8].

Parameter	Neonate Compared to adult	Parameter	Neonate Compared to adult
Heart rate	↑	Respiratory rate	↑
Mean arterial pressure	↓	Tidal volume (Vt)	↑
Systolic arterial pressure	↓	Minute ventilation (Vmin)	↑↑
Diastolic arterial pressure	↓	Partial pressure of oxygen (P_aO_2)	↓
Cardiac index	↑	Partial pressure of carbon dioxide (P_aCO_2)	↑

Table 64.2 Summary of relevant physiologic factors related to anesthetic management of the neonatal foal [2].

Cardiovascular system	Higher heart rate, CO dependent on heart rate Immature baroreceptor responses Lower SAP, MAP, DAP due to lower systemic vascular resistance Transition from fetal to neonatal circulation; risk of return to fetal circulation
Respiratory system	High respiratory rate, relatively low Vt High minute ventilation High O_2 consumption Immature responses of central chemoreceptors to CO_2 and O_2 blood levels Lower P_aO_2 first week of life Higher P_aCO_2 through first week of life
Nervous system	Greater permeability of BBB Immature central, peripheral, and autonomic nervous system function
Liver	Immature liver metabolic function first 4 weeks of life Limited glycogen stores at risk for hypoglycemia
Renal	Reduced concentrating ability
Thermoregulation	At risk of hypothermia: • High body surface area to weight • Lower total body fat • Limited subcutaneous fat • Heat generated by shivering or nonshivering activity is inhibited by anesthesia
Hematology/ biochemistry	Higher blood volume (13–15%) Higher total body water, increased ECF volume Total protein varies with colostrum intake, Albumin stable and similar to adult Serum enzymes may be elevated (CK, GGT, SDH, AST)=> interpret in light of clinical signs

SAP, Systolic arterial pressure; MAP, Mean arterial pressure; DAP, Diastolic arterial pressure; Vt, Tidal volume, BBB, Blood–brain barrier; ECF, Extracellular fluid; CK, Creatine kinase; GGT, Gamma glutamyl transferase; SDH, Sorbitol dehydrogenase; AST, Aspartate aminotransferase.

artery to the aorta; at this stage blood flow is right to left [2, 9, 10].

Gas exchange is abruptly transferred from the placenta to the lungs at birth. During passage through the birth canal, the chest is compressed, squeezing fluid out of the airways. As the lungs inflate, surfactant contributes to clearance of fluid, alveolar stability, and lung inflation [11]. Upon initial expansion of the lungs, a dramatic decrease in pulmonary vascular resistance occurs, allowing blood from the pulmonary artery to enter the pulmonary vasculature rather than passing through the DA to the aorta. Simultaneously, there is an increase in systemic vascular resistance (SVR) and cessation of placental blood flow [11]. As the pressure in the left atrium increases relative to the right atrium, flow through the FA decreases, although complete closure may take several weeks [12, 13]. Closure of the DA occurs in response to increased oxygen tension and decreased circulating prostaglandins; blood now flows preferentially to the lungs. Blood flow may be observed within the DA upon echocardiography and is left to right. Closure of the DA is initially physiologic due to constriction of the vessels and then becomes anatomic as the muscle contribution occurs. Complete fibrosis occurs within several weeks of birth, but partial reopening is possible up until that time [2]. Perinatal hypoxemia and acidosis, which can be associated with peri-anesthetic hypoventilation and atelectasis, can increase pulmonary vascular resistance sufficient to delay or reverse DA closure, resulting in reversion or persistent fetal circulation and severe hypoxemia [10, 14]. Blood flow through the shunt is typically left (high pressure) to right (low pressure); right-to-left shunting is rare and only occurs when the pulmonary artery pressure is higher than systemic pressure [10, 15].

Heart sounds and flow murmurs are much louder in neonates than adults due to their thin chest wall. Holosystolic murmurs are common, but most are innocent flow murmurs unless accompanied by clinical signs such as ascites, pleural effusion and jugular distension [1, 9]. A murmur associated with a persistent patent ducutus arteriosus (PDA) may be heard for up to 3–5 days, even in healthy foals [1, 2, 9, 11]. Definitive differentiation requires echocardiography, however some clinical differences may be used to distinguish flow murmurs from PDA. Flow murmurs have normal pulse quality; they are usually systolic murmurs with a point of maximal intensity at the aortic valve [1]. A murmur due to a PDA is typically a continuous systolic murmur, which extends into diastole (machinery murmur) with the point of maximal intensity dorsal and caudal to the aortic valve over the left heart base at the third intercostal space; a precordial thrill may be present, along with bounding pulses [1, 16]. Murmurs persisting beyond 7 days of age or any murmur accompanied by signs of cardiac disease (poor growth, cyanosis, lethargy, exercise intolerance) should be investigated with echocardiography. Auscultation of both sides of the thorax is important, as right-sided cardiac murmurs are a feature of several congenital cardiac anomalies [16].

Cardiac output (CO) is an indicator of global tissue perfusion and is defined by heart rate (HR) multiplied by stroke volume (SV). Cardiac index (CI) is CO adjusted for weight and expressed as ml/min/kg. Due to their high metabolic requirements, the CI of foals 2 hours, days, and weeks old are 155 ± 11.5, 204 ± 35.4, and 222 ± 43.2 ml/min/kg, respectively [17]. This is approximately two to three times that of adult horses [18, 19]. The neonatal ventricle has lower compliance and strength of contraction, limiting the ability to increase SV. Stroke volume is about one-third that of adult horses, thus requiring significantly higher HR in order to maintain CO [2, 7, 20]. Changes in preload and afterload may be poorly tolerated by neonatal foals. Significant dependence on HR for CO is typical for pediatric patients of many species and deserves consideration when choosing drug protocols, especially since many anesthetic drugs, especially α-2 agonists will decrease HR.

Foals have late maturation of the hypothalamic–pituitary-axis leading to underdeveloped baroreceptor responses resulting in decreased SVR, vasomotor tone and significantly lower systemic arterial blood pressure (BP) in the first few days of life compared to adult horses. This may put neonatal foals at special risk of hypotension, especially during anesthesia. Vagal influence predominates in the neonate; both sympathetic innervation and the response to adrenergic drugs is diminished. By 1 month of age, foals have a lower HR and CI but higher mean arterial pressure (MAP) due to higher SV and maturation of the sympathetic nervous system responses [2, 11].

Respiratory System

Functional residual capacity (FRC; volume of air in the lung after normal expiration) and tidal volume are decreased in the neonate compared to adult horses. Foals compensate with a much higher respiratory rates in order to maintain their significantly higher metabolic oxygen demand. The newborn can have respiratory rates up to 60–80 breaths/minute, which decrease to 40–50 breaths/min by 1 week, 30–40 breaths/min by 4–6 weeks and then to adult values after approximately 4 months of age [2, 20]. Arterial oxygen is low at birth (~40–50 mmHg) but increases to 85–90 mmHg by 1 week and then to 90–100 mmHg after the first week of life. Arterial carbon dioxide (CO_2) is significantly higher after birth (~50 mmHg) and remains at the high end of normal adult values through the first 4 weeks of life [2, 11, 16]. The high minute ventilation (V_{min}) and low FRC in neonatal foals allows for rapid changes in inhalant anesthetic depth. These factors, in conjunction with lower sensitivity of the respiratory centers to arterial CO_2 and oxygen make them at greater risk for hypoventilation and hypoxemia in the peri-anesthetic period.

Nervous System

Although the nervous system of the foal has substantial development to undergo, the cerebellum is well developed, allowing foals to stand within 30 minutes of birth, and nurse and ambulate soon thereafter. Smaller neurons and neuroglia differentiate later, and myelination may be incomplete at birth. Hence, transmission of nerve signals from the peripheral to CNS is slower than in the adult and the ability to localize stimuli may be decreased [2]. The palpebral reflex is present shortly after birth, but the pupillary light response may be slow. The menace response does not develop fully for several weeks, although the foal will move its head away from a menacing gesture [21]. Foals are a sentient species with mature neural mechanisms at birth and capable of perceiving pain in response to noxious stimuli immediately after birth. Foals respond more abruptly and profoundly to pain compared to adult horses. Even during general anesthesia, they may be hyper-responsive to the initial nociceptive stimulus at the start of surgery. Early pain experiences may have negative consequences on pain responses later in life due to altered sensory processing and negative pain-related memories. Therefore, adequate analgesia is indicated whenever the foal has a painful condition or will be exposed to noxious stimuli.

The autonomic nervous system also undergoes maturation after birth including the responsiveness of myocardial contractility and vasomotor tone. Parasympathetic activity predominates at birth while sympathetic nervous system innervation of the heart and vasculature remains immature leading to low SVR and prevalence of bradyarrhythmias associated with hypoxemia and hypothermia. Immaturity of the CNS as a whole and increased permeability of the blood-brain barrier (BBB) are likely responsible for differences in anesthetic drug responses between neonates and older foals or adults.

Liver and Renal Function

Drug metabolism generally converts lipid soluble drugs to more hydrophilic compounds that are either inactive or have reduced activity and can be readily excreted in the urine. Most anesthetic drugs are primarily metabolized in the liver; however, other organs such as the lung, kidneys, or intestine may contribute. Phase I reactions include oxidation (CYP450), reduction, and hydrolysis; Phase II reactions consist of conjugation, typically with glucuronic acid or less frequently with sulfate, glycine, glutamate, glutathione, acetylation, or methylation. The cytochrome P450 oxidation pathway and glucuronide conjugation are the principal pathways responsible for converting lipophilic compounds to more water soluble and inactive metabolites that are subsequently excreted by the kidneys [22]. Metabolic pathways differ depending on the specific drug and species; thus, it is not always accurate to transpose pharmacologic data between species.

The foal's functional capacity of the liver is still maturing at birth. Therefore, the capacity to metabolize endogenous and exogenous substances such as bilirubin or anesthetic drugs is significantly lower than adult horses. As blood flow to the liver increases after birth, enzyme induction occurs with exposure to various endogenous and exogenous substances. In general, metabolic pathways mature more quickly in horses (which are herbivores) than in dogs and cats which are omnivores or carnivores. Microsomal enzyme activity increases rapidly during the first 3–4 weeks of life and, although conjugation processes have a more gradual maturation, hepatic metabolic pathways are fully functioning by 6–12 weeks after birth [22]. Newborn foals have less glycogen stores in the liver and muscle compared to other species and are especially vulnerable to hypoglycemia. The risk diminishes somewhat from 2–4 weeks of age and onward.

Newborn foals have a glomerular filtration rate and renal plasma flow comparable to adult horses; however, they have a reduced renal concentrating ability. Due to their milk diet, foals produce a large volume of urine relative to their body weight. Normal urine output in neonatal foals is approximately 6 ml/kg/hr (5–10 times >adult horses). The high water intake and urine excretion leads to hyposthenuria (urine specific gravity of 1.001–1027) [2, 16].

The circulating blood and plasma volumes are approximately double that of adult horses. Total body water in foals is approximately 75% of body weight compared with 50–60% in adult horses. This difference is primarily due to a much higher extracellular fluid volume (ECF) in the neonate, which is about 43% in week-old foals compared to 22% in adults; this results in a higher volume of distribution of many drugs [23]. These factors should be accounted for when planning for peri-anesthetic fluid therapy and intravascular volume replacement. Maintenance fluid rates vary but are considerably higher than adult horses; 3.5–5.0 ml/kg/hr for foals up to 1 month of age [24, 25].

Normal rectal temperature is 99–102 °F during the first 4 days of life, which is approximately 1 °F above the adult range. Foals have a much higher body surface area to weight ratio and much lower total body fat compared to adult horses. These factors contribute to increased environmental heat loss and increased vulnerability to peri-anesthesia hypothermia.

Hematologic Values

Detailed information regarding clinical pathology findings in foals is in Chapters 42 and 44; parameters relevant to anesthesia are discussed here. As noted, blood volume is approximately 13–15% of total body weight and decreases to near adult levels (8–10%) by 12 weeks of age. Packed cell volume (PCV) and hemoglobin reach maximal levels at the time of birth (40–52%), decrease to 32–46% after colostrum and milk intake, and gradually decline to adult levels by 1–3 months of age [2, 16]. The decline in PCV is accelerated in foals with neonatal isoerythrolysis and is accompanied by icterus. Marked bilirubinemia is common in the first week of life due to breakdown of neonatal RBCs and immature liver function. Total protein (TP) values will vary widely as it increases following colostrum intake, however, albumin stays relatively constant.

Serum enzymes may be elevated in the first few days to weeks of life and should be interpreted carefully in conjunction with clinical signs. Creatine kinase (CK) may be elevated in the newborn due to muscle trauma during parturition. Alkaline phosphatase (ALP) is increased for the first few months of life due to a combination of high metabolic bone activity, intestinal pinocytosis, and hepatic maturation. Gamma glutamyl transferase (GGT), sorbitol dehydrogenase (SDH), and aspartate aminotransferase (AST) may be elevated in the first few weeks after birth due to hepatic maturation [1, 2, 16].

Pharmacologic Considerations

Differences between neonatal and adult animals in drug effects can be attributed to differences in drug distribution, metabolism, or excretion. Compared to adult horses, foals have a higher basal metabolic rate, larger percentage of body water and more permeable BBB leading to differences in pharmacokinetics and pharmacodynamics of drugs. General characteristics of the neonatal period include less drug binding to plasma proteins, increased apparent volume of distribution of drugs that are distributed in the ECF, and slower elimination (i.e. longer half-life) of many drugs [22].

Fasting

Neonatal foals are solely nursing the mare and do not require prolonged pre-anesthetic fasting. Preventing nursing for 15–30 minutes prior to anesthesia is sufficient in foals <1 month of age since regurgitation or aspiration are uncommon in the absence of gastrointestinal (GI) obstruction. Neonatal foals are usually able to maintain blood glucose for short anesthetic procedures (<2 hours). However, sick foals may not be nursing adequately and are at risk for dehydration and hypoglycemia. Blood glucose levels should be measured prior to sedation/anesthesia and approximately every hour during anesthesia. If blood glucose is low (<70 mg/dl), 2.5% dextrose can be added to the crystalloid IV fluids.

Sedation of the Mare

The mare and foal should be kept together and led to the induction stall to allow both to remain calm, facilitating a smoother induction of anesthesia. The mare is sedated prior to handling of the foal for IV catheterization, sedation, and induction. The mare should have a physical examination prior to administration of sedation. Consideration should be given to the level of sedation required to keep the mare calm and the length of time the foal will be separated from the mare.

Suggested protocols for mare sedation:

- Acepromazine (0.02–0.05 mg/kg IV/IM) alone or in combination with an α-2 agonist
- Detomidine (5.0–10.0 ug/kg IV/IM) or Xylazine (0.2–0.3 mg/kg IV)
- Once the mare is sedated and the foal is sedated or induced, the mare can be returned to her stall. The mare is returned to the recovery stall once the foal is recovered from anesthesia and then returned together to their stall.

Sedatives and Tranquilizers

Sedatives/tranquilizers may be used for diagnostic or minor procedures or before induction of general anesthesia. They are used to calm the patient, ease handling, reduce stress, decrease doses of induction and inhalant anesthetic drugs, and smooth induction and recovery. Drug selection and dose depends on the underlying disease and physical status of the patient, along with the age and temperament of the foal. Analgesics and local anesthetic techniques should accompany sedation and general anesthesia protocols. Oxygen supplementation is provided if sedation results in recumbency. Commonly used sedatives/tranquilizers used in equine patients include acepromazine, α-2 agonists, and benzodiazepines (Table 64.3).

Acepromazine

Acepromazine is a phenothiazine that provides sedation via central blockade of dopaminergic (D_2) receptors reducing activity in the basal ganglia, limbic, and reticular activating system. It also blocks peripheral α-1 adrenoreceptors leading to vasodilation, hypotension, and hypothermia [19, 26]. Hematologic effects include decreases in PCV, TP, and platelet aggregation. Side effects and duration of action are dose dependent, with acepromazine usually lasting 1–2 hours. There is no reversal agent, although the hypotensive effects

Table 64.3 Anesthetic management of neonatal foals.

Drug	<7 days	>7 days
Premedication/sedation		
Benzodiazepines	Midazolam 0.02–0.1 mg/kg IV or IM (typical IV dose 0.1 mg/kg) Diazepam 0.02–0.1 mg/kg IV	Midazolam 0.05–0.2 mg/kg IV or IM (typical IV dose 0.1 mg/kg) Diazepam 0.05–0.2 mg/kg IV
Opioids	Butorphanol 0.05 mg/kg, IV for sedation, 0.1 mg/kg, IV for analgesia Buprenorphine 0.01–0.02 mg/kg, IV or IM Hydromorphone 0.02–0.05 mg/kg, IV or IM[a] Fentanyl 2–4ug/kg bolus, 2–4ug/kg/hour CRI Morphine 0.05–0.2 mg/kg, IV or IM (typical dose 0.1 mg/kg)[a] Methadone 0.2–0.5 mg/kg IV[b]	Butorphanol 0.05 for sedation, 0.1 mg/kg, IV for analgesia Buprenorphine 0.01–0.02 mg/kg IV or IM Hydromorphone 0.02–0.05 mg/kg, IV or IM[a] Fentanyl 2–4ug/kg bolus, 2–4ug/kg/hour CRI Morphine 0.05–0.2 mg/kg, IV or IM (typical dose 0.1 mg/kg)[a] Methadone 0.2–0.5 mg/kg IV[b]
α-2 agonists	Xylazine 0.1–0.2 mg/kg, IV or IM[c]	Xylazine 0.1–0.5 mg/kg, IV or IM[d] Detomidine 0.002–0.08 mg/kg, IV or IM[d]
Phenothiazines	Not recommended	Acepromazine 0.01–0.02 mg/kg, IV or IM
Induction	**Dose**	**Comments**
Ketamine	2.0 mg/kg after midazolam premed 2.0 mg/kg + 0.1 mg/kg midazolam	 Mix in same syringe give ¼ to 1/2 at a time to effect
Propofol	2-4 mg/kg	Administer slowly to effect @1.0 mg/kg/min
Ketofol	2 mg/kg propofol +2 mg/kg ketamine 0.5 mg/kg propofol +1.5 mg/kg ketamine	Mix in same syringe, give slowly to effect @1.0 mg/kg/min
Alphaxalone	2 to 3 mg/kg	Administer slowly @0.5–1.0 mg/kg/min

[a] Adult dose, use low end of dose for foals.
[b] Adult dose.
[c] Use only for procedural sedation or if other sedatives are not effective, avoid in sick foals or as premedication for general anesthesia.
[d] Use higher end doses for IM administration.

can be reversed in standing healthy adult horses with norepinephrine (1.0 μg/kg/min) [27]. Acepromazine provides mild sedative effects and generally requires co-administration of an opioid to allow diagnostic or minor procedures to be performed. Due to the long duration of action, lack of reversal agent, and systemic effects of decreased SVR leading to hypotension and hypothermia, acepromazine is generally avoided as an anesthetic premedication in neonatal foals.

α-2 Agonists

Alpha-2 agonists such as xylazine and detomidine are reliable and effective sedatives in adult horses. They decrease CNS release of norepinephrine and dopamine resulting in sedation, analgesia, and muscle relaxation. Intravenous administration results in an initial increase in arterial BP, followed by a longer decrease. Increased BP is attributed to stimulation of α-2 receptors on vascular smooth muscle resulting in vasoconstriction and baroreceptor mediated bradycardia. Subsequent hypotension is caused by the decrease in CNS norepinephrine release resulting in peripheral vasodilation and bradycardia. Alpha-2 agonists also increase pulmonary vascular resistance, which could potentially cause reopening of fetal circulation, right-to-left shunting and severe hypoxemia and therefore are generally avoided in foals less than 7–10 days of age. Alpha-2 agonists can provide reliable sedation in healthy foals >7–10 days of age. Ataxia and recumbency should be expected. Heart rate is significantly decreased and BP displays a typical biphasic response. Respiratory rate and minute volume is significantly decreased and respiratory noise along with upper airway obstruction may occur [28].

Benzodiazepines

Benzodiazepines are unreliable sedatives in adult horses and are rarely used as a sole agent, but they are particularly effective in neonatal foals. Clinical doses (0.05–0.1 mg/kg) of diazepam or midazolam have minimal cardiorespiratory effects in adult horses. Respiratory rate, tidal volume, blood gas variables, HR, CO, and MAP do not change, but ataxia, muscle fasiculations, and recumbency may be observed.

Ataxia and recumbency can be seen with doses greater than 0.1 mg/kg [29].

Benzodiazepines exert their pharmacologic effects at $GABA_A$ receptors. They do not activate the receptor directly, but allosterically enhance the affinity of the receptors for GABA. This causes greater frequency of channel openings, increased chloride conductance, and hyperpolarization of the postsynaptic cell membrane, leading to less excitation of the postsynaptic neurons. Hyperpolarization and resistance to excitation is the presumed mechanism by which benzodiazepines produce anxiolysis, sedation, amnesia, anticonvulsant, and skeletal muscle relaxant effects [30]. Midazolam is generally preferred due to its solubility profile, lack of propylene glycol as carrier agent, and shorter plasma half-life. Flumazenil can be used to reverse the sedative, muscle relaxant and respiratory depression effects of benzodiazepines. It is highly selective and has a strong affinity but minimal intrinsic activity. Both benzodiazepines can be reversed with 0.01–0.025 mg/kg of flumazenil IM or IV. Dilution in saline and slow titration IV can help obtain the desired level of reversal of sedative/respiratory depression while avoiding potential excitement.

Analgesics

The use of opioids in horses has historically been limited due to minimal information and concern regarding side effects such as excitement and decreased GI motility. Most studies in horses indicate that opioids exert either negligible or minimum alveolar concentration (MAC)-increasing effect with considerable individual variation. Additionally, it is difficult to demonstrate the analgesic properties of opioid analgesics in horses under experimental conditions due to small study groups, individual variability, and/or flawed pain models. More recent pharmacokinetics and pharmacodynamics studies involving opioids in adult horses and foals have begun to change this stance and increase clinical usage. Increased awareness of pain management and the relationship between adequate treatment of pain and the overall well-being of patients has led to more common use of opioids in horses.

Butorphanol

Butorphanol is an opioid agonist–antagonist frequently used in adult horses and foals. It has antagonist activity at the mu receptor and agonist activity at the kappa receptor. Administration of 0.5 mg/kg IV or IM in neonatal pony foals did not cause a significant difference in HR or locomotor activity, minimal decrease in respiratory rate and GI motility, and increased rectal temperature [31]. Behavioral effects included sedation, ataxia, and increased nursing but no increase in locomotor activity. The sedative effects were subjectively classified as moderate and included inactivity, lowering of the head, relaxation of the front limbs, decreased response to external stimuli and recumbency and occurred within 3–15 minutes of administration and lasted 20–40 minutes. Pharmacokinetics in neonatal foals differ from adult horses and include a greater volume of distribution (3.86 vs 1–1.13 l/kg), faster clearance (31 vs 21 ml/kg/min), and longer elimination half-life (IV = 2.1 hours; IM = 0.94 for foals vs. IV = 0.74 hours; IM = 0.57 hour for adult horses) [31]. Butorphanol also has a higher absorption after IM administration in foals (66%) compared to adult horses (37%). The measured plasma levels after 0.05 mg/kg IV or IM did not reach the proposed analgesic plasma concentration for visceral analgesia in adult horses (20–30 ng/ml) [31, 32]. However, in one study, butorphanol dosed at 0.1 mg/kg IV produced thermal nociception in neonatal pony foals, whereas, a 0.05 mg/kg dose did not produce significant antinociceptive effects [33]. A dose of 0.05 mg/kg IV or IM may be used for sedation for nonpainful procedures, alone or administered with a benzodiazepine; the higher dose of 0.1 mg/kg is used for foals with painful underlying conditions or undergoing painful procedures.

Buprenorphine

Buprenorphine is a mu-receptor partial agonist. It has agonist activity at the mu receptor, but there is a "ceiling effect" for analgesia and other side effects. It has been studied extensively in adult horses and in neonatal foals to a lesser degree. The plasma half-life after IV doses of 0.005–0.006 mg/kg are approximately 4–6 hours in adult horses [34–36] and the anti-nociceptive effect has a duration of 6–12 hours [36–38]. Buprenorphine can cause opioid-mediated adverse behavioral and physiological effects when administered alone to non-painful adult horses, including increased locomotor activity, restlessness, head nodding, vocalization, decreased GI sounds, increased respiratory rate, increased BP and CI, and variable changes in HR. [34, 35, 39, 40] Increased locomotor activity is purported to be caused by activation of dopaminergic pathways, and these responses are ameliorated with concurrent administration of sedatives such as acepromazine (0.05 mg/kg), detomidine (10–20 μg/kg) or xylazine (0.5 mg/kg) [41–46]. When co-administered with detomidine, buprenorphine has been shown to provide reliable sedation and analgesia for a variety of minor procedures and standing laproscopy [44, 45, 47]. When used as part of a balanced anesthesia/analgesia protocol, it provides good surgical conditions and superior analgesia compared to butorphanol for equine castration [38, 48].

In neonatal foals 2–11 days of age, buprenorphine (0.01 mg/kg IM), provides anti-nociceptive effects as measured via nociceptive withdrawal reflex 90 minutes after administration [49]. This study did not measure the duration of the nociceptive effect, but a published case report indicated a clinical duration of approximately 12 hours when dosed at 0.006 mg/kg in a 5-month-old foal [50]. Foals may exhibit similar signs as adult horses, including increased locomotor activity and tachypnea but can also become sedate [49]. Physiologic and behavioral changes include tachypnea, tachycardia, increased body temperature, increased time spent nursing, increased motor activity, and decreased time spent recumbent, but foals typically do not display overt excitement, and physical exam parameters are not outside of normal limits and similar to that seen after IM butorphanol [31, 49, 51].

Following IV administration, neonatal foals have a larger volume of distribution (6.46 ± 1.54 l/kg) and a higher total clearance (55.83 ± 23.75 ml/kg/min) compared to adult horses (3.01–3.16 l/kg and 6.13–7.97 ml/kg/min, respectively) [34, 35]. Foals also have a shorter elimination half-life (1.95 ± 0.7 hours) compared to adult horses (3.58–5.79 hours) [34, 35]. Thus, despite foals having a larger volume of distribution, they also have a much higher clearance rate, leading to a shorter half-life compared to adult horses. Higher body water content, differences in plasma protein binding, and a more permeable BBB may contribute to the increased volume of distribution in foals. Clearance of some drugs is faster in foals than in adult horses, including butorphanol [31]. Foals that received 0.02 mg/kg IV achieved plasma concentrations above 0.6 ng/ml, which is considered an analgesic plasma concentration in other veterinary species, but only for 2–4 hours [51]. This differs from adult horses where, following administration of 0.005 mg/kg of buprenorphine IM or IV, plasma concentrations were above 0.6 ng/ml for 8 and 12 hours, respectively.

Sublingual administration provides a convenient, less-invasive method of analgesic administration in foals and was purported to provide approximately 12 hours of analgesia in a 5-month-old foal [50]. Pharmacokinetic studies indicate that buprenorphine has a bioavailability of approximately 25% after sublingual administration of 0.02 mg/kg in foals, whereas plasma concentrations were undetectable in adult horses following sublingual administration [35, 51]. Plasma concentrations did not reach concentrations that are noted to provide analgesia in other species after sublingual administration.

Buprenorphine IM or IV (0.001–0.002 mg/kg) in neonatal foals can provide systemic analgesia with less behavioral and physiological side effects noted in adult horses, thus not requiring concomitant sedative administration. However, patients should be assessed for adequacy of analgesia as the duration of action may be significantly shorter than the 8–12 hours in adult horses.

Transdermal Fentanyl

Transdermal fentanyl (fentanyl patch) has been studied in neonatal foals. The advantage of transdermal fentanyl is that it provides minimally invasive, continuous analgesia delivery without the frequent dosing. Four 8-day-old foals had a 100 μg (Mylan brand) matrix fentanyl patch applied to the proximal antebrachium, corresponding to a fentanyl dose of 1.4–1.8 μg/kg/hr. Maximal fentanyl concentrations were reached at 8–24 hours (14.3 ± 7.6) but were highly variable 0.1–28.7 ng/ml (6.9 ± 10.9). No significant adverse effects were noted. HR and RR remained within physiologic range for neonatal foals along with no significant change in appetite, urination/defecation or locomotion; however, rectal temperature did increase in most foals [52]. Although there is minimal information on analgesic plasma levels in veterinary patients, plasma levels of 0.6, 1.4, and 3.0 ng/ml correspond to slight, 50% reduction and profound, respectively, analgesia in people [53]. Extrapolating human analgesic plasma levels to fentanyl plasma levels in neonatal foals with transdermal patches indicates that some foals do not achieve even slight analgesic plasma levels and other foals achieve plasma levels well above the profound analgesia levels in people. Alternative analgesia is also required until plasma levels are achieved, keeping in mind the opioid receptor specificity and activity of alternative opioid analgesics (i.e. butorphanol is a mu-antagonist and therefore would interfere with the efficacy of the fentanyl patch). Due to the high variability of plasma concentrations, clinicians should continue to assess pain and adequacy of analgesia and supplement or have an alternative plan for cases where adequate plasma concentrations and therefore analgesic levels are not achieved.

Fentanyl

Fentanyl is a mu-opioid receptor agonist that is approximately 200 times more potent than morphine. It has rapid clearance and short elimination half-life in adult horses; however, use has been limited due to CNS excitation and increased locomotor activity. Two studies evaluated the use of injectable fentanyl in foals. One evaluated escalating doses of IV fentanyl in foals 5–13 days of age. Fentanyl was administered at doses of 2, 4, 8, 16, and 32 μg/kg every 10 minutes for a cumulative dose of 62 μg/kg at 40 minutes [54]. Another study administered 4.0 μg/kg of fentanyl IV to the same foals at 6–8, 20–22, and 41–42 days of age and evaluated pharmacokinetic and pharmacodynamic changes as foals aged [55]. The average volume of distribution was highest in 6- to 8-day-old foals and decreased with age. The elimination half-life of fentanyl in neonatal foals (aged 5–13 and 6–8 days) is approximately 49 minutes after a single IV dose of 4 μg/kg and 44 minutes after escalating doses over 40 minutes with a cumulative dose of 62 μg/kg; both are shorter compared to adult horses [54, 55].

The elimination half-life is prolonged in foals 6–8 days of age compared to older foals, however, there is a large variability between individuals within each age group [55].

As with adult horses, foals (5–13 days of age) exhibited dose-dependent behavior changes [54]. Foals were mostly unaffected at a dose of 2 μg/kg, however, most foals exhibited sedative-like effects following a dose of 4.0 μg/kg, regardless of age [54, 55]. No significant changes in HR, rhythm or GI motility were noted at 4.0 μg/kg. As the dose increased to 8 and 16 μg/kg, foals exhibited muscle rigidity (flexion of head, rigidity of neck musculature) and signs of excitation including increased HR and locomotor activity. At 32 μg/kg, most foals were heavily sedated, with several requiring reversal with naloxone. The dose and plasma concentration associated with different behaviors varied widely suggesting a large degree of variability between individual foals with respect to drug response at a given concentration [54]. Sedation after 4.0 μg/kg had a rapid onset but was short lived (5–15 minutes) with individual variation across different ages of foals 1–6 weeks of age.

There are both age-related and individual variation in the production of the major metabolite of fentanyl (N-(1phenethyl-4piperidyl) malonanilinic acid (PMA) indicating differences in metabolic capability; these differences are related to the clinical and behavioral effects of fentanyl [54, 55]. Foals (6–8 days of age) produce significantly less PMA than older foals and have a significantly longer elimination half-life [55]. The fentanyl dose of 4.0 μg/kg seems to provide sedation in the majority of neonatal foals 1–6 weeks of age while minimizing unwanted side effects. However, analgesic concentrations have not been established for foals and therefore fentanyl doses should be tailored based on individual patient's clinical status and pain assessment. To date, there are no studies evaluating the use of fentanyl in anesthetized neonatal foals; thus the anesthetist should pay particular attention to titration of inhalant levels, monitoring of HR, and the adequacy of ventilation via capnography.

Hydromorphone

Although hydromorphone has not been studied in neonatal foals, there have been studies in adult horses [56–59]. Intravenous and intramuscular hydromorphone has a rapid clearance, short terminal half-life, and a large volume of distribution. The rapid clearance of hydromorphone exceeds normal hepatic blood flow, suggesting either extra-hepatic metabolism and/or an opioid induced increase in CO [56, 57]. IV and IM doses of 0.04 mg/kg have average terminal half-lives of approximately 19–34 and 26 minutes, respectively. Intramuscular administration has a high bioavailability. Despite the relatively short half-life, thermal nociceptive threshold was significantly increased for up to 8–12 hours, indicating that the presumed analgesic effects persist beyond the plasma half-life. The major metabolite, hydromorphone-3-glucuronide (H-3-G) has a much longer half-life (~4 hours) and has been identified as an active metabolite in other species. The antinociceptive effect was accompanied by CNS excitation and associated physiologic effects including increased HR, BP, respiratory rate, and rectal temperature. Behavioral side effects are also dose dependent and include excitement, pacing, and vocalization. Transient decrease in abdominal borborygmi and decreased defecation frequency has been reported, but no significant difference in fecal output was associated with hydromphone administration [56–59]. Hydromorphone may provide a viable alternative for long-lasting IM or IV mu-agonist analgesia in neonatal foals. However, more studies are needed to delineate the effects of immature liver glucuronidation on drug clearance and formation of the active metabolite H-3-G presumably responsible for the prolonged thermal anti-nociception.

Morphine

Morphine is a mu-receptor agonist. It is the natural reference opioid and has been used to produce analgesia, varying degrees of sedation and reduce the MAC of inhalant anesthetics. In horses, regardless of analgesic efficacy, opioid use remains limited in part because of concerns regarding adverse effects, such as excitement, increased locomotor activity, cardiovascular stimulation and decreased GI motility, especially at higher doses. The effects have been attributed to the release of endogenous catecholamines, activation of dopaminergic receptors and species differences in distribution and density of opioid receptors in the CNS. Consequently mu-agonist opioids are either withheld from horses or administered in conjunction with α-2 agonists or phenothiazines, both of which are typically avoided in neonatal foals.

Morphine has been studied extensively in adult horses, both experimentally in healthy horses and in clinical cases undergoing surgery. Morphine administered at doses of 0.25 or 2.0 mg/kg in horses under isoflurane anesthesia resulted in variable effects on the MAC of isoflurane, but the MAC increased in the majority of the horses (50–66%) regardless of dose. Some horses had no change in MAC and 1/6 horses in each dose group had a decrease in MAC. Heart rate, BP, and P_aCO_2 significantly increased in a dose-dependent manner. Recoveries were poor to the point of unacceptable in horses receiving the high dose of morphine [60]. Morphine (0.1 mg/kg or 0.2 mg/kg IV) also does not contribute further to MAC sparing in halothane anesthetized horses [61].

The majority of studies note a decrease in GI borborygmus, although few horses demonstrated outward signs of abdominal pain or colic. Retrospective studies of clinical cases examining the effects of morphine on postoperative colic have found conflicting results. Senior et al. noted that morphine was associated with a fourfold increase in risk of colic compared to use of butorphanol or no opioid in approximately 500 equine orthopedic surgical cases [62]. However, Anderson et al. found no increased risk of post anesthetic colic risk associated with morphine administration in 553 surgical and MRI cases [63]. Multiple doses may exacerbate GI effects of morphine. Boscan et al. administered morphine (0.5 mg/kg) twice daily for 6 days; horses had decreased propulsive motility and GI moisture content, which may predispose to the development of ileus or constipation [64]. Another study administered morphine (0.1 mg/kg IV) three times 4 hours apart; abdominal US revealed a significant decrease in contractions of duodenum, cecum and right and left ventral colons. Food and water consumption significantly increased and the size of the stomach significantly increased with a cumulative effect with repeated doses. The authors suggested that patients receiving multiple doses of morphine should be monitored for signs of colic especially gastric distension [65].

When morphine is used in clinical surgical cases, cardiorespiratory values are generally not significantly different from patients not receiving morphine and side effects are minimal [66]. Recovery scores from anesthesia are better in clinical cases undergoing surgical procedures that receive morphine compared to those who do not [67, 68]. Recoveries in horses receiving morphine have fewer attempts to attain sternal recumbency and standing and a shorter time from first movement to time of standing [69]. However, the quality of recovery can deteriorate at higher doses [70]. The quality of sedation, surgical conditions and recovery were better with butorphanol (0.5 mg/kg) compared to morphine (0.1 mg/kg) for field castration of ponies [71].

Pharmacokinetic studies indicate a short terminal half-life of morphine. One study noted that IM morphine (0.1 mg/kg) had a terminal half-life of 1.5 hours. Only 70% of horses reached a plasma level ≥16 ng/ml (plasma level associated with postoperative analgesia in humans) in the first hour and in the second hour only 35% had adequate plasma morphine concentrations. The authors suggest that a dose of 0.2 mg/kg would result in plasma levels >16 ng/ml in all horses for first hour and 20/26 horses for second hour [72].

Pharmacokinetic studies of IV morphine demonstrate a short terminal half-life; a dose of 0.1 mg/kg IV had a $t_{1/2}$ life of 1.6 hours and mean plasma levels <10 ng/ml within 4 hours [73]. Different doses of IV morphine (0.05, 0.1, 0.2, 0.5 mg/kg) noted the average alpha half-life of morphine was 8.7 minutes, average beta half-life was 1.36 hours (metabolism half-life) and gamma half-life was 11 hours (elimination half-life). The two major metabolites were morphine-3-glucuronide (M3G), which is associated with neuroexcitation and morphine-6-glucuronide (M6G), which is associated with analgesia [74]. There is a correlation between increasing doses of morphine and increases in M3G concentrations and adverse effects including CNS excitation, increased locomotion, and decreased GI borborygmi [75]. The horse makes approximately twice the amount of M3G compared to people, potentially explaining the increase in neuroexcitement in this species. The only study evaluating anti-nociciptive effects of morphine noted no decrease in response to thermal or electrical noxious stimuli in horses administered 0.05 or 0.1 mg/kg IV or IM despite attaining plasma concentrations corresponding to analgesic levels in dogs and humans [76].

There are currently no studies evaluating the use of morphine in neonatal foals. Based on pharmacokinetic studies in adult horses a dose of 0.1–0.2 mg/kg IV or IM is recommended. Due to the short terminal half-life consideration should be given to following the loading dose with a constant rate infusion (CRI, 0.1 mg/kg/hr). In adult horses, morphine is quickly metabolized to its two major metabolites M3G and M6G. It is postulated that M3G may be responsible for the neuroexcitatory effects of morphine in horses, however M6G is involved in the analgesic effects. These metabolic reactions require glucuronidation, which has a more gradual maturation in neonatal foals and may not be fully functioning until 6–12 weeks of age [13]. The effect on pharmacokinetics of morphine in neonatal foals and/or efficacy or side effects is unclear.

Intra-Articular (IA) Morphine

Opioid receptors are located on the peripheral nerve terminals in the synovium, and are upregulated during inflammatory conditions. They have been identified in the equine synovial membrane, thus making IA administration of opioids an alternative to systemic administration to provide analgesia and anti-inflammatory effects. The analgesic effects of opioids are mediated by depression of cyclic AMP formation, activating inwardly directed potassium currents leading to cell hyperpolarization. The result is decreased neuronal excitability at peripheral sensory nerve endings. Peripheral anti-inflammatory effects are mediated through inhibition of calcium-dependent release of excitatory pro-inflammatory mediators from peripheral sensory-nerve endings. Studies evaluating potential toxic or pathologic effects in IA morphine on IA cartilage indicate only mild alterations to healthy synovium and cartilage, comparable to that caused by saline alone [77, 78].

Studies in adult horses using a lipopolysaccharide-induced synovitis model documented strong analgesic and anti-inflammatory effects of IA morphine [79–83]. The onset of action is 30–40 minutes and lasts

~24 hours [79, 83]. IA morphine levels are detectable for 24 hours while systemic plasma levels of morphine and its major metabolite M6G remain very low [82, 83]. Horses administered IA morphine had significantly lower clinical lameness scores compared to saline control or IV morphine. Decreased joint swelling, better kinematic variables, and more favorable behavioral parameters (i.e. less time spent recumbent, more limb loading at rest, time spent eating) were also noted when compared to saline placebo. Joints treated with IA morphine also had lower total nucleated cells, white blood cells, TP, prostaglandin E2, and bradykinin reflecting its anti-inflammatory effects [79–83].

Doses used in studies range from 40 mg diluted in 4 ml of saline to 0.05 mg/kg and 120 mg. To date there are no pharmacokinetic/pharmacodynamics studies relating dose with effectiveness or duration of action nor are there studies in foals with naturally occurring joint sepsis. Local anesthetics would not be recommended for IA analgesia in foals with septic arthritis since they may lose their effectiveness in inflamed tissue due to pH differences and may be contraindicated due to the chondrocyte toxicity effects. Therefore, IA morphine may be an effective alternative to provide localized, long-lasting analgesia without systemic side effects in foals with joint sepsis.

Morphine may also be added to intravenous regional limb perfusion (IVRLP) in cases where administration by direct joint injection is not deemed appropriate. In a study in standing sedated adult horses, the addition of 0.1 mg/kg of morphine to IVRLP resulted in mean peak synovial morphine concentrations of 3903 ± 4881 ng/ml and peak plasma morphine concentrations of 11–63 ng/ml at 2 hours. Thus, IVRLP with morphine may have greater analgesic and anti-inflammatory potential for treatment of synovial pain in the distal aspect of the limbs than systemic morphine. Of note, synovial concentrations of gentamicin were not affected when co-administered with morphine [84].

Methadone

Methadone is a mu-agonist opioid. It has additional mechanisms of action that enhance its analgesic properties, including N-methyl-D-aspartate (NMDA) antagonism and serotonin- and norepinephrine-reuptake inhibition. To date, there are no studies evaluating the use of methadone in neonatal foals, however, it has been studied extensively in adult horses. Adult horses administrated the injectable formulation orally at doses of 0.1, 0.15, 0.2, 0.4, and 0.5 mg/kg, or IV administration of 0.15 mg/kg did not demonstrate signs of excitement, increased locomotor activity nor cardiopulmonary or GI motility changes [85–88]. Although plasma concentrations exceeded the effective analgesic levels documented in humans, no thermal, electrical, or mechanical antinociceptive effects were produced [85, 87, 88]. Methadone (0.25 mg/kg bolus followed by 0.25 mg/kg/hr CRI) used in an experimental model of carpal synovitis did show a marked decrease in lameness in affected horses [89].

Methadone (0.5 mg/kg, IV) provided short acting anti-nociception using thermal and electrical nociceptive thresholds, however severe adverse behavioral effects and ataxia limit its clinical use. Methadone at a dose of 0.2 mg/kg IV did not provide thermal or electrical nociception. However, it potentiates and prolongs anti-nociception provided by detomidine (5–10 μg/kg) or acepromazine (0.05 mg/kg) without adverse effects [90, 91]. Nociception was of similar intensity but shorter duration when methadone was combined with 5.0 μg/kg of detomidine compared with 10 μg/kg. Horses were less sedated and GI motility better preserved [92]. The combination of detomidine and methadone can also be used as a CRI for standing surgeries in adult horses using loading doses of detomidine (5.0 μg/kg IV) and methadone (0.2 mg/kg IV) followed by CRI of 12.5 μg/kg/hr and 0.05 mg/kg/hr, respectively [93, 94]. Methadone (0.1 mg/kg IV) can also be combined with acepromazine (0.05 mg/kg IV) or detomidine (20 μg/kg IV) as a premedication prior to dissociative anesthesia induction in adult horses [95].

To date, methadone has not been shown to provide anti-nociception to thermal, electrical, or mechanical stimuli when used alone in adult horses at any studied doses or route of administration. There is a requirement for the co-administration of detomidine or acepromazine to potentiate analgesic effects. Since these drugs have significant cardiovascular depressant effects in neonatal foals, the usefulness of methadone is questionable at this time.

Epidural

Caudal epidural anesthesia and analgesia is an effective technique for management of moderate to severe pain of the hindlimbs, caudal aspect of the body, and in some cases up to the thoracic limbs and is extensively reviewed elsewhere [96, 97]. Epidural administration of different drugs has been studied and clinically applied including opioids, local anesthetics, α-2 agonists, dissociatives, and various combinations of each. The combination of epidural drugs offers the advantage of improved anesthesia/analgesia due to synergism between drugs and the ability to decrease the doses of individual medications thereby decreasing the incidence and severity of side effects. The choice of specific drugs or combination depends on the area of the body requiring anesthesia and/or analgesia and the duration of action desired. The dose and volume of epidural drugs affects the onset, duration, intensity, and spread of anesthesia/analgesia. The extent of cranial spread determines the level of dermatomal coverage and therefore, which regions are affected. A volume of 0.02 ml/kg is used to provide regional coverage of the coccygeal, perineal, and sacral regions. Higher volumes should be avoided when using local anesthetics as severe ataxia and recumbency can occur due to cranial spread affecting the motor nerves of the pelvic limbs [96, 97]. If more cranial analgesia is desired, volumes of 0.15–0.2 ml/kg containing opioids alone or in combination with α-2 agonists may provide analgesia up to the thoracic limbs [96, 97]. Epidural catheters may be placed for repeated dosing for longer-term analgesia. Although experimental and clinical studies and application have focused on adult horses, these techniques can be used in foals for nonsurgically related painful conditions and as an adjunct to general anesthesia to reduce general anesthetic requirements and provide effective perioperative pain control.

NSAIDs are reviewed in Chapter 63.

Sedatives/Premedication

The most common sedative/premedication for foals <7–10 days old are benzodiazepines such as midazolam or diazepam and an opioid. This combination provides good sedation, has minimal cardiovascular effects and both are reversible if necessary. Oxygen supplementation via face mask, nasal cannula or endotracheal tube at 50–100mL/kg/min should be provided if sedation causes recumbency. The negative cardiovascular effects of acepromazine and α-2 agonists make both poor options in neonatal foals <7 days of age.

Induction

Historically, inhalant anesthetics have been used for induction via tight-fitting mask or nasotracheal intubation, ostensibly to avoid prolonged recovery due to injectable barbiturates in neonatal foals with limited metabolic capacity [3, 6, 7]. The advantage lies in the ability to titrate the inhalant agent and rely on respiration rather than hepatic metabolism for elimination from the body. Disadvantages include the necessity of high levels of inhalant to achieve an appropriate level of anesthesia for intubation and the procedure and increased stress in handling the foal during induction. Furthermore, mortality is higher in “inhalant only” protocols in neonatal foals [4]. A balanced anesthetic regimen that uses a combination of injectable and inhalant agents may offer a safer alternative. Newer, shorter acting injectable anesthetics make it possible to use injectable anesthetics for induction of anesthesia, but there are few studies comparing different induction regimens in neonatal foals (Table 64.3).

Ketamine-Benzodiazepine

Ketamine is a dissociative agent with sedative, anesthetic, and analgesic effects via NMDA receptor antagonism. Although ketamine has direct depressant effects on myocardial contractility, these are usually masked by stimulation of the sympathetic nervous system resulting in increases in HR and BP. The depressant effects of ketamine may become apparent in patients with little to no catecholamine reserves. Neonatal foals can be induced with ketamine following premedication with a benzodiazepine and opioid or ketamine can be co-administered with a benzodiazepine after opioid premedication. A study comparing diazepam (0.2 mg/kg) versus xylazine (0.8 mg/kg) premedication prior to ketamine (2.0 mg/kg) induction in 1- to 2-week-old pony foals and then at 2–4 weeks of age indicated HR, SAP, MAP, DAP, and CI were significantly lower in foals receiving xylazine compared to those receiving diazepam [98]. Premedication with diazepam prior to induction of anesthesia with ketamine and maintenance with isoflurane resulted in significantly less hemodynamic depression than that observed when xylazine was used as the premedication [98]. Although the differences in cardiopulmonary effects were less marked in the older foals, premedication with diazepam continued to offer hemodynamic advantages over xylazine prior to ketamine and isoflurane maintenance. Most foals that received xylazine premedication had MAP values <60–65 mmHg, regardless of age. There was no significant difference in quality of induction, MAC reduction of isoflurane and recovery quality [98].

Propofol

Propofol has the pharmacokinetic advantage of rapid clearance, allowing quick recovery from anesthesia. Although there are no studies in neonatal foals, propofol has been studied as an induction agent in premedicated and unpremedicated adult horses [99–105]. Evaluation of doses of 2–8 mg/kg reveal that the quality of induction and recovery are dose-related. Induction quality is highly variable with lower doses of propofol (≤2 mg/kg) failing to produce recumbency and inducing an excitatory response characterized by muscle fasiculations and rigidity. Horses that become recumbent often have increased locomotor activity with stiffening of the shoulder and neck muscles, attempts to raise their head, nystagmus, and vocalization. Although the addition of midazolam and various doses of xylazine and detomidine improved induction in some cases and allowed use of lower induction doses, the quality of induction was still highly variable. With the addition of 5% guafenesin (average dose 72 mg/kg) followed propofol (average 2.5 mg/kg), anesthesia induction proceeded without adverse induction events, although all horses maintained palpebral reflexes [105]. Recovery is good to excellent across studies regardless of premedication but tends to worsen at higher induction doses.

Propofol is a negative inotrope and decreases SVR leading to dose-dependent hypotension in many species, but HR and arterial BP seem to be better preserved in horses [99–104]. However, propofol causes significant respiratory depression and hypoxemia (P_aO_2 <60 mmHg) when administered as a bolus; thus, oxygen supplementation and ventilatory support should be available. Although propofol is of questionable acceptability in adult horses due to poor induction conditions, putting the safety of patient and personnel at risk, this is less of a concern in neonatal foals who are smaller in size and more easily controlled during induction and recovery. Doses of 1–4 mg/kg have been used in neonatal foals by the author depending on the physical status and level of sedation from premedication. In dogs, the induction dose is decreased by approximately half and the incidence of post-induction apnea (PIA) is decreased from 100% to 25% when propofol is administered at a rate of 1.0 mg/kg/min rather than 4.0 mg/kg/min [106]. Therefore, propofol should be titrated slowly to decrease the overall induction dose and presumably limit the severity of respiratory depression and incidence of PIA. Oxygen supplementation and a means of ventilatory support should be available during induction.

Propofol-Ketamine

The co-administration of propofol and ketamine has been studied and used in cats, dogs, and humans with the intention of counteracting the adverse cardiovascular side effects of propofol alone [107–109]. In dogs, induction with the combination of propofol and ketamine resulted in a higher HR and arterial BP than when propofol was used alone and the quality of induction, intubation, and recovery were consistently good [109]. The combination of propofol and ketamine has been studied in adult horses to improve the quality of induction and recovery and investigate a substitute for benzodiazepines during a nationwide shortage in the United States. Wagner et al. compared eight different induction protocols in adult horses and found that the combination of ketamine (1.5 mg/kg) and propofol (0.5 mg/kg) afforded the best behavioral quality for induction and recovery [110]. A retrospective analysis of 100 client-owned horses (6 months to 30 years old) that were anesthetized for a variety of procedures with propofol (0.5 mg/kg) and ketamine (3.0 mg/kg) after xylazine premedication noted that none of the horses experienced postinduction apnea or other adverse events during induction, although 6 horses required additional ketamine. The majority (79%) of horses had a "smooth" recovery [111]. A study comparing co-administration of propofol (0.5 mg/kg) versus midazolam (0.1 mg/kg) with ketamine (3.0 mg/kg) found that the number of attempts to stand was significantly lower and quality of recovery was significantly better with propofol compared to midazolam in adult horses. There was no significant difference in induction quality. All horses required CV support with dobutamine to maintain BP at 75–85 mmHg. Plasma drug concentrations were also significantly lower as a percentage of induction dose in horses that received propofol compared to midazolam. Propofol may be advantageous in horses undergoing short anesthetic procedures (<60 minutes) [112].

The physical and chemical stability of the ketamine/propofol combination (1 : 1 mg ratio) has been confirmed and the two drugs may be mixed in the same syringe for administration [113]. Although administered as a bolus in adult horses, the mixture can be titrated more closely to effect in foals due to their less dangerous size and behavior. The optimal combination of ketamine and propofol has not been established in neonatal foals, but doses range from that used in small animal veterinary patients (2 mg/kg each of propofol and ketamine) to that used in adult horses (1.5 mg/kg ketamine and 0.5 mg/kg propofol).

Alfaxalone

Alphaxalone has been used for induction and short-term anesthesia in neonatal foals. In one study, 12-day-old foals were premedicated with butorphanol and induced with 3.0 mg/kg of alphaxalone IV administered slowly over one minute [114]. Compared to adult horses, neonatal foals have a smaller volume of distribution (1.6 vs 0.6 l/kg, respectively), comparatively lower clearance (37.1 vs. 19.9 ml/min/kg, respectively) and shorter terminal half-life (33.4 vs 22.8 minutes, respectively) [114, 115]. The time from induction to first movement/extubation and standing was 20 and 40 minutes, respectively, although foals were not stimulated surgically. Foals exhibited mild generalized muscle twitching but HR did not differ significantly from baseline, no arrhythmias were observed, and MAP remained >70 mmHg. Postinduction apnea was not observed; however, respiratory rates decreased, foals were hypercapnic, and several experienced moderate to severe hypoxemia (P_aO_2 =44–68 mmHg). Supplemental oxygen should be provided during induction and for short procedures. In dogs, the rate of administration affects the total dose requirement of alphaxalone and the incidence of PIA. When alphaxalone is administered at 0.5 mg/kg/min rather than the suggested rate of 2.0 mg/kg/min, the induction dose is decreased by approximately half and the incidence of PIA is decreased from 100% to 25%. Therefore, when possible, alphaxalone should be administered slowly to decrease the induction dose and incidence of PIA [106].

Maintenance of Anesthesia

The inhalants isoflurane and sevoflurane are the most common agents used for maintenance of anesthesia. All inhalant anesthetics cause dose-dependent cardiopulmonary depression due to decreasing myocardial contractility and vasodilation both leading to hypotension. Respiratory depression is due to decreased responsiveness of central respiratory centers to blood pH and P_aCO_2 leading to hypoventilation. Horses as a species, and foals in particular, are more sensitive to the respiratory depressant effects of inhalant anesthetics and commonly have arterial/end-tidal carbon dioxide concentrations >60 mmHg, requiring ventilation support at concentrations around MAC [116]. Isoflurane is the most widely used volatile inhaled anesthetic in equine anesthesia, since it is least expensive. The median effective concentration for inhaled anesthetics is expressed as the MAC. Isoflurane has a MAC of 1.3%, making it more potent than sevoflurane (MAC of 2.3%). However, sevoflurane has less blood solubility and therefore quicker anesthetic equilibration between the alveoli and CNS and quicker elimination during recovery. Approximately 2–5% of sevoflurane undergoes hepatic metabolism, whereas only 0.17% of isoflurane undergoes hepatic metabolism. During positive pressure ventilation, sevoflurane may preserve CO better than isoflurane [117, 118]. It is important to monitor BP and capnography and have a plan and means for intervention, including positive pressure ventilation and positive inotropes/vasopressors.

Positioning and Padding

Foals should be positioned with padding to evenly distribute their weight. Halters should be removed, limbs supported, and head placed in a neutral position without extreme extension. The eyes should be protected and lubricated every 30–120 minutes depending on the product used.

Intubation

Endotracheal (ET) intubation secures the airway and allows delivery of oxygen, inhalant anesthetic, and intermittent positive pressure ventilation (IPPV) in cases of hypoventilation or apnea. Intubation is performed blindly with the patient in lateral recumbency and head extended. Appropriately sized cuffed endotracheally tubes are typically 10–16 mm internal diameter (ID). The anesthetist should have a variety of lubricated ET tubes available, with the cuffs appropriately checked for leaks by fully inflating the cuff and setting aside for 5–10 minutes to allow identification of slow leaks. The ET cuffs are deflated immediately prior to premedication and induction. Although neonatal foals are typically only nursing, the mouth should be flushed with water, using a 60 mL catheter tip syringe prior to induction to avoid introducing foreign material (e.g. bedding, wood shavings) into the trachea during intubation. Flow by oxygen and capability to administer IPPV should be available. When using a demand valve, an airway pressure manometer should be placed between the ET tube and the end of the demand valve to allow the anesthetist to keep airway pressure ≤20 cmH_2O (Figure 64.1). The manometer is also helpful when inflating the ET cuff; the anesthetist

(a) (b)

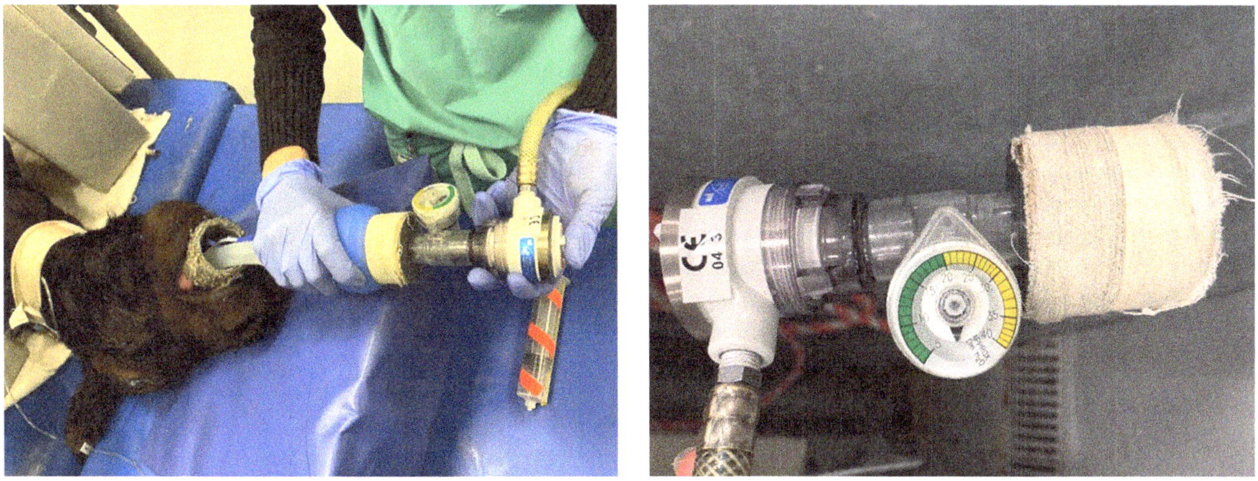

Figure 64.1 (a) Foal is intubated and positive pressure ventilation supplied via a demand valve. (b) The airway pressure manometer allows the anesthetist to limit the airway pressure to 20 cmH_2O or less to avoid barotrauma in young neonatal foals.

inflates the cuff while administering a positive pressure ventilation breath up to a pressure of 20 cmH_2O until any leak is dissipated.

Monitoring and Support

Monitoring during anesthesia provides information regarding the physical status of the patient and warns the anesthetist in order to allow appropriate intervention so that anesthetic emergencies or fatal consequences can be avoided. This is especially important in the equine neonate with limited physiologic reserves and immature cardiovascular responses. Variables monitored include anesthetic depth, cardiovascular and respiratory function, body temperature as well as parameters such as blood glucose, blood gas analysis, and electrolytes, depending on the underlying disease process and physical status of the foal. Multiparameter monitors developed for veterinary patients are readily available, as are refurbished human monitors, which may be more economically feasible. These multiparameter monitors include ECG, BP (invasive and noninvasive), pulse oximetry, capnography, and body temperature; an additional option is a multigas analyzer, which can measure inspired and expired inhalant gas and oxygen concentrations. However, monitors cannot replace a trained and attentive anesthetist, and the benefit of direct, hands-on interaction with the patient should not be overlooked. A veterinarian or a trained veterinary technician under veterinary supervision should be dedicated to continuously monitoring the patient thoroughout anesthesia and recovery. A plan for intervention should be devised and discussed prior to anesthetizing the patient should parameters stray outside acceptable values.

Foals undergoing only sedation may be monitored using techniques such as pulse palpation, cardiac auscultation, capillary refill time (CRT), mucous membrane color, and counting chest excursions for respiratory rate. Foals under heavy sedation or short-term injectable anesthesia who are laterally recumbent should have oxygen supplementation. Portable pulse oximeters can provide SpO_2% and an audible signal for pulse rate. All but the very briefest of procedures (<10–15 minutes) should entail more extensive monitoring.

Anesthetic Depth

Anesthetic depth should be assessed repeatedly and often and the level of anesthesia closely titrated to the needs and status of the patient and procedure. Anesthetic drugs, especially inhalant anesthetics, are dose dependent cardiovascular and respiratory depressants, therefore, patients that have excessive anesthetic depth will experience cardiorespiratory depression predisposing to anesthetic complications and patient morbidity/mortality. Conversely, inadequate anesthetic depth and analgesia may result in arousal during surgical stimulation and an increased likelihood of patient movement, increased stress to the patient, contamination of the surgical field and injury to themselves or personnel.

Physical attributes give the anesthetist an overall assessment of patient anesthetic depth and include: movement of patient, position of the eye globe, presence/absence of nystagmus, degree of depression of protective eye reflexes (palpebral, corneal), swallowing reflex, and response to surgical stimulus. Physiologic parameters such as HR, respiratory rate, and BP are less reliable indicators of anesthetic depth, as they are depressed at a surgical plane of anesthesia. Indications of a light plane of anesthesia include shivering, tightening of the neck muscles, or stretching. Lateral nystagmus, tear production, and spontaneous blinking are eye signs indicative of a light plane of anesthesia. The eyeball rotates ventromedially and returns to a central position as anesthesia deepens.

The palpebral reflex is elicited by stroking the cilia of the eye, resulting in closure of the eyelids. The palpebral reflex varies from a rapid response with closure of the eyelids and becomes progressively more depressed as depth of anesthesia increases and is sluggish or absent at a surgical plane of anesthesia. Patients induced with ketamine maintain active palpebral reflexes, a centrally positioned globe, lacrimation, and blinking, which progressively decreases as the patient transitions to inhalant anesthesia. The corneal reflex is elicited by applying pressure to the cornea resulting in closure of the eyelids and should always be present. Absence of the corneal reflex indicates excessive anesthetic depth and CNS depression. Due to the possibility of iatrogenic damage to the cornea, this reflex should only be used in emergent situations. The anal reflex is elicited by stimulating the anus, resulting in contraction of the anal sphincter, and serves as a crude indicator of anesthetic depth if the head is inaccessible. All reflex responses become more depressed as anesthetic depth increases and become less reliable as anesthesia time progresses.

Multiparameter patient monitors commonly have multigas/agent modules that allow measurement of inspired and end-tidal concentrations of inhalant anesthetics, which serve as indicators of the partial pressure of inhalant anesthetic in the alveoli and brain, respectively. Relating these concentrations to the known MAC values of inhalant anesthetics used can give the anesthetist an additional tool to gauge anesthetic depth as these values will be more precise and accurate than the vaporizer setting (Figure 64.2).

Effects on the Cardiovascular System

Delivery of oxygen to tissues is the key to patient survival and depends on adequately functioning cardiovascular and respiratory systems. Monitoring of cardiovascular function includes HR and rhythm, arterial BP, and subjective clinical

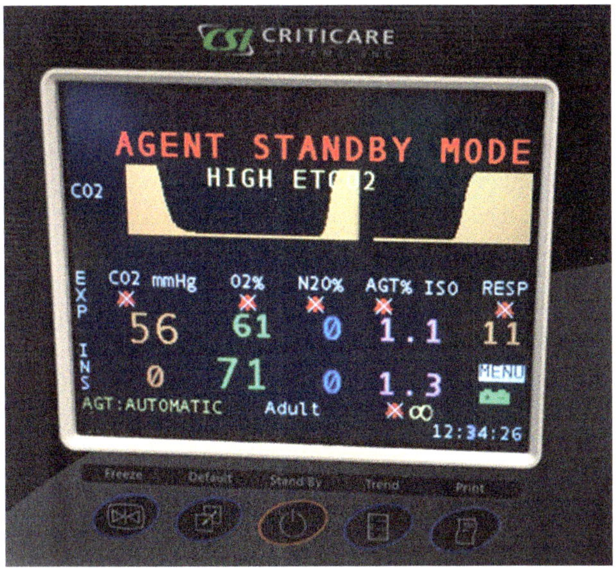

Figure 64.2 Multi-gas analyzer displaying inspired agent (isoflurane) concentration (1.3%) and expired agent (isoflurane) concentration (1.1%). The inspired % reflects the inhalant concentration in the alveoli and the expired % reflects the inhalant concentration in the brain. Both can be related to the MAC of isoflurane. Note: Vaporizer was set at 2%.

indicators of perfusion. Simple clinical techniques include palpation of peripheral pulses, auscultation of the chest, evaluation of CRT, and mucous membrane color. However, CRT and mucous membrane color can be affected by anesthetic drugs and pulse pressure only gives an indication of the difference between systolic and diastolic pressures and not MAP. Clinical techniques can be used, along with pulse oximetry for short (<10 minutes) sedation or general anesthesia. Flow by oxygen supplementation (50–100 ml/kg/min) should be available and delivered via face mask, nasal cannula or endotracheal tube. In humans, postanesthetic acute kidney injury (AKI) is associated with MAP 55–60 mmHg for as short as 10–20 minutes [119], therefore, procedures longer than 10 minutes should have more intensive monitoring including ECG, arterial BP, capnography (±gas analysis), and body temperature.

Monitoring of arterial BP provides a measure of adequacy of blood flow to vital organs and can be measured directly or indirectly (Table 64.4). Direct arterial BP measurement is most accurate and allows for continuous monitoring, however, it requires an arterial catheter which can be technically difficult in neonates. The facial, transverse facial, auricular, or metatarsal arteries can be used for direct BP monitoring depending on the positioning of the foal and procedure being performed. The catheter is then connected to a transducer or aneroid manometer. Indirect BP measurement is measured with a Doppler and syphingomanometer or oscillometric device. Oscillometric techniques have the advantage of providing measurement of mean and diastolic BP in addition to systolic and are generally more accurate than indirect methods in adult horses [120]. Mean arterial, rather than systolic or diastolic pressure, is a measure of the true driving pressure for systemic blood flow and organ perfusion and is the recommended measurement upon which clinical decisions and interventions should be made.

Table 64.4 Summary of treatment strategy for hypotension and cardiovascular stimulant drug categories.

Treatment strategy for hypotension
Decrease anesthetic depth/inhalant concentration
Fluid therapy
Cardiovascular stimulant drugs
Cardiovascular stimulant drugs
Chronotropes
Inotropes
Vasopressors

Accuracy of oscillometric BP compared to direct measurement depends on the specific commercially available monitor and cuff placement. From a clinical perspective and by standards used by the American Association of Advancement of Medical Instrumentation, both the Cardell and Dinamap monitors with cuffs placed over either the coccygeal or dorsal metatarsal arteries provide acceptable MAP measurement in foals [120]. Another study using a different oscillometric monitor found good agreement between mean and diastolic, but not for systolic BP between oscillometric measurement at the coccygeal artery compared to direct BP measurement at the greater metatarsal artery. A cuff placed around the base of the tail with a bladder width to tail girth ration of 1 : 2 to 1 : 3 provides the best agreement between indirect MAP and DAP direct arterial BP measurement from the metatarsal artery in neonatal foals [121].

A review of noninvasive BP in animals reviewed existing studies and evaluated performance based on the American College of Veterinary Internal Medicine Hypertension Consensus Panel and Veterinary Blood Pressure Society Recommendations (AHCP-VBPS) [122]. This study confirmed findings of two studies in anesthetized and conscious foals that oscillometry provided an acceptable estimate of MAP when measured from the tail in comparison to direct MAP measured from the metatarsal artery regardless of the monitor used (ProPaq Encore, Cardell, or Dinamap) [120–122]. The lowest bias (−1.07 mmHg) and narrowest limits of agreement (−9.39 to 7.25 mmHg) were found for the ProPaq Encore monitor, although all three monitors were clinically acceptable [122].

Reported MAP in conscious neonatal foals is 80–100 mmHg [2, 16]. Young foals rarely develop postanesthetic myopathy, but it is vital to maintain a minimum MAP of 60–65 mmHg to provide adequate cerebral, renal, and coronary blood flow. When hypotension occurs, the anesthetist should attempt to distinguish between decreased circulating volume, CO, or SVR, as treatment strategies include fluid therapy, decreasing inhalants, and cardiovascular support drugs (positive inotropes, vasopressors). Circulating volume can be assessed based on physical exam and underlying disease process and clinically with pulse quality, mucous membrane color, CRT, skin turgor, and PCV/TS. IV fluids restore circulating volume and improve venous return and cardiac preload. Decreased CO may be caused by bradycardia or decreased myocardial contractility caused by anesthetic drugs. Decreased SVR can also be caused by anesthetic drugs, especially inhalants. Sepsis and immaturity of vasomotor reflexes in neonatal foals also contribute to decreased SVR. Optimization of BP during anesthesia begins with appropriate preoperative patient stabilization, including rehydration and correction of electrolyte and acid/base abnormalities. Surgical efficiency and limiting anesthesia time will also help decrease cardiopulmonary depression.

The rate of IV fluid administration depends on patient status, underlying condition, and type and duration of procedure. Maintenance fluid rates during anesthesia are 5–10 ml/kg/hr using a balanced crystalloid solution (i.e. Lactated Ringer's, plasmalyte). Colloids, including synthetic solutions and plasma, may be required if albumin, TP, and colloid oncotic pressure are decreased or to supplement crystalloid fluid therapy in the hypotensive patients. Although use of synthetic colloids is controversial due to associated coagulopathy and AKI, newer formulations have lower molecular weight and molar substitution and are associated with less adverse effects.

A bolus dose of 20 ml/kg of tetrastarch (130/0.4) in 0.9% NaCl (Vetstarch®) has been shown to increase oncotic pressure in neonatal foals for up to 3 hours with no changes in clotting times, coagulation factors, platelet count fibrinogen, or urinary indices [123]. Hetastarch can be administered as a slow bolus or as a supplement or replacement to crystalloid fluids. An initial slow bolus of 2–10 ml/kg can be followed by an infusion of 0.5–2.0 ml/kg/hr or maintained on 2.0 ml/kg/hr. Synthetic colloids as a class are dosed up to 20 ml/kg/day, but tetrastarch (130/0.4) has been dosed up to 50 ml/kg/day in people [124].

Hydration status and PCV/TS should be monitored to prevent overhydration, particularly for procedures lasting >2 hours. Neonates have a large central compartment and tend to accumulate fluids in the interstitial space. This, along with decreased renal function due to immaturity and effects of anesthesia lead to retention of infused fluids for a longer time. IV fluids should be administered with a fluid pump to ensure accuracy and the foal should be monitored for serous nasal discharge, nasal edema, chemosis, and pulmonary crackles [2, 19]. Blood glucose should be monitored every 1–2 hours and 2.5% dextrose added to IV fluids if blood glucose is <70 mg/dl.

Inhalant anesthetics are direct myocardial depressants and potent vasodilators. Besides fluid therapy, strategies for prevention and treatment of cardiovascular depression and hypotension include reduction of anesthetic depth and use of cardiovascular stimulant drugs. Titration of inhalant anesthetic requires the use of balanced anesthesia and analgesia techniques; this entails use of lesser doses of multiple drugs and techniques to minimize adverse effects. In contrast to other species, opioids have little or no MAC-sparing effects on inhaled anesthetic potency in horses at clinically relevant doses [60, 125]. However, in contrast to adult horses, sedation has been reported with opioids buprenorphine and fentanyl in neonatal foals. Ketamine, lidocaine, and multiple opioids have been studied in adult horses as adjunct analgesia and inhalant sparing during general anesthesia, but little information is available in foals. Thus, caution should be exercised when extrapolating adult horse doses to neonates due to differences in volume of distribution of drugs, immature liver metabolic capacity, and changes in liver blood flow during anesthesia. The author has used CRIs of ketamine (0.6 mg/kg/hr), lidocaine (1.5–3.0 mg/kg/hr), and fentanyl (5–10 μg/kg/hr) in neonatal foals, allowing use of lower inhalant levels without clinical evidence of delayed or prolonged recovery.

The benefits of local-regional anesthesia/analgesia should also be considered for neonates to help decrease nociceptive stimuli from reaching the CNS. Depending on the anatomic location and the procedure performed, peripheral nerve blocks for the lower limbs or oral cavity, incisional or transversus abdominus plane blocks for abdominal surgeries, and epidurals for caudal abdominal or hindlimb procedures can be considered.

In situations where decreasing inhalant anesthetic and adequate fluid therapy are ineffective in maintaining MAP >60 mmHg, cardiostimulant drugs are indicated. In general, bradycardia resulting in hypotension is treated with chronotropes, decreased myocardial contractility with inotropes, and decreased SVR (vasodilation) with vasopressors.

The HR in awake neonatal foals is 80–100 beats per minute (bpm) within the first week of life. Since neonatal foals are more dependent on HR to maintain CO, efforts should be made to keep HR >50 bpm. If bradycardia occurs, steps should be taken to increase HR, including decreasing anesthetic depth and judicious use of anti-cholinergics (hyoscine 0.05–0.2 mg/kg, glycopyrrolate 0.0025–0.005 mg/kg, or atropine 0.005–0.01 mg/kg, IV). Hyoscine is a belladonna alkaloid related to atropine and has a shorter duration of action with regard to chronotropy and inhibitory effects on

GI motility [126–128]. Treatment of reflex bradycardia due to α-2 agonists with an anti-cholinergic can result in severe hypertension without an increase in CI, resulting in substantial increases in myocardial oxygen consumption and potential myocardial hypoxia due to a mismatch between myocardial oxygen delivery and consumption. Therefore, anti-cholinergics should only be administered when bradycardia is accompanied by hypotension. A low dose of hyoscine (0.05 mg/kg) increased HR from 18–40 beats/min and MAP from 65 to 85 mmHg in an anesthetized adult Thoroughbred [126]. Using the lower end of the dose may avoid causing typical anti-cholinergic side effects of tachycardia and hypertension.

Cardiovascular support dugs include inotropes and vasopressors and are reviewed elsewhere (Chapter 11) [129, 130]. Inotropes increase CO and MAP primarily by increasing myocardial contractility and SV. Vasopressors increase BP through vasoconstriction and increasing SVR. Most drugs have varying degrees of inotropy and pressor activity; the order of decreasing inotropy and increasing vasopressor effects of the CV support drugs commonly available are: dobutamine, dopamine, ephedrine, norepinephrine, and phenylephrine.

Dobutamine is a positive inotrope commonly used to treat hypotension in horses. It is primarily a β-1 agonist that increases CO and BP by increasing myocardial contractility. It has some β-2 activity leading to peripheral vasodilation; however, this is balanced with a mild α-1 effect. Lower doses (0.5–1.0 μg/kg/min) increase BP without increasing CO. Higher doses (2.5–5 μg/kg/min) increase both BP and CO, whereas doses of 10 μg/kg/min often result in tachycardia and ventricular arrhythmias [130]. The actual clinical effect in individual horses likely depends on the prevailing autonomic nervous system activity, HR and BP. Dobutamine is used extensively to support CV function in critically ill foals during hypotension caused by depressive effects of inhalant anesthesia. Dobutamine preserves muscle blood flow better than agents with more vasopressor activity such as dopamine and phenylephrine [131].

Calcium salts (calcium gluconate, calcium chloride) can be used to increase circulating calcium levels, thereby enhancing calcium availability to the contractile apparatus, resulting in positive inotropic effects and increased SV and CO. [130] The usefulness of calcium salts and the effects observed in individual patients varies with health status, cardiovascular status, and ionized calcium concentrations. Treatment with calcium salts tends to be most useful in patients with decreased ionized calcium levels.

Dopamine has dose-dependent effects, and the dose at which different receptors are activated depend not only on dose, but the patient's clinical status and preexisting level of sympathetic activity. In general, at low doses (<2–4 μg/kg/min) there is a predominance of stimulation of DA1 and DA2 receptors increasing renal blood flow and glomerular filtration rate. Intermediate doses (3–5 μg/kg/min) have a predominant β-1 effect of positive inotropy. Higher doses (>5–10 μg/kg/min) result in mainly α-adrenergic effects; arrhythmias including sinus tachycardia and ventricular ectopic activity increasingly possible [129, 130].

Ephedrine has both direct and indirect α and β adrenergic activity. It increases contractility, HR, CO, SV, and BP. It has more prolonged effects (duration of action ~15 minutes) and therefore is used more often as a bolus rather than CRI. Repeated dosing can result in tachyphylaxis due to depletion of norepinephrine stores in sympathetic neurons [130]. Ephedrine can be used in cases where dobutamine is less effective in increasing BP.

Norepinephrine is a β1-agonist and very potent α-agonist and thus functions primarily as a vasopressor. It increases myocardial contractility but CO may actually decrease due to substantial increase in SVR. A dose of 0.1 μg/kg/min was ineffective in increasing urine output or creatinine clearance in Thoroughbred foals, however a dose of 0.3 μg/kg/min was effective in pony foals [132, 133]. Norepinephrine (0.3 and 1.0 μg/kg/min) increased arterial BP, CI, SVR and delivery of oxygen to tissues (DO_2) but decreased the oxygen extraction ratio. However, the increase in CI and DO_2 were less pronounced compared to dobutamine administration [134]. Norepinephrine increases MAP and urine output in critically ill hypotensive foals that are non-responsive to fluid therapy and dobutamine [135]. Norepinephrine has arrhythmogenic properties as myocardial oxygen consumption is increased. Due to generalized vasoconstriction, renal, visceral, GI, and skeletal muscle may experience decreases in blood flow even though MAP increases.

Arginine vasopressin (AVP) is used for the management of vasodiliatory shock and cardiac arrest. It is involved in maintenance of blood osmolality and circulating volume due to its antidiuretic effects on the kidney and control of BP through vasoconstriction. AVP has only a minor role in BP regulation under normal conditions but is released from the neurohypophysis in response to hypotension. As septic shock progresses, either decreased concentration or responsiveness results in the loss of vasomotor tone seen with this condition. The release of AVP is increased early in septic shock and eventually results in exhaustion of AVP stores in the neurohypophysis and a subsequent decrease in circulating vasopressin [129]. An advantage of AVP is the nitric oxide mediated vasodilation that occurs in the pulmonary and coronary vascular beds, which differs from the generalized vasoconstriction associated with NE.

Phenylephrine is a selective α1-adrenergic agonist that has negligible effect on β-receptors. It increases arterial BP and PCV but also greatly increases SVR leading to a decrease in CO and reflex bradycardia, along with decreases in splanchnic and renal perfusion [130].

There are limited studies of the use of cardiostimulant drugs in neonatal foals. Valverde et al. reported that dobutamine and norepinephrine were superior to AVP for improving cardiovascular function in healthy foals under deep inhalant anesthesia. Although all three drugs increased MAP, only dobutamine and norepinephrine improved CI and DO_2. This was a low CO model of hypotension rather than decreased SVR seen with sepsis. Furthermore, foals in this study were healthy and therefore would not be expected to respond to exogenous administration of AVP. The authors concluded that dobutamine and norepinephrine are good choices to treat neonatal foals with inhalant-induced hypotension due to the resultant improvement in MAP, CI, and DO_2 [134]. However, plasma concentrations of endogenous AVP are depleted and inappropriately low in hypotensive patients due to septic shock. Therefore, the use of AVP may be more effective in restoring CV function in septic patients that are refractory to treatment with dobutamine and/or norepinephrine.

Norepinephrine can be effective in increasing MAP through its α-adrenergic effects in foals that are refractory to treatment with dobutamine. However, drugs with vasopressor activity can increase MAP without improving CI or even cause a decrease in CI due to the negative effects of increasing SVR and cardiac work. Although CI gives a more accurate assessment of overall cardiac function, arterial BP is the clinically monitored parameter since it is more easily measured. CI and MAP have been shown to be poorly correlated; therefore, assessing cardiovascular status and instituting treatment based on arterial BP alone may not be entirely appropriate.

A retrospective analysis of the use of pressor treatment in critically ill neonatal foals found that AVP was associated with a significant increase in MAP and urinary output and decrease in HR, whereas norepinephrine was associated with an increase in MAP only. Both agents are recommended for treatment of hypotension in critically ill foals that are refractory to treatment with dobutamine. Although norepinephrine and AVP both increase MAP, the combination may be a better choice as it decreases the norepinephrine requirement and may improve patient outcome [135, 136]. An algorithm for treatment of hypotension in neonatal foals is found in Figure 64.3.

Effective use of cardiovascular support drugs is dependent on the underlying cause(s) of hypotension (Table 64.5). Cardiovascular depression due to anesthetic drugs is best treated with a positive inotrope such as dobutamine. Dopamine at mid-range doses (2.5–10 μg/kg/min) is an alternative; lower doses may have minimal effects whereas higher doses may be arrhythmogenic [130]. The addition of the vasopressors norepinephrine, AVP or a low dose combination of the two agents can be added if the patient is septic and/or non-responsive to fluid therapy and positive inotropy. The use of combinations is advantageous in that

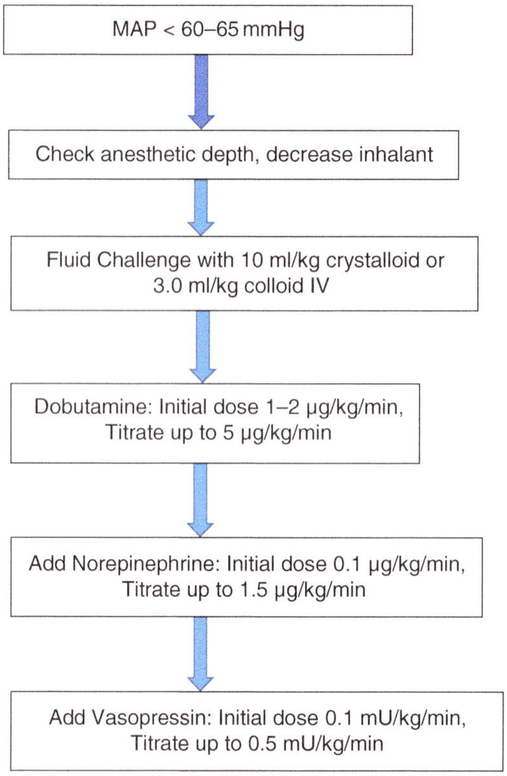

Figure 64.3 Algorithm for approaching hypotension in the anesthetized neonatal foal.

Table 64.5 Medications used to support cardiovascular system in the foal.

Agent	Dose	Comments
Dobutamine	1–5 μg/kg/min	β1 agonist, increases myocardial contractility
Dopamine	0.5–5.0 μg/kg/min	Mixed β and α effects depending on dose, patient status and sympathetic nervous system (SNS) activity
Ephedrine	0.03–0.06 mg/kg	IV bolus, can be repeated once
Calcium gluconate (10%)	10–50 mg/kg (0.1–0.5 ml/kg)	Administer slowly over 20–30 min, monitor ECG
Norepinephrine	0.05–1.5 μg/kg/min	Primarily vasopressor, increases SVR and arterial BP
Vasopressin	0.1–0.5 mU/kg/min	
Phenylephrine	0.25–2.0 μg/kg/min	Increases SVR and arterial BP

different agents exert different effects or exert similar effects but through different mechanisms of action. This strategy also allows use of lower doses of each individual drug, thereby potentially decreasing unwanted side effects. Examples of drug combinations include (each individual drug titrated to desired effect):

- Dopamine + Norepinephrine for vasodilatory shock
- Dopamine + Dobutamine for low CO states
- Dobutamine + Norepinephrine
- Norepinephrine + Arginine vasopressin – in critically ill hypotensive foals refractory to dobutamine
- Dobutamine + Phenylephrine – used instead of mixed inotrope/vasopressor drugs

Effects on the Respiratory System

Neonatal foals are susceptible to hypoventilation and hypoxemia associated with sedation and general anesthesia. Oxygenation is subjectively assessed via mucous membrane color and CRT, but cyanosis is a late sign of hypoxemia, occurring at a P_aO_2 of approximately 40 mmHg. Pulse oximetry noninvasively measures the percent of arterial hemoglobin saturated with oxygen (S_pO_2) and is related to P_aO_2 by the oxyhemoglobin dissociation curve. A limitation of pulse oximetry relates to the sigmoid shape of the curve where there is no difference in S_pO_2 whether the P_aO_2 is 100 mmHg versus 500 mmHg. In patients breathing 100% oxygen during anesthesia, S_pO_2 reads as 100% despite significant differences in P_aO_2. Therefore, arterial blood gas analysis is recommended to establish a baseline P_aO_2. Subsequent arterial blood gas analysis should be performed if alterations in ventilator parameters are instituted or every hour of general anesthesia to monitor for changes in ventilatory or oxygenation status.

Since hypoventilation can lead to hypoxemia when patients are breathing room air, supplemental oxygen should be supplied during induction and recovery as well as during sedation and short general anesthetic procedures. Subjective measures of ventilation include respiratory rate and pattern; these parameters only confirm the presence of ventilation but cannot give an assessment of the adequacy of ventilation. End-tidal carbon dioxide ($ETCO_2$) monitoring with capnomety or capnography is a more accurate method of assessing the adequacy of ventilation and also provides information regarding metabolism, perfusion and technical problems. Causes of high $ETCO_2$ include increase production of CO_2 (fever, malignant hyperthermia, treatment with sodium bicarbonate, tourniquet release), increase in pulmonary perfusion (increase in BP or CO after a period of low BP or CO) and decreased alveolar ventilation (hypoventilation). Capnography can also alert the anesthetist of technical issues such as exhausted soda lime or faulty one-way valves (Figures 64.4 and 64.5). Causes of decreased $ETCO_2$ include decreases in metabolism (hypothermia), decreased pulmonary perfusion (decreased CO, pulmonary embolism, cardiac arrest), and increased alveolar ventilation (hyperventilation, partial airway obstruction). Absence of a waveform alerts the anesthetist to respiratory apnea. Technical errors resulting in low $ETCO_2$ or absent waveform include patient disconnect, esophageal intubation, and leaks in the sampling line.

Hypoventilation is defined as $ETCO_2$ >45 mmHg. Permissive hypercarbia allows $ETCO_2$ to increase up to 60 mmHg; above this, blood pH can become excessively academic (<7.2). Neonatal foals are unlikely to ventilate adequately during general anesthesia, so IPPV should be readily available. Ideally, mechanical ventilation should be instituted either immediately after induction or after securing BP monitoring as IPPV is likely to decrease venous return and CO, especially in critically ill or compromised patients. Target tidal volume should be ~10–15 ml/kg, but airway pressure generated during manual or mechanical PPV should not exceed 20 cm H_2O. Adequacy of ventilation is monitored via capnography and arterial blood gases.

Although capnography is an invaluable noninvasive monitoring tool, its limitations should be understood. The difference between P_aCO_2 and $ETCO_2$ increases with

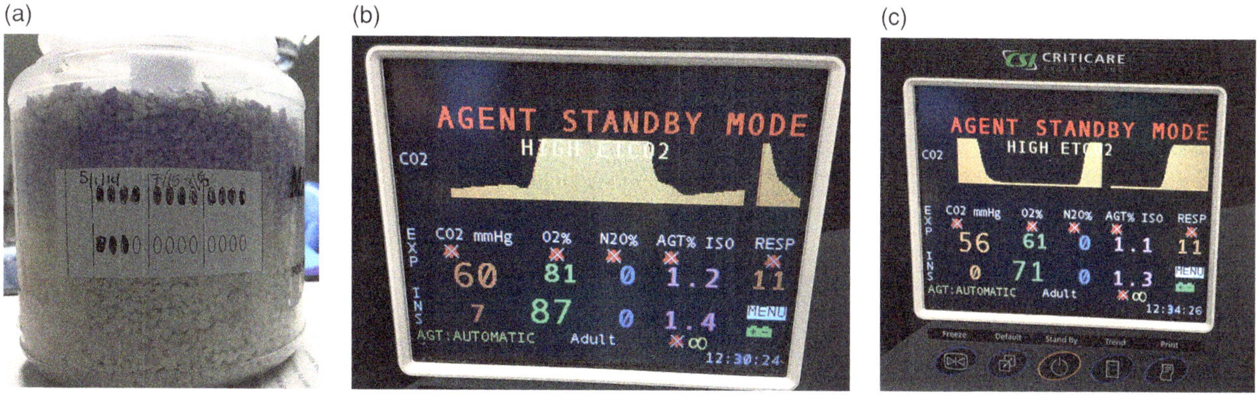

Figure 64.4 (a) Exhausted sodalime resulting in high inspired and expired CO_2 (b). (c) After changing the sodalime, baseline returns to normal and $ETCO_2$ decreases to an acceptable range for general anesthesia.

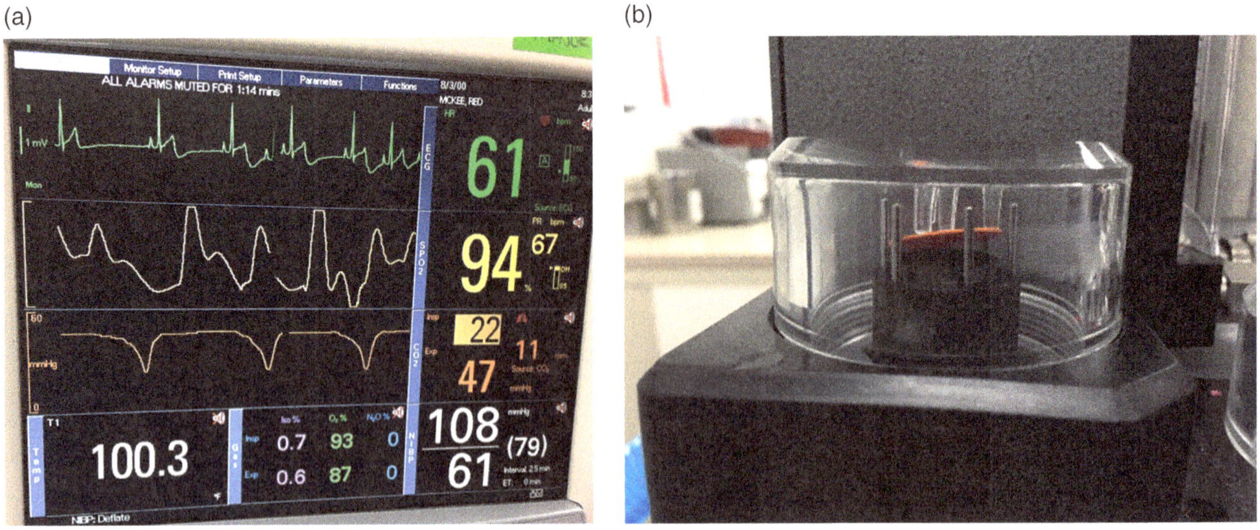

Figure 64.5 (a) High inspired CO_2 (inspired CO_2 = 22 mmHg and capnogram does not return to baseline) due to (b) faulty one-way valve in circle system.

increased physiologic dead space and the mismatch of pulmonary ventilation and perfusion (V/Q). V/Q mismatch can result from increased or constant alveolar ventilation with decreased perfusion, constant or increased perfusion with decreased ventilation, or a combination of both. The difference in P_aCO_2 and $ETCO_2$ increases over time in spontaneously breathing neonatal foals under inhalant anesthesia [137]. Therefore, due to the margin of error in predicting P_aCO_2 from a single $ETCO_2$ value, it is not recommended that $ETCO_2$ be used alone for making clinical judgments regarding ventilatory status in anesthetized neonatal foals. Baseline arterial blood gas analysis should be obtained soon after initiating inhalant anesthesia and the P_aCO_2–$ETCO_2$ difference used as a measure of accuracy of $ETCO_2$. Thereafter, arterial blood gas monitoring should occur every hour to monitor the P_aCO_2–$ETCO_2$ difference and accuracy of $ETCO_2$ readings.

Hypothermia

The normal rectal temperature of foals is 99–101.5 °F and hypothermia defined as <98 °F [1]. Neonatal foals are more susceptible to hypothermia due to their lack of subcutaneous fat, high surface area-to-body-weight ratio, decreased hypothalamic control of thermoregulation, lack of muscle activity and shivering to maintain/produce body heat and vasodilatory effects of anesthesia [2]. Consequences of hypothermia include altered pharmacokinetics of drugs, dysfunction of organ systems, increased susceptibility to infection, decreased wound healing, coagulation dysfunction and prolonged recovery [138, 139]. Ideally, core body temperature should be monitored continuously or intermittently every 5–10 minutes using an electronic temperature probe connected to a multi-parameter monitor. Heat loss is most dramatic in the first hour of anesthesia due to redistribution of blood volume, therefore, limiting anesthesia time is an important strategy in controlling hypothermia. Additionally, active warming devices can be used [138].

Treatment

Techniques for minimizing heat loss during anesthesia can be categorized as passive or active. Passive techniques include materials that function as an insulator to trap heat near the body of the patient such as towels and reflective blankets (Space All-Weather Blanket, REI, www.REI.com; PrimaCare Emergency Thermal blanket,. They reduce heat loss by counteracting convective and conductive heat loss [139]. Passive techniques are less effective than active techniques [139, 140]. Active heating techniques work through applying heat to the patient and include forced warm air blankets, resistive polymer electric blankets, warm water blankets, and IV fluid warmers. Forced-air warming blankets are the most efficacious method for patient warming whereas resistive polymer blankets can be as efficacious or less so depending on conditions of use [139]. IV fluid warmers and warm water blankets have minimal efficacy in preventing or treating hypothermia. Forced-air warming heating units are attached to specifically designed blankets, which allow warm air to be circulated around the patient. There are several units used in veterinary medicine (Figures 64.6 and 64.7) including: Bair Hugger® (3M Company, Maplewood, MN), WarmAir® (Cincinnati Sub-Zero, Cincinnati, OH), Baja®(Animal Hospital Supply, Flowery Branch, GA), and Equator® (SurgiVet, St Paul, MN). Single-use blankets are available to use with each unit or reusable washable blankets are also available through vendors (warming blankets, Jorvet, Loveland, CO; washable warming blankets, Avante Animal Health, Louisville, KY; Everlast, Animal Hospital Supply, Flowery Branch, GA).

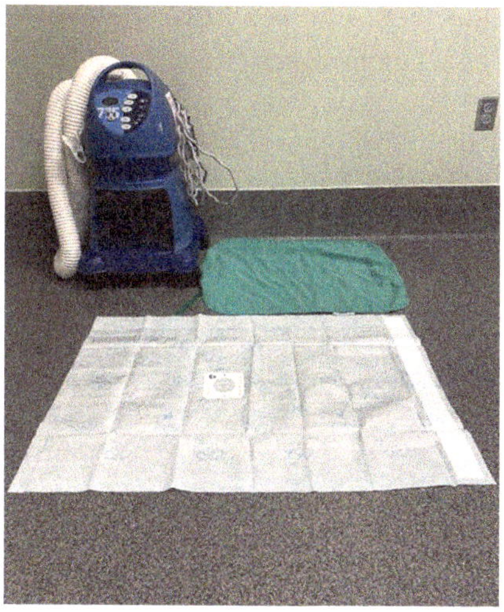

Figure 64.6 Bair Hugger (3M Company, Maplewood, MN) may be used with disposable, single-use blankets or reusable and washable warming blankets that are more economical and environmentally friendly. (Disposable warming blankets: 3M Health Care, St. Paul, MN; Jorvet, Loveland, CO, Animal Hospital Supply; Flowery Branch, Georgia. Washable warming blankets: Animal Hospital Supply, Flowery Branch, Georgia; Avante Animal Health, Louisville, KY; Everlast reusable canvas woven blankets for use with Baja forced-warm-air unit).

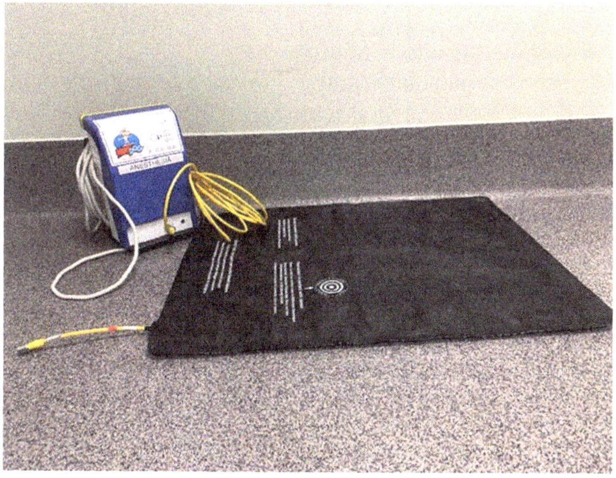

Figure 64.7 HotDog (Augustine Biomedical and Design, Eden Prairie, MN) with a medium-size blanket (five sizes available). The black side of the blanket should be exposed to the patient with the patient's body over the sensor.

Forced-air heating units should always be used with a blanket to avoid burns and the patient should be fully draped for surgery before turning on the unit to reduce contamination of the surgical site.

Conductive fabric warmers are resistive polymer heating systems that have a control box that attaches to a semiconductive polymeric blanket and are available in various sizes (HotDog®, Augustine Biomedical, Eden Prairie, MN). The patient should be positioned over the heat sensor, which is located on the black side of the blanket. Care should be taken with patient positioning, limiting pressure points and time in a single position to avoid the risk of thermal injury.

Recovery

The foal should be either weaned from the mechanical ventilator prior to moving into recovery or a means of PPV should be available to assist with ventilation until return to spontaneous ventilation. Once spontaneous ventilation has returned, the foal should have oxygen supplementation at 50–200 ml/kg/min [141] until returned to the dam or as long as tolerated by the foal. The foal can be placed in lateral recumbency on a padded surface with continued active heat support. Shivering significantly increases metabolic oxygen demand and should be avoided in the peri-anesthetic period. Propping the foal in sternal recumbency helps improve pulmonary gas exchange and allows for reinflation of atelectic lung. Once the foal begins exhibiting swallowing motions, the endotracheal cuff can be deflated and the tube removed; alternatively, the ET tube can be secured in place and removed after the foal is standing. Unlike adult horses, sedation in recovery is usually not needed. However, appropriate analgesia should be provided. The foal will typically remain recumbent and then can be assisted to standing (one person on the head and one on the tail). The mare can be returned to the recovery stall, reunited with the foal and the foal encouraged to nurse and then walked back to the stall. Alternately, if the mare is calm and facilities allow physical separation, the foal may recover in the mare's presence.

Anesthesia for Specific Conditions

Nonemergent indications for anesthesia in the neonate may be related to congenital abnormalities such as angular limb deformities, cleft palate, nonstrangulating hernias or brachygnathism. In these cases, the foal is otherwise healthy but still prone to anesthetic considerations associated with young age. More emergent or life-threatening indications for anesthesia include uroabdomen, septic arthritis, trauma, or colic. These patients can be of particularly high risk due to associated physical abnormalities such as dehydration, electrolyte, and acid–base abnormalities, sepsis, and pulmonary dysfunction.

Anesthesia for Healthy Neonatal Foals (American Society of Anesthesiologists (ASA)) Status 1–2

Anesthesia for orthopedic surgery in foals is managed similar to adults, as they are generally healthy. A primary consideration is provision of adequate pre-, intra-, and post-op analgesia. The anesthetist should consider balanced anesthesia/analgesia techniques, including opioids, CRI, and local-regional, including epidural.

Ruptured Urinary Bladder and Uroabdomen

Foals with a ruptured bladder/uroperitoneum typically present at 1–3 days after birth. This is a common disease entity and understanding the pathophysiology and importance of appropriate pre-operative stabilization is critical to successful outcome. Rupture is thought to occur during parturition as the foal's bladder is compressed during passage through the pelvic canal with male foals at higher risk. Clinical signs include lethargy, decreased mentation, decreased nursing, stranguria, abdominal pain, and distension. These foals are hypovolemic, hyperkalemic, hyponatremic, hypocholoremic, and uremic and typically have a metabolic acidosis. Signs suggestive of sepsis or infection are present in many of these patients [142]. These cases are considered medical emergencies and require stabilization prior to anesthesia and surgical correction. Preoperative management of fluid and electrolyte balance is the priority to decrease the risk of general anesthesia. Fluid accumulation can cause increased intra-abdominal pressure leading to abdominal compartment syndrome resulting in decreased pulmonary compliance and venous return to the heart [143, 144].

Circulating blood volume should be restored prior to anesthesia and electrolyte abnormalities corrected. This is accomplished by crystalloid IV fluid therapy and sequential drainage of fluid from the abdominal cavity. Serum potassium (K^+) needs to be decreased to 5.0–5.5 mEq/l prior to anesthesia, otherwise there is a risk of life-threatening cardiac arrhythmias [19]. Classic ECG changes associated with hyperkalemia include tented T waves, prolonged P-R interval, flattened or absent p waves and widening of the QRS complex. Cardiac arrhythmias can also occur with hyperkalemia and include bradycardia and second degree AV block; more malignant arrhythmias such as ventricular fibrillation and asystole can occur as increasing extracellular K^+ levels decrease the resting membrane potential across the cell membrane. Hyponatremia, acidosis, and other factors such as increased intra-abdominal pressure may contribute to the cardiotoxic effects associated with uroperitoneum as cardiac arrhythmias may develop even in normokalemic foals [142].

Hyperkalemia is treated with IV fluid therapy with a balanced crystalloid solution. Although 0.9% NaCl has been recommended historically due to the lack of K^+, Lactated Ringer's or plasmalyte are suitable substitutes since they are less likely to exacerbate the patient's metabolic acidosis. Urine should be repeatedly drained from the abdomen to relieve abdominal distension as diuresis is taking place. Ideally, as much fluid as possible is drained from the abdomen while the foal is awake as an overly distended abdomen significantly compromises ventilation and further predisposes the foal to hypoventilation and hypoxemia. Drainage of abdominal fluid in patients with increased abdominal pressure causes an expansion of the abdominal vasculature, decreasing SVR and contributing to a relative hypovolemia. This can result in a precipitous drop in arterial BP potentially leading to ventricular fibrillation or asystole. Therefore, fluid should be drained from the abdomen slowly, whether it is performed in the awake foal or during general anesthesia [143, 144].

Fluid therapy supplemented with 2.5% glucose promotes insulin production and intracellular uptake of K^+. Alternatively, insulin (0.1–0.3 IU/kg) can be administered directly. Sodium bicarbonate (1–2 mEq/kg slowly over 15 minutes) can be administered which stimulates extracellular release of hydrogen ions and uptake of K^+, maintaining electroneutrality and lowering serum K^+. Calcium gluconate (4 mg/kg, or 0.3–0.5 ml/kg of 10% IV slowly over 10–20 minutes) provides an indirect cardioprotective effect by increasing the threshold voltage to restore the normal resting membrane potential that is increased by hyperkalemia. β-2 adrenergic agonists such as terbutaline or albuterol can also be used to decrease serum K^+ by stimulation of the Na^+/K^+-ATPase pump [145].

Oxygen supplementation should be provided during induction and balanced anesthesia techniques should be used to limit inhalant effects on myocardial contractility and vasodilation. Foals should be placed on IPPV. Due to the critical patient status, the anesthetist should have an intervention plan for hypotension, monitoring and treatment of cardiac arrhythmias including calculation and availability of resuscitation emergency drugs.

Sepsis

Neonatal foals with sepsis can be particularly challenging due to the pathophysiology involving the release of cytokines and inflammatory mediators causing vasodilation and damage to the vascular endothelium resulting in hypotension and hypovolemia that may be minimally responsive to fluid therapy. This leads to hypoperfusion, lactic acidosis, and organ hypoxia. Preoperative stabilization efforts often need to continue into the anesthetic period as sedation or general anesthesia may be necessary to assist with underlying causes such as flushing of septic joints or removal of infected umbilical remnants. Additional IV catheters are advantageous to accommodate fluid therapy, CRIs for balanced anesthesia, and cardiostimulant drugs. Serial lactate, electrolyte, blood glucose, and arterial blood gas analyses can help gauge adequacy of fluid resuscitation, oxygenation and ventilation, and physical status of the patient. Cardiostimulant drugs are often necessary to maintain arterial BP, and the anesthetist is advised to follow the algorithm in Figure 64.3. Dobutamine is typically the first-line drug to increase myocardial contractility in anesthetized foals. If BP remains below 60 mmHg, norepinephrine or vasopressin or a combination of the two should be added as a vasopressor. The use of the combination of a positive inotrope such as dobutamine has been shown to preserve splanchnic perfusion more effectively than use of vasopressors alone [129].

Conclusion

The anesthetic management of neonatal foals presents significant challenges for even the most experienced anesthetist. Limited published information pertaining specifically to neonates adds to this challenge as direct extrapolation from adult horses is not appropriate in most cases. Knowledge and awareness of the unique neonatal physiology, careful drug selection, anticipation and preparation for possible complications and attentive monitoring contribute to successful patient outcome and decreased morbidity and mortality.

References

1. Bernard, W.V. and Reimer, J.M. (2018). Physical examination. In: *Equine Pediatric Medicine* (ed. W.V. Bernard and B.S. Barr), 1–15. Boca Raton, FL: CRC Press, Taylor Francis Group.
2. Driessen, B. (2019). Anesthesia and analgesia for foals. In: *Equine Surgery*, 5e (ed. J.A. Auer and J.A. Stick), 313–332. St. Louis, MO: Elsevier.
3. Dunlop, C. (1994). Anesthesia and sedation of foals. *Vet. Clin. North Am. Equine Pract.* 10: 67–85.
4. Johnston, G.M., Eastment, J.K., Wood, J.L.N. et al. (2002). The confidential enquiry into peroperative equine fatalities (CEPEF): mortality results of phases 1 and 2. *Vet. Anaesth. Analg.* 29: 159–170.
5. Johnston, G.M., Taylor, P.M., Holmes, M.A. et al. (1995). Confidential enquiry of peroperative equine fatalities (CEPEF-1): preliminary results. *Equine Vet. J.* 27: 193–200.
6. Tranquilli, W.J. (1990). Management of anesthesia in the foal. *Vet. Clin. North Am. Equine Pract.* 6: 651–663.
7. Klein, L. (1985). Anesthesia for neonatal foals. *Vet. Clin. North Am. Equine Pract.* 1: 77–90.
8. Stewart, J.H., Rose, R.J., and Barko, A.M. (1984). Echocardiography in foals from birth to three months old. *Equine Vet. J.* 16: 332–341.
9. Marr, C.M. (2015). The equine neonatal cardiovascular system in health and disease. *Vet. Clin. North Am.* 31: 545–565.
10. Doherty, T. and Valverde, A. (2006). Management of sedation and anesthesia. In: *Manual of Equine Anesthesia and Analgesia*, 219. Oxford, UK, Ames, IA and Victoria, Australia: Blackwell Publishing.
11. McKenzie HC. (2018). Disorders of foals. In: *Equine Internal Medicine* (ed. S.M. Reed, M. Bayly Warwick, and D.C. Sellon), 1367–1368. St. Louis, MO: Elsevier.
12. Marr, C.M. (2010). Cardiac murmurs: congenital heart disease. In: *Cardiology of the Horse* (ed. M. Cm and I.M. Bowen), 193–206. Edinburgh Scotland: Saunders Elsevier.
13. MacDonald, A., Fowden, A.L., Silver, M. et al. (1988). The foramen ovale of the foetal and neonatal foal. *Equine Vet. J.* 20: 255–260.
14. Cottrill, C., O'connor, W.N., Cudd, T. et al. (1987). Persistence of foetal circulatory pathways in a newborn foal. *Equine Vet. J.* 19: 252–255.
15. Dufouni, A., Decloedt, A., De Clercq, D. et al. (2018). Reversed patent ductus arteriosus and multiple congenital malformations in an 8-day-old Arabo-Friesian foal. *Equine Vet. Educ.* 30: 315–321.
16. Lester, G.D. and Axon, J.E. (2019). Assessment of the newborn foal. In: *Large Animal Internal Medicine* (ed. B.P. Smith, D. Van Metre, and N. Pusteria), 247–260. Mosby.
17. Thomas, W.P., Madigan, J.E., Backus, K.Q. et al. (1987). Systemic and pulmonary haemodynamics in normal neonatal foals. *J. Reprod. Fertil. Suppl.* 35: 623–628.
18. Schwarzwald, C.C., Bonagura, J.D., and Muir, W.W. (2009). The cardiovascular system. In: *Equine Anesthesia Monitoring and Emergency Therapy*, 2e (ed. W.W. Muir and J.A.E. Hubbell), 54. St. Louis, MO: Saunders Elsevier.
19. Fischer, B. and Clark-Price, S. (2015). Anesthesia of the equine neonate in health and disease. *Vet. Clin. North Am. Equine Pract.* 31: 567–585.
20. Sinclair, M. (2014). Sedation and anesthetic management of foals. In: *Robinson's Current Therapy in Equine Medicine* (ed. K.A. Spayberry and N.E. Robinson), 766–771. Saunders.
21. Bernard, W.V. (2018). Neurologic disorders. In: *Equine Pediatric Medicine* (ed. W.V. Bernard and B.S. Barr), 187. Boca Raton, FL: CRC Press, Taylor Francis Group.
22. Baggot, J.D. (1994). Drug therapy in the neonatal foal. *Vet. Clin. North Am. Equine Pract.* 10: 87–107.
23. Kami, G., Merrit, A.M., and Duelly, P. (1984). Preliminary studies of plasma and extracellular fluid volume in neonatal foals. *Equine Vet. J.* 16: 356–358.
24. Sanchez, C., Smith, R.L., Axon, J.E. et al. (2019). Manifestations and management of disease in neonatal foals. In: *Large Animal Internal Medicine*. G.D. Lester, consulting editor (ed. B.P. Smith, D. Van Metre, and N. Pusteria), 247–260. Mosby.
25. Magdesian, K.G. and Madigan, J.E. (2003). Volume replacement in the neonatal ICU: crystalloids and colloids. *Clin. Tech. Equine Pract.* 2: 20–30.

26 Sams, R.A. and Muir, W.W. (2009). Principles of drug disposition and drug interaction in horses. In: *Equine Anesthesia Monitoring and Emergency Therapy*, 2e (ed. W.W. Muir and H. JAE), 187. St. Louis, MO: Saunders Elsevier.

27 Pequito, M., Amory, H., de Moffarts, B. et al. (2013). Evaluation of acepromazine-induced hemodynamic alterations and reversal with norepinephrine infusion in standing horses. *Can. Vet. J.* 54: 150–156.

28 Carter, S.W., Robertson, S.A., Steel, C.J. et al. (1990). Cardiopulmonary effects of xylazine sedation in foals. *Equine Vet. J.* 22: 384–388.

29 Hubbell, J.A., Kelly, E.M., Aarnes, T.K. et al. (2013). Pharmacokinetics of midazolam after intravenous administration to horses. *Equine Vet. J.* 45: 721–725.

30 Rathmell, J.P. and Rosow, C.E. (2015). Intravenous sedatives and hypnotics. In: *Stoelting's Pharmacology and Physiology* (ed. P. Flood, J.P. Rathmell, and S. Shafer), 171–182. Philadelphia, PA: Wolters Kluwer.

31 Arguedas, M.G., Hines, M.T., Papich, M.G. et al. (2008). Pharmacokinetics of butorphanol and evaluation of physiologic and behavioural effects after intravenous and intramuscular administration in neonatal foals. *J. Vet. Intern. Med.* 22: 1417–1426.

32 Sellon, D.C., Monroe, V.L., Roberts, M.C. et al. (2001). Pharmacokinetics and adverse effects of butorphanol administerd by single intravenous injection or continuous intravenous infusion in horses. *Am. J. Vet. Res.* 62: 183–189.

33 McGowan, K.T., Elfenbein, J.R., Robertson, S.A. et al. (2013). Effect of butorphanol on thermal nociceptive threshold in healthy pony foals. *Equine Vet. J.* 45: 503–506.

34 Davis, J.L., Messenger, K.M., LaFevers, D.H. et al. (2011). Pharmacokinetics of intravenous and intramuscular buprenorphine in the horse. *J. Vet. Pharmacol. Ther.* 35: 52–58.

35 Messenger, K.M., Davis, J.L., LaFevers, D.H. et al. (2011). Intravenous and sublingual buprenorphine in horses: pharmacokinetics and influence of sampling sits. *Vet. Anaesth. Analg.* 38: 374–384.

36 Love, E.J., Pelligand, L., Taylor, P.M. et al. (2015). Pharmacokinetic-pharmacodynamic modelling of intravenous burprenorphine in conscious horses. *Vet. Anaesth. Analg.* 42: 17–29.

37 Taylor, P.M., Hoare, H.R., DeVries, A. et al. (2016). A multicentre, prospective, randomised, blinded clinical trial to compare some perioperative effects of buprenorphine or butorphanol premedication before equine elective general anaesthesia and surgery. *Equine Vet. J.* 48: 442–450.

38 Love, E.J., Taylor, P.M., Whay, H.R. et al. (2013). Postcastration analgesia in ponies using buprenorphine hydrochloride. *Vet. Rec.* 172: 635.

39 Carregaro, A.B., Teixeira Neto, F.J., Beier, S.L. et al. (2006). Cardiopulmonary effects of buprenorphine in horses. *Am. J. Vet. Res.* 67: 1675–1680.

40 Carregaro, A.B., Luna, S.P.L., Mataqueiro, M.I. et al. (2007). Effects of buprenorphine on nociception and spontaneous locomoter activity in horses. *Am. J. Vet. Res.* 68: 246–250.

41 van Dijk, P., Lankveld, D.P.K., Rijkenhuizen, A.B.M. et al. (2003). Hormonal, metabolic and physiological effects of laparoscopic surgery using a detomidine-buprenorphine combination in standing horses. *Vet. Anaesth. Angl.* 30: 71–79.

42 Love, E.J., Taylor, P.M., Murrell, J. et al. (2012). Effects of acepromazine, butorphanol and buprenorphine on thermal and mechanical nociceptive thresholds in horses. *Equine Vet. J.* 44: 221–225.

43 Love, E.J., Taylor, P.M., Murrell, J. et al. (2011). Assessment of the sedative effects of buprenorphine administered with 10ug/kg detomidine in horses. *Vet.Rec.* 168: 379.

44 Love, E.J., Taylor, P.M., Murrell, J. et al. (2011). Assessment of the sedative effects of buprenorphine administered with 20ug/kg detomidine in horses. *Vet. Rec.* 168: 409.

45 Taylor, P., Coumbe, K., Henson, F. et al. (2014). Evaluation of sedation for standing clinical procedures in horses using detomidine combined with buprenorphine. *Vet. Anaesth. Analg.* 41: 14–24.

46 Cruz, F.S.F., Carregaro, A.B., Machado, M. et al. (2011). Sedative and cardiopulmonary effects of buprenorphine and xylazine in horses. *Can. J. Vet. Res.* 75: 35–41.

47 Potter, J., MacFarlane, P.D., Love, E.J. et al. (2016). Preliminary investigation comparing a detomidine continuous rate infusion combined with either morphine or buprenorphine for standing sedation in horses. *Vet. Anaesth. Analg.* 43: 189–194.

48 Rigotti, C., De Vries, A., and Taylor, P.M. (2014). Buprenorphine provides better anaesthetic conditions than butorphanol for field castration in ponies: results of a rendomised clinical trial. *Vet. Rec.* 175: 623.

49 Risberg, A., Spadavecchia, C., Hendrickson, E.H.S. et al. (2015). Antinociceptive effect of buprenorphine and evaluation of the nociceptive withdrawal reflex in foals. *Vet. Anaesth. Analg.* 42: 329–338.

50 Walker, A.F. (2007). Sublingual administration of buprenorphine for long-term analgesia in the horse. *Vet. Rec.* 160: 808–809.

51 Grubb, T.L., Kurkowski, D., Sellon, D.C. et al. (2019). Pharmacokinetics and physiologic/behavioral effects of buprenorphine administered sublingually and intravenously to neonatal foals. *J. Vet. Pharmacol. Ther.* 42: 26–36.

52 Eberspacher, E., Stanley, S.D., Rezende, M. et al. (2008). Pharmacokinetics and tolerance of transdermal fentanyl administration in foals. *Vet. Anaesth. Analg.* 35: 249–255.

53 Peng, P.W. and Sandler, A.N. (1999). A review of the use of fentanyl analgesia in the management of acute pain in adults. *Anesthesiology* 90: 576–599.

54 Knych, H.K., Steffey, E.P., Casbeer, H.C. et al. (2015). Disposition, behavioural and physiological effects of escalating doses of intravenously administered fentanyl to young foals. *Equine Vet. J.* 47: 592–598.

55 Knych, H.K., Steffey, E.P., Mitchell, M.M. et al. (2015). Effects of age on the pharmacokinetics and selected pharmacodynamics of intravenously administered fentanyl in foals. *Equine Vet. J.* 47: 72–77.

56 Reed, R., Barletta, M., Mitchell, K. et al. (2019). The pharmacokinetics and pharmacodynamics of intravenous hydromorphone in horses. *Vet. Anaesth. Analg.* 46: 395–404.

57 Reed, R.A., Knych, H.K., Barletta, M. et al. (2020). Pharmacokinetics and pharmacodynamics of hydromorphone after intravenous and intramuscular administration in horses. *Vet. Anaesth. Analg.* 47: 210–218.

58 Martins, F.C., Keating, S.C.J., Clark-Price, S.C. et al. (2020). Pharmacokinetics and pharmacodynamics of hydromorphone hydrochloride in healthy horses. *Vet. Anaesth. Analg.* 47: 509–517.

59 Skrzypzak, H., Reed, R., Barletta, M. et al. (2020). A retrospective evaluation of the effect of perianesthetic hydromorphone administration on the incidence of postanesthetic signs of colic in horses. *Vet. Anaesth. Analg.* 47: 757–762.

60 Steffey, E.P., Eisele, J.H., and Baggot, J.D. (2003). Interactions of morphine and isoflurane in horses. *Am. J. Vet. Res.* 64: 166–175.

61 Bennett, R.C., Steffey, E.P., and Kollias-Baker, C. (2004). Influence of morphine sulfate on the halothane sparing effect of xylazine hydrochloride in horses. *Am. J. Vet. Res.* 65: 519–526.

62 Senior, J.M., Pinchbeck, G.L., Dugdale, A.H.A. et al. (2004). Retrospective study of the risk factors and prevalence of colic in horses after orthpaedic surgery. *Vet. Rec.* 155: 321–325.

63 Andersen, M.S., Clark, L., Dyson, S.J. et al. (2006). Risk factors for colic in horses after general anaesthesia for MRI or nonabdominal surgery: absence of evidence of effect from perianesthetic morphine. *Equine Vet. J.* 38 (4): 368–374.

64 Boscan, P., Van Hoogmoed, L.M., Farver, T.B. et al. (2006). Evaluation of the effects of the opioid agonist morphine on gastrointestinal tract function. *Am. J. Vet. Res.* 67: 992–997.

65 Tessier, C., Pitaud, J.P., Thorin, C. et al. (2019). Systemic morphine administration causes gastric distension and hyperphagia in healthy horses. *Equine Vet. J.* 51: 633–657.

66 Clark, L., Clutton, R.E., Blissitt, K.J. et al. (2005). Effects of peri-operative morphine administration during halothane anaesthesia in horses. *Vet. Anaesth. Analg.* 32: 10–15.

67 Mircica, E., Clutton, R.E., Kyles, K.W. et al. (2003). Problems associated with perioperative morphine in horses: a retrospective case analysis. *Vet. Anaesth. Analg.* 30: 147–155.

68 Love, E.J., Lane, J.G., and Murison, P.F. (2006). Morphine administration in horses anaesthetized for upper airway respiratory tract surgery. *Vet. Anaesth. Analg.* 33: 179–188.

69 Clark, L., Clutton, R.E., Blissitt, K.J. et al. (2008). The effects of morphine on the recovery of horses from halothane anaesthesia. *Vet. Anaesth. Analg.* 35: 22–29.

70 Chesnel, M.A. and Clutton, R.E. (2013). A comparison of two morphine doses on the quality of recovery from general anaesthesia in horses. *Res. Vet. Sci.* 95: 1195–1200.

71 Corletto, F., Raisis, A.A., and Brearley, J.C. (2005). Comparison of morphine and butorphanol as pre-anaesthetic agents in combination with romifidine for field castration in ponies. *Vet. Anaesth. Analg.* 32: 16–22.

72 Devine, E.P., KuKanich, B., and Beard, W.L. (2013). Pharmacokinetics of intramuscularly administered morphine in horses. *J. Am. Vet. Med. Assoc.* 243: 105–112.

73 Combie, J.D., Nugent, T.E., and Tobin, T. (1983). Pharmacokinetics and protein binding of morphine in horses. *Am. J. Vet. Res.* 44: 870–874.

74 Knych, H.K., Steffey, E.P., and McKemie, D.S. (2014). Preliminary pharmacokinetics of morphine and its major metabolites following intravenous administration of four doses to horses. *J. Vet. Pharmacol. Ther.* 37: 374–381.

75 Hamamoto-Hardman, B.D., Steffey, E.P., Weiner, D. et al. (2019). Pharmacokinetics and selected pharmacodynamics of morphine and its active metabolites in horses after intravenous administration of four doses. *J. Vet. Pharmacol. Ther.* 42: 401–410.

76 Figueiredo, J.P., Muir, W.W., and Sams, R. (2012). Cardiorespiratory, gastrointestinal, and analgesic effects of morphine sulfate in conscious healthy horses. *Am. J. Vet. Res.* 73: 799–808.

77 Raikallio, M., Taylor, P.M., Johnson, C.B. et al. (1996). The disposition and local effects of intra-articular morphine in normal ponies. *J. Vet. Anaesth.* 23: 23–26.

78 Tulamo, R.M., Raekallio, M., Taylor, P. et al. (1996). Intra-articular morphine and saline injections induce release of large molecular weight proteoglycans into equine synovial fluid. *J. Vet. Med. A Phys. Pathol. Clin. Med.* 43: 147–153.

79 Santos, L.C.P., Nunes de Moraes, A., and Saito, M.E. (2009). Effects of intraarticular ropivacaine and morphine on lipopolysaccharide-induced synovitis in horses. *Vet. Anaesth. Analg.* 36: 280–286.

80 Lindegaard, C., Thomsen, M.H., Larsen, S. et al. (2010). Analgesic efficacy of intra-articular morphine in experimentally induced radiocarpal synovitis in horses. *Vet. Anaesth. Analg.* 37: 171–185.

81 Lindegaard, C., Gleerup, K.B., Thomsen, M.H. et al. (2010). Anti-inflammatory effects of intra-articular administration of morphine in horses with experimentally induced synovitis. *Am. J. Vet. Res.* 71: 69–75.

82 Lindegaard, C., Frost, A.B., Thomsen, M.H. et al. (2010). Pharmacokinetics of intra-articular morphine in horses with lipopolysaccaharide-induced synovitis. *Vet. Anaesth. Analg.* 37: 186–195.

83 Van Loon, J.P.A.M., De Grauw, J.C., Van Dierendonick, M. et al. (2010). Intra-articular opioid analgesia is effective in reducing pain and inflammation in an equine LPS induced synovitis model. *Equine Vet. J.* 42 (5): 412–419.

84 Hunter, B.G., Parker, J.E., Wehrman, R. et al. (2015). Morphine synovial fluid concentrations after intravenous regional limb perfusion in standing horses. *Vet. Surg.* 44: 679–686.

85 Linardi, R.L., Stokes, A.M., Barker, S.A. et al. (2009). Pharmacokinetics of the injectable formulation of methadone hydrochloride administered orally in horses. *J. Vet. Pharmacol. Ther.* 32: 492–497.

86 Linardi, R.L., Stokes, A.M., and Andrews, F.M. (2012). The effect of P-glycoprotein on methadone hydrochloride flux in equine intestinal mucosa. *J. Vet. Pharmacol. Ther.* 36: 43–50.

87 Linardi, R.L., Stokes, A.M., Keowen, M.L. et al. (2012). Bioavailability and pharmacokinetics of oral and injectable formulation of methadone after intravenous, oral and intragastric adminstration in horses. *Am. J. Vet. Res.* 73: 290–295.

88 Crosignani, N., Luna, S.P., Dalla Costa, T. et al. (2017). Pharmacokinetics and pharmacodynamics of the injectable formulation of methadone hydrochloride and methadone in lipid nanocarriers administered orally to horses. *J. Vet. Pharmacol. Ther.* 40: 398–405.

89 Carregaro, A.B., Freitas, G.C., Ribeiro, M.H. et al. (2014). Physiological and analgesic effects of continuous rate infusion of morphine, butorphanol, tramadon or methadone in horses with lipopolysaccharide (LPS)-induced carpal synovitis. *BMC Vet. Res.* 10: 966.

90 De Oliveira, F.A., Pignaton, W., Teixeira-Neto, F.J. et al. (2014). Antinociceptive and behavioral effects of methadone alone or in combination with detomidine in conscious horses. *J. Equine Vet. Sci.* 34: 380–386.

91 Lopes, C., Luna, S.P.L., Rosa, A.C. et al. (2016). Antinociceptive effects of methadone combined with detomidine or acepromazine in horses. *Equine Vet. J.* 48: 613–618.

92 Gozalo-Marcilla, M., Luna, S.P.L., Crosignani, N. et al. (2017). Sedative and antinociceptive effects of different combination of detomidine and methadone in standing horses. *Vet. Anaesth. Analg.* 44: 1116–1127.

93 Gozalo-Marcilla, M., Luna, S.P.L., Gasthuys, F. et al. (2019). Clinical applicability of detomidine and methadone constant rate infusions for surgery in standing horses. *Vet. Anaesth. Analg.* 46: 325–334.

94 Gozalo-Marcilla, M., De Oliveira, A.R., Fonseca, M.W. et al. (2019). Sedative and antinociceptive effects of different detomidine constant rate infusions, with or without methadone in standing horses. *Equine Vet. J.* 51: 530–536.

95 Carregaro, A.B., Ueda, G.I., Censoni, J.B. et al. (2020). Effect of methadone combined with acepromazine or detomidine on sedation and dissociative anesthesia in healthy horses. *J. Equine Vet. Sci.* 86: 1–5.

96 Ronnow Kjoerulff, L.N. and Lindegaard, C. (2021). A narrative review of caudal epidural anaesthesia and analgesia in horses. Part 1: Safety and efficacy of epidural drugs. *Equine Vet. Educ.* Early view: https://doi.org/10.1111/eve.13488.

97 Ronnow Kjoerulff, L.N. and Lindegaard, C. (2021. Early view). A narrative review of caudal epidural anaesthesia and analgesia in horses. Part 2: clinical indications and techniques. *Equine Vet. Educ.* https://doi.org/10.1111/eve.13489.

98 Kerr, C.L., Boure, L.P., Pearce, S.G. et al. (2009). Cardiopulmonary effects of diazepam-ketamine-isoflurane or xylazine-ketamine-isoflurane during abdominal surgery in foals. *Am. J. Vet. Res.* 70: 574–580.

99 Mama, K.R., Steffey, E.P., and Pascoe, P.J. (1995). Evaluation of propfol as a general anesthetic for horses. *Vet. Surg.* 24: 188–194.

100 Mama, K.R., Steffey, E.P., and Pascoe, P.J. (1996). Evaluation of propfol as a general anesthetic in premedicated horses. *Am. J. Vet. Res.* 57: 512–517.

101 Frias, A.F.G., Marsico, F., Gomez de Segura, I.A. et al. (2003). Evaluation of different doses of propofol in xylazine pre-medicated horses. *Vet. Anaesth. Analg.* 30: 193–201.

102 Oku, K., Yamanaka, T., Ashihara, N. et al. (2003). Clinical observations during induction and recovery of xylazine-midazolam propofol anesthesia in horses. *J. Vet. Med. Sci.* 65: 805–808.

103 Muir, W.W., Lerche, P., and Erichson, D. (2009). Anaesthetic and cardiorespiratory effects of propofol at 10% for induction and 1% for maintenance of anaesthesia in horses. *Equine Vet. J.* 41 (6): 578–585.

104 Rezende, M.L., Boscan, P., Stanley, S.C. et al. (2010). Evaluation of cardiovascular, respiratory and biochemical effects, and anesthetic induction and recovery behavior in horses anesthetized with 5% micellar microemulsion propofol formulation. *Vet. Anaesth. Analg.* 37: 440–450.

105 Brosnan, R.J., Steffey, E.P., Escobar, A. et al. (2011). Anesthetic induction with guaifenesin and propofol in adult horses. *Am. J. Vet. Res.* 72: 1569–1575.

106 Bigby, S.E., Beths, T., Bauquier, S. et al. (2017). Effect of rate of administration of propofol or alfaxalone on induction dose requirements and occurrence of apnea in dogs. *Vet. Anaesth. Analg.* 44: 1267–1275.

107 Lerche, P. and Am, N. (2000). Comparative study of propofol or propofol and ketamine for the induction of anaesthesia in dogs. *Vet. Rec.* 146: 571–574.

108 Ravasio, G., Gallo, M., Beccaglia, M. et al. (2012). Evaluation of a ketamine-propofol drug combination with or without dexmedetomidine for intravenous anesthesia in cats undergoing ovariectomy. *J. Am. Vet. Med. Assoc.* 241: 1307–1313.

109 Martinez-Taboada, F. and Leece, E. (2014). Comparison of porpofol with ketofol, a propofol-ketamine admixture, for induction of anaesthesia in healthy dogs. *Vet. Anaesth. Analg.* 41: 575–582.

110 Wagner, A.E., Mama, K.R., Steffey, E.P. et al. (2002). Behavioral responses following eight anesthetic induction protocols in horses. *Vet. Anaesth. Analg.* 29: 207–211.

111 Posner, L.P., Kasten, J.I., and Kata, C. (2013). Propofol with ketamine following sedation with xylazine for routine induction of general anaesthesia in horses. *Vet. Rec.* 173: 550.

112 Jarrett, M.A., Bailey, K.M., Messenger, K. et al. (2018). Recovery of horses from general anesthesia after inductin with propofol and ketamine versus midazolam and ketamine. *J. Am. Vet. Med. Assoc.* 253: 101–107.

113 Donnelly, R.F., Willman, E., and Andolfatto, G. (2008). Stability of ketamine-propofol mixtures for procedural sedition and analgesia in the emergency department. *Can. J. Hosp. Pharm.* 61: 426–430.

114 Goodwin, W., Keates, H., Pasloske, K. et al. (2012). Plasma pharmacokinetics and pharmacodynamics of alfaxalone in neonatal foals after an intravenous bolus of alfaxalone following premedication with butorphanol tartrate. *Vet. Anaesth. Analg.* 39: 503–510.

115 Goodwin, W.A., Keates, H., Pasloske, K. et al. (2011). The pharmacokinetics and pharmacodynamics of the injectable anaesthetic alfaxalone in the horse. *Vet. Anaesth. Analg.* 38: 431–438.

116 Brosnan, R.J. (2013). Inhaled anesthetics. *Vet. Clin. North Am.* 29: 69–87.

117 Steffey, E.P. and Howland, D. (1980). Comparison of circulatory and respiratory effects of isoflurane and halothane anesthesia in horses. *Am. J. Vet. Res.* 41: 821–825.

118 Steffey, E.P., Mama, K.R., Galey, F.D. et al. (2005). Effects of sevoflurane dose and mode of ventilation on cardiopulmonary function and blood biochemical variables in horses. *Am. J. Vet. Res.* 66: 606–614.

119 Sun, L.Y., Wijeysundera, D.N., Tait, G.A. et al. (2015). Association of Intraoperative hypotension with acute kidney injury after elective noncardiac surgery. *Anesthesiology* 123: 515–523.

120 Giguere, S., Knowles, H.A., Valverde, A. et al. (2005). Accuracy of indirect measurement of blood pressure in neonatal foals. *J. Vet. Intern. Med.* 19: 571–576.

121 Nout, Y.S., Corley, K.T.T., Donaldson, L.L. et al. (2002). Indirect oscillometric and direct blood pressure measurements in anesthetized and conscious neonatal foals. *J. Vet. Emerg. Crit. Care* 12: 75–50.

122 Skelding, A. and Valverde, A. (2020). Review of non–invasive blood pressure measurement in animals: part 2 — evaluation of the performance of non-invasive devices. *Can. Vet. J.* 61: 481–498.

123 Hepworth-Warren, K.L., Wong, D.M., Hay Kraus, B.L. et al. (2015). Effects of administration of a synthetic low molecular weight/low molar substitution hydroxyethyl starch solution in healthy neonatal foals. *Can. Vet. J.* 56: 1069–1074.

124 Zoetis (2013). Vetstarch™: 6% hydroxyethyl starch 130/0.4 in 0.9% sodium chloride injection. https://www.zoetisus.com/contact/pages/product_information/msds_pi/pi/vetstarch.pdf (accessed 23 March 2023).

125 Thomasy, S.M., Steffey, E.P., Mama, K.R. et al. (2006). The effects of IV fentanyl administration on the minimum alveolar concentration of isoflurane in horses. *Br. J. Anaesth.* 97: 232–237.

126 Loomes, K. (2020). The use of hyoscine N-butylbromide to treat intraoperative bradycardia during isoflurane anaesthesia in a thoroughbred horse. *Vet. Anaesth. Analg.* 47: 847–849.

127 Pimenta, E.L., Teixeira Neto, F.J., Sa, P.A. et al. (2011). Comparative study between atropine and hyoscine-N butylbromide for reversal of detomidine induced bradycardia in horses. *Equine Vet. J.* 43: 332–340.

128 Marques, J.A., Teixeira Neto, F.J., Campbell, R.C. et al. (1998). Effect of hyoscine-N butylbromide given before romifidine in horses. *Vet. Rec.* 142: 166–168.

129 Corley, K.T.T. (2004). Inotrope and vasopressors in adults and foals. *Vet. Clin. North Am. Equine Pract.* 20: 77–106.

130 Schauvliege, S. and Gasthuys, F. (2013). Drugs for cardiovascular support in anesthetized horses. *Vet. Clin. North Am. Equine Pract.* 29: 19–49.

131 Lee, Y.H., Clarke, K.W., Alibhai, H.I. et al. (1998). Effects of dopamine, dobutamine, dopexamine, phenylephrine and saline solution on intramuscular blood flow and other cardiopulmonary variables in halothane anesthetized ponies. *Am. J. Vet. Res.* 59: 1463–1472.

132 Ar, H., Ousey, J.C., Palmer, L. et al. (2006). Effects of norepinephrine and a combined norepinephrine and dobutamine infusion on systemic hemodynamics and indices of renal function in normotensive neonatal thoroughbred foals. *J. Vet. Intern. Med.* 20: 1437–1442.

133 Hollis, A.R., Ousey, J.C., Palmer, L. et al. (2008). Effects of norepinephrine and combined norepinephrine and fenoldopam infusion on systemic hemodynamics and indices of renal function in normotensive neonatal foals. *J. Vet. Intern. Med.* 22: 1210–1215.

134 Valverde, A., Giguere, S., Sanchez, C. et al. (2006). Effects of dobutamine, norepinephrine and vasopressin on cardiovascular function in anesthetized neonatal foals with induced hypotension. *Am. J. Vet. Res.* 67: 1730–1737.

135 Corley, K.T., McKenzie, H.C., Amoroso, L. et al. (2000). Initial experience with norepinephrine infusion in hypotensive critically ill foals. *J. Vet. Emerg. Crit. Care* 10: 267–275.

136 Dickey, E.J., McKenzie, H.C., Johnson, A. et al. (2010). Use of pressor therapy in 34 hypotensive critically ill neonatal foals. *Aust. Vet. J.* 88: 472–477.

137 Geiser, D.R. (1992). Use of end-tidal CO_2 tension to predict arterial CO_2 values in isoflurane-anesthetized equine neonates. *Am. J. Vet. Res.* 53 (9): 1617–1621.

138 Baldo, C. and Palmer, D. (2018). Temperature regulation and monitoring. In: *Veterinary Anesthetic and Monitoring Equipment* (ed. K.G. Cooley and R.A. Johnson), 285–302. Hoboken, NJ: John Wiley & Sons.

139 Clark-Price, S. (2015). Inadvertent perianesthetic hypothermia in small animal patients. *Vet. Clin. North Am. Small Anim.* 45: 983–994.

140 Clark-Price, S.C., Dossin, O., Jones, K.R. et al. (2013). Comparison of three differenct methods to prevent heat loss in healthy dogs undergoing 90 minutes of general anesthesia. *Vet. Anaeth. Analg.* 40: 280–284.

141 Wong, D.M., Alcott, C.J., Wang, C. et al. (2010). Physiologic effects of nasopharyngeal administration of supplemental oxygen at various flow rates in healthy neonatal foals. *Am. J. Vet. Res.* 71: 1081–1088.

142 Dunkel, B., Palmer, J.E., Olson, K.N. et al. (2005). Uroperitoneum in 32 foals: influence of intravenous fluid therapy, infection and sepsis. *J. Vet. Intern. Med.* 19: 889–893.

143 Love, E.J. (2011). Anaesthesia in foals with uroperitoneum. *Equine Vet. Educ.* 23: 508–511.

144 Haga, H.A., Risberg, A., and Strand, E. (2011). Resuscitation of an anaesthetized foal with uroperitoneum and ventricular asystole. *Equine Vet. Educ.* 23: 502–507.

145 Marolf, V., Mirra, A., Fouche, N. et al. (2018). Advanced atrio-ventricular blocks in a foal undergoing surgical bladder repair: first step to cardiac arrest? *Front. Vet. Sci.* 5: article 96. https://doi.org/10.3389/fvets.2018.00096.

Chapter 65 Necropsy Examination and Sample Submission of the Fetus, Fetal Membranes, and Foal

Rebecca Ruby

Necropsy examination of the equine fetus, placenta, and deceased neonates is indicated in many cases. The primary goal of the examination is to determine the cause of fetal loss or neonatal morbidity or mortality. Equine abortion may be caused by many factors, including maternal illness, fetal malformation, infectious agents (contagious and non-contagious), genetic diseases, twinning, and idiopathic conditions. In all cases, examination of the placenta is indicated, both from an uneventful parturition and in cases of fetal loss. Farm personnel are often well trained in examination of the placenta to ensure complete passage as well as identify any potential abnormalities. If irregularities are noted or there are concerns about the health of the neonate, then submission of the placenta from a live foaling to a diagnostic laboratory is warranted. In cases of abortion, the intent is to determine if a definitive cause of abortion can be identified, and if this cause has implications that affect the remaining broodmares, horses on the farm, mare's future breeding potential, or herd management strategies. In all cases of abortion, the ideal sample is the fresh, intact fetus and placenta. If this is not possible, then a complete set of formalin fixed tissues should be collected as well as fresh fetal and placental tissues.

Complete information should be provided when submitting samples including the length of gestation, maternal clinical signs, treatment and vaccination history, prior maternal illness and/or reproductive loss, history of geographic movement, number of other pregnant mares on the farm, other horses affected, if the placenta is known to be incomplete and any other concerns. Standard diagnostic testing varies between laboratories. When possible, ensure that the diagnostic laboratory routinely evaluates equine samples and has appropriate tests for common infectious causes of equine abortion.

Tissue Examination

Examination of the placenta or fetus in cases of abortion should take place in an area that can be easily disinfected with proper biosecurity measures. The offending mare should be isolated from other mares until the results of infectious disease testing are available.

Sample sets should include:

- *Formalin fixed* (10% buffered formalin in a 10 : 1 formalin : tissue ratio): placenta, liver, lung, spleen, kidney, adrenal gland, heart, thymus, gastrointestinal tract sections, and skeletal muscle. Formalin fixed placenta should be collected from the middle of each horn, the body, cervical star, amnion and umbilical cord, as well as any sites, which appear abnormal. Additional tissues may be submitted if there is suspicion of abnormalities.
- *Fresh tissue* (sent individually bagged and chilled): liver, lung, spleen, adrenal gland, kidney, and placenta. Fetal heart blood is collected into a serum separator (red top) tube and maternal blood into EDTA and serum separator tubes. Fetal stomach contents are collected aseptically by needle aspiration and often yield valuable information following bacterial culture. A combination of tissues and placenta may be submitted for testing for EHV-1, Leptospirosis, Equine Arteritis Virus and bacterial or fungal culture. Ideally, multiple pieces, typically three of each, will expedite laboratory processing. In some cases, such as an EHV-1 abortion, a respiratory swab, and EDTA blood and serum from the mare may be included.

Placental examination involves the evaluation of the chorionic surface, allantoic surface, umbilical cord, and amnion (Figure 65.1).

Equine Neonatal Medicine, First Edition. Edited by David M. Wong and Pamela A. Wilkins.

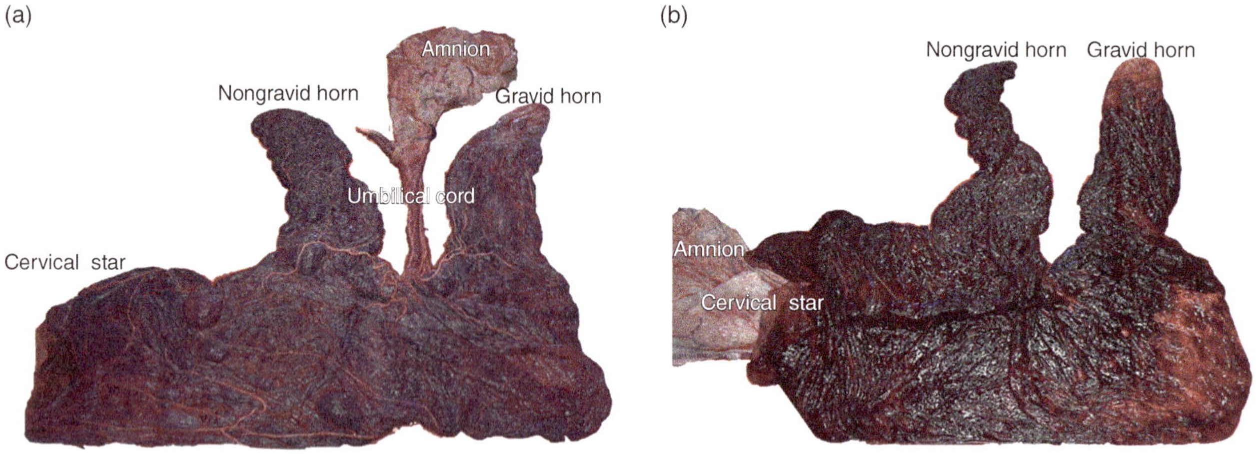

Figure 65.1 The allantoic surface of the equine placenta (a). The allantoic side is evaluated for vasculature, plaques, and areas of thickening but is rarely the site of primary pathology. The umbilical cord is best assessed on this side. (b) The chorionic surface of the equine placenta. The chorionic surface should be examined for areas of thickening, mucoid material, avillous regions or necrosis.

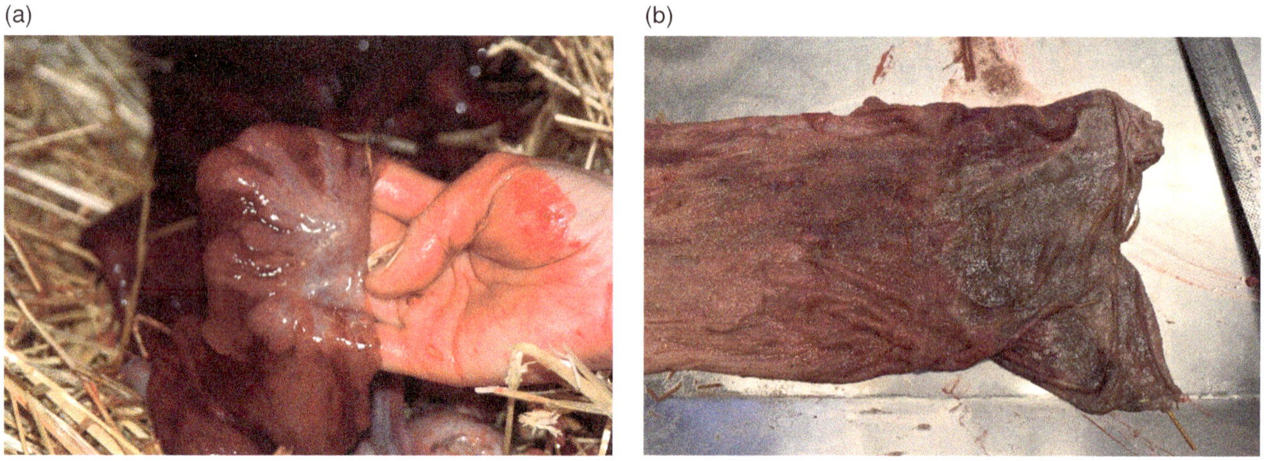

Figure 65.2 Normal (a) and abnormal (b) appearance of the cervical star region of the fetal membranes. (b) Cervical pole necrosis with a sharply delineated area of abnormal, thin, tan-brown chorioallantois involving the cervical star and pole.

Placenta

The placenta is weighed and checked for completeness with special attention to the presence of the tips of both horns. Normal placental weight at term is approximately 11% of foal weight. If possible, this weight should be obtained on farm to avoid dehydration or contamination. To avoid excessive environmental contamination samples for bacterial culture should be collected first. A common location of bacterial and fungal placentitis is the cervical star. In cases of peracute infection, inflammation may only be present on a microscopic level and even if this site looks normal, it should be sampled for bacterial culture and histopathologic evaluation. In one study, approximately one third of cases of placentitis were only diagnosed microscopically with no gross abnormalities observed. If grossly normal, the site for culture is from the folds in the area of the cervical star [1]. Samples may be collected as a fresh $3\,cm^3$ section or swabbed. At this time, the location of fetal expulsion is identified to determine if the cervical star (Figure 65.2) is intact (red bag delivery) or ruptured (normal site of expulsion). The remainder of the chorionic surface is examined for areas of exudate, thickening, lack of villi and completeness. The gravid horn is thicker and frequently more edematous than the non-gravid horn with many placentas having a focal site of tan discoloration and thickening at the tip of the gravid horn. This is known as the fetal pad and is presumed to develop due to chronic contact with the fetal hooves. The placenta is then inverted, most easily achieved by grasping the tips of the horns and lifting the chorionallantois; the allantoic surface is examined for plaques, cysts, and vascular abnormalities [2]. When examining fetal membranes, autolytic changes may appear pathologic, particularly in cases of retained fetal membranes. All areas that are suspected to be abnormal

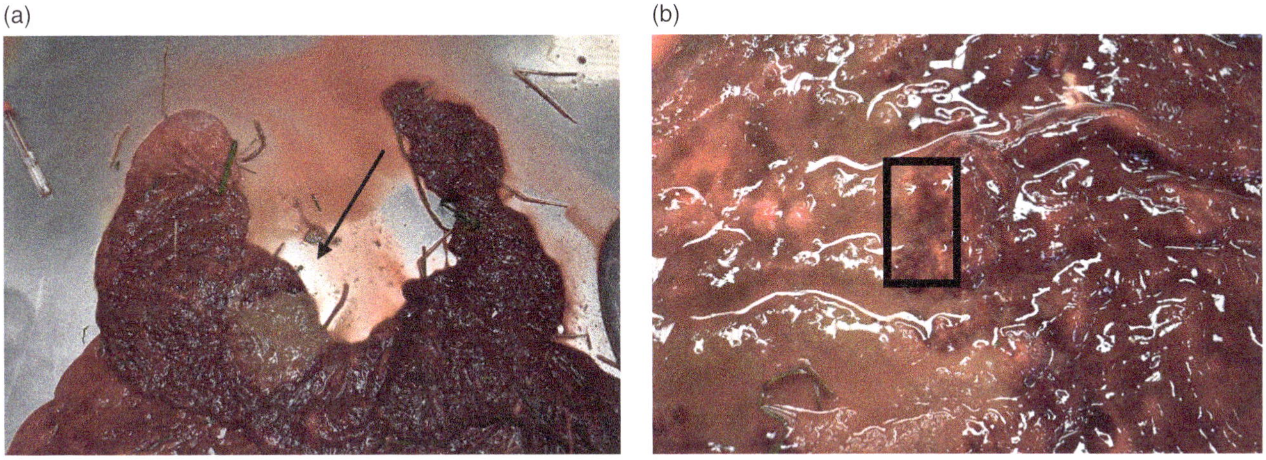

Figure 65.3 (a) Focal mucoid placentitis (arrow), in this case caused by *Crossiella equi*. (b) The site to collect tissue for formalin, bacterial culture, and PCR is the area of raised, red-tan chorion, indicated in the box in the second figure.

should be sampled for formalin fixation as well as for bacterial and/or fungal culture. Samples from areas of interest may be labeled by the submitter if correlation with pathology is desired. If the entire placenta is not submitted to a diagnostic laboratory, then photographs of all surfaces should be obtained.

In cases of focal mucoid placentitis (Figure 65.3), commonly associated with *Nocardioform sp* of bacteria, the abnormal chorion, rather than the mucoid material, is the sample of choice. Locate a section of the chorion which has a raised, irregular tan-gray appearance and aggressively swab the section for bacterial culture and PCR. These sections are most commonly at the edge of the lesion where there is still active bacterial growth. This is the same section that should be taken for formalin fixed tissue.

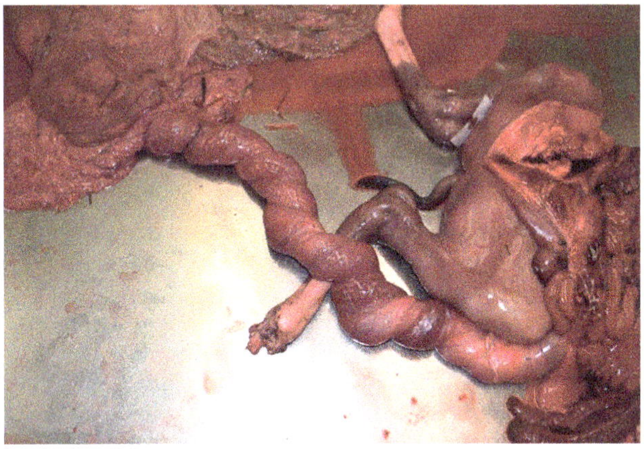

Figure 65.4 Umbilical cord torsion in a midgestation fetus. Note the edematous, thickened appearance of the umbilical cord, and alternating regions of pallor and reddening.

Umbilical Cord

The umbilical cord is examined for the presence of twists (Figure 65.4), urachal sacculation and inflammation. In Thoroughbred foals the mean umbilical cord length is approximately 66 cm. The upper limit for normal foals has been reported to be from 137 to 183 cm depending on the study. Umbilical cords generally greater than 85 cm are considered abnormally long. Normal values for a variety of breeds have been published in recent years. The significance of a long umbilical cord is not well understood in the absence of umbilical or fetal pathology. Long umbilical cords have been associated with cervical pole necrosis, body pregnancy, and umbilical cord torsion, but the presence of a long umbilical cord without lesions has been observed in aborted and term healthy foals [3]. Interestingly, the caseload of equine abortions in Newmarket was dominated by conditions associated with a long umbilical cord, suggesting an association with fetal demise. The presence of twists in the umbilical cord with areas of blanching, hemorrhage, thrombosis, and edema, is consistent with an umbilical cord torsion [4]. Twists should appear tight and are often difficult to completely reduce. Additional signs of significant umbilical cord torsion include distention of the fetal urinary bladder or enlargement of the umbilical structures at the body wall.

Amnion

The amnion is examined for thickness, discoloration, rents, and other pathology. Thickened sections or those that appear to have plaque-like raised areas should be sampled to include the junction between normal and abnormal appearing tissue. It may be helpful to distend the amnion with water if a tear or rent is suspected, as these will frequently contract and may be difficult to identify.

Several nonspecific changes may occur and the significance of these are not yet understood. Placental edema may be dramatic but the significance in most cases is not known. Correlation with clinical information to determine the presence of hydrops, fescue exposure, or maternal disease is useful. Typically, there is no evidence of fetal renal disease or fetal edema. Cystic allantoic hyperplasia may become pronounced but is considered a secondary change in a variety of processes rather than a primary cause of abortion.

When the fetus is available a complete internal and external examination is performed followed by collection of the tissue sets mentioned earlier. Changes observed in aborted fetus may include fetal diarrhea, characterized by meconium staining of the amnion and fetus, meconium aspiration in fetal lungs, and histopathologic evidence of chronic irritation of the amnion. This is considered an indicator of *in utero* fetal stress rather than a primary cause of abortion. However, the degree of inflammation in some cases may become severe enough that this likely contributes to fetal expulsion. There is overlap between abnormal findings in the late-term fetus and perinate in regard to fetal hypoxia, meconium staining, rib fractures, and several other potential causes of death. Late-term abortions may present as dystocia or, alternatively, dystocia may result in death of the perinate. For this reason, examination of near-term or term deaths may still yield important information.

In cases of neonatal disease or death, a necropsy examination may help identify infectious etiologies or underlying conditions. Each neonate is examined for evidence of infection, inflammation, malformations, necrosis, and trauma. Particular attention is paid to the presence of fractured ribs, pulmonary consolidation, passage of meconium, and patency of the intestinal tract as well as cardiac anatomy. Aerobic culture of the lung, liver, kidney, and spleen is often performed to demonstrate bacteriemia or sepsis. Common causes of death include sepsis, pneumonia, acute respiratory distress syndrome, EHV-1, neonatal maladjustment syndrome, neonatal isoerythrolysis, Tyzzer's disease, fractured ribs and associated hemorrhage or cardiac damage, hemorrhagic/clostridial enteritis, trauma, and congenital disease. All clinical concerns should be addressed at the time of necropsy or listed on the submission form (i.e. specific joints where there is a concern of sepsis, pneumonia, renal disease), as this might affect the order in which portions of the necropsy are performed. If done in a field setting, photographs taken after opening the thoracic and abdominal cavity but before manipulation of internal organs will aid a pathologist in interpretation of field necropsy results.

Summary

Examination of the fetal membranes, abortus, or neonate is generally a worthwhile endeavor and often yields valuable information. Initial examination of many placental units by farm personnel and veterinarians will help in identifying both pathology as well as variations of normal. In cases of abortion, lesions typically fall into one of three categories:

1) Findings that correspond with a cause of fetal death/abortion. These include positive laboratory testing and associated lesions of Equine Herpes Virus 1 and 4; Leptospirosis, Potomac Horse Fever, Equine Arteritis Virus, placentitis, cervical pole necrosis, umbilical cord torsion, and fetal malformations incompatible with life.
2) Findings that might contribute to fetal demise. This category includes placental edema, *in utero* fetal meconium passage, premature placenta separation, and a long umbilical cord (without evidence of associated lesions).
3) Findings that are likely reactive changes rather than evidence of primary disease. This category includes placental vascular mineralization and cystic allantoic hyperplasia.

References

1 Hong, C.B., Donahue, J.M., Giles, R.C. et al. (1993). Etiology and pathology of equine placentitis. *J. Vet. Diagn. Invest.* 5: 56–63.

2 Schlafer, D.H. (2004). Postmortem examination of the equine placenta, fetus, and neonate: methods and interpretation of findings. In: *Proc Ann Conv Am Assoc Equine Pract*, 144–161. Denver, CO: American Association of Equine Practitioners.

3 Foote, A.K., Ricketts, S.W., and Whitwell, K.E. (2012). A racing start in life? The hurdles of equine feto-placental pathology. *Equine Vet. J.* 44: 120–129.

4 Laugier, C., Foucher, N., Sevin, C. et al. (2011). A 24-year retrospective study of equine abortion in Normandy (France). *J. Equine Vet. Sci.* 31: 116–123.

Chapter 66 Special Considerations for the Neonatal Donkey and Mule Foal

Francisco Mendoza and Ramiro E. Toribio

Abbreviations

ACTH	Adrenocorticotropic hormone
AHV	Asinine herpesvirus
ALP	Alkaline phosphatase
AST	Aspartate aminotransaminase
BUN	Blood urea nitrogen
CK	Creatine kinase
CTUP	Combined thickness of the uterus and placenta
EHV	Equine herpesvirus
EVA	Equine viral arteritis
FTPI	Failure of transfer of passive immunity
GGT	Gamma-glutamyl transferase
GI	Gastrointestinal
IgG	Immunoglobulin G
IMHA	Immune-mediated hemolytic anemic
IMTP	Immune-mediated thrombocytopenia
LDH	Lactate dehydrogenase
NE	Neonatal encephalopathy
NI	Neonatal isoerythrolysis
NSAIDs	Nonsteroidal anti-inflammatory drugs
PCR	Polymerase chain rection
WBC	White blood cell
WMD	White muscle disease

Compared to the equine neonate, physiological, pathophysiological and pharmacological information in donkey and mule foals is scarce, reducing our ability to understand, diagnose and treat many of their disorders during the perinatal period [1]. This lack of information forces clinicians to extrapolate from equine foals, which in most instances is valid. However, it can also increase the risk of misdiagnosis, inappropriate drug use, potential side effects, and unnecessary expenses. There are anatomic, hematologic, metabolic, pharmacologic, and endocrine differences between adult donkeys and horses, and we can assume that these differences exist in the neonatal period. This paucity of information is even more evident for mule foals [2, 3]. Depending on the geographic region, mortality of donkey foals is higher than in equine foals, mainly from financial limitations, but also from reduced access to veterinary care, minimal preventative care, poor hygienic conditions, unsupervised pregnancies and foaling, and lack of knowledge. This chapter provides an overview on asinine neonatology, including unique aspects of this species in the perinatal period, differences with equine foals, and clinical considerations.

Gestational Factors Affecting Fetal Viability

Pregnancy in donkeys is longer than in horses (average 370 days; 331–421 days), which is important when planning delivery – to determine prematurity or postmaturity, but also to decide when to induce foaling [4, 5]. Gestation is longer in spring-bred (374 ± 8.7 days) compared to summer-bred (359.6 ± 5.8 days) and fall-bred (360.4 ± 9.2 days) jennies [5]. The effect of fetal sex on gestation length is minimal, although longer gestations have been reported in males fetuses [5, 6]. Jennies have an epitheliochorial diffuse microcotyledonary placenta with more complex microcotyledons than mares [7, 8]. The probability of twin pregnancy is higher in jennies than mares, likely due to the high frequency of multiple ovulations and higher microcotyledon and villi number per area [4, 8–10].

Despite longer gestation in jennies, the ratios between the newborn and mother's body weight (9.4%) and placenta to newborn body weight (12%) are similar to mares [7]. Based on these ratios and surface of fetomaternal contact per weight of the foal, it has been proposed that the conceptus-placental unit in the jenny is less efficient than in mares [7, 8]. While this could be valid, it could also be an evolutionary adaptation to harsh environments, food scarcity and unknown factors. This notion can be further

Equine Neonatal Medicine, First Edition. Edited by David M. Wong and Pamela A. Wilkins.

challenged considering that jennies are more likely to have viable twin foals than mares. Evaluation of the fetal membranes is not different for jennies than mares. In Martina Franca jennies, placental weight was 2.2 ± 0.6 kg [7, 11].

Care of the donkey neonate should start in the preterm period. Age and body condition of the jenny are important factors to consider before breeding because they can influence fertility rate, gestation, gestational complications, parturition, fetal maturation, and health of the neonate and mother. A negative energy balance predisposes jennies to metabolic problems such as hyperlipemia. Obesity, which is more common in donkeys in developed countries, also carries complications during pregnancy, including dystocia, dyslipidemias, and laminitis. In addition, disorders during pregnancy (e.g. insulin dysregulation, laminitis, placental disease, gastrointestinal [GI] disease) can result in abortion, prematurity, early lactation, reduced colostrum quantity and quality, and increased risk of perinatal infections. Information on the effect of diet on the development of donkey and mule embryos is lacking but assumed to be similar to mares. Ingestion of endophyte-infested fescue can lead to placental dysfunction, congenital disorders, insufficient mammary gland development, and lack of colostrum, with higher risk of foal diseases. Drugs with teratogenic potential to equine fetuses (e.g. fenbendazole, sulfonamides, pyrimethamine, enrofloxacin) may affect donkey fetuses but information is scarce.

Ruptures of the prepubic tendon and hydramnios have been reported in jennies but are rare conditions. There is minimal information on the prevalence of placental disease [4]. However, management of these conditions is similar to mares. Depending on the drugs used, it is important to consider pharmacologic differences with horses [12]. Jennies with placental disease can have premature udder development and vaginal discharge, although these abnormalities often go unnoticed. Jennies with poor vulvar conformation are predisposed to ascending uterine infections and the placenta should be evaluated throughout gestation. Ultrasonography is used to assess the combined thickness of the uterus and placenta (CTUP), uterine edema, presence of exudate, fetal viability, and properties of fetal fluids. The echogenicity of fetal fluids increases with gestation length [9].

Like horses, increased fetal mobility can be an indicator of fetal stress with reduced activity suggesting fetal compromise. Most fetal activity occurs at 6–8 months of gestation when uterine space allows for motion [9, 13]. The CTUP can be measured transabdominally and transrectally by 12 weeks of gestation depending on the size of the jenny. The CTUP measures 6–8 mm at 6 months, with rapid growth until month 12 (10–12 mm) [5, 9, 11, 13]. Like mares, a CTUP over 12 mm and presence of intracervical exudate are indicators of placentitis. Uterine edema does not indicate placentitis and can be observed in healthy jennies with normal pregnancies and deliveries. This is likely due to longer gestation length or decreased placental function [7, 9, 11].

The diagnosis and treatment of placentitis in jennies are beyond the scope of this chapter but treatment goals are to control bacterial infections, reduce inflammation, promote uterine quiescence, maintain uterine blood flow, and ultimately obtain a healthy foal with minimal complications to the jenny. Use of oral antimicrobials (e.g. sulfonamides/trimethoprim) combined with nonsteroidal anti-inflammatory drugs (NSAIDs; e.g. flunixin meglumine), progestogens (e.g. altrenogest), and estrogens (e.g. estradiol cypionate) is common in mares with placentitis and becoming routine in jennies [13].

Abortion in Jennies

Epidemiological information on causes of abortion in donkey and mule fetuses is scant. Infectious causes of abortion and neonatal disease include asinine herpesviruses (AHV), equine herpesvirus-1 (EHV-1), -4 (EHV-4), equine arteritis virus (EVA), *Leptospira* spp., *Taylorella asinigenitalis*, *Brucella abortus*, *Salmonella abortus equi*, *Pseudomonas* spp., *Streptococcus* spp., and *Trypanosoma* spp. Noninfectious causes include congenital (e.g. umbilical cord torsion, fetal anomalies), placental (e.g. insufficiency), and maternal (e.g. systemic disorders, toxicities) [14–17]. Gross and microscopic lesions from AHV, EHV-1 and EHV-4 aborted fetuses and fetal membranes are similar to those described for equine fetuses, including pulmonary congestion and septal edema, pleural effusion, and hepatic, renal, adrenal and thymic necrosis, and petechiation in multiple organs. Characteristic intranuclear inclusion bodies can be present in the liver, lung, kidney, adrenal gland, and lymphoid tissues. If abortion occurs at the end of pregnancy, aborted fetuses tend to be fresh or with minimal autolysis, and gross placental lesions may not be evident [18]. EHV-7 and EHV-8 were recently isolated from aborted donkey fetuses [19, 123].

Protocols to identify causes of equine abortion are not different for donkeys. Briefly, fresh fetal tissues and membranes must be processed taking biosecurity measures and sent to the laboratory for pathogen identification (culture and PCR) and histopathologic evaluation.

Vaccines used in donkeys are formulated for horses because no vaccine have been developed for donkeys. Vaccination principles to horses apply to donkeys (e.g. pregnant jennies vaccinated against EHV-1 and EHV-4 at 5, 7, and 9 months of pregnancy) as well as other pathogens depending on the region (e.g. rotavirus at 8, 9, and 10 month). There is effective transfer of antibodies against EHV-1 to donkey foals from vaccinated jennies [20].

Readiness of Birth and Foal Delivery

Due to management practices, foaling in donkeys is often missed. Methods to assess readiness to birth and impending foaling can be valuable. Accurate reproductive and breeding records are central to estimate delivery date and routine evaluation of jennies during pregnancy is important. Evaluation of mammary secretion and detection devices can be used.

One study in 17 multiparous (5–18 years old) Martina Franca jennies showed a steady increase in mammary secretion concentrations of calcium (>10 mmol/l) and potassium (>34.5 mmol/l) and a decrease in sodium concentrations (<19 mmol/l) and the sodium/potassium ratio starting 8–10 days before delivery. These changes were more evident 2 days before foaling, when reversal of the sodium/potassium ratio occurred, and was the best parameter associated with delivery [21]. Calcium is not a good predictor of when foaling will occur but is a better predictor that it will not occur [21, 22]. Magnesium also starts increasing 5 days (0.4 mmol/l) before delivery (1 mmol/l) [22]. Kits used to determine mammary secretion calcium in mares work well for jennies. More accurate measurements can be obtained using chemistry analyzers. Another study in 37 pregnant Dezhou jennies (9–12 years old) showed that a decrease in mammary secretion pH had good sensitivity (90%) and specificity (76%) to predict foaling, with a pH <6.4 being the best predictor of foaling within 24 hours [22]. Changes in mammary secretion pH seem to be slower in jennies (0.1 unit/d) compared to mares (0.5 unit/d).

Calcium concentrations in mammary secretions have been used to assess fetal maturity [7, 22]. However, dimensions of fetal structures, including chest, abdominal, stomach, eyeball, and aorta diameters are preferred to assess fetal development in donkeys (Table 66.1) [5, 9, 13]. Orbit diameter provides the best assessment of fetal development and expected delivery time [5]. One study found a strong association between fetal eyeball diameter and gestational age [5]. This is likely influenced by donkey breed.

Table 66.1 Fetal measurements from Amiata, Provencal, Martina Franca, Ragusa donkey breeds and crosses (3–18 years old, weighing 250–350 kg) [9, 13].

	Gestation length	
	22 weeks	52–53 weeks
Chest (mm)	80	180
Eyeball (mm)	20	25
Aorta (mm)	5	15
Fetal heart rate (bpm)	150	80

Similar to mares, phase I of parturition takes 65 minutes (20–135 minutes), with variable signs, including behavior changes, hyperactivity, lying down, frequent urination and defecation, looking at the flanks, and Flehmen reflex [6]. Term jennies have udder development and vulvar edema. Phase II (expulsion) in most jennies lasts 20 minutes (10–30 minutes) and phase III around 60 minutes (10–175 minutes) [6].

Adverse foaling events are not different between jennies and mares [23–25]. Dystocias are more frequent in miniature jennies due to narrow pelvic canal and domed head of the foal. In mules and hinnies this is more evident when a large stallion is used [17]. Principles of dystocia management for mares apply to jennies, including criteria for fetotomy and C-section.

Fetal membranes must be passed within 3 hours of foaling; beyond this point it is considered a retained placenta and proper preventative and therapeutic measures should be implemented to reduce the risk of metritis and associated complications, including endotoxemia and laminitis. These measures include uterine flushes with isotonic solutions, administration of oxytocin or prostaglandin, antimicrobial drugs, NSAIDs, polymyxin B, pentoxifylline, and feet cryotherapy. Measures to facilitate placenta detachment include knotting on itself or use of the Burns technique [4, 26]. Care should be taken when adding weight on the fetal membranes.

The Healthy Donkey and Mule Foal

Evaluation of donkey and mule foals is similar to horse foals. After birth, the donkey foal should stand within 1 hour, nurse within 2 hours, and pass meconium (and the jenny expulses fetal membranes) by 3 hours [6]. Time to first urination (8.5 hours) is similar to foals, with no sex differences [27]. In average-size donkey breeds, the umbilical cord weighs 0.15 ± 0.1 kg, is 62–63.5 cm in length, and ruptures at 15.9 ± 5.2 minutes [6, 7, 11], with earlier rupture occurring in foals that stand and nurse sooner. Contact with the neonate stimulates maternal oxytocin release, milk letdown, and uterine contractions, which favors placental expulsion. The Apgar score has been evaluated in donkey foals to assess the transition from birth, sternal position, standing, and nursing [27]. Higher Apgar scores were reported for donkey and mule compared to equine foals [27, 28].

Donkey foals born to high-risk jennies or from complicated deliveries should be monitored closely and receive a complete physical evaluation, clinicopathologic assessment, and measurement of serum immunoglobulin G (IgG) concentrations. Heart and respiratory rates are not different from equine foals [27], and rectal temperature should be 37–38.5 °C (98.6–101.3 °F). The Apgar score was associated with heart rate, respiratory rate, and rectal temperature; the lower these parameters, the lower the score, increasing the risk of illness and therefore, requiring prompt attention [27]. Donkey foals have a denser haircoat but are more prone to hypothermia than equine foals, regardless of breed, management, and health status [29]. It is a misconception that they are more tolerant to low temperatures. Therefore, it is important to protect them against cold conditions [30].

In the first week of age, healthy donkey foals nurse 5–6 times/hour (1–2 minutes each time) and consume approximately 20% of their body weight. Mare's milk replacers can be used to feed orphan donkey or mule foals without affecting daily weight gain [31]. Milk consumption peaks at 2 months of age then declines rapidly [32]. Mean weaning age is 6 months. Donkey foals can be fed milk starter at 2% bodyweight by 1 day of age, showing higher weekly and weaning growth compared with those just allowed to nurse [32]. This is more important for jennies with insufficient milk production or increased energy demands that can lead to other problems. Daily weight gain varies per breed and could be as high as 0.5 kg/d for Martina Franca foals [33]. There is minimal information on daily energy needs for growing donkey foals and in most instances is extrapolated from equine foals – in particular, in sick foals receiving enteral or parenteral nutrition. Information on daily energy requirements of pregnant and lactating jennies is described elsewhere [34, 35].

Hematology and Serum Biochemistry Profile

Hematological and biochemical differences exists between adult donkeys and horses as well as their foals [36–39]. Attention to these differences has become evident in recent years, especially in endangered donkey breeds [40]. These age and breed differences should be considered when evaluating donkey breeds. It is also important to note that donkey foals have thicker skin compared to equine foals.

Red cell series parameters decrease in the first week of life to values closer to adults (Table 66.2). This could be a result of increased erythrocyte destruction, reduced erythrocyte production, or a dilutional effect. The hematocrit and hemoglobin concentration are higher in donkey foals compare to horse foals [43]. No differences in white blood cell (WBC) count were noted between equine and donkey foals of the Amiata and Martina Franca breeds (Table 66.2) [43], but WBC count was lower in Amiata compared to Martina Franca donkey foals [41, 42]. Similar to equine foals [43], WBC count increases in the first 4 days of life reaching adult values by 1 week of age. In one study, neutrophil and monocyte counts were lower while lymphocyte, eosinophil, and basophil counts were higher in donkey compared to horse foals of similar age [43]. Of note, these studies were carried out at different geographic locations using different analytical systems. Platelet indices change minimally in the first week of age (Table 66.2). From birth to 7 days of age Martina Franca donkeys had platelet counts similar to newborn foals, but lower counts than Amiata donkey foals [41, 43]. These differences are unlikely to have clinical relevance.

Serum total protein and albumin concentrations remain unchanged in the first week of life and values are similar to equine foals (Table 66.3) [41, 42]. Low total protein concentrations in an otherwise healthy donkey foal is suggestive of failure of transfer of passive immunity (FTPI). Serum glucose concentrations in Martina Franca and Amiata foals were higher than values in equine foals at birth and higher than in adult donkeys (Table 66.3) [41, 42], but again, analytical methods should be considered. Lower glucose concentrations were reported in mule compared to equine foals at birth, but values were higher in mule foals at 12 and 24 hours, with no difference thereafter [44]. Like equine foals [45], blood urea nitrogen (BUN) and creatinine concentrations are higher at birth and steadily decrease over the first 48–72 hours of life to normal values [41, 42]. Abnormally high creatinine concentrations that remain elevated longer than expected suggests placental insufficiency, volume depletion, or renal injury. An increase in aspartate aminotransaminase (AST) activity in the first 3 days of life has been observed in donkey foals, but the explanation is unclear [41, 42]. Gamma-glutamyl transferase (GGT) and lactate dehydrogenase (LDH) activities change minimally in the first week of life, but an increase in GGT activity was noted in the first 24 hours of life in Amiata donkey and horse foals (Table 66.3) [41, 46]. Alkaline phosphatase (ALP) activity, as any mammalian neonate, is high at birth to decrease with aging [45], and inter-breed differences have been observed [41].

Serum triglyceride concentrations increase from birth (34.8 mg/dl [0.39 mmol/l]) to the first week of life (60.6 mg/dl [0.68 mmol/l]), remaining steady until adulthood, with no differences to horse foals or adult donkeys [41]. Serum triglyceride concentrations are higher in donkey foals receiving milk replacer, but no changes in serum glucose, cholesterol, and nonesterified fatty acid concentrations have been observed [32].

In the immediate postpartum period, serum sodium, chloride, potassium, and calcium concentrations are similar to adult donkeys and horse foals (Table 66.4) [41, 42]; serum phosphorus concentrations are higher in donkey foals than adults, peak by 48 hour of age, remain elevated for the first month, to decrease steadily to adult values by 6–12 months.

Table 66.2 Hemograms of healthy donkey foals at birth, 24 and 48 hours of life [41, 42].

Time from birth	RBC ($\times 10^6/\mu l$)	Hb (g/dl)	Hct (%)	MCV (fl)	MCH (pg)	MCHC (%)	RDW (%)	WBC ($\times 10^3/\mu l$)	Neu ($\times 10^3/\mu l$)	Lym ($\times 10^3/\mu l$)	Mono ($\times 10^3/\mu l$)	Eos ($\times 10^3/\mu l$)	Baso ($\times 10^3/\mu l$)	PLT ($\times 10^3/\mu l$)	MPV (fl)	PDW (%)	PCT (%)
0–10 min	9.8	17.4	48.2	48.8	17.8	36.3	17	6.5	5.2	1.4	0.10	0.09	0.08	288	8	24	0.2
24 h	8.8	15.3	41.8	48.3	17.5	36.4	17.8	7.3	4.9	2.0	0.13	0.07	0.05	280	7	25	0.2
48 h	8.1	14.5	39.8	47.8	17.4	36.7	17.8	8.1	5.9	1.8	0.22	0.07	0.04	288	8	23	0.2

Data expressed as mean. Baso, basophils; Eos, eosinophils; Hb, hemoglobin; Hct, hematocrit; Lym, lymphocytes; MCH, mean corpuscular hemoglobin; MCHC, mean corpuscular hemoglobin concentration; MCV, mean corpuscular volume; Mono, monocytes; MPV, medium platelet volume; Neu, neutrophils; PCT, plateletcrit; PDW, platelet distribution width; PLT, platelet count; RDW, red blood cell distribution width; RBC, red blood cell count; WBC, white blood cell count.

Table 66.3 Serum biochemical analytes in healthy donkey foals at birth, 24 and 48 hours of life [41, 42].

Time from birth	Glucose (mg/dl)	BUN (mg/dl)	Creatinine (mg/dl)	Total proteins (g/dl)	Albumin (g/dl)	Total bilirubin (mg/dl)	AST (IU/l)	GGT (IU/l)	CK (IU/l)	LDH (IU/l)	ALP (IU/l)
0–10 min	111	36.1	2.0	4.4	3.1	0.3	116	23.7	103	284	972
24 h	130	33.3	1.4	4.8	3.0	0.3	222	36.7	64	379	1015
48 h	134	26.5	1.2	5.0	3.1	0.3	250	34.1	70	348	745

Data expressed as mean. ALP, alkaline phosphatase; AST, aspartate aminotransferase; CK, creatine kinase; GGT, gamma glutamyl transferase; LDH, lactate dehydrogenase.

Table 66.4 Serum electrolyte concentrations in healthy donkey foals at birth, 24 and 48 hours of life [41, 42].

Time from birth	Sodium (mEq/l)	Chloride (mEq/l)	Potassium (mEq/l)	Total calcium (mg/dl)	Total magnesium (mg/dl)	Phosphorus (mg/dl)
0–10 min	135	101	4.4	11.4	1.8	4.4
24 h	136	136	4.2	11.2	1.9	4.9
48 h	135	135	4.5	11.4	1.9	6.1

Data expressed as mean.

Table 66.5 Blood gas parameters and serum lactate concentrations in healthy donkey foals from birth to 96 hours of life [42, 47].

Time from birth (h)	Sample	pH	PCO_2 (mmHg)	TCO_2 (mmol/l)	PO_2 (mmHg)	SO_2 (%)	HCO_3^- (mmol/l)	BE (mmol/l)	Lactate (mmol/l)
0–10 min	Arterial	7.39	41	27	60	85	25	−0.1	3.8
	Venous	7.37	44	27	34	61	26	0.3	4.7
12	Arterial	7.45	39	28	71	95	27	3.0	2.4
	Venous	7.46	39	28	40	75	27	2.6	2.4
24	Arterial	7.44	40	29	73	95	27	3.0	2.1
	Venous	7.44	40	29	39	74	28	2.8	1.8
48	Arterial	7.45	40	29	70	94	27	3	1.6
	Venous	7.44	43	30	36	71	28	4	1.4
96	Arterial	7.44	39	28	71	95	26	2	1.8
	Venous	7.43	41	28	36	70	27	3	1.6

Data expressed as mean. BE, base excess; HCO_3^-, bicarbonate; PCO_2, partial pressure of CO_2; PO_2, partial pressure of O_2; SO_2, oxygen saturation; TCO_2, total CO_2.

Information regarding blood gas analysis is noted in Table 66.5. Donkey foals are born with a lower pH than adult donkeys but similar to horse foals. This may be due to the hypoxic intrauterine environment [42, 47, 48]. PCO_2 decreases to adult values in the first 12 hours, similar to equine foals [49]. At birth, PaO_2 was similar but PvO_2 was lower than horse foals, increasing in the first 24 hours of life [49, 50]. HCO_3^- concentrations are similar to adult donkeys [42, 48] and horse foals [49]. Donkey foals are born with high lactate concentrations that reach normal values by 24 hours [42, 47, 51], which is similar to horse foals [52, 53].

Oxidative parameters (thiobarbituric acid reactive substances, lipid hydroperoxides, protein carbonyl concentrations) were higher in donkey foals fed milk replacer compared to natural nursing [32]. Based on differences in reactive oxygen metabolites and antioxidant potential between jennies and their foals [51], it has been proposed that like equine foals [54], the antioxidant system in donkey foals is not very effective at birth [51]. It also has been suggested that the placenta in equids is responsible for protecting the fetus against oxidative injury [51].

Even though differences in blood parameters between donkey breeds have been published, which could be real, they could also be attributed to different experimental conditions, methodologies, and analyzers.

Similar to equine foals, mule foals are born with high progestogen, androgen and glucocorticoid concentrations [55]. Newborn donkey foals also display a comparable steroid profile in the immediate postpartum period (R. E. Toribio, personal communication).

Maturity Disorders

Studies investing disorders of maturity in donkey or mule foals are lacking, but information from equine foals applies. Definitions of prematurity, dysmaturity, and postmaturity must be adjusted to gestation length in jennies (mean: 370 days; 331–421 days) as well as duration of previous pregnancies. Mares carrying mule pregnancies have similar gestation length (340 days), behavior, and duration of foaling stages to mares carrying equine pregnancies [4]. Due to the wide range in gestation length in jennies, donkey foals must be evaluated for evidence of dysmaturity. Assessment can be more challenging in donkeys managed under field conditions and incomplete breeding records.

Predisposing factors that interfere with maturity include maternal disease (e.g. hyperlipemia, colitis, laminitis, pneumonia), placental disease (e.g. placentitis, placental insufficiency), and fetal disorders (e.g. congenital defects, fetal disease, micromineral deficiency). Signs of prematurity/dysmaturity include weakness, inability to stand, domed head, floppy ears, fuzzy haircoat (for a donkey foal), delayed hoof cornification, incomplete ossification of cuboidal bones, tendon laxity, pulmonary atelectasis, GI intolerance to feeding, and abnormal glucose homeostasis. Laboratory abnormalities for premature equine foals applies to premature donkey foals, including hematologic (e.g. neutrophils<lymphocytes ratio) and biochemical abnormalities (e.g. hypoglycemia, azotemia, hyperlactatemia).

The diagnostic approach to premature/dysmature donkeys is similar to equine foals. A clinical history and physical examination are initial steps to assess maturity. Imaging and laboratory methods provide further confirmation. Radiographs of the carpus and tarsus are valuable to assess ossification of the cuboidal bones, and thoracic radiography is used to assess the pulmonary parenchyma for maturity, atelectasis, pneumonia, and rib fractures. Thoracic, abdominal, and umbilical ultrasonography is recommended. Hematology and blood chemistry provide an assessment of the systemic inflammatory and metabolic status of the foal and aid in therapeutic decisions and prognostication. The serum IgG concentrations should also be evaluated for FTPI. Due to the potential immune incompetent status of these animals and risk of bacterial translocation, antimicrobial therapy is highly indicated. Other therapeutic and support measures depend on clinical findings and disease progression. A warm environment is crucial due to their susceptibility to hypothermia compared to equine foals [29].

Failure of Transfer of Passive Immunity

Serum IgG concentrations in newborn donkey foals should be measured after 12 hours of age. Insufficient ingestion of colostrum or poor-quality colostrum results in FTPI predisposing to neonatal infections, in particular sepsis. Methods used to measure IgG concentrations in donkey foals are the same as equine foals [56]. Single radial immunodiffusion is the gold standard [57]. Immunoturbidometry provides accurate quantitative values for equine serum [57, 58]. Semiquantitative methods that work well in the donkey foal include glutaraldehyde coagulation test, zinc sulfate turbidity test, ammonium sulfate precipitation (immunocrit ratio), enzyme linked immunosorbent assay (ELISA), and latex agglutination.

Information on the association between IgG concentrations and disease severity in donkey and mule foals is lacking, but the principles of IgG categorization for equine foals should be used. IgG concentrations >800 mg/dl are considered adequate IgG transfer, 400–800 mg/dl as partial FTPI, and <400 mg/dl as total FTPI [58, 59]. Maximum IgG concentrations in donkey foals are measured at 24 hours [60, 61]. Serum IgG concentrations were higher in Amiata compared to Martina Franca foals, but IgG concentrations were measured with different methods [60, 61]. In mule foals, median serum IgG concentrations at 24 hours were 910 mg/dl (670–1100 mg/dl) [62]. Serum IgG concentrations decrease rapidly between 14 and 28 days.

The prevalence of FTPI in donkey foals is 30% [63]. Predisposing factors for low IgG and neonatal disease include maternal (poor udder development, premature lactation and colostrum loss, maternal diseases, maternal rejection), placental (placentitis, placental separation), neonatal (congenital, disorders that impair nursing [e.g. dysmaturity, neonatal encephalopathy, musculoskeletal, GI]), and environmental (management, hygiene, infectious agents in premises) factors. Equine neonates must consume 2–4% of body weight of good quality colostrum to achieve adequate IgG concentrations. Maiden or feral jennies could reject their foals in the period when they need to nurse sufficient colostrum [64].

Colostrum from the jenny or previously frozen colostrum should be administered to newborn foals that do not nurse or nurse incompletely within 3 hours. In breeding farms, it is recommended to freeze colostrum from multiparous jennies. The volume to be stored depends on the breed and amount of colostrum produced, which ranges from 200 to 500 ml. After 12 hours of age, in foals that did not ingest or that ingested insufficient amount of colostrum, administration of donkey plasma is recommended. Colostrum should be considered, although administration after 12 hours of birth has minimal effect on IgG concentrations. Equine plasma can also be used, but it is important to monitor for complications such immune-mediate hemolytic anemia (IMHA) and immune-mediate thrombocytopenia (IMTP).

Colostrometers estimate colostrum quality; in mares, a colostrum density >1.060 is consistent with good quality colostrum and the same principle likely applies to jennies. Brix refractometry can also be used to assess colostrum quality with values of 14–17% and >17% in jennies considered adequate or very good, respectively [60, 65]. In contrast, higher Brix values of 20–30% (50–80 g/l) and 30% (>80 g/l) in mares were considered adequate or very good, respectively [66]. This difference between jennies and mares likely reflects different experimental and analytical conditions as well as differences in colostrum and milk composition between species. In one study, Brix refractometry showed a decrease in colostrum quality from birth ($17.6 \pm 2.9\%$) to 24 hours post-foaling ($10.2 \pm 1.1\%$) [60].

When donkey colostrum is not available, equine colostrum should be considered, ideally from the same or nearby farms. Equine colostrum works well in donkey and mule foals; however, it is important to monitor foals for immune-mediated disorders (IMHA, IMTP). For a 25–45 kg foal, 100–300 ml of colostrum should be administered and repeated within few hours until a total of 4% of body weight is provided (ideally before of 12 hours of age). Smaller and more frequent volumes are ideal to mimic nursing and allow time for intestinal IgG absorption.

After 24 hours of age colostrum absorption is minimal and IV plasma transfusion is necessary. Locally produced plasma is cheaper but carries higher risk of complications. Plasma from the mother or a castrated donkey is a good option. If equine plasma will be used, mares with no history of having mule foals or foals with neonatal isoerythrolysis (NI) or a gelding are ideal. Commercial plasma is better because it is free of pathogens and donors have been tested against major equine incompatibility antigens, including donkey factor. Approximately 250 ml (miniature donkeys) to 1–1.5 l (25–45 kg donkey foals) of plasma may be needed to adequately increase the serum IgG. Of note, it is not unusual for donkey or mule foals that received equine plasma to develop thrombocytopenia (R. Toribio, personal communication) or hemolytic anemia. Therefore, a CBC is recommended 24–48 hours after administration. In addition to immune and nutritional factors, colostrum contains bacterial and fungal byproducts that can be detected in circulation of donkey foals. These factors are likely important to prime their immune system [67].

Sepsis

Sepsis is a main cause of mortality of newborn donkey and mule foals. Infections can occur in utero from placentitis or ascending infections, but more often are consequence of FTPI. The GI tract is the main route for bacterial translocation into systemic circulation and hematogenous dissemination. Bacterial entry also can occur from the respiratory tract or umbilicus. Foals born to dystocia, with maturity disorders, FTPI or neonatal encephalopathy (NE) have higher risk of sepsis and should be monitored closely.

Early diagnosis is central to implement therapies to improve survival. The stoic nature of sick donkey foals can be misleading. It is important to perform a complete physical evaluation in the first 24–48 hours of age, including measurement of serum IgG concentrations. History of previous gestations and foaling is relevant because it points out at higher-risk foals. Ischemic events and neonatal encephalopathy can favor bacterial translocation due to intestinal hypoxia, disorientation, and reduced colostrum intake. In addition, placental disease often results in premature lactation and colostrum loss. These foals are frequently born prematurely, further complicating their outcome.

Clinical signs of sepsis are similar to equine foals and might include fever, lethargy, anorexia, organ dysfunction (dyspnea, tachypnea, diarrhea, azotemia, liver injury, seizures, uveitis, umbilical infections, lameness, septic arthritis, physitis, osteomyelitis, and meningitis), recumbency, and sudden death.

The diagnosis of sepsis is based on clinical findings and laboratory and ancillary methods. The sepsis score developed for foals can be used but it has not been validated for donkey or mule foals [68]. In equine foals, a score >11 has >93% likelihood of sepsis [68]. The Apgar score can be useful to assess overall health, and it has been evaluated in Amiata donkey and mule foals [27, 28]; however, its clinical value remains to be determined. Blood cultures are used to identify the etiologic agent and guide proper antimicrobial selection and prognosis.

Common etiologic agents isolated in blood culture include *Escherichia coli*, *Actinobacillus* spp., *Enterobacter* spp., *Salmonella* spp., *Streptococcus* spp., and *Enterococcus* spp. Viruses such as AHV, EHV-1, EHV-4, and EVA, and fungal agents can also be involved. Treatment of septic donkey or mule foals is similar to equine foals, considering species variations. Differences on the pharmacokinetics of some antimicrobials and NSAIDs have been documented between adult donkeys and horses, but information in donkey and mule foals is lacking. Therefore, caution must be taken with doses. In addition, attention must be paid to energy homeostasis due to their propensity to develop hyperlipemia. See Chapter 34 for further discussion of sepsis.

Neonatal Isoerythrolysis (NI)

NI is a form of IMHA and occurs in donkey and mule foals [69, 70], with higher incidence in mule foals, in particular those born to mares that previously had mule foals. The incidence of NI in mule foals is approximately 10%, which is higher than the incidence in equine foals (incidence unknown in donkey foals) [71]. The high incidence of NI in mule foals is attributed to major antigenic differences between donkeys and horses, in particular to the donkey factor that sensitizes mares to produce antibodies that are passed in colostrum to the neonate. It is recommended to either test mares that had mule foals for anti-donkey antibodies or simply discard their colostrum and provide colostrum from either mares that have not been bred to donkeys [72] or from jennies. Alternatively, plasma transfusion can be considered. After 24 hours, the foal can nurse from the mare. Information on blood types in donkeys and mules is scant [73].

Clinical signs of NI include lethargy, anorexia, recumbency, icterus, pale mucous membranes, tachycardia, tachypnea, and pigmenturia. The diagnosis of NI in donkey and mule foals is made using the same principles of equine foals, including clinical and laboratory findings [74]. The Coombs test to detect agglutinating antibodies on the surface of erythrocytes can be confirmatory, but a negative test is unlikely to change the therapeutic plan, in particular when there is clinical and laboratory evidence of NI.

Treatment of NI is centered on fluid therapy and blood transfusion. Ideally, a mule foal should receive washed red blood cells from the mare or whole blood from a gelding that has tested negative for donkey factor. This also carries a risk due to equine-asinine antigenic differences, including IMTP and IMHA, which are complications of mule and donkey foals receiving equine plasma. Donkey foals with NI should receive red blood cells from the jenny or blood from a castrated donkey. Blood from a gelding should be considered in extreme circumstances. Pre-emptive treatment with dexamethasone may reduce severity of hypersensitivity reactions and oxygen insufflation (5–10 l/min) should be initiated in severe cases. Polymerized bovine hemoglobin (5 ml/kg) has been proposed for NI, although it may not be practical or commercially available [75]. Caution must be taken with the use of NSAIDs due to the risk of exacerbating renal injury. Foals with severe hypoxia (secondary to anemia) are at risk of sepsis due to intestinal bacterial translocation, and antimicrobial drugs should be considered. The prognosis is good with prompt treatment.

Other causes of hemolysis in neonates such as piroplasmosis and leptospirosis depend on geographical location. Hemolysis in these animals does not occur in the immediate postpartum period but days to weeks later. In areas endemic to piroplasmosis donkey foals may be protected up to 2 months of age when colostral antibodies decline [76]. Hemophilia linked to X-chromosome glucose-6-phosphate dehydrogenase has been documented in donkey, mule, and hinny foals [77].

Neonatal Alloimmune Thrombocytopenia

Newborn donkey and mule foals can develop alloimmune thrombocytopenia, which can also occur with NI [70, 78]. In other species the presence of both conditions is known as Evans syndrome. The pathogenesis of this type of IMTP is similar to NI, with colostral antibodies mediating platelet removal or destruction. These antibodies could also interfere with platelet function, further impairing clotting [78]. As previously mentioned, a similar phenomenon may also occur in donkey and mule foals after receiving equine plasma. Therefore, evaluation of a CBC is recommended 24 hours after transfusion (R. Toribio, personal communication). The diagnosis is often suspected based on clinical abnormalities (e.g. petechiations), supported by CBC evaluation, and confirmed by other methods (flow cytometry, immunofluorescence). Flow cytometry is the preferred method to demonstrate antibodies coating the platelets. Considerations for transfusion are similar to blood, but platelet-rich plasma is preferred [75]. Under a premise comparable to NI, donkey and mule foals receiving equine plasma should be pretreated with a fast-acting glucocorticoid.

Gastrointestinal (GI) Disorders

Differences in GI disorders between donkey, mule, and horse foals are minimal, with similar clinical presentations and laboratory findings. The same pathogens cause GI disease. Congenital anomalies (atresia coli, atresia ani) have been documented in donkey and mule foals [79, 80].

Causes of colic in donkey and mule foals are listed in Table 66.6. Most common include meconium impaction, enteritis, enterocolitis, and small intestine strangulation. Donkey foals are stoic, and signs of colic may not be evident. They can be standing, minimally active, and occasionally lie down. Rolling is not characteristic, but some may roll with severe abdominal pain. This has clinical implications for severe lesions that may require surgery. Transabdominal ultrasonography and abdominocentesis are important diagnostic tools. Depending on the age of the animal, abdominal radiography can be useful to diagnose meconium retention, atresia coli (with barium contrast), or foreign bodies. Medical and surgical therapeutic principles apply equally to equid neonates.

Diarrhea can be infectious (viral, bacterial) and noninfectious (lactose intolerance, microbiota changes,

Table 66.6 Gastrointestinal disturbances and causes in donkey and mule foals.

Diarrhea		Colic	
Noninfectious causes	**Infectious causes and parasites**	**Strangulating causes**	**Nonstrangulating causes**
Antibiotic-induced diarrhea Foal heat Lactose intolerance Necrotizing enterocolitis Nutritional dysbiosis Pancreatitis Peritonitis Sand accumulation Uroperitoneum	*Clostridium perfringens* *Clostridioides difficile* Coronavirus *Cryptosporidium parvum* *Giardia* spp. *Lawsonia intracellularis* *Parascaris equorum* *Rhodococcus equi* Rotavirus *Salmonella* spp. *Strongyloides* spp.	Colon displacement Inguinal hernia Intussusception Small and large intestine volvulus	Congenital abnormalities: atresia ani and coli Foreign bodies Gastroduodenal ulcers Ileus Meconium retention (impaction)

parasites, sand accumulation). Infectious diarrhea is more evident in farms with high animal density. A recent outbreak of rotavirus in China affected 119 of 206 donkey foals (≤4 months) in two intensive donkey farms. The highest morbidity occurred in foals of 1–3 months of age but fatality was the highest (45.5%) in foals <1 month of age [81].

Diagnostic methods to identify GI pathogens in equine neonates apply to donkey and mule foals and include fecal culture, PCR, and ELISA. Main bacteria causing diarrhea in donkey and mule foals include *Clostridium perfringens*, *Clostridioides difficile*, and *Salmonella* spp. The role of *E. coli* as a cause of diarrhea in donkey and equine foals remains unclear. Viral causes include rotavirus and coronavirus (Table 66.6) [81–83].

Hemoconcentration, leukocytosis or leukopenia, neutrophilia or neutropenia, and toxic changes may be observed on CBC. Frequent biochemical abnormalities include azotemia, hypoglycemia, hyperlactatemia, as well as acid-base and electrolyte disturbances. Often serum triglyceride concentrations are high. Serum IgG concentrations could be low [84, 85]. Most of these animals are septic.

Treatment of diarrhea includes hemodynamic support, restoring organ function, correction of acid-base and electrolyte abnormalities, provision of energy/nutrition, control of inflammation, and antimicrobials. Donkey foals with proximal GI disease (infectious or noninfectious) often develop lactose intolerance, leading to osmotic diarrhea. They can benefit from oral lactase supplementation in addition to fluid therapy. Foals with heat diarrhea, nutritional imbalances, or antibiotic-induced diarrhea have good prognosis.

Antimicrobial selection depends on clinical presentation, laboratory abnormalities, and the suspect pathogen(s). Newborn foals with GI disease often become septic. Broad-spectrum combinations such as penicillins and aminoglycosides are frequently used. Third-generation cephalosporins are also an option. In foals with enteritis or enterocolitis, metronidazole should be considered. For some drugs there are pharmacokinetic differences between donkeys and horses, but also between neonates and adults. For metronidazole, equine foals require lower doses less frequently compared to horses, but there is no pharmacokinetic information for donkey foals. It is important to keep in mind that metronidazole can cause anorexia, which is relevant in sick animals at risk of or with ongoing hyperlipemia. Bacterial resistance can be a problem. In one study, 19 donkey and a mule foals had diarrhea from *Salmonella enterica* that was resistant to sulfonamides, tetracyclines, fluoroquinolones, and cephalosporins [84]. Resistance patterns are regional, and caution must be taken when extrapolating antimicrobial selection.

Treatment of parasitic diarrhea depends on age of the foal, target parasite, and evidence of resistance. Imidazoles (e.g. fenbendazole) are considered safe while avermectins (e.g. ivermectin) and milbemycins (e.g. moxidectin) should be avoided in foals <6 months of age, in particular if they are in poor body condition. Praziquantel can be used to treat tapeworms, but usually in older animals due to the long life cycle of these parasites. Deworming jennies in the last trimester of pregnancy is recommended [86].

There use of probiotics is controversial. Based on studies in equine foals they may increase the risk of diarrhea and should be avoided [87], at least until controlled studies demonstrate their benefits. Regarding the microbiome, predominant phyla in donkey foals were Firmicutes in the foregut and Firmicutes and Bacteroidetes in the hindgut, similar to adult donkeys and horses [88, 89], but different to equine foals [90]. By 7 months of age, the microbiome between donkey foals and adults is similar [91].

The use of NSAIDs should be considered for specific conditions aimed at reducing inflammation, pain, and pyrexia and to ameliorate the effects of endotoxemia. Flunixin meglumine and ketoprofen are frequently used NSAIDs in foals. Cyclooxygenase-2 inhibitors such as meloxicam and firocoxib are preferred by some clinicians as they have less side effects; a meloxicam study showed that is equally effective against the systemic effects of endotoxemia in donkeys [92].

Other drugs used in donkey foals with GI disease include gastric acid reducers and protectants (e.g. omeprazole, pantoprazole, sucralfate, ranitidine), prostaglandin E analogs (e.g. misoprostol) and intestinal adsorbents (e.g. smectite, activated charcoal, bismuth subsalicylate, kaolin). Other measures will depend on the systemic status of the foal including nutrition, blood or plasma transfusion, and supportive care.

Gastric ulcers can occasionally be diagnosed in newborn donkey foals, but its prevalence and clinical relevance remain undetermined. Like equine foals, caution must be taken on the preemptive use of gastric acid reducers unless NSAIDs are used, because they can increase the risk of diarrhea. Biosecurity protocols in animals suspect of infectious diarrhea must be implemented, including use of protective equipment, disinfection, and isolation.

Respiratory Disorders

Donkey, mule, and horse foals develop the same respiratory disorders, although epidemiological information is scarce. Inciting causes can be respiratory or extra-respiratory, infectious, noninfectious, acquired, or congenital (Table 66.7). Congenital conditions include rostral displacement of the palatopharyngeal arch, collapse of arytenoid cartilages, choanal atresia, and cleft palate [93, 94]. Clinical signs do not differ from equine foals, although they could be missed due to foal behavior or because they are often in the field.

Infectious pneumonia ensues from aspiration or hematogenous bacterial dissemination, in particular in septic foals. They can develop acute respiratory distress syndrome. Fungal pneumonia was documented in five Albino Asinara donkey foals (20–30 days old) that died suddenly and were housed in the same paddock [95]. This unusual presentation suggested that these foals were immunocompromised. In acquired conditions, clinical signs can be present immediately after birth or become evident days later.

Depending on the condition, clinical signs include dyspnea, coughing (poor reflex in newborns), mucopurulent nasal discharge, milk coming out of the nostrils after nursing, tachypnea, and respiratory distress. Foals with congenital heart conditions can resemble some of these signs. Older foals can develop coughing from ascarid migration or bacterial pneumonia (e.g. *Rhodococcus equi*). Lungworms rarely cause evident pulmonary disease in donkey foals. Some animals may develop respiratory signs before parasites become patent. This is more evident in horse or mule foals.

Table 66.7 Respiratory and extra-respiratory causes of respiratory disease in donkey and mule foals.

Respiratory causes		Extra-respiratory causes	
Congenital	**Acquired**	**Congenital**	**Acquired**
Choanal atresia	Bacterial pneumonia:	Cardiac disease	Acid–base imbalances
Cleft palate	**Neonate foal:** *Streptococcus* spp., *Actinobacillus* spp., *Klebsiella* spp.	Diaphragmatic hernia	Botulism
Epiglottis hypoplasia	**Older foals:** *Rhodococcus equi* and *Streptococcus equi equi* and *zooepidemicus*	Neonatal encephalopathy	Cardiac disease
Laryngeal deformity	Viral pneumonia: AHV EHV-1, EHV-4, EVA, equine influenza virus	Rib deformity	Diaphragmatic hernia
Lung immaturity	Fungal pneumonia: *Aspergillus fumigatus, Pneumocystis carinii*		Dysphagia
Rostral displacement of palatopharyngeal arch	Acute respiratory distress syndrome		Fever, abdominal distension, etc.
Surfactant deficiency	Foreign bodies		Meningoencephalitis
Tracheal collapse	Guttural pouch empyema		Neonatal encephalopathy
Wry noise	Meconium or milk aspiration		Pulmonary hypertension
	Pneumothorax		Rib fractures
	Pulmonary edema		Tetanus
	Secondary surfactant deficiency: sepsis, pneumonia, edema, etc.		Volume overload
	Sinusitis		White muscle disease
	Tracheal rupture		
	Trauma		

AHV, asinine herpesvirus; EHV, Equine herpesvirus; EVA, equine viral arteritis.

Diagnostic methods include hematology, blood biochemistry, imaging (endoscopy, ultrasonography, radiography), evaluation of ventilation (arterial blood gas, oximetry), transtracheal wash, and bronchoalveolar lavage. Evaluation of cardiovascular function, including electrocardiography and echocardiography, may be indicated in some cases. In older foals (>3 months of age), bronchoalveolar lavage may be indicated to diagnose lungworms [96].

Treatment focuses on maintaining tissue oxygenation and perfusion, controlling inflammation, fever, and pain, providing hydration, supplying energy, and implementing other support measures. Broad-spectrum antimicrobials should be initiated in most sick donkey foals, whether the initial cause is infectious or noninfectious. Oxygen insufflation is often required. Drugs to control inflammation include NSAIDs (e.g. flunixin meglumine and meloxicam) and glucocorticoids (e.g. dexamethasone). Diuretics may be considered when pulmonary edema is present (e.g. furosemide). Expectorants (e.g. acetylcysteine, bromhexine) and cough suppressants are occasionally used, but their efficacy is unknown. Congenital conditions may require surgical correction and carry a guarded to grave prognosis, depending on underlying process.

Neurological Disorders

Observing the behavior of the newborn donkey foal and jenny is important to identify problems early, including their interactions [97]. Some jennies reject their foals or are aggressive to them, in particular maidens. Others just need time, but in the interim the foal needs to nurse. Foals lying down for prolonged period or showing no interest in nursing might suggest a perinatal disorder (sepsis, neonatal encephalopathy); alternatively, this could be a protective mechanism from an aggressive mother. Insufficient milk production from the jenny is another cause.

Donkey foals are very susceptible to tetanus, not in the immediate postpartum period but days to weeks later. Newborn donkey foals can also develop toxicoinfectious botulism (shaker foal syndrome). In North America, type B and C are the most common forms of botulism. Clinical signs include weakness, muscular tremors, inability to stand for long periods, dysphagia, weak eyelid, tongue and tail tone, mydriasis, tachycardia, constipation, and dysuria. Colic might also be observed although signs may be difficult to assess. If untreated, the disease progresses to respiratory muscle failure and death by asphyxia. Forage poisoning and wound botulism are rare conditions in donkey foals, although adult donkeys are equally or more susceptible to forage poisoning than horses. Other disorders such as hypocalcemia, electrolyte imbalances, selenium deficiency, and meningitis could have similar signs. Other uncommon neurologic disorders include congenital abnormalities [98, 99] and ivermectin toxicosis in donkey and mule foals [100].

Urogenital Disorders

Umbilical arteries and vein diameter in healthy newborn donkey foals is 0.6–0.7 cm, even smaller in miniature donkey foals [7, 101]. Umbilical disorders include omphalitis, omphaloarteritis, omphalophlebitis, and omphalourachitis that can lead to bacterial entry and sepsis. The diagnosis is based on physical examination and ultrasonography. In addition to pain, heat, and umbilical stump enlargement, some foals may develop a patent urachus. Occasionally, due to infection and necrosis of the urachus, some donkey foals can develop uroabdomen. Foals with uroabdomen or ruptured bladder have free anechoic or hypoechoic abdominal fluid and azotemia along with hyperkalemia and hyponatremia. Congenital conditions such as hypospadias and hydronephrosis have been documented in this species [80].

Renal dysfunction can be primary or secondary to a number of infectious and noninfectious pathologies. Milk deprivation due to rejection, insufficient milk production, or the foal not having interest due to physical limitations or illness can result in dehydration. This is common with sepsis, prematurity, and neonatal encephalopathy. Treatment is similar to equine foals and includes restoring blood volume and tissue perfusion. In foals with evidence of renal injury, nephrotoxic drugs such as NSAIDs and aminoglycosides should be avoided or used with caution.

Cardiovascular Disorders

There is limited cardiovascular information in newborn donkeys. Congenital disorders documented in equine foals also occur in donkey foals. These include septal defects, tetralogy of Fallot, patent ductus arteriosus, truncus arteriosus, and pseudotruncus arteriosus [102, 103]. Acquired disturbances are not different between equine, donkey, and mule foals [104].

Metabolic and Endocrine Disorders

Endocrine disorders documented in critically ill equine foals occur in sick donkey and mule foals. In donkey foals with a negative energy balance, hyperlipemia is a concern that can lead to complications including liver and renal dysfunction, tissue fatty infiltration, dysrhythmias, and diarrhea [105]. Hypoglycemia is frequent in sick donkey and mule foals, which often have normal or low insulin concentrations, supporting an appropriate response to energy deprivation. Information on most energy-regulating hormones in donkey foals is minimal. Hypocalcemia and hypomagnesemia are common in septic donkey and mule foals, although published information on their prevalence or on calcium-regulating hormones is scarce. This is more evident in those with GI disease. Critically ill donkey foals with hyperlipemia or receiving parenteral nutrition may develop hypomagnesemia, hypokalemia, and hypophosphatemia. Therefore, in addition to calcium treatment, some may require intravenous magnesium, phosphorus, and potassium supplementation (e.g. magnesium sulfate, potassium chloride, sodium or potassium phosphate).

Most critically ill donkey foals have an appropriate response to stress by releasing adrenocorticotropic hormone (ACTH) and cortisol, which is similar to equine foals; however, some can develop adrenal insufficiency characterized by inappropriately low cortisol concentrations with normal or high ACTH concentrations.

Musculoskeletal Disorders

Congenital musculoskeletal conditions in newborn donkey foals are not different to equine foals, including digital dysgenesis, patellar luxation, brachygnathism, osteopetrosis, incomplete ossification of cuboidal bones, and vertebral malformation [106–108]. Acquired disorders are the same of equine foals ranging from angular and flexural deformities to infections (septic arthritis, physitis, osteomyelitis). Risk of orthopedic infections in the immediate postpartum period is higher with low IgG concentrations.

Diagnosis can be simple or require ancillary methods including imaging, cytology, and bacterial culture. Management of angular and flexural deformities in donkey foals depends on the type of condition, size, and age of the foal. Due to anatomical and radiographical differences with equine foals, particular consideration must be taken with this species [109]. Orthopedic support (splints, bandages), toe extension, corrective shoeing, and intravenous oxytetracycline administration may be necessary. Severe cases may require surgery [110, 111]. Foals with musculoskeletal infections require systemic antimicrobials as well as local treatment, including arthrocentesis, joint lavage, debridement, arthroscopy, and intravenous regional limb perfusion with antimicrobials.

Donkey and mule foals born in selenium-deficient areas can develop white muscle disease (WMD). Endemic areas tend to be arid or volcanic with acid soils, and often jennies are fed poor-quality forage [112]. This occurs in some areas of the US and South America (R. Toribio, personal communication). Selenium or selenium activity via glutathione peroxidase as well as vitamin E (α-tocopherol) concentrations should be evaluated in suspect cases. Lower selenium concentrations were reported in donkey foals (0.05 μg/ml) than adult donkeys (0.11 μg/ml) [113], and horses [114]. Vitamin E concentrations were similar between donkeys and horses, but lower in donkey foals (5.9 μmol/l) than adult donkeys (7.7–8.9 μmol/l) [113]. It is important to use age-specific reference ranges. In endemic areas or where WMD has been diagnosed, pregnant jennies must be supplemented with selenium in their diet or with parenteral formulations. Recommended selenium daily intake is 0.1–0.15 mg/100 kg [115]. Administration of selenium (0.03 mg/kg/IM) in the last trimester of pregnancy should be considered. Some formulations have selenium and vitamin E. Verbascoside, a plant polyphenol with antimicrobial, anti-inflammatory and antioxidant properties was shown to increase serum and milk vitamin E concentrations in jennies, as well as their foals [116].

Esteatitis and myonecrosis have been described in donkey foals [117–120]. Whether these changes were due to vitamin E and selenium deficiency remains unclear. Clinical signs were nonspecific, including lethargy, anorexia, subcutaneous edema, fever, tachycardia, and focal pain over the nuchal ligament. Diagnosis is based on physical examination, increased muscle enzyme activity, low serum vitamin E and selenium concentrations, and histopathology. Muscle biopsy could be helpful to assess tissue degeneration, fibrosis, necrosis, inflammatory infiltration and lipopigment (ceroid) accumulation consistent with oxidative injury. Treatment includes vitamin E and selenium administration intramuscularly, followed of oral administration. Anti-inflammatory drugs are helpful to control pain and systemic inflammation.

Pharmacological Considerations

Differences in pharmacokinetics and pharmacodynamics for a number of drugs exist between adult donkeys and horses [12, 121, 122], which calls for proper adjustment of dosing and frequency to avoid under- or overdosing, as well as potential side effects [12, 36]. Pharmacologic information in donkey foals is lacking but is anticipated to parallel that of equine foals and horses. Differences are due to metabolic activities, plasma protein, and water content in the extracellular compartment. Until information is available for donkey foals, it is recommended to use that of equine foals (Table 66.8).

Table 66.8 Medications used in donkey and mule foals *

	Dose	Route	Interval
	Antimicrobials		
Amikacin	25 mg/kg	IV	24 h
	125-1000 mg	IVRLP	24 h
Ampicillin sodium	20-50 mg/kg	IV	6-8 h
Azithromycin	10 mg/kg	PO	24 h for 5 days, then every 48 h
Cefepime	11 mg/kg	IV	8 h
Cefotaxime	40-50 mg/kg	IV	6 h
Cefpodoxime	10 mg/kg	PO	6-12 h
Cefquinome	1-2.5 mg/kg	IV, IM	6-12 h
Ceftazidime	40-50 mg/kg	IV	6 h
Ceftiofur sodium	4-10 mg/kg	IV, IM	6-12 h
Ceftriaxone	25 mg/kg	IV	12 h
Clarithromycin	7.5 mg/kg	PO	12 h
Chloramphenicol	50-60 mg/kg	IV, PO	6 h
Doxycycline	10 mg/kg	PO	12 h
Gentamicin sulfate	10-12 mg/kg	IV	12-24 h
Imipenem and cilastatin §	10–20 mg/kg	IV	6-12 h
Meropenem §	5-10 mg/kg	IV	8-12 h
Metronidazole	10-15 mg/kg	IV, PO	8-12 h
Oxytetracycline #	6.6 mg/kg	IV	12 h
Penicillin K or Na	22,000-44,000 IU/kg	IV	6 h
Penicillin procaine	22,000-44,000 IU/kg	IM	12-24 h
Rifampin	5-10 mg/kg	PO	12-24 h
Sulfonamide/trimethoprim	20-30 mg/kg	PO	12 h
	Non-steroidal and steroidal anti-inflammatory drugs		
Acetaminophen (paracetamol)	10-20 mg/kg	IV, PO	12-24 h
Carprofen	0.5-0.7 mg/kg	PO	24 h
Dexamethasone	0.05-0.2 mg/kg	IV, IM, PO	12-24 h
Diphenhydramine hydrochloride	0.5-2 mg/kg	IV, IM	
Dipyrone (metamizole)	10-22 mg/kg	IV, IM	8-12 h
Firocoxib	0.1 mg/kg	IV	12-24 h
Flunixin meglumine	0.25-1.1 mg/kg	IV	8-12 h
Ketoprofen	1.1-2.2 mg/kg	IV	12-24 h
Meloxicam	0.6 mg/kg	IV	12-24 h
Prednisolone	0.5-2 mg/kg	PO	24 h
	Gastric acid reducers and protectants, and absorbent		
Activated charcoal	CJ	PO	CJ
Bismuth subsalicylate	CJ	PO	CJ
Famotidine	2-4 mg/kg	PO	8-12 h
	0.5-1 mg/kg	IV	8-12
Kaolin	CJ	PO	CJ
Lactase	2000-4000 IU/foal	PO	4-6 h
Misoprostol	1-4 μg/kg	PO	8-24 h
Omeprazole	0.5 mg/kg	IV	24 h
	1-2 mg/kg	PO (prevention)	24 h
	2-4 mg/kg	PO (treatment)	24 h
Pantoprazole	1-1.5 mg/kg	IV, PO	24 h

Table 66.8 (Continued)

	Dose	Route	Interval
Psyllium	CJ	PO	CJ
Ranitidine[¶]	0.9-1.5 mg/kg	IV, IM, PO	6-8 h
Smectite	CJ	PO	CJ
Sucralfate	20-40 mg/kg	PO	6-8 h
	Respiratory tract drugs		
Caffeine	10 mg/kg	PO (loading dose)	12 h
	2-5 mg/kg	PO (maintenance)	24 h
Clenbuterol	0.5-5 µg/kg	PO, IV, INH	12 h
Doxapram hydrochloride	0.5 mg/kg	IV	As needed
	0.02-0.05 mg/kg/h	CRI	
Fluticasone	100-500 µg/50 kg	INH	12-24 h
Furosemide	0.5-2 mg/kg	IV, CRI	4-6 h
Oxygen therapy	5-10 L/min	INH	CJ
	Neurologic and musculoskeletal treatments		
Dimethyl sulfoxide	0.5-1 g/kg as a solution <10%	IV	24 h, Use as <10% solution, slowly
Magnesium sulfate	20-50 mg/kg	IV (loading dose)	CJ
	10-25 mg/kg/h	CRI	
Mannitol	0.25-0.5 g/kg over 30 min	IV (oliguria)	24 h
	0.5-2 g/kg over 30-60 min	IV (cranial/spinal trauma)	Use as 20% solution, slowly
Selenium	1-2 mg	IM	Once
Thiamine	1-10 mg/kg	IV, IM	12-24 h
Vitamin C	30-50 mg/kg	IV	12-24 h
Vitamin E	6.6 IU/kg	IM	24 h for 3 days
	10-20 IU/kg	PO	24 h
	Anticonvulsants, sedatives and tranquilizers		
Acepromazine	0.02-0.1 mg/kg	IV, IM	
Butorphanol	0.02-0.1 mg/kg	IV, IM	
Detomidine	0.02-0.04 mg/kg	IV, IM	
Diazepam	0.02-0.4 mg/kg	IV, IM	CJ
Flumazenil	0.01-0.02 mg/kg	IV slowly	
Ketamine[†]	0.5-1 mg/kg	IV (loading dose)	CJ
	0.4-0.8 mg/kg/h	CRI	
Midazolam	0.02-0.2 mg/kg	IV, IM	CJ
	0.04 to 0.1 mg/kg/h	CRI	
Phenobarbital[‡]	2-10 mg/kg	IV	8-12 h
Romifidine	0.05-0.1 mg/kg	IV, IM	
Xylazine	0.5-1.1 mg/kg	IV	
	1-2 mg/kg	IM	

CJ, clinician judgment or manufacturer recommendation; CRI, continuous rate infusion; IM, intramuscular; INH, inhaled; IV, intravenous; IVRLP, IV regional limb perfusion; PO, per os, orally.

Some of these drugs are rarely used in equine practice or may not be available depending on the country. These doses are extrapolated from equine foals, adult donkeys and horses.

[*] Doses adapted from equine foals and from authors' experience

[§] Carbapenems are last resort antimicrobials in human medicine and should only be used when other antimicrobials are not effective or carbapenem sensitive multidrug resistant pathogens are identified. It is important to practice antimicrobial stewardship.

[#] Oxytetracycline is rarely used in newborn foals but could be used in older ones affected by *Lawsonia intracellularis* or rickettsial organisms (e.g. *Anaplasma phagocytophilum*). Information on the use of high doses of oxytetracycline to induce tendon relaxation in donkey or mule foals is lacking.

[¶] Currently discontinued in the US and Europe

[†] Higher or more frequent IV doses are required for anesthesia

[‡] Use when foal is no responsive to other drugs. It has a longer half-life in foals. It may induce severe neurologic and respiratory depression.

References

1 Aronoff, N. (2010). The donkey neonate. In: *Veterinary Care of Donkeys* (ed. N.S. Matthews and T.S. Taylor). International Veterinary Information Service https://www.ivis.org/library/veterinary-care-of-donkeys.

2 Ryder, O.A., Chemnick, L.G., Bowling, A.T. et al. (1985). Male mule foal qualifies as the offspring of a female mule and jack donkey. *J. Hered.* 76: 379–381.

3 Kay, G. (2003). A foal from a mule in Morocco. *Vet. Rec.* 152: 92.

4 Canisso, I.F., Panzani, D., Miró, J. et al. (2019). Key aspects of donkey and mule reproduction. *Vet. Clin. North Am. Equine Pract.* 35: 607–642.

5 Magalhaes, H.B. and Canisso, I.F. (2022). Transrectal ultrasonography of the caudal placental pole and fetal eyeball diameter and associations with the season, duration of gestation, placental weight, sex of the foal, and birthweight in donkeys. *J. Equine Vet. Sci.* 113: 103936.

6 Carluccio, A., Gloria, A., Veronesi, M.C. et al. (2015). Factors affecting pregnancy length and phases of parturition in Martina Franca jennies. *Theriogenology* 84: 650–655.

7 Carluccio, A., Panzani, S., Tosi, U. et al. (2008). Morphological features of the placenta at term in the Martina Franca donkey. *Theriogenology* 69: 918–924.

8 Veronesi, M.C., Villani, M., Wilsher, S. et al. (2010). A comparative stereological study of the term placenta in the donkey, pony and Thoroughbred. *Theriogenology* 74: 627–631.

9 Nervo, T., Bertero, A., Poletto, M. et al. (2019). Field ultrasound evaluation of some gestational parameters in jennies. *Theriogenology* 126: 95–105.

10 Deng, L., Shi, S., Li, J. et al. (2020). A cross-sectional survey of foaling-related parameters of jennies (*Equus asinus*) under smallholder farm conditions in Northeast China. *J. Equine Vet. Sci.* 87: 102928.

11 Carluccio, A., Noto, F., Parrillo, S. et al. (2016). Transrectal ultrasonographic evaluation of combined utero-placental thickness during the last half of pregnancy in Martina Franca donkeys. *Theriogenology* 86: 2296–2301.

12 Mendoza, F.J., Perez-Ecija, A., and Toribio, R.E. (2019). Clinical pharmacology in donkeys and mules. *Vet. Clin. North Am. Equine Pract.* 35: 589–606.

13 Crisci, A., Rota, A., Panzani, D. et al. (2014). Clinical, ultrasonographic, and endocrinological studies on donkey pregnancy. *Theriogenology* 81: 275–283.

14 Ramina, A., Dalla Valle, L., De Mas, S. et al. (1999). Detection of equine arteritis virus in semen by reverse transcriptase polymerase chain reaction-ELISA. *Comp. Immunol. Microbiol. Infect. Dis.* 22: 187–197.

15 Tewari, S.C., Verma, P.C., and Bhargava, D.N. (1994). Experimetnal equine herpes virus-1 infection of fetus in a pregnant donkey mare. *Indian Vet. J.* 71: 213–214.

16 Matsuda, M. and Moore, J.E. (2003). Recent advances in molecular epidemiology and detection of Taylorella equigenitalis associated with contagious equine metritis (CEM). *Vet. Microbiol.* 97: 111–122.

17 Tibary, A., Sghiri, A., Bakkoury, M. et al. (2006). Reproductive patterns in donkeys. In: *Congress of World Equine Veterninary Association*, 311–319. Marrakech, Morocco: WEVA.

18 Ali, A.A., Refat, N.A., Algabri, N.A. et al. (2020). Fetal lesions of EHV-1 in equine. *An. Acad. Bras. Cienc.* 92: e20180837.

19 LeCuyer, T.E., Rink, A., Bradway, D.S. et al. (2015). Abortion in a Mediterranean miniature donkey (*Equus asinus*) associated with a gammaherpesvirus similar to equid herpesvirus 7. *J. Vet. Diagn. Investig.* 27: 749–753.

20 Di Francesco, C.E., Smoglica, C., De Amicis, I. et al. (2020). Evaluation of colostral immunity against Equine Herpesvirus Type 1 (EHV-1) in Martina Franca's foals. *Front. Vet. Sci.* 7: 579371.

21 Carluccio, A., De Amicis, I., Panzani, S. et al. (2008). Electrolytes changes in mammary secretions before foaling in jennies. *Reprod. Domest. Anim.* 43: 162–165.

22 Magalhaes, H.B., Canuto, L.E.F., and Canisso, I.F. (2021). Electrolytes and pH of mammary gland secretions assessments to detect impending parturition and associations with placental and neonate features in donkeys. *J. Equine Vet. Sci.* 102: 103636.

23 Dubbin, E.S., Welker, F.H., Veit, H.P. et al. (1990). Dystocia attributable to a fetal monster resembling schistosomus reflexus in a donkey. *J. Am. Vet. Med. Assoc.* 197: 605–607.

24 Mungai Chacur, M.G., de Ruediger, F.R., and Yamasaki, L.P. (2014). Bilateral hydranencephaly in a hybrid foal: obstetric case. *Semina-Cienc. Agrar.* 35: 1389–1394.

25 Prada Torres, J.A., Molina, V.M., Jaramillo Morales, C. et al. (2016). Separación prematura de placenta en una hembra asnal (*Equus asinus*) y síndrome de mal ajuste neonatal: reporte de caso. *CES Med. Vet. Zootecnia* 11: 116–123.

26 Canisso, I.F., Rodriguez, J.S., Sanz, M.G. et al. (2013). A clinical approach to the diagnosis and treatment of retained fetal membranes with an emphasis placed on the critically ill Mare. *J. Equine Vet. Sci.* 33: 570–579.

27 Bonelli, F., Nocera, I., Conte, G. et al. (2020). Relation between Apgar scoring and physical parameters in 44 newborn Amiata donkey foals at birth. *Theriogenology* 142: 310–314.

28 Alonso, M.A., Boakari, Y.L., Riccio, A.V. et al. (2023). Behavior and perinatal parameters of mule and equine foals: similarities and differences. *J. Vet. Behav.* 63: 31–35.
29 Osthaus, B., Proops, L., Long, S. et al. (2018). Hair coat properties of donkeys, mules and horses in a temperate climate. *Equine Vet. J.* 50: 339–342.
30 Stephen, J.O., Baptiste, K.E., and Townsend, H.G. (2000). Clinical and pathologic findings in donkeys with hypothermia: 10 cases (1988–1998). *J. Am. Vet. Med. Assoc.* 216: 725–729.
31 De Palo, P., Maggiolino, A., Milella, P. et al. (2016). Artificial suckling in Martina Franca donkey foals: effect on in vivo performances and carcass composition. *Trop. Anim. Health Prod.* 48: 167–173.
32 De Palo, P., Maggiolino, A., Albenzio, M. et al. (2018). Survey of biochemical and oxidative profile in donkey foals suckled with one natural and one semi-artificial technique. *PLoS One* 13: e0198774.
33 Carluccio, A., Contri, A., Gloria, A. et al. (2021). Study of postnatal growth of mule and donkey foals sired by the same jackass. *Large Anim. Rev.* 27: 165–173.
34 Raspa, F., Cavallarin, L., Mc Lean, A.K. et al. (2019). A review of the appropriate nutrition welfare criteria of dairy donkeys: nutritional requirements, farm management requirements and animal-based indicators. *Animals* 9: 315.
35 Salari, F., Licitra, R., Altomonte, I. et al. (2020). Donkey feeding during maintenance, pregnancy, and lactation: effects on body weight, Milk production, and foal growth. *J. Equine Vet. Sci.* 91: 103131.
36 Mendoza, F.J., Toribio, R.E., and Perez-Ecija, A. (2018). Aspects of clinical relevance in donkeys. In: *Equine Internal Medicine*, 4e (ed. S.M. Reed, W.M. Bayly, and D.C. Sellon), 1513–1524. Elsevier.
37 Perez-Ecija, A. and Mendoza, F.J. (2017). Characterisation of clotting factors, anticoagulant protein activities and viscoelastic analysis in healthy donkeys. *Equine Vet. J.* 49: 734–738.
38 Mendoza, F.J., Estepa, J.C., Gonzalez-De Cara, C.A. et al. (2015). Energy-related parameters and their association with age, gender, and morphometric measurements in healthy donkeys. *Vet. J.* 204: 201–207.
39 Mendoza, F.J., Perez-Ecija, R.A., Toribio, R.E. et al. (2013). Thyroid hormone concentrations differ between donkeys and horses. *Equine Vet. J.* 45: 214–218.
40 Perez-Ecija, A., Gonzalez-De Cara, C.A., Aguilera-Aguilera, R. et al. (2014). Comparison of donkey hemogram using the LaserCyte hematology analyzer, an impedance system, and a manual method. *Vet. Clin. Pathol.* 43: 525–537.
41 Sgorbini, M., Bonelli, F., Rota, A. et al. (2013). Hematology and clinical chemistry in Amiata donkey foals from birth to 2 months of age. *J. Equine Vet. Sci.* 33: 35–39.
42 Veronesi, M.C., Gloria, A., Panzani, S. et al. (2014). Blood analysis in newborn donkeys: hematology, biochemistry, and blood gases analysis. *Theriogenology* 82: 294–303.
43 Harvey, J.W., Asquith, R.L., McNulty, P.K. et al. (1984). Haematology of foals up to one year old. *Equine Vet. J.* 16: 347–353.
44 Boakari, Y.L., Alonso, M.A., Riccio, A.V. et al. (2021). Evaluation of blood glucose and lactate concentrations in mule and equine foals. *J. Equine Vet. Sci.* 101: 103369.
45 Bauer, J.E., Harvey, J.W., Asquith, R.L. et al. (1984). Clinical chemistry reference values of foals during the first year of life. *Equine Vet. J.* 16: 361–363.
46 Patterson, W.H. and Brown, C.M. (1986). Increase of serum gamma-glutamyltransferase in neonatal Standardbred foals. *Am. J. Vet. Res.* 47: 2461–2463.
47 Carluccio, A., Contri, A., Gloria, A. et al. (2017). Correlation between some arterial and venous blood gas parameters in healthy newborn Martina Franca donkey foals from birth to 96 hours of age. *Theriogenology* 87: 173–178.
48 Bonelli, F., Laus, F., Briganti, A. et al. (2019). Evaluation of two handheld point-of-care blood gas analyzers in healthy donkeys. *J. Equine Vet. Sci.* 79: 94–99.
49 Hodgson, D.R. (1987). Blood gas and Acid-Base changes in the neonatal foal. *Vet. Clin. North Am. Equine Pract.* 3: 617–629.
50 Hackett, E.S., Traub-Dargatz, J.L., Knowles, J.E. Jr. et al. (2010). Arterial blood gas parameters of normal foals born at 1500 metres elevation. *Equine Vet. J.* 42: 59–62.
51 Sgorbini, M., Bonelli, F., Percacini, G. et al. (2021). Maternal and neonatal evaluation of derived reactive oxygen metabolites and biological antioxidant potential in donkey mares and foals. *Animals* 11: 2885.
52 Kitchen, H. and Rossdale, P.D. (1975). Metabolic profiles of newborn foals. *J. Reprod. Fertil. Suppl.* 705–707.
53 Pirrone, A., Mariella, J., Gentilini, F. et al. (2012). Amniotic fluid and blood lactate concentrations in mares and foals in the early postpartum period. *Theriogenology* 78: 1182–1189.
54 Sgorbini, M., Bonelli, F., Marmorini, P. et al. (2015). Maternal and neonatal evaluation of derivated reactive oxygen metabolites (d-ROMs) and biological antioxidant potential in the horse. *Theriogenology* 83: 48–51.
55 Boakari, Y.L., Legacki, E., Alonso, M.A. et al. (2022). Postnatal dynamics of circulating steroid hormones in mule and equine neonates. *Vet. Sci.* 9: 598.
56 Turini, L., Bonelli, F., Nocera, I. et al. (2021). Evaluation of different methods to estimate the transfer of immunity in donkey foals fed with colostrum of good IgG quality: a preliminary study. *Animals* 11: 507.
57 Ujvari, S., Schwarzwald, C.C., Fouché, N. et al. (2017). Validation of a point-of-care quantitative equine IgG

turbidimetric immunoassay and comparison of IgG concentrations measured with radial immunodiffusion and a point-of-care IgG ELISA. *J. Vet. Intern. Med.* 31: 1170–1177.

58 Liepman, R.S., Dembek, K.A., Slovis, N.M. et al. (2015). Validation of IgG cut-off values and their association with survival in neonatal foals. *Equine Vet. J.* 47: 526–530.

59 Sanctuary, T.D. (2018). The care of the foal. In: *The Clinical Companion of the Donkey* (ed. J. Duncan), 172–182. Matador Books.

60 Turini, L., Bonelli, F., Nocera, I. et al. (2020). Evaluation of jennies' colostrum: IgG concentrations and absorption in the donkey foals. A preliminary study. *Heliyon* 6: e04598.

61 Veronesi, M.C., Dall'Ara, P., Gloria, A. et al. (2014). IgG, IgA, and lysozyme in Martina Franca donkey jennies and their foals. *Theriogenology* 81: 825–831.

62 Baptista, V.D.S., Guttmann, P.M., Rusca, A.C. et al. (2020). Evaluation of acquired passive immunity in mule foals up to 60 days of age. *J. Equine Vet. Sci.* 31: 1–4.

63 Nervo, T., Bertero, A., Donato, G.G. et al. (2021). Analysis of factors influencing the transfer of passive immunity in the donkey foal. *Ital. J. Anim. Sci.* 20: 1947–1956.

64 Houpt, K.A. and Antczak, D. (1998). Abnormal maternal behavior in a donkey as a consequence of neophobia. *Appl. Anim Behav. Sci.* 60: 259–262.

65 Turini, L., Nocera, I., Bonelli, F. et al. (2020). Evaluation of brix refractometry for the estimation of colostrum quality in jennies. *J. Equine Vet. Sci.* 92: 5.

66 Cash, R.S.G. (1999). Colostral quality determined by refractometry. *Equine Vet. Educ.* 11: 36–38.

67 Lippolis, V., Asif, S., Pascale, M. et al. (2020). Natural occurrence of Ochratoxin a in blood and milk samples from jennies and their foals after delivery. *Toxins* 12.

68 Brewer, B.D. and Koterba, A.M. (1988). Development of a scoring system for the early diagnosis of equine neonatal sepsis. *Equine Vet. J.* 20: 18–22.

69 Brumpt, E. (1947). Jaundice in newly born mule foals not caused by babesia infections. *Ann. Parasitol. Hum. Comp.* 22: 5–10.

70 Traub-Dargatz, J.L., McClure, J.J., Koch, C. et al. (1995). Neonatal isoerythrrolysis in mule foals. *J. Am. Vet. Med. Assoc.* 206: 67–70.

71 McClure, J.J., Koch, C., and Traub-Dargatz, J. (1994). Characterization of a red blood cell antigen in donkeys and mules associated with neonatal isoerythrolysis. *Anim. Genet.* 25: 119–120.

72 Brion, A., Richard, G., and Laffolay, B. (1951). Prevention of haemolytic disease of mule foals. *Bull. Acad. Vet. Fr.* 24: 165–169.

73 Podliachouk, L. and Eyquem, A. (1953). Blood groups in Equidae. III. Blood groups in donkey. *Ann. Inst. Pasteur* 84: 966–968.

74 Saint-Martin, A. (1952). Prevention and treatment of haemolytic disease of mule foals. *Rev. Med. Vet.* 103: 263–268.

75 Boyle, A.G., Magdesian, K.G., and Ruby, R.E. (2005). Neonatal isoerythrolysis in horse foals and a mule foal: 18 cases (1988–2003). *J. Am. Vet. Med. Assoc.* 227: 1276–1283.

76 Kumar, S., Kumar, R., Gupta, A.K. et al. (2008). Passive transfer of Theileria equi antibodies to neonate foals of immune tolerant mares. *Vet. Parasitol.* 151: 80–85.

77 Trujillo, J.M., Walden, B., O'Neil, P. et al. (1965). Sex-linkage of glucose-6-phosphate dehydrogenase in the horse and donkey. *Science* 148: 1603–1604.

78 Ramirez, S., Gaunt, S.D., McClure, J.J. et al. (1999). Detection and effects on platelet function of anti-platelet antibody in mule foals with experimentally induced neonatal alloimmune thrombocytopenia. *J. Vet. Intern. Med.* 13: 534–539.

79 Teixeira, L.G., Spasiani, J.P., Meirelles, A.E.W.B. et al. (2010). Rectal atresia in a newborn donkey. *Equine Vet. Educ.* 22: 434–437.

80 Nelson, B.B., Ferris, R.A., McCue, P.M. et al. (2015). Surgical management of atresia ani and perineal hypospadias in a miniature donkey foal. *Equine Vet. Educ.* 27: 525–529.

81 Dong, J., Liu, G., Gao, N. et al. (2022). A reassortant G3P 12 rotavirus A strain associated with severe enteritis in donkeys (*Equus asinus*). *Equine Vet. J.* 54: 114–120.

82 Haq, I., Durrani, A.Z., Khan, M.S. et al. (2017). A study on causes of pathogenic diarrhea in foals in Punjab, Pakistan. *J. Equine Vet. Sci.* 56: 88–92.

83 Haq, I., Durrani, A.Z., Khan, M.S. et al. (2018). Identification of bacteria from diarrheic foals in Punjab, Pakistan. *Pakistan J. Zool.* 50: 381–384.

84 Haq, I., Durrani, A.Z., Khan, M.S. et al. (2017). Study of antimicrobial resistance and physiological biomarkers with special reference to Salmonellosis in diarrheic foals in Punjab, Pakistan. *Acta Trop.* 176: 144–149.

85 Ijaz, M., Farooqi, S.H., Rahmatullah et al. (2019). Effect of diarrhea on hematocrit and serum biochemical profile in foals. *Pakistan J Zoo* 51: 383–386.

86 Mengistu, A., Smith, D.G., Yoseph, S. et al. (2005). The effect of providing feed supplementation and anthelmintic to donkeys during late pregnancy and lactation on live weight and survival of dams and their foals in Central Ethiopia. *Trop. Anim. Health Prod.* 37: 21–33.

87 Schoster, A., Staempfli, H.R., Abrahams, M. et al. (2015). Effect of a probiotic on prevention of diarrhea and *Clostridium difficile* and *Clostridium perfringens* shedding in foals. *J. Vet. Intern. Med.* 29: 925–931.

88 Liu, G., Bou, G., Su, S. et al. (2019). Microbial diversity within the digestive tract contents of Dezhou donkeys. *PLoS One* 14: e0226186.

89 Kauter, A., Epping, L., Semmler, T. et al. (2019). The gut microbiome of horses: current research on equine enteral microbiota and future perspectives. *Anim. Microbiome* 1: 14–14.

90 Schoster, A., Staempfli, H.R., Guardabassi, L.G. et al. (2017). Comparison of the fecal bacterial microbiota of healthy and diarrheic foals at two and four weeks of life. *BMC Vet. Res.* 13: 144.

91 Xing, J., Liu, G., Zhang, X. et al. (2020). The composition and predictive function of the fecal microbiota differ between young and adult donkeys. *Front. Microbiol.* 11: 596394.

92 Mendoza Garcia, F.J., Gonzalez-De Cara, C., Aguilera-Aguilera, R. et al. (2020). Meloxicam ameliorates the systemic inflammatory response syndrome associated with experimentally induced endotoxemia in adult donkeys. *J. Vet. Intern. Med.* 34: 1631–1641.

93 Barton, A.K. and Ohnesorge, B. (2009). Concurrent unilateral choanal atresia and congenital laryngeal deformity in a miniature donkey. *Vet. Rec.* 164: 93–94.

94 Shaw, S.D., Norman, T.E., Arnold, C.E. et al. (2015). Clinical characteristics of horses and foals diagnosed with cleft palate in a referral population: 28 cases (1988–2011). *Can. Vet. J.* 56: 756–760.

95 Stefanetti, V., Marenzoni, M.L., Lepri, E. et al. (2015). Five fatal cases of primary pulmonary aspergillosis in albino Asinara donkey foals. *J. Equine Vet. Sci.* 35: 76–79.

96 Vitale, V., Bonelli, F., Briganti, A. et al. (2021). Bronchoalveolar lavage fluid cytological findings in healthy Amiata donkeys. *Vet. J.* 11: 160–164.

97 Mazzatenta, A., Veronesi, M.C., Vignola, G. et al. (2019). Behavior of Martina Franca donkey breed jenny-and-foal dyad in the neonatal period. *J. Vet. Behav.* 33: 81–89.

98 Chacur, M., Ruediger, F., and Yamasaki, L. (2014). Bilateral hydranencephaly in a hybrid foal: obstetric case. *Semina Ci. Agr.* 35: 1389–1394.

99 Sek, M. (1989). Anencephaly in an aborted miniature donkey. *Equine Pract.* 11: 32–33.

100 Plummer, C.E., Kallberg, M.E., Ollivier, F.J. et al. (2006). Suspected ivermectin toxicosis in a miniature mule foal causing blindness. *Vet. Ophthalmol.* 9: 29–32.

101 Vitale, V., Nocera, I., Sgorbini, M. et al. (2021). Ultrasonography evaluation of umbilical structures in clinically healthy donkey foals during the first week of life. *Animals* 11: 1650.

102 Lowe, J.S. (1972). Patent ductus arteriosus in a donkey foal. *N. Z. Vet. J.* 20: 15.

103 Dyson, D.A. (1975). Cardiac myopathy in a donkey foal. *Vet. Rec.* 97: 295–296.

104 Marr, C.M. (2015). The equine neonatal cardiovascular system in health and disease. *Vet. Clin. Equine* 31: 545–565.

105 Mendoza, F.J., Toribio, R.E., and Perez-Ecija, A. (2019). Metabolic and endocrine disorders in donkeys. *Vet. Clin. Equine* 35: 399–417.

106 Robbe, D., Carluccio, A., Gloria, A. et al. (2012). Digital Agenesia in Martina Franca donkey foal: a case report. *J. Equine Vet. Sci.* 32: 844–847.

107 Williamson, A.J., Stent, A.W., Milne, M. et al. (2016). Osteopetrosis in a neonatal donkey. *Aust. Vet. J.* 94: 358–361.

108 Abu-Seida, A.M. and Shamaa, A.A. (2022). Treatment of a congenital lateral patellar luxation by recession trochleoplasty in a donkey foal. *Equine Vet. Educ.* 34: 35–39.

109 Van Thielen, B., Willekens, I., Van der Schicht, A. et al. (2018). Radiography of the distal extremity of the Manus in the donkey foal: Normal images and quantitative characterization from birth to 2 years of age: a pilot study. *Anat. Histol. Embryol.* 47: 71–83.

110 Daniels, L.E., Conine, T.A., and Jackson, D.A. (1990). A rehabilitation team approach to correct flexural deformities in a donkey foal. *Can. Vet. J.* 31: 297–299.

111 Eggleston, R.B., Mueller, P.O.E., Chambers, J.N. et al. (2000). Use of an external ring fixator for correction of an acquired angular limb deformity in a donkey. *J. Am. Vet. Med. Assoc.* 217: 1186.

112 Quaresma, M., Marín, C., Bacellar, D. et al. (2021). Selenium and vitamin E concentrations in Miranda jennies and foals (*Equus asinus*) in Northeast Portugal. *Animals* 11: 1772.

113 Bazzano, M., McLean, A., Tesei, B. et al. (2019). Selenium and vitamin E concentrations in a healthy donkey population in Central Italy. *J. Equine Vet. Sci.* 78: 112–116.

114 Shawaf, T., Almathen, F., Meligy, A. et al. (2017). Biochemical analysis of some serum trace elements in donkeys and horses in eastern region of Kingdom of Saudi Arabia. *Vet. World* 10: 1269–1274.

115 Hosnedlova, B., Kepinska, M., Skalickova, S. et al. (2017). A summary of new findings on the biological effects of selenium in selected animal species-a critical review. *Int. J. Mol. Sci.* 18: 2209.

116 D'Alessandro, A.G., Casamassima, D., Jirillo, F. et al. (2014). Effects of Verbascoside administration on the blood parameters and oxidative status in jennies and their suckling foals: potential improvement of milk for human use. *Endocr. Metab. Immune Disord. Drug Targets* 14: 102–112.

117 Vanselow, B.A. and McCausland, I.P. (1981). Steatitis in 2 donkey foals. *Aust. Vet. J.* 57: 304–305.

118 Dixon, R.J., Nuttall, W.O., and Carthew, D.A. (1983). A case of steatitis and myonecrosis in a donkey foal. *N. Z. Vet. J.* 31: 62–63.

119 de Bruijn, C.M., Kroeze, E., and van Oldruitenborgh-Oosterbaan, M.M.S. (2006). Yellow fat disease in equids. *Equine Vet. Educ.* 18: 38–44.

120 Paulussen, E., Lefere, L., Bauwens, C. et al. (2019). Yellow fat disease (steatitis) in 20 equids: description of clinical and ultrasonographic findings. *Equine Vet. Educ.* 31: 321–327.

121 Grosenbaugh, D.A., Reinemeyer, C.R., and Figueiredo, M.D. (2011). Pharmacology and therapeutics in donkeys. *Equine Vet. Educ.* 23: 523–530.

122 Lizarraga, I., Sumano, H., and Brumbaugh, G.W. (2004). Pharmacological and pharmacokinetic differences between donkeys and horses. *Equine Vet. Educ.* 16: 102–112.

123 Wang, T,. Hu, L., Wang, Y., et al. (2022). Identification of equine herpesvirus 8 in donkey abortion: a case report. *Virol. J.* 19(1):10. doi: 10.1186/s12985-021-01738-2.

Part III

The Periparturient Mare

Chapter 67 Colic in the Periparturient Mare

Julie Dechant

Colic is a common presenting complaint in the peripartum mare. While some cases respond to minimal medical treatment, other cases require intensive management or surgical intervention. In most situations, the health and well-being of two lives (mare and fetus or foal) are intertwined and management of the sick periparturient mare can have implications on the survival of the fetus or foal.

Assessment of Abdominal Discomfort in the Periparturient Mare

Colic in the periparturient mare is a diagnostic and therapeutic challenge for the equine veterinarian. Prompt and accurate diagnosis leading to rapid and appropriate therapeutic management is crucial in many cases to maximize outcome and prevent irreversible deterioration. The differential diagnosis list is lengthy due to the added complications associated with the reproductive tract in the periparturient period. Unlike colic complaints in the general horse population, nongastrointestinal causes must be considered equally in peripartum mares with gastrointestinal causes of colic.

In the pregnant mare, the presence of a large gravid uterus, which confounds rectal, ultrasonographic, and abdominocentesis evaluation of the abdomen; overlap between normal and abnormal prepartum behavior in the mare; and the presence of two patients, one of which intimately dependent on the other for survival, complicates the diagnostic approach [1–4]. Similarly, in the postpartum mare, it can be difficult to differentiate signs of abdominal discomfort from normal behavior or more serious complications [1, 5, 6]. The postpartum mare may show signs of colic related to normal oxytocin release and uterine contractions, but many other serious problems and complications may present with similar clinical signs [1, 5, 6].

Important historical information to determine as part of the evaluation includes any history of previous foalings, breeding date, history of dystocia (past pregnancies or current birth, if postpartum), status of fetal membranes (if postpartum), possible exposure to stress, toxins (endophyte-infected fescue), or infectious agents, and preventative care and nutrition, including supplements [1, 3, 7]. When presented with a pregnant mare, the owner should be asked if the life of the mare or the foal is more important because that information may guide certain decision-making. Despite the owner's preferences, the clinical status and health of the pregnant mare needs to be the focus of the evaluation during an abdominal crisis, because she is the primary patient. The health and maturity of the fetus must be considered because its status may direct or alter the therapeutic management of the mare. The pregnant mare's life must be a priority even if the owner is focused on the life of the foal, because the mare is a better incubator for the fetus than any neonatal intensive care unit.

Normal pregnant mares should have cardiovascular, respiratory, and neurological parameters that are similar to non-pregnant mares, with the exception that mild tachycardia and mild tachypnea can be normal in the late-gestation mare due to increased cardiac output and reduced functional residual lung capacity associated with pregnancy, respectively [3, 7]. Hematologic, serum biochemistry, and peritoneal fluid analysis in the normal periparturient mare should generally approximate reference ranges for nonbreeding animals [2, 8–13], and alterations from normal should be attributed to a systemic or gastrointestinal abnormality [4, 6, 13]. In the postpartum mare, recent (<48 hours) dystocia can cause peritoneal fluid parameters to be moderately elevated (total nucleated cell count 15 000 cells/μl, neutrophil percentage 80%, total protein 3.0 g/dl) compared to typical reference

Equine Neonatal Medicine, First Edition. Edited by David M. Wong and Pamela A. Wilkins.

ranges [13], although further elevations in a single parameter (total nucleated cell count, neutrophil percentage, or total protein) may not be clinically significant [13]. Simultaneous elevations in two peritoneal fluid parameters are more likely to be associated with clinical disease [13]. The presence of degenerative neutrophils on peritoneal fluid cytology should prompt closer assessment of the integrity of the urogenital and gastrointestinal tracts [6]. Sanguineous peritoneal fluid is associated with periparturient hemorrhage, although concurrent involvement of the gastrointestinal or urogenital tract cannot be ruled out [6].

The clinical examination of the pregnant mare must include an evaluation of fetal health and well-being [2, 3, 7, 14–16]. This evaluation is dependent on ultrasound examination of the fetus and gravid uterus. Abnormal findings elevate the concern for a successful pregnancy; however, normal findings do not guarantee a successful outcome [7]. In emergency situations, this examination is typically abbreviated to include assessment of fetal viability (heart rate and movement), fetal stress (heart rate), and uterine environment (uteroplacental thickening, and integrity, quantity and turbidity of amniotic/allantoic fluid) [2, 7, 17]. The normal fetus has a heart rate between 70–110 beats/min with a regular rhythm, exhibits periods of activity for 50% of the examination, and is surrounded by anechoic fetal fluids of <13 cm depth [2, 3, 7]. Heart rate can be assessed intermittently with transabdominal ultrasound or continuously with a fetal ECG [7]. The uteroplacental thickness should be <13 mm [2, 14, 15, 17]. Fetal bradycardia is usually an adaptation to hypoxia or other in utero stressors [3, 7, 14]. Persistent tachycardia is a sign of fetal distress and more severe fetal compromise [2, 3, 7, 14].

Fetal maturity is best estimated by consideration of the mare's gestation length, in conjunction with evaluation of milk (mammary secretion) electrolytes [2, 7, 14, 18, 19]. Equine fetal maturity is correlated with a rise in milk calcium greater than 10 mmol/l and inversion of the sodium-potassium ratio (increased potassium, decreased sodium) [2, 18, 19]. While these criteria are fairly reliable for predicting impending parturition in the normal, multiparous mare, they may be less useful for maiden mares or abnormal pregnancies. Biometric measurements of the fetus using ultrasound can be used to estimate gestational age when breeding date is unknown, but these measurements currently lack sufficient precision when determining fetal maturation and readiness for birth [20]. Another application of these measurements would be to assess fetal growth when gestational age is known to detect evidence of intrauterine growth retardation [3, 20]. Regardless of the accuracy of these predictors, unless the mare has a poor prognosis for survival, the fetus's survival is best ensured by maintaining the pregnancy [2, 7].

Gastrointestinal Causes of Colic in the Pregnant Mare

It can be difficult to differentiate signs of abdominal discomfort from normal behavior or more serious complications [2]. Pregnant mares may be uncomfortable in late pregnancy due to movements of the fetus and the weight of the gravid uterus [1]; however, there are numerous complicating conditions that may cause abdominal pain. Prompt and accurate diagnosis leading to rapid and appropriate therapeutic management is crucial in many cases to maximize outcome and prevent irreversible deterioration. Challenges in examining late pregnant mares are that the gravid uterus physically obscures and prevents full assessment of intra-abdominal structures by transrectal palpation and transrectal or transabdominal ultrasound [1–3]. All diagnostic modalities should be utilized with the caveat that absence of abnormal findings does not rule out disease [1, 3]. Studies have shown that hematologic and peritoneal fluid analysis in pregnant mares should be within general references ranges, and alterations from normal should be attributed to a systemic or gastrointestinal abnormality [9–11].

When multiple case series describing colic in pregnant mare are collated, approximately half of presentations were treated medically [21–24]. Of those treated surgically, the most common diagnostic categories were strangulating large intestinal lesions (62%), nonstrangulating large intestinal lesions (17%), and strangulating small intestinal lesions (16%) [4, 21–25]. Nonstrangulating small intestinal lesions (11%) and other gastrointestinal lesions (1%) accounted for the remaining gastrointestinal diagnoses [22–24]. To compare prevalence, uterine torsion and preparturient hemorrhage were diagnosed in approximately 5% of pregnant mares with colic [22–25].

One cause of colic that has been described to be prevalent in pregnant mares and postpartum mares is entrapment of small intestine within a mesenteric rent, typically near the caudal duodenal flexure and with fibrotic margins indicating some chronicity [4, 26]. The prevalence in multiparous broodmares is attributed to previous mesenteric injury by movements of the foal, and during pregnancy, restriction of space within the ventral abdomen as the gravid uterus progressively enlarges throughout pregnancy causes displacement of the intestine toward the rent [26]. Immediate resolution of the entrapment, following by open or laparoscopic closure of the rent has been described [4, 26–28].

Survival of broodmares with gastrointestinal causes of colic is negatively associated with elevated blood lactate and hematocrit [2, 23] and lower arterial oxygen content [29], as well as diagnoses of strangulating large intestinal disease, small intestinal lesions (both strangulating and nonstrangulating), and gastrointestinal rupture [23].

Survival rates in broodmares with colic overall were mildly, but significantly, lower to not significantly different when compared to general colic population [23, 29]. Recurrent colic appears to be more prevalent in pregnant mares than reported in other mixed colic populations [23]. Recurrent colic was associated with Thoroughbred breed and younger age [23].

Gastrointestinal Causes of Colic in the Postpartum Mare

Gastrointestinal causes of medical colic in the postpartum mare include impaction, ileus, and bruising of the abdominal organs or pelvic inlet [1, 5, 30, 31]. Treatment is supportive and symptomatic, and may include nonsteroidal anti-inflammatory drugs (NSAIDs), laxatives, and fluid therapy.

During late gestation and parturition, movements of the foal and/or entrapment of the intestine between the uterus and the pelvis have been theorized to be the cause of trauma to the gastrointestinal tract [1, 30, 32]. The clinical signs vary with the location and severity of the intestinal injury. Cecal rupture is the second leading cause of death in postpartum mares [33]. Other intestinal segments that can be found to be ruptured in postpartum mares include stomach, small colon, large colon, small intestine, or rectum [1, 5, 6, 32]. A ruptured viscus presents with a rapid onset of colic, peracute peritonitis, and rapid deterioration [1, 5, 6, 32]. Small colon mesentery rupture or avulsion may occur during parturition or secondary to a Type III or IV rectal prolapse (Table 67.1; Figure 67.1) [1, 32, 34].

Table 67.1 Classification of Rectal Prolapse

Classification	Description	Clinical Signs
Type I	Prolapse of rectal mucosa through anal sphincter	Circumferential protrusion of swollen mucosa at anal sphincter
Type II	Prolapse of all layers of all or part of rectal wall	Asymmetric circumferential protrusion (thicker ventrally than dorsally) of swollen mucosal covered tissue at anal sphincter
Type III	Type II prolapse with intussusception of small colon into rectum	External appearance similar to Type II with internal intussusception
Type IV	Intussusception of rectum and small colon exiting from anal sphincter	Mucosal covered tubular tissue protruding from anal sphincter

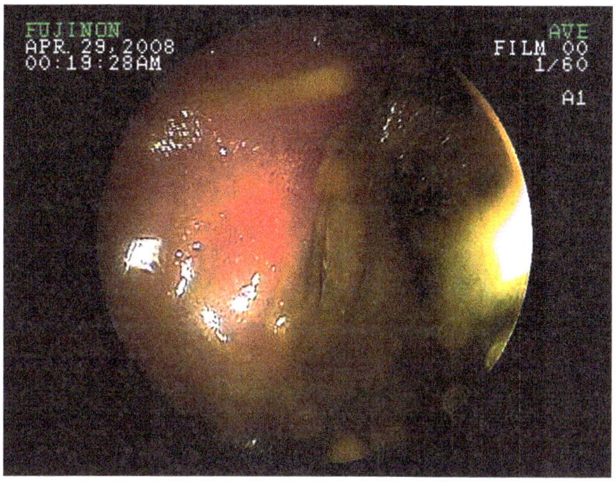

Figure 67.1 Rectal endoscopic image of a postpartum mare presenting for obtundation, fever, and colic after a type 4 rectal prolapse. A palpable demarcation in the mucosal texture was evident on transrectal palpation and correlated with the line of demarcation between viable and nonviable mucosa. Peritoneal fluid analysis was consisted with septic peritonitis. Necropsy examination confirmed thrombosis of the small colon mesentery and devitalization of the associated small colon.

Mesenteric injury disrupts the small colon blood supply and as the affected small colon becomes devitalized, clinical signs include failure to pass feces, followed by fever, colic, and bloating (Figure 67.2). If the vasculature is not injured, mesenteric rents may not initially produce clinical signs; however, the intestine can subsequently herniate through these mesenteric rents, causing colic and signs of intestinal obstruction or strangulation. Similarly, jejunal rents or mesenteric avulsions can occur, presumably due to foal movements or becoming entrapped between the uterus and bony structures or within prolapsed viscera (uterus,

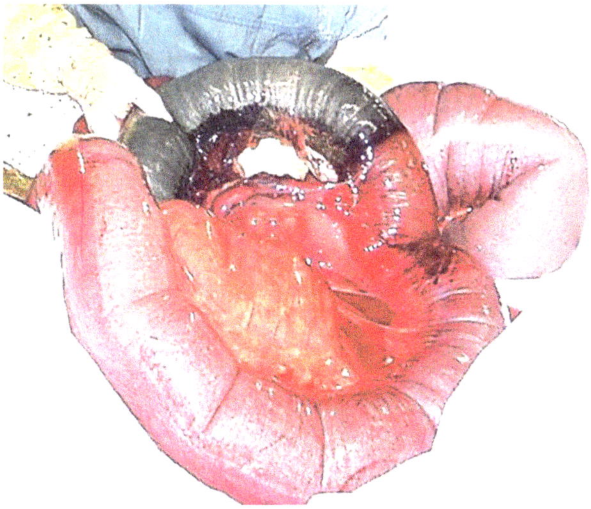

Figure 67.2 Intraoperative appearance of devitalized small colon secondary to mesenteric avulsion.

bladder) [1, 5, 6, 32]. Diaphragmatic hernias can occur with the extreme intra-abdominal pressure of foaling [1, 32]. Respiratory distress may be present, but colic signs are more typically seen with diaphragmatic hernia associated with displacement of abdominal organs into the thoracic cavity. Except for a ruptured viscus, which necessitates euthanasia, treatment of these cases is typically surgical, with the success of treatment depending on specific location of the lesion and condition of the patient.

Although any type of displacement may occur in the periparturient mare, broodmares in the early postpartum period (within 3 months of foaling) appear predisposed to large colon volvulus [1, 30, 32, 35, 36]. The reason for this predisposition to large intestinal displacement or volvulus may be related to the large void within the abdominal cavity following foaling, combined with the nutritional and metabolic changes associated with lactation [1, 30, 37]. Longitudinal studies of Thoroughbred broodmares have identified higher serum nonesterified fatty acids and lower ionized calcium, as well as changes in the fecal microbiota, in mares that colicked post foaling compared to mares that did not colic after foaling [37–39]. Genetic studies in Thoroughbreds suggested that large colon volvulus is moderately heritable [40].

Clinical signs of large colon volvulus include rapid progression of severe abdominal pain, abdominal distension, and cardiovascular shock [1, 30, 32]. The classic findings of a distended, edematous large colon via transrectal examination and transabdominal ultrasound can confirm the clinical suspicion; however, absence of these findings or inability to complete these diagnostic assessments in a severely painful horse should not delay surgical treatment [1, 30, 41]. Abdominocentesis is not necessary to confirm the diagnosis and may be contraindicated due to the risk to personnel and the potential for enterocentesis [30]. Blood lactate, complete blood count, and serum biochemistry have prognostic value and can better direct stabilization of the patient [42–44]. Because of the presence of a strangulating lesion, rapid surgical correction and intensive postoperative management is required to save the mare [1, 30, 32, 42]. Success of treatment depends on early diagnosis and prompt surgical correction; duration of colic greater than 4 hours is associated with 12 times lower survival than horses with duration of colic <2 hours [42]. Prognosis depends on the degree of intestinal damage, and large colon resection may be used to try to save the life of the mare if the colon is devitalized. There is approximately 15% chance of recurrence after the first episode, but after a recurrence, there is an 80% chance of a third episode [42]. Surgical treatments, such as colopexy and large colon resection, can be used to reduce the risk of recurrence, but they are not typically considered until the second episode of large colon volvulus.

Abortion

Abortion is always a concern for owners of pregnant mares with colic. Abortion is a differential diagnosis in a pregnant mare that presents with signs of colic [45]. Pregnancy loss in normal broodmares has been reported to be up to 15% [21]. In two separate studies, the risk of abortion in pregnant mares with either medical or surgical colic was not significantly different, with an overall abortion rate of 16–18% [21, 22]. A 2021 study found a 21.5% negative pregnancy outcome in pregnant mares treated with any type of colic [23]. However, a 2009 study found that the risk of abortion was significantly greater in mares treated surgically for colic (46%) than mares treated medically for colic (22%) [24]. Risk factors for pregnancy loss in the colicky pregnant mare include <40 days gestation [25], maternal age >15 years [25], duration of colic >5 hours [25], strangulating small intestinal disease [23], development of sustained endotoxemia or evidence of systemic inflammatory response syndrome [21–23], diarrhea [23], intraoperative hypoxemia [21, 22], intraoperative hypotension [24], and prolonged anesthetic time [24, 25]. Abortion following a colicky episode is frequently due to fetal death. Because the fetus cannot position itself properly for delivery, post-colic abortion is associated with a risk of dystocia.

Abortion in the pregnant mare with colic is best prevented by prompt and appropriate treatment of the mare to manage systemic and local derangements. If there is any concern for placentitis, systemic antimicrobials that achieve good penetration of the placental-uterine barrier should be used, such as trimethoprim sulfonamide (15–30 mg/kg, PO, q12h) or penicillin (22,000 iu/kg, IV, q6h or 22,000 iu/kg, IM, q12h) with gentamicin (6.6 mg/kg, IV, q24h) [2, 3, 14]. If there is evidence of placental dysfunction, intranasal oxygen supplementation (10–15 L/min, intranasally) of the mare may improve oxygen delivery to the foal [3, 7, 14]. Antiprostaglandins, most commonly flunixin meglumine (0.25 mg/kg, IV or PO, q8h to 1.1 mg/kg IV or PO, q12h), may be useful to counteract the effects of endotoxin or other pathogen-associated molecular pathogens and reduce uterine contractions [2, 3, 7, 14]. Pentoxifylline (8–10 mg/kg, PO, q12h) may be beneficial through its anti-inflammatory effect, and through its potential to improve blood flow to the uterus [2, 14]. Use of supplemental progestagens (0.088 mg/kg, PO, q24h) may be used at clinician discretion but is controversial in late gestation due to experimental data suggesting negative effects on the foal [14, 46, 47]. In one retrospective study, use of progestin/altrenogest in pregnant mares with colic was associated with improved pregnancy outcomes [23]. Tocolytic agents, such as clenbuterol, do not appear to be beneficial [3, 14]. Oral vitamin E (10 iu/kg, PO, q24h) may be useful as an antioxidant and neuroprotective agent [3, 7, 14].

Hydrops

Hydropsical conditions are very rare in the horse, but they do represent a life-threatening emergency [2, 48–52]. Hydrallantois is the accumulation of fluid in the allantoic space and is hypothesized to be caused by abnormal placental angiogenesis [48, 50, 53], placentitis [54], umbilical cord torsion, or genetic factors [51, 55]. It tends to develop quite rapidly during mid- to late gestation and accounts for 90% of hydropsical conditions [56]. Hydramnios is the accumulation of fluid in the amniotic space, thought to be associated with fetal abnormalities, although birth of a live foal has been reported [57]. It tends to be slower in development and is much less prevalent than hydrallantois. Hydropsical conditions are life-threatening to the mare due to complications resulting from this massively fluid-distended gravid uterus, such as intra-abdominal hypertension or abdominal compartment syndrome, respiratory compromise, hypovolemic shock, uterine rupture, and body wall disruption (Figure 67.3) [2, 48, 49, 51, 52, 55, 56, 58].

Hydrallantois should be suspected if there is a sudden increase in abdominal distension with accompanying discomfort and distress [2, 48–51, 55]. Differential diagnoses include twin pregnancies, abdominal wall disruption, ascites, and other causes for ventral abdominal edema [2, 48–50, 55, 56]. Diagnosis is made by transrectal palpation of a turgid, fluid-filled uterus bulging above the pelvic floor and transrectal or transabdominal ultrasonographic detection of excessive amniotic or allantoic fluid (>13 cm depth) [16, 48–52, 56, 58].

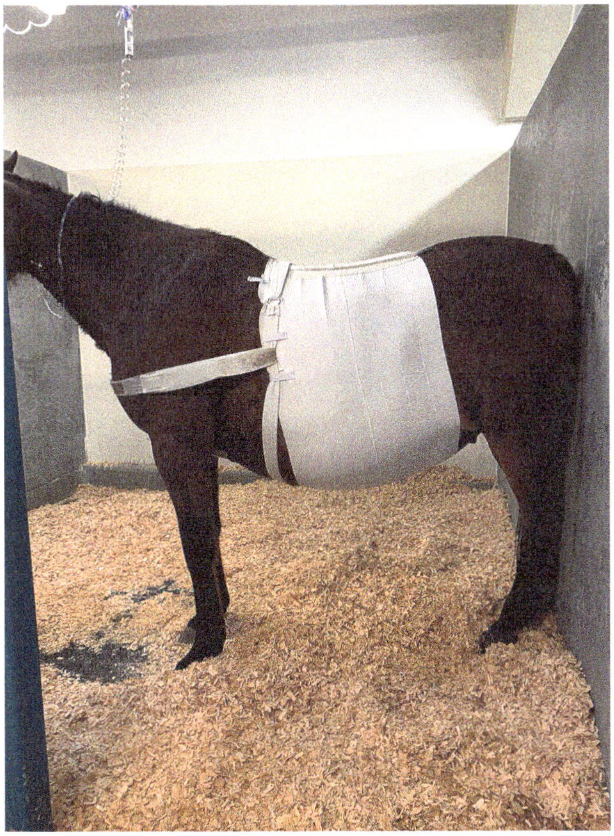

Figure 67.3 Abdominal support bandages for an 8-month gestation mare diagnosed with hydrops and associated disruption of the abdominal wall.

Treatment is typically directed at saving the mare, not the foal, because these conditions typically occur in mid- to late gestation when the fetus is not yet viable ex utero [48–52, 55]. Occasionally, hydropsical conditions occurs in late gestation, and treatment has resulted in birth of live foals surviving long term [52, 57, 58]. Treatment is initiated by controlled drainage of the uterine fluids via a 12–24 French Argyle chest tube or small nasogastric tube while providing intravenous fluid therapy to support the vascular system, and termination of the pregnancy [48–50, 52, 55, 58]. An initial intravenous bolus of 20 ml/kg balanced polyionic fluids should be administered, followed by continuous intravenous fluids at a rate equivalent to approximately 25% volume of the drained fetal fluids [49, 50, 55]. The mare should be monitored continuously, and drainage slowed or temporarily stopped, and intravenous fluid support increased if the heartrate increases by 10 beats/min or the mare becomes unsteady or develops muscle fasiculations [49, 50, 55]. Once most of the fetal fluid has been drained, oxytocin can be administered to promote expulsion of the fetus [49–53, 56]. Dystocia and retained fetal membranes are common due to the uterine size and flaccidity and weakened abdominal wall [48–52, 55, 56, 58]. The mare should be maintained on intravenous fluids, antimicrobials, and abdominal support bandages, as well as appropriate treatment for retained fetal membranes [49, 50, 55, 56]. The mare should be monitored closely for the next couple of days for signs of shock, laminitis, abdominal wall rupture, peritonitis, and organ dysfunction. Mares can be rebred after hydropsical pregnancies without recurrence [48, 58], or if complications of abdominal wall disruption or uterine injury occur, the mares may be used as an embryo or oocyte donor if permitted or desired to salvage genetics [50].

Abdominal Wall Disruption

Rupture of the ventral body wall and prepubic tendon can occur during late gestation [2, 3, 55, 59–62]. Draft breeds are thought to be predisposed to these conditions [3, 55, 59], but abdominal wall disruptions can be seen in any breed during normal or abnormal pregnancies [55, 60]. Other predisposing factors include older mares, twin pregnancies, hydrops, presence of ventral edema, or history of abdominal trauma [2, 3, 55, 59–61]. The most common clinical sign is abdominal pain caused by disruption and tearing of the abdominal support structures [61, 62]. The colic signs can be differentiated from colic of gastrointestinal causes by the presence of swelling and abnormal abdominal contour associated with the abdominal wall injury or failure [2, 3, 55, 59–61].

Ventral body wall rupture and prepubic tendon rupture have been reported to be difficult to differentiate from each other (Figure 67.4) [20, 60]. While the clinical presentation of ventral abdominal swelling is similar between the two conditions, differences have been described [55, 59, 61, 62]. Mares with prepubic tendon ruptures are described as being reluctant to walk, the pelvis is tilted cranioventrally, and the mammary gland is displaced cranioventrally (Figure 67.5) [3, 55, 59, 61]. Bloody mammary secretions are more typically associated with prepubic tendon rupture than ventral body wall disruption [2, 55]. In contrast, mares with ventral hernias may have less reluctance to move than mares with prepubic tendon rupture, and the pelvis and mammary glands are in a normal position and orientation (Figure 67.6).

Treatment of mares with abdominal wall disruption can be challenging. Partial tears or rupture of the abdominal wall or prepubic tendon may respond to stall confinement, NSAID treatment, and abdominal support wraps (Figure 67.7) [2, 3, 55, 59–61]. Parturition should

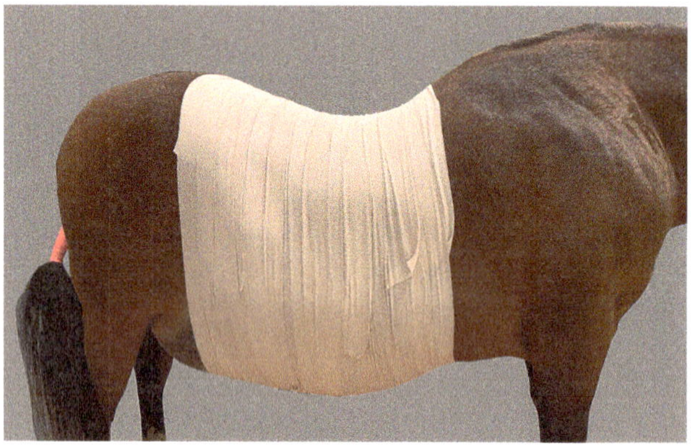

Figure 67.4 Abdominal support bandage in a late gestation mare with abdominal wall disruption.

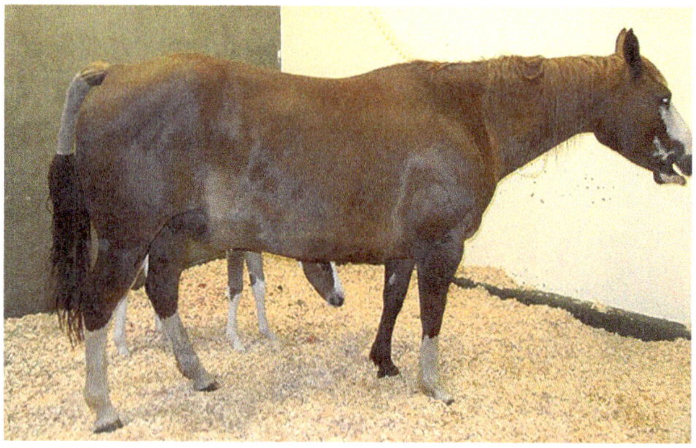

Figure 67.6 Abnormal abdominal wall contour in a postpartum mare with bilateral abdominal wall disruption.

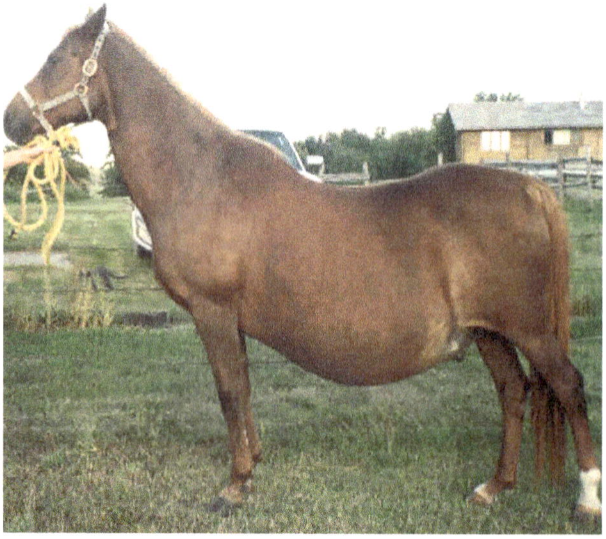

Figure 67.5 Appearance of a pregnant mare with abdominal wall disruption with the characteristic appearance, stance, and mammary gland displacement associated with prepubic tendon rupture.

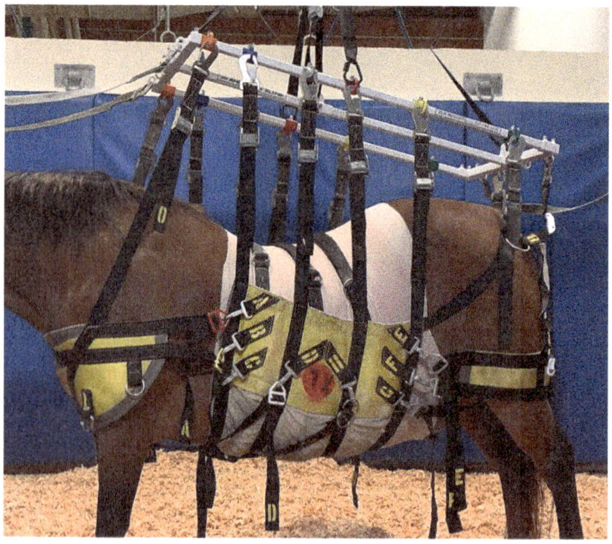

Figure 67.7 Abdominal support for a late gestation mare with abdominal wall disruption provided by an abdominal support bandage and the Large Animal Anderson sling.

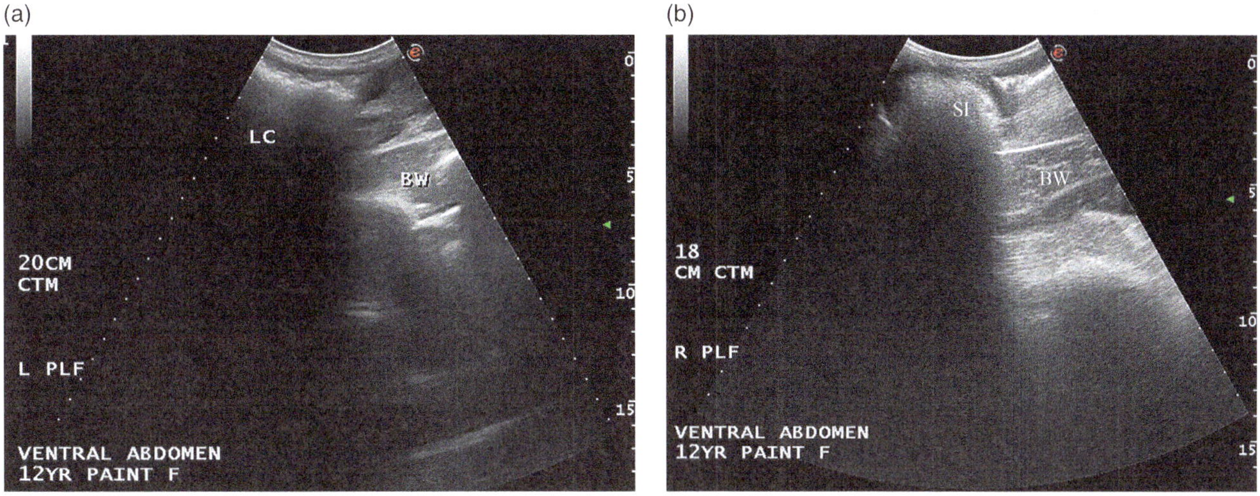

Figure 67.8 (a) Transcutaneous ultrasound for the mare pictured in Figure 67.6 showing the abdominal wall defect in the left ventral abdomen 20 cm cranial to the mammary gland showing large colon (LC) herniating through the abdominal wall defect (BW) to lie in the subcutaneous space. (b) Transcutaneous ultrasound for the mare pictured in Figure 67.6 showing the abdominal wall defect in the right ventral abdomen 18 cm cranial to the mammary gland showing small intestine (SI) herniating through the abdominal wall defect (BW) to lie in the subcutaneous space.

be attended because these mares may lack sufficient abdominal press to deliver the foal [2, 3, 55, 59]. Impending complete, severe disruption of the body wall may necessitate emergency caesarian section, terminal caesarian section, or euthanasia [55, 60]. Colic may develop if bowel becomes entrapped in the hernia (Figure 67.8a,b) [3, 61]. Ventral abdominal hernias have been surgically repaired after a fibrous hernia ring has formed 3–4 months after injury [61], but successful surgical repair of prepubic tendon rupture has not been reported in the horse.

Prognosis for survival of mare and foal with conservative management is fair to good [60, 61]; prognosis for survival of the foal if premature delivery is needed is poor [2, 60]. Recumbency, rupture of large vessels, intractable pain, and death are complications of these conditions, despite all efforts to manage the patient and support the abdomen [59, 62]. Rebreeding to carry a foal is not recommended if the mare survives the pregnancy; however, the reproductive potential of the mare may be salvaged if used as an embryo or oocyte donor [61].

Uterine Torsion

Uterine torsions in mares typically occur between 8 months gestation to term [1, 55, 63–65]; although uterine torsion has been described as early as 5 months gestation [66]. Unlike cattle, less than 50% of uterine torsions occur at parturition [55, 63, 64, 66–68]. Chronic uterine torsions have also been described [69–71]. It has been suggested that rolling or falling of the mare, fetal movements and a large fetus may predispose to development of a uterine torsion [55, 63, 64]. In a recent study, uterine torsion was diagnosed in 4% of all pregnant mare presenting for colic at a tertiary referral hospital [23].

Presence of a uterine torsion should be suspected in any third trimester pregnant mare exhibiting signs of colic [1, 55, 63–65]. The severity of signs and systemic compromise vary dependent on the degree of torsion, uterine damage, and gastrointestinal involvement [55, 63–65]. Gastrointestinal involvement, such as entrapment/strangulation of jejunum or small colon within the uterine torsion or concurrent intestinal displacement or volvulus, has been reported in up to 50% of cases [55, 66, 72]. Early diagnosis and treatment increase the likelihood of maternal and fetal survival. Rectal palpation of the broad ligaments is key to diagnosing uterine torsion [1, 55, 63–65]; vaginal examination is typically unrewarding because the torsion is typically cranial to the cervix and vaginal involvement is uncommon [1, 63, 64]. Uterine torsion is diagnosed by evaluating the orientation of the broad ligaments of the uterus (Figure 67.9). The ligament on the side toward which the uterus is torsed will be more caudal (palpated first) and palpated as a tight vertical band [63, 64]. The opposite ligament crosses horizontally over the top of the uterus cranial to the vertically palpated band before coursing ventrally. There is an approximately equal distribution of clockwise and counterclockwise directions for uterine torsion in mares [63, 66–68, 72]. Transabdominal ultrasound is useful to evaluate fetal viability, uterine damage, and concurrent gastrointestinal involvement [1, 55, 63, 64].

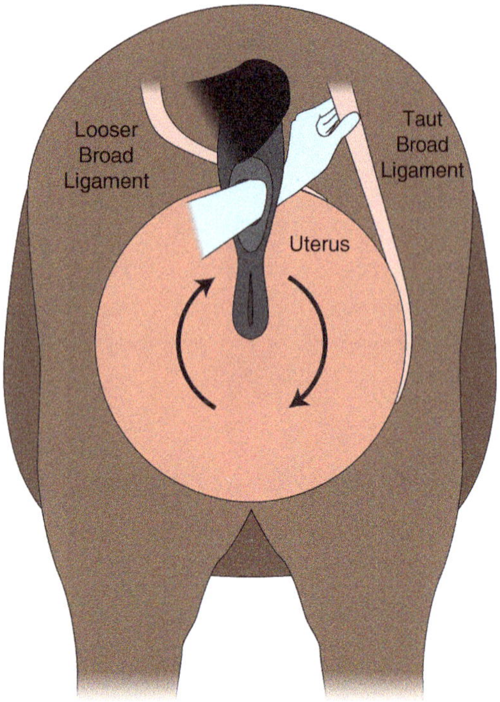

Figure 67.9 Diagram illustrating palpation of the uterine broad ligaments per rectum in a mare with a clockwise uterine torsion. The right broad ligament in a clockwise uterine torsion will be more caudal than the left broad ligament and will be taut and vertically oriented. The left broad ligament in a clockwise uterine torsion will be located more cranially than the right broad ligament, will be more horizontally oriented over the uterus, and will have less tension than the right broad ligament, although the degree of tension will vary with the severity of the uterine torsion.

Treatment of uterine torsion requires detorsion of the uterus. Detorsion of the uterus can be achieved by derotation of the fetus per vaginum in the term mare with a sufficiently dilated cervix [1, 55, 63, 64], rolling the mare under general anesthesia [1, 55, 63, 64, 68, 72], or surgical correction through a standing flank laparotomy [1, 55, 63, 64, 67, 68, 72], or ventral midline celiotomy (general anesthesia) [1, 55, 63, 64, 66, 68, 72]. Treatment selection depends on condition of the mare, degree of uterine compromise or damage, stage of gestation, economic considerations for the owner, available facilities, and clinician preference [1, 55, 63–65]. In general, ventral midline celiotomy is indicated during late gestation or if there are complicating factors (uterine rupture or compromise, gastrointestinal involvement, or intractable pain) [55, 68, 72], whereas flank laparotomy has significantly better mare and foal survival than ventral midline celiotomy if performed <320 days [68, 72].

Rolling of the mare can be performed in the field under injectable general anesthesia. It may be considered as an option in light breed mares prior to 320 days gestation, without evidence of gastrointestinal involvement, and especially if surgical management is not an option [55, 63–65]. Risks of rolling for uterine torsion include failure to correct the torsion, uterine rupture, placental separation, and fetal death [55]. It is imperative that the direction of uterine torsion can be confidently identified prior to considering a rolling procedure. The anesthetized mare is positioned in lateral recumbency on the side towards which the uterus is torsed (left lateral recumbency for a counterclockwise torsion and right lateral recumbency for a clockwise torsion) [55, 63–65]. A plank or board is then placed on the mare's abdomen from her dorsum at the level of the paralumbar fossa [55, 63–65]. The mare is then rolled over her dorsum to the opposite recumbency while one person sits on the plank to stabilize and hold steady the gravid uterus (the idea is to roll the mare to catch up with the uterus) [55, 63–65]. Failure to correct the uterine torsion within 2 attempts indicates that another treatment modality should be considered [55]. Rolling can be successful in ideal candidates with the survival rate dropping to <50% if ideal circumstances do not exist. [72].

Mare survival following treatment for uterine torsion is approximately 85–90% [68, 72], with mortality resulting from uterine necrosis or rupture, postoperative shock, and gastrointestinal complications. The live birth rate for foals is reported to be up to 80% [68]. Both mare and foal survival are significantly associated with stage of gestation, with improved survival if <320 days gestation [68, 72].

Periparturient Hemorrhage

Hemorrhage from the uterine arteries is a common cause of periparturient colic signs and death in older, multiparous mares; however, any age and parity can be affected [1, 6, 30, 73–76]. Signs typically occur within 24 hours after foaling but may occur before parturition or even days after foaling [74, 75, 77–79]. Uterine artery rupture is the leading cause of death in postpartum mares [33]. In a recent paper, preparturient hemorrhage accounted for 6% of pregnant mares presenting for colic at a tertiary referral hospital [23].

Clinical signs vary with the location and severity of hemorrhage. Affected mares may show signs of colic, severe shock, or be found dead [1, 30, 73–78]. It is important to be mindful that shocky mares can decompensate unpredictably, and safety of personnel (and the newborn foal, if possible) should be prioritized [30, 73, 78]. Diagnosis can be difficult and is supported by by clinical (depressed mentation, tachycardia, tachypnea, pale mucous membranes, weak peripheral pulses, cool extremities) and laboratory (anemia, hyperlactatemia, azotemia, hemoconcentration) evidence of severe hemorrhagic shock, identification of an enlarged broad ligament or uterine hematoma on physical examination, transrectal

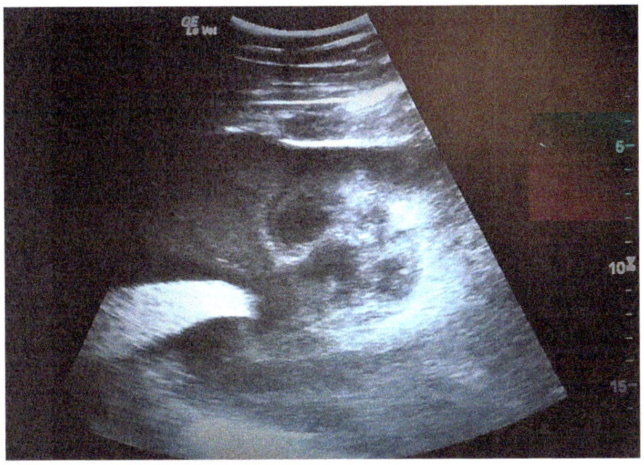

Figure 67.10 Transcutaneous abdominal ultrasound appearance of hemoperitoneum. This still image shows marked, echogenic peritoneal effusion with the characteristic smoke-swirl pattern associated with hemoperitoneum.

palpation or ultrasound, transabdominal ultrasound, and/or identification of hemoperitoneum on transabdominal ultrasound and/or abdominocentesis (Figure 67.10) [30, 41, 73–76]. Rectal palpation to aid diagnosis is controversial because it is argued that palpation may further agitate the mare or disrupt a blood clot [30, 75, 76].

Treatment of periparturient hemorrhage can be difficult as the damage to the affected artery can be extensive and not subject to self-correction via the coagulation cascade and clot formation (Figure 67.11) [1, 30, 73, 75, 77, 78]. This problem requires a surgical solution, but surgery is difficult because of the unstable patient and inaccessibility of the arterial rupture [30, 73, 76]. Therapy is based on keeping the mare quiet and comfortable, and maintaining perfusion to support adequate tissue oxygenation without increasing blood pressure so that blood clots are dislodged. Judicious administration of intravenous crystalloid fluids is the mainstay of treatment, and many horses will require whole blood transfusion to support oxygen-carrying capacity [30, 73–76, 78]. Analgesia is provided by use of NSAIDs (flunixin meglumine), alpha-2 agonists, and opioids [30, 73–75, 78]. The mare should be kept in a quiet environment with her foal nearby, but safely separated from her to ensure the foal's safety [30, 73]. After the mare has been stabilized, additional therapies should include anti-fibrinolytics (aminocaproic acid or tranexamic acid), broad-spectrum antimicrobial therapy, low-dose oxytocin, and adequate nutrition [30, 73–75, 78]. Intravenous formalin (40-50 ml 10% buffered formalin in 1 L isotonic fluids, IV), conjugated estrogens (0.6 mg/kg, IV or IM, q24h for 5 days), or Yunnan baiyao (8 mg/kg, PO, q6h or 15 mg/kg, PO, q12h) to promote hemostasis and naloxone (8–32 mg/450 kg in 500 ml isotonic fluids, IV) to counteract endogenous opiate responses, which may exacerbate shock or corticosteroids for management of shock have been

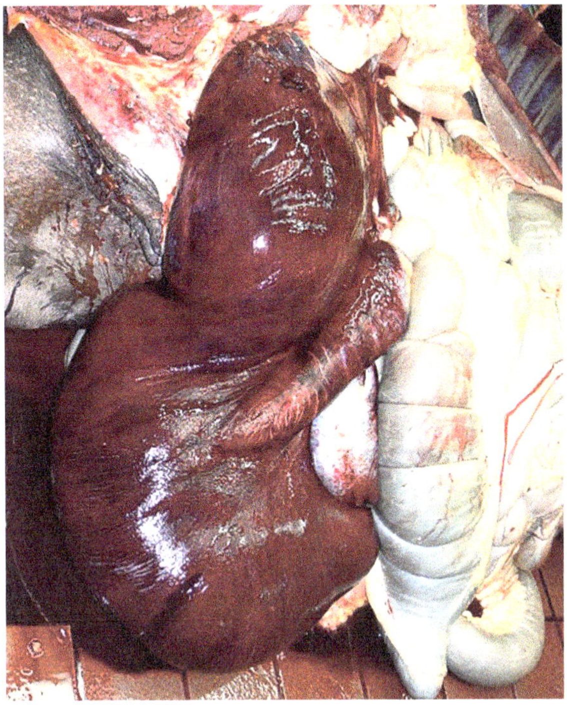

Figure 67.11 Necropsy image of a uterine hematoma in a postpartum mare diagnosed with periparturient hemorrhage that did not respond to supportive care, including anxiolytics, blood transfusion, procoagulants, anti-fibrinolytics, etc.

suggested by some authors, but objective data to prove efficacy is lacking [30, 74–76, 80–82].

Despite the mortality associated with these cases, many broodmares can survive episodes of periparturient hemorrhage and 82–88% survival rates have been reported [5, 6, 74]. Prognosis for survival has been negatively associated with tachycardia (heart rate >100 beats/min) and bleeding into the vagina [74]. If a mare has a history of periparturient hemorrhage, it is generally thought that there is a risk of recurrence with subsequent pregnancies [1]; however, recurrent periparturient hemorrhage has not recognized to be a major concern in Thoroughbred broodmare populations [30, 74].

Uterine Prolapse

Uterine prolapse is an uncommon complication of parturition or dystocia in horses. The diagnosis of a complete uterine prolapse or eversion of the uterus is visually obvious by the presence of a large, red, corrugated organ hanging from the vulva in the postpartum (or post abortion) mare [1, 83, 84]. This complication needs to be addressed immediately by replacement of the prolapse, because uterine prolapse applies tension on the broad ligaments and can cause rupture of the uterine arteries and can cause fatal hemorrhage [1, 30, 76, 82–85]. Uterine prolapse should be corrected by supporting and elevating the cleansed uterus in the standing or anesthetized mare and using the flat of the palm or closed fist to gently kneed the prolapsed uterus into the vagina and through the cervix [30, 84]. Incomplete prolapse of the uterus into the vagina or partial inversion of a uterine horn can occur, and will cause signs of abdominal pain and straining [1, 30, 76]. Sequela of untreated partial uterine prolapse or inversion of a uterine horn include complete uterine prolapse or necrosis of the inverted tip [1, 76, 84]. Similarly, when treating a uterine prolapse, it is essential to make sure that the tips of both uterine horns are fully everted during replacement [30, 76, 83, 84]. Other situations that could result in uterine prolapse are any causes of tenesmus in the postpartum mare or positioning of the anesthetized postpartum mare into dorsal recumbency for surgery [30, 76, 84, 85].

Metritis

Metritis involves the postpartum accumulation of fluid within the uterine lumen that may progress to systemic inflammatory response syndrome and sepsis [30, 86]. Metritis is often associated with dystocia [5, 86], but uterine atony and retained fetal membranes are predisposing factors too [30, 32, 83]. Clinical signs are most commonly inappetence, obtundation, and fever, which may be interpreted as abdominal discomfort [30, 32]. Laminitis is a common sequalae and may be the first sign recognized by owners [30, 32, 83].

Diagnosis is confirmed by physical examination and transrectal or transabdominal ultrasonographic identification of a fluid-filled uterus [30, 32, 83, 86]. Evaluation of a CBC is a relatively sensitive indicator of metritis as affected mares can be profoundly leukopenic and neutropenic, and moreover peritoneal fluid cytology may be indicative of peritonitis [5, 83]. Mainstays of treatment include broad-spectrum systemic antimicrobial therapy, uterine lavage (q 8–12h) and oxytocin to evacuate the septic uterine fluid, and NSAIDs [30, 32, 83, 86]. Laminitis prevention (solar support, digital cryotherapy, pentoxifylline, anti-endotoxin treatments) should be instituted concurrently due to the prevalence and life-threatening nature of this complication [30, 32, 86]. Prognosis with prompt and aggressive treatment is good, assuming that laminitis does not develop or is not associated with displacement of the distal phalanx [30, 86]. Severe laminitis with third phalanx rotation or sinking can occur quickly and may warrant euthanasia [30, 86].

Uterine Tear or Rupture

Uterine tears or ruptures can occur during dystocia, but they can occur after a normal parturition (Figure 67.12) or during the prepartum period, as a complication of hydrops

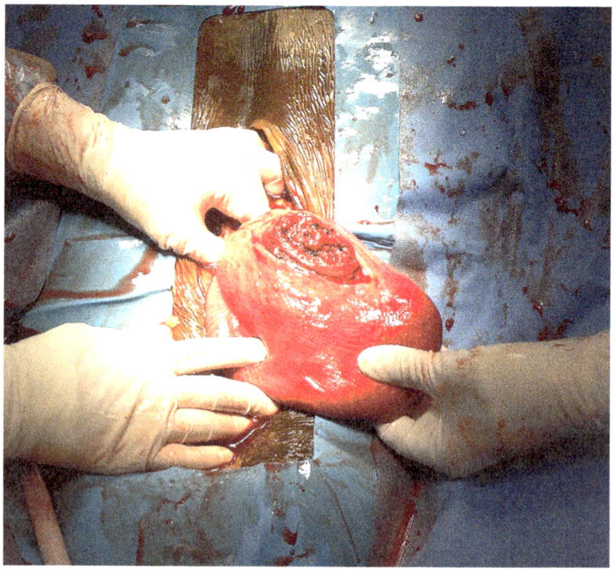

Figure 67.12 Intraoperative appearance of a uterine tear that was present in the nongravid horn of a postpartum mare.

or uterine torsion [1, 30, 76, 83, 87–90]. Uterine tears are the third leading cause of death in postpartum mares [33]. Unless a uterine tear is diagnosed during a post-foaling examination of the reproductive tract [86], clinical signs relate to the development of peritonitis [1, 5, 30, 76, 83, 87–90]. Within 24–48 hours of the tear occurring, the mare demonstrates signs of abdominal pain, depression, fever, and leukopenia caused by peritonitis [1, 30, 83, 87–90]. Diagnosis is made by evaluation of clinical signs, abdominocentesis, and occasionally palpation of the tear during transrectal or vaginal examination [1, 30, 76, 83, 87–90]. Peritoneal fluid is usually serosanguinous to sanguineous with septic inflammatory changes [5, 6, 30, 76, 88].

Although medical management has been described for some uterine tears [30, 83, 87–91], they are best repaired surgically, usually under general anesthesia (Figure 67.13) [1, 30, 76, 83, 87, 89, 90], although transvaginal repair or repair after prolapsing the uterus may be possible in selected cases [1, 76, 90]. Treatment must be undertaken for peritonitis and to promote uterine involution, including antimicrobial coverage, NSAIDs, oxytocin, peritoneal lavage, and abdominal drains (Figure 67.14) [1, 30, 83, 87–90]. Survival rates for uterine tears vary from 25% to 73% for medical management and 63–80% for surgical management [87–90]. Prognosis for survival has been negatively associated with delayed treatment, gastric reflux, higher heart rate, greater anion gap, hypocapnia, and leukopenia [1, 5, 76, 88–90].

Urogenital Trauma

Urogenital trauma (not including vaginal trauma, rectovaginal fistulas, or perineal lacerations) that can cause

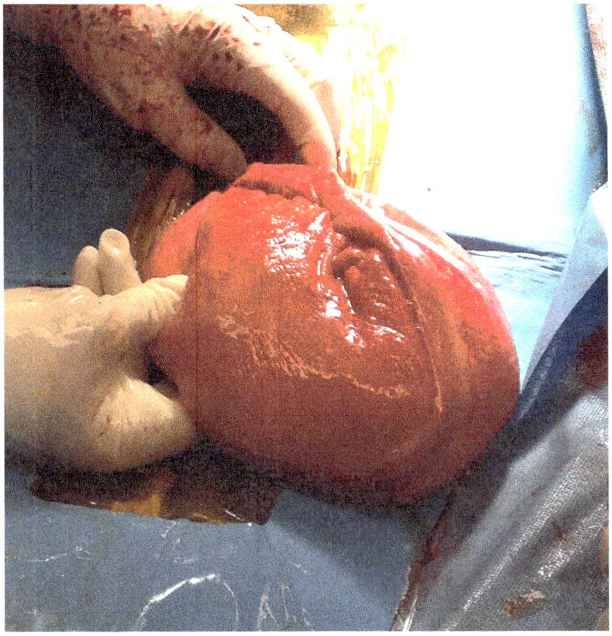

Figure 67.13 Intraoperative appearance of a repaired uterine tear in a postpartum mare (tear seen in Figure 67.12).

abdominal pain include bladder prolapse, bladder eversion, and bladder rupture. Bladder prolapse is extrusion of the bladder, exposing the serosal surface, through a vaginal tear [76]. In bladder prolapse, the serosal surface of the bladder is evident, and the bladder becomes increasingly distended with urine because kinking of the urethra prevents micturition [76]. This is in contrast to bladder eversion, which is invagination of the bladder through the urethra into the vaginal vault [76]. This is differentiated from bladder prolapse by the exposure of the mucosal surface on the everted organ and dribbling of urine from exposure of the ureteral openings at the trigone of the bladder [76]. It is not uncommon that a segment of intestine may be herniated and strangulated inside the everted bladder. This possibility should be investigated by transvesicular or transvaginal ultrasonographic assessment of the everted bladder, and if present, ventral midline celiotomy should be performed after replacement of the bladder to evaluate intestinal viability [76].

Bladder rupture or bladder wall necrosis can also occur in mares following parturition [1, 6, 76, 92, 93]. Clinical signs of bladder rupture may be delayed until uroperitoneum induces sufficient azotemia and electrolyte derangements to cause obtundation and inappetance [1, 76, 92–95]. Diagnosis is confirmed by cystoscopy to inspect the rent, peritoneal: blood creatinine ratios exceeding 2:1, and identification of peritoneal effusion and characteristic serum biochemistry abnormalities [1, 76, 92–95]. Treatment of bladder rupture in broodmares requires stabilization of the electrolyte derangements and fluid imbalance, peritoneal drainage and lavage, and conservative or surgical (either standing sedation vs general anesthesia) treatment of the bladder defect, as applicable to the individual case [1, 76, 92–95].

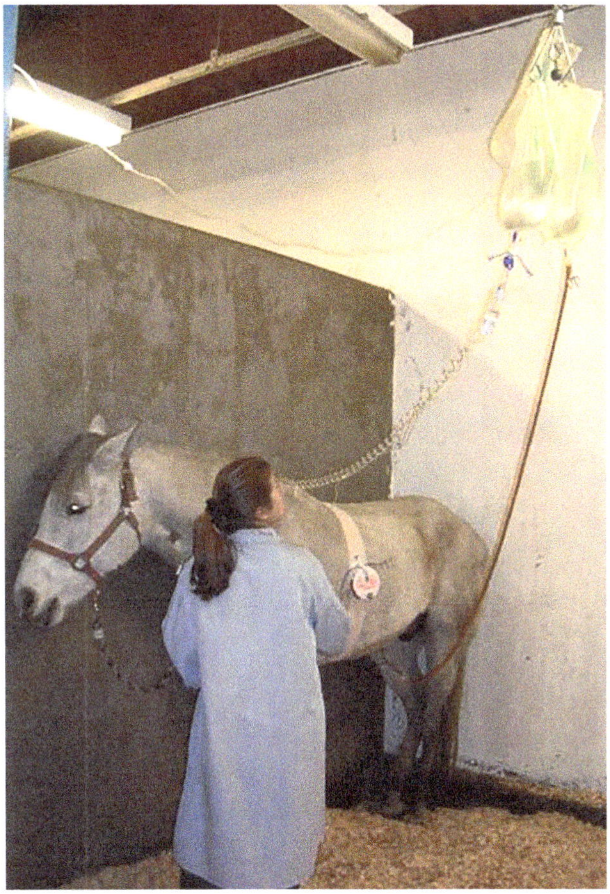

Figure 67.14 Peritoneal lavage in a horse. A partially fenestrated Jackson-Pratt drain has been placed intraperitoneally with the nonfenestrated portions exiting the abdomen. The external segments of the drain have been connected to sterile balanced electrolyte fluids via sterile tubing to allow ingress of fluids. After instillation of the desired amount of fluid (typically 10 l in a full-sized horse), the tubing is clamped, and the horse is walked for 5–10 minutes. Then the tubing is unclamped, and the intraperitoneal fluids are allowed to egress into the empty fluid bags by gravity flow. Once the egress fluid rate has slowed, the abdominal drains are reconnected to a collection cannister that provides a continuous negative pressure and a closed collection system.

Lactation Tetany

Although extremely rare, clinical signs of lactation tetany or postpartum eclampsia may be interpreted as colic by owners. Clinical signs include restlessness, tachypnea, trembling or muscle fasciculations, and synchronous diaphragmatic flutter, and can progress to recumbency [76]. Diagnosis is confirmed by identification of hypocalcemia, and treatment requires titrated administration of diluted intravenous calcium gluconate (recommend 250–500 ml 23% calcium gluconate for a 500 kg horse in 5 L isotonic fluids IV administered over at least 15 minutes and recheck ionized blood calcium) [76].

References

1 Steel, C.M. and Gibson, K.T. (2002). Colic in the pregnant and periparturient mare. *Equine Vet. Educ.* 5: 5–15.
2 Macpherson, M.L. (2007). Identification and management of the high-risk pregnant mare. *Proc. Am. Assoc. Equine Pract.* 53: 293–304.
3 Wilkins, P. (2006). High-risk pregnancy. In: *Equine Neonatal Medicine: A Case-Based Approach* (ed. M.R. Paradis), 13–29. Philadelphia, PA: Elsevier.
4 Slone, D.E. (1993). Treatment of pregnant mares with colic: practical considerations and concerns. *Compend. Contin. Educ. Pract. Vet.* 15: 117–120.
5 Dolente, B.A., Sullivan, E.K., Boston, R. et al. (2005). Mares admitted to a referral hospital for postpartum emergencies: 163 cases (1992–2002). *J. Vet. Emerg. Crit. Care* 15: 193–200.
6 Offer, K.S., Russell, C.M., Carrick, J.B. et al. (2022). Peritoneal fluid analysis in equine post-partum emergencies admitted to a referral hospital: a retrospective study of 110 cases. *Equine Vet. J.* 54: 1023–1030.
7 Wilkins, P.A. (2003). Monitoring the pregnant mare in the ICU. *Clin. Tech. Equine Pract.* 2 (2): 212–219.
8 Bazzano, M., Giannetto, C., Fazio, F. et al. (2014). Physiological adjustments of haematological profile during the last trimester of pregnancy and the early post partum period in mares. *Anim. Reprod. Sci.* 149: 199–203.
9 Faramarzi, B., Rich, L.J., and Wu, J. (2018). Hematological and serum biochemical profile values in pregnant and non-pregnant mares. *Can. J. Vet. Res.* 82: 287–293.
10 Mariella, J., Pirrone, A., Gentilini, F. et al. (2014). Hematologic and biochemical profiles in Standardbred mares during peripartum. *Theriogenology* 81: 526–534.
11 Van Hoogmoed, L., Snyder, J.R., Christopher, M. et al. (1996). Peritoneal fluid analysis in peripartum mares. *J. Am. Vet. Med. Assoc.* 209 (7): 1280–1282.
12 Taylor-MacAllister, C., MacAllister, C.G., Walker, D. et al. (1997). Haematology and serum biochemistry evaluation in normal postpartum mares. *Equine Vet. J.* 29 (3): 234–235.
13 Frazer, G., Burba, D., Paccamonti, D. et al. (1997). The effects of parturition and peripartum complications on the peritoneal fluid composition of mares. *Theriogenology* 48: 919–931.
14 Dobbie, T. (2014). Monitoring the pregnant mare. In: *Equine Emergencies, Treatments and Procedures*, 4e (ed. J.A. Orsini and T.J. Divers), 497–503. St. Louis, MO: Elsevier.
15 Bucca, S. (2014). Use of ultrasonography in fetal development and monitoring. In: *Atlas of Equine Ultrasonography* (ed. J.A. Kidd, K.G. Lu, and M.L. Frazer), 341–350. Ames, IA: Wiley.
16 Reef, V.B. (1998). Fetal ultrasonography. In: *Equine Diagnostic Ultrasound* (ed. V.B. Reef), 425–445. Philadelphia, PA: WB Saunders.
17 Vincze, B., Baska, F., Papp, M. et al. (2019). Introduction of a new fetal examination protocol for on-field and clinical equine practice. *Theriogenology* 125: 210–215.
18 Ousey, J.C., Dudan, F., and Rossdale, P.D. (1984). Preliminary studies of mammary secretions in the mare to assess foetal readiness for birth. *Equine Vet. J.* 16 (4): 258–263.
19 Korusue, K., Murase, H., Sato, F. et al. (2013). Comparison of pH and refractometry index with calcium concentrations in preparturient mammary secretions of mares. *J. Am. Vet. Med. Assoc.* 242: 242–248.
20 Renaudin, C.D., Kass, P.H., and Bruyas, J.-F. (2022). Prediction of gestational age based on foetal ultrasonographic biometric measurements in light breed horses. *Reprod. Domest. Anim.* 57: 743–753.
21 Santschi, E.M., Slone, D.E., Gronwall, R. et al. (1991). Types of colic and frequency of postcolic abortion in pregnant mares: 105 cases (1984–1988). *J. Am. Vet. Med. Assoc.* 199: 374–377.
22 Boening, K.J. and Leendertse, I.P. (1993). Review of 115 cases of colic in the pregnant mare. *Equine Vet. J.* 25: 518–521.
23 Douglas, H.F., Stefanovksi, D., and Southwood, L.L. (2021). Outcomes of pregnant broodmare treated for colic at a tertiary care facility. *Vet. Surg.* 50: 1579–1591.
24 Chenier, T.S. and Whitehead, A.E. (2009). Foaling rates and risks factors for abortion in pregnant mares presenting for medical or surgical treatment of colic: 153 cases (1993–2005). *Can. Vet. J.* 50: 481–485.
25 Drumm, N.J., Embertson, R.M., Woodie, J.B. et al. (2013). Factors influencing foaling rate following colic surgery in pregnant Thoroughbred mares in Central Kentucky. *Equine Vet. J.* 45: 346–349.
26 Lawless, S.P., Werner, L.A., Baker, W.T. et al. (2017). Duodenojejunal mesenteric rents: survival and complications after surgical correction in 38 broodmares (2006–2014). *Vet. Surg.* 46: 367–375.
27 Sutter, W.W. and Hardy, J. (2004). Laparoscopic repair of a small intestinal mesenteric rent in a broodmare. *Vet. Surg.* 33: 92–95.

28 Cypher, E.E., Blackford, J., Snowden, R.T. et al. (2020). Surgical correction of entrapment of the large colon and caecum through a mesoduodenal rent with standing laparoscopic repair in a mare. *Equine Vet. Educ.* 32: 185–188.

29 Klein, C.E., Stefanovski, D., Gardner, A.K. et al. (2022). A multicenter retrospective case-cohort study on the prevalence of incisional morbidities in late pregnant mares following exploratory celiotomy (2014–2019): 579 cases. *J. Vet. Emerg. Crit. Care* 33: 59–69.

30 Lu, K.G. and Sprayberry, K.A. (2021). Managing reproduction emergencies in the field, part 2: parturient and periparturient conditions. *Vet. Clin. Equine* 37: 367–405.

31 Hillyer, M.H., Smith, M.R.W., and Milligan, P.J.P. (2008). Gastric and small intestinal ileus as a cause of acute colic in the post partum mare. *Equine Vet. J.* 40: 368–372.

32 Frazer, G.S. (2003). Postpartum complications in the mare. Part 2: fetal membrane retention and conditions of the gastrointestinal tract, bladder, and vagina. *Equine Vet. Educ.* 15: 118–128.

33 Dwyer, R. (1993). Postpartum deaths of mares. *Equine Dis. Quart.* 2: 5.

34 Ragle, C.A., Southwood, L.L., Galuppo, L.D. et al. (1997). Laparoscopic diagnosis of ischemic necrosis of the descending colon after rectal prolapse and rupture of the mesocolon in two postpartum mares. *J. Am. Vet. Med. Assoc.* 210: 1646–1648.

35 Suthers, J.M., Pinchbeck, G.L., Proudman, C.J. et al. (2013). Risk factors for large colon volvulus in the UK. *Equine Vet. J.* 45: 558–563.

36 Moore, J.N., Dreesen, D.W., and Boudinot, D.F. (1991). Colonic distension, displacement, or torsion in Thoroughbred broodmares: results of a two-year study. *Proc. Equine Colic Symp.* 4: 23–25.

37 Holcombe, S.J., Embertson, R.M., Kurtz, K.A. et al. (2016). Increased serum nonesterified fatty acid and low ionised calcium concentrations are associated with post partum colic in mares. *Equine Vet. J.* 48: 39–44.

38 Salem, S.E., Hough, R., Probert, C. et al. (2019). A longitudinal study of the faecal microbiome and metabolome of periparturient mares. *Peer J.* 7: e6687. https://doi.org/10.7717/peerj.6687.

39 Weese, J.S., Holcombe, S.J., Embertson, R.M. et al. (2015). Changes in the faecal microbiota of mares precede the development of post partum colic. *Equine Vet. J.* 47: 641–649.

40 Petersen, J.L., Lewis, R.M., Embertson, R. et al. (2019). Preliminary heritability of complete rotation large colon volvulus in Thoroughbred broodmares. *Vet. Rec.* 185: 269–271.

41 Morresey, P.R. (2014). Ultrasonography of the post-foaling mare. In: *Atlas of Equine Ultrasonography* (ed. J.A. Kidd, K.G. Lu, and M.L. Frazer), 351–363. Ames, IA: Wiley.

42 Hackett, E.S., Embertson, R.M., Hopper, S.A. et al. (2015). Duration of disease influences survival to discharge of Thoroughbred mares with surgically treated large colon volvulus. *Equine Vet. J.* 47: 650–654.

43 Suthers, J.M., Pinchbeck, G.L., Proudman, C.J. et al. (2013). Survival of horses following strangulating large colon volvulus. *Equine Vet. J.* 45: 219–223.

44 Orr, K.E., True Baker, W., Lynch, T.M. et al. (2020). Prognostic value of colonic and peripheral venous lactate measurements in horses with large colon volvulus. *Vet. Surg.* 49: 472–479.

45 Mueller, P.O.E., Peroni, J.F., and Moore, J.N. (2014). Colic in the late-term pregnant mare. In: *Equine Emergencies, Treatments and Procedures*, 4e (ed. J.A. Orsini and T.J. Divers), 216–219. St. Louis, MO: Elsevier.

46 Neuhauser, S., Palm, F., Ambuehl, F. et al. (2008). Effect of altrenogest treatment of mares in late pregnancy on parturition and on neonatal viability. *Exp. Clin. Endocrinol. Diabetes* 116: 423–428.

47 Neuhauser, S., Palm, F., Ambuehl, F. et al. (2009). Effect of altrenogest-treatment of mares in late gestation on adrenocortical function, blood count and plasma electrolytes in their foals. *Equine Vet. J.* 41 (6): 572–577.

48 Govaere, J.L.J., De Schauwer, C., Hoogewjs, M.K. et al. (2013). Hydrallantois in the mare—a report of five cases. *Reprod. Domest. Anim.* 48: e1–e6.

49 Slovis, N.M., Lu, K.G., Wolfsdorf, K.E. et al. (2013). How to manage hydrops allantois/hydrops amnion in a mare. *Proc. Am. Assoc. Equine Pract.* 59: 34–39.

50 Diel de Amorium, M., Chenier, T.S., Card, C. et al. (2018). Treatment of hydropsical conditions using transcervical gradual fetal fluid drainage in mares with or without concurrent abdominal wall disease. *J. Equine Vet. Sci.* 64: 81–88.

51 Waelchli, R.O. (2011). Hydrops. In: *Equine Reproduction*, 2e (ed. A.O. McKinnon, E.L. Squires, W.E. Vaala, and D.D. Varner), 2368–2372. Ames, IA: Wiley.

52 Mitchell, A.R.M., Delvescovo, B., Tse, M. et al. (2019). Successful management of hydrallantois in a Standardbred mare at term resulting in the birth of a live foal. *Can. Vet. J.* 60: 495–501.

53 Dini, P., Carossino, M., Loynachan, A.T. et al. (2020). Equine hydrallantois is associated with impaired angiogenesis in the placenta. *Placenta* 93: 101–112.

54 Shanahan, L.M. and Slovis, N.M. (2011). Leptospira interrogans associated with hydrallantois in two pluriparous thoroughbred mares. *J. Vet. Intern. Med.* 25: 158–161.

55 Sprayberry, K.A. and Lu, K.G. (2021). Managing reproduction emergencies in the field, part 1: injuries in stallions, injury of the external portion of the reproductive tract and gestational conditions in the mare. *Vet. Clin. Equine* 37: 339–366.

56 Stich, K.L. and Blanchard, T.L. (2003). Hydrallantois in mares. *Compend. Contin. Educ. Pract. Vet.* 25: 71–75.

57 Christensen, B.W., Troedsson, M.H.T., Murchie, T.A. et al. (2006). Management of hydrops amnion in a mare resulting in birth of a live foal. *J. Am. Vet. Med. Assoc.* 228: 1228–1233.

58 Lemonnier, L.C., Wolfsdorf, K.E., Kreutzfeldt, N. et al. (2022). Factors affecting survival and future foaling rates in Thoroughbred mares with hydrops. *J. Equine Vet. Sci.* 113: 103941. https://doi.org/10.1016/j.jevs.2022.103941.

59 Wolfsdorf, K.E. (2003). Ventral abdominal hernia and prepubic tendon rupture. In: *Current Therapy in Equine Medicine 5* (ed. N.E. Robinson), 310–311. Philadelphia, PA: WB Saunders Co.

60 Ross, J., Palmer, J.E., and Wilkins, P.A. (2008). Body wall tears during late pregnancy in mares: 13 cases (1995–2006). *J. Am. Vet. Med. Assoc.* 232: 257–261.

61 Rodgerson, D.H. (2011). Prepubic and abdominal wall rupture. In: *Equine Reproduction*, 2e (ed. A.O. McKinnon, E.L. Squires, W.E. Vaala, and D.D. Varner), 2428–2430. Ames, IA: Wiley.

62 Hanson, R.R. and Todhunter, R.J. (1986). Herniation of the abdominal wall in pregnant mares. *J. Am. Vet. Med. Assoc.* 189: 790–793.

63 Vasey, J.R. and Russell, T. (2011). Uterine torsion. In: *Equine Reproduction*, 2e (ed. A.O. McKinnon, E.L. Squires, W.E. Vaala, and D.D. Varner), 2435–2440. Ames, IA: Wiley.

64 Frazer, G.S. (2003). Uterine torsion. In: *Current Therapy in Equine Medicine 5* (ed. N.E. Robinson), 311–315. Philadelphia, PA: WB Saunders Co.

65 Yorke, E.H., Caldwell, F.J., and Johnson, A.K. (2012). Uterine torsion in mares. *Compend. Contin. Educ. Pract. Vet.* 34 (12): E1–E7.

66 Jung, C., Hospes, R., Bostedt, H. et al. (2008). Surgical treatment of uterine torsion using a ventral midline laparotomy in 19 mares. *Aust. Vet. J.* 86: 272–276.

67 Pascoe, J.R., Meagher, D.M., and Wheat, J.D. (1981). Surgical management of uterine torsion in the mare: a review of 26 cases. *J. Am. Vet. Med. Assoc.* 179: 351–354.

68 Spoormakers, T.J.P., Graat, E.A.M., Ter Braake, F. et al. (2016). Mare and foal survival and subsequent fertility of mares treated for uterine torsion. *Equine Vet. J.* 48: 172–175.

69 Barber, S.M. (1995). Complications of chronic uterine torsion. *Can. Vet. J.* 36: 102–103.

70 Doyle, A.J., Freeman, D.E., Sauberli, D.S. et al. (2002). Clinical signs and treatment of chronic uterine torsion in 2 mares. *J. Am. Vet. Med. Assoc.* 220: 349–353.

71 Lopez, C. and Carmona, J.U. (2010). Uterine torsion diagnosed in a mare at 515 days' gestation. *Equine Vet. Educ.* 22: 483.

72 Chaney, J.P., Holcombe, S.J., LeBlanc, M.M. et al. (2007). The effect of uterine torsion on mare and foal survival: a retrospective study, 1985–2005. *Equine Vet. J.* 39: 33–36.

73 Byars, T.D. and Divers, T.D. (2011). Periparturient hemorrhage. In: *Equine Reproduction*, 2e (ed. A.O. McKinnon, E.L. Squires, W.E. Vaala, and D.D. Varner), 2517–2532. Ames, IA: Wiley.

74 Arnold, C.E., Payne, M., Thompson, J.A. et al. (2008). Periparturient hemorrhage in mares: 73 cases (1998–2005). *J. Am. Vet. Med. Assoc.* 232: 1345–1351.

75 Britt, B.L. (2003). Postpartum hemorrhage. In: *Current Therapy in Equine Medicine 5* (ed. N.E. Robinson), 327–330. Philadelphia, PA: WB Saunders Co.

76 Frazer, G.S. (2003). Postpartum complications in the mare. Part 1: conditions affecting the uterus. *Equine Vet. Educ.* 15: 45–54.

77 Rossdale, P.D. (1994). Differential diagnosis of periparturient hemorrhage in the mare. *Equine Vet. Educ.* 6: 135–136.

78 Lofstedt, R. (1994). Haemorrhage associated with pregnancy and parturition. *Equine Vet. Educ.* 6: 138–141.

79 Williams, N.M. and Bryant, U.K. (2012). Periparturient arterial rupture in mares: a postmortem study. *J. Equine Vet. Sci.* 32: 281–284.

80 Scroggin CF and McCue PM. (2007). How to assess and stabilize a mare suspected of periparturient hemorrhage in the field. *Proc. Am. Assoc. Equine Pract.* 53: 342–348.

81 Wong DM, Brockus C, Alcott C, Sponseller B. (2009). Modifying the coagulation cascade: available medications. *Comp. Cont. Educ. Vet. Pract.* 31(6): 224–235.

82 Moreno CR, Delph KM, Beard WL. (2021). Intravenous formalin for treatment of haemorrhage in horses. *Equine Vet. Educ.* 33: e460–e465.

83 Perkins, N.R. and Frazer, G.S. (1994). Reproductive emergencies in the mare. *Vet. Clin. North Am. Equine Pract.* 10 (3): 643–670.

84 Spirito, M.A. and Sprayberry, K.A. (2011). Uterine prolapse. In: *Equine Reproduction*, 2e (ed. A.O. McKinnon, E.L. Squires, W.E. Vaala, and D.D. Varner), 2431–2434. Ames, IA: Wiley.

85 Boye, J.K., Bulkeley, E.A., and Dujovne, G.A. (2022). Good prognosis for survival to hospital discharge in a group of horses with uterine prolapse treated at a veterinary medical teaching hospital. *J. Am. Vet. Med. Assoc.* 260 (S2): S80–S86. https://doi.org/10.2460/javma.20.11.0615.

86 Blanchard, T.L. (2011). Postpartum metritis. In: *Equine Reproduction*, 2e (ed. A.O. McKinnon, E.L. Squires, W.E. Vaala, and D.D. Varner), 2530–2533. Ames, IA: Wiley.

87 Sutter, W.W., Hopper, S., and Embertson, R.M. (2003). Diagnosis and surgical treatment of uterine lacerations in mares (33 cases). *Proc. Am. Assoc. Equine Pract.* 49: 357–359.

88 Javsicas, L.H., Giguere, S., Freeman, D.E. et al. (2010). Comparison of surgical and medical treatment of 49 postpartum mares with presumptive or confirmed uterine tears. *Vet. Surg.* 39: 254–260.

89 Hooper, R.N., Schumacher, J., Taylor, T.S. et al. (1993). Diagnosing and treating uterine ruptures in mares. *Vet. Med.* 88: 263–270.

90 Fischer, A.T. and Phillips, T.N. (1986). Surgical repair of a ruptured uterus in five mares. *Equine Vet. J.* 18: 153–155.

91 Hassel, D.M. and Ragle, C.A. (1994). Laparoscopic diagnosis and conservative treatment of a uterine tear in a mare. *J. Am. Vet. Med. Assoc.* 205: 1531–1533.

92 Rodgerson, D.H., Spirito, M.A., Thorpe, P.A. et al. (1999). Standing surgical repair of cystorrhexis in two mares. *Vet. Surg.* 28: 113–116.

93 Higuchi, T., Nanao, Y., and Senba, H. (2002). Repair of urinary bladder rupture through a urethrotomy and urethral sphinterotomy in four postpartum mares. *Vet. Surg.* 31: 344–348.

94 Peitzmeier, M.F., McNally, T.P., Slone, D.E. et al. (2016). Conservative management of cystorrhexis in four adult horses. *Equine Vet. Educ.* 28: 631–635.

95 Pye, J.L., Collins, N.M., and Adkins, A.R. (2018). Transurethral endoscopic-guided intraluminal closure of multiple urinary bladder tears in a standing mare. *Equine Vet. Educ.* 30: 127–131.

Chapter 68 Cesarean Section

Annette M. McCoy

Cesarean section is most commonly performed as an emergency procedure to relieve dystocia, although it has occasionally been reported as an elective procedure in select cases when vaginal birth is deemed unlikely to be successful (e.g. due to maternal pelvic canal abnormalities) [1, 2]. The priority when electing cesarean section is delivery of a live foal; if the fetus is dead at the time of presentation, a fetotomy is more likely to be elected as mare survival and fertility after this procedure is typically good [3]. To achieve a positive outcome, however, rapid decision-making and a well-prepared team are paramount. A coordinated dystocia management protocol (CDMP) has been proposed and suggests that it should take no more than 30 minutes after hospital admission to decide that a cesarean section is necessary, with clipping and rough preparation of the surgery site occurring during attempts at controlled vaginal delivery (CVD) [4].

Once the decision to proceed with a cesarean section has been made, preparation of patient and surgical personnel is the same as for a routine midline laparotomy, with the caveat that the incision will be made more caudal when compared to an exploratory procedure. A ventral midline incision is made starting 10 cm caudal to the umbilicus and extending 35–40 cm cranially such that the gravid uterine horn, typically containing the hind limbs, can be identified and exteriorized. In the case that the foal is in transverse presentation, exteriorization of the uterus may not be possible and abdominal contamination is a major concern. In a normal fetal presentation, once the uterine horn is exteriorized it is held in place by an assistant, with or without the use of stay sutures based on surgeon preference. The uterine horn is isolated with an additional layer of impermeable drapes to help reduce the risk of abdominal contamination. Subsequently, the uterine wall and chorioallantois are incised from the fetal hocks to the feet, the amniotic membrane is incised, and the foal is removed from the uterus hind-limbs first. Elevation of the foal out of the uterus can be challenging because of the weight of the foal and typically involves both the surgeon and an additional sterile assistant. The umbilicus is clamped, and the foal is transferred to a resuscitation team for care while the surgeon completes the surgical procedure.

Briefly, the chorioallantois is separated from the uterine wall for 3–4 cm around the circumference of the incision; if vaginal removal of the placenta in its entirety is possible, then this option is preferred, but this situation is uncommon. Subsequently, a hemostatic suture may be placed around the circumference of the uterine incision [5] (Figure 68.1a) prior to a two-layer inverting closure of the uterus (Figure 68.1b). The efficacy of a hemostatic suture at preventing postoperative anemia and hemorrhage has been called into question [6] and therefore its use is largely a matter of surgeon preference, with some choosing to individually ligate bleeding vessels prior to hysterotomy closure in addition to, or in lieu of, the hemostatic suture [7]. The uterus generally begins to contract during closure; this is promoted by the administration of 20 IU intravenous oxytocin. Stay sutures, if present, are removed, the extra draping discarded, and the uterus is replaced into its normal position in the abdomen. The surgical team may elect to change gowns and gloves prior to abdominal lavage and routine closure of the midline incision.

Rapid evaluation of a foal born via cesarean section will determine whether resuscitation efforts are needed. Even if the foal appears to be nonviable on initial examination, resuscitation is generally attempted for several minutes unless an obvious severe congenital malformation or other abnormality is present. Basic life support in foals includes intubation to establish an airway, ventilation, and rapid continuous chest compressions (100 per minute or more) [8, 9]. Respiratory arrest typically occurs before cardiac arrest in foals secondary to dystocia; therefore, ventilation should be prioritized, preferably through a nasotracheal tube [9]. Chest compressions should be instituted

Equine Neonatal Medicine, First Edition. Edited by David M. Wong and Pamela A. Wilkins.

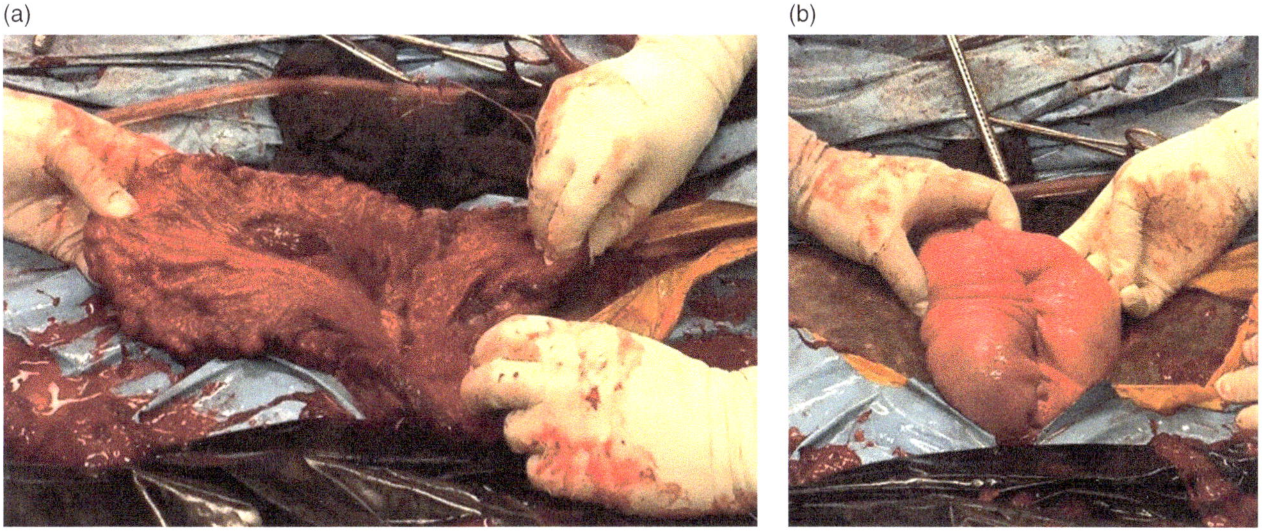

Figure 68.1 (a) Intra-operative exteriorization of the uterus with surgeon placing hemostatic suture around the circumference of the uterine incision. (b) Two-layer inverting suture pattern to close uterus after extraction of fetus.

30 seconds after ventilation has started if the heartbeat is <40 beats/min [9]. Vascular access should also be established as rapidly as possible so that resuscitative drugs (epinephrine, vasopressin, etc.) can be administered. Either an intravenous or intraosseous route is effective in neonates [8]. Cardiopulmonary resuscitation is discussed in detail in Chapter 2.

Unfortunately, even with optimal surgical management and resuscitation efforts, foal survival after emergency cesarean section is poor. Reports range from 20% to 35% survival to discharge [4, 10, 11]. Foal survival after elective cesarean section is better (up to 90% [2]), although accurate estimation of fetal maturity is crucial for success. Duration of dystocia has repeatedly been reported to be a key factor in foal survival [12], and it is likely that the comparatively longer time to deliver a foal via cesarean section accounts for at least some of the differences in foal survival when compared to other methods of assisted delivery. It is worth noting that there has been a single report of cesarean section in a field setting using a low-flank approach under heavy sedation and local/regional anesthesia, similar to what is commonly done in small ruminants. This approach was elected in seven miniature horse and pony mares, each with a dead malpositioned fetus, in lieu of a fetotomy or euthanasia and good outcomes were reported [13] although the utility of this surgical approach in standard-sized horses is likely limited to terminal procedures.

Prognosis for a mare after cesarean section is generally good unless the procedure was performed due to an acute injury or other underlying pathology (e.g. colic), with reported survival rates of 84–91% [2, 10, 11, 14]. There are conflicting reports on whether longer duration of dystocia is associated with mare mortality [2, 10, 14]. Death or euthanasia of mares undergoing cesarean section has been attributed to complications during anesthetic recovery (e.g. paresis/paralysis, fracture), intraabdominal hemorrhage, peritonitis/sepsis, uterine tear, gastrointestinal complications (e.g. intestinal ischemia, colitis), and incisional complications [2, 10, 14]. Postoperative care is similar to any exploratory celiotomy, with the duration of use of perioperative antibiotics and analgesia/anti-inflammatory medications dictated by the level of abdominal contamination and tissue trauma (typically 3–5 days). Intravenous fluids are used as needed to correct electrolyte imbalances or if oral fluids cannot be administered due to transient postoperative ileus. Feed is typically offered the first day after surgery, and a laxative diet may be preferred initially to reduce the risk of an impaction. If a live foal resulted from the cesarean section, the author prefers to maintain an abdominal bandage for up to 2 weeks postoperatively to reduce the risk of the foal contaminating the surgery site, but this is not a universal practice.

If the placenta has not passed within 2–3 hours after delivery, a dose of oxytocin is administered (40 IU in 1 l Lactated Ringer's solution given over 30–60 minutes). The rate of administration may be slowed if the mare develops signs of abdominal pain. Additional doses of oxytocin (20–80 IU q4–6 hours) may be administered as needed. Uterine lavage is typically performed daily for 3–4 days postoperatively, or longer if indicated. Retained placenta has been reported in 56–100% of mares undergoing cesarean section, with elective procedures at higher risk for this complication [2, 10].

The prognosis for breeding soundness after cesarean section is favorable, although pregnancy and foaling rates are lower for breedings performed in the season immediately after surgery than in subsequent years [10, 11]. In one study, mares had a foaling rate of 41% in the year following surgery, 61% in year 2, and 58% in year 3, although this number may have been skewed downward by the number of older mares (≥16 years) in the study cohort [10]. Another study reported a 60% foaling rate the year after cesarean section, and a cumulative postsurgery foaling rate of 72% [11]. These compare favorably with presurgery foaling rates of 77–84% in the study populations [10, 11]. Owners should be advised to wait at least 6 weeks after surgery before attempting to breed a mare; thus, depending on the timing of the dystocia, it may be better to wait until the next season if an early spring foal is desirable [11].

References

1 Watkins, J.P., Taylor, T.S., Day, W.C. et al. (1990). Elective cesarean section in mares: eight cases (1980–1989). *J. Am. Vet. Med. Assoc.* 197: 1639–1645.

2 Freeman, D.E., Hungerford, L.L., Schaeffer, D. et al. (1999). Caesarean section and other methods for assisted delivery: comparison of effects on mare mortality and complications. *Equine Vet. J.* 31: 203–207.

3 Carluccio, A., Contri, A., Tosi, U. et al. (2007). Survival rate and short-term fertility rate associated with the use of fetotomy for resolution of dystocia in mares: 72 cases (1991–2005). *J. Am. Vet. Med. Assoc.* 230: 1502–1505.

4 Lynch Norton, J., Dallap, B.L., Johnston, J.K. et al. (2007). Retrospective study of dystocia in mares at a referral hospital. *Equine Vet. J.* 39: 37–41.

5 Vandeplassche, M. (1980). Obstetrician's view of the physiology of equine parturition and dystocia. *Equine Vet. J.* 12: 45–49.

6 Freeman, D.E., Johnston, J.K., Baker, G.J. et al. (1999). An evaluation of the haemostatic suture in hysterotomy closure in the mare. *Equine Vet. J.* 31: 208–211.

7 Embertson, R.M. (1999). Dystocia and caesarean sections: the importance of duration and good judgement. *Equine Vet. J.* 31: 179–180.

8 Palmer, J.E. (2007). Neonatal foal resuscitation. *Vet. Clin. North Am. Equine Pract.* 23: 159–182.

9 Jokisalo, J.M. and Corley, K.T. (2014). CPR in the neonatal foal: has RECOVER changed our approach? *Vet. Clin. North Am. Equine Pract.* 30: 301–316, vii.

10 Abernathy-Young, K.K., LeBlanc, M.M., Embertson, R.M. et al. (2012). Survival rates of mares and foals and postoperative complications and fertility of mares after cesarean section: 95 cases (1986–2000). *J. Am. Vet. Med. Assoc.* 241: 927–934.

11 Byron, C.R., Embertson, R.M., Bernard, W.V. et al. (2003). Dystocia in a referral hospital setting: approach and results. *Equine Vet. J.* 35: 82–85.

12 Wilkins, P.A. (2015). Prognostic indicators for survival and athletic outcome in critically ill neonatal foals. *Vet. Clin. North Am. Equine Pract.* 31: 615–628.

13 Gandini, M., Iotti, B., and Nervo, T. (2013). Field caesarean section in seven miniature horses and ponies (2009–2012). *Reprod. Domest. Anim.* 48: e49–e51.

14 Rioja, E., Cernicchiaro, N., Costa, M.C. et al. (2012). Perioperative risk factors for mortality and length of hospitalization in mares with dystocia undergoing general anesthesia: a retrospective study. *Can. Vet. J.* 53: 502–510.

Chapter 69 The High-Risk Pregnancy

Pamela A. Wilkins and David Wong

This chapter will cover common causes of threats to pregnancy, both maternal and fetal. It is important to remember that in cases of critical maternal illness, the fetus cannot survive if the dam does not. Medical problems such as placentitis, body wall tears, critical illness of the dam, and repeated production of abnormal foals are discussed and diagnostic options, treatment choices, and development of plans for parturition are presented. This chapter is not exhaustive, and the reader is referred to other sources more directly associated with reproduction specialists for additional details and more complete information.

High-risk pregnancies are best managed by a team that includes theriogenologists, internists and, potentially, surgeons, particularly if Caesarian section is part of a potential intervention plan. Consultation with an anesthesiologist should be considered for the benefit of the fetus/foal following delivery as reversal of anesthetic medications that were administered to the mare might be provided to the newborn foal. Clinicians and the mare's owner must clearly communicate; sometimes it is necessary to determine if the life of the dam or that of the fetus is paramount.

Pregnant mares are considered at high risk of a poor outcome when they have a history of problems during past pregnancies or have a new problem during the current pregnancy (Table 69.1). As such, these cases are classified as either recurrent (historical or reemergent) problems or new/current problems resulting in a pregnancy being classified as high risk.

Determination of current or recurrent threats to pregnancy aids in assessment and development of a plan for that pregnancy. It is important that the team that manages the pregnancy, parturition, and post-parturient care of the dam and foal be in place early and that the desires of the owner are made clear. It is not unusual for the owner of the dam to explicitly value one over the other, and knowledge of any preference for survival of the dam or foal by the owner is important to help direct decisions regarding management. A decision maker for the patient needs to be identified, along with reliable contact information for that individual. This information should be clearly marked and readily available.

Threats to the Fetus

Any problems exhibited by the mare should be viewed in terms of how it threatens not only the dam but also fetal or neonatal well-being. After understanding the risks to both, the clinician must devise and implement a plan to minimize or eliminate those risks. For example, critical illness in the dam puts the fetus at tremendous risk, and the converse may also be true, for a compromised or dead fetus may complicate the clinical course of a critically ill dam.

Important physiologic changes occur with pregnancy, primarily associated with the mare's cardiovascular and respiratory systems. Late-term pregnant mares have reduced functional residual capacity (FRC) in their lungs accompanied by increased minute volume, resulting in increased respiratory rates at rest that, when combined with increased alveolar ventilation, produces chronic respiratory alkalosis. Cardiac output during pregnancy increases 30–50% and is associated with higher resting heart rates and stroke volumes. Fifty percent of this increased output goes to the uterus, with the remainder perfusing the skin, gastrointestinal tract, and kidneys to compensate for the increased demands of pregnancy. During the last trimester, blood flow to the placenta increases tremendously in parallel with fetal growth because the late-term fetus has a much higher oxygen demand, which is needed to support growth. A high rate of placental perfusion must occur for the fetus to receive enough oxygen, making pregnant mares at risk for severe complications should blood loss or hypovolemia occur.

Late-term pregnant mares have an increased plasma volume and a relative (physiologic) anemia. The enlarged

Equine Neonatal Medicine, First Edition. Edited by David M. Wong and Pamela A. Wilkins.

Table 69.1 Medical conditions associated with high-risk pregnancy.

Recurrent problems		
▪ Placentitis	▪ Abortion	
▪ Premature placental separation	▪ Premature birth	
▪ Recurrent dystocia	▪ Prolonged pregnancies	
▪ Recurrent abnormal foals	▪ Uterine artery hemorrhage	
▪ Premature termination of pregnancy		
Current problems		
Reproductive	**Musculoskeletal**	**Neurologic**
▪ Precious udder development	▪ Fractures	▪ Ataxia
▪ Placentitis	▪ Laminitis	▪ Weakness
▪ Twin pregnancy	▪ Lameness	▪ Seizures
▪ Premature placental separation	▪ Body wall hernia	
▪ Over term relative to past gestations	▪ Recent abdominal surgical incision	
▪ Hydrops allantois, hydrops amnion		
Miscellaneous		
▪ Endotoxemia		
▪ Systemic Inflammatory Response Syndrome (SIRS)	▪ Granulomatous disease	
▪ Colic, colitis, pleuropneumonia, others	▪ Hypoparathyroidism	
▪ Recent hypotension, hypoxemia, cardiac disease	▪ Recent hemorrhage	
▪ Pituitary pars intermedia dysfunction (PPID)	▪ Any critical illness in the dam	
▪ Lymphosarcoma, other cancers	▪ Innumerable other problems	
▪ Melanoma in pelvic canal		

uterus limits lung expansion, contributing to the reduction in FRC and ventilation-perfusion mismatching. The reduction in oxygen reserve and higher rate of oxygen consumption (20–25% increase compared with nonpregnant mares) results in intolerance of apnea and a propensity for hypoxemia.

Uterine blood flow is not autoregulated and is directly proportional to the mean perfusion pressure and inversely proportional to uterine vascular resistance. Blood gas transport is largely independent of diffusion distance in the equine placenta, particularly in late gestation, and is more dependent on blood flow. Information from other species cannot be extrapolated to the equine placenta because of its diffuse epitheliochorial nature and the arrangement of the maternal and fetal blood vessels within the microcotyledons. For example, umbilical venous PO_2 is 50–54 mmHg in the horse fetus, compared with 30–34 mmHg in the sheep, whereas the maternal uterine vein to umbilical vein PO_2 difference is near zero. Also, unlike sheep, in the mare the umbilical venous PO_2 values decrease 5–10 mmHg in response to maternal hypoxemia and increase in response to maternal hyperoxemia.

Another important variable to consider regarding provision of fetal nutrients is that the dam has complete control of the fetal environment; that is, the fetus is entirely dependent on the dam for life and must receive all nutritional support and oxygen from the dam. Unfortunately, there are no feedback mechanisms for the fetus to communicate its changing needs directly to the mare. The fetus can compensate for some changes brought about by disturbances in maternal homeostasis, but always at the cost to the fetus. Some threats to fetal well-being include lack of placental perfusion, lack of oxygen delivery, nutritional threats, placentitis/placental dysfunction, loss of fetal-maternal coordination of maturation, interaction with other fetuses (multiple pregnancy), and iatrogenic factors (e.g. drugs or other substances given to the dam, early termination of pregnancy via induced delivery). Discussion regarding some of these threats follows.

Lack of Placental Perfusion

Poor placental perfusion can be compensated for only in the short-term through redistribution of fetal blood flow; however, the margin of safety in late-term pregnancy is small. Whenever maternal perfusion is compromised, placental circulation and oxygen delivery may be compromised, thereby resulting in a significant threat to the fetus.

Lack of Oxygen Delivery to the Fetus

Reduced oxygen delivery to the fetus can arise from decreased placental perfusion, maternal anemia, or maternal hypoxemia. In the horse, alignment of fetal and maternal vessels results in a counter-current flow pattern. In this arrangement, the blood vessels are parallel to each other and the blood flows are in opposite directions. The venous side of the fetal capillary bed is aligned with the arterial side of the maternal capillary bed so that the gradient of oxygen and other nutrients is the highest possible. This creates the most efficient pattern for transfer of oxygen and nutrients and removal of waste products. However, consequences of this counter-current flow pattern in the horse can have a substantial impact on the foal. For example, changes in maternal PaO_2 significantly changes fetal PO_2. Thus, maternal hypoxia or hypoxemia can have a profound effect on the fetus. Hypoxia and hypoxemia may predispose the foal to hypoxic-ischemic asphyxial disease and/or neonatal maladjustment syndrome. When maternal PaO_2 is increased with inhaled oxygen, umbilical PO_2 increases substantially, and the driving force increases, allowing more efficient transport of dissolved oxygen to the fetus.

Maternal hypoxia/hypoxemia should be addressed rapidly to improve the mare's health and facilitate improved oxygen delivery to the fetus. If the mare is hypovolemic, an initial treatment goal is rapid volume replacement. The mare should also be supplemented with intranasal administration of humidified oxygen (10–15 l/min); this will increase oxygen delivery to the fetus and might help when there is fetal hypoxemia. Serious consideration should be given to blood transfusion therapy in the care of anemic mares to prevent fetal hypoxia. Loss of red cell mass impacts oxygen content of blood much more than does hypoxemia. Of note, administration of blood transfusions to a broodmare may predispose the mare to produce antibodies against foreign blood groups, putting future foals at risk for neonatal isoerythrolysis. This should be included in discharge instructions so future decision makers are aware of the risk.

Placentitis/Placental Dysfunction

The percentage of placenta affected is not a predictor of the outcome of the pregnancy; a foal born with widespread placental lesions may be better off than a foal with a focal placental lesion. The presence of placentitis, no matter how extensive, is predictive of a serious problem because approximately 80% of foals born with placentitis are abnormal in some clinically detectable way. Placentitis is a common cause of late-term abortion in mares and is perhaps the most common cause of a mare displaying clinical signs of a high-risk pregnancy, such as precocious udder development, premature lactation, cervical softening, and vaginal discharge. The cause is generally considered to be ascending infection that enters the uterus via the cervix, although hematogenous spread of some bacterial and viral agents (equine herpesvirus-1 and equine viral arteritis in particular) is possible. Mares with poor perineal conformation, abnormal cervical anatomy (sometimes resulting from a previous birth trauma), a history of vaginal/cervical examination performed late in pregnancy, or a history of being placed in dorsal recumbency while pregnant are at increased risk of placentitis, although for many there is no identified underlying cause. Table 69.2 provides a summary of causes of placental dysfunction in the mare.

Common bacteria isolated in equine placentitis/abortions include *Streptococcus equi* (subspecies *zooepidemicus*), *Escherichia coli, Pseudomonas aeruginosa, Klebsiella pneumoniae,* and nocardioform species. Fetal loss and premature delivery resulting from placentitis is not fully understood. Studies, however, suggest that infection of the chorioallantois results in increased expression of inflammatory mediators that, in addition to other local effects, alters myometrial contractility. Combined, these observations suggest that fetal loss can occur because of a compromised fetus, increased myometrial contractility, or both.

Ultrasonographic evaluation of the uterus and conceptus per rectum and transabdominally can provide valuable information, particularly regarding placental thickness if placentitis is a concern. Fetal fluids can be evaluated, and fetal size can be estimated from the size of the fetal eye later in gestation (see biophysical profile below).

All cases of suspected or proven bacterial placentitis/placental dysfunction should be treated, and all cases of premature onset of lactation should be managed as such until proved otherwise. Specific therapeutics include administration of broad-spectrum antimicrobial agents. Trimethoprim-sulfa drugs appear to cross the placental/uterine barrier; and recently, using microdialysis,

Table 69.2 Placental diseases that occur in late-term pregnancy.

- Premature placental separation
- Placental infection/infectious placentitis
- Ascending pathogens (bacteria, fungi)
- Hematogenous spread of pathogens (viruses, bacteria, Ehrlichia, fungi)
- Noninfectious inflammation
- Placental degeneration (placental edema)
- Hydrops allantois, hydrops amnion

Table 69.3 Commonly drugs used in high-risk pregnancy mares.

Medication	Dose	Reason for use
▪ Trimethoprim-sulfonamide	25 mg/kg PO, q12h	Antimicrobial
▪ Flunixin Meglumine	0.25 mg/kg PO or IV, q8h	Anti-inflammatory
▪ Altrenogest	0.44 mg/kg PO, q24h	Tocolytic
▪ Isoxsuprine	0.4–0.6 mg/kg PO, q12h	Tocolytic
▪ Clenbuterol	0.8 mg/kg PO, as needed	Tocolytic
▪ Pentoxifylline	8.5 mg/kg PO, q12h	Anti-inflammatory
▪ Vitamin E	5000–10 000 IU/d PO	Antioxidant

gentamicin, and penicillin were measured in the allantoic fluid after administration to mares (Table 69.3). If culture and sensitivity results are available, directed therapy should be instituted toward the specific organism. Recently enrofloxacin has been evaluated and also appears to be a potentially appropriate antimicrobial choice. Nonsteroidal anti-inflammatory agents, such as flunixin meglumine, are used to combat alterations in prostaglandin balance that may be associated with infection and inflammation.

Pentoxifylline has been used for its rheologic effect, potentially improving blood flow within the placenta, and for its general anti-inflammatory effects. However, absorption of orally administered pentoxifylline is reportedly quite variable in horses [1, 2]. Tocolytic agents and agents that promote uterine quiescence have been used and include altrenogest (Regumate), isoxsuprine, and clenbuterol. The efficacy of isoxsuprine as a tocolytic in the horse is unproven, and bioavailability of orally administered isoxsuprine appears to be highly variable [3]. Clenbuterol may be indicated during management of dystocia in preparation for assisted delivery or Cesarean section because, given IV, it has been shown to decrease uterine tone for up to 120 minutes [4]. Chronic use of clenbuterol results in changes in receptor density and activity and the drug becomes less effective over time.

Other strategies that can be considered in the management of mares in high-risk pregnancy situations include provision of intranasal oxygen supplementation (insufflation) in efforts to improve oxygen delivery to the fetus (10–15 l/min). Some clinicians advocate for administration of vitamin E (tocopherol) to high-risk mares as it may serve as an antioxidant for placental/uterine inflammation and as a neuroprotectant strategy for the fetus. Recent evidence suggests that large (>5000 IU/d) vitamin E doses do not increase maternal vitamin E concentration more than smaller (1000 IU/d) doses. Nutritional needs should also be considered in high-risk pregnancy mares, especially if they are anorectic or held off feed because of a specific medical condition. These mares are at particular risk for fetal loss because of their lack of feed intake, which alters prostaglandin metabolism. Therefore, IV dextrose (0.5–2 mg/kg/min) can be given to these patients. Of note, few of the strategies described are specifically aimed at the fetus, but rather focus on maintaining the pregnancy.

Recently, evidence reported that prenatal administration of adrenocorticotropic hormone (ACTH) or corticosteroids may be beneficial in advancing the maturity of the fetus [5]. In one study, pregnant Thoroughbred mares were administered 100 mg of dexamethasone intramuscularly at 315, 316, and 317 days of gestation. In this study, dexamethasone administration significantly reduced gestation length in mares without apparent adverse effects. The authors of that study suggested that dexamethasone stimulates precocious fetal maturation and delivery in late-term pregnant mares and could potentially improve foal viability in mares at risk of preterm delivery [5]. In a compromised pregnancy in which clinical signs of early delivery do not regress with treatment, these therapies may be considered to increase the chances of fetal survival.

Ventral Body Wall Tear and Hydrops Allantois/Hydrops Amnion

Any late-pregnant mare that has a rapidly enlarging abdomen and an area of painful edema in the flank region that advances to the ventral abdominal wall could be suffering from rupture of the abdominal musculature, the rectus abdominis muscle, or the prepubic tendon [6]. These can occur together or separately in pregnant mares. Together, these specific defects can be referred to as ventral ruptures and "body wall tears" and automatically categorizes the mare as a high-risk pregnancy. Hydrops allantois/hydrops amnion are a primary cause leading to rupture of the body wall. Other conditions such as twin pregnancies (increased uterine weight) or trauma in late pregnancy are less associated with body wall tears; trauma appears to be more common in older, unfit mare. Moreover, likely due to their size, Draft breeds are predisposed to body wall tears, but there may not be an obvious predisposing cause for this condition.

Hydrops allantois is an emergency condition requiring attention in a short time interval to ensure the health of the mare because secondary complications associated with intraabdominal hypertension may develop, potentially leading to abdominal compartment syndrome, including respiratory compromise, hypovolemic shock at delivery, and body wall hernia. This condition is often detected by the owner as sudden onset of abdominal distention, with progressive lethargy and anorexia, and possibly dyspnea. Diagnosis is made by rectal palpation, which reveals an enlarged fluid-filled uterus and is confirmed by sonographic examination per rectum showing a large amount of allantoic or amnionic fluid. Similar to body wall hernias and prepubic tendon rupture, hydrops is usually detected by the owner as an abrupt change in the contour of the abdominal wall and lethargy and anorexia in the mare. Mares with ventral ruptures may have ventral edema from the udder to the xiphoid cartilage of the sternum or only in the flank region initially. Signs of pain and intermittent colic may be observed. If the pain is severe, tachycardia and tachypnea can be present. Affected mares are generally reluctant to move or lay down.

Ultrasonographic examination of the posterior aspect of the ventral abdomen and flank regions may be useful to detect the presence of tears or a hernia. Any defect in the abdominal musculature may be complicated by bowel incarceration. All examinations are less than satisfactory because of the fetal presence and edema of the body wall. The udder may be displaced cranially and ventrally because of loss of its caudal attachment to the pelvis, and the plaque of edema can almost obliterate the outline of the mammary gland. Ventral body wall defects may easily lead to rupture of the blood supply to the mammary gland, disruption of its attachment to the body wall, and hemorrhage of the adjacent musculature. Blood may also be detectable in the milk. Together with the reluctance to walk and lie down, these signs are strongly indicative for rupture of the ventral body wall.

Treatment for suspected or confirmed body wall tears is aimed at stabilizing the horse by restricting activity. Box stall confinement is mandatory, and it is important to closely monitor for signs of blood loss, which can be significant. Decreased fecal production can be seen and the development of further discomfort can suggest progression of the tear. Anti-inflammatory drugs such as phenylbutazone or flunixin meglumine may help relieve discomfort and use of a strong bandage around the abdominal wall, acting as an abdominal sling, may provide support for the ventral abdominal wall. Any abdominal bandage must be well padded to avoid pressure necrosis along the dorsum. The possibility of bowel entrapment and strangulation should be investigated; surgical correction might be necessary if bowel strangulation has occurred. Repeated ultrasonographic evaluation of any entrapped bowel may be necessary. In a few cases, because of rapidly changing clinical parameters, the mare gains little from supportive treatment and induction of parturition (or termination of the pregnancy in mares earlier in gestation) must be performed. Pregnancy termination may be desirable in some mares with hydrops conditions, or twins, presenting well before their anticipated parturition date, even if ventral body wall tears have not yet occurred. Induction of parturition or Cesarean section not required to save the life of the dam has been associated with poorer outcomes for the fetus because of lack of readiness for birth. The best outcomes for the fetus seem to be achieved with conservative management and assistance at the time of parturition.

The clinician should assume that assistance with parturition will be necessary because the mare may be reluctant to lie down and/or may experience difficulty developing sufficient abdominal pressure during active labor. Equipment needed for assistance with parturition and resuscitation of the delivered foal should be readily at hand. Establishment of clear communication with the owner regarding whether the mare or the fetus is the priority is important because this crucial choice could determine the decisions made as the case progresses. Edema usually resolves quickly after foaling, and the mare can suckle the foal normally. Supplementation with colostrum or plasma may be indicated in cases in which the mare has leaked colostrum before delivery.

Poor Maternal Nutritional States

Pregnant mares require an adequate diet to sustain and develop a healthy fetus. The clinician should be cognizant of the fact that maternal malnutrition can impact growth of the fetus. Chronic conditions such as lack of intake (e.g. lack of opportunity), malabsorption, tumor cachexia, and other conditions that result in chronic conditions of malnutrition can negatively impact the growth of the fetus, especially in the last 3 months of gestation. Ideally, pregnant mares should enter late gestation in a body condition score of 6 to have available energy stores to buffer periods of scarce resources during late gestation [7]. During early and mid-gestation, the fetus is very small (approximately 2% of mare's body weight) and energy and caloric needs are likely met from adequate amounts of forage fed (2–2.5% body weight daily); however, it is possible that the diet may be deficient in key minerals such as copper, zinc, selenium, calcium, and phosphorus. Thus, diet balancers or mineral supplements should be considered [7]. During mid-gestation, there is increased caloric requirements for the development of the placental tissue and the requirement for protein and energy is increased above maintenance in the fifth month of gestation and continues to increase till term [7]. During late pregnancy, the fetus gains approximately 80% of its birth weight and the mare's requirements for calories, protein, and vitamins and minerals increases significantly. At birth, the foal's birth weight is estimated to be 10% of the mare's non-pregnant weight and over the entire pregnancy, mares gain approximately 10–15% of their non-pregnant weight.

Conversely, acute fasting that might occur with elective surgical procedures or treatment of colic in the pregnant mare can impact the nutritional delivery to the fetus. It is important to note that 30–48 hours of complete fasting in the late-term mare decreases glucose delivery to the fetus and increases circulating plasma free fatty acids, resulting in an increase in prostaglandin production in the maternal and fetal placenta [8]. Maternal and fetal placenta and fetal fluids contain a complex mix of prostaglandins, which seem to be important in maintaining pregnancy and may have a role in initiation of parturition. The risk of preterm delivery increases within 1 week of an anorectic episode; the foal often appears premature and not ready for delivery.

Treatment of pregnant mares in poor nutritional states includes supporting the mare's feed intake by providing adequate caloric intake, encouraging the mare to stay on a high plane of nutrition, and avoiding acute fasting. Fiber is the foundation of the mare's diet, and when good quality, should meet some of the mare's requirements from conception to parturition. However, during late gestation, mares have a more limited capacity for feed intake due to the fetus and fetal fluids compressing the digestive tract. Because of this physical limitation, mares are unable to consume sufficient forage necessary to meet energy and nutrient requirements (further compounded if poor-quality forage is provided). In late gestation, more energy-dense and nutrient-dense feeds should be provided, and meals can be provided in smaller volumes of highly digestible fiber. Concentrate feed can be offered as well throughout pregnancy. If the mare must be fasted, or becomes completely anorexic, provision of IV glucose supplementation (0.5–2 mg/kg/min) is recommended and will negate the changes in prostaglandins and greatly decreases the risk of early delivery [9]. When periodically anorectic mares are refractory to consuming more calories, the clinician can consider administering flunixin meglumine (0.25 mg/kg IV q8h).

Fetal Assessment and Monitoring

Fetal Heart Rate Monitoring

Monitoring of the fetal heart rate (FHR) is another method of assessing fetal viability and compromise and can be accomplished via transabdominal ultrasound of fetal ECG. While ultrasound evaluation of the FHR is typically easier to obtain, long-term measurements are not generally recorded, and the results may be misleading. The fetal ECG can serve as a companion to transabdominal ultrasonography. One can evaluate fetal ECGs measured continuously using telemetry or obtain recordings using more conventional techniques several times throughout the day (see Chapter 1, Section 1). Electrodes are placed on the skin of the mare in locations aimed at maximizing the magnitude of the fetal ECG but, because the fetus frequently changes position, multiple sites may be needed in any 24-hour period. Begin with an electrode placed dorsally in the area of the sacral prominence with two electrodes placed bilaterally in a transverse plane in the region of the flank. The fetal ECG maximal amplitude is low, usually 0.05–0.1 mV, and can be lost in artifact or background noise, so it is common to move electrodes to new positions to maximize the appearance of the fetal ECG.

The normal FHR during the last months of gestation ranges from 65 to 115 beats/min, a fairly wide distribution. The range of heart rate of an individual fetus can be narrow, however. Recordings should be made over a 10- to 20-minute period and repeated several times daily if conventional techniques are used. If telemetry is used, paper recordings should be obtained at approximately 2-hour intervals to allow for calculation of FHR and observation of rhythm. Bradycardia in the fetus is an adaptation to in utero stress, most usually thought to be hypoxia. By slowing the heart rate, the fetus prolongs exposure of fetal blood to maternal blood, increasing the time for equilibration of dissolved gas across the placenta and improving the oxygen content of the fetal blood. The fetus also alters the distribution of its cardiac output in response to hypoxia, centralizing blood distribution. Tachycardia in the fetus can be associated with fetal movement, and brief periods of tachycardia should occur in a 24-hour period. Persistent tachycardia is a sign of fetal distress and represents more severe fetal compromise than bradycardia. Tachycardia followed by severe bradycardia can be observed terminally in some feti. Dysrhythmias have been recognized in the challenged fetus, most commonly believed to be atrial fibrillation, but also apparent runs of ventricular tachycardia.

During the last weeks of pregnancy, fetal foals usually have a baseline heart rate between 60 and 75 beats/min with a low heart rate in the range of 40–75 beats/min and high heart rate in the range of 83–250 beats/min. Eighty percent have a low FHR < 70 beats/min; 55%, low FHR < 60 beats/min; and 14%, low FHR < 50 beats/min. Eighty-six percent have a high FHR > 100 beats/min; 50%, high FHR > 120 beats/min; and 20%, high FHR > 200 beats/min. Of note, transient low heart rates <60 beats/min are common and should not be considered ominous unless they are consistent with no accelerations. Also, FHR transiently may be >200 beats/min. Transient FHR > 120 beats/min is not threatening unless it is persistent and does not return to baseline levels.

If the FHR is <60 or >120 beats/min throughout an observation period, the clinician should repeat assessment within 24 hours or less. Beat-to-beat variability generally ranges from 0.5 to 4 mm, with most in the range of 1 mm. This beat-to-beat variability requires an intact central nervous system and functioning sympathetic and parasympathetic systems. When measuring the variation, periods when the heart rate is not accelerating or decelerating should be used for an accurate observation. The finding of no beat-to-beat variation in the absence of maternal drug therapy that may sedate the fetus is an indication of loss of fetal central nervous system input into cardiac function, and repeat observations are indicated.

Biophysical Profile

Transabdominal ultrasonography and determining FHR is a simple method to determine that the fetus is alive, but a biophysical profile of the fetus can be generated from fetal monitoring in the late-term fetus to help determine fetal well-being. Useful measurements that can be collected to form a biophysical profile of the fetus include fetal aortic diameter, FHR and activity, fetal fluid depth and consistency, utero-placental thickness and contact, fetal position and presentation, and the presence of fetal breathing movements and activity (Table 69.4) [11]. At present, there is a limited number of large prospective trials that have evaluated the use of a biophysical profile as a test of fetal well-being in high-risk pregnancies in women or horses. In women a normal biophysical profile performed close to the time of parturition confers a high probability of perinatal survival and lack of acidosis. However, a normal biophysical profile does not guarantee a normal foal, nor does an abnormal profile always accurately predict an abnormal foal.

In a large retrospective case study, Reimer examined 122 mares with complicated pregnancies (e.g. premature lactation, vaginal discharge, history of still born foals, prolonged gestation, excessive abdominal size, abdominal pain, severe systemic illness, or signs of hemorrhage); of these mares examined via transabdominal ultrasound, 61% of pregnancies were considered ultrasonographically normal; subsequently, 70% of these pregnancies resulted in the birth of a normal foal and 16% resulted in foals that were stillborn, died, or were euthanized within 48 hours of birth [12]. Reef et al. [13, 14] also proposed a biophysical profile in pregnant mares using variables such as FHR, aortic diameter, fetal activity level, utero-placental thickness, uteroplacental contact, and maximal fetal fluid depth. A score of 2 (normal) and 0 (abnormal) was assigned to each variable, and the six variables are summed to give a biophysical profile score (range 0–12). A fetal score of ≤8 was assured of a negative outcome but a maximal score was not an assurance of a healthy foal [13, 14]. More recently, a prospective study evaluated the original biophysical profile scoring system using the six variables noted above as well as a second abbreviated scoring system (rapid examination protocol [REP]) in 129 late-term pregnant mares [10]. In the REP, only the FHR (marker of acute hypoxia), aortic diameter (marker of chronic hypoxia), and combined thickness of the uteroplacental unit (marker of placentitis) were measured. In this study, 27 of 129 foals did not survive the first 6 weeks of life (12 abortions, 15 weak or stillborn foals). The results of this study (Tables 69.5 and 69.6) suggested that both scoring systems might be useful for diagnosis of fetal abnormalities but did not reach the high accuracy of human surveillance tests [10].

The sonogram is performed through the acoustic window present from the udder to the xiphoid ventrally and laterally to the skinfolds of the flank. Imaging of the fetus requires a low-frequency (3.5-MHz) probe, whereas examination of the placenta and endometrium usually requires a higher-frequency (7.5-MHz) probe. Imaging the fetal heart generally requires a 2.5-MHz probe and depth of at least

Table 69.4 Measurements of fetal and maternal parameters in the 11th month of gestation [10].

Parameter	Mean ± SD (range)	Reference value
Fetal heart rate (BPM)	90 ± 11 (62–102)	57–104
Aortic diameter (mm)	20.5 ± 1.6 (19–24)	18–27
Fetal activity	2.4 ± 0.8 (1–3)	1–3
Fetal fluid depth (cm)		
Allantoic fluid	4.5 ± 2.7 (1.3–10.6)	4.7–22.1
Amniotic fluid	2.7 ± 1.7 (1.2–4.4)	0.8–14.9
Combined thickness of uteroplacental unit (mm)	13 ± 3 (9–16.5)	7–20

Table 69.5 Results of two fetal biophysical profile scores (original equine biophysical profile and rapid examination protocol) used to evaluate 129 pregnant mares [10]. In this study, 29 of 129 foals did not survive beyond 6 weeks of age.

	Equine biophysical profile (six parameters evaluated)			
Foals	**Score ⩽ 8**	**Score 10**	**Score 12**	**Total**
Compromised	20	7	0	27
Healthy	0	40	62	102
Total	20	47	62	129
	Rapid examination protocol (three parameters evaluated)			
	Score ⩽ 4	**Score 6**	**Total**	
Compromised	23	4	27	
Healthy	13	89	102	
Total	36	93	129	

Table 69.6 Comparison of statistical results regarding the diagnostic value of the equine biophysical profile and rapid examination protocol used to evaluate 129 pregnant mares [10].

Test	**Equine biophysical profile**	**Rapid examination protocol**
Statistical parameter	**Value (95% confidence interval)**	**Value (95% confidence interval)**
Sensitivity	81.5% (62–94%)	85.2% (66–96%)
Specificity	83.3% (75–90%)	87.3% (79–93%)
Positive predictive value	56.4% (45–67%)	63.9% (51–75%)
Negative predictive value	94.4% (88–97%)	95.7% (90–98%)
Accuracy	82.9% (75–89%)	86.8% (80–92%)
Positive likelihood ratio	4.89 (3.06–7.82)	6.68% (3.93–11.37)
Negative likelihood ratio	0.22 (0.1–0.49)	0.17% (0.07–0.42)
Disease prevalence	20.9% (13–29%)	20.9% (14–29%)

30 cm. The fetal heart is visualized within the fetal thorax and is generally the only beating object observed. If the heart is not beating, careful examination, ensuring that the entire fetal thorax has been seen, is usually necessary to be positive of fetal death in utero. A complete description of this examination is beyond the scope of this chapter, but the reader can find complete descriptions of the technique and normal values for specific gestation lengths in the relevant veterinary literature. The utility of this type of examination lies in its repeatability and low risk to the dam and fetus. Sequential examinations over time allow the clinician to follow the pregnancy and identify changes as they occur.

References

1 Liska, D.A., Akucewich, L.H., Marsells, R. et al. (2006). Pharmacokinetics of pentoxifylline and its 5-hydroxyhexyl metabolite after oral and intravenous administration of pentoxifylline to healthy adult horses. *Am. J. Vet. Res.* 67: 1621–1627.

2 Crisman, M.V., Wilcke, J.R., Correll, L.S. et al. (1993). Pharmacokinetic disposition of intravenous and oral pentoxifylline in horses. *J. Vet. Pharmacol. Ther.* 16: 23–31.

3 Erkert, R.S. and Macallister, C.G. (2002). Isoxsuprine hydrochloride in the horse: a review. *J. Vet. Pharmcol. Ther.* 25: 81–87.

4 Card, C.E. and Wood, M.R. (1995). Effects of acute administration of clenbuterol on uterine tone and equine fetal and maternal heart rates. *Biol. Reprod.* 52: 7–11.

5 Ousey, J.C., Kolling, M., Kindahl, H. et al. (2011). Maternal dexamethasone treatment in late gestation induces precocious fetal maturation and delivery in healthy Thoroughbred mares. *Equine Vet. J.* 43: 424–429.

6 Ross, J., Palmer, J.E., and Wilkins, P.A. (2008). Body wall tears during late pregnancy in mares: 13 cases (1995–2006). *J. Am. Vet. Med. Assoc.* 232 (2): 257–261.

7 Mitchell, B. (2015). Feeding the pregnant mare. *Equine Health* 26: 12–15.

8 Wilkins, P.A. (2003). Monitoring the pregnant mare in the ICU. *Clin. Tech. Equine Pract.* 2: 212–219.

9 Hardy, J. (2003). Nutritional support and nursing care of the adult horse in intensive care. *Clin. Tech. Equine Pract.* 2: 193–198.

10 Vincze, B., Baska, F., Papp, M. et al. (2019). Introduction of a new fetal examination protocol for on-field and clinical equine practice. *Theriogenology* 125: 210–215.

11 McGladdery, A.J. (1999). Ultrasonographic diagnosis and management of fetal abnormality in the mare in late gestation. *Pferdeheikunde* 15: 618–621.

12 Reimer, J.M. (1997). Use of transcutaneous ultrasonography in complicated latter-middle to late gestation pregnancies in the mare: 122 cases. *AAEP Proc.* 43: 259–261.

13 Reef, V.B., Vaala, W.E., Worth, L.T. et al. (1995). Ultrasonographic evaluation of the fetus and intrauterine environment in healthy mares during late gestation. *Vet. Radiol. Ultrasound* 36: 533–541.

14 Reef, V.B., Vaala, W.E., Worth, L.T. et al. (1996). Ultrasonographic assessment of fetal wellbeing during late gestation: development of an equine biophysical profile. *Equine Vet. J.* 28: 200–208.

Chapter 70 Poor Maternal Behavior, Induction of Lactation, and Foal Grafting

Theresa Beachler

The time surrounding parturition can be wrought with multiple complications, including primary agalactia or insufficient milk production, and insufficient milk production due to maternal illness or death, all of which may necessitate the need for alternative sources for neonatal nutrition. Foal rejection or poor maternal behavior, ranging from avoidance behavior and prevention of nursing to outright aggression, can also complicate care for the neonatal foal and require close monitoring to aggressive intervention. This chapter discusses how the clinician can modify poor maternal behavior, induce lactation, and facilitate foal grafting.

Normal Peripartum Behavior

The early peripartum period, especially the first 4–12 hours following parturition, is critical for establishing a healthy maternal-neonatal bond [1]. Most mares give birth between 9 p.m. and 5 a.m., with many mares preferring dark, quiet, and calm environments [2–4]. After periods of rest for both the newborn foal and dam postparturition, most mares will begin to vocalize and nicker to the foal and begin exhibiting sniffing and licking behavior. Visual, auditory, and olfactory cues assist in the establishment of the normal maternal-neonatal bond, with olfactory cues appearing to play a primary role in the establishment and recognition of the foal's identity through the licking behavior and olfactory stimulant of amniotic fluid [1, 5]. Once the bond is established, maternal behavior is maintained through suckling and auditory cues [1, 6].

Poor Maternal Behavior and Foal Rejection

Poor maternal behavior is not uncommon, with conduct ranging in a continuum from common early behaviors in primiparous mares to outright aggression and abandonment. Avoidance or reluctance to allow nursing is most commonly seen in primiparous mares but can also be observed in cases of mammary discomfort or engorgement [6, 7]. Additionally, other causes of postpartum pain can contribute to inappropriate initial maternal behavior and interfere with establishment of the maternal-neonatal bond [7]. While foal rejection can occur in any breed, it is most commonly described in Arabians and maiden mares or first-time mothers [7, 8]. In Arabian mares experiencing rejection, an imbalance of postpartum hormones might be involved, with mares experiencing rejection demonstrating a significant decrease in prolactin concentrations from days 1 to 3 immediately after parturition [9].

Treatment Recommendations

Mares exhibiting signs of poor maternal behavior or foal rejection should be monitored closely for at least the first 48–72 hours following parturition, if not longer, on a case-by-case basis. Avoidance to allow nursing or "over mothering" behaviors that may be more commonly seen in primiparous or maiden mares can be managed initially by restraining the mare and/or providing a distraction via provision of supplemental or additional hay or grain. Periodic sedation can be provided through the administration of xylazine, detomidine, butorphanol, or acepromazine (Table 70.1) [10, 11]. Use of anxiolytic medications such as diazepam, alprazolam, or trazadone have also been described to help quiet the anxious or aggressive mare; sedation can be observed with these medications and if observed/undesired, the dose can be decreased [1, 12–14]. Caution must be taken as some horses administered sedatives may become overstimulated, hypersensitive, and aggressive to external stimuli.

Careful application of a twitch, nose or lip chain, hobbles, crossties, or placement of mares in stocks or nursing chutes

Equine Neonatal Medicine, First Edition. Edited by David M. Wong and Pamela A. Wilkins.

Table 70.1 Medications that can be administered to mares with poor maternal behavior toward their foals.

Sedatives	
Xylazine	0.2–1 mg/kg, IV
Detomidine	0.01–0.02 mg/kg, IV
	0.02–0.04 mg/kg, IM
Butorphanol	0.01–0.03 mg/kg, IV or IM
Tranquilizer	
Acepromazine	0.02–0.05 mg/kg, IV or IM
Anxiolytics	
Diazepam	0.05 mg/kg, IV
Alprazolam	0.1 mg/kg, PO (loading dose); 0.04 mg/kg, PO (maintenance dose)
Trazadone	4–10 mg/kg, PO, q24h

may also be considered [9]. Application of muzzles may additionally be utilized in mares who have shown overt aggressive behaviors while trying to bite either their foals or individuals assisting in their care. In mares where discomfort appears to be a primary source of untoward behaviors, administration of an anti-inflammatory such as flunixin meglumine (1.1 mg/kg IV, q12h) may be helpful [10]. Administration of altrenogest (0.044–0.088 mg/kg po q24h) has also been used in an attempt to modify maternal behavior with varied clinical success [10]. In primates, canines, and cattle, administration of intranasal atomized oxytocin has been utilized to stimulate appropriate social and maternal behavior and as an anxiolytic; however, to the author's knowledge, this has not yet been studied on an experimental or clinical basis in horses [15–17]. Continued close monitoring following initiation of treatment with any of the above-described therapies remains critical for monitoring of success or for regression and return of inappropriate behaviors. When treatment fails, or in cases of true overt unresponsive aggression, administration of prostaglandins as part of the concaveation (i.e. sensitizing the dam to the foal) method or reprogramming may be considered (described below). These protocols are also frequently utilized when introducing nurse mares for adopting or grafting orphan foals.

In situations where the mare fully rejects her foal, is unable to produce milk, or dies in the initial postpartum period, the orphan foal must be supplemented by alternative sources of nutrition, including nasogastric administration of mare's milk or milk replacer, bucket training, bottle feeding, or grafting onto a nurse mare. Nurse mares classically include mares who have recently weaned their natural foal, mares whose natural foal has recently died, or mares who are commercially leased to raise orphans [18]. Commercial nurse mare farms are located throughout the United States and either have mares that are bred to be available to adopt orphans or are brought into lactation pharmacologically for the same purpose. Raising an orphan foal with a nurse mare has additional benefits outside of a simple source of nutrition, including companionship, normal bonding, and establishment of normal social behaviors to other horses and humans involved in their care [18].

Induction of Lactation

Over the last 20 years, protocols have been developed to induce lactation in barren or open mares. Some commercial nurse mare farms have utilized these protocols to have mares available for serving as nurse mares and avoid ethical concerns of creating an unwanted pregnancy and separating a neonate from its natural mother. They additionally can be utilized to bring a mare, owned by the orphan foal, into lactation, thus avoiding the financial burden of pursuing a commercial nurse mare.

Initially, protocols used to induce lactation involved the administration of vaginal pessaries containing the synthetic progestin altrenogest and estradiol benzoate with subsequent treatment with either oxytocin and the dopamine antagonist sulpiride or domperidone, with most mares responding and beginning lactation 7–12 days following initiation of treatment [19, 20]. Dopamine antagonists increase prolactin secretion from the pituitary gland and subsequently cause and increase milk production. Domperidone is currently labeled for treating agalactia in mares affected by fescue toxicosis [21]. Clinically, many clinicians attempt to increase milk production in mares who are agalactic or dysgalactic at dose of 1.1 mg/kg PO, q12–24h.

Protocols for the induction of lactation have been refined over time and commonly involve the administration of a combination of synthetic progestin (altrenogest), estradiol, dopamine antagonist (domperidone or sulpiride), and prostaglandin, as described by Daels and colleagues [22–24]. Common protocols (for the average-sized 450–500 kg mare) consist of the administration of prostaglandin $F_2\alpha$ (5 mg IM), estradiol benzoate (50 mg IM), altrenogest (44 mg PO), and domperidone (1.1 mg/kg PO, q12h) on day 1. On days 2 through adoption, mares are administered estradiol benzoate (10 mg IM, q24h), altrenogest (44 mg PO, q24h), and domperidone (1.1 mg/kg PO, q12h). Domperidone is then continued for 7–10 days after successful adoption (1.1 mg/kg PO, q12h) [22, 23]. Another protocol utilizing sulpiride consists of the administration of estradiol benzoate (50 mg IM, once on day 1), altrenogest (22 mg IM, q24h, days 1–7), and sulpiride (1 mg/kg IM, q12h, days 1 until 5–7 days after adoption) [23].

Mares selected for lactation induction ideally should be open or not pregnant, in good body condition, in good general health with no systemic disease, gentle, easy to handle, and good-natured. Previous experience foaling and raising a foal is also ideal [22–24]. Some clinicians recommend keeping the mare and foal adjacent to each other or in visual contact during the induction protocol; however, this may not be necessary when utilizing subsequent grafting procedures as described below [23, 25]. General response in mammary development and milk production can be seen within 4 to 7 days following initiation of an induction protocol. Milking may be instituted upon the onset of secretion production or at the time of adoption, depending on preference [22]. Milking may be performed by hand, with commercialized milking devices, or using milking machines designed for sheep and goats. Small ruminant milking machines, when used, should be set to 120 aspirations/min; vacuum, 22 cmHg; and alternation vacuum/rest, 50/50 [19, 20, 22, 23]. When milk production has reached 3–5 l/d for the average 500 kg mare, readiness for adoption is typically indicated [22]. Some mares have been noted to produce good-quality colostrum following lactation induction, but this is not uniformly observed [19, 24]. Inducing lactation in an early pregnant mare has also been described using domperidone (1.1 mg/kg po q24h for 4 days) followed by sulpiride (1 mg/kg IM q12h) until day 10 [26].

Foal Grafting

Fostering a foal onto a nurse mare is another period that may be wrought with stress for the mare, foal, and individuals managing adoption. As described above, sedation and physical restraint methods should be utilized at the clinician's discretion. As mares rely on olfactory stimulation for recognition of their natural foal in addition to sight, placement of a blanket from a recently deceased foal or from the foal removed from a commercial nurse mare onto the adoptive foal has been utilized [1, 4, 5, 24]. Masking of the adopted foal's natural smell can also be considered by applying an odiferous ointment (camphor) into the adoptive mare's nostrils and onto the foal's coat [1, 4, 27]. Finally, topical administration of the mare's own milk or sweat onto the foal's coat following prostaglandin administration, as described below, might also be effective [1, 26].

Before introducing the orphan foal to the adoptive mare, clinicians can consider performing vaginal-cervical stimulation, the concaveation method, or a combination of both. Each of these methods aims to mimic neuroendocrine signals that occur at the time of parturition. Vaginal and cervical stimulation consists of vigorous massage to induce Ferguson's reflex following aseptic preparation of the mare's perineum. Massage of the internal vagina and external cervix is performed for 2–3 minutes, twice, in 10-minute intervals with the foal held at the mare's head or side [23, 28]. In one study, adoption took longer in mares who did not receive vaginal-cervical stimulation compared to those that did [28].

In the concaveation method, high doses of prostaglandins are administered to cause a release of oxytocin from the central nervous system [25, 26, 29]. Administration of systemic intramuscular and intravenous oxytocin has not been found to be effective [25, 26, 29]. Three to four times the typical luteolytic dose of prostaglandin are used (750–1000 μg of cloprostenol IM, or 15–25 mg of dinoprost IM, in the average-size light horse) [25, 26]. Over the next 15–20 minutes post-administration, the mare is monitored for signs of appropriate strong side effects, including sweating, restlessness, soft manure, abdominal discomfort, or mild colic (Figure 70.1) [30]. At this point, the foal is then introduced to the mare.

When introducing the foal, it is recommended to first bring the foal to the mare's head and monitor for signs of maternal behavior, including nickering, licking, and smelling of the foal. The foal is then gradually moved to the mare's flank, allowed, and stimulated as needed to latch and nurse from the mare's mammary gland. Continued maternal behavior is closely monitored for acceptance before leaving the pair unobserved, which may take 4–24 hours [18]. If acceptance is not complete or signs of aggression are noted upon introduction, consider allowing the pair to rest (either separated or within each other's sight) and repeating the protocol 12–24 hours later [25].

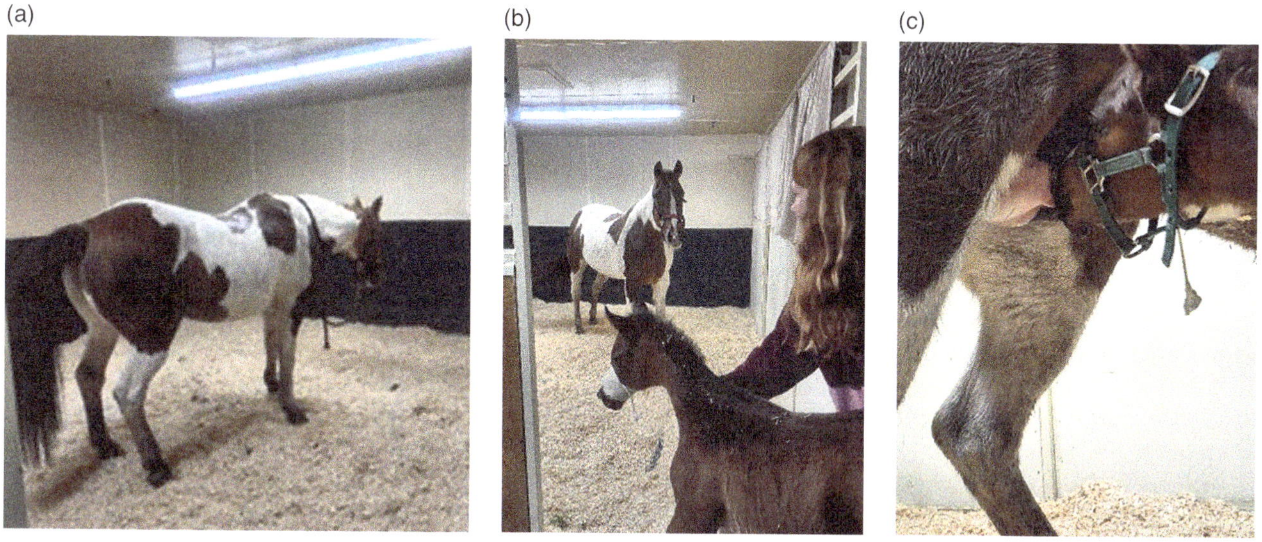

Figure 70.1 Induction of lactation in a Paint mare followed by grafting of an orphan foal to the mare. (a) Medications were administered for 7 days to the mare to induce lactation (as described in chapter). When udder development was present, grafting of an orphan foal to the mare was initiated. In this image, the mare received a high dose of prostaglandins; the mare subsequently displayed physical signs of sweating and mild colic. (b) 15 minutes post-prostaglandin administration, a 5-day-old orphan Thoroughbred foal was introduced to the mare. (c) Within 30–45 minutes post-prostaglandin administration, the mare allowed the foal to nurse and developed a maternal-neonatal bond.

References

1 Chavatte, P. (1991). Maternal behaviour in the horse; theory and practical applications to foal rejection and fostering. *Equine. Vet. Educ.* 3: 215–220.

2 Rossdale, P.D. and Short, R.V. (1967). The time of foaling of Thoroughbred mares. *J. Reprod. Fertil.* 13: 341–343.

3 Bain, A.M. and Howey, W.P. (1975). Observations on the time of foalings in Thoroughbred mares in Australia. *J. Reprod. Fertil. Suppl.* 23: 545.

4 Naylor, J.M. and Bell, R.J. (1987). Feeding the sick or orphaned foal. In: *Current Therapy in Equine Medicine*, 2e (ed. E. Robinson), 205–209. Philadelphia, PA: WB Saunders.

5 Keverne, E.B. (1988). Central mechanisms underlying the neural and neuroendocrine determinants of maternal behaviour. *Psychoneuroendocrinology* 13: 127–141.

6 Crowell-Davis, S.L. (1986). Developmental behaviour. *Vet. Clin. North Am. Equine Pract.* 2: 573–590.

7 Crowell- Davis, S.L. (1986). Maternal behaviour. *Vet. Clin. North Am. Equine Pract.* 2: 557–571.

8 Berlin, D., Steinman, A., and Raz, T. (2018). Post-partum concentrations of serum progesterone, oestradiol and prolactin in Arabian mares demonstrating normal maternal behaviour and Arabian mares demonstrating foal rejection behaviour. *Vet. J.* 232: 40–45.

9 Juarbe-Díaz, S.V., Houpt, K.A., and Kusunose, R. (1998). Prevalence and characteristics of foal rejection in Arabian mares. *Equine Vet. J.* 30: 424–428.

10 McCue, P.M. (2021). Foal rejection. In: *Equine Reproductive Procedures*, 2e (ed. J. Dascanio and P. McCue), 719–721. Hoboken, NJ: Wiley.

11 Hubbell, J.A.E. (2009). Practical standing chemical restraint of the horse. *Proc. Annu. Conv. Am. Assoc. Equine. Pract.* 55: 1–6.

12 Massey, R.E. (1991). Feeding and socializing orphed foals. *Vet. Med.* 86: 518–526.

13 Wong, D.M., Davis, J.L., Alcott, C.J. et al. (2014). Pharmacokinetics and physiologic effects of alprazolam after a single oral dose in healthy mares. *J. Vet. Pharmacol. Therap.* 38: 301–304.

14 Davis, J.L., Schirmer, J., and Medlin, E. (2018). Pharmacokinetics, pharmacodynamics and clinical use of trazodone and its active metabolite m-chlorophenyl-piperazine in the horse. *J. Vet. Pharmacol. Therap.* 41: 393–401.

15 Mason, S. (2016). The use of intranasal oxytocin therapy for bitches post caesarean section. In: *Proceedings of the Australian Reproduction Veterinarians Seminar, Treatment Updates for Specific Disease Conditions.*, 9–10. Surfers Paradise, Queensland: Australian Reproductive Veterinians.

16 Parker, K.J., Buckmaster, C.L., Schatzberg, A.F. et al. (2005). Intranasal oxytocin administration attenuates the ACTH stress response in monkeys. *Psychoneuroendocrinology* 30: 924–929.

17 Houpt, K.A. (2012). Small animal maternal behavior and its abberations. In: *Recent Advances in Companion Animal Behavior Problems* (ed. K.A. Houpt). Ithaca, NY: International Veterinary Information Service https://www.ivis.org/library/recent-advances-companion-animal-behavior-problems/small-animal-maternal-behavior-and-its.

18 Paradis, M.R. (2012). Feeding the orphan foal. *Proc. Annu. Conv. Am. Assoc. Equine Pract.* 58: 402–406.

19 Chavatte-Palmer, P., Arnaud, G., Duvaux-Ponter, C. et al. (2002). Quantitative and qualitative assessment of milk production after pharmaceutical induction of lactation in the mare. *J. Vet. Intern. Med.* 16: 472–477.

20 Guillaume, D., Chavatte-Palmer, P., Combarnous, Y. et al. (2003). Induced lactation with a dompamine antagonist in mares: different responses between ovariectomized mares and intact mares. *Reprod. Domest. Anim.* 38: 394–400.

21 Redmond, L.M., Cross, D.L., Strickland, J.R. et al. (1994). Efficacy of domperidone and sulpiride as treatments for fescue toxicosis in horses. *Am. J. Vet. Res.* 55: 722–729.

22 Daels, P.F., Ducham, P., and Porter, D. (2002). Induction of lactation and adoption of foals by non-parturient mares. *Proc. Annu. Conv. Am. Assoc. Equine Pract.* 48: 68–71.

23 Daels, P.F. and Bowers-Lepore, J. (2007). How to induce lactation in a mare and make her adopt an orphan foal: what 5 years of experience have taught us. *Proc. Annu. Conv. Am. Assoc. Equine Pract.* 53: 349–353.

24 Paradis, M.R. (2012). Feeding the orphan foal. *Proc. Annu. Conv. Am. Assoc. Equine Pract.* 58: 401–406.

25 Daels, P.F. and Dini, P. (2021). Fostering a foal onto a nurse mare. In: *Equine Reproductive Procedures*, 2e (ed. J. Dascanio and P. McCue), 723–724. Hoboken, NJ: Wiley.

26 Podico, G., Migliorisi, A.C., Wilkins, P.A. et al. (2022). Successful induction of lactation, foal grafting and maintenance of pregnancy in a nonparturient Thoroughbred mare. *Equine. Vet. Educ.* 34: e1–e10.

27 Rossdale, P.D. and Ricketts, S.W. (1980). Orphan foals. In: *Equine Stud Farm Medicine*, 2e, 372–343. London: Balliere Tindall Co.

28 Porter, R.H., Duchamp, G., Nowak, R. et al. (2002). Induction of maternal behavior in non-parturient adoptive mares. *Phisol. Behav.* 77: 151–154.

29 Fuchs, A. (1987). Prostaglandin F2alpha and oxytocin interactions in ovarian and uterine function. *J. Steroid Biochem.* 27: 1073–1080.

30 Coffman, E.A. and Pinto, C.R. (2016). A review on the use of prostaglandin F2α for controlling the estrous cycle of mares. *J. Equine Vet. Sci.* 40: 34–40.

Chapter 71 Maternal Complications Associated with Parturition

Giorgia Podico and Pamela A. Wilkins

Maternal complications associated with parturition are common in the mare and, at times, can be quite serious. While the attention is frequently focused on the newborn foal, a thorough physical examination of the mare, particularly of the reproductive tract, is a prudent measure to help ensure maternal health and future reproductive abilities. This chapter discusses some of the common postpartum medical concerns that can be observed.

Metritis

Metritis is one of the most common postpartum complications in the horse and is characterized by inflammation of all three layers of the uterus and by the presence of a systemic inflammatory response [1]. It most frequently occurs in the first 24–72 hours after foaling but may also occur up to 10 days post-foaling. While it is more common after dystocia, and retained fetal membranes (RFM), it can also develop after normal foaling. Draft horses seem more predisposed to metritis [2]; this also is observed by the authors, who have seen a considerably high number of Belgian mares presented for metritis from the nearby Amish communities. Due to their breed predisposition for RFM, Friesians are also considered more predisposed to metritis [3].

The pathogenesis of metritis is multifactorial and involves bacterial contamination and poor uterine clearance, worsened by a disruption in the endometrium that allows for the absorption of bacteria, endotoxins, and other pathogen associated molecular patterns (PAMPs). Metritis is most often characterized by mixed bacterial infections [4, 5] with *E. coli* and *S. zooepidemicus* being the most common isolates [6]. Anaerobes are involved only in rare cases [5].

Predisposing factors include variables that affect the integrity of the endometrium or increase the uterine bacterial load, such as dystocia and RFM (Figure 71.1) [7]. Additionally, conditions that affect uterine involution and clearance also predispose to metritis; in the author's experience, mares that have sick and hospitalized foals are at higher risk of metritis due to the lack of exercise/movement and the endogenous release of oxytocin from the foal suckling. As in other species, the integrity of the epithelial lining of the uterus is crucial to the development of toxic metritis; for example, uterine infusion of *E. coli* endotoxin in the postpartum uterus of healthy ponies did not lead to toxic metritis in one study [7, 8].

Clinical signs of metritis include depression, anorexia, and fever. One of the earliest detected signs is decreased milk production, evidenced by a foal that is continuously nursing. Other common signs include purulent vulvar discharge, lameness (e.g., laminitis), and abdominal contractions due to RFM (Figure 71.2). In cases of severe metritis, possible sequela includes the systemic inflammatory response syndrome (SIRS), laminitis, and death [7]. Other comorbidities that can present with metritis include cervicitis, vaginitis, and peritonitis [7].

Suspicion of metritis is based on physical examination that reveals congested mucous membranes, tachycardia, tachypnea, fever, and, potentially, increased digital pulses. Additional diagnostic tests include CBC, which commonly shows leukopenia with a degenerative left shift, and the assessment of acute phase proteins such as fibrinogen and serum amyloid A (SAA), which are increased in the presence of metritis. However, the clinician should be aware that in normal post-foaling mares, increased concentrations of fibrinogen and SAA can be present without metritis being present. A reproductive examination generally reveals purulent vulvar discharge and potential trauma due to parturition or dystocia (hematoma, bruises, vulvar lacerations); during transvaginal examination, different degrees of uterine involution, low uterine contractility, and a variable amount of intrauterine fluid (brownish to

Equine Neonatal Medicine, First Edition. Edited by David M. Wong and Pamela A. Wilkins.

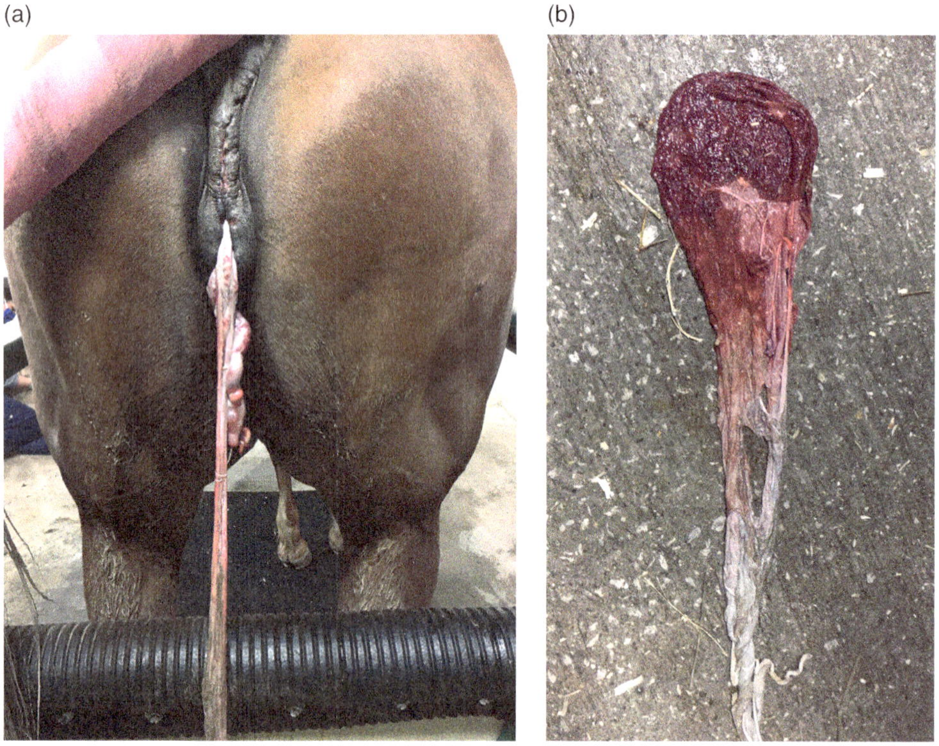

Figure 71.1 Retained fetal membranes predispose mares to metritis. The placenta can be retained (a) entirely or (b) partially.

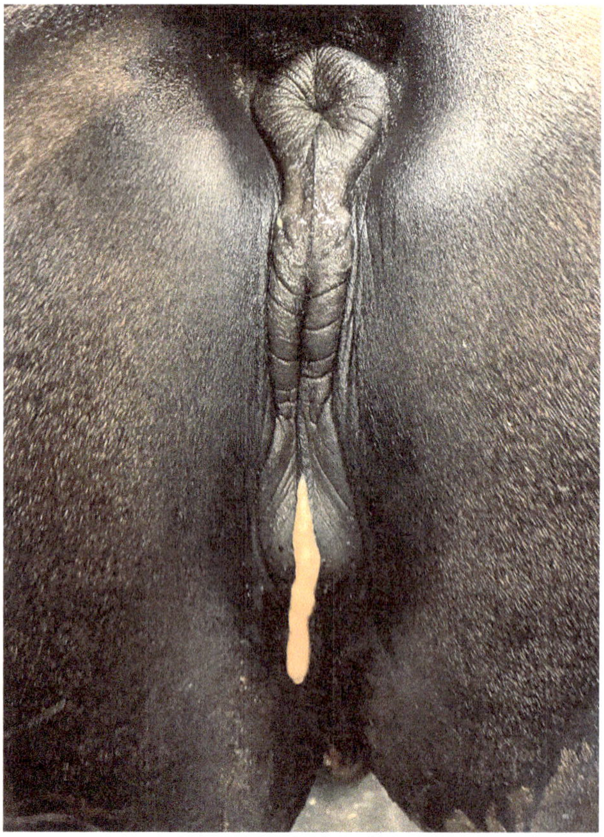

Figure 71.2 Postpartum mare with purulent vulvar discharge.

purulent) with varying viscosity are identifiable (Figure 71.3). The presence of pieces of the placenta, uterine tears, or roughening of the endometrium may also be found and support a diagnosis of metritis. Samples of uterine fluid should be submitted for culture, sensitivity testing, and cytology. Daily cytologic evaluation of recovered uterine fluid can be performed to monitor the efficacy of the treatments by assessing the pattern of the inflammatory cells present. Noteworthy, mares with uncomplicated puerperium had inflammatory cells and red blood cells (RBCs) in their lochia, but the amounts significantly decrease 4 days following foaling [9].

Treatment of metritis includes systemic and uterine therapies with broad-spectrum antibiotics as the first line of therapy. The choice of antibiotics follows principles for judicious use of antimicrobials; however, due to time constraints, treatments are often decided empirically prior to availability of culture results. The most commonly used antibiotic therapies are a combination of β-lactams and aminoglycosides or oral sulfonamides; metronidazole can also be selected in more severe cases and when anaerobic contribution is suspected. Of note, one study showed that the combination of penicillin G procaine and gentamicin was effective against bacteria isolated from 65% of the mares included in the study and from 48.8% of mares for trimethoprim/sulfonamide [6]. Intrauterine antibiotics are not often used due to concerns for lower efficacy in

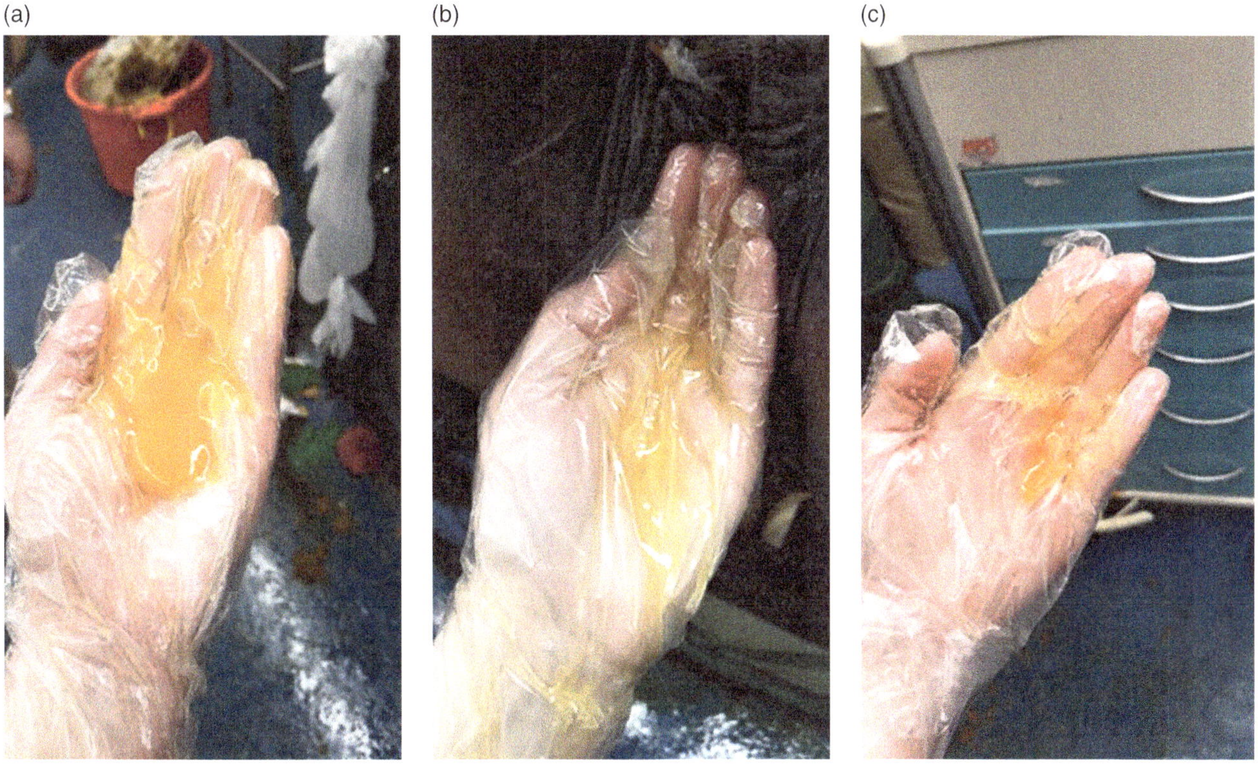

Figure 71.3 Macroscopic changes in the fluid recovered from a mare treated for metritis over the course of three days (a–c).

the presence of lochia, which has extreme variations in pH and the presence of purulent material [10]. While this appears true for ceftiofur, the efficacy of the combination of gentamicin and procaine penicillin G was not altered in the presence of lochia in an in vitro study [11]. Based on the author's experience, a key treatment component is local lavage; removal of any RFM and mechanical removal and dilution of uterine fluid to decrease the bacterial load and PAMPs present in the uterus appears to be the most effective therapy. Uterine lavage is performed using a large bore nasogastric tube and a large volume of fluid to fully distend the entire uterus[12]. Homemade saline or Lactated Ringer's solution can be used as the lavage fluid. The authors use distilled water supplemented with 45 g of table salt (NaCl) per gallon and iodine solution until it is roughly the same color as diluted tea (Figure 71.4). The fluid can be placed in robust obstetric sleeves, with the first bag having no iodine solution, and it is recovered in clear sleeves to be able to fully evaluate the character of the recovered fluid (Figure 71.5). Uterine lavage may be repeated 2-4 times per day, depending on the severity of the metritis and any underlying conditions such as RFM. Other clinicians might avoid the use of frequent uterine lavages containing iodine solution due to concerns that these solutions may alter blood flow and permeability of the uterus, potentially translating to increased PAMP absorption.

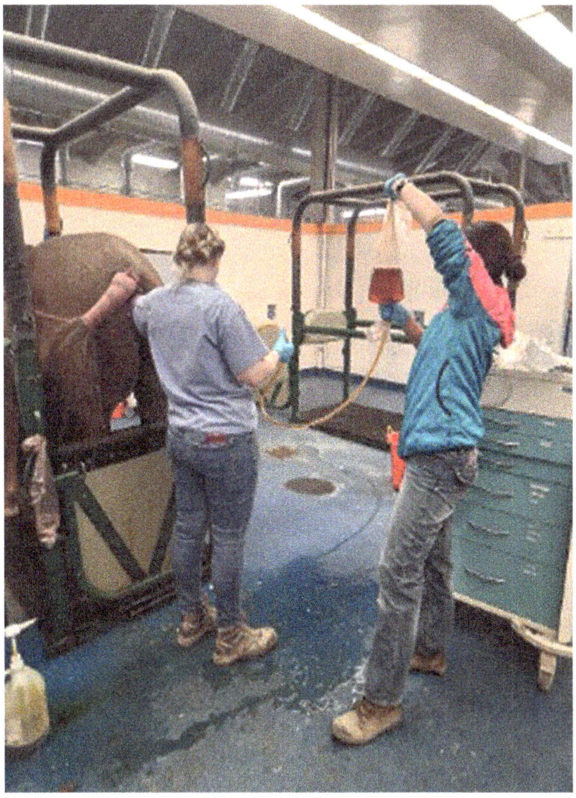

Figure 71.4 Large-volume uterine lavage in a mare with metritis. The clinician guides the tube transvaginally into the uterus to distend it with fluid before recovering back into the sleeve.

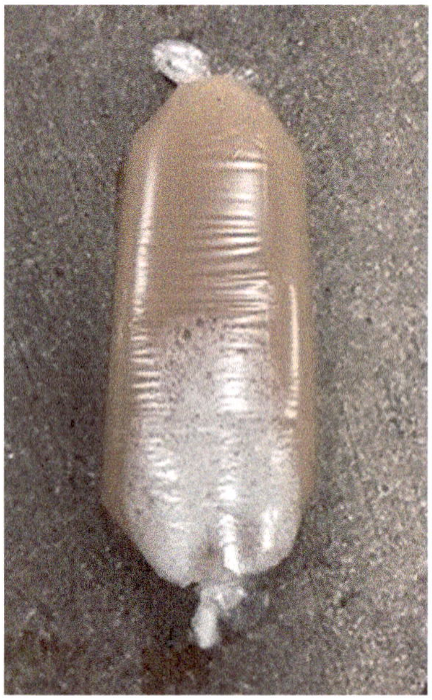

Figure 71.5 Effluent from the first uterine lavage performed in a mare with metritis.

Sedation can be used to modulate abdominal contractions and discomfort during lavage and improve safety as it is not unusual to perform these procedures with the mares restrained and standing in a stall doorway. The administration of ecbolics to promote uterine fluid clearance includes oxytocin (2–20 IU) as frequent IM or IV boluses (2-4 times per day) or as a continuous IV infusion with other fluids and calcium borogluconate. Prostaglandin F2α (e.g. cloprostenol sodium 250 µg IM) may be given in cases where only twice-a-day injections are possible. Drugs to support lactation are also recommended (sulpiride 1 mg/kg q12h, IM or PO; domperidone 1 mg/kg q24h, PO). IV fluids may be given if required by the overall condition of the mare, particularly if systemic illness is recognized. Anti-inflammatory medications commonly used include flunixin meglumine and acetaminophen (dosage adjusted based on severity of metritis). Medication to prevent gastric ulcers (omeprazole 1 mg/kg q24h PO) should be considered. Uterine contractility also benefits from exercise, but exercise should be avoided if there are signs of laminitis; it is common in the author's institution to bring the mare for a 10- to 15-minute walk after the uterine lavage and oxytocin administration. Exercise is commonly limited in cases where the foal is sick and hospitalized. Laminitis and endotoxemia, if present, are considered medical emergencies and require immediate attention.

Prevention of metritis points back to the peripartum and immediate post-foaling periods. Proper foaling detection and assistance and timely treatment of peripartum conditions (e.g. RFM, dystocia) are important predisposing factors of metritis and go a long way toward prevention. Hygiene in the foaling stall is paramount because ascending contamination can worsen the bacterial load and introduce opportunistic bacteria into the uterus through the open cervix. A post-foaling examination should be performed on every mare to evaluate for predisposing factors or early signs of metritis. An innovative approach was proposed by a research group from Kentucky that used a product based on Mycobacterium cell wall fraction to stimulate the uterine immune system and hasten postpartum involution. Noteworthy, the bacterial growth was lower in mares that were treated with Mycobacterium cell wall fraction and had a negative uterine culture three days earlier than control mares [13].

Retained Fetal Membranes

RFM occur in up to 10% of normal foalings and up to 54% of foalings in predisposed breeds such as the Friesian; they are considered a medical emergency due to the potentially severe consequences on the mare [3, 14]. The horse has a diffuse, epitheliochorial, microcotiledonary placentation that forms around 40–50 days of gestation and is arranged in tight interdigitations with the crypts present in the endometrium; it has been reported that older mares have deeper crypts and, thus, are more predisposed to RFM (Figure 71.6). The allantochorion membrane is the portion of fetal membranes that is entirely or partially retained during this condition [14, 15]. The expulsion of the amnion occurs during stage 2 together with the fetus as it is the membrane that directly surrounds it, whereas the expulsion of the allantochorion should occur and be completed during stage 3 of parturition within 3 hours of its onset [14–16]. The detachment and expulsion of the placenta requires highly coordinated inflammatory and immunologic cascades that lead to the release of the microvilli from the endometrial crypts and its passage adjuvanted by synchronized myometrial contractions [14, 17]. The exact pathogenesis of RFM in the mare is not fully elucidated; a higher amount of fibrotic tissue and adhesions and a different profile of the metalloproteinases responsible for the remodeling of the extracellular matrix has been found in draft horses that experience RFM [18, 19]. In cows with RFM, studies have demonstrated a reduced number of macrophages and proinflammatory molecules at the interface with the caruncular tissue; a similar mechanism remains unproven in mares [20]. A breed predisposition was found in Friesian horses, which appears to be linked to a lower level of serum calcium concentration [3]. Other risk factors for RFM include placental diseases, dystocia, prolonged gestation, peripartum hemorrhage, induction of parturition, and previous history of RFM [21–24].

Mares with RFM can present with no clinical signs other than pieces of fetal membranes protruding from the

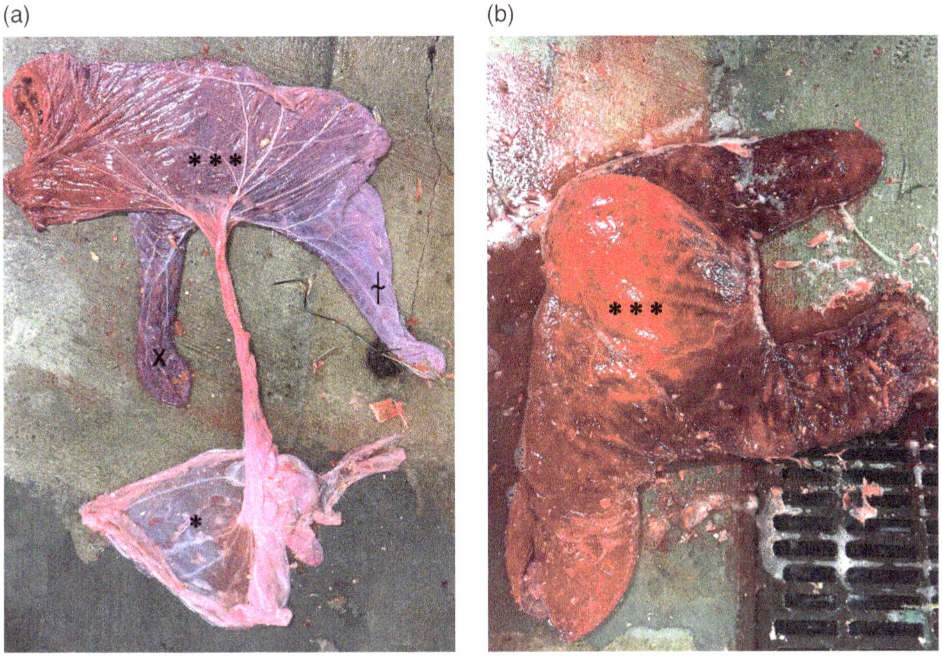

Figure 71.6 Normal and intact placenta recovered after parturition in a mare. Note the amniotic (*) and chorioallantoic membranes (***) (a, allantoic surface; b, chorionic surface). The portion of the uterine horn most often involved in retained fetal membranes is the gravid horn (✝), which is recognizable for the physiological presence of edema at its tip.

vulva; alternatively, mare can present with clinical signs of the common complications, metritis and laminitis. Thus, they present with fever, anorexia, purulent vulvar discharge, lameness, and other signs of endotoxemia (Figure 71.7) [14]. In some cases, RFM only causes mild endometritis, and tags of placenta can, in rare cases, be found as an incidental finding during the post-foaling examination [14]. The mare may also show signs of trauma to the caudal reproductive tract due to the occurrence of dystocia and its treatment (Figure 71.7) [24]. Diagnosis is established via physical examination and a thorough reproductive examination. Tags of retained membranes can vary in size and can be detected by palpation via transvaginal examination of the reproductive tract (Figure 71.8); during this procedure, the presence and features of the uterine content should also be evaluated to estimate the severity of the inflammatory process and gauge the intensity of treatments required. Ultrasound examination of the uterus can also help localize portions of retained membranes as hyperechoic structures in the lumen or adhering to the folds.

Additional diagnostic tests to determine the extent of the systemic inflammatory process and laminitis (e.g. CBC, radiography) should be pursued pending the severity of the case. The postpartum evaluation of the placenta ensures the earliest diagnosis as it allows the clinician to determine if it is intact and infer its morphology and the presence of pathological conditions that could affect the mare and the foal (Figure 71.6).

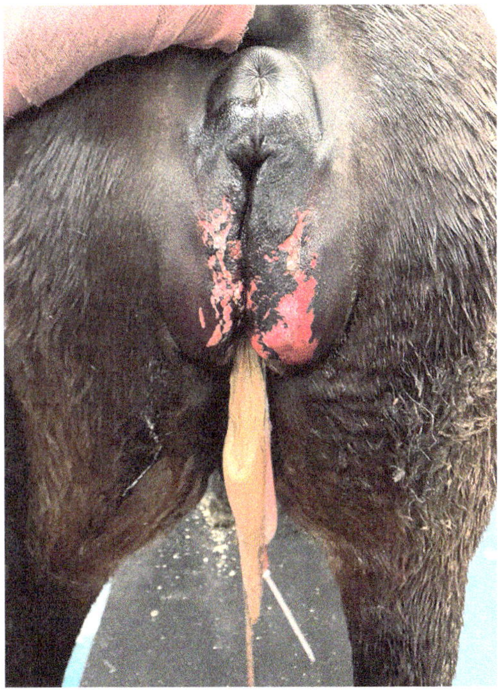

Figure 71.7 Portion of the chorioallantois is visibly protruding from the vulva. Mares presenting for retained fetal membranes often have lacerations, hematomas, and bruises linked to the dystocia and its correction.

One of the first treatment goals is removing the membrane portions still present in the uterus, which represent a constant source of bacteria and endotoxins. The degree of

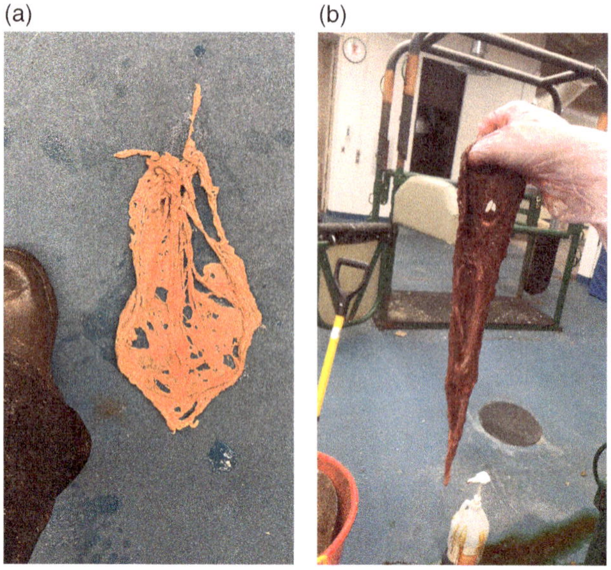

Figure 71.8 (a) and (b). Placental tags may differ greatly in size.

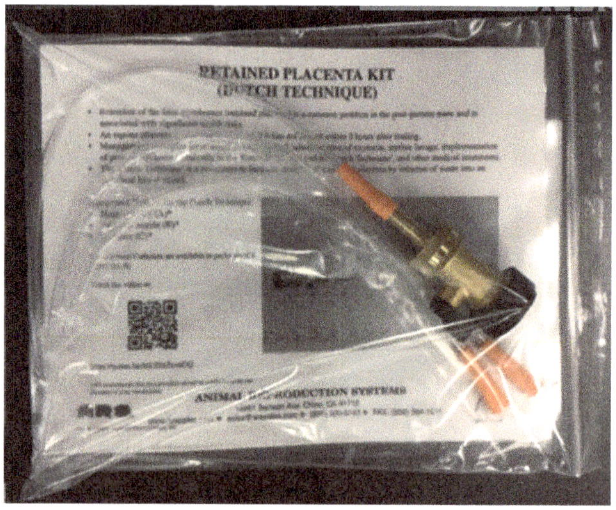

Figure 71.9 Commercial kit with adapter for the garden hose coupled to a stallion catheter to be used in mares with retained fetal membranes. *Source:* www.arsequine.com.

the treatment depends on the severity of the clinical signs shown by the mare, and in more severe cases, it is necessary to refer the mare to a facility with an intensive care unit [25]. Infusing the umbilical vessels with fluid is the most effective technique when the placenta is not yet necrotic and is entirely present in the uterus [26]. This technique ("Dutch technique") was first developed in the Netherlands on Friesian horses using a garden hose connected to a catheter to infuse water into the umbilical vessels of the placenta; a commercial kit is now available in the United States (Figure 71.9) [26]. The water infused through the umbilical vessels distends the chorionic vessels and helps with the mechanical distension and release of the membrane from the crypts of the endometrium.

One of the authors (GP) uses the Dutch technique with tap water and povidone-iodine solution (0.05–0.1%) that is infused using an stomach pump through a stallion catheter or a 16FR uterine flush catheter with a bullet-tip in one of the umbilical vessels. The author's clinical experience suggests that it is highly effective in 30–40 minutes and can be safely used on mares after dystocia and fetotomy. The management of RFM after cesarean section is controversial; some clinicians prefer to defer the removal of the placenta through either medical or mechanical means until a few days after the surgery with the concerns of bleeding, excessive contractions, and risk for evisceration. However, a recent study on a limited number of mares demonstrated that the Dutch technique could be safely applied immediately after C-section [27].

Another technique that could be used when the uterine body portion is protruding from the cervix or vagina is the Burns technique, where a large amount of fluid (tap water with table salt [45 g NaCl per gallon of water] with 0.05–0.1% povidone-iodine) is infused into the allantoic cavity until complete or semi-complete distension, and then kept in place for 10–15 minutes; the distension and weight of the distended membranes causes detachment from the endometrial crypts and stimulates uterine contractions [28].

Ecbolics and uterotonics may be administered simultaneously to increase the success of the above procedures [12]. Using an external pulling force on the placenta by adding weight to it, (e.g. bag of grain or water) is still made in the field, mostly by breeders; however, this method might cause further endometrial edema, postpone the release of the placenta, and sever the placenta into smaller pieces [24]. When there are only small pieces or a portion of the uterine horn (i.e. the nongravid horn), a uterine lavage may be performed 2-4 times per day using a large-bore nasogastric tube and a large volume of fluid. Ringer's lactate solution or saline made with distilled water and table salt (45 g of table salt per gallon of water) can be used; the author (GP) uses povidone-iodine (0.05–0.1%) in both types of fluid. The uterine lavage may be repeated based on the uterine content features and the mare's clinical status (i.e. fever, lameness) [12, 29].

There is no consensus about the active detachment and removal of the placenta from the uterus either after normal foaling or in the case of RFM [30]. Indeed, many clinicians consider those maneuvers risky, predisposing the mare to hemorrhage, uterine horn intussusception, uterine prolapse, delayed uterine involution, uterine scarring, and fibrosis. In the author's (GP) experience, the gentle detachment of the chorion from the endometrium using the fingertips during the uterine lavage does not pose harm and allows a quicker release of the retained membranes; if strong abdominal contractions start or there is a bloody recovery from the uterine lavage, then the detachment process should be discontinued immediately and the lavage should be completed without more manipulation on the membranes.

Ecbolics and uterotonics are used to promote and sustain uterine contractility. Oxytocin may be given as frequent boluses (2–20 IU, q6–12h, IM or IV), as a continuous rate infusion (1 U/min for 1h, q6h), or together with calcium borogluconate (60 IU oxytocin, 450 ml calcium borogluconate in 1 l of saline over 1 hour) [3, 15, 24]; some mares in the first 24–36 hours after parturition, especially in certain more sensitive breeds like Arabians, can show signs of colic, and the dose of ecbolics should be adjusted based on clinical signs [24]. Prostaglandin F2α (cloprostenol 250 µg q12h, IM) can also be used, but its efficacy for the treatment of RFM has not been investigated. In nonpregnant cycling mares, prostaglandin F2α causes uterine contractions of longer duration than oxytocin, and its administration can be advantageous in the field where more frequent administrations are not feasible [31]. Broad-spectrum antibiotics should be started following a regimen similar to that described in the metritis section. The use of an anti-inflammatory/analgesicmedication such as flunixin meglumine, is recommended for its anti-endotoxic effect at a lower dose (0.25 mg/kg q8h, IV) or its higher analgesic dose (1 mg/kg q12h, IV) to be used for the treatment of pain due to dystocia [32]. Hydration level and renal function must be monitored because of the nephrotoxicity side effects of nonsteroidal anti-inflammatory drugs (NSAIDs) and aminoglycosides; IV fluid therapy is recommended in case of dehydration and endotoxemia [33]. Tetanus toxoid should be administered in mares with unknown vaccination history. Managing laminitis as a complication of RFM is paramount for the prognosis; refer to Hood [34] for further details. The reproductive prognosis after RMF is good for uncomplicated cases but is not favorable in every case, depending on the severity of the metritis, chronic endometritis, and concomitant laminitis.

Trauma to the Caudal Reproductive Tract

The three barriers of the reproductive tract are the cervix, the vestibular sphincter, and the vulva. Conservation of their functional anatomy is paramount to avoid aspiration of air and contaminants that lead to inflammation and reproductive tract infections. Traumatic lesions to these barriers occur most often during parturition and dystocia [35]. Trauma is more common in maiden mares or during an abortion because the tissues are not properly relaxed and ready for delivery. Occasionally, trauma can be iatrogenic (e.g. mare left to foal with a vulvoplasty [Caslick's] in place; Figure 71.10).

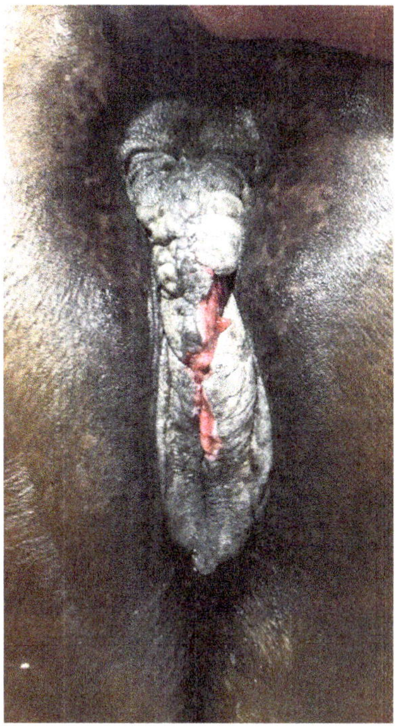

Figure 71.10 Perineal lacerations in a mare that foaled with an unopened Caslick's.

Any part of the birth canal could be damaged during delivery of the fetus, but the cervix, the vestibule, and the vulva are more prone to lacerations and contusions, whereas the vagina is more distensible and is less prone to trauma. Necrotic vaginitis has been reported in mares after prolonged dystocia and fetotomy [36]. Lacerations of the perineum are classified by their severity and the tissues involved. First-degree perineal lacerations affect only the mucosa of the vestibule and the skin of the dorsal vulvar commissure (Figure 71.11a); second-degree perineal lacerations also involve the muscle of the perineal body (Figure 71.11b), and third-degree perineal lacerations affect the vestibule dorsal wall, perineal body, rectum, and anal sphincter (Figure 71.11c) [37]. First- and second-degree perineal lacerations are common in normal foaling, especially with large-size foals; third-degree perineal lacerations occur primarily during unassisted dystocia or when the foal is presenting with a foot-nape posture (i.e. front legs crossed above the head) and result in the formation of a common cavity between the rectum and vagina.

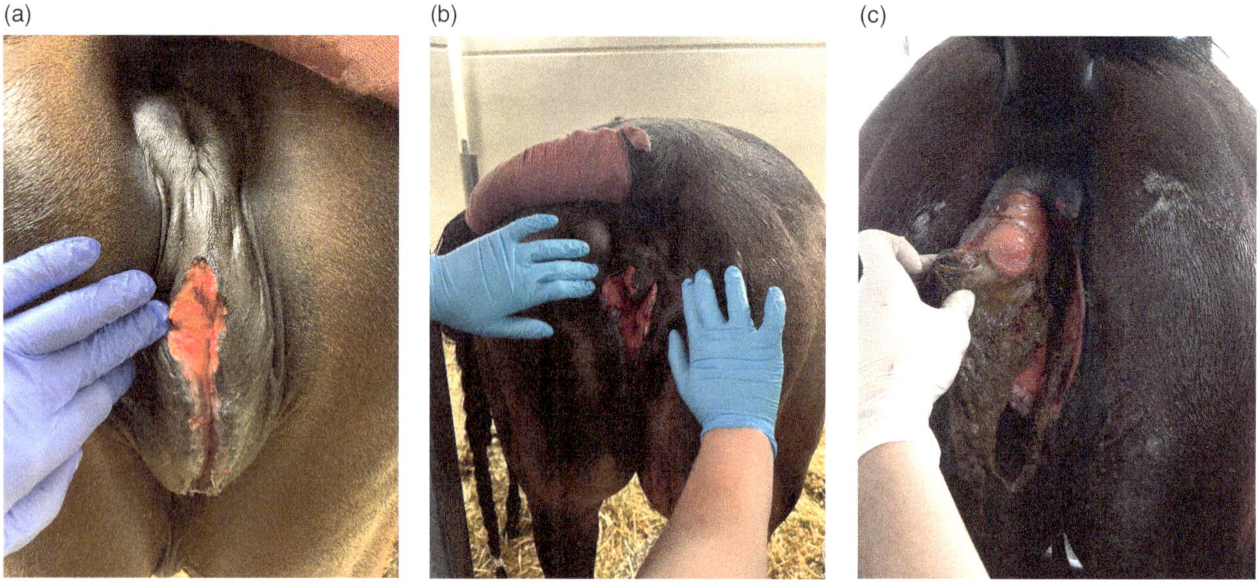

Figure 71.11 Perineal lacerations in postpartum mares: (a) first-degree; (b) second-degree; and (c) third-degree.

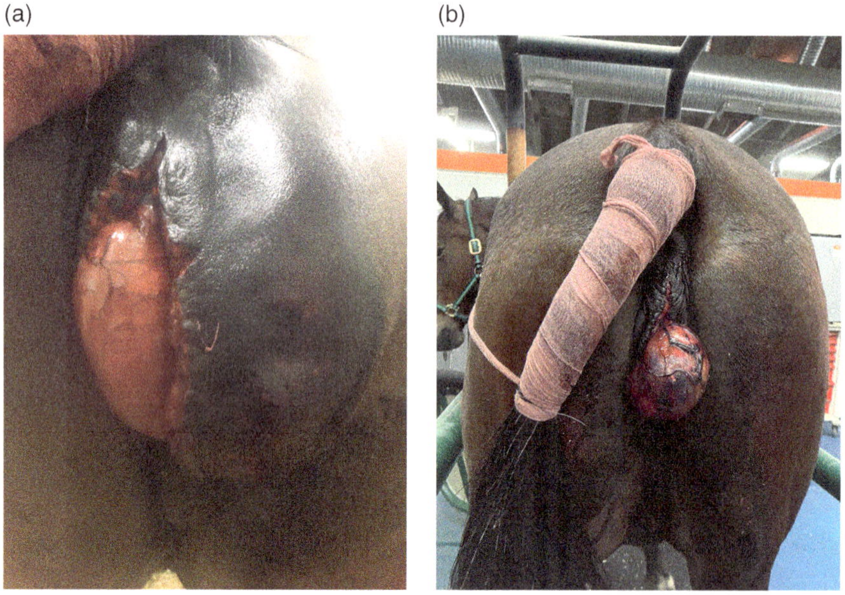

Figure 71.12 (a) A large-size hematoma involving the vulva and vestibule in a mare after dystocia; (b) A pedunculated hematoma with origin in the left side of the vestibule wall that was protruding from the vulva.

Hematomas are another birth-induced lesion; they commonly involve the vulva and vestibule but can also involve any of the soft tissue in and around the birth canal (Figure 71.12). Large hematomas may dissect along the fascial plane and arrive at the pelvic and abdominal cavity, causing internal bleeding [36]; another complication is abscess formation.

During dystocia and its correction, contusions and lacerations of the vestibule are also possible; unfortunately, one of the most common complications of dystocia is the formation of adhesions that sometimes preclude the possibility of rebreeding the mare and predispose the mare to pyometra (Figure 71.13) [36]. The diagnosis is simple and based on direct observation of the lesions on the external genitalia. The extent of the trauma can be better evaluated with a vaginal examination; the clinician can gently reach into the vagina to detect tears and other abnormalities or use a speculum. A transrectal ultrasound exam can

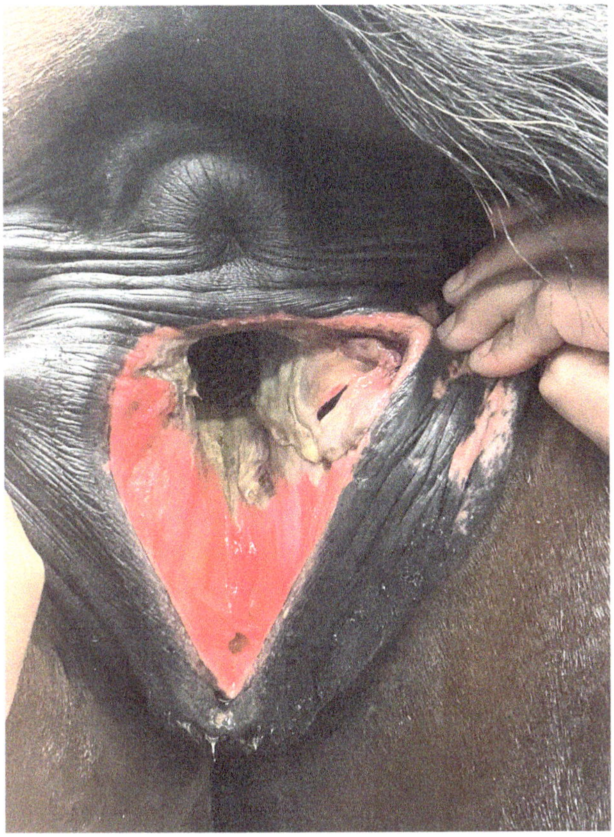

Figure 71.13 Necrotizing lesions in the vestibule of a mare after dystocia and fetotomy.

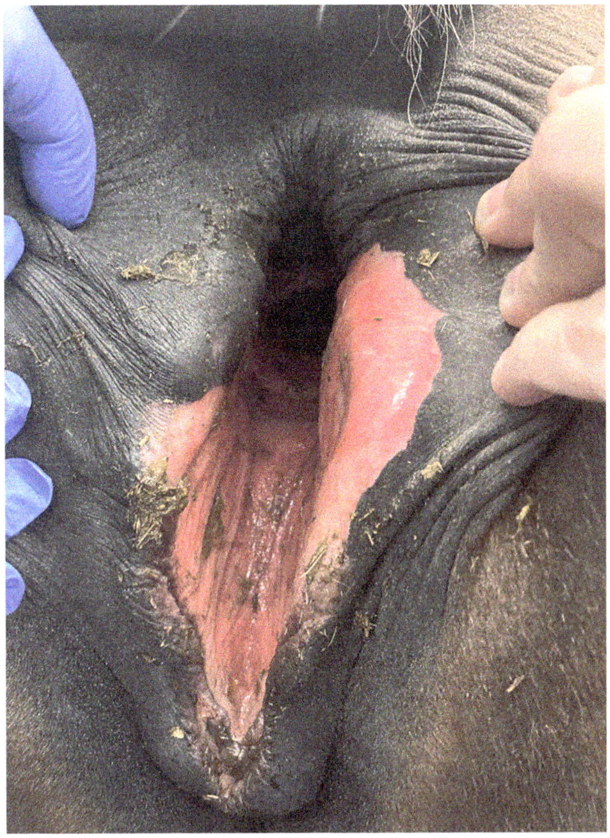

Figure 71.14 Mare with a third-degree perineal laceration ready for reconstructive surgery.

be performed to determine the extent of lesions such as hematomas in the soft tissues around the vagina and broad ligaments.

Although surgical correction of most perineal lacerations are postponed for 4–6 weeks post-foaling, medical therapy should be started immediately to prevent short- and long-term consequences, including hemorrhages, abscesses, and adhesions. Many times, mares with these types of injuries are already receiving antibiotics due to other concomitant conditions such as metritis or RFM; however, the need for antimicrobial administration should be evaluated based on the severity of the injury and signs of infections. Use of antimicrobials that are effective against anaerobes should be considered due to the nature and location of the trauma. If the vaccination history is unknown, tetanus toxoid should be administered.

Lesions of the caudal reproductive tract are very painful, especially in young maiden mares, and can cause discomfort, anorexia, and lethargy. Pain should be mitigated via NSAIDs (flunixin meglumine 1.1 mg/kg q12–24h, IV) or opioids (butorphanol 0.01–0.02 mg/kg q6–8h, IM or IV) in more severe cases. Perineal pain can also a cause fecal and urine retention; therefore, manual evacuation of feces 3–4 times per day and bladder catheterization may be necessary in severe cases. Feed that promotes softer stools (e.g. soaked pellets/mashes) and decreases straining to defecate also reduces discomfort. The inability to urinate due to vaginitis and vaginal masses has been described as a cause of bladder paralysis and atony in a postdystocia mare [38].

These lesions should be examined and treated daily to remove excess necrotic tissue and promote granulation tissue formation and reepithelization. Surgical correction is usually postponed until complete healing (Figure 71.14) [37]. If a hematoma is present, ice can be applied to the area multiple times per day; the authors fill a rectal sleeve with crushed ice and wrap it under the tail so that it applies to the hematoma when the tail is resting.

Prevention of birth-induced trauma is attempted by assisting the foaling and ensuring rapid correction of any malpositioning of the fetus. The prognosis of perineal lacerations on mare fertility depends on the degree and on the presence of concomitant lesions (i.e. cervical tears); surprisingly, endometritis followed by third-degree perineal lacerations can resolve within 2 weeks once the laceration is surgically treated [39].

Peripartum Hemorrhage in Mares

Peripartum hemorrhage is an important cause of perinatal death in broodmares and is also an important cause of peripartum morbidity. Sources of hemorrhage in mares include arterial rupture – more specifically, rupture of arterial vessels that supply the uterus and related structures. Excellent reviews exist but, overall, there is a paucity of information related to incidence in the field and appropriate/effective treatment [40]. One report from central Kentucky for the 1992–1993 foaling seasons found that, of 98 necropsy records, the majority (57/98) of deaths were associated with the reproductive tract or due to reproductive complications [41]. The risk of death was higher in older mares (>15 years of age more likely to die) [42, 43].

Three primary sources of hemorrhage are recognized: direct hemorrhage from a ruptured vessel into the peritoneal cavity; hemorrhage confined to the broad ligament or uterine serosa resulting in a hematoma; and hemorrhage into the uterine lumen. Of these, the most acutely life-threatening is direct hemorrhage into the peritoneal cavity that can rapidly lead to fatal hemorrhagic shock. Hemorrhage into the broad-ligament or uterine serosa results in clinical signs of abdominal pain and a degree of shock, but due to the hemorrhage being somewhat confined, bleeding might stop before the situation becomes life-threatening. Bleeding within the uterine lumen is less likely to involve rupture of a large vessel and, while potentially dramatic, is generally manageable.

Clinical signs of significant postpartum hemorrhage, regardless of origin, have been well-described. In brief, severe episodes resemble hemorrhagic shock, but can be confused with gastrointestinal conditions, most commonly large colon volvulus. Less severe episodes can be clinically silent or resemble mild to moderate colic. Measuring the packed cell volume (PCV) and total protein (TP) in the immediate postpartum period in all mares allows for the comparison of subsequent measurements in cases of hemorrhage. Mares presenting with compromised or sick foals should, at a minimum, have a PCV and TP documented and a brief physical examination at presentation. Recognition of clinically significant hemorrhage in adult horses is typically straightforward as they demonstrate signs of shock, including tachycardia, tachypnea, pale mucous membranes, delayed capillary refill time, agitation or depression, sweating, and cold extremities. It is important to remember that PCV may remain within normal values for up to 12 hours after onset of acute hemorrhage if IV fluids are not administered or if the mare does not drink water and make endocrine and renal adjustments to conserve volume. Measurement of serum L-lactate can also be easily performed stall-side to assess the degree of tissue hypoxia. Transabdominal ultrasonographic examination can help identify internal hemorrhage, which appears as mixed echogenicity effusion, often with a swirling or "snow globe" appearance. Abdominocentesis can confirm intraperitoneal hemorrhage, although the specific source can be difficult to identify. A hematoma in the broad ligament or blood in the uterine lumen can sometimes be identified ultrasonographically. Regardless of the source of blood loss, treatment takes precedence over lengthy diagnostic testing as additional testing can be performed once the mare is stable.

Management

Determining the most appropriate treatment for mares with postpartum hemorrhage can be challenging. Many approaches have been described, some directly contradictory, with scant evidence supporting choices made for treatment. Information available from peer-reviewed literature can be biased, as reports primarily originate from large private or university-based referral hospitals. Unfortunately, there are no large breeding farm population-based studies or studies directly comparing treatments [44]. Most common treatment protocols include flunixin meglumine (or other NSAID), IV polyionic crystalloid fluids, aminocaproic acid (or other promoters of coagulation), and whole blood/plasma transfusion.

The clinician should ensure that the mare and foal are in a quiet environment and that the mare can be controlled. Deciding whether to leave the foal with the mare or remove it from the stall should be based on balancing how fractious the mare becomes if the foal is removed against safety concerns for the foal and personnel.

Pain relief is a first-line treatment (e.g. flunixin meglumine 1.1 mg/kg, IV). There are arguments for and against the use of most tranquilizers and sedatives available. Butorphanol tartarate (0.02 mg/kg, IV) can relieve both anxiety and pain. Xylazine and detomidine can be used but carry a risk of initial hypertension with IV administration. Conversely, administration of acepromazine can induce a brief period of decreased blood pressure, either contributing to shock or decreasing the risk of further bleeding. Similar to the choice of sedative/tranquilizers, consider whether it is appropriate to give IV fluids (and if so, what type and rate). Regardless of the decision for or against fluid administration, it is prudent to place a large-bore catheter in a jugular vein, accompanied by a large bore extension.

Treatment

Crystalloid Fluids

Isotonic crystalloid fluids with a normal strong ion difference are used to restore circulating blood volume, especially in cases of hemorrhagic shock. However, administration of large volumes of crystalloid fluids can dilute platelets and coagulation factors, resulting in impaired clot formation. Synthetic colloids, such as hetastarch, have a similar negative effect on hemostasis through hemodilution [45]. "Hypotensive resuscitation," or initial conservative administration of crystalloid fluids, is the goal until definitive hemostasis can be established and maintained with other forms of blood loss, but this approach generally does not apply to postpartum mares in hemorrhagic shock because bleeding is almost always uncontrollable. Rather, a 20 ml/kg "shock dose" of IV crystalloid fluid can be administered. It is important to keep in mind in these severe cases that the red cell loss is not what kills the mare initially – it is the hypovolemic shock. The mare is reassessed after the initial fluid bolus, with administration of additional fluids if no improvement is noted.

Blood and Blood Products

An important consideration when attending to a mare with acute hemorrhage is whether – or when – to initiate a blood transfusion. Clinical indications to consider a transfusion include suspected or known large volume blood loss with signs of shock and decreasing total solids, acute blood loss and a PCV <20% (the PCV decrease will not be evident initially until fluids get into the vascular space), and increased L-lactate (>4 mmol/l) despite volume replacement (indicates tissue hypoxia/mitochondrial injury). Fresh whole blood is the ideal choice to replace acute volume loss (hypovolemic anemia) in bleeding mares. The volume to be administered should be determined based on the estimated volume lost, but this is almost impossible to predict in the mare that is bleeding into the peritoneal space. If the mare presents with acute blood loss and signs of shock, blood volume loss can be estimated at 20–30% (8–12 l in a 500 kg mare). Blood transfusion volume should aim at replacing 25–50% of the estimated volume lost (3–6 l in a 500 kg mare). Remaining blood volume loss will be compensated by fluid shifts after transfusion, with assistance from IV crystalloid fluid administration. In the case of blood loss into the peritoneal space, up to 75% of RBCs will be autotransfused within 1–3 days. The volume to administer can also be calculated from the donor and patient PCV (e.g. volume to be transfused = body weight recipient [kg] × 0.08 × PCV desired-PCV recipient/PCV donor), remembering that the initial PCV may very well be normal in acute hemorrhage. The maximum volume that can be collected from most blood donor horses is 8 l (16 ml/kg body weight), and the volume donated should be replaced in the donor with crystalloid fluids.

The initial blood transfusion can be performed without cross-matching. Only 2 of the 26 equine blood types are strongly antigenic (Qa and Aa), and horses usually do not develop antibodies until after exposure to an antigenic blood type, although anti-horse antibodies can spontaneously arise. However, broodmares may be sensitized to other blood types during pregnancy and parturition, and are therefore predisposed to adverse reactions, similar to how neonatal isoerythrolysis develops. Blood should initially be administered at a slow drip (0.3 ml/kg over the first 10–20 minutes) and the patient monitored for adverse reaction, including but not limited to increased temperature, pulse, and respiratory rate. Vital parameters (temperature, heart rate, respiratory rate) should be measured and recorded every 5 minutes for the first 20 minutes of transfusion, and every 15 minutes thereafter. If there are no signs of an adverse reaction, the rate can be increased for the remainder of the transfusion. If the mare is hypovolemic, increase the rate of 20–40 ml/kg/h (10–20 l/h for a 500 kg horse); practically, this equates to an open bolus on most blood administration sets. As a caveat, blood transfusion sets may develop clogged filters after a few liters and may need to be changed several times during a transfusion. Adverse reactions occur in 16% of blood transfusions [46]. Mild adverse reactions, including hives, fever, and tachypnea. If a mild adverse reaction is observed, administration of flunixin meglumine (1.1 mg/kg IV) with or without administration of an antihistamine (diphenhydramine 0.5–1 mg/kg IM, tripelennamine, 1.1 mg/kg IM, or hydroxazine 0.5–1 mg/kg PO) can be considered. Acute anaphylaxis is reported in 2% of transfusions and should be treated with epinephrine (0.01–0.02 ml of 0.1 mg/ml solution IV).

Plasma transfusion can be used to address clotting factor deficiency that occurs with whole blood loss. Fresh frozen plasma contains immunoglobulins, coagulation factors, and anticoagulant proteins such as antithrombin, protein C, and protein S. The recommended dose of plasma to support coagulation homeostasis is 4 ml/kg body weight (2 l in a 500 kg mare). Initial administration of plasma should be slow with careful monitoring for signs of reaction, as described above. During recovery, proteins, along with RBCs, may be autotransfused from the peritoneal space if the hemorrhage involves the abdominal cavity. If there is no protein rebound, plasma can also be used to correct significant hypoproteinemia/hypoalbuminemia at later stages.

Hemostatic Agents

Many hemostatic agents have been used in attempts to control or stop bleeding during peripartum hemorrhage. None have been shown effective in clinical trials with actual cases, which may be in part due to the source of blood loss in these cases. Free bleeding into the peritoneal cavity is very difficult to locate and control even with surgical exploration, while bleeding into a confined space, such as the broad ligament, will eventually become controlled, similar to most hematomas. Despite his, it is not without reason to attempt use of some of these products and therapies.

One commonly used hemostatic agent is aminocaproic acid (40 mg/kg or 20 g/500 kg) diluted in 1 l of isotonic saline and administered IV over 20 minutes [40]. Aminocaproic acid has been reported to be an inhibitor of fibrinolysis because of its inhibitory effects on plasminogen-activator substances. It is thought to have a similar action in horses, encouraging formation and stabilization of blood clots. This medication is primarily used in referral hospitals, but treatment could be initiated in a well-stocked large breeding farm with on-site veterinary care. Alternatively, tranexamic acid, has a similar mechanism of action and is purportedly more potent than aminocaproic acid. Tranexamic acid has been administered twice daily at a dose of 20 mg/kg, IV diluted in 1 liter of saline.

Yunnan baiyao, a Chinese herb product, has been used to help control hemorrhage in horses. The medication is administered as an orally administered paste, according to package instructions, and requires gastrointestinal absorption to be effective. Therefore, it should be administered as soon as peripartum bleeding is recognized. The mechanism of action is currently unknown. Yunnan baiyao has been shown to decrease template bleeding time in healthy halothane-anesthetized ponies and, anecdotally, practitioners in large breeding farms have had favorable comments regarding its efficacy [47].

Conflicting reports exist on the use of formalin in the treatment of horses with severe hemorrhage. While an early study reported an approximate 75% decrease in coagulation time after treatment with various doses and concentrations of formalin [48], another study was unable to determine a significant difference in coagulation parameters or template bleeding times between normal horses treated with formalin and control animals [49]. The dose is 30–150 ml of 10% buffered formalin in 1 l of isotonic fluids, IV [45].

Naloxone is a pure opioid antagonist; administration leads to binding of opioid receptors, thereby preventing binding of endogenous or exogenous opioids. It is not, in fact, a medication that encourages clot formation or maintenance, but rather produces a relative reduction in physiologic hypertension if present. There are not studies showing efficacy in postpartum hemorrhage and, due to it mechanism of action, should not be used in combination with opioids. Naloxone's popularity has waned in recent years.

Additional Therapies

Mares experiencing clinically apparent postpartum or peripartum hemorrhage frequently receive additional therapies, including those for pain management and broad-spectrum antimicrobials. While use of these medications may be warranted, mares that have suffered significant volume and red cell mass loss will experience some degree of organ injury due to hypoperfusion and, if severe enough, tissue hypoxia. Medication with a propensity for renal injury (NSAIDs, aminoglycoside antimicrobials) should be used with caution and the mare's renal function monitored appropriately.

Oxygen Therapy

Intranasal oxygen insufflation has been advocated by some in the treatment of periparturient hemorrhage in mares. The largest consideration is how well the mare will tolerate the treatment; the clinician must make a cost-benefit analysis of this therapy. The cost is how the mare tolerates the treatment, some will be quite upset by both the tube in their nose and by the feeling of rapid air flow in the nasopharynx. The benefit is in fact quite small, even at high flow rates. Considering that oxygen content of the blood is largely dominated by the amount of oxygen bound to hemoglobin and that oxygen dissolved in the blood provides a minimal contribution, there may be little to no benefit to the treatment. While it won't hurt, if the mare tolerates it, it may not help. Significant tissue hypoxia, recognized by increased L-lactate concentrations in the blood, is due to both decreased red cell mass and hypoperfusion secondary to hypovolemia.

Monitoring

Physical examination and improvement in heart rate, temperature of extremities, pulse pressure, CRT, and anxiety, among other clinical signs, is the first line for monitoring. There are several quick assessment/point-of-care (POC) tests available that might be of benefit. PCV/TS, blood gas analyses and viscoelastic coagulation testing device are readily available on the veterinary medical device market and might be considered in these cases. In particular, POC viscoelastic coagulation testing[1] (VCM Vet™) may be of

1 VCM Vet Entegrion, Durham, NC, USA.

benefit in severe cases to monitor the ability of the mare to both form and maintain clots during the initial episode and as follow-up to various treatment. Significant coagulation abnormalities can be recognized and inform both the need for and efficacy of treatment.

Outcome

Overall, survival of mares presented to referral institutions is quite good, ranging from 84% to 87% where those data could be gleaned from manuscripts, excluding case reports. This may, in the authors opinion, be related to the stability of the mare, location of the bleed associated with the reproductive tract, and the ability of the mare to survive the initial hemorrhage and transportation to a referral facility. There is no information available related to treatment at a farm location, the incidence of postpartum hemorrhage over the general population of broodmares, or survival of affected mares related to the general population [1, 22, 44].

References

1 Dolente, B.A., Sullivan, E.K., Boston, R., and Johnston, J.K. (2005). Mares admitted to a referral hospital for postpartum emergencies: 163 cases (1992–2002). *J. Vet. Emerg. Crit. Care* 15: 193–200.

2 Aoki, T., Yamakawa, K., and Ishii, M. (2014). Factors affecting the incidence of postpartum fever in heavy draft mares. *J. Equine Vet. Sci.* 34 (5): 719–721.

3 Sevinga, M., Barkem, H.W., and Hesselink, J.W. (2002). Serum calcium and magnesium concentrations and the use of a calcium-magnesium borogluconate solution in the treatment of Friesian mares with retained placenta. *Theriogenology* 57: 941–947.

4 Blanchard, T.L. (2011). Postpartum metritis. In: *Equine Reproduction*, vol. 2 (ed. A.O. McKinnon, E.L. Squires, W.E. Vaala, and D.D. Varner), 2530–2539. New Delhi, India: Wiley-Blackwell.

5 Blanchard, T.L. and Macphearson, M.L. (2007). Postparturient abnormalities. In: *Current Therapies in Equine Reproduction*, 1e (ed. J.C. Samper, J.F. Pycock, and A.O. McKinnon), 465–475. Missouri, USA: Saunders Elsevier.

6 Ferrer, M.S. and Palomares, R. (2018). Aerobic uterine isolates and antimicrobial susceptibility in mares with post-partum metritis. *Equine Vet. J.* 50: 202–207.

7 Blanchard, T.L., Vaala, W.E., Straughn, A.J. et al. (1987). Septic/toxic metritis and laminitis in a postpartum mare. *J. Equine Vet. Sci.* 7: 32–34.

8 Blanchard, T.L., Elmore, R.G., Kinden, D.A. et al. (1985). Effect of intrauterine infusion of E. coli endotoxin in postpartum pony mares. *Am. J. Vet. Res.* 46: 2157–2162.

9 Krohn, J., Eilenberg, R.D., Gajewski, Z. et al. (2019). Lochial and endometrial cytological changes during the first 10 days post-partum with special reference to the nature of foaling and puerperium in equine. *Theriogenology* 139: 43–48.

10 Wagner, C., Sauermann, R., and Joukhadar, C. (2006). Principles of antibiotic penetration into abscess fluid. *Pharmacology* 78 (1): 1–10.

11 Von Dollen, K.A., Jones, M., Beachler, T. et al. (2019). Antimicrobial activity of ceftiofur and penicillin with gentamicin against Escherichia coli and Streptococcus equi subspecies zooepidemicus in an ex vivo model of equine postpartum uterine disease. *J. Equine Vet. Sci.* 79: 121–126.

12 Brinsko, S.P. (2001). How to perform uterine lavage: indications and practical techniques. *Proc. Am. Assoc. Equine Pract.* 47: 407–411.

13 Fedorka, C.E., Murase, H., Loux, S.C. et al. (2020). The effect of mycobacterium cell wall fraction on histologic, immunologic, and clinical parameters of postpartum involution in the mare. *J. Equine Vet. Sci.* 90: 103013.

14 Vandeplassche, M., Spincemaille, J., and Bouters, R. (1971). Aetiology, pathogenesis and treatment of retained placenta in the mare. *Equine Vet. J.* 3: 3144–3177.

15 Threlfall, W.R. (2011). Retained fetal membranes. In: *Equine Reproduction*, vol. 2 (ed. A.O. McKinnon, E.L. Squires, W.E. Vaala, and D.D. Varner), 2520–2529. New Delhi, India: Wiley-Blackwell.

16 Lopate, C., Leblanc, M., Pascoe, R.R., and Knottenbelt, D.C. (2003). Parturition. In: *Equine Stud Farm Medicine and Surgery* (ed. D.C. Knottenbelt, M. Leblanc, and R.R. Pascoe), 269–324. Edinburgh: Saunders.

17 Rapacz-Leonard, A., Leonard, M., Chmielewska-Krzesińska, M. et al. (2018). Major histocompatibility complex class I in the horse (Equus caballus) placenta during pregnancy and parturition. *Placenta* 15 (74): 36–46.

18 Rapacz, A., Pazdizior, K., Ras, A. et al. (2012). Retained fetal membrane in heavy draft mares associated with histological abnormalities. *J. Equine Vet. Sci.* 32: 38–44.

19 Rapacz-Leonard, A., Kankofer, M., Leonard, M. et al. (2015). Differences in extracellular matrix remodeling in the placenta of mares that retain fetal membranes and mares that deliver fetal membranes physiologically. *Placenta* 36 (10): 1167–1177.

20 Miyoshi, M., Sawamukai, Y., and Iwanaga, T. (2002). Reduced phagocytotic activity of macrophages in the

bovine retained placenta. *Reprod. Domest. Anim.* 37 (1): 53–56.

21 Provencer, R., Threlfall, W.R., Murdick, P.W., and Wearly, W.K. (1988). Retained fetal membranes in the mare: a retrospective study. *Can. Vet. J.* 29: 903–910.

22 Arnold, C.E., Payne, M., Thompson, J.A. et al. (2008). Periparturient hemorrhage in mares: 73 cases (1998–2005). *J. Am. Vet. Assoc.* 232: 1345–1351.

23 Troedsson, M.H.T., Spensley, M.S., and Fahning, M.L. (1997). Retained fetal membranes. In: *Current Therapy in Equine Medicine*, 4e (ed. N.E. Robinson), 560–562. Philadelphia, PA: WB Saunders.

24 Canisso, I.F., Rodriguez, J.S., Sanz, M.C., and Coutimho da Silva, M.A. (2013). A clinical approach to the diagnosis and treatment of retained fetal membranes with an emphasis placed on the critically ill mare. *J. Equine Vet. Sci.* 33: 570–579.

25 Warnakulasooriya, D.N., Marth, C.D., McLeod, J.A. et al. (2018). Treatment of retained fetal membranes in the mare-a practitioner survey. *Front. Vet. Sci.* 5: 128.

26 Mejier, M., MacPherson, M.L., and Dijkman, R. (2015). How to use umbilical vessel water infusion to treat retained fetal membranes in mares. *Proc. Am. Vet. Pract. Assoc.* 61: 478–484.

27 Neto, M.E., Curcio, B.R.D., Pivato, G.M. et al. (2023). Efficiency of umbilical vessel water infusion in the management of retained fetal membranes after elective C-section in mares. *J. Equine Vet. Sci.* 125: 104813. Abstract.

28 Burns, S.J., Judge, N.G., Martins, J.E., and Adamas, L.G. (1977). Management of retained placenta in mares. *Proc. Am. Assoc. Equine Pract.* 23: 381–387.

29 Hospes, R. and Huchzermeyer, S. (2004). Treatment of retained placenta in broadmares in a 4-step-routine - review of 36 cases. *Pferdeheilkunde* 20: 498–504.

30 Cuervo-Arango, J. and Newcombe, J.R. (2009). The effect of manual removal of placenta immediately after foaling on subsequent fertility parameters in the mare. *J. Equine Vet. Sci.* 29: 771–774.

31 Troedsson, M.H.T., Liu, I.K.M., Ing, M., and Pascoe, J. (1995). Smooth muscle electrical activity in the oviduct and the effect of oxytocin, prostaglandin F2alpha, prostaglandin E2 on the myometrium and the oviduct of cyclic mares. *Biol. Reprod. Monogr.* 1: 475–488.

32 Semrad, S. and Moore, J. (1987). Effects of multiple low doses of flunixin meglumine on repeated endotoxin challenge in the horse. *Prostaglandins Leukot. Med.* 27: 169–181.

33 Lohman, K.L. and Barton, M.H. (2010). Endotoxemia. In: *Equine Internal Medicine*, 3e (ed. S.M. Reed, W.M. Bayly, and D.C. Sellon), 802–823. Saint-Louis, MO: Saunders Elsevier.

34 Hood, D.M. (1999). Laminitis in the horse. *Vet. Clin. North Am. Equine Pract.* 15 (2): 287–294.

35 McKinnon, A.O. and Jalim, S.L. (2011). Surgery of the caudal reproductive tract. In: *Equine Reproduction*, vol. 2 (ed. A.O. McKinnon, E.L. Squires, W.E. Vaala, and D.D. Varner), 2545–2263. New Delhi, India: Wiley-Blackwell.

36 Parkinson, T.J. and Noakes, D.E. (2019). Injuries and diseases consequent upon parturition. In: *Veterinary Reproduction and Obstetrics*, 10e (ed. D.E. Noakes, T.J. Parkinson, and G.C.W. England), 333–348. Saint-Louis, MO: Saunders Elsevier.

37 Tibary, A. and Pearson, L.K. (2012). Medical problems in the immediate postpartum period. *Proc. Am. Vet. Pract. Ass.* 58: 362–369.

38 Morley, S., Rodriguez, J., and Pearson, L. (2010). Post-dystocia paralysis and cystitis in a mare: medical management and outcome. *Clin. Theriogenol.* 2: 401.

39 Schumacher, J. and Blanchard, T. (1992). Comparison of endometrium before and after repair of third-degree rectovestibular lacerations in the mare. *J. Am. Vet. Med. Assoc.* 200: 1336–1338.

40 Scoggins, C.F. and McCue, P.M. (2007). How to assess and stabilize a mare suspected of periparturient hemorrhage in the field. *AAEP Proc.* 53: 342–348.

41 Dwyer, R. and Harrison, L. (1993). Postpartum deaths of mares. *Equine Dis. Q.* 2: 5.

42 Rooney, J.R. (1964). Internal hemorrhage related to gestation in the mare. *Cornell Vet.* 54: 11–17.

43 Pascoe, R.R. (1979). Rupture of the utero-ovarian or middle uterine artery in the mare at or near parturition. *Vet. Rec.* 104: 77.

44 Wilkins, P.A. What is the best treatment for mares with post-partum haemorrhage? *Equine Vet. J.* https://doi.org/10.1111/eve.12876.

45 Jones, W. IV (1998). Formalin to control hemorrhage. *J. Equine Vet. Sci.* 18: 581.

46 Hurcombe, S.D., Mudge, M.C., and Hinchcliff, K.W. (2007). Clinical and clinicopathologic variables in adult horses receiving blood transfusions: 31 cases (1999–2005). *J. Am. Vet. Med. Assoc.* 231 (2): 267–274.

47 Graham, L., Farnsworth, K., Cary, J. (2002). The effect of Yunnan baiyao on the template bleeding time and activated clotting time in healthy halothane anesthetized ponies. *8th Intl Vet Emer Crit Care Soc Symposium,* 790.

48 Roberts, S.J. (1943). The effects of various intravenous injections on the horse. *Am. J. Vet. Res.* 4: 226–239.

49 Sellon, D.C., Taylor, E.L., Wardrop, J. et al. (1999). The effects of intravenous formaldehyde on hemostasis in normal horses, in proceedings. *Am. Assoc. Equine Pract.* 45: 297–298.

Chapter 72 Anesthesia of the Late-Term Mare

Danielle Strahl-Heldreth and Graeme M. Doodnaught

Equine anesthesia inherently carries a higher risk than that for other domesticated animals, with reported mortality rates ranging from 0.08% to 1.8% [1]. The addition of comorbidities including pregnancy can further exacerbate those risks for the maternal patient as well as increase fetal mortality, depending on stage of pregnancy. These risks are elucidated by the survival rates for mares presenting with dystocia are about 90% and for foals between 10% and 40% [2, 3]. Anesthetic drug selection, delivery, and monitoring techniques for gravid mares undergoing an anesthetic episode are similar to those used for the nonpregnant horse. However, changes in maternal physiology and concerns for fetal viability impact the anesthetist drugs selection and mode of delivery. When anesthetizing a pregnant mare, the anesthetist faces the added challenge of assuring a good outcome for both the mare and the fetus.

A basic requirement of anesthetic drugs is their ability to achieve unconsciousness through their effects on the central nervous system, necessitating their ability to cross the blood-brain barrier (BBB). The downside to this quality is that these drugs easily pass through blood-tissue barriers such as the placenta. Thus, the majority of anesthetic agents reach the fetus, albeit, at varying rates and concentrations. Pregnancy also results in various physiologic and anatomic changes in the mare that influence anesthetic management. Therefore, it is prudent for the anesthetist to consider the physiological changes of the dam, teratogenic effects of the drugs, perfusion and oxygen delivery to the fetus, and cardiopulmonary depression in the neonate when choosing sedative, analgesic, and anesthetic drugs for the pregnant mare. Adding to the complexity of these cases, pregnant mares requiring anesthesia often present emergently. These cases therefore require decisiveness, weighing the cost and benefits for the mare and fetus. This chapter discusses current knowledge regarding the physiological changes during pregnancy, the anesthetic approach specific to the pregnant mare, and brief comments on neonatal resuscitation of the foal.

Physiologic Changes During Pregnancy

Maternal Physiology

Mares are pregnant for an average of 320–370 days. Within that time, several physiologic and anatomic adaptations are created to sustain the mare and fetus until foaling. These alterations in the dam are associated with the increase in metabolic demands imposed by the increase to uterine mass and the growing fetus within. Many of these adaptations impact the overall anesthetic management of the pregnant mare, particularly when it comes to planning for and managing concerns related to the cardiovascular, hematological, respiratory, gastrointestinal, renal, and central nervous systems. The most notable adaptations are outlined in this chapter (Table 72.1).

Cardiovascular Physiology

Changes to the cardiovascular system occur early in pregnancy in order to meet the increased metabolic demands of the mare and the added demands of the fetus. The effects of these changes peak during the last trimester and slowly return to prepartum values after foaling. The most notable changes are summarized in Table 72.1. In general, as metabolic demand increases during pregnancy, so does oxygen consumption, which increases by 20–25% in the late-term mare [4]. In order to appropriately meet the increase in demands, cardiac output increases 30–40% during pregnancy and increases further during labor and delivery by 75–100% [4]. Accompanying the increase in cardiac output is an increase in heart rate (increases 55%) and stroke

Equine Neonatal Medicine, First Edition. Edited by David M. Wong and Pamela A. Wilkins.

Table 72.1 Physiologic changes associated with pregnancy.

System	Increased	Decreased
Cardiovascular	Cardiac output (30–50%)	Vascular tone
	Systemic and pulmonary vascular resistance (20–30%)	Arterial blood pressure
	Fractional shortening and stroke volume (~20–30%)	Packed cell volume
	Resting heart rate (20–30%)	
	Plasma volume (~40% in women)	
	Red blood cell mass (~20%)	
	Ventricular and-diastolic volume and wall thickness	
	Procoagulant activity	
Respiratory	Metabolic rate and oxygen consumption	Functional residual capacity (~20%)
	Minute ventilation (~70%)	$PaCO_2$ *increase pH and normal PaO_2
	Tidal volume	
	Respiratory rate	
	Closing volume	
Gastrointestinal	Intragastric pressure	Lower esophageal sphincter pressure
	Gastrin production	Gastrointestinal motility
Renal	Blood flow	
	Glomerular filtration rate	
Central nervous	Progesterone and endogenous opioids	Minimum alveolar concentration (MAC) by 16–40%
Reproductive (uterus)	Blood flow	
	Altered vascular response to catecholamines	

$PaCO_2$, partial pressure of carbon dioxide in arterial blood; PaO_2, partial pressure of oxygen in arterial blood.

volume and a decrease in vascular tone and arterial blood pressure (decreases approximately 10%) [5, 6]. The blood flow to reproductive organs such as the uterus and mammary glands also increase by up to 40 times greater than that seen in the nongravid female.

Hematologic Physiology

There are several changes that occur hematologically in pregnant animals. The increase in fetal weight is supported by an increase in plasma volume. While the exact increase in blood volume is unknown in the pregnant mare, in beagles there is a 23% increase in blood volume an up to a 35% increase in the blood volume in pregnant women [6]. In a 2011 study in Spanish mares, the increase in plasma volume was described to be related to an increase in activity of the renin-angiotensin-aldosterone system (RAAS) and may be considered a natural physiological phenomenon during the first and second trimesters in the pregnant mare [7]. Red blood cell count, hematocrit, and hemoglobin concentrations can be significantly lower during pregnancy in the mare [8]. This relative pregnancy-associated anemia, hemodilution, and reduced blood viscosity is suspected to improve blood flow to the placenta and thus increase the delivery of nutrients and oxygen to the growing fetus [9]. Albumin, and thus total protein, significantly decreases during the second trimester in the pregnant mare [8]. This decrease, whether due to reduced synthesis or an increased catabolism, further decreases oncotic pressure and contributes to a general decrease in protein binding of anesthetic drugs [10].

The hemostatic profile varies during pregnancy in several species. In a 2014 study by Bazzano et al., pregnant mares showed a few differences in parameters related to hemostasis, specifically platelet count, fibrinogen, and prothrombin time. Platelet count remained unchanged throughout pregnancy, but significantly increased at parturition, returning to baseline 3 weeks later. This is likely due to splenic contraction releasing platelets into circulation following hemorrhage associated with parturition. Fibrinogen increased starting 2 months before and peaking at parturition. Numerous theories have been proposed as to why fibrinogen increases, but as an acute phase protein, physiologic stress can cause increases in fibrinogen and cause hypercoagulable states. Prothrombin time started to shorten a month before, reaching a peak at parturition. Activated partial thromboplastin time was unchanged throughout pregnancy. Presumably, these alterations are a result of the biological preparation for or result of blood loss associated with parturition [11].

Respiratory Physiology

The respiratory system undergoes several changes during pregnancy. A progressive increase in tidal volume, respiratory rate, and minute ventilation is seen in pregnant women, leading to a shift in $PaCO_2$ to 28–32 mmHg (contrary to normocapnia in nonpregnant patients of 35–45 mmHg) due to hyperventilation thus leading to a respiratory alkalosis [4]. At the same time, there is a decrease in reserve volumes, including functional reserve capacity, due to an increase of intrabdominal pressure and subsequent compressive atelectasis of lung tissues. Overall, these changes lead to a decrease in oxygen reserve capacity in the lungs. Arterial oxygen levels thus remain similar to the nonpregnant patient. However, due to lack of oxygen reserve in the lungs and the overall increase in oxygen consumption, any ventilatory depression including apnea under anesthesia can be detrimental due to an immediate decrease arterial oxygen concentration.

Gastrointestinal Physiology

The gravid uterus increases the intraabdominal pressure and can cause changes in gastrointestinal function. There is an increase in intragastric pressure and an overall decrease in GI motility in pregnant mares. In addition to decreased aboral flow, the increase in pregnancy-related hormones such as progesterone causes a decrease in lower esophageal sphincter tone, resulting in a greater risk of regurgitation and potential aspiration of gastric contents peri-anesthetically.

Renal Physiology

Pregnant mares have an increase in renal blood flow, glomerular filtration rate and plasma volume. These changes often lead to a decreased serum blood urea nitrogen (BUN) and creatinine.

Central Nervous System Physiology

As mentioned previously, circulating progesterone is more concentrated in pregnancy. The increase in circulating progesterone concentration, accompanied by a release in endorphins have been shown to contribute to a decrease in minimum alveolar concentration (MAC) by 16–40% in humans [12]. This effect on MAC is postulated to be conserved across species.

Uterine Blood Flow

Uterine blood flow is not autoregulated. Determinants of uterine blood flow are proportional to mean perfusion pressure (MPP) and inversely proportional to uterine vascular resistance pressure (UVR). Uterine blood flow is increased in pregnancy and there is an alteration in uterine vascular control. If uterine blood flow and subsequent blood flow to the fetus is compromised, there is an increased risk of fetal death, abortion, or premature delivery of the foal.

Anesthetic Concerns of the Pregnant Mare

Anesthesia in the horse is associated with complications such as systemic hypotension, reduced cardiac output, hypoventilation, hypoxemia, and impaired gas exchange, myopathy, neuropathy, and complications accompanying anesthetic recovery. When anesthetizing a pregnant mare, these concerns are not only present for the mare but can lead to detrimental effects on the fetus. Systemic hypotension and reduced cardiac output can result in reduced uterine blood flow. These complications are further exacerbated in the pregnant mare due to compression of the vena cava by the gravid uterus. Additionally, hypoventilation resulting from anesthetic drug effects and recumbency, is compounded by the weight of a gravid uterus and fetal tissues compressing the diaphragm, thereby further reducing thoracic volume and compliance. The risk of myopathy and neuropathies is increased with body mass in the nonpregnant horse. The increase in body mass associated with pregnancy, increased potential for reduced cardiac output, and hypoxemia all contribute to a greater risk of myopathy and neuropathies in the pregnant mare.

Pharmacokinetics and Pharmacodynamics of Pregnancy

Maternal and Placental Factors

While there are a few exceptions, most anesthetic agents cross the placenta and enter fetal circulation. Factors affecting drug disposition during equine pregnancy include plasma concentration of the drug, the degree of ionization, molecular weight, tissue blood flow, and lipid solubility. These same factors influence the rate of drug transfer through the BBB and are thus unavoidable when it comes to anesthesia.

The increase in cardiac output and overall increase in plasma volume in the pregnant mare influence the distribution of both injected and inhaled anesthetic agents. With the increase in cardiac output, there is a reduction in injectable agents being delivered to the brain, as well as a reduction of inhalant agent concentration in the blood. Anesthetic drugs that are weakly basic (opioids, benzodiazepines, local anesthetics) become more highly ionized at a pH lower than their pKa. The nonionized form of these drugs is present in the maternal circulation and readily crosses the placenta into the fetal circulation.

However, the pH within the fetus and fetal blood is approximately 0.1 units lower than the maternal blood, so weak bases become more ionized within the more acidic fetal environment and are less able to cross back to the maternal circulation. These drugs, particularly local anesthetics and benzodiazepines, undergo "ion trapping" within the fetus [13]. In addition, a decrease in serum albumin increases the unbound or free fraction or protein bound drug concentration.

Fetal Factors

Several factors within fetal circulation affect drug disposition within the developing fetus. The fetus has an albumin concentration that is greater than, or equal to, that of the mare (2.3–4.2 mg/dl). This can serve as a depot effect for highly protein bound drugs. In the equine fetus, the ductus venosus is lost early in development. As a result, all umbilical venous blood flows through the liver before reaching the right ventricle. Thus, some drugs can be metabolized, or filtered in the fetal liver prior to reaching general circulation. Anesthetics are further diluted prior to reaching the fetal brain through admixture with the left ventricular blood through the patent ductus arteriosus. The fetal BBB is immature, which allows for the direct assess of drugs to the brain.

Specific Anesthetic Agents

A full physical exam, with particular attention paid to the auscultation of the heart and lungs should be performed prior to administration of sedative or anesthetic agents (Table 72.2).

Table 72.2 Sedative and anesthetic agents and doses for the pregnant mare.

Drug **Sedatives**	Dose (mg/kg)	CRI	Duration of action
Acepromazine	0.01–0.05	—	≥360
Xylazine	0.2–1.0	0.2–1 mg/kg/h	20–30
Detomidine	0.002–0.04	0.01–0.04 mg/kg/h	30–60
Dexmedetomidine	1–5 ug/kg	0.25–2 ug/kg/h	25–45
Opioids			
Butorphanol	0.01–0.05	0.01–0.02 mg/kg/hr	45–75
Morphine	0.05–0.2	0.025–0.1 mg/kg/hr	120–240
Anesthetic agents			
Ketamine	2–3 mg/kg	0.03–4 mg/kg/hr	20–30
Muscle Relaxants (co-induction agents)			
Midazolam/Diazepam	0.02–0.1	0.05–0.15 mg/kg/hr	20–30
GGE (5%)	25–50	25–100 mg/kg/hr	15–25
Propofol	0.5	0.05–0.2 mg/kg/hr	5–10
Total Intravenous protocols			
Xylazine	0.5 mg/ml	0.25–2 mg/kg/hr	0.5–4 ml/kg/hr
Ketamine	2 mg/ml	1–8 mg/kg/hr	
GGE	50 mg/ml (5%)	25–200 mg/kg/hr	
Detomidine	0.02 mg/ml	0.01–0.08 mg/kg/hr	0.5–4 ml/kg/hr
Ketamine	2 mg/ml	1–8 mg/kg/hr	
GGE	50 mg/ml (5%)	25–200 mg/kg/hr	
Propofol	10 mg/ml (1%)	50–250 ug/kg/min	

CRI, Continuous rate infusion; GGE, Guaifenesin/glyceryl guaicolate ether

Sedation and Premedication

Acepromazine

Acepromazine is a centrally acting phenothiazine derivative that exerts its effects through dopamine receptor antagonism. While the use of acepromazine has been noted to improve recoveries from general anesthesia in horses, it is not recommended for concomitant use during general anesthesia with the pregnant or periparturient mare due to its long duration of action (>3 hours), lack of reversibility, and potential for profound hypotension via α-1 receptor blockade in the peripheral vasculature. Acepromazine should be used only for standing chemical restraint in pregnant mares.

α-2 Agonists

The use of α-2 agonists is essential for safe induction of general anesthesia of horses. However, the necessity of their use does not equate to safety for the fetus. The vasoconstrictive effect combined with the reduction of cardiac output can reduce placental perfusion leading to fetal acidosis. While no studies on the safety of various α-2 agonists exist in the pregnant horse, in parturient dogs, xylazine is associated with an increase in neonatal mortality [14]. However, in a more recent study evaluating medetomidine, where neonatal puppies were immediately administered atipamezole (reversal agent for α-2 agonists), reported survival up to 7 days was >90% [15]. While speed of delivery is often prioritized, a recent study in dogs showed that momentary delays to allow for drug clearance is associated with better neonatal outcomes [16]. Thus, when using α-2 agonists in the pregnant mare, the anesthetist must consider the physiologic impact to the fetus and consider early use of α-2 antagonists when resuscitating neonates. This is particularly important when these sedatives have been recently administered. It is likely prudent to use the minimally effective dose for standing sedation or as a pre-anesthetic agent.

Opioids

The administration of opioids to the pregnant mare results in placental transfer to the fetus. The extent of this transfer appears to be opioid dependent in the dog and cat [17]. For instance, the lower lipid solubility and higher molecular weight of morphine delays and restricts its placental transfer. While significant neurological and cardiorespiratory depression can be seen in newborn foals, naloxone can be administered early in the resuscitation of neonates to reverse these effects. The epidural route of administration of morphine minimizes systemic absorption, while providing a good degree of analgesia. A case report noted no adverse effects from prolonged use of epidural morphine in a pregnant mare 2 months before parturition for both the mare and foal [18].

Nonsteroidal Anti-inflammatory Drugs

Flunixin meglumine blocks the release of prostaglandin-$F_2\alpha$ and thus helps prevent fetal loss after uterine manipulation. However, caution should be taken with administering any nonsteroidal anti-inflammatory drug (NSAID) to a near-term mare, as these drugs might mediate premature closure of the ductus arteriosus, which can lead to pulmonary hypertension in the neonatal foal.

Induction

Ketamine

Ketamine is a dissociative anesthetic and remains the most common induction agent in equine anesthesia. It has minimal to no cardiovascular effect in the mare or fetus. Studies in pregnant ewes show evidence that this drug readily crosses the placenta and builds in concentration within the fetal circulation. In a 2004 study in bitches in which midazolam/ketamine was used for induction, there was a significant depressive effect of neurological reflexes compared to puppies of which the dams were administered propofol and epidural anesthesia [19]. In human mothers, where ketamine was used in the anesthetic protocol, there was some degree of drug-induced neonatal depression characterized by a decreased responsiveness and muscle rigidity seen in neonates at birth [20]. No similar studies have been performed in horses. Given the practicality of inductions and anesthesia in the horse and the necessity for the use of ketamine, judicious use is warranted. Resuscitation and support of the neonate immediately after parturition should consider the recency of ketamine administration.

Benzodiazepines

Benzodiazepines such as diazepam and midazolam are potent muscle relaxants that have minimal cardiovascular side effects. They cross the placenta readily due to their high lipid solubility and start out in the unionized form in maternal circulation. In prepartum infants, diazepam causes profound muscle relaxation, depression, and hypothermia in the neonate and contributes to low APGAR scores. However, in a 2008 study by Bidwell et al., the authors evaluated diazepam concentrations in foals after dystocia birth and noted detectable levels of diazepam in the foals, averaging 50% of the mare values; the levels did not seem to negatively affect the outcome of these cases [21]. Midazolam is considered preferable to diazepam since it has lower fetal-to-maternal plasma concentrations in the neonate but may also contribute to depression in the neonate. Administration of flumazenil in the early neonatal resuscitation phase can reverse these effects.

Guaifenesin

Guaifenesin is a centrally acting muscle relaxant. It can cause a decrease in systemic vascular resistance in both the pregnant and nonpregnant animals and readily crosses the placenta. However, it has been used in total intravenous anesthesia (TIVA) for controlled vaginal delivery of viable foals and in induction and maintenance for cesarean procedures.

Maintenance

Inhalational Anesthetics

Inhalational anesthetics have an increased potency in a variety of pregnant animals. For example, the potency of halothane and isoflurane are 25% and 40%, respectively, increased in pregnant sheep [22]. This change in anesthetic requirement is shown to be conserved across several different species and is also presumed to be true in the horse. With the increase in potency of inhalation anesthetics and the physiological changes of increased respiratory minute volume and reduction in FRC, the speed of induction of inhalation anesthesia is seemingly increased. However, the increase in cardiac output, particularly during labor and delivery, tends to slow inhalational induction.

Total Intravenous Anesthetics

While inhalational anesthesia is usually the anesthetic maintenance of choice, in certain scenarios, TIVA may be advantageous for short-term anesthesia in the pregnant mare. Advantages versus volatile anesthesia may be due to hospital-specific considerations, equipment availability, and the speed and simplicity of TIVA administration. Guaifenesin-ketamine-xylazine (GKX) is one of the most common TIVA choices in horses. This combination has been described in dystocias and neonatal survival in a case series as 1 in 4, though notably mortality of the other neonates was unrelated to anesthesia [23]. TIVA using the combination of detomidine, ketamine, and guaiphenesin (DKG) has been shown to be a suitable alternative for maintenance of general anesthesia in pregnant ponies undergoing laparotomy, but not dystocia [24]. The DKG combination produced a smooth anesthetic episode while preserving cardiovascular function in the mare and the fetus by maintaining maternal blood pressure and uterine blood flow. The use of propofol as a TIVA agent has been characterized in pregnant ponies and may be used as a suitable alternative for short-term anesthesia in pregnant equids, [25] however it may be cost prohibitive in larger patients. Dosing and concentrations of TIVA options are included in Table 72.2.

Adjunctive Lidocaine

The effects of systemic lidocaine are poorly understood in pregnant horses. Lidocaine CRIs administered during anesthesia of horses with colic are used to provide additional systemic analgesia, a MAC-sparing effect, presumed anti-inflammatory properties, and presumed prokinetic effect on the gastrointestinal system. While all these properties have not been investigated in the horse, lidocaine (50 μg/kg/min) has been shown to reduce isoflurane requirements by approximately 25% without negatively affecting physiologic and metabolic parameters or increases in stress-related hormones [26]. Lidocaine CRIs in horses undergoing colic surgery have shown reductions in the requirement for not only isoflurane but also dobutamine and phenylephrine [27].

Minimizing stress and maintaining blood pressure is vitally important in the pregnant mare. Some anesthetists advocate against its use, with concerns regarding pharmacology of lidocaine [28]. For example, lidocaine is moderately (~67%) protein bound. Thus, in patients with hypoproteinemia (as is common in pregnancy, especially with colic), there may be a greater proportion of free (active) drug. Additionally, lidocaine is a weak base that can lead to ion-trapping and sequestration of the drug in the more acidic fetal circulation. As is the case in any horse, lidocaine is often discontinued 20–30 minutes before the end of anesthesia to minimize the risk of paresis in recovery. Certainly, in the multiparous, potentially weak mare, this should be carefully considered before adding it to any anesthetic plan. Thus, lidocaine should not be administered to all pregnant mares. The anesthetist must identify those mares in which the benefits of lidocaine outweigh the risks. The considerations include the status of the mare, condition of the fetus, analgesic requirement during surgery, potential improvement in cardiovascular status with isoflurane reductions, and its impact on anesthetic recovery.

Anesthetic Monitoring

Anesthetic monitoring requirements are no different in the pregnant mare compared to a non-gravid horse undergoing an anesthetic episode. Direct arterial blood pressure measurement should be performed via cannulation of a peripheral artery. The mean arterial blood pressure should be maintained above 70 mmHg to ensure sufficient pressure for uterine perfusion. Similar to other anesthetized equids, it is vital to tailor anesthetic depth, fluid therapy, ionotropic therapy, and vasopressor administration to the individual patient. Maternal ventilation should be measured via end-tidal capnography and arterial blood gas analysis should be performed, when possible, to assess arterial oxygen and carbon dioxide tensions. These measurements are important to ensure optimal uteroplacental oxygen delivery. Hypoxemia and hypercarbia can induce a sympathetic nervous system response, leading to uterine artery constriction. However, it is important to avoid hyperventilating the mare, as hypocarbia can decrease cardiac output and increase uterine vascular resistance.

If available, electrocardiography should be instituted as it allows for detection of arrhythmias, which could lead to decreased cardiac output and compromised uterine blood flow. Arrhythmias may be associated with major electrolyte derangements. Thus, blood electrolyte analysis should be performed on pregnant mares, particularly laboring or dystotic mares undergoing general anesthesia and appropriate supplementation should be implemented. Fetal heart rate (FHR) is often monitored during pregnancy and labor in women to detect signs of fetal distress. In mares, FHR can be reliably assessed through fetomaternal electrocardiography from day 173 of gestation to foaling [29]. While this might aid in the prediction of foaling, within 30 minutes, and pre- and post-anesthetic readings may be informative of fetal status, this may not always be practical in the anesthetized mare.

Blood Pressure Support

Care should be taken to assess the mare's hydration status prior to anesthesia. Any blood loss during uterine surgery should be quantified and supplemented with goal directed fluid therapy. There is not a current consensus on best pharmaceutical treatment of hypotension during anesthesia of the pregnant mare. In the nonpregnant horse, a positive inotropic drug such as a dobutamine CRI is often recommended over vasoconstrictive agents to maintain peripheral perfusion [30]. However, in pregnant sheep that display epidurally induced hypotension, ephedrine has shown to improve cardiac output and effectively maintain uterine and placental perfusion when compared to phenylephrine [31]. In people, ephedrine and phenylephrine are commonly used agents for the treatment of hypotension secondary to epidural/spinal anesthesia during cesarean sections. This is to balance the vasodilatory effect of these neuraxial techniques. Of the two drugs, phenylephrine might be a better option as it reduces the likelihood of fetal acidosis during cesarean section [32]. Phenylephrine was also less likely than norepinephrine to cause fetal acidosis as well [33]. High epidurals with local anesthetic, which cause a similar degree of vasodilation, are contraindicated in the horse. Debilitated mares or those with significant blood loss under volatile anesthesia could behave similarly. As such, the anesthetist should manage systemic vascular resistance with adequate volume therapy and vasopressors, while supporting cardiac output with inotropes such as dobutamine. Care should be taken when using vasopressors to not "overconstrict" and potentially induce fetal acidosis.

Recovery

The heavily pregnant, periparturient, unfit, or older mare may need assistance when recovering from general anesthesia. Following controlled vaginal delivery or cesarean section, attention should be paid to drying the mare and recovery stall floor of obstetric lubricant and amniotic fluids. Hypoxemia is often associated with rough or poor-quality recoveries and is sometimes profound in postdystotic mares. Oxygen supplementation should be continued via demand valve and/or nasal insufflation at 15 l/min as a suggested flow rate to increase PaO_2 [34]. Mares that are unfit or have been laboring for a prolonged period prior to anesthesia will be exhausted and might need human assistance to get up. Multiparous mothers may display increased anxiety as they emerge from anesthesia and may rise quickly to search for their foal. While there is no consensus regarding the best method for recovering these patients, many anesthetists advocate for the use of assisted recovery systems such as head and tail ropes, air mattresses, tilt-tables, or a hydro-pool [35].

An important step in the recovery of these animals is the introduction of the mare and newborn foal. As normal maternal-fetal bonding is often disrupted by sedation/anesthesia, mares can be quite excitable during this phase, potentially risking trauma for the foal from kicks and/or bites. Thus, experienced handlers should restrain both mare and foal during introduction, and the two should be constantly monitored until both dam and neonate are well acquainted and relaxed.

Perioperative Pain Management

Epidural Anesthesia

Sacrococcygeal or intercoccygeal epidurals can be valuable analgesic techniques in periparturient mares for perivulvar obstetric procedures or pelvic/abdominal analgesia (Figure 72.1) [36]. Although epidural and spinal anesthesia can be the foundation of analgesic plans for cesarean sections in dogs, cats, small ruminants, and other species, the pregnant mare may not lend itself to this technique. The importance of time from the first signs of parturition to delivery of the foal and the necessity for rectal and uterine palpation during dystocias limits these techniques to planned elective procedures and postoperative analgesia in the horse. Additionally, the use of morphine can take up to 6 hours to achieve its effect when administered epidurally in horses; thus, the limitations of delaying delivery outweigh the benefits of preemptive epidural administration [37].

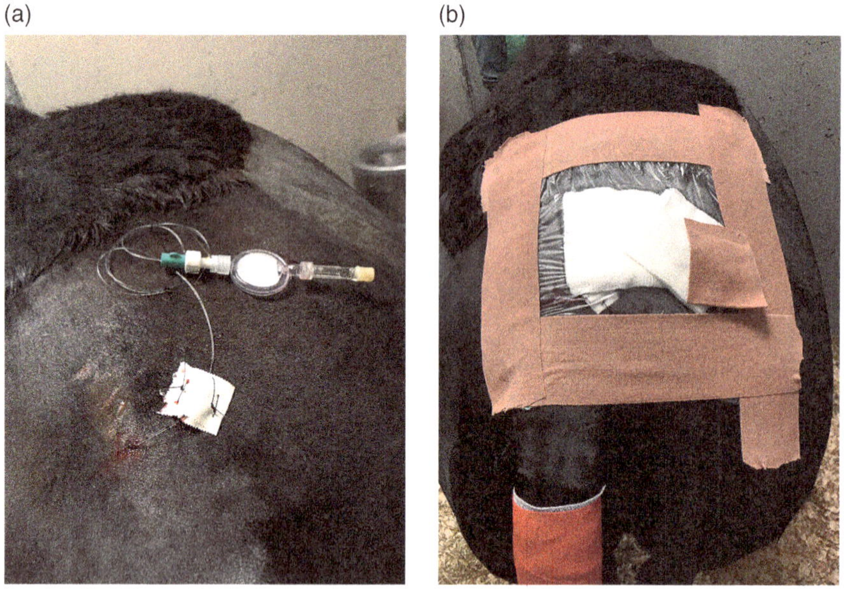

Figure 72.1 Sacrococcygeal epidural catheter placement in the horse. (a) Epidural catheter in situ after placement with aseptic preparation and sterile technique. (b) A sterile-occlusive bandage is placed over-top of the epidural catheter to protect the catheter from contamination.

Postoperatively, it is common that mares may require multiple rectal and vaginal palpations/treatments in addition to treatments administered to relieve the pain they may be experiencing due to delivery or cesarean section. Though the delay in onset (6 hours) is not ideal, the benefit is the long duration of action of epidural morphine (8–12 hours). Given that analgesia is likely to be required longer than this time frame, epidural catheters can be useful in providing good-quality analgesia while minimizing systemic side effects and avoiding the necessity to repeatedly sedate and re-administer epidurals two to three times per day.

For perivulvar obstetric procedures, commonly administered epidural agents include morphine (0.1 mg/kg), xylazine (0.17 mg/kg), detomidine (0.02 mg/kg), and local anesthetics (5 ml of either: Lidocaine 2%, Mepivacaine 2% or Bupivacaine 0.5%). Volume of injectate is critical in achieving effect with epidurals. However, in the horse, it is important not to exceed 10 ml in a 500 kg adult horse to prevent paresis/paralysis of the pelvic limbs when using local anesthetics. Additionally, ketamine can be used in epidurals but can have local anesthetic-like effects; therefore, careful use is also warranted to avoid paresis/paralysis.

Anesthetic Management for the Pregnant Mare for Nonobstetric Procedures

Anesthetizing a pregnant mare for elective surgery should be avoided if possible. If general anesthesia must be performed, the safest time window for mare and fetus is the middle trimester (114–220 days of gestation). This timing follows the initial differentiation and development of the fetus but before the added burdens of rapid growth.

The anesthetic goals for a pregnant mare undergoing a nonobstetric emergency surgery/procedure should take the added concern for the fetus into account. Thus, the anesthetist should strive to maintain maternal homeostasis to ensure appropriate uterine blood flow and subsequent fetal oxygenation. Nonobstetric emergencies include abdominal surgery for colic and surgery for traumatic injuries. Just as in a non-pregnant mare, intestinal emergencies can be fatal. While the short-term survival rate of pregnant and non-pregnant mares is not significantly different (61% and 65% respectively), there is a 30.7% prevalence of negative pregnancy outcome following treatment for colic in pregnant mares [38]. Factors including surgical intervention for colic, long duration of anesthesia (>3 hours), and intraoperative hypotension all contribute to negative pregnancy outcomes [38].

Anesthetic Management of the Pregnant Mare for Dystocia and Cesarean Delivery

Dystocia is a life-threatening emergency for both mare and foal. Early detection as well as rapid and appropriate interventions are critical to foal survival. While the speed of presentation is oftentimes out of the hands of the anesthetist, the anesthetic team must make efforts to minimize time between intake and induction of the mare. A hospital that admits pregnant horses and treatment for dystocia should have all equipment ready before arrival. While much of this includes materials for manipulation of the foal, anesthetic drugs should be readily available and anesthetic equipment assembled and prepared to prevent delays. It is helpful to have a generalized plan for sedation and anesthetic protocols to provide appropriate muscle relaxation and comfort to the mare so that fetal manipulation may be attempted.

Sedation and anesthetic protocols should assume that the foal is alive, unless there is definitive proof of fetal death, and that any drugs administered to the mare enter fetal circulation. Therefore, the anesthetist should select a protocol comprising short-acting or reversible drugs. Parturition adds several complicating factors to an anesthetic episode. The elevation of circulating hormones such as oxytocin contribute to further vasodilation in the peripheral vasculature, leading to hypotension. The weight of the gravid uterus and displaced abdominal viscera apply increased pressure on the diaphragm leading to further exacerbated hypoventilation and increase ventilation/perfusion (V/Q) mismatch, and there is a relaxation of lower esophageal sphincter tone, which contributes to a raised risk of regurgitation and aspiration.

On presentation, a mare in dystocia often shows signs of pain, agitation, tachycardia, and hemoconcentration with or without acid-base and electrolyte derangements [39]. Initial management of these patients should include assessment of physical examination, hematologic and biochemical parameters, and acid-base status. Based on these results, administration of analgesics and sedatives can be administered as required. Fluid resuscitation should be rapid if necessary. Often, two jugular catheters and the use of hypertonic saline can prevent delays to anesthetic induction and the process of delivery while providing significant improvement in volume status of the patient. If antibiotics are to be administered, it is ideal they are given before induction of anesthesia rather than during anesthesia. Much of this process will overlap into anesthetic induction, and any medications administered at this step often serve as all or part of the premedication.

Anesthetic induction in the horse is typically performed with a combination of ketamine (2.2 mg/kg IV) and a benzodiazepine such as diazepam or midazolam (0.02–0.1 mg/kg IV). In canine and feline patients, the induction of anesthesia for cesarean section is often performed with propofol, as it has shown to result in better neurological reflexes in neonates following cesarean section [19]. While similar studies have not been performed in the horse, induction quality with combinations of propofol and guaifenesin or propofol and ketamine is smooth in this species [40, 41]. Further research is needed to determine if a propofol combination for induction offers a favorable outcome in mares with dystocia.

If fetal manipulation is elected after induction (e.g. controlled vaginal delivery), the mare is placed in Trendelenburg position (Figure 72.2). This is most easily accomplished by moving the mare onto a padded mattress and hoisting the hind legs while the front half remains semilateral on the mattress. While the manual manipulation of the fetus takes place, the mare should be monitored continuously, and subsequent ventilation should be provided. Personnel not directly involved in the monitoring of the mare or in the manipulation of the fetus should clip and aseptically prepare the abdomen for potential surgery.

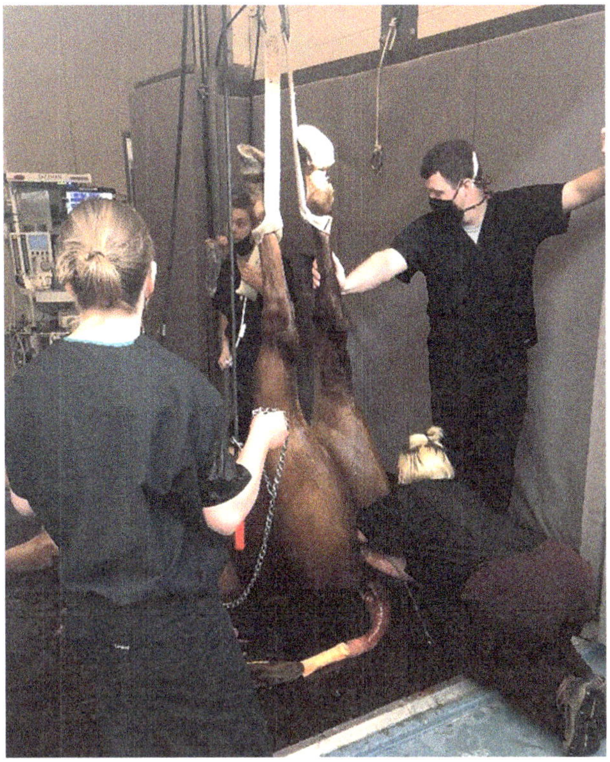

Figure 72.2 Controlled vaginal delivery in a mare with dystocia. Note the mare is anesthetized and the hindlimbs are elevated with a hoist to facilitate fetal manipulation.

It is important for the team to constantly communicate, and if manipulation of the fetus lasts longer than 20 minutes or the live fetus is showing signs of distress, a cesarean section is recommended.

If vaginal delivery attempts fail and cesarean section is elected, the mare should be moved onto the surgical table and into the operating room. As stated previously, there is likely a decrease in MAC for inhalational anesthetics in the pregnant mare. However, the decrease in MAC may not be noticed when a mare in dystocia undergoes cesarean section since supplemental anesthetics are avoided in many cases prior to the foal being removed. Local-regional techniques and epidurals should be considered.

Following the delivery of the foal, via assisted vaginal or cesarean means, the administration of oxytocin helps increase uterine vascular tone and increase uterine involution. This helps control uterine bleeding and reduces blood loss during uterine closure. The administration of oxytocin should be performed slowly (IM or IV over 30 minutes), as to not induce hypotension. Hypotension may result from maternal peripheral vasodilation leading to a decrease in systemic vascular resistance and a subsequent decrease in venous return and cardiac output.

Recovering the periparturient mare from anesthesia is not without risks. A mare that has undergone prolonged labor is often weak so a rope-assisted recovery is recommended. If there is evidence of electrolyte derangements, particularly hypocalcemia, or severe muscle weakness, the mare should be empirically treated. Recovery should be done in a padded recovery box, and particular attention should be paid to the footing within this environment. If obstetric lubricant was used, it is prudent to remove any lubricant from the mare and the floor to prevent slippage. In many cases, these mares do not require additional sedation during their recovery and are often quiet and take their time prior to attempting to stand.

Resuscitation of the Neonatal Foal

Following traumatic birth or cesarean section, the newborn foal is often severely depressed and may require resuscitation. In addition to prolonged labor, depressed mentation of the newborn is often secondary to anesthetic agents used in the dam and their depressive effects on the cardiopulmonary and central nervous systems. Prompt resuscitative therapy is necessary to ensure a positive outcome. Initial focus should be on providing a dry, warm environment, and stimulating the newborn to breathe. Resuscitative efforts should be tailored to the neonate based initial assessment of the heart rate, respiratory rate and character, and neuromuscular tone. Monitoring should be placed on the neonate regardless of their status. As a minimum this should include ECG, pulse oximetry, and end-tidal carbon dioxide ($EtCO_2$; if intubated).

Basic life support (CPR, intubation, and ventilation) should be provided if the foal is: [42]

- Gasping for longer than 30 seconds
- Absent respiratory movements or heartbeat
- Heart rate is <50 beats/min
- Obvious dyspnea/apnea

Table 72.3 Reversal agents and doses for the neonatal foal.

Drug	Dose (mg/kg), IV	Reversal agent for:
Flumazenil	0.01	Benzodiazepines
Naloxone	0.04	Opioids
Tolazoline	2.0 (IM or slow IV)	α2 agonists
Atipamezole	0.1–0.2 (IM or slow IV)	α2 agonists

For advanced life support, IV access is rapidly made with an 18–20 gauge catheter placed in the jugular vein. It is important to note that bradycardia is typically associated with hypoxemia in neonates, and intubation and ventilation are a more appropriate treatment than atropine in these cases. Ventilation does not require 100% oxygen; the use of an ambubag and room air is adequate. These recommendations have been made for the neonatal foal based on meta-analyses in human infants [42, 43]. During advanced life support of the neonatal foal, epinephrine (0.01 mg/kg IV, q3–5 min) is the drug primarily used. Additionally, any reversal agents that may be needed should be readily available (Table 72.3). The authors advocate calculating the dose and volume of any drugs before delivery of the neonate to minimize delay in administration. The choice of reversal agents depends on the anesthetic protocol selected by the anesthetist and considers administration timing of anesthetic drugs and time to delivery. See Chapter 2 for further information regarding CPR.

References

1 Dugdale, A.H., Obhrai, J., and Cripps, P.J. (2016). Twenty years later: a single-centre, repeat retrospective analysis of equine perioperative mortality and investigation of recovery quality. *Vet. Anaesth. Analg.* 43: 171–178.
2 Byron, C.R., Embertson, R.M., Bernard, W.V. et al. (2003). Dystocia in a referral hospital setting: approach and results. *Equine Vet. J.* 35: 82–85.
3 Norton, J.L., Dallap, B.L., Johnston, J.K. et al. (2007). Retrospective study of dystocia in mares at a referral hospital. *Equine Vet. J.* 39: 37–41.
4 Wilson, D.V. (1994). Anesthesia and sedation for late-term mares. *Vet. Clin. North Am. Equine. Pract.* 10: 219–236.
5 Camann, W.R. and Ostheimer, G.W. (1990). Physiological adaptations during pregnancy. *Int. Anesth. Clin.* 28: 2–10.
6 Brooks, V. and Keil, L. (1994). Hemorrhage decreases arterial pressure sooner in pregnant compared with nonpregnant dogs: role of baoreflex. *Am. J. Phys.* 266: H1610–H1619.
7 Satué, K. and Domingo, R. (2011). Longitudinal study of the renin angiotensin aldosterone system in purebred Spanish broodmares during pregnancy. *Theriogenology* 75: 1185–1194.
8 Faramarzi, B., Rich, L.J., and Wu, J. (2018). Hematological and serum biochemical profile values in pregnant and non-pregnant mares. *Can. J. Vet. Res.* 82: 287–293.
9 Chandra, S., Tripathi, A.K., Mishra, S. et al. (2012). Physiological changes in hematological parameters during pregnancy. *Ind. J. Hematol. Blood Trans.* 28: 144–146.
10 Frederiksen, M.C. (2001). Physiologic changes in pregnancy and their effect on drug disposition. *Semin. Perinatol.* 25: 120–123.
11 Bazzano, M., Giannetto, C., Fazio, F. et al. (2014). Hemostatic profile during late pregnancy and early postpartum period in mares. *Theriogenology* 81: 639–643.
12 Gin, T. and Chan, M.T.V. (1994). Decreased minimum alveolar concentration of isoflurane in pregnant humans. *Anesthesiology* 81: 829–832.
13 Goodger, W.J. and Levy, W. (1973). Anesthetic management of the Cesarean section. *Vet. Clinics North Am.* 3: 85–99.

14 Moon, P.F., Erb, H.N., Ludders, J.W. et al. (2000). Perioperative risk factors for puppies delivered by cesarean section in the United States and Canada. *J. Am. Anim. Hosp. Assoc.* 36: 359–368.
15 De Cramer, K.G., Joubert, K.E., and Nöthling, J.O. (2017). Puppy survival and vigor associated with the use of low dose medetomidine premedication, propofol induction and maintenance of anesthesia using sevoflurane gas-inhalation for cesarean section in the bitch. *Theriogenology* 96: 10–15.
16 Schmidt, K., Feng, C., Wu, T. et al. (2021). Influence of maternal, anesthetic, and surgical factors on neonatal survival after emergency cesarean section in 78 dogs: a retrospective study (2002 to 2020). *Can. Vet. J.* 62: 961.
17 Mathews, K.A. (2008). Pain management for the pregnant, lactating, and neonatal to pediatric cat and dog. *Vet. Clin. North Am. Small Anim. Pract.* 38: 1291–1308.
18 Mirra, A., Birras, J., Diez Bernal, S. et al. (2020). Morphine plasmatic concentration in a pregnant mare and its foal after long term epidural administration. *BMC Vet. Res.* 16: 1–5.
19 Luna, S.P., Cassu, R.N., Castro, G.B. et al. (2004). Effects of four anaesthetic protocols on the neurological and cardiorespiratory variables of puppies born by caesarean section. *Vet. Rec.* 154: 387–389.
20 Mahomedy, M.C., Downing, J.W., Jeal, D.E. et al. (1976). Ketamine for anaesthetic induction at caesarean section. *South Afr. Med. J.* 50: 846–848.
21 Bidwell, L., Embertson, R., Bone, N. et al. (2008). Diazepam levels in foals after dystocia birth. *Porc. Annu. Conv. Am. Assoc. Equine Pract.* 54: 286–287.
22 Daunt, D.A., Steffey, E.P., Pascoe, J.R. et al. (1992). Actions of isoflurane and halothane in pregnant mares. *J. Am. Vet. Med. Assoc.* 201: 1367–1374.
23 Lin, H.C., Wallace, S.S., Robbins, R.L. et al. (1994). A case report on the use of guaifenesin-ketamine-xylazine anesthesia for equine dystocia. *Cornell Vet.* 84: 61–66.
24 Taylor, P.M., Luna, S.P., White, K.L. et al. (2001). Intravenous anaesthesia using detomidine, ketamine and guaiphenesin for laparotomy in pregnant pony mares. *Vet. Anaesth. Analg.* 28: 119–125.
25 Taylor, P.M., White, K.L., Fowden, A.L. et al. (2001). Propofol anaesthesia for surgery in late gestation pony mares. *Vet. Anaesth. Analg.* 28: 177–187.
26 Dzikiti, T.B., Hellebrekers, L.J., and Van Dijk, P. (2003). Effects of intravenous lidocaine on isoflurane concentration, physiological parameters, metabolic parameters and stress-related hormones in horses undergoing surgery. *J. Vet. Med. A* 50: 190–195.
27 Bubb, L., Drissen, B., and Staffieiri, F. (2008). The isoflurane-sparing effect of intravenous lidocaine administered to horses undergoing exploratory celiotomy. *Proc. Vet. Emerg. Crit. Care.*
28 Miller, L., Gozalo-Marcilla, M., Pollock, P.J. et al. (2021). Anesthetic management of a pregnant broodmare with gastrointestinal colic. *Vlaams Diergeneeskd. Tijdschr.* 90: 29–36.
29 Nagel, C., Aurich, J., and Aurich, C. (2010). Determination of heart rate and heart rate variability in the equine fetus by fetomaternal electrocardiography. *Theriogenology* 73: 973–983.
30 Schauvliege, S. and Gasthuys, F. (2013). Drugs for cardiovascular support in anesthetized horses. *Vet. Clin. Equine Prac.* 29: 19–49.
31 Erkinaro, T., Mäkikallio, K., Kavasmaa, T. et al. (2004). Effects of ephedrine and phenylephrine on uterine and placental circulations and fetal outcome following fetal hypoxaemia and epidural-induced hypotension in a sheep model. *Brit. J. Anaesth.* 93: 825–832.
32 Xu, C., Liu, S., Huang, Y. et al. (2018). Phenylephrine vs ephedrine in cesarean delivery under spinal anesthesia: a systematic literature review and meta-analysis. *Int. J. Surg.* 60: 48–59.
33 Mohta, M., Garg, A., Chilkoti, G.T. et al. (2019). A randomised controlled trial of phenylephrine and noradrenaline boluses for treatment of postspinal hypotension during elective Caesarean section. *Anaesthesia* 74: 850–855.
34 McMurphy, R.M. and Cribb, P.H. (1989). Alleviation of postanesthetic hypoxemia in the horse. *Can. Vet. J.* 30: 37.
35 Loomes, K. and Louro, L.F. (2022). Recovery of horses from general anaesthesia: a systematic review (2000–2020) of risk factors and influence of interventions during the recovery period. *Equine Vet. J.* 54: 201–218.
36 Robinson, E.P. and Natalini, C.C. (2002). Epidural anesthesia and analgesia in horses. *Vet. Clin. Equine Pract.* 18: 61–82.
37 Natalini, C.C. and Robinson, E.P. (2000). Evaluation of the analgesic effects of epidurally administered morphine, alfentanil, butorphanol, tramadol, and U50488H in horses. *Am. J. Vet. Res.* 61: 1579–1586.
38 Chenier, T.S. and Whitehead, A.E. (2009). Foaling rates and risk factors for abortion in pregnant mares presented for medical or surgical treatment of colic: 153 cases (1993–2005). *Can. Vet. J.* 50: 481.
39 Rioja, E., Cernicchiaro, N., Costa, M.C. et al. (2012). Perioperative risk factors for mortality and length of hospitalization in mares with dystocia undergoing general anesthesia: a retrospective study. *Can. Vet. J.* 53: 502–510.
40 Brosnan, R.J., Steffey, E.P., Escobar, A. et al. (2011). Anesthetic induction with guaifenesin and propofol in adult horses. *Am. J. Vet. Res.* 72: 1569–1575.
41 Posner, L.P., Kasten, J.I., and Kata, C. (2013). Propofol with ketamine following sedation with xylazine for routine induction of general anaesthesia in horses. *Vet. Rec.* 173: 550.
42 Jokisalo, J.M. and Corley, K.T. (2014). CPR in the neonatal foal: has RECOVER changed our approach? *Vet. Clin. Equine Pract.* 30: 301–316.
43 Saugstad, O.D., Vento, M., Ramji, S. et al. (2012). Neurodevelopmental outcome of infants resuscitated with air or 100% oxygen: a systematic review and meta-analysis. *Neonatology* 102: 98–103.

Appendix Formulary for Equine Neonatal Medications

Drug Formulary. Although some of the medications noted in this formulary have undergone pharmacokinetic and pharmacodynamic studies in foals, several of the medications noted have only been documented from case reports and anecdotal use. Therefore, this formulary should be used as a guide as many medications noted have had minimal or no formal pharmacokinetic and pharmacodynamic studies performed in neonatal foals. IV, intravenous; IM, intramuscular; PO, per os; PR, per rectum, CRI, continuous rate infusion.

Drug	Dosing information	Comments/Indications
Acepromazine	0.03–0.06 mg/kg, IV or IM	Phenothiazine derivative that acts as a dopamine receptor antagonist. Used for sedation or premedication for general anesthesia. Anecdotal use (0.01 mg/kg, IV) in foals with stranguria and/or urinary dyssynergy to promote urination. Use with caution in sick or septic foals due to possible hypotension.
Acetaminophen	20–40 mg/kg, PO, q12–24h	Analgesic and antipyretic via interactions with serotonergic, opioid, nitric oxide, and cannabinoid pathways as well as effects on central prostaglandin production. Efficacy and safety in foals not determined.
Acetazolamide	2.2–4.4 mg/kg, PO, q12h	Carbonic anhydrase inhibitor used to prevent/control episodes of hyperkalemic periodic paralysis which, in foals, can present as a myopathy, respiratory stridor, and/or dysphagia [1, 2]. Diuretic for potassium and bicarbonate. Also used to treat glaucoma as it decreases production of aqueous humor and lowers intraocular pressure.
Acetylcysteine	Per rectum: 200 ml of 4% solution administered via foley catheter; leave in rectum for 20 minutes before allowing foal to evacuate rectum. Typically requires foal to be sedated prior to enema. Nebulization: 4–8 mg/kg q6h as a 20% solution	Mucolytic drug. Per rectum administration is used for treatment of meconium impaction. Enemas are commercially available (EZ-pass, Animal Reproductive Systems, Chino, CA) or can be made by combining 20 g of sodium bicarbonate (baking soda) and 8 g of acetylcysteine in 200 ml of water; produces a 4% acetylcysteine solution with a pH of 7.6 (increased pH enhances mucolytic activity). Alternatively, dilute 40 ml of a 20% acetylcysteine solution with 160 ml of water and 20 g of sodium bicarbonate to create 4% solution. Nebulization is used for treatment of meconium aspiration to decrease the viscosity of inhaled meconium. Typical volumes for nebulization are 3–10 ml [3].

Equine Neonatal Medicine, First Edition. Edited by David M. Wong and Pamela A. Wilkins.

Drug	Dosing information	Comments/Indications
Activated charcoal	1–4 g/kg, PO (via NG tube) in water (approximately 1 g/5 ml), q4–6h or as needed	Intestinal adsorbent for ingested toxins; sometimes used to combat endotoxemia secondary to colitis. Do not administer at same time as other oral medications as they may decrease bioavailability [4].
Acyclovir	10 mg/kg, IV, q12h over 60 minutes or 20 mg/kg, PO, q6–8h	Synthetic nucleoside analogue antiviral drug used in horses as a treatment for equine herpes virus. Doses derived from adult horses [5, 6].
Albuterol	1–10 μg/kg, nebulized, q6–8h or 0.8–2 μg/kg metered dose inhaler, q6h	β-2 receptor agonist drug that promotes bronchodilation; variable benefit in foals with respiratory disease [7–9].
Allopurinol	40 mg/kg, PO	Xanthine oxidase inhibitor used as an antioxidant to combat neonatal encephalopathy; best if given within 4 hours of injury to foals that are at high risk of developing neonatal encephalopathy [10]. Efficacy unknown.
Alfaxalone	2–3 mg/kg, IV (induction) 6 mg/kg/h CRI (maintenance)	Neuroactive steroid and anesthetic induction agent; administer slowly at 0.5–1 mg/kg/min [11]. Often combined with an α2 agonist and an opioid for induction.
Alprazolam	**MARES:** 0.1 mg/kg, PO (loading dose), followed by 0.04 mg/kg, PO, q12h (maintenance dose)	Benzodiazepine drug that acts via potentiation of gamma-aminobutyric acid (GABA) mediated inhibitory effects in the CNS. Oral drug used for sedative and anxiolytic effects. Has been given to postpartum mares that show aggression toward their newborn foal to facilitate maternal acceptance of foal [12]. Decrease dose or interval if excessive/unwanted sedation occurs.
Altrenogest	**MARES:** 0.044–0.088 mg/kg, PO, q24h	Synthetic progesterone is used to regulate estrus and for behavior modification to help reduce libido and aggression in stallions. Used to help maintain pregnancy in early gestation when concerned of a dysfunctional corpus luteum. May help maintain pregnancy in mares with endotoxemia at higher doses (0.088 mg/kg). Gloves should be worn during handling and administration.
Amikacin	Foals: 25–30 mg/kg, IM or IV, q24h	Aminoglycoside antimicrobial drug with excellent spectrum against Gram-negative pathogens and *Staphylococci*. Increased dose required for foals due to their larger volume of distribution. Evaluation of urinalysis and serum creatinine during treatment are recommended. Therapeutic drug monitoring should target serum values at 30 min ≥53–60 μg/ml or 60 min ≥40 μg/ml; trough values at 20 hours should be <2 μg/ml [13].
Aminocaproic acid	3.5 mg/kg/min for 15 minutes (loading dose), then 0.25 mg/kg/min CRI [14] 40 mg/kg dilute in 1 l of saline, IV, over 30–60 minutes (loading dose), then 20 mg/kg, IV, diluted in 1 l of saline over 30–60 minutes q6h (maintenance dose). 100 mg/kg, IV [15]	Antifibrinolytic drug that binds to plasminogen and thereby blocks the binding of plasminogen to fibrin and its activation of plasmin; this in turn reduces fibrinolysis. Used to help control or stop acute hemorrhage. Doses derived from adult horses. Therapeutic plasma concentrations of aminocaproic acid may be lower in horses than humans [16].
Aminophylline	5–12 mg/kg, IV, q6–12h slowly or 5–15 mg/kg, PO, q6–12h. Dosage should be diluted in at least 100 ml of D5W or normal saline.	Methylxanthine phosphodiesterase inhibitor drug that promotes bronchodilation and diuresis [17]. Aminophylline is a 2 : 1 complex of theophylline and ethylenediamine; doses described provide approximately 3.95–9.44 mg/kg based on theophylline content. Due to risk for serious adverse CNS effects, typically reserved for cases refractory to more common treatments.

(*Continued*)

Drug	Dosing information	Comments/Indications
Amiodarone	5 mg/kg, IV 5 mg/kg/h CRI for 1h (loading dose) followed by 0.83 mg/kg/h for 23h (maintenance dose)	Class III anti-arrhythmic drug that blocks potassium channels; used in people (suggested in foals) during CPR for ventricular tachycardia and ventricular fibrillation that is unresponsive to defibrillation. Doses derived from adult horses; drug not investigated in foals for this use [18, 19].
Ampicillin sodium	10–30 mg/kg, IV, q6–8h 10–22 mg/kg, IM, q12h	Aminopenicillin antimicrobial drug. Doses at the higher end of the dose range should be used for anaerobic infections. Doses up to 25–40 mg/kg q6–8h have been used for refractory infections. Resistance among Gram-negative organisms is high, therefore ampicillin should be combined with an aminoglycoside for broader spectrum treatment of neonatal sepsis [20, 21].
Ampicillin trihydrate suspension	6.6–22 mg/kg, IM, q12–24h	As above, marketed as Polyflex®. Intravenous administration of another appropriate antimicrobial is preferred in septic neonatal foals.
Amoxicillin	10–30 mg/kg, IV or IM, q6h 20–30 mg/kg, PO, q8–12h	Aminopenicillin antimicrobial drug. Oral bioavailability decreases rapidly within the first few months of life; therefore, this route should not be used in older foals [21].
Amoxicillin/clavulanic acid	15–25 mg/kg, IV, q6–8h 30 mg/kg, PO, q6–8h	Beta-lactam aminopenicillin antimicrobial drug combined with a beta-lactamase inhibitor [22]. Can be used as an oral broad-spectrum antimicrobial for foals up to 4 months of age [23].
Arginine vasopressin (aka vasopressin; anti-diuretic hormone)	0.25–1.0 mU/kg/min, CRI	Agonist drug at V1a receptors in peripheral vasculature causing vasoconstriction and V2 receptors in collecting tubule of nephron to enhance water resorption [24, 25]. Used for treatment of vasodilatory shock and can be combined with other pressor agents. Store refrigerated.
Aspirin	25 mg/kg, PO, q12h initially, then 10 mg/kg, PO, q24h 10 mg/kg, PO, q48h	Nonsteroidal anti-inflammatory drug that works as a nonselective cyclooxygenase inhibitor. Most commonly used as an anti-coagulant to reduce platelet aggregation, which occurs at lower doses and lasts for a prolonged period [26]. Higher doses are needed for providing analgesic and antipyrexic effects [27]. Higher doses are considered highly ulcerogenic.
Atipamezole	50–160 μg/kg, IV or IM	α-2 adrenergic antagonist used as reversal agent for α-2 agonists (detomidine, xylazine, romifidine, medetomidine) [28, 29].
Atropine	0.005–0.01 mg/kg, IV	Parasympatholytic (anti-cholinergic) drug used to increase heart rate during anesthesia or as a bronchodilator in cases of respiratory distress. Topical ophthalmic formulations are used as a long-acting mydriatic. Repeated use may cause gastrointestinal ileus and colic.
Azithromycin	10 mg/kg PO, q24h for 5–7 days, then q48h for subsequent dosing	Macrolide antimicrobial drug. Doses are based on treatment of predominantly intracellular organisms, including *Rhodococcus equi* and *Lawsonia intracellularis* [20, 30]. Keep foal out of sunlight and excess heat to prevent possible hyperthermia. Diarrhea has been seen in older foals and weanlings, anecdotally associated more with compounded formulations.

Drug	Dosing information	Comments/Indications
Bethanechol	0.025 mg/kg, SC, once then 0.35 mg/kg PO, q8h or 0.22–0.45 mg/kg, PO, q6–8h	Parasympathomimetic (cholinergic) drug that promotes gastric emptying in cases of gastroduodenal ulcers/stricture, gastric outflow obstruction and gastroesophageal reflux. Also used to treat postoperative ileus or bladder atony [31].
Bismuth subsalicylate	0.5–4 ml/kg, PO, q6–24h	Used as gastroprotectant and may help reduce bowel inflammation [4]. The subsalicylate portion is a nonsteroidal anti-inflammatory drug and can be associated with adverse GI and renal effects; do not combine with other NSAIDs.
Bretylium	5–10 mg/kg, IV bolus	Class III anti-arrhythmic drug. Used as a chemical treatment of ventricular fibrillation (limited success with chemical defibrillation); may no longer be commercially available.
Buprenorphine	0.01–0.02 mg/kg, IV or oral transmucosal	Partial μ agonist opioid analgesic drug that can be administered sublingual or oral transmucosal [32]. Due to partial agonist effects, should only be used for mild to moderate pain, but adverse effects are rare.
Butorphanol tartrate	0.005–0.05 mg/kg, IV or IM, as needed (sedation) up to 0.1 mg/kg, IV or IM, as needed (analgesia)	κ agonist, μ antagonist, opioid analgesic drug. May decrease cough reflex and cause respiratory depression [33].
Caffeine	10 mg/kg, PO (loading dose), followed by 2.5–5 mg/kg, PO or PR, q24h (maintenance dose)	Methylxanthine derivative drug used as a central respiratory stimulant in foals with hypercapnia, typically secondary to neonatal encephalopathy [34].
Calcium gluconate (23%)	150–250 mg/kg, diluted, slow IV to effect	Intravenous calcium supplement used to prevent or treat hypocalcemia. Dilute in 0.9% saline, give slowly.
Carprofen	0.7 mg/kg, IV, q24h	Nonsteroidal anti-inflammatory drug that works via inhibition of cyclooxygenase [35]. Slightly COX-2 selective in horses.
Cefadroxil	20–40 mg/kg, PO, q8–12h	First generation cephalosporin antimicrobial drug. Bioavailability decreases from 99.6% in 2-week-old foals to 14.5% in 5-month-old foals [21, 36].
Cefalexin	25 mg/kg, PO, q6h 30 mg/kg, PO, q8h	First generation cephalosporin antimicrobial drug [21, 37, 38].
Cefazolin	10–22 mg/kg, IV, q6–8h	First generation cephalosporin antimicrobial drug. May have some efficacy against Gram-negative organisms involved in neonatal sepsis but should be combined with an aminoglycoside for improved Gram-negative spectrum [38].
Cefepime	11 mg/kg, IV, q8h	Fourth-generation cephalosporin antimicrobial drug. Active against many Gram-negative bacteria that are resistant to third-generation cephalosporins. Crosses the blood-CSF-barrier [39].
Cefoperazone	30 mg/kg, IV, q8h, slow infusion	Third-generation cephalosporin antimicrobial drug. Doses derived from adult horses [40].
Cefotaxime	40 mg/kg, IV, q6h 40 mg/kg, IV (loading dose) then 6.7–8.3 mg/kg/h CRI	Third-generation cephalosporin antimicrobial drug. Crosses the blood-CSF-barrier. CRI dosing may provide optimal time that cefotaxime concentration exceeds MIC for common pathogens [41]. Monitor fecal consistency and for development of antibiotic associated colitis.
Cefoxitin	20 mg/kg, IV or IM, q4–6h	Second-generation cephalosporin antimicrobial drug. Often used for its increased anaerobic spectrum, including many strains of *Bacteroides fragilis* [38].

(*Continued*)

Drug	Dosing information	Comments/Indications
Cefpodoxime proxetil	10 mg/kg, PO, q6–12h	Third-generation cephalosporin antimicrobial drug. More frequent dosing (q6–8h) should be used for *Salmonella* or *Escherichia coli* infections [20, 42].
Cefquinome	1 mg/kg, IV or IM, q12h 2.5–4.5 mg/kg, IV, q12h	Fourth-generation cephalosporin antimicrobial drug. Higher dose regimen is recommended for treatment of bacteria with MICs of 0.125–0.5 μg/ml [38, 43, 44].
Ceftazidime	20–50 mg/kg, IV, q6h slow infusion	Third-generation cephalosporin antimicrobial drug [38, 45].
Ceftiofur sodium	5–10 mg/kg, IV or IM, q6–12h CRI: 5 mg/kg loading dose, then 0.42 mg/kg/h	Third-generation cephalosporin antimicrobial drug. Higher doses should be given slowly. CRI dose can be increased up to 20 mg/kg/d depending on MIC [38, 46, 47]. Does not cross blood-CSF-barrier.
Ceftiofur crystalline free acid	13.2 mg/kg, SC or IM, repeat once in 48h, then q72h	Third-generation cephalosporin antimicrobial drug. The initial dose should be repeated at 48 hours and then q72h afterwards. Weanling age foals can follow recommendations for adult dosing (6.6 mg/kg, IM, repeated at 96 hours). A loading dose of ceftiofur sodium can be administered to achieve more rapid therapeutic concentrations. This formulation is not recommended for severely ill foals [46, 48].
Ceftizoxime	20–50 mg/kg, IV, q6h slow infusion	Third-generation cephalosporin antimicrobial drug [38, 49].
Ceftriaxone	25–50 mg/kg, IV or IM, q12h	Third-generation cephalosporin antimicrobial drug. Crosses blood-CSF-barrier and has excellent penetration into most body tissues (pleural fluid, peritoneal fluid, bile, bone) [50].
Cefuroxime	30 mg/kg, PO, q8–12h	Second-generation cephalosporin antimicrobial drug [20, 38].
Cephalexin	30 mg/kg, PO, q8h	First-generation cephalosporin antimicrobial drug [20, 38].
Cephalothin	10–20 mg/kg, IV, q6h	First-generation cephalosporin antimicrobial drug [38].
Chloramphenicol	40–50 mg/kg, PO, q12h (1–2 days of age), q8h (3–5 days of age)	Broad-spectrum antimicrobial drug with excellent penetration into abscesses. Age-dependent pharmacokinetics documented; prematurity may result in severe prolongation of half-life. Wear gloves when handling [38, 51].
Cimetidine	15–25 mg/kg, PO, q8h 6.6 mg/kg, IV, q6h	Histamine type 2 (H_2) receptor antagonist drug used to treat or prevent gastric ulceration [52, 53]. Absorption is variable and there is a potential for drug–drug interactions, not used commonly.
Cisapride	0.1 mg/kg, IV or IM	Serotonin receptor type 4 (5-HT_4) agonist and 5-HT_3 antagonist that promotes gastric and/or small intestinal motility, used for treatment of post-operative ileus [54]. Injectable formulations must be compounded.
Clarithromycin	7.5 mg/kg PO, q12h	Macrolide antimicrobial drug. Doses are based on treatment of predominantly intracellular organisms, including *R. equi* [55]. Keep treated foals out of sunlight and excess heat to prevent hyperthermia.
Clenbuterol	0.8–3.2 μg/kg, PO, q12h	β-2 receptor agonist drug used for bronchodilation (foal) or uterine relaxation (pregnant mare) [56, 57]. Increases in dose for nonresponders should be done slowly in a stepwise fashion up to the maximum label dose.

Drug	Dosing information	Comments/Indications
Deferoxamine mesylate	20 mg/kg, SC, q12h	Iron chelating agent; potentially used in foals requiring multiple blood transfusions. In experimental study, medication was given at noted dose for 14 days [58].
Detomidine	0.01–0.04 mg/kg, IV	α-2 receptor agonist drug used for sedation and analgesia. Can cause cardio-respiratory depression; use with extreme caution in sick foals. Have reversal agents available.
Dexamethasone	0.05–0.2 mg/kg, IV, IM, or PO	Long-acting glucocorticoid drug used for immunosuppression and anti-inflammatory effects. Oral absorption not investigated in foals [59].
Diazepam	0.1–0.2 mg/kg, IV 1–3 mg/kg/h CRI	Benzodiazepine drug that acts via potentiation of gamma-aminobutyric acid (GABA) mediated inhibitory effects in the CNS. Used for sedation or seizure control in neonatal foals; do not use in patients with hepatic encephalopathy as it can worsen encephalopathy [60].
Diclofenac	7.3 mg (1.27 cm strip), topically, q12h	Nonspecific topical cyclooxygenase inhibitor used for local control of pain or inflammation [61].
Dimethyl Sulfoxide (DMSO)	0.2–1 g/kg diluted to ≤10% solution in 0.5–1 l of sterile isotonic fluid, IV, q12–24h	Solvent drug with proposed antioxidant and free radical scavenger effects. Used in foals for disease processes such as neonatal encephalopathy and intestinal adhesions secondary to intestinal ischemia or abdominal surgery. Efficacy unknown. Concentrations higher than 10% associated with red blood cell lysis. Wear gloves when handling.
Diphenhydramine	0.5–1 mg/kg, IV or IM	Histamine type-1 receptor antagonist drug used as an adjunctive therapy for transfusion reactions or anaphylaxis [62].
Dipyrone	20–30 mg/kg, IV or IM, q12h	Nonopioid, atypical nonsteroidal anti-inflammatory drug used for its antipyretic and analgesic effects [63, 64]. Mechanism of action not fully elucidated but likely involves both prostaglandin dependent and prostaglandin independent actions.
Dobutamine hydrochloride	2–5 μg/kg/min, CRI initial dose, titrated up to 10 μg/kg/min, CRI if necessary	β1-receptor adrenergic agonist with less affinity for β2- and α-adrenergic receptors. Used as a cardiac inotrope for shock; dose can be titrated to effect [25]. To prepare, mix 250 mg of dobutamine in 500 ml 5% dextrose or 0.9% saline to yield a solution of 500 μg/ml; incompatible with LRS and fluids containing bicarbonate.
Domperidone	**MARES**: 1.1 mg/kg, PO, q24h	Dopamine-2 receptor antagonist used for the treatment for agalactia or prolonged gestation, particularly in mares with fescue toxicity. Begin administration 10 days prior to expected foaling date and continue up to parturition [65].
Dopamine hydrochloride	1–5 μg/kg/min, CRI (vasodilation of renal, splanchnic, cerebral vessels) 5–10 μg/kg/min, CRI (inotropic activity) 10–15 μg/kg/min, CRI (vasopressor activity)	Has complex activity and binds with α-1, α-2, β-1, and dopamine-1 receptors depending on administered dose. Dose can be titrated to effect. To prepare, mix 200 mg of dopamine in 500 ml 5% dextrose or 0.9% saline to yield a solution of 400 μg/ml. Incompatible with LRS and fluids containing bicarbonate.
Doxapram hydrochloride	0.02–0.05 mg/kg/h, IV, CRI or 0.5 mg/kg, IV, repeated as needed up to 3 total doses at 5-minute intervals	Central-acting respiratory stimulant that acts via blockade of potassium channels on carotid body chemoreceptors resulting in an increased sensitivity to CO_2. CRI dose used to combat hypercapnia in some foals with neonatal encephalopathy; bolus dose used in resuscitative efforts [34]. Monitor for CNS/cardiovascular excitement, sweating and convulsions.

(Continued)

Drug	Dosing information	Comments/Indications
Doxycycline	10 mg/kg, PO, q12h	Oral tetracycline antimicrobial drug. Do not administer IV. Combining with rifampin may result in anemia and liver disease. May cause tendon laxity [20, 66].
Enrofloxacin	8 mg/kg, PO or IV, q24h	Fluoroquinolone antimicrobial drug reserved for cases when culture dictates and no other options are available due to potential severe, crippling cartilage toxicity. If used, strict stall rest during and after treatment is required [67].
Epinephrine	0.01–0.02 mg/kg, IV or IM, q3–5 min until return of spontaneous circulation. 0.1–0.2 mg/kg, intratracheal administration 0.1 mg/kg, IM	Nonspecific α- and β-adrenergic receptor agonist drug used as a cardiac inotrope during resuscitation and anaphylaxis [68]. Typical foal dose is 0.5–1 ml of 1 : 1000 (1 mg/ml), or 5–10 ml of 1 : 10 000 (0.1 mg/ml) IV during cardiopulmonary resuscitation; can repeat every 3–5 minutes; avoid SC administration. Higher dose can be used if no response is seen with lower doses.
Erythromycin estolate	25 mg/kg PO, q6–8h	Oral macrolide antimicrobial drug; must be administered as a salt as the erythromycin base degrades rapidly in gastric acid [69]. Highest risk for development of hyperthermia and diarrhea (particularly in older foals and mares).
Erythromycin lactobionate	0.5–2 mg/kg, IV, q6h in 1 l saline over 45 minutes	Intravenous macrolide antimicrobial drug used only as a prokinetic to stimulate motilin receptors and promote gastric and small intestinal motility associated with postoperative ileus [70]. Higher (antimicrobial) doses associated with severe diarrhea.
Esomeprazole	0.5–1 mg/kg, IV, q24h 1–2 mg/kg, PO, q24h	Proton pump inhibitor used to treat or prevent gastric ulceration. Intravenous formulation can be used to treat foals that are unable to receive oral formulation [71, 72].
Famotidine	0.3 mg/kg, IV, q12h 2.8 mg/kg, PO, q12h	H_2 receptor antagonist drug used to treat or prevent gastric ulceration [73].
Fenoldopam mesylate	0.04–0.05 μg/kg/min, CRI	Dopamine type-1 receptor agonist drug used as a diuretic to increase renal blood flow and urine output [74].
Fentanyl	100 μg/h transdermal patch, changed q72h	μ agonist opioid analgesic; 80–100× more potent than morphine. Efficacy with transdermal patches may be low due to variable absorption and often used in conjunction with other analgesic drugs [75].
Firocoxib	0.1–0.2 mg/kg, IV or PO, q12–24h	Highly COX-2 specific nonsteroidal anti-inflammatory drug. Despite specificity, adverse effects are still reported and firocoxib should not be co-administered with other NSAIDs. Pharmacokinetics and doses recommended are different in neonatal foals [76, 77].
Flunixin Meglumine	0.5 mg/kg q12h, IV or PO 1.1 mg/kg q24h, IV or PO 1.1–1.65 mg/kg, IV or PO, q24–36h	Nonselective nonsteroidal anti-inflammatory drug. Use judiciously in dehydrated foals or foals that are receiving other nephrotoxic medications. Pharmacokinetics differ in neonatal foals, suggesting lower doses or longer dosing intervals are needed to prevent adverse effects. Low dose may be used to counter endotoxin-induced inflammation, higher doses are necessary for analgesia [78, 79].

Drug	Dosing information	Comments/Indications
Furosemide	1–2 mg/kg, IV, q12–24h or 0.12 mg/kg, IV loading dose, 0.12 mg/kg/h, IV, CRI	Highly effective but short acting loop diuretic [80, 81]. Foals treated with furosemide should be monitored for dehydration and electrolyte imbalances.
Gabapentin	5–20 mg/kg, PO, q12h	Calcium channel blocker used as an analgesic and anticonvulsant; used for neuropathic pain in horses. Doses derived from adult horses. Doses of 40 mg/kg and 120 mg/kg were administered q12h for 14 days in adult horses with no observed side effects [82, 83].
Gamithromycin	6.6 mg/kg, IM, once a week	Macrolide antimicrobial drug. Dosing is presumed to be effective for *R. equi* and *Strep. zooepidemicus*. To avoid injection site reactions, drug can be diluted using 0.4 ml/kg qs to 50 ml in distilled water and injected in multiple sites [84].
Ganciclovir	2.5 mg/kg, IV, q8h for 24h (loading dose), 2.5 mg/kg, IV, q12h (maintenance dose)	Synthetic nucleoside analogue antiviral drug used in horses as a treatment for equine herpes virus; doses derived from adult horses [5, 85].
Gentamicin	12–14 mg/kg, IV or IM, q24–36h	Aminoglycoside antimicrobial drug with excellent spectrum against Gram-negative pathogens and staphylococci. Increased dose is required for foals due to the larger volume of distribution. Evaluation of urinalysis and serum creatinine during treatment are recommended. Therapeutic drug monitoring should target values at 30 minutes ≥30–40 μg/ml or 60 minutes ≥20 μg/ml; trough values at 20 hours < 1 μg/ml [86].
Glycopyrrolate	0.0025–0.005 mg/kg, IV or IM	Synthetic parasympatholytic (anti-cholinergic) drug used to increase heart rate during anesthesia or as a bronchodilator in cases of respiratory distress. Repeated use may cause gastrointestinal ileus and colic.
Granulocyte colony-stimulating factor (recombinant human) Neupogen® rhG-CSF	3–10 μg/kg, SC	Cytokine that promotes bone marrow to increase proliferation, differentiation, and activation of neutrophil-granulocyte line. Used in a sparse number of case reports involving foals with persistent leukopenia. Adjust dose based on neutrophil count/response; response should be observed within 24–48 hours [87].
Heparin-low-molecular-weight	100 IU/kg, SC, q24h (Dalteparin®, foal study) 40 or 100 IU/kg, SC, q24h (Enoxaparin®, adult horse study)	Anticoagulant drug used for thromboprophylaxis, treatment of thromboemboli, or hyercoagulable conditions. Neonatal foals might require higher dose (100 IU/kg) to achieve prophylactic plasma anti-factor-Xa activity compared to the adult horse dose (50 IU/kg) [88, 89].
Heparin-unfractioned	100 IU/kg, IV 80 IU/kg, SC, q12h	Anticoagulant drug used for renal replacement therapy in 2 foals (100 IU/kg) and as a preventative for development of abdominal adhesions (80 IU/kg). True dose unknown in foals [90–92]. May cause an abrupt decrease in red blood cell counts due to rouleaux formation.
Hydrocortisone	1.3 (range 1–3) mg/kg/d, IV divided q4h	Short-acting corticosteroid drug with both glucocorticoid and mineralocorticoid activity. May improve hypotension that is not responsive to fluid and vasopressor therapy in foals with critical illness related corticosteroid insufficiency [59, 93].
Hydromorphone	0.02–0.05 mg/kg, IV or IM	μ agonist opioid sedative and analgesic. Doses derived from adult horses; use low end of dose for foals.

(*Continued*)

Drug	Dosing information	Comments/Indications
Hyoscine butylbromide (N-butylscopolamine)	0.05–0.2 mg/kg, IV	Parasympatholytic; nonselective muscarinic antagonist drug used to increase heart rate during anesthesia; alternative to atropine [94].
Imipenem-cilastatin	15 mg/kg, IV, q6–8h or 0.4–0.8 mg/kg/h, IV, CRI	Broad spectrum carbapenem antimicrobial drug combined with cilastatin to decrease risk of nephrotoxicity. Use only when indicated by culture for highly resistant infections [20]. Pharmacokinetics studied in adult horses but not foals [95].
Imipramine	0.55 mg/kg, IM or IV, q12h	Tricyclic antidepressant drug used for cataplexy and narcolepsy [96].
Insulin – regular	0.01–0.07 IU/kg/h, CRI, initial dose. Can be increased incrementally every 2 hours until glucose stabilizes. 0.1–0.2 IU/kg IM or SC q4h	Hormone used to regulate blood glucose in foals with insulin resistance, particularly septic foals that become hyperglycemic with parenteral nutrition. Onset, peak, and duration of action are derived from other species. Regular insulin is an immediate onset formulation when administered IV; duration of action 1–4 hours. This is the only insulin formulation that should be given IV.; Insulin may bind to plastic tubing in IV lines and should be primed to allow equilibration. Following IM administration, onset 10–30 minutes, peak 1–4 hours, duration 3–8 hours. Following SC administration, onset 10–30 minutes, peak 1–5 hours, duration of action 4–10 hours. Intensive glucose monitoring is required during administration of IV insulin and until the optimum dose for other parenteral administrations is found.
Insulin – protamine zinc	0.4 IU/kg, IM or SQ, q24h	Long-acting formulation; onset 1–4 hours, peak 4–8 hours, duration 6–24 hours in dogs. See above for more information.
Ketamine hydrochloride	2.2 mg/kg, IV	Dissociative general anesthetic used to induce anesthesia after premedication (e.g. xylazine, diazepam) [60]. Avoid in foals with a history of head trauma.
Ketoprofen	2.2–3.6 mg/kg, IV or IM, q24h	Nonselective nonsteroidal anti-inflammatory drug with antipyretic, analgesic, and anti-inflammatory activity. Less ulcerogenic than either flunixin meglumine or phenylbutazone [97].
Levetiracetam	32 mg/kg, IV or PO, q12h	Anticonvulsant drug. Pharmacokinetic data available in healthy foals but efficacy is unknown [98].
Lidocaine	1.3 mg/kg, IV bolus (loading dose administered over 15 minutes), followed by 0.05 mg/kg/min, CRI (maintenance dose)	Sodium channel blocking local anesthetic drug potentially used for general ileus, postoperative ileus, and possible analgesic effects [99].
Magnesium sulfate	50 mg/kg/h (loading dose for first hour), followed by 25 mg/kg/h, CRI (maintenance dose)	Blocks NMDA receptors; potential therapy for neonatal encephalopathy by reducing excitotoxicity. Possible treatment for ventricular tachycardia, can act as a muscle relaxant for rhabdomyolysis and can be used for replacement therapy in foals with hypomagnesemia.
Mannitol	0.5–2.0 g/kg as 20% solution over 20 minutes, IV q12–24h	Osmotic diuretic used to reduce CNS edema or promote urine production. Do not use in anuric renal failure, use with caution in cases of suspected intracranial bleeding.

Drug	Dosing information	Comments/Indications
Marbofloxacin	2–4 mg/kg, PO, q24h	Fluoroquinolone antimicrobial drug reserved for cases when culture dictates and no other options are available as drug has potential to induce cartilage toxicity. If used, strict stall rest during and after treatment is recommended [20, 100].
Meloxicam	0.6 mg/kg, IV, IM or PO q12–24h	Slightly COX-2 selective nonsteroidal anti-inflammatory drug with antipyretic, analgesic, and anti-inflammatory activity [101]. Pharmacokinetics and doses differ in neonatal foals.
Meropenem	15 mg/kg, IV, q6h or 10–30 μg/kg/min, CRI	Broad spectrum carbapenem antimicrobial drug. Use only when indicated by culture; doses derived from adult horses [20, 38, 102].
Methadone	0.15–0.5 mg/kg, IV	μ, κ, δ opioid agonist drug used as alternative to morphine. Doses derived from adult horses.
Methocarbamol	5–55 mg/kg, IV slowly 25–100 mg/kg, PO, q12h	Centrally acting muscle relaxant used for neonatal myopathy or tetanus. Doses derived from adult horses [103].
Metoclopramide	0.1 mg/kg, IV, q6h diluted in 1 l saline over 1h 0.02–0.04 mg/kg/h, IV, CRI 0.6 mg/kg, PO, q4–6 h 0.1–0.2 mg/kg, SC, q6h	Prokinetic medication via 5-HT_4 agonist, 5-HT_3 antagonist, and dopaminergic antagonist activity that promotes gastric and small intestinal motility. Used for postoperative ileus [4, 21].
Metronidazole	10–15 mg/kg, PO or IV, q12h	Antimicrobial commonly used for susceptible anaerobes and some protozoa. Due to alterations in drug clearance in 1- to 2.5-day-old foals, the lower dose should be used for the first 2 weeks of life [38, 104]. Intravenous dosing given as slow IV bolus over at least 20 minutes to prevent neurotoxicity.
Midazolam	0.04–0.2 mg/kg, IV or IM, as needed or 0.02–0.06 mg/kg/h, CRI	Benzodiazepine drug that acts via potentiation of gamma-aminobutyric acid (GABA) mediated inhibitory effects in the CNS. Used for sedation or to control seizure controls in neonatal foals; do not use in patients with hepatic encephalopathy as it can worsen encephalopathy [105]. CRI solution made with 100 ml bag of 0.9% saline; remove 10 ml of saline and add 10 ml of 5 mg/ml (50 mg total) midazolam to bag to create solution of 0.5 mg/ml. Administer at a rate of 2–6 ml/h (1–3 mg/h) to 50 kg foal.
Minocycline	4 mg/kg, PO, q12h	Oral tetracycline antimicrobial drug used for susceptible pathogens [106].
Morphine	0.1–0.2 mg/kg (range 0.05–0.2 mg/kg), IV. Consider following above dose with CRI at 0.1 mg/kg/h	μ agonist opioid analgesic drug [107]. When used, monitor for the development of ileus, CNS excitement and possible histamine release.
Naproxen	10 mg/kg, PO, q12h	Nonselective nonsteroidal anti-inflammatory drug with antipyretic, analgesic, and anti-inflammatory activity; Doses derived from adult horses [108].
Neostigmine	0.005–0.06 mg/kg, SC or 1 mg/50 kg foal SC, q1–8h, IV for severe colonic distension	Parasympathomimetic, indirect-acting cholinergic drug that works via inhibition of acetylcholinesterase. Used to enhance cecal and colonic motility, relieves abdominal tympany (e.g. meconium impaction) [4].
Norepinephrine	0.05–2.0 μg/kg/min, CRI	Nonselective sympathomimetic adrenergic receptor agonist drug that binds to α-1, α-2, and β-1 receptors, but has greatest affinity for α-1. Used as vasopressor to support blood pressure [25, 109].

(Continued)

Drug	Dosing information	Comments/Indications
Nitazoxanide	25 mg/kg, PO, q24h × 7 days	Anti-parasitic medication used to treat rotaviral diarrhea in children; doses derived from adult horses [110]. Equine-specific formulation removed from US market due to an unacceptable risk of adverse GI effects.
Omeprazole	4 mg/kg, PO, q24h (treatment dose) 1 mg/kg, PO, q24h (preventative dose)	Proton pump inhibitor used to treat or prevent gastric ulcers; no adjustment to diet needed in foals on milk diet to accommodate feed-induced decrease in bioavailability noted in adult horses; older foals on roughage should have drug administered after a brief overnight fast and 30–60 minutes prior to feeding [111, 112]. Compounded formulations not recommended.
Oxytetracycline	50–70 mg/kg, IV diluted in 500 ml 0.9% saline, 2 doses given 24h apart (for tendon relaxation) 6.6 mg/kg, IV, q12h (antimicrobial dose)	Injectable tetracycline antimicrobial drug. Higher dose is used for treatment of contracted tendons, in combination with splinting of the limb [113]. Lower dose has been reported in cases of *L. intracellularis* in foals [114].
Oxytocin	**MARES**: 20 IU, IV or IM (evacuation of uterine fluid) **MARES**: 30–100 IU diluted in 1 l normal saline, IV over 30 minutes or 10–120 IU, IM or 10–40 IU, IV bolus (expulsion of fetal membranes)	Hypothalamic hormone that induces or enhances uterine contractions at parturition, treats postpartum retained fetal membranes, and can be used to encourage milk letdown post-foaling. May cause severe uterine contractions and premature labor.
Pantoprazole	1.5 mg/kg, IV, q24h	Intravenous proton pump inhibitor used to treat gastric ulcers in foals that are unable to receive oral formulation [115].
Penicillin G	Sodium or potassium salts: 22 000–44 000 U/kg IV, q6h Procaine: 22 000–44 000 U/kg IM, q12h	Bactericidal beta-lactam antimicrobial drug with multiple formulations. Spectrum covers streptococci and most anaerobic bacteria. When administered IV formulations, give slowly [20]. Use appropriate technique to avoid IV injection with procaine formulations. Avoid formulations that contain benzathine penicillin.
Pentobarbital	2–10 mg/kg, IV	Barbiturate sedative/anesthetic used for refractory seizures; titrate dose to effect using small incremental boluses over 20 minutes. Anecdotal reports suggest a dose of 7–8 mg/kg/h (diluted in 0.9% saline) as a CRI to induce barbiturate coma for intractable seizures [10].
Pentoxifylline	8.5 mg/kg, IV, q8h 8.5–10 mg/kg, PO, q8–12h	Methylxanthine, phosphodiesterase inhibitor drug. Increases erythrocyte flexibility and may attenuate some effects of sepsis/endotoxemia. Inhibits TNF-α production in equine blood and cultured equine macrophages. Stimulates production of anti-inflammatory cytokine IL-10, suppresses neutrophil activation, inhibits NF-KB in other species [116]. Oral absorption is variable in horses and doses may need to be increased with repeated administration.
Phenazopyridine	4 mg/kg, PO, q8–12h	Urinary tract anesthetic drug for bladder irritation or urethritis; stains urine [117].
Phenobarbital	2–20 mg/kg, IV diluted in 50 ml of 0.9% saline over 15 minutes, then 5 mg/kg, PO q12h; 3–10 mg/kg, PO, q12h	Barbiturate anticonvulsant; sedative; anesthetic. Adjust dose to desired effect and/or measure serum concentrations [118]. Therapeutic range (people) is serum concentration of 15–40 µg/ml. Side effects include respiratory depression and hypotension.

Drug	Dosing information	Comments/Indications
Phenoxybenzamine	0.2–0.6 mg/kg, PO, q6h	Sympatholytic α-adrenergic receptor antagonist with possible anti-diarrheal properties; used in adults for severe nonresponsive diarrhea, doses derived from adult horses [119].
Phenylbutazone	2.2 mg/kg, IV or PO, q12–24h	Nonselective nonsteroidal anti-inflammatory used for its antipyretic, anti-inflammatory, and/or analgesic properties [120]. Pharmacokinetics differ in neonatal foals, suggesting lower doses or longer dosing intervals are needed to prevent adverse effects.
Phenylephrine	0.25–2.0 μg/kg/min, CRI	Sympathomimetic α-adrenergic receptor agonist drug used to increase systemic vascular resistance and arterial blood pressure in patients with severe hypotension and shock after adequate volume replacement.
Phenylpropanolamine	**MARES:** 1–2 mg/kg, PO, q8–12h	Nonselective sympathomimetic agonist drug used to treat urethral sphincter hypotonus and incontinence in the postpartum mare. Doses derived from other species [121].
Polymyxin B	6000 IU/kg, IV, q8–12h	Polymyxin antimicrobial drug. Used at subtherapeutic doses to attenuate some effects of sepsis/endotoxemia; potential for renal or neurologic toxicity [122].
Potassium bromide (KBr)	Loading dose: 100–150 mg/kg, PO, for 5 days followed by maintenance dose of 25 mg/kg, PO, q24h	Anticonvulsant drug used in combination therapy for seizures refractory to monotherapy (e.g. combined with phenobarbital) [117]. Doses derived from adult horses [123, 124].
Prazosin	0.1–1.2 mg/kg, PO, daily (divide into q8h dosing) used in dogs. 0.01 mg/kg, PO, q8h (anecdotal reports in foals)	Sympatholytic α-adrenergic receptor antagonist drug that blocks receptors of the trigone and urethral smooth muscle. Anecdotal use in foals with stranguria and/or urinary dyssynergy to treat functional urethral obstruction and promote urination [125]. Doses derived from other species.
Prednisolone sodium succinate (Solu-Delta-Cortef®)	0.8–5 mg/kg, IV, q8–24h	Short-acting corticosteroid drug used in CNS/spinal trauma, shock, immune-medicated disease (e.g. ulcerative dermatitis, thrombocytopenia, neutropenia in neonatal foal), acute lung injury (ALI) and acute respiratory distress syndrome (ARDS) [59, 126, 127].
Propionibacterium acnes	1 ml per 114 kg, IV, q48–72h for 3 treatments	Immunostimulant drug that may induce macrophage activation, lymphokine production and increase natural killer cell activity and enhance cell-mediated immunity [128]. Unknown efficacy in foals.
Propofol	2 mg/kg, IV (induction) 0.2 mg/kg/min, CRI (to maintain anesthesia)	Short-acting anesthetic drug used for induction following premedication (e.g. xylazine, opioid) and/or performing short procedures in foals [60].
Ranitidine	6.6 mg/kg, PO, q6–8h 1.5–2 mg/kg, IV, q6–8h	H_2 receptor antagonist drug used to treat or prevent gastric ulceration [129].
Rifampin	5–10 mg/kg, PO, q12h	Rifamycin antimicrobial drug; used in chronic infections, typically in combination with other compatible antimicrobial drugs; will alter the pharmacokinetics of concurrently administered macrolide drugs [130]. Stains urine.
Romifidine	40–120 μg/kg, IV	α-2 receptor agonist drug used for sedation and analgesia [131]. Can cause cardio-respiratory depression; use with extreme caution in sick foals. Have reversal agents available.

(Continued)

Drug	Dosing information	Comments/Indications
Selenium	0.06 mg/kg, IM, repeat 3 days later and at 8–10 days	Supplement for treatment of selenium deficiency or nutritional myodegeneration (white muscle disease) in foals. Divide dose into 2 separate sites if large dose [132].
Sildenafil	0.5–2.5 mg/kg, PO, q6–24h	Specific phosphodiesterase V inhibitor resulting in vasodilation. Used for the treatment of persistent pulmonary hypertension of the newborn (PPHN) [133]. Very limited information of its use in foals [134].
Sucralfate	10–40 mg/kg, PO, q6–8h	Aluminum salt that acts as mucosal barrier protectant used to treat gastric/intestinal ulcers [135].
Tissue-plasminogen activator (t-PA)	1 mg/kg, IV, over 30 minutes, as needed	Enzyme that induces lysis of intravascular thrombi by activating plasminogen to plasmin [136]. Urokinase has also been used at a dose of 4000 units/min for 60 minutes in a case report involving thrombosis of the digital artery of a foal [137].
Theophylline	5–15 mg/kg, PO, q12h (immediate release) 15 mg/kg, PO, q24h (extended release)	Methylxanthine phosphodiesterase inhibitor that promotes bronchodilation and diuresis. Doses derived from adult horses [57, 138, 139]. Due to risk for serious adverse CNS effects, typically reserved for cases refractory to more common treatments.
Ticarcillin-clavulanic acid	50 mg/kg, IV, q6h 8–16 mg/kg/h, CRI	Broad-spectrum beta-lactam antimicrobial drug combined with clavulanate to block penicillinase. One of the few treatment options for *Pseudomonas* sp. Administer dilute infusion slowly or via CRI [20, 38].
Tolazoline	4 mg/kg, IV	α-2 adrenergic antagonist drug used as reversal agent for α-2 agonists (detomidine, xylazine, romifidine, medetomidine) [28].
Tramadol	3 mg/kg, IV 5 mg/kg PO q6–12h	Serotonin and norepinephrine reuptake inhibitor with weak μ opioid agonist activity. The O-desmethyl tramadol metabolite has stronger μ opioid agonist activity. Potential for use as an analgesic agent used for acute and chronic pain management [140]. Efficacy and exact oral dose not determined in foals.
Trazodone	**MARES:** 4–10 mg/kg, PO, q24h	Serotonin receptor antagonist and reuptake inhibitor used as an anxiolytic in mares demonstrating aggression or hyperexcitability toward foal. Can also be used as a sedative to promote stall rest when a mare is accompanying an ill foal. Sedation, muscle fasciculations, and ataxia can occur in some horses as well as transient arrhythmias at higher doses (10 mg/kg dose) [141, 142].
Tranexamic acid	20 mg/kg, IV, q12h 5–25 mg/kg, IV, q12h	Antifibrinolytic drug that blocks the action of plasminogen; used in acute hemorrhage. Approximately 10 times more potent than aminocaproic acid. Doses derived from adult horses [16, 143–145].

Drug	Dosing information	Comments/Indications
Trimethoprim-sulfonamide combinations	20–30 mg/kg, PO, q12h	Potentiated sulfonamide antimicrobial drugs; resistance among Gram-negative organisms is high and this combination should be reserved for nonlife-threatening infections. Efficacy in vivo is less than in vitro for anaerobic infections, and purulent infections or abscesses. Trimethorpim-sulfadiazine and trimethoprim-sulfamethoxazole combinations are most commonly used in foals.
Valacyclovir	40 mg/kg, PO, q8h [146] 27 mg/kg, PO, q9h for 2d then 18 mg/kg, PO, q12h for 1–2 weeks [5]	Synthetic nucleoside analogue antiviral drug used in horses as a treatment for equine herpes virus; doses derived from adult horses [5]. Valacyclovir is a prodrug of acyclovir with improved oral absorption.
Vancomycin	7.5 mg/kg, IV, q8–12h	Glycopeptide antimicrobial drug known for activity against methicillin resistant Staphylococci, Clostridia, and Enterococci [20, 147]. Use should be reserved for resistant bacteria when culture denotes it is the only option. Administer slowly IV; older formulations in particular are associated with severe histamine-like reactions.
Vasopressin	See Arginine Vasopressin	
Vitamin B_1 (Thiamine)	5–20 mg/kg, IV or SC, q12–24h	Antioxidant; potential benefit in foals with neonatal encephalopathy. Foals with critical illness can develop hypovitaminosis B_1 and might benefit from supplementation [148, 149].
Vitamin C (Ascorbic acid)	50–100 mg/kg, IV or PO, q24h	Antioxidant; potential benefit in foals with neonatal encephalopathy. Foals with critical illness can develop hypovitaminosis C and might benefit from supplementation. Optimal dose in foals is unknown [148, 149].
Vitamin E (α-tocopherol)	6.67–20 IU/kg, PO, q24h	Antioxidant; potential benefit in foals with neonatal encephalopathy. Use natural (or d-) α- tocopherol. Use water dispersible formulations (e.g. EMCELLE Tocopherol, Stuart Products, Bedford, TX) [150].
Vitamin E/Selenium	1 ml/100 pounds, IV or IM; Can be repeated at 5- to 10-day intervals	Supplement for the prevention and treatment of myositis caused by deficiency. Doses are based on equine combination product (E-SE®). Administration IV should be performed slowly to prevent possible anaphylaxis. Intramuscular administration should be done using deep injection and splitting the dose into multiple sites.
Xylazine	0.2–1.1 mg/kg, IV	α-2 receptor agonist drug used for sedation and analgesia. Can cause cardiorespiratory depression; use with extreme caution in sick foals. Have reversal agents available [130].
Yohimbine	0.075–0.125 mg/kg, IV (to reverse xylazine) 0.2 mg/kg IV (to reverse detomidine)	α-2 adrenergic antagonist drug used as reversal agent for α-2 agonists (detomidine, xylazine, romifidine, medetomidine) [28].

Inopressors (From Chapter 11, Section 5, Table 11.1): Inotrope and vasopressor receptor affinities of various drugs for neonatal foals.

Drug	Adrenergic				Dopaminergic		V1a receptor	Starting Dosage (titrate carefully to effect)
	β_1	β_2	α_1	α_2	1	2		
Dobutamine	+++	++	+	+	0	0	0	3–5 μg/kg/min (range 2–10 μg/kg/min)
Dopamine	++	+	++	(+)	+++	++	0	5–10 μg/kg/min (affinity varies with dose)
Epinephrine	+++	+++	+++	+++	0	0	0	Mainly for CPR; primarily β_1 at low doses
Norepinephrine	++	0	+++	++	0	0	0	0.05–2.0 μg/kg/min
Phenylephrine	(+)	0	+++	+	0	0	0	
Vasopressin	0	0	0	0	0	0	+++	0.1–0.5 mU/kg/min

strong affinity +++; moderate affinity ++; weak affinity +; possible weak affinity (+); no affinity 0.

Rule of 6 for calculating how much drug should be added to infusion fluids.

6 × body weight (kg) = number of milligrams of drug that is added to 100 ml of infusion fluids.

- Each 1 ml/h infusion the foal will receive 1 μg/kg/min of drug
- Example: Dobutamine dose of 5 μg/kg/min to a 50 kg foal
  - 6 × 50 kg = 300 mg dobutamine added to 100 ml of infusion fluids = concentration of 3 mg/ml (3000 μg/ml)
  - Dobutamine dose: 5 μg × 50 kg/min = 250 μg/min (for 50 kg foal)
    - Each 1 ml/h infusion results in foal receiving 1 μg/kg/min; if desired dose is 5 μg/kg/min then the rate would be 5 ml/h (total dose is 5 ml/h × 3 mg/ml = 15 mg/h [15000 μg/h] ÷ 60 min/h = 250 μg/min)

For drugs with infusion rate in the range of 0.1–1 μg/kg/min of drug, 0.6 should replace 6.

- Each 1 ml/h infusion the foal will receive 0.1 μg/kg/min of drug.
- Example: Norepinephrine 0.5 μg/kg/min to 50 kg foal
  - 0.6 × 50 kg = 30 mg norepinephrine added to 100 ml of infusion fluids = concentration of 0.3 mg/ml (300 μg/ml)
  - Norepinephrine dose: 0.5 μg × 50 kg/min = 25 μg/min (for 50 kg foal)
    - Each 1 ml/h infusion results in foal receiving 0.1 μg/kg/min; if desired dose is 0.5 μg/kg/min, then the rate would be 5 ml/h (total dose is 5 ml/h × 0.3 mg/ml = 1.5 mg/h [1500 μg/h] ÷ 60 min/h = 25 μg/min)

Ophthalmic Medications (From Chapter 53, Table 53.3): Commonly used medications in ophthalmic examination and treatment of the horse.

Medication	Dosage	Comments
Anesthetics		
▪ Lidocaine	2% s/c	Local anesthesia and akinesia
▪ Mepivicaine	2% s/c	Local anesthesia and akinesia
▪ Proparacaine	0.5% topically	Topical anesthesia; may induce minor superficial corneal irregularities; may decrease tear production
▪ Tetracaine	0.5% topically	Topical anesthesia; may induce minor superficial corneal irregularities; may decrease tear production
Antibiotics		
▪ Bacitracin–neomycin–polymyxin B	o/o topically q2–8h	Broad-spectrum bactericidal
▪ Chloramphenicol	1% o/o topically q2–8h	Gram-positive spectrum

Medication	Dosage	Comments
▪ Ciprofloxacin	0.3% o/s topically q2–8h	Broad-spectrum bactericidal fluoroquinolone; reserve for treatment of severe infections by sensitive organisms
▪ Gatifloxacin	0.3% topically q2–8h	Fourth-generation fluoroquinolone
▪ Gentamicin	0.3% o/s topically q2–8h	Bactericidal aminoglycoside; Gram-negative spectrum, some Gram-positive aerobes
▪ Moxifloxacin	0.5% topically q2–8h	Fourth-generation fluoroquinolone
▪ Ofloxacin	0.3% o/s topically q2–8h	Broad-spectrum antibiotic with better Gram-positive spectrum and less topical irritation than ciprofloxacin
▪ Tobramycin	0.3% o/s topically q2–8h	Gram-negative spectrum; restrict use to severe corneal infections, particularly *Pseudomonas aeruginosa*
Anticollagenolytics		
▪ Acetylcysteine	10% o/s topically q1–4h	
▪ EDTA	0.05% o/s topically	
▪ Serum	Topically q2–6h	Contains α-macroglobulins; inhibits matrix metallo-proteases, serine proteases; collect new autogenous sample every 7 days
Antifungals		
▪ Amphotericin B	1.5% o/s topically	Broad-spectrum polyene; poor intraocular penetration when given parenterally; poor corneal penetration topically
▪ Fluconazole	0.2% o/o topically q4–8h; 1 mg/kg PO, q12h	Imidazole
▪ Itraconazole	1% o/o topically q4–8h;	Imidazole; high corneal concentration; compounded in ointment with 30% dimethylsulfoxide
	3 mg/kg PO, q12h	
▪ Miconazole	1% o/s topically q4–8h	Imidazole; excellent corneal penetration; also active against Gram-positive cocci
▪ Natamycin	5% o/s topically q4–8h	Only commercially available antifungal
▪ Povidone–iodine	2% solution topically	Antibacterial, antiviral, antiprotozoal
▪ Voriconazole	1% o/s q4–8h	Triazole; effective against Aspergillus
Anti-inflammatories		
▪ Dexamethasone	0.05–0.1 mg/kg IV, q24h	Corticosteroid
	0.1% o/o or o/s topically	
▪ Diclofenac	0.1% o/s topically	Nonsteroidal anti-inflammatory
▪ Dimethylsulfoxide	30% o/o topically	Topical ointment compounded with itraconazole
▪ Flurbiprofen	0.03% o/s topically	Nonsteroidal anti-inflammatory
▪ Prednisolone acetate	1% o/s topically	Corticosteroid
▪ Flunixine meglumine	1 mg/kg, IV or PO q12–24h	Nonsteroidal anti-inflammatory; can cause GI ulceration
▪ Phenylbutazone	2.2–4.4 mg/kg, PO/IV, q12–48h	Nonsteroidal anti-inflammatory; can cause GI ulceration
▪ Dipyrone:	10–20 mg/kg, q12–24h, IV	Nonsteroidal anti-inflammatory

(*Continued*)

Medication	Dosage	Comments
▪ Firocoxib:	0.1 mg/kg, PO, q 24h	Nonsteroidal anti-inflammatory
▪ Ketoprofen:	2 mg/kg, q12–24h, IV	Nonsteroidal anti-inflammatory
▪ Methylprednisolone:	1–3 mg/kg, q12–24h, IV	Steroid
▪ Prednisolone sodium succinate:	1.0–2.5 mg/kg, q6–24h, IV	Steroid
▪ Pentoxifylline:	7.5–10 mg/kg, PO/IV, q8–12h Anti-tumor necrosis factor-α	
Mydriatic/Cycloplegics		
▪ Atropine	1% o/o or o/s topically	Parasympatholytic mydriatic, cycloplegic; use q8–12h until pupil dilates, then according to clinical needs
▪ Tropicamide	1% o/s topically	Shorter duration than atropine

o/o, ophthalmic ointment; o/s, ophthalmic solution.

Reference Intervals for **Hematology Parameters** (From Chapter 42, Table 42.2): For Foals at 1, 2, 7, 14, 30, and 90 days of age.

Parameter	Day 1	Day 2	Day 7	Day 14	Day 30	Day 90	Adult
WBC ($\times10^3/\mu l$)	6.2–13.0	6.8–8.1	9.5–10.9	8.8–10.4	8.4–9.8	11.6–13.1	5.4–14.3
Neutrophil ($\times10^3/\mu l$)	4.1–9.6	5–6.4	6.6–7.8	5.5–6.5	5.1–5.9	5.4–7.1	2.3–8.6
Lymphocyte ($\times10^3/\mu l$)	1.3–3.1	1.6–1.9	2.3–2.7	2.7–3.2	2.5–3.3	4.8–5.7	1.5–7.7
Monocyte ($\times10^3/\mu l$)	0.4–0.8	0.1–0.2	0.3–0.4	0.3–0.4	0.3–0.3	0.4–0.5	0–1.0
Eosinophil ($\times10^3/\mu l$)	0	0–0.1	0–0.1	0.1–0.1	0.1–0.1	0.1–0.2	0–1.0
Basophil ($\times10^3/\mu l$)	0–0.9	0–0	0–0.1	0–0.1	0–0	0–0.1	0–0.29
RBC ($\times10^6/\mu l$)	9.1–11.9	9.3–10.3	8.9–9.9	9.1–10	9.3–9.9	10.1–11.1	6.8–12.9
Hemoglobin (mg/dl)	12.9–15.5	13.3–14.8	12.3–13.8	12.2–13.3	11.4–12.5	12.2–13.2	11.9–19.0
Packed cell volume (%)	38.4–45.6	34.2–39.8	34.2–39.8	31.3–38.7	34.7–41.3	39.9–42.1	0–0.43
MCV (fl)	36–44	41–43	41–42	40–41	36–38	34–36	42.6–47.4
MCH (pg)	13–15	14–14.6	14–14.3	13.3–14	12.4–12.9	12–12.3	15.7–17.5
MCHC (%)	32–36	33–35	34–35	33–34	34–35	34–35	25.2–49.2
Platelet ($\times10^3/\mu l$)	163–369	189–213	162–195	217–243	233–274	177–210	95–183

WBC, white blood cell count; RBC, red blood cell count; MCV, mean corpuscular volume; MCH, mean corpuscular hemoglobin; MCHC, mean corpuscular hemoglobin concentration.

Reference Intervals for Serum Biochemistry Parameters (From Chapter 44, Table 44.3): Foal serum enzyme activity and organic molecules related to the liver at various ages.

Age Bilirubin	ALP Bilirubin	GGT Bilirubin	SDH	AST	ALT	Total	Conj.	Unconj.	Cholesterol Triglyceride Bile Acids		
<12 hours	152–2835	13–39	0.2–4.8	97–315	0–47	0.9–2.8	0.3–0.6	0.8–2.5	111–432	24–88	21.7–81.7
Days											
1	861–2671	18–43	0.6–4.6	146–340	0–49	1.3–4.5	0.3–0.7	1.0–3.8	110–562	30–193	26.0–74.3
3	283–1462	9–40	0.6–3.7	80–580	0–52	0.5–3.9	0.2–0.8	0.2–3.3	142–350	63–342	
5	156–1294	8–89	0.8–5.3	—	—	1.2–3.6	0.1–0.7	0.8–2.8	127–361	52–340	
7	137–1169	14–164	0.8–5.2	237–620	4–50	0.8–3.0	0.3–0.7	0.5–2.3	139–445	30–239	16.7–29.4
14	182–859	16–169	0.6–4.3	240–540	1–9	0.7–2.2	0.3–0.6	0.5–1.6	164–287	39–200	11.3–30.6
21	146–752	16–132	1.0–8.4	226–540	0–45	0.5–1.6	0.2–0.5	0.2–1.1	74–276	34–124	7.2–18.4
28	210–866	17–99	1.2–5.9	252–440	5–47	0.5–1.7	0.1–0.6	0.4–1.2	83–233	45–155	9.0–17.1
Months											
2	201–741	8–38	1.1–4.6	282–484	7–57	0.5–2.0	0.2–0.5	0.3–1.5	98–242	10–148	
3	206–458	0–27	1.1–3.9	282–480	8–65	0.4–2.0	0.1–0.7	0.4–1.4	110–226	28–151	
4	124–222	0–27	1.5–4.4	280–520	8–65	0.3–1.0	0.1–0.6	0.2–0.4	91–207	14–148	
5	105–239	0–30	1.3–4.8	225–420	0–65	0.3–1.8	0.1–0.7	0.1–1.1	51–137	14–57	
6	155–226	0–26	0.3–3.3	300–620	7–20	0.3–1.3	0.1–0.7	0.1–0.6	83–173	35–76	
9	158–232	0–26	0.3–3.3	246–728	4–27	0.3–1.1	0.1–0.7	0.2–0.6	11–187	38–86	
12	—	—	—	283–720	5–20	0.4–1.4	0.1–1.0	0.2–0.6	—	—	
Adult	64–214	5–28	0.5–3.0	149–267	4–10	0.5–1.8	0.2–0.7	0.3–1.0	58–109	6–44	4–11.5
Units	IU/l	IU/l	IU/l	IU/l	IU/l	mg/dl	mg/dl	mg/dl	mg/dl	mg/dl	µmol/l

ALP, alkaline phosphatase; GGT, gamma-glutamyl transferase; SDH, sorbital dehydrogenase; AST, aspartate aminotransferase; ALT, alanine aminotransferase; Conj, conjugated; Unconj, unconjugated.

Reference Intervals for Various Serum Biochemistry Parameters (From Chapter 44, Table 44.4): Organic molecules related to the kidney and electrolyte concentrations (mean ± SD) at various ages in the foal.

Age	BUN	Creatinine	Na^+	K^+	Cl^-	CO_2	HPO_4^-	Ca^{++}	Mg^{++}	Anion gap
<12 hours	12–27	1.7–4.2	148 ± 15	4.4 ± 1.0	105 ± 12	25 ± 5	4.7 ± 1.6	12.8 ± 2.0	1.5 ± 0.8	21 ± 12
Days										
1	9–40	1.2–4.3	141 ± 18	4.6 ± 10	102 ± 12	27 ± 6	5.6 ± 1.8	11.7 ± 2.0	2.4 ± 1.8	16 ± 8
3	2–29	0.4–2.1	142 ± 19	4.8 ± 1.4	101 ± 11	28 ± 12	6.4 ± 2.6	12.1 ± 4.4	2.1 ± 0.9	23 ± 4
5	—	—							2.2 ± 2.0	—
7	4–20	1.0–1.7	142 ± 12	4.8 ± 1.0	102 ± 8	28 ± 4	7.4 ± 2.0	12.5 ± 1.2	2.0 ± 0.6	17 ± 8
14	6–13	0.9–1.8	143 ± 8	4.6 ± 0.8	103 ± 6	26 ± 7	7.8 ± 1.8	12.4 ± 1.2	2.1 ± 1.1	18 ± 6
21	6–14	0.6–2.0	144 ± 8	4.3 ± 1.0	104 ± 11	27 ± 6	7.6 ± 0.8	12.3 ± 1.0	2.3 ± 3.0	18 ± 8
28	6–21	1.1–1.8	145 ± 9	4.6 ± 0.8	103 ± 6	27 ± 5	7.1 ± 2.2	12.2 ± 1.2	2.0 ± 1.1	19 ± 6
Months										
2	6–11	1.1–2.1	148 ± 12	4.8 ± 1.0	105 ± 12	27 ± 5	7.4 ± 1.4	12.3 ± 0.6	2.0 ± 0.8	21 ± 10
3	7–20	0.7–2.2	148 ± 8	4.6 ± 1.2	106 ± 4	27 ± 3	7.3 ± 1.0	12.2 ± 1.0	2.2 ± 0.6	20 ± 8
4	9–25	1.3–2.1	147 ± 12	4.8 ± 1.0	105 ± 11	27 ± 4	6.7 ± 1.8	12.3 ± 1.6	2.4 ± 0.7	21 ± 8
5	11–33	1.2–2.1	145 ± 12	4.5 ± 1.4	107 ± 7	27 ± 5	6.3 ± 1.6	11.8 ± 1.4	2.4 ± 0.6	16 ± 10
6	15–30	1.2–2.1	143 ± 10	4.2 ± 1.4	105 ± 7	26 ± 4	6.2 ± 1.4	11.8 ± 1.6	2.4 ± 0.7	17 ± 8
9	16–26	1.1–2.2	143 ± 5	3.7 ± 1.0	102 ± 6	28 ± 4	6.0 ± 1.4	12.0 ± 1.2	2.3 ± 0.4	16 ± 8
12	15–24	1.3–2.1	146 ± 12	3.8 ± 1.6	104 ± 5	29 ± 2	6.0 ± 0.8	12.7 ± 1.4	—	17 ± 12
Adult	12–24	0.9–2.0	139 ± 8	4.2 ± 1.0	101 ± 6	26 ± 4	4.5 ± 1.4	12.0 ± 1.2	2.2 ± 0.6	18 ± 8
Units	mg/dl	mg/Dl	mEq/l	mEq/l	mEq/l	mEq/l	mg/dl	mg/dl	mg/dl	mEq/l

Reference Intervals for Various Serum Biochemistry Parameters (Chapter 44, Table 44.8): Miscellaneous organic molecules at various ages in the foal.

Age	Glucose	CK	AST	Venous L-Lactate	SAA	Total Protein	Albumin	Total Globulin
Birth				1.9–5.7				
<12 hours	108–190	65–380	97–315	1.5–4.1		4.0–7.9	2.7–3.9	1.1–4.8
Days								
1	121–233	40–909	146–340	1.3–2.9	12.3[a]	4.3–8.1	2.5–3.6	1.5–4.6
2				1.1–2.3	36.6[a]			
3	101–226	21–97	80–580	1.2–2.6	27.1[a]	4.4–7.6	2.8–3.7	1.6–4.5
5	—	29–208						
7	121–192	52–143	237–620			4.4–6.8	2.7–3.4	1.6–3.9
14	137–205	46–208	240–540			4.8–6.7	2.6–3.3	2.0–3.5
21	130–240	44–210	226–540			4.7–6.5	2.6–3.2	1.7–3.6
28	130–216	81–585	252–440			5.0–6.7	2.7–3.4	1.8–3.7
Months								
2	119–204	50–170	282–484			5.2–6.5	2.7–3.5	1.9–3.8
3	88–170	57–204	282–480			5.5–7.0	2.8–3.5	2.6–4.1
4	113–196	60–266	280–520			5.7–7.3	2.8–3.7	2.7–3.9
5	95–210	60–125	225–420			6.0–6.9	2.9–3.4	2.7–4.0
6	110–210	97–396	300–620			6.0–6.9	3.0–3.5	2.8–3.7
9	104–207	97–396	246–728			5.6–6.7	3.0–3.6	2.2–3.1
12	106–165	—	283–720			5.8–6.6	3.1–3.8	2.2–3.5
Adult	57–96	69–272	149–267	< 2.5	0.5–20[J]	5.5–7.9	2.8–4.8	1.9–3.8
Units	mg/dl	mg/dl		mmol/l	mg/l	g/dl	g/dl	g/dl

[a] 95% percentile.

Reference Intervals for Various Blood Gas Analysis and Ventilation Parameters (Chapter 44, Table 44.9): Arterial blood gas values and ventilation parameters at various ages in the foal.

Age	pH	P_aCO_2	P_aO_2	HCO_3	V_E	V_T	VO_2	Breaths	Weight
Minutes of age									
Birth	7.41 ± 0.02	60.7 ± 1.5	32.7 ± 2.5	24.0 ± 0.8	418 ± 32	6.1 ± 0.50	7.8 ± 0.8	71 ± 6	44 ± 2.7
2	7.31 ± 0.02	54.1 ± 2.0	56.4 ± 2.3	24.0 ± 1.2					
15	7.32 ± 0.03	50.4 ± 2.7	57.5 ± 3.6	24.4 ± 1.6	463 ± 65	8.1 ± 0.76	10.5 ± 1.7	58 ± 5	44 ± 2.7
30	7.35 ± 0.01	51.5 ± 1.5	57.0 ± 1.8	25.3 ± 0.7	376 ± 37	7.1 ± 0.72	7.7 ± 1.0	53 ± 4	44 ± 2.7
60	7.36 ± 0.01	47.3 ± 2.2	60.9 ± 2.7	25.3 ± 1.0	349 ± 38	8.9 ± 0.95	7.4 ± 1.0	40 ± 3	44 ± 2.7
Hours of age									
2	7.36 ± 0.01	47.7 ± 1.7	66.5 ± 2.3	25.0 ± 0.9					
4	7.35 ± 0.02	45.0 ± 1.9	75.7 ± 4.9	23.6 ± 1.1	380 ± 46	6.7 ± 0.57	6.6 ± 0.9	57 ± 6	44 ± 2.7
12	7.36 ± 0.02	44.3 ± 1.2	73.5 ± 3.0	23.2 ± 1.6	245 ± 37	6.8 ± 0.52	5.2 ± 1.1	32 ± 5	25 ± 2.9
24	7.39 ± 0.01	45.5 ± 1.5	67.6 ± 4.4	26.2 ± 1.1	260 ± 22	6.4 ± 0.46	4.8 ± 0.6	42 ± 4	46 ± 2.9
Days									
2	7.37 ± 0.01	46.1 ± 1.1	74.9 ± 3.3	25.7 ± 0.6	271 ± 56	6.0 ± 0.45	4.6 ± 0.6	44 ± 7	47 ± 3.1
4	7.40 ± 0.01	45.8 ± 1.1	81.2 ± 3.1	23.2 ± 2.1	284 ± 31	6.1 ± 0.40	5.7 ± 0.8	46 ± 4	50 ± 2.9
7	7.37 ± 0.01	46.7 ± 1.1	86.9 ± 2.2	25.6 ± 0.8	320 ± 28	8.1 ± 1.21	7.0 ± 0.6	42 ± 5	54 ± 3.1
Units	—	mmHg	mmHg	mEq/l	ml/kg/min	ml/kg	ml/kg/min	per min	kg

P_aCO_2, partial pressure of carbon dioxide in arterial blood; P_aO_2, partial pressure of oxygen in arterial blood; HCO_3, bicarbonate; V_E, minute respiratory volume; V_T, tidal volume, VO_2, oxygen consumption.

Reference Intervals for Various Coagulation Parameters (From Chapter 44, Table 44.11): Coagulation parameters reported from healthy foals.

Diagnostic test	<7 hours	<24 hours	48 hours	4–7 days	10–14 days	25–30 days	Adult
PT (sec)	10.4 ± 0.4	10.9 ± 0.6	11.1 ± 1.8	9.6 ± 0.6	9.5 ± 0.4	9.4 ± 0.4	9.5 ± 0.3
aPTT (sec)	52.8 ± 8.1	56.8 ± 6.3	55.6 ± 10.4	39.8 ± 4.0	39.9 ± 4.8	40.8 ± 6.0	42.0 ± 8.9
Fibrinogen (mg/dl)	226.4 ± 57.3	116.8 ± 39.1	316.8 ± 42.8	196.8 ± 26.6	199.6 ± 50.0	221.1 ± 48.0	195 ± 54
Platelets ($\times 10^3/\mu l$)	381.6 ± 58.9	243 ± 170	222.2 ± 60.6	181 ± 60	218 ± 57	245 ± 59	153 ± 49
FDPs $(\mu g/ml + 1)^{1/2}$	—	8.2 ± 2.7	—	5.6 ± 3.4	4.5 ± 3.1	3.5 ± 2.6	1.8 ± 0.6
Antithrombin (%)	147.6 ± 15.0	107 ± 41	133.0 ± 20.7	164 ± 35	170.9 ± 40.9	166.5 ± 40.6	202 ± 82
D-dimers (ng/ml)	—	101 (36–270)	220 (140–472)	—	453 (304–716)	—	677 ± 119
TBT (min)	—	4 ± 2	—	4 ± 2	4 ± 2	4 ± 2	4 ± 2
ACT (min)	—	5.8 ± 1.3	—	5.8 ± 1.3	5.8 ± 1.3	5.8 ± 1.3	2.6 ± 0.5
Thrombin Time (sec)	—	—	—	—	—	—	13.5 ± 5.5
Protein C antigen (%)	—	63.5 ± 11.9	—	—	93.4 ± 10.6	—	98.9 ± 9.0
Protein C activity (%)	—	113 ± 23	—	—	84.6 ± 12.0	—	86.5 ± 17.6
Plasminogen (%)	—	82.3 ± 15.8	—	99.2 ± 16.1	98.1 ± 14.4	102 ± 14.4	114 ± 14
α-2 antiplasmin (%)	—	197 ± 40	—	207 ± 47.8	175 ± 55.5	174 ± 50.7	209 ± 43.6
TPA (U/ml)	—	2.2 ± 1.3	—	—	5.4 ± 4.6	8.9 ± 5.5	2.8 ± 1.9
PAI (U/ml)	—	39.0 ± 25.8	—	—	22.0 ± 10.3	10.0 ± 12.2	8.2 ± 2.5

TBT, Template Bleeding Time; ACT, Activated Clotting Time; TPA, tissue plasminogen activator; PAI, plasminogen activator inhibitor;

References

1 Beech, J. and Lindborg, S. (1995). Prophylactic efficacy of phenytoin, acetazolaminde and hydrochlorathiazide in horses with hyperkalemic period paralysis. *Res. Vet. Sci.* 59: 95–101.

2 Traub-Dargatz, J.L., Ingram, J.T., Stashak, T.S. et al. (1992). Respiratory stridor associated with polymyopathy suspected to be hyperkalemic periodic paralysis in four quarter horse foals. *J. Am. Vet. Med. Assoc.* 201: 85–89.

3 Morresey, P.R. (2008). How to deliver respiratory treatments to neonates by nebulization. *Proc. AAEP Conf.* 54: 520–526.

4 Slovis, N.M. (2003). Gastrointestinal failure. *Clin. Tech. Equine* 2: 79–86.

5 Maxwell, L.K., Bentx, B.G., Bourne, D.W.A. et al. (2008). Pharmacokinetics of valacyclovir in the adult horse. *J. Vet. Pharmacol. Ther.* 31: 312–320.

6 Wong, D.M., Belgrave, R.L., Williams, K.J. et al. (2008). Multinodular pulmonary firbosis in five horses. *J. Am. Vet. Med. Assoc.* 232: 898–905.

7 Giguere, S. and Prescott, J.F. (1997). Clinical manifestations, diagnosis, treatment, and prevention of *Rhodococcus equi* infections in foal. *Vet. Microbiol.* 56: 313–334.

8 Vander Werf, K.A., Beard, L.A., and McMurphy, R.M. (2010). Urinothorax in a quarter horse filly. *Equine Vet. Educ.* 22: 239–243.

9 Migliorisi, A.C., Metcalfe, L., and Gilsenan, W.F. (2023). Perinatal foreign body aspiration in a Thoroughbred foal. *Equine Vet. Educ.* 35: 28–31.

10 Wong, D.M., Wilkins, P.A., Bain, F.T. et al. (2011). Neonatal encephalopathy in foals. *Compend. Equine* E1–E10.

11 Goodwin, W., Keates, H., Pasloske, K. et al. (2012). Plasma pharmacokinetics and pharmacodynamics of alfaxalone in neonatal foals after an intravenous bolus of alfaxalone following premedication with butorphanol tartrate. *Vet. Anaesth. Analg.* 39: 503–510.

12 Wong, D.M., Davis, J.L., Alcott, C.J. et al. (2015). Phamracokinetics and physiologic effects of alprazolam after a single oral dose in healthy mares. *J. Vet. Pharmacol. Ther.* 38: 301–304.

13 Bucki, E.P., Giguere, S., Macpherson, M. et al. (2004). Pharmacokinetics of once-daily amikacin in healthy foals and therapeutic drug monitoring in hospitalized equine neonates. *J. Vet. Intern. Med.* 18: 728–733.

14 Ross, J., Dallap, D.L., Dolente, B. et al. (2007). Pharmacokinetics and pharmacodynamics of aminocaproic acid in horses. *Am. J. Vet. Res.* 68: 1016–1021.

15 Heidmann, P., Tornquist, S.J., Qu, A. et al. (2005). Laboratory measures of hemostasis and fibrinolysis after intravenous administration of epsilon-aminocaproic acid in clinically normal horses and ponies. *Am. J. Vet. Res.* 66: 313–318.

16 Fletcher, D.J., Brainard, B.M., Epstien, K. et al. (2013). Therapeutic plasma concentrations of epsilon aminocaproic acid and tranexamic acid in horses. *J. Vet. Intern. Med.* 27: 1589–1595.

17 Cotrill, C.M., O'Connor, W.N., Cudd, T. et al. (1987). Persistence of foetal circulatory pathways in a newborn foal. *Equine Vet. J.* 19: 252–255.

18 Javsicas, L.H. and Giguere, S. (2008). How to perform cardiopulmonary resuscitation in neonatal foals. *AAEP Proc.* 54: 513–519.

19 Corley, K.T.T. and Axon, J.E. (2005). Resuscitation and emergency management for neonatal foals. *Vet. Clin. Equine* 21: 431–455.

20 Corley, K.T.T. and Hollis, A.R. (2009). Antimicrobial therapy in neonatal foals. *Equine Vet. Educ.* 21: 436–448.

21 Magdesian, K.G. (2015). Foals are not just mini horses. In: *Equine Pharmacology* (ed. C. Cole, B. Bentz, and L. Maxwell), 99–117. Wiley.

22 Brumbaugh, G.H. (1999). Clinical pharmacology and the pediatric patient. *45th Annual AAEDP Convention 1999.*

23 Love, D.N., Rose, R.J., Martin, I.C. et al. (1981). Serum levels of amoxycillin flowing its oral administration to Thoroughbred foals. *Equine Vet. J.* 13L53–13L55.

24 Corley, K.T.T. (2004). Inotropes and vasopressors in adults and foals. *Vet. Clin. Equine* 20: 77–106.

25 Valverde, A., Giguere, S., Sanchez, L.C. et al. (2006). Effects of dobutamine, norepinephrine, and vasopressin on cardiovascular function in anesthetized neonatal foals with induced hypotension. *Am. J. Vet. Res.* 67: 1730–1737.

26 Brumbaugh, G.H., Lopez, G.H., and Sepulveda, L.H. (1999). The pharmacologic basis for the treatment of laminitis. *Vet. Clin. North Am. Equine* 15: 345–362.

27 Jenkins, W.L. (1987). Pharmacologic aspects of analgesic drgus in animals: an overview. *J. Am. Vet. Med. Assoc.* 191: 1231–1240.

28 Hubbell, J.A.E. and Muir, W.W. (2006). Antagonism of detomidine sedation in the horse using intravenous tolazoline or atipamezole. *Equine Vet. J.* 38: 238–241.

29 Jones, T., Bracomonte, J.L., Ambros, B. et al. (2019). Total intravenous anestheisa with alfaxalone, dexmedetomidine and remifentanil in healthy foals undergoing abdominal surgery. *Vet. Anaesth. Analg.* 46: 315–324.

30 Jacks, S., Giguere, S., Gronwall, R. et al. (2001). Pharmacokinetics of azithromycin and concentration in body fluids and bronchoalveolar cells in foals. *Am. J. Vet. Res.* 62: 1870–1875.

31 Booth, T.M., Howes, D.A., and Edwards, G.B. (2000). Behanechol-responsive bladder atony in a colt foal after cystorrhaphy for cystorrhexis. *Vet. Rec.* 147: 306–308.

32 Grubb, T.L., Kurkowski, D., Sellon, D.C. et al. (2019). Pharmacokinetics and physiologic/behavioral effects of buprenorphine administered sublingually and intravenously to neonatal foals. *J. Vet. Pharmacol. Ther.* 42: 26–36.

33 Arguedas, M.G., Hines, M.T., Papich, M.G. et al. (2008). Pharmacokinetics of butorphanol and evaluation of physiologic and behavioral effects after intravenous and intramuscular administration to neonatal foals. *J. Vet. Intern. Med.* 1417–1426.

34 Giguere, S., Slade, J.K., and Sanchez, L.C. (2008). Retrospective comparison of caffeine and doxapram for the treatment of hypercapnia in foals with hypoxic-ischemic encephalopathy. *J. Vet. Intern. Med.* 22: 401–405.

35 Boado, A., Clutton, E., and Booth, T.M. (2007). Repair of a Salter–Harris type II fracture of the calcaneus of a foal. *Vet. Rec.* 161: 350–352.

36 Duffee, N.E., Stang, B.E., and Schaeffer, D.J. (1997). The pharmacokinetics of cefadroxil over a range of oral doses and animal ages in the foal. *J. Vet. Pharmacol. Ther.* 20: 427–433.

37 Ladaga, G.J.B., Lezica, F.P., Barboni, A.M. et al. (2011). Pharmacokinetics of a single oral administration of cefalexin in mares and foals. *Vet. Rec.* 168: 431A.

38 Magdesian, K.G. (2017). Antimicrobial pharmacology for the neonatal foal. *Vet. Clin. Equine* 33: 47–65.

39 Gardner, S.Y. and Papich, M.G. (2001). Comparison of cefepime pharmacokinetics in neonatal foals and adult dogs. *J. Vet. Pharmacol. Ther.* 24: 187–192.

40 Soraci, A.L., Mestorino, O.N., and Errecalde, J.O. (1996). Pharmacokinetics of cefoperazone in horses. *J. Vet. Pharmacol. Ther.* 19: 39–43.

41 Hewson, J., Johnson, R., Arroyo, L.G. et al. (2013). Comparison of continuous infusion with intermittent bolus administration of cefotaxime on blood and cavity fluid drug concentrations in neonatal foals. *J. Vet. Pharm. Ther.* 36: 68–77.

42 Carrillo, N.A., Giguere, S., Gronwall, R.R. et al. (2005). Disposition of orally administered cefpodoxime proxetil in foals and adult horses and minimum inhibitory concentration of the drug against common bacterial pathogens of horses. *Am. J. Vet. Res.* 66: 30–35.

43 Rohdich, N., Zschiesche, E., Heckeroth, A. et al. (2009). Treatment of septicaemia and severe bacterial infections in foals with a new cefquinome formulation: a field study. *Dtsch. Tierarztl. Wochenschr.* 116: 316–320.

44 Uney, K., Altan, F., Altan, S. et al. (2017). Plasma and synovial fluid pharmacokinetics of cefquinome following the administration of multiple doses in horses. *J. Vet. Pharmacol. Ther.* 40: 239–247.

45 McNeal, C.D., Ryan, C.A., Berghaus, L.J. et al. (2021). Plasma disposition of ceftazidime in healthy neonatal foals following intravenous and intramuscular administration. *J. Vet. Pharmacol. Ther.* 44: 560–567.

46 Hall, T.L., Tell, L.A., Wetzlich, S.E. et al. (2011). Pharmacokinetics of ceftiofur sodium and ceftiofur crystalline free acid in neonatal foals. *J. Vet. Pharmacol. Ther.* 34: 403–409.

47 Meyer, S., Giguere, S., Rodriguez, R. et al. (2009). Pharmacokinetics of intravenous ceftiofur sodium and concentration in body fluids of foals. *J. Vet. Pharmacol. Ther.* 32: 309–316.

48 Pusterla, N., Hall, T.L., Wetzlich, S.E. et al. (2017). Pharmacokinetic parameters for single- and multi-dose regimens for subcutaneous administration of a high-dose ceftiofur crystalline-free acid to neonatal foals. *J. Vet. Pharmacol. Ther.* 40: 88–91.

49 Theelen, M.J.P., Wilson, W.D., Byrne, B.A. et al. (2019). Initial antimicrobial treatment of foals with sepsis: do our choices make a difference? *Vet. J.* 243: 74–76.

50 Ringger, N.C., Brown, M.P., Kohlepp, S.J. et al. (1998). Pharmacokinetics of ceftriaxone in neonatal foals. *Equine Vet. J.* 30: 163–165.

51 Adamson, P.J., Wilson, W.D., Baggot, J.D. et al. (1991). Influence of age on the disposition kinetics of chloramphenicol in equine neonates. *Am. J. Vet. Res.* 52: 426–431.

52 Clark, E.S. and Becht, J.L. (1987). Clinical pharmacology of the gastrointestinal tract. *Vet. Clin. North Am. Equine Pract.* 3: 101–122.

53 Lewis, S. (2003). Gastric ulceration in an equine neonate. *Can. Vet. J.* 44: 420–421.

54 Wong, D.M., Davis, J.L., and White, N.A. (2011). Motility of the equine gastrointestinal tract: physiology and pharmacotherapy. *Equine Vet. Educ.* 23: 88–100.

55 Jacks, S., Giguere, S., Gronwall, R.R. et al. (2002). Disposition of oral clarithromycin in foals. *J. Vet. Pharmacol. Ther.* 25: 359–362.

56 Card, C.E. and Wood, M.R. (1995). Effects of acute administration of clenbuterol on uterine tone and equine fetal and maternal heart rates. *Biol. Reprod.* 52: 7–11.

57 Baggot, J.D. (1994). Drug therapy in the neonatal foal. *Vet. Clin. North Am. Equine Pract.* 10: 87–107.

58 Elfenbein, J.R., Giguere, S., Meyer, S.K. et al. (2010). The effects of deferoxamine mesylate on iron elimination after blood transfusion in neoantal foals. *J. Vet. Intern. Med.* 24: 1475–1482.

59 Castagnetti, C. and Mariella, J. (2015). Anti-inflammatory drugs in equine neonatal medicine. Part II: Corticosteroids. *J. Equine Vet. Sci.* 35: 547–554.

60 Matthews, N. (2011). Foal anesthesia. *ACVS Vet. Symp.* 608–610.

61 Barnett, S.E., Sellon, D.C., Hines, M.T. et al. (2017). Randomized, controlled clinical trial of safety and plasma concentrations of diclofenac in healthy neonatal foals after repeated topical application of 1% diclofenac sodium cream. *Am. J. Vet. Res.* 78: 405–411.

62 Hardefeldt, L.Y., Keuler, N., and Peek, S.F. (2010). Incidence of transfusion reactions to commercial equine plasma. *J. Vet. Emerg. Crit. Care* 29: 421–425.

63 Le Corre, S., Janes, J., and Slovis, N.M. (2021). Multiple extra-pulmonary disorders associated with *Rhodococcus equi* infection in a 2-month-old foal. *Equine Vet. Educ.* 33: e231–e238.

64 Morresey, P.R., White, G.W., Poole, H.M. et al. (2019). Randomized blinded controlled trial of dipyrone as a treatment for pyrexia in horses. *Am. J. Vet. Res.* 80: 294–299.

65 Cross, D.L., Reinemeyer, C.R., Prado, J.C. et al. (2012). Efficacy of domperidone gel in an induced model of fescue toxicosis in periparturient mares. *Theriogenology* 78: 1361–1370.

66 Womble, A., Giguere, S., and Lee, E.A. (2007). Pharmacokinetics of oral doxycycline and concentrations in body fluids and bronchoalveolar cells of foals. *J. Vet. Pharmacol. Ther.* 30: 187–193.

67 Bermingham, E.C., Papich, M.G., and Vivrette, S.L. (2000). Pharmacokinetics of enrofloxacin administered intravenously and orally to foals. *Am. J. Vet. Res.* 61: 706–709.

68 Jokisalo, J.M. and Corley, K.T.T. (2014). CPR in the neonatal foal. Has RECOVER changed our approach? *Vet. Clin. Equine* 30: 301–316.

69 Lakritz, J., Wilson, W.D., March, A.E. et al. (2000). Pharmacokinetic of erythromycin estolate and erythromycin phosphate after intragastric administration to healthy foals. *Am. J. Vet. Res.* 61: 914–919.

70 Barr, B.S. (2006). Duodenal stricture in a foal. *Vet. Clin. North Am. Equine* 22: 37–42.

71 Camacho-Luna, P., Buchanan, B., and Andrews, F.M. (2018). Advances in diagnostics and treatments in horses and foals with gastric and duodenal ulcers. *Vet. Clin. Equine* 34: 97–111.

72 Videla, R., Sommardahl, C.S., Elliot, S.B. et al. (2011). Effects of intravenously administered esomeprazole sodium on gastric juice pH in adult female horses. *J. Vet. Intern. Med.* 25: 558–562.

73 Magdesian, K.G. (2005). Neonatal foal diarrhea. *Vet. Clin. Equine* 21: 295–312.

74 Hollis, A.R., Ousey, J.C., Palmer, L. et al. (2006). Effects of fenoldopam mesylate on systemic hemodynamics and indices or renal function in normotensive neonatal foals. *J. Vet. Intern. Med.* 20: 595–600.

75 Eberspächer, E., Stanley, S.D., Rezende, M. et al. (2008). Pharmacokinetics and tolerance of transdermal fentanyl administration in foals. *Vet. Anaesth. Analg.* 35: 249–255.

76 Hovanessian, N., Davis, J.L., McKenzie, H.C. 3rd et al. (2014). Pharmacokinetics and safety of firocoxib after oral administration of repeated consecutive doses to neonatal foals. *J. Vet. Pharmacol. Ther.* 37: 243–251.

77 Wilson, K.E., Davis, J.L., Crisman, M.V. et al. (2017). Pharmacokinetics of firocoxib after intravenous administration of multiple consecutive doses in neonatal foals. *J. Vet. Pharmacol. Ther.* 40: e23–e29.

78 Crisman, M.V., Wilcke, J.R., and Sams, R.A. (1996). Pharmacokinetics of flunixin meglumine in healthy foals less than twenty-four hours old. *Am. J. Vet. Res.* 57: 1759–1761.

79 Semrad, S.D., Sams, R.A., and Ashcraft, S.M. (1993). Pharmacokinetics of serum thromboxane suppression by flunixin meglumine in healthy foals during the first month of life. *Am. J. Vet. Res.* 54: 2083–2087.

80 Divers, T.J. and Perkins, G. (2003). Urinary and hepatic disorders in neonatal foals. *Clin. Tech. Equine Pract.* 2: 67–78.

81 Divers, T.J. (2003). Urine production, renal failure, and drug monitoring in the equine intensive-care unit. *Clin. Tech. Equine Pract.* 2: 188–192.

82 Gold, J.R., Grubb, T.L., Green, S. et al. (2020). Plasma disposition of gabapentin after intragastric administration of escalating doses to adult horses. *J. Vet. Intern. Med.* 34: 933–940.

83 Gold, J.R., Grubb, T.L., Cox, S. et al. (2022). Pharmacokinetics and pharmacodynamics of repeated dosing of gabapentin in adult horses. *J. Vet. Intern. Med.* 36: 792–797.

84 Berlin, S., Wallstabe, S., Scheuch, E. et al. (2018). Intestinal and hepatic contributions to the pharmacokinetic interaction between gamithromycin and rifampicin after single-dose and multiple-dose administration in healthy foals. *Equine Vet. J.* 50: 525–531.

85 Carmichael, R.J., Whitefield, C., and Maxwell, L.K. (2013). Pharmacokinetics of ganciclovir and valganciclovir in the adult horse. *J. Vet. Pharmacol. Ther.* 36: 441–449.

86 Burton, A.J., Giguere, S., Warner, L. et al. (2013). Effect of age on the pharmacokinetic of a single daily dose of gentamicin sulfate in healthy foals. *Equine Vet. J.* 45: 507–511.

87 Wong, D.M., Alcott, C.J., Clark, S.K. et al. (2012). Alloimmune neonatal neutropenia and neonatal isoerythrolysis in a Thoroughbred colt. *J. Vet. Diagn. Investig.* 24: 219–226.

88 Armengou, L., Monreal, L., Delgado, M.A. et al. (2010). Low-molecular-weight heparin dosage in newborn foals. *J. Vet. Intern. Med.* 24: 1190–1195.

89 Schwarzwald, C.C., Feige, K., Wunderli, H. et al. (2002). Comparison of pharmacokinetic variables for two low-molecular-weight heparins after subcutaneous

administration of a single dose to horses. *Am. J. Vet. Res.* 63: 868–873.

90 Wong, D.M., Ruby, R.E., Eatroff, A. et al. (2017). Use of renal replacment therapy in a neoantal foal with postresuscitation acute renal failure. *J. Vet. Intern. Med.* 31: 593–597.

91 Sullins, K.E., White, N.A., Lundrin, C.S. et al. (2004). Prevention of ischaemia-induced small intestinal adhesions in foals. *Equine Vet. J.* 36: 370–375.

92 Vivrette, S., Cowgill, L.D., Pascoe, J. et al. (1993). Hemodialysis for treatment of oxytetracycline induced acute renal failure in a neonatal foal. *J. Am. Vet. Med. Assoc.* 203: 105–107.

93 Hart, K.A. and Barton, M.H. (2011). Adrenocortical insufficiency in horses and foals. *Vet. Clin. Equine* 27: 19–34.

94 Pimenta, E.L.M., Neto, F.J., and Pignaton, W. (2011). Comparative study between atropine and hyoxcine-N-butylbromide for reversal of detomidine induced bradycardia in horses. *Equine Vet. J.* 43L332–43L340.

95 Orsini, J.A., Moate, P.J., Boston, R.C. et al. (2005). Pharmacokinetics of imipenem-cilastatin following intravenous administration in healthy adult horses. *J. Vet. Pharmacol. Ther.* 28: 355–361.

96 Lunn, D.P., Cuddon, P.A., Shaftoe, S. et al. (1993). Familial occurrence of narcolepsy in miniature horses. *Equine Vet. J.* 25: 433–487.

97 Wilcke, J.R., Crisman, M.V., Scarratt, W.K. et al. (1998). Pharmacokinetics of ketoprofen in healthy foals less than twenty-four hours old. *Am. J. Vet. Res.* 59: 290–292.

98 MacDonald, K.D., Hart, K.A., Davis, J.L. et al. (2018). Pharmacokinetics of the anticonvulsant levetiracetam in neonatal foals. *Equine Vet. J.* 50: 532–536.

99 Ohmes, C. (2014). *The Disposition of Lidocaine during a 6-Hour Intravenous Infusion to Young Foals*, 67. Manhattan, KS: Department of Clinical Sciences, College of Veterinary Medicine, Kansas State University.

100 Carretero, M., Rodriguez, C., San Andres, M.I. et al. (2002). Pharmacokinetics of marbofloxacin in mature horses after single intravenous and intramuscular administration. *Equine Vet. J.* 34: 360–365.

101 Raidal, S., Edwards, S., Pippia, J. et al. (2013). Pharmacokinetics and Safety of Oral Administration of Meloxicam to Foals. *J. Vet. Intern. Med.* 27.

102 Langston, V.C., Fontenot, R.L., Byers, J.A. et al. (2019). Plasma and synovial fluid pharmacokinetics of a single intravenous dose of meropenem in adult horses. *J. Vet. Pharmacol. Ther.* 42: 525–529.

103 Van Galen, G., Saegermann, C., Rijckaert, J. et al. (2017). Retrospective evaluation of 155 adult equids and 21 foals with tetanus in western, northern, and central Europe (2000–2014). Part 1: description of history and clinical evolution. *J. Vet. Emerg. Crit. Care* 27: 684–696.

104 Swain, E.A., Magdesian, K.G., Kass, P.H. et al. (2014). Pharmacokinetics of metronidazole in foals: influence of age within the neonatal period. *J. Vet. Pharmacol. Ther.* 38: 227–234.

105 Wilkins, P.A. (2005). How to use midazolam to control equine neonatal seisures. *AAEP Proc.* 51: 279–280.

106 Giguere, S., Burton, A.J., Berghaus, L.J. et al. (2017). Comparative pharmacokinetics of minocycline in foals and adult horses. *J. Vet. Pharmacol. Ther.* 40: 335–341.

107 Combie, J.D., Nugent, T.E., and Tobin, T. (1983). Pharmacokinetics and protein binding of morphine in horses. *Am. J. Vet. Res.* 44: 870–874.

108 Rocca, G.D., Salvo, A.D., Cagnardi, P. et al. (2014). Naproxen in the horse: pharmacokinetics and side effects in the elderly. *Res. Vet. Sci.* 96: 147–152.

109 Corley, K.T.T., McKenzie, H.C., Amoroso, L.M. et al. (2000). Initial experience with norepinephrine infusion in hypotensive critically ill foals. *J. Vet. Emerg. Crit. Care* 10: 267–276.

110 Magdesian, K.G., Dwyer, R.M., and Arguedas, M.G. (2014). Viral diarrhea. In: *Equine Infectious Diseases* (ed. D.C. Sellon and M.T. Long), 198–203. St. Louis, Missouri: Saunders.

111 Javsicas, L.H. and Sanchez, L.C. (2008). The effect of omeprazole paste on intragastric pH in clinically ill neonatal foals. *Equine Vet. J.* 40: 41–44.

112 Sanchez, L.C., Murray, M.J., and Merritt, A.M. (2004). Effect of omeprazole paste on intragastric pH in clinically normal neonatal foals. *Am. J. Vet. Res.* 65: 1039–1041.

113 Madison, J.B., Garber, J.L., Rice, B. et al. (1994). Effect of oxytetracycline on metacarpophalangeal and distal interphalangeal joint angles in newborn foals. *J. Am. Vet. Med. Assoc.* 204: 246–249.

114 Sampieri, F., Hinchcliff, K.W., and Toribio, R.E. (2006). Tetracycline therapy of *Lawsonia intracellularis* enteropathy in foals. *Equine Vet. J.* 38: 89–92.

115 Ryan, C.A., Sanchez, L.C., Giguere, S. et al. (2005). Pharmacokinetics and pharmacodynamics of pantoprazole in clinically normal neonatal foals. *Equine Vet. J.* 37: 336–341.

116 Moore, J.N. and Barton, M.H. (2003). Treatment of endotoxemia. *Vet. Clin. Equine* 19: 681–695.

117 Abuja, G.A., Garcia-Lopez, J.M., Doran, R. et al. (2010). Pararectal cystotomy for urolith removal in nine horses. *Vet. Surg.* 39: 654–659.

118 Aleman, M., Gray, L.C., Colette Williams, D. et al. (2006). Juvenile idiopathic epilepsy in Egyptian Arabian foals: 22 cases (1985–2005). *J. Vet. Intern. Med.* 20: 1443–1449.

119 Hood, D.M., Stephens, K.A., and Bowen, M.J. (1982). Phenoxybenzamine for the treatment of severe nonresponsive diarrhea. *J. Am. Vet. Med. Assoc.* 180: 758.

120 Wilkie, J.R., Crisman, M.V., Sams, R.A. et al. (1993). Pharmacokinetics of phenylbutazone in neonatal foals. *Am. J. Vet. Res.* 54: 2064–2067.

121 Byron, J.K., March, P.A., Chew, D.J. et al. (2007). Effect of phenylpropanolamine and psuedoephedrine on the urethral pressure profile and continence scores of incontinent female dogs. *J. Vet. Intern. Med.* 21: 47–31.
122 Wong, D.M., Sponseller, B.A., Alcott, C.J. et al. (2013). Effects of intravenous administration of polymyxin B in neonatal foals with experimental endotoxemia. *J. Vet. Intern. Med.* 874–881.
123 Raidal, S.L. and Edwards, S. (2005). Pharmacokinetics of potassium bromide in adult horses. *Aust. Vet. J.* 83: 425–430.
124 Fielding, C.L., Magdesian, K.G., Elliot, D.A. et al. (2003). Pharmacokinetics and clinical utility of sodium bromide (NaBr) as an estimator of extracellular fluid volume in horses. *J. Vet. Intern. Med.* 17: 213–217.
125 Barnes, K.H., Aulakh, K.S., and Liu, C. (2019). Retrospective evaluation of prazosin and diazepam after thoracolumbar hemilaminectomy in dogs. *Vet. J.* 253: 105377.
126 Perkins, G.A., Miller, W.H., Divers, T.J. et al. (2005). Ulcerative dermatitis, thrombocytopenia, and neutropenia in neonatal foals. *J. Vet. Intern. Med.* 19: 211–216.
127 Dunkel, B. (2005). Acute lung injury/actue respiratory distress syndrome in 15 foals. *Equine Vet. J.* 35: 435–440.
128 Rush, B.R. and Flaminio, M.J.B.F. (2000). Immunomodulation in horses. *Vet. Clin. North Am. Equine* 16: 183–197.
129 Sanchez, L.C., Lester, G.D., and Merritt, A.M. (2001). Intragastric pH in critically ill neonatal foals and the effect of ranitidine. *J. Am. Vet. Med. Assoc.* 218: 907–911.
130 Giguere, S., Jacks, S., Roberts, G.D. et al. (2004). Retrospective comparison of azithromycin, clarithromycin, and erythromycin for the treatment of foals with *Rhodococcus equi* pneumonia. *J. Vet. Intern. Med.* 18: 568–573.
131 Naylor, J.M., Garven, E., and Fraser, L. (1997). A comparison of romifidine and xylazine in foals: the effects on sedation and analgesia. *Equine Vet. Educ.* 9: 329–334.
132 Lofstedt, J. (1997). White muscle disease of foals. *Vet. Clin. North Am. Equine* 13: 169–185.
133 Baquero, H., Soliz, A., Neira, F. et al. (2006). Oral sildenafil in infants with persistent pulmonary hypertension of the newborn: a pilot randomized blinded sguty. *Pedaitrics* 117: 1077–1083.
134 Palmer, J.E. (2005). Ventilatory support of the critically ill foal. *Vet. Clin. Equine* 21: 457–486.
135 Ryan, C.A. and Sanchez, L.C. (2005). Nondiarrheal disorders of the gastrointestinal tract in neonatal foals. *Vet. Clin. Equine* 21: 313–332.
136 Baumer, W., Herrling, G.M., and Feige, K. (2013). Pharmacokinetics and thrombolytic effects of the recombinant tissue-type plasminogen activator in horses. *BMC Vet. Res.* 9: 1–6.
137 Forrest, L.J., Cooley, A.J., and Darien, B.J. (1999). Digital arterial thrombosis in a septicemic foal. *J. Vet. Intern. Med.* 13: 382–385.
138 Ingvast-Larsson, C., Kallings, P., Persson, S. et al. (1989). Pharmacokinetics and cardio-respiratory effects of oral theophylline in exercised horses. *J. Vet. Pharmacol. Ther.* 12: 189–199.
139 Goetz, T.E., Munsiff, I.J., and McKiernan, B.C. (1989). Pharmacokinetic disposition of an immediate-release aminophylline and a sustained-release theophylline formulation in the horse. *J. Vet. Pharmacol. Ther.* 12: 369–377.
140 Knych, H.K., Steffey, E.P., White, A.M. et al. (2016). Effects of age on the pharmacokinetics of tramadol and its active metabolite, O-desmethyltramadol following intravenous administration to foals. *Equine Vet. J.* 48: 65–71.
141 Knych, H.K., Mama, K.R., Steffey, E.P. et al. (2017). Pharmacokinetics and selected pharmacodynamics of trazodone following intravenous and oral adminsitration to horses underoing fitness training. *Am. J. Vet. Res.* 78: 1182–1192.
142 Davis, J.L., Schirmer, J., and Medlin, E. (2018). Pharmacokinetics, pharmacodynamics and clinical use of trazodone and its active metabolite m-chlorophenylpiperazine in the horse. *J. Vet. Pharmacol. Ther.* 41: 393–401.
143 Gray, S.N., Dechant, J.E., LeJeune, S.S. et al. (2015). Identification, management and outcome of postoperative hemoperitoneum in 23 horses after emergency exploratory celiotomy for gastrointestinal disease. *Vet. Surg.* 44: 379–385.
144 Rodriguez, A.C. and de Grauw, J. (2022). Spontaneous pulmonary hemorrhage in a standing sedated horse. *Vet. Rec.* 10: e319.
145 Wong, D.M., Brockus, C.W., Alcott, C.A. et al. (2009). Modifying the coagulation cascade: available medications. *Compend. Equine* 4: 224–236.
146 Garre, B., Baert, K., Nauwynck, H. et al. (2009). Multiple oral dosing of valacyclovir in horses and ponies. *J. Vet. Pharmacol. Ther.* 32: 207–212.
147 Orsini, J.A., Snooks-Parsons, C., Stine, L. et al. (2005). Vancomycin for the treatment of methicillin-resistant staphylococcal and enterococcal infections in 15 horses. *Can. J. Vet. Res.* 69: 278–286.
148 Vaala, W.E. (2009). Perinatal asphyxia syndrome in foals. *Compend. Equine* 134–140.
149 Wong, D.M., Young, L., and Dembek, K.A. (2021). Blood thiamine (vitamin B1), ascorbic acid (vitamin C), and cortisol concentrations in healthy and ill neonatal foals. *J. Vet. Intern. Med.* 35: 1988–1994.
150 Finno, C.J., Estell, K.E., Katzman, S. et al. (2015). Blood and cerebrospinal fluid tocopherol and selenium concentrations in neonatal foals with neuroaxonal dystrophy. *J. Vet. Intern. Med.* 29: 1667–1675.

Index

Equine Neonatal Medicine, First Edition. Edited by David M. Wong and Pamela A. Wilkins.

b

C

f

g

h

j

k

m

P